Volume 1

ROCKWOOD AND GREEN'S
Fractures in Adults

EIGHTH EDITION

EDITORS

Charles M. Court-Brown, MD, FRCS Ed (Orth)
Professor of Orthopaedic Trauma
Royal Infirmary of Edinburgh
Edinburgh, United Kingdom

James D. Heckman, MD
Editor-in-Chief
The Journal of Bone & Joint Surgery
Needham, Massachusetts
Clinical Professor of Orthopaedic Surgery
Harvard Medical School
Visiting Orthopaedic Surgeon
Department of Orthopaedic Surgery
Massachusetts General Hospital
Boston, Massachusetts

Margaret M. McQueen, MD, FRCS Ed (Orth)
Professor of Orthopaedic Trauma
The University of Edinburgh
Edinburgh, United Kingdom

William M. Ricci, MD
Professor and Chief
Orthopaedic Trauma Service
Department of Orthopaedic Surgery
Washington University School of Medicine
St. Louis, Missouri

Paul Tornetta III, MD
Professor and Vice Chairman
Department of Orthopaedic Surgery
Boston University School of Medicine
Director of Orthopaedic Trauma
Boston Medical Center
Boston, Massachusetts

ASSOCIATE EDITOR

Michael D. McKee, MD, FRCS(C)
Professor
Upper Extremity Reconstructive Service
Department of Surgery
Division of Orthopaedics
St. Michael's Hospital and the University of
Toronto
Toronto, Canada

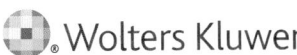
. Wolters Kluwer

Philadelphia • Baltimore • New York • London
Buenos Aires • Hong Kong • Sydney • Tokyo

Acquisitions Editor: Brian Brown
Product Development Editor: David Murphy
Production Project Manager: David Orzechowski
Design Coordinator: Joan Wendt
Manufacturing Coordinator: Beth Welch
Prepress Vendor: Aptara, Inc.

8th edition

Two Commerce Square
2001 Market Street
Philadelphia, PA 19103 USA
LWW.com

Not authorised for sale in United States, Canada, Australia, New Zealand, Puerto Rico, or U.S. Virgin Islands.

9 8 7 6 5 43 2 1

Printed in China

Library of Congress Cataloging-in-Publication Data

Rockwood and Green's fractures in adults / [edited by] Charles M. Court-Brown, James D. Heckman, Margaret M. McQueen, William Ricci, Paul Tornetta III; associate editor, Michael McKee. – Eighth edition.
   p. ; cm.
  Fractures in adults
  Includes bibliographical references and index.
   ISBN 978-1-4511-9508-8 (hardback : alk. paper)
  I. Court-Brown, Charles M., editor. II. Heckman, James D., editor. III. McQueen, Margaret M., editor. IV. Ricci, William M., editor. V. Tornetta, Paul, III, editor. VI. McKee, Michael D., editor. VII. Title: Fractures in adults.
  [DNLM: 1. Fractures, Bone. 2. Adult. 3. Dislocations. WE 175]
  RD101
  617.1'5—dc23
                                            2014016563

ROCKWOOD AND GREEN'S
Fractures in Adults

EIGHTH EDITION

We dedicate this Eighth Edition of Rockwood and Green's: Fractures in Adults to Charles A. Rockwood, Jr, MD, and David P. Green, MD, who served as our inspiration and mentors for carrying on the revision and update of this textbook.

To Susan for her patience and understanding during my 30-year tenure on the editorial board.

JDH

To the future: Emily, Jessica, and Rosie.

CCB

To my children Sacha, Tyler, Robbin, and Everett for enriching my life every day, and my partner Niloofar for her love and support.

MMcK

To Caroline, Elizabeth, and William without whom life would be easier but much less fun.

MMcQ

To Ann, Michael, and Luke, my reasons for being, for their patience, love, and support.

WMR

To my mother Phyllis, who found the best in people, had compassion for all, and whose insight, guidance, and love have always made me believe that anything is possible.

PT3

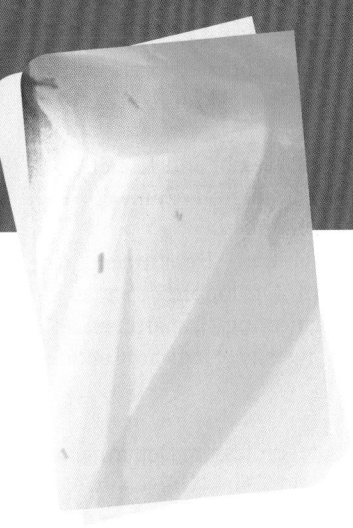

Contributors

Adewale O. Adeniran, MD   Resident, Department of Surgery, Dartmouth-Hitchcock Medical Center, Lebanon, New Hampshire

Animesh Agarwal, MD   Professor and Chief, Department of Orthopaedics, Division of Orthopaedic Trauma, University of Texas Health Science Center, Director of Orthopaedic Trauma, University Hospital, San Antonio, Texas

Devendra Agraharam, DNB   Associate Consultant in Trauma, Ganga Hospital, Coimbatore, India

Romney C. Andersen, MD   Clinical Assistant Professor of Orthopaedics, University of Maryland Medical Center, Baltimore, Maryland

George S. Athwal, MD, FRCSC   Associate Professor of Surgery, Western University, Consultant, Roth-McFarlane Hand and Upper Limb Centre, St Joseph's Health Care, Ontario, Canada

Roger M. Atkins, MA, MB, BS, DM, FRCS   Consultant Orthopaedic Surgeon, Bristol Royal Infirmary, Bristol, England

David P. Barei, MD, FRCSC   Associate Professor, Department of Orthopaedics, Harborview Medical Center, University of Washington, Seattle, Washington

Jan Bartoníček MD, DSc   Professor and Chairman, Department of Orthopaedic Trauma, 1st Faculty of Medicine of Charles University Prague and Central Military Hospital Prague, Department of Anatomy, 1st Faculty of Medicine of Charles University Prague, Prague, Czech Republic

Daphne M. Beingessner, BMath, BSc, MSc, MD, FRCSC   Associate Professor, Department of Orthopaedics and Sports Medicine, University of Washington, Orthopaedic Traumatology, Harborview Medical Center, Seattle, Washington

Mohit Bhandari, MD, PhD, FRCSC   Professor and Head, Division of Orthopedic Surgery, Associate Chair, Research, Department of Surgery, Canada Research Chair in Musculoskeletal Trauma, Associate Faculty, Department of Clinical Epidemiology and Biostatistics, McMaster University, Ontario, Canada

Leela C. Biant, BSc(hons), MBBS, AFRCSEd, FRCS (Tr & Orth), MS(res)Lond   Consultant Trauma & Orthopaedic Surgeon, The Royal Infirmary of Edinburgh, Honorary Senior Lecturer, The University of Edinburgh, NRS Career Clinician Scientist Fellow, Edinburgh, United Kingdom

Aaron J. Bois, MD, MSc, FRCSC   Section of Orthopaedic Surgery, Department of Surgery, University of Calgary, Alberta, Canada

Brett Bolhofner, MD   Director, Orthopaedic Trauma Services, Bayfront Medical Center, Clinical Assistant Professor, University of South Florida College of Medicine, Saint Petersburg, Florida

Christopher M. Bono, MD   Associate Professor, Department of Orthopaedic Surgery, Brigham and Women's Hospital, Harvard Medical School, Boston, Massachusetts

Christina Boulton, MD   Assistant Professor of Orthopaedics, Department of Orthopaedics, R Adams Cowley Shock Trauma Center, Department of Orthopaedics, University of Maryland School of Medicine, Baltimore, Maryland

Mark R. Brinker, MD   Director of Acute and Reconstructive Trauma, Co-Director, The Center for Problem Fractures and Limb Restoration, Texas Orthopedic Hospital, Fondren Orthopedic Group, Houston, Texas, Clinical Professor, Department of Orthopaedic Surgery, Tulane University School of Medicine, New Orleans, Louisiana, Clinical Professor, Joseph Barnhart Department of Orthopedic Surgery, Baylor College of Medicine, Clinical Professor Department of Orthopedic Surgery, The University of Texas Medical School at Houston, Houston, Texas

Kate E. Bugler, BA, MRCS   Specialty Registrar, Clinical Research Fellow, Orthopaedic Trauma Unit, Royal Infirmary of Edinburgh, Edinburgh, United Kingdom

Harvey Chim, MBBS   Hand Surgery Fellow, Department of Orthopedic Surgery, Division of Hand Surgery, Mayo Clinic, Rochester, Minnesota

David Ciceri, MD   Assistant Professor of Anesthesiology, Director, Surgical Intensive Care, Scott & White HealthCare, Texas A&M Health Science Center, Temple, Texas

Michael P. Clare, MD   Director of Fellowship Education, Foot & Ankle Fellowship, Florida Orthopaedic Institute, Tampa, Florida

Nicholas D. Clement, MRCSEd   Orthopaedic Research Fellow, Department of Trauma and Orthopaedic Surgery, Royal Infirmary of Edinburgh, Edinburgh, United Kingdom

Cory A. Collinge, MD   Director of Orthopaedic Trauma, Harris Methodist Fort Worth Hospital, Clinical Staff, John Peter Smith Hospital, Fort Worth, Texas

Marlon O. Coulibaly, MD   Assistant Professor, Department of General and Trauma Surgery, Rhur-University Bochum, Attending Orthopaedic Surgeon, Department of General and Trauma Surgery, Berufsgenossenschaftliches Universitäklinikum Bergmannshiel GmbH, Bochum, Germany

Charles M. Court-Brown, MD, FRCS Ed (Orth)   Professor of Orthopaedic Trauma, Royal Infirmary of Edinburgh, Edinburgh, United Kingdom

Anthony DeGiacomo, MD   Orthopaedic Surgery Resident, Boston University, Boston, Massachusetts

J. Dheenadhayalan, MS   Senior Consultant in Trauma and Upper Limb Service, Ganga Hospital, Coimbatore, India

Douglas R. Dirschl, MD   Professor and Chairman, Department of Orthopaedic Surgery, University of Chicago Medicine and Biological Sciences, Chicago, Illinois

Paul J. Dougherty, MD   Residency Program Director, Detroit Medical Center, Detroit, Michigan, Associate Professor, Residency Director, Department of Orthopaedic Surgery, University of Michigan, Ann Arbor, Michigan

Andrew D. Duckworth, MSc, MRCSEd   Edinburgh Orthopaedic Trauma Unit, Royal Infirmary of Edinburgh, Edinburgh, United Kingdom

Anil K. Dutta, MD   Associate Professor, Fred G. Corley, MD Distinguished Professorship in Orthopaedics, Shoulder and Elbow Surgery, Department of Orthopaedics, University of Texas Health Science Center, San Antonio, Texas

Cory Edgar, MD, PhD,   Assistant Professor and Team Physician, University of Connecticut, Farmington, Connecticut

Thomas A. Einhorn, MD   Chairman, Department of Orthopaedic Surgery, Professor of Orthopaedic Surgery, Biochemistry and Biomedical Engineering, Department of Orthopaedic Surgery, Boston University Medical Center, Boston, Massachusetts

William J. J. Ertl, MD   Associate Professor, Department of Orthopaedics and Rehabilitation, The University of Oklahoma, Oklahoma City, Oklahoma

Michael J. Gardner, MD   Associate Professor, Department of Orthopedic Surgery, Washington University School of Medicine, St. Louis, Missouri

Christos Garnavos, MD, PhD   Consultant Orthopaedic Surgeon, Department of Orthopaedics, Evangelismos General Hospital, Athens, Greece

Peter V. Giannoudis, MD, FRCS   Professor of Trauma & Orthopaedic Surgery, School of Medicine, University of Leeds, Leeds General Infirmary University Hospital, Leeds, United Kingdom

George J. Haidukewych, MD   Director of Orthopedic Trauma, Chief of Complex Joint Replacement, Academic Chairman for the Orthopedic Faculty Practice, Professor, University of Central Florida College of Medicine, Orlando, Florida

Mark H. Henry, MD   Hand & Wrist Center of Houston, Houston, Texas

Martin F. Hoffman, MD   Assistant Professor, Department of General and Trauma Surgery, Rhur-University Bochum, Attending Orthopaedic Surgeon, Department of General and Trauma Surgery, Berufsgenossenschaftliches Universitätsklinikum Bergmannshiel GmbH, Bochum, Germany

Andrew Jawa, MD   Assistant Professor of Orthopedic Surgery, Boston University School of Medicine, Boston, Massachusetts

Mark Jo, MD   Huntington Orthopedics, Pasadena, California

Leo Joskowicz, PhD   Professor, School of Engineering and Computer Science, The Hebrew University of Jerusalem, Jerusalem, Israel

Christopher C. Kaeding, MD The Ohio State University Sports Medicine Center, Judson Wilson Professor, Department of Orthopaedics, Co-Medical Director, Sports Medicine Center, Head Team Physician, Department of Athletics, The Ohio State University, Columbus, Ohio

Michael S. Kain, MD Director, Resident Education, Department of Orthopaedics, Lahey Hospital & Medical Center, Burlington, Massachusetts

Sanjeev Kakar, MD, MRCS Assistant Professor, Department of Orthopaedic Surgery, Mayo Clinic, Rochester, Minnesota

Kerry M. Kallas, MD Musculoskeletal Radiologist, Center for Diagnostic Imaging, Sartell, Minnesota

Matthew D. Karam, MD Assistant Professor of Orthopaedic Surgery, The University of Iowa, Iowa City, Iowa

Madhav A. Karunakar, MD Associate Professor, Orthopaedic Traumatologist, Department of Orthopaedic Surgery, Carolinas Medical Center, Charlotte, North Carolina

John F. Keating, MPhil, FRCS(Ed) (Orth) Consultant Orthopaedic Surgeon, Royal Infirmary of Edinburgh, Edinburgh, United Kingdom

Christopher K. Kepler, MD Department of Orthopaedic Surgery, Thomas Jefferson University, Philadelphia, Pennsylvania

Hubert T. Kim, MD, PhD Associate Professor and Vice Chairman, Department of Orthopaedic Surgery, University of California, Director, Department of Orthopaedic Surgery, UCSF Cartilage Repair and Regeneration Center, UCSF Orthopaedic Institute, San Francisco, California

Graham J.W. King, MD, MSc, FRCSC Professor, Departments of Surgery and Biomedical Engineering, Western University, Director, Roth McFarlane Hand and Upper Limb Centre, St. Joseph's Health Centre, London, Ontario, Canada

Erik N. Kubiak, MD Associate Professor, Department of Orthopaedics, University of Utah Medical Center, Salt Lake City, Utah

Joshua Langford, MD Orthopedic Traumatologist, Level One Orthopedics at Orlando Health, Orlando, Florida

Meir Liebergall, MD Professor of Orthopaedic Surgery, Hebrew University, Chairman, Department of Orthopaedic Surgery, The Hadassah-Hebrew University Medical Center, Jerusalem, Israel

Mark J. Lemos, MD Associate Professor of Orthopaedic Surgery, Boston University School of Medicine, Vice Chair, Department of Orthopaedic Surgery, Director of Sports Medicine, Lahey Hospital & Medical Center, Burlington, Massachusetts

Bruce A. Levy, MD Professor, Department of Orthopedics and Sports Medicine, Mayo Clinic, Rochester, Minnesota

Ralph Marcucio, PhD Associate Professor, Department of Orthopaedic Surgery, University of California, Director, Laboratory for Skeletal Regeneration, Orthopaedic Surgery, UCSF/SFGH Orthopaedic Trauma Institute, San Francisco General Hospital, San Francisco, California

J. L. Marsh, MD The Carroll B. Larson Professor of Orthopaedic Surgery, The University of Iowa, Iowa City, Iowa

Augustus D. Mazzocca, MS, MD Professor, Department of Orthopaedic Surgery, UConn Health Center, Director, Department of Orthopaedic Surgery, Division of Clinical Biomechanics, Director, Bioskills Laboratory, Farmington, Connecticut

Michael D. McKee, MD, FRCS(C) Professor, Upper Extremity Reconstructive Service, Department of Surgery, Division of Orthopaedics, St. Michael's Hospital and the University of Toronto, Toronto, Canada

Margaret M. McQueen, MD, FRCS Ed (Orth) Professor of Orthopaedic Trauma, The University of Edinburgh, Edinburgh, United Kingdom

J. Stuart Melvin, MD OrthoCarolina, Charlotte, North Carolina

Theodore Miclau III, MD Professor and Vice Chair, Department of Orthopaedic Surgery, University of California, Chief of Service, Director, UCSF/SFGH Orthopaedic Trauma Institute, Department of Orthopaedic Surgery, San Francisco General Hospital, San Francisco, California

Timothy L. Miller, MD Team Physician for The Ohio State University Track and Field and Cross-Country Teams, Assistant Director of The Ohio State University Medical Center Endurance Medicine Team, The Ohio State University Sports Medicine Center, Columbus, Ohio

Sohail K. Mirza, MD Professor of Orthopaedic Surgery, Professor of the Dartmouth Institute, Dartmouth-Hitchcock Medical Center, Lebanon, New Hampshire

Berton Moed, MD Professor and Chairman, Department of Orthopaedic Surgery, Saint Louis University School of Medicine, St. Louis, Missouri

Thomas Moore Jr, MD   Assistant Professor, Department of Orthopaedics, Emory University School of Medicine, Grady Health Systems, Orthopaedic Clinic, Atlanta, Georgia

Steven L. Moran, MD   Professor of Orthopedics, Professor of Plastic Surgery, Departments of Orthopaedic and Plastic Surgery, Mayo Clinic, Rochester, Minnesota

Rami Mosheiff   Professor of Orthopedic Surgery, Faculty of Medicine, The Hadassah-Hebrew University, Head of Orthopedic Trauma Unit, Department of Orthopedic Surgery, The Hadassah-Hebrew University Medical Center, Jerusalem, Israel

Soheil Najibi, MD, PhD   Senior Staff Orthopaedic Surgeon, Henry Ford Hospital, Detroit, Michigan

Sean E. Nork, MD   Associate Professor, Department of Orthopaedic Surgery, Harborview Medical Center, Seattle, Washington

Carol North, MD   The Nancy and Ray L. Hunt Chair in Crisis Psychiatry, Professor, Departments of Psychiatry and Surgery/Division, Emergency Medicine/Section on Homeland Security, The University of Texas Southwestern Medical Center, Dallas, Texas

Daniel P. O'Connor, PhD   Associate Professor, Laboratory of Integrated Physiology, University of Houston, Houston, Texas

Robert V. O'Toole, MD   Associate Professor of Orthopaedics, R Adams Cowley Shock Trauma Center, Department of Orthopaedics, University of Maryland School of Medicine, Baltimore, Maryland

Hans Christoph Pape, MD   Professor of Trauma & Orthopaedic Surgery, Department of Orthopaedic Trauma Surgery, University Clinic Aachen, RWTH University Aachen, Aachen, Germany

Adam M. Pearson, MD   Assistant Professor, Department of Orthopaedic Surgery, Dartmouth-Hitchcock Medical Center, Lebanon, New Hampshire

R. Perumal, DNB   Associate Consultant in Trauma Ganga Hospital, Coimbatore, India

Rodrigo F. Pesántez, MD   Chief of Orthopaedic Trauma, Departamento de Ortopedia y Traumatología, Fundación Santa Fe de Bogotá, Universidad de los Andes, Bogotá, Colombia

J. Whitcomb Pollock, MD, MSc, FRCSC   Assistant Professor, Department of Surgery, University of Ottawa, Ontario, Canada, The Ottawa Hospital General Campus, Ontario, Canada

Robert Probe, MD   Professor of Surgery, Chairman, Department of Orthopaedic Surgery, Scott & White Health-Care, Texas A&M Health Science Center, Temple, Texas

Robert H. Quinn, M.D.   Professor and Chairman, Residency Program Director, John J. Hinchey M.D. and Kathryn Hinchey Chair in Orthopaedic Surgery, Orthopaedic Oncology, Department of Orthopaedics, University of Texas School of Medicine, San Antonio, Texas

Rajiv Rajani, MD   Assistant Professor, Department of Orthopaedics, University of Texas School of Medicine, San Antonio, Texas

S. Rajasekaran, MS, FRCS, MCh, DNB, PhD   Chairman, Department of Orthopaedic & Spine Surgery, Ganga Hospital, Coimbatore, India

Stuart H. Ralston, MB ChB, MD, FRCP, FRSE   Arthritis Research UK Professor of Rheumatology, Institute of Genetics and Molecular Medicine, Western General Hospital, University of Edinburgh, Edinburgh, United Kingdom

Nalini Rao, MD, FACP, FSHEA   Clinical Professor of Medicine and Orthopedics, University of Pittsburgh School of Medicine, Chief, Division of Infectious Diseases (Shadyside Campus), UPMC Presbyterian Shadyside, Medical Director, Infection Control, UPMC Shadyside, Southside and Braddock, Pittsburgh, Pennsylvania

Mark C. Reilly, MD   Associate Professor and Chief Orthopaedic Trauma Service, Department of Orthopaedic Surgery, New Jersey Medical School, Newark, New Jersey

Eric T. Ricchetti, MD   Staff, Department of Orthopaedic Surgery, Orthopedic and Rheumatologic Institute, Cleveland Clinic, Cleveland, Ohio

William M. Ricci, MD   Professor, Chief, Orthopaedic Trauma Service, Department of Orthopaedic Surgery, Washington University School of Medicine, St. Louis, Missouri

David Ring, MD, PhD   Chief, Hand and Upper Extremity Service, Director of Research, Hand and Upper Extremity Service, Massachusetts General Hospital, Associate Professor of Orthopaedic Surgery, Harvard Medical School, Boston, Massachussets

Charles A. Rockwood, Jr, MD Professor and Chairman Emeritus of Orthopaedics, Director, Shoulder Service, University of Texas Health Science Center, San Antonio, Texas

Thomas P. Rüedi, MD, FACS Professor Dr med, FACS, Founding Member of the AO Foundation, Davos, Switzerland

Thomas A. Russell, MD Professor of Orthopaedic Surgery, Department of Orthopaedic Surgery, University of Tennessee and Campbell Clinic, University of Tennessee Center for the Health Sciences, Elvis Presley Trauma Center and Regional Medical Center, Memphis, Tennessee

Joaquin Sanchez-Sotelo, MD PhD Associate Professor of Orthopaedic Surgery, Department of Orthopedic Surgery, Mayo Clinic, Rochester, Minnesota

David W. Sanders, MD, MSc, FRCS(C) Associate Professor, Victoria Hospital, Western University, Ontario, Canada

Roy W. Sanders, MD Director, Orthopaedic Trauma Service, Florida Orthopaedic Institute, Chief, Department of Orthopaedic Surgery, Tampa General Hospital, Tampa, Florida

Adam A. Sassoon, MD Department of Orthopaedic Surgery, Orlando Regional Medical Center, Orlando, Florida

Thomas A. Schildhauer Clinical Professor, Department of General and Trauma Surgery, Rhur-University Bochum, Medical Director and Chairman, Department of General and Trauma Surgery, Berufsgenossenschaftliches Universitäklinikum Bergmannshiel GmbH, Bochum, Germany

Andrew H. Schmidt, MD Professor, Department of Orthopaedic Surgery, University of Minnesota, Director of Clinical Research, Department of Orthopedic Surgery, Hennepin County Medical Center, Minneapolis, Minnesota

Andrew J. Schoenfeld, MD Assistant Professor, Department of Orthopaedic Surgery, Texas Tech University Health Sciences Center, William Beaumont Army Medical Center, El Paso, Texas

Michael Schüetz, FRACS, FAOrthA, Dr. med. (RWTH Aachem) Dr. med. habil (HU Berlin) Professor and Chairman in Trauma, Science and Engineering Faculty, Institute of Health and Biomedical Innovation, Queensland University of Technology, Director of Trauma, Department of Surgery, Princess Alexandra Hospital, Queensland, Australia

Jesse Slade Shantz, MD, MBA Orthopaedic Trauma Fellow, Department of Orthopaedic Surgery, University of California, Orthopaedic Trauma Fellow, UCSF/SFGH Orthopaedic Trauma Institute, San Francisco General Hospital, San Francisco, California

Alexander Y. Shin, MD Professor and Consultant of Orthopaedic Surgery, Department of Orthopedic Surgery, Division of Hand Surgery, Mayo Clinic, Rochester, Minnesota

Sarina K. Sinclair, PhD Orthopaedics - Research Instructor, University of Utah School of Medicine, Salt Lake City, Utah

Wade R. Smith, MD, FACS Professor of Orthopaedic Surgery, University of Colorado School of Medicine, Orthopaedic Trauma Surgeon, HCA Healthone Clinical Services, Mountain Orthopaedic Trauma Surgeons at Swedish, Englewood, Colorado

Adam Starr, MD Professor, Department of Orthopaedic Surgery, University of Texas Southwestern Medical Center, Dallas, Texas

Scott P. Steinmann, MD Professor of Orthopaedic Surgery, Department of Orthopedic Surgery, Mayo Clinic, Rochester, Minnesota

Philipp N. Streubel, MD Assistant Professor, Hand and Upper Extremity Surgery, Department of Orthopaedic Surgery and Rehabilitation, University of Nebraska Medical Center, Omaha, Nebraska

S. R. Sundararajan, MS Senior Consultant in Trauma and Arthroscopy Ganga Hospital, Coimbatore, India

Allan F. Tencer, PhD Professor Emeritus, Department of Orthopaedics and Sports Medicine, University of Washington, Seattle, Washington

Paul Tornetta III, MD Professor and Vice Chairman, Department of Orthopaedic Surgery, Boston University School of Medicine, Director of Orthopaedic Trauma, Boston Medical Center, Boston, Massachusetts

Alexander R. Vaccaro, MD, PhD Everrett J. and Marion Gordon Professor of Orthopaedic Surgery, Professor of Neurosurgery, Thomas Jefferson University, Vice Chairman, Department of Orthopaedic Surgery, Co-Director, Regional Spinal Cord Injury Center of the Delaware Valley, Co-Director of Spine Surgery and the Spine Fellowship program, Thomas Jefferson University Hospital, Philadelphia, Pennsylvania

Eric Wagner, MD   Research Fellow, Department of Orthopaedics, Mayo Clinic, Rochester, Minnesota

J. Tracy Watson, MD   Professor Orthopaedic Surgery, Chief, Orthopaedic Traumatology Service, Department of Orthopaedic Surgery, Saint Louis University School of Medicine, St. Louis University Health Sciences Center, St. Louis, Missouri

Daniel B. Whelan, MD, MSc, FRCSC   Assistant Professor, University of Toronto Sports Medicine Program, Division of Orthopaedic Surgery, St. Michael's Hospital, Ontario, Canada

Timothy. O. White, MD, FRCSEd(Orth)   Consultant Orthopaedic Trauma Surgeon, Edinburgh Orthopaedic Trauma Unit, Royal Infirmary of Edinburgh, Edinburgh, Scotland

Michael A. Wirth, MD   Professor/Charles A. Rockwood Jr., M.D. Chair, Shoulder Service, Department of Orthopaedics, University of Texas Health Science Center, Division of Orthopaedics, Audie Murphy Veterans Hospital, San Antonio, Texas

Donald A. Wiss, MD   Director of Orthopaedic Trauma, Cedars-Sinai Medical Center, Los Angeles, California

Bruce H. Ziran, MD   Director of Orthopaedic Trauma, Orthopaedic Residency Program, Atlanta Medical Center, Atlanta, Georgia

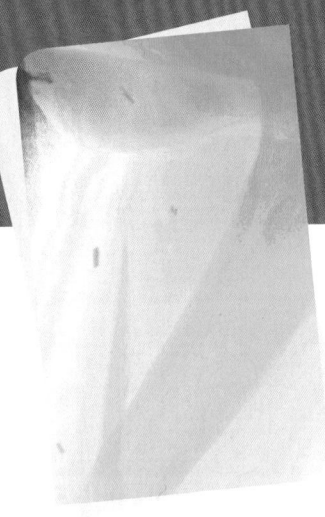

Preface

The eighth edition of *Rockwood and Green's: Fractures in Adults* continues with the changes that were instituted in the seventh edition. In this edition there are two more chapters and 61 new authors drawn from three continents and 11 different countries. In addition, many of the new authors represent the next generation of orthopedic trauma surgeons who will be determining the direction of trauma management over the next two or three decades.

Orthopedic trauma continues to be an expanding discipline, with change occurring more quickly than is often realized. When Drs. Rockwood and Green published the first edition in 1975, there were virtually no orthopedic trauma specialists in most countries, fractures were usually treated nonoperatively, and mortality following severe trauma was considerable. In one generation the changes in orthopedic surgery, as in the rest of medicine, have been formidable. We have worked to incorporate these changes in this edition. There is expanded coverage in this edition of the inevitable complications that all orthopedic surgeons have to deal with, and we have included chapters on geriatric trauma and the psychological aspects of trauma. The other area of orthopedic trauma that is expanding quickly, particularly in the developed countries, is the treatment of osteoporotic (or fragility) fractures. These fractures are assuming a greater medical and political importance, and orthopedic implants are now being designed specifically to treat elderly patients. It is likely that this trend will continue over the next few decades; many of the chapters in this edition reflect this change in emphasis.

The changes in the eighth edition include major changes in its chapter structure. Each of the clinical chapters now follows a specific template beginning with the physical examination, classification, and additional studies used in the diagnosis of each problem. This is followed by a description of the outcome measures used to evaluate patients for the specific injury they sustained. The indications and contraindications for each treatment method, including nonoperative and operative methods are highlighted in tables, as are the technical aspects of the surgeries. Old favorites such as pitfalls and problems are also listed in tables with solutions. Finally, the author's preferred treatment is now presented in the form of an algorithm, allowing the reader to understand the thought process of the expert writer in deciding on the treatment for the multiple subtypes of injuries described in each chapter. We believe that this will make it easy to get the most out of each chapter.

Finally, we are proud to introduce a new electronic format that should allow for easier access across platforms, a change that is overdue! Video supplementation is also available for the majority of the clinical problems.

We are indebted to the efforts of the experts who have taken the time to share their knowledge and experience with our broad readership and hope that this new edition will contribute to the care of patients.

Charles M. Court-Brown, MD, FRCS Ed (Orth)
James D. Heckman, MD
Margaret M. McQueen, MD, FRCS Ed (Orth)
William M. Ricci, MD
Paul Tornetta III, MD

Contents

ROCKWOOD AND GREEN'S
Fractures in Adults

EIGHTH EDITION

General Principles

1

BIOMECHANICS OF FRACTURES AND FRACTURE FIXATION

Mark J. Jo, Allan F. Tencer, and Michael J. Gardner

INTRODUCTION TO BIOMECHANICS OF FRACTURES AND FRACTURE FIXATION

"Biomechanics" is a complex and encompassing term that applies to many aspects related to orthopedic surgery, and specifically to fractures and fracture fixation. The application of biomechanical principles and concepts is essential to understand how the fracture occurred, how to best treat the injury, and how to avoid mechanical failures of the fixation construct. One must first understand the fundamental terms and concepts related to mechanical physics. This establishes the foundation that will be used to apply these concepts to the field of orthopedic surgery. The biomechanical properties of bone as well as the biomechanics of fracture healing are also essential to understand how bone is injured and how to best restore its function. Finally, understanding the biomechanical properties of common implants and failures seen with their application helps the clinician to a thorough understanding that aids in patient care.

In the study of biomechanics as it relates to fracture fixation, the fundamental mechanical question remains: Is the fixation system stable and strong enough to allow the patient early mobility before bony union is complete? This must occur without delaying healing, creating bone deformity, or damaging the

implant, and yet be flexible enough to allow transmission of force to the healing fracture to stimulate union. The common adage in orthopedics is that, "Fracture healing is a race between bony union and implant failure." A thorough understanding of the biomechanical concepts as they relate to bone, fracture, and implants is essential for the proper treatment of patients with fractures.

BASIC CONCEPTS

Before describing the performance of fracture fixation systems, some basic concepts used in biomechanics must be understood. A *force* causes an object to either accelerate or decelerate. It has *magnitude* (strength) and acts in a specific direction, which is termed a *vector*. However complex the system of forces acting on a bone, each force may be separated into its vector components (which form a 90-degree triangle with the force). Any of several components, acting in the same or different directions, can be added to yield the net or *resultant force*. As seen in Figure 1-1, a simplified example of the hip joint shows that the forces acting about the hip include the body weight, joint reactive force, and the hip abductors. As the hip in this example is at rest, the net force must be zero; therefore, if the body weight and hip abductor forces are known, the joint reactive

1

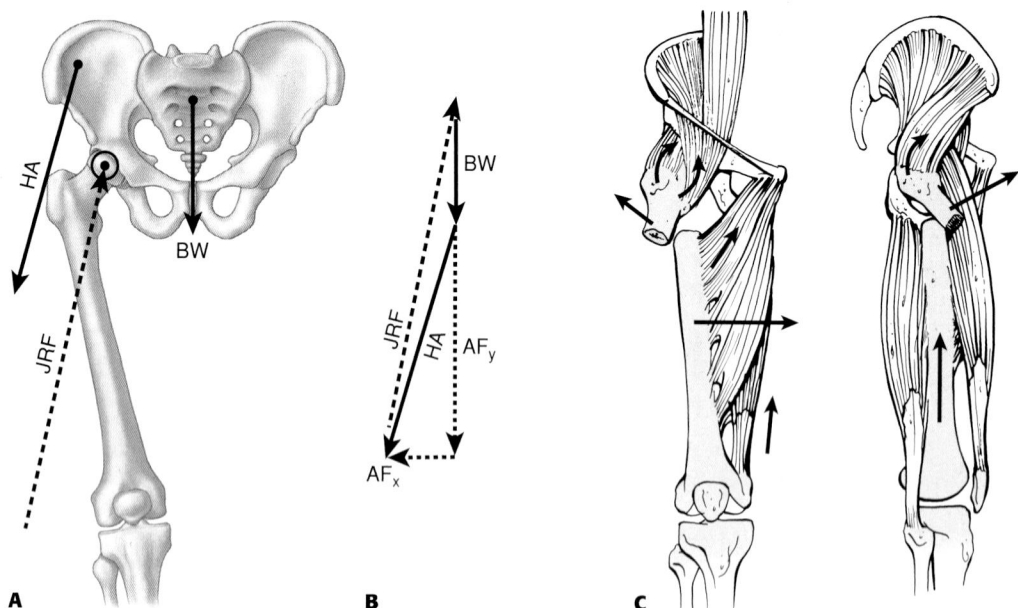

FIGURE 1-1 The force vectors acting on different parts of the body are a culmination of muscle, tendons, ligaments, and external forces. **A:** A simplified example of the force vectors acting on the hip joint. HA, hip abductors; BW, body weight; JRF, joint reactive force. **B:** Using the x and y vector components of the forces about the hip the joint reactive force (JRF) can be calculated because if the hip is at rest, the sum of all the forces should equal zero. AF_y (vertical component of HA force) AF_x (horizontal component of HA force). **C:** Understanding the forces that are applied about a fracture can help the surgeon understand the deforming forces and assist in reduction and fixation strategies.

force can be calculated using the x and y components of all the forces. Also, understanding the forces about a fracture help the surgeon to understand the deforming forces, the reduction maneuvers, as well as the proper application of implants to best stabilize the injury. Both the design of the implants as well as the application by the surgeon must be done with these concepts in mind so that they can withstand the mechanical loads applied without failure.

The two major loads acting on a long bone are those that cause it to displace in a linear direction (translation) and those that cause it to rotate around a joint center. Muscles typically cause a bone to rotate (e.g., the biceps causes the forearm to flex and supinate, the anterior tibialis causes the foot to dorsiflex). When a force causes rotation, it is termed a *moment* and has a *moment arm*. The moment arm is the lever arm against which the force acts to cause rotation. It is the perpendicular distance of the muscle force from the center of rotation of the joint. As shown in Figure 1-2, the moment or rotary force is affected not only by the magnitude of the force applied, but also by its distance from the center of rotation. In the example, two moments act on the outstretched arm. The weight carried in the hand as well as the weight of the hand and forearm rotate the arm downward, while the balancing muscle force rotates the forearm upward. Equilibrium is reached by balancing the moments so that the forearm does not rotate and the weight can be carried. Note that to achieve this, the muscle force must be eight times as large as the weight of the object, forearm, and hand because its moment arm or distance from the center of the joint is only one-eighth as long.

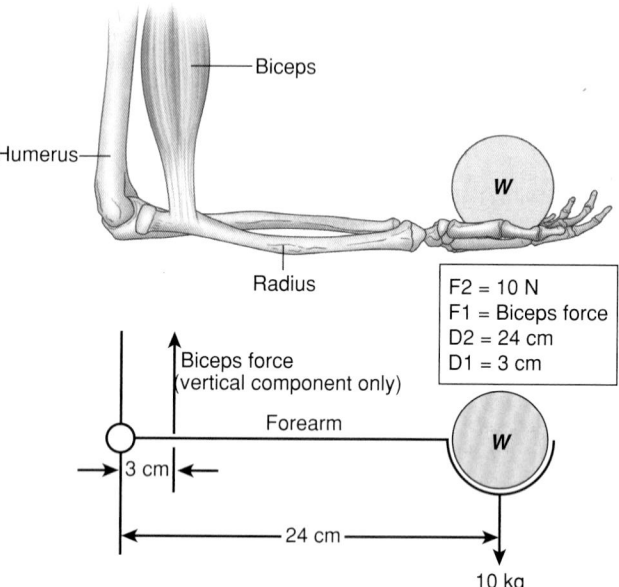

F2 = 10 N
F1 = Biceps force
D2 = 24 cm
D1 = 3 cm

FIGURE 1-2 In this simplified example of a free body diagram, the outstretched arm is a lever and is at rest. The rotational force, or the moment, is centered about the elbow. This moment is defined as the product of the weight (object + forearm + hand) (F_2) and the distance from the elbow (d_2). This moment must be counteracted by a moment in the opposite direction. In this example the vertical component of the biceps force (F_1) is the counteractive force. The lever arm of this force is the distance from the elbow to the insertion of the biceps (d_1). The biceps force is calculated from $10 \text{ kg} \times 24 \text{ cm} = F_1 \times 3 \text{ cm}$. Thus $F_1 = 80$ N. The biceps force is much greater than the weight of the object, arm, and hand because its lever arm is smaller.

The basic forces—compression, tension, torsion, and bending—cause the bone to behave in predictable ways. A *compressive force* (Fig. 1-3) results in shortening the length of the bone, whereas *tension* elongates it. *Torsion* causes twisting of a bone about its long axis, whereas *bending* causes it to bow at the center. When these forces are great enough to cause the bone to fracture, it results in characteristic fracture patterns that can be recognized on radiographs. Understanding these forces

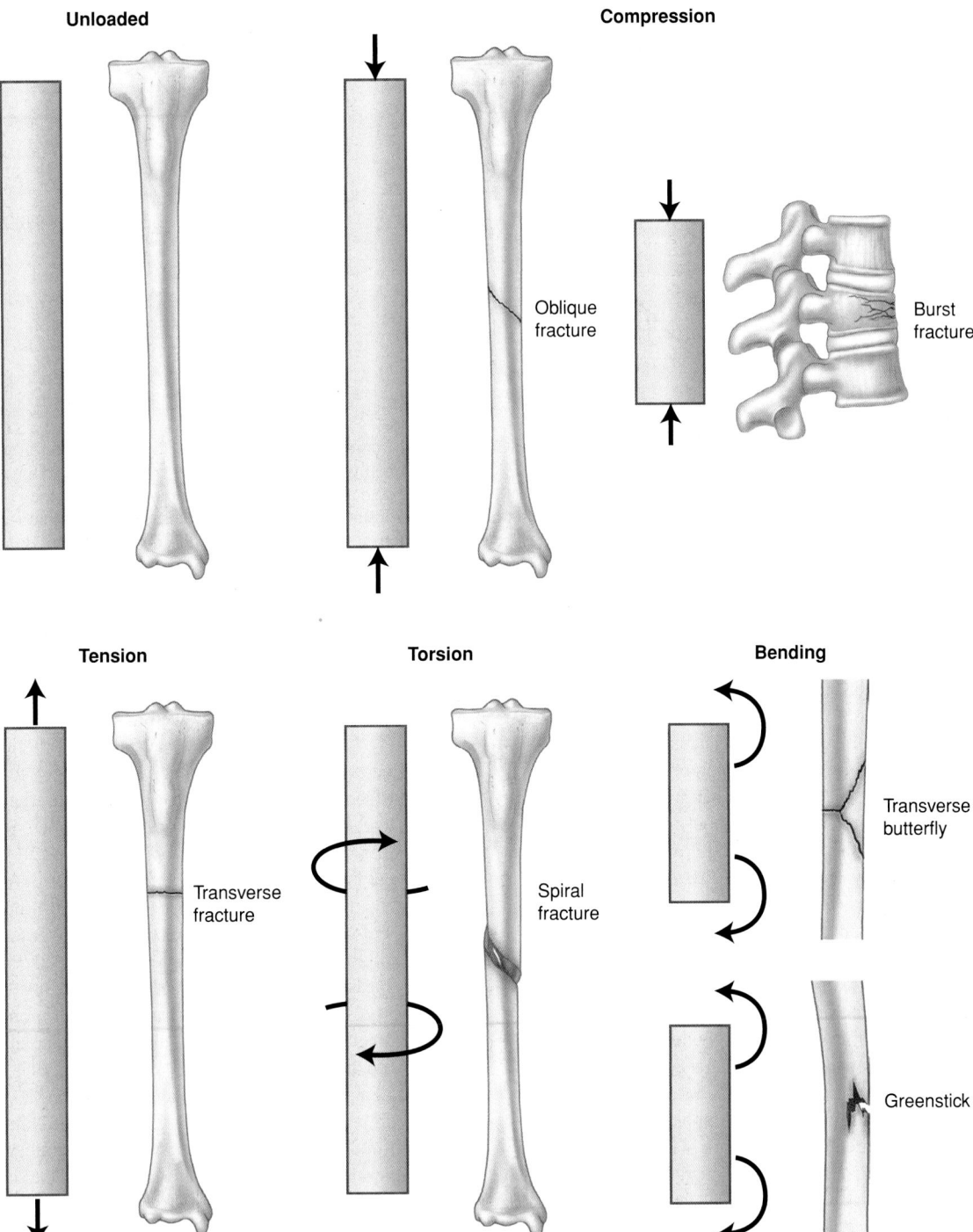

FIGURE 1-3 Basic forces: Unloaded; compression shortens length and can lead to an oblique fracture line or comminution; tension can lead to a transverse fracture. Torsional forces usually cause a spiral pattern. Bending forces cause compressive forces on one side and tensile forces on the other. This can result in a transverse fracture on the tensile side and comminution in a classic butterfly pattern on the compressive side. Bending forces can also result in incomplete or "greenstick" fractures in the pediatric population.

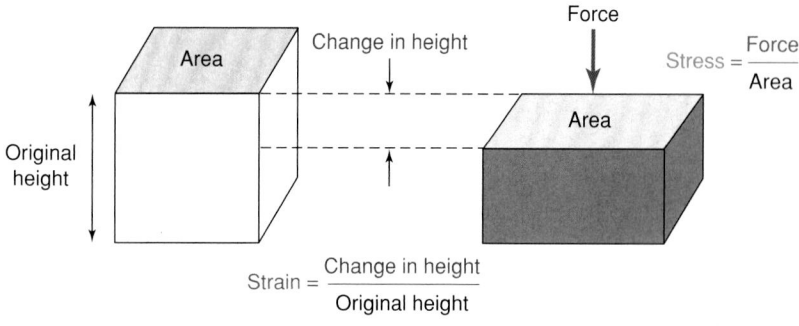

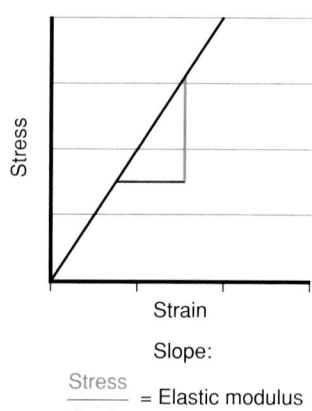

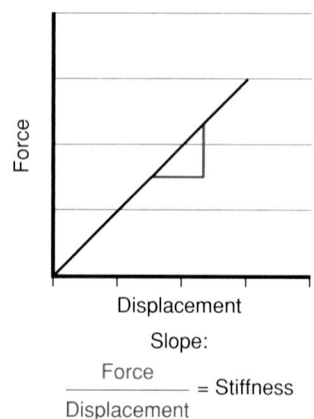

FIGURE 1-4 The stress is defined as the force acting on a surface divided by the area over which it acts. Strain is the change in the height or length of the object (displacement) under load divided by its original height or length. Stiffness is defined as the slope of a force versus displacement graph. Elastic modulus is the corresponding slope, but of a stress versus strain graph. Note the corresponding colors.

can help to understand the circumstances of the forces that occurred at the time of the fracture. Compressive forces can cause oblique fracture lines or can result in comminution and fragmentation of the bone. *Tensile* forces usually cause transverse fracture lines, whereas torsion can cause spiral fractures. Bending forces cause compressive stress on one side and tensile stress on the other side. Bending forces can also cause plastic deformation of immature or flexible bone or result in partial fractures. These partial fractures are also known as "greenstick" fractures and are usually seen in the pediatric population. In a more rigid bone, the tensile forces result in a transverse fracture line and the compressive forces cause comminution, usually in the characteristic butterfly fragment. In many cases an injury is caused by a combination of these forces and the fracture pattern may have a combination of patterns.

Stress, as shown in Figure 1-4, is simply the force divided by the area on an object over which it acts. This is a convenient way to express how the force affects a material locally. For example, when an equal force (hammer blow) is applied to both a sharp and a dull osteotome, the sharp osteotome will concentrate the same force over a smaller surface area than a dull osteotome because of the sharp edge. Therefore, the sharp osteotome will create a greater stress at the osteotome–bone interface, resulting in cutting of the bone. Just as stress is a normalized force (force per unit area), changes in length can also be normalized. *Strain* is simply the change in height or length that a material undergoes during loading, divided by its original height or length. If two plates of different lengths are both subjected to loads that lengthen the plate by 1 cm, the shorter of the two plates will

be subjected to more strain as change in length is spread over a shorter distance than it is for the longer plate.

Mechanical testing is used extensively to analyze the properties of different constructs as well as new implant designs.[67] The testing usually consists of a natural or synthetic fractured bone fixed with a certain implant in different configurations. This construct is then loaded into an apparatus that applies a specific load in either a constant or cyclic manner. Sensors can measure the forces applied to the bone as well as any deformity or eventual failure (Fig. 1-5). Depending on the purpose of the experiment the data can be collected measuring the *structural properties* of the bone–fixation construct; that is, the properties of the fixation device and the bone combined. Alternatively, the data can measure the *material properties* which relate to the properties of the substances that make up each component (bone, stainless steel, titanium). In this example, the material properties of the plate are being tested using a fracture model. The corresponding graph represents the data measured in this experiment plotted on a stress–strain graph. The force and displacement are measured and normalized to stress and strain. The initial deformation is termed *elastic* because when the load is removed, the plate will return to its original shape. This is represented by the linear portion of the graph, termed the elastic region. At some load, however, the construct becomes overloaded, entering the *plastic* range. If the load is released after loading in the plastic range but before failure, some *permanent deformation* remains in the construct. The point at which elastic behavior changes to plastic is termed the *yield point.* As previously mentioned, the slope of the stress–strain curve is the elastic (Young's) modulus.

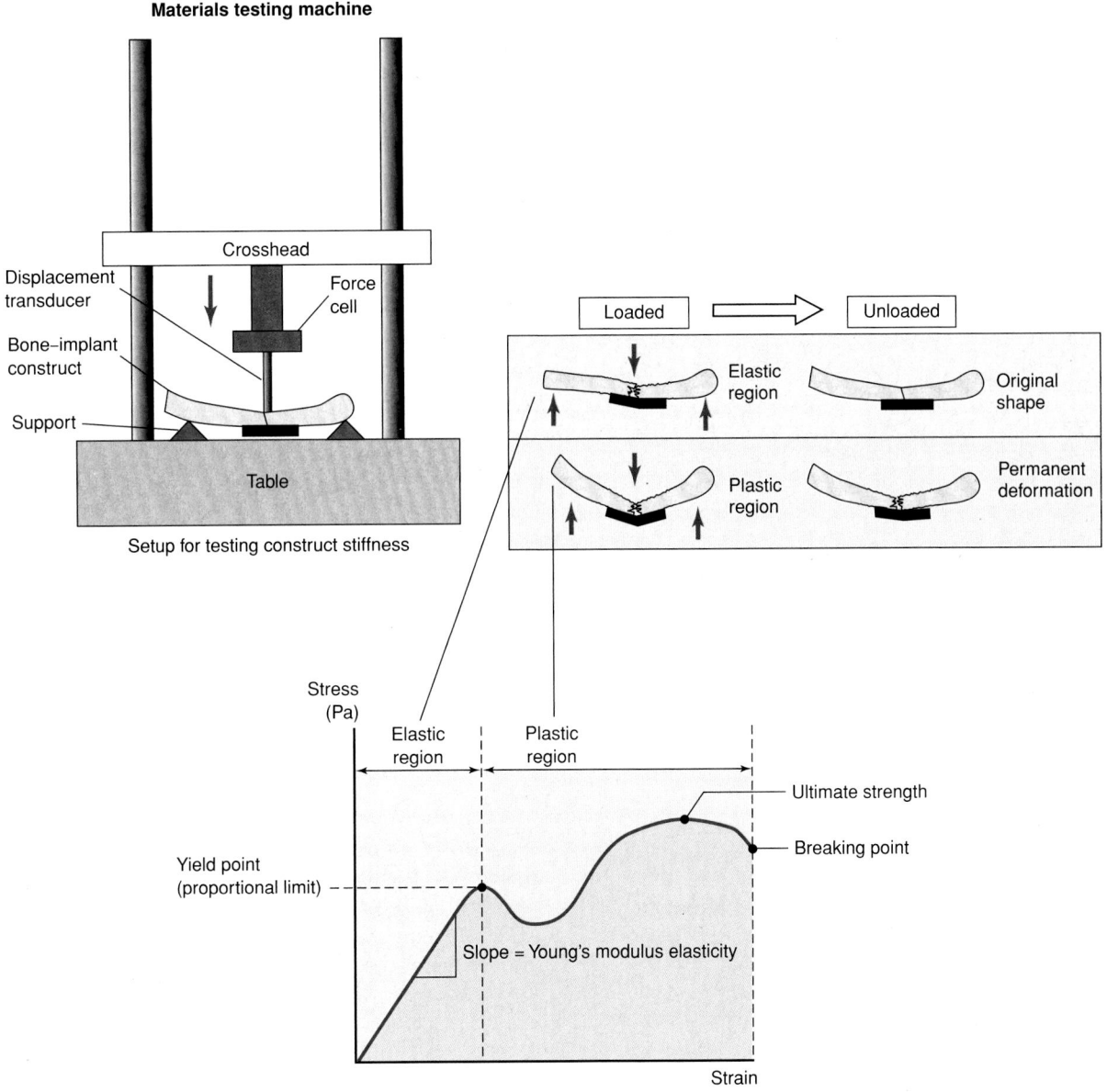

FIGURE 1-5 Top left: A fixation construct setup in a mechanical testing machine. In this example, a long bone is fixed with a plate and subjected to bending. **Top right:** The construct during loading in the elastic region and plastic region. **Bottom:** The resulting measurements from the testing machine, which measures stress and strain at the point of the applied load. The graph demonstrates the elastic region, in which the plate acts like a spring, returning to its original shape after the load is released; the plastic region, in which the plate may have permanent deformity; and the failure load, in which the plate fails. The area beneath the curve *(pink area)* is the toughness of the material, or the amount of energy that a material can absorb before failure.

The area under the stress–strain curve is termed the strain energy which is the energy absorbed. *Toughness* is the amount of energy that a material can absorb before failure.

The elastic range represents the working range for the fixation construct. In this region the plate is able to withstand the forces applied to it without losing its shape. The yield point defines the safe maximum functional load before the plate is permanently deformed. A third very important property, fatigue, will be discussed later.

Note that a fixation construct may have different yield points and stiffnesses for loads acting in different directions. An example is a half-pin external fixator construct applied to a tibia, with the pins oriented anteriorly–posteriorly. The stiffness is much greater in anterior–posterior (flexion/extension) bending than medial–lateral (varus/valgus) bending for this construct. Another property to consider is the *work done* in deforming a fixation construct. The product of the force applied and the distance the construct bends is defined as the work done, and is represented by the area under

TABLE 1-1	Basic Engineering Properties of Common Biologic and Implant Materials			
Material	Ultimate Strength Tensile (MPa)	Ultimate Strength Compressive (MPa)	Yield Strength 0.2% Offset (MPa)	Elastic Modulus (MPa)
Muscle	0.2			
Skin	8			50
Cartilage	4	10		20
Fascia	10			
Tendon	70			400
Cortical bone	100	175	80	15,000
Cancellous bone	2	3		1,000
Plaster of Paris	70	75	20	
Polyethylene	40	20	20	1,000
PTFE Teflon	25			500
Acrylic bone cement	40	80		2,000
Titanium (pure, cold worked)	500		400	100,000
Titanium (Al-4V) (alloy F 136)	900		800	100,000
Stainless steel (316 L) (annealed)	>500		>200	200,000
Stainless steel (cold worked)	>850		>700	200,000
Cobalt chrome (cast)	>450		>50	20,000
Cobalt chrome (wrought, annealed)	>300		>300	230,000
Cobalt chrome (wrought, cold work)	1,500		1,000	230,000
Super alloys (CoNiMo)	1,800		1,600	230,000

(Ultimate tensile strength or maximum force in tension, yield strength at 0.2% offset, the strength at which the strain in the material [change in length/original length] is 0.2%, a usual standard for metals, elastic modulus, or stress/strain.)

the force–displacement graph of Figure 1-4. A material may be flexible and tough (e.g., rubber, or a child's bone that deforms but is difficult to break) or stiff but brittle (e.g., glass, elderly bone), if it cannot absorb much deformation without fracturing.

The factors that govern stiffness and yield point are the material from which the fixation device is made and its shape. A construct made of higher elastic modulus materials will be stiffer (e.g., stainless steel is stiffer than titanium) (Table 1-1). The stiffness of a construct is found by dividing the force applied by the deformation that the construct exhibited. The *elastic* (or *Young's*) modulus is determined by dividing the stress applied by the resulting strain (Figs. 1-4 and 1-5). The moduli of some common orthopedic materials are given in Table 1-1. As shown, the elastic modulus of titanium alloy is about one-half that of stainless steel; so, given two plates of the same size and shape, the titanium plate has about one-half the stiffness of the stainless steel plate. This can be important to consider when using new devices made of different materials.

Another concept is how the shape and size of an implant influences the load it can support. As shown in Figure 1-6, a typical plate used in fracture fixation is wider than it is thick. Thus, the plate is actually stiffer when the load is placed against the edge rather than the broad surface of the plate. This is because when the load is applied on the edge of the plate, the material of the plate resisting the load is distributed further away from the center (note that in this example, the mate-

rial of the plate did not change, just its orientation relative to the load applied). This concept of distribution of material is reflected in the shape property, *moment of inertia*. The moment of inertia provides a measure of how the material is distributed in the cross section of the object relative to the load applied to it. The farther away the material is from the center of the beam, the greater its stiffness. Steel I-beams were developed to take advantage of this concept; that is, gaining greater stiffness for the same amount of material. For solid cylindrical objects like rods, pins, or screws, their stiffness is related to the fourth power of their radius. As shown in Figure 1-6, for rods made of the same materials, a 16-mm diameter intramedullary (IM) rod is 1.7 times as stiff as a 14-mm rod ($[8/7]^4 = 1.7$).

A third important property of a fracture fixation construct is its ability to resist *fatigue* under cyclic loading. Load can be applied that remains below the yield point of the construct, yet creates a crack that progressively grows. This lowers the yield point of the material and the local stresses will eventually exceed the yield point and the construct will fail (Fig. 1-7). Some materials have an *endurance limit* such that they can support a certain level of load indefinitely without failure. An important aspect of fatigue performance of a fixation construct is the effect of a *stress riser*. In completely uniform materials, the stresses will be almost identical throughout the material. But typical fixation devices have holes, screw threads, and other features in which the shape changes and leads to a change of

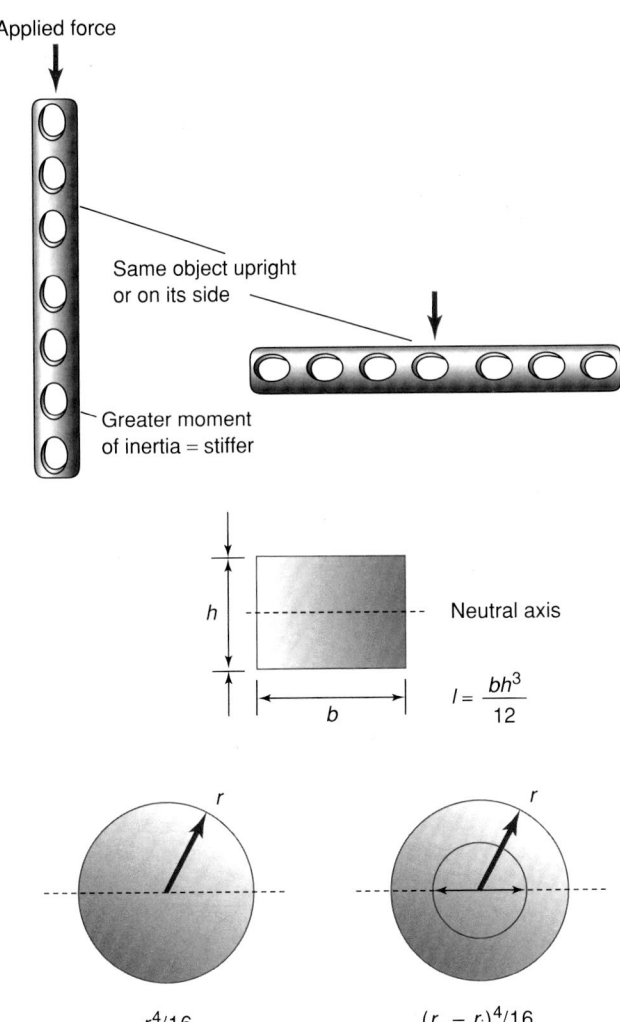

FIGURE 1-6 The concept of moment of inertia or the effect of the geometry of an object on its stiffness. **Top:** Looking at a typical plate used in fracture fixation, when the load is applied on the broader surface the plate is less stiff than when the load is applied to the narrower edge. This is because the distribution of the material is farther from the load applied. **Bottom:** The moment of inertia is a term used to describe how the material is distributed within an object. For a solid rectangular object such as a plate, the moment of inertia (I) and the stiffness increase directly with the width (b) of the plate and the cube of its height (h). For a solid cylinder, such as a pin or a screw, the moment of inertia increases with the fourth power of its radius (r). Therefore a 16-mm diameter IM rod is 1.7 times as stiff as a 14-mm rod, and 2.3 times as stiff as a 13-mm rod, if all the rods are made of the same material. For a hollow cylinder such as an intramedullary nail, the radius of the inner diameter (r_i) is subtracted from the radius of the outer diameter (r_o). The moment of inertia still increases by the fourth power.

$$I = \frac{bh^3}{12}$$

$$r^4/16 \qquad (r_o - r_i)^4/16$$

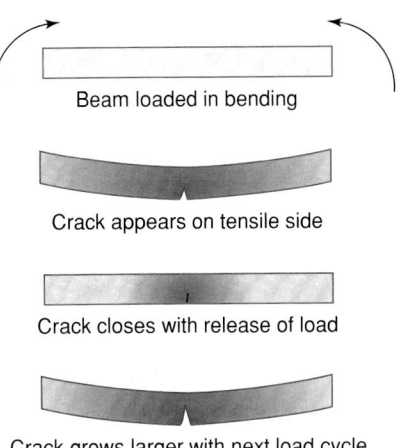

FIGURE 1-7 A stress concentrator is a region of an object in which stresses are higher than in the surrounding material. Taking the example of a fracture plate subjected to bending, the bottom surface elongates under load. In the region of highest tensile forces, a scratch starts to grow into a crack that closes when the load is released, then reopens slightly larger with the next load cycle, eventually growing to a point at which the plate fails. Crack growth is accentuated by stress corrosion, poor bone-to-bone contact at the fracture, and by loads applied by heavier patients.

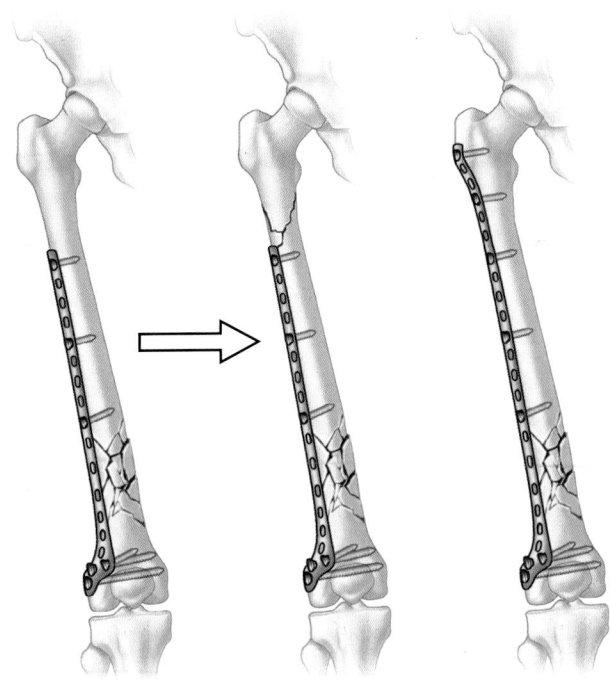

FIGURE 1-8 A stress riser at the end of a fracture construct can cause problems if it is in a region of high stress. In this example, a femoral shaft fracture is fixed using a lateral plate. If the end of the plate is in the high-stress subtrochanteric region, there is a risk that the stress riser can contribute to a periprosthetic fracture. To avoid this, a longer plate can be used to bypass the high-stress area.

the material properties. It is the transition points which create a stress riser. One must also take into account the interface at the end of a fixation construct. The end of the plate or rod creates an abrupt transition between the metal and bone creating a stress riser. Although this cannot always be avoided, placing the end of the implant in a high-stress area such as the subtrochanteric region of the femur can lead to periprosthetic fractures (Fig. 1-8). These fractures can be secondary to another

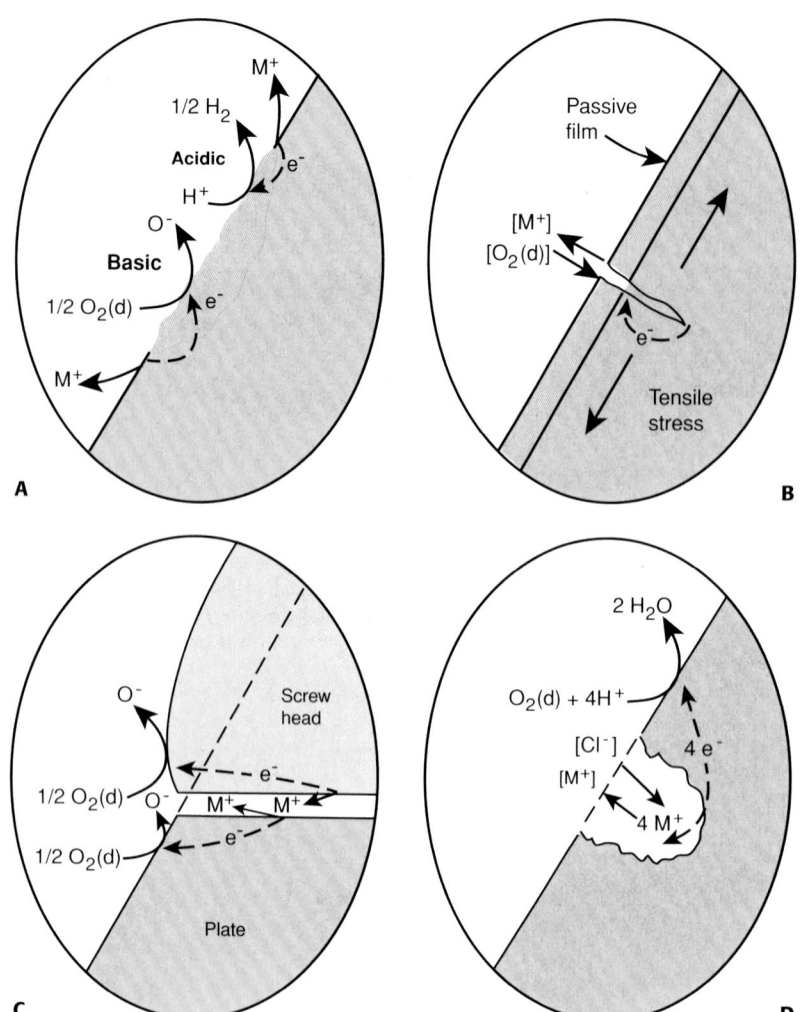

A

B

C

D

FIGURE 1-9 A: Illustration of crevice corrosion, with a local galvanic cell caused by an impurity in the surface of a plate and ions, M^+, being released, resulting in loss of material and formation of a crevice. **B:** Stress corrosion occurs by a local galvanic cell setup between the material at the tip of the crack, which just opened and has not oxidized, and the remaining oxidized surface of the plate. The released ions enhance crack growth occurring from loading. **C:** Fretting corrosion caused by the loss of the oxide layer on the surface of a plate caused by rubbing of the base of the screw against the plate. **D:** Galvanic corrosion around a scratch or pit in the plate.[26]

traumatic event or can be caused by cyclical loading and fatigue failure at the stress riser. Thus, in this situation a longer plate should be used to bypass the high-stress area, particularly in areas of poor bone quality.

A scratch can also cause a local small stress concentrator. When immersed in the saline environment of the body, *stress corrosion* can occur. Stress corrosion combines the effects of the local growth of the crack resulting from cyclic loading with galvanic corrosion. A *galvanic cell* describes a local environment in which electrons flow from the more negative to the more positive material when immersed in a liquid conductor (saline, in this case) (Fig. 1-9). Material is actually removed from the more negative electrode, such as the surface of the plate during galvanic corrosion. In a fixed fracture, the dissimilar materials are the surface of the plate (e.g., stainless steel), which creates an oxide surface coating, and the same material exposed by the fatigue crack that has not yet developed the oxide film. The conductive fluid is the blood and saline found in the surrounding tissues. Galvanic corrosion can accelerate the failure of an implant, even when the implant is loaded well below its yield point, by increasing the rate at which the crack grows. This occurs because in addition to the mechanical propagation at the

site of the crack, material at the crack is being removed by the corrosion process. Another mechanism of corrosion, termed *fretting*, results when the surfaces of two implants rub together, such as the head of a screw against the surface of the plate through which it passes. *Crevice corrosion*, which is not common in modern orthopedic materials, results from small galvanic cells formed by impurities in the surface of the implant, causing crevices as the material corrodes.[26]

Another basic property is *viscoelasticity* (Fig. 1-10). Biologic materials do not act as pure springs when load is applied to them. A spring deforms under load and then returns to its original shape when the load is released. For example, if a load is applied to a tendon, and the load is maintained for a period of time, the tissue will continue to deform or *creep*. This is the basic principle behind stretching exercises. Under a constant load, a metal fixation plate will deform and remain at that deformation until the load is removed (elastic behavior). In contrast, the tendon both deforms elastically and creeps, exhibiting both viscous and elastic behavior. This property has important implications for certain types of fixation, especially those that rely on loading of soft tissues, such as in certain types of spinal fixation (to be discussed later).

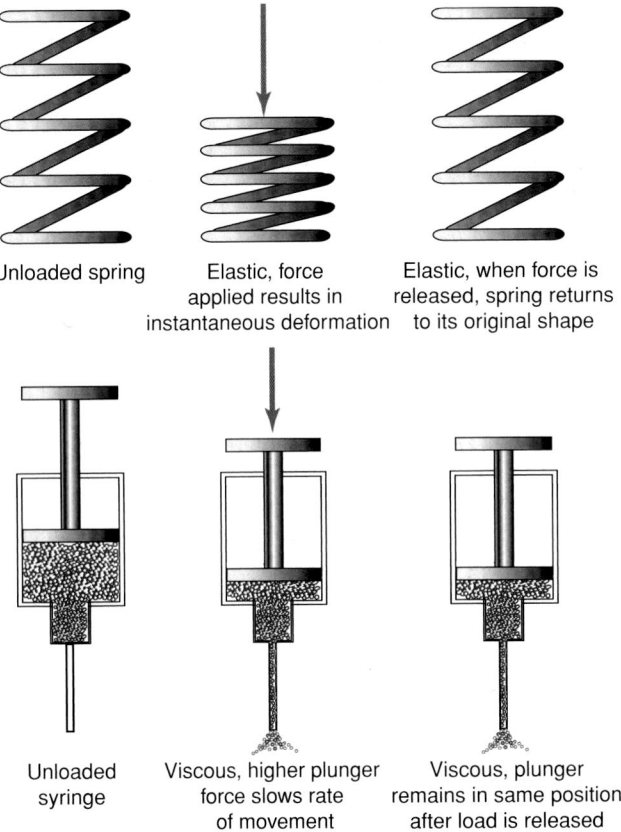

Unloaded spring   Elastic, force applied results in instantaneous deformation   Elastic, when force is released, spring returns to its original shape

Unloaded syringe   Viscous, higher plunger force slows rate of movement   Viscous, plunger remains in same position after load is released

FIGURE 1-10 Viscoelastic response in a biologic tissue can be explained by considering and combining the properties of two devices, a simple spring and a fluid-filled syringe. The elastic or spring component instantly compresses when a load is applied to it. When the load is released, the spring returns to its original shape. When a load is applied to the viscous component, represented by the syringe, fluid is forced out of the needle. If the load is released, the plunger does not return, but remains in its final position, representing the creep property of the tissue. Further, if the force is applied to the plunger more rapidly, there is greater resistance to motion, explaining the increased stiffness of tissue to increased rates of loading. Combinations of these simple components can be used to describe the mechanical properties of biologic tissues.

A second characteristic of viscoelastic behavior is *loading rate dependence*. In simple terms, stretching a soft tissue can be thought of as stretching two components, an elastic one and a viscous one, which make up that tissue. For example, consider a spring connected in series to the handle of a syringe. When a compressive force is applied, the spring instantly compresses, representing the elastic response of the tissue. The syringe plunger starts to displace and continues as it pushes fluid through the orifice. If the force is held constant, the plunger will continue to move, representing the viscous creep of the tissue. If the compressive force is applied slowly, the syringe handle offers little resistance. As the rate of force application increases, the resistance of the syringe to motion increases. This represents the increase in stiffness of the tissue at higher loading rates. Simply put, the stiffness of the tissue depends upon the rate at which the load is applied.

A well-known example of loading rate dependence relates to the failure of ligament and bone. At low loading rates, the ligament is weaker than the bone and the ligament generally fails in the midsubstance. At higher loading rates, the ligament becomes stiffer, and failure may occur by avulsion of the bony attachment of the ligament. *Stress relaxation* occurs if the applied force, instead of increasing, is held constant. As the fluid flows out of the syringe, without further movement of the plunger, the internal force decreases. These three properties—creep, stress relaxation, and load rate dependence—make up the basic tissue viscoelastic properties. It should be appreciated that the model used in this discussion is a simple linear series model, for explanation purposes only. Nevertheless, more complex models using combinations of these basic components have successfully described the observed properties of tissues. Another example of tissue viscoelasticity, besides tendon and other soft tissues, is found in trabecular bone (e.g., as found in vertebrae). In this case, the trabecular structure acts as the spring component, whereas forcing the interstitial fluid through the porous matrix as the trabeculae deform represents the viscous component. Under higher loading rates, there is resistance to flow, increasing the internal pressure and therefore the stiffness of the structure. These effects have been observed at high loading rates, such as during fracture (Fig. 1-11).[34]

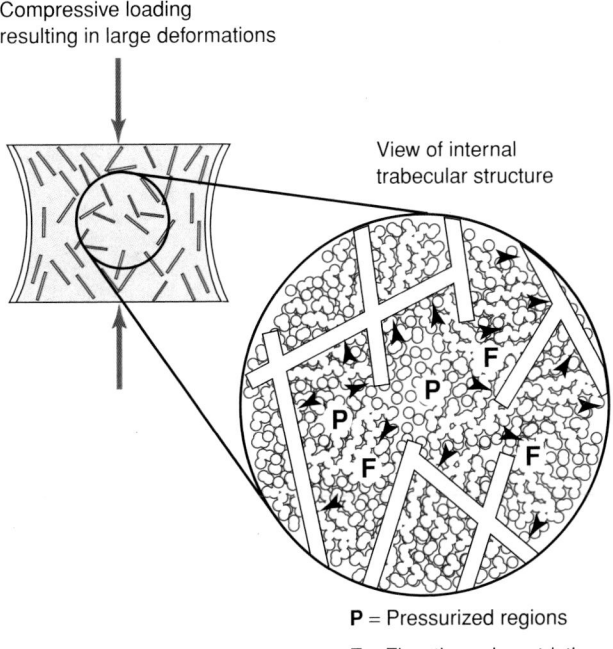

Compressive loading resulting in large deformations

View of internal trabecular structure

P = Pressurized regions

F = Flow through restrictions

FIGURE 1-11 The trabecular bone possesses some features of the spring and syringe viscoelastic model described in Figure 1-10, although it should be appreciated that this is an idealized model. The trabecular structure acts as the spring element. At higher loading rates, the interstitial fluid resists flowing through the trabecular spaces, causing increased internal pressure and greater bone stiffness. This anatomical feature allows vertebrae and the metaphyseal ends of long bones to resist dynamic loads caused by rapidly applied forces.[34]

TABLE 1-2	**Definitions of the Units Used to Describe the Basic Properties of Fracture Constructs**

Force, newtons (N) 1 N = 0.2246 lbs

Displacement, millimeters (mm)

Stress, pressure, modulus, megapascals (MPa) with 1 MPa = force of 1 N / area of 1 mm^2

Modulus = stress / strain, in which stress units are MPa; strain has no units

Strain (no units); strain = change in length (mm) / original length (mm)

In summary, bones and joints can be subjected to various forces, but these forces can be resolved into basic components that create tension, compression, shearing, twisting, and bending. These forces cause internal, compressive, tensile, and shear stresses in the tissue. The stiffness of a fixation construct used to stabilize a fracture describes how much it deforms under a given load acting in a specific direction. Stiffness may vary with direction and is highly dependent on the shape of the fixation construct. The effect of shape is described by the moment of inertia. In combination with the moment of inertia, the elastic modulus of the material describes how stiff the fixation will be under load, and its ability to withstand the forces of, for example, the patient's weight during ambulation. Failure of fixation results not only from loading above a construct's yield point but also as a result of repetitive stress. Repetitive loading can cause the growth of a crack at a stress concentrator, and can be significantly accentuated by corrosion when the implant is immersed in bodily fluids. Biologic tissues behave viscoelastically, that is, they creep under constant load, stress–relax when the elongation is fixed, and increase in stiffness as the rate of load application increases. In this chapter, these mechanical properties are described in basic units of measurements, defined in Table 1-2.

BIOMECHANICS OF INTACT AND HEALING BONE

Bone has a hierarchical structure. As shown in Figure 1-12, the lowest level of the structure consists of single collagen fibrils with embedded apatite crystals. At this level of structure, changing the collagen-to-mineral ratio has a significant effect on the elastic modulus of the bone,[32,34,41] which decreases with loss of minerals (Fig. 1-13). This is important from a fracture-healing perspective because mineralizing healing callus goes through phases of increasing mineral density and corresponding increased modulus as healing occurs. At the next level of structural organization, the orientation of the collagen fibrils is important.[9–12,57–59] As demonstrated in Figure 1-14, the orientation of its fibers affects the ability of the bone to support loads in specific directions. During fracture healing, the callus initially starts as a disorganized random array of fibers, which progressively reorganize to become stiffest along the directions of the major applied loads (body weight and muscle forces) to which the bone is exposed. At the next level, the density of the haversian systems affects bone strength. It has been repeatedly demonstrated that a power law relationship

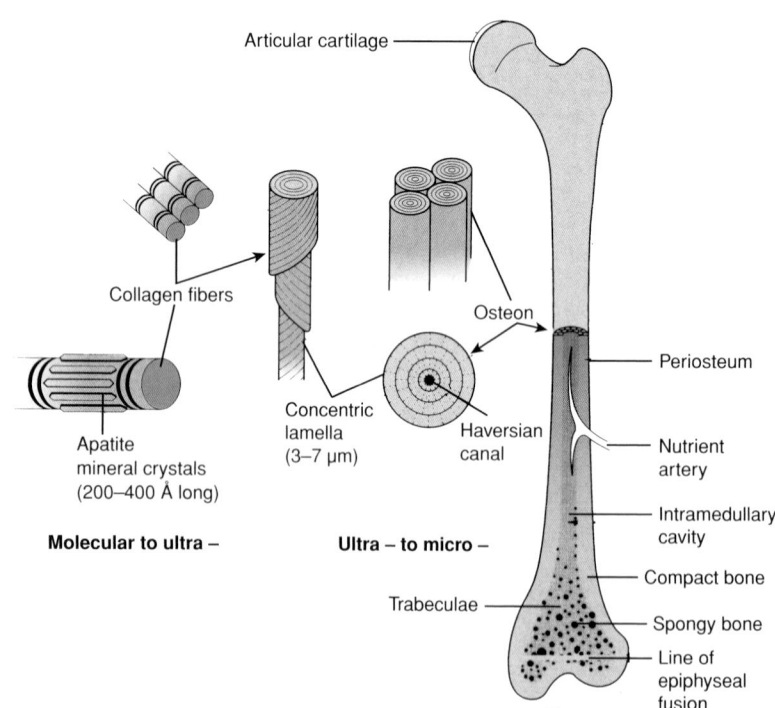

Articular cartilage

Collagen fibers

Osteon

Periosteum

Concentric lamella (3–7 μm)

Haversian canal

Nutrient artery

Apatite mineral crystals (200–400 Å long)

Molecular to ultra –

Ultra – to micro –

Intramedullary cavity

Compact bone

Trabeculae

Spongy bone

Line of epiphyseal fusion

Macro

FIGURE 1-12 The hierarchical structure of bone is demonstrated. At the lowest level of organization, the ratio of mineral crystals to collagen fibrils determines the elastic modulus of the combined material, as shown in Figure 1-13. At the next level, the fiber orientation is important in determining the difference in strength of bone in different directions. At the final level, the lamella of bone fibers form haversian systems that, particularly in cortical bone, are oriented in the direction of the major loads the bone must support.

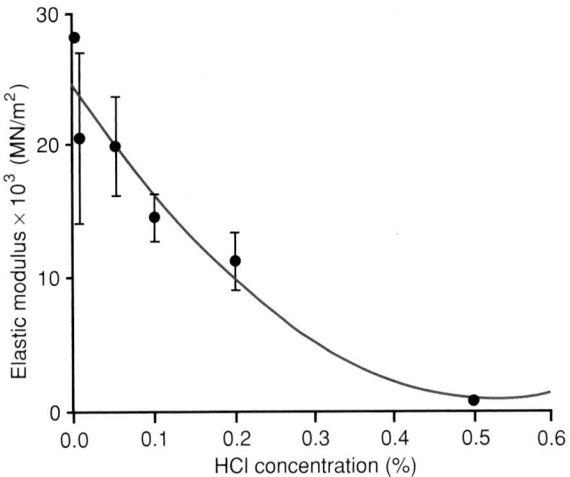

FIGURE 1-13 Elastic modulus of bone samples tested in tension after exposure to different concentrations of HCl. Greater HCl concentration progressively demineralizes bone, ultimately leaving only collagen. This diagram illustrates the contribution of bone mineral to the tensile elastic modulus of the whole bone.[32]

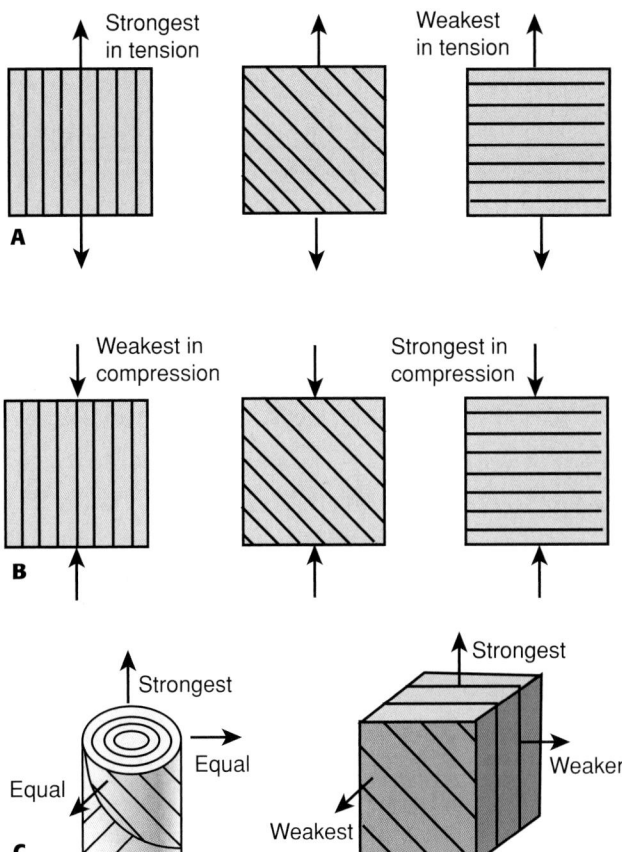

FIGURE 1-14 Effects of collagen fiber direction on the resistance to loads applied in different directions. **A:** Under tensile loading, the strongest arrangement is having the collagen fibers parallel to the load. **B:** Under compressive loading, the strongest arrangement is having the collagen fibers perpendicular to the load. **C:** In bone that must accommodate different loading directions, the arrangement of the haversian system produces one strongest direction along the axis, with approximately equal strengths in other directions.[58]

exists between bone density and strength at this level of structure (Fig. 1-15). This means that as bone density decreases, its strength decreases as the square of its density (as density decreases by half, strength decreases by a factor of four). This forms the basis for predicting changes in bone strength as a result of conditions such as osteoporosis. Similarly, the modulus changes with bone density by a power of between two and three.[20,22,31,37,64] Noninvasive measures of bone density such as quantitative computed tomography (QCT) have been shown to have a significant predictive relationship with bone strength.[2,45,46,108]

Several additional factors can affect the strength of the bone. As discussed previously, bone is a viscoelastic material

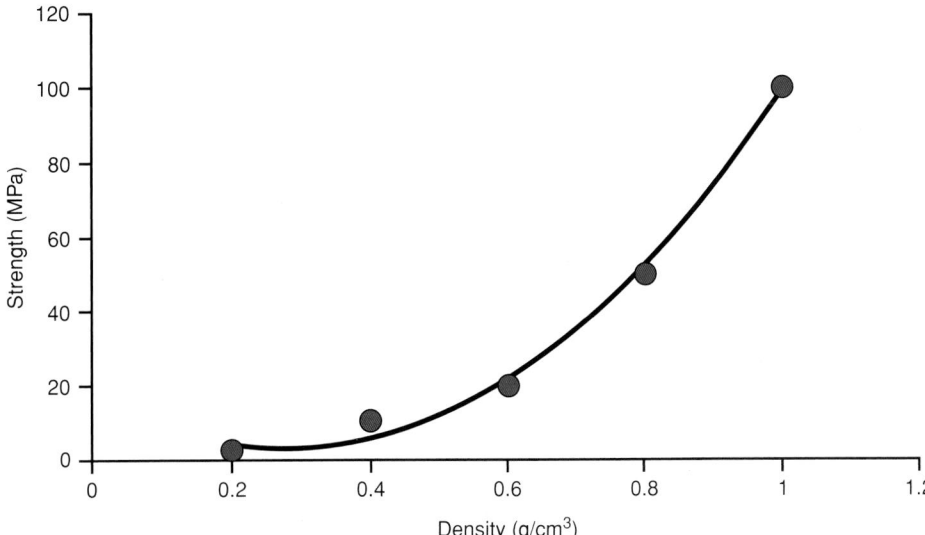

FIGURE 1-15 The relationship of trabecular bone density to compressive strength and modulus demonstrates a power law relationship, so that these properties decrease by a factor of about four when density decreases by half.[34]

whose strength and modulus both increase as loading rate increases (e.g., in fracture impact loading as compared with normal ambulation).[31,40,44,42,112,172] The geometry of bone, specifically the size of the cross section and thickness of the cortex, affects its moment of inertia and therefore its strength.[130] Age also affects bone properties. The bending strength and modulus increase as bone mineralizes and matures from childhood to adulthood and slowly decrease thereafter,[44,45,166] and the capacity to absorb impact energy decreases with age[43] as bone becomes more brittle. Defects or holes in bone (e.g., from drilling for screws) also affect its strength.[29,32,49,102,111] The torsional strength of bone decreases as the diameter of the hole or defect increases (Fig. 1-16). As the hole increases in size to 30% of the diameter of the bone, bone strength decreases

to about 50% of that of the bone without a defect. An important consideration, applicable in the resection of bone (such as in the removal of a tumor), is the shape of the hole or defect left after tumor removal. Leaving a hole with square corners significantly decreases bone strength compared with the same hole with rounded corners, because the square corner is a large stress concentrator. Oval or circular holes, although themselves still stress risers, do not contribute the additional effect of the sharp corner.[36] Table 1-3 summarizes the strength of cortical and cancellous bone material as well as the ultimate strengths of various whole bones.

As a fracture heals, its strength is affected by changes in its mineral content, callus diameter, and fiber organization, as discussed previously. The initial callus forms from the periosteal

TABLE 1-3 Mechanical Properties of Bone Material and Whole Bones in Different Loading Directions

Bone Type	Load Type	Elastic Modulus ($\times 10^9$ N/m²)	Ultimate Stress ($\times 10^6$ N/m²)	Reference
Cortical	Tension	11.4–19.1	107–146	57 58 93 172
	Compression	15.1–19.7	156–212	44
	Shear		73–82	
Cancellous	Tension	~0.2–5	~3–20	
	Compression	0.1–3	1.5–50	34 166 64
	Shear		6.6 ± 1.7	157

Bone Type	Loading Direction and Type	Ultimate Strength	Reference
Cervical spine	Axial compressive impact	980–7,400 N	93
	Extension	57 N m	
	Flexion	120 N m	
	Lateral bending	54 N m	
Lumbar spine	Axial compressive impact	1,400–9,000 N	22 37
Sacroiliac joint	Axial compressive impact	3,450–3,694 N	
Femoral neck	Lateral to medial at trochanter	1,000–4,000 N	
	Vertical impact at femoral head	725–10,570 N	2 103 155
Femur	Torsion	183 N m	
	From impact at knee along axis	6,230–17,130 N	
	Three-point bending, posterior	21.2–31.3 N m	
Patella	Impact perpendicular to anterior	6,900–10,012 N	
Tibia	Axial torsion	101 ± 35 Nm	
Foot and ankle	Impact perpendicular to sole	4,107–6,468 N	15 63

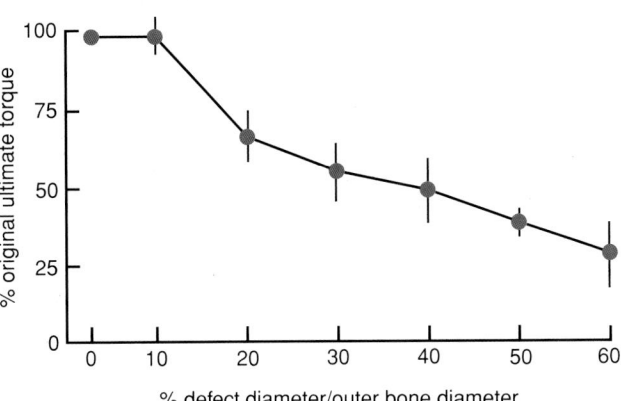

FIGURE 1-16 The relationship of ultimate torque (failure torque) of a long bone to the diameter of the hole divided by the outer diameter of the bone. There is no change in ultimate torque until the defect size increase beyond greater than 10% of the diameter of the bone.[49]

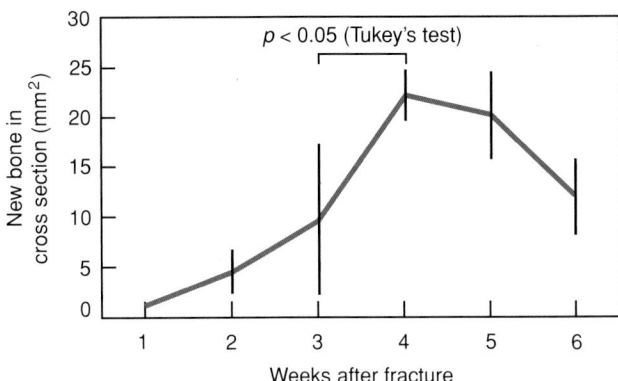

FIGURE 1-18 Changes in the cross-sectional area of a healing femoral fracture, which peaks and slowly decreases. There is a similar increase in the mineral content. (The data come from rats, which heal more rapidly than humans, indicated by the 4-week time to peak mineralization.)[8]

surface outward, which is beneficial mechanically, because as the outer diameter of the healing area enlarges, its moment of inertia and therefore its initial stiffness both increase, as shown in Figure 1-17.[128] The cross-sectional area increases progressively as shown in Figure 1-18, as does the mineral content of the callus.[8] The mechanical results of these bony changes (as the fracture heals) are shown in Figure 1-19. From torsional tests of healing rabbit long bones, progressive increases were observed in stiffness and peak torque to failure with time.[168] Interestingly,

in that experiment, the stiffness appeared to reach normal values before the peak torque to failure, showing that stiffness and strength are related, but not directly. Figure 1-19 shows that beyond 4 weeks (in rats, whose bones heal rapidly), the cross-sectional area starts to decrease as the bone remodels to normal shape, whereas the bone tissue continues to mineralize.

Age also plays a very important role in the healing of bone. Increased osteoclast activity, as well as less robust osteoid and vascular proliferation, impairs the healing process.[116]

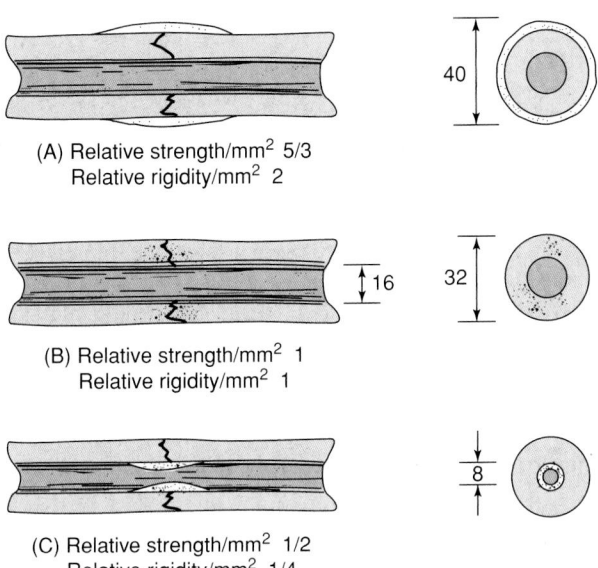

FIGURE 1-17 A comparison of the moments of inertia and resulting strengths when fracture callus is located **(A)** on the outer surface, **(B)** on the bone surfaces, or **(C)** in the medullary canal. The strength and rigidity are significantly increased when the callus is located over the periosteal surface, compared to within the medullary canal.[124]

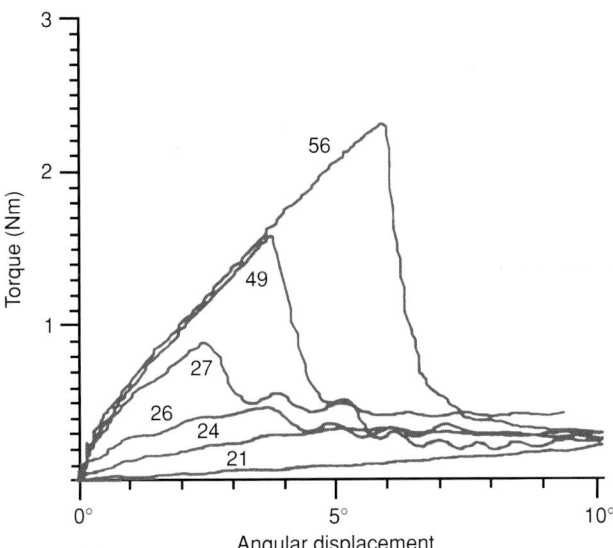

FIGURE 1-19 A comparison of superimposed torque–angular displacement plots taken from experimental long bones at different stages of healing shows the significant increase in both stiffness and peak torque to failure with increased duration of healing. Numerical values are time in days post fracture in rabbits.[168]

Although the development of modern orthopedic implants and techniques help to increase bony fixation and mechanical stiffness, which can improve healing results, the biology of aging is the main culprit.

The mechanical environment created by the fixation system along with the available blood supply affects the type of tissue formed in a healing fracture. The theory of interfragmentary strain attempts to relate the types of tissues formed to the amount of strain experienced by the tissue between the healing bone fragments.[128] This theory is a simple representation and cannot describe the complex stresses that the tissue is exposed to during actual healing. Nonetheless, within the limitations of the theory, when large strains occur in the tissues between the healing bone surfaces, granulation tissue is formed. Intermediate-level strains produce cartilage and small strains result in primary bone healing or direct deposition of bone tissue with limited callus formation.

Among the limitations of this theory, one should recognize that zero strain does not correlate with maximum bone formation. Load and some resulting strain are necessary within the healing fracture to stimulate bone formation. In a study in which controlled daily displacements in compression were applied to healing long bones using an external fixator, and the bone mineral content of the healing fracture was measured with time, there was an optimal displacement above or below which less mineral was created in the fracture callus (Fig. 1-20).[167] Furthermore, compression, rather than tension, is the preferred direction of loading.[16] Fracture fixation constructs of different stiffnesses within a certain range produce healed fractures with similar mechanical properties, although they may reach this endpoint by different biologic routes. In a study of femoral fixation using IM rods of either 5% or 50% of the torsional stiffness

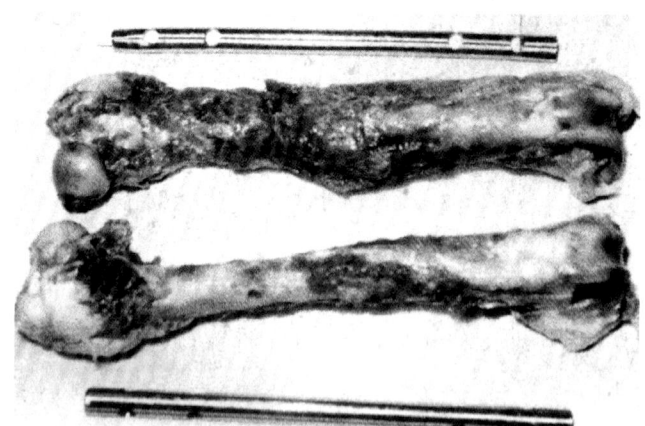

FIGURE 1-21 A comparison of the different healing responses of dog femurs with midshaft fractures fixed with **(top)** IM rods of 5%, or **(bottom)** 50% of the torsional stiffness of the intact femur. The femurs fixed with rods of lower stiffness produced more callus as additional stabilization against functional loads, but there was ultimately no difference in the mechanical properties between the femurs fixed with rods of different stiffnesses.[171]

of the intact femur, the femora fixed with the lower stiffness rods produced an abundance of stabilizing callus, as opposed to the femora with more rigid fixation; see Figure 1-21. In both cases, however, the mechanical properties of the healed fractures were ultimately similar.[171] With the development of newer implant designs and advent of locked plating the question of excessive construct stiffness has been raised. Although compression at the fracture site, coupled with rigid fixation, is desirable in the case of anatomical reduction, for comminuted fractures rigid fixation may lead to the development of non-union. The overzealous use of locking implants to combat the poor fixation in weak bone may also cause the implant–fracture construct to be too stiff for optimal healing. Finding the correct amount of stiffness of the construct, which will in turn maximize fracture healing, is still an active area of research.[27,65,66]

In summary, several factors affect the strength of bone and healing fractures. Increasing mineral content increases fracture stiffness. Callus that forms on the periosteal surface is beneficial in increasing the moment of inertia and therefore the stiffness of the fractured region. Healing fractures exhibit several stages, with the return of stiffness followed later by peak load to failure normalizing. Bone will heal within a range of mechanical environments. To a certain extent, healing bone will compensate for more flexible fixation by forming a greater quantity of fracture callus; however, there is a range of loading of a healing callus sufficient to stimulate bone formation, which increases as the callus matures.

BIOMECHANICS OF BONE FRACTURE

To appreciate why bone fractures in certain patterns, one must understand that, as shown in Table 1-3, the bone is weakest in tension and strongest in compression. Therefore, when a force creates tensile stresses in a particular region of a loaded bone, failure will generally occur first in that region. The simplest example, shown in Figure 1-22, is the transverse

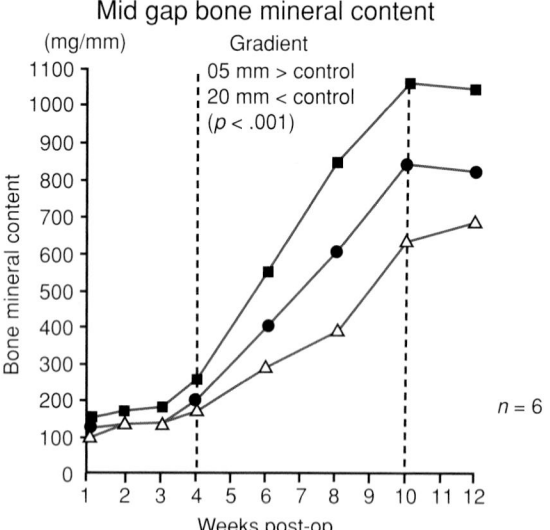

FIGURE 1-20 The effect on bone mineral of different cyclic displacements applied daily within a healing fracture (upper curve, 0.5 mm; middle curve, 1 mm; lower curve, 2 mm for 500 cycles/day). This shows that some displacement (in this experiment, 0.5 mm) stimulates bone formation, but that greater displacements (1 mm and 2 mm) do not enhance bone formation. These results point to an optimal range of displacements for maximum bone formation.[167]

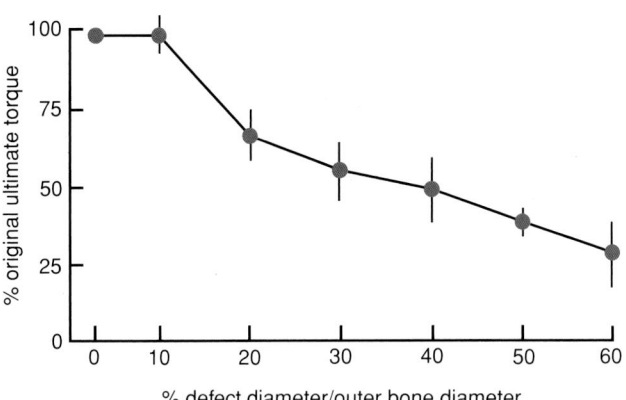

FIGURE 1-16 The relationship of ultimate torque (failure torque) of a long bone to the diameter of the hole divided by the outer diameter of the bone. There is no change in ultimate torque until the defect size increase beyond greater than 10% of the diameter of the bone.[49]

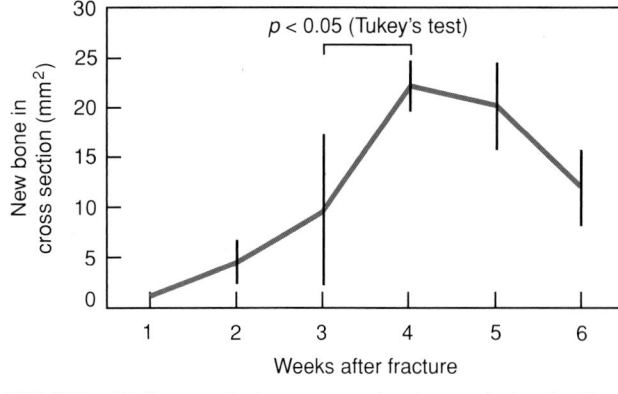

FIGURE 1-18 Changes in the cross-sectional area of a healing femoral fracture, which peaks and slowly decreases. There is a similar increase in the mineral content. (The data come from rats, which heal more rapidly than humans, indicated by the 4-week time to peak mineralization.)[8]

surface outward, which is beneficial mechanically, because as the outer diameter of the healing area enlarges, its moment of inertia and therefore its initial stiffness both increase, as shown in Figure 1-17.[128] The cross-sectional area increases progressively as shown in Figure 1-18, as does the mineral content of the callus.[8] The mechanical results of these bony changes (as the fracture heals) are shown in Figure 1-19. From torsional tests of healing rabbit long bones, progressive increases were observed in stiffness and peak torque to failure with time.[168] Interestingly,

in that experiment, the stiffness appeared to reach normal values before the peak torque to failure, showing that stiffness and strength are related, but not directly. Figure 1-19 shows that beyond 4 weeks (in rats, whose bones heal rapidly), the cross-sectional area starts to decrease as the bone remodels to normal shape, whereas the bone tissue continues to mineralize.

Age also plays a very important role in the healing of bone. Increased osteoclast activity, as well as less robust osteoid and vascular proliferation, impairs the healing process.[116]

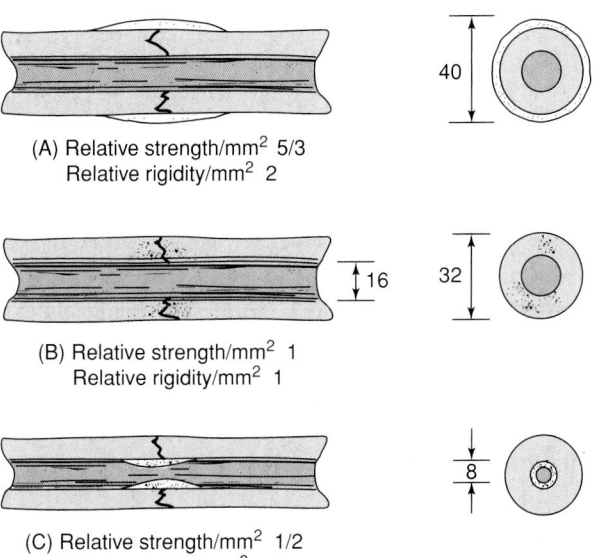

FIGURE 1-17 A comparison of the moments of inertia and resulting strengths when fracture callus is located **(A)** on the outer surface, **(B)** on the bone surfaces, or **(C)** in the medullary canal. The strength and rigidity are significantly increased when the callus is located over the periosteal surface, compared to within the medullary canal.[124]

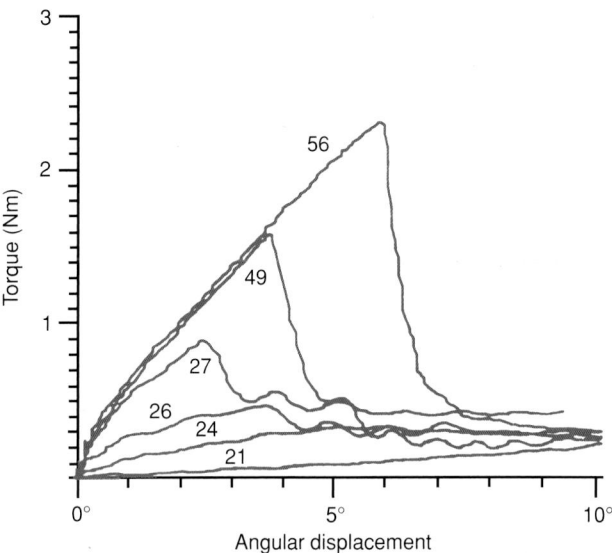

FIGURE 1-19 A comparison of superimposed torque–angular displacement plots taken from experimental long bones at different stages of healing shows the significant increase in both stiffness and peak torque to failure with increased duration of healing. Numerical values are time in days post fracture in rabbits.[168]

Although the development of modern orthopedic implants and techniques help to increase bony fixation and mechanical stiffness, which can improve healing results, the biology of aging is the main culprit.

The mechanical environment created by the fixation system along with the available blood supply affects the type of tissue formed in a healing fracture. The theory of interfragmentary strain attempts to relate the types of tissues formed to the amount of strain experienced by the tissue between the healing bone fragments.[128] This theory is a simple representation and cannot describe the complex stresses that the tissue is exposed to during actual healing. Nonetheless, within the limitations of the theory, when large strains occur in the tissues between the healing bone surfaces, granulation tissue is formed. Intermediate-level strains produce cartilage and small strains result in primary bone healing or direct deposition of bone tissue with limited callus formation.

Among the limitations of this theory, one should recognize that zero strain does not correlate with maximum bone formation. Load and some resulting strain are necessary within the healing fracture to stimulate bone formation. In a study in which controlled daily displacements in compression were applied to healing long bones using an external fixator, and the bone mineral content of the healing fracture was measured with time, there was an optimal displacement above or below which less mineral was created in the fracture callus (Fig. 1-20).[167] Furthermore, compression, rather than tension, is the preferred direction of loading.[16] Fracture fixation constructs of different stiffnesses within a certain range produce healed fractures with similar mechanical properties, although they may reach this endpoint by different biologic routes. In a study of femoral fixation using IM rods of either 5% or 50% of the torsional stiffness

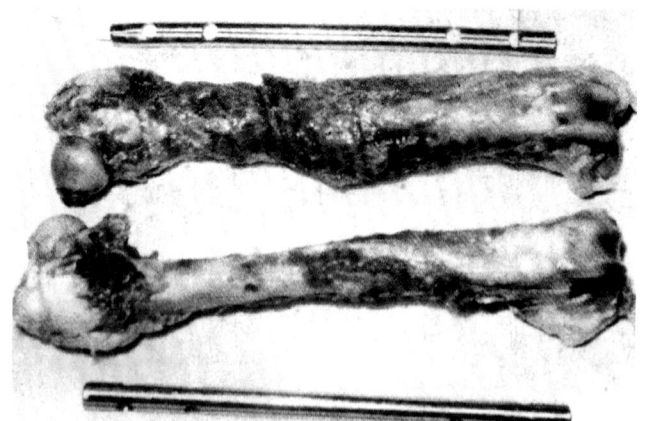

FIGURE 1-21 A comparison of the different healing responses of dog femurs with midshaft fractures fixed with **(top)** IM rods of 5%, or **(bottom)** 50% of the torsional stiffness of the intact femur. The femurs fixed with rods of lower stiffness produced more callus as additional stabilization against functional loads, but there was ultimately no difference in the mechanical properties between the femurs fixed with rods of different stiffnesses.[171]

of the intact femur, the femora fixed with the lower stiffness rods produced an abundance of stabilizing callus, as opposed to the femora with more rigid fixation; see Figure 1-21. In both cases, however, the mechanical properties of the healed fractures were ultimately similar.[171] With the development of newer implant designs and advent of locked plating the question of excessive construct stiffness has been raised. Although compression at the fracture site, coupled with rigid fixation, is desirable in the case of anatomical reduction, for comminuted fractures rigid fixation may lead to the development of nonunion. The overzealous use of locking implants to combat the poor fixation in weak bone may also cause the implant–fracture construct to be too stiff for optimal healing. Finding the correct amount of stiffness of the construct, which will in turn maximize fracture healing, is still an active area of research.[27,65,66]

In summary, several factors affect the strength of bone and healing fractures. Increasing mineral content increases fracture stiffness. Callus that forms on the periosteal surface is beneficial in increasing the moment of inertia and therefore the stiffness of the fractured region. Healing fractures exhibit several stages, with the return of stiffness followed later by peak load to failure normalizing. Bone will heal within a range of mechanical environments. To a certain extent, healing bone will compensate for more flexible fixation by forming a greater quantity of fracture callus; however, there is a range of loading of a healing callus sufficient to stimulate bone formation, which increases as the callus matures.

BIOMECHANICS OF BONE FRACTURE

To appreciate why bone fractures in certain patterns, one must understand that, as shown in Table 1-3, the bone is weakest in tension and strongest in compression. Therefore, when a force creates tensile stresses in a particular region of a loaded bone, failure will generally occur first in that region. The simplest example, shown in Figure 1-22, is the transverse

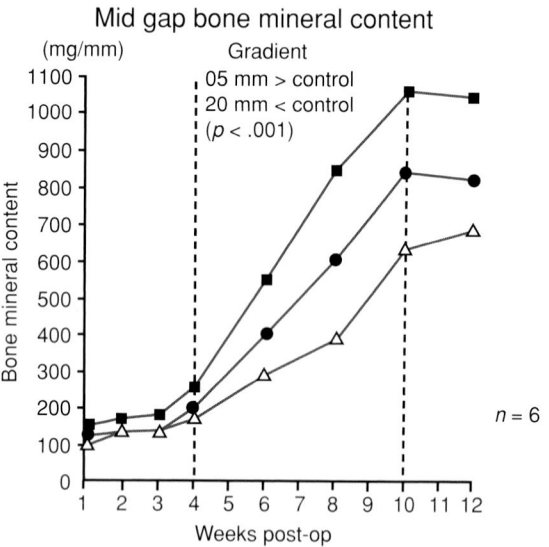

FIGURE 1-20 The effect on bone mineral of different cyclic displacements applied daily within a healing fracture (upper curve, 0.5 mm; middle curve, 1 mm; lower curve, 2 mm for 500 cycles/day). This shows that some displacement (in this experiment, 0.5 mm) stimulates bone formation, but that greater displacements (1 mm and 2 mm) do not enhance bone formation. These results point to an optimal range of displacements for maximum bone formation.[167]

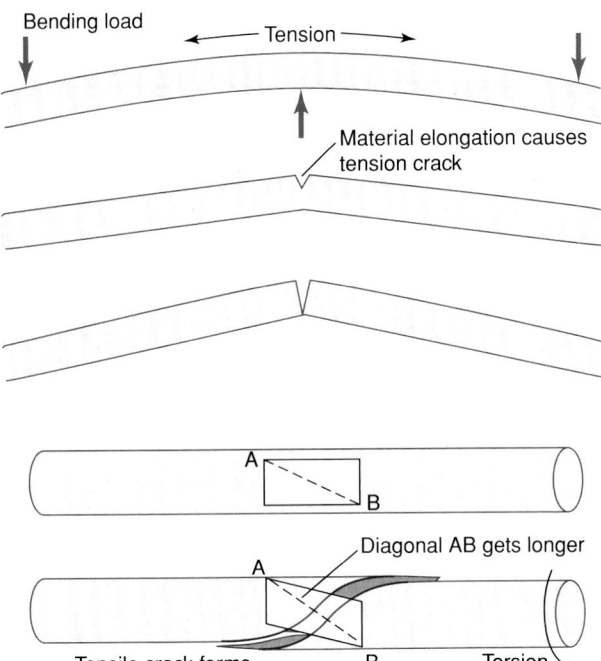

Bending load — Tension →

Material elongation causes tension crack

A / B
Diagonal AB gets longer

A
Tensile crack forms   B   Torsion

FIGURE 1-22 **Top:** A transverse fracture is created by the progressive tensile failure of bone material starting from the convex surface in which elongation, and therefore, stress is greatest, with the crack progressing to the concave side. **Bottom:** A spiral fracture is created by progressive failure in the tension of fibers on the bone surface along the diagonal that elongates as the material on the surface distorts when torque is applied. (A rectangle on the surface becomes a parallelogram, with one diagonal elongating. The fracture will be transverse to the diagonal.)

fracture created in a long bone subjected to pure bending. In this example, the upper, convex surface undergoes the greatest elongation and is subjected to the largest tensile stresses and subsequent failure, indicated by a cortical crack. The crack then progresses transversely through the material, and layers just below the outer layer become subjected to high tensile stress until they fail as well. In this manner, the crack progresses through the bone transversely until a complete fracture occurs. The concave surface is subjected to compression, so the crack does not initiate there. A second example is the fracture line or crack that occurs when a bone is subjected to torsion or axial twisting. In those cases, a spiral fracture results. Consider, as shown in Figure 1-22, a rectangular area on the surface of a long bone that is loaded in torsion. The rectangle distorts as the bone twists, with one diagonal of the rectangle elongating and the other shortening, depending on the direction of the twist. A crack will form perpendicular to the diagonal that is elongating (or under tension), and progresses around the perimeter of the bone resulting in a spiral fracture. The region of the bone with the smallest diameter is usually the least stiff region, resulting in the greatest distortion of the surface and is generally the location of the fracture. This explains why torsional fractures of the tibia often occur in the narrow distal third.

A compressive load results in the failure of cortical bone by shear, indicated by slippage along the diagonal, because

the bone is weaker in shear than in compression (Fig. 1-23). At very high loads, such as during impact fractures, crushing or comminution of bone also occurs, especially at the weaker metaphyseal ends of a long bone. The trabecular bone at the metaphyseal ends is weaker in compression than the diaphyseal cortical bone is in shear. Because of this, it is unlikely that shearing failure will occur in the diaphysis caused by pure compressive forces. The butterfly fracture (Fig. 1-23) results from combined bending and compression. Bending load causes the fracture to start to fail in tension producing a transverse crack, but as the crack progresses and the remaining intact bone weakens, it starts to fail in compression, causing an oblique (shear) fracture line. As the ends of the failing bone are driven together, a third fragment—the butterfly—may result as the oblique fragment splits off. The production of a butterfly fragment probably depends on the timing and magnitude of the two basic applied loads: compression and bending.

Aging, especially with osteoporotic changes, alters both the force required to fracture the bone and the types of fractures that occur. As shown in Figure 1-15, trabecular bone's stiffness varies with the cube (third power) of its density and its strength approximately with the square of its density.[34] Bone mass normally peaks around age 25 to 30 years and decreases up to 1% annually thereafter. If the density of the trabecular bone is decreased by 30% in a 60- to 70-year-old as a result of osteoporosis, the bone compressive strength is about half of that of a 30-year-old. Typically, fractures as a result of osteoporosis occur in the vertebrae, the distal radius, and the femoral neck. In addition, osteoporosis changes the cross-sectional shape of long bones, decreasing the thickness by increasing the endosteal diameter while causing the periosteal diameter to increase. If cortical outer diameter—for example, in the femur—increased and cortical thickness decreased at the same rate, the moment of inertia of the bone cross section would be larger. That is why large-diameter thin tubing can be substituted for smaller-diameter thicker tubing in structures (e.g., sailboat masts), saving weight, while not sacrificing strength. However, in the femur, the inner surface of the cortex also becomes more irregular and porous, decreasing its material strength. A common result of loss of femoral bone mass combined with other factors, such as poor balance, is a hip fracture (usually resulting from a fall).[1]

Auto crashes are a common cause of high-energy fractures, and some particular mechanisms have been observed over time. Fracture of the calcaneus, talus, or pilon can occur through a combination of the foot being forced against the brake pedal by the weight of the occupant during a high-speed frontal collision, or in combination with the floor pan of the auto crushing into the space in which the foot resides.[134] Drivers who were braking during a crash were shown to be much more likely to injure their right foot compared with their left foot.[15] If the Achilles tendon applies load to resist the forced dorsiflexion of the foot on the brake pedal, the combination of these two loads may cause three-point bending loading of the calcaneus, with the posterior facet of the talus as the fulcrum. A crack initiates on the plantar or tensile side of the calcaneus and a tongue-type calcaneus fracture can occur. Inversion or eversion, in which

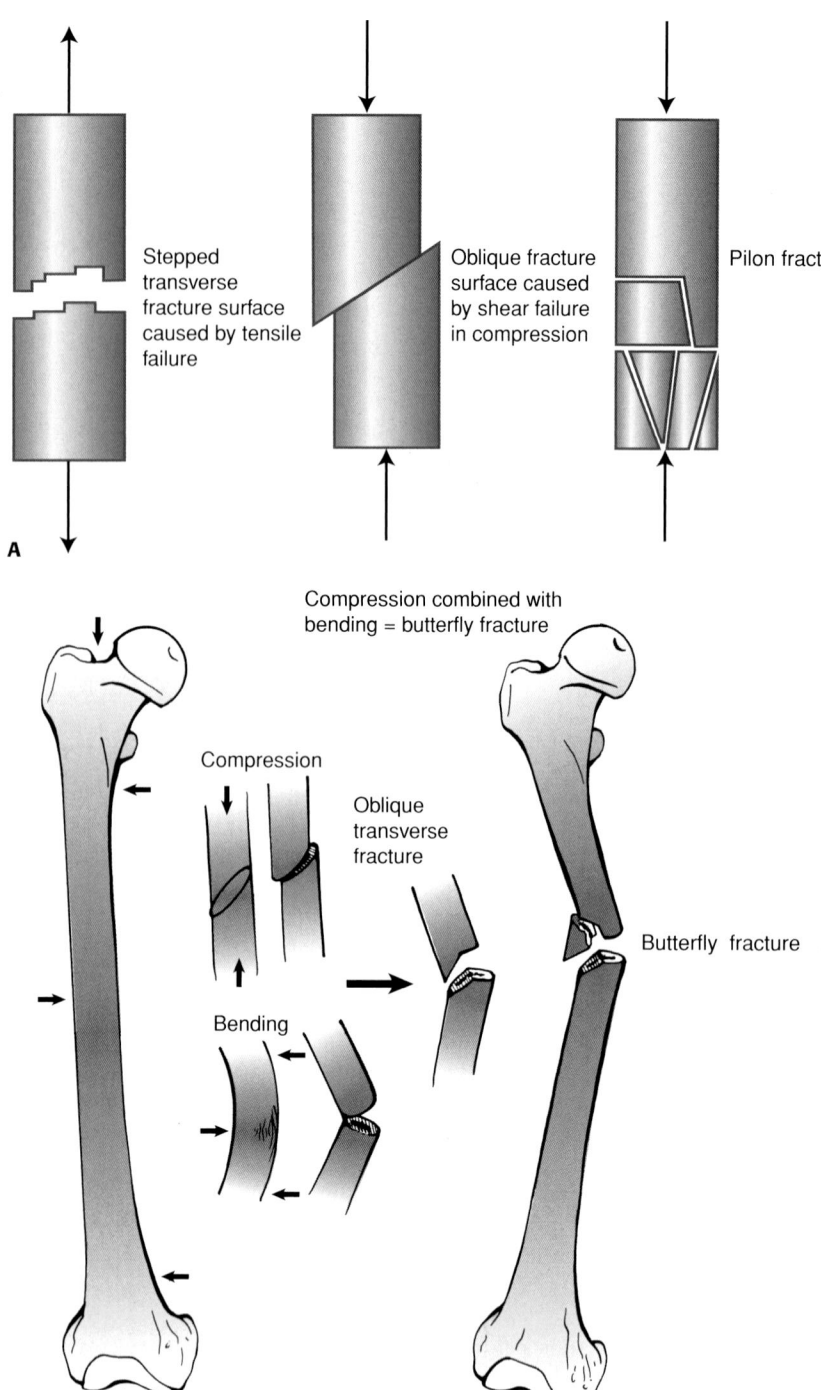

FIGURE 1-23 **A: Left:** Tensile fracture causes a stepped surface as fibers pull apart. The crack progresses, then steps to an adjacent region in which failure continues. **Right:** Pure compression of cortical bone results in failure by shearing or sliding along oblique surfaces. In reality, pure compression of a long bone (e.g., in a fall) results in crushing of the much weaker metaphyseal trabecular bone, such as with a tibial pilon or plateau fracture. **B:** Some fractures that combine bending and compression demonstrate transverse cracking as a result of bending followed by an oblique crack characteristic of compressive failure. The butterfly fracture with additional splitting of the fragment secondary to the initial fracture is an example.

the foot is not securely planted on the brake pedal and rotates with compression, is likely to result in a malleolar fracture,[63] although the combinations of forces causing these high-energy fractures are not entirely predictable.

A major mechanism of midshaft femur fractures is impact with the dashboard of the vehicle in a frontal collision, especially for unrestrained drivers who submarine or slide forward in the seat.[163] Tensing the quadriceps and hamstrings muscles during a crash applies significant additional compression along the femur.[163] The anterior bow of the femur causes the external compressive force from contact of the knee with the dashboard, and internal muscle forces bend the femur, resulting in bending and transverse or oblique fractures. If the femur of the occupant hits the dashboard in an adducted orientation, the femur can be displaced from the acetabulum, causing a fracture of the posterior wall of the acetabulum and dislocation of the hip joint. Pelvic fractures can result from loading in side-impact crashes, in which the door punches inward against the hip and pelvis. The actual fracture pattern of the posterior pelvis (sacrum, sacroiliac joint, or both) is probably the result of the specific alignment of the pelvis with the applied loads at impact. Some pelvic fracture classifications are based on the presumed mechanism of injury and specific forces applied.[147,148,175,176] Bilateral hip fractures have been found to occur in crashes in which the vehicle has a large center console that tends to trap the pelvis as force is also applied on the hip opposite that which contacts the door. Upper extremity injuries in auto crashes have been found to be related to airbag deployment and entrapment of the arm in the steering wheel.[70]

BIOMECHANICS OF FRACTURE IMPLANTS

Avoiding Mechanical Problems with Fracture Fixation Devices

When fracture implants fail prior to fracture union, a variety of underlying problems may be present, but in general, they can be divided into one of two categories: biologic or mechanical. Biologic causes of delayed union and fixation failure may be related to the patient's systemic biology, such as smoking, chronic diseases such as diabetes, medications such as steroids, and many other causes. Although some biologic etiologies of fixation failure are only minimally under the surgeon's control, others can be directly affected by the physician. The surgeon should make every effort to preserve soft tissue, respect the zone of injury, and preserve vascularity. Meticulous surgical technique, wound closure, and appropriate perioperative antibiotic therapy can all reduce the risk of infection and decrease the risk of treatment failure. When failure occurs acutely or prior to the expected time that fracture healing would occur, a mechanical issue is usually the primary culprit. Understanding the mechanical principles underlying stable fixation and fixation failure can help the surgeon determine the appropriate investigation and intervention.[67]

Screw Breakage by Shearing During Insertion

A screw is a mechanical device that is used to convert rotary load (torque) into compression between a plate and a bone or between bone fragments. The basic components of a screw are shown in Figure 1-24. As shown in Figure 1-25, the thread of a screw, if unwound from the shaft, is really a ramp or inclined plane that pulls the underlying bone toward the fixation plate, causing compression between them.[129] To achieve this effect, the screw head and shaft should be free to turn in the plate; otherwise, the compressive force generated may be limited (Fig. 1-26). Locking screws thread into the plate holes, and although this fixed interface can be beneficial in certain clinical circumstances, it precludes compression between the plate and the bone.

Tapping is necessary in cortical bone so that the torque applied by the surgeon is converted into compression instead of cutting threads and overcoming friction between the screw thread and the bone (F_t in Figure 1-25) that it is being driven into (Fig. 1-27).[80] In some cases such as screw insertion into dense bone or the insertion of smaller diameter screws, the use of a separate tap followed by screw insertion can facilitate screw advancement into the bone. Most modern screw designs have self-tapping screw tips that cut the path for the threads as the

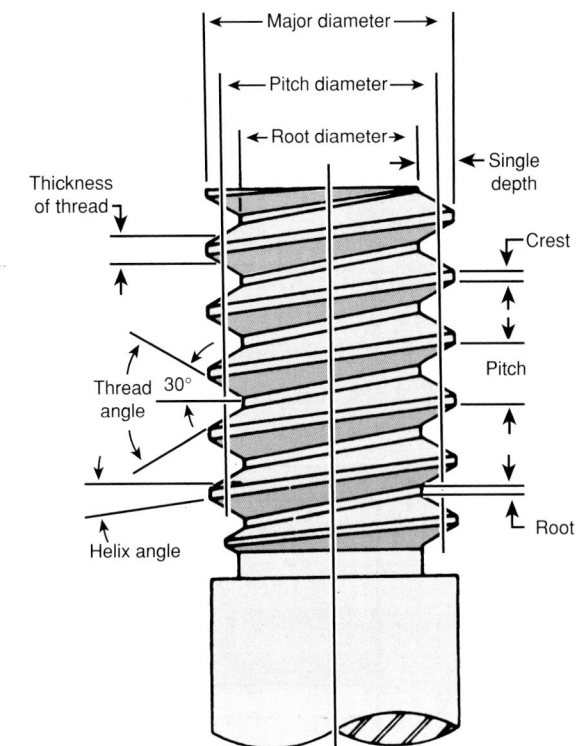

FIGURE 1-24 Nomenclature of screws. The root diameter is the inner diameter of the screw and the pitch defines the distance between threads.

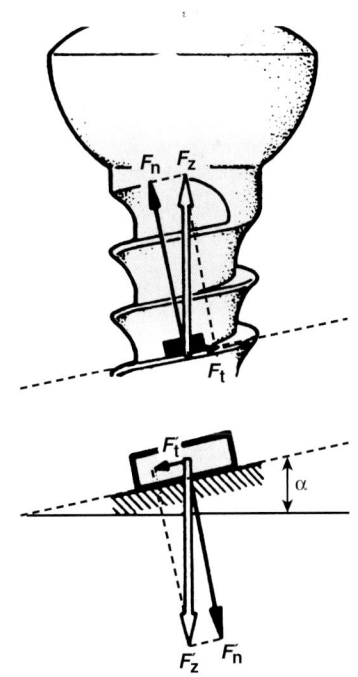

FIGURE 1-25 A screw is a mechanical device that converts torque into compression between objects. The screw thread is actually an inclined plane that slowly pulls the objects it is embedded into together. (F_n, normal or compressive force acting against the screw head; F_t, tangential or frictional force acting along the screw thread; F_z, resultant of the two forces; α, angle of the screw thread. The smaller the angle α [finer thread] the lower the frictional force.)

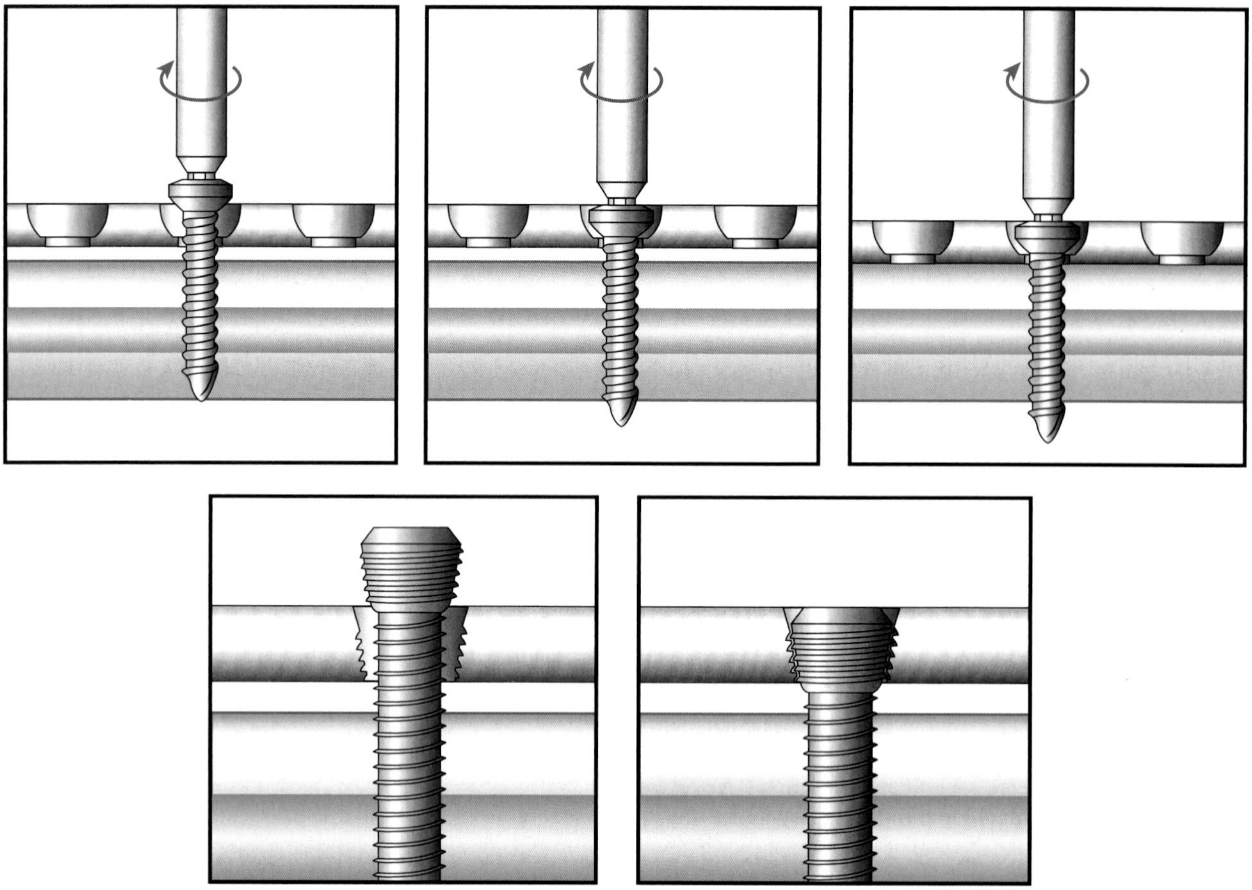

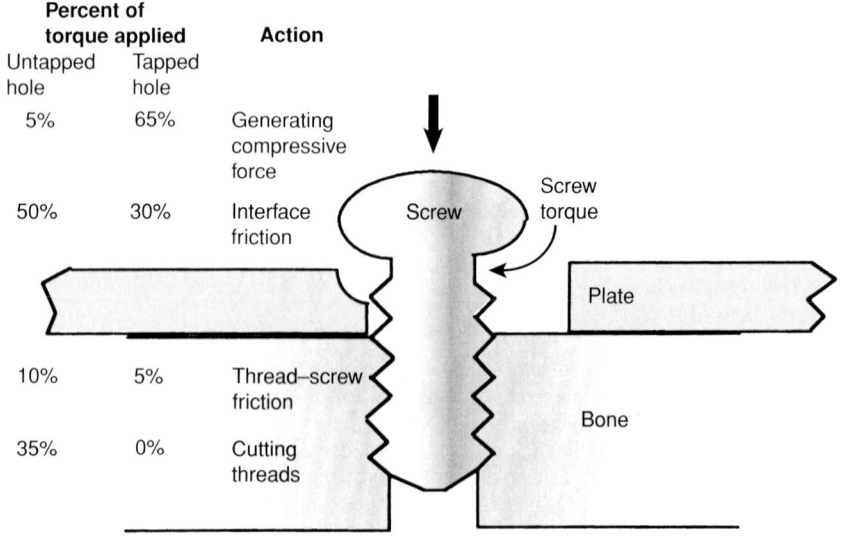

FIGURE 1-26 A comparison of cortical and locking screws. **Top:** Compression screw. As the screw is inserted, the head of the screw is free to rotate within the plate hole and thus allows for compression of the plate to the bone as the screw threads continue to drive the screw deeper into the bone. **Bottom:** Locking screw. As the screw is driven into the bone, the threads in the head of the screw engage and become fully threaded into the plate. Thus the screw is unable to apply a compression force to pull the plate and bone together.

Percent of torque applied

Untapped hole	Tapped hole	Action
5%	65%	Generating compressive force
50%	30%	Interface friction
10%	5%	Thread–screw friction
35%	0%	Cutting threads

Screw

Screw torque

Plate

Bone

FIGURE 1-27 Schematic diagram showing the approximate distribution of torque acting on a screw placed into cortical bone. With a pre-tapped hole, about 65% of the applied torque goes to produce compression and 35% to overcome the friction associated with driving the screw. When the hole is not tapped, only about 5% of the torque is used to produce compression, the rest going to overcome friction and to cut threads in bone. These observations do not apply in cancellous bone.

screw is inserted. Screws with multiple cutting flutes at the tip of the screw appeared to be the easiest to insert and had greater holding power.[174] Tapping is less advantageous in cancellous bone as it may decrease the pull-out strength of the screw in cancellous bone.[157] In some cases, tapping the cancellous bone may be beneficial. A clinical example would be when treating femoral neck fractures in a physiologically older patient versus a younger patient; one may need to use a tap to create the threads in the denser bone of a younger patient. The reason to use the tap in the dense bone is to prevent the frictional forces causing rotation of the femoral head during screw insertion with resulting malreduction. In particularly hard bones the frictional forces become so great that it becomes difficult to advance the screw.

One problem during screw placement is shear failure of the screw, typically the head twisting off, leaving the shaft embedded in bone and difficult to remove. This can occur especially when not using a tap before insertion, or when inserting smaller (less than 4-mm diameter) screws in dense bone. The stiffness and strength of a screw are related to the fourth power of its radius (the effect of moment of inertia for screws of the same material). A 6-mm diameter screw is approximately five times as stiff as a 3-mm diameter screw and 16 times as resistant to shear failure by overtorquing the screw during insertion. The junction of the screw head and threaded portion of the screw is a transition point in shape and size. Therefore, it acts as a stress concentrator and is usually the location of the screw breakage.

Screw Pullout

Particularly in cancellous bone, the maximum force that a screw can withstand along its axis, the pullout force, depends upon the size of the screw and the density of the bone it is placed into. As shown in Figure 1-28, when the force acting on the screw exceeds its pullout strength, the screw will pull or "strip" out of the hole, carrying the sheared bone within its threads, greatly decreasing the holding power and fixation strength. The pullout force increases with larger screw diameter, a greater number of threads per unit length, a longer embedded length of screw shaft, and a greater density of the bone it is placed into.[35,47,59,142] The diameter and length of the embedded screw can be thought of as defining the outer surface of a cylinder along which the screw shears. Given a maximum stress that bone of a particular density can withstand, increasing the surface area of the screw cylinder increases the pullout force (because force = stress multiplied by the area over which it acts). To enhance screw purchase, consider embedding the largest-diameter screw possible into the bone of the greatest density over as long a purchase length as possible.[35,47] Clinically, however, there are downsides to placing the largest-diameter screw possible. Larger screws can occupy a large volume in small fracture fragments, limit the number of fixation sites possible, and propagate adjacent fracture lines.

In cancellous bone, screw pullout becomes a more significant problem because the porosity of cancellous bone reduces its density and therefore its shear strength.[157] Hole preparation, specifically drilling, but not tapping, improves the pullout strength of screws placed into cancellous bone (such as pedicle screws in the vertebral body).[35] The reason that tapping reduces strength in cancellous bone, as shown in Figure 1-29,

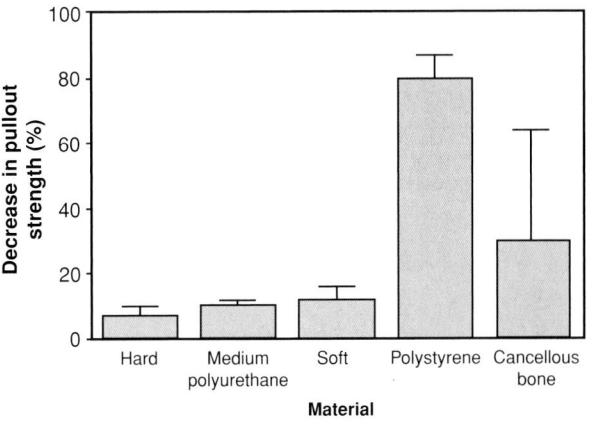

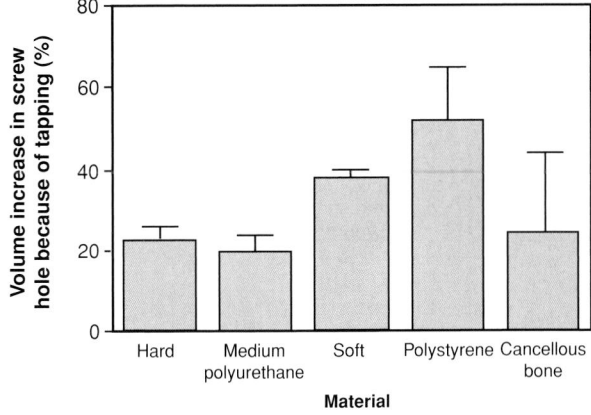

FIGURE 1-29 **Top:** The decrease in pullout strength in various types of foam used to test bone screws demonstrating the percentage decrease in pullout strength between screws placed into holes that were either drilled only or drilled and tapped. **Bottom:** The percentage increase in volume comparing holes that were drilled only and those that were drilled and tapped. Tapping in cancellous bone increases hole volume, which decreases pullout strength.[35]

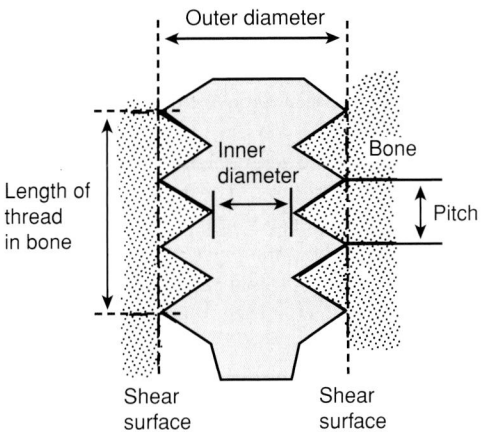

FIGURE 1-28 The factors that determine the pullout strength of a screw are its outer diameter and length of engagement (this defines the dimensions of a cylinder of bone that is carried in the threads and is sheared out as the screw is pulled out of bone) and the shear strength of bone at the screw–bone interface, which is directly related to its density. A finer pitch screw produces a small gain in purchase.[35]

is that running the tap in and out of the hole removes the bone, effectively increasing the diameter of the hole and reducing the amount of bone material that interacts with the screw threads. Tapping has a more detrimental effect as bone density decreases and can reduce the pullout strength from 8% to 27%.[35] Pullout strength can also be related to the time after insertion. As the bone heals, it can remodel around the screw, potentially doubling its initial pullout strength.[142]

Recent research has focused on whether pullout strength is an appropriate measure of screw performance in cancellous bone.[131] In a nonlocking plate and screw construct, much of the stability of the construct is from the friction generated from compression between the plate and the bone. As a screw is inserted into the bone, if it is able to generate high values of insertional torque, this will result in increased compression of the plate to the bone and increased stability. As the maximum insertional torque is reached and then exceeded, the screw will then "strip out" and lose its purchase in the bone. Although a relationship exists between maximum insertional torque, screw pitch, and compression forces, in this study, pullout strength was found to have no correlation with either the maximum insertional torque or screw pitch. Thus, this may be a better way to measure screw performance and optimize screw characteristics.

Screw Breakage by Cyclic Loading

Once screws are successfully inserted and the construct is finalized, screws become subject to cyclic bending forces as the patient begins to mobilize (Fig. 1-30). Ideally, a nonlocking screw is initially tightened against the plate to achieve the maximal torque possible, which is converted to the maximal

compressive force between the plate and the bone (Fig. 1-27). The screw holds the plate against the bone partly by frictional contact, which depends on the frictional force generated between the undersurface of the plate and the bone. The frictional force is directly dependent on the compressive force generated by the screws. If any sliding occurs between the plate and the bone, the bending load will be transferred from the head of the screw into the plate, where screw–plate contact occurs. Bending loads perpendicular to the axis of the screw, along with possible stress corrosion and fretting corrosion, may cause the screws to fail rapidly in fatigue. Zand et al.[177] showed that screws tightened against a plate with 10% to 15% less than the maximum force failed in less than 1,000 loading cycles by bending fatigue, compared with fully tightened screws that were able to sustain over 2.5 million loading cycles. This emphasizes the clinical importance of ensuring screw tightness during plate fixation.

Screws that lock into the plate reduce this problem as it is less subjective when threaded screw heads are fully tightened into the plate hole. Small-fragment screws (3.5- to 4-mm outer diameter) can fatigue because their core diameters are small. The trade-off in the use of locking screws is that a screw with a larger core diameter and shallower thread reduces the possibility of fatigue failure, but a smaller core diameter and deeper thread can increase purchase strength in the bone.[117] Screws with smaller core diameters fatigue and fail more rapidly than screws with larger diameters. The fatigue strength of the screw must be weighed against the purchase power of the screw as well as the size of the screw in relation to the size of the bone fragment. In some cases the decision must be made between a screw with a large core diameter with shallower thread, which maximizes fatigue strength or a smaller core diameter screw with deeper threads, which maximizes purchase power.

Cannulated screws are used for fixation when the insertion of a guide wire is helpful to guide the future path of the screw. However, drilling precision for the guide wire is decreased with increasing density of bone and the use of longer- and smaller-diameter guide wires.[79] Cannulated screws follow the same mechanical principles as solid screws, but material must be removed from the center of the screw to accommodate the channel for the guide wire. Manufacturers commonly increase the core diameter (the diameter of the screw at the base of the thread) to accommodate for the loss of this central material. The same-size cannulated screws usually have less thread depth compared with solid screws. The result—depending on the screw size—is less pullout strength. For 4-mm diameter screws, cannulated screws of the same outside diameter had about 16% less pullout strength.[160] Alternatively, to keep the same thread depth, the outer diameter of the screw may be increased. An additional consideration is that cannulated screws are significantly more expensive than solid screws.

Fully Threaded Lag Screws

The lag screw is a very effective device for generating large compressive forces across fracture fragments and the fracture site. The head and upper part of the shaft of the screw must be allowed to glide in the near fracture fragment so that it pulls the far fracture fragment toward it to create compression across

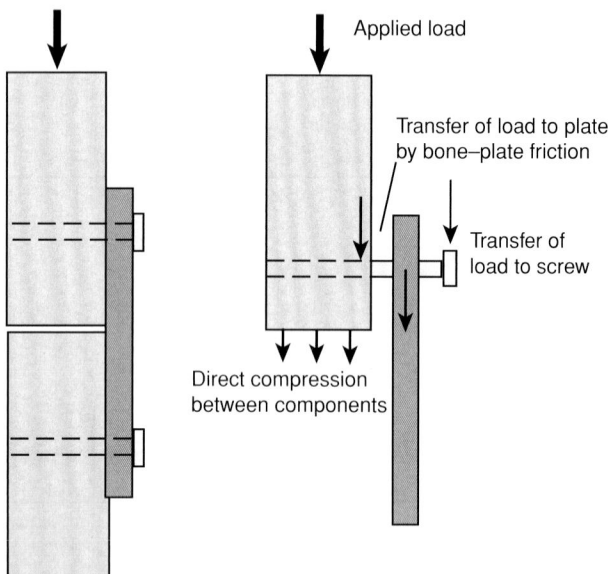

FIGURE 1-30 A mechanism for rapid failure of screws in cyclic bending occurs when the screw has not been tightened sufficiently to keep the plate from sliding along the bone surface (the plate–bone gap shown here is exaggerated for clarity). The result is that bending loads are applied transverse to the long axis of the screw, which in combination with fretting corrosion caused by the screws rubbing against the plate results in early failure of the screw.

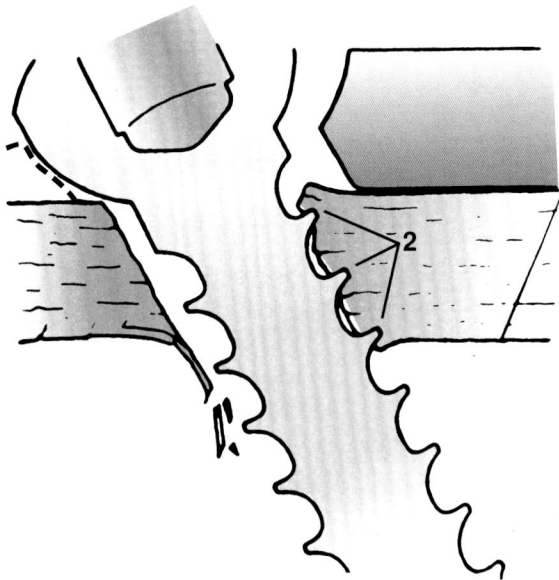

FIGURE 1-31 Using a fully threaded lag screw causes the threads to engage in bone on both sides of the fracture. This inhibits the screw from compressing the bone fragments together.[91]

the fracture surface. As shown in Figure 1-31, a fully threaded lag screw can block the gliding action between the two fracture fragments. Comparing the compressive forces across the fracture site using fully and partly threaded lag screws demonstrated that the average compressive force at the opposite cortex (i.e., the force in the screw itself) was about 50% greater when a partly threaded screw was used.[91]

Breakage of Fracture Fixation Plates

Fracture fixation plates can be used for several different functions, depending on how they are applied. One common application is for use as a "compression plate" in an attempt to achieve rigid stability. In this mode, the fracture fragments are driven together, compressing them. This is beneficial to fracture healing because it improves stability, allows primary

bone healing with minimal callus formation, and enhances the resistance of the plate to bending fatigue failure. Observing the cross section of an oval hole in a dynamic compression fracture plate, Figure 1-32 shows that one border of the hole actually has a cup-shaped inclined surface. When the head of the screw advances downward toward the bone surface, the screw and the fragment of bone it is attached to slide toward the center of the plate. This action, which occurs in both fracture components, causes the fracture surfaces to be driven together[4] and creates significant compressive forces across the ends of the fracture.[39] Compressing the ends of the fracture significantly improves the stability of the construct and reduces bending and torsional stresses applied to the plate, increasing its durability. Stability is improved because the bone ends resist bending forces that close the fracture gap, and torsional loads are resisted by the frictional force and interlock between the ends of the fracture components. Also, the fracture gap that must be healed is smaller.

It is important to appreciate that the plate is vulnerable to bending failure, because plates are relatively thin and easy to bend (compared with bone), and have low moments of inertia. When used to apply compressive force to the ends of the fracture, the stabilized bone can then resist the bending loads applied during functional use. If a gap is left on the side opposite the plate (Fig. 1-33), as when a bridge plating technique is used, the fracture site can become a fulcrum around which the plate bends under combined compressive and bending loads such as those which occur with axial loads. Gapping can also occur when a segment of bone is missing at the fracture site, or if the plate is not properly contoured during application. Figure 1-34 demonstrates how a flat, noncontoured plate tightened against a flat bone surface will cause a gap to appear on the opposite cortex.[124] This is why a plate should be slightly overcontoured to create an initial gap between it and the bone surface it will be applied to.[73,125,143] Gapping at the fracture also occurs when the plate is applied to the predominantly compressive side instead of the tensile side of a long bone during functional loading that causes bending. Figure 1-35 demonstrates that placing the plate on the compressive side will cause a gap to open under load.

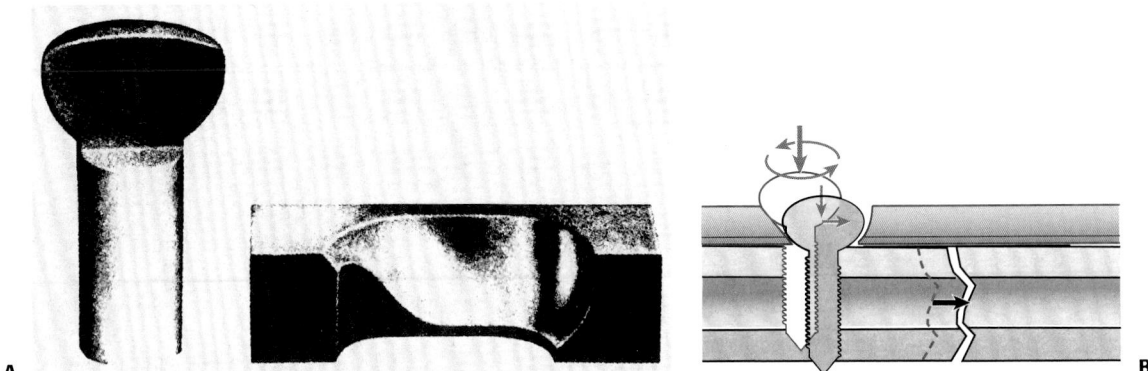

A

B

FIGURE 1-32 A: Cross section through the head of a bone screw and the hole in a fracture plate showing the geometry. B: As the screw is tightened, the head slides down the inclined border of the plate, which displaces the screw sideways, and therefore, the screw and the bone fragment to which the screw is attached are displaced toward the opposite fragment.

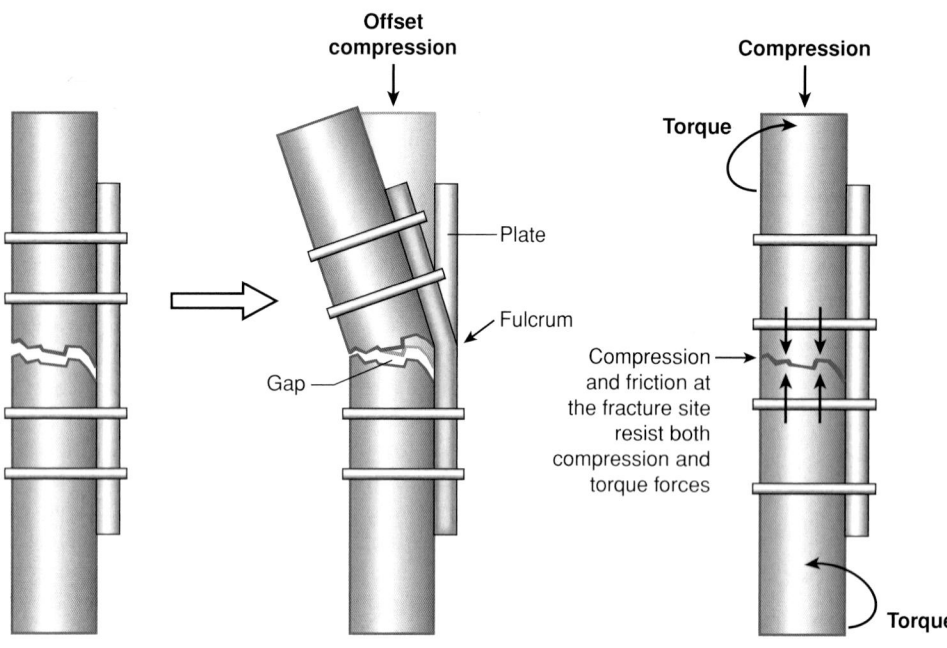

FIGURE 1-33 **Left:** When a gap is left on the cortex opposite that to which the plate is attached, bending of the plate at the fracture site can cause the plate to fail rapidly in bending. **Right:** Compressing the fracture surfaces not only allows the bone cortices to resist bending loads but the frictional contact and interdigitation help resist torsion.

Plate stresses are significantly increased by gapping at the fracture.[14] In comminuted fractures in which it is difficult to approximate the fracture ends, bridge plating can be performed, and screws should be placed as close as possible across the fracture gap and spread over a long plate length to reduce strains in the plate.[55] Torsional and bending stiffness of a fracture construct can be significantly increased, and therefore, plate strain reduced, by increasing the length of the plate itself.[141] While increasing the number of cortices of fixation also increases the stiffness, as shown in Figure 1-36, the number of screws is not the sole determinant of construct stiffness.[56] Figure 1-37 shows several interesting aspects related to plate fixation with screws. First, plate strains are highest at the two holes adjacent to the fracture gap and become very small five holes away. Second, this occurs regardless of whether the screws were placed near the fracture (locations 2, 3, 4, and 5), far from the fracture

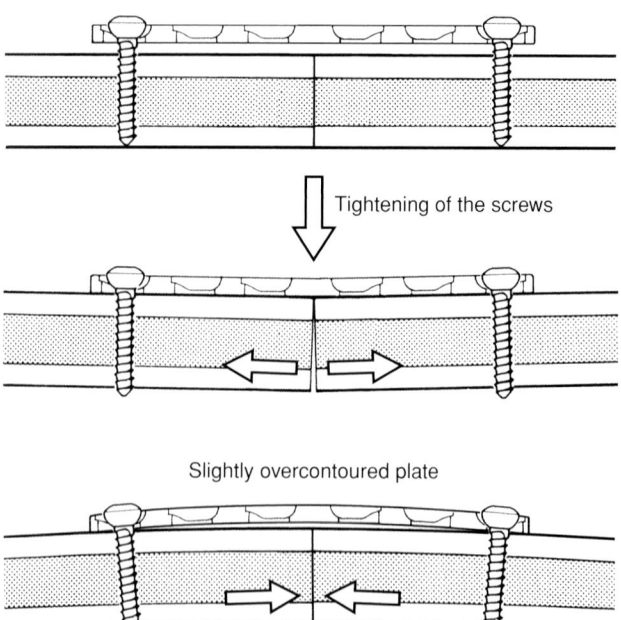

FIGURE 1-34 A demonstration of the gapping that occurs on the opposite cortex when a flat plate is applied to a flat bone surface. Slightly prebending the plate causes the ends of the opposite cortices to be driven together when the plate is applied.[124]

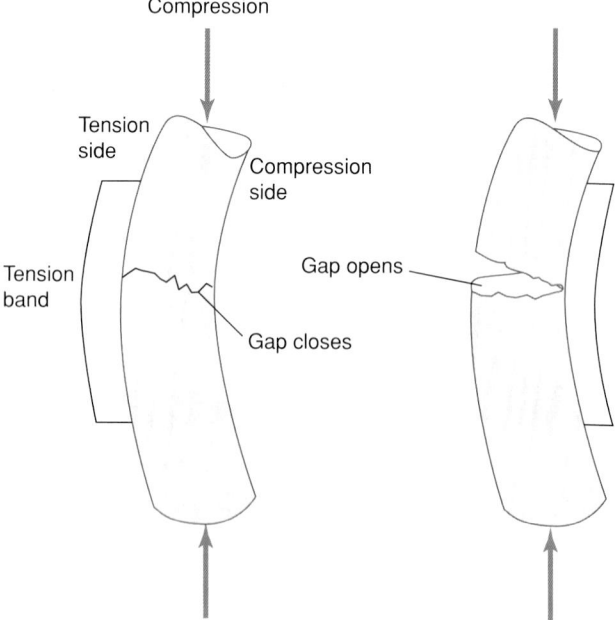

FIGURE 1-35 The application of a plate on the compressive as opposed to the tensile side of a bone subjected to bending causes a gap to open on the opposite side of the plate during functional loading.

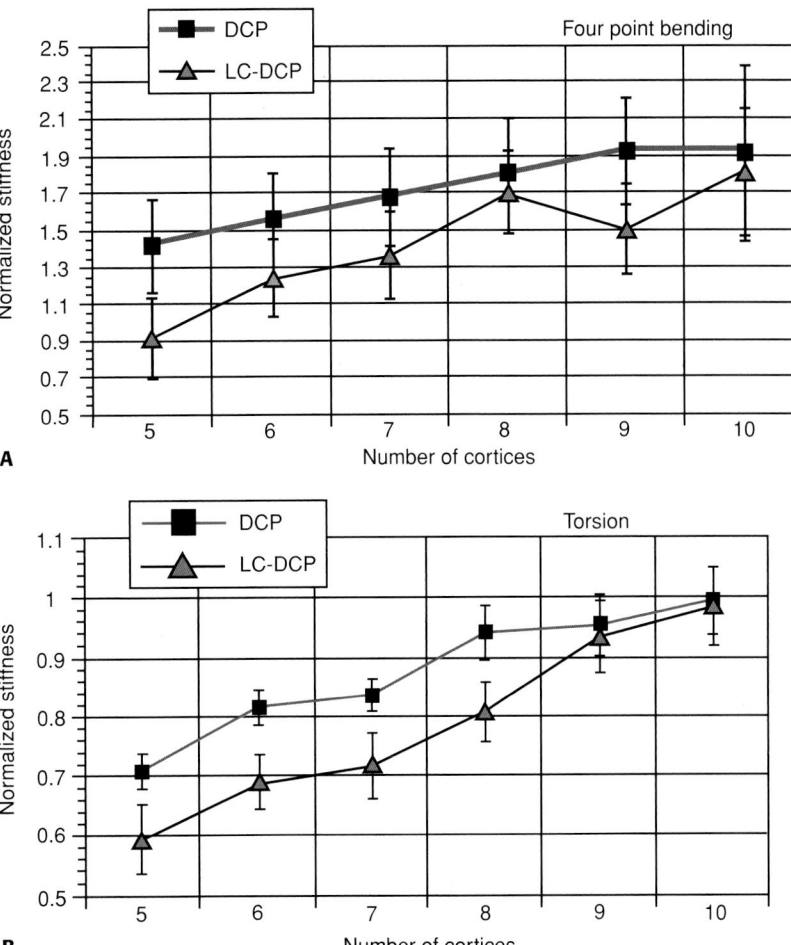

FIGURE 1-36 Relative stiffness of a plate–bone construct in **(A)** torsion and **(B)** bending as a function of the number of cortices through which screws have been placed (DCP, dynamic compression plate; LC-DCP, limited contact dynamic compression plate).[54]

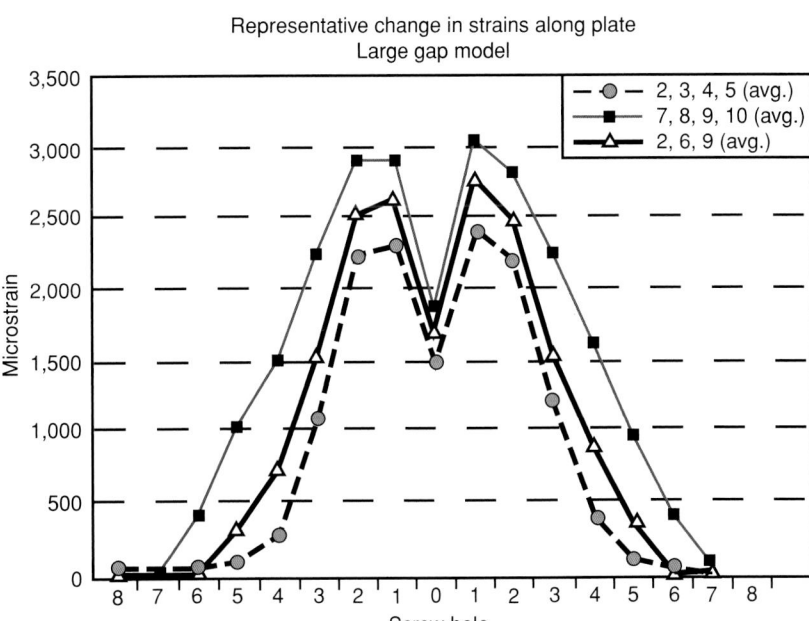

FIGURE 1-37 Distribution of strain (measured in microstrain or strain × 10⁻⁶) at various locations along a plate regardless of placement of the screws in different locations (holes 2, 3, 4, 5), (holes 7, 8, 9, 10), or holes (2, 6, 9).[56]

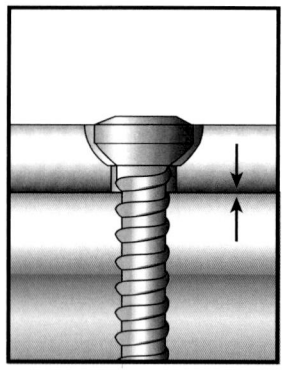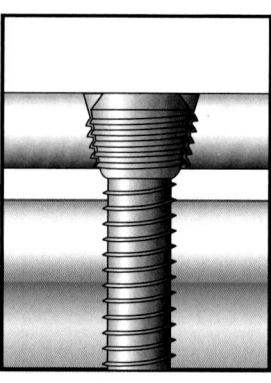

FIGURE 1-38 The difference between the conventional screw and locking screws are shown. The conventional screw has a smooth screw head that allows for compression between the plate and bone. The locking screw has a threaded screw head that engages the plate and "locks." It does not allow for compression between the plate and bone. The locking screw also has a finer screw pitch and a larger core diameter to increase resistance against bending forces.

(locations 7, 8, 9, and 10), or mixed (locations 2, 6, and 9).[55] This data also indicate that not all holes of the plate need to be filled with screws to provide similar fixation stiffness.

Locking Screws and Plates

Locking screws and plates are newer types of implants that can be used in the treatment of fractures. Most locking screws have threads machined into the screw heads, which can thread into the plate, thus locking with the plate and creating a fixed angle device (Fig. 1-38). In addition, the screws have been designed with a finer thread and larger core diameter, as torque generation during insertion is less of a priority, and resistance to bending forces is paramount.[55] As stated above, the bending stiffness of the screw is related to the radius to the fourth power. Locking plates function differently biomechanically compared with nonlocking plates. Nonlocking plates are compressed against the bone fragments by the screws and require bone-to-plate contact to produce a stable fracture construct. When the frictional forces of the bone–plate interface are greater than the load applied, a stable construct results. When the frictional force generated is less than the load applied, the construct becomes unstable (Fig. 1-39).

Locking plates and screws are rigidly connected to the plate which creates a fixed angle device that acts like an external fixator (Figs. 1-40 and 1-41).[62] Because each screw acts as a fixed implant they do not rely on bone quality as much as conventional screws. Conventional screws need good bony purchase to create the compression needed to secure the construct, whereas locking screws act as fixed angle devices that rely on the plate–screw interface, shear strength of the screw, and the compression strength of the bone for stability of the construct (Fig. 1-42).

Conventional screw constructs fail differently when compared with locking screw constructs (Fig. 1-43). When conventional constructs fail, it is usually because of loss of bony purchase of the screw and sequential pull out of the screws. Because the locking screw creates multiple fixed angle devices,

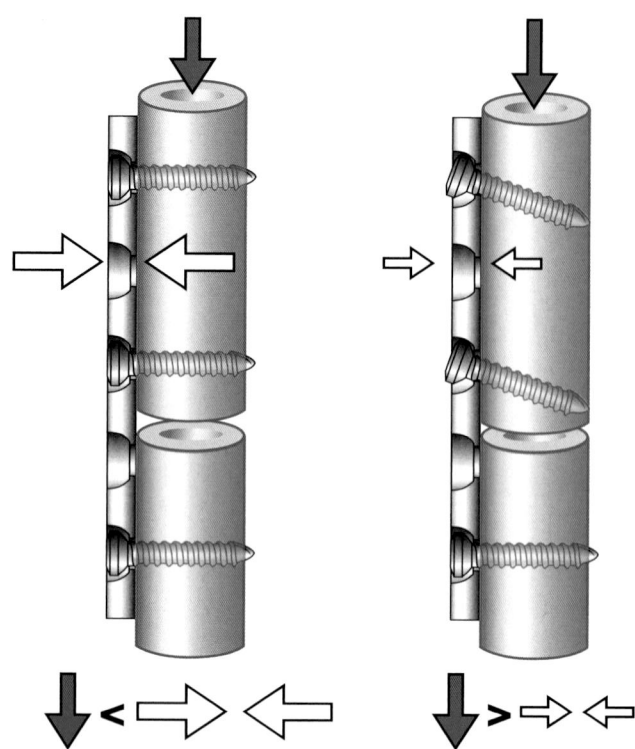

FIGURE 1-39 The function of a conventional plate and screw construct relies on frictional forces between the plate and bone to resist the applied force. When the frictional forces are greater than the load applied, the construct is stable. If the load applied is greater than the frictional forces the construct can fail.

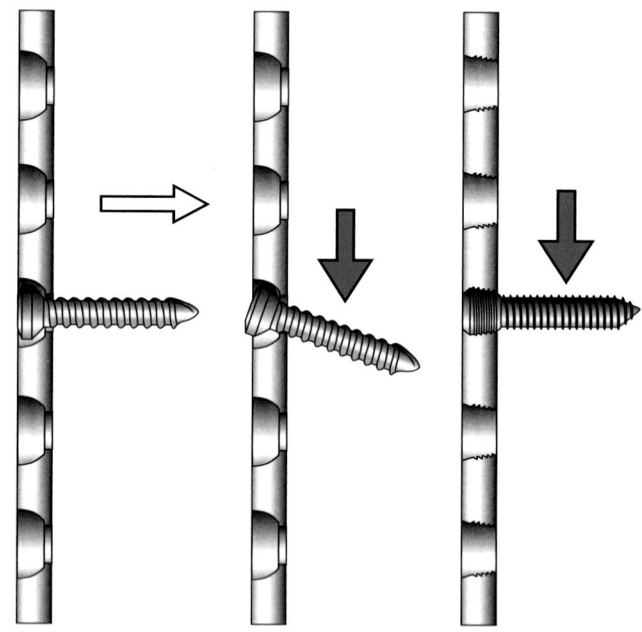

FIGURE 1-40 Because the conventional screw does not engage the plate when load is applied the screw has no angular stability, Thus it relies on the frictional forces between the plate and bone for stability. The locking screw engages into the plate and is able to resist the load because of the screwhead threading into the plate; thus, it is a fixed angle device.

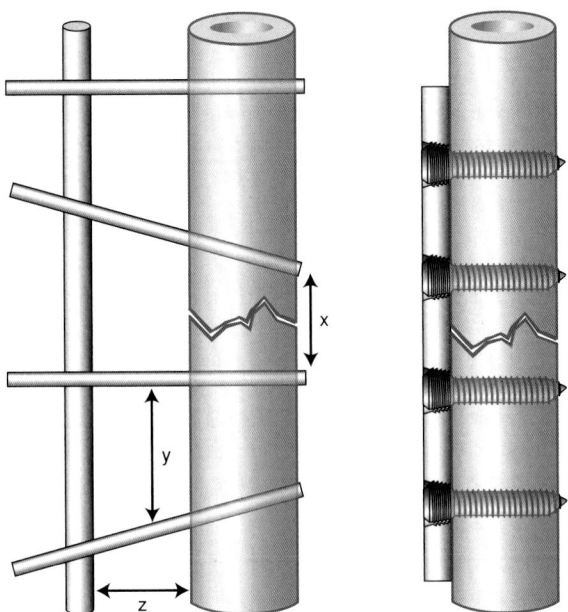

FIGURE 1-41 Locking plate–screw construct fuctions as an internal fixator. Decreasing the value of x, y and z (X - pin to fracture distance, y - pin to pin distance, z - bar to bone distance) will increase the stiffness in a fixed angle construct. A locking plate helps to do that by reducing z. The values of x and y can be modulated by the surgeon and how the pins or screws are placed.

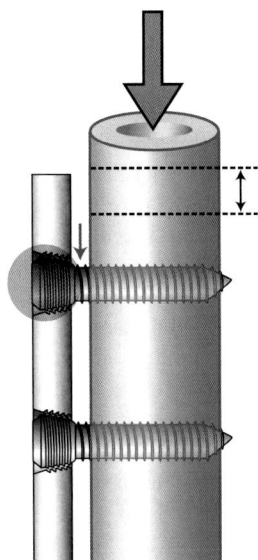

FIGURE 1-42 When load is applied (*red arrow*) to a locking construct, the load is resisted by the plate–screw interface (*orange circle*) acting as a fixed angle device. Also the screw shaft (*arrow*) exposed between the plate and bone resists the shear forces. And because of the fixed angle construct, the forces applied are also resisted by compression of the bone (*orange rectangle*).

the screws must all fail simultaneously and the entire construct ultimately fails only after compressive failure of the bone. As stated previously the bone is weakest in tension and strongest in compression.

The locking construct does not rely on compression between the plate and bone; therefore, the plate does not have to sit directly on the bone. This can preserve the soft tissue envelope and periosteum, and cause less interference with the biologic processes of fracture healing. Also, locking plates provide more stability in comminuted fractures[151] in which cortical apposition and compression are difficult to achieve and fracture mechanical stability occurs mainly from the implant.[52]

Conventional screw construct

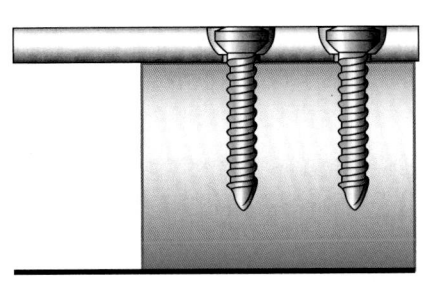

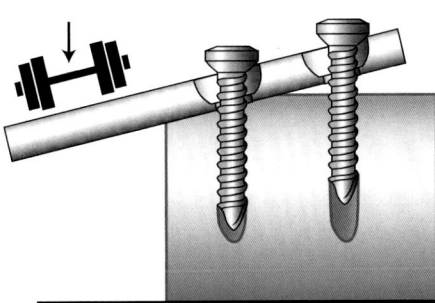

Locking construct

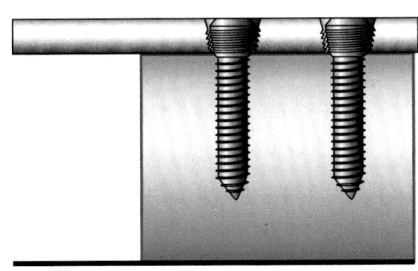

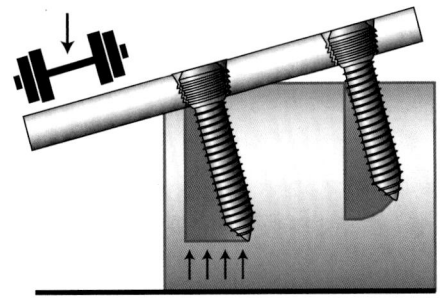

FIGURE 1-43 The conventional screw construct fails when the screws lose purchase in the bone and pull out of the bone. Note the screws fails sequentially. The locking construct acts as a fixed angle device and failure results when the bone fails in compression and all the screws fail simultaneously.

However, locking screws cannot create compression at the fracture site and thus rely on relative stability.

Dynamic fatigue testing has shown that locking plates have fatigue strengths similar to other systems and are able to support loads comparable to one body weight for two million cycles, which should be sufficient for normal fracture healing. Since screw pullout strength is related directly to the length of screw purchase in bone cortex, unicortical screws used in some systems have lower pullout strength than bicortical screws and should be avoided. As with other systems, locking plates have mechanical sensitivities. For example, accurate placement of the locking screws is important. As Figure 1-44 shows, angulation of the screw causes incomplete engagement of the thread at the screw–plate interface and, therefore, lower mechanical stability of the construct. In fact, comparatively, the bending stability of a 4.5-mm locking plate was reduced to 63% and 31%, respectively, with 5- or 10-degree axis deviation of the locking screw insertion vector.[86] Although some of the newer systems do allow for variable angle locking trajectories, deviating from the design parameters will result in loss of mechanical stability of the screw–plate interface.

Plate Failure Through a Screw Hole

Many plates have multiple screw holes to provide many fixation options depending on the specific requirements of the fracture pattern and bone quality. It is not necessary to place screws in every hole in the plate,[48] but the effects of screw placement on fixation stiffness should be understood. An empty screw hole

is an area of elevated stress on the plate, unless the plate is made thicker near the holes to compensate, as is the case with some implants. The plate material around the holes will have higher material stresses than occur in the solid regions of the plate. Around the holes, the force acts through a smaller cross-sectional area, so the material stresses must be higher. A second consideration related to multihole plates is that separating the screws, so that there is a greater distance between them across the fracture site, that is, increasing the "working length" of the construct, results in lower stiffness of the plate–fracture construct.[67] With an increased working length, a given applied load is distributed over a longer segment of plate, decreasing the amount of stress per unit length of the plate. This may have beneficial biologic ramifications as well, as fracture site motion is distributed to more of the comminuted fragments, decreasing strain at each fragment, and increasing the likelihood of callus formation.

Femoral Splitting as a Result of Intramedullary Nail Insertion

Insertion of an IM nail into the femur can lead to difficulties because the femur has a significant anterior curvature,[178] shown in Figure 1-45. Current femoral nails have radii of curvature that range from 186 to 300 cm, compared with an average of 120 ± 36 cm for a large sample of human femora. Therefore, current femoral nails are considerably straighter than the average human femur, especially in older individuals where anterior femoral bowing may be increased.[51] The nail, which has a curved shape to accommodate the femoral bow, must also conform to the curvature of the femur as insertion progresses. Placing a nail, which is essentially a curved spring, down the femoral canal causes the nail to bend slightly, because the femur is generally much stiffer than the nail (Fig. 1-46). In fact, the nail must conform not only to an anterior–posterior bow but also canal curvature medially and laterally.[53] Figure 1-47 demonstrates that nail contact with the internal surfaces of the femur generates forces which resist insertion. These nail–femur contact forces or "hoop stresses" directed perpendicular to the

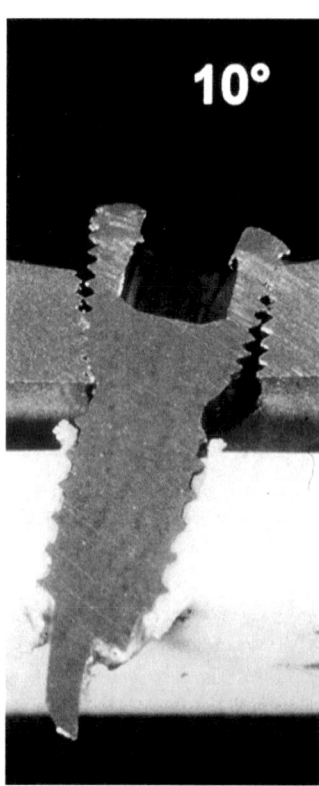

FIGURE 1-44 A demonstration of the importance of accurate placement of locking screws into the plate.[86]

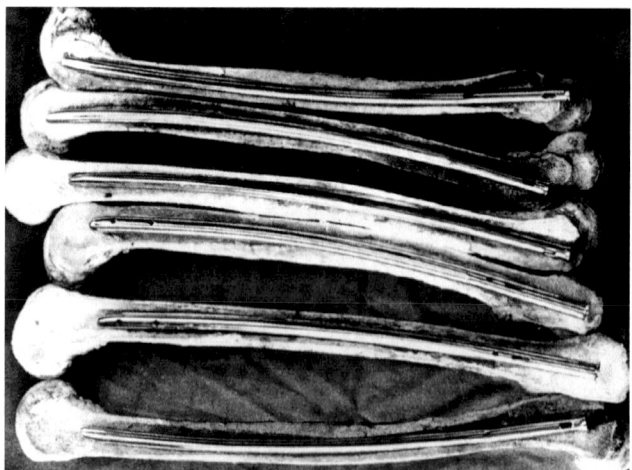

FIGURE 1-45 Cross sections of various femora demonstrate the curvature that an IM rod must conform to when it is fully inserted.[178]

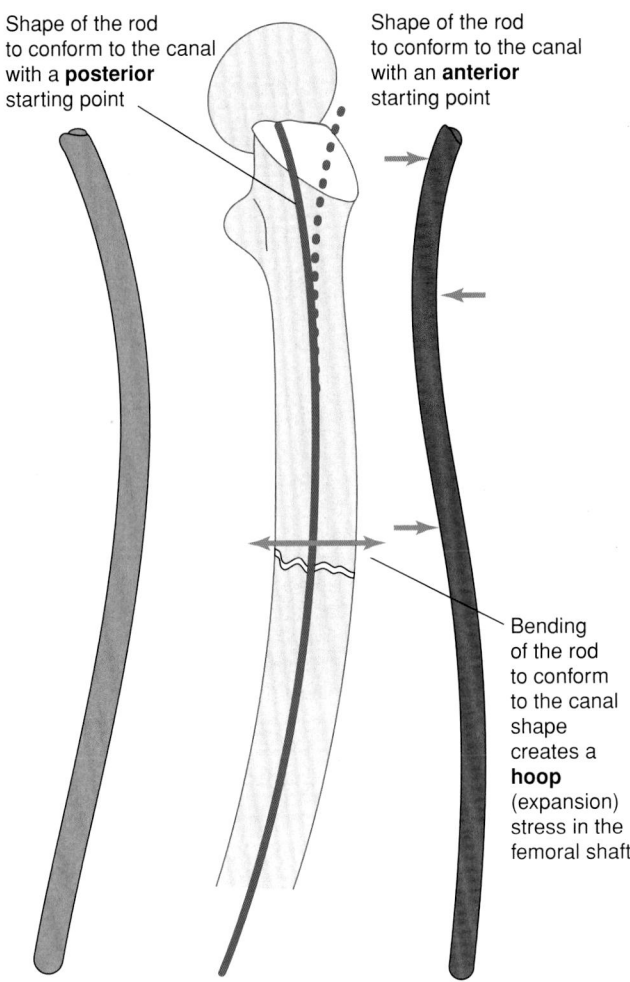

Shape of the rod to conform to the canal with a **posterior** starting point

Shape of the rod to conform to the canal with an **anterior** starting point

Bending of the rod to conform to the canal shape creates a **hoop** (expansion) stress in the femoral shaft

FIGURE 1-46 Mismatch of the curvature between the IM rod and the medullary canal results in bending stresses that could cause splitting of the femur during insertion.[85]

surface of the medullary canal cause the femur to expand and will result in splitting or fissuring if they become too large.[85]

The factors that govern the amount of bending of the nail during insertion and the resulting internal forces acting within the femur are the proximal start position, the length of the proximal fragment, the initial curvature of the IM nail compared with the curvature of the femur, and the bending stiffness of the nail. Nail stiffness can vary considerably, and depends heavily on diameter and material.[139] Many currently used nails are titanium, which is a less stiffer metal than stainless steel. Figure 1-47 demonstrates examples in which malposition of the proximal start point resulted in femoral splitting during nail insertion.[85] Some newer IM nails employ a valgus bend to be used with a femoral trochanteric entry portal.[126] The optimal entry point for retrograde nailing was found to be about 1.2 cm anterior to the femoral origin of the posterior cruciate ligament and at the midpoint of the intracondylar sulcus.[96]

IM Nail and Locking Screw Breakage

Fractures of IM nails and locking screws occur occasionally during healing. The most demanding mechanical situation for

IM nail fixation of the femur or tibia occurs when the fracture is very distal. Figure 1-48 compares the forces acting on idealized femora with more proximal and more distal fractures. For a specific location of the external load (muscle load or body weight), the more distal fracture results in a longer moment arm (the perpendicular distance from the load to the fracture site), creating a greater moment, and therefore higher stresses in the implant. The highest stresses in the nail occur near the fracture site. With a distal fracture, in addition to the greater moment, the locking holes—which are significant stress risers—are usually located just distal to the fracture site. It has been shown that the maximum stresses acting in the nail increase rapidly once the distance between the fracture and the most superior of the distal screw holes is reduced to less than about 4 cm.[30] Cyclic loading of nails used to fixed distal fractures, with peak loading of about one body weight, confirm that titanium alloy nails can survive more than one million loading cycles when the more proximal of the distal locking screws is more than 3 cm from the fracture site.[7] In addition, placing the distal locking screws can be difficult because they must be inserted freehand under fluoroscopic guidance. Sometimes, the corner of the screw hole of the nail can be nicked by the drill or while driving the screw, creating an additional stress riser that can accentuate the fatigue process. Awareness of these potential problems has led to design changes such as closing the proximal section of the nail, increasing material thickness around the screw holes, and cold forming, which increases the strength of the material.

Screw bending and breakage can also occur. When distal screws are placed into the bone with relatively low bone density, the screw is supported mostly by the cortices. The distal end of the femur widens rapidly (Fig. 1-49), so the unsupported length of the screw between the cortices can be quite variable. For the same diameter and material, the stiffness and strength of a screw subjected to bending decreases with the third power of its unsupported length (the distance between cortices, assuming no support from the trabecular bone). If the unsupported length of one screw is twice as long as that of another, and assuming that the trabecular bone does not contribute to support of the screw, one can expect the stiffness and strength of the screw with the longer unsupported length to be one-eighth that of the screw with the shorter length between cortical supports, and therefore, the deformation will be eight times greater under the same load. This does create a trade-off in fixation of these fractures with respect to screw placement. If the screws are too close to the fracture, the stresses in the nail increase, whereas if they are located within the flair of the metaphysis, with poor trabecular bone, their unsupported length increases, decreasing stiffness and strength. The fatigue life of the distal locking screws is directly related to the diameter of the root of the thread and the resulting moment of inertia, so it has been proposed to remove the threads to increase fatigue life by 10 to 100 times.[78] Stresses on interlocking screws are also significantly increased in comminuted fractures, where no load can be borne by the cortices at the fracture site, as is the case with simple transverse or short oblique fracture patterns.

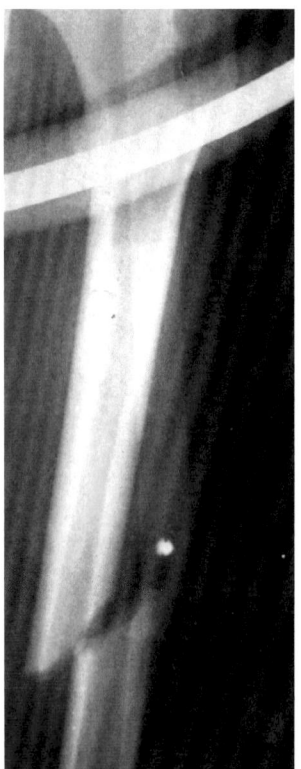 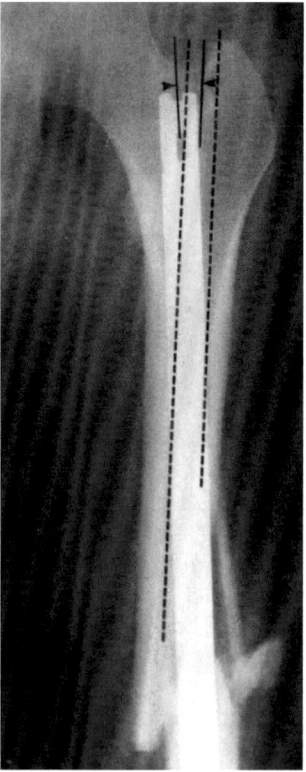 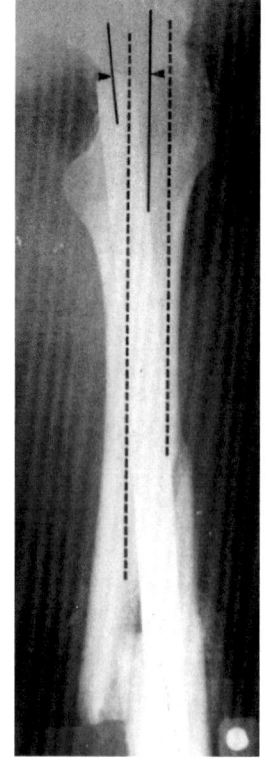

FIGURE 1-47 The starting position selected for rod entry into the medullary canal affects the degree to which it must bend and the internal forces generated in the femur. A starting position offset from the axis of the medullary canal, coupled with a stiff rod and a longer proximal segment that requires the rod to bend more during insertion, generate higher insertion forces and internal femoral forces. In this example of a midshaft femoral fracture **(left)**, the starting hole was selected medial relative to the axis of the medullary canal **(middle)** and posterior **(right)**. The medullary canal is outlined in dashed lines. Therefore the rod must bend both medially and posteriorly as it is inserted into the canal and has created internal stresses which have split the distal end of the proximal femoral segment.[85]

Loosening of External Fixator Pins

Loosening of fixator pins in bone is thought to result from several causes. The shape of the end of the pin itself, because it is self-tapping, can affect the local heat generated in the bone

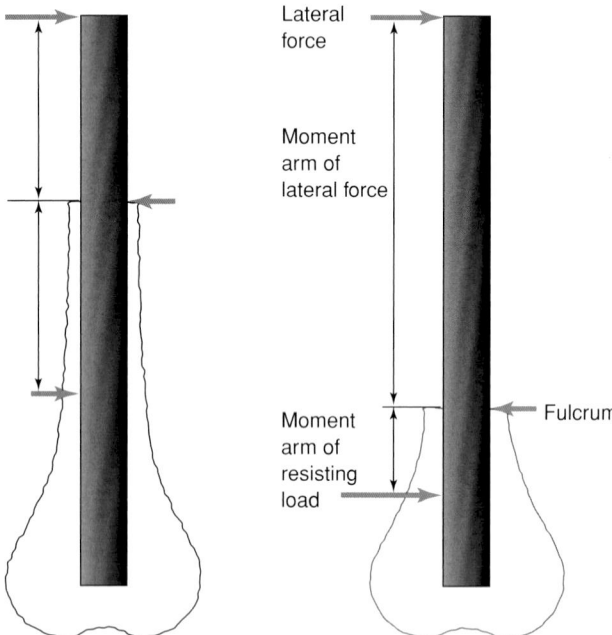

FIGURE 1-48 If the same force acts on IM rods placed in femora with more proximal **(left)** or more distal **(right)** fractures, the moment arm of the force will be longer in the case of the more distal fracture and therefore the moment acting at the fracture site on the implant will be larger. For the more distal fracture, the high-stress region close to the fracture site is also significantly closer to the distal locking screw holes which are significant stress risers.

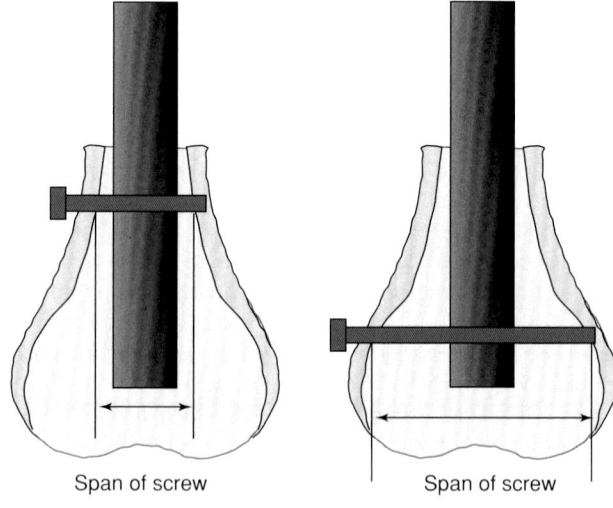

FIGURE 1-49 Because the distal end of the femur flares rapidly, the length of the locking screw required to crosslock the rod can be quite variable. If the screw is not well supported by trabecular bone but mainly by cortex, then its stiffness and strength decrease with the third power of its length between cortices. If the screw length doubles, the deformation of the screw under the same load increases by a factor of eight.

during insertion, potentially causing thermal necrosis around the pin hole site,[169] along with bone microfracturing. In addition, high local stresses can occur in the pins and bone if the hole through which the pin is inserted is undersized.[82] A third mechanism, shown in Figure 1-50, is micromotion, which induces bone resorption at the pin–bone interface if the pin is a loose fit in the hole. To reduce these problems, slight undersizing of the bone hole by about 0.1 mm in diameter has been advocated. If the bone hole is undersized by 0.3 mm in diam-

eter, the yield strength of bone may be exceeded when the pin is inserted, resulting in fracture.[124]

Excessively Flexible External Fixation

An external fixator is an assembly of pins attached to bone fragments, along with clamps and sidebars that couple the pins. This assembly allows considerable variation in construction of a frame to accommodate the fracture. The optimal stiffness of a fixator necessary to stabilize the fracture and induce healing changes as the fracture consolidates is not specifically known. It must be rigid enough to support the forces applied by the patient during ambulation without causing malalignment of the fracture. However, it should not be so stiff that the fracture is shielded from the motion required to stimulate healing by callus formation. Some basic mechanical guidelines in the construction of the frame, explained below, will ensure that frames are adequately constructed for the loads they are subjected to. Figure 1-51 demonstrates that when the diameter of a pin or sidebar increases, its stiffness and strength increase to the fourth power of the relative change in diameter (actually the ratio of the larger to the smaller diameter). As its length (the distance between bone surface and sidebar) decreases, stiffness and strength increase to the third power of the length change. This principle also holds for the pins spanning the fracture, which affect the unsupported length of the sidebar across the fracture.

In the construction of a frame, it is beneficial to decrease the sidebar-to-bone distance (which decreases the unsupported lengths of the pins), increase the pin diameter, and decrease the distance between the pins which span the fracture. Similarly, increasing the number of pins applied also increases frame stiffness. In terms of actual effects on bending strength, doubling the sidebar distance from bone decreases frame stiffness by approximately 67%, doubling the separation distance of the pins across the fracture decreases stiffness by 50%, and decreasing pin diameter by 1 mm (e.g., from 6 to 5 mm) decreases frame stiffness by about 50%.[161] Using a partly threaded pin and burying the pin thread completely within the cortex enhances the stiffness of the pin because the smaller diameter of the root of the pin thread is not exposed. Also, using hydroxyapatite-coated external fixation pins to enhance the screw–bone interface[123] has been shown to improve fixation and pin longevity.

The comments above pertain to uniplanar fixators, which are constructed to resist the major loads of axial compression and anterior–posterior bending that act on a long bone such as the tibia during walking. To resist torsion and out-of-plane (medial–lateral) bending, the fixator can be assembled with additional pins and sidebars in other planes. A comparison of the relative stiffnesses of different fixator assemblies is given in Figure 1-52. The unilateral half-pin frame with sidebars mounted at right angles provides the greatest overall resistance to bending, compression, and torsional loads.[21] Hybrid fixation devices have adopted components of both unilateral bar fixators and ring fixators with transfixing small-diameter wires. Both axial compression and torsional stiffnesses have been found to increase significantly with increases in the number and diameter of the transfixing wires, and pretensioning the wires.[33] More anterior placement of wires, or addition of an anteromedial half

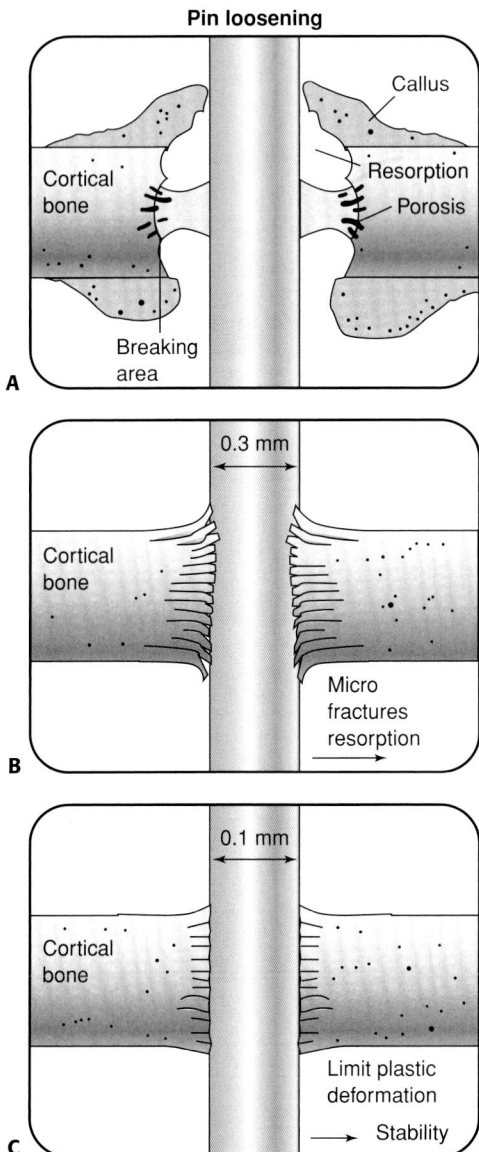

Pin loosening

FIGURE 1-50 A proposed mechanism for loosening of external fixation pins involves under- or oversizing the diameter of the pin relative to the bone hole. **A:** If the pin and bone hole are of the same diameter, micromotion can occur with bone resorption. **B:** If the pin is more than 0.3 mm smaller in diameter than the hole in the bone, microfracture may occur during insertion. **C:** If the bone hole diameter is about 0.1 mm smaller than the pin diameter, the bone is prestressed but does not fracture, micromotion is eliminated, and pin stability is maintained.[124]

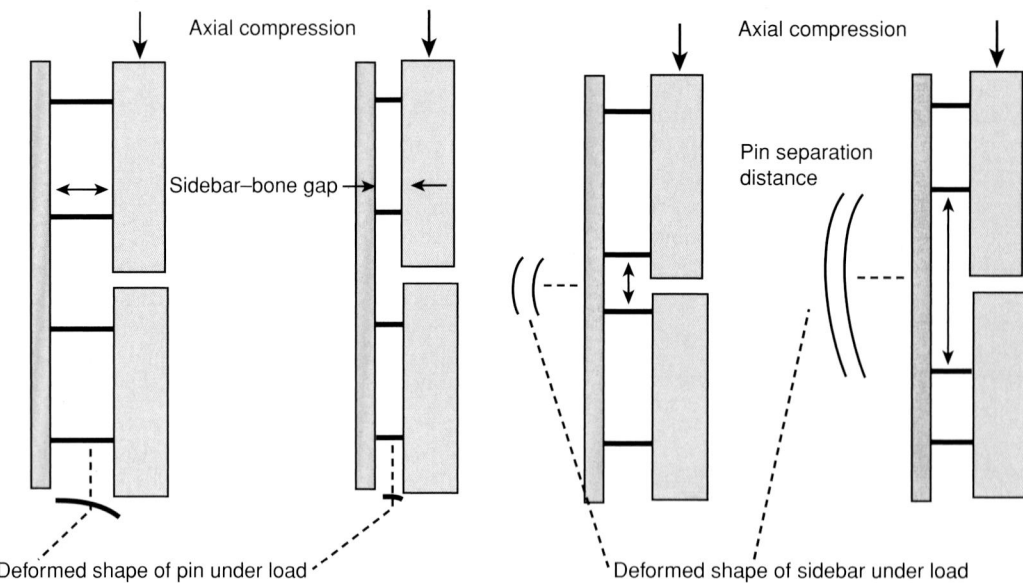

FIGURE 1-51 To produce more rigidity in the construction of an external fixator, the basic principles that should be considered are that for pin- and rod-type sidebars, stiffness increases with the fourth power of the cross-sectional area (the moment of inertia, Fig. 1-7) and decreases with the third power of their span or unsupported length (Fig. 1-44). This explains why it is beneficial to decrease the sidebar to bone distance, increase pin diameter, place pins as close together across the fracture site, and use larger diameter or multiple sidebars in frame construction.[82,161]

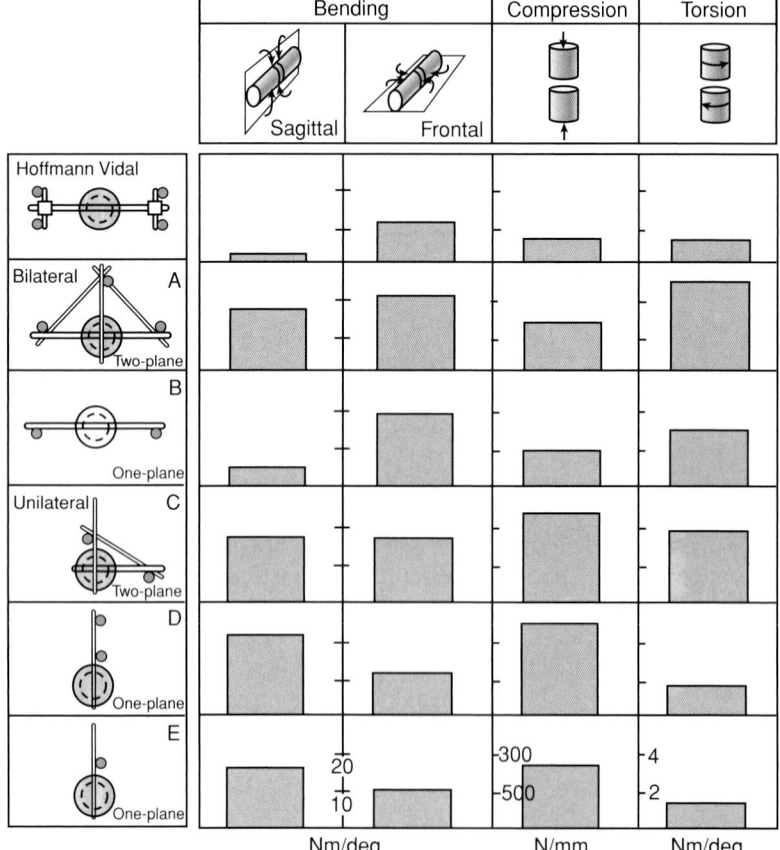

FIGURE 1-52 A comparison of the bending, compression, and torsional stiffnesses of different external fixation constructs for multiplane load resistance.[21]

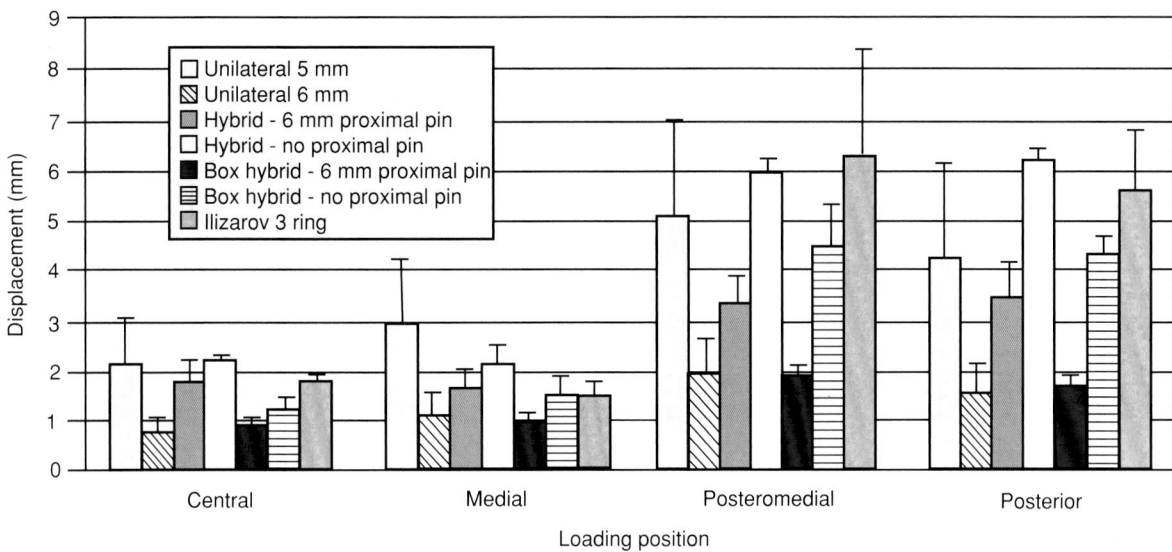

FIGURE 1-53 A comparison of displacement of the proximal fragment in a simulated tibia fracture under 100-N load with various unilateral and hybrid external fixators (the box type uses both a large unilateral frame connecting bar and two smaller diameter connecting rods).[135]

pin have been found to increase anterior–posterior bending stiffness.[68] Testing of several different configurations (Fig. 1-53) revealed that the box type (two rings above and two below the fracture, along with anterior half pins, two connecting rods, and a unilateral bar) was the stiffest configuration, compared with a unilateral frame alone or a unilateral frame with rings only proximal to the fracture site. The addition of an anterior half pin significantly increased fixation stiffness.[135]

Fixation in Osteoporotic Bone

The attachment strength of a fixation device to bone (e.g., a screw) is directly related to the local bone density. Since a dominant mechanical characteristic of osteoporotic bone is low den-

sity, several strategies to improve fixation strength can be used when osteoporotic bone is encountered. These include cortical buttressing by impaction; wide buttressing, which spreads the load over a larger surface area; long splintage; improved anchoring; and increasing the local bone density by injection of a denser substance such as hydroxyapatite or polymethylmethacrylate (PMMA); Figure 1-54.[76] Impaction strategies can be applied in fractures of the distal radius, femoral neck, and lumbar vertebrae. The dynamic hip screw is an example of a device which allows controlled impaction of the fracture of the femoral neck. An angled blade plate applied to supracondylar femur fractures, as compared with a condylar screw, provides wider buttressing—that is, a larger surface area of contact with

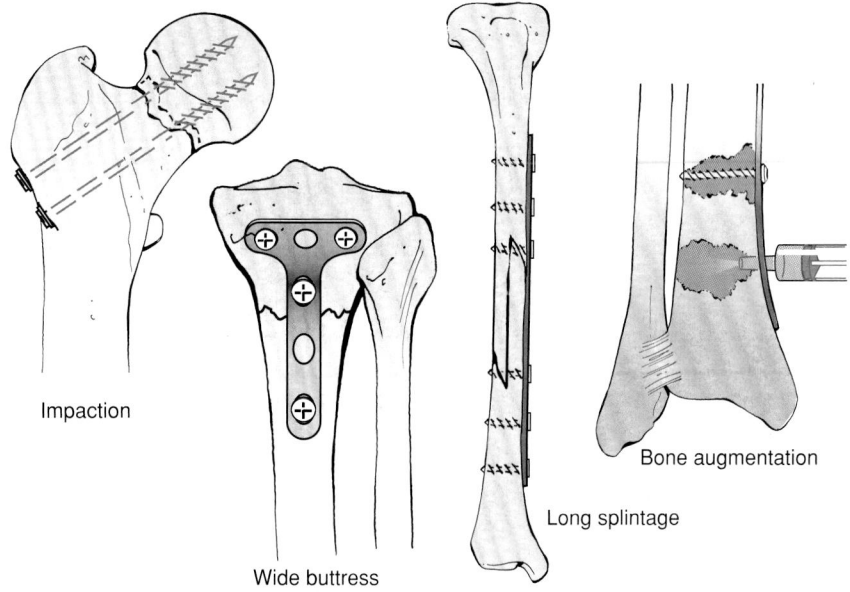

FIGURE 1-54 Some basic strategies to augment fixation strength in osteoporotic bone include impaction of the fracture components using a device that allows sliding, buttressing with a wide plate, increasing the plate length, and augmenting the bone locally by injection of methylmethacrylate or a calcium phosphate cement.[76]

the bone. Splinting with a longer plate has been applied in humeral and forearm fractures, and the interlocked IM rod is another example of long splinting. A periarticular locking plate, which permits placement of multiple points of angle-stable fixation, is another example of the application of this principle.[23] The locking plate, in which the screws are threaded into the plate and fixed so they cannot rotate or translate, can be particularly useful in stabilizing osteoporotic fractures when cortical buttressing is not practical because of low bone density, and the fixation hardware must support most of the load. Hydroxyapatite-coated external fixation pins have been shown to enhance the stability of the screw–bone interface.[123] Interlocking screws, in which a standard screw has a 45-degree hole drilled into the shaft to accept an interlocking pin, can be used to reduce screw backout.[114] Newer designs of IM nails also allow "angle-stable" interlocking screws that thread into the nail and create a fixed angle interface, which may improve fixation in osteoporotic bone.

Enhancement of local bone density using either PMMA or, more recently, calcium phosphate cements has been studied, particularly in relation to fixation of femoral and vertebral osteoporotic fractures. PMMA injection has been widely employed in vertebroplasty through a transpedicular approach[106] and has been shown to restore the stiffness of fractured vertebrae to that of intact vertebrae. Biomechanical studies have shown significantly improved strength of the fixation of femoral neck fractures up to 170%,[154] and similar findings, including decreased shortening and greater stability, were noted when hydroxyapatite cement was applied to unstable three-part intertrochanteric fractures fixed with a dynamic hip screw.[54] Calcium phosphate cements used in vertebroplasty instead of PMMA also restored the stiffness of fractured vertebrae to intact levels.[107] Calcium phosphate cement injection into the pedicle has been shown to improve the bending stiffness of pedicle screws by up to 125%.[18] Calcium phosphate cements have also been shown to support elevated metaphyseal fracture fragments (i.e., in the tibial plateau) in a variety of settings in randomized clinical trials of fracture care.[138]

Cerclage Wire Breakage

Cerclage wiring has been used less and less frequently for primary fracture fixation because of the negative effects of circumferential periosteal compression. However, this modality is still used occasionally, and understanding its mechanical behavior is important to avoid fixation failures. The tensile strength of surgical wire has been shown to increase directly with its diameter,[159] and when twisted, the optimal number of turns is between four and eight.[140] However, solid wire is very sensitive to notches or scratches. Testing shows that notches as small as 1% of the diameter of the wire can reduce its fatigue life by 63%.[140] For this reason, a cable has been introduced for cerclage applications. Cable has significantly better fatigue performance compared with wire, as shown in Figure 1-55.[69] Since cables consist of multiple strands of single thin wires, damage to any particular strand does not result in catastrophic failure of the entire cable. Single loops of suture such as Ethibond are about 30% as strong as 18-gage stainless steel wire in tension, and Mersilene tape is approximately 50% as strong. Four loops of Ethibond have a tensile strength equivalent to stainless steel wire.[75]

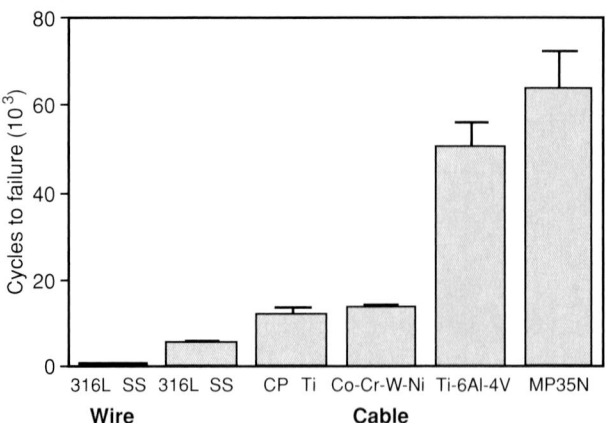

FIGURE 1-55 A comparison of the fatigue resistance of wire and cables made of the indicated materials. Wire, 316L SS (stainless steel), cable Co-Cr-W-Ni, cobalt chrome Ti-6Al-4V, titanium alloy, MP35N, nickel alloy.[69]

Biomechanical Aspects of Fracture Fixation in Specific Locations

In the previous discussion, problems such as screw pullout and plate breakage common to fracture fixation, mainly in the long bones, were discussed. In this section, the focus is placed on specific challenging problems in fixation, including the femoral neck, tibial plateau, pelvis, and spine.

Fixation in the Proximal Femur

Fixation of fractures of the proximal femur is particularly challenging because the compressive force acting through the femoral head can range from four to eight times the body weight during normal activities.[127] This force acts through a significant moment arm (the length of the femoral neck), which imposes large bending loads on the fixation hardware. In addition, many of these fractures occur in the elderly, who are likely to have trabecular bone of low density and poor mechanical quality.[103] Also, it is generally not possible to gain screw purchase in the cortical bone of the femoral head.

The major force acting in a basicervical fracture of the femoral neck, fixed with a sliding hip screw, is the joint reaction force through the femoral head, which derives from body weight and forces generated by muscle action during ambulation. The joint reaction force can be divided into two components. One component (Fig. 1-56) is perpendicular to the axis of the sliding screw and causes shearing of the fracture surfaces along the fracture line, which results in inferior displacement and varus angulation of the femoral head, and increases the resistance of the screw to sliding. The other component is parallel to the screw, driving the surfaces together and enhancing stability by friction and mechanical interlocking of the fracture. Therefore, the goal of femoral neck fixation systems is to utilize the component of the joint force parallel to the femoral neck to encourage the fracture surfaces to slide together. This is the basic principle behind selection of a higher angle hip screw when possible.

When using the compression (or sliding) hip screw, or a nail with a sliding lag screw, it is important to ensure that the screw

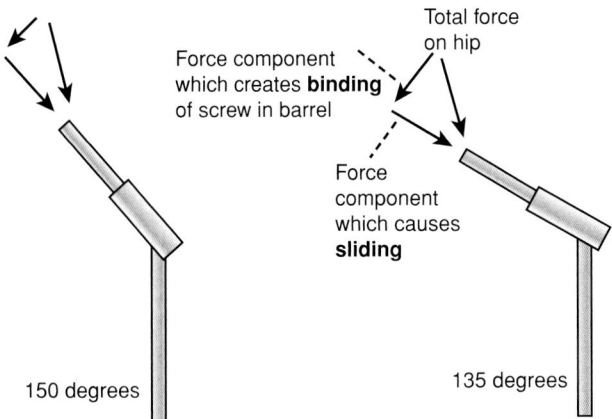

FIGURE 1-56 The joint reaction force in the femoral head can be divided into two major components. The one parallel to the axis of the femoral neck produces sliding and impaction of the fracture components and the other, transverse to the femoral neck, causes the screw component of the femoral hip screw to bind, resisting sliding. The higher-angle hip screw has a screw axis more closely aligned with the joint reaction force so the force component that produces sliding is larger whereas the transverse force component resisting sliding is smaller.

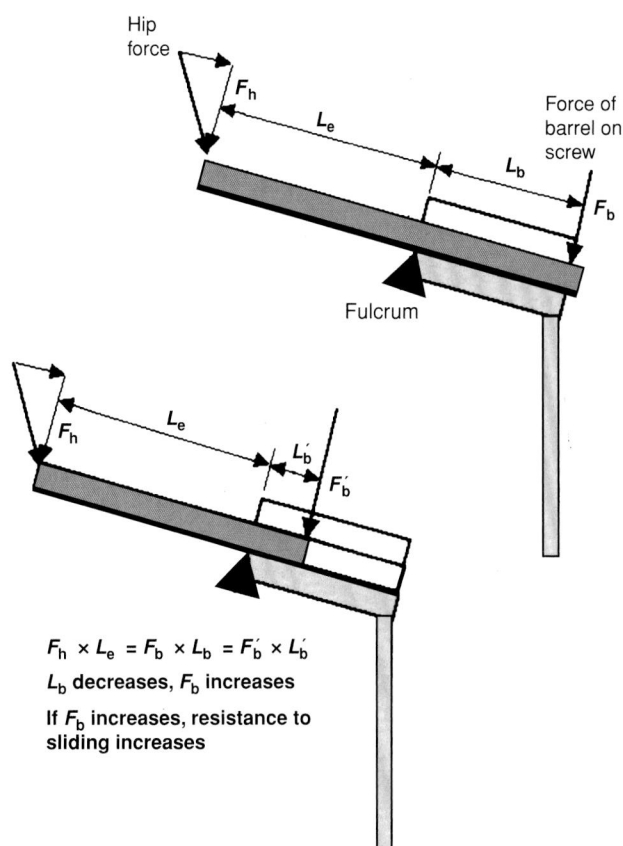

$$F_h \times L_e = F_b \times L_b = F_b' \times L_b'$$

L_b decreases, F_b increases

If F_b increases, resistance to sliding increases

FIGURE 1-57 The greater the length of the sliding screw within the barrel, the lower its resistance to sliding. In this diagram F_h is the component of the joint reaction force perpendicular to the axis of the screw. The inferior edge of the proximal end of the barrel is the location of the fulcrum in bending. An internal force, F_b, from the surface of the barrel acts against the screw to counteract F_h. For equilibrium, the moments produced by F_h ($F_h \times L_e$) and F_b ($F_b \times L_b$) must be equal. If L_b, the distance from the point of application of internal force F_b to the fulcrum, decreases, F_b must increase to produce the same moment. If F_b is larger, the frictional force and therefore the resistance to screw sliding will increase. (L_e is the length of the screw beyond the barrel).[98]

can slide freely in the barrel of the side plate or the hole in the nail. The following points related to sliding hip screw devices apply to nail/lag screw constructs as well. When screw sliding occurs, the screw is supported by the barrel against inferior bending of the femoral head because the construct is buttressed by fracture interdigitation. Adherence to two basic mechanical principles will enhance the ability of the screw to slide in the bore of the side plate or nail. As mentioned above, the higher angle hip screw is more effective at accommodating sliding. Also, the screw should be engaged as deeply as possible within the barrel. For the same force acting at the femoral end of the screw, the internal force where the screw contacts the barrel is increased if less of the screw shaft remains in the barrel. This occurs because the moment (bending load) caused by the force transverse to the axis of the screw (F_h in Fig. 1-57) at the femoral head acts over a longer moment arm or perpendicular distance, L_e (force × perpendicular distance to the edge of the barrel, which is the fulcrum). The balancing moment arm, L_b, is shorter because less of the screw remains in the barrel. Because F_h acts over a longer moment arm while F_e acts over a shorter moment arm, F_b increases. The internal force, F_b, where the screw contacts the barrel causes a greater frictional resistance force, which requires more force to overcome friction and permit sliding.[98] Sliding hip screws with either two- or four-hole side plates appear to provide equivalent resistance to physiologic compressive loading.[115]

Several factors affect the strength of femoral neck fixation using multiple screws, but the number of screws used (three or four) is not a significant factor.[164] Factors that increase the strength of this type of fixation include a more horizontal fracture line with respect to the long axes of the screws,[50] placement of the screws in areas of greater femoral head bone density,[155,158] fractures with less comminution,[136] and a shorter moment arm

for the joint load (shorter distance from the center of the femoral head to the fracture line).[155] However, the most important factor has been found to be the quality of the reduction because of the importance of cortical buttressing in reducing fracture displacement.[152] Under physiologic load, several mechanisms of failure of fixation have been observed (Fig. 1-58). In some cases the screws bend inferiorly, especially if buttressing of the fracture surfaces inferior to the screws is not possible because of comminution of the fracture. The screw heads, if no washers are used to distribute the screw load against bone, have been found to pull through the cortex near the greater trochanter when the cortex is thin. Finally, if the screws are not well supported inferiorly where they cross the fracture, they may rotate inferiorly carrying the femoral head into a varus orientation.[155] Supporting at least one screw against the inferior cortex, which is an established clinical technique, may help prevent this from occurring.

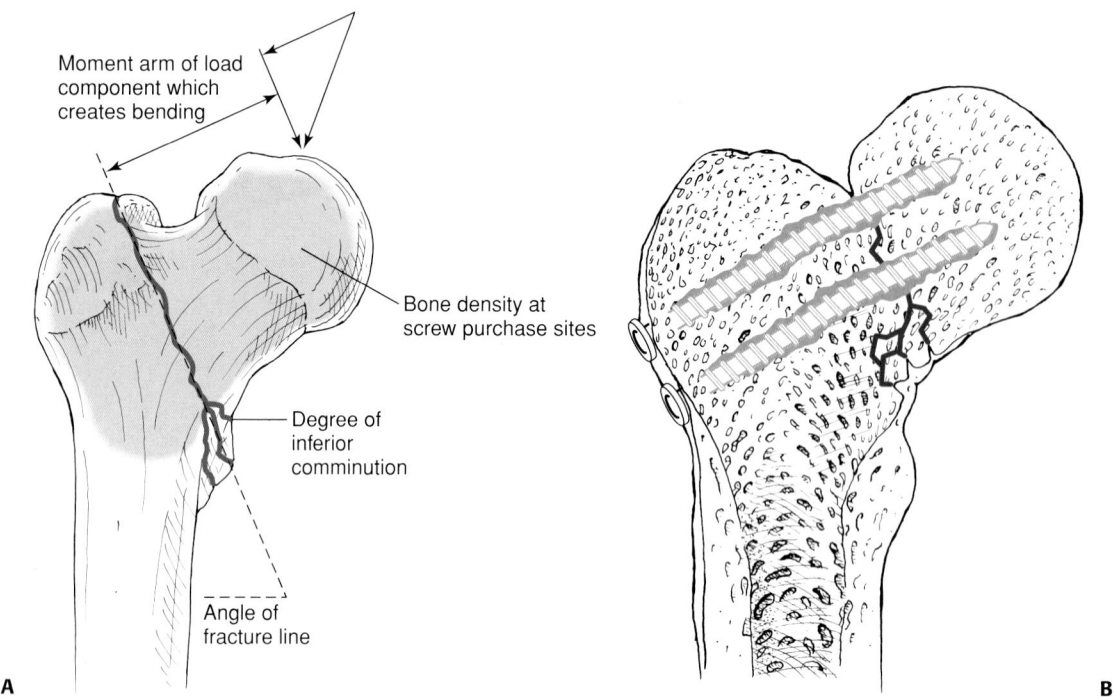

FIGURE 1-58 **A:** Some factors that decrease the strength of femoral neck fracture fixation include decreased bone density, a more vertical fracture surface (which facilitates sliding of the fracture components), comminution at the inferior cortex (which reduces buttressing against bending), and a longer moment arm or distance of the center of the femoral head to the fracture line. **B:** Observed mechanisms of failure of femoral neck fixation using screws include bending of the pins, displacement of the screw heads through the thin cortex of the greater trochanter, especially if washers are not used, and rotation of the screws inferiorly through the low-density cancellous bone of the Ward triangle area until they settle against the inferior cortex.[155]

With respect to the biomechanical performance of different devices, the actual stiffness provided by the sliding hip screw, the reconstruction nail, and multiple pin constructs are quite similar, except for significantly greater torsional stiffness of the reconstruction nail because of its tubular shape.[71,137] New techniques applied to proximal fracture fixation include the femoral locking plate and percutaneous compression plating. In fixation of the challenging vertical shear fracture of the proximal femur, the proximal femoral locking plate was found to produce considerably stiffer constructs than cannulated screws, a dynamic hip screw, or a dynamic condylar screw.[6] However, clinical series describing the use of the proximal femoral locking plate have demonstrated unacceptably high rates of failure, illustrating the dangers of relying solely on biomechanical data when choosing an implant.[19,156] Percutaneous compression plating has been found to provide adequate bending and torsional stability[97] and was equivalent to the trochanteric antegrade nail in fracture site stability, though it failed at about 2,100 N (about three times the body weight) compared with the antegrade nail at 3,200 N.[72]

Fixation Around the Metaphyseal Region of the Knee

Both supracondylar femur and tibial plateau fractures are challenging to stabilize because they often involve fixation of multiple small fragments of primarily cancellous bone. Supracondylar fixation alternatives that have been compared mechanically include condylar plates, plates with lag screws across the fracture site, and blade plates. All devices tested appeared to provide similar construct stiffnesses. The most important factor identified for plate fixation was maintaining contact at the cortex opposite to which the fixation device was applied. Fixation constructs without cortical contact were only 20% as stiff as those with cortical buttressing.[61,149] Using a retrograde IM supracondylar nail was found to produce constructs that were 14% less stiff in axial compression and 17% less stiff in torsion, compared with a fixed angle side plate.[118] However, longer nails (36 cm) enhanced fixation stability compared with shorter nails (20 cm).[153] Several newer fixation systems have been described for femoral supracondylar fracture stabilization. The less invasive stabilization system (LISS) uses a low-profile plate with monocortical screws distally, which also lock to the plate. LISS plates produced constructs with more elastic deformation and less subsidence than those with a condylar screw or buttress plate.[110,165]

Tibial plateau fractures are challenging to stabilize. Considering patient outcomes, risk factors for loss of reduction have been shown to include patients aged greater than 60 years old, premature weight bearing, fracture comminution, and severe osteoporosis.[3] Different methods of fixation include wires or

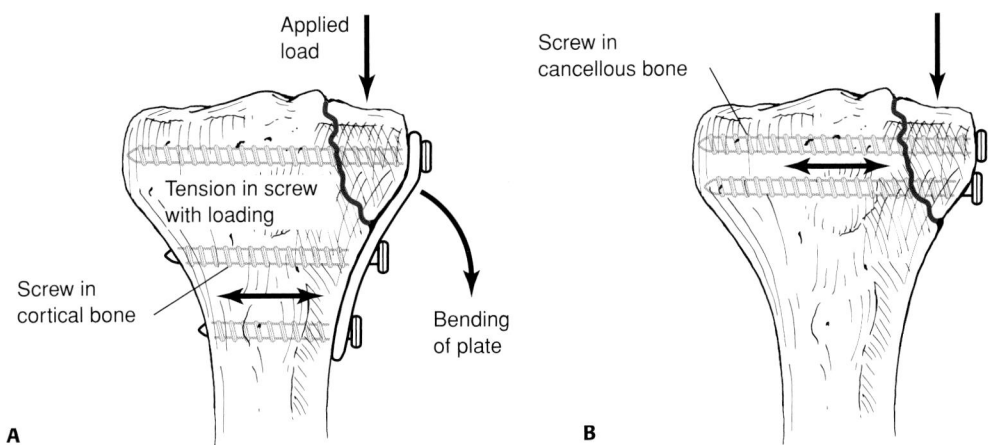

FIGURE 1-59 Two alternative methods of fixation of tibial plateau fractures: **(A)** transverse screws combined with a buttress plate and **(B)** transverse screws alone. The buttress plate provides additional support in bending as the tibial fracture component is loaded in an inferior direction and allows the screws to engage the thicker, more distal cortical bone.

screws alone (Fig. 1-59) or screws placed through an L- or T-shaped plate, buttressing the cortex. Various configurations of wires have been tested[25] and show that the stiffness of the construct increases with the number of wires, regardless of their specific orientations. As Figure 1-59 shows, fixation with screws alone requires that the screws resist bending forces as the tibial fragment is loaded distally in compression through the joint. With the addition of a plate, not only is the load distributed to the plate, but also additional screws can be placed in the stronger cortical bone distal in the metaphyseal region of the tibia. One disadvantage of a buttress plate is the soft tissue stripping required for application with potential for blood supply compromise. Fixation with T plates and screws showed the greatest resistance to an axial compressive load,[48] regardless of the specific configuration of the screws.[89] Investigations of different plate configurations found that for bicondylar tibial plateau fractures, dual (lateral and medial) side plating reduced subsidence under axial loading by about 50% compared with single-sided lateral locking plating.[77] For medial plateau fractures, the medial buttress plate, which supports the load directly, is significantly superior mechanically to a lateral locked plate.[133] A new alternative is a short proximal tibial nail with multiple interlocking screws. In combined axial loading, bending and rotation, the nail provided stability equivalent to that of double plating and was greater than constructs with a locking plate, external fixator, or conventional unreamed tibial nail.[74] This device may be applicable for cases without significant proximal (joint) comminution.

Fixation of the Spine

The halo apparatus is an external fixation device for cervical spine injuries that are stable in compression. It stabilizes the injured cervical spine mainly in bending but not in compression. Factors that affect its mechanical performance include (Fig. 1-60) the fit of the jacket on the torso and the frictional characteristics of the lining. High friction linings decrease slip

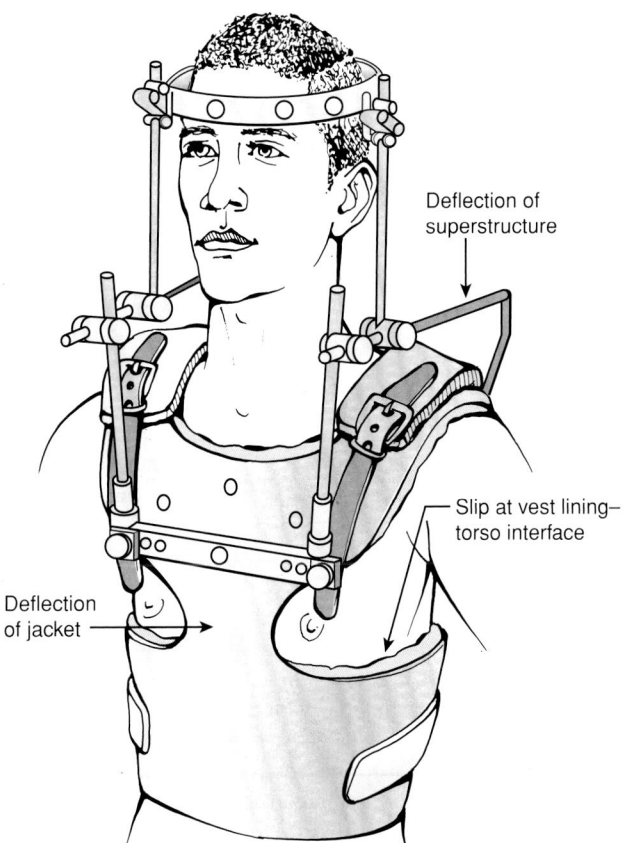

FIGURE 1-60 A schematic diagram showing possible sources of deformation in the halo apparatus. The large distance from the vest to chest contact points to the cervical injury site results in relatively large motions at the injury site for small motions of the vest.[120]

at the vest lining/torso interface, more rigid vests reduce deflection under loads, and less flexible superstructures all decrease cervical spine motion at the injury level. Although stiffening the vest enhances its ability to stabilize the injury, this property must be balanced with enough flexibility to provide reasonable comfort for the wearer and to accommodate expansion and contraction of the chest. Since the injured cervical segment is relatively distant from the vest, small motions of the vest can result in relatively large displacements at the injury site.[120] A very rigid halo superstructure attaching the vest to the halo ring may not increase injury stability if connected to a poorly fitting vest.

Several methods are available to reconstruct cervical spine injuries. The major differences between them relate to the location of the fixation device itself on the vertebra—anterior, lateral, or posterior—and to the method by which the fixation is attached to the bone. Generally, the most rigid fixation is the one with the longest moment arm from the center of rotation of the injured segment. For a specific applied moment, such as flexion, a posteriorly located fixation, being located farther from the center of rotation, results in greater rigidity. Figure 1-61 shows the approximate locations of the centers of rotation at different cervical spine levels when the posterior elements have been disrupted.[5] After corpectomy, biomechanical testing has shown that posterior rods provide the greatest stability, which is unchanged after augmentation with an anterior plate, whereas anterior plating alone offers the least stability.[150] Similarly, another test showed that after corpectomy, sagittal plane motion was most rigid after supplementation with lateral mass plates, less rigid with an anterior plate alone, and least with strut grafting alone.[90] Anterior plates provide relatively similar stability, especially if augmented with a bone graft; however, with multilevel corpectomy, anterior plate constructs were more prone to fatigue loosening than single-level corpectomies.[84] Newer semiconstrained anterior plates, most of which offer devices to lock the screws to prevent back out, allow screw rotation which results in more load sharing with the graft.[131] By comparison, the compressive load estimated to be transmitted through the graft increased from 40% with a fully constrained device to 80% when a semiconstrained device was used.[131] Wiring or plating with lateral mass screws generally reduces anterior–posterior motion across the fixed segment by 20% to 70%, so none of these techniques can be considered as entirely rigid.[119]

The type of attachment of the fixation system to the vertebra is fundamental to its performance. Wires, hooks, screws, or combinations, all produce different types of force transfer between the fixation and the vertebra (Fig. 1-62).[38] A wire can resist only tension, whereas a screw can resist forces in all directions (tension, compression, bending transverse to the axis of the screw) except for rotation about its longitudinal axis. A hook only resists forces that drive the surface of the hook against the bone, and depends on the shape of the hook and the bone surface it rests against. For this reason, screws are biomechanically superior to other forms of vertebral attachments.

In general, pedicle screws resist pullout in the same manner as bone screws described elsewhere. Therefore the pull-

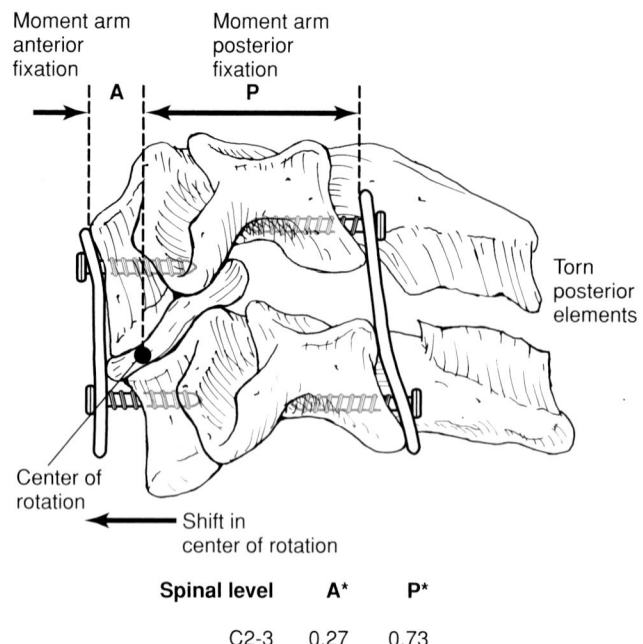

Spinal level	A*	P*
C2-3	0.27	0.73
C3-4	0.32	0.68
C4-5	0.36	0.64
C5-6	0.39	0.61
C6-7	0.44	0.56

*In % of anterior–posterior diameter of vertebra

FIGURE 1-61 The ratios, in terms or anterior–posterior diameter or the vertebra, of the location of the center of rotation at each vertebral level, from the anterior and posterior surfaces. A fixation device must resist bending moments caused by flexion, extension, lateral bending, and torsion. The resisting moment in the fixation is the product of the force acting in the fixation (e.g., at the screw–plate junction) and the distance of that point on the fixation to the center of rotation of the motion segment. The longer the moment arm for the same bending load, the smaller the force on the fixation components. Posterior fixation, by its location, will have lower moments in its components.[5]

out strength increases with increasing density of the bone it is embedded into,[35,109,170,173] a greater depth of insertion,[100] engagement of the anterior cortex,[121] and a larger screw diameter. Single screws placed into pedicles and loaded in a caudal–cephalad direction (which occurs during flexion and extension of the vertebra) are vulnerable to toggling, and eventual loosening, even under relatively small forces. As demonstrated in Figure 1-63, the screw tends to toggle about the base of the pedicle, which is the stiffest region as it mainly comprises cortical bone. Toggling tends to enlarge the screw hole in a "windshield wiper" fashion.[13,100] Toggling can be reduced if the screw head is locked to the plate or rod, and the plate or rod contacts the vertebra over a wide area.[100]

Some fundamental principles should be considered when applying lumbar spinal fixation. Longer fixation, attached to more vertebrae, reduces forces acting on the screws because of the effect of the greater lever arm of a longer plate or rod. A longer fusion, although biomechanically advantageous, is

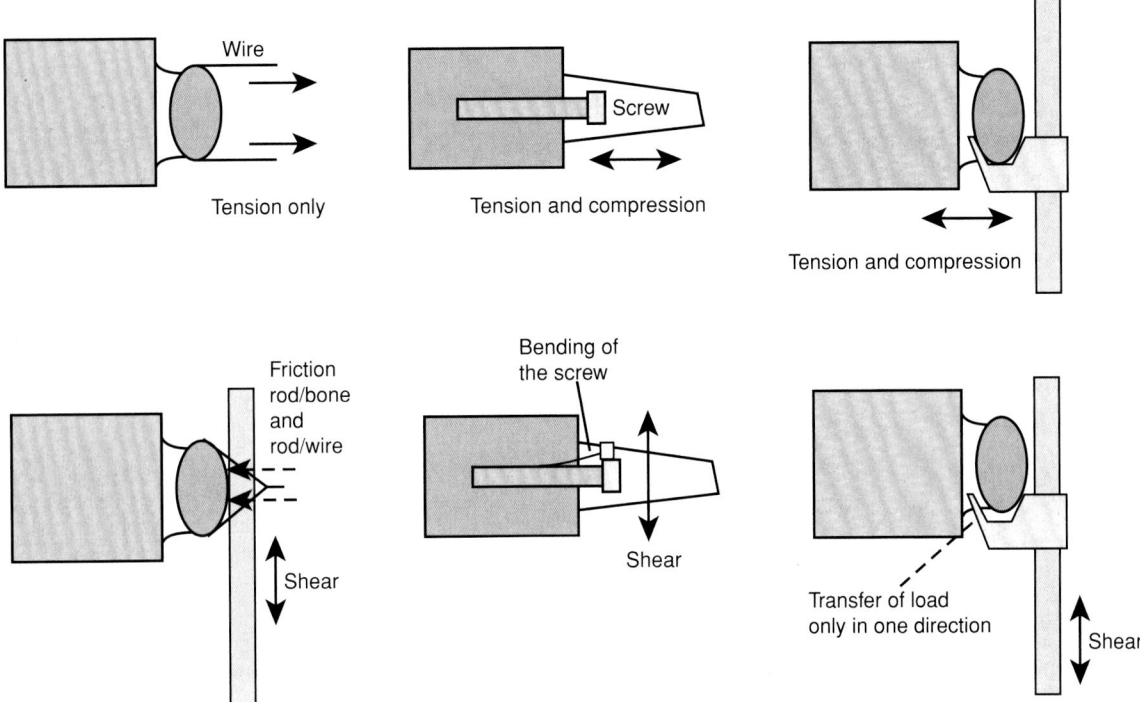

FIGURE 1-62 Comparisons of the forces that can be resisted by different methods of attachment of the fixation to the vertebra. A sublaminar wire resists only tension, whereas a screw can resist forces in all directions except for rotation about its long axis. A hook resists only forces that drive it against the bone surfaces.

not necessarily beneficial from a clinical perspective because the remaining spinal motion is significantly reduced. Adding an anterior strut graft or a fusion cage is important because it buttresses a posterior fixation system against flexion moments, reducing forces in the fixation.[94] Coupler bars, which connect the fixation rods to form an H configuration, prevent the rods from rotating medially or laterally when torsion is applied to the motion segment, as shown in Figure 1-64. This significantly enhances the torsional and lateral bending stability of the implant.[77]

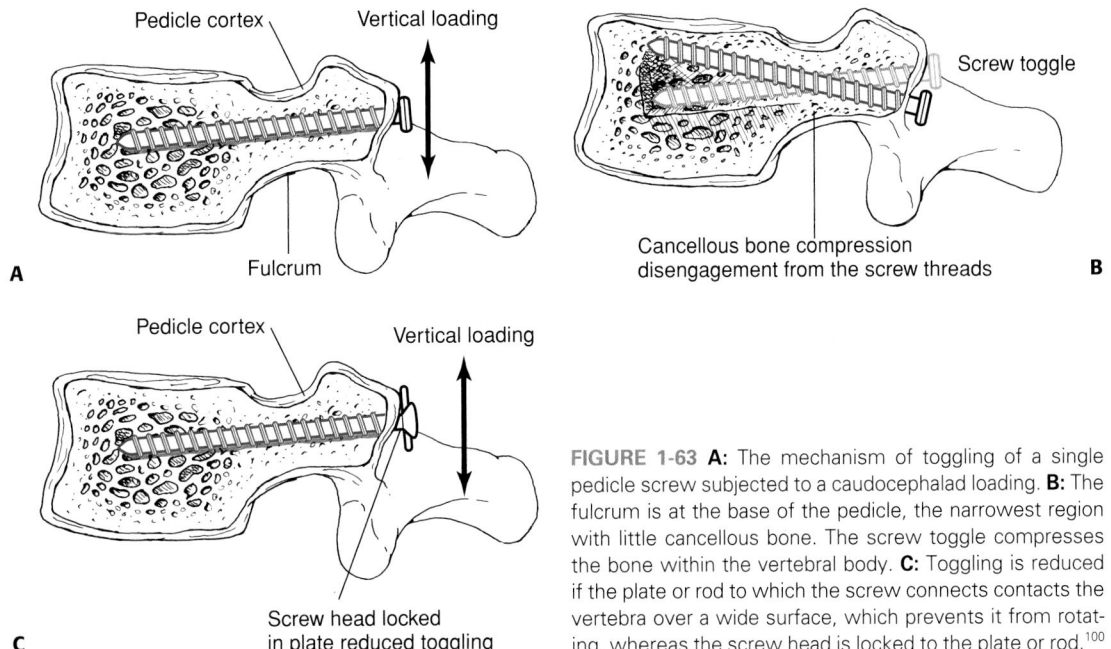

FIGURE 1-63 A: The mechanism of toggling of a single pedicle screw subjected to a caudocephalad loading. B: The fulcrum is at the base of the pedicle, the narrowest region with little cancellous bone. The screw toggle compresses the bone within the vertebral body. C: Toggling is reduced if the plate or rod to which the screw connects contacts the vertebra over a wide surface, which prevents it from rotating, whereas the screw head is locked to the plate or rod.[100]

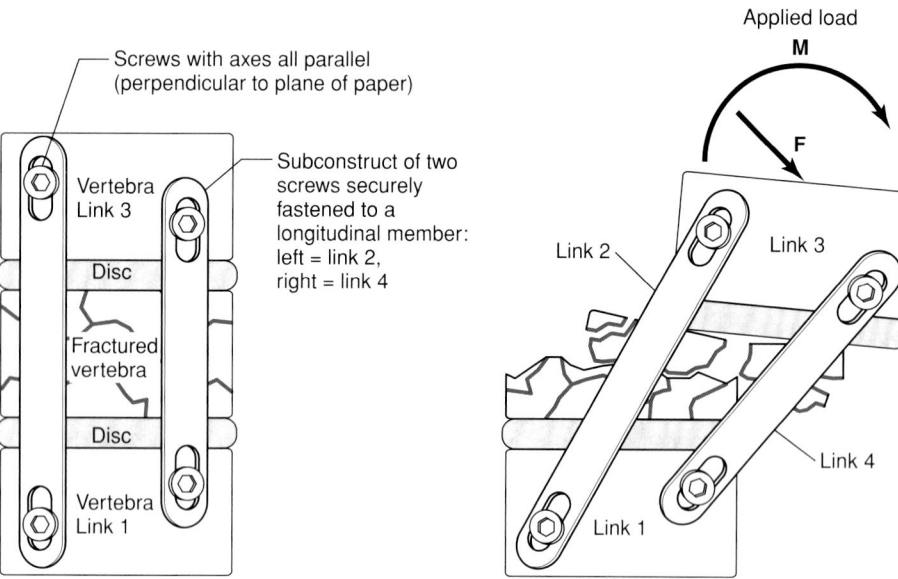

FIGURE 1-64 Without a coupler bar between two longitudinal rods **(left)**, they can rotate when a lateral moment or axial torsion is applied **(right)**. A coupler connecting the rods to form an H configuration reduces this effect.[77]

Extensive testing has been performed on various posterior and anterior thoracolumbar fixation devices as they continue to be developed. Testing of anterior fixation systems with and without an augmented strut graft showed that load sharing with the graft ranged from 63% to 89% for six systems tested, three being plates and three based on locked rods. These tests demonstrated the significant effect of the graft in sagittal plane stability. The most rigid systems relied on either a thick rigid plate or large rods, although this may not correlate with clinical performance.[28] In cases of delayed or nonunion, the cyclic performance of the implant can be very important, more so than its static stiffness or maximum load to failure. A comparison test of 12 fixation systems showed that only three could withstand two million load cycles with 600 N of compressive force. The two constructs with the greatest bending strength did not fail after cycling. However, there was no correlation between bending strength and cyclic failure for the other 10 systems, indicating that particular design aspects could cause fatigue failure regardless of static strength.[93] Three devices failed in less than 10,000 cycles. Currently, most posterior devices use essentially the same principles, including pedicle screws with an interface clamp to the rod that allows variable orientation of the screw, a low-profile assembly, and crosslinks. They provide similar fixation stiffness. Lumbosacral fixation using sacral screws was most rigid and demonstrated the least screw strain when supplemented with iliac screws, and was more effective than using screws at S1 supplemented with screws at S2.[101]

The biomechanical properties of fusion cages have been investigated. A fusion cage is a hollow threaded insert that can be applied from anterior, lateral, or posterior directions in single or double units. Various fusion cages are available for the cervical spine. The devices fall into one of three categories: screw designs with a horizontal cylinder and external threads, box shapes, and vertical cylinders. In general, all cage designs increased flexion stiffness by 130% to 180%. Only a few box or cylinder designs increased extension stiffness, and box designs were most effective in increasing axial rotation and lateral bending stiffnesses, ranging from 140% to 180% of intact values.[87] Testing of lumbar fusion cages has shown that placement of cages in lateral, posterolateral, or posterior orientations had little effect on stiffness. The exception was for torsional loading with posterior cage placement because posterior insertion damaged the lamina or facets, thus reducing the inherent torsional stability of the motion segment. Fixation with cages alone did not significantly increase lumbar motion segment stability, so augmentation with posterior fixation in cases of motion segment instability is necessary. Because cage fixation relies on the combination of distraction of the soft tissues and the strength of the vertebral cancellous bone, the properties of these tissues will have a significant effect on the performance of cage implant constructs.[162]

Fixation of the Humerus

Proximal humerus fractures fixed with locking plates provided greater stability against torsional loading, but were similar to blade plate constructs in bending, because both fixation devices are loaded as tension bands in bending.[122,145,146] In comparing different types of blade plate constructs, the stiffest construct employed an eight-hole, low-contact dynamic compression plate, contoured into a blade configuration, and fixed with a diagonal screw that triangulates with the end of the blade. This arrangement was considerably stiffer than other blade plates or T plate and screw constructs.[105] One potential problem is penetration of the screws through the subchondral bone in osteoporotic patients. Because of the stiffness of the locking plate–screw construct, if there is any "settling" of the fracture site the locking screws may penetrate into the joint. The incidence of intra-articular screw penetration with proximal humeral locking plates is considerably higher than with conventional implants.[52]

SUMMARY

Effective fracture fixation requires a biomechanical appreciation of the forces applied to a damaged bone or joint and the basic mechanisms by which these loads are transferred through the bridging fixation and the implant–bone interface. In particular, the importance of the contribution of cortex-to-cortex contact across the fracture site in resisting both compressive and bending forces must be emphasized. This contact creates a buttress that contributes significantly to the stability of the construct and the functional life of the implant. Many of the observations used to formulate these basic principles have been made using cadaveric bone in experimental laboratory simulations, and conclusions are based on comparisons of the most rigid mechanical construct. Other aspects such as the compromise of blood flow or the extent of the incision during installation should also be considered. Further, even if one construct is more rigid than another, within a certain range of mechanical stiffness, both may perform equally well in producing fracture healing with anatomic alignment. It is important to correlate biomechanical information with clinical observations of the performance of the implant during fracture healing.

REFERENCES

1. Aharonoff GB, Dennis MG, Elshinawy A, et al. Circumstances of falls causing hip fractures in the elderly. *Clin Orthop Rel Res.* 1998;348:10–14.
2. Alho A, Husby T, Hoiseth A. Bone mineral content and mechanical strength. An exvivo study on human femora at autopsy. *Clin Orthop Rel Res.* 1988;227:292–297.
3. Ali AM, El-Shafie M, Willett KM. Failure of fixation of tibial plateau fractures. *J Orthop Trauma.* 2002;16:323–329.
4. Allgower M. Cinderella of surgery-fractures? *Surg Clin North Am.* 1978;58:1071–1093.
5. Amevo B, Aprill C, Bogduk N. Abnormal instantaneous axes of rotation in patients with neck pain. *Spine.* 1992;17:748–756.
6. Aminian A, Gao F, Fedoriw WW, et al. Vertically oriented femoral neck fractures: Mechanical analysis of four fixation techniques. *J Orthop Trauma.* 2007;21:544–548.
7. Antekeier SB, Burden RL, Voor MJ, et al. Mechanical study of the safe distance between distal femoral fracture site and distal locking screws in antegrade intraduallary nailing. *J Orthop Trauma.* 2005;19:693–697.
8. Aro HT, Wippenman BW, Hodgson SF, et al. Prediction of properties of fracture callus by measurement of mineral density using microbone densitometry. *J Bone Joint Surg Am.* 1989;71A:1020–1030.
9. Ascenzi A, Bonucci E. The tensile properties of single osteons. *Anat Rec.* 1967;158:375–386.
10. Ascenzi A, Bonucci E. The compressive properties of single osteons. *Anat Rec.* 1968;161:377–392.
11. Ascenzi A, Bonucci E. The shearing properties of single osteons. *Anat Rec.* 1972;172:499–510.
12. Ascenzi A, Bonucci E, Simkin A. An approach to the mechanical properties of single osteonic lamellae. *J Biomech.* 1973;6:227–235.
13. Ashman RB, Galpin RD, Corin JD, et al. Biomechanical analysis of pedicle screw instrumentation in a corpectomy model. *Spine.* 1989;14:1398–1405.
14. Askew MJ, Mow VC, Wirth CR, et al. Analysis of the intraosseus stress field due to compression plating. *J Biomech.* 1975;8:203–212.
15. Assal M, Huber P, Rohr E, et al. Are drivers more likely to injure their right or left foot in a frontal car crash: A car crash and biomechanical investigation. *46th Annual Proceedings, Association for the Advancement of Automotive Medicine.* 2002:273–288.
16. Augat P, Merk J, Wolf S, et al. Mechanical stimulation by external application of cyclic tensile strains does not effectively enhance bone healing. *J Orthop Trauma.* 2001;15:54–60.
17. Ayerby SA, Ehteshami JR, McLain RF. Offset laminar hooks decrease bending moments of pedicle screws during in situ contouring. *Spine.* 1997;22:376–381.
18. Bai B, Kummer FJ, Spivak J. Augmentation of anterior vertebral body screw fixation by an injectable biodegradable calcium phosphate bone substitute. *Spine.* 2001;24:2679–2683.
19. Berkes MB, Little MT, Lazaro LE, et al. Catastrophic failure after open reduction internal fixation of femoral neck fractures with a novel locking plate implant. *J Orthop Trauma.* 2012;26:e170–e176.
20. Bartley MH Jr, Arnold JS, Haslam RK, et al. The relationship of bone strength and bone quantity in health, disease, and aging. *J Gerontol.* 1996;21:517–521.
21. Behrens F, Johnson WD. Unilateral external fixation methods to increase and reduce frame stiffness. *Clin Orthop Rel Res.* 1989;241:48–56.
22. Bell GH, Dunbar O, Beck JS, et al. Variations in strength of vertebrae with age and their relation to osteoporosis. *Calcif Tissue Res.* 1967;1:75–86.
23. Benirschke SK, Swiontkowski MF. Knee. In: Hansen ST, Swiontkowski MF, eds. *Orthopedic Trauma Protocols.* New York, NY: Raven Press, 1993.
24. Benjamin J, Bried J, Dohm M, et al. Biomechanical evaluation of various forms of fixation of transverse patellar fractures. *J Orthop Trauma.* 1987;1:219–222.
25. Beris AE, Glisson RR, Seaber AV, et al. Load tolerance of tibial plateau depressions reinforced with a cluster of K-wires. Paper presented at: 34th Annual Meeting of the Orthopedic Research Society; March 7–10, 1988; Atlanta, CA.
26. Black J. *Orthopedic Biomaterials in Research and Practice.* New York, NY: Churchill Livingstone; 1988.
27. Bottlang M, Lesser M, Koerber J, et al. Far cortical locking can improve healing of fractures stabilized with locking plates. *J Bone Joint Surg Am.* 2010;92(7):1652–1660.
28. Brodke DS, Gollogly S, Bachus KN, et al. Anterior thoracolumbar instrumentation: Stiffness and load sharing characteristics of plate and rod systems. *Spine.* 2003:1794–1801.
29. Brooks DB, Burstein AH, Frankel UH. The biomechanics of torsional fractures. *J Bone Joint Surg Am.* 1970;52A:507–514.
30. Bucholz RW, Ross SE, Lawrence KL. Fatigue fracture of the interlocking nail in the treatment of fractures of the distal part of the femoral shaft. *J Bone Joint Surg Am.* 1987;69A:1391–1399.
31. Burstein AH, Reilly DL, Martens M. Aging of bone tissue: Mechanical properties. *J Bone Joint Surg Am.* 1976;58A:82–86.
32. Burstein AH, Zika IM, Heiple KG, et al. Contribution of collagen and mineral to the elastic-plastic properties of bone. *J Bone Jt Surg Am.* 1975;57A:956–961.
33. Calhoun JH, Li F, Ledbetter BR, et al. Biomechanics of Ilizarov for fracture fixation. Paper presented at: 37th Annual Meeting of the Orthopedic Research Society; March 4–7, Anaheim, CA.
34. Carter DR, Hayes WC. The compressive behavior of bone as a two-phase porous structure. *J Bone Joint Surg Am.* 1977;59A:954–962.
35. Chapman JR, Harrington RM, Lee KM, et al. Factors affecting the pullout strength of cancellous bone screws. *ASME J Biomech Eng.* 1996;118:391–398.
36. Clark CR, Morgan C, Sonstegard DA, et al. The effect of biopsy-hole shape and size on bone strength. *J Bone Joint Surg Am.* 1977;59A:213–217.
37. Cody DD, Goldstein SA, Flynn MJ, et al. Correlations between vertebral regional bone mineral density (rBMD) and whole bone fracture load. *Spine.* 1991;16:146–154.
38. Coe JD, Herzig MA, Warden KE, et al. Load to failure of spinal implants in osteoporotic spines; a comparison of pedicle screws, laminar hooks, and spinous process wires. Paper presented at: 35th Annual Meeting of the Orthopedic Research Society; March 1–4, Las Vegas, NV.
39. Cordey J, Florin P, Klaue K, et al. Compression achieved with the dynamic compression plate: Effects of the inclined sloping cylinder and inclination of the screw. In: Uthhoff HK, ed. *Current Concepts of Internal Fixation of Fractures.* Berlin: Springer-Verlag; 1980:192–200.
40. Crowninshield RD, Pope MH. The response of compact bone in tension at various strain rates. *Ann Biomed Eng.* 1974;2:217–225.
41. Currey JD. The mechanical consequences of variation in the mineral content of bone. *J Biomech.* 1969;2:1–11.
42. Currey JD. The effects of strain rate, reconstruction, and mineral content on some mechanical properties of bovine bone. *J Biomech.* 1975;8:81–86.
43. Currey JD. Changes in the impact energy absorption of bone with age. *J Biomech.* 1979;12:459–469.
44. Currey JD. *The Mechanical Adaptation of Bones.* Princeton, NJ: Princeton University Press; 1984.
45. Currey JD, Butler G. The mechanical properties of the bone tissue in children. *J Bone Joint Surg Am.* 1975;57A:810–814.
46. Dalen N, Hellstrom LG, Jacobson B. Bone mineral content and mechanical strength of the femoral neck. *Acta Orthop Scand.* 1976;47:503–508.
47. DeCoster TA, Heetderks DB, Downey DJ, et al. Optimizing bone screw pullout force. *J Orthop Trauma.* 1990;4:169–174.
48. Denny LD, Keating EM, Engelhardt JA, et al. A comparison of fixation techniques in tibial plateau fractures. Paper presented at: 30th Annual Meeting of the Orthopedic Research Society; February 6–9, Atlanta, GA..
49. Edgarton BC, An K-A, Morrey BF. Torsional strength reduction due to cortical defects in bone. *J Orthop Res.* 1990;8:851–855.
50. Edwards WT, Lewallen DG, Hayes WC. The effect of pin number and fracture pattern on immediate mechanical fixation of a subcapital hip fracture model. Paper presented at: 31st Annual Meeting of the Orthopedic Research Society; February 19–22, Las Vegas, NV.
51. Egol KA, Chang EY, Cvitkovic J, et al. Mismatch of current intramedullary nails with the anterior bow of the femur. *J Orthop Trauma.* 2004;18:410–415.
52. Egol KA, Kubiak EN, Fulkerson E, et al. Biomechanics of locked plates and screws. *J Orthop Trauma.* 2004;18:488–493.
53. Ehmke LW, Polzin BMI, Madey SM, et al. Femoral nailing through the trochanter: The reamer pathway indicates a helical shaped nail. *J Orthop Trauma.* 2006;20:668–674.
54. Elder S, Frankenberg E, Yetkilner DN, et al. Biomechanical evaluation of calcium phosphate cement augmented fixation of unstable intertrochanteric fractures. Paper presented at: 43rd Annual Meeting of the Orthopedic Research Society; March 16–19, New Orleans, LA.
55. Ellis T, Bourgeault CA, Kyle RF. Screw position affects dynamic compression plate strain in an in vitro fracture model. *J Orthop Trauma.* 2001;15:333–337.
56. El Maraghy AW, Elmaraghy MW, Nousiainen M, et al. Influence of the number of cortices on the stiffness of plate fixation of diaphyseal fractures. *J Orthop Trauma.* 2001;15:186–191.
57. Evans FG. Relations between the microscopic structure and tensile strength of human bone. *Acta Anat.* 1958;35:285–301.
58. Evans FG, Bang S. Differences and relationships between the physical properties and the structure of human femoral, tibial, and fibular cortical bone. *Am J Anat.* 1967;120:79–88.
59. Evans FG, Vincentelli R. Relation of collagen fiber orientation to some mechanical properties of human cortical bone. *J Biomech.* 1969;2:63–71.
60. Finlay JB, Jarada I, Boune RB, et al. Analysis of the pull-out strength of screws and pegs used to secure tibial components following total knee arthroplasty. *Clin Orthop Rel Res.* 1989;247:220–231.

61. Frankenburg EP, Robinson AP, Urquhart AG, et al. Supracondylar femur fractures: A biomechanical analysis of four fixation devices. Paper presented at: 38th Annual Meeting of the Orthopedic Research Society; February 17–20, Washington, DC.
62. Frigg R, Appenzeller A, Christensen R, et al. The development of the distal femur Less Invasive Stabilization System (LISS). *Injury.* 2001;32:S-C-24–S-C-31.
63. Funk JR, Tourret LJ, George SE, et al. The role of axial loading in malleolar fractures. *SAE Transactions.* 2000–01–0155, 2000.
64. Galante J, Rostoker W, Ray RD. Physical properties of trabecular bone. *Calcif Tissue Res.* 1970;5:236–246.
65. Gardner MJ, Nork SE, Huber Pet al. Stiffness modulation of locking plate constructs using near cortical slotted holes: A preliminary study. *J Orthop Trauma.* 2009;23(4):281–287.
66. Gardner MJ, Nork SE, Huber P, et al. Less rigid stable fracture fixation in osteoporotic bone using locked plates with near cortical slots. *Injury.* 2010;41(6):652–656.
67. Gardner MJ, Silva MJ, Krieg JC. Biomechanical testing of fracture fixation constructs: variability, validity, and clinical applicability. *J Am Acad Orthop Surg.* 2012;20:86–93.
68. Geller J, Tornetta P III, Tiburzi D, et al. Tension wire position for hybrid external fixation of the proximal tibia. *J Orthop Trauma.* 2000;14:502–504.
69. Georgette FS, Sander TW, Oh I. *The fatigue resistance of orthopedic wire and cable systems.* Washington, DC: Second World Congress on Biomaterials; 1984:146.
70. Goldman MW, MacLennan PA, McGwin G, et al. The association between restraint system and upper extremity injury after motor vehicle collisions. *J Orthop Trauma.* 2005;19:529–534.
71. Goodman SB, Davidson JA, Locke L, et al. A biomechanical study of two methods of internal fixation of unstable fractures of the femoral neck. *J Orthop Trauma.* 1992;6:66–72.
72. Gotfried Y, Cohen B, Rotem A. Biomechanical evaluation of the percutaneous compression plating system for hip fractures. *J Orthop Trauma.* 2002;16:644–650.
73. Gotzen L, Hutter J, Haas N. The prebending of AO plates in compression osteosynthesis. In: Uhthoff HK, ed. *Current Concepts of Internal Fixation of Fractures.* Berlin: Springer-Verlag; 1980:201–210.
74. Hansen M, Mehler D, Hessmann MH, et al. Intramedullary stabilization of extra-articular proximal tibial fractures: A biomechanical comparison of intramedullary and extramedullary implants including a new proximal tibial nail (PTN). *J Orthop Trauma.* 2007;21:701–709.
75. Harrell RM, Tong J, Weinhold PS, et al. Comparison of the mechanical properties of different tension band materials and suture techniques. *J Orthop Trauma.* 2003;17:119–122.
76. Hertel R, Jost B. Basic principles and techniques of internal fixation in osteoporotic bone. In: Yhu An, ed. *Internal Fixation in Osteoporotic Bone.* New York, NY: Thieme; 2002:108–115.
77. Higgans TF, Klatt J, Bachus KN. Biomechanical analysis of bicondylar tibial plateau fixation: How does lateral locking plate fixation compare to dual plate fixation? *J Orthop Trauma.* 2007;21:301–306.
78. Hou S-H, Wang J-L, Lin J. Mechanical strength, fatigue life, and failure analysis of two prototypes and five conventional tibial locking screws. *J Orthop Res.* 2002;16:701–708.
79. Hufner T, Geerling J, Oldag G, et al. Accuracy study of computer assisted drilling: The effect of bone density, drill bit characteristics, and use of a mechanical guide. *J Orthop Trauma.* 2005;19:317–322.
80. Hughes AN, Jordan BA. The mechanical properties of surgical bone screws and some aspects of insertion practice. *Injury.* 1972;4:25–38.
81. Huiskes R, Chao EYS. Guidelines for external fixation frame rigidity and stresses. *J Orthop Res.* 1986;4:68–75.
82. Huiskes R, Chao EYS, Crippen TE. Parametric analyses of pin-bone stresses in external fracture fixation. *J Orthop Res.* 1985;3:341–349.
83. Hungerford DS, Barry M. Biomechanics of the patellofemoral joint. *Clin Orthop Rel Res.* 1979;144:9–15.
84. Isomi T, Panjabi MM, Wang J-L, et al. Stabilizing potential of anterior cervical plates in multilevel corpectomies. *Spine.* 1999;24:2219–2223.
85. Johnson KD, Tencer AF, Sherman MC. Biomechanical factors affecting fracture stability and femoral bursting in closed intramedullary nailing of femoral shaft fractures, with illustrative case presentations. *J Orthop Trauma.* 1987;1:1–11.
86. Kaab MJ, Frenk A, Schmeling A, et al. Locked internal fixator, sensitivity of screwplate stability to the correct insertion angle of the screw. *J Orthop Trauma.* 2004;18:483–487.
87. Kandziora F, Pflugmacher R, Schafer J, et al. Biomechanical comparison of cervical spine interbody fusion cages. *Spine.* 2001;26:1850–1857.
88. Karnezis IA, Miles AW, Cunningham JL, et al. Biological internal fixation of long bone fractures: A biomechanical study of a noncontact plate system. *Injury.* 1998;29:689–695.
89. Karunaker MA, Egol KA, Peindl R, et al. Split depression tibial plateau fractures: A biomechanical study. *J Orthop Trauma.* 2002;16:172–177.
90. Kirkpatrick JS, Levy JA, Carillo J, et al. Reconstruction after multilevel corpectomy in the cervical spine. *Spine.* 1999;24:1186–1191.
91. Klaue K, Perren SM, Kowalski M. Internal fixation with a self-compressing plate and screw: Improvements of the plate hole and screw design. I. Mechanical investigation. *J Orthop Trauma.* 1991;5:280–288.
92. Korner J, Diederichs G, Arzdorf M, et al. A biomechanical evaluation of methods of distal humerus fracture fixation using locking compression plates versus conventional reconstruction plates. *J Orthop Trauma.* 2004;18:286–293.
93. Kotani Y, Cunningham BW, Parker LM, et al. Static and fatigue biomechanical properties of anterior thoracolumbar instrumentation systems. *Spine.* 1999;24:1406–1413.
94. Krag MH. Biomechanics of thoracolumbar spinal fixation. A review. *Spine.* 1991;16:S85–S98.
95. Krag MH, Beynnan BD, Pope MH, et al. An internal fixator for posterior application to short segments of the thoracic, lumbar, or lumbosacral spine. Design and testing. *Clin Orthop Rel Res.* 1986;203:75–98.
96. Krupp RJ, Malkani AL, Goodin RA, et al. Optimal entry point for retrograde femoral nailing. *J Orthop Trauma.* 2003;17:100–105.
97. Kubiak EN, Bong M, Park SS, et al. Intramedullary fixation of unstable intertrochanteric hip fractures. *J Orthop Trauma.* 2004;18:12–17.
98. Kyle RF, Wright TM, Burstein AH. Biomechanical analysis of the sliding characteristics of compression hip screws. *J Bone Joint Surg Am.* 1980;62A:1308–1314.
99. Laurence M, Freeman MA, Swanson SA. Engineering considerations in the internal fixation of fractures of the tibial shaft. *J Bone Joint Surg Am.* 1969;51B:754–768.
100. Law M, Tencer AF, Anderson PA. Caudo-cephalad loading of pedicle screws: Mechanisms of loosening and methods of augmentation. *Spine.* 1993;18:2438–2443.
101. Lebwohl NH, Cunningham BW, Dmitriev A, et al. Biomechanical comparison of lumbosacral fixation techniques in a calf spine model. *Spine.* 2002;27:2312–2320.
102. Leggon RE, Lindsey RW, Panjabi MM. Strength reduction and the effects of treatment of long bones with diaphyseal defects involving 50% of the cortex. *J Orthop Res.* 1988;6:540–546.
103. Leicher I, Margulies JY, Weinreb A, et al. The relationship between bone density, mineral content, and mechanical strength in the femoral neck. *Clin Orthop Rel Res.* 1982;163:272–281.
104. Leighton RK, Waddell JP, Bray TJ, et al. Biomechanical testing of new and old fixation devices for vertical shear fracture of the pelvis. *J Orthop Trauma.* 1991;5:313–317.
105. Lever JP, Aksenov SA, Zdero R, et al. Biomechanical analysis of plate osteosynthesis systems for proximal humerus fractures. *J Orthop Trauma.* 2008;22:23–29.
106. Liebschner MAK, Rosenberg WS, Keaveny TM. Effects of bone cement volume and distribution on vertebral stiffness after vertebroplasty. *Spine.* 2001;26:1547–1554.
107. Lim TH, Breback GT, Renner SM, et al. Biomechanical evaluation of an injectable calcium phosphate cement for vertebroplasty. *Spine.* 2002;27:1297–1302.
108. Lotz JC, Gerhart TN, Hayes WC. Mechanical properties of trabecular bone from the proximal femur by single-energy quantitative computed tomography. *J Comput Assist Tomogr.* 1990;14:107–114.
109. Mann KA, Bartel DL. A structural analysis of the fixation of pedicle screws to vertebrae. Paper presented at: 36th Annual Meeting of the Orthopedic Research Society; February 5–8, New Orleans, LA.
110. Marti A, Fankhauser C, Frenk A, et al. Biomechanical evaluation of the less invasive stabilization system for the internal fixation of distal femur fractures. *J Orthop Res.* 2001;15:482–487.
111. McBroom, RJ, Cheal EJ, Hayes WC. Strength reductions from metastatic cortical defects in long bones. *J Orthop Res.* 1988;6:369–378.
112. McElhaney JH. Dynamic response of bone and muscle tissue. *J Appl Physiol.* 1966;21:1231–1236.
113. McElhaney JH, Alem NM, Roberts VL. A porous block model for cancellous bone. *Am Soc Mech Eng.* 1970;70-WA/BHF-2:1–9.
114. McKoy BE, Conner GS, An YH. An interlocking screw for fixation in osteoporotic bone. In: An YH, ed. *Internal Fixation in Osteoporotic Bone.* New York, NY: Thieme; 2002: 237–241.
115. McLoughlin SW, Wheeler DL, Rider J, et al. Biomechanical evaluation of the dynamic hip screw with two and four-hole side plates. *J Orthop Trauma.* 2000;14:318–323.
116. Mehta M, Strube P, Peters A, et al. Duda Influences of age and mechanical stability on volume, microstructure, and mineralization of the fracture callus during bone healing: Is osteoclast activity the key to age-related impaired healing? *Bone.* 2010;47(2):219–228.
117. Merk BR, Stern SH, Cordes S, et al. A fatigue life analysis of small fragment screws. *J Orthop Trauma.* 2001;15:494–499.
118. Meyer RW, Plaxton NA, Postak PD, et al. Mechanical comparison of a distal femoral side plate and a retrograde intramedullary nail. *J Orthop Trauma.* 2000;14:398–404.
119. Mihara H, Cheng BC, David SM, et al. Biomechanical comparison of posterior cervical fixation. *Spine.* 2001;26:1662–1667.
120. Mirza SK, Moquin RR, Anderson PA, et al. Stabilizing properties of the halo apparatus. *Spine.* 1997;22:727–733.
121. Misenhimer GR, Peek RD, Wiltze LL, et al. Anatomic analysis of pedicle canal and cancellous diameter related to screw size. *Spine.* 1989;14:367–372.
122. Molloy S, Jasper LE, Elliott DS, et al. Biomechanical evaluation of intramedullary nail versus tension band fixation for transverse olecranon fractures. *J Orthop Trauma.* 2004;18:170–174.
123. Moroni A, Aspenberg P, Toksvig-Larsen S, et al. Enhanced fixation with hydroxapatite coated pins. *Clin Orthop Rel Res.* 1998;346:171–177.
124. Muller ME, Allgower M, Schneider R, et al. *Manual of Internal Fixation.* Berlin: Springer-Verlag; 1979:85–96.
125. Nunamaker DM, Perren SM. A radiological and histological analysis of fracture healing using prebending of compression plates. *Clin Orthop Rel Res.* 1979;138:167–174.
126. Ostrum RF, Marcantonio A, Marburger R. A critical analysis of the eccentric starting point for trochanteric intramedullary femoral nailing. *J Orthop Trauma.* 2005;19:681–686.
127. Paul JP. Approaches to design, force actions transmitted by joints in the human body. *Proc Roy Soc London.* 1976;192:163–172.
128. Perren SM. Physical and biological aspects of fracture healing with special reference to internal fixation. *Clin Orthop Rel Res.* 1975;138:175–194.
129. Perren SM, Cordey J, Baumgart F, et al. Technical and biomechanical aspects of screws used for bone surgery. *Int J Orthop Trauma.* 1992;2:31–48.
130. Pierce MC, Valdevit A, Anderson L, et al. Biomechanical evaluation of dual energy A-ray absorptiometry for predicting fracture loads of the infant femur for injury investigation: An in vitro porcine model. *J Orthop Trauma.* 2000;14:571–576.
131. Rapoff AJ, Conrad BP, Johnson WM, et al. Load sharing in Premier and Zephir anterior cervical plates. *Spine.* 2003;28:2648–2651.
132. Ricci WM, Tornetta P III, Petteys T, et al. A Comparison of Screw Insertion Torque and Pullout Strength. *J Orthop Trauma.* 2010;24:374–378.
133. Ratcliff JR, Werner FW, Green JK, et al. Medial buttress versus lateral locked plating in a cadaver medial tibial plateau fracture model. *J Orthop Trauma.* 2007;21:444–448.
134. Richter M, Thermann H, Wippermann B, et al. Foot fractures in restrained front seat car occupants: A long-term study over 23 years. *J Orthop Trauma.* 2001;15:287–293.
135. Roberts CS, Dodds JC, Perry K, et al. Hybrid external fixation of the proximal tibia: Strategies to improve frame stability. *J Orthop Trauma.* 2003;17:415–420.
136. Rubin R, Trent P, Arnold W, et al. Knowles pinning of experimental femoral neck fractures: A biomechanical study. *J Trauma.* 1981;21:1036–1039.

137. Russell TA, Dingman CA, Wisnewski P. Mechanical and clinical rationale for femoral neck fracture fixation with a cephalomedullary interlocking nail. Paper presented at: 37th Annual Meeting of the Orthopedic Research Society; February 17–20, Washington, DC.
138. Russell TA, Leighton RK, Alpha-BSM Tibial Plateau Fracture Study Group. Comparison of autogenous bone graft and endothermic calcium phosphate cement for defect augmentation in tibial plateau fractures. A multicenter, prospective, randomized study. *J Bone Joint Surg Am.* 2008;90:2057–2061.
139. Russell TA, Taylor JC, LaVelle DG, et al. Mechanical characterization of femoral interlocking intramedullary nailing systems. *J Orthop Trauma.* 1991;5:332–340.
140. Sander TW, Treharne RW, Baswell I, et al. Development of a new orthopedic wire tester. *J Biomed Mat Res.* 1983;17:587–596.
141. Sanders R, Haidukewych GJ, Milne T, et al. Minimal versus maximal plate fixation techniques of the ulna: The biomechanical effect of number of screws and plate length. *J Orthop Res.* 2002;16:166–171.
142. Schatzker J, Sanderson R, Murnaghan JP. The holding power of orthopedic screws in vivo. *Clin Orthop Rel Res.* 1975;108:115–126.
143. Schawecker F. *The Practise of Osteosynthesis. A Manual of Accident Surgery.* Chicago, IL: Yearbook Medical Publishers; 1974.
144. Schildhauer TA, LeDoux WR, Chapman JR, et al. Triangular osteosynthesis and iliosacral screw fixation for unstable sacral fractures: A cadaveric and biomechanical evaluation under cyclic loads. *J Orthop Trauma.* 2003;17:22–31.
145. Schuster I, Korner J, Arsdorf M, et al. Mechanical comparison in cadaver specimens of three different 90-degree double-plate osteosyntheses for simulated C2-type distal humerus fractures with varying bone densities. *J Orthop Trauma.* 2008;22:113–120.
146. Siffri PC, Peindl RD, Coley ER, et al. Biomechanical analysis of blade plate versus locking plate fixation for a proximal humerus fracture: Comparison using cadaveric and synthetic humeri. *J Orthop Trauma.* 2006;20:547–554.
147. Simonian PT, Routt ML, Harrington RM, et al. The unstable iliac fracture: A biomechanical evaluation of internal fixation. *Injury.* 1997;28:469–475.
148. Simonian PT, Schwappach JR, Routt MLC Jr, et al. Evaluation of new plate designs for symphysis pubis internal fixation. *J Trauma.* 1996;41:498–502.
149. Simonian PT, Thomson GT, Emley W, et al. Angled screw placement in the lateral condyle buttress plate for supracondylar femur fractures. Paper presented at: 43rd Annual Meeting of the Orthopedic Research Society; March 16–19, New Orleans, LA.
150. Singh K, Vaccaro AR, Kim J, et al. Biomechanical comparison of cervical spine reconstructive techniques after a multilevel corpectomy of the cervical spine. *Spine.* 2003;28:2352–2358.
151. Snow M, Thompson G, Turner PG. A mechanical comparison of the locking compression plate (LCP) and the low contact dynamic compression plate (DCP) in an osteoporotic bone model. *J Orthop Trauma.* 2008;22:121–125.
152. Spangler L, Cummings P, Tencer AF, et al. Biomechanical factors and failure of transcervical hip fracture repair. *Injury.* 2001;32:223–228.
153. Spears BR, Ostrum RF, Litsky AS. A mechanical study of gap motion in cadaver femurs using short and long supracondylar nails. *J Orthop Trauma.* 2004;18:354–360.
154. Stankewich CJ, Swiontkowski MF, Tencer AF, et al. Augmentation of femoral neck fracture fixation with an injectable calcium-phosphate bone mineral cement. *J Orthop Res.* 1996;14:786–793.
155. Stankewitz CJ, Chapman J, Muthusamy R, et al. Relationship of mechanical factors to the strength of proximal femur fractures fixed with cancellous screws. *J Ortho Trauma.* 1996;10:248–257.
156. Streubel PN, Moustoukas MJ, Obremskey WT. Mechanical failure after locking plate fixation of unstable intertrochanteric femur fractures. *J Orthop Trauma.* 2013;27:22–28.
157. Stone JL, Beaupre GS, Hayes WC. Multiaxial strength characteristics of trabecular bone. *J Biomech.* 1983;16:743–752.
158. Swiontkowski MF, Harrington RM, Keller TS, et al. Torsion and bending analysis of internal fixation techniques for femoral neck fractures: The role of implant design and bone density. *J Orthop Res.* 1987;5:433–444.
159. Taitsman J, Saha S. Tensile properties of reinforced bone cement. *J Bone Joint Surg Am.* 1976;59A:419–425.
160. Tencer AF, Asnis SE, Harrington RM, et al. Biomechanics of cannulated and noncannulated screws. In: Asnis SE, Kyle RF, eds. *Cannulated Screw Fixation, Principles, and Operative Techniques.* New York, NY: Springer-Verlag; 1996.
161. Tencer AF, Claudi B, Pearce S, et al. Development of a variable stiffness fixation system for stabilization of segmental defects of the tibia. *J Orthop Res.* 1984;l:395–404.
162. Tencer AF, Hampton D, Eddy S. Biomechanical properties of threaded inserts for lumbar interbody spinal fusion. *Spine.* 1995;20:2408–2414.
163. Tencer AF, Kaufman R, Ryan K, et al. Estimating the loads in femurs of occupants in actual motor vehicle crashes using frontal crash test data. *Accident Analysis and Prevention.* 2002;34(1):1–11.
164. Van Audekercke R, Martens M, Mulier JC, et al. Experimental study on internal fixation of femoral neck fractures. *Clin Orthop Rel Res.* 1979;141:203–212.
165. Watford KE, Kregor PJ, Hartsock LA. LISS plate fixation of periprosthtic supracondylar femur fractures. In: An YH, ed. *Internal Fixation in Osteoporotic Bone.* New York, NY: Thieme; 2002:271–278.
166. Weaver JK, Chalmers J. Cancellous bone: Its strength and changes with aging and an evaluation of some methods for measuring its mineral content 1. Age changes in cancellous bone. *J Bone Joint Surg Am.* 1966:48A:289–299.
167. White AA III, Panjabi MM, Southwick WO. Effects of compression and cyclical loading on fracture healing—a quantitative biomechanical study. *J Biomech.* 1977A;10:233–239.
168. White AA III, Panjabi MM, Southwick WO. The four biomechanical stages of fracture repair. *J Bone Joint Surg Am.* 1977B;59A:188–192.
169. Wikenheiser MA, Lewallen DG, Markel MD. In vitro mechanical, thermal, and microstructural performance of five external fixation pins. Paper presented at: 38th Annual Meeting of the Orthopedic Research Society; February 17–20, Washington, DC.
170. Wittenberg RH, Shea M, Swartz DE, et al. Importance of bone mineral density in instrumented spinal fusions. *Spine* 1991;16:648–652.
171. Woodard Pl, Self J, Calhoun JH, et al. The effect of implant axial and torsional stiffness on fracture healing. *J Orthop Trauma.* 1987;l:331–340.
172. Wright TM, Hayes WC. Tensile testing of bone over a wide range of strain rates: Effects of strain rate, microstructure, and density. *Med Biol Eng.* 1976;14:671–680.
173. Wu S-S, Edwards WT, Zou D, et al. Transpedicular vertebral screws in human vertebrae: Effect on screw-vertebra interface stiffness. Paper presented at: 38th Annual Meeting of the Orthopedic Research Society; February 17–20, Washington, DC.
174. Yerby S, Scott CC, Evans NJ, et al. Effect of cutting flute design on cortical bone screw insertion torque and pullout strength. *J Orthop Trauma.* 2001;15:216–221.
175. Yinger K, Scalise J, Olson SA, et al. Biomechanical comparison of posterior pelvic ring fixation. *J Orthop Trauma.* 2003;17:481–487.
176. Young JWR, Burgess AR, Brumback RJ. Lateral compression fractures of the pelvis; the importance of plain radiographs in the diagnosis and surgical management. *Skeletal Radiol.* 1986:15:103–109.
177. Zand MS, Goldstein SA, Matthews LS. Fatigue failure of cortical bone screws. *J Biomech.* 1983;16:305–311.
178. Zuber K, Schneider E, Eulenberger J, et al. Form und Dimension der Markhöhle menschlicher Femora in Hinblick auf die Passung von Marknagelimplantaten. *Unfallchirurg.* 1988;91:314–319.

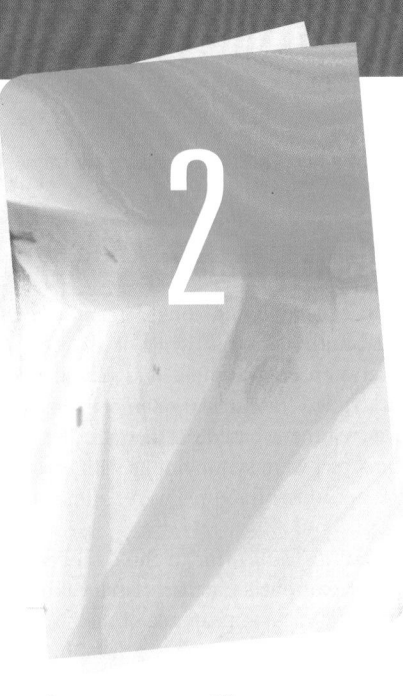

2

CLASSIFICATION OF FRACTURES

Douglas R. Dirschl

INTRODUCTION

Fracture classification systems have been in existence for nearly as long as people have identified fractures; they certainly pre-date the advent of radiography. Even in the earliest written surviving medical text, the Edwin Smith Papyrus, there was a rudimentary classification of fractures. If a fracture could be characterized as "having a wound over it, piercing through"—in other words, an open fracture—it was determined to be an "ailment not to be treated." This early form of one of the earliest systems of fracture classification served both to characterize the fracture and to guide the treatment—these are two goals of modern classification systems as well.

Throughout the ages, all systems of fracture classification have served numerous purposes: To characterize fractures according to certain general and specific features, to guide fracture treatment, and to predict outcomes of fracture care. This chapter will review the purposes and goals of fracture classification, the history of the use of such systems, and the general types of fracture classification systems in common use today. This chapter will also provide a critical analysis of the effectiveness of fracture classification systems, as well as some of the limitations of these systems. Finally, it will comment on the possible future of fracture classification systems.

PURPOSES OF FRACTURE CLASSIFICATION SYSTEMS

Taxonomy, or the naming and categorization of things, is not unique to orthopedics or to fractures. Taxonomy is a universal phenomenon that occurs in all fields of science and art. One example is the division of life in the natural world into three kingdoms: Animals, plants, and bacteria (Fig. 2-1). This simple taxonomy is a perfect example of the sorts of classification that permeate the world of arts and sciences, as well as of the first general purpose of classification systems—to name things.

A second purpose of classification systems is to provide a hierarchy of characteristics and to describe things according to those characteristics. Common descriptors are created so that individual items can be segmented into various groups. Groups are then ordered into a hierarchy according to a definition of complexity. A simple example of this is the phylogeny used to describe the animal kingdom; this system describes and groups animals according to common characteristics, and then orders those groups in a hierarchy of complexity of the organism. This is, in principle, analogous to many fracture classification systems, which group fractures by a series of descriptors, then order the groups according to complexity.

A third purpose of classification systems is to guide action or intervention. This feature of classification systems is not universally seen, and it is generally present only in classification

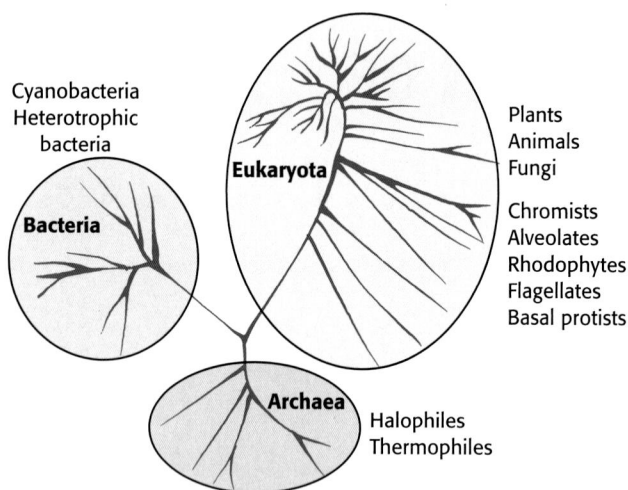

Cyanobacteria
Heterotrophic
bacteria

Bacteria

Eukaryota

Plants
Animals
Fungi

Chromists
Alveolates
Rhodophytes
Flagellates
Basal protists

Archaea
Halophiles
Thermophiles

FIGURE 2-1 Balloon diagram of taxonomy of the natural world.

systems that are diagnostic in nature. This introduces one of the key distinctions among classification systems—that between systems used for description and characterization and those used to guide actions and/or predict outcomes. For example, the classification system for the animal kingdom names and classifies animals, but it is descriptive only—it does not guide the observer to any suggested action. In orthopedic practice, however, physicians use fracture classification systems to assist in making treatment decisions. In fact, many fracture classification systems were designed specifically for the purpose of guiding treatment. We should have higher expectations of the validity and integrity of systems that are used to guide actions than those used purely as descriptive tools, since there can be consequences of actions taken, while there are none for merely describing something.

The fourth purpose of classification systems is to assist in predicting outcomes of an intervention or treatment. The ability to reliably predict an outcome from a fracture classification alone would be of tremendous benefit, for it would allow physicians to counsel patients, beginning at the time of injury, about the expected outcome—all from the fracture classification at the time of injury. This ability would also assist greatly in clinical research, as it would allow the comparison of the results from one clinical study of a particular fracture to that of another. It should be clear to the reader that, for a classification system to reliably predict outcome, a rigorous analysis of the reliability and validity of the classification system is necessary. Table 2-1 summarizes the purposes of classification systems,

TABLE 2-1	Purposes of Classification Systems	
To Name	High validity and reliability not required	
To Describe and Compare		
To Guide Action to	High validity and reliability recommended	
Predict Outcomes		

along with the level of reliability and validity necessary for high performance of the system.

HISTORY OF FRACTURE CLASSIFICATION

Fracture classifications have existed much longer than have radiographs. The Edmund Smith Papyrus, while it did not make a clear distinction between comminuted and noncomminuted fractures, clearly classified fractures as open or closed, and provided guidelines for treatment based on that classification. Open fractures, for example, were synonymous with early death in the Ancient Egypt, and these fractures were "ailments not to be treated."

In the 18th and 19th centuries, still prior to the discovery of radiographs, there were in existence fracture classification systems that were based on the clinical appearance of the limb. The Colles fracture of the distal radius, in which the distal fragment was displaced dorsally—causing the dinner fork deformity of the distal radius—was a common fracture. Any fracture with this clinical deformity was considered a Colles fracture and was treated with correction of the deformity and immobilization of the limb.[15] The Pott fracture, a fracture of the distal tibia and fibula with varus deformity, was likewise a fracture classification that was based only on the clinical appearance of the limb.[65] These are but two examples of fracture classifications that were accepted and used successfully prior to the development of radiographic imaging.

After the advent of radiography, fracture classification systems expanded in number and came into common usage. Radiography so altered the understanding of fractures and the methods of fracture care that nearly all fracture classification systems in use today are based on a characterization of the fracture fragments on plain radiographs. Most modern fracture classification systems are based on a description of the location, number, and displacement of fracture lines viewed on radiographs, rather than on the clinical appearance of the fractured limb. While countless fracture classification systems based on radiographs have been described in the past century for fractures in all parts of the skeleton, only the most enduring systems remain in common usage today. Examples of these enduring classification systems are the Garden[31] and Neer[56] classification systems of proximal femoral and proximal humeral fractures, respectively. These and other commonly used classification systems will be discussed in more detail in a later part of this chapter.

Nearly all fracture classification systems in use today are based upon having observers—usually orthopedic physicians—make judgments and interpretations based on the analysis of plain radiographs of the fractured bone. Usually, anteroposterior (AP) and lateral radiographs are used, although some fracture classification systems allow for or encourage the use of additional x-ray views, such as oblique radiographs, or internal and external rotation radiographs. It should be evident that each decision made in the process of classifying a fracture is based on a human's interpretation of the often complex patterns of shadows on a plain radiograph of the fractured limb. This, then, requires that the observer have a detailed and fundamental understanding of the osteology of the bone being imaged and of the fracture being classified. The observer must have the ability to accurately and completely identify all of the fracture lines, understand the origin and nature of all of the fracture fragments, and delineate the relationship of all of the fracture fragments to one another. Finally, the procedure of fracture classification requires that the observer accurately quantify the amount of displacement or angulation of each fracture fragment from the location in which it should be in the nonfractured situation.

More recently, computed tomography (CT) scanning has been added by many observers to assist in classifying fractures. In most cases, the CT scan data has been used and applied to a classification system that was devised for use with plain radiographs alone. There are a few classification systems, however, that are specifically designed for use with CT imaging data. The most well-known example of such a system is the Sanders classification system for fractures of the calcaneus,[67] which was designed for use with a carefully defined semicoronal CT sequence through the posterior facet of the subtalar joint.

Most fracture classification systems until very recently relied solely on radiographic images to classify the fracture, guide treatment, and predict outcomes. It is becoming increasingly appreciated, however, that nonradiographic factors such as the extent of soft tissue injury when there are other injuries (skeletal or nonskeletal), medical comorbidities, and various other nonradiographic factors have a large effect on treatment decisions and on the outcomes of fracture treatment.[23,42] These factors, however, are not accounted for in radiographic systems for fracture classification.

In reviewing a radiograph of a fracture, it is difficult to fully appreciate the extent of soft tissue damage that has occurred, and the image provides no information about the patient's medical history. For example, if one views a radiograph of a spiral tibial shaft fracture shown in Figure 2-2, one may conclude that this is a simple, low-energy injury. In this example, however, the fracture occurred as a result of very high energy,

and the patient sustained extensive soft tissue damage. In addition, the patient was an insulin-dependent diabetic with severe peripheral neuropathy and skin ulcerations on the fractured limb. There is no way, from view of the plain radiographs or application of a fracture classification based on radiographs alone, to account for these additional factors. The patient in this example required amputation, a treatment that would not be predicted by review of the radiographs alone. Some discussion of the role of classifying the soft tissue injury in characterizing fractures will take place later in this chapter.

TYPES OF FRACTURE CLASSIFICATION SYSTEMS

Classification systems used to characterize fractures can be grouped into three broad categories: (i) those that are fracture specific, which evolved around and were generated for the classification of a single fracture in a single location in the skeleton; (ii) classification of fractures in all parts of the human skeleton; and (iii) those that attempt to classify the soft tissue injury. It is beyond the scope of this chapter to discuss individually all the fracture classification systems now in common usage, but it is important for the reader to understand the differences between the general types of classification systems. For that reason, some examples of each of the three types of fracture classification systems will be discussed.

Examples of Fracture-Specific Classification Systems

The Garden classification of femoral neck fractures[31] is a long-standing fracture classification system that describes the displacement and angulation of the femoral head on AP and lateral radiographs of the hip (see Fig. 47-2). The classification is essentially a descriptive one, describing the location and displacement of the fractured femoral neck and head. The fracture types are ordered, however, to indicate increasing fracture severity, greater fracture instability, and higher risk of

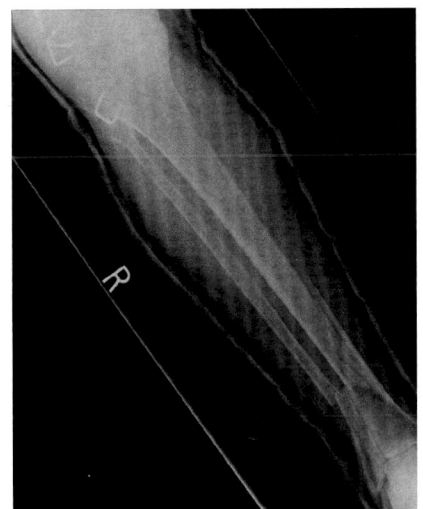
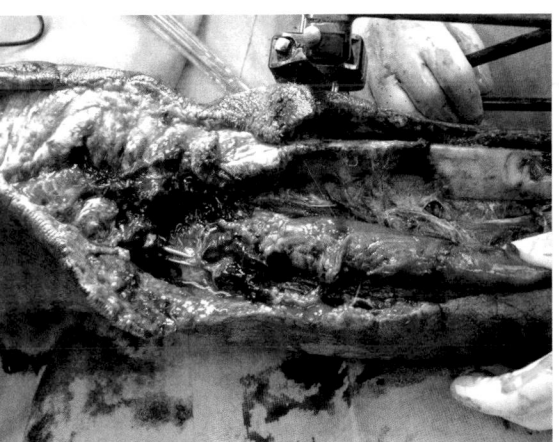

A   **B**

FIGURE 2-2 Tibial fracture as seen on radiograph **(A)** and intraoperatively **(B)**. The x-ray appearance greatly underestimates the overall severity of the injury.

complications with attempts at reduction and stabilization of the fracture. This feature of ordering fracture types by severity takes the classification system from a nominal system to an ordinal system. Garden types 1 and 2 fractures are considered to be stable injuries and are frequently treated with percutaneous internal fixation. Garden types 3 and 4 fractures have been grouped as unstable fracture patterns and, while closed reduction and internal fixation are used in some circumstances, most Garden types 3 and 4 fractures in elderly patients are treated with arthroplasty.

The Schatzker classification of proximal tibia fractures[68,69] is an example of another descriptive classification system that has been widely utilized and is based on the location of the major fracture line in the proximal tibia and the presence or absence of a depressed segment of the articular surface of the proximal tibia (see Fig. 53-9). This fracture classification is not dependent on the amount of displacement or depression of the articular fractures, but only on the location of the fracture lines. The Schatzker classification seems very simple, but it also demonstrates some of the areas of confusion that can result from fracture classifications. For example, the Schatzker VI fracture group includes fractures classified as types C1 and C3 by the AO/OTA system (described below), thus demonstrating an area of inconsistency between two commonly used but different systems for classifying the same fracture that can lead to confusion among observers.

The Neer classification system for proximal humeral fractures[56] is a descriptive fracture classification system that has been widely utilized and widely taught (Fig. 2-3). It is based on how many fracture "parts" there are—a part is defined as a fracture fragment that is either displaced more than 1 cm or angulated more than 45 degrees. The Neer classification groups fractures into nondisplaced (one-part), two-part, three-part, or four-part fractures. Nondisplaced fractures in the Neer system may have several fracture lines, but none of them meet the displacement or angulation criteria to be considered a "part." Two-part fractures in the Neer system can represent either a fracture across the surgical neck of the humerus or a greater or lesser tuberosity fracture that is displaced. Three-part fractures classically involve the humeral head, with a greater tuberosity fragment that is displaced or angulated. Four-part fractures involve displacement or angulation of the humeral head and greater and lesser tuberosities. The reader should note that, in addition to correct identification of the fracture fragments, this classification system requires the observer to make careful and accurate measurements of fragment displacement and angulation to determine if a fragment constitutes a part.

The Lauge-Hansen classification of malleolar fractures of the ankle[42] is an example of a widely used system that is based primarily on the mechanism of injury. The system makes use of the fact that particular mechanisms of injury to the ankle will result in predictable patterns of fracture to the malleoli. The appearance of the fracture on the radiographs, then, is used to infer the mechanism of the injury. The injuries are classified according to the position of the foot at the time of injury and the direction of the deforming force at the time of fracture. The position of the foot is described as pronation or supination, and the deforming force is categorized as external rotation, inversion, or eversion. This creates six general fracture types, which are essentially nominal—they are not ordered into increasing injury severity. Within each fracture type, however, there is an ordinal scale, with varying degrees of severity being assigned to each type (1 to 4) according to the fracture pattern. With this classification system, correct determination of the fracture type can guide the manipulations necessary to affect fracture reduction—the treating physician must reverse the direction of the injuring forces to achieve a reduction. For example, internal rotation is required to achieve reduction of a supination external rotation fracture pattern and abduction to reduce a supination adduction injury.

Generic or Universal Classification Systems

The AO/OTA (Orthopaedic Trauma Association) fracture classification[48,62] is essentially the only generic or universal system in wide usage today. It is universal in the sense that the classification system can be applied to any bone in the body. This classification system was devised through a consensus panel of orthopedic traumatologists who were members of the OTA and is based upon a classification system initially developed and proposed by the AO/ASIF group in Europe.[53-55] The OTA believed there was a need for a detailed universal system for classification of fractures to allow for standardization of research and communication among orthopedic surgeons.

In applying the OTA fracture classification system, there are five questions that must be answered for each fracture.

1. *Which bone?* The major bones in the body are numbered, with the humerus being no. 1, the forearm no. 2, the femur no. 3, the tibia no. 4, and so on (Fig. 2-4).

2. *Where in the bone is the fracture?* The answer to this question identifies a specific segment within the bone. In most long bones, the diaphyseal segment (2) is located between the proximal (1) and distal (3) segments. The dividing lines between the shaft segment and the proximal and distal segments occur in metaphysis of the bone. The tibia is assigned a fourth segment, which is the malleolar segment. An example of the application of answering the first two questions of the AO/OTA classification is that a fracture of the midshaft of the femur will be given a numeric classification of 32 (3 for femur, 2 for the diaphyseal segment) (Fig. 2-4).

3. *Which fracture type?* The fracture type in this system can be A, B, or C, but these three types are defined differently in diaphyseal fractures and fractures at either end of the bone. For diaphyseal fractures, the type A fracture is a simple fracture with two fragments. The type B diaphyseal fracture has some comminution, but there can still be contact between the proximal and distal fragments. The type C diaphyseal fracture is a highly comminuted or segmental fracture with no contact possible between proximal and distal fragments. For proximal and distal segment fractures, type A fractures are considered extra-articular, type B fractures are partial articular (there is some continuity between the shaft and some portion of the articular surface), and type C fractures involve complete disruption of the articular surface from the

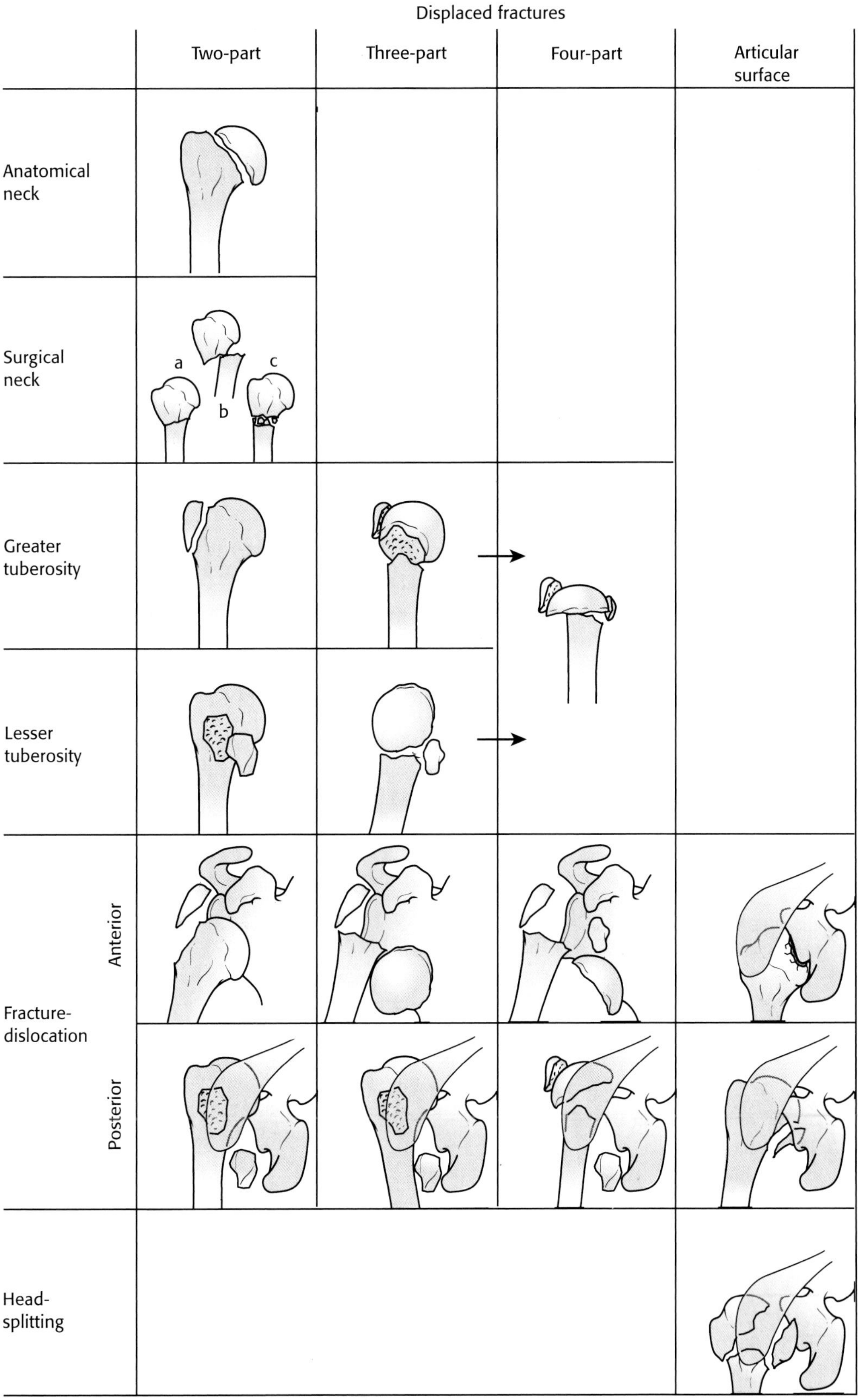

Displaced fractures

FIGURE 2-3 The Neer four-part classification of proximal humerus fractures. A fracture is displaced if the fracture fragments are separated 1 cm or greater, or if angulation between the fracture fragments is more than 45 degrees. A displaced fracture is either a two-, three-, or four-part fracture. (Adapted from: Neer CS. Displaced proximal humeral fractures: I. classification and evaluation. *J Bone Joint Surg.* 1970;52A:1077–1089, reprinted with permission from Journal of Bone and Joint Surgery.)

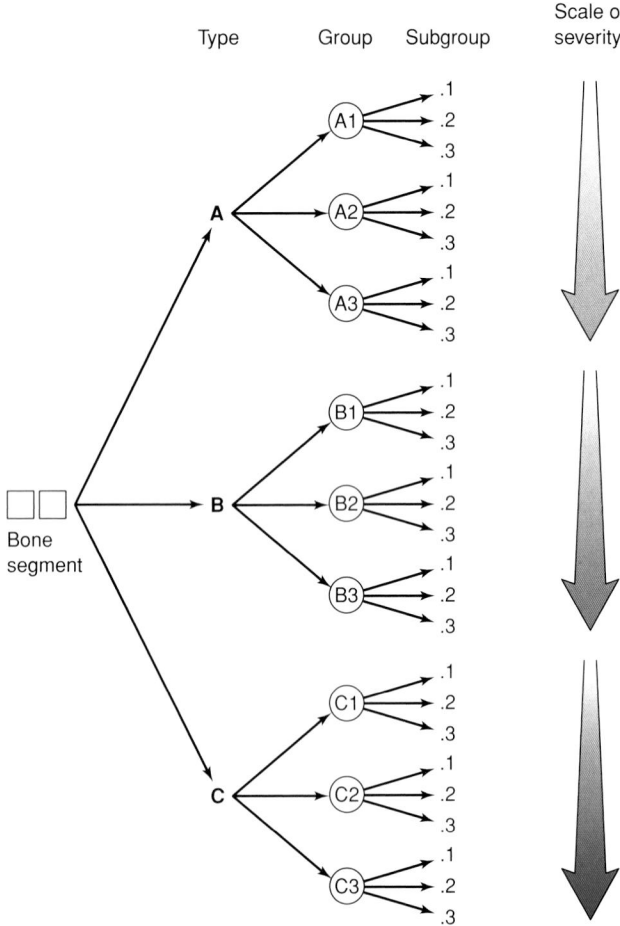

Type   Group   Subgroup   Scale of severity

FIGURE 2-4 The AO/ASIF comprehensive long bone classification applied to proximal humeral fractures. This system describes three types of proximal humerus fractures (types A, B, and C). Type A fractures are described as unifocal extra-articular (two-segment) fractures, type B as bifocal extra-articular (three-segment) fractures, and type C as anatomic neck or articular segment fractures. Each type includes three fracture patterns, with nine subgroups for each type of fracture. The subgroup classification indicates the degree of displacement. (Adapted from: Muller ME, Allgower M, Schneider R, et al. *Manual of Internal Fixation.* New York, NY: Springer-Verlag; 1991, with permission.)

diaphysis. An example of this portion of the classification system is shown in Figure 2-4.

4. *Which group do the fractures belong to?* Grouping further divides the fractures according to more specific descriptive details. Fracture groups are not consistently defined; that is, fracture groups are different for each fracture type. Complete description of the fracture groups is beyond the scope of this chapter.

5. *Which subgroup?* This is the most detailed determination in the AO/OTA classification system. As is the case with groups, subgroups differ from bone to bone and depend upon key features for any given bone in its classification. The intended purpose of the subgroups is to increase the precision of the classification system. An in-depth discussion of this fracture

classification is beyond the scope of this chapter, and the reader is referred to the references for a more detailed description of this universal fracture classification system.

The AO/OTA classification system is an evolving system. It is continually evaluated by a committee of the OTA, and is open for change where appropriate. The reader should note that the AO/OTA classification system of fractures, and its precursor, the AO/ASIF system, were designed for delineation and recording of the maximum possible amount of detail about the individual fracture pattern and appearance on radiographs. The assumption made during the development of these classification systems is that with specific definitions/diagrams and a high degree of detail will come greater accuracy and a superior fracture classification system that could be applied by any orthopedic surgeon. It was believed such a system could potentially result in better prognostic and research capabilities. As will be discussed later in the chapter, greater specificity and detail in a fracture classification system does not necessarily correlate well with good performance of the classification system.

Classifications of Soft Tissue Injury Associated with Fractures

The skin and soft tissue represent an organ system. The energy of the injury may be reflected in the soft tissue damage to the extremity involved. If one sees a radiograph demonstrating a comminuted fracture, it is often thought that it is a high-energy injury. However, there may be other patient factors that come into consideration and may lead to a comminuted fracture from a lower-energy mechanism. This may be evident in an elderly patient with a ground-level fall who has a significantly comminuted distal humerus fracture. The energy of the injury itself resulted only from a ground-level fall, but led to a complex fracture type as a result of underlying osteoporotic bone. Some of the value in the soft tissue classification system is in planning the treatment as well as in predicting the outcome.

The clearest example of a fracture with an associated soft tissue injury is the open fracture. Early classification systems for open fractures focused only on the size of the opening in the skin. With time, however, it was recognized that the extent of muscle injury, local vascular damage, and periosteal stripping are also of paramount significance. Gustilo et al.[33,34] developed the classification system now used by most North American orthopedists to describe open fractures. This classification system takes into account the skin wound, the extent of local soft tissue injury and contamination, and the severity of the fracture pattern (see Table 12-2). The Gustilo classification system originally included type 1, type 2, and type 3 fractures. However, this system was modified later to expand the type 3 open fractures into subtypes A, B, and C. It is important to note that the type 3-C fracture is defined as any open fracture in which there is an accompanying vascular injury that *requires repair*. The Gustilo classification system has been applied to open fractures in nearly all long bones. It is important to recognize that this classification system only can be applied fully after surgical debridement of the open fracture has been performed. This system has proven useful in predicting risk of infection in open tibial fractures.[33]

Interobserver agreement in grading open tibial fractures according to the classification of Gustilo was investigated by Brumback and Jones,[10] who presented radiographs and videotapes of surgical debridements to a group of orthopedic traumatologists who classified the fractures. They reported an average interobserver agreement of 60%. The range of agreement, however, was wide, ranging from 42% to 94%. Percentage agreement was best for the most severe and the least severe injuries, and was poorer for fractures in the middle range of the classification system. That the classification system did not have similar reliability across the spectrum of injury severity has been a criticism of this classification system as a prognostic indicator for any but the least severe and most severe injuries.

Recently, the Open Fracture Study Group of the OTA published a novel approach to classification of open fractures. A systematic literature review to identify factors felt to be important in treatment or prognosis for open fractures, followed by a prioritization of these factors by a panel of experience orthopedic trauma surgeons, followed by review, discussion, and consensus by the Open Fracture Study Group resulted in identification of five essential categories of open fracture severity assessment.[61] These categories, skin injury, muscle injury, arterial injury, contamination, and bone loss, were each assigned three levels of severity (1, 2, or 3) (Table 2-2). The result is an open fracture classification that does not assign an overall grade or number to the injury, but instead assigns a severity to each of the five essential factors. The system was tested prospectively by the study group for content validity and ease of use with good results. The system is believed to focus on the factors felt most essential by experts to guide treatment and predict outcome. Studies of interobserver reliability and predictive value in broad

clinical practice are currently underway. The use of this system was recently compared to the Gustilo classification and demonstrated a large disparity of injuries being grouped together in the Gustilo grades.[52]

The classification of Oestern and Tscherne can be used to characterize the severity of closed fractures (Table 2-3).[59] This system remains the only published classification system for the soft tissue injury associated with closed fractures. Fractures are assigned one of four grades, from 0 to 3. Figure 2-5 is an example of a patient with a Tscherne Grade 2 closed tibial plateau fracture. Deep abrasions of the skin, muscle contusion, fracture blisters, and massive soft tissue swelling, as in this patient, may lead the surgeon away from immediate articular stabilization and toward temporary spanning external fixation. No studies have been done to determine the interobserver reliability of the Tscherne system for the classification of the soft tissue injury associated with closed fractures.

The value of a classification system is greatly enhanced if it can assist in predicting outcome. A prospective study completed by Gaston et al.[32] assessed various fracture classification

TABLE 2-2 The Orthopaedic Trauma Association Classification of Open Fractures

Essential Factor	Severity
Skin	1. Can be approximated 2. Cannot be approximated 3. Extensive degloving
Muscle	1. No muscle in area or no appreciable necrosis 2. Loss of muscle, intact function, localized necrosis 3. Dead muscle, loss of function
Arterial	1. No injury 2. Artery injury without ischemia 3. Artery injury with distal ischemia
Contamination	1. None or minimal contamination 2. Surface contamination 3. Imbedded in bone or deep tissues
Bone Loss	1. None 2. Bone mission or devascularized, but still contact between proximal and distal segments 3. Segmental bone loss

TABLE 2-3 Oestern and Tscherne Classification of Closed Fractures

Grade	Soft Tissue Injury	Bony Injury
Grade 0	Minimal soft tissue damage Indirect injury to limb	Simple fracture pattern
Grade 1	Superficial abrasion/contusion	Mild fracture pattern
Grade 2	Deep abrasion with skin or muscle contusion Direct trauma to limb	Severe fracture pattern
Grade 3	Extensive skin contusion or crush Severe damage to underlying muscle Subcutaneous avulsion Compartmental syndrome may be present	Severe fracture pattern

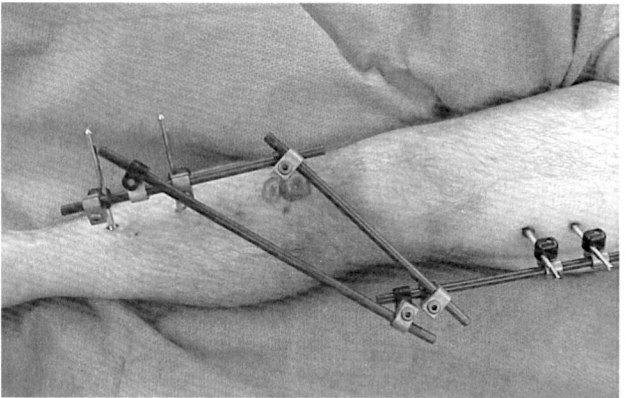

FIGURE 2-5 Example of a Tscherne II fracture of the proximal tibia.

schemes against several validated functional outcome measures in patients with tibial shift fractures. The Tscherne classification system of closed fractures was more predictive of outcome than the other classification systems used. The Tscherne system was most strongly predictive of time to return to prolonged walking or running.

Limitations of Fracture Classification Systems

To be successful and valuable as a predictive tool, a classification system must be both reliable and valid.[11,30,47] Reliability reflects the ability of a classification system to return the same result for the same fracture radiographs over multiple observers or by the same observer when viewing the fracture on multiple occasions. The former is termed interobserver reliability, or the agreement between different observers using the classification system to assess the same cases. The latter is termed intraobserver reproducibility—the agreement of the same observer's assessment, using the classification system, for the same cases on repeated occasions. There has been discussion over the appropriate use of the terms "agreement" and "accuracy" in reference to the performance of fracture classification systems, as well as which of these terms is the best measure of a system's performance. The term "accuracy" implies that there is a correct answer or a gold standard against which comparisons can be made, validated, and determined to be true or false. However, the term "agreement" indicates that there is no defined gold standard and that unanimous agreement among all observers that might classify a given fracture is the highest measure of performance of a classification system. These two terms are not congruent and they are not interchangeable. Each is tested by a vastly different statistical method and to optimize each would require a radically different method for generating and validating a fracture classification system. It has been unclear at times whether those developing and applying classification systems today are expecting the classification to serve as a gold standard or they are attempting to develop the classification to achieve optimal agreement among observers.

In the late 1980s and early 1990s, studies began to appear in the orthopedic literature assessing the interobserver reliability of various fracture classifications systems.[2,3,29,39,58,66,73,79] In a controversial editorial published in 1993, *Fracture Classification Systems: Do They Work and Are They Useful,* Albert Burstein, PhD, arrayed some important issues and considerations for fracture classification systems.[11] He stated that classification systems are tools, and that the measure of whether such a tool works is if it produces the same result, time after time, in the hands of anyone who employs the tool. Dr. Burstein went on to say that "any classification scheme, be it nominal, ordinal, or scalar, should be proved to be a workable tool before it is used in a discriminatory or predictive manner." He emphasized that the key distinction for a classification system was between its use to describe and characterize fractures and its use to guide treatment or predict outcomes. It is the latter use that requires a system to be proven to be a valid tool; the minimum criteria for acceptable performance of any classification system should be a demonstration of a high degree of interobserver reliability and intraobserver reproducibility.

Numerous studies have been published since Dr. Burstein's editorial appeared, and nearly all have concluded that fracture classification systems have substantial interobserver variability. Classification systems for fractures of the proximal femur,[2,29,58,63,70,79,81] proximal humerus,[7,9,39,44,45,73,74] ankle,[16,57,66,70,71,79] distal tibia,[22,47,77] and tibial plateau[12,26,35,46,50,82–84] among others, were all shown to have poor to slight interobserver reliability. The earliest of these studies looked only at the observed percentage of agreement—the percentage of times that individual pairs of observers categorized fractures into the same category. Subsequent studies, however, have most frequently used a statistical test known as the kappa statistic, a test that analyzes pair-wise comparisons between observers applying the same classification system to a specific set of fracture cases. The kappa statistic was originally introduced by Cohen in 1960,[13] and the kappa statistic and its variants are the most recognized and widely used methods for measuring reliability for fracture classification systems. The kappa statistic adjusts the proportion of agreement between any two observers by correcting for the proportion of agreement that could have occurred by chance alone. Kappa values can range from +1 (perfect agreement) to 0 (chance agreement) to –1 (perfect disagreement) (Table 2-4).

The original kappa statistic is appropriate when there are only two choices of fracture categories or when the fracture classification system is nominal—all categorical differences are equally important. In most situations, however, there are more than two categories into which a fracture can be classified, and fracture classification systems are ordinal—the categorical differences are ranked according to injury severity, treatment method, or presumed outcome. In these cases, the most appropriate variant of the kappa statistic to be used is the weighted kappa statistic, described by Fleiss,[27,28] in which some credit is given to partial agreement and not all disagreements are treated equally. For example, in the Neer classification of proximal humeral fractures, disagreement between a nondisplaced and a two-part fracture has fewer treatment implications than disagreement between a nondisplaced and a four-part fracture. By weighting kappa values, one can account for the different levels of importance between levels of disagreement. However, the most appropriate use of the weighted kappa statistic should include a clear explanation of the weighting scheme selected, since the results of the kappa statistic will vary—even with the same observations—if the weighting scheme varies.[30] Thus, without specific knowledge of the weighting scheme used, it is difficult to compare the results of fracture classification system reliability across different studies.

In most studies, the guidelines proposed by Landis and Koch[40] have been used to categorize kappa values; values less

TABLE 2-4 Range of the Kappa Statistic

Value of Kappa Statistic	Level of Agreement
+1.00	Perfect agreement
0.00	Agreement equal to chance
–1.00	Perfect disagreement

than 0.00 indicate poor reliability, 0.01 to 0.20 indicate slight reliability, 0.21 to 0.40 indicate fair reliability, 0.41 to 0.60 indicate moderate reliability, 0.61 to 0.80 indicate substantial reliability, and 0.81 to 1.00 indicate nearly perfect agreement. Although these criteria have gained widespread acceptance, the values were chosen arbitrarily and were never intended to serve as general benchmarks. A second set of criteria, also arbitrary, have been proposed by Svanholm et al.[75]: Less than 0.50 indicate poor reliability, 0.51 to 0.74 indicate good reliability, and greater than 0.75 indicate excellent reliability.

Observer variability, using the kappa statistic, has been found to be a limitation of many fracture classification systems. Many studies have documented only fair to poor intraobserver reliability for a wide range of fracture classification systems. Systems tested have included, among others, the Neer fracture classification system of proximal humeral fractures,[7,8,39,44,45,73] the Garden classification systems of proximal femoral fractures,[2,29,58,63,70] the Ruedi and Allgower and AO classification systems of distal tibial fractures,[22,49,77] the Lauge-Hansen and Weber classification of malleolar fractures,[16,57,78,79] and the Schatzker and AO fracture classification system of proximal tibial fractures.[12,26,35,46,50,82–84] In addition, studies have shown observer variability in classifying various other orthopedic injuries, such as fractures of the acetabulum,[6,63,80] the distal radius,[1,3,37] the scaphoid,[20] the spine,[5,60] the calcaneus,[36,41] and gunshot fractures of the femur.[72]

More recent studies have attempted to isolate the sources of this variability, but the root cause for the variability has not been identified. It remains unknown if any system for the classification of fractures can perform with excellent intraobserver reliability when it will be used by many observers. A methodology for validation for fracture classification systems has been proposed, but it is highly detailed and extremely time consuming and it is unknown if it can be practically applied.[4]

The use of the weighted kappa statistic in studies assessing the reliability of fracture classification systems should clearly state the weighting scheme used. Methodologic issues such as this were evaluated in a systematic review of 44 published studies assessing the reliability of fracture classification systems.[4] Various methodologic issues were identified, including a failure to assure that the study sample of fracture radiographs was representative of the spectrum and frequency of injury severity seen for the particular fracture in 61% of the studies, a failure to justify the size of the study group in 100% of the studies, and inadequate statistical analysis of the data in 61% of the studies. While the authors of this study used very rigid and, some would argue, unfairly rigorous criteria to evaluate these studies, the authors' conclusion that reliability studies of fracture classification cannot be easily compared to one another is valid and appropriate. The development and adoption of a systematic methodologic approach to the development and validation of new fracture classification systems seems appropriate and is needed.

Only one study to date has attempted to validate whether a fracture classification scheme correlates well with outcomes following fracture care.[76] In a prospective, multicenter study, 200 patients with unilateral isolated lower-extremity fractures (acetabulum, femur, tibia, talus, or calcaneus) underwent various functional outcome measurements at 6 and 12 months, including the Sickness Impact Profile and the AMA Impairment rating. The AO/OTA fracture classification for each of these patients was correlated with the functional outcome measures. While the study indicated some significant differences in functional outcome between type C and type B fractures, there was no significant difference between type C and type A fractures. The authors concluded that the AO/OTA code for fracture classification may not be a good predictor of 6- and 12-month functional performance and impairment for patients with isolated lower-extremity fractures.

Additional, deeper research has attempted to elucidate some of the reasons for interobserver variation in the classification of fractures. These studies have generally focused on a few specific variables or tasks involved in the fracture classification process. Some of those which have been investigated are discussed in the following paragraphs.

Quality of Fracture Radiographs

The quality of the radiographs varies normally in clinical practice and may affect the observer's ability to accurately or reproducibly identify and classify the fracture. Many have attributed observed intraobserver variability in fracture classifications systems to variations in the quality of radiographs.[1,7,29,38,39,73] Studies looking specifically at this variable, however, have not demonstrated it to be a significant source of intraobserver variability.[16,22] In one such study involving classification of tibial plafond fractures using the Ruedi and Allgower system, observers were asked to classify the fractures, but also asked to make a determination of whether the radiographs were of adequate quality to classify the fracture.[22] In that study, observers agreed less on the quality of the radiographs (mean kappa, 0.38 + 0.046) than on the classification of the fractures themselves (mean kappa, 0.43 + 0.048). In addition, the extent of interobserver agreement on the quality of the radiographs had no correlation with the extent of agreement in classifying the fractures. The authors concluded that, based on the results of their investigation, it appeared that improving the quality of plain radiographic images would be unlikely to improve the reliability of classification of fractures of the tibial plafond.

Further studies using advanced imaging modalities, such as CT or magnetic resonance imaging (MRI) scanning, in which high-quality images should always be obtained, have generally not demonstrated improved intraobserver reliability over studies that have used plain radiographs alone. Bernstein et al.[7] found that CT scans did not improve interobserver agreement for the Neer classification of proximal humerus fractures. Chan et al.,[12] in a study of the impact of a CT scan on determining treatment plan and fracture classification for tibial plateau fractures, found that viewing the CT scans did not improve interobserver agreement on classification, but did increase agreement regarding treatment plan. Two studies investigating the effect of adding CT information to plain radiographs on the interobserver agreement in classifying fractures of the tibial plateau and tibial plafond failed to show a significant improvement in agreement after the addition of CT scan information.[12,50,51]

Beaule et al.,[6] studying fractures of the acetabulum and came to the same conclusion; CT did not improve inter- or intraobserver agreement in classification of the fractures. Humphrey et al.,[36] studying fractures of the distal radius, found the addition of a CT scan occasionally resulted in changes in treatment plans and also increased agreement among observers on the surgical plan in treating these injuries. A study investigating the use of three-dimensional CT scanning in distal humeral fractures concluded that three-dimensional CT did not improve interobserver reliability over plain radiographs or two-dimensional CT scans, but that it did improve intraobserver reproducibility.[25] Two studies investigating the addition of three-dimensional CT imaging to the classification of tibial plateau fractures had conflicting results; one study reported the advanced imaging improved interobserver reliability,[35] while the other reported no improvement.[26] The differences in these reports may be that the numbers of observers and fractures evaluated were larger in the latter study; it is statistically much easier to demonstrate better interobserver agreement with a smaller number of observers and cases rated. It appears that CT scan information may be a useful adjunct in surgical planning for a severe articular fracture, but is probably not required for the purpose of fracture classification.

Some contradictory data was recently published in Germany.[18] Thirty-five distal radius fractures that had been classified as AO/OTA A2 and A3 (extra-articular types) after radiographic review underwent CT scanning. The scans revealed that 57% of the fractures had an intra-articular component and had been inappropriately classified as AO/OTA type A fractures. The reader should note that this study did not attempt to determine interobserver reliability of the classification, but simply that a single observer reviewing the CT scans disagreed with the original fracture classification in 57% of cases. It remains unproven whether CT scanning is a useful adjunct to improve interobserver agreement in the classification of fractures.

One study reported on the impact of MRI scanning on the interobserver reliability of classification of tibial plateau fractures according to the Schatzker classification system.[84] Three orthopedic trauma surgeons classified tibial plateau fractures first with plain radiographs, and then with either the addition of a CT and an MRI scan. Kappa values averaged 0.68 with plain radiographs alone, 0.73 with the addition of a CT scan, and 0.85 with addition of an MRI scan. No statistical analysis was reported to indicate whether the addition of CT and MRI information resulted in a statistically significant improvement in reliability.

Difficulty Identifying Fracture Lines on Radiographs

All fracture classification systems require the use of a diagnostic image, usually a radiograph, on which the observer must make observations, measurements, or both. Even with high-quality radiographs, however, overlapping osseous fragments or densities can make the accurate identification of each fracture fragment difficult. Osteopenia can also increase the difficulty in accurate classification of fractures. Osteopenic bone casts a much fainter "shadow" on radiographic films, making the delineation of fine trabecular or articular details a much more difficult task for the observer. Osteopenia represents a physiologic parameter that may affect treatment plans and outcomes, but is not mentioned in any classification system.

Periarticular fractures also may be difficult to accurately classify with plain radiographs. Articular fractures tend to occur in areas of the skeleton with complex three-dimensional osteology, may be highly comminuted, and the classification systems used for these fractures are predicated on the accurate identification of each fracture fragment and determination of its relationship to the other fragments and/or its position in the nonfracture situation. Observer variability in the identification of these small fracture fragments in complex fractures would be expected to lead to poorer interobserver reliability of the fracture classification system. Dirschl and Adams investigated the observers' ability to identify small articular fragments in classifying tibial plafond fractures according to the Ruedi and Allgower classification.[22] Observers classified 25 tibial plafond fractures on radiographs and then on line drawings that had been made from those radiographs by the senior author; interobserver reliability was no different in the two situations. At a second classification session, observers were asked to first mark, on the fracture radiographs, the articular fragments and then to classify the fractures; in a final session, the observers classified the radiographs after the fracture fragments had been premarked by the senior author. Having observers mark the fracture fragments resulted in no improvement in interobserver reliability of the fracture classification system. When identification of the articular fragments was removed from the fracture classification process; however, by having the fragments premarked by the senior author, the interobserver reliability was significantly improved (mean kappa value increased from 0.43 to 0.54, $p < 0.025$). The authors believed the results of this study indicated that observers classifying fractures of the tibial plafond have great difficulty identifying the fragments of the tibial articular surface on radiographs. They went on to postulate that fracture classification system predicated on the identification of the number and displacement of small articular fragments may inherently perform poorly on reliability analyses, because of observer difficulty in reliably identifying the fracture fragments.

Variability Making Measurements on Radiographs

The amount of displacement of fracture fragments, particularly articular fragments, has long been felt to be important in characterizing fractures and has been used by many to make decisions regarding treatment. In addition, some classification systems for fractures are predicated on the observer accurately identifying the amount of displacement and/or angulation of fracture fragments; the Neer classification system for proximal humeral fractures is an example. Finally, the quality of fracture care has frequently been judged by measuring the amount of displacement of articular fracture fragments on post-treatment radiographs.

Numerous studies have shown, however, that there is variability among observers in making measurements on radiographs and that this may be a source for variability in fracture classification. One such study assessed the error of measurement of articular incongruity of tibial plateau fractures.[51] In this study, five orthopedic traumatologists measured the maximum articular depression and the maximum condylar widening on 56 sets of tibial plateau fracture radiographs. For 38 of the cases, the observers also had a CT scan of the knee to assist in making measurements. The results of the study indicated that the 95% tolerance limits for measuring maximum articular depression were ±12 mm, and for measuring maximum condylar widening were ±9 mm. This result indicates that there is substantial variability in making these seemingly simple measurements.

Tolerance limits, of course, will decrease as the range of measurements decreases (the range of articular depression in the study above was 35 mm). Thus, it would be expected that lower tolerance limits would result from the measurement of reduced tibial plateau than those observed in the reported study, which measured injury films. However, in a study looking at the tolerance limits for measuring articular congruity in healed distal radial fractures, tolerance limits of ±3 mm were identified, when the range of articular congruity measurements was only 4 mm.[37]

It has been suggested that CT scanning may improve the reliability of measurement of articular fracture displacements. In one study of intra-articular fractures of the distal radius, there was poor correlation between measurement of gap widths or step deformities on plain radiographs as compared to CT scans.[14] Nearly one-third of measurements made from plain radiographs were significantly different than those made from CT scans. Another study extended these findings by examining known intra-articular displacements made in the hip joints of cadaveric specimens.[8] The authors observed that CT-generated data were far more accurate and reproducible than were data obtained from plain films. Moed et al.[53] reported on a series of posterior wall acetabular fractures treated with open reduction and internal fixation in which reduction was assessed on both plain radiographs and on CT scans. Of 59 patients who were graded as having an anatomic reduction based on plain radiographs and for whom postoperative CT scans were obtained, 46 had a gap or step-off greater than 2 mm. These results may not be characteristic of all fractures, since the posterior wall of the acetabulum may be more difficult to profile using plain radiographs than most areas of other joints.

From this work, it appears that there is significant observer variability in the routine measurement of articular incongruity on radiographs. It also seems highly unlikely that observers using plain radiographs can reliably measure small amounts of incongruity. This suggests that improvements in our ability to reliably assess the displacement of fracture fragments are necessary to reduce variability in articular fracture assessment.

Complexity of Decision Making in Applying a Fracture Classification

Some fracture classification systems are quite complex, requiring the observer to choose between many possible categories in characterizing a fracture. The AO/OTA system, for example, has up to 27 possible classifications for a fracture of a single-bone segment (there are three choices each for fracture type, group, and subgroup). It seems reasonable that observers would find it easier to classify a fracture if there were fewer choices to be made, and

studies of the AO/OTA fracture classification system have confirmed this. In nearly all cases, for various fractures, classification of type can be performed much more reliably than classification into groups or subgroups.[16,37,47,50,63,77,82] These studies concluded that, for optimal reliability, the use of this classification beyond characterization of type was not recommended.

It has also been proposed that limiting observers' choices to no more than two for any step in the classification of fractures would improve the ability of the observer to classify the fracture and would improve interobserver reliability. In 1996, the developers of the AO/ASIF comprehensive classification of fractures (CCF) modified to incorporate binary decision making.[55] The reasoning was that, if observers could answer a series of "yes or no" questions about the fracture, they could more precisely and reliably classify the fracture. The modification was planned, announced, and implemented without any sort of validation that the modification would achieve the desired outcomes or that binary decision making would improve reliability in fracture classification.

Two investigations of specific fracture types have evaluated whether binary decision making improves reliability in the classification of fractures. The first of these studies developed a binary modification of the Ruedi and Allgower classification of tibial plafond fractures and had observers classify 25 fractures according to the original classification system and the binary modification.[22] The binary modification was applied rigidly in fracture classification sessions that were proctored by the author; observers were forced to make binary decisions about the fracture radiographs, and not permitted to jump to the final fracture classification. The results of this study indicated that the binary modification of this classification system did not perform with greater reliability than the standard classification system (mean kappa 0.43 ± 0.048 standard and 0.35 ± 0.038 binary). Another investigation compared the interobserver reliability of classification of malleolar fractures of the tibia (segment 44) according to the classic and binary modification of the AO/ASIF CCF.[16] Six observers classified 50 malleolar fractures according to both the standard and binary systems, and no difference in interobserver reliability could be demonstrated between the two systems (mean kappa 0.61 standard and 0.62 binary). The authors concluded that strictly enforced binary decision making did not improve reliability in the classification of malleolar fractures according to the AO/ASIF CCF. The results of these two studies cast doubt on the effectiveness of binary decision making in improving interobserver reliability in the classification of fractures.

Another study tested the hypothesis that perhaps the amount of information provided an observer could be overwhelming and limit reliability of fracture classification.[36] This group tested the Sanders classification of calcaneal fractures and, rather than providing observers with the full CT scan data for each of the 30 cases, they provided each observer with only one carefully selected CT image from which to make a classification decision. The results indicated that the overall interobserver reliability was no better with only one CT cut than with the full series of CT cuts. The results clearly showed, however, that interobserver agreement was much better for the most and least severe fractures in the series and poorest for fractures in the midrange of severity. This finding is probably applicable to all classification schemes, in which observers are much better at differentiating the best from the worst than they are at cases in the middle of the spectrum of injury severity.

Categorization of a Continuous Variable

All fracture classification systems in common use today are categorical; regardless of the nature or complexity of the classification system, each group's fractures are grouped into discrete categories. Injuries to individual patients, however, occur on a continuum of energy and severity of injury; fractures follow this same pattern, occurring on a spectrum of injury severity. The process of fracture classification can therefore be said to be a process by which a continuous variable, such as fracture severity, is made a categorical one. This "categorization" of a continuous variable may be a source of intraobserver variability in fracture classification systems.[20,49] One study concluded that "it has become clear that these deficiencies are related to the fact that the infinite variation of injury is a continuous variable and to force this continuous variable into a classification scheme, a dichotomous variable, will result in the discrepancies that have been documented."[30] The authors further suggested that "multiple classifiers, blinded to the treatment selected and clinical outcomes, and consensus methodology should be used to optimize the utility of injury classification schemes for research and publication purposes."

In an effort to address this issue, some authors have proposed that, instead of classifying fractures, perhaps fractures should merely be rank ordered from the least severe to the most severe. This would serve as a means to preserve the continuum of fracture severity and has been proposed as a means of potentially improving interobserver reliability. An initial study using this methodology in tibial plafond fracture showed promise.[19] Twenty-five tibial plafond fractures were ranked by three orthopedic traumatologists from the least severe to the most severe, and the group demonstrated outstanding interobserver reliability, with a Cronbach alpha statistic[17] of 0.94 (nearly perfect agreement). In a subsequent study, the rank order concept was expanded and a series of 10 tibial plafond fractures were ranked by 69 observers.[21] The intraclass correlation coefficient (ICC) was 0.62, representing substantial agreement, but also represented some deterioration from the results with only three observers. Based on these results, which are superior to those of most categorical fracture classification systems that have been evaluated, further study of this sort of classification system appears to be warranted.

It has been postulated that one means of implementing a fracture classification system that ranks cases on a continuum of injury severity would be to approach the matter much in the same way as clinicians determine bone age in children.[21] A series of radiographs would be published that represent the spectrum of fracture severity, from the least severe to the most severe, and then an observer would simply review these examples and determine where the fracture under review lay on this spectrum of severity. This concept is markedly different from any scheme used to date to classify fractures, would be unlikely

to completely replace other systems of fracture classification, and may have weaknesses that have not yet been determined. Such a system will require extensive testing and validation before it could be widely used.

Poor Attention to Classification of Nonradiographic Factors

Measuring the injury severity and predicting the outcome following a fracture depends on much more than radiographic factors.[23,24,47] Recently, many have come to question whether any system for fracture classification that relies solely on radiographic data will be highly reliable or highly predictive of the outcome of severe fractures. There is strong evidence that the extent of injury to the soft tissues (cartilage, muscle, tendon, skin, etc.), the magnitude and durations of the patient's physiologic response to injury, the presence of comorbid conditions, and the patient's socioeconomic background and lifestyle may all play critical roles in influencing outcomes following severe fractures.

As an example, it is well recognized that injury to articular cartilage is a critical and significant contributor to the overall severity of an articular fracture, as evidenced by studies documenting poor outcomes after osteochondritis dissecans and other chondral injuries. The information present in the orthopedic clinical literature indicates that the severity of injury to the articular surface during fracture has an important bearing on outcome and the eventual development of post-traumatic osteoarthrosis. A better understanding of the impaction injury to the articular cartilage and the prognosis of such injury will be critical to improving our assessment and understanding of severe intra-articular fractures. Unfortunately, there are currently no imaging modalities that have been validated to indicate to the clinician the extent of injury to the cartilage of the articular surface and/or the potential for repair or the risk of post-traumatic degeneration of the articular cartilage. Plain radiographs and CT scans provide very little information about the current and future health of the articular cartilage in a joint with a fracture.

Inherent Variability in Human Observations

It is to be expected that human observers, no matter how well trained, will have some level of variability in applying any tool—no matter how reliable—in classifying fractures. The magnitude of the "baseline" level of inherent human variability in fracture classification is entirely unknown. As such, it is extremely difficult for investigators to know with precision what represents excellent interobserver reliability in fracture classification. There is disagreement over the best statistical analysis to use in assessing reliability or what level of agreement is acceptable in studies on fracture classification. Statistics such as the ICC are very good as indicators of when a laboratory test, such as the hematocrit or serum calcium level, has acceptable reliability and reproducibility. Whether the same threshold level of reliability should be applied to a process such as fracture classification is unknown. Similarly, the interpretation of the weighted kappa statistic for fracture classification is somewhat difficult, since there are few guidelines to aid in interpreting their results. Landis and Koch admit that their widely accepted reference intervals for the kappa statistic were chosen arbitrarily. In addition, a recent investigation seemed to indicate that using the kappa statistic with a small number of observers introduces the possibility of "sampling error" causing an increased variance in the kappa statistic itself.[4,64] Having many different observers causes stabilization of the kappa value around a "mean value" for the agreement among the population of observers. Invariably, however, using more observers results in a lower mean kappa value and indicated poorer interobserver reliability of the classification system being tested. Therefore, studies with a small amount of observers that reported excellent reliability in fracture classification systems may be reporting spuriously high results for the kappa statistic—results that would be much lower if more observers were used. Unfortunately, there are currently no better or more reliable methods for reporting and interpreting interobserver reliability than the use of the ICC or the kappa statistic.

CURRENT USEFULNESS OF FRACTURE CLASSIFICATION SYSTEMS

Fracture classification systems are highly useful for describing fractures; this has been one of the best uses for fracture classification systems. Using a well-known fracture classification to describe a fracture to an orthopedist or colleague who cannot immediately view the fracture radiographs immediately invokes in the orthopedist a visual image of the fracture. This visual image, even if it is not highly reliable to statistical testing, enhances communication between orthopedic physicians.

Fracture classification systems are also useful as educational tools. Educating orthopedic trainees in systems of fracture classification is highly valuable, for many systems are devised from the mechanism of injury or from the anatomical alignment of the fracture fragments. These are important educational tools to assist orthopedic trainees in better understanding the osteology of different parts of the skeleton and the various mechanisms of injury that can result in fractures. Educational systems using fracture classification methodologies can assist orthopedic trainees in formulating a context in which to make treatment decisions, and can also provide an important historical context of fracture care and fracture classification in orthopedics.

Fracture classification systems may be useful in guiding treatment, and it is clearly the intent of many fracture classification systems to do so. It is unclear, however, from much of the literature that has been published, whether fracture classification systems are valid tools to guide treatment. The fact that there is so much observer variability in fracture classification adds an element of doubt to comparative clinical studies that have used fracture classification as a guide to treatment.

Fracture classification systems have also been said to be useful in predicting outcomes following fracture care. The orthopedic literature to date, however, does not seem to clearly indicate that fracture classification systems can be used to predict patient outcomes in any sort of valid or reproducible way. The interobserver variability of many fracture classification systems is one of the key reasons that the literature cannot clearly show this correlation. One exception to this, however, is that most fracture classification systems have good reliability in characterizing the most severe and least severe injuries—those that correlate with the best and worst outcomes. It is in the midrange of injury severity that classification systems demonstrate the poorest reliability and the poorest ability to predict outcomes.

THE FUTURE OF FRACTURE CLASSIFICATION SYSTEMS

The future will bring a more comprehensive determination of injury severity than merely classifying a fracture according to plain radiographs. It has become clear in recent years that variables other than radiograph appearance of the fracture play a huge role in determining patient outcome, and these variables will be utilized in new systems of determining injury severity in patients with fractures. A simple example of this is the classification of open fractures published by the Open Fracture Classification Study Group of the OTA.[61] Instead of assigning an overall grade or number to the injury, this system assigns a severity to each of five essential factors (skin injury, muscle injury, arterial injury, contamination, and bone loss) determined by systematic analysis of the literature and consensus of experts. This system attempts to objectify important factors other than the radiographic appearance of the fracture. Objective measures of energy of injury include CT scans, finite-element models or volumetric measures, objective measures of the patient's physiologic reserve and response to injury, and serum lactate levels may also become part of fracture classification schemes. An assessment of overall health status and the existence of comorbid conditions are also ways that may be used, in combination with radiographs, to make more comprehensive the determination of fracture severity.

Better imaging modalities will also assist in better and more reliably determining and characterizing the injury severity in patients with fractures. Newer uses for CT scanning, MRI imaging, and ultrasound may be instrumental in providing the treating surgeon more information about the extent of soft tissue injury, the health of the bone and cartilage, and the biology at the fracture site. For example, it is possible with very high-energy MRI scans to determine the proteoglycan content of articular cartilage. Since articular cartilage is not imaged on CT or plain radiographic imaging, its health has been generally excluded from the classification of fractures. However, the long-term health of the articular cartilage is crucial to the patient's outcome following a severe articular injury. In the future, the ability to use advanced imaging modalities to better characterize the current health and predict the future health of the articular cartilage may greatly advance the ability to accurately classify fractures and to use fracture classification as a predictive measure.

Newer fracture classification schemes will be devised that will better assure that fractures can be measured and characterized on a continuum, which is how they occur. These new classification systems will better represent that injury severity occurs on a continuum than do systems in use today, many of which were based solely on anatomical consideration rather than on injury severity. Ideas such as rank-ordering fractures, putting fractures on a continuum, sending fractures to a fracture classification clearing house (for classification by one or just a few observers) are but a few possible future approaches to advancing and making more reproducible the classification of fractures.

There will be better agreement about what sort of process of validation a fracture classification system should undergo before becoming available for general use. Most classification systems in general use had no formal pre-hoc validation. Most of them have come into general use because of the reputation or influence of the person or group that devised them, or perhaps because the system has been in use so long that it has become part of the vernacular in fracture classification and fracture care. One study has proposed a formal, detailed, and very time-consuming methodology for the validation of all fracture classification systems, very similar to that which was performed for patient-based outcome measures, such as the short form 36 and the musculoskeletal functional assessment.[4] It is as of yet unclear whether such validation methods would improve the interobserver reliability of fracture classification systems. It is clear, however, that such methods would be exhaustive and very time consuming, and that many orthopedic surgeons do not believe that such detailed validation is necessary for fracture classification systems.

The use of image processing and analysis techniques will advance the understanding of and ability to classify fractures. Advances in image processing and image analysis, perhaps when coupled with neural nets and other learning technologies, may make it possible for computers to be taught to classify fractures with a high degree of reliability and reproducibility. One could envision a system by which digital images of a fracture are classified according to any of several classification systems automatically by a computer system at the time the radiographs are obtained, much as electrocardiograph (EKG) readings are currently generated by a computer at the time the patient's cardiac tracing is obtained. One rudimentary example of this is the computerized measurement of displacement of sacral fractures on CT scans, using a system that adjusts for pelvic rotation in three planes.[43]

Finally, there will be more rigorous validation of fracture classification systems. Rigorous statistical methods—or at least consensus statistical methodologies—will be developed and implemented that, while detailed, time consuming, and involved, will result in greatly improved validation of many fracture classification systems.

REFERENCES

1. Andersen DJ, Blair WF, Steyers CM, et al. Classification of distal radius fractures: An analysis of interobserver reliability and intraobserver reproducibility. J Hand Surg. 1996;21A:574–582.
2. Andersen E, Jorgensen LG, Hededam LT. Evans classification of trochanteric fractures: An assessment for the interobserver reliability and intraobserver reproducibility. Injury. 1990;21:377–378.
3. Anderson GR, Rasmussen JB, Dahl B, et al. Oldefs classification of Colle fractures: Good intraobserver and interobserver reproducibility in 185 cases. Acta Orthop Scan. 1991;62:463–464.
4. Audige L, Bhandari M, Kellam J. How reliable are reliability studies of fracture classifications? A systematic review of their methodologies. Acta Orthop Scand. 2004;75:184–194.
5. Barker L, Anderson J, Chesnut R, et al. Reliability and reproducibility of dens fracture classification with use of plain radiography and reformatted computer-aided tomography. J Bone Joint Surg Am. 2006;88:106–112.
6. Beaule PE, Dorey FJ, Matta JM. Letournel classification for acetabular fractures: Assessment of interobserver and intraobserver reliability. J Bone Joint Surg Am. 2003;85:1704–1709.
7. Bernstein J, Adler LM, Blank JE, et al. Evaluation of the Neer system of classification of proximal humeral fractures with computerized tomographic scans and plain radiographs. J Bone Joint Surg Am. 1996;78:1371–1375.
8. Borrelli J Jr, Goldfarb C, Catalano L, et al. Assessment of articular fragment displacement in acetabular fractures: A comparison of computed tomography and plain radiographs. J Orthop Trauma. 2002;16:449–456.
9. Brorson S, Bagger J, Sylvest A, et al. Low agreement among 24 doctors using the Neer classification; only moderate agreement on displacement, even between specialists. Int Orthop. 2002;26:271–273.
10. Brumback RJ, Jones AL. Interobserver agreement in the classification of open fractures of the tibia. J Bone Joint Surg Am. 1994;76:1162–1166.
11. Burstein AH. Fracture classification systems: Do they work and are they useful? J Bone Joint Surg Am. 1993;75:1743–1744.
12. Chan PSH, Klimkiewicz JJ, Luchette WT, et al. Impact of CT scan on treatment plan and fracture classification of tibial plateau fractures. J Orthop Trauma. 1997;11:484–489.
13. Cohen J. A coefficient of agreement for nominal scales. Educ Psych Meas. 1960;20:37–46.
14. Cole RJ, Bindra RR, Evanoff BA, et al. Radiographic evaluation of osseous displacement following intraarticular fracture of the distal radius: Reliability of plain radiographs versus computed tomography. J Hand Surg Am. 1997;22:792–800.
15. Colles A. On the fracture of the carpal extremity of the radius. Edinb Med Surg J. 1814;10:182–186.
16. Craig WL III, Dirschl DR. An assessment of the effectiveness of binary decision-making in improving the reliability of the AO/ASIF classification of fractures of the ankle. J Orthop Trauma. 1998;12:280–284.
17. Cronbach LJ. Coefficient alpha and the internal structure of tests. Psychometrika 1951;16:297–334.
18. Dahlen HC, Franck WM, Sabauri G, et al. Incorrect classification of extra-articular distal radius fractures by conventional x-rays: Comparison between biplanar radiologic diagnostics and CT assessment of fracture morphology. Unfallchirurg. 2004;107(6):491–498.
19. DeCoster TA, Willis MC, Marsh JL, et al. Rank order analysis of tibial plafond fracture: Does injury or reduction predict outcome? Foot Ankle Int. 1999;20:44–49.
20. Desai VV, Davis TRC, Barton NJ. The prognostic value and reproducibility of the radiological features of the fractured scaphoid. J Hand Surg Br. 1999;5:586–590.
21. Dirschl DR, Ferry ST. Reliability of classification of fractures of the tibial plafond according to a rank order method. J Trauma. 2006;61:1463–1466.
22. Dirschl DR, Adams GL. A critical assessment of methods to improve reliability in the classification of fractures, using fractures of the tibial plafond as a model. J Orthop Trauma. 1997;11:471–476.
23. Dirschl DR, Dawson PA. Assessment of injury severity in tibial plateau fractures. Clin Orthop Rel Res. 2004;423:85–92.
24. Dirschl DR, Marsh JL, Buckwalter JA, et al. Articular Fractures. J Am Acad Orthop Surg. 2004;12(6):416–423.
25. Doornberg J, Lindenhovius A, Kloen P, et al. Two-and three-dimensional computed tomography for the classification and management of distal humeral fractures. J Bone Joint Surg Am. 2006;88:1795–1801.
26. Doornberg JN, Rademakers MV, van den Bekerom MP, et al. Two-dimensional and three-dimensional computed tomography for the classification and characterization of tibial plateau fractures. Injury. 2011;42:1416–1425.
27. Fleiss JL. Statistical Methods for Rates and Proportions. 2nd ed. New York, NY: John Wiley & Sons; 1981:218.
28. Fleiss JL, Stakter MJ, Fischman SL, et al. Inter-examiner reliability in caries trials. J Dent Res. 1979;58:604–609.
29. Frandsen PA, Andersen E, Madsen F, et al. Garden classification of femoral neck fractures: An assessment of interobserver variation. J Bone Joint Surg Br. 1988;70:588–590.
30. Garbuz DS, Masri BA, Esdaile J, et al. Classification systems in orthopaedics. J Am Acad Orthop Surg. 2002;10:290–297.
31. Garden RS. Low-angle fixation in fractures of the femoral neck. J Bone Joint Surg Br. 1961;43:647–663.
32. Gaston P, Will R, Elton RA, et al. Fractures of the tibia: Can their outcome be predicted? J Bone Joint Surg. 1999;81B:71–76.
33. Gustilo RB, Anderson JT. Prediction of infection in the treatment of 1025 open fractures in long bones. J Bone Joint Surg. 1976;58A:453–458.
34. Gustilo RB, Mendoza RM, Williams DN. Problems in the management of Type III (severe) open fractures: A new classification of type III open fractures. J Trauma. 1984;24(8):742–746.
35. Hu YL, Ye FG, Ji AY, et al. Three-dimensional computed tomography imaging increases the reliability of classification systems for tibial plateau fractures. Injury. 2009;40:1282–1285.
36. Humphrey CA, Dirschl DR, Ellis TJ. Interobserver reliability of a CT-based fracture classification system. J Orthop Trauma. 2005;19:616–622.
37. Katz MA, Beredjiklian PK, Bozentka DJ, et al. Computed tomography scanning of intraarticular distal radius fractures: Does it influence treatment? J Hand Surg Am. 2001;26(3):415–421.
38. Kreder HJ, Hanel DP, McKee M, et al. Consistency of AO fracture classification for the distal radius. J Bone Joint Surg. 1996;78:726–731.
39. Kristiansen B, Andersen ULS, Olsen CA, et al. The Neer classification of fractures of the proximal humerus: An assessment of interobserver variation. Skeletal Radiol. 1988;17:420–422.
40. Landis JR, Koch GG. The measurement of observer agreement for categorical data. Biometrics. 1977;33:159–174.
41. Lauder AJ, Inda DJ, Bott AM, et al. Interobserver and intraobserver reliability of two classification systems for intra-articular calcaneal fractures. Foot Ankle Int. 2006;27:251–255.

42. Lauge-Hansen N. Fractures of the ankle. III: Genetic roentgenologic diagnosis of fractures of the ankle. *AJR.* 1954;71:456–471.
43. Lien J, Lee J, Maratt J, et al. Computed Tomographic Measurement of Pelvic Landmarks in Minimally Displaced Lateral Compression Sacral Fractures: Comparison to Radiographic Measurements. Poster presentation at the 28th Annual Meeting of the Orthopaedic Trauma Association, Minneapolis, MN, October 3–6, 2012.
44. Mahadeva D, Dias RG, Deshpande SV, et al. The reliability and reproducibility of the Neer classification system – digital radiography (PACS) improves agreement. *Injury.* 2011;42:339–342.
45. Majed A, MacLeod I, Bull A, et al. Proximal humeral fracture classifications systems revisted. *J Shoulder Elbow Surg.* 2011;20:1125–1132.
46. Maripuri SN, Rao P, Manoj-Thomas A, et al. The classification systems for tibial plateau fractures: How reliable are they? *Injury.* 2008;39:1216–1221.
47. Marsh JL, Buckwalter J, Gelberman RC, et al. Does an anatomic reduction really change the result in the management of articular fractures? *J Bone Joint Surg.* 2002;84-A:1259–1271.
48. Marsh JL, Slongo TF, Agel J, et al. Fracture and dislocation classification compendium—2007. *F Orthop Trauma.* 2007;21:S1–S160.
49. Martin JS, Marsh JL. Current classification of fractures; rationale and utility. *Radiol Clin North Am.* 1997;35:491–506.
50. Martin JS, Marsh JL, Bonar SK, et al. Assessment of the AO/ASIF fracture classification for the distal tibia. *J Orthop Trauma.* 1997;11:477–483.
51. Martin J, Marsh JL, Nepola JV, et al. Radiographic fracture assessments: Which ones can we reliably make? *J Orthop Trauma.* 2000;14(6):379–385.
52. Major Extremity Trauma Research Consortium. *Apples to Apples: Moving to the New OTA Fracture Severity Classification in Extremity Trauma Research.* Poster presentation at the 28th Annual Meeting of the Orthopaedic Trauma Association, Minneapolis, MN, October 3–6, 2012.
53. Moed RB, Carr SEW, Watson JT. Open reduction and internal fixation of posterior wall fractures of the acetabulum. *Clin Orthop and Rel Res.* 2000;377:57–67.
54. Muller ME. The comprehensive classification of fractures of long bone. In: Muller ME, Allgower M, Schneider R, et al., eds. *Manual of Internal Fixation: Techniques Recommended by the AO-ASIF Group.* 3rd ed. Heidelberg: Springer-Verlag; 1991.
55. Muller ME, Nazarian S, Kack P. *CCF: Comprehensive Classification of Fractures.* Bern: Maurice E Muller Foundation; 1996.
56. Neer CS. Displaced proximal humeral fractures. Part I: Classification and evaluation. *J Bone Joint Surg Am.* 1970;52:1077–1089.
57. Nielsen JO, Dons-Jensen H, Sorensen HT. Lauge-Hansen classification of malleolar fractures: An assessment of the reproducibility of 118 cases. *Acta Orthop Scand.* 1990;61:385–387.
58. Oakes DA, Jackson KR, Davies MR, et al. The impact of the Garden classification on proposed operative treatment. *Clin Orthop Relat Res.* 2003;409:232–240.
59. Oestern HJ, Txcherne H. Pathophysiology and classification of soft tissue injuries associated with fractures. In: Tscherne H, ed. *Fracture with Soft Tissue Injuries.* New York, NY: Springer-Verlag; 1984:1–9.
60. Oner FC, Ramos LMP, Simmermacher RKJ, et al. Classification of thoracic and lumbar spine fractures: Problems of reproducibility. *Eur Spine J.* 2002;11:235–245.
61. Orthopaedic Trauma Association: Open Fracture Study Group. A new classification scheme for open fractures. *J Orthop Trauma.* 2010;24:457–465.
62. Orthopaedic Trauma Association Committee for Coding and Classification. Fracture and dislocation compendium. *J Orthop Trauma.* 1996;10(suppl 1):1–154.
63. Pervez H, Parker MJ, Pryor GA, et al. Classification of trochanteric fracture of the proximal femur: A study of the reliability of current systems. *Injury.* 2002;33:713–715.
64. Petrisor BA, Bhandari M, Orr RD, et al. Improving reliability in the classification of fractures of the acetabulum. *Arch Orthop Trauma Surg.* 2003;123:228–233.
65. Pott P. *Some Few General Remarks on Fractures and Dislocations.* London: Hawes L, Clarke W and Collins R; 1765.
66. Rasmussen S, Madsen PV, Bennicke K. Observer variation in the Lauge-Hansen classification of ankle fractures: Precision improved by instruction. *Actat Orthop Scand.* 1993;64:693–694.
67. Sanders R. Displaced intra-articular fractures of the calcaneus. *J Bone Joint Surg Am.* 2000;82(2):225–250.
68. Schatzker J. Fractures of the tibial plateau. In: Schatzker M, Tile M, eds. *Rationale of Operative Fractures Care.* Berlin: Springer-Verlag; 1988:279–295.
69. Schatzker J, McBroom R. Tibial plateau fractures: The Toronto experience 1968–1975. *Clin Orthop Relat Res.* 1979;138:94–104.
70. Schipper IB, Steyerberg EW, Castelein RM, et al. Reliability of the AO/ASIF classification for peritrochanteric femoral fractures. *Acta Orthop Scand.* 2001;72:36–41.
71. Seigel G, Podgor MJ, Remaley NA. Acceptable values of kappa for comparison of two groups. *Am J Epidemiol.* 1992;135:571–578.
72. Shepherd LE, Zalavras CG, Jaki K, et al. Gunshot femoral shaft fractures: Is the current classification system reliable? *Clin Orthop Relat Res.* 2003;408:101–109.
73. Sidor JL, Zuckerman JD, Lyon T, et al. The Neer classification system for proximal humeral fractures: An assessment of interobserver reliability and intraobserver reproducibility. *J Bone Joint Surg Am.* 1993;75:1745–1750.
74. Siebenrock KA, Gerber C. The reproducibility of classification of fractures of the proximal end of the humerus. *J Bone Joint Surg Am.* 1993;75:1751–1755.
75. Svanholm H, Starklint H, Gundersen HJ, et al. Reproducibility of histomorphologic diagnoses with special reference to the kappa statistic. *APMIS.* 1989;97:689–698.
76. Swiontkowski JF, Agel J, McAndrew MP, et al. Outcome validation of the AO/OTA fracture classification system. *J Orthop Trauma.* 2000;14:534–541.
77. Swiontkowski JF, Sands AK, Agel J, et al. Interobserver variation in the AO/OTA fracture classification system for pilon fractures: Is there a problem? *J Orthop Trauma.* 1997;11:467–470.
78. Thomsen NOB, Olsen LH, Nielsen ST. Kappa statistics in the assessment of observer variation: The significance of multiple observers classifying ankle fractures. *J Orthop Sci.* 2002;7:163–166.
79. Thomsen NOB, Overgaard S, Olen LH, et al. Observer variation in the radiographic classification of ankle fractures. *J Bone Joint Surg Br.* 1991;73:676–678.
80. Visutipol B, Chobrangsin P, Ketmalasiri B, et al. Evaluation of Letournel and Judet classification of acetabular fracture with plain radiographs and three-dimensional computerized tomographic scan. *J Orthop Surg.* 2000;8:33–37.
81. Van Embden D, Roukema GR, Rhemrev SJ, et al. The Pauwels classification for intracapsular hip fractures: Is it reliable? *Injury.* 2011;42:1238–1240.
82. Walton NP, Harish S, Roberts C, et al. AO or Schatzker? How reliable is classification of tibial plateau fractures? *Arch Orthop Trauma Surg.* 2003;123:396–398.
83. Wicky S, Blaser PF, Blanc CH, et al. Comparison between standard radiography and spiral CT with 3D reconstruction in the evaluation, classification and management of tibial plateau fractures. *Eur Radiol.* 2000;10:1227–1232. (showed change in surgical plan in 59% of cases, but no diff in classification).
84. Yacoubian SV, Nevins RT, Sallis JG, et al. Impact of MRI on treatment plan and fracture classification of tibial plateau fractures. *J Orthop Trauma.* 2002;16:632–637.

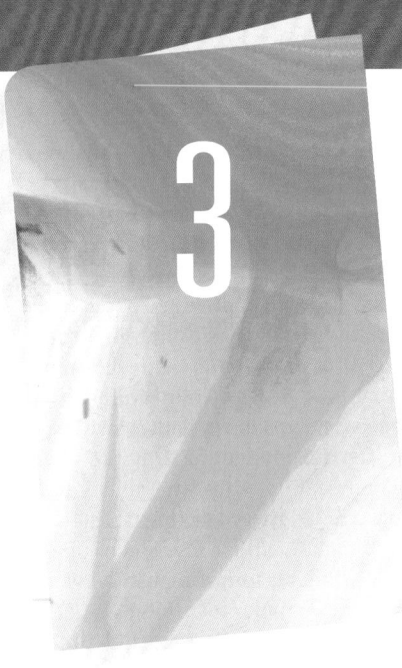

3

THE EPIDEMIOLOGY OF FRACTURES AND DISLOCATIONS

Charles M. Court-Brown

INTRODUCTION

In the seventh edition of Rockwood and Green[26] the epidemiology of fractures presenting to the Royal Infirmary of Edinburgh in a 1-year period in 2007 to 2008 was analyzed. This hospital is somewhat unusual in that it is the only hospital admitting orthopedic trauma from a large well-defined population living in the City of Edinburgh, Midlothian and East Lothian, in Scotland. It does not deal with pediatric fractures but it does act as a secondary referral center for complex fractures in the South East of Scotland. For the purposes of epidemiologic analysis these fractures have not been considered and the data in this chapter comes exclusively from the catchment area of the hospital. This provides an accurate analysis of the epidemiology of adult fractures in a developed country and the results will apply to other areas with a similar socioeconomic status. Obviously this does not include all parts of the world, but it is likely that our data is applicable to many areas. In this edition of Rockwood and Green the structure of the chapter has been altered. In the seventh edition of Rockwood and Green[26] the fracture epidemiology of the Royal Infirmary of Edinburgh

was compared with that of the R Adams Cowley Shock Trauma Center in Baltimore, USA in the belief that there would be a significant difference in fracture epidemiology between a large hospital dealing with all orthopedic trauma and a specialized Level 1 trauma center dealing mainly with severe trauma. In this edition adult fracture epidemiology has been examined more closely and the different factors that affect it have been defined. In addition to discussing the epidemiology of adult fractures in a specific year the epidemiology of adolescent fractures has been examined as has the epidemiology of open fractures. The epidemiology of dislocations has not received much attention in the literature and an analysis of dislocations over a 1-year period is presented.

The chapter will be based on the principle that fracture epidemiology is affected by gender and age, but is also influenced by a number of social and medical comorbidities which, as yet, have not been precisely defined. However it is likely that these comorbidities can be examined by looking at the effect of social deprivation on fracture epidemiology. This will also be undertaken in an attempt to provide a more complete epidemiologic analysis of fractures in adults.

HISTORY

Surgeons have treated fractures for several millennia but until the advent of radiographs the diagnosis of different fractures was based on knowledge of the human anatomy, clinical signs, and educated observation. However a number of surgeons did analyze fracture epidemiology in some detail a good example being Malgaigne[70] who analyzed 2,377 fractures in the Hôtel Dieu in Paris between 1806 and 1808 and 1830 and 1839. He analyzed these fractures according to age, gender, seasonality, and the location of the fracture. He observed that fractures were most commonly seen between 25 and 60 years of age. He understood the importance of calculating incidence and showed that while patients aged 25 to 30 and 55 to 60 had a similar prevalence of fractures the numbers of 55- to 60-year olds in the population was less than 50% that of 25- to 30-year olds. He stated that there were very few fractures in patients aged >60 years but there were very few people of that age left alive.

Malgaigne[70] stated that fractures in males exceeded fractures in females by a factor of 5:2 but that the factor varied with age. In children of 5 years or less females presented with twice as many fractures as males. The ratio changed with increasing age so that between 15 and 20 years there were eight male fractures for every female fracture. The ratio continued to change so that between 70 and 75 years of age the fracture rate was similar in males and females. Thereafter fractures were more commonly seen in females. Malgaigne did not agree with the previously stated view that fractures were more common in winter because cold weather made bones more fragile, and he actually recorded that fractures were more commonly seen in spring.

A review of the epidemiology of the fractures that Malgaigne[70] treated showed that 46.9% were upper limb fractures, 52% were lower limb fractures, and the remaining 1.1% were spinal or pelvic fractures. There was a high prevalence of humeral fractures (14.4%), femoral fractures (10.1%), and lower leg fractures (33.1%) and he recorded that 5.3% of the fractures were proximal femoral fractures and that 1.3% involved the proximal humerus. He, and his contemporaries were obviously aware that different fractures occurred at different ages and he observed that it had recently been stated that fractures of the diaphyses tended to occur in adulthood while intra-articular fractures occurred in old age. He thought that this observation was essentially correct and he stated that fractures of the "cervix femoris and cervix humeri" occurred in old age and that women sustained a large proportion of the fractures of "the carpal extremity of the radius."

More exact analyses of fracture epidemiology were undertaken by Stimson[95] in the Hudson Street Hospital, New York between 1894 and 1903 and by Emmett and Breck[37] of El Paso, Texas in three time periods between 1937 and 1956. To be strictly accurate these analyses cannot be compared with data from Edinburgh, Scotland as they simply report the workload of their particular institutions. However both hospitals dealt with a wide range of different patients and conditions and they treated many thousands of fractures. Thus their results are of

interest and there are, in fact, no better epidemiologic analyses to compare with modern data.

Table 3-1 shows a comparison of the prevalence of different fractures treated by Stimson and his colleagues[95] and by Emmett and Breck and their colleagues.[37] Both groups treated both children and adults and for comparative purposes their results have been compared to those of the Edinburgh Orthopaedic Trauma Unit in 2000 as both adult and childrens' fractures were examined that year. It is of course difficult to compare all the fractures accurately. This is particularly true of forearm fractures where proximal radial fractures are often combined with forearm diaphyseal fractures. In Table 3-1 all of Emmett and Breck's data on forearm fractures has been combined as it was difficult to analyze their assessment of the individual fractures. It is also difficult to distinguish between isolated fibular fractures and those fibular fractures associated with ankle fractures, tibial diaphyseal fractures, and proximal and distal tibial fractures. The overall figures do however point to changing trends in the epidemiology of fractures which reflect massive social, health, and economic changes in society.

A review of Table 3-1 shows that in 1894 to 1903, when motor vehicles were extremely rare and the life expectancy of both males and females might reasonably be expected to be about 50 years of age, there were many fractures that one would regard as high-energy injuries. There was a high prevalence of fractures of the scapula, tibia and fibula, and ankle and it seems likely that many of these fractures were work related as there would have been little workplace legislation. The prevalence of fractures of the tibia and fibula was particularly high in 1894 to 1903.

Unfortunately Stimson[95] did not separate proximal humeral and proximal femoral fractures from other fractures of the humerus and femur. But it seems likely that there was a much lower prevalence of fragility fractures in those days. This is confirmed by observing that the prevalence of distal radial fractures has doubled in the last 100 years or so and this must be largely because of the increase in numbers of elderly people in the population. Table 3-1 shows that the prevalence of proximal humeral and proximal femoral fractures has certainly increased since the period around the Second World War.

Another major difference in fracture epidemiology over the last 100 years or so is the decreased prevalence of fractures of the hand. Stimson found that 29.2% of the fractures that he treated involved the hand compared with 23.7% in Edinburgh in 2000. It seems likely that this is related to a safer work environment nowadays. It is also likely that Stimson's estimate of the prevalence of carpal fractures is an underestimate as radiographs were in their infancy at that time.

Table 3-1 shows that the epidemiology of fractures is changing and there is no doubt that it will continue to change. Recently many authors have commented on the increased incidence of fragility fractures but nothing is new and we should remember Malgaigne's[70] observation over 160 years ago that fractures of the proximal humerus, proximal femur, and distal radius were more common in the elderly and in women!

TABLE 3-1	**The Prevalence of Fractures in Three Time Periods Over the Last 100 Years**		
	Fracture Prevalence (%)		
	1894–1903[95]	**1937–1956[37]**	**2000[23,85]**
Clavicle	5.9	6.2	4.3
Scapula	0.7	0.7	0.2
Proximal humerus	5.7*	2.6	4.8
Humeral diaphysis	5.7*	2	1
Distal humerus	5.7*	5.2	2.5
Proximal ulna	1.1	21.2*	0.8
Proximal radius	9*	21.2*	3.8
Radius and ulnar diaphyses	9*	21.2*	2.3
Distal radius and ulna	11.2	21.2*	22.2
Carpus	0.2	2.4	2
Metacarpus	9.7	4.2	10.5
Finger phalanges	19.3	7.6	11.2
Pelvis	0.7	2.5	1.2
Proximal femur	4.7*	6.6	8.9
Femoral diaphysis	4.7*	2.5	0.9
Distal femur	4.7*	0.6	0.4
Patella	1.7	1.8	0.8
Proximal tibia	10.4*	7.3*	1
Tibia and fibula diaphyses	10.4*	7.3*	2
Distal tibia	10.4*	7.3*	1
Ankle	10.6	8.8	7.7
Tarsus	1.5	3.5	1.6
Metatarsus	2.8	4.1	6.4
Toe phalanges	3.1	4.4	2
Others	1.5	4.6	—
Fracture numbers	8,982	9,379	7,760

*Where it was impossible to separate the prevalence of individual fracture types in the same body area they have each been given the cumulative prevalence and marked with an asterisk.

FRACTURE INCIDENCE

It is surprisingly difficult to analyze the incidence of fractures accurately. In many parts of the world there are no facilities to allow accurate analysis of what is a common medical condition. However even in more affluent areas there is remarkably little accurate information about the incidence of fractures. One might think that the analysis of all fractures in a specific population during a specific time period would be relatively easy, but in many countries orthopedic trauma is treated in different types of institution with severe trauma being treated in Level 1 trauma centers, or their equivalent, whilst less severe trauma is often treated in community hospitals or by surgeons in private practice in the community. Thus few hospitals see the whole range of orthopedic trauma and as there is usually little com-munication between hospitals, it is often impossible to accurately analyze the incidence of fractures.

For this reason a number of different types of methodologies have been used to try to define fracture epidemiology in both adults and children. Table 3-2 shows the results of several analyses of fracture epidemiology in the United Kingdom,[23,31,32,56,85] Norway,[87] and the United States.[41] The difference in the results is striking! All the studies in Table 3-2 include both adults and children, but different methodologies have been used and this is likely to account for the wide variation in results.

Donaldson et al.,[31] in their early study, examined a geo-graphically well-defined population in England and looked at both the inpatient and outpatient fractures in the area. They observed that they might be missing some toe and spinal frac-tures, but they felt that they had missed relatively few fractures.

TABLE 3-2	Fracture Incidence Reported in Various Studies					
			Incidence (n/10⁵/yr)			
	Study Years	Country	Overall	Male	Female	
Donaldson et al.[31]	1980–1982	UK	9.1	10	8.1	
Johansen et al.[56]	1994–1995	UK	21.1	23.5	18.8	
Court-Brown and Caesar,[23] Rennie et al.[85]	2000	UK	12.6	13.6	11.6	
Donaldson et al.[32]	2002–2004	UK	36	41	31	
Sahlin[87]	1985–1986	Norway	22.8	22.9	21.3	
Fife and Barancik[41]	1977	USA	21	26	16	

To obtain the overall incidence in Scotland in 2000, the adult fractures reported by Court-Brown and Caesar[23] have been combined with the children's fractures reported by Rennie et al.[85]

A very similar methodology was employed by Court-Brown and Caesar[24] in the sixth edition of Rockwood and Green. They assessed all of the adult fractures treated in the Royal Infirmary of Edinburgh in 2000[23] from the same catchment area as in this study. The fractures admitted to the pediatric hospital in Edinburgh in the same year were also analyzed[83] and the incidence of fractures in the whole Edinburgh population is shown in Table 3-2. Given the 20-year gap between these two studies it would seem that both studies had very similar results.

Table 3-2 shows, however, that other studies have produced very different results. The studies by Johansen et al.[56] in Wales, Sahlin in Norway,[87] and Fife and Barancik[41] in the United States all record similar fracture incidences and it is interesting to observe that the diagnoses of the different fracture types were usually taken from the records of the local emergency departments. Many of these patients would not have been seen by an orthopedic surgeon and the diagnosis would have been made by an inexperienced junior doctor. This is in contrast to the Edinburgh study where all diagnoses were made by orthopedic trauma surgeons. In the United Kingdom much of the fracture data used in epidemiologic analysis is taken from the General Practice Research Database.[63,67] The diagnoses made by nonorthopedic surgeons, in the emergency departments of different hospitals, are relayed to local family physicians where they are recorded and then analyzed to produce epidemiologic information. This may lead to an incorrect estimation of the number of fractures in a community, particularly in those fractures that occur in areas where soft tissue injuries are relatively common such as the hand, wrist, ankle, and foot. An example of this problem is seen in the study by Johansen et al.[56] of fractures in the combined pediatric and adult population treated in South Wales in 1994. They stated that the overall incidence of fractures of the hand and foot, ankle and finger, thumb and hand were 2.41/1,000/year, 1.42/1,000/year, and 4.41/1,000/year, respectively. The combined pediatric and adult figures from Edinburgh in 2000 [24,85] for these fracture combinations were 1.3/1,000/year, 0.9/1,000/year, and 3/1,000/year carpal fractures, respectively suggesting that inexperienced doctors will overestimate the prevalence of fractures, many of which are seen on an outpatient basis. A good example of this is the "? scaphoid" soft tissue injury that is often documented as being a fracture.

The third type of methodology highlighted in Table 3-2 is that used by Donaldson et al.[32] in a later study. They asked patients to complete a questionnaire regarding whether they had had a fracture in a given time period. Table 3-2 shows that this methodology produces results that are about 300% greater than one would expect. If the incidences suggested in this study are applied to the United Kingdom population there would be about 2,200,000 fractures annually in the United Kingdom which is simply not the case. This problem is obviously methodologic as many patients will be told that recurrent or continuing pain may be secondary to undiagnosed fractures by family physicians, physiotherapists, nurses, osteopaths, or other paramedical professionals without there being any proof that this is the case.

Other methods have been employed to try to estimate fracture incidence. In countries with privatized medical systems insurance records have been used. These may be very large but they tend to present an unbalanced view of the population. Brinker and O'Connor[11] examined a large privately insured cohort of patients but the average age was 29 years for males and 28.7 years for females which is not representative of the population. However it explains why 57% of their population presented with fractures of the forearm, hand, and foot. In a cohort covering the whole population one would expect a figure of about 42% (Table 3-3). In a similar study Orces and Martinez[80] examined the incidence of wrist and forearm fractures in the United States. They looked at the records of a large number of emergency departments and concluded that the incidence of wrist and forearm fractures in males and females ≥50 years of age was 78.2/10⁵/year and 256.9/10⁵/year, respectively. It seems likely that these values should be much higher and ours are 154/10⁵/year and 642.6/10⁵/year. Clearly one must examine the whole population to get accurate figures. Bradley and Harrison[8] examined inpatients in Australia to provide fracture incidence figures but as about 55% to 60% of fractures are treated on an outpatient basis accurate figures cannot be obtained using this method.

TABLE 3-3	Epidemiology of Fractures Treated in a 1-Year Period						
	No.	%	n/10⁵/yr	Average Age (yrs)	≥65 yrs (%)	≥80 yrs (%)	M/F
Distal radius/ulna	1,221	17.5	235.9	58.4	41.8	18.1	28/72
Metacarpus	781	11.2	150.9	33.6	8.2	3.1	80/20
Proximal femur	753	10.8	145.5	80.7	90.6	63.7	27/73
Ankle	713	10.2	137.7	49	23.8	6	46/54
Finger phalanges	696	9.9	134.5	41.6	13.6	5.8	60/40
Proximal humerus	478	6.8	92.4	66.3	55.6	23	31/69
Metatarsus	465	6.6	89.8	44.6	17	5.2	37/63
Proximal forearm	378	5.4	73	45.6	17.2	5.8	46/54
Clavicle	257	3.7	49.7	44.5	21	9.7	70/30
Toe phalanges	248	3.5	47.9	35.7	3.9	1	59/41
Carpus	194	2.8	37.5	38	7.7	1.5	64/36
Pelvis	119	1.7	23	75.6	74.8	58.8	30/70
Femoral diaphysis	82	1.2	15.8	70.2	67.1	39	48/52
Humeral diaphysis	70	1	13.5	56.8	42.8	20	47/53
Tibial diaphysis	69	1	13.3	42.3	8.7	0	71/29
Calcaneus	65	0.9	12.6	41	9.2	3.1	74/26
Proximal tibia	59	0.8	11.4	54.5	30.5	11.9	52/48
Forearm diaphysis	55	0.8	10.6	48	27.3	16.4	69/31
Patella	49	0.7	9.5	64.8	55.1	28.6	41/59
Distal humerus	48	0.7	9.3	58.5	56.2	29.2	42/58
Distal tibia	42	0.6	8.2	41.7	17.7	4.4	67/33
Fibula	41	0.6	7.9	46.8	14.6	2.4	46/54
Scapula	37	0.5	7.1	54.8	32.4	16.2	76/24
Distal femur	36	0.5	7	67.3	52.8	38.9	17/83
Midfoot	28	0.4	5.4	39.4	7.1	0	61/39
Talus	12	0.2	2.3	30.1	0	0	83/17
	6,996	100	1,351.7	53.2	34	17.3	47/53

The numbers, prevalence, incidence, and gender ratios are shown together with the average ages and percentages of patients ≥65 yrs and ≥80 yrs of age.

The Incidence of Fractures in Adults

In this edition of Rockwood and Green a further year of inpatient and outpatient fractures presenting to the Royal Infirmary of Edinburgh has been prospectively analyzed. In the sixth edition[24] all fractures presenting to the hospital in 2000 were analyzed. In the seventh edition[26] a year of fractures between July 2007 and June 2008 was analyzed. In this edition a further year of fractures between September 2010 and August 2011 has been analyzed. The analysis has been confined to patients aged 16 years or older and the 2001 Scottish census[44] has been used to calculate fracture incidence, this being the last census that was undertaken. During this year soft tissue injuries and dislocations were not studied prospectively, but the chapter includes a retrospective analysis of dislocations which presented to the Trauma Unit in a 1-year period in 2008/9.

During the study all fractures were analyzed, including 104 spinal fractures that presented to the Orthopaedic Trauma Unit, but these spinal fractures have not been included in the epidemiology tables as in Edinburgh spinal fractures are also treated by neurosurgeons with spinal cord injuries being treated in the National Spinal Injuries Centre in Glasgow. However, spinal fractures have been included where they occurred in association with other fractures. All patients resident in and injured in the defined catchment area have been included as have those injured elsewhere but resident in our area. Patients resident outwith the area have not been included in the analysis. In this analysis the effect of gender, age, and social deprivation on fracture epidemiology has been studied and because of this fractures in males and females, and in the age ranges 16 to 35 years, 36 to 64 years, and ≥65 years, will be presented separately. Fractures in the very elderly will be discussed in Chapter 20.

The overall epidemiology of the fractures that presented during the year is shown in Table 3-3. It shows that there were 6,996 fractures during the year, giving an overall incidence of 1,351.7/10⁵/year. The average age was 53.2 years and 53% of

TABLE 3-4 **Epidemiology of Fractures in Males**

	No.	%	n/10^5/yr	Age (yrs)	≥65 yrs (%)	≥80 yrs (%)	Multiple Fractures (%)	Open Fractures (%)
Metacarpus	624	19	255.6	30.3	4	1.8	9.2	0.6
Finger phalanges	418	12.7	171.2	37.6	7.9	3.1	6.2	8.5
Distal radius/ulna	340	10.4	139.3	44.2	15.9	5.3	6.2	0.6
Ankle	330	10	135.2	42.4	14.2	3	3	0.3
Proximal femur	205	6.2	84	78.5	87.8	54.6	4.4	0
Clavicle	180	5.5	73.7	38.2	10.6	3.3	6.1	0
Proximal forearm	175	5.3	71.7	39.6	8.6	2.9	11	2.3
Metatarsus	170	5.2	69.6	36.6	6.5	1.8	8.2	0
Proximal humerus	149	4.5	61	59.7	39.6	16.8	9.4	0
Toe phalanges	146	4.4	59.8	37.1	1.4	0.7	5.5	8.2
Carpus	125	3.8	51.2	32.9	4.8	0.8	6.4	0
Tibial diaphysis	49	1.5	20	41.6	10.2	0	6.1	24.5
Calcaneus	48	1.5	19.7	37.5	4.2	0	32.6	6.2
Femoral diaphysis	39	1.2	16	63.9	51.3	30.8	18.9	5.1
Forearm diaphysis	38	1.1	15.6	40.3	10.5	7.9	7.9	7.9
Pelvis	36	1.1	14.7	65.2	55.5	36.1	22.2	2.8
Humeral diaphysis	33	1	13.5	51.5	30.3	18.2	3	0
Proximal tibia	31	0.9	12.7	49	25.8	9.7	12.9	3.2
Scapula	28	0.9	11.5	48.5	17.9	0	44.4	0
Distal tibia	28	0.9	11.5	35.2	7.1	0	29.6	17.9
Distal humerus	20	0.6	8.2	46.1	30	20	35	15
Patella	20	0.6	8.2	52.4	30	30	10	10
Fibula	19	0.6	7.8	38.3	15.8	15.8	0	0
Midfoot	17	0.5	7	36.5	0	0	30.8	5.9
Talus	10	0.3	4.1	28.5	0	0	40	10
Distal femur	6	0.2	2.5	55.3	50	50	0	0
	3,284	100	1,345.3	42.4	17.1	7.9	5.6	2.8

The numbers, prevalence, incidence, and gender ratios are shown together with the average ages and percentages of patients ≥65 yrs and ≥80 yrs of age. The prevalence of open fractures is also shown.

the fractures occurred in females. Overall 34% of the fractures occurred in patients ≥65 years of age and 17.3% in patients ≥80 years of age.

Gender and Age

The importance of gender and age to fracture epidemiology has been understood for many years. In their classic epidemiologic study Buhr and Cooke[13] highlighted the fact that men have a bimodal distribution of fractures and women have a unimodal distribution with a significant progressive increase in fracture incidence in the postmenopausal years. This is demonstrated in the overall fracture distribution curves shown in Figure 3-1. Analysis of the Edinburgh data shows that males between 16 and 19 years of age have a fracture incidence of 2,506.4/10^5/year which falls to 937.4/10^5/year in males aged between 50 and 59 years and then rises to 6,860.5/10^5/year in males

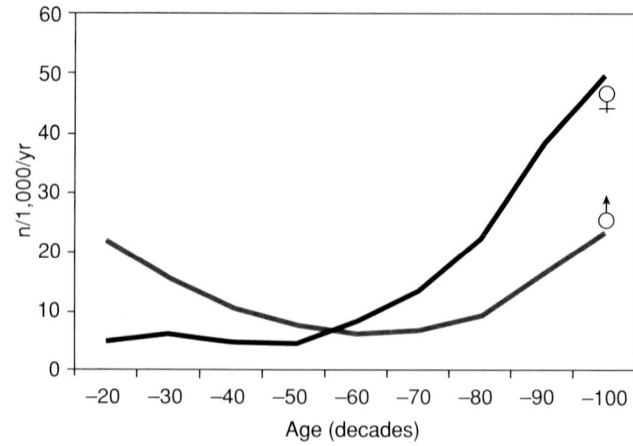

FIGURE 3-1 The overall age and gender fracture distribution curves.

aged 90 years or more. In females the equivalent values are 792.1/10^5/year, 1,398.5/10^5/year, and 7,769.8/10^5/year. This illustrates the considerable difference in the incidence of fractures between males and females.

The difference in fracture epidemiology between males and females is further highlighted by comparing Tables 3-4 and 3-5. Basic epidemiologic data for males is shown in Table 3-4 and for females in Table 3-5. In males the average age is 42.4 years and only 17.1% of fractures occurred in males ≥65 years of age. Fractures of the metacarpus, finger phalanges, distal radius, and ulna and ankles comprised 52.1% of all male fractures. In females the average age is 61.8 years and 48.8% of fractures occurred in patients ≥65 years of age. The obvious tendency for fragility fractures to be much more common in females is highlighted in Table 3-5 which shows that fractures of the distal radius and ulna and proximal femur make up

38.5% of all female fractures and if one includes ankle fractures and proximal humeral fractures the most common four fractures in females account for 57.7% of all fractures.

Tables 3-4 and 3-5 also contain an analysis of the prevalence of patients who presented with multiple fractures or with open fractures. Table 3-4 shows that 5.6% of male patients presented with multiple fractures. These will be discussed in more detail in the sections on individual fractures, but Table 3-4 shows that more than 20% of males who presented with fractures of the calcaneus, pelvis, scapula, distal tibia, distal humerus, midfoot, and talus had multiple fractures. Table 3-4 shows that at least 10% of fractures of the tibial diaphysis, distal tibia, distal humerus, patella, and talus in males were open. In females 4.4% of patients had multiple fractures (Table 3-5) but it was only in fractures of the scapula, midfoot, and talus that more than 20% of patients had multiple fractures. There were fewer

TABLE 3-5 Epidemiology of Fractures in Females

	No.	%	n/10^5/yr	Age (yrs)	≥65 yrs (%)	≥80 yrs (%)	Multiple Fractures (%)	Open Fractures (%)
Distal radius/ulna	881	23.7	322.2	63.9	51.8	23	5.6	0.9
Proximal femur	548	14.8	200.4	81.6	91.8	67	6.2	0
Ankle	383	10.3	140.1	54.7	32.1	8.6	2.9	1.6
Proximal humerus	329	8.9	120.3	69.3	63.2	26.1	7.6	0
Metatarsus	295	7.9	107.9	49.1	23.1	7.1	12.9	0
Finger phalanges	278	7.5	101.7	47.6	20.5	9.3	7.9	4.9
Proximal forearm	203	5.5	74.2	51.1	24.6	8.4	7.9	1.5
Metacarpus	157	4.2	57.4	46.8	24.8	8.3	9.4	1.3
Toe phalanges	102	2.7	37.3	33.6	2	0	3.9	4.9
Pelvis	83	2.2	30.4	79.8	83.1	68.7	12	0
Clavicle	77	2.1	28.2	79.8	45.5	24.7	3.9	1.3
Carpus	69	1.9	25.2	47.1	13	2.9	7.2	0
Femoral diaphysis	43	1.2	15.7	76	81.4	46.5	4.7	0
Humeral diaphysis	37	1	13.5	61.6	54.1	21.6	0	2.7
Distal femur	30	0.8	11	69.6	53.3	36.7	13.3	3.3
Patella	29	0.8	10.6	73.4	72.4	37.9	0	3.4
Proximal tibia	28	0.8	10.2	60.6	35.7	14.3	14.3	0
Distal humerus	28	0.8	10.2	67.4	75	35.7	10.7	0
Fibula	22	0.6	8	54.8	13.6	4.5	13.6	0
Tibial diaphysis	20	0.5	7.3	44.1	5	0	5	10
Calcaneus	17	0.5	6.2	51	23.5	11.8	11.8	0
Forearm diaphysis	17	0.5	6.2	65.1	64.7	35.3	5.9	0
Distal tibia	14	0.4	5.1	54.7	42.9	14.3	7.1	7.1
Midfoot	11	0.3	4	43.9	18.2	0	27.3	0
Scapula	9	0.2	3.3	74.5	77.8	66.6	22.2	0
Talus	2	0.05	0.7	37.5	0	0	50	0
	3,712	100	1,357.5	61.8	48.8	25.4	4.4	1.2

The numbers, prevalence, incidence, and gender ratios are shown together with the average ages and percentages of patients ≥65 yrs and ≥80 yrs of age. The prevalence of open fractures is also shown.

TABLE 3-6	Epidemiology of Fractures in Males Aged 16 to 35 Years					
	No.	%	n/10⁵/yr	Multiple Fractures (%)	Open Fractures (%)	Causes
Metacarpus	470	29.1	517.7	7.9	0.4	71.4% db/assault, 12.8% sport
Finger phalanges	237	14.7	261.2	5.5	6.3	44.7% sport, 35.9% db/assault
Distal radius/ulna	141	8.7	155.3	5	0	45.4% sport, 29.1% falls
Ankle	139	8.6	153.1	2.2	0.7	52.5% falls, 33.1% sport
Metatarsus	100	6.2	110.1	5.4	0	48% falls, 27.8% sport
Clavicle	98	6.1	107.9	3.1	0	51% sport, 23.5% falls
Proximal forearm	90	5.6	99.1	10.2	4.4	32.2% falls, 30% sport
Carpus	87	5.4	95.8	4.6	0	35.6% sport, 33.3% falls
Toe phalanges	78	4.8	85.9	0	11.5	50% db/assault, 40.6% sport
Calcaneus	26	1.6	28.6	39.1	7.7	76.9% fall height, 11.5% low falls
Tibial diaphysis	21	1.3	23.1	0	14.2	57.1% sport, 19% falls
Forearm diaphysis	19	1.2	20.9	0	0	57.9% sport, 15.8% db/assault
Proximal humerus	15	0.9	16.5	0	0	26.6% sport, 26.6% falls
Distal tibia	15	0.9	16.5	33.3	13.3	60% fall height, 13.3% MVA
Fibula	11	0.7	12.1	0	0	63.6% sport, 9.1% MVA
Humeral diaphysis	11	0.7	12.1	0	0	36.4% falls, 36.4% db/assault
Distal humerus	9	0.6	9.9	22.2	11.1	33.3% MVA, 22.2% sport
Proximal tibia	9	0.6	9.9	0	0	6.6% sport, 22.2% low falls
Talus	9	0.6	9.9	44.4	11.1	33.3% fall height, 33.3% sport
Midfoot	6	0.4	6.6	20	0	50% sport, 33.3% fall height
Femoral diaphysis	5	0.3	5.5	40	0	60% fall height, 20% MVA
Scapula	5	0.3	5.5	40	0	60% MVA, 20% fall height
Pelvis	4	0.2	4.4	50	0	50% fall height, 25% MVA
Patella	3	0.2	3.3	0	33.3	66.6% MVA, 33.3% sport
Proximal femur	3	0.2	3.3	33.3	0	33.3% MVA, 33.3% sport
Distal femur	2	0.1	2.2	0	0	50% sport, 50% MVA
	1,613	100	1,776.7	4.9	2.2	32.9% db/assault, 30.3% sport

The numbers, prevalence, and incidence of the different fractures are shown as are the prevalence of open fractures and patients with multiple fractures. The two commonest causes of each fracture are shown. (db = direct blow).

open fractures in females and only in fractures of the tibial diaphysis did 10% of patients present with open fractures.

The importance of age in the epidemiology of fractures in males is illustrated in Tables 3-6–3-8. Table 3-6 shows the fracture epidemiology for males aged 16 to 35 years with Table 3-7 dealing with males of 36 to 64 years and Table 3-8 with males aged ≥65 years. In addition to the numbers, prevalence, and incidence of each fracture the percentage of open fractures and patients with multiple fractures is also shown. Each table also gives the commonest two causes of each fracture.

Tables 3-6–3-8 show that age has a significant effect on fractures in males. Between 16 and 35 years of age fractures of the metacarpus and finger phalanges account for 43.8% of all male fractures and if one includes distal radius and ulna fractures and ankle fractures it can be seen that these four fractures comprise over 60% of all fractures in males aged 16 to 35 years.

Some of the high-energy fractures that are commonly associated with young males such as those of the femoral diaphysis, distal tibia, and hindfoot are in fact relatively uncommon, but when they do occur are associated with a high prevalence of open fractures and multiple fractures. The relatively low incidence of femoral diaphyseal fractures shown in Table 3-6 may be a surprise to some surgeons, but in recent years it has become clear that the femoral diaphyseal fracture is essentially a fragility fracture occurring mainly in older females. This is shown in Table 3-11.

As Figure 3-1 shows middle-aged males have a lower incidence of fractures and Tables 3-6–3-8 show that the incidence drops from 1,776.7/10⁵/year in the 16- to 35-year-old group to 977.5/10⁵/year in the 36- to 64-year-old group. They show that the incidence of metacarpal and finger phalangeal fractures falls markedly and there is also a slight drop in the incidence of

TABLE 3-7 **Epidemiology of Fractures in Males Aged 36 to 64 Years**

	No.	%	n/10^5/yr	Multiple Fractures (%)	Open Fractures (%)	Causes
Finger phalanges	146	13	127.3	5.8	14.1	47.4% db/assault, 21.5% falls
Distal radius/ulna	145	12.9	126.4	6.9	1.4	55.2% falls, 20% sport
Ankle	144	12.8	125.6	3.5	0	81.3% falls, 9.7% sport
Metacarpus	129	11.5	112.5	10.2	1.6	48.1% db/assault, 27.9% falls
Proximal humerus	75	6.7	65.4	8	0	65.3% falls, 10.7% sport
Proximal forearm	70	6.2	61	10.1	0	45.7% falls, 22.8% MVA
Clavicle	63	5.6	54.9	9.5	0	41.2% MVA, 33.3% falls
Toe phalanges	63	5.6	54.9	15.4	11.1	73.1% db/assault, 11.5% falls
Metatarsus	59	5.3	51.4	12.7	0	55.9% falls, 13.6% MVA
Carpus	32	2.8	27.9	12.5	0	62.5% falls, 12.5% MVA
Tibial diaphysis	23	2.1	20.1	8.7	30.4	52.2% falls, 17.4% MVA
Proximal femur	22	2	19.2	4.5	0	68.2% falls, 18.2% sport
Calcaneus	20	1.8	17.4	22.2	5	55% fall height, 25% low falls
Scapula	18	1.6	15.7	52.9	0	33.3% MVA, 22.2% falls
Forearm diaphysis	15	1.3	13.1	20	20	53.3% falls, 20% MVA
Femoral diaphysis	14	1.2	12.2	30.8	14.3	42.9% MVA, 28.6% falls
Proximal tibia	14	1.2	12.2	7.1	0	35.7% sport, 21.4% MVA
Pelvis	12	1.1	10.5	33.3	8.3	33.3% MVA, 33.3% falls
Humeral diaphysis	12	1.1	10.5	0	0	41.7% falls, 25% db/assault
Patella	11	1	9.6	18.2	9.1	45.5% falls, 27.3% MVA
Midfoot	11	1	9.6	37.5	9.1	45.5% fall height, 27.3% falls
Distal tibia	11	1	9.6	27.3	27.3	27.2% MVA, 27.2% falls
Distal humerus	5	0.4	4.4	60	40	40% falls, 40% MVA
Fibula	5	0.4	4.4	0	0	20% sport, 20% falls
Talus	1	0.09	0.9	0	0	100% fall height
Distal femur	1	0.09	0.9	0	0	100% falls
	1,121	100	977.5	6.2	4.7	45.5% falls, 17.1% db/assault

The numbers, prevalence, and incidence of the different fractures are shown as are the prevalence of open fractures and patients with multiple fractures. The two commonest causes of each fracture are shown. (db = direct blow).

fractures of the distal radius and ulna and ankle. The only fractures to show an increased incidence in middle-aged males are those of the proximal humerus, scapula, proximal femur, and femoral diaphysis. Much of the literature suggests that scapular fractures are simply high-energy injuries associated with motor vehicle accidents,[20] but Tables 3-7 and 3-8 show that this is not the case. Hindfoot fractures and fractures of the distal tibia decline in incidence in middle-aged males.

Despite the lowered incidence of male fractures in middle age, Table 3-7 shows that there is a higher prevalence of open fractures and more patients present with multiple fractures. Unsurprisingly the fractures that are associated with a high prevalence of open fractures and multiple fractures tend to be high-energy injuries. A high prevalence of open fractures is seen in fractures of the tibial diaphysis, forearm diaphyses, femoral diaphysis, distal tibia, and distal humerus. The fracture

associated with the highest prevalence of multiple fractures in middle-aged males is the scapula fracture, although fractures of the calcaneus, forearm diaphyses, femoral diaphysis, pelvis, patella, distal tibia, and distal humerus are associated with multiple fractures in at least 20% of middle-aged male patients.

Table 3-8 shows that there is a considerable change in the epidemiology of fractures in older males. Fractures of the metacarpus and finger phalanges are much less common and fractures of the proximal femur, proximal humerus, distal radius, and ulna and ankle account for over 60% of all the fractures in this age group. Fractures of the femoral diaphysis show a higher incidence, although none were associated with a high-energy injury. Pelvic fractures, humeral diaphyseal fractures, and patellar fractures are more commonly seen than fractures of the tibial diaphysis and hindfoot which are relatively rare. Overall the fracture incidence rises to 1,423.2/10^5/year

TABLE 3-8 Epidemiology of Fractures in Males Aged ≥65 Years

	No.	%	n/10⁵/yr	Multiple Fractures (%)	Open Fractures (%)	Causes
Proximal femur	180	32.7	465.8	3.9	0	92.2% falls, 3.9% low falls
Proximal humerus	59	10.7	152.7	13.6	0	94.9% falls, 1.7% low falls
Distal radius/ulna	54	9.8	139.7	9.3	0	94.4% falls, 3.7% MVA
Ankle	47	8.5	121.6	4.3	0	83% falls, 6.4% sport
Finger phalanges	35	6.4	90.6	13.8	3.1	59.4% falls, 18.7% db/assault
Metacarpus	25	4.5	64.7	41.2	0	72% falls, 12% sport
Pelvis	20	3.6	51.8	10	0	90% falls, 10% MVA
Femoral diaphysis	20	3.6	51.8	5	0	80% falls, 15% pathologic
Clavicle	19	3.5	49.2	10.5	0	63.2% falls, 10.5% MVA
Proximal forearm	15	2.7	38.8	20	0	80% falls, 6.6% MVA
Metatarsus	11	2	28.5	18.2	0	63.6% falls, 18.2% db/assault
Humeral diaphysis	10	1.8	25.9	10	0	100% falls
Proximal tibia	8	1.5	20.7	37.5	12.5	50% falls, 12.5% fall height
Distal humerus	6	1.1	15.5	33.3	0	66.6% falls, 16.7% fall height
Carpus	6	1.1	15.5	0	0	100% falls
Patella	6	1.1	15.5	0	0	83.3% falls, 16.6% low falls
Scapula	5	0.9	12.9	20	0	40% falls, 20% fall height
Toe phalanges	5	0.9	12.9	0	0	80% db/assault, 20% falls
Tibial diaphysis	5	0.9	12.9	20	40	60% falls, 40% MVA
Forearm diaphysis	4	0.7	10.4	0	0	75% falls, 25% sport
Fibula	3	0.5	7.8	0	0	33.3% falls, 33.3% db/assault
Distal femur	3	0.5	7.8	0	0	100% falls
Calcaneus	2	0.4	5.2	50	0	50% fall height, 50% low falls
Distal tibia	2	0.4	5.2	0	0	100% falls
Midfoot	0	0	0	0	0	
Talus	0	0	0	0	0	
	550	100	1,423.2	5.7	0.7	83.8% falls, 4% MVA

The numbers, prevalence, and incidence of the different fractures are shown as are the prevalence of open fractures and patients with multiple fractures. The two commonest causes of each fracture are shown. (db = direct blow).

which is in 16- to 35-year-old males. However, the incidence continues to rise with increasing age and in the 80+ male population the fracture incidence is 3,302.7/10⁵/year. The prevalence of open fractures is very low in this age group, although it is important to note that 5.7% of patients still presented with multiple fractures. This is related to osteoporosis in this elderly population.

A review of the causes of fractures in adult males shows that in younger males (Table 3-6) direct blows, assaults, and sports injuries account for almost two-thirds of all fractures although in 12 (46.1%) fracture types, motor vehicle accidents or falls from a height were one of the two main causes of fracture. In middle-aged males (Table 3-7) almost half the fractures were caused by falls from a standing height, although 17% were still caused by a direct blow or assault. Fifteen (57.6%) of the fracture types had a motor vehicle

accident or a fall from a height as one of the commonest causes. In older males (Table 3-8) 83.8% of fractures were caused by falls from a standing height, but it is interesting to note that motor vehicle accidents were still the second commonest cause of fracture.

Tables 3-9–3-11 illustrate the different fracture epidemiology in females of different ages. Table 3-9 shows that the overall incidence of fractures in females aged 16 to 35 years is 664.4/10⁵/year, this being 37% of the incidence in equivalently aged males. However, finger phalangeal fractures remain common in young females, although the incidence of metacarpal fractures is only 13% of that seen in males. Fractures of the finger phalanges, distal radius and ulna, metatarsus and toe phalanges comprise 56.1% of all fractures seen in young females. The prevalence of open fractures is very similar to that seen in young males, but only in tibial diaphyseal fractures were more

TABLE 3-9	Epidemiology of Fractures in Females Aged 16 to 35 Years					
	No.	%	n/10⁵/yr	Multiple Fractures (%)	Open Fractures (%)	Causes
Finger phalanges	97	15.5	102.8	3.5	5.4	37.8% db/assault, 34.1% falls
Distal radius/ulna	94	15	99.6	3.2	1.1	72.3% falls, 9.6% sport
Metatarsus	91	14.5	96.4	12.2	0	67% falls, 12.1% db/assault
Toe phalanges	70	11.1	74.1	0	5.7	55.2% db/assault, 40.9% falls
Ankle	69	11	73.1	1.4	1.4	78.3% falls, 15.9% sport
Metacarpus	65	10.3	68.9	1.5	1.5	50.8% db/assault, 26.2% falls
Proximal forearm	53	8.4	56.2	1.9	0	79.2% falls, 10.2% sports
Carpus	19	3	20.1	0	0	84.2% falls, 5.3% sport
Clavicle	17	2.7	18	5.9	0	29.4% MVA, 29.4% falls
Proximal humerus	10	1.6	10.6	0	0	60% falls, 20% sport
Tibial diaphysis	7	1.1	7.4	14.3	14.3	57.1% falls, 28.6% sport
Humeral diaphysis	6	1	6.4	0	0	66.6% falls, 16.6% sport
Midfoot	5	0.8	5.3	25	0	80% falls, 20% sport
Distal humerus	4	0.6	4.2	0	0	75% falls, 2050% stairs/low fall
Calcaneus	4	0.6	4.2	25	0	75% fall height, 25% sport
Forearm diaphysis	4	0.6	4.2	0	0	75% falls, 25% stairs/low falls
Distal tibia	3	0.5	3.2	33.3	0	66.7% fall height, 33.3 falls
Pelvis	2	0.3	2.1	50	0	50% MVA, 50% sport
Proximal tibia	2	0.3	2.1	50	0	50% fall height, 50% falls
Femoral diaphysis	1	0.2	1.1	100	0	100% fall height
Patella	1	0.2	1.1	0	0	100% falls
Fibula	1	0.2	1.1	100	0	100% fall height
Distal femur	1	0.2	1.1	0	0	100% fall height
Talus	1	0.2	1.1	0	0	100% sport
Proximal femur	0	0	0	0	0	
Scapula	0	0	0	0	0	
	627	100	664.4	3.8	2.1	56.2% falls, 18.6% db/assault

The numbers, prevalence, and incidence of the different fractures are shown as are the prevalence of open fractures and patients with multiple fractures. The two commonest causes of each fracture are shown. (db = direct blow).

than 10% of the fractures open. Only 3.8% of the young female patient group presented with multiple fractures, although the spectrum of multiple fractures was not dissimilar to that seen in young males (Table 3-6).

In middle-aged females (Table 3-10) the incidence of fractures is slightly higher than that seen in equivalently aged males (Table 3-7). The incidence of fractures in this age group is 162% higher than in the younger female age group, but the incidence of fractures of the distal radius and ulna rises by 275% and the incidence of ankle fractures by 216%. As with the younger female age group, most fractures are low-energy injuries and there is a very low prevalence of open fractures in middle-aged females, although the prevalence of multiple fractures is the same as seen in younger females.

In females aged ≥65 years (Table 3-11) the incidence of fractures rises by a further 284% to 3,063.3/10⁵/year. Fractures of

the proximal femur, distal radius and ulna, proximal humerus, and ankle account for 72.4% of all the fractures and the incidence of pelvic fractures increases by 1,200% compared with middle-aged females. It is interesting to monitor the increasing incidence of fragility fractures between Tables 3-9 and 3-10. The incidence of established fragility fractures of the distal radius and ulna, proximal femur, and proximal humerus rises very quickly, but the increased incidence of fractures of the humerus diaphysis, distal humerus, proximal forearm, femoral diaphysis, distal femur, patella, ankle, and pelvis should also be noted.

Predictably 94.3% of fractures in older females are caused by falls from a standing height with only 2.8% of fractures in this group of patients being caused by mechanisms other than a standing fall or a fall from a low height. The prevalence of female fractures caused by standing falls rises by approximately 20% in each age group shown in Tables 3-9–3-11.

TABLE 3-10 Epidemiology of Fractures in Females Aged 36 to 64 Years

	No.	%	n/10^5/yr	Multiple Fractures (%)	Open Fractures (%)	Causes
Distal radius/ulna	331	25.4	273.7	4.3	0	89.7% falls, 3.9% sport
Ankle	191	14.6	157.9	1.6	1	88.5% falls, 5.8% low falls
Metatarsus	136	10.4	112.5	9.9	0	89.7% falls, 4.4% db/assault
Finger phalanges	122	9.4	100.9	6.7	4.5	41% falls, 39.3% db/assault
Proximal humerus	111	8.5	91.8	5.4	0	88.3% falls, 5.4% low falls
Proximal forearm	100	7.7	82.7	7.1	1	80% falls, 12% MVA
Metacarpus	53	4.1	43.8	12.2	0	45.3% falls, 39.6% db/assault
Proximal femur	45	3.5	37.2	6.7	0	77.8% falls 8.9% pathologic
Carpus	41	3.1	33.9	9.8	0	87.8% falls, 4.9% sport
Toe phalanges	27	2.1	22.3	20	6.1	85.2% db/assault, 14.8% falls
Clavicle	25	1.9	20.7	0	3.7	44% falls, 32% MVA
Fibula	18	1.4	14.9	0	0	77.7% falls, 11.1% MVA
Proximal tibia	16	1.2	13.2	6.2	0	37.5% falls, 18.7% sport
Distal femur	13	1	10.7	18.2	0	100% falls
Pelvis	12	0.9	9.9	25	0	75% falls, 16.6% MVA
Tibial diaphysis	12	0.9	9.9	0	0	66.6% falls, 8.3% MVA
Humeral diaphysis	11	0.8	9.1	0	0	90.9% falls, 9.1% low falls
Calcaneus	9	0.7	9.1	0	0	44.4% falls, 22.2% fall height
Femoral diaphysis	7	0.5	5.8	0	0	85.7% falls, 14.2% sport
Patella	7	0.5	5.8	0	0	85.7% falls, 14.2% low falls
Distal tibia	5	0.4	4.1	0	0	80% falls, 20% fall height
Midfoot	4	0.3	3.3	50	0	50% falls, 25% low falls
Distal humerus	3	0.2	2.5	0	0	100% falls
Forearm diaphysis	2	0.2	1.7	0	0	50% sport, 50% low falls
Scapula	2	0.2	1.7	50	0	50% falls, 50% fall height
Talus	1	0.1	0.8	100	0	100% falls
	1,304	100	1,078.3	3.9	0.8	78.7% falls, 9% falls

The numbers, prevalence, and incidence of the different fractures are shown as are the prevalence of open fractures and patients with multiple fractures. The two commonest causes of each fracture are shown. (db = direct blow).

Social Deprivation

The other factor that undoubtedly affects the incidence of fractures is social deprivation. There is good evidence in the orthopedic literature that social deprivation correlates with musculoskeletal pain,[99] high-energy lower limb trauma,[69] Perthes disease,[83] and outcome after hip arthroplasty.[55] There is also evidence that social deprivation is associated with fractures in children,[10,91,93] adolescents,[75] and young adult males.[72] In adults it has been shown to be implicated in fractures of the tibial diaphysis[25] and hand,[52] but it has become clear that social deprivation is an important factor in determining the incidence of many fractures in adults.[27,29,76]

A study of the effect of social deprivation on the incidence of fractures was undertaken using the fractures treated in Edinburgh between July 2007 and June 2008[29] and analyzed in the seventh edition of Rockwood and Green.[26] In Scotland social deprivation is analyzed using the Carstairs score,[15] this being a Z-score created from each postcode which is based on overcrowding, male unemployment, household status, and car ownership. The Carstairs score has been successfully used for the analysis of deprivation in many branches of medicine including orthopedic surgery.[3,33,38,51] Using the Carstairs score the population can be divided into deciles with decile 1 being the most affluent and decile 10 the least affluent. Decile 10 contains the least affluent 10% of the population. Figure 3-2A shows the distribution of the population of the catchment area of the Royal Infirmary of Edinburgh according to the social deciles and Figure 3-2B shows the incidence of fractures within the different deciles in both males and females. It can be seen that there is a significant difference between the distribution of the population and their fractures. Statistical analysis shows that there is no significant difference in the incidence of fractures in either males

TABLE 3-11	Epidemiology of Fractures in Females Aged ≥65 Years					
	No.	%	n/10^5/yr	Multiple Fractures (%)	Open Fractures (%)	Causes
Proximal femur	503	28.2	865.2	6.2	0	96.8% falls, 1.8% low falls
Distal radius/ulna	456	25.6	784.3	7.1	1.5	95.6% falls, 2.9% low falls
Proximal humerus	208	11.7	357.8	9.2	0	93.8% falls, 5.3% low falls
Ankle	123	6.9	211.6	5.7	2.4	95.1% falls, 2.4% low falls
Pelvis	69	3.9	118.7	8.7	0	97.1% falls, 2.9% low falls
Metatarsus	68	3.8	117	20	0	91.2% falls, 4.4% low falls
Finger phalanges	59	3.3	101.5	18	3.6	72.9% falls, 15.3% db/assault
Proximal forearm	50	2.8	86	16	4	94% falls, 4% MVA
Metacarpus	39	2.2	67.1	17.6	2.6	92.3% falls, 2.4% low falls
Clavicle	35	2	60.2	5.7	0	91.4% falls, 5.7% MVA
Femoral diaphysis	35	2	60.2	2.9	0	88.6% falls, 5.7% pathologic
Distal humerus	21	1.2	36.1	14.3	0	100% falls
Patella	21	1.2	36.1	0	4.8	95.2% falls, 4.8% db/assault
Humeral diaphysis	20	1.1	34.4	0	5	85% falls, 10% pathologic
Distal femur	16	0.9	27.5	12.5	6.2	81.2% falls, 12.5% low falls
Forearm diaphysis	11	0.6	18.9	9.1	0	90.9% falls, 9.1% pathologic
Proximal tibia	10	0.6	17.2	20	0	70% falls, 20% low falls
Carpus	9	0.5	15.5	11.1	0	88.9% falls, 11.1% db/assault
Scapula	7	0.4	12	14.3	0	100% falls
Distal tibia	6	0.3	10.3	0	0	83.3% falls, 16.6% low falls
Toe phalanges	5	0.3	8.6	0	0	80% falls, 20% db/assault
Calcaneus	4	0.2	6.9	25	0	100% falls
Fibula	3	0.2	5.2	63.3	0	66.6% falls, 33.3% MVA
Midfoot	2	0.1	3.4	0	0	50% fall height, 50% sport
Tibial diaphysis	1	0.06	1.7	0	100	100% falls
Talus	0	0	0	0	0	
	1,781	100	3,063.3	5	1.2	94.3% falls, 2.9% low falls

The numbers, prevalence, and incidence of the different fractures are shown as are the prevalence of open fractures and patients with multiple fractures. The two commonest causes of each fracture are shown. (db = direct blow).

or females between deciles 1 and 8, but there is a significant difference in deciles 9 and 10 and it is clear that the effect of deprivation on fracture incidence is seen in the most deprived 10% of the population.

Table 3-12 shows the incidence of fractures when deprivation is taken into account. Once the figures are adjusted for age it can be seen that in males the overall incidence of fractures in the very socially deprived is about 4 times that of the rest of the population and in females the equivalent figure is about 3.5. The difference in incidences is statistically significant for both genders. Table 3-12 also shows which individual fractures show correlation between fracture incidence and significant deprivation.

The commonest fracture types in deprived males are those of the metacarpal, distal radius, and ulna and finger phalanges which constitute 55% of all fractures in the deprived population. This compares with 43% of the more affluent population.

Table 3-12 shows that the incidence of hand fractures is significantly higher in the deprived group than in the less deprived group, but it is salutary to note that while fractures of the hand and carpus constitute 35% of the more deprived group, they still constitute 30% of the less deprived population. Presumably testosterone and alcohol are an issue in all sectors of the male population!

It should be noted that proximal femoral fractures in males are only the sixth most common fracture in the socially deprived and are in fact less common than clavicle fractures. Further analysis shows that 15.3% of the most affluent male population in Edinburgh presented with proximal femoral fractures compared with only 8.6% of the least affluent. Analysis also shows that deprived patients present at a younger age and have a shorter life expectancy. It would seem that even in an affluent city such at Edinburgh, that many of the older socially deprived males do not live long enough to have a proximal femoral fracture.[27]

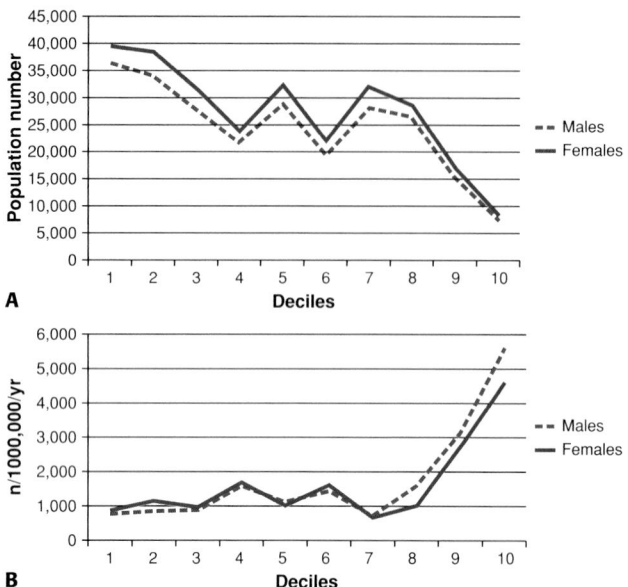

A

B

FIGURE 3-2 The population numbers in the different social deciles in the Edinburgh catchment area **(A)** and the fracture numbers in the same area **(B)**.

| TABLE 3-12 | The Effect of Social Deprivation on the Incidence of Fractures |

	Fracture Incidence (n/10^5/yr)			
	Males (1–8)	Males (9–10)	Females (1–8)	Females (9–10)
Distal radius/ulna	120.7	475.3	254.3	749.8[a]
Metacarpus	188.1	748.8[a]	44.1	153.1[a]
Proximal femur	80.8	219.7[a]	194.7	451.4[a]
Ankle	105.5	327.3[a]	103.3	345.5[a]
Finger phalanges	159.6	457.3[a]	78	219.8[a]
Proximal humerus	54.6	197.3	106.9	341.5[a]
Metatarsus	61.3	139[a]	78.8	251.2[a]
Proximal forearm	58	206.3[a]	58.4	172.7[a]
Clavicle	71.3	228.7[a]	24.5	78.5[a]
Toe phalanges	23.8	94.2[a]	18.8	47.1[a]
Carpus	48.5	179.3[a]	16.7	78.5[a]
Pelvis	18.5	58.3[a]	22.9	82.4
Femoral diaphysis	14.7	35.8[a]	13.9	66.7
Humeral diaphysis	11.9	44.8[a]	10.2	31.4
Tibial diaphysis	21.8	67.3[a]	5.7	7.8
Calcaneus	13.3	62.8[a]	4.1	7.8
Proximal tibia	8.1	89.7[a]	13.9	39.3[a]
Forearm diaphyses	20	62.8[a]	4.9	15.7
Patella	6.2	22.4	11	39.3
Distal humerus	4.3	40.4[a]	11.4	19.6
Distal tibia	12.8	35.9	6.5	11.8
Scapula	6.2	44.8[a]	8.6	31.4[a]
Distal femur	5.7	9[a]	7.3	31.4[a]
Midfoot	4.3	35.9	5.3	27.5[a]
Talus	7.6	17.9	4.1	7.8
	1,078	3,918.9[a]	1,096.9	3,317.1[a]

The population has been divided into deciles 1–8 and deciles 9–10 (see text).
[a]Fractures where there is statistical correlation between fracture incidence and social deprivation.

In females the incidence of distal radius and ulna fractures and proximal femoral fractures rose by 295% and 232%, respectively in the very deprived and Table 3-12 shows a similar increase in other fractures. The biggest increase in incidence in female fractures is in fact in the femoral diaphyseal fracture where there was a 480% increase in incidence in the very deprived population. The reason for this considerable increase is unknown. In males the proximal tibial fracture showed a rise of 1,107% with distal humeral fractures, midfoot fractures, and scapula fractures showing increases of 940%, 835%, and 723%, respectively. It would seem reasonable to assume that the overall effect of social deprivation is caused by a number of medical and social comorbidities which affect both males and females and will cause an increased rate of fractures, but in males more aggressive behavior may account for the greater difference in the incidence of a number of fractures.

There is evidence that a number of diseases are related to social deprivation and it has been shown that fracture incidence is affected by factors such as a rural or urban domicile,[74,88] education,[50] occupation,[35] type of residence,[39] marital status,[39] and smoking and alcohol.[4] There is also evidence that bone mineral density (BMD) is affected by social deprivation.[9] In recent years there has been interest in the effect of ethnicity on the incidence of fractures[17,94] and a number of authors have pointed to the different incidence of proximal femoral fractures in particular in different parts of the world.[30,59,94] It has been pointed out that in the United States, African American and Hispanic males who present with hip fractures are younger than White males.[94] Pressley et al.[84] drew attention to the paradox of African American males in the United States having a higher BMD, but also a higher incidence of fractures, than White males. It is likely that these findings relate to deprivation. Ethnicity is difficult to study in Scotland, but in other areas of medicine the relationship between ethnicity and deprivation has been shown[14,98] and it would seem likely to be important in the epidemiology of fractures.

Fracture Distribution Curves

The earliest fracture distribution curves, based on age and gender, were proposed by Buhr and Cooke.[20] They analyzed 8,539 fractures over a 5-year period in Oxford, England, and proposed five basic curves. Their type A curve affected young and middle-aged men and they referred to it as a "wage earners" curve. This is equivalent to our Type B curve (Fig. 3-3). They suggested that this occurred in patients who presented with fractures of the hand, medial malleolus, metatarsus, foot

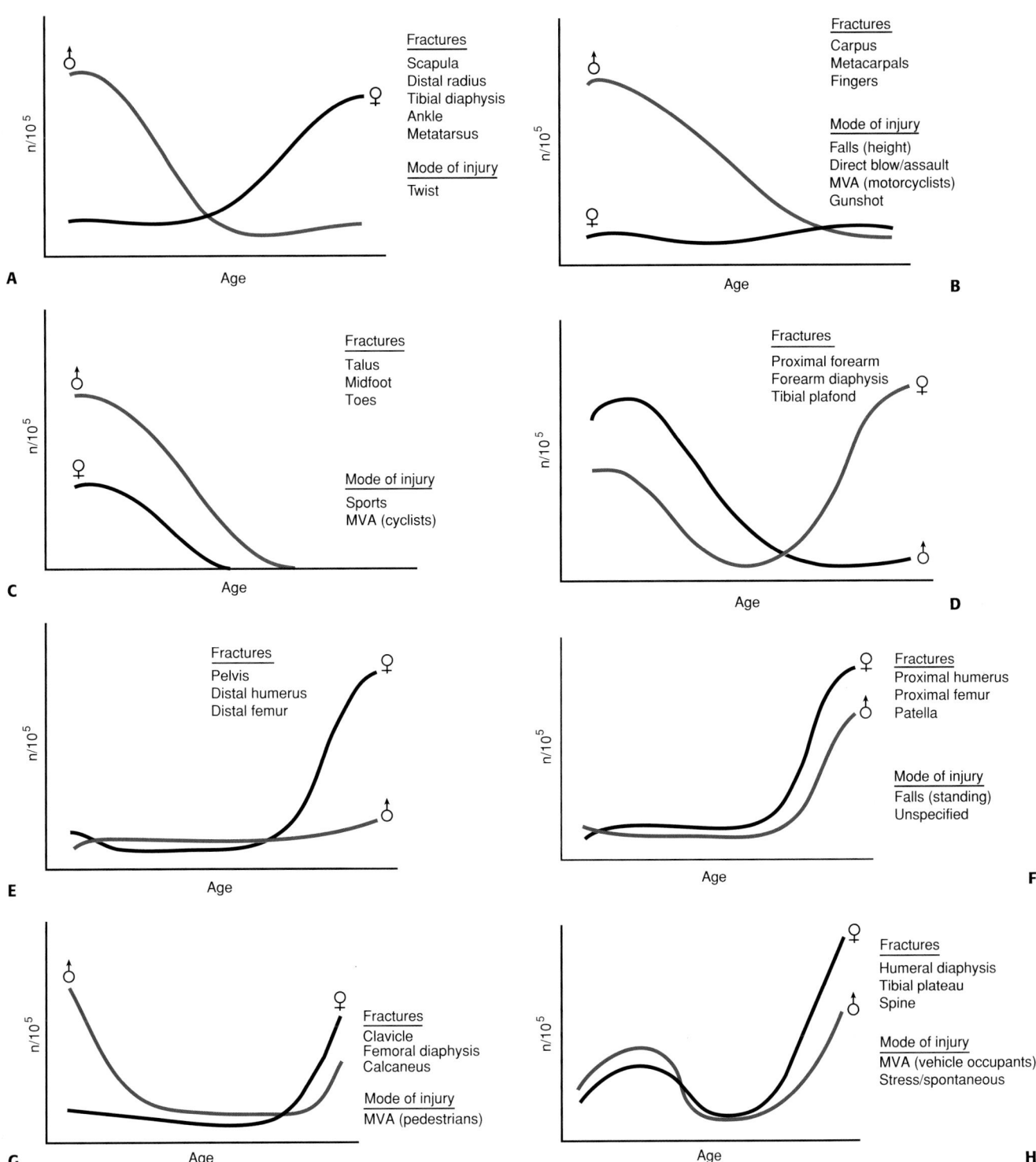

FIGURE 3-3 The eight fracture distribution curves. See Table 3-13 for list of distribution curves for different fractures.

phalanges, and spine. Their J-shaped curve affected older males and females and obviously it described fragility, or osteoporotic, fractures. It is equivalent to our type F curve (Fig. 3-3). They stated that fractures of the proximal humerus, humeral diaphysis, proximal femur, and pelvis together with bimalleolar ankle

fractures had a J-shaped curve. Buhr and Cooke's third curve was an L-shaped curve that affected younger males and females and was equivalent to our type C curve (Fig. 3-3). This was said to occur in distal humeral fractures, tibial diaphyseal fractures, and clavicular fractures. They also described two composite curves with either a bimodal male and unimodal female distribution or a unimodal male and bimodal female distribution. These are equivalent to our type D and G curves (Fig. 3-3). They said that these curves described fractures of the proximal and distal radius, femoral diaphysis, proximal tibia and fibula, and the lateral malleolus.

Later studies produced similar distribution curves. Knowelden et al.[64] analyzed patients in Dundee, Scotland and Oxford, England who were >35 years of age. They showed that fractures of the proximal humerus, pelvis, and proximal femur all demonstrated an osteoporotic type F curve (Fig. 3-3). It is interesting to note that they had a type A curve (Fig. 3-3) for femoral diaphyseal fractures, but they recorded that the highest incidence of femoral diaphyseal fractures occurred in the elderly. Donaldson et al.[31] constructed four curves for proximal femoral, proximal humeral, distal radial, and tibia and fibula diaphyseal fractures that are very similar to the curves shown in Figure 3-3. Johansen et al.[56] constructed eight curves covering different body areas, these being the hip, spine, upper limb, pelvis, forearm and wrist, ankle, hand, finger and thumb, and foot and toes. These are also very similar to the curves shown in Figure 3-3.

Analysis of incidence in different fracture types shows that there are eight basic fracture distribution curves which are shown in Figure 3-3. Most fractures have a unimodal distribution affecting either younger or older patients. Some fractures, however, have a bimodal distribution whereby younger and older patients are affected, but there is a lower incidence in middle age. If one analyzes males and females separately the distribution curves shown in Figure 3-3 can be constructed. It should be remembered that the curves shown in Figure 3-3 are diagrammatic. The relative heights of the peaks of the curves will vary, but the overall curve patterns remain appropriate for all fractures.

A type A curve is often thought of as a typical fracture curve with a unimodal distribution in younger males and in older females. Generally the younger male peak is higher than the older female peak, although this is not the case in all fractures. An example is the metatarsal fracture where the younger male peak and the older female peak are at a similar height. Type A curves are seen in fractures of the scapula, distal radius, tibial diaphysis, ankle, and metatarsus. In type B curves there is also a young male unimodal distribution, but fractures in females occur in relatively small numbers throughout the decades. Type B curves are generally seen in the hand and affect the carpus, metacarpus, and fingers. However, they are also characteristic of femoral head fractures.

In type C fractures both males and females show a unimodal distribution. These fractures are rare after middle age. These fractures tend to occur in the foot and affect the toes, midfoot, and talus. In type D fractures there is a young male unimodal distribution, but the female distribution is bimodal affecting younger and older females. Generally the second peak starts around the time of the menopause. Type D curves are seen in fractures of the proximal forearm, forearm diaphyses, and tibial plafond.

Type E fractures are the opposite of type B fractures. They show a unimodal female distribution affecting older females with a relatively constant, lower incidence of fractures in males

throughout the decades. The type E pattern is seen in pelvic fractures, distal humeral fractures, and distal femoral fractures. This may be surprising to orthopedic surgeons who see young male patients with these fractures after high-energy trauma. However, if the complete epidemiology of these fractures is analyzed across the community it is apparent that the high-energy injuries are relatively rare compared with the lower-energy injuries seen in later life.

Type F fractures are the opposite of type C fractures. In type F fractures both males and females show a unimodal distribution affecting older patients with the incidence being higher in females. This pattern is characteristic of fractures of the proximal humerus, proximal femur, and patella. There is some variation regarding when the rise in fracture incidence occurs. Generally it is earlier in females than males and usually occurs around the time of the menopause in proximal humeral fractures and patella fractures, but somewhat later in proximal femoral fractures.

In type G fractures females show a unimodal distribution affecting older females and males show a bimodal distribution affecting both younger and older males with the incidence being higher in younger males. This distribution is seen in calcaneal and clavicular fractures. It is also now seen in femoral diaphyseal fractures. Type H fractures are unusual in that both males and females show a bimodal distribution. This fracture pattern is seen in fractures of the humeral diaphysis, tibial plateau, and cervical spine.

One can use the system of eight curves shown in Figure 3-3 to define other fractures. Although Table 3-13 shows that ankle fractures have a type A distribution, analysis of the different types of ankle fractures shows that only lateral malleolar fractures have a type A distribution. Medial malleolar fractures have a type D distribution and suprasyndesmotic ankle fractures have a type C distribution. Both bimalleolar and trimalleolar fractures are fragility fractures showing a type E distribution. Similarly, proximal forearm fractures have a type D distribution when they are all considered together, but further analysis shows that radial neck fractures have a type A distribution, whereas radial head fractures have a type H distribution. Both olecranon fractures and fractures of the proximal radius and ulnar have a type F distribution and should be regarded as fragility fractures. The distribution curves for different fractures are listed in Table 3-13 which also shows the distribution curves for the different fracture types.

Changing Epidemiology

There is no doubt that fracture epidemiology is changing very quickly. This is due to multiple factors which reflect a massive change in the health and economic status of many countries. There has been a great deal of literature dealing with the increasing frequency of fragility fractures which is thought to be secondary to the improved health and longer life expectancies of the older members of the population.[5,48,57,61,62,73] However, the change in fracture epidemiology is much broader than this and reflects the important industrial and road safety legislation introduced in many countries since the Second World War. The changes are well illustrated in Table 3-1 and by comparing our

TABLE 3-13 The Distribution Curves Shown in Figure 3-3 Applied to Different Fractures

Fracture Location

Clavicle	G	Proximal femur	F
Medial	A	Head	B
Diaphyseal	G	Neck	F
Lateral	A	Intertrochanteric	F
Scapula	A	Subtrochanteric	F
Intra-articular	A	Femoral diaphysis	G
Extra-articular	A	Distal femur	E
Proximal humerus	F	Patella	F
Humeral diaphysis	H	Proximal tibia	H
Distal humerus	E	Tibia and fibular diaphysis	A
Proximal forearm	D	Tibial diaphysis	B
Radial head	H	Fibular diaphysis	A
Radial neck	A	Distal tibia	D
Olecranon	F	Ankle	A
Radius and ulna	F	Medial malleolus	D
Forearm diaphyses	D	Lateral malleolus	A
Radius	A	Bimalleolar	E
Ulna	H	Trimalleolar	E
Radius and ulna	A	Suprasyndesmotic	C
Distal radius/ulna	A	Talus	C
Distal ulna	A	Neck	C
Carpus	A	Body	C
Scaphoid	B	Calcaneus	G
Triquetrum	A	Intra-articular	B
Hamate	B	Extra-articular	G
Trapezium	B	Midfoot	C
Metacarpus	B	Metatarsus	A
Finger phalanges	B	Toe phalanges	C
Pelvis	E	Cervical spine	H
Acetabulum	G	Thoracolumbar spine	F

Fracture Types

Periprosthetic	F
Open	G
Multiple	A
Fatigue	C
Insufficiency	F

The curves of different fracture types are also shown. In this section the term "Multiple" applies to multiple fractures and not to multiple injuries.

epidemiology for 2010 and 2011 with that of Buhr and Cooke[13] who analyzed over 8,500 patients, between 1938 and 1956, in Oxford, England. They prefaced their paper by pointing out the changes in health they had encountered. They stated that smallpox, diphtheria, the enteric fevers, and rickets had practically been eliminated and had been replaced by new viral diseases, radiation hazards, and the diseases of degeneration. They noted that in the elderly population cardiovascular degeneration, strokes, diabetes, osteoarthritis, and fractures presented problems as pressing as the great infections of a few decades earlier. Buhr and Cooke[13] clearly recognized the problems that osteoporosis presented in the 1940s and 1950s. They pointed out the prevalence of proximal femoral fractures, particularly in

women, and they noted that in nonmalignant pathologic fractures a third were caused by "senile osteoporosis."

However, when one examines their results it is clear that the situation has changed dramatically. They defined five fracture distribution curves. Their type A, wage earners, curve was the equivalent of our type B curve affecting younger males. Their type L, prewage earners, curve was the equivalent of our type C curve affecting younger males and females, and their type J, postwage earners, curve is the same as our type F curve affecting older males and females. They also stated that there were two composite curves with bimodal distributions affecting males and females. These were the same as our type D and H curves.

They categorized 22 different fractures and a comparison of their distributions with ours indicates considerable social and medical differences between the two time periods. They classified carpal, metacarpal, finger phalangeal, medial malleolar, tarsal, metatarsal, toe phalangeal, and spinal fractures as being type B fractures. Table 3-13 shows that the intervening 50 to 60 years has altered things considerably and only metacarpal and finger phalangeal fractures still have a type B distribution. Surgeons now see many more females with the other fractures.

Their type F osteoporotic fractures were similar to ours. They felt that the humeral diaphyseal fracture was an osteoporotic fracture and if one compares the epidemiology of humeral diaphyseal fractures with distal radial and ulnar fractures shown in Table 3-3 it would seem that they were correct. They listed distal humeral and clavicle fractures as type C fractures and again a review of Table 3-11 shows that surgeons now expect to see many older women with these fractures. Thus the main difference between the two time periods is the numbers of fractures in females that are now seen, but were not seen in the 1940s and 1950s. This must reflect the changing role of women in society and the fact that successful medical and surgical treatment, including joint arthroplasty, now allows older women to sustain fractures that they could not have sustained in the past!

Other studies indicate that the increased incidence of fractures that is now seen is mainly because of a significant increase in the incidence of fractures in females. In a study carried out between 1954 and 1958 in Dundee, Scotland, and Oxford, England, Knowelden et al.[64] examined the incidence of fractures in patients aged >35 years and found that the incidences of the fractures listed in Table 3-3 in males and females in Dundee were $1,017.3/10^5$/year and $921.3/10^5$/year, respectively with the equivalent figures in Oxford being $811.4/10^5$/year and $871.5/10^5$/year. The equivalent incidences in Edinburgh in 2010 to 2011 were $1,062.5/10^5$/year and $1,711.6/10^5$/year. Thus in 50 to 55 years the incidence of fractures in Scottish males has risen by 4.4%, whereas the incidence of fractures in females has risen by 85.7%. The increased incidence in males is less but the spectrum of fractures in males has changed considerably over this period. There are now many fewer industrial fractures and many more fall-related fractures and consequently there are less hand and foot fractures in males.

The fact that the epidemiology of fractures has continued to change in recent years is illustrated by reference to Table 3-14. This shows the incidence, average age, and the prevalence of standing falls as a cause of fracture in six fractures treated in

| TABLE 3-14 | The Incidence, Average Age, and Prevalence of Fractures in Patients ≥15 Years Caused by Standing Falls for Six Common Fractures Treated in Three Time Periods | | | | | | |

	Incidence (n/10^5/yr)			Average Age (yrs)		Standing Falls (%)	
	Overall	Male	Female	Male	Female	Male	Female
Proximal Humerus							
1993	47.2	28.7	63.8	56	69.9	76.1	89.2
2000	65.1	41.4	86.3	57.4	68	71.3	84.7
2010/11	92.4	61	120.3	59.2	68.9	73.1	90.9
Distal Radius/ulna							
1991	158.3	87.3	221.5	42	64.2	54.4	83.5
2000	201.5	131.5	264	38	63.3	39.2	81.2
2010/11	235.9	139.3	322.2	43.7	63.4	50.6	91.3
Pelvis							
1991	21.6	16.3	26.3	46	73.6	28.9	73.9
2000	17.6	11.1	23.4	50.4	77.8	29.6	84.4
2010/11	22.9	14.7	30.4	64.7	80.4	56.4	91.6
Proximal Femur							
1991	143.8	57.4	220.8	71.9	80.2	86.6	91.2
2000	133.7	74.1	208.8	74.5	82.6	83.4	95.3
2010/11	145.5	84	200.4	78	81.1	88.3	95.3
Femur Diaphysis							
1991	8.9	8.6	9.2	39.5	62	25	54.2
2000	10.4	7.8	12.8	35.9	78.4	35	80
2010/11	8.3	8.6	8	63.4	75.6	42.8	86.4
Tibia Diaphysis							
1991	24.4	37.2	13	32.8	60.7	16.1	52.9
2000	18.5	24.6	11	35.8	49.5	18.3	50
2010/11	13.3	20.1	7.3	41	43.6	36.7	65

Edinburgh in three time periods. The results are taken from patients ≥15 years in three study years, over a 20-year period, using prospectively collected data from the same catchment area. Four of the fractures are the classic fragility fractures of the proximal humerus, distal radius and ulna, pelvis and proximal femur, and the other two fractures are the principal diaphyseal fractures of the lower limb, the femoral and tibial diaphyseal fractures. Table 3-14 shows that there are considerable differences in the epidemiology of all the fractures, but the changes vary between different fractures. It is quite clear that the overall incidence of proximal humeral and distal radial fractures has risen over the last 20 years in both males and females. This is not the case in pelvic fractures or in the overall incidence of proximal femoral fractures. However, Table 3-14 shows a marked increase in the incidence of proximal femoral fractures in males in the last 20 years, presumably because more males are living longer.

The comparison of the incidences of femoral and tibial diaphyseal fractures shows considerable differences in epidemiology. The femoral diaphyseal fracture has not changed in incidence, but the incidence of tibial diaphyseal fractures has decreased markedly in the last 20 years. The overall incidence has declined from 24.4/10^5/year to 13.3/10^5/year with a decline seen in both males and females. The difference is probably because the femoral diaphyseal fracture is essentially a fragility fracture, whereas the tibial diaphyseal fracture is not.

Examination of the age of the patients and the prevalence of fractures caused by a standing fall shows that there has been no major differences in proximal humeral or distal radial fractures in the last 20 years. However, the average age of patients presenting with pelvic fractures is rising in both males and females, although the rise in male age is more dramatic. This is because there are now fewer high-energy pelvic fractures and more lower-energy fractures in a male population which is living longer. This would seem to be confirmed by the increased number of pelvic fractures caused by standing falls. The average age of males presenting with proximal femoral fractures is also increasing, although no other differences were noted.

The differences noted in pelvic fractures are mirrored in the femoral diaphyseal fracture where there is clearly an increasing average age and a higher prevalence of fractures caused by standing falls. The same is seen in the tibial diaphyseal fracture, although this fracture is unique in that the average age of females presenting with tibial diaphyseal fractures is falling.

The tibial diaphyseal fracture is a very good example of the changing epidemiology of a nonfragility fracture. A review of the incidences of tibial diaphyseal fractures in Europe at different times shows that there has been a considerable decline. The literature is complicated by the fact that different age ranges of patients are often assessed and that children and adolescents are sometimes included. However, by calculating the incidences of equivalent age groups trends can be shown. Knowelden et al.[64] demonstrated an incidence of tibial diaphyseal fractures of 17.3/10⁵/year in patients aged >35 years in Dundee, Scotland, in 1954 to 1958. The equivalent incidence in Edinburgh in 1991 was 18/10⁵/year and in 2010 to 2011 it was 12.3/10⁵/year. Similar trends are also shown by examining the Swedish literature.[36,103] Emami et al.[36] compared the incidence of tibial diaphyseal fractures in 1971 to 1975 and 1986 to 1990. Their incidences in patients ≥20 years of age were 40.6/10⁵/year and 31.9/10⁵/year, respectively. In Edinburgh in 1991 the incidence of tibial diaphyseal fractures in patients aged ≥20 years was 24.7/10⁵/year. It is therefore clear that the incidence of tibial diaphyseal fractures has fallen since the Second World War and continues to fall.

A review of the epidemiology of tibial diaphyseal fractures in Edinburgh between 1990 and 2007 has shown a progressive decline in both males and females. In males the incidence fell from 43.6/10⁵/year to 25/10⁵/year and in females it fell from 15.8/10⁵/year to 6.2/10⁵/year. Analysis showed that there was a statistically significant decline in incidence in males aged 15 to 34 years and in both males and females ≥65 years. A review of the open fractures presenting between 1990 and 2007 also showed a statistically significant decline in incidence in both males and females with the greatest decline in incidence being seen in females ≥65 years. There was no decrease in incidence in Gustilo type I fractures, but there was in Gustilo type II and Gustilo type III fractures, with Gustilo type III fractures showing the greatest decrease in incidence.

A review of the causes of tibial diaphyseal fractures showed that there was a decline in standing fall–related fractures in females ≥65 years and in both sports-related fractures and motor vehicle accident fractures. The data showed that there was a significant decline in pedestrian tibial fractures in males aged 35 to 64 years and in females ≥65 years.

The various studies that have been quoted show that there has been a significant decline in tibial diaphyseal fractures since the Second World War.[36,103] Initially this was presumably related to industrial and workplace safety legislation, but more recently much of the decline must be due to a decline in motor vehicle accidents associated fractures. However, there is also a decline in sports-related tibial fractures, and in young males, the overall decline may simply relate to a more sedentary lifestyle. In older women the reduction in pedestrian fractures is presumably related to the reduction in age shown in Table 3-14. Tibial diaphyseal fractures are unusual in that there is a declining incidence in elderly women and presumably this relates to the fact that tibial fractures are not osteoporotic fractures and the causes of these fractures are changing.

The declining incidences of different fractures have had an effect on the distribution curves. Buhr and Cooke[13] defined tibial fractures as having a type C curve, but as females became more affected, it was changed to a type A curve. Tables 3-9–3-11 and Table 3-14 show a decline in elderly females and the distribution curve appears to be continuing to change and it may be that in the future a new curve will be required with a bimodal distribution in males and a unimodal distribution in younger women only.

Much has been written about the epidemiology of fragility fractures in the last 10 to 20 years. The assumption is that fragility fractures are increasing in incidence, but it is surprisingly difficult to know if this is actually the case and, if so, is it true for all fragility fractures or only for some. A good example of the confusion is seen in the proximal humeral fracture literature. There is no question of doubt that these have increased in frequency since the Second World War. Knowelden et al.,[64] in their analysis of patients >35 years in Dundee, Scotland in 1954 to 1958 quoted an incidence of 44/10⁵/year (32.8/10⁵/year in males and 52.2/10⁵/year in females). Table 3-14 shows the incidence of proximal humeral fractures in the population of Edinburgh over an 18-year period, but if patients >35 years are analyzed, the incidence of proximal humeral fractures in 1993 is 69.5/10⁵/year (39.9/10⁵/year in males and 94.1/10⁵/year in females). In 2010 to 2011 the incidence was 136.6/10⁵/year (88/10⁵/year in males and 178.2/10⁵/year in females). There has therefore been a progressive rise in the incidence of proximal humeral fractures in Scotland in the last 55 to 60 years. A review of the Swedish literature also shows a rise in incidence between 1950 and 1982,[5] although the incidence in the early 1950s was slightly higher than recorded by Knowelden et al.[64] However, Kannus et al.[62] in a study of proximal humeral fractures in females aged ≥80 years in Finland between 1970 and 2007, showed that the incidence in this age group was 88/10⁵/year in 1970 and 304/10⁵/year in 1995 but there was no further rise and in 2007 the incidence was 298/10⁵/year. It is interesting to note that the comparative figures for Edinburgh females ≥80 years were 285.5/10⁵/year in 1993 and 497.7/10⁵/year in 2010 to 2011. Thus our incidence in the 1990s was not dissimilar to the Finnish incidence, but our incidence of proximal humeral fractures continued to rise. Given the similarities between Finland and Scotland there is no obvious explanation for this difference but it seems likely that the incidence is rising.

The fracture that has received most attention in the epidemiologic literature is the proximal femoral fracture. There is no doubt that this fracture has also increased in incidence, but there is considerable variation in its current incidence throughout the world and there is also debate as to whether the incidence of proximal femoral fractures is now declining in developed countries.[19] The earliest incidences that are available are from Rochester, Minnesota in the United States where Melton et al.[73] studied the incidences of proximal femoral fractures in six time periods between 1928 and 1992. They looked at the incidences of proximal femoral fractures in the whole population and found that in the period 1928 to 1942 the incidences in males and females were 17.3/10⁵/year and 46.9/10⁵/year. They documented a rise in incidence in both males and females until 1963 to 1972 when the incidences were 69.3/10⁵/year and 125/10⁵/year, respectively. Thereafter the male incidence continued to rise until 1983 to 1992 when it was 82.2/10⁵/year, but the female incidence plateaued so that it was 115.2/10⁵/year in 1983 to 1992. However, Melton et al. also published the incidences of proximal femoral fractures in Olmsted County, Minnesota[74] and they stated that in males and females ≥35 years of age in 1989 to 1991 the incidences were 142/10⁵/year and 219/10⁵/year, respectively. The incidences appear to be different, but it may be that during the 1983 to 1992 period the incidences were rising. Knowelden et al.[64] stated that in 1954 to 1958 in Dundee, Scotland, the incidences of proximal femoral fractures in males and females >35 years were 43.4/10⁵/year and 105.4/10⁵/year, these being lower than the incidences in Rochester, Minnesota in a similar period. The current incidences of proximal femoral fractures in Edinburgh in males and females >35 years are 131.7/10⁵/year and 233.4/10⁵/year, respectively. This is about the same as in Olmsted County in 1989 to 1991. It is difficult to know why there should be a difference, but it may reflect better male health in Olmsted County.

Table 3-15 shows the incidence of proximal femoral fractures in different parts of the world at different times.[2,6,66,86] All of the studies looked at patients ≥50 years of age and all were carried out in Caucasian populations or were age adjusted for the Caucasian US population. The results encapsulate many of the problems that exist in defining hip fracture incidence. The Scandinavian studies[6,86] both show much higher incidences in males and females than in other parts of the world, but the two studies disagree about whether the fracture incidence in declining in Sweden. The incidence in Japanese males is very low[2] compared with the incidence in females and in general the incidence in males is highest in North Europe.[6,86]

There are many other studies of hip fracture incidence, but the age ranges are often different. Chang et al.[18] showed that the incidence of proximal femoral fractures in Australia in patients ≥60 years was 329/10⁵/year in males and 759/10⁵/year in females in 1989 to 2000, which is not dissimilar to the Swedish results in Table 3-15. Kanis et al.[59] undertook a systematic review of hip fracture incidence worldwide and standardized all the results with United Nations age data. They found a very wide difference in incidence from approximately 20/10⁵/year in South Africa to approximately 575/10⁵/year in Denmark. It is highly likely that in many countries data collection is poor, but the paper certainly highlights huge differences in the incidence of this fracture.

Clearly there are many other fractures in which the incidence is probably changing quite quickly, but these fractures serve to highlight the enormous changes in fracture epidemiology that have occurred in the last 50 to 60 years. There is no logical reason why the changing epidemiology should not continue in the future and surgeons should be aware that a number of fractures which are now not regarded as fragility fractures will probably be so in the next few decades.

Variation in Epidemiology

It has already been pointed out that the epidemiology of fractures varies widely. Some of the variations are undoubtedly accounted for by the different methods used to collect and to diagnose fractures. However, despite this there are significant differences in the incidence of fractures in different communities. These differences have mainly been studied in fragility fractures and the literature is consistent in pointing out that the population of Scandinavia[6,12,59,61,86] has the highest incidence of these fractures. The reason for this is unknown. However there is evidence that the incidence of fractures varies with racial type,[17,97,101] domicile,[46,48] season of the year,[54] and social deprivation.[25,75] The importance of social deprivation has already been discussed in this chapter, but clearly the reason for the variation in epidemiology is more complex. Scandinavian countries are relatively affluent and one would expect a lower incidence of fractures in more affluent countries. However, other factors such as life expectancy will clearly play a part in the epidemiology of fragility fractures. It seems likely that social deprivation accounts for some of the variation in fracture epidemiology attributed to ethnicity, particularly in the United States. Pressly et al.[84] pointed out the apparent contradiction of young Black males in the United States having a higher BMD, but also having a higher incidence of fracture. This is likely to represent deprivation. In a recent study Cauley[17] pointed out that despite increased bone density, Black women in the

TABLE 3-15	The Incidence of Proximal Femoral Fractures as Reported in Different Parts of the World		
	Incidence (n/10⁵/yr)		
Country	**Males**	**Females**	**Comments**
Sweden[6]			
1993–1996	390	706	Declining incidence except in females ≥90 yrs
2001–2005	317	625	
Sweden[86]			
1987 (rural)		710	Females only No change in incidence
1987 (urban)		750	
2002 (rural)		600	
2002 (urban)		690	
Hong Kong[66]	180	459	All 1997–1998
Singapore[66]	164	442	Age adjusted for US population
Malaysia[66]	88	218	
Thailand[66]	114	269	
Japan[2]			
1987–1988	59.2	245	Age adjusted for US population
2004	115.2	453.7	
Scotland			
1991	134.5	514.3	
2010–2011	224.7	494.4	

All studies[2,6,66,86] have reported on patients aged ≥50 yrs and all were carried out in Caucasian populations or age adjusted for the Caucasian US population.

United States were more likely to die after hip fracture, had longer hospital stays and were less likely to be ambulatory at discharge from hospital.

It has been suggested that there are racial differences in fracture incidences. This has mainly been studied in the Far East with Wang and Seeman[101] suggesting that in the Chinese population bone cortices are thicker and there is more mineralized bone matrix. However, it seems likely that racial differences, like most things in medicine, are multifactorial and will involve life expectancy, deprivation, and other social and medical comorbidities.

Open Fractures

In this study year 1.9% of the fractures were open. Further analysis shows that 66% of the fractures were Gustilo[47] type I fractures, 19.7% were Gustilo type II fractures, and the remaining 13.6% were Gustilo type III fractures. A review of the previous two editions of Rockwood and Green[24,26] show that in 2000 3.1% of the fractures were open, while in 2007 to 2008 2.6% were open. There also seems to have been a decline in the prevalence of Gustilo type III fractures with 22.8% being recorded in 2000, 19.9% in 2007 to 2008 and 13.6% in 2010 to 2011. It therefore seems likely that there is trend toward fewer and less severe open fractures. This would seem to be confirmed by examining the incidence of open tibial fractures in Edinburgh over the last 20 years. In 1991 34.7% of the tibial fractures were open giving an incidence of open tibial fractures of 8.5/10⁵/year ($8.5/10^5$/year) (13.8/10⁵/year in males and 3.8/10⁵/year in females). In 2010 to 2011 20.3% of the tibial fractures were open the incidence being 2.7/10⁵/year (4.9/10⁵/year in males and 0.7/10⁵/year in females). In 1991 42.9% of the open tibial fractures were Gustilo type III but by 2010 to 2011 this had fallen to 21.4%.

Tables 3-6–3-11 show the prevalence of open fractures in males and females of different ages, but given the relative infrequency of open fractures, particularly in older patients, it is difficult to analyze them meaningfully. For this reason all of the open fractures presenting to the Royal Infirmary of Edinburgh over a 15-year period between 1995 and 2009[28] have been analyzed. As many open fractures are associated with more severe injury, the injury severity score (ISS) for each patient was analyzed, in addition to creating a musculoskeletal index (MSI) which is the sum of all fractures and severe soft tissue injuries

such as ligament disruption, dislocations, nerve damage, vascular damage, and tendon injury. All were given the score of one and the total used to provide an assessment of the degree of musculoskeletal injury.

In the 15 years of the study 2,386 open fractures were treated, giving an incidence of 30.7/10⁵/year. They occurred in 2,206 patients with 2,079 (94.2%) presenting with a single open fracture and a further 127 (5.8%) presenting with between two and seven open fractures. The average age was 45.5 years. Analysis showed that 69.1% of the fractures occurred in males with an average age of 40.8 years and 30.9% occurred in females with an average age of 56 years. In males 10.2% of the fractures occurred in patients aged ≥65 years and 2.1% in patients aged ≥80 years. The equivalent figures for females were 42.9% and 18.6%, respectively.

The overall male and female fracture distribution curves for open fractures are different from those for all fractures shown in Figure 3-1. The curves for open fractures are shown in Figure 3-4. This shows that in adult males the highest incidence of open fractures occurs between 15 and 19 years and that there is an almost linear decline with increasing age. The incidence of open fractures in males aged 15 to 19 years was 54.5/10⁵/year compared with 23.3/10⁵/year in the 90+ age group. In females there is a unimodal distribution rising from 9.2/10⁵/year in the 15–19-year group to 14.6/10⁵/year in the 50–59-year group. Thereafter there is a rapid rise in incidence to 53/10⁵/year in the 80–89-year group. There were insufficient fracture numbers to calculate fracture curves for open fractures of the scapula, proximal radius, radial diaphysis, carpus, and proximal femur. Table 3-16 shows the fracture distribution curves for the different open fractures. It is clear that the overall fracture distribution is different from that of closed fractures. In open fractures it is younger males who are most affected and not infrequently they sustain their open fractures as a result of high-energy injuries. In females Figure 3-4 shows that the open fracture distribution curve is not dissimilar to the overall fracture distribution curve of females (Fig. 3-1), but there is one significant difference. The overall female distribution curve shows a marked increase in incidence in the 50–59-year group in the postmenopausal period. In open fractures this increase occurs one decade later and is therefore probably not just related to osteoporosis, but to increasing overall patient frailty

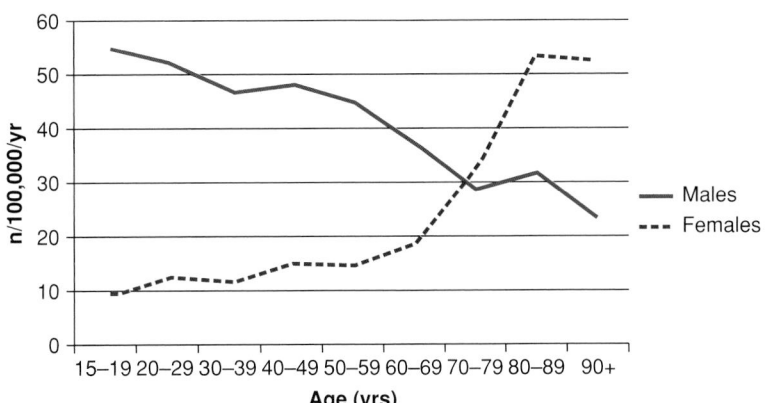

FIGURE 3-4 The age and gender distribution curves for open fractures.

TABLE 3-16	Fracture Distribution Curves for Different Open Fractures					
	Fracture Distribution Curves					
	Upper Limb			Axial Skeleton and Lower Limb		
	All Fractures	Open Fractures			All Fractures	Open Fractures
Clavicle	G	C		Pelvis	E	C
Proximal humerus	F	H		Femoral diaphysis	G	B
Humeral diaphysis	H	F		Distal femur	E	A
Distal humerus	E	G		Patella	F	A
Proximal ulna	F	H		Proximal tibia	H	A
Ulna diaphysis	H	D		Tibia and fibular diaphyses	A	A
Radius and ulna diaphyses	A	G		Distal tibia	D	D
Distal radius and ulna	A	E		Ankle	A	E
Metacarpus	B	A		Talus	C	C
Finger phalanges	B	A		Calcaneus	G	G
				Midfoot	C	B
				Metatarsus	A	A
				Toe phalanges	C	C
Modes of injury (Open fractures)						
Crush injuries	A			Direct blows or assaults	B	
Falls from standing height	F			Falls from height	C	
Road traffic accidents	G			Falls down stairs	F	
Cutting injuries	B			Sport	C	

The overall distribution curves are included for comparison. Distribution curves for the different modes of injuries that caused open fractures are also shown.

which affects the soft tissues as well as bone. It is also true that the ability to avoid dangerous situations is compromised in older patients. A review of the open fracture distribution curves shown in Table 3-16 indicates that in open fractures which are commonly caused by high-energy injuries such as fractures of the pelvis, femoral diaphysis, distal femur, patella, proximal tibia, distal humerus, and proximal ulna the distribution changes to one which highlights the increased frequency of open fractures in younger patients. Thus the distribution curve for femoral diaphyseal fractures changes from a type G curve to a type B curve showing that open femoral fractures are predominantly seen in young men. Other fractures such as those of the distal femur, patella and proximal tibia change from a curve showing a unimodal distribution affecting older patients to a bimodal distribution where younger patients are affected more commonly. In lower-energy open fractures it can be seen that there are a number of changes as more elderly patients are affected. Thus fractures of the metacarpals and finger phalanges change from a unimodal curve affecting younger patients to a bimodal curve where elderly females are also affected. In both distal radial and ankle fractures there is a change from a type A

curve in all fractures to a type E curve in open fractures emphasizing the frequency of open fractures in elderly females. Further analysis shows that 73.3% of open distal radial fractures and 20.8% of open ankle fractures occur in females aged ≥80 years. There are a number of fractures in which the distribution curve does not change. These tend to be fractures which mainly occur in young patients anyway. There is no change in the curves for the different foot fractures, although whilst closed talar fractures affect both young males and females, the open talar fracture seems mainly to occur in young males.

The basic epidemiologic data for all open fractures treated between 1995 and 2009 is shown in Table 3-17. This shows that almost half of all open fractures involve the fingers and that open fractures of the fingers, tibial diaphysis, distal radius, toes, and ankle accounted for about three quarters of all open fractures. Table 3-17 also shows that a number of open fractures are very rare with ten of the open fractures averaging less than one per year in a very busy trauma unit. In 15 years there were no open proximal radial fractures.

The severity of the different open fractures is shown in Table 3-18. The Gustilo grade has been used to define the

TABLE 3-17	The Epidemiology of Open Fractures					
	No.	%	Age (yr)	≥65 yrs (%)	≥80 yrs (%)	M/F
Finger phalanges	1,090	45.7	43.9	13.4	4.2	79/21
Tibial diaphysis	267	11.2	43.3	18	6.7	67/33
Distal radius	184	7.7	67	67.4	30.4	23/77
Toe phalanges	170	7.1	41.9	11.8	1.8	66/34
Ankle	126	5.3	56.7	42.9	14.3	43/57
Metacarpus	104	4.4	34.8	7.7	4.8	90/10
Proximal ulna	51	2.1	47.9	29.4	7.8	69/31
Metatarsus	49	2.1	42.2	14.3	8.2	80/20
Patella	46	1.9	36.5	10.9	4.3	72/28
Radius and ulna	44	1.8	40.9	20.5	6.8	74/26
Femoral diaphysis	43	1.8	31.8	4.7	2.3	77/23
Distal tibia	31	1.3	48.1	22.6	3.2	58/42
Proximal tibia	29	1.2	47.7	24.1	10.3	59/41
Distal femur	25	1	40.6	20	12	48/52
Ulna diaphysis	25	1	43.2	16	0	68/32
Calcaneus	18	0.8	43.7	22.2	0	78/22
Distal humerus	18	0.8	48.5	33.3	11.1	78/22
Humeral diaphysis	16	0.7	51.3	37.5	12.5	75/25
Proximal humerus	12	0.5	56	25	8.3	50/50
Clavicle	9	0.4	44	11.1	11.1	78/22
Pelvis	7	0.3	40.9	14.3	0	86/14
Talus	6	0.3	31.3	0	0	83/17
Radial diaphysis	5	0.2	44	20	0	80/20
Midfoot	5	0.2	28.2	0	0	100/0
Scapula	2	0.08	29.5	0	0	100/0
Proximal radius/ulna	2	0.08	71	50	50	50/50
Proximal femur	1	0.04	45	0	0	100/0
Carpus	1	0.04	20	0	0	100/0
Total	2,386	100	45.5	20.3	7.2	69/31

The number, prevalence, and gender ratios are shown as are the average ages and percentages of patients ≥65 yrs and ≥80 yrs.

severity of the fracture and the ISS and MSI have been used to define the overall injury suffered by the patient. Overall 75.9% of patients had an isolated open fracture with no other musculoskeletal injury with 81.3% of open upper limb fractures being isolated compared with 62.8% of open lower limb fractures. Overall 26.8% of open fractures were Gustilo type III with 18.6% of upper limb fractures being Gustilo type III compared with 42.6% of lower limb fractures. The overall average ISS was 7.2 with the average ISS of patients with upper and lower limb fractures being 5.1 and 11.1, respectively. Overall 7.2% of patients presented with an ISS of ≥16 with 2.5% and 13.8% of patients with upper and lower limb fractures having an ISS of ≥16.

Tables 3-17 and 3-18 show that open lower limb fractures tend to be more severe than open upper limb fractures. Open fractures of the femoral diaphysis, distal femur, patella, proxi-mal tibia, tibial diaphysis, distal tibia, talus, and calcaneus tend to be associated with the highest ISS and MSI and the highest prevalence of Gustilo III fractures. The majority of these fractures were caused by high-energy injuries such as motor vehicle accidents or falls from a height. The highest prevalence of Gustilo type III fractures is seen in fractures of the hindfoot and midfoot, although the incidence of these fractures is only 0.4/10⁵/year.

Analysis of the mode of injury showed that the commonest cause of open fractures was a crush injury with an incidence of 93.8/10⁵/year. Eighty-three percent of these open fractures were finger phalangeal fractures. The second commonest mode of injury was a fall from a standing height with an incidence of 59.4/10⁵/year. The average age of this group was 64.4 years and 60.9% were ≥65 years of age. Open fractures following falls

TABLE 3-18 **Severity of Open Fractures**

	Fracture Severity		Injury Severity Score		Soft Tissues	
	Isolated Fracture (%)	MSI	Average ISS	ISS ≥ 16	Gustilo Type III (%)	Principal Modes of Injury
Finger phalanges	84.5	1.3	2.9	0.5	24.9	55.4% crush, 31.5% cut
Tibia and fibula	71.9	1.7	13.5	15.3	44.6	46.1% mva
Distal radius	78.3	1.3	10.9	6.5	2.2	71.2% fall
Toe phalanges	67.6	1.8	3.3	3.5	17.1	45.3% crush
Ankle	86.5	1.3	12.6	5.5	47.6	54.8% fall
Metacarpus	45.2	1.7	5.7	1.9	10.6	55.8% direct blow or assault
Proximal ulna	82.3	1.5	11.3	5.9	13.7	43.1% fall
Metatarsus	22.4	3.6	7.6	0	57.1	40.8% crush, 36.7% mva
Patella	58.7	1.9	9.1	19.5	30.4	58.7% mva
Radius and ulna	86.4	1.2	10.8	6.8	4.5	43.2% fall, 25% mva
Femoral diaphysis	37.2	2.7	18.1	39.5	65.1	53.5% mva
Distal tibia	83.9	1.4	13.1	12.9	45.2	51.6% fall height
Proximal tibia	48.3	2.1	14.3	20.7	58.6	51.7% mva
Distal femur	25	2.7	18.6	40	72	80% mva
Ulna diaphysis	76	1.5	12	8	16	28% fall, 28% direct blow or assault
Calcaneus	22.2	2.7	15	50	77.8	72.2% fall height
Distal humerus	72.2	1.5	13.6	11.1	44.4	33.3% fall, 33.3% mva
Humeral diaphysis	62.5	1.8	17.5	37.5	18.7	50% mva
Proximal humerus	91.6	1.1	10.2	0	8.3	41.7% fall, 33.3% mva
Clavicle	77.8	1.7	6.4	11.1	0	33.3% fall
Pelvis	57.1	2	19	42.9	0	42.8% fall height
Talus	50	3	10.2	33.3	50	50% mva
Radial diaphysis	40	1.6	12.4	20	20	40% fall
Midfoot	20	5.8	14	40	80	40% mva , 40% fall height
Scapula	100	1	13	50	0	50% direct blow/assault, 50% fall height
Proximal radius/ulna	50	2	25.5	50	0	50% fall, 50% fall height
Proximal femur	0	2	10	0	0	100% mva
Carpus	0	6	8	0	0	100% cut
Total	75.9	1.5	7.2	6.5	26.8	

tended to be isolated and not particularly severe. Only 0.7% of patients who had an open fall-related upper limb fracture had an ISS of ≥16 and the average MSI was 1.2. Similar values were seen in open lower limb fractures where 1.1% had an ISS of ≥16 and the average MSI was 1.1. However 3.2% of the open upper limb fractures secondary to a standing fall were Gustilo type III in severity, compared with 31.1% of the open lower limb fractures.

It is often assumed that motor vehicle accidents cause the majority of open fractures, but this is not the case. In this study motor vehicle accidents caused 15.9% of the open fractures, giving an incidence of 48.8/10⁵/year. The average age of this group was 40 years of age and 14% were ≥65 years of age. Further analysis showed that 26.1% of these patients had an ISS of ≥16 and 50.7% of the fractures were Gustilo type III in severity.

Analysis of the multiple open fractures showed that 5.8% of patients presented with multiple open fractures. As one might expect, open lower limb fractures were associated with a higher prevalence of multiple open fractures. This was a particular problem with open fractures of the talus (50%), distal femur (44%), calcaneus (33.3%), patella (23.9%), proximal tibia (20.7%), and femoral diaphysis (14%). In the upper limb 12.5% of patients with humeral diaphyseal fractures, 9.1% of patients with distal humeral fractures and 3% of patients with distal radial fractures presented with multiple open fractures. Again this illustrates the greater severity of open lower limb fractures.

Multiple Fractures

Orthopedic surgeons will be aware that although most fractures present as isolated injuries, patients may present with more than one fracture and there are certain accepted patterns such as the association between calcaneal and spinal fractures in a fall from a height or the association between proximal femoral fractures and distal radial or proximal humeral fractures in elderly patients who fall from a standing height. It is often assumed that multiple fractures are the result of high-energy injuries but with increasing aging of the population it is likely that surgeons will be called on to treat an increasing number of patients who have multiple fractures.

Overall 4.8% of patients in the study year presented with multiple fractures and Tables 3-4 and 3-5 show that males had a higher prevalence of multiple fractures. The numbers of multiple fractures varied between two and eight with 77.3% of the patients with multiple fractures having two fractures, 16.1% having three fractures, and the remaining 6.5% having four or more fractures. Table 3-13 shows that multiple fractures have a Type A distribution curve and this emphasized by comparing the basic epidemiology of multiple fractures caused by falls from a standing height with those caused by falls from a height or motor vehicle accidents. Analysis shows that 5% of patients who were injured as a result of a standing fall presented with multiple fractures. Their average age was 63.5 years and the gender ratio was 25/75. In those patients injured by a fall from a height or in a motor vehicle accident 19.7% presented with multiple fractures. The average age was 41.6 years and the gender ratio was 83/17. The multiple fractures associated with each individual fracture are shown in the individual sections dealing with each fracture type.

Fragility Fractures

The importance of osteoporotic fractures has been highlighted by many authors but in a recent study Cauley et al.[16] compared the absolute risk of fractures with the risk of different cardiovascular events and breast cancer in women aged 50 to 79 years. They found that the projected number of women who would experience a fracture exceeded the combined number of women who would experience invasive breast cancer or a range of different cardiovascular events in all ethnic groups except Black women. They found that the annual incidence of fractures was greatest in White and American Indian women and lowest in Black women.

There has been some debate as to which fractures are osteoporotic fragility fractures. Traditionally four fractures have been regarded as osteoporotic or fragility fractures, these being fractures of the proximal femur, distal radius, proximal humerus, and the thoracolumbar spine. However it is self-evident that other fractures commonly occurring in osteopenic or osteoporotic bone should also be regarded as fragility fractures. Buhr and Cooke,[13] in 1959, indicated that humeral diaphyseal fractures, bimalleolar ankle fractures, and pelvic fractures had a type F distribution and they also demonstrated that proximal radial, femoral diaphyseal, proximal tibial, and lateral malleolar fractures had a bimodal distribution with a significant proportion of the fractures occurring in older women. Other workers have also suggested that there are a considerable number of fractures which should be regarded as fragility fractures.[23,57,64]

Kanis et al.[58] defined osteoporotic fractures as occurring at a site associated with low BMD that also increased after the age

TABLE 3-19	A List of Fractures which Should be Considered as Fragility Fractures
Proximal humerus	Femoral diaphysis
Humeral diaphysis	Distal femur
Distal humerus	Patella
Olecranon	Bimalleolar ankle
Proximal radius and ulna	Trimalleolar ankle
Distal radius	Pelvis
Proximal femur	Thoracolumbar spine

of 50 years. On the basis of this definition Johnell and Kanis[57] proposed that vertebral fractures, all femoral fractures, wrist and forearm fractures, humeral fractures, rib fractures, pelvic fractures, clavicular fractures, scapular fractures, and sternal fractures should be regarded as osteoporotic fractures. They also suggested that fractures of the tibial and fibular diaphyses should be regarded as osteoporotic fractures in women.

If Table 3-3 and Figure 3-3 are examined a list of the fragility fractures that may occur in osteopenic of osteoporotic bone can be drawn up. These are shown in Table 3-19. Table 3-3 shows that there are a further seven fractures where patients have a higher average age than that of patients with distal radial fractures, this fracture being widely accepted as a fragility fracture. If these fractures are combined with fractures that have Type E or F distribution curves and with those patients over 50 years of age who present with fracture types A, D, G, and H an estimate of the true scale of fragility fractures in a developed country can be obtained. All humeral and all femoral fractures, with the exception of the very rare femoral head fracture, should now be regarded as fragility fractures as should many long bone metaphyseal fractures. Based on the fractures shown in Table 3-19 and the patients who presented with Type A, D, G and H fractures and were over 50 years of age, Court-Brown and Caesar[23] estimated in 2000 that 30.1% of male fractures and 66.3% of female fractures were potentially fragility fractures. They also pointed out that in a large Orthopaedic Trauma Unit 34.7% of outpatient fractures and 70.4% of inpatient fractures were potentially fragility fractures. This illustrates the scale of the current problem. It seems likely that the problem will increase and with increasing aging of the population other fractures will be regarded as fragility fractures and will be added to the list shown in Table 3-19. The fact that Table 3-5 shows that only eight fracture types in women currently have an average age of <50 years illustrates the potential problem facing orthopedic surgeons in the future.

Mode of Injury

In this edition of Rockwood and Green the modes of injury have been divided into eight basic categories, these being falls from a standing height, falls from a low height, including stairs and slopes, and falls from a significant height, this being defined as above six feet. The other modes of injury are direct

| TABLE 3-20 | The Epidemiology of the Different Modes of Injury |

	Prevalence %	Incidence n/10⁵/yr	Average Age (yrs)			≥65 yrs	≥80 yrs	Multiple Fractures (%)	Open Fractures (%)	M/F (%)
			All	Males	Females					
Fall (standing)	62.5	836.4	62.3	54.3	65.7	38.9	20.6	1.5	0.5	30/70
Low fall	4.2	57	51.7	48.2	55.2	27.1	10.8	6.8	3.1	51/49
Fall (height)	2.3	31.6	36	37.5	30	8.1	2.5	33	10.6	88/12
Direct blow/ assault	13.6	182.6	33.3	31.1	40.1	3.6	1	5.7	5.8	75/25
Sport	11.1	149.2	31.3	30.4	35.5	3	0.3	2.1	0.6	82/18
MVA	5.2	69.6	42.6	41.7	45.8	10.2	3	17.4	6.4	78/22
Pathologic	0.4	4.8	67.3	63.5	70.3	60	24	0	0	44/56
Stress/ spontaneous	0.3	2.7	49.9	44.5	54	21.4	21.4	0	0	43/57

The prevalence, incidence, and gender ratios are shown as are the percentages of open fractures and patients with multiple fractures. The average ages and prevalence of patients ≥65 yrs and ≥80 yrs are also shown. Low falls include falls down stairs and slopes. Direct blows/assaults include crush injuries.

blows, assaults or crush injuries, sports injuries, motor vehicle accident injuries, pathologic fractures, and stress or spontaneous fractures. The epidemiologic parameters for these modes of injury are shown in Table 3-20. Gunshot injuries are very uncommon in Scotland and none were treated during the study year. In 0.4% of the patients the cause was unknown, usually because the patient was intoxicated.

The commonest cause of injury is a fall from a standing height which accounted for 62.5% of the fractures treated during the study year. These are commoner in older patients and are the most frequent cause of fragility fractures. The other common causes of fractures are direct blows, assaults or crush injuries which cause about 14% of all fractures and sports injuries which cause about 11% of all fractures. It is accepted that sports injuries are a combination of falls, direct blows, crushing injuries and falls from a height, but they are conventionally grouped together as sports injuries and this has been done. Both direct blows and assaults and sports injuries tend to occur in younger patients with only 3% to 4% of patients being ≥65 years of age. They are more common in males.

Motor vehicle accidents are often perceived to cause the majority of fractures, but Table 3-20 shows that this is not the case. In 2000 7.2% of all fractures in Edinburgh occurred as a result of motor vehicle accidents but it is now 5.2% and there is little doubt that the decline in motor vehicle accident fractures is partially responsible for the lower incidence of fractures such as those of the tibial diaphysis. The United Kingdom has one of the lowest mortalities from motor vehicle accidents in the world, but, as yet, does not have a formal trauma system such as seen in the United States, Germany, and other countries. This confirms the importance of accident prevention.

It is possible to construct age and gender curves for modes of injury in the same way as can be done for individual fractures and the eight curves shown in Figure 3-3 can be used to describe modes of injury.

Falls from a Standing Height

This is the commonest mode of injury and Tables 3-6–3-11 show that most fragility fractures occur as a result of standing falls. There seems no doubt that fractures as a result of standing falls are becoming more common and this is confirmed by comparing the 2000 study year data documented in the sixth edition of Rockwood and Green[24] with the current study year. In 2000 51.3% of fractures followed a standing fall or a twisting injury, compared with 62.5% in 2010 to 2011. However, the average age of the groups was the same. It seems likely that the incidence of fractures caused by standing falls will continue to rise.

Further analysis of fractures caused by standing falls shows that 40.7% of male fractures resulted from a standing fall, compared with 85.4% of female fractures. Table 3-20 shows that the average ages were very different and that about 40% of the patients were ≥65 years. A review of the incidence of fractures following a standing fall shows that the overall incidence in males and females is 530/10⁵/year and 1101.1/10⁵/year and that the incidence of fractures in the ≥65-year age group is 1182.6/10⁵/year and 2880.9/10⁵/year, illustrating that falls from a standing height is a particular problem in older patients. Overall fractures caused by falls from a standing height show a type F distribution (Fig. 3-3). However, falls from a standing height can cause fractures in younger patients. The data shows that in patients aged 16 to 35 years standing falls caused 22% of fractures in males and 55.2% of fractures in females. In the 36- to 64-year groups the equivalent figures are 44.5% and 78.3% and in the ≥65-year group they are 81.6% and 94.2%. As one would expect Tables 3-6–3-11 show that there is a relatively low prevalence of open fractures and patients who present with multiple fractures as a result of falls from a standing height.

Falls from a Low Height

In this edition of Rockwood and Green falls down stairs have been combined with falls from a low height and falls down slopes. Table 3-20 shows that these accounted for 4.2% of fractures in the study year and that they often affect older patients with about 27% of the patients being ≥65 years of age. The average age of males and females injured in low falls was 44.8 years and 54.4 years, respectively. The overall incidence of these fractures was 53.7/10^5/year in males and 51.6/10^5/year in females. If the population of patients ≥65 years of age is considered, the relative incidences are 44/10^5/year and 89.4/10^5/year indicating that there is only a small rise in incidence in females ≥65 years of age. Overall fractures that occur as a result of falls from a low height have a type F fracture distribution curve. Table 3-20 shows that there are other differences from fractures associated with falls from a standing height. Low falls are associated with a higher prevalence of open fractures and multiple fractures indicating that these falls are associated with higher-energy injuries than falls from a standing height.

Falls from a Height

Fractures caused by falls from a height are relatively infrequent accounting for only 2.3% of the fractures seen in the study year. They mainly affect young males and only 8% of the patients treated during the study year were ≥65 years of age. They therefore have a type B distribution (Fig. 3-3). The overall incidences of these fractures are 47.9/10^5/year in males and 5.9/10^5/year in females. This is the lowest incidence of fractures in females from any mode of injury, except for pathologic or stress fractures. There were only ten females injured in a fall from a height during the study year and none were aged ≥65 years of age. It is also interesting to note that the 117 male fractures occurred in 76 patients and that only ten (8.5%) occurred in patients ≥65 years of age.

Table 3-20 shows that falls from a height are associated with a higher prevalence of open fractures and multiple fractures than motor vehicle accidents. Unsurprisingly 70.6% of the open fractures were in the lower limb and 83.3% of these fractures were in the distal tibia, ankle, or foot. The number of multiple fractures varied between two and eight. Classically falls from a height are associated with hindfoot and spinal fractures and this was seen to be the case with 32.7% of the fractures being in the calcaneus. Although spinal fractures have not been included in the overall epidemiologic analysis, review of the data shows that 14 (11%) patients presented with a total of 28 thoracolumbar spine fractures, of which 32.1% were thoracic and 67.9% were lumbar. The commonest area to be fractured was the T12 to L1 area with 5 (17.8%) T12 fractures and 10 (35.7%) L1 fractures being seen in the study year.

Direct Blows, Assaults, or Crush Injuries

This mode of injury, like falls from a height, is commonest in young males and therefore has a type B distribution (Fig. 3-3). It is the second commonest mode of injury after falls from a standing height. It is accepted that it covers a number of different causes of fracture and that the patient's history may not always be accurate or honest. With that proviso, further analysis showed that 50.8% of the fractures followed a direct blow, 29.1% occurred in a fight or assault, 11.3% as a result of a crush and 7.3% as a result of a twisting injury. It is not surprising to see that 48.1% were metacarpal fractures and 27.5% were finger fractures. These are common fractures in adolescent males and

Table 3-12 shows that they are commonly associated with social deprivation. Indeed analysis of the incidence of metacarpal and finger phalangeal fractures in deciles 9 and 10 of the Edinburgh population showed it to be 959.5/10^5/year. The overall incidence of fractures caused by direct blows or assaults in males and females was 291.7/10^5/year and 85.2/10^5/year, respectively.

Table 3-20 shows that direct blows and assaults are associated with a relatively high rate of multiple and open fractures. This may be surprising to some surgeons given the low energy involved in most of these injuries. The fact that 5.7% of patients had multiple fractures relates to the fact that 7.6% of males had multiple metacarpal fractures. Interestingly, no female presented with multiple metacarpal fractures following a direct blow or assault. Four percent of males with a finger fracture following a direct blow or assault had multiple finger fractures, compared with 3.1% of females. Analysis of the open fractures caused by direct blows or assaults showed that 68.7% were finger fractures.

Sports

Sports injuries occur in a very heterogeneous group of patients who are injured by falls of different types, direct blows, and even motor vehicle accidents. In addition, there is an association between stress fractures and sport. In general sports fractures have a type C distribution affecting younger males and females, although as Table 3-20 shows many more young males are affected. Predictably there are very few patients ≥65 years of age and there are relatively few open fractures or multiple fractures.

It is self-evident that the epidemiology of sports-related fractures will vary throughout the world depending on the degree of affluence, availability of resources, and the popularity of different sports. Thus, analysis of sports in the United Kingdom will not include sports such as baseball, American football, ice hockey, or cross country skiing. However, many sports are universally popular and during the year football accounted for 39.5% of the fractures, rugby for 13%, cycling and mountain biking for 11.8%, and the different winter sports for 10.1%. The overall incidence of sports-related injuries in males was 258.9/10^5/year with 51.2/10^5/year being recorded in females. In the 16- to 34-year-old male group the incidence of fractures related to football was 594.9/10^5/year with 212.2/10^5/year, 106.1/10^5/year, and 72.5/10^5/year being recorded in rugby, cycling and mountain biking, and winter sports. In the 16 to 35 female group the highest incidence of fractures followed winter sports at 29.2/10^5/year with the incidence following football and rugby both being 20.6/10^5/year. Either ladies do not indulge in mountain biking or they are better at it than males as there were no fractures!

Motor Vehicle Accidents

The assumption is often made by the lay public that most fractures are caused by motor vehicle accidents. However, Table 3-20 shows that this is not the case. It is likely that the number of fractures caused by motor vehicle accidents will be greater in other parts of the world, but in the developed world improved automobile design, speeding restrictions, and improved alcohol legislation have caused a reduction in the incidence of fractures. Overall motor vehicle accident fractures have a type B distribution with a unimodal peak in young males and Table 3-20

TABLE 3-21	The Epidemiology of Fractures in the Different People Involved in Motor Vehicle Accidents					
	%	n/10⁵/yr	Average Age (yrs)	M/F (%)	Open Fractures (%)	Multiple Fractures (%)
Cyclist	46.7	32.5	40.2	81/19	6	8.6
Motorcyclist	21.7	15.1	41	90/10	10.3	21.3
Pedestrian	17.5	12.2	48.8	62/38	3.2	24.4
Vehicle driver	10.2	7.1	47.2	76/24	8.1	34.8
Vehicle passenger	2.2	1.5	29.6	50/50	0	16.7

The prevalence, incidence, average age, and gender ratios are shown as are the prevalence of open fractures and multiple fractures.

shows that the overall incidence of fractures is $69.6/10^5$/year. The prevalence of multiple fractures and open fractures is second to those associated with falls from a height. Further analysis of the incidence of fractures following motor vehicle accidents shows that the overall fracture incidence in males is $115.1/10^5$/year and in females it is $28.9/10^5$/year. Obviously the incidence of motor vehicle–related fractures will vary with the precise involvement of the patient. Table 3-21 shows the basic epidemiology of the different types of involvement in motor vehicle accidents.

Cyclists

Table 3-21 shows that the highest incidence of fractures as a result of motor vehicle accidents occurs in cyclists with an overall incidence of $32.5/10^5$/year. In males the incidence is $55.7/10^5$/year and in females it is $11.7/10^5$/year. Overall there is a type C distribution affecting younger males and females, but clearly the incidence in males is about five times that of females. A review of the fractures sustained by cyclists indicates that they are mostly upper limb fractures with the commonest fracture being the clavicle (20.8%), followed by the proximal radius (16.7%) and the distal radius and ulna (12.5%). Ninety percent of the open fractures caused by cycling occur in the upper limb.

Motor Cyclists

Motor cyclists present with the second highest incidence of motor vehicle accident associated fractures at $15.1/10^5$/year (Table 3-21). The overall distribution curve is a type B curve indicating that these fractures are most commonly seen in young men. The incidence of fractures in males is $28.9/10^5$/year, compared with $2.9/10^5$/year in females. Obviously many fractures in motor cyclists are very severe and may be fatal, but of the fractures that present to hospital the commonest in the study year was the distal radius and ulna at 17.9%. This was followed by the clavicle (14.1%). However, a review of the open fractures shows that 62.5% affected the lower limb with the patella (25%) and tibial diaphyses (25%) being the most common.

Pedestrians

Table 3-21 shows that pedestrians tend to be older and to present with fewer open fractures, but there are more patients with mul-

tiple fractures than in motor cyclists. At first sight this might seem unlikely, but review of Tables 3-6–3-11 shows that an increased prevalence of multiple fractures correlates with increasing age and osteopenia. The overall incidence of fractures in pedestrians is $12.2/10^5$/year, but it is higher in males ($16/10^5$/year) than in females ($8.8/10^5$/year). The commonest fractures seen in pedestrians were metatarsal fractures (23.8%), finger phalangeal fractures (11.1%), and tibial and fibular diaphyseal fractures (11.1%). The patients presenting with tibial and fibular diaphyseal fractures had an average age of 38.3 years and the gender ratio was 86/14. Overall pedestrians show a type G distribution of fractures with bimodal peaks in males and a unimodal peak in older females.

Vehicle Drivers

Surgeons may be surprised that vehicle occupants present with the lowest prevalence of fractures in road traffic accidents (Table 3-21). Overall 12.5% of the fractures occurring in motor vehicle accidents were in vehicle occupants and this in fact is higher than in the 2007 to 2008 study year presented in the sixth edition of Rockwood and Green[24] when the figure was 11.2%. Vehicle drivers, like pedestrians, have a higher average age and about a third of patients will present with multiple fractures. The rate of open fractures is also higher than that seen in pedestrians. The overall incidence of fractures in vehicle drivers was $7.1/10^5$/year, the incidence in males and females being $11.5/10^5$/year and $3.3/10^5$/year, respectively. The overall fracture distribution curve for all vehicle occupants is a type H curve with bimodal distributions in both males and females. This is also the case with vehicle drivers, but there are too few vehicle passengers to calculate a curve accurately. The two commonest fractures seen in vehicle drivers were the metacarpal fracture (16.2%) and the clavicle fracture (13.5%).

Vehicle Passengers

Fractures in vehicle passengers are surprisingly rare, which presumably is a testament to improved car design, seatbelts, and airbags. Only 2.2% of fractures in motor vehicle accidents occurred in vehicle passengers and Table 3-21 shows that they were in younger adults. The gender distribution was equal and there were no open fractures. The commonest fractures were spinal fractures (37.5%), followed by fractures of the distal radius and ulna (25%). All of the patients who presented with multiple fractures had spinal and distal radial fractures.

Pathologic Fractures

Table 3-20 shows that 0.4% of fractures in the study year were pathologic, being caused by the presence of metastases. Not unexpectedly, this group was older and there were no open fractures or multiple fractures. Further analysis showed that 76% of the fractures occurred in the femur with 57.9% of the femoral pathologic fractures being proximal in location and the remaining 42.1% being in the diaphysis. The remaining fractures occurred in the humeral diaphysis (8%), proximal humerus (4%), radial diaphysis (4%), spine (4%), and the distal tibia (4%). Pathologic fractures have a type F distribution.

Stress and Spontaneous Fractures

The remainder of the fractures that were seen during the study year were stress or insufficiency fractures where there was no obvious cause. Only 0.3% of fractures were stress or insufficiency fractures, giving an overall incidence of $2.7/10^5$/year. These fractures have a type H distribution with the stress fractures tending to occur in younger adults and the insufficiency fractures in the older population. In this group of patients 63.6% of fractures were metatarsal fractures with an average age of 34.4 years and two (18.2%) occurred in the proximal femur with an average age of 82.5 years. If stress and insufficiency fractures are considered separately, stress fractures have a type C distribution and insufficiency fractures a type F distribution.

Other Modes of Injury

During the study year 1.6% of patients either did not know or were not admitting to the cause of their fractures. The average age of this group was 39.1 years and the gender ratio was 57/43. It is interesting to note that 47.6% of the fractures were of the metacarpal or finger fractures where direct blows or assaults are common!

Gunshot Injuries

Civilian gunshot fractures are less common in Europe than in the United States. The North American literature suggests that they have a type B distribution and most commonly occur in young males.[49] In the last edition of Rockwood and Green[26] an analysis of gunshot wounds treated in the R Adams Cowley Shock Trauma Center in Baltimore, Maryland, was undertaken. In this very busy Level 1 trauma center 6.5% of all fractures were caused by gunshot wounds in 2007. The data confirmed the type B distribution with 93% of the patients being male with an average age of 28 years. There were also racial differences with 83% of patients being Black and 15% being Caucasian. The average ISS was 16 and the mortality was 5%. Analysis showed that 7% of patients had an injury to their central nervous system, 30% had a thoracic injury, 33% had an abdominal injury, and 22% had associated spinal injuries. Table 3-22 shows the distribution of the gunshot fractures. The most common fractures occurred in the tibia and fibula diaphyses, pelvis, and hand.

TABLE 3-22	The Numbers and Prevalence of Gunshot Fractures Presenting to the R Adams Cowley Shock Trauma Center in Baltimore in 2007	
	No.	**%**
Tibia and fibular diaphysis	24	9.8
Pelvis	23	9.4
Hand	23	9.4
Forearm diaphysis	16	6.6
Lumbar spine	15	6.1
Femoral diaphysis	13	5.3
Scapula	11	4.5
Distal humerus	10	4.1
Distal femur	10	4.1
Cervical spine	9	3.7
Skull	9	3.7
Thoracic spine	9	3.7
Proximal forearm	9	3.7
Humeral diaphysis	8	3.3
Proximal humerus	8	3.3
Foot	8	3.3
Proximal femur	8	3.3
Face	7	2.9
Acetabulum	5	2
Clavicle	5	2
Proximal tibia	5	2
Ankle	4	1.6
Calcaneus	1	0.4
Distal radius	1	0.4

Specific Fracture Types

Clavicle

Table 3-3 shows that clavicle fractures account for about 4% of all fractures. Overall they have a type G distribution mainly affecting younger and older males and older females. This is shown in Tables 3-6–3-11. If clavicle fractures are subdivided according to their location within the clavicle, fractures of the medial and lateral thirds of the clavicle have a type A distribution while middle third clavicle fractures show a type G distribution. Table 3-23 shows that fractures of the medial third of the clavicle are rare and it should be remembered that in younger patients these fractures may involve the proximal physis. In this study year there was a similar prevalence of fractures of the middle and lateral thirds, whereas in the 2007 to 2008 year published in the seventh edition of Rockwood and Green[26] there was a higher rate of fractures in the middle third. This is likely to be coincidental, but as lateral third fractures tend to occur in older patients it is possible that they will become more common in the future.

TABLE 3-23 The Basic Epidemiologic Characteristics of Clavicle Fractures

	Prevalence (%)	Average Age (yrs)	Male/ Female (%)
Medial third	2.7	51.6	86/14
Middle third	48.6	37.9	77/23
Lateral third	48.6	49.6	62/38
Common Modes of Injury			
Fall (standing height)	40.5	56	54/46
Sport	25.3	28	91/9
MVA	22.2	41.1	74/26
Associated Fractures			
Scapula	2.3		
Spine	1.9		
Metacarpal	1.2		

Table 3-23 shows that standing falls, sport, and motor vehicle accidents are the commonest causes of clavicular fractures. However, analysis of the different fracture locations shows that 56.8% of lateral third fractures resulted from a standing fall, compared with 24.8% of middle third fractures. The commonest cause of middle third clavicle fractures is sport (34.4%), followed by motor vehicle accidents (29.6%). Cycling or motorcycling are clearly important causes of clavicular fractures and if one combines all types of cycling, it is apparent that cycling causes about one-third (33.6%) of middle third clavicle fractures and 25.7% of all clavicle fractures. Tables 3-4 and 3-5 show that open clavicle fractures are very rare and few patients who have clavicle fractures present with multiple fractures. Table 3-23 shows that when patients do present with multiple fractures, the other fractures tend to be spinal or upper limb fractures with 2.3% of patients with clavicle fractures also have a coexisting scapular fractures.

Scapula

Tables 3-3–3-5 show that scapular fractures are rare and are more commonly seen in males. Much of the literature relating to scapular fractures has come from Level 1 trauma centers and has reinforced the view that scapular fractures are invariably high-energy fractures, mainly involving the scapula body.[20] This is in fact not the case and scapular fractures actually have a type A distribution affecting younger males and older females. Table 3-5 shows that the average age of female patients with scapular fractures is in fact 74.5 years and that 77.8% were ≥65 years of age. Thus in females, scapular fractures are unquestionably fragility fractures.

Scapular fractures are divided into fractures of the body and neck, glenoid, acromion, and coracoid. The epidemiology of these fractures is shown in Table 3-24. Fractures of the acromion and coracoid are clearly very rare and fractures of the glenoid are in fact commoner than fractures of the body and neck and are often associated with a dislocation. Table 3-24 shows

that patients who present with fractures of the glenoid and patients who present with fractures of the neck and body have a similar average age. Table 3-24 also shows that the commonest causes of scapular fractures are standing falls, motor vehicle accidents, and low falls. However, further analysis shows that 66.6% of glenoid fractures were caused by low-energy standing falls and falls from a low height, whereas 41.7% of body fractures resulted from motor vehicle accidents or falls from a height although a further 33.3% of scapula body fractures followed a standing fall. The average age of this latter group was 61.5 years.

Open scapular fractures are incredibly rare and none were seen in the 15-year study detailed in this chapter. It seems likely that open scapular fractures associated with blunt injuries are essentially unsurvivable. The fact that most scapular fractures in younger patients follow high-energy injuries and that low-energy scapular fractures are associated with advanced age means that many patients who present with scapular fractures, will also have multiple fractures. Tables 3-6–3-11 show that multiple fractures are mostly commonly seen in males aged 36 to 64 years. Table 3-24 shows that the overall distribution of the fractures associated with scapular fractures is not dissimilar to that of the clavicle with upper limb and spinal fractures being most commonly seen.

Proximal Humerus

These are common fractures accounting for about 7% of all fractures (Table 3-3). Tables 3-4 and 3-5 show that the incidence in females is twice that seen in males. Overall they have a type F distribution mainly affecting older males and females and Table 20-8 shows that in patients aged at least 80 years of age, they are the third most common fracture. Table 3-25 shows the epidemiology of proximal humeral fractures. They have been divided according to the OTA classification[43] into

TABLE 3-24 The Basic Epidemiologic Characteristics of Scapular Fractures

	Prevalence (%)	Average Age (yrs)	Male/ Female (%)
Acromion	8.1	52	100/0
Coracoid	2.7	71	100/0
Glenoid	56.7	56	67/33
Neck and Body	32.4	50.3	83/17
Common Modes of Injury			
Fall (standing height)	40.5	64.1	47/53
MVA	27	43.9	100/0
Low fall (stairs)	13.5	56	100/0
Associated Fractures			
Clavicle	16.2		
Spine	10.8		
Distal radius	8.1		

TABLE 3-25	The Basic Epidemiologic Characteristics of Proximal Humeral Fractures		
	Prevalence (%)	Average Age (yrs)	Male/ Female (%)
Unifocal, extra-articular	64.2	65.2	37/63
Bifocal, extra-articular	27.4	67.4	18/82
Intra-articular	8.4	65.3	27/73
Fall (standing height)	85.4	68.4	27/73
Low fall (stairs)	5.4	61.1	27/73
Sport	4.2	45.4	65/35
Associated Fractures			
Proximal femur	46.2		
Distal radius	17.9		
Scapula	5.1		

unifocal extra-articular (Type A), bifocal extra-articular (Type B), and intra-articular (Type C) fractures. About two-thirds of proximal humeral fractures are unifocal extra-articular fractures and only about 8% are intra-articular fractures.

The majority of proximal humeral fractures occur as a result of a fall from a standing height, although in younger patients sporting injuries can cause proximal humeral fractures. As with other fractures around the shoulder, 30% of sports-related proximal humeral fractures were caused by cycling.

Table 3-14 shows that proximal humeral fractures are increasing in incidence. In 1993 the overall incidence was $47.2/10^5$/year and in 2000 the incidence of proximal humeral fractures was $65.1/10^5$/year, whereas in this study it was $92.4/10^5$/year. The incidence in both males and females has increased similarly. In males it has increased from $28.7/10^5$/year to $61/10^5$/year and in females it has increased from $63.8/10^5$/year to $120.3/10^5$/year.

As one might expect with a low-velocity fragility fracture, open proximal humeral fractures are extremely rare and there were none recorded in the study year. As with other fragility fractures there is an increasing prevalence of multiple fractures with increasing age. This is shown in Tables 3-6–3-11. Tables 20-9 and 20-10 show that the prevalence of multiple fractures continues to increase in advanced old age. Table 3-25 shows that the two commonest associated fractures are the other common fragility fractures of the proximal femur and distal radius, but about 5% of patients who have multiple fractures with a proximal humeral fracture will also have a scapula fracture.

Humeral Diaphysis

Humeral diaphyseal fractures have a type H distribution curve with a bimodal distribution in both males and females. However, it is likely that the distribution of these fractures is changing. Analysis of these fractures in 2010 to 2011 shows that there was a low incidence in young females (Table 3-9)

and with increasing aging of the population it seems likely that humeral fractures will show a type G curve in years to come. Table 3-3 shows that patients who present with humeral diaphyseal fractures have a very similar average age to those that present with distal radius and ulna fractures. It also shows that there is a very similar prevalence of patients aged ≥65 years and ≥80 years and that humeral diaphyseal fractures should now be considered as fragility fractures. The age of the population who present with these fractures accounts for the fact that 71.4% of humeral diaphyseal fractures follow a standing fall.

Table 3-26 separates the humeral diaphyseal fractures according to their location within the humerus or whether the fracture was periprosthetic or not. Fractures in the upper third of the humeral diaphysis tend to occur in older patients with 77.3% being caused by a standing fall and 18.2% by a direct blow or assault. Fractures of the middle third of the humerus tend to occur in younger patients, although 71% were still caused by a standing fall, with 12.9% being caused by sport, of which 50% were caused by horse riding. Fractures of the distal humeral diaphysis occurred in the youngest group of patients with 64.7% following a simple fall and 17.6% following a direct blow or assault.

Table 3-26 shows that 5.7% of the humeral fractures were periprosthetic with 50% occurring around a shoulder prosthesis and 50% around a previously inserted plate. These occurred in older patients and all followed a standing fall. There was only one pathologic fracture during the study year, but it is likely that these will become more common in the future.

The fact that humeral diaphyseal fractures are mainly low-energy fractures occurring in older patients means that the prevalence of open fractures is low and only one open fracture was seen during the study year. The prevalence of multiple fractures was surprisingly low for a fragility fracture and only one humeral diaphyseal fracture was associated with a distal radial fracture.

TABLE 3-26	The Basic Epidemiologic Characteristics of Humeral Diaphyseal Fractures		
	Prevalence (%)	Average Age (yrs)	Male/ Female (%)
Upper third	30	67.7	57/43
Middle third	40	52.4	46/54
Lower third	24.3	45.8	41/59
Periprosthetic	5.7	78.3	25/75
Common Modes of Injury			
Fall (standing height)	71.4	62.7	38/62
Direct blow/assault	11.4	40.4	87/13
Sport	8.6	31.2	83/17
Associated Fractures			
Distal radius	1.4		

TABLE 3-27	The Basic Epidemiologic Characteristics of Distal Humeral Fractures		
	Prevalence (%)	Average Age (yrs)	Male/ Female (%)
Extra-articular	50	54.1	54/46
Partial articular	35.4	61.5	29/71
Complete articular	14.6	66	29/71
Common Modes of Injury			
Fall (standing height)	72.9	65.8	23/77
MVA	10.4	37.4	100/0
Sport	6.3	43.3	100/0
Associated Fractures			
Proximal ulna	20		
Proximal radius	20		
Distal radius/ulna	20		

Distal Humerus

Distal humeral fractures in adults are comparatively rare with Table 3-3 showing that only 0.7% of fractures in the study year involved the distal humerus. Overall they have a type E distribution which may surprise some surgeons as much of the literature has concentrated on high-energy intra-articular fractures in younger patients. However, Table 3-5 shows that in females the average age is 67.4 years and 75% of the fractures occurred in patients aged ≥65 years. Thus distal humeral fractures should be regarded as fragility fractures.

Table 3-27 shows that the majority of distal humeral fractures are actually OTA[43] type A extra-articular fractures with only 14.6% of the fractures being type C intra-articular fractures. Even in this group it is interesting to note that there is a relatively high average age of 66 years. In fact 57.1% of type C fractures followed a standing fall in patients with an average age of 76 years and the remaining 42.9% were caused by motor vehicle accidents or falls from a height, but even their age averaged 52.7 years, suggesting that many of these fractures occur in fitter older patients.

In recent years much of the literature about distal humeral fractures in the elderly has concerned the argument regarding replacement or reconstruction of type C fractures, but these are relatively rare. The commonest subtype seen is the A2.3 simple extra-articular metaphyseal fracture which accounted for 25% of all the distal humeral fractures seen in the study year. The average age of this group of patients was 74.3 years and 91.7% were caused by standing falls.

Table 3-27 shows that 10.4% of distal humeral fractures occurred as a result of a motor vehicle accident. All occurred in cyclists and 16% were B1.1 partial articular fractures. Analysis shows that 40% of distal humeral fractures caused by motor vehicle accidents were associated with multiple fractures and 40% were open. Tables 3-4 and 3-5 show that open fractures are more commonly seen in males than females, but that multiple fractures are fairly common in both genders. Table 3-27 shows that patients who present with distal humeral fractures and who have multiple fractures tend to have fractures in the proximal forearm or distal radius.

Proximal Forearm

Proximal forearm fractures are relatively common with Table 3-3 showing that they account for 5.4% of all fractures. They are evenly distributed between males and females and overall they have a type D distribution. However, a review of the four basic types of proximal forearm fractures shown in Table 3-13 indicates that the epidemiology of proximal radial fractures is somewhat different from that of proximal ulna fractures and fractures of both the proximal ulna and radius. Radial head fractures have a type H distribution and radial neck fractures have a type A distribution. The remaining two fracture types, the proximal ulna and the proximal radius and ulna, have a type F distribution and should be regarded as fragility fractures.

Proximal radial fractures accounted for 74.3% of all proximal forearm fractures. Overall 63.3% occurred as a result of a standing fall, 12.8% from a motor vehicle accident and 12.5% as a result of a sporting injury. The average ages of these groups were 46.4 years, 40 years, and 29.6 years, respectively. Table 3-28 shows that patients with proximal ulna fractures had the highest average age of all patients who presented with proximal forearm fractures. Overall 66.6% of proximal ulna fractures followed a fall with the average age of the patients being 62.5 years. A further 13.1% were caused by sporting injuries, with the patients' average age being 34.8 years. Further analysis of the proximal ulna fractures showed that 92.9% were olecranon fractures and only 7.1% were coracoid fractures. Patients

TABLE 3-28	The Basic Epidemiologic Characteristics of Proximal Radial and Ulnar Fractures		
	Prevalence (%)	Average Age (yrs)	Male/ Female (%)
Proximal ulna	22.2	54.2	50/50
Radial head	59.5	42.4	44/56
Radial neck	14.8	42.4	44/56
Proximal radius and ulna	3.4	50.1	38/62
Common Modes of Injury			
Fall (standing height)	64	50.4	30/70
Sport	13	31.6	76/24
MVA	10.8	40.4	76/24
Associated Fractures			
Distal radius/ulna	20.5		
Carpus	10.2		
Bilateral proximal forearm	10.2		

with coracoid fractures have an average age of 34.5 years and clearly coracoid fractures are not fragility fractures.

Fractures of both the proximal radius and ulna are relatively unusual with only 3.4% of proximal forearm fractures involving both bones. Analysis showed that 61.5% occurred following falls from a standing height and that they had an average age of 54.5 years.

Tables 3-4 and 3-5 show that open fractures are relatively unusual in both males and females, but 11% of males and 7.9% of females had multiple fractures. Table 3-28 shows that 10% of these were bilateral proximal forearm fractures and that the other two commonly associated fractures were distal radial and carpal fractures.

Forearm Diaphyses

When all fractures are considered it becomes apparent that forearm diaphyseal fractures are relatively uncommon. Table 3-3 shows that they accounted for only 0.8% of the fractures seen in the study year. Table 3-29 shows a similar prevalence for isolated ulnar and radial diaphyseal fractures. This is different from the 2007 to 2008 year documented in the seventh edition of Rockwood and Green.[26] In this year there were more radial diaphyseal fractures, although the prevalence of fractures of both forearm bones was very similar. Table 3-29 shows that the patients' average age and gender ratio was similar in the three types of forearm fracture. However, the distribution curves are different. The overall distribution curve for forearm fractures is a type D curve affecting younger males and females and older females. However, isolated ulnar fractures have a type H distribution, while isolated radial fractures show a type A distribution. There were few females with fractures of both the radius and ulna, but in the last edition of Rockwood and Green[26] it was recorded that fractures of the radial and ulnar diaphyses had a type A distribution. This is still likely to be the case.

| TABLE 3-29 | The Basic Epidemiologic Characteristics of Radius and Ulnar Diaphyseal Fractures |

	Prevalence (%)	Average Age (yrs)	Male/ Female (%)
Ulna diaphysis	43.6	45.8	67/33
Radial diaphysis	40	49.5	68/32
Radius and ulnar diaphyses	16.4	46.9	78/22
Common Modes of Injury			
Fall (standing height)	49.1	60	52/48
Sport	27.3	32.2	93/7
MVA	7.3	40.7	100/0
Associated Fractures			
Metacarpal	25		
Finger phalanx	25		
Proximal tibia	25		

The common causes of these fractures are listed in Table 3-29, but if one analyzes the three fracture types separately it is apparent that the causes are very similar with 50% of ulnar diaphyseal fractures, 50% of radial diaphyseal fractures, and 44.4% of both bone fractures occurring as a result of a standing fall. A further 25% of ulnar diaphyseal fractures, 36.4% of radial diaphyseal fractures, and 11.1% of both bone fractures occurred as a result of a sporting injury. The main difference was that 33% of both bone fractures were caused by motor vehicle accidents compared with 4.2% of ulnar diaphyseal fractures and no radial fractures.

Analysis of the fracture morphology shows that there were no OTA[43] type C fractures and this probably relates to the diminishing prevalence of fractures associated with motor vehicle accidents. In fact 83.6% of forearm diaphyseal fractures were OTA type A simple fractures and 16.4% were OTA type B wedge fractures. However, the average ages were very similar at 47.2 years and 48.3 years respectively, although the gender ratios were 33/67 and 22/78 respectively, suggesting that the type B fractures were associated with higher-energy injuries. This is confirmed by examining the prevalence of fall-related fractures which accounted for 52.2% of type A fractures and 33.3% of type B fractures.

Tables 3-4 and 3-5 show that all the open forearm diaphyseal fractures occurred in males with 66.6% occurring in motor vehicle accidents. Table 3-29 shows that the prevalence of multiple fractures was relatively low and most were in the upper limbs.

Distal Radius and Ulna

Distal radial fractures are the commonest fractures to be treated by orthopedic surgeons. Table 3-3 shows that there was an incidence of 235.9/10[5]/year and Tables 3-4 and 3-5 show that the incidence is considerably higher in females than males. Tables 3-6–3-8 show that in males the incidence is highest in 16- to 35-year-old males although it rises to 231.7/10[5]/year in males ≥80 years, whereas Tables 3-9–3-11 show that the incidence in females increases with age. The incidence rises in the very elderly and in females ≥80 years of age the incidence is 1174.4/10[5]/year.

A considerable number of studies have been undertaken to look at the incidence of distal radial fractures in different parts of the world. However, it is quite difficult to compare the results of these studies. Different methods of data collection are used and there seems little doubt that some studies have concentrated on hospital admissions thereby missing the majority of patients who are treated on an outpatient basis. Authors have also used different age ranges, but even when similar age ranges are extracted from the papers there are large differences in incidence which are difficult to explain. Most studies come from developed countries with similar standards of living and medical systems, but despite this there is considerable variation in the incidence of distal radial fractures. Sakuma et al.[89] recorded the incidence of distal radial fractures in a small population in Japan in 2004, the population being aged between 8 and 91 years. They recorded the incidence as 108.6/10[5]/year. Analysis of the overall adult and pediatric incidence of distal radial fractures in Edinburgh in 2000 showed an incidence of 277.6/10[5]/year and it seems unlikely that the Japanese incidence will be that much lower, particularly when one realizes that the Japanese have the longest life expectancy in the world.

Analysis of fracture incidence in patients aged ≥35 years varies from 89/10⁵/year and 368/10⁵/year for males and females, respectively in the United Kingdom in 1997 to 1998[79] to 104/10⁵/year and 295/10⁵/year in Rochester, Minnesota, USA in 1989 to 1991[74] with the equivalent for our study year being 131.7/10⁵/year and 441.2/10⁵/year in males and females. A recent study from Texas, USA[80] of forearm and wrist fractures occurring between 2001 and 2007 in patients ≥50 years of age gives the incidence of forearm and wrist fractures as 78.2/10⁵/year and 256.9/10⁵/year in males and females, respectively. This compares with 136.9/10⁵/year and 631.8/10⁵/year in Edinburgh and 141.6/10⁵/year and 676.7/10⁵/year in South Sweden in 2001.[12] It seems likely that the social conditions in Edinburgh, Texas, and Sweden are not too dissimilar and as has already been pointed out the changes in incidences in apparently similar populations may simply reflect the methods used in collecting the data.

Table 3-30 shows that the majority of distal forearm fractures are distal radial fractures with only 1.7% being isolated distal ulna fractures. Both have a type A distribution, but more males present with distal ulna fractures and the average age is less. This is reflected in the fact that while 80.8% of distal radial fractures follow a standing fall, 42.8% of distal ulna fractures are caused by a direct blow or assault and only 28.6% follow a standing fall. Given the low-energy nature of the majority of these fractures, it is not surprising that Tables 3-4 and 3-5 show that very few are open. Analysis of the open fractures showed that 80% of them were Gustilo[47] type I and the average age of the patients was 64.2 years.

As one would expect with a fragility fracture, Tables 3-6–3-11 show that the prevalence of multiple fractures increases with age. Table 3-30 shows that the commonest coexisting

TABLE 3-30 | **The Basic Epidemiologic Characteristics of Distal Radial and Ulnar Fractures**

	Prevalence (%)	Average Age (yrs)	Male/Female (%)
Distal radius ± ulna	98.3	58.2	27/73
Distal ulna	1.7	41.5	48/52
Common Modes of Injury			
Fall (standing height)	79.9	63	18/82
Sport	9.5	32.3	80/20
Low fall (stairs)	3.8	50.3	34/66
Associated Fractures			
Proximal femur	22.7		
Bilateral distal radius/ulna	14.8		
Metacarpus	13.3		

TABLE 3-31 | **The Basic Epidemiologic Characteristics of Carpal Fractures**

	Prevalence (%)	Average Age (yrs)	Male/Female (%)
Scaphoid	72.7	33.6	66/34
Triquetrum	22.7	50.8	57/43
Hamate	2.1	29.7	75/25
Pisiform	1.6	34	67/33
Trapezium	1	43	100/0
Common Modes of Injury			
Fall (standing height)	58.8	43.5	48/52
Sport	18.6	25.8	92/8
Direct blow/assault	9.8	28.7	84/16
Associated Fractures			
Distal radius/ulna	38.5		
Proximal radius	38.5		
Metacarpus	7.7		

fractures in patients who present with a distal radial fracture is a fracture of the proximal femur. However, ten patients presented with bilateral distal radial fractures. Analysis of this group showed that the average age was 65.4 years, 90% followed a standing fall and the gender ratio was 10/90. Thus bilateral distal radial fractures would seem to be a sign of increasing frailty.

Carpus

Carpal fractures are relatively common and accounted for 2.8% of all fractures during the study year. Table 3-31 shows that scaphoid and triquetral fractures account for about 95% of all carpal fractures and that fractures of the other carpal bones are rare, although fractures of the hamate, pisiform, and trapezium were seen during the study year. Overall the carpal bones have a type A distribution curve, although fractures of the scaphoid, hamate, and trapezium tend to occur in younger males and have a type B curve. Triquetral fractures are somewhat different. They show a type A distribution curve involving younger males and older females.

Table 3-31 shows that overall about 60% of all carpal fractures follow a standing fall, with most of the remaining fractures being caused by a sporting injury or a direct blow or assault. Analysis of scaphoid fractures shows that 56% followed a fall, 20.6% were caused by sporting injury and 12% by a direct blow or assault. The equivalent figures for triquetral fractures were 63.6%, 15.9% and none, suggesting that the older ladies with triquetral fractures have a rather more refined lifestyle! It is interesting to note that 5.7% of scaphoid fractures occurred in road traffic accidents compared with 11.4% of triquetral fractures.

There were no open carpal fractures during the study year and Tables 3-4 and 3-5 show that relatively few patients presented with multiple fractures, although when they did Table 3-31 shows that about 80% were in the distal or proximal radius.

Metacarpus

Table 3-3 shows that during the study year metacarpal fractures were the second most common fracture after distal radial fractures with 11.2% of all fractures occurring in the metacarpus. This is different from the 2007 to 2008 fractures examined in the seventh edition of Rockwood and Green[26] where proximal femoral fractures were the second most common fractures seen. The change may point to a reduction in the incidence of proximal femoral fractures as has been suggested by a number of authorities, but it is not known if this is in fact the case. It may also be related to increased deprivation which plays a significant role in the incidence of metacarpal fractures.[29]

Tables 3-4 and 3-5 confirm the considerable difference in the incidence of metacarpal fractures in males and females. The incidence in males is about 445% greater than the incidence in females and metacarpal fractures are by far the commonest fractures seen in males with about one-fifth of all male fractures being in the metacarpus. Table 3-4 shows that they are associated with the second youngest average age of all male fractures after talar fractures and that only 4% occur in the ≥65-year group. They therefore have a type B distribution.

Table 3-32 shows that metacarpal fractures are least common in the thumb metacarpal and become commoner as one moves toward the ulnar border of the hand such that 17% of metacarpal fractures occur in the ring finger metacarpal and 60% in the little finger metacarpal. The average age is highest in patients who present with thumb metacarpal fractures and more females present with fractures of the ring and little finger metacarpals.

Figure 3-5 shows the prevalence of metacarpal fractures according to their location within the metacarpus. The three commonest sites for metacarpal fractures are all in the little finger metacarpal with 36.1% of all the metacarpal fractures

	V	IV	III	II	I
Phalanges	32.8	26.0	14.3	9.1	18.4
Metacarpals	60.6	17.0	7.9	8.6	5.6

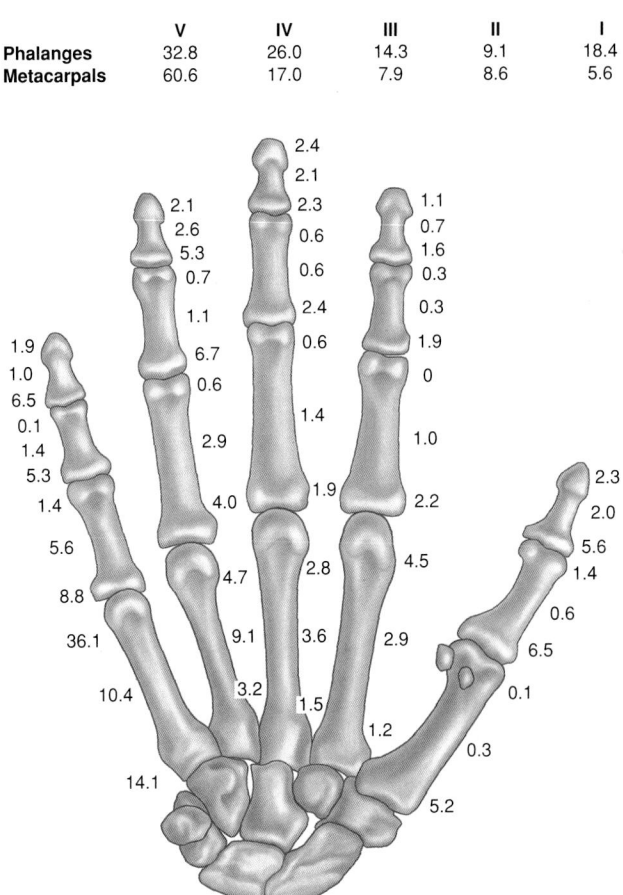

FIGURE 3-5 The prevalence of metacarpal and phalangeal fractures in the hand. They are divided into basal fractures, diaphyseal fractures, and fractures of the distal metacarpals and phalanges. The overall prevalences in each finger are also shown.

| TABLE 3-32 | **The Basic Epidemiologic Characteristics of Metacarpal Fractures** |

	Prevalence (%)	Average Age (yrs)	Male/ Female (%)
Thumb	5.8	39.7	87/13
Index	8.6	32	88/12
Middle	8.1	33.6	89/11
Ring	17	33.7	76/24
Little	60.6	32.4	78/22
Common Modes of Injury			
Direct blow/assault	58.1	26.8	88/12
Fall (standing height)	23.8	48.8	59/41
Sport	10.9	28	89/11
Associated Fractures			
Two metacarpals	62.7		
Three metacarpals	25.3		
Distal radius/ulna	11.9		

being "Boxers fractures" situated distally in the little finger metacarpal. There were 283 such fractures during the study year and Table 3-3 shows that if this fracture was regarded as a separate fracture type, it would be the ninth most common fracture to present to orthopedic surgeons. The commonest metacarpal fracture outwith the little finger is seen at the base of the thumb, although distal fractures of the index and ring fingers have similar prevalences.

Table 3-32 shows that 58% of metacarpal fractures are said to follow direct blows, although the prevalence may, of course, be higher. The mode of injury varies between metacarpals. In thumb metacarpal fractures 31.1% were caused by motor vehicle accidents and 31.1% by standing falls, with a further 20% following a direct blow or assault. In the little finger metacarpal 64.2% of the fractures followed a direct blow or assault, 23.6% followed a fall and 2.5% occurred as a result of a motor vehicle accident. The difference in the patient population is highlighted by comparing the average ages; 26.5 years for a little finger metacarpal fracture caused by a direct blow and 48.5 years for those fractures caused by a standing fall.

Tables 3-4 and 3-5 show that there is a very low rate of open fractures in both males and females. There is a similar prevalence of patients with multiple fractures, but most of the multiple fractures involve multiple metacarpals, although 11.9% of patients who presented with multiple fractures had distal radial and ulna fractures. Analysis of the 708 patients who presented with metacarpal fractures showed that 42 (5.9%) presented with two metacarpal fractures and six (0.8%) with three metacarpal fractures. By far the commonest location of the two metacarpal fractures was in the ring and little finger metacarpals with 26 (61.9%) of the double metacarpal fractures involving these two metacarpals. The average age of patients who presented with multiple metacarpal fractures was 39.4 years, compared with 31.7 years for those with single metacarpal fractures. The gender radios were 85/15 and 79/21, respectively. The causes of multiple metacarpal fractures were similar to those of single fractures with 56.2% of the multiple metacarpal fractures following a direct blow or assault, compared with 59.7% of the single fractures.

Finger Phalangeal Fractures

Table 3-3 shows that fractures of the finger phalanges account for about 10% of all fractures that are seen. They are the second most common fracture in males and overall they have a type B distribution because of the high incidence in young males. Tables 3-9–3-11 show that there is a fairly constant incidence of finger fractures in females of different ages. Table 3-33 shows an analysis of the epidemiology of fractures in the different fingers and as with metacarpal fractures (Table 3-32) it is apparent that the little and ring fingers are the most affected. The average age and gender ratio of the patients who present with fractures in the different fingers is not dissimilar and all have a type B distribution.

The causes of finger phalangeal fractures are very similar to that of metacarpal fractures, although more occur as a result of a sporting injury. Predictably the average age of the patients

injured by direct blows or sports injuries is lower than those injured by standing falls and more are male. The prevalence of fractures caused by direct blows or assaults is higher on the radial side of the hand with 34.3% and 33.9% of fractures of the little and ring fingers being caused by direct blows or assaults, compared with 47.4%, 50%, and 43.4% of fractures of the middle finger, index finger, and thumb, respectively. More fractures of the little and ring fingers were caused by falls and sports injuries.

Figure 3-5 shows a breakdown of the different fracture locations within each finger phalanx. It shows that 23.4% of finger phalangeal fractures are basal fractures of the proximal phalanxes. The average age of patients with these fractures was 56.3 years and 51.9% of them followed standing falls. A further 11.5% of fractures were diaphyseal fractures of the proximal phalanges. The average age of this group was 41.2 years and the most common cause of these fractures was a direct blow or assault which caused 39.3% of the fractures. Distal fractures of the proximal phalanges accounted for only 4% of the finger phalangeal fractures. The average age of this group was 41.6 years and 35.7% were caused by falls.

Analysis of the middle phalangeal fractures of the index, middle, ring, and little fingers shows that 16.3% of all the finger phalangeal fractures were basal fractures of the middle phalanges. The average age was 39.1 years and sport was the commonest cause (40.4%). Only 3.4% of phalangeal fractures were diaphyseal fractures of the middle phalanges. The average age of this group was 34.7 years. All followed a fall. Only 1.7% of finger phalangeal fractures were distal fractures of the middle phalanges. Again, all followed a fall, but the average age was 50.2 years. Fractures of the base of the distal phalanges of all five digits accounted for 21.3% of all the phalangeal fractures. The average age of the patients was 37.6 years and as one might expect with distal phalangeal fracture, a direct blow was the commonest cause accounting for 41% of the fractures. A further 8.4% of phalangeal fractures occurred in the diaphyses of the distal phalanges. The average age of this group was 43 years and 76.4% were caused by direct blows. The remaining 9.8% of phalangeal fractures were distal fractures of the distal phalanges. The average age of the patients was 35.5 years and 85.7% were caused by direct blows to the tips of the fingers.

Tables 3-4 and 3-5 show that open fractures of the phalanges are relatively common with the highest prevalence being seen in 36- to 64-year-old males. Unsurprisingly, the commonest site of the open fractures was the distal phalanges where 25.3% of the fractures were open.

Tables 3-6–3-11 show that in younger patients 6% to 9% of patients present with multiple fractures, although this rises with increasing age. The majority of the multiple fractures are upper limb fractures and Table 3-33 shows that about 55% of the other fractures are other phalangeal fractures. Eighteen (3.1%) of patients had two phalangeal fractures and seven (1.2%) had three phalangeal fractures. The average age of patients who presented with multiple phalangeal fractures was 55.4 years. The gender ratio was 50/50 and 50% sustained their multiple fractures following a fall with 41.6% occurring as a result of a direct blow.

TABLE 3-33 The Basic Epidemiologic Characteristics of Finger Phalangeal Fractures

Finger Phalanges	Prevalence (%)	Average Age (yrs)	Male/ Female (%)
Thumb	18.4	44.3	63/37
Index	9	38.9	58/42
Middle	14.3	39.3	64/36
Ring	25.8	38.9	60/40
Little	32.5	42.4	56/44
Direct blow/assault	39.1	39.1	61/39
Fall (standing height)	29.5	52.7	37/63
Sport	23.8	29.1	82/18
Associated Fractures			
Other finger fractures	55.8		
Distal radius/ulna	13.9		
Metacarpus	9.3		

Proximal Femur

There is considerable debate about the epidemiology of proximal femoral fractures in different parts of the world and this has already been outlined in the section on changing epidemiology. Table 3-15 illustrates some of the issues relating to the incidence of proximal femoral fractures in different countries. It highlights the different incidences in different parts of the world[2,19,66] and the higher incidences in Scandinavia.[6,59,86] As has already been discussed, it seems likely that some of the differences are attributable to different data collection techniques but there are also considerable differences in life expectancy, deprivation, and other medical and social comorbidities in different parts of the world. The worldwide differences in proximal femoral fracture incidence have recently been examined by Kanis et al.[59] Table 3-3 shows that proximal femoral fractures were the third most common fracture after distal radius and ulna and metacarpal fractures. The overall incidence was $145.5/10^5$/year, but Tables 3-4 and 3-5 show that the incidence varies considerably in both males and females and Tables 3-6– 3-11 show that they are the least common fractures in the 16- to 35-year age group but are the commonest fracture in the ≥65-year age group. Table 3-14 shows that the incidence in males has risen in the last 20 years as has the average age of males who present with proximal femoral fractures.

Table 3-34 shows that in the study year the majority of proximal femoral fractures were subcapital intracapsular fractures. The average age for subcapital and intertrochanteric fractures was similar although the average age for patients with greater trochanter fractures was lower and there were more males. Virtually all proximal femoral fractures are low-energy injuries and most are caused by a standing fall. Tables 3-4 and 3-5 show that some patients do present with multiple fractures and Table 3-34 shows that these are usually proximal humeral or distal radial fractures. Open fractures are extremely rare and will only be associated with high-energy injuries.

Overall proximal femoral fractures have a type F distribution and this is true of both intracapsular and extracapsular fractures. The very rare femoral head fracture is associated with hip dislocation and has a type B distribution. The section on dislocations indicates that four hip dislocations were admitted during the study year of which one (25%) had an associated femoral head fracture.

Femoral Diaphysis

There has been a considerable change in the epidemiology of femoral diaphyseal fractures in the last 100 years (Table 3-1). It was the femoral diaphyseal fracture that was largely responsible for the change in management of severely injured patients in a number of countries in the 1960s and 1970s. The mortality associated with nonoperative management of young people injured in motor vehicle accidents was unacceptable and new fracture techniques were adopted and specialized trauma centers were set up. As a result of this, it is still felt that the femoral diaphysis is mainly a young person's fracture, but this is simply not the case and in fact the femoral diaphyseal fracture is a fragility fracture. The change in epidemiology of femoral diaphyseal fractures is emphasized by comparing the age of the patients treated in our catchment area in 1991 with today's patients (Table 3-14).

In the previous two editions of Rockwood and Green[24,26] femoral diaphyseal fractures have been shown to have a type A distribution affecting younger males and older females, but the situation has undoubtedly changed and it is likely that these fractures now have a type G distribution. Tables 3-6– 3-11 show a higher incidence in younger males than younger females, but the incidence rises quickly with increasing age and Table 20-8 shows the incidence of femoral diaphyseal fractures in both patients aged ≥80 years. The incidence of femoral fractures in males aged 20 to 29 years in 2010 to 2011 was $8.5/10^5$/year but it would seem that this incidence is probably declining in many developed countries and it may well be that in years to come the femoral diaphyseal fracture will have a type F distribution.

Table 3-35 shows that femoral diaphyseal fractures have been divided according to whether they are subtrochanteric, diaphyseal, or periprosthetic. It shows that 69.5% of patients sustained their fractures in a standing fall, but if one simply looks at the subtrochanteric fractures, 76% were injured in a standing fall with a further 12% having a pathologic fracture. In the diaphyseal fractures 58.1% of the patients had a standing fall and 11.6% presented with a pathologic fracture. In the periprosthetic group 92.9% were injured as a result of a standing fall. Given the popular misconception that femoral diaphyseal fractures are mainly high-energy injuries, it is interesting that only 9.8% of the fractures resulted from motor vehicle accidents with 62.5% of them occurring in motorcyclists. The average age of this group was 47.6 years and all were male. An analysis of the periprosthetic fracture showed that all were around hip replacements and that 42.9% were in the proximal third of the femur with the remaining 57.1% being in the middle third.

TABLE 3-34	The Basic Epidemiologic Characteristics of Proximal Femoral Fractures		
	Prevalence (%)	Average Age (yrs)	Male/ Female (%)
Greater trochanter	0.9	64.8	57/43
Subcapital	59.1	79.9	30/70
Intertrochanteric	39.2	81.2	22/78
Periprosthetic	0.8	78	67/33
Common Modes of Injury			
Fall (standing height)	93.3	81.1	26/74
Low fall (stairs)	2.7	78.5	35/65
Pathologic	1.5	69.4	36/64
Associated Fractures			
Proximal humerus	41.8		
Distal radius/ulna	41.8		
Pelvis	4.7		

TABLE 3-35 The Basic Epidemiologic Characteristics of Femoral Diaphyseal Fractures	Prevalence (%)	Average Age (yrs)	Male/ Female (%)
Subtrochanteric	30.5	74.1	36/64
Diaphyseal	52.4	64.6	49/51
Periprosthetic	17.1	78.2	64/36
Common Modes of Injury			
Fall	69.5	77.6	35/65
Pathologic	9.8	65.1	75/25
MVA	9.8	47.6	100/0
Associated Fractures			
Pelvis	33.3		
Ankle	22.2		
Proximal humerus	22.2		

TABLE 3-36 The Basic Epidemiologic Characteristics of Distal Femoral Fractures	Prevalence (%)	Average Age (yrs)	Male/ Female (%)
Distal femur	72.2	63.8	15/85
Periprosthetic	27.8	74.4	20/80
Common Modes of Injury			
Fall (standing height)	86.1	70.5	13/87
Low fall (stairs)	5.5	79	0/100
MVA	3.6	26	100/0
Associated Fractures			
Bilateral distal femurs	50		
Ankle	25		
Proximal humerus	25		

The changing epidemiology of femoral fractures means that open fractures are now seen less frequently and there were none in females during the study year. Tables 3-6–3-8 show that in males the open fractures occurred in the 36- to 64-year group. Predictably multiple fractures associated with femoral diaphyseal fractures were much more common in males aged 16 to 64 years (Tables 3-6–3-8). Table 3-35 shows that patients who presented with multiple fractures most commonly had a pelvic fracture and two (2.4%) patients presented with bilateral femoral diaphyseal fractures.

Distal Femur

The distal femoral fracture should be regarded as the classic fracture of elderly ladies! Tables 3-3–3-5 show that they very rarely occur in males, but when they do it is usually in older patients. These fractures therefore have a type E distribution and should be regarded as fragility fractures. Nowadays, an increasing number of these fractures are periprosthetic and Table 3-36 shows that in 2010 to 2011 27.8% were periprosthetic fractures. This compares with 15.4% in 2007 to 2008. Review of the periprosthetic fractures shows that 70% occurred around knee prostheses with the remaining 30% occurring around long-stem hip prostheses. All periprosthetic fractures occurred as a result of a standing fall. Open fractures and multiple fractures are very rare. Tables 3-6–3-11 show that there were no open fractures or multiple fractures in males. Two (5.5%) older female patients had bilateral distal femoral fractures and only one (2.8%) female patient had an open fracture.

Patella

Patellar fractures are relatively rare with only 0.7% of the fractures in the study year occurring in the patella. Table 3-3 indicates that they are fragility fractures with an average age of 64.8 years and 55.1% occurring in patients ≥65 years. They have a

type F distribution. Table 3-37 shows that about three quarters result from a standing fall. There is a small male cohort in which patella fractures are caused by motor vehicle accidents. Analysis shows that 66.6% of these resulted from motorcycle or cycle injuries. In females 93.1% of patella fractures resulted from a standing fall. Intra-articular fractures accounted for 87.8% of all patella fractures.

Tables 3-4 and 3-5 show that open fractures of the patella are more common in males and 40% of the patella fractures caused by motor vehicle accidents were open. There was only one open patella fracture in a female injured in a fall. All the patients who presented with multiple fractures associated with a patella fracture were injured in motor vehicle accidents and Table 3-37 shows that most of the associated fractures were located in the lower limbs.

TABLE 3-37 The Basic Epidemiologic Characteristics of Patellar Fractures	Prevalence (%)	Average Age (yrs)	Male/ Female (%)
Extra/partial articular	12.2	47.2	67/33
Intra-articular	87.8	66.8	37/63
Common Modes of Injury			
Fall (standing height)	75.5	70.9	27/73
MVA	10.2	37.2	100/0
Low fall (stairs)	4.1	61	50/50
Associated Fractures			
Acetabulum	25		
Distal tibia	25		
Clavicle	25		

CHAPTER 3 The Epidemiology of Fractures and Dislocations   **97**

Proximal Tibia

Proximal tibia fractures accounted for 0.8% of the fractures seen in the study year. Tables 3-4 and 3-5 show a similar incidence in males and females, but an older average age in females. Proximal tibial fractures have a type H distribution with bimodal peaks in both males and females. The overall average age is 54.5 years which is similar to that of the distal radius and it is possible that in years to come, proximal tibial fractures will be regarded as fragility fractures. Table 3-38 shows that the majority of proximal tibial fractures were partial articular fractures, although the highest average age is seen in the complete articular fracture group. Table 3-38 shows that while standing falls in older patients were the commonest cause of proximal tibial fractures about a quarter were caused by sports injuries and occurred in younger adults. A variety of sports were involved but 33.3% of the fractures were caused by soccer.

Open fractures are relatively rare and there were none in females during the study year with the only open fracture being seen in a 67-year-old male. Multiple fractures were more commonly seen with 13.6% of the patients who presented with proximal tibial fractures having multiple fractures. The majority of multiple fractures (75%) resulted from high-energy injuries but two patients, with an average age of 75.5 years, sustained multiple fractures from a standing fall.

Tibial Diaphyseal Fractures

The changing epidemiology of tibial diaphyseal fractures has already been discussed in the section on changing epidemiology but a review of Table 3-14 emphasizes not only the declining incidence but also the increasing average age in males and the decreasing average age in females. It has also been pointed out that the declining incidence in of tibial fractures in older females will, in time, alter the distribution curve although the distribution curve has been kept as a type A.

TABLE 3-38 The Basic Epidemiologic Characteristics of Proximal Tibial Fractures

	Prevalence (%)	Average Age (yrs)	Male/Female (%)
Extra-articular	25.4	57.5	60/40
Partial articular	62.7	51.4	54/46
Complete articular	11.9	59.6	29/71
Common Modes of Injury			
Fall (standing height)	33.9	64.9	30/70
Sport	25.4	43	80/20
Low fall (stairs)	15.3	52.8	33/67
Associated Fractures			
Metacarpus	25		
Proximal humerus	12.5		
Femoral diaphysis	12.5		

TABLE 3-39 The Basic Epidemiologic Characteristics of Tibial Diaphyseal Fractures

	Prevalence (%)	Average Age (yrs)	Male/Female (%)
Simple	65.2	43.3	71/29
Wedge	24.6	42.1	70/30
Comminuted/Segmental	10.1	40	71/29
Common Modes of Injury			
Fall (standing height)	44.9	49.1	58/42
Sport	26.1	29.3	83/17
MVA	15.9	44.2	91/9
Associated Fractures			
Ankle	25		
Midfoot	25		
Femoral diaphysis	25		

Tibial diaphyseal fractures now account for only 1% of the fractures treated by orthopedic surgeons. Rapidly changing epidemiology means that the modes of injury are changing. In 1988 to 1990 37.5% of tibial diaphyseal fractures treated in our catchment area were caused by motor vehicle accidents, 30.9% by sports injuries, and 17.8% by falls from a standing height.[22] Table 3-39 shows that the situation is now radically different with 44.9% of patients now sustaining their tibial diaphyseal fracture as a result of a standing fall. However, sports injuries are still fairly common and further analysis shows that soccer was responsible for 44.4% of the sports-related tibial diaphyseal fractures in the study year. Open fractures of the tibia have always proved challenging to treat and they have been relatively common. As has already been pointed out, the prevalence of open tibial fractures is decreasing, although 20.2% of the tibial diaphyseal fractures in this study year were open. Tables 3-4 and 3-5 showed that there were fewer multiple fractures associated with tibial diaphyseal fractures than many surgeons might expect. This is because of the change in patterns of injury. Table 3-39 shows that when patients present with multiple fractures they tend to be in the lower limbs.

There is an important subgroup of tibial diaphyseal fractures, those with an intact fibula. In the seventh edition of Rockwood and Green[26] it was noted that they comprised 21.9% of the tibial fractures treated in 2007 to 2008. In the current study year only 11.6% of fractures had an intact fibula. These fractures have a type B distribution and generally occur in younger males.

Fibula

The isolated fibular fracture has received little attention in the orthopedic literature. These are fibular fractures that are not associated with a tibial diaphyseal fracture, a proximal or distal tibial fracture or an ankle fracture. They are relatively rare and accounted for only 0.6% of the fractures seen in the study

TABLE 3-40	The Basic Epidemiologic Characteristics of Fibular Fractures		
	Prevalence (%)	Average Age (yrs)	Male/ Female (%)
Proximal fibula	65.8	49.2	41/59
Fibular diaphysis	34.2	42	57/43
Common Modes of Injury			
Fall (standing height)	46.3	53.9	16/84
Sport	22	32.8	100/0
MVA	12.2	50.6	40/60
Associated Fractures			
Ankle	2.4		
Proximal tibia	2.4		
Femoral diaphysis	2.4		

TABLE 3-41	The Basic Epidemiologic Characteristics of Distal Tibial Fractures		
	Prevalence (%)	Average Age (yrs)	Male/ Female (%)
Extra-articular	33.3	58.9	50/50
Partial articular	45.2	31.3	68/32
Complete articular	21.4	36.8	89/11
Common Modes of Injury			
Fall (standing height)	38.1	56.8	38/62
Fall height	33.3	28.5	79/21
MVA	11.9	34.6	100/0
Associated Fractures			
Calcaneus	33.3		
Talus	22.2		
Ankle	22.2		

year. In the seventh edition of Rockwood and Green[26] they were defined them as having a type B distribution, but Tables 3-4 and 3-5 show that they actually occur in both younger males and older females and that they should be redefined as having a type A distribution.

There are two types of isolated fibular fracture with 65.8% being proximal fractures at or adjacent to the fibular neck. The remaining 34.2% are diaphyseal fractures. Table 3-40 shows that a fall from a standing height will cause fibular fractures in older females and 68.4% of the fractures caused by falls were in the fibular neck. This is very different from the sports-related fractures where 77.8% were fibular diaphyseal fractures which were probably caused by direct blows. All of the fibular fractures caused by motor vehicle accidents were located in the proximal fibula and 60% occurred in cyclists or motorcyclists. There were no open fractures and few multiple fractures, although those that did occur were in the lower limb.

Distal Tibia

Distal tibial fractures receive a lot of attention in the orthopedic literature, but they are comparatively rare, accounting for only 0.6% of all fractures. They have a type D distribution affecting younger males and older males and females. However, Table 3-41 indicates that the OTA[43] type B partial articular fracture tends to occur in younger patients with the OTA type A extra-articular fracture occurring in older patients.

As with other fractures, distal tibial fractures resulting from a standing fall tended to occur in older patients, with the higher-energy fractures resulting from motor vehicle accidents or falls from a height occurring in younger patients, most of whom are male. Seven (16.6%) of the distal tibial fractures were isolated posterior malleolar fractures. These patients had an average age of 29.4 years and a gender radio of 83/17. Four (57.1%) occurred following twisting injuries and three (42.9%) as a result of sporting accidents.

Tables 3-4 and 3-5 show that open fractures are relatively common particularly in males. Further analysis of the open

fractures showed that 83.3% occurred in males, 66.6% resulted from a fall from a height and 66.6% were OTA type C complete articular fractures. Tables 3-6–3-11 also show that multiple fractures are relatively common particularly in males and females aged 16 to 35 and in males aged 36 to 64. Table 3-41 shows that when present multiple fractures are commonly seen in the hindfoot and contralateral ankle.

Ankle

Ankle fractures are very common with Table 3-3 showing that they account for 10.2% of all fractures. Tables 3-4 and 3-5 show that the incidence is very similar in males and females, but the average ages are somewhat different with younger males and older females presenting with ankle fractures. They therefore have a type A distribution. However, different ankle fractures have different distributions curves. Lateral malleolar fractures have a type A distribution curve, whereas medial malleolar fractures have a type D distribution curve. Supra-syndesmotic fractures have a type C distribution curve and both bimalleolar and trimalleolar fractures have a type E distribution curve and should be regarded as fragility fractures. It is educational to note that Buhr and Cooke,[13] in 1959, drew attention to the number of bimalleolar and trimalleolar fractures in the elderly over 50 years ago.

It is likely that ankle fractures are increasing in incidence. In 2000 there was an incidence of $100.8/10^5$/year,[24] whereas it is now $137.7/10^5$/year. However Kannus et al.[61] have suggested that in Finland the incidence of ankle fractures is decreasing in the elderly, having reached a peak of $169/10^5$/year in 1997. They recorded an incidence of $137/10^5$/year in females and $100/10^5$/year in males in patients aged ≥60 years. Our figures for the incidence of ankle fractures in the ≥60-year group are $225.1/10^5$/year and $122.5/10^5$/year in females and males respectively, indicating a much higher incidence of ankle fractures in the elderly in Scotland than in Finland. The reason for these

TABLE 3-42	The Basic Epidemiologic Characteristics of Ankle Fractures		
	Prevalence (%)	Average Age (yrs)	Male/ Female (%)
Infrasyndesmotic	24.1	50.7	38/62
Transsyndesmotic	65.8	49.7	48/52
Suprasyndesmotic	10.1	40.2	51/49
Common Modes of Injury			
Fall (standing height)	79.8	51.9	40/60
Sport	11.2	32	78/22
Low fall (stairs)	4.3	45.5	42/58
Associated Fractures			
Metatarsus	23.8		
Calcaneus	14.2		
Spine	14.2		

TABLE 3-43	The Basic Epidemiologic Characteristics of Talar Fractures		
	Prevalence (%)	Average Age (yrs)	Male/ Female (%)
Avulsion, process, head	25	31	33/67
Neck	41.7	32.6	100/0
Body	33.3	24.5	100/0
Fall (standing height)	33.3	29	100/0
Sport	33.3	29	75/25
Direct blow/assault	16.6	17.5	100/0
Associated Fractures			
Midfoot	40		
Ankle	40		
Distal tibia	20		

differences is probably methodologic as the Finnish study only looked at inpatients.

Table 3-42 shows the ankle fractures divided according to the OTA classification.[43] It shows that type B transsyndesmotic fractures accounted for about two-thirds of all ankle fractures and that about 80% of all fractures occur as a result of a standing fall, although many of these fractures may well have occurred as a result of the twisting injury that preceded the fall. Overall 77.3% of Type A, 79.6% of Type B, and 68.1% of Type C fractures were caused by falls or twisting injuries. Examination of the Type C fractures shows that 20.8% were caused by sporting injuries. The average age of this group was 32.5 years and all were male. Tables 3-4 and 3-5 show that open ankle fractures and multiple fractures are relatively unusual. Table 3-42 shows that when multiple fractures occur they tend to be in the foot or the spine.

Talus

Talar fractures were the least common fractures seen in the study year, accounting for only 0.2% of the fractures (Table 3.3). This is less than in the 2007 to 2008 study year when 32 fractures were treated. There is no explanation for the difference which may simply be coincidental. Talar fractures are seen in young males and females and have a type C distribution. In Table 3-43 the talar fractures have been divided according to the OTA classification.[43] The avulsion fractures, process fractures, and head fractures have been combined together and the neck and body fractures have been recorded separately. Talar neck fractures are the most common and all fractures are seen in younger adults.

Talar neck and body fractures tend to be high-energy injuries with 44.4% occurring as a result of a fall from a height, although 33.3% were also caused by sports injuries. Given the severity of these fractures, it is not surprising that 8.3% were open fractures and that 41.6% of the patients presenting with talar fractures had multiple fractures. Table 3-43 shows that the multiple fractures were in the foot and distal tibia.

Calcaneus

Calcaneal fractures are relatively uncommon accounting for 0.9% of the fractures in the study year. Tables 3-4 and 3-5 show that they are more commonly seen in males, although there has been a recent increase of calcaneal fractures in older females and overall calcaneal fractures have a type G distribution. Buhr and Cooke,[13] in 1959, indicated that hindfoot fractures were "wage earners fractures" and mainly affected males. Kannus et al.[60] drew attention to the rising incidence of low-trauma fractures of the calcaneus and foot in Finnish patients aged ≥50 years, so it is clear that in the last 50 to 60 years more older patients have been getting calcaneal fractures.

In Table 3-44 calcaneal fractures have been divided into extra-articular tuberosity fractures, extra-articular body fractures,

TABLE 3-44	The Basic Epidemiologic Characteristics of Calcaneal Fractures		
	Prevalence (%)	Average Age (yrs)	Male/ Female (%)
Tuberosities	20	31.6	73/27
Extra-articular body	24.6	38.5	81/19
Intra-articular	55.4	45.6	71/29
Common Modes of Injury			
Fall height	56.9	33.1	86/14
Fall (standing height)	18.5	57.7	33/67
Low fall (stairs)	16.9	47	82/18
Associated Injuries			
Bilateral calcaneus	31.3		
Spine	31.3		
Ankle	12.5		

and intra-articular fractures, the latter being a fracture which has received considerable attention in the orthopedic literature in recent years. Because of this recent interest, the implication is that most calcaneal fractures are intra-articular, but Table 3-44 shows that extra-articular fractures are relatively common. Intra-articular and extra-articular calcaneal fractures have different distribution curves. Intra-articular fractures tend to present in younger males and they have a type B distribution. Extra-articular fractures have a type G distribution with older males and females also being affected.

The commonest mode of injury is a fall from a height. Tables 3-4 and 3-5 show that open fractures tend to occur in males and this study all open fractures were intra-articular fractures resulting from a fall from a height. As with other high-energy fractures, multiple fractures are not uncommon, particularly in males. Table 3-43 shows that patients who presented with multiple fractures usually had bilateral calcaneal fractures or spinal fractures. Five patients (8.3%) presented with bilateral calcaneal fractures. Their average age was 32.8 years, all were male and all had occurred as a result from a fall from a height.

Midfoot

Midfoot fractures are also comparatively rare and accounted for only 0.4% of fractures in the study year. Tables 3-6–3-11 show that they occur in younger patients and have a type C distribution. Table 3-45 shows that the cuboid bone had the highest prevalence of fractures and females were more commonly affected, with males presenting with more fractures of the cuneiforms and navicular. The overall modes of injury are shown in Table 3-45, but if one examines the bones separately, cuboid fractures were mainly caused by falls (27.3%) and sports injuries (27.3%), whereas navicular fractures were mainly caused by falls (50%) and cuneiform fractures by falls from a height (44.4%). Open fractures are rare, but Tables 3-4

TABLE 3-45	The Basic Epidemiologic Characteristics of Midfoot Fractures		
	Prevalence (%)	Average Age (yrs)	Male/ Female (%)
Cuboid	39.3	43	36/64
Cuneiforms	32.1	30.4	78/22
Navicular	28.6	42.6	75/25
Fall (standing height)	32.1	39.4	67/33
Fall height	25	32.3	100/0
Sport	17.9	32.3	60/40
Associated Fractures			
Metatarsus	57.1		
Multiple midfoot bones	42.9		
Talus	42.9		

TABLE 3-46	The Basic Epidemiologic Characteristics of Metatarsal Fractures		
	Prevalence (%)	Average Age (yrs)	Male/ Female (%)
Hallux	3.7	40.5	59/41
Second	8.2	41	39/61
Third	9.5	36.5	39/61
Fourth	9.7	43.8	36/64
Fifth	69	45.7	35/65
Fall (standing height)	71.6	47.4	26/74
Sport	8.8	26.9	73/27
Direct blow	8.6	37.7	50/50
Associated Injuries			
Other metatarsals	47.8		
Midfoot	8.7		
Ankle	8.7		

and 3-5 show that patients with midfoot fractures have a high prevalence of multiple fractures. Table 3-45 shows that these are usually fractures of the other midfoot bones, metatarsus, or talus.

Metatarsus

Metatarsal fractures are common and accounted for 6.6% of the fractures in the study year. Tables 3-4 and 3-5 show that they tend to occur in younger males and older females and therefore have a type A distribution. They are mostly commonly caused by a fall from a standing height with 83.1% of fractures in females being caused by a twist or a fall. This compares to 51.8% of male metatarsal fractures.

Table 3-46 shows that fractures of the hallux metatarsal were least commonly seen and only 17.6% of them were caused by a standing fall. A further 29.4% resulted from sport with 29.4% also being caused by direct blows or assaults. Metatarsal fractures become more common as one moves toward the lateral border of the foot and 69% of all metatarsal fractures affect the fifth metatarsal. The average age is higher and the majority occur in females. Further analysis shows that 78.8% of fifth metatarsal fractures follow a fall or a twisting injury. The average age of this group is 48.1 years and the gender ratio was 26/74.

The commonest site of a fifth metatarsal fracture is at the base of the metatarsal. There were 274 of these fractures, meaning that 58.9% of all metatarsal fractures and 87.7% of all fifth metatarsal fractures were basal fractures of the fifth metatarsal. This makes the fifth metatarsal base fracture one of the ten fractures mostly commonly seen by surgeons and they have a very similar incidence to distal fractures of the fifth metacarpal. Overall 81.2% are caused by twisting injuries or falls, the average age is 46 years and the gender ratio is 34/66.

Given the frequency with which metatarsal fractures occur, it is perhaps surprising that there were no open fractures.

Table 3-46 shows that the patients who presented with multiple fractures usually had multiple metatarsal fractures. Of these 31 patients, 11 (35.5%) had two fractures, 19 (61.3%) had three fractures, and one (3.2%) had four metatarsal fractures. The average age of the patients who presented with multiple metatarsal fractures was 43.6 years, the gender ratio was 24/76 and 61.3% had sustained a fracture following a twisting injury or a standing fall.

Toes

Toe fractures are relatively common accounting for about 3.5% of fractures in the study year. They have a type C distribution affecting younger males and females. Unsurprisingly, 61.8% were caused by direct blows.

Pelvis and Acetabulum

Fractures of the pelvis and acetabulum accounted for 1.7% of the fractures in the study year. There has been considerable interest in their management over the last 25 to 30 years and, as with some other fractures, the implication is that they occur as a result of high-energy trauma. Clearly some do, but Tables 3-6 and 3-9 show that the incidence of pelvic fractures in the 16- to 35-year age group is very low, although most were caused by high-energy injuries. The incidence rises with age such that pelvic fractures are the seventh most common fracture in males aged ≥65 years (Table 3-8) and the fifth most common fracture in females ≥65 years (Table 3-11). Overall pelvic fractures have a type E distribution, but if acetabular fractures are considered separately they have a type G distribution affecting younger males and females and older females.

Table 3-47 shows that in the study year about 86% of pelvic and acetabular fractures involved the pelvis and 14% the acetabulum. The average age of patients with acetabular fractures was slightly lower and the gender ratio of the two fracture types was markedly different. The modes of injury were as expected with the majority of fractures following standing falls, although

8.4% were caused by motor vehicle accidents. Tables 3-4 and 3-5 show that there is a high prevalence of patients with multiple fractures and these obviously usually occur in high-energy injuries. Table 3-47 shows that the associated fractures are usually lower limb fractures.

Tables 3-4 and 3-5 show that open pelvic fractures are rare with none being seen in females during the study year. They are high-energy injuries and are associated with a significant mortality. Data from a Level 1 Trauma Center in the United States[7] indicates that even in specialized trauma centers the prevalence of open pelvic fractures is low. In a 10-year study period they admitted 3,053 pelvic fractures, of which 52 (1.7%) were open. Of these 43 (82.7%) were in males. They commented that motorcycle injuries were the commonest cause of open pelvic fractures.

Spinal Fractures

The incidence of vertebral fractures during the study year was not analyzed because of the difficulty in retrieving them and the impossibility of producing accurate figures. It seems likely that spinal fractures are by far the commonest fracture that occurs because osteoporotic fractures of the spine are extremely common and the majority are never seen by a doctor as many elderly ladies merely accept a bit more back pain!

Table 3-48 shows an analysis of the spinal fractures that were admitted during the study year. Most were thoracolumbar and were caused by a fall from a height or a standing fall. The majority were seen in males, but as has already been stated many elderly females sustain thoracolumbar fragility fractures, but do not seek medical help. In Level 1 Trauma Centers thoracolumbar fractures have a Type A distribution but overall Table 3-13 shows a Type F distribution as there are so many elderly patients who have this fracture. Cervical spine fractures have a type H distribution. Open spinal fractures are extremely unusual and one must assume that open spinal fractures are often fatal. Overall 57.5% of the patients admitted with

TABLE 3-47	The Basic Epidemiologic Characteristics of Pelvic and Acetabular Fractures		
	Prevalence (%)	Average Age (yrs)	Male/ Female (%)
Pelvis	85.7	77.5	21/79
Acetabulum	14.3	64.5	88/12
Common Modes of Injury			
Fall (standing height)	82.4	81.3	22/78
MVA	8.4	51.4	70/30
Sport	3.4	37.5	50/50
Associated Injuries			
Femoral diaphysis	16.6		
Distal tibia	16.6		
Calcaneus	11.1		

TABLE 3-48	The Basic Epidemiologic Characteristics of Spinal Fractures		
	Prevalence (%)	Average Age (yrs)	Male/ Female (%)
Cervical	6.7	68.4	57/43
Thoracic	42.3	57.1	61/39
Lumbar	51	47	70/30
Common Modes of Injury			
Fall height	26.9	36	86/14
Fall (standing height)	23.1	69.7	71/29
Low fall	22.1	67	83/17
Associated Injuries			
Two spinal fractures	20.6		
Calcaneus	10.3		
Distal tibia	8.8		

spinal fractures had multiple fractures and Table 3-48 shows that these were usually multiple spinal fractures or fractures of the distal tibia and hindfoot.

Cooper et al.[21] estimated the age and gender-adjusted incidence of clinically diagnosed vertebral fractures, between 1985 and 1989, in the United States as 117/10^5/year. Grados et al.[45] analyzed the prevalence of vertebral fractures in elderly French women. They found that 22.8% of women with an average age of 80.1 years had a vertebral fracture. The prevalence and the number of fractures increased with age such that 41.4% of women aged ≥85 years had vertebral fractures. Recently attempts have been made to assess the frequency of vertebral fractures in postmenopausal females using radiologic techniques. El Moghraoui et al.[34] studied 228 postmenopausal women and showed that 25.6% had vertebral fractures. Ferrar et al.[40] undertook a similar study in premenopausal and postmenopausal women. They found vertebral fractures in 1.4% of the premenopausal women and in 6.8% of the postmenopausal women. A further 3% of the postmenopausal women developed vertebral fractures within 6 years. A Dutch study[100] showed that 30.7% of women ≥50 years had a previously undiagnosed vertebral fracture. Obviously these studies had different results, but if one assumes a 25% incidence of vertebral fractures in women ≥50 years, the overall incidence of these fractures is about 18 times the incidence of all other fractures in this segment of the population. Clearly further work is required!

Epidemiology of Adolescent Fractures

There is very little information available about adolescent fractures.[75] This is because the epidemiologic studies tend to concentrate on adults or pediatric fractures with a dividing age of 14, 16, or 18 years. Unfortunately, adolescent fractures are lost in the division. They are an important group because fractures in adolescent males in particular are common and the curves shown in Figure 3-2 do not emphasize this. To study adolescent fracture epidemiology, the epidemiologic data from the year 2000, which was presented in the sixth edition of Rockwood and Green,[24] was combined with the pediatric data from the same year,[85] Adolescent fractures were defined as being between 10 and 19 years of age. Table 3-49 shows the incidences of different fractures in the adolescent population. It can be seen that there is a significant rise in the incidence of adolescent fractures from 10 to 19 years of age compared with the incidences of fractures in children and adults. Male adolescents in 2000 had a fracture incidence of 3,830/10^5/year. There was a progressive decrease in fracture incidence in boys after 13 years and in girls after 11 years and at 19 years of age the fracture incidence in males was 3.6 times that in females. The overall incidence in adolescents in 2000 was 2,430/10^5/year and the gender ratio was 72/28.

Table 3-49 shows the incidence of the different fractures seen in children, adolescents, and adults in 2000. What is striking is the very high incidence of fractures of the distal radius, finger phalanges, metacarpus, clavicle, metatarsus, and ankle in adolescents. Some fractures have a lower incidence in adolescents. These tend to be fragility fractures although

TABLE 3-49 The Incidence of Fractures in Adolescents, Children, and Adults in 2000

	Adolescents (10–19 yrs)	Children (0–13 yrs)	Adults (≥14 yrs)
Distal radius	659	689.7	195.2
Finger phalanges	439.9	294.7	107.3
Metacarpus	405.3	111.8	130.3
Clavicle	139.8	137.9	36.5
Metatarsus	132.7	99.3	75.4
Ankle	118.6	60.6	100.8
Toe phalanges	110.1	63.7	39.6
Carpus	69.2	19.9	29.7
Forearm diaphysis	63.5	111.8	13.8
Proximal forearm	55.1	59.6	55.5
Tibial diaphysis	52.2	44.9	21.5
Distal tibia	35.3	33.4	7.9
Distal humerus	32.5	166.2	5.8
Proximal humerus	29.7	38.7	63
Spine	12.7	5.2	7.5
Proximal tibia	11.3	4.2	13.3
Humeral diaphysis	11.3	5.2	12.9
Patella	9.9	4.2	10.7
Pelvis	9.9	4.2	17
Femoral diaphysis	8.5	16.7	10.3
Calcaneus	7.1	2.1	13.7
Midfoot	5.7	4.2	5
Talus	5.7	1	3.2
Proximal femur	5.7	1	129.4
Distal femur	2.8	5.2	4.5
Scapula	2.8	0	3.2
	2,430.2	1,986.5	1,113.3

Data used in this Table is from Court-Brown and Caesar[24] and Rennie et al.[85] Incidence is n/10^5/year.

calcaneal fractures are also rare in the adolescent period. In other fractures such as distal humeral fractures the adolescent group is clearly midway between the high incidence seen in childhood and the lower incidence seen in adulthood. Menon et al.[75] divided the adolescents into male and female junior and senior adolescents of 10 to 14 years and 15 to 19 years. They examined the influence of social deprivation in these groups and showed a correlation between social deprivation and fracture incidence in senior male and female adolescents and junior male adolescents. They also found that social deprivation was an independent predictor of fractures of the hand in senior adolescent males, fractures of the upper limb in junior adolescent males and in fractures of the upper limb and distal radius in senior adolescent females.

THE EPIDEMIOLOGY OF DISLOCATIONS

Paul Hindle and Eleanor K. Davidson

This is the first edition of Rockwood and Green to discuss the overall epidemiology of dislocations. Obviously the assessment of their epidemiology is subject to the same methodologic considerations as were discussed in the section on the epidemiology of fractures. As with fractures there are relatively few hospitals with a captive, well-defined population that allows for accurate epidemiologic assessment. Thus surgeons have often employed an overview of emergency department admissions[102] or they have analyzed insurance company records[11] or, in the case of shoulder and knee dislocations, the records of the United States military.[53,81] Clearly this will define epidemiology in a particular, usually younger, subset of the population but not the whole population. To our knowledge no one has, as yet, attempted to assess the epidemiology of dislocations by postal questionnaire!

There are some other complications when assessing the epidemiology of dislocations that one is not faced with when estimating fracture epidemiology. It can be subjectively difficult to differentiate between a subluxation and a dislocation and one simply has to accept the surgeon's view. This is a particular problem in situations such as fracture dislocations of the ankle or finger joints where, because of the fracture, there may be a significant subluxation. The other issue which can prove impossible to resolve is whether the joint was dislocated before a well-meaning doctor, physical therapist, or bystander reduced it. Clearly some of the joints will have been dislocated but others will not have been.

In this assessment of the epidemiology of dislocations we have examined the incidence of dislocations in the Edinburgh catchment area in a 1-year period between November 2008 and October 2009. We have included both children and adults treated during the year. Unlike the fracture epidemiology assessment this was a retrospective study with the data being obtained from the three hospitals in the Edinburgh area that deal with adult and childhood trauma or provide an emergency minor injury service. The question of whether a dislocation was present prior to a prehospital reduction was resolved as best as it could be by careful analysis of the clinical records. However this is a persistent problem with the assessment of dislocations and we accept that there might be some errors.

It should be emphasized that there are very few studies of the overall epidemiology of dislocations. Yang et al.[104] studied the incidence of dislocations in Taiwan between 2000 and 2005 using data from their National Health Insurance Program. They analyzed a randomly selected 1 million people from the National database stating that the demographics of the selected population was similar to the overall Taiwanese population. They estimated the incidence of dislocations of the shoulder, elbow, wrist, fingers, hip, knee, ankle, and foot during each year between 2000 and 2005 and noted that the incidence rose annually. They also analyzed the dislocations to see if they were simple dislocations or fracture dislocations and they monitored the prevalence of recurrent dislocations. Their overall average incidence of dislocations was 42.1/10⁵/year which is relatively low and their reported incidence of dislocations of different joints is lower than that of many other studies. Thus, as with the incidence of fractures, one does not know if there is a different incidence of dislocations around the world or if the different methodologies used to assess epidemiology give different results.

Brinker and O'Connor,[11] in their insurance-based study in the United States looked at the common dislocations referred to orthopedic surgeons. They found that the commonest dislocation was the patellofemoral joint which accounted for 55% of their dislocations and that 78% of their dislocations involved the patellofemoral, shoulder, and acromioclavicular joints. In the section on the epidemiology of fractures it was pointed out that the average age of their capitated population was low and it seems unlikely that it represents the complete population.

The basic epidemiology of the dislocations treated in the 1-year study period is shown in Table 3-50. It shows that the overall incidence was 157.4/10⁵/year with an incidence of 188/10⁵/year in males and 128/10⁵/year in females. There were 50 dislocations in children and adolescents <15 years in the study giving an overall incidence of 48.9/10⁵/year for this group and an incidence of 53.6/10⁵/year in males and 44.1/10⁵/year in females. The overall incidence of dislocations in adults was 178.5/10⁵/year with 215.9/10⁵/year being recorded in males and 145.2/10⁵/year in females. Table 3-50 shows the numbers, prevalence, incidence, average age, and gender ratio for all dislocations in the population. The distribution curve for all dislocations is also shown as is the percentage of patients ≥65 years and ≥80 years. It should be noted that because dislocations of prosthetic hips are so common they have been included in the analysis. However if only dislocations of native joints are considered the overall incidence is 138.4/10⁵/year and the average age is 39.3 years. The percentage of patients ≥65 years is 15.5% with 5.1% of patients ≥80 years. The gender ratio changes to 62/38.

Shoulder Dislocations

Shoulder dislocations are the commonest dislocations that present to orthopedic surgeons. In the study year we had an overall incidence of 51.2/10⁵/year but this covered both primary and recurrent dislocations. The incidence in males was 63.1/10⁵/year and in females it was 40.2/10⁵/year. Table 3-50 shows that the distribution curve is Type H (Fig. 3-3) with bimodal peaks in both males and females. Table 3-50 shows that with the exception of dislocations of prosthetic hips shoulder dislocations have the highest prevalence of patients ≥80 years. A review of the fracture dislocations that occurred during the study year showed that they have a different distribution curve. These tend to occur in older patients and they have a Type F curve affecting older males and females (Fig. 3-3). It is well established that posterior dislocations are much less common than anterior dislocation and in the study year the incidence of posterior dislocations was 2.4/10⁵/year.

It is important to differentiate between primary and secondary or recurrent dislocations when considering the epidemiology. In the study year 58% of the shoulder dislocations were primary and the remaining 42% were recurrent. Thus the incidence of primary dislocations was 29.7/10⁵/year and the incidence of recurrent dislocations was 21.5/10⁵/year. These figures

TABLE 3-50 **The Prevalence, Incidence, and Epidemiologic Characteristics of Different Dislocation.**

Dislocation	No.	%	n/10⁵/yr	Average Age (yrs)	≥65 yrs (%)	≥80 yrs (%)	M/F	Distribution Curve
Shoulder	317	32.5	51.2	43	23.6	9.4	59/41	H
Hand (MCPJ, PIPJ, and DIPJ)	185	19	29.9	40.7	13.5	5.9	79/21	G
Patellofemoral	134	13.8	21.6	24.8	2.2	0	51/49	C
Prosthetic hip	114	11.7	19	75.9	87.7	35.1	30/70	F
Ankle	71	7.3	11.5	49.8	31	4.2	30/70	H
Acromioclavicular	55	5.6	8.9	37.1	5.4	0	87/13	B
Elbow	37	3.8	5.5	33.4	2.7	0	49/51	C
Toes (MTPJ, PIPJ, and DIPJ)	33	3.4	5.3	35.5	9.1	0	64/36	H
Carpometacarpal	9	0.9	1.5	27.2	11.1	0	67/33	C
Native Hip	4	0.4	0.6	22.5	0	0	75/25	C
Tarsometatarsal	4	0.4	0.6	25.5	0	0	75/25	C
Knee	3	0.3	0.5	43	0	0	67/33	C
Perilunate	3	0.3	0.5	25.7	0	0	100/0	B
Distal radioulnar	2	0.2	0.3	44	0	0	50/50	?
Sternoclavicular	2	0.2	0.3	15.5	0	0	50/50	?
Subtalar	1	0.1	0.2	47	0	0	0/100	?
	974	100	157.4	43	23.9	8.6	57/43	H

The distribution curves are shown in Figure 3-3

are very similar to those published by Liavaag et al.[68] who analyzed the incidence of shoulder dislocations in Oslo, Norway in 2009. They had an overall dislocation rate of 56.3/10⁵/year with a primary dislocation rate of 26.2/10⁵/year. Their male and female dislocation rates were a little different from ours at 82.2/10⁵/year and 30.9/10⁵/year, respectively.

Liavaag et al.[68] drew attention to the differences in the published rates of shoulder dislocation over the last 40 years. Some researchers have investigated specific groups in the population. An example is Owen et al.[81] who published an overall incidence of 435/10⁵/year in the United States military. However other authors have looked at their whole population. Simont et al.[92] published an incidence of 11.2/10⁵/year in males and 5/10⁵/year in females in Olmsted County, Minnesota in 1970 to 1979. Kroner et al.[65] published an incidence of 12.3/10⁵/year in 1989 and Zacchilli and Owens[105] reported an incidence of 23.9/10⁵/year in 2002 to 2009 using a randomized sample of US hospitals with emergency departments. They had fewer elderly patients with shoulder dislocations than seen in Oslo or Edinburgh. They were not able to document recurrence and they stated that only 2.1% of their dislocations were recurrent. This would seem to be an underestimate of the prevalence of recurrent dislocations but it may well be that they mainly recorded primary dislocation which would explain the lower incidence of dislocations.

It may well be that dislocations, like fractures, are increasing in incidence. There are an increasing number of older active

people in most communities and it therefore seems logical to assume that the rate of dislocations, such as shoulder dislocations, is rising. Simont et al.[92] in 1970 to 1979 noted that 15.2% of his patients were ≥40 years whereas Liavaag et al.[68] in 2009 found that 39.5% of his patients were ≥40 years of age. Presumably this trend will continue.

Sternoclavicular and Acromioclavicular Dislocations

There were only two sternoclavicular dislocations during the study year giving an incidence of 0.3/10⁵/year. However acromioclavicular dislocations are considerably more common and accounted for 5.6% of the dislocations. Type I dislocations were excluded from analysis as they are simply joint sprains. However we have included Type II subluxations as they are usually referred to as dislocations. The overall incidence was 8.9/10⁵/year and these dislocations have a Type B distribution being commoner in young males. Very few occur in females.

Analysis of the severity of the acromioclavicular dislocations during the study year shows that there were no Type VI dislocations but 28% of the dislocations were Type II, 37% were Type II, 2% were Type IV, and 33% were Type V.

Elbow Dislocations

Table 3-50 shows that elbow dislocations are relatively uncommon with an incidence of 5.5/10⁵/year. Overall we believe that simple dislocations of the elbow, which do not have an associated fracture, have a Type C distribution affecting young males and females. However in the study year we collected both simple fractures and fracture dislocations and the fracture dislocations had a Type G distribution with a bimodal distribution in males and a unimodal distribution in older females. Thus the fractures tend to occur in older patients. Of the 35 patients who had confirmatory radiographs 28 (80%) had a dislocation of both the humeroulnar and radiocapitellar joints with the remaining 7 (20%) simply having a dislocation of the radiocapitellar joint.

A review of the complete elbow dislocations involving both joints showed that in 2 (7.1%) there was anterior displacement with posterior displacement being seen in the other 26 (92.3%) dislocations. Fifteen (53.6%) of the elbow dislocations were associated with a fracture. Four (57.1%) of the radiocapitellar dislocations were associated with a fracture. Two (5.4%) of the elbow dislocations were open.

In a previous analysis of simple elbow dislocations over a period of 10 years in Edinburgh the overall incidence was noted to be 2.9/10[5]/year.[1] The average patient age was 38.8 years and the gender ratio was 54/46. The main causes of simple dislocations in males were a standing fall (46%) or sport (24%) with 71% of dislocations in females being caused by a standing fall. Stoneback et al.[96] analyzed the incidence of simple elbow dislocations in the United States. They had a slightly higher overall incidence at 5.21/10[5]/year and noted that the incidence was similar in males and females at 5.26/10[5]/year in males and 5.16/10[5]/year in females. Most of the dislocations occurred as a result of sports or gymnastic activity. Yang et al.[104] reported an incidence of 7.7/10[5]/year in Taiwan but it is likely that these included fracture dislocations.

Wrist and Hand Dislocations

Table 3-50 shows that dislocations of the wrist and hand are relatively common with an overall incidence of 32.2/10[5]/year. Dislocations of the fingers are by far the most common and it is surprising that there is comparatively little written about these injuries. In this study year there were only two dislocations of the distal radioulnar joint and little useful information could be gained from them. In the study year documented in the section on the epidemiology of fractures there were three Galeazzi fractures associated with distal radioulnar dislocation. All occurred in males with an average age of 29 years. The overall incidence of Galeazzi fractures is therefore 0.6/10[5]/year.

There were three perilunate dislocations giving an overall incidence of 0.5/10[5]/year although all occurred in adults and therefore the adult incidence was 0.6/10[5]/year. All were associated with carpal or distal radial fractures but it is well recognized that carpal dislocations can occur without an associated fracture. All occurred in young males and the distribution curve is therefore type B. There were nine complete carpometacarpal dislocations. Carpometacarpal subluxations are more commonly seen but these were not included. As with most hand injuries

these occurred in young adults and they had a type C distribution. Of the nine dislocations five (55.6%) were single and the remaining four involved two or three joint. Five (55.6%) had an associated fracture.

The second most common dislocation, after the shoulder dislocation is that of the joints of the fingers. The overall incidence of dislocations in all the metacarpophalangeal and interphalangeal joints is 29.9/10[5]/year with the incidence in males and females being 59.9/10[5]/year and 12.1/10[5]/year. There is a bimodal distribution in males and a unimodal distribution affecting older females. Hand dislocations therefore have a type G curve. Overall 6.4% of the dislocations occurred in patients <15 years and the overall incidence in this group was 11.8/10[5]/year with incidences of 13.4/10[5]/year and 10/10[5]/year being recorded in males and females. In patients ≥15 years the overall incidence was 35.7/10[5]/year with the incidences in males and females being 59.9/10[5]/year and 14.3/10[5]/year. There were 22 (11.9%) open injuries and 60 (32.4%) fracture dislocations giving fracture dislocations of the hand an overall incidence of 11.6/10[5]/year.

Figure 3-6 shows the prevalence of dislocations in the different joints of the hand. It can be seen that 59.4% of all the

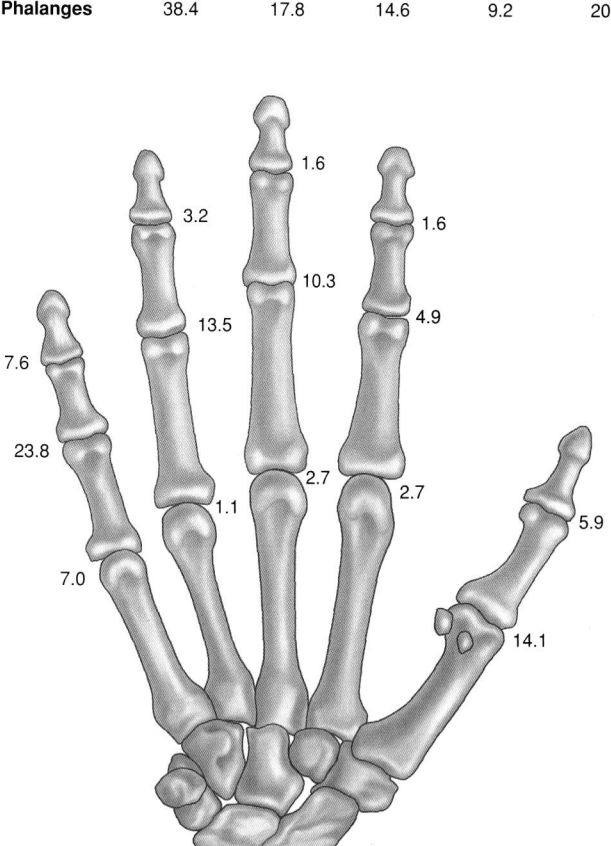

FIGURE 3-6 The prevalence of metacarpophalangeal and interphalangeal dislocations. The prevalences in each finger are also shown.

dislocations involved the joints of the thumb or little finger with the highest dislocation rates being in the proximal inter-phalangeal joint of the little finger, the metacarpophalangeal joint of the thumb and the proximal interphalangeal joint of the ring finger. Figure 3-6 shows that 58.4% of all hand dislo-cations affect the proximal interphalangeal joints of the fingers or the interphalangeal joint of the thumb, 27.6% occur in the metacarpophalangeal joints and 14% at the distal interphalan-geal joints. There was no significant difference in the average ages or the gender ratios of the patients relative to which digit was affected.

The incidence of dislocations in this study is considerable higher than that recorded by Yang et al.[104] in Taiwan between 2000 and 2005 who found in incidence of finger dislocations of $4.6/10^5$/year. Mall et al.[71] studied the incidence of dislocations in American football players and showed that subluxations or dislocations comprised 49% of all finger injuries. As in our series the commonest site of a finger dislocation was the proxi-mal interphalangeal joint.

Hip Dislocations

Hip dislocations tend to be high-energy injuries with the major-ity being caused by motor vehicle accidents although in the study year one dislocation occurred in a rugby match. There were four in the study year all of which occurred in adults giving an overall incidence in patients ≥15 years of $0.8/10^5$/year with an incidence in males and females of $1.2/10^5$/year and $0.4/10^5$/year, respectively. The condition has a Type C distribu-tion curve. Three (75%) of the hip dislocations were associated with fractures with one both column fracture, two posterior lip fractures, and one femoral head fracture being recorded.

Dislocations of prosthetic hips are much commoner and presumably are increasing in incidence. Obviously all occurred in adults and the overall incidence in patients aged ≥15 years was $22/10^5$/year with the incidence in adult males and females being $13.9/10^5$/year and $29.3/10^5$/year. They have a Type F distribution.

Knee Dislocations

Dislocation of the knee joint is very rare and is usually caused by high-energy injuries although, as with hip dislocations dur-ing the study year, one knee dislocation occurred as a result of playing rugby with the other two following motor vehicle accidents. All the dislocations occurred in adults and if the over-all incidence is calculated in the population aged ≥15 years it is $0.6/10^5$/year with the incidences in males and females being $0.8/10^5$/year and $0.4/10^5$/year. As with hip dislocations they have a Type C distribution curve. It is possible that the inci-dence of knee dislocations will rise in developed countries in the future. In a study from Finland, Peltola et al.[82] drew attention to the fact that knee dislocation usually followed a high-energy injury but they found a significant incidence of knee dislocation in obese patients following a fall. They estimated the incidence as $0.1/10^5$/year.

Dislocations of the patellofemoral joint are extremely diffi-cult to evaluate accurately. A significant number of dislocations

will have been reduced prior to attendance at an emergency department and patients will also have been told that they have had a knee dislocation without any good evidence that this is the case. It is also very difficult to separate an actual or per-ceived subluxation from a dislocation. Thus the best that can be done is to calculate the incidence from those patients who are believed to have had a dislocation but we accept that there may be inaccuracies.

Table 3-50 shows that the overall incidence for the whole population was recorded at $21.6/10^5$/year. The overall incidence for primary dislocators was $11.9/10^5$/year with $9.7/10^5$/year being recorded for secondary or recurrent dislocators. The over-all incidence of dislocations in males and females was $22.9/10^5$/year and $20.4/10^5$year, respectively. However this is a condi-tion that is common in children and adolescents and the male and female incidences in the <15-year groups were $21.1/105$/year and $16/10^5$/year, respectively. The equivalent incidences in the male and female ≥15-year groups were $23.8/10^5$/year and $20.8/10^5$/year. The distribution curve is Type C.

A review of the literature shows widespread variation in the results that have been published probably because of the prob-lems that have already been stated. Nielsen and Yde[77] examined the incidence of patellar dislocation in Denmark in 1986 and stated that the overall incidence was $30/10^5$/year with incidences of $20/10^5$/year in males and $50/10^5$/year in females. Nietosvaara et al.[78] investigated the incidence of patellar dislocation in chil-dren and adolescents <16 years of age in the early 1990s in Finland and documented an incidence of $43/10^5$/year. Fithian et al.[42] studied the condition between 1992 and 1997 in the United States in members of a health plan. The overall incidence of primary dislocators was $5.8/10^5$/year and for secondary dis-locators it was $3.8/10^5$/year. The incidence was age dependent, the highest incidence being reported in primary female disloca-tors aged 10 to 17 years. Hsiao et al.[53] investigated patellar dis-location in the United States military between 1996 and 2007. They reported an overall incidence of $69/10^5$/year with a higher incidence in females and in patients <20 years of age. A similar incidence of $77/10^5$/year was reported in males in the Finnish military[90] whereas Yang et al.[104] reported an incidence of $1.4/10^5$/year in Taiwan although they were not specific is to whether they were documenting both knee and patellofemoral disloca-tions. These results demonstrate the difficulty in assessing the incidence of patellar dislocations accurately.

Ankle and Foot Dislocations

An analysis of the literature indicates that most dislocations of the ankle are fracture dislocations and a review of the ankle dislocations during the study year confirmed this as only four (5.6%) dislocations were not associated with a fracture. Table 3-50 shows that the overall incidence of ankle fractures is $11.5/10^5$/year but the incidence of pure dislocations in adults is only $0.8/10^5$/year. The distribution curve for fracture disloca-tions is Type H, with bimodal distributions in both males and females, but for pure dislocations it is Type C with younger patients being affected. Table 3-50 shows that ankle fracture dislocations are more common in females and this is probably due to the osteoporotic nature of bimalleolar and trimalleolar fractures (Table 3-13). The overall incidence of all ankle dislocations in males is 7.2/10⁵/year compared with $15.5/10^5$/year in females. A review of the fractures associated with ankle dislocations showed that 54% were trimalleolar, 23% were bimalleolar, and 14% were lateral malleolar fractures. The remaining fractures were talar and distal tibial fractures. Six (8.5%) of the ankle dislocations were open.

Hindfoot dislocations are extremely rare and there is little information available about their epidemiology. There was only one subtalar dislocation in the study year which was associated with a talar neck fracture. There were no dislocations affecting Chopart's joint. Lisfranc injuries to the tarsometatarsal joint are more commonly seen although the true epidemiology is difficult to determine as a substantial number remain undiagnosed. There were four Lisfranc injuries all of which occurred in adults giving an overall incidence in the ≥15-year population of $0.8/10^5$/year. Three (75%) of the dislocations were associated with fractures Lisfranc dislocations have a Type C distribution curve.

Toe dislocations had an overall incidence of $5.3/10^5$/year. They have a Type H distribution curve with bimodal distributions in both males and females. The overall incidence in males and females is $7.1/10^5$/year and $3.7/10^5$/year, respectively. As with finger dislocations the first and fifth toes are most affected with 27% of the dislocations being in each toe. These were followed by the second (21%), third (15%), and the fourth (10%) toes. Again as with finger dislocations the proximal interphalangeal joints and the interphalangeal joint of the hallux were most affected (61%). A further 27% of the dislocations occurred in the metatarsophalangeal joints and the remaining 12% occurred in the distal interphalangeal joints. There were 8 (24.2%) fracture dislocation and one (3%) dislocation was open.

REFERENCES

1. Anakwe RE, Middleton SE, Jenkins PJ, et al. Patient-reported outcomes after simple dislocation of the elbow. *J Bone Joint Surg Am.* 2011;93:1220–1226.
2. Arakaki H, Owan I, Kudoh H, et al. Epidemiology of hip fractures in Okinawa, Japan. *J Bone Miner Metab.* 2011;29:309–314.
3. Barakat K, Stevenson S, Wilkinson P, et al. Socioeconomic differentials in recurrent ischaemia and mortality after acute myocardial infarction. *Heart.* 2000;85:390–394.
4. Baron JA, Farahmand BY, Weiderpass E, et al. Cigarette smoking, alcohol consumption and risk of hip fracture in women. *Arch Intern Med.* 2001;161:983–988.
5. Bengnér U, Johnell O, Redlund-Johnell I. Changes in the incidence of fracture of the upper end of the humerus during a 30-year period. *Clin Orthop.* 1988;231:179–182.
6. Bergström U, Jonsson H, Gustafson Y, et al. The hip fracture incidence curve is shifting to the right. A forecast of the age-quake. *Acta Orthopaedica.* 2009;80:520–524.
7. Black EA, Lawson M, Smith S, et al. Open pelvic fractures: The University of Tennessee medical center at Knoxville experience over ten years. *Iowa Orthop J.* 2011;31:193–198.
8. Bradley C, Harrison J. Descriptive epidemiology of traumatic fractures in Australia. Injury Research and Statistics Series Number 17. Adelaide AIHW(AIHW cat no INJ-CAT 57), 2004.
9. Brennan SL, Henry MJ, Wluka AE, et al. Socioeconomic status and bone mineral density in a population-based sample of men. *Bone.* 2010;46:993–999.
10. Bridgeman S, Wilson R. Epidemiology of femoral fractures in children in the West Midlands region of England 1991 to 2001. *J Bone Joint Surg Br.* 2004;86B:1152–1157.
11. Brinker MR, O'Connor DP. The incidence of fractures and dislocations referred for orthopaedic services in a capitated population. *J Bone Joint Surg Am.* 2004;86-A:290–297.
12. Brogren E, Petranek M, Atroshi I. Incidence and characteristics of distal radius fractures in a southern Swedish region. *BMC Musculoskelet Disord.* 2007;8:48.
13. Buhr AJ, Cooke AM. Fracture patterns. *Lancet* 1959;1(7072):531–536.
14. Byrd GS, Edwards CL, Kelkar VA, et al. Recruiting intergenerational African American males for biomedical research studies: A major research challenge. *J Natl Med Assoc.* 2011;103:480–487.
15. Carstairs V, Morris R. Deprivation and health in Scotland. *Health Bull.* 1990;48:162–175.
16. Cauley JA, Wampler NS, Barnhart JN. Incidence of fractures compared to cardiovascular disease and breast cancer: The Women's Health Observational study. *J Bone Min Res.* 2004;19(4):532–536.
17. Cauley JA. Defining ethnic and racial differences in osteoporosis and fragility fractures. *Clin Orthop.* 2011;469:1891–1899.
18. Chang KP, Center JR, Nguyen TV, et al. Incidence of hip and other osteoporotic fractures in elderly men and women: Dubbo osteoporosis epidemiology study. *J Bone Miner Res.* 2004;19(4):532–536.
19. Chevally T, Guilley E, Herrmann FR, et al. Incidence of hip fracture over a 10-year period (1991-2000): Reversal of a secular trend. *Bone.* 2007;40(5):1284–1289.
20. Cole PA, Gauger EM, Schroder LK. Management of scapular fractures. *J Am Acad Orthop Surg.* 2012;20:130–141.
21. Cooper C, Atkinson EJ, O'Fallon WM, et al. Incidence of clinically diagnosed vertebral fractures: A population-based study in Rochester, Minnesota, 1985–1989.
22. Court-Brown CM, McBirnie J. The epidemiology of tibial fractures. *J Bone Joint Surg Br.* 1995;77B:417–421.
23. Court-Brown CM, Caesar B. Epidemiology of adult fractures; A review. *Injury.* 2006;30(11):691–697.
24. Court-Brown CM, Caesar B. The epidemiology of fractures. In: Heckman JD, Buchholz RW, Court-Brown CM, eds. *Rockwood and Green's Fractures in Adults.* 6th ed. Philadelphia, PA: Lippincott, Williams and Wilkins; 2006:95–113.
25. Court-Brown CM, Brydon A. Social deprivation and adult tibial diaphyseal fractures. *Injury.* 2007;38:750–754.
26. Court-Brown CM, Aitken SA, Forward D, et al. The epidemiology of fractures. In: Bucholz RW, Court-Brown CM, Heckman JD, Tornetta P, eds. *Rockwood and Green's Fractures in Adults.* 7th ed. Philadelphia, PA: Lippincott, Williams and Wilkins; 2010:95–113.
27. Court-Brown CM, Aitken SA, Ralston SH, et al. The relationship of fall-related fractures to social deprivation. *Osteoporos Int.* 2011;22:1211–1218.
28. Court-Brown CM, Bugler KE, Clement ND, et al. The epidemiology of open fractures in adults. A 15-year review. *Injury.* 2012;43:891–897.
29. Court-Brown CM, Aitken SA, Duckworth AD, et al. The relationship between social deprivation and the incidence of adult fractures. *J Bone Joint Surg Am.* 2013;95(6):e321–e327.
30. Dhanwal DK, Dennison EM, Harvey NC, et al. Epidemiology of hip fracture: World-wide geographic variation. *Indian J Orthop.* 2011;45:15–22.
31. Donaldson LJ, Cook A, Thomson RG. Incidence of fractures in a geographically defined population. *J Epidemiol Community Health.* 1990;44(3):241–245.
32. Donaldson LJ, Reckless IP, Scholes S, et al. The epidemiology of fractures in England. *J Epidemiol Community Health.* 2008;62(2):174–180.
33. Dunn L, Henry J, Beard D. Social deprivation and adult head injury: A national study. *J Neurol Neurosurg Psychiatry.* 2003;74:1060–1064.
34. El Moghraoui A, Morjane F, Nouijai A, et al. Vertebral fracture assessment in Moroccan women: Prevalence and risk factors. *Maturitas.* 2009;62:171–175.
35. Elliot JR, Gilchrist NL, Wells JE. The effect of socioeconomic status on bone density in a male Caucasian population. *Bone.* 1996;18:371–373.
36. Emami A, Mjöberg B, Ragnarsson B, et al. Changing epidemiology of tibial shaft fractures. 513 cases compared between 1971-1975 and 1986-1990. *Acta Orthop Scand.* 1996;67:557–561.
37. Emmett JE, Breck LW. A review and analysis of 11,000 fractures seen in a private practice of orthopaedic surgery 1937–1956. *J Bone Joint Surg Am.* 1958;40A:1169–1175.
38. Evans JM, Newton RW, Ruta DA, et al. Socio-economic status, obesity and prevalence of type 1 and type 2 diabetes mellitus. *Diabet Med.* 2000;17:478–480.
39. Farahmand BY, Persson PG, Michaëlsson K, et al. Socioeconomic status, marital status and hip fracture risk: A population-based case-control study. *Osteoporos Int.* 2000;11:803–808.
40. Ferrar L, Roux C, Felsenberg D, et al. Association between incident and baseline vertebral fractures in European women: Vertebral fracture assessment in the Osteoporosis and Ultrasound Study (OPUS). *Osteoporos Int.* 2012;23:59–65.
41. Fife D, Barancik J. Northeastern Ohio Trauma Study III: Incidence of fractures. *Ann Emerg Med.* 1985;14(3):244–248.
42. Fithian DC, Paxton EW, Stone ML, et al. Epidemiology and natural history of acute patellar dislocation. *Am J Sports Med.* 2004;32:1114–1121.
43. Fracture and dislocation compendium (Orthopaedic Trauma Association Committee for coding and Classification). *J Orthop Trauma.* 1996;10(suppl 1):v–ix,1–154.
44. General Register Office for Scotland 2001 Census. Available at http://www.gro-scotland.gov.uk/census/censushm/index.html. Accessed May 18, 2012.
45. Grados F, Marcelli C, Dargent-Molina P, et al. Prevalence of vertebral fractures in French women older than 75 years from the EPIDOS study. *Bone.* 2004;34(2):362–367.
46. Guilley E, Chevally F, Herrmann D, et al. Reversal of the hip fracture secular trend is related to a decrease in the incidence of institution-dwelling elderly women. *Osteoporos Int.* 2008;19(12):1741–1748.
47. Gustilo RB, Mendoza RM, Williams DM. Problems in the management of type III (severe) open fractures. A new classification of type III open fractures. *J Trauma.* 1984;24(8):742–746.
48. Hagino H, Yamamoto K, Ohshiro H, et al. Changing incidence of hip, distal radius and proximal humerus fractures in Tottori Prefecture, Japan. *Bone.* 1999;24:265–270.
49. Hakanson R, Nussman D, Gorman RA, et al. Gunshot injuries: A medical, social and economic analysis. *Orthopaedics.* 1994;17:519–523.
50. Ho SC, Chen YM, Woo JLF. Educational level and osteoporosis risk in postmenopausal Chinese women. *Am J Epidemiol.* 2005;161:680–690.
51. Hole DJ, McArdle CS. Impact of socioeconomic deprivation on outcome after surgery for colorectal cancer. *Br J Surg.* 2002;89:586–589.
52. Horton TC, Dias JJ, Burke FD. Social deprivation and hand injury. *J Hand Surg Eur.* 2007;26:29–35.

53. Hsiao M, Owens BD, Burks R, et al. Incidence of acute traumatic patellar dislocation among active-duty United States military service members. *Am J Sports Med.* 2010;38:1997–2004.

54. Jacobsen SJ, Goldberg J, Miles TP, et al. Seasonal variation in the incidence of hip fracture among white persons aged 65 years or older in the United States, 1984-1987. *Am J Epidemiol.* 1991;133:996–1004.

55. Jenkins PJ, Perry PW, Ng CW, et al. Deprivation influences the functional outcome from hip arthroplasty. *Surgeon.* 2009;7:351–356.

56. Johansen A, Evans RJ, Stone MD, et al. Fracture incidence in England and Wales: A study based on the population of Cardiff. *Injury.* 1997;28:655–660.

57. Johnell O, Kanis J. Epidemiology of osteoporotic fractures. *Osteoporos Int.* 2005;16(suppl 2):S3–S7.

58. Kanis J, Oden A, Johnell O, et al. The burden of osteoporotic fractures: A method for setting intervention thresholds. *Osteoporsis Int.* 2001;12:417–427.

59. Kanis JA, Odén A, McCloskey EV, et al. A systematic review of hip fracture incidence and probability of fracture worldwide. *Osteoporos Int.* 2012;23(9):2239–2256.

60. Kannus P, Niemi S, Palvanen M, et al. Rising incidence of low-trauma fractures of the calcaneus and the foot among Finnish older adults. *J Gerontol A Biol A Sci Med Sci.* 2008;63:642–645.

61. Kannus P, Palvanen M, Niemi S, et al. Stabilizing influence of low-trauma ankle fractures in elderly people. Finnish statistics for 1970 to 2006 and prediction for the future. *Bone.* 2008;43:340–342.

62. Kannus P, Palvanen M, Niemi S, et al. Rate of proximal humeral fractures in older Finnish women between 1970 and 2007. *Bone.* 2009;44:656–659.

63. Kaye JA, Jick H. Epidemiology of lower limb fractures in general practice in the United Kingdom. *Inj Prev.* 2004;10:368–374.

64. Knowelden J, Buhr AJ, Dunbar O. Incidence of fractures in persons over 35 years of age. A report to the MRC working party on fractures in the elderly. *Brit J Prev Soc Med.* 1964;18:130–141.

65. Kroner K, Lind T, Jensen J. The epidemiology of shoulder dislocations. *Arch Orthop Trauma Surg.* 1989;108:288–290.

66. Lau EMC, Lee JK, Suriwongpaisal P, et al. The incidence of hip fracture in four Asian countries: The Asian osteoporosis study (AOS). *Osteoporos Int.* 2001;12:239–243.

67. Lawson DH, Sherman V, Hollowell J. The general practice research database. *Q J Med.* 1998;91:445–452.

68. Liavaag S, Svenningsen S, Reikerås O, et al. The epidemiology of shoulder dislocations in Oslo. *Scand Med Sci Sports.* 2011;21:3334–3340.

69. MacKenzie EJ, Bosse MI, Kellam JF, et al. Characterization of patients with high-energy lower extremity trauma. *J Orthop Trauma.* 2000;7:455–466.

70. Malgaigne JF. *A Treatise on Fractures.* Philadelphia, PA: JP Lippincott; 1859.

71. Mall NA, Carlisle JC, Matava MJ, et al. Upper extremity injuries in the national football league. *Am J Sports Med.* 2008;36:1938–1944.

72. Mattila VM, Jormanainen V, Sahi T, et al. An association between socioeconomic, health and health behavioural indicators and fractures in young adult males. *Ostoporos Int.* 2007;18:1609–1615.

73. Melton LJ, Therneau TM, Larson DR. Long-term trends in hip fracture prevalence: The influence of hip fracture incidence and survival. *Osteoporos Int.* 1998;8:68–74.

74. Melton LJ, Crowson CS, O'Fallon WM. Fracture incidence in Olmsted County, Minnesota: Comparison of urban with rural rates and changes in urban rates over time. *Osteoporos Int.* 1999;9:29–37.

75. Menon MRG, Walker JL, Court-Brown CM. The epidemiology of fractures in adolescents with reference to social deprivation. *J Bone Joint Surg Br.* 2008;90-B:1482–1486.

76. Navarro MC, Sosa M, Saavedra P, et al. Poverty is a risk factor for osteoporotic fractures. *Osteoporos Int.* 2009;20:393–398.

77. Nielsen AB, Yde J. Epidemiology of acute knee injuries: A prospective hospital investigation. *J Trauma.* 1991;31:1644–1648.

78. Nietosvaara Y, Aalto K, Kallio PE. Acute patellar dislocation in children: Incidence and associated ostechondral fractures. *J Pediatr Orthop.* 1994;14:513–515.

79. O'Neill TW, Cooper C, Finn JD, et al. Incidence of distal forearm fracture in British men and women. *Osteoporos Int.* 2001;12(7):555–558

80. Orces CH, Martinez FJ. Epidemiology of fall related forearm and wrist fractures among adults treated in US hospital emergency department. *Inj Prev.* 2011;17:33–36.

81. Owens BD, Dawson L, Burks R, et al. Incidence of shoulder dislocation in the united States military: Demographic considerations from a high-risk population. *J Bone Joint Surg Am.* 2009b:91:791–796.

82. Peltola EK, Lindahl J, Hietaranta H, et al. Knee dislocation in overweight patients. *AJR.* 2009;192:101–106.

83. Pillai A, Ativa S, Costigan PS. The incidence of Perthes' disease in Southwest Scotland. *J Bone Joint Surg (Br).* 2008;90B:1482–1486.

84. Pressley JC, Kendig TD, Frencher SK, et al. Epidemiology of bone fracture across the age span in blacks and whites. *J Trauma.* 2011;71:S541–S548.

85. Rennie L, Court-Brown CM, Mok JY, et al. The epidemiology of fractures in children. *Injury.* 2007;38:913–922.

86. Rosengren BE, Ahlborg HG, Gärdsell P, et al. Bone mineral density and incidence of hip fracture in Sweden urban and rural women 1987-2002. *Acta Orthopaedica.* 2010;81:453–459.

87. Sahlin Y. Occurrence of fractures in a defined population: A 1-year study. *Injury.* 1990;21:158–160.

88. Sanders KM, Nicholson GC, Ugoni AM, et al. Fracture rates lower in rural than urban communities: The Geelong osteoporosis study. *J Epidemiol Community Health.* 2002;56:466–470.

89. Sakuma M, Endo N, Oinuma T, et al. Incidence and outcome of osteoporotic fractures in 2004 in Sado City, Niigata Prefecture, Japan. *J Bone Miner Metab.* 2008;26:373–378.

90. Sillanpää P, Mattila VM, Livonen T, et al. Incidence and risk factors of acute traumatic primary patellar dislocation. *Med Sci Sports Exerc.* 2008;40:606–611.

91. Silversides JA, Gibson A, Glasgow JF, et al. Social deprivation and childhood injuries in North and West Belfast. *Ulster Med J.* 2005;74:22–28.

92. Simont WT, Melton LJ, Cofield RH, et al. Incidence of anterior shoulder dislocation in Olmsted County, Minnesota. *Clin Orthop.* 1984;186:186–191.

93. Stark AD, Bennet GC, Stone DH, et al. Association between childhood fractures and poverty: Population based study. *BMJ.* 2002;324:457.

94. Sterling RS. Gender and race/ethnicity differences in hip fracture incidence, morbidity, mortality, and function. *Clin Orthop Relat Res.* 2011;469:1913–1918.

95. Stimson LA. *A Practical Treatise on Fractures and Dislocations.* 4th ed. New York, NY, Philadelphia, PA: Lea Brothers & Co; 1905.

96. Stoneback JW, Owens BD, Sykes J, et al. Incidence of elbow dislocations in the United States population. *J Bone Joint Surg Am.* 2012;94:240–245.

97. Tracy JK, Meyer WA, Flores RH, et al. Racial differences in rate of decline in bone mass in older men: The Baltimore men's osteoporosis study. *J Bone Mine Res.* 2005;20:1228–1234.

98. Trauer T, Eagar K, Mellsop G. Ethnicity, deprivation and mental health outcomes. *Aust Health Rev.* 2006;30:310–321.

99. Urwin M, Symmons D, Allison T, et al. Estimating the burden of musculoskeletal disorders in the community: The comparative prevalence of symptoms at different anatomical sites, and the relation to social deprivation. *Ann Rheum Dis.* 1998;57:649–655.

100. van den Berg M, Verdiik NA, van den Bergh JP, et al. Vertebral fractures in women aged 50 years and older with clinical risk factors for fractures in primary care. *Maturitas.* 2011;70:74–79.

101. Wang X-F, Seeman E. Epidemiology and structural basis of racial differences in fragility fractures in Chinese and Caucasians. *Ostoporos Int.* 2012;23:411–422.

102. Waterman BR, Belmont PJ, Owens BD. Patellar dislocation in the United States: Role of sex, age, race, and athletic participation. *J Knee Surg.* 2012;25:51–57.

103. Weiss RJ, Montgomery SM, Ehlin A, et al. Decreasing incidence of tibial shaft fractures between 1998 and 2004: Information based on 10,627 Swedish inpatients. *Acta Orthop.* 2008;79:526–533.

104. Yang N-P, Chen H-C, Phan D-V, et al. Epidemiological survey of orthopedic joint dislocations based on nationwide insurance data in Taiwan, 2000-2005. *BMC Musculoskelet Disord.* 2011;12:253.

105. Zacchilli MA, Owens BD. Epidemiology of shoulder dislocations presenting to emergency departments in the United Stataes. *J Bone Joint Surg Am.* 2010;92A:542–549.

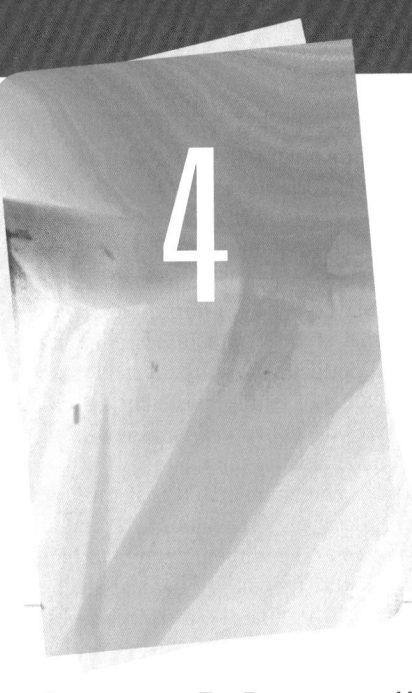

4 BONE AND CARTILAGE HEALING

Jesse Slade Shantz, Ralph Marcucio, Hubert T. Kim, and Theodore Miclau III

INTRODUCTION: THE RATIONALE FOR UNDERSTANDING THE BIOLOGY OF INJURY

Bone and cartilage healing are central to the practice of orthopedic surgery. Orthopaedic treatments should attempt to optimize the cells, scaffold, molecules, and blood supply required for healing. This chapter will describe the components required for successful healing, detail the role of each factor, and outline the complex interactions that occur during the healing processes of bone and cartilage. The cellular processes of bone and cartilage healing will also be examined in detail with a focus on the dynamic repair processes, and the disruptions that impair successful healing particularly as it relates to factors under a surgeon's control.

The clinical importance for understanding the principles of bone and joint healing can be realized when little evidence exists to guide a treatment decision. In the age of evidence-based medicine, surgeons may be obligated to base decisions on basic science rather than clinical evidence. The translation of basic science findings into clinical practice has been traditionally applied throughout the practice of fracture care, and can be appreciated in the works of Urist and McLean,[104] Young,[119] Perren,[82] and McKibbin.[66] These seminal findings still form the foundations for both clinical treatment and scientific understanding of bone and joint injuries.

COMPONENTS OF FRACTURE HEALING

Fracture healing is a complex and dynamic process. One of the unique characteristics of bone repair is that the bone heals with new tissue that is indistinguishable from its preinjured state. Further, bone repair occurs in the vast majority of cases, with most fractures, treated in a myriad of ways, progressing to union. However, delayed union and nonunion remain clinically significant issues, with nearly 10% of fractures having some degree of impaired healing.[29] It has been reported, for example, that 4.5% of tibia fractures exhibit delayed healing and overall 2.5% of tibia fractures fail to unite.[84] Fractures heal through the parallel processes of endochondral and intramembranous ossification, with most fractures exhibiting both types of healing. The fracture repair process is intimately influenced by the mechanical and biologic environments at the fracture site. While many of the factors that cause impaired healing are not within the control of the surgeon, it is increasingly appreciated that bone repair can be affected by surgical approaches. In order to best understand the healing response, surgeons should understand the basic components of cellular and molecular repair. These components can be categorized as cells and tissues, scaffold, blood supply, and molecules and their receptors (summarized in Table 4-1). Subsequent sections will further describe the coordination of these components in the process of fracture healing and how disruptions can negatively affect healing.

Cells and Tissues Involved in Fracture Healing

Progenitor Cells (Periosteum and Endosteum)

Bone surfaces are covered by tissue layers called the periosteum (outer layer) and the endosteum (inner layer), both of which are distinct fibrous layers rich in cells and blood vessels. It has been recognized for nearly a century that the periosteum responds to fracture through extensive cellular proliferation.[42] The resulting pluripotent cells differentiate into either osteoblasts or chondrocytes, depending on inflammatory signals and the local mechanical and vascular environment, with increased mechanical stability favoring osteogenic differentiation. It has been shown that the periosteum provides a supply of osteoblasts, and is the primary source of chondrocytes, during fracture healing.[21] In contrast, the endosteum is more restricted in its potential and appears to primarily give rise to osteoblasts during fracture healing.[41] The results of an early case-control study suggested that the integrity of the vascularity and the periosteum related to initial fracture displacement played a role in improving fracture healing.[67] Subsequent animal studies have investigated fracture healing following extraperiosteal or subperiosteal dissection, and found that the callus of extraperiosteally dissected osteotomy sites demonstrates decreased callus mineralization and inferior mechanical characteristics more similar to that of soft tissue.[110] Further work has demonstrated that the violation and elevation of the periosteal sleeve about the fracture site is associated with a decreased bending moment and bending rigidity in a rat femur fracture model.[41] In clinical practice, these studies have led to the belief that the disruption of the periosteum leads to failures of healing through the invasion of fibrous tissue and loss of fracture hematoma contents into the surrounding soft tissues. The emerging concept of biologic fracture fixation is aimed at reducing the potentially deleterious effects due to soft tissue stripping at the fracture site.[108]

Chondrocytes

Chondrocytes, while usually associated with articular cartilage, also play an important role in the healing of fractures. The function of chondrocytes is to produce extracellular matrix (ECM) proteins such as proteoglycans and collagen, and during fracture healing, hypertrophic chondrocytes participate in endochondral ossification through the synthesis of matrix and the deposition of intracellular calcium.[32] Early in the process, chondrocytes are identified by the expression of type II collagen and SOX-9, and the synthetic activity of chondrocytes is determined in vitro by quantifying proteoglycan and hydroxyproline production.[23]

TABLE 4-1	**The Essential Components of Fracture Healing**	
	Components	**Importance in Fracture Healing**
Cells	Inflammatory cells Progenitor cells Chondrocytes Osteoblast Osteoclast Muscle cells	Debride necrotic tissues Signal for upregulation of synthetic functions Form repair tissues Remodel healed bone for optimal strength/ weight ratio
Scaffold	Hematoma Collagen Noncollagenous proteins	Support cellular function Inflammatory cell chemotaxis Scaffold for mineralization
Blood Supply	Blood vessels Supporting cells (pericytes)	Supply inflammatory cells to injury site Deliver building blocks of repair tissues Reverse hypoxic environment
Molecules	Matrix-embedded proteins Locally produced factors Systemic hormones	Regulate cellular function and proliferation during fracture healing process

Morphologically, chondrocytes in fracture callus are ovoid cells surrounded by ECM. During fracture healing chondrocytes hypertrophy as they terminally differentiate and develop intracellular calcium deposits before undergoing apoptosis. Chondrocytes subsequently undergo apoptosis, leaving a bed of woven bone that is invaded by new blood vessels and remodeled by osteoblasts and osteoclasts.

Osteoblasts

An osteoblast is defined by its ability to produce osteoid, the organic component of bone composed primarily of type I collagen. Osteoblasts line the surfaces of bone where they perform their functions of forming bone matrix and regulating the process of bone turnover by influencing osteoclast activity. Differentiating cells in the periosteum and endosteum provide a local source of osteoblasts at the fracture site.

On histologic examination, osteoblasts appear basophilic as a result of the abundant endoplasmic reticulum contained in the cytoplasm. This reflects the major role these cells play in protein production. Osteoblasts primarily produce type I collagen, osteocalcin, bone sialoprotein, and other matrix proteins associated with bone.[16] In addition, osteoblasts express alkaline phosphatase, a membrane-bound enzyme responsible for dephosphorylation, an enzymatic activity that is often used as an assay for osteoblast activity in vitro.

Osteoclasts

Osteoclasts are the cell population responsible for the resorption of bone enabling the remodeling of fractures. Osteoclasts are derived from pluripotent hematopoietic stem cells of the macrophage/monocyte lineage. They are distinguished from other cells by the expression of tartrate-resistant acid phosphatase (TRAP) and cathepsin K.[27] Other proteins associated with osteoclasts are calcitonin receptor and receptor activator of nuclear factor-kappa beta ligand (RANKL).[12]

Histologically, osteoclasts are large, multinucleated cells that are formed by the fusion of mononuclear cells. Intracellular lysosomal vesicles and numerous mitochondria dot the cytoplasm of osteoclasts, and provide for the resorption of mineralized bone matrix. On bone surfaces, osteoclasts reside in Howship lacunae, or resorption pits in the bone surface.

Inflammatory Cells

Several inflammatory cell populations are associated with the cell-mediated and humoral responses to bone injury. Platelets, neutrophils, macrophages, and leukocytes are all found at the fracture site within the first hour after fracture.[96]

Platelets are small cell fragments that are derived from megakaryocytes and are present in circulating blood and the spleen. Platelets are activated after fracture by encountering injured epithelial cells with exposed collagen and von Willebrand Factor (vWF). The activation of these factors results in the aggregation of platelets, blood coagulation, and the excretion of granule contents, which include platelet-derived growth factor (PDGF),

vascular endothelial growth factor (VEGF), transforming growth factor beta (TGF-β), fibroblast growth factor (FGF), insulin-like growth factor-1 (IGF-1), and platelet-derived endothelial growth factor (PEGF). All of these trophic factors are putative mediators of the healing response and none of these factors alone has the synergistic effect of the myriad platelet-released growth factors.[5] Therefore, platelets have a role in both hemostasis and the early local fracture healing process.

Polymorphonuclear leukocytes (PMNs) or neutrophils are the most abundant form of granulocytes in the peripheral blood. Histologically, they are distinguished by a multilobed nucleus and cytoplasmic granules. Under normal conditions PMNs circulate in the bloodstream making up 75% of the white blood cell mass. After tissue trauma, PMNs arrive immediately, and their numbers continue to increase at 4 hours after injury.[96] PMNs invade traumatized tissues in response to chemotactic signals and vessel endothelium cell surface capture mechanisms at the site of injury, including selectins and integrins.[51] After activated PMNs have extravasated into the target tissue, their life span is only 1 to 2 days. Activated PMNs perform both phagocytic and degranulation functions at the site of trauma. Reducing the number of PMNs at the fracture site leads to reduced callus rigidity in a rat femur osteotomy model, suggesting neutrophil actions negatively impact endochondral ossification.[39] It may be that this effect is caused by an increase in reactive oxygen species at the fracture site.[37] Alternatively, PMNs could be providing an inhibitory cytokine signal to bone forming cells as fracture healing progresses, although the cytokines produced by PMNs, including C-C motif chemokine 2 and interleukin (IL)-6, are generally thought to enhance fracture repair.[115,117]

Macrophages and precursor monocytes closely follow PMNs, arriving at the fracture site after several hours. Resident tissue macrophages may even participate at the earliest stages of fracture healing given their location nearer the site of the fracture.[83] Macrophages and monocytes are derived from the hematopoietic stem cell lineage and are traditionally thought to play a role in the debridement of tissue injury sites. Macrophages also play a role in the activation of the adaptive immune system through the presentation of antigens on the cell surface and the secretion of cytokines. Resident tissue macrophages may also play a role in the regulation of bone formation and local tissue homeostasis.[4]

Lymphocytes, including various subpopulations of B-cells and T-cells, form the adaptive immune system. As granulation tissue develops at the fracture site about 7 days after fracture, the number of T-cells eclipses that of macrophages. The main contribution of lymphocytes to fracture healing appears to be the production of cytokines. This contribution appears to be inhibitory, as the ablation of the adaptive immune system leads to improved endochondral bone healing in a rat model.[102]

Mesenchymal Stem Cells

An area of intense clinical interest is the therapeutic potential of mesenchymal stem cells (MSCs) in fracture healing applications, such as nonunion and critical sized defects. MSCs were first identified as a population of marrow-derived, adherent cells capable of colony formation in vitro.[63] Subsequently, the definition of MSCs has tightened to include the requirement of differentiation of the cells into bone, cartilage, and adipose tissue in vitro.[26] Osteoblastic differentiation in cell culture is stimulated by the inclusion of dexamethasone, β-glycerol phosphate, and ascorbate-2-phosphate in the cell culture medium. Chondrogenic differentiation is encouraged by culturing cells in a pellet in the presence of dexamethasone, insulin-transferrin-sodium selenite (ITS), ascorbate-2-phosphate, sodium pyruvate, proline, and TGF-β3. Adipogenic differentiation requires a medium containing dexamethasone, isobutylmethylxanthine (IBMX), and insulin. MSCs reside in defined tissue reservoirs, or niches,[61] within the body, including bone marrow, adipose tissue, and the synovial lining. In addition, vascular pericytes[22] and muscle cells[94] exhibit the ability to express osteogenic markers given the appropriate stimulus and, although they may not be considered MSCs, they may also contribute to bone healing.

MSCs are identified histologically as fibroblast-like cells that grow to confluence in culture and express specific cell surface antigens.[85] MSCs participate in the healing of fractures by supplying a cell population capable of differentiating into chondrocytes or osteoblasts based on local cytokine queues and mechanical environments. MSCs are also present at the fracture site as they reside in adjacent bone marrow niches. Therefore, MSCs are not necessarily recruited to the fracture site, but rather resident MSCs may proliferate and differentiate in response to the evolving cytokine milieu of the fracture hematoma.

Despite claims of the therapeutic benefit of injected MSCs in the stimulation of fracture repair, experimental evidence suggests that circulating MSCs play a minor role, if any, in fracture healing. Circulating cells expressing markers of osteogenic potential have been identified.[28] However, the injection of ex vivo cultured MSCs expressing a green fluorescent protein (GFP) marker into a rabbit fracture model did not yield an accumulation of labeled cells at the fracture site.[97] In a more definitive study, a mouse constitutively expressing GFP and a mouse with a fracture shared a common circulation. During fracture healing, the callus had a large number of GFP-labeled cells but there was no evidence of GFP-derived osteoblasts or chondrocytes in the newly formed callus, suggesting that circulating MSCs did not significantly contribute to the cell population in the callus.[55]

Muscle

The envelope of muscle that surrounds most bones plays an important role in fracture healing. This fact is evidenced by the impaired healing seen in open fractures, where the surrounding muscle is disrupted or deficient. In vivo experimental work has demonstrated that the resection of muscles surrounding a femoral fracture reduces the mechanical characteristics of the fracture callus.[106] These experimental results are complemented by clinical results suggesting that early soft tissue coverage of severe open tibial fractures leads to faster union and a reduced number of secondary procedures.[46]

There has also been some interest in the contribution of muscle-derived cells to fracture healing. Although little evidence exists for the direct involvement of muscle satellite cells in fracture healing, there is a considerable body of evidence confirming the ability of muscle cells to express markers of bone formation in vitro and in vivo.[94] Future research must clarify the contribution of muscle to fracture healing to enhance our understanding of the interaction of fractures and the adjacent muscle.

Scaffold

Bone healing is a three-dimensional process that requires a scaffold to allow the cellular components of the healing process to perform their functions. This scaffold, or ECM, is responsible for conferring the structural properties of bone and cartilage as well as serving in some cell regulatory functions. The ECM of bone is composed primarily (60% to 70%) of inorganic material in the form of mineral crystals containing calcium, phosphate and other ions including sodium, magnesium, and carbonate. The organic portion of bone (30% to 40%) consists primarily of type I collagen (90%) with the remainder being made up of other types of collagen and several noncollagenous proteins. Important noncollagenous proteins involved directly in bone healing include osteocalcin, bone sialoprotein, proteoglycans, and matricellular proteins. When the organic phase of bone is not mineralized it is termed osteoid.

Immediately after fracture, the conversion of fibrinogen to fibrin creates a semisolid blood clot in the fracture site that provides the initial scaffold for inflammatory cell migration. During the rest of fracture repair, the ECM must be constantly remodeled to allow for the restoration of functional anatomy. An extreme example, endochondral ossification is a process where a cartilage scaffold rich in type II collagen is completely replaced by bone. In order to allow the rapid reorganization of tissue types in the ECM, matrix metalloproteinases (MMPs) such as collagenases, gelatinases, stromelysins, and other catabolic enzymes like cathepsins, are required to work in parallel with synthetic processes.[16] In fact, there is evidence that the absence of MMPs, particularly MMP9, results in nonunion associated with the failure to replace cartilage with osteoid at the fracture site.[20]

Blood Supply

The central role of the vasculature in fracture healing is well established.[24] When bone is fractured, local blood vessels are disrupted, creating a relatively avascular and hypoxic area within the fracture hematoma and the early fracture callus.[14] In the hypoxic environment hypoxia-inducible factor (HIF)-1 promotes the production of vascular endothelial growth factor (VEGF), promoting revascularization.[33] The absence of competent blood vessels crossing the fracture site necessitates angiogenesis during the process of bone repair. For vascular repair to proceed concurrently with bone healing, the newly forming matrix must be degraded in concert with the proliferation of endothelial cells. Mechanistically, it may be that the failure of MMP9 knockout mice to replace cartilage with bone is related to the failure of vascular invasion.[20]

TABLE 4-2	Molecules Important in the Fracture Healing Process		
	Source Cells	Effector Cells	Effect on Fracture Healing
Bone Morphogenetic Protein-2 (BMP-2)	Persistent cambial layer, macrophages, osteoprogenitors, bone, and cartilage matrix	Osteoblast and osteocytes in new woven bone	Stimulates differentiation of chondroprogenitor and osteoprogenitor cells in early fracture healing
Receptor Activator of Nuclear Factor-Kappa Beta Ligand (RANKL)	Osteoblast, lymphocytes	Osteoclast Precursors	Induces resorption of calcified cartilage and stimulates osteoclast activity
Insulin-like Growth Factor-1 (IGF-1)	Osteoprogenitor, bone matrix	Osteoprogenitor cells	Stimulates osteoblast proliferation and differentiation
Platelet-derived Growth Factor (PDGF)	Degranulating platelets, fracture hematoma macrophages	Chondroprogenitor and osteoprogenitor cells	Stimulates migration of progenitor cells and osteoblast
Transforming Growth Factor Beta (TGF-β)	Platelets, bone, and cartilage matrix	Chondroprogenitor and osteoprogenitor cells	Stimulates progenitor cell proliferation
Fibroblast Growth Factor (FGF)	Macrophages, chondrocytes, and osteoblast	Chondroprogenitor and osteoprogenitor cells	Stimulates progenitor cell proliferation
Parathyroid Hormone (PTH)	Parathyroid gland (chief cells)	Chondrocytes	Recruits and activates chondrocytes in the early fracture callus
Vascular Endothelial Growth Factor (VEGF)	Platelets, hypertrophic chondrocytes	Macrophages, endothelial cells and granulocytes	Angiogenesis, chemotactic for macrophages and endothelial cells and vasodilation

Molecules

Given the complexity of the healing response to a fracture, an intricate communication system is required to regulate the actions of participating cells. Cellular interactions are primarily mediated through the actions of molecules termed cytokines through receptors on effector cell surfaces. Although detailing all of the cytokine–receptor interactions at play during the healing of a fracture is beyond the scope of this chapter, there are several molecules that require a detailed explanation of the mechanism of action given their use in clinical applications or their future potential as targets to improve fracture healing and treat nonunion (Table 4-2).

Perhaps the molecules with the most controversial and clinically relevant role in fracture healing are the bone morphogenetic proteins (BMPs). The concept of osteoinduction and the role of BMPs in this process were discovered by Urist in 1965 when he observed that intramuscularly implanted demineralized bone induced the ectopic formation of bone.[104,105] The number of unique isoforms of BMP, all members of the TGF-β superfamily, has now surpassed 16. The BMPs act on cells during fracture healing through heterodimers of type I and type II transmembrane receptors, which are serine/threonine kinases. After the binding of BMPs, activated BMP receptors phosphorylate cytoplasmic proteins of the Smad family, which in turn regulate the expression of down-stream target genes that affect cellular processes such as proliferation and differentiation.[91]

BMPs are antagonized by noggin, a protein that binds BMP-2, BMP-4, and BMP-7, rendering them inactive. Noggin expression is increased in osteoblasts in response to BMP-2 receptor activation by BMP-2 suggesting that noggin and BMP-2 form a negative feedback loop.[1] In addition, in rodent models of nonunion the expression of chordin, another BMP antagonist,

is upregulated, suggesting that the balance between BMPs and BMP antagonists must be tightly regulated during fracture healing, possibly representing a therapeutic target for the enhancement of fracture healing.[78]

Activation of receptor activator of nuclear factor-kappa beta (RANK) by RANKL is the final signaling step in the production of osteoclasts from progenitor cells. Given the important role of osteoclasts in the remodeling of bone, this receptor–ligand pair has been a target for the treatment of osteoporosis. Experimental evidence suggests that antagonizing RANK signaling does not interfere with the early fracture healing process nor does it prevent the formation of bridging callus.[34] In that study, however, there was a marked delay in the mineralization of cartilage in unstable fractures. The authors proposed that the delay in mineralization was due to the reduced number of blood vessels in the callus. Others have found similar results and confirmed that inhibition of osteoclast differentiation by RANKL antagonism or inhibition of function through bisphosphonate treatment after fracture results in improved mechanical properties of the fracture callus despite delayed mineralization.[35]

With increasing interest in the clinical applications of platelet-rich plasma in musculoskeletal repair, the effects of PDGF on fracture repair have received some attention. PDGF is found in the fracture site of humans early in the fracture repair process.[8] On a cellular level, PDGF has been found to be associated with platelets, macrophages, fibroblasts, endothelial cells, and the bone matrix, suggesting a broad range of activities. The effects of PDGF on the bone healing process have also been investigated both in vitro and in vivo. These studies have shown that PDGF activates macrophages and stimulates angiogenesis,[90] attracts fibroblasts and enhances collagen synthesis,[64] and stimulates the proliferation of bone cells.[116]

The exogenous supplementation of PDGF at the fracture site has also been examined in a rabbit osteotomy model with the findings of increased mineralization and increased bending strength when compared to controls.[76] Another study in rats comparing the healing of tibia fractures after stabilization with control or PDGF-coated intramedullary wires showed accelerated radiographic union of fractures with PDGF, but the cellular rationale for these differences was not clear.[11] Therefore, PDGF remains an experimental therapy with future promise for clinical use.

The role of growth hormone (GH) and IGF-1 in fracture healing has been investigated given the clinical availability of GH for the treatment of short stature.[103] GH is released by the pituitary gland through the action of GH-releasing hormone. The main action of GH is to cause the systemic release of IGF, which has myriad biologic activities, including the stimulation of osteoblasts. Of particular interest is the paracrine activity of IGF-1 as a chemotactic factor for osteoblast migration. Employing a cell line of primary murine osteoblasts in culture, investigators demonstrated that an IGF-1 gradient enhanced the migration of osteoblasts.[74] Given that osteoblasts also produce IGF-1, this molecule may be an important regulator of cell trafficking at the fracture site. Animal work investigating the potential therapeutic roles of both local and systemic GH and IGF-1 has shown mixed results with some studies demonstrating enhancement of fracture healing and others suggesting no effect of exogenously applied GH and IGF-1.[9,18,95,111]

TGF-β has been shown previously to be expressed constantly during fracture healing.[112] Expressed in many tissues, TGF-β is a member of a protein superfamily that encompasses the BMPs, growth and differentiation factors (GDFs), activins, and inhibins.[62] TGF-β1 expression has been associated primarily with endochondral ossification, and it has a particularly high expression in the periosteum after fracture. In human fractures, it has been shown that serum TGF-β1 levels are significantly lower in patients with impaired healing than in those with normal healing, suggesting TGF-β1 may be a biomarker for an increased risk of nonunion.[121] Clinically, however, the broad effects of TGF-β limit the use of TGF-β1 for fracture healing enhancement due to fears of unforeseen side effects upon other tissues and cell populations.

FGFs are members of another family of signaling molecules that are expressed throughout the body. Acidic FGF (FGF-1) and basic FGF (FGF-2) are the proteins most relevant to the fracture healing process. Both proteins are known for their angiogenic and cell activating properties and there has been interest in their potential clinical application for the enhancement of fracture healing.[89] The actions of FGFs are transduced through transmembrane receptors. Mutations in these receptors have been identified as the genetic cause of several common skeletal dysplasias including achondroplasia, which involves a mutation in the FGF receptor-3 (FGFR-3) and severely affects endochondral ossification during skeletal development. During fracture healing, the local injection of recombinant human FGF-2 (rhFGF-2) accelerated early chondrocyte maturation and increased the proportion of intramembranous ossification in a study in beagles.[73] The time to remodeling was also decreased in rhFGF-2 treated animals, suggesting that treatment accelerated the entire process of fracture healing, including remodeling. One well-designed randomized controlled trial has been conducted using rhFGF-2 as an adjunct to closed tibial fracture treatment.[50] Although the authors did not show a difference in the rate of secondary procedures in this study, they did note an accelerated rate of union in fractures treated with a percutaneous injection of rhFGF-2. In addition, no adverse events were noted among the treated patients, suggesting the safety of the treatment, although further testing is necessary before there is widespread clinical acceptance of rhFGF-2 as an adjunct to fracture treatment.

TYPES OF BONE HEALING

Endochondral

During development, the process whereby a cartilaginous anlage is replaced by bone is referred to as endochondral ossification. This process typically occurs as the resident chondrocytes mature and senesce, and vessels invade the cartilage. In many ways fracture healing replicates this process of skeletal development.[32] In unstable fractures, cartilage is found during the early phase of fracture healing and, as stated previously, chondrocytes hypertrophy and are replaced by osteoblasts as vessels invade the cartilage callus (Fig. 4-1). In the past, the predominance of endochondral ossification was referred to as secondary bone healing, which proceeded through three sequential phases: soft callus, hard callus, and remodeling. This healing response was associated with motion at the fracture site, such as can occur with cast treatment or incomplete stability.

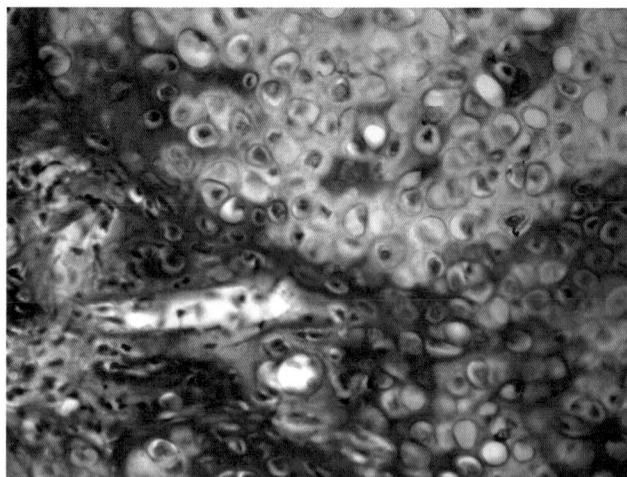

FIGURE 4-1 Ossification of the cartilage scaffold in endochondral ossification. In this Hall-Bryant quadruple stained section of a mouse tibia 10 days after fracture, the transition of cartilage callus to ossified tissue is demonstrated. In the upper right of the photomicrograph, typical chondrocytes can be seen. In the lower left, the red matrix denotes calcified tissue surrounding osteoblasts. Chondrocyte-like cells with calcium deposits in the cytoplasm can be visualized at the transition between the nonossified and the ossified cartilage scaffold.

Intramembranous

The process of direct bone formation without a cartilaginous intermediate is referred to as intramembranous ossification.[107] During skeletal development, intramembranous bone formation involves the direct deposition of osteoid by cells of mesenchymal origin. During fracture repair, intramembranous, or primary healing, results when the motion between two fracture surfaces is abolished through rigid internal fixation. Healing then progresses without the formation of visible fracture callus. Instead, fragments are united by the passage of osteoclast-led cutting cones across the fracture site along the long axis of the bone. The leading edge of the cutting cone is followed by osteoblasts that restore the lamellar architecture of cortical bone as evidenced by scant type I collagen at the fracture site.[101] Clinically, primary bone healing manifests as loss of the obvious fracture line with an absence of visible fracture callus on postoperative radiographs.[70]

These two forms of bone healing represent distinct processes. Modern fracture fixation techniques benefit from both types of healing in different circumstances. Neither form of bone repair can be regarded as inferior, with most fractures healing through a combination of the two types of healing. In addition, the time eventually required to restore the mechanical integrity of bones is not reduced by healing either through endochondral or intramembranous ossification. The influence of mechanical factors on the biology of fracture healing will be further elaborated below.

STAGES OF ENCHONDRAL FRACTURE REPAIR

A fracture results in a cascade of events aimed at restoring mechanical integrity to that unstable limb segment. The conventional way to define this process is through discrete stages of enchondral fracture healing including, inflammation, soft cal-

lus, hard callus, and remodeling (Figs. 4-2 to 4-4). These four stages, preceded by the early hematoma stage, will be presented in sequence here, although it is key to remember that they can overlap one another in time during the healing process, and different parts of any given fracture callus may exhibit different stages simultaneously, depending on the microenvironment to which individual cells are exposed (Fig. 4-5).

Hematoma Formation

The first consequence of fracture is a local structural disruption of the bone and the associated marrow, periosteum, surrounding muscle, and blood vessels (Fig. 4-2). These events lead to the accumulation of a fracture hematoma composed of the debris from these structures as well as platelets, erythrocytes, and immune cells extravasated from sheared blood vessels. Due to the lack of a vascular supply and increased cellular activity, the oxygen tension of a fracture hematoma is decreased significantly over the first 72 hours after fracture.[31]

The fracture hematoma is bioactive. The transplantation of a 4-day old fracture hematoma to a remote subperiosteal or intramuscular location in rats results in ectopic formation of bone and cartilage, whereas putting a peripheral blood clot there does not result in a similar response.[69] In addition, the removal of a fracture hematoma from a femoral fracture in a rat after 2 or 4 days resulted in mechanically inferior healing, and removal of the hematoma after 30 minutes has a similar result.[40]

Others have demonstrated the immunologic activity of the fracture hematoma.[45] As compared to the peripheral blood of fracture patients, the fracture hematoma contains seven-fold greater amount of membrane-bound tumor necrosis factor-alpha (TNF-α). The concentration of IL-6 and IL-8 in the fracture hematoma is also greatly elevated, whereas inflammatory cytokines are barely detectable in the plasma of these patients

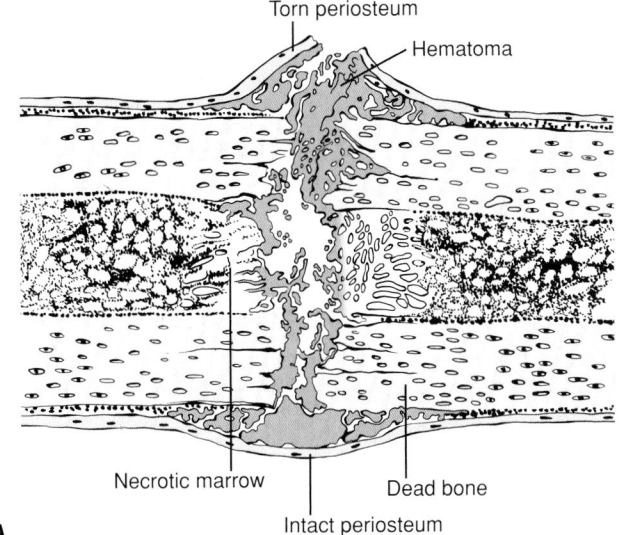

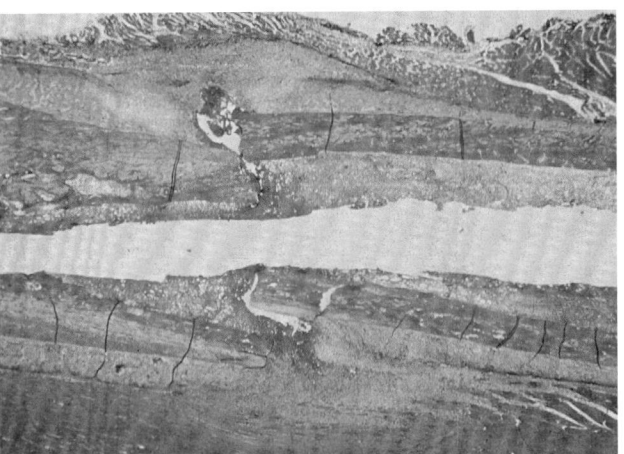

A   **B**

FIGURE 4-2 Initial events following fracture of a long bone diaphysis. **A:** Drawing showing that the periosteum is torn opposite the point of impact, and may remain intact on the other side. A hematoma accumulates beneath the periosteum and between the fracture ends. There is necrotic marrow and cortical bone close to the fracture line. **B:** A photomicrograph of a fractured rat femur 3 days after injury showing the proliferation of the periosteal repair tissue.

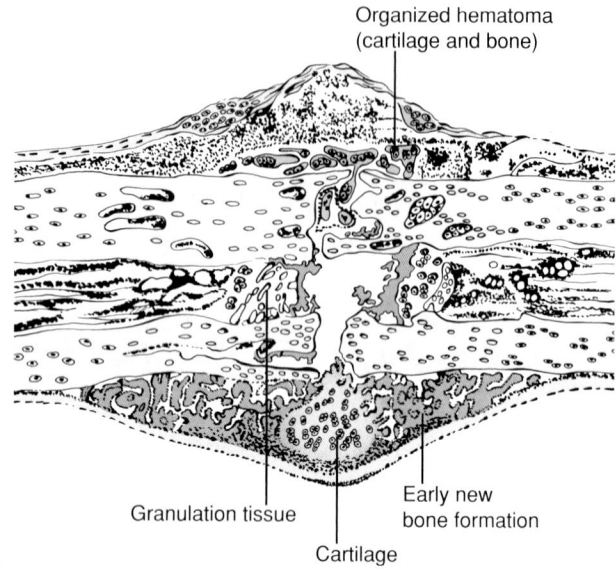

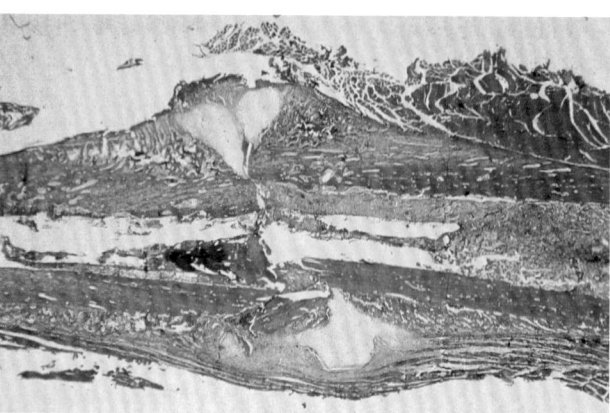

Organized hematoma
(cartilage and bone)

Granulation tissue

Early new
bone formation

Cartilage

A

B

FIGURE 4-3 Early repair of a diaphyseal fracture of a long bone. **A:** Drawing showing organization of the hematoma, early woven bone formation in the subperiosteal regions, and cartilage formation in other areas. Periosteal cells contribute to healing this type of injury. If the fracture is rigidly immobilized or if it occurs primarily through cancellous bone and the cancellous surfaces lie in close apposition, there will be little evidence of fracture callus. **B:** Photomicrograph of a fractured rat femur 9 days after injury showing cartilage and bone formation in the subperiosteal regions. (Reprinted from: Einhorn TA. The cell and molecular biology of fracture healing. *Clin Orthop Relat Res.* 1998;335(suppl):S7–S21, with permission.)

at 24 and 48 hours. These results support a role for the local inflammatory response in fracture repair, in contrast to the systemic response seen in polytraumatized patients. It is not clear what role the systemic inflammation plays upon the local environment during fracture repair.

Inflammation

The inflammatory stage of fracture repair dominates the cellular response during early healing. Although this response to injury often continues for a prolonged period, it is the initial pro-inflammatory environment that influences the progression

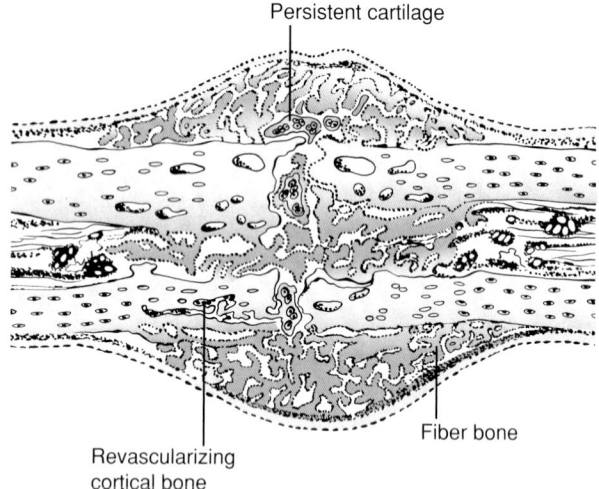

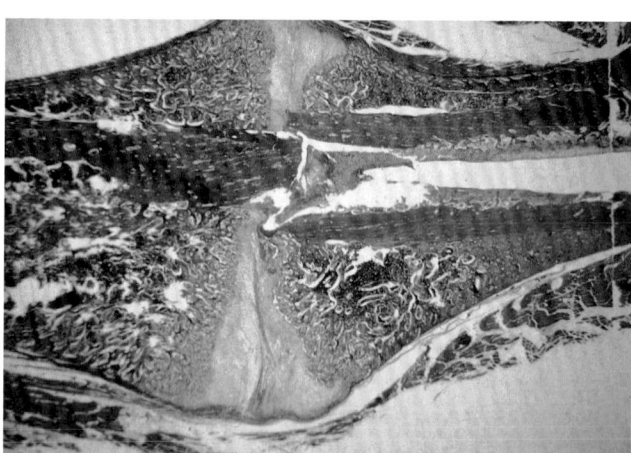

Persistent cartilage

Revascularizing
cortical bone

Fiber bone

A

B

FIGURE 4-4 Progressive fracture healing by fracture callus. **A:** Drawing showing woven or fiber bone bridging the fracture gap and uniting the fracture fragments. Cartilage remains in the regions most distant from ingrowing capillary buds. In many instances, the capillaries are surrounded by new bone. Vessels revascularize the cortical bone at the fracture site. **B:** Photomicrograph of a fractured rat femur 21 days after injury showing fracture callus uniting the fracture fragments. (Reprinted from: Einhorn TA. The cell and molecular biology of fracture healing. *Clin Orthop Relat Res.* 1998;335(suppl):S7–S21, with permission.)

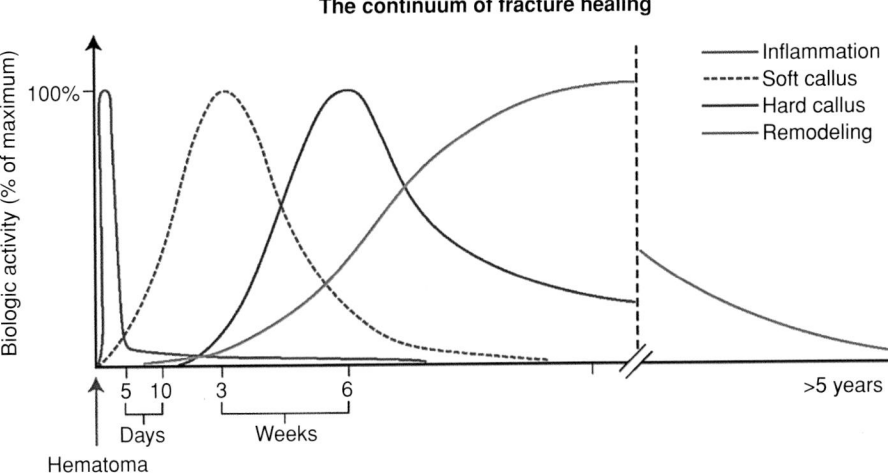

The continuum of fracture healing

FIGURE 4-5 The overlapping stages of fracture repair. Fracture healing cannot be separated into discrete phases of cellular activity, but should rather be looked at as a continuum. Although at any one time one phase may dominate, basic science research suggests that all processes are occurring simultaneously early in fracture healing. Remodeling continues for up to 6 years after the initial injury depending on the treatment modality.

of healing. As a result of the initial energy imparted during a fracture, there is extensive damage to bone and the surrounding tissues, shearing of local blood vessels, and a variable disruption of the integrity of the periosteum. As a result, the area immediately adjacent to the fracture site becomes relatively hypoxic and localized tissue necrosis occurs.[42]

The presence of cellular debris initiates an inflammatory response mediated by both local and infiltrating inflammatory cells, including platelets, polymorphonuclear cells (PMN), macrophages, and lymphocytes. These cells help orchestrate the subsequent healing process by phagocytosing necrotic tissue and by producing cytokines that influence the repair process. Neutrophils are the first cells to arrive at the fracture site, and are present at least as early as 3 hours after fracture.[13] Even at this early phase of fracture healing, markers of osteogenic differentiation can be detected at the site, reinforcing the concept that the various stages of fracture repair occur in continuum rather than as distinct steps.[52] Clinicians should note that surgical interventions typically occur during this early phase of fracture healing, and therefore they can disrupt the hematoma or inflammatory stages of fracture healing. Animal models have demonstrated that the removal of hematoma early during fracture repair (2 to 4 days) and repeated debridement of the fracture site (for the first 2 days) after fracture can result in both delayed union and nonunion.[40,52,80]

Soft Callus

The soft callus stage of fracture healing is heralded by the differentiation of progenitor cells into chondrocytes and osteoblasts (Fig. 4-3). This stage begins at the end of the first week after fracture in a murine model, and typically by 3 weeks in humans. Depending on the mechanical environment and the vascular supply to the fracture site, cartilage or osteoid becomes the predominant tissue in the callus, replacing the fibrous tissue and hematoma. Types I and II collagen are produced in order to form a matrix that restores stability to the bone ends. Mechanical testing of the fracture callus at this stage reveals the stability of soft tissue rather than a consolidated mass that

confers bone stability. Radiographically, the fracture site does not appear united at this stage, but a fluffy appearance of the early mineralizing callus may start to be detected.

Hard Callus

The hard callus stage is defined by the conversion of cartilage to a calcified cartilage matrix with terminal differentiation of the chondrocytes (Fig. 4-4). This occurs during the second week in murine tibia fracture models and several weeks after a fracture in humans. Concurrently, with the wave of calcification, hypertrophic chondrocytes senesce and blood vessels invade the callus. Given the reduction in the number of chondrocytes, the dominant cell types during the hard callus phase are the osteoblast and osteoclast. The woven bone deposited at this time by the osteoblasts further strengthens the callus, but does not follow the stress-induced pattern seen in the surrounding, intact bone. The reduction in strain that occurs at this point in the bridging bone appears to have a molecular effect on both bone cells and newly forming vessels. Clinically, this phase of healing is seen as the calcification and consolidation of the fracture callus on radiographs. During cast or traction treatment of fractures, the hard callus phase is also accompanied by a clinically evident reduction in pain and increased sense of stability at the fracture site.

Remodeling

The remodeling phase is the phase of bone healing that returns the previously damaged tissue nearer to its pre-injured state. During remodeling, the canalicular architecture of bone is reestablished, and the haversian system with its osteocytes is restored. This process starts in concert with bone consolidation and continues for months or years after a solid osseous union has been achieved. During remodeling, intricate communication between osteoblasts and osteoclasts leads to the creation of lamellar bone consistent with the mechanical stress imposed on the bone by loading, particularly weight bearing. This phenomenon, described by Wolff's law, involves the strengthening of the internal and cortical architecture of bones in response to applied

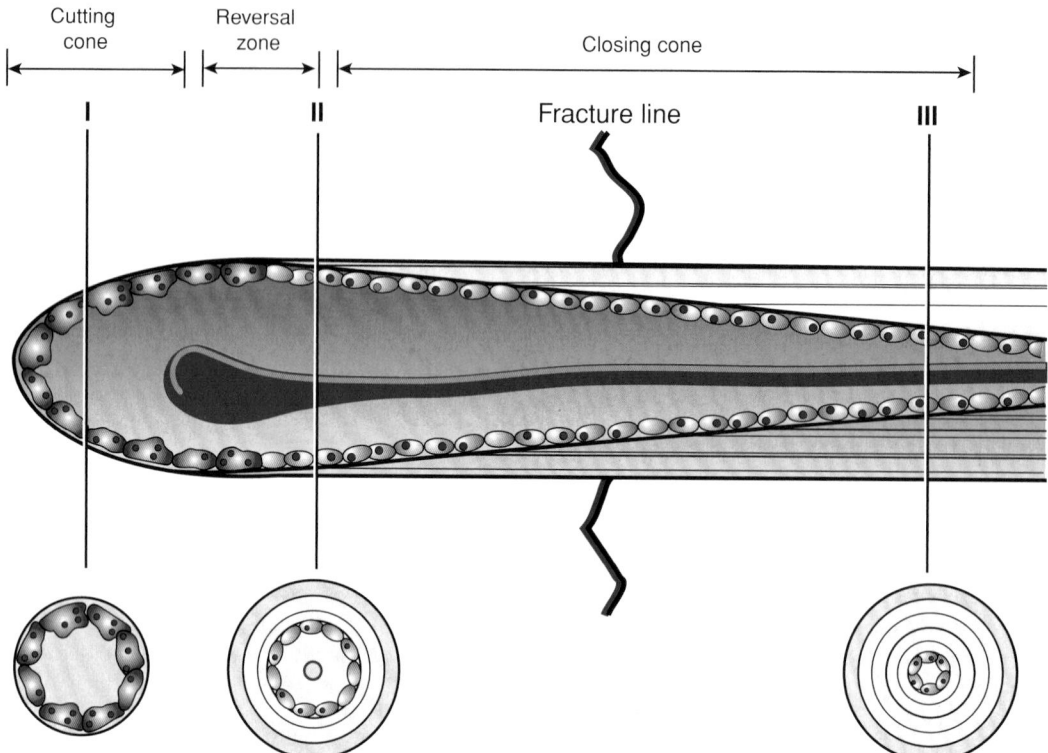

FIGURE 4-6 Primary bone healing utilizes an osteoclastic cutting cone crossing the fracture gap (*I*) followed by bone reconstitution by the trailing osteoblasts (*II, III*).

loads.[114] In order to accomplish the stress-induced remodeling of bone, the actions of osteoclasts and osteoblasts are coupled in the functional unit of bone remodeling—the cutting cone (Fig. 4-6). Cutting cones are formed by osteoclasts that first remove the disorganized woven bone. Then osteoblasts follow and lay down lamellar bone in an organized pattern around a central blood vessel. The activity of bone resorption by osteoclasts and bone formation by osteoblasts is linked through the actions of RANK, RANKL, and osteoprotegerin (OPG).[43] As RANKL exists primarily as a membrane-bound protein, binding to RANK is usually limited. The soluble RANKL concentration is increased by the presence of IL-1β, IL-6, TNF-α, vitamin D3, parathyroid hormone (PTH), and other cytokines, and the subsequent cleavage of membrane-bound RANKL by proteolytic processing or altered gene expression. Binding of RANKL to RANK results in the differentiation and activation of osteoclasts.[48] The role of OPG in this pathway is as a receptor decoy for RANKL. OPG competes for the binding of RANKL, thereby effectively reducing activity in osteoclasts and osteoclast progenitors and decreasing bone resorption.[118] Through this molecular connection, the balance of bone resorption and formation can be coordinated to restore the structural integrity of the damaged tissue.

MECHANICAL INFLUENCES ON BONE HEALING

Early clinical observations led to the belief that fracture stability influenced healing.[100] Subsequent experimental evidence demonstrates that the mechanical environment plays a role in determining the cellular events that define bone repair. Mechanical instability at the fracture site favors endochondral ossification (i.e., the formation of cartilage prior to ossification), whereas mechanical stability results in fracture healing through intramembranous ossification (i.e., direct or primary bone formation) (Fig. 4-7).[58] Classical teaching refers to the concepts of primary (direct) and secondary (indirect) bone healing.[113] Both primary and secondary bone healing have specific roles in the repair of specific fracture patterns and treatments.[81] Given the wide range of implant options now available for the treatment of fractures, it is important to understand the biologic implications of various forms of fixation.

In one study, a 10-day delay in the stabilization of fractures in rabbits was shown to enhance fracture healing.[30] However, a 4-day delay did not enhance fracture repair or callus mechanics in another study in mice.[30,68] The histologic examination of the fracture calluses demonstrated an increased predominance of cartilage 14 days after fracture when the fracture stabilization was delayed 24 hours or greater, suggesting that cell fate is determined early in the fracture healing process. When considering the closed management of fractures, one can appreciate that the cellular elements in the fracture hematoma have already acted on local progenitor cells at the time of treatment, and therefore, some degree of endochondral ossification should be expected and a callus should be seen on radiographs. After the open reduction and rigid internal fixation of fractures, the initial fracture hematoma typically has been removed, and

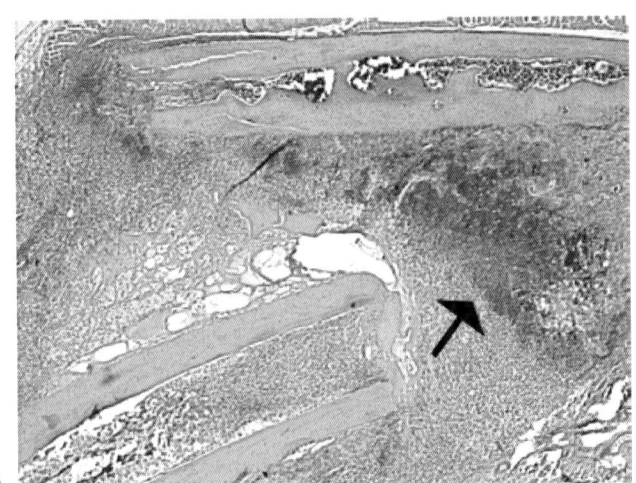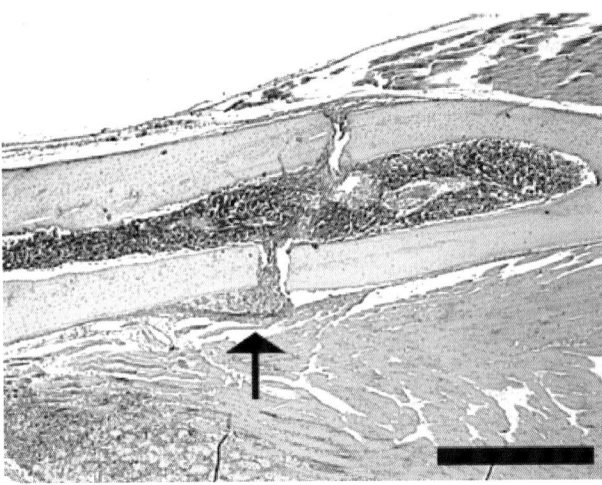

FIGURE 4-7 Fracture healing under unstable and stable conditions. Tibia fractures were created in C57 BL/6 mice by three-point bending. **A:** Fractures allowed to heal without stabilization demonstrate a large callus seven days after fracture. Cartilage can be seen forming around the fractured bone ends (*dark areas indicated by arrowhead*). **B:** Stabilized fractures heal without appreciable callus. No cartilage is present after seven days; however, osteoprogenitor cells from the periosteum and endosteum are seen in the fracture gap. The periosteal reaction is indicated by the arrowhead. (Reprinted from: Thompson Z, Miclau T, Hu D, et al. A model for intramembranous ossification during fracture healing. *J Orthop Res.* 2002;20(5):1091–1098, with permission.)

therefore a new population of progenitor cells responds to the altered fracture environment through intramembranous ossification, with the subsequent absence of visible callus on postoperative radiographs.

FAILURES OF HEALING—ETIOLOGIES AND OVERVIEW OF TREATMENT STRATEGIES

Failures of healing fall into two broad categories with associated cellular mechanisms: Biologic and mechanical failures. The two different nonunion etiologies are recognized clinically by the appearance of atrophic or hypertrophic nonunions, respectively. The natural history of failure of healing is nonunion, an ill-defined term meant to signify the failure of a fracture to achieve stability through bridging bone. Atrophic nonunion is defined by the absence of any visible bone formation on radiographs. Hypertrophic nonunion is defined by abundant bone formation without bone bridging the fracture site. Oligotrophic nonunion is defined as failure to bridge the fracture site with only a moderate amount of bone formation adjacent to a visible fracture line. Delayed union represents the situation where healing is prolonged compared to that expected for a given anatomic location.

Atrophic Nonunion

The major factors that contribute to atrophic nonunions include, infection, compromised nutrition, smoking, medications, and surgeon-controlled factors such as fracture vascularity. These modifiable risk factors for impaired fracture healing will be reviewed below.

Nutritional status remains an important component in the workup of patients presenting with an atrophic nonunion. Fracture healing is an anabolic process requiring molecular building blocks and substantial energy. Leung et al.[60] showed that the fracture callus in rabbits 2 weeks after fracture contains 1,000-fold more adenosine triphosphate than that of normal bone. Malnutrition can also lead to deficiencies in cofactors necessary to catalyze important reactions during fracture healing. Research has shown that up to 18% of hip fracture patients are clinically malnourished, and these malnourished patients stay in the hospital longer and are less likely to recover to pre-injury functional levels.[53] Poor nutrition is indicated by low serum albumin levels, low iron binding capacity, and decreased systemic lymphocyte counts. Failure to correct nutritional deficiencies can expose traumatized patients to an increased risk of impaired wound and fracture healing, and other complications.

The use of tobacco has been implicated in delays in open tibia fracture healing, and in the consolidation of osteotomies performed for hallux valgus deformity correction.[2,54] Tobacco in cigarettes contains over 4,000 chemicals, and the most prominent of these compounds is the cholinergic stimulant, nicotine. In animal studies, the administration of pure nicotine orally or subcutaneously has been shown to increase fracture callus strength and subcutaneous administration also showed an increase in bending stiffness in a rat femur fracture model.[44] Orally administered tobacco extract without nicotine, however, reduced strength, ultimate torque, and torque at yield point.[98] A recent review has postulated that the key to the delay in fracture healing seen in smokers may be through the cholinergic anti-inflammatory pathway and associated inhibition of TNF-α in smokers.[19] This divergence of opinion suggests that further clarification is needed to determine the effects of the individual components of tobacco products on fracture healing, and smokers should be counseled to abstain from smoking during the fracture healing process. However, it is still unclear if transdermal nicotine patches are contraindicated as an adjunct to cessation strategies in fracture patients who smoke.[98]

The chronic use of corticosteroids is known to have detrimental effects on bone mineral density after prolonged administration.[3] The cellular effects of corticosteroids include the inhibition of osteogenic differentiation of MSCs, osteoblast and osteocyte apoptosis, and a reduction in organic matrix synthesis.[79,109] Taken together, these effects of corticosteroids should interfere with processes central to fracture healing and increase individual susceptibility to fracture. However, mixed results have been found in animal studies on the effects of corticosteroids upon fracture healing.[86] At a minimum, alterations in bone quality after prolonged use do increase the difficulty in operatively treating corticosteroid-associated fractures, and the systemic effects of this class of therapeutic agents expose patients to higher rates of complications as a result of immunosuppression.

Nonsteroidal anti-inflammatory drugs (NSAIDs) are among the most commonly used medications. Given the pain and inflammation associated with musculoskeletal injuries, NSAIDs can be a useful addition to the analgesic armamentarium of physicians treating fractures. While the perioperative use of NSAIDs has been associated with impaired healing in spinal fusion patients,[92] a recent meta-analysis of available clinical trials failed to convincingly support the hypothesis that NSAID use increases the risk of nonunion.[25] NSAIDs reduce inflammation through the inhibition of cyclooxygenases (COX). The COX-2 isoform of the enzyme has been shown to stimulate bone formation through the action of prostaglandin E_2 (PGE_2) and the subsequent upregulation of Cbfa1 (or Runx2), a transcription factor necessary for osteoblastogenesis.[120] Despite the link between the genetic loss of COX-2 activity and impaired fracture healing, studies where animals with fractures are administered NSAIDs have not definitively demonstrated impaired healing with both nonspecific and COX-2–specific NSAIDs.[71] Therefore, current guidelines suggest that the clinician weigh the current theoretical risk of impaired fracture healing against the benefits of improved pain relief.[86]

Hypertrophic Nonunion

The development of a hypertrophic nonunion is generally related to a lack of adequate stability at the fracture site. As stated above, motion at the fracture site favors the differentiation of progenitor cells into chondrocytes. In addition, macroscopic movement of fracture fragments prevents normal vascular invasion and the associated senescence of chondrocytes and mineralization of the cartilage matrix seen in optimally stable fractures. Morphologically, hypertrophic nonunions are identified by a persistent fracture line with a large fusiform callus

that has been compared to the shape of two elephants' feet, sole-to-sole. With revision surgery to provide adequate stability, a hypertrophic nonunion typically goes on to heal uneventfully without the need to augment local biology with bone graft or growth factor stimulation.

SYSTEMIC PHARMACOLOGIC TREATMENTS INFLUENCING BONE HEALING

Bisphosphonates are a class of drug commonly used to decrease the risk of fracture in patients with low bone mineral density.[65] The molecular structure of bisphosphonates is similar to that of pyrophosphate, an essential component of the mineral phase of bone. Bisphosphonates are incorporated into the lattice structure of bone and inhibit osteoclast function, thereby limiting bone turnover in the steady state. After bone fracture, bisphosphonates do not appear to interfere with the early phases of repair, rather continued bisphosphonate use in one study resulted in a larger, stronger callus.[17] Although time-to-union was not affected, a marked delay in the completion of remodeling was seen, and the authors of this study proposed that the enlarged callus was an adaptation to this delay.

Parathyroid hormone (PTH), an endogenously occurring regulator of calcium, phosphate, and vitamin D homeostasis, has been shown in animal studies to enhance fracture healing when given intermittently.[10] Teriparatide, the 1 to 34 amino terminus of the 84 amino acid endogenous protein, has also been shown to possess biologic activity similar to the native protein and is FDA-approved for the treatment of osteoporosis.[47,77] In a rat femur fracture model teriparatide was found to increase the external callus volume and the ultimate load to failure of the femoral fracture callus while concurrently increasing bone mineral density in the opposite femur.[7] Although not completely elucidated, the mechanism of improved fracture healing with PTH treatment is felt to relate to the increase in chondroprogenitor and osteoprogenitor cells in the early fracture callus.[72] Further research has shown that the stimulatory effects on chondroprogenitor cell proliferation are noted early in the fracture healing process, with both proliferation rates and the expression of chondrocyte maturation-related genes (SOX-9, pro-1α (II) collagen, pro-1α (X) collagen, and osteopontin) normalizing by the soft callus phase of healing.[75] At a molecular level, the canonical Wnt pathway appears to drive the beneficial effects of teriparatide on fracture healing by accelerating the maturation of chondrocytes through the nuclear localization of β-catenins.[49]

CARTILAGE HEALING

Cartilage Healing Response to Isolated Chondral Injury

The body does not heal isolated cartilage damage effectively. This defective healing response is attributable to the lack of a blood supply necessary for the initiation and support of the repair process, a lack of sufficient stem cells to repopulate and repair the defect, and chondrocyte cell death in the surrounding cartilage which compromises tissue integrity and interferes with repair tissue integration. Viable chondrocytes near the injury may proliferate, form clusters of new cells, and synthesize new matrix, but chondrocytes cannot migrate readily through cartilage tissue to the site of the injury, and the matrix components they synthesize usually are not sufficient to fill the defect.

Cartilage Healing Response to Osteochondral Injury

Articular injuries that also disrupt the subchondral bone initiate the fracture healing process within the subchondral bone, and the repair tissue from the bone can fill the overlying cartilage defect. Cartilage healing then follows the sequence of inflammation, repair, and remodeling like that seen in bone or dense fibrous tissue. Blood from ruptured subchondral vessels fills the injury site with a hematoma that extends from the area of bony injury into the chondral defect. Inflammatory cells migrate through the clot followed by fibroblasts that begin to synthesize a collagenous matrix. Within the repair tissue, some of the cells assume a rounded shape and begin to synthesize a matrix that has some properties of articular cartilage.

Within a few weeks of injury, the repair tissue forming within the defect begins to undergo differentiation into cartilaginous and osseous tissues. This cartilage tissue is a mixture of fibrocartilage and variable amounts of hyaline-like cartilage. While the initial repair of an osteochondral injury typically follows a predictable course, subsequent changes in the cartilage repair tissue vary considerably among similar defects. In some chondral defects the production of a cartilaginous matrix continues, and the cells may retain the appearance and some of the functions of articular chondrocytes, including the production of some type II collagen and proteoglycans. However, the composition, structure, and organization of normal articular cartilage is never recreated. Instead, the end product is a fibrocartilaginous scar that may still provide clinically satisfactory joint function for many years. Unfortunately, in many injuries, the cartilage repair tissue deteriorates more rapidly. The cells lose the appearance of chondrocytes and appear to become more fibroblastic, and the fibrous matrix fibrillates and fragments (Fig. 4-8).

Factors Influencing Cartilage Healing

Gap: A primary objective of surgery is to close the diastasis between fracture fragments, and it is reasonable to expect that

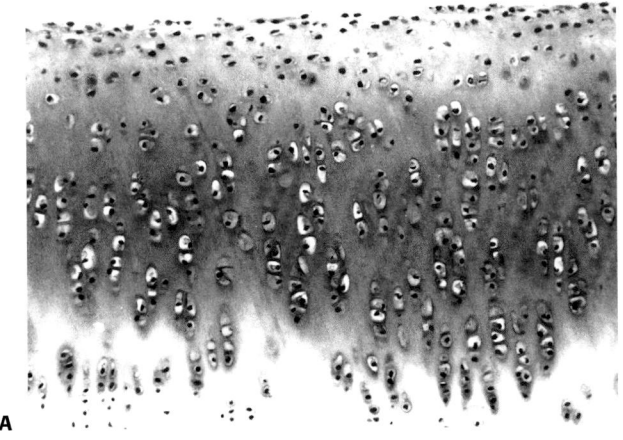
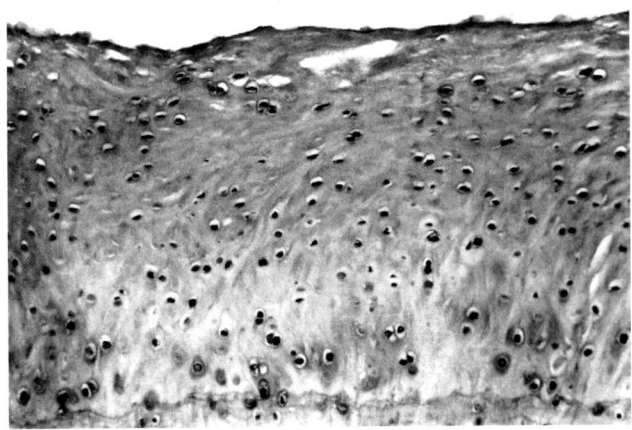
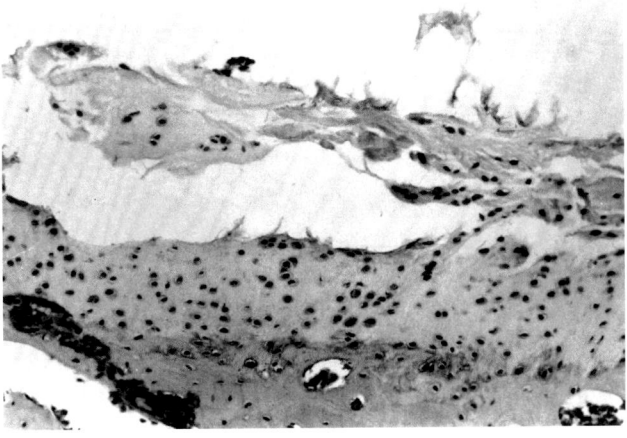

FIGURE 4-8 **A:** Normal rabbit articular cartilage showing the homogeneous extracellular matrix. The chondrocytes near the articular surface are relatively small and flattened, in which those in the middle and deeper zones of the articular cartilage have a more spherical shape. **B:** Well-formed fibrocartilaginous repair cartilage. Notice that the extracellular matrix is more fibrillar and the chondrocytes do not show the same organization as normal articular cartilage. Nonetheless, this repair cartilage does fill the defect in the articular surface. In most instances after osteochondral injury, this type of tissue forms within 6 to 8 weeks. **C:** Photomicrograph showing fibrillation and fragmentation of fibrocartilaginous repair tissue. Because fibrocartilaginous repair tissue lacks the mechanical properties of normal articular cartilage, it often degenerates over time. (Reprinted from: Buckwalter JA, Mow VC. Cartilage repair and osteoarthritis. In: Moskowitz RW, Howell DS, Goldberg VM, Mankin HJ, eds. *Osteoarthritis Diagnosis and Medical/Surgical Management*. 2nd ed. Philadelphia, PA: WB Saunders, 1992:86–87, with permission.)

minimizing the volume and surface area of a chondral defect would increase the probability of successful cartilage repair. Experimental work indicates that 1-mm or smaller defects tend to heal more successfully than larger defects. However, some residual separation of osteochondral fragments or the loss of segments of the articular surface may not always produce clinically significant disturbances of joint function or rapid cartilage deterioration.[36] The extent of tolerable loss of the articular surface has not been defined and may vary among joints.[36]

Step-off: Residual step-off of the articular surface can cause instability, locking, catching, and restricted range of motion. Some degree of step-off can be corrected through cartilage tissue remodeling; however, excessive articular step-off is associated with progressive deterioration of the articular cartilage, likely due to resulting supra-physiologic contact stresses on the more prominent areas. Abnormal contact stress is a key determinant of both cartilage repair and cartilage degeneration. A study of contact stress aberrations following imprecise reduction of simulated human cadaver tibial plateau fractures showed that, in general, peak local cartilage pressure increased with increasing step-off, but the results varied among specimens.[15] In most specimens, cartilage pressure did not increase significantly until the fragment step-off exceeded 1.5 mm. However, in some specimens incongruities of as little as 0.25-mm caused peak local pressure elevations, suggesting that results may vary even among individuals with the same degree of articular incongruity. The degree of joint step-off that can be tolerated without causing long-term joint deterioration differs from joint to joint. A common "rule of thumb" is that residual step-off should not exceed the thickness of the articular cartilage at the injury site, but this rule almost certainly overstates the amount of step-off that can be accepted without consequence.

Loading and Motion: Prolonged immobilization of a joint following intra-articular fractures can lead to adhesion formation as well as deterioration of the cartilage, resulting in poor joint function. Early motion during the repair and remodeling phases of healing can decrease or prevent adhesions and the immobilization-induced deterioration of cartilage. However, animal experiments have shown that early joint loading can also increase inflammation and lead to cartilage degeneration.[38] Cartilage repair tissue is particularly vulnerable to damage from excessive loading, so strict non–weight-bearing is typically maintained for at least 6 weeks. The role of continuous passive motion (CPM) remains a topic of debate, but its routine use after microfracture cartilage repair surgery and the results of some animal studies argues for its inclusion in the rehabilitation process after cartilage injury.[93]

Patient Age: The long-term results of traumatically induced articular cartilage injury may also depend on the age of the patient. Recent studies have demonstrated age-specific differences in the response of chondrocytes to mechanical injury, with immature cartilage being much more susceptible to mechanical

injury than mature cartilage.[56] On the other hand, older age is often associated with poorer results after treatment of intra-articular fractures, possibly due to age-related alterations that decrease the capacity to repair injuries or withstand alterations in loading caused by joint incongruity.[99]

RESPONSE OF CARTILAGE TO MECHANICAL INJURY

Cartilage damage associated with traumatic injuries is characterized by catastrophic disruption of cartilage matrix integrity and structure, extensive chondrocyte death in the area of cartilage injury, and expansion of this "zone of injury" which is facilitated by diffusible mediators such as nitric oxide. The initial damage can be worsened by persistent mechanical overload due to associated joint incongruity, instability, and/or limb malalignment.[57] Chondrocytes in the superficial zone of articular cartilage are at particular risk. In vitro data show that the extent of cartilage damage is related to both the peak stress and strain rate.[88] Injurious compression disrupts the collagen framework resulting in decreased load carrying capacity. Mechanical injury is also associated with proteoglycan loss, both from alterations to chondrocyte biosynthetic activity and from chondrocyte death. Mechanical overload causes chondrocytes to upregulate their expression of matrix degrading enzymes including ADAMTS family members and several MMPs, which may play a major role in subsequent cartilage degeneration.[59]

CONSEQUENCES OF CARTILAGE INJURY

Clinical outcomes after cartilage injury depend on many factors including the size and location of the injury. Small lesions and/or lesions outside of the main weight-bearing areas of the hip, knee, and ankle often are well tolerated. However, this is not universally true, and small lesions often progress over time, particularly if there are associated injuries to other structures such as menisci or the stabilizing ligaments. Furthermore, cartilage injuries, with or without fractures, are risk factors for the development of osteoarthritis. Although the development of post-traumatic osteoarthritis is a complex, multifactorial process, there appears to be a clear relationship between the severity of the injury to the subchondral bone and subsequent joint degeneration. This relationship is best exemplified by recent studies that used CT data to estimate the energy absorbed in tibial pilon fractures, and then correlated that data with the subsequent development of ankle arthritis.[6] There was 88% concordance of fracture energy and the development of arthritis, and linear regression analysis showed that fracture energy and articular comminution explained 70% of the variation in arthritis severity 2 years after injury.

MODIFIERS OF CARTILAGE DAMAGE

The acutely traumatized joint is a particularly hostile environment for articular cartilage, with the presence of multiple mediators of chondrocyte cell death, including: proinflammatory cytokines, reactive oxygen species, blood, and damaged matrix. Furthermore, surgical intervention poses additional risks of iatrogenic cartilage injury from mechanical damage associated with hardware insertion and cell death due to desiccation of exposed cartilage. Fortunately, some of these factors are easily addressed, while others are targets for emerging therapeutic approaches. At present, the most easily modified mediators of cartilage damage are joint hemarthrosis, which can be managed by evacuation and/or lavage, and cartilage desiccation, which is effectively managed by periodic rewetting of the joint surface intraoperatively.[87]

SUMMARY

The biology that underlies bone and cartilage healing involves complex processes. A basic understanding of these processes is essential to the rational treatment of fractures with a mind to optimizing the environment for uncomplicated healing. The main components essential to the healing of musculoskeletal tissues are: cells, ECM, bioactive molecule–receptor pairs, and blood supply. The cellular milieu is responsible for the creation of new tissues. ECM forms the scaffold on which these cells perform their synthetic function. Bioactive molecules allow communication between the various cell types described above. The blood supply provides fuel for this energy-intensive process. Thinking about the treatment of injuries with these components in mind will enhance the surgeon's ability to promote healing and avoid complications during the treatment of their patients.

REFERENCES

1. Abe E, Yamamoto M, Taguchi Y, et al. Essential requirement of BMPs-2/4 for both osteoblast and osteoclast formation in murine bone marrow cultures from adult mice: Antagonism by noggin. *J Bone Miner Res.* 2000;15(4):663–673.
2. Adams CI, Keating JF, Court-Brown CM. Cigarette smoking and open tibial fractures. *Injury.* 2001;32(1):61–65.
3. Adinoff AD, Hollister JR. Steroid-induced fractures and bone loss in patients with asthma. *N Eng J Med.* 1983;309(5):265–268.
4. Alexander KA, Chang MK, Maylin ER, et al. Osteal macrophages promote in vivo intramembranous bone healing in a mouse tibial injury model. *J Bone Miner Res.* 2011;26(7):1517–1532.
5. Alsousou J, Thompson M, Hulley P, et al. The biology of platelet-rich plasma and its application in trauma and orthopaedic surgery: A review of the literature. *J Bone Joint Surg Br.* 2009;91(8):987–996.
6. Anderson DD, Marsh JL, Brown TD. The pathomechanical etiology of post-traumatic osteoarthritis following intraarticular fractures. *Iowa Orthop J.* 2011;31:1–20.
7. Andreassen TT, Ejersted C, Oxlund H. Intermittent parathyroid hormone (1–34) treatment increases callus formation and mechanical strength of healing rat fractures. *J Bone Miner Res.* 1999;14(6):960–968.
8. Andrew JG, Hoyland JA, Freemont AJ, et al. Platelet-derived growth factor expression in normally healing human fractures. *Bone.* 1995;16(4):455–460.
9. Bak B, Jørgensen PH, Andreassen TT. The stimulating effect of growth hormone on fracture healing is dependent on onset and duration of administration. *Clin Orthop Relat Res.* 1991;(264):295–301.
10. Barnes GL, Kakar S, Vora S, et al. Stimulation of fracture-healing with systemic intermittent parathyroid hormone treatment. *J Bone Joint Surg Am.* 2008;90(suppl 1):120–127.
11. Bordei P. Locally applied platelet-derived growth factor accelerates fracture healing. *J Bone Joint Surg Br.* 2011;93(12):1653–1659.
12. Boyce BF, Xing L. Biology of RANK, RANKL, and osteoprotegerin. *Arthritis Res Ther.* 2007;9(suppl 1):S1.
13. Brighton CT, Hunt RM. Early histologic and ultrastructural changes in microvessels of periosteal callus. *J Orthop Trauma.* 1997;11(4):244–253.
14. Brighton CT, Hunt RM. Early histological and ultrastructural changes in medullary fracture callus. *J Bone Joint Surg Am.* 1991;73(6):832–847.
15. Brown TD, Anderson DD, Nepola JV, et al. Contact stress aberrations following imprecise reduction of simple tibial plateau fractures. *J Orthop Res.* 1988;6(6):851–862.
16. Buckwalter JA, Einhorn TA, O'Keefe RJ. *American Academy of Orthopaedic Surgeons. Orthopaedic Basic Science : Foundations of Clinical Practice.* 3rd ed. Rosemont, IL: American Academy of Orthopaedic Surgeons; 2007.
17. Cao Y, Mori S, Mashiba T, et al. Raloxifene, estrogen, and alendronate affect the processes of fracture repair differently in ovariectomized rats. *J Bone Miner Res.* 2002;17(12):2237–2246.
18. Carpenter JE, Hipp JA, Gerhart TN, et al. Failure of growth hormone to alter the biomechanics of fracture-healing in a rabbit model. *J Bone Joint Surg Am.* 1992;74(3):359–367.
19. Chen Y, Guo Q, Pan X, et al. Smoking and impaired bone healing: Will activation of cholinergic anti-inflammatory pathway be the bridge? *Int Orthop.* 2011;35(9):1267–1270.
20. Colnot C, Thompson Z, Miclau T, et al. Altered fracture repair in the absence of MMP9. *Development.* 2003;130(17):4123–4133.
21. Colnot C. Skeletal cell fate decisions within periosteum and bone marrow during bone regeneration. *J Bone Miner Res.* 2009;24(2):274–282.
22. Covas DT, Panepucci RA, Fontes AM, et al. Multipotent mesenchymal stromal cells obtained from diverse human tissues share functional properties and gene-expression profile with CD146+ perivascular cells and fibroblasts. *Exp Hematol.* 2008;36(5):642–654.
23. Dennis JE, Merriam A, Awadallah A, et al. A quadripotential mesenchymal progenitor cell isolated from the marrow of an adult mouse. *J Bone Miner Res.* 1999;14(5):700–709.
24. Dickson KF, Katzman S, Paiement G. The importance of the blood supply in the healing of tibial fractures. *Contemp Orthop.* 1995;30(6):489–493.
25. Dodwell ER, Latorre JG, Parisini E, et al. NSAID exposure and risk of nonunion: A meta-analysis of case-control and cohort studies. *Calcif Tissue Int.* 2010;87(3):193–202.
26. Dominici M, Le Blanc K, Mueller I, et al. Minimal criteria for defining multipotent mesenchymal stromal cells. The International Society for Cellular Therapy position statement. *Cytotherapy.* 2006;8(4):315–317.
27. Drake FH, Dodds RA, James IE, et al. Cathepsin K, but not cathepsins B, L, or S, is abundantly expressed in human osteoclasts. *J Biol Chem.* 1996;271(21):12511–12516.
28. Eghbali-Fatourechi GZ, Lamsam J, Fraser D, et al. Circulating osteoblast-lineage cells in humans. *N Engl J Med.* 2005;352(19):1959–1966.
29. Einhorn TA. Enhancement of fracture-healing. *J Bone Joint Surg Am.* 1995;77(6):940–956.
30. Ellsasser JC, Moyer CF, Lesker PA, et al. Improved healing of experimental long bone fractures in rabbits by delayed internal fixation. *J Trauma.* 1975;15(10):869–876.
31. Epari DR, Schell H, Bail HJ, et al. Instability prolongs the chondral phase during bone healing in sheep. *Bone.* 2006;38(6):864–870.
32. Ferguson C, Alpern E, Miclau T, et al. Does adult fracture repair recapitulate embryonic skeletal formation? *Mech Dev.* 1999;87(1–2):57–66.
33. Ferrara N, Gerber HP, LeCouter J. The biology of VEGF and its receptors. *Nat Med.* 2003;9(6):669–676.
34. Flick LM, Weaver JM, Ulrich-Vinther M, et al. Effects of receptor activator of NFkappaB (RANK) signaling blockade on fracture healing. *J Orthop Res.* 2003;21(4):676–684.
35. Gerstenfeld LC, Sacks DJ, Pelis M, et al. Comparison of effects of the bisphosphonate alendronate versus the RANKL inhibitor denosumab on murine fracture healing. *J Bone Miner Res.* 2009;24(2):196–208.
36. Giannoudis PV, Tzioupis C, Papathanassopoulos A, et al. Articular step-off and risk of post-traumatic osteoarthritis. Evidence today. *Injury.* 2010;41(10):986–995.
37. Göktürk E, Turgut A, Bayçu C, et al. Oxygen-free radicals impair fracture healing in rats. *Acta Orthop Scand.* 1995;66(5):473–475.
38. Green DM, Noble PC, Bocell JR Jr, et al. Effect of early full weight-bearing after joint injury on inflammation and cartilage degradation. *J Bone Joint Surg Am.* 2006;88(10):2201–2209.
39. Grøgaard B, Gerdin B, Reikerås O. The polymorphonuclear leukocyte: Has it a role in fracture healing? *Arch Orthop Trauma Surg.* 1990;109(5):268–271.
40. Grundnes O, Reikerås O. The importance of the hematoma for fracture healing in rats. *Acta Orthop Scand.* 1993;64(3):340–342.
41. Grundnes O, Reikerås O. The role of hematoma and periosteal sealing for fracture healing in rats. *Acta Orthop Scand.* 1993;64(1):47–49.
42. Ham AW. A histological study of the early phases of bone repair. *J Bone Joint Surg Am.* 1930;12(4):827–844.
43. Hanada R, Hanada T, Penninger JM. Physiology and pathophysiology of the RANKL/RANK system. *Biol Chem.* 2010;391(12):1365–1370.
44. Hastrup SG, Chen X, Bechtold JE, et al. Effect of nicotine and tobacco administration method on the mechanical properties of healing bone following closed fracture. *J Orthop Res.* 2010;28(9):1235–1239.
45. Hauser CJ, Zhou X, Joshi P, et al. The immune microenvironment of human fracture/soft-tissue hematomas and its relationship to systemic immunity. *J Trauma.* 1997;42(5):895–903; discussion 903–904.
46. Hertel R, Lambert SM, Müller S, et al. On the timing of soft-tissue reconstruction for open fractures of the lower leg. *Arch Orthop Trauma Surg.* 1999;119(1–2):7–12.
47. Hodsman AB, Bauer DC, Dempster DW, et al. Parathyroid hormone and teriparatide for the treatment of osteoporosis: A review of the evidence and suggested guidelines for its use. *Endocr Rev.* 2005;26(5):688–703.
48. Hsu H, Lacey DL, Dunstan CR, et al. Tumor necrosis factor receptor family member RANK mediates osteoclast differentiation and activation induced by osteoprotegerin ligand. *Proc Natl Acad Sci U S A.* 1999;96(7):3540–3545.

49. Kakar S, Einhorn TA, Vora S, et al. Enhanced chondrogenesis and Wnt signaling in PTH-treated fractures. *J Bone Miner Res.* 2007;22(12):1903–1912.
50. Kawaguchi H, Oka H, Jingushi S, et al. A local application of recombinant human fibroblast growth factor 2 for tibial shaft fractures: A randomized, placebo-controlled trial. *J Bone Miner Res.* 2010;25(12):2735–2743.
51. Klaus Ley, Carlo Laudanna, Myron I. Cybulsky & Sussan Nourshargh. *Nat Rev Immunol.* 2007;7:678–689.
52. Kolar P, Gaber T, Perka C, et al. Human early fracture hematoma is characterized by inflammation and hypoxia. *Clin Orthop Relat Res.* 2011;469(11):3118–3126.
53. Koval KJ, Maurer SG, Su ET, et al. The effects of nutritional status on outcome after hip fracture. *J Orthop Trauma.* 1999;13(3):164–169.
54. Krannitz KW, Fong HW, Fallat LM, et al. The effect of cigarette smoking on radiographic bone healing after elective foot surgery. *J Foot Ankle Surg.* 2009;48(5):525–527.
55. Kumagai K, Vasanji A, Drazba JA, et al. Circulating cells with osteogenic potential are physiologically mobilized into the fracture healing site in the parabiotic mice model. *J Orthop Res.* 2008;26(2):165–175.
56. Kurz B, Lemke A, Kehn M, et al. Influence of tissue maturation and antioxidants on the apoptotic response of articular cartilage after injurious compression. *Arthritis Rheum.* 2004;50(1):123–130.
57. Kurz B, Lemke AK, Fay J, et al. Pathomechanisms of cartilage destruction by mechanical injury. *Ann Anat.* 2005;187(5–6):473–485.
58. Le AX, Miclau T, Hu D, et al. Molecular aspects of healing in stabilized and non-stabilized fractures. *J Orthop Res.* 2001;19(1):78–84.
59. Lee JH, Fitzgerald JB, Dimicco MA, et al. Mechanical injury of cartilage explants causes specific time-dependent changes in chondrocyte gene expression. *Arthritis Rheum.* 2005;52(8):2386–2395.
60. Leung KS, Sher AH, Lam TS, et al. Energy metabolism in fracture healing. Measurement of adenosine triphosphate in callus to monitor progress. *J Bone Joint Surg Br.* 1989;71(4):657–660.
61. Li L, Xie T. Stem cell niche: Structure and function. *Annu Rev Cell Dev Biol.* 2005;21:605–631.
62. Lieberman JR, Daluski A, Einhorn TA. The role of growth factors in the repair of bone biology and clinical applications. *J Bone Joint Surg Am.* 2002;84(6):1032–1044.
63. Luria EA, Owen ME, Friedenstein AJ, et al. Bone formation in organ cultures of bone marrow. *Cell Tissue Res.* 1987;248(2):449–454.
64. Matsuda N, Lin WL, Kumar NM, et al. Mitogenic, chemotactic, and synthetic responses of rat periodontal ligament fibroblastic cells to polypeptide growth factors in vitro. *J Periodontol.* 1992;63(6):515–525.
65. McClung MR, Geusens P, Miller PD, et al. Effect of risedronate on the risk of hip fracture in elderly women. Hip Intervention Program Study Group. *N Engl J Med.* 2001;344(5):333–340.
66. McKibbin B. The biology of fracture healing in long bones. *J Bone Joint Surg Br.* 1978;60-B(2):150–162.
67. McNab I, de Haas WG. The role of periosteal blood supply in the healing of fractures of the tibia. *Clin Orthop Relat Res.* 1974;105:27–33.
68. Miclau T, Lu C, Thompson Z, et al. Effects of delayed stabilization on fracture healing. *J Orthop Res.* 2007;25(12):1552–1558.
69. Mizuno K, Mineo K, Tachibana T, et al. The osteogenetic potential of fracture haematoma. Subperiosteal and intramuscular transplantation of the haematoma. *J Bone Joint Surg Br.* 1990;72(5):822–829.
70. Morshed S, Corrales L, Genant H, et al. Outcome assessment in clinical trials of fracture-healing. *J Bone Joint Surg Am.* 2008;90(suppl 1):62–67.
71. Mullis BH, Copland ST, Weinhold PS, et al. Effect of COX-2 inhibitors and non-steroidal anti-inflammatory drugs on a mouse fracture model. *Injury.* 2006;37(9):827–837.
72. Nakajima A, Shimoji N, Shiomi K, et al. Mechanisms for the enhancement of fracture healing in rats treated with intermittent low-dose human parathyroid hormone (1–34). *J Bone Miner Res.* 2002;17(11):2038–2047.
73. Nakamura T, Hara Y, Tagawa M, et al. Recombinant human basic fibroblast growth factor accelerates fracture healing by enhancing callus remodeling in experimental dog tibial fracture. *J Bone Miner Res.* 1998;13(6):942–949.
74. Nakasaki M, Yoshioka K, Miyamoto Y, et al. IGF-I secreted by osteoblasts acts as a potent chemotactic factor for osteoblasts. *Bone.* 2008;43(5):869–879.
75. Nakazawa T, Nakajima A, Shiomi K, et al. Effects of low-dose, intermittent treatment with recombinant human parathyroid hormone (1–34) on chondrogenesis in a model of experimental fracture healing. *Bone.* 2005;37(5):711–719.
76. Nash TJ, Howlett CR, Martin C, et al. Effect of platelet-derived growth factor on tibial osteotomies in rabbits. *Bone.* 1994;15(2):203–208.
77. Neer RM, Arnaud CD, Zanchetta JR, et al. Effect of parathyroid hormone (1–34) on fractures and bone mineral density in postmenopausal women with osteoporosis. *N Engl J Med.* 2001;344(19):1434–1441.
78. Niikura T, Hak DJ, Reddi AH. Global gene profiling reveals a downregulation of BMP gene expression in experimental atrophic nonunions compared to standard healing fractures. *J Orthop Res.* 2006;24(7):1463–1471.
79. O'Brien CA, Jia D, Plotkin LI, et al. Glucocorticoids act directly on osteoblasts and osteocytes to induce their apoptosis and reduce bone formation and strength. *Endocrinology.* 2004;145(4):1835–1841.
80. Park S-H, Silva M, Bahk W-J, et al. Effect of repeated irrigation and debridement on fracture healing in an animal model. *J Orthop Res.* 2002;20(6):1197–1204.
81. Perren SM. Evolution of the internal fixation of long bone fractures. The scientific basis of biological internal fixation: Choosing a new balance between stability and biology. *J Bone Joint Surg Br.* 2002;84(8):1093–1110.
82. Perren SM. Physical and biological aspects of fracture healing with special reference to internal fixation. *Clin Orthop Relat Res.* 1979;(138):175–196.

83. Pettit AR, Chang MK, Hume DA, et al. Osteal macrophages: A new twist on coupling during bone dynamics. *Bone.* 2008;43(6):976–982.
84. Phieffer LS, Goulet JA. Delayed unions of the tibia. *J Bone Joint Surg Am.* 2006;88(1):205–216.
85. Pittenger MF. Multilineage potential of adult human mesenchymal stem cells. *Science.* 1999;284(5411):143–147.
86. Pountos I, Georgouli T, Blokhuis TJ, et al. Pharmacological agents and impairment of fracture healing: What is the evidence? *Injury.* 2008;39(4):384–394.
87. Pun SY, Teng MS, Kim HT. Periodic rewetting enhances the viability of chondrocytes in human articular cartilage exposed to air. *J Bone Joint Surg Br.* 2006;88(11):1528–1532.
88. Quinn TM, Allen RG, Schalet BJ, et al. Matrix and cell injury due to sub-impact loading of adult bovine articular cartilage explants: Effects of strain rate and peak stress. *J Orthop Res.* 2001;19(2):242–249.
89. Radomsky ML, Thompson AY, Spiro RC, et al. Potential role of fibroblast growth factor in enhancement of fracture healing. *Clin Orthop Relat Res.* [Research Support, Non-U.S. Gov't]. 1998(355 suppl):S283–S293.
90. Raines EW, Ross R. Platelet-derived growth factor. I. High yield purification and evidence for multiple forms. *J Biol Chem.* 1982;257(9):5154–5160.
91. Reddi AH. Initiation of fracture repair by bone morphogenetic proteins. *Clin Orthop Relat Res.* 1998(355 suppl):S66–S72.
92. Riew KD, Long J, Rhee J, et al. Time-dependent inhibitory effects of indomethacin on spinal fusion. *J Bone Joint Surg Am.* 2003;85-A(4):632–634.
93. Salter RB, Simmonds DF, Malcolm BW, et al. The biological effect of continuous passive motion on the healing of full-thickness defects in articular cartilage. An experimental investigation in the rabbit. *J Bone Joint Surg Am.* 1980;62(8):1232–1251.
94. Schindeler A, Liu R, Little DG. The contribution of different cell lineages to bone repair: Exploring a role for muscle stem cells. *Differentiation.* 2009;77(1):12–18.
95. Schmidmaier G, Wildemann B, Ostapowicz D, et al. Long-term effects of local growth factor (IGF-I and TGF-beta 1) treatment on fracture healing. A safety study for using growth factors. *J Orthop Res.* 2004;22(3):514–519.
96. Schmidt-Bleek K, Schell H, Kolar P, et al. Cellular composition of the initial fracture hematoma compared to a muscle hematoma: A study in sheep. *J Orthop Res.* 2009;27(9):1147–1151.
97. Shirley D, Marsh D, Jordan G, et al. Systemic recruitment of osteoblastic cells in fracture healing. *J Orthop Res.* 2005;23(5):1013–1021.
98. Skott M, Andreassen TT, Ulrich-Vinther M, et al. Tobacco extract but not nicotine impairs the mechanical strength of fracture healing in rats. *J Orthop Res.* 2006;24(7):1472–1479.
99. Tannast M, Najibi S, Matta JM. Two to twenty-year survivorship of the hip in 810 patients with operatively treated acetabular fractures. *J Bone Joint Surg Am.* 2012;94(17):1559–1567.
100. The classic. The aims of internal fixation. *Clin Orthop Relat Res.* 1979;(138):23–25.
101. Thompson Z, Miclau T, Hu D, et al. A model for intramembranous ossification during fracture healing. *J Orthop Res.* 2002;20(5):1091–1098.
102. Toben D, Schroeder I, El Khassawna T, et al. Fracture healing is accelerated in the absence of the adaptive immune system. *J Bone Miner Res.* 2011;26(1):113–124.
103. Trippel SB, Rosenfeld RG. Growth factor treatment of disorders of skeletal growth. *Instr Course Lect.* 1997;46:477–482.
104. Urist MR, McLean FC. Osteogenetic potency and new-bone formation by induction in transplants to the anterior chamber of the eye. *J Bone Joint Surg Am.* 1952;34-A(2):443–476.
105. Urist MR. Bone: Formation by autoinduction. *Science.* 1965;150(3698):893–899.
106. Utvåg SE, Iversen KB, Grundnes O, et al. Poor muscle coverage delays fracture healing in rats. *Acta Orthop Scand.* 2002;73(4):471–474.
107. Vu TH, Shipley JM, Bergers G, et al. MMP-9/gelatinase B is a key regulator of growth plate angiogenesis and apoptosis of hypertrophic chondrocytes. *Cell.* 1998;93(3):411–422.
108. Weber BG. *Minimax Fracture Fixation: Case Collection: Lower Leg, Ankle Joint, Nonunions, Autogenous Bone Transplantation.* 1st ed. New York, NY: Thieme; 2004.
109. Weinstein RS, Jilka RL, Parfitt AM, et al. Inhibition of osteoblastogenesis and promotion of apoptosis of osteoblasts and osteocytes by glucocorticoids. Potential mechanisms of their deleterious effects on bone. *J Clin Invest.* 1998;102(2):274–282.
110. Whiteside LA, Lesker PA. The effects of extraperiosteal and subperiosteal dissection. II. On fracture healing. *J Bone Joint Surg Am.* 1978;60(1):26–30.
111. Wildemann B, Lubberstedt M, Haas NP, et al. IGF-I and TGF-beta 1 incorporated in a poly(D,L-lactide) implant coating maintain their activity over long-term storage-cell culture studies on primary human osteoblast-like cells. *Biomaterials.* 2004;25(17):3639–3644.
112. Wildemann B, Schmidmaier G, Brenner N, et al. Quantification, localization, and expression of IGF-I and TGF-beta1 during growth factor-stimulated fracture healing. *Calcif Tissue Int.* 2004;74(4):388–397.
113. Willenegger H, Perren SM, Schenk R. [Primary and secondary healing of bone fractures]. *Chirurg.* 1971;42(6):241–252.
114. Wolff J. The classic: On the inner architecture of bones and its importance for bone growth. 1870. *Clin Orthop Relat Res.* 2010;468(4):1056–1065.
115. Xing Z, Lu C, Hu D, et al. Multiple roles for CCR2 during fracture healing. *Dis Model Mech.* 2010;3(7–8):451–458.
116. Yang D, Chen J, Jing Z, et al. Platelet-derived growth factor (PDGF)-AA: A self-imposed cytokine in the proliferation of human fetal osteoblasts. *Cytokine.* 2000;12(8):1271–1274.

117. Yang X, Ricciardi BF, Hernandez-Soria A, et al. Callus mineralization and maturation are delayed during fracture healing in interleukin-6 knockout mice. *Bone*. 2007;41(6): 928–936.
118. Yasuda H, Shima N, Nakagawa N, et al. Identity of osteoclastogenesis inhibitory factor (OCIF) and osteoprotegerin (OPG): A mechanism by which OPG/OCIF inhibits osteoclastogenesis in vitro. *Endocrinology*. 1998;139(3):1329–1337.
119. Young RW. Cell proliferation and specialization during endochondral osteogenesis in young rats. *J Cell Biol*. 1962;14:357–370.
120. Zhang X. Cyclooxygenase-2 regulates mesenchymal cell differentiation into the osteoblast lineage and is critically involved in bone repair. *J Clin Invest*. 2002;109(11): 1405–1415.
121. Zimmermann G, Henle P, Küsswetter M, et al. TGF-beta1 as a marker of delayed fracture healing. *Bone*. 2005;36(5):779–785.

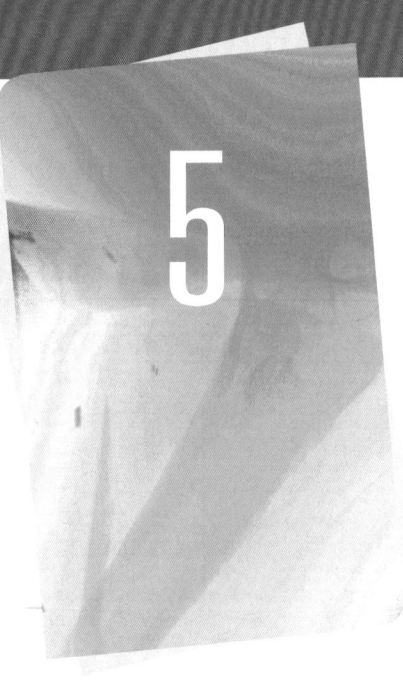

5

BIOLOGIC AND BIOPHYSICAL TECHNOLOGIES FOR THE ENHANCEMENT OF FRACTURE REPAIR

Eric Wagner, Thomas A. Einhorn, and Sanjeev Kakar

INTRODUCTION

Fracture repair is a well-orchestrated biologic process that includes multiple signaling pathways and is regulated by both local and systemic factors. However, any abnormality within this well-orchestrated cascade has the potential to impair healing, leading to between 5% and 10% of fractures failing to achieve complete union.[96] In many instances, the cause of the impairment is unknown and may be related to inadequate reduction, instability,[73] the systemic state of the patient,[97,215] or the nature and extent of energy associated with the traumatic insult itself.[245,326] In addition, the local environment or blood supply can predispose fractures to an abnormal or impaired healing process. For example, open fractures of the tibia have a wide range of delayed union rates of between 16% and 100% depending on the grade of injury.[135] In the scaphoid and femoral neck, fracture healing is dependent on an intact blood supply from a single vessel, and disruption of that vessel leads to high rates of nonunion.[83,137,255] Finally, the subtrochanteric region of the femur is at an increased risk since the mechanical loads occurring there are among the highest in the skeleton.[162]

While fracture healing typically occurs without incident, complications related to delayed union or nonunion can be severe with regard to patient morbidity and medical treatment costs. For example, Busse et al.[58] found that the direct costs associated with the treatment of a tibial nonunion are approximately $7,500, while this estimate can be over $17,000 when indirect costs, such as loss of work productivity, are taken into account. To improve and expedite repair, surgeons may consider the use of bone grafts, biologic agents, or physical stimulation. This chapter will review the current use and development of these approaches in the restoration of skeletal function.

TABLE 5-1	Properties of Types of Autologous Bone Grafts		
Property	Cancellous	Nonvascularized Cortical	Vascularized Cortical
Osteoconduction	+++	+	+
Osteoinduction	++[a]	+/–	+/–
Osteoprogenitor cells	+++	–	++
Immediate strength	–	+++	+++
Strength at months	++	++, +++	+++
Strength at a year	+++	+++	+++

[a]Although cancellous bone is widely believed to be osteoinductive, there is no evidence to critically demonstrate that inductive proteins and cytokines are active in autologous cancellous bone graft.

Reprinted with permission from: Finkemeier CG. Bone-grafting and bone graft substitutes. *J Bone J Surg Am.* 2002;84:454–464.

BONE GRAFTS AND BONE-GRAFT SUBSTITUTES

It is estimated that more than 2.2 million bone-graft procedures are performed worldwide each year, with over 200,000 performed within the United States.[147,201] Indications for their use include malunions, nonunions, arthrodesis, and reconstructive procedures.[239] Their successful incorporation depends on osteoinductive growth factors, an osteoconductive extracellular matrix, and osteogenic pluripotent stem cells residing in the bone marrow. *Osteoinduction* refers to the recruitment and differentiation of pluripotent mesenchymal stem cells (MSCs) into bone-forming osteoprogenitor cells, mediated by graft-derived growth factors such as bone morphogenetic protein (BMP).[308,329] *Osteoconduction* involves the creation of the bone scaffold that supports the ingrowth of blood vessels and perivascular tissue, as well as the attachment of osteoprogenitor cells. This occurs in an ordered sequence which is dependent on the three-dimensional structure of the graft, the local blood supply, and the biomechanical forces exerted on the graft and surrounding tissues.[308] *Osteogenesis* refers to the process of bone formation after the terminal differentiation of osteogenic progenitor cells into mature osteoblasts. These three processes create the signals, scaffolds and cells necessary for the initial phases of fracture healing (Table 5-1).[239,308]

Bone grafting stimulates a sequence of events similar to most tissue regeneration. After initial hematoma formation, there is a release of cytokines, including platelet-derived growth factors (PDGFs), transforming growth factor-betas (TGF-betas), and fibroblast growth factors (FGFs) that lead to the recruitment of circulating progenitor cells and the production of regenerative, angiogenic, and inflammatory factors.[42] The recruited cells then begin the process of graft incorporation, as osteoclasts resorb necrotic graft material. Pluripotential mesenchymal cells respond to local growth factors and differentiate into osteoblasts that produce osteoid. While osteoblasts and endosteal cells on the surface of the graft may survive the transplantation and contribute to the healing, the main contribution of the graft is to act as an osteoinductive and osteoconductive substrate. These properties provide the necessary mechanical and chemical requirements to support the attachment, prolifera-

tion, migration, and differentiation of bone forming cells. The final stages in the process involve mineralization of the osteoid, remodeling of the callus, and incorporation of the remaining graft. The process of remodeling of the callus (composed of woven bone) involves the coordinated activities of osteoblastic bone formation and osteoclastic bone resorption, with woven bone ultimately being replaced by lamellar bone.

Autogenous bone grafting is considered to be the "gold standard" as it utilizes osteoinductive growth factors, an osteoconductive matrix, and osteogenic stem cells to provide consistent results with regard to healing and integration.[38,198,285,305] However, the morbidity associated with graft harvesting, such as donor-site pain, nerve or arterial injury, and infection rates of between 8% and 10%,[23,111,134,317,349] as well as a limited number of donor sites and the increased operative time required for harvest, have prompted extensive research into alternatives. One alternative that avoids many of these limitations and complications is allograft bone.[53,88,138,153,291] However, allogeneic graft is limited by its lack of osteoinductive capabilities[32] and increased costs.[254] Furthermore, although perhaps unfairly as the current donor selection process has greatly reduced any risk, many patients and surgeons remain concerned regarding the risk of disease transmission.[24,156] As a result, there have been investigations into bone-graft substitutes and other tissue engineering strategies for fracture management.

Autologous Bone

Autologous bone grafting remains the gold standard to which all materials and technologies to enhance bone healing are compared. Possessing excellent osteoinductive, osteoconductive, and osteogenic potential, it is the ideal bone graft. Furthermore, graft versus host disease and any disease transmission risk are eliminated since it is the patient's own bone.

Either cancellous or cortical bone can be harvested depending on the procedure. In some cases, it is necessary to augment healing via a vascularized graft, usually from the fibula, rib, or distal femur. Careful planning is needed to ensure that the proposed harvest site will contain both the correct type and amount of graft. For example, a large segmental defect in the radius would need a large structural cortical graft,[105,231] whereas a tibia plateau fracture with a depressed fragment may require only a small amount of cancellous graft. The most common and best-described sources of autologous bone include the pelvis, the distal radius,[315] the fibula,[198] the proximal tibia,[248] the ribs,[208] the greater trochanter,[239] and the olecranon.[239]

Autologous Cancellous Bone Graft

Cancellous bone is the most commonly used bone-graft source, serving as an effective graft material for fractures that do not require immediate structural support from the graft. Instead, it serves as a scaffold for the attachment of host cells and it provides the osteoconductive and osteoinductive functions required for the laying down of new bone. However, it lacks immediate structural stability and strength and is therefore unable to support force transmission alone.

Although cancellous bone graft lacks mechanical strength, its main advantage lies in its tremendous biologic activity. Lining the trabeculae of the graft material are pluripotent progenitor cells capable of differentiating into multiple different lineages, including osteoid-producing cells.[294] Furthermore, the large surface area leads to immediate graft incorporation. In fracture healing, the initial phase involves progenitor cell recruitment and proliferation under the control of local cytokine release. As resorption ensues, more cytokines are released, leading to the formation of granulation tissue and neoangiogenesis, or the formation or new blood vessels. These cytokines also direct the differentiation of osteoprogenitor cells into mature bone forming cells. Within the first couple days, the graft appears to be completely vascularized, while bone formation occurs within weeks.[28,91]

The cancellous graft also serves as a scaffold to be resorbed as the mature osteogenic cells lay down a new osteoid matrix.[308] This begins the graft incorporation and can take many months to complete. When seen on x-ray, this phase represents the gradual loss of a clear delineation between the native bone and fracture lines or graft incorporation.[184] The mechanical properties begin to be restored after the initial weeks of graft incorporation. The process by which the graft is replaced by new bone is known as "creeping substitution"[306] and is usually complete within 1 year (Fig. 5-1, Table 5-1).

While cancellous graft does not provide structural support by itself, through impaction and aided by internal fixation, it is used for areas of bone loss. Examples of such use are in the treatment of bone loss associated with depressed tibial plateau fractures or revision hip and knee arthroplasty.[322,323] Excellent results have also been demonstrated with nonunions and arthrodeses, due to its rapid incorporation and osteogenic regeneration potential (Fig. 5-2).[47,90,250]

Autologous Cortical Bone Graft

Cortical bone can provide good structural support, but it has much weaker osteoconductive and osteoinductive properties. Its use is indicated when immediate structural support is necessary, but it has slightly limited long-term healing potential.[239] This is partly due to the thickness of the cortical matrix, limiting the diffusion of nutrients, and subsequent neovascularization and osteogenesis (Table 5-1).[81] This density also limits the

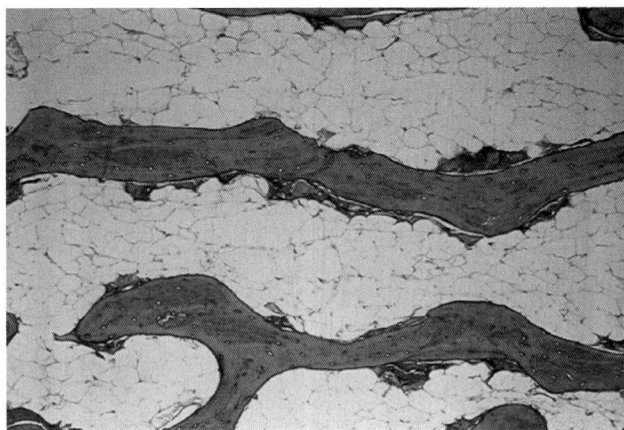

FIGURE 5-1 Low-power photomicrograph showing creeping substitution. Newly formed woven bone, containing osteoblasts with basophilic-staining nuclei, is laid down upon dead lamellar bone identified by the presence of empty osteocytic lacunae (hematoxylin and eosin stain, original magnification 10×).

remodeling process, with the bone incorporation relying on osteoclasts instead of osteoblasts. This resorption phase during the first 6 months leads to progressive mechanical weakness, which is eventually restored around a year after the procedure.[108,132] Remodeling proceeds and creeping substitution can require up to 2 years for completion.[56,104,295] Cortical bone grafts are usually harvested from the ribs, fibula, or crest of the ilium (as a so-called tricortical graft) and can be transplanted with or without a vascular pedicle (Table 5-1).

Vascularized bone-graft biology is different from its nonvascularized counterpart, not only in terms of the rate of repair but also in the way in which remodeling occurs.[81] Most of these grafts are harvested from the iliac crest with the deep circumflex artery, the fibula with peroneal artery branches, the medial femoral condyle with descending genicular artery branches, the distal radius with supraretinacular artery branches, or the ribs with the posterior intercostal artery.[51] Once implanted with its viable vascular pedicle, the independent blood supply leads to significant biologic activity and regeneration potential with retention of up to 90% of the graft's osteocytes.[108,239,247] Dell et al.[81] examined vascularized and nonvascularized grafts histologically and graded the amount of necrosis based on the presence or absence of osteocytes. At 2 weeks, the vascularized graft remained mostly viable, with the only area of necrosis noted at the periphery, while the nonvascularized grafts showed diffuse necrosis of the medullary cavity, taking up to 24 weeks to resemble the vascularized grafts. The increase in osteocyte survival and the early vascularity leads to a rapid incorporation of a vascularized bone graft.[130,295] The initial differences in strengths are due to the remodeling processes. While nonvascularized grafts are incorporated through creeping substitution, vascularized grafts do not induce a robust inflammatory and angiogenic response compromising the early mechanical strength.

In the treatment of critical-sized defects, or bone defects that will not heal without grafting, both vascularized and nonvascularized grafts are indicated. For defects up to 6 cm in length where immediate structural support is desired, nonvascularized

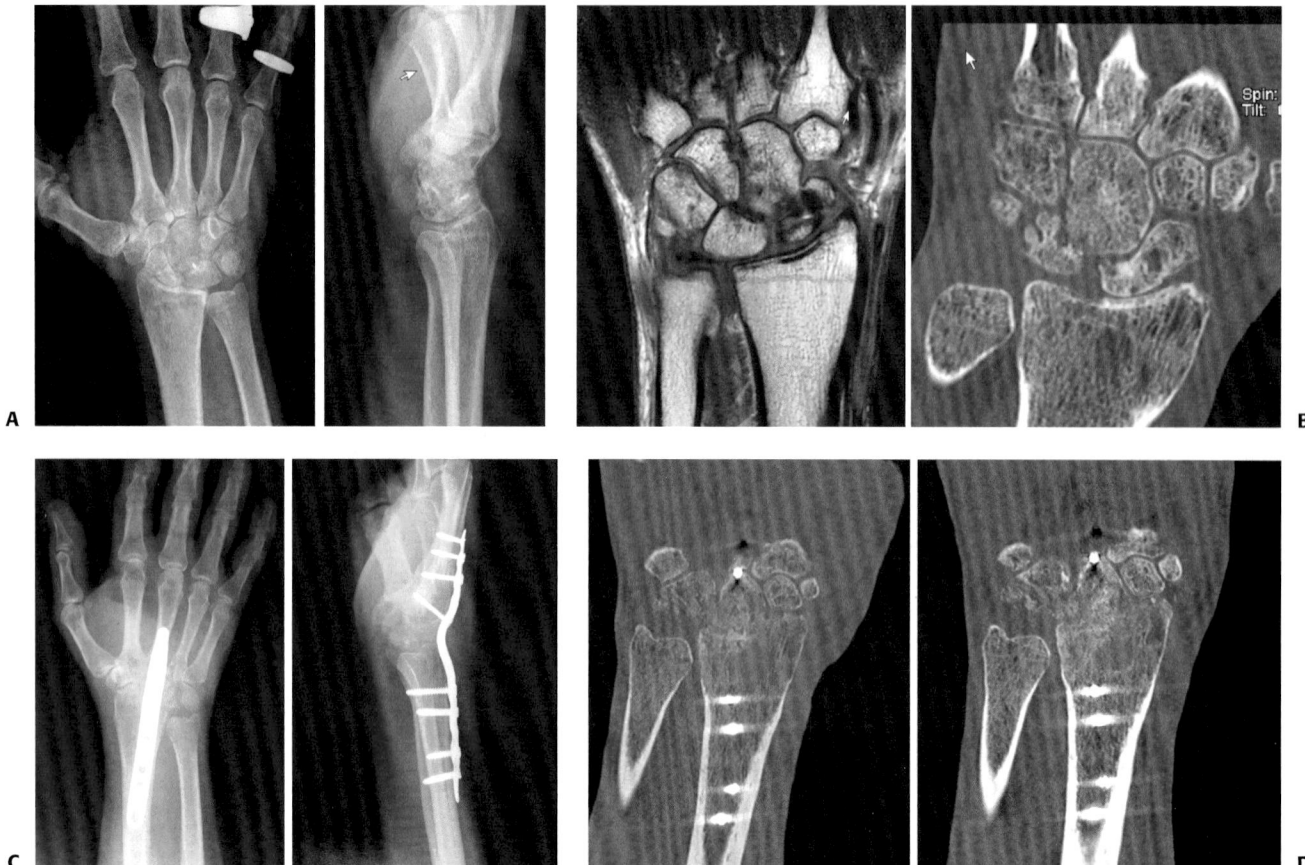

FIGURE 5-2 A 52-year-old laborer developed a scapholunate advanced collapse (SLAC) and scaphoid nonunion, which are shown in plain radiographs **(A)**, as well as on CT and MRI **(B)**. He underwent a total wrist arthrodesis augmented with iliac crest bone grafting and demonstrated good healing of the fusion at 6 months **(C)** and **(D)**.

cortical autografts can be used.[108] Controversy exists regarding the best alternative for defects between 6 and 12 cm, while defects greater than 12 cm are good candidates for vascularized grafting procedures.[81,105] Vascularized grafts are also indicated for reconstruction of defects where the microenvironment of the host is inadequate to initiate an effective biologic response. Examples include acute traumatic injuries with extensive soft tissue damage and impairment of blood supply, atrophic nonunions, and irradiated or severely scarred tissue.[81,105] For example, free vascularized medial femoral condyle flaps have been successfully used to treat many upper-extremity nonunions, including those of the distal radius, scaphoid, and humeral shaft (Fig. 5-3, Table 5-1).[65,172,173]

Complications of Autologous Grafting

In addition to longer operative times associated with harvesting autologous bone grafts, the morbidity associated with the donor sites is a significant concern. The most common donor site for harvesting autograft is the iliac crest.[239] Arrington et al.[15] reviewed 414 cases of iliac crest bone-graft harvesting and found that patients experienced multiple superficial hematomas and infections as well as a variety of more significant complications including 4 deep hematomas, 2 incisional hernias, 6 neurologic injuries, 3 vascular injuries, 2 iliac wing fractures, and 7 deep infections.

Another similar review of iliac crest grafting by Younger et al.[349] of 243 iliac crest harvests demonstrated 57 (24%) superficial complications, such as infection or hematoma, and 15 (6%) deep complications, such as deep hematomas and infections. Other reviews have demonstrated similar rates of adverse events, with deep major complications also including sacroiliac injury, ureteral injury, and vascular injury, in addition to deep hematomas, infections, and iliac crest fractures.[91,134,239] According to a review of the literature by Myeroff and Archdeacon,[239] superficial or minor complications occur in 7.1% to 39% of patients, while major or deep complications occur in 1.8% to 10% of patients.

Other common donor sites include the proximal and distal tibia, distal radius, greater trochanter, and medial femoral condyle. Postoperative pain and superficial hematomas are relatively common complications of harvest from these areas. Significant adverse events from proximal tibia graft harvesting include deep hematomas and infections, joint compromise or proximal tibial fracture, and permanent neurologic injury, occurring in 0.5% to 2% of patients.[117,120,123,239] The distal radius harvesting site is associated with de Quervain's tenosynovitis, superficial radial nerve injury and fracture through the donor site.[256]

A relatively new technique developed in 2005 to overcome the donor-site morbidity associated with autologous bone-graft harvesting is the use of the reamer-irrigator-aspirator (RIA).

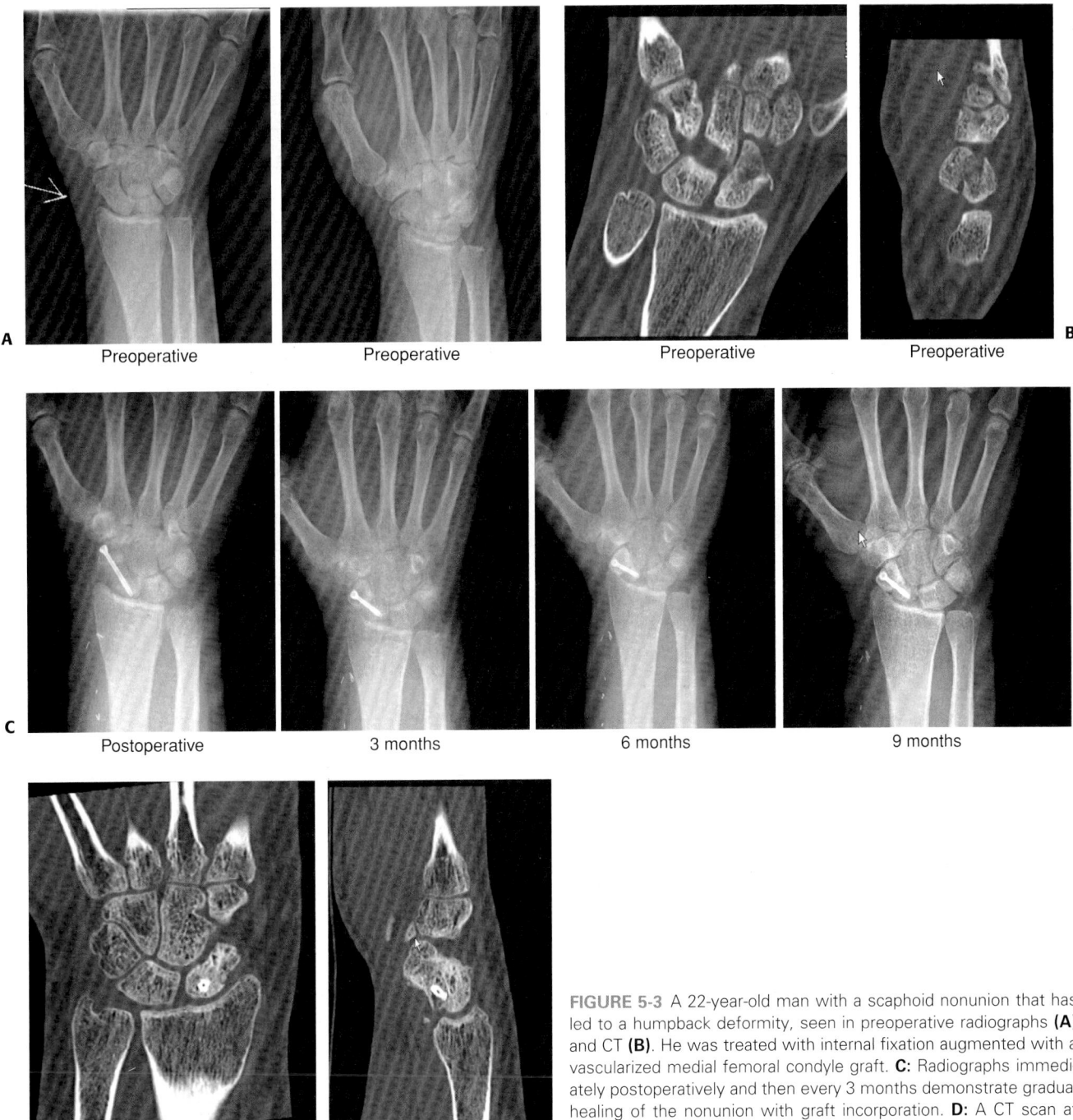

FIGURE 5-3 A 22-year-old man with a scaphoid nonunion that has led to a humpback deformity, seen in preoperative radiographs **(A)** and CT **(B)**. He was treated with internal fixation augmented with a vascularized medial femoral condyle graft. **C:** Radiographs immediately postoperatively and then every 3 months demonstrate gradual healing of the nonunion with graft incorporation. **D:** A CT scan at 1 year postoperatively demonstrates good healing of the nonunion and graft incorporation.

This is a novel intramedullary (IM)-reaming device that is used to irrigate and aspirate the bone marrow canal. Initially developed to reduce IM pressure and fat embolism associated with reaming, its indications have also begun to include autologous bone marrow and graft harvesting.[175,219,239] Overall, it appears to be a safe and effective method for autologous graft harvesting, leading to less persistent postoperative pain.[33,175,219,239] Belthur et al.[33] compared 41 patients who underwent either RIA of the femur or tibia, or iliac crest bone-graft harvest. The patients who underwent RIA had lower pain scores than the iliac crest group.

The average graft volume was 40.3 mL (25 to 75 mL) from the RIA system. Porter et al[261] demonstrated the aspirate obtained via RIA contains many osteogenic growth factors, including FGF-2, IGF-1, and TGF-β1, as well as multiple mesenchymal progenitor cells. Complications have been reported with its use, including fractures at the donor site (Fig. 5-4).[129,213,263]

In conclusion, autologous bone graft remains the gold standard in bone grafting due to its osteogenic, osteoinductive, and osteoconductive properties. However, it is associated with important complications that must be considered before

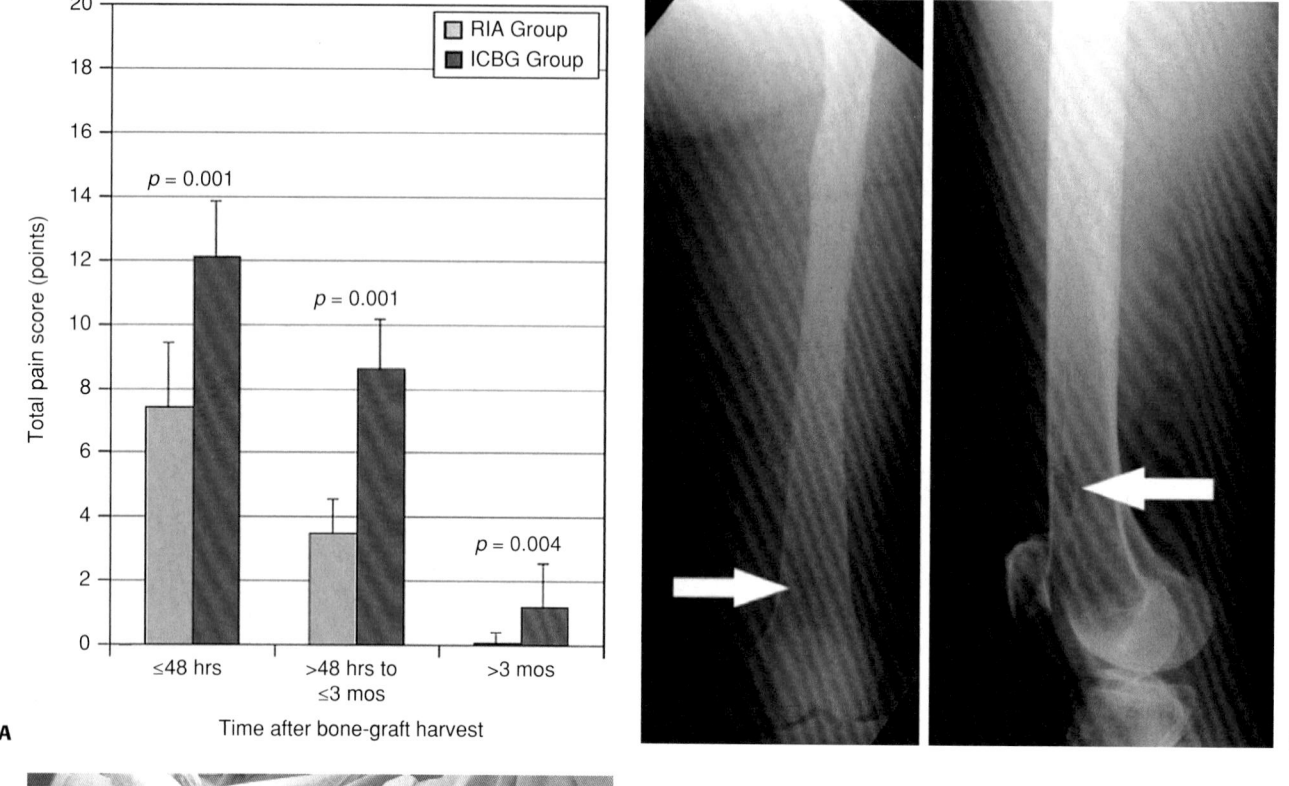

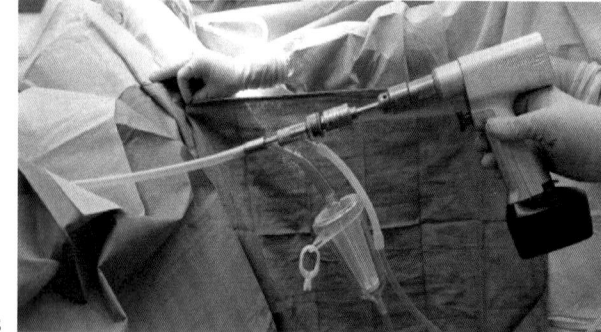

FIGURE 5-4 Reamer Irrigator Aspirator (RIA) system and its complications. **A:** Total pain scores reported by patients in the autograft and RIA groups. With RIA,the pain scores were substantially less immediately postoperatively and at long-term follow-up. **B:** The system consists of a reamer head, collection tube, drive shaft, and aspiration and irrigation ports. **C:** Anteroposterior and lateral radiographs demonstrate a perforation of the anterior femoral cortex from using the RIA. (Reprinted with permission from: Belthur MV, Conway JD, Jindal G, et al. Bone graft harvest using a new intramedullary system. *Clinic Orthop Relat Res.* 2008;466(12): 2973–2980).

proceeding with this technique. Use of the RIA is a relatively new technique that holds promise to reduce persistent postoperative pain associated with autograft harvesting. However, to date there have been insufficient studies to fully evaluate its efficacy and any associated adverse events.

Allogeneic Bone

Due to the morbidity associated with harvesting autogenous bone graft and the limited quantity available when attempting to fill large defects, alternatives such as allogeneic bone graft have gained popularity and shown significant promise.[71,153] The abundance of modern tissue banks and stringent measures to ensure safety have lead to the use of hundreds of thousands bone allografts each year.[321] They account for approximately one-third of the bone grafts performed in the United States. Cortical allografts are harvested from a number of sites including the pelvis, ribs, and fibula. Allografts are frequently used in spinal surgery,[87] joint arthroplasty,[103,232] and upper- and lower-extremity arthrodesis, including total wrist arthrodesis.[65]

Despite their widespread use in these elective procedures, only recently have they been investigated for use in the repair of fresh fractures or nonunions.

Many of the limitations of the efficacy of allogeneic bone as a bone-graft material are likely associated with its preparation. To decrease the risk of disease transmission, allograft bone is prepared and sterilized via freeze-drying, freezing, or irradiation. Freeze-drying, or lyophilization, via a removal of water and vacuum packing of the tissue significantly reduces immunogenicity.[115,351] For example, it reduces the osteoblast expression of the major histocompatibility complex (MHC) class I antigen, blunting the host immune response usually modified by MHC antigens.[115,154,351] Furthermore, Pelker et al.[258] demonstrated that such treatment of the graft reduces its mechanical integrity, thereby diminishing its load-bearing properties. Irradiation has a similar effect on the mechanical strength, decreasing it in a dose-dependent fashion.[169] In addition, both freeze-drying and irradiation reduce the osteoinductive potential of the allograft by inducing the death of its osteogenic cells.

Although slower than with autografts, allograft incorporation occurs through a process similar to autogenous graft incorporation.[131] The delayed incorporation is in part due to the paucity of donor progenitor cells, and partly due to an inhibitory host immune response to the allograft that inhibits osteoblastic differentiation.[184] Mononuclear cells have been demonstrated to line newly developing blood vessels. Thus, a limited initial revascularization, creeping substitution and ultimate remodeling lead to a higher incidence of early fractures.[55,106,309,319] Enneking and Mindell[106] reported the histologic evaluation of 73 retrieved allografts, 24 (33%) of which were obtained at autopsy or after amputation. The investigators found new vessel penetration rarely exceeded a depth of 5 mm within the first 2 years, and new bone apposition occupied no more than 20% of the graft. The depth of penetration after 2 years was typically less than 10 mm, with necrotic tissue remaining in the central aspects of the allograft throughout the remodeling process.

The biologic nature of the recipient host bed is a critical factor in facilitating allograft incorporation. Allograft bone incorporation occurs by sporadic appositional bone formation and is dependent on neoangiogenesis. A well-vascularized bed aids in the incorporation of the allograft through a combination of revascularization, osteoconduction, and remodeling.[182] However, poor vascularization, as seen in some large defects, leads to a prolonged incorporation process and significant mechanical weakness.

A technique first described by Wang and Weng[341] to combat the relative inertness of cortical allografts involves placing harvested autologous iliac crest at the allograft–host bone interface. They treated 13 patients with femoral nonunions via open reduction and internal fixation combined with deep-frozen cortical allograft struts. Seven unicortical, five bicortical, and one tricortical allografts, with an average length of 10 cm, were used. Autogenous bone grafts were inserted into the defect between the allograft and host femur. All nonunions united at an average of 5 months.

Demineralized Bone Matrix

Demineralized bone matrix (DBM) is produced by acid extraction of allograft bone.[330] Although it contains type I collagen, noncollagenous proteins, and osteoinductive growth factors, such as BMPs and TGF-betas, similar to allografts it provides little structural support.[214] However, the abundance of growth factors gives it more osteoinductive potential than allografts.[110] Numerous DBM formulations exist based on refinements of the manufacturing processes. They are available as a freeze-dried powder, granules, a gel, a putty, or strips. Recently, various companies have combined DBM with copolymers that become firm when warmed to body temperature.[184] Despite these many options, there is minimal clinical data to support each one's efficacy. Furthermore, donor-to-donor variability in the osteoinductive capacity of DBM exists, resulting in the requirement by the American Association of Tissue Banks and the U.S. Food and Drug Administration (FDA) that each batch of DBM be obtained from a single human donor.[19] Bae et al.[18] examined 10 production lots of a single DBM product, demonstrating significant variations in the BMP-2 and BMP-7 content, both of which have a large impact on fusion rates (Fig. 5-5).

Animal studies have demonstrated monocyte cell infiltration into the graft within 18 hours and cartilaginous differentiation of progenitor cells within the first week after DBM grafting. Cartilage mineralization ensues, followed by perivascular infiltration and the eventual formation of osteoblasts, leading to complete DBM resorption and bone formation.[308] In humans, multiple case series have demonstrated DBM to be a viable alternative in both acute and nonunion fracture care, arthrodesis, and implant fixation. Ziran et al.[352] followed 107 patients treated with DBM and cancellous allograft bone chips for the treatment of acute fractures with bone loss or atrophic nonunions, the majority (18 of 25) of which occurred in smokers. They found that 87 fractures healed at a mean of 32 months. Hatzokos et al.[142] treated 43 patients with an average tibial bone defect of 9.49 cm via distraction osteogenesis, filling the defects with either closed compression, autograft, or DBM and bone marrow. Although the closed compression site had a prolonged consolidation time, there were no differences between the autograft and DBM regarding the docking site healing time.

A prospective nonrandomized study comparing the use of autograft and human DBM (Grafton, Osteotech, Inc., Eatontown, NJ) in anterior cervical spine fusion found higher rates of pseudarthrosis and graft collapse with DBM, although the differences did not reach statistical significance.[7] Ziran et al.[353] retrospectively reviewed 41 patients with atrophic and oligotrophic nonunions treated with human DBM (AlloMatrix; Wright Medical Technologies, Memphis, TN). Postoperative complications were high, with 51% experiencing wound complications, of which 32% required operative debridement. Of the 41 treated patients, only 22 went on to heal the nonunion without the need for additional bone grafting. Bibbo and Patel[38] studied the use of human DBM and calcium sulfate compound (AlloMatrix Wright Medical, Arlington, TN) combined with vancomycin for the treatment of calcaneal fractures. Their results demonstrated that fractures treated with AlloMatrix and vancomycin healed at a mean of 8.2 weeks, compared with 10.4 weeks being needed for those that were not grafted. Of note, while the study was not randomized, the fractures that received DBM and calcium sulfate represented more significant injuries in that they had substantial bone loss and included six open fractures (Gustilo grade I). Hierholzer et al.[151] retrospectively reviewed the results of the treatment of 45 aseptic nonunions of the humerus treated with either autograft or DBM allograft (Grafton; Osteotech, Inc., Eatontown, NJ). The union rate in the 45 patients treated with autograft was 100%, which was similar to the 97% union rate in 33 patients treated with DBM. Donor-site pain was a significant problem in the patients treated with autograft, with 44% of the patients experiencing prolonged pain or paresthesias and one patient having an infection requiring operative debridement.

AUTHORS' PREFERRED METHOD OF TREATMENT

Autologous Cancellous Bone Graft

We prefer the autologous cancellous bone graft to be used for fractures associated with bone loss, nonunions, and small bone

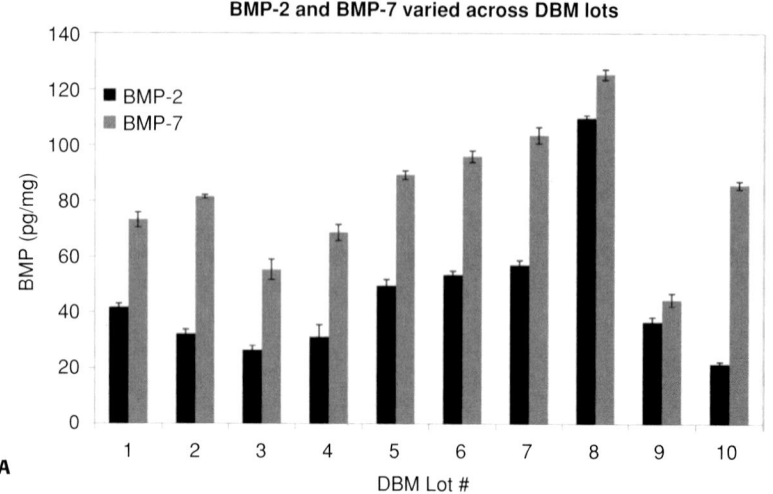

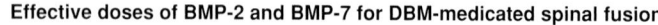

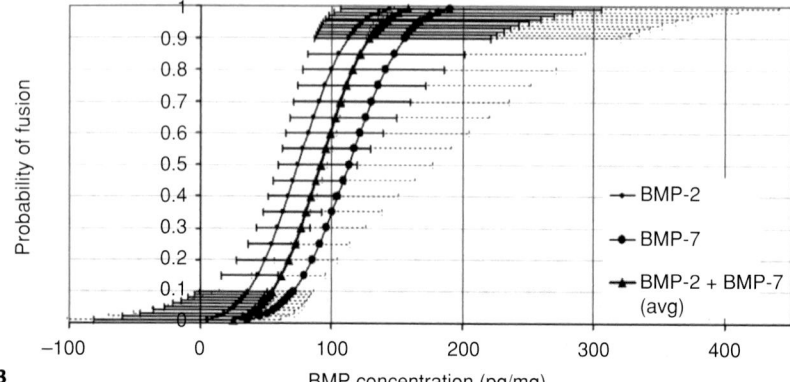

FIGURE 5-5 The content of bone morphogenetic protein (BMP) 2 and 7 across 10 production lots of a single demineralized bone matrix (DBM) product. **A:** The content of both BMP 2 and 7 in DBM varies significantly across multiple samples of DBM lots. The content of BMP 2 was positively correlated with BMP 7 ($p < 0.0001$), suggesting the osteoinductive capabilities of some products are significantly higher than others. **B:** The effective doses of BMP 2 and 7 in DBM as a predictive measure for fusion rates. The higher concentrations in the DBM lead to higher fusion rates. (Reprinted with permission from: Bae H, Zhao L, Zhu D, et al. Variability across ten production lots of a single demineralized bone matrix product. *J Bone Joint Surg Am.* 2010;92(2):427–435.)

defects (e.g., a metaphyseal or mid-diaphyseal cyst that has undergone curettage). Due to its osteoconductive, osteoinductive, and osteogenic properties, autologous graft material has a well-established history of successful augmentation of fracture healing. Up to 12-cm diaphyseal defects can be treated with nonvascularized autografts, while those over 12 cm are successfully augmented with vascularized grafts. However, there are significant complications associated with autograft harvesting, including deep infections and hematomas, neurologic or vascular injury, iatrogenic fractures, nonunions, and persistent postoperative pain. Use of the RIA is a new harvesting technique that has the potential to overcome some of these morbidities, but has not been extensively studied enough for us to make a recommendation.

Regarding allogeneic bone, there is limited information on its use in fresh fractures or nonunions. In combination with autologous graft, we recommend the use of allograft to augment the volume of graft material in the treatment of fractures associated with large volume loss or nonunions. Incorporation of allogeneic strut grafts may also be enhanced by the use of autogenous cancellous bone at the junction with the host bone.

The efficacy of human DBM as a graft material remains unclear. Although widely available and known to contain BMP,

we do not believe there is sufficient evidence demonstrating its efficacy when used alone in the treatment of fresh fractures or nonunions or in the reconstruction of bone defects. However, when used in conjunction with autologous cancellous bone, it has tremendous potential. We believe that DBM provides an osteogenic advantage and may enhance the ability of a fixed volume of autologous graft or bone marrow to be effective.

Bone-Graft Substitutes

An ideal osteoconductive scaffold should have the appropriate three-dimensional structure to promote osteoconduction, as well as allow for osteointegration and invasion by cells and blood vessels. In addition, it should also be biocompatible and biodegradable with biomechanical properties similar to those of the surrounding bone.

Calcium Phosphate Ceramics

The first clinical use of calcium phosphate ceramics for the repair of bony defects was reported by Albee in 1920[5] and repeated in several animal studies. Despite these early experiments, it was not until the 1970s that calcium phosphates, and in particular, hydroxyapatite (HA), were synthesized, characterized, and used clinically.[165,225,277] Calcium phosphate ceramics are osteoconductive materials produced by a process called sintering in which mineral salts are heated to over 1,000°C. Sintering reduces the amount of carbonated apatite, an unstable and weakly soluble form of HA, producing a solid, porous substance. Part of the osteoconductive potential of calcium phosphate depends on porosity and pore size, with the optimal size being greater than 150 μm.[79] Examples of calcium phosphate ceramics include HA, tricalcium phosphate (TCP), and calcium phosphate–collagen composite.

Hydroxyapatite

Calcium phosphate ceramics can be divided into slowly and rapidly resorbing ceramics. This is important with regard to whether the compound will need to provide long-term structural support or is acting as a void filler that will be quickly replaced.[108] HA is a slowly resorbing compound that is derived from several sources, both animal[218] and synthetic.[145,270] It is degraded by osteoclasts in 2 to 5 years.[41] Interpore (Interpore International, Irvine, CA) is a coralline HA and was the first calcium phosphate–based bone-graft substitute approved by the FDA. A hydrothermal treatment process converts it from its native coral state to the more stable HA form with pore diameters of between 200 and 500 μm, a structure very similar to human trabecular bone. Bucholz et al.[52] randomized 40 patients with tibial plateau fractures to be treated with either Interpore HA or autologous bone graft. After insertion of the graft, cortical fracture fragments were reduced, and a standard AO interfragmentary screw and plate fixation device was used to stabilize the reduction. With an average of 15.4 months for the autograft and 34.5 months for the Interpore-treated groups, radiographic and functional knee joint assessments revealed no differences between the two groups. However, attempts at using HA as a stand-alone implant for fixation in distal radius fractures did not show such promising results.[167] Compared with Kapandji wiring, those fractures treated with only HA showed substantial loss of reduction at 6, 12, and 26 weeks. Clinical parameters were also decreased for the HA-treated patients with regard to decreased grip strength and palmar flexion. Another commercial HA, Apapore 60, has shown promise in impaction grafting for acetabular defects. McNamara et al.[229] demonstrated a 100% clinical survival for acetabular total hip reconstructions at a mean of 5-year follow-up when using irradiated allograft bone combined with Apapore 60. Sixty percent showed radiographic signs of incorporation, while only 4% demonstrated cup migration prior to stabilization.

Tricalcium Phosphate

TCP undergoes partial resorption and some of it may be converted to HA once implanted in the body. The composition of TCP is very similar to the calcium and phosphate phase of human bone. This, combined with its porous nature appears to facilitate incorporation with host bone in both animals and humans by 24 months.[11,16]

Reports have demonstrated the efficacy of TCP as a bone-graft substitute. McAndrew et al.[225] investigated the suitability of TCP to treat bony defects in a series of 43 patients with 33 acute fractures and 13 nonunions. Patients were followed for an average of 1 year. Healing was demonstrated in 90% of the fracture patients and 85% of those with nonunions. Radiographic analysis showed complete resorption of the TCP between 6 and 24 months after implantation. Anker et al.[11] retrospectively reviewed 24 patients with 24 bone defects treated with TCP. Most of the defects were metaphyseal and located in the lower extremity. The average defect size was 43 cm^3, and the patients were followed for an average of 10 months. Full weight bearing in patients with a lower-extremity defect occurred at a mean of 7 weeks, and radiographic follow-up showed that the graft had completely resorbed in all defects smaller than 43 cm at 6 months.

Similar to HA, TCP has shown promise in acetabular grafting for revision hip surgery. Multiple biomechanical studies have demonstrated superior stability when HA/TCP composites are mixed with allograft bone when compared to allograft alone.[43,334] BoneSave is a biphasic ceramic composed 80% of TCP and 20% of HA. Blom et al.[39] examined the use of this composite combined with allograft bone for acetabular impaction grafting in revision total hip arthroplasty in 43 patients. At a mean of 2-year follow-up, there were no rerevisions and no radiographic evidence of implant migration. In a large animal spinal fusion study, Solchaga et al.[303] reported on the ability of Augment (Biomimetic Therapeutics, Inc., Franklin, TN), a material combining recombinant PDGF and TCP, to facilitate double-level fusion via an interbody spacer. The fusion rates with this growth factor–TCP combination were equivalent to those of autograft controls.

Calcium Phosphate Cements

Calcium phosphate cements (CPCs) can be used as bone-void fillers in the treatment of bony defects associated with acute fractures. Inorganic calcium and phosphate are combined to form an injectable paste that can be delivered into the fracture site. After injection the CPC hardens within minutes, achieving its maximum compressive strength after approximately 4 hours. This strength is comparable to intact cancellous bone. However, its strength is significantly diminished in torsion or shear and so it should be used as an adjunct, rather than as the primary method of fixation, in these cases.[196]

Sanchez-Sotelo et al.[284] conducted a randomized controlled study examining the use of a commercially available CPC, Norian Skeletal Replacement System (Norian SRS) (Norian Corporation, Cupertino, CA), in the treatment of distal radius fractures. One hundred and ten patients, who were between 50 and 85 years of age and who had sustained either an AO type A3 or C2 distal radius fracture, were followed for 12 months. Patients were prospectively randomized to receive either closed reduction with a short arm cast for 6 weeks or closed reduction and stabilization with Norian SRS and cast immobilization for 2 weeks. The results showed improved functional and radiographic outcomes in the patients treated with Norian SRS. In a subsequent randomized controlled study, Cassidy et al.[66] compared the use of Norian SRS and closed reduction to closed reduction and the application of a cast or external fixation in 323 patients with fractures of the distal radius. Significant clinical differences were seen at 6 to 8 weeks postoperatively, with better grip strength, wrist and digit range of motion, and hand function and less swelling in the patients treated with Norian SRS. By 1 year, these differences had disappeared.

In light of the promising results seen with distal radius fractures, Norian SRS has been used to treat other fractures. Schildhauer et al.[288] reported its use in the treatment of complex calcaneal fractures. Thirty-six joint depression fractures were treated with Norian SRS after standard open reduction and internal fixation. Patients were allowed to bear weight fully as early as 3 weeks postoperatively. Results demonstrated no statistical difference in clinical outcome scores in patients who bore full weight before or after 6 weeks postoperatively, suggesting that this cement may permit early full weight bearing after surgical treatment of this fracture. Another study by Thordarson and Bollinger, examined the treatment of 15 patients with intra-articular calcaneal fractures using the same CPC technique, with the walls of the defect impacted with a curette and filled with SRS cement. All fractures had less than 2 mm of step-off on postoperative CT which also showed complete filling of the bony defect with cement. Despite early weight-bearing protocols at 3 and 6 weeks, there was no demonstrated loss of reduction at an average of 13-month follow-up.[320]

CPC has also been used in the treatment of valgus-impacted proximal humerus fractures. Robinson and Page[273] demonstrated complete healing without any signs of osteonecrosis or loss of reduction in 29 patients with severely valgus-impacted proximal humerus fractures treated with screws or buttress plates augmented with CPC in the subchondral space. Egol et al.[94] examined the treatment of 92 patients with proximal humerus fractures treated via open reduction and internal fixation without augmentation, with cancellous bone chips, or with CPC. At 3-, 6-, and 12-month follow-ups, the CPC group had significantly less fracture settling and intra-articular screw penetration.

Tibial plateau fractures can displace due to the bone void underneath the articular surface. In order to promote early weight bearing without loss of reduction, these fractures may undergo operative fixation with grafting of the bone void to withstand significant compressive forces. Although such forces are not able to be withstood by autograft until the fracture has completely healed, multiple biomechanical studies have demonstrated that CPC possesses the necessary compressive strength to enable early weight bearing.[196,348] Furthermore, multiple animal studies have demonstrated its effectiveness in reducing tibial plateau subsidence at long-term follow-up after fracture fixation.[196,343]

Lobenhoffer et al.[210] used Norian SRS in the treatment of 26 tibial plateau fractures (OTA types B2, B3, and C3) followed for a mean of 19.7 months. Twenty-two fractures healed without any displacement or complications. Two cases required early wound revision secondary to sterile drainage, and two cases developed partial loss of fracture reduction between 4 and 8 weeks postoperatively requiring revision surgery. The high mechanical strength of the cement allowed earlier weight bearing after a mean postoperative period of 4.5 weeks. Similar results supporting the use of Norian SRS to fill metaphyseal defects in the treatment of displaced tibial plateau fractures have been reported by others.[155,178,343] Simpson and Keating[300] followed 13 tibial plateau fractures treated with either limited internal fixation and injectable Norian SRS or buttress plating

and cancellous autograft. At 1-year follow-up, the mean subsidence of the autograft-treated group was 4 mm, while the SRS-treated group had only subsided 0.7 mm. Russell and Leighton[280] performed a prospective, randomized multicenter examination of CPC versus autograft in acute, unstable tibial plateau fractures. There was a significantly higher rate of articular subsidence between 3- and 12-month follow-up in the autograft group compared to the CPC-treated fractures.

Although most intertrochanteric fractures are stable after internal fixation, CPC has shown promise in those patterns that possess inherent instability. Elder et al.[98] performed a biomechanical study of unstable intertrochanteric fractures with a detached lesser trochanter, comparing sliding hip screw alone to its combination with Norian SRS CPC. Fracture stiffness, stability, and ultimate strength were significantly increased by supplementation with CPC. Mattsson et al.[221] performed a prospective, multicenter study of 112 unstable trochanteric fractures with detached posteromedial fragments augmented with Norian SRS CPC compared to controls without augmentation. The patients were allowed to undergo early weight bearing after surgery. Augmentation with CPC improved the patient's postoperative pain, SF-36 lifestyle scores and ability to return to activities of daily living. A subset of these patients underwent a biomechanical analysis to show that CPC decreased fracture displacement and varus angulation.[223] CPC has also shown promise in augmenting femoral neck fracture fixation by stabilizing the threads of cannulated screws. A biomechanical study showed improved stability and screw pull out strength in those augmented with CPC.[307] However, this same group examined CPC augmentation of internal fixation of displaced femoral neck fractures and did not find any difference in the group augmented with CPC with regard to pain, quality of life, or reoperations.[222]

Bajammal et al.[21] conducted a meta-analysis of 14 randomized controlled trials that evaluated the use of CPC. The authors found that the use of CPC was associated with a lower incidence of pain compared with control subjects with no graft material used. They also found a 68% relative risk reduction in the loss of fracture reduction compared with fractures supplemented with autograft. Despite this, sterile serous drainage was reported in at least three of the papers.[209,220,331] The exact cause for the sterile drainage is not known but may be related to local reaction to cement particles or loose bodies secondary to hematoma formation before complete curing of the cement.

Calcium Sulfate

Calcium sulfate, or plaster of Paris, was first used as a bone filler in the early 1900s.[316] It acts as an osteoconductive material, which completely resorbs within 6 to 12 weeks as newly formed bone remodels and restores anatomic features and structural properties.[259]

Calcium sulfate alone and in combination with autologous bone graft has been shown to significantly augment fracture healing. In a prospective nonrandomized multicenter study, Kelly et al.[180] treated 109 patients with bone defects with calcium sulfate pellets alone or mixed with unconcentrated bone marrow aspirate, demineralized bone, or autograft. After 6 months, the radiographic results showed that 99% of the pellets were resorbed and 88% of the defects were filled with trabeculated bone. Borrelli et al.[45] treated 26 patients with persistent long-bone nonunions or osseous defects after an open fracture, with a mixture of autogenous iliac crest bone graft and medical-grade calcium sulfate. Twenty-two patients achieved healing after the primary surgery, while an additional two demonstrated union after a second procedure. Persistent nonunions were seen in two patients. Kim et al.[186] filled bony voids left after the treatment of 56 patients with various bone tumors with either injectable calcium sulfate or DBM with 28 patients in each group. Successful incorporation and fusion was seen in 24 patients in each group, with times to complete healing of 17.3 versus 14.9 weeks in the calcium sulfate and DBM groups, respectively. Yu et al.[350] treated 31 patients with tibial plateau fractures with an injectable calcium sulfate followed by early range of motion exercises. Although 3 were lost to follow-up, all 28 patients demonstrated complete fracture healing with radiographic evidence of cancellous bone incorporation by 6 months following surgery.

Despite these encouraging results, Jepegnanam and von Schroeder[166] reported on two cases of calcium sulfate failure following a corrective distal radius osteotomy for distal radius malunion. Both were elderly patients with poor underlying bone quality. The implant failures were thought to occur as the result of inadequate bone formation resulting from the resorption of the calcium sulfate graft. This highlights an important consideration for patients who lack inherent osteoinductive capabilities, such as is seen in many elderly patients.

Calcium sulfate is also available as an injectable cement. The cement (CSC) possesses good biocompatibility, is rapidly incorporated and is resorbed by 70 days.[179] In a prospective, randomized trial, McKee et al.[228] treated 30 patients with chronic osteomyelitis and nonunions with either antibiotic impregnated polymethylmethacrylate (PMMA) or calcium sulfate cement to fill the bone void. The involved bones included femurs, tibias, humeri, and one ulna. Infection was eradicated in 86% of patients in both groups who were treated for osteomyelitis. Seven of 8 patients achieved healing of their nonunion in the calcium sulfate group, while 6 of 8 patients achieved union in the PMMA group. The patients receiving PMMA cement had a significantly higher rate of reoperations ($p = 0.04$).

AUTHORS' PREFERRED METHOD OF TREATMENT

Calcium-Based Bone Graft Substitutes and Calcium Phosphate–Based Cement

The calcium-based bone-graft substitutes are best used as bone void fillers, especially when supplemented with autologous bone. It is preferable to use them in parts of the skeleton where tensile strains are low or nonexistent, as their compressive strength is comparable to cancellous bone.[126] Calcium sulfate, which is much more rapidly resorbed than the other calcium-based materials, must be used in parts of the skeleton where compressive strength is required for only short periods. These materials should not be used to bridge segmental diaphyseal defects or as onlay grafts where the majority of the surface is exposed to soft tissues.

Calcium phosphate–based cement has been tested in several randomized controlled clinical trials. Based on these data, its use to shorten the time in a cast during treatment of distal radius fractures or to shorten the time to loading such as weight bearing in the augmentation of tibial plateau, distal radius, proximal humerus, and calcaneal fractures is supported by clinical evidence, and this is a viable treatment options for these indications. Furthermore, it appears to lower postoperative pain levels when compared to no graft, as well as to decrease the risk of loss of fracture reduction when compared to autograft. It may be useful in other applications such as acetabular fractures and fractures of the hip, but sufficient evidence is not yet available for its use in these settings.

ENHANCEMENT OF FRACTURE HEALING WITH BIOLOGIC THERAPIES

Mesenchymal Stem Cells and Progenitor Cells

Adult MSCs and pluripotent progenitor cells are able to differentiate into multiple musculoskeletal cell lineages. The differentiation of these cells into mature osteoblasts is controlled by complex interactions involving systemic hormones, growth factors, and signaling molecules. In addition to differentiation, these factors are also critical in the regulation of cell growth and tissue repair. These molecules have autocrine, paracrine, or endocrine effects through actions on appropriate target cells. In addition to promoting cell differentiation, some have direct effects on cell adhesion, proliferation, and migration by modulating the synthesis of proteins, other growth factors, and receptors.[170]

Fracture repair requires that cells be present or recruited to the site of injury to provide a source to differentiate into chondroblasts and osteoblasts during endochondral and intramembranous bone formation. In the musculoskeletal system, MSCs are able to differentiate into a variety of bone and soft tissue lineages.[267] These cells play a critical role in fracture healing. However, in the elderly, the pool of available cells may be diminished, leading to delayed or possibly impaired fracture healing.[139,311]

Adult MSCs obtained from bone marrow have been shown to be a source of autologous graft material. When Muschler et al.[238] aspirated MSCs from the iliac crest, they noted that the mean prevalence of colony-forming units expressing alkaline phosphatase (CFU-APs), a marker of osteoblast progenitors, was 55 per 1 million nucleated cells. The investigators demonstrated an age-related decline in the number of progenitor cells for both men and women. When considered as graft material, these investigators showed that the volume of aspirate used for grafting can affect the number of CFU-APs. Although the numbers of CFU-APs increase as the aspirate volume increases, so does contamination of the sample by peripheral blood. For example, increasing the aspirate volume from 1 to 4 mL caused an approximate 50% decrease in the final concentration of CFU-APs.[237] These and other findings have resulted in the search for alternatives to standard autogenous bone marrow grafting, including the use of allogeneic MSCs and expansion of autogenous cells in vitro.

Early reports in patients with the use of unconcentrated bone marrow showed promising results.[150] Healey et al.[143] treated eight patients with nine nonunions after lower-extremity sarcoma resections using injections of freshly harvested, unconcentrated autologous bone marrow. The results showed that five of nine constructs had achieved union, with new bone formation evident in seven of the patients. Later, Hernigou et al.[147] aspirated autologous bone marrow from the iliac crest of patients and concentrated the progenitor cells via centrifuge. They injected 189 patients with the MSC concentrate during core decompression for avascular necrosis of the femoral head and found an increasing cell concentrate lead to improved overall results. In a later study, Hernigou et al.[149] studied percutaneous injection of concentrated autologous bone marrow aspirated from the iliac crest in 60 patients with established nonunions of the tibia. Analysis of the patients at 6 months found that bony union had occurred in 53 of the patients as determined by clinical and radiographic criteria. A retrospective analysis of the composition of the graft found that osteogenic progenitor cell concentration was significantly lower ($<1,000$ cells/cm^3) in the seven patients who failed to achieve union in comparison to the 53 who did heal. In light of these findings, the authors recommended the use of greater than 1,000 progenitors/cm^3 in the treatment of tibial nonunions.

In addition to adult stem cells, it has been hypothesized that embryonic stem cells are deposited during embryogenesis in various organs, including bone marrow, and may persist in these locations into adulthood as pluripotent stem cells.[122,193] These cells have the capability to both respond to a normal repair process in the body and participate in the repair of soft tissue and bone. Examples of such cells include very small embryonic-like (VSEL) cells, multipotent adult progenitor cells (MAPCs), MSCs, and marrow-isolated adult multilineage inducible (MIAMI) cells.[266] Although there is little known about the use of these cells for skeletal grafting, there is currently great interest in gaining a better understanding of their potential because the use of embryonic stems cells in other organ systems has yielded impressive results.[268] Undale et al.[327] compared the induction of fracture repair by embryonic and bone marrow–derived stem cells in a rat nonunion model. Following fixation, fractures supplemented with adult bone marrow stromal cells demonstrated higher torque and stiffness than those supplemented with embryonic stem cells. However both of the groups treated with cells induced more radiographic evidence of fracture healing than the control group.

The ability to derive progenitor cells from adult cells offers a promising source of stem cells. Kim et al.[185] isolated pluripotent stem cells from human adipose tissue and assessed their ability to induce osteogenic differentiation and produce osteoid matrix when supplemented with DBM in critical-sized calvarial defects. The adipocyte-derived stem cells were able to be induced into osteoprogenitor phenotypes, and when supplemented with DBM, demonstrated enhanced bone healing when compared to DBM alone.

Bone Morphogenetic Proteins

Since the discovery of the osteoinductive properties of BMP,[328] these proteins have been defined to play an important role in osteogenic development and bone repair.[72,170,271] BMPs are a group of noncollagenous glycoproteins that belong to the TGF-β superfamily. They exert their effects by autocrine and paracrine mechanisms. Fifteen different BMPs have been identified in humans and their genes have been cloned.[78] The two that have received approval for patient treatment by the FDA are BMP-2 and BMP-7 (also called OP-1). However, while BMP-2 has received full premarket approval for the treatment of open tibia fractures, OP-1 has only received a Humanitarian Device Exemption for the treatment of recalcitrant nonunions of long bones. This approval limits the sales of OP-1 to only 4,000 units per year and requires that the surgeon obtain Institutional Review Board approval in order to use it. The studies that led to these approvals are discussed below.

After promising results in bone development and regeneration in animal studies, as well as spine and other joint fusion studies, recent investigations have established the key role that BMPs play in fracture healing. Kloen et al.[188] established that human fracture callus contains multiple BMPs and their receptors. Tissue was obtained from the fracture site of malunions in five patients undergoing a corrective osteotomy. Immunohistochemical analysis was performed and results demonstrated consistent positive staining for all BMPs and BMP receptors, most intense for BMP-3 andBMP-7. More recently, Tsuji et al.[324] demonstrated the importance of BMP-2 in the fracture repair cascade. Tibia fractures were produced in transgenic mice in which BMP-2 was deleted in a limb-specific manner, before the onset of skeletal development. Mice heterozygous for this mutation were shown to have impaired healing during the earliest stages of repair with reduced periosteal reaction and decreased formation of other BMPs involved in the repair process (e.g., BMP-4 and BMP-7). However, in mice homozygous for this mutation, fracture healing was completely abolished. This study demonstrated that BMP-2 is essential for fracture healing.[324]

Several clinical investigations have tested the use of recombinant human (rh)BMPs (BMPs synthesized by recombinant gene technology using human BMP DNA) in the treatment of fractures and nonunions. In a large prospective randomized partially blinded, multicenter study, Friedlaender et al.[116] assessed the efficacy of rhBMP-7 (OP-1) versus iliac crest bone graft in the treatment of 122 patients with 124 tibial nonunions treated with IM nail fixation. Clinical assessment at 9 months indicated equivalent rates of union (81% of patients treated with BMP-7 and 85% of the 61 control autograft patients), while radiographic union was seen in 75% and 84% of these patients, respectively. As these results showed equivalent efficacy between OP-1 and autogenous bone graft, the authors concluded that OP-1 was a safe and effective alternative to bone graft in the treatment of tibial nonunions (Fig. 5-6).

Bong et al.[44] prospectively followed 23 patients with humeral nonunions treated with plate and screw or IM nail fixation in conjunction with various combinations of autograft, allograft, or DBM, in conjunction with rhOP-1. While all patients had healed at an average of 144.3 days, they concluded that OP-1 used in conjunction with allograft and/or DBM was equivalent to autograft for the treatment of humeral nonunions. These findings were supported by a prospective cohort study performed

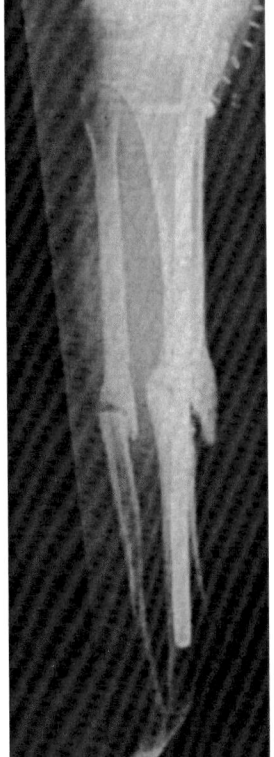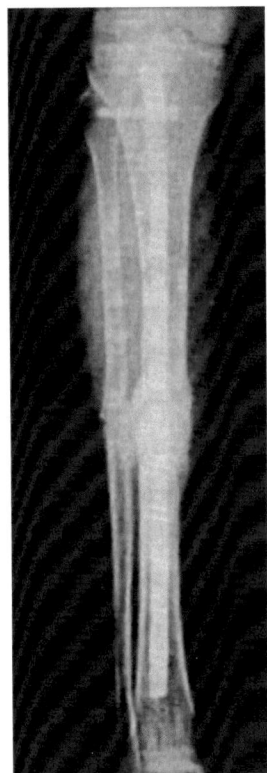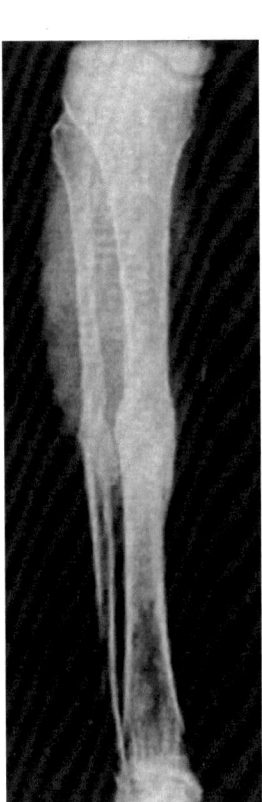

FIGURE 5-6 Sequential radiographs of a tibial nonunion treated with recombinant human OP-1 immediately postoperatively and at 9 months and 24 months after intramedullary nailing. Note the bridging callus and subsequent tibial union. (Reprinted with permission from: Friedlaender GE, Perry CR, Cole JD, et al. Osteogenic protein 1 (bone morphogenetic protein 7) in the treatment of tibial nonunions. *J Bone Joint Surg Am.* 2001;83:S151–S158).

by Dimitriou et al.[85] of 25 patients with 26 upper and lower-extremity nonunions that were treated with OP-1. Autologous bone grafting was also used in 10 of the 26 fractures. Twenty-four of 26 nonunions went on to union at an average of 4.2 months, with the 2 cases of persistent nonunion occurring in prior open fractures complicated by infection. Another prospective trial evaluated 45 patients with humeral, femoral, or tibial aseptic atrophic nonunions who underwent autologous bone grafting combined with BMP-7. Union was achieved in 100% of the nonunions, with the median time to union of 5 months and profoundly improved long-term pain and functional scores.[127]

Another TGF-β family member, BMP-2, has shown promise in the treatment of acute fractures in several human studies. The BMP-2 Evaluation in Surgery for Tibial Trauma (BESTT) Study Group reported on a large prospective randomized controlled multicenter trial evaluating the effects of rhBMP-2 in the treatment of open tibial fractures.[135] Four hundred and fifty patients with these injuries were randomized to receive irrigation and debridement followed by treatment either with IM nail fixation alone or IM fixation plus an implant containing either 0.75-mg/kg or 1.5-mg/kg rhBMP-2. The implant was placed over the fracture site at the time of wound closure. After 1 year, there were fewer secondary interventions (returns to the operating room for additional treatment) in the group treated with 1.5-mg/kg rhBMP-2. In addition, those patients treated with 1.5-mg/kg rhBMP-2 had accelerated times to union, improved wound healing, and reduced infection rates (Fig. 5-7). A subgroup analysis was performed on this cohort by Swiontkowski et al.,[313] who analyzed 113 patients with either type IIIA or type IIIB open fractures and included only patients who received placebo (65 patients)

or 1.5 mg/ml of rhBMP-2 (66 patients). The results showed that the treatment group required significantly fewer bone grafts to achieve union and had a lower incidence of infection. Another subgroup analysis by Jones et al.[171] compared the treatment of 30 patients with tibial shaft fractures and significant associated cortical defects with IM fixation augmented with either autograft or allograft and rhBMP-2. There were comparable rates of union and functional outcome scores, while the blood loss and operative time was significantly less in the rhBMP-2 group.

Despite numerous studies demonstrating the positive effects of BMPs in animal and human models of fracture and nonunion healing, results of the use of BMPs in many other clinical trials or reviews have been less impressive. For example, Aro et al.[12] performed a randomized control trial of 277 patients with Gustilo and Anderson[141] grade IIIB open tibial shaft fractures treated with either IM nail fixation alone or augmented with a collagen sponge containing 1.5 mg/ml of rhBMP-2. Initially there was a slight difference in healing at 13 weeks, with 60% of fractures in the rhBMP-2 group compared to 48% in the control group being healed; however, the healing rates had become equivalent at 20 weeks at 68% and 67%, respectively. Furthermore, 30% of those in the rhBMP-2 group underwent another procedure compared to 57% in the control group, but this and other adverse events differences were not statistically significant. One possible explanation for the conflicting results between studies might be related to the differential response of mesenchymal progenitor cells to BMPs. Diefenderfer et al.[84] cultured bone marrow cells from patients undergoing hip replacement with or without dexamethasone and treated with BMPs. The results demonstrated no significant osteogenic response to BMP-2, BMP-4, or BMP-7,

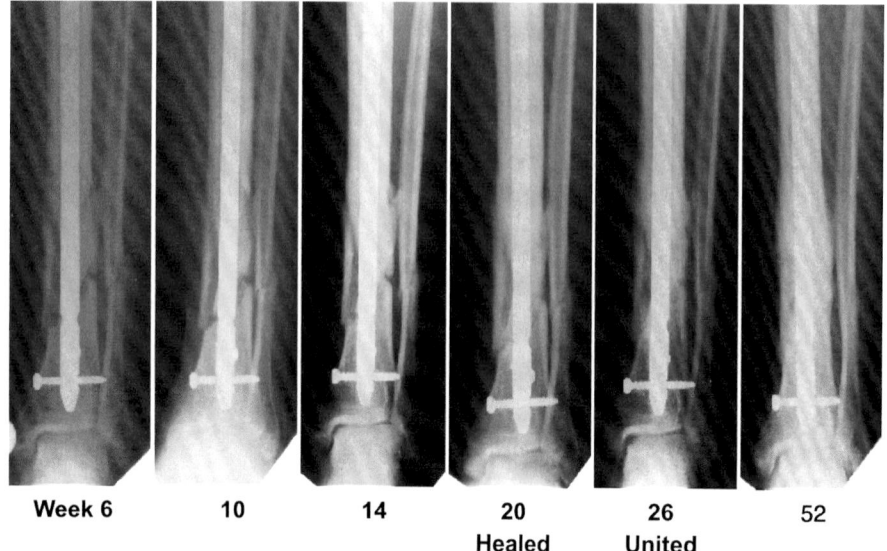

Week 6   10   14   20   26   52
Healed   United

FIGURE 5-7 Radiographs of a patient who had sustained an open fracture of the left tibia (Gustilo and Anderson type IIIB) and was treated with an unreamed intramedullary nail and 1.50 mg/mL recombinant human BMP-2. The fracture was considered to be clinically healed by 20 weeks and healed radiographically by 26 weeks. (Reprinted with permission from: Govender S, Csimma C, Genant HK, et al. Recombinant human bone morphogenetic protein 2 for the treatment of open tibial fractures. A prospective, controlled, randomized study of 450 patients. *J Bone Joint Surg Am.* 2002; 84:2123–2134).

unless the cells were pretreated with dexamethasone. Moreover, even when the cells were pretreated, the osteogenic response to BMPs was only about 50% of mouse bone marrow stromal cell cultures. Thus, the response to BMPs may differ between species, and even between individual patients.

Finally, BMP-2 must be administered in children with caution. There are no well-established dosing parameters, thus potentially exposing them to unwanted side effects not seen in the adult population. For example, Ritting et al.[272] reported on a case of a significantly enhanced inflammatory response and subsequent bone resorption in response to BMP-2 treatment of an ulnar nonunion in a child.

Wnt Proteins

The Wnt signaling pathway is critical in the regulation of osteogenesis and bone formation. The Wnt ligands are a secreted group of proteins that act by binding to the LRP 5/6 receptors. This leads to activation of a complex composed of multiple factors, including GSK3, that causes B-catenin translocation into the nucleus to induce the production of osteogenic differentiation-inducing factors.[1,54] The Wnt signaling cascade is responsible for the osteogenic effects of parathyroid hormone (PTH).[337]

The Wnt signaling cascade is regulated by the secreted proteins Dkk1 and sclerostin, which competitively bind to the LRP 5/6 receptors to inhibit bone formation (Fig. 5-8)[337] Animals deficient in sclerostin, or to a lesser extent Dkk1, exhibit increased bone mass and bone formation.[204,205,227,269] Antibodies to these Wnt inhibitors have been shown to enhance bone formation. Animal studies have shown antibodies to both Dkk1 and sclerostin increase bone mass, cortical and trabecular bone formation, and bone mineral density.[18,207] Furthermore, cultured cells from human nonunions were shown to have increased levels of Dkk1.[20] These antibodies have shown promise in fracture healing. Komatsu et al.[191] demonstrated mice with closed femur fractures treated with Dkk1 antibodies had increased fracture callus volume, bone mineral density and overall strength. Ominsky et al.[251] found that rats with closed femur fractures

and monkeys with fibular osteotomies treated with sclerostin antibodies had increased callus size, bone mass, and fracture strength. Other studies have demonstrated increased bone formation and enhanced proximal tibial metaphyseal fracture healing by antibodies to Dkk1 and sclerostin.[2,3,227,333] Both of these proteins are currently being evaluated in phase two clinical trials regarding fracture and nonunion healing.

Other Peptide Signaling Molecules
Transforming Growth Factor-β

TGF-β has a similar structure and function to the BMPs. It is known to influence a number of cell processes including the stimulation of MSC growth and differentiation, and the enhancement of collagen and other extracellular matrix protein synthesis. It also functions as a chemotactic factor for fibroblast and macrophage recruitment.[183]

Several studies have found dose-dependent effects of TGF-β improve fracture healing. Lind et al.[209] analyzed the use of TGF-β in rabbits with tibial defects treated with plate fixation, demonstrating that those treated with the low dose had improved stiffness, while both low and high doses increased callus formation. Critchlow et al.[77] established in a tibial defect healing model in rabbits that a low dose of TGF-β had an insignificant effect on callus development, whereas the higher dose resulted in a larger callus.

Although TGF-β appears to only have a modest, dose-dependent influence on fracture repair, a recombinant fusion protein with TGF-β, containing a collagen-binding domain, has been shown to induce osteogenic differentiation of bone marrow cells in rats.[8] Becerra et al.[29] presented a case report of a 69-year-old man with a proximal tibial defect from resection of long-standing osteomyelitis. Bone marrow cells were cultured in the presence of the TGF-β fusion protein and then placed in the tibial defect in conjunction with an HA carrier. Imaging at 90 days was consistent with new bone formation including bridging callus, and biopsy samples taken at 8 weeks showed new bone formation.

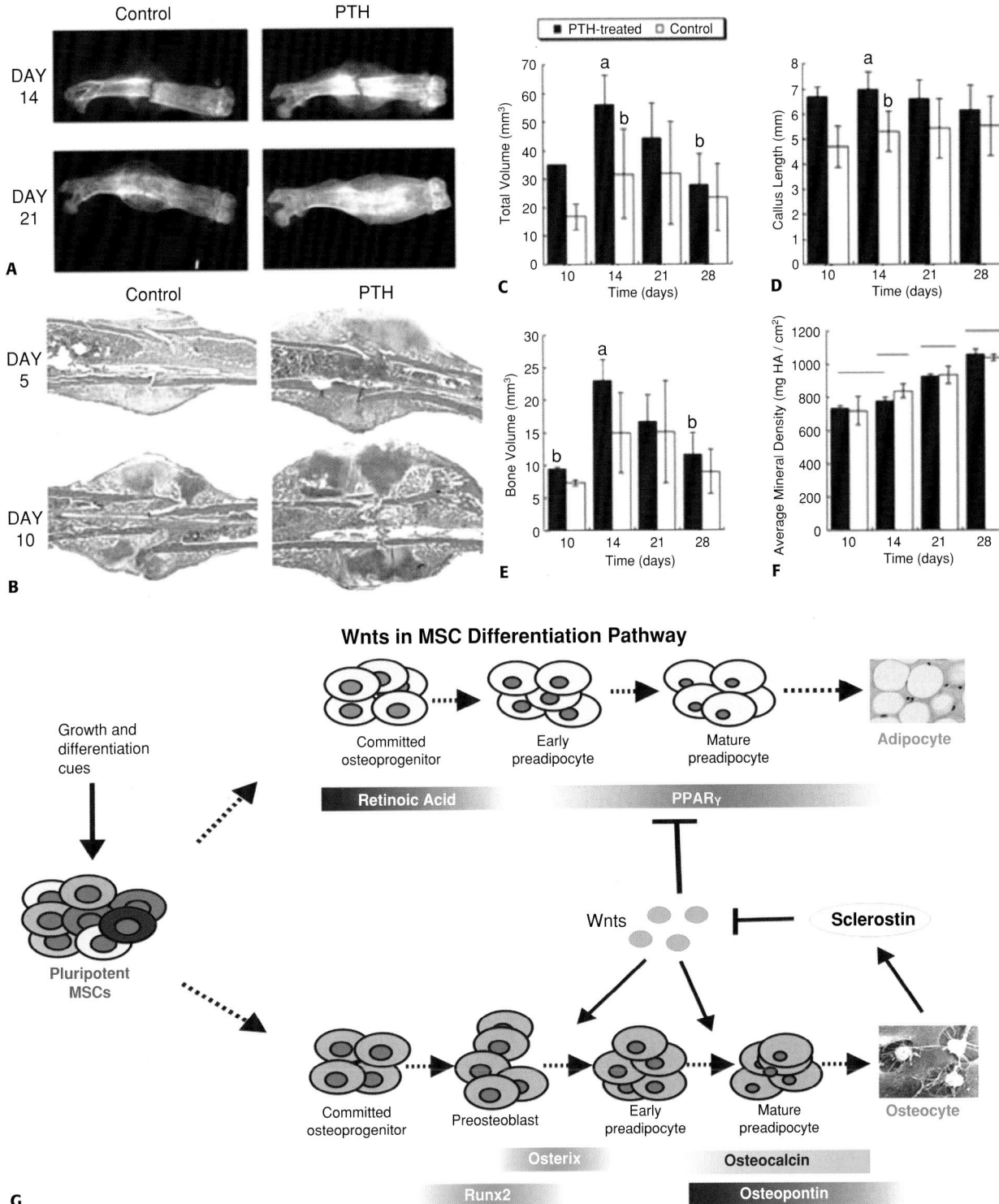

FIGURE 5-8 Parathyroid hormone induces fracture healing via modulation of the Wnt pathway. Total callus formation and chondrogenesis induction were increased in fractures in rats which were treated with daily injections of PTH (1–34) **(A)** Radiographs examining callus formation in the femurs of rats 2 and 3 weeks after injury. **B:** Safranin O staining of fracture slices 5 and 10 days after injury. Chondrogenic cells are stained red. **C, D, E,** and **F.** MicroCT analysis of callus and bone volume and mineral density. **G:** PTH exerts its effects through the Wnt pathway, inducing the osteogenic and hypertrophic chondrogenic differentiation of progenitor cells, while inhibiting the adipogenic lineage. These effects are modulated by the Wnt inhibitor, Sclerostin, which is secreted by osteocytes in a feedback loop. (Reprinted with permission from: Kakar, S, Einhorn TA, Vora S, et al. Enhanced chondrogenesis and Wnt signaling in PTH-treated fractures. *J Bone Miner Res.* 2007;22(12):1903–1912; and from: Wagner E R, Zhu G, Zhang BQ, et al. The therapeutic potential of the Wnt signaling pathway in bone disorders. *Curr Mol Pharmacol.* 2011;4(1):14–25.)

Vascular Endothelial Growth Factor

Angiogenesis is required for bone healing to occur, permitting cells to receive nutrients and oxygen. Early in the fracture repair process, vascular endothelial growth factor (VEGF) has been shown to be upregulated.[310] Eckardt et al.[92] tested the ability of rhVEGF to heal critical-sized defects in rabbits when compared to autograft controls. Biomechanical testing of the treated bones found that the ultimate strength and stiffness were significantly greater in the rhVEGF-treated animals than in controls and equivalent to autograft treatment. Micro-computed tomographic analysis showed abundant callus in both the rhVEGF-and autograft-treated groups, but absent callus in the control groups.

As noted earlier, remodeling of allograft bone is a slow process that occurs through creeping substitution. Surface healing can leave large central areas of necrotic bone that contributes to the 25% to 35% failure rate with this type of grafting.[36,212] Ito et al.[163] found that VEGF and receptor activator of nuclear factor–κB ligand (RANKL) were downregulated during allograft healing. They developed a method by which RANKL and VEGF were combined with a viral vector and attached to the surface of allografts. Theses allografts were then used in a mouse fracture model, where histologic analysis at 4 weeks showed periosteal resorption with new bone formation and medullary neovascularization that was not seen in untreated controls. These preliminary results demonstrate a novel way to increase allograft healing and warrant further study.

Fibroblast Growth Factor

Basic fibroblast growth factor (bFGF), also known as FGF-2, belongs to a class of growth factors that have an affinity for heparin.[164,187] It is one of the most potent stimulators of angiogenesis, partially through its influence on endothelial cell migration and upregulation of integrin expression.[187] Its mitogenic effects on osteoblasts, chondrocytes, and fibroblasts play a critical role during growth, wound healing, and fracture repair.[158,162]

During fracture repair, FGFs differ in their temporal and spatial expression.[279] In the early stages, FGF-1 and FGF-2 are localized to the proliferating periosteum. This expression is then limited to osteoblasts during intramembranous bone formation and to the chondrocytes and osteoblasts during endochondral bone formation. In light of their active involvement during fracture repair, investigators have studied the potential therapeutic roles of FGFs in bone formation. Chen et al.[68] demonstrated FGF-2 injections into tibial shaft fractures in rabbits increased bone density and fracture callus volume, with increased cellular proliferation markers. Kawaguchi et al.[177] performed a recent randomized control trial comparing 70 patients with tibial shaft fractures treated with IM nailing who were augmented with a gelatin hydrogel alone, or in combination with 0.8 mg or 2.4 mg of rhFGF-2 in the fracture site. The high-dose group demonstrated significantly higher rates of radiographic union compared to the placebo, and 0 compared to 4 nonunions, respectively. There were no differences in long-term weight bearing or functional outcomes measures. At this time, the status of the FGFs in the enhancement of fracture healing in patients is relatively unknown, but it appears to have a satisfactory safety profile.

Platelet-Derived Growth Factor

PDGF is a large polypeptide that consists of two chains that share 60% amino acid sequence homology.[304] Its potential role in bone healing is related to its mitogenic and chemotactic properties for osteoblasts.[60,63] A positive effect of PDGF on fracture healing was demonstrated in a rabbit tibial osteotomy model in which the fractures were injected with either 80 μg of PDGF in a collagen carrier or collagen alone.[242] Results showed an increase in callus formation, but no effects on the mechanical properties of the calluses compared with controls. A more recent study by Hollinger et al.[152] in a geriatric, osteoporotic rat model found significant gains in mechanical strength in fractures treated with PDGF combined with an injectable beta-TCP–collagen matrix. At 5 weeks after the initial injury, the torsion to failure in the PDGF-treated tibias was comparable to that of the uninjured extremity, while control and untreated fractures remained unhealed. These preclinical data and encouraging results from clinical studies of PDGF treatment of dental implants[244] and diabetic foot ulcers[345] suggest a potential role for PDGF in skeletal trauma.

Prostaglandin Modulators

Prostaglandins (PGs) comprise a group of unsaturated fatty acids that include PGE and PGF. These are known to have osteogenic effects when implanted into skeletal sites[203,253] or infused systemically.[325] The release of arachidonate from alkyl-arachidonyl phospholcholine produces the precursor of several proangiogenic and proinflammatory mediators. These factors are important in the early phases of bone formation, as they serve as osteogenic differentiation mediators of progenitor stem cells. Thus, inhibition of this cascade by drugs such as nonsteroidal anti-inflammatory drugs (NSAIDs) in the acute phase of fracture healing or bone formation can block inflammatory cell recruitment and stem cell differentiation.[233]

Arachidonic acid is converted to several types of PGs by two known PG synthases (cyclooxygenases): COX-1 or the inducible COX-2. These bind to one of four EP receptors, EP1, EP2, EP3, or EP4. In a study of rabbit tibial fractures, Dekel et al.[80] demonstrated that PGE_2 caused a dose-dependent stimulation of callus formation and an increase in total bone mineral content. Its effects were also shown to be greatest during the latter stages of fracture healing, suggesting that the primary effect may be to stimulate osteoblasts and osteoprogenitor cells as opposed to undifferentiated MSCs. The inhibition of lipoxygenase, an enzyme that converts arachidonic acid to leukotrienes, may enhance bone healing. Cottrell and O'Connor[76] administered 5-lipoxygenase inhibitors to rats with closed femoral fractures and noted callus proliferation and mineralization rate, as well as completion via endochondral ossification to be significantly enhanced. In addition, mice lacking 5-lipoxygenase have significantly enhanced fracture healing.[217]

Nonsteroidal Anti-Inflammatory Drugs

NSAIDs are effective and commonly used analgesics. They act by binding to and blocking the activity of the COX enzymes, which results in a suppression of PG synthesis.[195] These drugs can either selectively target COX-2 or nonselectively target both COX-1 and COX-2. Targeting the COX-2 enzyme with either selective or nonselective inhibitors leads to an inhibition of PGE_2 and $PGF_{2\alpha}$ thereby preventing their ability to activate osteoblasts.[35,233] Although the role of PGs in acute fracture healing is well established, the clinical evidence that inhibition of this pathway has a significant adverse effect has yet to be established.

Both selective and nonselective NSAIDs have been shown to delay acute fracture healing and increase the risk of nonunions.[50,195,236,269,312,344] For example, Simon et al. treated closed rat femoral fractures with varying concentrations and durations of the selective COX-2 inhibitor celecoxib.[236,297] They found early administration of celecoxib reduced the mechanical properties of the callus and increased the proportion of nonunions. Conversely, treatment with celecoxib preoperatively or 14 days postprocedure did not affect fracture healing. Other studies have confirmed this finding, demonstrating a decrease in mineralized callus and inhibition of haversian remodeling secondary to NSAID administration.[195,269,312,344] Another study in rats found NSAIDs administered during the acute phases of fracture healing caused a significant decrease in bone density, as well as a reduction in the bone's overall strength and stiffness.[335] COX-2 knockout mice were also found to have suppressed intrinsic capabilities in fracture healing.[336] In rabbits, multiple models have demonstrated COX-2 inhibitors impair fracture healing, bone ingrowth, and callus formation.[86,101,140,236]

There are a number of studies that provide conflicting data to the negative effects of NSAIDs on fracture healing.[30,133,176,211,262] Goodman et al.[133] implanted cylindrical titanium chambers called osseointegration centers into rabbit tibiae and administered rofecoxib (COX-2 inhibitor) for the first 2 weeks of fracture healing, weeks 5 and 6 of the repair process or continuously for 6 weeks postoperatively. These bone harvest devices contain an inner and out chamber that is able to measure the rate of bone ingrowth. The authors noted no difference in bone ingrowth or osseointegration for the initial or final 2 weeks, but did demonstrate less ingrowth if treated continuously for 6 weeks. Karachalios et al.[176] compared the administration of prednisolone, indomethacin, meloxicam, or rofecoxib for 5 days after right ulna mid-diaphyseal osteotomy. Although radiographic and biomechanical parameters were lower in the prednisolone, indomethacin, and meloxicam groups, the highly selective COX-2 inhibitor rofecoxib did not demonstrate a significant difference in fracture healing from the control group. Similarly, Long et al.[211] demonstrated that the rate of spinal fusions in rabbits was negatively affected by the nonselective COX inhibitor indomethacin, but not the COX-2 inhibitor celecoxib.

These conflicting results may be due to the effects of differing dosage regimes and subsequent local bioavailability of the NSAID. Bo et al.[40] examined the effect of treating closed, nonimmobilized femoral shaft fractures in rats with indomethacin at varying concentrations. They demonstrated the suppression of fracture healing when indomethacin was administered at doses >2 mg/kg/day. Many other studies have confirmed this effect from high-dose regimens of both selective and nonselective COX inhibitors.[86,101,102,125] However, similar to the timing of NSAID

administration, there appears to be controversy regarding the dose-dependent effects as many rodent trials have failed to demonstrate any significant suppression in fracture healing.[4,86,233] It also appears that after NSAID discontinuation, the PGE2 levels gradually return to normal and any effect on fracture healing diminishes. Gerstenfeld et al.[124] administered either ketorolac, valdecoxib, or a control dose to rats in a fracture-healing model for either 7 or 21 days. Although there was a trend for a higher rate of nonunions after the 7 and 21 days protocols, when each was discontinued for 14 days, the rate of nonunions and overall levels of PGE2 were comparable to the controls.

Considerable controversy exists as to the effect of NSAIDs in patients with acute fractures.[95] Giannoudis et al.[128] retrospectively examined the effect of NSAIDs in 32 patients with femoral nonunion compared to 67 patients with united femoral shaft fractures. The primary NSAIDs taken were ibuprofen and diclofenac. A larger portion of patients with fracture nonunions had taken the NSAIDs (62.4% vs. 13.4%) for a longer period of time (average of 21.2 weeks vs. 1 week). Burd et al.[57] examined 112 patients with acetabular fractures who also had concomitant long-bone fractures that were randomized to receive radiation therapy, high-dose indomethacin 25 mg three times a day for 6 weeks or no prophylaxis against heterotropic ossification. Those who received indomethacin had a significantly higher rate of nonunions of the long bones than those in either of the other groups ($p = 0.004$). Another study reviewed a cohort of 9,995 patients with humeral shaft fractures from the Medicare Database, and found that prescription of NSAID used within 90 days after the fracture was correlated to an increase in the incidence of nonunions.[37] In addition to the dose-dependent effects from the above studies, the authors noted an increase in nonunions among patients who took NSAIDs within the 61 to 90 days time period after the injury and not in the 1- to 30- or 31- to 60-day time periods.

Although there appears to be a trend toward a decreased rate of fracture healing from high-dose NSAID administration in animal studies, this relationship has not been demonstrated in clinical studies. Given the paucity of large prospective studies and inherent deficiencies with the existing retrospective body of literature, the exact role of NSAIDs during fracture healing remains unclear. Furthermore, the inhibitory effect of NSAIDs appears to be reversible and PGE levels return to normal about 1 to 2 weeks after discontinuation of NSAID use. Therefore, as noted by Kurmis et al.,[195] NSAID use as an analgesic appears to be safe in short durations (10 to 14 days) after fractures or spinal fusions, as long as they are stopped within a couple weeks.

AUTHORS' PREFERRED METHOD OF TREATMENT

Bone Morphogenetic Proteins

We recommend the use of OP-1 (BMP-7) for the treatment of recalcitrant nonunions of long bones and BMP-2 for the treatment of open tibia fractures and those with large cortical defects. Some of other molecules, including Wnt pathway modulators and FGF-2 have shown promising preclinical and early clinical study results, but there is not enough evidence to recommend for or against their use at this time.

Regarding freshly harvested bone marrow, we believe there is insufficient evidence to support its routine use in traumatic or reconstructive orthopedic surgery. Alternatively, multiple small aspirations from the iliac crest, with centrifuge-mediated concentration (bone marrow aspirate concentrate) has been able to optimize the concentration of the osteoprogenitor cells.[148,150] The senior author (TAE) has used this technique with success in several cases of long-bone nonunions.

While the role of NSAIDs in animal models appears to be well established, there is lack of scientifically rigorous clinical data for or against its effects in the acute phases of fracture healing. In addition, if there is an effect of NSAIDs on fracture healing, it appears to be dose-dependent and reversible, as it disappears after 7 to 10 days once the NSAID has been stopped. Therefore, we believe NSAIDs are safe to be used as an analgesic in short durations (10 to 14 days) after fractures or spinal fusions. However, we would recommend caution of their use in patients with comorbidities, such as smoking, glucocorticoid use, and diabetes.

Systemic Enhancement of Fracture Healing

Parathyroid Hormone

Calcium and phosphate homeostasis is a complex process that involves multiple signaling pathways and organ systems. The largest storage site of calcium and phosphate is the skeletal system, and the release of these ions is largely regulated by the coordinated stimulation and suppression of osteoblasts and osteoclasts. PTH is a major regulator of mineral homeostasis, exerting its effects by binding to a receptor on osteoblasts.[274,275] PTH is an 84-amino acid peptide that is produced in response to depressed serum calcium levels. Its major effects are in the kidneys, where it regulates phosphate diuresis and 1,25-dihydroxyvitamin D synthesis with its subsequent enhancement of gastrointestinal calcium and phosphate absorption.[264] The actions of PTH on bone metabolism can be both stimulatory and inhibitory. It has been found that continuous release of PTH leads to an increase in osteoclast numbers and activity,[206] while intermittent exposure results in increased bone formation in both rats and humans through osteoblast and osteoprogenitor cell recruitment.[82,243] This occurs through the activation of the Wnt signaling pathway within osteogenic differentiation.[261]

Teriparatide (PTH [1–34]) is currently an FDA-approved treatment for osteoporosis. Intermittent injections increase bone formation on all aspects of the bone, including the cortical and cancellous matrices.[54,114] Clinical trials using PTH (1–34) have shown an increase in bone mass in osteoporotic men and an increase in bone mineral density and a reduction of vertebral and other osteoporotic related fractures in postmenopausal women.[82,243] Neer et al.[243] assessed the efficacy of intermittent PTH (1–34) to improve bone mineral density in a clinical trial involving 1,673 postmenopausal women with prior non-traumatic vertebral fractures. Results demonstrated that PTH increased bone mineral density and reduced the risk of fracture. In addition, Saag et al.[282] demonstrated that teriparatide is more effective at treating glucocorticoid-induced osteoporosis and reducing vertebral fracture risk than the bisphosphonates raloxifene and alendronate.

Based on this anabolic effect of PTH on the skeleton, several animal studies have been conducted examining the effects of PTH on the repair of bone. All have demonstrated an enhancement of fracture healing when doses were given intermittently.[240,241] Kakar et al.[174] examined daily systemic PTH injections in the treatment of femoral shaft fractures in mice. The PTH injections increased callus volume and density, with a greater induction of chondrogenesis and chondrocyte hypertrophy, carried out through an induction of the canonical Wnt pathway (see Fig. 5-8). Manabe et al.[216] studied PTH in 17 female cynomolgus monkeys who underwent a femoral osteotomy with plate fixation, augmented with either low-dose (0.77 μg/kg) or high-dose (7.5 μg/kg) PTH or placebo, given twice weekly for 3 weeks. All groups healed by 26 weeks, with a larger callus size but a lower callus density in the control animals. The ultimate stress and elastic moduli of the healing osteotomy were significantly higher in PTH-treated animals. Alkhiary et al.[6] reported on the use of PTH (1–34) in the treatment of experimental femur fractures in Sprague-Dawley rats. Animals were treated with either 5- or 30-μg/kg/day PTH (1–34) for a total of 35 days beginning at the time of fracture creation. There were significant increases in strength and bone mineral content for the 30-μg/kg group as early as 3 weeks, and these differences were sustained at 85 days.

A clinical trial on the use of PTH (1–34) in the treatment of fractures of the distal radius in humans showed that the time to fracture healing was shorter in the PTH-treated patients.[6] Aspenberg et al.[17] performed a randomized double-blind placebo controlled trial of 102 postmenopausal women with distal radius fractures treated with teriparatide beginning within 10 days of the fracture and continuing for 8 weeks. Although a 40 mcg daily dosage did not significantly enhance fracture-healing times, it was noted that a lower dose of 20 mcg did shorten the time to complete fracture healing, although it was not quite statistically significant. Other case series have shown improved fracture healing from teriparatide treatment in patients with pelvic fragility fractures, as well as nonunions of the humeral shaft and sternum.[69,257] In a randomized control trial, Peichl et al.[257] treated 65 elderly osteoporotic patients with pelvic fragility fractures with either daily injections of PTH (1–84) or a placebo. These treatments reduced the time to fracture healing to 7.8 weeks, as compared to 12.6 weeks for the controls. These findings suggest that PTH (1–34), as well as other PTH fragments, may have a role in the clinical treatment of fractures, especially in osteoporotic bones.

Growth Hormone and Insulin-Like Growth Factor I

Growth hormone (GH) and insulin-like growth factors (IGFs) play an important role in skeletal development and remodeling. GH is currently used clinically to treat patients with short stature[249] because it stimulates endochondral ossification, periosteal bone formation, and linear growth. It mediates these effects through the IGF system including the ligands, receptors, IGF-binding proteins (IGFBPs), IGFBP proteases and activators, and inhibitors of IGFBP proteases. Through these mediators, it is able to induce osteogenic differentiation and upregulate bone formation.

Two IGFs have been identified: IGF-I (somatomedin C) and IGF-II. Although IGF-II is the most abundant growth factor in bone, IGF-I has the greater potency for promoting growth and has been localized in healing fractures of humans.[10,61,62] IGF-I and IGF-II promote bone matrix formation (type I collagen and noncollagenous matrix proteins) by fully differentiated osteoblasts, inhibit collagen degradation, and promote osteoblast maturation and replication.[64] Expression of the IGF-I increases with expression of GH,[265] and it is likely responsible for the anabolic effects of GH.

Several studies have reported moderate enhancement of skeletal repair using either GH[9,22,190] or IGF-I.[318] Mazziotti et al.[224] found increased spinal deformities in patients with a GH deficiency, and a reduced fracture risk after GH therapy administration. A recent randomized clinical trial was presented by Raschke et al.[265] in which 406 patients with tibia fractures were treated daily for 26 weeks with either placebo or gradually increasing concentrations of GH in an attempt to avoid adverse events, such as water retention, typically caused by GH. Although there was no difference in radiographic union rates in the open fractures, the relative risk for healing a closed fracture was greatest in the group treated with the highest dose of GH (60 µg/day; relative risk [RR], 1.44; 95% confidence interval [CI], 1.01 to 2.05; $p = 0.045$). While patients treated with 60-µg/day GH were able to bear full weight earlier, there was a higher number of adverse events: 58% in the 60-µg/day GH-treated group compared with 35% in controls. These adverse events included arthralgias, edema, and, to a lesser extent, wound infection. Two other prospective randomized controlled trials demonstrated that recombinant GH administration enabled an earlier return to prefracture activity and overall function in elderly patients with hip fractures or those undergoing total hip arthroplasties.[333,342] When considering GH treatment for fractures or other musculoskeletal pathologies, one must consider the risk associated with high or even moderate dose GH administration, as a higher mortality has been shown in critically ill patients who received GH treatments.[314]

Statins

Statins, HMG-CoA reductase inhibitors, are lipid-lowering drugs that block cholesterol synthesis through the inhibition of mevalonic acid production. The conversion of HMG-CoA to mevalonic acid occurs early in the pathway and also inhibits the production of farnesyl pyrophosphate (FPP) and geranylgeranyl pyrophosphate (GGPP). Small GTP-binding proteins such as Rho and Ras require GGPP and FPP, respectively, for translocation to the plasma membrane.[197] Inhibition of this process by statins may block osteoclast maturation and subsequent bone catabolism.[295] In addition, studies have shown that statins stimulate the BMP-2 promoter in osteoblasts leading to enhanced bone formation.[234]

In mice, Skoglund and Aspenberg[301] showed that daily injections of simvastatin had no effect on fracture healing, while a continuous systemic infusion and continuous local delivery improved the force to failure by 160% and 170%, respectively. However, Chissas et al.[70] treated 54 rabbits with low- or high-dose simvastatin, or a control group. The high-dose simvastatin reduced callus formation and decreased the fracture gap compared to the low dose or control groups. Local delivery of statins, such as with hydrogels or nanoparticle beads, has shown promise in enhancing fracture repair. Garrett et al.[121] used poly(lactic-coglycolide acid) nanoparticle beads containing various concentrations of lovastatin to augment femur fracture repair in rats. Their results showed at 4 weeks that doses of 1 and 1.5 µg/day significantly accelerated fracture healing as measured by the size of the fracture gap and biomechanical strength. Furthermore, Fukui et al.[119] found simvastatin conjugated gelatin hydrogel increased the healing of a femoral nonunion in rats. The success of local delivery also demonstrates that the effects of statins on fracture healing is likely a locally mediated induction, independent of the systemic cholesterol lowering effects of the drug.

In a recent meta-analysis of multiple cohorts and reviews, Bauer et al.[27] found that statins reduce fracture risk in the hip and to a lesser extent in the spine. This finding is likely due to the increased bone mineral density as the result of statin therapy, as demonstrated by Edwards et al.[93] in postmenopausal women. However, there remains a paucity of good prospective controlled trials analyzing the true effects of statins on fracture healing.

Bisphosphonates and Osteoclast Inhibitors

Bisphosphonates are commonly used for the treatment of osteoporosis. They act by binding to HA and inhibiting osteoclast-mediated bone resorption by inducing osteoclast apoptosis. Bone remodeling is subsequently inhibited, increasing the bone mineral density.

The role of bisphosphonates in fracture prevention and repair is less clear. Multiple animal studies have demonstrated bisphosphonates to enhance callus formation and bone mineral density; however, the remodeling and mineralization phases are delayed or completely inhibited.[54,202,226] Huang et al.[157] demonstrated a 50% delay in spinal fusion healing in rats treated with bisphosphonates. Furthermore, unlike the effects seen when administering PTH, Sloan et al.[302] found bisphosphonates to suppress fracture healing by a rate of 44% compared to the control. Interestingly in patients, Munns et al.[235] examined the effects of pamidronate therapy on pediatric patients with osteogenesis imperfecta. They noted a significant delay in long-bone osteotomy healing, but minimal delays in acute fracture healing. Rozental et al.[278] reviewed 196 patients who sustained a distal radius fracture, with 43 who were currently on bisphosphonate therapy at the time of injury. The fractures in the patients, treated both with operative and nonoperative management, who were taking bisphosphonates demonstrated a longer time to union.

One potential solution to the pitfalls seen with using bisphosphonates for fracture prevention or treatment could be to augment it with an anabolic agent, such as a BMP. Schindeler et al.[289] demonstrated significant increases in number and rates of unions in neurofibromatosis-1 (NF-1) deficient mice with tibial pseudarthrosis treated with both a BMP and bisphosphonate.

Another antiresorptive agent that has recently been approved for osteoporosis is the monoclonal antibody denosumab. This antibody binds to osteoblast-produced RANK ligand, preventing its association with the RANK receptors on osteoclasts. Although there have not been any clinical studies on fracture healing, this antibody has been shown to have a similar effect to bisphosphonates, by increasing callus formation and delaying remodeling.[15] However, unlike bisphosphonates, Denosumab increased bone mineral density within the callus, not just bone mineral content.

AUTHORS' PREFERRED METHOD OF TREATMENT

Although the above compounds all show some promise for the systemic enhancement of fracture healing, their lack of FDA approval would require off-label use in the setting of fracture treatment. Because of this, the authors cannot recommend their use at this time.

PHYSICAL ENHANCEMENT OF SKELETAL REPAIR

The mechanical environment has a direct impact on fracture healing. Direct mechanical perturbation and biophysical modalities such as electrical and ultrasound stimulation have been shown to affect fracture healing. To enhance fracture repair by these mechanical measures, it is necessary to develop a fundamental understanding of the ways by which the mechanical environment impacts cellular and molecular signaling.

Mechanical and Biophysical Stimulation

Mechanical forces play a crucial role in the healing process. Sarmiento et al.[286] found that early weight bearing accelerates the fracture-healing process. Early weight bearing in rats after standard nonrigid IM femoral fracture fixation demonstrated improved histologic, radiographic, and mechanical parameters of fracture healing. The authors attributed these findings to early mobilization facilitating the maturation of callus tissue produced by endochondral ossification.

The degree of stability at the fracture site has a direct impact on the repair process. Lewallen et al.[200] demonstrated compression plating–enhanced bone formation 120 days after injury when compared to external fixation. Those treated with the external fixators had significantly less intracortical and endosteal new bone formation, with more bone porosity compared to those treated with compression plates. Compression plating increased fixation stiffness in almost all modes. Thus, the authors concluded that the rigidity of the fixation is critical in early fracture remodeling. Furthermore, several investigators have attempted to show micromotion as seen with the compression plating actually modulates fracture healing. For example, in a prospective randomized clinical trial, Kenwright et al.[181] used a pneumatic pump to deliver a small cyclic amount of axial displacement in order to compare the effects of controlled micromotion on tibial diaphyseal fracture healing in patients treated with external fixation. The controlled micromotion significantly enhanced both clinical and mechanical healing compared with only rigid fixation, with no increase in complication rates.

Distraction Osteogenesis

Limb lengthening was first described by Codivilla[74] in 1904 for the treatment of limb length discrepancies. It was not until the work of Ilizarov et al.[160,161] 50 years later that the technique of distraction osteogenesis gained popularity as a method for enhancing bone regeneration in both orthopedic and maxillofacial operations.

Distraction osteogenesis is divided into three phases, latency, distraction, and consolidation. The latency phase begins immediately after the osteotomy and is related to the robust inflammatory response and recruitment of molecules involved in the early phases of fracture repair. The distraction phase occurs when the longitudinal stresses creating the gap lead to a central fibrous zone with chondrocytes and fibroblast progenitors along with columns of early mineralization.[14] This histologically resembles endochondral ossification in the early phases, but gradually becomes intramembranous ossification in the later stages.[14,107,283] Once the distraction phase ceases, the consolidation phase takes over with extensive bone matrix and osteoid production by osteoblasts.

Through the controlled distraction of bone fragments, the expression of various growth factors ensues, including those involved in angiogenesis. Pacicca et al.[252] demonstrated the expression of several of these molecules localized to the leading edge of the distraction gap. The greatest levels were seen during the active phase, consistent with the apposition of new bone matrix. Others have shown that robust angiogenesis and progenitor recruitment, under VEGF control, occurs during the active and consolidation phase.[199]

Several investigators have used the technique of distraction osteogenesis to stimulate new bone formation in the clinical setting. Kocaoglu et al.[189] treated 16 patients with hypertrophic nonunions with the Ilizarov distraction method. All patients had at least 1 cm of shortening, three patients had a deformity in one plane, and the remainder had a deformity in two planes. Distraction was begun on the first postoperative day at the rate of 0.25 mm/day and was left in place until at least three of four cortices showed bridging callus. All nonunions had healed at an average follow-up of 38.1 months, with correction of all preoperative length inequalities and limb angulation to normal alignment. A similar study of 17 patients with tibial nonunions associated with bone loss found an average treatment time of 8 months, with functional results being reported as excellent in 15 and good in 2.[292]

Open fractures have also been managed successfully with distraction osteogenesis. Sen et al.[293] managed 24 patients with Gustilo and Anderson[141] grade III open tibia fractures with compression–distraction osteogenesis using the Ilizarov-type circular external fixator. After an average of 30-month follow-up, results were excellent in 21 and good in 3 patients. Functional assessment scores were excellent in 19, good in 4, and fair in 1 patient.

However, not all studies have shown acceptable bone formation as the result of distraction osteogenesis. Many factors have been associated with increased fracture risk after the removal of the external fixators, including age, location of lengthening, and smoking.[13,159,299] Fracture rates can be as high as 8% to 9% after fixator removal and initiation of weight bearing.[299] Thus, there may be a need to augment the healing and bone formation with additional modalities, such as low-intensity pulsed ultrasound (LIPUS), pulsed electromagnetic field (PEMF), extracorporeal shockwave therapy (ESWT), or osteogenic-inducing agents.

Electrical Stimulation

Electrical potentials were first described in mechanically loaded bone by Fukada and Yasuda[118] in 1957. With this discovery, investigators began to study the influence that electrical current might have on the healing of bone. In 1971, Friedenberg et al.[113] found that the healing of nonunions could be affected by the use of direct current. Within 5 years, more than 119 articles had been published highlighting the use of electrical stimulation on bone growth and repair.[48] Its effects are thought to be carried out by stimulating the local production of osteogenic and mitogenic growth factors, including BMP-2 and BMP-4, as well as TGF-β.[67] These induce osteogenesis and recruit osteoprogenitors to facilitate bone formation.

There are currently three methods for the electrical stimulation of bone healing: (i) constant direct current (DC) stimulation with the use of percutaneous or implanted electrodes (invasive), (ii) capacitive coupling (noninvasive), or (iii) time-varying inductive coupling produced by a magnetic field (noninvasive; also known as PEMF stimulation). DC stimulation uses stainless steel cathodes placed in the tissues near the fracture site, stimulating new bone formation according to the level of applied current, with a threshold level above which cellular necrosis may occur.[112] With pulsed electromagnetic stimulation, externally applied coils produce an alternating current, leading to time-varying magnetic and electrical fields within the bone. In capacitively coupled electric fields (CCEFs), an electrical field is induced in bone through the use of an external capacitor—that is, two electrically charged metal plates placed on either side of a limb.[109]

Electrical stimulation has primarily been used in orthopedics for the treatment of nonunions. Brighton et al.[49] found DC for the treatment of 178 nonunions in 175 patients resulted in an 84% union rate regardless of the presence of metallic internal fixation devices. Interestingly, the investigators found that even in the presence of osteomyelitis the healing rate was nearly 75%. Although initially half of the patients received a lower dose of 10 μA, poor healing was noticed after 12 weeks and all patients were switched to receive the higher dose of 20 μA. When this study was expanded to include other centers, an additional 58 of 89 nonunions achieved similar results. Treatment failures were attributed to inadequate electricity, the presence of a synovial pseudarthrosis or infection, and dislodgment

of the electrodes. Complications were minor with the exception of patients with previous osteomyelitis. The authors concluded that given proper electrical parameters and cast immobilization, a rate of bone union comparable to that seen with bone-graft surgery could be achieved.

Scott and King[290] reported similar results in a prospective, double-blind trial using capacitive coupling in patients with established nonunions. In a population of 21 patients, healing was achieved in 60% of the patients who received electrical stimulation. Patients managed with the placebo unit showed a complete lack of bone formation.

Bassett et al.[26] reported on the use of PEMF in the treatment of 127 nonunited tibial diaphyseal fractures treated with long-leg plaster cast immobilization. Patients were treated with nonweight-bearing ambulation and a total of 10 hours of PEMF stimulation daily. Bony union occurred in 87% of the patients and was independent of patient age or sex, the number of previous operations, and the presence of infection or metal fixation. Later, Sharrard[296] conducted a double-blind, multicenter trial of the use of PEMFs in patients who had developed a delayed union of a tibial fracture. Forty-five tibial fractures that had not united for more than 16 weeks but less than 32 weeks were treated with immobilization in a plaster cast that incorporated the PEMF coils, with activation in only 20 of the 45 units. There was radiographic evidence of union in nine of the fractures that had been subjected to electromagnetic stimulation compared with only three of the fractures in the control group. Simonis et al.[298] performed a similar double-blind trial in 34 patients with tibial nonunions treated with an oblique fibular osteotomy and external fixator. The union rate for those treated with electrical stimulation was 89%, compared 50% in the control group.

Despite the promising results seen in patients with nonunions and delayed unions, the application of this technology to the treatment of fresh fractures has not been clearly defined. Although some studies have shown that PEMFs favorably influence fracture healing in experimental animals[112] and osteotomies in patients,[46,215] other studies have failed to demonstrate clinically significant effects.[26] Beck et al.[31] found no difference in healing time in 44 patients who were randomly assigned to either CCEF or placebo.

Mollon et al.[230] performed a meta-analysis of 11 randomized control trials evaluating the efficacy of electrical stimulation in fracture healing. The authors found electrical stimulation had a nonsignificant benefit in delayed unions or fracture nonunions ($p = 0.15$), as well as in callus formation in femoral intertrochanteric osteotomies. However, there was minimal to no benefit in limb-lengthening, nonoperative management of Colles fractures, tibial stress fractures, or operations for pseudarthrosis. Thus, while some studies have shown a potential benefit for this technology, there are methodologic limitations in the current literature without any unified consensus and therefore we are unable to determine the impact of electrical stimulation on fracture healing.

Ultrasound Stimulation

LIPUS has been shown to promote fracture repair and increase the mechanical strength of fracture callus in both animal[260,347] and clinical[144,192] studies. LIPUS increases the quantity of osteo-progenitors recruited to the fracture site in animal studies,[194] thus acting as an osteoinduction modulator.

In a prospective randomized double-blind trial, Heckman et al.[144] examined the use of LIPUS as an adjunct to conventional treatment with a cast in 67 patients with closed or open Gustilo and Anderson[141] grade I tibial shaft fractures. Thirty-three fractures were treated with the active device and 34 with the placebo. Using clinical and radiographic criteria, the authors noted that there was a statistically significant decrease in the time to union (86 ± 5.8 days in the LIPUS treatment group vs. 114 ± 10.4 days in the control group) and in the time to overall healing (96 ± 4.9 days in the ultrasound treatment group vs. 154 ± 13.7 days in the controls). There were no issues with patient compliance in the treatment group and no serious complications reported with its use.

In a subsequent multicenter prospective randomized double-blind study, Kristiansen et al.[192] evaluated the efficacy of LIPUS in the treatment of dorsally angulated distal radius fractures that had been treated with closed reduction and a cast. The time to union was significantly shorter for the fractures that were treated with LIPUS compared with the controls (61 ± 3 days vs. 98 ± 5 days). The authors further noted that treatment with LIPUS was associated with significantly less loss of reduction (20% ± 6% vs. 43% ± 8%) as determined by the degree of volar angulation as well as with a significant decrease in the mean time until the loss of reduction ceased (12 ± 4 days vs. 25 ± 4 days).

There are several known risks factors for delayed or nonunion, and one of the most common is tobacco use. Cook et al.[75] studied LIPUS for the treatment of acute tibial and distal radius fractures in smokers. Healing time in this patient population is typically delayed, with tibial and distal radius fractures requiring 175 ± 27 days and 98 ± 30 days, respectively, to achieve bony union. Treatment with LIPUS was able to reduce this time to 103 ± 8.3 days in the tibial fracture group and 48 ± 5.1 days in the patients with distal radius fractures. Treatment

with LIPUS also substantially reduced the incidence of delayed union in tibias in smokers and nonsmokers. These results are important because they suggest that LIPUS can override some of the detrimental effects that smoking has on fracture healing. Rutten et al.[281] prospectively analyzed 71 cases of tibial nonunion and found that treatment with LIPUS resulted in a healing rate of 73%, and that this was significantly higher than the rate of spontaneous healing. Within the subgroups analyzed, the rate of healing in smokers and nonsmokers was not found to be statistically significantly different. Multiple other studies have found LIPUS to be a successful treatment for nonunions, with union rates between 75% and 86% with important confounders including time from initial surgery, BMI, and smoking habits (Fig. 5-9).[146,168,246,276]

In contrast to these findings, the effects of LIPUS on fracture healing may be affected by the presence of fixation devices. Emami et al.[100] noted that ultrasound did not appear to have a stimulatory role on tibial fracture repair in a prospective randomized controlled double-blinded study to evaluate its effects in patients with fresh tibial fractures who were treated with a reamed and statically locked IM rod. Patients all underwent treatment with an ultrasound device for 20 minutes daily for 75 days without knowing whether it was active. LIPUS did not shorten the healing time compared to the inactive control. However, when combined with distraction osteogenesis, it does appear to improve healing time. In a randomized control trial of distraction osteogenesis alone or combined with LIPUS, Dudda et al.[89] found most healing indices were not significantly different, although LIPUS significantly reduced the fixator gestation period.

In a meta-analysis performed by Bashardoust Tajali et al.,[25] 23 prospective or cohort studies were identified examining LIPUS in acute fractures and nonunions. They found the time to fracture healing was significantly reduced in acute fractures by LIPUS. This was determined by an increase in periosteal reaction or density as seen on radiographs, as well as an earlier

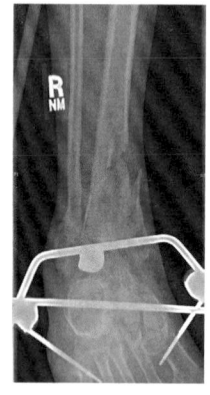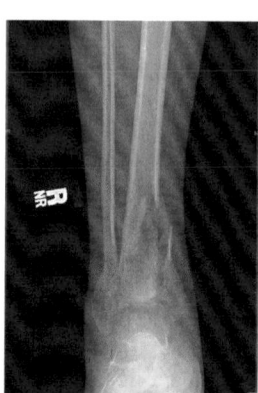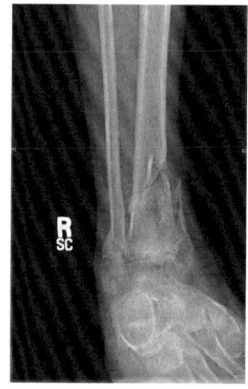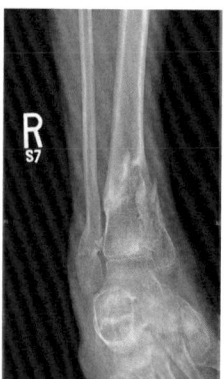

A, B   **C, D**

FIGURE 5-9 Sequential radiographs of a patient who sustained a grade II distal tibia fracture that underwent irrigation and debridement with placement of an external fixator. **A:** At 4 months, the external fixator was removed and the patient was believed to have a delayed union. Daily treatments with Exogen (Smith and Nephew, Memphis, TN) ultrasound stimulation was started. **B:** At 1 month of treatment, the patient progressed to partial weight bearing. **C:** At 2 months, radiographs showed continued progression of healing. **D:** At 6 months, the patient was bearing full weight without pain. (Courtesy Paul Tornetta III, MD.)

improvement in clinical outcome measures. Although they also found six out of seven studies of nonunions to have an increased rate of fracture healing stimulated by LIPUS, there was a paucity of uniform outcome measures and no definitive conclusions could be drawn. Another meta-analysis was performed by Griffin et al.[136] examining LIPUS for the treatment of acute fractures. Twelve randomized control trials were examined. They did not find a significant improvement with LIPUS in reducing the time to union in the initial treatment of the acute fractures. However, there were minimal complications associated with this therapy.

Extracorporeal Shock Wave Therapy

Extracorporeal shock wave therapy (ESWT) involves the production single high amplitude sound waves producing tension and forces on a focused area. This stimulates bone formation by increasing local and systemic inflammatory and osteogenic growth factors. The shock wave translates into a formation of membrane hyperpolarization and growth factor production. Wang et al.[340] found systemic concentrations of TGF-β1, VEGF, BMP-2, and nitric oxide after treatments of ESWT. These are in part stimulated by the creation of free radicals that induce this osteogenic response.[339]

Several studies have examined the effects of ESWT on non-unions. A prospective randomized control trial performed by Cacchio et al.[59] treated 126 patients with long-bone hypertrophic nonunion with either ESWT with an energy flux density of 0.4 or 0.7 mJ/mm(2), or surgery. At 6 months, 70% to 71% of the fractures had healed in the ESWT groups compared to 73% in the surgical group. However, at both 3 and 6 months after treatment, the ESWT groups had significantly improved pain and functional outcome scores compared to the surgical group. There was no difference by 1 year. In a retrospective review by Elster et al.[99] of 129 tibial nonunions treated with ESWT, 80% demonstrated complete healing with the average time to healing completion of 4 to 5 months. Multiple other studies have shown similar efficacies of ESWT in the treatment of nonunions.[287,332,346] Wang et al.[338] treated 72 patients with nonunions of long-bone fractures, and demonstrated an 80% union rate at 1-year follow-up. ESWT worked well for hypertrophic nonunions but was less optimal for atrophic nonunions. Although there are promising initial results in the treatment of nonunions, there have not been enough clinical studies to evaluate the efficacy of this relatively new technology.

AUTHORS' PREFERRED METHOD OF TREATMENT

Distraction Osteogenesis, Electrical Stimulation, Ultrasound Stimulation

The use of controlled micromotion to enhance fracture healing, as described by Easley et al.[90] has not been widely used and we have no experience with this method. The use of distraction osteogenesis for the treatment of nonunions for surgeons experienced in this technique is appropriate, but there is an established risk of fracture after the removal of external fixators.

There are data to support the use of electrical stimulation for the treatment of nonunions and delayed unions. DC, capacitive coupling, and PEMFs have all shown the potential to stimulate the healing of nonunions. PEMFs can also be used for the treatment of delayed unions. However, methodologic limitations and high between-study heterogeneity leave the impact of electromagnetic stimulation on fracture healing uncertain. There is no evidence that electrical stimulation of any type enhances the healing of fresh fractures.

Ultrasound stimulation can be used for the treatment of fresh closed fractures of the distal radius and tibia when treated in a cast or external fixation device. We have also had good results in the treatment of tibia fractures that show delayed union. While this therapy might not reduce the rate of reoperations, it appears to influence fracture-healing time and union rates. Until there is evidence to support the use of LIPUS in patients treated with fixation devices apart from distraction osteogenesis, we do not recommend the use of ultrasound in the treatment of fractures of patients who have undergone an operation in which fixation devices have been implanted.

ESWT is a relatively new technology whose potential in fracture healing does not have enough evidence to evaluate for or against its use.

CONCLUSIONS AND FUTURE DIRECTIONS

The repair of fractures is a predictable event for most skeletal injuries. There are, however, instances when fracture repair is delayed or fails to occur. With improved understanding of the intracellular and extracellular pathways involved in bone healing, our ability to successfully augment this repair process continuously evolves.

Currently, the ability to promote fracture healing is limited. Accepted options include returning to the operating room to perform an open procedure supplemented with some type of physiologic or synthetic graft, rhOP-1 or rhBMP-2, electrical or mechanical stimulation or the use of LIPUS. Systemic treatments, such as the use of statins or hormones, are still in the development stages. Current advances, including improved methods for obtaining autogenous and allogenic MSCs, development of delivery mechanisms for gene therapy, and improvements in synthetic bone-graft materials, may enhance the ability to improve fracture repair in the future.

REFERENCES

1. Agholme F, Aspenberg P. Wnt signaling and orthopedics, an overview. *Acta Orthop.* 2011;82(2):125–130.
2. Agholme F, Isaksson H, Kuhstoss S, et al. The effects of Dickkopf-1 antibody on metaphyseal bone and implant fixation under different loading conditions. *Bone.* 2011;48(5):988–996.
3. Agholme F, Isaksson H, Li X, et al. Anti-sclerostin antibody and mechanical loading appear to influence metaphyseal bone independently in rats. *Acta Orthop.* 2011;82(5):628–632.
4. Akman S, Gogus A, Sener N, et al. Effect of diclofenac sodium on union of tibial fractures in rats. *Adv Ther.* 2002;19(3):119–125.
5. Albee FH. Studies in bone growth: Triple calcium phosphate as a stimulus to osteogenesis. *Ann Surg.* 1920;71(1):32–39.
6. Alkhiary YM, Gerstenfeld LC, Krall E, et al. Enhancement of experimental fracture-healing by systemic administration of recombinant human parathyroid hormone (PTH 1-34). *J Bone Joint Surg Am.* 2005;87(4):731–741.

7. An HS, Simpson JM, Glover JM, et al. Comparison between allograft plus demineralized bone matrix versus autograft in anterior cervical fusion. A prospective multicenter study. *Spine.* 1995;20(20):2211–2216.

8. Andrades JA, Han B, Becerra J, et al. A recombinant human TGF-beta1 fusion protein with collagen-binding domain promotes migration, growth, and differentiation of bone marrow mesenchymal cells. *Exp Cell Res.* 1999;250(2):485–498.

9. Andreassen TT, Oxlund H. Local anabolic effects of growth hormone on intact bone and healing fractures in rats. *Calcif Tissue Int.* 2003;73(3):258–264.

10. Andrew JG, Hoyland J, Freemont AJ, et al. Insulinlike growth factor gene expression in human fracture callus. *Calcif Tissue Int.* 1993;53(2):97–102.

11. Anker CJ, Holdridge SP, Baird B, et al. Ultraporous beta-tricalcium phosphate is well incorporated in small cavitary defects. *Clin Orthop Relat Res.* 2005;(434):251–257.

12. Aro HT, Govender S, Patel AD, et al. Recombinant human bone morphogenetic protein-2: A randomized trial in open tibial fractures treated with reamed nail fixation. *J Bone Joint Surg Am.* 2011;93(9):801–808.

13. Aronson J. Limb-lengthening, skeletal reconstruction, and bone transport with the Ilizarov method. *J Bone Joint Surg Am.* 1997;79(8):1243–1258.

14. Aronson J, Good B, Stewart C, et al. Preliminary studies of mineralization during distraction osteogenesis. *Clin Orthop Relat Res.* 1990;(250):43–49.

15. Arrington ED, Smith WJ, Chambers HG, et al. Complications of iliac crest bone graft harvesting. *Clin Orthop Relat Res.* 1996;(329):300–309.

16. Artzi Z, Weinreb M, Givol N, et al. Biomaterial resorption rate and healing site morphology of inorganic bovine bone and beta-tricalcium phosphate in the canine: A 24-month longitudinal histologic study and morphometric analysis. *Int J Oral Maxillofac Implants.* 2004;19(3):357–368.

17. Aspenberg P, Genant HK, Johansson T, et al. Teriparatide for acceleration of fracture repair in humans: A prospective, randomized, double-blind study of 102 postmenopausal women with distal radial fractures. *J Bone Miner Res.* 2010;25(2):404–414.

18. Bae H, Zhao L, Zhu D, et al. Variability across ten production lots of a single demineralized bone matrix product. *J Bone Joint Surg Am.* 2010;92(2):427–435.

19. Bae HW, Zhao L, Kanim LE, et al. Intervariability and intravariability of bone morphogenetic proteins in commercially available demineralized bone matrix products. *Spine.* 2006;31(12):1299–1306; discussion 1307–1308.

20. Bajada S, Marshall MJ, Wright KT, et al. Decreased osteogenesis, increased cell senescence and elevated Dickkopf-1 secretion in human fracture non union stromal cells. *Bone.* 2009;45(4):726–735.

21. Bajammal SS, Zlowodzki M, Lelwica A, et al. The use of calcium phosphate bone cement in fracture treatment. A meta-analysis of randomized trials. *J Bone Joint Surg Am.* 2008;90(6):1186–1196.

22. Bak B, Jorgensen PH, Andreassen TT. The stimulating effect of growth hormone on fracture healing is dependent on onset and duration of administration. *Clin Orthop Relat Res.* 1991;(264):295–301.

23. Banwart JC, Asher MA, Hassanein RS. Iliac crest bone graft harvest donor site morbidity. A statistical evaluation. *Spine.* 1995;20(9):1055–1060.

24. Barriga A, Diaz-de-Rada P, Barroso JL, et al. Frozen cancellous bone allografts: Positive cultures of implanted grafts in posterior fusions of the spine. *Eur Spine J.* 2004;13(2):152–156.

25. Bashardoust Tajali S, Houghton P, MacDermid JC, et al. Effects of low-intensity pulsed ultrasound therapy on fracture healing: A systematic review and meta-analysis. *Am J Phys Med Rehabil.* 2012;91(4):349–367.

26. Bassett CA, Mitchell SN, Gaston SR. Treatment of ununited tibial diaphyseal fractures with pulsing electromagnetic fields. *J Bone Joint Surg Am.* 1981;63(4):511–523.

27. Bauer DC, Mundy GR, Jamal SA, et al. Use of statins and fracture: Results of 4 prospective studies and cumulative meta-analysis of observational studies and controlled trials. *Arch Intern Med.* 2004;164(2):146–152.

28. Bauer TW, Muschler GF. Bone graft materials. An overview of the basic science. *Clin Orthop Relat Res.* 2000;(371):10–27.

29. Becerra J, Guerado E, Claros S, et al. Autologous human-derived bone marrow cells exposed to a novel TGF-beta1 fusion protein for the treatment of critically sized tibial defect. *Regen Med.* 2006;1(2):267–278.

30. Beck A, Salem K, Krischak G, et al. Nonsteroidal anti-inflammatory drugs (NSAIDs) in the perioperative phase in traumatology and orthopedics effects on bone healing. *Oper Orthop Traumatol.* 2005;17(6):569–578.

31. Beck BR, Matheson GO, Bergman G, et al. Do capacitively coupled electric fields accelerate tibial stress fracture healing? A randomized controlled trial. *Am J Sports Med.* 2008;36(3):545–553.

32. Becker W, Becker BE, Caffesse R. A comparison of demineralized freeze-dried bone and autologous bone to induce bone formation in human extraction sockets. *J Periodontol.* 1994;65(12):1128–1133.

33. Belthur MV, Conway JD, Jindal G, et al. Bone graft harvest using a new intramedullary system. *Clin Orthop Relat Res.* 2008;466(12):2973–2980.

34. Beredjiklian PK, Hotchkiss RN, Athanasian EA, et al. Recalcitrant nonunion of the distal humerus: Treatment with free vascularized bone grafting. *Clin Orthop Relat Res.* 2005;(435):134–139.

35. Bergenstock M, Min W, Simon AM, et al. A comparison between the effects of acetaminophen and celecoxib on bone fracture healing in rats. *J Orthop Trauma.* 2005;19(10):717–723.

36. Berrey BH Jr, Lord CF, Gebhardt MC, et al. Fractures of allografts. Frequency, treatment, and end-results. *J Bone Joint Surg Am.* 1990;72(6):825–833.

37. Bhattacharyya T, Levin R, Vrahas MS, et al. Nonsteroidal antiinflammatory drugs and nonunion of humeral shaft fractures. *Arthritis Rheum.* 2005;53(3):364–367.

38. Bibbo C, Patel DV. The effect of demineralized bone matrix-calcium sulfate with vancomycin on calcaneal fracture healing and infection rates: A prospective study. *Foot Ankle Int.* 2006;27(7):487–493.

39. Blom AW, Wylde V, Livesey C, et al. Impaction bone grafting of the acetabulum at hip revision using a mix of bone chips and a biphasic porous ceramic bone graft substitute. *Acta Orthop.* 2009;80(2):150–154.

40. Bo J, Sudmann E, Marton PF. Effect of indomethacin on fracture healing in rats. *Acta Orthop Scand.* 1976;47(6):588–599.

41. Bohner M. Physical and chemical aspects of calcium phosphates used in spinal surgery. *Eur Spine J.* 2001;10(suppl 2):S114–S121.

42. Bolander ME. Regulation of fracture repair by growth factors. *Proc Soc Exp Biol Med.* 1992;200(2):165–170.

43. Bolder SB, Verdonschot N, Schreurs BW, et al. The initial stability of cemented acetabular cups can be augmented by mixing morsellized bone grafts with tricalciumphosphate/hydroxyapatite particles in bone impaction grafting. *J Arthroplasty.* 2003;18(8):1056–1063.

44. Bong MR, Capla EL, Egol KA, et al. Osteogenic protein-1 (bone morphogenic protein-7) combined with various adjuncts in the treatment of humeral diaphyseal nonunions. *Bulletin.* 2005;63(1–2):20–23.

45. Borrelli J Jr, Prickett WD, Ricci WM. Treatment of nonunions and osseous defects with bone graft and calcium sulfate. *Clin Orthop Relat Res.* 2003;(411):245–254.

46. Borsalino G, Bagnacani M, Bettati E, et al. Electrical stimulation of human femoral intertrochanteric osteotomies. Double-blind study. *Clin Orthop Relat Res.* 1988;(237):256–263.

47. Bradbury N, Hutchinson J, Hahn D, et al. Clavicular nonunion. 31/32 healed after plate fixation and bone grafting. *Acta Orthop Scand.* 1996;67(4):367–370.

48. Brighton CT, Friedenberg ZB, Mitchell EI, et al. Treatment of nonunion with constant direct current. *Clin Orthop Relat Res.* 1977;(124):106–123.

49. Brighton CT. Treatment of nonunion of the tibia with constant direct current (1980 Fitts Lecture A.A.S.T.). *J Trauma.* 1981;21(3):189–195.

50. Brown KM, Saunders MM, Kirsch T, et al. Effect of COX-2-specific inhibition on fracture-healing in the rat femur. *J Bone Joint Surg Am.* 2004;86-A(1):116–123.

51. Bruno RJ, Cohen MS, Berzins A, et al. Bone graft harvesting from the distal radius, olecranon, iliac crest: A quantitative analysis. *J Hand Surg Am.* 2001;26(1):135–141.

52. Bucholz RW, Carlton A, Holmes R. Interporous hydroxyapatite as a bone graft substitute in tibial plateau fractures. *Clin Orthop Relat Res.* 1989;(240):53–62.

53. Buecker PJ, Gebhardt MC. Are fibula strut allografts a reliable alternative for periarticular reconstruction after curettage for bone tumors? *Clin Orthop Relat Res.* 2007;461:170–174.

54. Bukata SV. Systemic administration of pharmacological agents and bone repair: What can we expect. *Injury.* 2011;42(6):605–608.

55. Burchardt H. Biology of bone transplantation. *Orthop Clin North Am.* 1987;18(2):187–196.

56. Burchardt H, Busbee GA 3rd, Enneking WF. Repair of experimental autologous grafts of cortical bone. *J Bone Joint Surg Am.* 1975;57(6):814–819.

57. Burd TA, Hughes MS, Anglen JO. Heterotopic ossification prophylaxis with indomethacin increases the risk of long-bone nonunion. *J Bone Joint Surg Br.* 2003;85(5):700–705.

58. Busse JW, Bhandari M, Sprague S, et al. An economic analysis of management strategies for closed and open grade I tibial shaft fractures. *Acta Orthop.* 2005;76(5):705–712.

59. Cacchio A, Giordano L, Colafarina O, et al. Extracorporeal shock-wave therapy compared with surgery for hypertrophic long-bone nonunions. *J Bone Joint Surg Am.* 2009;91(11):2589–2597.

60. Canalis E. Effect of platelet-derived growth factor on DNA and protein synthesis in cultured rat calvaria. *Metabolism.* 1981;30(10):970–975.

61. Canalis E, Centrella M, McCarthy TL. Regulation of insulin-like growth factor-II production in bone cultures. *Endocrinology.* 1991;129(5):2457–2462.

62. Canalis E, McCarthy T, Centrella M. Isolation and characterization of insulin-like growth factor I (somatomedin-C) from cultures of fetal rat calvariae. *Endocrinology.* 1988;122(1):22–27.

63. Canalis E, McCarthy TL, Centrella M. Effects of platelet-derived growth factor on bone formation in vitro. *J Cell Physiol.* 1989;140(3):530–537.

64. Canalis E, Pash J, Gabbitas B, et al. Growth factors regulate the synthesis of insulin-like growth factor-I in bone cell cultures. *Endocrinology.* 1993;133(1):33–38.

65. Carlson JR, Simmons BP. Wrist arthrodesis after failed wrist implant arthroplasty. *J Hand Surg Am.* 1998;23(5):893–898.

66. Cassidy C, Jupiter JB, Cohen M, et al. Norian SRS cement compared with conventional fixation in distal radial fractures. A randomized study. *J Bone Joint Surg Am.* 2003;85-A(11):2127–2137.

67. Chalidis B, Sachinis N, Assiotis A, et al. Stimulation of bone formation and fracture healing with pulsed electromagnetic fields: Biologic responses and clinical implications. *Int J Immunopathol Pharmacol.* 2011;24(1 suppl 2):17–20.

68. Chen WJ, Jingushi S, Aoyama I, et al. Effects of FGF-2 on metaphyseal fracture repair in rabbit tibiae. *J Bone Miner Metab.* 2004;22(4):303–309.

69. Chintamaneni S, Finzel K, Gruber BL. Successful treatment of sternal fracture nonunion with teriparatide. *Osteoporos Int.* 2010;21(6):1059–1063.

70. Chissas D, Stamatopoulos G, Verettas D, et al. Can low doses of simvastatin enhance fracture healing? An experimental study in rabbits. *Injury.* 2010;41(7):687–692.

71. Chmell MJ, McAndrew MP, Thomas R, et al. Structural allografts for reconstruction of lower extremity open fractures with 10 centimeters or more of acute segmental defects. *J Orthop Trauma.* 1995;9(3):222–226.

72. Cho TJ, Gerstenfeld LC, Einhorn TA. Differential temporal expression of members of the transforming growth factor beta superfamily during murine fracture healing. *J Bone Miner Res.* 2002;17(3):513–520.

73. Claes L, Augat P, Suger G, et al. Influence of size and stability of the osteotomy gap on the success of fracture healing. *J Orthop Res.* 1997;15(4):577–584.

74. Codivilla A. On the means of lengthening, in the lower limbs, the muscles and tissues which are shortened through deformity. 1904. *Clin Orthop Relat Res.* 1994;(301):4–9.

75. Cook SD, Ryaby JP, McCabe J, et al. Acceleration of tibia and distal radius fracture healing in patients who smoke. *Clin Orthop Relat Res.* 1997;(337):198–207.

76. Cottrell JA, O'Connor JP. Pharmacological inhibition of 5-lipoxygenase accelerates and enhances fracture-healing. *J Bone Joint Surg Am.* 2009;91(11):2653–2665.

77. Critchlow MA, Bland YS, Ashhurst DE. The effect of exogenous transforming growth factor-beta 2 on healing fractures in the rabbit. *Bone.* 1995;16(5):521–527.

78. Croteau S, Rauch F, Silvestri A, et al. Bone morphogenetic proteins in orthopedics: From basic science to clinical practice. *Orthopedics.* 1999;22(7):686–695; quiz 696–697.

79. Daculsi G, Passuti N. Effect of the macroporosity for osseous substitution of calcium phosphate ceramics. *Biomaterials.* 1990;11:86–87.

80. Dekel S, Lenthall G, Francis MJ. Release of prostaglandins from bone and muscle after tibial fracture. An experimental study in rabbits. *J Bone Joint Surg Br.* 1981;63-B(2):185–189.

81. Dell PC, Burchardt H, Glowczewskie FP Jr. A roentgenographic, biomechanical, and histological evaluation of vascularized and non-vascularized segmental fibular canine autografts. *J Bone Joint Surg Am.* 1985;67(1):105–112.

82. Dempster DW, Cosman F, Parisien M, et al. Anabolic actions of parathyroid hormone on bone. *Endocr Rev.* 1993;14(6):690–709.

83. Dias JJ, Wildin CJ, Bhowal B, et al. Should acute scaphoid fractures be fixed? A randomized controlled trial. *J Bone Joint Surg Am.* 2005;87(10):2160–2168.

84. Diefenderfer DL, Osyczka AM, Garino JP, et al. Regulation of BMP-induced transcription in cultured human bone marrow stromal cells. *J Bone Joint Surg Am.* 2003;85-A(suppl 3):19–28.

85. Dimitriou R, Dahabreh Z, Katsoulis E, et al. Application of recombinant BMP-7 on persistent upper and lower limb non-unions. *Injury.* 2005;36(suppl 4):S51–S59.

86. Dimmen S, Nordsletten L, Engebretsen L, et al. Negative effect of parecoxib on bone mineral during fracture healing in rats. *Acta Orthop.* 2008;79(3):438–444.

87. Dodd CA, Fergusson CM, Freedman L, et al. Allograft versus autograft bone in scoliosis surgery. *J Bone Joint Surg Br.* 1988;70(3):431–434.

88. Dolan CM, Henning JA, Anderson JG, et al. Randomized prospective study comparing tri-cortical iliac crest autograft to allograft in the lateral column lengthening component for operative correction of adult acquired flatfoot deformity. *Foot Ankle Int.* 2007;28(1):8–12.

89. Dudda M, Hauser J, Muhr G, et al. Low-intensity pulsed ultrasound as a useful adjuvant during distraction osteogenesis: A prospective, randomized controlled trial. *J Trauma.* 2011;71(5):1376–1380.

90. Easley ME, Trnka HJ, Schon LC, et al. Isolated subtalar arthrodesis. *J Bone Joint Surg Am.* 2000;82(5):613–624.

91. Ebraheim NA, Elgafy H, Xu R. Bone-graft harvesting from iliac and fibular donor sites: Techniques and complications. *J Am Acad Orthop Surg.* 2001;9(3):210–218.

92. Eckardt H, Ding M, Lind M, et al. Recombinant human vascular endothelial growth factor enhances bone healing in an experimental nonunion model. *J Bone Joint Surg Br.* 2005;87(10):1434–1438.

93. Edwards CJ, Hart DJ, Spector TD. Oral statins and increased bone-mineral density in postmenopausal women. *Lancet.* 2000;355(9222):2218–2219.

94. Egol KA, Sugi MT, Ong CC, et al. Fracture site augmentation with calcium phosphate cement reduces screw penetration after open reduction-internal fixation of proximal humeral fractures. *J Shoulder Elbow Surg.* 2011;21(6):741–748

95. Einhorn TA. Cox-2: Where are we in 2003? - The role of cyclooxygenase-2 in bone repair. *Arthritis Res Ther.* 2003;5(1):5–7.

96. Einhorn TA. Enhancement of fracture-healing. *J Bone Joint Surg Am.* 1995;77(6):940–956.

97. Einhorn TA, Bonnarens F, Burstein AH. The contributions of dietary protein and mineral to the healing of experimental fractures. A biomechanical study. *J Bone Joint Surg Am.* 1986;68(9):1389–1395.

98. Elder S, Frankenburg E, Goulet J, et al. Biomechanical evaluation of calcium phosphate cement-augmented fixation of unstable intertrochanteric fractures. *J Orthop Trauma.* 2000;14(6):386–393.

99. Elster EA, Stojadinovic A, Forsberg J, et al. Extracorporeal shock wave therapy for nonunion of the tibia. *J Orthop Trauma.* 2010;24(3):133–141.

100. Emami A, Petren-Mallmin M, Larsson S. No effect of low-intensity ultrasound on healing time of intramedullary fixed tibial fractures. *J Orthop Trauma.* 1999;13(4):252–257.

101. Endo K, Sairyo K, Komatsubara S, et al. Cyclooxygenase-2 inhibitor delays fracture healing in rats. *Acta Orthop.* 2005;76(4):470–174.

102. Endo K, Sairyo K, Komatsubara S, et al. Cyclooxygenase-2 inhibitor inhibits the fracture healing. *J Physiol Anthropol Appl Human Sci.* 2002;21(5):235–238.

103. Engh GA, Ammeen DJ. Use of structural allograft in revision total knee arthroplasty in knees with severe tibial bone loss. *J Bone Joint Surg Am.* 2007;89(12):2640–2647.

104. Enneking WF, Burchardt H, Puhl JJ, et al. Physical and biological aspects of repair in dog cortical-bone transplants. *J Bone Joint Surg Am.* 1975;57(2):237–252.

105. Enneking WF, Eady JL, Burchardt H. Autogenous cortical bone grafts in the reconstruction of segmental skeletal defects. *J Bone Joint Surg Am.* 1980;62(7):1039–1058.

106. Enneking WF, Mindell ER. Observations on massive retrieved human allografts. *J Bone Joint Surg Am.* 1991;73(8):1123–1142.

107. Fink B, Pollnau C, Vogel M, et al. Histomorphometry of distraction osteogenesis during experimental tibial lengthening. *J Orthop Trauma.* 2003;17(2):113–118.

108. Finkemeier CG. Bone-grafting and bone-graft substitutes. *J Bone Joint Surg Am.* 2002;84-A(3):454–464.

109. Fischgrund J, Paley D, Suter C. Variables affecting time to bone healing during limb lengthening. *Clin Orthop Relat Res.* 1994;(301):31–37.

110. Fleming JE Jr, Cornell CN, Muschler GF. Bone cells and matrices in orthopedic tissue engineering. *Orthop Clin North Am.* 2000;31(3):357–374.

111. Fowler BL, Dall BE, Rowe DE. Complications associated with harvesting autogenous iliac bone graft. *Am J Orthop.* 1995;24(12):895–903.

112. Friedenberg ZB, Andrews ET, Smolenski BI, et al. Bone reaction to varying amounts of direct current. *Surg Gynecol Obstet.* 1970;131(5):894–899.

113. Friedenberg ZB, Harlow MC, Brighton CT. Healing of nonunion of the medial malleolus by means of direct current: A case report. *J Trauma.* 1971;11(10):883–885.

114. Friedl G, Turner RT, Evans GL, et al. Intermittent parathyroid hormone (PTH) treatment and age-dependent effects on rat cancellous bone and mineral metabolism. *J Orthop Res.* 2007;25(11):1454–1464.

115. Friedlaender GE. Immune responses to osteochondral allografts. Current knowledge and future directions. *Clin Orthop Relat Res.* 1983;(174):58–68.

116. Friedlaender GE, Perry CR, Cole JD, et al. Osteogenic protein-1 (bone morphogenetic protein-7) in the treatment of tibial nonunions. *J Bone Joint Surg Am.* 2001;83-A (suppl 1 Pt 2):S151–S158.

117. Frohberg U, Mazock JB. A review of morbidity associated with bone harvest from the proximal tibial metaphysis. *Mund Kiefer Gesichtschir.* 2005;9(2):63–65.

118. Fukada E, Yasuda I. On the piezoelectric effects of bone. *J Phys Soc Japan.* 1957;12:1158.

119. Fukui T, Ii M, Shoji T, et al. Therapeutic effect of local administration of low dose simvastatin-conjugated gelatin hydrogel for fracture healing. *J Bone Miner Res.* 2012;27(5):1118–1131

120. Galano GJ, Greisberg JK. Tibial plateau fracture with proximal tibia autograft harvest for foot surgery. *Am J Orthop.* 2009;38(12):621–623.

121. Garrett IR, Gutierrez GE, Rossini G, et al. Locally delivered lovastatin nanoparticles enhance fracture healing in rats. *J Orthop Res.* 2007;25(10):1351–1357.

122. Garvin K, Feschuk C, Sharp JG, et al. Does the number or quality of pluripotent bone marrow stem cells decrease with age? *Clin Orthop Relat Res.* 2007;465:202–207.

123. Geideman W, Early JS, Brodsky J. Clinical results of harvesting autogenous cancellous graft from the ipsilateral proximal tibia for use in foot and ankle surgery. *Foot Ankle Int.* 2004;25(7):451–455.

124. Gerstenfeld LC, Al-Ghawas M, Alkhiary YM, et al. Selective and nonselective cyclo-oxygenase-2 inhibitors and experimental fracture-healing. Reversibility of effects after short-term treatment. *J Bone Joint Surg Am.* 2007;89(1):114–125.

125. Gerstenfeld LC, Einhorn TA. COX inhibitors and their effects on bone healing. *Expert Opin Drug Saf.* 2004;3(2):131–136.

126. Gheduzzi S, Webb JJ, Miles AW. Mechanical characterisation of three percutaneous vertebroplasty biomaterials. *J Mater Sci Mater Med.* 2006;17(5):421–426.

127. Giannoudis PV, Kanakaris NK, Dimitriou R, et al. The synergistic effect of autograft and BMP-7 in the treatment of atrophic nonunions. *Clin Orthop Relat Res.* 2009;467(12):3239–3248.

128. Giannoudis PV, MacDonald DA, Matthews SJ, et al. Nonunion of the femoral diaphysis. The influence of reaming and non-steroidal anti-inflammatory drugs. *J Bone Joint Surg Br.* 2000;82(5):655–658.

129. Giori NJ, Beaupre GS. Femoral fracture after harvesting of autologous bone graft using a reamer/irrigator/aspirator. *J Orthop Trauma.* 2011;25(2):e12–e14.

130. Goldberg VM, Shaffer JW, Field G, et al. Biology of vascularized bone grafts. *Orthop Clin North Am.* 1987;18(2):197–205.

131. Goldberg VM, Stevenson S. Natural history of autografts and allografts. *Clin Orthop Relat Res.* 1987;(225):7–16.

132. Goldberg VM, Stevenson S, Shaffer JW, et al. Biological and physical properties of autogenous vascularized fibular grafts in dogs. *J Bone Joint Surg Am.* 1990;72(6):801–810.

133. Goodman SB, Ma T, Mitsunaga L, et al. Temporal effects of a COX-2-selective NSAID on bone ingrowth. *J Biomed Mater Res A.* 2005;72(3):279–287.

134. Goulet JA, Senunas LE, DeSilva GL, et al. Autogenous iliac crest bone graft. Complications and functional assessment. *Clin Orthop Relat Res.* 1997;(339):76–81.

135. Govender S, Csimma C, Genant HK, et al. Recombinant human bone morphogenetic protein-2 for treatment of open tibial fractures: A prospective, controlled, randomized study of four hundred and fifty patients. *J Bone Joint Surg Am.* 2002;84-A(12):2123–2134.

136. Griffin XL, Smith N, Parsons N, et al. Ultrasound and shockwave therapy for acute fractures in adults. *Cochrane Database Syst Rev.* 2012;2:CD008579.

137. Griffith JF, Yeung DK, Tsang PH, et al. Compromised bone marrow perfusion in osteoporosis. *J Bone Miner Res.* 2008;23(7):1068–1075.

138. Grogan DP, Kalen V, Ross TI, et al. Use of allograft bone for posterior spinal fusion in idiopathic scoliosis. *Clin Orthop Relat Res.* 1999;(369):273–278.

139. Gruber R, Koch H, Doll BA, et al. Fracture healing in the elderly patient. *Exp Gerontol.* 2006;41(11):1080–1093.

140. Gurgel BC, Ribeiro FV, Silva MA, et al. Selective COX-2 inhibitor reduces bone healing in bone defects. *Braz Oral Res.* 2005;19(4):312–316.

141. Gustilo RB, Anderson JT. Prevention of infection in the treatment of one thousand and twenty-five open fractures of long bones: Retrospective and prospective analyses. *J Bone Joint Surg Am.* 1976;58(4):453–458.

142. Hatzokos I, Stavridis SI, Iosifidou E, et al. Autologous bone marrow grafting combined with demineralized bone matrix improves consolidation of docking site after distraction osteogenesis. *J Bone Joint Surg Am.* 2011;93(7):671–678.

143. Healey JH, Zimmerman PA, McDonnell JM, et al. Percutaneous bone marrow grafting of delayed union and nonunion in cancer patients. *Clin Orthop Relat Res* 1990;(256):280–285.

144. Heckman JD, Ryaby JP, McCabe J, et al. Acceleration of tibial fracture-healing by non-invasive, low-intensity pulsed ultrasound. *J Bone Joint Surg Am.* 1994;76(1):26–34.

145. Hee SL, Nik Intan NI, Fazan F. Comparison of hydroxyapatite powders derived from different resources. *Med J Malaysia.* 2004;59(suppl B):77–78.

146. Hemery X, Ohl X, Saddiki R, et al. Low-intensity pulsed ultrasound for non-union treatment: A 14-case series evaluation. *Orthop Traumatol Surg Res.* 2011;97(1):51–57.

147. Hernigou P, Beaujean F. Treatment of osteonecrosis with autologous bone marrow grafting. *Clin Orthop Relat Res.* 2002;(405):14–23.

148. Hernigou P, Mathieu G, Poignard A, et al. Percutaneous autologous bone-marrow grafting for nonunions. Surgical technique. *J Bone Joint Surg Am.* 2006;88(suppl 1 Pt 2):322–327.

149. Hernigou P, Poignard A, Beaujean F, et al. Percutaneous autologous bone-marrow grafting for nonunions. Influence of the number and concentration of progenitor cells. *J Bone Joint Surg Am.* 2005;87(7):1430–1437.

150. Hernigou P, Poignard A, Manicom O, et al. The use of percutaneous autologous bone marrow transplantation in nonunion and avascular necrosis of bone. *J Bone Joint Surg Br.* 2005;87(7):896–902.

151. Hierholzer C, Sama D, Toro JB, et al. Plate fixation of ununited humeral shaft fractures: Effect of type of bone graft on healing. *J Bone Joint Surg Am.* 2006;88(7):1442–1447.

152. Hollinger JO, Onikepe AO, MacKrell J, et al. Accelerated fracture healing in the geriatric, osteoporotic rat with recombinant human platelet-derived growth factor-BB and an injectable beta-tricalcium phosphate/collagen matrix. *J Orthop Res.* 2008;26(1):83–90.

153. Hornicek FJ, Zych GA, Hutson JJ, et al. Salvage of humeral nonunions with onlay bone plate allograft augmentation. *Clin Orthop Relat Res.* 2001;(386):203–209.

154. Horowitz MC, Friedlaender GE. Induction of specific T-cell responsiveness to allogeneic bone. *J Bone Joint Surg Am.* 1991;73(8):1157–1168.

155. Horstmann WG, Verheyen CC, Leemans R. An injectable calcium phosphate cement as a bone-graft substitute in the treatment of displaced lateral tibial plateau fractures. *Injury.* 2003;34(2):141–144.

156. Hou CH, Yang RS, Hou SM. Hospital-based allogenic bone bank–10-year experience. *J Hosp Infect.* 2005;59(1):41–45.

157. Huang RC, Khan SN, Sandhu HS, et al. Alendronate inhibits spine fusion in a rat model. *Spine.* 2005;30(22):2516–2522.

158. Hurley MM, Abreu C, Harrison JR, et al. Basic fibroblast growth factor inhibits type I collagen gene expression in osteoblastic MC3T3-E1 cells. *J Biol Chem.* 1993; 268(8):5588–5593.

159. Ilizarov GA. The tension-stress effect on the genesis and growth of tissues: Part II. The influence of the rate and frequency of distraction. *Clin Orthop Relat Res.* 1989; (239):263–285.

160. Ilizarov GA, Khelimskii AM, Saks RG. [Characteristics of systemic growth regulation of the limbs under the effect of various factors influencing their growth and length]. *Ortop Travmatol Protez.* 1978;(8):37–41.

161. Ilizarov GA, Pereslitskikh PF, Barabash AP. [Closed directed longitudino-oblique or spinal osteoclasia of the long tubular bones (experimental study)]. *Ortop Travmatol Protez.* 1978;(11):20–23.

162. Ingber DE, Folkman J. Mechanochemical switching between growth and differentiation during fibroblast growth factor-stimulated angiogenesis in vitro: Role of extracellular matrix. *J Cell Biol.* 1989;109(1):317–330.

163. Ito H, Koefoed M, Tiyapatanaputi P, et al. Remodeling of cortical bone allografts mediated by adherent rAAV-RANKL and VEGF gene therapy. *Nat Med.* 2005;11(3):291–297.

164. Itoh N, Ornitz DM. Evolution of the Fgf and Fgfr gene families. *Trends Genet.* 2004;20(11):563–569.

165. Jarcho M, Kay JF, Gumaer KI, et al. Tissue, cellular and subcellular events at a bone-ceramic hydroxylapatite interface. *J Bioeng.* 1977;1(2):79–92.

166. Jepegnanam TS, von Schroeder HP. Rapid resorption of calcium sulfate and hardware failure following corrective radius osteotomy: 2 case reports. *J Hand Surg Am.* 2012;37(3):477–480.

167. Jeyam M, Andrew JG, Muir LT, et al. Controlled trial of distal radial fractures treated with a resorbable bone mineral substitute. *J Hand Surg Br.* 2002;27(2):146–149.

168. Jingushi S, Mizuno K, Matsushita T, et al. Low-intensity pulsed ultrasound treatment for postoperative delayed union or nonunion of long bone fractures. *J Orthop Sci.* 2007;12(1):35–41.

169. Jinno T, Miric A, Feighan J, et al. The effects of processing and low dose irradiation on cortical bone grafts. *Clin Orthop Relat Res.* 2000;(375):275–285.

170. Johnson EE, Urist MR, Finerman GA. Repair of segmental defects of the tibia with cancellous bone grafts augmented with human bone morphogenetic protein. A preliminary report. *Clin Orthop Relat Res.* 1988;(236):249–257.

171. Jones AL, Bucholz RW, Bosse MJ, et al. Recombinant human BMP-2 and allograft compared with autogenous bone graft for reconstruction of diaphyseal tibial fractures with cortical defects. A randomized, controlled trial. *J Bone Joint Surg Am.* 2006;88(7):1431–1441.

172. Jones DB Jr, Moran SL, Bishop AT, et al. Free-vascularized medial femoral condyle bone transfer in the treatment of scaphoid nonunions. *Plast Reconstr Surg.* 2010;125(4):1176–1184.

173. Kakar S, Duymaz A, Steinmann S, et al. Vascularized medial femoral condyle corti-coperiosteal flaps for the treatment of recalcitrant humeral nonunions. *Microsurgery.* 2011;31(2):85–92.

174. Kakar S, Einhorn TA, Vora S, et al. Enhanced chondrogenesis and Wnt signaling in PTH-treated fractures. *J Bone Miner Res.* 2007;22(12):1903–1912.

175. Kanakaris NK, Morell D, Gudipati S, et al. Reaming irrigator aspirator system: Early experience of its multipurpose use. *Injury.* 2011;42(suppl 4):S28–S34.

176. Karachalios T, Boursinos L, Poultsides L, et al. The effects of the short-term administration of low therapeutic doses of anti-COX-2 agents on the healing of fractures. An experimental study in rabbits. *J Bone Joint Surg Br.* 2007;89(9):1253–1260.

177. Kawaguchi H, Oka H, Jingushi S, et al. A local application of recombinant human fibroblast growth factor 2 for tibial shaft fractures: A randomized, placebo-controlled trial. *J Bone Miner Res.* 2010;25(12):2735–2743.

178. Keating JF, Hajducka CL, Harper J. Minimal internal fixation and calcium-phosphate cement in the treatment of fractures of the tibial plateau. A pilot study. *J Bone Joint Surg Br.* 2003;85(1):68–73.

179. Kelly CM, Wilkins RM. Treatment of benign bone lesions with an injectable calcium sulfate-based bone graft substitute. *Orthopedics.* 2004;27(1 suppl):s131–s135.

180. Kelly CM, Wilkins RM, Gitelis S, et al. The use of a surgical grade calcium sulfate as a bone graft substitute: Results of a multicenter trial. *Clin Orthop Relat Res.* 2001;(382):42–50.

181. Kenwright J, Richardson JB, Goodship AE, et al. Effect of controlled axial micromovement on healing of tibial fractures. *Lancet.* 1986;2(8517):1185–1187.

182. Kerry RM, Masri BA, Garbuz DS, et al. The biology of bone grafting. *Instr Course Lect.* 1999;48:645–652.

183. Khan SN, Bostrom MP, Lane JM. Bone growth factors. *Orthop Clin North Am.* 2000;31(3):375–388.

184. Khan SN, Cammisa FP Jr, Sandhu HS, et al. The biology of bone grafting. *J Am Acad Orthop Surg.* 2005;13(1):77–86.

185. Kim HP, Ji YH, Rhee SC, et al. Enhancement of bone regeneration using osteogenic-induced adipose- derived stem cells combined with demineralized bone matrix in a rat critically-sized calvarial defect model. *Curr Stem Cell Res Ther.* 2012;7(3):165–172.

186. Kim JH, Oh JH, Han I, et al. Grafting using injectable calcium sulfate in bone tumor surgery: Comparison with demineralized bone matrix-based grafting. *Clin Orthop Surg.* 2011;3(3):191–201.

187. Klein S, Giancotti FG, Presta M, et al. Basic fibroblast growth factor modulates integrin expression in microvascular endothelial cells. *Mol Biol Cell.* 1993;4(10):973–982.

188. Kloen P, Di Paola M, Borens O, et al. BMP signaling components are expressed in human fracture callus. *Bone.* 2003;33(3):362–371.

189. Kocaoglu M, Eralp L, Sen C, et al. Management of stiff hypertrophic nonunions by distraction osteogenesis: A report of 16 cases. *J Orthop Trauma.* 2003;17(8):543–548.

190. Kolbeck S, Bail H, Schmidmaier G, et al. Homologous growth hormone accelerates bone healing–a biomechanical and histological study. *Bone.* 2003;33(4):628–637.

191. Komatsu DE, Mary MN, Schroeder RJ, et al. Modulation of Wnt signaling influences fracture repair. *J Orthop Res.* 2010;28(7):928–936.

192. Kristiansen TK, Ryaby JP, McCabe J, et al. Accelerated healing of distal radial fractures with the use of specific, low-intensity ultrasound. A multicenter, prospective, randomized, double-blind, placebo-controlled study. *J Bone Joint Surg Am.* 1997;79(7):961–973.

193. Kucia M, Machalinski B, Ratajczak MZ. The developmental deposition of epiblast/germ cell-line derived cells in various organs as a hypothetical explanation of stem cell plasticity? *Acta Neurobiol Exp (Wars).* 2006;66(4):331–341.

194. Kumagai K, Takeuchi R, Ishikawa H, et al. Low-intensity pulsed ultrasound accelerates fracture healing by stimulation of recruitment of both local and circulating osteogenic progenitors. *J Orthop Res.* 2012;30(9):1516–1521.

195. Kurmis AP, Kurmis TP, O'Brien JX, et al. The effect of nonsteroidal anti-inflammatory drug administration on acute phase fracture-healing: A review. *J Bone Joint Surg Am.* 2012;94(9):815–823.

196. Larsson S, Hannink G. Injectable bone-graft substitutes: Current products, their characteristics and indications, new developments. *Injury.* 2011;42(suppl 2):S30–S34.

197. Laufs U, Liao JK. Direct vascular effects of HMG-CoA reductase inhibitors. *Trends Cardiovasc Med.* 2000;10(4):143–148.

198. LeCroy CM, Rizzo M, Gunneson EE, et al. Free vascularized fibular bone grafting in the management of femoral neck nonunion in patients younger than fifty years. *J Orthop Trauma.* 2002;16(7):464–472.

199. Lee DY, Cho TJ, Kim JA, et al. Mobilization of endothelial progenitor cells in fracture healing and distraction osteogenesis. *Bone.* 2008;42(5):932–941.

200. Lewallen DG, Chao EY, Kasman RA, et al. Comparison of the effects of compression plates and external fixators on early bone-healing. *J Bone Joint Surg Am.* 1984;66(7):1084–1091.

201. Lewandrowski KU, Gresser JD, Wise DL, et al. Bioresorbable bone graft substitutes of different osteoconductivities: A histologic evaluation of osteointegration of poly(propylene glycol-co-fumaric acid)-based cement implants in rats. *Biomaterials.* 2000;21(8):757–764.

202. Li J, Mori S, Kaji Y, et al. Concentration of bisphosphonate (incadronate) in callus area and its effects on fracture healing in rats. *J Bone Miner Res.* 2000;15(10):2042–2051.

203. Li M, Ke HZ, Qi H, et al. A novel, non-prostanoid EP2 receptor-selective prostaglandin E2 agonist stimulates local bone formation and enhances fracture healing. *J Bone Miner Res.* 2003;18(11):2033–2042.

204. Li X, Ominsky MS, Niu QT, et al. Targeted deletion of the sclerostin gene in mice results in increased bone formation and bone strength. *J Bone Miner Res.* 2008;23(6):860–869.

205. Li X, Ominsky MS, Warmington KS, et al. Sclerostin antibody treatment increases bone formation, bone mass, bone strength in a rat model of postmenopausal osteoporosis. *J Bone Miner Res.* 2009;24(4):578–588.

206. Li X, Qin L, Bergenstock M, et al. Parathyroid hormone stimulates osteoblastic expression of MCP-1 to recruit and increase the fusion of pre/osteoclasts. *J Biol Chem.* 2007;282(45):33098–330106.

207. Li X, Warmington KS, Niu QT, et al. Inhibition of sclerostin by monoclonal antibody increases bone formation, bone mass, bone strength in aged male rats. *J Bone Miner Res.* 2010;25(12):2647–2656.

208. Lin CH, Wei FC, Levin LS, et al. Free composite serratus anterior and rib flaps for tibial composite bone and soft-tissue defect. *Plast Reconstr Surg.* 1997;99(6):1656–1665.

209. Lind M, Schumacker B, Soballe K, et al. Transforming growth factor-beta enhances fracture healing in rabbit tibiae. *Acta Orthop Scand.* 1993;64(5):553–556.

210. Lobenhoffer P, Gerich T, Witte F, et al. Use of an injectable calcium phosphate bone cement in the treatment of tibial plateau fractures: A prospective study of twenty-six cases with twenty-month mean follow-up. *J Orthop Trauma.* 2002;16(3):143–149.

211. Long J, Lewis S, Kuklo T, et al. The effect of cyclooxygenase-2 inhibitors on spinal fusion. *J Bone Joint Surg Am.* 2002;84-A(10):1763–1768.

212. Lord CF, Gebhardt MC, Tomford WW, et al. Infection in bone allografts. Incidence, nature, treatment. *J Bone Joint Surg Am.* 1988;70(3):369–376.

213. Lowe JA, Della Rocca GJ, Murtha Y, et al. Complications associated with negative pressure reaming for harvesting autologous bone graft: A case series. *J Orthop Trauma.* 2010;24(1):46–52.

214. Macey LR, Kana SM, Jingushi S, et al. Defects of early fracture-healing in experimental diabetes. *J Bone Joint Surg Am.* 1989;71(5):722–733.

215. Mammi GI, Rocchi R, Cadossi R, et al. The electrical stimulation of tibial osteotomies. Double-blind study. *Clin Orthop Relat Res.* 1993;(288):246–253.

216. Manabe T, Mori S, Mashiba T, et al. Human parathyroid hormone (1-34) accelerates natural fracture healing process in the femoral osteotomy model of cynomolgus monkeys. *Bone.* 2007;40(6):1475–1482.

217. Manigrasso MB, O'Connor JP. Accelerated fracture healing in mice lacking the 5-lipoxygenase gene. *Acta Orthop.* 2010;81(6):748–755.

218. Manjubala I, Sivakumar M, Sampath Kumar TS, et al. Synthesis and characterization of functional gradient materials using Indian corals. *J Mater Sci Mater Med.* 2000;11(11):705–709.

219. Masquelet AC, Benko PE, Mathevon H, et al. Harvest of cortico-cancellous intramedullary femoral bone graft using the Reamer-Irrigator-Aspirator (RIA). *Orthop Traumatol Surg Res.* 2012;98(2):227–232.
220. Matsumine A, Kusuzaki K, Matsubara T, et al. Calcium phosphate cement in musculoskeletal tumor surgery. *J Surg Oncol.* 2006;93(3):212–220.
221. Mattsson P, Alberts A, Dahlberg G, et al. Resorbable cement for the augmentation of internally-fixed unstable trochanteric fractures. A prospective, randomised multicentre study. *J Bone Joint Surg Br.* 2005;87(9):1203–1209.
222. Mattsson P, Larsson S. Calcium phosphate cement for augmentation did not improve results after internal fixation of displaced femoral neck fractures: A randomized study of 118 patients. *Acta Orthop.* 2006;77(2):251–256.
223. Mattsson P, Larsson S. Unstable trochanteric fractures augmented with calcium phosphate cement. A prospective randomized study using radiostereometry to measure fracture stability. *Scand J Surg.* 2004;93(3):223–228.
224. Mazziotti G, Bianchi A, Bonadonna S, et al. Increased prevalence of radiological spinal deformities in adult patients with GH deficiency: Influence of GH replacement therapy. *J Bone Miner Res.* 2006;21(4):520–528.
225. McAndrew MP, Gorman PW, Lange TA. Tricalcium phosphate as a bone graft substitute in trauma: Preliminary report. *J Orthop Trauma.* 1988;2(4):333–339.
226. McDonald MM, Dulai S, Godfrey C, et al. Bolus or weekly zoledronic acid administration does not delay endochondral fracture repair but weekly dosing enhances delays in hard callus remodeling. *Bone.* 2008;43(4):653–662.
227. McDonald MM, Morse A, Mikulec K, et al. Inhibition of sclerostin by systemic treatment with sclerostin antibody enhances healing of proximal tibial defects in ovariectomized rats. *J Orthop Res.* 2012;30(10):1541–1548.
228. McKee MD, Li-Bland EA, Wild LM, et al. A prospective, randomized clinical trial comparing an antibiotic-impregnated bioabsorbable bone substitute with standard antibiotic-impregnated cement beads in the treatment of chronic osteomyelitis and infected nonunion. *J Orthop Trauma.* 2010;24(8):483–490.
229. McNamara I, Deshpande S, Porteous M. Impaction grafting of the acetabulum with a mixture of frozen, ground irradiated bone graft and porous synthetic bone substitute (Apapore 60). *J Bone Joint Surg Br.* 2010;92(5):617–623.
230. Mollon B, da Silva V, Busse JW, et al. Electrical stimulation for long-bone fracture-healing: A meta-analysis of randomized controlled trials. *J Bone Joint Surg Am.* 2008;90(11):2322–2330.
231. Moore JR, Weiland AJ, Daniel RK. Use of free vascularized bone grafts in the treatment of bone tumors. *Clin Orthop Relat Res.* 1983;(175):37–44.
232. Moucha CS, Einhorn TA. Enhancement of skeletal repair. In: Browner BD, Jupiter JB, Levine AM, eds. *Skeletal Trauma; Basic Science Management, and Reconstruction.* 3rd ed. Philadelphia, PA: Saunders; 2003:639
233. Mullis BH, Copland ST, Weinhold PS, et al. Effect of COX-2 inhibitors and non-steroidal anti-inflammatory drugs on a mouse fracture model. *Injury.* 2006;37(9):827–837.
234. Mundy G, Garrett R, Harris S, et al. Stimulation of bone formation in vitro and in rodents by statins. *Science.* 1999;286(5446):1946–1949.
235. Munns CF, Rauch F, Zeitlin L, et al. Delayed osteotomy but not fracture healing in pediatric osteogenesis imperfecta patients receiving pamidronate. *J Bone Miner Res.* 2004;19(11):1779–1786.
236. Murnaghan M, Li G, Marsh DR. Nonsteroidal anti-inflammatory drug-induced fracture nonunion: An inhibition of angiogenesis? *J Bone Joint Surg Am.* 2006;88(suppl 3):140–147.
237. Muschler GF, Boehm C, Easley K. Aspiration to obtain osteoblast progenitor cells from human bone marrow: The influence of aspiration volume. *J Bone Joint Surg Am.* 1997;79(11):1699–1709.
238. Muschler GF, Nitto H, Boehm CA, et al. Age- and gender-related changes in the cellularity of human bone marrow and the prevalence of osteoblastic progenitors. *J Orthop Res.* 2001;19(1):117–125.
239. Myeroff C, Archdeacon M. Autogenous bone graft: Donor sites and techniques. *J Bone Joint Surg Am.* 2011;93(23):2227–2236.
240. Nakajima A, Shimoji N, Shiomi K, et al. Mechanisms for the enhancement of fracture healing in rats treated with intermittent low-dose human parathyroid hormone (1-34). *J Bone Miner Res.* 2002;17(11):2038–2047.
241. Nakazawa T, Nakajima A, Shiomi K, et al. Effects of low-dose, intermittent treatment with recombinant human parathyroid hormone (1-34) on chondrogenesis in a model of experimental fracture healing. *Bone.* 2005;37(5):711–719.
242. Nash TJ, Howlett CR, Martin C, et al. Effect of platelet-derived growth factor on tibial osteotomies in rabbits. *Bone.* 1994;15(2):203–208.
243. Neer RM, Arnaud CD, Zanchetta JR, et al. Effect of parathyroid hormone (1-34) on fractures and bone mineral density in postmenopausal women with osteoporosis. *N Engl J Med.* 2001;344(19):1434–1441.
244. Nevins M, Camelo M, Nevins ML, et al. Periodontal regeneration in humans using recombinant human platelet-derived growth factor-BB (rhPDGF-BB) and allogenic bone. *J Periodontol.* 2003;74(9):1282–1292.
245. Nicoll EA. Fractures of the tibial shaft. A survey of 705 cases. *J Bone Joint Surg Br.* 1964;46:373–387.
246. Nolte PA, van der Krans A, Patka P, et al. Low-intensity pulsed ultrasound in the treatment of nonunions. *J Trauma.* 2001;51(4):693–702; discussion 702-3.
247. Nusbickel FR, Dell PC, McAndrew MP, et al. Vascularized autografts for reconstruction of skeletal defects following lower extremity trauma. A review. *Clin Orthop Relat Res.* 1989;(243):65–70.
248. O'Keeffe RM Jr, Riemer BL, Butterfield SL. Harvesting of autogenous cancellous bone graft from the proximal tibial metaphysis. A review of 230 cases. *J Orthop Trauma.* 1991;5(4):469–474.
249. Ohlsson C, Bengtsson BA, Isaksson OG, et al. Growth hormone and bone. *Endo Rev.* 1998;19(1):55–79.
250. Olsen BS, Vaesel MT, Sojbjerg JO. Treatment of midshaft clavicular nonunion with plate fixation and autologous bone grafting. *J Shoulder Elbow Surg.* 1995;4(5):337–344.
251. Ominsky MS, Li C, Li X, et al. Inhibition of sclerostin by monoclonal antibody enhances bone healing and improves bone density and strength of nonfractured bones. *J Bone Miner Res.* 2011;26(5):1012–1021.
252. Pacicca DM, Patel N, Lee C, et al. Expression of angiogenic factors during distraction osteogenesis. *Bone.* 2003;33(6):889–898.
253. Paralkar VM, Borovecki F, Ke HZ, et al. An EP2 receptor-selective prostaglandin E2 agonist induces bone healing. *Proc Natl Acad Sci U S A.* 2003;100(11):6736–6740.
254. Parikh SN. Bone graft substitutes: Past, present, future. *J Postgrad Med.* 2002;48(2):142–148.
255. Parker MJ, Raghavan R, Gurusamy K. Incidence of fracture-healing complications after femoral neck fractures. *Clin Orthop Relat Res.* 2007;458:175–179.
256. Patel JC, Watson K, Joseph E, et al. Long-term complications of distal radius bone grafts. *J Hand Surg Am.* 2003;28(5):784–788.
257. Peichl P, Holzer LA, Maier R, et al. Parathyroid hormone 1-84 accelerates fracture-healing in pubic bones of elderly osteoporotic women. *J Bone Joint Surg Am.* 2011;93(17):1583–1587.
258. Pelker RR, Friedlaender GE, Markham TC, et al. Effects of freezing and freeze-drying on the biomechanical properties of rat bone. *J Orthop Res.* 1984;1(4):405–411.
259. Peters CL, Hines JL, Bachus KN, et al. Biological effects of calcium sulfate as a bone graft substitute in ovine metaphyseal defects. *J Biomed Mater Res A.* 2006;76(3):456–462.
260. Pilla AA, Mont MA, Nasser PR, et al. Non-invasive low-intensity pulsed ultrasound accelerates bone healing in the rabbit. *J Orthop Trauma.* 1990;4(3):246–253.
261. Porter RM, Liu F, Pilapil C, et al. Osteogenic potential of reamer irrigator aspirator (RIA) aspirate collected from patients undergoing hip arthroplasty. *J Orthop Res.* 2009;27(1):42–49.
262. Pountos I, Georgouli T, Blokhuis TJ, et al. Pharmacological agents and impairment of fracture healing: What is the evidence? *Injury.* 2008;39(4):384–394.
263. Quintero AJ, Tarkin IS, Pape HC. Technical tricks when using the reamer irrigator aspirator technique for autologous bone graft harvesting. *J Orthop Trauma.* 2010;24(1):42–45.
264. Raisz LG. Physiology and pathophysiology of bone remodeling. *Clin Chem.* 1999;45(8 Pt 2):1353–1358.
265. Raschke M, Rasmussen MH, Govender S, et al. Effects of growth hormone in patients with tibial fracture: A randomised, double-blind, placebo-controlled clinical trial. *Eur J Endocrinol.* 2007;156(3):341–351.
266. Ratajczak MZ, Machalinski B, Wojakowski W, et al. A hypothesis for an embryonic origin of pluripotent Oct-4(+) stem cells in adult bone marrow and other tissues. *Leukemia.* 2007;21(5):860–867.
267. Ratajczak MZ, Zuba-Surma EK, Machalinski B, et al. Bone-marrow-derived stem cells–our key to longevity? *J Appl Genet.* 2007;48(4):307–319.
268. Ratajczak MZ, Zuba-Surma EK, Shin DM, et al. Very small embryonic-like (VSEL) stem cells in adult organs and their potential role in rejuvenation of tissues and longevity. *Exp Gerontol.* 2008;43(11):1009–1017.
269. Reikeraas O, Engebretsen L. Effects of ketoralac tromethamine and indomethacin on primary and secondary bone healing. An experimental study in rats. *Arch Orthop Trauma Surg.* 1998;118(1-2):50–52.
270. Rhee SH. Synthesis of hydroxyapatite via mechanochemical treatment. *Biomaterials.* 2002;23(4):1147–1152.
271. Ripamonti U, Duneas N. Tissue morphogenesis and regeneration by bone morphogenetic proteins. *Plast Reconstr Surg.* 1998;101(1):227–239.
272. Ritting AW, Weber EW, Lee MC. Exaggerated inflammatory response and bony resorption from BMP-2 use in a pediatric forearm nonunion. *J Hand Surg Am.* 2012;37(2):316–321.
273. Robinson CM, Page RS. Severely impacted valgus proximal humeral fractures. *J Bone Joint Surg Am.* 2004;86-A(suppl 1 Pt 2):143–155.
274. Rouleau MF, Mitchell J, Goltzman D. Characterization of the major parathyroid hormone target cell in the endosteal metaphysis of rat long bones. *J Bone Miner Res.* 1990;5(10):1043–1053.
275. Rouleau MF, Mitchell J, Goltzman D. In vivo distribution of parathyroid hormone receptors in bone: Evidence that a predominant osseous target cell is not the mature osteoblast. *Endocrinology.* 1988;123(1):187–191.
276. Roussignol X, Currey C, Duparc F, et al. Indications and results for the Exogen ultrasound system in the management of non-union: A 59-case pilot study. *Orthop Traumatol Surg Res.* 2012;98(2):206–213.
277. Roy DM, Linnehan SK. Hydroxyapatite formed from coral skeletal carbonate by hydrothermal exchange. *Nature.* 1974;247(438):220–222.
278. Rozental TD, Vazquez MA, Chacko AT, et al. Comparison of radiographic fracture healing in the distal radius for patients on and off bisphosphonate therapy. *J Hand Surg Am.* 2009;34(4):595–602.
279. Rundle CH, Miyakoshi N, Ramirez E, et al. Expression of the fibroblast growth factor receptor genes in fracture repair. *Clin Orthop Relat Res.* 2002;(403):253–263.
280. Russell TA, Leighton RK. Comparison of autogenous bone graft and endothermic calcium phosphate cement for defect augmentation in tibial plateau fractures. A multicenter, prospective, randomized study. *J Bone Joint Surg Am.* 2008;90(10):2057–2061.
281. Rutten S, Nolte PA, Guit GL, et al. Use of low-intensity pulsed ultrasound for posttraumatic nonunions of the tibia: A review of patients treated in the Netherlands. *J Trauma.* 2007;62(4):902–908.
282. Saag KG, Zanchetta JR, Devogelaer JP, et al. Effects of teriparatide versus alendronate for treating glucocorticoid-induced osteoporosis: Thirty-six-month results of a randomized, double-blind, controlled trial. *Arthritis Rheum.* 2009;60(11):3346–3355.
283. Sailhan F. Bone lengthening (distraction osteogenesis): A literature review. *Osteoporos Int.* 2011;22(6):2011–2015.
284. Sanchez-Sotelo J, Munuera L, Madero R. Treatment of fractures of the distal radius with a remodellable bone cement: A prospective, randomised study using Norian SRS. *J Bone Joint Surg Br.* 2000;82(6):856–863.

285. Sanders RA, Sackett JR. Open reduction and internal fixation of delayed union and nonunion of the distal humerus. *J Orthop Trauma.* 1990;4(3):254–259.

286. Sarmiento A, Schaeffer JF, Beckerman L, et al. Fracture healing in rat femora as affected by functional weight-bearing. *J Bone Joint Surg Am.* 1977;59(3):369–375.

287. Schaden W, Fischer A, Sailler A. Extracorporeal shock wave therapy of nonunion or delayed osseous union. *Clin Orthop Relat Res.* 2001;(387):90–94.

288. Schildhauer TA, Bauer TW, Josten C, et al. Open reduction and augmentation of internal fixation with an injectable skeletal cement for the treatment of complex calcaneal fractures. *J Orthop Trauma.* 2000;14(5):309–317.

289. Schindeler A, Birke O, Yu NY, et al. Distal tibial fracture repair in a neurofibromatosis type 1–deficient mouse treated with recombinant bone morphogenetic protein and a bisphosphonate. *J Bone Joint Surg Br.* 2011;93(8):1134–1139.

290. Scott G, King JB. A prospective, double-blind trial of electrical capacitive coupling in the treatment of non-union of long bones. *J Bone Joint Surg Am.* 1994;76(6):820–826.

291. Segur JM, Torner P, Garcia S, et al. Use of bone allograft in tibial plateau fractures. *Arch Orthop Trauma Surg.* 1998;117(6–7):357–359.

292. Sen C, Eralp L, Gunes T, et al. An alternative method for the treatment of nonunion of the tibia with bone loss. *J Bone Joint Surg Br.* 2006;88(6):783–789.

293. Sen C, Kocaoglu M, Eralp L, et al. Bifocal compression-distraction in the acute treatment of grade III open tibia fractures with bone and soft-tissue loss: A report of 24 cases. *J Orthop Trauma.* 2004;18(3):150–157.

294. Sen MK, Miclau T. Autologous iliac crest bone graft: Should it still be the gold standard for treating nonunions? *Injury.* 2007;38(suppl 1):S75–S80.

295. Shaffer JW, Field GA, Goldberg VM, et al. Fate of vascularized and nonvascularized autografts. *Clin Orthop Relat Res.* 1985;(197):32–43.

296. Sharrard WJ. A double-blind trial of pulsed electromagnetic fields for delayed union of tibial fractures. *J Bone Joint Surg Br.* 1990;72(3):347–355.

297. Simon AM, O'Connor JP. Dose and time-dependent effects of cyclooxygenase-2 inhibition on fracture-healing. *J Bone Joint Surg Am.* 2007;89(3):500–511.

298. Simonis RB, Parnell EJ, Ray PS, et al. Electrical treatment of tibial non-union: A prospective, randomised, double-blind trial. *Injury.* 2003;34(5):357–362.

299. Simpson AH, Kenwright J. Fracture after distraction osteogenesis. *J Bone Joint Surg Br.* 2000;82(5):659–665.

300. Simpson D, Keating JF. Outcome of tibial plateau fractures managed with calcium phosphate cement. *Injury.* 2004;35(9):913–918.

301. Skoglund B, Aspenberg P. Locally applied Simvastatin improves fracture healing in mice. *BMC Musculoskelet Disord.* 2007;8:98.

302. Sloan AV, Martin JR, Li S, et al. Parathyroid hormone and bisphosphonate have opposite effects on stress fracture repair. *Bone.* 2010;47(2):235–240.

303. Solchaga LA, Hee CK, Aguiar DJ, et al. Augment bone graft products compare favorably with autologous bone graft in an ovine model of lumbar interbody spine fusion. *Spine.* 2012;37(8):E461-E467.

304. Solheim E. Growth factors in bone. *Int Orthop.* 1998;22(6):410–416.

305. Souter WA. Autogenous cancellous strip grafts in the treatment of delayed union of long bone fractures. *J Bone Joint Surg Br.* 1969;51(1):63–75.

306. Springfield DS. Massive autogenous bone grafts. *Orthop Clin North Am.* 1987;18(2):249–256.

307. Stankewich CJ, Swiontkowski MF, Tencer AF, et al. Augmentation of femoral neck fracture fixation with an injectable calcium-phosphate bone mineral cement. *J Orthop Res.* 1996;14(5):786–793.

308. Stevenson S. Biology of bone grafts. *Orthop Clin North Am.* 1999;30(4):543–552.

309. Stevenson S, Li XQ, Martin B. The fate of cancellous and cortical bone after transplantation of fresh and frozen tissue-antigen-matched and mismatched osteochondral allografts in dogs. *J Bone Joint Surg Am.* 1991;73(8):1143–1156.

310. Street J, Winter D, Wang JH, et al. Is human fracture hematoma inherently angiogenic? *Clin Orthop Relat Res.* 2000;(378):224–237.

311. Street JT, Wang JH, Wu QD, et al. The angiogenic response to skeletal injury is preserved in the elderly. *J Orthop Res.* 2001;19(6):1057–1066.

312. Sudmann E, Bang G. Indomethacin-induced inhibition of haversian remodelling in rabbits. *Acta Orthop Scand.* 1979;50(6 Pt 1):621–627.

313. Swiontkowski MF, Aro HT, Donell S, et al. Recombinant human bone morphogenetic protein-2 in open tibial fractures. A subgroup analysis of data combined from two prospective randomized studies. *J Bone Joint Surg Am.* 2006;88(6):1258–1265.

314. Takala J, Ruokonen E, Webster NR, et al. Increased mortality associated with growth hormone treatment in critically ill adults. *N Engl J Med.* 1999;341(11):785–792.

315. Tambe AD, Cutler L, Murali SR, et al. In scaphoid non-union, does the source of graft affect outcome? Iliac crest versus distal end of radius bone graft. *J Hand Surg Br.* 2006;31(1):47–51.

316. Tay BK, Patel VV, Bradford DS. Calcium sulfate- and calcium phosphate-based bone substitutes. Mimicry of the mineral phase of bone. *Orthop Clin North Am.* 1999;30(4):615–623.

317. Tessier P, Kawamoto H, Posnick J, et al. Complications of harvesting autogenous bone grafts: A group experience of 20,000 cases. *Plast Reconstr Surg.* 2005;116(5 suppl):72S–73S; discussion 92S–94S.

318. Thaller SR, Dart A, Tesluk H. The effects of insulin-like growth factor-1 on critical-size calvarial defects in Sprague-Dawley rats. *Ann Plast Surg.* 1993;31(5):429–433.

319. Thompson RC Jr, Pickvance EA, Garry D. Fractures in large-segment allografts. *J Bone Joint Surg Am.* 1993;75(11):1663–1673.

320. Thordarson DB, Bollinger M. SRS cancellous bone cement augmentation of calcaneal fracture fixation. *Foot Ankle Int.* 2005;26(5):347–352.

321. Tomford WW, Mankin HJ. Bone banking. Update on methods and materials. *Orthop Clin North Am.* 1999;30(4):565–570.

322. Toms AD, Barker RL, Jones RS, et al. Impaction bone-grafting in revision joint replacement surgery. *J Bone Joint Surg Am.* 2004;86-A(9):2050–2060.

323. Toms AD, McClelland D, Chua L, et al. Mechanical testing of impaction bone grafting in the tibia: Initial stability and design of the stem. *J Bone Joint Surg Br.* 2005;87(5):656–663.

324. Tsuji K, Bandyopadhyay A, Harfe BD, et al. BMP2 activity, although dispensable for bone formation, is required for the initiation of fracture healing. *Nat Genet.* 2006;38(12):1424–1429.

325. Ueda K, Saito A, Nakano H, et al. Cortical hyperostosis following long-term administration of prostaglandin E1 in infants with cyanotic congenital heart disease. *J Pediatr.* 1980;97(5):834–836.

326. Uhthoff HK, Rahn BA. Healing patterns of metaphyseal fractures. *Clin Orthop Relat Res.* 1981;(160):295–303.

327. Undale A, Fraser D, Hefferan T, et al. Induction of fracture repair by mesenchymal cells derived from human embryonic stem cells or bone marrow. *J Orthop Res.* 2011;29(12):1804–1811.

328. Urist MR. Bone: Formation by autoinduction. *Science.* 1965;150(3698):893–899.

329. Urist MR. Osteoinduction in undemineralized bone implants modified by chemical inhibitors of endogenous matrix enzymes. A preliminary report. *Clin Orthop Relat Res.* 1972;87:132–137.

330. Urist MR, Silverman BF, Buring K, et al. The bone induction principle. *Clin Orthop Relat Res.* 1967;53:243–283.

331. Uygur F, Ulkur E, Pehlivan O, et al. Soft tissue necrosis following using calcium phosphate cement in calcaneal bone cyst: Case report. *Arch Orthop Trauma Surg.* 2008;128(12):1397–1401.

332. Valchanou VD, Michailov P. High energy shock waves in the treatment of delayed and nonunion of fractures. *Int Orthop.* 1991;15(3):181–184.

333. Van der Lely AJ, Lamberts SW, Jauch KW, et al. Use of human GH in elderly patients with accidental hip fracture. *Eur J Endocrinol.* 2000;143(5):585–592.

334. van Haaren EH, Smit TH, Phipps K, et al. Tricalcium-phosphate and hydroxyapatite bone-graft extender for use in impaction grafting revision surgery. An in vitro study on human femora. *J Bone Joint Surg Br.* 2005;87(2):267–271.

335. Vane JR. Inhibition of prostaglandin synthesis as a mechanism of action for aspirin-like drugs. *Nat New Biol.* 1971;231(25):232–235.

336. Vuolteenaho K, Moilanen T, Moilanen E. Non-steroidal anti-inflammatory drugs, cyclooxygenase-2 and the bone healing process. *Basic Clin Pharmacol Toxicol.* 2008;102(1):10–14.

337. Wagner ER, Zhu G, Zhang BQ, et al. The therapeutic potential of the Wnt signaling pathway in bone disorders. *Curr Mol Pharmacol.* 2011;4(1):14–25.

338. Wang CJ, Chen HS, Chen CE, et al. Treatment of nonunions of long bone fractures with shock waves. *Clin Orthop Relat Res.* 2001;(387):95–101.

339. Wang CJ, Liu HC, Fu TH. The effects of extracorporeal shockwave on acute high-energy long bone fractures of the lower extremity. *Arch Orthop Trauma Surg.* 2007;127(2):137–142.

340. Wang CJ, Yang KD, Ko JY, et al. The effects of shockwave on bone healing and systemic concentrations of nitric oxide (NO), TGF-beta1, VEGF and BMP-2 in long bone non-unions. *Nitric Oxide.* 2009;20(4):298–303.

341. Wang JW, Weng LH. Treatment of distal femoral nonunion with internal fixation, cortical allograft struts, and autogenous bone-grafting. *J Bone Joint Surg Am.* 2003;85-A(3):436–440.

342. Weissberger AJ, Anastasiadis AD, Sturgess I, et al. Recombinant human growth hormone treatment in elderly patients undergoing elective total hip replacement. *Clin Endocrinol (Oxf).* 2003;58(1):99–107.

343. Welch RD, Zhang H, Bronson DG. Experimental tibial plateau fractures augmented with calcium phosphate cement or autologous bone graft. *J Bone Joint Surg Am.* 2003;85-A(2):222–231.

344. Wheeler P, Batt ME. Do non-steroidal anti-inflammatory drugs adversely affect stress fracture healing? A short review. *Br J Sports Med.* 2005;39(2):65–69.

345. Wieman TJ, Smiell JM, Su Y. Efficacy and safety of a topical gel formulation of recombinant human platelet-derived growth factor-BB (becaplermin) in patients with chronic neuropathic diabetic ulcers. A phase III randomized placebo-controlled double-blind study. *Diabetes care.* 1998;21(5):822–827.

346. Xu ZH, Jiang Q, Chen DY, et al. Extracorporeal shock wave treatment in nonunions of long bone fractures. *Int Orthop.* 2009;33(3):789–793.

347. Yang KH, Parvizi J, Wang SJ, et al. Exposure to low-intensity ultrasound increases aggrecan gene expression in a rat femur fracture model. *J Orthop Res.* 1996;14(5):802–809.

348. Yetkinler DN, McClellan RT, Reindel ES, et al. Biomechanical comparison of conventional open reduction and internal fixation versus calcium phosphate cement fixation of a central depressed tibial plateau fracture. *J Orthop Trauma.* 2001;15(3):197–206.

349. Younger EM, Chapman MW. Morbidity at bone graft donor sites. *J Orthop Trauma.* 1989;3(3):192–195.

350. Yu B, Han K, Ma H, et al. Treatment of tibial plateau fractures with high strength injectable calcium sulphate. *Int Orthop.* 2009;33(4):1127–1133.

351. Yu HB, Shen GF, Wei FC. Effect of cryopreservation on the immunogenicity of osteoblasts. *Transplant Proc.* 2007;39(10):3030–3031.

352. Ziran BH, Hendi P, Smith WR, et al. Osseous healing with a composite of allograft and demineralized bone matrix: Adverse effects of smoking. *Am J Orthop.* 2007;36(4):207–209.

353. Ziran BH, Smith WR, Morgan SJ. Use of calcium-based demineralized bone matrix/allograft for nonunions and posttraumatic reconstruction of the appendicular skeleton: Preliminary results and complications. *J Trauma.* 2007;63(6):1324–1328.

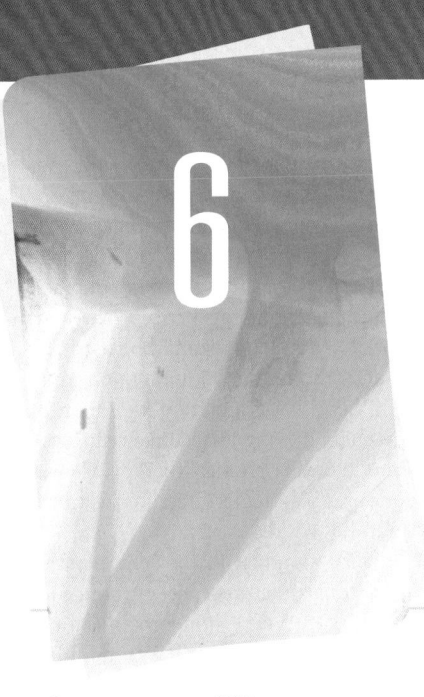

6 PRINCIPLES OF NONOPERATIVE FRACTURE TREATMENT

Charles M. Court-Brown

INTRODUCTION

Nonoperative fracture management was the only method of fracture management until about 1750. Since then there have been advances in operative fracture treatment, which accelerated considerably after World War II because of improved surgical techniques, better anesthesia and postoperative treatment, and the introduction of antibiotics. Even today, nonoperative management remains a very important tool in the armamentarium of the orthopedic trauma surgeon. The concentration of severe injuries into specialized trauma centers in many countries has unquestionably improved their treatment but has also caused surgeons to overestimate the role of operative treatment in the full spectrum of fractures. In fact, nonoperative fracture treatment remains the most common method of fracture management, although its role has changed significantly during the last 30 to 40 years. This chapter presents an epidemiologic analysis of nonoperative fracture management from a major trauma center, illustrates common nonoperative techniques, and discusses indications for their use.

HISTORY OF NONOPERATIVE FRACTURE TREATMENT

The ancient Egyptians were the first to document how fractures should be managed and to record the basic results of their management[69] The Edwin Smith Papyrus dates from 2800 to 3000 BC and was translated in 1930 in the United States.[12] It is composed of a series of case reports of specific injuries and their associated prognoses, good and bad. Case 37 describes a coexisting humeral fracture and wound over the upper arm. It suggests that if the two are not connected the arm should be splinted and the wound dressed. If the wound and fracture connect the prognosis is poor and the ailment should not be treated! In those days, splintage relied on bandaging over splints of wood and linen and using glue to stiffen the bandages.

There does not appear to have been any significant advance in fracture management until the Ancient Greek Empire, with Hippocrates being credited with many advances that were probably the results of clinical work of many doctors. Hippocrates described six different methods of applying roller bandages depending on the fracture location. The bandages were stiffened with cerate, which was an ointment consisting of lard or oil mixed with wax, resin, or pitch to essentially create a cast. It was customary to defer definitive management, usually fracture manipulation, until the swelling had diminished, which often took about 7 days. It is interesting to note that delayed management still remains popular in the treatment of some fractures. The Ancient Greeks also used mechanical aids to facilitate the reduction of fractures and dislocations, and Hippocrates is credited with the first audit of fracture healing time. However, he was either an optimist or the ancient Greeks had a superior genetic makeup because he said that femoral fractures and tibial fractures united in 50 and 40 days, respectively![45]

Further progress occurred in Ancient Rome and in Asia, but it is Albucasis, an Arabic physician, who is credited with advancing nonoperative fracture treatment and for acting as a conduit through which the philosophies of Ancient Rome and Greece could be transferred to Western Europe. Albucasis clearly upset his colleagues by suggesting that in femoral diaphyseal fractures the knee should be placed in full flexion.[69] His cast was a mixture of mill dust and egg whites or mixtures of grain, herbs, clay, and egg whites that were supported by bandages. He also introduced the somewhat radical practice of maintaining his casts for a longer period rather than changing them every few days, as had been done up to that time.

Following the introduction of gunpowder in 1338 AD, cannon shot in 1346 AD, and half-pound gunshot in 1364 AD, it was obvious that surgeons were going to be faced with many more open fractures than they had encountered before. As one would expect this stimulated innovation and surgeons began to challenge the views that open wounds should be encouraged to suppurate and that "laudable pus" was essential for wound healing. Paré and others demonstrated that wounds could be cleaned and sometimes closed primarily. Paré made the discovery that primary wound cleaning using a paste of oil of roses, turpentine, and egg yolk gave better results than the use of boiling oil. Paré's views were very influential, and the management of open wounds improved considerably.[2] He and others realized that devitalized bone fragments should be removed from open wounds but it was Desault and Larrey who introduced debridement at the l'Hotel Dieu in Paris at the end of the 18th century.[69]

Despite considerable progress being achieved in the management of open wounds, surgeons were essentially still left with the fracture treatment principles outlined by Albucasis around 1000 AD. Seutin,[87] a Belgian surgeon, had introduced a method of applying rigid dressings which could be left in position for a longer period, but it was the introduction of plaster of Paris bandages that revolutionized fracture treatment. These were introduced by Pirogov from Russia and Mathijsen from Holland in the early 1800s.[69] A better method of fracture management had become essential because of the carnage caused by the Napoleonic wars in Europe and the increased urbanization associated with the Industrial Revolution. While plaster of Paris bandages were not used during the American Civil War, Sayre[85] and Stimson[93] in New York together with Scudder[86] in Boston promoted the use of plaster of Paris bandages in the United States. Volkmann[103] was a particular enthusiast of the use of plaster of Paris in the management of fractures in Europe.

As with all new inventions, it took time for most surgeons to accept plaster of Paris bandaging, and the use of supportive splints such as the Thomas splint remained popular in the United Kingdom. They were strongly supported by Thomas[94] and Jones.[50] Eventually plaster casts became the routine method of managing most fractures and the arguments between surgeons centered around the amount of padding that should be used, the use of early weight bearing, and whether early joint motion could be allowed. Lorenz Böhler of Vienna[7] was a particular proponent of plaster of Paris cast treatment, believing in accurate reduction, the use of skintight casts, and intensive physical therapy. He was also very influential in developing a system of fracture treatment that was adopted throughout the world.

Sarmiento[80–84] was a particular advocate of nonoperative management, particularly of tibial fractures. He introduced a lower leg functional brace to permit early joint mobilization. Credit must be given to Sarmiento for continuing to popularize nonoperative management of diaphyseal fractures and for providing a counterargument to those surgeons who felt that operative management was always indicated. Sarmiento's tibial functional brace became popular but its introduction coincided with the explosion of interest in operative lower limb fracture treatment, which started in the 1960s.

The operative treatment of fractures first started around 1775 in France, and the first operative textbook detailing techniques of fracture fixation was published by Bérenger-Féraud in 1870.[6] He described six methods of fracture management, of which three are still in use today—cerclage wiring, interosseous sutures, and external fixation. In the 20th century operative management rapidly increased in popularity in both the United States and Europe. Pioneers such as Lambotte, Hey-Groves, Lane, Hoffman, Küntscher, Ilizarov, and Müller and his colleagues in Europe and Parkhill, the Rush brothers, and Sherman in the United States promoted internal and external fixation.[69] However, it was the introduction of antibiotics and the development of modern anesthesia and improved surgical techniques that altered the way orthopedic surgeons considered fracture management. The prevalence of operative fracture management has now increased significantly but it is not used in all fractures. It is instructive to review the current use of nonoperative fracture management and to compare it with 50 or 60 years ago, when many surgeons were beginning to think seriously about operative management for the first time.

EPIDEMIOLOGY OF NONOPERATIVE FRACTURE TREATMENT

There has been no previous study of the use of nonoperative management in a defined population of adults, although there have been studies of the use of nonoperative treatment in more specialized hospitals, which were not responsible for treating all fractures in an entire community.[31,39,59,95] These studies have mainly dealt with pediatric fractures[39,59,95] but in 1958 Emmett and Breck[31] published a paper detailing the treatment of almost 11,000 fresh fractures in El Paso, Texas. To analyze the current role of nonoperative management, a study of the primary treatment of 7,863 consecutive fractures in Edinburgh, Scotland, in 2000 was undertaken. To allow the examination of the role of nonoperative management in the complete population, the fractures in adults and children have been combined.

The data includes all inpatients and outpatients treated in the Royal Infirmary of Edinburgh and The Royal Hospital for Sick Children in Edinburgh. These two hospitals provide the only trauma care for a defined population in the East of Scotland. In 2000 the catchment population of the area was 643,702 patients. In the study all patients treated in the catchment area but residing outside were excluded, and all patients who had primary treatment outside the catchment area but were subsequently treated within the area were included. All inpatient and outpatient fractures were included except spinal fractures. As in other centers these are treated by both orthopedic surgeons and neurosurgeons in Edinburgh, with spinal cord injury patients being transferred to a specialized national center outside Edinburgh.

In this study manipulation under anesthesia was defined as nonoperative management but the soft tissue surgery inherent in the management of open fractures was defined as operative treatment regardless of whether fixation was used. Secondary procedures were not analyzed and the management of pure dislocations and soft tissue damage was not considered. In the study children were defined as being less than 16 years of age, with all patients 16 years and older being defined as adults. The basic demographic details of all patients were included in the database. Fracture location was defined using regional descriptors familiar to all orthopedic surgeons. The OTA classification[34] was used to classify all long-bone fractures and the Carstairs and Morris index[15] was used to define social deprivation. This index has been used extensively to investigate correlation between disease and social deprivation.[27,32] In this study, it was used to test whether social deprivation determined the choice of treatment method in different fractures. Several measures were used to analyze fracture severity and the subsequent decision to use operative treatment. Fracture severity was assessed using the OTA classification[34] in metaphyseal and intra-articular fractures of the long bones. OTA type A fractures are extra-articular, type B fractures are partial articular, and type C fractures are complete articular fractures. This system does not apply to proximal humeral, proximal forearm, or proximal femoral fractures, and fracture severity was therefore assessed in fractures of the distal humerus, distal radius, distal femur, proximal tibia, and distal tibia. Nowadays the degree of severity of diaphyseal fractures is often not a major factor in determining management. This is particularly true of lower limb diaphyseal fractures for which intramedullary nailing is now commonly used regardless of the degree of displacement, comminution, or soft tissue damage.

The type of fracture treatment was also assessed with reference to the mode of injury and the presence of multiple fractures. The seven most common modes of injury were examined to see if particular modes of injury were associated with a higher prevalence of operative treatment. These were motor vehicle accidents, twisting injuries, falls, falls down stairs or slopes, falls from a height, assaults or direct blows, and sporting injuries. The association between operative treatment and the presence of multiple fractures was also examined.

TABLE 6-1	**Number and Prevalence of Surgically Treated Adult Fractures Showing Gender and Regional Differences**		
		Operatively Treated	
	Total Number	Number	%
Adult fractures	**5,576**	**1,804**	**32.4**
Males	2,650	720	27.2
Females	2,926	1,084	37.0
Upper limb	**3,232**	**590**	**18.3**
Lower limb	**2,255**	**1,200**	**53.2**
Pelvis	**89**	**14**	**15.7**

Table 6-1 shows that, in adults, 67.6% of fractures were nonoperatively managed in 2000 with 63% of fractures in females and 72.8% of fractures in males being treated nonoperatively. There is a significant difference between upper and lower limb fractures, with 81.7% of upper limb fractures and 46.8% of lower limb fractures being treated nonoperatively. In addition, 84.3% of pelvic fractures were treated nonoperatively but most of these were pubic rami fractures occurring in elderly patients.

Age is an important predictor of the role of operative fracture treatment, as illustrated in Figure 6-1. To allow for a complete analysis of the relationship between age and the requirement for operative fracture treatment, the children's data from 2000 has been combined with the adult data. Figure 6-1 shows a gradual increase in operative treatment with age. Only 7.3% of patients younger than 5 years were treated operatively compared with 56.9% of patients aged 95 years or more. At about 80 years the prevalence of operative management overtakes nonoperative management and the highest prevalence of operative management is seen between 90 and 94 years of age when 67.4% of patients were treated operatively. Analysis of the equivalent results for males and females shows that both sexes have a similar distribution to the overall distribution shown in Figure 6-1.

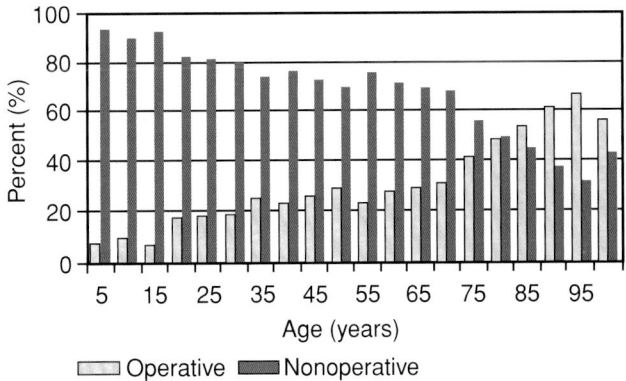

FIGURE 6-1 The prevalence of operatively and nonoperatively treated fractures according to patient age. The children's fracture data has been included and all patients have been divided into 5-year age bands.

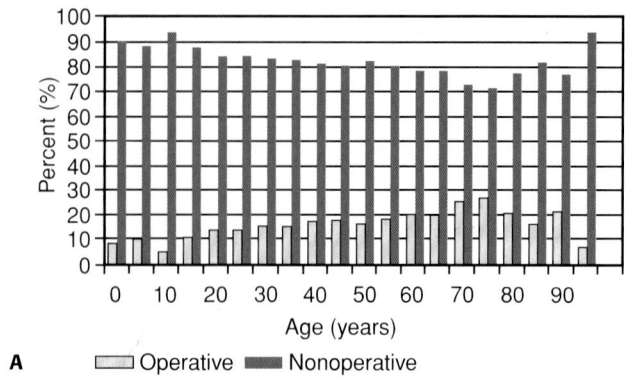

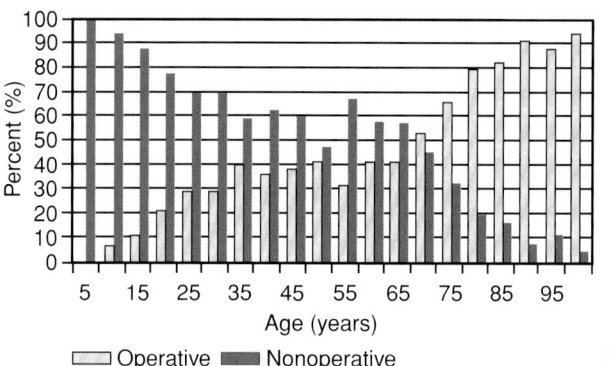

FIGURE 6-2 The prevalence of operatively and nonoperatively treated upper limb **(A)** and lower limb **(B)** fractures according to patient age. Patients are divided into 5-year age bands. The children's data has been added to the adult data.

Figures 6-2A and B shows the equivalent age-related curves for upper and lower limb fractures. These are very different from Figure 6-1 and from each other. In the upper limb (Fig. 6-2A) there is a progressive increase in surgery from 9.1% in patients aged less than 5 years to 27.9% in patients aged 70 to 75 years. Older patients show a gradual reduction in surgical treatment. In the lower limb (Fig. 6-2B) there was no surgery undertaken in patients less than 5 years old but in older patients there was a gradual increase in operative treatment up to 95.1% in patients aged 95 years or more. The prevalence of lower limb operative surgery overtakes nonoperative treatment between 65 and 70 years of age. Analysis of the gender-specific curves for upper and lower limb fractures shows no difference to the overall distribution curves shown in Figure 6-2.

When considering fracture treatment nowadays it is important to look carefully at the elderly. There has been an increase in the incidence of osteoporotic fractures[23,48] as well as an appreciation that many fractures that formerly occurred in younger patients now commonly occur in the elderly.[21] Figure 6-3A shows the prevalence of operative treatment in adults aged 80 years or more, and it can be seen that there is a gradual increase in the use of surgery to treat fractures in this group up to about 93 years of age, when the use of surgical management begins to decline. Figures 6-3B and C shows the relationship between old age and surgery in upper and lower limb fractures. In the upper limb, Figure 6-3B shows that 25% to 35% of adults in their early eighties who present with upper limb fractures are treated surgically, but the prevalence declines to the extent that

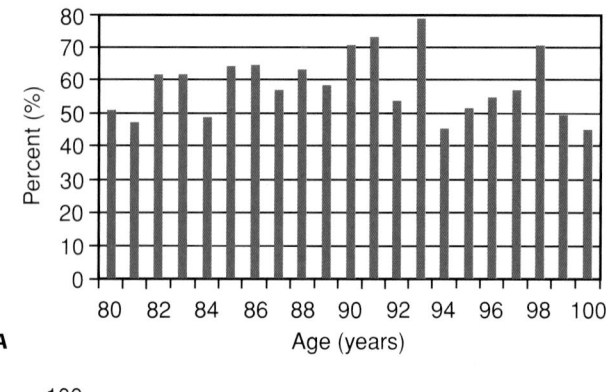

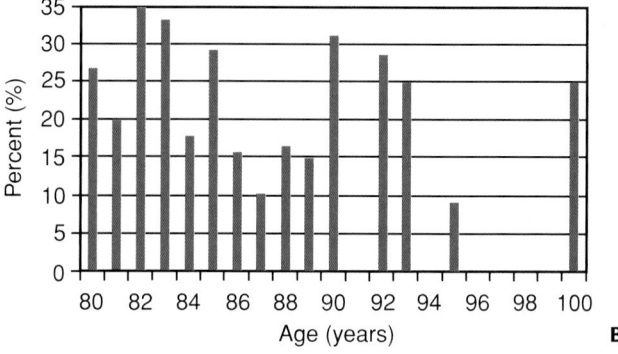

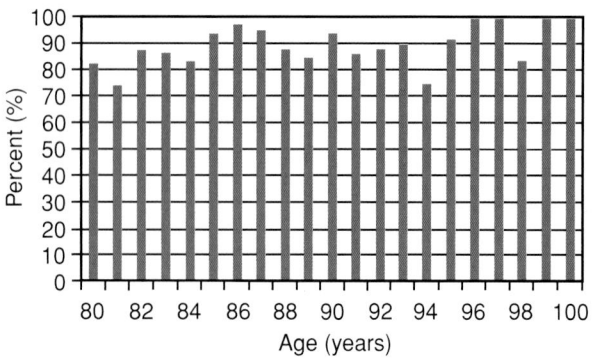

FIGURE 6-3 A: Prevalence of operative surgery in adults aged 80 years or more. **B, C:** Equivalent graphs for upper limb **(B)** and lower limb **(C)** fractures.

only 7.4% of upper limb fractures in patients aged 95 years or more were treated surgically. The situation is very different in lower limb fractures, and Figure 6-3C shows that the operative treatment of lower limb fractures gradually increases in the ninth and tenth decades of life.

Table 6-2 shows the prevalence of nonoperative management in different fractures. It indicates that virtually all proximal femoral, femoral diaphyseal, and tibial diaphyseal fractures are now treated operatively, with a very high prevalence of surgery in forearm diaphyseal fractures. There is a very low prevalence of surgery in proximal humeral, proximal radial, clavicular, metatarsal, and toe phalangeal fractures, and in this study no scapular surgery was undertaken—although obviously it is sometimes required. In the remaining fractures shown in Table 6-2, the prevalence of operative treatment varies between 11% and 71%, suggesting that both operative and nonoperative treatments are commonly used. In all fractures the surgeon clearly has to decide whether to treat the fracture operatively or nonoperatively based on many objective and subjective criteria, including the location and severity of the fracture and

TABLE 6-2 The Prevalence of Operatively Treated Fractures in Adults in Decreasing Order

| | | Fractures | | Average Age | | |
| | | Treated Operatively | | | | |
	Total	n	%	Surgery	Nonop	p
Proximal femur	693	676	97.5	80.4	79.7	Ns
Femoral diaphysis	54	51	94.4	67.9	89.0	Ns
Tibial diaphysis	102	96	94.1	42.0	62.7	0.022
Radius/ulna diaphyses	10	9	90.0	33.5	16.0	Ns
Radial diaphysis	11	9	81.2	46.2	54.5	Ns
Distal tibia	35	25	71.4	43.6	44.9	Ns
Proximal tibia	70	48	68.6	48.1	52.1	Ns
Proximal ulna	59	36	61.0	65.4	49.3	<0.001
Distal femur	23	14	60.9	61.7	65.0	Ns
Proximal radius/ulna	12	7	58.3	60.3	64.8	Ns
Talus	15	8	53.3	31.2	34.1	Ns
Distal humerus	28	14	50.0	60.5	61.1	Ns
Ankle	517	206	39.8	48.0	46.9	Ns
Humeral diaphysis	66	24	36.4	45.6	63.0	<0.001
Patella	56	20	35.7	55.1	58.5	Ns
Calcaneus	72	25	34.7	43.5	39.2	Ns
Ulnar diaphysis	38	12	31.6	32.2	43.0	Ns
Midfoot	27	8	29.6	48.0	46.9	Ns
Distal radius	977	285	29.2	61.8	56.9	<0.001
Pelvis	89	14	15.7	56.1	73.2	<0.001
Carpus	151	18	15.7	26.7	34.9	Ns
Finger phalanges	516	59	11.4	37.7	38.9	Ns
Metacarpus	626	69	11.0	28.8	32.1	Ns
Proximal humerus	336	25	7.4	61.5	65.0	Ns
Proximal radius	223	14	6.3	44.4	41.5	Ns
Clavicle	162	9	5.6	42.0	43.2	Ns
Metatarsus	381	15	3.9	42.0	44.4	Ns
Toe phalanges	209	8	3.8	37.6	35.8	Ns
Scapula	17	0	—	—	—	—
Sesamoid	1	0	—	—	—	—

The average age of patients treated operatively and nonoperatively is shown as is the probability of the age differences being significant.

any associated soft tissue damage; the age and medical condition of the patient; the ability to cooperate with a postoperative treatment regime; and any social habits such as smoking, drinking, and drug taking. Tables 6-1 and 6-2 both show that more surgical intervention is undertaken in lower limb fractures than in upper limb fractures. Table 6-2 also shows the five fractures for which multivariate analysis showed that age was an independent predictor of fracture management. In three fractures—those of the tibial diaphysis, humeral diaphysis, and the pelvis—increasing age was associated with the use of non-operative treatment but for fractures of the proximal ulna and the distal radius increasing age predicted surgical management.

Empirically it seems clear that there must be a relationship between the prevalence of operative surgery and the severity of the fracture that has been treated. It is quite difficult to define such a relationship in diaphyseal fractures, as Table 6-2 shows that most diaphyseal fractures tend to be treated operatively now regardless of how serious they are. This does not apply to isolated fractures of the ulnar diaphysis or to humeral diaphyseal fractures but femoral, tibial, and other forearm diaphyseal fractures are now usually treated by internal fixation. On the other hand, an analysis of the severity of the five metaphyseal or intra-articular fractures classified by the OTA[34] shows that fracture severity is an independent predictor of surgery (Table 6-3). The only fracture that does not appear to show such a relationship is the distal femoral fracture and many of the patients that present with this fracture are very elderly and frail. It is also interesting to note that ankle fractures show a relationship between fracture severity and the requirement for operative treatment, although the classification basis is different from the fractures listed in Table 6-3. In the 517 ankle fractures shown in Table 6-2, 12.3% of the OTA type A ankle fractures were operatively treated compared with 49.1% of type B fractures and 70% of type C fractures.

An analysis of the role of surgery in the treatment of patients who present with multiple fractures shows that 42.1% of fractures that occur in adults who present with multiple fractures were treated surgically. Statistical analysis showed that the presence of more than one fracture was an independent predictor of surgery in fractures of the midfoot, distal radius, and metatarsus. Table 6-4 shows the prevalence of surgical treatment for the seven most common modes of injury for those fractures in which multivariate analysis showed that the mode of injury was an independent predictor of surgical treatment. The seven modes of injury shown in Table 6-4 accounted for 93.4% of adult fractures. As one might expect, the highest prevalence of surgical fracture treatment is often, but not exclusively, related to motor vehicle accidents. Ankle fractures following falls were more commonly treated operatively than ankle fractures that occurred as a result of motor vehicle accidents, but further analysis showed a higher prevalence of OTA Type C fractures in the older population who sustained an ankle fracture as a result of a fall. The only fracture in which social deprivation independently determined treatment was the metacarpal. These fractures often occur in socially deprived male adolescents and in the Edinburgh study 46.3% followed a fight or an assault. As in many centers, these fractures were most frequently treated nonoperatively.

Many surgeons will probably be surprised that in 2000 67.6% of fractures were treated nonoperatively in a major trauma unit. One assumes that the prevalence of nonoperative management is declining, and almost certainly this is the case, but this study indicates that in fact nonoperative management is still the most common overall treatment method for fractures in general. However, the overall figure of 67.6% disguises the overall trends. Figures 6-2 and 6-3 show a difference between upper and lower limb fractures, particularly in the elderly. It would be interesting to know if the prevalence of surgery in different fractures is changing in response to a changing population and to improved treatment methods.

There is very little data by which the changing prevalence can be assessed. There has been no previous complete epidemiologic study in adults but in a remarkable paper Emmet and Breck[31] working in El Paso, Texas, before, during, and after World War II analyzed about 11,000 fresh fractures. They combined their pediatric and adult fractures and detailed the

---

TABLE 6-3 **Prevalence of Surgical Treatment in Different Severities of Metaphyseal and Intra-Articular Fractures**

	OTA Fracture Type			
	Type A Extra-Articular %	Type B Partial Articular %	Type C Complete Articular %	p
Distal humerus	15.4	88.9	66.7	0.002
Distal radius	28.0	10.7	51.8	<0.001
Distal femur	58.3	66.7	62.5	ns
Proximal tibia	18.2	78.0	77.8	<0.001
Distal tibia	30.0	76.9	100.0	0.001

The probability of increasing fracture complexity being a predictive factor for surgical treatment is shown.

TABLE 6-4	Prevalence of Surgical Treatment in Different Modes of Injury and the Probability of a Statistical Association							
	Twist	Fall	Fall Stairs	Fall Height	Assault/ Direct Blow	Sport	MVA	p
Adults								
Proximal humerus	—	5.1	22.2	25.0	25.0	7.1	10.5	0.01
Humeral diaphysis	—	23.1	—	60.0	50.0	100	100	0.003
Distal radius	0	28.2	39.4	32.0	11.1	21.9	56.1	0.001
Metacarpus	—	5.2	0	15.3	11.7	15.8	21.7	0.035
Distal tibia	0	66.6	50.0	88.9	0	100	100	0.005
Ankle	22.4	52.8	33.3	36.4	52.2	48.9	38.1	<0.001
Midfoot	0	—	0	37.5	0	66.0	100	0.003
Metatarsus	1.3	3.1	3.2	4.3	11.1	0	16.6	<0.001
Children								
Clavicle	—	0	0	0	0	0	10.0	0.011
Proximal radius	0	3.6	—	9.1	100	0	0	0.015
Proximal ulna	—	0	100	—	0	—	—	0.012
Distal radius	0	5.4	0	18.3	0	15.7	4.2	<0.001
Finger phalanges	50.0	0	0	0	0	4.6	0	<0.001

If the fracture is not listed there was no correlation between fracture treatment and mode of injury.

management of different fractures. The epidemiology of their population was different from the Edinburgh population, but they analyzed a very large number of fractures and it is interesting to compare their results between 1937 and 1955 with the Edinburgh results in 2000. To permit this the data from the pediatric fractures that were treated in Edinburgh in 2000 have been combined with the adult data.

Emmet and Breck categorized their fractures differently from the fractures listed in Table 6-2. They combined all of their tibial fractures, except for ankle fractures, and they also combined talar, calcaneal, and midfoot fractures as tarsal fractures. They separated forearm fractures into radius and ulna fractures as well as isolated radius and ulna fractures but they combined proximal and diaphyseal forearm fractures together. Using Emmet and Breck's fracture criteria the comparative data between 1937 and 1955 and 2000 are shown in Tables 6-5 and 6-6.

Table 6-5 shows those fractures in which there is an increased prevalence of surgery in 2000 and Table 6-6 shows those fractures for which there is no evidence that we now operate more frequently than surgeons in the early 1950s. Table 6-5 indicates that we operate on many more diaphyseal fractures than in the early 1950s. The only exception appears to be the isolated radial fracture (Table 6-6). It must be remembered that proximal radial fractures have been combined with radial diaphyseal fractures and if one looks at Table 6-2 it is obvious that we now operate on many more diaphyseal fractures than were operated on in the 1950s. Table 6-5 also

shows that we operate on four or five times the amount of distal radial fractures and this difference is undoubtedly greater if adults alone are examined.

It is probably more instructive to examine Table 6-6 and see which fractures we do not operate on any more frequently than in the 1950s. It would seem that we in fact treat fewer hand fractures nonoperatively, and this is presumably because of the beneficial effects of industrial legislation, which has significantly decreased the incidence of crushed hand injuries in many countries. However, in some parts of the world serious hand injuries are still relatively common and operative treatment will be more common.

One should consider that, with the possible exception of toe and patella fractures, surgeons now have access to better implants and techniques than surgeons in the 1950s. It is therefore interesting that the treatment of fractures of the clavicle and proximal humerus in particular seem to be much the same as 50 or 60 years ago. There are now studies suggesting that more of these fractures may be treated surgically in the future, but only time will tell if this occurs.[14,62] Many clavicle fractures have a relatively simple morphology and the early results of locked plating of proximal humeral fractures have not been as encouraging as was hoped[67] (see Chapter 20). Therefore, it seems likely that nonoperative management of the fractures listed in Table 6-6 will continue to be a popular treatment method. The fractures in Table 6-6 comprise 46.2% of all the fractures treated in Edinburgh in 2000 and this explains the relatively low overall operation rate for this year. The demographic

TABLE 6-5	Comparison of Edinburgh Data with Emmet and Breck, Fractures with an Increased Prevalence of Surgery in 2000			
	Emmett and Breck[21]			Edinburgh
	1937–1945 (%)	1946–1950 (%)	1951–1955 (%)	2000 (%)
Humeral diaphysis	22.2	10.6	20.8	33.3
Distal humerus	8.5	17.8	25.3	32.9
Radius and ulna	6.0	13.6	14.9	26.4
Ulna	20.7	17.7	19.8	38.3
Distal radius	6.0	4.2	4.6	20.3
Carpus	0	4.9	7.3	10.1
Proximal femur	47.1	72.3	73.3	97.4
Femoral diaphysis	27.5	41.8	52.1	76.1
Distal femur	50.0	26.1	36.0	65.5
Tibia and fibula	27.5	22.9	30.4	61.8
Ankle	13.0	20.4	22.5	35.8
Tarsus	4.3	5.9	17.4	35.2

The Edinburgh data have been adjusted to correspond with Emmet and Breck's fracture definitions. See text for details.

characteristics of nonoperative fracture treatment are summarized in Table 6-7.

TECHNIQUES OF NONOPERATIVE MANAGEMENT

Currently, we tend to use nonoperative techniques to treat stable fractures rather than to facilitate the reduction and stabilization of unstable fractures. It tends to be used to treat undisplaced or minimally displaced fractures or in patients who are elderly, frail, or who have significant medical or social comorbidities. However, in parts of the world with less access to operative fixation techniques, it remains an important treatment method for all fractures, and it is therefore important that surgeons understand the rationale behind the use of all nonoperative techniques.

TABLE 6-6	Comparison of Edinburgh Data with Emmet and Breck, Detailing the Fractures Without an Increased Prevalence of Surgery in 2000			
	Emmett and Breck[21]			Edinburgh
	1937–1945 (%)	1946–1950 (%)	1951–1955 (%)	2000 (%)
Clavicle	1.7	2.8	8.7	3.0
Scapula	0	0	3.0	0
Proximal humerus	2.9	7.9	9.6	6.9
Radius	5.5	8.8	10.6	10.4
Metacarpus	7.9	15.7	16.6	9.2
Finger phalanges	13.5	13.6	20.9	7.5
Patella	35.3	38.3	32.1	32.8
Metatarsus	0	6.2	8.5	3.6
Toe phalanges	0	8.4	7.6	3.2
Pelvis	0	22.2	18.2	15.7
Total (Tables 6-5–6-6)	12.2	17.1	21.6	25.4

The Edinburgh data have been adjusted to correspond with Emmet and Breck's fracture definitions. See text for details.

| TABLE 6-7 | **Essential Demographics of Nonoperative Management** |

Prevalence of Nonoperative Management (%)

	All Adults (>16 yrs)	Adults (>80 yrs)
Overall	67.6	59.5
Males	72.8	68.3
Females	63.0	57.9
Upper limb	81.7	78.4
Lower limb	46.8	12.2

Fractures Most Commonly Treated

Nonoperatively (>90%)	Operatively (>70%)
Scapula	Proximal femur
Toe phalanges	Femoral diaphysis
Metatarsus	Tibial diaphysis
Clavicle	Radius and ulnar diaphyses
Proximal radius	Radial diaphysis
Proximal humerus	Distal tibia

Factors Affecting Decision to Operate

Age

Severity of fracture (metaphyseal and intra-articular fractures)

Multiple fractures

Mode of injury (some fractures)

There have been several advances in nonoperative fracture management in the last 20 to 30 years, although the basic tenets of management remain unchanged. The use of plaster of Paris casts remains widespread as they are inexpensive and easy to apply. However, fiberglass casts are now more frequently used as they are lighter and more radiolucent. In addition, plastic orthoses, braces, and splints are now more frequently used. Their design has improved but their overall function remains unchanged.

Traction

The initial argument regarding the role of internal fixation of fractures after World War II centered on femoral diaphyseal fractures. Intramedullary nailing gradually grew more popular and essentially superseded traction as the treatment of choice for femoral fractures in the 1970s and 1980s, but traction is still used in parts of the world and surgeons should understand the rationale behind its use and complications. In addition to the treatment of femoral diaphyseal fractures, traction was used to treat acetabular fractures and fracture dislocations of the hip as well as comminuted fractures of the tibial diaphysis and distal tibia, although its role in the management of these fractures is now extremely limited and essentially confined to situations when internal and external fixation techniques are unavailable. It is still used for the acute management of cervical spine fractures.

There are six basic methods of skeletal traction that are shown in Figure 6-4. Most traction methods rely on a splint on

which the leg is placed. The proximal end or ring of the splint is placed in the patient's groin and traction is applied by placing a transosseous pin through the distal femur or proximal tibia. Fixed traction is undertaken when the pin is secured to the distal end of the splint by traction cords. In balanced traction the splint is suspended by a pulley system and a second pulley system is applied to the transosseous pin. Traction, using a variable weight, then alters the fracture position with countertraction being achieved by placing the patient head down and raising the end of the bed. Once traction is established the fracture alignment is checked radiologically and pads inserted appropriately to push the femur into correct alignment. A posterior pad under the distal femur is almost always required because of the posterior sag produced by the effect of gravity.

Many types of traction have been described but the six basic types are shown in Figure 6-4. The first of these is a Thomas splint with a Pearson knee piece attached to the splint (Fig. 6-4A). The Thomas splint supports the leg and balanced traction is applied. After 4 to 6 weeks the knee piece is applied and knee mobilization commenced. This was a commonly used traction apparatus.

A second type of traction is Braun traction and a weight and pulley system (Fig. 6-4B). This is a very simple traction system that permits traction in the longitudinal axis of the femur. Control of the femoral fragments was difficult. The system, using skin rather than skeletal traction, is still used for temporary traction prior to femoral diaphyseal surgery.

Another type of traction is Hamilton-Russell traction, which uses a one-pulley system to provide support for the femur and to apply traction (Fig. 6-4C). The mechanical advantage offered by two pulleys at the foot of the bed theoretically meant that the longitudinal pull was twice as great as the upward pull and the resulting traction was at an axis of 30 degrees to the horizontal, approximately in line with the femur. This method of traction does not adequately control the femoral fragments and it was sometimes used after a period of skeletal traction.

A fourth type of traction is Perkins traction (Fig. 6-4D). This is essentially a straight pull along the axis of the femur through a proximal pin but without a splint. The control of femoral alignment was poor and malunion was common. Perkins believed in early knee mobilization and advocated the use of a split bed later in the treatment of femoral diaphyseal fractures. In this system the patients sat on a bed with the knee flexed over the mattress and knee movement was encouraged while longitudinal traction was maintained.

A fifth variety of traction is Fisk traction (Fig. 6-4E). This consists of a short Thomas splint and a hinged knee piece. Traction in the axis of the femur was maintained using a proximal tibial transosseous pin but the patient could flex the hip and knee by pulling on a separate cord attached to the end of the thigh splint.

Finally, there is 90-90 traction (Fig. 6-4F). In this method, the thigh is pulled upward and both hip and knee are at 90 degrees. The advantage of this method is that gravity does not cause posterior sag of the femoral fragments. It was used for proximal femoral diaphyseal fractures when the proximal femoral fracture was flexed by the unopposed action of iliopsoas. The method is still used for pediatric femoral fractures.

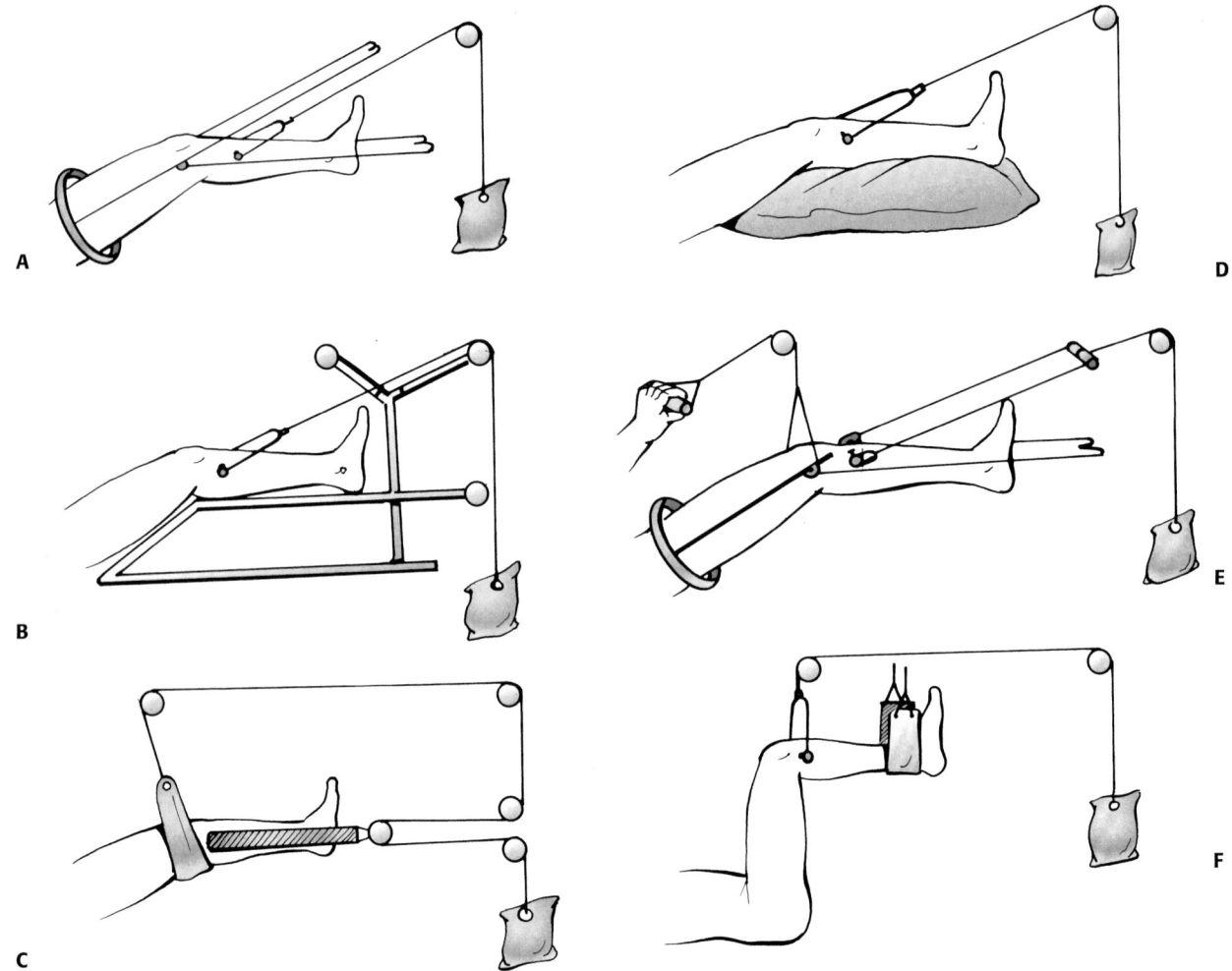

FIGURE 6-4 Six methods of skeletal traction. See text for explanation.

Treatment of femoral diaphyseal fractures by traction should be reserved for cases for which no other method is available. There is considerable morbidity associated with its use. The main complications are failure to maintain normal femoral alignment and significant knee stiffness. Charnley[16] documented 34 cases in patients between 20 and 45 years of age with middle and distal third diaphyseal fractures. On average, knee mobilization was commenced at 10 to 25 weeks and the final range of motion was 120 degrees. He also quoted very similar results from Massachusetts General Hospital stating that 44.4% of patients, with an average age of 37 years, had actually regained full knee function. Keep in mind that these were selected series of patients and Charnley's results were not matched by other surgeons. Connolly et al.[17] reported that the use of traction was associated with malunion and nonunion requiring operative treatment in 11% to 29% of cases. Shortening of more than 2 cm occurred in 14% to 30% of cases and refracture in 4% to 17% of cases. They pointed out that the most significant complication was knee stiffness, which occurred in 30% to 50% of cases and affected both elderly and younger patients. In addition to these complications, prolonged traction

is associated with significant medical problems and decubitus ulcers. Younger patients also suffered significantly with loss of employment and financial hardship. Psychological problems associated with prolonged bed rest were not uncommon.

To minimize these complications surgeons turned to the use of a cast brace, which is essentially a long-leg cast with knee hinges to facilitate knee mobilization. This was applied after a few weeks of bed rest but its use was far from problem free. If the surgeon used prolonged bed rest prior to the application of the cast, patients tended to have the problems associated with traction, and if they shortened the period of bed rest it was difficult to apply the cast and mobilize the patient without losing fracture alignment. Using a regime of early application of a cast brace and mobilization, Connolly et al.[17] documented a 0.7% prevalence of nonunion and malunion with 13% shortening of more than 2 cm and 5.4% symptomatic loss of knee motion, 2% refracture, and 3% pulmonary emboli. They found the method particularly useful for distal fractures, comminuted mid-diaphyseal fractures, and open fractures. Hardy[42] used a similar regime and quoted femoral malalignment in 72.2% of patients, significant knee disfunction in 7.4%, and knee instability in 35.2% of patients. As with femoral traction, the cast brace has now essentially disappeared and should only be used if surgical treatment is unavailable.

Tibial traction should not be used. It was used in cases of mid-diaphyseal comminution or if it was considered that a tibial plafond fracture was too complex to be treated surgically. Traction was applied through a transosseous calcaneal pin. Unfortunately, the use of excessive traction has been shown to increase the risk of compartment syndrome[88] and even if this complication does not occur, traction is associated with the same complications as femoral fractures, these being malalignment, joint stiffness, and nonunion. There is now no indication for tibial traction unless appropriate internal or external fixation techniques are unavailable.

Spinal Traction
Cervical Spine

Unlike skeletal traction spinal traction remains popular and is in widespread use for the management of cervical fractures and dislocations. It has been shown to be effective in various cervical fractures. Traction is commonly used to reduce a fracture or dislocation, thereby decompressing the neural elements and providing a degree of spinal stability. Spinal traction is rarely used for definitive management and it is usually changed to a halo-body cast or vest, or the surgeon may opt for later surgical stabilization. There are two principal types of cervical traction. These are cranial tongs, of which the best known are the Gardner-Wells tongs, and halo traction.

Cranial Tongs. Cranial tongs consist of a hemicircular frame with two spring-loaded angulated pins (Fig. 6-5) that are placed into the outer table of the skull at points about 1 cm posterior to the external auditory meatus and 1 cm superior to the pinna of each ear. Because this is below the widest diameter of the skull the upward pin angulation means that traction can be applied. Each spring-loaded pin is applied with an insertion torque of 6- to 8-inch pounds, and once the tongs are in position a simple pulley system can be set up with a weight hanging over the end of the frame or bed. Care must be exercised in applying weights in case overdistraction and neural damage occurs.

The weight required to reduce the spine varies with the position of the fracture, the degree of ligamentous damage, and the size of the patient. As a rule the surgeon should start with an initial weight of 10 pounds. Approximately 5 pounds per spinal

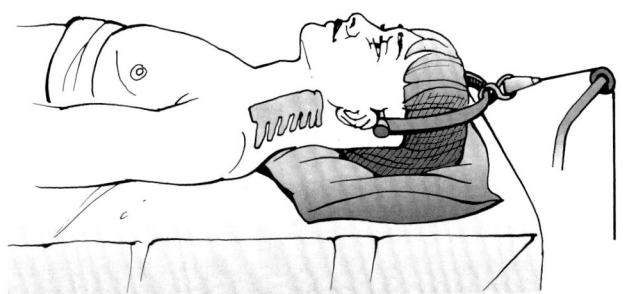

FIGURE 6-5 The use of cranial tongs to apply traction.

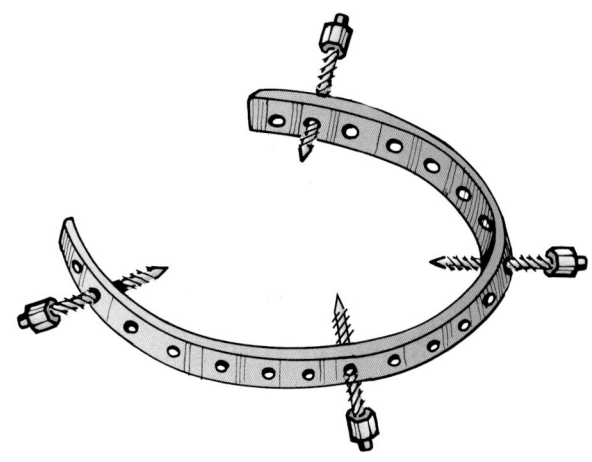

FIGURE 6-6 A halo ring.

segment are required to reduce the fracture in most patients, although this is only a guide. Thus a load of about 40 pounds will be required for a C5 to C6 injury although the exact weight varies and serial imaging is required to check the position as the load is increased. It is important to obtain a lateral radiograph or fluoroscopic image to visualize fracture reduction.

Halo Rings. Closed or open halo rings are now a more popular choice for cervical traction (Fig. 6-6) because they can tolerate higher loading than cranial tongs and can be incorporated into a cast or brace to allow definitive treatment. The halo is attached with four pins: two anterior and two posterior. The pins should be inserted below the widest diameter of the skull with two anterior pins being placed through stab incisions under local anesthetic about 1 cm above the lateral third of the orbital rim. In this location they are lateral to the supraorbital and supratrochlear nerves. The posterior pins are placed about 1 cm above the helix of the ear and to prevent skin necrosis they should not make contact with the ear. Opposing pins should be tightened at the same time to avoid pin displacement, with the pins then being retightened 24 to 48 hours after the initial application. If a pin loosens it can be retightened once to 8-inch pounds.

Halo-Body Fixation. The original halo-body device was a body cast attached to a halo. It was devised by Perry and Nickel.[70] Halo casts may still be useful if the appropriate bracing materials are not available or if the patient is uncooperative, but nowadays the halo is usually attached to a vest or orthosis (Fig. 6-7), which is made of plastic and tightened with buckles or straps. It is attached to the halo by two anterior and two posterior rods and it is worn until union occurs or a cervical brace is used.

Complications. As with skeletal traction, cervical traction is associated with several complications. It has been estimated that up to 31% of normal cervical spinal motion is permitted by halo-body orthoses and about 10% of patients lose fracture reduction.[53] Thus serial radiographs are essential during treatment. As with external skeletal fixation, pin track sepsis is a problem with it occurring in up to 20% of patients. As the fixation is unicortical, pin loosening is also a problem and rates

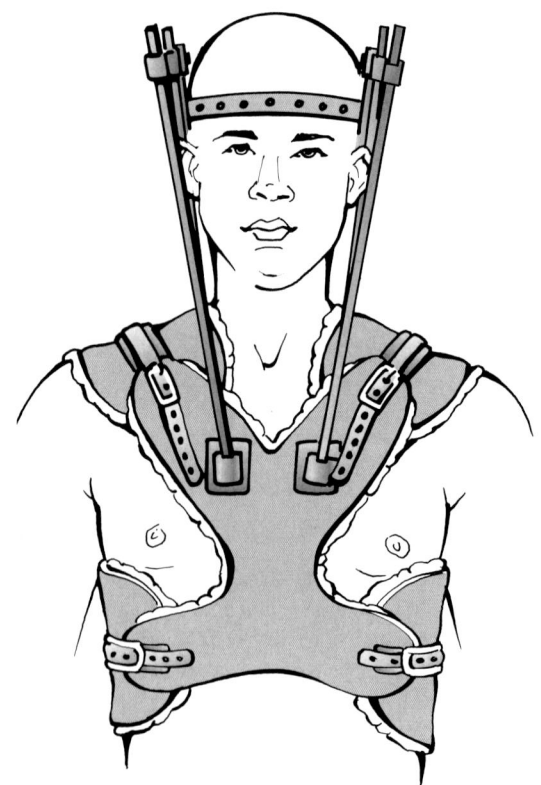

FIGURE 6-7 A halo vest.

of 36% to 60% have been recorded.[35,60] Nerve damage, dural puncture, skull perforation, and brain abscesses have all been reported, and when halo-body fixation is used in quadriplegic patients there is a high incidence of pressure sores, decubitus ulcers, and respiratory complications.[35,60] Dysphagia has also been reported.

Thoracolumbar Spine

Traction is not used for the definitive management of thoracolumbar fractures although prolonged bed rest is still used despite an increasing prevalence of surgical stabilization. Prolonged immobilization necessitates the use of a rotating bed, such as a Stryker bed, which is designed to facilitate skin care, physiotherapy, and personal hygiene. Complications include respiratory problems and decubitus ulcers, and intensive nursing is required. In less-severe thoracolumbar fractures the surgeon may opt for a short period of bed rest followed by surgical stabilization or the use of a thoracolumbar brace or orthosis.

The use of a short period of thoracolumbar traction is sometimes used as a method of reducing thoracolumbar and lumbar burst fractures prior to the application of a thoracolumbar cast.[97] This technique involves the use of a Cotrel frame for a few days to facilitate fracture reduction. At this time, this technique is not in widespread use.

Casts

Unlike skeletal traction, casts remain popular for fracture treatment and probably remain the most common method

of fracture treatment throughout the world. Figures 6-2 and 6-3 and Table 6-2 show that casts are more commonly used to treat upper limb fractures but Table 6-2 also indicates that many less-severe lower limb fractures continue to be treated with casts. Nowadays casts are less commonly used to control the position of a diaphyseal fracture after closed reduction but in some metaphyseal and intra-articular fractures, such as distal radial fractures and ankle fractures, this method of treatment is still widely used. Casts are often used for pain management and to facilitate mobilization in less-severe fractures. The decision between cast management and surgery is frequently subjective and influenced by the patient's age, physical condition, mental status, and degree of prefracture mobility. In decades to come, it is likely that this decision will become more difficult as the age of the patients increases and they get progressively less fit.

There are three principles that apply to the treatment of unstable fractures with a cast.

1. Utilization of intact soft tissues
2. Three-point fixation
3. Hydrostatic pressure

These are illustrated in Figure 6-8 with reference to a fracture of the tibia and fibula. In theory there will often be a hinge of intact soft tissue on one side of the fracture, which can be used to assist with fracture reduction. If three-point fixation is applied through the cast the fracture will be maintained in a reduced position. This theory is somewhat naive, although it may well work in the OTA A3.3 tibial fracture illustrated in Figure 6-8. However, many tibial fractures are not transverse, and obviously the theoretical concept of a soft tissue hinge will be less applicable in spiral, butterfly, segmental, or comminuted

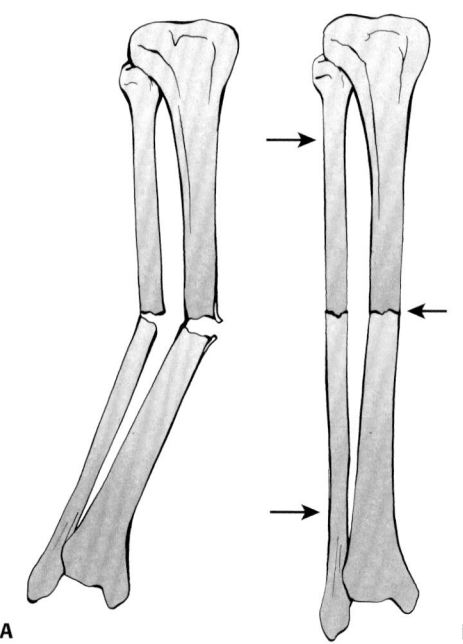

FIGURE 6-8 A: An OTA A3.3 fracture with valgus angulation. **B:** Three-point fixation, or pressure, will reduce fracture if a soft tissue hinge is present.

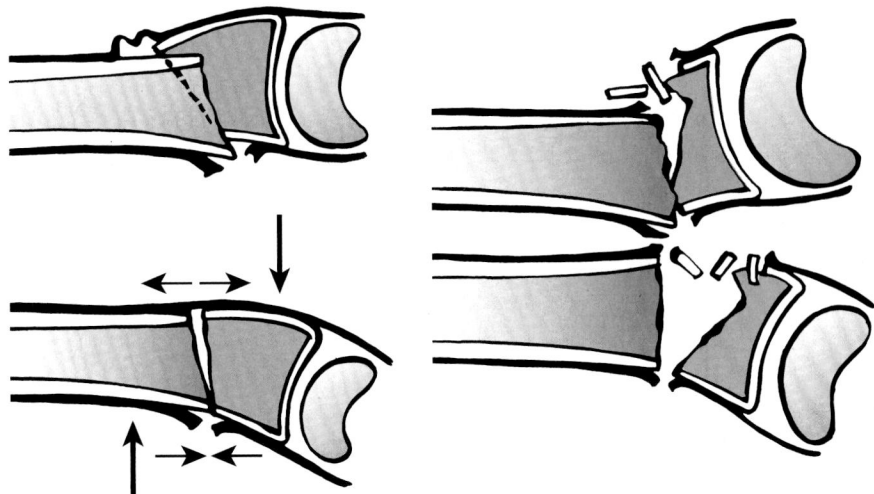

FIGURE 6-9 A: The use of an intact soft tissue hinge and three-point fixation in a distal radial fracture in a young patient. **B:** The same situation in an older patient with poor soft tissues and bone comminution.

fractures. In addition, there may well be soft tissue stripping from the diaphysis adjacent to the fracture and the fracture ends may overlap, which makes reduction more difficult. The last point to bear in mind is that while the soft tissue hinge may be intact in low-velocity fractures in younger patients, it is unlikely to be intact after high-energy injury or in older patients. The periosteum becomes thinner with increasing age and is more easily damaged. As many fractures occur in older patients, the fracture reduction concepts promoted by Charnley[16] and others are less applicable. This is illustrated in Figure 6-9. It shows the theoretical use of the soft tissue hinge in a metaphyseal distal radial fracture compared with the more common distal radial fracture in an older person, which is associated with metaphyseal comminution and a poor or absent soft tissue hinge.

The principle of hydrostatic pressure is illustrated in Figure 6-10. Hydrostatic pressure relies on the fact that the soft tissues and the diaphysis of the bone are not compressible. Thus, when they are encased in a complete cast or brace they essentially become rigid and maintain the position of the fracture. As with the soft tissue hinge, the explanation is somewhat simplistic and does not take into account active muscle contraction around the fracture.

Cast Application

All casts are applied in a similar manner no matter whether the traditional plaster of Paris or more modern fiberglass materials are used. Both types of cast material are frequently used as "slabs," which are often applied to a limb soon after injury to give temporary support. A full cast is rarely applied immediately after injury because of the potential of swelling associated with the injury to lead to compartment syndrome if the limb is encased in a rigid cast. Slabs are applied by using a layer of protective stockinette and layers of synthetic wool padding (Fig. 6-11). A slab of the appropriate length is then cut and, after soaking, applied to the limb. The location of the slab

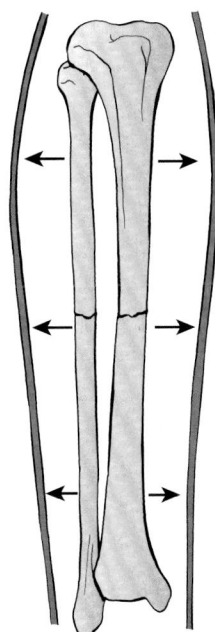

FIGURE 6-10 The principle of hydrostatic pressure in cast use. See text for explanation.

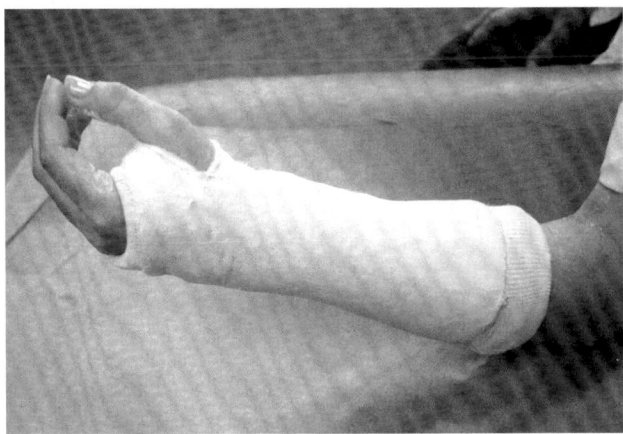

FIGURE 6-11 A forearm back slab used to treat an undisplaced distal radial fracture.

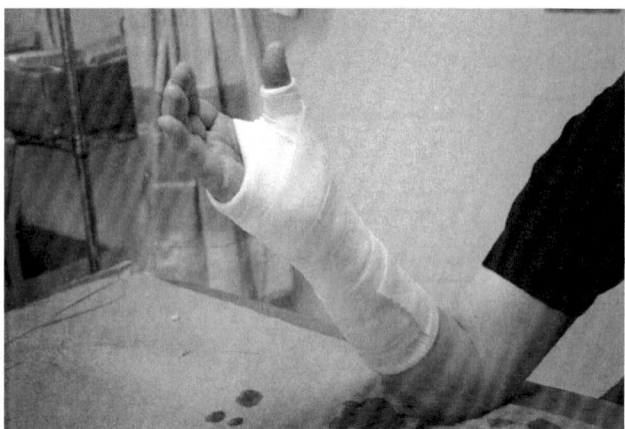

FIGURE 6-12 A fiberglass scaphoid cast.

depends on the fracture. In the lower limb, backslabs or dorsal slabs are usually used, these being applied to the posterior leg and calf to support the fracture until a full cast can be applied or surgery is undertaken. In the upper limb, humeral diaphyseal fractures are often supported with a laterally located slab, fractures around the elbow and forearm being supported with a posteriorly located backslab, and distal radial and carpal fractures with a dorsal slab.

Full casts are applied by wrapping plaster of Paris or fiberglass bandages around the limb after stockinette and synthetic wool have been applied (Fig. 6-12). Up to 30 years ago there was considerable debate regarding how much padding should be used, as surgeons recognized that too much padding permitted secondary fracture displacement but too little padding

caused skin problems and increased the risk of compartment syndrome. On the other hand, if the cast is being used to control the position of a reduced fracture, excessive padding should be avoided because redisplacement of the fracture may occur. Cast bandages should be applied carefully, keeping the bandages flat to avoid soft tissue damage. As the cast hardens the surgeon should manipulate the fracture, taking care not to indent the cast material, thereby compressing the underlying soft tissue. Care must be taken not to obstruct joint motion or, if a joint is encased by the cast, it should be placed in the correct position. Once the cast has been applied, radiographs should be obtained to confirm the fracture is in an acceptable position. Cast management of unstable fractures is very labor intensive. Follow-up must be assiduous until callus starts to stabilize the fracture, as it is easy to miss secondary fracture displacement. If this occurs, the position of the fracture must be corrected without undue delay as soft tissue contracture occurs fairly quickly and secondary reduction becomes progressively more difficult. If this occurs, it is important that the surgeon knows how to deal with it.

In diaphyseal fractures angular malalignment can be corrected by wedging the cast. In this technique (Fig. 6-13) radiographs, or preferably fluoroscopy, are used to identify the fracture site and the cast is cut leaving a hinge of 2 to 3 cm of the cast intact, the location of the hinge depending on the direction of the necessary correction. Thus if the fracture is in valgus a medial hinge is left and a varus force applied to the distal cast to open the window. Once opened, the position is maintained until more cast material can be applied to maintain the reduced position. In years gone by, plaster rooms would keep a jar of wooden dowling to insert into the cast window to

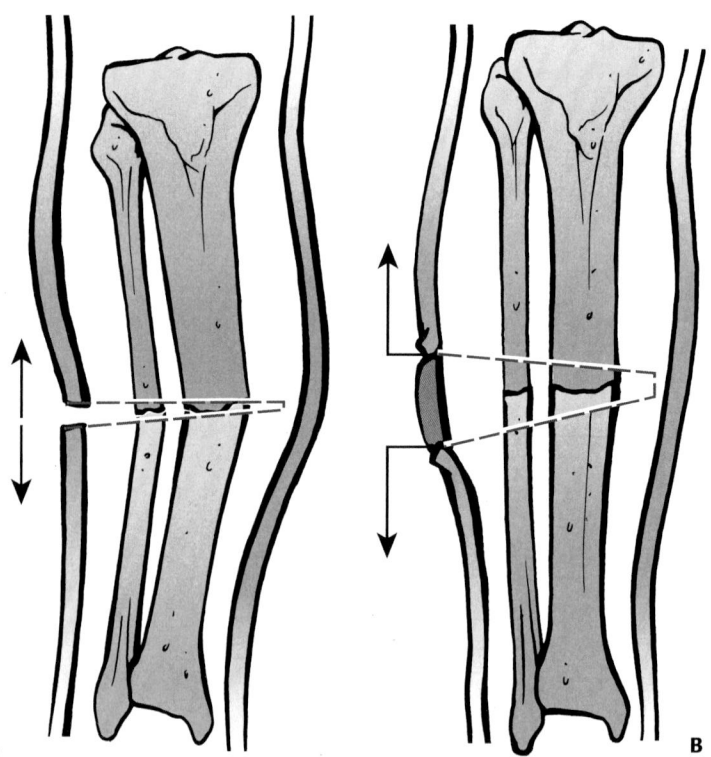

A   B

FIGURE 6-13 Wedging a cast to straighten a diaphyseal fracture of the tibia and fibula. **A:** The fracture is in valgus. The cast is cut at the level of the fracture to leave a medial hinge. **B:** The fracture is straightened and the gap in the cast kept open while the cast is completed.

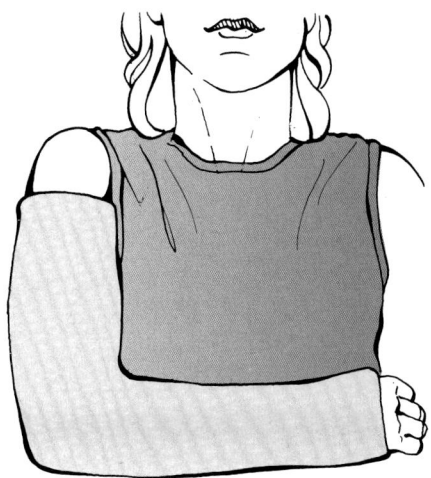

FIGURE 6-14 A long-arm cast.

maintain the reduced fracture position while the supplementary plaster of Paris dried. Theoretically, rotational deformity is also correctible by cutting the cast. Again a cut is made in the cast at the level of the fracture and the rotation is corrected, but it is easy to lose position and sometimes it is better to remove the cast and reapply it. Surgeons should be aware that it is difficult to maintain the position of an unstable fracture in a cast, and that is why earlier surgeons defined levels of "acceptable" malunion. If the fracture position is not maintained by the cast, consideration should be given to operative treatment.

Types of Cast
Upper Limb Casts
Long-Arm Cast. The classic long-arm cast with the elbow at 90 degrees and the wrist included in the cast (Fig. 6-14) is less commonly used now because forearm and elbow fractures

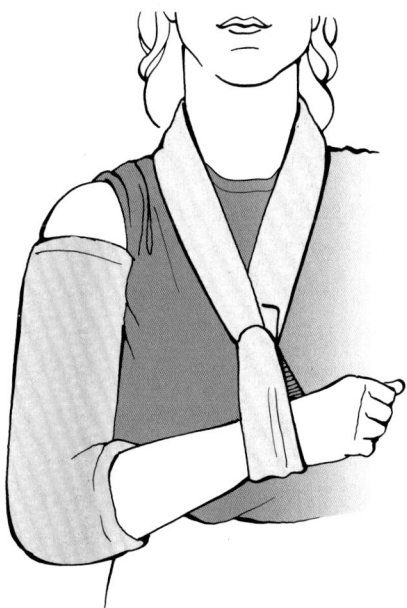

FIGURE 6-15 A hanging cast.

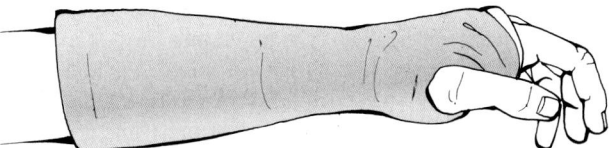

FIGURE 6-16 A Colles, or forearm, cast.

are often internally fixed, but it is still used for less-severe fractures. The cast is applied from just below the axilla to just proximal to the metacarpophalangeal joints of the digits but leaving the thumb free. The wrist is placed in 30 degrees of dorsiflexion and the elbow in 90 degrees of flexion. In more minor fractures the wrist may not be included and a full-arm cylinder is then applied.

Hanging Cast or U-Slab. These casts are routinely used to treat humeral diaphyseal fractures in the acute phase. The arm is placed over the lower chest with the elbow at 90 degrees. A collar and cuff support can be used to maintain the position. A cast is then applied as shown in Figure 6-15, so that the top of the humeral component of the cast is above the humeral fracture. Gravity is used to regain humeral length and the alignment of the fracture can be theoretically adjusted by altering the length of the cast between the neck and forearm. The shorter the cuff the more varus is applied to the fracture. An alternative to the hanging cast is the U-slab or sugar-tong splint, in which a plaster is placed from just below the axilla on the medial side of the arm down and around the elbow and then upward to just below the shoulder. The slab is then bandaged into position. In proximal humeral fractures the slab can be extended above the shoulder but surgeons should be aware that this will negate any beneficial reduction effects of gravity. These casts are often replaced at 2 to 4 weeks by a functional brace (Fig. 6-23).

Colles Cast (Forearm Cast). The Colles, or forearm cast, is the most widely used upper limb cast and is used for most distal radial and ulnar fractures as well as for some carpal injuries. The cast extends from below the elbow to just proximal to the metacarpal necks of the digits with the thumb left free (Fig. 6-16). The application of the Colles cast is frequently preceded by the use of a dorsal plaster slab, which is replaced by the cast once the swelling has reduced.

Scaphoid Cast. The scaphoid cast is commonly used to treat scaphoid fractures and pain in the anatomical snuff box on the radial border of the wrist when radiographs do not confirm the presence of a fracture. The wrist is held in slight dorsiflexion and the thumb is in abduction and slight flexion as if a glass is being held between the index finger and thumb (Fig. 6-17). The

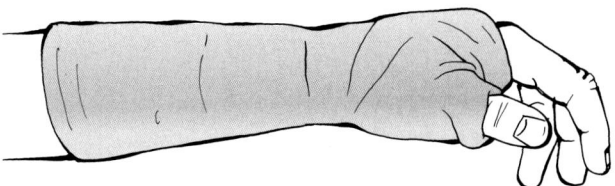

FIGURE 6-17 A scaphoid cast.

cast extends from just below the elbow to just proximal to the metacarpal necks of the digits. On the thumb the cast extends to just proximal to the interphalangeal joint. A modification of the scaphoid cast is the extended scaphoid cast, which may be used for fractures distal to the metacarpophalangeal joint of the thumb. In the extended scaphoid cast the whole thumb is included.

Bruner Cast. The Bruner cast is a variant of the extended scaphoid cast that is cut short to release the wrist joint. It is particularly useful for the treatment of ligamentous injuries of the thumb metacarpophalangeal joint but may be used to treat associated minor avulsion fractures.

Burkhalter Cast. This cast is used to treat metacarpal or phalangeal fractures. The wrist is placed in 40 degrees of extension and the metacarpophalangeal joints are placed in 70 to 90 degrees of flexion (Fig. 6-18). The cast relies on the intact dorsal hood of the fingers acting as a tension band or a soft tissue hinge. It is usually applied by placing a slab over the dorsum of the forearm and the hand, with the wrist and fingers in the correct position and then applying a forearm cast to secure the slab. Finger extension is not permitted by the dorsal slab but some flexion is allowed.

James Cast. In this cast the fingers are kept in the "position of function" of the hand. The wrist is maintained at 40 degrees of extension with the metacarpophalangeal joints at 90 degrees and the interphalangeal joints of the fingers at 70 to 90 degrees. In this position the collateral ligaments of the metacarpophalangeal joints and the interphalangeal joints are stretched maximally and thus contractures will not occur (Fig. 6-19). As with the Burkhalter cast, the James cast is in fact a combination of a slab and a cast. Initially a volar slab is applied to the forearm and hand with the joints in the correct position. A forearm cast is then applied.

Other Upper Limb Casts. Surgeons used to use shoulder spicas to treat factures around the shoulder girdle. These were mainly used for clavicle or proximal humeral fractures. Sometimes the shoulder was placed at 90 degrees of abduction with the elbow at 90 degrees of flexion and the forearm pronated in

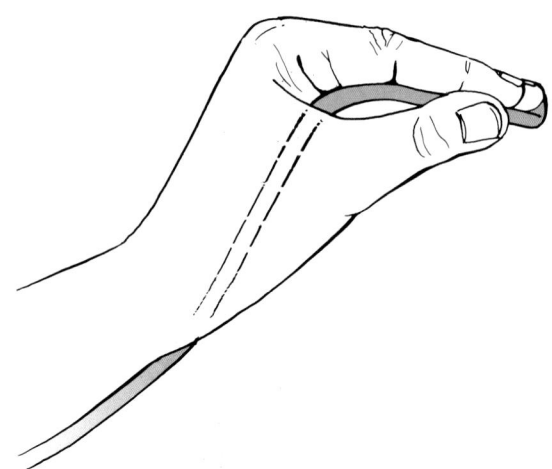

FIGURE 6-19 A James slab. This is volar slab that may be supplemented by a forearm cast.

the "policeman's halt position." These casts are now very rarely used with surgeons favoring operative management for the fractures that they were employed to treat.

Lower Limb Casts

Below-Knee Cast. This is the most common cast used for lower limb injury including ankle fractures, foot fractures, and soft tissue injuries. It is occasionally used to treat undisplaced lower tibial diaphyseal fractures or minor pilon fractures. The cast is applied from below the level of the fibular neck proximally to the level of the metatarsal heads distally with the ankle at 90 degrees and the foot in the plantigrade position (Fig. 6-20). The below-knee cast may be applied as a first stage in a long-leg cast used to treat an unstable tibial diaphyseal fracture.

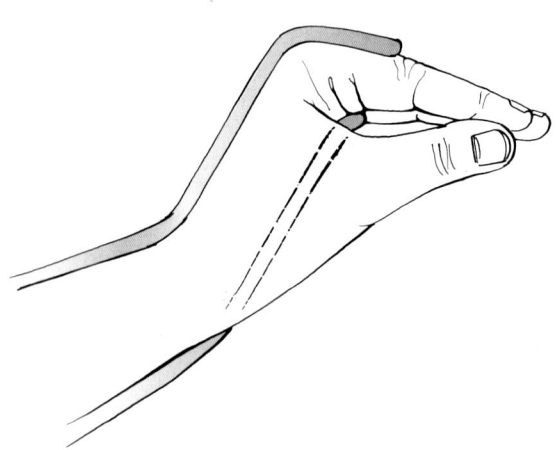

FIGURE 6-18 A Burkhalter cast. This is a combination of a forearm cast and a dorsal slab.

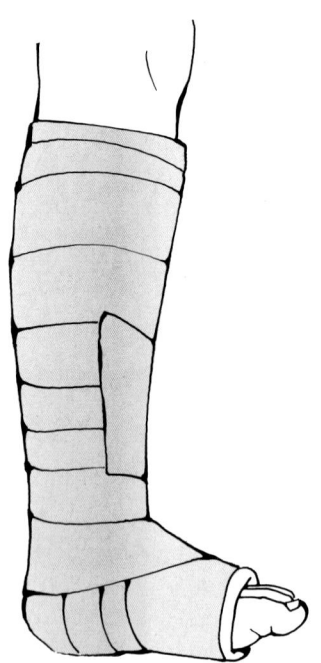

FIGURE 6-20 A below-knee cast.

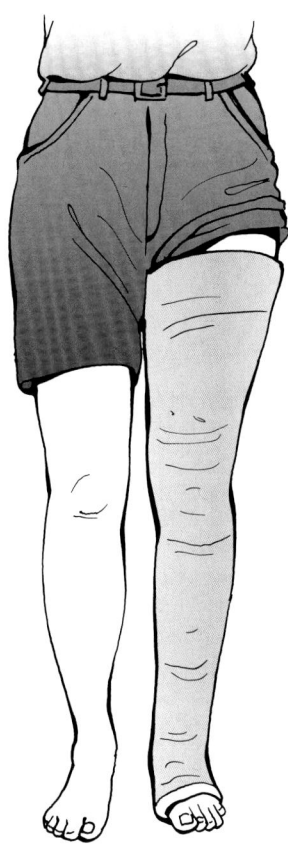

FIGURE 6-21 A long-leg cast.

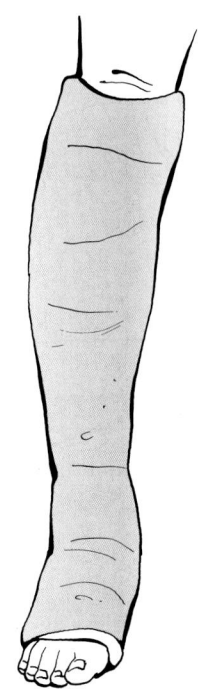

FIGURE 6-22 A patella tendon-bearing cast.

Long-Leg Cast. Surgeons usually use a long-leg cast to treat unstable tibial diaphyseal fracture in the acute phase changing to a patellar tendon-bearing cast after a few weeks. They may also be used to treat fractures around the knee. A long-leg cast is best constituted by applying a below-knee cast and then flexing the knee to about 10 degrees, following which the thigh extension is applied (Fig. 6-21).

Patellar Tendon-Bearing Cast. The other variant of the below-knee cast is the patellar tendon-bearing cast, which is usually used to treat tibial diaphyseal fractures after a few weeks in a long-leg cast. In this cast the proximal end of a below-knee cast is extended upward as far as the lower pole in the patella and moulded around the patellar tendon to provide a degree of rotational stability (Fig. 6-22). Care must be taken not to apply pressure over the common peroneal nerve running around the neck of the fibula.

Spinal Casts. Spinal casts are now rarely used. The basic cast is a plaster jacket that extends from the sternal notch to the symphysis pubis and is carefully moulded. If fractures lower than L3 are to be treated, the cast should be extended downward to include one thigh. If cervical fractures are treated in a cast, the cast is extended upward into a collar but the use of cervical casts is now extremely unusual and they would only be used if no other treatment method was available. Thoracolumbar casts are still used by some surgeons,[97] but the results are no better than those associated with spinal braces.

Braces
Limb Braces
Many different limb braces have been designed but they fall into four main types used to treat fractures of the humeral diaphysis, distal radius, metacarpus, and lower leg. Most braces are made of polyethylene or plastic and secured by Velcro, plastic straps, and buckles. Braces tend to be lighter than casts and are often used after a short period of cast immobilization once the fracture is more stable. Other advantages are that braces can be tightened as the soft tissue swelling decreases and they can be removed for personal hygiene and radiologic evaluation of the fracture.

Upper Limb
Humeral Brace. A simple polyethylene or plastic brace is often used to treat humeral diaphyseal fractures after the initial cast management. The brace fits around the arm and is usually wider laterally than medially to support the humerus proximally (Fig. 6-23).

Distal Forearm Brace. These are used to treat distal radial fractures and may be used after a period of cast immobilization or they may be applied primarily to the forearm. There are two basic types. Figure 6-24 shows a conventional distal forearm brace, which extends to the radiocarpal joint. Alternatively, the brace may have a dorsal extension to just proximal to the metacarpophalangeal joints of all digits except the thumb.

Metacarpal Brace. Metacarpal braces are usually either made up of a strap worn around the hand under which padding is placed to maintain fracture reduction or they take the form of a heat-molded plastic brace which is placed around the hand and then molded into an appropriate shape to maintain fracture reduction (Fig. 6-25). They can be used for the primary

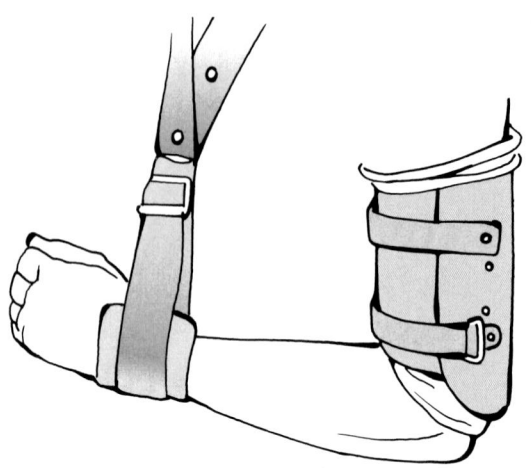

FIGURE 6-23 A humeral brace. The sling length can be altered to change the fracture position.

treatment of metacarpal fractures[40] or to protect the metacarpus after operative fracture treatment.[55] Skin necrosis has been reported.[36]

Lower Limb

Below-Knee Brace. The most popular lower limb brace is the equivalent of the below-knee cast. There are many available but all tend to be made of plastic and fasten with Velcro or straps (Fig. 6-26). They are used for the same indications as below-knee casts and may be used after an initial period of cast management. They are commonly used after internal fixation of ankle and foot fractures or to allow mobilization after a soft tissue injury to the ankle, hindfoot, or midfoot.

Patellar Tendon-Bearing Brace. This is the equivalent of the tendon-bearing cast but it permits ankle movement (Fig. 6-27). The plastic brace is fitted with an ankle hinge and a heel cup and can therefore be worn inside a shoe.

Knee Brace. This is the modern equivalent of the old cast brace but it is no longer used to treat femoral diaphyseal fractures. Now it is made from synthetic material and fitted with

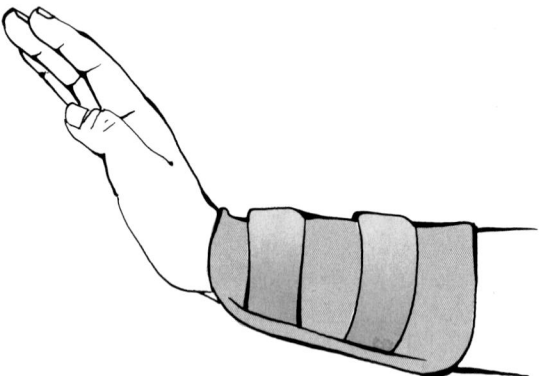

FIGURE 6-24 A distal forearm brace. A modification of this brace includes an extension to just proximal to the MCPJs, except the thumb.

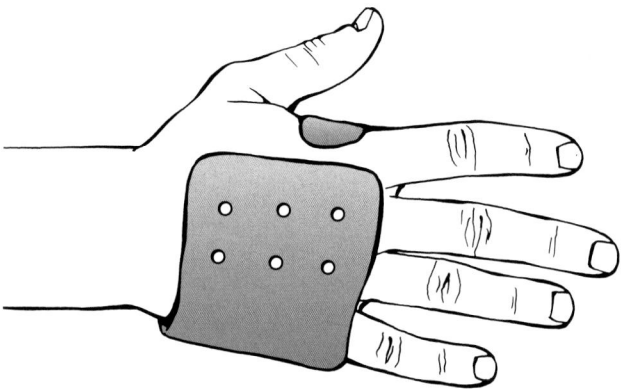

FIGURE 6-25 A metacarpal brace.

adjustable integral knee hinges (Fig. 6-28). These are often used to treat soft tissue injuries around the knee but may be used to facilitate mobilization after internal fixation of distal femoral or proximal tibial fractures. In some minor fractures around the knee they may be used for definitive treatment.

Spinal Braces

Cervical Braces. There are three types of cervical braces: Soft and hard collars, high cervicothoracic orthoses, and low cervicothoracic orthoses (Fig. 6-29A). Within these three types there are many different designs but they all have the same basic function. Standard soft and hard collars are not generally used for the treatment of acute cervical fractures or dislocations but they are useful for the treatment of minor soft tissue sprains and whiplash injuries. They allow up to 80% of normal cervical movement and therefore confer little stability to the cervical

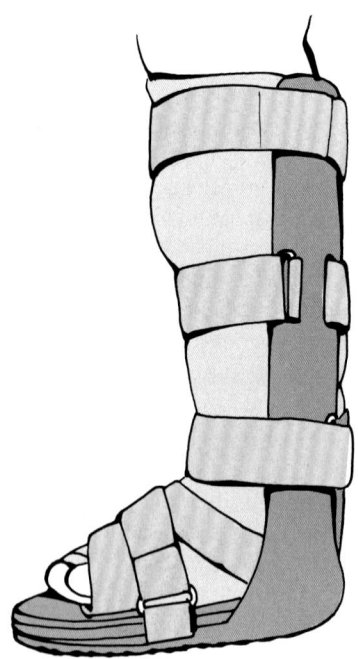

FIGURE 6-26 A below-knee brace.

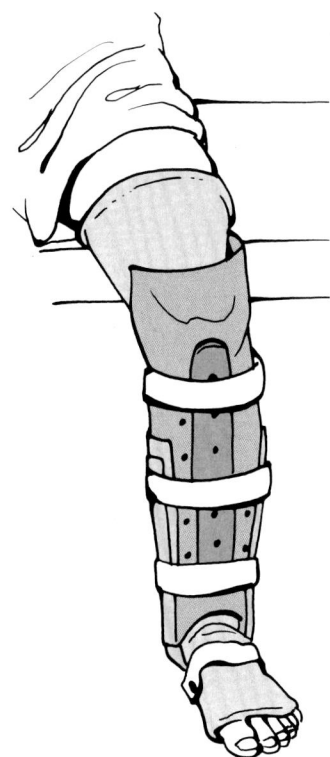

FIGURE 6-27 A patella tendon-bearing brace.

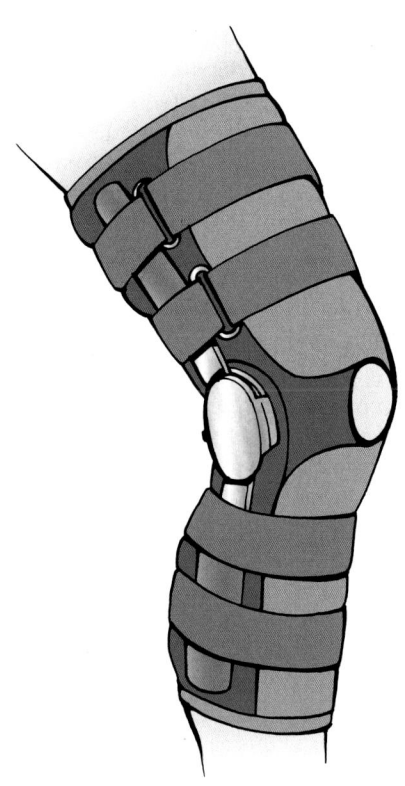

FIGURE 6-28 A knee brace.

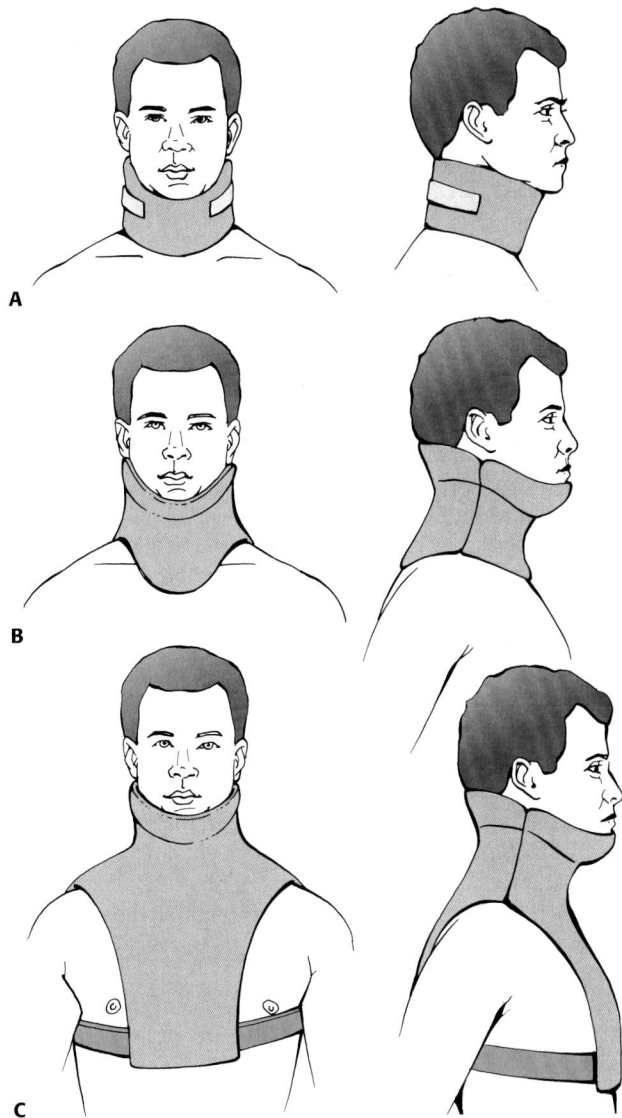

FIGURE 6-29 Different types of cervical braces. **A:** A cervical collar. **B:** A high cervicothoracic orthosis. **C:** A low cervicothoracic orthosis.

spine.[49,60] Their main function is to act as a proprioceptive stimulus to remind patients to take care. Rigid cervical collars may be used for emergency stabilization of the injured cervical spine but the most effective way of stabilizing the cervical spine is by strapping the chin and forehead to a rigid spinal board.

High cervicothoracic orthoses (Fig. 6-29B) have molded occipitomandibular supports that extend to the upper part of the thorax. The best-known example of this orthosis is the Philadelphia collar. Studies indicate that the Philadelphia collar resists 71% of normal cervical flexion and extension, 34% of lateral bending, and 54% of rotation.[60] Other similar orthoses show similar results. These types of braces are useful for the management of cervical sprains or to provide temporary immobilization during transport or after surgical stabilization of the cervical spine.

Low cervicothoracic orthoses have the same molded upper support but extend to the lower part of the thorax (Fig. 6-29C). Examples of these braces are the Minerva and SOMI (sternal–occipital–mandibular immobilizer) braces. Low cervicothoracic orthoses are better than high cervicothoracic orthoses in resisting cervical rotation and sagittal movement in the mid and lower cervical spine but they do not prevent all cervical movement. If any type of neck brace is used to treat an unstable or potentially unstable cervical fracture serial radiographs must be taken to check that fracture reduction is maintained until union.

The complications of cervical braces are essentially the same as those associated with limb braces. As cervical movement is not prevented, loss of fracture reduction may occur in unstable fractures. In addition, a poorly fitting brace may be uncomfortable and cause skin and soft tissue irritation and damage.[60]

Thoracic and Lumbar Braces. The role of thoracolumbar braces is to support the spine by limiting overall trunk motion, decreasing muscular activity, increasing the intra-abdominal pressure, resisting spinal loading, and limiting spinal motion. Several braces are available; the simplest is a lumbosacral corset and the most complex is an individually moulded thoracolumbar–sacral orthosis made from plastic and tightened by buckles and straps (Fig. 6-30). A useful intermediate brace is the Jewett brace (Fig. 6-31), which provides three-point fixation and permits spinal extension but not flexion.

Lumbar corsets, like cervical collars, are essentially proprioceptive and serve to remind the patient to take care. They are used in the management of low back pain but their only use in spinal injury is in the management of minor stable fractures or soft tissue injury. The Jewett brace is useful in the treatment of injuries between T6 and L3, which are unstable in flexion. Studies have shown that it reduces intersegmental motion and flexion at the thoracolumbar joint while lateral bending and axial rotation remain unaffected.[9] They are more effective in

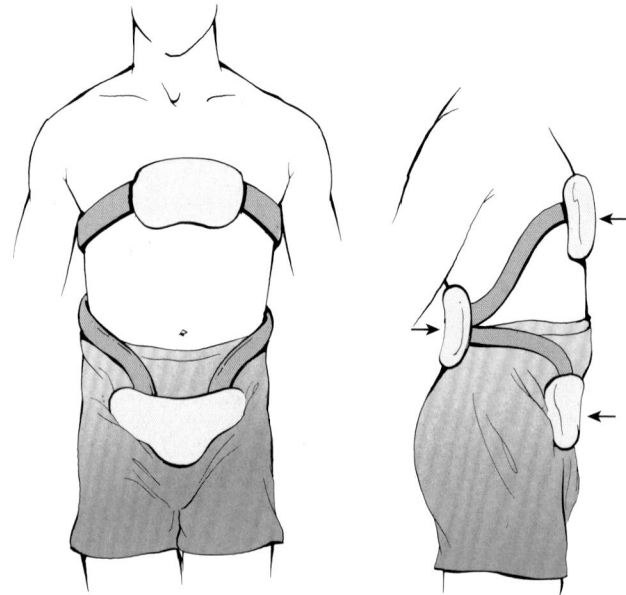
FIGURE 6-31 A Jewett brace.

the treatment of one- and two-column spinal fractures than in the treatment of three-column fractures. Thoracolumbar–sacral orthoses provide more stability but maintenance of reduction of unstable thoracolumbar fractures cannot be guaranteed and serial radiographs are required to confirm the maintenance of fracture reduction.

Casts or Braces?

There has been a lot of debate whether casts or braces are more useful and which gives better results. The debate is mainly centered on tibial diaphyseal fractures, distal radial fractures, and ankle fractures. In ankle fractures the debate has mainly concerned the management of internally fixed fractures in the postoperative phase, whereas in the other fractures surgeons have compared the use of casts and braces in nonoperatively managed patients.

Tibial Diaphyseal Fractures

The comparative usefulness of casts and braces in the treatment of tibial diaphyseal fractures was a subject of considerable debate until about 20 years ago, when intramedullary nailing became the treatment of choice for these fractures. The implication in the literature is that functional bracing produced better results, with Sarmiento and colleagues being particular proponents of functional bracing.[80–82] Table 6-8 shows a comparison of the results of tibial fractures treated with long-leg casts, patellar tendon-bearing casts, and functional bracing. It shows the results of the major papers published between 1965 and 1992, when patellar tendon-bearing casts and functional braces were popular. It must be remembered that the importance of functional outcome following tibial diaphyseal fracture became more widely recognized during this period, and several earlier papers extolled the virtues of their chosen method without analyzing functional outcome to any significant degree.

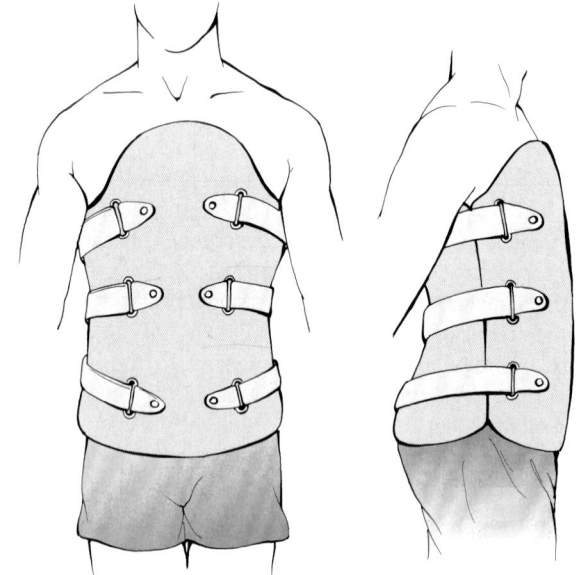
FIGURE 6-30 A thoracolumbarsacral orthosis.

TABLE 6-8	Comparison of Use of Long-Leg Casts, Patellar Tendon-Bearing Casts, and Functional Braces				
	No.	Open (%)	Union (wks)	Malunion (%)	Joint Stiffness (%)
Long-Leg Casts					
Nicoll[63]	674	22.5	15.9	8.6	25.0
Slatis and Rokkanen[90]	198	33.3	19.8	?	?
Karaharju et al.[51]	80	23.7	?	11.2	27.5
Steen Jensen et al.[91]	102	?	?	21.0	7.0
Van der Linden and Larsson[100]	50	12.0	17.0	50.0	24.0
Haines et al.[38]	91	36.3	16.3	25.3	33.0
Kay et al.[52]	79	22.8	19.1	9.1	?
Kyrö et al.[56]	165	21.0	13.7	30.0	42.0
Patellar Tendon-Bearing Casts					
Sarmiento[80]	69	0	13.6	?	?
Austin[4]	132	11.4	16.7	39.0	?
Bostmann and Hanninen[10]	114	16.0	15.3	40.0	?
Puno et al.[73]	141	17.0	16.7	4.4	?
Oni et al.[66]	100	0	?	21.0	43.0
Hooper et al.[46]	33	21.0	18.3	27.3	15.0
Bone et al.[8]	25	0	26.0	27.0	Yes
Functional Braces					
Sarmiento[80]	135	24.4	15.5	?	?
Sarmiento[81]	780	31.0	18.7	13.7	?
Digby et al.[25]	82	20.7	17.4	9.0	45.0
Den Outer et al.[24]	94	11.7	?	40.0	?
Pun et al.[72]	97	7.2	17.1	23.7	28.9
Alho et al.[1]	35	31.4	17.0	8.6	26.0

The papers shown in Table 6-8 that discuss the use of long-leg casts confirm that the method is associated with significant knee stiffness, particularly if used for complex fractures, open fractures, or in fractures that were associated with nonunion. Few modern surgeons would treat open tibial diaphyseal fractures with a long-leg cast but it is interesting to note that Nicoll[63] reported 60% delayed or nonunion in open tibial fractures managed in a long-leg cast in 1965. He also reported 25% joint stiffness rising to 70% in tibial nonunions associated with an open fracture. The results of the use of long-leg casts were reported as late as 1991, when Kyrö et al.[56] analyzed the use of long-leg casts in 165 consecutive tibial fractures. Traction was used in severe open fractures and a calcaneal pin was incorporated into the cast of 23% of the patients. They found that 26% of patients had impaired knee flexion and 9% had impaired knee extension. In addition, 42% had impaired ankle flexion and 37% had impaired toe movement. Only 21% of the patients thought that they had an excellent result. The other papers listed in Table 6-8 show the significant problems of malunion and joint stiffness associated with the use of long-leg casts.

There is no doubt that the use of patellar tendon-bearing casts and functional braces facilitated knee mobilization but it should be remembered that during the period when these methods of management were introduced surgeons had turned to operative treatment for open and more severe closed fractures, and thus the results presented in Table 6-8 for patellar tendon-bearing casts and functional braces may well have been achieved in more straightforward fractures than those treated by long-leg casts in earlier years. However, comparison of the results of tendon-bearing casts with long-leg casts shows a similar prevalence of malunion and probably joint stiffness. Functional braces were introduced to facilitate hindfoot mobility but again one must remember that the patients analyzed in these studies almost certainly had more benign fractures than those treated previously in long-leg casts. Sarmiento et al.[82] analyzed 780 patients treated with a functional brace but selected ambulatory patients and excluded fractures with excessive initial shortening and those that showed an increasing angular deformity in the initial cast. Their results were good but they did not assess malunion or joint stiffness. Table 6-8 shows that other studies have found significant levels of malunion and joint stiffness. Digby et al.[25]

reviewed 103 adult tibial fractures and reported that 11% had restricted ankle motion and 45% had reduced subtalar function. These results match those of the other papers listed in Table 6-8, and it is salutary to observe that a comparison of the three methods of casting and bracing does not show that functional bracing gives superior results, although long-leg casts are associated with greater knee stiffness.

Distal Radial Fractures

Stewart et al.[92] undertook a prospective study comparing a conventional Colles cast with an above-elbow cast brace and a below-elbow cast brace in the treatment of displaced distal radial fractures. In both the above-elbow and below-elbow cast brace they used a dorsal extension of the brace beyond the wrist joint, which extended as far as the metacarpophalangeal joints of the fingers. The brace only extended to the carpometacarpal joint of the thumb. The authors undertook a radiographic and functional analysis of the patients and found no statistical difference in either the radiographic or functional results between the three different methods of management. They also noted no difference in the prevalence of complications between the three groups of patients. They did comment that there was better patient tolerance of casts than braces with the main problem of bracing being pressure over the distal radial border and the head of the ulna. They felt that in most patients there was no reason to change from the traditional Colles cast.

In a later study, Tumia et al.[99] compared the traditional Colles cast with a forearm functional brace that did not have an extension beyond the wrist joint (Fig. 6-24). They treated both minimally displaced fractures, which did not require manipulation, and displaced fractures which did require manipulation. The results were assessed using a functional and anatomical scoring system. They found that the brace-treated patients had lower functional scores than the cast-treated group at 12 weeks, but the difference was not statistically significant. By 24 weeks the results were similar. Grip strength was initially higher in both manipulated and nonmanipulated brace-treated groups, but by 12 weeks there was no difference with cast-managed fractures. There was also more pain associated with the brace during the first 5 weeks, but this settled later. Their conclusion was that a brace could be used effectively in treating Colles fractures. In a similar study O'Connor et al.[65] compared a plastic cast with a lightweight removable splint in 66 patients with minimally displaced radial fractures. They also used both anatomical and functional evaluation systems and found no significant differences between the two groups, but patients tended to prefer the brace.

Ankle Fractures

There have been several studies comparing the use of casts and braces after operative management of ankle fractures. Tropp and Norlin[98] compared the use of a plaster cast for 6 weeks with an ankle brace applied 1 to 2 weeks after surgery. They permitted early weight bearing in both groups and showed that by 10 weeks there was improved function in the brace-managed group. This had disappeared by 12 months but they did report impaired dorsiflexion in the cast group, compared with the functional brace group.

DiStasio et al.[26] examined a group of U.S. military personnel with operatively treated ankle fractures. They compared the use of a nonweight-bearing cast for 6 weeks with the use of a nonweight-bearing removable orthosis, and showed that the orthosis group had better subjective scores for pain, function, cosmesis, and motion 3 and 6 months after injury, but there was no difference in objective assessment of function on return to duty. Simanski et al.[89] compared the use of a functional brace with early weight bearing with a standard cast without weight bearing after ankle fixation. Both groups did well and most of the patients achieved their preinjury level of activity. The authors of both these studies stated that braces were useful but emphasized the requirement of reliable, cooperative patients! In a prospective randomized study Lehtonen et al.[57] compared the use of a below-knee cast and a functional brace in Weber type A and B fractures treated operatively. There were no significant differences between the study groups in the final subjective and objective evaluations, but there were more wound complications in the brace-managed group. In all studies dealing with casts or braces in operatively managed ankle fractures, differences in outcome have been shown to be relatively minor.

The comparative results of the use of casts or braces in tibial diaphyseal fractures, distal radial fractures, and ankle fractures indicate that there is no advantage of either method. The studies suggest return of joint movement is slightly faster if a brace is used but there is no evidence that overall function is better with a brace. There is also some evidence that early complications are higher if a brace is used. The choice between a brace and a cast is determined by the surgeon and patient. Braces are obviously useful. Personal hygiene is easier, and physical therapy, if indicated, can be more easily undertaken, but braces are also more expensive and are not freely available in all countries. The decision should be based on these factors but also on the reliability of the patient. Casts have a great advantage in that they are difficult, although not impossible, to remove and are therefore advantageous in the treatment of many young males in particular!

Slings, Bandages, and Support Strapping

Several types of minor injuries, soft tissue sprains, and minor fractures are treated by support and analgesia with mobilization of the affected area encouraged after a relatively short period. Tubular elastic support bandages are frequently used to treat minor soft tissue injuries such as ankle and foot sprains, wrist sprains, or minor ligament damage in other joints. Several upper limb fractures are treated by the use of slings, which may be supplemented by bandaging.

Fractures of the clavicle, proximal humerus, and radial head and neck are often treated by sling support until the discomfort settles enough to allow joint movement. Several different methods of bandaging have been used to treat clavicle fractures in an effort to reduce pain and maintain fracture reduction. The figure-of-eight bandage remains popular in the treatment of clavicle fractures. This is placed anteriorly around both shoulders and crossed over at the level of the upper thoracic spine. Theoretically, tightening the bandage reduces and stabilizes the fracture, but unfortunately it loosens quickly and clinical evidence suggests that it is no better than a sling.[3] Fractures of

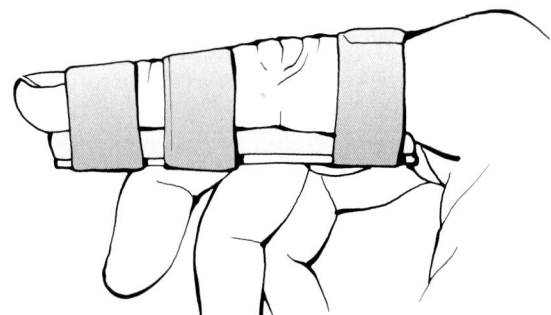

FIGURE 6-34 An aluminium foam-backed splint.

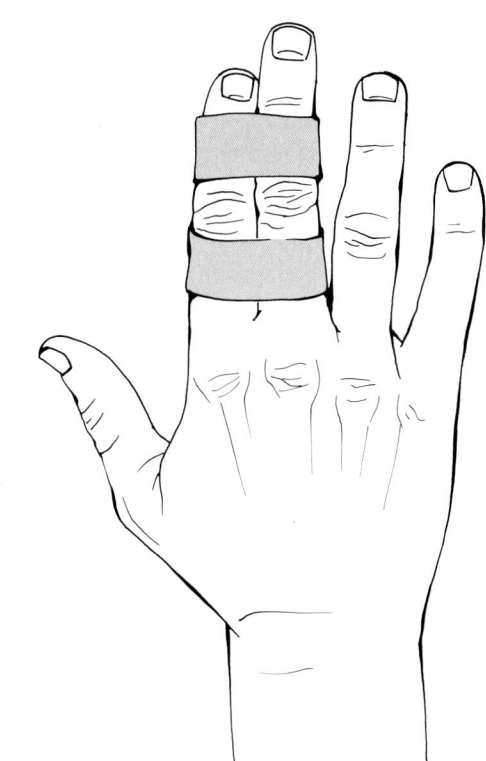

FIGURE 6-32 Buddy strapping.

the clavicle, proximal humerus, and proximal radius that are treated nonoperatively are best treated by the use of a sling for 2 weeks followed by mobilization of the affected joint.

Another area for which strapping is useful is in the management of stable undisplaced fractures of the phalanges of the hand and foot. These fractures can be treated by buddy strapping the affected digit to an adjacent digit (Fig. 6-32). Usually two strips of half-inch tape are placed around the proximal and middle phalanges with protective gauze between the fingers. The joints should be left free to permit mobilization. It should be remembered that this type of strapping loosens quickly and the patient, or companion, should be taught how to replace it.

The use of an elastoplast thumb spica (Fig. 6-33) may be helpful in treating sprains or minor tears of the collateral ligaments of the thumb. It can also be used for treating minor-associated avulsion fractures. These are constructed of elastoplast tape, which is placed around the thumb and extends down to the carpometacarpal area. As with buddy strapping, they tend to loosen quickly and need to be replaced. Neither buddy strapping nor elastoplast spicas should be used to treat unstable fractures.

Splints

Many different splints have been designed, usually for the treatment of metacarpal and phalangeal fractures. The two most popular splints are the aluminium foam-backed splint (Fig. 6-34) and the mallet finger splint (Fig. 6-35). Aluminium foam-backed splint are used for phalangeal fractures. They are commonly applied to the volar or dorsal aspects of the digits to immobilize fractures or joints after reduction of a dislocation. They are also useful for immobilizing the finger after soft tissue injuries, and a volar splint may be particularly helpful for maintaining extension after a volar plate injury. In more unstable fractures the surgeon may elect to use an aluminium foam-backed splint in the same way as a Burkhalter (Fig. 6-18) or James

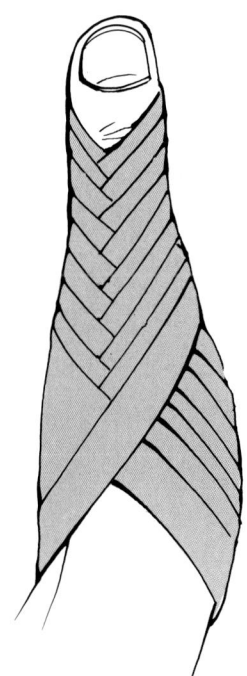

FIGURE 6-33 A thumb spica.

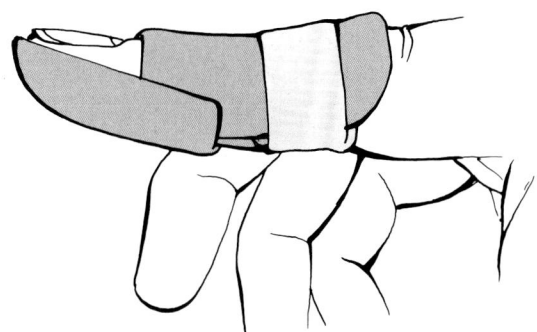

FIGURE 6-35 A mallet finger splint.

(Fig. 6-19) cast might be used. This is appropriate for a single digit fracture and the splint is extended across the wrist joint maintaining the position of the wrist as described for the Burkhalter or James splint.

Mallet fingers caused by either avulsion of the extensor tendons from the distal phalanx or by a fracture of the distal phalanx are well treated by the use of a Mallet finger splint (Fig. 6-35). An appropriately sized splint is applied to the digit with the distal interphalangeal joint in full extension. If this method of management is used the patient is taught that the distal interphalangeal joint must be kept extended for a period of 6 weeks. The main problem with the technique is failure of the patient to follow the treatment protocol, with the splint being removed too early.

SPECIFIC FRACTURES

Upper Limb

Suggested guidelines for the nonoperative management of upper limb fractures are shown in Table 6-9.

Shoulder Girdle

Clavicle. The management of clavicular fractures is described in detail in Chapter 38. Historically most clavicle fractures have been managed nonoperatively (Fig. 6-36A) and

Table 6-2 shows that this continues to be the case. However in recent years there has been considerable interest in primary internal fixation of clavicle fractures, with both plating and intramedullary pinning being used.[14,37,64] Not surprisingly, opinion continues to be divided regarding the best method of treatment. Nordqvist et al.[64] analyzed 225 consecutive clavicle fractures treated nonoperatively and showed that 185 were symptomatic, 39 had moderate pain, and 1 patient had a poor result. There were seven nonunions in displaced fractures. They advocated nonoperative management as did Grassi et al.,[37] who compared nonoperative treatment and intramedullary pinning in 80 clavicle fractures. They found no difference in the outcome scores between the two groups.

More recently the Canadian Orthopaedic Trauma Society[14] pointed out that several studies indicated there was a high prevalence of symptomatic malunion and nonunion after nonoperative management of midshaft clavicle fractures, and they undertook a prospective study comparing plate fixation with nonoperative management in displaced clavicle fractures. They found that the outcome scores were significantly improved in the operatively managed group at all time points and that there was a reduced union time and prevalence of nonunion in the operatively managed fractures. They advocated plate fixation of completely displaced midshaft clavicle fractures in active adult patients.

TABLE 6-9	Guidelines for Nonoperative Management for Different Upper Limb Fractures if Nonoperative Management is Chosen as the Treatment Method
Fracture Type	**Nonoperative Management**
Scapula	Sling and mobilize at 2 wks
Clavicle	Sling and mobilize at 2 wks
Proximal humerus	Sling and mobilize at 2 wks
Humeral diaphysis	Hanging U-slab or sugar-tong cast. Brace at 2–3 wks
Distal humerus	Long-arm cast for 4–8 wks
Olecranon	Long-arm cast for 6 wks
Proximal radius	Sling and mobilize at 2 wks
Forearm diaphysis	
Both bones (undisplaced)	Long-arm cast. Forearm cast at 4 wks
Radius only	Forearm cast 6 wks
Ulna only	Forearm cast 6 wks
Distal radius and ulna	Forearm cast or brace for 6 wks
Scaphoid	Scaphoid cast for 6–12 wks
Other carpal bones	Forearm cast for 3–6 wks
Metacarpal fractures	
Undisplaced	Mobilize
Displaced	Burkhalter or James splint. Mobilize at 3 wks
Phalangeal fractures	
Proximal and middle phalanges	
Undisplaced	Buddy strapping and mobilize
Displaced	Burkhalter, James, or aluminium splint. Mobilize at 3 wks
Distal phalanx	Mobilize or mallet splint

See relevant chapters for suggested management for different fractures.

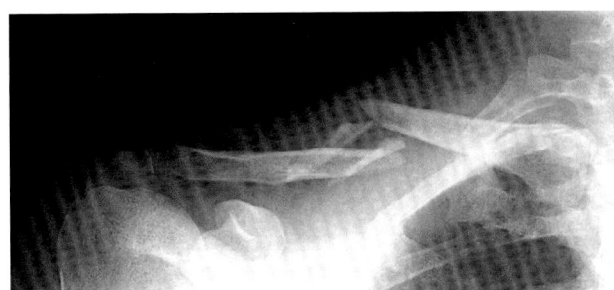
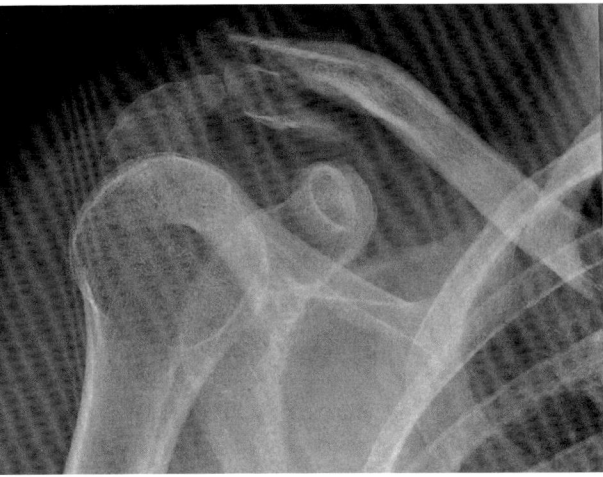

A   **B**

FIGURE 6-36 **A:** A clavicular fracture with a two large intermediate fragments but little shortening. There is debate about whether operative or nonoperative treatment is appropriate for these fractures, but in this case union and good function was successfully achieved with nonoperative management. **B:** A Neer Type I distal clavicle fracture which was treated nonoperatively. Good function was achieved.

It seems likely that more midshaft clavicle fractures will be treated by internal fixation in the future but clearly more work is required to establish the precise indications for operative treatment. As many clavicle fractures are undisplaced or minimally displaced nonoperative management will continue to be an important treatment method and it is important to review the alternative methods of nonoperative management.

Most surgeons use a sling when treating clavicle fractures nonoperatively. The sling is usually maintained for 2 weeks and then physical therapy is started. The historical alternative to the sling was the figure-of-eight bandage. The rationale behind the use of a figure-of-eight bandage was that the shoulders were extended and fracture reduction thereby facilitated, but comparative studies have shown no advantage of the figure-of-eight bandage over a simple sling. Andersen et al.[3] actually found that the sling caused less discomfort and fewer complications. If nonoperative management is used to treat a clavicle fracture, it is suggested that a sling should be worn for about 2 weeks and then a physical therapy regime instituted.

Approximately 28% of clavicle fractures occur in the distal third of the bone (Fig. 6-36B).[76] As with midshaft clavicle fractures, there has been debate about how lateral clavicular fractures should be treated, with interest concentrating on the Neer type 2 distal clavicle fractures associated with transection of the coronoid and trapezoid ligaments. The treatment of the condition will be discussed in detail in Chapter 38, but the literature suggests that nonoperative management is a good alternative for many lateral third clavicle fractures, particularly in middle-aged and elderly patients.[76,77] As with mid-diaphyseal clavicle fractures, if nonoperative management is chosen to treat a distal clavicle fracture a sling should be used for 2 weeks and a physical therapy regime then commenced.

Scapula Fractures. Scapula fractures are very rare and are predominantly treated nonoperatively. The implication is that they occur in high-energy injuries and they have been documented to occur in 7% of multiple-injured patients.[102] However, Chapter 3 shows that they actually have a type A distribution with a proportion of scapula fractures occurring in the elderly and, in general, nonoperative treatment will be used.

There are four basic types of scapula fractures: Intra-articular and extra-articular glenoid fractures, acromion fractures, coracoid fractures, and fractures of the scapula body (Fig. 6-37).

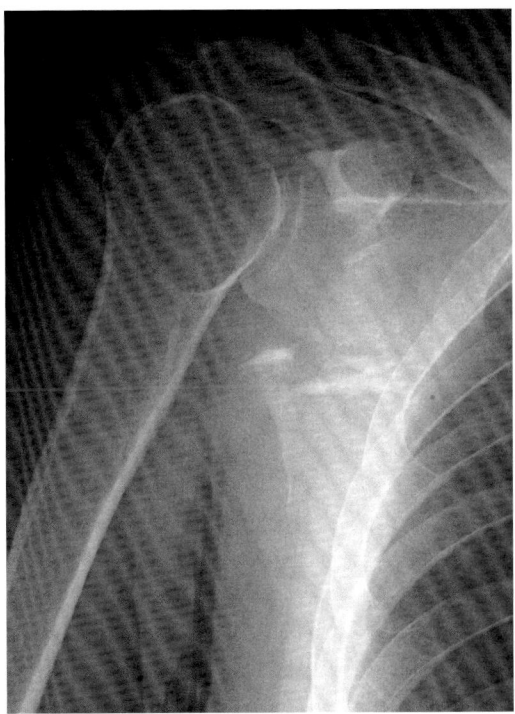

FIGURE 6-37 A fracture of the scapular body and neck in a 52-year-old male. Nonoperative management was used and the patient had a good result although he had some pain at the extremes of shoulder movement.

Most scapular fractures do not require operative management, the obvious exception being the displaced glenoid rim fracture associated with instability of the glenohumeral joint. Most coracoid and acromion fractures are undisplaced and few require surgical treatment. In addition, there is little evidence that scapular body fractures need operative treatment, with a meta-analysis of scapula fractures showing that 99% of body fractures were treated nonoperatively.[106] The same study also showed that the literature indicates that 83% of scapula neck fractures are treated nonoperatively.[106] Van Noort and van Kampen[101] examined 13 patients with scapula neck fractures and found an average Constant score[18] of 90 after nonoperative management with no correlation between functional outcome and malunion. Pace et al.[68] confirmed the good outcome associated with nonoperative management but pointed out that most patients had some activity-related pain and minor cuff tendinopathy which, they thought, related to glenoid neck malunion.

It is likely that most scapula fractures will continue to be treated nonoperatively and if this method of treatment is chosen, it is suggested a sling is used for about 2 weeks to provide pain relief, following which a physical therapy program should be instituted. Scapular fractures are discussed in detail in Chapter 39.

Floating Shoulder. The term "floating shoulder" is given to a combination of clavicle and scapular neck fractures. It was initially felt that clavicle stabilization would minimize scapular neck malunion[44] but later papers suggest that nonoperative treatment of the floating shoulder gives equivalent or better results. Egol et al.[29] compared operative and nonoperative management and showed no significant difference between the two methods. They did note that internal and external rotation was weaker in the operatively treated group although there was improved forward flexion in this group. Edwards et al.[28] reported similar results but stressed that more severely displaced fractures were associated with poorer results. Thus the literature suggests that most floating shoulders should be treated nonoperatively using a sling for 2 weeks followed by a course of physical therapy.

Proximal Humeral Fractures

Most proximal humeral fractures are treated nonoperatively (Fig. 6-38) and a comparison with the prevalence of surgery in the 1950s (Table 6-6) suggests that there was little change for a considerable period. The recent introduction of locking plates has increased the rate of surgical treatment but this must be balanced against the increasing age and infirmity of the elderly population who tend to present with this fracture. It seems logical to assume that most proximal humeral fractures will continue to be treated nonoperatively for the foreseeable future. The overall management of this fracture is discussed in Chapter 37.

The debate about the treatment of proximal humeral fractures is centered around three- and four-part fractures and fracture dislocations, which comprise about 12.5% of proximal humeral fractures.[20] Neer[61] stated that 85% of proximal humeral fractures were minimally displaced fractures, although a more recent study showed that 49% of proximal humeral

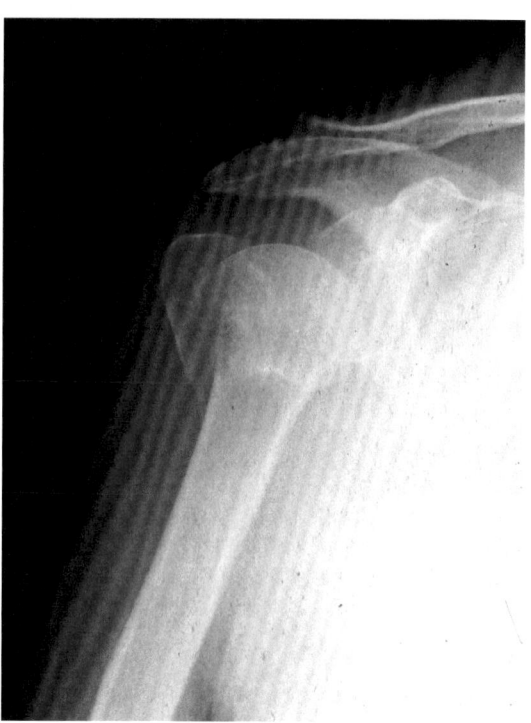

FIGURE 6-38 A three-part valgus impacted (OTA B1.1) proximal humeral fracture presenting in a 78-year-old female. This united and at 1 year the Neer score was 84 and the Constant score was 74.

fractures were minimally displaced.[19] The difference probably relates to the increased incidence of osteopenic and osteoporotic fractures in the population since Neer's study. These fractures should be managed nonoperatively. There is debate about the management of two-part fractures, particularly with the introduction of the locking proximal humeral plate, but these plates have only been partially successful[67] and it seems likely that many two-part fractures will continue to be managed nonoperatively. If further information about the results of nonoperative treatment of two-part proximal humeral fractures and fracture dislocations is required, the 1-year Neer[61] and Constant[18] scores of all two-part fractures classified according to the OTA classification has been published.[22] Figure 6-38 shows an impacted valgus three-part B1.1 fracture in a 78-year-old female who had a good result with nonoperative management.

Nonoperative management is undertaken by placing the patient in a sling for 2 weeks and then gradually introducing a program of physical therapy. The patient should be warned that progress is slow and that it is often more than 1 year before maximum shoulder motion is regained.

Humeral Diaphyseal Fractures

Table 6-2 shows that together with isolated ulnar diaphyseal fractures, humeral diaphyseal fractures are the only diaphyseal fractures that are now commonly treated nonoperatively. Table 6-2 also shows that there is a significant age difference between the patients treated operatively and those treated nonoperatively, with younger patients tending to be treated operatively.

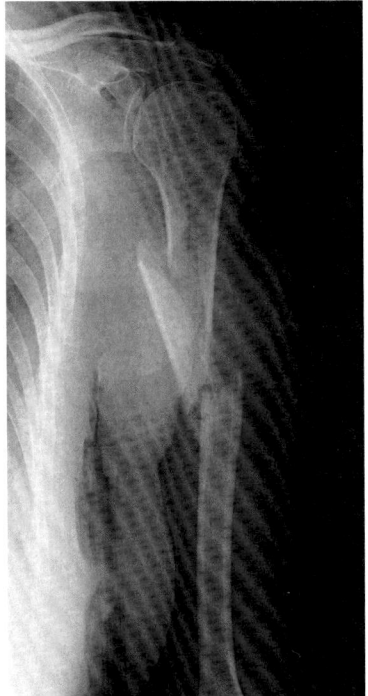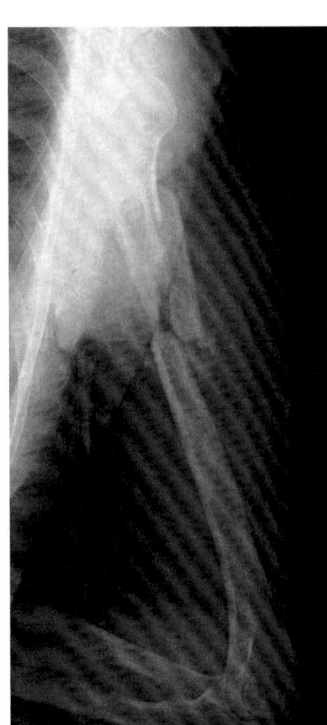

FIGURE 6-39 AP and lateral radiographs of an OTA B2.1 humeral diaphyseal fracture in a 68-year-old patient. The fracture extends into the proximal humerus. It was treated by the application of a U-slab followed by a brace and union occurred.

About two-thirds of patients with humeral diaphyseal fractures are treated nonoperatively (Fig. 6-39) and this figure is supported by an analysis of the literature. In 1988, Zagorski et al.[105] reported on the use of a functional brace in humeral diaphyseal fracture. They analyzed 170 patients and showed that 167 had excellent or good functional results. Since then, further studies[30,33,47,74,78,96] have accepted that nonoperative management gives good results but they have tried to analyze which fractures, if any, are better treated surgically. Clearly open fractures, irreducible fractures, pathologic fractures, fractures in the multiply injured, and floating elbows may well be treated surgically, but Ekholm et al.[30] also noted that OTA type A fractures seemed to have a high prevalence of nonunion and often required revision surgery. Ring et al.[74] took a similar view stating that spiral or oblique fractures that involved the middle or proximal third had a high rate of nonunion after treatment with a functional brace. Toivanen et al.[96] treated 93 consecutive fractures with a brace but found that 23% required surgery. Again they found a higher rate of nonunion in proximal third diaphyseal fractures.

The other disadvantage of nonoperative management that has been highlighted recently is impairment of shoulder function. Fjalestad et al.[33] reported that 38% of patients treated with a humeral brace lost external rotation of the shoulder, which they attributed to malrotation at the fracture site. Rosenberg and Soudry[78] analyzed 15 patients treated by bracing and showed that the Constant shoulder scores were significantly lower in the injured shoulder. The average age was only 43 years and only 40% of the patients returned to their previous professional activities.

There has been a particular interest in bracing fractures of the distal third of the humeral diaphysis. Fracture alignment can be difficult to maintain and there is concern about elbow stiffness.[47]

Sarmiento et al.[83] analyzed 85 distal third fractures, of which 15% were open. They recorded 96% union with no infections. In a recent study Jawa et al.[47] compared operative and nonoperative management and found very similar results between them, although they stated that operative treatment gives more predictable alignment and potentially a quicker return of function, although there was as risk of nerve damage and infection.

It seems likely that the prevalence of surgical treatment of humeral diaphyseal fractures will increase. As studies have become more refined it is becoming apparent that there are advantages to surgery in some fractures. Nonoperative management will probably continue to be an important method of management for reducible middle third closed fractures but other fracture types will probably be treated operatively more frequently than they are now. If nonoperative management is selected, it is suggested that a U-slab or sugar-tong cast is used for about 2 weeks and a functional brace then applied. The brace is usually used for 8 to 12 weeks with serial radiographs used to determine union. Active elbow motion is usually allowed by about 4 weeks. The treatment of humeral diaphyseal fractures is discussed in Chapter 36.

Distal Humeral Fractures

It is perhaps surprising to see that Table 6-2 shows that only 50% of distal humeral fractures were treated nonoperatively in a major trauma center in a 1-year period. However, Table 6-3 shows there is a considerable difference in surgery based on the OTA classification. A review of the OTA Type A extra-articular distal humeral fractures shows that nonoperative management was mainly reserved for undisplaced or minimally displaced epicondylar fractures or supracondylar fractures in the elderly (Fig. 6-40). Most OTA Type B and C fractures were treated

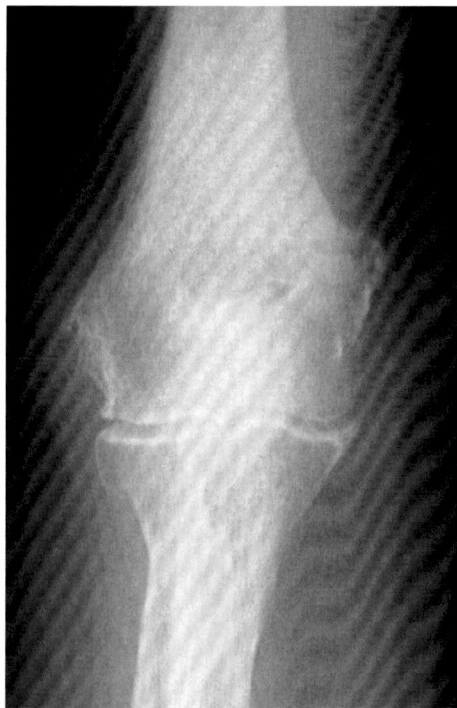
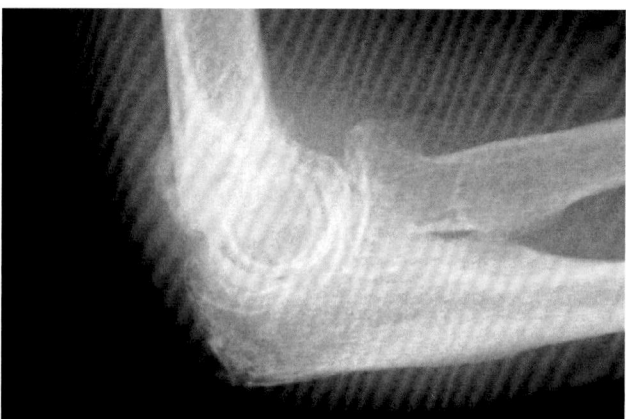

FIGURE 6-40 AP and lateral radiographs of an OTA A2.3 undisplaced supracondylar humeral fracture in an 89-year-old patient. Union occurred with nonoperative management but there is a high rate of nonunion in displaced supracondylar fractures.

operatively. The average age of the patients with Type C fractures who were treated nonoperatively was 92 years! Thus most displaced distal humeral fractures are treated operatively.

There is little literature dealing with type A extra-articular distal humeral fractures. A1 fractures affecting the epicondyle tend to occur in younger patients and A2 and A3 supracondylar fractures tend to occur in the elderly. There is debate about whether these should be managed nonoperatively as there is a relatively high rate of nonunion. However it is likely that undisplaced Type A distal humeral fractures will continue to be treated nonoperatively. If nonoperative management is used for A1 fractures, a long-arm cast should be used for 4 to 6 weeks. If an A2 or A3 fracture is treated in the elderly the cast may need to be worn for up to 8 weeks. Distal humeral fractures are discussed in Chapter 35.

Proximal Forearm Fractures

Proximal Radial Fractures. Table 6-2 shows that most radial head and neck fractures continue to be treated nonoperatively, and a review of Table 6-6 suggests that the treatment has changed little for many years. The 6.3% primary surgery listed in Table 6-2 related mainly to complex fracture dislocations of the elbow and the relatively uncommon OTA C2 and C3 fractures. Most surgeons accept that most proximal radial fractures should be treated nonoperatively. If nonoperative management is used, all that is required is a sling with joint movement being started as soon as pain permits.

Olecranon Fractures. Table 6-2 shows that most olecranon fractures are treated by internal fixation. It also shows

that those fractures treated nonoperatively tended to occur in younger patients. Nonoperative treatment is usually used for undisplaced fractures or if there is only a minor avulsion fracture from the tip of the olecranon. If nonoperative management is used for a potentially unstable olecranon fracture, a long-arm cast should be applied for 6 weeks following which a physical therapy regime is instituted. If there is a minor avulsion fracture from the tip of the olecranon treatment should be symptomatic and mobilization commenced about 2 weeks after fracture. The treatment of proximal forearm fractures is discussed in Chapter 34.

Forearm Fractures

Most forearm fractures are treated by internal fixation as detailed in Chapter 33. Table 6-2 shows that over 80% of isolated radial diaphyseal and 90% of radial and ulna diaphyseal fractures will be treated operatively. The only exceptions are stable undisplaced fractures, which can be treated in a cast or brace. Isolated ulna diaphyseal fractures are frequently treated nonoperatively, with Table 6-2 indicating that about 30% are treated operatively. Many isolated ulna diaphyseal fractures are undisplaced or minimally displaced and the use of a cast or brace will give good results. Sarmiento et al.[84] reported on 287 ulnar shaft fractures and recorded 99% union. They found that proximal third ulna fractures were associated with an average loss of pronation of 12 degrees but overall there were good or excellent results in 96% of patients. If nonoperative management is used for undisplaced fractures of the radius and ulna, a long-arm cast should be applied, which can be converted to a

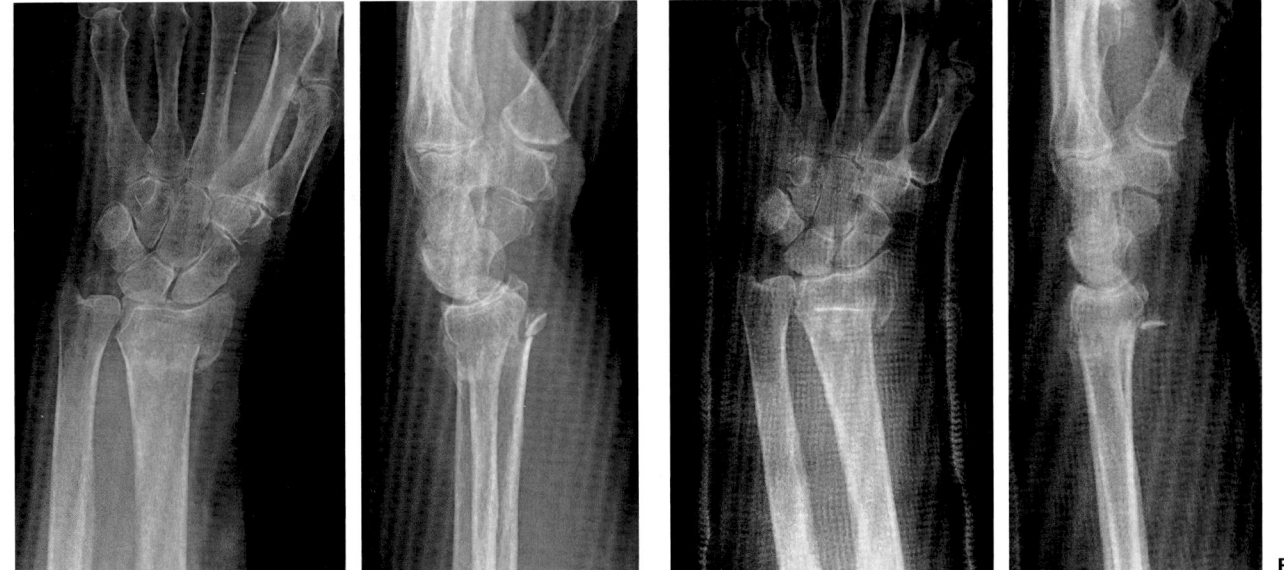

FIGURE 6-41 **A:** AP and lateral radiographs of a distal radial fracture in a frail 70-year-old female. Note the presence of dorsal and volar comminution. **B:** Closed manipulation was undertaken and AP and lateral radiographs at 6 weeks show that good alignment has been maintained although there is some radial shortening. Good function was achieved.

forearm cast or brace at about 6 weeks if further immobilization is required. For undisplaced isolated fractures of the radius, a forearm cast or brace can be used, usually for 6 weeks, and if isolated ulna fractures are to be treated nonoperatively a forearm cast or brace can be applied for 6 weeks.

Distal Radial Fractures

Table 6-2 shows that about 70% of distal radial fractures are treated nonoperatively (Fig. 6-41) and Table 6-5 shows that there has been an increase in operative management over the years. There is an increased appreciation of the importance of fracture reduction and carpal alignment and progressively more distal radial fractures are being treated operatively. The introduction of locked plates and different types of external fixation has altered the management of these fractures but a substantial proportion of distal radial fractures are stable and will continue to be managed nonoperatively. As with other osteopenic and osteoporotic fractures the epidemiology of distal radial fractures will change significantly in a rapidly aging population, who will present with more medical comorbidities. As a result of changing patient demographics it may well be that more distal radial fractures will be treated nonoperatively in the future. Distal radial fracture treatment is discussed in Chapter 32.

If a stable distal radial fracture is to be treated nonoperatively, a forearm cast or brace should be applied for 6 weeks, and following removal a physical education program instituted. If an unstable fracture is to be treated nonoperatively, reduction needs to be undertaken using a hematoma block, regional block, or general anesthetic. The classic reduction technique is to apply traction, flexion, and ulnar deviation and to check the fracture position on radiographs or fluoroscopy. If the fracture does not reduce, the Agee maneuver can be used (Fig. 6-42).

Once the fracture has been reduced a dorsal slab or short forearm cast is applied. The fracture must be x-rayed 7 to 10 days after the initial reduction to check that the reduction has been maintained. If it has not been maintained, the surgeon must

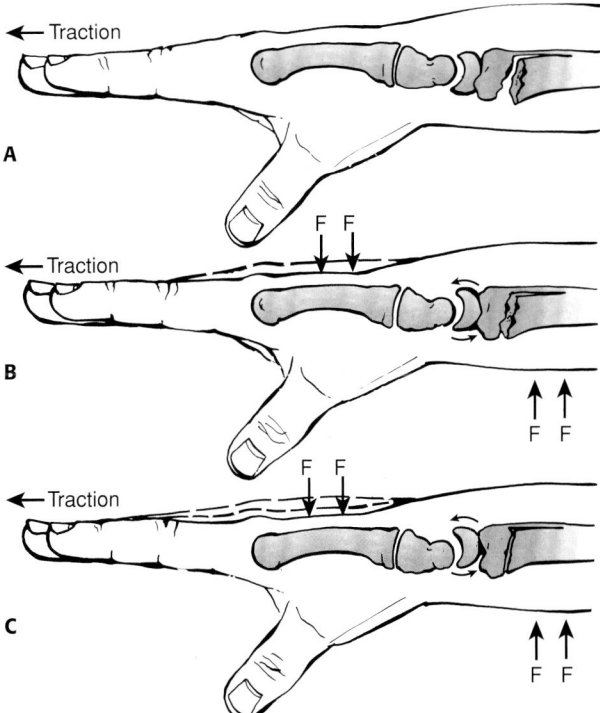

FIGURE 6-42 The Agee maneuver. This places a volar translation force on the distal radial fragment, which allows the lunate to tilt the distal fragment in a volar direction.

decide on further fracture management based on the age of the patient, his or her functional state, and the presence of medical comorbidities. Remanipulation is generally unsuccessful in older patients, and in most cases of redisplacement the surgeon will have to consider operative treatment, although in very elderly demented patients the fracture will often be left in the malreduced position. If the fracture position is maintained the cast or slab is completed and worn for 6 weeks. Alternatively, a functional brace can be used. Following removal of the cast or brace, a physical therapy regime should be instituted.

Carpal Fractures

Table 6-2 shows that about 15% of carpal fractures are treated surgically, and Table 6-5 indicates that the prevalence of operative treatment has recently increased. There has been increasing interest in primary scaphoid fixation after fracture and it seems likely that the number of scaphoid fractures treated surgically will increase. However, many scaphoid fractures are stable fractures and it is likely that nonoperative management will continue to be popular. A recent analysis[20] showed that scaphoid fractures comprise about 82% of carpal fractures suggesting that nonoperative management for carpal fractures will continue to be used. A further 9% of carpal fractures were triquetral fractures, which are also treated nonoperatively. Complex carpal fractures and dislocations do require surgical treatment but are relatively uncommon.

If nonoperative management is used a scaphoid cast is applied (Fig. 6-17). It usually needs to be worn for 6 to 8 weeks but union can be slow and the cast may need to be worn for up to 12 weeks. If other carpal fractures are treated a cast or brace is usually worn for 3 to 6 weeks, depending on the type of fracture. Flake fractures of the triquetrum usually require only 3 weeks in a forearm cast. The treatment of carpal fractures is discussed in Chapter 31.

Metacarpal Fractures

Metacarpal fractures are very unusual in that it would seem that they are more frequently treated nonoperatively than they were 60 years ago, despite the availability of screws, mini-plates and mini-fixators. Table 6-2 shows than only about 11% of metacarpal fractures had primary operative treatment in 2000 in a major trauma unit. It is likely that the reduction in operative treatment relates to improved industrial and workplace safety legislation in many countries. Crushed hands are much less common than in the post World War II period and an analysis of metacarpal fractures in 2000 shows that they are mainly low-energy fractures with about 50% being caused by a direct blow. About 60% of fractures affect the little finger metacarpal (Fig. 6-43) and 54% of these affect the metacarpal neck.[20]

Nonoperative treatment of isolated stable undisplaced or minimally displaced metacarpal fractures usually involves the use of buddy strapping and mobilization, although not infrequently no supportive strapping is actually required at all. If closed reduction is required, it can be achieved by flexing the metacarpophalangeal joint to 90 degrees and using the proximal phalanx to push the metacarpal head dorsally and to control rotation. This is known as the Jahss technique. The indications

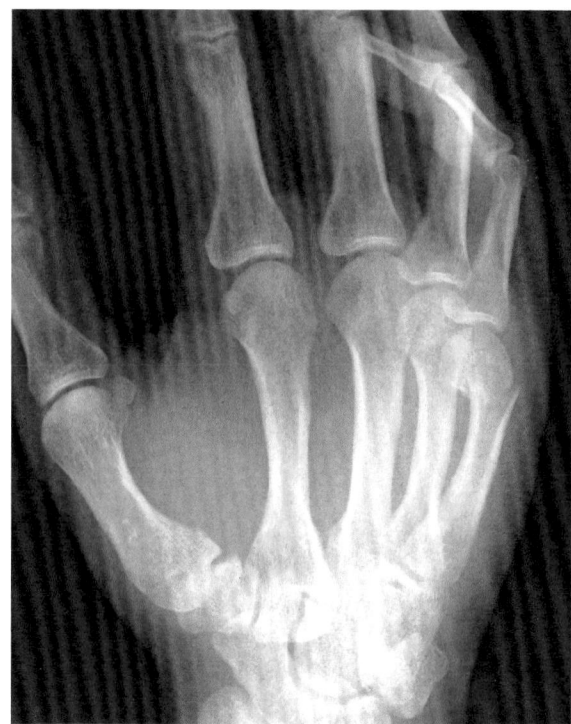

FIGURE 6-43 A fracture of the neck of the little finger metacarpal. Most of these fractures are treated nonoperatively.

for fracture reduction mainly relate to angulation, rotation, and shortening and are discussed in Chapter 30. Surgeons may elect to treat malreduced or unstable fractures operatively but if nonoperative management is undertaken a Burkhalter or James type of cast or splint should be used. These are usually maintained for about 3 weeks, following which a physical therapy regime is organized. Fractures of the neck, diaphyses, and bases of metacarpals are similarly treated but basal fractures or fracture dislocations of the thumb metacarpal may well be treated by the application of a Brunner cast, which may be maintained for 4 to 6 weeks.

Phalangeal Fractures

The prevalence of operative treatment of phalangeal fractures is similar to metacarpal fractures (Table 6-2) and, as with metacarpal fractures, comparison with Emmett and Breck's data from 60 years ago[31] shows that we seem to operate less now. Presumably, as with metacarpal fractures, this is because the incidence of crushed hands and severe hand injuries has declined mainly as a result of improved workplace legislation. As with metacarpal fractures, many phalangeal fractures are stable (Fig. 6.44) and require no more than buddy strapping or the application of an aluminium foam–backed splint to minimize pain and the possibility of secondary displacement. If phalangeal fractures are stable after reduction they can be treated by the application of a Burkhalter- or James-type splint, or by the use of a longer aluminium foam-backed splint bent to maintain the finger in the same position as achieved by the splint. Again the splint will be maintained for 2 to 3 weeks.

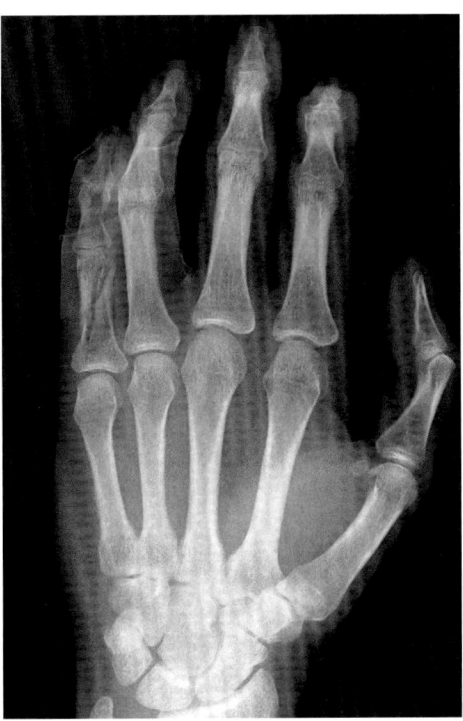

FIGURE 6-44 A comminuted fracture of the proximal phalanx of the little finger. This was treated with an aluminium foam-backed splint. Good alignment and function was achieved.

Fractures of the distal phalanges are frequently treated nonoperatively. Tuft fractures and closed diaphyseal fractures tend to be stable and are often treated by local splintage for pain relief. Basal fractures of the distal phalanx are often unstable but can frequently be treated in full extension on a splint for 4 weeks. Bony mallet injuries are treated similarly in a mallet splint. The treatment of phalangeal fractures is discussed in Chapter 30.

Lower Limb Fractures

Suggested guidelines for the nonoperative treatment of lower limb fractures are shown in Table 6-10.

Proximal Femoral Fractures

Table 6-2 indicates that proximal femoral fractures are treated operatively unless the patient's medical condition means that surgery is contraindicated. In undisplaced intracapsular femoral neck fractures, there is a higher prevalence of nonunion, avascular necrosis, and fracture displacement in nonoperatively treated fractures.[20] In addition, nonoperative management means that an elderly patient, often with significant medical comorbidities, is confined to bed for 4 to 6 weeks, which is clearly undesirable. The only proximal femoral fracture for which nonoperative management may be the treatment of choice is the greater trochanter fracture, when there may be little or no displacement. Even in these fractures, surgeons should be aware that there may be an intertrochanteric extension.

TABLE 6-10	Guidelines for Nonoperative Management for Different Lower Limb Fractures if Nonoperative Management is Chosen as the Treatment Method

Fracture Type	Nonoperative Management
Pelvis	
Insufficiency fracture (elderly patient)	Mobilize as pain permits
APC Type 1 and LC Type 1	Mobilize as pain permits
Undisplaced acetabulum (except trans-tectal type)	Mobilize as pain permits
Proximal femur	Not recommended
Femoral diaphysis	Not recommended
Distal femur (undisplaced)	Hinged knee brace for 6–8 wks
Patella (undisplaced)	Long-leg cylinder cast or brace. Mobilize at 4–6 wks
Proximal tibia (undisplaced)	Hinged knee brace for 6–8 wks
Tibial diaphysis	Long-leg cast. Patellar tendon-bearing cast or brace at 4–6 wks
Distal tibia (undisplaced)	Lower leg cast or brace for 6–8 wks
Ankle	Lower leg cast or brace for 6 wks
Talus	Lower leg cast or brace for 6 wks
Calcaneus	Lower leg cast or brace for 6 wks
Midfoot	Lower leg cast or brace for 4–6 wks
Metatarsus	Mobilize or lower leg cast or brace for 4–6 wks
Toes	Buddy strapping and mobilize

See relevant chapters for suggested management for different fractures.

Lesser trochanter fractures are very rare but may be treated nonoperatively. In older patients these fractures should be assumed to be metastatic fractures until proven otherwise. The treatment of proximal femoral fractures is discussed in Chapters 48 to 50.

Femoral Diaphyseal Fractures

Femoral diaphyseal fractures should no longer be treated non-operatively unless the patient is not fit for surgery or the facilities to allow operative treatment are unavailable. The results from nonoperative treatment are significantly inferior to operative management. If nonoperative management is used then one of the methods of traction illustrated in Figure 6-4 should be used. There is probably no other fracture in which there is such a strong consensus in favor of one treatment method, and intramedullary nailing is generally used for all femoral diaphyseal fractures. The management of femoral diaphyseal fractures in discussed in Chapter 52.

Distal Femoral Fractures

Table 6-2 shows that most distal femoral fractures are treated operatively, which is what one would expect, although in recent years there has been a significant change in the epidemiology of distal femoral fractures. These fractures now commonly occur in the elderly, with the epidemiologic review in Chapter 3 giving an average age of 55.3 years in males and 69.6 years in females for patients with this fracture. Many of the patients who present with distal femoral fractures have other medical comorbidities. A review of the 39.1% of distal femoral fractures that were treated nonoperatively as detailed in Table 6-2 shows that virtually all were undisplaced fractures in older or clinically unwell patients. Thus, nonoperative management is now mainly used for low-energy undisplaced fractures that usually occur in elderly patients. Nonoperative management will usually involve the application of a long-leg cast for about 4 weeks following which a hinged knee brace can be applied. As fractures treated nonoperatively are usually undisplaced, union may be fairly rapid. This is particularly true for OTA type B partial articular fractures (Fig. 6-45), which are not infrequently undisplaced or minimally displaced. Under these circumstances a cast or brace may well only need to be used for 6 to 8 weeks. The treatment of distal femoral fractures is detailed in Chapter 53.

Patella Fractures

Patella fractures are discussed in Chapter 54. Most occur in older patients as a result of a fall.[20] Therefore, undisplaced or minimally displaced patella fractures are relatively common and these are usually treated nonoperatively. Table 6-2 shows that about 35% to 40% of patella fractures are treated operatively, these being the more serious fractures. Nonoperative management usually involves the use of a long-leg cylinder cast or brace, which is worn for about 6 weeks. A physical therapy program is then instituted.

Proximal Tibial Fractures

Proximal tibial fractures have a somewhat unusual distribution with a bimodal distribution in both males and females (Chapter 3). About 48% of the fractures detailed in Table 6-2 were high-energy injuries that occurred in younger patients, which explains the higher incidence of operative treatment with

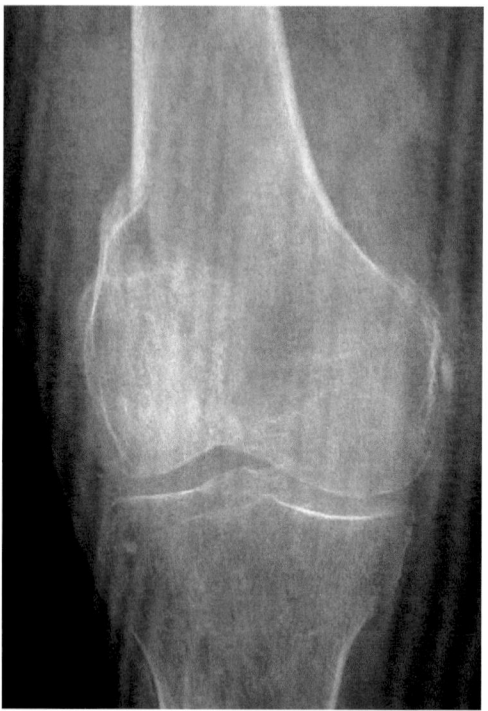
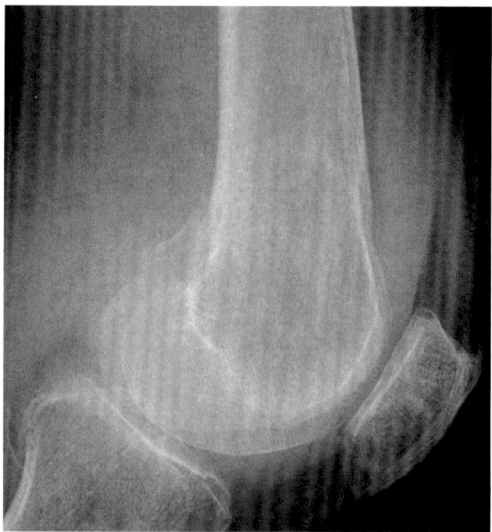

FIGURE 6-45 AP and lateral radiographs of an OTA B1.1 lateral condylar fracture in an 82-year-old female with significant medical comorbidities who did not mobilize. It was treated with a long-leg cast.

almost 70% of patients being treated operatively. As with distal femoral fractures, the patients treated nonoperatively tend to present with undisplaced or minimally displaced fractures. If nonoperative management is used for proximal tibial fractures, a hinged knee brace should be applied for 6 to 8 weeks. If this is unavailable a long-leg cylinder cast can be used. The treatment of proximal tibial fractures is discussed in Chapter 55.

Tibial Diaphyseal Fractures

The treatment of tibial diaphyseal fractures has changed considerably in the last 20 years. The treatment of these fractures was the subject of much debate until relatively recently. Long-leg casts, patellar tendon-bearing casts and functional braces have all been used to treat both closed and open tibial diaphyseal fractures (Table 6-8) but the results were relatively poor and intramedullary nailing has become the treatment of choice for these fractures. This is discussed in Chapter 57. Table 6-2 shows that about 94% of tibial diaphyseal fractures were treated operatively in Edinburgh, with nonoperative management being mainly reserved for stable OTA A3.1 transverse tibial fractures with an intact fibula that occur mainly in younger patients. These unite quickly and are treated in a below-knee cast.

If nonoperative management is to be used for an unstable tibial diaphyseal fracture it is recommended that a long-leg cast is applied initially and that a patellar tendon-bearing cast or brace be applied after 4 to 6 weeks. Serial radiographs will be required to determine when union has occurred and, therefore, when to remove the cast. Traction should not be used to stabilize tibial diaphyseal fractures as it is associated with increased intracompartmental pressure and the effects of prolonged bed rest. There is now no indication for traction. If internal fixation cannot be used to treat a tibial diaphyseal fracture, external fixation is usually possible.

Distal Tibial Fractures

Much of the literature dealing with distal tibial or pilon fractures concerns displaced high-energy fractures occurring in younger patients. These fractures are treated operatively as detailed in Chapter 58. Further analysis of the distal tibial fractures shown in Table 6-2 shows that about 40% of them were OTA type A extra-articular fractures and 31% were OTA type B partial articular fractures. Table 6-3 shows the prevalence of surgery in the different OTA fracture types, and it can be seen that while most type B and all type C fractures are treated operatively only 30% of type A fractures were treated surgically. Of these patients, 47% were 14 to 16 years of age and had physeal fractures, and the remaining 53% had an average age of 59 years and presented mainly with low-energy undisplaced or minimally displaced fractures. Thus, as with other lower limb fractures, there is a distinct difference in fracture treatment based on age, mode of injury, and fracture displacement. If nonoperative management is to be used for an undisplaced or a minimally displaced type A or type B pilon fracture, a nonweight-bearing below-knee cast or brace is adequate and it may need to be worn for 8 to 10 weeks depending on the speed of union. In younger patients with physeal fractures the use of a cast or brace for 4 to 6 weeks is adequate.

Ankle Fractures

Table 6-2 shows that overall about 40% of ankle fractures are treated operatively. As has already been pointed out, the prevalence of operative treatment of metaphyseal and intra-articular fractures varies with the degree of severity of the fracture as defined by the OTA classification (Table 6-3). This principle also applies to ankle fractures, although their OTA classification is somewhat different from the classifications of the fractures shown in Table 6-3. Further analysis of the ankle fractures shown in Table 6-2 shows that about 12% of type A infrasyndesmotic fractures were treated operatively, these mainly being isolated medial malleolar fractures. This compares with 49% of transsyndesmotic type B fractures and 70% of suprasyndesmotic type C fractures. Thus most type A and about half of type B fractures will be treated nonoperatively. A review of the patients who present with type C fractures but were treated nonoperatively shows that most had external rotation rather than abduction injuries and it was felt that the posterior tibiofibula ligaments were intact. They were considered to be stable after the application of a cast. If this method of management is chosen, serial radiographs must be undertaken to make sure there is no evidence of late syndesmotic widening.

Analysis of the type B fractures shows that 84.3% of the bimalleolar fractures and 94.3% of the trimalleolar fractures were treated operatively. A review of the lateral malleolar fracture associated with talar shift, the OTA B2.1 fracture, showed that 91.4% of fractures were treated operatively but an analysis of the prevalence of operative management in the common OTA B1.1 spiral lateral malleolar fracture caused by external rotation shows that only 16.8% of these fractures were treated operatively. It is important to realize that B1.1 fractures associated with 2 to 3 mm of displacement do not require operative treatment and that an excellent result can be obtained with cast or brace management (Fig. 6-46).[5,54] Care must be taken to be certain that the patient does not actually have an OTA B2.1 fracture with talar shift, and radiographs should be obtained after the application of the cast and at 2 weeks to check for this. If nonoperative ankle fracture treatment is undertaken a below-knee cast or brace is applied for 6 weeks. Many surgeons do not permit weight bearing for 6 weeks after cast application but there is no good evidence to support this regime[41] and weight bearing can be allowed in most ankle fractures. Ankle fractures are discussed in Chapter 59.

Talar Fractures

Fractures of the talus are relatively uncommon, but Table 6-2 shows that about 50% are treated operatively. A review of the epidemiology of talar fractures has shown that about 70% are body fractures and 30% are neck fractures.[20] Further analysis of the body fractures shows that about 42% are shear or crush injuries but 50% are fractures of the lateral or posterior processes, which are often treated nonoperatively. Undisplaced fractures of the talar body are relatively rare but can be treated nonoperatively (Fig. 6-47).

A review of the talar neck fractures showed that about 30% were Hawkins type I[43] fractures, which are also commonly treated

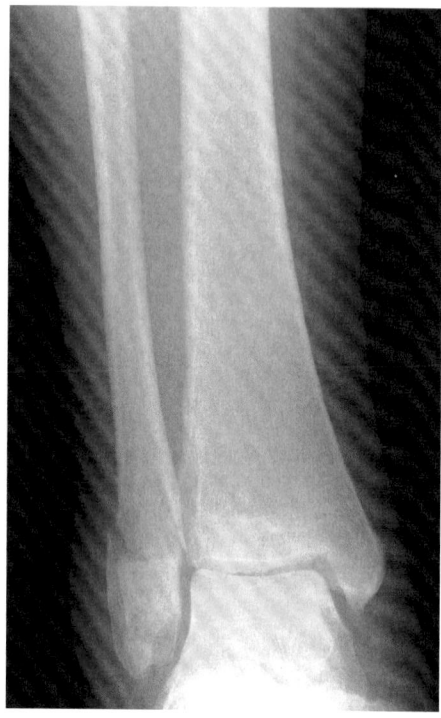
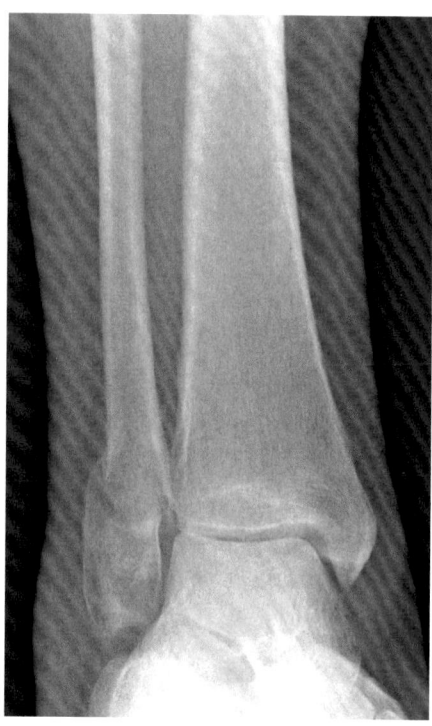

A

B

FIGURE 6-46 **A:** An OTA B1.1 ankle fracture in a 50-year-old female. Note the slight lateral translation of the distal fibula. **B:** Surgery is not required. Union occurred with good ankle function.

nonoperatively. Thus while displaced neck and body fractures will usually be treated operatively, there are several talar fractures that will be managed nonoperatively. If nonoperative management is to be undertaken, the use of a nonweight-bearing below-knee cast or brace for 6 to 8 weeks is recommended. Following

its removal a physical therapy regime should be instituted. Talar fractures are discussed in Chapter 60.

Calcaneal Fractures

There has been considerable recent discussion about the management of calcaneal fractures.[13,71] These are often displaced intra-articular fractures and as such should benefit from operative treatment. There is continued debate about the indications for surgery and many calcaneal fractures continue to be managed nonoperatively.[13] Table 6-2 shows that in a trauma unit where fracture fixation of intra-articular calcaneal fractures remains routine about 35% of fractures are treated by primary operative fixation. As with talar fractures, it is important to understand the epidemiology of calcaneal fractures in order to understand why only 35% of fractures are treated operatively. Analysis of the calcaneal fractures included in Table 6-2 shows that about 60% are intra-articular; the remaining 40% are extra-articular calcaneal body fractures or fractures of the anterior, medial, or lateral processes or of the posterior tuberosity.[20] Many of these fractures will be treated nonoperatively. Also, an analysis of types of intra-articular calcaneal fracture using the Sanders classification[79] shows that about 16% of intra-articular calcaneal fractures are undisplaced Sanders type 1 that do not require surgery (Fig. 6-48). In addition, there are other factors that affect the choice of management in calcaneal fractures. It is assumed that intra-articular calcaneal fractures occur in young patients and many do, but there has been an increasing prevalence of these fractures in older patients, with 12.7% of the calcaneal fractures included in Table 6-2 occurring in patients of at least 65 years of age. Surgeons often treat these patients nonoperatively.

If nonoperative treatment is used for calcaneal fractures it is suggested that a nonweight-bearing below-knee cast or brace

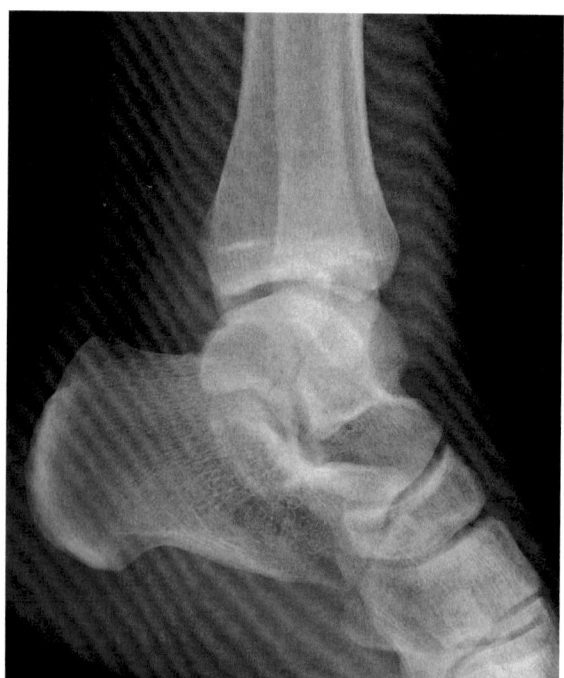

FIGURE 6-47 A lateral radiograph of an undisplaced fracture of the talar body in a 26-year-old male. It was treated in a below-knee cast with a good result being obtained.

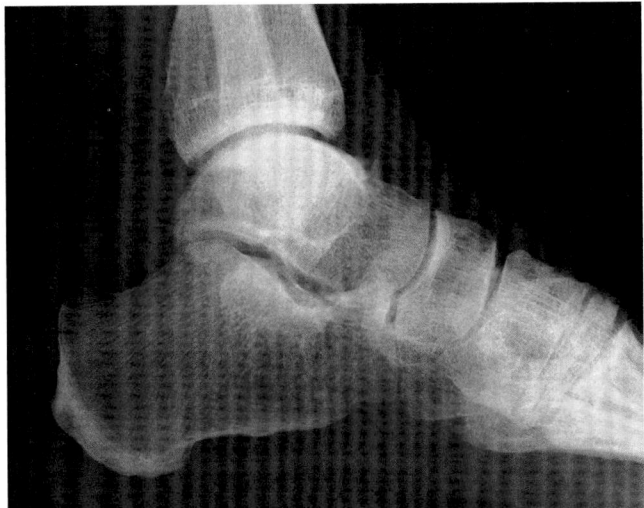
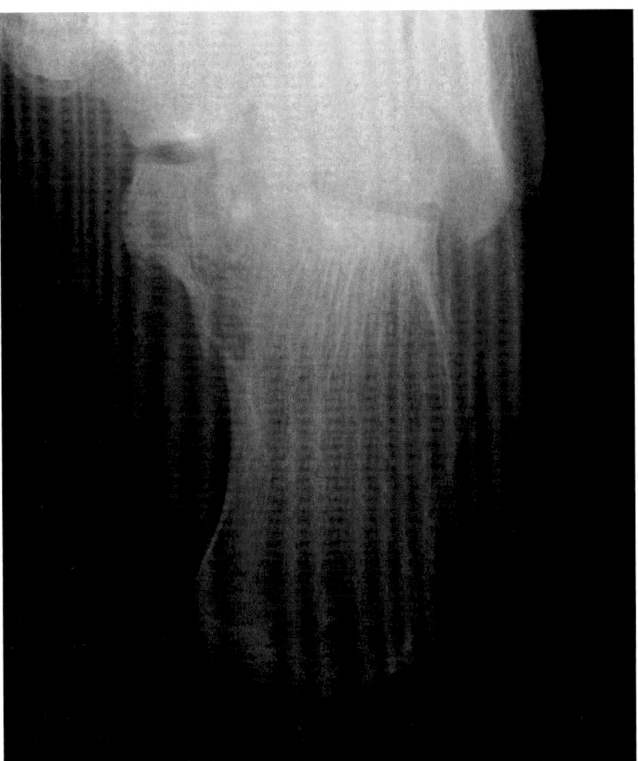

FIGURE 6-48 Axial and lateral radiographs of an undisplaced fracture of the calcaneus which does not require surgery.

be used for 6 weeks, and then weight bearing and a physical therapy regime instituted. Calcaneal fractures are discussed in Chapter 61.

Midfoot Fractures

Table 6-2 indicates that about 30% of midfoot fractures are treated operatively. A review of the epidemiology of midfoot fractures shows that there are four basic fracture types, these being avulsion fractures, shear fractures, uniarticular impaction fractures, and biarticular impaction fractures.[20] About 45% of midfoot fractures are avulsion fractures, which are generally treated nonoperatively. Operative treatment tends to be used mainly for shear fractures or for maintaining the length of the medial and lateral columns of the midfoot in more severe fractures or fracture dislocations. The other indication for operative treatment is if the fracture is associated with a Lisfranc dislocation of the tarsometatarsal joint. Thus, more severe midfoot injuries tend to be treated operatively. If nonoperative treatment is used it is usually for less-severe injuries and the use of a nonweight-bearing cast or brace for 6 weeks is adequate. Midfoot fractures are discussed in Chapter 62.

Metatarsal Fractures

Metatarsal fractures are relatively common but Table 6-2 shows that very few are treated operatively. About 90% of metatarsal fractures are isolated injuries, with about 70% to 75% affecting the fifth metatarsal.[20] Most are low-energy injuries and are treated nonoperatively (Fig. 6-49). Some multiple metatarsal

fractures or fractures associated with significant displacement or with a Lisfranc dislocation of the tarsometatarsal joint require operative treatment but these are frequently associated with high-energy injuries to the foot. Stress fractures of the metatarsal are not uncommon and are also treated nonoperatively. Treatment of metatarsal fractures is essentially symptomatic. No treatment is required if the patient can manage to mobilize without significant discomfort. If the fracture is painful, it is suggested that a below-knee cast or brace be applied for 3 weeks and then reapplied if the pain continues. Mobilization can be allowed when the patient can manage this. Metatarsal fractures are discussed in Chapter 62.

Toe Fractures

Table 6-2 shows that, as with metatarsal fractures, nonoperative treatment of toe fractures is very common. Analysis of the toe phalangeal fractures in Table 6-2 shows that about 20% involved the hallux, and that five of the eight fractures that were treated operatively were in the hallux. Surgical treatment of the other toes is rarely required. If nonoperative management is used, buddy strapping to the adjacent toe is usually all that is needed, although the treatment is usually symptomatic and frequently no treatment is actually required.

Pelvic and Acetabular Fractures

Table 6-2 shows that the prevalence of operative management of pelvic and acetabular fractures is relatively low. This may be surprising to surgeons working in Level I trauma centers but it

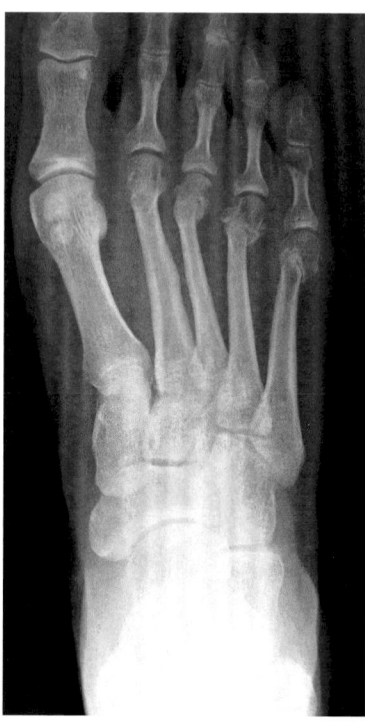

FIGURE 6-49 Minimally displaced fractures of the third, fourth and fifth metatarsal necks in a 43-year-old female. These should be managed nonoperatively.

must be remembered that most fractures involving the pelvis are insufficiency fractures of the pubic rami and occur in the elderly. In the last 30 years there has been an explosion of interest in the surgical treatment of pelvic and acetabular fractures. The pelvic fractures that occur in younger patients that are still frequently treated nonoperatively are anterior posterior compression type I injuries and the lateral compression[104] type I injuries. Treatment is restricted weight bearing depending on the degree of discomfort. Most acetabular fractures are treated operatively with nonoperative management reserved for undisplaced fractures with the exception of transtectal transverse fractures, which may displace later.[20] Treatment is restricted weight bearing for 10 to 12 weeks and a physical therapy program. Pelvic and acetabular fractures are discussed in Chapters 46 and 47.

Spinal Fractures

Very little is known about the prevalence of nonoperative management of all cervical and thoracolumbar fractures, but it is a very common method of treatment with many of the perceived advantages of spinal fixation not having been proven in clinical trials. The management of spinal fractures is discussed in detail in Chapters 43 to and 45.

SPECIFIC FRACTURE TYPES

Periprosthetic Fractures

Increasing longevity, with associated osteopenia and osteoporosis, together with an increased use of arthroplasty and frac-

ture fixation have lead to a rapid increase in the incidence of periprosthetic fractures. These usually occur in older patients and can be very difficult to treat. Many periprosthetic fractures will be treated operatively but there is a role for nonoperative management in certain circumstances. Most periprosthetic fractures associated with arthroplasty will occur in the femur following hip or knee replacement. The classification and management of these is detailed in Chapter 23 but if the Vancouver classification[11] of proximal femoral periprosthetic fractures is employed, most Type B and C fractures will be treated operatively with nonoperative treatment being reserved for stable Type A fractures (Fig. 6-50). The basic principle governing the use of nonoperative management is that the fractures should be undisplaced or minimally displaced and the implant should not be loose. If these conditions apply, type A proximal femoral periprosthetic fractures can be treated by a period of restricted weight bearing.

The same basic principle applies to periprosthetic fractures affecting the acetabulum or distal femur. Minor undisplaced perioperative acetabular fractures are sometimes caused by the insertion of hemiarthroplasty prosthesis in the treatment of proximal femoral fractures. These can be treated nonoperatively with a period of restricted weight bearing. More severe displaced acetabular fractures are usually treated operatively.

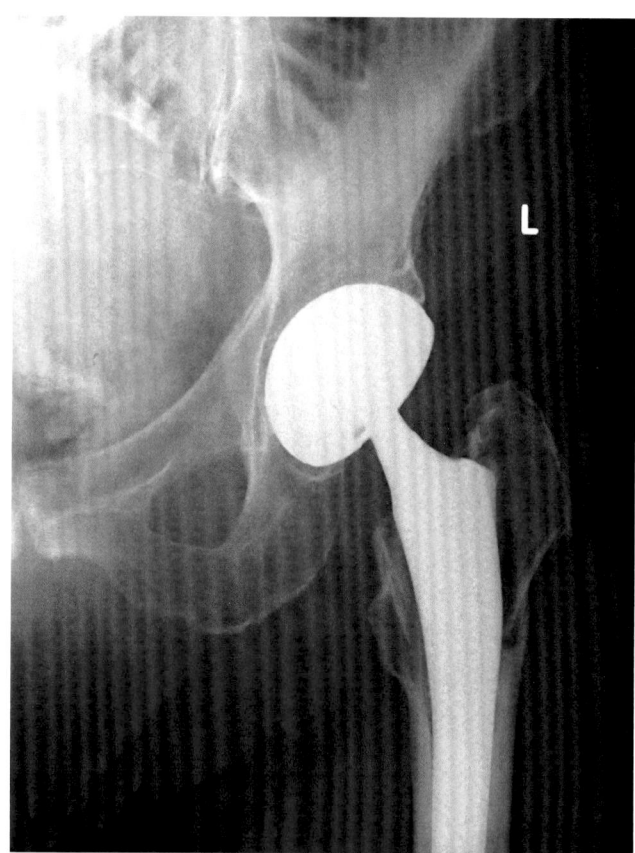

FIGURE 6-50 A Vancouver Type A fracture around the proximal stem of a stable bipolar prosthesis. This type of periprosthetic fracture generally does not need surgical treatment.

In the distal femur Lewis and Rorabeck[58] type I fractures can be treated nonoperatively as they are undisplaced and stable, but type II and III fractures are best treated operatively. Again a period of restricted weight bearing is used. The same principles are applied to periprosthetic patellar and proximal tibial fractures.

Humeral periprosthetic fractures can be very difficult to treat. They occur in elderly patients and analysis of implant failure has shown that loosening is relatively rare.[75] Thus the surgeon may be faced with a type B[104] periprosthetic fracture in osteopenic bone and a stable implant. An example of this is shown in Figure 6-51 in which there had been an earlier humeral diaphyseal fracture as well. Nonoperative management may be the only realistic option under these circumstances. Periprosthetic fractures associated with elbow or ankle arthroplasties are treated using the basic principles of fracture displacement and implant stability that have already been outlined.

In recent years there has been an increasing prevalence of femoral fractures associated with proximal femoral fracture fixation. These are most commonly associated with proximal femoral nails but may occur after the use of compression and dynamic hip screws. These fractures are usually displaced and there is little role for nonoperative management.

Stress Fractures

There are two types of stress fracture: Fatigue fractures and insufficiency fractures. They are discussed in Chapter 21. Fatigue fractures usually occur in younger patients and, with the exception of some fractures of the proximal femur, femoral diaphysis, distal femur, and tibial diaphysis they are usually undisplaced and are managed nonoperatively (Fig. 6-52). The general principles of management are the same as described for other fractures and the same treatment regimes outlined in Tables 6-9 and 6-10 should be followed. Insufficiency fractures occur in abnormal bone and obviously the most common causes for these fractures are osteopenia and osteoporosis. Many of these fractures are undisplaced and nonoperative management will be used. The treatments outlined in Tables 6-9 and 6-10 should be followed.

Metastatic Fractures

Metastatic fractures are discussed in Chapter 22. It is difficult to be prescriptive about the role of nonoperative treatment as it largely depends on the location of the fracture, the type of tumor, and the medical condition of the patient. Generally speaking, most metastatic fractures are treated operatively unless the patient has a very short life expectancy as surgical stabilization will diminish pain and improve the quality of the patient's remaining life.

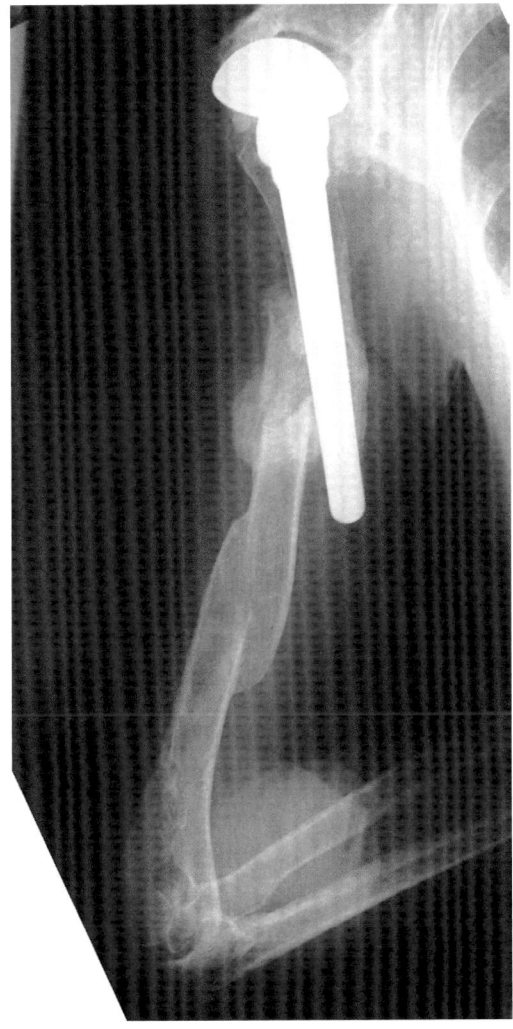

FIGURE 6-51 A periprosthetic fracture that is virtually impossible to treat surgically. A Vancouver Type B fracture in a humerus with an old nonoperatively managed diaphyseal fracture in an 89-year-old female. The shoulder was already very stiff.

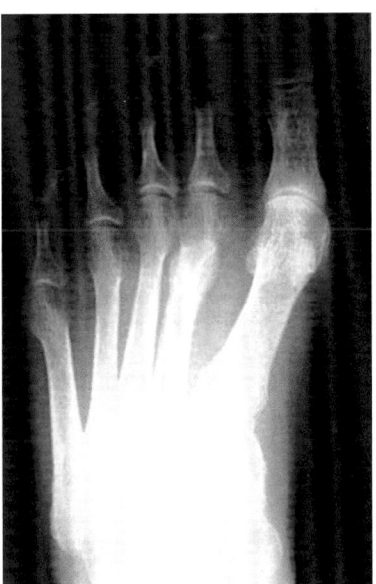

FIGURE 6-52 A stress fracture of the second metatarsal. The treatment is nonoperative.

THE FUTURE OF NONOPERATIVE FRACTURE TREATMENT

There are two principal competing factors that will determine the role of nonoperative management of fractures in the future. It is likely that fracture fixation techniques will become more sophisticated and fractures that we now treat nonoperatively may be shown in the future to have better results if treated operatively. It is certain that in many parts of the world the population that is going to present with fractures is the elderly population and it is highly likely that the patients who present with fractures in the future will be older and less fit than current patients. Future fracture research will need to determine the role of operative management in elderly patients who already have functional impairment and significant medical comorbidities. It seems likely that as we develop into a "super-elderly" population we will re-evaluate the role of nonoperative management in many fractures.

Surgeons have analyzed the properties of osteoporotic bone in the belief that better fixation methods will improve the outcome of fractures in the elderly, but it is also necessary to consider the effect of aging on soft tissues and their recovery after injury and surgery. It may well be that the effect of increasing age on muscles, tendons, ligaments, and other soft tissues will negate any advantages gained by improved operative fixation but only time will tell.

Overall it seems likely that the prevalence of operative treatment will rise, but probably not as quickly as has been the case in the last 30 to 40 years. Improved vehicle design together with enhanced industrial legislation, speed restrictions, and drinking and driving laws will continue to reduce the incidence of severe injuries but there is no doubt that orthopedic surgeons will be faced with an epidemic of less-severe fractures in the elderly.

REFERENCES

1. Alho A, Benterud JG, Hogevold HE, et al. Comparison of functional bracing and locked intramedullary nailing in the treatment of displaced tibial shaft fractures. Clin Orthop. 1992;277:243–250.
2. Ambroise Paré. The Apologie and Treatise of Ambroise Paré Geoffrey Keynes. London: Falcon; 1951.
3. Andersen K, Jensen PO, Lauritzen J. Treatment of clavicular fractures. Figure-of-eight bandage versus a simple sling. Acta Orthop Scand. 1987;58:71–74.
4. Austin RT. The Sarmiento tibial plaster: A prospective study of 145 tibial fractures. Injury. 1981;13:12–22.
5. Bauer M, Jonsson K, Nilsson B. Thirty-year follow-up of ankle fractures. Acta Orthop Scand. 1985;56:103–106.
6. Bérenger-Féraud LJB. Traité de l'immobilisation directe. Paris: Adrien Delahaye; 1870.
7. Böhler L. The Treatment of Fractures. New York, NY: Grune and Stratton; 1956.
8. Bone LB, Sucato D, Stegemann PM, et al. Displaced isolated fractures of the tibial shaft treated with either a cast or intramedullary nailing. J Bone Joint Surg Am. 1997;79A:1336–1341.
9. Bono CM, Rinaldi M. Thoracolumbar fractures and dislocations. In: Court-Brown CM, McQueen MM, Tornetta P, eds. Trauma. Philadelphia, PA: Lippincott Williams and Wilkins; 2006:226–237.
10. Böstmann O, Hänninen A. Tibial shaft fractures caused by indirect violence. Acta Orthop Scand. 1982;53:981–990.
11. Brady OH, Kerry R, Masri BA, et al. The Vancouver classification of periprosthetic fractures of the hip: a rational approach to treatment. Tech Orthop. 1999;14:107–114.
12. Breasted JF. The Edwin Smith Papyrus. Chicago, IL: University of Chicago Press; 1930.
13. Buckley R, Tough S, McCormack R, et al. Operative compared with nonoperative treatment of displaced intra-articular calcaneal fractures: A prospective, randomized, controlled multicenter trial. J Bone Joint Surg Am. 2002;84A:1733–1744.
14. Canadian Orthopaedic Trauma Society. Nonoperative treatment compared with plate fixation of displaced midshaft clavicular fractures. A multicenter, randomized clinical trial. J Bone Joint Surg Am. 2007;89:1–10.
15. Carstairs V, Morris R. Deprivation and health in Scotland. Health Bulletin. 1990;48:162–175.
16. Charnley J. The Closed Treatment of Common Fractures. 3rd ed. Edinburgh: E&S Livingstone; 1972.
17. Connolly JF, Dehne E, Lafollette B. Closed reduction and early cast-brace ambulation in the treatment of femoral fractures. Part II: Results in one hundred and forty-three fractures. J Bone Joint Surg Am. 1973;55A:1581–1599.
18. Constant CR. Age Related Recovery of Shoulder Function after Injury. Thesis. University College, Cork, 1986.
19. Court-Brown CM, Garg A, McQueen MM. The epidemiology of proximal humeral fractures. Acta Orthop Scand. 2001;72:365–371.
20. Court-Brown CM, McQueen MM, Tornetta P. Trauma. Philadelphia, PA: Lippincott Williams and Wilkins; 2006.
21. Court-Brown CM, Caesar B. The epidemiology of adult fractures: A review. Injury. 2006;37:691–697.
22. Court-Brown CM, McQueen MM. Two-part fractures and fracture dislocations. Nand Clin. 2007;23:397–414.
23. Dennison E, Cooper C. Epidemiology of osteoporotic fractures. Horm Res. 2000;54(suppl 1):58–63.
24. Den Outer AG, Meeuwis JD, Hermans J, et al. Conservative versus operative treatment of displaced noncomminute tibial shaft fractures. Clin Orthop. 1990;252:231–237.
25. Digby JM, Holloway GMN, Webb JK. A study of function after tibial cast bracing. Injury. 1993;14:432–439.
26. DiStasio AJ, Jaggears FR, DePasquale LV, et al. Protected early motion versus cast immobilization in postoperative management of ankle fractures. Contemp Orthop. 1994;29:273–277.
27. Dunn L, Henry J, Beard D. Social deprivation and adult head injury: A national study. J Neurol Neurosurg Psychiatry. 2003;74:1060–1064.
28. Edwards SG, Whittle AP, Wood GW. Nonoperative treatment of ipsilateral fractures of the scapula and clavicle. J Bone Joint Surg Am. 2000;82A:774–780.
29. Egol KA, Connor PM, Karunakar MA, et al. The floating shoulder: Clinical and functional results. J Bone Joint Surg (Am). 2001;83A:1188–1194.
30. Ekholm R, Tidermark J, Törnkvist H, et al. Outcome after closed functional bracing of humeral shaft fractures. J Orthop Trauma. 2006;20:591–596.
31. Emmett JE, Breck LW. A review and analysis of 11,000 fractures seen in a private practice of orthopaedic surgery 1937-1956. J Bone Joint Surg Am. 1958;40:1169–1175.
32. Evans JMM, Newton RW, Ruta DA, et al. Socioeconomic status, obesity, and prevalence of Type 1 and Type 2 diabetes mellitus. Diabetic Med. 2000;17:478–480.
33. Fjalestad T, Stromsoe K, Salvesen P, et al. Functional results of braced humeral diaphyseal fractures; why do 38% lose external rotation of the shoulder? Arch Orthop Trauma Surg. 2000;120:281–285.
34. Fracture and dislocation classification compendium. J Trauma. 2007;21:10(suppl).
35. Garfin SR, Botte MJ, Centeno RS, et al. Osteology of the skull as it affects halo pin placement. Spine. 1985;10:696–698.
36. Geiger KR, Karpman RR. Necrosis of the skin over the metacarpal as a result of functional fracture-bracing. J Bone Joint Surg Am. 1989;71:1199–1202.
37. Grassi FA, Tajana MS, D'Angelo F. Management of midclavicular fractures: Comparison between nonoperative treatment and open intramedullary fixation in 80 patients. J Trauma. 2001;50:1096–1100.
38. Haines JF, Williams EA, Hargadon ES, et al. Is conservative treatment of displaced tibial shaft fractures justified? J Bone Joint Surg Br. 1984;66B:84–88.
39. Hanlon CR, Estes WL. Fractures in childhood. A statistical analysis. Am J Surg. 1954;87:312–323.
40. Hansen PB, Hansen TB. The treatment of fractures of the ring and little metacarpal necks. A prospective randomized study of three different types of treatment. J Hand Surg Br. 1998;23B:245–247.
41. Harager K, Hviid K, Jensen CM, et al. Successful immediate weight-bearing of internally fixated ankle fractures in a general population. J Orthop Sci. 2000;5:52–54.
42. Hardy AE. The treatment of femoral fractures by cast-brace application and early ambulation. A prospective review of 106 patients. J Bone Joint Surg Am. 1983;65A:56–65.
43. Hawkins LG. Fractures of the neck of the talus. J Bone Joint Surg Am. 1970;52A:991–1002.
44. Herscovici D, Fiennes AG, Allgöwer M, et al. The floating shoulder: Ipsilateral clavicle and scapular neck fractures. J Bone Joint Surg Br. 1992;74B:362–364.
45. Hippocrates. The Genuine Works of Hippocrates Francis Adams, trans. Baltimore, MD: Williams and Wilkins; 1939.
46. Hooper GJ, Keddell RG, Penny ID. Conservative management or closed nailing for tibial shaft fractures. A randomized prospective trial. J Bone Joint Surg Br 1991;73B:83–85.
47. Jawa A, McCarty P, Doornberg J, et al. Extra-articular distal-third diaphyseal fractures of the humerus. A comparison of functional bracing and plate fixation. J Bone Joint Surg (Am). 2006;88A:2343–2347.
48. Johnell O, Kanis JA. An estimate of the worldwide prevalence and disability associated with osteoporotic fractures. Osteoporos Int. 2006;17:1726–1733.
49. Johnson RM, Hart DL, Simmons BF, et al. Cervical orthoses: A study comparing their effectiveness in restricting cervical movement in normal subjects. J Bone Joint Surg Am. 1977;59A:332–339.
50. Jones R. An orthopaedic view of the treatment of fractures. Am J Orthop. 1913;11:314.
51. Karaharju EO, Alho A, Neimenen J. Results of operative and nonoperative management of tibial fractures. Injury. 1979;7:49–52.
52. Kay L, Hansen BA, Raaschou HO. Fractures of the tibial shaft conservatively treated. Injury. 1986;17:P5–P11.
53. Koch RA, Nickel VL. The halo vest: An evaluation of motion and forces across the neck. Spine. 1978;3:103–107.
54. Kristensen KD, Hansen T. Closed treatment of ankle fractures. Stage II supinationeversion fractures followed for 20 years. Acta Orthop Scand. 1985;56:107–109.

55. Küntscher M, Blazek J, Bruner S, et al. Functional bracing after operative treatment of metacarpal fractures. *Unfallchirurg.* 2002;105:1109–1114.

56. Kyrö A, Tunturi T, Soukka A. Conservative treatment of tibial fractures. Results in a series of 163 patients. *Ann Chir Gynaecol.* 1991;80:294–300.

57. Lehtonen H, Järvinen TLN, Honkonen S, et al. Use of a cast compared with a functional ankle brace after operative treatment of an ankle fracture: A prospective, randomized study. *J Bone Joint Surg Am.* 2003;85A:205–211.

58. Lewis PL, Rorabeck CH. Periprosthetic fractures. In: Engh GA, Rorabeck CH, eds. *Revision Total Knee Arthroplasty.* Baltimore, MD: Wiliams and Wilkins; 1997.

59. Lichtenberg RP. A study of 2532 fractures in children. *Am J Surg.* 1954;87:330–338.

60. Lindsay RW, Pneumaticos SG, Gugala Z. Management techniques for spinal injuries. In: Browner BD, Jupiter JB, Levine AM, Trafton PG, eds. *Skeletal Trauma.* 3rd ed. Philadelphia, PA: WB Saunders; 2003:746–776.

61. Neer CS. Displaced proximal humeral fractures. I. Classification and evaluation. *J Bone Joint Surg Am.* 1970;52A:1077–1089.

62. Nho SJ, Brophy RH, Barker JU, et al. Management of proximal humeral fractures based on current literature. *J Bone Joint Surg.* 2007;89(suppl 3):44–58.

63. Nicoll EA. Fractures of the tibial shaft. A survey of 705 cases. *J Bone Joint Surg Br.* 1965; 46B:373–387.

64. Nordqvist A, Pettersson CJ, Redlund-Johnell I. Midclavicle fractures in adults: End result study after conservative treatment. *J Orthop Trauma.* 1998;12:572–576.

65. O'Connor D, Mullett H, Doyle M, et al. Minimally displaced Colles fractures: A prospective randomized trial of treatment with a wrist splint or a plaster cast. *J Hand Surg Br.* 2003;28:50–53.

66. Oni OOA, Hui A, Gregg PJ. The healing of closed tibial shaft fractures. *J Bone Joint Surg Br.* 1988;70B:787–790.

67. Owsley KC, Gorczyca JT. Fracture displacement and screw cutout after open reduction and locked plate fixation of proximal humeral fractures. *J Bone Joint Surg Am.* 2008;90:233–240.

68. Pace AM, Stuart R, Brownlow H. Outcome of glenoid neck fractures. *J Shoulder Elbow Surg.* 2005;14:585–590.

69. Peltier LF. Fractures. *A History and Short Iconography of their Treatment.* San Francisco: Norman Publishing; 1990.

70. Perry J, Nickel VL. Total cervical spine fusion for neck paralysis. *J Bone Joint Surg Am.* 1959;41A:37–60.

71. Poeze M, Verbruggen JP, Brink PR. The relationship between the outcome of operatively treated calcaneal fractures and institutional fracture load. A systematic review of the literature. *J Bone Joint Surg Am.* 2008;90A:1013–1021.

72. Pun WK, Chow SP, Fang D, et al. A study of function and residual joint stiffness after functional bracing of tibial shaft fractures. *Clin Orthop.* 1991;267:157–163.

73. Puno RM, Teynor JT, Nagano J, et al. Critical analysis of results of treatment of 201 tibial shaft fractures. *Clin Orthop* 1986;212:113–121.

74. Ring D, Chin K, Taghinia AH, et al. Nonunion after functional brace treatment of diaphyseal humerus fractures. *J Trauma.* 2007;62:1157–1158.

75. Robinson CM, Cairns DA. Primary nonoperative treatment of displaced lateral fractures of the clavicle. *J Bone Joint Surg.* 2004;86A:778–782.

76. Robinson CM, Page RS, Hill RM. Primary hemiarthroplasty for treatment of proximal humerus fractures. *J Bone Joint Surg Am.* 2003;85A:1215–1223.

77. Rokito AS, Zuckerman JD, Shaari JM, et al. A comparison of nonoperative and operative treatment of type II distal clavicle fractures. *Bull Hosp Jt Dis.* 2002;61:32–39.

78. Rosenberg N, Soudry M. Shoulder impairment following treatment of diaphyseal fractures of humerus by functional brace. *Arch Orthop Trauma Surg.* 2006;126: 437–440.

79. Sanders R, Fortin P, DiPasquale T, et al. Operative treatment in 120 displaced intraarticular calcaneal fractures: Results using a prognostic computed tomography scan classification. *Clin Orthop.* 1993;290:87–95.

80. Sarmiento A. A functional below-the-knee cast for tibial fractures. *J Bone Joint Surg.* 1967;49A:855–875.

81. Sarmiento A. A functional below-the-knee cast for tibial fractures. *J Bone Joint Surg Am.* 1970;52A:295–311.

82. Sarmiento A, Gersten LM, Sobol PA. Tibial shaft fractures treated with functional braces. Experience with 780 fractures. *J Bone Joint Surg Br.* 1989;71B:602–609.

83. Sarmiento A, Horowitch A, Aboulafia A, et al. Functional bracing for comminuted extra-articular fractures of the distal third of the humerus. *J Bone Joint Surg Br.* 1990; 72B:283–287.

84. Sarmiento A, Latta LL, Zych GA, et al. Isolated ulnar shaft fractures treated with functional braces. *J Orthop Trauma.* 1998;12:420–423.

85. Sayre LA. Report on fractures. *Trans Am Med Assoc.* 1874;25:301.

86. Scudder CL. The ambulatory treatment of fractures. *Boston Med Surg J.* 1898;138:102.

87. Seutin LJG. *Du traitement des fractures par l'appareil inamovible.* Bruxelles. 1835.

88. Shakespeare DT, Henderson NJ. Compartment pressure changes during calcaneal traction in tibial fractures. *J Bone Joint Surg Br.* 1982;64:498–499.

89. Simanski CJ, Maegele MG, Lefering R, et al. Functional treatment and early weightbearing after an ankle fracture: A prospective study. *J Orthop Trauma.* 2006;20:108–114.

90. Slatis P, Rokkanen P. Conservative treatment of tibial shaft fractures. *Acta Chir Scand.* 1967;134:41–47.

91. Steen Jensen J, Wang Hansen S, Johansen J. Tibial shaft fractures: A comparison of conservative treatment and internal fixation with conventional plates or AO compression plates. *Acta Orthop Scand.* 1977;48:204–212.

92. Stewart HD, Innes AR, Burke FD. Functional cast-bracing for Colles fractures. A comparison between cast-bracing and conventional plaster casts. *J Bone Joint Surg Br.* 1984;66B:749–753.

93. Stimson LA. *A Treatise on Fractures.* Philadelphia, PA: Henry C. Lea; 1883.

94. Thomas HO. *The Principles of the Treatment of Fractures and Dislocations.* London: HK Lewis; 1886.

95. Thompson GH, Wilber JH, Marcus RE. Internal fixation of fractures in children and adolescents. *Clin Orthop.* 1984;188:10–20.

96. Toivanen JAK, Niemenen J, Laine HJ, et al. Functional treatment of closed humeral shaft fractures. *Int Orthop.* 2005;29:10–13.

97. Tropiano P, Huang RC, Louis CA, et al. Functional and radiographic outcome of thoracolumbar and lumbar burst fractures managed by closed orthopaedic reduction and casting. *Spine.* 2003;28:2459–2465.

98. Tropp H, Norlin R. Ankle performance after ankle fracture: A randomized study of early mobilization. *Foot Ankle Int.* 1995;16:79–83.

99. Tumia N, Wardlaw D, Hallett J, et al. Aberdeen Colles brace as a treatment for Colles fracture. A multicenter, prospective, randomized, controlled trial. *J Bone Joint Surg Br.* 2003;85:78–82.

100. Van der Linden W, Larsson K. Plate fixation versus conservative treatment of tibial shaft fractures. A randomized trial. *J Bone Joint Surg Am.* 1979;61A:873–878.

101. Van Noort A, van Kampen A. Fractures of the scapula surgical neck: Outcome after conservative treatment in 13 cases. *Arch Orthop Trauma Surg.* 2005;125:696–700.

102. Veysi VT, Mittal R, Agarwal S, et al. Multiple trauma and scapula fractures: So what? *J Trauma.* 2003;55:1145–1147.

103. Volkmann R. Verletzungen der knochen (knochenbruchen und knochenwunden). In: Pithia, Billroth, eds. *Handbuch der Allemeinen und Speziellen Chirurgie.* vol 2. Erlangen: Ferdinand Enke; 1865.

104. Young JWR, Burgess AR, Brumback RJ, et al. Pelvic fractures: Value of plain radiography in early assessment and management. *Radiology.* 1986;160:445–451.

105. Zagorski JB, Latta LL, Zych GA, et al. Diaphyseal fracture of the humerus. Treatment with prefabricated braces. *J Bone Joint Surg Am.* 1988;70A:607–610.

106. Zlowodzki M, Bhandari M, Zelle BA, et al. Treatment of scapula fractures: Systematic review of 520 fractures in 22 case series. *J Orthop Trauma.* 2006;20:230–233.

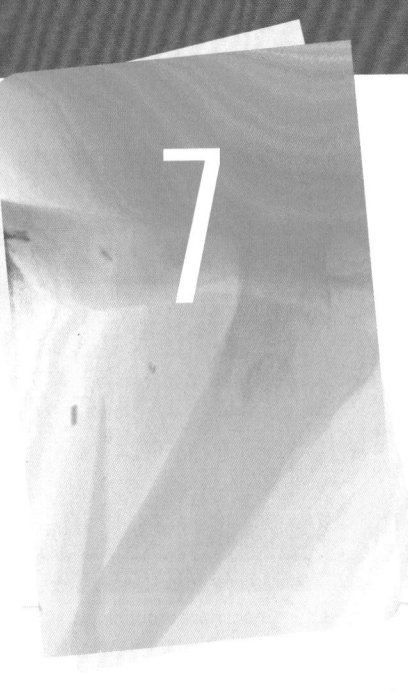

7

PRINCIPLES OF INTERNAL FIXATION

Michael Schütz and Thomas P. Rüedi

HISTORICAL BACKGROUND AND THE GOALS OF INTERNAL FIXATION

Already the ancient Egyptians of 3,000 BC knew that splinting of a fractured limb not only reduces pain but also supports the healing process. The first reports on modern techniques of internal fixation are however only about 100 years old. The brothers Elie and Albin Lambotte from Belgium have described in detail the essentials of what they called "osteosynthesis" of fractures with plates and screws, wire loops and external fixators. Albin Lambotte (1866 to 1955) highlighted the importance of anatomical reduction and stable fixation of articular fractures as the only way to regain good joint function. While he planned and drew every fracture in detail, he also emphasized the importance of careful soft tissue handling to preserve vascularity and prevent infection. His pupil Robert Danis (1880 to 1962) introduced the term of "soudure autogéne" or primary bone healing without visible callus, which he observed when the fracture was anatomically reduced and fixed with

his compression plate. In 1950 the 32-year-old Swiss orthopedic surgeon Maurice Müller spent 1 day only in the clinic of Danis and was deeply impressed by the patients he saw and the results of compression plating. Back in Fribourg, Switzerland Müller, got permission from his chief to treat a patient with the new technique and compression plates, which he soon modified and technically improved. Together with 13 other young Swiss surgeons he founded in 1958 the Arbeitsgemeinschaft für Osteosynthesefragen (AO) the main representatives being Martin Allgöwer, Walter Bandi, Robert Schneider, and Hans Willenegger.[55] The AO set as their goal to improve the outcome of the injured patient by defining guidelines of the surgical management of fractures. They agreed on and adhered to strict rules and principles of fracture surgery and thanks to a meticulous follow-up of every single fracture, they were able to document their results and learn from the mistakes and complications. In parallel to the Swiss AO, Gerhard Küntscher (1900 to 1972) in Germany had developed the technique of IM nailing, which soon revolutionized the treatment of diaphyseal fractures especially of the femur and tibia.[45] In contrast to the rigid fixation by interfragmentary compression, IM nailing was an internal splinting technique, which allowed for some motion at the fracture site and therefore healing by callus formation. Rigid fixation on one hand and the more elastic internal splinting on the other, have often been considered as competing techniques, while they are actually complementary, each having its pros and cons and specific indications.

The ultimate goal of operative fracture fixation is to obtain full restoration of function of the injured limb and the patient to return to his preinjury status of activities, as well as to minimize the risk and incidence of complications. The purpose of the use of implants is to provide a temporary support, to maintain alignment during the fracture healing, and to allow for a functional rehabilitation.

INFLUENCE OF BIOLOGY AND BIOMECHANICS ON FRACTURE HEALING

The biologic and biomechanical influences on fracture treatment will be considered in this chapter. Any procedure will alter the biologic and biomechanical environment for fracture healing, which every surgeon treating fractures should be familiar with. From mechanical and biologic points of view, a fractured bone needs a certain degree of immobilization, an optimally preserved blood supply and biologic or hormonal stimuli in order to unite. All three factors are important, the mechanical part is however the easiest to quantify. We may distinguish two types of mechanical stability, absolute and relative. Absolute stability is defined as rigid fixation that does not allow any micro motion between the fractured fragments under physiologic loading. It is best obtained by interfragmentary compression and is based on preload and friction. More elastic fixation as provided by internal or external splinting of the bone is defined as relative stability which allows limited motion at the fracture site under functional loading. The degree of stability determines the type of fracture healing which is either by primary or direct bone remodeling (Fig. 7-1) or by secondary or indirect healing with callus formation. Indirect fracture healing by callus can take place in a much wider spectrum of mechanical environments than primary or direct bone remodeling (Fig. 7-2). Callus will not form if there is no motion; however, if there is excessive movement, healing will equally be delayed.

The strain theory[13,64] describes, in a simplified manner, what occurs at a cellular level in a fracture gap. Strain is the deformation of a material (e.g., granulation tissue within a gap) when a given force is applied relative to its original form, thus it has no dimension. The amount of deformation a tissue can tolerate before it breaks varies greatly. The strain of normal intact bone until it breaks is "low," about 2%, while granulation tissue has a high-strain tolerance of 100%.[64] In a narrow fracture gap a defined distracting force will disrupt the few cells within it (Fig. 7-3). The same force applied to a wider gap filled with granulation tissue will however only deform this tissue and not cause any rupture (Fig. 7-3B). If we look at a specific fracture type we may appreciate, that in a simple transverse or short

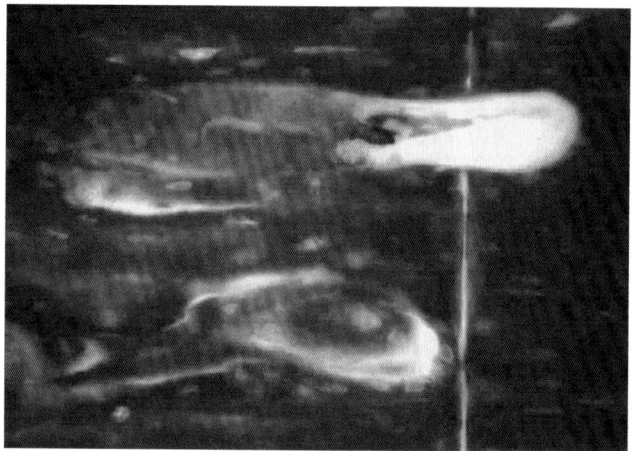

FIGURE 7-1 Direct or primary fracture healing as observed with absolute stability. A new Havers osteon transversing the osteotomy, thereby interdigitating across the osteotomy line.

oblique fracture any deforming force is acting very locally on the single fracture gap, corresponding to a concentration of stress, while in complex, multifragmentary fractures the same force will be distributed over a wide range of different fracture fragments or gaps (stress distribution). By applying the strain theory we may deduct that in a simple diaphyseal fracture we have a situation of "high strain." Therefore such a fracture is best reduced anatomically and fixed by interfragmentary compression (lag screw and plate), a method that produces a high degree or absolute stability (Fig. 7-4).

On the other hand a more complex, multifragmentary diaphyseal fracture corresponds to a "low strain" situation, which profits from correct axial and rotational alignment and less rigid fixation (locked intramedullary nail, bridge plate, or external fixator) providing relative stability (Fig. 7-5). It appears most important that in simple fracture types treated with rigid fixation that persistent gaps at the fracture site are avoided, while in complex fractures treated with less rigid fixation such gaps may be tolerated

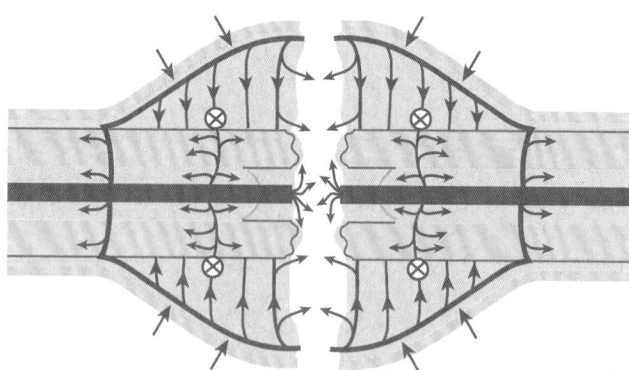

FIGURE 7-2 Secondary healing by callus as observed with relative stability. Schematic drawing of vessel ingrowth from the periphery to the fracture gap.

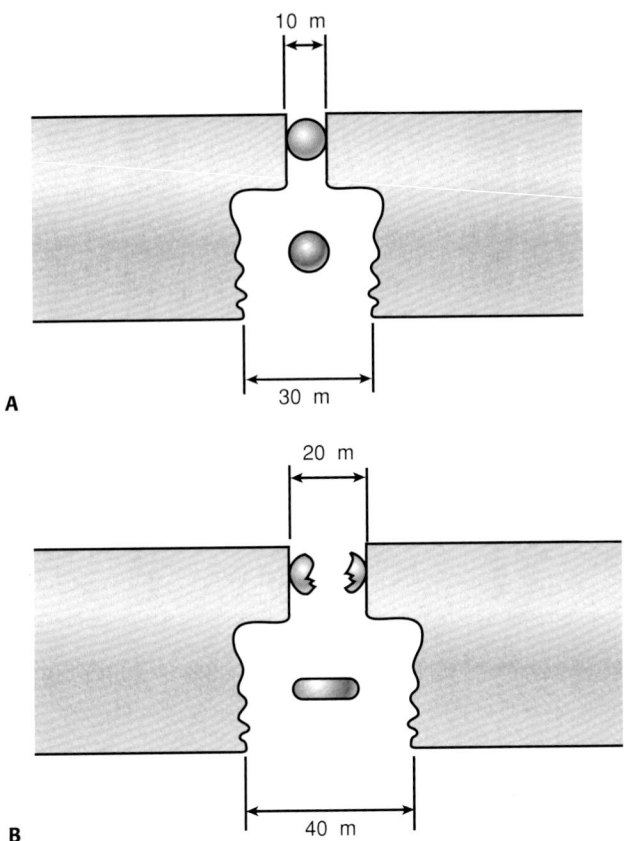

FIGURE 7-3 Strain theory by Perren. **A:** Within a narrow gap (10 μm) a single cell will rupture upon minimal distraction (high strain), **B:** In a wide gap (30 μm) with room for several layers of cells the same amount of distraction will only deform or stretch these cells (low strain).

(Table 7-1). Bhandari[71] and Audigé[2] have independently shown in large clinical series of surgically stabilized tibia shaft fractures that persistent fracture gaps of over about 2 mm were closely related or predictive for the development of a healing delay or nonunion.

In articular fractures the anatomical congruity of the joint surface must be restored and the fragments should be fixed rigidly by interfragmentary compression, while associated metaphyseal comminution or a diaphyseal extension of the fracture can be correctly aligned in all planes and bridged by an appropriate device (Fig. 7-30).

SOFT TISSUE INJURY AND FRACTURE HEALING

Every fracture is associated to a certain extent with an injury to the tissues surrounding the bone. The energy, direction, and concentration of forces inducing the fracture will determine the fracture type and the associated soft tissue lesions.[58] As a result of the displacement of the fragments, periosteal and endosteal blood vessels may be disrupted and the periosteum will be stripped.[74] There is the statement that "every fracture is a soft tissue injury, where the bone happens to be broken," which should emphasize the great importance of the soft parts, which unfortunately are still often not considered and respected enough.

The healing process of a fracture starts with the formation of granulation tissue within the fracture hematoma and is dependent on a preserved or restored blood supply to the area. The more extensive the zone of injury and the tissue destruction, the higher is the risk for a delay of the healing process or for other complications. Depending on the mecha-

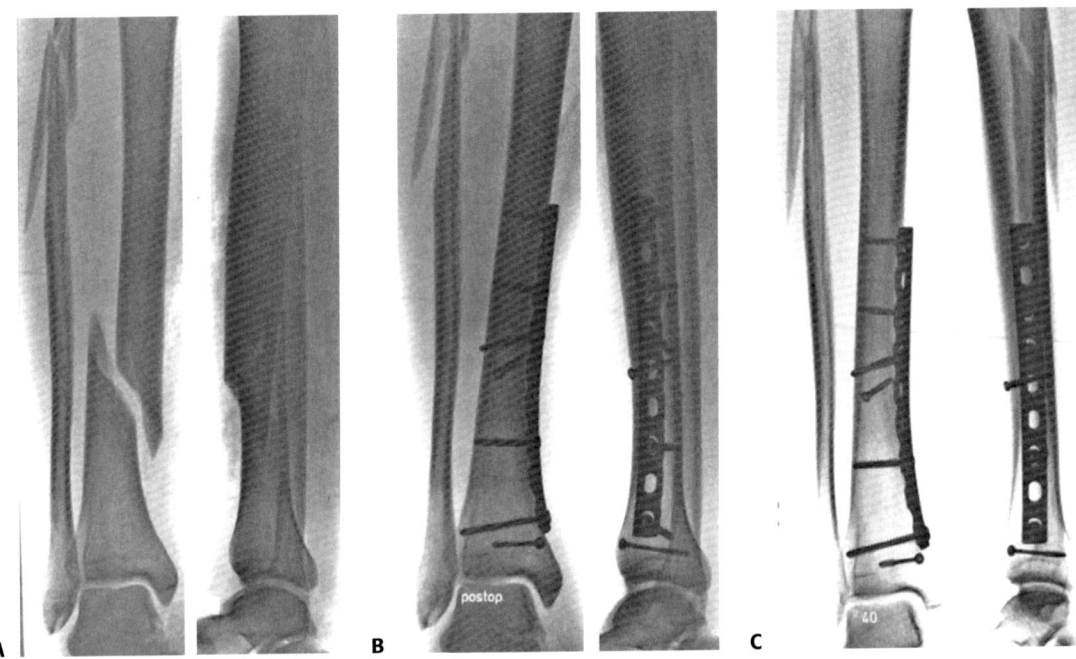

FIGURE 7-4 A simple tibia and fibula spiral fracture by indirect trauma **(A)** is reduced anatomically and fixed with interfragmentary compression (lag screw and protection plate) providing absolute stability **(B). C:** Healing occurs without callus formation, at 1-year follow-up.

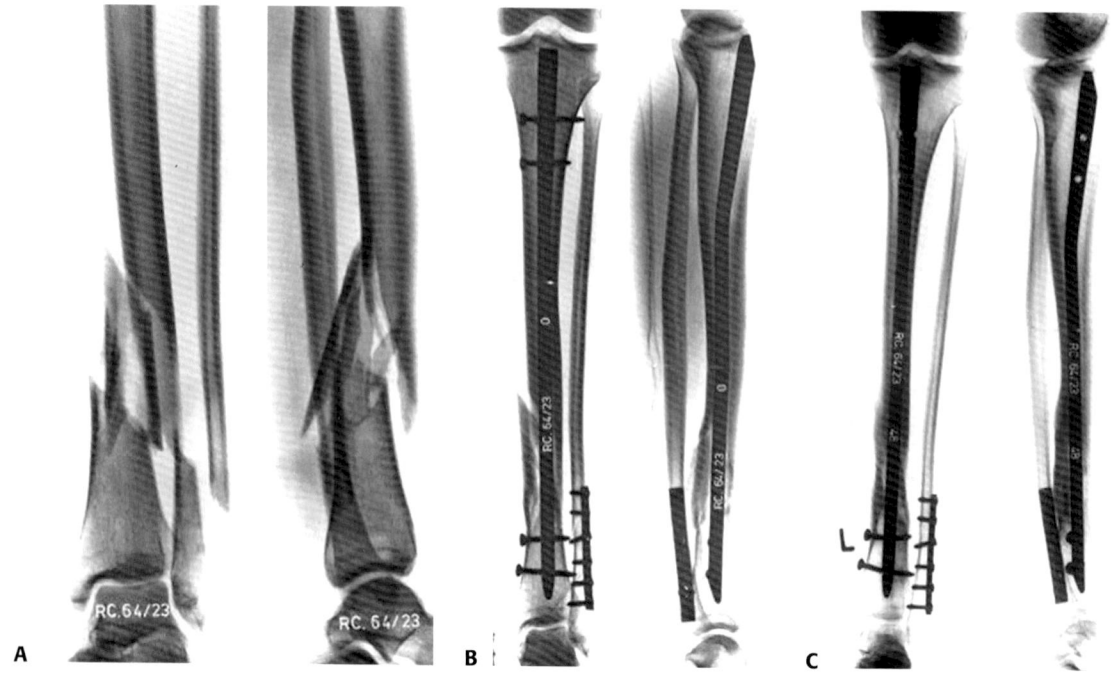

FIGURE 7-5 Complex, distal tibia and fibula fractures by direct trauma. **A:** Fixed after axial and rotational alignment with a locked intramedullary nail providing relative stability. **B:** Healing occurred after proximal dynamization with callus formation. **C:** The fibula fracture was fixed because of the vicinity to the ankle joint.

nism and the magnitude or energy of the insult that caused the bone to break, direct and indirect fracture mechanisms are distinguished, which can usually be deducted from the radiographic appearance of the fracture pattern. An indirect fracture mechanism like a rotation or bending will cause a spiral or butterfly fracture, respectively, with relatively little soft tissue injury. Adequately reduced and immobilized by nonoperative or operative means these fractures generally heal rather uneventfully (Fig. 7-4). In contrast a direct blow will induce, at a minimum, a local contusion of the skin, or more often will result in an open transverse or wedge type fracture with an extensive area of soft tissue injury (Fig. 7-6). In open fractures the severity or extent of the lesion is usually much more

evident than in closed fractures.[19] The latter may however also involve important neurovascular structures surrounding the bone. In closed fractures occult injuries are therefore more often missed.[52] A careful assessment, classification, and documentation of the fracture and the soft tissue injury is therefore of greatest importance in the planning and especially for correct timing of surgery. As a rule and if there are any doubts about the extent of the soft tissue injury, it is much safer to temporarily immobilize the zone of injury by traction or more adequately by an external fixator, postponing definitive fixation until the soft tissues have recovered (Fig. 7-6).

In open fractures with a soft tissue defect or an associated vascular injury, it may be advisable to perform emergency

TABLE 7-1	**Relation of the Stability of Fixation (Absolute vs. Relative), the Type of Fracture (Simple or Complex), and the Size of the Fracture Gap to Fracture Healing**	
	Fracture Gap	
	Simple Small (<2 mm)	Complex Large (>2 mm)
Relative stability	Bone resorption, healing delay, or nonunion	Secondary bone healing (callus)
Absolute stability	Primary bone healing, osteonal remodeling	Bone resorption, healing delay, or nonunion

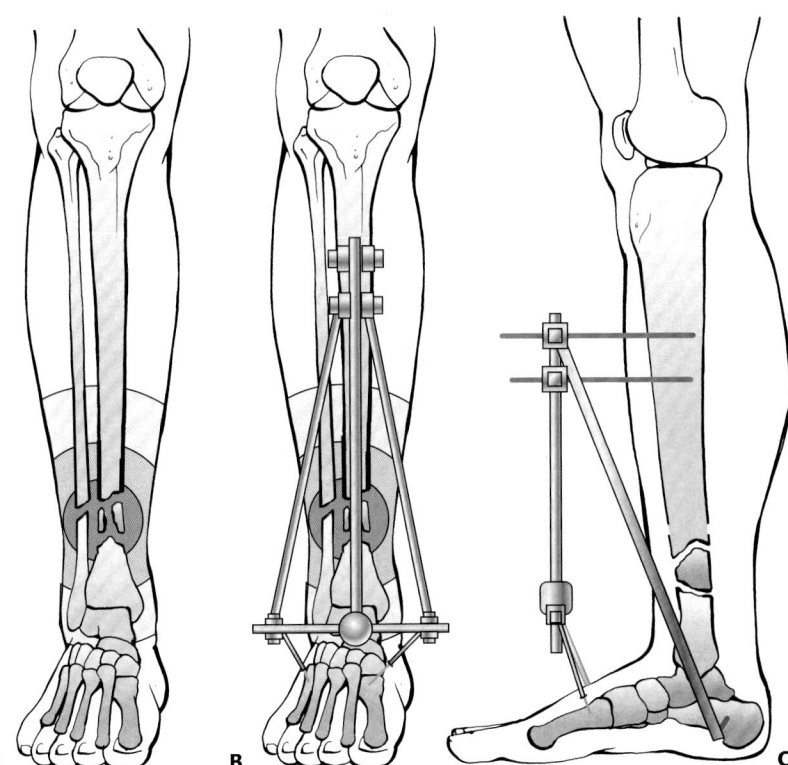

FIGURE 7-6 Zone of injury around a tibia and fibula fracture caused by direct trauma **(A)**. Bridging external fixator to protect the zone of injury in a severely contused distal tibia fracture **(B)** and **(C)**.

fixation of the bone, followed by vessel repair and immediate or early plastic reconstructive procedure to cover the tissue defect. Decision making under such circumstances requires much experience and it may be advisable to involve a senior surgeon or the entire team including a plastic-reconstructive surgeon (see also Chapter 10, Initial Management of Open Fractures).

As we cannot influence the extent of soft tissue lesions caused by the injury mechanism, we must do our best to limit any additional injury to the blood supply of the bone and surrounding structures. Minimally invasive surgical approaches without exposure of the fracture, indirect reduction techniques and fixation devices that do not additionally harm the blood supply to the bone should be used wherever possible.

PREOPERATIVE PLANNING

Every fracture needs a careful preoperative assessment and planning process, which is essential in order to obtain a predictable outcome and to prevent intraoperative problems, hazards and unnecessary delays.

The preoperative assessment should take into consideration the patient, the fracture, and the soft tissues. Planning includes the evaluation not only of the fracture and limb per se, but of the whole patient. Factors like the history and mechanism of the accident, the age of the patient, preexisting vascular and metabolic diseases, the use of drugs, alcohol, and nicotine all may greatly influence the outcome

and therefore must be included in the decision making. The expectations of the patient, their profession, and recreational activities should be known and discussed. The treatment plan is adapted accordingly.

For the fracture as such, plain x-rays are studied and additional imaging requested if considered necessary. CT scans with 2D or 3D reconstruction usually give more information,[12,48,60] while traction views may still be helpful in greatly displaced articular fractures. The classification of the fracture will help to communicate and discuss the type of treatment, to evaluate the problems, and to make a prognosis as to the outcome. The soft tissues and neurovascular conditions are then assessed carefully, as also closed fractures may have severe involvement of these structures. The timely diagnosis of a compartment syndrome and its correct treatment may save a critically injured limb. The assessment and classification of the soft tissue injury is often more difficult than that of the fracture per se and requires much experience.

The components of a preoperative plan include the following.

- Timing of surgery
- Surgical approach
- Reduction maneuvers
- Fixation construct
- Intraoperative imaging
- Wound closure/coverage
- Postoperative care
- Rehabilitation

PRE-, PERI-, AND POSTOPERATIVE CARE

While the anatomical location and pattern of a fracture may dictate a certain method of fixation, for example, a complete articular fracture will require open reduction and stable internal fixation; other fracture types may be approached by different fixation techniques or even by nonoperative treatment. The conditions of the soft tissue such as severe swelling or a skin contusion may preclude immediate surgery and make a staged procedure recommendable. Once the indication and best time for surgery has been established, the type of anesthesia, positioning of the patient, use of a tourniquet, the need for prophylactic antibiotics or a bone graft has to be communicated to the anesthesia and OR team as well as the method of fixation, approach, reduction aids, type of implant, and intraoperative imaging. The more complex the fracture and the procedure, the more detailed the planning must be. Drawing the outlines of a fracture on tracing paper will help to recognize the number, shape, position, and relationship of the different fragments. Thereby the character and challenges of a fracture will be appreciated and the experienced surgeon will be able to decide how to reduce and fix the fracture without additional damage to the most vulnerable blood supply of the area.

Planning Technique on Paper

Two good orthogonal x-rays of the injured and also the uninjured side including the adjacent joints, tracing paper, colored pens, templates of the implants, a set of goniometers, and an x-ray screen are needed for preoperative templating. Step one: The outlines of the intact bone(s) are drawn. Step two: The outlines of the fractured bone(s) are drawn, with the different fragments separated from each other. Step three: The main fragments and the intermediate pieces are reassembled on the drawing of the intact bones. To do so, the separate fragments can be copied on different pieces of drawing paper or cut with scissors. The restored fracture on paper helps indicate how to best reduce the fracture and which function of the fixation device, absolute or relative stability will be utilized (Fig. 7-7). The plan also indicates what size implant is needed and where and how to place or introduce it to minimize additional soft tissue injury. Finally, the reduced fracture with the implant in place is drawn, and the different steps of applying the fixation device are numbered. For an open fracture, the question of wound closure or coverage should be addressed. The OR team will be grateful if a list of the required equipment, instrument sets, reduction tools, intraoperative imaging, etc. is provided.

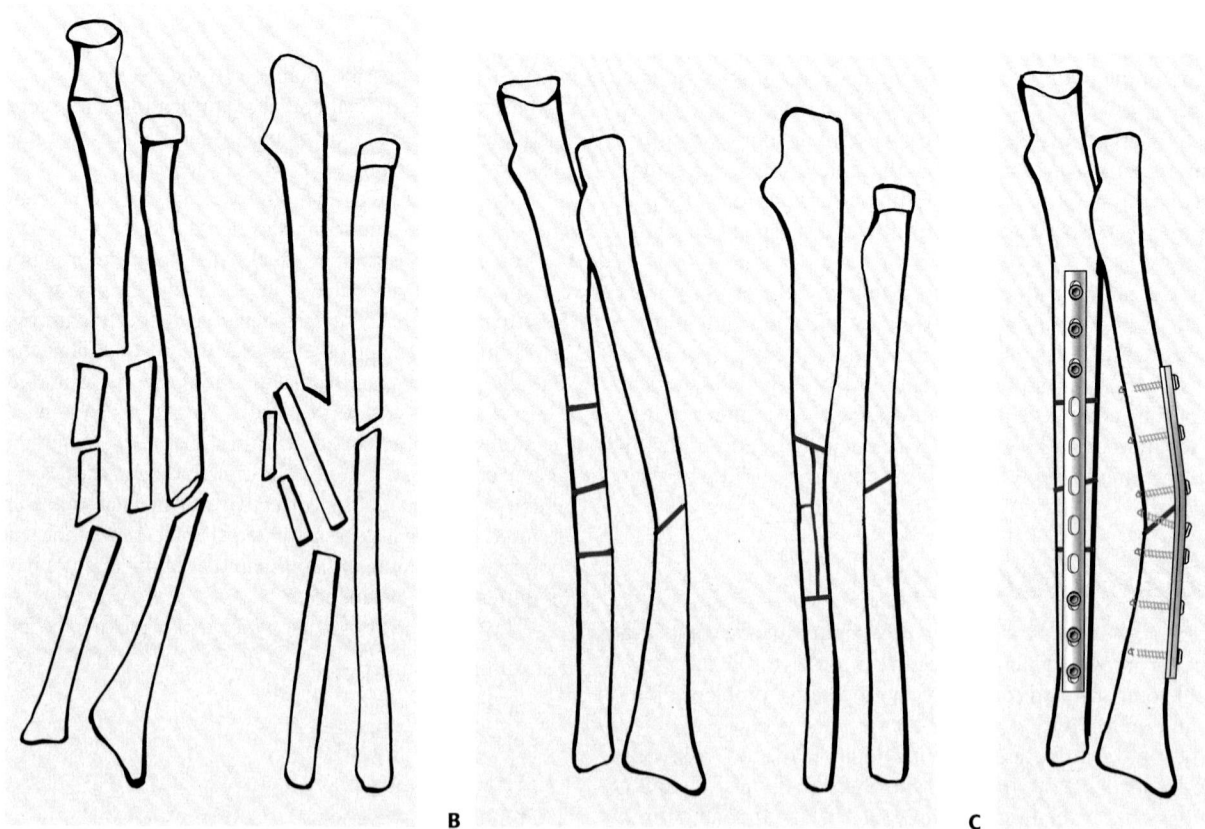

A   **B**   **C**

FIGURE 7-7 Planning on paper. **A:** First the different fracture fragments are drawn separately on tracing paper. **B:** They may be cut out with a scissor to be assembled again, or they may be copied onto the outlines of the intact bones of the opposite side. **C:** Finally, the implants are added in the correct position, length, and function providing absolute (compression) or relative (bridging) stability.

With digital x-ray imaging becoming standard equipment in most newer radiology departments, online planning tools and templates are under development and will soon be available, which hopefully will make the whole planning process on personal laptops more attractive, easier, and less time consuming. A good preoperative plan will reduce OR time, make a procedure more efficient and thus be beneficial to the patient.

Prophylactic Antibiotics and Thromboembolic Prophylaxis

While the use of prophylactic antibiotics in operative fracture fixation of open as well as closed fractures is an evidence-based standard treatment today,[8,60] discussion concerns the kind of antibiotic and the duration of application. As there is a large variation in the recommendations depending on national, regional and local factors, we suggest that the infectious disease specialist of a specific hospital should be consulted to determine a local standard. In general a second generation cephalosporin with a broad spectrum is recommended, applied as single dose 30 minutes before the start of surgery or for a period of a maximum of 24 to 48 hours postoperatively. Furthermore frequent wound irrigation with saline during surgery is recommended ("Keep the soft tissues wet and they will love you") to reduce the risk for infection.[4] The addition of antibiotics or antiseptics to irrigate solutions is however debatable and not proven to be effective. The detailed treatment of open fractures is discussed in Chapter 10.

The risk of venous thromboembolism depends on multiple factors including age, type of surgery, duration of immobilization, and pre-existing disposition. The incidence of deep vein thrombosis (DVT) is high in patients with fractures of the hip, pelvis, spine and lower extremity, while upper limb injuries are rarely the source of thrombosis. DVT has a considerable morbidity with significant complications and mortality. However and similar to the use of antibiotics, the recommendations for a thromboembolic prophylaxis vary greatly from one institution to the other. Early postoperative mobilization of the entire patient is probably the most effective prophylaxis but not always possible. Low molecular heparin, aspirin, intermittent compression devices applied to the feet as well as warfarin or cumarines are all recommended by some but also rejected by others, as there is no evidence of superiority of one single method.

Postoperative Care and Rehabilitation

The postoperative care starts with the wound bandage and/or splinting, positioning of the injured limb, and the initiating of physiotherapy exercises. A general goal is to move the joints, the injured limb as well as the whole patient as soon as possible, usually by 24 hours after surgery, provided the fixation of the fracture is stable and the soft tissues permit such an aggressive management. In the case of lower limb injuries and if the patient is considered compliant, a plan for early start of partial weight bearing should be made. In patients that are not compliant (old age, mental disturbances), the fixation must be able to tolerate early full weight bearing or the fracture has to be protected externally by a splint or cast.

FRACTURE REDUCTION

The gentle and atraumatic reduction of a fracture is not only one of the most important and most challenging steps in fracture management, operative as well as nonoperative, but probably also the most difficult part to teach and practice. The goal of reduction is to restore the anatomical relationship of the fractured bone and the limb by reversing the mechanism of fragment displacement during the injury. It seems a fact that due to the muscle insertions to the bone, a fracture tends to redisplace in the direction and degree of the original displacement. It is therefore important not only to assess imaging studies carefully, but also to appreciate the vectors and forces of fragment displacement by muscle pull (Fig. 7-8).

In the diaphysis and regardless of whether the fracture is simple, multifragmentary or has a bone defect the correct restoration of length, axial alignment, and rotation is considered an adequate reduction. In the epiphyseal segment however a meticulous, anatomical reconstruction of the articular surface and joint congruency is advocated in order to obtain a good functional result. Such ambitious aims are sometimes difficult to achieve without risks—such as long incisions and a wide exposure. A careful balance between a perfect reconstruction and the necessary respect for the soft tissue biology has to be

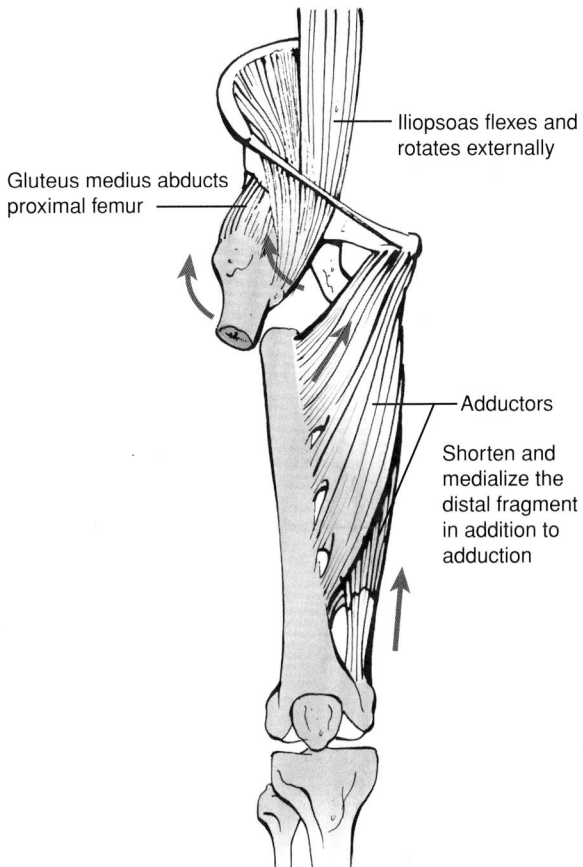

FIGURE 7-8 Typical displacement of a subtrochanteric fracture with external rotation, abduction, and flexion of the proximal and adduction of the distal fragment.

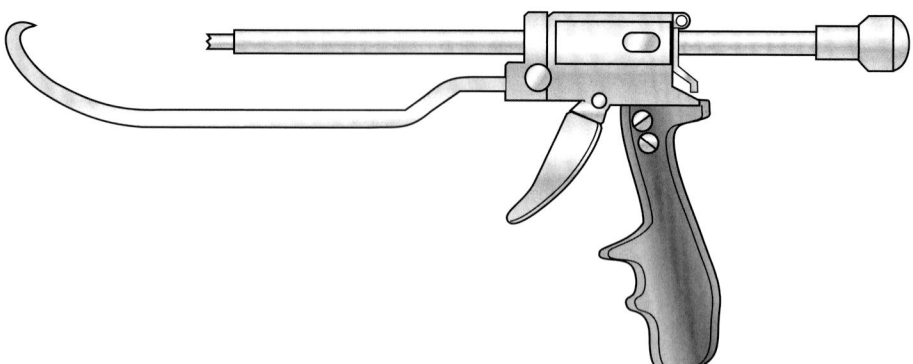

FIGURE 7-9 Collinear reduction clamp for minimally invasive approaches.

chosen. Furthermore, irreparable damage to the joint cartilage may be a limiting factor.

Mast et al.[49] created the term of "biologic fracture fixation" which refers not only to the method of fixation, but also to the reduction techniques. Accordingly, distinctions between direct and indirect as well as open and closed reduction will be made. Although direct and open reduction and indirect and closed techniques are usually associated, they are not necessarily synonymous. At the end, the essentials are that any reduction or fragment manipulation occurs atraumatic and gently, minimizing any additional harm to the vascularity of the already compromised fracture fragments and soft tissues envelope.

Direct Reduction

Direct reduction means that the fracture fragments are manipulated directly by the application of different instruments or hands, which usually requires an open exposure of the fracture site. Some newly developed instruments and devices may however also be applied directly to the bone through very small incisions and without wide exposure of the fracture such as joysticks, large pointed reduction forceps, the collinear clamp (Fig. 7-9), or new cerclage wire tools. The application of these

new techniques is called minimally invasive surgery (MIS) or when applied to plating, minimally invasive plate osteosynthesis (MIPO) inspite of the fact that thanks to the new instruments direct fragment manipulation has occurred.

The advantages of direct reduction are a precise restoration of anatomy; however, at the cost of more interference with bone and soft tissue biology. A higher risk of infection and possibly a delay in bony union that accompany striping of the soft tissues are further potential disadvantages.

Indirect Reduction

Indirect reduction means that the reduction and alignment of the fracture fragments is being achieved without exposing the fracture site as such by applying reduction forces indirectly—via the soft tissue envelope—to the main fragments by manual or skeletal traction, a distractor, or some other means. The classical example of indirect reduction is the "closed" insertion of an intramedullary nail on a fracture table (Fig. 7-10), where reduction has been obtained by traction on the lower leg, while the nail provides the final alignment of the fragments. The advantages of indirect reduction are that there is virtually no exposure of the fracture site which reduces the risk of additional damage to the vascularity of the tissues, as well as that

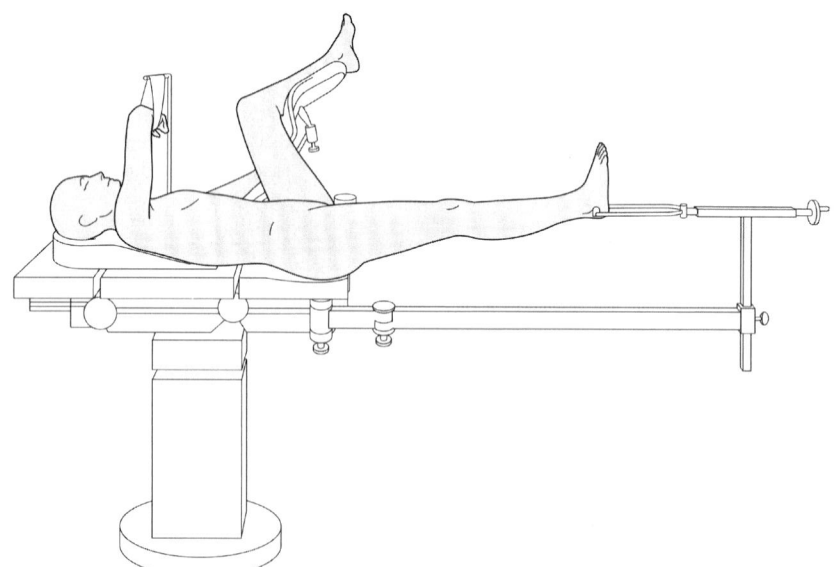

FIGURE 7-10 Fracture table with patient in supine position for femoral nailing. (Copyright by AO Foundation, Switzerland.)

of an infection. The disadvantages are that it is a demanding technique and that the correct overall alignment of the fracture is more difficult to assess, especially in rotation.

Open Reduction

Open reduction implies that the fracture site is exposed, allowing to watch and inspect the adequacy of reduction with our eyes. It is usually combined with direct manipulation of some fragments, but can also involve indirect techniques such as the use of a joint bridging distractor in an articular fracture.

Indications for open reduction are the following.

- Displaced articular fractures with impaction of the joint surface
- Fractures which require exact axial alignment (e.g., forearm fractures, simple metaphyseal fractures)
- Failed closed reduction due to soft tissue interposition
- Delayed surgery where granulation tissue or early callus has to be removed
- Where there is a high risk for harming neurovascular structures
- In cases of no or limited access to perioperative imaging to check reduction

Careful preoperative planning including adequate imaging is essential to choose the best approach, the tools for a gentle reduction and the appropriate implant. In articular fractures it is usually sufficient to be able to see into the joint, in order to carefully clear it from hematoma and debris and to judge the cartilage damage as well as the quality of reduction after the reconstruction. The periosteum and any soft tissue attachments must be preserved wherever possible, while separate stab incisions may help the placement of pointed reduction clamps, temporary K-wires or the insertion of lag screws.

Closed Reduction

Closed reduction relies entirely on indirect fragment alignment by ligamentotaxis or the pull of the soft tissue envelope. Longitudinal traction is the main force which may be modified by adduction or abduction, flexion, or extension and rotation as well as supporting bolsters, etc. These maneuvers may be quite demanding and usually require the presence of an image intensifier. Profound knowledge of the anatomy (location of muscle insertion and direction of muscle pull) as well as careful planning are prerequisites. Percutaneously applied joysticks, and special instruments may be helpful.[18,43] If correctly applied, the advantages of closed reduction are minimal additional damage to the soft tissues, safer, and more rapid fracture repair as well as lower risk of infection.

Indications for closed reduction are the following.

- Most diaphyseal fractures, where correct axial alignment, length, and rotation is considered sufficient for a good outcome.
- Minimally displaced articular fractures suited for percutaneous fixation.

- Geriatric femoral neck fractures, trochanteric fractures, subcapital humerus fractures, and certain distal radius fractures.

The size of an incision will not necessarily be indicative of the amount of damage done to the biology of a fracture. Much harm can be done through a short incision, but also little harm through a larger exposure. All that matters is the gentleness of the surgeon's hands and his skills in managing the reduction process.

TECHNIQUES AND INSTRUMENTS FOR FRACTURE REDUCTION

Traction and Distraction

Traction is the most common means to reduce a fracture. This can occur manually, with the help of a fracture table or by applying a distractor directly to the main fragments of a long bone or in an articular fracture across the joint (Fig. 7-11). While longitudinal traction will usually correct shortening, it may be difficult to align the fragments in both the sagittal and coronal planes. There are a number of tricks described to overcome the problem. The fracture table has the disadvantage that traction is usually applied across a joint and that there are limited possibilities to move the limb. The distractor on the other hand offers many possibilities and more freedom of movement, but it is quite demanding to manipulate and requires considerable practice (Fig. 7-12).[3,5]

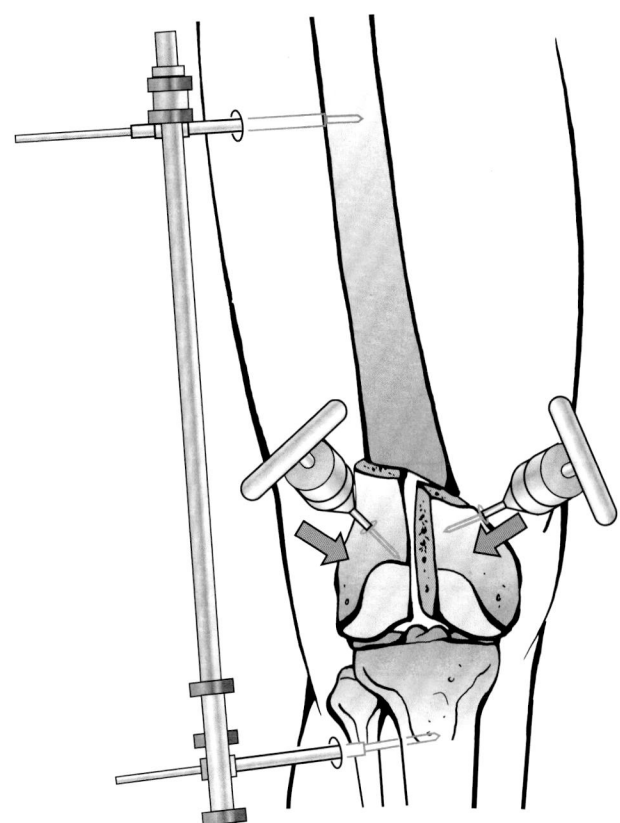

FIGURE 7-11 Joint bridging distractor to support reduction of a distal femur fracture with joysticks.

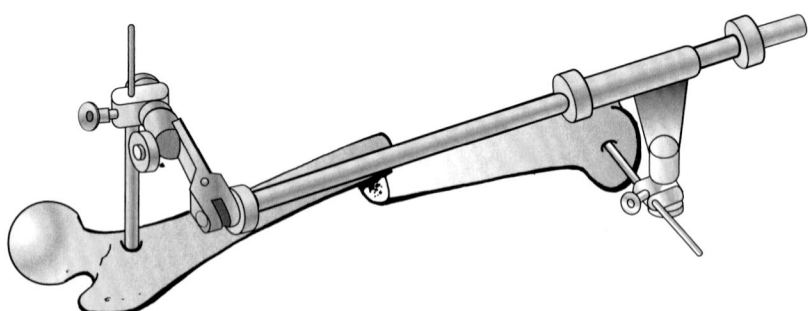

FIGURE 7-12 Femoral distractor applied in two planes to allow axial and rotational alignment such as for IM nailing or minimally invasive plating.

Reduction Forceps

There is a great variety of reduction forceps available, some for general use, others for rather specific applications (Table 7-2). The reduction forceps with sharp points (Weber forceps) (Fig. 7-13) is the most commonly used as it comes in many different dimensions. The points provide an excellent purchase on the fragments without stripping or squeezing the periosteum; in osteopenic bone they can however penetrate through the thin cortex. Occasionally a small hole, created with a drill or K-wire, is helpful to gain purchase for the tip. The forceps may be applied directly through a surgical wound or percutaneously through stab incisions.

Two special forceps (Faraboeuf and Jungbluth) have originally been developed for pelvic and acetabular fractures. Both are applied to the heads of two screws that are inserted on either side of a fracture (Fig. 7-14). The newest reduction forceps is the collinear forceps which is no longer based on a hinge between the two branches but on a sliding mechanism that allows a linear movement (Fig. 7-9). Thanks to this, the new reduction tool can be introduced through very short incisions or through narrow openings in the pelvis which makes it ideal for minimally invasive techniques.

Other reduction tools include joysticks (preferably Schanz screws), Hohmann retractors for intrafocal manipulation and cerclage wires, while every surgeon has additional tricks and tools in his personal armamentarium (Fig. 7-15).

There are furthermore situations where the implant, intramedullary nail, plate or modular external fixator, may be used for the reduction and fixation at the same time. Especially in conventional nonlocked plating, angle blade and precontoured plates can be used to reduce the fracture toward the plate.

Computer assisted surgery (CAS) with navigation software has promised to open completely new applications especially for hip and knee replacement, but appears at present to be still in an early stage for acute fracture reduction and management.[31,36]

Intra- and Postoperative Assessment of the Reduction

After the reduction of a fracture, the position of the fragments should be held reduced with temporary K-wires and/or a forceps and then the reconstruction and axial alignment must be carefully assessed in at least two planes preferably with the image intensifier. However, the resolution of the images is not as precise as that of x-rays, and the size of the field or picture is usually too small to allow to evaluate the longitudinal axis of a bone or its rotation. Another shortcoming of the image intensifier is the often prolonged exposure to radiation for the patient, surgeon, and staff. Several tricks have been described to overcome these drawbacks, some of them will be described in the chapter on IM nailing where axial and rotational alignment is particularly difficult. In articular fractures, inspection of the joint surface occurs best with our eyes or

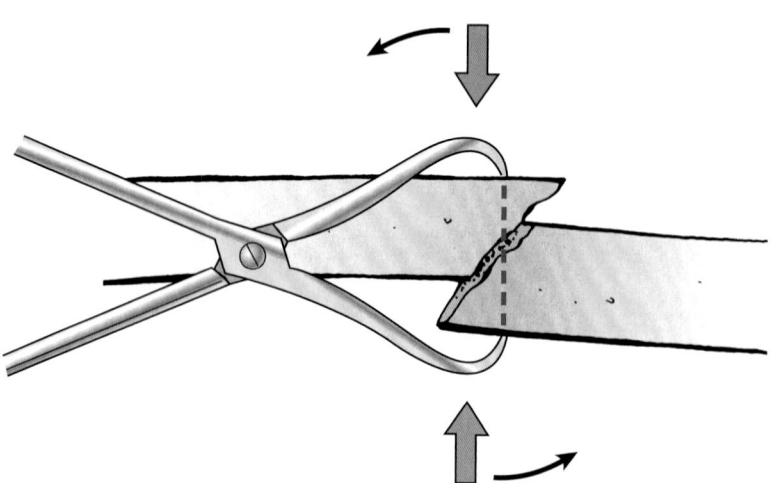

FIGURE 7-13 Pointed reduction forceps (Weber), which allows safe purchase of the bone without stripping of the periosteum. By manipulating the forceps (*arrows*) a simple oblique fracture can be easily reduced.

TABLE 7-2 Useful and Frequently Used Instruments for Reduction

Instrument	Image of Instrument	Description	Application Technique, Degrees of Freedom
Reduction forceps with points (Weber forceps)		Different sizes and angulations of the branches available, different mechanisms	One-forceps technique, two-forceps technique, three linear and two rotational degrees of freedom
Reduction forceps, toothed		Different sizes	Mainly used for alignment of a plate on a diaphyseal bone and reduction
Bone holding forceps, self-centering (Verbrugge forceps)		Four different sizes	
Bone spreader		Different sizes and angulations	Only for distraction, one linear degree of freedom
Collinear reduction forceps		Different insertable branches (hooks)	Only for compression, one linear degree of freedom
Pelvic reduction forceps with ballpoints ("King Tong," "Queen Tong")		Symmetric and asymmetric, two spikes and three spikes, spiked mountable washer	
Angled pelvic reduction forceps (Matta forceps)		Large and small	
Pelvic reduction forceps (Faraboeuf forceps)		Different sizes, 3.5- and 4.5-mm screws	
Pelvic reduction forceps (Jungbluth forceps)		Two different sizes, 3.5- and 4.5-mm screws	Can be used in different directions, as the screw directly links the forceps to the bone fragment
Periarticular reduction forceps with ball points ("Ice Tong," "King Kong")		Multiple sizes, spiked mountable washer	Mainly used for periarticular fractures, large radius prevents soft tissue crush

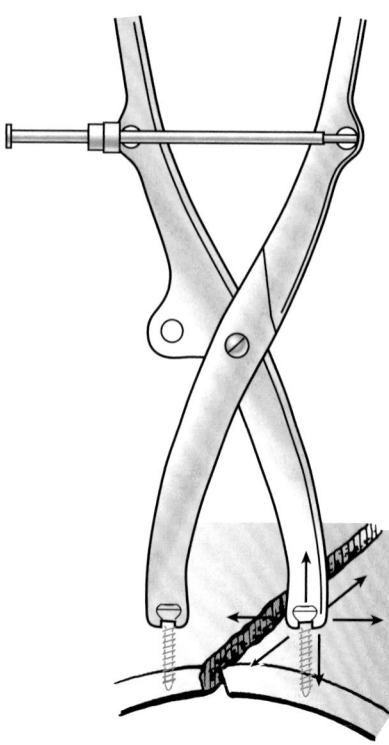

FIGURE 7-14 The Jungbluth forceps is applied with the help of the head of two screws that are inserted close to the fracture. Distraction as well as translation movements may be performed, which is helpful especially in the pelvis.

with the image intensifier. The most reliable way to assess an articular reconstruction is with a CT scan, which is becoming more available in the OR integrated into the new 2D and 3D fluoroscopes. Arthroscopy has also been advocated for minimally invasive surgical control of articular fractures.[30,50] It offers advantages to evaluate menisci and ligaments as well as the consistency of articular cartilage; however, for the judgment of axial alignment open reduction usually appears to be superior.

TECHNIQUES AND DEVICES FOR INTERNAL FIXATION

Operative fracture fixation can be performed with devices applied either externally (percutaneously) or internally (underneath the soft tissue cover). The former include the many different types of external fixators that will be described in Chapter 8. Internal fixation devices stabilize the bone from within the medullary canal (intramedullary nails) or are fixed to the exterior of the bone (conventional nonlocked screws and plates and locked plates as well as tension band wires).

Screws

Screws are the basic and most efficient tool for internal fixation especially in combination with plates. A screw is a powerful element that converts rotation into linear motion.

Most screws are characterized by some common design features (Fig. 7-16).

- A central core that provides strength.
- A thread which engages the bone and is responsible for the function and purchase.
- A tip that may be blunt or sharp, self-cutting or self-drilling and -cutting.
- A head that engages in bone or a plate.
- A recess in the head to attach the screw driver.

Screws are provided in different forms, sizes, and materials. They are typically named according to their design, function, or way of application.

- Design (partially or fully threaded, cannulated, self-tapping, etc.)
- Dimension of major thread diameter (most common used 1.5, 2, 2.4, 2.7, 3.5, 4.5, 6.5, 7.3 mm, etc.)
- Area of typical application (cortex, cancellous bone, bicortical, or monocortical)
- Function (lag screw, locking head screw [LHS], position screw, etc.)

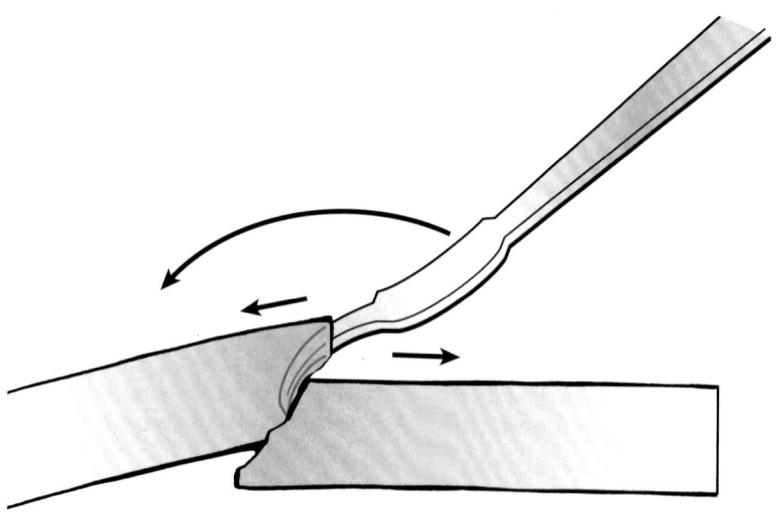

FIGURE 7-15 Hohmann retractor for direct reduction of a simple fracture.

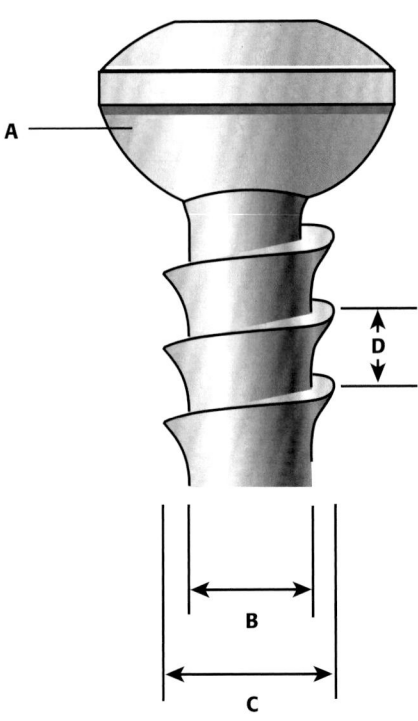

FIGURE 7-16 Schematic illustration of a conventional 4.5-mm cortex screw. **A:** Spherical screw head allowing a congruous fit in the plate hole. **B:** Core diameter (3.2 mm), **C:** Outer diameter (4.5 mm), and **D:** The thread pitch are commonly referenced screw design parameters.

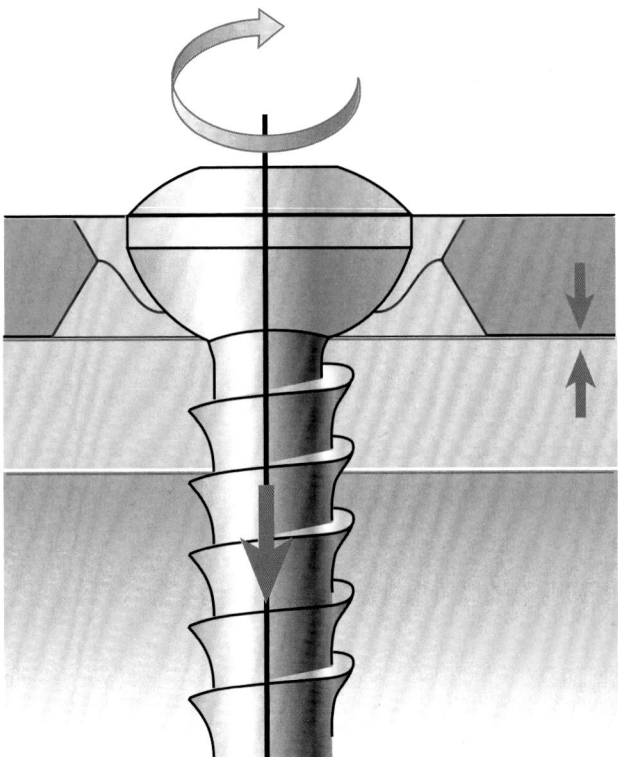

FIGURE 7-17 A conventional cortical screw applied as a plate screw. It presses the plate against the bone surface thereby creating friction and preload.

- One and the same screw can have different functions, which depend on the screw design and way of application. The two basic principles of a conventional screw are to compress a fracture plane (lag screw) and to fix a plate to the bone (plate screw). The more recent designed LHS provide angular stability between the implant and the bone (Figs. 7-17 and 7-18). The LHS have a head with a thread that engages with the reciprocal thread of the plate hole.[15] This creates a screw-plate device with angular stability. Locking screw tightening does not press plate against the bone surface. The load transfer occurs through the locking screws and the plate, similarly as with an external fixator, and not by friction and preload. As the locked plate lies underneath the soft tissues the principle of this purely locked construct has been termed internal fixator (Fig. 7-19). A more recent development offers the option of variable angular stability, which allows angulating locking screws within the plate hole to address specific fracture configurations (e.g., for complex comminuted metaphyseal fractures especially distal radius fractures).

Lag screws (Fig. 7-20) can be applied independently or through a plate hole. In both situations compression between two fragments or between the plate and the bone produces preload and friction, which oppose fragment displacement by other forces including shear. Interfragmentary compression is the basic element responsible for absolute stability of fracture fixation.

To insert a screw, a hole has to be drilled into the bone with a drill bit slightly larger in diameter than the minor diameter

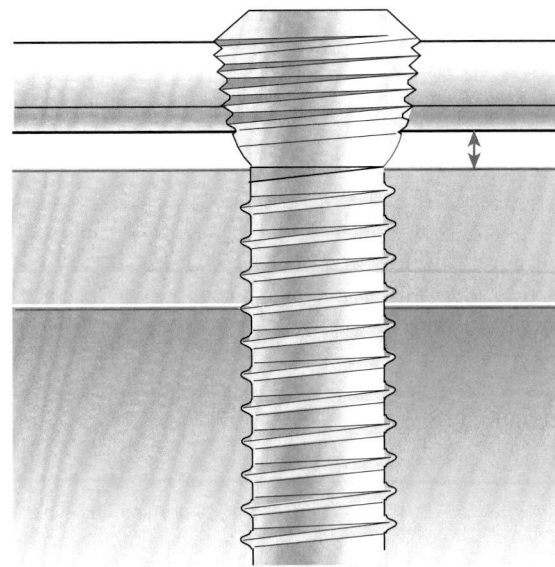

FIGURE 7-18 Locking head screw. The screw head is firmly locked in the screw hole without pressing the plate against the bone. It provides angular stability.

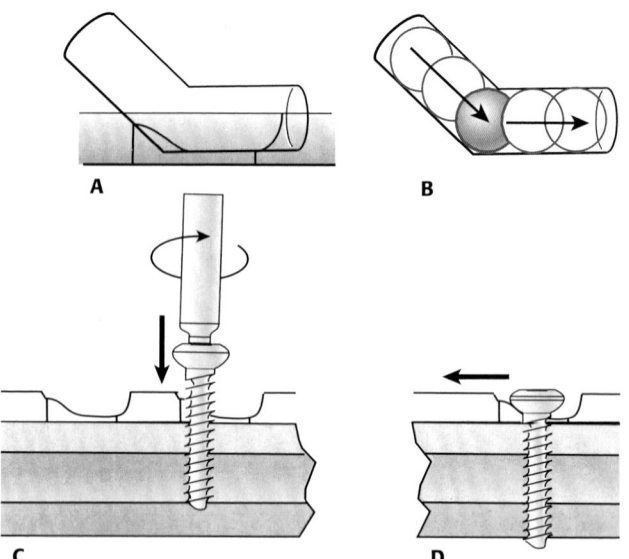

FIGURE 7-19 Dynamic compression principle: The holes of the DC-plate are shaped like an inclined and transverse cylinder **(A)**. Like a ball, the screw head slides down the inclined cylinder **(B)**. Due to the shape of the plate hole, the plate is being moved horizontally relative to bone when the screw is driven home **(C)** and **(D)**.

of the selected screw. To ensure safe purchase of the screw it is recommended to cut a thread with a matching tap before the screw is inserted especially in cortical as well as in hard cancellous bone in young patients. In bone of softer quality such as cancellous bone, screw insertion may be done without tapping. Alternatively there are also self-tapping screws, which reduce insertion time but require some practice. Turning the screw within the bone creates friction and thereby heat is generated, which may in turn cause thermal necrosis of the adjacent bone. The screw design and the technique of screw insertion influence the amount of damage done and ultimately the holding power of a screw. Thermal necrosis may also be caused by dull drill bits or by inserting pins and wires with a diameter larger than 2 mm without predrilling, leading to loosening, and ring sequester. It is the surgeon's responsibility to adequately prepare the holes.

In general, three different types of screws are differentiated as follows.

1. The cortex screw thread is designed for use in cortical bone (Fig. 7-16). It is typically fully threaded but maybe partially threaded and is commonly available in diameters from 1 to 4.5 mm. Each size has a pair of drill bits corresponding to the screws major and minor diameter and a tap. The drill

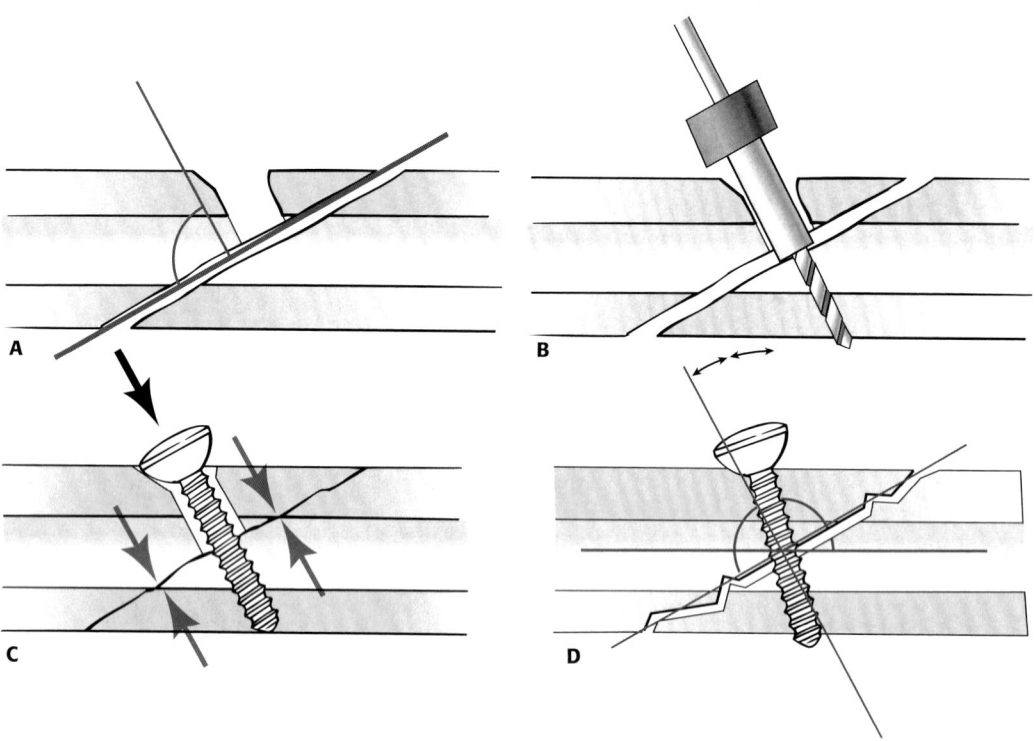

FIGURE 7-20 To insert a lag screw the first step consists of drilling the glide hole in the near cortex with a drill bit slightly larger than the major screw diameter **(A)**. Into this hole a drill sleeve is inserted to correctly centre the pilot or threaded hole in the opposite or far cortex, which is drilled with a drill bit the same size as the minor diameter of the screw **(B)**. After measuring the screw length with the depth gauge and tapping the thread in the far cortex, the cortex screw is inserted. Driving home the screw, the fracture surfaces will be compressed (interfragmentary compression) **(C)**. While the ideal screw direction to generate compression is at right angles to the fracture plane, this is only rarely possible. Therefore the screw is directed halfway between the perpendicular to the fracture plane and to that of the bone **(D)**.

corresponding to the major diameter is used for drilling the gliding hole for a lag screw while the drill corresponding to the minor diameter is used for drilling the threaded hole. Today self-tapping cortex screws are available and also recommended, except for hard cortical bone of the young adult. Some of the screws are also available in a cannulated version.

2. The cancellous bone screw has a deeper thread, a larger pitch, and typically a larger outer diameter (4 to 8 mm) than the cortex screws. They are indicated for meta-epiphyseal cancellous bone. The screw may be partially or fully threaded. Tapping is recommend to open the cortex and in dense bone of the young adult.

3. The LHS of locking plate systems (Fig. 7-18) are primarily characterized by the threaded screw head. They may have a larger core diameter and a relatively shallow thread with blunt edges. This increases the strength and interface between screw and cortical bone compared to conventional screws. Locking screws are used in combination with plates that have holes able to accommodate the threaded screw head. Variable angle locking screws follow the same locking principle, but offer in addition that the locking screws can be angulated to some degree. Certain comminuted metaphyseal fractures required the fixation of small fragments, still providing angular stability. This development has become more broadly available specially for complex unstable or displaced metaphyseal fracture fixation of the distal radius,[62] the proximal humerus,[40,81] distal femur,[22,59,84] and proximal tibia.[21,56] These types of screws certainly provide a greater versatility and flexibility in both screw and plate placement but may at the same time cause reduction of ultimate fatigue strength. Thus, for clinical use it needs to be taken in consideration that an increase in screw angulation can cause reduction of locking strength and thereby potential load failure.[29,84]

Different Functions of a Screw

Various different screw functions are listed in Table 7-3. Three examples are given in more depth due to their importance in daily operative fracture care.

Lag Screw. One of the basic principles of modern internal fixation is absolute stability thanks to interfragmentary compression as it is provided by a lag screw.[65] A fully threaded conventional cortex screw is acting as a lag screw when the thread engages only in the cortex opposite to the fracture line (far cortex) and not in the cortex close to the screw head (near cortex). This is obtained by first drilling a glide hole with a drill bit slightly larger than the major diameter of the cortex screw. Next a drill sleeve is inserted into the gliding hole to precisely centre the threaded or pilot hole in the opposite cortex collinear with the gliding hole, which is drilled with a smaller drill bit corresponding to the minor diameter of the screw. After measuring the screw length with a depth gauge, the thread in the far cortex

TABLE 7-3	**Various Screw Functions and Clinical Examples**	
	Function	
Name	**Mechanism**	**Clinical Example**
Nonlocked plate screw	Preload and friction is applied to create force between the plate and the bone	Forearm plating
Lag screw	The glide hole allows compression between bone fragments	Fixation of a butterfly or wedge fragment or medial malleolus fracture
Position screw	Holds anatomical parts in correct relation to each other without compression (i.e., thread hole only, no glide hole)	Syndesmotic screw
Locking head screw	Used exclusively with locked plates; threads in the screw head allow mechanical coupling to a reciprocal thread in the plate and provide angular stability	Complex metaphyseal fracture Osteoporotic
Variable locking screw	Used exclusively with special locked plates; same mechanical angular stability as locking head screw, but allows some variability in screw angulation within the plate hole	Complex comminuted metaphyseal fractures and periprosthetic fractures
Interlocking screw	Couples an intramedullary nail to the bone to maintain length, alignment, and rotation	Interlocked femoral or tibial intramedullary nail
Anchor screw	A point of fixation used to anchor a wire loop or strong suture	Tension band anchor in a proximal humerus fracture
Push–pull screw	A temporary point of fixation used to reduce a fracture by distraction and/or compression	Use of an articulated compression device
Reduction screw	Conventional screw used through a plate to pull fracture fragments toward the plate; the screw may be removed or exchanged once alignment is obtained	Minimally invasive plate osteosynthesis technique to reduce multifragmentary fracture onto the plate
Poller screw	Screw used as a fulcrum to redirect an intramedullary nail	Proximal tibial fracture during IM nailing

is cut with a tap or a self-tapping screw is inserted. As the screw advances in the threaded hole, the head will engage in the near cortex and create preload and compression between the two fragments. It is advisable to apply only about two-third of the possible torque to a lag screw corresponding to about 2,000 to 3,000 N.[68,75] The ideal direction of a lag screw, for generation of compressive force, is perpendicular to the fracture plane. As this is often not practical, an inclination halfway between the perpendiculars to the fracture and to the long axis of the bone is typically chosen (Fig. 7-20). The head of an independent lag screw should be countersunk in the underlying cortex, which increased the area of contact between the screw and the bone and reduces the risk of stress risers producing cracks. A further advantage of countersinking consists of reducing the protuberance of the large screw head underneath the skin (e.g., on the tibial crest).

The partially threaded cancellous bone screw will also produce interfragmentary compression, provided that the thread engages only in the fragment opposite to the fracture plane. A washer may prevent the screw head from sinking into the thin metaphyseal cortex (Fig. 7-21).

Plate Screws. Conventional nonlocked screws used to fix a plate to the bone are called plate screws. They are introduced with a special drill guide that fits into the plate hole either centrally or eccentrically depending on whether axial compression is demanded. The drill bit has the diameter of the minor diameter of the screw, which may be self-tapping or not. By driving home the plate screws the plate is pressed against the bone which produces preload and friction between the two surfaces.

Positioning Screw. A positioning screw is a fully threaded screw that joins two anatomical parts at a defined

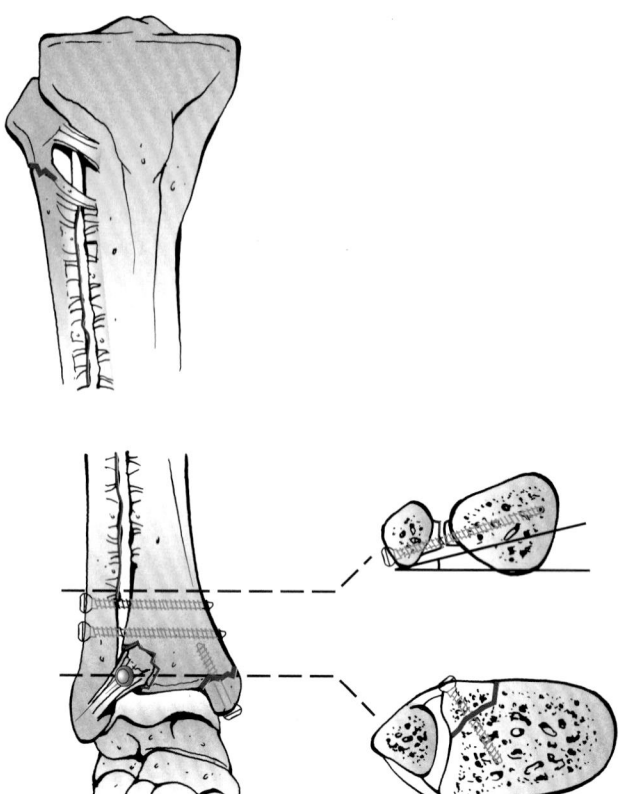

FIGURE 7-22 Example of a cortex screw in the function as a position screw between fibula and tibia to secure the ruptured syndesmosis. A thread is cut in every cortex thus preventing compression between the two bones.

distance without compression. The thread is therefore tapped in both cortices. An example is a screw placed between fibula and tibia in a malleolar fracture to secure the syndesmotic ligaments (Fig. 7-22).

Plates

Besides the lag screw as a basic principle of operative fracture fixation, conventional compression plating is the other principle providing absolute stability and inducing primary or direct bone healing without visible callus. Today the classical open reduction with considerable exposure of the fracture and internal fixation by plates and screws is being challenged by less invasive and more elastic fixation methods, so-called biologic techniques. Nevertheless plating with absolute stability still has its definitive place in operative fracture treatment, especially since we have learned to better protect the delicate soft tissues also during open approaches. Fractures of the forearm bones as well as simple metaphyseal fractures of other long bones are good indications for conventional nonlocked plating, so are mal- and nonunions. In articular fractures that require anatomical reduction and rigid fixation by interfragmentary compression, plates will often support lag screws and/or buttress the metaphysis. However, for most

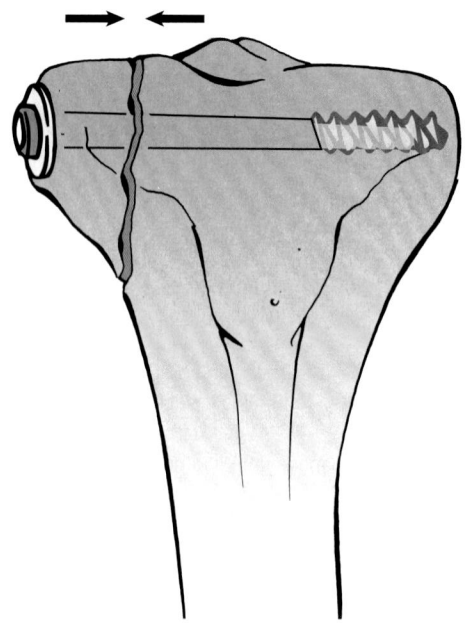

FIGURE 7-21 A partially threaded 6.5-mm cancellous bone screw will act as a lag screw, provided that the thread has its purchase opposite to the fracture line only.

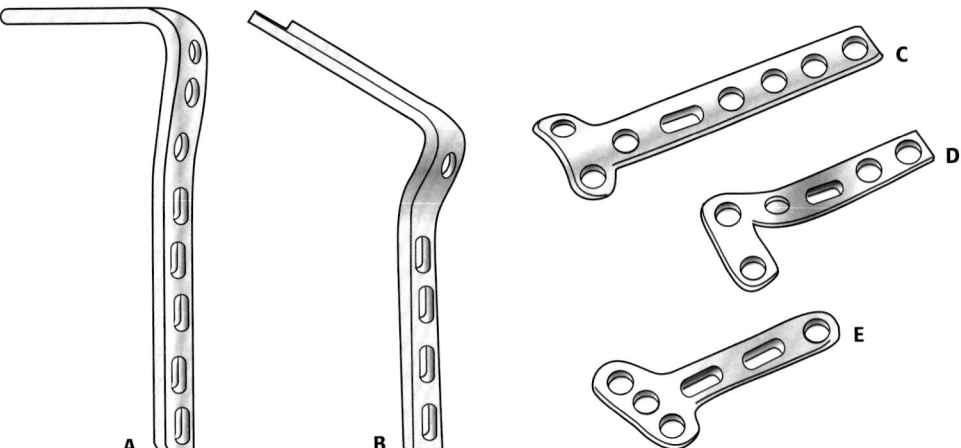

FIGURE 7-23 Different types and forms of early plates. **A:** 95-degree and **B:** 130-degree angle blade plates, **C:** T and **D:** L plates, and **E:** Small fragment 3.5 distal radius plate.

diaphyseal fractures of the femur and tibia IM nailing is the golden standard today.

Absolute stability results in direct fracture healing, which generally takes longer than healing by callus. Appearance of callus after attempted rigid plate fixation is unexpected and a sign of unplanned instability, which may lead to implant failure, healing delay or nonunion. The classical technique of compression plating relies on pressing the plate to the bone surface, which may disturb the blood flow to the underlying cortex, leading to local cortical necrosis. This so called footprint of the plate induces a slow cortical remodeling by creeping substitution and revascularization. What was considered as stress protection in former times is now interpreted as disturbed vascularity of the cortex and has been addressed by new plate designs with limited bone contact or more effectively by the internal fixator principle, where there is no direct compression between the plate and the bone.[67]

Plate Design

Early modern plates had round holes in which the conical screw head had a firm fit. Axial compression was obtained with a removable external device. In 1967 the dynamic compression plate (DCP) designed by Perren introduced a new principle of applying axial compression by leveraging the interaction of a spherical screw head and an inclined oval screw hole (Fig. 7-19). The oval hole also allowed angulation of the screw in different directions.[66] The use of special drill guides precisely placed the screws in relation to the plate hole in neutral or compression mode. These features of the DCP greatly extended and facilitated the possibilities of application of plates.

While the original plates were all straight and of two sizes only, 4.5 narrow and broad, soon smaller sizes followed and also different designs for special applications such as the angle blade plates for the proximal and distal femur, tubular plates, reconstruction plates, the sliding hip screw and dynamic condylar screws, and other form plates (Fig. 7-23).

A further advancement was the LC-DCP (limited contact-DCP) which featured a new design of the under surface reducing the area of contact between the plate and the bone to reduce the adverse effects of pressure and friction on bone vascularity (Fig. 7-24). This plate generation, designed with finite-element analysis displayed an even distribution of strength throughout its length and irrespective of the plate holes. All conventional plates usually had to be contoured to match the shape of the bone, as the plate was either pressed against the bone or the bone was pulled toward the plate.

The most recent and most revolutionary design changes to modern plates that also introduced a completely new principles of fixation, the internal fixators or locking plates, will be discussed later in a separate section of this chapter.

Plate Functions

While there are many different designs and dimensions of plates, the function that is assigned to a plate by the surgeon

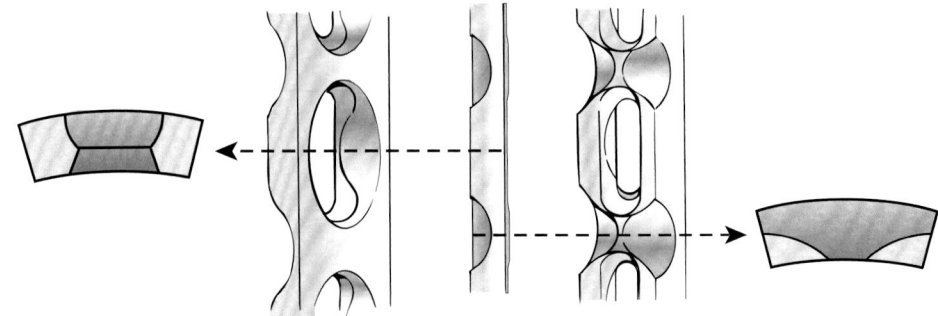

FIGURE 7-24 More recent plate designs (like the LC-DCP, limited contact-dynamic compression plate) feature the dynamic compression unit and have undercuts between the screw holes to reduce the area of contact between the plate and the bone. This plate design has uniform strength throughout.[69]

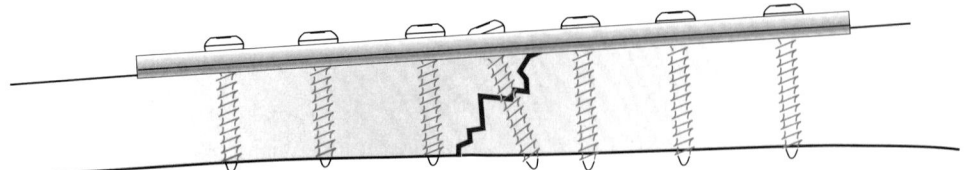

FIGURE 7-25 Protection or neutralization plate to protect a simple fracture of the radius. The oblique screw inserted through the plate is a lag screw crossing the fracture plane, which adds to the absolute stability of the fixation.

and how it is applied is decisive for the outcome. There are five key functions or modes any plate can have. In order to assign a specific function to a plate, the preoperative plan has to take into account the fracture pattern, its location, the soft tissues and biomechanical surrounding.

The five functions are the following.

- Neutralization or protection
- Compression
- Buttressing
- Tension band function
- Bridging

Neutralization or Protection Plate for Absolute Stability. A simple, torsion or butterfly fracture of the diaphysis or metaphysis, caused by indirect rotational forces, is best reduced anatomically and fixed by one or two lag screws providing interfragmentary compression. It is normally recommended to protect the lag screw fixation with the addition of a plate in order to protect it or to neutralize any shearing or rotational forces, thereby improving the stability (Fig. 7-25). This type of classical plate application can also be performed with minimal exposure of the fracture site and percutaneous reduction with the help of pointed reduction forceps.

Compression Plate. Axial compression of a transverse fracture of a forearm bone is best obtained by a compression plate. By slightly over bending the plate in relation the shape of the bone and by eccentric placement of the screws axial

compression is obtained. In short oblique fractures in addition to axial compression a lag screw inserted through the plate and across the oblique fracture plane will significantly increase the stability of the fixation. In oblique fractures the plate must be fixed first to the fragment with an obtuse angle, so that when compression is added on the opposite side of the fracture the fragment locks in the axilla between the plate and the bone (Fig. 7-26).

Buttress Plate (Antiglide Function). In articular fractures such as malleolar fractures, tibia plateau or distal radius fractures, we can observe how a large fragment has been displaced by shearing forces.[9] To counter act these forces and keep the reduced fragment in place, a plate is best applied in a position that locks the spike of the fragment back in place thereby preventing any further shearing or gliding of the fragment. Buttress plates are often combined with lag screws either through the plate or independently (Fig. 7-27).

Tension Band Plate. Certain bones such as the femur are loaded eccentrically. We know from the studies of Pauwels[63] that with weight bearing the concave, medial side of the femur is undergoing compressive forces, while the convex, lateral cortex is under tension. An eccentrically applied plate on the convex side of the bone will theoretically convert tensile forces into compression, provided the opposite medial cortex is stable. In a subtrochanteric fracture that is fixed with a plate, this implant will function as a tension band provided the medial cortex, opposite to the plate, has been reduced anatomically without any residual gap (Fig. 7-28).

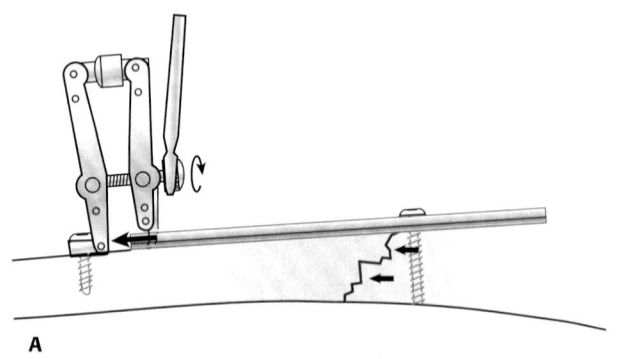

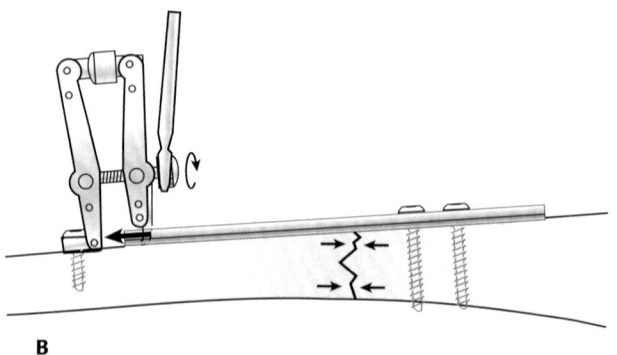

A **B**

FIGURE 7-26 Axial compression with a plate can be obtained with the removable, articulated tension device. The plate is first fixed on one side of the fracture and then compressed in the axial direction. In case of an oblique fracture **(A)** a lag screw across the fracture plane will increase stability and compress the opposite cortex. In order to obtain an equal compression of both cortices of a transverse fracture **(B)** the plate has to slightly over contoured before axial compression is applied.

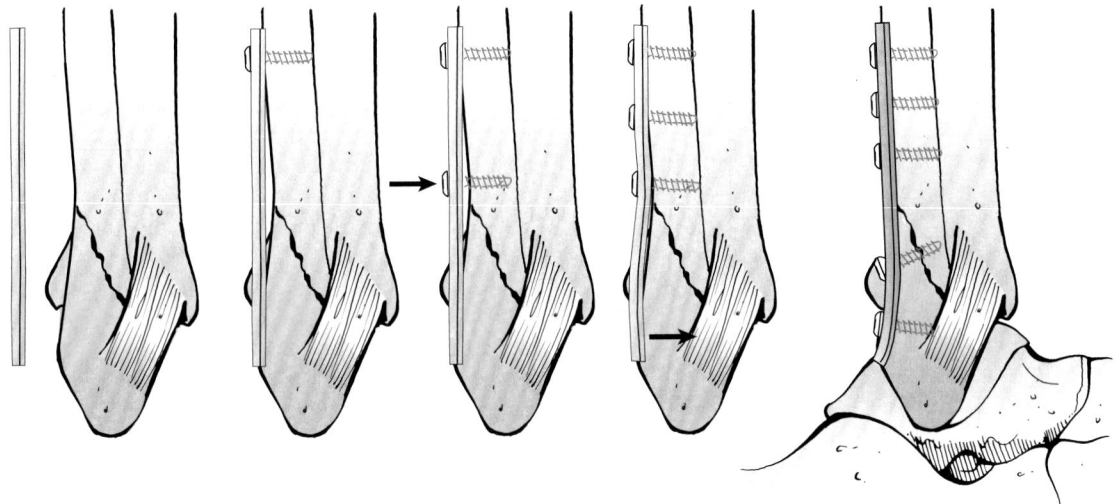

FIGURE 7-27 A buttress plate or antiglide plate has the function of preventing any secondary displacement of an oblique fracture in the metaphysis of a bone. The example shows the application in a malleolar fracture, where the plate is positioned on the posterolateral aspect of the distal fibula. The different steps and the sequence of introducing the screws are illustrated.

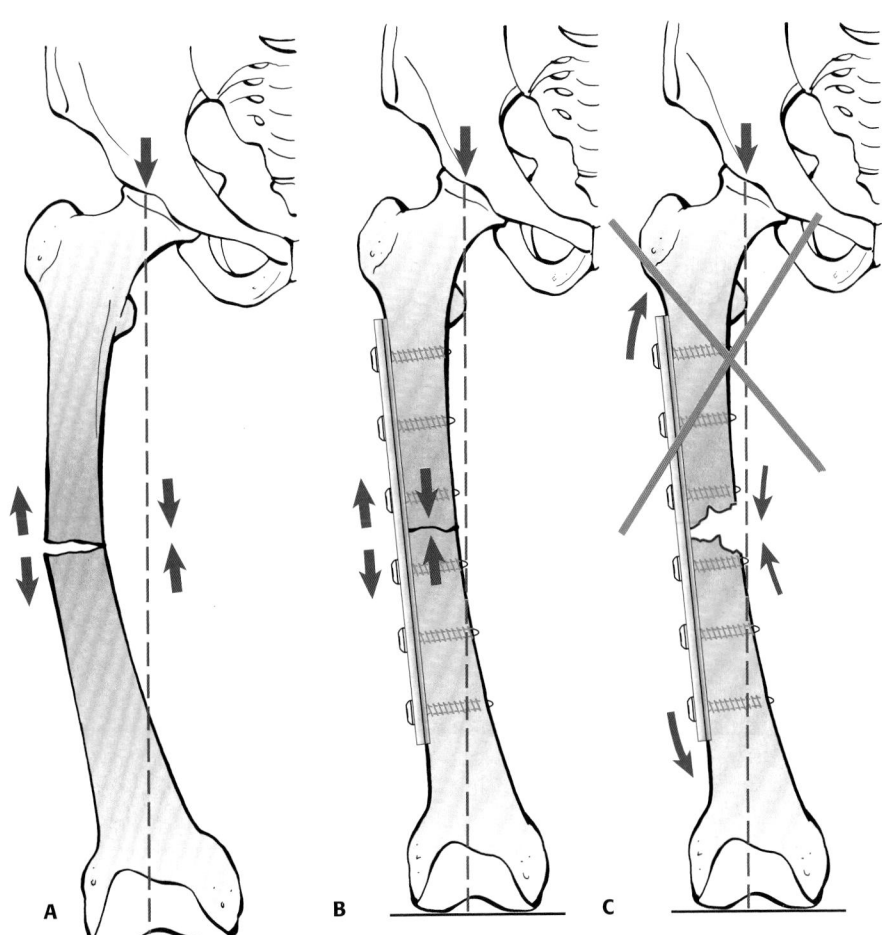

FIGURE 7-28 By placing the plate in a transverse femur fracture **(A)** to the lateral aspect of the femur **(B)** this implant will undergo tensile forces which are theoretically converted into compression at the fracture site. A precondition is however that the bone opposite to the plate has close contact to resist the compressive forces. If the essential medial support is missing, the plate is more likely to break due to fatigue **(C).**

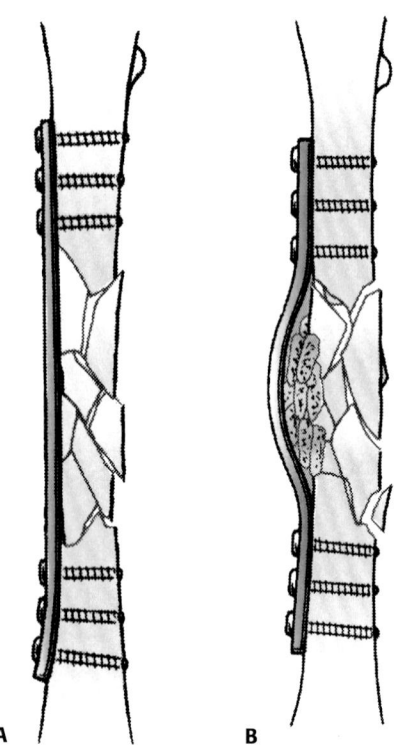

A   **B**

FIGURE 7-29 **A, B:** Bridge plating can be performed with any plate of the adequate length. Nevertheless, the new locking plate systems are considered ideally suited for bridge plating and simplify the technique of minimal invasive application. The bridging device should be about three times the length of the fracture zone providing relative stability.

Bridge Plate. Since the introduction of more biologic indirect reduction and minimally invasive techniques with less rigid or elastic fixations providing relative stability, a plate can also be applied as an internal bridging device, similar to an external fixator.[24,79] The best indications for bridge plating[9] are comminuted diaphyseal or metaphyseal fractures that are not suited for IM nailing. While we do not know precisely the ideal working length of a plate, it is recommended to choose a plate about three times as long as the fracture zone and to fix it with only a few firmly anchored screw proximally and distally (Fig. 7-29).

From Biologic to Minimally Invasive
Plate Fixation (MIPO)

Although the protagonists of modern operative fracture fixation or ORIF, starting with Albin Lambotte—stressed already 100 years ago the importance of gentle soft tissue handling and minimal stripping of the periosteum in order to preserve bone vascularity, the request for anatomical reduction seemed somehow in contradiction with this principle. In inexperienced hands too wide exposures and extensive denudation of bone occurred all too often, resulting in catastrophes such as delayed or nonunions or infections or the combination of the two. Mast et al.[49] described in detail the advantages of indirect reduction techniques without exposing the fracture fragments and

created the term of biologic plate fixation with long bridging angle blade or straight plates. In a study comparing a series of subtrochanteric fractures treated by conventional "open" technique with indirection and bridge plating demonstrated that in the latter group the time for union was shorter and predictable even without bone graft, the complication rate was lower and the functional outcome better.[37] An important prerequisite was however that the procedure was carefully planned and well performed.

We have learned from closed IM nailing with interlocking that in complex diaphyseal fractures correct axial and rotational alignment is all that is needed for early callus formation and that anatomical reduction of every fragment is not required.

Krettek et al.[44] have further developed these observations and ideas by minimizing the approaches to quite short incisions far away from the fracture focus and by inserting extra long plates via a bluntly prepared submuscular space close to the bone and across the fracture (Fig. 7-30). The screws were inserted through equally short incisions and straight through the muscles. In cadaver studies Farouk et al.[14] could show that the perforator vessels were not injured by these tunneling maneuvers. Similar to the rapid appearance of callus in IM nailing, the healing of these minimally exposed fractures fixed with only relatively stable bridge plates occurred very consistently with early callus formation.

The drawback of minimally invasive techniques is the higher incidence of axial and rotational malalignment just as in IM nailing,[77] especially of the femur. Furthermore the intraoperative radiation exposure of the patient and staff is higher, but may be reduced when navigation techniques are refined and used more in the future.

For high energy articular fractures of the distal femur, proximal and distal tibia that often show extensions into the diaphysis a combination of open anatomical reduction and stable fixation (ORIF) of the articular block with minimally invasive bridging fixation of the meta-diaphysis (MIPO) can be recommended (Fig. 7-31).

**LOCKED PLATING—INTERNAL
FIXATOR PRINCIPLE**

In an endeavor to further reduce or abolish the area of contact and friction between a plate and the bone surface Tepic and Perren[80] reported about a new principle of fracture fixation based on what they called the internal fixator (Fig. 7-32). The first development was the PC-Fix (point contact fixator), where every screw head was locked in the plate hole through a tight fit between the conical shape of the head and the plate hole (Fig. 7-33). The stability of the fixation was thereby not based on compressing the plate onto the bone nor on preload and friction, but depended on the stiffness of the plate screw construct. As the locked plate is not based on friction between the plate and the bone, there is no requirement for contact with the bone surface. Leaving a narrow free space between the implant and the bone preserves the periosteal blood flow

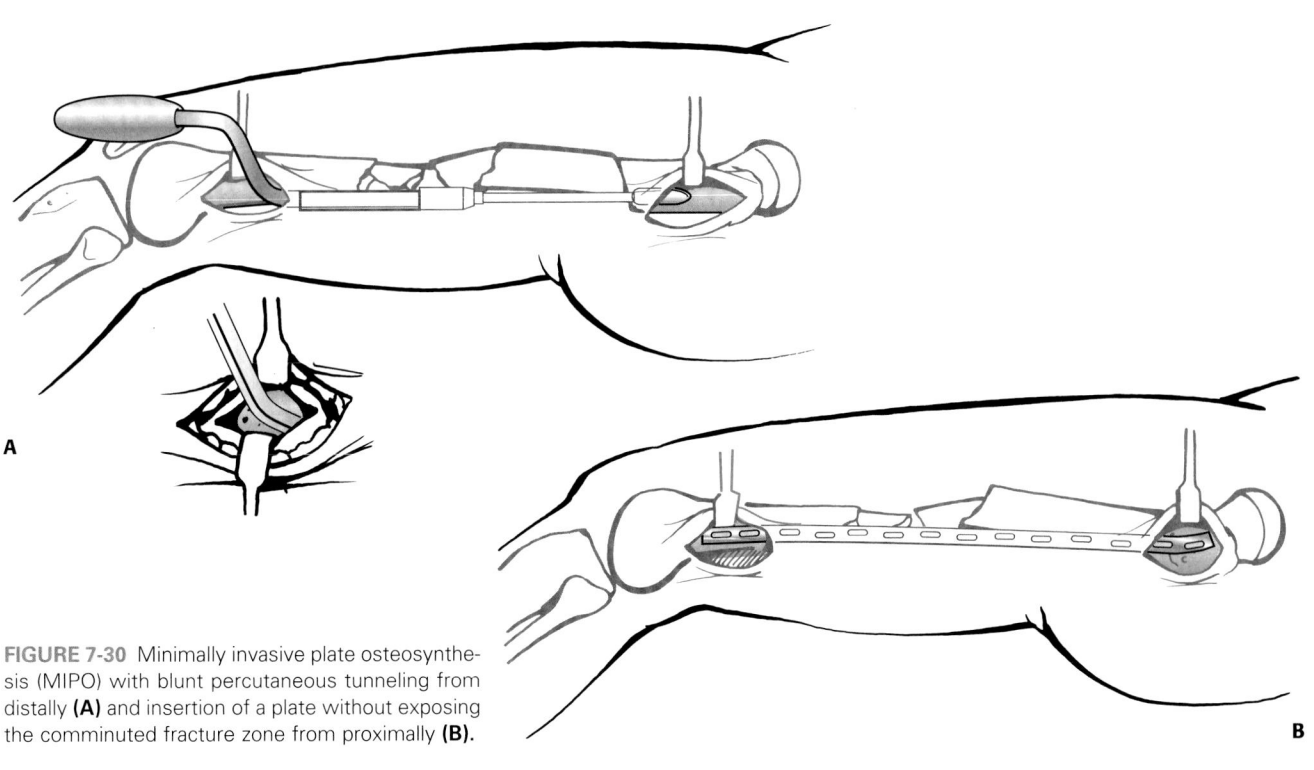

FIGURE 7-30 Minimally invasive plate osteosynthesis (MIPO) with blunt percutaneous tunneling from distally **(A)** and insertion of a plate without exposing the comminuted fracture zone from proximally **(B).**

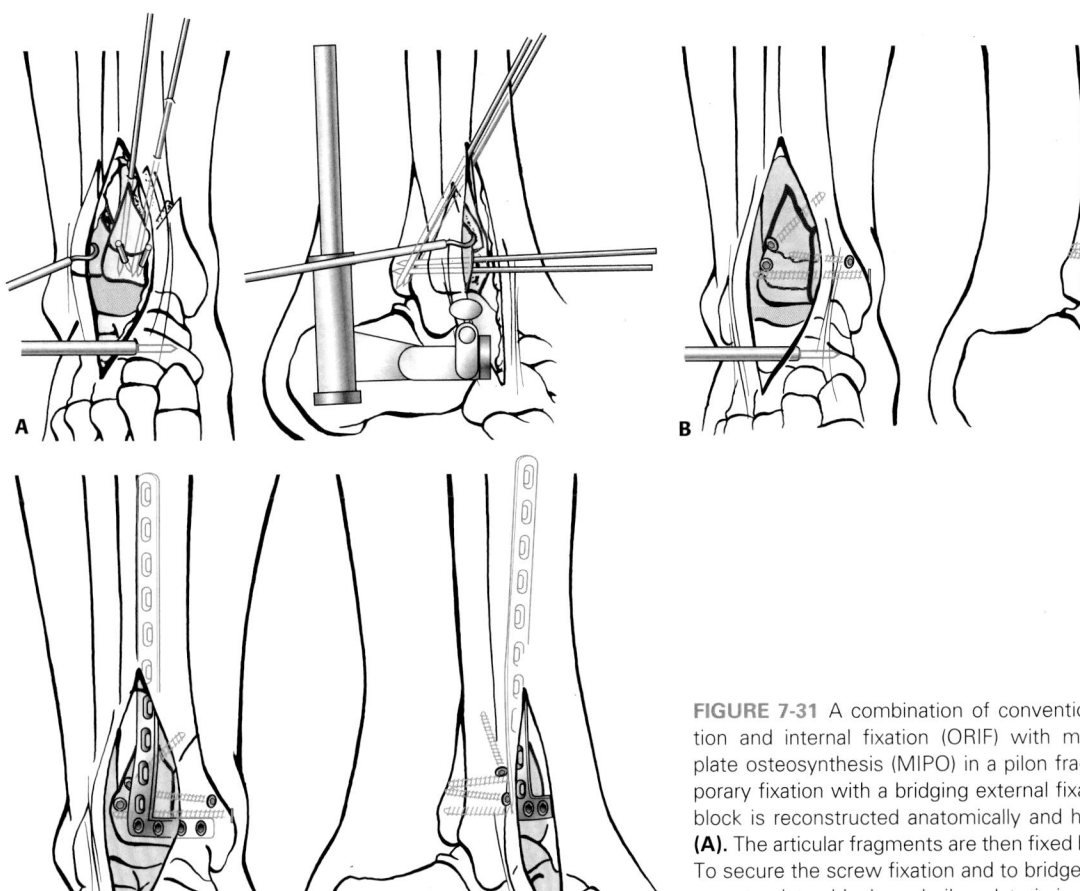

FIGURE 7-31 A combination of conventional open reduction and internal fixation (ORIF) with minimally invasive plate osteosynthesis (MIPO) in a pilon fracture. After temporary fixation with a bridging external fixator, the articular block is reconstructed anatomically and held with K-wires **(A).** The articular fragments are then fixed by lag screws **(B)** To secure the screw fixation and to bridge the metaphysis, an anterolateral L-shaped pilon plate is inserted percutaneously in MIPO technique **(C).**

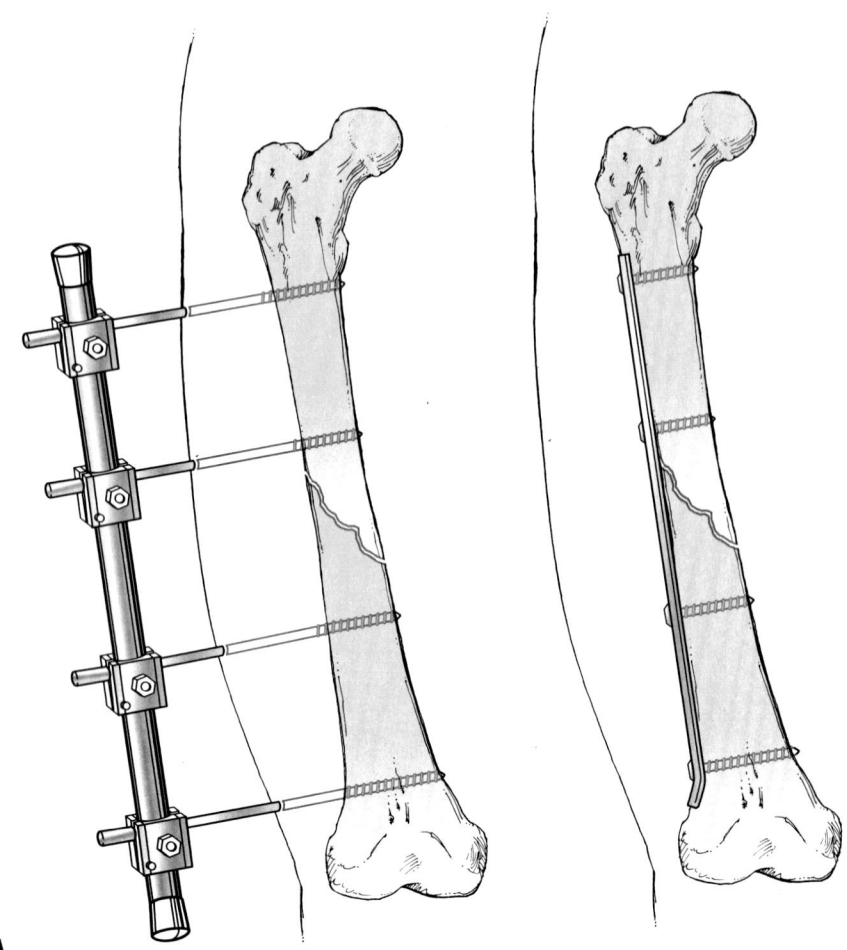

A

B

FIGURE 7-32 The principle of the "Internal Fixator" is based on moving an external fixator **(A)** close to the bone and underneath the soft tissue envelope **(B).** A plate replaces the longitudinal rod and the locking head screws (LHS) provide the angular stability of the clamps and Schanz screws.

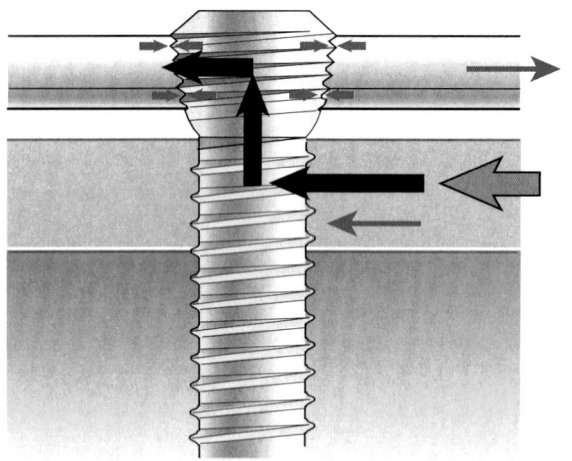

FIGURE 7-33 The force transfer in the internal fixator principle occurs primarily through the locking head screws (LHS) across the plate and fracture. It is not dependent on preload and friction as in conventional plating, but rather on the stiffness of the fixator device. The locked plate does not have to touch the bone surface and therefore interferes less with the periosteal blood flow.[82]

and the underlying cortex remains vital, which appears to increase resistance against infection.[1,80] Further features of the LHS are the angular stability of the construct, which prevents any secondary displacement or collapse of fixation. There is no need for a precise contouring of the plate to the shape of the bone with a pure locked plate construct, as plate is not pressed against bone as in conventional nonlocked plating. Last but not least the LHS often have a larger core diameter (4 vs. 3 mm), which increases their strength, while the thread may be shallow as it adds very little to the resistance to pull out. Thanks to the angular stability of the screws, any bending forces will have to displace and pull out the entire screw-plate construct together and not one screw after the other as in conventional plating (Fig. 7-34). This feature has proven most useful in poor quality or osteoporotic bone as well as in periprosthetic fractures, where often only monocortical screws can be inserted besides the shaft of a prosthesis.[33]

Advantages of the internal fixator due to angular stability of the construct are the following.

- No requirement for direct contact to the underlying bone, preservation of periosteal blood flow
- Improved construct stability in osteopenic bone

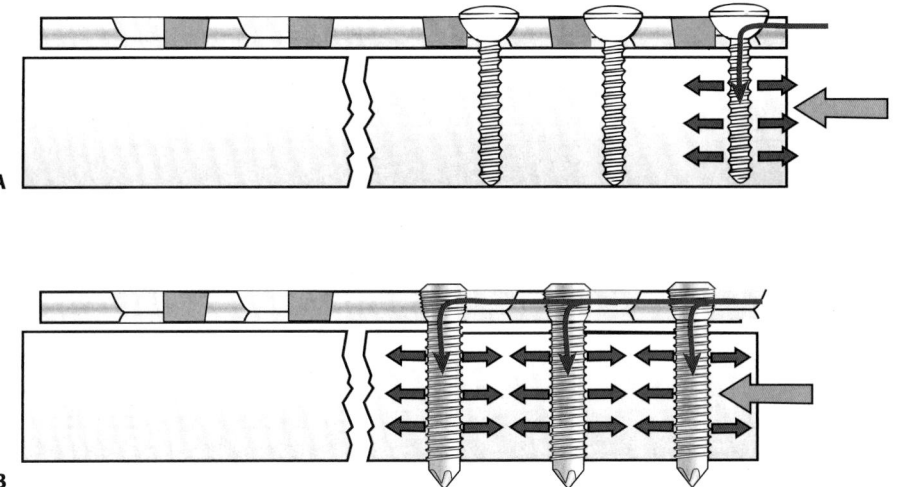

FIGURE 7-34 In conventional plating **(A)** the screw head is allowed to toggle under loading. This process of load concentration starts at the end screw and continues from one screw to the next until the plate is completely pulled out. In locked plates **(B)** the angular stable screws prevent a load concentration at a single bone screw interface, by distributing the load more evenly. To pull out a locked plate, much greater forces are needed as all screws have to be loosened at the same time.[17,71]

- Resistance to secondary collapse or screw displacement
- No need for precise plate contouring

About 10 years before Tepic and Perren[80] a group of Polish surgeons[70] had apparently developed a similar system with conventional plates and screws, which was applied to the medial aspect of the tibia but outside the skin and where the so-called "platform screws" were locked with some sort of washers in the screw holes (Fig. 7-35). In 1931 Paul Reinhold and in 1987 Wolter[85] had apparently already described the idea of angular stability or locked plating.

The clinical applicability and validity of the internal fixator principle was proven in a series of over 350 forearm fractures that were successfully fixed with the PC-Fix.[20]

The next development was the locked plate (less invasive stabilization system [LISS]) for the distal femur.[41] It combines the fixed angle device with the possibility of a minimally inva-

sive plate insertion technique (MIPO) using a special jig and monocortical, self-drilling and self-tapping screws that are introduced through short stab incisions. The advantages of the monocortical screws were seen in the precise, single-step insertion through stab incisions and a jig, as well as the fact that the endosteal blood supply is hardly disturbed. The LISS (Fig. 7-36

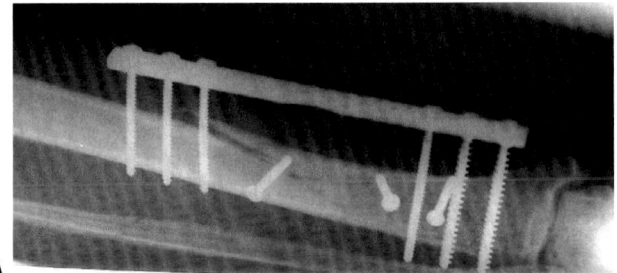

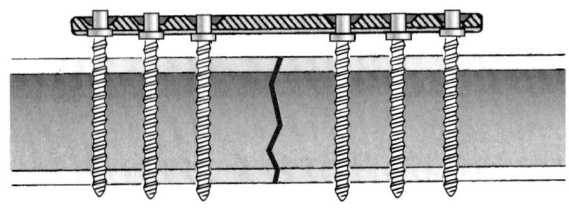

FIGURE 7-35 A locked plate as it was developed by the Polish Zespol Group in the 1980s, where the plate remains outside the skin cover **(A)**. The screws are locked with some sort of washers in the plate holes **(B)**.

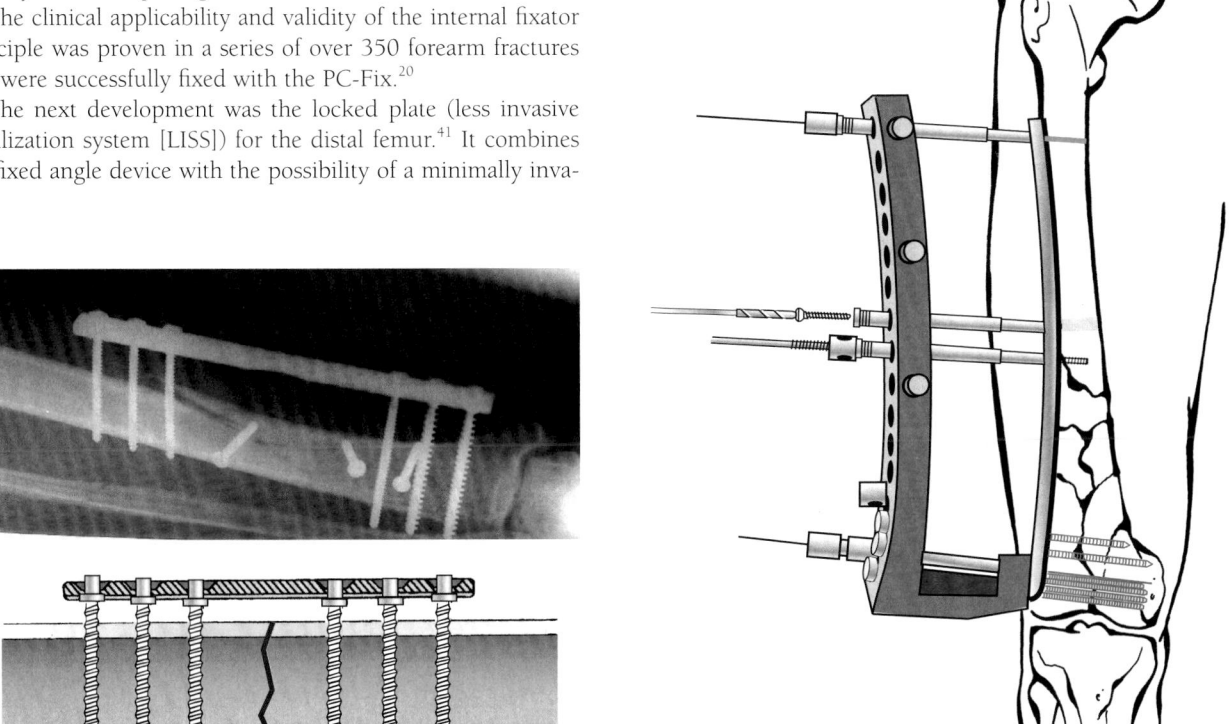

FIGURE 7-36 Locking plate (LISS) for distal femur fractures. After reconstruction and preliminary fixation of the articular fracture components under direct vision, the LISS can be inserted in a submuscular space with a special jig. The locking head screws (LHS) are introduced percutaneously through the jig.

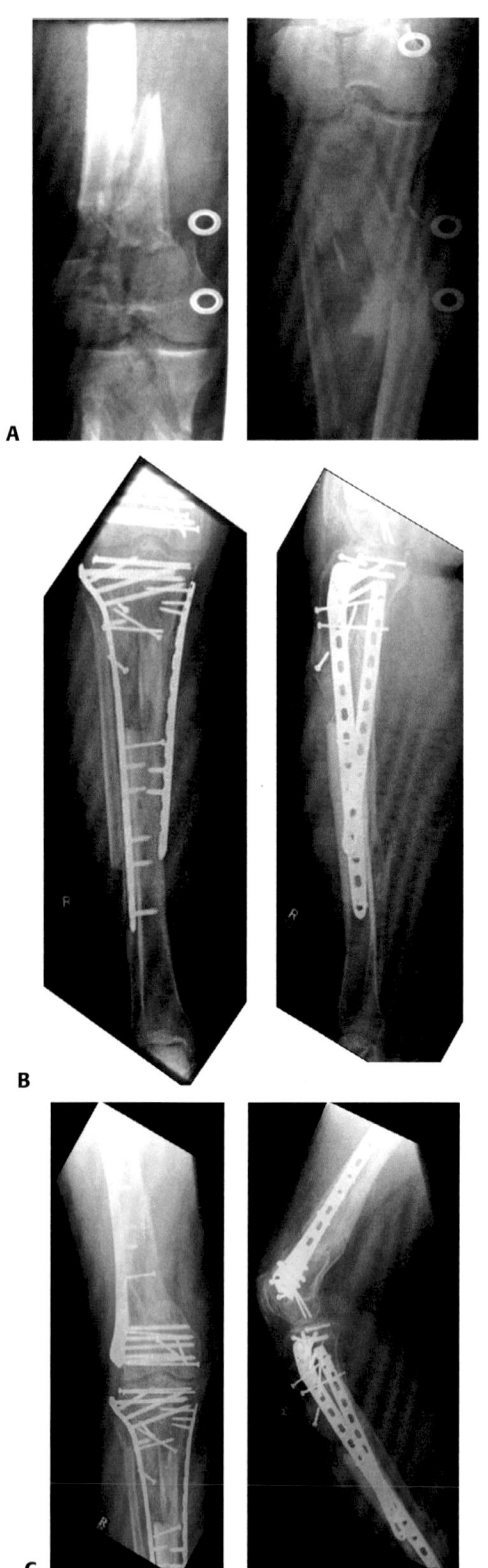

A

B

C

FIGURE 7-37 Clinical example of a "floating knee," proximal tibia combined with distal femur fractures, extending into both shaft and extensive open soft tissue injury **(A)**, fixed by locking plates **(B)**. After reconstruction of articular congruency with lag screws, the locking plates were placed percutaneously to the lateral aspect of the tibia. **C:** Follow-up after 1 year with good restitution of function.

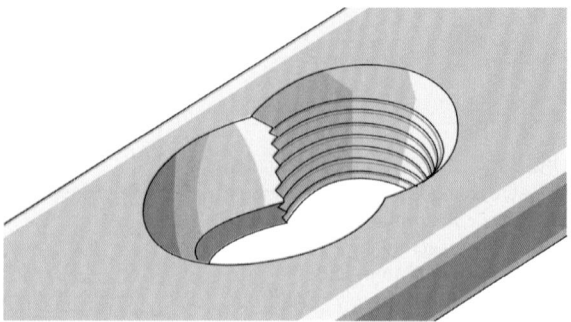

FIGURE 7-38 The combination hole of the LCP allows conventional screws in the smooth DC unit part of the hole and locking head screws (LHS) in the threaded part.

and 7-37) has advanced the surgical fixation of distal femur fractures by making the clinical results more reliable especially in complex fracture situations, osteoporotic and periprosthetic fractures.[41,43,44,77] While the LISS did only accept LHS, there was a rising demand for a possibility to also use conventional screws in this new plate. This led to the idea of the combination hole[43] which can accommodate either a smooth, conventional nonlocked screw or a threaded locking head screw (Fig. 7-38) and resulted in the dynamic locking plate (LCP).[15] With the further development of locked plates, more and more plates have become precontoured fitting the periarticular anatomical regions (Fig. 7-39).

Available plates now cover the full range of plate functions including the advantages of both locked and nonlocked plating.[23]

- Conventional compression-, protection-, or buttress plate with conventional nonlocked screws

- Pure locked plating with all LHS

- Hybrid plating with a combination of conventional nonlocked screws (to use plate as template for reduction) and locked screws (for advantages of fixed angle support of end segment fractures and improved fixation in osteoporotic bone)

When using hybrid plating technique, certain technical aspects have to be followed to avoid failures. Once a locking head screw has been inserted in a bone segment, no conventional screws should be added in the same segment, as this would create unwanted tension forces within the plate and bone. The sequence should be "lag first, lock second." A reduction screw may be used to approximate a fragment to the locked plate as an indirect reduction tool, it should however not be applied in a compression mode after a locked screw has been applied to the same fracture fragment, as this would counteract the bridging effect and bend the plate or crack the bone.

INTRAMEDULLARY FIXATION TECHNIQUES

Introduction and History

The medullary canal of a long bone offers itself to accept splinting devices of different designs and sizes. The major advantages are that any intramedullary implant is mostly with some bony

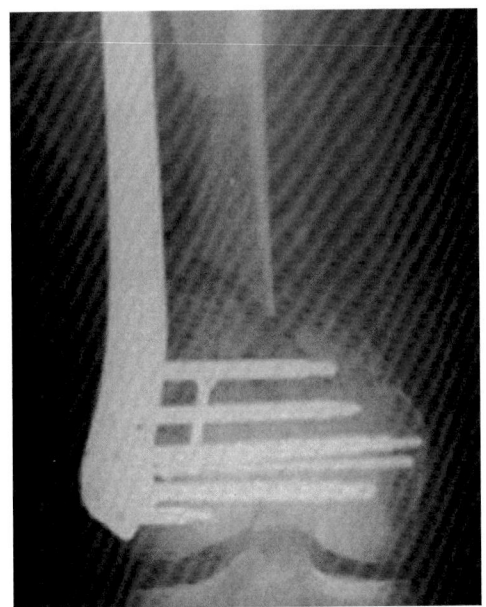
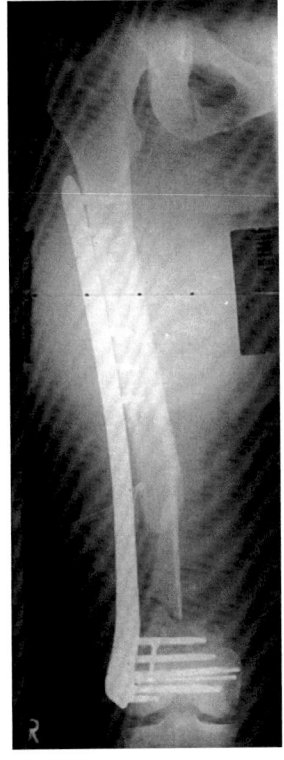
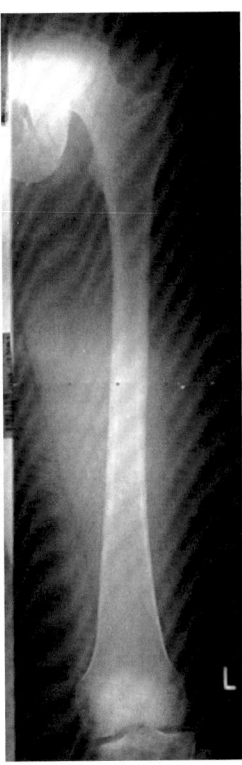

A   **B**   **C**

FIGURE 7-39 Precontoured implants, like the locking plate for the distal femur, can facilitate reduction in complex fracture situations **(A)**. This open fracture had significant metaphyseal bone loss. In accordance to the anatomical fit of the plate, the distal screws were placed parallel to the AP joint line of the distal femur. Following this intraoperative guideline the postoperative films **(B)** show a good alignment similar to the uninjured contralateral side **(C)** (further secondary bone graft was required to bridge the defect).

contact between the main fragments weight sharing and not weight bearing. Only in very comminuted shaft fractures the nail is a weight-bearing device, while no weight is transferred by the bony structures.

On the other hand a major problem is how to control axial displacement or to neutralize rotational forces. The interlocking techniques have helped to solve these drawbacks to a great extent. Depending on the anatomy, the insertion can usually occur closed, without exposure of the fracture focus, in an anteo or retrograde direction. A closed procedure would of course require the availability of an image intensifier in the operating room for reduction and interlocking.

Today intramedullary nails are the implant of choice for the femoral and tibial diaphysis and recently with new nail designs the spectrum of indications has been extended to even intra-articular fractures of these bones (Fig. 7-40). For the humeral shaft IM nails are an option competing with the still very popular and more versatile plating techniques. Flexible nails as used in pediatric fractures[46] have been advocated for the clavicle, while nailing of the forearm bones has not yet proved to be equal or superior for the fixation for ulna and radius fractures due to the difficulty of reliable locking systems, that can control the rotational forces.

Historically the first description of an intramedullary splinting with ivory pegs goes back to the 19th century[78] Hey-Groves[27]

used solid metal rods for femur fractures and pointed to the rapid healing, preservation of soft tissues and periosteum as well as the abolition of prolonged plaster cast immobilization. The Rush brothers[72] presented their technique with multiple flexible intramedullary pins in 1927. The most important contributions to intramedullary fixation came however from Küntscher (1900 to 1972)[45] who performed a number of animal experiments and perfected not only the nailing technique but also the implant shape and design. He requested a tight fit between nail and bone to achieve a higher stability and to allow compression of transverse fractures under load. To extend the area of contact within the medullary cavity he started to ream the canal in order to insert thicker, longer, and slotted cloverleaf nails. Herzog,[26] in 1950, introduced the tibia nail with a proximal bend and lateral slots at the distal end to accept antirotational wires. Shortly before his death Küntscher designed the "detensor nail" for comminuted femur fractures with a sort of interlocking device. This idea was further developed by Klemm and Schellmann[39] in Germany and Kempf et al.[35] in France and were precursors to today's interlocking nails.

Mechanics of IM Nailing

The original concept of Küntscher was based on the principle of elastic deformation or "elastic locking" of the nail within the medullary canal. To increase the elasticity, the hollow cloverleaf

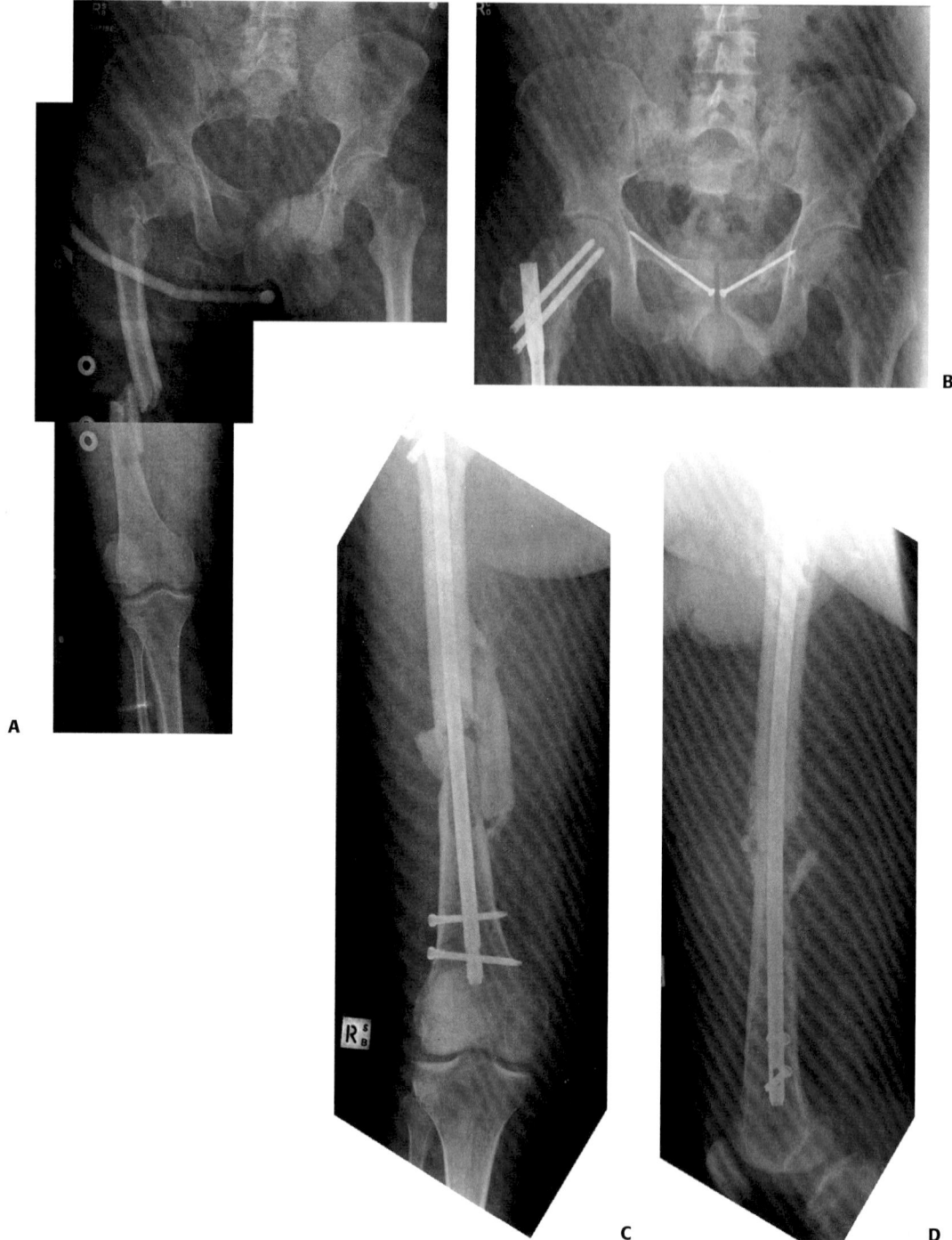

FIGURE 7-40 Intramedullary nailing (IM) systems offer possibilities to stabilize simultaneously ipsilateral trochanteric and shaft fractures. A 38-year-old multitrauma patient stabilized with an antegrade femoral with a retrograde locking **(A)**. The healing of both fractures was already reliable after 14 weeks **(B–D)**.

nail was slotted and reaming of the canal enlarged the area of contact and friction between the nail and the bone (working length). Nails with larger diameters had an increased bending and torsional stiffness. The weak point of the first nails remained the poor resistance to axial (telescoping) forces and rotation especially in comminuted fractures. The introduction of interlocking screws and bolts at the proximal and distal end of the nail addressed these issues rather well, there remains however the problem of the strength and purchase of the locking screws in the bone. This problem is not yet completely solved as twisted blades and an increase in screw diameter and number (larger and more holes) may weaken the nail ends. Based on the positive experience and data of Lottes[47] who presented very low infection rates in open tibia fractures with the use of solid nails that were introduced without reaming, thinner, solid tibia nails with holes for interlocking were developed. At the beginning those thin nails were to be inserted without reaming with mandatory interlocking as a temporary splint in open tibia fractures.[73] Animal experiments showed that after nail insertion the endosteal blood supply was not destroyed to the extent as after reaming and also that the resistance to infection was much higher if solid nails were compared with tubular ones.[51] The clinical experience as to the infection rate in open fractures was most encouraging however the time to union took longer, especially as in the majority of cases the original concept of secondary exchange nailing to a thicker nail was not followed. The enthusiasm for the new nails without reaming rapidly extended their indications and use also to closed and highly complex tibia and femur fractures. This resulted in a higher incidence of delayed and malunions due to a poorer mechanical stiffness of the construct especially in long bone fractures of the lower extremity.[11,73]

Pathophysiology of IM Nailing

Depending on the surgical technique, nail design, and anatomical region the use of intramedullary nails has both local and systemic effects, some of which may be beneficial, others however detrimental to the patient and fracture healing.

Local Effects

The insertion of a nail into the medullary canal is inevitably associated with damage of the endosteal blood supply, which was shown to be reversible within 8 to 12 weeks.[76] Experimental data have also shown that the cortical blood perfusion is significantly reduced after reaming of the medullary canal, if compared to a series without reaming.[38] Accordingly the return of cortical blood flow takes considerably longer after reaming than in the unreamed cases, which may have an influence on the resistance to infection especially in open fractures. Furthermore tight-fitting nails appear to compromise the cortical blood flow to a higher degree than loose fitting ones.[32] Reaming of a narrow medullary canal may be associated with a risk of heat necrosis of the bone and surrounding tissues especially if blunt reamers and/or a tourniquet are used.[57] On the other hand the bone debris produced during the reaming has been shown to act like an autogenous bone graft enhancing fracture healing.[16,28] Meta-analysis of current clinical studies found "gentle" reaming superior to the undreamed technique for reliable healing of long bone fractures in closed and low-degree open fractures.[11]

Systemic Response

Reaming of the medullary canal has been associated with pulmonary embolization, coagulation disorders, humoral, neural, immunologic, and inflammatory reactions. The development of post-traumatic pulmonary failure after early femoral nailing in the polytrauma patient with chest injury appears to be more frequent following reaming of the medullary canal than without it.[61] In clinical and experimental studies the passage of large thrombi into the pulmonary circulation has been demonstrated with intraoperative echocardiography especially during the reaming process and to lesser extent, already when introducing the reaming guide.[83] Measurements of the intramedullary pressure have shown values between 420 and 1,510 mm Hg during reaming procedures compared with 40 to 70 mm Hg when thin solid nails were inserted without reaming.[53,54] Nevertheless there is an ongoing controversy between the advocators of reamed nailing also in the multiply injured patient and those who are recommending the use of thinner solid or cannulated nails without reaming. Especially the young adult with a simple transverse femoral shaft fracture and a high ISS (>25) appears to have an increased risk for pulmonary complications, which is why there is the recommendation for a staged nailing procedure according to the concept of damage control surgery (DCS) under such circumstances. DCS starts as soon as possible with the stabilization of the femoral shaft fracture with an external fixator followed by a conversion to an intramedullary nail after 5 to 10 days (window of opportunity).[34] The described systemic responses of IM nailing of femoral shaft fractures seem to be much more critical than in tibial shaft fractures, where such effects have hardly ever been observed.

Implants for Nailing

There is a great variety of intramedullary nails and entire nailing systems available for the femur, tibia, and humerus. Forearm nails are also on the market, but until now they have not proven to be superior or as versatile as the fixation with plates. Originally intramedullary nails were offered in a tubular, usually slotted form, while today solid and especially cannulated nails are most popular. In children the elastic nails according to Ligier et al.[46] have become the implant of choice for long bone fractures. The implant material is either stainless steel or a titanium alloy. The holes or openings for interlocking devices are usually situated at either end of the implant and oriented in different directions, some nails have also locking possibilities throughout the entire nail length.

Accordingly the indications have increased from originally midshaft fractures to fractures involving the proximal and distal femur and tibia as well as the proximal humerus.

The nail design and the dimensions have to be adapted to the shape of the medullary cavity and the bone. The correct diameter and length of the nail should to be selected beforehand, unfortunately the accuracy of templates is rather poor. The best tool is probably a radiolucent ruler placed on the intact contralateral leg under C-arm control or the measurement with the intramedullary guidewire.

A very important issue is the correct entry point and starting trajectory of the nail, which varies from one type of nail to the other (Fig. 7-41).

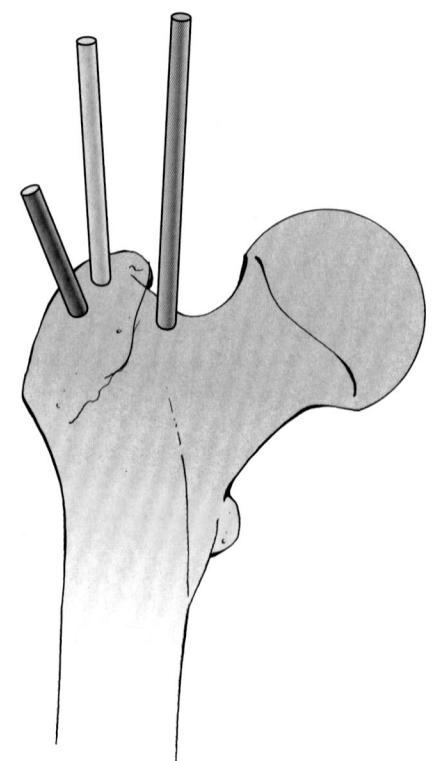

FIGURE 7-41 The correct entry point is crucial, but may vary from one type of nail to the other. (Always study the recommendations of the manufacturer as to the recommended nail entry point.)

A misplaced starting point may lead to axial and/or rotational malalignment, that is usually tricky to correct, and even additional stress fractures have been described. It is therefore advisable to study the technical guide of a specific type of nail carefully and to check the correct entry point and direction of the guidewire with the image intensifier preferably in two planes.

Positioning of the Patient for IM Nailing and Reduction

Every surgeon has his preferred way of how to nail a specific bone, with or without a fracture table, or with the help of a distractor, in a supine or in a lateral decubitus position, etc. As each way has its pros and cons, much depends on the experience of the OR team and the surgeon. It appears most important for any patient positioning that the nail entry point can be clearly seen in two projections with the C-arm and the same holds true for the distal locking procedure.

Reduction of fresh diaphyseal fractures is rarely a problem. The guidewire can usually be inserted easily into the opposite fragment, or a solid nail or reduction device can be used as a joystick. In metaphyseal fractures the correct alignment may be much more difficult especially in the proximal or distal tibia. Blocking or Poller screws[42] may be helpful to guide the nail in the right direction (Fig. 7-42). The technique of the Poller screws can be used to decrease the functional width of a wide metaphyseal cavity or to force and redirect the nail

into a particular direction for a better alignment or improved stabilization. The use of the screw can be temporary or definitive. This technique is especially helpful to steer the nail into another "right" direction, after it had been misplaced in the first attempt.

Locking Technique

Most nails are inserted with a special handle, which also serves as an aiming device for locking the driving end of the nail with bolts, blades, or more commonly locking screws. Placement of the far locking device is usually more difficult as during the insertion most nails are more or less distorted, so that the locking holes are not in the original alignment anymore. Far locking must therefore be done in a "free hand" technique or with the aid of aiming devices usually mounted on the drill. Tight-fitting nails tend to distract the fractures resulting in wide gaps, which may lead to increased compartment pressure as well as to delayed or nonunion.[6] It is therefore recommended to lock first at the far end, then to backslap the nail, and finally to lock the driving end. Finally locking can be done in a static or dynamic mode, while it is advisable to use at least two locking screws at either end of the nail to control rotation in a reliable way. Static locking is recommended for complex fractures to prevent telescoping, while dynamic locking is advisable in short oblique or transverse fracture, to allow fracture compression during weight bearing.

Assessment of Axial Alignment and Rotation in IM Nailing

In simple fractures axial alignment is not a problem. However in more complex, segmental, or comminuted fractures or in floating knee injuries it may be difficult to judge the correct axial alignment. The most useful intraoperative indicator of an acceptable coronal plane alignment is, when the nail entrance point is correct and the nail is centrally placed in the distal fragment (or proximal segment in retrograde nailing). In the lower extremity the long cable of electrocautery, a C-arm and the patient in supine position is helpful to judge the right direction. The cable is centered to the femoral head and distally to the middle of the ankle joint under x-ray view. At the level of the knee the cable should now run exactly through the centre of the joint as well. Any deviation indicates an axial malalignment in the coronal plane.

The clinical assessment of the rotation intraoperatively is more difficult and less accurate. There are several radiologic signs like the size of the diameter of two adjacent fragments or the projection of the greater trochanter in relation to the patella in the AP view, but they are all not very reliable. With the patient still on the OR table internal and external rotation can be performed to reliably check the rotation in comparison with the uninjured side. The most accurate evaluation is with a few CT slices through the knee and the hip joint allowing also a comparison with the uninjured side.[25]

The intramedullary nail to fix diaphyseal fractures of the long bones is the golden standard today. It is a minimally

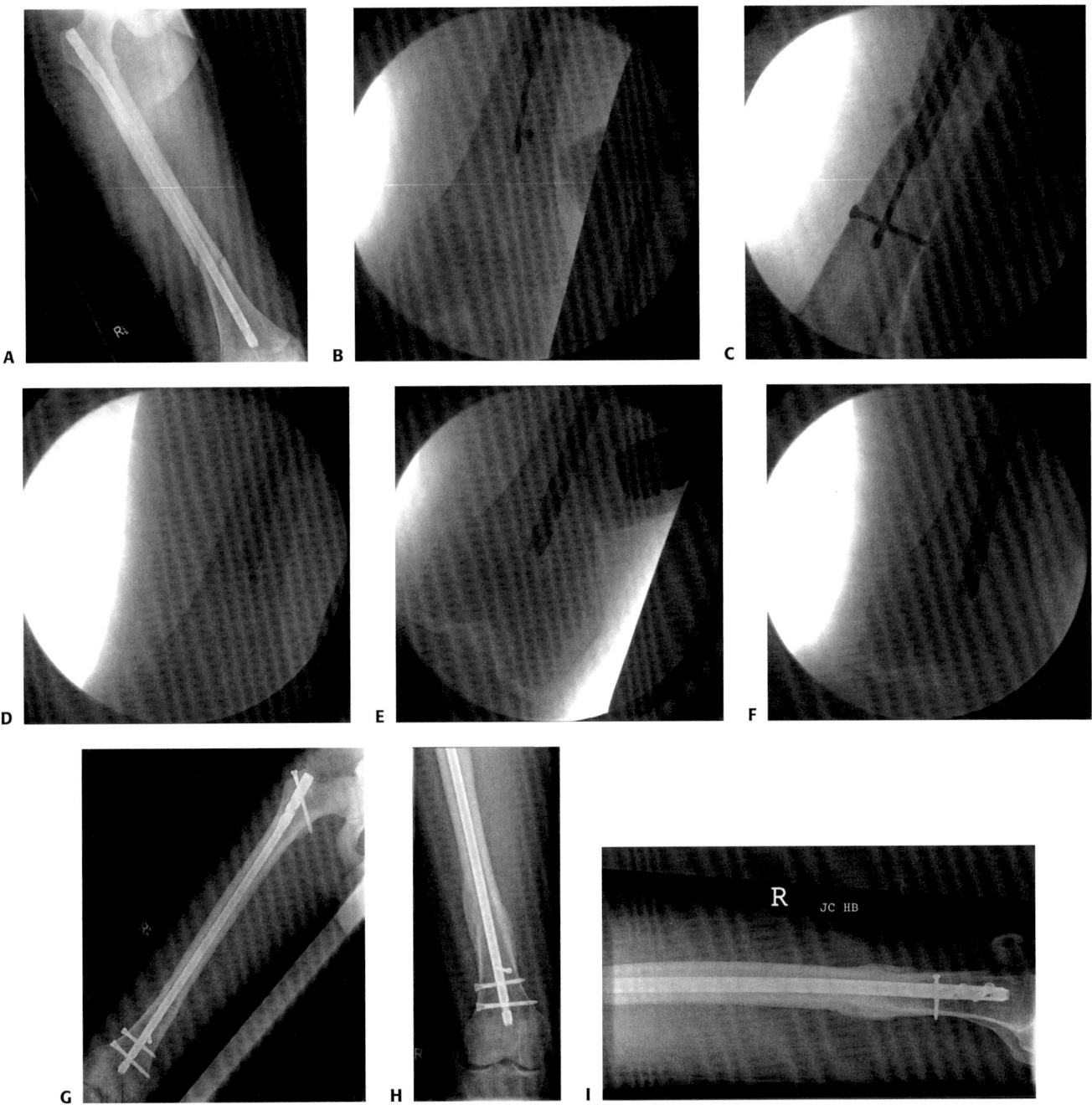

FIGURE 7-42 Example of Poller screws in the femur to correct a valgus malalignment of the distal fragment **(A).** After the nail was backed out, a 3.5-mm cortical screw was placed **(B, C)** to steer the nail into the appropriate position **(D–F).** Postoperative control and healing after 1 year **(G–I).** To correct valgus with a blocking screw, the screw must be placed lateral to the nail and near the fracture or medial to the nail and far from the fracture.

invasive procedure allowing early weight bearing and with a good chance of rapid and undisturbed fracture healing.

TENSION BAND PRINCIPLE

Pauwels was the one who observed that a curved tubular structure when subjected to an axial load, always presents a tension side on the convexity and a compression side on the concavity. The same occurs when a straight tube or bone is loaded eccentrically like in the femur, where we have tensile forces on the lateral and compression on the medial side. By applying a tension band device laterally these tensile forces are converted to compression forces provided the opposite side is stable and has good contact.

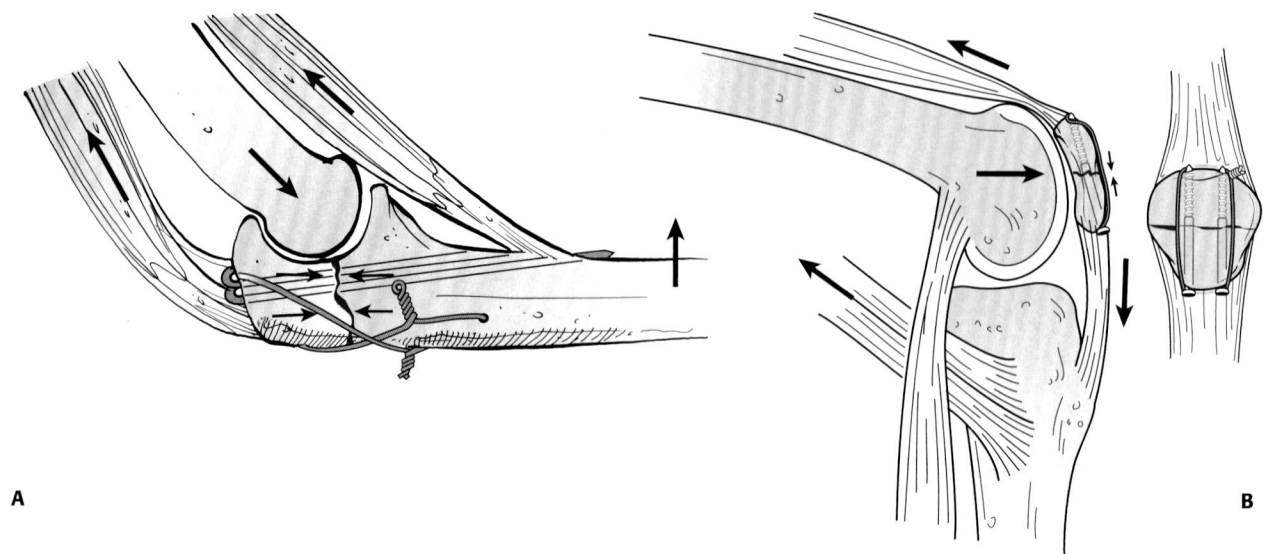

A

B

FIGURE 7-43 **A:** Atypical example of tension band fixation of the olecranon with two K-wires and a figure-of-eight tension band wiring. **B:** Tension band fixation of a transverse patella fracture with a tension band wire loop. Note that the tension band device must lie eccentrically on the tensile side of the bone and that this dynamic fixation is enhanced by flexion of the joint.

In fractures where muscle pull tends to displace fragments as in the olecranon, patella or the avulsion fracture of the greater tuberosity of the humerus, a tension band will neutralize the distraction forces and under flexion of the joint the fragments will be compressed (Fig. 7-43). We therefore speak of dynamic tension band providing absolute stability and encourage the patients with tension band fixation of one of these joints to regularly make flexion exercises.

In principle any fixation device, plate, wire loop and even an external fixator, if applied correctly to the tension of a fractured bone can act as a tension band. The tension band device must withstand tensile forces, while the bone must resist compressive forces, while the cortex opposite to the tension band must be exactly reduced without a gap.

The most commonly used 1.4- or 1.6-mm metal wire can be inserted through a drill hole in the bone, or it can be placed through the Sharpey fibers of a tendon insertion such as at the patella or it may be looped around a screw head or a K-wire. The wire loop should always be placed eccentrically to the load axis, for example, in front of the patella, and not around it (Fig. 7-43). Wire withstands tensile forces quite well; however, if bending forces are added it will easily break. The same is true for any type of plate.

In mal- and nonunions we often can observe an angular deformity. Any fixation device should therefore be applied to the convex side of the deformity, in such a way as to act as a tension band, which then automatically induces compression and enhances bony union (Fig. 7-44).

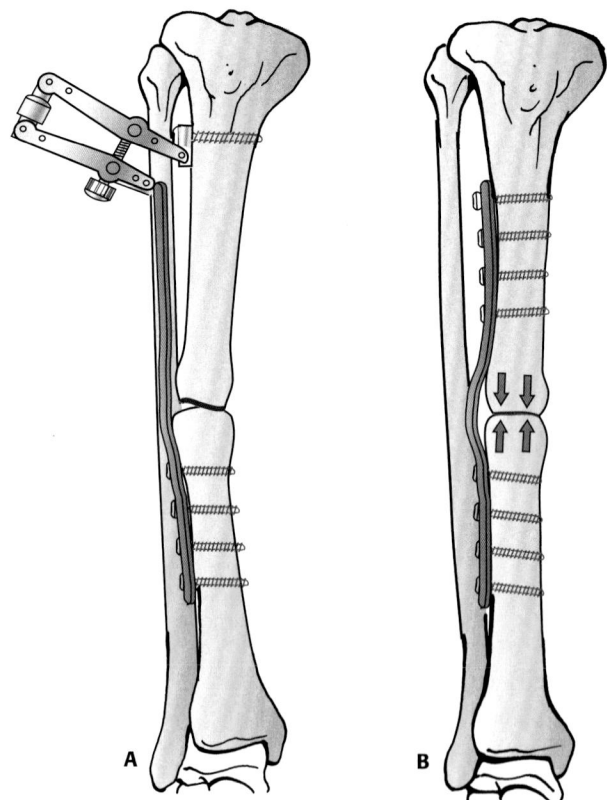

A

B

FIGURE 7-44 In a mal- and nonunions with deformity as the plate to the convex or tension side of the bone **(A)** acts as a tension and compresses the bone ends **(B)**.

REFERENCES

1. Arens S, Eijer H, Schlegel U, et al. Influence of the design for fixation implants on local infection: Experimental study of dynamic compression plates versus point contact fixators in rabbits. *J Orthop Trauma.* 1999;13(7):470–476.

2. Audigé L, Griffin D, Bhandari M, et al. Path analysis of factors for delayed healing and nonunion in 416 operatively treated tibial shaft fractures. *Clin Orthop Relat Res.* 2005;438:221–232.

3. Babst R, Hehli M, Regazzoni P. LISS Tractor. Kombination des less invasiven stabilisation systems (LISS) mit dem AO-Distraktor fuer distale Femur- und proximale Tibiafrakturen. *Unfallchirurg* 2001;104:530–535.

4. Badia JM, Torres JM, Tur C, et al. Saline wound irrigation reduces the postoperative infection rate in guinea pigs. *J Surg Res.* 1996;63(2):457–459.

5. Baumgaertel F, Dahlen C, Stiletto R, et al. Technique of using the AO-femoral distractor for femoral IM nailing. *J Orthop Trauma.* 1994;8:315–321.

6. Bhandari M, Guyatt GH, Tong D, et al. Reamed versus nonreamed IM nailing of lower extremity long bone fractures: A systematic overview and meta-analysis. *J Orthop Trauma.* 2000;14:2–9.

7. Bhandari M, Tornetta P 3rd, Sprague S, et al. Predictors of reoperation following operative management of fractures of the tibial shaft. *J Orthop Trauma.* 2003;17(5):353–361.

8. Boxma H, Broekhuizen T, Patka P, et al. Randomised controlled trial of singledose antibiotic prophylaxis in surgical treatment of closed fractures: The Dutch Trauma Trial. *Lancet.* 1996;347:1133–1137.

9. Brunner CF, Weber BG. Antigleitplatte. In: Brunner CF, Weber BG, eds. *Besondere Osteosynthesetechniken.* Berlin: Springer; 1981.

10. Brunner CF, Weber BG. Wellenplatte. In: Brunner CF, Weber BG, eds. *Besondere Osteosynthesetechniken.* Berlin: Springer; 1981.

11. Canadian Orthopedic Trauma Society. Nonunion following intramedullary nailing of the femur with and without reaming. Results of a multicenter randomized clinical trial. *J Bone Joint Surg Am.* 2003;85-A(11):2093–2096.

12. Chan PS, Klimkiewicz JJ, Luchetti WT, et al. Impact of CT scan on treatment plan and fracture classification of tibial plateau fractures. *J Orthop Trauma.* 1997;11(7):484–489.

13. Claes LE, Augat P, Suger G, et al. Influence of size and stability of the osteotomy gap on the success of fracture healing. *J Orthop Res.* 1997;15(4):577–584.

14. Farouk O, Krettek C, Miclau T, et al. Minimally invasive plate osteosynthesis: Does percutaneous plating disrupt femoral blood supply less than the traditional technique? *J Orthop Trauma.* 1999;13(6):401–406.

15. Frigg R. Locking compression plate (LCP). An osteosynthesis plate based on the dynamic compression plate and the point contact fixator (PC-Fix). *Injury.* 2001;32(suppl 2):63–66.

16. Frolke JP, Bakker FC, Patka P, et al. Reaming debris in osteotomized sheep tibiae. *J Trauma.* 2001;50:65–69.

17. Gautier E, Sommer C. Guidelines for the clinical application of the LCP. *Injury.* 2003;34(suppl 2):B63–B76.

18. Georgiadis GM, Burgar AM. Percutaneous skeletal joysticks for closed reduction of femoral shaft fractures during IM nailing. *J Orthop Trauma.* 2001;15:570–571.

19. Gustilo RB, Mendoza RM, Williams DN. Problems in the management of type III (severe) open fractures: A new classification of type III open fractures. *J Trauma.* 1984;24:742–746.

20. Haas N, Hauke C, Schutz M, et al. Treatment of diaphyseal fractures of the forearm using the Point Contact Fixator (PC-Fix): Results of 387 fractures of a prospective multicentric study (PC-Fix II). *Injury.* 2001;32(suppl 2):B51–B62.

21. Haidukewych G, Sems SA, Huebner D, et al. Results of polyaxial locked-plate fixation of periarticular fractures of the knee. Surgical technique. *J Bone Joint Surg Am.* 2008;90(suppl 2 pt 1):117–134.

22. Haidukewych G, Sems SA, Huebner D. Results of polyaxial locked-plate fixation of periarticular fractures of the knee. Surgical technique. *J Bone Joint Surg Am.* 2008;90(suppl 2 pt 1):117–134.

23. Haidukewych GJ, Ricci W. Locked plating in orthopaedic trauma: A clinical update. *J Am Acad Orthop Surg.* 2008;16(6):347–355.

24. Heitemeyer U, Kemper F, Hierholzer G , et al. Severely comminuted femoral shaft fractures: Treatment by bridging-plate osteosynthesis. *Arch Orthop Trauma Surg.* 1987;106:327–330.

25. Hernandez RJ, Tachdjian MO, Poznanski AK, et al. CT determination of femoral torsion. *AJR Am J Roentgenol.* 1981;137:97–101.

26. Herzog K. Die Technik der geschlossenen Marknagelung frischer Tibiafrakturen mit dem Rohrschlitznagel. *Chirurg.* 1958;29(11):501–506.

27. Hey-Groves EW. Ununited fractures with special reference to gunshot injuries and the use of bone grafting. *J Bone Joint Surg [Br].* 1918;6:203–228.

28. Hoegel F, Mueller CA, Peter R, et al. Bone debris: Dead matter or vital osteoblasts. *J Trauma.* 2004;56(2):363–367.

29. Hoffmeier KL, Hofmann GO, Mückley T. The strength of polyaxial locking interfaces of distal radius plates. *Clin Biomech.* 2009;24(8):637–641.

30. Holzach P, Matter P, Minter J. Arthroscopically assisted treatment of lateral tibial plateau fractures in skiers: Use of a cannulated reduction system. *J Orthop Trauma.* 1994;8(4):273–281.

31. Hüfner T, Gebhard F, Grützner PA, et al. Which navigation when? *Injury.* 2004;35(suppl 1):S-A30–34.

32. Hupel TM, Aksenov SA, Schemitsch EH. Cortical bone blood flow in loose- and tight-fitting locked unreamed IM nailing: A canine segmental tibia fracture model. *J Orthop Trauma.* 1998;12(2):127–135.

33. Kaab MJ, Stockle U, Schutz M, et al. Stabilisation of periprosthetic fractures with angular stable internal fixation: A report of 13 cases. *Arch Orthop Trauma Surg.* 2006;126(2):105–110.

34. Keel M, Trentz O. Pathophysiology of polytrauma. *Injury.* 2005;36(6):691–709.

35. Kempf I, Jaeger JH, North J, et al. L'enclouage centro-medullaire du femur et du tibia selon la technique de Kuntscher. Interet du verrouillage du clou. Etude experimentale. *Acta Orthop Belg.* 1976;42(suppl 1):29–43.

36. Kendoff D, Citak M, Gardner MJ, et al. Navigated femoral nailing using noninvasive registration of the contralateral intact femur to restore anteversion. Technique and clinical use. *J Orthop Trauma.* 2007;21(10):725–730.

37. Kinast C, Bolhofner BR, Mast JW, et al. Subtrochanteric fractures of the femur. Results of treatment with the 95 degrees condylar blade-plate. *Clin Orthop Relat Res.* 1989;(238):122–130.

38. Klein MP, Rahn BA, Frigg R, et al. Reaming versus non-reaming in medullary nailing: Interference with cortical circulation of the canine tibia. *Arch Orthop Trauma Surg.* 1990;109(6):314–316.

39. Klemm K, Schellmann WD. Dynamische und statische Verriegelung des Marknagels. *Monatsschr Unfallheilkd Versicher Versorg Verkehrsmed.* 1972;75(12):568–575.

40. Königshausen M, Kuebler L, Godry H, et al. Clinical outcome and complications using a polyaxial locking plate in the treatment of displaced proximal humerus fractures. A reliable system? *Injury.* 2012;43(2):223–231.

41. Kregor PJ, Hughes JL, Cole PA. Fixation of distal femoral fractures above total knee arthroplasty utilizing the less invasive stabilization system (L.I.S.S.). *Injury.* 2001;32(suppl 3):SC64–SC75.

42. Krettek C, Miclau T, Schandelmaier P, et al. The mechanical effect of blocking screws ("Poller screws") in stabilizing tibia fractures with short proximal or distal fragments after insertion of small-diameter IM nails. *J Orthop Trauma.* 1999;13(8):550–553.

43. Krettek C, Muller M, Miclau T. Evolution of minimally invasive plate osteosynthesis (MIPO) in the femur. *Injury.* 2001;32(suppl 3):SC14–SC23.

44. Krettek C, Schandelmaier P, Miclau T, et al. Transarticular joint reconstruction and indirect plate osteosynthesis for complex distal supracondylar femoral fractures. *Injury.* 1997;28(suppl 1):A31–A41.

45. Küntscher G. *Praxis der Marknagelung.* Stuttgart: Schattauer; 1962.

46. Ligier JN, Metaizeau JP, Prevot J, et al. Elastic stable intramedullary nailing of femoral shaft fractures in children. *J Bone Joint Surg [Br].* 1988;70(1):74–77.

47. Lottes JO. Medullary nailing of the tibia with the triflange nail. *Clin Orthop Relat Res.* 1974;(105):53–66.

48. Magid D, Michelson JD, Ney DR, et al. Adult ankle fractures: Comparison of plain films and interactive two- and three-dimensional CT scans. *AJR Am J Roentgenol.* 1990;154(5):1017–1023.

49. Mast J, Jakob R, Ganz R. *Planning and Reduction Technique in Fracture Surgery.* Berlin, Heidelberg: Springer-Verlag; 1996.

50. Mehta JA, Bain GI, Heptinstall RJ. Anatomical reduction of intra-articular fractures of the distal radius. An arthroscopically-assisted approach. *J Bone Joint Surg [Br].* 2000;82:79–86.

51. Melcher GA, Metzdorf A, Schlegel U, et al. Influence of reaming versus nonreaming in intramedullary nailing on local infection rate: Experimental investigation in rabbits. *J Trauma.* 1995;39(6):1123–1128.

52. Mubarak SJ, Hargens AR. Acute compartment syndromes. *Surg Clin North Am.* 1983;63(3):539–565.

53. Muller C, Frigg R, Pfister U. Effect of flexible drive diameter and reamer design on the increase of pressure in the medullary cavity during reaming. *Injury.* 1993;24(suppl. 3):S40–S47.

54. Muller C, McIff T, Rahn BA, et al. Influence of the compression force on the IM pressure development in reaming of the femoral medullary cavity. *Injury.* 1993;24(suppl 3):S36–S39.

55. Muller ME, Allgower M, Schneider R, et al. *Manual of Internal Fixation.* Heidelberg: Springer; 1991.

56. Nikolaou VS, Tan HB, Haidukewych G, et al. Proximal tibial fractures: Early experience using polyaxial locking-plate technology. *Int Orthop.* 2011;35(8):1215–1221.

57. Ochsner PE, Baumgart F, Kohler G. Heat-induced segmental necrosis after reaming of one humeral and two tibial fractures with a narrow medullary canal. *Injury.* 1998;29(suppl. 2):B1–B10.

58. Oestern HJ, Tscherne H. Pathophysiology and classification of soft tissue injuries associated with fractures. In: Tscherne H, Gotzen L, eds. *Fractures with Soft Tissue Injury.* Berlin, Heidelberg, New York: Springer; 1984.

59. Otto RJ, Moed BR, Bledsoe JG, et al. Biomechanical comparison of polyaxial-type locking plates and a fixed-angle locking plate for internal fixation of distal femur fractures. *J Orthop Trauma.* 2009;23(9):645–652.

60. Paiement GD, Renaud E, Dagenais G, et al. Double-blind randomized prospective study of the efficacy of antibiotic prophylaxis for open reduction and internal fixation of closed ankle fractures. *J Orthop Trauma.* 1994;8:64–66.

61. Pape HC, Giannoudis PV, Grimme K, et al. Effects of IM femoral fracture fixation: What is the impact of experimental studies in regards to the clinical knowledge? *Shock.* 2002;18:291–300.

62. Park JH, Hagopian J, Ilyas AM. Variable–angle locking screw volar plating of distal radius fractures. *Hand Clin.* 2010;26(3):373–380.

63. Pauwels F. *Biomechanics of the Locomotor Apparatus.* Berlin: Springer; 1980.

64. Perren SM, Cordey J. *The Concept of Interfragmentary Strain.* Berlin, Heidelberg, New York: Springer-Verlag; 1980.

65. Perren SM, Frigg R, Hehli M, et al. Lag screw. In: Rüedi TP, Murphy WM, eds. *AO principles of fracture management.* NewYork: Thieme; 2001.

66. Perren SM, Russenberger M, Steinemann S, et al. A dynamic compression plate. *Acta Orthop Scand Suppl.* 1969;125:31–41.

67. Perren SM. Evolution of the internal fixation of long bone fractures. The scientific basis of biological internal fixation: choosing a new balance between stability and biology. *J Bone Joint Surg Br.* 2002;84(8):1093–1110.

68. Perren SM. Force measurements in screw fixation. *J Biomech.* 1976;9:669–675.

69. Perren SM. The concept of biological plating using the limited contact-dynamic compression plate (LC-DCP). Scientific background, design and application. *Injury.* 1991;22(suppl. 1):1–41.

70. Ramotowski W, Granowski R. Das "Zespol"-Osteosynthesesystem: Mechanische Grundlage und klinische Anwendung. *Orthop Praxis.* 1984;9:750–758.
71. Ricci WM, Loftus T, Cox C, et al. Locked plates combined with minimally invasive insertion technique for the treatment of periprosthetic supracondylar femur fractures above a total knee arthroplasty. *J Orthop Trauma.* 2006;20(3):190–196.
72. Rush LV, Rush HC. A reconstruction operation for a comminuted fracture of the upper third of the ulna. *Am J Surg.* 1937;38:332–333.
73. Schandelmaier P, Krettek C, Tscherne H. Biomechanical study of nine different tibia locking nails. *J Orthop Trauma.* 1996;10:37–44.
74. Schaser KD, Zhang L, Haas NP, et al. Temporal profile of microvascular disturbances in rat tibial periosteum following closed soft tissue trauma. *Langenbecks Arch Surg.* 2003;388:323–330.
75. Schatzker J, Sanderson R, Murnaghan JP. The holding power of orthopedic screws in vivo. *Clin Orthop.* 1975;115–126.
76. Schemitsch EH, Kowalski MJ, Swiontkowski MF, et al. Cortical bone blood flow in reamed and unreamed locked IM nailing: a fractured tibia model in sheep. *J Orthop Trauma.* 1994;8:373–382.
77. Schutz M, Muller M, Krettek C, et al. Minimally invasive fracture stabilization of distal femoral fractures with the LISS: A prospective multicenter study. Results of a clinical study with special emphasis on difficult cases. *Injury.* 2001;32(suppl 3): SC48–SC54.
78. Stimson LA. *A Treatise on Fractures.* Philadelphia: H.C. Lea's son & co; 1883.
79. Sturmer KM. Die elastische Plattenosteo-synthese, ihre Biomechanik, Indikation und Technik im Vergleich zur rigiden Osteosynthese. *Unfallchirurg* 1996;99:816–829.
80. Tepic S, Perren SM. The biomechanics of the PC-Fix internal fixator. *Injury.* 1995;26(suppl 2):5–10.
81. Voigt C, Geisler A, Hepp P. Are polyaxially locked screws advantageous in the plate osteosynthesis of proximal humeral fractures in the elderly? A prospective randomized clinical observational study. *J Orthop Trauma.* 2011;25(10):596–602.
82. Wagner M. General principles for the clinical use of the LCP. *Injury.* 2003;34:31–42.
83. Wenda K, Runkel M, Degreif J, et al. Pathogenesis and clinical relevance of bone marrow embolism in medullary nailing: Demonstrated by intraoperative echocardiography. *Injury.* 1993;24(suppl 3):S73–S81.
84. Wilkens KJ, Curtiss S, Lee MA, et al. Polyaxial locking plate fixation in distal femur fractures: A biomechanical comparison. *J Orthop Trauma.* 2008;22(9):624–628.
85. Wolter D, Reckert L, Kortmann H-R, et al. Der Plattenfixateur interne zur Wirbelsäulenstabilisierung (Operationstechnik und erste Ergebnisse). *Langenbecks Archiv für Chirurgie.* 1987;372(1):926.

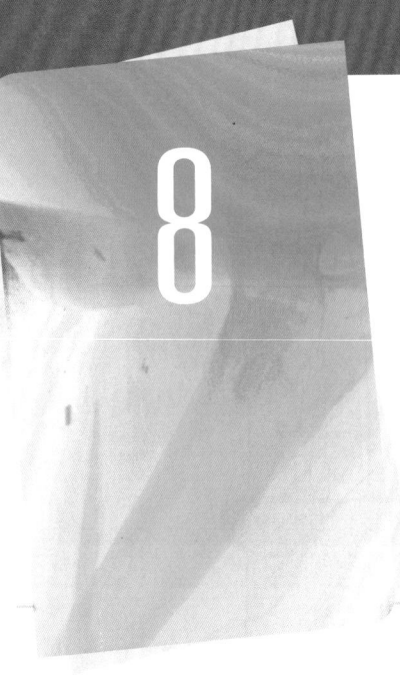

8 PRINCIPLES OF EXTERNAL FIXATION

J. Tracy Watson

HISTORICAL PERSPECTIVE

External fixation was described by Hippocrates almost 2,400 years ago, when he described a method to immobilize a fracture of the tibia, which also allowed inspection of the soft tissue injury. This was accomplished by wrapping the proximal and distal tibia with leather wraps, "such as are worn by persons confined for a length of time in large shackles, and they should have a thickened coat on each side, and they would be well stuffed and fit well, the one above the ankle, and the other below the knee. Four flexible rods, made of the cornel tree (European dogwood), of equal length should be placed between the knee and ankle wrap. If these things be properly contrived, they should occasion a proper and equable extension in a straight line. And the rods are commodiously arranged on either side of the ankle so as not to interfere with the position

of the limb; and the wound is easily examined and arranged" (Fig. 8-1).[133,229]

The history of modern external fixation dates back to the 19th century with Malgaigne's description of an ingenious mechanism consisting of a clamp that approximated four transcutaneous metal prongs for use in reducing and maintaining patellar fractures. This was described in 1843 a full 12 years before the introduction of plaster casting techniques.[116,229]

Origins of Monolateral External Fixation

The original description of the management of long bone fractures suggestive of an external fixator is attributed to a British surgeon, Keetley, in 1893.[34,118] In an effort to decrease malunion and nonunion in the femur, rigid pins were inserted percutaneously into the femur and attached to an external splint system.

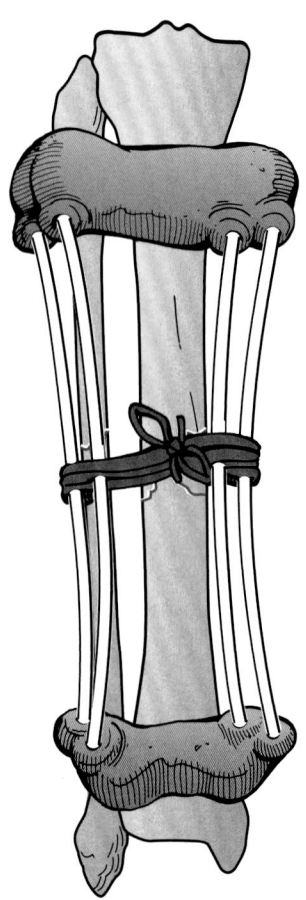

FIGURE 8-1 Hippocrates "shackle" external device for maintaining a tibia fracture at length.

"A carefully purified pin of thickly plated steel, made to enter through a puncture in the skin, cleansed with equal care" was passed through drill holes, one in each main fragment. The two horizontal arms of each device, suitably notched along the edges, were united by twists of wire, and the construct was then dressed with a wrapping of iodoform gauze (Fig. 8-2).

In 1897, Clayton Parkhill, a Denver surgeon and dean of the University of Colorado School of Medicine (1895 to 1897) reported on the results of nine patients treated with an exter-

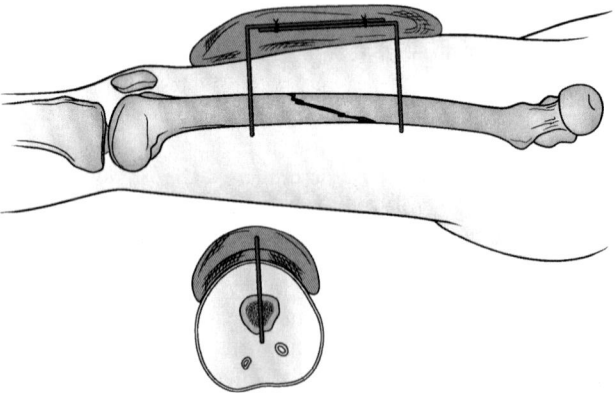

FIGURE 8-2 Keetley's fixator consisted of implanted pins connected by wire, then overwrapped with gauze.

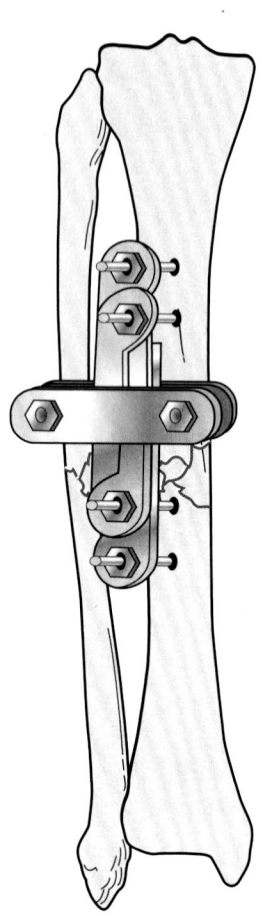

FIGURE 8-3 Parkhill's external fixator for tibia fractures.

nal device similar to a modern simple monolateral four-pin external fixator. His first case was performed in 1894, and his device consisted of four screws, two of which were inserted into each fragment above and below the fracture. The ends of the screws were fixed together by interlocking plates and bolts. He did require supplemental plaster immobilization to provide additional support to the construct (Fig. 8-3). He treated eight nonunions and one unstable tibial shaft fracture. Union of the fractures occurred in eight of the nine patients.[225,226] His career was unfortunately cut short when he died from appendicitis. Although himself a surgeon, he would not submit to surgery for his condition and died in Denver in 1902.

Leonard Freeman was a contemporary of Parkhill, as both were professors of surgery in the Medical Department of the University of Colorado. Freeman developed his own system of external fixation which he thought was much simpler than Parkhill's device. Single pins were inserted above and below the fracture or nonunion and were connected to each other using an external metal band with wooden plate liners firmly clamping the pin shafts (Fig. 8-4A). He was the first to develop a system of instrumentation to insert the pins applied through very small incisions, and he carefully reviewed the technique of "clean" insertion using a trocar and drill sleeve to protect the soft tissues during predrilling of the fixation holes. He also utilized a "T handle" to carefully insert the pins into the bone. He recommended that the pins

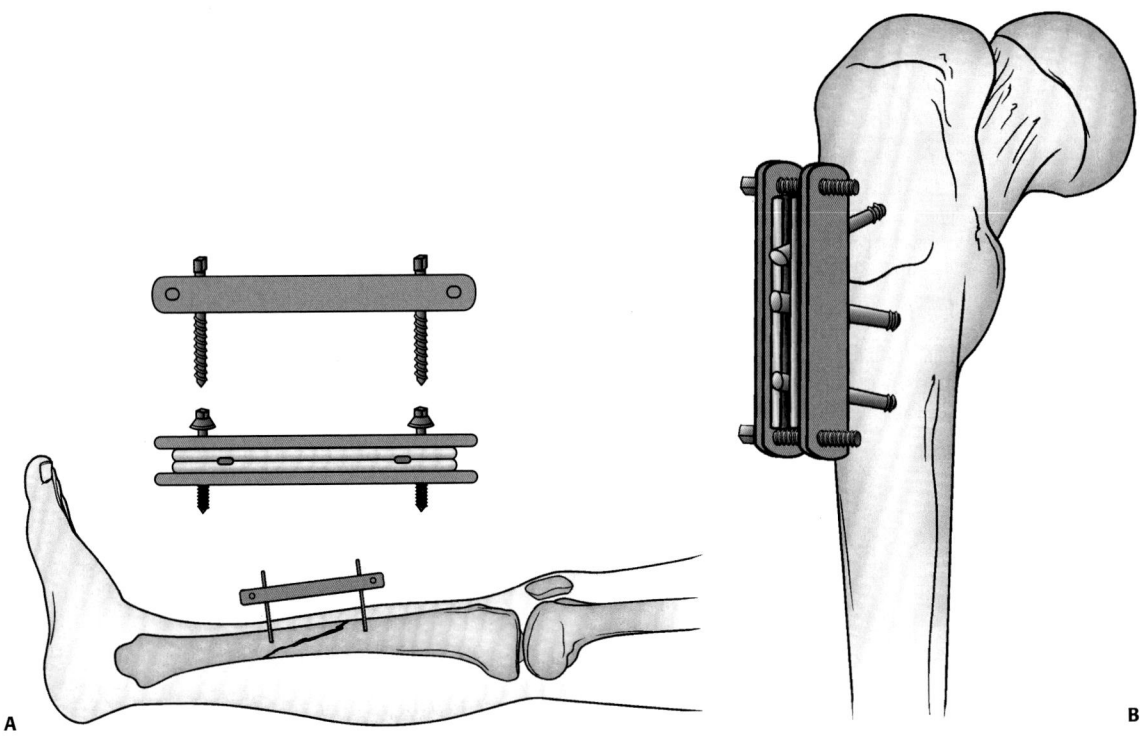

FIGURE 8-4 A: Freeman's fixator. **B:** Freeman device used to stabilize proximal femoral fractures and nonunions.

be inserted "at a distance from the fracture, perhaps in normal tissues, through small openings in the skin." In spite of the fact that he continually praised Parkhill's work, he felt that Parkhill's clamp, and "others which have appeared abroad are unnecessarily complicated and difficult of application, owing to the various wings, nuts, and adjustments with which they are hampered. This apparatus described...is so simple that it can always rapidly and easily be inserted."[100–104] He initially reported the treatment of a proximal femoral neck nonunion and two tibial nonunions with this technique (Fig. 8-4B).[100]

The Belgian surgeon Lambotte recognized Parkhill's work but was unable to obtain a copy of Parkhill's paper. In 1902 he expanded external fixation further and was the first to apply a simple unilateral frame in a systematic fashion. He recognized that the metal pins which penetrated the bone and protruded through the skin were remarkably well tolerated and could be connected to an external clamp device, which would allow for stabilization of these pins and the bone fragments they were attached to (Fig. 8-5).[172] Lambotte's concepts and design evolved and eventually allowed for frame adjustments to occur including compression and distraction at the fracture site.

In Europe, Lambotte's original concepts were expanded significantly and in 1938, Raul Hoffmann began tinkering with the external fixators of his era, whose shortcomings included the need for open reduction before fixator application. He developed his own technique for fracture fixation, which he termed "ostéotaxis," a Greek term meaning "to put the bones in place." Hoffmann was also a doctor of theology and a carpenter in his free time, and his external fixator incorporated a universal ball

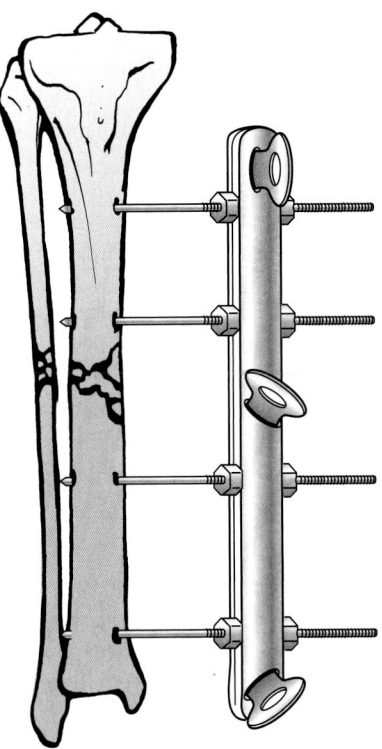

FIGURE 8-5 Lambotte's external fixator using simple pins and a clamp device.

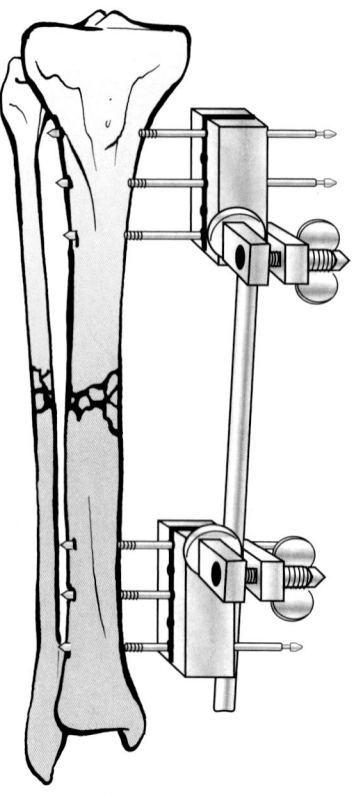

FIGURE 8-6 Hoffman's multipin clamp external fixator.

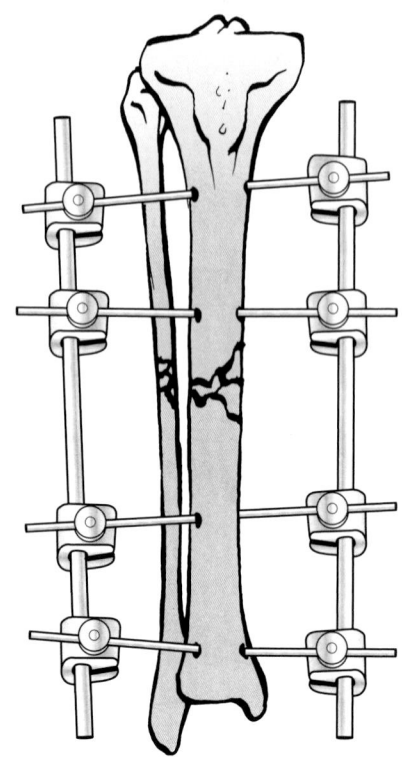

FIGURE 8-7 Anderson device with through-and-through transfixion pins.

joint connecting the external ball of the fixator to strong pin-gripping clamps. This universal joint permitted fracture reduction to occur in three planes while the fixator was in place. Hoffman could substitute a sliding compression—distraction bar connecting the pin-gripping clamps, and then interfragmentary compression or limb length restoration could be performed (Fig. 8-6).[134,135] In 1938, Hoffmann published his new technique and presented it to the French Congress of Surgery.[247]

In the United States, Roger Anderson devised an apparatus for the mechanical reduction of fractures utilizing transcutaneous pins connected to metal clamps. Anderson's early concept called for application of transfixion pins. This permitted multiplanar adjustment of the fracture fragments and also allowed compression at the fracture site. Following reduction, a cast was applied whereas the limb was still held by the external device.[7] After the cast was applied, the external device was removed and reused on additional patients. Later, Anderson extended this concept and designed an entire external system that connected transcutaneous pins to bars, eliminating the need for a plaster cast (Fig. 8-7).[115]

In 1937, Otto Stader devised a system of fracture management for use in his veterinary practice, which permitted stabilization of fractures and also allowed the independent reduction of fracture fragments to occur in three planes.[115,229] Stader's work was observed by surgeons from Bellevue Hospital in New York. They persuaded him to adapt his fixator for use in humans and thus the Stader device was refined and enlarged for use in human long bones. In 1942, Lewis and Breidenbach reported their experience with this device for treating 20

patients with long bone fractures at Bellevue Hospital They were encouraged by the frame's ability to achieve excellent alignment and early ambulation without the need for adjunctive casting. (Fig. 8-8).[184] They were the first to describe the technique of placing pins as far from the fracture as possible and avoiding pins directly near the site of fracture. This was done to improve the fixator's ability to gradually reduce a malaligned extremity by adjusting the device. They felt a wide pin spread increased the overall mechanical stability of the construct. They also were one of the first investigators along with Schanz, Riedel, and Anderson to point out the advantages of inserting the fixation pins at an angle to each other (not parallel) as a means of firmer control over the bone fragments.[184,229]

World War II Use of External Fixation

During World War II (WWII) there were initial favorable reports on the use of the Roger Anderson device in the European theatre where external fixation techniques were demonstrated at base hospitals. However, experience showed that the techniques were too specialized and time consuming for use in an active combat zone. Also, there was a high incidence of complications, including poor pin fixation, pin tract infection, and localized osteomyelitis. Indeed, the copious purulent drainage from the pin sites of Anderson device became so infamous that it was dubbed "Seattle serum," after the city in which he worked.[247] This technique fell into general disfavor because these complications were by and large attributed to the external fixation device and not necessarily to the problems of treating high-energy open fractures.[120] This resulted in a directive

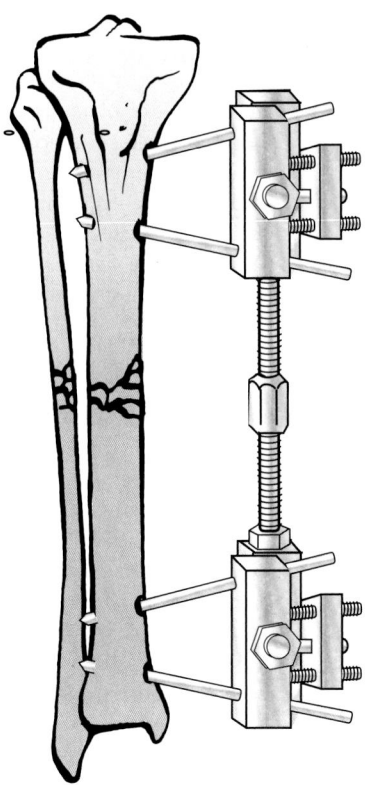

FIGURE 8-8 The Stader device.

issued to military surgeons of the United States Armed Forces to discontinue the use of external fixation in the European theatre of WWII conflict.[115]

However, excellent results were reported by the United States Navy, utilizing external fixation techniques in the Pacific conflict. These were documented by Shaar and Kreuz in their monograph outlining their use and results of the Stader splint.[266,267] They describe the use of this fixator for a wide variety of fractures including femur, tibia, humerus, forearm, and even facial and mandibular fractures. These procedures were primarily performed on evacuation hospital ships and away from the chaos of field hospitals.

Similar results were documented by the Canadian Armored Corps with their use of the Stader device beginning in 1942. They felt that pretraining with cadaver application and familiarity of the device was a crucial factor in their excellent results. They also discussed pin insertion technique extensively to avoid heat generation and the development of ring sequestra.[250]

In 1950, a study was commissioned by the Committee on Fracture and Trauma Surgery of the American Academy of Orthopaedic Surgeons (AAOS) to investigate the efficacy and indications for external fixation in clinical fracture management. The study was based on 3,082 questionnaires sent to practicing clinicians who were members of the AAOS, the American association for the surgery of trauma and the Iowa Medical Society. Only 395 replies were analyzed by the committee. In all, 28% of the respondents felt that external skeletal fixation had a definite place for fracture management, whereas 29.4% felt that external fixation was not inadvisable except in select rare

instances.[140] Over 43% of respondents had used external fixation at one time, but had abandoned it completely at the time of the survey. Based on the results of the survey and concerns that practitioners had with the potential mechanical difficulty associated with these frames, as well as the prospect of converting a closed fracture to an open fracture, the committee concluded that any physicians who contemplated the use of external skeletal fixation required special training under the supervision of a surgeon who had treated at least 200 cases by this method.[115,271] As a consequence, by 1950, the majority of American surgeons were not using this modality.

CONTEMPORARY MONOLATERAL EXTERNAL FIXATION EVOLUTION

From 1950 to 1970, external fixators were generally unpopular with American orthopedists, although the "pins and plaster" technique was still widely used for wrist and tibial fractures. In Europe, Vidal and his coworkers were the first to subject the various external fixator frames to mechanical testing. Vidal utilized Hoffman's equipment, but designed a quadrilateral frame to provide rigid stabilization of complex fracture problems. His biomechanical studies determined that the quadrilateral configuration was quite stable.[115,287]

Similarly, Franz Bernie continued with Dr. Hoffman's original concept of a unilateral frame utilizing a single connecting bar and half pins. His extensive clinical experience with a half-pin frame documented the success of this device when treating several large series of fractures.[40,41] This European experience in the late 60s and early 70s demonstrated that the use of external fixation could not only treat fractures, but could also be extended to the treatment of pseudoarthrosis, infections, and arthrodeses.

During the 70s, De Bastiani developed the "dynamic axial fixator" and Gotzen the "monofixator." These were simple four-pin frames with large pin clusters positioned at either ends of the bone. These were then connected to each other by a large-diameter telescoping tubular rod (Fig. 8-9). This innovation allowed the frames to be more patient-friendly compared with the complex fixators of Vidal-Adrey. These frames would promote axial loading with full weight bearing, accentuating micromotion, and dynamization at the fracture site to enhance healing.

The outstanding basic science work on external fixation and the promising clinical results emanating from Europe in the early 70s stimulated renewed interest in the use of these techniques in North America. This also coincided with the publication of the second edition of the Arbeitsgemeinschaft für Osteosynthesefragen (AO) Manual in 1977.[132] It was at this time that external fixation was recommended for the treatment of acute open fractures. Simultaneously, with the recommendations found in the second AO Manual was the production of a new tubular monolateral external fixation system. The tubular system of the Association for the Study of Internal Fixation (ASIF) gained wide acceptance very rapidly, because of improved pin design and frame biomechanics, as well as precise indications for their use. These factors contributed to many North American surgeons revisiting and adopting this technique, with good clinical results (Fig. 8-10).

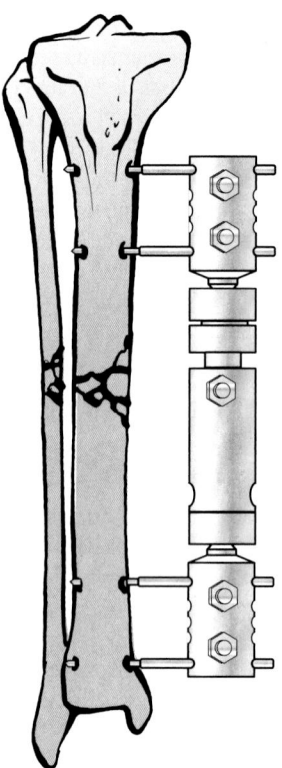

FIGURE 8-9 Large body monotube external fixator.

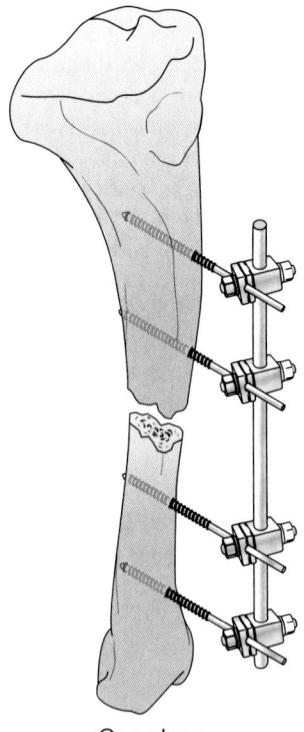

One-plane

FIGURE 8-10 The "simple monolateral" multicomponent external fixation system that helped renew interest in contemporary external fixation techniques.

External fixation has enjoyed a renaissance over the last 10 years with the adoption of damage control orthopedic (DCO) techniques and the concepts of temporary spanning external fixation for the treatment of complex periarticular injuries. These treatment methodologies emphasize the application of simplistic monolateral external fixators to facilitate the initial management of complex articular injuries, or long bone fractures in the polytraumatized patient.[234] Minimalistic frames combined with delayed skeletal reconstruction using locking plates and IM nails have become the standard of care for most centers treating these patients.

Circular External Fixation

The credit for establishing circular external fixation as a method for fracture reduction and limb lengthening has to be given to Joseph E. Bittner MD, a general surgeon from Yakima, Washington. He developed a system of circular rings with transfixion wires which were tensioned by expanding a hinged ring with the wire attached between the hinges. As the ring diameter was expanded, the tension increased in the wires (Fig. 8-11). He published his work in a German Science Journal in 1933 and patented his device 1 year later in 1934. This was followed by a plethora of Russian and European circular fixators initiated first by Pertsovsky in 1938, followed by other Russian surgeons including Gudushauri and Kalnberz. Their devices all resembled Bittner's original concept of circular rings with tensioned wires.[116,141]

External fixation as a modality for fracture treatment continued to remain viable in Russia following WWII. Instead of concentrating on half-pin and monolateral type configurations that were popular in the United States, their techniques continued to focus on the use of tensioned transfixion wires to maintain bone segment fixation. In 1948, Gavril Abramovich Ilizarov developed his version of a circular fixator, which permitted surgeons to stabilize bone fragments with distraction techniques and also made three-dimensional reconstructions possible. In 1950 Ilizarov moved to the city of Kurgan where he continued to explore ways to achieve improved results in bone healing and patented his device in 1954. By attaching these wires to separate rings, the rings could be individually manipulated to provide for three planes of correction, similar to the concepts pioneered by Hoffman, Bernie, Vidal, and Bittner. This ability to achieve precise ring positioning resulted in significant flexibility of the device (Fig. 8-12). Because of the success rate he reported for complex problems, devices similar to the Ilizarov circular frame began emerging in other areas of the USSR.[141] Gudushauri device was a half ring (bow) designed at the Central Institute of Traumatology and Orthopedics (CITO) in 1955. Later, the Gudushauri device was given the green light and became the "official" external device used in Moscow for many years. In the mid 1960s the central power structure in Moscow did not want to credit a simple "province" doctor from Siberia (Ilizarov) with these revolutionary concepts.[141]

Dr. Mstislav V. Volkoff, head of the CITO, was one of the prominent figures who actively worked against universal acceptance of the Ilizarov methodology in the USSR. Together with Dr. Oganesyan they patented a similar device and used their

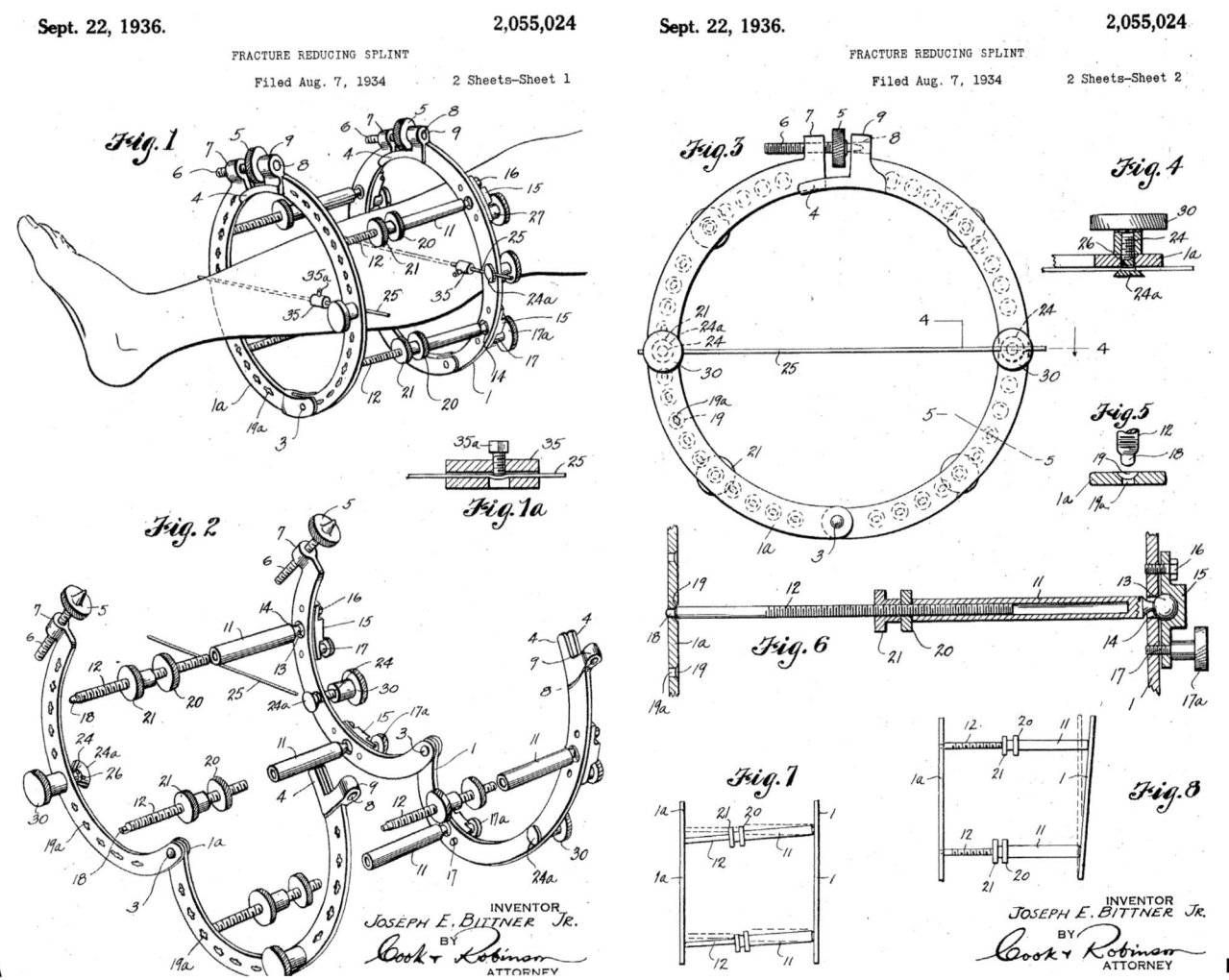

FIGURE 8-11 A, B: The original patent application for Bittner's circular external fixator with the principle of tensioned thin fixation wires.

prestige to promote their device for many years.[141] In 1975, Volkoff and Oganesyan published a series of patients treated with distraction arthroplasty at the knee and elbow utilizing small transfixion wires attached to ring fixators. Their work went largely unnoticed in North America even though it was published in the American Journal of Bone and Joint Surgery.[290]

Dr. David Fisher was exposed to Volkoff's circular apparatus and designed a circular type fixator of his own. Instead of using thin tensioned wires as with the Russian device, he designed a fixator construct which allowed for significant pin separation, deviation of pins at various angles, and a semicircular configuration using larger Schanz half pins. He determined that fracture site stability could be increased using these circular configuration concepts.[94,115]

As the traditional Soviet Ilizarov type devices were quite cumbersome and complex compared with the more straightforward A/O and Hoffman type fixators, Kroner, in 1978, refined and modified the Russian devices by employing plastic components and transfixion pins in place of the thin wires used by the Ilizarov technique.[1,115,140]

For many years, the Ilizarov method was restricted to the region of Kurgan in Siberia. In 1980, the technique was introduced in Western Europe thanks to the persistence of world famous Italian explorer, Carlo Mauri. Mauri traveled to Russia specifically for this technique, and was successfully treated for an infected psuedoarthrosis of the tibia by Ilizarov. His fracture had occurred 10 years earlier in a mountain climbing accident. Through the friendship established by Mauri with Professor Ilizarov, the technique was introduced to Mauri's initial treating surgeons, and subsequently, Ilizarov was invited to speak at the XXII Italian AO conference in Bellagio, Italy. This was the first clinical presentation that Ilizarov gave on his techniques outside of the "Iron Curtain." Italian surgeons realized the significance of his methods and brought the techniques back to Italy under the guidance of Professor Roberto Cattaneoto and his associates, Villa, Catagni, and Tentori. They began the first western clinical trials with transosseous osteosynthesis utilizing Ilizarov's fixator in Lecco, Italy, in 1981.[1,140,141]

When the political climate in the Soviet Union changed under different leadership in the 1980s, the possibilities of the

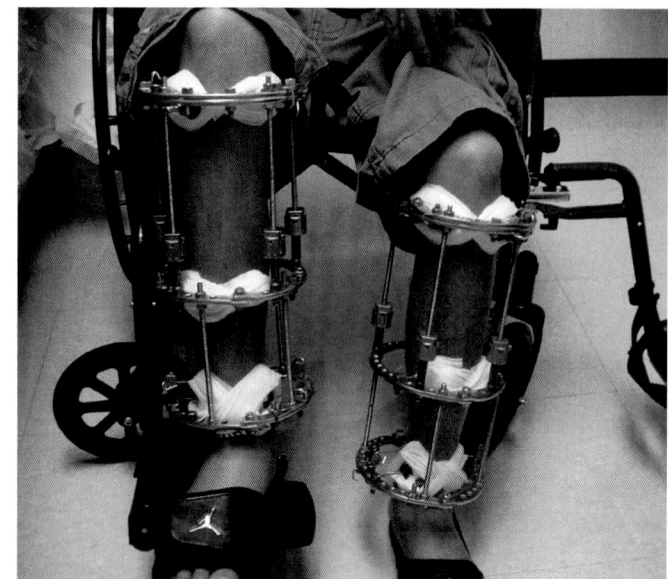
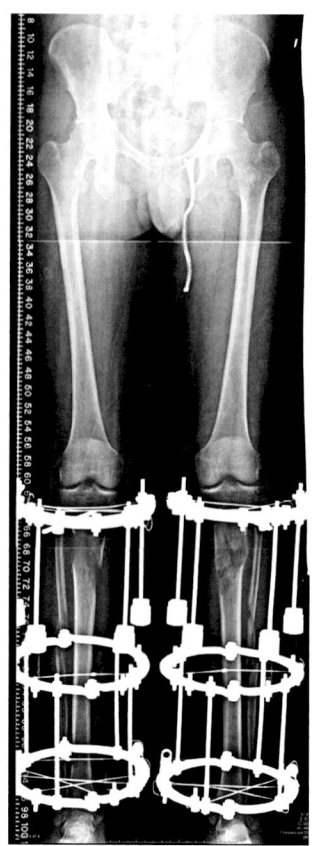

FIGURE 8-12 **A:** Ilizarov's circular fixators using small tensioned wires attached to individual rings. Note the pins wrapped with gauze to provide stabilization of the pin–skin interface. **B:** Radiographs demonstrating bilateral tibial lengthening using classic Ilizarov thin wire frames.

Ilizarov method that had previously been unrecognized in the West became more apparent. These techniques were presented at various orthopedic meetings in Italy and other centers in Western Europe in the early 1980s.[115,135,140,141] Victor H. Frankel (then president of the Hospital for Joint Diseases) saw the external device at a scientific exhibition while attending a meeting in Spain. He investigated further and eventually traveled to Kurgan to visit Ilizarov's center along with Dr. Stuart Green MD in 1987. This began a progression of North American surgeons, notably Victor Frankel, James Aronson, Dror Paley, and Stewart Green, who were exposed to Ilizarov's work. They recognized the potential of this methodology as applied to difficult contemporary orthopedic problems and all began clinical applications in the mid 1980s.[140,141] In 1989, Stewart Green, who had significant expertise in treating nonunions and osteomyelitis with external fixation techniques, was entrusted by Ilizarov to translate his original basic science work into English. This was published in Clinical Orthopaedics and Related Research in 1989.[1,138–141]

The North American experience was popularized by a small cadre of American surgeons in the late 1980s. In an effort to simplify and apply these techniques to traumatology, the tensioned ring concept was married to the unilateral fixator, and the hybrid external fixator was developed to address periarticular injuries with all the advantages of tensioned wires, while limiting the disadvantages of tethering large musculotendinous units with through-and-through transfixion wire constructs. (Fig. 8-13).[1,117] However, this "advancement" had a relatively short life span because of inferior biomechanics.

A significant innovation in deformity correction and precise fracture reductions was developed by Charles Taylor and others to correct complex deformities through the use of simple ring constructs using half-pin fixation. These "hexapod" fixators have rings interconnected and manipulated by a system of adjustable struts, which allow for six-axis correction of bone fragments (Fig. 8-14).[246,262,263] The development of this concept, as well as the ability to interface deformity correction with web-based software, has vastly simplified frame construction and is the basis for contemporary circular external fixation techniques in use at this time.

FRAME TYPES, BIOMECHANICS, AND COMPONENTS

External fixation systems in current clinical use can be categorized according to the type of bone anchorage utilized. This is accomplished by using either large threaded pins, which are screwed into the bone or by drilling small-diameter transfixion wires through the bone and then placing the wires under tension to maintain bone fragment position.

The pins or wires are then connected to one another through the use of longitudinal bars or circular rings. Thus the distinction is made between monolateral external fixation (longitudinal connecting bars) and circular external fixation (wires and/or pins connecting to rings). Circular fixation may use either threaded pins or small tensioned wires to attach the bone to the frame. Monolateral fixation is accomplished using

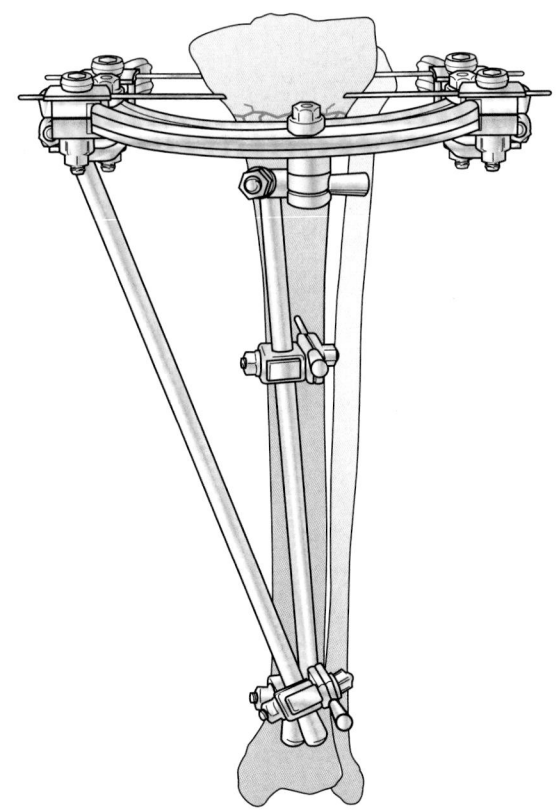

A

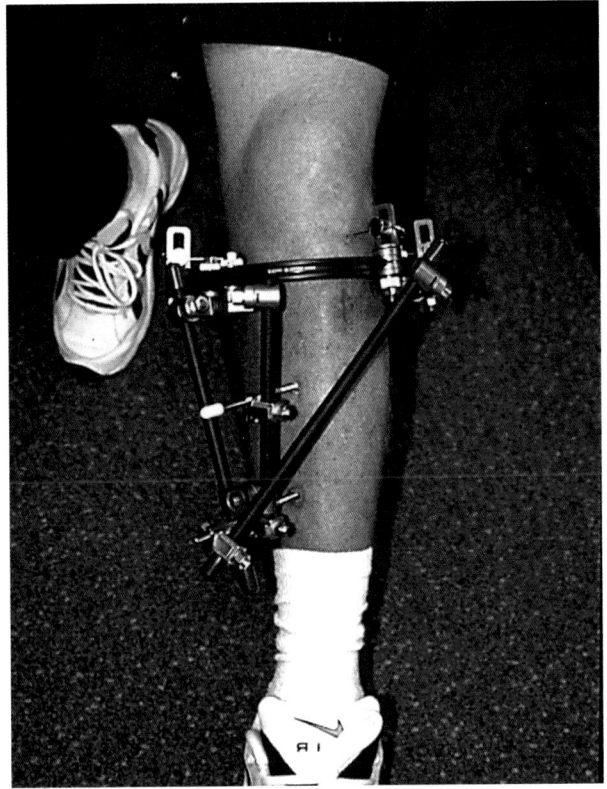

B

FIGURE 8-13 **A:** An early version of a hybrid external fixator which combines periarticular tensioned wires and diaphyseal half-pin configurations. **B:** Clinical picture of the same hybrid frame on a patient with a tibial plateau fracture.

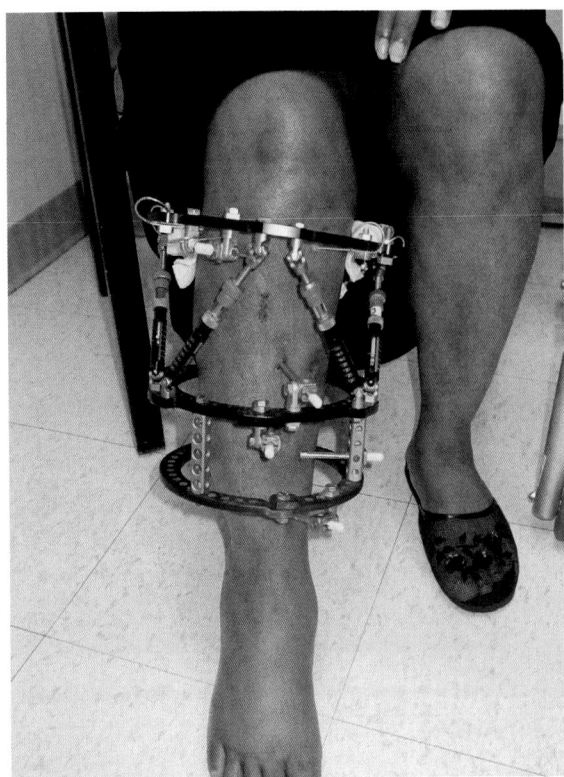

FIGURE 8-14 Hexapod external fixator with multiple oblique connecting struts through which the limb segments can be manipulated for simultaneous correction of multiple deformities.

various diameter threaded pins; however, these may occasionally involve the use of centrally threaded through-and-through transfixion pins.

Large Pin Fixation

Large pin fixator constructs are attached to the bone using various sizes of terminally threaded pins. The half pins have a wide range of diameter ranging from 2 to 6 mm with all intermediate sizes available. In addition, there are large-diameter pins with threads in the midportion of the device (centrally threaded pins), for use in transfixion-type constructs, that is, Hoffman-Vidal configurations (Fig. 8-15A–E).

The basic indications for large pin external skeletal fixation are numerous. The actual biomechanical function that a monolateral frame will perform is dependent upon the placement of the pins and orientation of the connecting bars applied. These factors, as well the inherent skeletal pathology treated, combine to impart a specific biomechanical function to the fixation construct. The ability to neutralize deforming forces is the most common mechanical principle exploited by external fixation. This is especially true for acute fractures accompanied by severe soft tissue damage. The use of monolateral fixation for the stabilization of acute fractures deals with the soft tissue compromise in the immediate posttrauma/postoperative period.[90] Following resolution of the soft tissue injury, secondary procedures such as bone grafting or delayed internal fixation are performed. The primary function of fixators used in this way is to provide

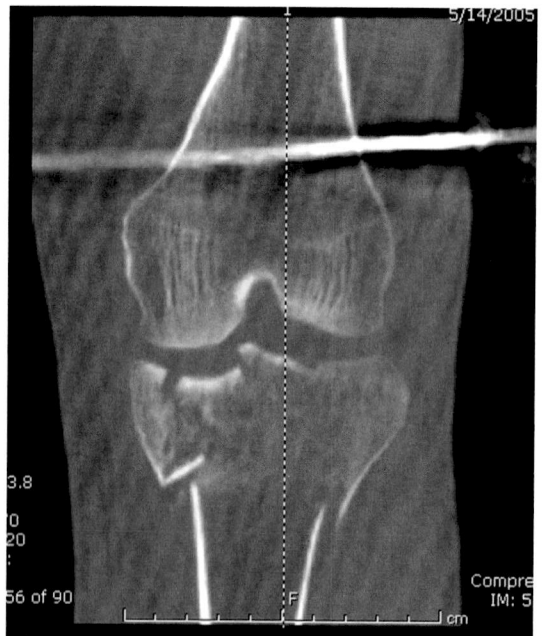

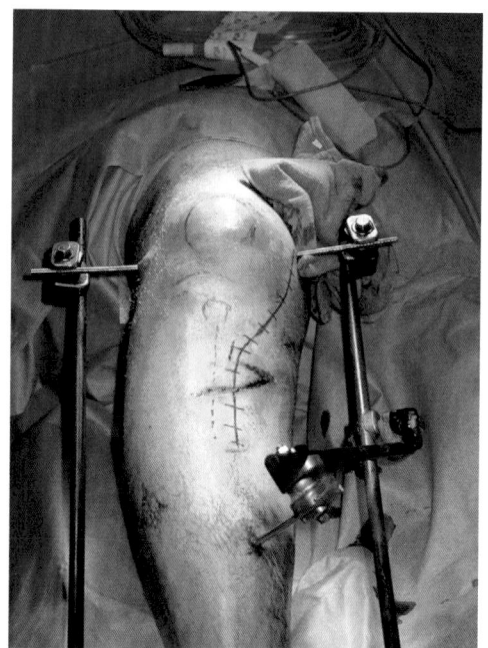

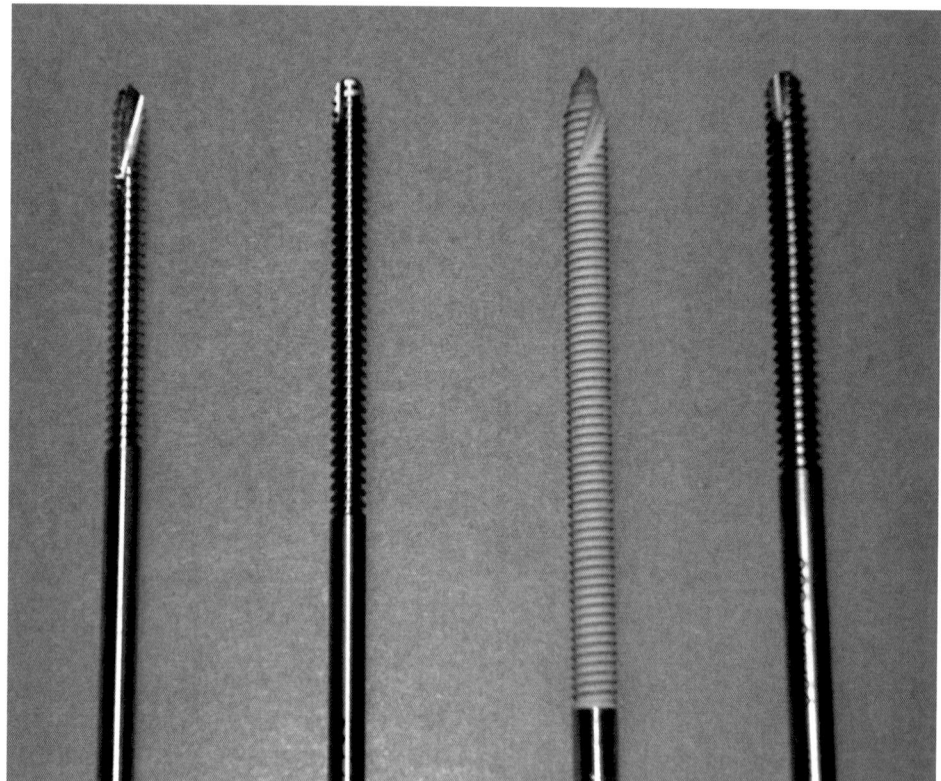

FIGURE 8-15 A: Large centrally threaded Schanz pin placed as a distal femoral transfixion pin in a temporary knee-spanning external fixator as seen on radiographs. Clinical image of proximal transfixion pin and quadrilateral spanning frame with intercalary half pin mid tibia. **B–E:** Multiple pin types; **(B)** 5-mm self-tapping predrilled pins with a short thread length, **(C)** 5-mm self-tapping predrilled pin with long threads, **(D)** 6-mm hydroxyapatite self-drilling pin, note self-drilling tip, and **(E)** 6-mm self-tapping predrilled titanium pin.

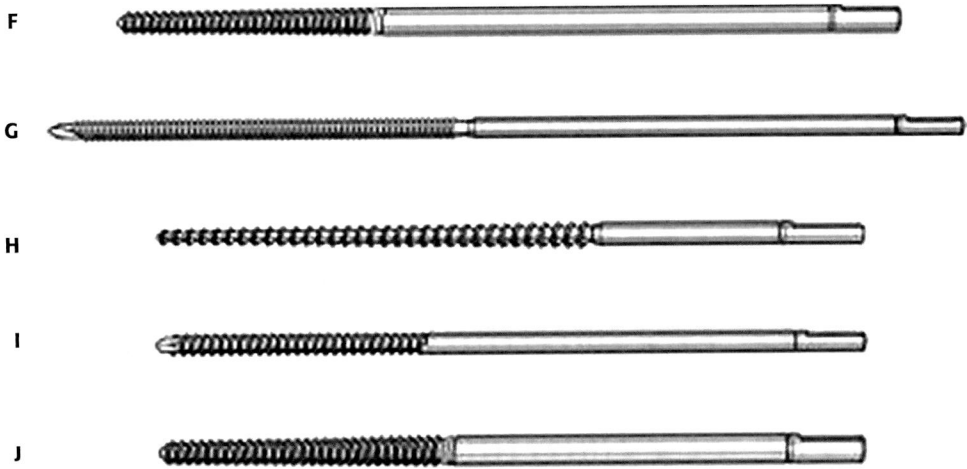

FIGURE 8-15 (*continued*) **F–J:** Multiple thread designs are used for specific purposes; **(F)** tapered pins facilitate subsequent pin removal, **(G)** self-drilling pins with drill-type pin tip; **(H)** pins with larger thread diameter suitable for cancellous bone insertion, **(I)** small pitch angle and narrow thread-diameter pins are applied in cortical bone, and **(J)** hydroxyapatite-coated pins improve the pin–bone interface by encouraging direct bone apposition and ingrowth.

relative stability to maintain temporary fracture reduction and length to avoid collapse of the fracture construct (Fig. 8-16). It should be noted, however, that this type of stabilization is reasonably "flexible." It is nearly impossible to achieve absolute rigidity to achieve primary bone healing utilizing monolateral external fixation.

Monolateral as well as circular frames can also be used to bring areas of metaphyseal or metadiaphyseal bone into close contact through the use of compression techniques. This may be useful in arthrodesis, osteotomy, or nonunion repair (Fig. 8-17).[187,221] Similarly, distraction forces can also be applied across pin groups to effect deformity correction, intercalary bone transport, or limb lengthening.

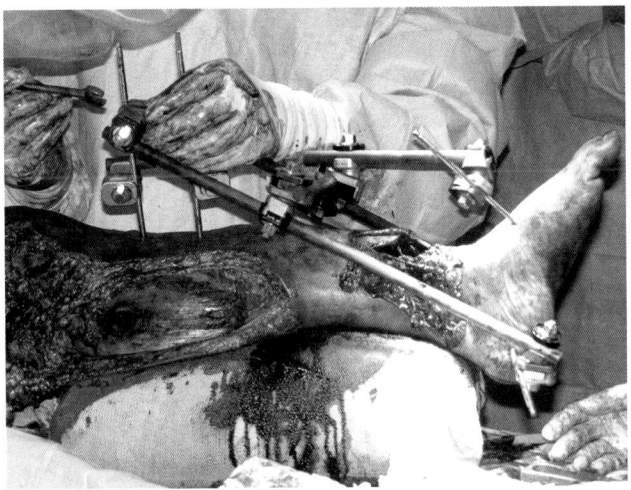

FIGURE 8-16 Simple triangular ankle-"spanning" fixator across a distal tibial injury, with a transfixion pin through the calcaneal tuberosity and two midtibial half pins. This maintains the reduction but is not "rigid" and requires additional temporary splinting.

Components

No matter what the biomechanical function of the frame type, the most important factor regarding the longevity and performance of the frame is the strength and competency of the pin–bone interface. Pin loosening with subsequent pin sepsis continues to be problematic. There are many biomechanical factors, which have been evaluated for the prevention of pin tract problems.[14,25,64,111,114,126]

1. Pin geometry and thread design
2. Pin biomaterials and biocompatibility
3. Pin insertion techniques and pin–bone interface mechanics

Pin Design

It has been determined that both the screw thread design and the type of cutting head have a significant effect on the holding power of screws. Screw diameter is crucial in determining the stiffness of the frame, as well as determining the risk of stress fracture at the pin site entry portal. The bending stiffness of the screw increases as a function of the pin's radius raised to the fourth power ($S = r^4$). Placing a screw hole greater than 20% or 30% of the bone's diameter will substantially increase the risk for pinhole fracture. It is important to match the pin diameter to the diameter of the bone being stabilized. In general, it is recommended to err on the side of using a smaller pin diameter.

Calculations have determined that in adult bone, a pin diameter of 6 mm is the maximum that can be used to achieve a stable implant without suffering the consequences of stress fracture through the pinhole itself.[47,232,265] This risk will resolve in 6 to 8 weeks through bone remodeling once the pin has been removed. However, the pin site does remain a stress riser until full remodeling of the pin site can occur.

In addition to the variable diameter of the pin, the screw thread may also have differing pitch angle and pitch height. The screw design must make allowances for the quality and

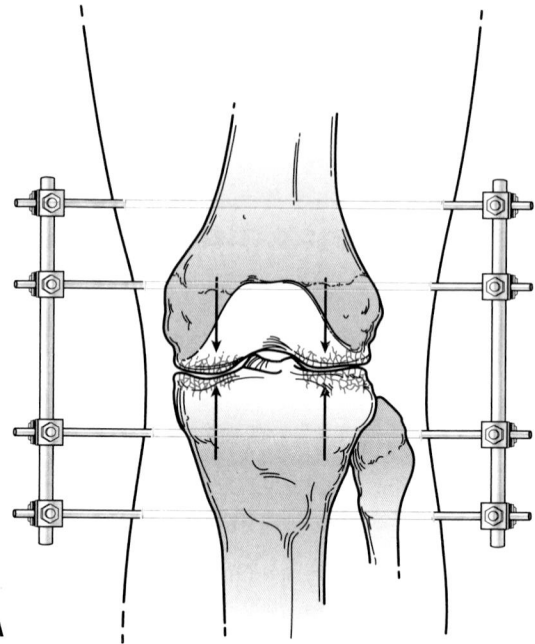

FIGURE 8-17 **A:** A simple "compression" monolateral system constructed to achieve arthrodesis of the knee. **B:** Complex ring external fixator to effect similar compression forces for an infected knee fusion below a pre-existing femoral nail. Solid arthrodesis was achieved following frame nail removal, debridement, and compression treatment.

A

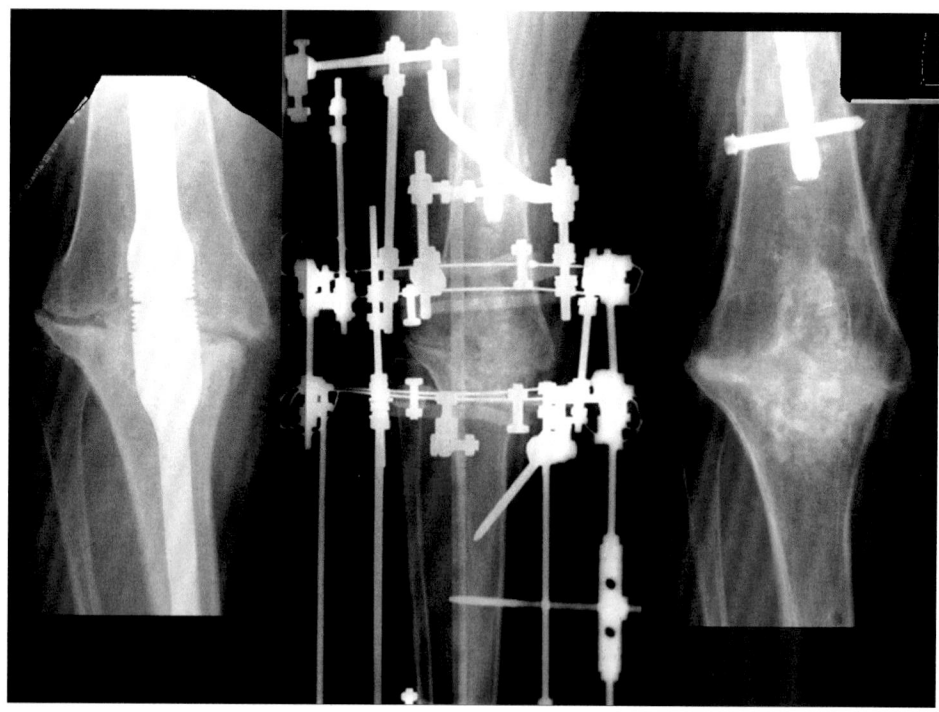

B

location of the bone to which the screw is applied. Pins with a small pitch height and low pitch angle are usually applied in regions of dense cortical bone, such as femoral and tibial diaphysis (Fig. 8-15F–J).

As the pitch vertex angle increases and the curvature and the diameter of the thread increases, the area captured by each individual thread is broader and more likely to be applied in cancellous bone rather than hard cortical bone. Conical pins have been designed so that the threads taper and increase in diameter from the tip of the pin to the shaft. This allows the pins to increase their purchase theoretically by cutting a

new larger path in the bone with each advance of the pin. This conical taper also produces a gradual increase in radial preload and thus the screw–bone contact is optimized (Fig. 8-15F–J). Micromotion typical of a straight cylindrical screw is avoided.[175,206,208]

Pin Biomaterials and Biocompatibility

Traditionally, external fixator pins have been composed of stainless steel offering substantial stiffness.[151] Finite element analyses of the near pin–bone interface cortex revealed stress values which were significantly increased by the use of deep threads and by the use of stainless steel as opposed to titanium pins. Titanium has a much lower modulus of elasticity. However, because of the better biocompatibility afforded with titanium and titanium alloys, there are some investigators who prefer the lower pin–bone interface stresses, as well as the better biocompatibility when using titanium, as they feel there is a lower rate of pin sepsis. Titanium alloy half pins had greater recoverable deformation and less stress concentration at the pin–bone interface. Micro-CT analysis also indicated a larger and higher quality of newly formed bone at the pin–bone interface in titanium alloy group when compared with a pin with a titanium core and a vanadium surface coat (TAV). Histology demonstrated that the newly formed bone integrated well into the threads of titanium alloy half pins. In contrast, there was a layer of necrotic tissue between the bone tissue and the vanadium half pin at the pin–bone interface in the TAV group. The extraction torque values of the titanium alloy half pins near the fracture line were significantly higher than the TAV pins. It appears that pins with a low elastic modulus and excellent biocompatibility can enhance osseointegration and reduce pin loosening.[322]

The perceived advantages of titanium in demonstrating excellent biocompatibility may be because of the oxide layer formed on titanium implants. Biocompatibility studies comparing the efficacy of pins coated with titanium dioxide (TiO_2) for inhibition of infection was compared with that of stainless steel control pins in an in vivo study. The bone–implant contact ingrowth ratio of the TiO_2-coated pin group was significantly higher (71.4%) than in the control pin group (58.2%). The TiO_2 was successful in decreasing infection both clinically and histomorphometrically.[161]

This improved performance may be because of many factors including an actual bone ingrowth phenomenon seen at the pin–bone interface.[186,201,202,206] A prospective trial examined 80 patients (320 pins) with unstable distal radius fractures who were treated with external wrist fixators. The ex-fix pins were either stainless steel or titanium alloy. The rate of premature fixator removal because of severe pin tract infection (5% vs. 0%) and the rate of pin loosening (10% vs. 5%) were higher in the stainless steel pin group. The authors concluded that the use of titanium alloy external fixator pins in distal radial fractures may reduce pin-related complications and significantly reduce pain levels compared with the stainless steel pin fixators.[232]

Among the many different techniques to enhance the pin–bone interface fixation, coating the pins with hydroxyapatite (HA) has been shown to be one of the most effective.[20,43,202]

Moroni et al.[205] demonstrated that HA-coated tapered pins improved the strength of fixation at the pin–bone interface, which corresponded to a lower rate of pin tract infection. The HA coating provides a significant increase in direct bone apposition with a decrease in the fibrous tissue interposition at the pin–bone interface. There is significantly less pin loosening in studies comparing HA-coated pins with other pin material groups.[256] These advantages provided by HA coating appear to be more relevant clinically when these pins are used in cancellous bone rather than in cortical bone (Fig. 8-15B–E).[43,203,204] In subsequent studies HA coating on fixator pins has been shown to be more important for optimal pin

fixation than the particular combination of design parameters used in each pin type (i.e., thread pitch, thread configuration, tapered, etc.).[200]

Pin Insertion Technique and Pin–Bone Interface Mechanics

Preloading the implant–bone interface has an effect on pin loosening. Radial preload is a concept that prestresses the pin–bone interface in a circumferential fashion rather than in just one direction.[30,78] Fixator pins are placed with a slight mismatch in the greater thread diameter versus the core diameter of the pilot hole. The small mismatch increases insertion and removal torque, with a decrease in signs of clinical loosening. There is a point at which insertion of pins with a mismatch of greater than 0.4 mm can result in significant microscopic structural damage to the bone surrounding the pin. High degrees of radial preload or large pilot hole thread diameter mismatch will exceed the elastic limit of cortical bone, with subsequent stress fracture. Thus, the use of oversize pins producing excessive radial preloads must be questioned.[30,105,149]

However, local bone yielding at the pin–bone interface of external fixation half pins has been known to initiate fixator loosening. Deterioration of bone properties because of aging and disease can lead to an increase in the risk of pin loosening. Finite element analysis has demonstrated that peri-implant bone resorption around pins increases three-fold comparing young with old-aged cases. The authors recommend fixator modifications when treating elderly patients such as the use of three, rather than two, half pins on either side of the fracture.[75]

Additional recommendations include the use of small tensioned wire constructs in severely osteopenic individuals as a means to avoid pin–bone resorption and subsequent loosening. The volume of resorped bone at all wire–bone interfaces decreased with an increase in wire pre-tension. The absence of continuous cortical thickness resorption offers an explanation for the clinical observation that Ilizarov ring-wire fixation can provide stable fracture fixation even in a bone with high porosity.[75,76]

Screw insertion technique also has an effect on the pin–bone interface. The pins typically come in two types, predrilled pins and self-drilling pins (Fig. 8-15B–E). Predrilled pins by their name require a drill to be used to produce a pilot hole *prior* to insertion of the pin. The pilot hole has a root diameter equal to or somewhat less than the core diameter of the pin itself.[137,265] As a better pilot hole is drilled with a precise cutting tip, the radial preload is also effected, which will also effect the overall pullout strength. The advantages of predrilling using very sharp drills for pilot holes minimizes the risk of thermal necrosis and subsequent bone damage.[78] The use of self-tapping cortical pins allows each thread to purchase bone as the pin is slowly advanced by hand (Fig. 8-15B–E).[57,64]

Self-drilling pins have a drill tip point and are driven under power into the bone to engage the threads in cortical or cancellous bone. There is some concern that when using self-drilling pins, the near cortex thread purchase may be stripped as the drill tip of the pin engages the far cortex. As the drill tip on the pin spins to cut the far cortex, the newly purchased bone

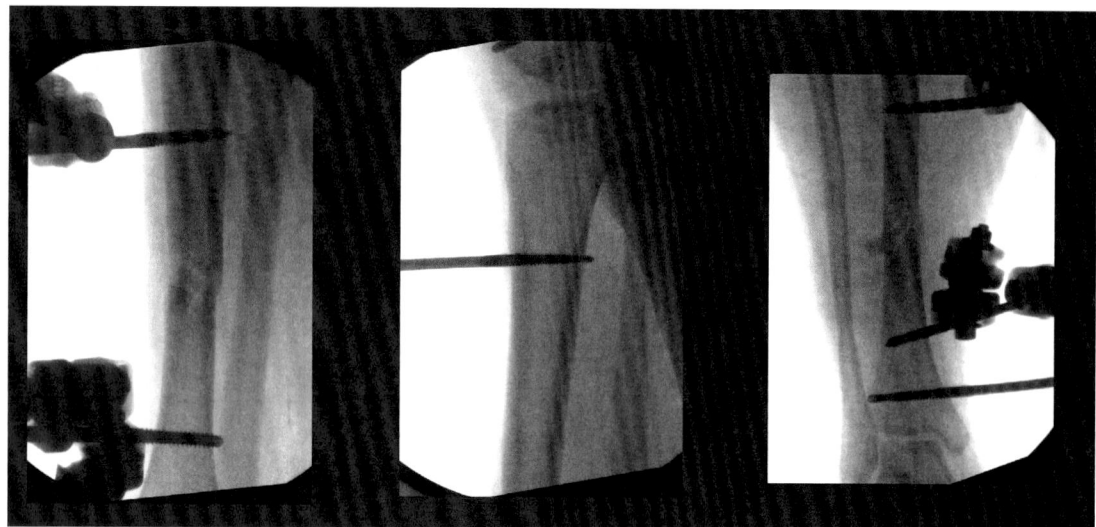

FIGURE 8-18 Pin insertion technique should include the evaluation of the far cortex–pin interface to determine the appropriate depth pin penetration. Excessive penetration can result in potential neurovascular injury if self-drilling pins "pull" the pin too far to gain adequate thread purchase. These pins are placed correctly and do not protrude excessively beyond the far cortex.

in the near threads is stripped and the pin stability compromised (Fig. 8-15F–J). Some studies indicate a 25% reduction in bone purchase of self-drilling, self-tapping pins compared with that of predrilled pins.[22] This is also accompanied by a marked increase in the depth of insertion required to achieve a similar pin purchase or pin "feel," when a self-drilling pin has a long sharp-tipped drilling portion adjacent to the actual threads.[190] To have both cortices engaged with full threads, the pin must be advanced through the far cortex enough to capture the fully threaded portion of the pin and avoid the tapered drill tip. This may leave the tip of the pin "proud" for 2 to 3 mm, which may be problematic in certain anatomic areas where neurovascular structures are directly adjacent to the bone (Fig. 8-18).

Reduction in the length of the drilling portion of the pin means that less of the pin tip needs to project through the far cortex before a firm grip is achieved on the bone. The flutes for tapping the bone run obliquely back down the shaft of the pin. The helical or spiral nature of the flutes steer the bone debris back along the pins and out into the soft tissue. The efficient removal of this bone is mandatory to avoid compacting and jamming the cutting flutes with bone debris and thus compromising their cutting ability, increasing the heat of insertion.[105]

The potential disadvantages of self-drilling pins are increased heat of insertion, increased microfracture at both cortices (specifically at the near cortex with increased bone resorption), and subsequent decreased pullout strength with decreased insertion and extraction torque.[57,206] Studies have noted elevations of temperature on heat of insertion with a direct drill technique, where temperatures in excess of 55°C can occur during insertion of self-drilling pins.[193] Temperatures that exceed 50°C can result in cell death leading to an increased risk for pin site loosening. The use of a water-cooled sharp drill at lower torque speeds can decrease the risk of thermal necrosis.[113,193] The complication of thermal necrosis with secondary loosening caused by the resorption of nonviable bone is a practical concern (Fig. 8-19). Clinically, however, an increased incidence of pin tract infection or other pin complications associated with the use of self-drilling pins has yet to be confirmed.[264]

Monolateral Frame Types

Monolateral frames are subdivided into those fixators that come with individual separate components, that is, separate bars, attachable pin bar clamps, bar-to-bar clamps, and separate Schanz pins. These "simple monolateral" frames allow for a wide range of flexibility with "build-up" or "build-down" capabilities. These components are available with various diameter connection bars as well as multiple clamp sizes and pin clamp configurations. These are often available in "mini" configurations as well for the stabilization of smaller areas of involvement such as for the fingers, wrist, and hand, as well as foot and ankle involvement (Fig. 8-20). As noted above, pin diameters should be undersized especially when stabilizing lesser diameter bones (Fig. 8-21). This allows the surgeon to apply a frame specific to the clinical and biomechanical needs of the pathology addressed (Fig. 8-22).

The other major category of monolateral frames is a more constrained type fixator which is supplied preassembled with a multi pin clamp at each end of a long rigid tubular body. The telescoping tube will allow for axial compression or distraction of this so-called "mono tube"-type fixator. "Simple monolateral fixators" have the distinct advantage of allowing individual pins to be placed at different angles and varying obliquities while still connecting to the bar. This is helpful when altering the pin position relative to the areas of soft tissue compromise. The advantage of the monotube-type fixator is its simplicity. Pin placement is predetermined by the multipin clamps. Loosening the universal

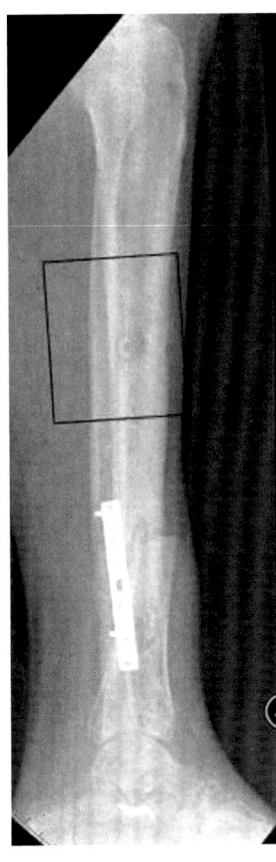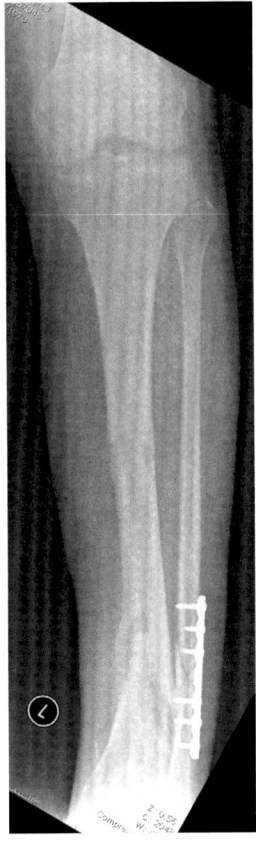

A, B

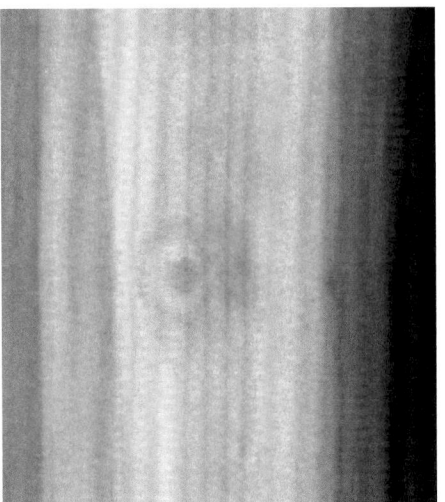

C

FIGURE 8-19 **A, B:** Distal tibial nonunion with varus deformity following failure of a hybrid external fixation. Self-drilling pins utilized in the diaphysis resulted in a ring sequestrum at the proximal pin site (black box). **C:** Sclerotic bone at prior pin location, with circumferential lucency characteristic of ring sequestrum. This complication required excision of the infected sequestrum.

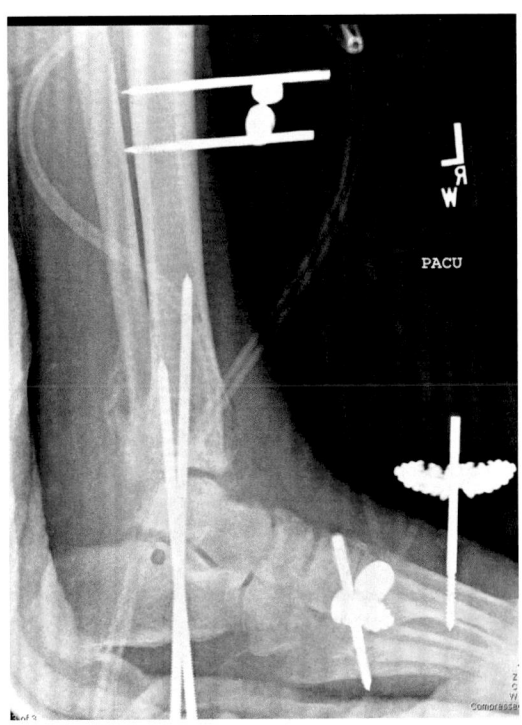

A   **B**

FIGURE 8-20 **A:** "Mini" monolateral frame used to span an ankle. **B:** 4-mm pins used to provide stabilization of the ankle to maintain neutral position.

(continues)

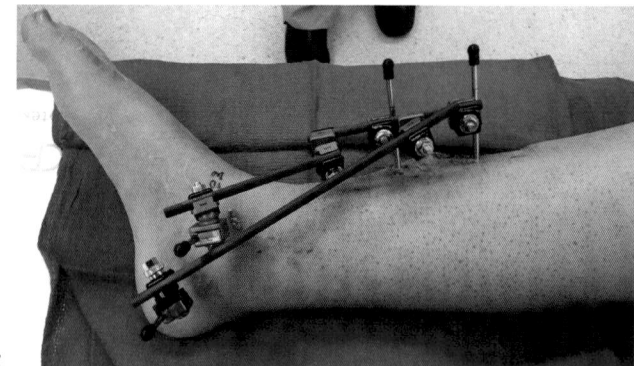

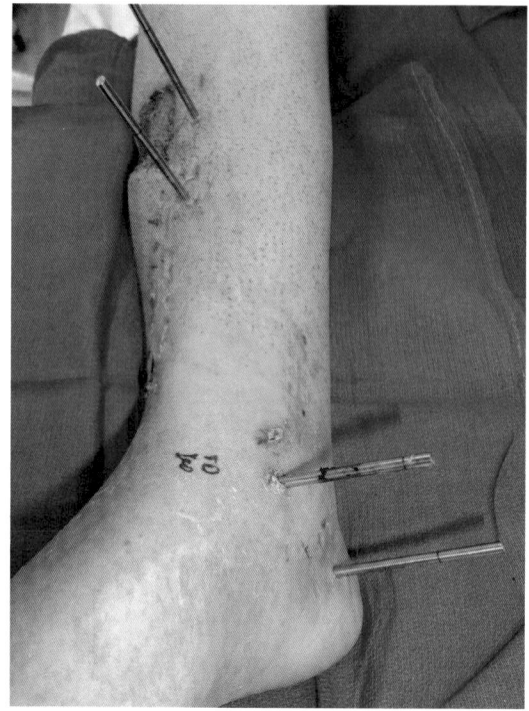

FIGURE 8-20 (*continued*) **C:** Mini fixator spanning into talar neck and calcaneous with mini connecting bars. **D:** Titanium 4-mm fixation pins at the time of frame removal; note excellent biocompatibility at pin–skin interface with the use of Ti pins.

articulations between the body and the clamps allows these frames to be easily manipulated to reduce a fracture. Similarly, compression (dynamization) or distraction can be accomplished by a simple adjustment of the monotube body (Fig. 8-9).

"Simple" Monolateral Fixators

The stability of all monolateral fixators is based on the concept of a simple "four-pin frame." Pin number, pin separation, and pin proximity to the fracture site, as well as bone–bar distance and

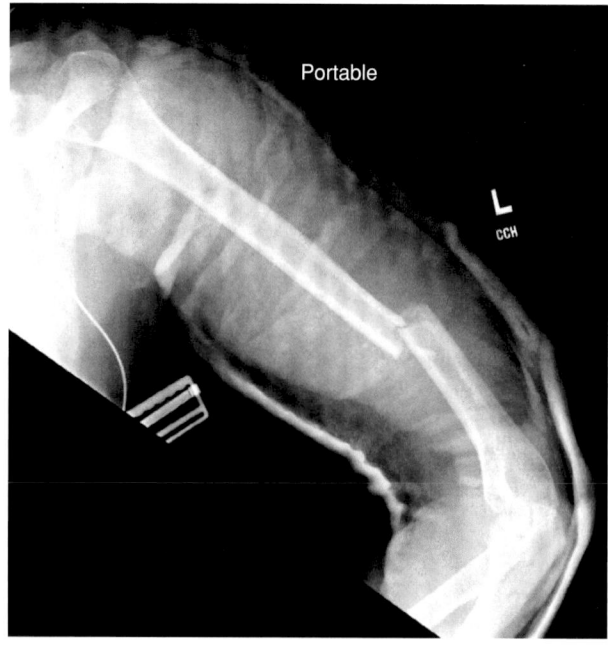

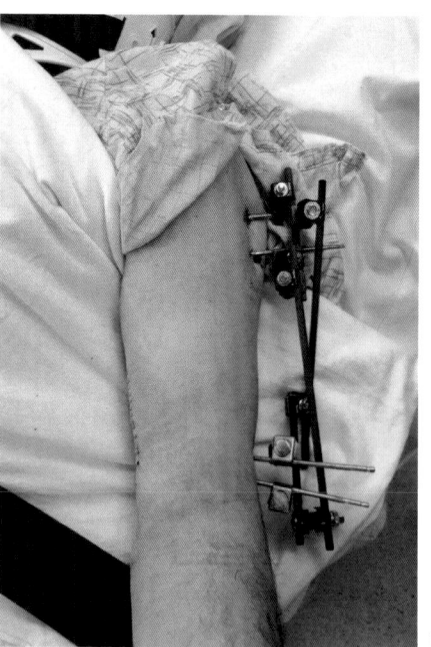

FIGURE 8-21 A: Small diameter humeral shaft, with fracture and arterial disruption. **B–D:** Fracture stabilized with mini fixator to allow for arterial repair. Diameter of pins used to match the small relative diameter of the humeral shaft.

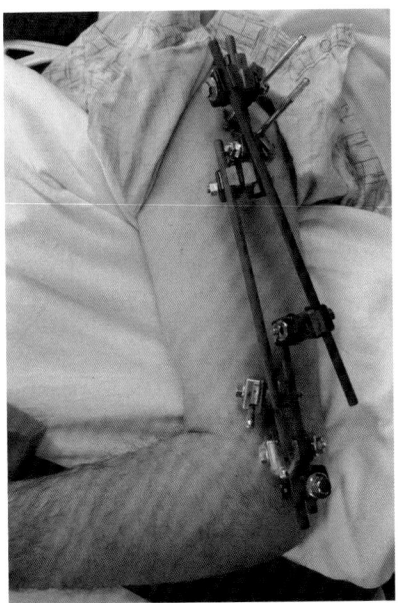 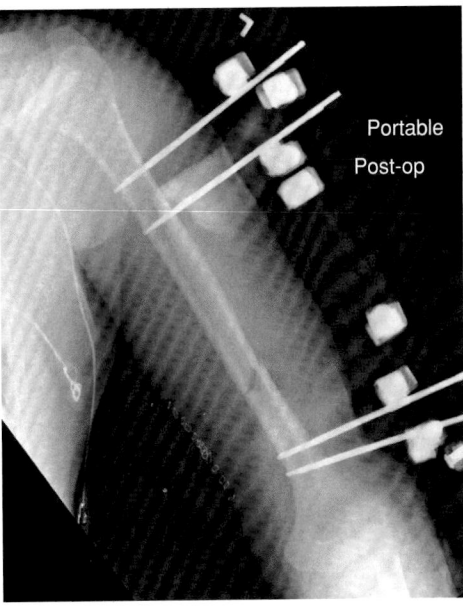 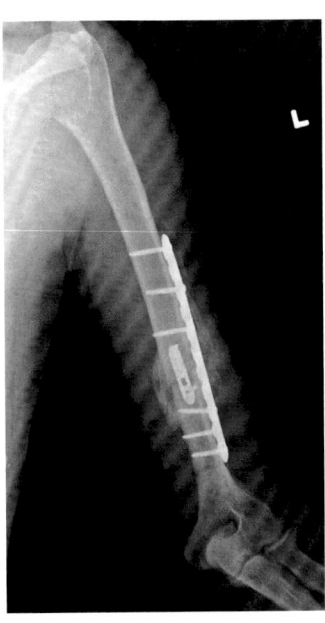

C, D

E

FIGURE 8-21 (*continued*) **E:** Following recovery of soft tissues and success of arterial repair, conversion of the fixator to a plate was carried out 7 days after initial injury with excellent healing.

the diameter of the pins and connecting bars, all influence the final mechanical stability of the external fixator frame (Fig. 8-23).

Most simple monolateral frames allow for individual placement of pins prior to the application of the connecting bars. This permits the surgeon to place pins out of the zone

of compromised skin or away from the fracture hematoma. The versatility of contemporary pin/bar clamps have multiple degrees of freedom built into the clamp which allows a single bar to attach to all four clamps while still retaining the ability to reduce the fracture. The pins do not have to be placed in

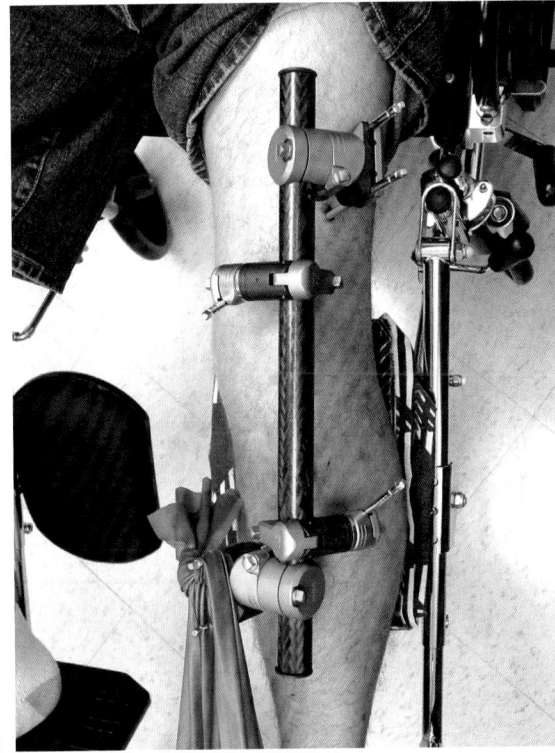 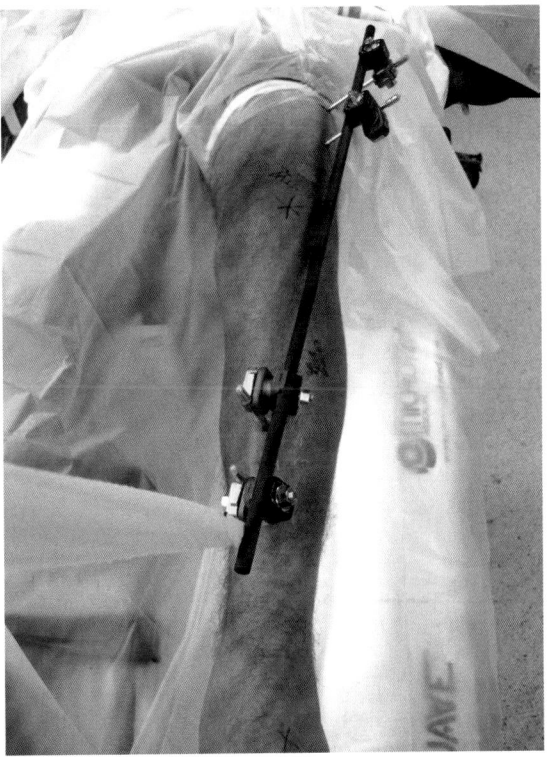

A

B

FIGURE 8-22 **A, B:** Two similar monolateral external fixators both used to span knee dislocations. Note similar components: Separate pin clamps and bars.

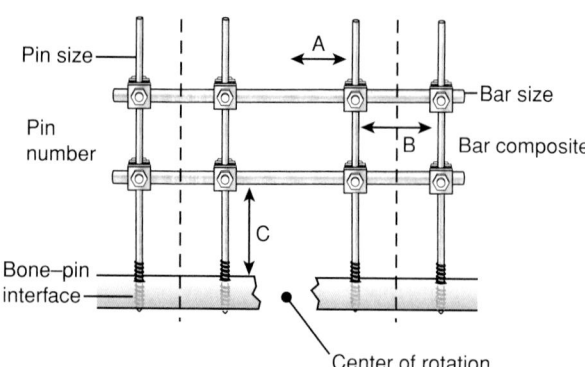

FIGURE 8-23 Factors affecting the stability of monolateral fixation include pin distance from fracture site, pin separation, bone–bar distance, connecting bar size and composition, pin diameter, pin number, and pin–bone interface. **A:** Pin to center of rotation; **(B)** pin separation; **(C)** bone–bar distance.

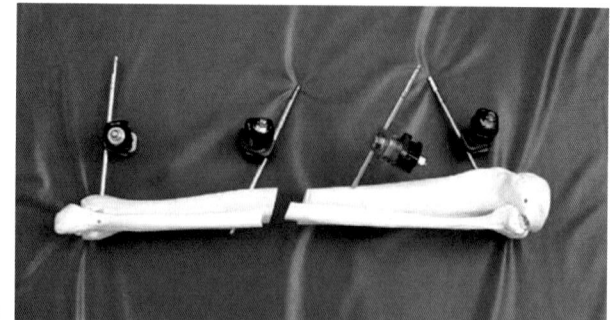

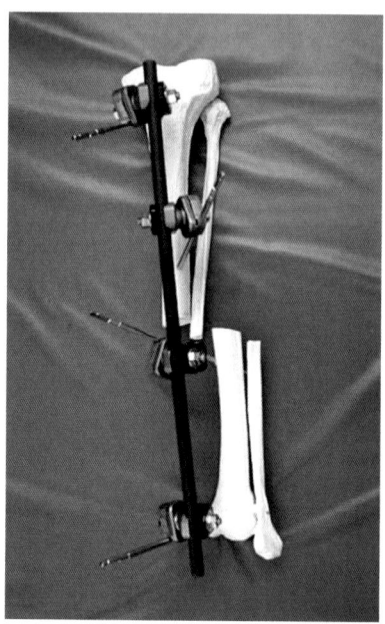

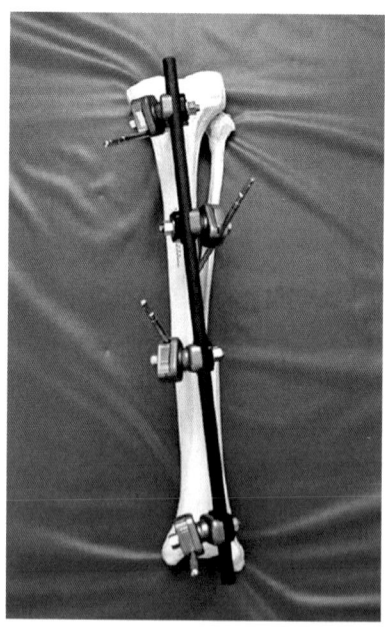

precise alignment as was required by earlier monolateral frame designs (Fig. 8-24). If aligned pin placement is contraindicated because of soft tissue or other concerns, the fractures can still be reduced by simply adding additional connecting bars and using the proximal and distal pin groupings as reduction handles. Once reduction is achieved, the bar-to-bar connecting clamp is tightened and reduction maintained (Fig. 8-25).

Simple four-pin system rigidity can be increased by maximizing pin separation distance on each side of the fracture site as well as the number of pins used. In the case of a four-pin system, two pins on each limb segment with maximal pin spread, and minimizing the bone-connecting bar distance also increases stability (Fig. 8-23).[215,216] Behrens demonstrated that unilateral configurations with stiffness characteristics similar to those of the most rigid two-plane constructs are easily built using the "four-pin frame" as a basic building block (Figs. 8-23 and 8-24).[25–27] Mechanically, most effective were the "delta" plane configurations, when two simple four-pin fixators are applied at 90-degree angles to each other and connected (Fig. 8-26). However, single and double stacked bar anterior four-pin frames have the best combination of clinical and mechanical features (Fig. 8-27).

The complex delta frames allow for gradual frame removal on a rational basis to slowly transfer more load to the bone. This stepwise frame reduction leads from the most rigid unilateral constructs to frames that allow the most complete force transmission across the fracture site while still providing adequate protection against sagittal bending movements.[25–27] Studies have shown that a unilateral biplanar delta frame without transfixion pins have an overall rigidity equal to a bilateral transfixion-type device.[280]

When the connecting bar to bone distance increases, implant stability decreases. This is clinically significant when dealing with patients who present with wide areas of soft tissue compromise, which may preclude the ability to place the connecting bar close to the subcutaneous border of the bone. To counteract this, a standard four-pin fixator should be augmented by increasing the number of pins applied in each fracture segment (Fig. 8-27).[36]

FIGURE 8-24 **A:** The versatility of a monolateral frame is demonstrated. Pins can be positioned out of plane with respect to each other. **B:** A solitary connecting bar is able to connect to all pin–bar clamps. **C:** Reduction can be accomplished by manipulating each limb segment and then tightening the clamps to lock the reduction in place.

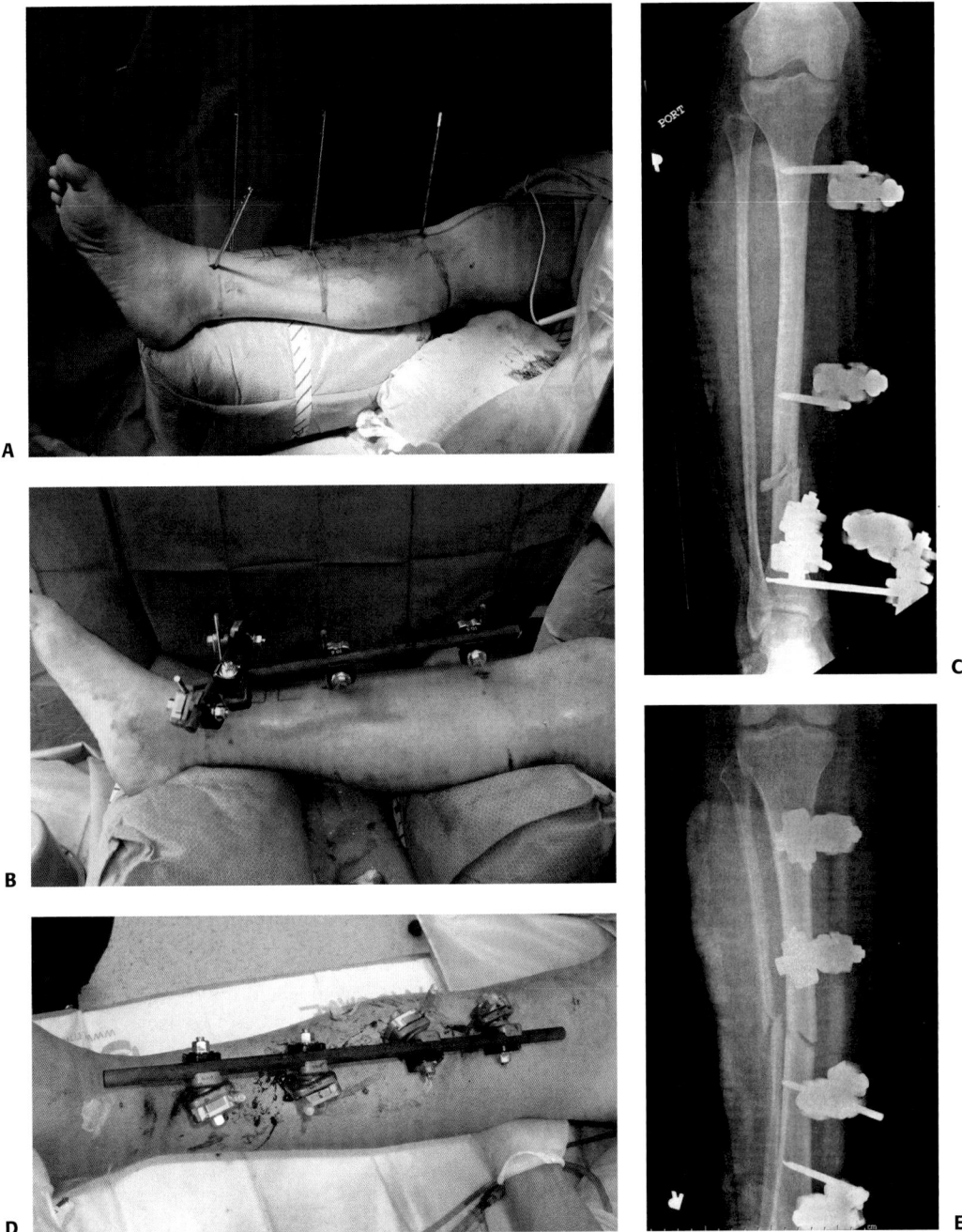

FIGURE 8-25 A: A tibia fracture is grossly reduced and two pins each placed above and below the fracture. **B:** Each two-pin segment is connected with a single bar. The reduction is fine-adjusted and the two bars are connected to each other to lock in the reduction. **C:** Final postreduction x-ray demonstrating two pins in each limb segment. **D:** Four-pin monofixator with pins out of plane to each other. **E:** Temporary reduction with four-pin frame.

The materials that the connecting bars are constructed of have a significant effect on overall frame stability. Kowalski et al.[162] demonstrated that carbon fiber bars were approximately 15% stiffer than stainless steel tubes, and that an external fixator with carbon fiber bars achieved 85% of the fixation stiffness compared with that achieved with stainless steel tubes. They felt that the loss of stiffness of the carbon fiber construct

was likely because of the clamps being less effective in connecting the carbon fiber rods to the pins.

The weakest part of the system is the junction between the fixator body and the clamp or between the fixator clamp and the Schanz pins. Insufficient holding strength on a pin by a clamp may result in a decrease in the overall fixation rigidity, as well as increased motion and cortical bone reaction at

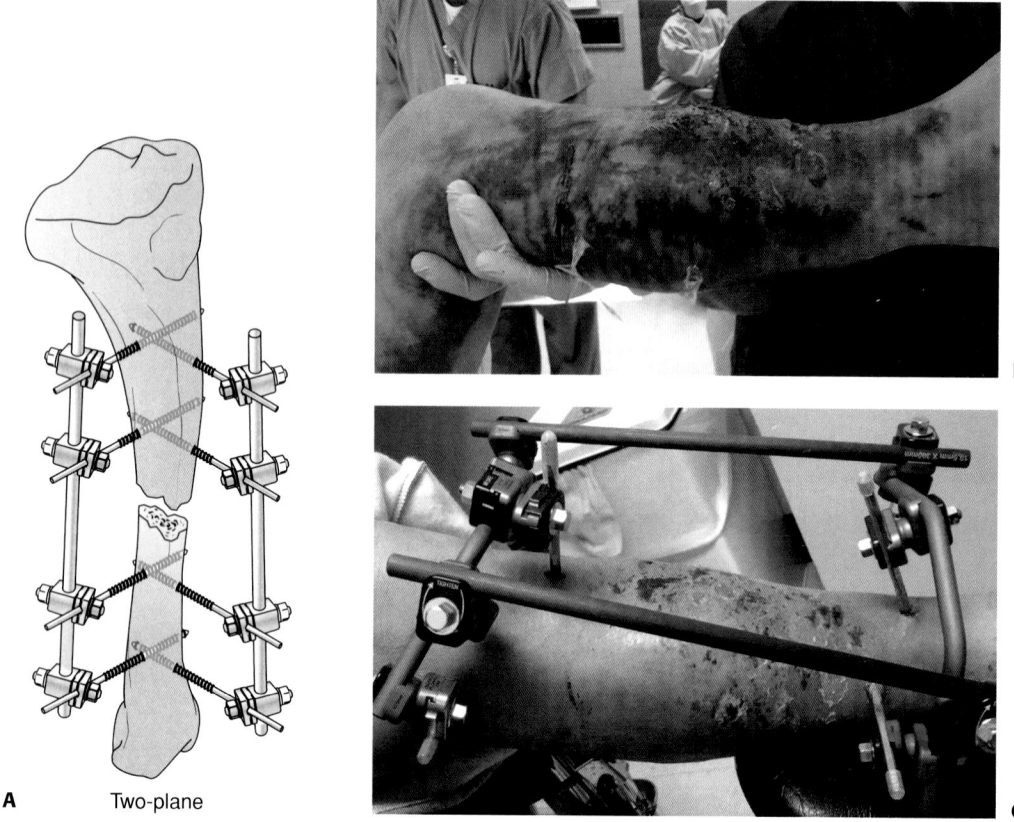

A Two-plane

FIGURE 8-26 **A:** A delta configuration is composed of two "simple" four-pin frames connected at 90 degrees to each other. **B:** Clinical examination of severe crush injury to tibia with soft tissue compromise. **C:** Fracture stabilized with modified delta configuration with two out-of-plane half pins on either side of the fracture and two connecting bars. Note soft tissue recovery afforded by the external fixator.

the pin–bone interface.[11] Cyclic loading of external fixators has been shown to loosen the tightened screws in the pin clamps. Thus, one needs to be aware of the mechanical yield characteristics of the clamps, bars, and pins throughout the course of treatment.[79]

Because of the gradual fatigue of components and loosening of pin-to-bar and bar-to-bar connections, the clinical practice of regular tightening of the device during the course of treatment should be routine.[79,126,313]

Monotube Fixators

Stability of the large monotube fixators is obtained in a distinctly different way compared with that of simpler monolateral fixators. Most monotube fixators have a fixed location for their pins mounted in pin clusters. These are connected to the body and thus the ability to vary pin location is substantially less when compared with simple monolateral fixators. Because the pin clusters are fixed at either end of the monotube body, the ability to maximize pin spread in relation to the fracture site is limited by the monotype body's length. There is little variability to lower the large monotube connection bar closer to the bone in an effort to increase stability. These frames are very stable and accomplish their inherent rigidity by having a large-

diameter monotube connecting body, which are typically three to four times the diameter of the simpler monolateral connecting bars. Because of the large body configuration, these devices offer higher bending stiffness, as well as equal torsional stiffness and variable axial stiffness when compared with standard Hoffman-Vidal quadrilateral frames with transfixion pins (Fig. 8-28).[36,51,131,145,147]

These frames have ball joints at either end connecting the large fixator bodies to their respective pin clamp configurations. There has been concern about the ability to achieve stability because of the ball locking mechanism. Chao determined that the ball joint locking cam and fixation screw clamp required periodic tightening during clinical application to prevent loss of frame stiffness under repetitive loading. However, frank clinical failure with these types of ball joint devices has not been demonstrated.[12,51,131]

In an attempt to provide the convenience of a multipin clamp, most monolateral manufacturers now provide a large clamp which can accommodate four to six Schanz pins applied directly through the clamp as a template. These clamps are then connected to the separate monolateral bars and other modular components. These frames attempt to combine the ease of pin insertion with excellent biomechanics. However, the exact

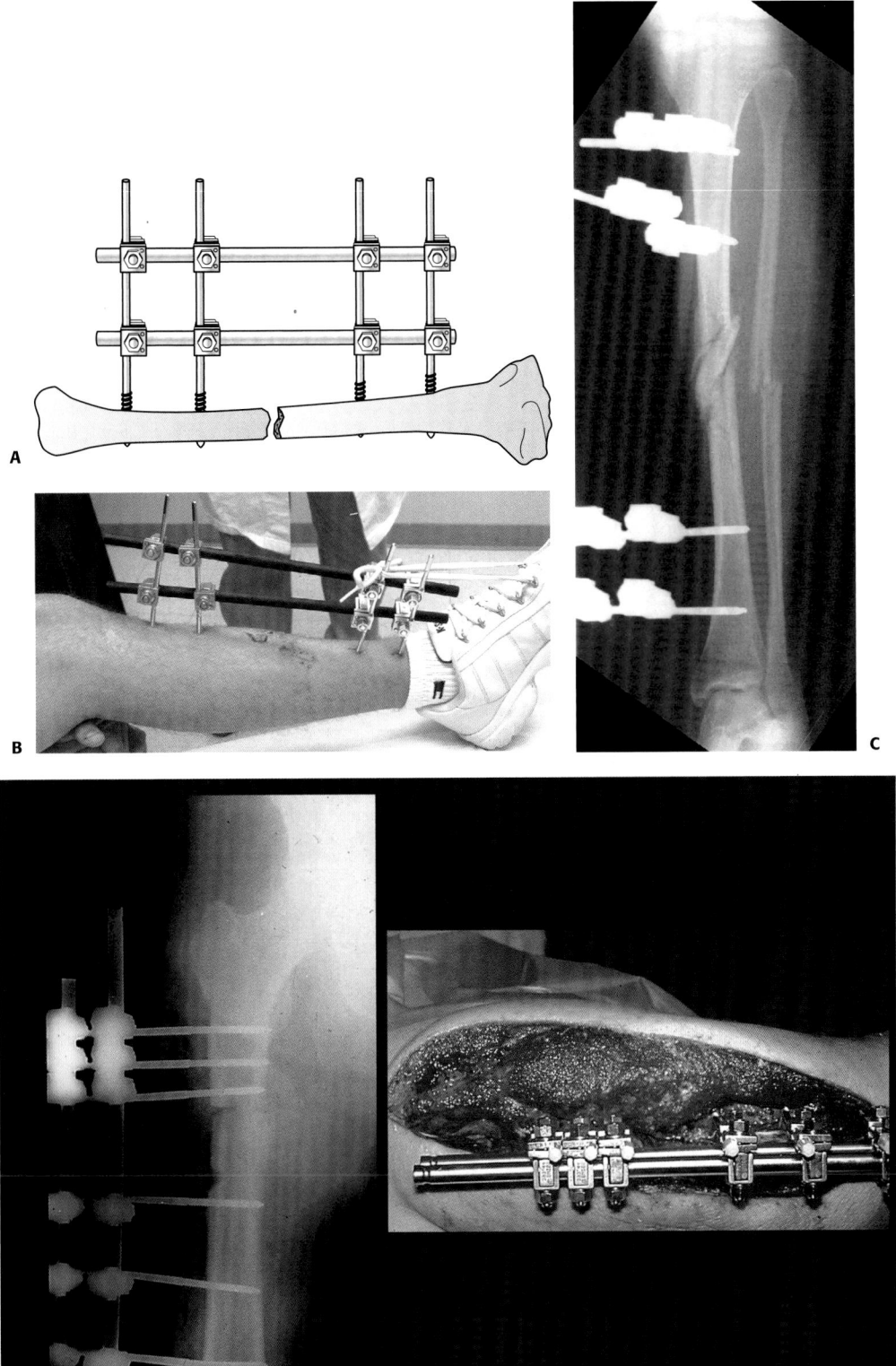

FIGURE 8-27 A: Stability of a "simple" four-pin frame can be increased by adding a second connecting bar. A "double-stacked" frame. **B:** The bone-connecting bar distance was increased to avoid soft tissue impingement on the bars. Because of the increased distance to the bone an additional connecting bar was added to increase the stability of the frame. **C:** Reduction maintained with "simple" four-pin double stack frame. Early consolidation is noted in this comminuted open fracture. **D:** Infected femur fracture with severe soft tissue injury and bone loss required additional pins (six) and a double stack frame to achieve the stability necessary to treat this injury.

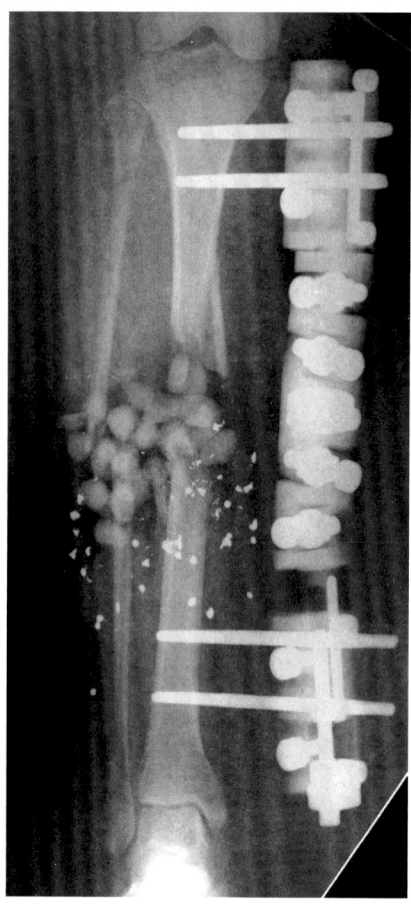

FIGURE 8-28 Large-pin "monotube" fixator. Device has fixed proximal and distal pin clamps and a large telescoping body.

mechanical performance of these frames has not been ascertained (Fig. 8-29).[219]

Insufficient holding strength on a pin within a constrained pin clamp may result in the diminution of the overall construct rigidity, as well as pin movement at the pin–bone interface. This is a distinct disadvantage compared with the single component simple monolateral frames where each pin has its own pin–bone clamp.[12] When using monotube fixators the use of six pins increased torsional rigidity, but the configuration failed at lower bending loads when compared with the four-pin configuration, reflecting the uneven holding strength of the pin clamp on three pins.[12]

Monolateral Pin Orientation and Frame Stability

The rigidity of a half-pin system is maximal in the plane of the pins and is minimal at right angles to this plane. Thus, a simple four-pin frame placed along the anterior border of the tibia will resist the anterior and posterior forces generated with normal stride, whereas this frame is weakest in mediolateral bending.[280,283,310] This demonstrates the biomechanical advantages of adding an additional two to four pins perpendicular (90 degrees) to the anterior pins (Figs. 8-25 and 8-26).

Stability is also improved when the pins are placed in a nonorthogonal position (i.e., not at 90 degrees to the long axis of the tibia).[316] If half the pins are oriented out of plane in relation to the remaining pins, this decreases the overall strength of the construct in the primary plane of the pins; however, this would be compensated for by increasing the strength of the construct in the plane at right angles.[26,27,268] Thus, overall frame rigidity would be improved.

Shear and Eagan demonstrated that a system in which the pins were placed at 60 degrees to each other offered substantial

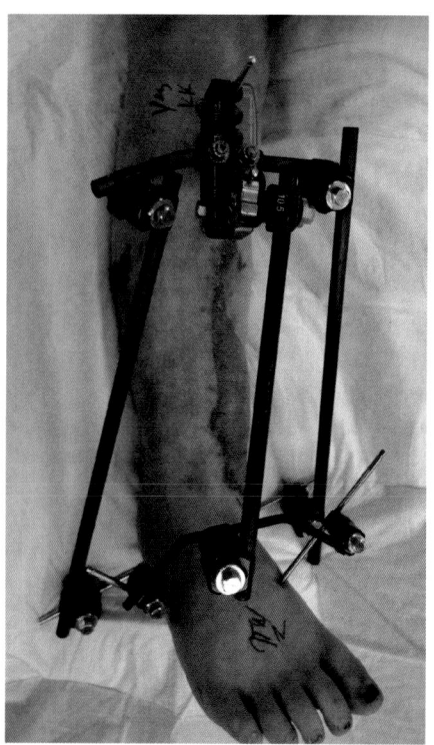
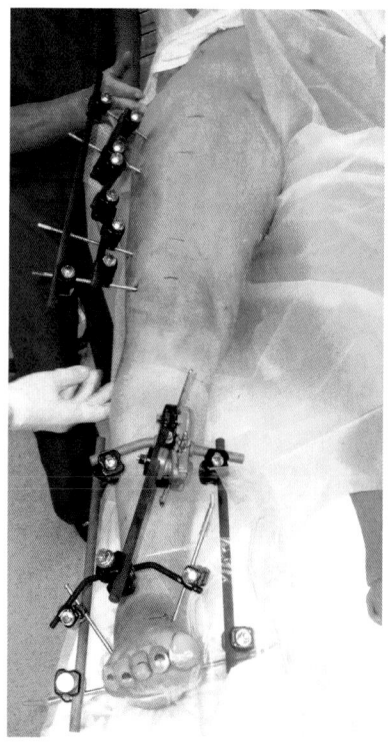

A
B

FIGURE 8-29 **A:** Monolateral ankle-spanning frame demonstrating a multipin clamp proximally, and mini fixator components at the foot. **B:** Polytrauma patient with double stack femoral frame for more stability. Ankle-spanning frame with proximal multipin clamp, mini fixator components spanning ankle and a "delta"-like configuration of connecting bars on tibial component.

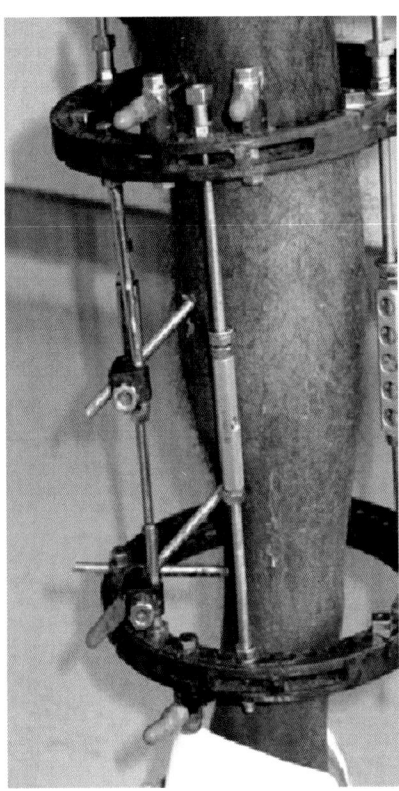

FIGURE 8-30 Frames with nonlinear pin placement neutralize forces similar to the normal forces developed in a tibia. This frame demonstrates pins out of plane to each other in the transverse and sagittal orientations. Six-millimeter HA-coated pins were utilized which gives this simple frame very stable mechanics requiring only three pins on each side of the fracture line.

advantages. This increase in torsional rigidity is maintained to 30 degrees of pin divergence angle, after which torsional stability rapidly decreases. With only a 10-degree separation between the pin angles, displacement and response to torsional stress was reduced by 97%. The effects on compressive forces are much less. When fixator pins are spread out, the fixator was 91% stronger for resisting angular displacements and torsion compared with the traditional monolateral orientation.[268] However, preferable to merely reducing rigidity in all planes is the production of a frame which more closely mimics the biomechanics of normal bone. An external fixator which allows an offset pin angle of 60 degrees demonstrates the ability to equalize forces in the sagittal and coronal planes, providing mechanical stimuli much closer to those normally encountered in the sagittal and coronal planes (Fig. 8-30).[52,198,215,216,260,268]

Many investigators are currently examining alternative pin placement as a way to achieve maximal fracture stability with relative frame simplicity.[26,27,198,280,283,310] A simplified two-ring circular frame utilizing three 6-mm half pins has been shown to increase circular frame stability compared with more complex ring constructs. The pins for these simple frames were applied at divergent angles of at least 60 degrees to the perpendicular. These divergent 6-mm half-pin frames demonstrated similar mechanical performance compared with standardized

multiple tensioned wire and 5-mm half-pin frames in terms of axial micromotion and angular deflection.[177]

A recent study evaluated the stiffness characteristics of a simple Taylor Spatial Frame (TSF) fixed with 1.8-mm transverse wires or HA-coated 6.5-mm half pins in 45-, 60-, 75-, and 90-degree divergence angles. There was an increase in axial and torsional stiffness with the increase in the divergence angle between the wires or pins ($p < 0.05$). The simple half pins provide greater stiffness to TSF frames and allowed for axial micromotion as well.[159] Thus the clinical decision making regarding the use of tensioned transverse wires in comparison to half pins when using a circular fixator can be based on soft tissue or boney constraints without fear of inferior biomechanics with half-pin frames.

Based on the available evidence, the mechanical performance of these simplified divergent half-pin frames are equivalent, if not superior, to the traditional transfixion wire frames. Surgeons can now reliably improve frame stability by simply placing pins out of plane to the long axis of the bone (Fig. 8-31).

Frame stability is most problematic when treating highly comminuted fractures or in fractures with significant fracture obliquity and increased shear stresses. Standard half pin application with pins placed perpendicular to the long axis of the bone fails to oppose the shear force vector directly, because the pins are placed oblique to the shear force vector, and thus do

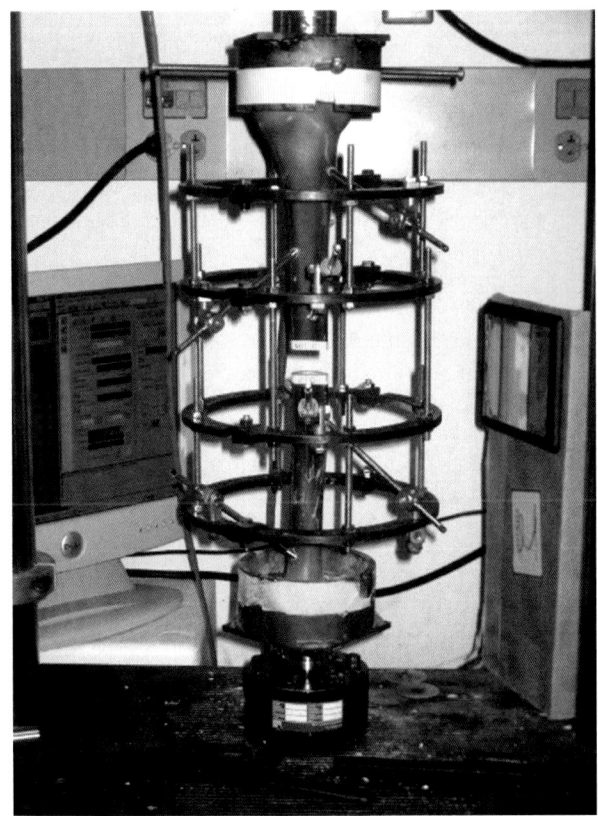

A

FIGURE 8-31 A: Oblique (out of plane) pin testing construct, which confirms oblique orientation of pins, allows for fewer pins to be used with no decrease in relative fixator stability.

(continues)

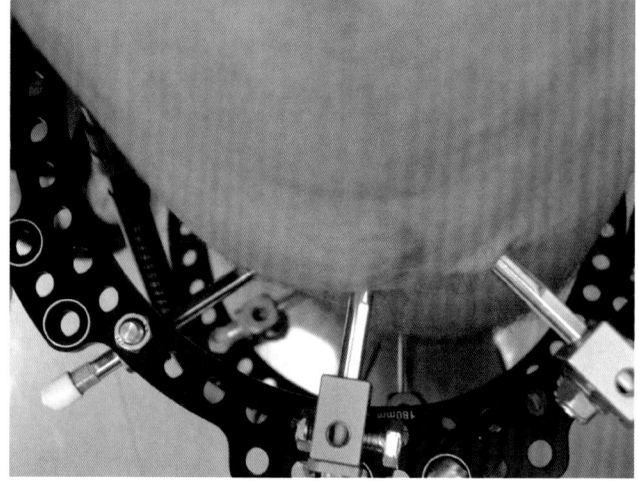

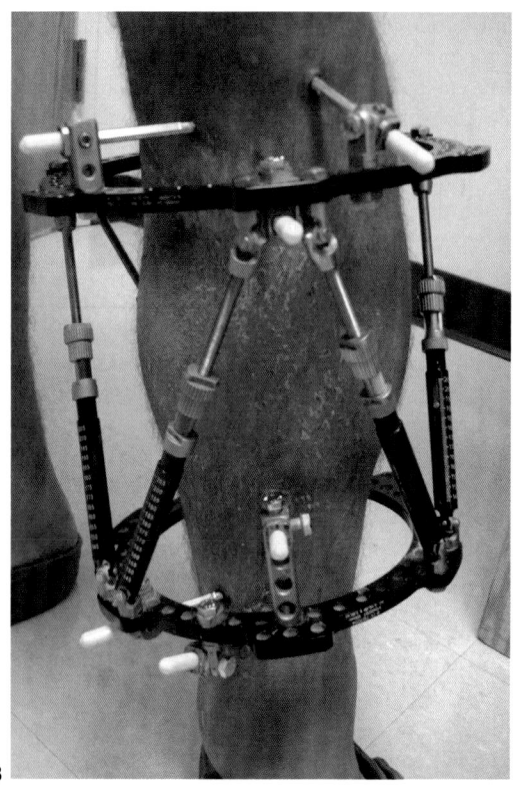

B

FIGURE 8-31 (*continued*) **B, C:** "Simple" construct with only 3- to 6-mm pins above and below the nonunion. All pins were placed out of plane to each other to affect larger pin spread and confer increased stability.

not neutralize the cantilever forces induced by this standard pin insertion angle.

When half pins are placed parallel to the fracture line, they are known as steerage pins. Steerage pins placed parallel to the fracture line are thus in direct opposition to the shear force vector. The shear force is actively converted into a dynamic compressive moment directed at to the edge of the fracture fragments. (Fig. 8-32). In this way, compression is *dependent* on axial load, and the shear phenomenon is dramatically reduced, thereby yielding nearly zero shear. For fracture obliquities less than or equal to 30 degrees, there is inherent stability such that standard modes of fixation can be utilized without undue concern.[132,185,316] However, at fracture obliquities greater than 30 degreesi nherent shear is present at the fracture ends with axial loading. Added steps should therefore be considered to help minimize this shear component, such as the application of the steerage pin concept. At fracture obliquities greater than 60 degrees, shear is a dominating force and one must be aware that even with steerage pins (pins placed parallel to the fracture lines), the forces may be extreme. Frames should be modified to perform strictly as a neutralization device as interfragmentary compression will be difficult to achieve even with the most complex devices (Fig. 8-32).[132]

An alternative method of monolateral external fixation has developed using anatomically-contoured metaphyseal locking compression plates as external fixators (Fig. 8-33). The locking plates are applied outside the soft tissue envelope following closed reduction. The plates function as external monolateral connecting bars, and the locking screws secure the bone to the external plate. The locking compression plates function well as external fixators, given their angular stable screw fixation, much

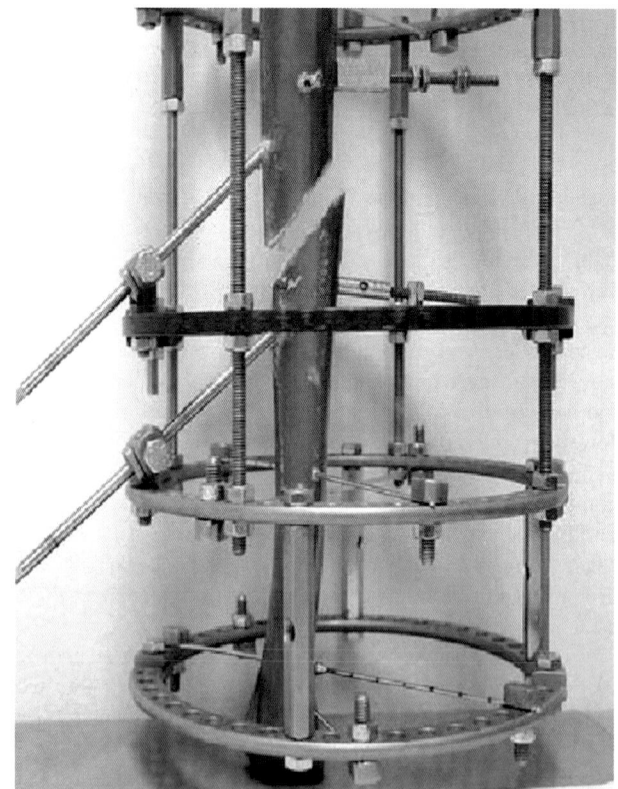

FIGURE 8-32 Steerage pin experimental set up demonstrating pins placed parallel to the major fracture line, dramatically reducing the shear forces and accentuating compressive forces with axial weight bearing. (Courtesy of David Lowenberg MD.)

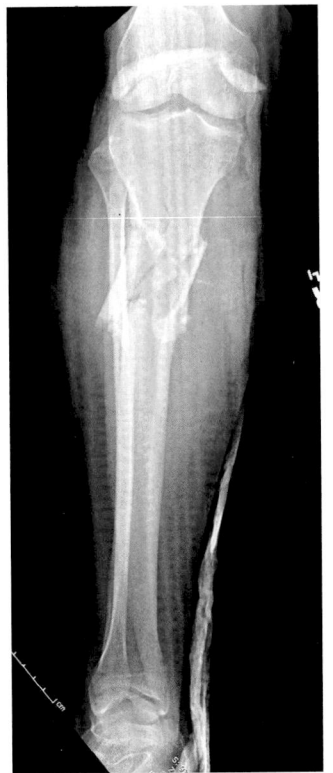
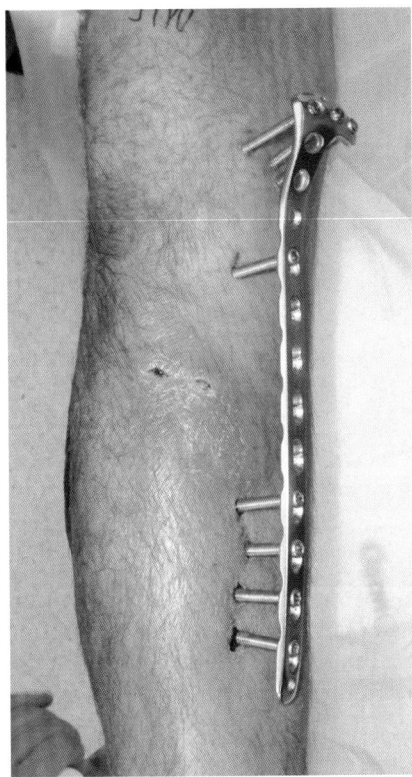
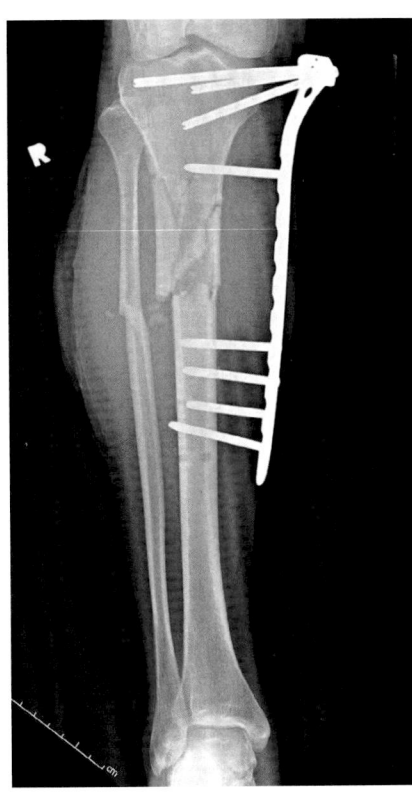

A

C, D

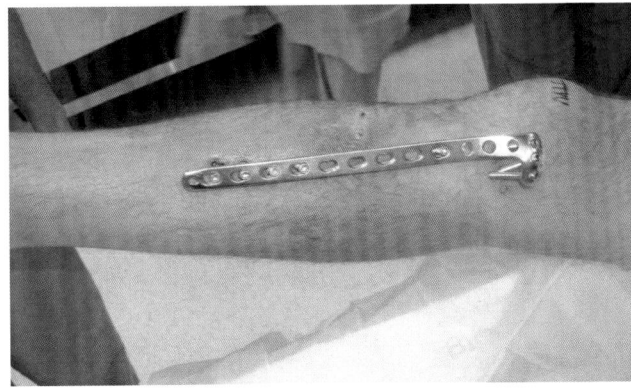

B

FIGURE 8-33 A: Comminuted, closed proximal tibial fracture with significant soft tissue concerns which precluded internal fixation. **B, C:** Use of proximal tibial locking plate as an external fixator. **D:** Plate (fixator) stabilizing comminuted fracture.

like Schanz pins, which are also locked into their connecting clamps. In a series of seven patients for acute or posttraumatic problems of the tibia ("supercutaneous plating") locking compression plate (LCP) external fixators facilitated mobilization and were more manageable and aesthetically acceptable than traditional bar-Schanz pin fixators.[160,286,312] The locking plates were applied outside the soft tissue envelope following closed reduction. The locking compression plates functioned well as external fixators, given their angular stable screw fixation.

Small Wire Circular Frame Fixation

A major advantage of a monolateral system is that it can be applied in a uniplanar fashion minimizing the transfixion of soft tissues. The ring-type systems have the disadvantage of transfixion-type wires tethering soft tissues, as the wires pass from one side of the limb to the other.[115,140] Because of the smaller

wire diameter, soft tissue trauma, bony reaction, and intolerance to the wires are minimized. Large-pin monolateral fixators rely on stiff pins for frame stability. Upon loading, these pins act as cantilevers and do produce eccentric loading characteristics. Shear forces are regarded to be inhibitory to fracture healing and bone formation, which may be accentuated with certain types of monolateral half pin stabilization, especially when the pins are aligned.[10,11,13,19,50,224,314] Circular or semicircular fixators allow for multiple planes of fixation which minimizes the harmful effects of cantilever loading and shear forces, while accentuating axial micromotion and dynamization.[94,185,194,216,233,310,311]

Components

Ring fixators are built with longitudinal connecting rods and rings to which the small-diameter tensioned wires are attached. Alternatively, the bone fragments may be attached to the rings by half pins. The connecting rods may incorporate universal joints, which give these frames their ability to produce gradual multiplanar angular and axial adjustments.

There are several component-related factors which can be manipulated to increase the stability of the ring fixation construct.

1. Increase wire diameter
2. Increase wire tension
3. Increase pin-crossing angle to approach 90 degrees
4. Decrease ring size (distance of ring to bone)
5. Increase number of wires
6. Use of olive wires/drop wires
7. Close ring position to either side of the fracture (pathology) site
8. Centering bone in the middle of the ring

Wires

Thin, smooth wires of 1.5, 1.8, and 2 mm are the most basic component used in a circular small wire fixator (Fig. 8-34A). Wire strength and stiffness increases as the square of the diameter of the wire ($S = d^2$). As these wires are tensioned, they provide increased stability. This occurs by increasing wire stiffness which simultaneously decreases the axial excursion of the wires during loading. The amount of tension in the wires directly affects the stiffness of the frame. Compression and bending resistance increases as a function of wire tension as it is gradually increased up to 130 kg. Beyond this threshold, further wire tensioning is difficult to accomplish because commercially available wire tensioning devices are unable to stop the slippage of the wire in the device as the wire is tensioned.[16,245]

Beaded wires (olive wires) perform many specialized functions. During insertion the beaded portion of the wire is juxtaposed onto the cortex. As the far side of the wire is tensioned, the bead is compressed into the near cortex. This allows olive wires to be inserted to perform interfragmentary compression, which may be useful in fracture applications (Fig. 8-35). These wires act as a source of additional transverse force to correct deformity in malunions or nonunions and provide additional support to a limb segment that a smooth wire cannot achieve.[140]

Wire Tension

During limb lengthening, tension in the wire will inherently be generated from the soft tissue forces achieved through distraction. This may generate tension in the wire up to as much as

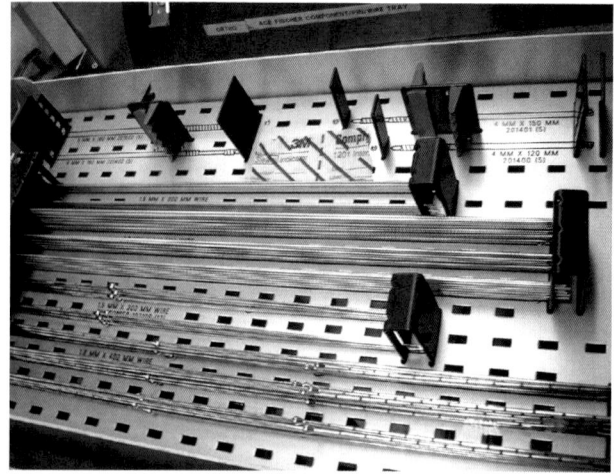
A

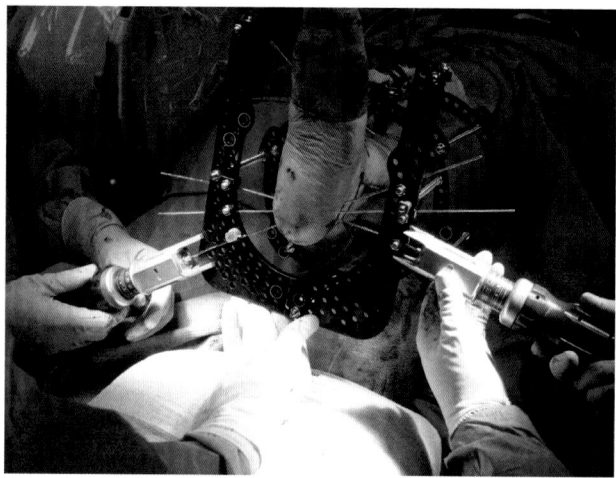
B

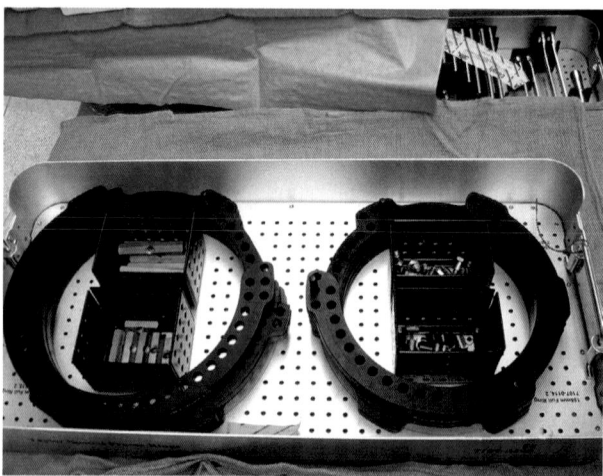
C

FIGURE 8-34 **A:** Smooth and beaded (olive) wires come in the common sizes of 1.5-, 1.8-, and 2-mm diameters. **B:** A wire tensioning device used to increase the overall rigidity of the frame construct. **C:** Multiple ring diameters are available to match the diameter of the applied extremity. Too large a ring increases the distance from bone to ring and thus makes the frame less rigid.

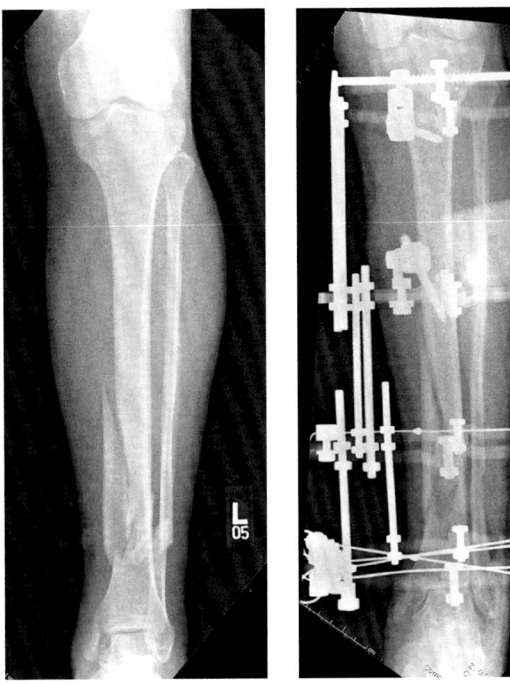

FIGURE 8-35 A: Fracture extending over distal one-third of tibia with large medial butterfly fragment is an ideal indication for a small-wire fixator. **B:** Olive wires were used as a "lag screw" to achieve additional stability of the medial butterfly fragment and distally in the metaphyseal region.

50 kg. If the patient is weight bearing, and the limb is loaded, then further wire deflection (tension) occurs. This generates additional tension in the wire. Additional rigidity of the entire construct is also demonstrated (the so called "self-stiffening effect of tensioned wires"). If the wire was initially tensioned to 130 kg and additional tension is added through lengthening and weight bearing, then the yield point of the wire may be approached with possible wire breakage occurring (Fig. 8-34B). A fracture frame is essentially a static fixator where additional wire tension will only occur through weight bearing. Thus the degree of initial wire tension should take into account the pathology being treated and the treatment forces being generated.[15,44,45,59]

Ring Diameter

The diameter of the ring also affects the stiffness of frame; as the diameter of the ring increases so does the distance of the ring to the bone, similar to the bone–bar distance described for half-pin monolateral fixators (Fig. 8-34C). Stability decreases as this distance increases. Ring diameter and wire tension have a dramatic effect on overall frame stability. As ring diameter increases, the effect of increasing wire tension on gap stiffness and gap displacement is also decreased. Decreased ring diameter has a greater affect on all variables compared with simply increasing wire tension. Although the effect of wire tension decreases as ring diameter increases, tensioning wires on frames with larger ring constructs is important because these constructs are inherently less stiff because of longer wires.[15,42,44,45,59]

Wire Orientation

Wires placed parallel to each other, and parallel to the applied forces, provide little resistance to deformation. The bone can slide along this axis much like a central axle in a wheel. In bending stresses, the frames are much less rigid because of bowing of the transverse wires and slippage of the bone along these wires. The most stable configuration occurs when two wires intersect at 90 degrees. The bending stiffness in the plane of the wire is decreased by a factor of two as the angles between the wires converge from 90 to 45 degrees (Fig. 8-36). Therefore, changing pin orientation to a less acute angle decreases the stiffness in anterior posterior (AP) bending, but has a lesser effect on lateral bending, torsion, and axial compression.[44,45,97,218]

Clinically, a wire divergence angle of at least 60 degrees should be attempted. Because this is not always possible because of anatomic constraints of passing transfixion wires, the use of olive wires or the addition of a wire at a distance from the primary ring (drop wires) significantly improves bending stiffness. The use of olive wires placed at the same level but from opposite directions improves resistance to shear forces by "locking" in the segment (Fig. 8-35).[44,45,97,119,140,233,300,301,305]

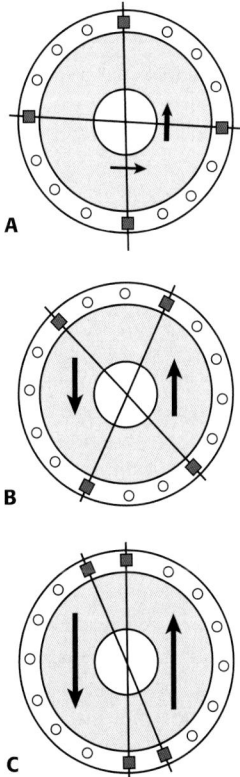

FIGURE 8-36 A: Wire-crossing angle of 90 degrees provides the most stable configuration with small mediolateral translations and a rigid frame. **B:** A wire convergence angle of 45 to 60 degrees allows acceptable amounts of translations to occur with satisfactory frame stability. **C:** As the convergence angle decreases, the translation increases dramatically to the point where the bone slides along a single axis. Parallel wires produce a grossly unstable frame configuration.

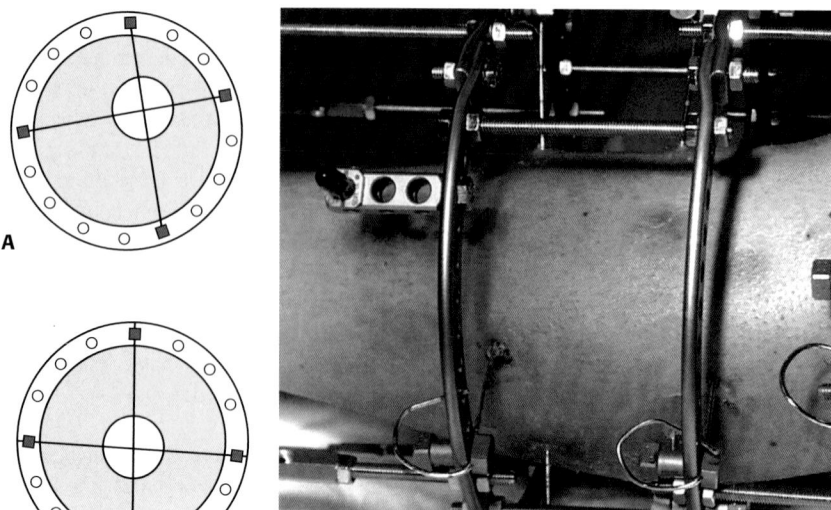

FIGURE 8-37 **A:** Eccentric bone location in the ring, simulating a tibial mounting. **B:** Center/center location of bone in the ring mounting simulating a femoral or humeral mounting. **C:** Central position of tibia in too small of a ring, results in posterior soft tissue impingement. A larger ring should have been used to center the bone within the ring and avoid soft tissue concerns.

Limb Positioning in the Ring

The location of the tibial bone in the limb is actually eccentric in nature compared with the humerus or the femur. This is important when placing the rings around the particular extremity. The center of the ring applied may not be located over the actual center of the bone. It may be positioned eccentrically with respect to the ring, affecting the overall stiffness of the frame. If the bone is located off center, this position provides greater stiffness to loading in axial compression, compared with a construct where the center of the ring is positioned exactly over the center of the bone. This center/center configuration demonstrates lowered axial stiffness at the fracture site during axial loading.[15,42,44,45,47,86,218] Clinically, since tibial frames are most common, this is usually not an issue because the bone is routinely eccentric in the ring as long as the ring is centered on the leg itself. The eccentric location of the muscular compartments ensures this offset bone position. To place a frame on a tibia with the center/center orientation, a very large ring would be needed. This would vastly increase the ring–bone distance and further decrease the frame stiffness (Fig. 8-37).

A typical three- or four-ring frame consists of eight crossed wires, two wires at each level and four rings with supporting struts connecting two rings on either side of the fracture (Fig. 8-12). When this circular frame was tested against the standard Hoffman-Vidal quadrilateral transfixion frame, the circular type frame was noted to be stiffer in compression. However, the circular fixators are less rigid than all other monolateral-type fixators in all modes of loading, most particularly in axial compression.[15,45,59] This may be clinically beneficial to allow for axial micromotion and facilitate secondary bone healing.[80] The Ilizarov fixator allowed significantly more axial motion at the fracture site during axial compression than the other fixators tested; however, the device controlled shear at the fracture site as well as other half-pin frames.[80,147] The overall stiffness and shear rigidity of the Ilizarov external fixator are similar to those of the half-pin fixators in bending and torsion.[95,140,158,194,233,258,311]

Wire Connecting Bolts

Mechanical slippage between wire and fixation bolt is the primary reason for loss of wire tension and thus frame instability. The change in wire stiffness can be explained mainly as a result of wire slippage, but plastic deformation and material yielding also contribute.[108] Studies demonstrate that when clamping a wire to the frame, the wire tension is reduced by approximately 7%.[260] This may be because of wire deformation by the bolts and as such can reduce wire tension during fixator assembly.[306,307] Slippage can be avoided by adequate torque on the fixation bolt, that is, greater than 20 N m. Material yield accompanied by some wire slippage through the clamps is responsible for the decreased tension at the pin–clamp interface (Fig. 8-38). The relatively simple modification made by roughening the wire–bolt interface resulted in improved holding capacity and wire stiffness and these fixation devices are

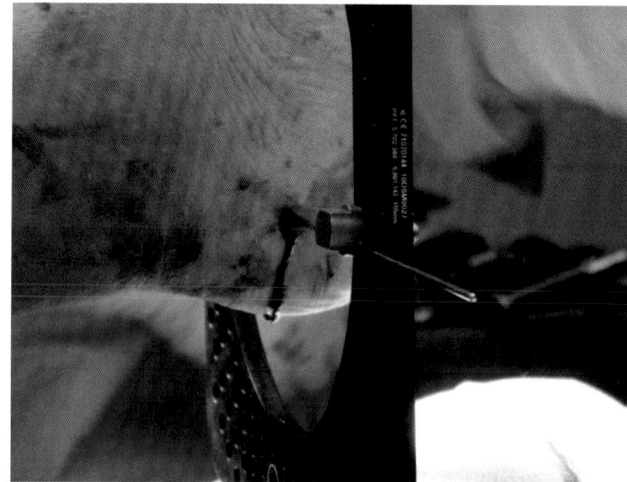

FIGURE 8-38 Wire fixation bolt that captures the wire and prevents "slippage" after tensioning has taken place.

FIGURE 8-39 "Hybrid" frame demonstrating mechanical instability with only two periarticular tensioned wires on the distal ring and two small monolateral bars connecting two diaphyseal half pins located at an extreme distance from the fracture. This unstable fixation resulted in fracture nonunion.

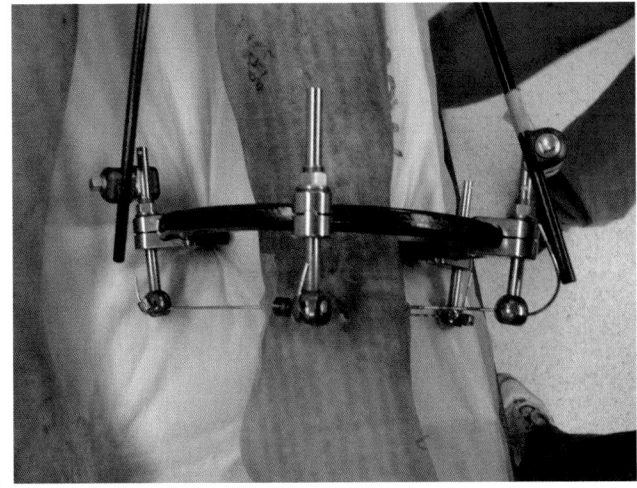

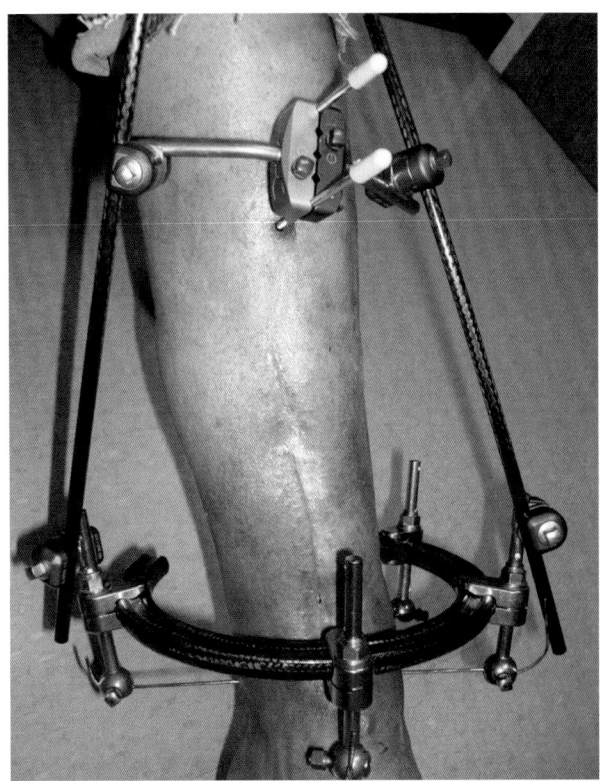

A   **B**

now clinically available.[108] Although the initial wire tension has an appreciable effect on the wire stiffness, it does not affect the elastic load range of the clamp wire system. To prevent yield of the clamp wire system in clinical practice, the fixator should be assembled with sufficient wires to ensure that the load transmitted to each wire by the patient does not exceed 15 N.[313] Adding additional wires will increase the frame stiffness directly proportional to the number of wires in the system. Stiffness of an Ilizarov frame is more dependent on bone preload than on wire number, wire type, or frame design. Preload stiffness can be increased simply by compressing the rings together and achieving bone-on-bone contact.[15,16,42,44,47,97]

Hybrid Fixators

Because of the complexity in the assembly of a full circular ring fixator, hybrid configurations were developed to take advantage of tensioned wires' ability to stabilize complex periarticular fractures. Early designs married a periarticular ring using few tensioned wires to a monolateral bar connected to the shaft using two to three half pins. Unfortunately, these simple frames were shown to be mechanically inferior in their abilities to resist cantilever loading with resultant malunion/nonunion (Fig. 8-13B).[158,236,237,246,301] Mechanical instability was especially pronounced when the frames were applied with specific errors in technique: (1) Insertion of only two transfixion wires in periarticular locations. Because of anatomic constrains the wires cannot be placed at 90 degrees to each other in most periarticular locations. As noted previously, if the two wires are not at 90 degrees then the bone can translate easily along the two wires. (2) Half pins placed too far from the site of pathology

placing significant strain on the connecting clamps to maintain frame stability (Fig. 8-39).

The term "hybrid" when applied to external fixation denotes the use of half pins and wires in the same frame mounting as well as using a combination of rings and monolateral connecting bars. Stable hybrid frames should include a ring incorporating multiple levels of fixation in the periarticular fragment. This is accomplished with a minimum of three tensioned wires and if possible, an additional level of periarticular fixation using adjunctive half pins.[5,6,15,38,158]

The use of a single bar connecting the shaft to the periarticular ring places significant stresses on the single connecting clamp and accentuates the harmful off-axis forces generated with weight bearing. Multiple connecting bars or a full circular frame is preferred with a minimum of four half pins attached to the shaft component.[5,6,42,236,237,246,311]

BIOLOGY OF EXTERNAL FIXATION AND DISTRACTION HISTOGENESIS

Basic Biology

The fracture repair process proceeds through constant physiologic stages depending on external forces imparted to the fracture site. There are four distinct types of fracture healing which have been identified. External fixation facilitates external bridging callous.

External bridging callous is largely under the control of mechanical and biologic factors and is highly dependent upon the integrity of the surrounding soft tissue envelope. The critical cells necessary for healing are derived from the surrounding soft tissues and from the revascularization response that occurs during the inflammatory phase of fracture healing.[39,138,139] This type of fracture healing has the ability to bridge large gaps and is very tolerant of movement. It results in the development of a large callous with the formation of cartilage because of the greater inflammatory response caused by increased micromovement of the fragments.[155,174] Migrating mesenchymal cells from the surrounding area reach the fracture ends where they differentiate into various cell types, primarily cartilage. The cartilage is formed in the well-vascularized granulation tissue because of its ability to repel vessels. These early cartilaginous elements undergo remodeling through endochondral bone formation. It is well known that this type of indirect bone healing occurs with less rigid interfragmentary stabilization.[154–156] The rate of this type of healing and the extent of callous in this type of repair can be modulated by mechanical conditions at the fracture site.[183] It has been shown that applying cyclic interfragmentary micromotion for short periods of time influences the repair process and leads to a larger area of callous formation compared with those fractures that are rigidly fixed.[10,11,56,80,110,111,123,147,154–156,224,230] Alternatively, efforts to reduce micromotion by increasing frame stiffness can cause a significant reduction in the rate of healing.[21,50,310,314]

Larger interfragmentary movements lead to more fibrocartilage, as well as an increase in the number of blood vessels.[56,292] However, as the amount of fibrocartilages increases, the ability for remodeling and bone formation is simultaneously decreased. There appears to be some threshold at which the degree of micromotion becomes inhibitory to the remodeling process and thus hypertrophic nonunion can result. It should be noted, however, that fractures requiring external fixation in general are usually more complex, which may result in an intrinsically higher rate of nonunion. Healing problems encountered in these severe injuries may reflect the severity of the local soft tissue and periosteal injury, and should not be attributed solely to the inherent features of the external fixation device.

Bony healing is not complete until remodeling of the fracture has been achieved. At this stage, the visible fracture lines in the callous decrease and subsequently disappear. The bone transmits mechanical forces to the encapsulating callous as the tissue differentiates from granulation tissue to collagen and hyaline cartilage, and then to woven intramedullary bone through the process of endochondral bone formation.[140,293]

Dynamization

Dynamization converts a static fixator which neutralizes all forces including axial motion to a construct that allows the passage of controlled forces across the fracture site. As the elasticity of the callous decreases, bone stiffness and strength increase and larger loads can be supported. Thus the advantages of axial dynamization help to restore cortical contact and produce a stable fracture pattern with inherent mechanical support. Aro described a uniform distribution of callous following dynamization and noted this as "secondary contact healing."[11,13] By increasing cortical contact, dynamization attempts to decrease the translational shear forces.[10,11,13] Shear forces are thought to

be the leading factor in producing a predominance of fibrous tissue at the fracture site with resultant delayed or nonunion.[19,26,42,52]

Frames are distinguished between static and dynamic fixators. Active dynamization occurs with weight bearing or with loading when there is progressive closure of the fracture gap. This usually occurs by making adjustments in the pin bar clamps with simple monolateral fixators. This is accomplished by loosening the clamp portion that attaches to the bar which then allows the bar to slide within the clamp. The pin portion is still tight and thus the fracture can "slide" and compress or dynamize, whereas the alignment is maintained by the pin portion still remaining securely attached. For large monotube fixators the telescoping body can be released and the tow portions allowed to compress across the fracture. Dynamization also decreases the pin–bone stresses and prolongs the lifetime of the frame.[147,154,192]

There is a race between the gradually increasing load-carrying capacity of the healing bone and failure of the pin–bone interface. In unstable fractures, very high stresses can occur at the pin–bone interface which may create localized yielding failure. In half-pin frames these high stresses are generated primarily at the entry cortex and stress-related pin–bone failures occur mainly in this location.[231] It is well accepted that the relative motion of the bone ends at the fracture site is a very important parameter in the healing of the fracture; however, the threshold at which this motion becomes deleterious is as yet unknown.[60,140]

Fracture Healing with Limited ORIF Combined with External Fixation

On occasion, it is advantageous to perform limited internal fixation in combination with an external fixator. Whereas this type of methodology is very useful in metaphyseal bone and has been demonstrated to work well in periarticular fractures, its use in diaphyseal regions must be questioned. The use of interfragmentary screws seeks to achieve direct bone healing through the use of constant compression. Primary cortical healing occurs only when mechanical immobilization is absolute and bony apposition is perfect. It is very intolerant of movement and is not dependent upon soft tissues. This type of healing is very slow and has no ability to cross gaps, as opposed to external bridging callous.[127,154] In many ways, it represents bone healing through gradual remodeling. Primary cortical healing is characterized by sequential cutting cones of osteoclasts crossing across the fracture line with subsequent re-establishment of new osteons. The vasculature develops from a budding process sprouting from the intramedullary blood vessels, which are very fragile and intolerant of motion. The external fixator does not entirely eliminate extraneous forces, but seeks to limit the degree of micromotion.[56,127,132,140,147,154,292] Therefore, because the bone is rigidly fixed with lag screws, very poor bridging callous develops. Because external fixators do not produce absolute rigidity, insufficient cortical healing occurs, demonstrating the worst of both biologic entities.[224] This technique has been abandoned for use in diaphyseal regions because of the increased incidence of pseudoarthrosis. A combination of internal and external fixation for diaphyseal fractures may at first appear to be desirable, but is in fact often disastrous and should be avoided.[274]

Biology of Distraction Osteogenesis

Distraction osteogenesis is the mechanical induction of new bone that occurs between bony surfaces that are gradually pulled apart. Ilizarov described this as "the tension stress effect."[138–140] Osteogenesis in the gap of a distracted bone takes place by the formation of a physis-like structure. New bone forms in parallel columns extending in both directions from a central growth region known as the *interzone* (Fig. 8-40A). Recruitment of the tissue-forming cells for the interzone originates in the periosteum.[15,16,140] Under the influence of tension stress, fibroblast-like cells found in the middle of the growth zone develop an elongated shape and are orientated along the tension stress vector during distraction. Surrounding the fibroblast-like cells are collagen fibers aligning parallel to the direction of the tension vector. The fibroblastic cells transform into osteoblasts which deposit osteoid tissue upon these collagen fibers. They further differentiate to become osteocytes within the bone matrix laid down upon the longitudinal collagen bundles. These cells will become incorporated into their own HA matrix as the collagen bundles are consolidated into bone. This tissue gradually blends into the newly formed bone trabeculae in the regions farthest away from the central interzone. Thus, newly formed bone grows both proximally and distally away from the middle of the distraction zone during elongation. These columns of

bone will eventually cross the fibrous interzone to bridge the osteogenic surfaces following distraction (Fig. 8-40B).[138–140]

With stable fixation, osteogenesis in the distraction zone proceeds by direct intramembranous ossification omitting the cartilaginous phase characteristic of endochondral ossification. Distraction osteogenesis also provides a significant neovascularization effect. The fibroblast precursors are concentrated around sinusoidal capillaries. The growth of these newly formed capillaries under the influence of tension stress proceeds very rapidly and in some instances overgrows development of bony distraction resulting in enfolding of this tremendous capillary response. This dense network of newly formed blood cells has a longitudinal orientation connecting to the surrounding soft tissue vessels by numerous arteries that perforate the regenerate bone. Thus the regenerate distraction gap is very vascular, with large vascular channels that surround each longitudinal column of distracted collagen. Neovascularization extends from each bone end surface toward the central fibrous interzone. This intense formation of new blood vessels under the influence of tension stress occurs not only in the bone, but also in the soft tissues. These vessels contain a thin lining of endothelial cells very similar to the neovascular response that occurs in a centripetal fashion during routine fracture healing (Fig. 8-40B).

The rate and rhythm of distraction are crucial in achieving viable tissue following distraction histogenesis. Histologic and biochemical studies have determined that a distraction rate of 0.5 mm per day or less leads to premature consolidation of the lengthening bone, whereas a distraction rate of 2 mm or greater

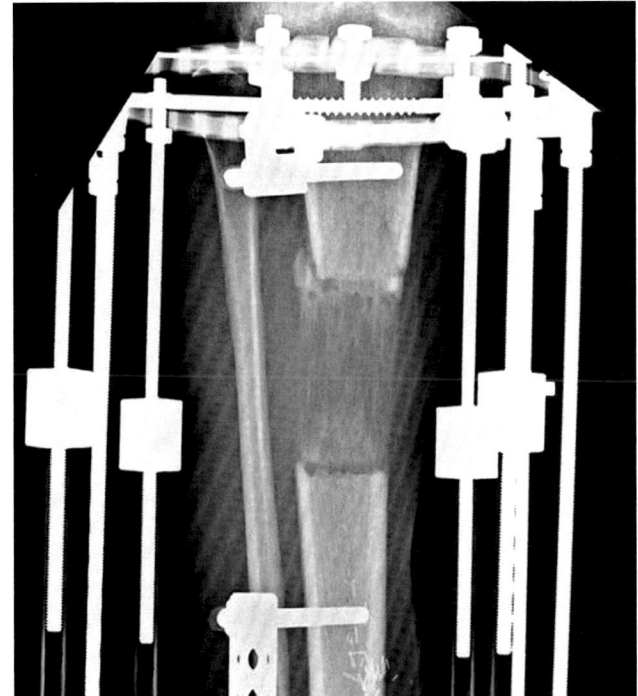
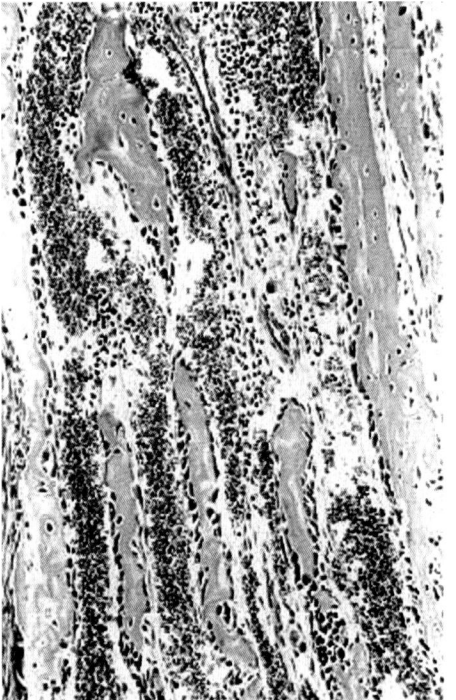

FIGURE 8-40 A: The interzone (dark "z" area midregenerate) is the central growth region involved in the genesis of new bone formation during distraction. **B:** Collagen fibrils line up along the vector of distraction. Osteoblasts line the collagen bundles forming new bone. There are large vascular channels surrounding each collagen bundle.

often results in undesirable changes within the distracted tissues. Faster rates of distraction will disrupt the small vascular channels and areas of cysts can occur inhibiting mineralization.[15,16,138–140] For osteogenesis to proceed more rapidly, optimum preservation of the periosteal tissues, bone marrow, and surrounding soft tissue blood supply at the time of osteotomy is mandatory.[140,299] The new bone and soft tissues are formed parallel to the tension vector even when the vector is perpendicular to the limb's overall mechanical axis.

Studies have documented that superior bone regenerate is formed when a very low energy osteoclasis technique is utilized to produce a corticotomy. This is achieved by osteotomizing the anterior, anterior lateral, and anterior medial cortices, and then performing a closed osteoclasis maneuver to the posterior cortex preserving the periosteal tissues as much as possible.[164] Ilizarov recommended a rate of 1-mm total distraction (*rate of distraction*) per day. The actual number of distractions (*rhythm of distraction*) should be at least four each day, achieving the total daily distraction in four divided doses. His work has also demonstrated that constant distraction over a 24-hour period produces a significant increase in the regenerate quality as compared to other variables.[138–140]

In this setting, when motion is present at the fracture site, bone resorption always occurs. The greater the interfragmentary motion at the site of the fracture, the greater the resorption of the fragment and slower the consolidation. The healing process depends on arterial revascularization and if the fracture fragments are excessively mobile, the local blood supply is traumatized by the moving bone ends.[56,212,292] Instability that introduces translational shear across the distraction gap will result in an atrophic fibrous nonunion with mixed cartilage and incomplete vascular channels, interspersed within the longitudinal collagen columns. In these areas of mechanical instability, intramembranous ossification is irregular with islands of endochondral ossification seen and if local vascularity is insufficient, mineralization will be inhibited leaving necrotic fibrous areas or vascular cysts.

Circular frames are able to limit the magnitude of abnormal forces when they are placed in compression.[15,16,80,158] This stabilizes the small blood vessels and allows for neutralization of the forces that are destructive to the neovascular region.[15,16] This allows endochondral bone remodeling to proceed.

Compression osteosynthesis with constant compression on the bone does not suppress the reparative process and does not cause damage or resorption of the bone tissues. Under conditions of both compression and distraction in the presence of stable fixation, bone is actively formed by cellular elements of the endosteum, bone marrow, and periosteum. The osteogenic activity of connective tissue is stimulated by tension stress when the tissue is stabilized. Soon after the end of distraction, the connective tissue is replaced by bone. Therefore compression or dynamization can facilitate healing of delayed or nonunions under this mechanical environment. Increase in axial loading is accompanied by enhanced blood supply that activates osteogenesis.[138–140,292] Many authors have demonstrated the positive benefit that axial loading combined with muscular activity has on new bone formation.[154–156,174]

As noted by Ilizarov, all tissues will respond to a slow application of prolonged tension with metaplasia and the differentiation into the corresponding tissue type. Bone responds best followed by muscle, ligament, and tendons in that order. Neurovascular structures will respond with gradual new vessels and some degree of nerve and vessel lengthening. However, they respond very slowly and are intolerant of acute distraction forces.[138–140,179]

Muscle growth results from the tension stress effect by increasing the number of myofibrils in pre-existing muscle. Muscle also responds by the formation of new muscle tissue through the increased numbers of muscle satellite cells, the appearance of myoblasts, and their fusion into myotubes. Within the newly formed muscle fibers active formation of myofibrils and sarcomeres also occurs.[138–140] Smooth muscle tissue and blood vessels walls are also stimulated by tension stress. Smooth muscle activity and proliferation are accompanied by an increase in the extent and number of intercellular contacts between myocytes and by the formation of new elastic structures. These morphologic changes in the ultra structure of arterial smooth wall muscle cells resemble the changes seen in the walls of arteries elongated during active prenatal and early postnatal growth.[138–140]

A similar response also occurs in the connective tissue of fascia, tendons, and dermis. The number of fibroblasts is increased during distraction and an increase in the density of intracellular junctions is multiplied, which is characteristic of fibroblasts in the developing connective tissue of embryos, fetuses, and newborn animals. The adventitial blood vessels in the epineurium and perineurium of major nerve trunks also undergo similar changes.[138–140]

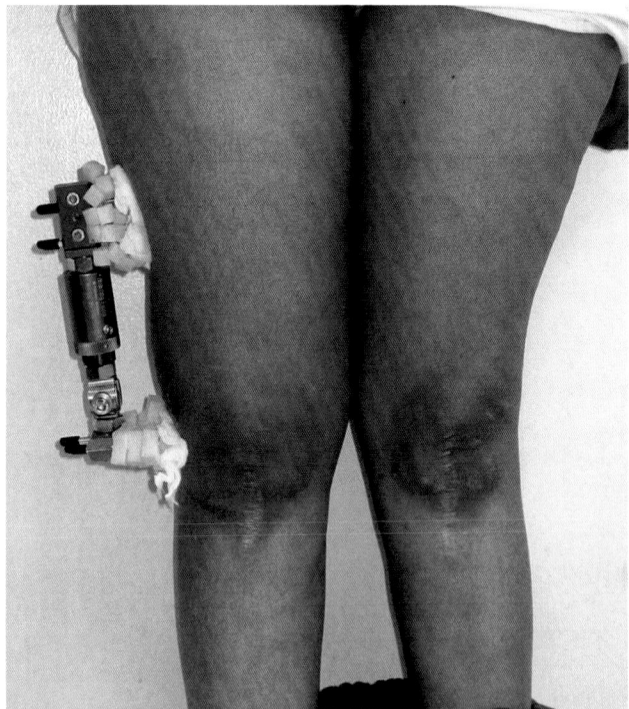

FIGURE 8-41 Monotube device used to correct valgus deformity of the right knee (compare with left knee). This is accomplished via gradual distraction across a distal femoral corticotomy.

Distraction, accomplished through the use of a ring fixator, or a stable monotube device, initiates the histogenesis of bone, muscle, nerves, and skin.[15,16,138–140,180] This facilitates the treatment of complex orthopedic diseases, including pathologic conditions such as osteomyelitis and fibrous dysplasia. Other conditions that have been historically refractory to standard treatments such as congenital pseudoarthrosis and severe hemimelias can also be addressed.[61,64,140,150,196,211,253,275,281]

Bone transport methodologies can replace large skeletal defects with normal healthy bone structure, which is well vascularized and is relatively impervious to stress fractures. The ability to correct significant angular, translational, and axial deformities simultaneously through relative percutaneous techniques, as well as perform these corrections in an ambulatory outpatient setting adds to the attractiveness of this methodology (Figs. 8-41 and 8-42).[55,81,118,119,140,148,187,220,257,258,285,295,298–300,302]

CONTEMPORARY EXTERNAL FIXATOR APPLICATIONS

Traditionally, external fixation has been used primarily for trauma applications, including the treatment of open fractures and closed fractures with high-grade soft tissue injury or compartment syndrome. In addition, external fixation has been used in critically ill patients with multiple long bone fractures as a method for temporary stabilization of these injuries.

Following the adoption of circular and hybrid techniques, indications have been expanded to include the definitive treatment of complex periarticular injuries which include high-energy tibial plateau and distal tibial pilon fractures. With the introduction of minimally invasive techniques, combined with locking plate technologies, the indications for use of circular fixation for the definitive fixation of periarticular fractures have narrowed. Circular fixator use in periarticular injuries is largely

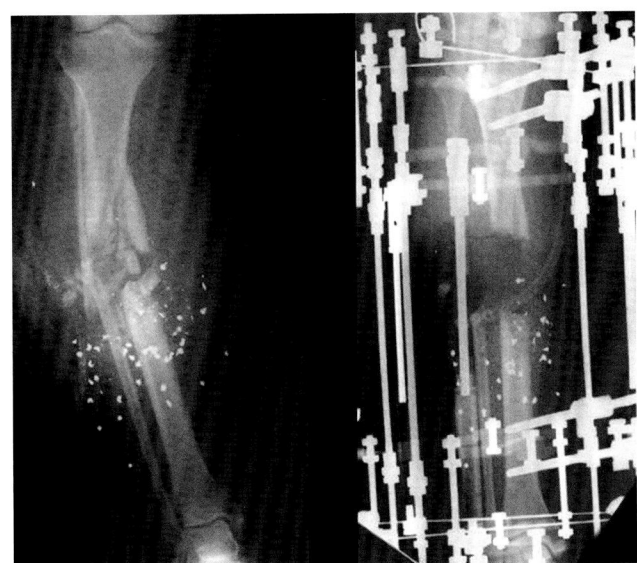

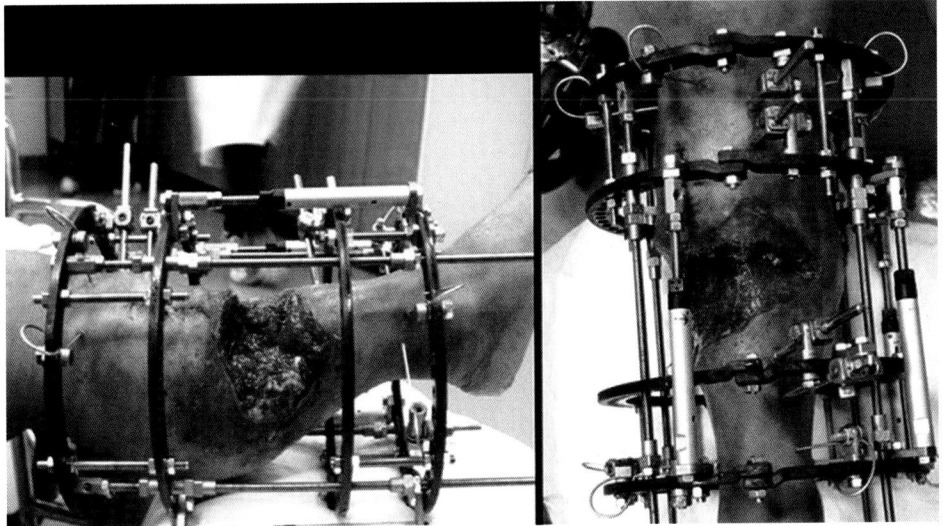

FIGURE 8-42 **A:** Severe bone and soft tissue loss stabilized with a ring fixator. **B:** Gradual compression across defect gradually closes down the defect via soft tissue transport. (*continues*)

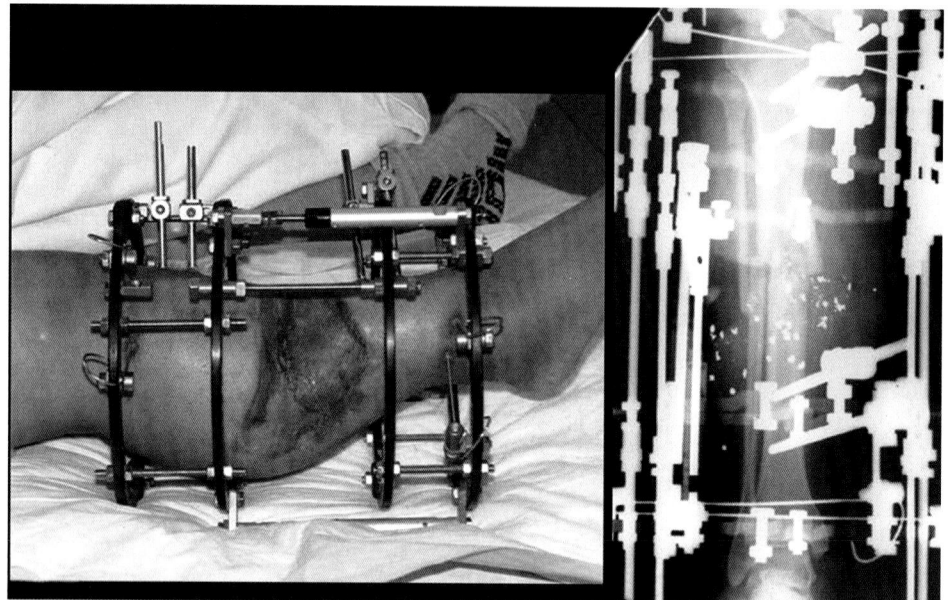

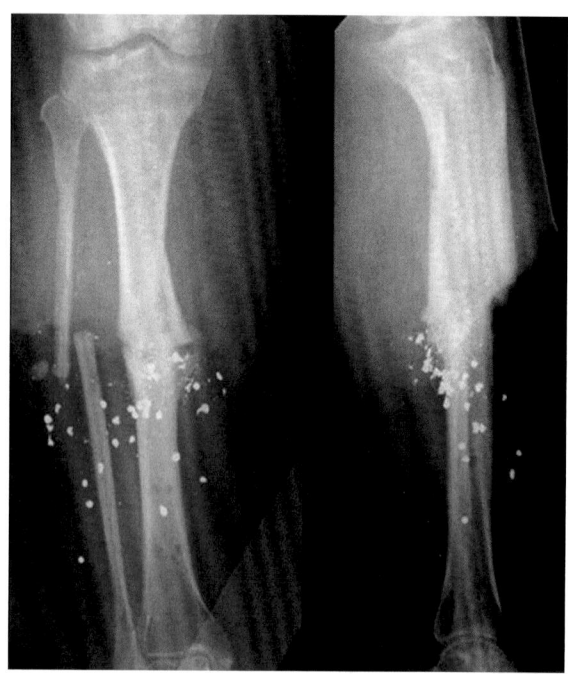

FIGURE 8-42 (*continued*) **C:** Skin grafting was performed over reconstructed soft tissues, once docking of the bone ends had been completed. **D:** Healed tibia later underwent limb lengthening.

restricted to the most severe fractures patterns with extensive comminution, bone loss, or critical soft tissue injury.

Given the mechanical and biologic advantages of external fixation, their use in reconstructive orthopedics has gained wider acceptance and is currently used for limb lengthening, osteotomy, fusion, and deformity correction, as well as bone transport for the reconstruction of bone defects.[37,119,170,221,246,298,300]

Damage Control External Fixation

The concept of temporary spanning fixation for complex articular injuries has become widely accepted. The ability to achieve an initial ligamentotaxis reduction substantially decreases the amount of injury-related swelling and edema by reducing deformity. It is important to achieve an early reduction, as a delay for more than a few days will result in an inability to disimpact displaced metaphyseal fragments. When definitive stabilization is attempted, reduction will be more difficult by indirect means and may require larger or more extensile types of incisions.[227,270,294,296,302,303] With temporary fixation in place, the patient is then able to have other procedures or tests performed while effective distraction is maintained and the soft tissues are put to rest (Fig. 8-43).

Many types of temporary "traveling traction" have been described. Most commonly used are the knee- or ankle-bridging constructs. This may be a simple quadrilateral frame, constructed by applying medial and lateral radiolucent external bars

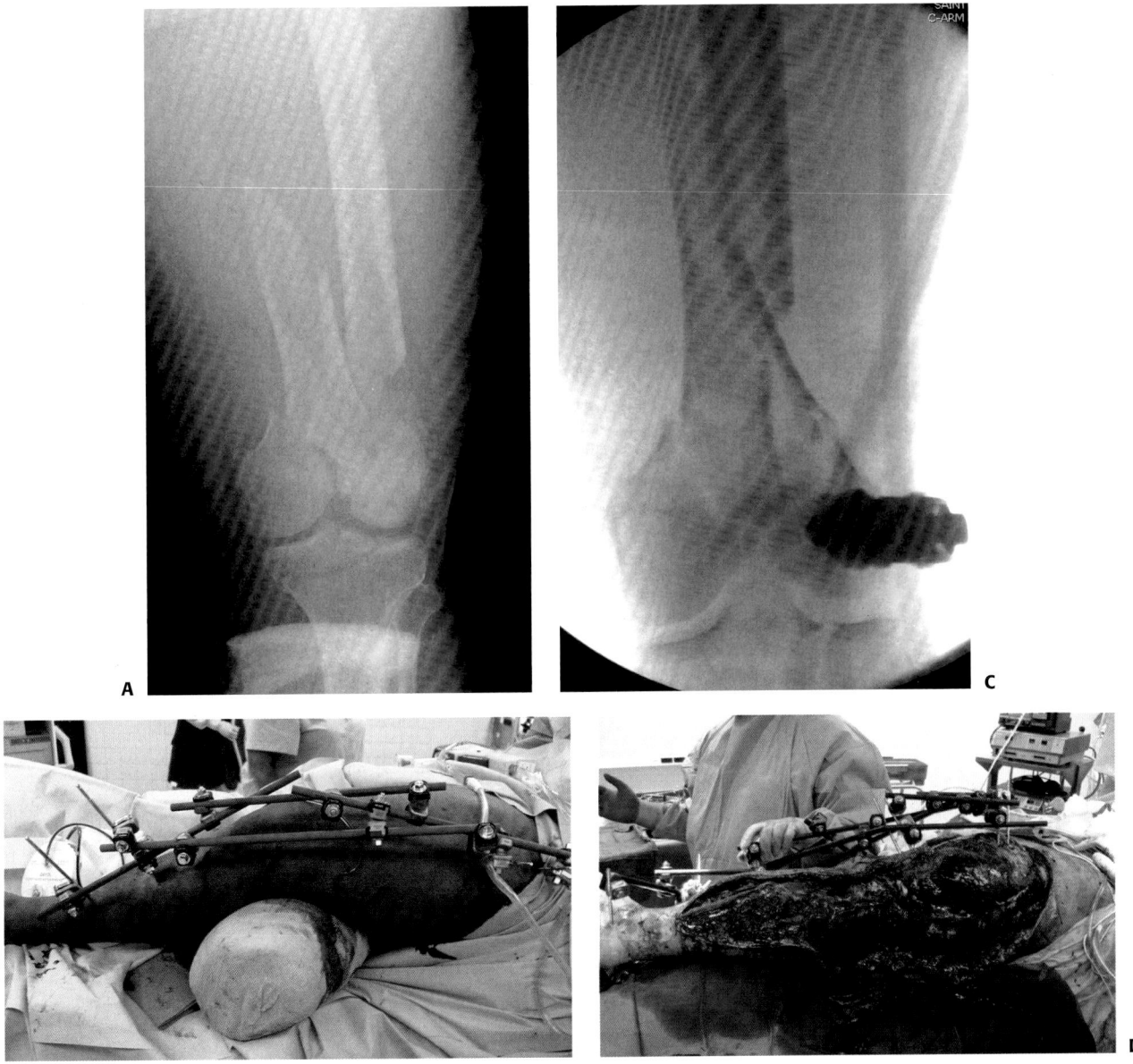

FIGURE 8-43 **A:** Polytrauma patient with a complex injury at the knee with a distal femur and proximal tibial fracture. **B:** Temporary knee-spanning frame placed on this patient. Note multiple connecting bars to compensate for this large patient. **C:** Knee fractures spanned out to length to await definitive reconstruction once patient's condition improves. **D:** Necrotizing fasciitis in another polytrauma patient who had sustained a severe crush injury to the entire lower extremity. The spanning fixator is spanning multiple ipsilateral fractures with an associated compartment syndrome. Entire limb was spanned to include the patient's knee and ankle.

to proximal and distal threaded transfixion pins placed across the respective joint. Manual distraction is carried out and a ligamentotaxis reduction achieved (Fig. 8-44). A simple anterior monolateral frame can be used to maintain similar reduction across the knee joint for temporizing the management of knee dislocations, complex distal femoral fractures, and tibial plateau fractures (Fig. 8-58).[227,270,294,296,297,303] A simple monolateral frame can be configured in a triangular-type construct about the distal tibial and ankle region in an effort to achieve relative stability. These are usually constructed with two or three pins in the mid-

to distal tibia and a single transversely placed centrally threaded calcaneal tuberosity pin. These tibia pins are then connected in a triangular fashion with distraction across the calcaneal pin effecting a ligamentotaxis reduction at the distal tibia (Figs. 8-44 and 8-45). This typical external fixator construct can obscure the site of injury on radiographs, and because the construct may rotate about the solitary pin calcaneal, many complications have been attributed to this unstable pin site. Pin tract infections, loosening of the calcaneal pin fixation, and heel ulcerations, have all been reported.[323] Strategies to prevent calcaneal complications have

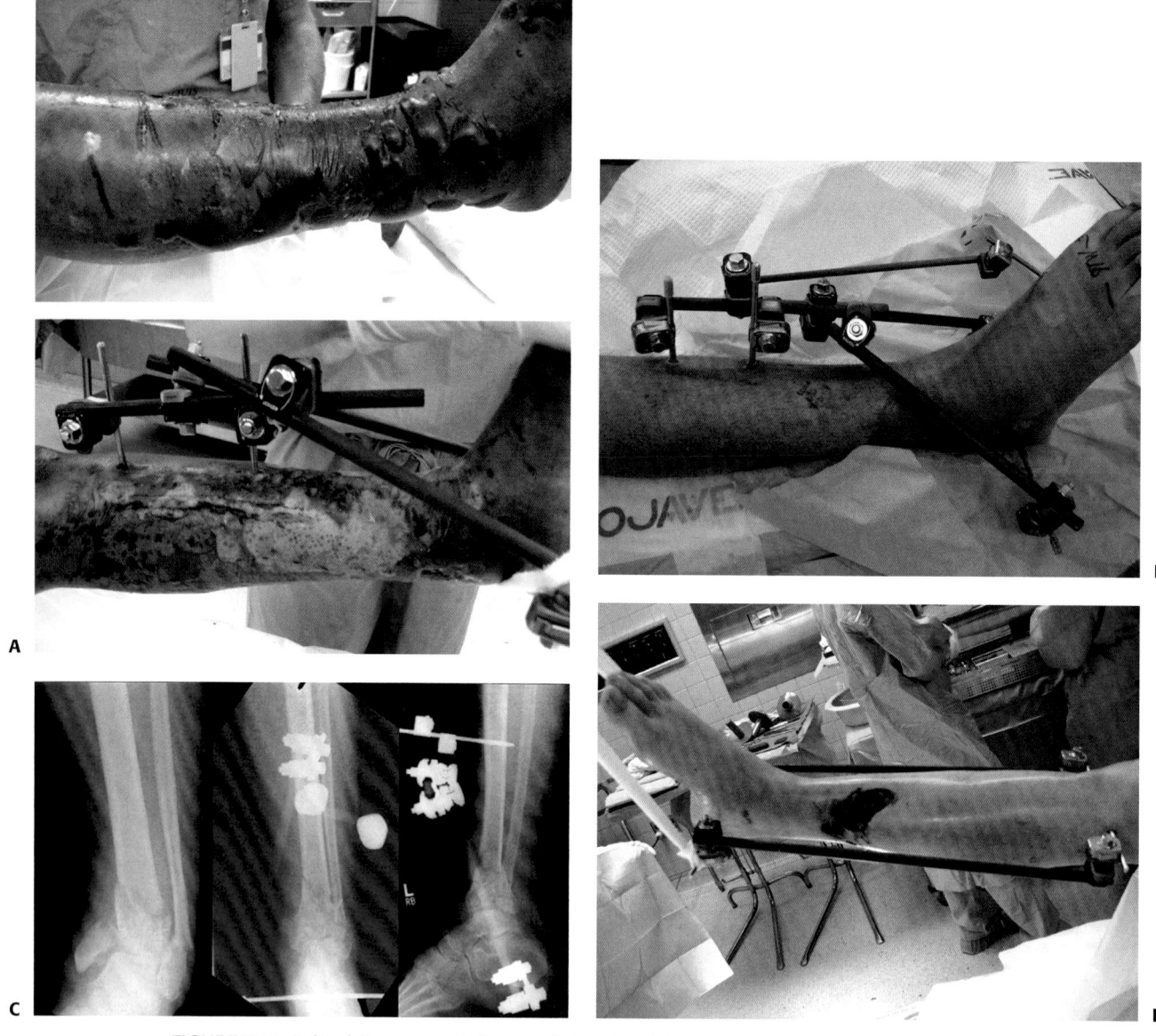

FIGURE 8-44 A: (top) A severe ankle fracture dislocation with compartment syndrome and significant soft tissue compromise was spanned with a triangular ankle-spanning external fixator. The reduction achieved with the simple frame facilitates the definitive reconstructive procedures once soft tissue recovery has occurred and the fasciotomy incisions have healed **(bottom). B:** A pilon fracture stabilized with an ankle-spanning frame. The forefoot was maintained in neutral with the addition of a metatarsal pin. **C:** A ligamentotaxis reduction maintained alignment and allowed definitive reconstruction once the soft tissues had recovered. **D:** Simple two-pin fixator spanning open tibia fracture to allow for staged debridement and eventual IM nailing, once the zone of injury has been defined.

included the placement of two longitudinal axis pins placed from posterior to anterior in the body of the calcaneous to prevent rotation. These are then connected to a U-tube bar around the posterior calcaneous. The calcaneous pin connecting the bar is then attached to the tibial shaft pin/bar couple with distraction performed at the ankle joint. Alternatively, application of forefoot pins and stabilization of the foot in neutral position not only prevents rotation with calcaneal pin loosening, but also maintains the foot in neutral and prevents the common complication of forefoot equinus (Fig. 8-46).[24]

Temporary column distraction is a useful technique for complex foot injuries. Mini–ex fix components are used to distract across medial column injuries such as complex "nut cracker" navicular fractures,[162] medial cuneiform fractures, and metatarsal base fractures/dislocations where the fracture morphology results in significant shortening of the medial column. Similarly, lateral column mini fixators can be used to maintain length in cases of comminuted cuboid, lateral cuneiform, and lateral metatarsal base fracture/dislocations. Simple two-pin mini fixators are placed with single 2.5-, 3-, or 4-mm Schanz

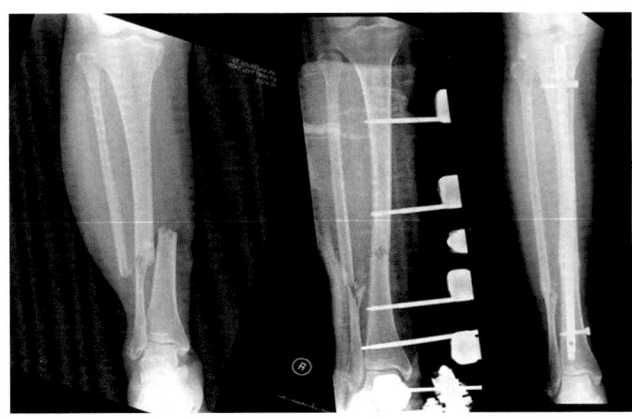 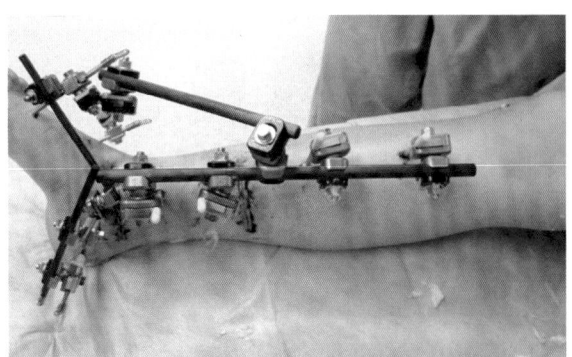

FIGURE 8-45 **A:** Open tibial shaft fracture with complex foot injury is temporarily stabilized with a spanning monolateral fixator. **B:** An anatomic reduction was achieved and maintained with the frame. Once soft tissues are recovered and the patient's condition stabilized, the frame was converted to an IM nail at 10 days post injury.

pins placed proximally (usually medially in the talar neck or in the lateral calcaneous), with distal fixation into the first or fifth metatarsal shafts and a simple distraction bar attached to maintain length (Fig. 8-47). Once the soft tissues have recovered then definitive reconstruction is carried out with the reduction accomplished and maintained early (Fig. 8-48).[32,49,71,217]

Application of these techniques in a polytraumatized patient is valuable when rapid stabilization is necessary for a critically injured or physiologically unstable patient, so-called DCOs. Simple monolateral or monotube fixators can be placed very rapidly across long bone injuries providing adequate stabilization to facilitate the management and resuscita-

tion.[121,279] Excessive traction across a joint should be avoided when applying these temporary joint-spanning frames. By overdistracting these extremities, the muscular compartments can become stretched effectively compressing the compartments and lead to late compartment syndrome.[84] However, the most common complication encountered when utilizing temporary spanning external fixation is the inability to re-establish length. As well, fixator "creep" or gradual loosening of the fixator components may occur prior to definitive reconstruction, causing the initial reduction and length to be lost. If correct length is not maintained, then when definitive reconstruction is undertaken many of the perceived advantages of

FIGURE 8-46 **A:** Ankle-spanning fixator placed to distract pilon fracture and place soft tissues at rest. Note excellent skin wrinkles denoting soft tissues' availability for surgery. **B:** Patient did not have any forefoot pins or adjunctive calcaneous fixation allowing the heel to rotate about the axis of the heel pin. This can result in early pin loosening and equinus positioning.

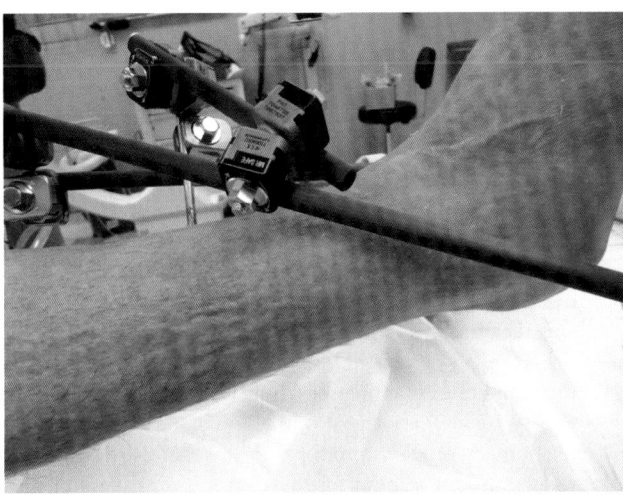 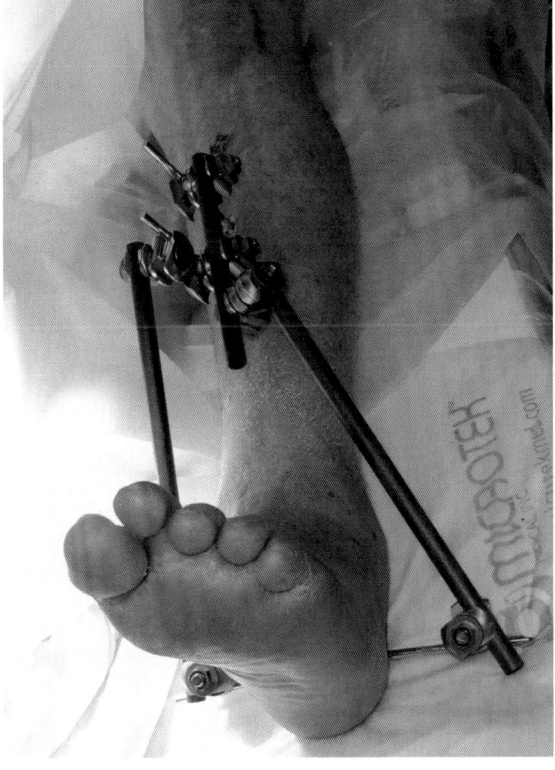

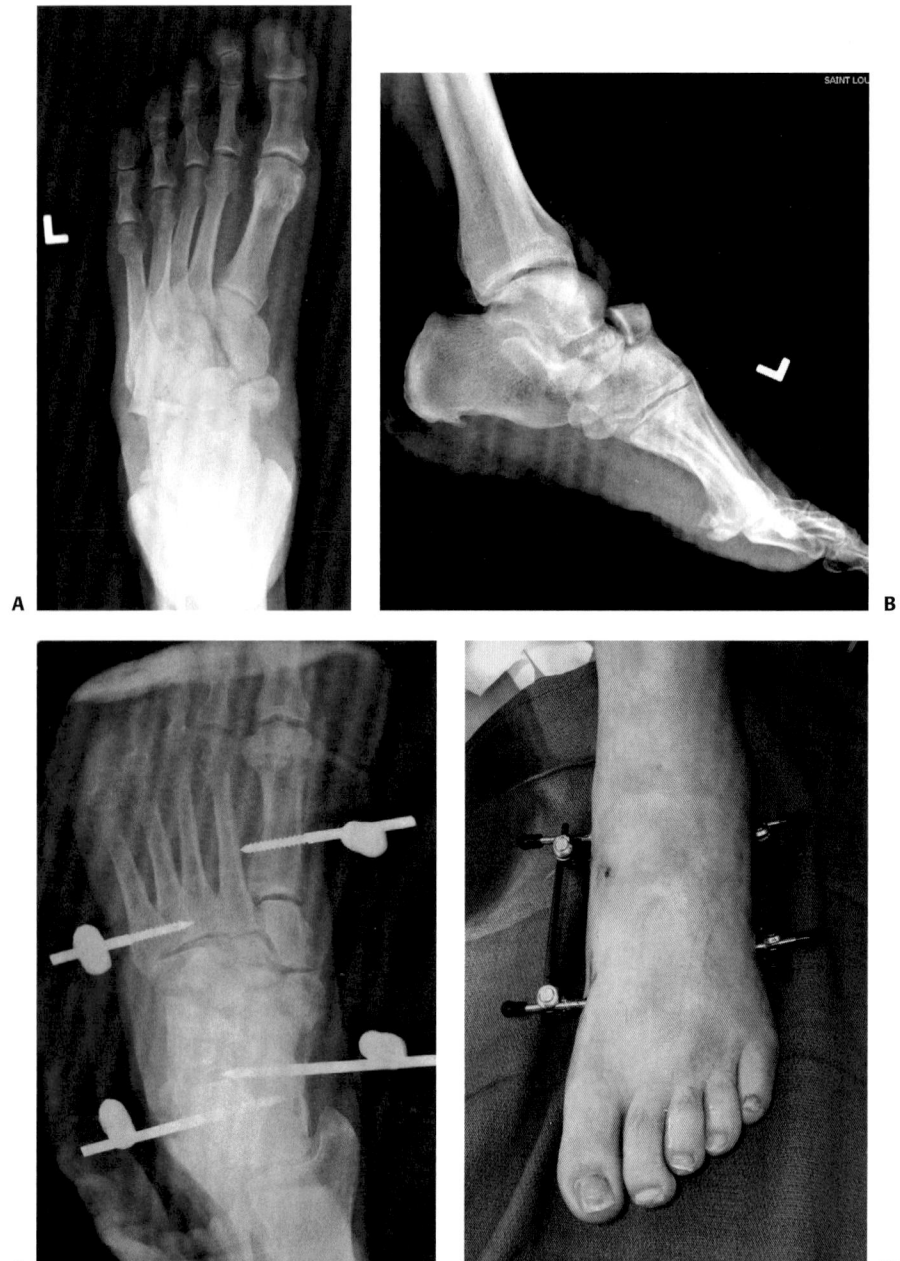

FIGURE 8-47 **A, B:** Complex forefoot injury with midfoot dislocation and navicular fracture. **C, D:** Medial and lateral column distraction accomplished with mini fixator components.

spanning external fixation are lost.[214] If a delay of more than a week is anticipated prior to definitive reconstruction, interim radiographs should be performed and repeat reduction performed if length has been lost.

For periarticular fractures, the decision to convert to definitive stabilization is usually based on the condition of the soft tissues. A latency period of at least 10 to 14 days is required to allow the soft tissues to recover to the extent where definitive fixation can be undertaken safely. Many series have demonstrated excellent results achieved with a staged approach consisting of early fracture stabilization using spanning external fixation. This is followed by careful preoperative planning based on traction CT scans and the judicious clinical evaluation of the soft tissue injury prior to definitive internal fixation.[4,181,223,227,270,303] When applying temporary spanning external fixation there was

concern that overlap of external fixation pins and the proposed definitive incision would increase infection rates and should be avoided. Investigators evaluated the overlap between temporary external fixator pins and definitive plate fixation correlates with infection in high-energy tibial plateau fractures.

There was no correlation seen between any deep plate-related infection and distance from pin to plate, pin–plate overlap distance, time in the external fixator, open fracture, classification of fracture, sex of the patient, age of the patient, or healing status of the fracture.[171] Fears of definitive fracture fixation site contamination from external fixator pins do not appear to be clinically grounded. Thus a temporary external fixation construct with pin placement that provides for the best reduction and stability of the fracture, regardless of plans for future surgery, is recommended (Fig. 8-49).

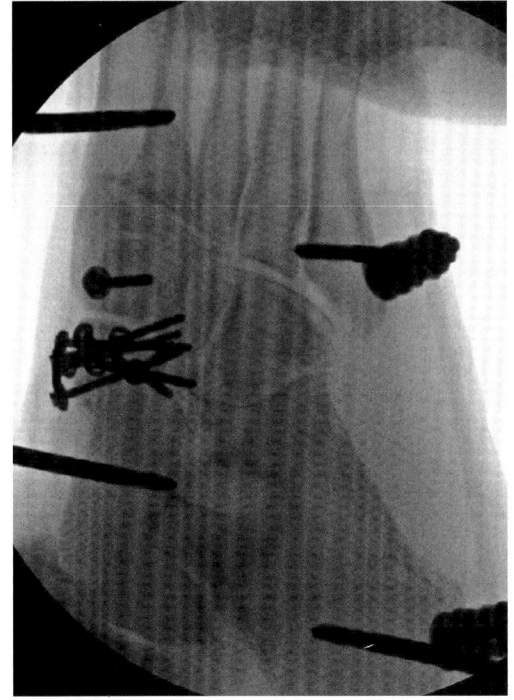

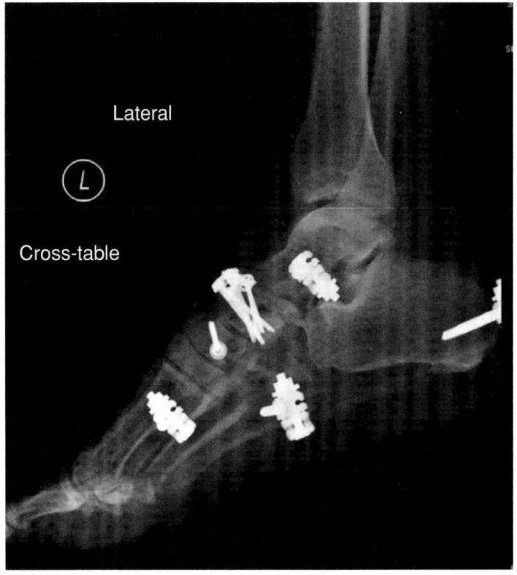

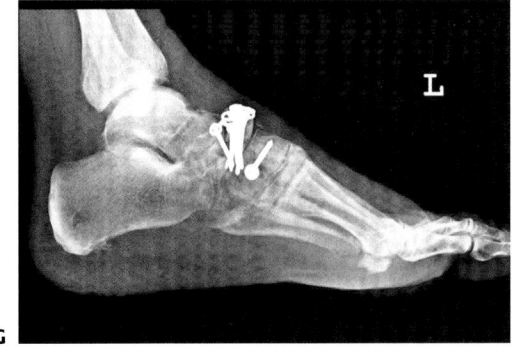

FIGURE 8-47 (continued) **E, F**: Fixator maintained during definitive reconstruction for additional stability postoperatively. **G**: Frames removed at approximately 3 weeks post ORIF.

The timing of conversion of a DCO external fixator to an intramedullary nail is determined by the condition of the soft tissues and the overall stability of the patient. With the temporary stabilization of long bone fractures, definitive conversion to intramedullary nailing has demonstrated variable success especially in the tibia.[67] Most authors would suggest early (within the first 2 to 3 weeks of frame application) conversion to intramedullary nailing to avoid colonization of the medullary canal by the external fixator pins. Increased infection rates have been documented when conversion is done after 2 weeks of external fixation. It has been shown that the longer the external fixator remains in place, the greater the risk of complications occurring following conversion to intramedullary devices, especially if the pins are removed and the nail exchanged at the same operative setting (Fig. 8-50).[143,196]

In the femur, conversion from external fixation to nailing has demonstrated good rates of success if the exchange is done when the patient's overall physical condition has improved. Acute conversion to an intramedullary device for the femur in a single procedure is preferred in patients without evidence of pin tract infection. Studies have shown that infection rates after DCO for femoral fractures are comparable to those after primary intramedullary nailing (IMN). One study suggested an increased risk for DCO femoral fractures treated with initial external fixation compared with those placed in traction.[259] Scannell et al.[259] found in a comparative study that the initial traction group of femoral fractures had a lower rate of sepsis (8.3% vs. 31.6%, $p = 0.0194$) and a shorter length of stay (26.5 days vs. 36.2 days, $p = 0.0237$) than the initial external fixation group. However, there appears to be no contraindication to the implementation of a damage control approach for severely injured patients with femoral shaft fractures initially subjected to general anesthesia for life-saving procedures when appropriate. Pin site contamination is more common when the femoral fixator is in place for more than 2 weeks. For patients treated by using a DCO approach, conversion to definitive fixation should be performed in a timely fashion.[29,128]

Stabilization of unstable pelvic fractures has been achieved by the rapid application of simple external fixation for use in the immediate resuscitative period. The application of an external frame affords significant reduction in the volume of the true pelvis, as well as stabilizing the movement of large bony cancellous surfaces along the posterior aspect of the pelvic ring. The

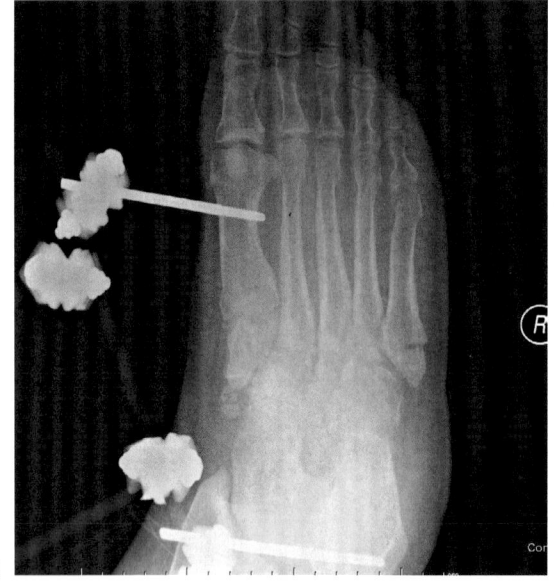

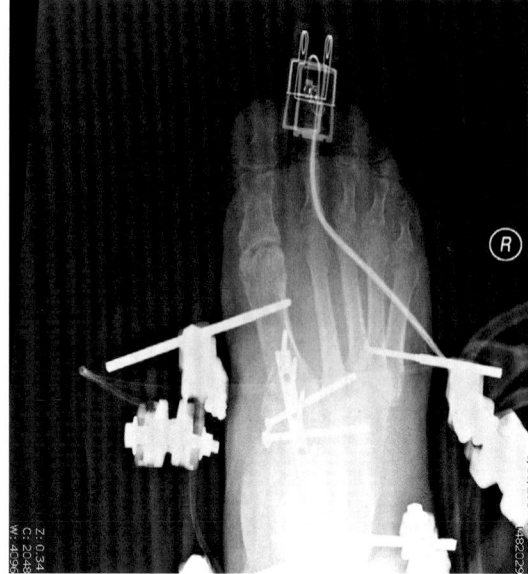

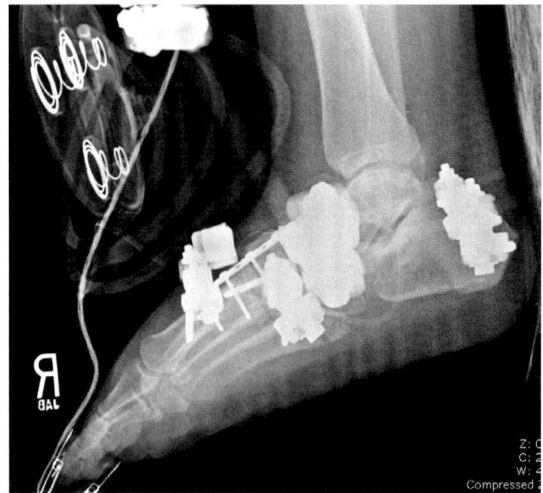

FIGURE 8-48 **A:** Complex Lisfranc fracture dislocation of forefoot stabilized initially with medial column distraction. **B, C:** Postoperative views of bridge plate fixation of medial column injury with the addition of a lateral column distractor to maintain the reduced position.

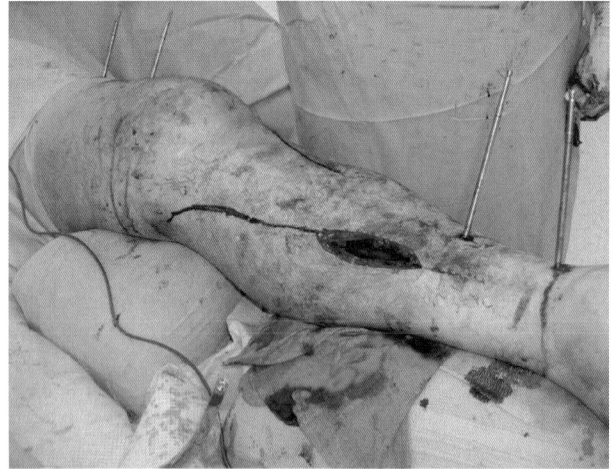

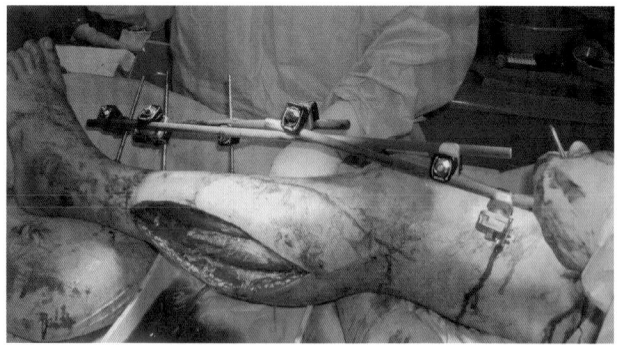

FIGURE 8-49 **A, B:** Complex bicondylar plateau fracture with associated compartment syndrome with medial and lateral fasciotomy wounds. Note the location of potential incisions for eventual ORIF have been marked on the skin medially and laterally. This is done to place pins and connecting bars out of the proposed fixation area.

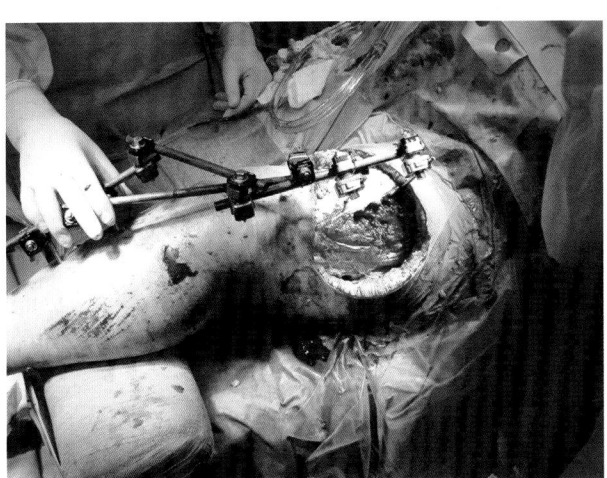
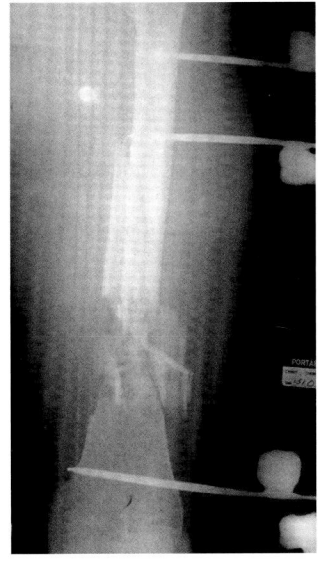
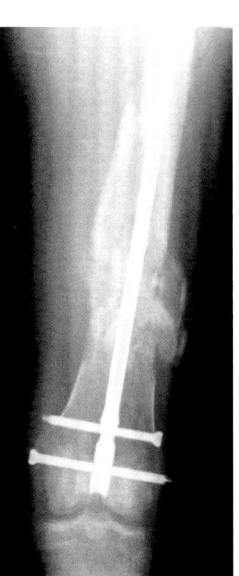

A, B   C

FIGURE 8-50 **A–C:** Severe soft tissue injury prevents acute IM nailing of the femoral shaft. Fracture. Stability required spanning across the knee to maintain reduction. Secondary conversion to IM occurred at 12 days post injury with no secondary infection noted.

ability to provide stabilization and decrease the pelvic volume allows the surgeon to control hemorrhage and has helped to contribute to the low mortality seen with these injuries.[63,153]

Anterior pelvic external fixator constructs provide excellent adequate fixation, and traditional constructs include single and multiple pin placements in several locations in each iliac crest.

However, anterior frame application, specifically the anterior superior iliac crest pins that course between the inner and outer iliac tables may be problematic. These frames may be difficult to apply in a large obese patient.[122] As well, these pins may loosen very rapidly because of the variable pin purchase in cancellous bone (Fig. 8-51).

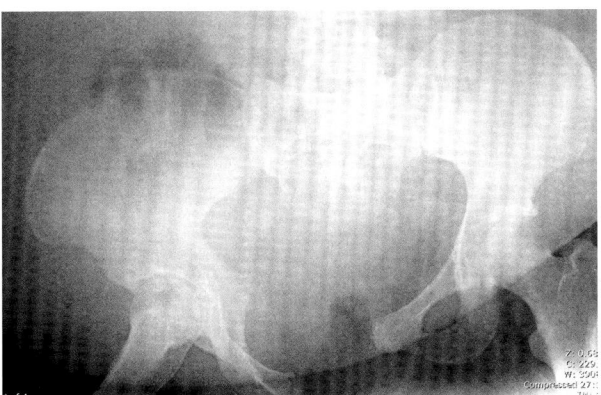

A

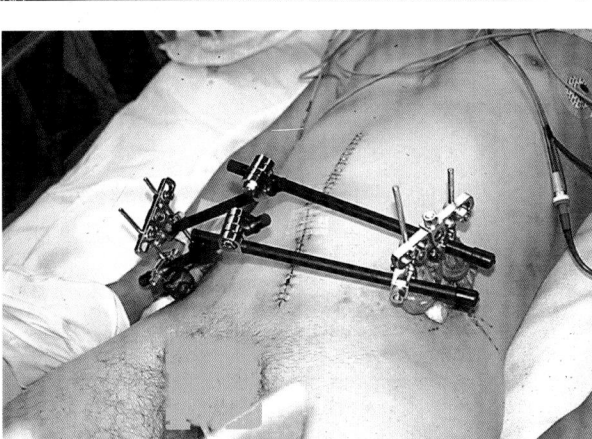

C

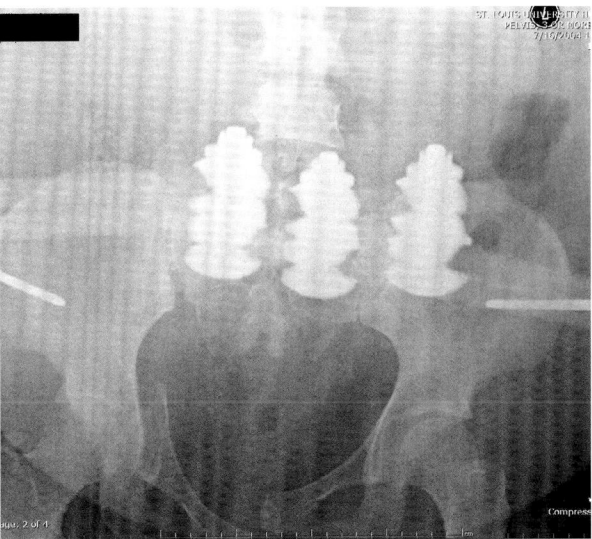

B

FIGURE 8-51 **A:** Pelvic injury with anterior and posterior disruption and hemodynamic instability. Note large abdominal pannus prohibiting supra-acetabular pin placement. **B:** Simple anterior frame applied to help in the resuscitation of the patient and provide temporary pelvic stabilization. **C:** Anterior iliac wing frames can be modified with additional crest pins and additional bars to increase stability.

A recent study compared the stability provided by a two-pin iliac crest fixator to the stability provided by a commercially available binder device (trauma pelvic orthotic device [T-POD]). Mechanical testing simulated log rolling the patient and performing bed transfers. The T-POD conferred more stability in all planes of motion, although this did not reach statistical significance. This study does document the equivalency of the T-POD devices and suggests that clinicians advocate acute, temporary stabilization of pelvic injuries with a binder device followed by early conversion to internal fixation when the patient's medical condition allows.[223]

Recent biomechanical and anatomic studies have focused on pin placement lower in the pelvis, specifically in the supra-acetabular region. Pins in this location are more stable biomechanically because of the improved purchase in the hard cortical bone of the posterior column (Fig. 8-52). This pin placement allows for pelvic reduction in the transverse plane of deformity and may allow improved reduction of the posterior elements. In addition, the location of the pins and frame can facilitate concurrent or subsequent laparotomy procedures.[106,178]

Pelvic frames are most useful in those fractures that are vertically stable.[195] Rotationally unstable fracture such as anterior–posterior compression and lateral compression injuries are best suited to application of an anterior pelvic frame.[63] At times, the application of an anterior frame may be complicated, cumbersome, and time consuming, and may be contraindicated as an emergency application. For this reason, a modification of pelvic external fixation, the C-clamp, can provide temporary stability in the patients with massive pelvic ring disruption and hemorrhage.

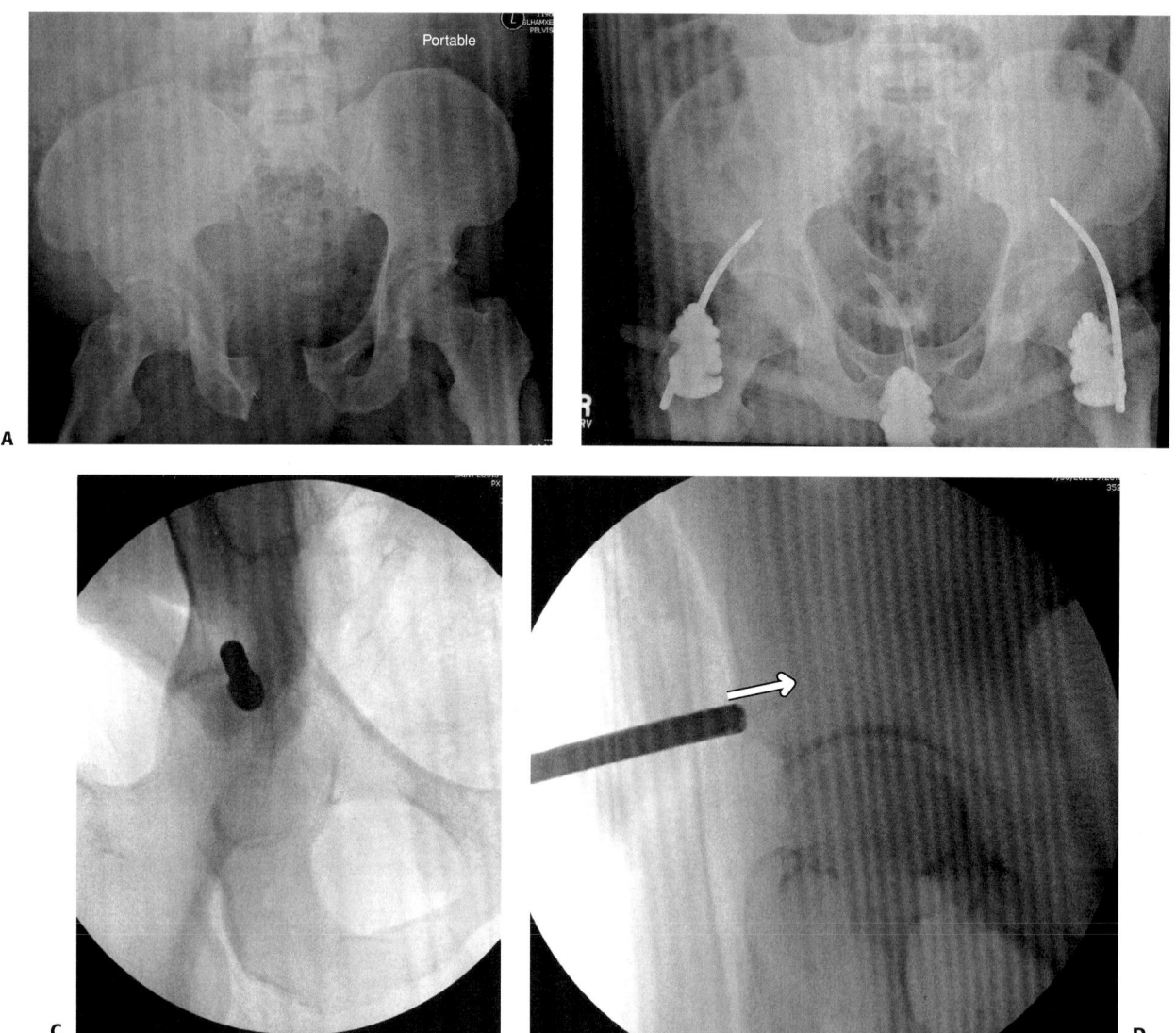

FIGURE 8-52 **A:** Severe pelvic injury with anterior and posterior injury. **B:** Supra-acetabular pins placed and pelvic volume decreased. Note significant bending of these pins needed to maintain symphysis reduction. **C, D:** Correct placement technique of supra-acetabular pins using a trocar and drill sheath to protect the anterior soft tissue structures during insertion. The pin trajectory should parallel the superior acetabular dome (*white arrow*).

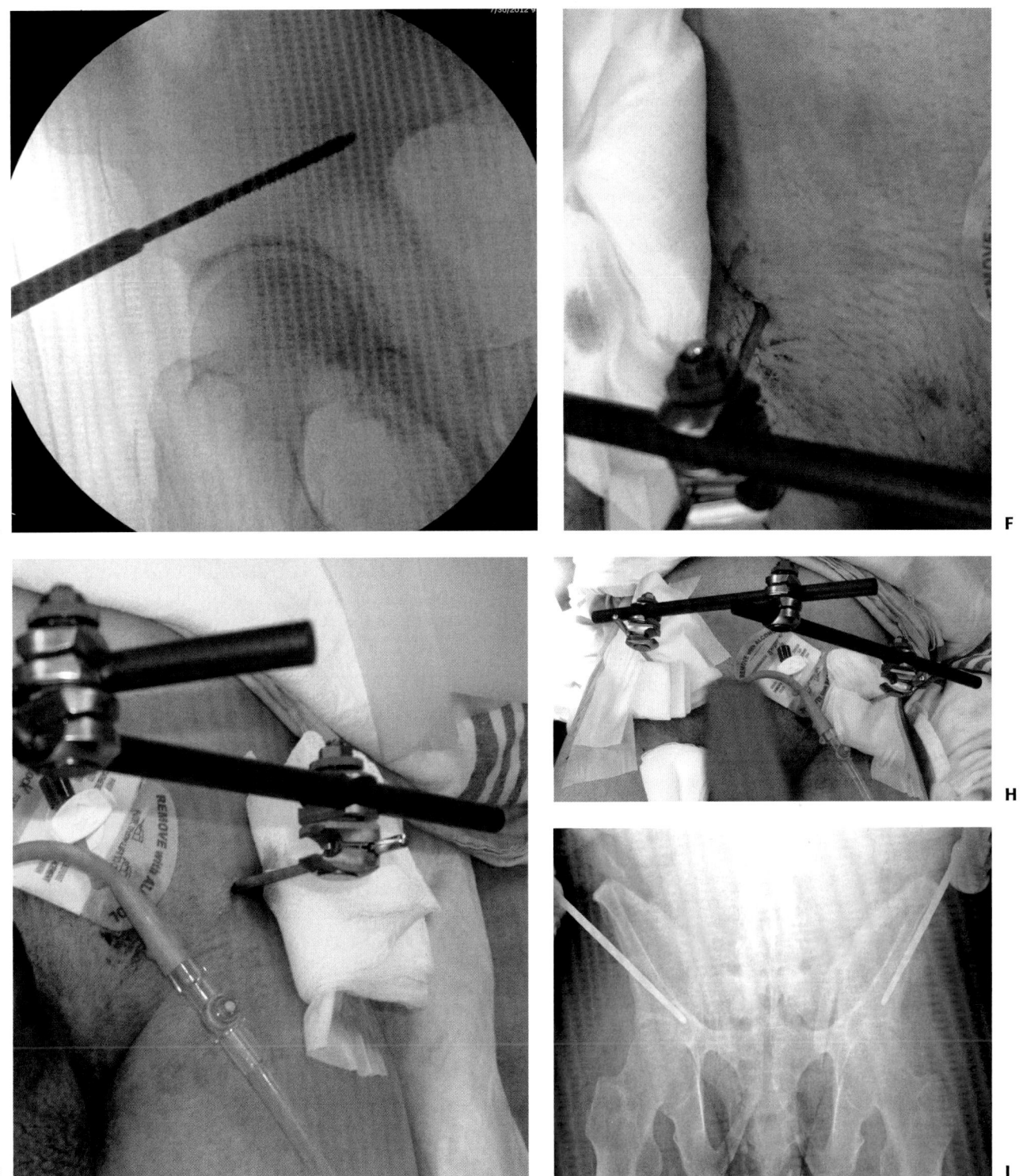

FIGURE 8-52 (*continued*) **E:** Pins traverse the area just superior to the dome of the hip joint and gain purchase in the dense cortical bone of the posterior column. **F, G:** Location of supra-acetabular pins placed using 1.5-cm incisions which are closed following insertion. **H:** The connecting bar is located low on the pins and does not impinge on the abdominal tissues. **I:** Pins perfectly located just above the acetabular domes on both hips with excellent reduction of symphysis achieved.

Specific Fracture Management Using External Fixation

The choice of external fixator type depends on the location and complexity of the fracture, as well as the type of wound present when dealing with open injuries. The less stable the fracture pattern, the more stable a frame needs to be applied to control motion at the bone ends. If possible, weight bearing should be promoted. If periarticular extension or involvement is present, the ability to bridge the joint with the frame provides satisfactory stability for both hard and soft tissues. It is important that the frame be constructed and applied to allow for multiple debridements and subsequent soft tissue reconstruction. This demands that the pins are placed away from the zone of injury to avoid potential pin site contamination with the open wound (Fig. 8-49). In this setting, ring fixators have a potential advantage for extra-articular injuries in that they allow for immediate weight bearing and can gradually correct deformity and malalignment, as well as achieve active compression or distraction at the fracture site.

Monolateral Applications

The largest indication for the use of monolateral frames for fracture management occurs in the distal radius and in the tibial shaft. This is followed closely by temporary application of trauma frames for complex femoral and humeral shaft injuries. Much less likely is the use of monolateral frames for forearm injuries.

Wrist External Fixation

Specific fixators have been designed for use in the distal radius, and may be either joint bridging or joint sparing. Following the restoration of palmar tilt by closed fracture manipulation, wrist position can be adjusted into neutral or extension to help avoid finger stiffness and carpal tunnel syndrome without compromising fracture reduction. For unstable fractures, it has been shown that augmentation of the fixator construct with multiple dorsal and radial percutaneous pins corrects the dorsal tilt and maintains the reduction in those fractures that are difficult to maintain with distraction ligamentotaxis alone (Fig. 8-53).[188,208]

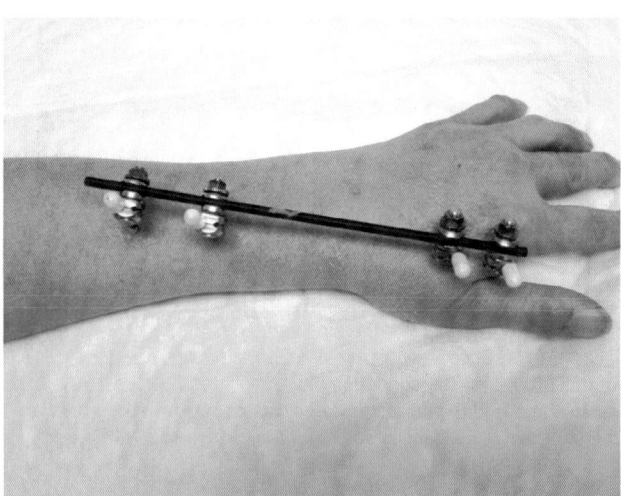

FIGURE 8-53 Simple wrist spanning (bridging) fixator with two pins in the second metacarpal and two pins in the distal radius.

The use of dynamic external fixation devices across the wrist allowing movement during fracture healing of unstable distal radial fractures has demonstrated mixed results. The concept was to achieve a ligamentotaxis reduction, and decrease the rate of stiffness by initiating early range of motion through uncoupling the device.[74,113,167] For distal radius fractures with metaphyseal displacement but with a congruous joint, there exists a trend for better functional, clinical, and radiographic outcomes when treated by immediate external fixation and optional K-wire fixation compared with most conservative approaches including pins and plaster and closed reduction and casting.

Adjuvant K-wire fixation is useful in cases with poor bone quality or in cases where the joint is highly comminuted with small articular fragments (Fig. 8-54). The K-wires are used as a buttress to maintain articular congruency, whereas the external fixator maintains the overall metaphyseal length and orientation.[228]

Though there is insufficient evidence to confirm a better functional outcome, external fixation reduces redisplacement, and gives improved anatomical results compared with pins and plaster and other conservative modalities. Most of the surgically related complications are minor, probably related to the meticulous technique of pin insertion.[124,165,182,276] External fixation devices function best when maintaining radial length alone.[208]

Joint-bridging external fixation allows the radial length to be restored with the fixator; however, the anatomic reduction of articular fragments and restoration of the normal volar tilt proves to be more difficult when using a joint spanning frame. A method of nonbridging external fixation combined with percutaneous pinning facilitates fracture reduction and allows for free wrist movements (Fig. 8-55). The cross K-wires capture and stabilize the larger fragments while buttressing the smaller fragments.

This technique has been modified and combines traditional cross-pin fixation of the distal fragments with a nonbridging external fixator. The cross K-wire configuration is constructed with pins in multiplanar and multiangle directions which creates a rigid construct. These cross pins are then attached an external strut locking them into position. Attaching the cross wires to an external fixator significantly improves fracture stability, allows for early mobilization of the wrist, and resumption of usual activities.[199] This technique is simple and most orthopedic surgeons are familiar with it. This method has demonstrated no clinical differences when used for both intra- and extra-articular distal radius fractures compared with wrist bridging fixation.[18,114,166,212] However, nonbridging fixation has been shown radiographically to reduce the risk of dorsal malunion compared with bridging external fixation.[130] Major complication rates are low and the technique is applicable to most unstable fractures of the distal radius. Most authors recommend that nonbridging external fixation be used in cases where there is space for the pins in the distal fragment. The ability to maintain the reduction and minimize the total load transmitted from the wrist joint to the fracture site is fixator-dependent, and will differ from manufacturer to manufacturer.[315]

There is no consensus on the surgical management of unstable distal radius fractures. In one systematic review and meta-analysis, data was pooled from trials comparing external fixation and open reduction and internal fixation (ORIF) for this

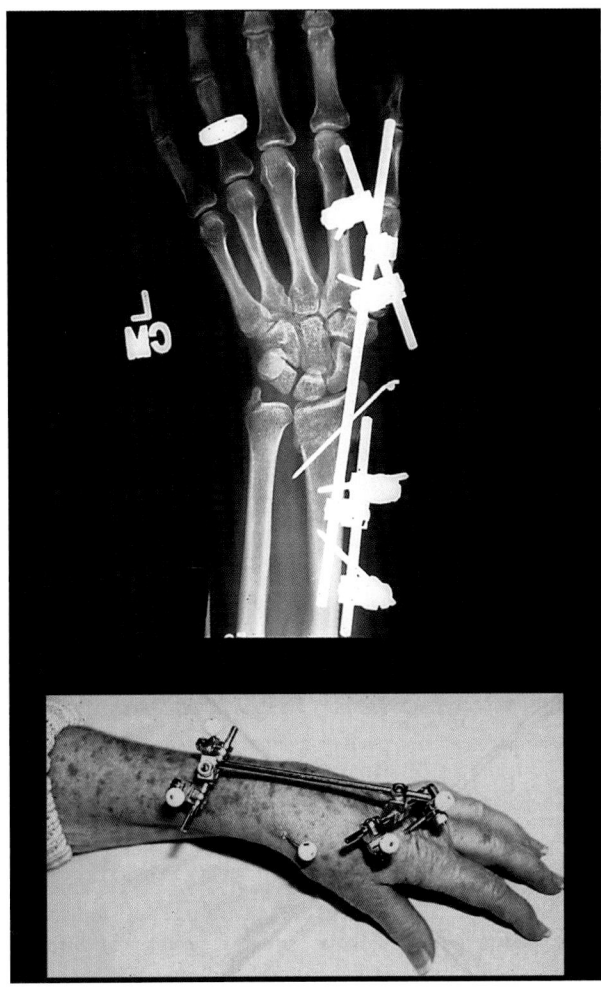

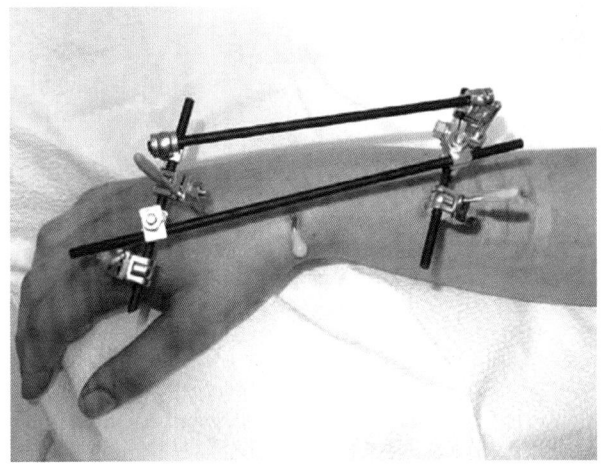

FIGURE 8-54 **A:** Mini fixator used in combination with percutaneous pins to maintain reduction of a distal radius fracture. Solitary connecting bar placed between the metacarpal and radial pins. **B:** Alternative configuration using quadrilateral frame construct with percutaneous pins.

injury. For unstable distal radius fractures, ORIF demonstrated significantly better functional outcomes, forearm supination, and restoration of anatomic volar tilt. However, external fixation resulted in better grip strength, wrist flexion, and remains a viable surgical alternative.[228,309]

Femoral External Fixation

The use of external fixation for the management of acute femur fractures is primarily limited to pediatric indications, fractures with significant soft tissue or neurovascular compromise, or to those severely injured patients who cannot tolerate more extensive

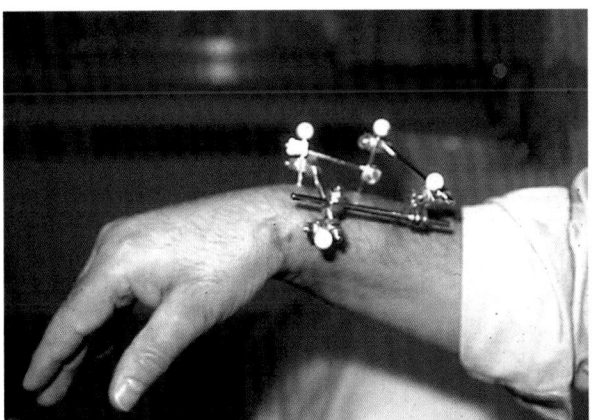

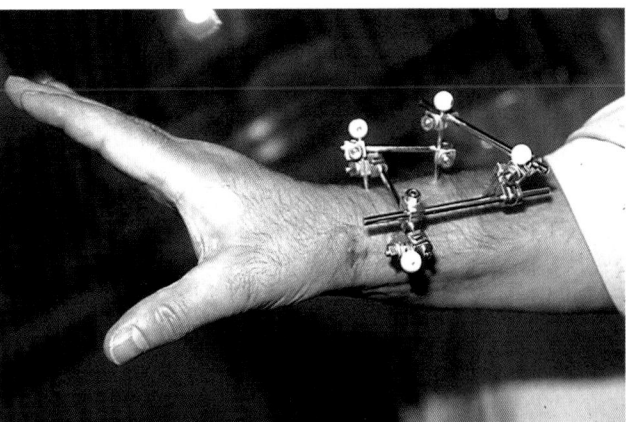

FIGURE 8-55 Fracture spanning (nonbridging) wrist fixator allows for range of motion with no loss in stability. This joint sparing configuration is indicated in certain select distal radius fractures that have a distal fragment of sufficient size.

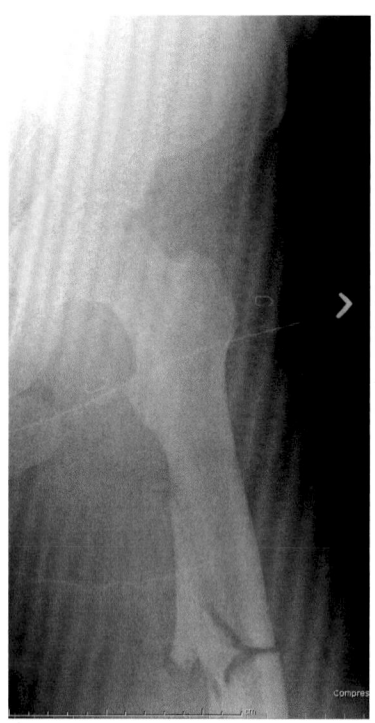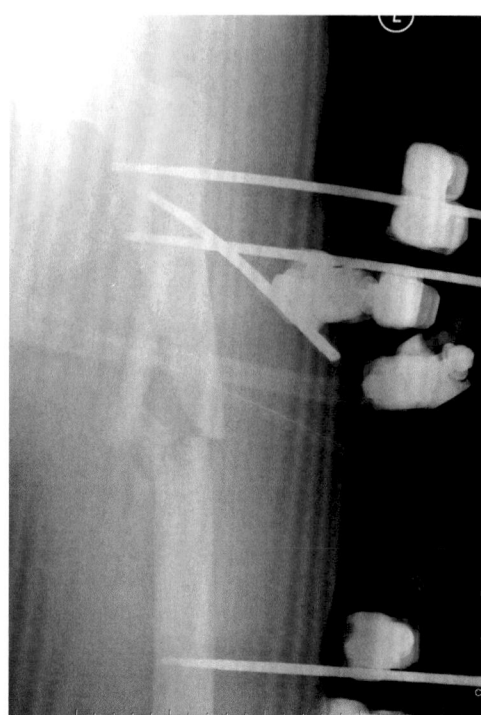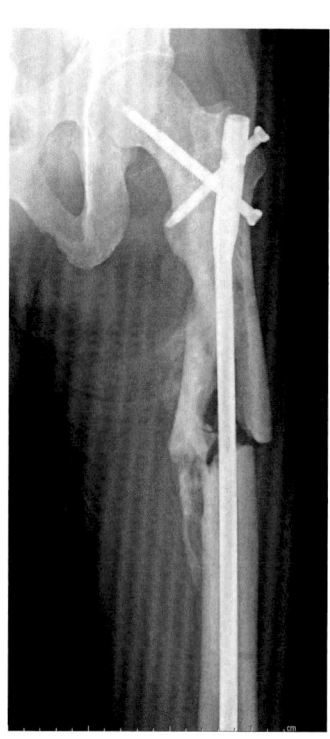

A, B   **C**

FIGURE 8-56 **A–C:** Proximal femoral shaft fracture in a polytrauma patient. Damage control measures were necessary for the overall management of the patient and a simple external fixator maintained length and alignment while the patient recovered from his other injuries. Successful IM nailing was carried out at 14 days from his initial injury.

surgery (DCO). Commonly, femoral applications include the use of a minimum of four pins placed along the anterolateral aspect of the femoral shaft. These simple monolateral frames have been shown to provide adequate stabilization for most complex femoral fracture patterns (Figs. 8-50 and 8-56).[6,31] Fixator constructs with independent pins placed out of plane relative to one another allow for safer pin insertion and demonstrate increased stability over monotube or simple monolateral frames where pins are placed in a straight line orientation.[33,77]

In many underdeveloped nations, external fixation of femoral shaft fractures is often the definitive treatment. Monolateral or monotube fixators are commonly utilized with four or six pin configurations (Fig. 8-57). A pin tract infection with occasional pin loosening is the most commonly reported complication. Pin tract infections, although a common occurrence, are not a major problem and can be treated by local wound care and antibiotic therapy, and pin removal when required. The most common problem is significant decrease in the range of motion of the knee which can be difficult to treat successfully and is the major drawback to using this technique as definitive fixation when other methods are available.[87,309] Other complications include the high rate of refracture following frame removal, especially when used in a pediatric population for definitive femoral shaft fracture treatment.[48,238]

Knee Dislocation

Knee dislocation is always a difficult topic mainly with regard to the structures that have been damaged and the best treatment

option. Knee dislocation in the polytrauma patient is also problematic in the context of open knee dislocations or dislocation in association with arterial disruption, or compartment syndrome.

In an effort to maintain the reduction and allow for arterial repair, compartmental release or the treatment of other injuries, spanning external fixation is a valuable option. Simple

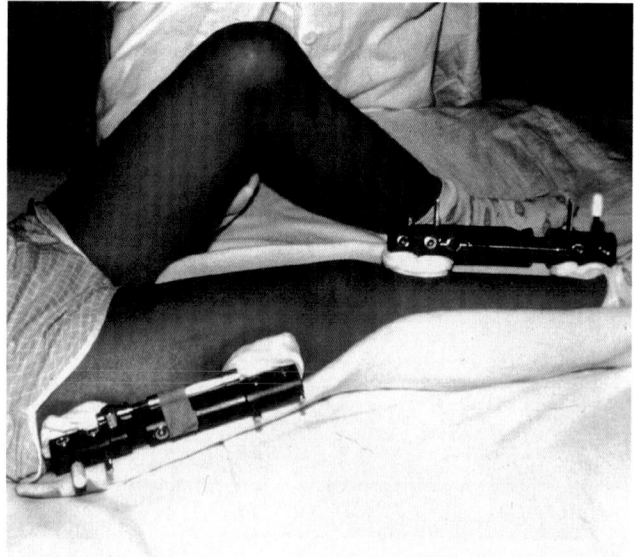

FIGURE 8-57 Pediatric patient with proximal femoral and tibial shaft fractures treated definitively with monotube large body fixators.

knee-spanning monolateral or monotube fixators can be easily applied with two pins above the knee located in the distal femur and two pins in the midtibia. The knee is reduced under fluoroscopy and the fixator locked, maintaining the reduction to facilitate other procedures and avoid the phenomenon of redislocation or subluxation that can occur when stabilizing these severe injuries with temporary splinting or casting (Fig. 8-58). In a biomechanical study, the stiffest construct for external fixation of a knee dislocation consisted of two anterolateral femoral pins and two monolateral rods connected to two tibial half pins (compared with a large monotube bar and a circular construct). This stiffer construct may provide a better clinical outcome and this frame configuration was recommended by the authors.[197]

Following definitive surgical repair of associated ligamentous injuries of the globally unstable knee, some investigators advocate the immediate application of an articulated hinged knee fixator. Articulated external fixation has been proposed as a method to protect ligament reconstructions while allowing aggressive and early postoperative rehabilitation after knee dislocation.[144,321] Mechanical studies have evaluated the additional stability afforded to knees by these monolateral or bilateral hinged knee frames.[273] Application of articulated external fixators to specimens with intact ligaments significantly reduced cruciate ligament forces for Lachman, anterior drawer, and posterior drawer tests, respectively. Thus, there is biomechanical evidence that articulated external fixation of the knee can reduce stresses in the cruciate ligaments after multiligament reconstructions and can decrease anteroposterior translation in the cruciate-deficient knee.[96]

Humeral External Fixation

External fixation is an infrequent treatment option for the management of acute humeral shaft fractures. Unlike the tibia in which fixator half pins can be placed perpendicular to the subcutaneous medial tibial face, external fixation in the humerus often involves transfixion of crucial musculotendinous units. Complications related to these frames may include pin track sequelae and an inhibition of shoulder and elbow motion. However, with contemporary fixation devices, the indications for use in the humerus continue to expand. In addition to their initial use for shaft injuries, many series now report the successful treatment of supracondylar and proximal humerus fractures treated with monolateral, circular, and hinge fixators.[53,120,191]

The most frequent indication for use in the humerus is for the stabilization of severely contaminated open fractures from blunt trauma or gunshot wounds that occur in association with vascular disruption (Figs. 8-21 and 8-59). Rapid application of a simple four-pin external fixator provides excellent stability such that the limb may be manipulated during subsequent vascular arterial repair without concern for disruption of the repair. External fixation together with radical debridement has reduced the incidence of chronic infection and improved the

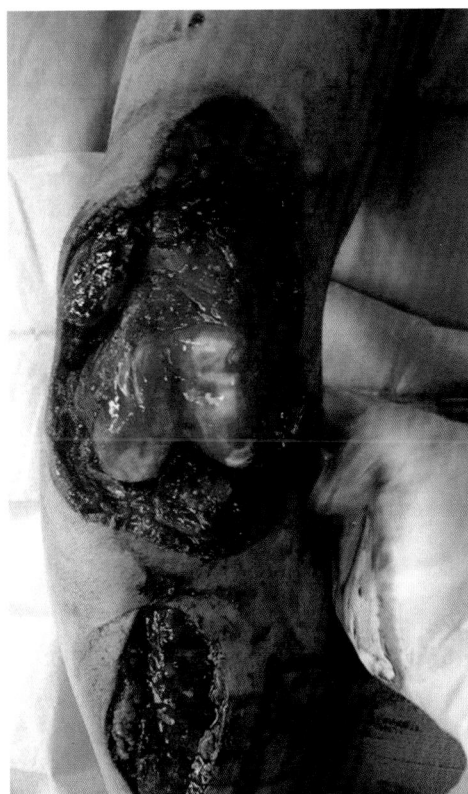
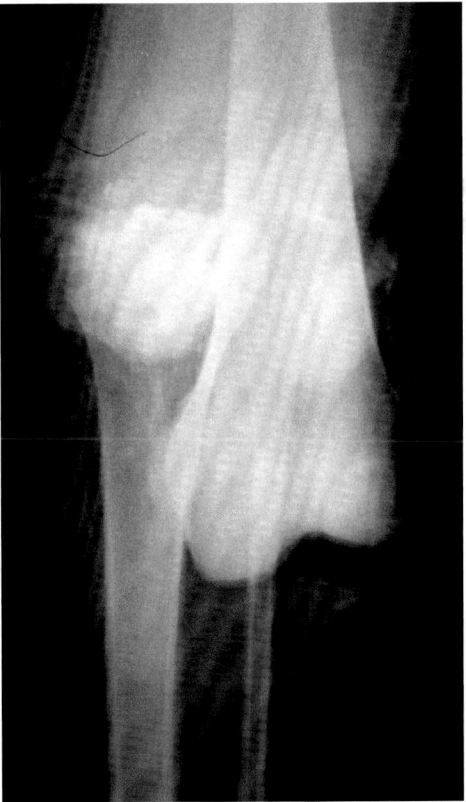

FIGURE 8-58 A, B: Severe open knee dislocation in conjunction with arterial disruption.

(continues)

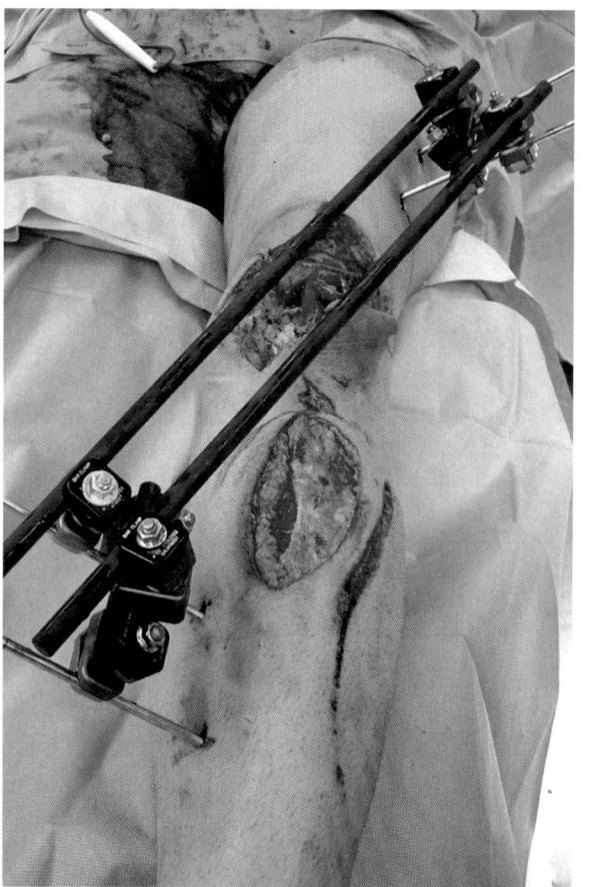
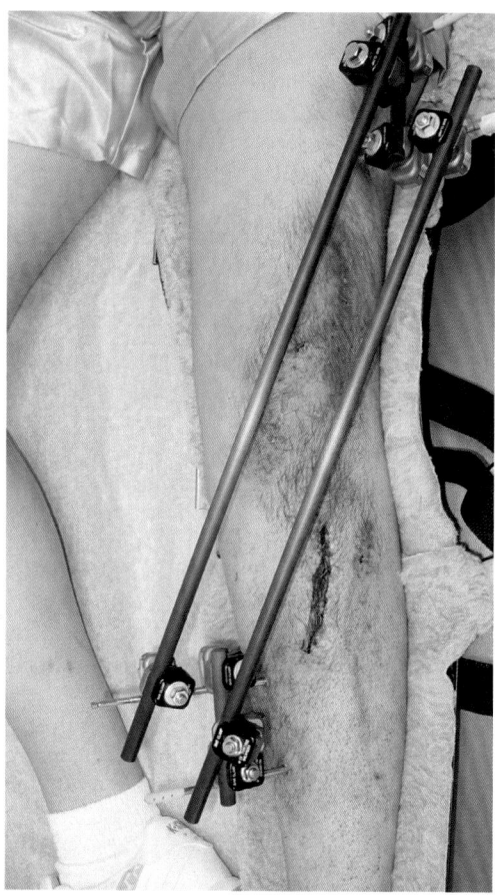

C

D

FIGURE 8-58 (*continued*) **C, D:** Emergent knee-spanning fixator was applied at the time of initial surgical management which included arterial repair and multiple debridements. Wound was eventually closed and the patient underwent delayed ligamentous reconstruction at 10 weeks post injury.

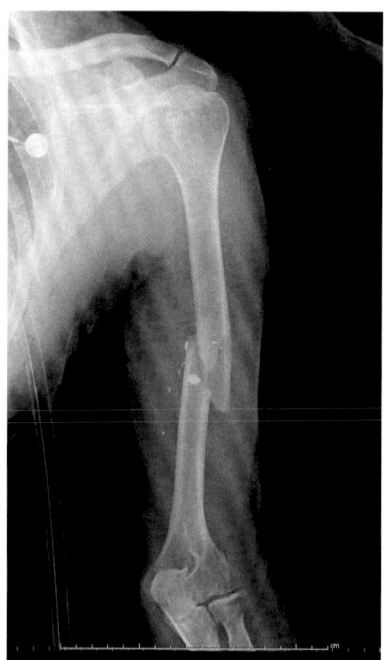
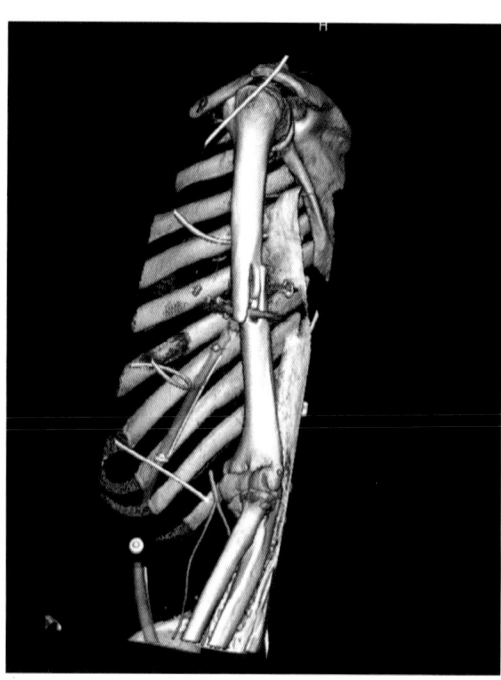

A

B

FIGURE 8-59 **A, B:** Gunshot wound humerus fracture in association with arterial injury.

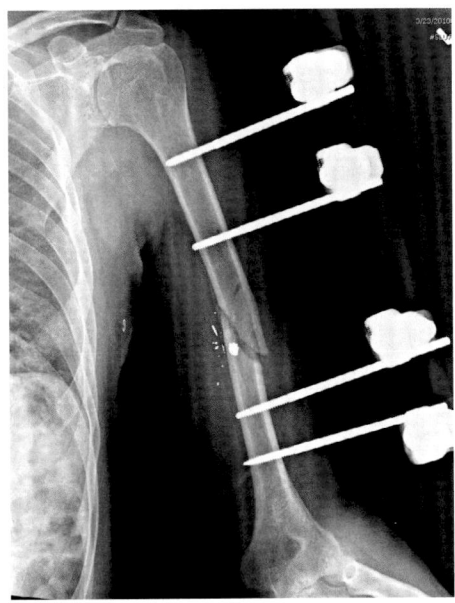
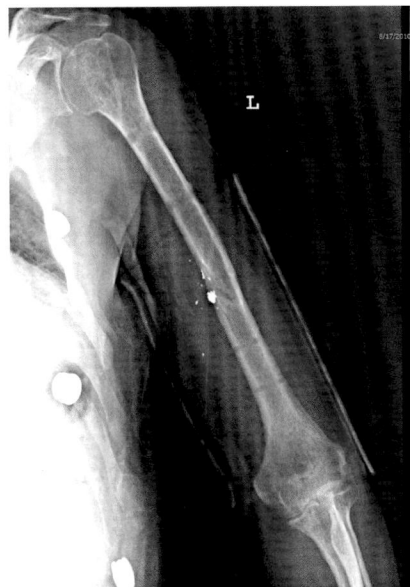
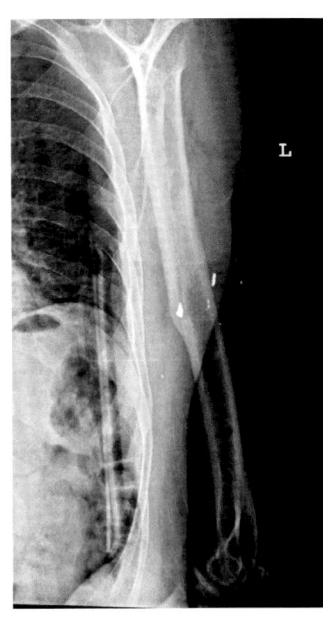

C, D   E

FIGURE 8-59 (*continued*) **C:** Humerus was emergently stabilized with a spanning external fixator and arterial repair was performed. **D, E:** Frame was removed at 11 weeks post injury with complete healing.

prognosis for the vascular repair (Fig. 8-60). Average fixator time is dependent upon associated extremity injures and has been reported to be an average 16 weeks for these severe injuries. Secondary surgical procedures for soft tissue and bony reconstruction are facilitated and reported rates of pin tract infection are relatively low.[207]

When treating polytrauma or multiply injured patients, immediate external fixation and planned conversion to internal fixation of humeral shaft fractures is an option in the treatment of associated severe soft tissue injuries and severely injured patients (Fig. 8-60). A recent review of this technique documented no systemic complications after conversion from external to internal fixation, with excellent rates of healing following plating. The authors suggested that planned conversion to plate

fixation within 2 weeks of external fixator application proved to be a safe and effective approach for the management of humeral shaft fractures in these selected patients.[278]

Patients with supracondylar, intracondylar, and other fracture/dislocations about the elbow can be temporized by the application of a provisional elbow-spanning fixator. This restores length with a generalized repositioning of the fragments and can maintain the reduction of a grossly unstable elbow dislocation. When the patients' status improves, or the soft tissues recover, definitive fixation of the injuries can be safely undertaken (Fig. 8-61).

In select severe elbow injuries which undergo internal fixation, the stability can be augmented by the application of a hinge-type elbow fixator or a static elbow-spanning fixator. The

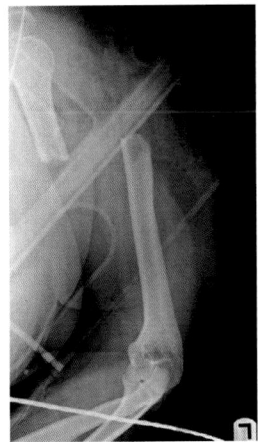
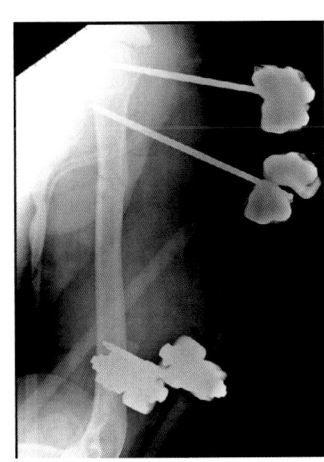
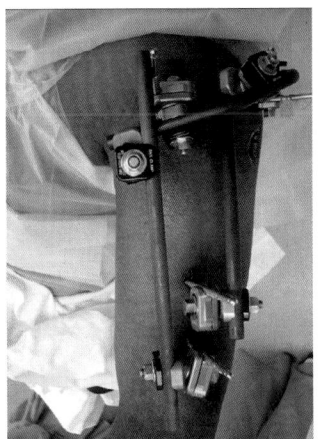
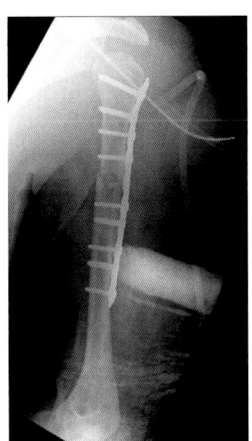

A, B   C, D

FIGURE 8-60 Multiply injured patient with proximal humerus fracture. Damage control measures included application of fracture-spanning external fixator. When the patient had recovered from initial injuries, definitive fixation was carried out at 9 days post injury.

FIGURE 8-61 **A, B:** Severe open elbow injury with substantial articular injury. Stability was maintained with an elbow-spanning fixator before and after definitive surgery. Fixator was removed 3 weeks post ORIF and range of motion initiated.

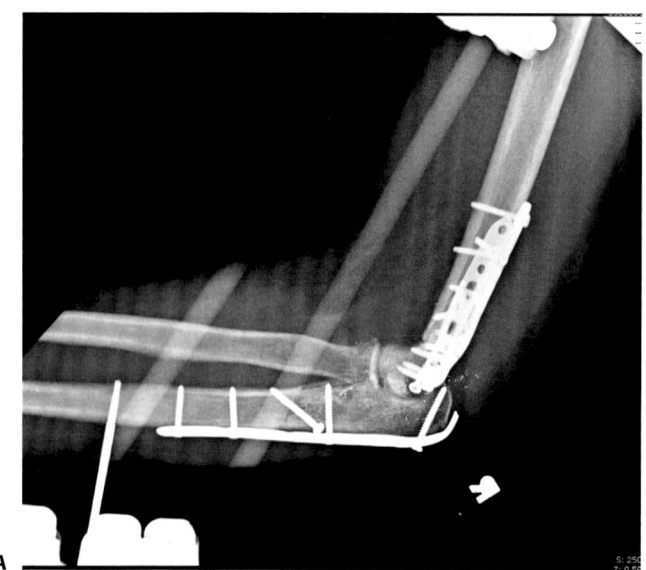

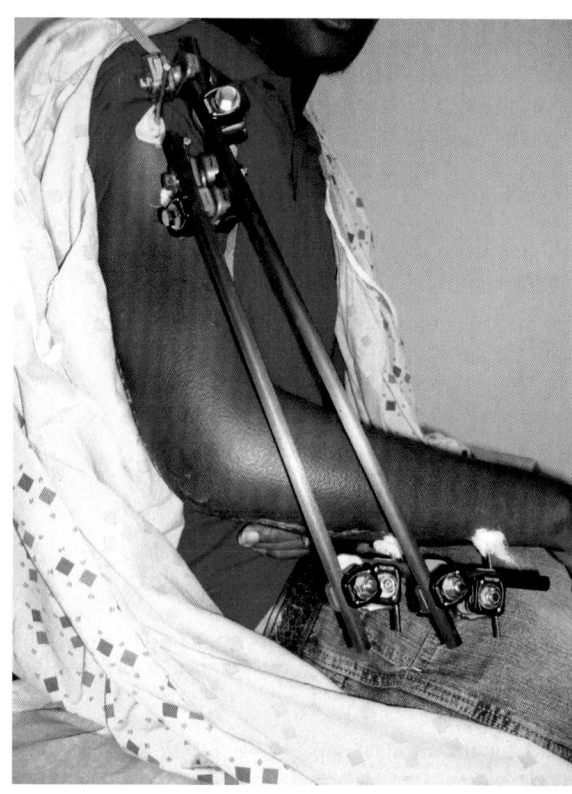

A

B

use of a hinged external fixator for supplemental fixation of distal humerus fractures may be effective in cases where internal fixation is severely compromised by comminution, bone loss, or in conjunction with an unstable elbow joint.[68] Other indications for application of an elbow hinge fixator are related to elbow instability as the primary pathology. This includes recurrent dislocation or subluxation of the elbow after repair or tenuous fixation of large coronoid fractures because of comminution or osteopenia (Fig. 8-62). The hinge fixator has also been used to augment the reconstruction of bony, capsuloligamentous, and/or musculotendinous stabilizers following open stabilization of the joint. A relative indication for use of an elbow hinge includes providing stability following fascial arthroplasty or debridement for infection, if the debridement destabilizes the elbow (Figs. 8-63 and 8-64).[210,242,243,319]

One of the difficulties encountered with the use of hinge fixators for the elbow is the ability to precisely position the center of rotation axis pin to accurately reproduce and preserve the concentric motion of the elbow once the fixator is applied. Recent works suggest that compared with the conventional free hand method of axis pin placement for an elbow fixator, two-dimensional guidance from virtual images (computer-assisted navigation) allows a reduction in the number of drilling attempts required. Furthermore, the accuracy in terms of AP angulation and lateral distance from a defined optimal placement is better when compared with that obtained with the conventional technique (Figs. 8-62 to 8-64).[83] Many investigators using hinge fixators document the restoration of stability and excellent motion after relocation of a chronic elbow disloca-

tion. Good results have also demonstrated its usefulness as a tool following the reconstruction of acute and chronic elbow instability or instability after fracture-dislocation (Fig. 8-64).

In some cases of nonunion of the humerus shaft, standard treatment options such as intramedullary nailing or compression plating and bone grafting may not be applicable or recommended, because of lingering infection, severe osteoporosis, poor soft tissue coverage, or other confounding variables. Many authors have advocated a one-stage debridement, with or without autogenous bone grafting, and application of an Ilizarov external fixator. Successful treatment of complex distal humeral and midshaft nonunions that have failed internal fixation have been reported with this technique.[37,239,284]

Tibial Fractures

Open tibial diaphyseal fractures are primarily treated with intramedullary nailing, but there are occasions when external fixation is indicated. External fixation is favored when there is significant contamination and severe soft tissue injury or when the fracture configuration extends into the metaphyseal/diaphyseal junction or the joint itself, making intramedullary nailing problematic. In these settings, monolateral external fixation allows for rapid reduction, which also helps to limit the amount of operative time and blood loss. In addition, it is useful in patients with multiple injuries or in the patients where prolonged anesthesia is contraindicated. A simple single or double bar unilateral system allows for independent pin placement, whereas the larger monotube frames facilitate rapid application with fixed pin couples.[29,54,82,91,94]

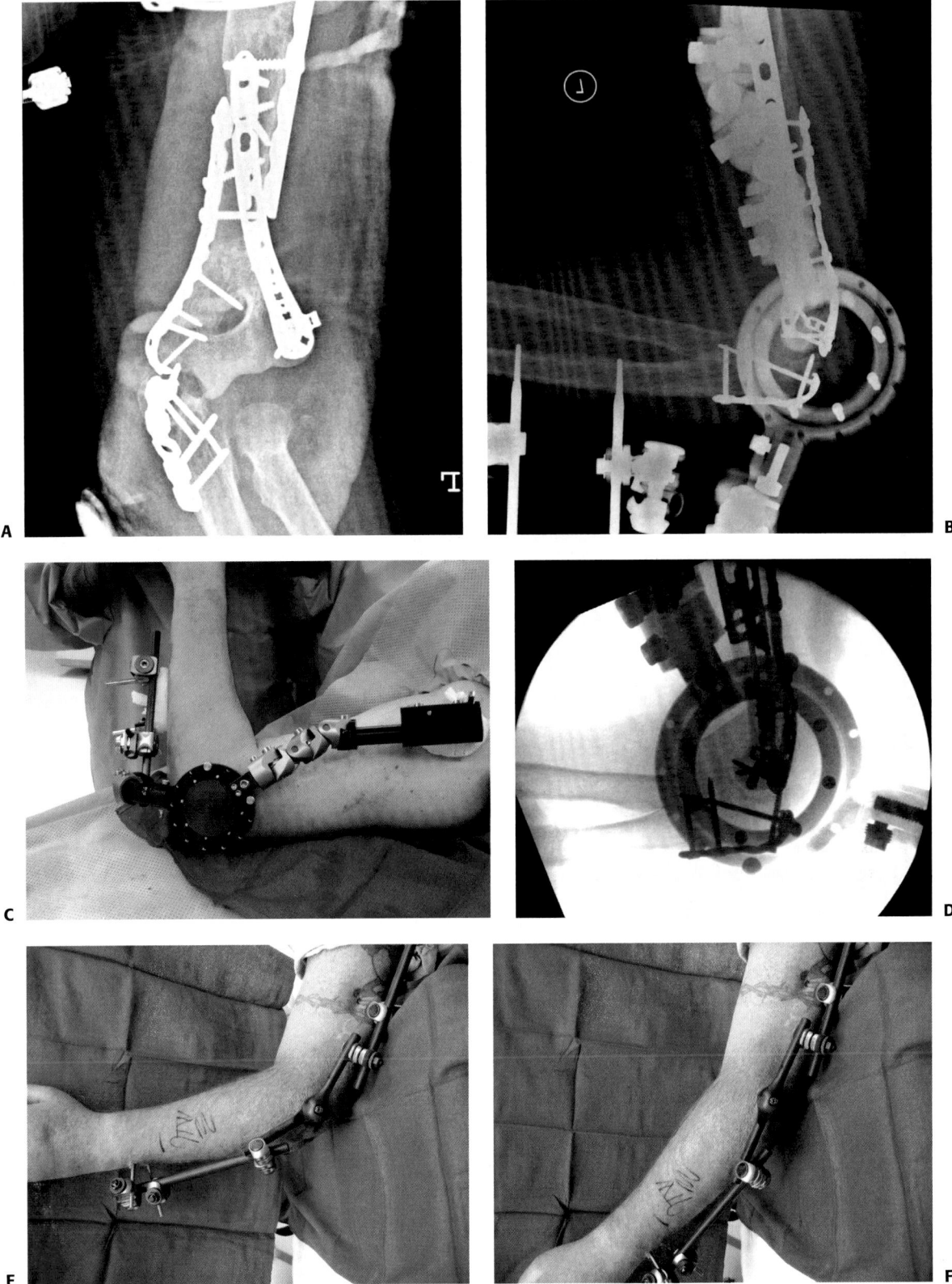

FIGURE 8-62 A, B: Complex fracture/dislocation with residual post-op instability. Hinge fixator applied to provide concentric stability and allow range of motion. **C, D:** Intra-op images demonstrating the precise nature of positioning the hinge exactly at the center of rotation of the elbow. **E, F:** A simple elbow fixator hinge attached to humeral and ulnar monolateral fixator components to provide stable range of motion.

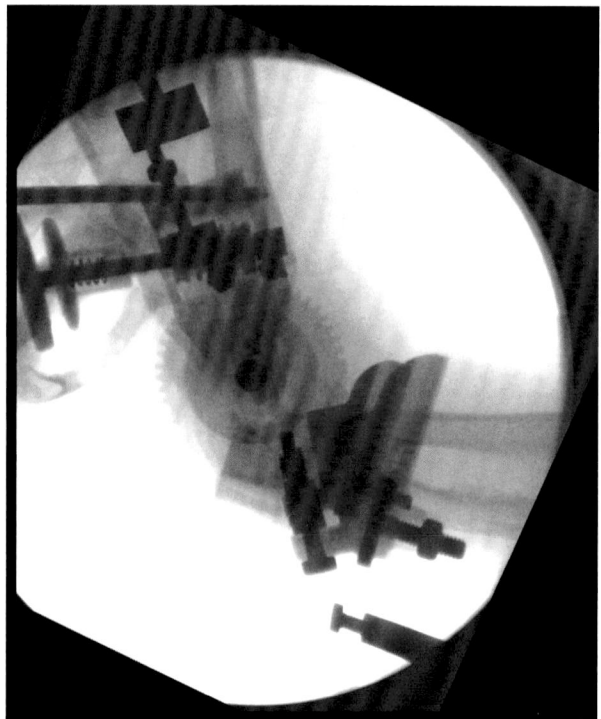 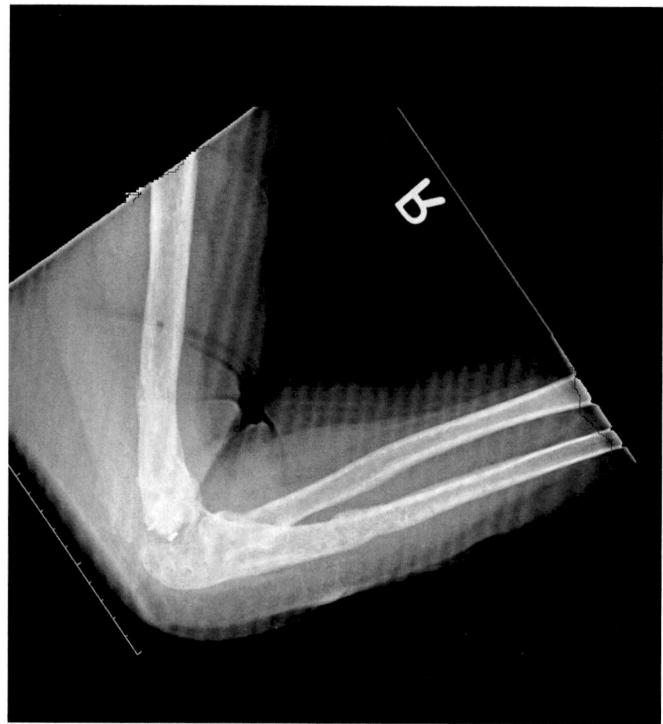

FIGURE 8-63 Hinge elbow fixator utilized to provide elbow stability and facilitate physical therapy following fascial arthroplasty of the elbow joint. Key to application is the precise location of the center of rotation pin as seen on fluoroscopy.

Contemporary simple monolateral fixators have clamps that allow independent adjustments at each pin–bar interface allowing wide variability in pin placement which helps to avoid areas of soft tissue compromise. In general, the most proximal and most distal pins are first inserted as far away from the fracture line as possible and the connecting rod attached. The rod is positioned close to the bone to increase the strength of the system. The intermediate pins can then be inserted using the multiaxial pin fixation clamps as templates with drill sleeves as guides. Upon placement of these two additional pins, the reduction can then be achieved with minimal difficulty (Figs. 8-24 and 8-25). Alternatively, the two proximal pins can be connected by a solitary bar and the two distal pins are connected to a solitary bar. Both proximal and distal bars are then used as reduction tools to manipulate the fracture into alignment. Once reduction has been achieved, an additional bar-to-bar construct between the two fixed pin couples is connected.

Use of the large monotube fixators facilitate rapid placement of these devices with the fixed pin couple acting as pin templates. Two pins are placed through the fixator pin couple proximal to the fracture and two pins placed through the pin couple distal to the fracture. Care must be taken to allow adequate length of the monotube frame prior to final reduction and tightening of the body (Fig. 8-65).

Most monotube bodies have a very large diameter which limits the amount of shearing, torsional, and bending movements of the fixation construct. Axial compression is achieved by releasing the telescoping mechanism. Dynamic weight bearing is initiated at an early stage once the fracture is deemed stable. In fractures that are highly comminuted, weight bearing is delayed until visible callous is achieved and sufficient stability has been maintained. The telescoping body allows for dynamic axial compression once weight bearing is initiated, and this serves to stimulate early periostel callous formation.[12–14]

External fixators offer the ability to compress actively across fracture fragments, and fracture gaps secondary to comminution and minimal bone loss can be closed directly by this maneuver. Fracture gaps secondary to malalignment can be corrected sequentially as bone union takes place. This can be accomplished with most circular and select monolateral fixators with three-dimensional adjustability.[13,14,220,241]

Closed tibial fractures treated with external fixation heal on an average in 4 to 5 months. In an effort to accelerate this rate, most proponents of external tibial fixation feel that early dynamization or gradual frame disassembly should be performed in an effort to effect load transfer to the fracture and promote secondary callous formation. Research and clinical studies have been inconclusive on the advantages of passive dynamization. However, dynamization does seem to facilitate fracture healing if it is utilized within the first 6 to 8 weeks following the fracture. Kenwright demonstrated significant improvement in the time to union with active dynamization.[153–155] If a major bone defect exists at the fracture site, dynamization may result in permanent shortening. If more than 1.5 to 2 cm of shortening will occur then dynamization is contraindicated. Most external fixators have bone transport capabilities as an option to regain limb length and skeletal continuity.[295,298–300,302]

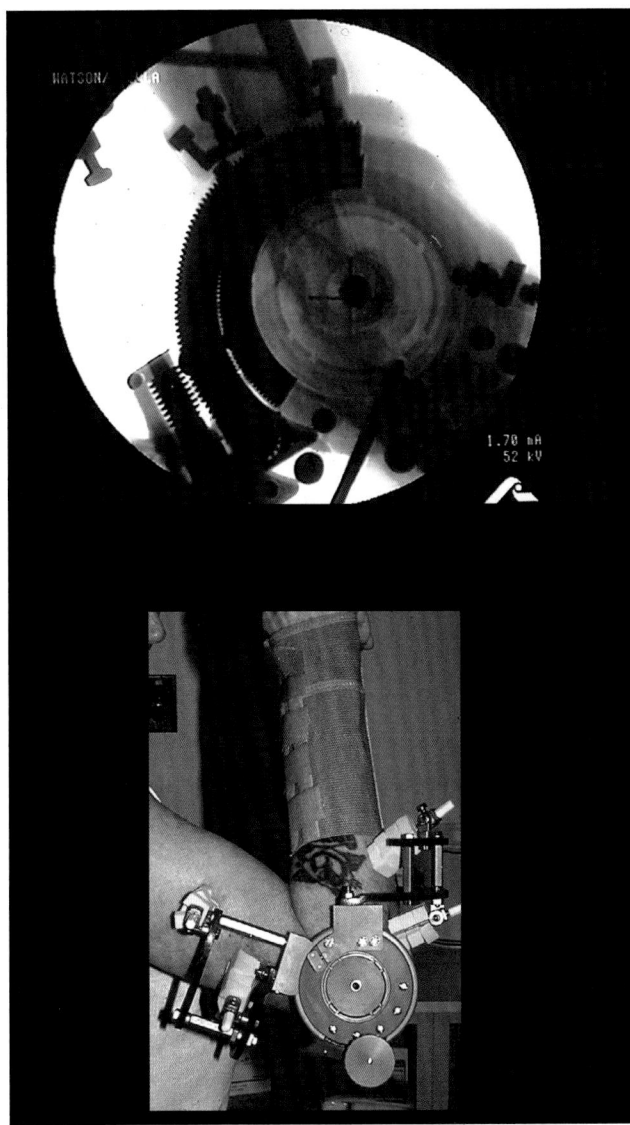

FIGURE 8-64 Elbow hinge placed to augment the repair of a chronically dislocated elbow. Hinge assists in providing concentric reduction while the repair heals. Patient is able to continue to perform therapy without fear of redislocation.

Tibia fractures with severe soft tissue injury may have concomitant foot injuries as well. These patients require multiple reconstructive procedures and are often initially treated with external fixation techniques such as a bridging frame. It is advantageous to extend these frames to the hind and forefoot to avoid the common complication of equinus deformity. This can develop over time specifically in those patients with a wide zone of injury, causing the posterior compartment and other tissues to contract (Figs. 8-29, 8-45, 8-46).

Small Wire External Fixation

Diaphyseal long bone injuries are best managed using half-pin techniques. This is readily accomplished when the fracture occurs in the mid portion of the long bone, allowing the diaphyseal bone above and below the fracture to be stabilized by half pins which achieve solid bicortical pin purchase. However, as many high-energy fractures involve the tibial metaphyseal regions, transfixion techniques using small tensioned wires are ideally suited to this area, as they demonstrate superior mechanical stability and longevity. The improved stability of these tensioned periarticular wires may eliminate the need to span the ankle or the knee joint. The small tensioned wires may be used in concert with limited open reduction if necessary. Olive wires can be used to achieve and maintain "tension compression fixation" across small metaphyseal fragments, similar to the effect achieved with small lag screws. Therefore, the combination of smooth and olive wires is used to neutralize deforming forces across the fracture lines and also help to achieve and maintain compression across the fracture lines (Fig. 8-66).[140]

Randomized prospective trails comparing circular external fixation with standard internal fixation for the treatment of bicondylar tibial plateau fractures have demonstrated excellent functional results comparable to traditional open methodologies. The major advantage of circular techniques was the reduction of soft tissue complications and infections that are traditionally associated with open procedures. In contrast to other hybrid techniques, a completely circular frame offers more adjustability and superior resistance to deformation from detrimental mechanical forces such as cantilever bending. The "hybrid" frame has evolved to include a traditional monolateral diaphyseal bar attached to a solitary circular periarticular ring. Full ring stabilization is preferable to monolateral shaft stabilization because of the cantilever loading accentuated with this construct. Specifically in the proximal tibia, this type of frame configuration functions similar to a diving board producing tremendous loads at the metaphyseal diaphyseal junction with the associated development of nonor malunion.[4–6,296,297,299,305,318] If monolateral adaptations are to be used, it is recommended that at least three divergent connecting bars be attached to the periarticular ring.[5] The bars should be oriented to achieve at least 270 degrees of separation to alleviate cantilever loading. An additional disadvantage of this "hybrid" construct is the inability to easily dynamize the fixator.[236,237,301,311]

Surgical application of a circular hybrid periarticular fixator can be performed with the patient on either a fracture or radiolucent table with calcaneal pin or distal tibial pin traction. Following a ligamentotaxis reduction of the metaphyseal fragments, olive wires or percutaneous small fragment screws can be used to achieve interfragmentary compression of these metaphyseal components. If necessary, limited incisions are used to elevate the depressed articular fragments as well as bone graft the subchondral defects. It has been shown that at least three periarticular wires are necessary to stabilize these injuries. Most authors using small wire techniques recommend that as many wires as can be inserted safely should be used for maximal stability.[6,88,289,303] Biomechanical data supports the use of tensioned wire fixation stabilizing complex fractures of the proximal tibia. The stability achieved with a four-wire fixation construct is comparable to that of dual plating for bicondylar tibial plateau fractures.[23,297,305]

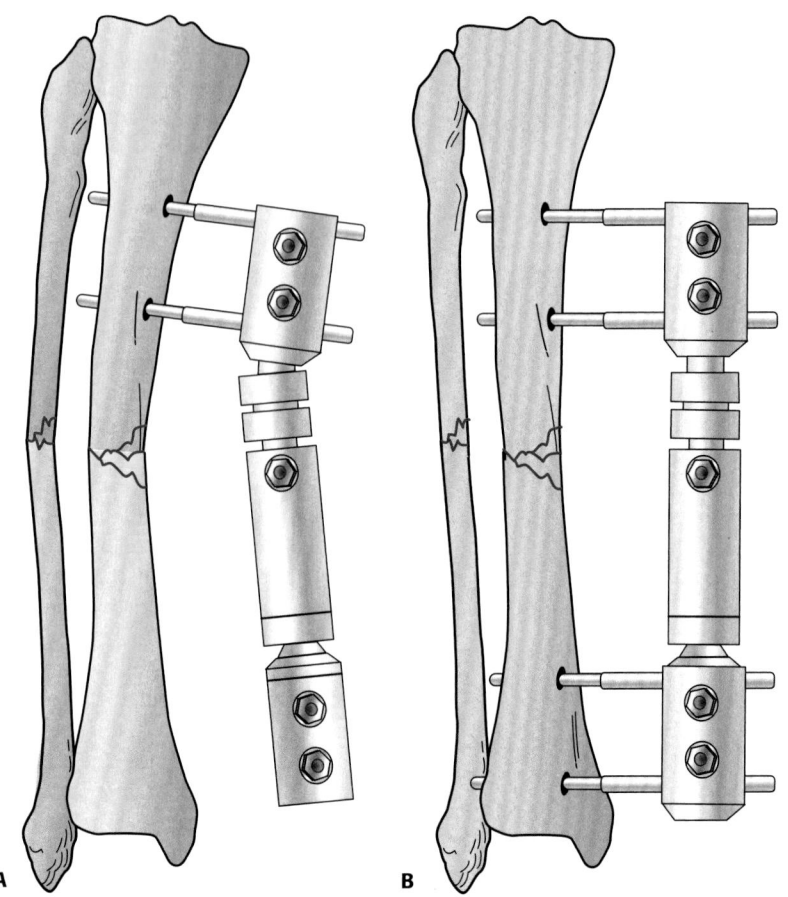

A   B

FIGURE 8-65 **A:** Monotube fixator allows rapid reduction and stabilization for complex tibia fractures. Fixed pin connectors act as templates to place proximal pins. **B:** Distal pins are then applied again through the distal pin clamp. The monotube allows for reduction in all three planes. Once reduction has been achieved the monotube is locked and reduction maintained.

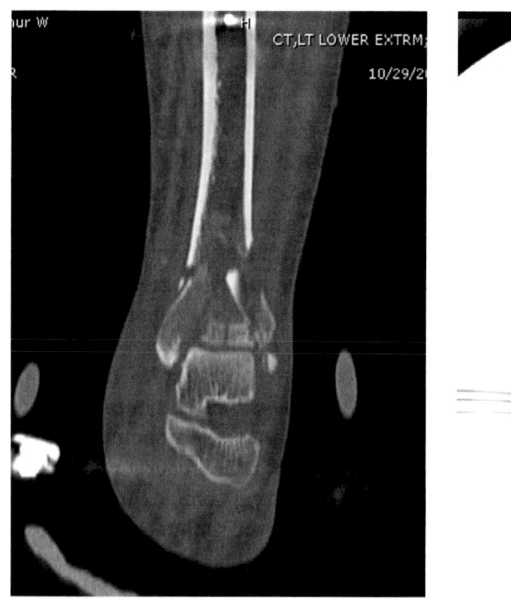

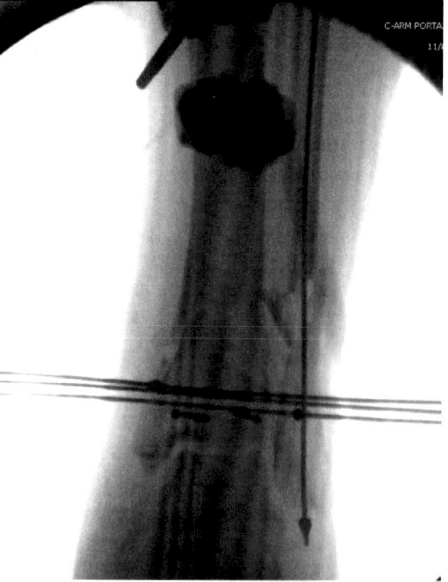

FIGURE 8-66 **A:** Comminuted pilon fracture with articular and metaphyseal involvement.

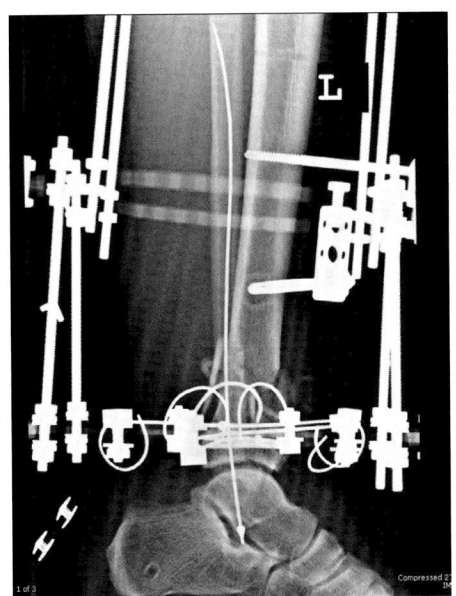
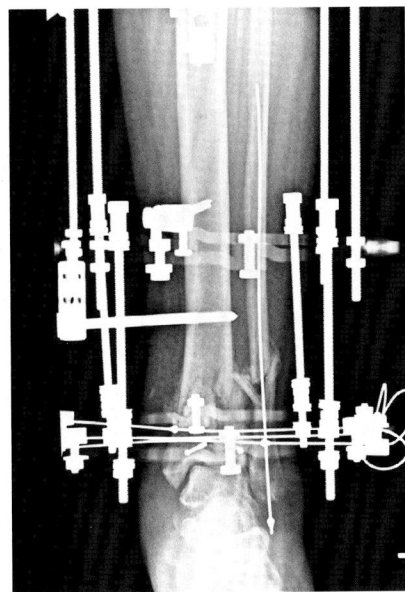
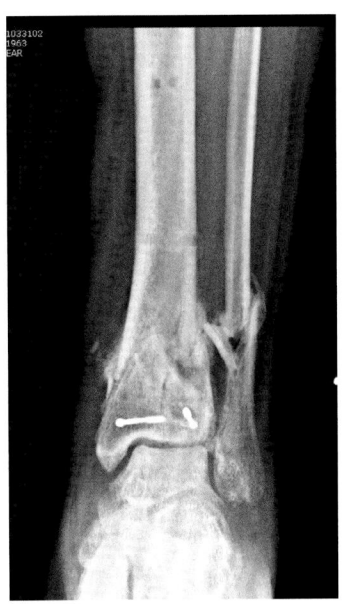

C, D   E

FIGURE 8-66 (*continued*) **B–D:** Distal ring construct using tensioned smooth and olive wires to stabilize small periarticular fracture fragments at the joint. The zone of injury is spanned with the proximal rings. **E:** Postframe with articular and metaphyseal healing noted.

When utilizing transfixion wires, care should be taken to avoid the proximal tibial capsular reflection and ankle joint capsule to avoid penetrating the capsule.[107,289,291] This maintains the wires in an extra-articular location and avoids secondary contamination of the joints which can result in knee or ankle sepsis (Fig. 8-67).

In certain situations a multiplane circular external fixator can be used to prevent further deformity while allowing weight bearing for a neglected diabetic ankle fracture. This technique may also be utilized for the management of complex diabetic ankle fractures that are prone to future complications and possible limb loss (Fig. 8-68).[70,91]

The treatment of tibial metaphyseal injuries has also included the use of monotube ankle bridging and simple

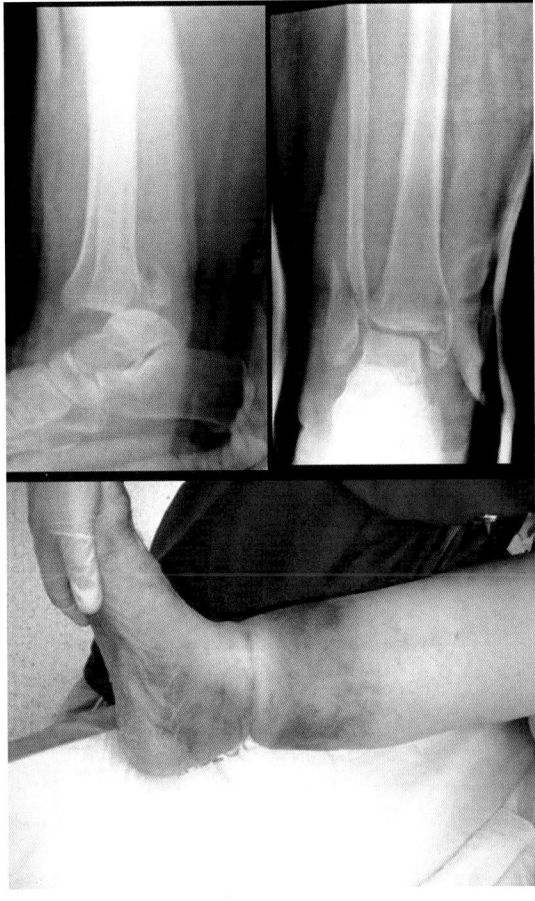

A

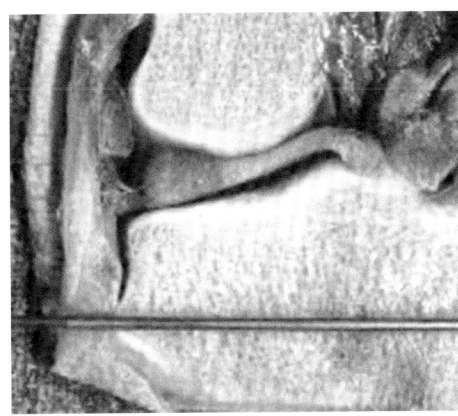

FIGURE 8-67 Anatomic specimen showing the capsular reflections around the knee joint. Care must be taken to avoid capsular penetration when placing periarticular wires around the knee. (Courtesy of Spence Reid, MD.)

FIGURE 8-68 **A:** Bimalleolar ankle fracture with poor soft tissues in a diabetic with early Charcot development. Reduction could not be maintained in a cast or splint.

(*continues*)

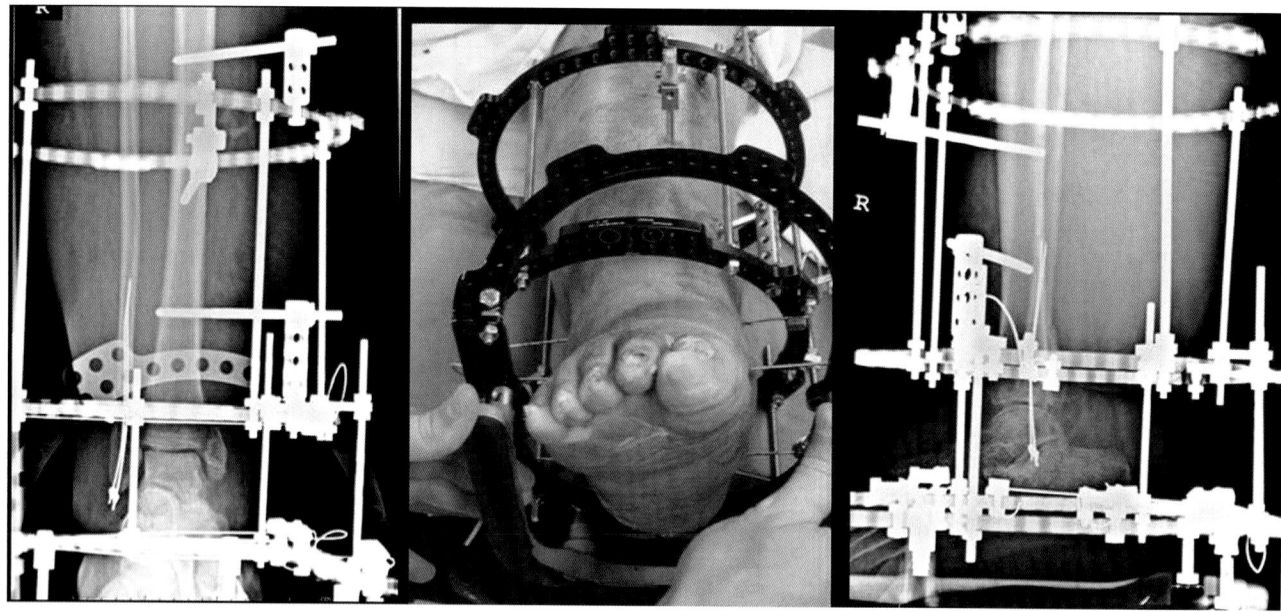

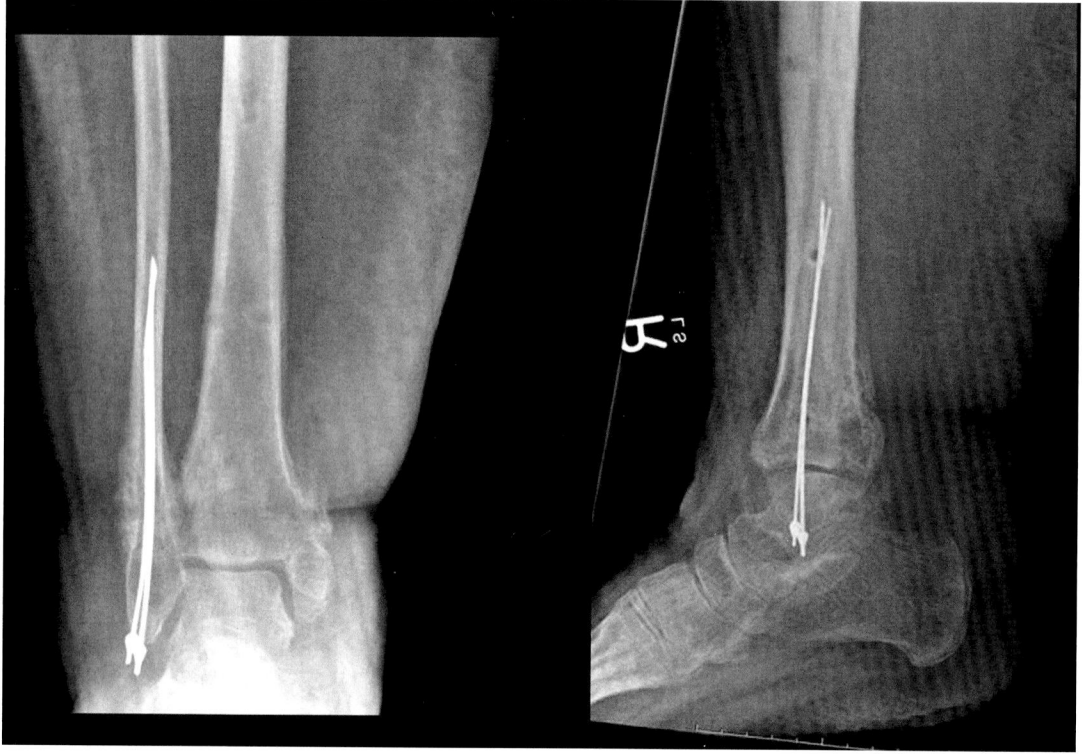

FIGURE 8-68 (*continued*) **B:** A circular frame was used in concert with percutaneous techniques to achieve reduction of the fractures and maintain stability while permitting weight bearing. **C:** Frame removed at 10 weeks with excellent joint congruency and ankle stability.

monolateral external fixator designs.[35,95] These are applied to achieve a distraction reduction across their respective joints, followed by limited ORIF (Figs. 8-69A,B). The advantage of using monotube constructs for either plateau or pilon fractures is that articular fixation is achieved and maintained without the use of small tensioned wires, and the potential for articular contamination is avoided (Fig. 8-69A).[236]

Bone Transport

Treatment of acute bone loss following severe tibial shaft fractures continues to be a complex reconstructive challenge. Many procedures have been devised to reconstitute bone stock, obtain fracture union, and provide a stable functional limb. Cancellous grafting whether placed directly into the defect or through

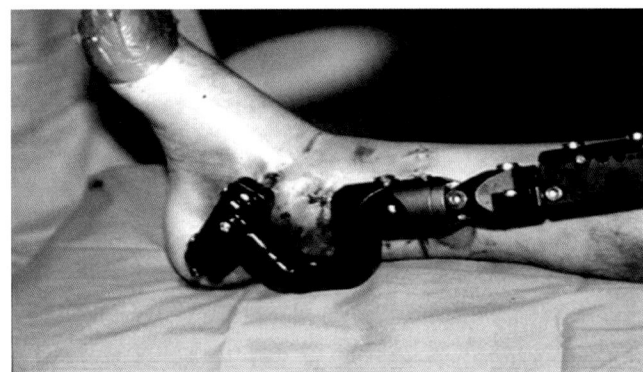
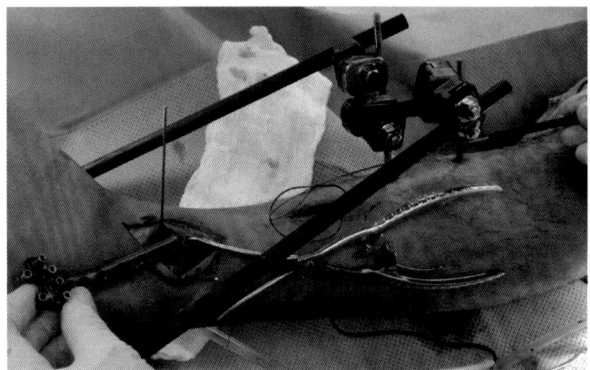

FIGURE 8-69 A: Monotube ankle bridging fixator used to provide distraction in combination with limited internal fixation for pilon fractures. **B:** Limited ORIF of a pilon fracture is carried out while a spanning fixator is in place maintaining the reduction during surgery.

a posterolateral approach has been the most common methodology; however, often, this technique requires numerous grafting procedures.[54,55,282] Fibular bypass, tibial fibular synostosis, ipsilateral direct fibular transfer, as well as free vascularized fibular transfer, have been used to reconstruct these large defects.[9,55,82,89] Internal bone transport has been developed as a primary method of bony reconstruction in acute tibial fractures with bone loss. This technique is indicated for reconstruction of defects greater than 4 cm.[17,55,69,119,140,148,220,252,295,298,299,302]

Bone transport can be carried out with a modified monotube monolateral fixator that has an intercalary sliding mechanism to transport the bone segment. Similarly, ring fixators can also be configured to perform successful intercalary bone transport.

The basic transport frame utilizing a ring fixator consists of three rings. A stable proximal and distal ring block is placed and at the level of the knee and ankle joints. A transport ring is placed in the midportion of the tibia. Orientation of the frame on the limb is crucial to ensure that the proposed docking site is aligned and will provide sufficient cortical contact for union to occur. Likewise, appropriate alignment utilizing a monotube construct is also critical to ensure docking site alignment. The intercalary transport component is attached to the bone using either transfixion wires or half-pin techniques. An antibiotic cement spacer is also placed across the defect. This block provides additional stability to the frame–bone construct and acts to maintain the transport space. This is very similar to the Masquelet technique allowing the development of a well-circumscribed soft tissue sleeve through which the transport segment can occur. The block remains in place until the final debridement, free flap procedure, or delayed primary closure of the wound (Figs. 8-70A–C).

At the time of definitive wound coverage, the antibiotic block spacer is removed and a solitary string of antibiotic cement beads is placed in the defect. The beads provide and maintain a "potential space" or fibrous tunnel through which the transport segment will travel. This space allows relative unencumbered movement of the transport segment underneath the flap. If no flap is needed, the wound is closed primarily and antibiotics beads are still used to maintain the potential space and prevent invagination of the intact soft tissue envelope

into the transport pathway (Figs. 8-70D–I).[118,119,140,258,298,299,302] In addition, this well-vascularized Masquelet-"like" transport sleeve facilitates the healing of the docking site.[281]

If soft tissue coverage is adequate then soft tissue transport in conjunction with the bone transport is possible.[55,69,138,139] Tissue loss that exposes bone is not amenable to combined soft tissue–bone transport without first addressing the exposed bone. This is accomplished through rotational or free tissue transfer. Alternatively, the bone should be resected until healthy soft tissue covers the bony segment.[198,250,298,299] At this time acute shortening or gradual shortening can be accomplished and the soft tissue defect allowed to heal without additional coverage procedures. Following soft tissue healing, lengthening or deformity correction can then be carried out through the use of the frame.

Transport is delayed for at least 3 weeks following free flap coverage. This allows for healing of the flap over the bony defect and neovascularization of the zone of injury. The delay also allows the free flap anastomosis site to become fully epithelialized which is then able to withstand the inevitable tension forces that it is subjected to during the bone transport process.[140] If no flap is utilized, corticotomy and transport can be undertaken immediately at the time of wound closure. The location of the transport Schanz pins should be in the inferior portion of the transport segment, so that it will "pull" the bone into docking position rather than "push" the transport segment, which occurs if the pins were located more proximally in the transport segment. This construct results in an unstable situation where the transport segment will have a tendency to deviate during transport.[118,119,140,299]

Following fixation of the transport segment, a proximal or distal corticotomy is performed. Following open tibial fractures, a wide zone of injury may be present and it is preferred that the corticotomy be performed away from this potentially compromised area. A latency period of 7 to 10 days is allowed prior to the initiation of transport. The initial rate of distraction begins slowly at 0.25 to 0.5 mm per day. A slower distraction rate is recommended initially because of the wide variability in injury patterns and vascularity of the limb. In more extensive fractures with a wide zone of injury, transport should be undertaken very slowly and only after the regenerate bone is visualized approximately

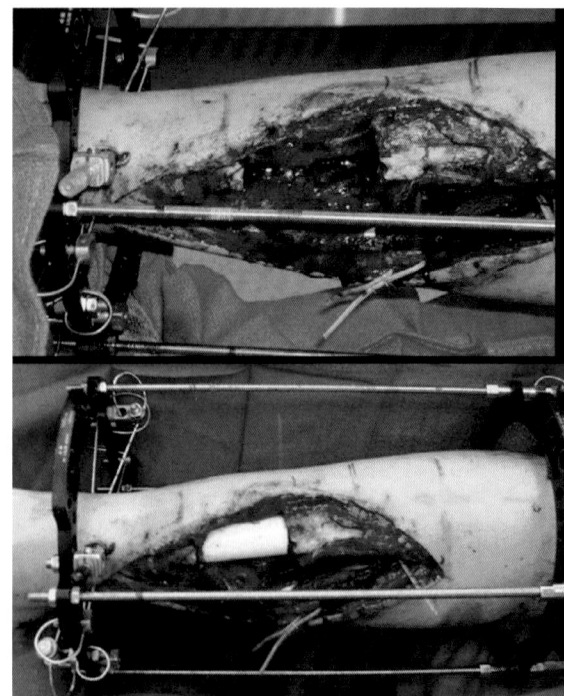
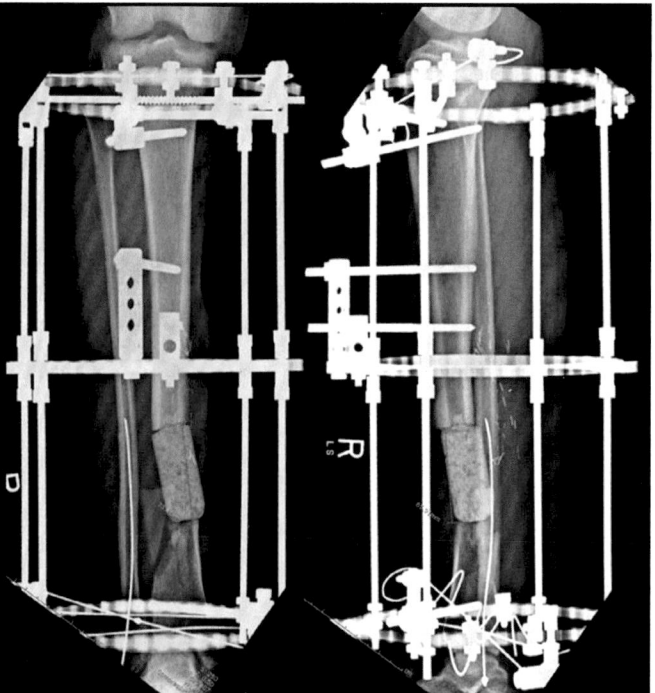
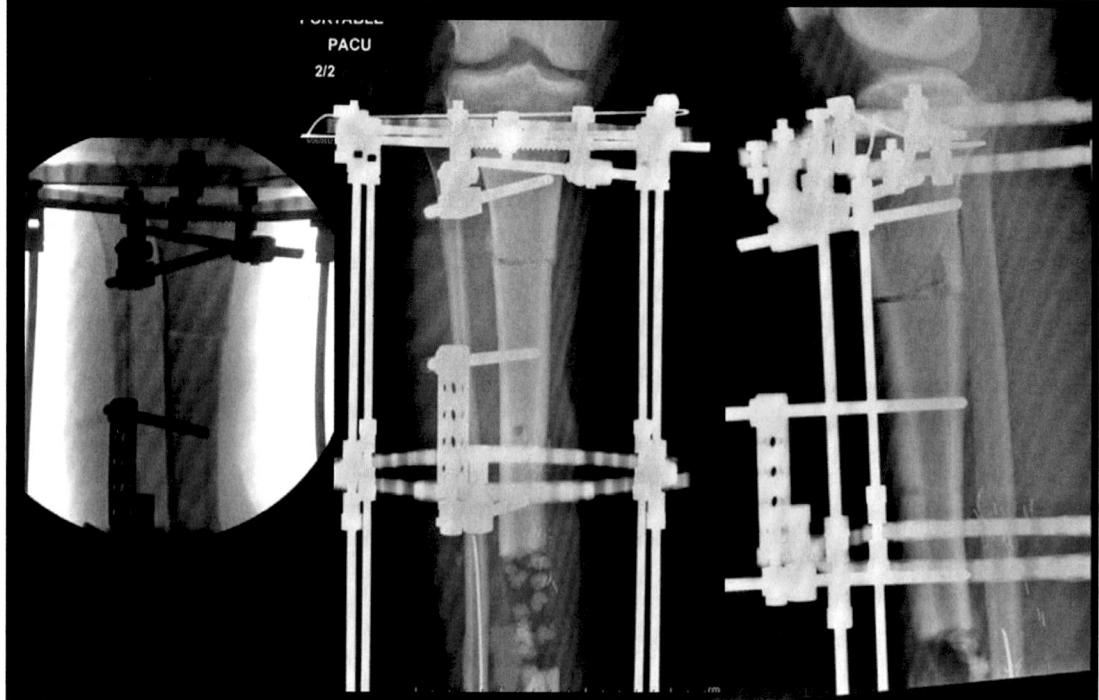

FIGURE 8-70 **A, B:** A transport frame spanning the segmental injury with the defect filled with an antibiotic spacer and the soft tissue deficiency treated with a free flap. The frame is attached to the bone using a combination of transfixion wires or half pins. **C:** Following flap maturation, the antibiotic spacer is removed and replaced with a small chain of antibiotic beads and a proximal corticotomy is performed.

2 to 3 weeks post corticotomy. The distraction rate can then be adjusted depending on the quality of the regenerative bone. Transport in the acute fracture proceeds at a much slower rate, 0.5 to 0.75 mm per day, as opposed to the standard rate of 1 mm a day typical for standard limb lengthening.

To decrease the transport distance, the limb can be shortened acutely at the time of frame application.[55,295,299,302] This shortening aids in soft tissue coverage by decreasing tension and gaps in the soft tissues. Shortening acutely can be accomplished safely for defects up to 3 to 4 cm in the tibia or humerus, and 5 to 7 cm in the femur. In some situations, it is advantageous to decrease the transport distance, and thus patient time, in the frame. Shortening aids in soft tissue coverage by decreasing tension and gaps in the open wound; this approach combined with vacuum-assisted closure (VAC) may allow wounds to be closed by delayed primary closure or healed by secondary intention or simple skin grafting. With this technique, one may avoid extensive free flap coverage.[55,69,138,139,209,254,295]

However, acute shortening greater than 4 cm is not recommended because of distortion of the neurovascular elements which results in the development of edema and inability of the musculotendinous units to function properly (Fig. 8-42).[295,299,302]

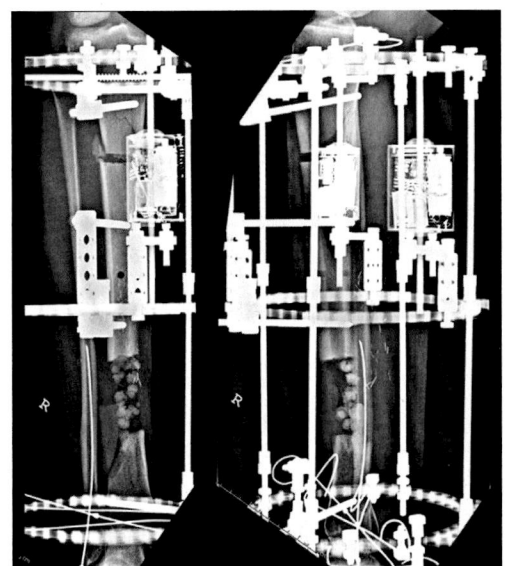
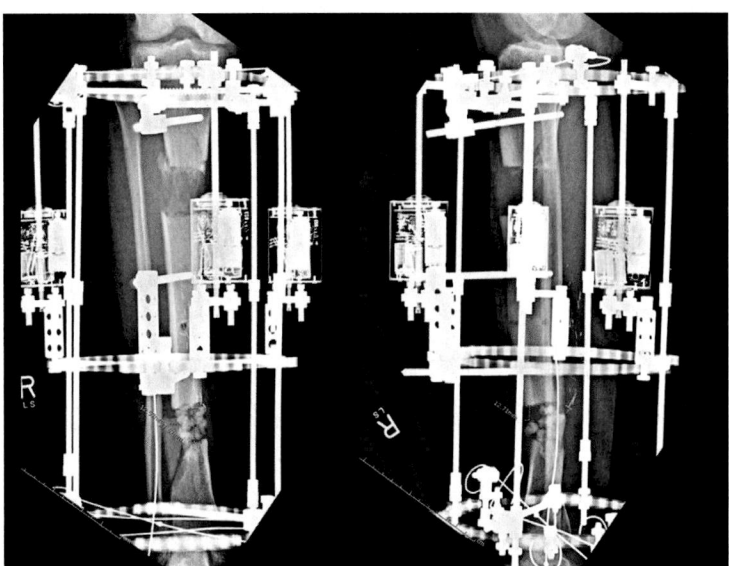
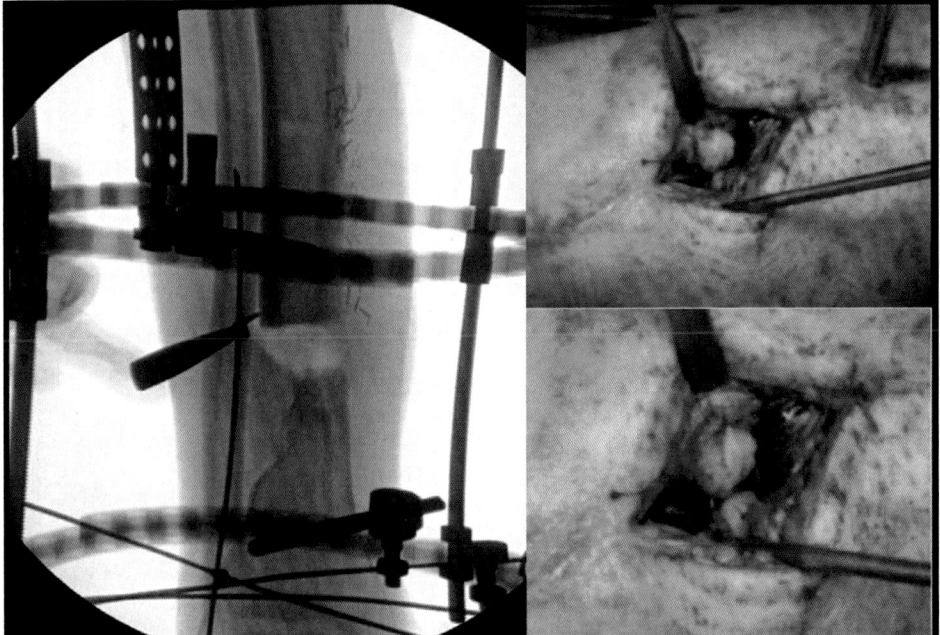

FIGURE 8-70 (continued) **D, E:** Transport is initiated using autodistractors. As distraction continues the docking site gradually shortens and compresses the beads. **F:** At near docking, the beads are removed and bone grafting to the docking site is carried out.

(continues)

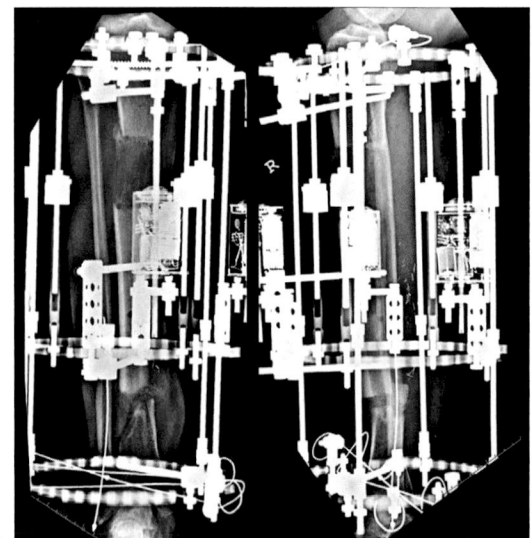
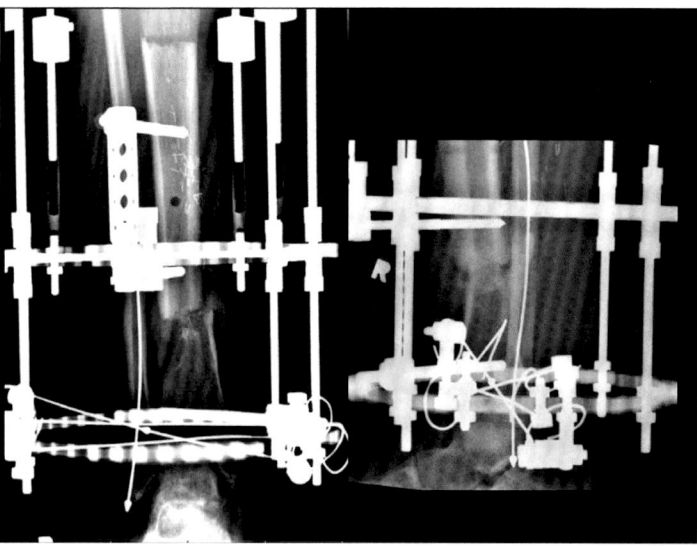

G

H

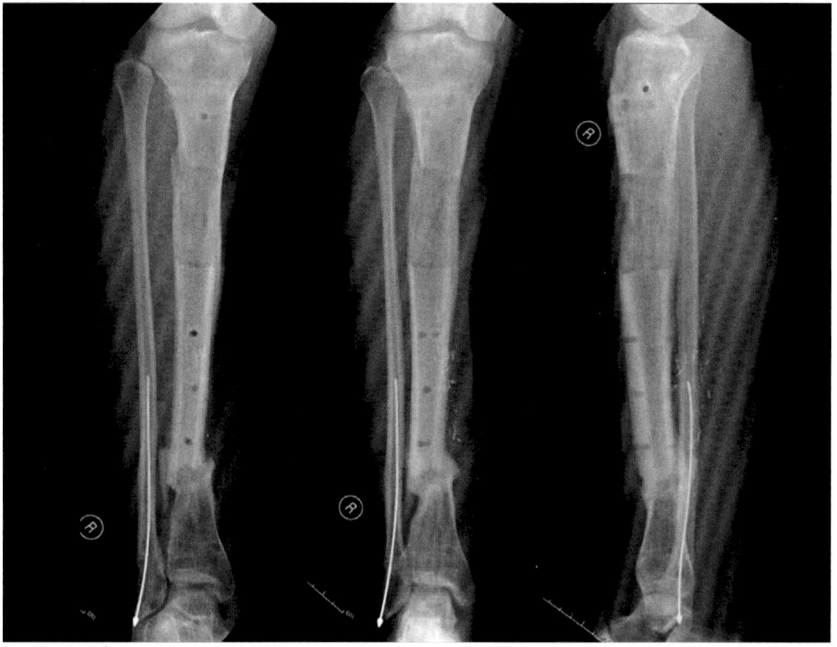

I

FIGURE 8-70 (*continued*) **G, H:** Transport is then continued, fully compressing the graft, achieving a stable docking site. **I:** The frame was successfully removed without docking site nonunion or late deformity of the regenerate.

Bone transport continues until the antibiotic beads have been compressed to the width of one bead. At this time, the patient is returned to surgery and the docking site exposed. The beads are removed and the bone ends freshened to achieve punctate bleeding surfaces. A high-speed burr can be used to fashion congruent surfaces on the ends of the proposed docking segments. This ensures maximal cortical contact and increases stability at the docking site. Autogenous iliac crest bone graft is placed directly into the docking site at this time and distal transport is resumed within 24 hours of the procedure (Figs. 8-70F–I).[55,118,119,295,298–300,302]

The docking site is impacted and gradually compressed 0.25 mm every 48 hours until the docking site is radiographically healed. Numerous authors have found that grafting the atro-phic docking site aids in the speed of union with a subsequent decrease in the overall time the patient must remain in the fixator.[55,118,119,295] Bone transport is a reliable technique; however, it is very time consuming and requires extreme patient compliance.

Other strategies have been developed to decrease the amount of fixator time the patient must undergo during these arduous reconstructions. Recently, bone segment transport for the treatment of large tibia bone defects was described by applying a locked bridge plate and transporting with a monolateral external fixation frame.[109] This technique allows correction of length and alignment, stabilizes the limb, and facilitates earlier frame removal. Rapid distraction is accomplished and once the defect has docked, the opportunity to additionally compress and stabilize the transported segment by additional nonlocking and/or locking screws through the plate is present. This technique has been modified to include rapid transport or lengthening of a limb segment and once the pathology has been corrected, insertion of a locked plate allows earlier removal of the external fixator during consolidation. Plate insertion is accomplished through a clean pin-free zone avoiding contamination, and before frame removal (Fig. 8-71).[125,142]

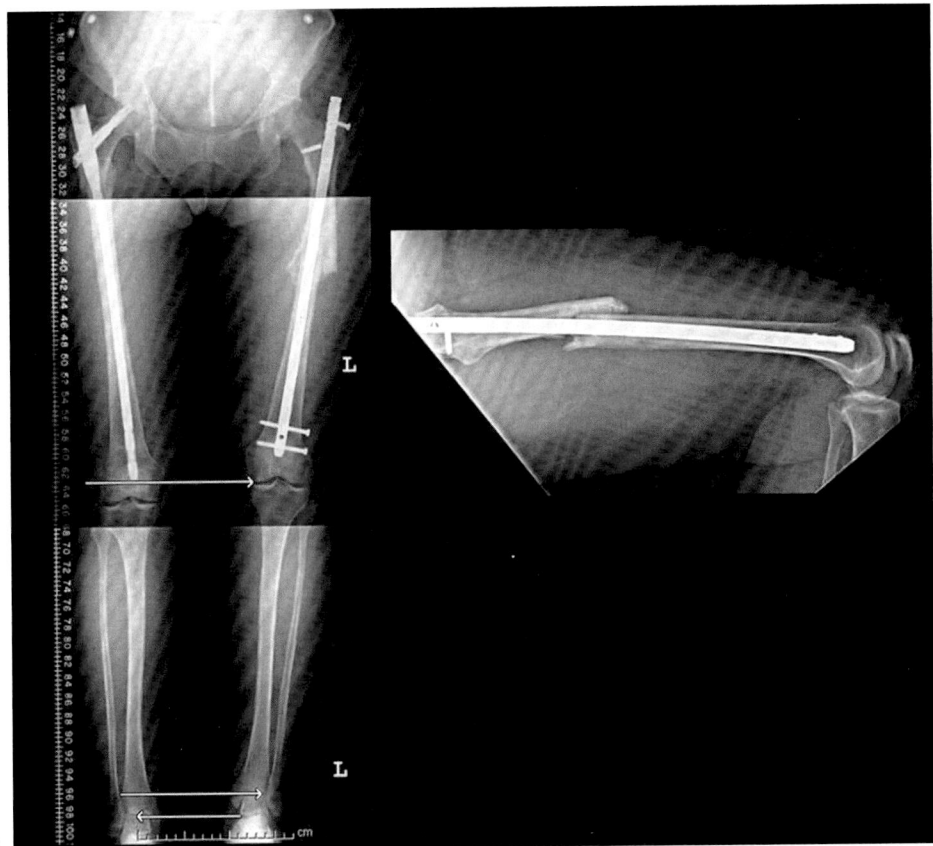

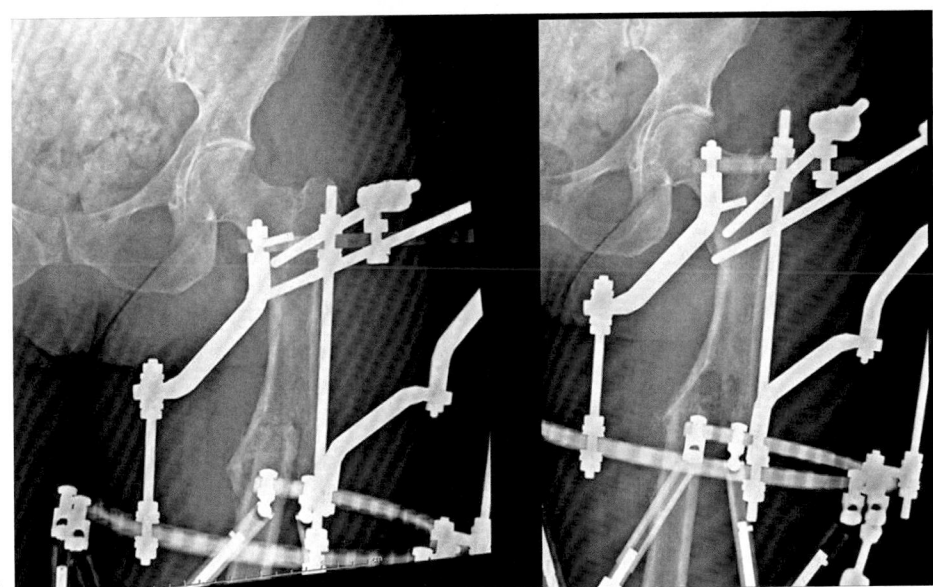

FIGURE 8-71 **A:** Bisphosphonate-related atypical femur fracture with resultant nonunion and 2 inches of shortening following locking screw failure. **B:** Gradual distraction is carried out following nail removal. Length was re-established slowly over 4 weeks.

(continues)

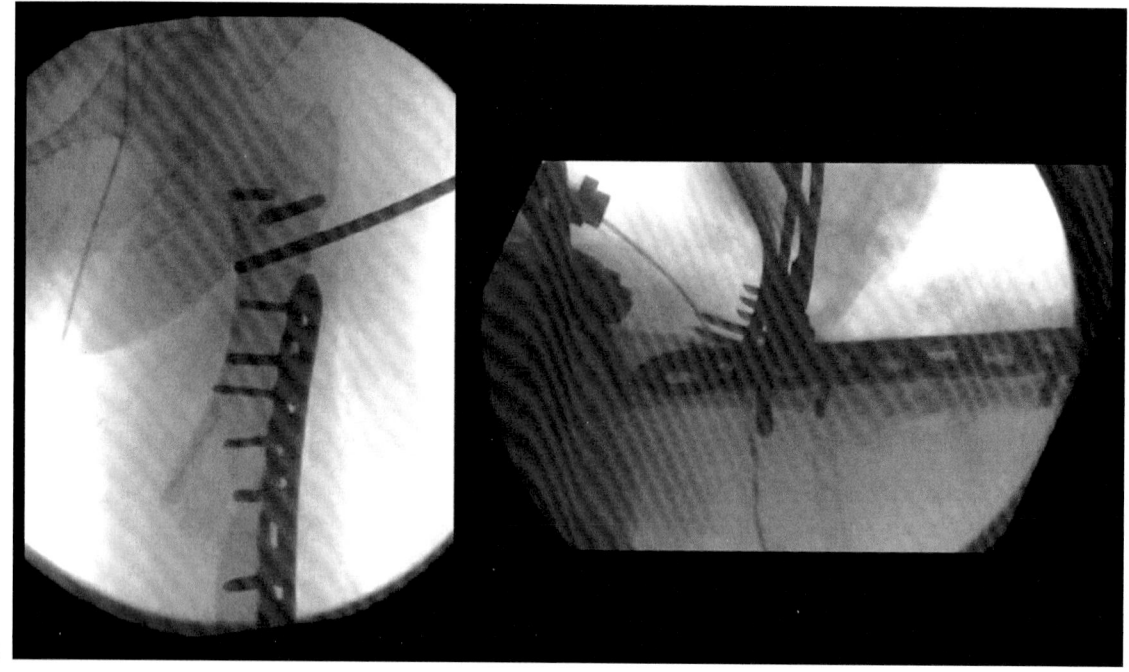

C

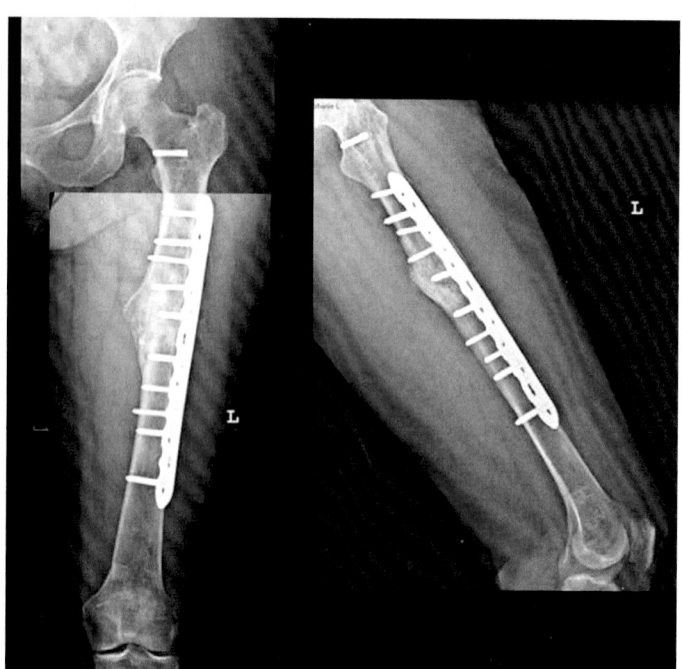

D

FIGURE 8-71 *(continued)* **C:** Percutaneous plating was carried out at the end of distraction (LOP [lengthening over plate]) and the frame is removed. **D:** Healed femur maintained at length with the plate.

Bone transport over intramedullary nails has also been employed for larger femoral and tibial defects.[213,240] The "monorail" technique is similar to transport over plates; however, the ability to compress the docking site is problematic and some authors have advocated applying a small compression plate to this area to avoid transport segment "rebound." This occurs when the transport segment retracts away from the docking site gradually once the distraction force has been removed. These hybrid transports using internal and external fixation combinations have limited applicability and published results are limited at best. Thus, use of these should be carried out with great caution and under ideal circum-stances. The combination of a circular fixator performing transport over a percutaneously applied locking plate demonstrates all the advantages that lengthening/transport over an intramedullary nail provides. However this technique eliminates the concern regarding deep infection that can occur in the medullary canal from the intramedullary nail. It also can be applied to virtually any bone in any age group of patients without any concern with regard to causing avascular necrosis, fat embolism, or physeal injury.[142] One should strictly adhere to the principles of transport which include a stable external fixation system above and below the defect, and a biologically sound wound at the transport location.

Hexapod Fixators

As external fixation devices and techniques have become more sophisticated, the ability to simultaneously correct a complex deformity with a simplistic device has become more attractive. The TSF was designed to allow simultaneous correction in six axes, that is, coronal angulation, translation, sagittal angulation and translation, rotation, and shortening. To achieve this with conventional frames a complex customized frame mounting would be required. In addition, the mounting of these traditional frames would be fairly difficult because of the fact that the rings need to be placed parallel to the respective reference joints, as well as perpendicular to the long axis of the limb. In cases of deformity or fracture, this can be very problematic. The hexapod-type frames allow the rings to be positioned in any orientation within their respective limb segment, that is, above the fracture site. It is not necessary that the rings be parallel with respect to joints or perpendicular to the long axis of the bones. This demanding technique has been vastly simplified using this six-axis "hexapod" concept.[262,263]

The hexapod is a ring fixator Ilizarov-type design with a configuration consisting of 6 distractors and 12 ball joints which allows for six degrees of freedom of bone fragment displacement. By adjusting the simple distractors, gradual three-dimensional corrections or acute reductions are possible without the need for complicated frame mechanisms.[263]

As a fixation device, it is unique in that deformity correction depends on the use of computer software. Once the rings are mounted, the deformity parameters are calculated with respect to angulation and translation, in both the coronal and sagittal planes. Additional information about rotational and axial malalignment is also entered. These deformity parameters are then placed into the software program along with the frame mounting parameters. The frame mounting parameters include data points such as height of the distance of the frame from the deformity or fracture site location. The overall length of the six struts is also a variable, which is entered into the software calculations. The program will then calculate the final strut lengths necessary to achieve a corrected limb alignment. In addition, daily strut adjustments can also be calculated to affect a very gradual correction over a specific time period that the surgeon wishes to achieve. The final alignment can be further adjusted using the same software applying similar deformity and strut parameters to the program.[249]

In the acute application, this frame allows emergent placement of a relatively simple frame. The frame can be attached using either transfixion wires or a minimum of three half pins on either side of the fracture. At this point, an approximate reduction can be achieved grossly at the time of surgery and the final reduction can be completed over a short period of time using the software program and gradual adjustment of the six struts (Figs. 8-72A,B). The hexapod frames and internet software offer the advantage of very accurate and precise control of multiple deformities without significant soft tissue dissection. A relatively straightforward and simple external device is applied to effect these corrections.

Studies now have documented the hexapod frames' ability to achieve gradual realignment of complex pediatric fractures, defor-

mities, and complex foot reconstruction procedures.[3,86,87,93,99,129,272] Traditional reconstructive surgical approaches involve large, open incisions to remove bone and the use of internal fixation to attempt to fuse dislocated joints. Such operations can result in shortening of the foot and/or incomplete deformity correction, fixation failure, incision healing problems, infection, and the long-term use of casts or braces. The ability to gradually reduce a chronically dislocated ankle or foot deformity in the setting of a severe diabetic and Charcot arthropathy without the need for extensive incisions is advantageous.[173] As extensive open reduction can frequently be contraindicated because of local skin conditions and contractures (Fig. 8-68).[173]

One can comprehensively approach tibial nonunions with the TSF. This is particularly useful in the setting of stiff hypertrophic nonunion, infection, bone loss, leg length discrepancy (LLD), and poor soft tissue envelope. Investigators have determined that previously infected nonunions have a higher risk of failure than noninfected cases, consistent with most studies on this topic.[238,239] What is unique is the hexapod frames' ability to resolve multiple deformities and restore leg length equality with a relatively simplistic frame application (Fig. 8-73).[92,251,254,263,290]

Correction of severe tibial deformity because of a nonunion of the tibia can be achieved by slow gradual correction, allowing the compromised tissues to adapt. Studies have demonstrated that patients with either a hypertrophic or oligotrophic nonunion of the tibia with deformity are the best candidates for TSF application. Similarly, patients with three-dimensional deformity and malunion can also be corrected through the use of select corticotomies and gradual distraction with a TSF.[251,254]

As noted previously in this chapter, acute shortening with a circular external fixator has been shown to be helpful in the treatment of open tibia fractures with simultaneous bone and soft tissue loss. This is especially true in cases of axial bone transport where longitudinal defects are closed by the soft tissue recruitment that accompanies the transport segment. However, in most cases the soft tissue defect considerably exceeds the bone loss and may require a concomitant soft tissue procedure. There are a number of potential difficulties with vascularized pedicle flaps and free tissue flaps, including anastomotic complications, partial flap necrosis, and flap failure in these cases. With the versatility of the TSF open fractures can be acutely deformed with regard to shortening and angulation to facilitate primary wound closure.[209] This limb distortion is temporary and does not require a concomitant soft tissue reconstructive procedure to achieve coverage (Figs. 8-72A,B). Once the wound is healed, the limb deformity and length are gradually corrected by distraction using the Direct Scheduler module of the web-based TSF software (Figs. 8-72C–E). A relatively simplistic (two-ring) frame has been described for the use of these techniques when treating complex tibial shaft fractures with concomitant soft tissue injuries.[6]

EXTERNAL FIXATOR FRAME MANAGEMENT

Secondary procedures are frequently required during treatment utilizing external fixators. These may include soft tissue

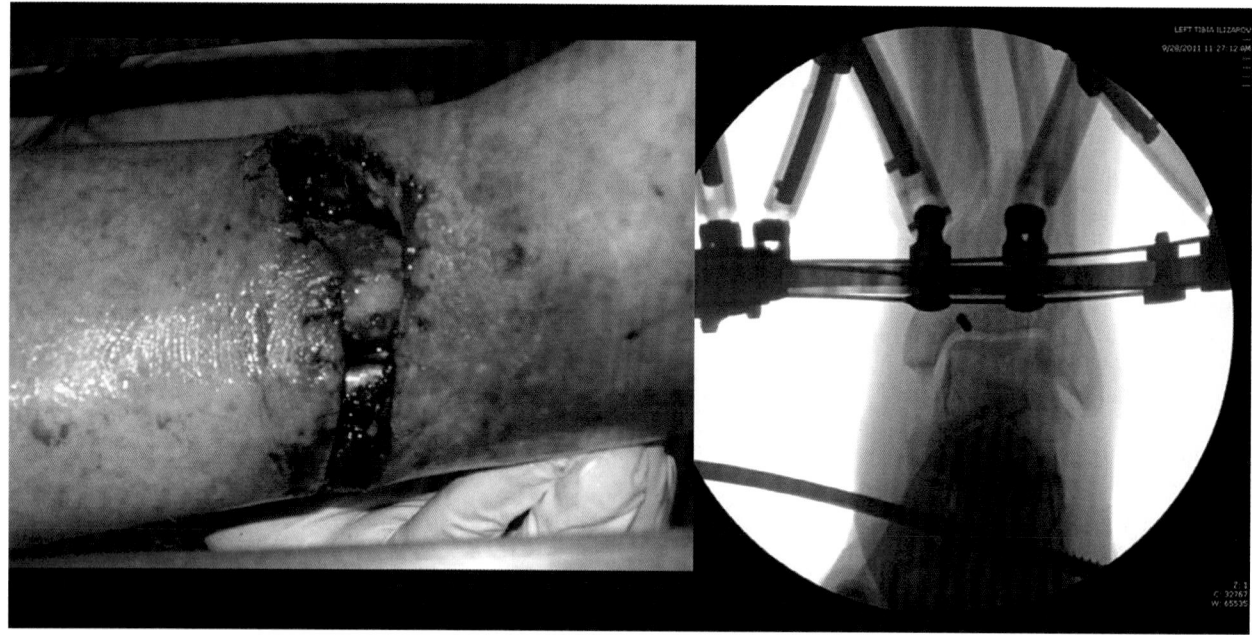

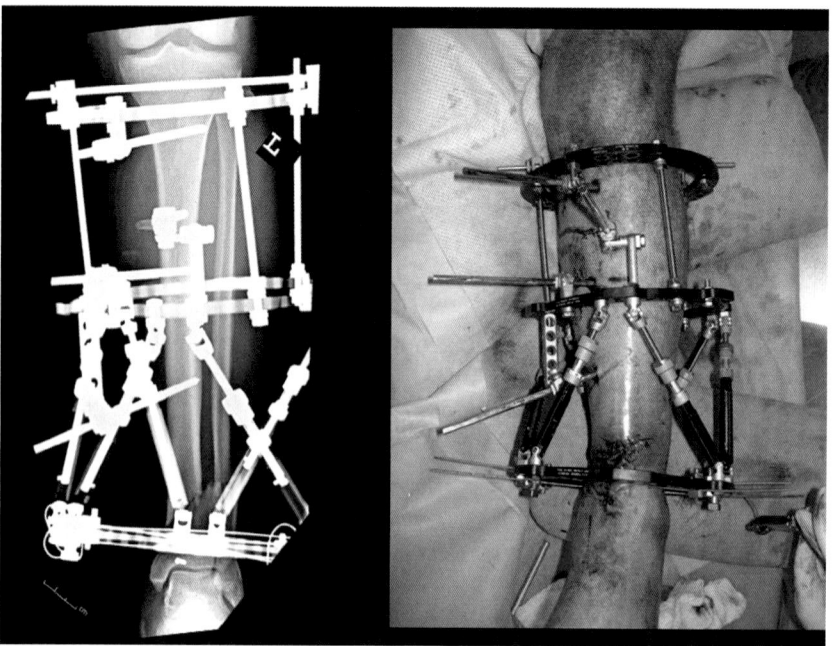

FIGURE 8-72 **A, B:** Complex open distal tibial fracture with large open wound potentially requiring free flap coverage. Acute management included conversion of the spanning fixator to a Taylor Spatial Frame, with intentional shortening and creation of varus deformity, to help achieve primary wound closure.

coverage procedures or delayed bone grafting. Most external fixator frames can be easily modified or placed out of the zone of injury. Most surgeons find it problematic to drape the fixator out of the operative field and maintain this unusually small area as sterile throughout an entire procedure. The benefits of safely prepping an external frame into the operative field include the ability to maintain reduction during secondary conversion procedures, and decreasing the time, material cost, and frustration of trying to drape a fixator safely out of the operative field. It has been shown that following a standardized protocol, including precleansing the external fixator frame, followed by an alcohol wash, sequential povidone-iodine prep, paint, and spray

with air drying followed by draping the extremity and fixator directly into the operative field, additional surgery can be safely performed without the risk of an increased rate of postoperative wound infection.[115,304] It is possible to perform free flaps and other soft tissue procedures directly around the external fixator pins as long as the pins do not communicate directly with the operative site.

Pin Insertion Technique

The integrity of the pin–bone interface is the critical link in the stability of the external fixation system. External fixation pins placed in cancellous metaphyseal bone frequently loosen with

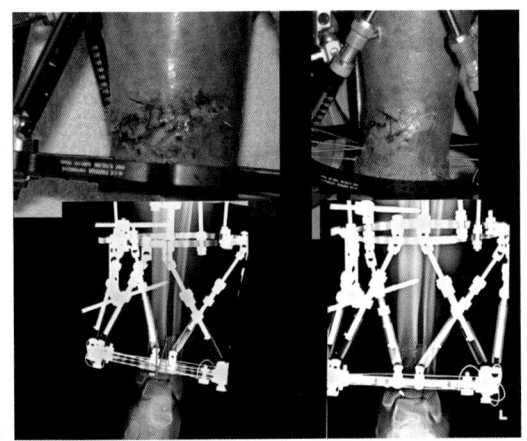
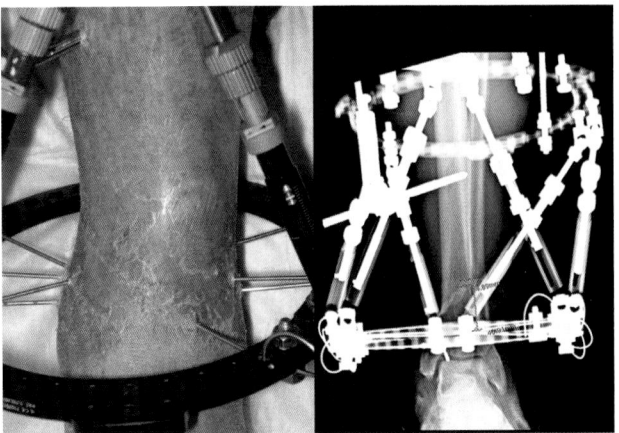

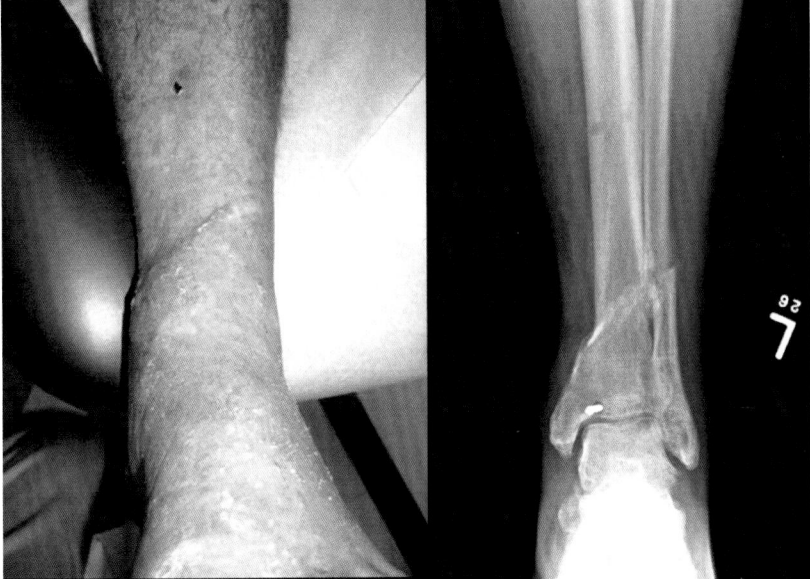

FIGURE 8-72 (*continued*) **C, D:** Once the wound has been stabilized, gradual correction of the induced deformity was gradually carried out. Complete healing of the wound is noted. **E:** Skin appears normal following frame removal and subsequent follow-up.

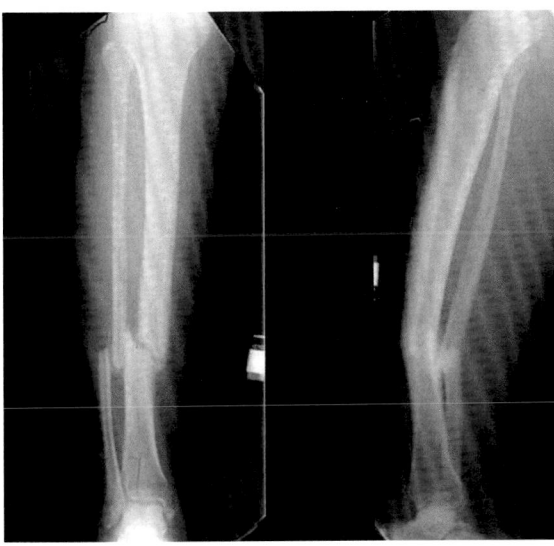
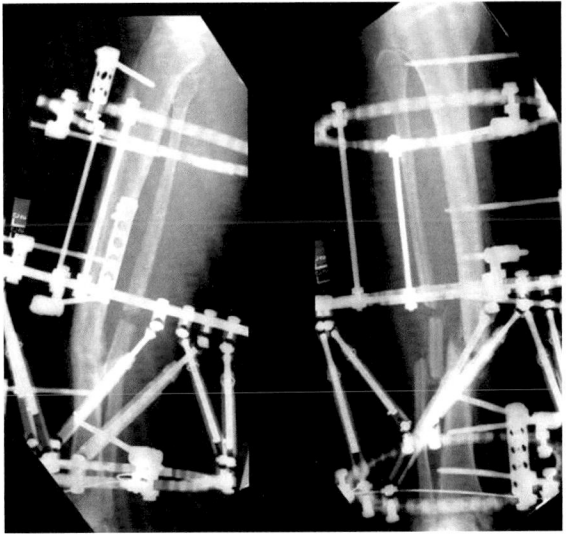

FIGURE 8-73 A: Complex tibial nonunion with malrotation, angulation, translation, and leg length discrepancy. **B:** Taylor Spatial Frame applied to limb using primarily half-pin attachments. Patient self-adjustment of the six oblique struts will gradually correct all deformity parameters.

(*continues*)

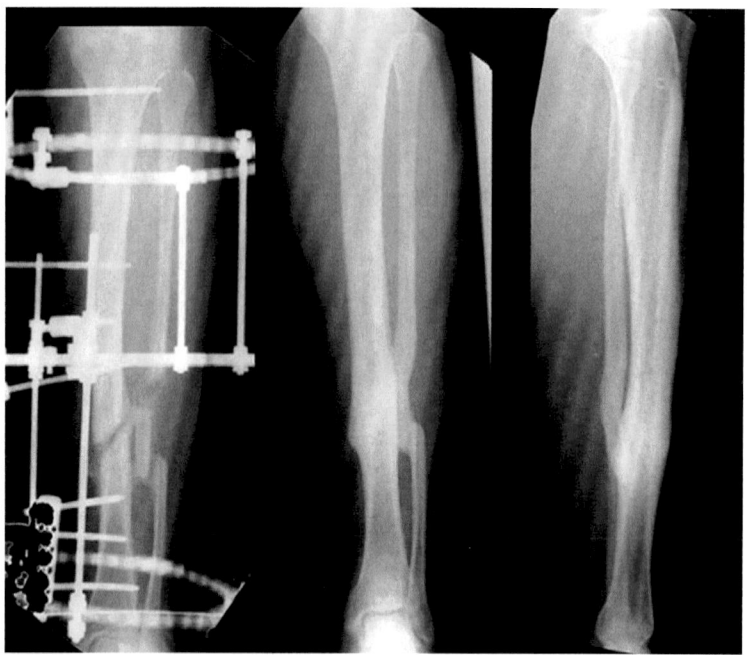

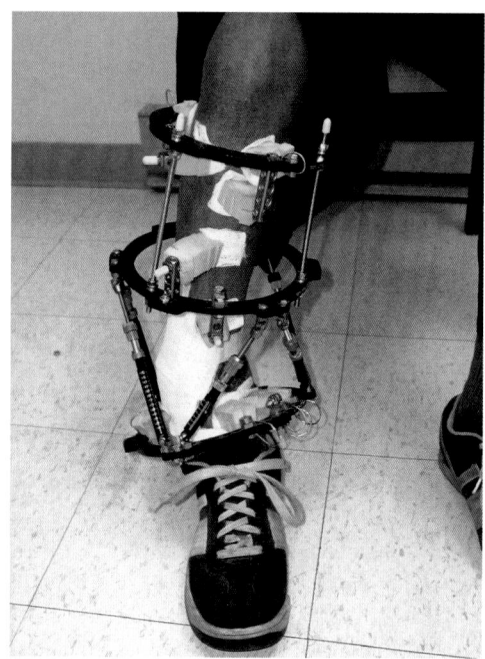

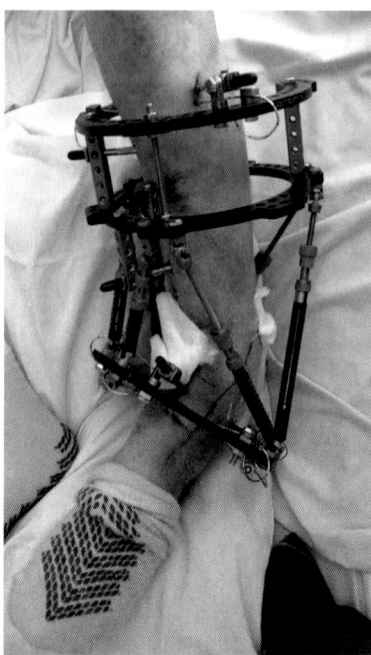

FIGURE 8-73 (*continued*) **C:** Complete realignment and consolidation via gradual distraction osteogenesis, no grafting was required to achieve these results. **D, E:** Clinical views of Taylor Spatial Frame applied to combined deformities, both consisting of varus, extension, lateral translation, and external rotation.

time resulting in fixation failure and increased risk for infection. The fixation pin in cortical/diaphyseal regions can remain intact and infection-free for extended periods of time. Thus each pin in the fixation construct should be continually evaluated for these potential problems to avoid an unstable fixator. The correct insertion technique involves incising the skin directly at the side of pin insertion. Following a generous incision, dissection is carried directly down to bone and the periosteum incised where anatomically feasible. A small Penfield-type elevator is used to gently reflect the periosteum off of the bone at the site of insertion. Extraneous soft tissue tethering and necrosis is avoided by minimizing soft tissue at the site of insertion. A trocar and drill

sleeve is advanced directly to bone, minimizing the amount of soft tissue entrapment that might be encountered during predrilling. The drill sleeve should be centered in the midportion of the medullary canal (Figs. 8-74A–D). One needs to ensure that the pin trajectory traverses the near cortex, then the medullary canal, and finally exits the far cortex. In this fashion a transcortical pin, which acts as a stress riser and can be a site of fracture once the frame has been removed, is avoided. A sleeve should also be used if a self-drilling pin is selected. Following predrilling, an appropriate size depth of pin is advanced to achieve bicortical purchase and any offending soft tissue tethering should be released with a small scalpel (Figs. 8-74D–I).[115]

Pin Care

There is no consensus in the literature as to the appropriate regimen for pin tract care and infection prevention. A recent intra-subject, randomized, prospective controlled trial comparing daily pin tract care with no pin tract care was undertaken. Outcome measures evaluated in this study included the pin/skin soft tissue interface integrity, stability of the pins including torsional stability as determined with a torque meter, presence of radiographic pin site osteolysis and presence of pin site pain. There were no statically significant differences between the two groups (pin care to no pin care) when comparing granulation tissue and pin site drainage (36% vs. 35%), pin stability (20 vs. 25 pins with loosening), osteolysis (7 vs. 6 pins), or torque on extraction (mean 0.75 Nm and maximum 3.05 Nm vs. mean 0.6 Nm and maximum

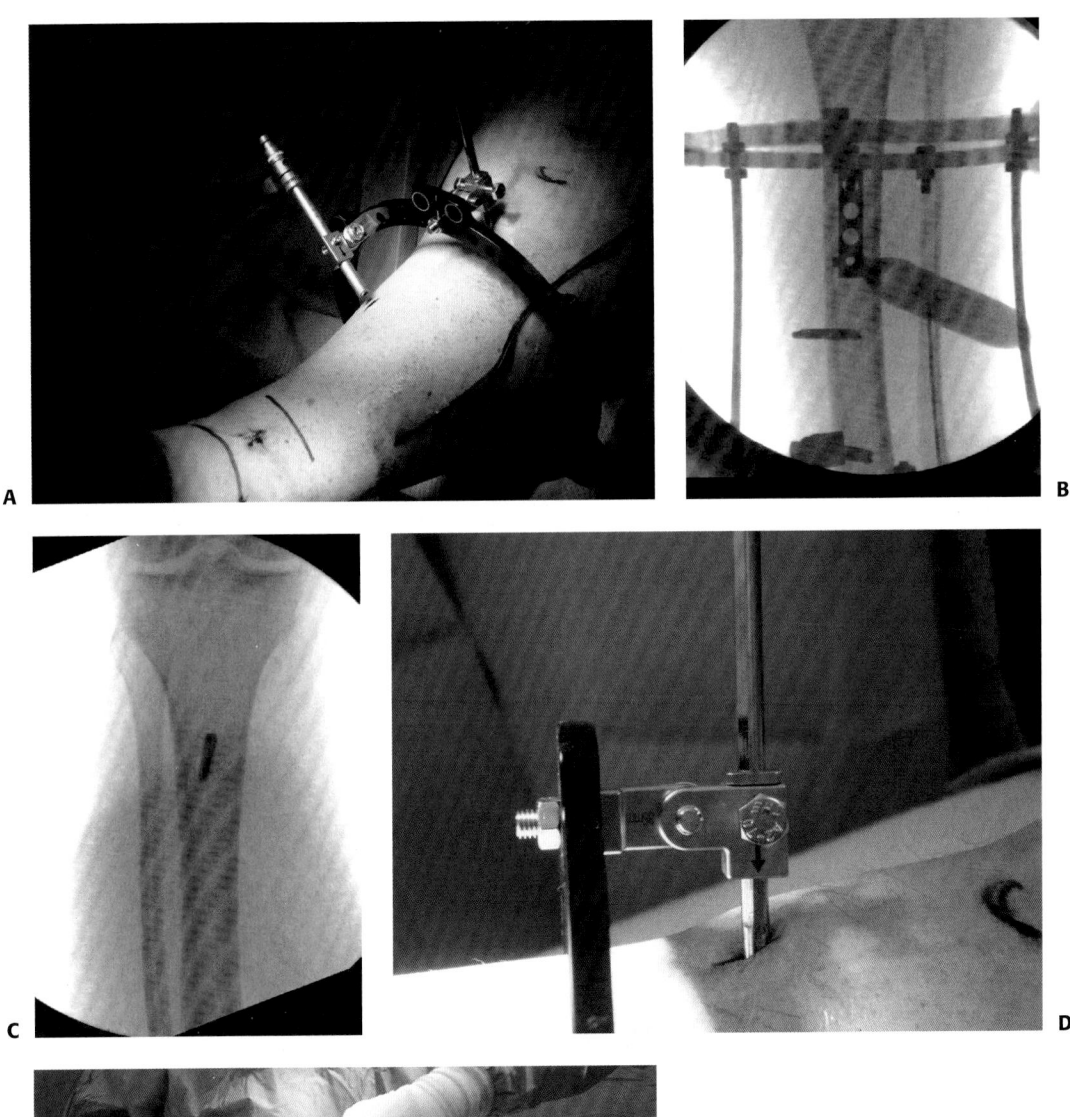

FIGURE 8-74 **A, B:** A trocar and drill sleeve is centered on the bone under fluroscopic control to ensure that the pin is not eccentrically located and traverses both cortices as well as bisects the medullary canal. **C:** The pin must engage the posterior cortex and be central in the bone to avoid postframe stress fracture through an errant transcortical pin tract. Note the central location of the diaphyseal pin. **D, E:** Following pin insertion there is some degree of soft tissue tethering. Because of this tissue encroachment, hand placement of the pins with a "T" handle limits any soft tissue damage during pin insertion.

(continues)

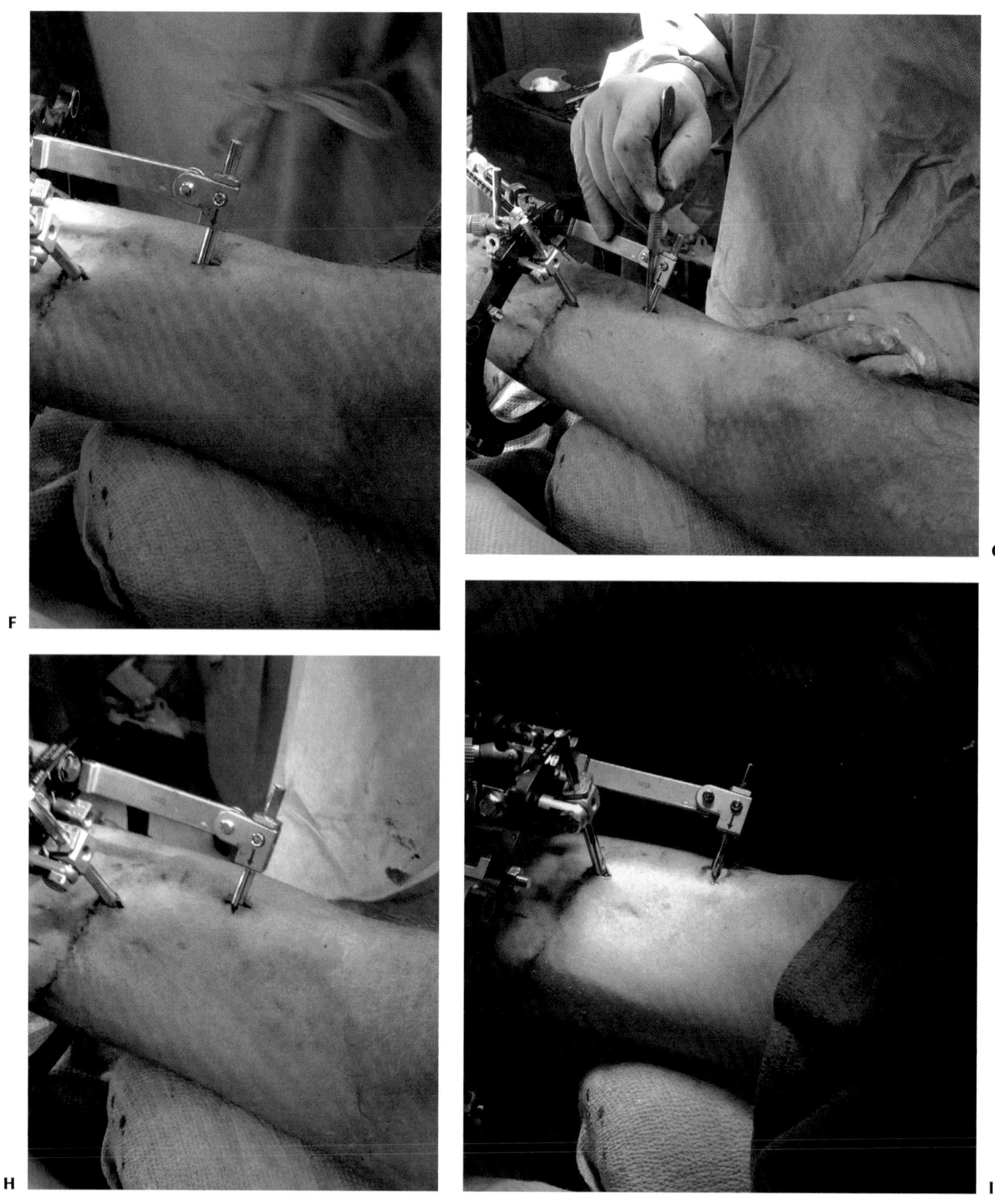

FIGURE 8-74 (*continued*) **F, G:** The skin can be released using a no. 11 blade scalpel. **H, I:** The tethering is relieved and a small suture can be used to loosely reapproximate the skin.

3.55 Nm). This study suggested that specific routine pin tract care is unnecessary as long as daily hygiene for the patient and frame is maintained.[46] Thus a universal standard for pin care has yet to be identified. Pin site recommendations are based more often on clinical preference rather than strict research findings.[94] It should be noted that correct pin site insertion technique removes most of the factors that cause pin site infection and subsequent pin loosening.[8,115,222] If appropriate insertion technique is utilized, the pin sites will completely heal around each individual pin, much like a pierced earring insertion site heals. Once healed, only showering without any other pin cleaning procedures is necessary.[307] The occasional removal of a serous crust around the pins using dilute hydrogen peroxide and saline may be beneficial.[28,112,116]

In general, recommendations include using normal saline as the cleansing agent in concert with dilute hydrogen peroxide.[112,116] A review of the Cochrane database with regard to the most effective pin care regime was performed, and all randomized controlled trials (RCTs) comparing the effect on infection and other complication rates of different methods of cleansing or dressing orthopedic percutaneous pin sites were evaluated. Three trials compared a cleansing regimen with no cleansing, two trials compared cleansing solutions, one trial compared identical pin site care performed daily or weekly, and four trials compared dressings. One of these trials reported that infection rates were lower (9%) with a regimen that included cleansing with half-strength hydrogen peroxide and application of Xeroform dressing when compared with other regimens.[180] Additional studies have recommended the use of polyhexamethylene biguanide, silver sulfadiazine, or 10% polyvinylpyrrolidone iodine (Polyod)-impregnated gauze pin wraps to reduce the risk of pin tract infection compared with pin gauze wraps soaked in normal saline.[58,65,176,320] However, the authors agree with the conclusions of other investigators that there is insufficient evidence for a single particular strategy of pin site care which minimizes infection rates.[85,180] Ointments are not recommended for postcleansing care, as these tend to inhibit the normal skin flora and can lead to superinfection or pin site colonization.[189] It is important to remove the buildup of crusted material, which will tend to stiffen the pin–skin interface and increase shear forces at the pin–bone interface (Fig. 8-75A). This leads to the development of additional necrotic tissues and fluid buildup around the pin.[58] Immediate postoperative compressive dressing should be applied to the pin sites to stabilize the pin–skin interface and thus minimize pin–skin motion, which can lead to additional necrotic debris. By "training" the skin, the pin site remains stable.[140] This allows the skin to heal around the pin undisturbed. Compressive dressings can be removed within 10 days to 2 weeks' time once the pin sites are healed (Figs. 8-75B,C). If pin drainage does develop, then providing pin care three times per day should be undertaken. This may also involve rewrapping and compressing the offending pin site in an effort to minimize the abnormal pin–skin motion (Figs. 8-12A, 8-75B,C).[140]

Review of large pin site registries has documented a significant difference in the rates of pin tract infection between large Schanz half pins and small transfixion wires. For acute fracture fixation fixators, patients with hybrid external fixators demonstrated a similar risk of pin tract infection as patients who had unilateral fixators. The infection rate in the ring fixator (using small transfixion wires) group was significantly lower than the hybrid external and unilateral fixator groups (using primarily Schanz half pins).[222] Pin registries evaluating the rates of pin tract infection for limb-lengthening procedures demonstrated similar results. The rate of half-pin site infection was significantly ($p < 0.05$) higher in half-pin fixators (100%) compared with hybrid fixators (78%) where a combination of thin wire and half pins was used. When half pins were compared exclusively with thin wires, a significantly ($p < 0.05$) higher incidence of half-pin site infection (78%) over fine-wire site infection (33%) was revealed.[8] These findings highlight the need to insert half pins with correct technique (as described above) to avoid excessive soft tissue impingement, incarceration, or development of necrotic tissue at the site of half-pin insertion. In general, it appears that a simple, inexpensive, and patient-friendly plan of pin site care is equal to more complex or costly plans.

Frame Removal

Definitive treatment with an external fixator demands close scrutiny of radiographs to ensure that the fracture or distraction site has completely healed prior to frame removal. Numerous authors have described various techniques including CT scans, ultrasound, and bone densitometry to determine the adequacy of fracture healing.[16,17,140] In general, the patient should be fully weight bearing with a minimal amount of pain noted at the fracture site. The frame should be fully dynamized such that the load is being borne by the patient's limb rather than by the external fixator (Fig. 8-76). For distraction osteogenesis, radiographs are visualized in the AP and lateral plane. It is necessary to see three out of four neocortices in the regenerate zone reconstituted to ensure that the bone is mechanically stable and able to tolerate frame removal (Fig. 8-77).[15,17,118,119] Late deformity following frame removal is very common and usually is the result of incomplete healing of the distraction regenerate.[140] In the tibia, this is because the subcutaneous border anteriorly has the least amount of soft tissue coverage, and thus, blood supply. However, mechanical stability requires only three out of four reconstituted cortices. With standard external fixation techniques, similar precautions should be adhered to in order to avoid refracture or the development of nonunion. Multiple x-ray views of the extremity should be obtained to determine the adequacy of fracture healing prior to frame removal. Out of plane ununited fracture lines may be present and may be overlooked if only orthogonal AP and lateral x-rays are obtained to confirm fracture healing. Oblique views should also be obtained in addition to standard views to help identify any residual fracture gaps.

Ease of frame removal in an outpatient or office setting is variable depending upon the type of fixator pins utilized. A study evaluated the ability to remove stainless steel pin fixators in the office setting without anesthesia. Removal of these particular external fixators without anesthesia was well tolerated by the great majority of patients. Inflammation at pin sites was associated with a higher degree of discomfort during external fixator removal. Despite the higher pain score, most patients with pin site inflammation report that they would repeat the procedure

(text continues on page 298)

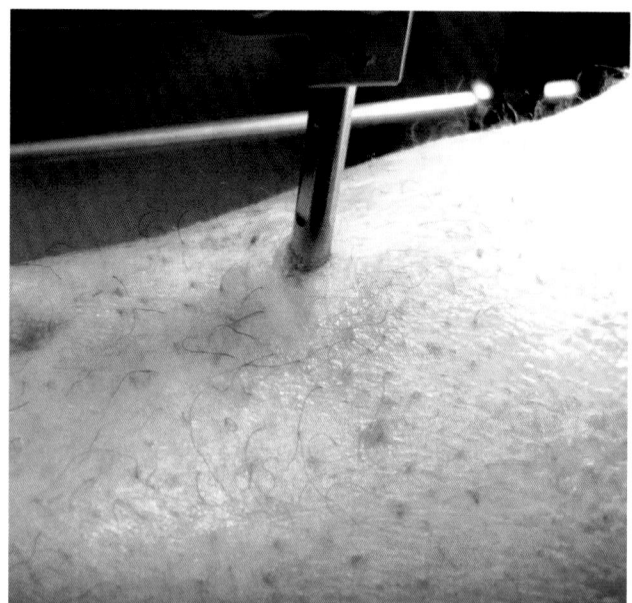

A

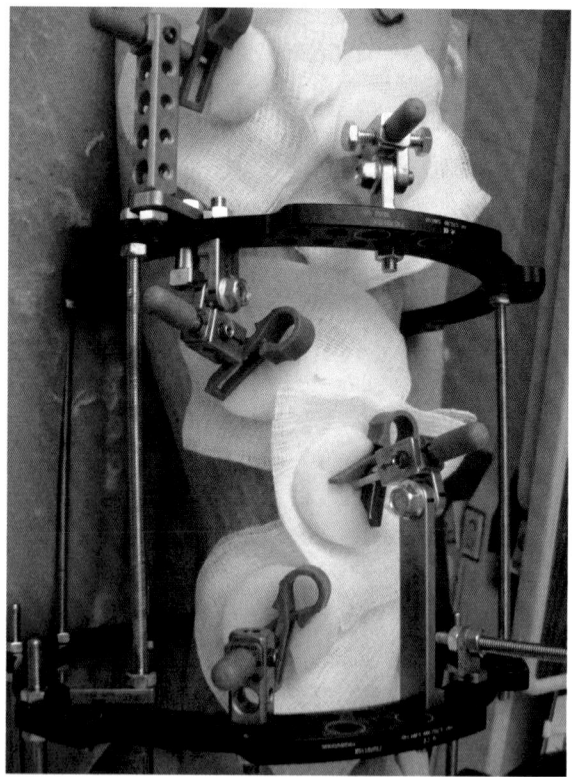

B

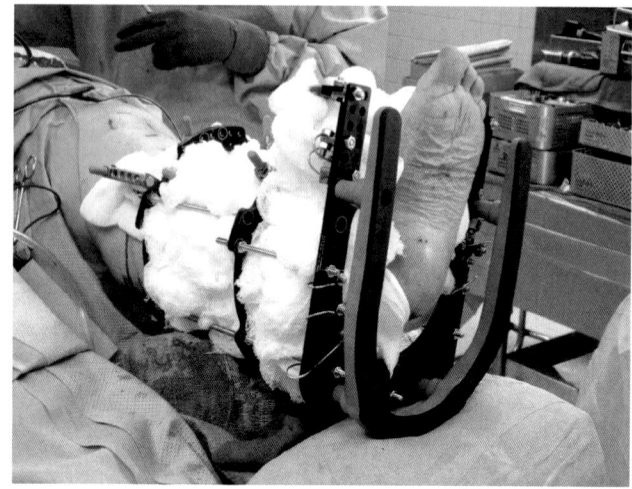

C

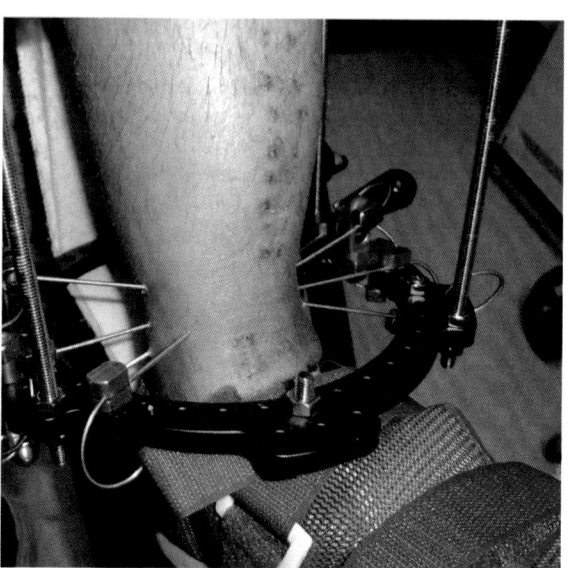

D

FIGURE 8-75 A: Whereas the pin sites are healing, serous fluid exudes at the pin site and develops crusting which should be removed with mild peroxide or mild soap and water. **B:** The pin–skin interface should be compressed and stabilized to minimize motion and subsequent development of any necrotic material. Gauze wraps around the pins or pin sponges can be used to provide stabilization following pin site healing. **C:** Immediate postoperative dressings should include compressive dressings around all pins to compress and stabilize the pin–skin interface. **D:** Healed pin sites require no special care other than mild soap and water. No ointments or antiseptics are required for the maintenance of a healed/sealed pin site.

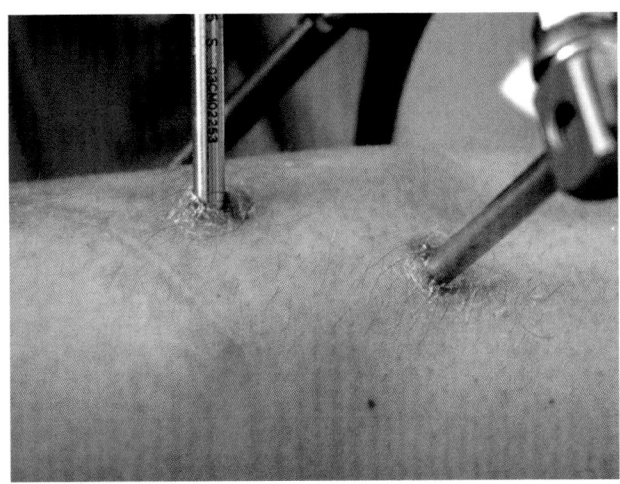

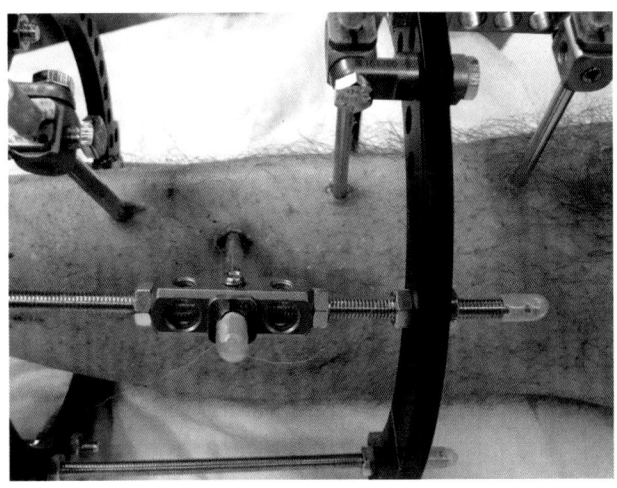

E   F

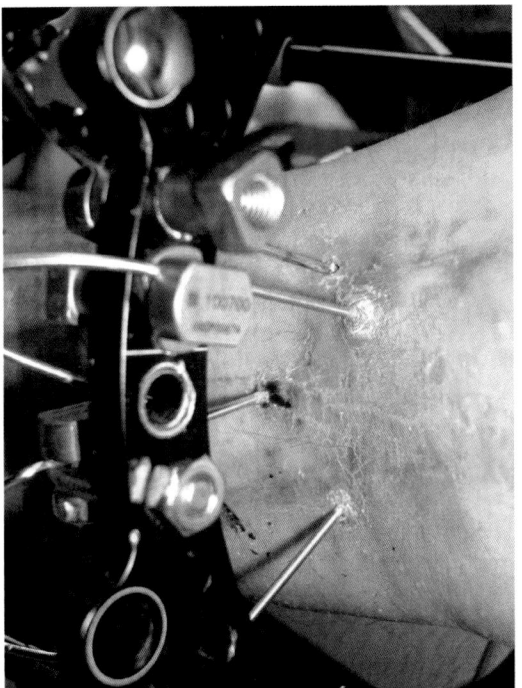

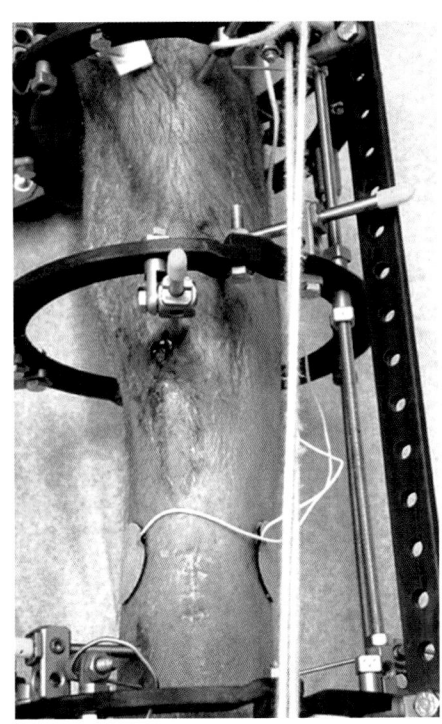

G   H

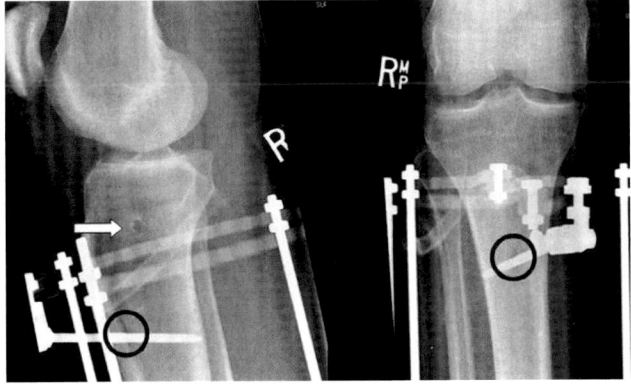

I

FIGURE 8-75 (*continued*) **E:** A mildly inflamed pin site with serous type discharge. At long term, these pins can develop painful hypertrophic keratosis surrounding the pin sites and should be excised at the time of pin removal. **F, G:** Grade IV pin tract infection with seropurulent drainage and redness requires vigorous pin care and antibiotics. **H:** Grade V pin tract infection with surrounding erythema, inflammation, and purulent drainage. Radiographs of this region must be examined for radiographic signs, suggestive of pin loosening. **I:** Radiographic evidence of pin sepsis and loosening includes pin sequestrum (*white arrow*) and cortical lucencies (*black circle*).

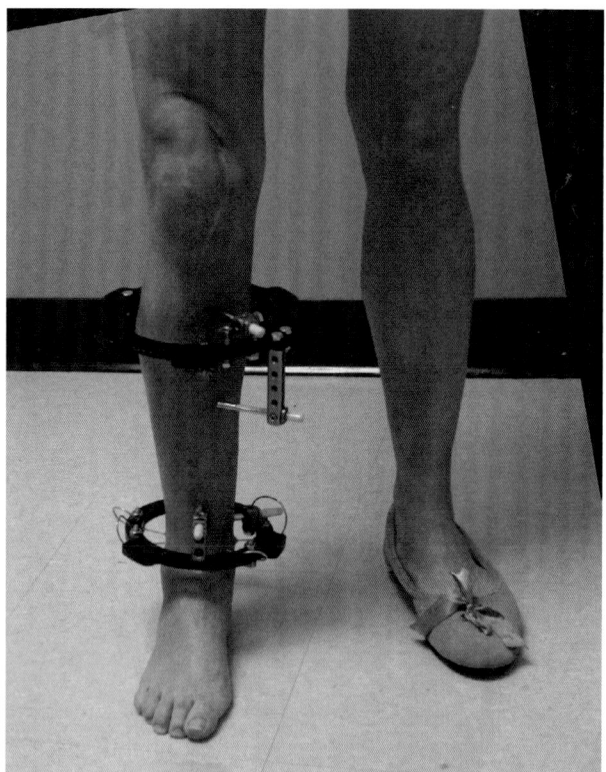

FIGURE 8-76 Prior to frame removal all the connecting rods were removed and only the rings remain. The frame has been fully dynamized and the patient allowed to ambulate full weight bearing. The patient is instructed to be aware of any signs of pain or deformity which would indicate incomplete healing. If this occurs, the connecting bars can easily be reapplied and the frame not removed at this time.

without anesthesia.[255] This study confirms the concept that stainless steel pins are usually easily removed; however, newer pin designs including titanium pins, as well as HA-coated pins are more problematic. With the biologic ingrowth nature of these biomaterials, pin removal is often difficult requiring sufficient force to loosen (break) the intact pin–bone interface. This may inflict a significant amount of pain which may preclude this procedure occurring in an office setting.[202,206,256] In patients whose treatment time has been prolonged, there is often a large overgrowth of heterotopic pin keratosis which has built up around the pin sites. This can leave an unsightly painful scar if not removed, and therefore should be excised at the time of pin removal (Fig. 8-78).

Frame Reuse

In this era of cost containment for health care, the practice of recycling external fixator components makes economic sense. Dirschl and Smith reported on a single center's experience with a reuse program. Components in good repair were returned to the operating room stock for reuse, whereas those showing signs of wear were discarded. No component was used more than three times. The institution charged patients a "loaner fee" equal to the hospital's cost for the inspection, processing, and recycling of fixator components. The mean hospital cost for a fixator decreased 34% as a result of this program. There were no differences in the rates of reoperation or complications before and after institution of the reuse program. No patient had mechanical failure of a new or reused component.[72,73,169] Many investigators have evaluated the mechanical properties of recycled fixator components.[72,73,136,169] A thorough examination of clinically removed frames, including static mechanical testing, has shown no reduction in performance or catastrophic

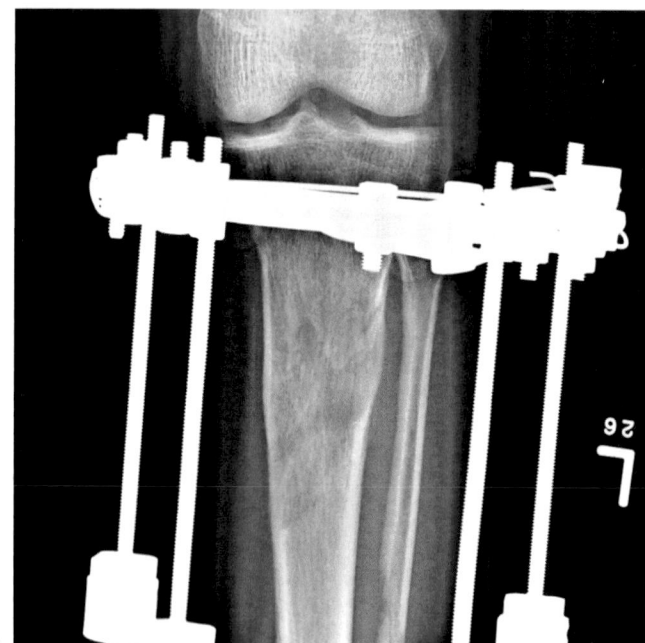
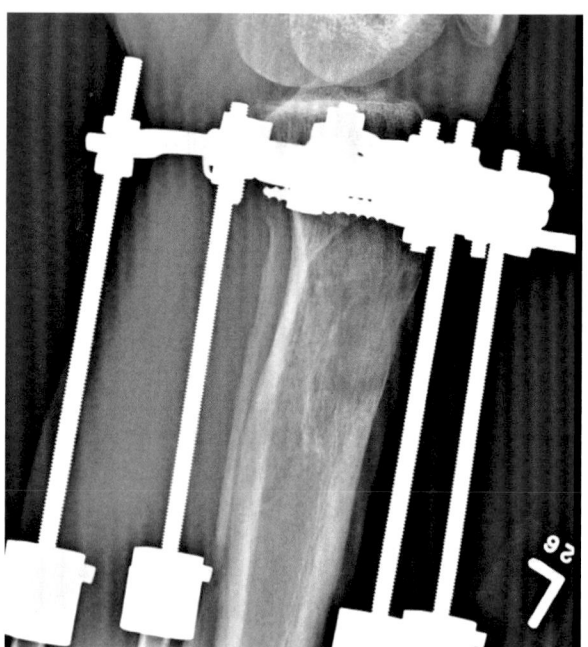

FIGURE 8-77 **A, B:** Reconstitution of both medial and lateral cortices on the AP view, as well as the anterior and posterior cortices on the lateral view, demonstrates complete healing of the regenerate and the fixator can be safely removed at this time.

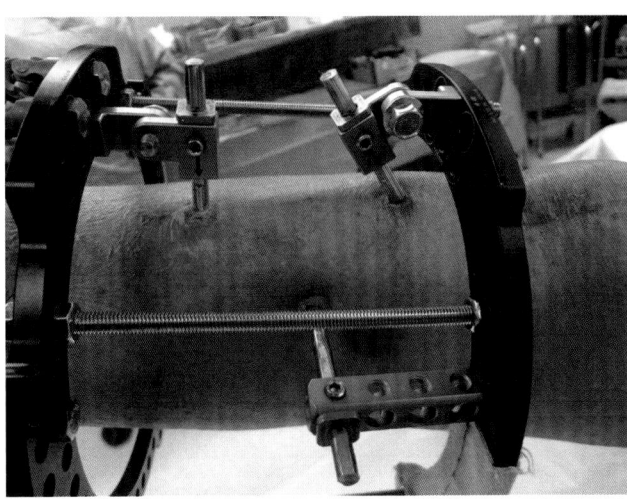

FIGURE 8-78 Hypertrophic pin site keratosis develops around pin sites with long-term fixator applications and should be excised sharply at the time of frame removal to avoid unsightly scarring.

mechanical failure of recycled parts that showed no visual signs of wear. A recent study from the U.S. Army evaluated reprocessed connecting bars from a commonly used external fixation system. The bending strength and stiffness of these rods was determined using four-point bending testing. The location of rod failure was noted. Testing conditions simulated those utilized by the manufacturer for release of new rods. There was no statistically significant difference in bending strength, but there was a 6% decrease in bending stiffness of the used rods compared with the new rods, the clinical significance of which is unknown. Thirteen total used/refurbished rods broke at locations of previous clamping.[244] Thus it is recommended that the rods undergo thorough examination for signs of notching or excessive wear prior to reuse. The potential cost savings, combined with the documented safety of recycled components, makes reuse of these devices attractive.

August 2000 marked a significant change for hospitals or companies that perform in-house reprocessing of single use medical devices (such as external fixator components) The U.S Food and Drug Administration (FDA) announced new guidelines for hospitals as well as third party reprocessing companies that now holds them to the same rigorous premarket submission requirements as manufacturers. For every device a hospital wants to reprocess, it must submit information to the FDA that demonstrates the safety and effectiveness of that device following reprocessing. This means that hospitals now face tough choices, with a wide range of factors to consider, such as cost liability, quality assurance, and device tracking. Since this ruling went into effect many hospitals have determined that they lack the resources to meet the arduous premarket submission requirements. (510K approval). Hospitals that performed their own reprocessing have been forced to decide whether to continue to recycle at great expense, stop using reprocessed devices, or outsource to a third party preprocessor. Many have decided to outsource the service.

Reprocessing, whether in-house or by a third party company, can result in cost savings over the purchase price of new fixator components. Data currently suggests that this does not compromise the standard of care or patient outcome. A recent study at Boston University evaluated reuse of reprocessed external fixator frames at the time of removal, for efficacy of function and potential complications.[277] The authors found no statistical differences in the incidence of pin tract infections, loss of fixation, or loosening of the components compared to those patients treated with new fixators. Their study demonstrated that this type of reuse program was safe and effective with a potential savings of 25% compared with the cost of all new frames.

Devices must be tested and recertified prior to redeployment in hospital stock. Horwitz et al.,[136] utilizing a conservative pass rate and the assumption of a maximum of three recertifications for each component, calculated the total potential hospital savings on external fixation components when this program was instituted. Components were returned back to the original manufacturer for reprocessing. The first pass rate was 76% for initial reprocessing. The second pass rate (i.e., the rate for components that had already been recertified once and had been sent for a second recertification) was 83%. On the basis of a conservative pass-rate estimate of 75%, the predicted average number of uses of a recyclable component was 2.7. The recertified components were sold back to their institution at 50% of the original price. Because carbon fiber bars and half pins were not recycled, 85% of the charges expended on new external fixation components were spent on portions of the system that were recyclable. The potential total savings on reusable components was found to be 32%, with a total savings of 27% for the whole external fixation system. The investigators noted that no recertified components failed in clinical use over the course of the study.

These studies demonstrate the real cost savings associated with a manufacturer-based testing and recertification program. However, issues of voluntary participation in reuse programs by the patient as well as informed consent of the use of reprocessed components, component ownership, and the impact of savings on patient charges, still need to be clarified.

FIXATOR-RELATED COMPLICATIONS

Infection

Wire and pin site complications include pin site inflammation, chronic infection, loosening, or metal fatigue failure. Most authors agree that infection rates from external fixation pins have steadily decreased, as pin technology has increased, but are still significant.[60] The rates of frank pin tract infection have been based on anecdotal accounts in many studies regarding external fixation. The major problem inherent in all external fixator studies has been the exact definition of an infected pin site. Histologic examination of the tissues surrounding the inflamed pin site might lead to the conclusion that almost every pin tract is infected. The most common wire and pin site complications are now graded by the classification as described by Dahl et al.[62] (Table 8-1).

The *Grade 0* pin site appears normal other than marginal erythema and requires only weekly pin care (Figs. 8-75D, E).

	DAHL Pin Site Classification			
TABLE 8-1				
Grade	**Inflammation**	**Drainage**	**X-ray Findings**	**Treatment**
0	None or marginal	None	None	Weekly care
1	Marginal inflammation	None	None	Frequent pin care with mild soap or half-strength peroxide
2	Inflamed	Serous	None	Same as for grade 1 plus oral antibiotics
3	Inflamed	Purulent	None	Same as grade 2 treatment
4	Inflamed with induration	Seropurulent	Osteolysis at near and far cortices	Pin removal local wound care
5	Inflamed with induration, tenderness, surrounding erythema	Gross purulent drainage	Sequestrum and medullary abscess	Formal surgical debridement with culture-specific antibiotics

Grade 1 infection does show marginal inflammation; however, no drainage is apparent and treatment requires more frequent pin care consisting of daily cleansing with mild soap or half-strength peroxide and saline solution.

Grade 2 pin tract infection consists of an inflamed pin site with serous type discharge. *Grade 3* pin tract infections consist of an inflamed pin site with purulent discharge (both *grade 2* and *grade 3* pin tract infections require placement of the patient on antibiotics and continued daily pin care).

Grade 4 pin tract infection consists of serous or seropurulent drainage in concert with redness, inflammation, and radiographs demonstrating osteolysis of both the near and far cortices (Figs. 8-75 F,G). Once osteolysis is visible demonstrating bicortical involvement, removal of the offending pin should be carried out immediately. Local soft tissue debridement of the pin tract with peroxide or other astringent irrigant should be performed. Formal surgical management is unnecessary as long as there are no obvious radiolucencies noted on radiographs.

Grade 5 pin tract inflammation consists of inflamed purulent drainage, osteolysis, as well as sequestrum noted around these abscesses within the medullary canal. Deep-seated infection is present and this requires formal irrigation and debridement procedures with delivery of culture-specific antibiotics (Figs. 8-75H,I). In an effort to avoid collapse of the external fixation construct and the establishment of biomechanical frame instability, pin exchange should be carried out in conjunction with the pin removal process.

Premature Consolidation and Refracture

In patients undergoing distraction osteogenesis techniques, the problem of premature consolidation is most commonly diagnosed as a failure of the corticotomy site to open and lengthen following initiation of distraction. In most instances, the problem is actually an incomplete osteotomy rather than the premature healing of the osteotomy site.[140,295] When this occurs in the tibia, it is often a failure to completely osteotomize the posterior lateral cortex. Most experienced surgeons perform the corticotomy and then manually distract the corticotomy site acutely for 1 to 2 mm under fluoroscopic control to ensure that the corticotomy is complete and can be distracted manually. Using the fixator pins above and below the corticotomy as joysticks, the limb segments can be counterrotated one against the other under fluoroscopy to ensure that a complete osteotomy has occurred.[117–119,140,295]

Premature consolidation does occur most commonly in a pediatric population where distraction must begin much sooner compared with a mature patient. It is usually because of a prolonged latency period allowing significant callous formation to bridge across the corticotomy site. This is seen clinically as excessive deflection of the wires or half pins with a concomitant lack of a distraction gap on radiographs. If this is recognized early in the treatment phase, continued slow distraction can be carried out until the premature area of consolidation ruptures.[140] The patient should be warned, however, that he may feel or hear an audible ache, snap, or pop in the limb with sudden pain and concomitant swelling. Should this occur, the patient should immediately reverse the distraction and compress the region until the pain has subsided. If the patient continues to distract following the fracture of the premature consolidation zone, significant diastasis in the distraction gap will be created causing rupture of the neovascular channels. This may result in the formation of cysts with incomplete regenerate formation and possible regenerate failure.[15,16,138–140,220] Should the slow distraction fail to achieve disruption of the premature consolidation, the patient should be returned to the operating room where closed manipulation can sometimes be successful in achieving complete corticotomy. Should this fail, a repeat corticotomy should be carried out.

The most common cause of incomplete regenerate healing includes disruption of the periosteum and soft tissues during corticotomy, too rapid a distraction, and frame instability.[15,16,138–140]

The rate and rhythm of distraction should be modulated in accordance with the radiographic visualization of the regenerate bone including the formation of the interzone and longitudinal orientation of trabecular bone. Any evidence of disruption or nonlinear orientation of the trabecular bone should be a clear sign that frame instability has occurred. Each pin, wire, and ring connection should be checked and if necessary, additional pins or wires added to assure adequate frame stability. This will help to avoid the formation of intercalary cartilaginous elements.

Regenerate refracture or late deformity following removal of the apparatus usually presents as a gradual deviation of the limb. This often occurs as a result of the patient and treating surgeon becoming "frame weary," which results in premature frame removal prior to complete healing of the regenerate or fracture.[140] The frame should remain on for an extended period of time to ensure that the fracture has healed. Refracture through a docking site is unusual and is typically the result of incomplete healing. What is more common is fracturing through an osteoporotic stress fracture or through a previous pin or wire hole site. When late deformity or regenerate collapse occurs, this usually leads to an unsatisfactory outcome unless collapse is detected early and the frame reapplied. Untreated, the resulting malunion requires secondary osteotomy procedures.

Pin- and wire site fracture, as well as docking site or fracture site refractures can usually be treated with a cast if detected early before significant malalignment occurs. However, in complex cases, frame reapplication is required.

Contractures

Muscle contractures usually result from excessive joint distraction, and occur when elastic tissues and contractile elements cannot accommodate changes in length. This can occur over an extended period of time such as the use of an ankle-bridging monotube fixator, or temporary traveling traction spanning the knee or ankle.[269] A common complication when using lower extremity external fixators is the development of equinus contractures of the foot and ankle. To prevent this, spanning the tibial frame to the forefoot in a neutral position can be performed.

As well, extension contracture of the knee can occur with femoral lengthening or impalement of the quadriceps mechanisms from prolonged monolateral external fixation. Knee flexion exercises to stretch the contracture with physical therapy can be effective but take a prolonged amount of time to work and place increased stress across the patellofemoral joint. An extension contracture can be corrected if manipulated early, utilizing general anesthesia. However, long-standing contracture can be corrected with limited open or formal quadricepsplasty.[157]

Contractures result when the resting muscle length becomes relatively short to that of the newly lengthened bone. Thus, tibial lengthening or bone transport can cause flexion contractures at the knee and equinus contractures of the ankle. Measures should be taken to prevent severe muscle contractures when dealing with correction of leg length discrepancy.[140] This also occurs during the correction of malunions or nonunions, where, following the deformity correction, relative length is restored. Preventive measures include avoiding transfixion of tendons and maximizing muscle excursion before placing transfixion wires or half pins. Physical therapy throughout the course of treatment is helpful as is splinting and maintaining a plantigrade foot in neutral and the knee in full extension when the patient is at rest.

CONCLUSION

The traditional complications of external fixation have been related to the complexity of the external devices, the prolonged treatment times in the frame, and suboptimal outcomes of nonunion, malunion, and pin-related infection. These have largely been eliminated because of advancements in contemporary pin design and frame constructs as a result of innovations in biomaterials and orthobiologics, and an improved understanding of fracture biomechanics. External fixation frames can now remain in place for prolonged periods of time without degradation of the pin–bone interface, and the stiffness of the frames can be adapted to match the clinical demands of the application at hand. Simplified frame mountings have extended the indications for use of these devices, not only for acute fracture management but also for the reconstruction of complex post-traumatic conditions. Advanced technologies such as web-based software interfacing with digital x-rays, uncomplicated frame adjustments, and automated distraction devices can now produce anatomic restoration of limbs that previously could not be achieved with external devices.[168] External fixation continues to provide a powerful means to treat a variety of challenging conditions as the ultimate noninvasive tool.

REFERENCES

1. A.S.A.M.I. Group; Maiocchi AB, Aronson J, eds "OPERATIVE PRINCIPLES OF ILIZAROV: Fracture Treatment, Nonunion, Osteomyelitis, Lengthening, Deformity Correction. Williams and Wilkins Baltimore; 1991.
2. Agee JM. External fixation. Technical advances based upon multiplanar ligamentotaxis. Orthop Clin North Am. 1993;24(2):265–274.
3. Ali AM, Burton M, Hashmi M, et al. Outcome of complex fractures of the tibial plateau treated with a beam-loading ring fixation system. J Bone Joint Surg Br. 2003;85(5):691–699.
4. Ali AM, Saleh M, Bolongaro S, et al. The strength of different fixation techniques for bicondylar tibial plateau fractures–a biomechanical study. Clin Biomech (Bristol, Avon). 2003;18(9):864–870.
5. Ali AM, Yang L, Hashmi M, et al. Bicondylar tibial plateau fractures managed with the Sheffield Hybrid Fixator. Biomechanical study and operative technique. Injury. 2001;32(Suppl 4):SD86–SD91.
6. Al-Sayyad MJ. Taylor Spatial Frame in the treatment of pediatric and adolescent tibial shaft fractures. J Pediatr Orthop. 2006;26(2):164–170.
7. Anderson R. An automatic method of treatment for fractures of the tibia and the fibula. Surg Gynecol Obstet. 1936;62:865–869.
8. Antoci V, Ono CM, Antoci V Jr, et al. Pin-tract infection during limb lengthening using external fixation. Am J Orthop. 2008;37(9):E150–E154.
9. Apard T, Bigorre N, Cronier P, et al. Two-stage reconstruction of post-traumatic segmental tibia bone loss with nailing. Orthop Traumatol Surg Res. 2010;96(5):549–553.
10. Arazi M, Yalcin H, Tarakcioglu N, et al. The effects of dynamization and destabilization of the external fixator on fracture healing: a comparative biomechanical study in dogs. Orthopedics. 2002;25(5):521–524.
11. Aro HT, Chao EY. Bone-healing patterns affected by loading, fracture fragment stability, fracture type, and fracture site compression. Clin Orthop Relat Res. 1993;(293):8–17.
12. Aro HT, Hein TJ, Chao EY. Mechanical performance of pin clamps in external fixators. Clin Orthop Relat Res. 1989;(248):246–253.
13. Aro HT, Kelly PJ, Lewallen DG, et al. The effects of physiologic dynamic compression on bone healing under external fixation. Clin Orthop Relat Res. 1990;(256):260–273.
14. Aro HT, Markel MD, Chao EY. Cortical bone reactions at the interface of external fixation half-pins under different loading conditions. J Trauma. 1993;35(5):776–785.
15. Aronson J, Harp JH Jr. Mechanical considerations in using tensioned wires in a transosseous external fixation system. Clin Orthop Relat Res. 1992;(280):23–29.
16. Aronson J, Harrison B, Boyd CM, et al. Mechanical induction of osteogenesis: the importance of pin rigidity. J Pediatr Orthop. 1988;8(4):396–401.
17. Aronson J, Johnson E, Harp JH. Local bone transportation for treatment of intercalary defects by the Ilizarov technique. Biomechanical and clinical considerations. Clin Orthop Relat Res. 1989;(243):71–79.
18. Atroshi I, Brogren E, Larsson GU, et al. Wrist-bridging versus non-bridging external fixation for displaced distal radius fractures: a randomized assessor-blind clinical trial of 38 patients followed for 1 year. Acta Orthop. 2006;77(3):445–453.
19. Augat P, Burger J, Schorlemmer S, et al. Shear movement at the fracture site delays healing in a diaphyseal fracture model. J Orthop Res. 2003;21(6):1011–1017.
20. Augat P, Claes L, Hanselmann KF, et al. Increase of stability in external fracture fixation by hydroxyapatite-coated bone screws. J Appl Biomater. 1995;6(2):99–104.
21. Augat P, Merk J, Wolf S, et al. Mechanical stimulation by external application of cyclic tensile strains does not effectively enhance bone healing. J Orthop Trauma. 2001;15(1):54–60.
22. Awndrianne Y, Wagenknecht M, Donkerwolcke M, et al. External fixation pin: an in vitro general investigation. Orthopedics. 1987;10(11):1507–1516.
23. Babis GC, Evangelopoulos DS, Kontovazenitis P, et al. High energy tibial plateau fractures treated with hybrid external fixation. J Orthop Surg Res. 2011;6:35–41.
24. Barrett MO, Wade AM, Della Rocca GJ, et al. The safety of forefoot metatarsal pins in external fixation of the lower extremity. J Bone Joint Surg Am. 2008;90(3):560–564.
25. Behrens F. General theory and principles of external fixation. Clin Orthop Relat Res. 1989;241:15–23.
26. Behrens F, Johnson W. Unilateral external fixation. Methods to increase and reduce frame stiffness. Clin Orthop Relat Res. 1989;(241):48–56.

27. Behrens F, Johnson WD, Koch TW, et al. Bending stiffness of unilateral and bilateral fixator frames. *Clin Orthop Relat Res.* 1983;178:103–110.
28. Bereton V. Pin-site care and the rate of local infection. *J Wound Care.* 1998;7(1):42–44.
29. Bhandari M, Zlowodzki M, Tornetta P 3rd, et al. Intramedullary nailing following external fixation in femoral and tibial shaft fractures. *J Orthop Trauma.* 2005;19(2):140–144.
30. Biliouris TL, Schneider E, Rahn BA, et al. The effect of radial preload on the implant–bone interface: a cadaveric study. *J Orthop Trauma.* 1989;3(4):323–332.
31. Blasier RD, Aronson J, Tursky EA. External fixation of pediatric femur fractures. *J Pediatr Orthop.* 1997;17(3):342–346.
32. Borrelli J Jr, De S, VanPelt M. Fracture of the cuboid. *J Am Acad Orthop Surg.* 2012; 20(7):472–477.
33. Bosse MJ, Holmes C, Vossoughi J, et al. Comparison of the Howmedica and Synthes military external fixation frames. *J Orthop Trauma.* 1994;8(2):119–126.
34. Bosworth DM. Skeletal distraction. *Surg Gynecol Obstet.* 1931;52:893.
35. Bottlang M, Marsh JL, Brown TD. Articulated external fixation of the ankle: minimizing motion resistance by accurate axis alignment. *J Biomech.* 1999;32(1):63–70.
36. Briggs BT, Chao EY. The mechanical performance of the standard Hoffmann-Vidal external fixation apparatus. *J Bone Joint Surg Am.* 1982;64(4):566–573.
37. Brinker MR, O'Connor DP, Crouch CC, et al. Ilizarov treatment of infected nonunions of the distal humerus after failure of internal fixation: an outcomes study. *J Orthop Trauma.* 2007;21(3):178–184.
38. Bronson DG, Samchukov ML, Birch JG. Stabilization of a short juxta-articular bone segment with a circular external fixator. *J Pediatr Orthop B.* 2002;11(2):143–149.
39. Broos PLO, Sermon A. From unstable internal fixation to biological osteosynthesis: A historical overview of operative fracture treatment. *Acta Chir Belg.* 2004;104:396–400.
40. Burny F. Elastic external fixation of fractures of the long bones. *Arch Putti Chir Organi Mov.* 1986;36:323–329.
41. Burny F, Bourgois R. [Biomechanical study of the Hoffman external fixation device]. *Acta Orthop Belg.* 1972;38(3):265–279.
42. Caja VL, Larsson S, Kim W, et al. Mechanical performance of the Monticelli-Spinelli external fixation system. *Clin Orthop Relat Res.* 1994;(309):257–266.
43. Caja VL, Piza G, Navarro A. Hydroxyapatite coating of external fixation pins to decrease axial deformity during tibial lengthening for short stature. *J Bone Joint Surg Am.* 2003; 85-A(8):1527–1531.
44. Calhoun JH, Li F, Bauford WL, et al. Rigidity of half-pins for the Ilizarov external fixator. *Bull Hosp Jt Dis.* 1992;52(1):21–26.
45. Calhoun JH, Li F, Ledbetter BR, et al. Biomechanics of the Ilizarov fixator for fracture fixation. *Clin Orthop Relat Res.* 1992;(280):15–22.
46. Camathias C, Valderrabano V, Oberli H. Routine pin tract care in external fixation is unnecessary: a randomised, prospective, blinded controlled study. *Injury.* 2012;43(11): 1969–1973.
47. Capper M, Soutis C, Oni OO. Pin-hole shear stresses generated by conical and standard external fixation pins. *Biomaterials.* 1993;14(11):876–878.
48. Carmichael KD, Bynum J, Goucher N. Rates of refracture associated with external fixation in pediatric femur fractures. *Am J Orthop.* 2005;34(9):439–444; discussion 444.
49. Chandran P, Puttaswamaiah R, Dhillon MS, et al. Management of complex open fracture injuries of the midfoot with external fixation. *J Foot Ankle Surg.* 2006;45(5):308–315.
50. Chao EY, Aro HT, Lewallen DG, et al. The effect of rigidity on fracture healing in external fixation. *Clin Orthop Relat Res Relat Res.* 1989;(241):24–35.
51. Chao EY, Hein TJ. Mechanical performance of the standard Orthofix external fixator. *Orthopedics.* 1988;11(7):1057–1069.
52. Chao EY, Kasman RA, An KN. Rigidity and stress analyses of external fracture fixation devices–a theoretical approach. *J Biomech.* 1982;15(12):971–983.
53. Chaudhary S, Patil N, Bagaria V, et al. Open intercondylar fractures of the distal humerus: Management using amini-external fixator construct. *J Shoulder Elbow Surg.* 2008;17(3):465–470.
54. Christian EP, Bosse MJ, Robb G. Reconstruction of large diaphyseal defects, without free fibular transfer, in grade IIIB tibial fractures. *J Bone Joint Surg.* 1989;71A:994–1002.
55. Cierny G, Zorn KE. Segmental tibial defects. Comparing conventional and Ilizarov methodologies. *Clin Ortho.* 1994;301:118–123.
56. Claes L, Eckert-Hubner K, Augat P. The effect of mechanical stability on local vascularization and tissue differentiation in callus healing. *J Orthop Res.* 2002;20(5):1099–1105.
57. Clary EM, Roe SC. In vitro biomechanical and histological assessment of pilot hole diameter for positive-profile external skeletal fixation pins in canine tibiae. *Vet Surg.* 1996; 25(6):453–462.
58. Clasper JC, Cannon LB, Stapley SA, et al. Fluid accumulation and the rapid spread of bacteria in the pathogenesis of external fixator pin track infection. *Injury.* 2001;32(5): 377–381.
59. Cross AR, Lewis DD, Murphy ST, et al. Effects of ring diameter and wire tension on the axial biomechanics of four-ring circular external skeletal fixator constructs. *Am J Vet Res.* 2001;62(7):1025–1030.
60. Cunningham JL, Evans M, Harris JD, et al. The measurement of stiffness of fractures treated with external fixation. *Eng Med.* 1987;16(4):229–232.
61. Dahl MT. The gradual correction of forearm deformities in multiple hereditary exostoses. *Hand Clin.* 1993;9(4):707–718.
62. Dahl MT, Gulli B, Berg T. Complications of limb lengthening a learning curve. *Clin Orthop Relat Res.* 1994;301:10–18.
63. Dahners LE, Jacobs RR, McKenzie EB, et al. Biomechanical studies of an anterior pelvic external fixation frame intended for control of vertical shear fractures. *South Med J.* 1986; 79(7):815–817.
64. Degernes LA, Roe SC, Abrams CF Jr. Holding power of different pin designs and pin insertion methods in avian cortical bone. *Vet Surg.* 1998;27(4):301–306.
65. DeJong ES, DeBerardino TM, Brooks DE, et al. Antimicrobial efficacy of external fixator pins coated with a lipid stabilized hydroxyapatite /chlorhexidine complex to prevent pin tract infection in a goat model. *J Trauma.* 2001;50(6):1008–1014.
66. De la Huerta F. Correction of the neglected clubfoot by the Ilizarov method. *Clin Orthop Relat Res.* 1994;(301):89–93.
67. Della Rocca GJ, Crist BD. External fixation versus conversion to intramedullary nailing for definitive management of closed fractures of the femoral and tibial shaft. *J Am Acad Orthop Surg.* 2006;14(10 Suppl):S131–S135.
68. Deuel CR, Wolinsky P, Shepherd E, et al. The use of hinged external fixation to provide additional stabilization for fractures of the distal humerus. *J Orthop Trauma.* 2007; 21(5):323–329.
69. D'Hooghe P, Defoort K, Lammens J, et al. Management of a large post-traumatic skin and bone defect using an Ilizarov frame. *Acta Orthop Belg.* 2006;72(2):214–218.
70. DiDomenico LA, Brown D, Zgonis T. The use of Ilizarov technique as a definitive percutaneous reduction for ankle fractures in patients who have diabetes mellitus and peripheral vascular disease. *Clin Podiatr Med Surg.* 2009;26(1):141–148.
71. DiGiovanni CW. Fractures of the navicular. *Foot Ankle Clin.* 2004;9(1):25–63.
72. Dirschl DR, Obremskey WT. Mechanical strength and wear of used EBI external fixators. *Orthopaedics.* 2002;25(10):1059–1062.
73. Dirschl DR, Smith IJ. Reuse of external fixator components: Effects on costs and complications. *J Trauma.* 1998;44(5):855–858.
74. Dodds SD, Cornelissen S, Jossan S, et al. A biomechanical comparison of fragment-specific fixation and augmented external fixation for intra-articular distal radius fractures. *J Hand Surg Am.* 2002;27(6):953–964.
75. Donaldson FE, Pankaj P, Simpson AH. Bone properties affect loosening of half-pin external fixators at the pin–bone interface. *Injury.* 2012A;43(10):1764–1770.
76. Donaldson FE, Pankaj P, Simpson AH. Investigation of factors affecting loosening of Ilizarov ring-wire external fixator systems at the bone-wire interface. *J Orthop Res.* 2012B; 30(5):726–732.
77. Dougherty PJ, Vickaryous B, Conley E, et al. A comparison of two military temporary femoral external fixators. *Clin Orthop Relat Res.* 2003;(412):176–183.
78. Doyle J, Hayes P, Fenlon G. Experimental analysis of effects of pin pretensioning on external fixator rigidity. *Arch Orthop Trauma Surg.* 1988;107(6):377–380.
79. Drijber FL, Finlay JB. Universal joint slippage as a cause of Hoffmann half-frame external fixator failure [corrected]. *J Biomed Eng.* 1992;14(6):509–515.
80. Duda GN, Sollmann M, Sporrer S, et al. Interfragmentary motion in tibial osteotomies stabilized with ring fixators. *Clin Orthop Relat Res.* 2002;(396):163–172.
81. Easley ME, Montijo HE, Wilson JB, et al. Revision tibiotalar arthrodesis. *J Bone Joint Surg Am.* 2008;90(6):1212–1223.
82. Edwards CC. Staged reconstruction of complex open tibial fractures using Hoffmann external fixation: clinical decisions and dilemmas. *Clin Orthop Relat Res.* 1983;178:130–161.
83. Egidy CC, Fufa D, Kendoff D, et al. Hinged external fixator placement at the elbow: navigated versus conventional technique. *Comput Aided Surg.* 2012;17(6):294–299.
84. Egol KA, Bazzi J, McLaurin TM, et al. The effect of knee-spanning external fixation on compartment pressures in the leg. *J Orthop Trauma.* 2008;22(10):680–685.
85. Egol KA, Paksima N, Puopolo S, et al. Treatment of external fixation pins about the wrist: a prospective, randomized trial. *J Bone Joint Surg Am.* 2006;88(2):349–354.
86. Eidelman M, Bialik V, Katzman A. Correction of deformities in children using the Taylor Spatial Frame. *J Pediatr Orthop B.* 2006;15(6):387–395.
87. Eidelman M, Keren Y, Katzman A. Correction of residual clubfoot deformities in older children using the Taylor spatial butt frame and midfoot Gigli saw osteotomy. *J Pediatr Orthop.* 2012;32(5):527–533.
88. El Hayek T, Daher AA, Meouchy W, et al. External fixators in the treatment of fractures in children. *J Pediatr Orthop B.* 2004;13(2):103–109.
89. Endres T, Grass R, Biewener A, et al. [Advantages of minimally invasive reposition, retention, and hybrid Ilizarov fixation for tibial pilon fractures with particular emphasis on C2/C3 fractures.] *Unfallchirurg.* 2004;107(4):273–284.
90. Enneking WF, Eady JL, Burchardt H. Autogenous cortical bone grafts in the reconstruction of segmental skeletal defects. *J Bone Joint Surg Am.* 1980;62(7):1039–1058.
91. Etter C, Burri C, Claes L, et al. Treatment by external fixation of open fractures associated with severe soft tissue damage of the leg. Biomechanical principles and clinical experience. *Clin Orthop Relat Res.* 1983;(178):80–88.
92. Facaros Z, Ramanujam CL, Stapleton JJ. Combined circular external fixation and open reduction internal fixation with pro-syndesmotic screws for repair of a diabetic ankle fracture. *Diabet Foot Ankle.* 2010;(1):13–19.
93. Feldman DS, Madan SS, Koval KJ, et al. Correction of tibia vara with six-axis deformity analysis and the Taylor Spatial Frame. *J Pediatr Orthop.* 2003;23(3):387–391.
94. Fischer DA. Skeletal stabilization with a multiplane external fixation device. Design rationale and preliminary clinical experience. *Clin Orthop Relat Res.* 1983;(180):50–62.
95. Fitzpatrick DC, Foels WS, Pedersen DR, et al. An articulated ankle external fixation system that can be aligned with the ankle axis. *Iowa Orthop J.* 1995;15:197–203.
96. Fitzpatrick DC, Sommers MB, Kam BC, et al. Knee stability after articulated external fixation. *Am J Sports Med.* 2005;33(11):1735–1741.
97. Fleming B, Paley D, Kristiansen T, et al. A biomechanical analysis of the Ilizarov external fixator. *Clin Orthop Relat Res.* 1989;(241):95–105.
98. Flinkkila T, Ristiniemi J, Hyvonen P, et al. Nonbridging external fixation in the treatment of unstable fractures of the distal forearm. *Arch Orthop Trauma Surg.* 2003;123(7):349–352.
99. Floerkemeier T, Stukenborg-Colsman C, Windhagen H, et al. Correction of severe foot deformities using the Taylor spatial frame. *Foot Ankle Int.* 2011;32(2):176–182.
100. Freeman L. The union of ununited fractures of the neck of the femur by open operation. *Ann Surg.* 1904;40(4):561–570.
101. Freeman L. "Discussion on surgical treatment of fractures." Surgical vol., Transactions of Amer. *Medical Assoc.* 1909;317.
102. Freeman L. The treatment of oblique fractures of the tibia and other bones by means of external clamps inserted through small openings in the skin. *Trans Am Surg Assoc.* 1911A; 28:70–93.
103. Freeman L. The treatment of oblique fractures of the tibia and other bones by means of external clamps inserted through small openings in the skin. *Ann Surg.* 1911B; 54(3):381–389.
104. Freeman L. The application of extension to overlapping fractures, especially of the tibia by means of bone screws and a turnbuckle, without open operation. *Ann Surg.* 1919; 70(2):231–235.

105. Gantous A, Phillips JH. The effects of varying pilot hole size on the holding power of miniscrews and microscrews. *Plast Reconstr Surg.* 1995;95(7):1165–1169.
106. Gardner MJ, Nork SE. Stabilization of unstable pelvic fractures with supra-acetabular compression external fixation. *J Orthop Trauma.* 2007;21(4):269–273.
107. Geller J, Tornetta P 3rd, Tiburzi D, et al. Tension wire position for hybrid external fixation of the proximal tibia. *J Orthop Trauma.* 2000;14(7):502–504.
108. Gessmann J, Jettkant B, Königshausen M, et al. Improved wire stiffness with modified connection bolts in Ilizarov external frames: a biomechanical study. *Acta Bioeng Biomech.* 2012;14(4):15–21.
109. Girard PJ, Kuhn KM, Bailey JR, et al. Bone transport combined with locking bridge plate fixation for the treatment of tibial segmental defects: A report of two cases. *J Orthop Trauma.* 2013;27:e220–e226.
110. Goodship AE, Cunningham JL, Kenwright J. Strain rate and timing of stimulation in mechanical modulation of fracture healing. *Clin Orthop Relat Res.* 1998;355(Suppl):S105–S115.
111. Goodship AE, Watkins PE, Rigby HS, et al. The role of fixator frame stiffness in the control of fracture healing. An experimental study. *J Biomech.* 1993;26(9):1027–1035.
112. Gordon JE, Kelly-Hahn J, Carpenter CJ, et al. Pin site care during external fixation in children: results of nihilistic approach. *J Pediatr Orthop.* 2000;20(2):163–165.
113. Goslings JC, DaSilva MF, Viegas SF, et al. Kinematics of the wrist with a new dynamic external fixation device. *Clin Orthop Relat Res.* 2001;(386):226–234.
114. Gradl G, Jupiter JB, Gierer P, et al. Fractures of the distal radius treated with a nonbridging external fixation technique using multiplanar k-wires. *J Hand Surg Am.* 2005;30(5): 960–968.
115. Green SA. *Complications of External Skeletal Fixation: Causes, Prevention, and Treatment.* Charles C Thomas, Springfield IL; 1981.
116. Green SA. Book review: external fixation joint deformities and bone fractures. *Techniques in Orthop.* 1988;3(2):87–88.
117. Green SA. The Ilizarov method: Rancho technique. *Orthop Clin North Am.* 1991;22(4): 677–688.
118. Green SA. Skeletal defects: A comparison of bone grafting and bone transport for skeletal defects. *Clin Orthop Relat Res.* 1994;310:111–117.
119. Green SA, Jackson JM, Wall DM, et al. Management of segmental defects by the Ilizarov intercalary bone transport method. *Clin Orthop Relat Res.* 1992;280:136–142.
120. Haasper C, Jagodzinski M, Krettek C, et al. Hinged external fixation and closed reduction for distal humerus fracture. *Arch Orthop Trauma Surg.* 2006;126(3):188–191.
121. Haidukewych GJ. Temporary external fixation for the management of complex intra- and periarticular fractures of the lower extremity. *J Orthop Trauma.* 2002;16(9):678–685.
122. Haidukewych GJ, Kumar S, Prpa B. Placement of half-pins for supra-acetabular external fixation: an anatomic study. *Clin Orthop Relat Res.* 2003;(411):269–273.
123. Hampton OP, ed. Orthopaedic Surgery in the Mediterranean theatre of Operations (Washington, D.C.: Office of the Surgeon General, Department of the Army, 1957), 203–210: Charles Bradford and Phillip D Wilson, "Mechanical Skeletal fixation in War Surgery, with a Report of 61 Cases," SGO 75 (1942): 486–76.
124. Handoll HH, Huntley JS, Madhok R. Different methods of external fixation for treating distal radial fractures in adults. *Cochrane Database Syst Rev.* 2008;(1):CD006522.
125. Harbacheuski R, Fragomen AT, Rozbruch SR. *Does lengthening and then plating (LAP) shorten duration of external fixation? Clin Orthop Relat Res Relat Res.* 2012;470(6):1771–1781.
126. Harer T, Hontzsch D, Stohr E, et al. [How much are external fixator nuts tightened in general practice]. *Aktuelle Traumatol.* 1993;23(4):212–213.
127. Hart MB, Wu JJ, Chao EY, et al. External skeletal fixation of canine tibial osteotomies. Compression compared with no compression. *J Bone Joint Surg Am.* 1985;67(4):598–605.
128. Harwood PJ, Giannoudis PV, Probst C, et al. The risk of local infective complications after damage control procedures for femoral shaft fracture. *J Orthop Trauma.* 2006;20(3): 181–189.
129. Hassan A, Letts M. The management of the neglected congenital foot deformity in the older child with the Taylor spatial frame. *J Pediatr Orthop.* 2012;32(1):85–92.
130. Hayes AJ, Duffy PJ, McQueen MM. Bridging and non-bridging external fixation in the treatment of unstable fractures of the distal radius: a retrospective study of 588 patients. *Acta Orthop.* 2008;79(4):540–547.
131. Hein TJ, Chao EY. Biomechanical analysis of the Orthofix axial external fixator. *Biomed Sci Instrum.* 1987;23:39–42.
132. Hierholzer G, Ruedi Th, Allgower M, Schatzker J, eds. *Manual on the AO/ASIF Tubular External Fixator.* Berlin: Springer-Verlag; 1985.
133. Hippocrates. An abridged report on external skeletal fixation. *Clin Orthop Relat Res.* 1989; 241:3–4.
134. Hoffmann R. Closed osteosynthesis with special references to war surgery. *Acta Chir Scand.* 1942;86:255–261.
135. Hoffman R. *Osteotaxis: Transcutaneous Osteosynthesis by Means of Screws and Ball and Socket Joints.* Paris, Gead; 1953.
136. Horwitz DS, Schabel KL, Higgins TF. The economic impact of reprocessing external fixation components. *J Bone Joint Surg Am.* 2007;89(10):2132–2136.
137. Hutchinson DT, Bachus KN, Higgenbotham T. External fixation of the distal radius: to predrill or not to predrill. *J Hand Surg Am.* 2000;25(6):1064–1068.
138. Ilizarov GA. The tension-stress effect on the genesis and growth of tissues: Part II. The influence of the rate and frequency of distraction. *Clin Orthop Relat Res.* 1989A;(239):263–285.
139. Ilizarov GA. The tension-stress effect on the genesis and growth of tissues. Part I. The influence of stability of fixation and soft-tissue preservation. *Clin Orthop Relat Res.* 1989B;(238): 249–281.
140. Ilizarov GA. Transosseous Osteosynthesis. In: Stuart Green ed. *Theoretical and Clinical Aspects of the Regeneration and Growth of Tissue.* Berlin: Springer Verlag;1992.
141. Ilizarov S. The Ilizarov method: History and scope. In: Rozbruck SR, Ilizarov S. Informa, eds. *Limb Lengthening and Reconstructive Surgery.* New York, NY: 2007:1–18.
142. Iobst CA, Dahl MT. Limb lengthening with submuscular plate stabilization: a case series and description of the technique. *J Pediatr Orthop.* 2007;27(5):504–509.
143. Jackson M, Topliss CJ, Atkins RM. Fine wire frame-assisted intramedullary nailing of the tibia. *J Orthop Trauma.* 2003;17(3):222–224.
144. Jagodzinski M, Haasper C, Knobloch C, et al. [Treatment of chronic knee dislocation with an external fixator]. *Unfallchirurg.* 2005;108(7):597–600.
145. Jaskulka RA, Egkher E, Wielke B. Comparison of the mechanical performance of three types of unilateral, dynamizable external fixators. An experimental study. *Arch Orthop Trauma Surg.* 1994;113(5):271–275.
146. Johnson HF, Stovall SL. External fixation of fractures. *J Bone Joint Surg.* 1950;32A:466–471.
147. Juan JA, Prat J, Vera P, et al. Biomechanical consequences of callus development in Hoffmann, Wagner, Orthofix and Ilizarov external fixators. *J Biomech.* 1992;25(9): 995–1006.
148. Kabata T, Tsuchiya H, Sakurakichi K, et al. Reconstruction with distraction osteogenesis for juxta-articular nonunions with bone loss. *J Trauma.* 2005;58(6):1213–1222.
149. Karnezis IA, Miles AW, Cunningham JL, et al. Axial preload in external fixator half-pins: a preliminary mechanical study of an experimental bone anchorage system. *Clin Biomech (Bristol, Avon).* 1999;14(1):69–73.
150. Kashiwagi N, Suzuki S, Seto Y, et al. Bilateral humeral lengthening in achondroplasia. *Clin Orthop Relat Res.* 2001;(391):251–257.
151. Kasman RA, Chao EY. Fatigue performance of external fixator pins. *J Orthop Res.* 1984; 2(4):377–384.
152. Keetley CB. On the prevention of shortening and other forms of malunion after fracture, by the use of metal pins passed into the fragments subcutaneously. *Lancet.* 1893; 10:137.
153. Kellam JF. The role of external fixation in pelvic disruptions. *Clin Orthop Relat Res.* 1989;(241):66–82. Review.
154. Kenwright J, Gardner T. Mechanical influences on tibial fracture healing. *Clin Orthop Relat Res.* 1998;355(Suppl):S179–S190.
155. Kenwright J, Goodship AE. Controlled mechanical stimulation in the treatment of tibial fractures. *Clin Orthop Relat Res.* 1989;(241):36–47.
156. Kenwright J, Richardson JB, Cunningham JL, et al. Axial movement and tibial fractures. A controlled randomised trial of treatment. *J Bone Joint Surg Br.* 1991;73(4):654–659.
157. Khakharia S, Fragomen AT, Rozbruch SR. Limited quadricepsplasty for contracture during femoral lengthening. *Clin Orthop Relat Res.* 2009;467(11):2911–2917.
158. Khalily C, Voor MJ, Seligson D. Fracture site motion with Ilizarov and "hybrid" external fixation. *J Orthop Trauma.* 1998;12(1):21–26.
159. Khurana A, Byrne C, Evans S, et al. Comparison of transverse wires and half pins in Taylor Spatial Frame: a biomechanical study. *J Orthop Surg Res.* 2010;5:23–31.
160. Kloen P. Supercutaneous plating: use of a locking compression plate as an external fixator. *J Orthop Trauma.* 2009;23(1):72–75.
161. Koseki H, Asahara T, Shida T, et al. Clinical and histomorphometrical study on titanium dioxide-coated external fixation pins. *Int J Nanomedicine.* 2013;8:593–599.
162. Kowalski TC, Mader K, Siedek M, et al. Minimal invasive treatment of a comminuted os naviculare body fracture using external fixation with limited open approach. *J Trauma.* 2008;65(6):E58–E61.
163. Kowalski M, Schemitsch EH, Harrington RM, et al. Comparative biomechanical evaluation of different external fixation sidebars: stainless-steel tubes versus carbon fiber rods. *J Orthop Trauma.* 1996;10(7):470–475.
164. Krawczyk A, Kuropka P, Kuryszko J, et al. Experimental studies on the effect of osteotomy technique on the bone regeneration in distraction osteogenesis. *Bone.* 2007;40(3): 781–791. Epub 2006 Nov 30.
165. Kreder HJ, Agel J, McKee MD, et al. A randomized, controlled trial of distal radius fractures with metaphyseal displacement but without joint incongruity: closed reduction and casting versus closed reduction, spanning external fixation, and optional percutaneous K-wires. *J Orthop Trauma.* 2006;20(2):115–121.
166. Krishnan J, Wigg AE, Walker RW, et al. Intra-articular fractures of the distal radius: a prospective randomized controlled trial comparing static bridging and dynamic non-bridging external fixation. *J Hand Surg Br.* 2003;28(5):417–421.
167. Krukhaug Y, Ugland S, Lie SA, et al. External fixation of fractures of the distal radius: a randomized comparison of the Hoffman compact II non-bridging fixator and the Dynawrist fixator in 75 patients followed for 1 year. *Acta Orthop.* 2009;80(1):104–108.
168. Kucukkaya M, Karakoyun O, Armagan R, et al. Calculating the mounting parameters for Taylor Spatial Frame correction using computed tomography. *J Orthop Trauma.* 2011; 25(7):449–452.
169. Kummer FJ, Frankel VH, Catagni MA. *Reuse of Ilizarov frame components: A potential cost savings? Contemp Orthop.* 1992;25(2):125–128.
170. Lai D, Chen CM, Chiu FY, et al. Reconstruction of juxta-articular huge defects of distal femur with vascularized fibular bone graft and Ilizarov's distraction osteogenesis. *J Trauma.* 2007;62(1):166–173.
171. Laible C, Earl-Royal E, Davidovitch R, et al. *Infection after spanning external fixation for high-energy tibial plateau fractures: is pin site-plate overlap a problem? J Orthop Trauma.* 2012;26(2):92–97.
172. Lambotte A. The operative treatment of fractures: report of fractures committee. *Br Med J.* 1912;2:1530.
173. Lamm BM, Gottlieb HD, Paley D. A two-stage percutaneous approach to Charcot diabetic foot reconstruction. *J Foot Ankle Surg.* 2010;49(6):517–522.
174. Larsson S, Kim W, Caja VL, et al. Effect of early axial dynamization on tibial bone healing: a study in dogs. *Clin Orthop Relat Res.* 2001;(388):240–251.
175. Lavini FM, Brivio LR, Leso P. Biomechanical factors in designing screws for the Orthofix system. *Clin Orthop Relat Res.* 1994;(308):63–67.
176. Lee CK, Chua YP, Saw A. Antimicrobial gauze as a dressing reduces pin site infection: a randomized controlled trial. *Clin Orthop Relat Res.* 2012;470(2):610–615.
177. Lenarz C, Bledsoe G, Watson JT. Circular External Fixation Frames with Divergent Half Pins: A pilot biomechanical Study. *Clin Orthop Relat Res relat Res.* 2008;466(12): 2933–2939.
178. Lerner A, Fodor L, Keren Y, et al. External fixation for temporary stabilization and wound management of an open pelvic ring injury with extensive soft tissue damage: case report and review of the literature. *J Trauma.* 2008;65(3):715–718.
179. Lerner A, Ullmann Y, Stein H, et al. Using the Ilizarov external fixation device for skin expansion. *Ann Plast Surg.* 2000;45(5):535–537.

180. Lethaby A, Temple J, Santy J. Pin site care for preventing infections associated with external bone fixators and pins. *Cochrane Database Syst Rev.* 2008;(4):CD004551.
181. Leung F, Kwok HY, Pun TS, et al. Limited open reduction and Ilizarov external fixation in the treatment of distal tibial fractures. *Injury.* 2004;35(3):278–283.
182. Leung F, Tu YK, Chew WY, et al. Comparison of external and percutaneous pin fixation with plate fixation for intra-articular distal radial fractures. A randomized study. *J Bone Joint Surg Am.* 2008;90(1):16–22.
183. Lewallen DG, Chao EY, Kasman RA, et al. Comparison of the effects of compression plates and external fixators on early bone-healing. *J Bone Joint Surg Am.* 1984;66(7):1084–1091.
184. Lewis KM, Breidenbach L, Stader O. The Stader reduction splint for treating fractures of the shafts of the long bones. *Ann Surg.* 1942;116:623–631.
185. Lowenberg DW, Nork S, Abruzzo FM. Correlation of shear to compression for progressive fracture obliquity. *Clin Orthop Relat Res Relat Res.* 2008;466(12):2947–2954.
186. Magyar G, Toksvig-Larsen S, Moroni A. Hydroxyapatite coating of threaded pins enhances fixation. *J Bone Joint Surg Br.* 1997;79(3):487–489.
187. Manzotti A, Pullen C, Deromedis B, et al. Knee arthrodesis after infected total knee arthroplasty using the Ilizarov method. *Clin Orthop Relat Res.* 2001;(389):143–149.
188. Markiewitz AD, Gellman H. Five-pin external fixation and early range of motion for distal radius fractures. *Orthop Clin North Am.* 2001;32(2):329–335, ix.
189. Marotta JS, Coupe KJ, Milner R, et al. Long-term bactericidal properties of a gentamicin-coated antimicrobial external fixation pin sleeve. *J Bone Joint Surg Am.* 2003;85-A(Suppl 4):129–131.
190. Marti JM, Roe SC. Biomechanical comparison of the trocar tip point and the hollow ground tip point for smooth external skeletal fixation pins. *Vet Surg.* 1998;27(5):423–428.
191. Martin C, Guillen M, Lopez G. Treatment of 2- and 3-part fractures of the proximal humerus using external fixation: a retrospective evaluation of 62 patients. *Acta Orthop.* 2006;77(2):275–278.
192. Matsushita T, Nakamura K, Ohnishi I, et al. Sliding performance of unilateral external fixators for tibia. *Med Eng Phys.* 1998;20(1):66–69.
193. Matthews LS, Green CA, Goldstein SA. The thermal effects of skeletal fixation-pin insertion in bone. *J Bone Joint Surg.* 1984;66A:1077–1083.
194. McCoy MT, Chao EY, Kasman RA. Comparison of mechanical performance in four types of external fixators. *Clin Orthop Relat Res Relat Res.* 1983;(180):23–33.
195. Mears DC, Rubash HE. External and internal fixation of the pelvic ring. *Instr Course Lect.* 1984;33:144–158.
196. Menon DK, Dougall TW, Pool RD, et al. Augmentative Ilizarov external fixation after failure of diaphyseal union with intramedullary nailing. *J Orthop Trauma.* 2002;16(7):491–497.
197. Mercer D, Firoozbakhsh K, Prevost M, et al. Stiffness of knee-spanning external fixation systems for traumatic knee dislocations: a biomechanical study. *J Orthop Trauma.* 2010;24(11):693–696.
198. Metcalfe AJ, Saleh M, Yang L. Techniques for improving stability in oblique fractures treated by circular fixation with particular reference to the sagittal plane. *JBJS Br.* 2005;87B:868–872.
199. Mirza A, Jupiter JB, Reinhart MK, et al. Fractures of the distal radius treated with cross-pin fixation and a nonbridging external fixator, the CPX system: a preliminary report. *J Hand Surg Am.* 2009;34(4):603–616.
200. Moroni A, Cadossi M, Romagnoli M, et al. A biomechanical and histological analysis of standard versus hydroxyapatite-coated pins for external fixation. *J Biomed Mater Res B Appl Biomater.* 2008;86B(2):417–421.
201. Moroni A, Caja VL, Maltarello MC, et al. Biomechanical, scanning electron microscopy, and microhardness analyses of the bone-pin interface in hydroxyapatite coated versus uncoated pins. *J Orthop Trauma.* 1997;11(3):154–161.
202. Moroni A, Faldini C, Marchetti S, et al. Improvement of the bone–pin interface strength in osteoporotic bone with use of hydroxyapatite-coated tapered external-fixation pins. A prospective, randomized clinical study of wrist fractures. *J Bone Joint Surg Am.* 2001;83-A(5):717–721.
203. Moroni A, Faldini C, Pegreffi F, et al. Fixation strength of tapered versus bicylindrical hydroxyapatite-coated external fixation pins: an animal study. *J Biomed Mater Res.* 2002;63(1):61–64.
204. Moroni A, Faldini C, Pegreffi F, et al. Dynamic hip screw compared with external fixation for treatment of osteoporotic pertrochanteric fractures. A prospective, randomized study. *Bone Joint Surg Am.* 2005;87(4):753–759.
205. Moroni A, Heikkila J, Magyar G, et al. Fixation strength and pin tract infection of hydroxyapatite-coated tapered pins. *Clin Orthop Relat Res.* 2001;(388):209–217.
206. Moroni A, Vannini F, Mosca M, et al. State of the art review: techniques to avoid pin loosening and infection in external fixation. *J Orthop Trauma.* 2002;16(3):189–195.
207. Mostafavi HR, Tornetta P 3rd. Open fractures of the humerus treated with external fixation. *Clin Orthop Relat Res.* 1997;(337):187–197.
208. Nakata RY, Chand Y, Matiko JD, et al. External fixators for wrist fractures: a biomechanical and clinical study. *J Hand Surg Am.* 1985;10(6 Pt 1):845–851.
209. Nho SJ, Helfet DL, Rozbruch SR. Temporary intentional leg shortening and deformation to facilitate wound closure using the Ilizarov/Taylor spatial frame. *J Orthop Trauma.* 2006;20(6):419–424.
210. Nolla J, Ring D, Lozano-Calderon S, et al. Interposition arthroplasty of the elbow with hinged external fixation for post-traumatic arthritis. *J Shoulder Elbow Surg.* 2008;17(3):459–464.
211. Noonan KJ, Price CT. Pearls and pitfalls of deformity correction and limb lengthening via monolateral external fixation. *Iowa Orthop J.* 1996;16:58–69.
212. Ochman S, Frerichmann U, Armsen N, et al. [Is use of the fixateur externe no longer indicated for the treatment of unstable radial fracture in the elderly?]. *Unfallchirurg.* 2006;109(12):1050–1057.
213. Oh CW, Song HR, Roh JY, et al. Bone transport over an intramedullary nail for reconstruction of long bone defects in tibia. *Arch Orthop Trauma Surg.* 2008;128(8):801–808.
214. Oh JK, Hwang JH, Sahu D, et al. Complication rate and pitfalls of temporary bridging external fixator in periarticular communited fractures. *Clin Orthop Relat Res Surg.* 2011;3(1):62–68.
215. Oni OO, Capper M, Soutis C. A finite element analysis of the effect of pin distribution on the rigidity of a unilateral external fixation system. *Injury.* 1993;24(8):525–527.
216. Oni OO, Capper M, Soutis C. External fixation of upper limb fractures: the effect of pin offset on fixator stability. *Biomaterials.* 1995;16(3):263–264.
217. Ooi KS, Tang HM, Yap V. Management of talonavicular fracture dislocation with external fixator. *ANZ J Surg.* 2011;81(6):492.
218. Orbay GL, Frankel VH, Kummer FJ. The effect of wire configuration on the stability of the Ilizarov external fixator. *Clin Orthop Relat Res.* 1992;(279):299–302.
219. Orsak JE, Watson JT. Biomechanics of external fixation. In: Cooper P, Polyzios, Zgonis T, eds. *External Fixators of the Foot and Ankle.* Philadelphia, PA: KW/Lippincott Williams and Wilkins; 2013:33–40.
220. Paley D, Catagni MA, Argnani F, et al. Ilizarov treatment of tibial nonunions with bone loss. *Clin Orthop Relat Res.* 1989;(241):146–165.
221. Paley D, Lamm BM, Katsenis D, et al. Treatment of malunion and nonunion at the site of an ankle fusion with the Ilizarov apparatus. Surgical technique. *J Bone Joint Surg Am.* 2006;88(Suppl 1 Pt 1):119–134.
222. Parameswaran AD, Roberts CS, Seligson D, et al. Pin tract infection with contemporary external fixation: how much of a problem? *J Orthop Trauma.* 2003;17(7):503–507.
223. Parekh AA, Smith WR, Silva S, et al. Treatment of distal femur and proximal tibia fractures with external fixation followed by planned conversion to internal fixation. *J Trauma.* 2008;64(3):736–739.
224. Park SH, O'Connor K, McKellop H, et al. The influence of active shear or compressive motion on fracture-healing. *J Bone Joint Surg Am.* 1998;80(6):868–878.
225. Parkhill C. A new apparatus for the fixation of bones after resection and in fractures with a tendency to displacement. *Trans Am Surg Assoc.* 1897;15:251–256.
226. Parkhill C. Further observations regarding the use of the bone clamp in ununited fractures, fractures with malunion and recent fractures with tendency to displacement. *Ann Surg.* 1898;27:553–570.
227. Patterson MJ, Cole JD. Two-staged delayed open reduction and internal fixation of severe pilon fractures. *J Orthop Trauma.* 1999;13:85–91.
228. Payandeh JB, McKee MD. External fixation of distal radius fractures. *Hand Clin.* 2010;26(1):55–60.
229. Peltier LM. External skeletal fixation for the treatment of fractures. In: Peltier LM, ed. *Fractures: A History and Iconography of their Treatment.* Novato, CA: Norman Publishing; 1990:183–196.
230. Pettila MH, Sarna S, Paavolainen P, et al. Short-term external support promotes healing in semirigidly fixed fractures. *Clin Orthop Relat Res.* 1997;(343):157–163.
231. Pettine KA, Chao EY, Kelly PJ. Analysis of the external fixator pin–bone interface. *Clin Orthop Relat Res.* 1993;(293):18–27.
232. Pieske O, Geleng P, Zaspel J, et al. Titanium alloy pins versus stainless steel pins in external fixation at the wrist: a randomized prospective study. *J Trauma.* 2008;64(5):1275–1280.
233. Podolsky A, Chao EY. Mechanical performance of Ilizarov circular external fixators in comparison with other external fixators. *Clin Orthop Relat Res Relat Res.* 1993;(293):61–70.
234. Possley DR, Burns TC, Stinner DJ, et al. Temporary external fixation is safe in a combat environment. *J Trauma.* 2010;69(Suppl 1):S135–S139.
235. Prasarn ML, Horodyski M, Conrad B, et al. Comparison of external fixation versus the trauma pelvic orthotic device on unstable pelvic injuries: a cadaveric study of stability. *J Trauma Acute Care Surg.* 2012;72(6):1671–1675.
236. Pugh KJ, Wolinsky PR, Dawson JM, et al. The biomechanics of hybrid external fixation. *J Orthop Trauma.* 1999;13(1):20–26.
237. Pugh KJ, Wolinsky PR, Pienkowski D, et al. Comparative biomechanics of hybrid external fixation. *J Orthop Trauma.* 1999;13(6):418–425.
238. Ramseier LE, Bhaskar AR, Cole WG, et al. Treatment of open femur fractures in children: comparison between external fixator and intramedullary nailing. *J Pediatr Orthop.* 2007;27(7):748–750.
239. Raschke M, Khodadadyan C, Maitino PD, et al. Nonunion of the humerus following intramedullary nailing treated by Ilizarov hybrid fixation. *J Orthop Trauma.* 1998;12(2):138–141.
240. Raschke MJ, Mann JW, Oedekoven G, et al. Segmental transport after unreamed intramedullary nailing. Preliminary report of a "Monorail" system. *Clin Orthop Relat Res Relat Res.* 1992;(282):233–240.
241. *Redento Mora Nonunion of the Long Bones: Diagnosis and Treatment with Compression-distraction Techniques preface.* Milan berlin, Heidelberg new York: Springer;2006:1.
242. Ring D, Hotchkiss RN, Guss D, et al. Hinged elbow external fixation for severe elbow contracture. *Bone Joint Surg Am.* 2005;87(6):1293–1296.
243. Ring D, Jupiter JB. Compass hinge fixator for acute and chronic instability of the elbow. *Oper Orthop Traumatol.* 2005;17(2):143–157.
244. Robbins J, Gerlinger TL, Ward JA. *Can the carbon fiber rods for the Hoffmann II external fixation system be reused? Am J Orthop (Belle Mead NJ).* 2012;41(12):551–553.
245. Roberts CS, Antoci V, Antoci V Jr, et al. The accuracy of fine wire tensioners: a comparison of five tensioners used in hybrid and ring external fixation. *J Orthop Trauma.* 2004;18(3):158–162.
246. Roberts CS, Dodds JC, Perry K, et al. Hybrid external fixation of the proximal tibia: strategies to improve frame stability. *J Orthop Trauma.* 2003;17(6):415–420.
247. Rochman R, Jackson Hutson J, Alade O. Tibiocalcaneal arthrodesis using the Ilizarov technique in the presence of bone loss and infection of the talus. *Foot Ankle Int.* 2008;29(10):1001–1008.
248. Rödl R, Leidinger B, Böhm A, et al. [Correction of deformities with conventional and hexapod frames–comparison of methods]. *Z Orthop Ihre Grenzgeb.* 2003;141(1):92–98.
249. Rogers MJ, McFadyen I, Livingstone JA, et al. Computer hexapod assisted orthopaedic surgery (CHAOS) in the correction of long bone fracture and deformity. *J Orthop Trauma.* 2007;21(5):337–342.
250. Ross JW. O.B.E., E.D. External Fixation In Fractures. *Can Med Assoc J.* 1944;51:543–546.
251. Rozbruch SR, DiPaola M, Blyakher A. Fibula lengthening using a modified Ilizarov method. *Orthopedics.* 2002;25(11):1241–1244.
252. Rozbruch SR, Fragomen AT, Ilizarov S. Correction of tibial deformity with use of the Ilizarov-Taylor spatial frame. *J Bone Joint Surg Am.* 2006;88(Suppl 4):156–174.

253. Rozbruch SR, Pugsley JS, Fragomen AT, et al. Repair of tibial nonunions and bone defects with the Taylor Spatial Frame. *J Orthop Trauma*. 2008;22(2):88–95.

254. Rozbruch SR, Weitzman AM, Watson JT, et al. Simultaneous treatment of tibial bone and soft-tissue defects with the Ilizarov method. *J Orthop Trauma*. 2006;20(3):197–205.

255. Ryder S, Gorczyca JT. Routine removal of external fixators without anesthesia. *J Orthop Trauma*. 2007;21(8):571–573.

256. Saithna A. The influence of hydroxyapatite coating of external fixator pins on pin loosening and pin track infection: a systematic review. *Injury*. 2010;41(2):128–132.

257. Sakurakichi K, Tsuchiya H, Uehara K, et al. Ankle arthrodesis combined with tibial lengthening using the Ilizarov apparatus. *J Orthop Sci*. 2003;8(1):20–25.

258. Saleh M, Rees A. Bifocal surgery for deformity and bone loss after lower-limb fractures. Comparison of bone-transport and compression-distraction methods. *J Bone Joint Surg Br*. 1995;77(3):429–434.

259. Scannell BP, Waldrop NE, Sasser HC, et al. Skeletal traction versus external fixation in the initial temporization of femoral shaft fractures in severely injured patients. *J Trauma*. 2010;68(3):633–640.

260. Schuind FA, Burny F, Chao EY. Biomechanical properties and design considerations in upper extremity external fixation. *Hand Clin*. 1993;9(4):543–553.

261. Schwechter EM, Swan KG. Raoul Hoffmann and his external fixator. *J Bone Joint Surg Am*. 2007;89(3):672–678.

262. Seide K, Wolter D. [Universal 3-dimensional correction and reposition with the ring fixator using the hexapod configuration]. *Unfallchirurg*. 1996;99(6):422–424.

263. Seide K, Wolter D, Kortmann HR. Fracture reduction and deformity correction with the hexapod Ilizarov fixator. *Clin Orthop Relat Res Relat Res*. 1999;(363):186–195.

264. Seitz WH Jr, Froimson AI, Brooks DB, et al. External fixator pin insertion techniques: biomechanical analysis and clinical relevance. *J Hand Surg Am*. 1991;16(3):560–563.

265. Seligson D, Donald GD, Stanwyck TS, et al. Consideration of pin diameter and insertion technique for external fixation in diaphyseal bone. *Acta Orthop Belg*. 1984;50(4):441–450.

266. Shaar CM, Kreuz FP, (eds). Manual of fractures. *Treatment by External Skeletal Fixation*. Philadelphia, PA: WB Saunders; 1943:1–300.

267. Shaar CM, Kreuz FP, Jones DT. End results of treatment of fresh fractures by the use of the Stader apparatus. *J Bone Joint Surg*. 1944;26:471–474.

268. Shearer J, Egan J. Computerized analysis of pin geometry. In: Coombs R, Green SA, Sarmeinto A, eds. *External Fixation and Functional Bracing*. Orthotext, London; 1989: 129–135.

269. Simpson AH, Cunningham JL, Kenwright J. The forces which develop in the tissues during leg lengthening. A clinical study. *J Bone Joint Surg Br*. 1996;78(6):979–983.

270. Sirkin M, Sanders R, DiPasquale T, et al. A staged protocol for soft tissue management in the treatment of complex pilon fractures. *J Orthop Trauma*. 1999;13:78–84.

271. Sisk DT. External fixation. Historical review, advantages, disadvantages, complications and indications. *Clin Orthop Relat Res*. 1983;180:15–22.

272. Sluga M, Pfeiffer M, Kotz R, et al. Lower limb deformities in children: two-stage correction using the Taylor spatial frame. *J Pediatr Orthop B*. 2003;12(2):123–128.

273. Sommers MB, Fitzpatrick DC, Kahn KM, et al. Hinged external fixation of the knee: intrinsic factors influencing passive joint motion. *J Orthop Trauma*. 2004;18(3):163–169.

274. Spiegel PG, VanderSchilden JL. Minimal internal and external fixation in the treatment of open tibia fractures. *Clin Orthop Relat Res*. 1983;(178):96–102.

275. Stanitski DF, Dahl M, Louie K, et al. Management of late-onset tibia vara in the obese patient by using circular external fixation. *J Pediatr Orthop*. 1997;17(5):691–694.

276. Strauss EJ, Banerjee D, Kummer FJ, et al. Evaluation of a novel, nonspanning external fixator for treatment of unstable extra-articular fractures of the distal radius: biomechanical comparison with a volar locking plate. *J Trauma*. 2008;64(4):975–981.

277. Sung JK, Levin R, Siegel J, et al. Reuse of external fixation components: a randomized trial. *J Orthop Trauma*. 2008;22(2):126–301.

278. Suzuki T, Hak DJ, Stahel PF, et al. Safety and efficacy of conversion from external fixation to plate fixation in humeral shaft fractures. *J Orthop Trauma*. 2010;24(7):414–419.

279. Taeger G, Ruchholtz S, Zettl R, et al. Primary external fixation with consecutive procedural modification in polytrauma. *Unfallchirurg*. 2002;105(4):315–321.

280. Tencer AF, Claudi B, Pearce S, et al. Development of a variable stiffness external fixation system for stabilization of segmental defects of the tibia. *J Orthop Res*. 1984;1(4):395–404.

281. Tetsworth KD, Paley D. Accuracy of correction of complex lower-extremity deformities by the Ilizarov method. *Clin Orthop Relat Res*. 1994;(301):102–110.

282. Thakur AJ, Patankar J. Open tibial fractures. Treatment by uniplanar external fixation and early bone grafting. *J Bone Joint Surg Br*. 1991;73(3):448–451.

283. Thordarson DB, Markolf KL, Cracchiolo A 3rd. External fixation in arthrodesis of the ankle. A biomechanical study comparing a unilateral frame with a modified transfixion frame. *J Bone Joint Surg Am*. 1994;76(10):1541–1544.

284. Tomić S, Bumbasirević M, Lesić A, et al. Ilizarov frame fixation without bone graft for atrophic humeral shaft nonunion: 28 patients with a minimum 2-year follow-up. *J Orthop Trauma*. 2007;21(8):549–556.

285. Tsuchiya H, Uehara K, Abdel-Wanis ME, et al. Deformity correction followed by lengthening with the Ilizarov method. *Clin Orthop Relat Res*. 2002;(402):176–183.

286. Tulner SA, Strackee SD, Kloen P. Metaphyseal locking compression plate as an external fixator for the distal tibia. *Int Orthop*. 2012;36(9):1923–1927.

287. Vidal J. External fixation. *Clin Orthop Relat Res*. 1983;180:7–14.

288. Viskontas DG, MacLeod MD, Sanders DW. High tibial osteotomy with use of the Taylor Spatial Frame external fixator for osteoarthritis of the knee. *Can J Surg*. 2006;49(4):245–250.

289. Vives MJ, Abidi NA, Ishikawa SN, et al. Soft tissue injuries with the use of safe corridors for transfixion wire placement during external fixation of distal tibia fractures: an anatomic study. *J Orthop Trauma*. 2001;15(8):555–559.

290. Volkov MV, Oganesian OV. Restoration of function in the knee and elbow with a hinge-distractor apparatus. *J Bone Joint Surg Am*. 1975;57(5):591–600.

291. Vora AM, Haddad SL, Kadakia A, et al. Extracapsular placement of distal tibial transfixation wires. *J Bone Joint Surg Am*. 2004;86-A(5):988–993.

292. Wallace AL, Draper ER, Strachan RK, et al. The vascular response to fracture micromovement. *Clin Orthop Relat Res*. 1994;(301):281–290.

293. Wang ZG, Peng CL, Zheng XL, et al. Force measurement on fracture site with external fixation. *Med Biol Eng Comput*. 1997;35(3):289–290.

294. Watson JT. High energy fractures of the tibial plateau. *Ortho Clin of N Amer*. 1994;25: 723–752.

295. Watson JT. Bone transport. *Techniques in Orthopaedics*. 1996A;11(2):132–143.

296. Watson JT. Tibial pilon fractures. *Techniques in Orthopaedics*. 1996B;11(2):150–159.

297. Watson JT. Hybrid external fixation for tibial plateau fractures. *Am J Knee Surg*. 2001; 14(2):135–140.

298. Watson JT. Distraction osteogenesis. *Journal of AAOS*. 2006;14(10):168–174.

299. Watson JT. Nonunion with extensive bone loss: Reconstruction with Ilizarov techniques and orthobiologics. *Op Tech in Orthop*. 2009;18(2):95–107.

300. Watson JT, Anders M, Moed BR. Bone loss in tibial shaft fractures: Management strategies. *Clin Ortho*. 1995;316:1–17.

301. Watson JT, Karges DE, Cramer KE, et al. Analysis of failure of hybrid external fixation techniques for the treatment of distal tibial pilon fractures. Abstract Procedings 16th Annual Meeting Orthopaedic Trauma Association San Antonio, TX Oct. 12–14, 1999.

302. Watson JT, Kuldjanov D. Bone Defects. Rozbruck SR, Ilizarov S eds. Book Chapter in: *Limb Lengthening and Reconstructive Surgery*. Informa, New York: 2007:184–202.

303. Watson JT, Moed BR, Karges DE, et al. Pilon fractures: Treatment protocol based on severity of soft tissue injury. *Clin Orthop Relat Res*. 2000;375:78–90.

304. Watson JT, Occhietti M, Parmar V. Rate of Postoperative Wound Infections in Patients with Pre-existing External Fixators Treated with Secondary Open Procedures. Abstract Procedings 15th Annual Meeting Orthopaedic Trauma Association Charlotte, North Carolina Oct. 22–24, 1999.

305. Watson JT, Ripple S, Hoshaw SJ, et al. Hybrid external fixation for tibial plateau fractures: clinical and biomechanical correlation. *Orthop Clin North Am*. 2002;33(1):199–209.

306. Watson MA, Mathias KJ, Maffulli N, et al. The effect of clamping a tensioned wire: implications for the Ilizarov external fixation system. *Proc Inst Mech Eng H*. 2003;217(2): 91–98.

307. Watson MA, Matthias KJ, Maffulli N, et al. Yielding of the clamped-wire system in the Ilizarov external fixator. *Proc Inst Mech Eng H*. 2003;217(5):367–374.

308. W-Dahl A, Toksvig-Larsen S, Lindstrand A. No difference between daily and weekly pin site care: a randomized study of 50 patients with external fixation. *Acta Orthop Scand*. 2003;74(6):704–708.

309. Wei DH, Poolman RW, Bhandari M, et al. External fixation versus internal fixation for unstable distal radius fractures: A systematic review and meta-analysis of comparative clinical trials. *J Orthop Trauma*. 2012;26(7):386–394.

310. Williams EA, Rand JA, An KN, et al. The early healing of tibial osteotomies stabilized by one-plane or two-plane external fixation. *J Bone Joint Surg Am*. 1987;69(3):355–365.

311. Windhagen H, Glockner R, Bail H, et al. Stiffness characteristics of composite hybrid external fixators. *Clin Orthop Relat Res*. 2002;(405):267–276.

312. Woon CY, Wong MK, Howe TS. LCP external fixation–external application of an internal fixator: two cases and a review of the literature. *J Orthop Surg Res*. 2010;5:19.

313. Wosar MA, Marcellin-Little DJ, Roe SC. Influence of bolt tightening torque, wire size, and component reuse on wire fixation in circular external fixation. *Vet Surg*. 2002;31(6): 571–576.

314. Wu JJ, Shyr HS, Chao EY, et al. Comparison of osteotomy healing under external fixation devices with different stiffness characteristics. *J Bone Joint Surg Am*. 1984;66(8): 1258–1264.

315. Yamako G, Ishii Y, Matsuda Y, et al. Biomechanical characteristics of nonbridging external fixators for distal radius fractures. *J Hand Surg Am*. 2008;33(3):322–326.

316. Yang W, Watson JT, Zheng Y, et al. Optimizing Half Pin Placement of Mono-lateral External Fixation Frames for Superior Stability. Paper presentation. In Abstracts: The Seventh International Congress of Chinese Orthopaedic Association, November 15–18, 2012, Beijing, China.

317. Yasui N, Nakase T, Kawabata H, et al. A technique of percutaneous multidrilling osteotomy for limb lengthening and deformity correction. *J Orthop Sci*. 2000;5(2):104–107.

318. Yildiz C, Atesalp AS, Demiralp B, et al. High-velocity gunshot wounds of the tibial plafond managed with Ilizarov external fixation: a report of 13 cases. *J Orthop Trauma*. 2003; 17(6):421–429.

319. Yu JR, Throckmorton TW, Bauer RM, et al. Management of acute complex instability of the elbow with hinged external fixation. *J Shoulder Elbow Surg*. 2007;16(1):60–67.

320. Yuenyongviwat V, Tangtrakulwanich B. Prevalence of pin-site infection: the comparison between silver sulfadiazine and dry dressing among open tibial fracture patients. *J Med Assoc Thai*. 2011;94(5):566–569.

321. Zaffagnini S, Iacono F, Lo Presti M, et al. A new hinged dynamic distractor, for immediate mobilization after knee dislocations: Technical note. *Arch Orthop Trauma Surg*. 2008; 128:1233–1237.

322. Zheng K, Li X, Fu J, et al. Effects of Ti2448 half-pin with low elastic modulus on pin loosening in unilateral external fixation. *J Mater Sci Mater Med*. 2011;22(6):1579–1588.

323. Ziran BH, Morrison T, Little J, et al. A new ankle spanning fixator construct for distal tibia fractures: optimizing visualization, minimizing pin problems, and protecting the heel. *J Orthop Trauma*. 2013;27(2):e45–e49.

324. Zlowodzki M, Prakash JS, Aggarwal NK. External fixation of complex femoral shaft fractures. *Int Orthop*. 2007;31(3):409–413. Epub 2006 Aug 15.

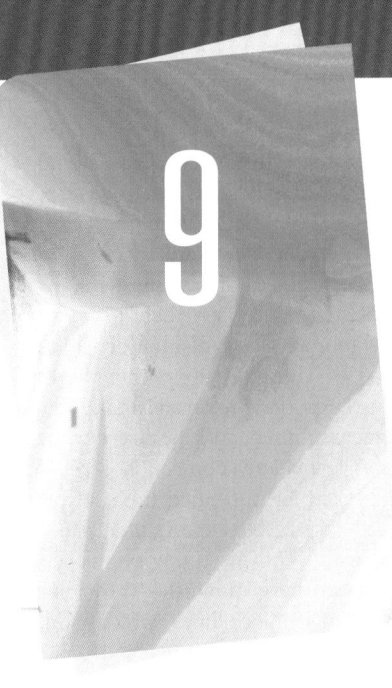

9

MANAGEMENT OF THE MULTIPLY INJURED PATIENT

Hans Christoph Pape and Peter V. Giannoudis

EPIDEMIOLOGY OF POLYTRAUMA

Incidence and Mortality

Trauma is a major cause of death and disability worldwide that mainly affects young adults.[427] According to the World Health Organization (WHO) 2nd Global Status Report on Road Safety, which involved 178 countries, over 1.2 million people die each year worldwide because of road traffic injuries.[440,441] However, only 10% of these fatalities occur in high-income countries. The WHO predicts that the rate of fatal injuries will increase in the next few decades. In addition, between 20 and 50 million patients are injured on the world's roads every year. Severe injuries have an especially large impact on society and health systems. Trauma registries in western countries have been established to document the epidemiology, pattern, and causes of death, thereby enhancing the quality of trauma care systems.

The definition of multiple trauma varies among surgeons from different specialties and between different centers and countries. This variation has led to the development of standardized scoring systems to allow comparable stratification of injuries between centers and to aid prediction of morbidity and mortality.

Polytrauma is a term describing injured patients who have sustained injuries to more than one body region or organ system of which at least one is life threatening. The cumulative severity of this trauma load on the injured patients' anatomy and physiology is usually expressed using the injury severity score (ISS) with polytrauma being defined as an ISS of ≥16 or ≥18.[5,383] Trentz emphasized the pathophysiologic systemic impact of multiple trauma defining polytrauma as "a syndrome of multiple injuries exceeding a defined severity (ISS ≥ 17) with sequential systemic reactions (systemic inflammatory response syndrome (SIRS) for at least 1 day) that may lead to dysfunction or failure of remote organs and vital systems, which have not themselves been directly injured."[199,415]

About 30 years ago, the concept of a trimodal distribution of deaths was introduced by Trunkey.[417] Deaths occurred at the scene of the accident, within 60 minutes, in the emergency department or operating room, within 1 to 4 hours, or later after 1 week. Severe brain injury and exsanguination were documented as the leading causes of death within the first 1 to 6 hours. However recent epidemiologic studies from the Trauma Registry of the German Society of Trauma Surgery (TR-DGU) and the Trauma Audit and Research Network (TARN, UK) show a bimodal distribution of mortality with a first and a second peak occurring within 0 to 6 hours and 1 to 6 days, respectively. Massive hemorrhage and severe brain injury remain the commonest causes of death in the first 6 hours. Later deaths are associated with advanced age and complications such as sepsis and organ failure.

The TR-DGU was established in 1993 and documents data from 367 participating clinics from 7 European countries.[220] The recently published annual report from 2011 included epidemiologic evaluation of 67,782 trauma patients. The potential need for intensive care treatment and admission from the trauma bay were the main inclusion criteria. A typical multiply injured trauma patient is male (71.5%) with a mean age of 43.4 years.[221] Blunt trauma accounts for 95.2% of all cases and motor-vehicle-traffic–related injuries account for 57.3% of all cases. These were followed by falls (>3 meters = 16.3%; <3 meters = 15.1%) and suicides (5.1%). The analysis of the injury distribution according to the body region using the abbreviated injury scale (AIS) ≥2 demonstrates that craniocerebral injuries and thoracic trauma are present in 60.7% and 61.9%, respectively. Injuries of the upper extremity (34.7%), lower extremity (31.8%), pelvis (22%), and spine (34.2%) were less common.

Recent data show that the time period from the initial injury to emergency department admission was approximately 70 minutes (a mean of 20 minutes to arrival + 30 minutes on site + 20 minutes for patient transport to the hospital).[451] The initial focused abdominal sonography in trauma (FAST) was performed within an average of 6 minutes after admission. The mean time interval to the first chest and pelvis x-rays was

13 minutes and 17 minutes, respectively. Computed tomography (CT) of the head and a whole-body CT scan were performed after 24 minutes and 28 minutes from the time of arrival. Emergency surgical intervention was initiated approximately 79 minutes after arrival at the trauma room.

According to the TR-DGU trauma registry there has been a continuous decrease in the mortality rate of multiply injured patients in the past decades.[352] The mortality within the first 24 hours after admission was 7% and approximately 13.2% died during the hospital stay. Demographic changes in society can also be observed in this database. The elderly population is becoming increasingly active. The mean age increased from 38 years in 1990 to 43 years in 2011 and 25% of the trauma patients were older than 65 years of age.[221] This increasing prevalence is important since the elderly often have diminished physiologic reserve and associated significant comorbidities, which require special consideration. The distribution of injuries and type of injury mechanism is likely to be different in a population with a high incidence of osteoporosis. Elderly patients can become multiply injured following low-energy trauma and these injuries may have worse outcomes. For example, while falls have been reported to account for only 9% to 11% of injury-related deaths in the general population, they comprise more than 50% of trauma deaths in persons over 65 years of age.[10] Patients with limited mental or physical capacity are also more likely to be involved in accidents as they are slower to identify and respond to dangerous situations.[195,213] One must also consider the likelihood of a medical emergency such as a myocardial infarction (MI) or stroke precipitating an accident, making it necessary to treat this pathology as well as the patient's injuries.

Effects of Legislation

In 1997, in the United States, motor-vehicle accidents resulted in 41,967 deaths (16/100,000/yr) and 3.4 million nonfatal injuries (1270/100,000/yr).[94] Motor-vehicle–related injuries were the leading cause of death among persons aged 1 to 24 years.[94]

Between 1982 and 2001, in a review of 858,741 traffic deaths in the United States, five risk factors were noted to contribute to mortality: (a) alcohol use by drivers and pedestrians (43%), (b) not wearing a seat belt (30%), (c) lack of an air bag (4%), (d) not wearing a motorcycle helmet (1%), and (e) not wearing a bicycle helmet (1%).[82] Over the 20-year period, mortality rates attributed to each risk factor declined due to legislation. There were: (1) 153,168 lives saved by decreased drinking and driving, (2) 129,297 by increased use of seat belts, (3) 4,305 by increased air bag prevalence, (4) 6,475 by increased use of motorcycle helmets, and (5) 239 by increased use of bicycle helmets.

Research has shown the effectiveness of lower blood alcohol laws for young and inexperienced drivers and of intervention training programs for servers of alcoholic beverages.[444] All the 50 states and the District of Columbia have laws defining it as a crime to drive with a blood alcohol concentration (BAC) at or above 0.08%.

Seat belts stop the occupant with the car and therefore prevent the body from being ejected when the car stops. Deceleration energy is spread over more energy absorbing parts of the body such as the pelvis, chest, and shoulders. Safety belts are the single most effective means of reducing fatal and nonfatal injuries in motor-vehicle crashes and primary enforcement seat belt laws, where the police are allowed to stop a driver and issue a ticket for the sole reason of not wearing a seat belt, are likely to be more effective than secondary laws, which allow nonbelted occupants or drivers to be ticketed only after being stopped for another moving violation.[287,340,379,380] According to the National Highway Traffic Safety Administration (NHTSA)[286] seat belt use nationwide was 82% in 2007, ranging from 63.8% in New Hampshire to 97.6% in Hawaii. Twenty-eight states had primary enforcement seat belt laws. However, almost 70% of the 16- to 34-year-old passenger vehicle occupant fatalities killed during night time hours were unrestrained.[286] All states have child passenger protection laws. These vary widely in age and size requirements as do the penalties for noncompliance. Child-restraint use in 1996 was 85% for children aged less than 1 year and 60% for children aged 1 to 4 years. Since 1975, deaths among children aged less than 5 years have decreased by 30% to 3/100,000/yr, but the rate of deaths in the 5 to 15 years group has declined by only 11% to 13%.[285] In a study reviewing accidents involving 4,243 children aged 4 to 7 years between 1998 and 2002, injuries occurred among 1.81% of all 4- to 7-year olds, including 1.95% of those in seat belts and 0.77% of those in belt-positioning booster seats. The odds of injury were 59% lower for children in belt-positioning boosters than in seat belts. Children in booster seats sustained no injuries to the abdomen, spine, or lower extremities, while children in seat belts alone had injuries to all body regions.[99,100]

Motor-Vehicle Design/Passive Car Safety and Prevention

Driver air bags have been shown to reduce mortality by 8%, whether the driver was belted or not. However, seat belts provide much greater protection, with seat belt use reducing the risk of death by 65% (or by 68% in combination with an air bag).[81] No differences in the risk of frontal crash deaths were observed between adult occupants with sled-certified and first-generation air bags. Together with reports of decreases in air bag–related deaths, significant reductions in frontal deaths among children seated in the right-front position in sled-certified vehicles have also been reported.[40] Air bags have been reported to be associated with reduced in-hospital mortality and decreased injury severity.[442] In a systematic review, helmets have been shown to reduce the risk of death by 42% and the risk of head injury by roughly 69% in motorcycle riders.[231]

Current evidence supports the view that reduced speed limits, speed-camera networks, and speed calming substantially reduce the number of road deaths, a trend that is apparent in the United Kingdom, Australia, France, and other countries.[336] There is also evidence that speed enforcement detection devices are a promising method for reducing the number of road traffic injuries and deaths.[444] It is of note however that in the United States, there are no speed-camera networks.[336]

With regard to pedestrians, cars and light trucks (vans, pick-ups, and sport utility vehicles) are responsible for most of the pedestrian deaths (85.2%) in the United States. Heavy trucks, buses, and motorcycles are responsible for the remainder.[318] Buses kill eight times as many pedestrians as cars per mile of vehicle travel. Vehicle characteristics such as mass, front end design, visibility,[66] and degree of interaction with pedestrians probably determine their risk per mile.[318] Therefore, one option to reduce pedestrian fatalities might be the modification of motor vehicles. However, every type of motor vehicle has to be evaluated on an individual basis. Lowering the front end of light trucks, and consequently the point of impact with a pedestrian's body, might reduce the likelihood of serious head and chest injuries.[64]

In order to investigate the relationship between changes in the mechanism and pattern of injury for vehicular trauma victims with modern vehicle design, restrained car occupants, bicyclists, and pedestrians injured between 1973 and 1978, and between 1994 and 1999 in a specific region in Germany were compared.[337] Lower average ISSs (5.0 vs. 12.1), lower rates of polytrauma (4.5% vs. 15 %), and lower mortality rates (3.4% vs. 14%) were measured for all groups during the later period. Analysis showed that the crash severity was unchanged between the two periods and the reductions were related to improvements in vehicle design and not just seat belt use.[337]

ECONOMIC IMPACT ON SOCIETY

Trauma Care Systems

Organized civilian trauma care in the United States has its origins in the late 1960s when it was stated that the quality of civilian trauma care in the United States was below the standard in combat zones in Vietnam: "If seriously wounded, the chances of survival would be better in the zone of combat than on the average city street." A trauma system provides the full range of coordinated care to all injured patients in a defined geographic area. It includes injury prevention, pre- and in-hospital care as well as rehabilitation. The concepts of organized trauma care[320] have proven to be one of the most important advances in the care of the injured patient over the last 30 years.[170,226] The number of states with a trauma system increased from 7 in 1981 to 36 in 2002.[377] Nevertheless, in 2000 approximately 40% of the US population still lived in states without a trauma system.[281]

Using an established trauma system network also might facilitate the care of victims of natural disasters[307] or terrorist attacks.[180] The performance of hospitals and health providers in a trauma system is subjected to review from both within and without the system.[247,276,321] Research and constant re-evaluation are necessary for continuous assessment of the system and improvement of its outcomes and efficiency.[227,377] According to a systematic review of published evidence[245] of the effectiveness of trauma systems in the United States, until 1999 the implementation of trauma systems decreased hospital mortality of patients who were severely injured to approximately 15%.[48,193,239,245,275] The relative risk of death due to motor-vehicle accidents was 10% lower in states with organized systems of trauma care than in states without such systems.[281] However it took about 10 years to establish an organized system of trauma care that was effective in reducing mortality. Nathens et al. concluded that this is consistent with the maturation and development of trauma triage protocols, interhospital transfer agreements, organization of trauma centers, and ongoing quality assurance.[280] Counties with 24-hour availability of surgical specialties, CT scanners, and operating rooms have a lower motor-vehicle–collision–related mortality, compared with counties without these resources. Counties with designated trauma centers have lower motor-vehicle–related mortality rates.[257] Recently published, prospectively collected, data comparing mortality in trauma centers to nontrauma centers showed a 25% mortality reduction in patients under 55 years of age when treated in a trauma center.[236] Outcome results obviously depend on every single part of the chain in the trauma system, as well as on the interplay of these elements and there is a lack of evidence in the understanding of the contribution of individual components on the efficacy of the system. However, pre-hospital notification protocols and performance improvement programs appear to be most associated with decreased risk-adjusted odds of death.[226] With regard to pre-hospital trauma care, there are ongoing national and international debates and studies as to which system is best[39,95] and how pre-hospital trauma care could be improved.[47,68,108,138,328] Analysis shows that worldwide there are three different types of organized pre-hospital trauma care systems. These are:

1. Basic life support (BLS) systems

   • noninvasive supportive care to trauma patients by emergency medical technicians (splinting)

   • transport trauma patients rapidly to a medical care facility

2. Paramedic advanced life support (PARAALS) systems

   • undertake invasive procedures such as intubation and intravenous (IV) fluid therapy, administer drugs

3. Physician advanced life support (PHYSALS) systems

The pre-hospital trauma system in the United States results from the experience in the Vietnam war, where trained paramedical personnel were responsible for initial treatment in the combat zone, whereas physicians were thought to best contribute in a hospital setting.[279] Extensive medical care at the scene was almost impossible due to combat, so that "load and go" or "scoop and run" was favored. In contrast, Franco-German[95] emergency medical systems are physician directed and in most cases prefer longer periods at the scene of the accident ("stay and play") to stabilize the patient before transport to an appropriate hospital.

An international study comparing these systems[279] by using shock rate at the Emergency Department (ED shock rate) and early trauma fatality rate as outcome parameters to assess pre-hospital outcomes found out that the ED shock rate did not vary significantly between PHYSALS and PARAALS systems. The early trauma fatality rate was significantly lower in PHYSALS systems compared to PARAALS systems. Therefore a physician at the scene may be associated with lower early trauma fatality rates. However, often there is a lack of data to allow proper comparisons of outcomes between the emergency medical systems of different countries.[95]

Several other studies and reviews focusing on pre-hospital trauma care systems however have concluded that there is no evidence supporting advanced pre-hospital trauma care (ALS). Almost all of these studies used hospital trauma fatality as the main outcome parameter and only compared ALS with BLS

| TABLE 9-1 | A Comparison of the Mean Time to Definitive Treatment of Major Fractures in Patients with Multiple Injuries in the United States and Germany |

Duration Until Definitive Treatment	USA n = 77	GERMANY n = 93	p-value
All fractures	5.5 ± 4.2 d	6.6 ± 8.7 d	n.s
Humerus fractures	5 ± 3.7 d	6.6 ± 6.1 d	n.s
Radius fractures	6 ± 4.7 d	6.1 ± 8.7 d	n.s
Femur fractures	7.9 ± 8.3 d	5.5 ± 7.9 d	n.s
Tibia fractures	6.2 ± 5.6 d	6.2 ± 9.1 d	n.s
Pelvis fractures	5 ± 2.8 d	7.1 ± 9.6 d	n.s

d = days

Schreiber V, Tarkin IS, Hildebrand F, et al. The timing of definitive fixation for major fractures in polytrauma—a matched pair comparison between a US and European level I centers: analysis of current fracture management practice in polytrauma. *Injury.* 2011;42(7):650–654.

systems.[51,224,225,349] One further study also compared PARA-ALS in Montreal to PHYSALS in Toronto and BLS in Quebec using in-hospital mortality as the outcome parameter.[225] The PHYSALS system was not associated with a reduction in risk of in-hospital death, so that the conclusion was that in urban centers with highly specialized level I trauma centers, there is no benefit in having on-site ALS for the pre-hospital management of trauma patients.[225]

Moreover, it has been questioned whether the trauma system dictates the surgical priorities in trauma care. In a recently published study, the timing and management of major fractures in multiply injured patients were compared between level I trauma centers in the United States and Germany. This matched pair analysis demonstrated that the timing of fracture fixation is comparable between a cohort treated at a level I trauma center in the United States and the German Trauma Registry (Table 9-1).[314,368]

Reimbursement and Development of Costs

Trauma is a global problem and continues to have a major impact on health systems. Trauma-associated expenses have been calculated by numerous study groups.[19,78,146,255,290,327] However, due to the heterogeneity of the health and trauma systems and methodologic differences the comparison of these calculations is difficult. Studies have emphasized the importance of cost calculation in trauma care by indicating that it allows not only the estimation of the national burden of injury, but it also enables the identification of inefficient treatment strategies and assessment of the development of costs.[19,78,146,255,290,327] Standardized analyses have been suggested in order to compare different trauma systems. This data can be crucial for political decision making. The expenses of trauma care in developed countries have been shown to be similar to the costs of cancer and stroke.[254] Due to an aging society an immense increase of trauma-associated expenses is expected. Injury burden in the United States exceeds $400 billion in medical care costs, but 80% of these costs were related to loss of productivity.[78] It has been suggested that productivity and the ability to work be used as long-term outcome parameters in patients with multiple injuries. Occupation and financial independence have been shown to be associated with superior long-term quality of life.[78] Therefore, the health economics issue is currently an important topic of debate in every National Health System around the world. In patients with multiple injuries, the issue of reimbursement is still unresolved and has been the focus of considerable discussion lately.

Most of the health systems continue to be in deficit as a result of their disproportionate funding and inadequacy of reimbursement policies.[146,203,327,348,363,383,388] Before, however, one decides to evaluate the real cost of treatment of a specific procedure to the National Health System, one must be familiar with the elements that a thorough economic analysis should include. A thorough economic analysis of any medical condition measures direct, indirect, and intangible costs.[196,403] It incorporates both fixed and variable costs; the direct monetary expenses and the indirect expenses associated with the duration of therapy, the final functional outcome, disability payments, and the monetized quality of life aspects.[85,200,330]

Fixed costs are related to the hospital's overhead and are those where the clinician has the least control. The variable costs are mostly related to clinical practice and thus they have been more extensively studied. Direct medical and nonmedical costs are easier to record, compared to the indirect costs, and most of the existing literature focuses on these. The indirect and intangible costs are considered to be more difficult to estimate and they require longer follow-up of the patients. However they can be significantly larger than the direct costs. Thus, a large deficit of the existing health economics studies evidence is their lack of an "all-inclusive cost analysis."

The health economics of orthopedic trauma rely heavily on resources and expertise that span the entire trauma system, including pre-hospital, in-hospital, and post-hospital care. The financial implications are very diffuse and not easily assessed.

In polytrauma patients a complete economic evaluation is even more difficult. It involves expenses related to the pre-hospital and emergency services, the intensity of the medical and nursing staff workload that varies with individual patient and the element of "trauma readiness."[103] "Trauma readiness" is related to the ongoing evolution of the personnel's expertise, the infrastructure's effectiveness, and the efficacy of the trauma team coordination. The expense of maintaining a dedicated trauma team on a 24-hour-a-day schedule has been proven to be the most difficult economic parameter to assess and reimburse.[402] Over the years several authors have attempted to address the trauma and polytrauma cost issues.[80,164,191,206,261,291,382,430] In all these studies it was evident that conventional cost accounting tools were inadequate despite the recent advances in "operations management" and health economics. The necessary components of an all-inclusive economic analysis of a trauma system were first outlined in the Model Trauma Care Systems Plan published by the U.S. Bureau of Health Resources Development in 1992.[101] Table 9-2 presents a description of the different aspects of trauma-related health economics.

Allowing for the difficulties in undertaking cost estimations, medical spending on injuries in the United States in 1987 was $64.7 billion. In 2000 it accounted for 10.3% of the total medical expenditure and had reached $117.2 billion. The considerable increase in the expense of trauma can also be seen in studies from the United Kingdom, Germany, Switzerland, and the rest of Europe.[18,114,135,278,294,295,299,353,398]

Taking the above issues into consideration one can easily appreciate the reasons why providing a service for these cases is not sustainable. The issue of reimbursement is still unresolved and has been the focus of recent discussion. Most health care organizations and trauma systems apply a predetermined charge for their trauma services, which does not relate to each injured patient's direct or indirect medical and nonmedical costs. It is no surprise therefore, that especially for complex cases and polytrauma patients, cost estimation has been proven

TABLE 9-2 The Different Aspects of Health Economics that Need to be Evaluated in an All-Inclusive Financial Profile of the Management of Trauma

Direct Costs		Indirect Costs	Intangible Costs
Medical	**Nonmedical**		
Personnel costs	Transportation	Lost productivity	Quality of life (pain, suffering, grief)
Supplies costs	Lodging of patients	Lost earnings	
Length of hospitalization	and relatives	Impairment	QALY evaluation (quality-adjusted life years lost)
Diagnostic interventions		payments	
Medications		Residential and	Psychosocial parameters
		nursing care	
Surgical interventions		Insurance costs	
Outpatient attendances		Legal costs	
Rehabilitation			
Pre-hospital costs			
Trauma readiness			
Trauma training			

to be inadequate and inaccurate. The overall comparison of the actual direct costs of polytrauma and the relative reimbursement resulted in a negative balance of 80% to 900% across the different health systems.[383] Moreover, the absence of a single formal trauma network and the existence of many small informal networks centered upon teaching or large general hospitals, almost certainly hinders the efforts to achieve a thorough financial assessment of the trauma services that are provided. Without an accurate assessment of the overall provided services, reimbursement and justification of adequate resources are hampered.

The workload of the trauma hospitals in these networks varies significantly; and is often unrecognized, and under-funded by the authorities. These units often function under significant pressure. The continuous and intense utilization of the infrastructure's resources (operating room time, intensive care unit [ICU] beds, etc.) for trauma and polytrauma patients, prolongs the waiting lists, and limits the level of services provided to local patients for the more rewarding and better reimbursed routine elective treatments.[83,90,185,316] Thus these centers often present a less "healthy" profile, according to strict financial and managerial criteria, in comparison to smaller hospitals with a reduced trauma workload. In the United Kingdom, the National Health Service (NHS) revenues from elective orthopedic cases have been shown to be more than those of acute trauma cases, again highlighting the problem of inadequate, trauma tariffs.[24] Unfortunately, as the number of trauma cases grows the administrative focus is directed more to the government imposed targets on elective waiting lists and is therefore reducing the resources of specialist trauma services such as pelvic or spine units[24] despite the fact that pelvic fractures are the third most common cause of death after motor-vehicle accidents.[198]

The health economics of patients with pelvic trauma was evaluated in 2004.[24] The authors identified that one of the main reasons for the financial difficulties inherent in treating pelvic trauma and polytrauma, in tertiary centers in the United Kingdom, was the establishment of an out of area transfer system (OATS) in 1999. According to the analysis, the acquired reimbursement covered only 60% of the treated cases due to the fact that it was calculated in a retrospective manner and referred to trauma workloads of previous years. The increasing numbers of trauma cases in such centers requires a more accurate and up-to-date estimation of the actual volume of the trauma care services and their costs.

It is of note that currently a comprehensive and complete evaluation of the financial implications of polytrauma does not exist. The assessment of the cost effectiveness of any trauma system must be correlated with the return of trauma victims to a productive life. The complexity and multiplicity of the different aspects of treatment and rehabilitation in these patients is the main reason for the deficiency of the contemporary health economics literature. However, the necessity for good health economics literature cannot be overstressed in order to develop and monitor the provided services, and assess the deficiency of the associated financial frameworks. Trauma centers must identify and understand their cost structure not only to improve their efficiency, but also to survive. In this context, medical and

financial researchers must focus on all the different aspects of the polytrauma expenses. More specifically, the following recommendations can be made:

(1) The direct medical costs should include all the diagnostic and therapeutic procedures and interventions in these patients and avoid the limitations of the "polytrauma tariff." The target should be to achieve an accurate assessment of all the expenses of the trauma hospital services in order to claim a satisfactory reimbursement.

(2) The concept of "trauma readiness" is of particular importance to the in-hospital personnel and services. The variability and intensity of the trauma workload cannot be compared with that of any other medical service. The 24-hour-a-day availability of a trauma team and the financial implications of this have to be included at any trauma economic analysis and then reimbursed.

(3) The costs of pre-hospital services related to trauma and polytrauma should also be assessed on a prospective and all-inclusive basis taking into account the aspects of "readiness" and also the secondary transportation of individual polytrauma patients to tertiary specialized centers with established pelvic and spine units.

(4) The health authorities should assess the tertiary referral trauma centers using different criteria and financial algorithms than the referring hospital centers. The "waiting list targets" and "length of hospital stay" of these hospitals should be compared with those of similar trauma centers with a proportionate trauma workload and multidisciplinary readiness, and not with those of hospitals which provide services of a more elective nature.

(5) The difficulties of evaluating the more difficult factors such as the monetized quality of life and the psychosocial costs of trauma and polytrauma should not discourage the researchers. A prospective study following up these patients so that their final outcome is known should be initiated as soon as possible. It would provide all the necessary information to the Health Service administration of the real and unrecognized socioeconomic burden of contemporary trauma. This could then be used to justify requests for increased resources to the policy-making authorities.

(6) The multi-fragmentation of health services and trauma networks should be also avoided. The conclusions and the decisions made after an all-inclusive assessment of the financial implications should include all the health care providers that are involved with polytrauma care.

PATHOPHYSIOLOGY AND IMMUNE RESPONSE TO TRAUMA

Local and Systemic Inflammatory Response

A fracture is associated with damage to bone, periosteum, and adjacent soft tissues such as muscle and connective tissue. Adjacent blood vessels bleed into the affected area and cause a hematoma. Bone marrow content in the form of stem and precursor cells then gains access to the hematoma. Limited oxygenation and restricted nutrient supply induce necrosis of the surrounding tissue. The analysis of fracture hematoma has been studied numerous times but its content is not completely understood. It is clear that fracture hematoma plays a crucial role in bone and tissue regeneration.[208] The removal of fracture hematoma is associated with prolonged fracture healing.[147,264,317] In contrast, the implantation of it into tissue remote to the fracture leads to new bone formation.[147,264,317] It is known that local tissue damage stimulates the liberation of damage-associated molecular patterns (DAMPs), chemokines, and alarmins which lead to systemic spill over and activation of the systemic immune response.[199,249] The additional activation of the complement cascade initiates the chemotaxis of leukocytes and neutrophil cells.[282] Surprisingly, studies have shown that human skin and muscle tissue demonstrate limited activation (cytokine expression [IL-1β, IL-6, and TNF-α] and neutrophil cell migration) as a result of adjacent blunt femoral fracture.[421] In contrast, pronounced pro- and anti-inflammatory immune response was identified in adipose tissue.[421] The authors postulated that cytokines are mainly produced by adipose tissue surrounding the fracture after blunt trauma. Thus, it is feasible to trigger the local and systemic inflammatory response after trauma. If muscle tissue is injured, cellular composition of muscle hematoma appears to have discrepancies compared with fracture hematoma.[364] The initial rate of neutrophil cell migration was reduced in fracture hematoma when compared to levels measured in muscle hematoma.[364] Moreover, fracture hematoma was associated with higher percentages of CD4+ T helper cells and reduced rates of CD8+ cytotoxic cells.[364] Whether these differences affect the local and systemic immune response could not be deduced from these studies.

During the past century the physiologic response to injury was described as showing 3 phases: (a) a hypodynamic ebb phase (shock) where our body initially attempts to limit the blood loss and to maintain perfusion to the vital organs; (b) a hyperdynamic flow phase lasting for up to 2 weeks, characterized by increased blood flow, in order to remove waste products and to allow nutrients to reach the site of injury for repair; and (c) a recuperation phase, lasting for months, to allow the human body to attempt to return to its pre-injury level.[118] However, with the knowledge accumulated during the past 20 years, it soon became clear that the physiologic response to injury was not as simplistic as it was initially thought but rather it represents a complex phenomenon involving the immune system and even today is still not fully understood. With the advances made in every field of medicine and particularly in the disciplines of molecular biology and molecular medicine, it is now possible to characterize and quantify the cellular elements and molecular mediators involved in this dynamic physiologic process.

The first physiologic reaction after injury involves the neuroendocrine system leading to an adrenocortical response characterized by the increased release of adrenocorticosteroids and catecholamines.[55] Subsequently, the work of Hans Selye further illustrated the importance of this neuroendocrine response to trauma by pointing out that this was involved in what he named "the general adaptation syndrome."[374] This is considered nowadays as a forerunner to the SIRS.[30] This activation of the neuroendocrine system is responsible for the increase in heart rate, respiratory rate (RR), fever, and leukocytosis observed in trauma patients after major injury. Besides trauma, SIRS can be induced by other insults such as burns, infection or major surgery and is defined as being present when two or more of the criteria apply (body temperature: >38 or <36°C; heart rate: >90/min; RR: >20/min or $PaCO_2$ < 32 mm Hg; white blood cell count: >12,000 or <4,000/mm^3 or >10% band forms).[30]

The activation of the immune system following a traumatic insult is necessary for hemostasis, protection against invading microorganisms, and for the initiation of tissue repair and tissue healing. Restoration of homeostasis is dependent on the magnitude of the injury sustained and the vulnerability of the host who may possess an abnormal or defective local and systemic immune response and fail to control the destructive process. Multiple alterations in inflammatory and immunologic functions have been demonstrated in clinical and experimental situations following trauma and hemorrhage, suggesting that a cascade of abnormalities that ultimately leads to adult respiratory distress syndrome (ARDS) and multiple organ dysfunction syndrome (MODS) is initiated in the immediate postinjury period.[126,130,132,133,159] Blood loss and tissue damage caused by fractures and soft tissue crush injuries induce generalized hypoxemia in the entire vascular bed of the body. Hypoxemia is the leading cause of damage as it causes all endothelial membranes to alter their shape. Subsequently, the circulating immune system, namely the neutrophil and macrophage defense systems, identify these altered membranes. The damaged endothelial cell walls, by trying to seal the damaged tissue, induce activation of the coagulatory system (Fig. 9-1). This explains why these patients develop a lowered platelet count. Further cascade mechanisms, such as activation of the complement system, the prostaglandin system, the specific immune system, and others, are set in motion.

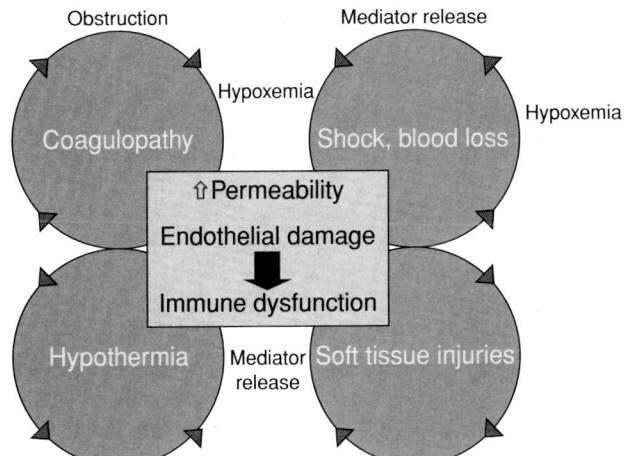

FIGURE 9-1 Four cycles demonstrate the pathophysiologic cascades associated with the development of post-traumatic immune dysfunction and endothelial damage. The exhaustion of the compensatory mechanisms results in development of complications such as ARDS/MODS.

The release of mediators of both pro-inflammatory and anti-inflammatory nature is dependent primarily on the severity of the "first hit phenomenon" (accidental trauma) and secondarily on the activation of the various molecular cascades during therapeutic or diagnostic interventions, surgical procedures, and post-traumatic/postoperative complications ("second" or "third" hits).[119,127] The mediators that are involved in the sequelae of post-traumatic events are released from the cellular populations locally at the site of injury and subsequently systemically. The sequestration and the activation mainly of the polymorphonuclear granulocytes (PMN), the monocytes, and the lymphocytes trigger a multifocal molecular and pathophysiologic process. The pathomechanism of complement activation, leukostasis, and macrophage activation has been associated with the concept of the "low flow syndrome"[332] and more recently with endothelial and PMN leukocyte activation.[168,223] The cells interact and adhere to the endothelium via adhesion molecules like L-selectin, ICAM-1, and integrin β2 (representatives of the selectin, immunoglobulin, and integrin superfamilies, respectively). After firm adhesion, PMN leukocytes can extravasate and by losing their autoregulatory mechanisms can release toxic enzymes causing remote organ injury in the form of ARDS, MODS.[127,159]

If the systemic immune response is not able to restore the integrity of the host, dysregulation of the immune system will occur leading initially to an exaggerated systemic inflammation and at a later stage to immune paralysis.[31] However, recent studies analyzing the genome expression of leukocytes in the postinjury period support the idea of simultaneous induction of the innate and suppression of the adaptive immune systems[452] (Fig. 9-2). The analysis of the genomic response to trauma has shown a "genomic storm" with activation of more than 5,136 genes.[452] Trauma has stimulated the expression of genes involved in innate immunity, microbial recognition, or inflammation. In contrast, the expression was decreased in genes for T-cell function and antigen presentation. Moreover, a comparable genetic response was registered after severe blunt trauma, severe burns, and low-dose endotoxemia. These results indicate that the initiation of the immune response following both trauma and sepsis starts through common pathways (e.g., TLR-4). In addition, this study revealed that the gene expression between patients with complicated versus uncomplicated clinical recovery is not qualitative, but rather quantitative. Patients with uncomplicated recovery were associated with a down regulation of genes within 7 to 14 days after trauma.[452]

The availability of techniques to measure molecular mediators has allowed different research groups to search for inflammatory markers which could detect patients in a borderline condition and who are at risk of developing post-traumatic complications. Appropriate treatment may then prevent the onset of adverse sequelae. Serum markers of immune reactivity can be selectively grouped into markers of acute phase reactants, mediator activity, and cellular activity (Table 9-3).[122,256,284,312,397]

Interleukin-6 (IL-6) has perhaps been the most useful and widely employed of these mediators, partly due to its more consistent pattern of expression and plasma half life.[315] A measurement of >500 pg/dL in combination with early surgery has been associated with adverse outcome.[315] Clinical parameters are also useful in such an assessment with the SIRS score having been developed for such a purpose.[243] Though both systems have previously been correlated with injury severity, with early elevation being associated with adverse outcome,[343] little work examining in detail the relationship between these two assessments exists. In a recent study it was found that in the early phase both IL-6 and SIRS are closely correlated with the new injury severity score (NISS) and each other. A cut-off value of 200 pg/dL was shown to be significantly diagnostic of an "SIRS state." Significant correlations between adverse events and both the IL-6 level and SIRS state were demonstrated.[121]

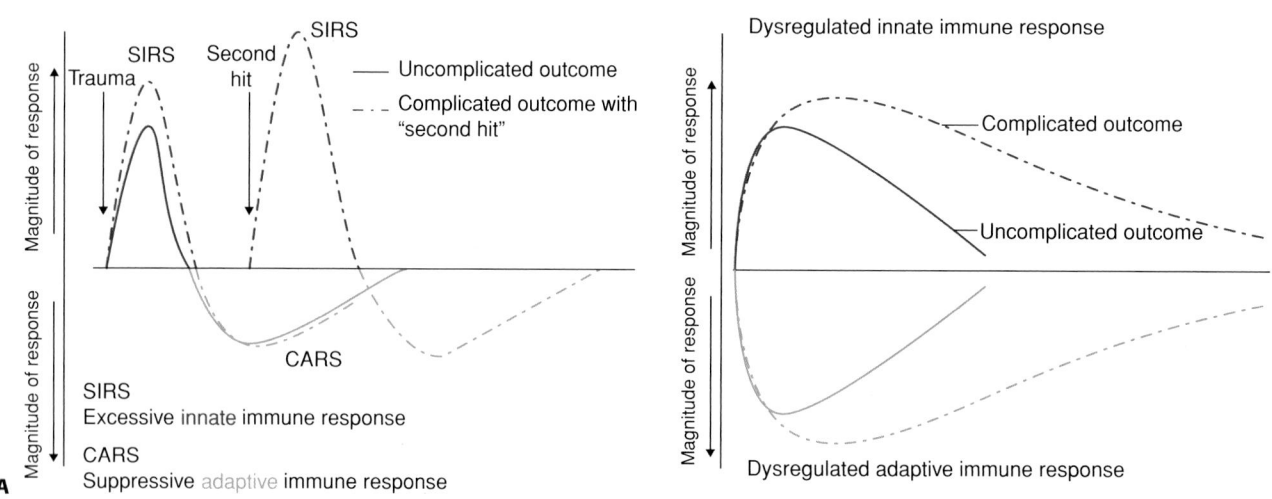

FIGURE 9-2 A: Current paradigm shows initial pro-inflammatory response associated with the development of systemic inflammatory response syndrome and delayed immunosuppression also known as compensatory anti-inflammatory response syndrome (CARS). **B:** New data shows a simultaneous induction of pro- and anti-inflammatory genes and suppression of adaptive immune system following trauma (Xiao W, Mindrinos MN, Seok J, et al. A genomic storm in critically injured humans. *J Exp Med.* 2011;208(13):2581–2590.).

TABLE 9-3	Serum Pro- and Anti-Inflammatory Markers[314]	
Pro-Inflammatory Cytokines	**Cellular Sources**	**Function in Inflammation**
TNF	Monocytes/macrophages, mast cells, T lymphocytes epithelial cells	Stimulates upregulation of endothelial adhesion molecules. Induction of other cytokines, chemokines, and NO secretion. The inducer of acute phase response. Induce fever. Short half life, not useful marker of the inflammatory response after trauma.
IL-1	Monocytes/macrophages, T lymphocytes endothelial cells, some epithelial cells	Similar to TNF.
IL-6	Monocytes/macrophages, T lymphocytes, endothelial cells	Inducer of acute-phase response. Stimulate proliferation of T and B lymphocytes. Long half life, the best prognostic marker of complications after trauma(SIRS, sepsis, MOF).
Chemokines (IL-8)	Macrophages, endothelial cells, T lymphocytes, mast cells	The function of chemoattractant, leukocytes activation. Useful for diagnostic markers of ARDS.
Anti-Inflammatory Cytokines	**Cellular Sources**	**Function in Inflammation**
IL-10	Monocytes/macrophages, T lymphocytes	Inhibit pro-inflammatory cytokines secretion, oxygen radical production, adhesion molecule expression, and Th-1 lymphocyte proliferation. Enhance B lymphocyte survival, proliferation, and antibody production. IL-10 levels are correlated with severity of injury and the risk of development of sepsis, ARDS, and MOF.
IL-6	See the Table of anti-inflammatory cytokines.	Reduction of TNF and IL-1 synthesis. Regulate the release of IL-1Ra and sTNF-Rs.

Lately, the quest to discover new biomarkers of immune reactivity has led to the discovery of signaling substances termed alarmins, so named because they are danger signals.[22] The alarmins are endogenous molecules capable of activating innate immune responses as a signal of tissue damage and cell injury. In this group of endogenous triggers belong molecules such as the high mobility group box 1 (HMGB1), heat shock proteins (HSPs), defensins, cathelicidin, eosinophil-derived neurotoxin (EDN), as well as others. These structurally diverse proteins function as endogenous mediators of innate immunity, chemoattractants, and activators of antigen presenting cells (APCs).[300] HMGB1 is a nuclear protein which influences nuclear transactions and plays a role in signaling after tissue damage. In contrast to alarmins, the so-called pathogen-associated molecular patterns (PAMPs) represent inflammatory molecules of a microbial nature being recognized by the immune system as foreign due to their peculiar molecular patterns. Both PAMPS and alarmins are currently considered to belong to the larger family of DAMPs.[22] PAMPs and DAMPs are being recognized by our immune system by the expression of multiligand receptors such as the Toll-like receptors (TLRs).[453] Overall, the above molecules represent a newly documented superfamily of danger signals being capable of activating innate immune responses after trauma. The number of molecules being categorized in this superfamily is expanding but their pathophysiologic contribution in trauma-related induced systemic activation is still under investigation.

The evolution of molecular biology has allowed scientists to monitor different variables related to the endothelial cell activation and interaction process. We can now achieve characterization and quantification of the endothelial response to the initial trauma and to the subsequent stress events, thus monitoring the clinical course of the patient.[110,228] It is now becoming clear that the problem of managing patients with multiple injuries has shifted from early and effective resuscitation to the treatment of the host response to injury. The quantification of the resulting activity of the variety of the circulating mediators may predict a potential disaster but does not necessarily contribute to the salvage of the patient at risk. Too much or too little immune response? Which one of the two opposites is worse or better? Can we intervene and if so at what stage, in which direction, and in which of the affected individuals? The real question may well be whether all these markers and molecules are just epiphenomena or related to the outcome. Currently, research is attempting to better understand all the processes and the cascade of events that regulate these responses. Research has aimed to describe responses to surgery at the molecular level and to develop and evaluate techniques to modify surgical stress responses. The release mechanisms of the surgical stress response as well as the factors that could amplify the response should be considered by the surgeons. The severity of the injury, type of anesthesia, administration of adequate pain relief, the type of surgical procedure, the timing and length of surgery, the preexisting comorbid conditions, any genetic influences that will cause an adverse outcome, the expertise of the theatre staff, and the expertise of the surgeon are some of the important factors to be taken into account.

Genetics and Trauma

It has been our observation that there are still patients who do not "obey" the roles set by the predictive parameters following trauma. Some patients fare worse and some others fare better than predicted. In the early 1990s it was recognized that these differences in the clinical course of the patients and outcome are subject to biologic variation in the context of trauma or surgery.[148] This biologic variation is highly dependent on the genetic constitution and the importance of genes as cause of diseases or as predisposing factors has become indisputable. The observed polymorphisms are of different types. Some of them are mutations located within endonuclease restriction sites whereas others are SNPs, or consist of insertions or deletions of larger fragments, as detected by the polymerase chain reaction technique.[131] The polymorphism can be located within the gene or in the promoter region. Polymorphisms are different alleles, none of which is predominant in the population. A specific polymorphism variation can be associated with a genetic disease. The polymorphism can also interact with the environment and then exert detrimental actions.

With the availability of molecular diagnostic techniques, there has been an increased interest in conducting "disease-gene association" studies determining the role of genetic variations in the inflammatory response to injury and infection. The existence of susceptible genotypes for postoperative sepsis is no longer a myth. A growing body of evidence suggests now that genetic susceptibility influences the development of surgical sepsis and its sequelae of ARDS and MODS. The identification of functional polymorphisms in several cytokine genes and other important molecules provides a potential mechanism whereby these variations may exist. Several studies have reported the relationship between different polymorphic variants and the risk of developing post-traumatic complications.[137,139,194,232,334,369,435]

However, when investigating genetic polymorphisms, it is not enough just to determine the presence of a polymorphism. One has to take several criteria into account. Patients do show evidence of different genetic constitutions. Investigating polymorphisms linked to disease can be blurred by the existing genetic variation. Therefore, it is necessary to determine the overall genetic constellation of the population under investigation. Furthermore, the power of the study has to be sufficient to be able to have specific results. One has to consider whether other genes may be involved. These genes might be the actual cause for the differences that are being investigated. The investigated gene is then just an epiphenomenon. It is therefore important to study family genetics at the same time. The family constitution can tell more about underlying genes involved in the disease process. If differences in disease outcome are linked to one or more genetic polymorphisms, one has to perform a subsequent study in another cohort. This cohort has to show similar linkage of genes to outcome. Currently, the abovementioned studies, and others,[232,341,369] have indicated the influence of specific polymorphic variants of important genes in the development of post-traumatic sepsis. However, most of the published studies have been undertaken in small populations, with geographic, but not necessarily ethnic, differences. This makes the interpretation of the results more difficult. Because of the limited groups examined and the fact that not all studies have adhered to specific genetic association criteria, application of genetic information to random patients will need multicenter and multinational studies.

Future research should focus on a broad array of genes. Single nucleotide polymorphism (SNP) genotyping assays can do that and categorize the patients. Early identification of patients at risk would allow direct interventions with biologic response modifiers in an attempt to improve morbidity and mortality rates. Early results appear to have been achieved in septic patients. In these patients, goal-directed therapy, low-dose steroid supplementation, blood glucose control, and activated protein C therapy appear to be associated with an improved outcome after sepsis.[84,341,342] Hopefully, similar achievements can be made in patients with acute trauma in the future.

Scoring Systems

Trauma patients are a very heterogeneous population. The need for comparative analysis of the injury-, management-, and outcome-related parameters among the different patient groups, hospitals, trauma management strategies, and health systems has stimulated the development of many trauma scoring systems and scales over the last 40 years.[11,38,42,59,205,439]

These scoring systems represent a means of quantifying the injuries that have been sustained together with multiple other independent parameters such as comorbidities, age, and mechanism of injury. They serve as a common language between clinicians and researchers. Initially, they were designed for the purpose of field triage and in that regard they needed to be simple and user friendly. Subsequently, they have evolved to more complex and research-focused systems. Their concept is based on converting many independent factors into a one-dimensional numeric value that ideally represents the patient's degree of critical illness. They are often based on complex mathematical models derived from large data sets and registries such as the major trauma outcome study (MTOS) or the TARN.[61,413]

Ideally, a complete trauma scoring system should reflect the severity of the anatomic trauma, the level of the physiologic response, the inherent patient reserves in terms of comorbidities and age, and as proven recently, should incorporate immunologic aspects and genetic predisposition parameters.[15,117,128,129,131,132,386] The variety of the potential applications of such scoring systems ranges from the basic pre- and inter-hospital triage and mortality prediction to other prognostic parameters such as the length of hospital stay and risk of disability. These systems can be used as a tool for comparison of diagnostic or therapeutic methods as well as for the auditing of trauma management.

The existing injury scoring systems can be classified into scales based on anatomic parameters. Examples of these are the AIS,[9] the injury severity score (ISS),[11] the maximum abbreviated injury severity scale (MAIS),[9] the NISS,[301] the anatomic profile (AP),[77] the modified anatomic profile (mAP),[355] the organ injury scale (OIS),[4] and the ICD-9 injury severity score (ICISS) (ICISS).[354] Other scoring systems are based on physiologic parameters. Examples of these are the trauma score (TS),[62] the revised trauma score (RTS),[63] the acute physiology and chronic health evaluation (APACHE).[456] Some scoring systems are based on combinations of these parameters. Examples are the trauma and injury severity score (TRISS),[42] a severity characterization of trauma (ASCOT),[205] and the physiologic trauma score (PTS).[214]

Numerous studies have assessed the accuracy, reliability, and specificity of the different trauma scores (TSs).[60,202]

Anatomical-Based Scales and Scoring Systems

The AIS was initially introduced in 1971.[73] It has been revised a number of times and is continuously monitored and evolved by a committee of the Association of Advancements of Automotive Medicine (AAAM).[131] Its latest version was published in 2005,[116] but the most used versions in the current literature are the AIS90 and AIS98. In general, the AIS is an anatomically based consensus-derived, global severity scoring system that classifies each injury by body region according to its relative significance. All the different anatomic injuries are matched with a different seven digit number code. They are classified by (1) the affected body region (first digit, with body region 1 = head, 2 = face, 3 = neck, 4 = thorax, 5 = abdomen, 6 = spine, 7 = upper extremities, 8 = pelvis and lower extremities, and 9 = external and thermal injuries); (2) the type of anatomic structure (second digit, ranges from 1 to 6); (3) the specific anatomic structure (third and fourth digits, range from 02 to 90); and (4) the level of the injury (fifth and sixth digits, range from 00 to 99). The last digit of each 7-digit AIS-code follows a dot and represents the injury severity of the specific injury on a scale of 1 to 6 (1 = minor, 2 = moderate, 3 = serious, 4 = severe, 5 = critical, and 6 = maximal currently untreatable injury). This last severity digit has been developed by a consensus of many experts and is continuously monitored by the committee.

The ISS was introduced by Baker et al. in 1974.[11] Each injury in the patient is allocated an AIS code and then the codes are grouped in six ISS-body regions: head and neck, face, chest, abdomen, extremities and pelvis, and external. Only the highest AIS severity score (post dot digit—seventh digit of the AIS code) in each ISS body region is used. The ISS is the sum of the squared AIS scores from the three most severely injured ISS-body regions. It can take values from 1 to 75. A value of 75 can be assigned either by the sum of three AIS severities of 5 in three different ISS-body regions, or by the presence of at least one AIS severity of 6. Any patient with an AIS severity of 6 in any body region is automatically given an ISS of 75 independent of any other injuries. The ISS score is virtually the only anatomical scoring system in widespread use. It has been validated on numerous occasions and it has been shown to have a linear correlation with mortality, morbidity, hospital stay, and other measures of injury severity. Currently, it represents the gold standard of anatomic trauma scoring systems.[36,238,258] However, it has certain weaknesses as any error in AIS coding or scoring increases the ISS error. In addition, it is not weighted over the different body regions and injury patterns and it often underestimates the overall anatomic injury particularly in penetrating trauma, or in multiple injuries of one body region. The ISS is not a useful triage tool as a full description of the patient's injuries is not initially available.

The MAIS is another anatomic injury score often used in daily clinical practice and research, which also originates from the AIS. It is the highest AIS code in a multitrauma patient, and is used by researchers to describe the overall injury to a particular body region and to compare frequencies of specific injuries and their relative severity.[184,262]

In order to address some of the disadvantages of the ISS Osler et al.[301] described the new ISS (NISS) in 1997. This is calculated as the sum of the squares of the highest three AIS severity scores regardless of the ISS-body regions. It has been found to be better than the ISS especially for orthopedic trauma and penetrating injuries.[13,14,158,181] However, it has still not extensively evaluated and has the disadvantage of requiring an accurate injury diagnosis before a precise calculation can be made.

The AP[76,117] was also introduced to address the weaknesses of the ISS. It was described as one of the components of the ASCOT and includes all the serious injuries (AIS severity ≥3) of all the body regions. It is also weighted more toward the head and the torso. All serious injuries are grouped into four categories (A = head and spine, B = thorax and anterior neck, C = all remaining serious injuries, and D = all nonserious injuries). The square root of the sum of squares of the AIS-scores of all the injuries in each of the four categories is computed and by logistic regression analysis a probability of survival is calculated. The AP has been proven to be superior to the ISS in discriminating survivors from nonsurvivors. However, its complex computational model has restricted its applications and limited its use.

A mAP[355] has subsequently been introduced. This is a four number characterization of the injury. These four numbers are the MAIS severity across all body regions, and the modified A, B, C component scores of the original AP (mA = head and spine, mB = thorax and neck, and mC = all other serious injuries).[76] The mAP component score values (A, B, C) are equal to the square root of the sum of the squares of the AIS values for all serious injuries (AIS 3 to 6) in the specified body region groups. This leads to an AP score, a single number defined as the weighted sum of the four mAP components. The coefficients are derived from logistic regression analysis of 14,392 consecutive admissions to four level I trauma centers of the MTOS.[61]

The OIS is a scale of anatomic injury within an organ system or body structure. It was originally designed in 1987. The OIS offers a common language between trauma surgeons, but it is not designed to correlate with patient outcomes. The organ injury scaling committee of the American Association for the Surgery of Trauma (AAST) is responsible for revising and auditing the OIS tables that can be found on the AAST web site.[4] The severity of each organ injury may be graded from 1 to 6 using the severity subcategories of the AIS. The injuries can also be divided by mechanism such as blunt or penetrating or by anatomic description such as hematoma, laceration, contusion, or vascular.

Recently, another anatomical injury scoring system was introduced based on the well-accepted and popular coding system of international classification of diseases (ICD)-9 instead of that of the AIS. The ICD-9 is a standard taxonomy used by most hospitals and health care providers. The ICISS[354] utilizes survival risk ratios (SRRs) calculated for each ICD-9 discharge diagnosis. The SRRs are calculated by relating the number of survivors of each different ICD-9 code to the total number of patients with such an injury. The product of all the different SRRs of a patient's injuries produces the ICISS. Neural networking has been employed to further improve ICISS accuracy. ICISS has been shown to be better than ISS and to outperform TRISS in identifying outcomes and resource utilization. However, in several studies the mAP scores, AP and NISS appear to outperform ICISS in predicting hospital mortality.[156,269,270,396]

Physiology-Based Scores

Initially, the trauma scoring systems based on physiology parameters were introduced as field triage tools. The basic characteristic of these physiology-based scores is that they are comparatively simple but also time dependent. In 1981, Champion et al.[62] hypothesized that early trauma deaths are associated with one of the three basic systems: the central nervous, cardiovascular, and respiratory systems. They designed a scoring system, the trauma score (TS), based on a large cohort of trauma patients, which focused on five parameters these being the Glasgow coma scale (GCS), the unassisted RR, respiratory expansion, the systolic blood pressure (SBP), and capillary refill. All contributed equally in the calculation of this score. It was proven to be useful in predicting survival outcomes, with good inter-rater reliability, but was shown to underestimate head injuries and it also incorporated parameters, such as respiratory expansion and capillary refill, which were difficult to assess in the field.[63]

Consequently a revised trauma score (RTS) was developed 8 years later[63] by the same authors. This was internationally adopted and is still in clinical use as both a field triage and a clinical research tool. It includes three variables (GCS, RR, SBP), and a coded value from 0 to 4 can be assigned to each (Table 9-4). An RTS score may range from 0 to 12 with lower scores representing a more critical status. In its initial validation this physiologic scoring system identified 97% of the fatally injured as those having an RTS ≤11. It also indicated certain weaknesses which suggested that it should be used in combination with an anatomic-based score.[271,347] Currently, the threshold of 11 is used as a decision-making tool for transferring an injured patient to a dedicated trauma center.

The RTS is used in its weighted form in clinical research, auditing, and accurate outcome prediction and is called coded RTS (RTSc). It is calculated with the following mathematical formula that allows weighting of the three contributing parameters (GCS, RR, SBP) and their significance.

$$RTSc = 0.9368\ GCS + 0.2908\ RR + 0.7326\ SBP$$

The RTSc emphasizes the significance of head trauma and ranges from 0 to 7.8408 with lower values representing worse physiologic derangement. The threshold for transfer to dedicated trauma centers for the RTSc is 4. Besides the obvious calculation difficulties that this formula may impose, the use of the RTS or the RTSc is compromised by the fact that the GCS cannot be estimated in intubated and mechanically ventilated patients or in intoxicated patients. Also the calculated value may vary with the physiologic parameters, which often change rapidly. It may also underestimate the severity of trauma in a well-resuscitated patient.

The APACHE was introduced in 1981[207] and its latest revision in 2006 (APACHE IV) represents the most modern scoring system utilized in the demanding environment of ICU and therefore also in intensive trauma units (ITU). The evaluated parameters include the age of the injured patient, any chronic health comorbidities, several physiologic elements required for the calculation of the acute physiology score (APS),[456] previous length of ITU stay, emergency surgery, admission source, and diagnosis on admission to ITU. These parameters are responsible for both the complexity of the APACHE score as well as for its superior prognostic accuracy.

Combined Scores

The individual deficiencies of the anatomic scales and the physiology-based TSs led researchers to develop combined approaches to more accurately translate the overall injury load of a trauma victim to a single score or value. The TRISS[38] uses both the ISS and the RTS as well as the patient's age to predict survival. The probability for survival (Ps) is expressed using the formula Ps = $1/(1 + e^{-b})$, where e is a constant (approximately 2.718282) and b = $b_0 + b_1(RTS) + b_2(ISS) + b_3$(age factor). The b coefficients are derived by regression analysis from the MTOS database.[61] The probability of survival according to this model ranges from 0 to 1.000 for a patient with a 100% expectation of survival. TRISS has been used in numerous studies.[34,35,50,93,241,298,389,433] Its value as a predictor of survival or death has been shown to be from 75% to 90% depending on the patient data set used. However, the deficiencies that govern the ISS and the RTS were also found in their derivative, the TRISS. In particular, the inability to account for multiple injuries in the same anatomic region, the variability of the RTS value, the inability to calculate a value in intubated patients, because of the inaccuracy of the GCS, and RR, the difficulty of assessing comorbidities, and the physiologic reserve of the injured patient encouraged the researchers to continue their quest for a better TS.

In 1990, another more inclusive trauma scoring system was introduced. ASCOT[59] attempts to incorporate anatomic (AP) and physiology (RTS) parameters as well as the patient's age in a more efficient way than TRISS. The ASCOT score is derived from the same formula (Ps = $1/(1 + e^{-b})$) as the TRISS but has different coefficients for blunt and penetrating injuries. The principal claimed advantage of ASCOT was the use of the AP instead of the ISS, which better reflected the cumulative anatomic injury load of the patient. However, while the predictive performance of the ASCOT was marginally better than that of the TRISS its complexity is considerably greater.[155,246,302]

TABLE 9-4	Unweighted Revised Trauma Score as Used in Field Triage		
GCS	**RR (per Minute)**	**SBP (mm Hg)**	**Coded Value**
13–15	10–29	>89	4
9–12	>29	76–89	3
6–8	6–9	50–75	2
4–5	1–5	1–49	1
3	0	0	0

GCS, Glasgow coma scale; RR, respiratory rates; SBP, systolic blood pressure.

In 2002, the physiologic trauma score (PTS) was described. This incorporated the SIRS score on admission (range 0 to4, one point for the presence of each of the following: T > 38° or < 36°C; HR > 90/min; RR > 20/min; neutrophil count >12,000 or <4000/mm^3, or the presence of 10% bands), the age, and the GCS into a simple calculation to predict mortality. This new statistical model appeared to be accurate and comparable with the TRISS, or the ICISS in subsequent studies.[214]

Despite the considerable effort that has gone into designing these different assessment methodologies and mathematical models, it is very difficult to translate the multifactorial problems inherent in an injured patient into a single number or score and all scoring systems will have advantages and disadvantages. In the future additional factors are likely to be evaluated and incorporated into future trauma scoring systems. Obvious examples are the immunologic responses to trauma and possibly genetic predisposition. Until the development of an "ideal" scoring model, we should be cautious in our conclusions regarding the existing systems and the prediction of outcome of the injured patient.

INITIAL EVALUATION AND MANAGEMENT OF THE MULTIPLY INJURED PATIENT

Principles of ATLS

The management of a polytrauma patient can be divided into the pre-hospital phase and the in-hospital phase. The chance of survival and the extent of recovery are highly dependent on the medical care that follows the injury. The speed with which lethal processes are identified and halted makes the difference between life and death and between recovery and disability. Time is an independent and cynical challenger of any physician managing multiply injured patients. Thus the adopted approach to this peculiar clinical setting should be based on getting most things right and very few things wrong. Due to the inherent imperfections of the human nature of medical personnel, this approach should be based on simple, well-organized and standardized principles.

Starting from the pre-hospital phases of extrication and transfer to the hospital the initial evaluation and management, despite its inherent limitations due to lack of time and means, has been proven to be decisive for the severely injured patient.[304] The effect on survival of early extrication,[443] the initial management from trained emergency personnel whether they are physicians or paramedics,[189,375,407] and equally importantly, fast transfer to designated trauma centers[338,405] has been evaluated and highlighted in numerous studies. The concept of advanced trauma life support (ATLS) was initially introduced by an orthopedic surgeon in cooperation with the University of Nebraska in 1978.[7,57] After having an airplane crash with his family he recognized that there were serious deficiencies in medical education and inconsistencies in the delivery of trauma care in the United States at that time. This initiative encouraged surgeons and doctors in Nebraska to develop a regional training course including lectures and lifesaving demonstrations. One year later the American College of Surgeons Committee of Trauma adopted this course and

developed it further to create a practically orientated educational program. The main purpose of this course was to train doctors in order to standardize the process of care of injured patients. In particular, an effective approach to initial assessment and the clinical skills required for good initial management should be taught to surgeons early in their training.

The concept of ATLS was kept very simple. The ABCDE rule allows a standardized and ordered evaluation of patients.[6] The greatest threats to life should be identified first and addressed in an efficient and adequate manner. The definitive diagnosis is not immediately important and should never impede the application of required treatment. Necessary critical interventions should be performed early. Therefore, required clinical skills are taught in "skill stations" where several emergency scenarios are simulated. During the primary survey the following sequential steps should be addressed.

A: Airway Maintenance with Cervical Spine Protection

The assessment of the airway should be performed first. Airway obstruction due to facial fractures, foreign bodies, or bleeding should be identified as soon as possible. In patients with severe head injuries (GCS < 8), or who are unconsciousness, definitive management is usually required. During the initial assessment the immobilization of the cervical spine should be accomplished and maintained to avoid further spinal cord injuries.

B: Breathing and Ventilation

Injuries of the lung, chest wall, and diaphragm may compromise gas exchange. Therefore, clinical and radiologic examination, with a chest radiograph, should be performed as soon as possible in order to identify injuries that can impair ventilation, these commonly being tension pneumothorax, flail chest with pulmonary contusion, massive hemothorax, and open pneumothorax. Adequate and effective treatment of the respiratory disorder has to be initiated immediately.

C: Circulation with Hemorrhage Control

Hemorrhagic shock is a common cause of death in severely injured patients. Hidden bleeding is most likely in the chest, abdomen, pelvis, or long bones. In patients with clinical signs or radiologic signs of thoracic or abdominal bleeding IV volume resuscitation, using crystalloids or blood products, has to be initiated and the patient investigated in case they need surgery to control the bleeding. In the case of unstable pelvic injuries pelvic stabilization can be achieved with pelvic binders in the trauma bay.

D: Disability (Neurologic Evaluation)

Hemodynamic and respiratory stable patients should be evaluated for the presence of neurologic deficits. In trauma victims suspected of having brain injury repeated evaluation of pupillary size and level of consciousness is required. Decreased level of consciousness might be a clinical sign of reduced cerebral perfusion or direct cerebral trauma. Therefore, unconscious patients should be re-evaluated for airway maintenance and adequate oxygenation, ventilation and circulation status.

E: Exposure/Environmental Control

Patients should be completely undressed in order to identify clinical signs of hidden injuries. Rewarming of patients with warm blankets avoids the development of hypothermia and associated complications such coagulopathy, circulatory dysfunction, inadequate oxygenation, and the appearance of cardiac arrhythmias.

If the patient demonstrates vital functions and the primary survey is completed a secondary survey can be started within 12 to 24 hours after injury. During the secondary survey a complete examination from head-to-toe should be performed including the evaluation of the complete history, where this is possible, medication, allergies, and past illnesses. In particular, the presence of hidden injuries should be actively sought.

Following these principles and the structured initial diagnostic evaluation of the traumatized patient, the priorities of the airway, breathing, circulation, and disability (neurologic deficit) have proven to be the gold standard. Together with direct triage to the appropriate health center, protection of the spine, early aggressive pre-hospital resuscitation, modern telemedicine and informatics, advances in transportation, and the rationalization of the location of the trauma centers have resulted in minimizing pre-hospital mortality and reaching mortality rates that are lower than those of the predicting mathematical models (TRISS, ASCOT).[47,303,358] With reference to the pre-hospital period in the course of trauma management some of the important subjects of current debate are

(i) the management of the airway

  a. pre-hospital endotracheal intubation (ETI) or not[45,87,96]

  b. the use of neuromuscular blocking agents[86,88]

  c. effect of hyperventilation, which is common in the pre-hospital setting, on the outcome of patients in shock[244] or with head trauma[71])

(ii) the control of the hemorrhage and circulatory resuscitation

  a. control of external hemorrhage with modern dressings[283]

  b. appropriate pre-hospital fluid resuscitation endpoints—limited fluid resuscitation versus standard aggressive strategy,[23,65] the optimal type of resuscitation fluids.[46,75,140,142,344,428] Standard crystalloid fluids (N/S 0.9%, R/L) versus hypertonic fluids (N/S 7.5% ± 6%) Dextran 70 versus polymerized hemoglobin blood substitutes)

(iii) the management of potential spinal injuries

  The universally accepted guidelines are that the spine should be protected if any suspicion of spinal injury is raised by the mechanism of injury or the clinical findings. However, recently some concerns regarding the liberal use of these guidelines have been reported.[20,43,160] However, the lack of strong evidence promoting the liberal pre-hospital protection of the spine currently supports the more conservative and traditional approach.

(iv) Improved triage

  With current financial restrictions and a demand for optimal management of resources and facilities,[123] the role of transfer of each trauma victim to the most appropriate hospital according to the injury load and the patient-related reserves, is crucial. The basic tool to accomplish this task is the different triage scales and scores.[236] The use of models combining physiology-based data together with patient-related and mechanism-of–injury–related parameters is of considerable interest.[74,174,175]

Respiratory Function Assessment

Airway obstruction has been shown to be usually due to the following injuries or problems.

1. Mid-facial fractures with obstruction of the nasopharynx

2. Mandibular fractures with the obstruction of the pharynx by the base of the tongue

3. Direct laryngeal or tracheal injury

4. Blood or vomit aspiration

5. Foreign bodies (e.g., dentures)

Treatment should prioritize removal of any airway obstruction. If the obstruction is sub-glottic, emergency cricothyroidotomy or tracheostomy can be lifesaving. Obstruction of the trachea in the region of the mediastinum can cause severe respiratory impairment. This can lead to severe mediastinal emphysema and perforation of the endotracheal tube.

The next priority is to maintain respiration, which can be compromised by thoracic or central nervous dysfunction. Disorders of the respiratory system can be diagnosed clinically from symptoms and signs including dyspnea, cyanosis, stridor, depressed conscious level, abnormal chest expansion, and the presence of major thoracic injuries. Thoracic injury can cause acute respiratory derangement, including lung contusion, tension pneumothorax, and hemothorax. Tension pneumothorax is a life-threatening condition and represents an acute life-threatening condition. The management of pneumothorax and hemothorax should include the insertion of a chest drain to decompress the chest.

Pulmonary edema can be caused by cardiac dysfunction and can occur as a consequence of direct cardiac trauma[419] or secondary MI. Alternatively, isolated blunt thoracic trauma may cause high-pressure edema, which has also been observed following thoracic compression. Management of these two conditions differs—one requiring fluid replacement therapy and the other the use of diuretics. However, the initial management of both types of edema involves continues suction and the use of positive end expiratory pressures (PEEPs).

Severe head injury can cause central respiratory impairment and severe shock may result in severe cerebral hypoxia and subsequent respiratory impairment. It is important that the emergency physician does not underestimate the effect of hemorrhagic shock. Continuous observation of the spontaneously breathing patient with minor injuries can be justified in these cases. In the severely or multiply injured patient, immediate intubation and ventilation for adequate oxygenation is indicated. The tidal volume of 8 to 10 mL/kg of body weight, PEEP of 5 mL, and 50% O_2 saturation of the air are prerequisite for adequate ventilation.

Assessment of Volume Status

Using a parallel approach it is usual to start the immediate management of post-traumatic shock while full evaluation of respiratory, neurologic, and cardiovascular status is ongoing. Prolonged shock can lead to further post-traumatic complications and therefore impact negatively on the patient's prognosis. Two large bore IV cannulae should be inserted during the preclinical phase and rapid fluid replacement therapy should commence as soon as possible. The cannulae are usually placed in the antecubital fossa and fastened securely to prevent them being dislodged.

On arrival to the emergency room, further IV lines can be inserted as appropriate. Single internal jugular or subclavian vein lines have the disadvantage of being too long and narrow to allow rapid transfusion of large amounts of fluid. If the lines in the peripheral veins are not feasible a venous cut down can be undertaken using the long saphenous vein at the ankle.

The choice of fluid for trauma resuscitation remains a controversial issue.[268] Historically, crystalloid solutions were considered unsuitable, as they were rapidly lost from circulation, with plasma or serum being preferred. In the 1960s, it was discovered that resuscitation with crystalloid solutions was associated with lower rates of renal impairment and mortality. It was considered that losses into the interstitial space occurred due to edema formation that required additional fluid replacement. Therefore infusion of a combination of crystalloid and blood in a 3:1 ratio was recommended. The application of these principles, particularly in military conflicts, coincided with the emergence of "adult respiratory distress syndrome" or shock lung as a clinical entity in survivors of major trauma. Whether this was a consequence of large volume crystalloid infusion was unclear. Interest in the use of colloid products was therefore renewed. However, early results were conflicting, partly due to shortcomings in trial design. Meta-analyses of these smaller studies revealed no overall difference in the rate of pulmonary insufficiency following resuscitation with either fluid type. Moreover, when final mortality was considered, particularly in the subgroup of trauma patients, a significant improvement in the overall survival rate was observed in the group administered crystalloid.[67,362] Crystalloid fluid is therefore considered to be the first treatment choice in most centers and is particularly favored in US trauma centers. Ringer's lactate has various theoretical advantages over isotonic saline though clinical trials have not shown differences in outcome. Research into fluid selection for resuscitation is ongoing, particularly as much early evidence is based on the use of albumin as a colloid. More recently, newer products with higher molecular weights have become available that should be more efficient in maintaining fluid in the intravascular space. There is further evidence however that in cases of severe hemorrhagic shock, increased capillary permeability allows these molecules to leak into the interstitium, worsening tissue edema and oxygen delivery.[268]

Animal studies demonstrating that small bolus administration of hypertonic saline was as effective as large volume crystalloid infusions have provoked considerable interest with regard to potential clinical applications.[267] This effect was enhanced by combination with dextran.[384] Though improvements in microvascular circulation were observed, this also appeared to increase bleeding. A meta-analysis of early clinical trials revealed that hypertonic saline offered no advantage over standard crystalloid resuscitation although hypertonic saline dextran might.[428] This effect was particularly striking in patients with closed head injury and further animal studies have revealed that hypertonic saline can increase cerebral perfusion while decreasing cerebral edema.[376]

Damage control using hypotensive resuscitation is a new concept in controlling hemorrhage in injured patients. This concept has evolved from military experience and is based on the argument that aggressive resuscitation leads to dislodgement of clot, dilutional coagulopathy, and consequently more bleeding. The modern approach to damage control resuscitation refers to prevention of iatrogenic resuscitation injury (hypotensive resuscitation) followed by correction of hypercoagulopathy and the surgical control of the bleeding (i.e., minimizing the blood loss prior to surgical intervention). This is accomplished by maintaining a blood pressure lower than normal and utilizing transfusion of red blood cells, plasma, and platelets in a 1:1: 1 ratio together with coagulation factors such as the recombinant factor VIIIa, fibrinogen concentrates, and cryoprecipitate.

Frequent Sources of Hemorrhage

External blood loss is usually obvious though the volume lost prior to admission is usually unclear. Furthermore, the identification of external sites of hemorrhage should not distract from a rigorous search for internal bleeding, the identification of which can be more problematic. Internal blood loss should be suspected in all patients, particularly where shock is recalcitrant. This usually occurs in the thorax, abdomen, or pelvis. Differentiation of the site of internal bleeding can usually be made by using a combination of clinical judgment, thoracic and pelvic AP radiographs, and abdominal ultrasonography. Abdominal ultrasound should be conducted in the first few minutes of the patient's arrival to the emergency room, where this is available. Increasingly, emergency department and trauma personnel are being trained in ultrasound examination and appropriate equipment is being made available.

Endpoints of Volume Therapy

An adequate clinical response includes improvement of the pulse, blood pressure, capillary refill, and urine output. In the severely injured or complex patient, invasive techniques including invasive arterial monitoring and central venous or pulmonary artery pressure recording should be considered at an early stage. Though controversy still exists in specific situations, current goals include normalization of vital signs and maintenance of the central venous pressure between 8 and 15 mm Hg. Serial recording of acid–base parameters, the base excess and serum lactate in particular, have been shown to be particularly useful in assessing response to therapy and detecting the presence of occult hypoperfusion in apparently stable patients.[26,69,259] Ongoing requirement for blood transfusion should be monitored by regular measurement of the hemoglobin concentration. This value can be rapidly estimated where necessary using the majority of bedside arterial blood gas analyzers. Ongoing excessive fluid or blood requirement should always prompt a further search for sources of hemorrhage. Shock treatment is a dynamic process and in cases where there is ongoing bleeding, surgical intervention is often indicated.

More recently several methods for improved monitoring of cardiovascular status have been introduced including gastric tonometry, near infrared spectroscopy, transthoracic impedance, cardiography, central venous oximetry, and skeletal muscle acid–base estimation. Many of these techniques remain experimental and they are currently not available on a widespread basis. They may be available in certain centers and expert advice is essential.

Replacement of Blood and Coagulation Products

Secondary to maintaining intravascular volume, preservation of the patient's oxygen carrying capacity is essential. In cases of massive hemorrhage this will inevitably require the replacement of red blood cells. Furthermore, lost, depleted, and diluted components of the coagulation cascade will also require replacement. However, it should be noted that it is becoming increasingly apparent that, particularly in young healthy trauma victims, much lower hemoglobin concentrations than previously thought optimal are tolerated and indeed may be beneficial.[150] Not only is blood a precious resource, but transfusion also carries the risk of various complications including the transmission of infectious agents. Traditionally, target hemoglobin concentrations of 10 g/L have been advocated, but it has recently been shown that concentrations as low as 5 g/L are acceptable in normovolemic healthy volunteers.[437] Randomized trials in selected normovolemic intensive care patients showed that maintenance of hemoglobin concentrations between 7 and 9 g/L resulted in equivalent and perhaps superior outcomes to maintenance of hemoglobin concentrations above 10 g/L[166,242] and transfusion requirement has been shown to constitute an independent risk factor for mortality in trauma.[165] This may be related to the potential of blood products to cause an inflammatory response in the recipient.[3,165]

In cases with severe blood loss, there is no clear point where continued administration becomes futile.[423] Ideally, fully cross-matched blood should be used but in an emergency universal donor O-negative blood can be utilized immediately. A sample should be drawn for cross-match prior to administration as the transfusion of O-negative blood can interfere with subsequent analysis. The blood bank should be able to deliver type-specific blood within 15 to 20 minutes of the patient's arrival in the emergency room. This blood is not fully cross-matched and therefore still carries a relative risk of transfusion reaction. Cross-matched blood should be available within 30 to 40 minutes in most cases. Administration of platelets, fresh frozen plasma, and other blood products should be guided by laboratory results and clinical judgment. Expert hematologic advice is often required.[92,157] Procoagulant therapy for severe coagulopathy remains experimental, though early results are promising.

The costs and potential adverse effects of autologous blood transfusion are becoming increasingly relevant, but so far no convincing evidence has been found that tetrameric polymerized human hemoglobin can be used on a routine basis.[268] Instead, the use of Factor VII appears to be a promising alternative in patients who present with uncontrollable coagulopathy if there is no surgical source of bleeding.[248,367]

Differential Diagnosis of Hemorrhagic Shock

Hemorrhagic shock should be distinguished from other causes like cardiogenic and neurogenic shock. The presence of flat jugular veins might indicate the presence of hemorrhagic shock. An elevated jugular venous pressure (JVP) can be diagnostic of cardiogenic shock, caused by coronary heart disease, MI, cardiac contusion, tension pneumothorax, or cardiac tamponade. To establish this diagnosis the insertion of a pulmonary artery catheter may be necessary.

(a) *Neurogenic Shock:* Relative hypovolemia is the cause of neurogenic shock. This is usually due to spinal injury. Loss of autonomic supply leads to a decrease in vascular tone with blood pooling in the periphery. This pooling can occur without significant blood loss. The resultant increase in skin perfusion leads to warm peripheries and a decrease in central blood flow. This type of shock may be difficult to distinguish from hypovolemia.

(b) *Cardiogenic Shock:* Cardiogenic shock requires immediate attention and often immediate surgical intervention. The heart can be impaired by cardiac tamponade, tension pneumothorax, and hemothorax or in rare cases by intra-abdominal bleeding. These pathologies may necessitate immediate surgical intervention including placement of a chest drain, pericardiocentesis, or emergency thoracotomy. If there is indirect impairment of cardiac function, medical treatment should be introduced and normovolemia should be restored. An elevated jugular venous pressure in cardiogenic shock may be the result of right-sided heart failure. This should be confirmed through measurement of the central venous pressure. Impaired right heart function may result in blood pooling in the pulmonary vasculature. This can be difficult to distinguish from peripheral blood loss. The two can co-exist and may impair cardiac function. These conditions include cardiac tamponade, tension pneumothorax, MI, and cardiac contusion.

The presence of penetrating cardiac trauma associated with an elevated central pressure and a decreased peripheral systemic pressure should alert the treating doctor to the possibility of cardiac tamponade. A normal chest x-ray may not rule out this possibility, but ultrasound can provide an immediate diagnosis. The treatment of this condition should include emergency pericardiocentesis. Following aspiration of 10 mL of fluid from the pericardial sac, an immediate improvement of the heart stroke volume is seen with an increase in the peripheral systemic perfusion. Emergency thoracotomy is rarely indicated. If required it can be performed through an incision between the fourth and fifth ribs on the left side, followed by opening the pericardium in a craniocaudal direction to avoid injury to the phrenic nerve. One or two transmural stitches allow temporary cardiac closure and cardiac massage can then be conducted.

Tension pneumothorax causes rapidly increasing cyanosis and a rapid deterioration of respiratory function. It can also cause acute right ventricular failure. As the condition progresses, raised intrathoracic pressure causes reduced right-sided venous return to the heart. As mediastinal shift occurs, kinking or obstruction of the vena cava can lead to complete obstruction resulting in cardiac arrest. Rapid diagnosis followed by immediate decompression is a lifesaving measure.

Cardiac failure may cause MI independent of the trauma. This diagnosis should be considered in elderly people following road traffic accidents. In these patients MI may have been caused by hypovolemia, hypoxia, or the acute release of catecholamines at the time of the accident. Alternatively, MI may have occurred incidentally causing the accident. A diagnosis of MI can be confirmed from acute changes on the ECG and an increase of blood markers. The treatment of MI should include medical therapy to control arrhythmias. Patients with MI should be treated in the ICU with continued monitoring from the medical team.

Cardiac contusion can be difficult to differentiate from MI. Contusion is usually seen following a blunt anterior thoracic wall trauma associated with fracturing of the sternum. Differentiating this condition from MI in the acute setting is of secondary importance to the initial management as both diagnoses require similar management, including control of cardiac arrhythmias and heart failure, with continuous invasive monitoring.

Assessment of Neurologic Status

If a patient has to be intubated and sedated it is important for the emergency doctor to evaluate their neurologic status fully. The size and reaction of the pupils are important indicators of the presence of any central impairment. The light reflex reflects the function of the second and third cranial nerves, the oculocephalic reflex depends on the integrity of the third and fourth cranial nerves and the corneal reflex represents intact fifth and seventh cranial nerves. The GCS also provides important information regarding the neurologic status of patients, particularly where serial measurements are possible. It can provide a useful aid in clinical decision making: It has been argued that CT should be performed if the GCS is less than 10, and if GCS is less than 8, continuous intracranial pressure monitoring may be necessary. These indications are only estimates and the severity of impact and the clinical condition of the patient should also be used for evaluation.

Staging of the Patient's Physiologic Status

Once the initial assessment and intervention is complete patients should be placed into one of the four categories in order to guide the subsequent approach to their care. This categorization is done on the basis of overall injury severity, the presence of specific injuries, and the current hemodynamic status as detailed above (Table 9-5).[133] Three out of the four parameters must be met to allow a patient to be classified in a particular category. Patients who respond to resuscitation can be managed with early definitive fracture care as long as prolonged surgery is avoided.

Any deterioration in the patient's clinical state or physiologic parameters should prompt rapid reassessment with adjustment of the management approach as appropriate. Achieving the endpoints of resuscitation is of paramount importance for the stratification of the patient into the appropriate category.

TABLE 9-5 **Classification Systems for Clinical Patient Assessment**

	Parameter	Stable (Grade I)	Borderline (Grade II)	Unstable (Grade III)	In Extremis (Grade IV)
Shock	Blood pressure (mm Hg)	100 or more	80–100	60–90	<50–60
	Blood units (2 h)	0–2	2–8	5–15	>15
	Lactate levels	Normal range	Around 2.5	>2.5	Severe acidosis
	Base deficit (mmol/L)	Normal range	No data	No data	>6–8
	ATLS classification	I	II–III	III–IV	IV
Coagulation	Platelet count (µg/mL)	>110	90–110	<70–90	<70
	Factor II and V (%)	90–100	70–80	50–70	<50
	Fibrinogen (g/dL)	1	Around 1	<1	DIC
	D-dimer	Normal range	Abnormal	Abnormal	DIC
Temperature		<33°C	33–35°C	30–32°C	30°C or less
Soft Tissue Injuries	Lung function; PaO$_2$/FiO$_2$	350–400	300–350	200–300	<200
	Chest trauma scores; AIS	AIS 1 or 2	AIS 2 or more	AIS 2 or more	AIS 3 or more
	Chest trauma score; TTS	0	I–II	II–III	IV
	Abdominal trauma (Moore)	< or = II	< or = III	III	III or > III
	Pelvic trauma (AO class.)	A type (AO)	B or C	C	C (crush, rollover abd.)
	Extremities	AIS I–II	AIS II–III	AIS III–IV	Crush, rollover extrem.

Endpoints of resuscitation include stable hemodynamics, stable oxygen saturation, lactate level <2 mmol/L, no coagulation disturbances, normal temperature, urinary output >1mL/kg/hr and no requirement for inotropic support.

Stable

Stable patients have no immediately life-threatening injuries, they respond to initial therapy and they are hemodynamically stable without inotropic support. There is no evidence of physiologic disturbances such as coagulopathy or respiratory distress nor ongoing occult hypoperfusion which will present as abnormalities of acid–base status. They are not hypothermic. These patients have the physiologic reserve to withstand prolonged operative intervention where this is appropriate and they can be managed using an early total care (ETC) approach, with reconstruction of complex injuries.

Borderline (Patients at Risk)

Borderline patients have stabilized in response to the initial resuscitative attempts but they have clinical features or combinations of injury, which are often associated with poor outcome and put them at risk of rapid deterioration. These have been defined as follows.

- ISS >40
- Hypothermia below 35°C
- Initial mean pulmonary arterial pressure >24 mm Hg or a >6 mm Hg rise in pulmonary artery pressure during intramedullary nailing or other operative intervention
- Multiple injuries (ISS >20) in association with thoracic trauma (AIS >2)
- Multiple injuries in association with severe abdominal or pelvic injury and hemorrhagic shock at presentation (systolic BP <90 mm Hg)
- Radiographic evidence of pulmonary contusion
- Patients with bilateral femoral fracture
- Patients with moderate or severe head injuries (AIS 3 or greater)

This group of patients can be initially managed using an ETC approach but this should be undertaken with caution and careful thought given to the operative strategy should the patient require a rapid change of treatment. In addition, invasive monitoring should be instituted and provision made for ICU admission. A low threshold should be used for conversion to a damage control approach to management at the first sign of deterioration.

Unstable

Patients who remain hemodynamically unstable, despite initial intervention, are at a greatly increased risk of rapid deterioration, subsequent multiple organ failure, and death. Treatment in these cases has evolved to utilize a "damage control" approach. This entails rapid, essential lifesaving surgery and timely transfer to the ICU for further stabilization and monitoring. Temporary stabilization of fractures using external fixation, hemorrhage control, and exteriorization of gastrointestinal injuries where possible is advocated. Complex reconstructive procedures should be delayed until stability is achieved and the acute immuno-inflammatory response to injury has subsided. This rationale is intended to reduce the magnitude of the "second hit" of operative intervention or at least delay it until the patient is physiologically equipped to cope.

In Extremis

These patients are very close to death having suffered severe injuries and they often have ongoing uncontrolled blood loss. They remain severely unstable despite ongoing resuscitative efforts and are usually suffering the effects of a "deadly triad" of hypothermia, acidosis, and coagulopathy. A damage control approach is certainly advocated. Only absolutely lifesaving procedures are attempted in order to avoid exhaustion of their biologic reserve. The patients should then be transferred directly to intensive care for invasive monitoring and advanced hematologic, pulmonary, and cardiovascular support. Orthopedic injuries can be stabilized rapidly in the emergency department or ICU using external fixation and this should not delay other therapy. Any reconstructive surgery is again delayed and can be performed if the patient survives.

Staging of the Patient's Management Periods

The in-hospital period in which the evaluation and management of the trauma patient is undertaken is divided into four different periods. These are:

1. Acute "reanimation" period (1 to 3 hours)
2. Primary "stabilization" period (1 to 48 hours)
3. Secondary "regeneration" period (2 to 10 days)
4. Tertiary "reconstruction and rehabilitation" period (weeks)

This division allows surgeons to anticipate potential problems and undertake sensible decision making regarding the timing of surgical interventions using a systematic approach.

Acute "Reanimation" Period

This phase covers the time from admission to the control of the acute life-threatening conditions. Rapid systematic assessment is performed to immediately identify potentially life-threatening conditions. Diagnosis should be followed by prioritized management of the airway and any breathing disorders followed by circulatory support as set down in ATLS. This is followed by the "secondary survey," a complete acute diagnostic "checkup," but this should only be undertaken if there is no acute life-threatening situation, which would make immediate surgery necessary. In these cases this secondary assessment is intended to identify all the injuries in which definitive treatment should be delayed until the patient is properly stabilized.

Primary "Stabilization" Period

This phase begins when any acute life-threatening situation has been remedied and there is complete stability of the patient's respiratory, hemodynamic, and neurologic systems. This is the usual phase where major extremity injuries are managed, including acute management of fractures associated with arterial injuries or the treatment of acute compartment syndrome. Fractures can be temporarily stabilized with external fixation and the compartments released where appropriate. The primary period lasts about 48 hours.

Secondary "Regeneration" Period

In this phase the general condition of the patient is stabilized and monitored. It is vital to regularly re-evaluate the constantly evolving clinical picture to avoid any harmful impact from intensive care treatment or any problems associated with complex operative procedures. Unnecessary surgical interventions should not be performed during the acute response phase following trauma. Physiologic and intensive care scoring systems may be employed to monitor clinical progress. In the presence of systemic inflammation and MODS, appropriate supportive measures should be undertaken in an ICU.

Tertiary "Reconstruction and Rehabilitation" Period

This final rehabilitation period is when any necessary surgical procedures, including final reconstructive measures, should be undertaken. Only when adequate recovery is demonstrated should complex surgical procedures be contemplated. Such interventions include the definitive management of complex mid-face fractures, spinal or pelvic fractures, or joint reconstruction.

The acute period of "reanimation" originally included the initial 1 to 3 hours from admission, but due to the improvement of the pre-hospital trauma care it is now considered to extend from the arrival of the emergency services at the scene until the acute problems are controlled. This first period of trauma management is governed, in a large number of countries, by the ATLS principles.[422] The concept of a dedicated trauma team coordinated by someone who is experienced in trauma and emergency management has been adopted in most trauma centers.[141,297,331] Rapid primary assessment and simultaneous interventions to control the airway and the cervical spine, to facilitate respiration, and to maintain the circulation are started immediately. After establishing a nonacute life-threatening situation the secondary survey is undertaken and a thorough examination aims to identify all injuries and clinically relevant conditions.

During this treatment clinicians should use appropriate diagnostic tests to assist the decision-making process.[162,216,230,333,426,449] The use of standardized diagnostic and therapeutic protocols has been shown to improve timing, quality, and the overall clinical outcome of the therapeutic process.[457] It has been shown that the use of predefined and validated algorithms helps inexperienced personnel and reduces mortality, particularly in moderately severe polytrauma patients (ISS 20–50).[25] The primary goal of the initial management is to rapidly diagnose and immediately treat all life-threatening conditions, including airway obstruction or any injury, such as laryngeal trauma, that causes asphyxia, tension pneumo/hemothorax, cardiac tamponade, open thoracic trauma or flail chest, and massive internal or external hemorrhage. The acute management of these conditions may necessitate an urgent transfer to the operating room thereby delaying the use of diagnostic algorithms and the

secondary survey. An example would be the neglect of an intra-abdominal or pelvic hemorrhage, while attempting to deal with a severe extremity injury. Of particular importance is the fact that the condition of a polytrauma patient is dynamic and may become unstable at any moment. The continuous awareness of this by the treating team and the flexibility to change the management process is essential.[44,70,136,346,391]

The initial evaluation of multiply injured patients has continued to evolve as has the debate about the ATLS protocols. Continuous monitoring of the blood pressure, electrocardiography, the use of pulse oximetry to monitor oxygen saturation, assessment of the ventilatory rate, the insertion of urine and/or gastric catheters, the assessment of the initial full blood count and arterial blood gases, and cross-matching of the patient have been generally accepted as important objectives of the acute phase. There is more debate regarding the usefulness of radiographs and imaging in the first stages of the patient's evaluation and management. The current ATLS manual recommends AP chest, AP pelvis, and lateral cervical spine x-rays, and the use of deep peritoneal lavage (DPL) or abdominal ultrasonography.

The introduction of modern imaging modalities such as multislice computed tomography (MSCT)[27] and total-body digital x-rays[28] has caused a change in the initial radiographic assessment protocols in many trauma centers and a degree of confusion between the trauma and emergency personnel. The necessity for the AP pelvis x-ray[201,293] and the lateral cervical spine x-ray[197,424] has been disputed by the advocates of these new imaging techniques. However, studies[105,109,329,381] demonstrate promising results from these new imaging modalities, and it appears that despite their additional costs, their expected benefits in improving the effectiveness of trauma management will be significant. The advantages and disadvantages of these new modalities still have to be fully evaluated and compared with current practice.

IMAGING

The use of MSCT has revolutionized early diagnostic radiology in most level I trauma centers. Nowadays, the availability of such imaging is the standard of care in these institutions. Nevertheless, many other diagnostic tools are available to give a complete picture of all injuries. While clinical examination and judgment still provide the fundamental basis of contemporary trauma management, the role of emergency radiology continues to expand.

In the current trauma and emergency setting the 24-hour-a-day availability and immediate proximity of emergency radiology units (ERU) to the accident and emergency (A&E) departments is considered essential. The architectural design and the infrastructure planning demand the close coordination of the four components of acute trauma services these being the resuscitation room, the ERU, the trauma operating room, and the ITU.[106,446]

Conventional Radiography—Plain X-rays

Conventional radiography is currently used in most of the institutions that have adopted the ATLS concept. It consists of the standard three x-rays (AP chest, AP pelvis, and a lateral cervical spine) that are usually taken with portable bedside machines during the primary survey. This is followed by abdominal ultrasound and, in many cases, by a CT scan and additional plain x-rays of the extremities. This standard protocol is accepted in all trauma centers and in general hospitals that treat trauma.

The initial bedside lateral cervical spine x-ray is considered necessary in case an urgent intubation is required and the patient's GCS does not allow a clinical screening. It is considered accurate enough to diagnose severe or unstable fractures or fracture dislocations but it is less effective in identifying more subtle fractures, or clearing the thoracocervical area.[212,306]

The supine chest x-ray remains the most important of the three initial bedside x-rays. Its sensitivity is very high (>95%) for identifying a large hemothorax, flail chest, pneumothorax, hemomediastinum, pulmonary contusions, and lacerations. However, its specificity is quite low and a number of injuries, such as diaphragm ruptures and small hemothoraces are likely to be missed.[52,371,390]

The routine use of the AP pelvis x-ray, in the first phase of trauma evaluation and management, has received some criticism. Pelvic trauma can be used as a paradigm of polytrauma[120] because it reflects the severity of injury in a multiply injured population with potential hemodynamic compromise. After the use of the CT scan in the secondary survey of moderately or severely injured trauma patients become common it was considered that the routine bedside pelvic x-ray for hemodynamically stable patients might be abandoned. However in hemodynamically unstable patients it is still considered to be a useful screening tool to allow for early notification of the orthopedic team and the interventional radiologist. It also facilitates the use of techniques such as pelvic binders, plain sheet rapping and keeping the lower extremities adducted in internal rotation, to reduce the disrupted pelvis.[311,335]

The introduction of digital x-ray imaging appears to offer certain advantages even in the resuscitation room.[52] Recently, the use of total-body x-rays in the acute evaluation of multiply injured patients was introduced. Despite the increasing role of modern CTs this new technology appears to offer additional quick and vital information in the resuscitation room. It is based on an enhanced linear slot-scanning device that produces high-quality radiographic biplane whole-body images of any size in seconds. It has been evaluated in a number of centers[17,274] and its usefulness is expected to be confirmed in the near future.

Ultrasonography

The ultrasound scan has a significant role in the acute trauma setting, and it is now considered a vital tool in the hands of the trained emergency physician or trauma surgeon.[351] Although it is operator dependent, its advantages are its flexibility, speed, noninvasiveness, and ease of repetition.

The focused assessment with sonography for trauma (FAST) scan, introduced in 1990, offers a quick, comprehensive, and sensitive method of detecting free intra-abdominal fluid or a pericardial effusion. It includes:

(a) A transverse subxiphoid view (pericardial effusion, left liver lobe)

(b) A longitudinal right upper quadrant view (right liver lobe, right kidney, free fluid at Morrison's pouch)

(c) A longitudinal left upper quadrant view (spleen, left kidney, free fluid)

(d) Transverse and longitudinal suprapubic views (bladder, free fluid at Douglas pouch)

(e) Bilateral longitudinal thoracic views (pleural effusions)

The reported sensitivity for intra-abdominal free fluid is high (70% to 98%), but it is highly dependent on the volume of the free fluid, and on the completion of scanning in all areas.[41,204,209]

The sensitivity of FAST is poor for the diagnosis of solid organ injuries (45% to 85%).[289] However, its specificity for either free fluid or visceral injuries is high (86% to 100%).[41,204] It has been shown to be more sensitive in the diagnosis of pneumothorax than plain x-rays[387] and its efficacy is recorded as excellent (97% to 100%) in the detection of cardiac injuries and pericardial collections.[350] Its limitations are mostly in the identification of solid organ injuries. However, it should be noted that it is highly operator dependent[58] and there is a need for free access to the previously described anatomic areas. In addition, movement of the patient may affect its accuracy.[277,360]

Computed Tomography (CT Scan)

Since the generalized use of CT scanning in trauma management became common in the 1980s its contribution has been immense. CT is the basic adjunct of the ATLS secondary survey and is the gold standard for head, spinal, chest, and abdominal imaging. Its disadvantages are the time that is required to transfer the patient, undertake the scan, and assess the images, its inaccuracy in noncompliant patients, and its radiation dose.[445] Currently, in certain trauma centers its use is moving to even earlier phases of acute trauma management. The use of IV contrast enhancement, the advances of modern software and the image reconstruction ability of modern scanners have significantly enhanced the quality and considerably shortened the duration of a whole-body scan undertaken for trauma. Contemporary MSCT is capable of producing high-quality whole-body images in only a few minutes.[438]

Compared with MSCT, the traditional techniques of acute diagnostic evaluation for blunt trauma have certain disadvantages. The fundamental clinical examination has a diagnostic accuracy for abdominal trauma of about 60% to 65%.[240,373] DPL, despite its high sensitivity, had a low specificity and was replaced by FAST because it provided an overview of the intra-abdominal trauma and not an accurate diagnosis. Whole-body scanning gives diagnostic information regarding head, spinal, pelvic, and chest trauma. MSCT minimizes the time to accurate diagnosis, particularly for hemodynamically stable patients.[167] The advantages of this new CT-scanning modality can also be employed after a more traditional approach and it can be done after an initial bedside chest x-ray, a FAST scan, the initial resuscitation of the unstable patient, or even after urgent surgery of the patients in extremis.[310,345] The existing evidence related to the new MSCT-based protocols is encouraging especially for intubated, sedated, and hemodynamically stable patients. Nevertheless further proof from well-designed randomized prospective trials is needed before radically changing the established ATLS protocols.

Angiography

CT angiography has assumed a central role in the diagnosis and management of injured patients. It is the best method for detecting traumatic aortic and vascular injuries. In addition to the detection of these life-threatening injuries, in the presence of trained vascular radiologist, it offers the possibility of intervening to stop hemorrhage.[112,154] Its inherent disadvantages are the necessary infrastructure, allergic reactions to the contrast, the difficulty of finding an experienced vascular radiologist, given the inconsistent time schedule of trauma, and most importantly its duration because of the time it takes to transfer the injured patient to the angiographic suite, perform the investigation, and undertake any intervention that is required.

Initially, the indication for angiography and subsequent intervention was in stable hemodynamic patients.[152,370] Subsequently, the indications expanded to include the "transient responders" to fluid resuscitation,[153] and lately also to include those cases where hemodynamic instability persists even after laparotomy, thoracotomy, or packing have been undertaken as a salvage procedure.[356,409] Its successful use is often associated with pelvic trauma,[414,425] arterial vessel injury,[149,322,414] and abdominal solid organ injuries.[21,229,266,366,385]

The available radiologic interventional practices that are employed in acute trauma management are either embolization of moderate to small vessels and injured solid organs, using gelfoam slurry or coils, or percutaneous endovascular balloon-expandable stenting of larger vessels. They are considered to be minimal risk procedures especially in the setting of trauma management where they represent potentially lifesaving interventions. Currently, the angiographic protocols, with or without radiologic intervention, differ significantly between the different centers and trauma care systems. The main controversial issues relate to the difficulty and expense of providing a 24-hour vascular radiology service and in providing evidence that it is a worthwhile service.

PRIORITIES FOR LIFESAVING SURGERIES

In patients with polytrauma the decision as to which injury to address first can be lifesaving. Among the emergent operative treatments that do not permit prolonged diagnostic procedures are the treatment of cardiac tamponade, arterial injuries to major vessels, and head trauma with imminent herniation. Furthermore, injuries to cavities associated with severe hemorrhage and shock must be addressed promptly. In a multidisciplinary approach close communication is therefore crucial.

Chest Trauma
Hemothorax

Hemothorax is usually easily diagnosed from the chest x-ray, although in the presence of extensive lung contusion or atelectasis the diagnosis can be difficult. Ultrasound examination can identify free thoracic fluid though CT remains the gold standard and often reveals the source of bleeding.[1]

Significant bleeding into the pleural cavity with a resultant hemothorax is treated during the primary survey by the insertion of a chest tube. Usually, the decision is made following a review of the chest x-ray and only occasionally are clinical findings the sole indication for chest tube insertion, as a chest x-ray can usually be performed very rapidly. Standard surgical practice is to insert the chest tube in the mid-axillary line at the fifth intercostal space. Lower insertion risks injury to the diaphragm or intra-abdominal organs. The use of blunt dissection should prevent structural injury and it is important to use blunt dissection even where the operator is confident of positioning as intra-abdominal injuries may lead to increased intra-abdominal pressure and diaphragmatic elevation or even rupture. A traditional chest tube of least 28 gauge should be used to drain a hemothorax. The modern percutaneous drains used in thoracic medicine should not be used. The larger diameter reduces the danger of coagulation, allows rapid blood evacuation and the surgeon can be relatively confident that the drained contents are representative of thoracic blood loss. It is usual to direct the tube caudally to drain blood and cranially in the presence of a pneumothorax.

The presence of a hemothorax is not diagnostic of major thoracic hemorrhage. In most cases, bleeding is the result of injury to one intercostal vessel and this will usually stop spontaneously. Indications for emergency department thoracotomy remain controversial although recognized indications include traumatic arrest and recalcitrant profound hypotension in penetrating trauma, rapid exsanguination (>1500 mL initially or 250 mL/hr) and unresponsive hypotension in blunt thoracic trauma. As a last resort it can be used to control catastrophic sub-diaphragmatic hemorrhage by cross-clamping the aorta. These interventions are useless in patients with blunt thoracic trauma, in cardiac arrest where there has been no witnessed cardiac output and in patients with severe head injuries. There is recent evidence that increased caution should be employed before undertaking emergency thoracotomy in blunt trauma patients for all indications, particularly in the emergency department, due to the relatively high rate of nontherapeutic procedures and poor outcome.[12,178]

Mediastinal Hemorrhage and Thoracic Aortic Injury

Mediastinal hemorrhage due to injury to the thoracic aorta is commonly misdiagnosed due to the poor quality chest radiographs that are often obtained in emergency situations. Mediastinal enlargement observed on chest x-ray is nonspecific. In this context, one should pay careful attention to the presence of dilated jugular veins which help differentiate cardiac from aortic injuries. Nonetheless, further imaging should be rapidly obtained in the hemodynamically stable patient with contrast enhanced thoracic CT. Though traditional CT scanning sometimes lead to false positive results, and angiography is often regarded as providing the best diagnosis, many centers feel that contrast enhanced high resolution spiral CT is preferable.[56,97,365]

Rupture of the thoracic aorta is exceedingly rare in patients surviving long enough to reach the emergency room alive. In most cases, the adventitia is preserved and further intra-thoracic blood loss is prevented by the parietal pleura. Furthermore there is increasing evidence that repair can be delayed in the presence of other life-threatening injuries and occasionally conservative management can be successful.[176,218,401] These patients should, however, always be treated in a center with an acute thoracic surgical service. Nonoperative treatment of incomplete aortic ruptures in hemodynamically stable patients consists of permissive hypotension or active reduction of blood pressure while controlling for a difference in blood pressure between the upper and lower body parts. Indications for immediate intervention include the development of hemodynamic instability without an alternative explanation, hemorrhage via the chest tubes (>500 mL/hr) or a blood pressure gradient between upper and lower extremities leading to an impaired perfusion of the lower limbs (difference of mean blood pressure >30 mm Hg). Given the high mortality of emergency repair in cases of traumatic aortic injury there is increasing interest in the use of endovascular stenting in such situations.[182,217,357]

If the clinical situation arouses the suspicion of cardiac injury in the presence of radiologic mediastinal abnormality the diagnosis is generally cardiac tamponade. Pericardiocentesis should be performed. If there is acute decompensation, an emergent thoracocentesis is indicated. Further diagnostic tests are too time consuming in this immediately life-threatening situation. If the patient is still hemodynamically stable, a very sensitive and readily available test is the transthoracic echocardiogram.

The thoracic trauma severity score (TSS) is a standardized method for evaluation of thoracic injuries.[169] This CT-independent scoring system evaluates anatomical and physiologic parameters at the time of admission (Table 9-6). The TTS score ranges from 0 to 25 and includes the following parameters: PaO_2:FiO_2 ratio (0 to 5 points), presence of rib fractures (0 to 5 points), pulmonary contusion (0 to 5 points), lung lesions (hemothorax/pneumothorax) (0 to 5 points), and patient age (0 to 5 points).

Abdominal Trauma

Exsanguinating Abdominal Hemorrhage Versus Expanding Intracranial Hematoma

There is controversy over how this difficult combination of injuries should be treated. There is increasing evidence for conservative management of abdominal injuries, except in the most unstable patients, and it should be remembered that apparent intra-abdominal hemorrhage is often pelvic in origin. Evacuating an intracranial hematoma if the patient exsanguinates is obviously futile. However, there is equally little, and some would say less, benefit in saving a patients life if the result is profoundly disabling brain injury or death from tentorial herniation. Once compensatory autoregulatory mechanisms are overwhelmed, intracranial pressure rapidly increases. There is evidence that in people with head injury, mortality from extracranial causes alone is unusual. In a study of almost 50,000 trauma patients 70% of deaths were attributed to the head injury alone and only 7% to extracranial trauma, with the rest caused by a combination of both.[115] However, craniotomy should not be undertaken, without imaging to confirm an operable lesion, except in the rarest of circumstances. CT scanning is time consuming and can cause a significant delay in treatment. This time might be better spent attempting rapid hemodynamic stabilization. There is also evidence that in hypotensive patients undergoing head CT emergency laparotomy is required far more frequently than craniotomy (21% vs. 2.5%).[447] Furthermore, poorer outcomes have been demonstrated in head injured patients with shock, suggesting that early correction of hypotension may minimize secondary brain injury.[429]

It is clear that in these patients rapid complex management decisions must be made and clinical experience is essential. Thankfully, it would appear that such dilemmas seldom occur. In a review of 800 patients with significant head and abdominal injuries, 52 required craniotomy, 40 laparotomy, and only 3 required both.[406]

Pelvic Trauma

Pelvic fractures are often seen in conjunction with multi-system trauma and they can lead to rapid occult hemorrhage. Treatment should be seen as part of the resuscitative effort and early intervention can be lifesaving (Fig. 9-3).[125] Bleeding is commonly from multiple small sites rather than injured major vessels and in severe cases, due to the large volume of the retroperitoneum, spontaneous arrest is unusual.[145] Furthermore, it is common for the retroperitoneum to be breached during the injury further decreasing the barrier to ongoing hematoma expansion. Treatment with a pneumatic antishock garment or pelvic belt straps can give some temporary stabilization[432] but

TABLE 9-6	Thoracic Trauma Severity Score					
Grade	PO$_2$/FiO$_2$	Rib Fractures	Pulmonary Contusion	Pleural Lesion	Age (years)	Points
0	>400	0	None	None	<30	0
I	300–400	1–3 unilateral	1 lobe unilateral 1 lobe bilateral	Pneumothorax	30–40	1
II	200–300	4–6 unilateral	2 lobes unilateral	Hemothorax/hemopneumothorax unilateral	41–54	2
III	150–200	>3 bilateral	<2 lobes bilateral ≥2 lobes bilateral	Hemothorax/hemopneumothorax bilateral	55–70	3
IV	<150	Flail chest		Tension pneumothorax	>70	5

Described by Hildebrand F, van Griensven M, Garapati R, et al. Diagnostics and scoring in blunt chest trauma. *Eur J Trauma Emerg Surg.* 2002;28(3):157–167.

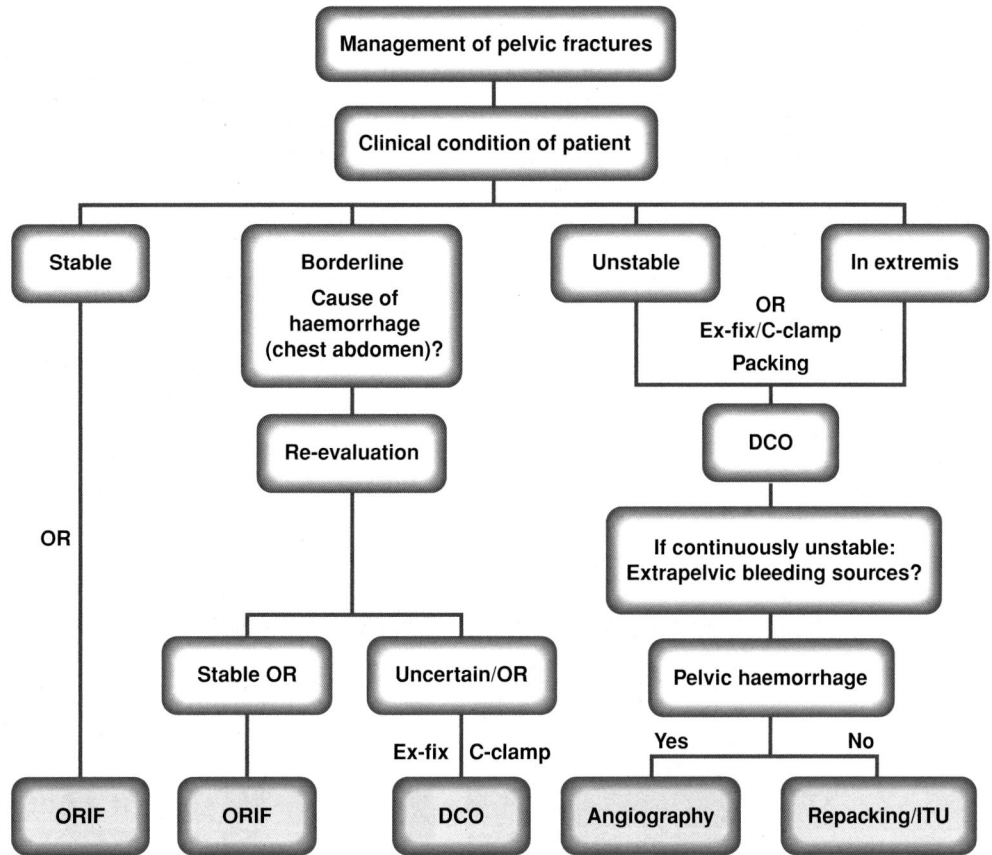

FIGURE 9-3 Treatment algorithm for patients with pelvic fractures and hemodynamic instability.

results are inconclusive and severe complications have been reported in relation to their use.

Although there has been increasing interest in the use of selective angiography in these cases to embolize bleeding vessels this intervention is often time consuming to organize and perform. Patients must be relatively stable and careful selection is crucial. Embolization can be used as an adjunct to other interventions where continued arterial hemorrhage is suspected. In severe injuries with profound hemodynamic instability, external fixation, pelvic C-clamps, and open tamponade with packing is recommended.[395,404] With the patient supine preparation from the sub-costal margin to the pubic symphysis is performed with the abdomen and pelvis completely exposed. If a C-clamp has already been applied for posterior pelvic instability it should be rendered mobile. In vertical pelvic instability (C type injury), the appropriate lower extremity should be accessible to allow reduction where necessary.

If there is prior evidence of free intraperitoneal fluid following application of an external fixation device a midline laparotomy should be performed and the intra-abdominal organs examined for bleeding following standard management protocols for blunt abdominal trauma. If, however, initial diagnostic imaging has shown no evidence of intra-abdominal fluid and a major source of pelvic hemorrhage is suspected a lower midline laparotomy can be employed. Initial attention should be directed to the retroperitoneum. Following the skin inci-

sion ruptured pelvic soft tissues are usually readily visible. Any hematoma is evacuated and the paravesical space explored for bleeding sources. Large bleeding vessels should be ligated where possible. In diffuse bleeding well-directed packing with external stabilization is recommended (Fig. 9-4).

If hemorrhage is obviously originating from a deep dorsal source, particularly in cases of posterior pelvic instability, attempts at further extraperitoneal exploration should be made in the presacral region. Large bleeding sources can be identified and treated appropriately. In cases of catastrophic arterial hemorrhage, temporary control can be achieved by cross-clamping the aorta. Often in venous hemorrhage, no single bleeding source is identifiable. Usually, bleeding originates from disruption of the presacral venous plexus or the fracture site itself. Again, well-directed packing can often adequately control hemorrhage. Recent studies have reported mortalities rates between 25% and 30% following pelvic packing in unstable patients.[79,411]

Following this intervention, temporary abdominal closure is performed and correction of physiologic derangements should be undertaken without delay, with particular regard being given to coagulopathy and hypothermia. Packing is left in situ and changed routinely at 24 to 48 hours, though in cases of suspected ongoing hemorrhage and recalcitrant shock earlier re-intervention should be considered. During planned revision the cavity should be debrided as required. Any residual hematoma should be removed and it should be thoroughly examined for

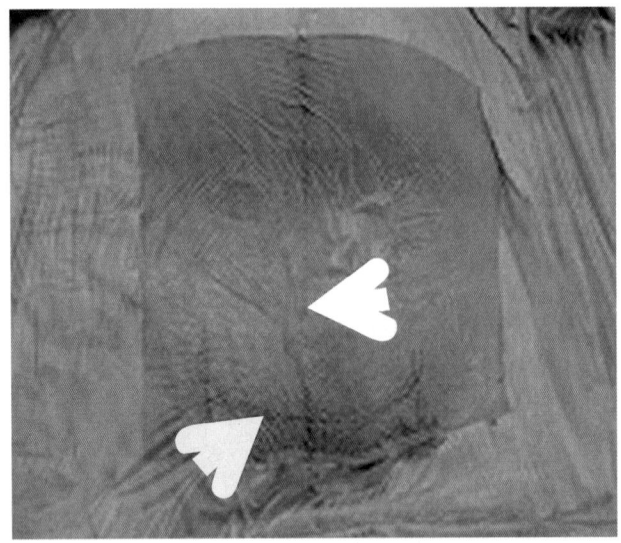

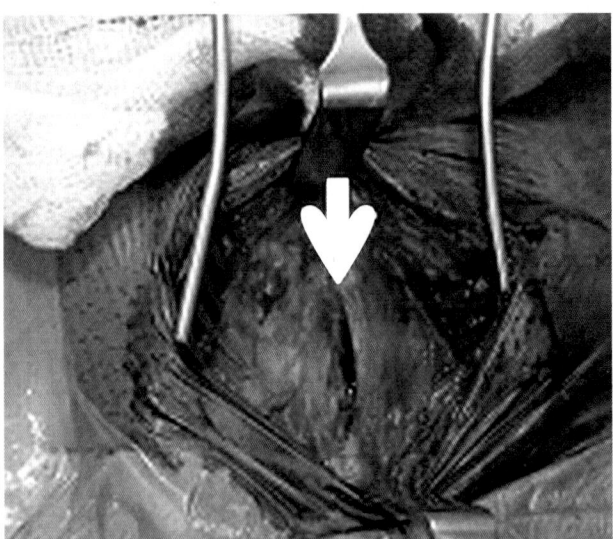

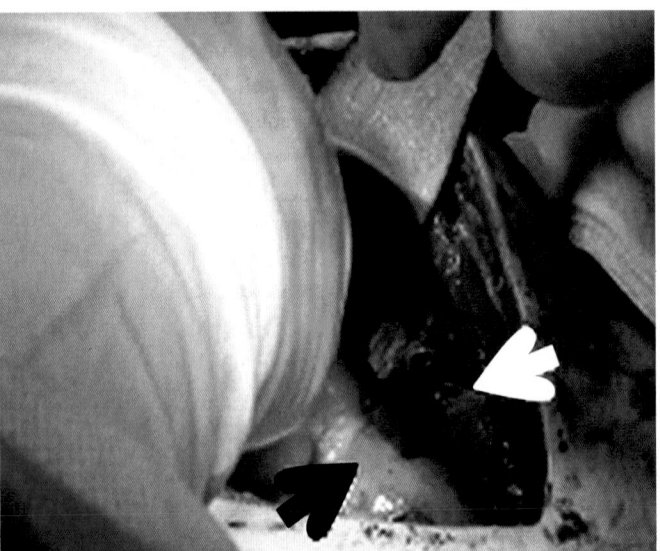

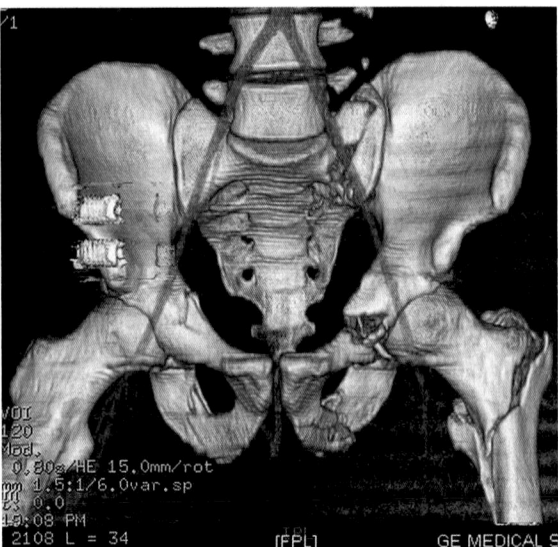

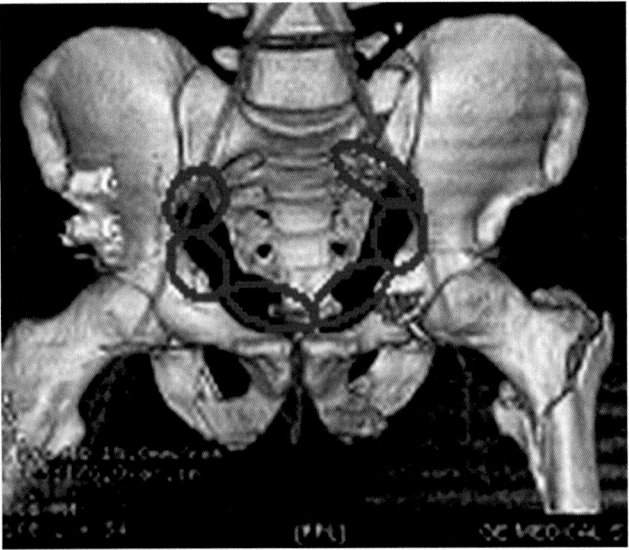

FIGURE 9-4 Retroperitoneal packing of the pelvis. **A:** Midline vertical incision (*white arrow*) is demonstrated (*yellow arrow* represents lower abdominal transverse incision). **B:** Incision of linea alba (*white arrow*). **C:** Retraction of the bladder to one side (*black arrow*) and placement of unfolded lap sponges in to the true pelvis (*white arrow*). Note that the first lap sponge is placed adjacent to the sacroiliac joint and the next should be placed anteriorly to the middle of the pelvic brim and the retropubic space. **D:** CT pelvic image revealing a lateral compression fracture pattern. **E:** Schematic representation of the position of the packs around the pelvic floor.

sites of ongoing hemorrhage. Further bleeding points can be dealt with, but if diffuse hemorrhage persists further packing should be used and later surgical revision undertaken.

TIMING OF DEFINITIVE STABILIZATION OF MAJOR FRACTURES: INDICATIONS FOR EARLY DEFINITIVE FIXATION

Before fracture fixation in polytrauma patients was routinely performed patients did poorly and the mortality rate secondary to fat embolism syndrome and organ failure was high. The major fear of surgeons treating these patients was the development of fat embolism syndrome. Pulmonary dysfunction is the hallmark of this problem, and develops several days after trauma. Once the fat embolism syndrome becomes full blown treatment is often unsuccessful and mortality rates of about 50% have been reported.[16]

The syndrome was found to be caused by fat and intramedullary contents liberated from an unstabilized fracture. It was therefore concluded that fixation of major fractures could prevent this complication in addition to minimizing soft tissue damage and ongoing blood loss. Multiple authors reported dramatic improvements in the clinical condition when fracture fixation was performed routinely.[188,339,418]

A decrease in the incidence of pneumonia and ARDS, a shorter stay in the ICU, and better survival rates were reported. The first prospective, randomized trial by Bone et al.[29] demonstrated the advantages of early fracture stabilization, now referred to as ETC. Patients with delayed fracture stabilization had a prolonged duration of ventilatory therapy and stayed longer in both critical care and hospital.[29,339] It was therefore accepted that a major aim in the treatment of the multiple trauma patient with fractures was rapid stabilization of the pelvic and extremity injuries. An essential prerequisite for ETC was optimization of retrieval conditions and a reduction of the retrieval time. Furthermore, the improvements in intensive care medicine with improved cardiovascular monitoring and facilities for prolonged ventilatory support facilitated the development of a more aggressive surgical approach.

The strict application of ETC even in patients with a high ISS, brain injury, or severe chest trauma limited discussion about the best management for these polytraumatized patients. As it became evident that these specific subgroups of polytraumatized patients do not benefit from ETC, the borderline patient was identified. These patients were demonstrated to be at particular risk of a poor late outcome. The clinical and laboratory characteristics of the borderline patient have been previously described.[133]

The concept of damage control orthopedics (DCO) provided a solution to the management of these borderline patients together with patients in an unstable or extremis condition. The term damage control was initially described by the US Navy as the capacity of the ship to absorb damage and maintain mission integrity. In the polytraumatized patient, this concept of surgical treatment intends to control but not to definitively repair the trauma-induced injuries early after trauma. After restoration of normal physiology (core temperature, coagulation, hemodynamics, respiratory status), definitive management of

injuries is performed.[378] The damage control concept consists of three separate components:

(a) Resuscitative surgery for rapid hemorrhage control

(b) Restoration of normal physiologic parameters

(c) Definitive surgical management

Within the DCO framework, the first stage involves early temporary stabilization of unstable fractures and the control of hemorrhage. The second stage consists of resuscitation of the patients in the ICU and optimization of their condition. Finally, the third stage involves delayed definitive fracture management when the patient's condition allows. The favorite tool of the trauma surgeon to achieve temporary stabilization of the fractured pelvis or a long bone is the external fixator. External fixation is a quick and minimally invasive method of providing stabilization and it can be used very efficiently to accomplish early fracture stabilization and it postpones the additional biologic stresses posed by prolonged surgical procedures. The delayed definitive procedure to stabilize long bone fractures, in particular the femur, is usually intramedullary nailing which is carried out when the condition of the patient allows. Recent studies have reported that the DCO approach was a safe treatment method for fractures of the shaft of the femur in selected multiply injured patients.[288,313,361] The application of DCO in the multiply injured patients is illustrated in Figure 9-5.

In patients with additional severe injuries to the head, chest, and pelvis with life-threatening hemorrhage an acute change in the clinical condition may rapidly occur. The EAST evidence-based workgroup conducted a systematic review of the literature regarding the timing of fracture fixation in different subsets of patients with multiple trauma.[98] Specifically, this group concluded that there is no compelling evidence that early long bone stabilization neither enhances nor worsens the outcome in patients with severe head injury or in patients with associated pulmonary trauma. While the available data suggests that early fracture fixation may reduce associated morbidity in certain patients with polytrauma the workgroup stopped short of recommending early fixation for all patients. An algorithm for the treatment of these patients is shown in Figure 9-6.

The practice of delaying definitive surgery in DCO attempts to reduce the biologic load of surgical trauma on the already traumatized patient. This hypothesis was assessed in a prospective randomized study by means of measuring pro-inflammatory cytokines. Clinically stable patients with an ISS >16 and a femoral shaft fracture were randomized to ETC (primary intramedullary nailing of the femur within 24 hours) and DCO (initial temporary stabilization of the femur with external fixator and subsequent intramedullary nailing). A sustained inflammatory response (higher levels of IL-6) was measured after primary (<24 hours) intramedullary femoral instrumentation, but not after initial external fixation or after secondary conversion to an intramedullary implant. The authors concluded that DCO surgery appears to minimize the additional surgical impact induced by the acute stabilization of the femur.[312]

Other issues that have been discussed with regard to the DCO concept include the ideal timing at which to perform the secondary definitive surgery and whether it is safe to convert

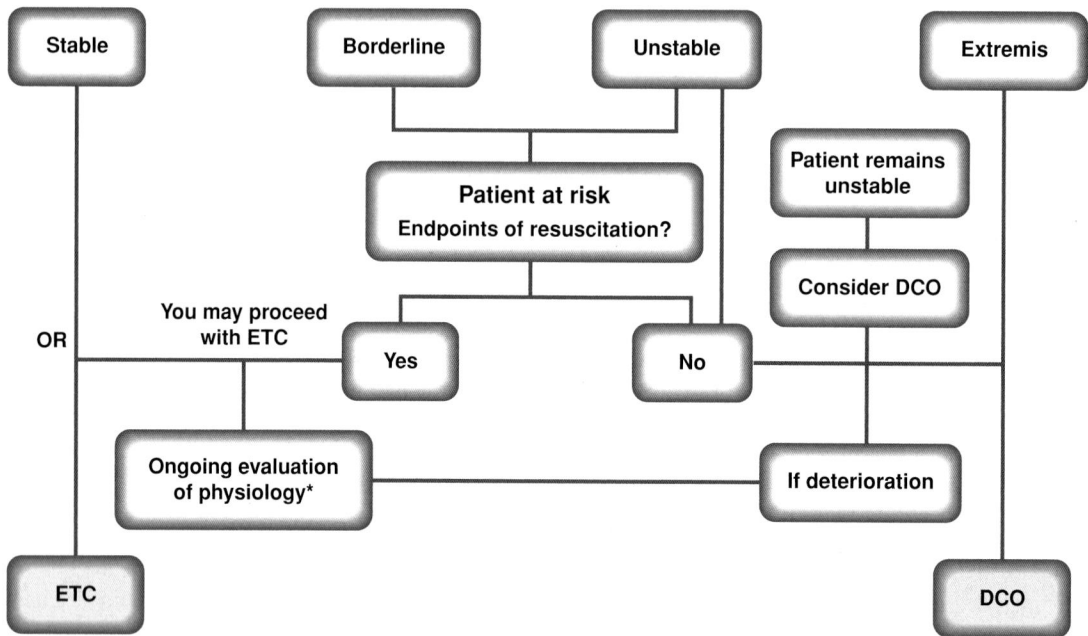

*Lactate, blood pressure, urine output, oxygenation, temperature, coagulation profile.

FIGURE 9-5 Treatment of severely injured patients with damage control orthopedics (DCO) algorithm. Early total care (ETC) with definitive stabilization of fractures can be used in stable patients. Unstable patients require a damage control orthopedic strategy with temporary external fixation of fractures. "Patients at risk" are patients with a high injury severity score (ISS), hypovolemia, lactate over 2.5 mmol/L, and associated chest and abdominal injuries. These patients need aggressive resuscitation and repeated evaluation as to whether DCO or ETC is indicated.

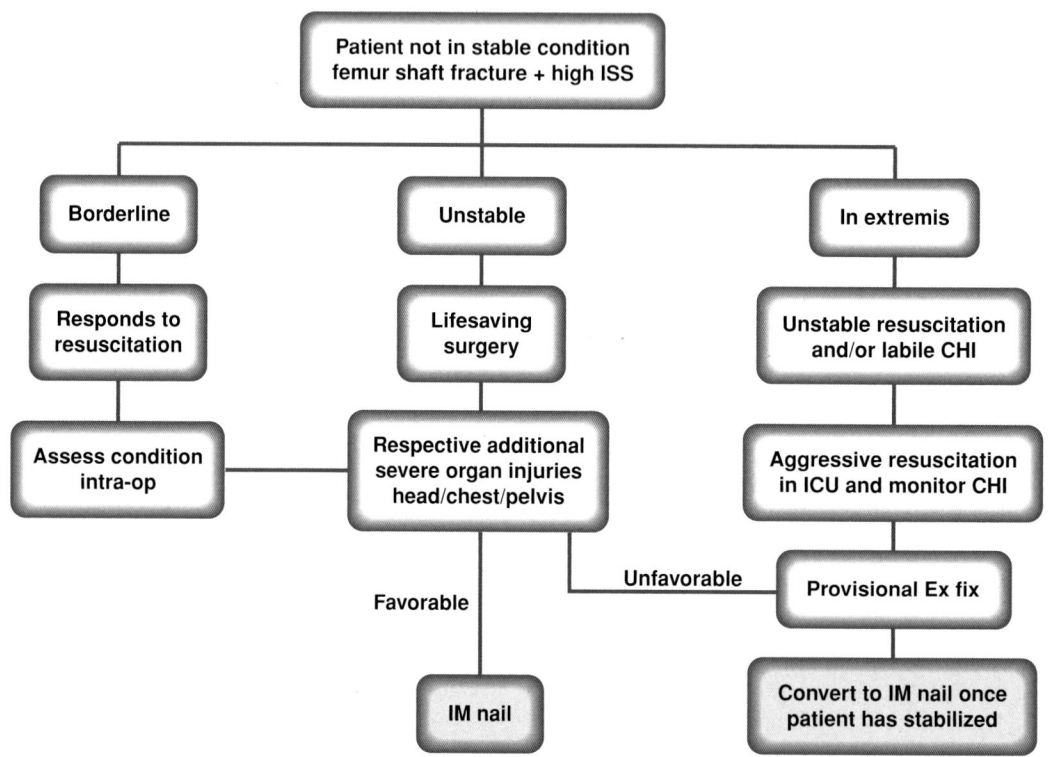

FIGURE 9-6 Management of orthopedic injuries in patients with associated injuries (e.g., traumatic brain injury).

TABLE 9-7 Indications for Early Total Care

Stable hemodynamics
No need for vasoactive/inotropic stimulation
No hypoxemia, no hypercapnia
Lactate <2 mmol/L
Normal coagulation
Normothermia
Urinary output >1 mL/kg/h

an external fixator to an intramedullary nail or is this associated with an unacceptably high infection rate? It has been shown that days 2 to 4 do not offer optimal conditions for definitive surgery. In general during this period, marked immune reactions are ongoing and enhanced generalized edema is observed.[436] Nevertheless, these patients represent a highly diverse group and individual clinical judgment is more reliable, especially when combined with information from the newer laboratory tests. In a retrospective analysis of 4,314 patients treated in our clinic, it was found that a secondary procedure lasting more than 3 hours was associated with the development of MODS. Also the patients who developed complications had their surgery performed between days 2 and 4, whereas patients who did not go on to develop MODS were operated on between days 6 and 8 ($p < 0.001$).[309]

With regard to the issue of whether external fixation can be converted safely to intramedullary nailing, the infection rates reported in the literature are low ranging from 1.7% to 3%.[288,361] According to these reports conversion of the external fixator to a nail should be done within the first 2 weeks as this minimizes the risk of developing deep sepsis.

In general terms, the measurement of inflammatory mediators has been shown to be sensitive in predicting the clinical course, morbidity, and mortality in trauma patients.[72,183,219] Based on the latest available studies, the following recommendations can be made in terms of patient selection for ETC and DCO (Tables 9-7 and 9-8).

STANDARD OF CARE FOR THE TREATMENT OF SKELETAL INJURIES

The sequence of fracture treatment in multiply injured patients with multifocal injuries to an extremity is a crucial part of the

TABLE 9-8 Indications for "Damage Control" Surgery

1. Physiologic criteria
   - Blunt trauma: hypothermia, coagulopathy, shock/blood loss, soft tissue injury = Four vicious cycles
   - Penetrating trauma: hypothermia, coagulopathy, acidosis = "Lethal Triad"
2. Complex pattern of severe injuries—expecting major blood loss and a prolonged reconstructive procedure in a physiologically unstable patient

management concept. Some parts of the body are prone to progressive soft tissue damage because of their anatomy. Therefore, the recommended sequence of treatment is tibia, femur, pelvis, spine, and upper extremity.

In this context the simultaneous treatment of different extremity injuries should be considered. Initially, trauma surgeons must undertake the shortest possible interventions in these patients to minimize the "second hit phenomenon,"[117,118] The simultaneous employment of different surgical approaches and different surgical specialties, whenever this is feasible, minimizes the risks and facilitates the transfer of the unstable patient to the controlled environment of the ITU as early as possible. Even in the later reconstructive phase of treatment it may be possible to undertake simultaneous operations at different anatomic sites. This is straightforward if there are contralateral fractures of the upper and lower extremities, or a combination of facial, thoracic, and lower extremity trauma. These combinations of injuries allow two different teams such as orthopedic and plastic surgeons or maxillofacial and thoracic surgeons to work together thereby minimizing the duration of anesthesia, the surgical stress on the injured patient, and at the same time optimizing the operating room time, and the costs of treatment.[118,123,311]

As the main goal in any trauma system is to offer definitive, specialized care for the injured patient in the shortest possible time the preservation of high standards of acute trauma care requires complex clinical capabilities, particular infrastructure logistics, and, even more importantly, algorithms facilitating simultaneous activities in diagnosis and therapy.

Unfortunately, the existing evidence about the role of simultaneous surgery for polytraumatized patients is not of adequate quality and quantity to justify generalized conclusions. However, it is anticipated that in the future there will be further research which will better define its role. It is also important to realize that the type of osteosynthesis used in multiply injured patients not only depends on the state of the bone and soft tissues but much more so on the general, pulmonary, and hemodynamic status of the patient.

Management of Unilateral Fracture Patterns

In multifocal injuries of the upper extremity, the surgeon should be aware of the overall fracture distribution rather than consider each fracture as an isolated problem. Even though an early definitive osteosynthesis would be preferred in all fractures, often the general state of the multiply injured patient or the local fracture conditions do not permit this. In these cases it is recommended that careful immobilization of diaphyseal fractures is the first phase of fracture management. If there are periarticular fractures of the large joints and urgent open reduction and fixation is impossible transarticular external fixation (TEF) should be performed. In any case with a concomitant vascular injury or any evidence of a developing compartment syndrome, fasciotomies should be undertaken.

In multifocal injuries of the lower extremity such as ipsilateral distal femoral and proximal tibial fractures, known as a floating knee, similar flexible but nonetheless structured and priority-oriented management protocols should be applied.

The overall status of the patients is crucial to the concept. If the floating knee occurs in a stable patient, a retrograde femoral nail can be inserted through a small incision at the knee joint which is flexed at 30 degrees. An antegrade tibial nail can then be inserted through the same incision. The same fracture pattern in an unstable patient is best treated using a transarticular external fixator to span both fractures. A secondary definitive osteosynthesis can then be done when the patient has recovered from the initial, potentially life-threatening injuries. It is very important that there is good communication between the anesthesiologist and the surgeon since the procedure may have to be adapted to any change in the patient's vital parameters.

In metaphyseal and periarticular fractures, the priorities of treatment are often dictated by the state of the soft tissues. A high priority is given to femoral head and talar fractures. Other periarticular fractures have a lower priority unless complicated by factors such as vascular dysfunction, compartment syndrome, or an open wound. Apparently minor fractures to the hand, fingers, tarsus, and toes should not be overlooked. They should be considered in the overall management concept and treated appropriately.

Management of Bilateral Fracture Patterns

In bilateral fractures, simultaneous treatment is ideal. This is particularly true in bilateral tibial fractures where both legs are surgically cleaned and draped at the same time. However, the operative procedure is performed sequentially because of the problems inherent in the use of fluoroscopy. If the vital signs of the patient deteriorate during the operation the second leg may be temporarily stabilized using an external fixator. The definitive osteosynthesis then may be delayed until the general status of the patient is stabilized again. The priorities in the treatment of bilateral fracture patterns follow the evaluation of the injury severity with more severe injuries being treated first.

Upper Extremity Injuries

The management of upper extremity fractures in multiply injured patients is usually undertaken secondary to the treatment of injuries of the head, trunk, or lower extremity. If there is a closed fracture of the upper extremity without any associated injury, such as vascular or nerve damage or compartment syndrome, proximal fractures of the shoulder girdle, proximal humerus, and humeral shaft can be stabilized by a shoulder body bandage. If definitive osteosynthesis is required it may be performed during the secondary management phase, possibly after further imaging. External fixation is an alternative for the temporary stabilization of humeral diaphyseal fractures and TEF may be used to stabilize fractures about the elbow if definitive stabilization has to be delayed. Primary management of fractures of the forearm, wrist, and hand is often with a cast but temporary external fixation may be used.

Lower Extremity Injuries

Our experience suggests that long bone fractures associated with a severe head injury or chest trauma require a specially modified strategy. We strongly recommend the expanded monitoring of respiratory function, ventilation (capnography), and pulmonary hemodynamics. In addition, intracranial pressure monitoring is mandatory in patients with severe head injury.[48]

Unstable Pelvic Injuries

The management of the rare unstable pelvic injury is much easier if a standardized protocol is followed. A thorough clinical and radiologic examination is essential for the assessment of pelvic injuries. This assessment is usually done during the initial examination phase. Following this examination it may only be possible to arrive at an approximate classification of the pelvic injury. However, sophisticated classifications of pelvic injuries in this context are not of much use. Instead, the simple AO classification, the A B C system (Fig. 9-7), can assist in the decision-making process.[273] In this classification, type A injuries include stable fractures such as fractures of the pelvic rim, avulsion fractures and undisplaced anterior pelvic ring fractures. The posterior rim is not injured at all. Type B injuries comprise fractures with only partially intact posterior structures and rotational dislocations may be possible. Sometimes, this injury may

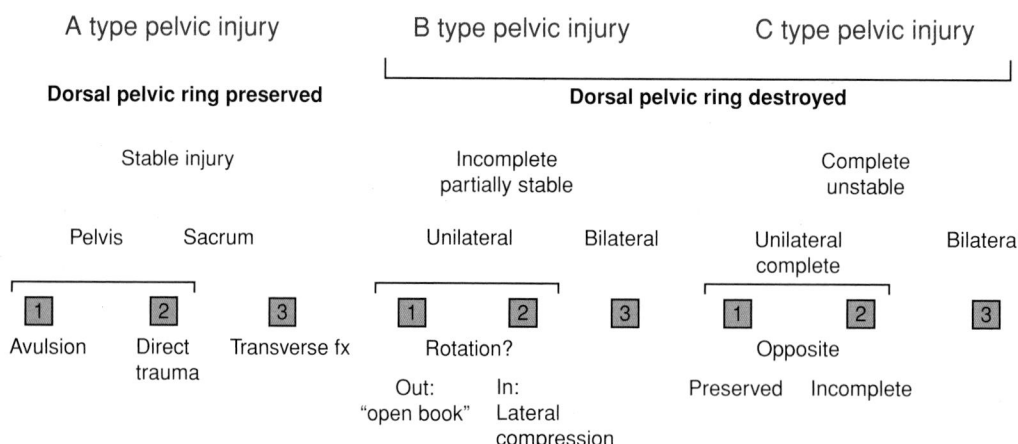

FIGURE 9-7 Classification of pelvic ring fractures in A, B, and C type fractures similar to the AO classification.

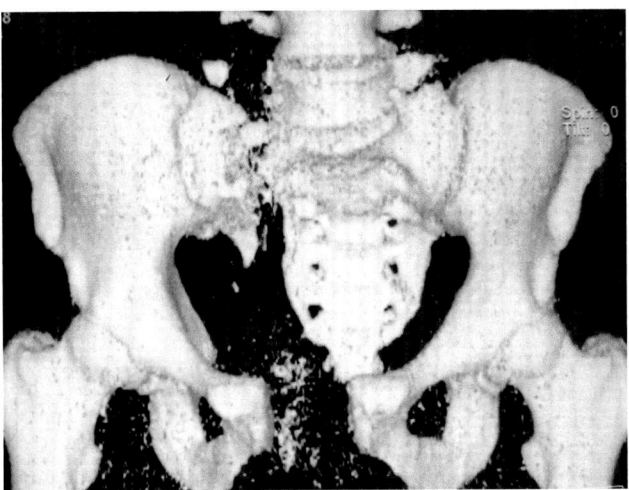

FIGURE 9-8 Type C pelvic fracture. Three-dimensional computed tomography scan.

initially be an internal rotation dislocation resulting in marked bone compression and stabilization of the pelvis. However these injuries are associated with a high risk of intra-abdominal damage. If the injury results in an open book type of fracture with both alae being externally rotated urogenital lesions and hemorrhagic complications are much more common.

Since the differentiation of AO type B and C injuries may be difficult, a CT scan of the pelvis is strongly recommended. If there is no CT available diagonal inlet and outlet x-rays may serve as an alternative. In C type injuries, the pelvis shows translational instability of the dorsal pelvic ring, because the stabilizing structures are all divided (Fig. 9-8). One or both hemipelves are separated from the trunk. This injury is associated with an extremely high rate of hemorrhagic complications and other pelvic injuries. The simple AO classification has significant therapeutic implications. In type A injuries operative treatment is generally not required whereas in type B injuries adequate stabilization is obtained by osteosynthesis of the anterior pelvic ring only. Type C injuries require anterior and posterior osteosynthesis to gain adequate stability.

The differentiation of several sectors of injury has also proved useful. Transsymphyseal, transpubic, transacetabular, and transiliacal fractures are differentiated from transiliosacral and transsacral fractures. This process is easy to memorize and requires a careful analysis of the x-rays. For each of the injured regions we have standardized the recommendations for osteosynthesis. Thus an adequate management plan is available for the small numbers of unstable pelvic fractures that will be seen. Since more than 80% of unstable pelvic injuries are associated with multiple injuries, stabilization techniques that can be undertaken with the patient in the supine position are much preferred during the primary period. In addition, the supine position facilitates reconstruction of symphyseal and iliosacral ruptures. Generally speaking, we recommend that fractures of the pelvic ring be stabilized as soon as possible to avoid ongoing blood loss and to simplify ICU care and promote early ambulation.[125]

Complex Pelvic Injuries

Pelvic injuries associated with any other injury to local pelvic organs are called complex pelvic injuries.[32] These injuries comprise about 10% of pelvic injuries and they are associated with a significantly higher mortality of between 30% and 60% in comparison with simple pelvic injuries. During the early phase hemorrhage is the most common cause of death. Later ARDS and MODS occur because of the blood loss.

During the acute treatment phase, only immediate priority-guided management protocols save the lives of these severely injured patients and improve their prognosis. A variety of methods for hemorrhage control in pelvic injuries are discussed in the literature. Along with these techniques several complex therapeutic protocols have been developed. Our own experience has resulted in a rather simple algorithm requiring three decisions to be made within the first 30 minutes after admission. The therapeutic goal is based on a combined strategy of intensive shock treatment, early stabilization of the pelvic ring, and potential operative hemorrhage control and packing rather than a single treatment option. Once hemorrhage control has been achieved the associated urogenital and intestinal injuries should be treated expeditiously to avoid septic complications.

In urogenital injuries reliable drainage of the urine is the primary goal. During the first laparotomy intraperitoneal ruptures of the bladder are repaired. In injuries of the urethra, it is recommended that the urethra be splinted with a transurethral catheter in the acute phase and that a definitive reconstructive procedure be undertaken during the secondary period to reduce the incidence of late strictures. If early realignment is not possible, then a suprapubic catheter should be inserted.

In open pelvic fractures with injuries to the rectum or anus a temporary colostomy of the transverse colon generally guarantees proper excretion and safeguards the healing process in the pelvis. At the end of the procedure, an extensive antegrade wash-out of the distal colon is assumed to reduce the microbial load. Any potential muscular or skin necrosis is radically debrided to reduce the risk of infection.

Unstable Injuries of the Spine

In general, operative treatment of unstable spine injuries in multiply injured patients is mandatory, if only for intensive care nursing purposes. Nonoperative treatment using a plaster jacket or a halo-body fixator is unsuitable for multiply injured patients because the immobilization is associated with a high risk of complications. Not only are the intensive care nursing procedures much easier after internal stabilization, but also the period of immobilization and the period of intensive care stay are significantly reduced. Spinal fractures associated with neurologic dysfunction are usually stabilized at the same time as the spinal cord is decompressed. However in recent years there has been a move toward stabilizing more unstable injuries of the spine in patients who present without neurologic symptoms for the same reasons. It is our experience that after diagnosing an unstable injury of the spine in a patient who does not have neurologic symptoms a closed reduction should be undertaken if there is a fracture of the cervical spine or an AO type C rotational injury of the lower thoracic or lumbar spines. In any other injury, the reduction is performed in the operating room just before the actual procedure. It is important to understand that even if there is a slight suspicion that a fracture fragment or a protruding intervertebral disc may narrow the spinal canal after closed reduction, further diagnostic imaging with a CT or MRI scan should be carried out preoperatively.

In multiply injured patients in particular closed reduction may be difficult because of co-existing extremity injuries. In these cases correct axial and rotational alignment should be obtained intraoperatively. If there is interposition of a bone fragment or an intervertebral disc, open reduction is indicated to avoid spinal cord compression.

We routinely use the anterior approach for operative management of the upper (C1 to C3) and lower (C4 to C7) cervical spine. The patient's head is fixed to a special reduction apparatus using the rim of the halo fixator. In thoracic or lumbar spine injuries associated injuries to the chest and abdomen have to be considered. Nonetheless, in our experience, injuries requiring posterior and anterior stabilization may usually be fixed with a posterior internal fixator in the acute management period. Depending on the general status of the patient, the anterior stabilization may be performed secondarily. Even intrathoracic or intra-abdominal injuries are not necessarily a contraindication to the use of the prone position which is required for posterior instrumentation. The prone position can even be used successfully in patients with severe lung injury.

Assessment of Fracture Severity

Closed Fractures. Fractures in polytrauma patients managed either with the ETC or the DCO approach must be stabilized before being admitted to the ITU. Stabilized fractures not only reduce pain but also minimize the release of intramedullary material into the circulation and secondary damage to the soft tissues. Furthermore, nursing is easier and early functional treatment can be initiated.

Assessment of the degree of soft tissue damage in closed fractures is often difficult. A skin contusion over an otherwise closed fracture may present more therapeutic and prognostic problems than an inside-out puncture wound in an open fracture. Although the skin wound may not be particularly impressive, this type of blunt injury can lead to significant skin damage. As necrosis is the main complication of a skin contusion secondary infection can occur, particularly in the ICU. This issue has been addressed by the development of a classification system which allows the clinician to decide the appropriate therapeutic approach that would be beneficial to the patient's overall condition. The Tscherne classification of closed fractures is detailed in Table 9-9.[296]

Open Fractures. In polytrauma patients prompt evaluation and treatment of open fractures is of paramount importance. It involves careful assessment of the damage to the soft tissues, radical debridement, extensive irrigation, and stable fracture fixation. Careful assessment of the injury severity is the first step in the development of a treatment strategy. The time and mechanism of injury, the energy of the causative force and

TABLE 9-9	Classification of Soft Tissue Injury in Closed Fractures

Closed fracture C0: No injury or very minor soft tissue injury. The C0 classification covers simple fractures caused by indirect mechanisms of injury.

Closed fractures C1: Superficial abrasions or contusions from internal fragment pressure. Simple to moderate fracture types are included.

Closed fractures C2: Deep, contaminated abrasions or local dermal and muscular contusions. An incipient compartment syndrome is also classified as a C2 fracture. These injuries are usually caused by direct forces, resulting in moderate to severe fracture types. The closed segmental tibia diaphyseal fracture is a good illustration of a C2 fracture.

Closed fractures C3: Extensive skin contusions or muscular damage, subcutaneous degloving and clinical compartment syndrome in any closed fracture are graded as C3 fractures. Severe and comminuted fractures occur in this subgroup.

Closed fractures C4: The same injuries as listed in the C3 fracture classification but the C4 group are associated with significant vascular requiring operative treatment.

Oestern HJ, Tscherne H. *Pathophysiology and Classification of Soft Tissue Injuries Associated with Fractures.* Berlin: Springer-Verlag; 1984.

the severity of the fracture should be considered. The extent of any co-existing vascular and nerve damage and the general condition of the patient are also of great importance. In high-energy trauma the soft tissues may be severely damaged and may require careful evaluation and extensive debridement during the initial assessment.

Open fractures resulting from low-energy trauma are usually associated with less soft tissue damage and may almost be treated like closed injuries. After the initial debridement, the fracture may be appropriately stabilized. Open fractures resulting from high-energy trauma often have extensive soft tissue damage combined with significant bone destruction. This injury requires a sequential program of management. The treatment plan consists of an adequate debridement, initial temporary stabilization followed by definitive secondary stabilization and wound closure. Our experience with this type of injury indicates that each fracture has almost unique characteristics which require individual management. In multiply injured patients the overall injury severity has to be considered as has the degree of shock and the initial blood loss. Once these factors have been taken into account a clear therapeutic plan should be established for each patient. Open fractures are discussed further in Chapters 10, 11 and 12.

Classification of Soft Tissue Damage. Several classifications have been proposed over the years for the grading of open fractures but the standard system of classifying the soft tissue component of a fracture remains that of Gustilo and Anderson.[151] Despite the doubts which have been raised over its reliability, it seems likely to remain in common usage as it is straightforward to remember and to apply.

In multiply injured patients a thorough assessment of soft tissue damage is even more crucial. In this group, the prognosis for the soft tissue damage depends on a multitude of parameters including tissue hypoxia, acidosis, and hypoperfusion of the extremities due to hemorrhagic shock. All these factors should be taken into account in clinical decision making and planning.

Reconstruction Versus Amputation? With advances in free tissue transfer and microsurgical techniques and a better appreciation of the usefulness of the Ilizarov technique of limb preservation, especially in Gustilo grade IIIb and IIIc fractures of the lower extremity reconstruction is more commonly attempted nowadays. Reconstructive bone and soft tissue surgery usually requires repeated operations, long-term hospital stays and prolonged periods of treatment. The surgeon must appreciate that this is very difficult for the patient and his or her family and there are often significant social and economic consequences. Several authors have therefore looked into criteria to help guide surgeons in their decision between reconstruction and amputation of a severely injured extremity. From the surgical point of view an attempt to preserve the limb often seems to be the best decision for the patient. However from a socioeconomic point, multiple prolonged hospital stays may have a deleterious effect on the patient. The financial loss for the patient from prolonged hospital stays and time off work may prove to be higher than that associated with a primary amputation and not infrequently multiple attempts at reconstruction leave patients incapable of earning their living for more than 2 years.[372] In addition, it should be remembered that many patients with reconstructed limbs often find it difficult to return to their occupations at all.

If a severely injured patient survives after a primary amputation the question that arises is whether the amputation was unavoidable or whether reconstruction was possible. If the patient dies the question is whether the severity of the injuries was underestimated initially and would an early amputation have saved the patient's life? Lastly, if the patient survives after primary reconstruction but suffers from complications requiring prolonged treatment, the question is whether the bad outcome justified the resources that were expended.

Several classification systems have been developed in order to help surgeons in this decision-making process.[143,163,179] Recently, McNamara et al. evaluated the mangled extremity severity Score (MESS) by retrospectively studying 24 patients with Gustilo IIIc fractures. The results confirmed high predictability. To improve the predictive value nerve damage and a detailed assessment of the bone and soft tissue damage were included. The new score that resulted from this is called the nerve injury, ischemia, soft tissue injury, skeletal injury, shock and age (NISSSA) score. It has been shown to have a sensitivity of 81.8% and a specificity of 92.3%.[252] Amputations are discussed further in Chapter 14.

Debridement. After deciding to salvage the limb, a careful extensive debridement is the first step in the operative treatment plan. All soft tissues have to be considered. If the debridement is overcautious this may lead to a deterioration of the patient's condition and even organ failure. Adequate surgical exposure of the injury is essential to both assess and treat the soft tissue damage. In multiply injured patients there is a high risk of late

soft tissue necrosis secondary to impaired soft tissue perfusion which may occur with post-traumatic edema, increased capillary permeability, massive volume resuscitation, and an unstable circulation. Therefore, in many patients regular operative explorations need to be undertaken. These second look surgeries allow for continuous assessment of the soft tissues. This strategy enables the surgeon to undertake re-debridement procedures every 48 hours if required. Once debridement is complete fracture stabilization and soft tissue repair should be planned and undertaken.

Operative Strategy Depending on the Overall Injury Severity. Clearly, the ability of the multiply injured patient to tolerate reconstructive surgery depends mainly on the overall condition of the patient and the extent of any co-existing injuries. Any lengthy reconstruction or reimplantation procedure may potentially harm the patient and induce a life-threatening situation. Attention also has to be paid to the long-term prognosis of an open injury in the multiply injured patient. All these variables need to be considered when constructing a therapeutic plan.

Patients with an ISS of 1 to 15 or 16 to 25 and Gustilo Grade IIIa, b, or c Soft Tissue Injuries. In this subgroup of multiply injured patients reconstruction is indicated. The surgical process is now largely standardized. After a radical debridement, the second step consists of vascular repair, if this is required. This may necessitate the use of an interposition vein graft. Following this the fractures should be stabilized, ideally using intramedullary osteosynthesis. Intramedullary implants are much less damaging to the soft tissues than direct osteosynthesis. There is less soft tissue stripping and only minimal impairment of the circulation of the bone.[211]

The closure of any associated soft tissue defect depends on the extent of the injury. In most cases, the wound will be temporarily covered with synthetic skin grafts or vacuum systems, before final closure using plastic reconstructive surgery techniques. This is discussed further in Chapter 15. In general, the expected result of a reconstructive limb saving strategy should be better than that of amputation.

Patients with an ISS of 1 to 15 or 16 to 25 with Complete or Incomplete Amputations. The surgical management of these injuries is very similar. The option of reimplantation has to be considered and this may require referral to a specialized center. If reimplantation is anticipated appropriate preparations must be made. Hemorrhage should be stopped by elevation and application of a pressure bandage. The treatment of the amputated limb follows clear emergency medicine guidelines.[399]

Patients with an ISS of 26 to 50 Points or >50 Points. In recent years level I trauma centers have improved their critical care and fracture management techniques and they now succeed in saving most severely traumatized extremities. However, unfortunately these limbs still sometimes require secondary amputation.[187] In very severely injured patients with extremity injuries the preservation of the extremity should not be attempted at all. The principle "life before limb" should hold true and the indications for amputation are generous. If the decision to amputate a limb is made the actual procedure should ideally be performed quickly through healthy tissue using a guillotine method. Under these circumstances primary closure is associated with an extremely high rate of complications because the overall extent of the soft tissue damage and post-traumatic edema cannot be adequately estimated.

Open Intra-Articular Fractures. A two-step strategy has been advocated for the management of open intra-articular fractures. Initially, the injury is debrided and the joint surface is reconstructed using a minimal invasive osteosynthesis technique. The joint is then immobilized by bridging, or transarticular, external fixation. The definitive osteosynthesis is carried out secondarily following soft tissue healing. In this procedure, the previously reconstructed articular segment is attached to the metaphysis. Sometimes bone shortening has to be accepted, at least temporarily, to close potential bony or soft tissue defects. The Ilizarov frame is often used under these circumstances. This is discussed further in Chapter 15.

The Timing of Soft Tissue Defect Reconstruction

In many multiply injured patients primary wound closure represents bad practice. The relative hypoxia of the tissues may lead to impaired and delayed wound healing associated with a higher risk of wound infection. In small soft tissue injuries, we recommend secondary closure of the wound after covering the wound with artificial skin until the swelling decreases. An absolute prerequisite for wound closure is to completely cover implants with well-perfused soft tissues. In these defects, artificial skin cover is used primarily and the wound is secondarily closed later over a period of several days. In some selected cases, continuous wound closure may also be an option. This is discussed further in Chapter 10.

In medium-sized soft tissue defects secondary closure is often achieved by local soft tissue transposition following appropriate mobilization of the soft tissues. In extensive soft tissue defects, associated with exposure of bone, with significant periosteal damage the soft tissues used to cover the defect require to be very well perfused. Soft tissue reconstruction should be undertaken within 72 hours of the trauma or there is danger of further damage.

Large post-traumatic soft tissue defects are very challenging for the surgeon and require a well-defined therapeutic strategy. The overall concept of soft tissue coverage depends on the extent of uncovered bone, tendons, and nerves. For bone associated with significant periosteal stripping, damaged neurovascular structures and injuries involving open joints soft tissue cover with well-perfused tissues is essential. To achieve satisfactory results timely communication and continuous cooperation between trauma and plastic surgeons is essential.

Soft Tissue Reconstruction

There are numerous local and distant flaps described in the literature to cover soft tissue defects. See chapter 15.

Local Flaps. Rotational flaps are used to cover small- and medium-sized soft tissue defects. These flaps consist of different combinations of muscle, fascia, and skin. They are very adaptable but are associated with a number of disadvantages.

In multiply injured patients it may be difficult to use local flaps because of co-existing injuries to the adjacent soft tissues. Meticulous preoperative planning is mandatory. Local flaps are discussed in more detail in Chapter 15.

Distant Flaps. For the reasons stated earlier distant flaps are commonly used in multiply injured patients. However the choice of flap is often difficult. On the one hand the patient may need urgent soft tissue closure but on the other hand a prolonged procedure may be contraindicated. Careful planning is essential (see Chapter 15).

SPECIAL SITUATIONS
Geriatric Trauma

The incidence of severely injured elderly patients is expected to increase in the near future. This is related to increasing life expectancy and to a more healthy and active lifestyle in people of advanced age. In addition, physiologic changes associated with the aging process including muscle atrophy, cardiovascular and neurovascular diseases, osteoporosis, and alterations in senses, vision and hearing, make the elderly patients prone to more severe injuries even after low-energy trauma. There is an increasing incidence of hypertension, obesity, diabetes mellitus, and heart disease among patients aged 55 years and older.[107,272] However, it must be kept in mind that the aging process is a subject of considerable individual variation. Thus, the chronologic age might not be reflected in the biologic age. The distribution of injuries and the injury mechanisms are different from those in young trauma victims.[215] Elderly patients more frequently fall and are involved in motor-vehicle injuries either as drivers or pedestrians.[215] The prevalence of severe (AIS $\geq$ 3) chest, abdominal, and extremity injuries has been shown to decrease with the age, in contrast to an increase of head injuries in older patients.[215]

The primary evaluation of multiply injured elderly patients can be very challenging. It has been suggested that early invasive monitoring and prompt adequate treatment be done in designated trauma centers to avoid complications.[215] The principles of initial assessment are similar to those in younger patients. Several characteristics of aged patients should be considered and are summarized below.

Airway Maintenance with Cervical Spine Protection

The airway should be examined in order to avoid airway obstruction. The presence of age-related neurologic disorders or dementia may be associated with the loss of protective airway reflexes. Liquids or vomit may be aspirated into the lung and lead to pneumonia and respiratory complications. It should be remembered that dentures may act as foreign bodies in the oral cavity. The immobilization and protection of the cervical spine is crucial. Chronic degenerative disease may facilitate fractures in the cervical spine.

Breathing and Ventilation

The aging process in the lung is characterized by loss of elasticity, decreased pulmonary compliance and alveolar loss.[251]

Pre-existing pulmonary diseases, such as chronic obstructive pulmonary disease or emphysema, limit the gas exchange within the lung. Blunt chest trauma frequently results in multiple fractures related to osteoporosis and chest rigidity in the aged population and this may significantly compromise mechanical ventilation and oxygenation of the patient.

Circulation with Hemorrhage Control

Younger patients compensate for blood loss by increasing the heart rate and myocardial contractility. Stiffness of the myocardium and reduction of the pump function in elderly patients reduces the cardiac reserve and the response to hypovolemia. Circulatory decompensation can therefore rapidly occur. Furthermore, clinical signs of hypovolemia may be masked by β-blockers or other heart medications.

Disability (Neurologic Evaluation)

Brain injuries are often present in elderly trauma patients and are the leading cause of death. Patients develop intracranial bleeding because of the increasing vulnerability of brain vessels with advanced age. This injury can be compounded by anticoagulation therapy. Repeated re-evaluation of the neurologic status and invasive monitoring is crucial. In the case of neurologic deficits it is important to distinguish whether these might be related to pre-existing conditions, such as stroke or dementia, or to the trauma itself.

Orthopedic Injuries

In patients with fractures, muscle atrophy and osteoporosis should be considered when considering the treatment strategy. Implants from earlier fractures, joint prostheses, and the presence of arthritis can make fracture treatment very challenging. In addition, alterations of the immune system, decreased circulation of the skin and pre-existing metabolic diseases may affect wound healing.

In stable patients a complete head-to-toe assessment should be undertaken. This secondary survey allows the surgeon to identify any missed injuries and any clinical signs of prior operations or diseases. The re-evaluation of medications, allergies, and any relevant medical history is critical in elderly patients and should be performed as soon as possible.

INTENSIVE CARE UNIT

One of the most important aspects of the clinical pathway of the polytrauma patient during the phase when survival is critical is management in the ICU environment. This is when the patients' vital organs require support and pharmacologic treatment strategies are implemented in order to regulate the hosts' response to injury.

Ventilation Strategies

Multiple trauma patients often present with blunt thoracic trauma and suffer from a variable degree of respiratory insufficiency. Management strategies for these patients should begin upon arrival at the trauma center. The objective is to initiate treatment early in order to minimize the risk of development of atelectasis and/or parenchymal damage. Mechanical ventilation should facilitate alveolar recruitment and enhance intrapulmonary gas distribution. Modern ventilation strategies with low tidal volume (4 to 8 mL/kg), best PEEP, low airway pressures (<35 cm H_2O) and an inspiratory oxygen concentration of 55% to 60% are often ideal. Hypercapnia may be allowed up to a certain degree. This is known as permissive hypercapnia (PHC).[420] It is well tolerated in patients with ARDS and a pCO_2 of 60 to 120 mm Hg. Clinical experience shows that pressure controlled ventilation with inverse ratio ventilation (I:E [1:1 to 4:1]), low tidal volumes (4 to 8 mL/kg), frequencies of 10 to 15/min, PHC ($pCO_2 \sim 70$ mm Hg) an individual PEEP of 5 to 12 cm H_2O, a high oxygen concentration ($FiO_2 < 0.5$) and a high airway pressure can prevent the lung from further ventilation damage.[448] Early experiences using other ventilation strategies, such as bilevel positive airway pressure (BIPAP), demonstrate that they are also feasible, although there may be problems with BIPAP in cases where long-term sedation is required. One of the most recent concepts developed for the prevention of pulmonary failure is the recruitment of alveoli by a temporary increase in positive end expiratory pressure (open-lung concept).[2] It does not cause sustained cardiovascular side effects and also does not lead to the development of bronchopleural fistulae. However the clinical relevance of this new concept has still to be proven in larger series.[263]

Recently, a new study compared an established low–tidal-volume ventilation strategy with an experimental strategy based on the original "open-lung approach," combining low tidal volume, lung recruitment maneuvers, and high positive end expiratory pressure. The authors concluded that for patients with acute lung injury and acute respiratory distress syndrome (ARDS), a multifaceted ventilation strategy designed to recruit and open the lung resulted in no significant difference in hospital mortality or barotrauma compared with an established low–tidal-volume ventilation strategy. This "open-lung" strategy did appear to improve secondary endpoints related to hypoxemia and the use of rescue therapies.[253]

Adult Respiratory Distress Syndrome

Acute lung injury can be caused by severe pneumonia or trauma and ARDS is its most critical form. In ARDS, the lungs become swollen with water and protein, and breathing becomes impossible, leading to death in 3% to 40% of the cases. Activated blood cells, cytokines, toxins, cell debris, and local tissue damage facilitate endothelial cell damage leading to decompensation of lymph drainage and pulmonary interstitial edema. Patients with ARDS have higher hospital mortality rates and reduced long-term pulmonary function and quality of life. ARDS is treated with mechanical ventilation, which can provide life support but often at the expense of further lung injury. Ventilation that employs a low tidal volume inhaled in each breath reduces the risk of death in patients who are critically ill with ARDS. The use of steroids has been controversial despite the fact that published trails support the administration of low to moderate dose corticosteroids in the treatment of early and late phase ARDS.[89] The impact of clinical risk factors in the conversion from acute lung injury to acute ARDS in severe multiple trauma patients has also been evaluated. It has been shown that the impact of pulmonary contusion, the APACHE II score and disseminated intravascular coagulation may help to predict the conversion of acute lung injury to ARDS in severe multiple trauma.[450] Historically, three phases of ARDS have been differentiated, the third leading to a state of scarring of pulmonary tissue and often irreversible loss of organ function. Currently, we believe that the formation of scar tissue is often the result of high intra-alveolar pressures due to inadequate ventilation techniques. Because of the improved ventilation strategies described above, the later form is usually no longer seen.[323]

Multiple Organ Dysfunction Syndrome

MODS is the result of an inappropriate generalized inflammatory response of the host to a variety of insults. Currently, it is believed that in the early phase of MODS, circulating cytokines cause universal endothelium injury in organs. In the later phase of MODS overexpression of inflammatory mediators in the interstitial space of various organs is considered a main mechanism of parenchymal injury. The difference in constitutive expression and the upregulation of adhesion molecules in vascular beds and the density and potency of intrinsic inflammatory cells in different organs are the key factors determining the sequence and severity of organ dysfunction.[411] The sequence of organ failure is variable. The most commonly reported sequence is pulmonary failure followed by hepatic and intestinal failure.[91,102]

Rehabilitation

The aftercare of polytrauma patients has to start during the immediate postoperative period. This requires mobilization of the extremities during the course of the intensive care treatment. Passive continuous motion may be used but mobilization of all major joints must be performed and should be part of a standardized rehabilitation program. Once the patient has been returned to the normal ward these measures must be maintained and they may be accompanied by active exercises by the patient. These should be performed under the supervision of a trained physical therapist. The modes of mobilization and the degree of weight bearing should be carefully discussed between the treating surgeon and the physical therapist. Patients tend to be cautious about mobilization and there is often a particular fear about weight bearing. This can often be explained by the severe psychological impact induced by the traumatic insult. Reassurance of the patient is an important additional factor if adequate mobilization is going to be achieved. These factors are important not only with regard to the maintenance of joint mobility, but also to prevent osteoporosis induced by immobility. It is crucial that patients realize the importance of muscular activity, joint mobility, and weight bearing with reference to neuromuscular function and the maintenance of an optimal osseous microstructure.

Patients with Head Trauma

When treating patients who have had significant head trauma special care must be taken to avoid the development of secondary brain damage. These patients also benefit from early rehabilitation measures. An appropriate transfer to a rehabilitation center is advisable. Although it may be considered appropriate to commence treatment in the primary center the patients are often still under the influence of sedative drugs or undergoing withdrawal symptoms from these drugs. In this situation a thorough work-up cannot be performed and cognitive training is useless. In an ideal situation, transfer to a specialized facility may overlap with the normalization of the withdrawal symptoms and thus forms the basis of a timely beginning of the rehabilitation program.

LATE OUTCOME AFTER POLYTRAUMA

Evaluation of the effectiveness of trauma care was traditionally focused on mortality rates, the incidence of preventable deaths, complication rates, in-hospital morbidity, and length of hospital stay.[38,354] However, due to the advances of acute trauma management and the increased survival rates over the last few decades, the long-term functional recovery, health-related quality of life, return to work, and patient satisfaction have been added to the classic trauma evaluation endpoints.

The long-term outcome of major trauma reflects the result of multiple phases and factors including diagnostic procedures, therapeutic interventions, inherent characteristics of the patient, and the effectiveness of the trauma services over a long period of time this being from the time of the accident until rehabilitation or even later. It is the end result of this multifactorial and complicated system that is of most concern to the patient. In the last two decades the importance of the patient's point of view and their perception of health outcomes has been acknowledged, and has led to the development of a large number of functional and patient-related outcome scores.[37]

However, the increasingly high priority of assessing the long-term functional outcome of trauma cannot only be based on patients' concerns as proper assessment facilitates the development and improvement of management guidelines, discharge and rehabilitation planning, and the optimal allocation of resources. In addition, the long-term outcome of trauma management has significant social and economic implications.[37]

Recovery following polytrauma is often prolonged and thus the appropriate time interval for assessment of long-term outcomes is usually longer than the customary time frame of 2 years. In particular, social rehabilitation including return to work or hobbies and change of occupation or retirement appears to be a long-term process. This suggests that the evaluation of the functional outcome following polytrauma should be based on a lengthened follow-up period by which time surgical outpatient review is sporadic if it is still occurring at all. This fact together with the complexity of parameters associated with the outcome of polytrauma explains the difficulty of long-term assessment and the scarcity of comprehensive clinical studies and adequate data.

Currently, the long-term outcome evaluation of trauma care encompasses parameters related to quality of life, return-to-work or sports, persistent physical or psychological complaints, and restrictions and acquired disabilities. The term "quality of life" entered Index Medicus in 1977.[144,455] In order to apply its concept in the specific clinical setting of trauma four basic areas should be considered these being physical function, psychological function, social function, and symptoms.[416] The unique character of this outcome assessment is that it relies largely on subjective variables judged by the patients themselves.

A large number of validated scoring systems are used to quantify outcome after mainly isolated injuries in almost all anatomic areas. In the case of polytrauma they are often utilized to objectively quantify the anatomical and physical components of the final outcome. Examples are the Lysholm and Merle d'Aubigne scores. For patients with multiple musculoskeletal disorders patient-assessed scales have been developed that describe self-reported complaints and subjective parameters. In addition, numerous scoring systems have been developed to determine psychological outcome after trauma.

In most of the large series it is musculoskeletal injuries of the lower extremity below the knee[372,412,435] together with injuries of the spine,[124,161,221] the pelvis[308,410] and brain injury[222,237] that are identified as those most influencing the long-term functional outcome of polytrauma patients.[393] According to most published series, they seem to determine a major proportion of the patient's quality of life with respect to functional status and pain.

Predictors of disability such as mechanism of injury, gender, injury severity, sociodemographic status, social support, and psychological sequelae have also been reported.[49,173,177] Clinically relevant psychological impairments such as anxiety, depression, and post-traumatic stress disorder have been reported especially within the first year after injury when they have a prevalence of 30% to 60%. In succeeding years the prevalence drops and has been reported to be 7% to 22%.[260] The importance of psychological outcomes, particularly post-traumatic stress disorder (PTSD), has been highlighted in many series.[359,394] It is described as an anxiety disorder that can develop after exposure to a terrifying event or ordeal in which grave physical harm occurred or was threatened.

Upper Extremity Injuries

Publications addressing the long-term outcome of upper extremity injuries are rare. Usually studies focus on isolated upper extremity fractures.[104] These results are likely to be different from those of multiply injured patients who have sustained high-energy trauma. Superior long-term results were reported in patients with upper extremity injuries in contrast to outcomes after lower extremity fractures.[53,235] However studies show that associated vascular and neurologic injuries negatively affect the long-term functional outcome.[190] An analysis of the musculoskeletal recovery after 5 years in 158 multiply injured patients treated between 1989 and 1990 has shown that approximately 50% of patients with shoulder girdle injuries had functional impairment and persistent disability.[265] In addition, 45% of trauma victims with shoulder girdle fractures and 62% of patients with upper extremity fractures reported chronic pain.[265] Displaced and intra-articular fractures, or a combination of shoulder girdle and diaphyseal fractures, were associated with poor long-term results. In the Hannover Rehabilitation Study a total of 637 multiply injured patient (ISS >15) were evaluated with a follow-up of 10 years (mean 17.5 years).[227] This study showed worse long-term results in patients who had combined intra-articular and diaphyseal upper extremity fractures. One possible explanation for this might be the complexity inherent in the reconstruction of intra-articular and multiple trauma. Moreover, concomitant injuries may interfere with the rehabilitation process and deleteriously affect the long-term outcome.

Pelvic Fractures

Pelvic injuries are usually the result of high-energy trauma and are often associated with multiple co-existing injuries.[113,408] Whether it is the accompanying injuries or the pelvic injuries that mainly lead to the poor long-term results is difficult to know. Research has shown that the presence of associated injuries and the stability or instability of pelvic fractures contribute to poor long-term outcomes.[325] In particular chronic pain and neurologic impairment have been shown to influence outcome.[326] Pohlemann et al.[324–326] have documented chronic pain in all pelvic fracture classification groups. They showed that 45% of patients with type A fractures had chronic pain compared with 59% of patients with type B fractures and 63% of patients with type C fractures. Furthermore, neurologic sequelae such as peripheral nerve lesions, incontinence, and sexual dysfunction have been shown to correlate with poor long-term results and were identified as a principal reason for work disability.[400]

Lower Extremity Fractures

Fractures of the lower extremity are often associated with significant long-term impairment and loss of function.[53,372] Trauma patients with these injuries have been shown to have the lowest rates of full recovery and overall satisfaction.[265,292] In the LEAP study, a prospective multicenter lower extremity assessment project[33,233,234] the long-term functional outcome of 601 patients with high-energy trauma below the distal femur was studied. The results demonstrated comparable outcomes in patients who had limb salvage and those who had an amputation. Only 58% of those working prior to their injury were able to return to work within 7 years. There was also no significant improvement in outcomes at the 7-year follow-up when compared to the 2-year follow-up.

The Hannover Rehabilitation Study, in a 10-year follow-up, has shown that 30% to 50% of patients have chronic pain and 10% to 30% report impaired range of motion. Patients with femoral shaft fractures had superior long-term results compared with those who had intra-articular fractures and proximal femur fractures.[319] Patients who sustained fractures below the knee had worse results compared with patients with fractures above the knee joint. The thin soft tissue envelope and restricted blood supply were suggested as possible factors leading to an inferior outcome (Table 9-10).[453]

Notwithstanding the differences in injury pattern, severity of injury, trauma management practices, and rehabilitation there is strong evidence that the quality of life and overall outcome is significantly impaired after major trauma. In the past, the principal aim of treatment was the prevention of late organ failure and death. In contrast, nowadays the ultimate goal of trauma care is to restore patients to their previous functional status and role in society. The exact measurement of functional outcome still lacks accuracy but the results of a number of studies reporting on the functional outcome after multiple trauma are shown in Table 9-11.[8,111,171,172,192,210,305,316] The commonly used functional outcome scores are shown in Table 9-12.[134,186,392,434] We anticipate that in the near future there will be better assessment of the outcome of the treatment of the multiply injured patient.

TABLE 9-10	Functional Long-Term Outcome of the Lower Extremities' Fractures Following Polytrauma				
	Acetabulum N = 20 (%)	Prox. Femur N = 20 (%)	Femoral Shaft N = 107 (%)	Knee[a] N = 48 (%)	Tibial Shaft N = 34 (%)
Persistent pain	50	45	32.7	43.8	26.5
Abnormal gait	35[b,c]	20[b]	3.7	8.3	14.7[b]
Work disability	27.8[b,d,e]	10	7.6	19.8	8.8
Successful rehabilitation	70	60[b]	80.4	56.3[b]	67.7

[a]Knee: Including fractures of the distal femur and proximal tibia.
[b]Significantly worse outcome versus femoral shaft fractures ($p < 0.05$).
[c]Significantly worse outcome versus injuries at the knee joint ($p < 0.05$).
[d]Significantly worse outcome versus fractures of the proximal femur ($p < 0.05$).
[e]Significantly worse outcome versus tibial shaft fractures ($p < 0.05$).
Pfeifer R, Zelle B, Kobbe P, et al. Impact of isolated acetablar and lower extremity fractures on long-term outcome. *J Trauma Acute Care Surg*. 2012;72(2):467–472.

TABLE 9-11	Studies Focused on Long-Term Outcome of Major Trauma Patients			
Authors, Origin, Year	Number of Patients	ISS—Follow-up	Outcome Parameters	Conclusions
Bull,[125] Birmingham, UK, 1975	1,268	N/a—on discharge	• Disability—5-point scale	• Of the 1,268 cases 264 suffered some residual disability • The ISS rating may be a useful measure of likely disabilities when applied to groups of cases, but should be used with great caution in forecasting the outcome of an individual patient
MacKenzie et al.,[429] Baltimore, USA, 1986	473	N/a—6 months	• Activities of daily living (ADL) • Instrumental activities of daily living (IADL) • Mobility	• AIS of the most severe extremity and spinal cord injury carry considerably more weight when predicting functional status than do the AIS scores of injuries to any other body region
Horne and Schemitsch,[145] Wellington, New Zealand, 1989	90	Mean ISS 23.3— mean 3.2 years	• Modified Glasgow scale	• Correlation between outcome and the severity of brain injury, the severity of skeletal injuries and the ISS • ISS < 24 no physical impairment • ISS of 25–30 slight impairment • ISS > 30 at least one moderate impairment
Gaillard et al.,[16] Creteil, France, 1990	250	Mean ISS 25— minimum 2 years	• Long-term survey	• There was no parallelism between objective sequelae and duration of work stop and gravity of lesions ISS
Jurkovich et al.,[339] Seattle, Baltimore, Nashville, USA, 1995	329	N/a—12 months	• Sickness impact profile (SIP)	• 48% had some form of disability even at 12 months • Disability was present for a wide spectrum of activities of daily life, including ambulation, psychosocial health, sleep, home management, and return to work and leisure activities • Need for psychological intervention and social support long into the recovery period of patients who might not at first seem to require them

TABLE 9-11 **Studies Focused on Long-Term Outcome of Major Trauma Patients** (continued)

Authors, Origin, Year	Number of Patients	ISS—Follow-up	Outcome Parameters	Conclusions
Ott et al.,[188] Nurnberg, Germany, 1996	73	PTS ≥ 40—range 1–13 years	• Aachen Long-term Outcome Score (ALOS) • Spitzer index (SI) • Self-assessment. • Return to work	• Predominantly, handicaps resulted from permanent physical disability, in particular the lower extremities • Head injuries, extremity trauma, severity of injury and increasing age correlated with worse outcome
Anke et al.,[416] Oslo, NOR, 1997	69	Mean ISS 25 (range 17–50)— 35 ± 4 months	• Checklist on social network • Occurrence of impairments and disabilities	• (74%) had physical impairments, about one-third (32%) of the subjects had cognitive impairments. • significant correlation between ISS and degrees of impairments • high prevalence of impairments after severe multiple trauma
Holbrook et al.,[29] San Diego, USA, 1999	780	Mean ISS 13 +/– 8.5—18 months	• Quality of well-being (QWB) scale • Functional disability score • Center for Epidemiologic Studies Depression (CES-D) scale • Impact of events scale	• Depression, post-traumatic stress disorder and serious extremity injury play an important role in determining outcome • A prolonged and profound level of functional limitation after major trauma was identified at 12-month and 18-month follow-up
Korosec-Jagodic et al.,[378] Celje, Slovenia, 2000	98	APACHE II 14.3 ± 6.6—2 years	• EuroQol 5D questionnaire • Health-related quality of life (HRQOL)	• Trauma patients had a tendency toward anxiety and depression • Survival and quality of life after critical illness are independent
Holbrook et al.,[361] San Diego, USA, 2001	1,048	Mean ISS 13.5— 18 months	• Quality of well-being (QWB) scale • Center for Epidemiologic Studies Depression (CES-D) scale • Impact of events scale	• Gender may play a strong and independent role in predicting functional outcome and quality of life after major trauma • Functional outcome and quality of life were markedly lower in women compared with men, as measured by the QWB scale
Stalp et al.,[406] Hannover, Germany, 2002	254	Mean ISS 24 ± 6— mean 2.1 years ± 0.1	• Hannover score for polytrauma outcome (HASPOC) • Musculoskeletal function assessment (MFA) • 12-item health survey (SF-12) • Functional independence measurement (FIM) • Glasgow outcome scale • Evaluation of specific body regions	• The most severe impairment in functional outcome occurs after injuries of the lower extremities, spine and pelvis • The main problems in patients with multiple injuries with skeletal injuries 2 years after trauma were secondary to injuries of the lower extremity below the knee, the spine, and the pelvis
Tran and Thordarson,[401] Los Angeles, USA, 2002	24	Mean ISS 17— minimum 12 months	• 36-item health survey (SF-36) • AAOS lower limb • Foot and ankle score	• Significant negative impact on outcome in multiply injured patients who have also sustained a foot injury • Multiply injured patients with foot injuries had significantly more limitations in physical and social activities, increased bodily pain

(continues)

TABLE 9-11 **Studies Focused on Long-Term Outcome of Major Trauma Patients (continued)**

Authors, Origin, Year	Number of Patients	ISS—Follow-up	Outcome Parameters	Conclusions
Zelle et al.,[365] Hannover, Germany, 2005	637	Mean ISS 20.7 ± 9.7—mean 17.5 (range 10–28)	• Hannover score for polytrauma outcome (HASPOC) • 12-item health survey (SF-12) • Self-reported require-ment for medical aids and devices • Self-reported requirement for inpatient rehabilitation • Self-reported length of rehabilitation • Retired because of injury	• Psychosocial factors play a major role for the recovery following polytrauma • Workers' compensation patients were significantly more likely to use medical aids and devices, be retired because of their injury, and have inpatient rehabilitation • The workers' compensation status has a significant impact on the long-term subjective and objective outcome following polytrauma
Zelle et al.,[176] Hannover, Germany, 2005	389	Mean ISS 20.2 ± 4.3 mean PTS 29.5 ± 13.3—mean 17.3 ± 4.8 years	• Lower extremity specific outcome measurements • The Hannover score for polytrauma outcome (HASPOC) • 12-item health survey (SF-12) • Tegner activity score • The inability to work	• Injuries below the knee have a major impact on the functional recovery following polytrauma • The analysis of general outcome and lower extremity specific out-come measurements suggests that patients' fractures above the knee joint achieve superior outcomes than patients with fractures below the knee joint
Pape et al.,[411] Hannover, Germany, 2006	637	Mean ISS 20.7 (range 4–54)—mean 17.5 years (range 0–28)	• Lower extremity specific outcome measurements • General outcome mea-surements • 12-item health survey (SF-12) • Inability to work • Subjective outcome ques-tionnaires	• The injury most often responsible for physical disability was head trauma, followed by injuries to the lower extremities • A high percentage of patients can be recruited for follow-up even after 10 years after polytrauma

TABLE 9-12 **Commonly Used Functional Outcome Scores in the Clinical Setting of Polytrauma**

Name—*Abbreviation*	Characteristics	Range of Values	Studies Where Used
Quality of well-being scale— QWB scale	1 symptom scale and 3 function scales (mobility, physical activity, social activity)	0–1.0 Death—asymptomatic full function	29,361
Glasgow Outcome Score— GOS	5 item score	1–5 Dead—good recovery	145,288,406
Activities of daily living scale— ADL scale	21 items of basic capacities of self-care (BADL) and higher levels of performance (IADL)	0–21 Worst–best	418,429
Sickness impact Profile—SIP	12 categories physical and psychosocial	0–210 Worst–best	313,339
Functional independence measurement—FIM	13 motor items and 5 cognitive items	1–7 Total assist–complete independence	406
Hannover score for polytrauma outcome—HASPOC score	Part 1 (113 questions) patient questionnaire (HASPOC-subjective) and Part 2 (191 questions) physical examination (HASPOC-objective)	5–411 points Best–worst	98,176,406
Health survey short form 36 or 12 item—SF-36/12	36/12 health related aspects	0–100 points	176,411,436
EuroQol 5D questionnaire— EQ-5D	Part I—descriptive system Part II—visual-analogue scale Part III—EuroQol 5D Index	−0.11–1 Worse than death–perfect health	378

REFERENCES

1. Abboud PA, Kendall J. Emergency department ultrasound for hemothorax after blunt traumatic injury. *J Emerg Med.* 2003;25(2):181–184.
2. Agro F, Barzoi G, Doyle DJ, et al. Reduction in pulmonary shunt using the Open Lung Concept. *Anaesthesia.* 2004;59(6):625–626.
3. Aiboshi J, Moore EE, Ciesla DJ, et al. Blood transfusion and the two-insult model of post-injury multiple organ failure. *Shock.* 2001;15(4):302–306.
4. American Association for the Surgery of Trauma O-A. Organ Injury Scale. http://www.aast.org. 2008.
5. American College of Surgeons Committee on Trauma 2005. American College of Surgeons (Committee of Trauma. National Trauma Data Bank Annual Report 2005).
6. American College of Surgeons Committee on Trauma 2008. *Advanced Trauma Life Support for Doctors.* 8th ed. Chicago, IL: 2008.
7. American College of Surgeons. Trauma Programs. History of the ATLS Program. http://www.facs.org/trauma/atls/history.html. 2012.
8. Anke AG, Stanghelle JK, Finset A, et al. Long-term prevalence of impairments and disabilities after multiple trauma. *J Trauma.* 1997;42(1):54–61.
9. Association of Advancements of Automotive Medicine. http://www.aaam.org
10. Baker SP, Harvey AH. Fall injuries in the elderly. *Clin Geriatr Med.* 1985;1(3):501–512.
11. Baker SP, O'Neill B, Haddon W Jr, et al. The injury severity score: a method for describing patients with multiple injuries and evaluating emergency care. *J Trauma.* 1974;14(3):187–196.
12. Balkan ME, Oktar GL, Kayi-Cangir A, et al. Emergency thoracotomy for blunt thoracic trauma. *Ann Thorac Cardiovasc Surg.* 2002;8(2):78–82.
13. Balogh Z, Offner PJ, Moore EE, et al. NISS predicts postinjury multiple organ failure better than the ISS. *J Trauma.* 2000;48(4):624–627.
14. Balogh ZJ, Varga E, Tomka J, et al. The new injury severity score is a better predictor of extended hospitalization and intensive care unit admission than the injury severity score in patients with multiple orthopaedic injuries. *J Orthop Trauma.* 2003;17(7):508–512.
15. Barber RC, Chang LY, Purdue GF, et al. Detecting genetic predisposition for complicated clinical outcomes after burn injury. *Burns.* 2006;32(7):821–827.
16. Beck J, Colins J. Theoretical and clinical aspects of post traumatic fat embolism syndrome. *AAOS Instr Course letters.* 1973;22:38–44.
17. Beningfield S, Potgieter H, Nicol A, et al. Report on a new type of trauma full-body digital X-ray machine. *Emerg Radiol.* 2003;10(1):23–29.
18. Berg J, Tagliaferri F, Servadei F. Cost of trauma in Europe. *Eur J Neurol.* 2005;12(suppl 1):85–90.
19. Berg J. Economic evidence in trauma: a review. *Eur J Health Econnom.* 2004;(suppl 1):S84–S91.
20. Bernhard M, Gries A, Kremer P, et al. Spinal cord injury (SCI)–prehospital management. *Resuscitation.* 2005;66(2):127–139.
21. Bessoud B, Duchosal MA, Siegrist CA, et al. Proximal splenic artery embolization for blunt splenic injury: clinical, immunologic, and ultrasound-Doppler follow-up. *J Trauma.* 2007;62(6):1481–1486.
22. Bianchi ME. DAMPs, PAMPs and alarmins: all we need to know about danger. *J Leukoc Biol.* 2007;81(1):1–5.
23. Bickell WH, Wall MJ Jr, Pepe PE, et al. Immediate versus delayed fluid resuscitation for hypotensive patients with penetrating torso injuries. *N Engl J Med.* 1994;331(17):1105–1109.
24. Bircher M, Giannoudis PV. Pelvic trauma management within the UK: a reflection of a failing trauma service. *Injury.* 2004;35(1):2–6.
25. Bishop M, Shoemaker WC, Avakian S, et al. Evaluation of a comprehensive algorithm for blunt and penetrating thoracic and abdominal trauma. *Am Surg.* 1991;57(12):737–746.
26. Blow O, Magliore L, Claridge JA, et al. The golden hour and the silver day: detection and correction of occult hypoperfusion within 24 hours improves outcome from major trauma. *J Trauma.* 1999;47(5):964–969.
27. Boehm T, Alkadhi H, Schertler T, et al. [Application of multislice spiral CT (MSCT) in multiple injured patients and its effect on diagnostic and therapeutic algorithms]. *Rofo.* 2004;176(12):1734–1742.
28. Boffard KD, Goosen J, Plani F, et al. The use of low dosage X-ray (Lodox(Statscan) in major trauma: comparison between low dose X-ray and conventional x-ray techniques. *J Trauma.* 2006;60(6):1175–1181.
29. Bone LB, Johnson KD, Weigelt J, et al. Early versus delayed stabilization of femoral fractures. A prospective randomized study. *J Bone Joint Surg Am.* 1989;71(3):336–340.
30. Bone RC, Balk RA, Cerra FB, et al. Definitions for sepsis and organ failure and guidelines for the use of innovative therapies in sepsis. The ACCP/SCCM Consensus Conference Committee. American College of Chest Physicians/Society of Critical Care Medicine. *Chest.* 1992;101(6):1644–1655.
31. Bone RC. Toward a theory regarding the pathogenesis of systemic inflammatory response syndrome: What we do and do not know about cytokine regulation. *Crit Care Med.* 2008;24:163–172.
32. Bosch U, Pohlemann T, Tscherne H. [Primary management of pelvic injuries]. *Orthopade.* 1992;21(6):385–392.
33. Bosse MJ, MacKenzie EJ, Kellam JF, et al. An analysis of outcomes of reconstruction or amputation after leg-threatening injuries. *N Engl J Med.* 2002;347(24):1924–1931.
34. Bothig R. [TRISS–a method of assessment of the prognosis in multiple trauma patients]. *Zentralbl Chir.* 1991;116(14):831–844.
35. Bouamra O, Wrotchford A, Hollis S, et al. A new approach to outcome prediction in trauma: A comparison with the TRISS model. *J Trauma.* 2006;61(3):701–710.
36. Bouillon B, Lefering R, Vorweg M, et al. Trauma score systems: Cologne Validation Study. *J Trauma.* 1997;42(4):652–658.
37. Bouillon B, Neugebauer E. Outcome after polytrauma. *Langenbecks Arch Surg.* 1998;383(3–4):228–234.
38. Boyd CR, Tolson MA, Copes WS. Evaluating trauma care: the TRISS method. Trauma Score and the Injury Severity Score. *J Trauma.* 1987;27(4):370–378.
39. Braver ER, Kyrychenko SY, Ferguson SA. Driver mortality in frontal crashes: comparison of newer and older airbag designs. *Traffic Inj Prev.* 2005;6(1):24–30.
40. Braver ER, Scerbo M, Kufera JA, et al. Deaths among drivers and right-front passengers in frontal collisions: redesigned air bags relative to first-generation air bags. *Traffic Inj Prev.* 2008;9(1):48–58.
41. Brenchley J, Walker A, Sloan JP, et al. Evaluation of focussed assessment with sonography in trauma (FAST) by UK emergency physicians. *Emerg Med J.* 2006;23(6):446–448.
42. Brenneman FD, Boulanger BR, McLellan BA, et al. Measuring injury severity: time for a change? *J Trauma.* 1998;44(4):580–582.
43. Brouhard R. To immobilize or not immobilize: that is the question. *Emerg Med Serv.* 2006;35(5):81–86.
44. Bruns B, Lindsey M, Rowe K, et al. Hemoglobin drops within minutes of injuries and predicts need for an intervention to stop hemorrhage. *J Trauma.* 2007;63(2):312–315.
45. Bulger EM, Copass MK, Maier RV. An analysis of advanced prehospital airway management. *J Emerg Med.* 2002;23(2):183–189.
46. Bulger EM, Jurkovich GJ, Nathens AB, et al. Hypertonic resuscitation of hypovolemic shock after blunt trauma: a randomized controlled trial. *Arch Surg.* 2008;143(2):139–148.
47. Bulger EM, Maier RV. Prehospital care of the injured: what's new. *Surg Clin North Am.* 2007;87(1):37–53.
48. Bulger EM, Nathens AB, Rivara FP, et al. Management of severe head injury: institutional variations in care and effect on outcome. *Crit Care Med.* 2002;30:1870–1876.
49. Bull J. The Injury Severity Score of road traffic casualties in relation to mortality, time of death, hospital treatment time and disability. *Accid Anal Prev.* 1975;7:249–255.
50. Bull JP, Dickson GR. Injury scoring by TRISS and ISS/age. *Injury.* 1991;22(2):127–131.
51. Bunn F, Kwan I, Roberts IRW. Effectiveness of prehospital trauma care. *Cochrane Injuries Group.* 2001.
52. Burger C, Zwingmann J, Kabir K, et al. [Faster diagnostics by digital X-ray imaging in the emergency room: a prospective study in multiple trauma patients]. *Z Orthop Unfall.* 2007;145(6):772–777.
53. Butcher JL, MacKenzie EJ, Cushing B, et al. Long-term outcomes after lower extremity trauma. *J Trauma.* 1996;41(1):4–9.
54. Cales RH. Trauma mortality in Orange County: the effect of implementation of a regional trauma system. *Ann Emerg Med.* 1984;13(1):1–10.
55. Cannon W. The emergency function of the adrenal medulla in pain and the major emotions. *Am J Physiol.* 1914;356–372.
56. Cardarelli MG, McLaughlin JS, Downing SW, et al. Management of traumatic aortic rupture: a 30-year experience. *Ann Surg.* 2002;236(4):465–469.
57. Carmont M. The Advanced Trauma Life Support Course: a history of its development and review of related literature. *Postgrad Med J.* 2005;81:87–91.
58. Catalano O, Siani A. Focused assessment with sonography for trauma (FAST): what it is, how it is carried out, and why we disagree. *Radiol Med.* 2004;108(5–6):443–453.
59. Champion HR, Copes WS, Sacco WJ, et al. A new characterization of injury severity. *J Trauma.* 1990;30(5):539–545.
60. Champion HR, Copes WS, Sacco WJ, et al. Improved predictions from a severity characterization of trauma (ASCOT) over Trauma and Injury Severity Score (TRISS): results of an independent evaluation. *J Trauma.* 1996;40(1):42–48.
61. Champion HR, Copes WS, Sacco WJ, et al. The Major Trauma Outcome Study: establishing national norms for trauma care. *J Trauma.* 1990;30(11):1356–1365.
62. Champion HR, Sacco WJ, Carnazzo AJ, et al. Trauma score. *Crit Care Med.* 1981;9(9):672–676.
63. Champion HR, Sacco WJ, Copes WS, et al. A revision of the Trauma Score. *J Trauma.* 1989;29(5):623–629.
64. Chawla A, Mohan D, Sharma V. Safer truck front design for pedestrian impacts. *J Crash Prev Inj Cont.* 2000;33–43.
65. Chesnut RM, Marshall SB, Piek J, et al. Early and late systemic hypotension as a frequent and fundamental source of cerebral ischemia following severe brain injury in the Traumatic Coma Data Bank. *Acta Neurochir Suppl (Wien).* 1993;59:121–125.
66. Choi CB, Park P, Kim YH, et al. Comparison of visibility measurement techniques for forklift truck design factors. *Appl Ergon.* 2009;40(2):280–285.
67. Choi PT, Yip G, Quinonez LG, et al. Crystalloids vs. colloids in fluid resuscitation: a systematic review. *Crit Care Med.* 1999;27(1):200–210.
68. Ciesla D, Sava JA, Street JH III, Jordan MH. Secondary overtriage: a consequence of an immature trauma system. *J Am Coll Surg.* 2008;206(1):131–137.
69. Claridge JA, Crabtree TD, Pelletier SJ, et al. Persistent occult hypoperfusion is associated with a significant increase in infection rate and mortality in major trauma patients. *J Trauma.* 2000;48(1):8–14.
70. Cocchi MN, Kimlin E, Walsh M, et al. Identification and resuscitation of the trauma patient in shock. *Emerg Med Clin North Am.* 2007;25(3):623–642.
71. Coles JP, Minhas PS, Fryer TD, et al. Effect of hyperventilation on cerebral blood flow in traumatic head injury: clinical relevance and monitoring correlates. *Crit Care Med.* 2002;30(9):1950–1959.
72. Collighan N, Giannoudis PV, Kourgeraki O, et al. Interleukin 13 and inflammatory markers in human sepsis. *Br J Surg.* 2004;91(6):762–768.
73. Committee on Medical Aspects of Automotive Safety. Rating the severity of tissue damage. *JAMA.* 1971;215:277–280.
74. Cooke WH, Salinas J, Convertino VA, et al. Heart rate variability and its association with mortality in prehospital trauma patients. *J Trauma.* 2006;60(2):363–370.
75. Cooper DJ, Myles PS, McDermott FT, et al. Prehospital hypertonic saline resuscitation of patients with hypotension and severe traumatic brain injury: a randomized controlled trial. *JAMA.* 2004;291(11):1350–1357.
76. Copes WS, Champion HR, Sacco WJ, et al. Progress in characterizing anatomic injury. *J Trauma.* 1990;30(10):1200–1207.
77. Copes WS, Champion HR, Sacco WJ, et al. The Injury Severity Score revisited. *J Trauma.* 1988;28(1):69–77.

78. Corso P, Finkelstein E, Miller T, et al. Incidence and lifetime costs of injuries in the United States. *Injury Prevention.* 2006;12:212–218.

79. Cothren CC, Osborn PM, Moore EE, et al. Preperitonal pelvic packing for hemodynamically unstable pelvic fractures: a paradigm shift. *J Trauma.* 2007;62(4):834–839.

80. Cummings G, O'Keefe G. Scene disposition and mode of transport following rural trauma: a prospective cohort study comparing patient costs. *J Emerg Med.* 2000;18(3):349–354.

81. Cummings P, McKnight B, Rivara FP, et al. Association of driver air bags with driver fatality: a matched cohort study. *BMJ.* 2002;324(7346):1119–1122.

82. Cummings P, Rivara FP, Olson CM, et al. Changes in traffic crash mortality rates attributed to use of alcohol, or lack of a seat belt, air bag, motorcycle helmet, or bicycle helmet, United States, 1982–2001. *Inj Prev.* 2006;12(3):148–154.

83. Curtis K, Zou Y, Morris R, et al. Trauma case management: improving patient outcomes. *Injury.* 2006;37(7):626–632.

84. Dahabreh Z, Dimitriou R, Chalidis B, et al. Coagulopathy and the role of recombinant human activated protein C in sepsis and following polytrauma. *Expert Opin Drug Saf.* 2006;5(1):67–82.

85. Dahabreh Z, Dimitriou R, Giannoudis PV. Health economics: a cost analysis of treatment of persistent fracture non-unions using bone morphogenetic protein-7. *Injury.* 2007;38(3):371–377.

86. Davis DP, Ochs M, Hoyt DB, et al. Paramedic-administered neuromuscular blockade improves prehospital intubation success in severely head-injured patients. *J Trauma.* 2003;55(4):713–719.

87. Davis DP, Stern J, Sise MJ, et al. A follow-up analysis of factors associated with head-injury mortality after paramedic rapid sequence intubation. *J Trauma.* 2005;59(2):486–490.

88. Davis DP, Valentine C, Ochs M, et al. The Combitube as a salvage airway device for paramedic rapid sequence intubation. *Ann Emerg Med.* 2003;42(5):697–704.

89. Deal EN, Hollands JM, Schramm GE, et al. Role of corticosteroids in the management of acute respiratory distress syndrome. *Clin Ther.* 2008;30(5):787–799.

90. DeBritz JN, Pollak AN. The impact of trauma centre accreditation on patient outcome. *Injury.* 2006;37(12):1166–1171.

91. Deitch EA. Multiple organ failure. *Adv Surg.* 1993;26:333–356.

92. Deloughery TG. Coagulation defects in trauma patients: etiology, recognition, and therapy. *Crit Care Clin.* 2004;20(1):13–24.

93. Demetriades D, Sofianos C. Penetrating trauma audit–TRISS analysis. *S Afr J Surg.* 1992;30(4):142–144.

94. Department of Transportation NHTSA. (NHTSA), U. D. o. T. N. H. T. S. A.: Traffic Safety Facts 1997. Washington, DC: 1998.

95. Dick WF. Anglo-American vs. Franco-German emergency medical services system. *Prehosp Disaster Med.* 2003;18(1):29–35.

96. Doran JV, Tortella BJ, Drivet WJ, et al. Factors influencing successful intubation in the prehospital setting. *Prehosp Disaster Med.* 1995;10(4):259–264.

97. Downing SW, Sperling JS, Mirvis SE, et al. Experience with spiral computed tomography as the sole diagnostic method for traumatic aortic rupture. *Ann Thorac Surg.* 2001;72(2):495–501.

98. Dunham CM, Bosse MJ, Clancy TV, et al. Practice management guidelines for the optimal timing of long-bone fracture stabilization in polytrauma patients: the EAST Practice Management Guidelines Work Group. *J Trauma.* 2001;50(5):958–967.

99. Durbin DR, Elliott MR, Winston FK. Belt-positioning booster seats and reduction in risk of injury among children in vehicle crashes. *JAMA.* 2003;289(21):2835–2840.

100. Durbin DR, Runge J, Mackay M, et al. Booster seats for children: closing the gap between science and public policy in the United States. *Traffic Inj Prev.* 2003;4(1):5–8.

101. Durham R, Pracht E, Orban B, et al. Evaluation of a mature trauma system. *Ann Surg.* 2006;243(6):775–783.

102. Durham RM, Moran JJ, Mazuski JE, et al. Multiple organ failure in trauma patients. *J Trauma.* 2003;55(4):608–616.

103. Eastman AB, Bishop GS, Walsh JC, et al. The economic status of trauma centers on the eve of health care reform. *J Trauma.* 1994;36(6):835–844.

104. Ekholm R, Tidermark J, Törnkvist H, et al. Outcome after closed functional treatment of humeral shaft fractures. *J Orth Trauma.* 2006;20:591–596.

105. Exadaktylos AK, Benneker LM, Jeger V, et al. Total-body digital X-ray in trauma. An experience report on the first operational full body scanner in Europe and its possible role in ATLS. *Injury.* 2008;39(5):525–529.

106. Finefrock SC. Designing and building a new emergency department: the experience of one chest pain, stroke, and trauma center in Columbus, Ohio. *J Emerg Nurs.* 2006;32(2):144–148.

107. Ford E, Giles W, Dietz W. Prevalence of the metabolic syndrome among US adults: findings from the third National Health and Nutrition Examination Survey. *JAMA.* 2002;287:356–359.

108. Frink M, Probst C, Hildebrand F, et al. [The influence of transportation mode on mortality in polytraumatized patients. An analysis based on the German Trauma Registry]. *Unfallchirurg.* 2007;110(4):334–340.

109. Fung Kon Jin PH, Goslings JC, Ponsen KJ, et al. Assessment of a new trauma workflow concept implementing a sliding CT scanner in the trauma room: the effect on workup times. *J Trauma.* 2008;64(5):1320–1326.

110. Furst DE, Breedveld FC, Kalden JR, et al. Updated consensus statement on biological agents, specifically tumour necrosis factor {alpha} (TNF{alpha}) blocking agents and interleukin-1 receptor antagonist (IL-1ra), for the treatment of rheumatic diseases, 2005. *Ann Rheum Dis.* 2005;64(suppl 4):iv2–iv14.

111. Gaillard M, Pasquier C, Guerrini P, et al. [Short- and long-term outcome of 250 patients admitted in surgical intensive care units after multiple injuries]. *Agressologie.* 1990;31(9):633–636.

112. Gansslen A, Giannoudis P, Pape HC. Hemorrhage in pelvic fracture: who needs angiography? *Curr Opin Crit Care.* 2003;9(6):515–523.

113. Gansslen A, Pohlemann T, Paul C, et al. Epidemiology of pelvic ring injuries. *Injury.* 1996;27(suppl 1):S13–S20.

114. Ganzoni D, Zellweger R, Trentz O. [Cost analysis of acute therapy of polytrauma patients]. *Swiss Surg.* 2003;9(6):268–274.

115. Gennarelli TA, Champion HR, Sacco WJ, et al. Mortality of patients with head injury and extracranial injury treated in trauma centers. *J Trauma.* 1989;29(9):1193–1201.

116. Gennarelli TA, Wodzin E. AIS 2005: a contemporary injury scale. *Injury.* 2006;37(12):1083–1091.

117. Giannoudis PV, Abbott C, Stone M, et al. Fatal systemic inflammatory response syndrome following early bilateral femoral nailing. *Intensive Care Med.* 1998;24(6):641–642.

118. Giannoudis PV, Dinopoulos H, Chalidis B, et al. Surgical stress response. *Injury.* 2006;37(suppl 5):S3–S9.

119. Giannoudis PV, Fogerty S. Initial care of the severely injured patient: predicting morbidity from sub-clinical findings and clinical proteomics. *Injury.* 2007;38(3):261–262.

120. Giannoudis PV, Grotz MR, Tzioupis C, et al. Prevalence of pelvic fractures, associated injuries, and mortality: the United Kingdom perspective. *J Trauma.* 2007;63(4):875–883.

121. Giannoudis PV, Harwood PJ, Loughenbury P, et al. Correlation between IL-6 levels and the systemic inflammatory response score: can an IL-6 cutoff predict a SIRS state? *J Trauma.* 2008;65(3):646–652.

122. Giannoudis PV, Hildebrand F, Pape HC. Inflammatory serum markers in patients with multiple trauma. Can they predict outcome? *J Bone Joint Surg Br.* 2004;86(3):313–323.

123. Giannoudis PV, Kanakaris NK. The unresolved issue of health economics and polytrauma: the UK perspective. *Injury.* 2008;39(7):705–709.

124. Giannoudis PV, Mehta SS, Tsiridis E. Incidence and outcome of whiplash injury after multiple trauma. *Spine (Phila Pa 1976).* 2007;32(7):776–781.

125. Giannoudis PV, Pape HC. Damage control orthopaedics in unstable pelvic ring injuries. *Injury.* 2004;35(7):671–677.

126. Giannoudis PV, Pape HC. Trauma and immune reactivity: too much, or too little immune response? *Injury.* 2007;38(12):1333–1335.

127. Giannoudis PV, Smith RM, Banks RE, et al. Stimulation of inflammatory markers after blunt trauma. *Br J Surg.* 1998;85(7):986–990.

128. Giannoudis PV, Smith RM, Perry SL, et al. Immediate IL-10 expression following major orthopaedic trauma: relationship to anti-inflammatory response and subsequent development of sepsis. *Intensive Care Med.* 2000;26(8):1076–1081.

129. Giannoudis PV, Smith RM, Windsor AC, et al. Monocyte human leukocyte antigen-DR expression correlates with intrapulmonary shunting after major trauma. *Am J Surg.* 1999;177(6):454–459.

130. Giannoudis PV, Tosounidis TI, Kanakaris NK, et al. Quantification and characterisation of endothelial injury after trauma. *Injury.* 2007;38(12):1373–1381.

131. Giannoudis PV, van GM, Tsiridis E, et al. The genetic predisposition to adverse outcome after trauma. *J Bone Joint Surg Br.* 2007;89(10):1273–1279.

132. Giannoudis PV. Current concepts of the inflammatory response after major trauma: an update. *Injury.* 2003;34(6):397–404.

133. Giannoudis PV. Surgical priorities in damage control in polytrauma. *J Bone Joint Surg Br.* 2003;85(4):478–483.

134. Gilson BS, Gilson JS, Bergner M, et al. The sickness impact profile. Development of an outcome measure of health care. *Am J Public Health.* 1975;65(12):1304–1310.

135. Goldfarb MG, Bazzoli GJ, Coffey RM. Trauma systems and the costs of trauma care. *Health Serv Res.* 1996;31(1):71–95.

136. Goldschlager T, Rosenfeld JV, Winter CD. 'Talk and die' patients presenting to a major trauma centre over a 10 year period: a critical review. *J Clin Neurosci.* 2007;14(7):618–623.

137. Gong MN, Zhou W, Williams PL, et al. -308GA and TNFB polymorphisms in acute respiratory distress syndrome. *Eur Respir J.* 2005;26(3):382–389.

138. Gonzalez RP, Cummings GR, Phelan HA, et al. Does increased emergency medical services prehospital time affect patient mortality in rural motor vehicle crashes? A statewide analysis. *Am J Surg.* 2009;197(1):30–34.

139. Gordon AC, Lagan AL, Aganna E, et al. TNF and TNFR polymorphisms in severe sepsis and septic shock: a prospective multicentre study. *Genes Immun.* 2004;5(8):631–640.

140. Gould SA, Moore EE, Hoyt DB, et al. The life-sustaining capacity of human polymerized hemoglobin when red cells might be unavailable. *J Am Coll Surg.* 2002;195(4):445–452.

141. Green SM, Steele R. Mandatory surgeon presence on trauma patient arrival. *Ann Emerg Med.* 2008;51(3):334–335.

142. Greenburg AG, Kim HW. Hemoglobin-based oxygen carriers. *Crit Care.* 2004;8(suppl 2):S61–S64.

143. Gregory RT, Gould RJ, Peclet M, et al. The mangled extremity syndrome (M.E.S.): a severity grading system for multisystem injury of the extremity. *J Trauma.* 1985;25(12):1147–1150.

144. Grieco A, Long CJ. Investigation of the Karnofsky Performance Status as a measure of quality of life. *Health Psychol.* 1984;3(2):129–142.

145. Grimm MR, Vrahas MS, Thomas KA. Pressure-volume characteristics of the intact and disrupted pelvic retroperitoneum. *J Trauma.* 1998;44(3):454–459.

146. Grotz M, Schwermann T, Lefering R, et al. [DRG reimbursement for multiple trauma patients—a comparison with the comprehensive hospital costs using the German trauma registry.] *Unfallchirurg.* 2004;107(1):68–75.

147. Grundnes O, Reikeras O. The importance of the hematoma for fracture healing in rats. *Acta Orthop Scand.* 1993;64:340–342.

148. Guillou PJ. Biological variation in the development of sepsis after surgery or trauma. *Lancet.* 1993;342(8865):217–220.

149. Gunn M, Campbell M, Hoffer EK. Traumatic abdominal aortic injury treated by endovascular stent placement. *Emerg Radiol.* 2007;13(6):329–331.

150. Gunter P. Practice guidelines for blood component therapy. *Anesthesiology.* 1996;85(5):1219–1220.

151. Gustilo RB, Mendoza RM, Williams DN. Problems in the management of type III (severe) open fractures: a new classification of type III open fractures. *J Trauma.* 1984;24(8):742–746.

152. Haan J, Scott J, Boyd-Kranis RL, et al. Admission angiography for blunt splenic injury: advantages and pitfalls. *J Trauma.* 2001;51(6):1161–1165.
153. Hagiwara A, Murata A, Matsuda T, et al. The efficacy and limitations of transarterial embolization for severe hepatic injury. *J Trauma.* 2002;52(6):1091–1096.
154. Hagiwara A, Murata A, Matsuda T, et al. The usefulness of transcatheter arterial embolization for patients with blunt polytrauma showing transient response to fluid resuscitation. *J Trauma.* 2004;57(2):271–276.
155. Hannan EL, Mendeloff J, Farrell LS, et al. Validation of TRISS and ASCOT using a non-MTOS trauma registry. *J Trauma.* 1995;38(1):83–88.
156. Hannan EL, Waller CH, Farrell LS, et al. A comparison among the abilities of various injury severity measures to predict mortality with and without accompanying physiologic information. *J Trauma.* 2005;58(2):244–251.
157. Hardy JF, de MP, Samama M. Massive transfusion and coagulopathy: pathophysiology and implications for clinical management. *Can J Anaesth.* 2004;51(4):293–310.
158. Harwood PJ, Giannoudis PV, Probst C, et al. Which AIS based scoring system is the best predictor of outcome in orthopaedic blunt trauma patients? *J Trauma.* 2006;60(2): 334–340.
159. Harwood PJ, Giannoudis PV, van GM, et al. Alterations in the systemic inflammatory response after early total care and damage control procedures for femoral shaft fracture in severely injured patients. *J Trauma.* 2005;58(3):446–452.
160. Hauswald M, Ong G, Tandberg D, et al. Out-of-hospital spinal immobilization: its effect on neurologic injury. *Acad Emerg Med.* 1998;5(3):214–219.
161. Hebert JS, Burnham RS. The effect of polytrauma in persons with traumatic spine injury. A prospective database of spine fractures. *Spine (Phila Pa 1976).* 2000;25(1): 55–60.
162. Heinzelmann M, Imhof HG, Trentz O. [Shock trauma room management of the multiple-traumatized patient with skull-brain injuries. A systematic review of the literature]. *Unfallchirurg.* 2004;107(10):871–880.
163. Helfet DL, Howey T, Sanders R, et al. Limb salvage versus amputation. Preliminary results of the Mangled Extremity Severity Score. *Clin Orthop Relat Res.* 1990;(256):80–86.
164. Helling TS, Watkins M, Robb CV. Improvement in cost recovery at an urban level I trauma center. *J Trauma.* 1995;39(5):980–983.
165. Hensler T, Heinemann B, Sauerland S, et al. Immunologic alterations associated with high blood transfusion volume after multiple injury: effects on plasmatic cytokine and cytokine receptor concentrations. *Shock.* 2003;20(6):497–502.
166. Herbert P, Wells G, Blajchmann M. A multicenter randomised controlled clinical trial of transfusion requirements in critical care. *N Engl J Med.* 1999;54(5):898–905.
167. Herzog C, Ahle H, Mack MG, et al. Traumatic injuries of the pelvis and thoracic and lumbar spine: does thin-slice multidetector-row CT increase diagnostic accuracy? *Eur Radiol.* 2004;14(10):1751–1760.
168. Hildebrand F, Pape HC, Krettek C. [The importance of cytokines in the posttraumatic inflammatory reaction]. *Unfallchirurg.* 2005;108(10):793–803.
169. Hildebrand F, van Griensven M, Garapati R, et al. Diagnostics and scoring in blunt chest trauma. *Eur J Trauma Emerg Surg.* 2002;28(3):157–167.
170. Hoff WS, Schwab CW. Trauma system development in North America. *Clin Orthop Relat Res.* 2004;5(422):17–22.
171. Holbrook TL, Anderson JP, Sieber WJ, et al. Outcome after major trauma: 12-month and 18-month follow-up results from the Trauma Recovery Project. *J Trauma.* 1999; 46(5):765–771.
172. Holbrook TL, Hoyt DB, Anderson JP. The importance of gender on outcome after major trauma: functional and psychologic outcomes in women versus men. *J Trauma.* 2001;50(2):270–273.
173. Holbrook TL, Hoyt DB, Stein MB, et al. Gender differences in long-term posttraumatic stress disorder outcomes after major trauma: women are at higher risk of adverse outcomes than men. *J Trauma.* 2002;53(5):882–888.
174. Holcomb JB, Niles SE, Miller CC, et al. Prehospital physiologic data and lifesaving interventions in trauma patients. *Mil Med.* 2005;170(1):7–13.
175. Holcomb JB, Salinas J, McManus JM, et al. Manual vital signs reliably predict need for life-saving interventions in trauma patients. *J Trauma.* 2005;59(4):821–828.
176. Holmes JH, Bloch RD, Hall RA, et al. Natural history of traumatic rupture of the thoracic aorta managed nonoperatively: a longitudinal analysis. *Ann Thorac Surg.* 2002;73(4):1149–1154.
177. Horne G, Schemitsch E. Assessment of the survivors of major trauma accidents. *Aust N Z J Surg.* 1989;59(6):465–470.
178. Hoth JJ, Scott MJ, Bullock TK, et al. Thoracotomy for blunt trauma: traditional indications may not apply. *Am Surg.* 2003;69(12):1108–1111.
179. Howe HR Jr, Poole GV Jr, Hansen KJ, et al. Salvage of lower extremities following combined orthopedic and vascular trauma. A predictive salvage index. *Am Surg.* 1987; 53(4):205–208.
180. Hoyt DB, Coimbra R. Trauma systems. *Surg Clin North Am.* 2007;87(1):21–35, v–vi.
181. Husum H, Strada G. Injury Severity Score versus New Injury Severity Score for penetrating injuries. *Prehosp Disaster Med.* 2002;17(1):27–32.
182. Iannelli G, Piscione F, Di TL, et al. Thoracic aortic emergencies: impact of endovascular surgery. *Ann Thorac Surg.* 2004;77(2):591–596.
183. Iba T, Gando S, Murata A, et al. Predicting the severity of systemic inflammatory response syndrome (SIRS)-associated coagulopathy with hemostatic molecular markers and vascular endothelial injury markers. *J Trauma.* 2007;63(5):1093–1098.
184. Ivarsson BJ, Crandall JR, Okamoto M. Influence of age-related stature on the frequency of body region injury and overall injury severity in child pedestrian casualties. *Traffic Inj Prev.* 2006;7(3):290–298.
185. Jameson S, Reed MR. Payment by results and coding practice in the National Health Service. The importance for orthopaedic surgeons. *J Bone Joint Surg Br.* 2007;89(11): 1427–1430.
186. Jennett B, Snoek J, Bond MR, et al. Disability after severe head injury: observations on the use of the Glasgow Outcome Scale. *J Neurol Neurosurg Psychiatry.* 1981;44(4):285–293.
187. Johansen K, Daines M, Howey T, et al. Objective criteria accurately predict amputation following lower extremity trauma. *J Trauma.* 1990;30(5):568–572.
188. Johnson KD, Cadambi A, Seibert GB. Incidence of adult respiratory distress syndrome in patients with multiple musculoskeletal injuries: effect of early operative stabilization of fractures. *J Trauma.* 1985;25(5):375–384.
189. Jones JH, Murphy MP, Dickson RL, et al. Emergency physician-verified out-of-hospital intubation: miss rates by paramedics. *Acad Emerg Med.* 2004;11(6):707–709.
190. Joshi V, Harding GE, Bottoni DA. Determination of functional outcome following upper extremity arterial trauma. *Vasc Endovascular Surg.* 2007;41:111–114.
191. Joy SA, Lichtig LK, Knauf RA, et al. Identification and categorization of and cost for care of trauma patients: a study of 12 trauma centers and 43,219 statewide patients. *J Trauma.* 1994;37(2):303–308.
192. Jurkovich G, Mock C, MacKenzie E, et al. The Sickness Impact Profile as a tool to evaluate functional outcome in trauma patients. *J Trauma.* 1995;39(4):625–631.
193. Jurkovich GJ, Mock C. Systematic review of trauma system effectiveness based on registry comparisons. *J Trauma.* 1999;47(suppl 3):S46–S55.
194. Kahlke V, Schafmayer C, Schniewind B, et al. Are postoperative complications genetically determined by TNF-beta NcoI gene polymorphism? *Surgery.* 2004;135(4):365–373.
195. Kallin K, Jensen J, Olsson LL, et al. Why the elderly fall in residential care facilities, and suggested remedies. *J Fam Pract.* 2004;53(1):41–52.
196. Kanakaris NK, Giannoudis PV. The health economics of the treatment of long-bone non-unions. *Injury.* 2007;38(suppl 2):S77–S84.
197. Kanz KG, Korner M, Linsenmaier U, et al. [Priority-oriented shock trauma room management with the integration of multiple-view spiral computed tomography]. *Unfallchirurg.* 2004;107(10):937–944.
198. Katsoulis E, Giannoudis PV. Impact of timing of pelvic fixation on functional outcome. *Injury.* 2006;37(12):1133–1142.
199. Keel M, Trentz O. Pathophysiology of polytrauma. *Injury.* 2005;36(6):691–709.
200. Kelsey JL, White AA III, Pastides H, et al. The impact of musculoskeletal disorders on the population of the United States. *J Bone Joint Surg Am.* 1979;61(7):959–964.
201. Kessel B, Sevi R, Jeroukhimov I, et al. Is routine portable pelvic X-ray in stable multiple trauma patients always justified in a high technology era? *Injury.* 2007;38(5):559–563.
202. Kim Y, Jung KY, Kim CY, et al. Validation of the International Classification of Diseases 10th Edition-based Injury Severity Score (ICISS). *J Trauma.* 2000;48(2):280–285.
203. Kinzl L, Gebhard F, Arand M. [Polytrauma and economics]. *Unfallchirurgie.* 1996; 22(4):179–185.
204. Kirkpatrick AW, Sirois M, Laupland KB, et al. Prospective evaluation of hand-held focused abdominal sonography for trauma (FAST) in blunt abdominal trauma. *Can J Surg.* 2005;48(6):453–460.
205. Kirkpatrick JR, Youmans RL. Trauma index. An aide in the evaluation of injury victims. *J Trauma.* 1971;11(8):711–714.
206. Kizer KW, Vassar MJ, Harry RL, et al. Hospitalization charges, costs, and income for firearm-related injuries at a university trauma center. *JAMA.* 1995;273(22):1768–1773.
207. Knaus WA, Zimmerman JE, Wagner DP, et al. APACHE-acute physiology and chronic health evaluation: a physiologically based classification system. *Crit Care Med.* 1981; 9(8):591–597.
208. Kolar P, Gaber T, Perka C, et al. Human early fracture hematoma is characterized by inflammation and hypoxia. *Clin Orthop Rel Res.* 2011;469:3118–3126.
209. Korner M, Krotz MM, Degenhart C, et al. Current Role of Emergency US in Patients with Major Trauma. *Radiographics.* 2008;28(1):225–242.
210. Korosec JH, Jagodic K, Podbregar M. Long-term outcome and quality of life of patients treated in surgical intensive care: a comparison between sepsis and trauma. *Crit Care.* 2006;10(5):R134.
211. Krettek C, Schandelmaier P, Rudolf J, et al. [Current status of surgical technique for unreamed nailing of tibial shaft fractures with the UTN (unreamed tibia nail)]. *Unfallchirurg.* 1994;97(11):575–599.
212. Kristinsson G, Wall SP, Crain EF. The digital rectal examination in pediatric trauma: a pilot study. *J Emerg Med.* 2007;32(1):59–62.
213. Krueger PD, Brazil K, Lohfeld LH. Risk factors for falls and injuries in a long-term care facility in Ontario. *Can J Public Health.* 2001;92(2):117–120.
214. Kuhls DA, Malone DL, McCarter RJ, et al. Predictors of mortality in adult trauma patients: the physiologic trauma score is equivalent to the Trauma and Injury Severity Score. *J Am Coll Surg.* 2002;194(6):695–704.
215. Kuhne CA, Ruchholtz S, Kaiser GM, et al. Mortality in severely injured elderly trauma patients—when does age become a risk factor? *World J Surg.* 2005;29:1476–1482.
216. Kuhne CA, Ruchholtz S, Sauerland S, et al. [Personnel and structural requirements for the shock trauma room management of multiple trauma. A systematic review of the literature]. *Unfallchirurg.* 2004;107(10):851–861.
217. Kwok PC, Ho KK, Chung TK, et al. Emergency aortic stent grafting for traumatic rupture of the thoracic aorta. *Hong Kong Med J.* 2003;9(6):435–440.
218. Langanay T, Verhoye JP, Corbineau H, et al. Surgical treatment of acute traumatic rupture of the thoracic aorta a timing reappraisal? *Eur J Cardiothorac Surg.* 2002;21(2):282–287.
219. Lausevic Z, Lausevic M, Trbojevic-Stankovic J, et al. Predicting multiple organ failure in patients with severe trauma. *Can J Surg.* 2008;51(2):97–102.
220. Lefering R, DGU. Trauma Register DGU: Jahresbericht 2011. 2011.
221. Lefering R, Paffrath T. [Reality of care based on the data from the Trauma Registry of the German Society of Trauma Surgery]. *Unfallchirurg.* 2012;115(1):30–32.
222. Lehmann U, Gobiet W, Regel G, et al. [Functional, neuropsychological and social outcome of polytrauma patients with severe craniocerebral trauma]. *Unfallchirurg.* 1997;100(7):552–560.
223. Leone M, Boutiere B, Camoin-Jau L, et al. Systemic endothelial activation is greater in septic than in traumatic-hemorrhagic shock but does not correlate with endothelial activation in skin biopsies. *Crit Care Med.* 2002;30(4):808–814.
224. Liberman M, Branas C, Mulder DS. Advanced versus basic life support in the prehospital setting—the controversy between the scoop and run and the stay and play approach to the care of the injured patient. *Int J Disaster Med.* 2004;2:1–9.
225. Liberman M, Mulder D, Lavoie A, et al. Multicenter Canadian study of prehospital trauma care. *Ann Surg.* 2003;237(2):153–160.

226. Liberman M, Mulder DS, Jurkovich GJ, et al. The association between trauma system and trauma center components and outcome in a mature regionalized trauma system. *Surgery.* 2005;137(6):647–658.
227. Liberman M, Mulder DS, Lavoie A, et al. Implementation of a trauma care system: evolution through evaluation. *J Trauma.* 2004;56(6):1330–1335.
228. Lin E, Calvano SE, Lowry SF. Inflammatory cytokines and cell response in surgery. *Surgery.* 2000;127(2):117–126.
229. Lin WC, Chen YF, Lin CH, et al. Emergent transcatheter arterial embolization in hemodynamically unstable patients with blunt splenic injury. *Acad Radiol.* 2008;15(2):201–208.
230. Lindner T, Bail HJ, Manegold S, et al. [Shock trauma room diagnosis: initial diagnosis after blunt abdominal trauma. A review of the literature]. *Unfallchirurg.* 2004;107(10):892–902.
231. Liu BC, Ivers R, Norton R, et al. Helmets for preventing injury in motorcycle riders. *Cochrane Database Syst Rev.* 2008;(1):CD004333.
232. Lowe PR, Galley HF, Abdel-Fattah A, et al. Influence of interleukin-10 polymorphisms on interleukin-10 expression and survival in critically ill patients. *Crit Care Med.* 2003;31(1):34–38.
233. MacKenzie EJ, Bosse MJ, Pollak AN, et al. Long-term persistence of disability following severe lower-limb trauma. Results of a seven-year follow-up. *J Bone Joint Surg Am.* 2005;87(8):1801–1809.
234. MacKenzie EJ, Bosse MJ. Factors influencing outcome following limb-threatening lower limb trauma: Lessons learned from the Lower Extremity Assessment Project (LEAP). *J Am Acad Orthop Surg.* 2006;14:S205–S210.
235. MacKenzie EJ, Morris JA, Jurkovich GJ, et al. Return to work following injury: the role of economic, social, and job-related factors. *Am J Public Health.* 1998;88:1630–1637.
236. MacKenzie EJ, Rivara FP, Jurkovich GJ, et al. A national evaluation of the effect of trauma-center care on mortality. *N Engl J Med.* 2006;354(4):366–378.
237. MacKenzie EJ, Shapiro S, Moody M, et al. Predicting posttrauma functional disability for individuals without severe brain injury. *Med Care.* 1986;24(5):377–387.
238. MacKenzie EJ, Steinwachs DM, Shankar B. Classifying trauma severity based on hospital discharge diagnoses. Validation of an ICD-9CM to AIS-85 conversion table. *Med Care.* 1989;27(4):412–422.
239. MacKenzie EJ. Review of evidence regarding trauma system effectiveness resulting from panel studies. *J Trauma.* 1999;47(suppl 3):S34–S41.
240. Mackersie RC, Tiwary AD, Shackford SR, et al. Intra-abdominal injury following blunt trauma. Identifying the high-risk patient using objective risk factors. *Arch Surg.* 1989;124(7):809–813.
241. Maimaris C, Brooks SC. Monitoring progress in major trauma care using TRISS. *Arch Emerg Med.* 1990;7(3):169–171.
242. Malone DL, Dunne J, Tracy JK, et al. Blood transfusion, independent of shock severity, is associated with worse outcome in trauma. *J Trauma.* 2003;54(5):898–905.
243. Malone DL, Kuhls D, Napolitano LM, et al. Back to basics: validation of the admission systemic inflammatory response syndrome score in predicting outcome in trauma. *J Trauma.* 2001;51(3):458–463.
244. Manley GT, Hemphill JC, Morabito D, et al. Cerebral oxygenation during hemorrhagic shock: perils of hyperventilation and the therapeutic potential of hypoventilation. *J Trauma.* 2000;48(6):1025–1032.
245. Mann NC, Mullins RJ, MacKenzie EJ, et al. Systematic review of published evidence regarding trauma system effectiveness. *J Trauma.* 1999;47(suppl 3):S25–S33.
246. Markle J, Cayten CG, Byrne DW, et al. Comparison between TRISS and ASCOT methods in controlling for injury severity. *J Trauma.* 1992;33(2):326–332.
247. Markovchick VJ, Moore EE. Optimal trauma outcome: trauma system design and the trauma team. *Emerg Med Clin North Am.* 2007;25(3):643–654.
248. Martinowitz U, Holcomb JB, Pusateri AE, et al. Intravenous rFVIIa administered for hemorrhage control in hypothermic coagulopathic swine with grade V liver injuries. *J Trauma.* 2001;50(4):721–729.
249. Matsuda N, Hattori Y. Systemic inflammatory response syndrome (SIRS): molecular pathophysiology and gene therapy. *J Pharmacol Sci.* 2006;101(3):189–198.
250. McLain RF. Functional outcomes after surgery for spinal fractures: return to work and activity. *Spine (Phila Pa 1976).* 2004;29(4):470–477.
251. McMahon D, Schwab CW, Kauder DR. Comorbidity and the elderly trauma patient. *World J Surg.* 1996;20:1113–1120.
252. McNamara MG, Heckman JD, Corley FG. Severe open fractures of the lower extremity: a retrospective evaluation of the Mangled Extremity Severity Score (MESS). *J Orthop Trauma.* 1994;8(2):81–87.
253. Meade MO, Cook DJ, Guyatt GH, et al. Ventilation strategy using low tidal volumes, recruitment maneuvers, and high positive end-expiratory pressure for acute lung injury and acute respiratory distress syndrome: a randomized controlled trial. *JAMA.* 2008;299(6):637–645.
254. Meerding WJ, Bonneux L, Polder JJ, et al. Demographic and epidemiological determinants of healthcare costs in Netherlands: costs of illness study. *BMJ.* 1998;317(7151):111–115.
255. Meerding WJ, Mulder S, van Beek EF. Incedence and costs of injures in the Netherlands. *Eur J Publ Health.* 2006;16(3):271–277.
256. Meisner M, Adina H, Schmidt J. Correlation of procalcitonin and C-reactive protein to inflammation, complications, and outcome during the intensive care unit course of multiple-trauma patients. *Crit Care.* 2005;10(1):R1.
257. Melton SM, McGwin G Jr, Abernathy JH III, et al. Motor vehicle crash-related mortality is associated with prehospital and hospital-based resource availability. *J Trauma.* 2003;54(2):273–279.
258. Meredith JW, Evans G, Kilgo PD, et al. A comparison of the abilities of nine scoring algorithms in predicting mortality. *J Trauma.* 2002;53(4):621–628.
259. Meregalli A, Oliveira RP, Friedman G. Occult hypoperfusion is associated with increased mortality in hemodynamically stable, high-risk, surgical patients. *Crit Care.* 2004;8(2):R60–R65.
260. Michaels AJ, Michaels CE, Moon CH, et al. Psychosocial factors limit outcomes after trauma. *J Trauma.* 1998;44(4):644–648.
261. Miller TR, Levy DT. The effect of regional trauma care systems on costs. *Arch Surg.* 1995;130(2):188–193.
262. Miltner E, Wiedmann HP, Leutwein B, et al. Technical parameters influencing the severity of injury of front-seat, belt-protected car passengers on the impact side in car-to-car side collisions with the main impact between the front and rear seats (B-pillars). *Int J Legal Med.* 1992;105(1):11–15.
263. Miranda DR, Gommers D, Papadakos PJ, et al. Mechanical ventilation affects pulmonary inflammation in cardiac surgery patients: the role of the open-lung concept. *J Cardiothorac Vasc Anesth.* 2007;21(2):279–284.
264. Mizuno K, Mineo K, Tachibana T, et al. The osteogenetic potential of fracture haematoma. Subperiosteal and intramuscular transplantation of the haematoma. *J Bone Joint Surg Br.* 1990;72(5):822–829.
265. Mkandawire NC, Boot DA, Braithwaite IJ, et al. Musculoskeletal recovery 5 years after severe injury: long term problems are common. *Injury.* 2002;33:111–115.
266. Mohr AM, Lavery RF, Barone A, et al. Angiographic embolization for liver injuries: low mortality, high morbidity. *J Trauma.* 2003;55(6):1077–1081.
267. Moore EE. Hypertonic saline dextran for post-injury resuscitation: experimental background and clinical experience. *Aust N Z J Surg.* 1991;61(10):732–736.
268. Moore FA, McKinley BA, Moore EE. The next generation in shock resuscitation. *Lancet.* 2004;363(9425):1988–1996.
269. Moore L, Lavoie A, Bergeron E, et al. Modeling probability-based injury severity scores in logistic regression models: the logit transformation should be used. *J Trauma.* 2007;62(3):601–605.
270. Moore L, Lavoie A, Le SN, et al. Consensus or data-derived anatomic injury severity scoring? *J Trauma.* 2008;64(2):420–426.
271. Moore L, Lavoie A, LeSage N, et al. Statistical validation of the Revised Trauma Score. *J Trauma.* 2006;60(2):305–311.
272. Morris J, McKenzie E, Damiano A. Mortality in trauma patients: the interaction between host factor and severity. *J Trauma.* 1990;30:1476–1482.
273. Mueller M, Allgower M, Schneider R, et al. *Manual of Osteosynthesis.* Heidelberg, New York, NY: Springer-Verlag; 1970.
274. Mulligan ME, Flye CW. Initial experience with Lodox Statscan imaging system for detecting injuries of the pelvis and appendicular skeleton. *Emerg Radiol.* 2006;13(3):129–133.
275. Mullins RJ, Mann NC. Population-based research assessing the effectiveness of trauma systems. *J Trauma.* 1999;47(suppl 3):S59–S66.
276. Mullins RJ. A historical perspective of trauma system development in the United States. *J Trauma.* 1999;47(suppl 3):S8–S14.
277. Myers J. Focused assessment with sonography for trauma (FAST): the truth about ultrasound in blunt trauma. *J Trauma.* 2007;62(suppl 6):S28.
278. Nast-Kolb D, Ruchholtz S, Waydhas C, et al. [Is maximum management of polytrauma patients financially assured?]. *Langenbecks Arch Chir Suppl Kongressbd.* 1996;113:323–325.
279. Nathens AB, Brunet FP, Maier RV. Development of trauma systems and effect on outcomes after injury. *Lancet.* 2004;363(9423):1794–1801.
280. Nathens AB, Jurkovich GJ, Cummings P, et al. The effect of organized systems of trauma care on motor vehicle crash mortality. *JAMA.* 2000;283(15):1990–1994.
281. Nathens AB, Jurkovich GJ, Rivara FP, et al. Effectiveness of state trauma systems in reducing injury-related mortality: a national evaluation. *J Trauma.* 2000;48(1):25–30.
282. Neher M, Weckbach S, Flierl M, et al. Molecular mechanisms of inflammation and tissue injury after major trauma—is complement the "bad guy"? *J Biomed Science.* 2011;18(90):1–16.
283. Neuffer MC, McDivitt J, Rose D, et al. Hemostatic dressings for the first responder: a review. *Mil Med.* 2004;169(9):716–720.
284. Neumaier M, Scherer MA. C-reactive protein levels for early detection of postoperative infection after fracture surgery in 787 patients. *Acta Orthop.* 2008;79(3):428–432.
285. (NHTSA), U. D. o. T. N. H. T. S. A.: Research note. National occupant protection use survey, 1996-controlled intersection study. Washington DC: 1997.
286. (NHTSA), U. D. o. T. N. H. T. S. A.: Traffic Safety Facts. Seat Belt Use in 2007—Use Rates in the States And Territories. Washington, DC: 2008.
287. nh-Zarr TB, Sleet DA, Shults RA, et al. Reviews of evidence regarding interventions to increase the use of safety belts. *Am J Prev Med.* 2001;21(suppl 4):48–65.
288. Nowotarski PJ, Turen CH, Brumback RJ, et al. Conversion of external fixation to intramedullary nailing for fractures of the shaft of the femur in multiply injured patients. *J Bone Joint Surg Am.* 2000;82(6):781–788.
289. Nural MS, Yardan T, Guven H, et al. Diagnostic value of ultrasonography in the evaluation of blunt abdominal trauma. *Diagn Interv Radiol.* 2005;11(1):41–44.
290. O'Donnell ML, Creamer M, Elliott P, et al. Health costs following motor vehicle accidents: The role of posttraumatic stress disorder. *J Trauma Stress.* 2005;18(5):557–561.
291. O'Kelly TJ, Westaby S. Trauma centres and the efficient use of financial resources. *Br J Surg.* 1990;77(10):1142–1144.
292. O'Toole RV, Castillo RC, Pollak AN, et al. Determinants of patient satisfaction after severe lower-extremity injuries. *J Bone Joint Surg Am.* 2008;90:1206–1211.
293. Obaid AK, Barleben A, Porral D, et al. Utility of plain film pelvic radiographs in blunt trauma patients in the emergency department. *Am Surg.* 2006;72(10):951–954.
294. Obertacke U, Neudeck F, Wihs HJ, et al. [Emergency care and treatment costs of polytrauma patients]. *Langenbecks Arch Chir Suppl Kongressbd.* 1996;113:641–645.
295. Oestern HJ, Schwermann T. [Quality and economy—contradictory demands]. *Kongressbd Dtsch Ges Chir Kongr.* 2002;119:937–940.
296. Oestern HJ, Tscherne H. *Pathophysiology and Classification of Soft Tissue Injuries Associated with Fractures.* Berlin: Spinger-Verlag; 1984.
297. Oestern HJ. [Management of polytrauma patients in an international comparison]. *Unfallchirurg.* 1999;102(2):80–91.
298. Offner PJ, Jurkovich GJ, Gurney J, et al. Revision of TRISS for intubated patients. *J Trauma.* 1992;32(1):32–35.
299. Oppe S, De Charro FT. The effect of medical care by a helicopter trauma team on the probability of survival and the quality of life of hospitalised victims. *Accid Anal Prev.* 2001;33(1):129–138.

300. Oppenheim JJ, Yang D. Alarmins: chemotactic activators of immune responses. *Curr Opin Immunol.* 2005;17(4):359–365.
301. Osler T, Baker SP, Long W. A modification of the injury severity score that both improves accuracy and simplifies scoring. *J Trauma.* 1997;43(6):922–925.
302. Osterwalder JJ, Riederer M. [Quality assessment of multiple trauma management bu ISS, TRISS or ASCOT?]. *Schweiz Med Wochenschr.* 2000;130(14):499–504.
303. Osterwalder JJ. Can the "golden hour of shock" safely be extended in blunt polytrauma patients? Prospective cohort study at a level I hospital in eastern Switzerland. *Prehosp Disaster Med.* 2002;17(2):75–80.
304. Osterwalder JJ. Mortality of blunt polytrauma: a comparison between emergency physicians and emergency medical technicians—prospective cohort study at a level I hospital in eastern Switzerland. *J Trauma.* 2003;55(2):355–361.
305. Ott R, Holzer U, Spitzenpfeil E, et al. [Quality of life after survival of severe trauma]. *Unfallchirurg.* 1996;99(4):267–274.
306. Padayachee L, Cooper DJ, Irons S, et al. Cervical spine clearance in unconscious traumatic brain injury patients: dynamic flexion-extension fluoroscopy versus computed tomography with three-dimensional reconstruction. *J Trauma.* 2006;60(2):341–345.
307. Papadopoulos IN, Kanakaris N, Triantafillidis A, et al. Autopsy findings from 111 deaths in the 1999 Athens earthquake as a basis for auditing the emergency response. *Br J Surg.* 2004;91(12):1633–1640.
308. Papakostidis C, Kanakaris NK, Kontakis G, et al. Pelvic ring disruptions: treatment modalities and analysis of outcomes. *Int Orthop.* 2009;33(2):329–338.
309. Pape H, Stalp M, Griensven M, et al. [Optimal timing for secondary surgery in polytrauma patients: an evaluation of 4,314 serious-injury cases]. *Chirurg.* 1999; 70(11):1287–1293.
310. Pape HC, Giannoudis P, Krettek C. The timing of fracture treatment in polytrauma patients: relevance of damage control orthopedic surgery. *Am J Surg.* 2002;183(6):622–629.
311. Pape HC, Giannoudis PV, Krettek C, et al. Timing of fixation of major fractures in blunt polytrauma: role of conventional indicators in clinical decision making. *J Orthop Trauma.* 2005;19(8):551–562.
312. Pape HC, Grimme K, van GM, et al. Impact of intramedullary instrumentation versus damage control for femoral fractures on immunoinflammatory parameters: prospective randomized analysis by the EPOFF Study Group. *J Trauma.* 2003;55(1):7–13.
313. Pape HC, Rixen D, Morley J, et al. Impact of the method of initial stabilization for femoral shaft fractures in patients with multiple injuries at risk for complications (borderline patients). *Ann Surg.* 2007;246(3):491–499.
314. Pape HC, Sanders R, Borrelli J. *The Poly-Traumatized Patient with Fractures - A Multi-Disciplinary Approach.* Heidelberg, New York, NY: Springer, 2011.
315. Pape HC, van GM, Rice J, et al. Major secondary surgery in blunt trauma patients and perioperative cytokine liberation: determination of the clinical relevance of biochemical markers. *J Trauma.* 2001;50(6):989–1000.
316. Pape HC, Zelle B, Lohse R, et al. Evaluation and outcome of patients after polytrauma—can patients be recruited for long-term follow-up? *Injury.* 2006;37(12):1197–1203.
317. Park S, Silva M, Bahk W, et al. Effect of repeated irrigation and debridement on fracture healing in an animal model. *J Orthop Res.* 2002;20:1197–1204.
318. Paulozzi LJ. United States pedestrian fatality rates by vehicle type. *Inj Prev.* 2005;11(4):232–236.
319. Pfeifer R, Zelle B, Kobbe P, et al. Impact of isolated acetablar and lower extremity fractures on long-term outcome. *J Trauma Acute Care Surg.* 2012;72(2):467–472.
320. Physicians ACoE. Guidelines for trauma care systems. *Ann Emerg Med.* 1987;16:459–463.
321. Physicians ACoE. Trauma care systems development, evaluation, and funding. *Ann Emerg Med Clin North Am.* 1999;34:308.
322. Pitton MB, Herber S, Schmiedt W, et al. Long-term follow-up after endovascular treatment of acute aortic emergencies. *Cardiovasc Intervent Radiol.* 2008;31(1):23–35.
323. Plotz FB, Slutsky AS, van Vught AJ, et al. Ventilator-induced lung injury and multiple system organ failure: a critical review of facts and hypotheses. *Intensive Care Med.* 2004;30(10):1865–1872.
324. Pohlemann T, Bosch U, Gansslen A, et al. The Hannover experience in management of pelvic fractures. *Clin Orthop Relat Res.* 1994;(305):69–80.
325. Pohlemann T, Gansslen A, Schellwald O, et al. [Outcome evaluation after unstable injuries of the pelvic ring]. *Unfallchirurg.* 1996;99(4):249–259.
326. Pohlemann T, Tscherne H, Baumgartel F, et al. [Pelvic fractures: epidemiology, therapy and long-term outcome. Overview of the multicenter study of the Pelvis Study Group]. *Unfallchirurg.* 1996;99(3):160–167.
327. Polinder S, Meerding WJ, van Baar ME, et al. Cost estimation of injury-related hospital admissions in 10 European countries. *J Trauma.* 2005;59(6):1283–1291; discussion 1290–1291.
328. Probst C, Hildebrand F, Frink M, et al. [Prehospital treatment of severely injured patients in the field: an update]. *Chirurg.* 2007;78(10):875–884.
329. Prokop A, Hotte H, Kruger K, et al. [Multislice CT in diagnostic work-up of polytrauma]. *Unfallchirurg.* 2006;109(7):545–550.
330. Puleo D. Biotherapeutics in orthopaedic medicine: accelerating the healing process? *Bio Drugs.* 2003;17(5):301–314.
331. Rainer TH, Cheung NK, Yeung JH, et al. Do trauma teams make a difference? A single centre registry study. *Resuscitation.* 2007;73(3):374–381.
332. Redl H, Schlag G, Hammerschmidt DE. Quantitative assessment of leukostasis in experimental hypovolemic-traumatic shock. *Acta Chir Scand.* 1984;150(2):113–117.
333. Regel G, Bayeff-Filloff M. [Diagnosis and immediate therapeutic management of limb injuries. A systematic review of the literature]. *Unfallchirurg.* 2004;107(10):919–926.
334. Reid CL, Perrey C, Pravica V, et al. Genetic variation in proinflammatory and anti-inflammatory cytokine production in multiple organ dysfunction syndrome. *Crit Care Med.* 2002;30(10):2216–2221.
335. Rice PL Jr, Rudolph M. Pelvic fractures. *Emerg Med Clin North Am.* 2007;25(3):795–802.
336. Richter ED, Berman T, Friedman L, et al. Speed, road injury, and public health. *Annu Rev Public Health.* 2006;27:125–152.

337. Richter M, Pape HC, Otte D, et al. Improvements in passive car safety led to decreased injury severity–a comparison between the 1970s and 1990s. *Injury.* 2005;36(4):484–488.
338. Ringburg AN, Spanjersberg WR, Frankema SP, et al. Helicopter emergency medical services (HEMS): impact on on-scene times. *J Trauma.* 2007;63(2):258–262.
339. Riska EB, von BH, Hakkinen S, et al. Primary operative fixation of long bone fractures in patients with multiple injuries. *J Trauma.* 1977;17(2):111–121.
340. Rivara FP, Thompson DC, Cummings P. Effectiveness of primary and secondary enforced seat belt laws. *Am J Prev Med.* 1999;16(suppl 1):30–39.
341. Rivers EP, Nguyen HB, Huang DT, et al. Early goal-directed therapy. *Crit Care Med.* 2004;32(1):314–315.
342. Rivers EP. Early goal-directed therapy in severe sepsis and septic shock: converting science to reality. *Chest.* 2006;129(2):217–218.
343. Rixen D, Siegel JH, Friedman HP. "Sepsis/SIRS," physiologic classification, severity stratification, relation to cytokine elaboration and outcome prediction in posttrauma critical illness. *J Trauma.* 1996;41(4):581–598.
344. Rizoli SB. Crystalloids and colloids in trauma resuscitation: a brief overview of the current debate. *J Trauma.* 2003;54(suppl 5):S82–S88.
345. Roberts CS, Pape HC, Jones AL, et al. Damage control orthopaedics: evolving concepts in the treatment of patients who have sustained orthopaedic trauma. *Instr Course Lect.* 2005;54:447–462.
346. Rockswold GL, Leonard PR, Nagib MG. Analysis of management in thirty-three closed head injury patients who "talked and deteriorated". *Neurosurgery.* 1987;21(1):51–55.
347. Rodenberg H. Effect of aeromedical aircraft on care of trauma patients: evaluation using the Revised Trauma Score. *South Med J.* 1992;85(11):1065–1071.
348. Rogers FB, Osler TM, Shackford SR, et al. Financial outcome of treating trauma in a rural environment. *J Trauma.* 1997;43(1):65–72.
349. Roudsari BS, Nathens AB, Cameron P, et al. International comparison of prehospital trauma care systems. *Injury.* 2007;38(9):993–1000.
350. Rozycki GS, Feliciano DV, Schmidt JA, et al. The role of surgeon-performed ultrasound in patients with possible cardiac wounds. *Ann Surg.* 1996;223(6):737–744.
351. Rozycki GS. Surgeon-performed ultrasound: its use in clinical practice. *Ann Surg.* 1998;228(1):16–28.
352. Ruchholtz S, Lefering R, Paffrath T, et al. Reduction in mortality of severely injured patients in Germany. *Dtsch Arztebl Int.* 2008;105(13):225–231.
353. Ruchholtz S, Nast-Kolb D, Waydhas C, et al. [Cost analysis of clinical treatment of polytrauma patients]. *Chirurg.* 1995;66(7):684–692.
354. Rutledge R, Osler T, Emery S, et al. The end of the Injury Severity Score (ISS) and the Trauma and Injury Severity Score (TRISS): ICISS, an International Classification of Diseases, ninth revision-based prediction tool, outperforms both ISS and TRISS as predictors of trauma patient survival, hospital charges, and hospital length of stay. *J Trauma.* 1998;44(1):41–49.
355. Sacco WJ, MacKenzie EJ, Champion HR, et al. Comparison of alternative methods for assessing injury severity based on anatomic descriptors. *J Trauma.* 1999;47(3):441–446.
356. Sadri H, Nguyen-Tang T, Stern R, et al. Control of severe hemorrhage using C-clamp and arterial embolization in hemodynamically unstable patients with pelvic ring disruption. *Arch Orthop Trauma Surg.* 2005;125(7):443–447.
357. Sam A, Kibbe M, Matsumura J, et al. Blunt traumatic aortic transection: endoluminal repair with commercially available aortic cuffs. *J Vasc Surg.* 2003;38(5):1132–1135.
358. Sanson G, Di BS, Nardi G, et al. Road traffic accidents with vehicular entrapment: incidence of major injuries and need for advanced life support. *Eur J Emerg Med.* 1999;6(4):285–291.
359. Sayer NA, Chiros CE, Sigford B, et al. Characteristics and rehabilitation outcomes among patients with blast and other injuries sustained during the Global War on Terror. *Arch Phys Med Rehabil.* 2008;89(1):163–170.
360. Scalea T, Rodriguez A, Chiu W, et al. Focused Assessment with Sonography for Trauma (FAST): results from an international consensus conference. *J Trauma.* 1999;46(3):466–472.
361. Scalea TM, Boswell SA, Scott JD, et al. External fixation as a bridge to intramedullary nailing for patients with multiple injuries and with femur fractures: damage control orthopedics. *J Trauma.* 2000;48(4):613–621.
362. Schierhout G, Roberts I. Fluid resuscitation with colloid or crystalloid solutions in critically ill patients: a systematic review of randomised trials. *BMJ.* 1998;316(7136):961–964.
363. Schmelz A, Ziegler D, Beck A, et al. [Costs for acute, stationary treatment of polytrauma patients]. *Unfallchirurg.* 2002;105(11):1043–1048.
364. Schmidt-Bleek K, Schell H, Kolar P, et al. Cellular composition of the initial fracture hematoma compared to a muscle hematoma: a study in sheep. *J Orthop Res.* 2009; 27(9):1147–1151.
365. Schoder M, Prokop M, Lammer J. Traumatic injuries: imaging and intervention of large arterial trauma. *Eur Radiol.* 2002;12(7):1617–1631.
366. Schonholz CJ, Uflacker R, De Gregorio MA, et al. Stent-graft treatment of trauma to the supra-aortic arteries. A review. *J Cardiovasc Surg (Torino).* 2007;48(5):537–549.
367. Schreiber MA, Holcomb JB, Hedner U, et al. The effect of recombinant factor VIIa on coagulopathic pigs with grade V liver injuries. *J Trauma.* 2002;53(2):252–257.
368. Schreiber V, Tarkin HI, Hildebrand F, et al. The timing of definitive fixation for major fractures in polytrauma—a matched pair comparison between a US and European level I centers: analysis of current fracture management practice in polytrauma. *Injury.* 2011;42(7):650–654.
369. Schroder O, Laun RA, Held B, et al. Association of interleukin-10 promoter polymorphism with the incidence of multiple organ dysfunction following major trauma: results of a prospective pilot study. *Shock.* 2004;21(4):306–310.
370. Sclafani SJ, Weisberg A, Scalea TM, et al. Blunt splenic injuries: nonsurgical treatment with CT, arteriography, and transcatheter arterial embolization of the splenic artery. *Radiology.* 1991;181(1):189–196.
371. Sears BW, Luchette FA, Esposito TJ, et al. Old fashion clinical judgment in the era of protocols: is mandatory chest X-ray necessary in injured patients? *J Trauma.* 2005;59(2):324–330.

372. Seekamp A, Regel G, Bauch S, et al. [Long-term results of therapy of polytrauma patients with special reference to serial fractures of the lower extremity]. *Unfallchirurg.* 1994; 97(2):57–63.

373. Self ML, Blake AM, Whitley M, et al. The benefit of routine thoracic, abdominal, and pelvic computed tomography to evaluate trauma patients with closed head injuries. *Am J Surg.* 2003;186(6):609–613.

374. Selye H. The general adaptation syndrome and the diseases of adaptation. *Am J Med.* 1951;10:549–555.

375. Sethi D, Kwan I, Kelly AM, et al. Advanced trauma life support training for ambulance crews. *Cochrane Database Syst Rev.* 2001;(2):CD003109.

376. Shackford SR. Effect of small-volume resuscitation on intracranial pressure and related cerebral variables. *J Trauma.* 1997;42(suppl 5):S48–S53.

377. Shafi S, Nathens AB, Elliott AC, et al. Effect of trauma systems on motor vehicle occupant mortality: A comparison between states with and without a formal system. *J Trauma.* 2006;61(6):1374–1378.

378. Shapiro MB, Jenkins DH, Schwab CW, et al. Damage control: collective review. *J Trauma.* 2000;49(5):969–978.

379. Shults RA, Elder RW, Sleet DA, et al. Primary enforcement seat belt laws are effective even in the face of rising belt use rates. *Accid Anal Prev.* 2004;36(3):491–493.

380. Shults RA, Nichols JL, nh-Zarr TB, et al. Effectiveness of primary enforcement safety belt laws and enhanced enforcement of safety belt laws: a summary of the Guide to Community Preventive Services systematic reviews. *J Safety Res.* 2004;35(2):189–196.

381. Siebers C, Stegmaier J, Kirchhoff C, et al. [Analysis of failure modes in multislice computed tomography during primary trauma survey]. *Rofo.* 2008;180(8):733–739.

382. Siegel JH, Mason-Gonzalez S, Dischinger PC, et al. Causes and costs of injuries in multiple trauma patients requiring extrication from motor vehicle crashes. *J Trauma.* 1993;35(6):920–931.

383. Sikand M, Williams K, White C, et al. The financial cost of treating polytrauma: implications for tertiary referral centres in the United Kingdom. *Injury.* 2005;36(6):733–737.

384. Smith GJ, Kramer GC, Perron P, et al. A comparison of several hypertonic solutions for resuscitation of bled sheep. *J Surg Res.* 1985;39(6):517–528.

385. Smith HE, Biffl WL, Majercik SD, et al. Splenic artery embolization: Have we gone too far? *J Trauma.* 2006;61(3):541–544.

386. Smith RM, Giannoudis PV. Trauma and the immune response. *J R Soc Med.* 1998; 91(8):417–420.

387. Soldati G, Testa A, Sher S, et al. Occult traumatic pneumothorax: diagnostic accuracy of lung ultrasonography in the emergency department. *Chest.* 2008;133(1):204–211.

388. Southard PA. Trauma economics: realities and strategies. *Crit Care Nurs Clin North Am.* 1994;6(3):435–440.

389. Spence MT, Redmond AD, Edwards JD. Trauma audit—the use of TRISS. *Health Trends.* 1988;20(3):94–97.

390. Sriussadaporn S, Luengtaviboon K, Benjacholamas V, et al. Significance of a widened mediastinum in blunt chest trauma patients. *J Med Assoc Thai.* 2000;83(11):1296–1301.

391. Stafford RE, Linn J, Washington L. Incidence and management of occult hemothoraces. *Am J Surg.* 2006;192(6):722–726.

392. Stalp M, Koch C, Regel G, et al. [Development of a standardized instrument for quantitative and reproducible rehabilitation data assessment after polytrauma (HASPOC)]. *Chirurg.* 2001;72(3):312–318.

393. Stalp M, Koch C, Ruchholtz S, et al. Standardized outcome evaluation after blunt multiple injuries by scoring systems: a clinical follow-up investigation 2 years after injury. *J Trauma.* 2002;52(6):1160–1168.

394. Stein DJ, Seedat S, Iversen A, et al. Post-traumatic stress disorder: medicine and politics. *Lancet.* 2007;369(9556):139–144.

395. Stein DM, O'Toole R, Scalea TM. Multidisciplinary approach for patients with pelvic fractures and hemodynamic instability. *Scand J Surg.* 2007;96(4):272–280.

396. Stephenson SC, Langley JD, Civil ID. Comparing measures of injury severity for use with large databases. *J Trauma.* 2002;53(2):326–332.

397. Strecker W, Gebhard F, Perl M, et al. Biochemical characterization of individual injury pattern and injury severity. *Injury.* 2003;34(12):879–887.

398. Sturm JA. [Polytrauma and the hospital structure]. *Langenbecks Arch Chir Suppl Kongressbd.* 1997;114:123–129.

399. Sudkamp N, Haas N, Flory PJ, et al. [Criteria for amputation, reconstruction and replantation of extremities in multiple trauma patients]. *Chirurg.* 1989;60(11):774–781.

400. Suzuki T, Shindo M, Soma K, et al. Long-term functional outcome after unstable pelvic ring fracture. *J Trauma.* 2007;63(4):884–888.

401. Symbas PN, Sherman AJ, Silver JM, et al. Traumatic rupture of the aorta: immediate or delayed repair? *Ann Surg.* 2002;235(6):796–802.

402. Taheri PA, Butz DA, Lottenberg L, et al. The cost of trauma center readiness. *Am J Surg.* 2004;187(1):7–13.

403. Task Force on Principles for Economic Analysis of Health Care Technology. Economic analysis of health care technology. A report on principles. *Ann Intern Med.* 1995; 123:61–70.

404. Thannheimer A, Woltmann A, Vastmans J, et al. [The unstable patient with pelvic fracture]. *Zentralbl Chir.* 2004;129(1):37–42.

405. Thomas SH. Helicopter emergency medical services transport outcomes literature: annotated review of articles published 2000–2003. *Prehosp Emerg Care.* 2004;8(3):322–333.

406. Thomason M, Messick J, Rutledge R, et al. Head CT scanning versus urgent exploration in the hypotensive blunt trauma patient. *J Trauma.* 1993;34(1):40–44.

407. Timmermann A, Russo SG, Hollmann MW. Paramedic versus emergency physician emergency medical service: role of the anaesthesiologist and the European versus the Anglo-American concept. *Curr Opin Anaesthesiol.* 2008;21(2):222–227.

408. Tornetta P III, Matta JM. Outcome of operatively treated unstable posterior pelvic ring disruptions. *Clin Orthop Relat Res.* 1996;(329):186–193.

409. Totterman A, Dormagen JB, Madsen JE, et al. A protocol for angiographic embolization in exsanguinating pelvic trauma: a report on 31 patients. *Acta Orthop.* 2006;77(3):462–468.

410. Totterman A, Glott T, Soberg HL, et al. Pelvic trauma with displaced sacral fractures: functional outcome at one year. *Spine (Phila Pa 1976).* 2007;32(13):1437–1443.

411. Totterman A, Madsen JE, Skaga NO, et al. Extraperitoneal pelvic packing: a salvage procedure to control massive traumatic pelvic hemorrhage. *J Trauma.* 2007;62(4):843–852.

412. Tran T, Thordarson D. Functional outcome of multiply injured patients with associated foot injury. *Foot Ankle Int.* 2002;23(4):340–343.

413. Trauma Audit & Research Network T. Available at: http://www.tarn.ac.uk. 2008.

414. Travis T, Monsky WL, London J, et al. Evaluation of short-term and long-term complications after emergent internal iliac artery embolization in patients with pelvic trauma. *J Vasc Interv Radiol.* 2008;19(6):840–847.

415. Trentz OL. *Polytrauma: Pathophysiology, Priorities, and Management.* Stuttgart, New York, NY: Thieme; 2007.

416. Troidl H. Quality of life: definition, conceptualization and implications—a surgeon's view. *Theor Surg.* 1991;6:138–142.

417. Trunkey DD, Lim RC. Analysis of 425 consecutive trauma fatalities. *J Am Coll Emerg Phys.* 1974;3:368–371.

418. Tscherne H, Oestern HJ, Sturm J. Osteosynthesis of major fractures in polytrauma. *World J Surg.* 1983;7(1):80–87.

419. Tsoukas A, Andreades A, Zacharogiannis C, et al. Myocardial contusion presented as acute myocardial infarction after chest trauma. *Echocardiography.* 2001;18(2):167–170.

420. Tuxen DV. Permissive hypercapnic ventilation. *Am J Respir Crit Care Med.* 1994;150(3):870–874.

421. van der Laan N. *Acute Lical Inflammation After Blunt Trauma.* University Groningen, 2001.

422. Various A. *ATLS, Advanced Trauma Life Support, Student's Manual.* Chicago, IL: American College of Surgeons; 1997.

423. Vaslef SN, Knudsen NW, Neligan PJ, et al. Massive transfusion exceeding 50 units of blood products in trauma patients. *J Trauma.* 2002;53(2):291–295.

424. Velmahos GC, Theodorou D, Tatevossian R, et al. Radiographic cervical spine evaluation in the alert asymptomatic blunt trauma victim: much ado about nothing. *J Trauma.* 1996;40(5):768–774.

425. Velmahos GC, Toutouzas KG, Vassiliu P, et al. A prospective study on the safety and efficacy of angiographic embolization for pelvic and visceral injuries. *J Trauma.* 2002;53(2):303–308.

426. Voggenreiter G, Eisold C, Sauerland S, et al. [Diagnosis and immediate therapeutic management of chest trauma. A systematic review of the literature]. *Unfallchirurg.* 2004;107(10):881–891.

427. W.H.O. World Health Statistics World Health Organisation - WHO 2006. (Last accessed 9 January 2008). www.who.int/whosis. 2006.

428. Wade CE, Kramer GC, Grady JJ, et al. Efficacy of hypertonic 7.5% saline and 6% dextran-70 in treating trauma: a meta-analysis of controlled clinical studies. *Surgery.* 1997;122(3):609–616.

429. Wald SL, Shackford SR, Fenwick J. The effect of secondary insults on mortality and long-term disability after severe head injury in a rural region without a trauma system. *J Trauma.* 1993;34(3):377–381.

430. Waller JA, Payne SR, McClallen JM. Trauma centers and DRGs–inherent conflict? *J Trauma.* 1989;29(5):617–622.

431. Wang H, Ma S. The cytokine storm and factors determining the sequence and severity of organ dysfunction in multiple organ dysfunction syndrome. *Am J Emerg Med.* 2008;26(6):711–715.

432. Ward LD, Morandi MM, Pearse M, et al. The immediate treatment of pelvic ring disruption with the pelvic stabilizer. *Bull Hosp Jt Dis.* 1997;56(2):104–106.

433. Wardrope J. Traumatic deaths in the Sheffield and Barnsley areas. *J R Coll Surg Edinb.* 1989;34(2):69–73.

434. Ware J Jr, Kosinski M, Keller SD. A 12-Item Short-Form Health Survey: construction of scales and preliminary tests of reliability and validity. *Med Care.* 1996;34(3):220–233.

435. Watanabe E, Hirasawa H, Oda S, et al. Cytokine-related genotypic differences in peak interleukin-6 blood levels of patients with SIRS and septic complications. *J Trauma.* 2005;59(5):1181–1189.

436. Waydhas C, Nast-Kolb D, Trupka A, et al. Posttraumatic inflammatory response, secondary operations, and late multiple organ failure. *J Trauma.* 1996;40(4):624–630.

437. Weiskopf RB, Viele MK, Feiner J, et al. Human cardiovascular and metabolic response to acute, severe isovolemic anemia. *JAMA.* 1998;279(3):217–221.

438. Weninger P, Mauritz W, Fridrich P, et al. Emergency room management of patients with blunt major trauma: evaluation of the multislice computed tomography protocol exemplified by an urban trauma center. *J Trauma.* 2007;62(3):584–591.

439. West TA, Rivara FP, Cummings P, et al. Harborview assessment for risk of mortality: an improved measure of injury severity on the basis of ICD-9-CM. *J Trauma.* 2000;49(3):530–540.

440. WHO. 2nd Global Status Report on Road Safety. 2012.

441. WHO. Global status report on road safety: time for action. 2009.

442. Williams RF, Fabian TC, Fischer PE, et al. Impact of airbags on a Level I trauma center: injury patterns, infectious morbidity, and hospital costs. *J Am Coll Surg.* 2008;206(5):962–968.

443. Wilmink AB, Samra GS, Watson LM, et al. Vehicle entrapment rescue and pre-hospital trauma care. *Injury.* 1996;27(1):21–25.

444. Wilson C, Willis C, Hendrikz JK, et al. Speed enforcement detection devices for preventing road traffic injuries. *Cochrane Database Syst Rev.* 2006;19(2):CD004607.

445. Winslow JE, Hinshaw JW, Hughes MJ, et al. Quantitative assessment of diagnostic radiation doses in adult blunt trauma patients. *Ann Emerg Med.* 2008;52(2):93–97.

446. Wintermark M, Poletti PA, Becker CD, et al. Traumatic injuries: organization and ergonomics of imaging in the emergency environment. *Eur Radiol.* 2002;12(5): 959–968.

447. Wisner DH, Victor NS, Holcroft JW. Priorities in the management of multiple trauma: intracranial versus intra-abdominal injury. *J Trauma.* 1993;35(2):271–276.

448. Wolter TP, Fuchs PC, Horvat N, et al. Is high PEEP low volume ventilation in burn patients beneficial? A retrospective study of 61 patients. *Burns.* 2004;30(4):368–373.

449. Woltmann A, Buhren V. [Shock trauma room management of spinal injuries in the framework of multiple trauma. A systematic review of the literature]. *Unfallchirurg.* 2004;107(10):911–918.

450. Wu JS, Sheng L, Wang SH, et al. The impact of clinical risk factors in the conversion from acute lung injury to acute respiratory distress syndrome in severe multiple trauma patients. *J Int Med Res.* 2008;36(3):579–586.

451. Wutzler S, Westhoff J, Lefering R, et al. [Time intervals during and after emergency room treatment. An analysis using the trauma register of the German Society for Trauma Surgery]. *Unfallchirurg.* 2010;113(1):36–43.

452. Xiao W, Mindrinos MN, Seok J, et al. A genimic storm in critically injured humans. *J Exp Med.* 2011;208(13):2581–2590.

453. Zedler S, Faist E. The impact of endogenous triggers on trauma-associated inflammation. *Curr Opin Crit Care.* 2006;12(6):595–601.

454. Zelle BA, Brown SR, Panzica M, et al. The impact of injuries below the knee joint on the long-term functional outcome following polytrauma. *Injury.* 2005;36(1):169–177.

455. Zelle BA, Panzica M, Vogt MT, et al. Influence of workers' compensation eligibility upon functional recovery 10 to 28 years after polytrauma. *Am J Surg.* 2005;190(1): 30–36.

456. Zimmerman JE, Kramer AA, McNair DS, et al. Acute Physiology and Chronic Health Evaluation (APACHE) IV: hospital mortality assessment for today's critically ill patients. *Crit Care Med.* 2006;34(5):1297–1310.

457. Zintl B, Ruchholtz S, Nast-Kolb D, et al. [Quality management in early clinical multiple trauma care. Documentation of treatment and evaluation of critical care quality]. *Unfallchirurg.* 1997;100(10):811–819.

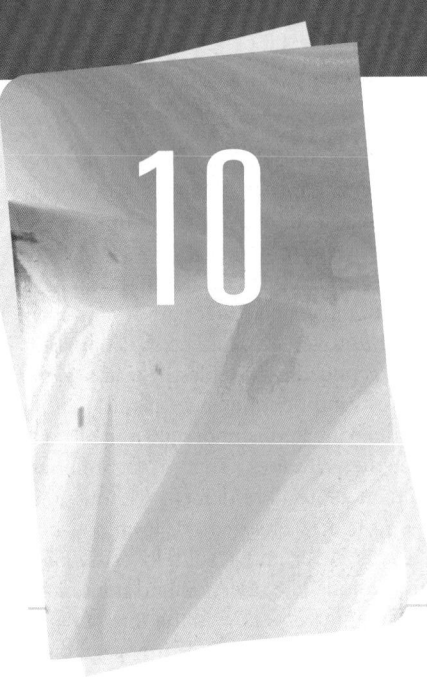

10 INITIAL MANAGEMENT OF OPEN FRACTURES

S. Rajasekaran, A. Devendra, R. Perumal, J. Dheenadhayalan, and S.R. Sundararajan

INTRODUCTION

An open fracture is defined as an injury where the fracture and the fracture hematoma communicate with the external environment through a traumatic defect in the surrounding soft tissues and overlying skin. It should be emphasized that the skin defect may not lie directly over the fracture site and may lie at a distant site. It may communicate with the fracture under degloved skin. Hence any fracture associated with a wound in the same region must be considered to be an open injury until proven otherwise by surgical exploration.

Open fractures are often high-energy injuries and are frequently associated with life-threatening polytrauma. They are best managed by a team approach in centers that have appropriate facilities for resuscitation and multispecialty care.[48,95,121,171,181] Apart from severe bone and soft tissue involvement, these injuries have other risk factors such as skin degloving, soft tissue crushing, contamination with dirt and debris and injury to neurovascular structures. Hence they are associated with a high risk of complications, including amputation. Recent developments such as advances in the management of polytrauma, the availability of powerful antibiotics, refinement of the techniques of radical debridement, bone stabilization, and early soft tissue reconstruction have helped to improve the outcome considerably. The present challenge of the trauma surgeon is not simply salvage of the limb but the restoration of maximal function. Patients with a disfigured or painful limb are often very dissatisfied with the results of treatment and may opt for amputation at the end of a prolonged treatment regime.

The principles of treatment of open injuries have gradually evolved over the centuries and many advances have come from the experience gained in treating war injuries. Tscherne[186] has grouped the developments into four eras of life preservation, limb preservation, infection prevention, and functional restoration. The problem of contamination was recognized in the 16th century by Ambroise Pare who emphasized the need for cleaning wounds of all foreign matter and necrotic tissue and leaving the wound open.[110,146] The term *"debridement"* was coined by Desault in the 18th century to describe a procedure that involved surgical extension of the wound and the removal of all necrotic and contaminated tissue.[88,189] In the absence of antibiotics and aseptic surgical techniques, the incidence of mortality and amputation following infection was very high. "Lose a Limb to save a Life" was an accepted dictum of management as gross infection of open injuries often led to gangrene, septicemia, and death. In the Franco-Prussian War of 1870, more than 13,000 therapeutic amputations were performed.[194] Billroth (1829–1894) reported a mortality of 39% following open injuries which led him to comment, "Perhaps the treatment of no other condition gives me as much satisfaction as that of a successfully treated open injury."[18]

World War I saw the successful beginning of the *"Era of Life Preservation"* as mortality was considerably reduced as a result of the application of the principles of good resuscitation, thorough debridement, stabilization, and avoiding closing the wounds. Survival continued to improve as sulfonamides and other antibiotics became available in World War II with more antibiotics being used during the Korean War.

The 1970s saw major advances in both orthopedic and plastic surgery and the *"Era of Limb Preservation"* was introduced. The refinement of the principles and techniques of external fixation allowed rapid and effective stabilization of the skeleton in the presence of complex fracture patterns. The advent of bone transport and ring fixators led to the possibility of successful bone regeneration even in the presence of major bone loss. Simultaneous advances in plastic surgery with the evolution of numerous flaps in different regions of the body together with the development of microvascular free tissue transfer made reconstruction of composite tissue loss possible. These advances made limb reconstruction a technical possibility, even in challenging situations.

The availability of antibiotics and the understanding of the need for aggressive debridement and early soft tissue cover helped to control infection bringing in the *"Era of Infection Control."* Meanwhile the principles of treatment were being constantly refined. Gustilo and Anderson[84,85,80] published their landmark classification scheme for open fractures that brought attention to the importance of the wound and the need for early soft tissue cover. The seminal work of Godina clearly emphasized the advantages of early soft tissue cover.[72–74] The source of the infection was frequently identified to be from the hospital environment and the principle of "Fix and Flap" and the indications and advantages of primary skin suturing were developed. The huge variability in presentation and the challenges inherent in the management of Gustilo IIIb injuries led to the development of the Ganga Hospital Open Injury Score (GHOIS) with specific guidelines for salvage and reconstruction in IIIb injuries.[154] Recently, the availability of vacuum foam dressings

(VFD) using negative pressure wound therapy (NPWT) has also proved to be very useful in wounds that cannot be covered early. It acts as a bridge between the index procedure and the definitive soft tissue cover procedure.

The understanding that open fractures are not in the domain of any single specialty and must be treated by a combined approach has helped to improve results. The "Orthoplastic approach"[25,43] where the orthopedic and plastic teams work together from the stage of wound debridement onward is now recognized as the standard of care and is undertaken in all centers which regularly treat these injuries. This protocol allows surgeons to undertake a meticulous debridement without concern about the problems of late reconstruction. It emphasizes the need for early soft tissue cover and results in better outcomes by reducing complications like infection and nonunion.

The management of open injuries is now in the *"Era of Functional Restoration."* Functional restoration is aided by aggressive wound debridement, early definitive fracture stabilization and early wound closure or cover to achieve bone and soft tissue healing as soon as possible. Surgeons have now realized that success in treatment of open injuries is not merely salvage and they should not succumb to the "triumph of technique over reason." Patients are often dissatisfied if they are left with a deformed or painful lower limb at the end of the treatment and often opt for a secondary amputation. The future will focus on identifying and understanding factors that affect healing of bone and soft tissues at the molecular and genetic level so that the treatment can be tailored to each patient and secondary amputations avoided. There will also be a focus on the development of safe protocols for reconstruction that will facilitate better function and cosmesis in the shortest possible period of time.

PATHOPHYSIOLOGY

Long bone open fractures have been quoted to occur with a frequency of 11.5 per 100,000 persons per year.[39,44,57,99] The incidence must be much higher in developing countries where road traffic and work place accidents are abundant and increasing every day. In many countries motor cycle accidents are the commonest cause of open long bone fractures with more fractures occurring in the lower limbs than in the upper limbs.[74] Open tibial diaphyseal fractures are the commonest open long bone fracture but open femoral diaphyseal, distal femoral, and proximal tibial fractures occur frequently. Open fractures of the upper limb are usually associated with less severe soft tissue damage and fewer associated musculoskeletal injuries. Figure 10-1 shows the spectrum of open fractures presenting to our Unit.

Open fractures can occur in low-velocity injuries due to the sharp ends of the fractured bone piercing the skin and soft tissues but more often they are the result of high-energy injuries. The amount of energy absorbed by the injured limb is determined by the equation $KE = MV^2/2$, where KE is the kinetic energy absorbed, M is the mass, and V is the speed.[37,78] Examples of energy absorbed in different energy mechanisms are shown in Table 10-1. The bone and soft tissues of the limb absorb the energy but when the threshold is exceeded there is significant comminution of the bone with periosteal stripping

Total open injuries 1554

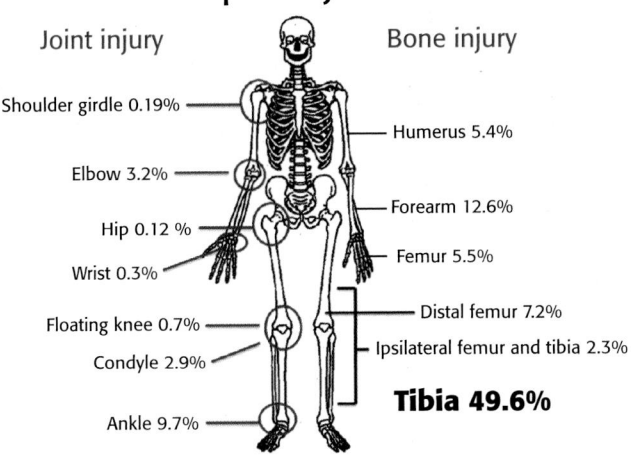

FIGURE 10-1 The distribution of open injuries in 1,554 consecutive cases treated in our unit. Lower limb injuries are more common with open injuries of tibia accounting for nearly 50% of all open injuries.

TABLE 10-1	Energy Transmitted by Injury Mechanism (ft–lb)[37]	
• Fall from curb		100
• Skiing injury		300–500
• High-velocity gunshot wound (single missile)		2000
• 20-mph bumper injury (assumes bumper strikes fixed target)		100,000

and soft tissue damage. The sharp comminuted bone fragments are frequently devoid of all soft tissue attachments and may be displaced with a velocity that results in additional damage to the soft tissues and neurovascular structures. When the skin is torn a temporary vacuum can be created that sucks in all adjacent foreign material. This dirt and debris may be deposited in the depths of the wound in the deep intermuscular planes and is often deposited in the intramedullary cavity of the bone. This fact should be borne in mind during the wound debridement where meticulous examination of all possible areas of contamination must be done.

A few facts require emphasis. The size and nature of the external wound may not reflect the damage to the deeper structures (Fig. 10-2). Frequently small lacerated wounds are associated with extensive occult degloving with severe soft tissue damage and bone comminution. Open injuries may damage one or more compartments of the limb, but the severe swelling may result in compartment syndrome of the other intact compartments of the same limb.[128] It must be remembered that the presence of an open wound does not preclude the occurrence of a compartment syndrome in the injured limb. One must also be aware that the extent of injury to the soft tissues and bone may not be fully exposed on day 1 and the actual "zone of injury" may be revealed only over the next few days. This has important implications in choosing the timing and nature of soft tissue reconstruction. It should also be understood that an open injury is just not a simple combination of a fracture and a wound. Additional factors such as contamination with dirt and debris and devitalization of the soft tissues increase the risk of infection and other complications.

FIGURE 10-2 The severity of the skin wound often has no bearing on the extent of damage to deeper tissues. An open tibial diaphyseal fractures with a small skin wound **(A)** was associated with significant bone **(B, D)** and soft tissue **(C)** damage. The wound ultimately required a free fibula graft **(E)** and a soft tissue flap **(F)**.

(continues)

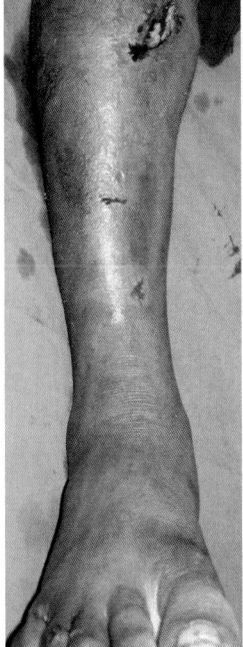 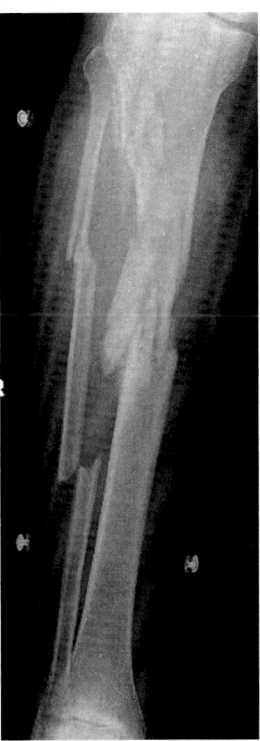 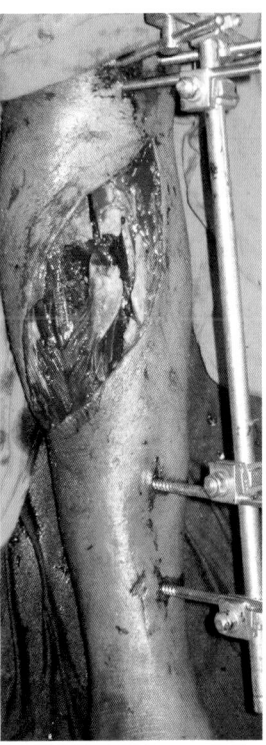

A, B   **C**

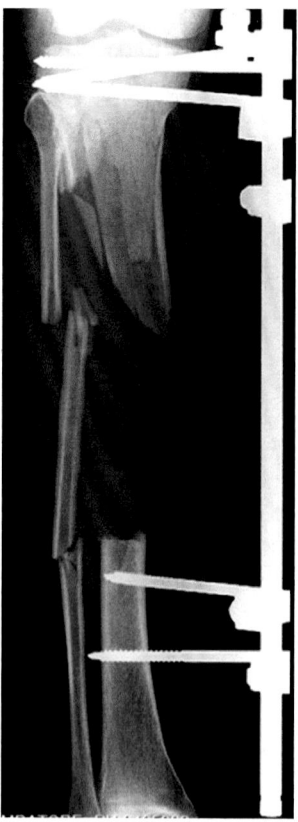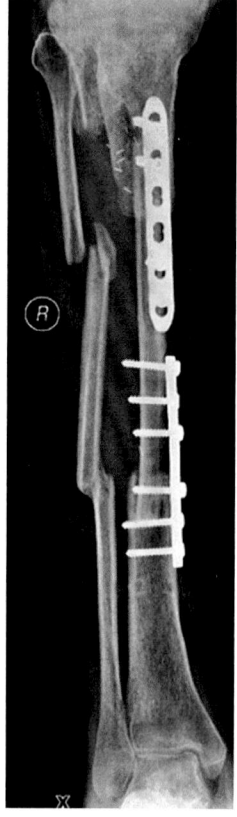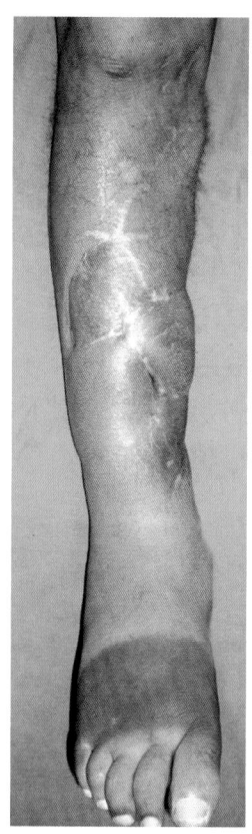

D, E   **F**   **FIGURE 10-2** *(continued)*

ASSESSMENT

Initial Evaluation

Every open injury is an orthopedic emergency and the success of treatment depends on a thorough initial evaluation and management that starts at the emergency room.

An open injury always presents dramatically and has the capacity to distract the untrained person from assessing the more serious occult injuries which may be life threatening (Fig. 10-3). Thirty percent of patients with open injuries have more than one injury and the temptation to focus attention on the bleeding wound must be avoided. The emergency room doctor must not restrict his or her attention to the obvious injury but undertake a thorough evaluation as per ATLS protocols. The patient must be thoroughly assessed for airway, breathing, and circulation. There may be a number of injuries that are missed and there is a role for fast whole-body CT scanning which helps to identify injuries to the head, neck, spine, chest, and pelvis.

An estimate of the blood loss must be undertaken quickly and, if necessary, resuscitation measures immediately instituted. Inadequate resuscitation is an important cause of avoidable deaths and later comorbidities such as infection, delayed wound healing, and pulmonary complications. Acidosis, hypothermia, and coagulopathy, the deadly triad in injured patients, are often present in patients with open injuries and these must be identified and corrected quickly.[27,106,169] It is now understood that simply monitoring the vital signs may be insufficient to determine the adequacy of resuscitation and treatment regimes that simply target vital signs may be harmful in the setting of polytrauma.[53,136,167] Surgeons should consider damage control orthopedics as a part of the resuscitation process.[94,141,179] This is discussed in Chapter 9.

Once the patient is stabilized it is important that the circumstances of the accident and the patient's history are meticulously documented. Documentation starts with a thorough history which includes details of the accident, the time of injury, any loss of consciousness, and other evidence of head injury, temporary or partial paralysis, the probable velocity of injury, the use of seat belts and helmets, and emergency medical attention received at the site of accident. Witnesses and accompanying family members may provide useful information regarding the nature of the injury. Information about the condition of the patient and the resuscitative measures undertaken at the scene of the accident, and the condition of the patient during transport to the hospital must be obtained from the emergency medical attendants. The type of injuries sustained by accompanying passengers in the vehicle will also provide information about the circumstances of the accident.

Special attention should be paid to documenting any comorbidities of the patient as they may significantly influence treatment decisions and the final outcome.[155,154] (Fig. 10-4). Any systemic illness, history of smoking, medications, and pertinent allergies should be documented. Illnesses such as diabetes mellitus, rheumatoid arthritis, and connective tissue disorders which are associated with osteoporosis and bleeding disorders should

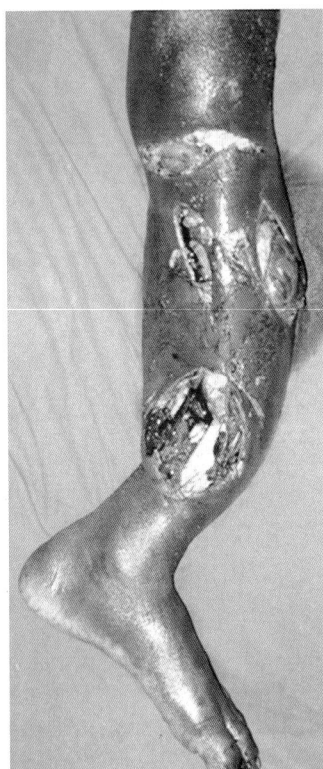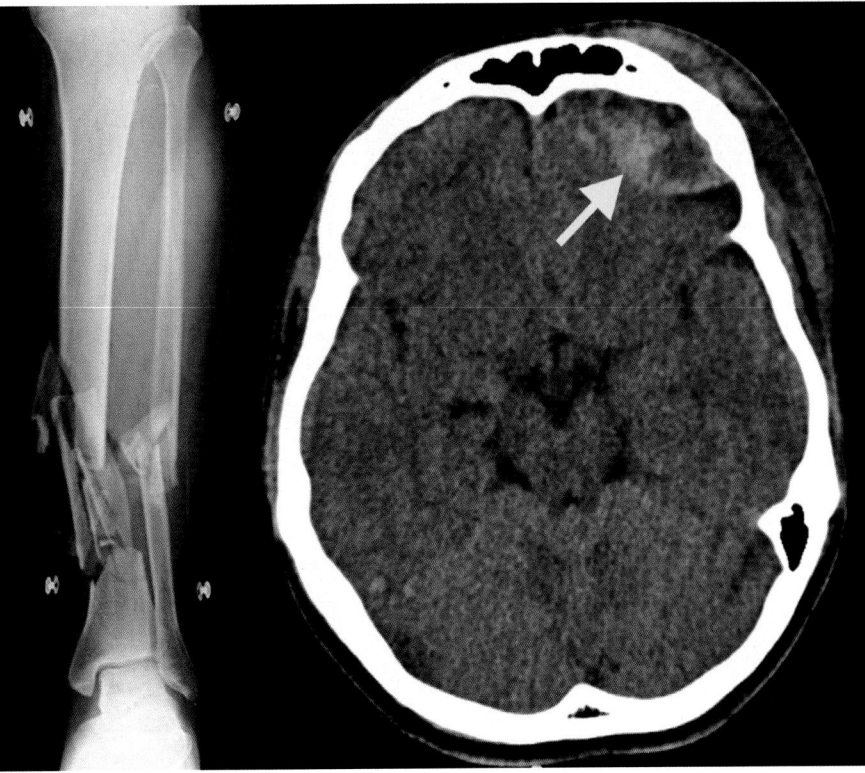

FIGURE 10-3 Open fractures are often high-energy injuries and have a variable amount of damage to the skin, soft tissues, and bone **(A, B).** They are often associated with serious life-threatening injuries such as the intracranial bleeding seen in this patient **(C).**

be recorded as should the use of drugs such as phenytoin which may cause osteomalacia or osteoporosis. Any history of previous surgery must also be documented. Smoking is associated with an increased rate of flap failure, delayed union, and nonunion and this must be documented. Patients who are smoking must be urged to stop smoking during the treatment process.[2,35]

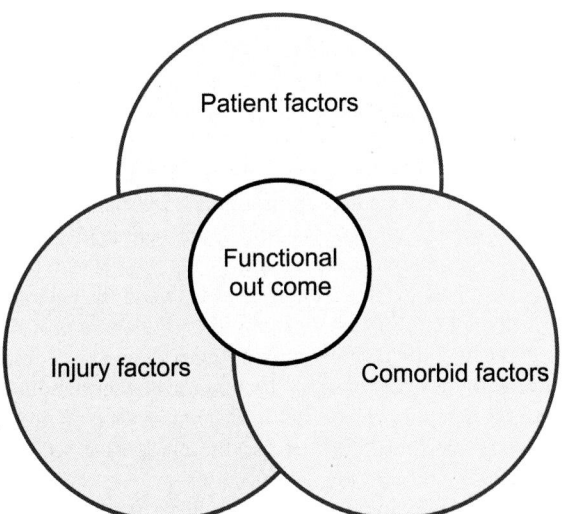

FIGURE 10-4 The functional outcome in a Type IIIb injury depends on a triad of factors related to the patient, any comorbidities that may be present and the severity of injury.

Examination

A thorough physical examination of the patient is important. The patient should be adequately undressed so that any bruising and contusions in other parts of the body that might indicate more significant injury can be seen. This is especially important in patients who are not fully conscious or under the influence of alcohol. All constrictive clothing must be removed and the vascularity and movements of all four limbs must be examined. An injured limb that is grossly deformed or shortened must be gently reduced and splinted so that vascularity is not compromised. Tenting of the skin by sharp bone fragments or dislocated joints may lead to avascularity and further loss of skin and these fractures must be considered as impending open fractures even when no wound is present (Fig. 10-5). Persistent dislocation of the joints, especially the knee and ankle joints, may also cause vascular compromise and these joints require urgent reduction in the emergency room. The limb must also be examined for any signs of compartment syndrome (see Chapter 29).

The size and severity of the wound and the relationship of the wound to the fracture must be carefully examined. Although most open fractures, especially Gustilo Type III fractures, expose one or both ends of the fractured bone, the wound may be distant and there may be no direct exposure of the fracture (Fig. 10-6). Any wound, no matter how small or distant from the fracture, must still be considered indicative of an open fracture. Communication with the actual fracture site due to disruption of the fascia and degloving of the skin is

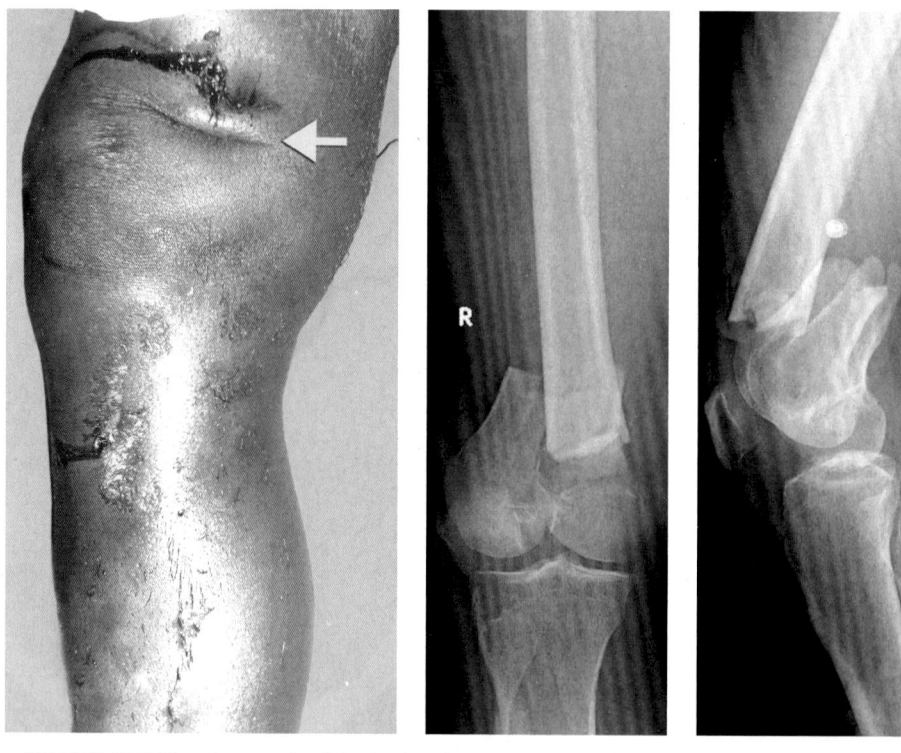

FIGURE 10-5 The sharp ends of the broken bone may cause skin tethering jeopardizing its vascular supply **(A)**. The bone ends may also cause pressure on local neurovascular structures resulting in distal avascularity. In this patient the flexed distal fragment **(B, C)** caused local vascular pressure resulting in absent distal pulses. Distal vascularity was established once the bone was reduced by gentle traction.

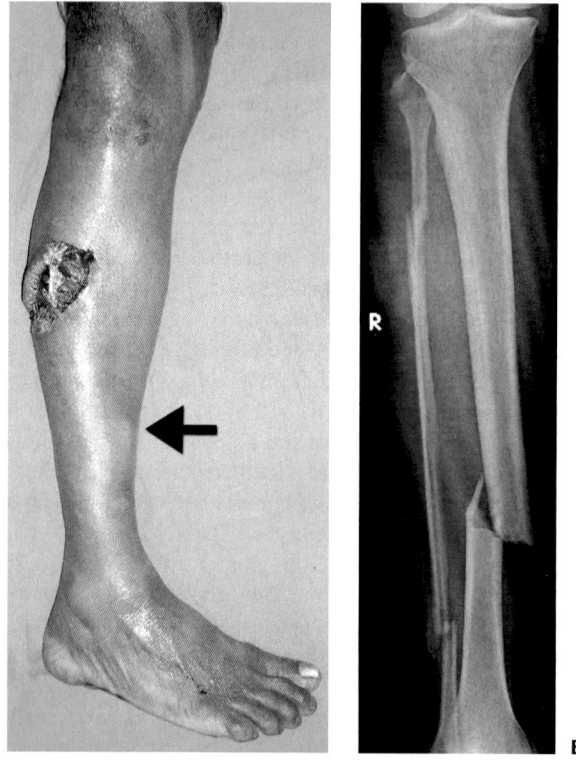

FIGURE 10-6 The skin wound in this patient, although located proximal to the fracture **(A),** communicated with it under degloved skin **(B)**.

often obvious during the debridement. Persistent oozing from a small laceration, especially if it carries fat globules indicates a discharging fracture hematoma.

In the emergency room examination of the wound should include the size and location of the wound, the orientation of the wound, to define if it is longitudinal, transverse or irregular, the depth of the wound and whether bone, tendons, and muscle are exposed. Attention should be paid to the status of the skin adjacent to the wound. If there is extensive damage or contusions to the skin around the wound there may be significant skin avascularity and therefore skin loss during debridement (Fig. 10-7).

Photographic documentation of the wound should ideally be undertaken. This is important as a good visual documentation surpasses any written description and will be of immense value during follow-up examinations and for research purposes.[132] A digital camera should be available in the emergency room where open injuries are received.[174] Following the initial assessment and documentation, the wound must be quickly covered with a sterile dressing. Probing or further handling of the wound may in fact be disadvantageous as it may provoke unnecessary bleeding and increase the chances of secondary contamination and nosocomial infections.

Significant bleeding may be controlled by application of a compression dressing and firm bandages with elevation of the limb. This will be sufficient to arrest the bleeding in the majority of patients. The surgeon should not attempt to blindly

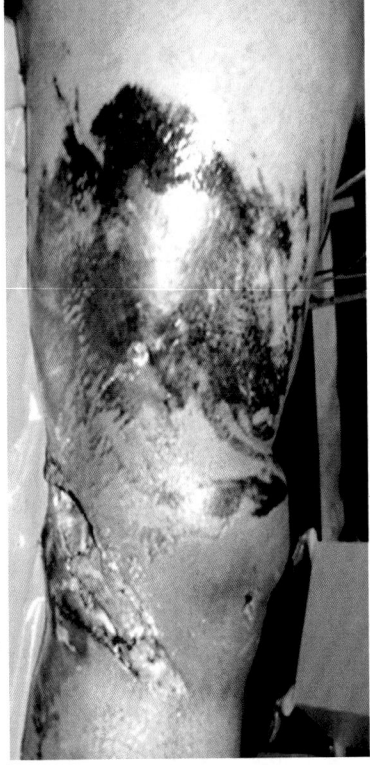
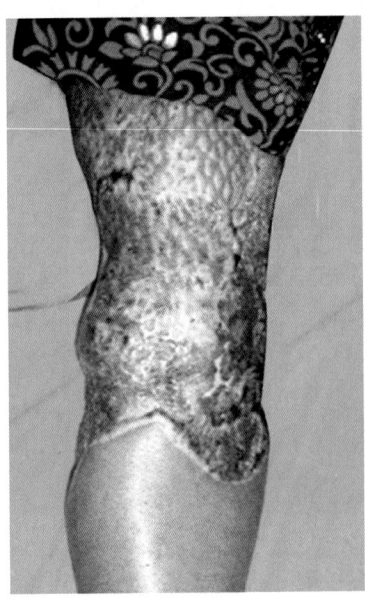

FIGURE 10-7 Closed degloving is a major risk factor for extensive skin avascularity. In this case there was a large skin defect after debridement of nonviable skin **(A)**. This required to be covered with a skin graft **(B)**.

clamp a bleeding vein or artery in the emergency room as this may result in the inadvertent clamping of an adjacent major neurovascular structure and lead to permanent and irreversible neurologic deficit. Uncontrollable bleeding from a wound can be arrested with the help of a tourniquet. The patient should then be taken to the operating room as quickly as possible.

Establishing and documenting intact vascularity in all fractured limbs, and especially in severely mangled limbs, is crucial. Signs of vascular injury are listed in Table 10-2. Apart from the presence of a positive pulse examination, adequate filling of the veins and a positive capillary refill sign, a warm and normally colored distal limb is also indicative of an intact circulation. If pulses are absent, one must reexamine the limb after the limbs are anatomically aligned and splinted as shortening and angulation of the fractured skeleton may result in kinking and

occlusion of the vessels. If the pulses are still absent, a vascular injury must be suspected unless proven otherwise. A diagnosis of vascular spasm should not be made as the inevitable loss of time in initiating treatment may result in amputation. Additional investigations such as arterial doppler or a CT angiogram may be necessary. CT angiograms are particularly useful as apart from indicating the location and type of the block, they reveal the status and adequacy of the collateral circulation (Fig. 10-8). The disadvantage, however, is that they are time consuming and not available in all centers. The high dose of contrast required may also cause renal damage in a patient in severe shock and precipitate acute renal failure.

Although a thorough neurologic examination may be difficult in the emergency room setting due to pain, documentation of the distal neurologic status is the next step. Both touch sensation and pinprick testing can be used to examine distal dermatomes and motor movements can also be tested. Determination of the exact power of the muscle groups may be difficult. If for any reason testing of specific muscle groups is not possible, it should be documented so that a proper evaluation can be done later as soon as possible.

The surgeon should look for wounds over the thorax, abdomen, or pelvis. These may be associated with a very poor prognosis if not recognized and treated properly as they may represent communications with the body cavities. In the pelvis, a laceration of the rectum, vagina, or urinary tract represents an open fracture of the pelvis and a colostomy is required to prevent fecal contamination. Overlooking these wounds and delaying treatment is a frequent cause of increased mortality and morbidity.

TABLE 10-2 **Signs of Vascular Injury**

Hard Signs
- Absent or significant difference in pulsations compared to normal side.
- Severe hemorrhage from the wound.
- Expanding and pulsatile hematoma.
- Bruit or thrill.

Associated Signs
- Associated numbness and neurologic deficit.
- Difference in skin temperature distal to injury.
- Absence of venous filling.
- Absence of pulse-oximeter reading. No capillary blanching.

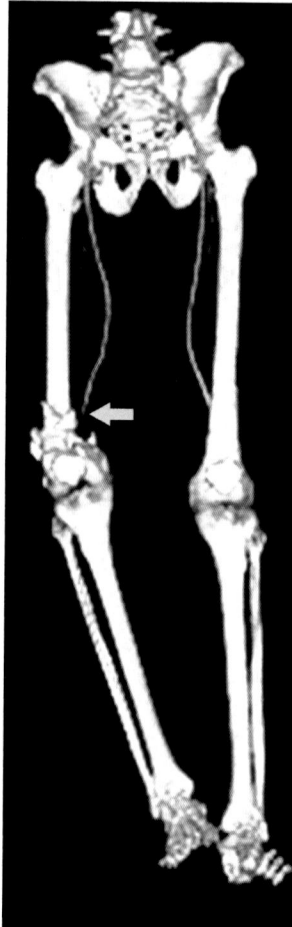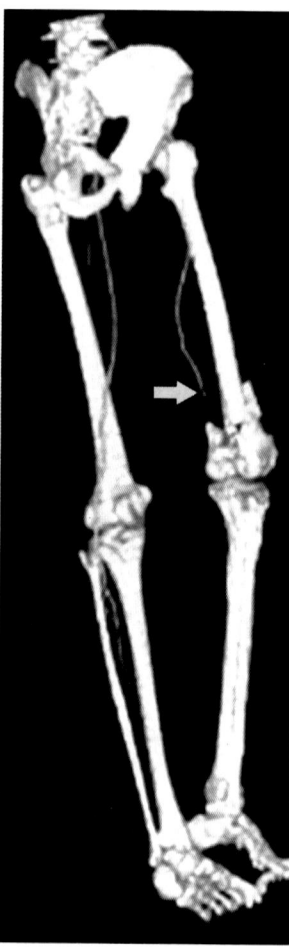

FIGURE 10-8 In the absence of the distal pulses, if there is no contraindication to undertaking it, a CT angiogram will not only show the level and severity of the block but will also show the status of the collateral vessels. Here there is a complete block of the artery due to a supracondylar fracture of the femur with poor collateral blood supply.

Role of Cultures in the Emergency Room

Infection is the major complication that leads to the need for secondary procedures, nonunions, failure of flaps, and even amputations. This fact stimulated surgeons to try to identify the bacteria that cause wound contamination. However studies have shown poor correlation between the presence of positive cultures and subsequent rate of clinical infection.[131] There is disparity between the organisms grown on the initial wound swabs and the organisms grown subsequently[129,192] after the development of wound infection The commonly isolated organisms from established infection are *Staphylococcus aureus, Pseudomonas,* and *Escherichia coli*.[148] These organisms are frequently due to hospital contamination[34] and are never isolated from the environment where the accidents occur. The practice of obtaining routine cultures from the wound either pre- or post-debridement is no longer advocated.[111,116,138,188] It is now understood that in addition to contamination, infection is influenced by various factors related to the wound, host, and environment.

Antibiotics

Once the limb is properly splinted, bleeding has been controlled and the wound is covered with a wet saline dressing appropriate intravenous antibiotics should be administered The antibiotic therapy should be considered therapeutic and not prophylactic and it must be instituted as early as possible[26,148,179] as all open fractures are contaminated to a varying extent.[72,87,81,82] In the absence of organic or sewage contamination intravenous first or second generation cephalosporins are typically given before the patient leaves the emergency room.[77,81,137,162,184,185] An aminoglycoside is added in Gustilo Type III injuries. Penicillin, with or without metronidazole, should be given to patients with gross organic contamination. Recommendations for the administration of intravenous antibiotics are given in Table 10-3. In addition, the patient's tetanus status must be documented and supplementary injections given if necessary. It should be remembered that the prolonged use of antibiotics is not indicated and will lead to the development of resistant organisms.[71] Guidelines for the use of intravenous antibiotics are shown in Table 10-4.

Radiographic Imaging and Other Diagnostic Studies

Plain radiographs are sufficient in the majority of cases to identify the extent of injury and plan treatment. An anteroposterior and lateral radiograph of the injured bone with inclusion of the joints above and below is the minimum that is required. Open injuries are often high-velocity injuries and the fracture may extend into the adjacent joints or there could be associated injuries of the articular surfaces. Hence radiographs including the adjacent joints are essential. In high-energy injuries involving the femur, radiographs of the pelvis which depict the status

---

TABLE 10-3 **Intravenous Antibiotic Therapy for Open Fractures[26]**

Latest British Orthopaedic Association online recommendations (Open fractures of lower limb—September 2009)

- Give antibiotics as soon as possible (within 3 hours).
- Agent of choice co-amoxiclav (1.2 g 8 hourly), or a cephalosporin (e.g., cefuroxime 1.5 g 8 hourly), continued until first debridement (excision).
- At the time of first debridement, co-amoxiclav (1.2 g) or a cephalosporin (such as cefuroxime 1.5 g) and gentamicin (1.5 mg/kg) should be administered and co-amoxiclav/cephalosporin continued until soft tissue closure or for a maximum of 72 hours, whichever is sooner.
- Gentamicin 1.5 mg/kg and either vancomycin 1 g or teicoplanin 800 mg should be administered on induction of anesthesia at the time of skeletal stabilization and definitive soft tissue closure. These should not be continued postoperatively. Ideally start the vancomycin infusion at least 90 minutes before surgery.
- True penicillin allergy (anaphylaxis) clindamycin (600 mg IV pre-op/qds) in place of co-amoxiclav/cephalosporin. Lesser allergic reaction to penicillin (rash, etc.) a cephalosporin is considered to be safe and is the agent of choice.

TABLE 10-4 Intravenous Antibiotic Therapy[71]

Evidence Supports
- Intravenous antibiotics at the earliest, preferably in the emergency room.
- Use of metronidazole and aminoglyosides in severely contaminated wounds.
- Equivalent efficacy of oral to parenteral antibiotics during the follow-up (when necessary).

Evidence Does Not Support
- Prolonged and continuous use of antibiotics.
- Continuing antibiotics as long as the drains are in.
- Continuation of the empirical antibiotic regime till wound drainage is present.
- Prophylactic antibiotics to prevent pin tract infections.
- Antibiotic therapy as a substitute for debridement in presence of necrotic and contaminated material.

of the sacroiliac joints, pubic symphysis, and both hips are important (Fig. 10-9). Radiographic clearance of the cervical and thoracolumbar spines must be undertaken when necessary.

The presence of air in the subcutaneous tissues, intramuscular planes, and joint cavities and the visualization of foreign bodies are indicative of open injuries. The presence of air in the subcutaneous tissues in puncture wounds or small lacerations indicates severe degloving of the skin. Radiographic evidence of severe mud contamination, shattered glass, or metal pieces suggests significant contamination (Fig. 10-10). In patients presenting late the presence of radiographic gas shadows in the muscular planes should arose suspicion of an established infection by gas producing organisms such as *Clostridium perfringens* or *Escherichia coli*.[29,157]

In the absence of life-threatening injuries, a CT scan may prove helpful particularly in intra-articular fractures of the ankle and knee joint. It will identify the three dimensional orientation of the fracture planes and any distortion of the articular margins. This will facilitate fracture reduction and skeletal stabilization following debridement during the index surgery. If the state of the patient does not permit a CT scan temporary external fixation may be undertaken during the index procedure and a detailed CT scan of the joints can be performed later. The role of an MRI of the limb or the whole body is minimal in the acute setting and it is rarely performed.

Role of Biochemical Markers

Major injuries activate multiple humoral and cellular cascade mechanisms involving the inflammatory mediators and complex mechanisms of host defense.[10,63,67,140] These include an increase in capillary damage and permeability, multiple organ dysfunction syndrome (MODS), and even mortality. The value of markers in identifying the presence of systemic inflammatory response syndrome (SIRS) and in predicting outcomes is being investigated[20,69,143–145] (Table 10-5). Identification of a single ideal marker in trauma has been elusive and may in fact be impossible given the wide diversity of injured patients and the wide range of underlying injuries and comorbidities.

The following markers are being investigated.[63,65,182]

(1). CRP

The CRP is commonly used in clinical practice and is widely available. However it has the disadvantage of being unable to distinguish infection and inflammation and it does not exhibit a proportionate increase to the injury thereby being unable to predict outcome. It is still however used widely as a high level of CRP may indicate either

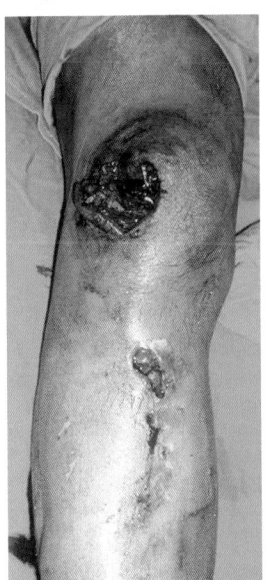
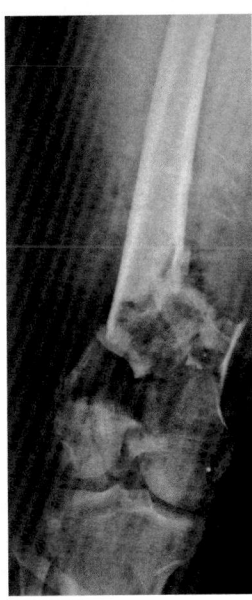
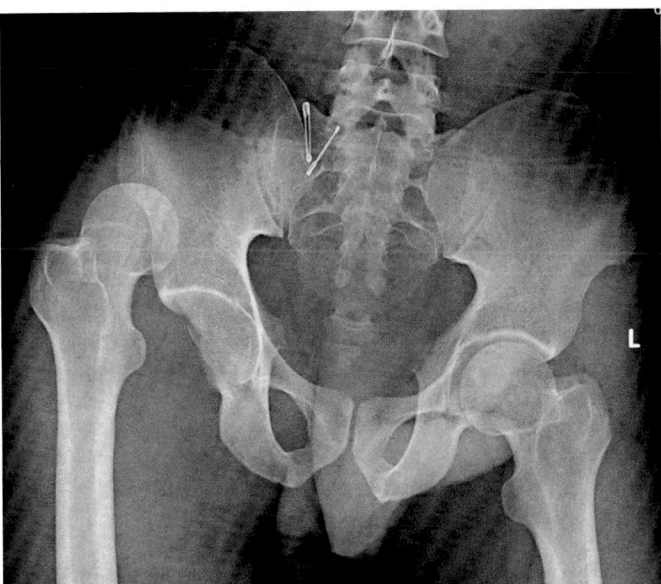

A, B **C**

FIGURE 10-9 Radiographs of a severely injured limb must include the joints on both sides of a fracture. Here, an open injury of the knee joint **(A, B)** was associated with an undiagnosed dislocation of the right hip **(C)** which was detected only after a delay of 48 hours.

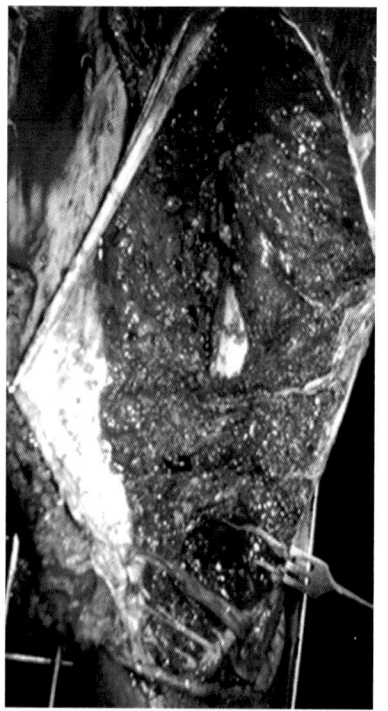
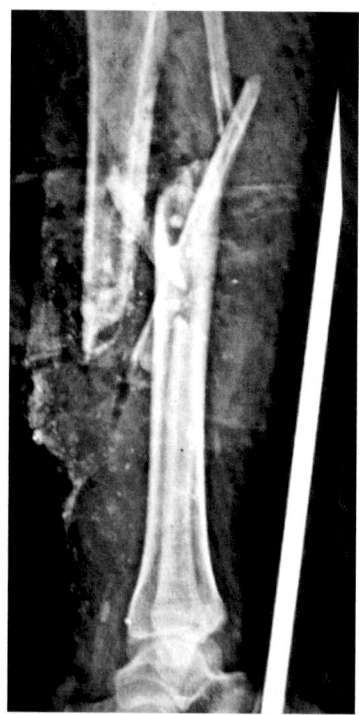
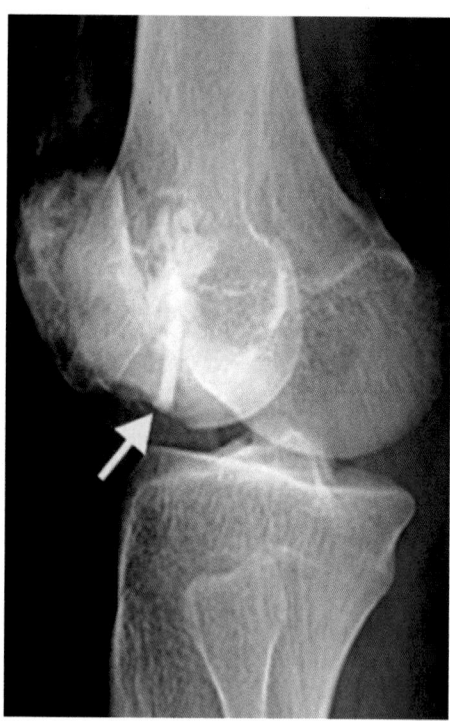

A, B

C

FIGURE 10-10 Major open injuries often carry contamination deep into the wound. This may be seen on radiographs. In this case a Type IIIb open fracture of the tibia and fibula had extensive contamination of mud and dirt in the intramuscular planes **(A, B)**. Glass fragments and air in the joint can also be identified on radiographs **(C)**.

infection or severe inflammation, both of which have important implications in deciding future reconstruction.

(2). Interleukins

Many interleukins have been investigated for their relevance to major trauma and IL-6 has been identified to be a reliable and consistent marker of systemic inflammation.[68,102,103,156] IL-6 is a cytokine with both pro- and anti-inflammatory properties and its increase in the peripheral blood is an early marker of the severity of injury following trauma. Although in the acute phase of inflammatory

TABLE 10-5   Biochemical Markers used in Trauma[63]

	Normal Levels	Significant Levels	Uses	Disadvantages
Serum lactate	0.5–2 22 mmol/L	>2.5 mmol/L	• High levels indicate cellular hypoxia with hypoperfusion and anaerobic metabolism • Delay in return to normal indicates poor prognosis. • Persistent continuous elevation in spite of resuscitation indicates high chances of MODS and mortality.	Serial estimation
Interleukin-6	<7 pg/mL	>200 pg/mL	• High levels in initial stages indicate presence of SIRS. • High levels indicate an inappropriate situation for definitive reconstruction surgery. • High levels indicate a high risk of mortality.	• Has bimodal initial proinflammatory action and downregulatory' action in late stages. • Exact use in isolated limb injury is not yet defined. • Not easily available in all centers. • Expensive, serial estimations are required.
C-reactive protein	<3 ug/mL	>30 ug/mL	• Easily available. • Less expensive. • Raised in both inflammatory and infective conditions.	• Cannot distinguish inflammatory and infective conditions.

TABLE 10-6	Gustilo and Anderson's Classification[84,85]			
Type	Wound	Level of Contamination	Soft Tissue Injury	Bone Injury
I	<1 cm long	Clean	Minimal	Simple, minimal comminution
II	>1 cm long	Moderate	Moderate; some muscle damage	Moderate comminution
III A	Usually >10 cm	High	Severe with crushing	Usually comminuted; soft tissue coverage of bone possible
III B	Usually >10 cm	High	Very severe loss of cover	Bone cover poor; usually requires soft tissue reconstructive surgery
III C	Usually >10 cm	High	Very severe loss of cover and vascular injury requiring repair	Bone cover poor; usually requires soft tissue reconstructive surgery

response, its proinflammatory properties dominate, later its anti-inflammatory properties dominate as it downregulates proinflammatory responses of tumor necrosis factor TNF-α and IL-1.[65,69,117]

Stensballe et al.[177] concluded that early systemic inflammatory response measured with serum IL-6 and IL-10 correlated well with injury severity and 30-day mortality following trauma. The detection limit (minimum detectable dose) of IL-6 was 0.039 pg/mL and 0.5 pg/mL for IL-10 and it requires serial estimation at 6, 12, 24 hours following injury.[2,3,6]

Tschoeke et al.[187] studied the early second hit in trauma management with respect to the proinflammatory response in multiple injuries and concluded that immediate surgical treatment causes additional surgical stress which might promote post-traumatic complications. The exact implications of a raised IL-6 are still not clear but current studies have confirmed a significant association between altered levels and mortality and morbidity. Current interest concerns whether the level of IL-6 would provide information to identify safe windows for secondary soft tissue reconstruction in open injuries especially when associated with other major injuries.[153]

(3). Serum Lactate

Another approach to identify ongoing physiologic insult is the estimation of products of tissue hypoperfusion and anaerobic metabolism such as lactic acidosis.[1,112,122] Serum lactate is a good screening method for occult hypoperfusion and both a high and persistent lactate level is predictive of organ failure and increasing mortality. The time needed to normalize lactate following resuscitation is also an important prognostic indicator and a persistent or increasing lactate level may be one of the earliest signs of MODS.[9,89,127] Studies have revealed higher mean lactate levels in nonsurvivors as compared with survivors in patients with trauma and major sepsis.

Although the above studies have all concentrated on the importance of these changes in polytrauma, the relevance of these markers in isolated major injuries has not been extensively reported. In a preliminary study involving 285 patients with Gustilo IIIb injuries done in our Unit, it was found that there is a proportionate increase in both serum lactate and IL-6 even in isolated injuries of limbs when the severity was measured by the Ganga Hospital Score. The clinical implication of this phenomenon needs to be further investigated.

Classifications and Scores for Open Fractures

Gustilo and Anderson proposed a classification for open injuries in 1976 which still is the most commonly followed classification worldwide.[84] Open injuries were divided into three types. Type I injuries were associated with minimal soft injury, Type II with moderate injury, and Type III injuries were severe injuries which exposed the fracture site and were associated with muscle damage and periosteal stripping. In 1984, Type III open fractures were subdivided again into three types, depending upon the nature and size of the skin wound, degree of muscle damage, extent of contamination, amount of periosteal stripping, and the presence of arterial injury.[85] The classification is listed in Table 10-6.

Gustilo's contribution was a milestone in the management of open injuries as it brought into focus the importance of soft tissue injury and wound contamination. Gustilo reported that the infection rate was 1.9% in Type I injuries, 8% in Type II injuries but it increased to 41% in Type III injuries.[86] Their work emphasized the need for early coverage of wounds and the requirement for early plastic surgery intervention.

However, many disadvantages have been exposed in the routine use of Gustilo and Anderson's classification. These are listed in Table 10-7. A classification system is useful in routine

TABLE 10-7	Disadvantages of Gustilo and Anderson's Classification

- Definition has undergone many modifications and does not have uniformity in application.
- Includes wide spectrum of injuries in Type IIIB injuries.
- Mainly depends on size of the skin wound.
- Does not evaluate the severity of injury to skin, bone and musculotendinous units separately.
- Does not address the question of salvage.
- Poor interobserver reliability.

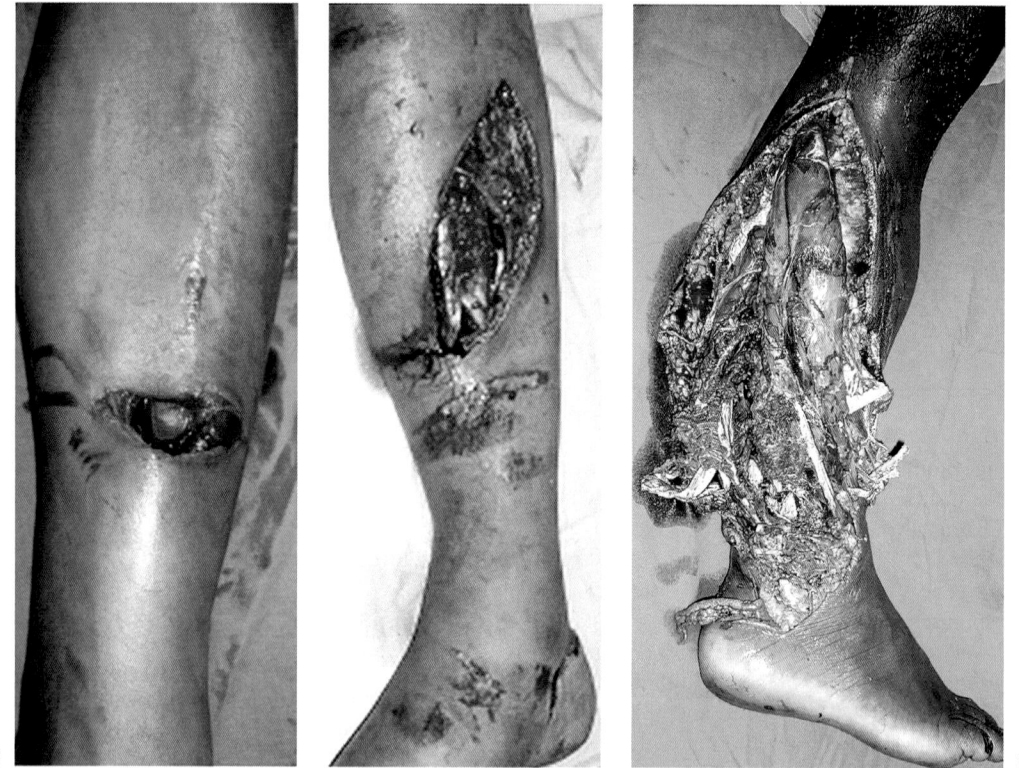

A, B

C

FIGURE 10-11 Gustilo Type IIIb fractures include a wide variety of fractures. By definition fractures **A, B,** and **C** are all Type IIIb injuries. However their severity varies between the easily treatable and the barely salvageable.

practice only if it is capable of consistently and reliably grouping injuries according to their severity. It should form a basis on which guidelines for treatment can be formed, predict the ultimate outcomes, and promote research by allowing comparison of results from different units. Gustilo's classification is deficient in many of the above[22,151–155] and the following deficiencies have been noted.

(a) From the time of its original description, the classification has undergone many modifications which have led to different interpretations by various authors, resulting in loss of uniformity in its global application.

(b) Type IIIb injuries, by definition, include a wide spectrum of easily manageable to barely salvageable injuries (Fig. 10-11). Hence it cannot offer uniform guidelines in management nor allow comparison of published results from different units.

(c) Gustilo originally proposed the classification on the basis of the severity of the wound but the description is now frequently based on treatment. In North America any wound, irrespective of its size and nature, is Type IIIA if it is closed and Type IIIB, if treated by a flap. So rather than guiding treatment it has become a retrospective classification.

(d) The classification is based more on the nature and size of the wound and does not address equally the severity of the injuries to the musculotendinous and skeletal structures. In practice, injury to the muscles, nerves, and bones are often

more crucial than the nature of the wound in predicting function and deciding whether limb salvage is worthwhile (Fig. 10-12).

(e) The classification does not provide for scoring of the comorbid factors which influence the timing and safety of major reconstructive procedures.

(f) The system relies on subjective description such as "significant periosteal stripping" and "extensive soft tissue damage," and this leads to significant variation of interpretation and evaluation among surgeons. There are two major studies which have both reported a low interobserver agreement rate of only 60%. Agreement varied widely depending upon the experience of the surgeon and the type of injury as some of these injuries were inherently difficult to classify.[30,83,98,184]

(g) Being a classification and not a score, Gustilo's classification does not address and provide guidelines for salvage.

It is now accepted that a more accurate and objective method for the assessment of these challenging injuries is needed.

Many injury severity scores such as the Mangled Extremity Severity Score (MESS),[104] the limb salvage index,[161] the predictive salvage index,[100] the nerve injury, ischemia, soft tissue injury, skeletal injury, shock and age patient (NISSSA) score[126] and the Hannover fracture scale[180] have since been proposed. The components of different lower-extremity injury scoring systems are listed in Table 10-8. These scores have attempted to evaluate the degree of injury to different tissues separately and

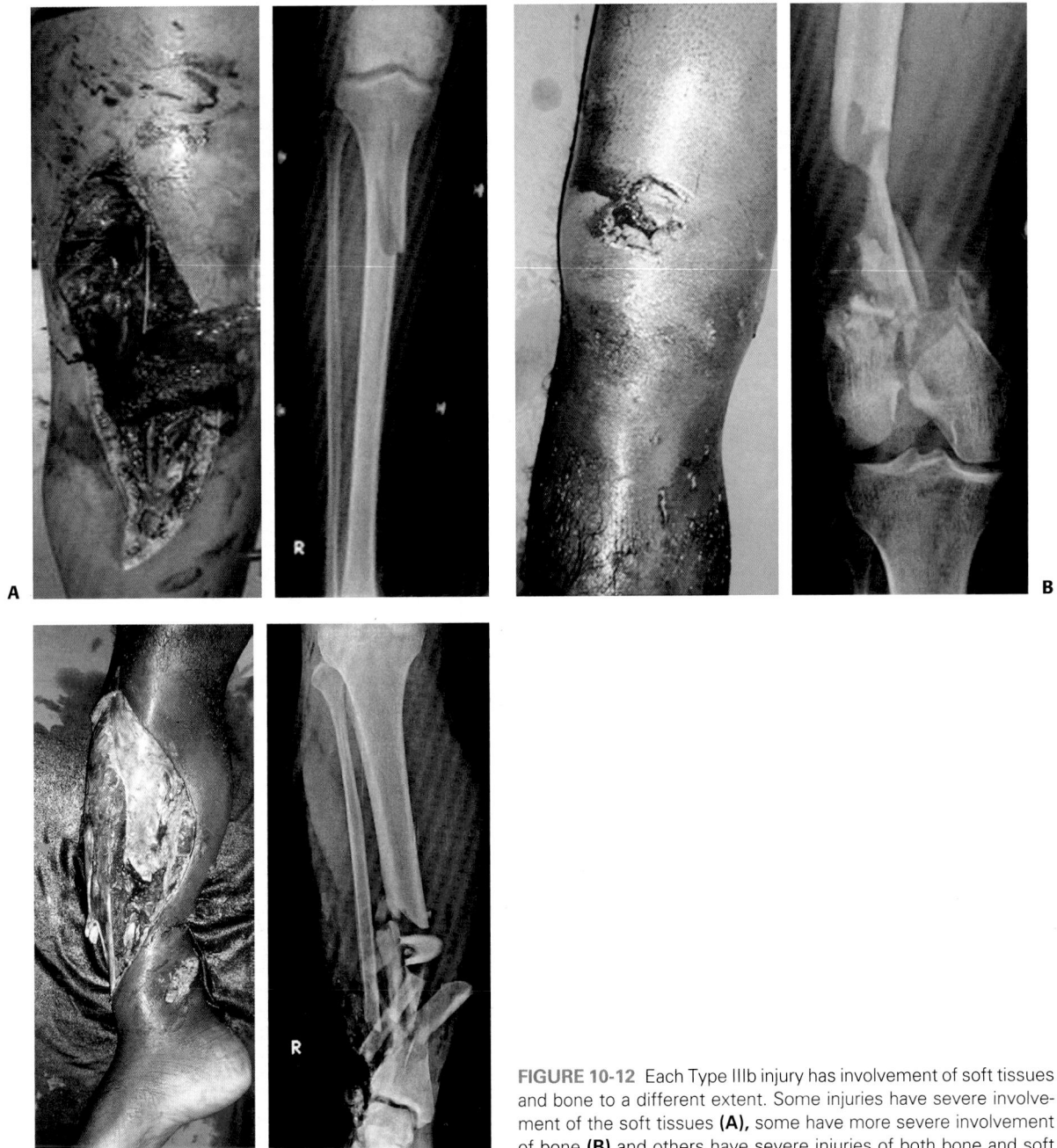

FIGURE 10-12 Each Type IIIb injury has involvement of soft tissues and bone to a different extent. Some injuries have severe involvement of the soft tissues **(A)**, some have more severe involvement of bone **(B)** and others have severe injuries of both bone and soft tissues **(C).**

include a few external factors which influence the outcome.[168] Retrospective design, small sample sizes, and a bias of the score designers in the selection of the component and weighting of the indices have been identified as disadvantages in these scores.[21,22,55,114] These scores also have been designed to address limbs which have combined orthopedic and vascular injuries and they are not suitable for evaluating Gustilo IIIb injuries. A severely injured limb with large bone loss and crushing of the soft tissues, which will be a poor choice for salvage, will be grossly underweighted by the above scores if it does not have a vascular injury. This flaw in design will guide the treating

surgeon toward attempts at salvage and lead to a higher incidence of secondary amputation.[155] A prospective evaluation of their clinical use documented poor performance when applied to Gustilo IIIb injuries. These scores are also not easily applied and therefore not regularly used in practice.

Mangled Extremity Severity Score

The MESS,[104] although originally designed to address limbs with vascular damage, is frequently used to predict the likelihood of amputation in Gustilo IIIb injuries. The system is based on four criteria these being the energy of trauma that decides

TABLE 10-8 Components of Lower-Extremity Injury Severity Scoring Systems[22,168]

	Scoring Systems[a]					
	MESS	LSI	PSI	NISSSA	HFS-97	GHOIS
Age	X			X		X
Shock	X			X	X	X
Warm ischemia time	X	X	X	X	X	X
Bone injury		X	X		X	X
Muscle injury		X	X			X
Skin injury		X			X	X
Nerve injury		X		X	X	
Deep-vein injury		X				
Skeletal/Soft tissue injury	X			X		
Contamination				X	X	X
Time to treatment			X			
Comorbid conditions						X

[a]MESS, mangled extremity severity score; LSI, limb salvage index; PSI, predictive salvage index; NISSSA, nerve injury, ischemia, soft tissue injury, skeletal injury, shock and age of patient score; HFS-97, Hannover fracture scale (1997 version); GHOIS, Ganga Hospital open injury score.

the extent of skeletal and soft tissue injury, the presence and duration of limb ischemia, the presence of shock, and the age of the patient (Table 10-9). A score of >7 has been reported to predict amputation accurately in both retrospective and

TABLE 10-9 Mangled Extremity Severity Score (MESS)[104]

Type	Definition	Points
A	**Skeletal/soft tissue injury**	
	• Low energy (stab;simple fracture; "civilian" GSW)	1
	• Medium energy (open or multiple fractures; dislocation)	2
	• High energy (close-range shotgun or "military" GSW; crush injury)	3
	• Very high energy (above and gross contamination; soft tissue avulsion)	4
B	**Limb ischemia** (*Score doubled for ischemia >6 hours)	
	• Pulse reduced or absent but perfusion normal	1*
	• Pulseless; paraesthesia; diminished capillary refill	2*
	• Cool; paralysed; insensate; numb.	3*
C	**Shock**	
	• Systolic BP always >90 mm Hg	0
	• Hypotensive transiently	1
	• Persistent hypotension	2
D	**Age (years)**	
	• <30	0
	• 30–50	1
	• >50	2

prospective studies.[104] However it has not been duplicated in other prospective series in which an overall sensitivity rate of 46%, increasing to 72% when only ischemic limbs are considered, has been reported.[22] Our experience with this score has been the same. In the absence of a vascular deficit, severely injured limbs which are barely salvageable often score below 7 prompting attempts at salvage. This may increase the number of patients requiring secondary amputation.[168]

Ganga Hospital Open Injury Score

The GHOIS was described in 2005 by Rajasekaran et al.[154] to specifically address the issue of salvage and reconstruction pathways in Type IIIb injuries. It is shown in Table 10-10. The basis of the score is that the three components of a limb—covering tissues (skin), structural tissues (bone), and functional tissues (muscles, tendons, and nerves) are injured to different severity in every Type III injury and hence are graded separately by points ranging from one to five (Figs. 10-13 to 10-15). In addition, seven comorbidities that are known to influence the outcomes are given two points each. The total score is used to assess the need for amputation and the individual scores provide guidelines for management such as the need for a flap or the requirement for bone transport. The scoring involves a detailed assessment of the degree of injury of the different components of the limb and hence must be done after debridement.

In an initial study of 109 consecutive Type IIIb injuries, all limbs with a score of 14 and below were salvaged successfully. All limbs with a score of 17 and above required an amputation.[154] The injuries with a score of 15 and 16 were categorized to be in a gray zone. The unique feature of GHOIS was to recognize that there could not be a single cut off score in a complex clinical situation such as an open injury. The authors,

TABLE 10-10	Ganga Hospital Open Injury Score (GHOIS)[154]

Covering Structures: Skin and Fascia

• Wound with no skin loss and not over the fracture site	1
• Wound with no skin loss and over the fracture site	2
• Wound with skin loss and not over the fracture site	3
• Wound with skin loss and over the fracture site	4
• Wound with circumferential skin loss	5

Functional Tissues: Musculotendinous and Nerve Units

• Partial injury to musculotendinous unit	1
• Complete but repairable injury to musculotendinous units	2
• Irreparable injury to musculotendinous units, partial loss of a compartment, or complete injury to posterior tibial nerve	3
• Loss of one compartment of musculotendinous units	4
• Loss of two or more compartments or subtotal amputation	5

Skeletal Structures: Bone and Joints

• Transverse or oblique fracture or butterfly fragment <50% circumference	1
• Large butterfly fragment >50% circumference	2
• Comminution or segmental fractures without bone loss	3
• Bone loss <4 cm	4
• Bone loss >4 cm	5

Comorbid Conditions: Add Two Points for Each Condition Present

- Injury leading to debridement interval >12 hours
- Sewage or organic contamination or farmyard injuries
- Age >65 years
- Drug-dependent diabetes mellitus or cardiorespiratory diseases leading to increased anesthetic risk
- Polytrauma involving chest or abdomen with injury severity score >25 or fat embolism
- Hypotension with systolic blood pressure <90 mm Hg at presentation
- Another major injury to the same limb or compartment syndrome

---

- Injuries with a score equal to 14 or below are advised salvage.
- Injuries with score 17 and above usually end up in amputation.
- Injuries with score 15 and 16 fall into gray zone where decision is made on patient to patient basis.

while recommending salvage in all injuries with a score of <14 and that amputation should be considered in injuries with a score of >17 emphasized that there was a gray zone of scores 15 and 16 where the decision to salvage or amputate must be based on factors such as associated injuries, the expertise of the treating team, the social, educational, and cultural background of the patient, the personality of the patient and considerations of the cost where this was applicable.

In practice GHOIS has many advantages over both the Gustilo classification and MESS. These are listed in Table 10-11. At a threshold score of 14 the score was found to be more accurate than MESS in predicting the need for amputation and avoidance of secondary amputations.[155] The individual scores of the GHOIS were found to predict the need for soft tissue cover and the requirement for complex flap procedures.[155]

Ninety-five percent of patients with a skin score of <3 were treated successfully by simple wound management either by primary skin closure or skin grafting. In comparison, 92% of patients with a score of ≥4 required flap cover. The skeletal score was useful in predicting the nature of the reconstruction procedures that were required.[155] Injuries with a score of ≤2 were found to have a high rate of union without the need for bone grafting. Injuries with a bony score of 4 and 5 had a prolonged time to union and required additional surgical procedures. Injuries with a bone score of 4 may be treated with bone grafting alone as the defect was less than 4 cm whereas injuries with a bone score of 5 will require either a bone transport procedure or a free fibular graft procedure as the defect too large to manage by grafting alone.

Salvage or Amputation?

The decision to amputate or salvage a severely injured limb is an important, but often difficult, decision that requires experience.[90,91,190] Availability of advanced soft tissue reconstruction techniques using microsurgery and skeletal reconstruction devices has made limb salvage technically possible even in extreme cases. If not carefully chosen, the patient may be subjected to prolonged attempts at reconstruction with multiple surgeries but finally have a secondary amputation.[22,23,68,92,190,196] Every attempt must be made to avoid the "*triumph of technique over reason*" and a decision regarding the probability of amputation should be made during the index procedure or at least before the definitive soft tissue reconstruction procedure is attempted.

The need for primary amputation may be obvious in certain instances (Table 10-12). However many injured limbs fall into a gray zone where the availability of an objective assessment criteria would be helpful. The GHOIS, unlike the other scores that have been described for combined orthopedic and vascular injuries, has a better sensitivity and specificity for predicting amputation in Type IIIb injuries.[154,155] It must be remembered that no score is infallible and the final decision should depend on a combination of factors including severity of injury, the overall health status of the patient, the technical expertise of the treating team, and the suitability of the patient for prolonged surgical procedures. The patient and his or her family must also be actively involved in the decision at all stages.

TREATMENT OPTIONS

Debridement and Lavage

Thorough debridement is important if the risk of infection is to be minimized. Debridement is an active surgical procedure and not just wound washing. All foreign material and tissues that are contaminated or suspected to be avascular are systematically removed so that whatever is left behind is vascularized living tissue, devoid of contamination. A secondary aim of debridement is also to minimize risk factors for infection such as dead space or hematoma so that the incidence of infection is reduced.

Debridement should be done as soon as possible after injury and the traditional teaching was that it preferably be completed (*text continues on page 371*)

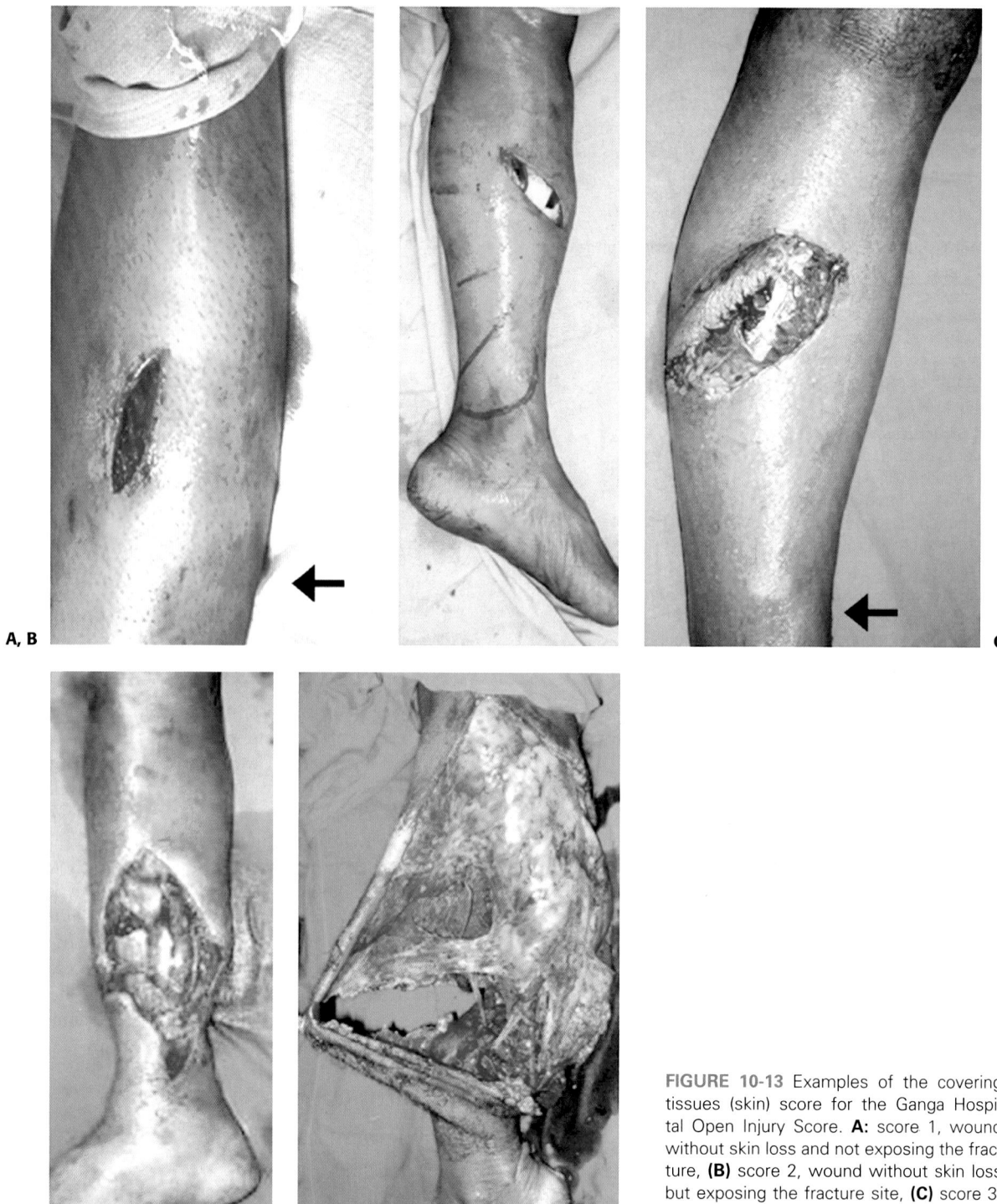

A, B

C

D

E

FIGURE 10-13 Examples of the covering tissues (skin) score for the Ganga Hospital Open Injury Score. **A:** score 1, wound without skin loss and not exposing the fracture, **(B)** score 2, wound without skin loss but exposing the fracture site, **(C)** score 3, wound with skin loss and not over the fracture site, **(D)** score 4, wound with skin loss and over the fracture site, and **(E)** score 5, circumferential wound with bone circumferentially exposed.

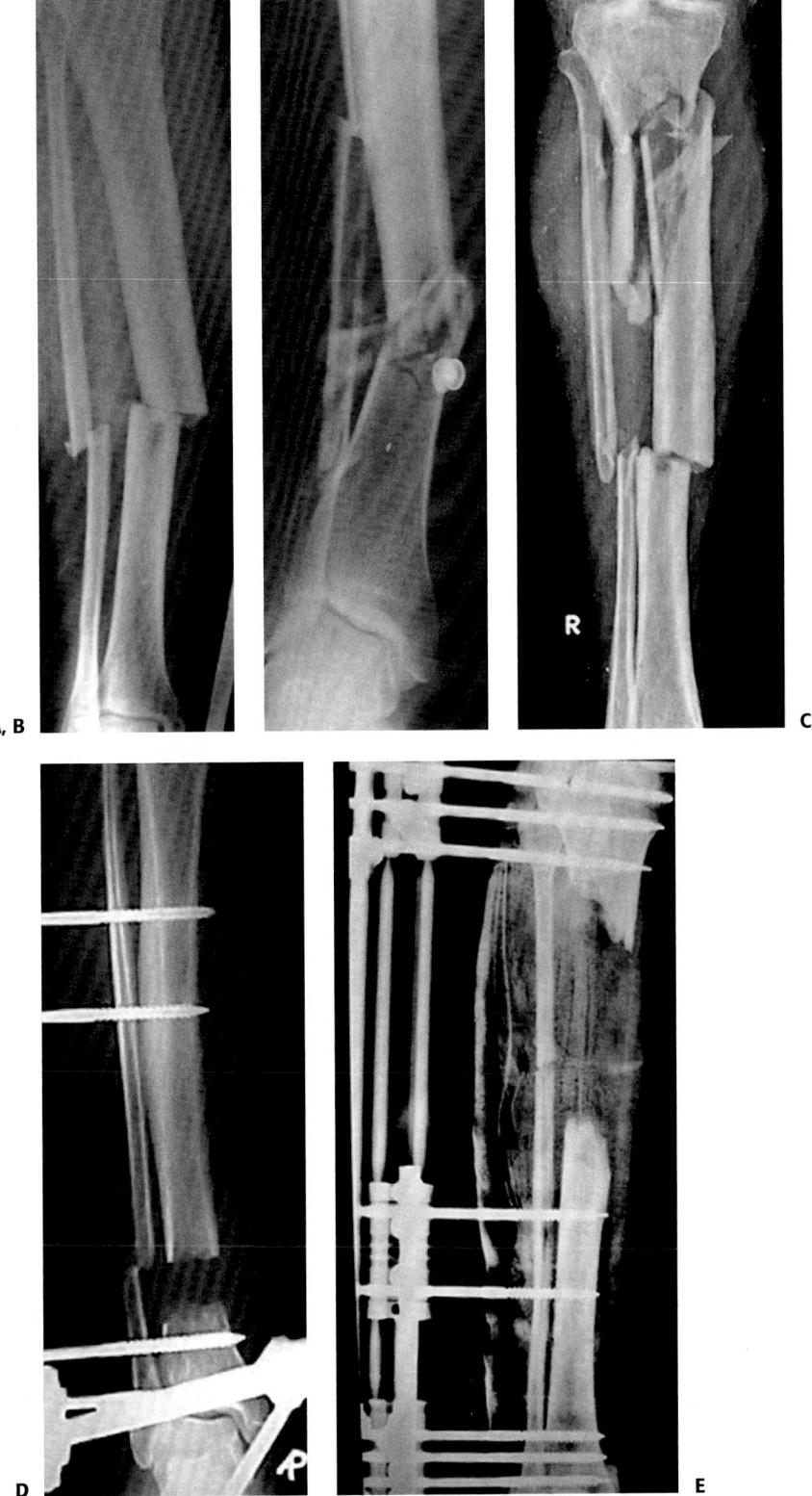

FIGURE 10-14 Examples of the structural tissues (bone) score for the Ganga Hospital Open Injury Score. **A:** score 1, transverse or oblique fractures or a butterfly fragment involving less than 50% of the circumference. **B:** score 2, the presence of a large butterfly fragment involving more than 50% of the circumference **(C)** score 3, extensively comminuted or segmental fractures without loss of bone. **D:** score 4, primary or secondary loss of bone of less than 4 cm **(E)** score 5 loss of more than 4 cm.

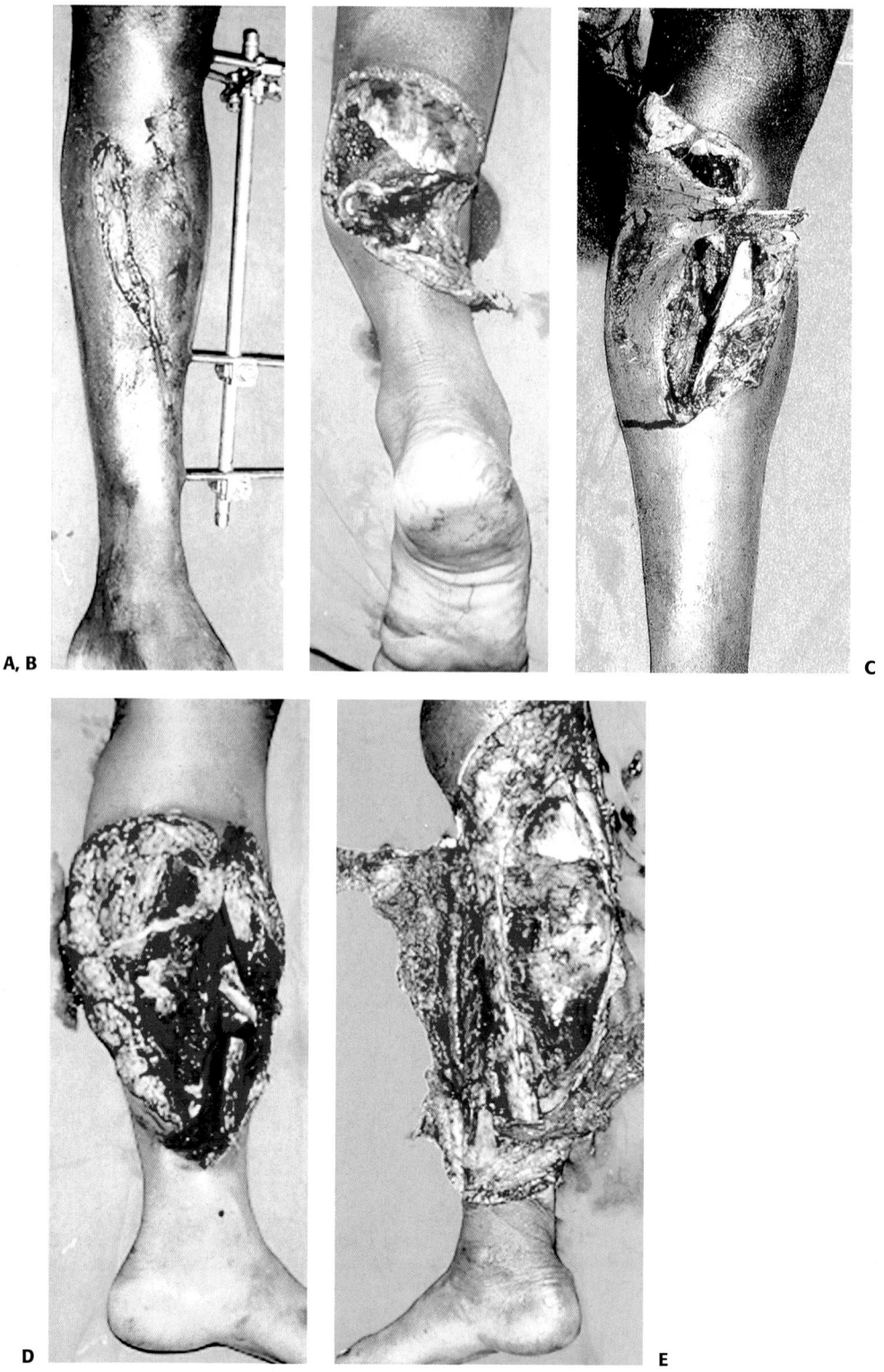

FIGURE 10-15 Examples of the functional tissues (muscles, tendons, and nerves) score for the Ganga Hospital Open Injury Score **(A)** score 1, partial injury to musculotendinous units, **(B)** score 2, complete but repairable injury to musculotendinous units, **(C)** score 3, irreparable injury to musculotendinous units involving one or more muscles in a compartment or complete injury to the posterior tibial nerve, **(D)** score 4, loss of one entire compartment **(E)** score 5, loss of two or more compartments or subtotal amputation.

TABLE 10-11	Advantages of Ganga Hospital Open Injury Score

- Specifically designed for Type IIIb injuries.
- Assesses severity of injury to skin, muscle, bone separately.
- Total score predicts amputation.
- Individual score provides guidelines for reconstruction.
- Scoring includes comorbidities which influences outcome.
- Better intra- and interobserver agreement compared to Gustilo classification.

within 6 hours. The aim was to prevent contamination from becoming infection and early debridement will prevent colonization of the bacteria within the tissues. The basis of the 6-hour rule was animal studies where a threshold of 10^3 organisms was found to be critical to establish infection.[159] This limit was achieved in 5.17 hours. Others have also documented that a colony count of this level can overrun the immune defenses and lead to infection.[42] This led to the practice of debridement being done even in the middle of the night when an experienced work force was often not available. The 6-hour rule has been challenged by many recent studies.[32,45,149,164,183] Current literature suggests no obvious advantage in performing debridement within 6 hours compared to debridement performed between 6 and 24 hours after injury.[45] The effect of delaying debridement >24 hours is however not yet clear.[193] Although debridement must be done as soon as safely possible, the thoroughness of debridement seems to be more important than the timing. There are also other local and systemic factors that influence infection and wound healing. These are listed in Table 10-13.

Debridement should be done by an experienced team of both orthopedic and plastic surgeons. An "Orthoplastic approach" involving the plastic surgeon right from the time of debridement has numerous advantages. The combined experience of both specialists in the assessment of soft tissue and skeletal injury will improve debridement and favor early reconstruction without compromising further reconstruction.[25,43] In heavily contaminated wounds, thorough washing with copious amounts of saline is advisable before draping the limb. We

TABLE 10-12	Indications for Primary Amputation

- Warm ischemia time over 8 hours and the limb is completely nonviable.
- Vascular injury which is nonrepairable with no collateral flow seen in arteriograms.
- Limb is severely crushed with minimal viable tissue.
- Presence of severe and debilitating systemic diseases where lengthy surgical procedures to preserve the limb will endanger life.
- Presence of severe multisystem injuries with an injury severity score of 25 or more where salvage may lead to MODS and death.
- Damage is so severe that ultimate function will be less satisfactory than with a prosthesis.
- Ganga hospital open injury severity score 17 and above.

TABLE 10-13	Factors Increasing Risk for Infection

Local Factors
- Organic, farm yard, or sewage contamination.
- Poor debridement with retention of foreign debris and nonviable tissues.
- Inadequate skeletal stabilization.
- Presence of dead space.
- Debridement later than 24 hours.

Systemic Factors
- Presence of shock and ARDS
- Comorbid factors like age above 65 years, metabolic disorders like diabetes mellitus, history of smoking.
- Compartment syndrome and hypovascular tissues.
- Prolonged hospital stay and exposure to resistant organisms.
- Poor nutrition.

utilize specially made trolleys for washing the wound before draping and mesh trays of different sizes with outlet tubing for lavage after draping. A soft brush may be used to aid cleaning of dirt particles and debris. It is preferable to apply a tourniquet to the limb before washing. This will allow quick control of severe hemorrhage which may occur rarely during the stage of lavage either by displacement of a clot or from an injury to an exposed, partially damaged vein.

Lavage

Lavage is used before and after debridement as it clears the debris and hematoma and provides optimal exposure and reduces contamination and the bacterial count.[6,4,46,108,134,158] Adequate quantity of lavage fluid must be used for cleaning on the principle that the "solution for pollution is dilution." Typically more than 9 L of fluid is required in Type IIIb injuries. Evidence supporting the use of lavage in open injuries is given in Table 10-14. There has been considerable debate

TABLE 10-14	Wound Lavage in Open Injuries

Evidence Supports
- Adequate quantity of fluid must be used for lavage. Typically at least 9 L of fluid are used for Type III B fractures.
- Lavage clears blood clot, nonviable tissues and debris from tissue planes and dead spaces.
- Lavage reduces bacterial population.
- No advantage in adding antiseptic solutions or antibiotics to lavage fluid.
- Use of hydrogen peroxide, alcohol solution, povidone iodine, and other chemical agents may impair osteoblast function, inhibit wound healing and cause cartilage damage.
- High pressure pulsatile lavage can reduce bacterial load by 100-fold but has a disadvantage of microscopic damage to the bone, considerable soft tissue damage and may push the bacteria contamination to deeper tissue plane.
- Low-pressure pulsatile lavage (14 psi @ 550 pulsations per minute) is equally effective as high pressure pulsatile lavage (70 psi @ 1,050 pulsation per minute) and has less harmful effects on tissues.

regarding the use of soap solutions,[5,41] the addition of antibiotics to the lavage fluid[52,160] and the use of high and low-pressure lavage.[12,15,28,51,54,115] Current evidence indicates that normal saline should be routinely used as there is no advantage in adding any soap, antiseptic, or antibiotic to the fluid.[46] The use of betadine has also no advantage but has the disadvantage of staining the tissues and obscuring contamination and small dirt particles.[24,70,120] It is also possibly toxic to tendon sheaths, cartilage, and periosteum. High-pressure lavage, which was once popular, is now not used as it has not shown any advantage. It may also have the disadvantage of damaging tissues such as periosteum and tendon sheaths and it may also push dirt and debris deeper into the tissues. At present, low-pressure lavage with normal saline is preferred.[46] Debridement must be done in a systematic fashion with proper attention to the thorough removal of devitalized tissues. It is outlined in Table 10-15.

TABLE 10-15 **Principles of Debridement**

Debridement Principles
- Must be performed by an experienced team and as early as possible.
- Orthoplastic approach with involvement of plastic surgeons even at the time of index surgery.

Steps
- Pre-debridement photographs are taken in different angles.
- Use of tourniquet allows a clear, bloodless field.

Skin and Fascia
- Wounds must be longitudinally extended to provide adequate visualization of deeper structures.
- Margins must be trimmed to bleeding dermis to create a clean wound edge.
- Gentle handling of the skin and prevention of degloving are essential.
- All avascular fascia must be excised.

Muscles
- All muscles in the compartment must be evaluated for viability ("4 C" Color, Consistency, Contractility, Capacity to bleed) and debrided.

Bone
- Bone ends and medullary cavity must be carefully examined for impregnated paint, mud, and organic material.
- All fragments without soft tissue attachment must be excised.

Lavage
- Adequate quantity of fluid with low-pressure pulsatile lavage is preferable.

Completion
- Deflate tourniquet and evaluate viability of all retained structures.
- Assess loss of tissues and document with photograph for future reference and planning.
- Decide on method and timing of wound closure or coverage and bone stabilization.
- Document sequence of reconstruction.
- In very severe tissue loss VAC may be used as a bridging procedure till the patient is fit for flap cover.

The Use of Tourniquets

There is controversy regarding the use of a tourniquet during debridement. The traditional teaching is not to use a tourniquet during debridement as it may injure the already hypoxic tissues and will also interfere with the assessment of muscle viability.[166] However, our experience is the opposite and we routinely use a tourniquet as it improves the thoroughness of debridement and prevents unnecessary blood loss. In a limb without vascular deficit there is no proof that application of a tourniquet for the period of debridement, which ranges from 30 to 60 minutes, has any deleterious effects on the retained viable tissues. Without a tourniquet, the injured tissues bleed easily if touched and this disturbing bleeding often hampers the surgeon's vision and hides contamination, especially in the deeper muscular planes. In contrast, a bloodless field helps to identify contamination, protect the vital structures, explore the joint cavities and also save unnecessary blood loss in a patient who may already be in shock. At the end of the debridement, the tourniquet is released and the viability of all retained tissues can be ascertained reliably. Viable muscles appear pale while under tourniquet and blush immediately on release, whereas avascular muscles appear dark red even while under tourniquet with no change after release of the tourniquet. With experience we have found that it is much easier to identify nonviable muscles under tourniquet than in a bloody field. We attribute our high success rate of early reconstruction with low infection to our routine protocol of performing debridement under tourniquet. The use of loupes also facilitates the identification of dirt and contamination and helps to improve the quality of debridement.

Superficial Debridement

Debridement of the skin begins with assessment of the orientation of the wound, its margins, the quality of the skin surrounding the wound, and the presence of any flaps or closed degloving. Irrespective of the initial orientation, wounds must be extended using extensile incisions for proper inspection of the deeper tissues. The length of incision depends upon the nature of injury. Typically longer incisions are required for more severely contaminated wounds and wounds over a joint to allow proper inspection of all parts of the joint. Extension of skin incisions must be done without separating the skin from the deep fascia as this may decrease viability and increase hematoma formation. Debridement of the skin must be undertaken without a tourniquet as the extent of skin resection is usually decided by the presence of bleeding skin edges. All nonviable, shredded, and irregular margins of the skin must be gradually trimmed so that only healthy skin remains. Although nonviable skin must not be retained, indiscriminate removal of skin flaps must be avoided. Viable skin flaps can cover exposed bone and help to limit the extent of soft tissue reconstruction that is required. Distally based skin flaps have less vascularity than proximally based skin flaps but flaps with a large base often have sufficient vascularity to allow good healing (Fig. 10-16). Whenever the viability of a flap is in doubt, it is better to retain the skin for debridement during the secondary procedure. Special attention must be paid to debridement of the fascia as retaining nonviable

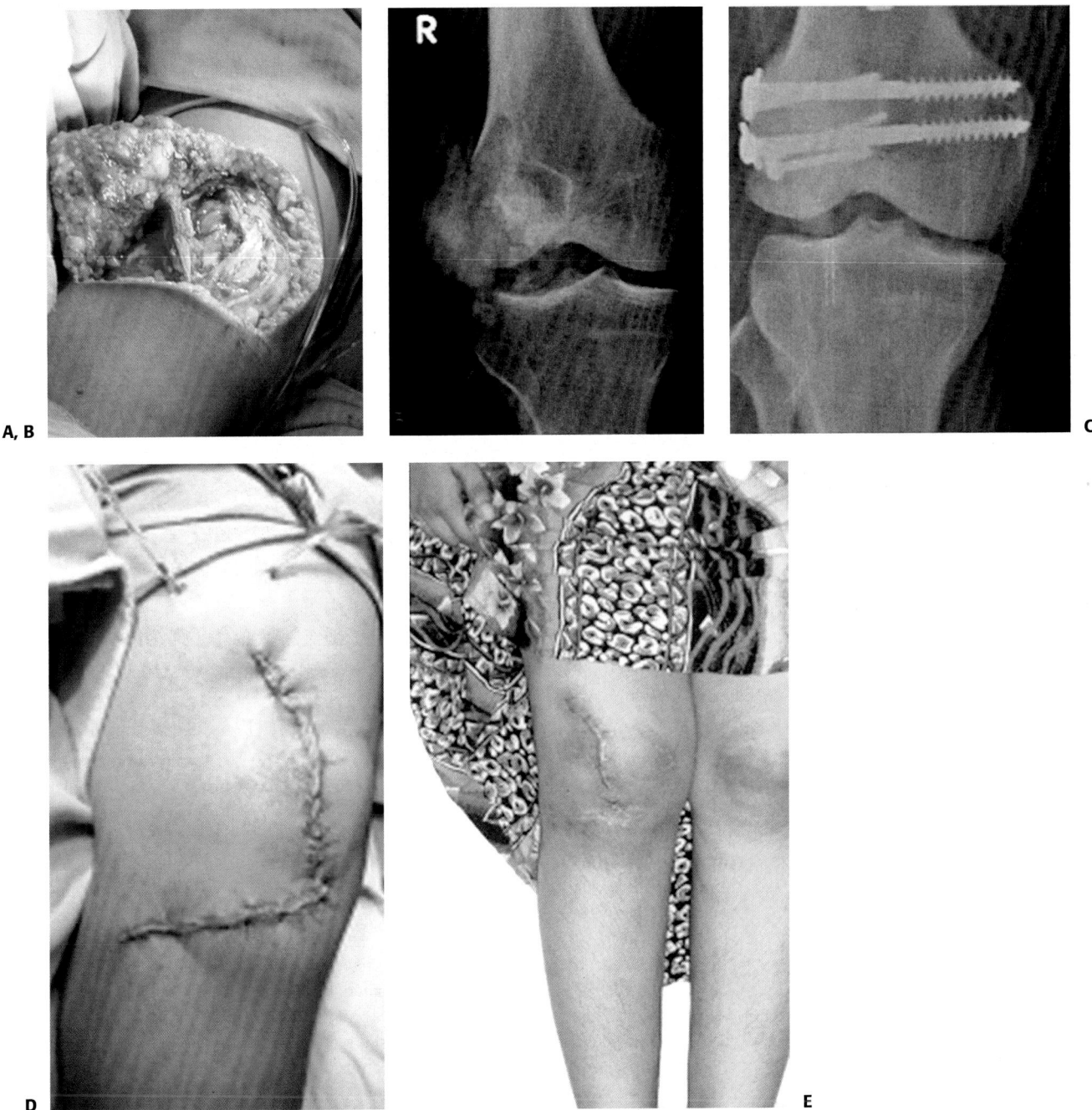

FIGURE 10-16 Large skin flaps, especially over the joints, may be viable and can be retained with great benefit. Here, an open injury of the lower end of the femur has a large flap **(A, B)** which satisfied the requirements for primary closure which was done after suitable internal fixation **(C, D)**. Primary healing of both the skin **(E)** and bone were achieved.

fascia often causes infection. Fascia which is detached, shredded, or even doubtfully nonviable must be excised.

Deep Debridement

Debridement of the muscles and deeper structures must be done with great care. An aggressive approach to muscle debridement must be adopted as retained necrotic muscle is a major growth medium for bacteria and greatly increases the risk of

anaerobic infection. Classically muscle viability is assessed by the four C's: Contractability, Color, Consistency, and Capacity to bleed.[148] Different authors have reported differently on the relative importance of these four parameters. We feel that accurate judgment comes with experience but where there is doubt it is better to excise than retain dubiously vascularized muscle. If a tourniquet is used, viable muscles appear pale while under tourniquet and blush immediately on release, whereas

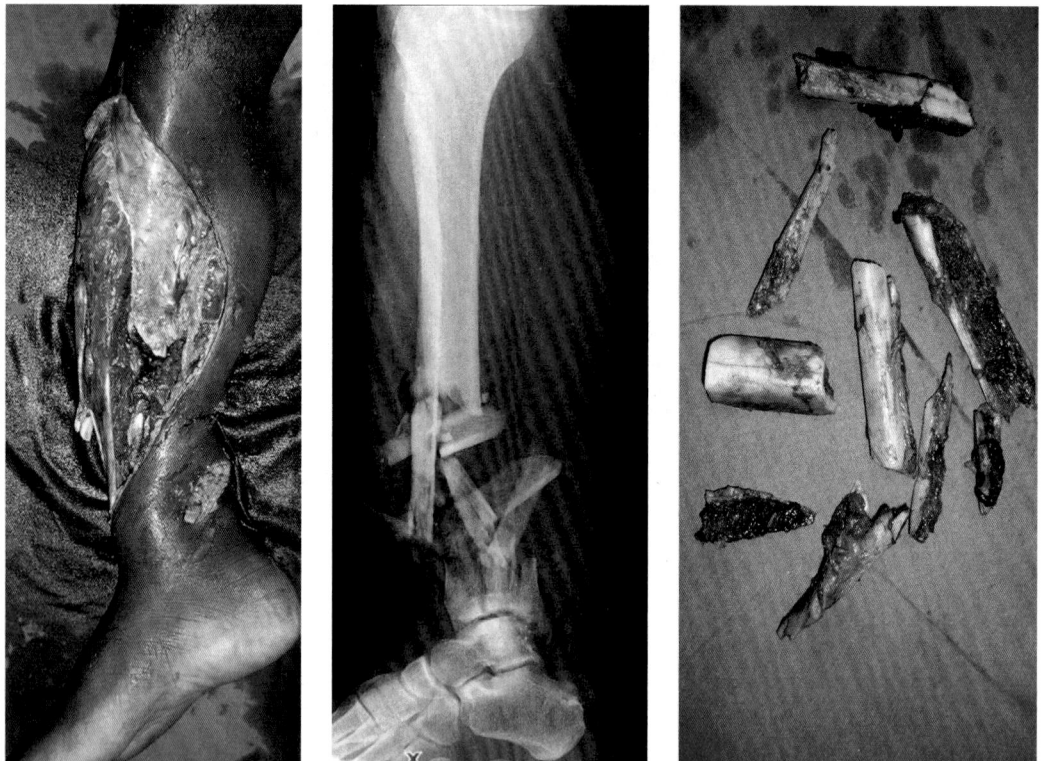

A, B   **C**

FIGURE 10-17 Comminuted cortical bone fragments without soft tissue attachments are avascular and nonviable. **(A, B)** They must be removed **(C)** as retaining them may result in infection.

avascular muscles appear dark red even while under tourniquet with no change after release of the tourniquet.

Muscles may be damaged quite extensively even in the presence of a small external wound. Careful examination of all muscles of the different compartments is required to rule out occult muscle damage. Proximal avulsion of entire muscle bellies with complete devascularization of the muscles is common in the forearm and this should be recognized. This will require the excision of the entire muscle bellies but the tendons can be retained and tethered to intact muscles in a later reconstructive procedure. However, the tendons and tendon sheaths are highly susceptible to drying and desiccation and care must be taken to protect them under skin flaps or bury them under muscles.

Bone

Bone damage varies considerably with the site of the injury and may be independent of the damage to the soft tissues. The decision to retain or discard damaged bone is done on the basis of vascularity and whether the fragments are from the diaphysis, metaphysis, or the articular margins. Retained avascular bone is a rich source of infection and diaphyseal fragments, regardless of their size, which are devoid of soft tissue attachments must be removed (Fig. 10-17). It is not clear how much soft tissue attachment is required for viability but pieces with less than 50% soft tissue attachment should be considered to have poor viability. If preserved, they should be carefully examined during subsequent relook surgery to reassess their viability. Large bone fragments may be used temporarily to achieve length and align-

ment after thorough cleaning. Once stabilization is complete, they can then be discarded. In contrast to diaphyseal bones, metaphyseal bones, which are purely cancellous, have a higher capacity for revascularization and integration and can be preserved if not grossly contaminated. Cancellous bone involving the articular surface is usually retained so that reconstruction of the joint surface is possible.[139] (Fig. 10-18). In the ankle, foot and carpal regions, entire tarsal and carpal bones may sometimes be extruded. We have frequently retained such bones, if not severely contaminated, with good results. If there is metaphyseal comminution adjacent to a joint, the retained bone fragments must be stably fixed so that the complications of secondary loss of bone, joint incongruity ,and infection are reduced.

In injuries where the fractured ends of the bones have been exposed, there may be deep impregnation of paint, mud, and other organic material in the fractured bone ends. This is often difficult to completely remove by cleaning and ideally the contaminated bone should be resected to clean the bone. In sports and farmyard injuries, there can be considerable mud and dirt inside the medullary canal which should be carefully curetted and cleaned. If necessary, the bone ends must be delivered out of the wound for proper inspection and cleaning. Otherwise, fulminant deep infection can ensue which may lead to amputation.

It is important that during debridement, the surgical team should focus only on adequacy of debridement without being concerned about the ease of reconstruction. Modern methods of microvascular soft tissue reconstruction and bone transport allow successful reconstruction but only in the absence

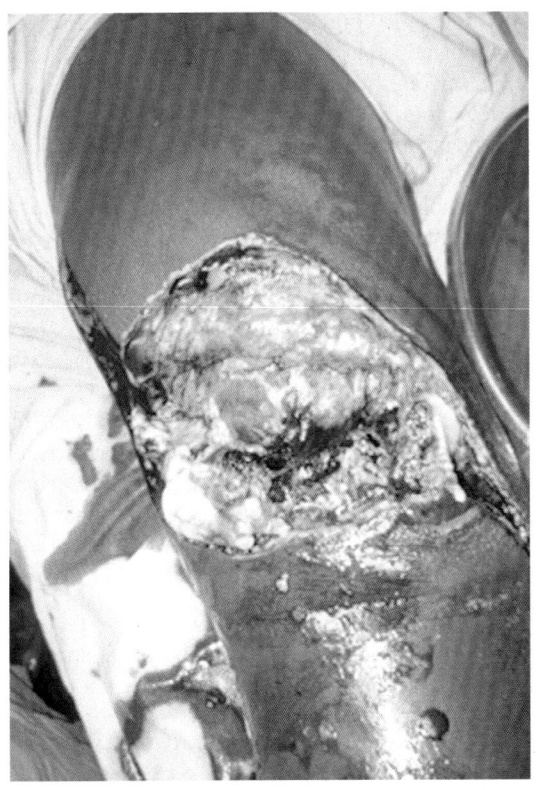
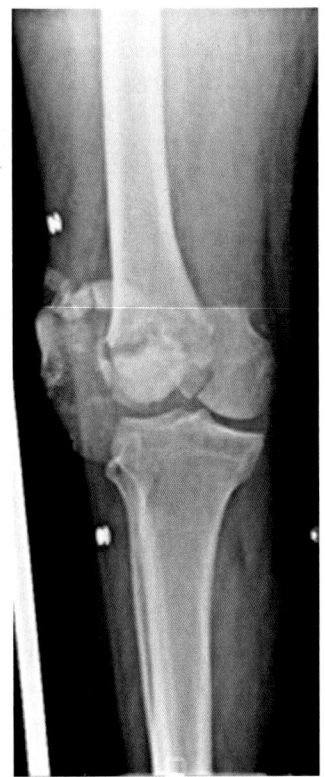

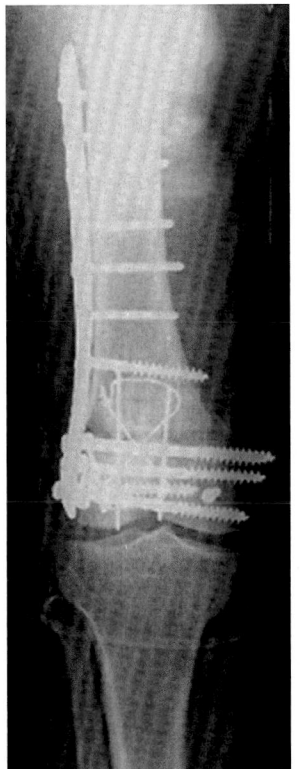
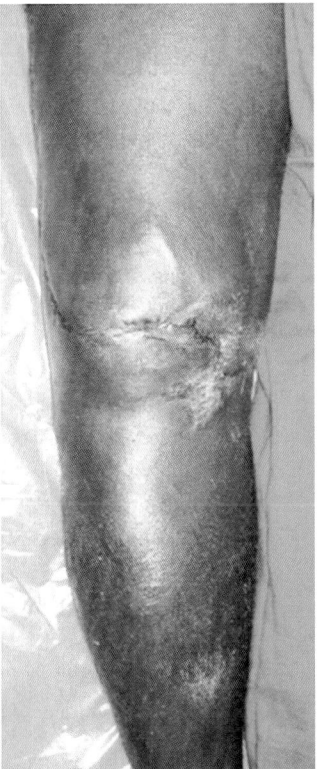

FIGURE 10-18 Metaphyseal fragments, with attached articular surfaces, can be retained even if they are devoid of soft tissue attachments. In this case the femoral condylar fragments were found to be freely floating without soft tissue attachments **(A, B).** The lower end of femur was reconstructed and primary skin closure undertaken. Both bone and soft tissue healing were achieved **(C, D).**

of infection. A large, clean wound has a higher chance of successful reconstruction than a smaller but inadequately debrided wound. Errors of judgment by the less experienced at this stage are an important cause of complications and failure.

Skeletal Stabilization

It is good practice to discard the instruments and table that are utilized during debridement and use a separate set of fresh instruments for skeletal stabilization so that contamination is avoided. In cases of severe organic contamination, it is also advisable to redrape the limb and for the surgical team to rescrub before reconstruction is undertaken.

Stable skeletal stabilization must be achieved as it helps to alleviate pain and prevent further soft tissue damage. During skeletal stabilization the length of the limb must be restored as this restores the correct tension to the soft tissues and this decreases swelling, improves circulation, and aids venous and lymphatic return. It also increases the comfort of the patient during wound inspection and facilitates early rehabilitation and movement of joints.

Skeletal stabilization should be undertaken quickly especially in the setting of vascular deficit and it must be designed to allow future soft tissue reconstruction. A variety of stabilization methods are available and the choice depends on the morphology of the fracture and the planned reconstructive procedures. In high-energy injuries associated with contamination, our preference is to use a temporary external fixator device followed by secondary internal fixation at a later operation.

In situations where there is a good soft tissue envelope as in upper limb and femoral fractures or in situations where soft tissue cover could be achieved within 48 to 72 hours primary internal fixation can be considered. The choice of plate or nailing depends on the location of injury. As a general rule, we have found that plate fixation is preferable for all open upper limb injuries and periarticular injuries with or without articular surface involvement. Lower limb diaphyseal fractures are usually treated by IM nailing either as a primary or secondary procedure. However there are many exceptions to these rules and individual decisions need to be done on a patient to patient basis.

Plaster Casts and Traction

Plaster casts and traction are now rarely used in open injuries. Wound inspection and dressing is very difficult and cast contamination can be unpleasant and increase the risk of infection. Casts also compromise the early detection of compartment syndrome, skin blistering, and skin necrosis. Puno et al.[150] reported an infection rate of >15% and a malunion rate of up to 70% in tibial fractures treated with plaster cast immobilization. Skeletal traction can be used in open pelvic fractures in addition to external fixation or in open femoral fractures for a short time till definitive treatment is planned.

External Skeletal Fixation

External fixation, especially half pin unilateral frames, is the workhorse for skeletal stabilization in open fractures as it provides a swift versatile method of providing stability without the need for additional exposure or periosteal striping even in demanding situations.[11] Ilizarov ring fixators and other ring fixators are used mainly in juxta-articular fractures with soft tissue injury and in fractures with bone loss.

External fixators are mainly used as temporary stabilizers with conversion to internal fixation being undertaken at an appropriate time. They can be used as a definitive treatment when a stable fracture configuration with good reduction and circumferential contact is achieved (Fig. 10-19). A meta-analysis of the treatment of open tibial diaphyseal fractures by Giannoudis et al.[66] reported a union rate of 94% at a mean of 37 weeks and an overall infection rate of 16.2%. Chronic osteomyelitis developed in 4.2% of fractures. External fixators also have a high rate of complications[62,172] the most common being pin loosening, infection, and malunion. Pin tract infection is the most frequent complication with external fixation and occurs in up to 32% of patients. This can lead to chronic osteomyelitis and make future conversion to IM nailing difficult. Utmost care should be exercised in the placement of the pins and during follow-up.[62]

The following points need emphasis.

(1) Whenever external fixation has to be maintained for a long period, pre-drilling should be done to minimize thermal necrosis as this may lead to pin loosening and infection.[33,197]

(2) The pins must be judiciously placed to allow further soft tissue reconstruction. The availability of a plastic surgeon at the time of debridement is valuable to plan the soft tissue reconstruction and place the pins suitably.

(3) Pins should be placed through intact soft tissues rather than through the open wound.[118]

(4) In the presence of degloving, further debridement may lead to further secondary loss of skin and the need to change pin sites.

(5) External fixators must be applied with good reduction of the fracture. When the fracture is distant from the open wound small pin incisions may be made in consultation with the plastic surgeons.

(6) Whenever conversion to internal fixation is planned in advance, care must be taken to avoid placing the pins in the line of future surgical incisions.

(7) In fractures with articular surface involvement, especially in fractures around the knee and elbow, joint congruity must be achieved on day 1 with appropriate internal fixation as late reconstruction of the joint surface is often not possible.

(8) Pins must be placed with a thorough knowledge of the regional anatomy so that injuries to the neurovascular structures are avoided.

(9) Pins should avoid joints and the capsular reflections of joints as any infection will lead to septic arthritis.[101] For example, proximal tibial pins should be placed 14 mm distal to the articular surface to avoid intra-articular placement.

(10) Muscle and tendon impalement must be avoided as entrapped musculotendinous units restrict movement

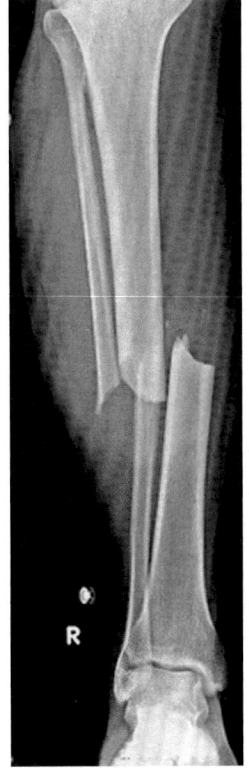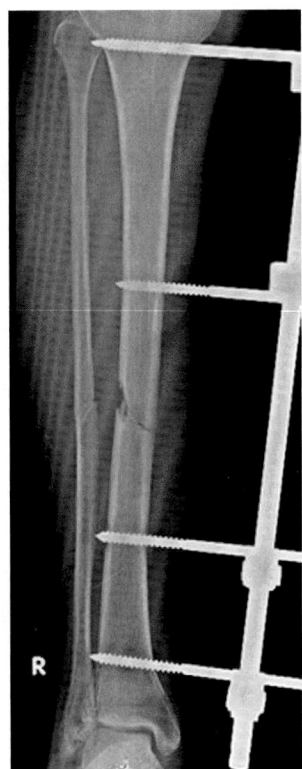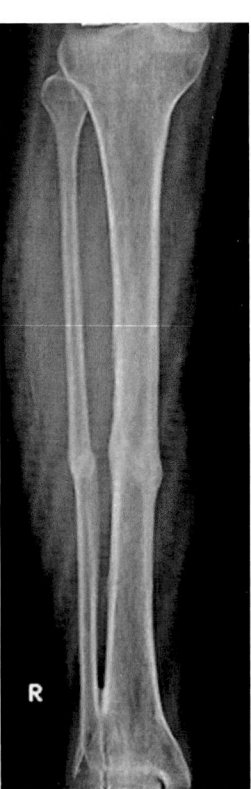

FIGURE 10-19 In patients where there is good circumferential bone contact, with a stable reduction, external fixation can be maintained until bone union is achieved.

and cause pain and discomfort.[56] Drill sleeves should be used and appropriate dissection of the soft tissues must be done to avoid critical soft tissue impalement.

Meticulous care of pin tracts is very important to avoid infection. The pin tracts must be cleaned with hydrogen peroxide and dressed every day with chlorhexidine solution or povidone iodine. Even a few days of neglect may result in a deep pin tract infection which will complicate the management of the fracture and delay the process of reconstruction.

Conversion to internal fixation, when needed, must be performed early provided there are no contraindications. In our experience[152,154,155] definitive internal fixation either by an interlocking nail or a plate is ideally performed before the stage of definitive soft tissue cover. Once a flap is performed, conversion has to be postponed to accommodate the flap settling time which may be between 3 and 4 weeks. There is a high chance of colonization of bacteria through the pin tracts at this time.[7,19,123–125] In a meta-analysis[16] it was demonstrated that conversion of external fixation to IM nailing in open tibial and femoral fractures within 28 days resulted in a reduced rate of infection of only 3.7% compared to 22% when performed later. In late conversions, an interval of 10 to 14 days between removal of the external fixator and internal fixation has also been advised.

Primary Internal Fixation

Primary internal fixation was considered unacceptable[38,165] even two decades ago due to the fear of increased infection and damage to the blood supply during the process of fixation. However, with refinement of the techniques of debridement, primary bone stabilization by interlocking nails and plate fixations are being increasingly performed with good results.[61,107] As a general rule, plate fixation is ideal for fractures of the upper limb. The choice between a locking nail and a plate for the lower limb bones is made depending on the fracture morphology, the instrumentation that is available and the surgeon's preference.

Plate Fixation

Internal fixation using plates[40,8] has the disadvantages of needing increased soft tissue exposure and periosteal stripping but these can be largely minimized by experience and careful technique. Plate fixation is the method of choice in most open upper limb fractures, femoral fractures involving the periarticular and articular regions, all intra-articular and juxta articular fractures, and in open injuries with vascular involvement (Fig. 10-20). If plate fixation is performed, a critical factor to maximizing the chances of success is achieving wound cover within 3 days. Locking plates provide internal fixation with greater stability but it should be stressed there are no large series reporting the outcome or superiority of locking plates.

Intramedullary Nails

Intramedullary nails are often the first choice for fixation of lower limb diaphyseal fractures as they provide superior biomechanical conditions and also maintain the length and rotation of the limb (Fig. 10-21). They are ideally suited for Gustilo Type I and II injuries and even in Type III injuries where contamination is

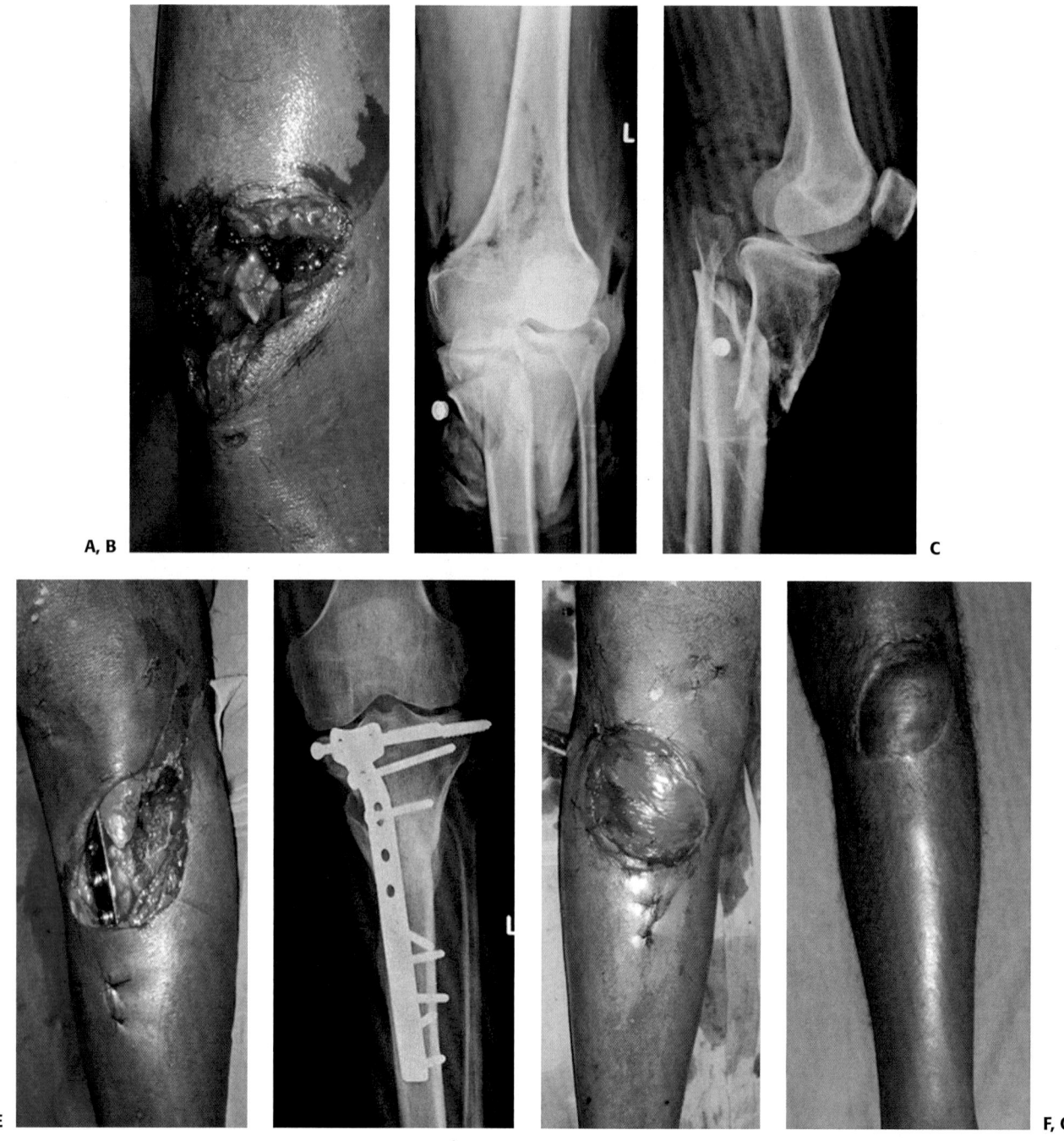

FIGURE 10-20 Plate fixation is the preferred form of skeletal stabilization in metaphyseal and articular fractures of both the femur and tibia. The figure shows a Type IIIb open fracture of the proximal tibia **(A, B, C)** which was stabilized with a plate **(D, E)**. A medial gastrocnemius flap was used for soft tissue cover **(F, G)**.

minimal and effective debridement has been performed. Giannoudis et al.[66] found a union rate of 95% for unreamed nails and 97% for reamed nails in open tibial fractures proving the safety and superiority of this method of skeletal fixation even in open injuries. Analysis showed that 15.5% of patients required bone grafting and 32% required an additional procedure to achieve bone union. The overall infection rate was 6% to 7%. Kakar and Tornetta[105] reported a very low rate of infection of only

3% and there are now many studies proving the advantages of primary nail fixation in open injuries.[79,105,119]

The decision to use reamed or unreamed nails was debated but now there are many studies which show the superiority of the reamed nail.[75] Some of the stated advantages and disadvantages are listed in Table 10-16. Unreamed nails appear more biologic[64] as they cause less devascularization,[163] are quicker to perform and have lower incidence of fat embolism and thermal

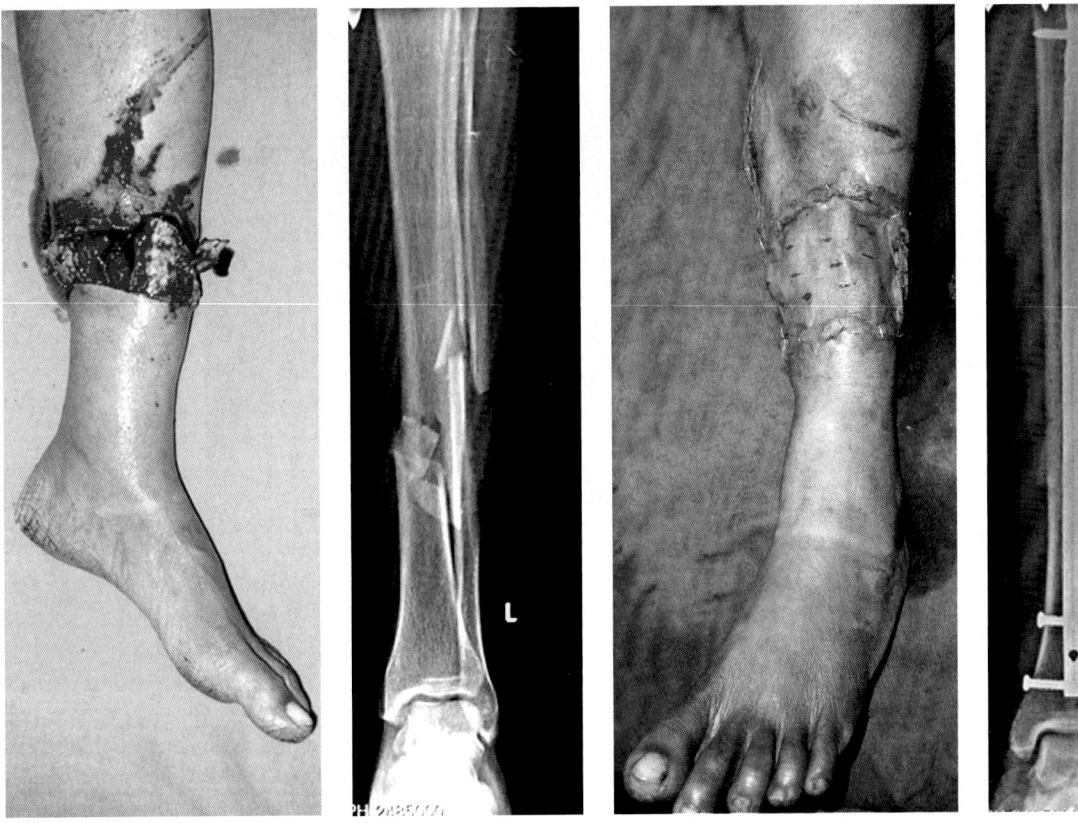

A, B

C, D

FIGURE 10-21 Tibial diaphyseal fractures are ideally stabilized with interlocking nails as they provide both longitudinal and rotational stability. In this case a comminuted Type IIIb fracture **(A, B)** has been treated with a locking nail and a rotational flap **(C, D).**

necrosis.[142] But they have the disadvantage of an increased rate of implant failure with screw and nail breakages, fracture disruption during surgery and a higher rate of nonunion and malunion. The general consensus is toward the use of reamed nailing, but over-reaming must be avoided to prevent thermal necrosis and infection. Adequate careful reaming allows the use of larger diameter nails that give better stability with reduced rates of hardware failure. The reamed products also stimulate osteogenesis at the fracture site which augments fracture healing. In a canine study, Klein et al.[109] documented damage to cortical blood flow of up to 70% in reamed nails but only 31% in unreamed nails. However, many trials including the SPRINT

trial[13] and different meta-analyses[14] have not proved any significant superiority of unreamed over reamed nailing in achieving bony union.

Acute Management of Bone Loss

Bone loss of varying degrees can occur due to primary bone loss at the time of accident or during primary or secondary debridement. Considerable experience is often required regarding the retention of comminuted bone fragments as there is no clear indication as to how much soft tissue attachment is required to maintain viability of the fragments. Although a low threshold is advised for retaining cortical fragments, metaphyseal fragments with cancellous bone and fragments containing articular margins are usually retained after adequate cleaning even when there is no soft tissue attachment. Although large bone gaps may tilt the balance toward amputation in many cases, the dictum that a larger bone gap without infection is a preferable to a smaller gap with nonviable bone must also be remembered.

Bone gaps in the upper limb can generally be managed by bone shortening followed by bone grafting. Whenever there is bone loss, the ends of the bone can be trimmed suitably so that there is a good contact for stable fixation. In the humerus, it is our experience that patients cope with shortening of even 4 cm very easily. There is rarely any residual weakness after adequate therapy. In the forearm, bone shortening must be very carefully

TABLE 10-16 Reamed versus Unreamed Nailing

Reamed Nailing
- Reamings function as autologous bone graft
- Induces a sixfold increase in periosteal blood flow
- Shorter union time with fewer nonunions
- Allows insertion of larger nails with increased stability.

Unreamed Nailing
- Higher rate of secondary interventions
- Patello-femoral complications are more common
- Smaller diameter nails with decreased stability
- Shorter operating time

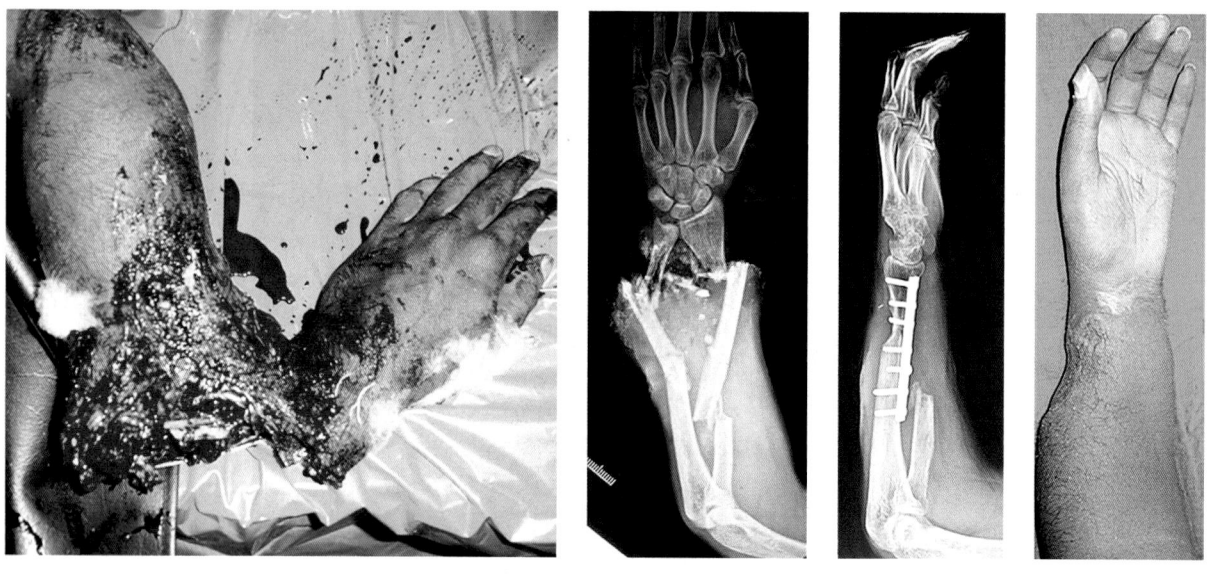

FIGURE 10-22 This patient presented with a severe mangled injury of the forearm and major bone loss involving both the radius and ulna **(A, B)**. A one-bone forearm reconstruction procedure was undertaken and a good result was achieved **(C, D)**.

done because of the presence of two bones. A differential loss of up to 2 cm in one bone can be easily managed by bone grafting the defect. If there is a very severe loss of either the radius or the ulna, reconstruction to create a single bone forearm is a viable option. In many mangled extremities, this option has not only allowed us quick and early reconstruction but has also made salvage possible avoiding amputation (Fig. 10-22).

In the lower limb, the extent of bone loss determines reconstruction options. A loss of less than 2 cm is well tolerated and

primary shortening can be safely done. When the loss is due to the removal of a large comminuted fragment, or when the circumferential loss is less than 3 cm, iliac crest bone grafting will usually suffice. The timing of bone grafting is determined by the status of the soft tissue bed and the soft tissue cover. Early or even immediate bone grafting has been reported to give good results depending upon the timing of soft tissue cover. When the loss exceeds 4 cm, a decision is made between primary bone shortening and subsequent lengthening (Fig. 10-23) or

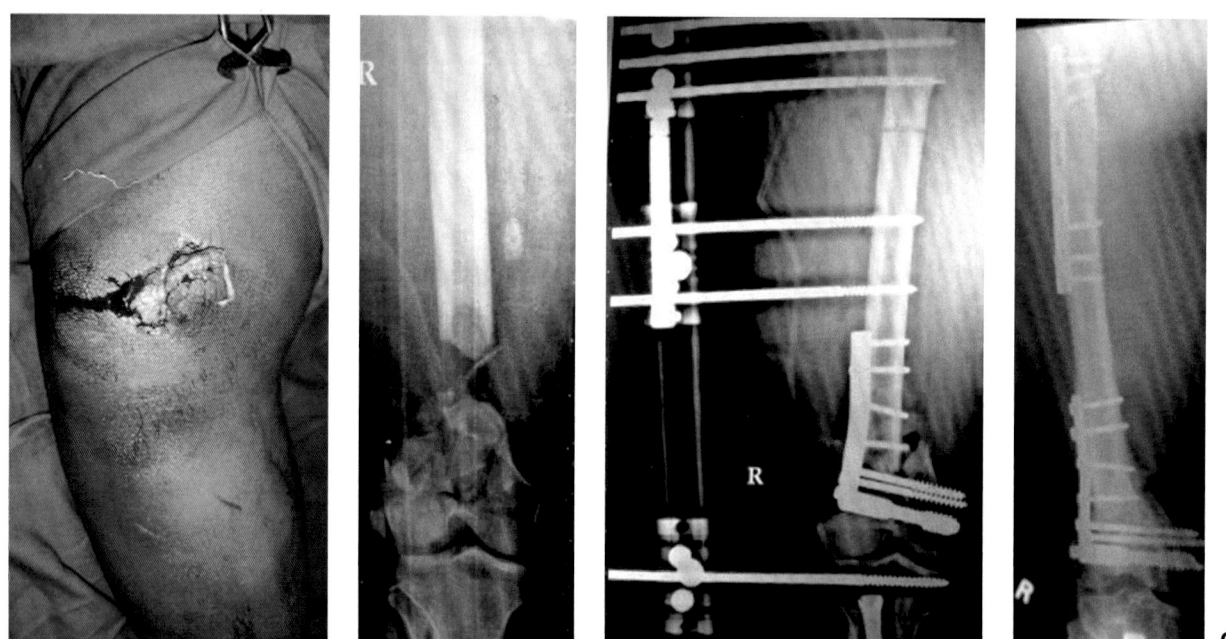

FIGURE 10-23 Acute bone shortening and lengthening. This patient presented with a Type IIIb open supracondylar femoral fracture with primary bone loss **(A, B)**. The patient was treated with acute shortening with lengthening at the subtrochanteric region **(C, D)**.

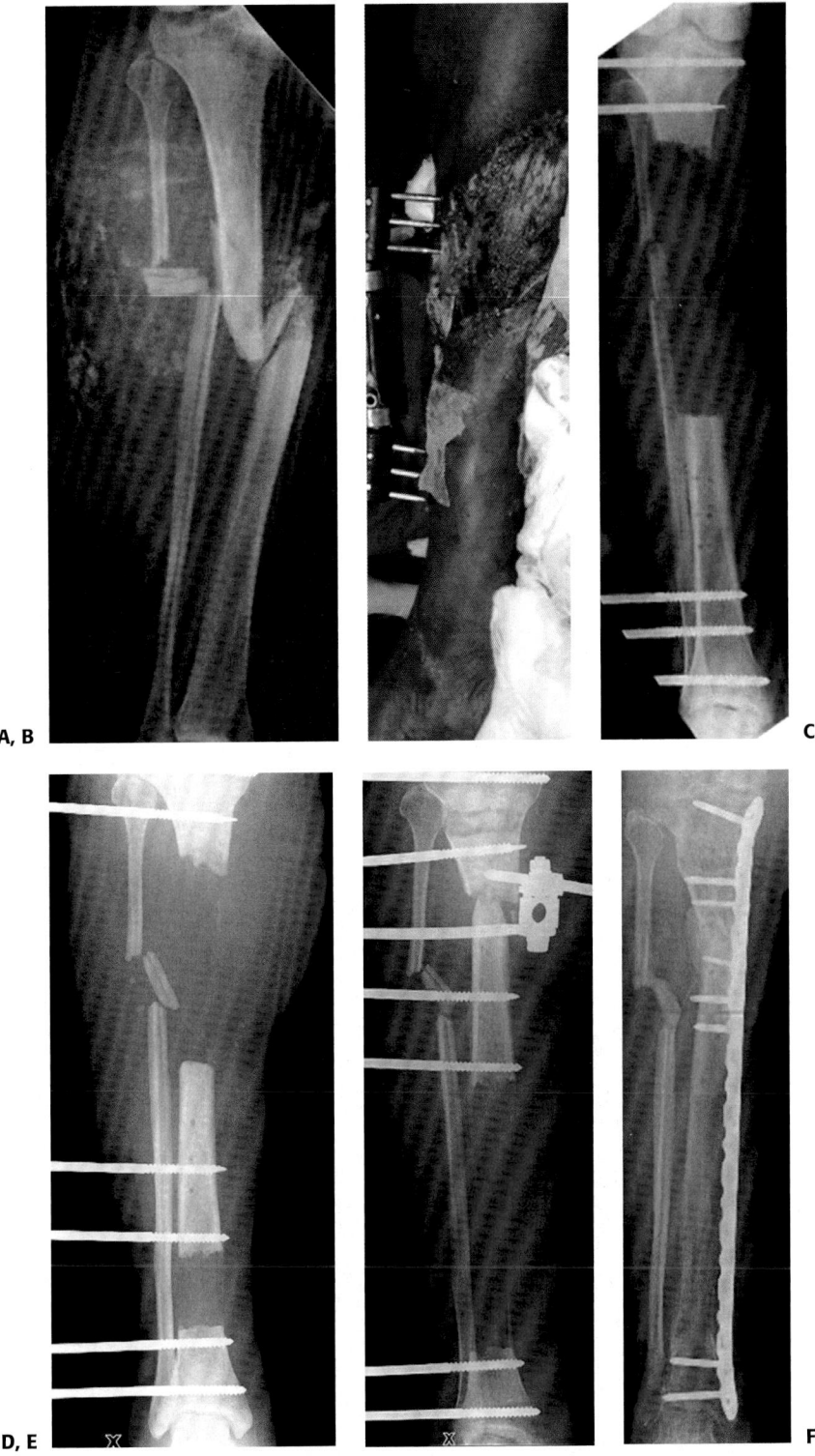

A, B

C

D, E

F

FIGURE 10-24 Large bone gaps of more than 4 cm cannot be treated by acute shortening. They are ideally treated by bone transport. This patient presented with a Type IIIb fracture with extensive soft tissue loss and fracture comminution **(A, B)**. Following debridement there was a considerable bone defect **(C)**. This was treated by bone transport **(D, E)** and subsequent plating **(F)**.

bridging the gap by bone transport (Fig. 10-24). Although ring fixators undoubtedly provide excellent stability and versatility of bone transport, they are not usually the primary choice in the acute phase. Loading a frame in the acute setting can be time consuming and cumbersome and can also interfere with future plastic surgical procedures. Unilateral limb reconstruction systems not only offer the advantages of ease and speed of application but they are also more patient and surgeon friendly and are equally effective in bone transport. (See Chapter 15 for further information about the management of bone defects.)

WOUND COVER

Primary Closure of Wounds

Although controversial, good results are being increasingly reported after primary skin closure[31,36,50,58,72,76,93,96,130,166,173,184] a concept that was advocated as early as 1948. Hope and Cole[97] in a series of tibial fractures in children reported an infection rate of 7.8% with primary closure compared with 14.6% with secondary closure. Cullen et al.[47] reviewed the records of 83 children with open fractures of the tibial metaphysis and diaphysis in which 57 wounds were closed primarily. Only two children developed superficial infection.

Recently Rajasekaran et al.[152] reported the results of immediate primary skin closure in Type III injuries using strict inclusion and exclusion criteria which are listed in Table 10-17. They have reported excellent results with only 3% deep infection rate. They emphasized that a GHOIS skin score of 1 or 2, a total score of less than 10, the presence of bleeding wound margins which could be opposed without tension and stable skeletal fixation were important (Fig. 10-25). Successful immediate closure was possible in 32% of the patients but they advised that the wounds be left open whenever there was doubt regarding the fitness for closure.

If primary closure is to be successful, the following points have to be kept in mind.

TABLE 10-17 Primary Closure of Open Wounds[155]

Indications
- Type I and II open injuries and III A and B injuries of limbs without vascular deficit.
- Wounds without primary skin loss or secondary skin loss after debridement.
- Ganga Hospital skin score of 1 or 2 and a total score of 10 or less.
- Injury to debridement interval less than 12 hours.
- Presence of bleeding wound margins which can be apposed without tension.
- Stable fixation achieved either by internal or external fixation.

Contraindications
- Type IIIC injuries.
- Ganga Hospital skin score of 3 or more and a total score of >10.
- Wounds in patients with severe polytrauma involving and an injury severity score >25.
- Sewage or organic contamination/farmyard injuries.
- Peripheral vascular diseases/thromboangiitis obliterans.
- Drug-dependent diabetes mellitus/connective tissue disorders/peripheral vasculitis.

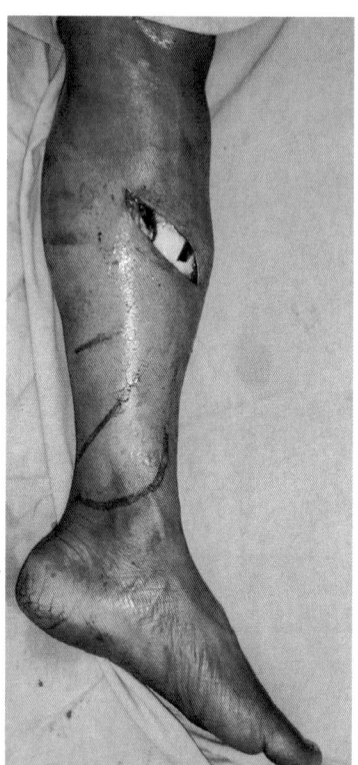
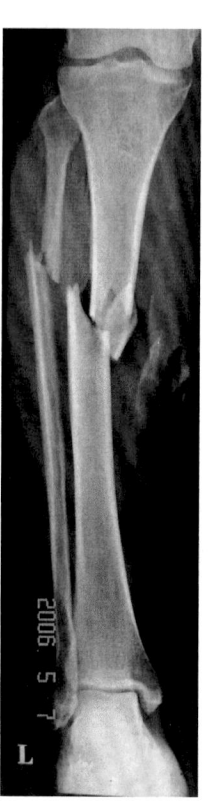
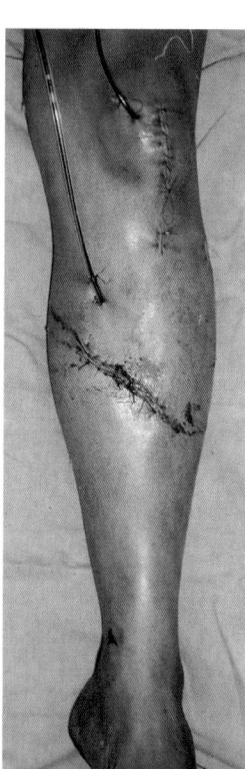
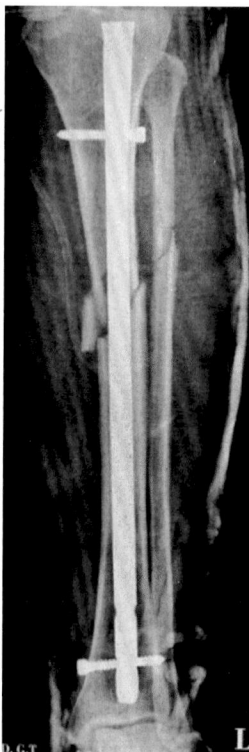

A, B　　　　　　　　　　　　　　　　　　　　　　　　　　　　　**C, D**

FIGURE 10-25 An open tibial fracture with a GHIOS score of 6 (skin 2, bone 2, and MTS 2) **(A, B)** which has been treated by primary closure and interlocking nail at the index procedure **(C, D)**. A good functional outcome was achieved without any complications **(E, F)**.

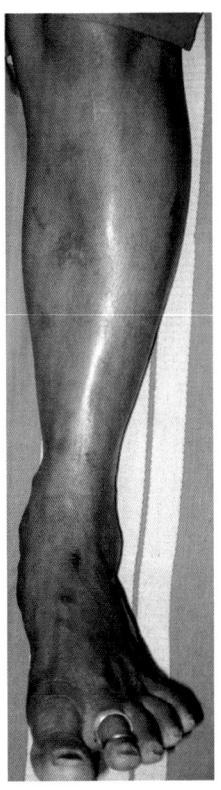
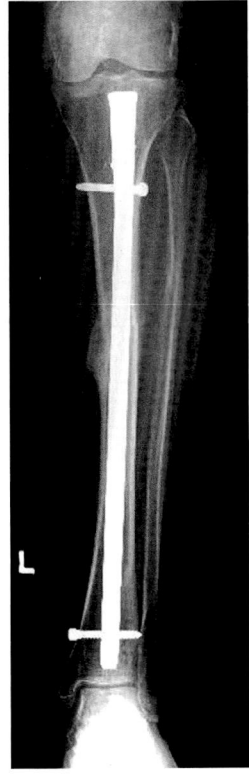

E   **F**

FIGURE 10-25 (*continued*)

1. When the patient initially presents in the emergency room, almost all open injuries appear to have skin loss. Because of shortening or angulation at the fracture site, the lacerated wound often gapes open exposing deeper structures and bone. In many cases, the margins will oppose easily when the fracture is reduced and limb length restored. (Fig. 10-26). Hence the assessment of skin and the ability to oppose the skin without tension should be done only after fracture reduction.

2. The length of the wound does not correlate with the ease with which the wound can be closed by primary closure. Lacerated wounds without skin loss can be closed, irrespective of the size of the wound, provided the skin can be opposed without tension (Fig. 10-27).

3. A GHOIS of ≥10 denotes a high-energy injury possibly with a crushing component. The zone of injury may not be obvious on day 1 or during the index procedure. These limbs have a tendency to swell up in the next few days and therefore are not suitable for primary closure.

4. Careful judgment is required in the presence of skin flaps. Flaps are common especially in wounds around the joints where there is loose skin on the extensor aspect. When the joint is flexed, these flaps retract making the wound appear very large. Many of these flaps, if viable, can be managed by primary closure when the joint is extended.

5. Flaps must be differentiated from closed degloving as the viability of the skin over degloved tissue is very poor.

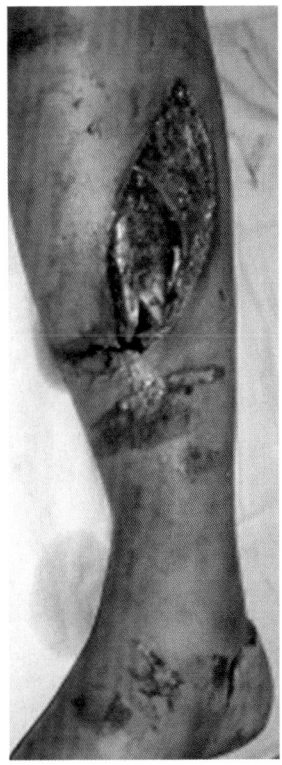
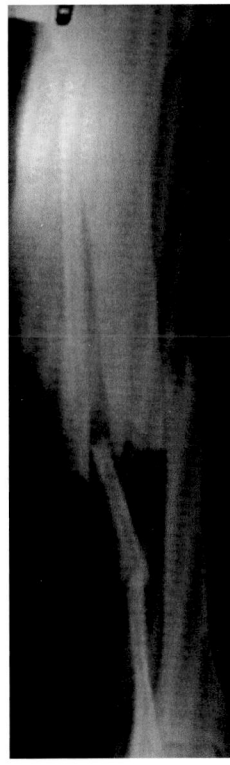
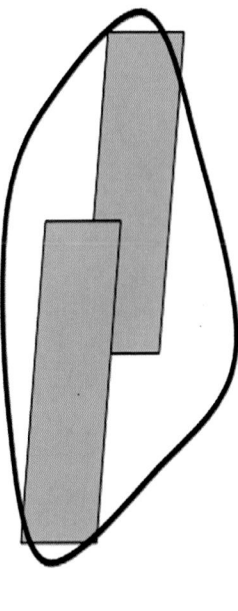

FIGURE 10-26 Assessment of skin loss requires experience and must be done after the skeletal length is restored. In the emergency room and during debridement, all lacerated wounds appear to have skin loss as they gape due to bone shortening and angulation **(A).**

(*continues*)   **A**

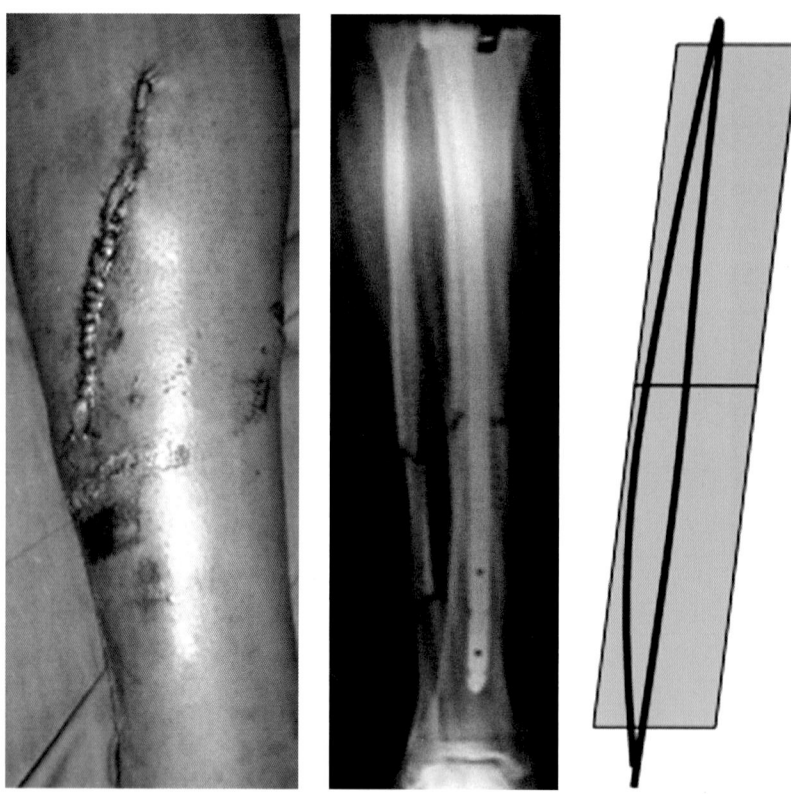

B

FIGURE 10-26 (*continued*) Once fracture reduction is achieved, the wound margins usually come together and primary closure is possible in nearly one-third of injuries **(B).**

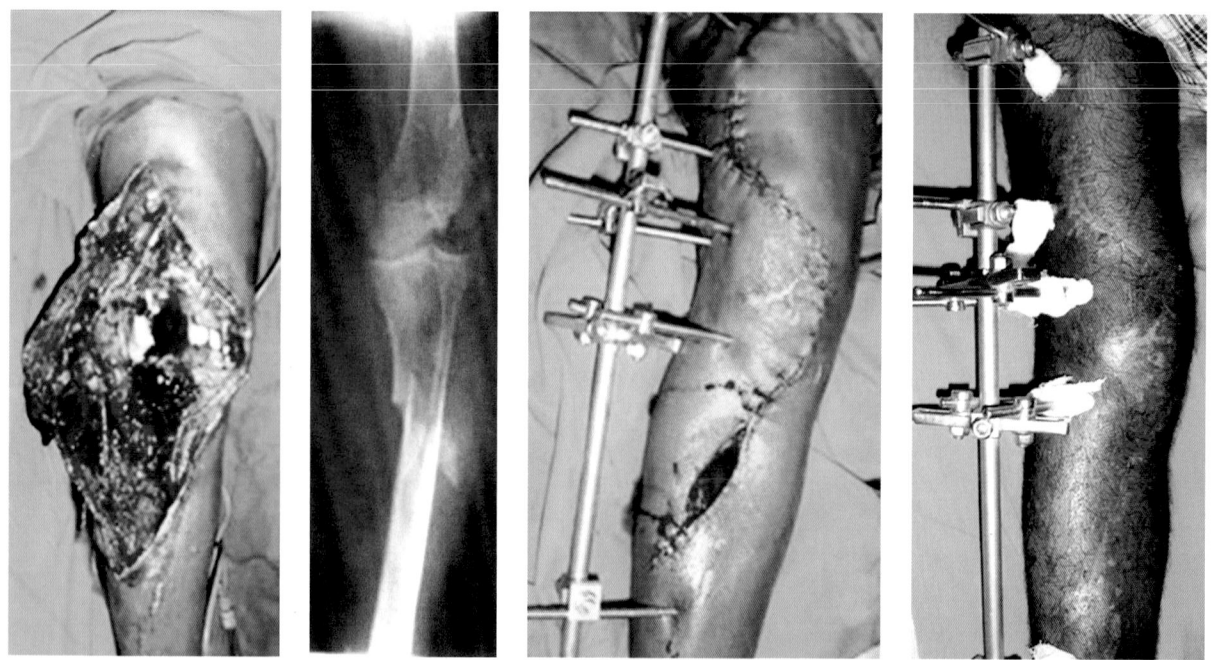

A, B

C, D

FIGURE 10-27 An open fracture with tibial comminution and exposure of the articular surfaces **(A, B).** Although the wound measured 31 cm, there was no loss of skin and bleeding viable skin margins could be opposed without tension **(C).** Primary wound healing was achieved **(D).** Leaving the wound open would have carried the risk of severe joint infection and desiccation of the articular cartilage. Soft tissue reconstruction using a flap would have also involved a complicated procedure.

TABLE 10-18	**Need for Second Look Debridement**

- High-energy blast injuries
- Severe contamination, farmyard, and sewage contamination
- Delayed presentation >12 hours
- Evidence of infection during debridement
- Initial debridement considered unsatisfactory

TABLE 10-19	**Timing of Wound Closure**

- **Primary Closure:** Wound closed by direct skin suturing during the index procedure.
- **Immediate Cover:** Soft tissue cover performed within 48 hours.
- **Early Cover:** Soft tissue cover performed within 1 week.
- **Delayed Cover:** Soft tissue cover performed within 3 weeks.
- **Staged Reconstruction:** Soft tissue reconstruction done after 3 weeks.

Lacerations adjacent to closed degloving or associated with extensive bruising of the skin are not suitable for primary closure.

6. Wounds treated with primary closure should have a deep drain inserted so that an underlying hematoma is avoided. They should be observed carefully for early infection to facilitate early intervention if this is required.

7. A useful policy is "whenever in doubt, do not close." Whenever in doubt, delayed primary closure where the decision to close the wound is postponed to the second look surgery 48 to 72 hours later is preferable. Indications for a second look are listed in Table 10-18.

Timing of Wound Cover

After debridement and appropriate skeletal stabilization, the most important factor that determines outcome is the timing and method of wound coverage. Adequate cover of the exposed wound by viable skin or soft tissue at the earliest possible time is essential. Exposure and desiccation can quickly lead to necrosis of many important deeper structures such as periosteum, articular cartilage, paratenon, and fascia. Delay also increases the chances of contamination and infection which can deleteriously affect the reconstruction process and even result in amputation. However there is still considerable controversy regarding the ideal timing and method of wound cover with different definitions being used by different authors. Suggested definitions are given in Table 10-19. It is important to understand the concept of the zone of injury and the sources of infection before discussing the timing of wound cover.

Zone of Injury

Blunt and open injuries with a crushing element have a larger area of impact and tissue destruction than penetrating injuries.[74,76,88] The extent of damage, especially to the deeper tissues, may be much wider than it initially appears. This has given rise to the concept of the zone of injury (Fig. 10-28). Three typical zones of injury are described. The direct trauma contact area is the central zone or "zone of necrosis" and is directly beneath

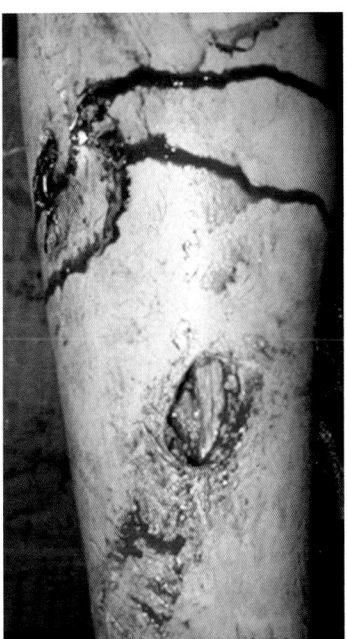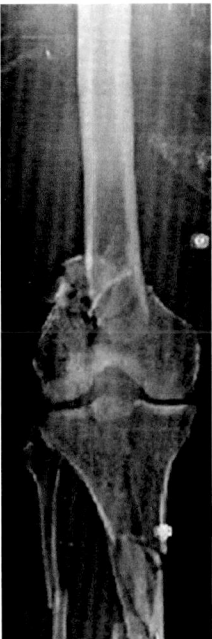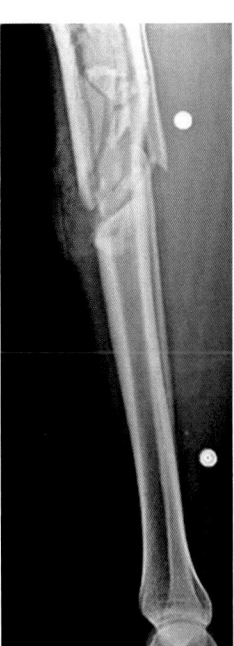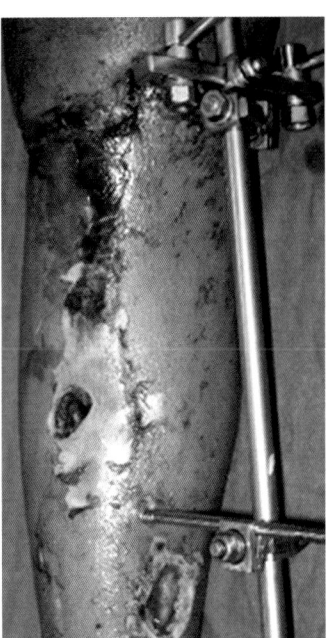

A, B   **C, D**

FIGURE 10-28 This case demonstrates the concept of "zone of injury." The injury resulted in a comminuted fracture of the femur and tibia. On presentation, the wound was deceptively small **(A, B, C).** There was extensive skin and tissue over the next 3 days as the zone of injury slowly revealed itself **(D).**

(*continues*)

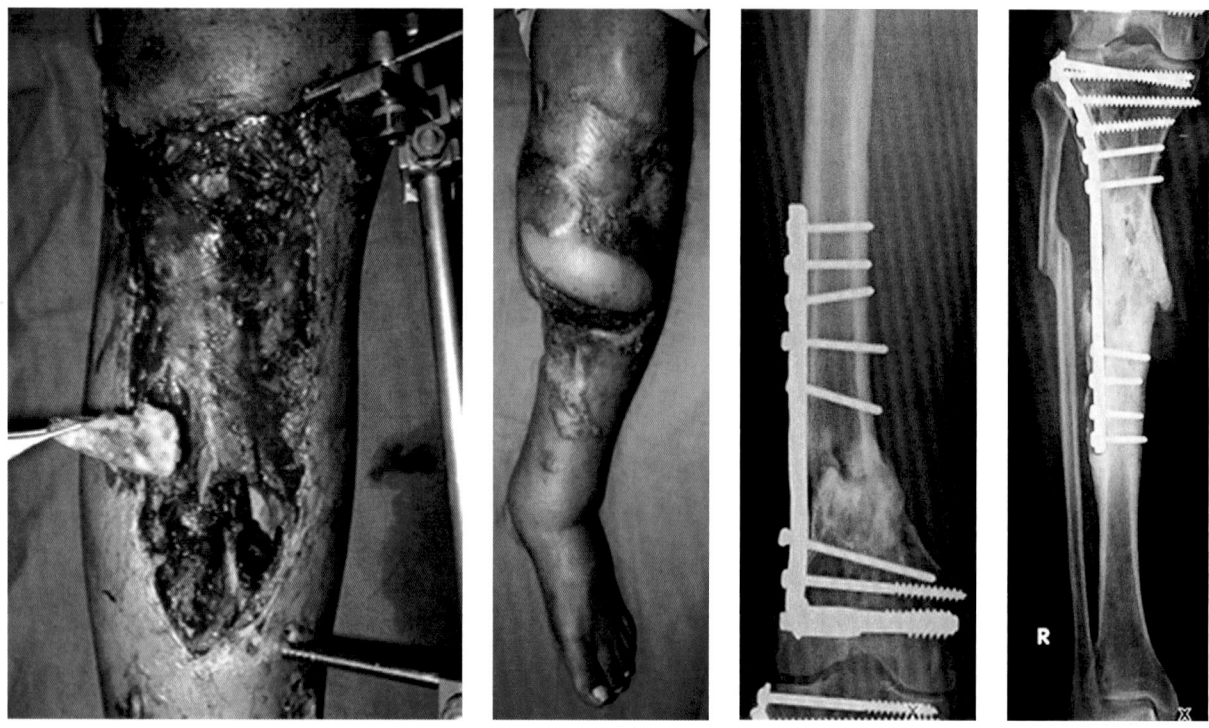

E, F   **G, H**

FIGURE 10-28 (*continued*) This required secondary debridement **(E)** and the defect required a latissimus dorsi free flap **(F).** The fractures were treated by primary plate fixation **(G, H).**

the wound. Surrounding this zone is the "zone of injury" which extends into the peripheral uninjured viable zone. The extent of these zones depends on the amount of energy imparted to the tissues at the time of impact and also on the anatomy of the area of impact. This zone of injury is characterized by inflammatory edematous soft tissue with disturbed microcirculation. Following a severe impact, the zone may appear viable at the initial debridement but may show evidence of partial or complete nonviability and loss of tissue over the next few days. It is often difficult to clearly distinguish the zone from adjacent healthy tissues immediately after trauma and during the initial debridement. This has considerable clinical importance because the vascular pedicles of flaps which are based in this zone of injury or microvascular anastomoses performed in this area are associated with an increased rate of failure. Failure to recognize this phenomenon will result in failure of soft tissue reconstruction failures and may make further reconstruction impossible.

Wherever there is suspicion of a severe crush element it is better to stage any soft tissue reconstruction so that the zone of injury will reveal itself over the next few days and all soft tissue reconstruction procedures can then be planned when the extent of the healthy zone is known. In our experience whenever GHOIS is >9, it is preferable to stage the soft tissue reconstruction.

Source of Infection in Open Injuries

Although infection does result from wound contamination especially if the debridement has been poor, there is now firm evidence that most acute infections after open injuries are the result of pathogens acquired in the hospital rather than from the site of injury.[3,13,14,130,155] In a prospective study of 326 open fractures, Gustilo et al.[85] reported that eight patients developed infection of which five were acquired secondarily in the hospital. They concluded that "during the long intervals when such wounds were open, secondary infection usually with gram-negative organisms may be a problem since these organisms are usually difficult to control by antibiotics alone." In a prospective study, Patzakis et al.[147] found that only 18% of infections were caused by the organism which was initially isolated in the perioperative period. Since the site of the fracture and soft tissue wound are probably most sterile after an adequate debridement by an experienced surgeon this is an opportune time to provide soft tissue cover.

The Timing of Soft Tissue Cover

The optimal timing of soft tissue reconstruction in open injuries still remains imprecise, and to date, there are no Level 1 studies that have looked into the timing of soft tissue cover. Traditionally, the protocol in a majority of units is to limit the initial surgical procedure to debridement and skeletal stabilization. The definitive soft tissue and bony reconstruction is postponed to a later date. The argument favoring staged procedures centers around the need for a second look debridement as any uncertainty about the presence of traumatized and devascularized tissue necessitates a second look to allow adequate resection. Godina[72–74] initiated the trend toward early soft tissue cover and reported a significant difference between wounds reconstructed within 72 hours of injury and those reconstructed later. The rates of infection (1.5%) and free-flap failure (0.75%) in wounds where microvascular reconstruction was performed within 72 hours of injury were significantly lower than the rates (2% infection, 12% flap failure) for wounds reconstructed between 72 hours and 3 months after injury. Recently, the "Fix and Flap" protocol has been described where wounds were reconstructed with muscle flaps as early as within 72 hours of injury.[76] In a review of early debridement and muscle flap cover, patients undergoing soft cover within 72 hours had a deep infection rate of only 6%. This was significantly lower than the 29% deep infection rate in patients undergoing soft tissue cover after 72 hours. There is considerable support in the literature for early soft tissue reconstruction. Hertel et al.[93] reported on the results of 29 consecutive open tibial fractures (24 Type IIIB and 5 Type IIIC) of which 14 were reconstructed immediately and 15 were reconstructed with a mean delay of 4.4 days (range: 1 to 9 days). In the delayed reconstruction group the time to full unprotected weight bearing ($p = 0.021$), the time to definitive union ($p = 0.004$), the number of reoperations ($p = 0.0001$), and the infection rate ($p = 0.037$) were significantly higher. The better outcome in all parameters was related to the fact that bone infection did not occur in the immediate reconstruction group. They advocated that whenever possible and where the condition of the patient allowed, a "zero delay protocol" might be useful to maximize results.

The practice of debridement that retains only viable tissues and the facility to cover large soft tissue and bone defects by modern microsurgical soft tissue and bone transport procedures have allowed early reconstruction. As Godina[73] stated, "Wide, early, experienced debridement to clearly healthy tissue and early rotational or free muscle flap cover may be better in experienced hands than sequential debridement and delayed closure."

Type of Cover

In patients with established skin loss there are many options for providing skin cover over the fracture site from releasing incisions to microvascular free tissue transfer. Traditionally it is viewed as a reconstructive ladder starting from simple split skin grafts and progressing to fasciocutaneous flaps, rotational muscle flaps, and free muscle flaps (Fig. 10-29). Each step of the ladder provides a wound cover option of increasing complexity and the traditional advice was to choose the simplest option as the first choice for soft tissue cover. However, this approach has been questioned recently because of extensive advances in microsurgery. Free flaps are now undertaken with a high success rate and they have the advantage of providing versatile skin cover with vascular tissue. Hence, it has been suggested that the reconstructive ladder concept should be replaced by the "reconstructive elevator" concept as the ladder's top step option is often the one that provides the best wound healing. Rather than adopting a stepwise algorithm for wound cover, surgeons now choose the appropriate method (Fig. 10-30). Recently, a "revised reconstructive ladder"[195] has been advocated where newer developments such as vacuum-assisted closure (VAC) therapy, acute bone shortening, and bone transport are incorporated.

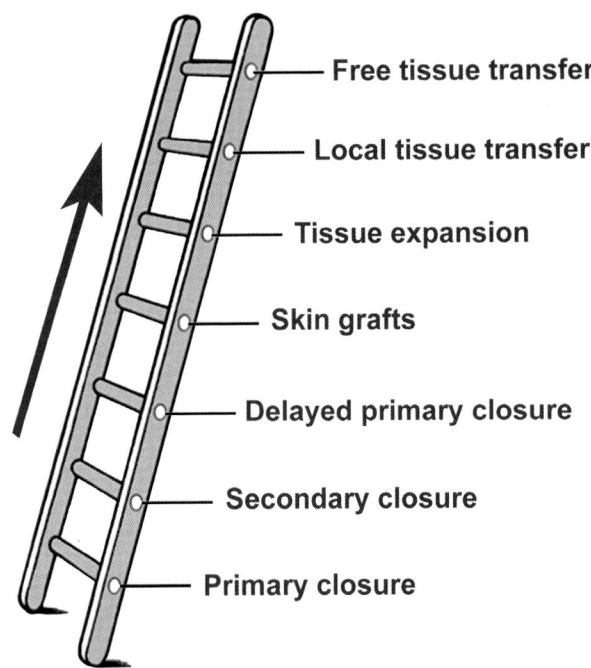

The Reconstructive Ladder

FIGURE 10-29 The traditional reconstructive ladder proposes a plan for reconstruction where each step of the ladder denotes a reconstruction of increasing complexity starting from primary closure. It was originally suggested that the surgeon must choose the lowest possible step that will suit the defect. However, this concept is not followed now.

Type III injuries are associated with wounds of varying size and complexity. Reconstruction should be tailored to the wound and also the surgeon's expertise. Every surgeon has certain preferences in reconstruction techniques but the following guidelines generally hold true. Lacerated wounds without skin loss, which can be opposed without tension, can be primarily sutured. In small linear vertical wounds, lying over bone, with minimal soft tissue loss cover can be achieved using a parallel releasing skin incision which will allow direct closure of the laceration. The releasing skin incision should be over a good muscle bed or fascia so that it will allow skin grafting of the defect. Wounds which are not directly over the bone and which have a healthy muscle bed can usually be treated by split skin grafting with good results. Small defects in the skin which are directly over bone and are exposing implants can be successfully covered with rotational fasciocutaneous flaps which may have either a proximal or a distal base (Fig. 10-31). The commonly seen defect over the subcutaneous surface of the tibia can be treated by a rotational flap, provided there is no degloving and the zone of injury is not extensive. A distally based flap is commonly performed for a defect in the anterior part of the leg as it creates a donor area over healthy calf muscles that take skin grafts well. Larger defects and injuries exposing the bone and tendons require to be covered with vascularized tissue and the best option is a muscle flap covered with split skin graft. A good example of this is the rotational

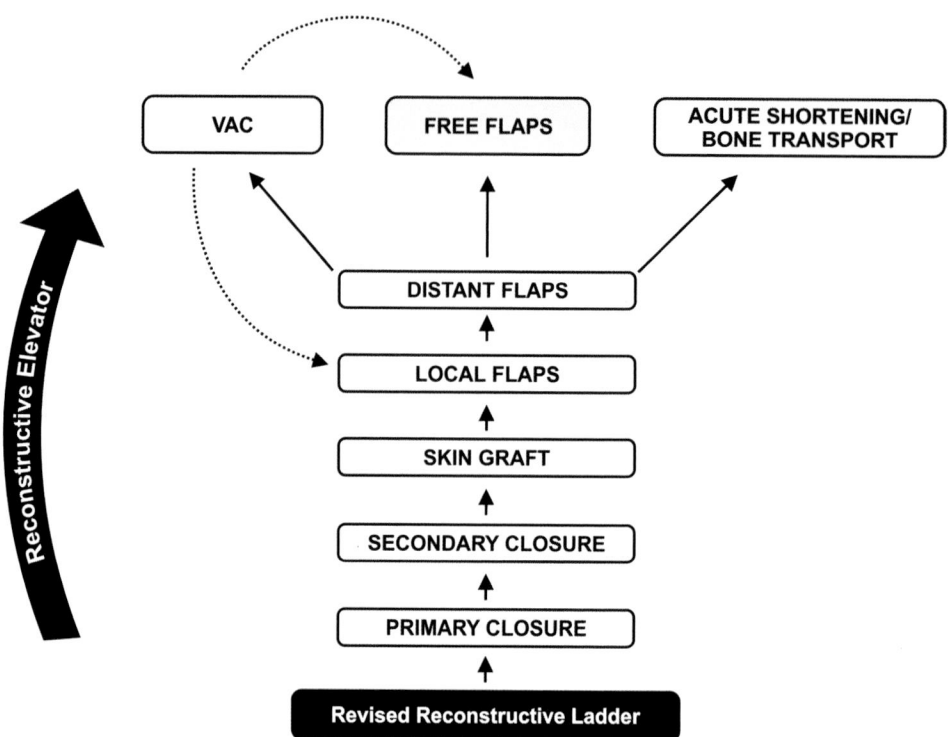

FIGURE 10-30 The revised reconstructive ladder includes the newer methods of reconstruction such as NPWT and acute shortening/bone transport. The "reconstructive elevator" concept is more popular now where the most appropriate and effective method of cover is chosen as the primary choice, however complex it may be.

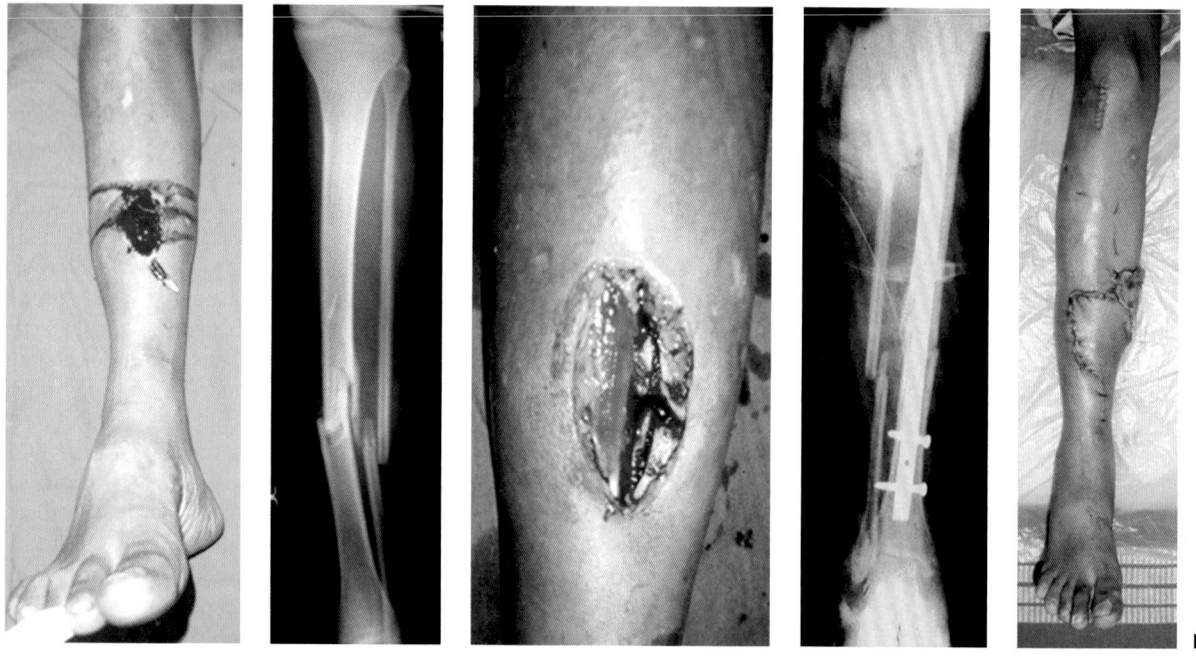

FIGURE 10-31 An open tibial fracture with soft tissue loss and exposure of the fracture site, and a GHIOS score of 8 **(A, B, C)**. This was nailed and an early fasciocutaneous flap was undertaken **(D, E)**. A low total score allowed successful early flap cover.

gastrocnemius flap which is used for injuries around the proximal tibia. The medial gastrocnemius is especially useful as it has a good blood supply from the superior branch of the popliteal artery which is usually uninjured in fractures of the tibia. Even in patients who require an amputation due to severe crushing of the soft tissues in the calf the gastrocnemius is usually viable and can be utilized effectively to cover the amputation stump. Failure of a gastrocnemius flap is very uncommon unless there is an injury to the popliteal vessels or the pedicle blood supply is damaged during dissection. Wounds in which a pedicle flap is not suitable or which are too large to be treated with a pedicle flap require free microvascular tissue transfer (Fig. 10-32). Although demanding and requiring the availability of an experienced microvascular surgeon, it is frequently the best option in complex injuries and may make the difference between amputation and salvage. The workhorse for lower limb injuries is the free latissimus dorsi flap followed by rectus and gracilis flaps. The choice is made depending on the dimensions of the wound and the size of the muscle that is required. Further information on soft tissue reconstruction can be found in Chapter 15.

Negative Pressure Wound Therapy

A useful treatment option in all injuries where soft tissue cover is not immediately possible is Vacuum-assisted wound closure (VAC) using NPWT. NPWT has largely replaced wet dressing therapy in most centers that treat a large number of open injuries. Wet dressings have to be changed frequently this being labor intensive and costly. Repeated dressings lead to increased exposure and susceptibility to the risk of nosocomial infection. From the time of the first clinical report of NPWT in 1993 by Fleischmann et al.,[59,60] its mechanism and beneficial effects in the management of different soft tissue defects, with and without infection, have been reported.[178]

Although there are numerous commercially available NPWT systems the basic components include an open pore sponge, a semi occlusive dressing, and a negative pressure source. The commercially available sponges are either made of polyvinyl alcohol or polyurethane ether. The sponges are cut to the correct shape and then secured by adhesive drapes which seal the wound and allow the creation of an effective vacuum. These drapes also stop protein loss, minimize wound desiccation, and prevent additional contamination from the hospital environment. In practice, iodophor-impregnated surgery drapes are useful as they can be cut to accommodate soft tissue defects of various dimensions and also seal wounds around external fixation devices.

The negative pressure is supplied by commercially available vacuum pumps which allow regulation of the magnitude and duration of the negative pressure. In animal models, it has been shown that a pressure of -125 mm Hg, applied for 5 minutes at intervals of 7 minutes, has the most beneficial effect on the formation of granulation tissue and it increases the blood flow in the surrounding tissues by almost fourfold. Continuous negative pressure increases granulation tissue by only 63% compared to 103% with intermittent negative

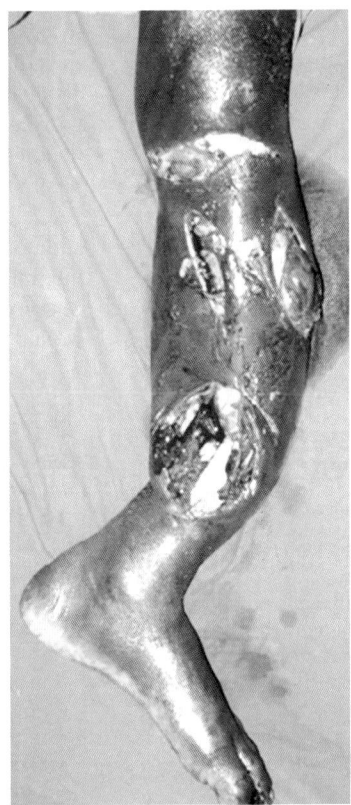
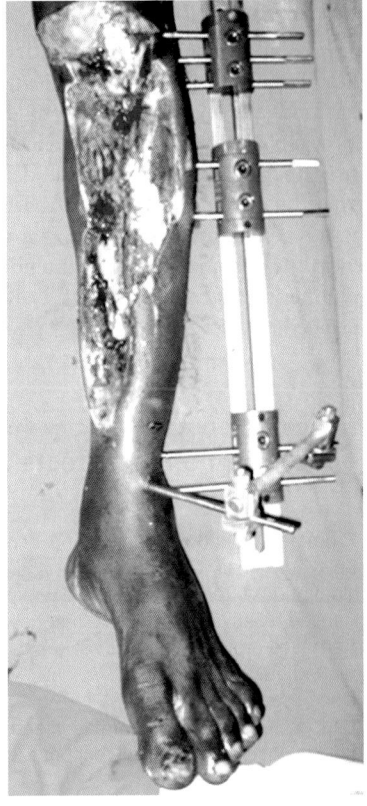

FIGURE 10-32 A severe open injury of leg with a GHIOS score of 13. There was significant soft tissue loss during debridement **(A, B)**.

(continues)   **A**

B

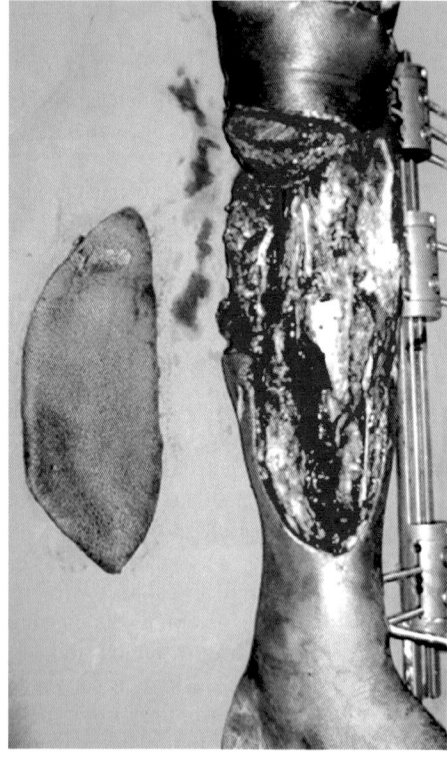
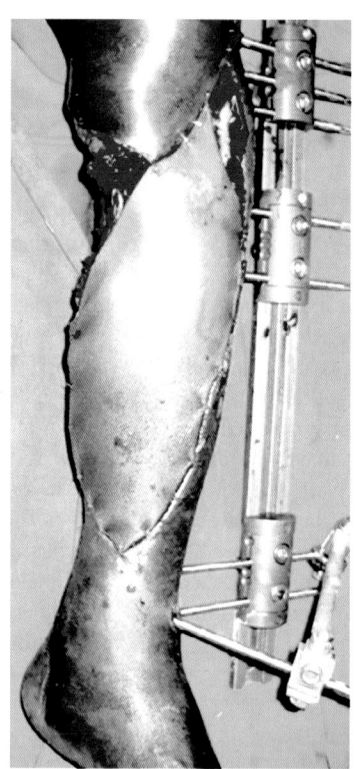

C

D

FIGURE 10-32 (*continued*) This was managed by secondary debridement and a delayed free flap performed at 1 week **(C, D)**. A score of 10 or more indicates a very severe injury to all compartments of the limb and immediate soft tissue reconstruction is contraindicated.

pressure. The numerous beneficial effects of NPWT are listed in Table 10-20.[178]

Application of NPWT Device

Before the application of the VAC device, the FDI guidelines and the indications and contraindications for NPWT must be understood[178] (Table 10-21). It should be emphasized that VAC is not a replacement for good surgical principles. The wound must be thoroughly debrided of all debris and infected tissues and bleeding should be well controlled before the application of negative pressure. Application of a VAC may be contraindicated in the presence of exposed tendons, surgical anastomosis of a nerve or a vessel or when heavy bleeding or oozing is anticipated.

The sponge is usually pressed against the wound and a template is created on the sponge by the wound exudate or blood. The sponge is then cut to size, applied over the wound and held in place by applying the adhesive dressing in small strips to minimize creases (Fig. 10-33). Keeping the skin dry helps the adhesive drapes to get a firm hold. Circumferential application of the adhesive drapes must be avoided to prevent a tourniquet effect. A 1.5 to 2 cm hole is then cut in the center of the dressing over the sponge and the suction track pad is firmly secured over the hole. The track pad is then connected to the VAC device and any residual leaks are addressed by applying additional adhesive strips. If patients complain of pain with the intermittent suction protocol continuous suction can be used. The VAC device is left in place for 2 or 3 days after which the wound can be inspected and suction continued.

TABLE 10-20 **Beneficial Effects of VAC Therapy[178]**

- Promotes wound contraction and increases the chance of delayed primary closure.
- Continuously removes excess edematous fluid.
- Causes reactive increase in blood flow and promotes healing.
- Removes proteins and electrolytes that are harmful for wound healing.
- Decreases bacterial burden.
- Causes cellular microdeformation and favorable electrical fields which stimulate cell response and growth factors.

TABLE 10-21 **VAC Therapy[178]**

Indications
- Severely crushed injuries not amenable for immediate soft tissue cover.
- Wounds which require dead space management
- Exposed bone with degloved skin
- Exposed Tendons and ligaments
- Open joint injuries with soft tissue loss

Contraindications
- Presence of necrotic skin with eschar.
- Untreated osteomyelitis
- Exposed neurovascular bundle.
- Exposed vascular anastomosis

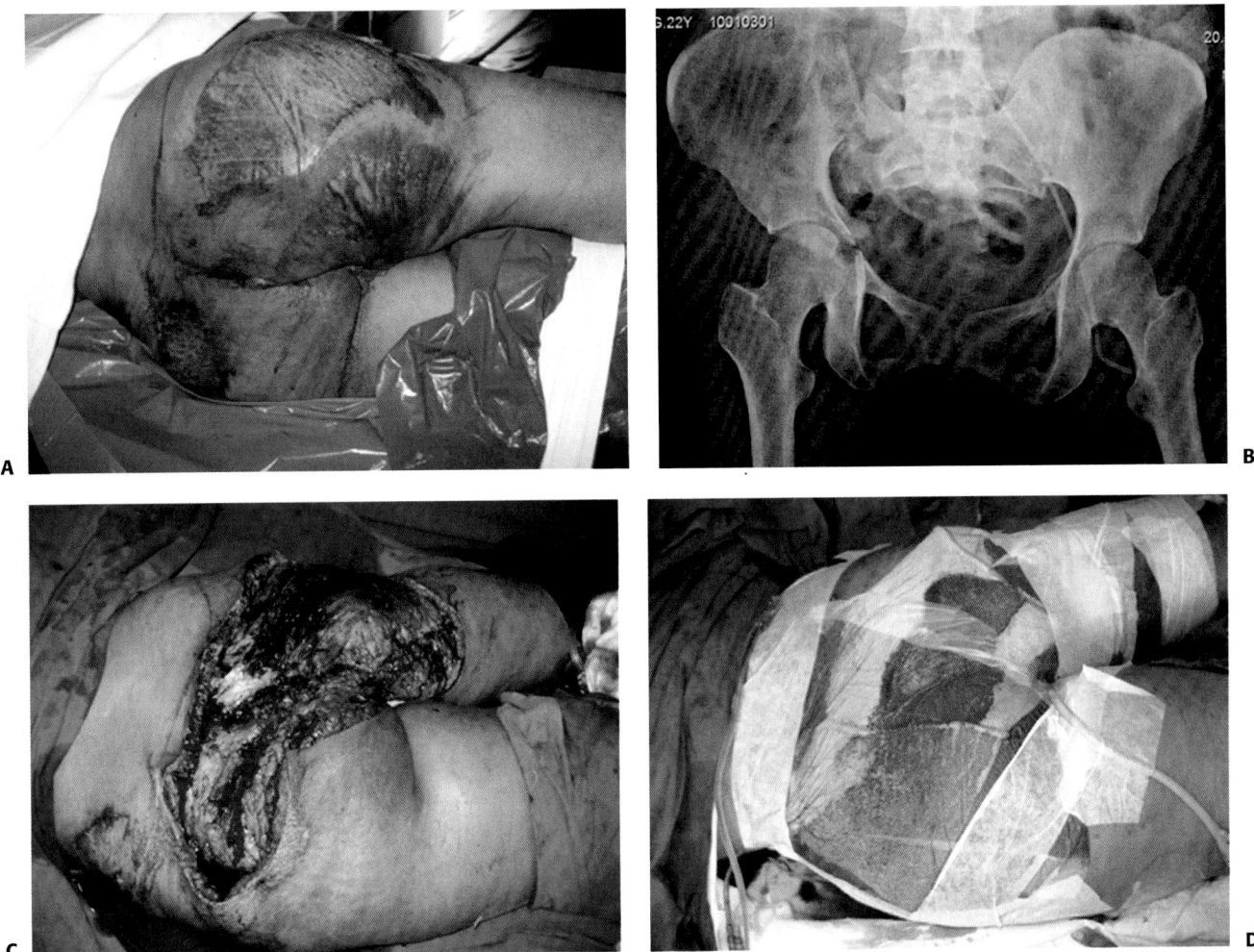

FIGURE 10-33 An extensive degloving injury of the buttocks **(A)** with a pelvic fracture **(B)** had a large defect following debridement **(C)**. Such large defects are amenable to immediate VAC therapy **(D)** which facilitated early granulation and treatment by skin grafting.

Clinical Effects

Several studies have reported the beneficial effects of NPWT and NPWT has been compared with standard wet dressing in a randomized controlled trial.[175] Fractures treated with NPWT needed 0.8 days less to achieve definitive closure status than those treated with standard dressings. Furthermore the infection rate in the NPWT group was only 5.4% compared to 28% in the controlled group this being significantly different. Mouës et al.[135] performed a randomized study in 54 patients with full-thickness wounds. They analyzed the time taken for the wound to form a clean granulating wound bed which was "ready for surgical therapy" as determined by an examiner who was not blinded to the treatment modality. No significant difference was observed between the two groups. However, patients in the NPWT group had a wound surface reduction of 3.8% compared to only 1.7% in the control group. This was statistically significant. However it should be noted that the examiner was not blinded to the treatment modality. In another recent study by Dedmond et al.[49] reporting on 50 Type III open tibial fractures man-

aged by NPWT superficial infection occurred in four patients (8%) and deep infection occurred in 10 patients (20%). The prevalence of infection in Type IIIA, IIIB, and IIIC injuries was 8.3%, 45.8%, and 50% respectively which is similar to studies which did use NPWT. Reduction of bacterial wound colonization and clearance of bacteria from the wound are frequently cited as benefits of NPWT. However the literature does not present a uniform view. A few studies have shown a decrease in the bacterial load[133] but others have found no difference or an overall increase in the bacterial load.[113,135,191]

The rate of infection appears to be related to the timing of coverage as delay affects the capacity of NPWT to reduce infection rates. In a retrospective analysis of 38 patients, patients who underwent definitive cover less than 7 days post injury, had an infection rate of only 12.5% compared to 57% in patients in whom definitive cover was performed after 7 days.[17] However studies by Steiert[176] and Fleischmann[60] did not find the same difference in infection rate. The usage of NPWT should be kept to a minimum and early flap coverage should be performed in a physiologic stable patient. If surgical delay is required for any reason, NPWT can then be continued safely till delayed cover is possible.

Although there are many encouraging reports, there is no conclusive evidence supporting the superiority of NPWT over standard wet dressings in avoiding wound infection and the requirement for flap cover. There are also no studies that have compared NPWT with other treatment methods such as the use of antibiotic bead pouches which have also been reported to be useful. The overall outcome is affected by the nature of the wound, the adequacy of debridement, the presence of comorbidities, and the health status and nutrition of the patient.

Complications

Twelve deaths have been reported related to the use of NPWT due to bleeding when used in wounds near the groin or pre-sternal region or when used over vascular grafts.[170] NPWT is also contraindicated in patients taking anticoagulants and in those who have significant adhesions between the wound bed and dressings when dressings are removed. Bleeding can be reduced by the use of a nonadherent dressing or polyvinyl alcohol sponges placed in the base of the wound.

Loss of suction and failure of the VAC system to maintain a vacuum will increase the risk of wound infection. The adhesive dressing must be applied to dry skin to permit adequate sealing and maintenance of suction. Puncture of the occlusive dressing and clogging of the sponge or tubing can result in failure of the suction and therefore continuous monitoring NPWT system is essential.

TABLE 10-22 Definitive Limb Reconstructive Pathway[155]

- "Fix and close" protocol
- "Fix, bone graft and close" protocol.
- "Fix and flap" protocol
- "Fix and delayed flap" protocol
- "Stabilize, observe, assess and reconstruct" protocol

AUTHOR'S PREFERRED TREATMENT[151–155]

Our Unit treats more than 300 Type IIIb injuries every year and our choice of reconstruction pathway is guided by the GHOIS. In an analysis of 965 injuries treated in a 3-year period, we found that the limb reconstruction pathway that was selected followed one of a number of options which are shown in Table 10-22. It must be stressed that an essential requirement for success is a thorough debridement by an experienced "Orthoplastic" team. Bone stabilization is tailored to the fracture requirements and the skin cover is undertaken as early as possible. The individual skin score is used to choose the method of wound cover and the total score guides the time of treatment (Fig. 10-34).

Fix and Primary Closure

Injuries with a skin Score of 1 and 2 have no skin loss at injury or during debridement. When contamination is low and there has been a satisfactory debridement, these patients are suitable for direct suturing. The total score must be <9 as this indicates

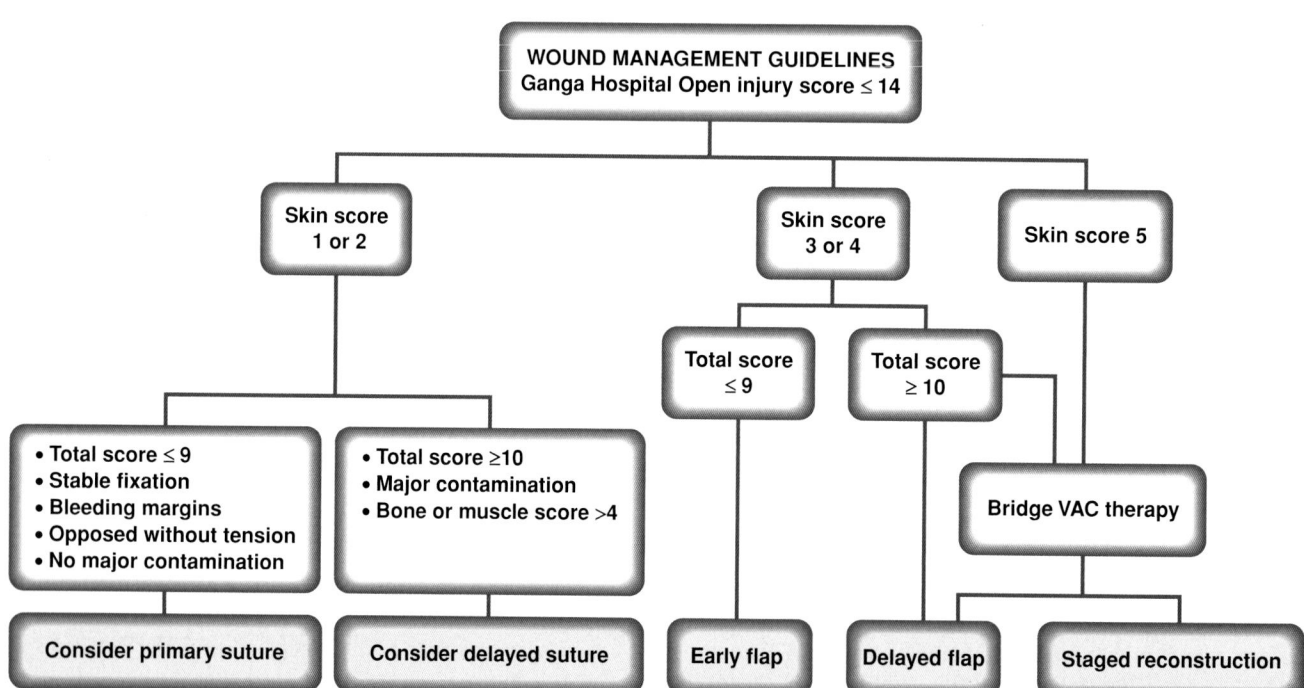

FIGURE 10-34 Treatment algorithm for wound management derived from the Ganga Hospital Open Injury Score. The algorithm assumes that a satisfactory meticulous debridement and stable skeletal fixation has been achieved to allow soft tissue reconstruction.

low-energy violence and the chances of postoperative swelling or compartment syndrome are low. Stable skeletal fixation and bleeding skin margins which are opposed without tension are the prerequisites for primary closure. It should be noted that the length of the wound is not a criterion (Fig. 10-33).

Fix and Delayed Closure

Injuries with skin score of 1 or 2, but with either a total score of >9 or with moderate or severe contamination are not treated by primarily closure. A higher score of >9 indicates high-energy violence and a reassessment at 48 or 72 hours is necessary. A delayed closure is performed if the wound characteristics at a second look debridement allow closure. If additional debridement is required at the time of the second look leading to further skin and soft tissue resection, the patient is managed by a staged flap protocol.

Fix and Skin Grafting

A skin score of 3 indicates skin loss either at injury or during debridement. In skin score 3 the wound either does not expose the fracture site or there is adequate soft tissue cover. A classic example is open fractures of femur where good soft tissue cover is usually present after skeletal stabilization. Here simple wound management by split skin grafting possible.

Fix and Early Flap

A skin score of 3 or 4 indicates skin loss either at injury or during debridement. If the wound exposes bone, articular cartilage, tendons, or a vascular anastomosis site, a flap is necessary. The type of the flap will be determined by the location and size of the defect and the structures that are exposed. Again timing is guided by the total score of GHOIS. An early flap can be done if the total score is less than 9. This indicates a lower-energy injury and a more definable zone of injury.

We do not favor the traditional reconstructive ladder philosophy but rather would choose the most appropriate procedure that best suits the injury as defined by the bone and soft tissue defect. Often a well-performed free tissue transfer gives better functional results and can even make the difference between salvage and amputation.

Fix and Delayed Flap

A fix and delayed flap protocol is performed whenever there is severe contamination or the total score is >10. The duration of delay will depend on the condition of the wound, the swelling of surrounding soft tissues and the presence of infection. If, during the relook procedure, the wound is not suitable for flap cover the use of NPWT following another debridement is an attractive option.

Staged Reconstructions

A score of 5 in any of the tissue scores and a total score of >9 indicates a limb that is not suitable for immediate or even early reconstruction. These limbs have considerable associated bony and soft tissue injury or loss. Often the wound may not be ready for reconstruction even after a few weeks. Here the option

of immediate or early application of NPWT at the initial procedure must be seriously considered. The expertise of a skilled plastic surgical team with microsurgical reconstruction capability and an orthopedic team capable of bone reconstruction and regeneration techniques is essential. If this is not available, patients must be expeditiously transferred to a center where such facilities are available. The choice and timing of the reconstruction method must be made on an individual patient basis.

REFERENCES

1. Abramson D, Hitchcock R, Trooskin S, et al. Lactate clearance and survival following injury. *J Trauma.* 1993;35:584–588.
2. Adams CI, Keating JF, Court-Brown CM. Cigarette smoking and open tibial fractures. *Injury.* 2001;32:61–65.
3. Al-Arabi YB, Nader M, Hamidian-Jahromi AR, et al. The effect of the timing of antibiotics and surgical treatment on infection rates in open long-bone fractures: A 9-year prospective study from a district general hospital. *Injury.* 2007;38:900–905.
4. Anglen JO. Wound irrigation in musculoskeletal injury. *J Am Acad Orthop Surg.* 2001; 9:219–226.
5. Anglen JO. Comparison of soap and antibiotic solutions for irrigation of lower-limb open fracture wounds. A prospective, randomized study. *J Bone Joint Surg Am.* 2005;87: 1415–1422.
6. Anglen JO, Apostoles PS, Christensen G, et al. Removal of surface bacteria by irrigation. *J Orthop Res.* 1996;14:251–254.
7. Antich-Adrover P, Marti-Garin D, Murias-Alvarez J, et al. External fixation and secondary intreamdullary nails of open tibial fractures. A Randomised, prospective trial. *J Bone Joint Surg Br.* 1997;79:433–437.
8. Bach AW, Hansen ST Jr. Plates versus external fixation in severe open tibial shaft fractures. A randomized trial. *Clin Orthop Relat Res.* 1989;241:89–94.
9. Bakker J, Gris P, Coffernils M, et al. Serial blood lactate levels can predict the development of multiple organ failure following septic shock. *Am J Surg.* 1996;171:221–226.
10. Baue AE. Multiple organ failure, multiple organ dysfunction syndrome, and the systemic inflammatory response syndrome-where do we stand? *Shock.* 1994;2: 385–397.
11. Behrens F, Searls K. External fixation of the tibia. Basic concepts and prospective evaluation. *J Bone Joint Surg Br.* 1986;68:246–254.
12. Bhandari M, Adili A, Lachowski RJ. High pressure pulsatile lavage of contaminated human tibiae: An in vitro study. *J Orthop Trauma.* 1998;12:479–484.
13. Bhandari M, Guyatt G, Tornetta P 3rd, et al. Randomized trial of reamed and unreamed intramedullary nailing of tibial shaft fractures. Study to prospectively evaluate reamed intramedullary nails in patients with tibial Fracture. *J Bone Joint Surg Am.* 2008;90:2567–2578.
14. Bhandari M, Guyatt GH, Swiontkowski MF, et al. Treatment of open fractures of the shaft of the tibia. *J Bone Joint Surg Br.* 2001;83:62–68.
15. Bhandari M, Schemitsch EH, Adili A, et al. High and low pressure pulsatile lavage of contaminated tibial fractures: An in vitro study of bacterial adherence and bone damage. *J Orthop Trauma.* 1999;13:526–533.
16. Bhandari M, Zlowodzki M, Tornetta P 3rd, et al. Intramedullary nailing following external fixation in femoral and tibial shaft fractures. *J Orthop Trauma.* 2005;19:140–144.
17. Bhattacharyya T, Mehta P, Smith M, et al. Routine use of wound vacuum-assisted closure does not allow coverage delay for open tibia fractures. *Plast Reconstr Surg.* 2008;121:1263–1266.
18. Billroth. *Clinical Surgery.* London: The new Sydenham Society; 1881.
19. Blachut PA, Meek RN, O'Brien PJ. External fixation and delayed intramedullary nailing of open fractures of tibial shaft. A sequential protocol. *J Bone Joint Surg Am.* 1990;72:729–735.
20. Blow O, Magliore L, Claridge JA, et al. The golden hour and the silver day: Detection and correction of occult hypoperfusion within 24 hours improves outcome from major trauma. *J Trauma.* 1999;47:964–969.
21. Bonanni F, Rhodes M, Lucke JF. The futility of predictive scoring of mangled lower extremities. *J Trauma.* 1993;34:99–104.
22. Bosse MJ, MacKenzie EJ, Kellam JF, et al. A prospective evaluation of the clinical utility of the lower-extremity injury-severity scores. *J Bone Joint Surg Am.* 2001;83-A:3–14.
23. Bosse MJ, MacKenzie EJ, Kellam JF, et al. An analysis of outcomes of reconstruction or amputation after leg-threatening injuries. *N Engl J Med.* 2002;347:1924–1931.
24. Brennan SS, Leaper DJ. The effect of antiseptics on the healing wound: A study using the rabbit ear chamber. *Br J Surg.* 1985;72:780–782.
25. British Orthopaedic Association and British Association of Plastic Surgeons. The Early Management of Severe Tibial Fractures: The Need for Combined Plastic and Orthopaedic Management: A Report by the BOA/BAPS Working Party on Severe Tibial Injuries, 1993; London.
26. British Orthopaedic Association recommendations (Open fractures of lower limb). Online Recommendations September 2009.
27. Brohi K, Cohen MJ, Davenport RA. Acute coagulopathy of trauma: Mechanism, identification and effect. *Curr Opin Crit Care.* 2007;13:680–685.
28. Brown LL, Shelton HT, Bornside GH Jr. Cohn I. Evaluation of wound irrigation by pulsatile jet and conventional methods. *Ann Surg.* 1978;187:170–173.
29. Brown PW, Kinman PB. Gas gangrene in a metropolitan community. *J Bone Joint Surg Am.* 1974;56:1445–1451.

30. Brumback RJ, Jones AL. Interobserver agreement in the classification of open fractures of the tibia. The results of a survey of two hundred and forty-five orthopaedic surgeons. *J Bone Joint Surg Am.* 1994;76:1162–1166.
31. Byrd HS, Spicer TE, Cierney G 3rd. Management of open tibial fractures. *Plast Reconstr Surg.* 1985;76:719–730.
32. Calhoun JH. Optimal timing of operative debridement: A known unknown: commentary on an article by Mara L. Schenker, MD, et al.: "Does timing to operative debridement affect infectious complications in open long-bone fractures? A systematic review". *J Bone Joint Surg Am.* 2012;94:e90.
33. Carroll EA, Koman LA. External fixation and temporary stabilization of femoral and tibial trauma. *J Surg Orthp Adv.* 2011;20:74–81.
34. Carsenti-Etesse H, Doyon F, Desplaces N, et al. Epidemiology of bacterial infection during management of open leg fractures. *Eur J Clin Microbiol Infect Dis.* 1999;18:315–323.
35. Castillo RC, Bosse MJ, MacKenzie EJ, et al. Impact of smoking on fracture healing and risk of complications in limb-threatening open tibia fractures. *J Orthop Trauma.* 2005; 19:151–157.
36. Caudle RJ, Stern PJ. Severe open fractures of the tibia. *J Bone Joint Surg Am.* 1987; 69-A:801–807.
37. Chapman M. Role of bone stability in open fractures. *Instr Course Lect.* 1982;31:75–87.
38. Chapman MW. The use of immediate internal fixation in open fractures. *Orthop Clin North Am.* 1980;11:579–591.
39. Chung KC, Saddawi-Konefka D, Haase SC, et al. A cost-utility analysis of amputation versus salvage for Gustilo IIIB and IIIC open tibial fractures. *Plast Reconstr Surg.* 2009;124:1965–1973.
40. Clifford RP, Beauchamp CG, Kellam JF, et al. Plate fixation of open fractures of the tibia. *J Bone Joint Surg Br.* 1988;70:644–648.
41. Conroy BP, Anglen JO, Simpson WA, et al. Comparison of castile soap, benzalkonium chloride, and bacitracin as irrigation solutions for complex contaminated orthopaedic wounds. *J Orthop Trauma.* 1999;13:332–337.
42. Cooney WP, Fitzgerald RH Jr, Dobyns JH, et al. Quantitative wound cultures in upper extremity trauma. *J Trauma.* 1982;22:112–117.
43. Court-Brown CM, Cross AT, Hahn DM, et al. *The Management of Open Tibial Fractures.* in BOA/BAPS Working Party September 1997: London.
44. Court-Brown CM, Rimmer S, Prakash U, et al. The epidemiology of open long bone fractures. *Injury.* 1998;29:529–534.
45. Crowley DJ, Kanakaris NK, Giannoudis PV. Debridement and wound closure of open fractures: the impact of the time factor on infection rates. *Injury.* 2007;38:879–889.
46. Crowley DJ, Kanakaris NK, Giannoudis PV. Irrigation of the wounds in open fractures. *J Bone Joint Surg Br.* 2007;89:580–585.
47. Cullen MC, Roy DR, Crawford AH, et al. Open fracture of the tibia in children. *J Bone Joint Surg [Am].* 1996;78-A:1039–1047.
48. Dabezies EJ, D'Ambrosia RD. Treatment of the multiply injured patient: Plans for treatment and problems of major trauma. *Instr Course Lect.* 1984;33:242–252.
49. Dedmond BT, Kortesis B, Punger K, et al. The use of negative-pressure wound therapy (NPWT) in the temporary treatment of soft-tissue injuries associated with high-energy open tibial shaft fractures. *J Orthop Trauma.* 2007;21:11–17.
50. DeLong W, Born CT, Wei SY, et al. Aggressive treatment of 119 open fracture wounds. *J Trauma.* 1999;46:1049–1054.
51. Di Pasquale DJ, Bhandari M, Tov A, et al. The effect of high and low pressure pulsatile lavage on soft tissue and cortical blood flow: a canine segmental humerus fracture model. *Arch Orthop Trauma Surg.* 2007;127:879–884.
52. Dirschl DR, Wilson FC. Topical antibiotic irrigation in the prophylaxis of operative wound infections in orthopedic surgery. *Orthop Clin North Am.* 1991;22:419–426.
53. Dollery W, Driscoll P. Resuscitation after high energy polytrauma. *Br Med Bull.* 1999; 55:785–805.
54. Draeger RW, Dahners LE. Traumatic wound debridement: A comparison of irrigation methods. *J Orthop Trauma.* 2006;20:83–88.
55. Durham RM, Mistry BM, Mazuski JE, et al. Outcome and utility of scoring systems in the management of the mangled extremity. *Am J Surg.* 1996;172:569–573.
56. Edwards CC, Simmons SC, Browner BD, et al. Severe open tibial fractures. Results treating 202 injuries with external fixation. *Clin Orthop Relat Res.* 1988:98–115.
57. Emami A, Mjoberg B, Ragnarsson B, et al. Changing epidemiology of tibial shaft fractures. 513 cases compared between 1971–1975 and 1986–1990. *Acta Orthop Scand.* 1996;67:557–561.
58. Fischer MD, Gustilo RB, Varecka TF. The timing of flap coverage, bone-grafting, and intramedullary nailing in patients who have a fracture of the tibial shaft with extensive soft-tissue injury. *J Bone Joint Surg Am.* 1991;73:1316–1322.
59. Fleischmann W, Becker U, Bishoff M, et al. Vacuum sealing: Indication, technique and results. *Eur J Orthop Surg Traumatol.* 1995;5:37–40.
60. Fleischmann W, Strecker W, Bombelli M, et al. Vacuum sealing as treatment of soft tissue damage in open fractures. *Unfallchirurg.* 1993;96:488–492.
61. Franklin JL, Johnson KD, Hansen ST. Immediate internal fixation of open ankle fractures. Report of thirty-eight cases treated with a standard protocol. *J Bone Joint Surg Am.* 1984;66:1349–1356.
62. French B, Tornetta P 3rd. High energy tibial shaft fractures. *Orthop Clin North Am.* 2002; 33:211–230.
63. Giannoudis PV. Current concepts of the inflammatory response after major trauma: An update. *Injury.* 2003;34:397–404.
64. Giannoudis PV, Furlong AJ, MacDonald DA, et al. Reamed against unreamed nailing of the femoral diaphysis: A retrospective study of healing time. *Injury.* 1997;28:15–18.
65. Giannoudis PV, Hildebrand F, Pape HC. Inflammatory serum markers in patients with multiple trauma. Can they predict outcome? *J Bone Joint Surg Br.* 2004;86: 313–323.
66. Giannoudis PV, Papakostidis C, Roberts C. A review of the management of open fractures of the tibia and femur. *J Bone Joint Surg Br.* 2006;88:281–289.
67. Giannoudis PV, Perry S, Smith RM. Systemic response to trauma. *Curr Orthop.* 2001;15: 176–183.
68. Giannoudis PV, Smith MR, Evans RT, et al. Serum CRP and IL-6 levels after trauma. Not predictive of septic complications in 31 patients. *Acta Orthop Scand.* 1998;69: 184–188.
69. Giannoudis PV, Smith RM, Banks RE, et al. Stimulation of inflammatory markers after blunt trauma. *Br J Surg.* 1998;85:986–990.
70. Gilmore OJ, Sanderson PJ. Prophylactic interparietal povidone-iodine in abdominal surgery. *Br J Surg.* 1975;62:792–799.
71. Glass GE BS, Sanderson F, Pearse MF, et al. The microbiological basis for a revised antibiotic regimen in high-energy tibial fractures: Preventing deep infections by nosocomial organisms. *J Plast Reconstr Aesthet Surg.* 2011;64:375–380.
72. Godina M. Early microsurgical reconstruction of complex trauma of the extremities. *Plast Reconstr Surg.* 1986;78:285–292.
73. Godina M. The tailored latissimus dorsi free flap. *Plast Reconstr Surg.* 1987;80: 304–306.
74. Godina M, Arnez ZM, Lister GD. Preferential use of the posterior approach to blood vessels of the lower leg in microvascular surgery. *Plast Reconstr Surg.* 1991;88:287–291.
75. Gopal S, Giannoudis PV. Prospective randomized study of reamed versus unreamed femoral intramedullary nailing: An assessment of procedures. *J Orthop Trauma.* 2001;15:458–460.
76. Gopal S, Majumder S, Batchelor AG, et al. Fix and flap: The radical orthopaedic and plastic treatment of severe open fractures of the tibia. *J Bone Joint Surg Br.* 2000;82:959–966.
77. Gosselin RA, Roberts I, Gillespie WJ. Antibiotics for preventing infection in open limb fractures. *Cochrane Database Syst Rev.* 2004;(1):CD003764.
78. Gregory CF, Chapman MW, Hansen ST. Open fractures. In: Rockwood CA, Green DP eds. *Fractures in Adults.* Philadelphia, PA: J.B. Lippincott; 1984: 169–218.
79. Grosse A, Christie J, Taglang G, et al. Open adult femoral shaft fracture treated by early intramedullary nailing. *J Bone Joint Surg Br.* 1993;75:562–565.
80. Gustilo RB. Management of open fractures. An analysis of 673 cases. *Minn Med.* 1971;54:185–189.
81. Gustilo RB. Use of antimicrobials in the management of open fractures. *Arch Surg.* 1979;114:805–808.
82. Gustilo RB. Management of infected fractures. *Instr Course Lect.* 1982;31:18–29.
83. Gustilo RB. Interobserver agreement in the classification of open fractures of the tibia. The results of a survey of two hundred and forty-five orthopaedic surgeons. *J Bone Joint Surg Am.* 1995;77:1291–1292.
84. Gustilo RB, Anderson JT. Prevention of infection in the treatment of one thousand and twenty-five open fractures of long bones: Retrospective and prospective analyses. *J Bone Joint Surg Am.* 1976;58:453–538.
85. Gustilo RB, Mendoza RM, Williams DN. Problems in the management of type III (severe) open fractures: A new classification of type III open fractures. *J Trauma.* 1984;24:742–746.
86. Gustilo RB, Corpuz V, Sherman RE. Epidemiology, mortality and morbidity in multiple trauma patients. *Orthopedics.* 1985;8:1523–1528.
87. Gustilo RB, Gruninger RP, Davis T. Classification of type III (severe) open fractures relative to treatment and results. *Orthopedics.* 1987;10:1781–1788.
88. Guthrie HC, Clasper JC. Historical origins and current concepts of wound debridement. *J R Army Med Corps.* 2011;157:130–132.
89. Guyette F, Suffoletto B, Castillo JL, et al. Prehospital serum lactate as a predictor of outcomes in trauma patients: A retrospective observational study. *J Trauma.* 2011;70: 782–786.
90. Hansen ST Jr. The type-IIIC tibial fracture. Salvage or amputation. *J Bone Joint Surg Am.* 1987;69:799–800.
91. Hansen ST Jr. Overview of the severely traumatized lower limb. Reconstruction versus amputation. *Clin Orthop Relat Res.* 1989:17–19.
92. Has B, Nagy A, Pavic R, et al. External fixation and infection of soft tissues close to fracture localization. *Mil Med.* 2006;171:88–91.
93. Hertel R, Lambert SM, Muller S, et al. On the timing of soft tissue reconstruction for open fractures of the lower leg. *Arch Orthop Trauma Surg.* 1999;119.
94. Hildebrand F, Giannoudis PV, Kretteck C, et al. Damage control: Extremities. *Injury.* 2004;35:678–689.
95. Hoff WS, Reilly PM, Rotondo MF, et al. The importance of the command-physician in trauma resuscitation. *J Trauma.* 1997;43:772–777.
96. Hohmann E, Tetsworth K, Radziejowski MJ, et al. Comparison of delayed and primary wound closure in the treatment of open tibial fractures. *Arch Orthop Trauma Surg.* 2007;127.
97. Hope PG, Cole WG. Open fractures of the tibia in children. *J Bone Joint Surg Br.* 1992;74-B:546–553.
98. Horn BD, Rettig ME. Interobserver reliability in the Gustilo and Anderson classification of open fractures. *J Orthop Trauma.* 1993;7:357–360.
99. Howard M, Court-Brown CM. Epidemiology and management of open fractures of the lower limb. *Brit J Hosp Med.* 1997;57:582–587.
100. Howe HR Jr, Poole GV Jr, Hansen KJ, et al. Salvage of lower extremities following combined orthopedic and vascular trauma. A predictive salvage index. *Am Surg.* 1987;53:205–208.
101. Hyman J, Moore T. Anatomy of the distal knee joint and pyarthrosis following external fixation. *J Orthop Trauma.* 1999;13:241–246.
102. Jawa RS, Anillo S, Huntoon K, et al. Interleukin 6 in Surgery, Trauma, and Critical Care–Part II: Clinical Applications. *J Intensive Care Med.* 2010.
103. Jawa RS, Anillo S, Huntoon K, et al. Analytic review: Interleukin-6 in surgery, trauma, and critical care: part I: basic science. *J Intensive Care Med.* 2011;26:3–12.
104. Johansen K, Daines M, Howey T, et al. Objective criteria accurately predict amputation following lower extremity trauma. *J Trauma.* 1990;30:568–572.
105. Kakar S, Tornetta P 3rd. Open fractures of the tibia treated by immediate intramedullary tibial nail insertion without reaming: A prospective study. *J Orthop Trauma.* 2007;21:153–157.
106. Kashuk JL, Moore EE, Millikan JS, et al. Major abdominal vascular trauma–a unified approach. *J Trauma.* 1982;22:672–679.

107. Ketenjian AY, Shelton ML. Primary internal fixation of open fractures: A retrospective study of the use of metallic internal fixation in fresh open fractures. *J Trauma.* 1972;12:756–763.

108. Klein MB, Hunter S, Heimbach DM, et al. The Versajet water dissector: A new tool for tangential excision. *J Burn Care Rehabil.* 2005;26:483–487.

109. Klein MP, Rahn BA, Frigg R, et al. Reaming versus non-reaming in medullary nailing: Interference with cortical circulation of the canine tibia. *Arch Orthop Trauma Surg.* 1990;109:314–316.

110. Kocher MS. Early limb salvage: Open tibia fractures of Ambroise Pare (1510-1590) and Percivall Pott (1714-1789). *World J Surg.* 1997;21:116–122.

111. Kreder HJ, Armstrong P. The significance of perioperative cultures in open pediatric lower-extremity fractures. *Clin Orthop Relat Res.* 1994:206–212.

112. Krishna U, Joshi SP, Modh M. An evaluation of serial blood lactate measurement as an early predictor of shock and its outcome in patients of trauma or sepsis. *Indian J Crit Care Med.* 2009;13:66–73.

113. Lalliss SJ, Stinner DJ, Waterman SM, et al. Negative pressure wound therapy reduces pseudomonas wound contamination more than Staphylococcus aureus. *J Orthop Trauma.* 2010;24:598–602.

114. Lange RH. Limb reconstruction versus amputation decision making in massive lower extremity trauma. *Clin Orthop Relat Res.* 1989:92–99.

115. Lee EW, Dirschl DR, Duff G, et al. High-pressure pulsatile lavage irrigation of fresh intraarticular fractures: Effectiveness at removing particulate matter from bone. *J Orthop Trauma.* 2002;16:162–165.

116. Lee J. Efficacy of cultures in the management of open fractures. *Clin Orthop Relat Res.* 1997:71–75.

117. Lenz A, Franklin GA, Cheadle WG. Systemic inflammation after trauma. *Injury Int J Care Injured.* 2007;38:1336–1345.

118. Lethaby A, Temple J, Santy J. Pin site care for preventing infections associated with external bone fixators and pins. *Cochrane Database Syst Reviews.* 2008;(4):CD004551.

119. Lhowe DW, Hansen ST. Immediate nailing of open fractures of the femoral shaft. *J Bone Joint Surg Am.* 1988;70:812–820.

120. Lineaweaver W, McMorris S, Soucy D, et al. Cellular and bacterial toxicities of topical antimicrobials. *Plast Reconstr Surg.* 1985;75:394–396.

121. Lu WH, Kolkman K, Seger M, et al. An evaluation of trauma team response in a major trauma hospital in 100 patients with predominantly minor injuries. *The Aust N Z J Surg.* 2000;70:329–332.

122. Manniks P, Jankowski S, Zhang H, et al. Correlation of serial lactate levels to organ failure and mortality after trauma. *Am J Emerg Med.* 1995;13:619–622.

123. Marshall PD, Saleh M, Douglas DL. Risk of deep infection with intramedullary nailing following the use of external fixators. *J Roy Coll Surg Edin.* 1991;36:268–271.

124. Maurer DJ, Merkow RL, Gustilo RB. Infection after intramedullary nailing of severe open tibial fractures initially treated with external fixation. *J Bone Joint Surg Am.* 1989;71:835–828.

125. McGraw JM, Lim EV. Treatment of open tibial-shaft fractures. External fixation and secondary intramedullary nailing. *J Bone Joint Surg Am.* 1988;70:900–911.

126. McNamara MG, Heckman JD, Corley FG. Severe open fractures of the lower extremity: A retrospective evaluation of the Mangled Extremity Severity Score (MESS). *J Orthop Trauma.* 1994;8:81–87.

127. McNelis J, Marini CP, Jurkiewicz A, et al. Prolonged lactate clearance is associated with increased mortality in the surgical intensive care unit. *Am J Surg.* 2001;182:481–485.

128. McQueen MM, Gaston P, Court-Brown CM. Acute compartment syndrome: Who is at risk? *J Bone Joint Surg Br.* 2000;82:200–203.

129. Merritt K. Factors increasing the risk of infection in patients with open fractures. *J Trauma.* 1988;28:823–827.

130. Moola F, Jacks D, Reindl R, et al. Safety of primary closure of soft tissue wounds in open fractures. *J Bone Joint Surg Br.* 2008;90-B:94.

131. Moore TJ, Mauney C, Barron J. The use of quantitative bacterial counts in open fractures. *Clin Orthop Relat Res.* 1989:227–230.

132. Morgan BW, Read JR, Solan MC. Photographic wound documentation of open fractures: An update for the digital generation. *Emerg Med J.* 2007;24:841–842.

133. Morykwas MJ, Argenta LC, Shelton-Brown EI, et al. Vacuum-assisted closure: A new method for wound control and treatment. Animal studies and basic foundation. *Ann Plast Surg.* 1997;38:553–562.

134. Mosti G, Iabichella ML, Picerni P, et al. The debridement of hard to heal leg ulcers by means of a new device based on Fluidjet technology. *Int Wound J.* 2005;2:307–314.

135. Mouès CM, Vos MC, van den Bemd GJ, et al. Bacterial load in relation to vacuum-assisted closure wound therapy: A prospective randomized trial. *Wound Repair Regen.* 2004;12:11–17.

136. Murray MJ. We can't go home again: Advances in the resuscitation of patients with polytrauma. *Anesth Analg.* 2012;115:1263–1264.

137. Nusem I, Otremski I. Prophylactic antibiotics in orthopedic practice. Part II: Closed and open fractures. *Harefuah.* 1999;136:316–317.

138. Okike K, Bhattacharyya T. Trends in the management of open fractures. A critical analysis. *J Bone Joint Surg Am.* 2006;88:2739–2748.

139. Olson SA, Schemitsch EH. Open fractures of the tibial shaft: An update. *Instr Course Lect.* 2003;52:623–631.

140. Pape HC, Griensven MV, Hildebrand FF, et al. Systemic inflammatory response after extremity or truncal fracture operations. *J Trauma.* 2008;65:1379–1384.

141. Pape HC, Grimme K, Van Griensven M, et al. Impact of intramedullary instrumentation versus damage control for femoral fractures on immunoinflammatory parameters: Prospective randomized analysis by the EPOFF Study Group. *J Trauma.* 2003;55:7–13.

142. Pape HC, Regel G, Dwenger A, et al. Influences of different methods of intramedullary femoral nailing on lung function in patients with multiple trauma. *J Trauma.* 1993;35:709–716.

143. Pape HC, Schmidt RE, Rice J, et al. Biochemical changes after trauma and skeletal surgery of the lower extremity: Quantification of the operative burden. *Critical Care Med.* 2000;28:3441–3448.

144. Pape HC, Tornetta P 3rd, Tarkin I, et al. Timing of fracture fixation in multitrauma patients: The role of early total care and damage control surgery. *J Am Acad Orthop Surg.* 2009;17:541–549.

145. Pape HC, van Griensven M, Rice J, et al. Major secondary surgery in blunt trauma patients and perioperative cytokine liberation: Determination of the clinical relevance of biochemical markers. *J Trauma.* 2001;50:989–1000.

146. Paré A. *The Works of That Famous Chirurgion Ambrose Paré.* London; 1634.

147. Patzakis MJ, Bains RS, Lee J, et al. Prospective, randomized, double-blind study comparing single-agent antibiotic therapy, ciprofloxacin, to combination antibiotic therapy in open fracture wounds. *J Orthop Trauma.* 2000;14:529–533.

148. Patzakis MJ. Orthopedics-epitomes of progress: The use of antibiotics in open fractures. *West J Med.* 1979;130:62.

149. Pollak AN. Timing of debridement of open fractures. *J Am Acad Orthop Surg.* 2006;14:S48–S51.

150. Puno RM, Teynor JT, Nagano J, et al. Critical analysis of results of treatment of 201 tibial shaft fractures. *Clin Orthop Relat Res.* 1986;212:113–121.

151. Rajasekaran S. Early versus delayed closure of open fractures. *Injury.* 2007;38:890–895.

152. Rajasekaran S, Dheenadhayalan J, Babu JN, et al. Immediate primary skin closure in type-III A and B open fractures: Results after a minimum of five years. *J Bone Joint Surg Br.* 2009;91:217–224.

153. Rajasekaran S, Giannoudis PV. Open injuries of the lower extremity: issues and unknown frontiers. *Injury.* 2012;43:1783–1784.

154. Rajasekaran S, Naresh Babu J, Dheenadhayalan J, et al. A score for predicting salvage and outcome in Gustilo type-IIIA and type-IIIB open tibial fractures. *J Bone Joint Surg Br.* 2006;88:1351–1360.

155. Rajasekaran S, Sabapathy SR. A philosophy of care of open injuries based on the Ganga hospital score. *Injury.* 2007;38:137–146.

156. Raman R, Pape HC, Giannoudis PV. Cytokines in orthopaedic practice: A review. *Curr Orthop.* 2003;17.

157. Raunest J, Derra E. Clostridium perfringens infection following intramedullary nailing of an open femur shaft fracture. *Aktuelle Traumatol.* 1990;20:254–256.

158. Rennekampff HO, Schaller HE, Wisser D, et al. Debridement of burn wounds with a water jet surgical tool. *Burns.* 2006;32:64–69.

159. Robson MC, Duke WF, Krizek TJ. Rapid bacterial screening in the treatment of civilian wounds. *J Surg Res.* 1973;14:426–430.

160. Rosenstein BD, Wilson FC, Funderburk CH. The use of bacitracin irrigation to prevent infection in postoperative skeletal wounds. An experimental study. *J Bone Joint Surg Am.* 1989;71:427–430.

161. Russell WL, Sailors DM, Whittle TB, et al. Limb salvage versus traumatic amputation. A decision based on a seven-part predictive index. *Ann Surg.* 1991;213:473–480.

162. Saveli CC, Belknap RW, Morgan SJ, et al. The role of prophylactic antibiotics in open fractures in an era of community-acquired methicillin-resistant Staphylococcus aureus. *Orthopedics.* 2011;34:611–616.

163. Schemitsch EH, Turchin DC, Kowalski MJ, et al. Quantitative assessment of bone injury and repair after reamed and unreamed locked intramedullary nailing. *J Trauma.* 1998;45:250–255.

164. Schenker ML, Yannascoli S, Baldwin KD, et al. Does timing to operative debridement affect infectious complications in open long-bone fractures? A systematic review. *J Bone Joint Surg Am.* 2012;94:1057–1064.

165. Schmidt AH, Swiontkowski MF. Pathophysiology of infections after internal fixation of fractures. *J Am Acad Orthop Surg.* 2000;8:285–291.

166. Scully RE, Artz CP, Sako Y. An evaluation of the surgeon's criteria for determining the viability of muscle during debridement. *Arch Surg.* 1956;73:1031–1035.

167. Shafi S, Kauder DR. Fluid resuscitation and blood replacement in patients with polytrauma. *Clin Orthop Relat Res.* 2004:37–42.

168. Shanmuganathan R. The utility of scores in the decision to salvage or amputation in severely injured limbs. *Indian J Orthop.* 2008;42:368–376.

169. Shapiro MB, Jenkins DH, Schwab CW, et al. Damage control: Collective review. *J Trauma.* 2000;49:969–978.

170. Silver S. Update on Serious Complications Associated With Negative Pressure Wound Therapy Systems. US Food and Drug Administration: FDA Safety Communication February 24, 2011.

171. Simons R, Eliopoulos V, Laflamme D, et al. Impact on process of trauma care delivery 1 year after the introduction of a trauma program in a provincial trauma center. *J Trauma.* 1999;46:811–815.

172. Sims M, Saleh M. Protocols for the care of external fixator pin sites. *Prof Nurse.* 1996;11:261–264.

173. Sinclair JS, McNally MA, Small JO, et al. Primary free-flap cover of open tibial fractures. *Injury.* 1997;28:581–587.

174. Solan MC, Calder JD, Gibbons CE, et al. Photographic wound documentation after open fracture. *Injury.* 2001;32:33–35.

175. Stannard JP, Robinson JT, Anderson ER, et al. Negative pressure wound therapy to treat hematomas and surgical incisions following high-energy trauma. *J Trauma.* 2006;60:1301–1306.

176. Steiert AE, Gohritz A, Schreiber TC, et al. Delayed flap coverage of open extremity fractures after previous vacuum-assisted closure (VAC) therapy: Worse or worth? *J Plast Reconstr Aesthet Surg.* 2009;62:675–683.

177. Stensballe J, Christiansen M, Tonnesen E, et al. The early IL-6 and IL-10 response in trauma is correlated with injury severity and mortality. *Acta Anaesthesiol Scand.* 2009;53:515–521.

178. Streubel PN, Stinner DJ, Obremskey WT. Use of negative-pressure wound therapy in orthopaedic trauma. *J Am Acad Orthop Surg.* 2012;20:564–574.

179. Stubig T, Mommsen P, Krettek C, et al. Comparison of early total care (ETC) and damage control orthopedics (DCO) in the treatment of multiple trauma with femoral shaft fractures: Benefit and costs. *Unfallchirurg.* 2010;113:923–930.

180. Suedkamp NP, Barbey N, Veuskens A, et al. The incidence of osteitis in open fractures: an analysis of 948 open fractures (a review of the Hannover experience). *J Orthop Trauma.* 1993;7:473–482.
181. Sugrue M, Seger M, Kerridge R, et al. A prospective study of the performance of the trauma team leader. *J Trauma.* 1995;38:79–82.
182. Svoboda P, Kantorova I, Ochmann J. Dynamics of interleukin 1, 2, and 6 and tumor necrosis factor alpha in multiple trauma patients. *J Trauma.* 1994;36:336–340.
183. Swiontkowski MF. Commentary on an article by Christopher J. Lenarz, MD, et al.: "Timing of wound closure in open fractures based on cultures obtained after debridement". *J Bone Joint Surg Am.* 2010;92:e12.
184. Templeman DC, Gulli B, Tsukayama DT, et al. Update on the management of open fractures of the tibial shaft. *Clin Orthop Relat Res.* 1998:18–25.
185. Tkachenko SS, Rabinovich IM, Poliak MS, et al. Use of antibiotics in open fractures of the bones of the extremities. *Voen Med Zh.* 1975:20–23.
186. Tscherne H. [Management of open fractures]. *Hefte zur Unfallheilkunde.* 1983;162: 10–32.
187. Tschoeke SK, Hellmuth M, Hostmann A, et al. The early second hit in trauma management augments the proinflammatory immune response to multiple injuries. *J Trauma.* 2007;62:1396–1403; discussion 1403–1404.
188. Valenziano CP, Chattar-Cora D, O'Neill A, et al. Efficacy of primary wound cultures in long bone open extremity fractures: Are they of any value? *Arch Orthop Trauma Surg.* 2002;122:259–261.
189. Wangensteen O, Wangensteen S. *The Rise of Surgery from Empiric Craft to Scientific Discipline.* Minneapolis: University of Minnesota Press; 1978.
190. Webb LX, Bosse MJ, Castillo RC, et al. Analysis of surgeon-controlled variables in the treatment of limb-threatening type-III open tibial diaphyseal fractures. *J Bone Joint Surg Am.* 2007;89:923–928.
191. Weed T, Ratliff C, Drake DB. Quantifying bacterial bioburden during negative pressure wound therapy: Does the wound VAC enhance bacterial clearance? *Ann Plast Surg.* 2004;52:276–280.
192. Weitz-Marshall AD, Bosse MJ. Timing of closure of open fractures. *J Am Acad Orthop Surg.* 2002;10:379–384.
193. Werner CM, Pierpont Y, Pollak AN. The urgency of surgical debridement in the management of open fractures. *J Am Acad Orthop Surg.* 2008;16:369–375.
194. Yannascoli S. The Urgency of Surgical Debridement and Irrigation in Open Fractures: A Systematic Review of the 6-hour Rule. *University of Pennsylvania Orthopaedic Journal (UPOJ).* 2011;21.
195. Yehuda U, et al. The Revised Reconstructive Ladder and its applications for high energy injuries to the extremities. *Ann Plast Surg.* 2006;56:401–405.
196. Yokoyama K, Uchino M, Nakamura K, et al. Risk factors for deep infection in secondary intramedullary nailing after external fixation for open tibial fractures. *Injury.* 2006;37:554–560.
197. Ziran BH, Smith WR, Anglen JO, et al. External fixation: how to make it work. *J Bone Joint Surg Am.* 2007;89:1620–1632.

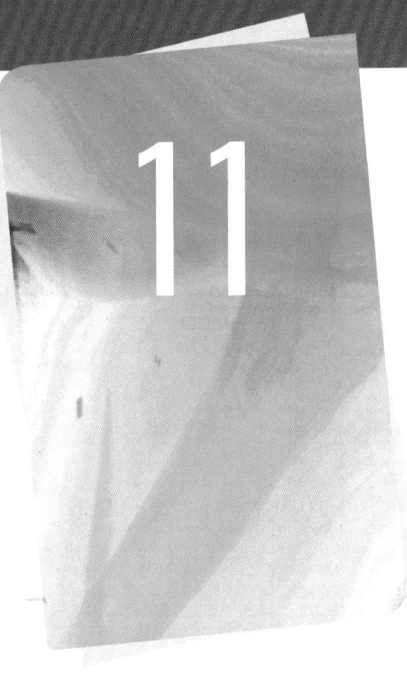

11

GUNSHOT AND WARTIME INJURIES

Paul J. Dougherty, Romney C. Andersen, and Soheil Najibi

INTRODUCTION

Gunshot injuries remain a significant part of the workload for some urban trauma centers in the United States and are also common in war-torn regions throughout the world. The purpose of this chapter is to review the epidemiology, pathophysiology, and treatment of gunshot wounds and war injuries. This chapter is intended not only to assist those who evaluate gunshot wounds as a major part of their practice but also orthopedic surgeons who occasionally see patients with such injuries.

NONMILITARY AND MILITARY WEAPONS

Weapons that are used in nonmilitary and military settings differ. Firearms seen in nonmilitary settings include handguns,

rifles, and shotguns.[8,33,81,83,142] Conventional military weapons can be divided into the categories of small arms and explosive munitions. *Small arms* consist of pistols, rifles, and machine guns. *Explosive munitions* consist of artillery, grenades, bombs, mortars, land mines, and improvised explosive devices (IEDs). Armored vehicle crew casualties represent a special subgroup of injuries seen in those who work and fight in and around armored vehicles.

Small Arms

Small arms are weapons that fire a bullet from a rifled barrel to a target. The bullet is usually contained in a cartridge consisting of powder, a primer, and a cartridge case all in one unit

(Fig. 11-1). Handguns and rifles are classified by the diameter (size) of the barrel (9 mm, 0.45 inch, 7.62 mm). Handguns used by the military are the same as used those by civilian police and others in regard to size, shape, and caliber. They are usually semiautomatic, which means a bullet is fired every time the trigger is pulled and as long as there is ammunition in the weapon's magazine.[8,33,81]

Handguns are the most common firearms associated with nonmilitary injuries. A handgun is intended to be fired over a short range and is small. Two types of handguns are most commonly seen: Pistols and revolvers (Fig. 11-2A). A pistol has a magazine that contains cartridges, which are fed (or *cycled*) into the barrel every time the trigger is pulled (Fig. 11-2B). Revolvers contain cylinders with chambers that contain cartridges. The cylinder rotates so that a cartridge is aligned to the barrel when the trigger is pulled.[81,142]

Rifles are shoulder-fired weapons that are intended to strike a target farther away from the shooter than a handgun or shotgun can (Fig. 11-3). In general, the barrel is longer and has rifling to impart a spin on the bullet. Rifling consists of spiral grooves that line the barrel, engaging the bullet and causing it to spin on the longitudinal axis lending gyroscopic stability in air. The bullets fired from rifles are more aerodynamic in shape than those fired from pistols, leading to more accurate bullet flight. Bullets for nonmilitary rifles may have an open tip or "soft nose" to allow for expansion of the bullet when striking the target. Military bullets have complete metal jacketing to limit deformation or fragmentation, which decreases wound damage. Machine guns are intended to fire in the full automatic mode; this occurs when repeated shots are fired as long as the trigger is held down, as opposed to the semiautomatic fire described earlier. Machine guns generally weigh more than rifles and are installed onto vehicles and aircraft.[86,142]

Modern military rifles are most often "assault rifles" and have the ability to fire in both fully automatic and semiautomatic

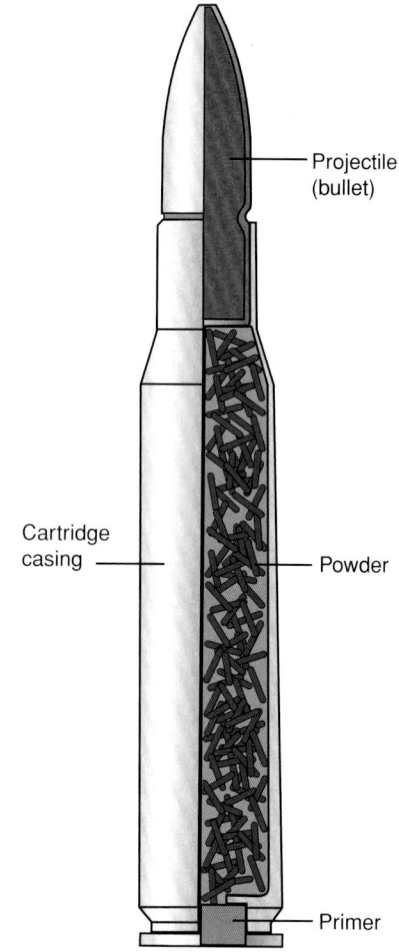

FIGURE 11-1 Schematic drawing of a cartridge. An entire cartridge is made up of the cartridge case, the bullet, a primer, and powder. When struck, the primer initiates powder burning, generating the pressure to propel the bullet in flight.

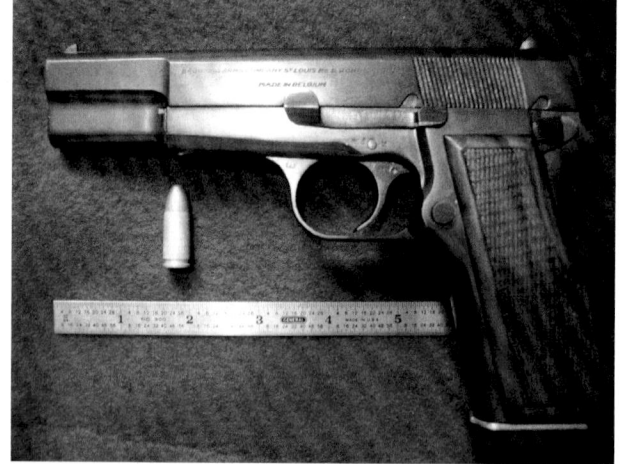
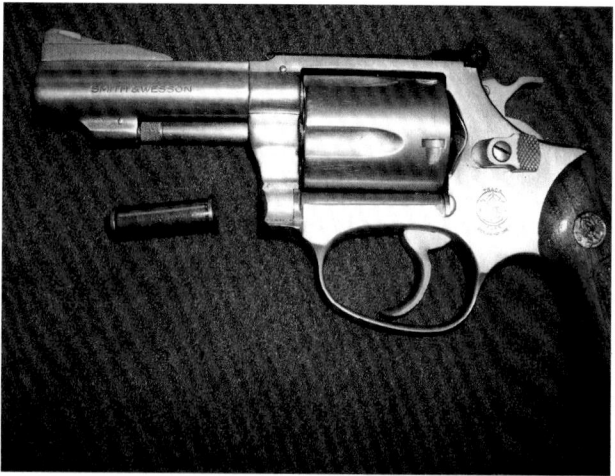

FIGURE 11-2 Types of handgun. **A:** A 9-mm Browing P-35 pistol used in several countries as the military handgun. It is also available to the nonmilitary market. This firearm was first produced in the 1930s. **B:** Revolver; the cylinder rotates to align with the barrel for each cartridge.

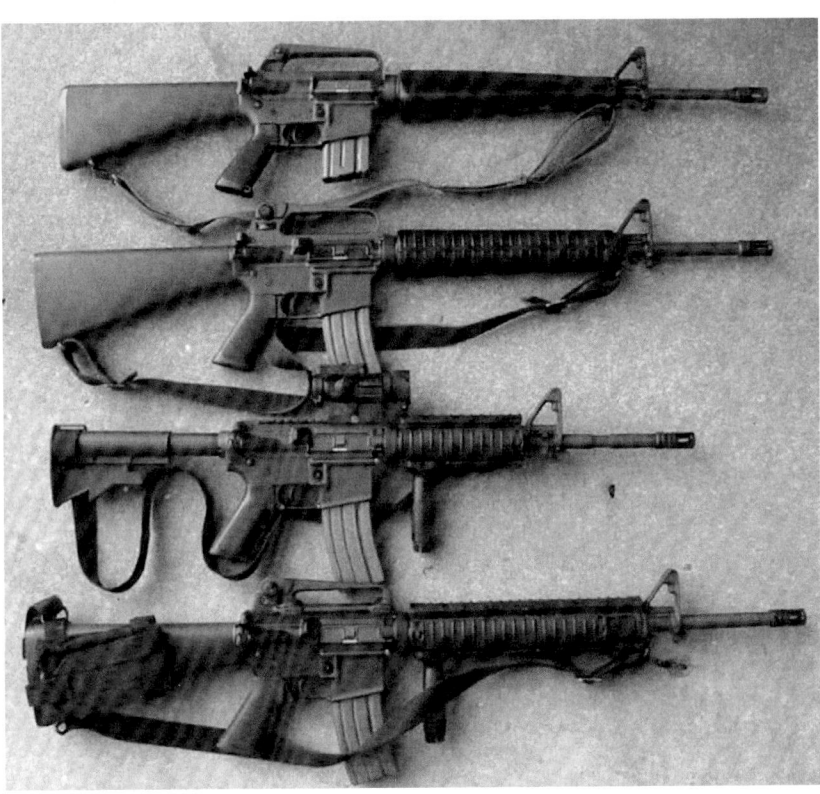

FIGURE 11-3 M16 series military rifles (from **top** to **bottom**): M16A1, M16A2, M4A1, and M16A4.

modes. In an effort to reduce recoil, cartridges used in these weapons are not the full-powered rifle cartridges seen in civilian hunting rifles or in military weapons of the first half of the 20th century.[130,142] Shotguns are shoulder-fired weapons that have a smooth barrel (Fig. 11-4). Shotgun gauge sizes are inversely proportional to the diameter of the barrel. The gauge expresses the inverse of the size of a lead sphere able to be fired from the shotgun. For example, a 12-gauge shotgun can shoot a 1/12-lb lead sphere, while a 20-gauge shotgun can shoot a 1/20-lb lead sphere. This is why it is not intuitive that a "12-gauge" shotgun is more lethal than a "20-gauge" shotgun. Although shotguns are able to fire a solid lead sphere and a number of other types of rounds most often shotguns fire multiple projectiles, called pellets, which vary in size from 0.012 to 0.36 inch. The pellets are often contained in a cup or wad that keeps them together and pushes the shot out of the barrel (Fig. 11-5). The pellets begin to spread the farther they move as they exit the barrel.[83,136] The spread of the pellet shot over a given distance is dependent on the size of the shot, the length of the barrel, and the degree of "choke" on the barrel. Choke is a constriction at the end of the barrel that will cause less spread of the shot over a given distance. A standard measure of choke is the amount of pellets that are put into a circle at 40 yards. A full choke should put 70% of its pellets into the circle, whereas an "improved cylinder" choke should put 50%. When within a few feet of the barrel, the spread of the shot is negligible.[8,83]

Explosive Munitions

Explosive munitions include artillery, grenades, mortars, land mines, bombs, and IEDs.[8,34] They are the most common agents

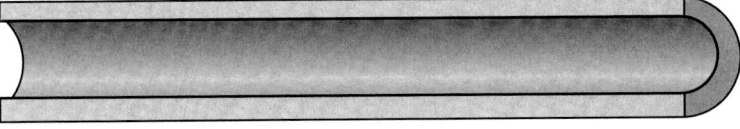

Smooth barrel shotgun

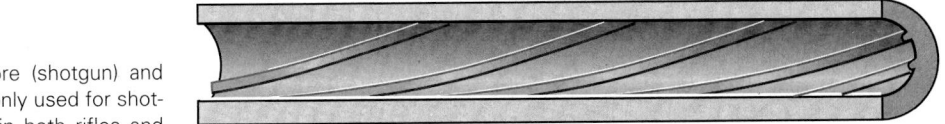

Rifled barrel

FIGURE 11-4 Barrel types: Smoothbore (shotgun) and rifled. The smoothbore barrel is commonly used for shotguns, whereas a rifled barrel is used in both rifles and handguns.

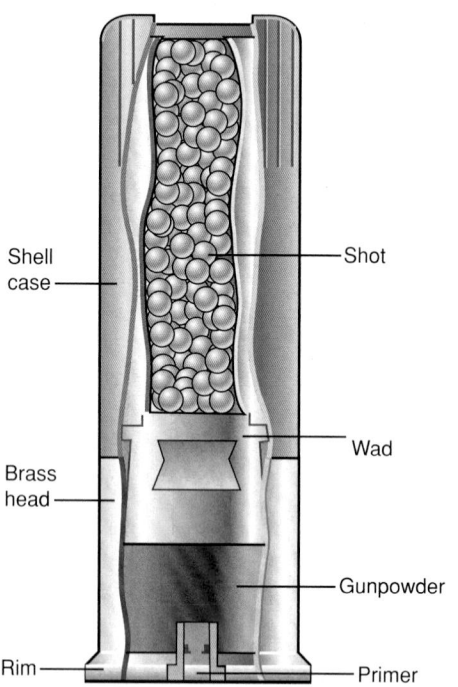

Shell case — **Shot**

Brass head — **Wad**

Rim — **Gunpowder**

— **Primer**

FIGURE 11-5 Shotgun shell. A shotgun shell consists of the primer, powder, wad, and shot. All of this is contained in the shell casing. When powder burning is initiated by the primer, the wadding propels the shot down the barrel and into free flight.

for wounding soldiers on a battlefield, beginning with World War I (1914 to 1918), when artillery became more common on the battlefield. Table 11-1 describes the relative proportion of different types of weapons that generated casualties on the battlefield from various wars during the 20th and 21st centuries.

Explosive munitions wound via one or more of four mechanisms: Ballistic, blast, thermal, or translational (Fig. 11-6). *Ballistic injuries* occur from fragments of exploding munitions or from material around the explosive device. *Blast injuries* occur because of a transient blast wave caused by the exploding munitions. *Thermal injuries* are caused by a transient increase in local temperature as a result of the explosion. *Translational* injuries are caused by a person being propelled and sustaining

blunt trauma due to the explosion. Patients often sustain closed injuries as the result of these translational injuries.

Explosive, ballistic, and thermal injuries are similar to those seen with civilian injuries; however, the blast mechanism is unique to military injuries. The blast and thermal effects occur relatively close to the exploding munitions, whereas ballistic injuries can also occur farther from the device.[12,34,118] The distances from the munitions that the various effects may be seen (ballistic, blast, thermal) will vary with the type of device and the environment. An explosion in a confined space, for example, will increase the effects of blast overpressure. Someone who is wounded closer to the exploding munitions may have combined ballistic, thermal, and blast effects compared with someone farther away. A typical mortar shell, when detonated in an open area, might have thermal effects within a few feet of detonation. The blast or pressure wave may cause ear injury within 30 feet. Fragments; however, can still cause injury at greater than 100 yards from detonation.

Blast injuries tend to have large soft tissue wounds associated with fractures. The rate of infection is significantly higher in blast-induced injuries than blunt injuries. This is due to the "outside in" mechanism of a blast versus the typical "inside out" mechanism of a blunt injury. In blunt fractures, the bone frequently breaks and the sharp edge of the bone lacerates the skin exposing the fracture to contamination—"inside out." A blast injury on the other hand has significant amounts of foreign material deposited deep into tissue both surrounding and at the fracture site—"outside in."

Artillery includes cannons that fire large projectiles for a greater range. The projectiles may be antivehicle, contain white phosphorus, or be explosive filled. The diameter of US military artillery cannon barrels ranges in size from 105 mm to 8 inches. The explosive-filled projectiles are most often used against infantry soldiers. When detonated, they produce fragments of varying shape and size, which cause wounds. The fragments produced depend on the casing of the artillery round. Modern artillery casings break up to produce more uniform fragments over a given area. The fragments may range from a few milligrams to several grams in weight. After detonation, fragments may initially travel at several thousand meters per second. This initial velocity rapidly decreases because of the irregular shape of the fragments.[8,12,34,118]

TABLE 11-1 Casualty Generation by Weapon

Wounding Agent	World War I	Bougainville Campaign, Solomon Islands (World War II)	Vietnam Conflict (Wound Data and Munitions Effectiveness Team [WDMET])	Wars in Afghanistan and Iraq
Bullet	28.06%	34%	30%	12.8%
Mortar	NR	39.5%	19%	NR
IED/Booby trap/land mine	NA	1.9%	17%	74.3%
Hand grenade	1.21%	12.7%	11%	0.2%
Artillery	70.4%	11%	3%	8.3%
RPG[a]	NA	NA	12%	4.4%

NA, not available; NR, not reported; RPG, rocket propelled grenade.

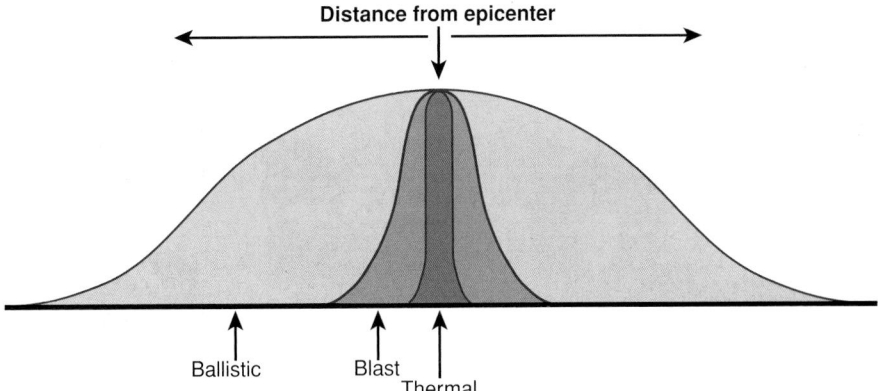

FIGURE 11-6 Mechanisms of injury explosive munition. The three mechanisms of injury are ballistic, blast, and thermal. The ballistic effects take place much farther away from the explosion compared with blast or thermal effects.

Grenades are small explosive-filled devices that may be thrown or fired from a special launcher (Fig. 11-7). Grenades may produce smoke for signaling or be designed to disable destroy tanks or soldiers. As with artillery shells, the type of fragment produced is dependent on the composition of the container. Most modern grenades have a notched or prefragmented casing that produces fragments of a uniform size when detonated.[8,12,34,118]

Mortars are weapons that have barrels aimed at a high arc to produce indirect fire. Projectiles fired from mortars may produce smoke, white phosphorus, or explosive fragments. These weapons are smaller and are more limited in range compared

with the cannon. As with the other weapons described earlier, fragments produced by the explosive shells vary with the composition of the shell's casing.[8,9,12]

Land mines may be one of two major types: Antipersonnel or antivehicle. *Antipersonnel* land mines are those intended to injure individual soldiers. *Antivehicle* land mines are intended to destroy or disable vehicles, such as tanks. Antipersonnel land mines are classified by the US Army as static, bounding, or horizontal spray (Fig. 11-8). Another category, unconventional or improvised devices, will be handled separately in this section. Currently, there is much concern about land mines

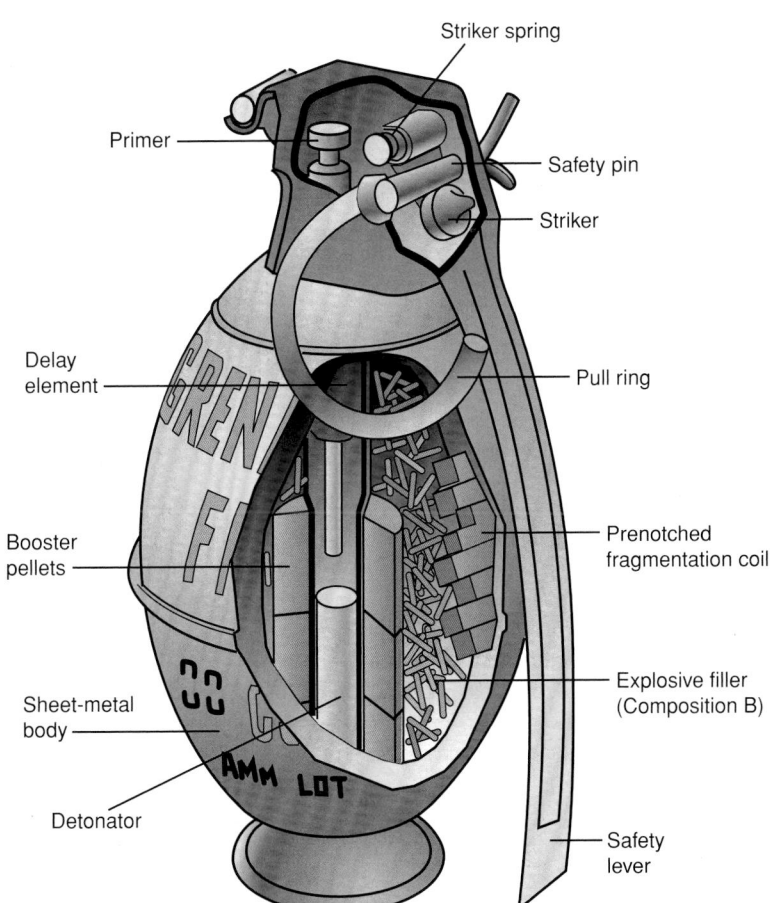

FIGURE 11-7 Grenade. This cutaway illustrates the casing, which is composed of notched wire, producing fragments when detonated. The powder is stored in the casing and is ignited by the detonator.

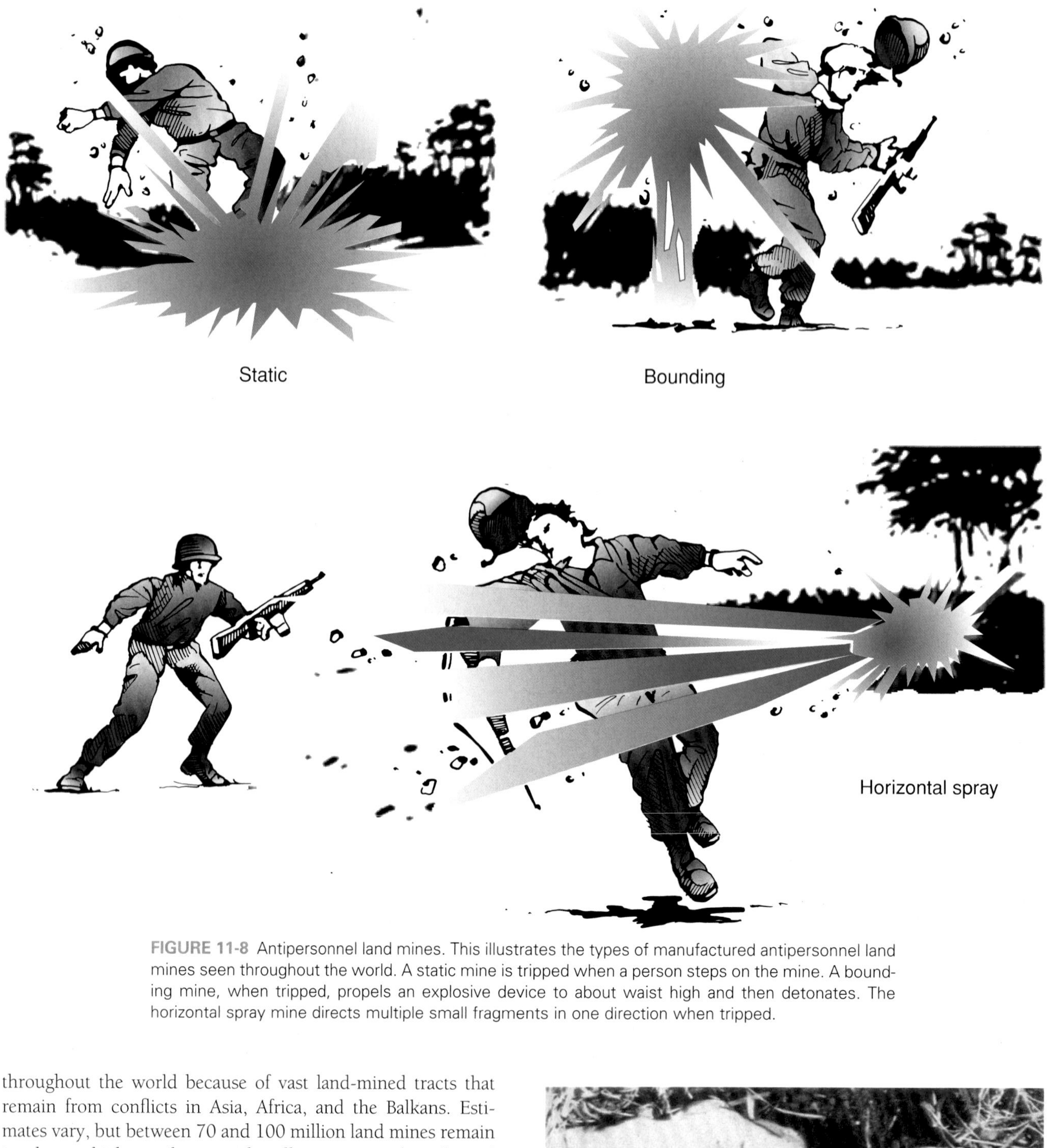

Static

Bounding

Horizontal spray

FIGURE 11-8 Antipersonnel land mines. This illustrates the types of manufactured antipersonnel land mines seen throughout the world. A static mine is tripped when a person steps on the mine. A bounding mine, when tripped, propels an explosive device to about waist high and then detonates. The horizontal spray mine directs multiple small fragments in one direction when tripped.

throughout the world because of vast land-mined tracts that remain from conflicts in Asia, Africa, and the Balkans. Estimates vary, but between 70 and 100 million land mines remain in place, which, until removed, will continue to be a hazard to those living or working in the area (Fig. 11-9).[1,7,8,12,34,110,118]

Static land mines are those that are laid on top of the ground or buried in soil and are detonated when someone steps on the device, and are the most common type of mine. They contain a small amount of explosive (100 to 200 g) and produce a characteristic pattern of injury (Fig. 11-10).[110] Soviet surgeons obtained considerable experience with land mines during the war in Afghanistan (1979 to 1988), which prompted them to conduct both laboratory and clinical investigations on the

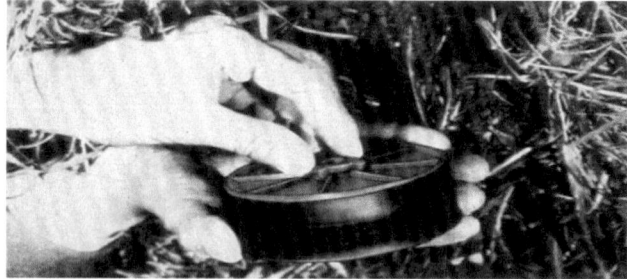

FIGURE 11-9 Small static land mine. Note the small size of this land mine compared with a hand. These are usually made of minimal metal components to avoid detection.

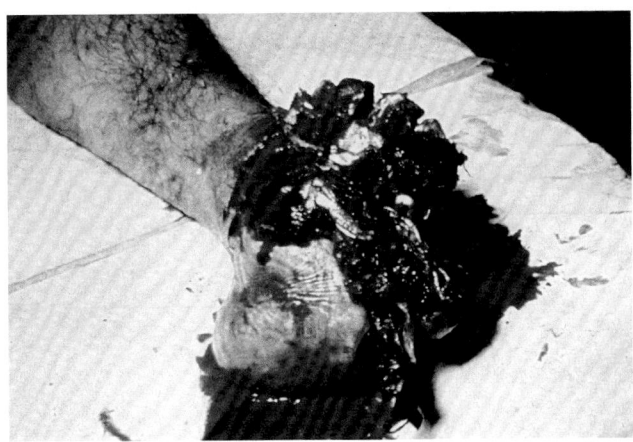

FIGURE 11-10 This photograph is of a foot injured by a small planted land mine. The mine was under the forefoot and the patient had footwear.

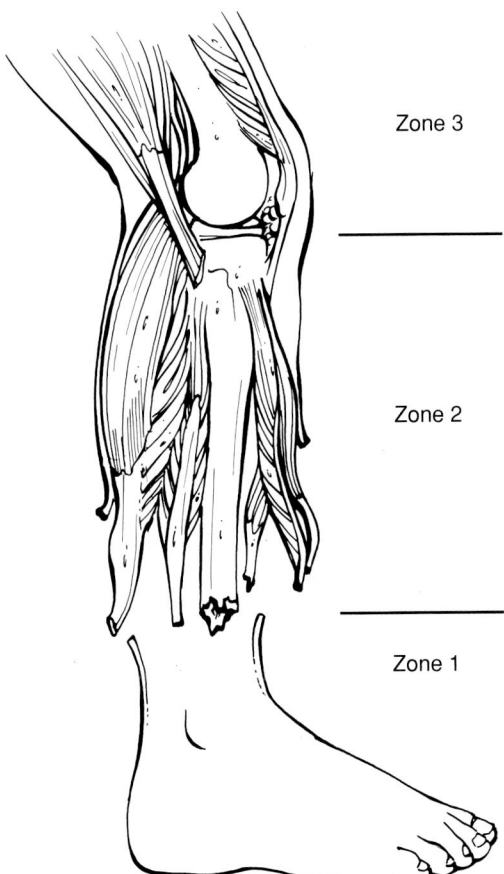

Zone 3

Zone 2

Zone 1

FIGURE 11-11 Small static land mine injury. This illustrates the three areas of injury sustained from a small static land mine. First, there is an area of avulsion or amputation; second, there is an area of soft tissue stripping where tissue may or may not survive. Third, proximal to this area, there may be fragment wounds from debris or the land mine, or injury from the fast translation of being propelled upward from the land mine itself.

mechanism of injury. Injuries produced by static land mines are primarily to the lower extremity (Fig. 11-11). There are three areas of injury—there is an area of *mangling* or *avulsion (traumatic amputation),* which occurs at the midfoot or distal tibia. There is a second area in which the *soft tissues are separated* from bone along fascial planes in the leg (brisant). This area is a tidewater area in terms of tissue survival; the tissue is compromised, but it may heal. Third, more proximally at or above the knee, injuries may occur from *fragments* or *debris* propelled from the land mine but not necessarily from direct effects of the blast itself. The degree of injury is dependent on the size and shape of the individual's limb, the type of footwear and clothing worn, the amount and type of soil overlying the land mine, and the size of the land mine.[1,110]

Bounding mines are land mines that, when tripped, propel a small grenade-like device to about 1 to 2 m in height. The device then explodes, producing multiple small fragment wounds similar in nature to those produced by grenades.[110]

Horizontal spray land mines are mines that, when tripped, fire fragments in one direction. These land mines may be used to protect a perimeter or during an ambush. The Claymore mine is an example of this type of mine. It fires about 700 steel balls that weigh 10 grains each in one direction. The weapons produce multiple fragment wounds to exposed personnel nearby (Fig. 11-12).[110]

Unconventional or *improvised devices* are another category of land mine. These mines are fabricated out of another piece of ordnance, such as a grenade or mortar shell. They are designed to detonate when a person steps on the device, a person pulls a tripwire, or the device is triggered remotely by radio or control wires. These devices may be made out of locally available materials as well. They vary in construction from smaller antipersonnel devices to large explosive devices with several kilograms of explosive to disable or destroy vehicles (Fig. 11-13).

The majority of explosive devices used in Afghanistan and Iraq conflicts are IEDs. One of the larger antipersonnel mines used against civilians is the *suicide bomber.* This is a term given to an individual who carries a large explosive charge and detonates it

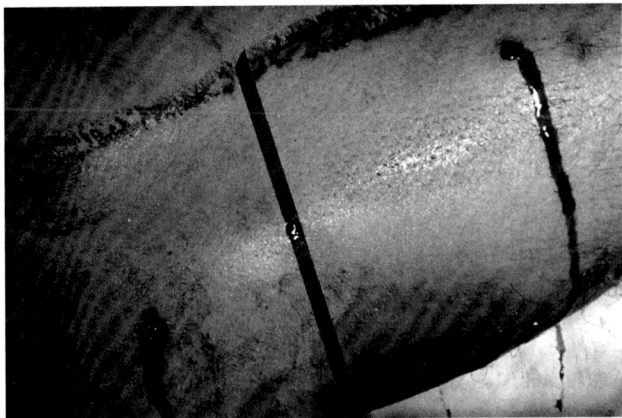

FIGURE 11-12 Claymore mine injury. This photograph illustrates multiple small fragment wounds of a thigh from a patient injured by a Claymore mine.

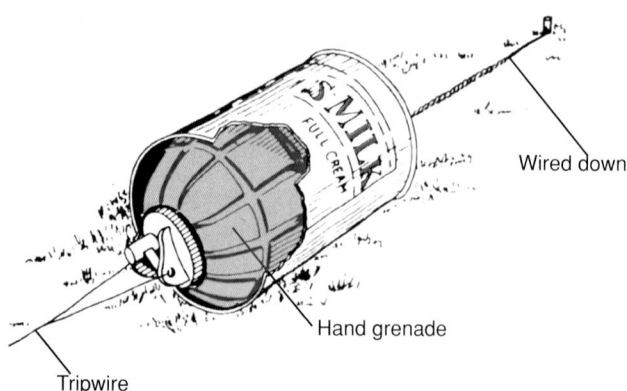

FIGURE 11-13 Improvised explosive device (IED). This illustrates an IED ("booby trap") made from a grenade that is inserted into a can. When the wire is tripped, the grenade explodes. This drawing is taken from a World War II British Commando manual. IEDs are the most common type of land mine or booby trap seen in the Vietnam, Iraq, and Afghanistan conflicts.

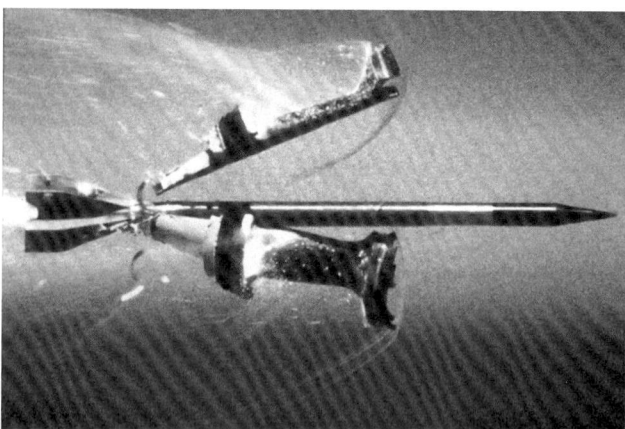

FIGURE 11-14 Kinetic energy armor piercing round. This illustration shows the dense metal penetrator, shaped like an arrow and the "petals" of the sabot surrounding the penetrator falling away.

in location of a crowd or building to achieve maximum casualties. One of the more common constructs for such a bomb is in the form of a vest containing explosive along with material for fragments. The fragments increase the wounding potential of the device and consist of items such as ball bearings or nails. Large antivehicle land mines have made transportation and troop movements difficult.[1,8,34,126,127] Bombs are explosive devices that are dropped from aircraft. They may consist of one large explosive device or may carry submunitions that are distributed more uniformly over a target area. Cluster bombs are an example of the latter device.[9,12,118]

ARMORED VEHICLE CREW CASUALTIES

Most of the world's armies have tanks, infantry fighting vehicles, and armored reconnaissance vehicles within their inventory. Injuries to crewmembers occur both in and around vehicles. Those injured outside of the vehicle have injuries similar to infantrymen. Two types of weapons are used to perforate the armored vehicle's envelope to cause injury to the crewmen (antitank land mines may be considered a third type).

First, there is the kinetic energy round (Fig. 11-14). This consists of a hard piece of metal, such as tungsten or depleted uranium, which is fired out of a cannon at a high velocity. The projectiles used today are long and narrow and cause a high concentration of pressure over a very small cross-sectional area to defeat the armor plate. If the round penetrates to the crew compartment, injuries may be caused by the penetrating round itself, debris knocked off from the inside of the vehicle itself, or armor debris. Because the penetrating rounds are large, injuries to individuals tend to be catastrophic.[33]

Shaped charges are the other type of weapon seen on the battlefield (Fig. 11-15). They consist of an explosive-filled war head that is packed around a reverse cone-shaped piece of metal (copper or aluminum). When detonated, the liner collapses and a jet is produced, which travels at up to 10,000 feet per second.

The jet produces an area of high temperature and pressure over a very small cross-sectional area. When the jet penetrates the armor, it produces two areas of under armor debris. First, there is the jet of the shaped charge. The jet produces catastrophic wounds when it directly hits one of the crewmen. Second, there is an area of under armor debris called *spall*, which is material knocked off from the inside face of the armored plate itself. Many of today's armored vehicles have liners that do not allow spall debris to form.[33,110]

A variation on the shaped charge is the "explosively formed projectile (EFP)" (Fig. 11-16). This device has a shallow concavity for the liner and forms a "slug" rather than a fully developed jet to penetrate vehicles. The "slug" is less affected by intermediate targets, such as dirt and debris, than the jet of the shaped charge. Although it is considered to be a new innovation, this technology has been present since at least the 1930s.[2]

EPIDEMIOLOGY

Nonmilitary Gunshot Wounds

Gotsch et al.[55] reported estimates of gunshot injuries in the United States for 1993 through 1998. The authors estimated that during this period, there were approximately 180,533 fatal gunshot wounds and about 411,000 nonfatal gunshot wounds for the 6-year period. Over the course of the study there was a decline in the annual nonfatal rate by 40% (from 40.5 to 24 per 100,000 population) and in the fatal rate by 21.1% (from 15.4 to 12.1 per 100,000 population). This decline corresponded with the overall decrease in violent crime of 21%. During the study period, the average annual number of self-inflicted fatalities exceeded those from assault (18,227 vs. 15,371 per year).[55]

From 1998 through 2006, there has been a further decline in violent crime from 566.4 to 473.5 per 100,000 population (16.5%) and in murder from 6.3 to 5.7 per 100,000 population (9.5%).[77] Deaths caused by firearms in the United States also decreased from 35,957 (13.5 per 100,000) to 29,569 (10.5 per 100,000).[125]

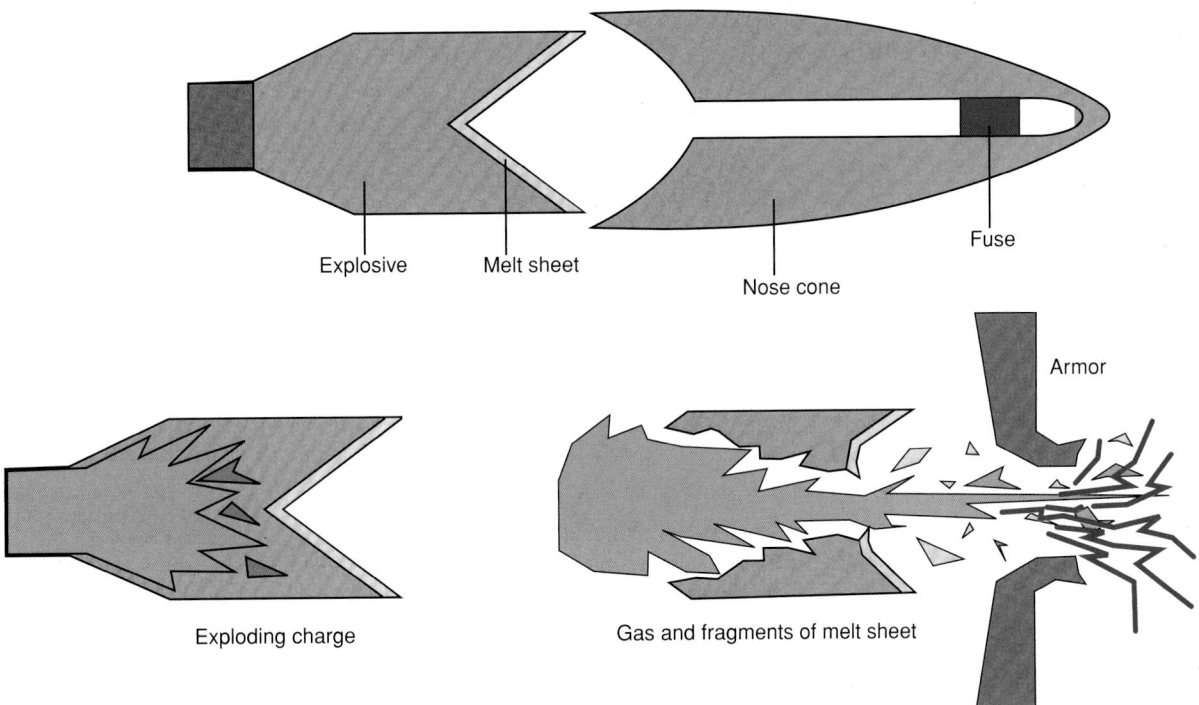

FIGURE 11-15 Shaped charge or high-explosive anti-tank (HEAT) round. Explosive is packed around a reverse cone-shaped metal liner called a melt sheet. When detonated, it generates a jet of high temperature and pressure that defeats armor through plastic or elastic deformation.

Gotsch et al.[55] also found that males were seven times more likely to receive a firearm injury than females. Black men aged 20 to 24 years had the highest annual firearm-related injury rate for both fatal and nonfatal groups (166.7 and 690 per 100,000 population, respectively). This compared unfavorably to the firearm injury rate of 13.4 per 100,000 (fatal) and 30.1 per 100,000 (nonfatal) for the entire population. These demographics also explain why the concentration of patients with gunshot wounds is higher in trauma centers for cities with a higher black population such as Detroit, Los Angeles, Philadelphia, Chicago, and New Orleans.[55,60,77]

There is an economic, as well as a human, cost in caring for patients with gunshot wounds.[23,60,154] Hakanson et al.[60] reported that the average cost of treating a gunshot orthopedic injury is $13,108 per patient. Brown et al.[23] reported on orthopedic patients treated for gunshot wounds in New Orleans at an inner-city Level I trauma center. They found that patients with gunshot wounds represented 24% of all admissions and 26% of all orthopedic trauma surgical cases. The most common locations for nonfatal gunshot wounds are in the extremities (Table 11-2). Gotsch et al.[55] reported that extremity wounds represented 46% of nonfatal wounds caused by assault and 71.8% of unintentional wounds. A series from Cordoba, Argentina, found that 63% of gunshot victims had injuries to the upper or lower extremities.[14] A review of records at Henry Ford Hospital in Detroit, MI, from 2001 through 2006 found that 42.4% of all patients admitted with a diagnosis of gunshot wounds had extremity wounds. This figure increases to 50.2% if pelvic and spine injuries are included.

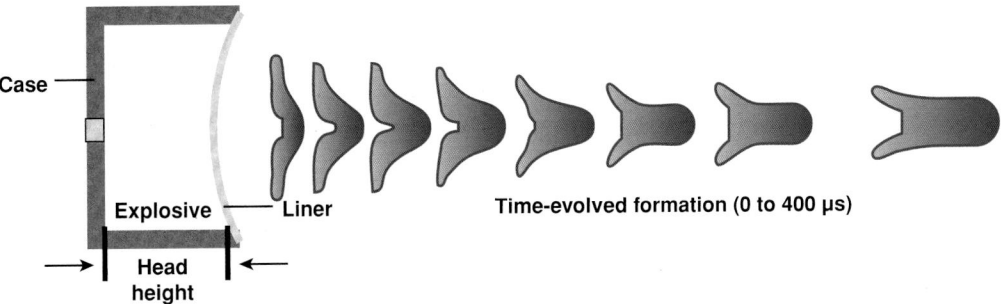

FIGURE 11-16 Explosively formed projectile (EFP). A modification of the shaped charge, the liner has a shallow concavity that propels a "slug" at high velocity. The slug is less likely to be disturbed by intermediate targets or debris compared with the jet of the shaped charge.

TABLE 11-2	Anatomic Distribution of Gunshot Wounds	
	Henry Ford Hospital Detroit, MI (%) ($n = 1,505$)	Cordoba, Argentina ($n = 1,326$)
Head, ears, eyes, nose, throat	11.7	12%
Chest	16	12%
Abdomen/pelvis	24	13%
Upper extremity	16.2	18%
Lower extremity	26.2	45%
Spine	5	Not reported

Many patients with gunshot wounds are also treated in emergency departments without admission.[21,55,116] Estimates for the number of patients with gunshot wounds who are treated on an outpatient basis range from 45% to 60%.[13,116,122,125]

Overview of Battle Casualties

Two prospective epidemiologic studies concerning battle casualties have been done (one during World War II and the second during the Vietnam War), collecting data on the tactical nature surrounding casualty wounding, the type of weapon, the anatomic locations of wounds, and mortality.[9,118] The first was conducted during the Bougainville campaign in the Solomon Islands during World War II to assess patient injuries based on the weapon and tactical circumstances.[118] There were 1,569 casualties who were followed through their initial surgical care to look at outcome. A second study was performed during the Vietnam Conflict to assess 7,964 casualties during an 18-month period during the conflict. The patients in this study (Wound Data and Munitions Effectiveness Team [WDMET]) were evaluated in terms of the tactical situation, the weapons used, the injuries produced, and the patient outcome.[9] A retrospective review of service members wounded in Operation Iraqi Freedom/Operation Enduring Freedom (OIF/OEF)[119] from 2001 to 2005 showed 54% percent of injuries were extremity injuries with 82% of those being open fractures.

The anatomic distribution of wounds among the war injured is relatively constant, probably because wounds produced on the battlefield tend to be a random event (Table 11-3). Between 60% and 70% of wounded patients admitted to a medical treatment facility have wounds to the extremities, and about 21% of those admitted have fractures. The use of body armor to protect soldiers and airmen was studied in World War II and the Korean Conflict and was found to reduce thoracic and abdominal wounds.[13,37,72,99,119,122,127]

The proportion of casualties caused by various weapons from World War I, the Bougainville campaign in World War II, the Vietnam Conflict, and the Global War on Terrorism is shown in Table 11-1.[9,99,118,119] The proportion of injuries caused by bullets has been relatively constant from conflict to conflict. Recently, fragment producing explosive munitions have accounted for an increasing proportion of casualties seen from the battlefield. This trend is expected to continue.

The *lethality* of a weapon is defined as the probability of death following a hit from that weapon (Table 11-4). The Bougainville and WDMET data showed the lethality of a bullet wound was approximately 0.33. Fragments from grenades, mortars, and artillery ranged from 0.05 to 0.10. Death from tripping a land mine has been shown to be approximately 33%.[7,9,97,98,118,148]

MEDICAL EVACUATION

Wounded soldiers from the battlefield must be simultaneously treated and moved through the evacuation chain (Fig. 11-17). All major armies throughout the world have made some provisions to care for wounded soldiers. The first treatment of a wounded soldier on the battlefield consists of self-care or buddy care. The first step may be to take cover from hostile fire. Treatment for extremity wounds consists of stopping the bleeding, applying a dressing, and splinting. The next step is care provided by a medic, who evaluates the patient and adjusts the dressings and splint. The medic also has the capability of providing pain relief, administering antibiotics, and arranging for further evacuation. A battalion aid station may be the first physician contact for a wounded soldier. Here, the patient is further evaluated, splints and dressings are adjusted, and the patient is triaged. If the casualty load is light, patients are treated as they arrive. If the casualty load is heavy, patients must be triaged to allocate the resources of evacuation and surgical care. Ideally, the triage takes place along the entire evacuation chain. If a patient's condition worsens, his or her priority may increase.[97,98]

A more established medical setting is typically the next echelon of care in the evacuation scheme. This facility has the capability of providing blood transfusions and has limited

TABLE 11-3	Percentage Anatomic Distribution of Wounds (Living Wounded US Soldiers)				
Anatomic Area	US Civil War	World War I	World War II	Bougainville Campaign	OIF/OEF
Head, Face, Neck	9.1%	11.4%	16.1%	**20.7%**	30%
Chest	11.7%	3.6%	9.8%	12.4%	6%
Abdomen	6.0%	3.4%	5.6%	5.7%	11%
Upper Extremity	36.6%	36.2%	28.3%	27.4%	54% upper and lower
Lower Extremity	36.6%	45.4%	40.3%	33.8%	

TABLE 11-4 **Lethality by Weapon**

Weapon	Bougainville Campaign	Vietnam Conflict WDMET
Bullet	0.32	0.39
Mortar	0.12	0.13
Grenade	0.05	0.13
Artillery	0.11	0.25
Land mine	0.38	0.31

radiographic capability. This unit is the first level of care with any bed holding capability. Adjacent to the medical company may be the forward surgical team (FST) that provides the first possible surgical support near the battlefield. The purpose of this unit is to provide surgical care of those patients whose outcome would be compromised by being evacuated farther for surgical care. Examples of patients who should have surgery at the FST are those with penetrating abdominal wounds who are in shock and those with major traumatic amputations. Because of the mission to treat emergent patients, the FST is staffed with one orthopedic surgeon and two general surgeons. Having an orthopedic surgeon is important to make decisions concerning amputations as well as caring for those with multiple injuries. Often those with multiple injuries have major extremity wounds. Because the FST has no bed holding capability, it must be collocated with a medical company to complete its mission. Goals of surgery are to stabilize the patients and prepare them for evacuation. The next echelon of care on the battlefield is a permanent structure with inpatient beds and includes intensive care unit capability, operating rooms, laboratory capability, and it is staffed by orthopedic surgeons in addition to general surgeons, internists, and emergency physicians. This type of facility is the first surgical echelon for the majority of battlefield patients, including those with orthopedic injuries. Goals of care at this hospital (which is ideally located near the battlefield) are to stabilize the patients and to prepare them for evacuation out of the combat zone. Examples of care for patients arriving at this point include the treatment of soft tissues, fracture stabilization via casting or external fixator application, and treatment of a partial or complete amputation. Patients may be moved to one of these surgical facilities directly from the battlefield depending on the severity of the injury and if the tactical situation permits. In more stationary situations, such as during the Vietnam Conflict, this occurs more frequently.[117,146] During the Vietnam Conflict, the US military controlled the airspace and had little geographic movement of hospitals or troops, such as occurred during World War II. Because of this, overflight of facilities in the evacuation chain occurred to bring patients promptly to a permanent facility that could provide more care.

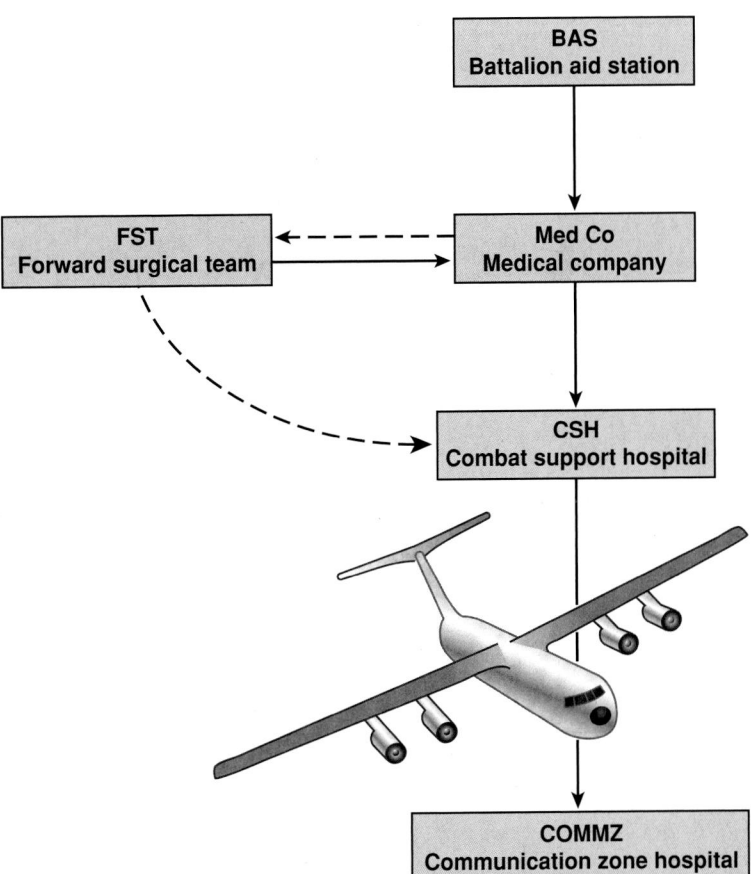

FIGURE 11-17 Military medical evacuation. This shows the present scheme of evacuation for wounded soldiers used by the modern armed forces. Surgical care by orthopedic surgeons takes place at the forward surgical team (FST), combat support hospital (CSH), or communication zone hospitals (COMMZ).

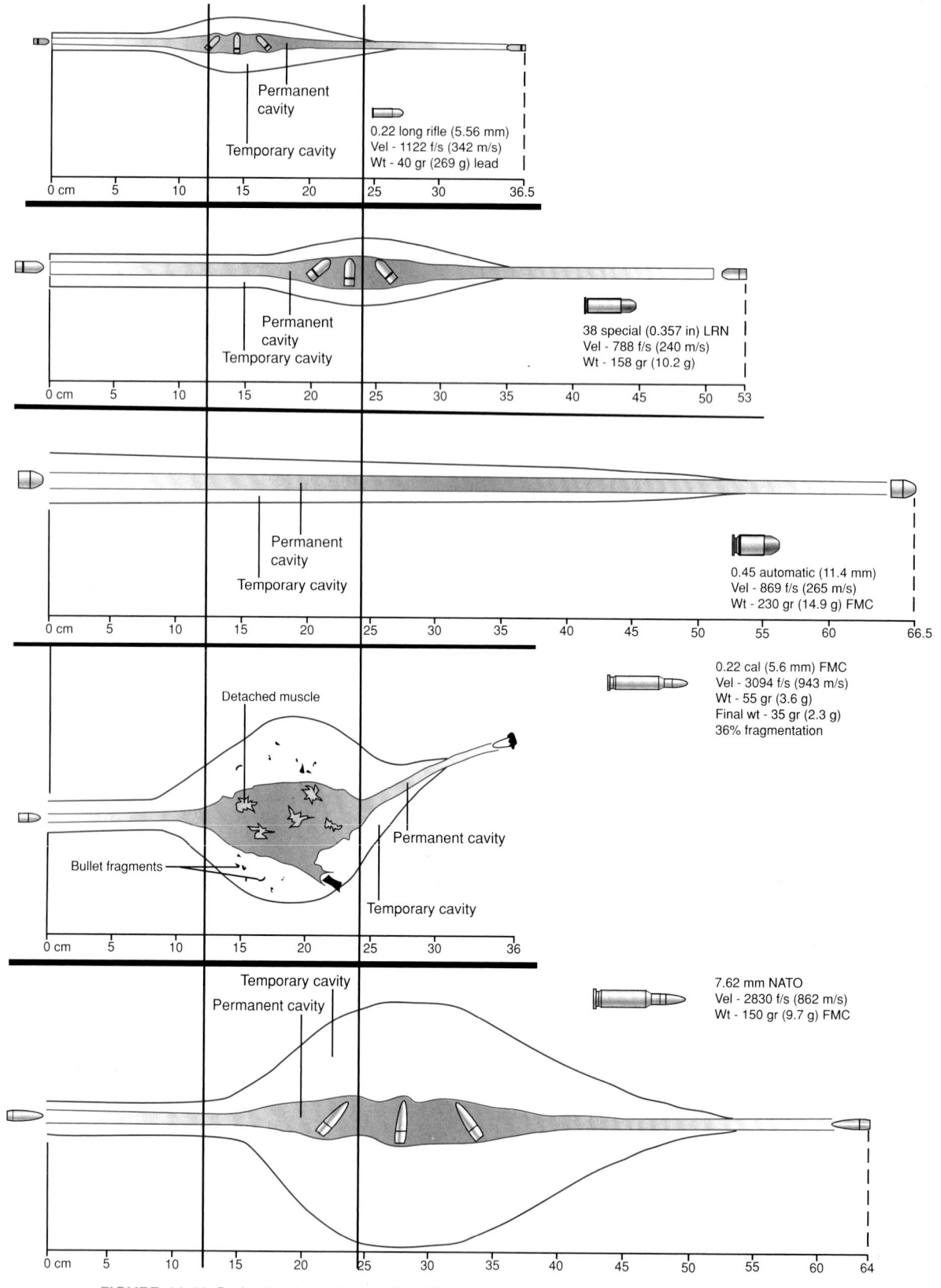

FIGURE 11-18 Projectile tissue interaction. Three areas can be measured in the projectile tissue interaction: The sonic wave, the temporary cavity, and the permanent track. The temporary cavity is caused by a transient lateral displacement of tissue (stretch), whereas the permanent track is made by passage of the projectile, crushing tissue. The sonic wave, although measurable, has not been shown to cause tissue injury.

WOUND BALLISTICS

Wound ballistics is the science that studies the effects of penetrating projectiles on the body.[27,35,36,38,40,41,43,45,46,56,57,65–68,77,88,102,105,131] Three observable phenomena occur when a bullet strikes tissue. First, tissue is crushed by the projectile as it passes through, leading to a localized area of cell necrosis that is proportional to the size of the projectile. This area of the projectile's path is called the permanent track or permanent cavity (Fig. 11-18).

There is a second area in which elastic tissue is stretched, causing a temporary cavity.[35,36,45,75,78,88,102] The stretch results from a lateral displacement of tissue that occurs after the passage of the projectile. There is a transient increase in pressure of 4 to 6 atmospheres (atm) for a few milliseconds' duration. This transient lateral displacement of elastic tissue, such as skeletal muscle, vessels, and nerves, appears as blunt trauma, whereas inelastic tissue, such as bone, may fracture.

A third component, known as the shock wave, is a pressure wave that travels at the speed of sound preceding the bullet in tissue. This pressure wave is only a few microseconds, but may generate pressures up to 100 atm in magnitude.[45,65,66] The shock wave has not been shown to cause tissue injury.

The two mechanisms of injury (crush and stretch) have differing effects on skin just as with other tissues.[35,36,66,68,77,88,102] When a projectile strikes skin and creates a permanent cavity, it produces a small amount of necrosis that is proportional to the size of the projectile. The temporary cavity splits the skin, which produces a larger opening of tissue. Grundfest et al.[56] used cadaver skin stretched over a frame to test threshold velocities for penetration. The authors used steel ball bearings from 1/16 to 1/4 inch in size as well as 11/64-inch lead spheres fired from an air rifle. They found that increasing the size of the projectile also required increasing the velocity needed to perforate the skin.

Fackler et al.[41] studied healing of soft tissue using a large porcine animal model. These investigators used a solid nondeforming 5.56-mm bullet and fired it into the thighs of the animals. The authors found larger exit wounds compared with the entrance wounds as a result of splits in the skin caused by the larger temporary cavity produced as the bullet yawed in tissue. The larger wound allowed for better exposure of the wound path and freer drainage of wounds. Also, the authors found skin vasospasm, which produces blanching, soon after wounding. This area did not revascularize for several hours. If the loss of blood supply is a criterion for excision, the transitory nature of the blanching shows that viable tissue would be sacrificed in this area if evaluated soon after wounding.

In another study, Fackler et al.[39] found that projectile shape was important in determining the appearance of a skin wound. The authors fired a solid nondeforming bullet point first and then base first, noting the different appearance of the skin wound in each case. The bullets were fired at over 5,000 fps. For the projectile going base first, large skin splits were produced by an early temporary cavity. No such effect was seen with the bullets going point first through the skin.

Injury to skeletal muscle has been studied using animal models by Harvey et al.,[66] Dziemian et al.,[36,102] Mendelson and Glover,[102] Fackler et al.,[45] Brien et al.,[20] and Fackler.[45,48] Muscle

that is touched by the projectile in the permanent tract has a microscopic rim of tissue that is actually necrotic. This tissue, if the blood supply to the muscle remains intact, can heal over time without surgical intervention. The area of cell death sloughs and, as long as the wound can drain, will heal spontaneously.

Surrounding the path is an area damaged by the stretch causing the temporary cavity, which may split along fascial planes. This area appears grossly as bruised or contused tissue. Microscopically, there are disrupted skeletal muscle fibers and capillaries. After a period, there is leukocyte infiltration followed by inflammation and healing.[35,44,48,65,102]

When a bullet fragments, many permanent paths are formed; thus, the region stretched by the temporary cavity is perforated in multiple places. Tissue weakened by these tiny perforations is often split by the temporary cavity stretch, and pieces between perforations become detached. This often greatly increases the size of the permanent cavity.[45]

If the muzzle of a firearm is in contact with a living body when it is fired, the high-pressure gas that pushes the projectile out of the barrel will pass into the tissues through the hole formed by the projectile—often causing greatly increased tissue displacement and disruption.

Bone injury is common with gunshot wounds to the extremities.[27,57,75,76,105,131] Fractures may occur via two mechanisms, directly when the projectile strikes bone (Fig. 11-19) or, rarely,

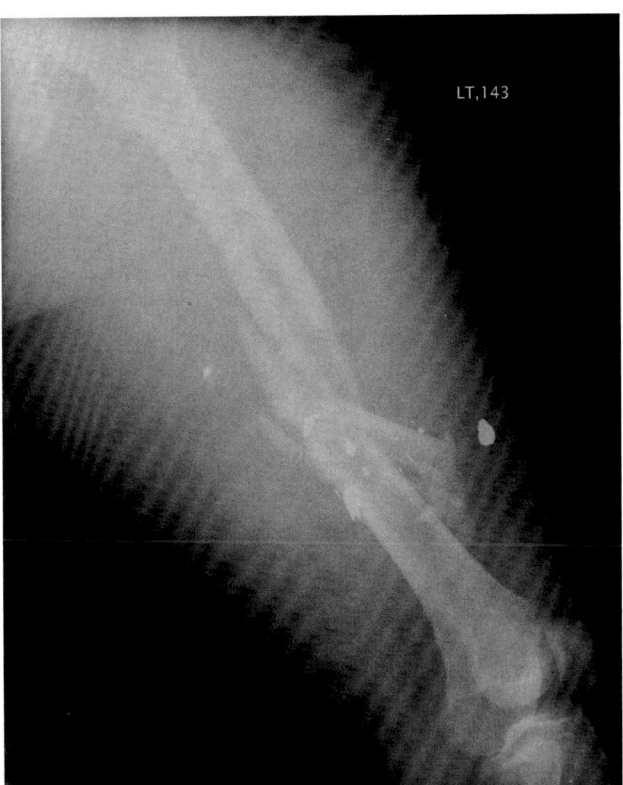

FIGURE 11-19 Direct fracture. Cortical bone is very dense, so when a projectile strikes, fracture lines propagate away from the bullet's path, causing comminution. The temporary cavity may cause further displacement.

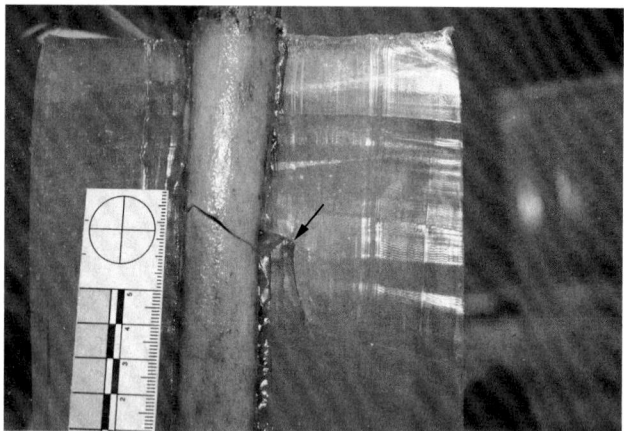

FIGURE 11-20 Indirect fracture. A fracture may occur without the bullet striking the bone. This illustrates a bullet path *(arrow)* 8 mm away from the edge of the bone. The path of the bullet is perpendicular to the plane of the page, with the bullet path going away from the reader. A simple fracture occurred from the effects of the temporary cavity.

indirectly by the temporary cavity. Due to the density and relative inelastic behavior of bone, fracture line propagation may occur well beyond the area crushed by the projectile itself, leading to bone comminution and the production of secondary missiles from the bone itself. Because the secondary missiles of bone disrupt tissue before it is stretched by the temporary cavity, this has the effect of increasing comminution around the bullet path, and can cause increased soft tissue disruption, reminiscent of the previously mentioned synergism between bullet fragmentation and temporary cavity stretch.

Indirect fractures (Fig. 11-20) may occur when a projectile passes close to the bone in soft tissue and a strain occurs to such a degree as to cause a fracture. Indirect fractures are almost always simple in pattern (Fig. 11-20). Clinically, indirect fractures to bone are rare compared with those formed when bone is struck directly by the projectile.[3,47,70,74,99] Figure 11-20 illustrates the shot path 8 mm from the edge of the diaphyseal bone in ordnance gelatin, showing how indirect fractures appear. The bullet path is perpendicular to the page, going away from the reader.

Clasper et al.[27] used sheep femora and hind limbs to study contamination of both direct and indirect fractures. The authors fired through fluorescein-soaked gauze placed on the surface of the skin to determine the amount of fracture site contamination that occurred with each shot. The authors found massive fluorescein contamination with the direct fractures; however, only 3 of 14 bones with indirect fractures had medullary fluorescein contamination. Periosteal contamination was less with indirect fractures compared with the direct fractures.

Rose et al.[131] proposed a classification of incomplete fractures because of gunshot wounds, describing "drill hole" and "divot" fractures. The "drill hole" fractures are seen with bullet perforation of both cortices yet minimal comminution surrounding the bullet tract. They occur in metaphyseal bone. The "divot" fracture was described as an eccentric perforation of a diaphyseal long bone usually producing a unicortical defect. More extensive injury may be present than apparent on plain

radiographs, and the "divot" injury may be an occult complete fracture of diaphyseal bone. Such fractures should be treated as complete fractures unless other radiographic measures, such as a CT scan, show an incomplete fracture.

There are common misconceptions about wound ballistics.[48] First, some authors have exaggerated the effects of velocity to include it as being the sole criterion for increased injury or as a means to classify gunshot wounds. Velocity is one of several factors involved with the production of the wound. The introduction of the M16 rifle during the Vietnam Conflict was heralded as producing equivalent wounds or causing equivalent "incapacitation" because of the weapon's higher muzzle velocity of an advertised 3,200 fps. Later testing in the laboratory found that the increased severity of wounds sometimes seen with the M16A1 was the result of bullet fragmentation, not the modest 10% increase in velocity. In fact, the greatest increase in muzzle velocity for military rifles occurred in the late 19th century when the armed services of several nations, changed to a full metal-jacketed bullet from a solid lead one: This doubled muzzle velocity. This resulted in an increase of muzzle velocity from about 1,000 to 2,000 fps.[48] The change in firearms; however, resulted in decreased wound severity because bullet deformation was limited by the jacketing.

A second common misconception[48] is the idea that "kinetic energy" or "energy deposit" is directly proportional to wound severity. Kinetic energy is the amount of potential energy available for work. "Energy deposit" is a description of how much energy is lost or "deposited" in tissue. While one can measure the projectile's velocity and weight as it enters and exits a body or tissue medium, it does not describe how this potential energy is used. The potential energy may be used for the crush or stretch, but it may also be consumed in mechanics that may not cause any tissue injury. Examples where energy may be consumed, but not cause tissue damage, include the shock wave, bullet heating, and bullet deformation.

SOFT TISSUE WOUND MANAGEMENT
Patient Evaluation
Initial evaluation of a patient with any gunshot wound should include a thorough history and physical examination. The extremity should be inspected for both entrance and exit wounds after all clothing has been removed. The limb should also be inspected for swelling, deformity or shortening, and ecchymosis. The limb should be palpated for crepitus. Examination for distal pulses should be done to assess vascular status. In an awake patient, assessment should also be done to assess the patient's motor and sensory status distal to the injury. If the patient is not able to comply, this fact should be documented with a note to recheck if the patient's condition improves: The routine practice of writing "neurovascular intact" for a patient who cannot be properly examined is to be discouraged.

Biplanar radiographs should be taken of the injured limb covering the path of the bullet. Standard long bone radiographs, including both the joint above and below, should be done if included in the bullet's path. If a joint wound is suspected, standard views should be taken of the joint.

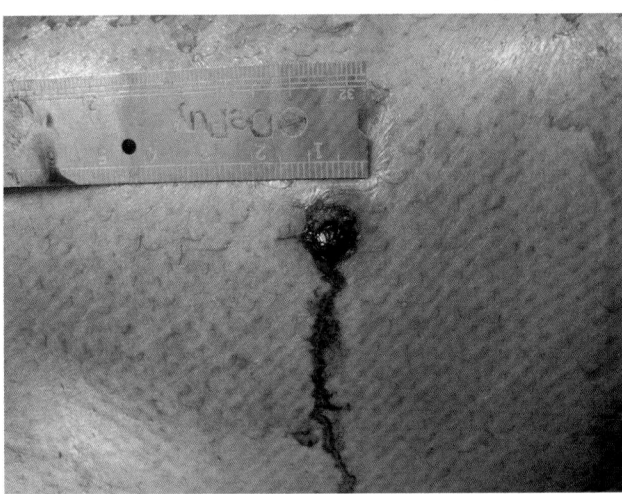

FIGURE 11-21 Simple perforating wound. This shows a simple wound caused by perforation of the bullet.

The most common injuries by gunshot wound are to the soft tissues of skin, subcutaneous fat, and the skeletal muscle.

Skin Injuries

Gunshot skin wounds have three general patterns. First, there is a punctate wound the size of the penetrating bullet (Fig. 11-21). Second, there is a wound that contains splits in the skin but has negligible skin loss and can eventually be closed without resorting to more extensive skin grafting or flap coverage (Fig. 11-22). Third, there is a wound in which there is skin loss, which requires the use of partial-thickness skin grafting or flap coverage (Fig. 11-23).

Perforating nonarticular wounds without a fracture or vascular injury may be candidates for outpatient treatment.[25,118] Under controlled circumstances, simple perforating wounds have been shown to heal uneventfully with simple dressing changes.[49,67,102] Successful treatment with local wound care has

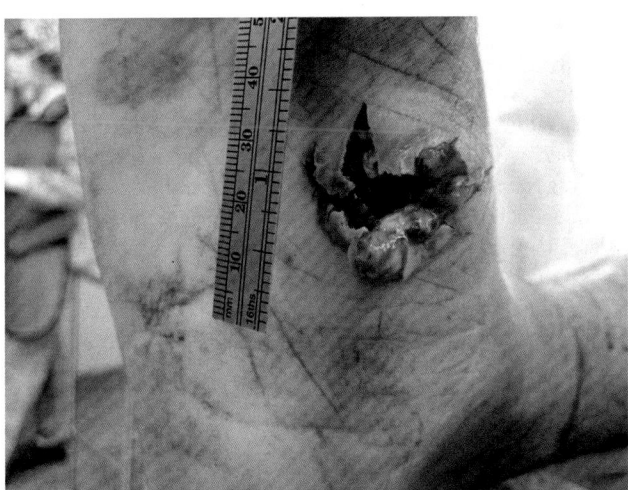

FIGURE 11-22 Skin splits. Splits in the skin may be caused by bone fragments, debris, or the stretch of the temporary cavity.

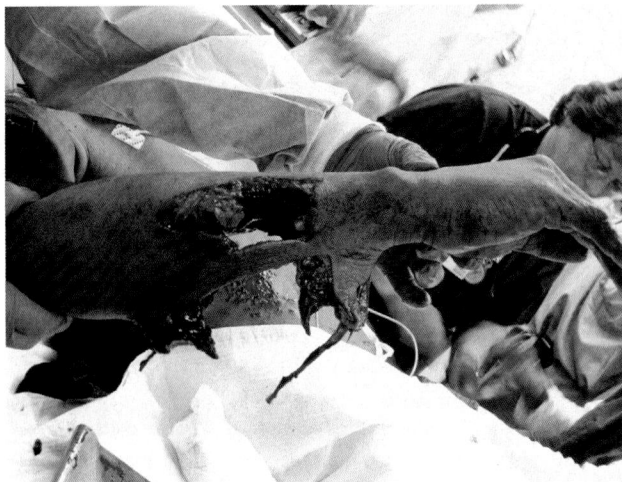

FIGURE 11-23 Skin defect. A skin defect may occur from secondary missiles created by bone fragments or by multiple fragments or projectiles. This case illustrates a shotgun wound from close range.

been reported by several authors.[25,31,62,100,108] Likewise, successful treatment of simple fractures associated with minimal soft tissue disruption have also been treated with local wound care and fracture stabilization in a cast or splint.[85,92,100,158]

Simple splits in the skin are produced from dilation resulting from the temporary cavity, from a projectile that is traveling sideways and presenting the long axis of the bullet to the skin, or from bone becoming a secondary missile, causing a more extensive wound. The splits produce an exit wound that will allow for free drainage of the wound, preventing the formation of an abscess or a hematoma.

More extensive wounds with skin loss may be produced from shotgun pellets, bullets, or bone fragmentation. Initial treatment of the more extensive wounds should be done in the operating room. Longitudinal incisions of the skin and underlying fascia to relieve pressure, remove hematoma and debris, and expose the underlying muscle should be done. Surgical removal of skin is rarely indicated for the initial surgery, other than trimming irregular edges. As described earlier, blanching may give a false impression of nonviable skin if seen soon after injury and lead the surgeon to excise viable skin.

In contrast, fragment wounds are the most common types seen in wartime. Injuries range from single fragment wounds to multiple fragment wounds with extensive soft tissue loss (Fig. 11-24). Often, a person has multiple fragment wounds of the extremity skin, subcutaneous fat, and skeletal muscle, yet without significant injury to bone, vascular, or nerve structures.[9,118,148] In certain controlled circumstances, small fragment wounds may be treated nonoperatively.[17,77]

The use of negative pressure wound therapy (NPWT) for the initial management of more extensive wounds has been suggested to reduce the size of defect needing coverage, promote local growth factors, and remove debris and nonviable tissue from the wound. A randomized study comparing NPWT to standard dressing changes in "high-risk" fracture patients demonstrated a decreased incidence of wound dehiscence and total infections in the NPWT group.[91,117,143]

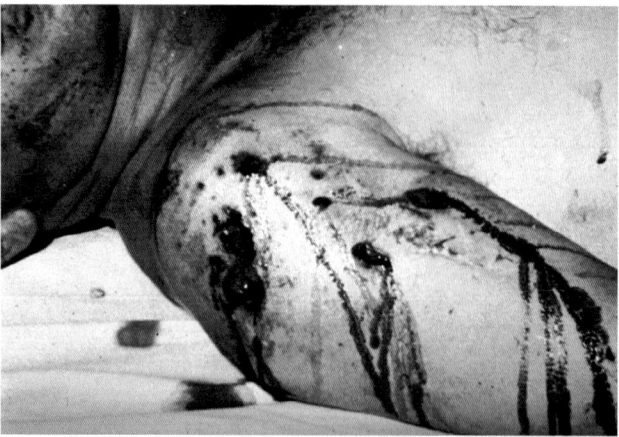

FIGURE 11-24 Multiple fragment wounds. This illustrates multiple small skin wounds that occur with many exploding munitions. They are often of the skin, subcutaneous fat, and skeletal muscle only.

Large soft tissue injury deficits that cannot be closed primarily can be treated with split-thickness skin grafting if there is adequate muscle to support the graft. Areas where tendon or bone are exposed generally require tissue transfers; however, some success has been achieved with the use of dermal substitutes followed by skin grafting.[70] An early consultation should be made with a plastic surgeon or a hand surgeon who is skilled in extremity soft tissue coverage. Before soft tissue coverage, the wound should be stable.

Skeletal Muscle Injuries

One of the most controversial aspects in caring for gunshot wounds is the treatment of skeletal muscle. Mendelson and Glover,[102] Brien et al.,[20] Dziemian and Herget,[35] Fackler,[46] Harvey et al.,[66] and Helgeson et al.[70] all demonstrated that a relatively minimal margin of necrosis occurs in skeletal muscle if the blood supply remains intact. Excision of tissue has been recommended for dead skeletal muscle but identification of tissue that needs to be excised remains imprecise. Artz et al.[3] and Heitmann et al.[69] evaluated 60 biopsy samples taken from the initial wound excision of 12 war wounds during the Korean Conflict. The surgery took place between 3 and 8 hours from the time of injury. The samples were graded by the surgeon as to the presence of the four "C's": Color, consistency, contractility, and circulation (bleeding). The samples were then evaluated by a pathologist who graded the degree of muscle fiber damage. The authors found correlation of microscopic damage to consistency, contractility, and bleeding. Color was not found to correlate to the degree of soft tissue damage. Also, time was not found to be a factor in determining tissue viability.

For wounds in which there is a simple perforation of the limb, there is a small rim of cell death that will heal uneventfully if the wounds are allowed to drain.[41,67,102] For wounds in which there is more extensive skeletal muscle injury, a more formal exploration of the wound is warranted. The wound may be enlarged through the use of longitudinal skin incisions as described earlier. Macroscopic evaluation of skeletal muscle helps determine what tissue needs to be removed. A simple analogy for surgeons is, "muscle that looks like hamburger should be excised, muscle that looks like steak should stay."

The term *debridement* is derived from the French verb *débrider,* which means "to unbridle or release."[29,47,52,65,74,94] As noted by Harvey et al.[65] and Fackler,[47] the original translation of works from the Napoleonic Wars by Larrey and Desault showed that incision, to allow for free drainage of the wound and to relieve swelling (compartment pressure), was the technique used by these surgeons for extremity wounds.

Hampton had a similar description: "Debridement of any wound is designed to relieve the area of excessive tension, rid it of dead tissue and massive hematoma and provide excellent drainage. *Perhaps relief of tension is the most important contribution of wound debridement.*"[62]

Compartment syndrome occurs when there is swelling inside a relatively closed space, such as the anterior compartment of the leg, which is surrounded by fascia and bone. The swelling occurs because of direct trauma, hemorrhage, hematoma, or ischemia, and the diagnosis of compartment syndrome remains primarily clinical.

Compartment syndrome associated with gunshot wounds has been reported in the forearm,[37,107] leg,[151] and thigh.[11,52] Forearm compartment syndrome has been well documented and is present in up to 10% of patients with GSW's to the forearm.[107] Longitudinal incisions to release pressure within a compartment and to expose tissue has been recommended by military surgeons since the time of the Napoleonic Wars.[47]

The amount of swelling present in a compartment after a gunshot wound may range from minimal to that involving the entire compartment. Involvement of the entire compartment is rare, but it does occur when patients have extensive soft tissue injury or vascular injury causing ischemia. With the initial evaluation, patients with a large hematoma, vascular injury, or excess swelling are candidates for formal operative release of the fascia.

WOUND INFECTION

Infection has been documented in 1.5% to 5% for those who sustain gunshot injury. Bullet wounds are contaminated wounds. Bullets themselves, when fired, do not become "sterile" because of the heating and friction encountered in the barrel. LaGarde[89] created contaminated wounds by firing bullets contaminated with anthrax into an animal model. The animals developed an anthrax infection. Dziemian and Herget[35] placed barium sulfate dye on the surface of an ordnance gelatin block. After shooting through the surface into the gelatin, the dye coated the entire path of the projectile's path, showing that surface material is brought into the wound.

Simchen et al.[138] and Simchen and Sacks[139] evaluated 420 wounded Israeli soldiers following the 1973 October War. They found an overall infection rate of 22% for all wounded. Wounds from explosive munitions have a higher rate of infection than those from gunshot wounds alone. Eight of 20 (40%) soldiers with femur fractures developed infection. In addition to femur fractures, the authors found burns of greater than 25% body surface area and penetrating abdominal wounds of the colon were risk factors.

Simchen et al.[138] further evaluated risk factors in war wounds after the 1982 War in Lebanon. The authors compared 1 month of hospital admissions for wounded Israeli soldiers during the 1973 and 1982 wars. They found the overall infection rates were similar between the two groups (31.5% and 30.4%, respectively). Risk factors for fracture site infections were found to be the presence of open drains, amputations, multisystem injury, and a fractured femur.

The discovery of penicillin in 1929 by Sir Alexander Fleming led to its use in caring for the wounded during World War II. Fisher et al.[51] compared 3,471 wounded soldiers with 436 soldiers who had wounds "at risk" for the development of gas gangrene (open fractures, more extensive soft tissue injury, long delay to care, wounds to the buttock or thigh). Those with wounds at risk were treated with penicillin, whereas those without at-risk wounds were not. Infection developed in 28 of 3,471 (5 with gas gangrene) untreated wounds and in 2 of 436 (0 with gas gangrene) penicillin-treated wounds.

In a recent series of military long bone fractures treated with intramedullary fixation an infection rate of 40% was found, with osteomyelitis in 17%. Blast injuries were found to have a significantly higher number of infections. In a recent series of open tibia fractures treated with circular ring external fixation the infection rate was 8%.[82]

Patzakis et al.[121] divided 310 patients with open fractures (78 due to gunshot wounds) into one of three treatment groups: No antibiotics, penicillin and streptomycin, and cephalothin. Four of 78 wounds (5%) became infected, one with osteomyelitis. The authors attributed the infection to severity of injury in three of the patients who had shotgun wounds with extensive soft tissue damage. A fourth infection occurred in the no-antibiotic group.

Hansraj et al.[63] compared the use of a one dose of 1-g intravenous ceftriaxone to a 1-g intravenous dose of cefazolin given three times a day for 3 days for gunshot fractures with minimal soft tissue disruption (<1-cm wound) that were treated nonoperatively. There were 50 patients in each group with a follow-up of 59%. The authors reported no infections based on the cultures taken in the emergency department and concluded that the single 1-g dose of ceftriaxone regimen was more cost effective than the 3-day cefazolin regimen.

Knapp et al.[85] reported a prospective study at their institution of 186 patients with 218 gunshot fractures. All fractures were treated nonoperatively and were considered to be "low velocity" based on the appearance of the wound and history. Wounds larger than 1 cm associated with fractures were excluded. The authors compared the use of oral antibiotics (ciprofloxacin 750 mg twice a day) to the use of intravenous antibiotics (cephapirin sodium 2 g every 4 hours and gentamicin 80 mg every 8 hours). There were two infections reported in each group. All infections were associated with fractures of the distal tibia.

The prevalence of infected gunshot wounds in the nonmilitary setting is low. These studies showed no difference in infection rates with any particular antibiotic regimen; rather, it was the use of antibiotics that helped reduce infection. Infection rates from war wounds remain higher than those associated with nonmilitary gunshot wounds alone due to multiple factors including higher velocity gunshot wounds, explosive munitions, and delayed care because of medical evacuation.[53,59,161]

AUTHORS' PREFERRED METHOD OF TREATMENT

Antibiotic Recommendations for Nonmilitary Gunshot Wounds

The authors' current antibiotic recommendations (Table 11-5) for nonmilitary gunshot wounds are dependent on injury severity. Isolated perforating wounds of the soft tissue only without vascular injury, or those patients with isolated simple fractures, may be treated initially with a first-generation cephalosporin. This applies to those who are treated as either inpatients or outpatients. Those with more extensive injuries with soft tissue loss may benefit from the addition of an aminoglycoside. For patients who are allergic to penicillin, clindamycin or vancomycin is used.

TABLE 11-5	Recommended Antibiotic Regimen	
Location	**Antibiotic**	**Dosing**
Soft tissue	First-generation cephalosporin	1 g IV in ED, then followed by PO if outpatient
Soft tissue (shotgun) with defect	First-generation cephalosporin; consider aminoglycoside for similar time	Check renal function
Joint	First-generation cephalosporin	1 g IV q8h for 48 h
Joint with soft tissue defect	First-generation cephalosporin; consider aminoglycoside for similar time	Check renal function
Long bone fracture; minimally displaced with minimal soft tissue injury, outpatient	First-generation cephalosporin or oral fluoroquinolones	1 g IV kefzol followed by cephalexin 500 mg PO TID or ciprofloxacin 750 mg BID
Long bone fracture with internal fixation	First-generation cephalosporin	1 g IV q8h for 48 h
Long bone plus extensive soft tissue injury	First-generation cephalosporin; consider aminoglycoside	Check renal function

If cephalosporin or penicillin allergy, consider clindamycin (600 mg IV BID) or vancomycin (dosing per individual patient).

JOINT INJURY

Gunshot injuries of the joint are associated with a high morbidity compared with other gunshot wounds. Intra-articular injuries may result in arthritis secondary to trauma as well as through the degenerative effects of lead itself if there is a retained intra-articular bullet fragment. While elevated serum lead levels may be present with extra-articular gunshot wounds, the most common reports are with intra-articular retained bullet fragments.[95,136]

Pathophysiology of Lead Toxicity

Lead is soluble in synovial fluid and has been shown to induce lead synovitis and degenerative arthritis.[15,64,93,95,136] Retained intra-articular bullets not only cause lead synovitis and arthritis but also can cause systemic lead poisoning. Animal studies have demonstrated significant articular degeneration with implantation of lead into rabbit knees compared with controls.[15] Early changes (1 to 2 weeks) include synovial hyperplasia, mild inflammation, and articular surface slit formation. Late changes (3 to 6 weeks) include giant cells and foreign particles (lead and bone fragments) in the synovium, focal chondrocyte proliferation, duplication of the tidemark, and chondrocyte columnar disorganization.[15,164] Implantation of lead pellets into rabbit knees induces significantly greater degeneration in the femoral and tibial articular surfaces; medial and lateral menisci; and synovium at 4, 6, 10, and 14 weeks.[15,64,93,95,136]

The normal blood lead level for adults is 0 to 19 μg/dL. Nearly 95% of the lead storage in the body occurs in bone. The half-life of lead in the blood stream is less than 2 months compared with 20 to 30 years in the bone.[95]

Principles of Management

Lead is still the major component of both rifle and handgun bullets, and it may be a potential source of lead poisoning. Steel shot has replaced lead in many areas of the world in an attempt to reduce the lead burden on wildlife. Bismuth shot is also being used as a lead replacement in Canada. Modern shotguns may therefore be firing steel rather than lead shot. Regardless of whether the projectile is known to be lead, trauma from a bullet, pellet, or fragment will still have adverse consequences for the joint and most intra-articular projectiles should be removed. Through irrigation and debridement of the joint cavity is necessary to remove all the foreign material, including fragments of skin and clothing.

A perforating wound through a joint cavity, even with the absence of fracture, should undergo surgery. Clothing and other debris from the outside may be left entrapped in the joint. Cartilage damage is common despite the normal radiographic appearance of the joint.[149]

Arthroscopy has been described as a technique for treating patients with intra-articular bullet injures of the shoulder, elbow, hip, and knee. Advantages of this technique include better visualization of the joint surface and the ability to more easily repair osteochondral fragments, ligament tears, or meniscal damage. Disadvantages include increased[146] operative and setup time as well as potential compartment syndrome from extravasation of lavage fluid, particularly if a pressure pump is used. Care must be taken with using this technique to ensure the equipment is available and the surgeon is familiar with its use.

Shoulder Injuries

Gunshot injury to the entire shoulder region is relatively common, with one series reporting an incidence of 9%.[117] Injuries involving the shoulder joint itself, however, range from 1% to 2% of an overall series.[24,29,109,116,117,146] Associated injuries are common with penetrating injuries of the shoulder region, including arterial, venous, and nerve injuries. Vascular injury is present in 15% of these cases. The risk of vascular injury in the shoulder is four times higher in patients with a major fracture than in those without a major fracture.[158,161] Nerve injuries are the most important determinant of long-term function of the limb. The literature supports the use of either arthroscopy or open surgical techniques for removal of the bullet or its fragments from the shoulder joint and the subacromial space.[24,29,116,117,146] In cases where the joint capsule is violated by the bullet and the bullet has traversed the joint, clothing fragments, skin, and other debris may be driven into the joint. Even in the absence of intra-articular bullet fragments, irrigation and debridement of the joint is warranted.

Fractures that are nondisplaced or easily reducible may be stabilized with arthroscopic techniques. Small and nonviable fragments should be removed.[26] Unstable fractures and those involving the articular surface require open reduction and internal fixation. Large osteochondral fragments can be stabilized with bioabsorbable pins, headless screws, or a combination of these devices (Fig. 11-25). In the presence of intra-articular fracture displacement, comminution, and metaphyseal–diaphyseal dissociation, an open technique with a deltopectoral approach is used to reconstruct the joint surface. Fractures of the surgical neck and shaft can be addressed with internal fixation using a locked plate and screws. Hemiarthroplasty is an option in nonreconstructable fractures.

Brachial plexus and nerve injuries can occur with gunshot wounds to the shoulder region.[144] In a series of 58 patients with penetrating injury to the brachial plexus, there were 6 ulnar nerve injuries, 12 median nerve injuries, 2 radial nerve injuries, 5 musculocutaneous nerve injuries, 1 axillary nerve injury, and 3 suprascapular nerve injuries. In the same cohort, there were 13 fifth cervical, 10 sixth cervical, 10 seventh cervical, 5 eighth cervical, and 10 first thoracic root injuries. There were 8 lateral cord, 6 medial cord, and 10 posterior cord injuries. The trunk injuries included seven upper trunk, three middle trunk, and three lower trunk injuries. In this series, 24% of the patients had associated vascular injuries. One or more elements of the plexus were repaired in 36 of the 58 patients in this series. There were 3 good (8%), 23 useful (64%), and 8 (22%) poor results.[144] The main complications include stiffness, infection, and pain.

Elbow Injuries

The incidence of gunshot wounds to the elbow may be underestimated in the literature.[18,24,30,78,101,141] Associated injuries include periarticular fractures, nerve injuries, and arterial and venous injuries.[24,115] In rare cases of an isolated bullet or pellet retained in the elbow joint, irrigation and debridement and bullet removal can be achieved with the use of the arthroscope.[78]

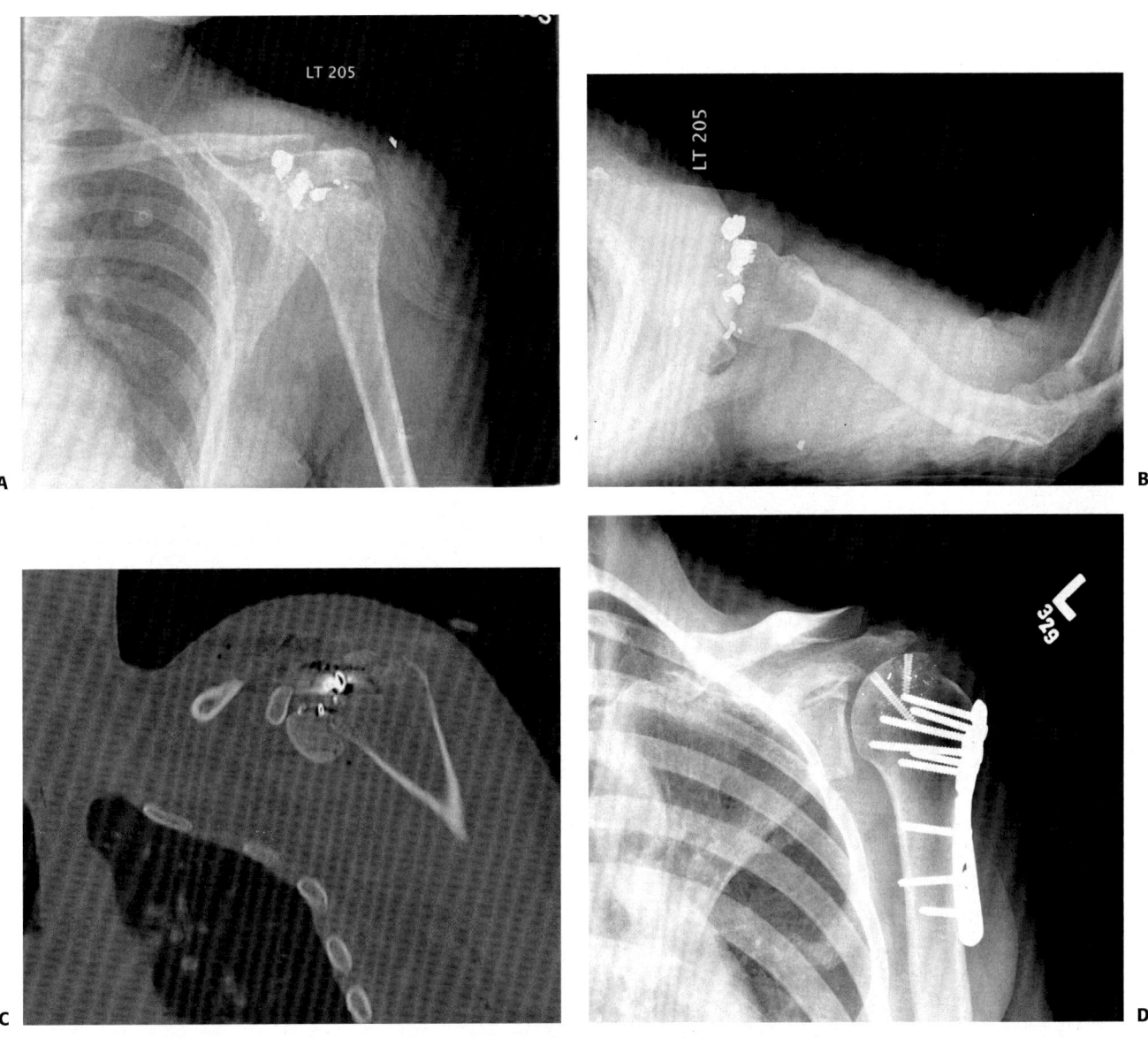

FIGURE 11-25 Preoperative anteroposterior **(A)** and lateral **(B)** radiographs and computed tomography scan **(C)** of the shoulder showing intra-articular injury from gunshot. **D:** Postoperative radiograph showing reduction with plate and screws and removal of intra-articular bullet fragments. Headless screws were used for the articular fragments.

Authors' Preferred Method of Treatment

Recommended Treatment for a Suspected Elbow Joint Injury

Recommended treatment for patients with a suspected elbow joint injury from a gunshot wound is open irrigation and debridement of the joint, and removal of foreign material, bullet fragments, or small loose bone fragments, if present. Initial stabilization of the elbow following a fracture of the distal humerus, the proximal radius, or proximal ulna can be done with a splint. With more comminuted fractures, use of external fixation spanning the elbow can be utilized temporarily. After stabilization, CT will aid in assessment of the fracture and the elbow joint for definitive fracture fixation (Fig. 11-26A–D). In unstable fracture-dislocations, urgent internal fixation of the fractures may be necessary, alone or in addition to spanning external fixation of the joint.[18]

Definitive treatment may involve a combination of various techniques, including internal fixation and/or hinged external fixation (Fig. 11-26E–F). Salvage of a severely injured joint may be achieved with compression plate arthrodesis of the elbow[101] or, in elderly low demand patients arthroplasty could be used.[30] Young and active patients are not good candidates for elbow arthroplasty. In one study, intermediate-range follow-up of 8 to 12 years postarthroplasty showed a five of seven (71%)

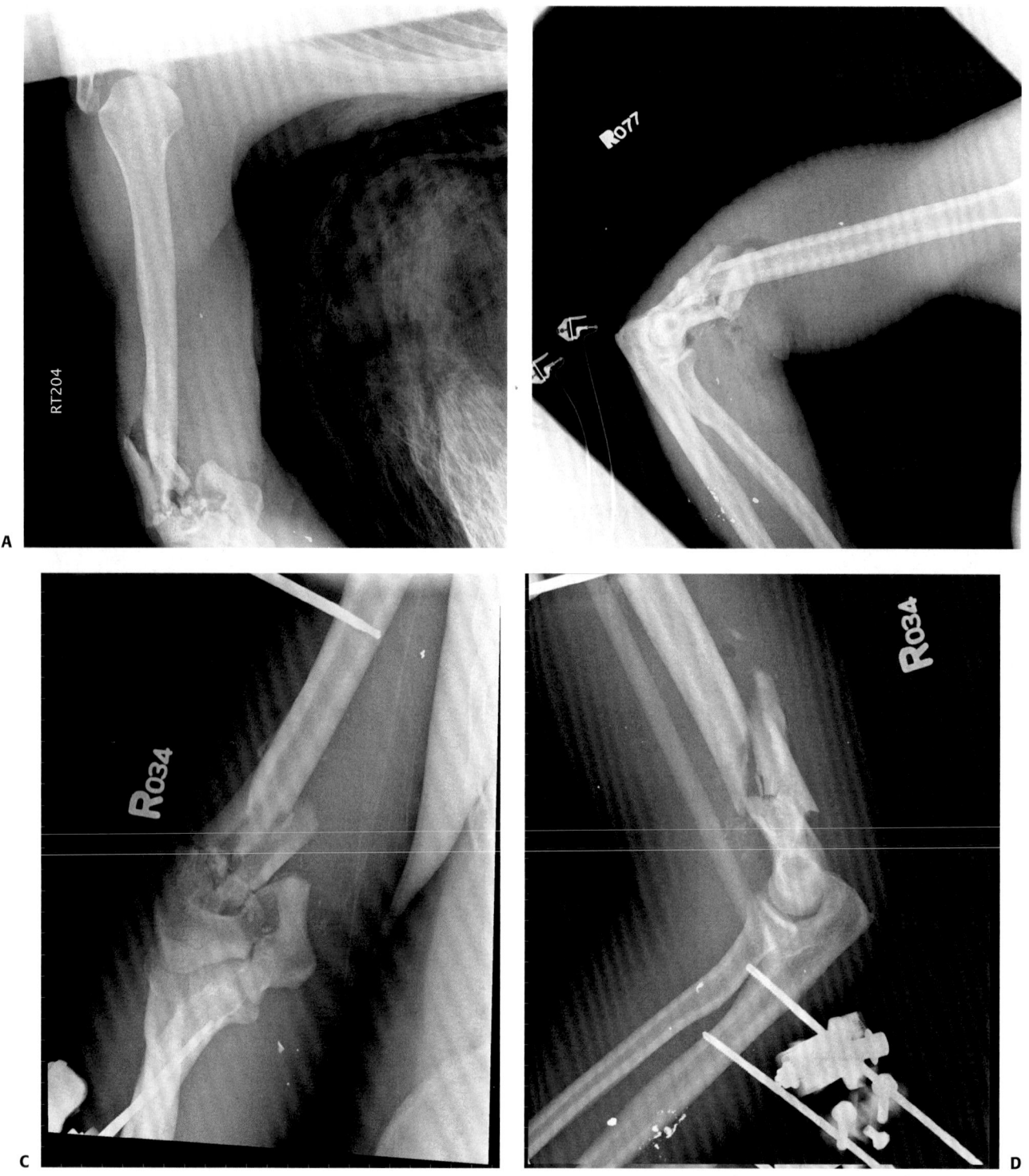

FIGURE 11-26 Anteroposterior **(A)** and lateral **(B)** preoperative views of a distal humerus fracture with intra-articular extension. **C, D:** Computed tomography scan shows the lateral femoral condyle fracture at that both CT scans shown are of the distal femur at multiple levels.

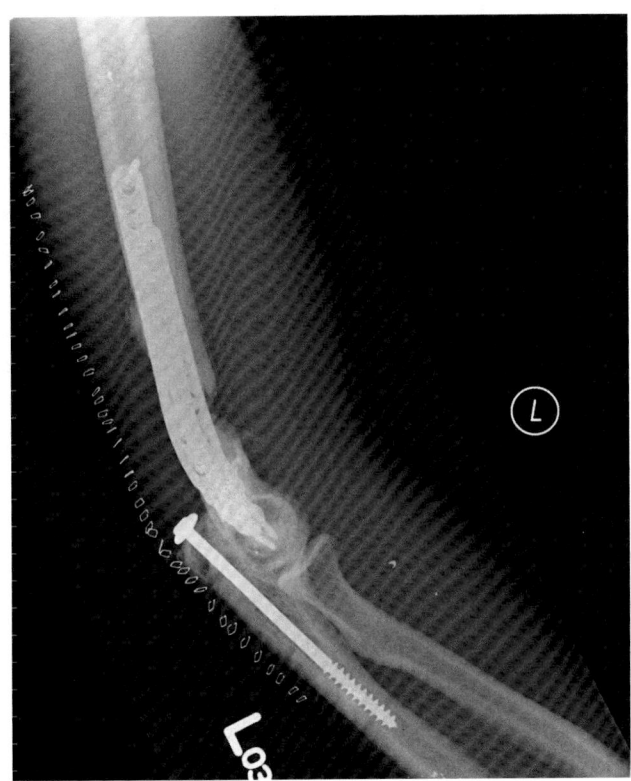
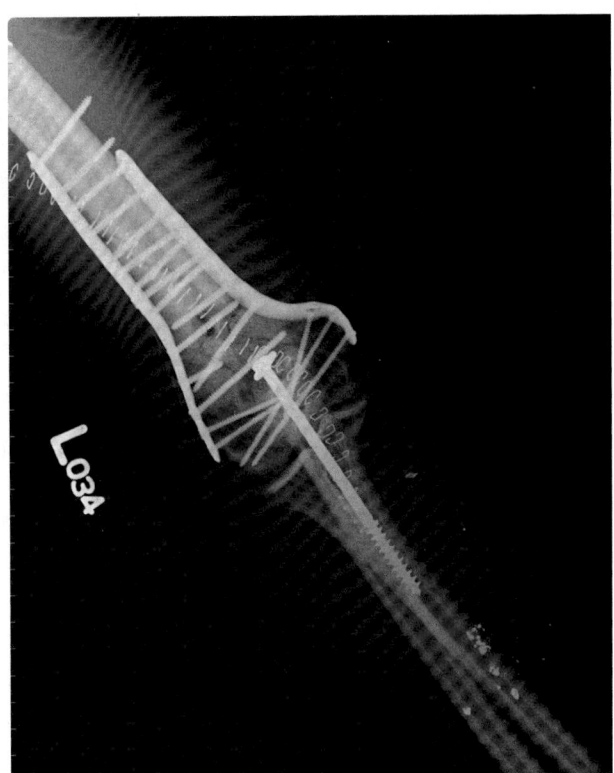

FIGURE 11-26 (*continued*) **E, F:** An external fixator was applied, followed by bicolumnar plate fixation after the swelling of the limb subsided. The external fixator pins should be placed outside the (1) zone of injury and (2) the anticipated operative field.

failure rate. Arthrodesis may be indicated for a nonsalvagable elbow joint in which there is good distal limb function. This is particularly true if the patient is young, has reasonable bone stock, poor soft tissue coverage, and is free of infection.[101] Complications of elbow gunshot wounds include stiffness, malunion, nonunion, infection, and nerve injury.[115] In a cohort of 44 patients at the author's institution, 4 died of other injuries and 6 were lost to follow-up. Of the remaining 34 patients, 19 (56%) patients had nerve injuries. The nerve injuries included 8 ulnar, 11 radial, and 2 median nerve injuries. Two patients had combined injuries. Two nerves (one radial and one ulnar) were repaired with partial return of function. Two complete radial nerve injuries were treated with tendon transfers. Four patients (12%) had brachial artery injury that required repair. Four patients (12%) developed deep infections requiring irrigation and debridement in the operating room. Three patients required secondary bone grafting to achieve bony union of the fracture.

Hip Injuries

In our series (Table 11-2), the prevalence of gunshot wounds to the hip joint was 2% of all extremity gunshot wounds and 4% of lower extremity gunshot wounds. The prevalence of gunshot wounds to the hip region (femoral neck, peritrochanteric region), was 9% of all extremity gunshot wounds and 17% of lower extremity gunshot wounds.

The diagnosis of hip joint violation is an important step in management of these injuries. The trajectory of the bullet or its fragments can traverse the abdomen, bowel, and/or bladder before violating the hip joint. The projectile may enter the hip capsule without causing a fracture of the acetabulum or the proximal femur, or enter through the acetabulum. In the absence of a fracture, the diagnosis of hip joint violation can be difficult.

The diagnosis is based on radiographic and CT scan findings. In the absence of fractures, or when radiographs are inconclusive, a fluoroscopically assisted arthrogram is the most sensitive test to detect joint violation.[20,96] Documentation is important to determine the need for surgery to lavage the joint. A negative arthrogram eliminates the need for surgery due to joint contamination.

Transabdominal gunshot wounds to the hip joint carry a high risk of infection and should be treated with emergent arthrotomy, irrigation, and debridement. Bowel and bladder injuries should be managed by general surgeons and urologists with either direct repair or diverting colostomy and diversion procedures for the urinary tract respectively.[6,20,32]

Bullet removal can be achieved via arthrotomy or arthroscopy.[28,54,96,103,104,106,140,147,163] Hip arthroscopy requires special equipment and experience with the technique. The use of a fracture table and fluoroscopy aids in arthroscopy of the hip. Hip arthroscopy carries the risk of intra-abdominal fluid extravasation and abdominal compartment syndrome.[6] In the presence of acetabular fractures, extreme care must be taken to measure the arthroscopy fluid inflow and outflow. If the inflow and outflow

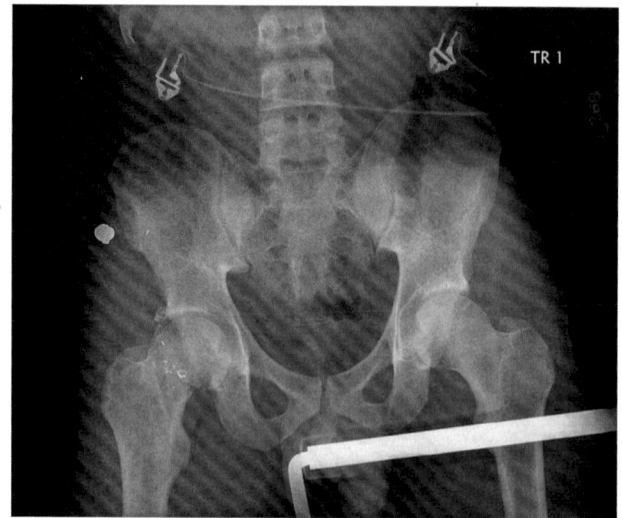
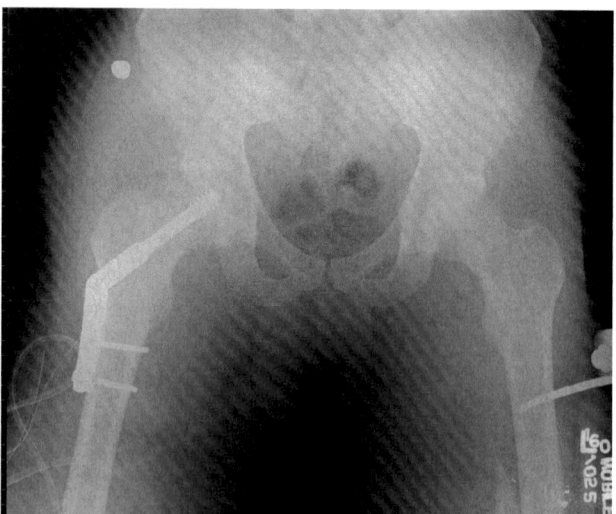

FIGURE 11-27 Anteroposterior preoperative **(A)** and postoperative **(B)** radiographs of a femoral neck fracture caused by a gunshot. Femoral neck fractures caused by gunshots tend to be comminuted.

are mismatched, fluid is likely extravasating into the pelvis and abdomen and can cause cardiopulmonary arrest.[96]

Recommended treatment of associated fractures is by open reduction and internal fixation. For acute fractures of the femoral neck, use of standard techniques such as a compression screw and side plate may be used for fractures with minimal comminution (Fig. 11-27). Comminuted fractures of the femoral neck may be treated by using fixed-angle devices such as a locking plate or blade plate.

Patients with more extensive injury to the articular surface of the femoral head or acetabulum represent difficult clinical problems. Hip arthroplasty or arthrodesis in the acute setting is not recommended.[109,112] These procedures are reserved as elective salvage procedures. In the presence of severe comminution when inadequate bone is available for internal fixation, resection arthroplasty may be performed in the acute setting. Complications of gunshot wounds to the hip include arthrosis, infection, fistula formation,[115,132] nonunion, malunion, and osteonecrosis.

Knee Injuries

Gunshot wounds to the knee region, including the distal femur and proximal tibia, are relatively frequent in reported series of gunshot wounds.[9,24,120,122–124,149] Perry et al.[122] and Guo and Chiou-Tan[58] described on gunshot-related 67 fractures to the knee: 37 sustained intra-articular fractures and 27 sustained extra-articular fractures. There were 29 femoral, 29 tibial, and 9 patellar fractures. Twenty-three patients had arteriograms for suspected vascular injury; six were positive. Five limbs required vascular repair: One each of the common popliteal artery, a branch of the common femoral artery, both the peroneal and posterior tibial arteries, and the superficial femoral artery. Two patients had a common peroneal nerve injury. There were also two reported infections: One superficial and one deep.

The diagnosis of an open knee joint injury in the absence of radiographic evidence of intra-articular debris, air, or presence of fractures can be difficult. A saline arthrogram or dye arthrogram can aid in diagnosis if the test is positive although large volumes of saline (75 to 100 mL) may be required. However, these tests traditionally have a low sensitivity of around 40% and a negative arthrogram does not rule out an open joint injury.[128,148] More recent studies have revealed higher sensitivities with increased volumes of saline injected.[87]

Goals of initial surgical treatment are to prevent infection and stabilize the limb. In the presence of severely comminuted and unstable fractures, spanning external fixation of the joint is recommended. Delayed reconstruction of the joint may be undertaken once the limb is stable. For larger fractures, an arthrotomy should be used in treating major fractures with open reduction and internal fixation (Fig. 11-28).

In the presence of unstable fractures, or other associated injuries, acute reconstruction of ligaments is not recommended. In these cases, a delayed reconstruction after fracture healing and rehabilitation may be undertaken. Meniscal tears, ligament tears with bony avulsions, and large osteochondral fragments may be fixed acutely.

The role of arthroscopy in managing gunshot wounds of the knee has been studied by Tornetta and Hui[149] and Nowotarski and Brumback.[114] In a review of 33 gunshot wounds to the knee without radiographic evidence of injury, arthroscopy showed 5 chondral injuries, 14 meniscal injuries, and 5 cases with intra-articular debris not seen on radiographs. Based on these findings, diagnostic arthroscopy and arthroscopic-assisted bullet removal and irrigation and debridement are recommended for gunshot wounds through the knee.

Ankle Injuries

In our series, the prevalence of gunshot wounds to the ankle is 0.5% of those to the lower extremity. Associated injuries include fractures and nerve, vascular, and tendon injuries.[16,160] Treatment is based on the personality of the fracture, ranging from spanning external fixation and/or internal fixation for a low-velocity injury. For patients with more severe soft tissue or

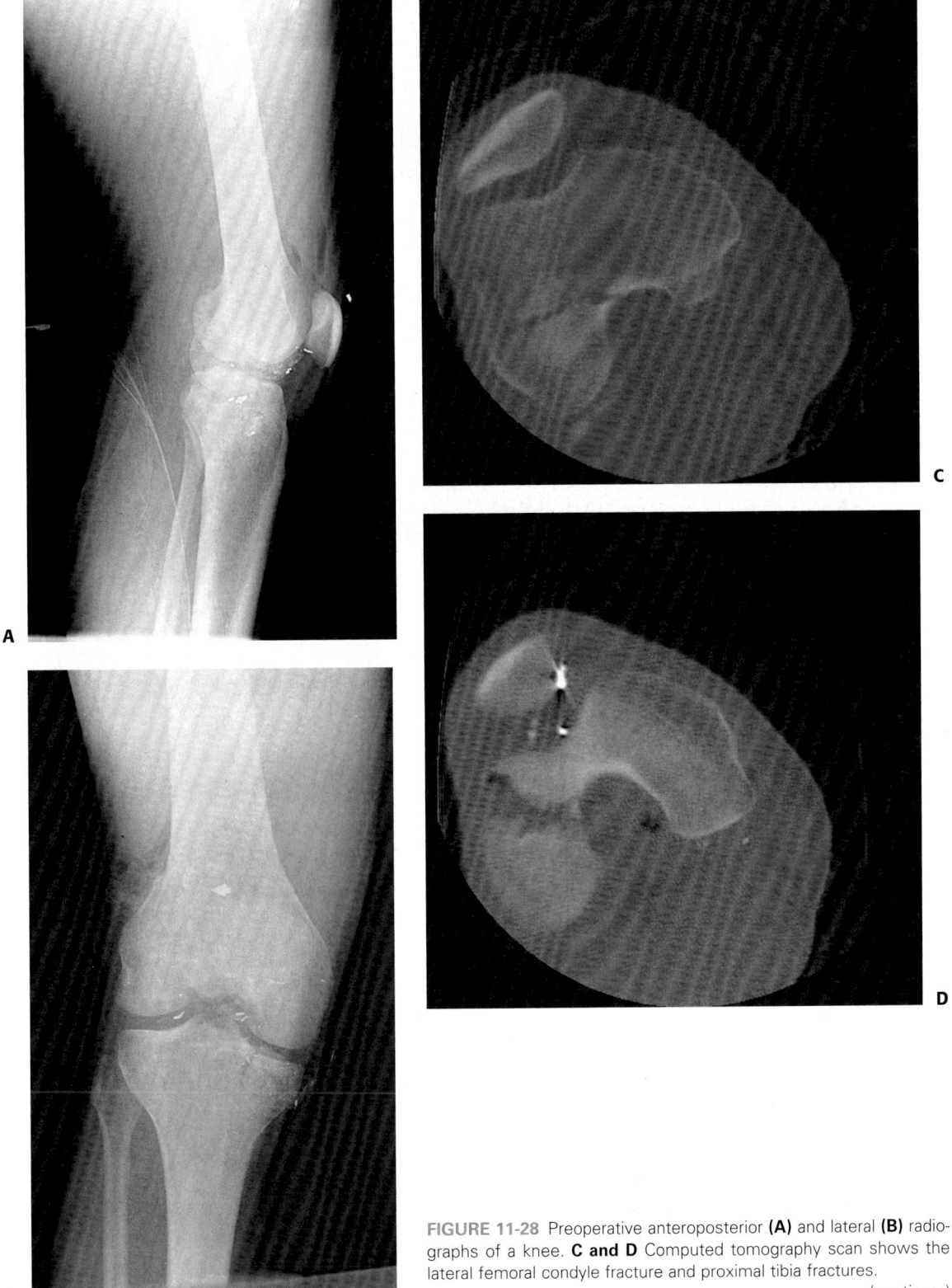

FIGURE 11-28 Preoperative anteroposterior **(A)** and lateral **(B)** radiographs of a knee. **C and D** Computed tomography scan shows the lateral femoral condyle fracture and proximal tibia fractures.

(continues)

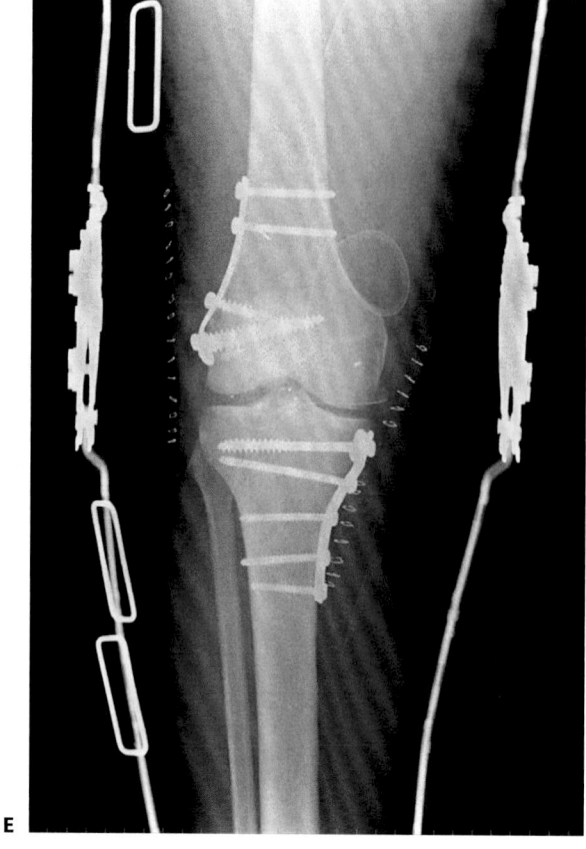

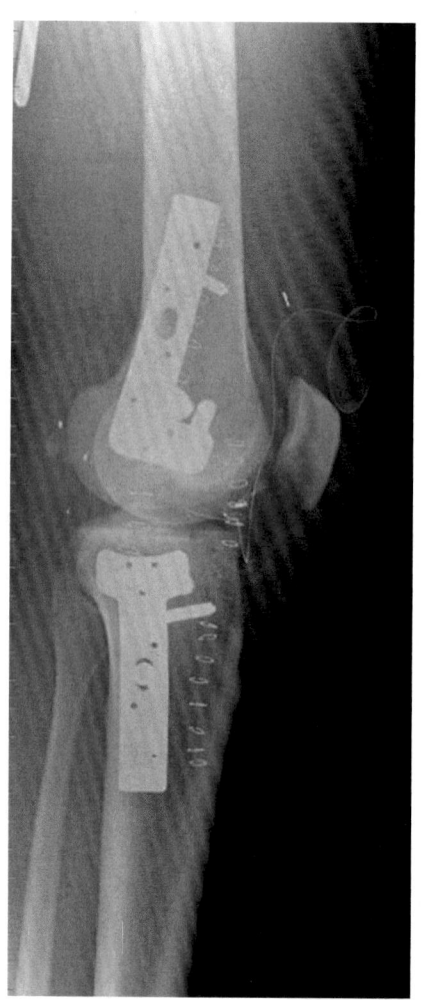

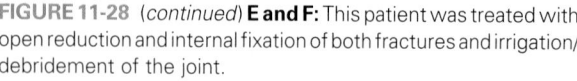

FIGURE 11-28 (*continued*) **E and F:** This patient was treated with open reduction and internal fixation of both fractures and irrigation/debridement of the joint.

bone injury, arthrodesis or even amputation should be considered. Arthroscopy is of limited use because of the confined ankle space, good access through conventional incisions, and the prevalence of fracture necessitating open debridement or repair.

LONG BONE FRACTURES

Long bone fractures caused by gunshot wounds still pose a significant clinical problem for orthopedic surgeons in war or peace. On the battlefield, caring for patients involves both transportation and treatment. The evacuation of patients may involve long distances, aircraft flight, and delayed definitive care. Initial treatment of gunshot fractures in this setting involves temporary stabilization with subsequent evacuation, followed by definitive fixation once the patient arrives in a stable hospital environment. Temporary stabilization involves the use of an external fixator to span the fracture segment.

In the nonmilitary setting, patients are usually seen and cared for at the same institution, in a stable medical environment without the complexity of patient transportation through multiple echelons of care. Immediate definitive stabilization for patients with isolated long bone gunshot fractures is the standard of care in most civilian settings.

Humerus Fractures

Upper extremity long bone fractures are less prevalent than lower extremity long bone fractures, with gunshot diaphyseal humerus fractures generally being the third most common shaft fracture. Complication such as nerve injuries[58,115,137] are relatively common with patients who sustain gunshot wounds of the humerus. There is an increased prevalence of nerve injury associated with the distal humerus compared with more proximal injuries.[4,5,61,79,80,84,86,132,133,155,162]

Treatment of humeral fractures in either war or peace is controversial. Reported methods of care include fracture brace, external fixation, and internal fixation. There are no prospective studies comparing the various methods of treatment for patients with gunshot wounds.[5,80,84,132,133,155,162]

The fracture brace or coaptation splint is appropriate when there is minimal soft tissue injury and the fracture can be held in alignment by this means. Proximal or very distal fractures are often not amenable to this method of care.[5,132,133]

External fixation has been reported for use in patients with more extensive soft tissue injuries, such as with military wounds. Zinman et al.[162] reported on 26 Israeli war casualties who had external fixation applied for treatment of open humerus fractures. They applied monolateral external fixators to obtain union in 15 patients (57.7%). Conversion to compression plates (five patients) or a cast (six patients) was used for the other patients. Five delayed unions were identified, four of which were treated with plating and bone grafting. Fifteen patients had a total of 20 nerve injuries. One of the nerve injuries was caused by a distal, lateral pin placement that injured the radial nerve. There were four brachial and two radial artery repairs. Of 23 patients with 6.5 years of follow-up there were excellent results in 14 patients, good results in 4, fair results in 3, and poor results in 2. All fractures did eventually heal. The authors felt that external fixation was the best means for stabilizing fracture and allowing access to wounds for wound care. For the distal humerus, the authors recommended open pin placement if lateral pins are to be used or placing the pins from a posterior direction.

In 1995, the Red Cross evaluated the treatment of refugees who sustained gunshot fractures of the humerus. Keller[84] studied 37 patients who were treated at a Red Cross Hospital on the Sudanese border. Patients were seen an average of 9.5 days after injury, at which time 89% of the wounds were found to be infected. Nerve palsy secondary to injury was present in eight patients in this series. Twenty-three patients received a functional brace with plaster of Paris and splint, and seven patients received external fixation skeletal traction. Those treated with the splint had an average time of immobilization of 35.8 days, and 90% obtained adequate alignment. The authors also reported eight reoperations on four patients. The seven patients treated with external fixation had the frame applied for an average of 46.3 days, and 60% obtained adequate angulation. The authors also reported a 71.5% nonunion rate and 11 reoperations in five of the patients. Traction was used in seven patients as well, with an average immobilization of 27.7 days, with five patients obtaining union, and six reoperations on three of the patients. Although the best results were obtained in patients who were treated with splinting, the authors reported that those who had external fixation and traction had the more severe injuries.

Keller et al.[84] reported on 37 patients who sustained gunshot humerus fractures and were treated at a Red Cross Hospital on the Sudanese border. The patients were seen late (average 9.5 days after injury) and nearly 90% were infected. There were three treatment methods: (1) functional brace (n = 23, average 35 days treatment), (2) external fixation (n = 7, average 46.3 days treatment), and (3) skeletal traction (n = 7, average treatment 28 days). The authors reported the best results were obtained with functional bracing, but noted the more severely injured were treated with external fixation and traction.

Hall and Pankovich[61] treated 89 humerus fractures with Ender nails, of which 22 were caused by gunshot wounds (4 shotgun wounds). The authors reported good results with these patients using this technique. We know of no reports using Ender nails since this 1987 report. This technique has been superseded by other methods.

For simple fractures with minimal soft tissue disruption, use of a functional brace following a coaptation splint seems to yield acceptable results for both initial and definitive care.[5,132,133] For patients with more extensive injuries, such as a shotgun blast at close range, we recommend the use of a spanning external fixator to provide initial stabilization for the patient.[80,86,155,162]

Use of the spanning external fixator is more common with distal fractures. When both the limb and the patient are stable, planning for fracture stabilization and soft tissue coverage can be done.

Definitive treatment of severe bone or soft tissue defects may be challenging. Dressing changes, as well as maintaining fracture alignment, are difficult with bracing/splinting. With extensive comminution and soft tissue injury, use of a small pin fixator has been reported with good success.[4,141] For skeletal defects, use of a cage with allograft[4] or a fibular osteoseptocutaneous flap[69] has been described.

Forearm Fractures

There are relatively few reports describing treatment and results of gunshot wounds to the forearm.[37,42,53,59,71,129,130,159] There is a high reported rate of nerve injury associated with gunshot wounds to this region, and a 10% rate of compartment syndrome.[37,59,107] The goals of fracture care are to restore the length, alignment, and radial bow of the forearm. Care for diaphyseal forearm fractures depends on the severity of both the soft tissue and bone injury, just as with open forearm fractures not associated with firearms.[37,42,53,59,71,107,129,130,144,159] Patients with isolated relatively stable fractures of the ulna from a gunshot wound and associated minimal soft tissue trauma may be treated by application of a cast after appropriate wound treatment. Displaced fractures should be treated with open reduction and plate fixation when soft tissues permit.

For patients with bone loss, initial stabilization with external fixation should be done when both forearm bones are involved.[53,59] If just the radius or ulna is involved, only splinting may be required. Use of a soft tissue antibiotic-impregnated spacer may be used for initial care of the void.[53] A second, staged procedure to reconstruct bone defects should then be done once the limb is stable. Use of autologous bone graft has been described to fill defects. Use of allograft and bioactive substances, such as bone morphogenetic protein (BMP) or demineralized bone matrix, has yet to be described.

Femur Fractures

Diaphyseal femur fractures are the most common long bone fractures associated with gunshot wounds.[10,19,26,73,111,112,114,128,134,150,152,156] Within the past 50 years, balanced skeletal traction has been the mainstay of care for femur fractures in war or peace.[150,152] Temporary stabilization with balanced skeletal traction may still be used today as a means of stabilization until more definitive care can be provided, particularly for patients who are not able to withstand more extensive, definitive procedures in the operating room.[135,156]

External fixation has been used for open fractures on the battlefield. Reis et al.[128] reported on 19 femur fractures that were intended to be treated with external fixation to union. Six were converted to cast brace because of pin track infection and a further five femurs underwent open reduction internal fixation (one for refracture). Fourteen of the femurs were treated with bone grafting. The authors noted that further procedures were not done until the limb was free of obvious infection. Average time to union was 19 weeks.

Recently, external fixation been used for patients who are physiologically unable to undergo a more extensive surgery.[114,134,135] The concept of using temporary external fixation as a bridge from injury to definitive fracture stabilization has become the standard to initially stabilize a patient's fracture. Recently, Scannell et al.[135] reviewed 79 patients who sustained femur fractures due to blunt trauma with an Injury Severity Score ≥17. Nineteen of the patients were treated with external fixation while 60 were initially treated with skeletal traction as a temporizing measure prior to intramedullary rodding of the femur. The authors concluded that unless the patient was going to the operating room for other reasons, balanced skeletal traction offered a safe means to temporize the patient.[135]

The use of intramedullary nailing for complex femur fractures or malunion, nonunion, and infection associated with gunshot wounds became widespread after World War II, influenced by the pioneering work of Küntscher.[26,101]

Hollman and Horowitz[73] reviewed 26 patients who sustained fractures because of "low-velocity" gunshot wounds that were treated with intramedullary nailing an average of 9 days after injury. Nineteen of the patients were followed to union, which occurred an average of 4.5 months after injury. Two patients had open nailing and the remaining 17 had closed nailing.

Bergman et al.[10] reviewed a series of 65 patients with gunshot femur fractures at Kings County Hospital Center in Brooklyn, New York. The patients were treated with reamed intramedullary nailing an average of 2 days (range, 0 to 14 days) after injury and were followed an average of 2 years after injury (range, 9.5 months to 6 years). The authors found all fractures healed at an average of 18 weeks (range, 13 to 31 weeks). Two patients had persistent drainage, which resolved with a course of oral antibiotics at 2 and 3 weeks.

Tornetta and Tiburzi[150] reviewed 38 of 55 patients with gunshot femur fractures treated with intramedullary nailing who were followed an average of 2 years (range, 14 to 36 months). Average time to union was 8.6 weeks (range, 5 to 22 weeks). Nicholas and McCoy[111] reviewed 12 patients with 14 femur fractures treated with immediate (within 8 hours) intramedullary nailing. Three patients had vascular repairs and two patients had sciatic nerve injuries. Average time to union was 5.5 months (range, 3 to 8 months). None of the patients developed an infection. Wiss et al.[156] performed a retrospective review of 77 patients who sustained gunshot femur fractures, of which 56 had adequate records for follow-up. The patients were initially treated with skeletal traction for 10 to 14 days, with intramedullary nailing done when the wound tracks healed. No deep wound infections were reported. Average time to union was 23 weeks (range, 14 to 40 weeks), and average follow-up was 16 months (range, 12 to 29 months). Five patients had limb length discrepancy of greater than 1 cm, and one patient had angulation of 15 degrees.

This review shows that antegrade reamed, locked intramedullary nails may be safely used for gunshot-induced diaphyseal femur fractures. This procedure may be done immediately or on a delayed basis, depending on the patient's condition and the degree of soft tissue injury. More proximal fractures, such as subtrochanteric fractures, may do best with using reconstruction nails to obtain more proximal fracture stabilization (Fig. 11-29).

Retrograde nailing has become a popular technique in caring for diaphyseal femur fractures, particularly those near the knee. Initially, it was believed that an open fracture would be too great of a risk for knee sepsis to permit using retrograde nails. Our group recently reported on our series of 196 gunshot femur fractures, of which 56 were treated with retrograde nailing (Fig. 11-30). There was no increased infection rate associated with this method of treatment, at either the fracture site or the knee joint. Therefore, use of retrograde nailing for diaphyseal gunshot femur fractures does not appear to result in an increased infection rate compared to antegrade nailing.

Complications

Wiss et al.[156] reported 5 of 56 patients requiring vascular repair in addition to the treatment of the femur fracture. He also reported three associated sciatic nerve injuries, one with full recovery, one with partial recovery, and one with no recovery. Two patients had peroneal nerve palsies, one of which recovered. Infection of patients is infrequent in the civilian setting following gunshot femur fractures. Wiss et al.[156] reported no deep infections with 56 patients at follow-up. Hollman and Horowitz[73] reported no patients with infection after intramedullary nailing. Bergman et al.[10] reported two patients with persistent drainage, and Nicholas and McCoy[111] reported that none of their 14 patients with immediate nailing were infected.

Compartment syndrome is an infrequent complication of femoral shaft fractures. We found the 3 of 102 patients treated for diaphyseal gunshot wounds from 2001 through 2006 at Henry Ford Hospital had the diagnosis of thigh compartment syndrome. The patients were treated with compartment release of the anterior and lateral thigh compartments via one incision at the time of their initial surgery.

Malunion is infrequent with the use of intramedullary nailing. Wiss et al.[156] reported angulation deformity of 15 degrees for one of 56 patients, rotational deformity reported in one patient, and five patients with a leg length discrepancy of greater than 1 cm.

Immediate intramedullary nailing is now routine in many hospitals that treat nonmilitary gunshot wound femoral fractures on a routine basis. Intramedullary nailing allows for better alignment, less limb length discrepancy, and earlier return to ambulation without an increased rate of infection. The use of temporary external fixation to initially care for patients with more extensive soft tissue wounds, severe systemic injuries, or fractures sustained in austere environments, allows for the patient to be stabilized before undergoing more extensive surgery. Skeletal traction is an option for the short-term stabilization of a fracture before more definitive care.

Treatment of femur fractures during the recent Iraq and Afghanistan conflicts has been with the staged management of care. For Coalition soldiers, the fracture is stabilized with an external fixator and the patient transported to a site of definitive care, where fixation by intramedullary nailing is performed secondarily.

FIGURE 11-29 Anteroposterior preoperative **(A)** and postoperative **(B–D)** views of a subtrochanteric fracture. The patient was treated with a reconstruction nail and had good callus formation in the zone of injury at 6 months. The periosteal sleeve and soft tissue envelope, if left relatively undisturbed, will allow for rapid bone formation despite the lack of anatomic reduction of the same fragments.

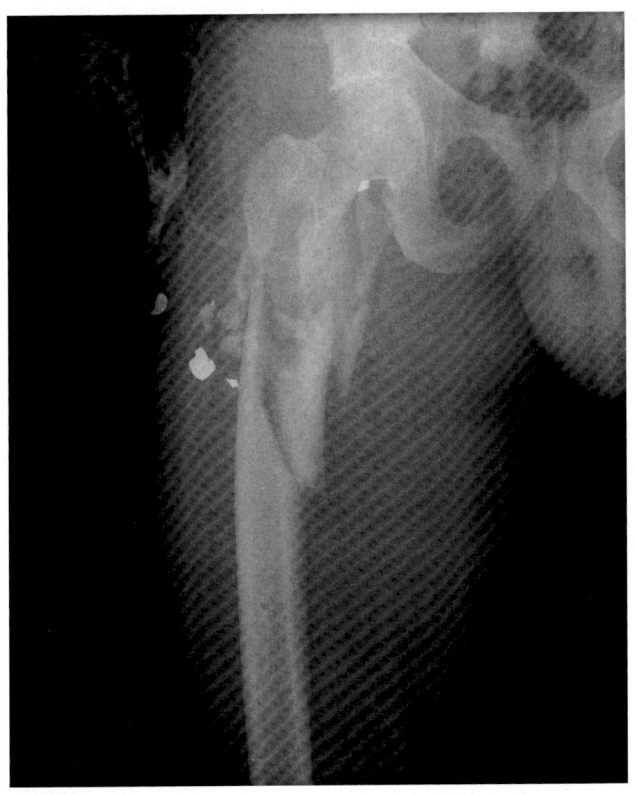

A

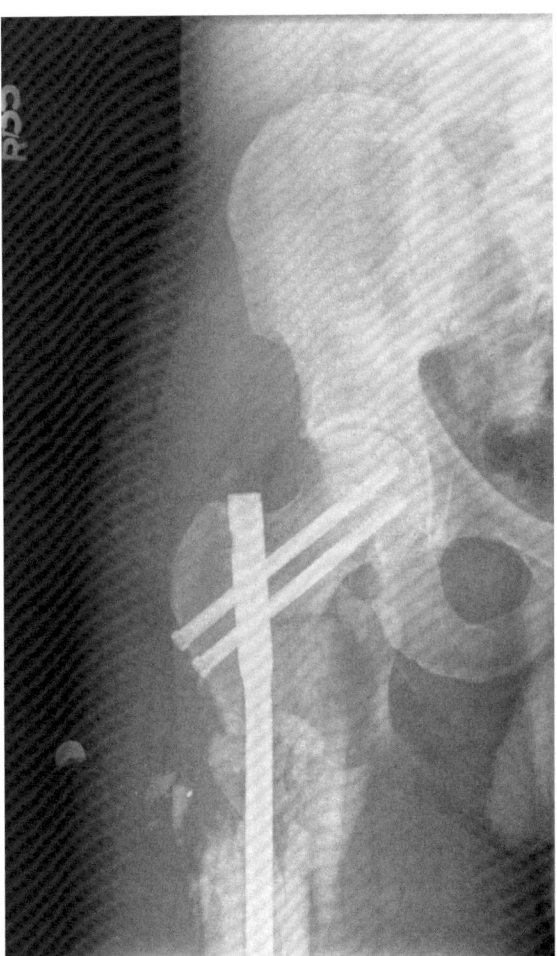

B

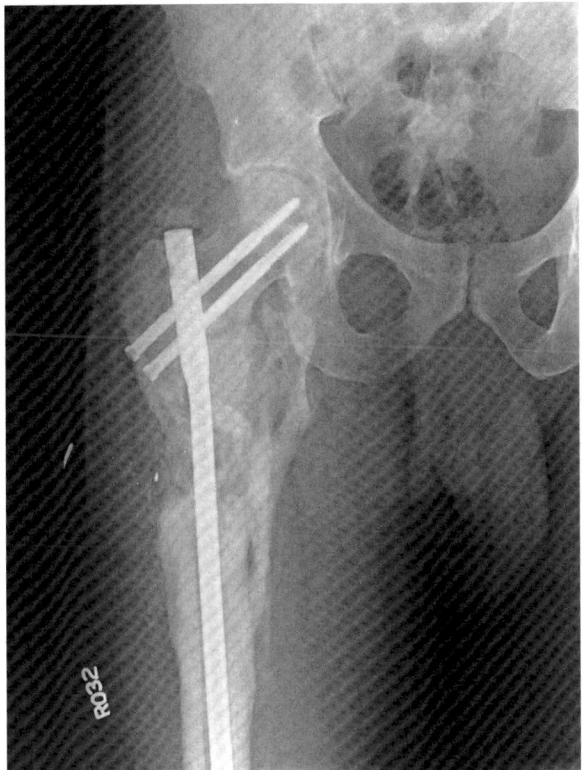

C

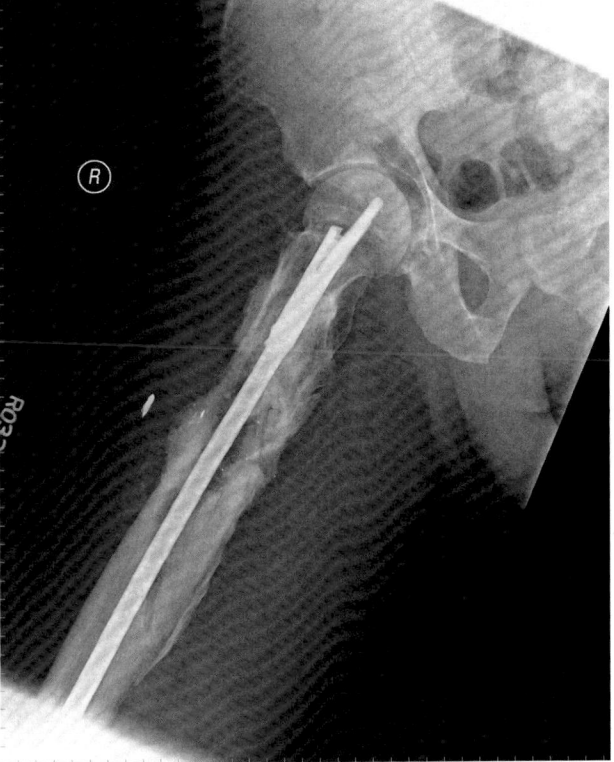

D

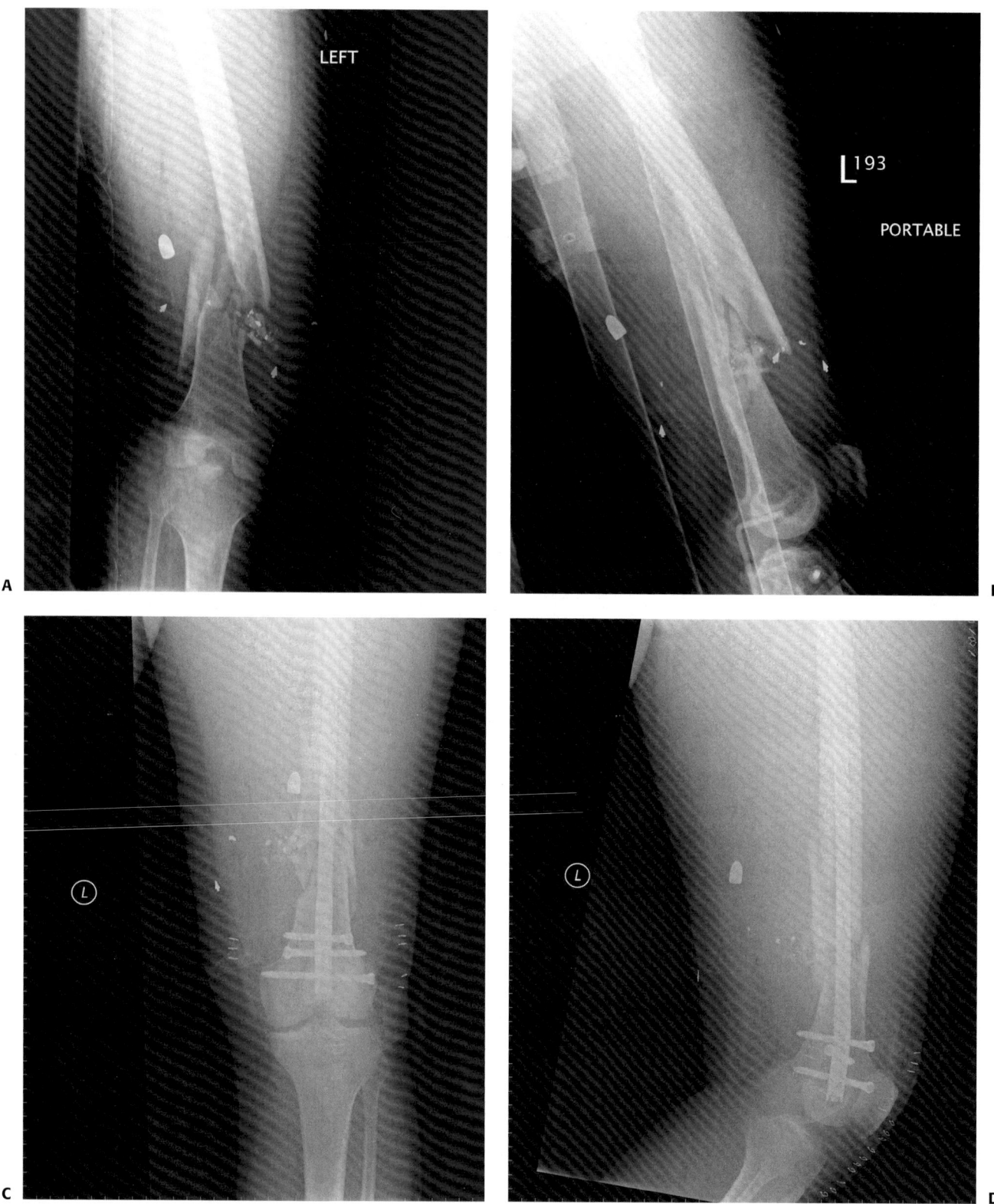

FIGURE 11-30 Preoperative **(A and B)** and postoperative **(C and D)** radiographs of a distal femur fracture that resulted from a "low-velocity" gunshot. The patient was treated with an immediate retrograde intramedullary nail, with excellent restoration of length, angulation, and rotation.

Tibia Fractures

The tibia is the second most frequent long bone fractured by gunshot, following the femur.[21,22,50,90,157] A variety of treatment methods have been reported for fracture care, including the use of cast or fracture brace, external fixation, and intramedullary nailing.

Witschi and Omer[157] reported on the ambulatory treatment in a cast and then fracture brace of 84 patients who sustained tibia fractures secondary to missile injuries. All of the fractures in this series had some comminution. Despite this, the authors reported less than 1 cm of shortening in 48 of 58 patients with isolated injury and an additional three patients with 1 cm of shortening. Seven patients were reported to have osteomyelitis, which prolonged the time to union. Brown and Urban[22] reported on 63 fractures in 60 patients who were also injured by war wounds and were treated in a similar manner. The fractures in this series healed at an average of 19 weeks. Shortening averaged 9 mm, ranging from 2 to 38 mm, compared with the contralateral limb. Twenty-seven of the fractures had no shortening. Four of the 63 patients had persistent drainage. Sarmiento reported on 32 tibia fractures caused by gunshot wounds treated with a fracture brace. The average time to union was 17.5 weeks, with one nonunion, and little residual deformity.

Leffers and Chandler[90] conducted a retrospective review of 40 patients with 41 tibia fractures caused by gunshot wounds. Thirty-five fractures were treated by casting followed by fracture brace. An additional five fractures were treated with external fixation because of injury severity, followed by a functional brace within the first 2 months. One patient had pins and plaster. Those treated by casting healed at an average of 12 weeks, whereas those treated by external fixation healed at an average of 21 weeks. Eight patients had persistent wound drainage, with two undergoing a surgical procedure to care for the wound. This study was limited in that it reported follow-up of only 27% of the total number of patients seen with this diagnosis at the institution.

Ferraro and Zinar[50] reported a retrospective review of 90 of 133 patients with tibia fractures caused by gunshot wounds treated at Harbor/UCLA Medical Center. Fracture stabilization was a long leg cast for 58, external fixation for 17, and unreamed intramedullary nailing for 15 patients. The authors found that fractures classified as Winquist 0, 1, or 2 healed within 12 to 14 weeks and those with Winquist 3, 4, or 5 and treated with intramedullary nailing healed at an average of 18 weeks; those treated with external fixation averaged 27 weeks to union.

Present treatment of gunshot fractures of the tibial shaft depends on the amount of bone comminution and degree of soft tissue injury. Patients with tibia shaft fractures having minimal comminution, soft tissue injury, displacement, and angulation may be successfully treated with local wound care in the emergency department and application of a cast, followed by a functional brace. More comminuted fractures are better cared for with intramedullary nailing. If there is major soft tissue injury requiring a soft tissue transfer, consideration should be given to external fixation until the soft tissues are reconstructed and stable, at which point the fixator may be removed and an intramedullary nail is inserted. Because of concerns about pin site sepsis, external fixation should be used for a limited period of time, generally less than 2 weeks if definitive fixation with an intramedullary rod is anticipated.

Foot Injuries

Injuries to the foot are infrequent with nonmilitary gunshot wounds. Foot and ankle injuries accounted for only 39 of 2,277 (1.7%) injuries in 1,505 patients with gunshot wounds seen at Henry Ford Hospital between 2001 and 2006. Gunshot toe and metatarsal injuries vary in the degree of both soft tissue and bone injury. Minimally displaced fractures, particularly when isolated, may be treated without surgical stabilization. After treatment of the soft tissues, a period of using a hard-soled postoperative shoe with dressing changes allows for a good result.

Patients with multiple metatarsal fractures or those with bone loss are candidates for surgical stabilization. Kirschner wires or external fixation may be used for initial surgical stabilization in these patients.[16,153] Midfoot injuries tend to be more comminuted than metatarsal injuries and as a consequence require surgical stabilization. For acute injuries with bone loss, external fixation is used to span the fracture defect, followed by reconstruction of the bone with plates when the limb is stable. Talus and calcaneus fractures are less likely to require surgical stabilization unless bone loss is present. Treatment for isolated fractures should be dependent on the degree of bone and soft tissue injury. With minimal soft tissue and bone disruption, treatment of the soft tissues followed by casting gives the best results. Infection is more common with foot injuries than other anatomic regions. Boucree et al.[16] reported that 12 of 101 patients with gunshot foot wounds had an infection; this is a higher incidence than reported with other anatomic regions.

Foot injuries in wartime are common injuries, most often resulting from mine explosions. Nikolic et al.[113] reported that 250 of 1,860 war casualties (13.4%) treated at the authors' facility in the former Republic of Yugoslavia had foot injuries. Amputations were performed in 76 (26.5%) of the feet.

Severe closed fractures are reported in patients inside vehicles struck by a large mine. This "behind armor blunt trauma" is similar to injuries seen with severe motor vehicle accidents and may be treated with the same definitive care.[110]

CONCLUSIONS

Gunshot injuries remain a major clinical problem in both war and peace. Caring for patients in war-torn regions of the world remains challenging. Patients are often initially managed under austere circumstances before and during transport for definitive care. Gunshot injuries are a significant part of the health care problem for inner-city hospitals around the world. The orthopedic surgeon should be knowledgeable about the clinical course and outcome of patients with gunshot wounds to provide the complete, thorough, and efficient care within the context of his or her medical system.

AUTHORS' PREFERRED METHOD OF TREATMENT (MILITARY-RELATED INJURIES)

Blast injuries and combat-related gunshot wounds are generally more contaminated than similar injuries seem in the civilian sector and an increased focus on adequate debridement is necessary. Blast injuries in particular are much more highly contaminated as significant quantities of foreign material is driven deep into the soft tissues. The Emergency War Surgery Handbook specifically recommends early aggressive debridement and advises against early closure of wounds. The nature of the blast injury frequently makes tissue friable and wounds tend to progress for many days after the initial injury. Frequent debridements every other day until wounds are stable and clean are the mainstay of treatment. Long bone fixation in an austere setting is also avoided and external fixation should be used not only for damage control but rather as a stabilizing frame to aid in transfer of rewounded soldier to a stable medical environment. Definitive stabilization varies little from civilian standards; however, higher grade tibia fractures are less likely to become infected when utilizing circular external fixation.[82] Soft tissue management is also frequently a challenge requiring large soft tissue transfers. Not infrequently the extremity injury is so great that patients choose elective amputation. As prosthesis improves and the care of the amputee has improved, small improvements in outcomes have been seen with amputation compared to limb salvage.[145]

REFERENCES

1. Aboutanos MB, Baker SP. Wartime civilian injuries: Epidemiology and intervention strategies. J Trauma. 1997;43(4):719–726.
2. Anonymous. Improvised Explosive Device/Booby Trap. 2008.
3. Artz CP, Sako Y, Scully RE. An evaluation of the surgeon's criteria for determining the viability of muscle during debridement. AMA Arch Surg. 1956;73(6):1031–1035.
4. Attias N, Lehman RE, Bodell LS, et al. Surgical management of a long segmental defect of the humerus using a cylindrical titanium mesh cage and plates: A case report. J Orthop Trauma. 2005;19(3):211–216.
5. Balfour GW, Marrero CE. Fracture brace for the treatment of humerus shaft fractures caused by gunshot wounds. Orthop Clin North Am. 1995;26(1):55–63.
6. Bartlett CS, DiFelice GS, Buly RL, et al. Cardiac arrest as a result of intra-abdominal extravasation of fluid during arthroscopic removal of a loose body from the hip joint of a patient with an acetabular fracture. J Orthop Trauma. 1998;12(4):294–299.
7. Bellamy RF, Zajtchuk R, eds. Assessing the effectiveness of conventional weapons. Conventional Warfare: Ballistic Blast and Burn Injuries. Washington, DC: Borden Institute, Office of the Surgeon General; 1991:53–82.
8. Bellamy RF, Zajtchuk R. The weapons of conventional land warfare. In: Conventional Warfare: Ballistic Blast and Burn Injuries. Washington, DC: Borden Institute, Office of the Surgeon General; 1991:1–52.
9. Bellamy RF. Combat trauma overview. In: Zajtchuk R, ed. Anesthesia and Perioperative Care of the Combat Casualty. Washington, DC: Borden Institute, Office of the Surgeon General; 1995.
10. Bergman M, Tornetta P, Kerina M, et al. Femur fractures caused by gunshots: Treatment by immediate reamed intramedullary nailing. J Trauma. 1993;34(6):783–785.
11. Best IM, Bumpers HL. Thigh compartment syndrome after acute ischemia. Am Surg. 2002;68(11):996–998.
12. Beyer JC, Arima JK, Johnson DW. Enemy ordnance material. In: Beyer JC, ed. Wound Ballistics. Washington, DC: Office of the Surgeon General; 1962: 1–90.
13. Beyer JC, Enos WF, Holmes RH. Personal protective armor. In: Beyer JC, ed. Wound Ballistics. Washington, DC: Office of the Surgeon General; 1962.
14. Biasutto SN, Moral AL, Bella JA. Firearm-related injuries: Clinical considerations on 1326 cases. Int Surg. 2006;91(1):39–43.
15. Bolanos AA, Vigorita VJ, Meyerson RI, et al. Intra-articular histopathologic changes secondary to local lead intoxication in rabbit knee joints. J Trauma. 1995;38(4):668–671.
16. Boucree JB Jr, Gabriel RA, Lezine-Hanna JT. Gunshot wounds to the foot. Orthop Clin North Am. 1995;26:191–197.
17. Bowyer GW, Cooper GJ, Rice P. Small fragment wounds: Biophysics and pathophysiology. J Trauma. 1996;40(3 suppl):S159–S164.
18. Brannon JK, Woods C, Chandran RE, et al. Gunshot wounds to the elbow. Orthop Clin North Am. 1995;26(1):75–84.
19. Brav EA. Further evaluation of the use of intramedullary nailing in the treatment of gunshot fractures of the extremities. J Bone Joint Surg Am. 1957;39-A(3):513–520.
20. Brien EW, Brien WW, Long WT, et al. Concomitant injuries of the hip joint and abdomen resulting from gunshot wounds. Orthopedics. 1992;15(11):1317–1319; discussion 1319–1320.
21. Brien WW, Kuschner SH, Brien EW, et al. The management of gunshot wounds to the femur. Orthop Clin North Am. 1995;26(1):133–138.
22. Brown PW, Urban JG. Early weight-bearing treatment of open fractures of the tibia. An end-result study of sixty-three cases. J Bone Joint Surg Am. 1969;51(1):59–75.
23. Brown TD, Michas P, Williams RE, et al. The impact of gunshot wounds on an orthopaedic surgical service in an urban trauma center. J Orthop Trauma. 1997;11(3):149–153.
24. Burkhalter A, Ballard WE, eds. Orthopedic surgery in Vietnam. In: Medical Department, United States Army, Surgery in Vietnam. Washington, DC: Office of the Surgeon General and Center for Military History; 1994.
25. Byrne A, Curran P. Necessity breeds invention: A study of outpatient management of low velocity gunshot wounds. Emerg Med J. 2006;23(5):376–378.
26. Carr CR, Turnipseed D. Experiences with intramedullary fixation of compound femoral fractures in war wounds. J Bone Joint Surg Am. 1953;35-A(1):153–171.
27. Clasper JC, Hill PF, Watkins PE. Contamination of ballistic fractures: An in vitro model. Injury. 2002;33(2):157–160.
28. Cory JW, Ruch DS. Arthroscopic removal of a .44 caliber bullet from the hip. Arthroscopy. 1998;14(6):624–626.
29. Davis GL. Management of open wounds of joints during the Vietnam war. A preliminary study. Clin Orthop Relat Res. 1970;68:3–9.
30. Demiralp B, Komurcu M, Ozturk C, et al. Total elbow arthroplasty in patients who have elbow fractures caused by gunshot injuries: 8- to 12-year follow-up study. Arch Orthop Trauma Surg. 2008;128(1):17–24.
31. Depage A. The peace lessons of war surgery. Br Med J. 1919;2(3077):820–821.
32. DiGiacomo JC, Schwab CW, Rotondo MF, et al. Gluteal gunshot wounds: Who warrants exploration? J Trauma. 1994;37(4):622–628.
33. Dougherty P. Armored vehicle crew casualties. Mil Med. 1990;155:417–420.
34. Dougherty PJ, Hetz SP, Fackler ML. Weapons and weapons effects. In: Lounsbury DE, ed. Emergency War Surgery Handbook. 4th ed. Washington, DC: Office of the Surgeon General; 2004.
35. Dziemian AJ, Herget CM. Physical aspects of primary contamination of bullet wounds. Mil Surg. 1950;106:294–299.
36. Dziemian AJ, Mendelson JA, Lindsey D. Comparison of the wounding characteristics of some commonly encountered bullets. J Trauma. 1961;1:341–353.
37. Elstrom JA, Pankovich AM, Egwele R. Extra-articular low-velocity gunshot fractures of the radius and ulna. J Bone Joint Surg Am. 1978;60(3):335–341.
38. Fackler M. Missile-caused wounds. In: Bowen TF, Bellamy RF, eds. Emergency War Surgery. 2nd Am. Rev. Washington, DC: Office of the Surgeon General; 1988:13–34.
39. Fackler ML, Bellamy RF, Malinowski JA. A reconsideration of the wounding mechanism of very high velocity projectiles—importance of projectile shape. J Trauma. 1988;28(1 suppl):S63–S67.
40. Fackler ML, Bellamy RF, Malinowski JA. The wound profile: Illustration of the missile-tissue interaction. J Trauma. 1988;28(1 suppl):S21–S29.
41. Fackler ML, Breteau JP, Courbil LJ, et al. Open wound drainage versus wound excision in treating the modern assault rifle wound. Surgery. 1989;105(5):576–584.
42. Fackler ML, Burkhalter WE. Hand and forearm injuries from penetrating projectiles. J Hand Surg Am. 1992;17(5):971–975.
43. Fackler ML, Dougherty PJ. Theodor Kocher and the scientific foundation of wound ballistics. Surg Gynecol Obstet. 1991;172(2):153–160.
44. Fackler ML, Malinowski JA. Internal deformation of the AK-74; a possible cause for its erratic path in tissue. J Trauma. 1988;28(1 suppl):S72–S75.
45. Fackler ML, Surinchak JS, Malinowski JA, et al. Bullet fragmentation: A major cause of tissue disruption. J Trauma. 1984;24(1):35–39.
46. Fackler ML, Surinchak JS, Malinowski JA, et al. Wounding potential of the Russian AK-74 assault rifle. J Trauma. 1984;24(3):263–266.
47. Fackler ML. Misinterpretations concerning Larrey's methods of wound treatment. Surg Gynecol Obstet. 1989;168(3):280–282.
48. Fackler ML. Wound ballistics. A review of common misconceptions. JAMA. 1988;259(18):2730–2736.
49. Ferguson LK, Brown RB, Nicholson JT, et al. Observations on the treatment of battle wounds aboard a hospital ship. US Nav Med Bull. 1943;41:299–305.
50. Ferraro SP Jr, Zinar DM, Management of gunshot fractures of the tibia. Orthop Clin North Am. 1995;26(1):181–189.
51. Fisher GH, Florey ME, Adelaide. M. B, et al. Penicillin in clostridial infections. Lancet. 1945;245(6344):395–399.
52. Foster RD, Albright JA. Acute compartment syndrome of the thigh: Case report. J Trauma. 1990;30(1):108–110.
53. Georgiadis GM, DeSilva SP. Reconstruction of skeletal defects in the forearm after trauma: Treatment with cement spacer and delayed cancellous bone grafting. J Trauma. 1995;38(6):910–914.
54. Goldman A, Minkoff J, Price A, et al. A posterior arthroscopic approach to bullet extraction from the hip. J Trauma. 1987;27(11):1294–1300.
55. Gotsch KE, Annest JL, Mercy JA, et al. Surveillance for fatal and nonfatal firearm-related injuries: United States, 1993–1998. MMWR Morb Mortal Wkly Rep. 2001;50:1–31.
56. Grundfest H, Korr IM. McMillen JH, et al. Ballistics of the Penetration of Human Skin by Small Spheres. Washington, DC: Office of Scientific Research and Development; 1945.
57. Grundfest H. Penetration of Steel Spheres into Bone. Washington, DC: Office of Scientific Research and Development; 1945.

58. Guo Y, Chiou-Tan FY. Radial nerve injuries from gunshot wounds and other trauma: Comparison of electrodiagnostic findings. *Am J Phys Med Rehabil.* 2002;81(3): 207–211.
59. Hahn M, Strauss E, Yang EC. Gunshot wounds to the forearm. *Orthop Clin North Am.* 1995;26(1):85–93.
60. Hakanson R, Nussman D, Gorman RA, et al. Gunshot fractures: A medical, social, and economic analysis. *Orthopedics.* 1994;17(6)519–523.
61. Hall RF Jr, Pankovich AM. Ender nailing of acute fractures of the humerus. A study of closed fixation by intramedullary nails without reaming. *J Bone Joint Surg Am.* 1987;69(4):558–567.
62. Hampton OP Jr. The indications for debridement of gunshot (bullet) wounds of the extremities in civilian practice. *J Trauma.* 1961;1:368–372.
63. Hansraj KK, Weaver LD, Todd AO, et al. Efficacy of ceftriaxone versus cefazolin in the prophylactic management of extra-articular cortical violation of bone due to low-velocity gunshot wounds. *Orthop Clin North Am.* 1995;26:9–17.
64. Harding NR, Lipton JF, Vigorita VJ, et al. Experimental lead arthropathy: An animal model. *J Trauma.* 1999;47(5):951–955.
65. Harvey EN, Korr IM, Oster G, et al. Secondary damage in wounding due to pressure changes accompanying the passage of high velocity missiles. *Surgery.* 1947;21(2): 218–239.
66. Harvey EN, Mcmillan JH, Butler EG. Mechanism of wounding. In: Beyer JC, ed. *Wound Ballistics.* Washington, DC: Office of the Surgeon General; 1962:143–235.
67. Harvey EN. Studies on wound ballistics. In: Andrus EC, Keefer CS, et al. eds. *Advances in Military Medicine.* Boston, MA: Little, Brown, and Co; 1948:191–205.
68. Harvey EN. The mechanism of wounding by high velocity missiles. *Proc Am Philos Soc.* 1948;92(4):294–304.
69. Heitmann C, Erdmann D, Levin LS. Treatment of segmental defects of the humerus with an osteoseptocutaneous fibular transplant. *J Bone Joint Surg Am.* 2002;84-A(12):2216–2223.
70. Helgeson MD, Potter BK, Evans KN, et al. Bioartificial dermal substitute: A preliminary report on its use for the management of complex combat-related soft tissue wounds. *J Orthop Trauma.* 2007;21(6):394–399.
71. Hennessy MJ, Banks HH, Leach RB, et al. Extremity gunshot wound and gunshot fracture in civilian practice. *Clin Orthop Relat Res.* 1976(114):296–303.
72. Herget CM, Coe GB, Beyer JC. Wound ballistics and body armor in Korea. In: Beyer JC, ed. *Wound Ballistics.* Washington, DC: Office of the Surgeon General; 1962:691–767.
73. Hollmann MW, Horowitz M. Femoral fractures secondary to low velocity missiles: Treatment with delayed intramedullary fixation. *J Orthop Trauma.* 1990;4(1): 64–69.
74. Hoover NW, Ivins JC. Wound debridement. *Arch Surg.* 1959;79:701–710.
75. Huelke DF, Harger JH, Buege LJ, et al. An experimental study in bio-ballistics femoral fractures produced by projectiles. *J Biomech.* 1968;1(2):97–105.
76. Huelke DF, Harger JH, Buege LJ, et al. An experimental study in bio-ballistics: Femoral fractures produced by projectiles–II. Shaft impacts. *J Biomech.* 1968;1(4):313–321.
77. Investigation, F.B.o. *Uniformed crime reports.* 2012.
78. Jamdar S, Helm AT, Redfern DR. Arthroscopic removal of a shotgun pellet from the elbow joint. *Arthroscopy.* 2001;17(7):E30.
79. Johnson EC, Strauss E. Recent advances in the treatment of gunshot fractures of the humeral shaft. *Clin Orthop Relat Res.* 2003;408:126–132.
80. Joshi A, Labbe M, Lindsey RW. Humeral fracture secondary to civilian gunshot injury. *Injury.* 1998;29(suppl 1):SA13–SA17.
81. Josserand MH, Stevenson J. *Pistols, Revolvers, and Ammunition.* New York, NY: Bonanza Books; 1972.
82. Keeling JJ, Gwinn DE, Tintle SM, et al. Short-term outcomes of severe open wartime tibial fractures treated with ring external fixation. *J Bone Joint Surg Am.* 2008;90(12): 2643–2651.
83. Keith E. *Shotguns.* Harrisburg, PA: Stackpole Books; 1950.
84. Keller A. The management of gunshot fractures of the humerus. *Injury.* 1995;26(2): 93–96.
85. Knapp TP, Patzakis MJ, Lee J, et al. Comparison of intravenous and oral antibiotic therapy in the treatment of fractures caused by low-velocity gunshots. A prospective, randomized study of infection rates. *J Bone Joint Surg Am.* 1996;78(8):1167–1171.
86. Kömürcü M, Yanmiş I, Ateşalp AS, et al. Treatment results for open comminuted distal humerus intra-articular fractures with Ilizarov circular external fixator. *Mil Med.* 2003;168(9):694–697.
87. Konda SR, Howard D, Davidovitch RI, et al. The saline load test of the knee redefined: A test to detect traumatic arthrotomies and rule-out periarticular wounds not requiring surgical intervention. *J Orthop Trauma.* 2013;27(9):491–497. [Epub ahead of print].
88. Krause M. Studies in wound ballistics: Temporary cavity effects in soft tissues. *Mil Med.* 1957;121:221–231.
89. LaGarde L. Poisoned wounds by the implements of warfare. *JAMA.* 1903;40:984–1067.
90. Leffers D, Chandler RW. Tibial fractures associated with civilian gunshot injuries. *J Trauma.* 1985;25(11):1059–1064.
91. Leininger BE, Rasmussen TE, Smith DL, et al. Experience with wound VAC and delayed primary closure of contaminated soft tissue injuries in Iraq. *J Trauma.* 2006; 61(5):1207–1211.
92. Lenihan MR, Brien WW, Gellman H, et al. Fractures of the forearm resulting from low-velocity gunshot wounds. *J Orthop Trauma.* 1992;6(1):32–35.
93. Leonard MH. The solution of lead by synovial fluid. *Clin Orthop Relat Res.* 1969;64: 255–261.
94. Lewis DD. Debridement. *JAMA.* 1919;73:377–383.
95. Linden M, Manton W, Stewart R, et al. Lead poisoning from retained bullets. Pathogenesis, diagnosis, and management. *Ann Surg.* 1982;195(3):305–313.
96. Long WT, Brien EW, Boucree JB, et al. Management of civilian gunshot injuries to the hip. *Orthop Clin North Am.* 1995;26:123–131.
97. Lounsbury DE. Levels of medical care. In: Lounsbury DE, ed. *Emergency War Surgery.* 4th ed. Washington, DC: Borden Institute, Office of the Surgeon General; 2004:1–11.
98. Lounsbury DE. *Triage.* In: Lounsbury DE, ed. *Emergency War Surgery.* 4th ed. Washington D C: Borden Institute, Office of the Surgeon General; 2004:1–17.
99. Love AG. *Statistics.* The Medical Department of the United States in the World War. Vol 15. Washington, DC: Office of the Surgeon General; 1925.
100. Marcus NA, Blair WF, Shuck JM, et al. Low-velocity gunshot wounds to extremities. *J Trauma.* 1980;20(12):1061–1064.
101. McAuliffe JA, Burkhalter WE, Ouellette EA, et al. Compression plate arthrodesis of the elbow. *J Bone Joint Surg Br.* 1992;74(2):300–304.
102. Mendelson JA, Glover JL. Sphere and shell fragment wounds of soft tissues: Experimental study. *J Trauma.* 1967;7(6):889–914.
103. Meyer NJ, Thiel B, Ninomiya JT. Retrieval of an intact, intra-articular bullet by hip arthroscopy using the lateral approach. *J Orthop Trauma.* 2002;16(1):51–53.
104. Mineo RC, Gittins ME. Arthroscopic removal of a bullet embedded in the acetabulum. *Arthroscopy.* 2003;19(9):E121–E124.
105. Ming L, Yu-Yuan M, Rong-Xiang F, et al. The characteristics of the pressure waves generated in the soft target by impact and its contribution to indirect bone fractures. *J Trauma.* 1988;28:s104–s109.
106. Miric DM, Bumbasirevic MZ, Senohradski KK, et al. Pelvifemoral external fixation for the treatment of open fractures of the proximal femur caused by firearms. *Acta Orthop Belg.* 2002;68(1):37–41.
107. Moed BR, Fakhouri AJ. Compartment syndrome after low-velocity gunshot wounds to the forearm. *J Orthop Trauma.* 1991;5(2):134–137.
108. Morgan MM, Spencer AD, Hershey FB. Debridement of civilian gunshot wounds of soft tissue. *J Trauma.* 1961;1:354–360.
109. Najibi S, Dougherty PJ, Morandi M. Management of gunshot wounds to the joints. *Techniques in Orthopaedics.* 2006;21(3):200–204.
110. Nechaev EA, Gritsanov AI, Fomin, NF, et al. *Mine blast trauma. Experience from the war in Afghanistan.* Stockholm: Falths Tryckeri; 1995.
111. Nicholas RM, McCoy GF. Immediate intramedullary nailing of femoral shaft fractures due to gunshots. *Injury.* 1995;26(4):257–259.
112. Nikolić D, Jovanović Z, Turković G, et al. Subtrochanteric missile fractures of the femur. *Injury.* 1998;29(10):743–749.
113. Nikolic D, Jovanovic Z, Vulovic R, et al. Primary surgical treatment of war injuries of the foot. *Injury.* 2000;31(3):193–197.
114. Nowotarski P, Brumback RJ. Immediate interlocking nailing of fractures of the femur caused by low- to mid-velocity gunshots. *J Orthop Trauma.* 1994;8(2):134–141.
115. Omer GE Jr. Injuries to nerves of the upper extremity. *J Bone Joint Surg Am.* 1974; 56(8):1615–1624.
116. Ordog GJ, Wasserberger J, Balasubramanium S, et al. Civilian gunshot wounds–outpatient management. *J Trauma.* 1994;36(1):106–111.
117. Otero F, Cuartas E. Arthroscopic removal of bullet fragments from the subacromial space of the shoulder. *Arthroscopy.* 2004;20(7):754–756.
118. Oughterson AW, Hull HC, Sutherland FA, et al. Study on wound ballistics: Bougainville campaign. In: Beyer JC, ed. *Wound Ballistics.* Washington, DC: Office of the Surgeon General; 1962: 281–436.
119. Owens BD, Kragh JF Jr, Macaitis J, et al. Characterization of extremity wounds in Operation Iraqi Freedom and Operation Enduring Freedom. *J Orthop Trauma.* 2007; 21(4):254–257.
120. Parisien JS, Esformes I. The role of arthroscopy in the management of low-velocity gunshot wounds of the knee joint. *Clin Orthop Relat Res.* 1984(185):207–213.
121. Patzakis MJ, Harvey JP Jr, Ivler D. The role of antibiotics in the management of open fractures. *J Bone Joint Surg Am.* 1974;56(3):532–541.
122. Perry DJ, Sanders DP, Nyirenda CD, et al. Gunshot wounds to the knee. *Orthop Clin North Am.* 1995;26(1):155–163.
123. Petersen W, Beske C, Stein V, et al. Arthroscopical removal of a projectile from the intra-articular cavity of the knee joint. *Arch Orthop Trauma Surg.* 2002;122(4):235–236.
124. Pool EH, Lee BJ, Dineen PA. Surgery of the soft parts, bones, and joints, at a front hospital. *Surg Gynecol Obstet.* 1919:289–311.
125. Prevention, C.C.f.D.C.a. *WISQARS fatal injuries: Mortality reports.* 2012; http://webappa.cdc.gov/sasweb/ncipc/mortrate.html.
126. Ramasamy A, et al. Blast mines: Physics, injury mechanisms and vehicle protection. *J R Army Med Corps.* 2009;155(4):258–264.
127. Ramasamy A, Hill AM, Clasper JC. Improvised explosive devices: Pathophysiology, injury profiles and current medical management. *J R Army Med Corps.* 2009;155(4):265–272.
128. Reis ND, Zinman C, Besser MI, et al. A philosophy of limb salvage in war: Use of the fixateur externe. *Mil Med.* 1991;156(10):505–520.
129. Robert RH. Gunshots to the hand and upper extremity. *Clin Orthop Relat Res.* 2003; 408:133–144.
130. Rodrigues RL, Sammer DM, Chung KC. Treatment of complex below-the-elbow gunshot wounds. *Ann Plast Surg.* 2006;56(2):122–127.
131. Rose SC, Fujisaki CK, Moore EE. Incomplete fractures associated with penetrating trauma: Etiology, appearance, and natural history. *J Trauma.* 1988;28(1):106–109.
132. Sarmiento A, Latta L. The evolution of functional bracing of fractures. *J Bone Joint Surg Br.* 2006;88(2):141–148.
133. Sarmiento A, Zagorski JB, Zych GA, et al. Functional bracing for the treatment of fractures of the humeral diaphysis. *J Bone Joint Surg Am.* 2000;82(4):478–486.
134. Scalea TM, Boswell SA, Scott JD, et al. External fixation as a bridge to intramedullary nailing for patients with multiple injuries and with femur fractures: Damage control orthopedics. *J Trauma.* 2000;48(4):613–621.
135. Scannell BP, Waldrop NE, Sasser HC, et al. Skeletal traction versus external fixation in the initial temporization of femoral shaft fractures in severely injured patients. *J Trauma.* 2010;68(3):633–640.
136. Sclafani SJ, Vuletin JC, Twersky J. Lead arthropathy: Arthritis caused by retained intra-articular bullets. *Radiology.* 1985;156(2):299–302.
137. Shao YC, Harwood P, Grotz MR, et al. Radial nerve palsy associated with fractures of the shaft of the humerus: A systematic review. *J Bone Joint Surg Br.* 2005;87(12): 1647–1652.

138. Simchen E, Raz R, Stein H, et al. Risk factors for infection in fracture war wounds (1973 and 1982 wars, Israel). *Mil Med.* 1991;156(10):520–527.

139. Simchen E, Sacks T. Infection in war wounds: Experience during the 1973 October War in Israel. *Ann Surg.* 1975;182(6):754–761.

140. Singleton SB, Joshi A, Schwartz MA, et al. Arthroscopic bullet removal from the acetabulum. *Arthroscopy.* 2005;21(3):360–364.

141. Skaggs DL, Hale JM, Buggay S, et al. Use of a hybrid external fixator for a severely comminuted juxta-articular fracture of the distal humerus. *J Orthop Trauma.* 1998;12(6):439–442.

142. Smith WHB. *Small Arms of the World.* Harrisburg, PA: Stackpole Books; 1983.

143. Stannard JP, Volgas DA, McGwin G 3rd, et al. Incisional negative pressure wound therapy after high-risk lower extremity fractures. *J Orthop Trauma.* 2012;26(1):37–42.

144. Stewart MP, Birch R. Penetrating missile injuries of the brachial plexus. *J Bone Joint Surg Br.* 2001;83(4):517–524.

145. Stinner DJ, Burns TC, Kirk KL, et al. Prevalence of late amputations during the current conflicts in Afghanistan and Iraq. *Mil Med.* 2010;175(12):1027–1029.

146. Tarkin IS, Hatzidakis A, Hoxie SC, et al. Arthroscopic treatment of gunshot wounds to the shoulder. *Arthroscopy.* 2003;19(1):85–89.

147. Teloken MA, Schmietd I, Tomlinson DP. Hip arthroscopy: A unique inferomedial approach to bullet removal. *Arthroscopy.* 2002;18(4):E21.

148. Tornetta P 3rd, Boes MT, Schepsis AA, et al. How effective is a saline arthrogram for wounds around the knee? *Clin Orthop Relat Res.* 2008;466(2):432–435.

149. Tornetta P 3rd, Hui RC. Intra-articular findings after gunshot wounds through the knee. *J Orthop Trauma.* 1997;11(6):422–424.

150. Tornetta P 3rd, Tiburzi D. Anterograde interlocked nailing of distal femoral fractures after gunshot wounds. *J Orthop Trauma.* 1994;8(3):220–227.

151. Turen CH, Burgess AR, Vanco B. Skeletal stabilization for tibial fractures associated with acute compartment syndrome. *Clin Orthop Relat Res.* 1995;(315):163–168.

152. Urist MR, Quigley TB. Use of skeletal traction for mass treatment of compound fractures; a summary of experiences with 4,290 cases during World War II. *AMA Arch Surg.* 1951;63(6):834–844.

153. Verheyden CN, McLaughlin B, Law C, et al. Through-and-through gunshot wounds to the foot: The "Fearless Fosdick" injury. *Ann Plast Surg.* 2005;55(5):474–478.

154. Weaver LD, Hansraj KK, Idusuyi OB, et al. Gunshot wound injuries. Frequency and cost analyses in south central Los Angeles. *Orthop Clin North Am.* 1995;26(1):1–7.

155. Wisniewski TF, Radziejowski MJ. Gunshot fractures of the humeral shaft treated with external fixation. *J Orthop Trauma.* 1996;10(4):273–278.

156. Wiss DA, Brien WW, Becker V Jr. Interlocking nailing for the treatment of femoral fractures due to gunshot wounds. *J Bone Joint Surg Am.* 1991;73(4):598–606.

157. Witschi TH, Omer GE Jr. The treatment of open tibial shaft fractures from Vietnam War. *J Trauma.* 1970;10(2):105–111.

158. Woloszyn JT, Uitvlugt GM, Castle ME. Management of civilian gunshot fractures of the extremities. *Clin Orthop Relat Res.* 1988;(226):247–251.

159. Wu CD. Low-velocity gunshot fractures of the radius and ulna: Case report and review of the literature. *J Trauma.* 1995;39(5):1003–1005.

160. Yildiz C, Ateşalp AS, Demiralp B, et al. High-velocity gunshot wounds of the tibial plafond managed with Ilizarov external fixation: A report of 13 cases. *J Orthop Trauma.* 2003;17(6):421–429.

161. Zellweger R, Hess F, Nicol A, et al. An analysis of 124 surgically managed brachial artery injuries. *Am J Surg.* 2004;188(3):240–245.

162. Zinman C, Norman D, Hamoud K, et al. External fixation for severe open fractures of the humerus caused by missiles. *J Orthop Trauma.* 1997;11(7):536–539.

163. Zura RD, Bosse MJ. Current treatment of gunshot wounds to the hip and pelvis. *Clin Orthop Relat Res.* 2003;(408):110–114.

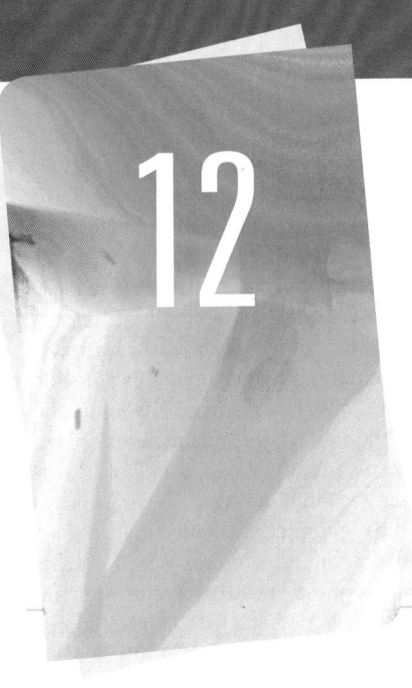

12

PRINCIPLES OF MANGLED EXTREMITY MANAGEMENT

Sarina K. Sinclair and Erik N. Kubiak

INTRODUCTION

The term "mangled extremity" refers to an injury to an extremity so severe that the viability of the limb is often questionable and loss of the limb a likely outcome. The mangled extremity has been previously defined as a complex fracture with additional involvement of at least two of the following: artery, tendon, nerve, or soft tissue (skin, fat, and muscle).[35,43] This injury is always a result of high-energy trauma caused by some combination of crush, shear, and/or blast. Associated fractures usually verify the high-energy forces of the mechanism of injury by exhibiting extensive comminution patterns frequently a result of a combination of three-point bending, axial load, and torsional forces imparted to the extremity. The skin is often degloved with large areas of loss secondary to avulsion or ischemia and the fascial compartments are typically incompletely opened by explosion or tear. Muscles are typically damaged at both local and regional levels by direct as well as indirect injury. Furthermore, soft tissue planes are usually extensively disrupted and, when present, contaminants generally infiltrate all of these tissue planes (Fig. 12-1). Not only are the

injury patterns themselves complex, but the medical, psychological, and socioeconomic impacts that these injuries have on the patient make their management a difficult task, even in the most experienced of hands.

Although most of the advances that have taken place in the management of the mangled extremity have occurred during times of war, the majority of limb-threatening injuries seen in practice today are the result of high-speed motor vehicle collisions. Injuries to the lower and upper extremities occur more frequently than head injuries in motorcycle crashes.[59] Modification of passenger restraints, vehicle safety engineering, and the legislation of seatbelt and air bag protection appear to be decreasing the mortality rate associated with motor vehicle crashes. As a result, the incidence of severe lower extremity trauma may be increasing. In the United States, injuries to the lower extremity account for over 250,000 hospital admissions annually for patients 18 to 54 years of age. It is estimated that over half of these admissions result from high-energy mechanisms.[45] An analysis of the largest available registry of trauma patients in the United States, the National Trauma Data Bank, found that 1% of

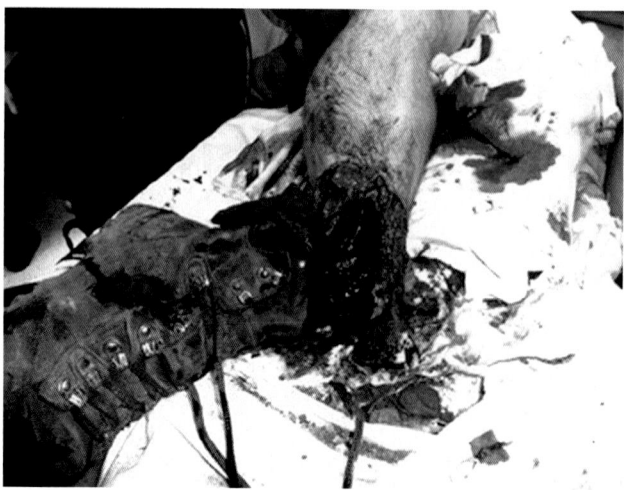

FIGURE 12-1 Soft tissue injury demonstrating gross contamination in multiple tissue planes. Caution should be used in making viability determinations prior to debridement and irrigation in the controlled setting of the operating room.

all trauma patients sustained an amputation between 2000 and 2004.[7] Although less frequent than the lower extremity, 90% of upper extremity amputations are a result of trauma.[6] It is evident from these reported figures that a large population of extremity trauma patients do not undergo amputation and must endure long-term treatment with the goal of functional restoration to preinjury levels. Orthopedic surgeons providing emergency department trauma coverage need to understand the historical concepts surrounding the care for these complex injuries as well as recent modifications of these concepts based on numerous advances in technology combined with a better understanding of the long-term clinical outcomes of these injury patterns.

HISTORICAL BACKGROUND

From the time of Hippocrates, the management of the limb-threatening lower extremity injury has plagued patients and surgeons alike. Until the implementation of amputation, most severe open fractures resulted in sepsis and these injuries were often fatal.[4] Historically, amputation itself was associated with high mortality rates, often from hemorrhage or sepsis. Amputations performed during the Franco-Prussian War and American Civil War carried mortality rates ranging from 26% to as high as 90%.[28,112] As amputation techniques improved, so did our understanding of the concepts of bacterial contamination and infection. By the mid 1880s, through the pioneering works of Pasteur, Koch, and Lister on bacterial contamination and infection, there was a rapid increase in the use of antiseptic agents, soon followed by the introduction of aseptic methods, and then mortality rates rapidly declined.[150] Subsequently, topical sulfa agents were introduced just before World War I and systemic antibiotics became available during World War II and the Korean War.[112,114] Because of advances in surgical technique, as well as through a better understanding of microbial prophylaxis and treatment, extremity injuries that were once considered to be life threatening have now been rendered, at the very least, survivable.[39]

Despite the relative success of amputation surgery in reducing mortality in the treatment of patients with a life- or limb-threatening injury of the extremity, many patients and physicians have historically perceived amputation as a failure of therapy and have fought aggressively to salvage the mangled limb. Although a pioneer in the field of amputation, Ambroise Paré knowingly risked his own life over limb when he insisted on conservative management of his own open tibia fracture rather than amputation. Not only did he survive the injury, but also his documentation of the conservative treatment of a potentially limb- and life-threatening injury serves as one of the first known documented cases of "limb salvage."[119] Nevertheless, for the years to come, most complex extremity injuries were routinely treated with amputation. After World War II, medical and surgical training became more specialized and numerous developments in the civilian medical arena led to a revolution in the management of limb-threatening battlefield injuries, which dictates our treatment today. Arterial repair and bypass were attempted on a wide scale during the Korean and Vietnam Wars, subsequently reducing the amputation rates in extremities with vascular injuries from 50% to 13%.[69,70,71,112,126] On the battlefields of Iraq and Afghanistan, body armor, the widespread use of tourniquets, and in-theater resuscitation techniques have saved a higher percentage of combat casualty victims than in any previous US military conflicts;[120] however, because of the nature of body armor coverage, the extremities are often left exposed. The high energy explosive mechanism of injury resulting from improvised explosive devices (IEDs) has led to a high prevalence of "mangled" extremities with severe damage to the hard and soft tissues. Subsequently, the incidence of amputations within the United States military population has doubled during the most recent conflicts compared to previous wars.[127] Soldiers with strong wishes to return to active duty following their injury have driven the strong interest in limb salvage.[121] Advances in all aspects of wound and fracture management have improved our ability to reconstruct the severely injured extremity. Limbs that would have required an amputation over 25 years ago are now routinely entered into complex reconstruction protocols. The development of second- and third-generation antibiotics, microsurgical tissue transfers,[18,81,133,146] and the use of temporary intraluminal vascular shunts,[74] wound irrigation strategies, and tissue-friendly fracture fixation methods have combined to make initial limb salvage, at the very least, feasible in most cases. Furthermore, by using massive autogenous grafts and/or osteoinductive materials,[26,44,54,77,83] as well as through the technique of bone transport,[32,105,118,128] delayed large-segment bone defect reconstruction has become routine. Although limb salvage has become technically feasible, the initial assessment and management of the patient and the injury are paramount in determining whether salvage is advisable.

PRINCIPLES OF MANAGEMENT

Initial Evaluation

Most limb-threatening injuries are very impressive on presentation and can often be distracting to the treating surgeon and the medical team. Because these injuries are usually the result of a high-energy mechanism, routine trauma protocols should be followed that first address the patient as a whole and not just the injured extremity, because 10% to 17% of these patients will have an associated life-threatening injury.[22,88] Evaluation should begin by following the principles of Advanced Trauma Life Support (ATLS). Once the patient has been stabilized and the primary and secondary trauma surveys have been completed, a thorough orthopedic evaluation is mandatory (Table 12-1).

The mechanism of injury, age of the patient, and the presence of any other social or medical comorbidities should also be determined. Prophylactic antibiotics should be administered as soon as possible and tetanus prophylaxis should be administered

as indicated. The injured extremity should first be evaluated for adequate vascular perfusion and, if a vascular injury is suspected, vascular surgery consultation should be obtained. A determination of the time of injury is of great importance to assess the duration of limb ischemia. The soft tissue wound should be inspected and the pattern of soft tissue injury and contamination should be noted. If possible, a cursory removal of any gross contamination via irrigation should be performed before dressing the wounds and immobilizing the extremity, especially if a fracture reduction or joint reduction is thought to be necessary before transporting to the operating room for initial wound debridement. A detailed motor and sensory examination should be performed

---

TABLE 12-1	The Current Algorithmic Approach to Mangled Extremity Decision Making as Defined by the Orthopaedic Trauma Association Open Fracture Committee 2012[2]

Management of the Mangled Extremity

Criteria for Immediate Amputation

- Life-threatening injury to the extremity
- Hemodynamic instability
- Prolonged limb ischemia (>6 hr lower extremity, >8 hr upper extremity)
- Severe soft tissue loss without option for free flap reconstruction
- Nonreconstructable bone injury
- Muscle loss affecting more than two lower leg compartments
- Bone loss involving more than one-third of the length of the tibia

Management Steps After Patient Stabilization

- Debridement and stabilization by senior surgeon
  - Zones of injury: central, marginal stasis, minimally injured
  - Serial debridements will be required
  - Be conservative with muscle on first debridement
- Document injury in photographs
- Evaluation of five major areas of concern:

Discussion with Patient

- Present all objective information and recommendation
- Discuss outcome data of amputation vs. salvage
- Psychosocial factors to consider: type of employment, support system, access to medical and rehabilitation facilities
- Self efficacy

Limb Salvage

- Multiple procedures
- 30–50% usefully employed at 2 years if successful
- 30% rate of late amputation

Amputation

- Beneficial in short term
- Permanent
- Lifelong issues with prosthetic device
- Most distal level possible
- Preserve as much viable tissue as possible

Important that patient makes final treatment decision

Major Areas of Concern

1. **Skin**
   - Pattern of soft tissue injury
   - Extent of damage
   - Availability of tissue for reconstruction
   - Reconstruction needs to be performed within 14 days
2. **Muscle**
   - Muscle necrosis (Four Cs)
   - Amount of muscle function
   - Muscle-tendon unit
3. **Arterial**
   - Vessel injury with or without distal ischemia
   - Duration of ischemia:
     Lower extremity limits
       Cold > 10 hr
       Warm > 6 hr
     Upper extremity limits
       Warm > 8 hr
   - Observe for hard and soft signs of vascular injury
   - Arterial pressure indices <0.9 or absent distal pulse should consult with vascular surgery
4. **Contamination**
   - Surface versus embedded in tissues
   - From high-risk environment (i.e., fecal)
5. **Bone Loss**
   - Size of defect
   - Is critical-sized defect too great for grafting or transplant?

and documented, both before and after any manipulation of the extremity. The presence of an associated compartment syndrome, which occurs at a rate of 1% to 10% in open fractures,[84] should be considered and ruled out. Radiographic evaluation should include two orthogonal views of any involved joints or long bones, as well as the joint above and below any confirmed fractures. Photographs of the extremity should be obtained whenever possible with permission of the patient or legal representative if possible. These can provide invaluable documentation of the extent of the initial injury and, during the course of treatment, serve as a visual record of progress to or away from a functional salvaged extremity,[37] as long as the patient's right to privacy is not violated.

Not only should the orthopedic examination include the extremity in question, but a comprehensive musculoskeletal examination should be performed to rule out any concomitant musculoskeletal injuries. In the case of a polytrauma patient with a mangled extremity, the initial diagnostic workup and treatment of any life-threatening injuries can often be time consuming and precede the management of the injured limb; therefore, a sterile dressing should be applied to all wounds and the limb immobilized as soon as possible to prevent any ongoing soft tissue damage until proper debridement and stabilization procedures can be performed in the controlled setting of the operating room.

Vascular Assessment

Limb-threatening injuries are often associated with vascular insult. Arterial injuries usually present with either hard or soft signs suggestive of injury. Examples of hard signs that should be documented and investigated include pulsatile bleeding, the presence of a rapidly expanding hematoma, a palpable thrill, or audible bruit, as well as the presence of any of the classic signs of obvious arterial occlusion (pulselessness, pallor, paresthesia, pain, paralysis, poikilothermia). Soft signs of arterial injury include a history of arterial bleeding, a nonexpanding hematoma, a pulse deficit without ischemia, a neurologic deficit originating in a nerve adjacent to a named artery, and the proximity of a penetrating wound, fracture, or dislocation near to a named artery.[109] In addition to observing for these hard and soft signs of vascular injury, a formal vascular examination should be conducted. The skin color and time required for capillary refilling of the skin of the distal extremity should be compared with and documented against that of the uninjured contralateral side. The distal extremity should be evaluated for the presence of palpable peripheral pulses and/or Doppler signal. The limb with gross deformity secondary to fracture or dislocation with questionably palpable pulses or reduced Doppler audible flow should undergo immediate gentle reduction of the deformity and immobilization of the reduced limb in an effort to relieve possible kinking or compression of the vascular structures. Subsequently, pulse assessment of the distal extremity should again be performed and documented after any reduction maneuvers. Arterial pressure indices (APIs) should also be obtained in the presence of a history of pulselessness in the extremity or if the vascular status of the distal extremity remains unclear even after reduction attempts have been made to restore reasonable alignment to the extremity. APIs are obtained by first identifying the dorsalis pedis and posterior tibial arteries of the injured extremity using a Doppler probe. Next, a blood pressure cuff is placed proximal to the level of injury and then inflated to a suprasystolic level causing cessation of the normal Doppler signal. The cuff is then slowly deflated and the pressure at which the Doppler signal returns identifies the ankle systolic pressure to the injured limb. This procedure should then be repeated on the contralateral extremity as well as in the arm (brachial pressures). The pressure in the injured extremity is then compared with the pressure in the arm or the unaffected extremity and reported as a ratio of the normal systolic pressure (e.g., if the brachial systolic pressure is equal to 120 mm Hg and the systolic pressure in the injured limb is equal to 90 mm Hg, then API is reported as 0.75). If the API is lower than 0.9 or distal pulses remain absent despite reduction, angiography and/or vascular surgery consultation is indicated.

Once the location of an arterial injury has been identified, treatment should first address restoration of arterial inflow and skeletal stabilization. In the patient with a pulseless but perfused limb, the priority and sequence of vascular and orthopedic repair depend primarily on the experience and availability of both the orthopedic and vascular teams. At times, if the fracture is relatively stable and will require little manipulation, immediate arterial repair should precede bony stabilization. However, if the fracture is excessively comminuted, displaced, or shortened, rapid bony stabilization should be performed before any attempts at vascular repair. Not only will this aid in the exposure of the vascular injury, but doing so brings the limb out to its proper resting length, ensuring the vascular repair is of sufficient length to allow for further manipulation and reduction of the extremity with less risk of vascular complications after the repair has been completed.[73]

In the patient who has undergone a period of prolonged ischemia, the restoration of arterial inflow should be the highest priority and consideration should be given to temporary intraluminal vascular shunting of the extremity.[74,36,111] The insertion of an intraluminal shunt can rapidly restore arterial inflow and allow for a more detailed examination to better determine the extent of the injury and whether the limb is indeed salvageable. Because the shunt will hold up to fairly vigorous manipulation, it will also allow for a more thorough debridement and appropriate stabilization of the bone and soft tissues. Once the debridement has been completed and the bony injury temporarily or definitively stabilized, formal vascular repair can then either proceed immediately or in a delayed fashion if the patient remains in extremis.

A compartment syndrome is not uncommon after restoration of arterial inflow to an ischemic and traumatized limb. The diminished arterial inflow during the ischemic period combined with the "reperfusion injury" that occurs after arterial repair can result in interstitial fluid leakage and elevated compartment pressures. Fasciotomies should be performed after any revascularization procedure in the mangled extremity.[88,90,103] Whereas most vascular and general surgeons are adequately trained to perform decompressive fasciotomies, ideally, these should be performed by or under the supervision of the orthopedic surgeon to ensure adequate compartment decompression as well as appropriate fasciotomy placement that will not compromise later bony and soft tissue reconstructive procedures.

Operative Debridement and Stabilization

Once the extremity has been evaluated in the emergency department and photographs have been taken for the medical record, any open wounds should be gently rinsed with a copious amount of normal saline and dressed with sterile gauze.[29] The dressings should be left in place until the patient reaches the operating room for definitive debridement.

In the operating room, a sterile tourniquet should be placed to prevent the possibility of exsanguination, unless tourniquet placement restricts prepping of the limb. It should not be inflated unless absolutely necessary to avoid further ischemic injury to the extremity. Once the tourniquet is in place, the splint and dressings can be removed and the extremity again examined for perfusion. Although typically referred to as "irrigation and debridement," the first and most important step is a thorough debridement of the wound. (Fig. 12-2) This should be done in a methodical manner to ensure adequate removal of any contaminating material and devitalized tissues. The skin and subcutaneous tissue should be addressed first. Whereas the initial open skin wounds are obvious, the energy imparted at the time of injury typically produces a shock wave that causes stripping of the soft tissues and typically results in so-called zones of injury. A gradient of energy extends peripherally from the site of impact, variably damaging tissues along its path. A central zone of necrotic tissue exists at and around the point of impact and greatest injury. These tissues are typically nonviable regardless of the intervention. Surrounding this area lies a zone of marginal stasis. This ischemic penumbra consists of tissue that is variably injured and may or may not survive despite appropriate intervention. Finally, at the periphery of the injury exists a zone of noninjured or minimally injured tissue that, while not subject to the primary injury, could be at risk from the delayed physiologic responses to the primary area of injury.[56,90] To address these zones of injury, the open wounds should be extended or separate extensile incisions should be performed to adequately assess and debride the wound. These incisions should be axially aligned and thoughtfully placed so as not to create "at-risk" flaps or preclude any later reconstructive efforts.

Once the skin wounds have been extended, all necrotic muscle, fat, fascia, skin, and other nonviable tissue within the central zone of injury should be removed. Muscle should be tested for viability based on its contractility, consistency, color, and capillary bleeding (the four Cs), and if it is found to be obviously nonviable, it should be debrided, regardless of the expected functional loss. Marginally questionably viable muscle should be preserved during the initial debridement. Although the amount of tissue damage seen on the initial debridement can be quite extensive, the quantity of tissue necrosis from the delayed response to the injury within the zone of marginal stasis can far exceed the loss and destruction caused by the initial traumatic injury. Because the exact degree of expected tissue loss and necrosis cannot be determined easily at the time of initial debridement, serial debridements will be required until the identification and removal of all nonviable tissue has been achieved and wound homeostasis obtained.

Skeletal Stabilization

Skeletal stabilization is an extremely important tenant in the initial management of the limb at risk. Stabilization of the bony skeleton prevents ongoing soft tissue damage, promotes wound healing, and is thought to protect against infection. In an animal study, Worlock et al.[159] examined the rate of infection and osteomyelitis associated with stable and unstable skeletal fixation. They reported that the infection rate in the unstable group was nearly double than that in the skeletal stabilization group.

The choice of skeletal stabilization is dependent on the location of the bony injury, the degree of soft tissue injury, and the overall condition of the patient at the time of initial operative management. Stabilization options range from splint immobilization or skeletal traction to internal or external fixation. Whereas no one technique has proved to be superior to all others in all clinical situations, in general, the more severe

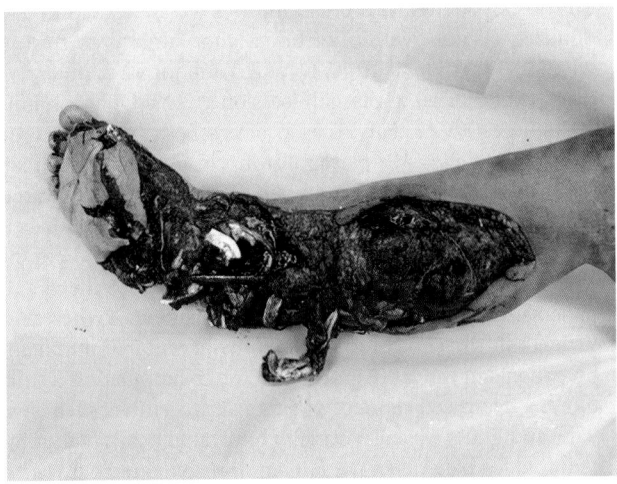
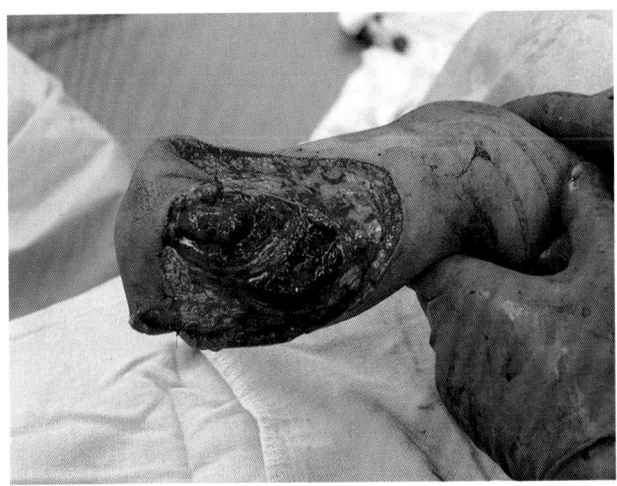

FIGURE 12-2 An 8-year-old child slipped and fell under a lawn mower sustaining extensive soft tissue injury with severe contamination **(A)**. After extensive debridement as much soft tissue as possible was preserved **(B)** and then secondary closure with skin grafting was performed in a delayed fashion.

the injury, the greater is the need for direct skeletal fixation to provide improved access to the traumatic wound. Immediate intramedullary stabilization or plate fixation of type I, II, and IIIA open fractures remains an accepted treatment strategy. However, most limb-threatening injuries present as type IIIB or type IIIC open fractures. These injuries are perhaps most judiciously managed with temporizing external fixation. External fixation in this setting offers many advantages. It can be applied relatively quickly and without the use of fluoroscopy while still providing excellent stability and alignment of the limb until definitive fixation can be performed. External fixation also allows for redisplacement of the fracture fragments for a more thorough evaluation and debridement of the soft tissues during any repeat procedures. Once wound homeostasis has been obtained, conversion to definitive internal fixation can be performed on a delayed basis with good results.[5,136,137] External fixation can also be chosen as the form of definitive fixation for diaphyseal fractures, but multiple studies have found this approach to have slightly higher complication rates and poorer outcomes when directly compared with intramedullary fixation. (Fig. 12-3). Henley et al.[63] prospectively compared unreamed intramedullary nailing with external fixation in patients with type II, IIIA, and IIIB open fractures of the tibial shaft. Both groups underwent identical soft tissue management before and after skeletal fixation. Their study showed that those patients in the intramedullary nail fixation group had significantly fewer incidences of malalignment and underwent fewer subsequent procedures than did those in the external fixation group. Tornetta et al.[151] also reported on the early results of a randomized, prospective study comparing external fixation with the use of nonreamed locked nails in type IIIB open tibial fractures. Again, both groups had the same initial management, soft tissue procedures, and early bone grafting. They found that the intramedullary nail treatment group had slightly better knee and ankle motion and less final angulation at the fracture site. They also concluded that the nailed fractures were consistently easier to manage, especially in terms of soft tissue procedures and bone

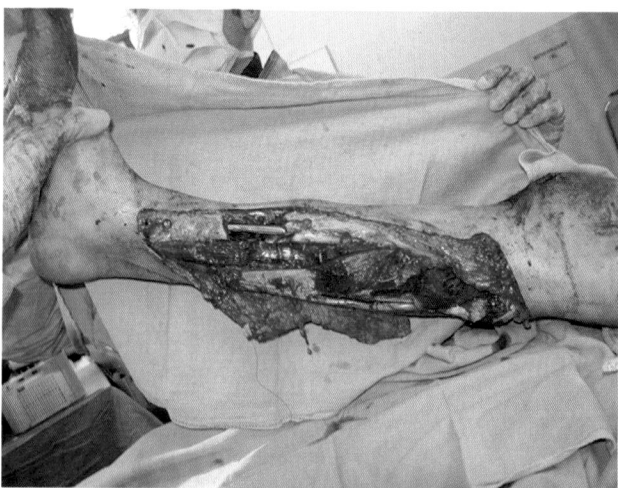

FIGURE 12-3 An intramedullary nail can be used for both provisional and definitive stabilization of the tibia during the multiple phases of limb salvage.

grafting. Furthermore, they thought that intramedullary nailing was preferred by their patients and that it did not require the same high level of patient compliance as external fixation. Using data obtained through the Lower Extremity Assessment Project (LEAP), Webb et al.[156] reviewed 156 patients with the combination of a fractured tibia in association with a mangled lower extremity. One hundred and five patients with 17 type IIIA, 84 type IIIB, and 4 type IIIC tibial fractures had follow-up to 2 years. The authors found that definitive treatment with a nail yielded better outcomes than definitive treatment with external fixation. In their series, the external fixation patients had a significantly increased likelihood of both infection and nonunion.

Hyperbaric Oxygen

Hyperbaric oxygen (HBO) allows patients to breathe 100% oxygen in a chamber under increased barometric pressure. This results in a supraphysiologic arterial oxygen saturation level, creating an expanded radius of diffusion for oxygen into the tissues that results in increased oxygen delivery at the periphery of certain wounds. As a result, HBO is thought to enhance oxygen delivery to injured tissues affected by vascular disruption, thrombosis, cytogenic and vasogenic edema, and cellular hypoxia as a result of trauma to the extremity.

This improved oxygen delivery is believed to be most beneficial in the peripheral zone of injury where tissue that is variably injured may or may not survive despite other appropriate interventions. Injured but viable cells in this area have increased oxygen needs at the very time when oxygen delivery is decreased by disruption of the microvascular supply.[72,117] As such, HBO can be applied in an effort to mitigate this process of secondary injury in extremity trauma and minimize the resultant tissue loss at different points in both the pathologic and recovery processes.[56]

Most clinical reports on HBO therapy in the treatment of extremity trauma are observational with fairly anecdotal reports on its efficacy. However, in 1996, Bouachour et al.[15] performed a randomized placebo-controlled human trial of HBO as an adjunct to the management of crush injuries to the extremity. Thirty-six patients with crush injuries were assigned in a randomized fashion, within 24 hours after surgery, to treatment with HBO (session of 100% O_2 at 2.5 atm for 90 minutes, twice daily, over 6 days) or placebo (session of 21% O_2 at 1.1 atm for 90 minutes, twice daily, over 6 days). Both treatment groups (HBO group, $n = 18$; placebo group, $n = 18$) were similar in terms of age; risk factors; number, type, or location of vascular injuries, neurologic injuries, or fractures; and type, location, or timing of surgical procedures. The authors found complete wound healing without tissue necrosis in 17 of the 18 HBO patients and in 10 of the 18 control patients. Whereas two patients in the control group eventually required amputation, no patients in the HBO group went on to amputation. Furthermore, a decreased number of surgical procedures such as skin flaps and grafts, vascular surgery, or eventual amputation were required for patients in the HBO group compared with the placebo group. A subgroup analysis of patients matched for age and severity of injury showed that HBO was especially effective in patients older than 40 with severe soft tissue injury. They concluded that HBO improved wound healing and reduced the number of additional surgical procedures required for treatment of the injury, and that it could be considered a useful adjunct in the management of severe crush injuries of the limbs, especially in patients over 40 years old.

To date, controlled animal experiments, select human case series, and a small number of randomized studies seem to suggest a potential benefit of HBO therapy as an adjunct to the management of the severely traumatized limb. However, if efficacious, HBO use in the mangled extremity patient will be selective as many patients are critically ill and are often unable to travel to receive and to tolerate HBO therapy. At this time, more data and stringent clinical investigations are needed to determine the exact indications for, optimal timing of, and appropriate duration and dosage of HBO therapy before it can be recommended in the routine management of complex injuries of the limb. An international multicenter, randomized control trial is currently being conducted to study repair of open tibia fracture involving severe soft tissue injury with or without a concurrent course of HBO treatments (Clinical Trials Identifier NCT00264511). Patients randomized to the experimental (HBO) group will receive a course of HBO therapy in addition to normal trauma care for a total of 12 sessions over 8 days to measure the incidence of acute complications after injury as the primary endpoint. The findings of this trial could offer better insight into the use of this technology in mangled extremity treatment.

Soft Tissue Coverage

Wound closure and soft tissue reconstruction are covered in more depth in Chapter 15. However, a few principles are worth discussing here. The first addresses the type of soft tissue coverage selected in the reconstruction pathway. Whereas multiple options for coverage exist, such as skin grafts, local flaps, or free flaps, complications will occur with each. Pollak et al.[123] found that 27% of high-energy tibia injuries requiring soft tissue reconstruction had at least one wound complication within the first 6 months after injury. They also found that the rate of complication differed based on the type of flap coverage. For limbs with the most severe osseous injury (OTA type C fractures), treatment with a rotational flap was 4.3 times more likely to lead to an operative wound complication than was treatment with a free flap. The rate of complications for the limbs with less severe osseous injury did not differ significantly based on soft tissue coverage selection. Based on this information, one should be very cautious when selecting a local flap in the setting of high-energy trauma as the flap, although originally healthy in appearance, may have indeed been included in the initial zone of injury.

A second and perhaps more controversial principle is the timing of the soft tissue reconstructive procedure. The primary argument for early soft tissue reconstruction is to reduce the risk of nosocomial contamination because of repeated exposures of the vulnerable wound to the hospital environment. Some more recent data have brought into question the efficacy of early soft tissue reconstruction. When analyzing a subset of patients with open tibial fractures in association with a mangled extremity, Webb et al.[156] failed to observe any advantages related to the performance of early muscle flap wound coverage within the first 72 hours after the injury. In contrast, multiple authors have shown that early reconstruction (within 72 hours) reduces postoperative infection, flap failure, and nonunion rates as well as the risk for the development of osteomyelitis.[46,51,53,64] Others have recommended muscle flap coverage on a more delayed basis (7 to 14 days).[160] Recently, with the advent of negative pressure wound therapy (NPWT) and the decreasing availability of surgeons trained in rotational flaps and free tissue transfer, there seems to be a trend toward increased delays until definitive soft tissue reconstructive procedures are performed. While NPWT can be a very effective tool in the initial soft tissue management of high-energy open fractures, its routine use in open tibia fractures has not been found to reduce the overall infection rates compared with historical controls nor has it been shown to reduce the need for free tissue transfer or rotational muscle flap coverage in these injuries.[34] Bhattacharyya et al.[8] evaluated whether the use of NPWT could allow for a delay of flap coverage for open tibia fractures without a subsequent increase in the infection rate. They concluded that despite the routine use of NPWT before definitive soft tissue reconstruction in patients with Gustilo type IIIB fractures, patients who underwent definitive soft tissue coverage within 7 days had significantly decreased infection rates compared with those who underwent soft tissue coverage at 7 days or more after injury (12.5% versus 57%).

Despite best efforts, delays in soft tissue reconstruction are often inevitable; however, based on a preponderance of evidence, it still appears that soft tissue coverage should be performed as early as possible once both the patient and the wound bed appear stable enough for such a procedure.

PATIENT ASSESSMENT AND DECISION MAKING

In 1943, US Army Major General NT. Kirk, a leader at the field of amputation during World War I and World War II, wrote, "Injury, disability, or deformity incompatible with life and function indicates amputation. The surgeon must use his judgment as to whether the amputation is indicated and at what level it can safely be done."[82] Since that time, numerous physicians caring for the patient with a mangled extremity have delineated a multitude of clinical factors to help better guide in the decision-making process in the setting of a potentially salvageable versus an unsalvageable limb injury (Table 12-2).[89]

In 2002, factors that influenced the mangled extremity treatment decision process were studied by Swiontkowski[147] and the LEAP Study Group. Orthopedic and general trauma surgeons caring for the mangled limbs were surveyed to determine the factors they typically used to make a reconstruction or amputation treatment decision. More than 33% of 52 orthopedic surgeons indicated that plantar sensation was the most important determinant for limb salvage. The severity of the soft tissue injury (17%) and limb ischemia (15%) followed in importance. No orthopedic surgeon ranked the patient's Injury Severity Score (ISS) as a critical factor. In contrast, 33 general trauma surgeons from the same centers ranked the ISS as the

| TABLE 12-2 | Limb Salvage Decision-Making Variables |

Patient Variables

Age
Underlying chronic diseases (e.g., diabetes)
Occupational considerations
Patient and family desires

Extremity Variables

Mechanism of injury (soft tissue injury kinetics)
Fracture pattern
Arterial/venous injury (location)
Neurologic (anatomic status)
Injury status of ipsilateral foot
Intercalary ischemic zone after revascularization

Associated Variables

Magnitude of associated injury (Injury Severity Score)
Severity and duration of shock
Warm ischemia time

sensation were the factors considered to be most important at the time to predict amputation. Patient characteristics and the experience level of the surgeon did not appear to influence the decision-making process. Of important note, the orthopedic surgeon was responsible for the initial treatment decision in all cases. General trauma surgeons participated in the decision-making process 58% of the time and plastic surgeons contributed to the process 26% of the time. Although all of these variables play a key role in decision making by the orthopedic surgeon and the trauma team, a few of these warrant further discussion, as new evidence suggests that we should reconsider their importance. In the final analysis limb salvage is dependent on the reconstructability of the soft tissue envelope which is both provider and patient resource dependent as the bone is almost always reconstructable. Provider resources include, but are not exclusive to, the availability of appropriately trained personnel for soft tissue management. Patient resources include, but are not exclusive to, the intrinsic physiologic and psychological reserves of the patient.

Survivability

Often, the decision to amputate a severely injured limb can be a long, drawn-out, and difficult decision for both the patient and the treating surgeon. However, on rare occasions, the decision for amputation can be quite simple (Fig. 12-4). Amputation is generally the only treatment option in cases of a

most critical determinant (31%), followed by limb ischemia (27%) and plantar sensation (21%). An analysis of the patient, injury, and surgeon characteristics determined that the soft tissue injury (i.e., the extent of muscle injury, deep vein injury, skin defects, and contamination) and the absence of plantar

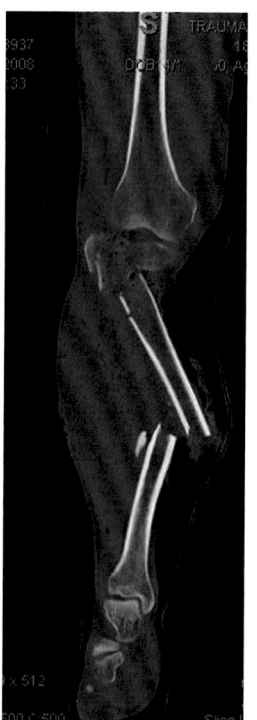
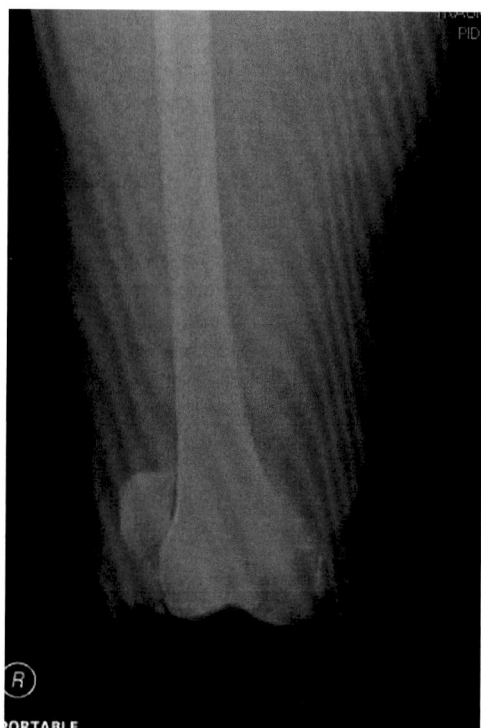
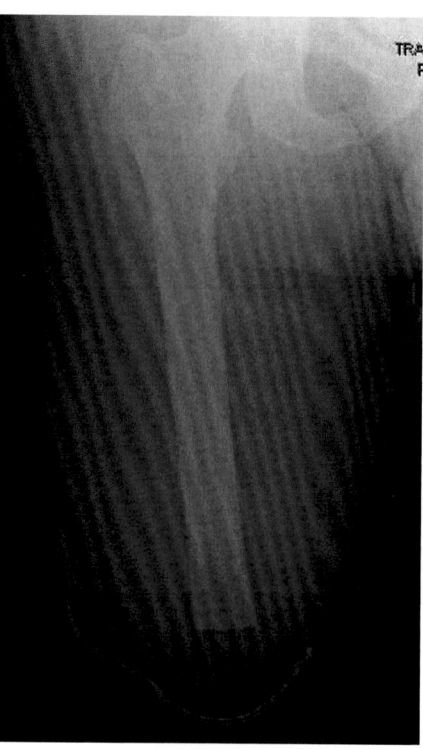

A, B

C

FIGURE 12-4 A 38-year-old woman was involved in a rollover motor vehicle accident (MVA) and presented *in extremis* with her blood pressure only transiently responsive to IV fluid administration. A CT scan demonstrates an unstable comminuted segmental tibia fracture **(A)**. Because of extensive soft tissue damage to the leg and the hemodynamic instability a through-knee amputation **(B)** was performed at the time of crash laparotomy to control intra-abdominal bleeding. An above knee amputation **(C)** was performed later as the definitive procedure.

severely injured extremity with an irreparable vascular injury or in the setting of prolonged warm ischemia (longer than 6 hours for a lower extremity and 8 hours for an upper extremity).[88] In some instances, when the patient's life would be threatened by attempts to save the limb, the dictum of "life over limb" supersedes the feasibility issue of limb salvage, and amputation should be the only option despite the presence of a potentially salvageable limb. Immediate amputation should also be considered in patients critically injured with significant hemodynamic instability, coagulopathy, or an injury constellation that would preclude the multiple surgeries required for limb salvage.[88,89] In these cases, an immediate open amputation (as opposed to a "guillotine" amputation which is no longer performed) is performed to minimize the soft tissue wound area. In the leg, the initial amputation is performed 2 to 3 cm distal to the distal-most extent of the gastrocnemius muscle, if possible, leaving the bone long and not transecting muscle bellies. This amputation is then revised to a formal closure once the patient's condition is improved.

Plantar Sensation

The origin of the concept that initial plantar sensation is critical to the salvage of an extremity is difficult to trace. Although the LEAP Study Group's[147] decision-making analysis supported the inclusion and perceived importance of plantar sensibility, the fact that this was an established treatment axiom at the time of that study may have driven a self-fulfilling prophesy phenomenon. Because surgeons believed that absent plantar sensation was a reason to amputate a limb, they acted accordingly. Indeed, the literature before 1980 warns of neuropathic ulcers and chronic complications associated with absent plantar sensation. Johansen et al.,[75] Howe et al.,[68] and Russell et al.[130] however, describe a *confirmed* avulsion or complete transection of the tibial nerve as the definition of absent plantar sensation in their limb salvage algorithms. Lange et al.[88] considered complete tibial nerve disruption in adults to be an absolute indication for amputation.

In most clinical scenarios, however, the assessment of the limb is performed in the emergency department. Once in the operating room, additional dissection of the deep posterior compartment to assess the tibial nerve is usually considered unwise, as surgical exploration of the nerve within the zone of injury is contraindicated because doing so can cause additional soft tissue injury. Therefore, in many centers, the absence of initial plantar sensation has been considered the same as a physiologic disruption of the nerve. Ischemia, compression, contusion, and stretch can temporarily affect the function of the tibial nerve. Once these factors resolve, nerve function typically returns. Furthermore, in the face of no sensory return, orthopedic surgeons have successfully demonstrated the ability to care for the insensate foot in other conditions (diabetes or incomplete spine lesions) through education and shoe modifications. Furthermore, the orthopedic oncology literature has documented cases of limb salvage in the face of tumor with acceptable results after sciatic, peroneal, or tibial nerve resection.[9,16]

In an effort to better understand the true importance of plantar sensation in the mangled extremity, Bosse et al.[14] used the variations in physician practice patterns to explore the outcomes of patients admitted to the LEAP study with absent plantar sensation. They examined the outcomes of a subset of 55 subjects without plantar foot sensation at the time of initial presentation. The patients were divided into two groups depending on their hospital treatment (i.e., insensate amputation group [n = 26] and insensate salvage group, the study group of primary interest [n = 29]). In addition, a control group was constructed from the parent cohort so that a comparison could also be made to a group of patients in whom plantar sensation was present and whose limbs were reconstructed. The sensate control group consisted of 29 subjects who were matched to the 29 insensate salvage subjects on four limb injury severity characteristics (i.e., severity of muscle, venous, and bony injury as well as the presence of an associated foot injury). Patient and injury characteristics and functional and health-related quality of life outcomes at 12 and 24 months after injury were compared between subjects in the insensate salvage and the other study groups.

The insensate salvage patients did not report or exhibit significantly worse outcomes at 12 or 24 months after injury compared with subjects in the insensate amputation or the sensate control cohort. Among those with a salvaged limb (insensate salvage and sensate control groups), equal proportions (55%) had normal foot sensation at 2 years after injury regardless of whether plantar sensation was reported as intact (sensate control group) or absent (insensate salvage group) on admission. Pain, weight-bearing status, and the percentage of patients who had returned to work were similar for subjects in the insensate salvage group compared with subjects in the insensate amputation and the sensate control groups. Furthermore, there were no significant differences noted in the overall, physical, or psychosocial Sickness Impact Profile (SIP) scores between subjects without plantar sensation whose limbs were salvaged (insensate salvage group) and subjects who had undergone amputation (insensate amputation group) or subjects with intact sensation whose limbs were salvaged (sensate control group). More than one-half of the patients initially presenting with an insensate foot and treated with limb reconstruction had regained normal sensation at 2 years. At 2 years, only two patients in the insensate salvage group and one patient in the sensate control group had absent plantar sensation. In this cohort, initial plantar sensation was not found to be prognostic of long-term plantar sensory status or functional outcomes. Based on these data, the authors concluded that plantar sensation should not be included as a factor in the decision making for limb salvage in lower extremity trauma.

Decision-Making Protocols and Limb Salvage Scores

Because the decision to amputate or salvage a severely injured lower extremity is difficult, several researchers have attempted to enumerate certain indications for amputation or quantify the severity of the trauma to establish numerical guidelines for the decision to amputate or salvage a limb. These lower extremity injury scoring systems (ISSs) all vary in terms of the factors considered relevant to limb salvage and the relative weights assigned to each element. These scoring systems were validated by the developers and demonstrated a high sensitivity and specificity in predicting limb salvage at the time of their design. It is impossible to achieve 100% accuracy using a scoring system in a clinical setting and any metric evaluation must be weighed carefully in conjunction with knowledge of the surgical skills of the clinician, the technical facilities available, and subjective factors that can impact the overall success of the treatment.

In 1985, Lange et al.[88] proposed a decision-making protocol for primary amputation in type IIIC open tibial fractures. They suggested that the occurrence of one of two absolute indications (complete tibial nerve disruption in an adult or a crush injury with a warm ischemia time of longer than 6 hours) or at least two of three relative indications (serious associated polytrauma, severe ipsilateral foot trauma, or a projected long course to full recovery) warranted amputation. This protocol, however, presented several limitations in that only a minority of cases could be resolved based on the absolute indications and that the relative indications were quite subjective. Furthermore, this protocol did not address individual patient variables such as age, medical comorbidities, or occupational and other psychosocial factors that can have a significant effect on the overall outcome, and no subsequent clinical studies were performed to validate this protocol.

Beginning in 1985, research teams reported attempts to quantify extremity injury severity with scoring systems. Over a 10-year period, six scoring systems were published that valued different injury components as critical to the treatment decision (Table 12-3).[57,62,68,75,106,130,145] These components were assigned arbitrary weights and the summation scores were used to establish "cutoffs" for limb salvage or amputation.

Gregory et al.[57] published the first grading system for the mangled extremity, the Mangled Extremity Syndrome Index (MESI) . In this study, the authors included 17 patients over a 3-year period who met their criteria of a mangled extremity syndrome (defined by three of four organ/tissue systems—integument, nerve, vessel, bone—injured in the same extremity). These patients' charts were retrospectively reviewed and their injuries classified according to a point system based on the degree of integumentary, nervous, vascular, and osseous

injury. Additional scoring schemes were also included to address patient age, the time lag to treatment, pre-existing medical comorbidities, and the presence or absence of shock. In their series, they found that 100% of patients with an MESI score of greater than 20 underwent either primary or secondary amputation. From their data, they suggested that if applied prospectively, the MESI could have been used to identify those patients in their series who ultimately underwent amputation and guide their treatment at the time of initial evaluation. They suggested that their scoring system could help better identify the salvageable versus the unsalvageable extremity. Unfortunately, the MESI had numerous faults, and 5 of the 17 cases studied were injuries to the upper extremity. The system can also be both cumbersome and somewhat subjective in nature, making it prone to interobserver variability and difficult to apply during the initial evaluation of the patient. These factors prevented its widespread acceptance and application in orthopedic practice.

The Predictive Salvage Index (PSI)[68] was introduced in 1987 as another scoring system to help predict amputation versus salvage in patients with combined musculoskeletal and vascular injuries of the lower extremity. The PSI ascribes points based on information from four key categories (level of arterial injury, degree of bone injury, degree of muscle injury, and interval from injury to treatment). In the initial retrospective analysis, all 12 patients in the salvage group had PSI scores of less than 8, while 7 of 9 in the amputation group had scores of 8 or higher. The authors concluded that the PSI determined the likelihood of amputation with a sensitivity of 78% and a specificity of 100%. Although less complex than the MESI, it still had similar faults in that many of the scores attributed were subjective in nature and thus prone to interobserver variability. And as with the MESI, the information necessary to complete the scoring can be difficult to ascertain readily during the patient's initial evaluation.

In 1990, Johansen et al.[75] and Helfet et al.[62] proposed and reported on the utility of the Mangled Extremity Severity Score (MESS) (Table 12-4). Like the PSI, the MESS system is also based on four clinical criteria (skeletal/soft tissue injury,

TABLE 12-3 Index Domains

MESI	PSI	MESS	LSI	NISSSA	HFS 98
Injury Severity Score	Ischemia	Ischemia	Ischemia	Ischemia	Ischemia
Bone	Bone	Bone/tissue	Bone	Bone	Bone
Age	Muscle	Age	Muscle	Muscle	Muscle
Integument injury	Timing	Shock	Skin	Skin	Skin
Nerve			Nerve	Nerve	Nerve
Lag time to operation			Vein	Age	Contamination
Pre-existing disease				Shock	Bacteria
Shock					Onset of treatment

MESI, Mangled Extremity Syndrome Index; MESS, Mangled Extremity Severity Score; NISSSA, Nerve injury, Ischemia, Soft tissue injury, Skeletal injury, Shock, and Age of patient Score; HFS 98, Hanover Fracture Scale 98; PSI, Predictive Salvage Index; LSI, Limb Salvage Index.

TABLE 12-4 Mangled Extremity Severity Scoring System (MESS)

Criterion	Score
Skeletal/Soft Tissue Injury	
Low energy	1
Medium energy	2
High energy	3
Very high energy	4
Limb Ischemia	
Pulse reduced or absent but normal perfusion	1[a]
Pulseless, diminished capillary refill	2[a]
Cool, paralyzed, insensate, numb	3[a]
Shock	
SBP always >90 mm Hg	0
SBP transiently <90 mm Hg	1
SBP persistently <90 mm Hg	2
Age (yr)	
<30	0
30–50	1
>50	2

[a]Double value if duration of ischemia exceeds 6 hours.
SBP, systolic blood pressure.

shock, ischemia, and patient age), and it was developed through the retrospective review of 26 severe lower extremity open fractures with vascular compromise. It was then validated in a prospective trial involving 26 patients at two separate trauma centers. In both the prospective and retrospective studies, all salvaged limbs had scores of 6 or lower and an MESS score of 7 or greater had a 100% positive predictive value for amputation.

Shortly after the MESS scoring system had been published, Russell et al.[130] proposed the Limb Salvage Index (LSI). In this study, the authors performed a 5-year retrospective review of 70 limbs in 67 patients. Their proposed index was slightly more complex in that it quantified the likelihood of salvage according to the presence and severity of arterial injury, nerve injury, bone injury, skin injury, muscle injury, and venous injury as well as the presence and duration of warm ischemia. They reported that all 59 limbs with an LSI score of less than 6 were able to undergo successful limb salvage, whereas all 19 patients with an LSI score of 6 or greater had amputations. Criticisms of the LSI are that it is very detailed and requires a thorough operative evaluation to complete the initial scoring. Furthermore, because accurate scoring of the skin category requires a prior knowledge of the treatment and final outcome, the LSI is essentially ineffective during the initial phases of treatment.

In 1994, McNamara et al.[106] modified the MESS by including nerve injury in the scoring system and by separating soft tissue and skeletal injury. Their modification was named the NISSSA (Nerve Injury, Ischemia, Soft tissue Injury, Skeletal Injury, Shock, and Age of patient) scoring system. Subsequently, the authors applied the MESS and the NISSSA to retrospective data of 24 patients previously treated for limb-threatening

injuries. The authors found both the MESS and the NISSSA to be highly accurate in predicting amputation. The NISSSA was also found to be more sensitive (81.8% versus 63.6%) and more specific (92.3 versus 69.2%) than the MESS in their patient population. Despite the improved statistical outcomes when comparing the NISSSA to the MESS, it inherently retains all the faults of the MESS scoring system while increasing its complexity. The NISSSA has also not been validated in prospective clinical trials.

Lastly, a version of the Hanover Fracture Scale (HFS) was first published in 1980 that consisted of 13 weighted variables that included a analysis of the bacterial colonies present in the wound and was weighted toward vascular injuries.[40,134] It was later simplified to only include eight domains by Krettek et al.[85] and renamed the HFS 98. The HFS 98 was found to have higher sensitivity and equivalent specificity when compared to the NISSSA and MESS scales when prospectively applied to 87 open long-bone fractures.[85]

Although the introduction of these scoring systems has helped highlight certain key factors considered relevant to limb salvage, each system, in and of itself, is not without its own limitations. First, although these scoring systems were validated by the developers and demonstrated a high sensitivity and specificity in predicting limb salvage in their respective studies, the development of the lower extremity ISSs has been flawed by retrospective designs and small sample sizes. In each study, with the exception of the small prospective series in which the MESS system was validated, each proposed classification system was applied retrospectively to patients with known outcomes, rather than prospectively to patients with unknown outcomes. Another important flaw in the development of the scoring systems lies in the fact that component selection and weighting in all of the indices were affected by the clinical bias of the index developers. The NISSSA and LSI include the result of the initial plantar neurologic examination. Age, the presence of shock, severity of contamination, and time to treatment are included in some of the other scoring strategies. Whereas each of these factors plays a key role in decision making, strict reliance on certain criteria with disregard to others via strict adherence to a scoring system might lead to premature amputation in an otherwise salvageable situation. As an example, the commonly cited MESS assigns an additional point if the patient is above the age of 29, a point for normal perfusion but with a diminished pulse, and points for transient or persistent hypotension without qualifying cause or response to treatment. The suggested MESS threshold score for amputation is 7. Thus using the MESS, for example, in a 30-year-old patient (1 point) with a high-energy open tibia fracture (3 points), with normal perfusion but a diminished pulse secondary to spasm or compression (1 point), who has persistent hypotension before laparotomy related to a spleen injury (2 points) would undergo amputation at the conclusion of the laparotomy despite the fact that the limb perfusion will likely return to normal and splenectomy and appropriate resuscitation will resolve the patient's hypotension.

Since the time of their initial publication, various other authors have attempted to validate several of the proposed scoring systems. In a later study Lin et al.[91] suggested attempted salvage should be done for MESS scores of ≤9 because of improvements that have been made in clinical techniques and patient care. Support for the higher score cut-off was recently provided by Soni et al.[143] in a 15-year retrospective study of patients with Gustilo type III fractures that also found the MESS score was a positive predictor of functional outcomes.

Roessler et al.[129] and Bonanni et al.[10] both attempted to apply the MESI retrospectively to each of their patient populations. Both authors determined that the MESI inaccurately predicted amputation versus salvage. Furthermore, they found that MESI scores were often only approximate at best because many of the variables required surgical intervention for accurate determination of the scores, which negated its usefulness as a prediction tool in the acute phase of assessment and treatment.

Bonanni et al.[10] also evaluated the MESS, LSI, and PSI limb salvage score strategies. They retrospectively applied each limb salvage scoring system to 58 lower limb salvage attempts over a 10-year period. Failure of the reconstruction effort was defined as an amputation or functional failure at 2 years. A limb was considered to be a functional failure based on the ability to walk 150 feet without assistance, climb 12 stairs, or independently transfer. Based on their data, they were not able to support the use of any of the three scores to determine limb treatment.

In an attempt to further clarify the clinical utility of any of the limb salvage scores, the LEAP study prospectively captured all of the elements of the MESS, LSI, PSI, NISSSA, and the HFS[145] at the time of each patient's initial assessment and critical decision making.[13] The elements were collected in a fashion so as to not provide the evaluator with a "score" or

impact on the decision-making process. The analysis did not validate the clinical utility of any of the lower extremity ISSs. The high specificity of the scores did, however, confirm that low scores could be used to predict limb salvage potential. The converse was not true, though, and the low sensitivity of the indices failed to support the validity of the scores as predictors of amputation (Table 12-5). The authors concluded that lower extremity ISSs at or above the amputation threshold should be used cautiously by surgeons deciding the fate of a mangled lower extremity.

Ideally, a trauma limb salvage index would be 100% sensitive (all amputated limbs will have scores at or above the threshold) and 100% specific (all salvaged limbs will have scores below the threshold). In the decision to amputate, high specificity is important to ensure that only a small number (ideally, none) of salvageable limbs are incorrectly assigned a score above the amputation decision threshold. A high sensitivity is also important to guard against inappropriate delays in amputation when the limb is ultimately not salvageable. Unfortunately, few clinical scoring systems perform ideally and the limb salvage scoring systems have proved to be no exception.

Ultimately it falls to the treating physicians in consultation with the patient and their family to come to a decision regarding when to salvage and when to amputate. We have historically relied on multiple physicians in multiple specialties (vascular, general surgery trauma, orthopedics, and/or plastics) to concur in those circumstances where the injury is life threatening. In those circumstances where the injury is not immediately life threatening, we have found the provisional fixation (external fixator or intramedullary nail) and serial debridements

TABLE 12-5	**Clinical Usefulness of Limb Salvage Scores**		
Score	All Gustilo Type III Fractures (*n* = 357)[a]	Gustilo Type IIIB Fractures (*n* = 214)[a]	Gustilo Type IIIC Fractures (*n* = 59)[a]
MESS			
Sensitivity	0.45 (0.35–0.55)	0.17 (0.1–0.3)	0.78 (0.64–0.89)
Specificity	0.93 (0.9–0.95)	0.94 (0.89–0.97)	0.69 (0.39–0.91)
PSI			
Sensitivity	0.47 (0.37–0.57)	0.35 (0.22–0.51)	0.61 (0.45–0.75)
Specificity	0.84 (0.79–0.88)	0.85 (0.79–0.9)	0.69 (0.39–0.91)
LSI			
Sensitivity	0.51 (0.41–0.61)	0.15 (0.10–0.28)	0.91 (0.79–0.98)
Specificity	0.97 (0.94–0.99)	0.98 (0.95–1)	0.69 (0.39–0.91)
NISSSA			
Sensitivity	0.33 (0.24–0.43)	0.13 (0.05–0.25)	0.59 (0.43–0.73)
Specificity	0.98 (0.96–1)	1 (0.98–1)	0.77 (0.46–0.95)
HFS-97			
Sensitivity	0.37 (0.28–0.47)	0.1 (0.04–0.23)	0.67 (0.52–0.81)
Specificity	0.98 (0.95–1)	1 (0.97–1)	0.77 (0.46–0.95)

[a]95% confidence intervals given in parentheses.
MESS, Mangled Extremity Severity Scoring System; PSI, Predictive Salvage Index; LSI, Limb Salvage Index; NISSSA, Nerve Injury, Ischemia, Soft tissue Injury, Skeletal Injury, Shock, and Age of Patient; HFS-97, Hanover Fracture Scale.

combined with ongoing patient counseling is the best means by which to determine whether or not a prolonged limb salvage attempt can succeed.

Concomitant Foot and Ankle Injuries

When discussing the mangled extremity or massive lower extremity trauma, the prototypical injury is the severe open tibial fracture. However, in reality these injuries often occur in conjunction with severe crushing type injuries to the ankle, hindfoot, and forefoot and this factor should also be carefully considered when opting for salvage versus amputation. Myerson et al.[110] and others[155,157] have shown that despite successful salvage and treatment of crush injuries to the foot, a substantial proportion of these patients will continue to have pain, often neuropathic in nature, and poor functional outcomes.

Turchin et al.[153] also assessed the effect of foot injuries on functional outcomes in the multiply injured patient. They matched 28 multiply injured patients with foot injuries against 28 multiply injured patients without foot injuries and compared their outcomes using the Short Form-36 (SF-36), the Western Ontario and McMaster Universities Arthritis Index (WOMAC), and the modified Boston Children's Hospital Grading System. They found that the outcome of the multiply injured patients with foot injuries was significantly worse than that of the patients without foot injuries when using any of the three outcome measures. Postinjury evaluation also showed that not only were the physical scores affected in the patients with associated foot injuries, but also the pain and social and emotional health perceptions were dramatically reduced compared with a control population of trauma patients without foot injuries. When using the SF-36, the patients in their study were similar to patients with well-recognized chronic debilitating conditions such as congestive heart failure, ischemic heart disease, or chronic obstructive pulmonary disease. In a similar study, Tran and Thordarson,[152] using validated outcome instruments such as the SF-36, the American Academy of Orthopaedic Surgeons (AAOS) lower limb core questionnaire, and the AAOS foot and ankle questionnaire,[76,116] found that the multiply injured patients with associated foot injuries in their study had dramatically lower Physical Function (38.9 versus 80.7), Role Physical (a perception of their physical function, 41.1 versus 87.5), Bodily Pain (50.6 versus 81.8), and Social Function (67.9 versus 96.6) compared with the control group of multiply injured patients without associated foot injuries. By use of the AAOS questionnaire, their study also addressed specific lower extremity musculoskeletal endpoints. All five of these scales also showed significantly lower scores for factors such as pain, treatment expectations, satisfaction with symptoms, and shoe comfort in those patients with associated foot injuries.

Armed with this information and the knowledge of the severity of injury to the ipsilateral foot, one should proceed cautiously when recommending salvage in the face of severe crush injuries to the foot. In this situation, a given tibial injury or "mangled" lower limb with concomitant severe injuries to the foot might preclude achieving reasonable limb function despite the feasibility of salvage, and amputation may indeed be a better long-term option.

The Mangled Foot

Severe mangled foot injuries are rare in civilian patients and these injuries have not been widely studied.[41,80,135] Both civilian and military clinicians have determined that the extent of the soft tissue injury is the major deciding factor for salvage versus amputation of the mangled foot. Keeling et al.[80] suggested that an assessment by at least two surgeons with limb salvage experience is the most consistent way to decide whether a limb has the potential to be saved. Ellington et al.[41] reported on 174 open severe hindfoot or ankle injuries that were part of the prospective LEAP study, of which 116 were salvaged and 58 had a below-knee amputation (BKA). Using the SIP as the major outcome measure at 2 years, patients with foot injuries that required flaps or ankle fusions did significantly worse than the BKA patients.[41] Shawen et al.[135] also noted that foot injuries requiring free flaps and patients whose pain management require large doses of narcotics or nerve blocks had the worst clinical outcomes.

There is insufficient literature to determine what is salvageable in the foot and at what level the amputation should be performed. In our hands, most patients with mangled feet with severe soft tissue injuries rarely undergo free flap coverage. The most common reason for this is the low success rates of microvascular anastomosis in the distal lower extremity. Because of the high rates of infection in the setting of a severe unreconstructable soft tissue envelope of the foot many patients end up with BKAs.

Smoking

Not only is cigarette smoking a marker for potential medical comorbidities such as coronary heart disease and chronic obstructive pulmonary disease in a patient with a potentially limb threatening injury, but also it also can be used early as a prognostic variable to help inform the patient of potential long-term treatment complications and perhaps better guide treatment recommendations. Both basic science and clinical studies have consistently documented links between cigarette smoking and complications of the fracture healing process. Several studies have provided preliminary evidence of a link between smoking and delayed bone healing and nonunion,[1,12,17,25,27,58,61,87,102,113,132] infection,[48,102,148] and osteomyelitis.[48,138] Laboratory studies have also shown that nicotine reduces vascularization and inhibits bone cell metabolism at bone healing sites, and this is associated with delayed healing in animal models.[31,67,78,154] Smoking has also been associated with decreased immune function.[79,92,139]

A concern with many of the current clinical studies has been the presence of many potential confounding variables that may have also affected the outcomes, thus refuting the overall impact of smoking on such negative outcomes as delayed union, nonunion, and infection. Patient age, education, and socioeconomic status have all been shown to have deleterious effects on overall health status, access to treatment, treatment compliance, and other health behaviors, which may have affected the higher complication rates seen in some of the smoking cohorts. In an effort to address these issues, Castillo et al.[19] used data from the

LEAP project to determine if cigarette smoking increased the risk of complications in patients with a limb-threatening open tibial fracture, while adjusting for the previously mentioned confounders. They were able to demonstrate that current smoking and even a previous smoking history independently placed the patient at an increased risk for nonunion and infectious complications. Current smokers and previous smokers were 37% and 32%, respectively, less likely to achieve union than nonsmokers. Current smokers were also more than twice as likely to develop an infection and 3.7 times more likely to develop osteomyelitis than were nonsmokers. Furthermore, previous smokers were also 2.8 times more likely to develop osteomyelitis than were patients without a prior history of tobacco use.

Not only has cigarette smoking been shown to correlate with increased bone healing complications in the patient with a limb-threatening injury, but also smoking can significantly threaten the likelihood of success of the soft tissue portion of the reconstructive effort. Smoking is associated with a significant reduction in peripheral blood flow. Sarin et al.[131] have shown that blood flow to the hand is reduced by as much as 42% after smoking just one cigarette. Cigarette use has also been shown to negatively affect peripheral blood flow in free transverse rectus abdominus flaps.[11] Microsurgeons have reported poor outcomes after digital replantation in smokers. Chang et al.[24] noted that approximately 80% to 90% of cigarette smokers will lose their replanted digits if tobacco use has occurred within 2 months before their surgery. Cigarette use has been shown to lead to increased local flap and full-thickness graft necrosis compared with nonsmoking status.[52] Smoking has also been shown to adversely affect the success and complication rates associated with microvascular free tissue transfer. Reus et al.[125] studied the incidence of free tissue transfer survival and complications in nonsmokers, active smokers, and patients who had discontinued smoking before surgical intervention. In their series, they found that complications occurred more often in active smokers, with these complications often occurring at the interface between the flap and its bed or an overlying skin graft. They also found that smokers required more secondary surgical procedures at the recipient site to accomplish ultimate wound closure. Lovich and Arnold[93] examined the effect of smoking on various muscle transposition procedures. They performed a retrospective review of 300 pedicled muscle flap procedures and determined that active smokers had a significantly higher complication rate than nonsmokers and smokers who had previously quit. Not only is smoking associated with an increased complication rate at the recipient site, but also smokers have been shown to have an increased rate of complications at the donor site.[23]

Clearly, both a history of previous cigarette use and current cigarette smoking places the patient with a limb-threatening injury at increased risk for both osseous and soft tissue complications These factors must be discussed at length and weighed very carefully with the patient before embarking on a prolonged course to salvage a mangled limb.

Patient Characterization

Successful treatment of the mangled extremity and the return of the patient to as close to a preinjury level of performance and social interaction as possible are dependent on the interaction of the patient, the patient's environment, the injury, and the treatment course. Understanding the potential impact of elements outside of the surgeon's control—the patient and the patient's environment—is critical to the development of an effective care plan. Through data obtained by the LEAP Study Group, Mackenzie et al.[98] were able to characterize and help provide the medical community with a better understanding of the type of patients who face the challenge of amputation versus salvage in the face of a limb-threatening injury. In that study, most of the patients were male (77%), white (72%), and between the ages of 20 and 45 years (71%). These patients were often less educated, as only 70% were high school graduates versus a national rate of 86%. Significantly, more of the patients (25%) lived in households with incomes below the federal poverty line compared with the national rate (16%). This patient cohort also had significantly higher rates of uninsured individuals (38%) and had double the national average of heavy drinkers. Not only do these patients typically present with socioeconomic challenges, but many will have psychological and psychosocial issues, which can make the treatment plan and recovery even more of a challenge. Patients in this study were also found to be slightly more neurotic and extroverted and less open to new experiences compared with the general population. No significant differences were detected between the characteristics of patients entered into the reconstruction or amputation groups. Interestingly, in a thorough review of LEAP study-related publications, Higgins et al.[66] conclude that the single most important characteristic of patient success following treatment for a mangled limb is the patient's "self-efficacy" and ability to handle change.[66]

Although the LEAP study is still considered the most comprehensive study on the topic of mangled extremity trauma, it was conducted more than 15 years ago and was limited to level I trauma centers. de Mestral et al.[35] performed a retrospective analysis of lower limb trauma patients from the National Trauma Database, which is inclusive of a wide range of Level I and II trauma centers in the United States, between 2007 and 2009.[35] A total of 1,354 patient records were examined for information on the frequency and timing of amputation, which occurred at nearly equal rates: early (<24 hours), 9% and late (>24 hours), 11%. Characterization of the early amputees in this cohort found that limb injury factors (i.e., higher energy mechanism, shock in the emergency department, severe head injury) were the strongest determinants of early amputation, whereas age was not.[35]

These findings are important to surgeons planning to care for patients with mangled lower extremities. Compared with the general population, patients with limb-threatening injuries have fewer resources, which can potentially limit their access to rehabilitation services and affect their ability to accommodate to residual disability. These patients are typically employed in more physically demanding jobs, which may impede efforts to return to work, and they have poorer health habits, which may complicate recovery. The personality traits identified in this population could also predispose these patients to a more difficult recovery.

OUTCOMES: AMPUTATION VERSUS LIMB SALVAGE

The clinical challenge faced in every case is deciding, as early as possible, the correct treatment pathway for the patient. The surgeon must weigh the fact that, in most cases, limb reconstruction is possible given the appropriate application of current techniques and counterbalance the expected result of salvage against that which is possible with amputation. Prosthetic bioengineering innovations have significantly improved the function and comfort of lower extremity amputees. Most series reporting on the results of limb salvage or amputation are single center, small, and retrospective. Their conclusions provide a glimpse into the complexity of the clinical decision-making process, but these studies alone should not be used to guide clinical decisions.

Several of these series have supported amputation as the optimal treatment option in the setting of the mangled extremity. Georgiadis et al.[50] retrospectively compared the functional outcomes of 26 patients with successfully reconstructed grade IIIB open tibia fractures with the outcomes of 18 patients managed with early BKA. Five patients in the reconstruction group required a late amputation to treat infection complications. The reconstruction patients had more operations, more complications, and longer hospital stays than did patients treated by early amputation. The functional outcomes of the 16 successful reconstructions were compared with the outcomes of the early amputation patients. They found that the reconstruction patients took more time to achieve full weight bearing and were less willing or able to return to work. Validated outcomes instruments were used to assess the quality of life for a subset of the patients. Significantly more limb salvage patients considered themselves to be severely disabled and impaired for both occupational and recreational activities. The authors concluded that early BKA resulted in a quicker recovery with less long-term disability. Ly et al.[94] attempted to use the previously described limb scoring systems (MESS, LSI, PSI, NISSSA, HFS-98) as predictors of functional outcome status. Using a cohort of 407 limb salvage subjects from the LEAP study who had successful outcomes at 6 months, physical SIP scores were compared to the limb salvage scores at 6 and 24 months. It was determined that the injury scores were not able to predict the functional recovery of patients who undergo successful limb reconstruction.[94]

Francel et al.,[49] in a retrospective review of 72 acute grade IIIB open tibia fractures requiring soft tissue reconstruction from 1983 to 1988, also showed that although limb salvage can be successful, over 50% of the patients in the salvage group had severe limitations in the salvaged limb by objective motion measurements, and 48% of the patients in the salvage group at least intermittently required the use of an assistive device for ambulation after complete healing. They also found that in the salvage group, the long-term employment rate was 28% and no patient returned to work after 2 years of unemployment. In contrast, 68% of trauma-related lower extremity amputees from their institution over the same time period returned to work within 2 years.

Based on these studies, proponents of early amputation claim that patients undergoing amputation often have shorter initial hospital stays, decreased initial hospital costs, and a higher likelihood of resuming gainful employment, thus decreasing the financial burden of this life-altering injury.

Hertel et al.[65] also retrospectively compared below-knee amputees with patients receiving complex reconstructions after a grade IIIB or IIIC open tibial fracture. They also concluded that for the first 4 years after injury, amputation resulted in lower mean annual hospital costs than reconstruction, and amputation patients required 3.5 interventions and 12 months of rehabilitation compared with an average of 8 interventions and 30 months of rehabilitation for the reconstruction patients. However, amputation patients were reported as having a higher dollar cost to society, a figure that was inflated by adding the amounts of permanent disability assigned to an amputee compared to a reconstruction patient. Despite this fact, the authors eventually concluded that functional outcome based on pain, range of motion, quadriceps wasting, and walking ability was better in the reconstruction group than in the amputation group, and therefore, limb reconstruction was advisable (although the data to support this conclusion was soft and no patient-based outcome measures were used).

Dagum et al.[33] also touted reconstruction as the preferred option in the management of the mangled extremity. They retrospectively evaluated 55 grade IIIB and IIIC tibia fractures cared for over a 12-year period. The SF-36 was used as the primary outcomes measure. Although both groups had SF-36 (physical component) outcomes scores as low as or lower than those of many serious medical illnesses, successful salvage patients had significantly better physical subscale scores than did amputees. Both groups had psychological subscores similar to a healthy population. Furthermore, 92% of their patients preferred their salvaged leg to an amputation at any stage of their injury, and none would have preferred a primary amputation. Based on their findings, the authors suggested that a BKA was an inferior option to a successfully reconstructed leg.

Whereas some authors have found that amputation may be less costly in the short term, reconstruction may be more cost effective compared with amputation when lifelong prosthetic costs are taken into account. Smith et al.[141] reviewed hospital and prosthetist records for 15 of 20 patients who survived initial trauma and eventually underwent isolated BKA from 1980 through 1987. Using the medical record and the billing records of the prosthetist, they calculated the number of prostheses fabricated and the overall prosthetic charges since the initial amputation. They found that during the first 3 years, the mean number of prostheses acquired per patient was 3.4 (range 1 to 5), with an average total prosthetic charge of $10,829 (range $2,558 to $15,700). Over the first 5 years, the mean number of prostheses acquired per patient increased to 4.4 (range 2 to 8), with average total prosthetic charges of $13,945 (range $6,203 to $20,070). Williams[158] also compared hospital costs and professional fees of 10 patients with Ilizarov limb reconstruction to the hospital costs, professional fees, and prosthetic costs of 3 patients with acute and 3 patients with delayed lower extremity amputation. The average treatment time was higher in the Ilizarov reconstruction group. The hospital costs and professional fees for the amputation group averaged $30,148 without prosthetic costs, whereas the total cost of the Ilizarov limb reconstruction averaged $59,213. However, with projected lifetime prosthetic costs included, the average long-term cost for the amputee was estimated to be $403,199. Thus, he concluded that Ilizarov limb reconstruction is a more cost-effective treatment option than amputation when long-term prosthetic costs are considered.

The issue of the health care cost of amputation versus limb reconstruction has best been analyzed through information collected via the LEAP study. MacKenzie et al.[100] compared the 2-year direct health care costs and projected lifetime health care costs associated with both treatment pathways. The calculated patient costs included the initial hospitalization, all rehospitalizations for acute care related to the limb injury, any inpatient rehabilitation, outpatient physician visits, outpatient physical and occupational therapy, and the purchase and maintenance of any prosthetic devices. When the costs associated with rehospitalizations and postacute care were added to the cost of the initial hospitalization, the 2-year costs for reconstruction and amputation were similar. However, when prosthesis-related costs were added, there was a substantial difference between the two groups ($81,316 for patients treated with reconstruction and $91,106 for patients treated with amputation). Furthermore, the projected lifetime health care cost for the patients who had undergone amputation was three times higher than that for those treated with reconstruction ($509,275 and $163,282, respectively). Based on these estimates, they concluded that efforts to improve the rate of successful reconstructions have merit and that not only is reconstruction a reasonable goal, but also it may result in lower lifetime costs to the patient.

Whereas most of the conclusions reached in the previous studies offer important insight into the various arguments for amputation or salvage of the mangled extremity, they are also somewhat contradictory, which is likely a result of the retrospective design and small sample sizes in many of the series. The research teams could not adequately assess or control for the injury, treatment, patient, and patient environment variables that could influence the outcome.

The LEAP study prospectively compared the functional outcomes of a large cohort of patients from eight level I trauma centers who underwent reconstruction or amputation following an open tibial shaft fracture. The hypothesis was that after controlling for the severity of the limb injury, the presence and severity of other injuries, and patient characteristics, amputation would prove to have a better functional outcome than reconstruction. Detailed patient, patient environment, injury, and treatment (hospital and outpatient) data were collected for each patient.[97] The SIP was used as the primary outcome measurement. The SIP is a multidimensional measure of self-reported health status (scores range from 0 to 100, scores for the general population average 2 to 3, and scores of greater than 10 represent severe disability). Secondary outcomes included the limb status and the presence or absence of a major complication that required rehospitalization. Five hundred and sixty nine patients were followed over 2 years. No significant difference was detected at 2 years in the SIP scores between the amputation and the reconstruction patients. After adjustment

TABLE 12-6	Predictors of Poor Outcome Found in the LEAP Study After Adjusting for Extent of Injury

- Major complication
- High school education or less
- Nonwhite
- Low income and no private insurance
- Current smoker
- Low self-efficacy and social support
- Involvement with legal system

for the characteristics of the patients and their injuries, patients who underwent amputation had outcomes that were similar to those who underwent limb reconstruction.[12,60,66,95,124]

The analysis of all patient, injury, treatment, and environmental variables in the LEAP study also identified a number of predictors of poorer SIP scores. Negative factors included the rehospitalization of a patient for a major complication, a low education level, nonwhite race, poverty, lack of private health insurance, a poor social support network, a low self-efficacy (the patient's confidence in being able to resume life activities), smoking, and involvement with disability-compensation litigation (Table 12-6). To underscore the combined influence of these multiple factors on outcome, adjusted SIP scores were estimated for two subgroups of patients. A patient with a high school education or less, poor social support, and rehospitalization for a major complication had a mean adjusted SIP score of 15.8. A comparable score for a patient with some college education, strong social support, and an uncomplicated recovery was 8.3. Although patients with substantial economic and social resources and no complications could not function at the level of a healthy adult of similar age and gender (SIP typically less than 4), they were still significantly better off than those without such resources.

The study also found that patients who underwent reconstruction were more likely to be rehospitalized than were those who underwent amputation (47.6% versus 33.9%). Nonunion and wound infection were the most common complications reported.[60] Osteomyelitis develop in 7.7% of the LEAP cases. The limb salvage group displayed a higher risk of complication. At 2 years, nonunion was present in 10.9% of the reconstruction patients and 9.4% had developed osteomyelitis. Additional operations were required for 14.5% of the amputation patients to revise the stump, and the reconstruction patients required twice as many operations.[60] The levels of disability, as measured by the SIP, were high in both groups. More than 40% of the patients had an SIP score of greater than 10, reflecting severe disability. Except for scores on the psychosocial subscale, there was significant improvement in the scores over time in both treatment groups. Return to work success was disappointing. At 24 months, only 53% of the patients who underwent amputation and 49.4% of those who underwent reconstruction had returned to work.

Subsequent to the publication of the original LEAP data, MacKenzie et al.[99] re-examined the outcomes of patients originally enrolled in the study to determine whether their outcomes improved beyond 2 years and whether differences according to the type of treatment emerged. A total of 397 of the 569 patients who had originally undergone amputation or reconstruction of the lower extremity were interviewed by telephone at an average of 84 months after the injury. Functional outcomes were assessed using the physical and psychosocial subscores of the SIP and were compared with the scores obtained at 24 months. On average, physical and psychosocial functioning deteriorated between 24 and 84 months after the injury. At 84 months, half of the patients had a physical SIP subscore of 10 or more points, which is indicative of substantial disability, and only 34.5% had a score typical of the general population of similar age and sex. There were few significant differences in the outcomes of the two groups according to the type of treatment, with two exceptions. Compared with patients treated with reconstruction for a tibial shaft fracture, those with only a severe soft tissue injury of the leg were 3.1 times more likely to have a physical SIP subscore of 5 points and those treated with a through-knee amputation were 11.5 times more likely to have a physical subscore of 5 points. There were no significant differences in the psychosocial outcomes according to the treatment group. At 7-year follow-up, patient characteristics that were significantly associated with poorer outcomes included older age, female sex, nonwhite race, lower education level, living in a poor household, current or previous smoking, low self-efficacy, poor self-reported health status before the injury, and involvement with the legal system in an effort to obtain disability payments. Except for age, predictors of poor outcome were similar at 24 and 84 months after the injury. These results confirmed the previous conclusion of the LEAP study that limb reconstruction results in functional outcomes equivalent to those of amputation. The results also showed that regardless of the treatment option, long-term functional outcomes are likely to be poor.

CLINICAL PRACTICE CONSIDERATIONS

Generalization of the findings of the LEAP study beyond level I trauma centers must be cautioned against. In the level I trauma center, surgeons should advise their patients with mangled lower limbs that the functional results of reconstruction are equivalent to amputation. The reconstruction process requires more operations and more hospitalizations and is associated with a higher complication rate. At 2 years, both patient groups were significantly disabled, and only 48% had returned to work. Both patient groups show evidence of lingering psychosocial disability. Given the "no outcome difference" at 2 years, patients and surgeons can be comfortable recommending or selecting limb-preservation surgery. Efforts to minimize complications and hastened fracture union might improve the outcome of the reconstruction patients (Fig. 12-5).

The results of the LEAP study also suggest that major improvements in outcome might require greater emphasis on nonclinical interventions such as early evaluation by vocational rehabilitation counselors. The study also confirms previous research that found both self-efficacy and social support to be important determinants of outcome.[42,101] Interventions aimed at improving support networks and self-efficacy may benefit patients facing a challenging recovery. Surgeons also need to acknowledge the long-term psychosocial disability associated with the mangled extremity, regardless of the treatment. Post-traumatic stress disorder screening and appropriate referral of patients for therapy should become a proactive part of the postoperative treatment plan.[104,107,108,144]

For patients undergoing limb amputation, the LEAP study also identified a number of clinical issues that can be used by the surgeon in planning amputation level and stump coverage. There were no significant differences between above-knee amputations and BKAs in return to work rates, pain, or SIP scores. Patients with through-knee amputations had SIP scores

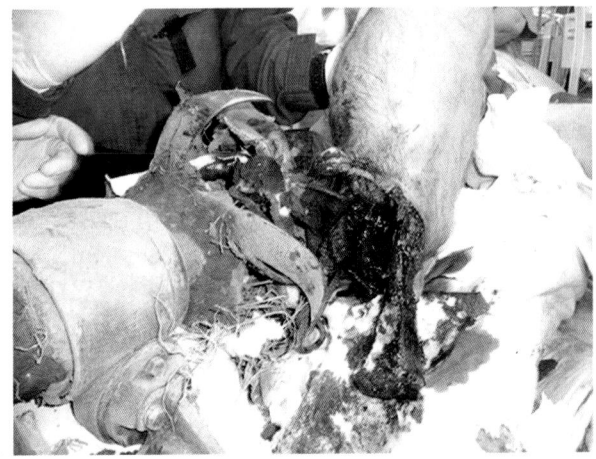 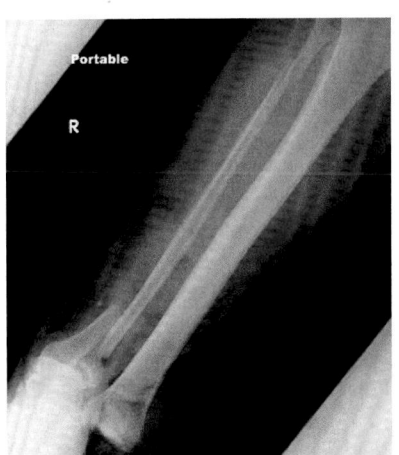

A B

FIGURE 12-5 A 54-year-old man caught his leg in a rotor tiller blade. The blade was removed from the machine and the patient was transferred for definitive care to a regional facility where the limb was extracted from the tiller blade **(A)**. Radiographs demonstrate a relatively simple ankle fracture and do not adequately reflect the extensive soft tissue injury **(B)**.

(continues)

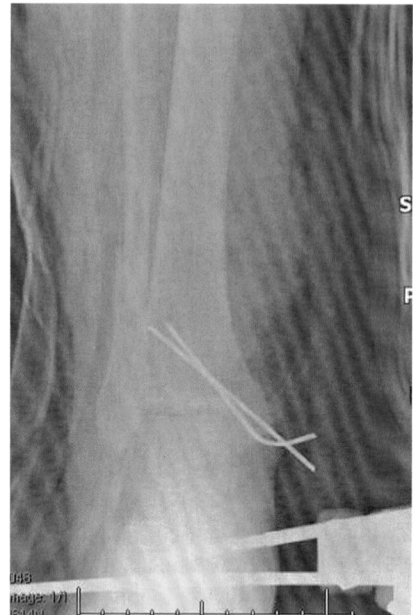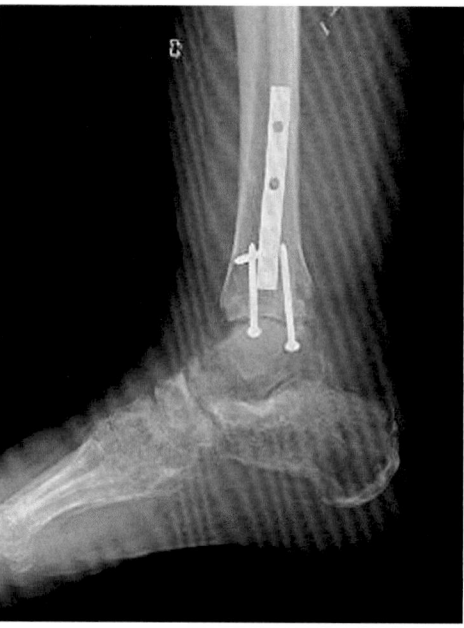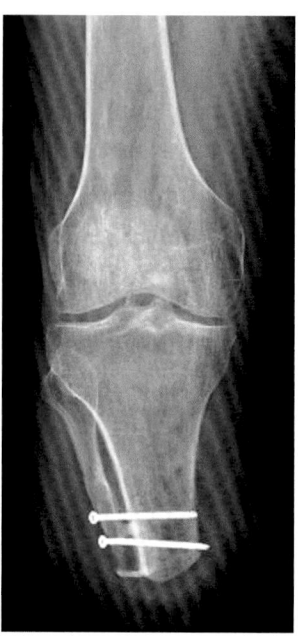

C   D, E

FIGURE 12-5 (continued) Initial spanning external fixation and provisional pin fixation of the medial malleolus were performed (C). After counseling with the family and the patient a plan was made to proceed with limb salvage. Definitive fixation of the fractures was performed 10 days from the initial injury and at the same time a latissimus free flap was placed to provide anterior soft tissue coverage (D). Over the next 2 years he had three deep infections requiring debridement and intravenous antibiotics and at that point he elected to proceed with a below-knee amputation (E).

that were 40% worse than those patients who received either a BKA or an above-knee amputation. Patients with through-knee amputations also demonstrated significantly lower walking speeds. Physicians were less satisfied with the clinical, cosmetic, and functional recovery of through-knee amputations compared with above-knee and below-knee amputation. Thus, as a generality, in the adult trauma population, a through-knee amputation should be avoided whenever possible.

Atypical wound closures, skin grafts, and flaps did not adversely affect the outcome in this study, suggesting that efforts to preserve the knee are worthwhile.[96] Furthermore, patient outcomes were not affected by the technical sophistication of the prosthesis, although patients with higher-technology prostheses were more satisfied. These findings will challenge the physician who currently fits a patient with a sophisticated (and expensive) prosthesis and the results underscore the need for controlled studies that examine the relationships between the type of prosthetic device, the fit of the device, and its functional outcomes.[30,96]

PSYCHOLOGICAL CONSIDERATIONS

Most studies related to management options for the mangled extremity have centered on functional outcomes and the complications that are associated with each procedure. While these are the most obvious areas of concern for clinicians, the psychological well being of the patient must also be explored when considering the best approach. Data on depression, anxiety, and

pain were also collected from patients enrolled in the LEAP study using a psychological self-report symptom scale. Patients were categorized as having normal (58.4%), moderate (15.8%), or severe (25.7%) depression or anxiety at the 3-month follow-up.[21] Patients in the latter category were found to be at highest risk (40%) for suffering from chronic pain at 7 years post discharge after adjusting for pain intensity at 3 months ($p <$ 0.001). The authors suggested that early referral to psychological intervention for patients found to be at moderate and severe levels of anxiety or depression within 3 months of injury could be beneficial in reducing the risk of prolonged suffering from pain. Two years after injury, the LEAP study participants were also surveyed regarding their satisfaction with the treatment of their lower extremity.[115] The level of satisfaction was found to be independent of the details of the injury, treatment option, patient demographics, or psychological profile of the patient. O'Toole et al.[115] listed physical function, pain intensity, the absence of depression, and the ability to return to work at 2 years as the most important factors affecting patient satisfaction.

A systematic meta-analysis of 11 peer-reviewed studies centered around amputation versus limb salvage in the mangled lower limb was performed by Akula et al.[3] with the goal of comparing the two treatments based on the patient perspective of quality of life. The analysis only included studies that administered the widely validated SF-36 and SIP to establish which injury treatment method yields better psychological outcomes. The 11 studies were compiled to include 1,138 cases involving unilateral lower limb trauma, of which there were

CHAPTER 12 Principles of Mangled Extremity Management

769 amputations and 369 limb salvage cases. Findings from this unique analysis supported the previous conclusion that there was no significant difference in physical recovery between the two treatment modalities; however, limb reconstruction patients fared better than the amputees when comparing psychological outcomes. The results of these studies highlight the importance of using a systematic approach to patient treatment that is concerned with both the physical and mental aspects of patient recovery.

MILITARY TRAUMA CARE

It is a harsh reality that military conflicts lead to advancements in the field of trauma care. A specific subgroup of mangled extremity patients has emerged from the most recent conflicts experiencing combat blast injuries. Most soldiers who are fortunate to survive an attack by an IED sustain a mangled extremity, which comprise 54% to 71% of all traumatic combat injuries.[47] The systematic process by which these patients are stabilized in the field and evacuated to level V facilities has led to reconstruction being a viable option in many cases. Limb salvage is approached in the same way as in the civilian populations, although in many cases less tissue is available for reconstruction increasing the need for bone grafts, graft substitutes and nontraditional material options during repair. When reconstruction is not an option, guillotine amputations are avoided with the goal of preserving as much viable tissue as possible.[47] The military hospital system of care for the combat casualty patient population is unmatched in the civilian community.[55] Care for these extremity trauma patients includes prolonged stays on the medical campus and intensive nursing, therapy (mental and physical) interventions, and the provision of the best orthotic and prosthetic devices available. A unique aspect of the military treatment of extremity trauma is that the majority of care is done in group treatment facilities. A comprehensive team of physicians, prosthetists, and physical and occupational therapists work together using a standardized five-phase protocol that has been developed to manage amputees: (1) Acute management and wound healing; (2) introduction to prosthetic training; (3) intensive prosthetic training; (4) advanced functional training; and (5) discharge planning.[142] Different therapies are introduced within each phase to meet the individual needs and progress each soldier to occupational therapy. Pain management and psychological support are also important aspects of the military protocol.

The Military Extremity Trauma Amputation/Limb Salvage (METALS) study was a comprehensive retrospective cohort study of US service members or reservists who sustained a major limb injury while serving in Afghanistan or Iraq between 2003 and 2007 to compare the two treatment options.[38] Doukas et al.[38] reported the findings for 324 lower limb patients that were included in the METALS study. The levels of disability in the military patients were at levels comparable to those found in the LEAP civilian study; however, unlike the LEAP study, a significantly higher level of function was reported for military amputee patients when compared to those that underwent limb salvage procedures ($p < 0.01$). The military amputees were

2.6 times more likely to be at high levels of activity compared to the reconstructed group. These results may be indicative of the intensive rehabilitation program that military amputees are subjected to as quickly as possible following the procedure and their access to state-of-the-art prosthetic devices and care. Military limb salvage patients are not exposed to the same organized rehabilitation protocols and have longer recovery times, which may have contributed to their lower function outcomes at 2-year follow-up.

REHABILITATION OF THE MANGLED EXTREMITY

The civilian sector does not currently have a system in place to require a specific amount of inpatient rehabilitation for patients following severe extremity trauma. There are still questions about the effectiveness of rehabilitation, and there is great variability in the methods and outcome measures used in studies that have examined this issue. A secondary analysis of the LEAP subjects found that physical therapy was beneficial for the patients and that those subjects identified as having an unmet need by a physical therapist had statistically significantly less improvement overtime in five measures of physical impairment.[20] Pezzin et al.[122] examined the effect of inpatient rehabilitation on lower limb traumatic amputees from the University of Maryland Shock Trauma Center between 1984 and 1994. Using a retrospective chart review and administering the SF-36 ($n = 78$, 68% response rate), it was determined that inpatient rehabilitation significantly improved outcomes in terms of return to work rates and functional and vocational prospects. Factors that influenced the discharge to rehabilitation at the level I trauma center included age, gender, and ethnicity; however, these findings did not translate to the larger statewide results for Maryland, where these factors where found to not affect discharge to inpatient rehabilitation. Insurance status was not found to be a factor in determining how much inpatient rehabilitation was provided. These independent studies in conjunction with the recent advances made within the military trauma patient population suggest a need for improved standards for prescribing rehabilitation therapies in civilian medical centers.

UPPER EXTREMITY

Whereas traumatic injuries to the upper extremity do not occur as frequently, they are the leading cause of amputations in the civilian population.[124,142] Prasarn et al.[124] discussed some important differences between the upper and lower extremities in terms of trauma care. The critical ischemic time is longer for the arms at 8 to 10 hours versus 6 hours for the lower extremity. Nerve reconstruction has been more successful in the upper extremity and shortening of the limb has less of an effect on successful postoperative function than it does in the lower extremity.[39,142] Limb salvage for the upper extremity has a different set of considerations than the lower extremity since an upper limb with severe limitations of motor and/or sensory function may still be more useful to the patient than a prosthetic device. The same advancements have not been made in

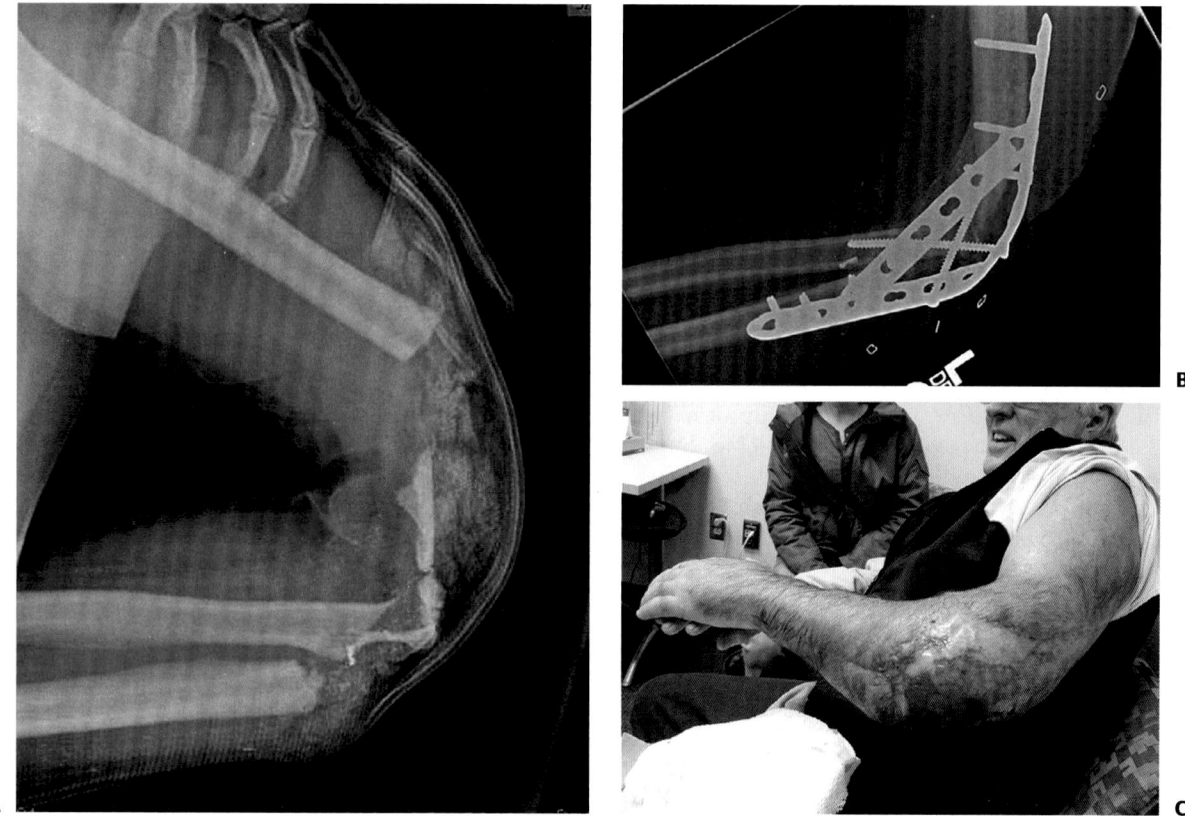

FIGURE 12-6 A 51-year-old man sustained an open-fracture dislocation of the left elbow in a motor vehicle crash **(A).** Sixteen months after the initial injury the lateral radiograph **(B)** demonstrates a fused elbow and the clinical image of the hand and forearm **(C)** demonstrates excellent soft tissue coverage.

upper extremity prosthetic systems as have been achieved in the lower extremity systems, and attachment and wearability of the devices are still a major issue for this patient population.[39] Kumar et al.[86] reported a low infection rate (8%) and a high flap success rate (96%) in a set of 26 mangled upper extremity military patients with wounds necessitating soft tissue coverage by means of flap reconstruction (pedicled or free tissue transfer). Their "Bethesda limb salvage protocol" stressed the importance of vascularized coverage of a clean wound over the specific type of flap used, and they achieved 100% coverage without amputation. Patients underwent an average of six debridements and/or wound washouts before reconstruction was attempted and all had early (≤ 5 days) occupational hand therapy treatment in addition to physical therapy (supervised active and passive postoperative splint protocols), physical medicine, and prosthetics evaluations within 30 days.

Although it was originally devised to assess injuries to the lower limb, Slauterbeck et al.[140] applied the MESS to high-energy injuries of the upper extremity. In their series, they retrospectively reviewed the data of 37 patients with 43 mangled upper extremities and found that all nine upper extremity injuries with an MESS of greater than or equal to 7 were amputated and 34 of 34 with an MESS of less than 7 were successfully salvaged. Based on their findings, they concluded that the MESS system was an accurate predictor of amputation versus salvage

when applied to the upper extremity. Conversely, Togawa et al.[149] also retrospectively applied the MESS to patients with severe injuries of the upper extremity with associated arterial involvement. In their series, they successfully salvaged two of three upper extremity injuries with an MESS score of 7 or higher with good functional outcomes. They concluded that because of the decreased muscle mass in the upper extremity compared with the lower extremity and the increased collateral circulation and tolerance to ischemia seen in the upper extremity, the MESS score was inappropriate for application to the upper limb.

At our institution we will attempt to salvage all mangled upper extremity injuries. Vascular repair takes precedence over nerve and bone repair which can be performed in a staged manner. The microvascular (hand/plastics) service is enlisted early on in the management of these injuries as tendon transfers, nerve grafts, and soft tissue transfers are frequently necessary to recreate a functional hand (Fig. 12-6). In many circumstances, a partially functional hand that can be used for positioning objects and grasping is more functional than prosthesis.

SUMMARY

The decision to amputate or salvage a severely injured lower extremity is a difficult one, which relies not only on the expertise of the orthopedic surgeon but also on the input of subspecialty colleagues (general trauma surgeons, vascular surgeons, and plastic surgeons) as well as the patient. The decision to reconstruct or amputate an extremity cannot depend on limb salvage scores, as all have proved to have little clinical utility. Using current technology and level I trauma center orthopedic clinical experience, combined with multispecialty support, current data appear to suggest that the results of limb reconstruction are equal to those of amputation following severe lower extremity trauma, and this observation should encourage the continued efforts to reconstruct severely injured limbs. Ideally, the patient with a mangled extremity should be directed to an experienced limb injury center, where strategies to minimize complications, address related posttraumatic stress disorder, improve the patient's self-efficacy, and target early vocational retraining may improve the long-term outcomes in patients with these life-altering injuries.

REFERENCES

1. Adams CI, Keating JF, Court-Brown CM. Cigarette smoking and open tibial fractures. *Injury*. 2001;32:61–65.
2. Agel J, Evans AR, Marsh JL, et al. The OTA open fracture classification: a study of reliability and agreement. *J Orthop Trauma*. 2013;27:379–384.
3. Akula M, Gella S, Shaw CJ, et al. A meta-analysis of amputation versus limb salvage in mangled lower limb injuries–the patient perspective. *Injury*. 2011;42:1194–1197.
4. Aldea PA, Shaw WW. The evolution of the surgical management of severe lower extremity trauma. *Clin Plast Surg*. 1986;13:549–569.
5. Antich-Adrover P, Marti-Garin D, Murias-Alvarez J, et al. External fixation and secondary intramedullary nailing of open tibial fractures. A randomized, prospective trial. *J Bone Joint Surg Br*. 1997;79:433–437.
6. Atroshi I, Rosberg HE. Epidemiology of amputations and severe injuries of the hand. *Hand Clin*. 2001;17:343–350.
7. Barmparas G, Inaba K, Teixeira PG, et al. Epidemiology of post-traumatic limb amputation: a National Trauma Databank analysis. *Am Surg*. 2010;76:1214–1222.
8. Bhattacharyya T, Mehta P, Smith M, et al. Routine use of wound vacuum-assisted closure does not allow coverage delay for open tibia fractures. *Plast Reconstr Surg*. 2008;121:1263–1266.
9. Bickels J, Wittig JC, Kollender Y, et al. Sciatic nerve resection: is that truly an indication for amputation? *Clin Orthop*. 2002;399:201–204.
10. Bonanni F, Rhodes M, Lucke JF. The futility of predictive scoring of mangled lower extremities. *J Trauma*. 1993;34:99–104.
11. Booi DI, Debats IB, Boeckx WD, et al. Risk factors and blood flow in the free transverse rectus abdominis (TRAM) flap: smoking and high flap weight impair the free TRAM flap microcirculation. *Ann Plast Surg*. 2007;59:364–371.
12. Bosse MJ, MacKenzie EJ, Kellam JF, et al. An analysis of outcomes of reconstruction or amputation after leg-threatening injuries. *N Engl J Med*. 2002;347:1924–1931.
13. Bosse MJ, MacKenzie EJ; the LEAP Study Group. A prospective evaluation of the clinical utility of the lower-extremity injury severity scores. *J Bone Joint Surg*. 2001;83:3–14.
14. Bosse MJ, McCarthy ML, Jones AL, et al. The insensate foot following severe lower extremity trauma: an indication for amputation? *J Bone Joint Surg Am*. 2005;87A:2601–2608.
15. Bouachour G, Cronier P, Gouello JP, et al. Hyperbaric oxygen therapy in the management of crush injuries: a randomized double-blind placebo-controlled clinical trial. *J Trauma*. 1996;41:333–339.
16. Brooks AD, Gold JS, Graham D, et al. Resection of the sciatic, peroneal, or tibial nerves: assessment of functional status. *Ann Surg Oncol*. 2002;9:41–47.
17. Brown CW, Orme TJ, Richardson HD. The rate of pseudarthrosis (surgical nonunion) in patients who are smokers and patients who are nonsmokers: a comparison study. *Spine*. 1986;11:942–943.
18. Byrd HS, Spicer TE, Cierney G III. Management of open tibial fractures. *Plast Reconstr Surg*. 1985;76:719–730.
19. Castillo RC, Bosse MJ, MacKenzie EJ, et al. Impact of smoking on fracture healing and risk of complications in limb-threatening open tibia fractures. *J Orthop Trauma*. 2005;19:151–157.
20. Castillo RC, MacKenzie EJ, Archer KR, et al. Evidence of beneficial effect of physical therapy after lower-extremity trauma. *Arch Phys Med Rehabil*. 2008;89:1873–1879.
21. Castillo RC, MacKenzie EJ, Wegener ST, et al. Prevalence of chronic pain seven years following limb threatening lower extremity trauma. *Pain*. 2006;124:321–329.
22. Caudle RJ, Stern PJ. Severe open fractures of the tibia. *J Bone Joint Surg Am*. 1987;69A:801–807.
23. Chang DW, Reece GP, Wang B, et al. Effect of smoking on complications in patients undergoing free TRAM flap breast reconstruction. *Plast Reconstr Surg*. 2000;105:2374–2380.
24. Chang LD, Buncke G, Slezak S, et al. Cigarette smoking, plastic surgery, and microsurgery. *J Reconstr Microsurg*. 1996;12:467–474.
25. Chen F, Osterman AL, Mahony K. Smoking and bony union after ulna-shortening osteotomy. *Am J Orthop*. 2001;30:486–489.
26. Christian EP, Bosse MJ, Robb G. Reconstruction of large diaphyseal defects, without free fibular transfer, in Grade-IIIB tibial fractures. *J Bone Joint Surg Am*. 1989;71A:994–1004.
27. Cobb TK, Gabrielsen TA, Campbell DC, et al. Cigarette smoking and nonunion after ankle arthrodesis. *Foot Ankle Int*. 1994;15:64–67.
28. Colton C. The history of fracture treatment. In: Browner BD, Jupiter JB, Levine AM, Trafton PG, eds. *Skeletal Trauma*. Philadelphia, PA: Saunders; 2003:3–28.
29. Crowley DJ, Kanakaris NK, Giannoudis PV. Irrigation of the wounds in open fractures. *J Bone Joint Surg Br*. 2007;89B:580–585.
30. Cyril JK, MacKenzie EJ, Smith DG, et al. Prosthetic device satisfaction among patients with lower extremity amputation due to trauma. Toronto, Ontario, Canada:Orthopaedic Trauma Association 18th Meeting Abstracts. 2002.
31. Daftari TK, Whitesides TE Jr, HellerJG, et al. Nicotine on the revascularization of bone graft. An experimental study in rabbits. *Spine*. 1994;19:904–911.
32. Dagher F, Roukoz S. Compound tibial fractures with bone loss treated by the Ilizarov technique. *J Bone Joint Surg Br*. 1991;73B:316–321.
33. Dagum AB, Best AK, Schemitsch EH, et al. Salvage after severe lower-extremity trauma: are the outcomes worth the means? *Plast Reconstr Surg*. 1999;103:1212–1220.
34. Dedmond BT, Kortesis B, Punger K, et al. The use of negative-pressure wound therapy (NPWT) in the temporary treatment of soft-tissue injuries associated with high-energy open tibial shaft fractures. *J Orthop Trauma*. 2007;21:11–17.
35. de Mestral C, Sharma S, Haas B, et al. A contemporary analysis of the management of the mangled lower extremity. *J Trauma Acute Care Surg*. 2013;74:597–603.
36. Ding W, Wu X, Li J. Temporary intravascular shunts used as a damage control surgery adjunct in complex vascular injury: collective review. *Injury*. 2008;39(9):970–977.
37. Dirschl DR, Dahners LE. The mangled extremity: when should it be amputated? *J Am Acad Orthop Surg*. 1996;4:182–190.
38. Doukas WC, Hayda RA, Frisch HM, et al. The Military Extremity Trauma Amputation/Limb Salvage (METALS) study: outcomes of amputation versus limb salvage following major lower-extremity trauma. *J Bone Joint Surg Am*. 2013;95:138–145.
39. Durham RM, Mistry BM, Mazuski JE, et al. Outcome and utility of scoring systems in the management of the mangled extremity. *Am J Surg*. 1996;172:569–573.
40. Durrant CA, Mackey SP. Orthoplastic classification systems: the good, the bad, and the ungainly. *Ann Plast Surg*. 2011;66:9–12.
41. Ellington JK, Bosse MJ, Castillo RC, et al. The mangled foot and ankle: results from a 2-year prospective study. *J Orthop Trauma*. 2013;27:43–48.
42. Ewart CK, Stewart KJ, Gillilan RE, et al. Self-efficacy mediates strength gains during circuit weight training in men with coronary artery disease. *Med Sci Sports Exerc*. 1986;18:531–540.
43. Feliciano D. Management of the Mangled Extremity. American College of Surgeons Committee on Trauma. In Trauma ACoSCo ed. Online Publications, 2001.
44. Finkemeier CG. Bone-grafting and bone-graft substitutes. *J Bone Joint Surg Am*. 2002;84A:454–464.
45. Finklestein EA, Corso PS, Miller TR, Associates. *Incidence and Economic Burden of Injuries in the United States*. New York, NY: Oxford University Press; 2006.
46. Fischer MD, Gustilo RB, Varecka TF. The timing of flap coverage, bone-grafting, and intramedullary nailing in patients who have a fracture of the tibial shaft with extensive soft-tissue injury. *J Bone Joint Surg Am*. 1991;73A:1316–1322.
47. Fleming ME, Watson JT, Gaines RJ, et al. Evolution of orthopaedic reconstructive care. *J Am Acad Orthop Surg*. 2012;20(Suppl 1):S74–S79.
48. Folk JW, Starr AJ, Early JS. Early wound complications of operative treatment of calcaneus fractures: analysis of 190 fractures. *J Orthop Trauma*. 1999;13:369–372.
49. Francel TJ, Vander Kolk CA, Hoopes JE, et al. Microvascular soft-tissue transplantation for reconstruction of acute open tibial fractures: timing of coverage and long-term functional results. *Plast Reconstr Surg*. 1992;89:478–487.
50. Georgiadis GM, Behrens FF, Joyce MJ, et al. Open tibial fractures with severe soft-tissue loss. Limb salvage compared with below-the-knee amputation. *J Bone Joint Surg Am*. 1993;75A:1431–1441.
51. Godina M. Early microsurgical reconstruction of complex trauma of the extremities. *Plast Reconstr Surg*. 1986;78:285–292.
52. Goldminz D, Bennett RG. Cigarette smoking and flap and full-thickness graft necrosis. *Arch Dermatol*. 1991;127:1012–1015.
53. Gopal S, Majumder S, Batchelor AG, et al. Fix and flap: the radical orthopaedic and plastic treatment of severe open fractures of the tibia. *J Bone Joint Surg Br*. 2000;82B:959–966.
54. Govender S, Csimma C, Genant HK, et al. Recombinant human bone morphogenetic protein-2 for treatment of open tibial fractures. *J Bone Joint Surg*. 2002;84:2123–2134.
55. Granville R, Menetrez J. Rehabilitation of the lower-extremity war-injured at the center for the intrepid. *Foot Ankle Clin*. 2010;15:187–199.
56. Greensmith JE. Hyperbaric oxygen therapy in extremity trauma. *J Am Acad Orthop Surg*. 2004;12:376–384.
57. Gregory RT, Gould RJ, Peclet M, et al. The mangled extremity syndrome (M.E.S.): a severity grading system for multisystem injury of the extremity. *J Trauma*. 1985;25:1147–1150.
58. Hak DJ, Lee SS, Goulet JA. Success of exchange reamed intramedullary nailing for femoral shaft nonunion or delayed union. *J Orthop Trauma*. 2000;14:178–182.
59. Hanna R, Austin, R. Lower-Extremity Injuries in Motorcycle Crashes. In Mathematical Analysis Division NCfSaA, NHTSA. ed. Washington, DC, 2008.
60. Harris AM, Althausen PL, Kellam J, et al. Complications following limb-threatening lower extremity trauma. *J Orthop Trauma*. 2009;23:1–6.
61. Harvey EJ, Agel J, Selznick HS, et al. Deleterious effect of smoking on healing of open tibia-shaft fractures. *Am J Orthop*. 2002;31:518–521.
62. Helfet DL, Howey T, Sanders R, et al. Limb salvage versus amputation. Preliminary results of the Mangled Extremity Severity Score. *Clin Orthop Relat Res*. 1990;(256):80–86.
63. Henley MB, Chapman JR, Agel J, et al. Treatment of type II, IIIA, and IIIB open fractures of the tibial shaft: a prospective comparison of unreamed interlocking intramedullary nails and half-pin external fixators. *J Orthop Trauma*. 1998;12:1–7.
64. Hertel R, Lambert SM, Muller S, et al. On the timing of soft-tissue reconstruction for open fractures of the lower leg. *Arch Orthop Trauma Surg*. 1999;119:7–12.
65. Hertel R, Strebel N, Ganz R. Amputation versus reconstruction in traumatic defects of the leg: outcome and costs. *J Orthop Trauma*. 1996;10:223–229.

66. Higgins TF, Klatt JB, Beals TC. Lower Extremity Assessment Project (LEAP)—the best available evidence on limb-threatening lower extremity trauma. *Orthop Clin North Am.* 2010;41:233–239.
67. Hollinger JO, Schmitt JM, Hwang K, et al. Impact of nicotine on bone healing. *J Biomed Mater Res.* 1999;45:294–301.
68. Howe HR Jr, Poole GV Jr, Hansen KJ, et al. Salvage of lower extremities following combined orthopedic and vascular trauma. A predictive salvage index. *Am Surg.* 1987;53:205–208.
69. Hughes CW. Acute vascular trauma in Korean War casualties; an analysis of 180 cases. *Surg Gynecol Obstet.* 1954;99:91–100.
70. Hughes CW. The primary repair of wounds of major arteries; an analysis of experience in Korea in 1953. *Ann Surg.* 1955;141:297–303.
71. Hughes CW. Arterial repair during the Korean war. *Ann Surg.* 1958;147:555–561.
72. Hunt TK, Pai MP. The effect of varying ambient oxygen tensions on wound metabolism and collagen synthesis. *Surg Gynecol Obstet.* 1972;135:561–567.
73. Iannacone WM, Taffet R, DeLong WG Jr, et al. Early exchange intramedullary nailing of distal femoral fractures with vascular injury initially stabilized with external fixation. *J Trauma.* 1994;37:446–451.
74. Johansen K, Bandyk D, Thiele B, et al. Temporary intraluminal shunts: resolution of a management dilemma in complex vascular injuries. *J Trauma.* 1982;22:395–402.
75. Johansen K, Daines M, Howey T, et al. Objective criteria accurately predict amputation following lower extremity trauma. *J Trauma.* 1990;30:568–572.
76. Johanson NA, Liang MH, Daltroy L, et al. American Academy of Orthopaedic Surgeons lower limb outcomes assessment instruments. Reliability, validity, and sensitivity to change. *J Bone Joint Surg Am.* 2004;86A:902–909.
77. Jones AL, Bucholz RW, Bosse MJ, et al. Recombinant human BMP-2 and allograft compared with autogenous bone graft for reconstruction of diaphyseal tibial fractures with cortical defects. A randomized, controlled trial. *J Bone Joint Surg Am.* 2006;88A:1431–1441.
78. Kallala R, Barrow J, Graham SM, et al. The in vitro and in vivo effects of nicotine on bone, bone cells and fracture repair. *Expert Opin Drug Saf.* 2013;12:209–233.
79. Kalra R, Singh SP, Savage SM, et al. Effects of cigarette smoke on immune response: chronic exposure to cigarette smoke impairs antigen-mediated signaling in T cells and depletes IP3-sensitive Ca(2+) stores. *J Pharmacol Exp Ther.* 2000;293:166–171.
80. Keeling JJ, Hsu JR, Shawen SB, et al. Strategies for managing massive defects of the foot in high-energy combat injuries of the lower extremity. *Foot Ankle Clin.* 2010;15:139–149.
81. Khouri RK, Shaw WW. Reconstruction of the lower extremity with microvascular free flaps: a 10-year experience with 304 consecutive cases. *J Trauma.* 1989;29:1086–1094.
82. Kirk NT. The classic amputations. *Clin Orthop Relat Res.* 1989;(243):3–16.
83. Kobbe P, Tarkin IS, Frink M, et al. [Voluminous bone graft harvesting of the femoral marrow cavity for autologous transplantation: an indication for the "Reamer-Irrigator-Aspirator" (RIA-) technique.]. *Unfallchirurg.* 2008;111:469–472.
84. Kostler W, Strohm PC, Sudkamp NP. Acute compartment syndrome of the limb. *Injury.* 2004;35:1221–1227.
85. Krettek C, Seekamp A, Köntopp H, et al. Hannover Fracture Scale '98–re-evaluation and new perspectives of an established extremity salvage score. *Injury.* 2001;32:317–328.
86. Kumar AR, Grewal NS, Chung TL, et al. Lessons from the modern battlefield: successful upper extremity injury reconstruction in the subacute period. *J Trauma.* 2009;67:752–757.
87. Kyro A, Usenius JP, Aarnio M, et al. Are smokers a risk group for delayed healing of tibial shaft fractures? *Ann Chir Gynaecol.* 1993;82:254–262.
88. Lange RH, Bach AW, Hansen ST Jr, et al. Open tibial fractures with associated vascular injuries: prognosis for limb salvage. *J Trauma.* 1985;25:203–208.
89. Lange RH. Limb reconstruction versus amputation decision making in massive lower extremity trauma. *Clin Orthop Relat Res.* 1989;(243):92–99.
90. Langworthy MJ, Smith JM, Gould M. Treatment of the mangled lower extremity after a terrorist blast injury. *Clin Orthop Relat Res.* 2004;(422):88–96.
91. Lin CH, Wei FC, Levin LS, et al. The functional outcome of lower-extremity fractures with vascular injury. *J Trauma.* 1997;43:480–485.
92. lister-Sistilli CG, Caggiula AR, Knopf S, et al. The effects of nicotine on the immune system. *Psychoneuroendocrinology.* 1998;23:175–187.
93. Lovich SF, Arnold PG. The effect of smoking on muscle transposition. *Plast Reconstr Surg.* 1994;93:825–828.
94. Ly TV, Travison TG, Castillo RC, et al. Ability of lower-extremity injury severity scores to predict functional outcome after limb salvage. *J Bone Joint Surg Am.* 2008;90:1738–1743.
95. MacKenzie EJ, Bosse MJ. Factors influencing outcome following limb-threatening lower limb trauma: lessons learned from the Lower Extremity Assessment Project (LEAP). *J Am Acad Orthop Surg.* 2006;14:S205–S210.
96. MacKenzie EJ, Bosse MJ, Castillo RC, et al. Functional outcomes following trauma-related lower-extremity amputation. *J Bone Joint Surg Am.* 2004;86A:1636–1645.
97. MacKenzie EJ, Bosse MJ, Kellam JF, et al. Characterization of patients with high-energy lower extremity trauma. *J Orthop Trauma.* 2000;14:455–466.
98. MacKenzie EJ, Bosse MJ, Kellam JF; LEAP Study Group. Characterization of the patients undergoing amputation versus limb salvage for severe lower extremity trauma. *J Orthop Trauma.* 2000;14:455–466.
99. MacKenzie EJ, Bosse MJ, Pollak AN, et al. Long-term persistence of disability following severe lower-limb trauma. Results of a 7-year follow-up. *J Bone Joint Surg Am.* 2005;87A:1801–1809.
100. MacKenzie EJ, Jones AS, Bosse MJ, et al. Health-care costs associated with amputation or reconstruction of a limb-threatening injury. *J Bone Joint Surg Am.* 2007;89A:1685–1692.
101. MacKenzie EJ, Morris JA Jr, Jurkovich GJ, et al. Return to work following injury: the role of economic, social, and job-related factors. *Am J Public Health.* 1998;88:1630–1637.
102. Marsh DR, Shah S, Elliott J, et al. The Ilizarov method in nonunion, malunion, and infection of fractures. *J Bone Joint Surg Br.* 1997;79B:273–279.
103. McCabe CJ, Ferguson CM, Ottinger LW. Improved limb salvage in popliteal artery injuries. *J Trauma.* 1983;23:982–985.
104. McCarthy ML, MacKenzie EJ, Edwin D, et al. Psychological distress associated with severe lower-limb injury. *J Bone Joint Surg Am.* 2003;85A:1689–1697.
105. McKee MD, Yoo DJ, Zdero R, et al. Combined single-stage osseous and soft tissue reconstruction of the tibia with the Ilizarov method and tissue transfer. *J Orthop Trauma.* 2008;22:183–189.
106. McNamara MG, Heckman JD, Corley FG. Severe open fractures of the lower extremity: a retrospective evaluation of the Mangled Extremity Severity Score (MESS). *J Orthop Trauma.* 1994;8:81–87.
107. Michaels AJ, Michaels CE, Moon CH, et al. Psychosocial factors limit outcomes after trauma. *J Trauma.* 1998;44:644–648.
108. Michaels AJ, Michaels CE, Moon CH, et al. Posttraumatic stress disorder after injury: impact on general health outcome and early risk assessment. *J Trauma.* 1999;47:460–466.
109. Modrall JG, Weaver FA, Yellin AE. Diagnosis of vascular trauma. *Ann Vasc Surg.* 1995;9:415–421.
110. Myerson MS, McGarvey WC, Henderson MR, et al. Morbidity after crush injuries to the foot. *J Orthop Trauma.* 1994;8:343–349.
111. Nichols JG, Svoboda JA, Parks SN. Use of temporary intraluminal shunts in selected peripheral arterial injuries. *J Trauma.* 1986;26:1094–1096.
112. Noe A. Extremity injury in war: a brief history. *J Am Acad Orthop Surg.* 2006;14:S1–S6.
113. Nolte PA, van der KA, Patka P, et al. Low-intensity pulsed ultrasound in the treatment of nonunions. *J Trauma.* 2001;51:693–702.
114. Olson SA, Willis MD. Initial management of open fractures. In: *Rockwood and Green's Fractures in Adults.* 6th ed. Philadelphia, PA: Lippincott Williams & Wilkins;2006:390–391.
115. O'Toole RV, Castillo RC, Pollak AN, et al. Determinants of patient satisfaction after severe lower-extremity injuries. *J Bone Joint Surg Am.* 2008;90:1206–1211.
116. Outcomes instruments and information: lower extremity instruments. American Association of Orthopaedic Surgeons web site. Retrieved February 24,. 2009, from http://www.aaos.org/research/outcomes/outcomeslower.asp.
117. Pai MP, Hunt TK. Effect of varying oxygen tensions on healing of open wounds. *Surg Gynecol Obstet.* 1972;135:756–758.
118. Paley D, Maar DC. Ilizarov bone transport treatment for tibial defects. *J Orthop Trauma.* 2000;14:76–85.
119. Pare A. *Dix Livres de la Chirurgie avec la Magasin des instruments Necessaires a Icelle.* 7, Chapter 13. Paris: Jean le Royer; 1564.
120. Pasquina PF. Guest Editorial: Optimizing care for combat amputees: Experiences at Walter Reed Army Medical Center. *J Rehabil Res Dev.* 2004;41:vii-xii.
121. Patzkowski JC, Blanck RV, Owens JG, et al. Comparative effect of orthosis design on functional performance. *J Bone Joint Surg Am.* 2012;94:507–515.
122. Pezzin LE, Dillingham TR, MacKenzie EJ. Rehabilitation and the long-term outcomes of persons with trauma-related amputations. *Arch Phys Med Rehabil.* 2000;81:292–300.
123. Pollak AN, McCarthy ML, Burgess AR. Short-term wound complications after application of flaps for coverage of traumatic soft-tissue defects about the tibia. The Lower Extremity Assessment Project (LEAP) Study Group. *J Bone Joint Surg Am.* 2000;82A:1681–1691.
124. Prasarn ML, Helfet DL, Kloen P. Management of the mangled extremity. *Strategies Trauma Limb Reconstr.* 2012;7:57–66.
125. Reus WF III, Colen LB, Straker DJ. Tobacco smoking and complications in elective microsurgery. *Plast Reconstr Surg.* 1992;89:490–494.
126. Rich NM, Baugh JH, Hughes CW. Acute arterial injuries in Vietnam: 1,000 cases. *J Trauma.* 1970;10:359–369.
127. Robbins CB, Vreeman DJ, Sothmann MS, et al. A review of the long-term health outcomes associated with war-related amputation. *Mil Med.* 2009;174:588–592.
128. Robert RS, Weitzman AM, Tracey WJ, et al. Simultaneous treatment of tibial bone and soft-tissue defects with the Ilizarov method. *J Orthop Trauma.* 2006;20:197–205.
129. Roessler MS, Wisner DH, Holcroft JW. The mangled extremity. When to amputate? *Arch Surg.* 1991;126:1243–1248.
130. Russell WL, Sailors DM, Whittle TB, et al. Limb salvage versus traumatic amputation. A decision based on a seven-part predictive index. *Ann Surg.* 1991;213:473–480.
131. Sarin CL, Austin JC, Nickel WO. Effects of smoking on digital blood-flow velocity. *JAMA.* 1974;229:1327–1328.
132. Schmitz MA, Finnegan M, Natarajan R, et al. Effect of smoking on tibial shaft fracture healing. *Clin Orthop Relat Res.* 1999;184–200.
133. Seyfer AE, Lower R. Late results of free-muscle flaps and delayed bone grafting in the secondary treatment of open distal tibial fractures. *Plast Reconstr Surg.* 1989;83:77–84.
134. Shanmuganathan R. The utility of scores in the decision to salvage or amputation in severely injured limbs. *Indian J Orthop.* 2008;42:368–376.
135. Shawen SB, Keeling JJ, Branstetter J, et al. The mangled foot and leg: salvage versus amputation. *Foot Ankle Clin.* 2010;15:63–75.
136. Siebenrock KA, Gerich T, Jakob RP. Sequential intramedullary nailing of open tibial shaft fractures after external fixation. *Arch Orthop Trauma Surg.* 1997;116:32–36.
137. Siebenrock KA, Schillig B, Jakob RP. Treatment of complex tibial shaft fractures. Arguments for early secondary intramedullary nailing. *Clin Orthop Relat Res.* 1993;269–274.
138. Siegel HJ, Patzakis MJ, Holtom PD, et al. Limb salvage for chronic tibial osteomyelitis: an outcomes study. *J Trauma.* 2000;48:484–489.
139. Singh SP, Kalra R, Puttfarcken P, et al. Acute and chronic nicotine exposures modulate the immune system through different pathways. *Toxicol Appl Pharmacol.* 2000;164:65–72.
140. Slauterbeck JR, Britton C, Moneim MS, et al. Mangled extremity severity score: an accurate guide to treatment of the severely injured upper extremity. *J Orthop Trauma.* 1994;8:282–285.
141. Smith DG, Horn P, Malchow D, et al. Prosthetic history, prosthetic charges, and functional outcome of the isolated, traumatic below-knee amputee. *J Trauma.* 1995;38:44–47.
142. Smurr LM, Gulick K, Yancosek K, et al. Managing the upper extremity amputee: a protocol for success. *J Hand Ther.* 2008;21:160–175.
143. Soni A, Tzafetta K, Knight S, et al. Gustilo IIIC fractures in the lower limb: our 15-year experience. *J Bone Joint Surg Br.* 2012;94:698–703.
144. Starr AJ, Smith WR, Frawley WH, et al. Symptoms of posttraumatic stress disorder after orthopaedic trauma. *J Bone Joint Surg Am.* 2004;86A:1115–1121.
145. Suedkamp NP, Barbey N, Veuskens A, et al. The incidence of osteitis in open fractures: an analysis of 948 open fractures (a review of the Hannover experience). *J Orthop Trauma.* 1993;7:473–482.

146. Swartz WM, Mears DC. Management of difficult lower extremity fractures and nonunions. *Clin Plast Surg.* 1986;13:633–644.
147. Swiontkowski MF, MacKenzie EJ, Bosse MJ, et al. Factors influencing the decision to amputate or reconstruct after high-energy lower extremity trauma. *J Trauma.* 2002;52:641–649.
148. Thalgott JS, Cotler HB, Sasso RC, et al. Postoperative infections in spinal implants. Classification and analysis—a multicenter study. *Spine.* 1991;16:981–984.
149. Togawa S, Yamami N, Nakayama H, et al. The validity of the mangled extremity severity score in the assessment of upper limb injuries. *J Bone Joint Surg Br.* 2005;87B:1516–1519.
150. Toledo-Pereyra LH, Toledo MM. A critical study of Lister's work on antiseptic surgery. *Am J Surg.* 1976;131:736–744.
151. Tornetta P III, Bergman M, Watnik N, et al. Treatment of grade-IIIb open tibial fractures. A prospective randomised comparison of external fixation and nonreamed locked nailing. *J Bone Joint Surg Br.* 1994;76B:13–19.
152. Tran T, Thordarson D. Functional outcome of multiply injured patients with associated foot injury. *Foot Ankle Int.* 2002;23:340–343.
153. Turchin DC, Schemitsch EH, McKee MD, et al. Do foot injuries significantly affect the functional outcome of multiply injured patients? *J Orthop Trauma.* 1999;13:1–4.
154. Ueng SW, Lee SS, Lin SS, et al. Hyperbaric oxygen therapy mitigates the adverse effect of cigarette smoking on the bone healing of tibial lengthening: an experimental study on rabbits. *J Trauma.* 1999;47:752–759.
155. Vora A, Myerson MS. Crush injuries of the foot in the industrial setting. *Foot Ankle Clin.* 2002;7:367–383.
156. Webb LX, Bosse MJ, Castillo RC, et al. Analysis of surgeon-controlled variables in the treatment of limb-threatening type-III open tibial diaphyseal fractures. *J Bone Joint Surg Am.* 2007;89A:923–928.
157. Westphal T, Piatek S, Schubert S, et al. [Quality of life after foot injuries.]. *Zentralbl Chir.* 2002;127:238–242.
158. Williams MO. Long-term cost comparison of major limb salvage using the Ilizarov method versus amputation. *Clin Orthop Relat Res.* 1994;156–158.
159. Worlock P, Slack R, Harvey L, et al. The prevention of infection in open fractures: an experimental study of the effect of fracture stability. *Injury.* 1994;25:31–38.
160. Yaremchuk MJ, Brumback RJ, Manson PN, et al. Acute and definitive management of traumatic osteocutaneous defects of the lower extremity. *Plast Reconstr Surg.* 1987;80:1–14.

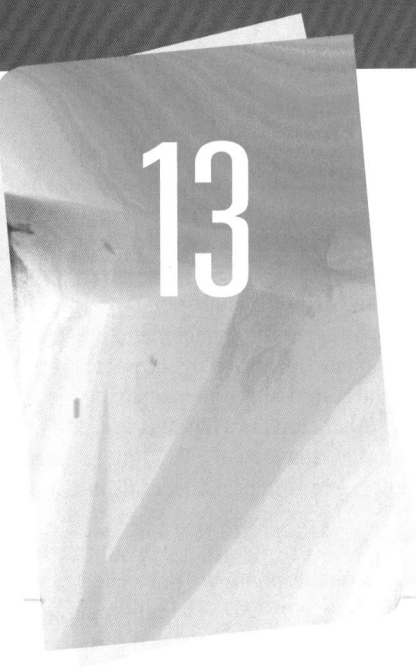

13

POST-TRAUMATIC STRESS DISORDER

Thomas Moore, Jr., Carol North, and Adam Starr

INTRODUCTION

Post-traumatic stress disorder (PTSD) has evolved as a diagnosis both in name and in its description of signs and symptoms. Its first formal diagnostic criteria came in the third edition of the Diagnostic and Statistical Manual of Mental Disorders (DSM-III; American Psychiatric Association, 1980), which detailed characteristic psychiatric symptoms following exposure to a traumatic event. The evolution of this diagnosis can be traced back to physicians describing acute combat reactions ranging from sleep disturbances to loss of appetite to palpitations. In 1678, Norwegian physicians called this constellation of symptoms *nostalgia*. PTSD has also been called neurasthenia, combat exhaustion, gross stress reaction, irritable heart syndrome, shell shock, and stress response syndrome, and this condition has been suspected in many historical and literary figures. This psychiatric disorder was well documented in World War II and Vietnam combat forces, but more recently PTSD has also been recognized in association with noncombat-related traumatic events, including motor vehicle collisions and other orthopedic traumas.

The DSM-IV[1] criteria for the diagnosis of PTSD describe symptoms following an experienced or directly witnessed event that involves actual or threatened death or serious injury or a threat to the physical integrity of oneself or others. The individual's response to this traumatic event is fear, helplessness, or horror. In addition, specific manifestations of the disorder from three symptom groups are required for the diagnosis of PTSD. The first symptom group is intrusive re-experience, including recurrent dreams, a sense of reliving the traumatic experience (such as flashbacks), and psychological distress in response to reminders of the traumatic event. The second symptom group is avoidance and numbing, involving efforts to avoid activities, places, memories, or thoughts associated with the traumatic event. The third symptom group is hyperarousal, including sleep difficulties, irritability, poor concentration, and exaggerated startle response. After exposure to a qualifying traumatic event, PTSD may be diagnosed in individuals who develop one or more intrusion symptoms, three or more avoidance/numbing symptoms, and two or more hyperarousal symptoms in association with the event, with the symptoms continuing for more than a month and resulting in impairment of social or occupational life or clinically significant distress.

Although the formal inclusion of the diagnosis of PTSD in official diagnostic criteria is relatively recent, possible examples of PTSD can be found throughout history. In the Old Testament, the book of Job tells of a man in mental agony after being tested by Satan, and many believe this story describes the characteristic signs and symptoms of PTSD.[17] Also, in Jonathan Shay's book *Achilles in Vietnam, Combat Trauma and the Undoing of Character,* the similarity between "the wrath of Achilles" in the *Iliad* and the experience of many Vietnam veterans with PTSD is described. Achilles' grief after Hector kills his friend Patroclus and his reaction of finding, killing, and defiling Hector's body are also postulated examples of post-traumatic emotional responses including PTSD.[39]

The diagnosis of PTSD was established with the combat experiences of soldiers and war veterans, but there are also examples of noncombat-related PTSD in history as well. The author Charles Dickens had what many people think is PTSD after a train he was on derailed, killing 10 people and injuring many more. He tended to the dead and injured, later describing the scene as "unimaginable"; he recollected his "presence of mind...and steady hand" during the incident. Afterward, when writing about the incident, he explains "I am not quite right within, but believe it to be an effect of the railway shaking... I am getting right, though still low in pulse and very nervous." Dickens developed a phobia of railway traveling, and wrote after the incident, "I am curiously weak—weak as if I were recovering from a long illness." This affected his occupation and productivity, which is known to occur in patients with PTSD.[43]

The stereotypical image of a person with PTSD is a war veteran struggling with nightmares and flashbacks after returning home, as portrayed by countless Hollywood motion pictures. Approximately 15% of Vietnam War veterans were found to meet diagnostic criteria for combat-related PTSD.[19] A more recent study estimates PTSD rates in soldiers returning from the war in Iraq as between 12% and 20%.[18] The burden of PTSD on military veterans is immense.

Traumatic incidents experienced by orthopedic trauma patients represent life-changing events not only in time lost due to hospitalization, surgery, or rehabilitation, but also in the loss of ability to function and work. Orthopedic trauma patients commonly have injuries in multiple organ systems, including the brain, abdomen, and genitourinary tract, often leading to chronic pain, sexual dysfunction, disability, and psychological distress. There is a wide range of emotional reactions to traumatic events and pain, and people vary in their ability to cope with these events. Those who struggle to cope may have unrecognized symptoms of PTSD.

PTSD is a diagnosis in evolution partly because it is a relatively new disorder and also because of the complexity of the components of the diagnosis. The definition of a traumatic event, how it is experienced, and related symptoms have all changed throughout the different editions and text revisions of the DSM since the first inclusion of the diagnosis. At the same time, orthopedic trauma care is evolving as well. Psychological distress, including PTSD, is being increasingly recognized in these patients, and efforts to improve the diagnosis, treatment, and even prevention of psychopathology in these patients are ongoing.

MAGNITUDE OF THE PROBLEM

Orthopedic surgeons are not specifically trained to identify PTSD in their patients and are therefore unlikely to treat it. The focus of attention of orthopedic surgeons is on the physical injury and tissue damage, and recognizing psychiatric illness such as PTSD is often difficult. The focus on the visual (or palpable) is apparent even in the early descriptions of traumatized populations. During a historical period of rapid increases in mass transit and railroad injuries, there was a rise in cases of "railway spine disorder." Later called Erichson disease, this syndrome was considered a neurologic injury, and it could persist long after other physical injuries had healed. Its manifestations varied, but had many similarities to those of current descriptions of PTSD.[14] A disorder known as "shell shock" in military personnel was initially attributed to neurologic injury sustained during proximity to an explosive detonation. Myers[28] wrote about shell shock in 1940, suggesting that it stemmed from a psychological insult rather than from physical or neurologic injury.

Biologic explanations for this psychological condition have been proposed. Understanding the chemical processes and brain functions involved in the development of PTSD can help to elucidate treatment options and possibly even help prevent the disorder. Yehuda et al.[47] suggested that PTSD represents an aberrant physiologic response to stress or trauma that is rooted in "disruptions in the normal cascade of the fear response and its resolution." These researchers found lower cortisol levels and a higher heart rate both in the emergency room and 1 week later among patients who eventually developed PTSD.[47] They proposed that aberrations in the hypothalamic–pituitary–adrenal (HPA) axis may play a pivotal role in the development of PTSD. Highly stressful events precipitate the release of cortisol and epinephrine, which act to heighten arousal and prepare for action in a "fight-or-flight response." Alterations in HPA axis functioning are thought to be central in the pathology of PTSD, but research to date has not demonstrated a consistent model of disturbance in this system.

From an anatomic standpoint, the parts of the brain involved in the fear conditioning response are postulated to be involved in the pathophysiology of PTSD. The amygdala and other paralimbic structures, including the prefrontal cortex and anterior cingulate cortex, have been shown to be involved in the emotional response and are also dysregulated in PTSD. Positron emission tomography (PET) scans, functional MRI, and single photon emission CT scans have been used to identify active or hypoactive areas of the brain in patients with PTSD, confirming that the amygdala is involved in emotional memory in the development of PTSD. Reduced MRI hippocampal volume has been demonstrated in patients with pretraumatic vulnerability to PTSD, though this finding is nonspecific and can be found in many diverse conditions.[16]

Proinflammatory processes have also been suggested as having a role in PTSD development. A study comparing inflammatory markers in the serum of patients with PTSD and healthy individuals showed that IL-1β and TNF-α, both proinflammatory markers, were elevated in PTSD patients. In addition, levels of IL-4, an anti-inflammatory cytokine, were found to be lower in PTSD patients compared to healthy individuals.[45]

Genetic predispositions have also been postulated in PTSD. For example, a family history study of 6,744 male twins from the Vietnam era found that the risk of exposure to traumatic events was associated with family history of mood disorder, pre-existing mood disorder, or a history of substance abuse. The study also showed that risk for PTSD after exposure to a traumatic event did not follow a family history of PTSD, but PTSD was instead related to a lack of education and a history of conduct disorder, generalized anxiety disorder, or major depression.[20] Thus there is a complex interplay between other psychiatric disorders and PTSD, and the specific neurobiologic pathways and genetic contributors that lead specifically to PTSD have not been entirely elucidated. Genetic predisposition to PTSD has also been suggested in altered gene expression patterns in the HPA axis. For example, lower levels of the glucocorticoid signaling proteins, FKBP5 and STAT5B, and certain major histocompatibility complex type II proteins have been found in patients with PTSD compared to healthy controls suggesting heightened genetically expressed sensitivity of glucocorticoid receptors in PTSD.[48]

PTSD symptoms and psychological distress have been found to be quite prevalent among orthopedic trauma patients, as illustrated in a brief review of the literature summarized in Table 13-1. Estimates of PTSD prevalence in trauma patients

TABLE 13-1 Psychiatric Problems in Orthopedic/Trauma Patients

Study	Patient Population	Assessment Tool	Prevalence	Psychological Effect on Outcome
Adult Samples				
Zatzick et al. (2002)	73 trauma patients	PTSD checklist	30% had elevated PTSD symptoms at 1 yr	Screening positive for PTSD was the strongest predictor of adverse SF-36 outcome measure
Michaels et al. (1999)	100 trauma patients	Civilian Mississippi Scale for PTSD, BSI	42% had elevated PTSD symptoms at 6 mos	Screening positive for PTSD was independently and inversely related to general health outcome as measured by SF-36
Feinstein and Dolan (1991)	48 patients with femur, tibia, or fibula fracture	Impact of Event Scale, PTSD Checklist	14% screened positive for PTSD at 6 mos	Not studied
Starr et al. (2004)	580 orthopedic trauma patients	Revised Civilian Mississippi Scale for PTSD	51% (295/580) screened positive for PTSD at 1 y	Not studied
METALS Doukas et al. (2013)	324 military service members with severe lower-extremity trauma	PTSD Checklist—military version	18% had PTSD symptoms and 38% had depressive symptoms	Not studied
NSCOT Zatzick et al. (2008)	2,707 trauma surgical inpatients across the United States	PTSD Checklist	21% had screened positive for PTSD and 7% screened positive for depression at 12 mos	Odds ratio for not returning to work was 3.2 in patients with positive PTSD screen and 5.6 in those with positive depression screen
Crichlow et al. (2006)	161 orthopedic trauma patients	Beck Depression Inventory	45% screened positive for depression at 3–12 mos	Positive depression screen was related to poorer functional outcomes
LEAP study McCarthy et al. (2003)	385 severe lower-extremity trauma patients	BSI	20% had severe phobic anxiety and 42% had a positive screen for a likely psychological disorder at 24 mos	Not studied
Daubs et al. (2010)	400 patients presenting to tertiary care spine center	Distress and Risk Assessment Method	64% had psychological distress	Not studied
Pediatric Samples				
Wallace et al. (2012)	76 pediatric trauma patients or patients with isolated upper extremity fractures	Child PTSD Symptom Scale	33% had high levels of PTSD symptoms	Children who screened positive for PTSD had significantly more functional impairment than those without PTSD
Sanders et al. (2005)	400 pediatric orthopedic patients	Child PTSD Symptom Scale	33% had high levels of PTSD symptoms	Not studied
Onen et al. (2005)	49 pediatric patients with posterior urethral rupture due to pelvic trauma	Diagnostic Psychiatric Interview	43% with psychiatric disorder at 12 yrs post injury on average. PTSD in 12% and major depression in 4%	Not directly assessed
Subasi et al. (2004)	55 pediatric patients treated nonoperatively for unstable pelvic fractures	Diagnostic Psychiatric Interview	56% with psychiatric disorder at 7.4 yrs post injury on average. PTSD in 11% and major depression in 7% of patients	Not directly assessed

PTSD, post-traumatic stress disorder; METALS, Military Extremity Trauma Amputation/Limb Salvage; NSCOT, national study of the costs and outcomes of trauma; BSI, Brief Symptom Inventory; SF-36, Short Form Health survey.

has been found to range from 15% to 42% at 6 months post trauma[15,26] and from 21% to 51% at 1-year post trauma.[41,49,51] These studies all used self-reported symptom measures which are known to overestimate PTSD prevalence; studies are needed with full diagnostic assessment methods to provide more definitive prevalence estimates.

In a study of major lower limb trauma among combat personnel returning from Afghanistan and Iraq, 18% screened positive for PTSD and 38% screened positive for depression.[12] Patients who received amputations were 57% less likely to screen positive for PTSD and were almost three times more likely to be engaged in vigorous sports or recreational activity than patients who underwent limb salvage. The emphasis on inpatient rehabilitation in the military and a structured and readily available prosthetics program may help explain why the amputees fared better than those who underwent limb salvage.

Pediatric trauma patients represent a separate category of trauma patients who have been studied separately from adult trauma patients because their PTSD prevalence and risk factors may differ from those in adults. About one-third of pediatric trauma patients screened positive for PTSD in two studies using symptom scales.[35,46] Pediatric trauma patients did not differ in post-traumatic symptom levels from children with isolated nonoperative upper extremity fractures.[46] Hospital admission for injuries has been found to represent an independent risk factor for post-traumatic symptoms in pediatric patients.[35]

Mental health consequences of trauma can come in different forms, and several studies have documented evidence of high rates of depressive and other psychiatric disorders after trauma as well as PTSD. In one study, 45% of orthopedic trauma patients screened positive for depression on a symptom scale[10] and another study of lower extremity orthopedic trauma using a symptom scale estimated that 42% of patients had a psychological disorder 24 months post injury.[24] Two studies of pediatric patients with pelvic fractures estimated that 43% and 56%, respectively, had a psychiatric disorder based on diagnostic psychiatric interviews.[33,42] These studies have demonstrated that PTSD often coexists with major depression, substance abuse problems, sleep disturbances, and other psychiatric conditions in trauma patients. Multiple psychiatric disorders compound the overall morbidity, with more severe psychopathology and worse psychiatric and medical outcomes than in patients with only one psychiatric disorder.

The studies to date of orthopedic trauma patients with PTSD have all investigated PTSD in early post-trauma time frames. Delayed-onset PTSD in orthopedic patients has not yet been studied. The duration of PTSD may vary, but it generally tends to follow a chronic course in most orthopedic trauma studies. The time course of PTSD has been studied in populations exposed to disasters.[31] A study of survivors of the Oklahoma City bombing found that PTSD symptoms developed on the day of the bombing in 76%, within the first week in 94%, and within the first post-bombing month in 98% of directly exposed survivors.[30] Research studies of combat-related PTSD and adult survivors of sexual abuse have found that these populations may be more likely to have delayed-onset PTSD (defined by DSM-IV as PTSD with symptoms beginning more than 6 months after the incit-

ing event), but the definitions of delayed-onset and other methodologic aspects of these studies have varied and may not be directly comparable to the findings from disaster studies.

The research reviewed above has demonstrated that the prevalence of PTSD, major depression, and other psychiatric illness after orthopedic trauma is substantial. The occurrence of these disorders has often not been well appreciated in orthopedic practice, and consequently the orthopedist's ability to detect psychiatric illness in patients has historically been lacking.[11] The exact pathophysiologic underpinnings of psychiatric disorders in orthopedic trauma patients are not yet fully understood, but now there is a concerted effort to understand, identify, and treat these disorders as they apply to the care of orthopedic trauma patients.

IMPACT OF THE PROBLEM

PTSD is not only surprisingly prevalent in orthopedic trauma patients, but it is also associated with functional disability and significant medical and mental health care utilization that has not been well recognized in the orthopedic treatment literature. Common orthopedic outcome measures include ability to return to work and perform activities of daily living (ADL) and pain scores. These orthopedic outcome measures do not directly measure psychological distress, but these outcome measures are adversely affected in patients with PTSD. Not only is the prevalence of PTSD in orthopedic trauma patients higher than previously recognized, but also the impact of this disorder on functional outcomes is substantial. Psychiatric illness such as major depression and PTSD have been found to correlate strongly with health-related quality of life in trauma patients,[2] even more than injury severity, presence of chronic medical conditions, age, or history of alcohol abuse.[49]

PTSD in orthopedic trauma patients has been demonstrated to be one of the most predictive variables of functional outcome following orthopedic injury.[51] In the National Study on the Costs and Outcomes of Trauma (NSCOT) by Zatzick et al.,[51] PTSD was prospectively found to be associated with a 3.2 times higher odds of not returning to work. PTSD was also associated with functional impairment 12 months post trauma in ability to eat, bathe, toilet, grocery shop, prepare meals, and pay bills. Functional impairments in ADLs and instrumental ADLs, high musculoskeletal pain scores, and general health dysfunction are also found in patients with PTSD.[34,51] A meta-analysis by Pacella et al.[34] found that PTSD symptoms were associated with general health symptoms, cardiorespiratory symptoms, pain frequency and severity, and gastrointestinal upset. A study of VA health care utilization of patients with and without PTSD found a significantly higher general medical and mental health service utilization in patients with PTSD.[9]

PTSD and pain problems often co-occur, as demonstrated by a study of musculoskeletal pain complaints in association with PTSD in military veterans[25] and a prospective study of trauma patients predicting PTSD at 4 to 8 months from pain symptoms at 24 to 48 hours.[29] Other studies have yielded conflicting results related to the association of PTSD and pain.[27] Cognitive behavioral therapy has been shown to improve PTSD severity, neck disability, and physical, emotional, and social functioning in patients with chronic whiplash and PTSD even in the absence of documented changes in pain sensitivity or intensity.[13] Treatment of PTSD has not been demonstrated to improve pain in orthopedic patients.

Ultimately, patient-derived outcome measures rely on more than just objective physical examination findings. A patient's emotional state is important in the interpretation of his or her own outcome. For example, a patient involved in a motor vehicle collision who has nightmares about the accident and a phobia of traveling may not perceive his or her outcome as good, even if the fractures unite in an anatomic position with functional soft tissue healing. The orthopedic surgeon is often the only physician managing these patients after their injury, representing the sole opportunity to recognize the psychiatric sequelae of trauma exposure that are highly pertinent to the patient's functional outcome.

ADDRESSING THE PROBLEM

Interventions for trauma-related syndromes including PTSD have varied through history. They have ranged from outright neglect to herbal medications and from the placement of clinical psychiatrists at the front lines of battle to berating those affected. General Patton, visiting a military hospital in Sicily, asked a patient about his injuries, and after hearing, "It's my nerves," he slapped him across the face and called him a coward. This response clearly reflected a lack of understanding of emotional difficulties following trauma exposure at the time. Similarly, during the Vietnam War, if a soldier had "stress response syndrome" lasting longer than 6 months, it was deemed pre-existing and therefore the diagnosis was not service-connected.[38] This mindset persisted until a better understanding of PTSD and more successful ways of treating it were available.

Addressing PTSD can be accomplished through efforts directed toward prevention and treatment. A long-standing approach to prevention of post-traumatic psychological problems among trauma survivors is the practice of psychological debriefing. Psychological debriefing has not been shown to be effective for the prevention or treatment of PTSD and has the potential to harm those with PTSD.[7] In a randomized controlled trial examining road traffic accident victims, psychological debriefing was shown to be ineffective in reducing PTSD symptoms, and at a 3-year follow-up, intrusive and avoidance symptoms were found to be worse in those who underwent psychological debriefing.[22]

Identifying patients at risk for PTSD can aid the development of early prevention strategies. Risk factors for PTSD in traumatized populations include trauma severity and intensity of exposure, female gender, low socioeconomic status, lack of social support, and pre-existing psychopathology including polysubstance abuse.[6,32,37] Higher Injury Severity Scores (ISS) in orthopedic trauma patients have not reliably been found to correlate with the eventual development of PTSD, but rather patients with early post injury emotional distress and greater physical pain have been found to be susceptible to PTSD symptoms.[50]

Identifying patients at risk for PTSD and diagnosis of the disorder are important aspects of the management of ortho-

pedic patients with PTSD. This process can begin with the application of symptom-screening questionnaires. In a study of patients undergoing spine surgery, use of a questionnaire identified more patients with psychological distress than when ordinary clinical observation alone was employed.[11] A clinical tool for identification of psychiatric problems in orthopedic trauma patients is how much patients agree with the statement, "The emotional problems caused by the injury have been more difficult than the physical problems." A study by Starr et al.[41] found a 78% probability that patients with potential PTSD had high scores on a 5-point Likert scale to this question. Although screening tools are helpful for identifying PTSD risk, the diagnosis of PTSD requires careful determination of the presence of the criteria for PTSD according to current diagnostic criteria by a qualified mental health professional.

Although the literature on the treatment of orthopedic trauma patients with PTSD is scant, the more general psychiatric literature contains many treatment options for PTSD. Selective serotonin reuptake inhibitors (SSRI) medications such as paroxetine and sertraline, which are FDA approved for the indication of PTSD, have been shown to reduce PTSD symptoms in patients suffering from PTSD.[5,23] Psychotherapy with cognitive behavioral therapy, exposure therapy, and supportive therapy has been shown to significantly reduce PTSD symptom levels.[3,4,8] Exposure therapy is a method of desensitizing patients to aspects of the traumatic event in a controlled fashion. Cognitive behavioral therapy helps patients to develop more adaptive responses to fear and thoughts of previous traumatic events. These treatment strategies are administered over time by a mental health professional. Therefore, appropriate referral to a mental health professional is an important intervention in the care of patients with PTSD.

Other medications used to augment the treatment of certain PTSD symptoms include prazosin to treat post-traumatic nightmares,[21] α-2 agonists, α-1 antagonists, anticonvulsants, and lithium in the augmentation of the treatment of PTSD. There have also been studies investigating pharmacologic prevention of PTSD in the immediate postinjury period to prevent or dampen the physiologic cascade of events leading to PTSD, using medications such as β-blockers, SSRIs, benzodiazepines, and corticosteroids to provide "inoculation" or "molecular debriefing" with varying degrees of success.[36,40,44]

Psychiatric problems among orthopedic trauma patients are well established in this population. Psychiatric illness in these patients is associated with adverse medical outcomes, yet few orthopedic surgeons have the training or inclination to try to identify and address psychiatric illness in their patients. Attention to the signs, symptoms, and risk factors of PTSD as delineated in this chapter can help physicians to recognize patients at risk for PTSD and other psychiatric disorders among their orthopedic patients, and can affect all aspects of patient care.

REFERENCES

1. American Psychiatric Association. *Diagnostic and Statistical Manual of Mental Disorders.* 4th ed, text revision. Washington DC: American Psychiatric Association; 2000.
2. Bhandari M, Busse JW, Hanson BP, et al. Psychological distress and quality of life after orthopedic trauma: An observational study. *Can J Surg.* 2008;51:15–22.

3. Bisson JI, Shepherd JP, Joy D, et al. Early cognitive behavioral therapy for posttraumatic stress symptoms after physical injury. Randomised controlled trial. *Br J Psychiatry.* 2004;184:63–69.

4. Blanchard E, Hickling E, Devineni T, et al. A controlled evaluation of cognitive behavioral therapy for posttraumatic stress in motor vehicle accident survivors. *Behav Res Ther.* 2003;41(1):79–96.

5. Brady K, Pearlstein T, Asnis GM, et al. Efficacy and safety of sertraline treatment of posttraumatic stress disorder: A randomized controlled trial. *JAMA.* 2000;283:1837–1844.

6. Brewin CR, Andrews B, Valentine JD. Meta-analysis of risk factors for posttraumatic stress disorder in trauma-exposed adults. *J Consult Clin Psychol.* 2000;68(5):748–766.

7. Bryant RA. Early intervention for post-traumatic stress disorder. *Early Interv Psychiatry.* 2007;1(1):19–26.

8. Bryant RA, Harvey AG, Dang ST, et al. Treatment of acute stress disorder: A comparison of cognitive-behavioral therapy and supportive counseling. *J Consult Clin Psychol.* 1998; 66:862–866.

9. Calhoun PS, Bosworth HB, Grambow SC, et al. Medical service utilization by veterans seeking help for posttraumatic stress disorder. *Am J Psychiatry.* 2002;159(12): 2081–2086.

10. Crichlow RJ, Andres PL, Morrison SM, et al. Depression in orthopaedic trauma patients. Prevalence and severity. *J Bone Joint Surg Am.* 2006;88:1927–1933.

11. Daubs MD, Patel AA, Willick SE, et al. Clinical impression versus standardized questionnaire: The spinal surgeon's ability to assess psychological distress. *J Bone Joint Surg Am.* 2010;92(18):2878–2883.

12. Doukas CR, Hayda CR, Frisch HM, et al. The Military Extremity Trauma Amputation/Limb Salvage (METALS) Study: Outcomes of amputation versus limb salvage following major lower-extremity trauma. *J Bone Joint Surg Am.* 2013;95(2):138–145.

13. Dunne RL, Kenardy J, Sterling M. A randomized controlled trial of cognitive-behavioral therapy for the treatment of PTSD in the context of chronic whiplash. *Clin J Pain.* 2012; 28(9):755–765.

14. Erichsen J. *On Railway and other Injuries of the Nervous System.* Philadelphia, PA: Henry C. Lea; 1867.

15. Feinstein A, Dolan R. Predictors of post-traumatic stress disorder following physical trauma: An examination of the stressor criterion. *Psychol Med.* 1991;21:85–91.

16. Gilbertson MW, Shenton ME, Ciszewski A, et al. Smaller hippocampal volume predicts pathologic vulnerability to psychological trauma. *Nat Neurosci.* 2002;5(11):1242–1247.

17. Haughn C, Gonsiorek J. The Book of Job: Implications for construct validity of posttraumatic stress disorder diagnostic criteria. *Mental Health, Religion, & Culture.* 2009; 12(8):833–845.

18. Hoge CW, Castro CA, Messer SC, et al. Combat duty in Iraq and Afghanistan, mental health problems, and barriers to care. *N Engl J Med.* 2004;351(1):13–22.

19. Jordan BK, Schlenger WE, Hough R, et al. Lifetime and current prevalence of specific psychiatric disorders among Vietnam veterans and controls. *Arch Gen Psychiatry.* 1991;48(3):207–215.

20. Koenen KC, Harley R, Lyons MJ, et al. A twin registry study of familial and individual risk factors for trauma exposure and posttraumatic stress disorder. *J Nerv Ment Dis.* 2002;190(4):209–218.

21. Kung S, Espinel Z, Lapid MI. Treatment of nightmares with prazosin: A systematic review. *Mayo Clin Proc.* 2012;87(9):890–900.

22. Mayou RA, Ehlers A, Hobbs M. Psychological debriefing for road traffic accident victims: Three-year follow-up of a randomized controlled trial. *Br J Psychiatry.* 2000;176: 589–593.

23. Marshall RD, Beebe KL, Oldham M, et al. Efficacy and safety of paroxetine treatment for chronic PTSD: A fixed-dose, placebo-controlled study. *Am J Psychiatry.* 2001;158: 1982–1988.

24. McCarthy ML, MacKenzie EJ, Edwin D, et al. Psychological distress associated with severe lower-limb injury. *J Bone Joint Surg Am.* 2003;85:1689–1697.

25. Magruder KM, Yeager DE. Patient factors relating to detection of posttraumatic stress disorder in Department of Veterans Affairs primary care settings. *J Rehabil Res Dev.* 2008;45(3):371–381.

26. Michaels AJ, Michaels CE, Moon CH, et al. Posttraumatic stress disorder after injury: Impact on general health outcome and early risk assessment. *J Trauma.* 1999;47:460–466.

27. Moeller-Bertram T, Keltner J, Strigo IA. Pain and post traumatic stress disorder – Review of clinical and experimental evidence. *Neuropharmacology.* 2012;62:586–597.

28. Myers CS. *Shell-Shock in France 1914-1918.* Based on a War Diary kept by C. S. Myers. Cambridge: Cambridge University Press; 1940.

29. Norman SB, Stein MB, Dimsdale JE, et al. Pain in the aftermath of trauma is a risk factor for post-traumatic stress disorder. *Psychol Med.* 2008;38:533–542.

30. North CS, Nixon SJ, Shariat S, et al. Psychiatric disorders among survivors of the Oklahoma City bombing. *JAMA.* 1999;282(8):755–762.

31. North CS, Oliver J. Analysis of the longitudinal course of PTSD in 716 survivors of 10 disasters. *Soc Psychiatry Psychiatr Epidemiol.* 2013;48(8):1189–1197.

32. North C, Yutzy S. Goodwin and Guze's psychiatric diagnosis. 6th ed. New York, NY: Oxford University Press; 2010.

33. Onen A, Subasi M, Arslan H, et al. Long-term urologic, orthopaedic, and psychological outcome of posterior urethral rupture in children. *Urology.* 2005;66(1):174–179.

34. Pacella ML, Hruska B, Delahanty DL. The physical health consequences of PTSD and PTSD symptoms: A meta-analytic review. *J Anxiety Disord.* 2013;27(1):33–46.

35. Sanders MB, Starr AJ, Frawley WH, et al. Posttraumatic stress symptoms in children recovering from minor orthopaedic injury and treatment. *J Orthop Trauma.* 2005;19(9): 623–628.

36. Schelling G, Briegel J, Roozendaal B, et al. The effect of stress doses of hydrocortisone during septic shock of posttraumatic stress disorder in survivors. *Biol Psychiatry.* 2001; 50:978–985.

37. Schnyder U, Moergeli H, Klaghofer R, et al. Incidence and prediction of posttraumatic stress disorder symptoms in severely injured accident victims. *Am J Psychiatry.* 2001;158(4):594–599.

38. Scott WJ. *Vietnam Veterans Since the War: The Politics of PTSD, Agent Orange, and the National Memorial.* Norman: University of Oklahoma Press; 2004.

39. Shay J. *Achilles in Vietnam: Combat Trauma and the Undoing of Character.* New York, NY: Touchstone; 1995.

40. Stahl SM. Can psychopharmacologic treatments that relieve symptoms also prevent disease progression? *J Clin Psychiatry.* 2002;63(11):961–962.

41. Starr AJ, Smith WR, Frawley WH, et al. Symptoms of posttraumatic stress disorder after orthopaedic trauma. *J Bone Joint Surg Am.* 2004;86:1115–1121.

42. Subasi M, Arslan H, Necmioglu S, et al. Long-term outcomes of conservatively treated paediatric pelvic fractures. *Injury.* 2004;35:771–781.

43. Trimble MR. *Post-traumatic Neurosis.* Chicester: Wiley; 1981.

44. Vaiva G, Ducrocq F, Jezequel K, et al. Immediate treatment with propranolol decreases posttraumatic stress disorder two months after trauma. *Biol Psychiatry.* 2003;54(9): 947–949.

45. von Känel R, Hepp U, Kraemer B, et al. Evidence for low-grade systemic proinflammatory activity in patients with posttraumatic stress disorder. *J Psychiatr Res.* 2007; 41(9):744–752.

46. Wallace M, Puryear A, Cannada LK. An evaluation of posttraumatic stress disorder and parent stress in children with orthopaedic injuries. *J Orthop Trauma.* 2013;27(2):e38–e41.

47. Yehuda R, MacFarlane A, Shalev A. Predicting the development of posttraumatic stress disorder from the acute response to a traumatic event. *Biol Psychiatry.* 1998;44(12): 1305–1313.

48. Yehuda R, Cai G, Golier JA, et al. Gene expression patterns associated with posttraumatic stress disorder following exposure to the World Trade Center attacks. *Biol Psychiatry.* 2009;66(7):708–711.

49. Zatzick DF, Jurkovich GJ, Gentilello L, et al. Posttraumatic stress, problem drinking, and functional outcomes after injury. *Arch Surg.* 2002;137:200–205.

50. Zatzick DF, Rivara FP, Nathens AB, et al. A nationwide US study of post-traumatic stress after hospitalization for physical injury. *Psychol Med.* 2007;37(10):1469–1480.

51. Zatzick D, Jurkovich GJ, Rivara FP, et al. A national US study of posttraumatic stress disorder, depression, and work and functional outcomes after hospitalization for traumatic injury. *Ann Surg.* 2008;248(3):429–437.

14

AMPUTATIONS

William J. J. Ertl

INTRODUCTION

This chapter is written to provide the orthopedic fracture and trauma surgeon a foundation for amputation surgery. Amputation surgery is one of the oldest known surgical procedures but has, in the past generation of surgeons, been given decreased importance particularly with regard to the proper surgical handling of residual limbs. This may be due to the stigma that is attached to amputations as a procedure of failure, namely failure of vascular reconstruction, joint reconstruction, or limb salvage. Amputation should be regarded as a reconstructive procedure restoring limb function with the prosthesis serving as an extension of the limb, not the limb solely being an attachment site for the prosthesis. It is my hope with this chapter to instill renewed interest in amputation surgery in the traumatized patient.

HISTORICAL BACKGROUND

Amputation as a surgical technique has its roots dating back to prehistoric times. The earliest known documentation of an amputation as a ritualistic act was noted on cave wall drawings dating back to approximately 5000 BC. Archeologists noted that a Neanderthal skeleton found in present-day Iraq provides evidence that the individual had survived an above-elbow amputation.[56] Indications for amputation were extended by Hippocrates and Celsus to include the treatment of infection, a reduction in invalidism, removal of useless limbs, and as a

life-saving procedure in selected circumstances. It was not until later when the ancient surgeons Archigenes and Heliodorus expanded the indications to include traumatic injuries and the utilization of proximal tight bandages for hemorrhage control, akin to the modern tourniquet.[56] During the 1500s, Paré reintroduced the importance of ligatures for hemorrhage control and Clowes is credited with performing the first successful transfemoral amputation. With the introduction of projectile weaponry in the mid-1300s, battlefield injuries became more severe and maiming, requiring a renewed interest in treating limb injuries with amputation. During the late 1700s and into the early 1800s, the British surgeon George Guthrie and the French surgeon Dominique Jean Larrey challenged the practice of delaying amputations for battlefield injuries for 3 weeks by advocating rapid primary amputation for these injuries. This change in practice resulted in fewer deaths from severe limb injury. Larrey also promoted the rapid transport of wounded soldiers from the field with his "flying ambulance."

The development of amputation techniques has centered on armed conflicts. As a consequence of improvements in armaments, soldiers who survived other injuries often sustained significant limb injuries requiring amputation. Having emphasized expeditious transport and rapid amputation, attention was placed on reconstructive efforts of the residual limb. This was due in part to effective developments in anesthetics, aseptic surgery, antibiotics, the understanding of the basic physiology of the lower extremity, and prosthetic devices. A primary goal of amputation reconstruction was to preserve length and maintain the end-bearing capabilities of the residual limb as emphasized by Chopart and Lisfranc at the midfoot level and Pirogoff, Boyd, and Syme at the ankle level. During the late 1800s, Bier attempted osteoplastic reconstruction by placing a bony block between the tibia and the fibula secured with screw fixation. The only transtibial amputation capable of end bearing was developed by Ertl.[18–20] End bearing was accomplished by combining the concepts of bony reconstruction (osteoplasty) with soft tissue reconstruction (myoplasty) to create an osteomyoplastic amputation for the transtibial level. The same concepts of reconstructive surgery have also been applied to the transmetatarsal level and the transfemoral level. Ertl[20] was able to apply his reconstructive techniques to approximately 13,000 patients over the years from World War I to World War II. Dederich continued to promote soft tissue stabilization, showing the advantages of restoring normal vascularity to the limb after myoplastic amputation at the transfemoral level.[13] Gottschalk et al.[23,24] further elucidated the importance of myoplastic reconstruction by characterizing improved alignment and gait at the transfemoral level when using this technique.

With new unique materials and engineering principles, the prosthetic field has rapidly advanced the art and science of prosthetic manufacturing and is now able to fit many patients with poorly performed amputations with a functional prosthesis. As a result, the emphasis on proper surgical technique and focusing on amputation as a reconstructive procedure has slowly faded over time. The remainder of the chapter will serve to re-emphasize the need for sound surgical handling of the residual limb and review various surgical approaches and outcomes.

Goals of Amputation

The ultimate goal of amputation is to restore and provide function to the patient. Surgery is not and should not be the only focus. The surgeon should be cognizant of the effect that limb loss will have on the patient and be able to provide the patient all resources necessary to regain maximum function. This will require a team approach with the patient at the center of attention.[39] The team will include the patient, surgeon, prosthetist, rehabilitation expert, peer support, family, and even psychological support. Burgess[9] believed that the residual limb should function as an end organ. To this end, the surgeon responsible for the patient should strive for total comprehensive care.

Injured Limb Scoring Systems

As orthopedic and vascular surgical techniques improved over the last couple of decades, there has been renewed interest in salvaging traumatized limbs. However, our ability to predict which limb can be salvaged and which patients would benefit from early amputation remains very subjective and is quite limited. Gregory et al. first attempted to create a scoring system, the mangled extremity syndrome (MES), in a retrospective review of 60 patients. Utilizing this scoring system, they felt patients could be identified preoperatively for salvage or amputation.[25] A second scoring system, the mangled extremity severity score (MESS) was employed by Johansen et al.[30] and was felt to be simple and predictive. Helfet et al.[27] then applied this scoring system prospectively and found it to be simple and accurate in determining limbs that could be salvaged and those that should undergo primary amputation. The American College of Surgeons[1] simplified the definition of a mangled limb as one with "high energy transfer or crush causing a combination of injuries to the artery, bone, tendon, nerve, and/or soft tissue." Other scoring systems also have been developed, including the predictive salvage index (PSI),[28] The limb salvage index (LSI),[54] the nerve injury, ischemia, soft tissue injury, skeletal injury, shock, and age of patient (NISSA) score,[40] and the Hannover Fracture Scale (HFS).[61] Each scoring system placed emphasis on different components of the limb and developed various criteria for amputation or salvage. At this point, the most widely system utilized in the United States is the MESS.

Although ease and applicability have been touted for each scoring system, questions regarding sensitivity and specificity have arisen. Robertson's[52] review of 152 patients suggested poor sensitivity of the MESS as some patients with scores below the amputation threshold eventually went on to an amputation. Bonanni et al. retrospectively reviewed a 10-year experience of attempted limb salvage on 58 limbs utilizing the mangled extremity severity index (MESI), MESS, PSI, and LSI. Their review suggested poor predictive utility for limb salvage for all four scoring systems in their patient population.[3] Poole et al. attempted to predict limb salvage of extremities with combined osseous, soft tissue, and vascular injuries independent of a named scoring system. The severity of soft tissue and nerve injury was highly interrelated but soft tissue injury did not correlate with the severity of the osseous injury. Further, limb salvage or amputation could not be accurately predicted by any variable or group of variables studied. Due to the dynamic changes that can occur in these patients these authors suggested initial limb salvage to observe the limb and then perform delayed amputation when indicated.[50] Dirschl and Dahners comprehensively reviewed the MESI, MESS, NISSA, LSI, and PSI. No scoring system was predictive of salvage or amputation. They proposed that scoring systems be used for documentation and as guides in clinical decision making, not as absolute indicators for salvage or amputation.[14] Durham et al. assessed the MESI, MESS, PSI, and LSI retrospectively over a 10-year period. Although there was significant variability in predicting amputation versus salvage, no scoring system was able to predict functional outcome.[16] Thuan et al.[58] showed that no injury severity score could predict functional outcome in patients who underwent limb salvage. Bosse et al. (the LEAP group) prospectively evaluated the utility of multiple scoring systems: MESS, LSI, PSI, NISSA, and HFS-97. The overall analysis showed that lower scores had specificity for limb salvage potential but the low sensitivity of these scoring systems did not validate them as predictors of amputation. The authors recommended caution in using these scoring systems at or above the amputation threshold.[4] In comparison, Krettek et al. re-evaluated the HFS naming it the

HFS-98 and applied the new scoring system prospectively to 87 open long bone fractures. They concluded that the HFS-98 was a reliable extremity salvage scoring system.[31]

Lower extremity trauma is unique to each individual patient. The spectrum of injury to each organ system, namely the skin and subcutaneous tissue, the muscle, the neurovascular structures, and the bone, is varied. No scoring system has been shown to be predictive of amputation, outcome, or function. Scores that are predictive of salvage may be helpful but caution is stressed with regard to identifying a specific amputation threshold. Scoring systems may be used as a documentation tool and as a tool to facilitate communication between surgeons. In most cases, initial limb salvage attempts should be instituted first allowing a complete assessment of the patient, informing the patient of potential surgical options, and allowing the patient to become involved in decision making regarding salvage versus amputation. Although patients undergoing salvage of a severely injured limb may require frequent rehospitalizations, 2- and 7-year results of amputation compared to limb salvage demonstrate similar outcomes as measured by the Sickness Impact Profile.[5,37] However, projected lifetime costs for patients having undergone an amputation are estimated to be three times greater than those for limb salvage patients due to costs of prosthetic devices.[35]

CLINICAL ASSESSMENT OF THE PATIENT REQUIRING AMPUTATION

Urgent Evaluation

In the emergent setting, assessment of the traumatized limb and patient begins with as detailed a history and as complete a physical examination as possible using the American College of Surgeons Advanced Trauma Life Support ABC algorithm. Once the primary survey is completed and the injury inventory is complete, a secondary survey should be performed and repeated every 4 to 6 hours, especially in the obtunded and/or intubated patient. Additional information can be gained by questioning first responders regarding the initial presentation of the patient, the time required for extrication, exposure to the elements, the amount of blood loss at the scene, the potential degree of wound contamination, resuscitation efforts, and the total time lapsed from the scene to the hospital. This information may provide a much more comprehensive clinical assessment of the patient, guiding the surgeon in his/her decision making. Once the patient has been assessed, life-threatening injuries addressed and resuscitation instituted, a focused examination of the limb can be undertaken. Overall inspection of the limb should take into account its appearance and the presence of any and all open wounds. Closed soft tissue wounds can be quite severe and should be graded using the Tscherne classification[60] and open wounds in association with a fracture should be classified using the Gustilo/Anderson open fracture wound classification system.[26,44] Peripheral pulses should be monitored closely and documented after any reduction maneuver. Dislocations and fractures should be reduced and held reduced with an appropriate splint. Motor and sensory function should also be documented as thoroughly as

possible both before and after manipulating the limb. If there are no palpable pulses, a simple Doppler examination of the entire extremity should be performed. A complete Doppler examination may identify occult injuries remote from the main zone of injury that are impacting perfusion and threatening viability of the limb. With diminished or absent distal pulses, an ankle-brachial index (ABI) should be determined in the following manner: A blood pressure cuff is placed around the calf of the extremity in question. The cuff is inflated until no audible Doppler pulse is appreciated. The cuff pressure is then slowly released and once a pulse is heard, the blood pressure value is noted. The same is then done for the upper extremity and a ratio of the lower extremity pressure to the upper extremity pressure is created. The ratio obtained should be 0.9 or greater if no vascular injury is present. A value below 0.9 is suggestive of a vascular injury that may require further workup (e.g., angiography) or intervention. This simple test has shown value in patients with knee dislocation and high-energy tibial plateau fractures.[43] Further, simple duplex Doppler examination of the arterial system can be performed prior to angiography. Angiography should be reserved to determine the exact location of an arterial injury and guide potential intervention such as intraluminal stenting. If a specific vascular injury is diagnosed, revascularization should be performed to preserve limb viability. If the limb is unstable due to a fracture or ligamentous injury, a simple uniplanar external fixator can be applied quickly to maintain the length and alignment of the limb and provide provisional stability during revascularization.[21] Definitive skeletal stabilization can then be staged when deemed appropriate.

Elective Evaluation

In patients who present with delayed or nonemergent indications for amputation, a detailed physical examination is imperative. Often these patients are functionally impaired, have significant pain and have a desire to re-enter societal participation.[51] These patients may present with progressive soft tissue necrosis and infection (Fig. 14-1). Overall inspection of the wounds to determine the extent of potential superficial and/or deep infection is needed as this may determine the ultimate level of amputation. Further, noninvasive vascular assessment should be performed. An ABI of less than 0.45 suggests that distal healing is unlikely.[15] However, in patients with calcific arteriosclerosis, these values may be falsely high and caution should be used when evaluating this test in these patients. Other useful tests include the duplex Doppler examination of the arterial system and transcutaneous oxygen tension (TcPO$_2$) measurements. Duplex Doppler tests will characterize the arterial anatomy and TcPO$_2$ measurements will aid in determining the healing potential of surgical wounds. TcPO$_2$ values below 20 mm Hg are indicative of nonhealing and values of 40 mm Hg or greater are indicative of healing. Between these values, the surgeon should take into account the patient's pre-existing comorbidities, arterial anatomy, and nutritional status. In my experience, in a patient who has undergone a distal vascular bypass below the knee, a below-knee amputation usually will fail due to the single vessel dominance of the lower limb. The goal of this workup is to provide both the patient and

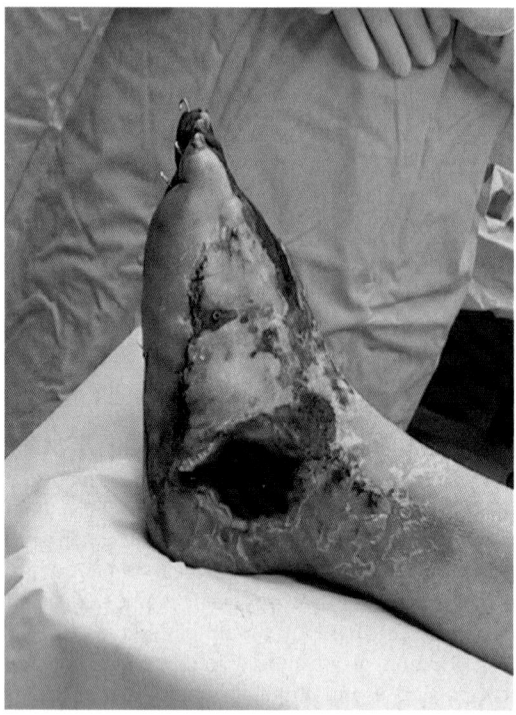

FIGURE 14-1 Depicted is the end-point of wound deterioration following a crush injury to the foot. This patient sustained multiple metatarsal fractures that were treated with percutaneous pin fixation. The foot remained with a pulse and the wounds were closed; however, the soft tissue envelope did not survive and a transtibial amputation was eventually performed.

the surgeon information that can be used to determine the optimal level of amputation to facilitate prosthetic planning and to estimate rehabilitation demands. A combination of tests should be used to determine amputation level as no one test has been shown to be specific or sensitive enough to predict amputation level.

SURGICAL TECHNIQUES

Upper Extremity

Temporizing Versus Immediate Amputation

Patients who present with a complete amputation of the limb rarely are able to undergo successful replantation, usually because the underlying soft tissue injury is so severe compared to the bony injury (Fig. 14-2). Traumatized limbs with segmental injuries, significant vascular injury, significant soft tissue loss, and/or near amputation may be best treated with an immediate open amputation (Fig. 14-3). Traumatized limbs with a nonreconstructible vascular injury will require amputation. The most important factor regarding limb salvage versus amputation will be the severity of the soft tissue injury.[36] These patients often have an obvious constellation of nonreconstructible injuries. When immediate amputation is preferred, all viable soft tissue should be maintained as it can be used later for definitive wound closure. Obviously, ischemic, devitalized tissue should be aggressively and thoroughly debrided. Osseous structures

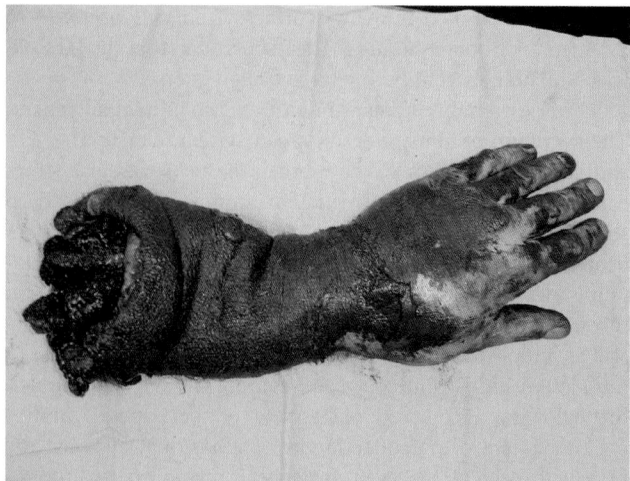

FIGURE 14-2 An oil well driller sustained a traumatic amputation during a drilling operation. Significant soft tissue contamination and extensive degloving precluded replantation. The radius and ulna both remained attached to the arm while the hand and forearm soft tissue envelope was completely degloved.

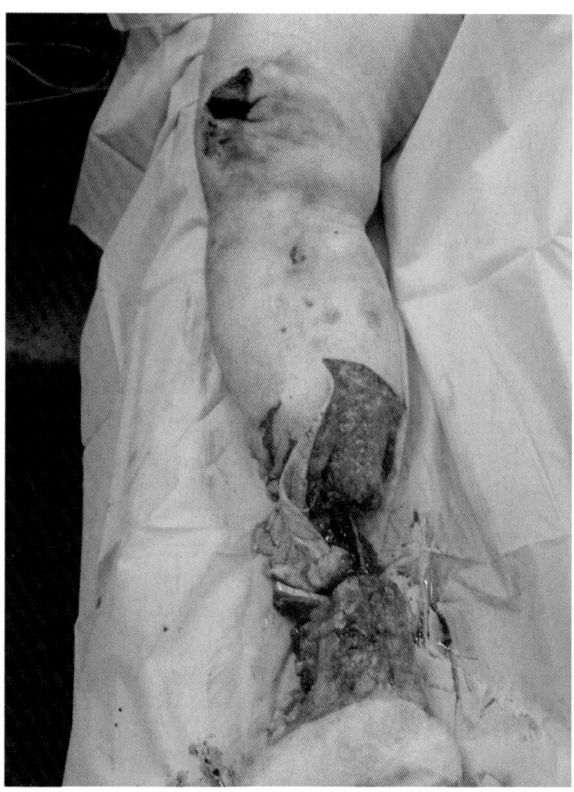

FIGURE 14-3 A motorcyclist sustained severe injuries to the lower leg. There was segmental bone loss and extensive soft tissue loss, and the foot was pulseless. Vascular reconstruction was not feasible. Injuries such as this one should be treated with staged amputation. An open amputation preserving as much length as possible should be performed first. Following intensive wound care, a definitive amputation is performed when the wound bed seems stable.

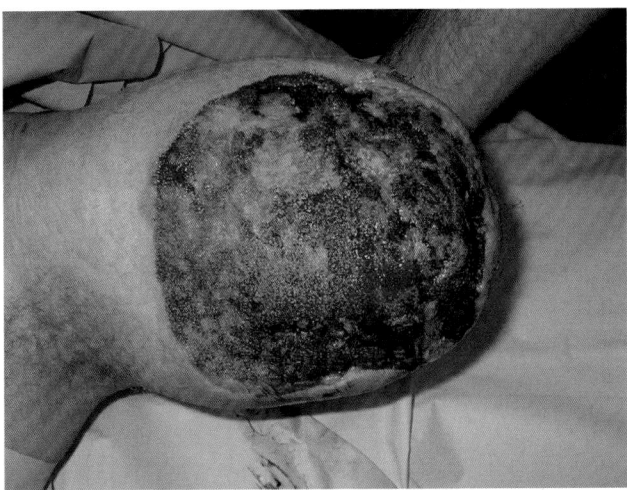

FIGURE 14-4 Negative pressure wound therapy is a powerful adjunctive tool to create healthy granulation tissue and a stable wound bed. In this transhumeral amputation, length was preserved by maintaining muscle coverage over the humerus and applying negative pressure wound therapy until a healthy granulation tissue bed was created. Then a split-thickness skin graft was successfully applied and the patient was ultimately fitted with a myoelectric prosthesis.

should be resected initially to the level of soft tissue resection. Wound care should then be instituted with serial debridements until a stable wound bed is achieved. Negative pressure wound therapy may play an adjunctive role in creating granulation tissue that may aid in wound healing (Fig. 14-4). During this time period, patient education and prosthetic consultation should be employed to maintain patient involvement in their treatment course. Further, the clinical workup should be continued to determine the optimum level of amputation, similar to the patient undergoing a nonemergent amputation.

Patients who present with no clear-cut evidence for immediate amputation should undergo early temporizing treatment. This may include the utilization of temporary external fixation and serial wound debridements. The primary focus of initial temporizing treatment is to obtain and maintain perfusion of the limb prior to extensive and exhausting reconstructive procedures. If limb viability cannot be maintained or reconstruction/salvage is deemed unfeasible, then an elective amputation should be undertaken.

Below-Elbow Amputation

Preserving a functional elbow joint is vital as this joint serves to position the hand in space. Maintaining limb length and a functional elbow joint will substantially increase functional outcome at this level of amputation. If possible, preserving the pronator quadratus allows the patient to maintain two-thirds of active forearm rotation, and thus a body-powered prosthesis can be applied to this level. If a myoelectric prosthesis in utilized, the optimum length will be at the junction of mid- and distal thirds of the forearm. The soft tissue reconstruction must be stable and can be accomplished with myodesis (muscle sutured to bone) or a combination of a myodesis of the deeper layer and myoplasty

(antagonistic muscles sutured together) of the superficial layer (using a pants-over-vest technique). This will provide adequate soft tissue coverage distally with volar and dorsal flaps and allow the residual musculature to be active and dynamic, providing a strong myoelectric signal. Although not routinely performed, a Krukenberg procedure splits the radius and ulna to create a pincers mechanism. It has been recommended for blind patients with bilateral below-elbow amputations or in third world countries where prosthetic resources are limited.[56]

Transhumeral Amputation

If the elbow joint cannot be preserved, then a transhumeral amputation is performed. An amputation through the elbow is a difficult level both for prosthetic fitting and appearance as the prosthetic elbow will be more distal than the contralateral native elbow, therefore this amputation level is rarely selected. The ideal length of the humerus for a body-powered prosthesis is just proximal to the distal metaphyseal–diaphyseal junction. However, for a myoelectric prosthesis the humerus will need to be transected at the midshaft to allow for adequate fitting of this prosthesis. Achieving soft tissue stabilization again is important to provide distal bony coverage and to provide the residual limb with dynamic muscle function. This can be accomplished by securing the deeper layer via myodesis and the superficial layer with a myoplasty using a pants-over-vest technique.

The rate of overall prosthetic use and satisfaction with a transhumeral amputation is much lower than it is for a below-elbow amputation.[15] Recently, targeted nerve reinnervation has shown promise in improving myoelectric prosthetic function.[32,33,41] This technique employs selective nerve implantation into various muscles to improve myoelectric signaling to the prosthesis. It has been applied to a limited number of patients and continues to evolve, providing hope for improved prosthetic function in the proximal upper extremity amputee.

Lower Extremity
Ankle Disarticulation

Ankle disarticulation was developed as a method to preserve the end-bearing capabilities of the limb. The best known is the Syme amputation (Fig. 14-5) but variations include the Pirogoff amputation involving a calcaneotibial arthrodesis,[49] the Boyd amputation (similar to the Pirogoff),[7] the Lefort-Neff modification of the Pirogoff method,[56] and the Camilleri modification of the Pirogoff method.[10] A requirement for this level of amputation is an intact plantar soft tissue flap that will be able to provide stable coverage and wound closure. This may not be feasible in a patient with compromised soft tissue as the result of an old injury. Further, prosthetic fitting may be challenging in this patient, and prosthetic options are limited when compared to those available for a below-knee amputation. A potential limitation of the Syme amputation is migration of the heel pad after surgery which may occur in 7.5% to 45% of patients.[57] Tenodesing the Achilles tendon to the distal tibia with sutures placed through drill holes was shown to be successful in eliminating this problem in a series of 10 out of 11 patients.[57]

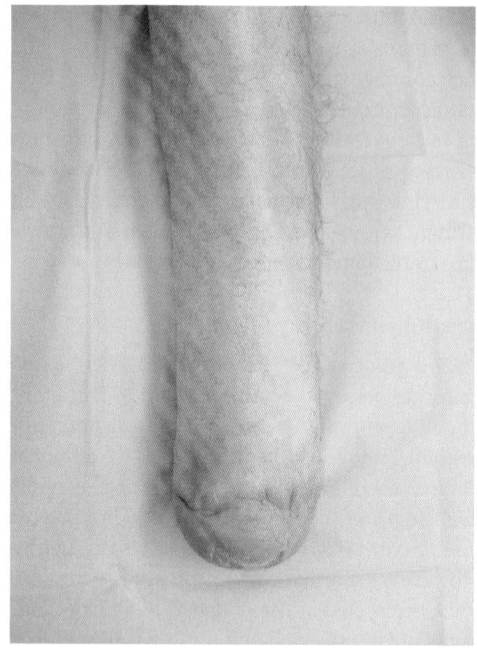

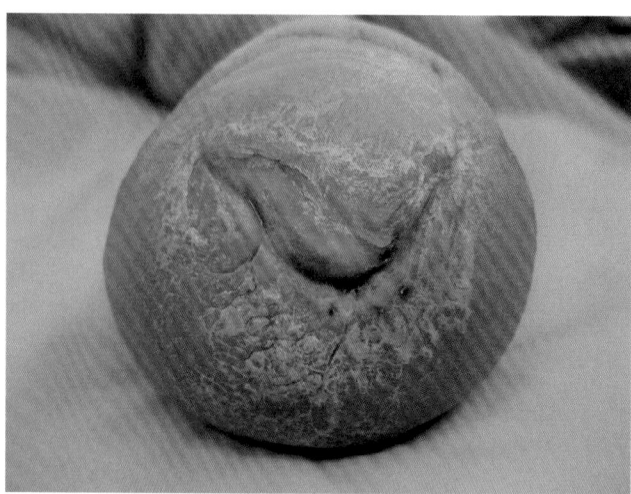

FIGURE 14-5 A: A frontal picture of a patient with a mature Syme amputation demonstrates the regional soft tissue atrophy that can occur over time and the instability of the heel pad that has occurred. The distal tibia became very prominent and painful in the prosthesis. **B:** The distal end of this Syme amputation demonstrates a hypertrophic callous with fissuring that developed as a result of the unstable heel pad.

The surgical approach for a Syme amputation is based on the comprehensive description provided by Smith et al.[56] An incision is marked out transversely across the anterior ankle joint 1 cm distal to the malleoli and stopping 1 cm anterior to them. Then a vertical incision is carried distally from each malleolus to the plantar aspect of the foot, anterior to the heel pad. The long extensor tendons are transected and the peroneal nerves are isolated, transected and cut, allowing them to retract into the wound bed. The anterior vascular structures should be isolated and controlled with a suture ligature. The foot is then plantarflexed, the collateral ligaments are transected, and the flexor hallucis longus tendon is isolated. The calcaneus is then stripped of soft tissue attachments and the Achilles tendon is found and carefully detached from the calcaneal tuberosity. Care should be taken to avoid penetration of the posterior soft tissues at the Achilles insertion. The plantar fascia origin is then transected and the foot is disarticulated. The malleoli should be thinned to reduce the potential for a bulbous-shaped distal limb. Closure should be meticulous and the heel pad must be secured to the distal tibia to ensure soft tissue stability. Achilles tendon tenodesis has also been recommended to achieve heel pad stability.[57]

Transtibial Amputation

The most common method of transtibial amputation is with a posterior myocutaneous flap. Historically, this approach was first proposed by Verduyn in 1696 to provide better distal coverage over the residual distal tibia. Bickel is credited with utilizing this amputation in the United States in 1943 and through the educational efforts of Burgess, this technique gained wide acceptance throughout the United States.[8,56] Transtibial amputation has seen multiple variations proposed: Posterior flap,[8] extended posterior flap,[2] symmetric anterior/posterior flaps,[17] symmetric medial/lateral (sagittal) flaps,[46] skewed sagittal flaps,[53] medial flap,[29] and distal end bearing via a tibia-fibular synostosis.[19,20] With a well-constructed amputation, patients have predictable outcomes with favorable prosthetic use.[55] The selection of amputation level follows guidelines similar to those described earlier for the urgent or elective workup, utilizing TcPO$_2$ measurements and characterizing the vascular anatomy with duplex Doppler arterial ultrasonography. Staged treatment of the traumatized limb may be needed to allow a determination of the optimum level of amputation. This may not be possible until the soft tissue envelope has stabilized which may take several weeks.[2] Preserving the knee joint should always be the goal and many patients can function well with a short residual below-knee stump. A variety of surgical techniques (as listed above) may need to be employed to salvage a below-knee amputation level. Finally, the overall goal is to provide the patient with a cylindrical, (not conical), residual limb that has a stable soft tissue envelope and adequate sensation and perfusion, which can then accept and support a prosthesis to maximize function.

After observing the regenerative potential of periosteum in craniofacial reconstruction,[18] Ertl[19,20] applied the concept of osteoperiosteal flaps to the amputation surgery, combining bony reconstruction (osteoplasty—creating a synostosis between the tibia and the fibula distally) with soft tissue reconstruction (myoplasty). This effectively created the osteomyoplastic amputation, combining two procedures into one. To create the synostosis, osteoperiosteal flaps are raised from all surfaces of the tibia and the fibula distal to the planned level of resection of each bone. This may only require up to 3 cm of bone to be resected as the distance from the medial tibial cortex to the lateral fibular cortex is approximately 5 to 6 cm. In primary amputations, the tibial periosteum is quite thick and the surgeon can utilize only tibial osteoperiosteal flaps to create the synostosis. This will only require up to 6 cm of tissue and not unduly shorten the limb.[1] The tibia and the fibula are then transected at the same level, and the anterior cortex of the tibia is beveled to reduce its prominence. The osteoperiosteal flaps are then sewn together to create a synostosis between the tibia and the fibula. Over time, this flap regenerates bone, and the bony bridge matures with progressive weight bearing. Alternative approaches have utilized a segment of fibula incorporated into the osteoperiosteal sleeve hinged on its periosteal tissue, a full section of fibula placed between the tibia and the fibula, and screw fixation of the fibular graft.[11,45,47,48] Stress shielding is a concern with screw fixation, and removal of the screw has been advocated once the synostosis has formed. A modified technique was applied to a group of military amputees using a segment of fibula and various internal fixation methods. There was noted to be a 32% bone bridge complication rate,[59] raising the question of the need to alter the original technique described by Ertl.

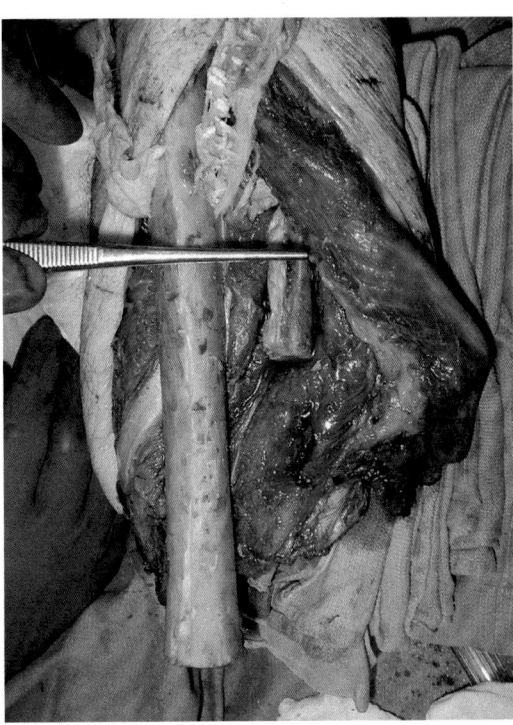

FIGURE 14-7 A primary osteomyoplastic amputation. The forceps demonstrate the level of planned tibial and fibular transection. Note the osteoperiosteal flaps that have been elevated from all surfaces of the tibia. If a portion of the fibula is used, it should be transected about 2 to 2.5 cm below the level of the tibial cut. The fibula can then be osteotomized at the level of the tibial transection, hinged on its medial periosteal sleeve, and incorporated into the osteoperiosteal flaps that create the synostosis.

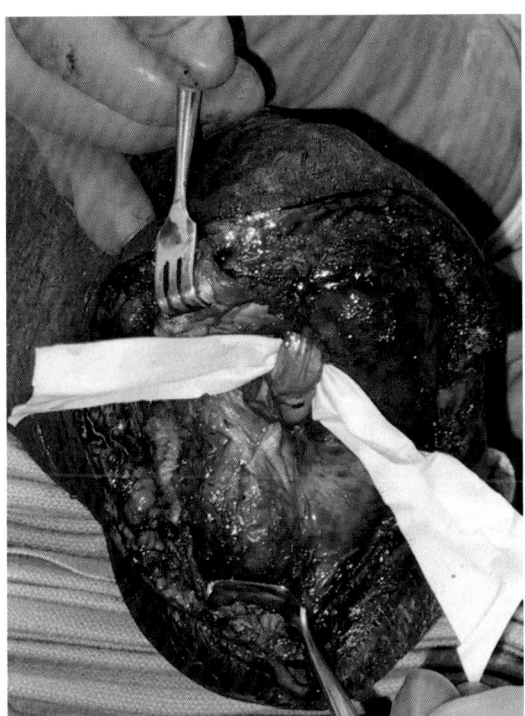

FIGURE 14-6 A revision transtibial amputation demonstrating the tibial nerve which originally was buried directly into the end of the residual tibia. The patient experienced exquisite neurogenic pain with ambulation. Transected nerves should not be buried, placed on tension, or compressed as doing so will promote the development of a postoperative neuroma. They should simply be transected sharply and allowed to retract into the soft tissues proximally.

Soft tissue stabilization is then performed to provide distal coverage over the residual osseous structures. Nerve handling should be meticulous with care being taken to resect the sural, saphanous, deep, and superficial peroneal and tibial nerves proximally and allowing them to retract away from any potential external compressive force. Burying the nerves places them on tension and may produce a neuroma (Fig. 14-6). A meticulous-layered closure should be performed, removing any and all redundant tissue and dog-ears. The resultant residual limb then assumes a cylindrical shape (Figs. 14-7 to 14-10).[34]

The posterior flap technique of transtibial amputation relies on the superficial posterior compartment for distal soft tissue coverage (Figs. 14-11 to 14-14). An incision is marked on the limb with an anterior reference point 10 to 15 cm distal to the knee joint. The width of the limb from anterior to posterior is then measured. At the junction of the anterior one-third and posterior two-thirds of the limb, the posterior flap is drawn extending distally down the leg for this measured distance with 1 cm being added for a traditional posterior flap or 5 cm for the extended posterior flap technique. At the anterior reference point, a partial transverse incision is made to the line extending distally and then the incision is carried distally to the planned end of the flap. The anterior and lateral compartments are exposed and the muscles are transected. Large vessels should be ligated. Nerves

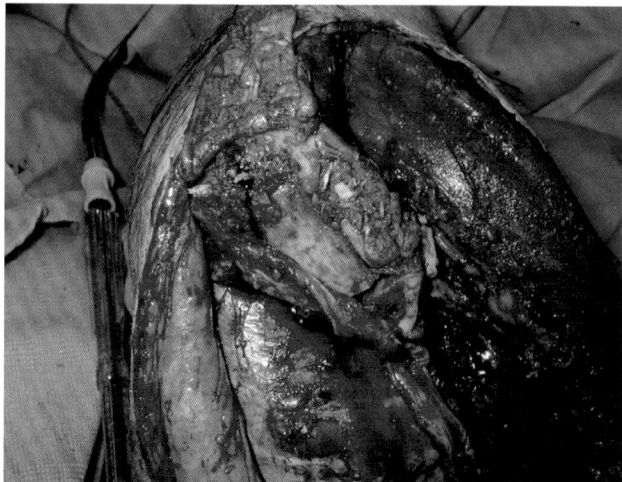

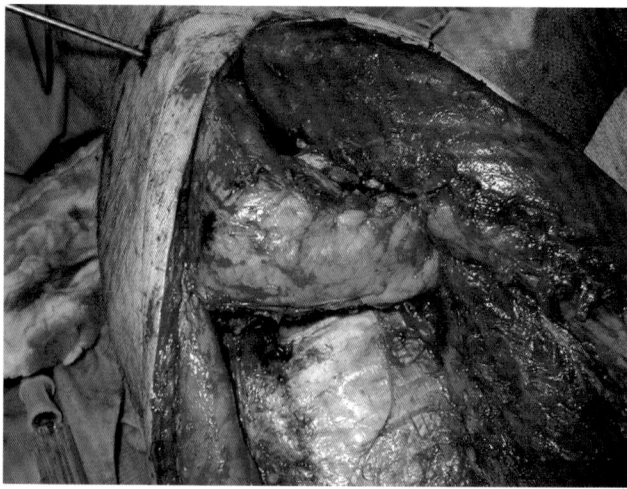

FIGURE 14-8 Bridge formation is created by suturing the tibial osteoperiosteal flaps to the fibula. The fibular portion can be incorporated into the flap. Cancellous bone can be placed into the created synostosis as an autogenous graft. The cut ends of the osteoperiosteal flaps should be imbricated to prevent exostosis formation from the cambium layer.

FIGURE 14-9 Completed bridge formation between the tibia and the fibula.

should be resected sharply and allowed to retract proximally. The tibia is transected and the fibula should be transected no higher than 1.5 to 2 cm proximal to the cut edge of the tibia. This will assure maintenance of a cylindrical residual limb. A fibula which is too short in relation to the tibia will result in a conical limb, and one which is too long will result in distal

irritation of the soft tissue envelope and discomfort with the prosthesis. This will also lead to challenges in prosthetic fitting. The interval between the deep and superficial compartments is then defined and the deep posterior compartment muscles are transected. The posterior compartment vessels are also tied off with suture ligatures. The plane between the two posterior compartments is developed and the superficial posterior compartment is then transected. Multiple vascular perforators cross from the deep compartment to the superficial compartment, and they may also require suture ligature for hemostasis. The

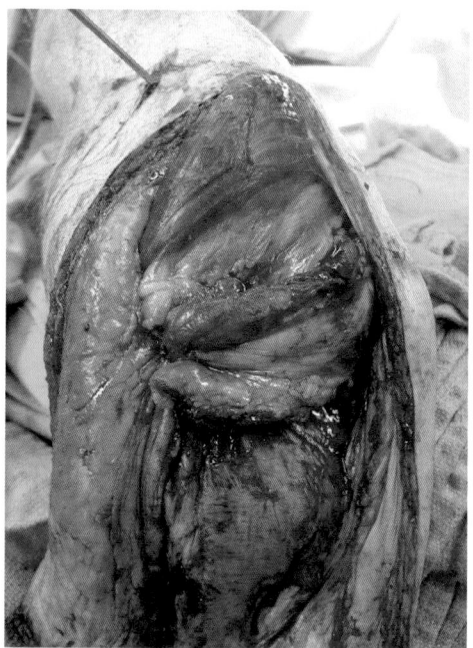

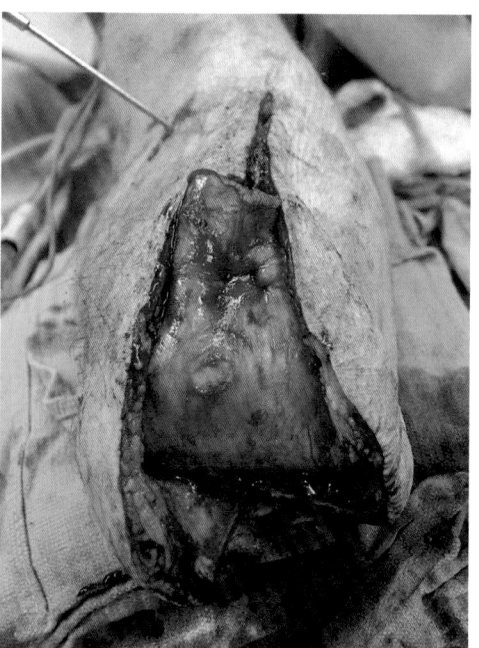

A

B

FIGURE 14-10 A: Soft tissue stabilization for the osteomyoplastic amputation is begun by suturing the anterior and lateral compartments into the deep fascia, providing anterior and distal soft tissue coverage. B: After debulking the deep posterior compartment, the superficial posterior compartment is brought over the end of the residual limb and secured with sutures. Final closure is performed by closing the fascia over the myoplasty, excising redundant skin and performing a meticulous skin closure.

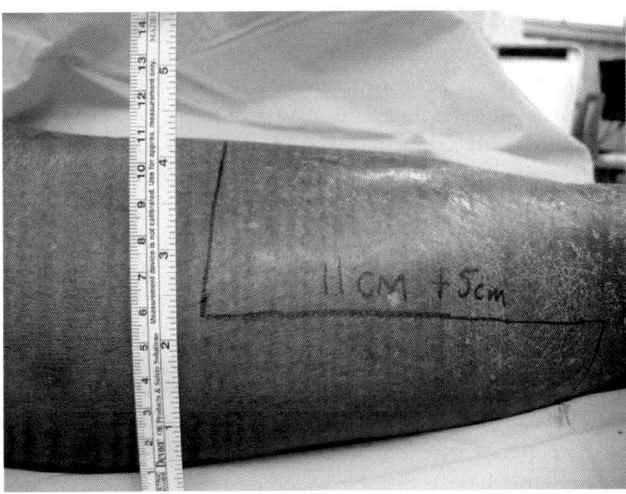

FIGURE 14-11 An extended long posterior flap transtibial amputation. The anterior–posterior distance of the limb is measured at the level of tibial transection and lines are drawn distally to equal the anterior–posterior distance of 11 cm plus 5 cm.

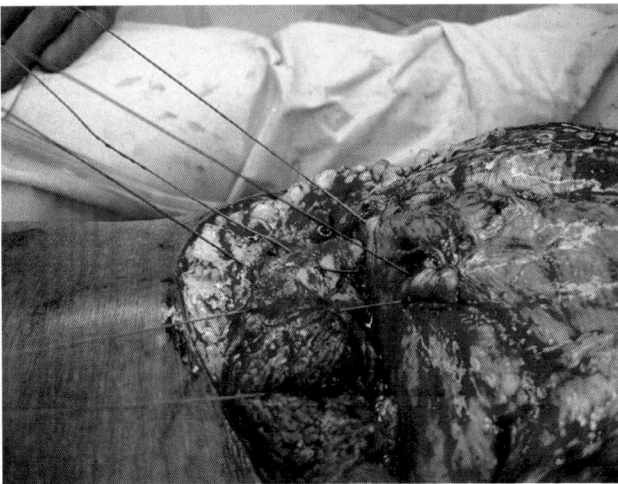

FIGURE 14-13 Drill holes are placed into the anterior tibial cortex such that sutures can be passed through them to anchor the deep fascia of the posterior flap.

anterior cortex of the tibia should be beveled to avoid any bony prominence. Drill holes are placed in the tibia, and deep soft tissue stabilization of the posterior flap is performed by anchoring its deep fascia with sutures placed through these drill holes. A meticulous-layered closure is then performed taking care to remove any and all redundant tissue to provide a cylindrical shape to the limb. With the extended posterior flap technique, the anterior aspect of the limb will appear substantially bulky but will atrophy over time.

Through-Knee Amputation

A through-knee amputation or knee disarticulation maintains the end-bearing capabilities of the femur and will maintain mechanical and anatomic alignment of the femur. Knee

disarticulation has been indicated for the dysvascular patient, children, bedbound/nonambulatory patients and in traumatic amputations. In the nonambulatory patient, the long lever arm of the residual limb can be of assistance in transfers. Caution should be used in the traumatic amputee as the functional result with a through the knee amputation is less than that of either the transtibial amputation or transfemoral amputation.[35]

The surgical approach utilizes either sagittal flaps as described by Wagner[63] or a long posterior myofasciocutaneous flap.[6] Employing the posterior flap technique (Figs. 14-15 to 14-17), at the level of the knee joint, a transverse anterior incision is made to the midcoronal line medially and laterally. The skin incision is then carried distally to the junction of the conjoined portion of the gastrocnemius and soleus muscles. Anteriorly, dissection

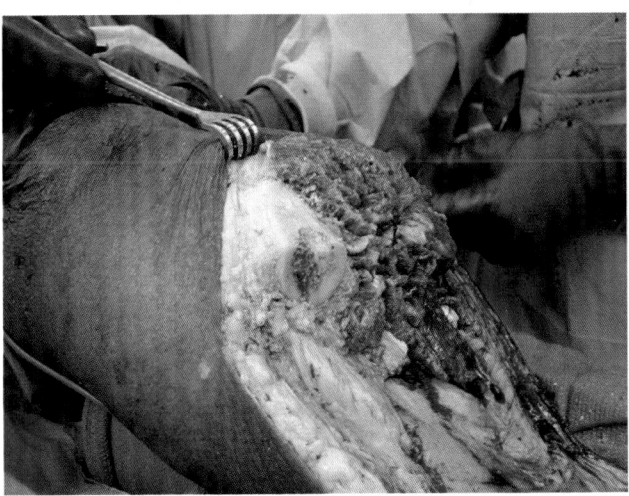

FIGURE 14-12 The extended posterior flap provides an adequate myofasciocutaneous flap for closure and anterior coverage. The anterior cortex of the tibia should always be beveled.

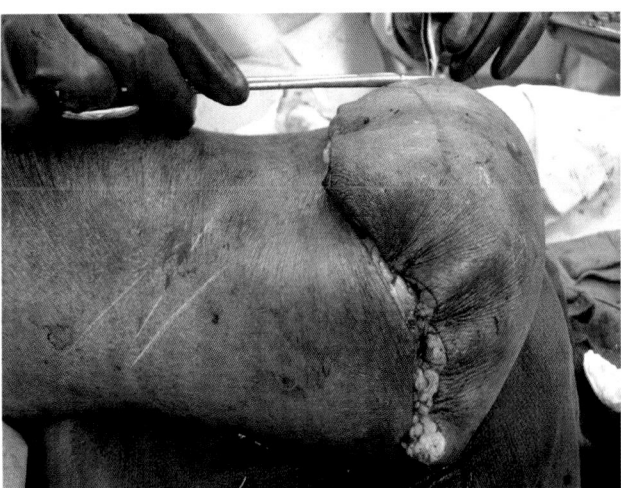

FIGURE 14-14 The remainder of the extended posterior flap is then closed in a layered fashion. This will initially provide a bulky appearance to the distal end of the residual limb but this tissue will atrophy over time, providing adequate soft tissue protection to the anterior tibia.

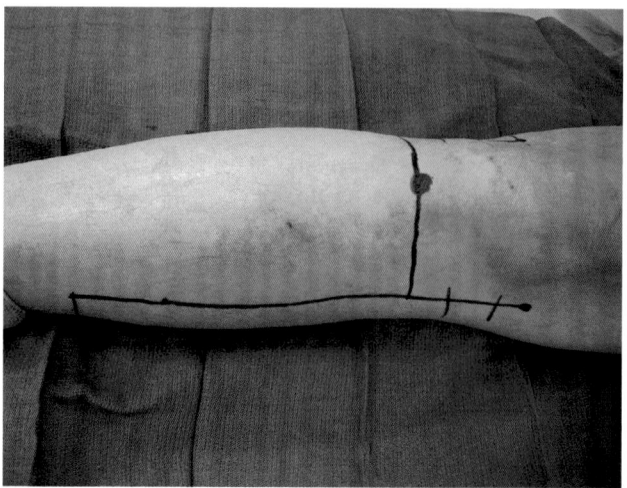

FIGURE 14-15 The basic landmarks for a knee disarticulation with a long posterior flap are the tibial tubercle anteriorly and the medial and lateral epicondyles on either side of the distal femur. The incision should not extend much more proximal than the epicondyles. Doing so will create large dog-ears that will be difficult to control surgically.

is carried down to the tibial plateau and a full thickness anterior flap is made. The knee joint is entered and the collateral and cruciate ligaments are transected. Posterior dissection then transects the capsule and the medial and lateral hamstrings, exposing the neurovascular structures. The vessels are isolated and tied off with suture ligatures. The tibial and peroneal nerves should be isolated, transected and allowed to retract proximally into the soft tissue bed. The interval between the gastrocnemius and deep posterior compartment muscles should be developed and carried distally. Deep vascular perforators may need to be controlled with suture ligatures. A posterior transverse incision distally then allows the lower leg to be removed en bloc. The patella may be retained or removed. Removing the patella creates additional length for the quadriceps which should be sutured to the remnants of the cruciate ligaments and the posterior capsule. Both the medial and lateral hamstrings can be sutured to the capsular remnants to maintain their function as hip extensors. The posterior flap is then brought over the distal end of the residual femur in a pants-over-vest fashion. The anterior flap skin can be removed to accommodate the length of the posterior flap. The sural nerve should be identified and transected as high as possible to reduce the risk of postsurgical neuroma formation.

Transfemoral Amputation

The key to transfemoral amputation is restoring mechanical and anatomic alignment of the residual femur.[23,24] A long medial flap[22] or equal anterior/posterior flaps can be utilized or occasionally in the trauma setting, the surgeon may have to utilize any viable residual soft tissue uniquely for wound closure (Fig. 14-18). In general, soft tissue flaps should be kept as long as possible to reduce the potential for undue tension at closure and to prevent the need to shorten the femur because of inadequate flap length. A proper soft tissue reconstruction creates a dynamic residual extremity, improves the vascularity

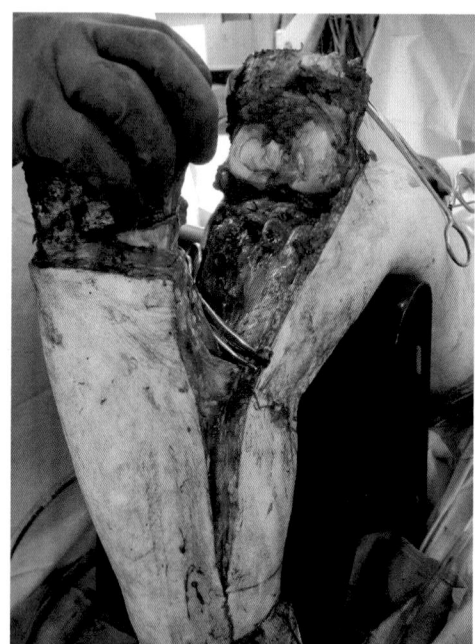
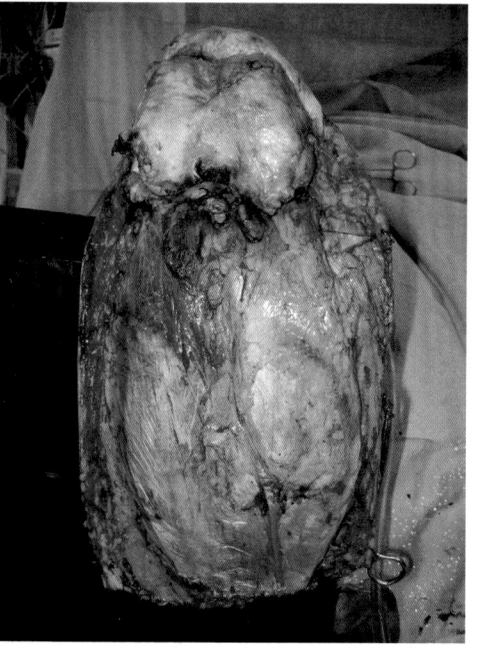

FIGURE 14-16 **A:** An anterior flap which includes the extensor mechanism has been elevated and the dissection is carried into the knee joint. The cruciate and collateral ligaments are transected, the vessels are ligated and the nerves sharply transected. A plane between the gastrocnemius and soleus muscles should be developed as depicted here. This plane should be extended as far distally as possible. **B:** With removal of the distal limb, a long posterior myofasciocutaneous flap is created.

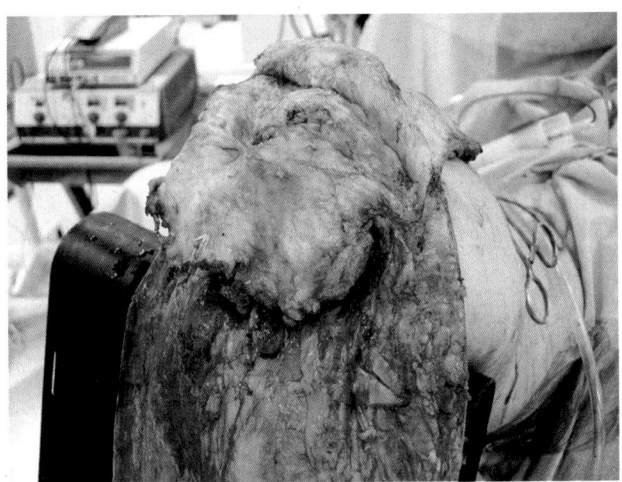
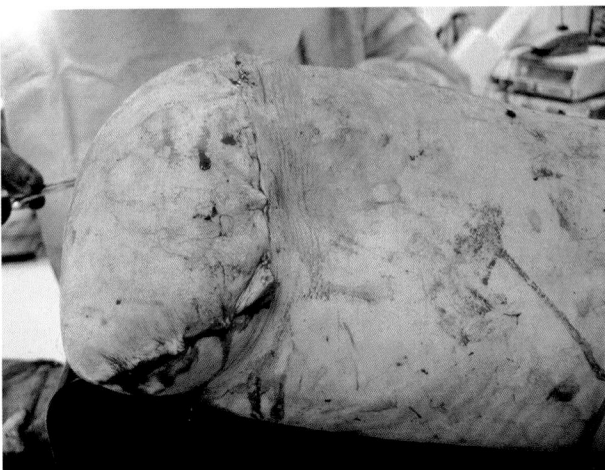

FIGURE 14-17 A: The quadriceps should be anchored with sutures to the remnants of the cruciate ligaments. **B:** Final closure results in an abundant distal soft tissue envelope.

of the residual limb, and will help to maintain alignment of the residual femur which in turn improves gait.[12,13,19,20,23,24]

During a primary transfemoral amputation, a knee disarticulation can be performed first. This will preserve the soft tissues needed for closure. In the traumatic setting, all viable tissue should be preserved for wound closure. The three muscle groups (adductors, quadriceps, and hamstrings) are each isolated and reflected proximally to expose the distal femur. Vascular structures are isolated and tied off with suture ligatures, preferably double suture ligatures. The distal femur is then transected to a level that will allow for proper prosthetic fitting. In general, the minimum space required to achieve symmetric knees is 5 cm (2 in) from the end of the residual limb. Therefore, depending on the technique chosen, the surgeon will need to take into account the amount of space the soft tissue reconstruction will require and add it to the amount of femur removed. The sciatic and obturator nerves should be isolated, transected proximally, and allowed to retract into the soft tissue bed. Nerves should never be buried into bone or tethered for this may create chronic tension and neuroma formation (Fig. 14-19). Soft tissue reconstruction begins with securing the adductor musculature to the distal end of the femur, typically with suture passed through drill holes, thus restoring proper anatomic and mechanical alignment of the residual limb. The quadriceps can also be secured distally to the end of the femur with the hip in extension with sutures passed through additional drill holes. Finally, the hamstrings are secured posteriorly. A meticulous-layered closure should then be performed to create a cylindrical shape to the residual limb.

Ertl[19,20] described an alternative method of treatment for the femur. Osteoperiosteal flaps are elevated off of the femur. After shortening the femur to an appropriate level, the osteoperiosteal flaps are sewn over the end of the femur closing the medullary canal (Figs. 14-20 and 14-21). Soft tissue reconstruction is then performed as described above.

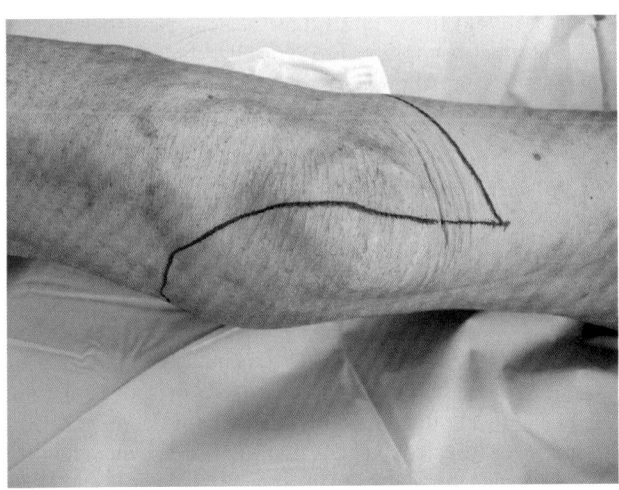
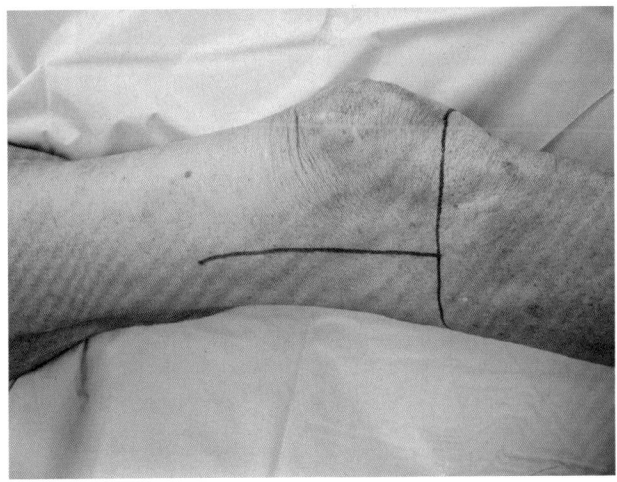

FIGURE 14-18 A: A medial-based flap for a transfemoral amputation as described by Gottschalk. **B:** Equal anterior and posterior flaps for a transfemoral amputation.

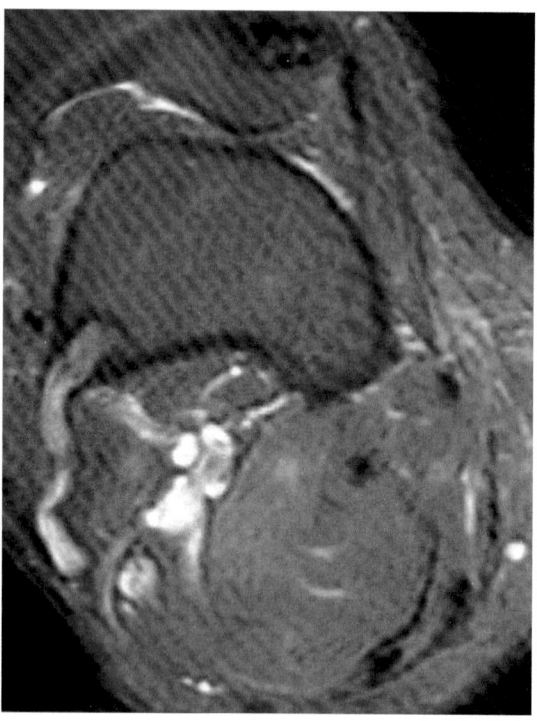

FIGURE 14-19 MRI demonstrating a nerve buried into the posterior femoral cortex and an enlarged neuroma.

PATIENT-ORIENTED THERAPY

Following amputation, full recovery must include a comprehensive rehabilitation program to restore function maximally.

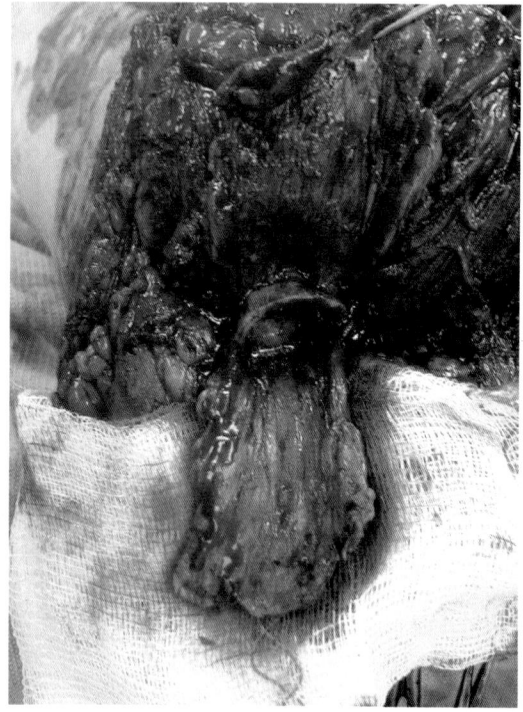

FIGURE 14-20 Osteoperiosteal flaps elevated for the osteomyoplastic transfemoral amputation.

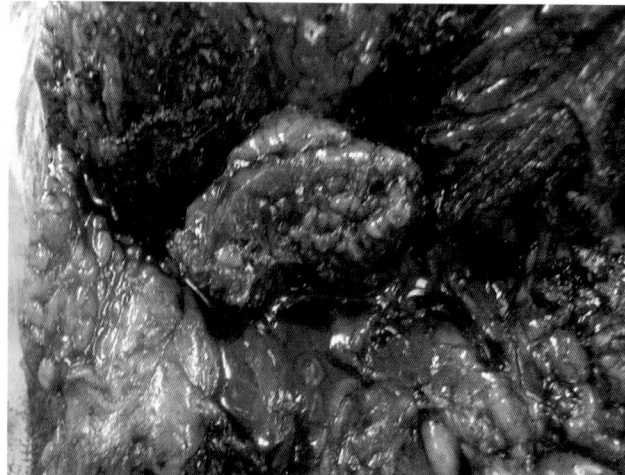

FIGURE 14-21 Medullary canal closure in the osteomyoplastic amputation is accomplished by suturing the osteoperiosteal flaps over the end of the residual femur. The femoral canal can also be packed with cancellous bone graft to augment closure with the osteoperiosteal flaps.

The primary goal of the rehabilitation program is to return the patient back to a functional status in everyday society. The combination of a sound surgical procedure, proper prosthetic application, and comprehensive rehabilitation is essential. In the acute phase, pain control is paramount and can be accomplished via oral or intravenous narcotics, peripheral nerve blocks, patient-controlled analgesia (PCA) or epidural catheter delivery of analgesic medication. Acute phase physical therapy includes wound care, basic mobilization, swelling control, joint mobilization and prevention of contractures, desensitization, upper extremity strengthening, and isometric muscle training of the residual limb.

The patient may want to visit with their prosthetist, if they have not done so prior to surgery, regarding their prosthesis and develop a timeline for its fabrication and application, usually about 6 weeks after surgery. Once the swelling has decreased and the wounds have healed, the patient is evaluated for socket application. Typically, the patient will have a preparatory prosthesis constructed to begin physical therapy and gait training.

It is not simply enough to tell the patient to start walking; rather, a qualified physical therapist is required to teach the patient proper body mechanics and posture during gait and how to employ a program of core strengthening. Balance training and confidence with balance may be challenging in amputees and varies with the level of amputation and the indication for amputation.[42] After the acute phase, advanced therapy should be instituted to educate the patient beyond basic functions, in preparation to return to work or sport. All patients with a limb amputation will also require in-depth occupational therapy for instructions on activities of daily living and the use of assistive technology. Finally, cognitive therapy and psychological support should be considered for all amputees, especially the posttraumatic amputee.

SUMMARY

Amputation resulting from trauma should not be thought of as a failure of intervention. Following severe limb trauma the surgeon should plan a dynamic, functional amputation that can accept a prosthesis and improve the functionality and mobility of the patient. Amputation should be reconstructive with a strong emphasis placed on the rehabilitative potential of the patient.

ACKNOWLEDGMENTS

The author would like to acknowledge and thank Janos P. Ertl, MD, FAAOS, and Christian W. Ertl, MD, FACS, for their suggestions on surgical techniques and Carol Dionne, PT, PhD, OCS, Cert MDT, and Jonathan Day, CPO, for their insightful suggestions regarding amputee rehabilitation and prosthetic application.

REFERENCES

1. American College of Surgeons Committee on Trauma. *Advanced Trauma Life Support Courses.* Chicago, IL: American College of Surgeons; 1985.
2. Assal M, Blanck R, Smith DG. Extended posterior flap for transtibial amputation. *Orthopedics.* 2005;28(6):542–546.
3. Bonanni F, Rhodes M, Lucke JF. The futility of predictive scoring of mangled lower extremities. *J Trauma.* 1993;34(1):99–104.
4. Bosse MJ, MacKenzie EJ, Kellam JF, et al. A prospective evaluation of the clinical utility of the lower-extremity injury-severity scores. *J Bone Joint Surg Am.* 2001;83-A(1):3–14.
5. Bosse MJ, MacKenzie EJ, Kellam JF, et al. An analysis of outcomes of reconstruction or amputation after leg-threatening injuries. *N Engl J Med.* 2002;347(24):1924–1931.
6. Bowker JH, San Giovanni TP, Pinzur MS. North American experience with knee disarticulation with use of a posterior myofasciocutaneous flap: Healing rate and functional results in seventy-seven patients. *J Bone Joint Surg Am.* 2000;82-A(11):1571–1574.
7. Boyd HB. Amputations of the foot with calcaneotibial arthrodesis. *J Bone Joint Surg.* 1939;21(4):997–1000.
8. Burgess EM. The below-knee amputation. *Bull Prosthet Res.* 1968;10:19–25.
9. Burgess EM. The stabilization of muscles in lower extremity amputations. *J Bone Joint Surg.* 1968;50A(7):1486–1487.
10. Camilleri A, Anract P, Missenard G, et al. Apurations et désarticulations des members: Membre inférieur. In: *Encyclopédie Médico-Chirurgicale.* Paris, France: Scientifiques et Médicales Elsevier, SAS; 2000:6–8.
11. DeCoster TA, Homedan S. Amputation osteoplasty. *Iowa Orthop J.* 2006;26:54–59.
12. Dederich R, Van De Weyer KH. [Arteriographic studies of muscle plastic surgery in amputation stump correction]. *Arztl Wochensch.* 1959;14(11):208–211 (German).
13. Dederich R. Plastic treatment of the muscles and bone in amputation surgery. A method designed to produce physiologic conditions in the stump. *J Bone Joint Surg Br.* 1963;45-B:60–66.
14. Dirschl DR, Dahners LE. The mangled extremity: When should it be amputated? *J Am Acad Orthop Surg.* 1996;4(4):182–190.
15. Dirschl DR, Tornetta P III, Sims SH. Amputations and prosthetics (Chapter 15). In: Koval KJ, ed. *Orthopaedic Knowledge Update.* Rosemont, IL: American Academy of Orthopaedic Surgeons; 2002.
16. Durham RM, Mistry BM, Mazuski JE, et al. Outcome and utility of scoring systems in the management of the mangled extremity. *Am J Surg.* 1996;172(5):569–573.
17. Epps CH. Amputation of the lower limb. In: Evarts SM, ed. *Surgery of the Musculoskeletal System.* 2nd ed. New York, NY: Churchill Livingstone; 1990.
18. Ertl J. *Die Chirurgie der Gesichts – und Kieferdefekte.* Berlin/Wien: Urban & Schwarzenberg; 1918.
19. Ertl J. *Regeneration. Ihre Ahnwendung in der Chirurgie.* Leipzig: Ambrosius Barth; 1939.
20. Ertl J. Über Amputationstümpfe. *Chirurgie.* 1949;20:218–224.
21. Ertl W, Henley MB. Provisional external fixation for periarticular fractures of the tibia. *Tech Orthop.* 2002;12(2):135–144.
22. Gottschalk F. Transfemoral amputation: Biomechanics and surgery. *Clin Orthop.* 1999;361:15–22.
23. Gottschalk FA, Kouroush S. Stills M, et al. Does socket configuration influence the position of the femur in above-knee amputation? *J Prosthet Orthot.* 1989;2:94–102.
24. Gottschalk FA, Stills M. The biomechanics of trans-femoral amputation. *Prosthet Orthot Int.* 1994;18:12–17.
25. Gregory RT, Gould RJ, Peclet M, et al. The mangled extremity syndrome (M.E.S.): A severity grading system for multisystem injury of the extremity. *J Trauma.* 1985;25(12):1147–1150.
26. Gustilo RB, Anderson JT. Prevention of infection in the treatment of 1025 open fractures of long bones. *J Bone Joint Surg Am.* 1976;58-A:453–458.
27. Helfet DL, Howey T, Sanders R, et al. Limb salvage versus amputation. Preliminary results of the Mangled Extremity Severity Score. *Clin Orthop Relat Res.* 1990;(256):80–86.
28. Howe HR Jr, Poole GV Jr, Hansen KJ, et al. Salvage of lower extremities following combined orthopedic and vascular trauma. A predictive salvage index. *Am Surg.* 1987;53:205–208.
29. Jain AS, Stewart CP, Turner MS. Trans-tibial amputations using a medially based flap. *J R Coll Surg Edinb.* 1995;40:263–265.
30. Johansen K, Daines M, Howey T, et al. Objective criteria accurately predict amputation following lower extremity trauma. *J Trauma.* 1990;30(5):568–572.
31. Krettek C, Seekamp A, Köntopp H, et al. Hannover Fracture Scale '98–re-evaluation and new perspectives of an established extremity salvage score. *Injury.* 2001;32(7):611.
32. Kuiken TA, Dumanian GA, Lipschutz RD, et al. The use of targeted muscle reinnervation for improved myoelectric prosthesis control in a bilateral shoulder disarticulation amputee. *Prosthet Orthot Int.* 2004;28(3):245–253.
33. Kuiken TA, Li G, Lock BA, et al. Targeted muscle reinnervation for real-time myoelectric control of multifunction artificial arms. *JAMA.* 2009;301(6):619–628.
34. Loon HE. Biological and biomechanical principles in amputation surgery. In: *International Prosthetics Course, Second Proceedings. Committee on Prosthesis, Braces, and Technical Aids.* Copenhagen; 1960:41–58.
35. MacKenzie EJ, Bosse MJ, Castillo RC, et al. Functional outcomes following trauma-related lower-extremity amputation. *J Bone Joint Surg Am.* 2004;86-A(8):1636–1645.
36. MacKenzie EJ, Bosse MJ, Kellam JF, et al. Factors influencing the decision to amputate or reconstruct after high-energy lower extremity trauma. *J Trauma.* 2002;52(4):641–649.
37. MacKenzie EJ, Bosse MJ, Pollak AN, et al. Long-term persistence of disability following severe lower-limb trauma. Results of a seven year follow-up. *J Bone Joint Surg Am.* 2005;87(8):1801–1809.
38. MacKenzie EJ, Jones AS, Bosse MJ, et al. Health-care costs associated with amputation or reconstruction of a limb-threatening injury. *J Bone Joint Surg Am.* 2007;89(8):1685–1692.
39. Malone JM, Moore W, Leam JM, et al. Rehabilitation for lower extremity amputation. *Arch Surg.* 1981;116:93–98.
40. McNamara MG, Heckman JD, Corley FG. Severe open fractures of the lower extremity: A retrospective evaluation of the Mangled Extremity Severity Score (MESS). *J Orthop Trauma.* 1994;8:81–87.
41. Miller LA, Stubblefield KA, Lipschutz RD, et al. Improved myoelectric prosthesis control using targeted reinnervation surgery: A case series. *IEEE Trans Neural Syst Rehabil Eng.* 2008;16(1):4–50.
42. Miller WC, Speechley M, Deathe AB. Balance confidence among people with lower-limb amputations. *Phys Ther.* 2002;82(9):856–865.
43. Mills WJ, Barei DP, McNair P. The value of the ankle-brachial index for diagnosing arterial injury after knee dislocation: A prospective study. *J Trauma.* 2004;56(6):1261–1265
44. Oestern HJ, Tscherne HJ. Pathophysiology and classification of soft tissue injuries associated with fractures. In: Tscherne H, Gotzen L, eds. *Fractures with Soft Tissue Injuries.* Berlin, Germany: Springer-Verlag; 1984:1–19.
45. Okamoto AM, Sangeorzan R, Coelho RF, et al. The use of bone bridges in transtibial amputations. *Rev Hosp Clin Fac Med Sao Paulo.* 2000;55(4):1–13.
46. Persson BM. Sagittal incision for below-knee amputation in schaemic gangrene. *J Bone Joint Surg Br.* 1974;56:110–114.
47. Pinto MA, Harris WW. Fibular segment bone bridging in trans-tibial amputation. *Prosthet Orthot Int.* 2004;28(3):220–224.
48. Pinzur MS, Pinto MA, Schon LC, et al. Controversies in amputation surgery. *Instr Course Lect.* 2003;52:445–451.
49. Pirogoff NI. Osteoplastic elongation of the bones of the leg in amputation of the foot. *Voyenno Med J.* 1854;68:83.
50. Poole GV, Agnew SG, Griswold JA, et al. The mangled lower extremity: Can salvage be predicted? *Am Surg.* 1994;60(1):50–55.
51. Quon DL, Dudek NL, Marks M, et al. A qualitative study of factors influencing the decision to have an elective amputation. *J Bone Joint Surg Am.* 2011;93:2087–2092.
52. Robertson PA. Prediction of amputation after severe lower limb trauma. *J Bone Joint Surg Br.* 1991;73-B(5):816–818.
53. Robinson K. Skew flap myoplastic below-knee amputation: A preliminary report. *Br J Surg.* 1982;69:554–557.
54. Russell WL, Sailors DM, Whittle TB, et al. Limb salvage verses traumatic amputation. A decision based on a seven-part predictive index. *Ann Surg.* 1991;213:473–481.
55. Smith DG, Horn P, Malchow D, et al. Prosthetic history, prosthetic charges, and functional outcome of the isolated traumatic below-knee amputation. *J Trauma.* 1995;38:44–47.
56. Smith DG, Michael JW, Bowker JH, eds. *Atlas of Amputations and Limb Deficiencies.* 3rd ed. Rosemont, IL: American Academy of Orthopaedic Surgeons. 2004.
57. Smith DG, Sangeorzan BJ, Hansen ST Jr, et al. Achilles tendon tenodesis to prevent heel pad migration in the Syme's amputation. *Foot Ankle Int.* 1994;15(1):14–17.
58. Thuan VL, Travison TG, Castillo RC, et al. Ability of lower-extremity injury severity scores to predict functional outcome after limb salvage. *J Bone Joint Surg Am.* 2008;90(8):1738–1743.
59. Tintle SM, Keeling JJ, Forsberg JA, et al. Operative complications of combat-related transtibial amputations: A comparison of the modified burgess and modified Ertl tibiofibular synostosis techniques. *J Bone Joint Surg Am.* 2011;93:1016–1021.
60. Tscherne H, Gotzen L. *Fractures with Soft Tissue Injuries.* Berlin, Germany: Springer-Verlag; 1984.
61. Tscherne H, Oestern HJ. [A new classification of soft-tissue damage in open and closed fractures]. *Unfallheilkunde.* 1982;85:111–115 (German).
62. Varnell RM, Coldwell CM, Sangeorzan BJ, et al. Arterial injury complicating knee disruption. *Am Surg.* 1989;55(12):699–704.
63. Wagner FW Jr. Management of the diabetic-neuropathic foot: Part II. A classification and treatment program for diabetic, neuropathic, and dysvascular foot problems. *Instr Course Lect.* 1979;28:143–165.

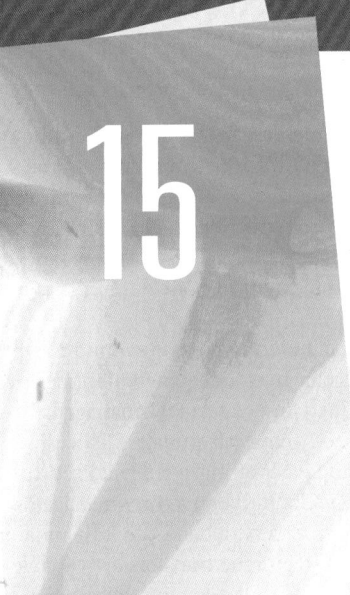

15

BONE AND SOFT TISSUE RECONSTRUCTION

Harvey Chim, Steven L. Moran, and Alexander Y. Shin

INTRODUCTION

Open fractures and their associated soft tissue injuries are difficult to treat and often require a multidisciplinary approach for wound management. These injuries place a significant financial burden on the patient and society because of prolonged patient disability. Despite the great diversity among the individuals who sustain open fractures, a majority of these patients are typically young active adults who tend to be injured in automobile or motorcycle collisions or while engaged in sporting activities.[66]

Successful management of these open fractures and soft tissue wounds requires treatment of the bone as well as soft tissue injuries. Advances in microsurgical techniques and our knowledge of the vascular anatomy of the extremities have led to novel advances in wound coverage that can allow for rapid coverage of these wounds and replacement of injured bone, nerve, and muscle. In this chapter, we will review a multidisciplinary approach for the management of bone and soft tissue defects, which includes a combination of orthopedic surgery, neurosurgery, and plastic surgery expertise, in addition to providing the reader with a variety of reconstructive options for upper and lower extremity open fracture management.

HISTORY

Advances in vascular reconstruction, external and internal fixations, and antimicrobial agents have maximized the rate of limb salvage after severe injuries to the extremities. Continuing advances in the field of microsurgery, including refinement and development of new perforator flaps for free tissue transfer as well as a better understanding of wound pathophysiology have improved surgeons' ability to obtain rapid wound coverage, allowing patients to return to ambulation and the workforce. However, many challenges remain and the patient may still succumb to local infection or other soft tissue or bony complications requiring amputation after major limb trauma.

COMPLEX MUSCULOSKELETAL INJURIES

The open wound should be inspected carefully and the wound pattern and any contamination documented. Photographic documentation is tremendously helpful when available. Wounds should not be explored in the emergency department setting. Instead, exploration should be performed whenever possible in the sterile conditions of an operating room. With polytrauma patients, where the workup of other injuries takes priority over treatment of the open fracture/soft tissue injuries, careful packing of the wound with a sponge moistened with saline and dilute antiseptic solution (Betadine or chlorhexidine) prevents desiccation of the exposed bone and soft tissues until they can be addressed formally in the operating suite.

INITIAL MANAGEMENT OF COMPLEX MUSCULOSKELETAL INJURIES

Decision Making

Open fractures are by definition a multisystem injury, and the management of the soft tissue is often as important as the treatment of the fracture itself.[338] Historically, the outcome of the treatment of open fractures was typically determined by the soft tissue defect. In 1966, Carpenter[41] stated, "If the soft tissues overlying the tibia are not preserved, any hope of primary

healing of the underlying fracture is lost forever." Although Carpenter was referring to the tibia, the importance of the soft tissue envelope to bone healing is real and applicable throughout the body. If soft tissue reconstruction is successful in these injuries, the bone often becomes the problematic area, and the final outcome depends on the extent of bone devascularization and contamination.[132]

Often the fear of not being able to cover a wound has prevented the orthopedic surgeon from adequately debriding the soft tissues. This has resulted in "expectant" management of the soft tissues, an approach that unfortunately still prevails in some surgeons' minds today. Waiting for devitalized tissue to "declare itself" prolongs definitive fracture management, increases the risk of infection, and attenuates the inflammatory response. Pedicled flaps and free tissue transfers are capable of covering large soft tissue defects, thus allowing the surgeon the freedom to perform a wide and thorough initial debridement. Early multidisciplinary collaboration and communication with surgeons skilled in these techniques is crucial for successful outcomes.

The basic principle of complex musculoskeletal injury management begins with application of Advanced Trauma Life Support (ATLS) protocols.[5] Once the basics of ATLS are satisfied, a complete assessment of each wound can be made. Understanding the mechanism of injury and the patient's unique medical and social history are imperative. When possible, the reconstructive options should be discussed with the patient and family.

Principles of Management

During the management of any complex musculoskeletal injury there are several principles one should keep in mind to expedite patient care and maximize patient outcome (Table 15-1).

Principle 1

The first principle is to *prevent further injury.* After understanding the mechanism of injury, one must determine whether a compartment syndrome[107] may be an issue or if ongoing vascular compromise is present. Any salvage of the extremity is dependent on the prevention of further injury or the neutralization of ongoing injury including chemical, mechanical, or traumatic injury.

Principle 2

When debridement of injured tissue is undertaken, an aggressive tumor-like *debridement of all necrotic and nonviable tissue,* including bone, is essential.[111] This is often considered the most important single step in the management of soft tissue trauma and will be further discussed later in this chapter. Often reconstructive plans impede adequate soft tissue debridement, as the surgeon is afraid to lose further soft tissues, which would make the reconstruction more complicated or difficult.

Principle 3

Once adequate debridement of soft tissue and bone has been accomplished, *bone stability* should be achieved. Bone stability

TABLE 15-1	The Eight General Principles of Management of Soft Tissue Injuries Associated with Fractures
Principle 1:	Prevent further injury.
Principle 2:	When debridement of injured tissue is undertaken, an aggressive tumor-like debridement of all necrotic and nonviable tissues, including bone, is essential.
Principle 3:	Achieve bone stability.
Principle 4:	Strive for early bone coverage when possible.
Principle 5:	Do not ignore secondary reconstructive needs when addressing initial bone coverage (i.e., plan for future reconstructive procedures).
Principle 6:	Replace damaged tissues with similar tissues when possible (replace like with like).
Principle 7:	Know when a salvage procedure, such as an amputation, may be the better reconstructive option.
Principle 8:	Know when you have taken on too much and seek assistance and advice.

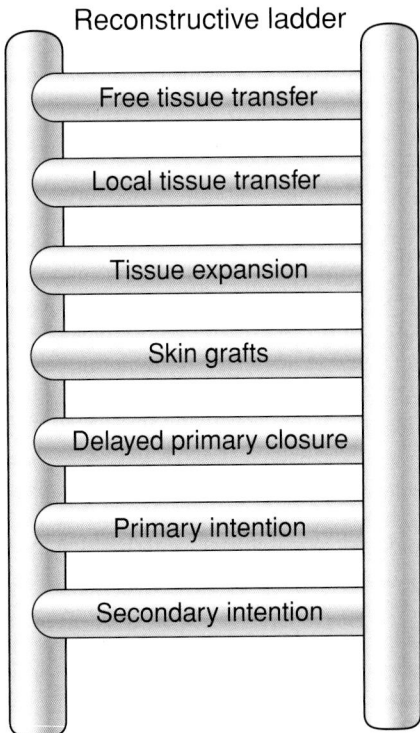

Reconstructive ladder

- Free tissue transfer
- Local tissue transfer
- Tissue expansion
- Skin grafts
- Delayed primary closure
- Primary intention
- Secondary intention

FIGURE 15-1 The reconstructive ladder.

can be achieved with external fixation, internal fixation, or a combination of both. In highly contaminated wounds or wounds that have poor soft tissue coverage, external fixation is often preferred. In wounds that are adequately debrided with good soft tissue coverage of the bone, internal fixation can be used.

Principle 4

When *soft tissue coverage* is needed, *acute coverage* should be considered. Use of the reconstructive ladder[163,204] can be helpful in reconstructing the injured extremity (Fig. 15-1). When soft tissue coverage is considered, a surgeon should evaluate the simplest type of procedure needed to achieve wound coverage, and increase in the complexity only as needed. The reconstructive ladder progresses as follows: *Primary closure, skin grafting, local cutaneous flaps, fasciocutaneous transposition flaps, island fascial or fasciocutaneous flaps, local or distant one-stage muscle or myocutaneous transposition, distant temporary pedicle flaps, and microvascular free tissue transfer.* When evaluating the wound for possible coverage options, it is imperative to consider patient factors; defect genesis; the location, size, and depth of the defect; exposed structures; structures needing reconstruction; the degree of contamination; and the quality of the surrounding tissues.

The concept of achieving wound coverage within 72 hours was popularized by Godina.[118] Although the data presented by Godina is compelling, achieving wound coverage within 72 hours can be difficult secondary to both hospital system issues (operating room and surgeon availability) and patient factors. With advances in wound management with vacuum-assisted closure (VAC) devices (Fig. 15-2) and antibiotic bead pouches, wound coverage can occur later than the 72 hours initially recommended without untoward complications.[111]

Principle 5

When the initial task at hand is to cover the wound, *secondary reconstructive needs* are often ignored. It is important to determine these needs before the soft tissue coverage and the initial reconstructive procedure are undertaken. If nerve grafts need to be placed in the future, the vascular pedicle of the free flap should be placed as far away from the nerve graft sites whenever possible. If future bone grafting (vascularized

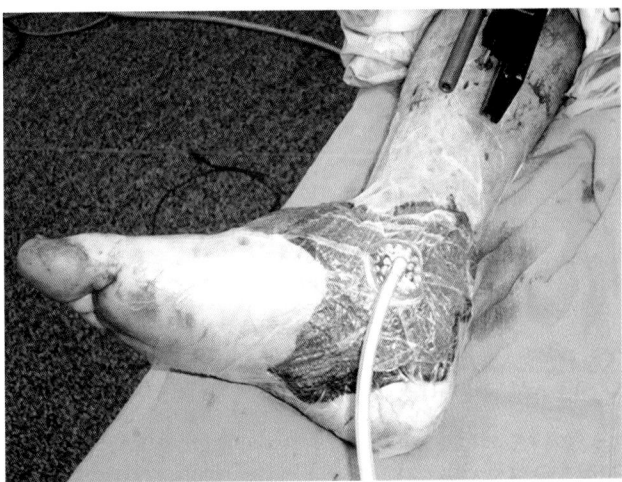

FIGURE 15-2 A vacuum-assisted closure device properly placed on a wound after debridement.

or conventional) or tendon work needs to be performed, planning of the location of the free flap or pedicled flap needs to occur early to prevent future injury to the vascular supply of the flap, potentially compromising its survival or soft tissue coverage.

Principle 6

When composite soft tissue loss occurs, *composite soft tissue reconstruction* should be considered. Composite reconstruction refers to the use of flaps that contain more than one type of tissue. Such an example is an osteocutaneous flap, such as a free fibula, which may contain bone, skin, and muscle. This piece of composite tissue can then be used to replace segmental defects of the tibia and replace any overlying skin loss at the same time. The concept of replacing like tissue with like when possible can be applied to upper extremity injuries as well. As a general rule when there is a need for bone, muscle, and skin, one should always consider the possibility of reconstructing the defect with a composite flap.

Principle 7

A *salvage procedure,* such as an amputation, may be a reasonable solution in selected situations. Although technically feasible, some heroic efforts to reconstruct a limb can lead to prolonged recovery times with loss of gainful employment, psychological problems, and increased morbidity for the patient.

Principle 8

The surgeon should know when he or she has taken on too much and should *seek assistance and advice.* This is the most humbling of the principles, but can be one of the most important. Collaboration with other surgeons may be extremely helpful in difficult cases. A different perspective can often drastically change the patient's outcome.

Patients with open or closed fractures associated with severe soft tissue injury are typically polytrauma patients with multiple organ systems affected. As such, their fractures and soft tissue injuries must be considered in the context of the polytrauma, recognizing the patient as a whole. Care of these patients and their injuries progresses in three phases: Acute stabilization, reconstruction, and rehabilitation. The *acute phase* includes wound debridement, fracture stabilization, soft tissue reconstruction, and initiating muscle function and joint mobility. The *reconstructive phase* addresses indirect sequelae of injury, such as nonunions, infections, and malunions. Finally the *rehabilitative phase* focuses on returning the patient to society.

TO RECONSTRUCT OR NOT: AMPUTATION VERSUS LIMB SALVAGE

In complex extremity injuries, the treating physician must make two critical decisions early within the reconstructive process. The first is to determine if it is technically possible to save the injured extremity and the second is to determine whether salvaging the limb is in the best interest of the patient. An insen-

sate, painful, or chronically unstable leg may provide no benefit over a prosthesis. Many factors have historically come into play when making these decisions, such as patient age, comorbid injuries, and preinjury ambulation status. Several algorithms have been designed to aid the surgeon in this decision-making process.[197,244]

Absolute indications for amputation of the lower extremity in an adult include sciatic nerve transection and irreparable vascular injury. Relative indications for amputation include life-threatening multisystem trauma, a warm ischemia time of greater than 6 hours, an insensate plantar foot, a crushed foot with fracture comminution, extensive bone loss, and multiple joint disruption with multilevel injury, advanced peripheral vascular disease, and rehabilitation concerns.[149,167,233]

Before an amputated limb is discarded, the salvage of uninjured soft tissues should be considered with the goal of maintaining maximum limb length and functioning joints, because this will minimize energy expenditure during ambulation. For example, the glabrous sole of the foot can provide durable stump coverage and an intact ankle joint can be rotated to simulate a missing knee joint.[175,380] Often these salvaged parts may be transferred without microsurgery if their sensory and vascular supply remains intact.

Some investigators have suggested that the function of a salvaged extremity is often poorer than can be achieved with early amputation and prosthetic fitting.[69,95,104,316] The Lower Extremity Assessment Project (LEAP) was a multicenter prospective study of severe lower extremity trauma in the United States civilian population designed to answer this question. The investigators collected prospective outcome data on patients with Gustilo grade IIIB and grade IIIC open fractures. Patient outcomes were evaluated through the use of the Sickness Impact Profile, which is a self-reported health status questionnaire. At 2 and 7 years after injury, patients who underwent amputation had functional outcomes that were similar to those who underwent reconstruction. Predictors of poor outcome after reconstruction included a low education level, nonwhite race, poverty, lack of private health insurance, smoking status, a poor social support network, and involvement in disability compensation litigation. Approximately 50% of the patients in each group were able to return to work at 2 years.[29,217]

An additional finding from this study suggested that sensation within the injured extremity had no bearing on long-term outcome. Patients with an insensate extremity at the time of presentation did not demonstrate significantly worse outcomes at 2 years when compared with patients who presented with a sensate foot. Approximately 55% of those with absent or abnormal plantar sensation had recovered normal sensation at 2 years after injury. This study also suggested that initial plantar sensation is not a prognostic factor for long-term plantar sensation and should not be used as a component of the limb salvage decision algorithm.[30]

Overall the study's findings seemed to indicate that outcome is more significantly affected by the patient's economic, social, and personal resources than by the bony injury or the level of amputation. If the patient is still adamant about limb salvage and understands the long-term potential for future surgery;

however, we still remain aggressive in our attempts to salvage the severely injured extremity.

BONE RECONSTRUCTION

When bone defects are present there are three basic reconstruction options: Distraction osteogenesis (Ilizarov technique), nonvascularized bone grafting, or vascularized bone grafting. The specific technique employed is dependent on the size of the defect, the quality of the soft tissue envelope, and the location of the defect.

Distraction Osteogenesis (Ilizarov Technique)

Distraction osteogenesis was popularized by Ilizarov, who in the western Siberian city of Kurgan, discovered that normal tissue could be generated under carefully applied tension.[156–159] The tension-stress effect on bone resulted in neovascularization, increased metabolic activity, and cellular proliferation, similar to but not identical to normal endochondral ossification at the physis. The resulting fibrous tissue in between the distracted bone segments ossifies in an orderly fashion, resulting in structurally sound bone. The soft tissues concomitantly grow linearly in response to the applied tension.[162]

The Ilizarov technique employs a modular system of rings that are held in place by fine wires that are crossed and secured to the ring. The wires are tensioned to between 60 and 130 kg. A series of rings are constructed and bridged together with threaded posts, each with a distraction or compression device that can be adjusted every several hours. Many modifications to this system have been described.

When applied to bone loss, the defect of long bones can be filled with one of the two methods: acutely shortening the bone and then gradually lengthening it to restore the original bone length; or transporting bone from either proximal or distal to the bone defect to gradually fill in the defect.[51,78,79,123]

In addition to application of the external ring fixator device, a free tissue transfer can be performed to address complex lower extremity bone injury with associated significant soft tissue defects. In the acute setting, the external ring fixator or modifications of the fine-wire fixators can be applied as the primary management of the fracture. When these devices are applied it is imperative that if soft tissue coverage is required, discussions between the microsurgeon and the orthopedic surgeon occur early in the care of the injured extremity. The presence of a ring fixator can make microsurgery extremely challenging, and it is preferable that straight external fixators are used instead.[51]

Nonvascularized Bone Grafts

Nonvascularized bone grafts include autografts as well as allografts. They are ideal for small defects and voids and can be obtained from a number of anatomic locations and are typically cancellous or corticocancellous in composition. Autografts are superior in general to allograft material. For most bone defects of less than 6 cm with a well-vascularized bed, adequate soft tis-

sue coverage and absence of infection, a conventional cancellous or corticocancellous bone graft is generally recommended.[26] The most common areas for nonvascularized autograft bone harvest include the iliac crest (anterior or posterior), distal radius, and olecranon.[372] Cancellous bone has greater inductive capacity than cortical bone and should be used unless mechanical stability is required.

The process of bone graft incorporation is by "creeping substitution," a process in which vascular ingrowth gradually occurs with resorption and replacement of the necrotic bone graft with viable bone.[156] Creeping substitution results in rapid revascularization in small cancellous grafts, but is slow and incomplete in cortical bone. As much as 40% to 50% of lamellar bone remains necrotic, and the revascularization process that does occur causes significant mechanical weakening because of bone resorption at 6 to 12 months.[26,35,315] Allografts, like autografts, must also be replaced by living bone. They are replaced more slowly and less completely, and they invoke a local and systemic immune response that reduces the stimulus of new bone formation. This effect may be diminished by freezing, freeze drying, irradiating, or decalcifying the graft; or eliminated with the use of immunosuppressive drugs.[119,120,151,161,264,265,308,372] Structural nonvascularized grafts of all types have substantial problems with fatigue fracture, even years after implantation. Successful grafting requires a well-vascularized bed, adequate immobilization, and protection from excessive stress by rigid internal fixation.[91]

Vascularized Bone Grafts

Unlike conventional bone grafts, the cellular elements of a vascularized bone graft remain alive and dynamic in its new site. Because of its preserved circulation, cell viability is greater than in conventional grafts,[10,23] obviating the need for the gradual creeping substitution of living bone into nonvascularized bone.[26,35,170] During healing, extensive osteopenia is not seen with vascularized bone grafts as it is in conventional bone grafts.[68] Vascularized grafts have improved strength, healing and stress response as compared with nonvascularized bone grafts.[24,43,86,114,199,304,379,382] The incidence of stress fracture is lower than in massive structural autografts or allografts.[134,268,317,355] Finally, union is more rapid, and bone hypertrophy in response to applied stress may occur with time.[109] Bone healing is more likely in difficult circumstances including scarred or irradiated beds, or in an avascular bone bed.[105,106]

In addition to superior cell survival, maintained circulation, and better mechanical properties, vascularized grafts have other significant advantages over conventional grafts. These include the possibility to restore longitudinal growth by inclusion of the growth plate,[235,335,378] revascularize necrotic bone,[154,203,221,229,280,307,324,340,341] improve local blood flow in scarred soft tissue beds,[269,299] and reconstruct composite tissue loss in one procedure by the inclusion of skin, muscle, tendon, nerve, and other tissues with the bone graft.

Vascularized Bone Graft Indications

Based on the information reported in the preceding, it would seem that vascularized autografts would be ideal for grafting under most circumstances. Their use as free tissue transfers is technically demanding however, and pedicle grafts are often more limited in dimension and pedicle length and hence their indications are limited. Prolonged operative times and extensive dissection increase the risk of complications, and donor site morbidity may be significant. Therefore, for bone defects of less than 6 to 8 cm with normal soft tissues, conventional techniques remain the method of choice under many circumstances.

Iliac crest can be used as a pedicled vascularized bone graft. The principal advantages of a vascularized autogenous iliac crest graft are its largely cancellous nature and the large amount of soft tissue that may be raised with the bone as a combined osteomusculocutaneous flap. In such flaps, a more reliable skin flap may be obtained with inclusion of both superficial and deep circumflex iliac vessels. The advantages of this osteocutaneous flap include the ability to (i) supply vascularized bone to what is frequently a poor recipient bed for a bone graft, (ii) reconstruct both soft tissue and bony defects simultaneously, and (iii) be used in facilities without a capability for microvascular surgery when used as a pedicle flap for the upper extremity.[278] It may also be used for smaller defects.

Segmental Bone Loss

Vascularized transfer is indicated in segmental bone defects larger than 6 to 8 cm due to tumor resection,[1,59,87,115,202,237,245,276,331,370] traumatic bone loss,[27,93,155,208,220,255,258,362] osteomyelitis, or infected nonunion.[27,141,142,171,173,238,246]

Vascularized transfer in smaller defects is reasonable in cases in which "biologic failure" of bone healing is likely or has already occurred.[250] Examples include persistent nonunion after conventional treatment, poorly vascularized bone and/or its soft tissue bed because of scarring, infection or irradiation, and congenital pseudarthrosis.[6,228,259,343,356]

Other indications include osteonecrosis, composite tissue loss requiring complex reconstruction, joint arthrodesis in exceptional circumstances, and the need for longitudinal growth with physeal transfer.

Fibula

The fibula is the most commonly used vascularized bone graft because its structure and shape are appropriate for diaphyseal reconstruction (Fig. 15-3). A long, straight segment of 26 to 30 cm in length can be harvested, and osteosynthesis can be securely obtained to the recipient bone. The blood supply to the fibula, as to other long bones, is derived normally from a nutrient artery via radially oriented branches that penetrate the cortex and anastomose with the periosteal vessels. The resulting blood flow is centrifugal from the medullary cavity to the cortex. This arrangement is the norm for the fibula, which has a single nutrient vessel entering its middle third from the peroneal artery. Additional periosteal branches from the peroneal and anterior tibial arteries also supply the diaphysis.[360] The proximal epiphysis is supplied by an arcade of vessels, of which the lateral inferior genicular vessel is the most important.[235] This vessel must be anastomosed if physeal growth is desired after transfer of the fibular head.[106,235]

The vascularized bone may be transferred with a fasciocutaneous skin paddle of up to 10 to 20 cm. This is possible because a series of fasciocutaneous or myocutaneous perforators from the peroneal artery typically pierce the soleus muscle adjacent to the lateral intermuscular septum.[189,377] The location of the perforators may be determined in the operating room prior to skin incision with the use of a Doppler ultrasound probe. Osteomuscular flaps including the flexor hallucis longus (FHL) muscle or portions of the soleus or peroneal muscles may also be raised using the same peroneal artery pedicle.[25,49,361] The peroneal pedicle has a length of 6 to 8 cm and an arterial diameter of 1.5 to 3 mm.

Multiple series have reported the successful salvage in the upper and lower extremities with the use of the free fibula flap in cases of osteomyelitis,[352] pathologic fracture,[296] and segmental bone loss of the femur,[352] tibia,[363] radius and ulna,[3,368] humerus,[368] and pelvis (Fig. 15-4).[2] The bone is capable of hypertrophy over time through a process of fracture and callus healing.[248] In addition, single or multiple osteotomies may be made in the bone as long as one preserves a periosteal sleeve and the nutrient vessel. This then allows for double fibular strut reconstruction in cases of segmental bony injuries.[47,352]

The flap is typically harvested under tourniquet control through a lateral approach with the patient in the supine or lateral position. Preoperative vascular studies, although controversial in the literature, have been very useful to us in preoperative planning in cases of posttraumatic reconstruction and in patients with peripheral vascular disease.[84,216] We obtain a CT angiogram in all patients in preparation for free fibular transfer. Unlike a formal angiogram, a CT angiogram has no additional morbidity while providing information on inflow and outflow vessels in both legs. In 10% of the population the peroneal artery is the dominant arterial supply to the leg, and is referred to as the peroneal arteria magna; in such cases the contralateral leg should be considered for flap harvest.[84,216]

The incision is centered over the posterior margin of the fibula in a line running from the fibular head to the lateral malleolus. We have found it helpful to always include a skin paddle in the flap design; it facilitates closure as well as postoperative flap monitoring. Inclusion of a cuff of soleus muscle or FHL muscle can improve the reliability of the skin paddle if skin perforators are small. Dissection is initiated between the plane of the soleus and peroneal muscles. Once the fibula is visualized laterally, the peroneal nerve is identified and protected as dissection then continues superficial to the periosteum in a medial direction (Fig. 15-5). The interosseous membrane is incised. The bone is then divided proximally and distally with the use of a Gigli saw or sagittal saw, taking care to protect the surrounding neurovascular structures. Six centimeters of the distal fibula must remain intact to stabilize the ankle. In the skeletally immature patients, we always perform a synostosis at the lateral malleolus after fibula harvest.[251] Six centimeters of fibula bone is also preserved proximally (below the head of the fibula) to preserve the stability of the knee. This is achieved by maintaining the attachment of the tibia to the fibula, and the attachments of the biceps femoris muscle and the fibular collateral ligament to the head of the fibula. The proximal part of the fibula hosts parts of the origins of the peroneus longus, the extensor digitorum longus, the extensor hallucis longus, the soleus, and the tibialis

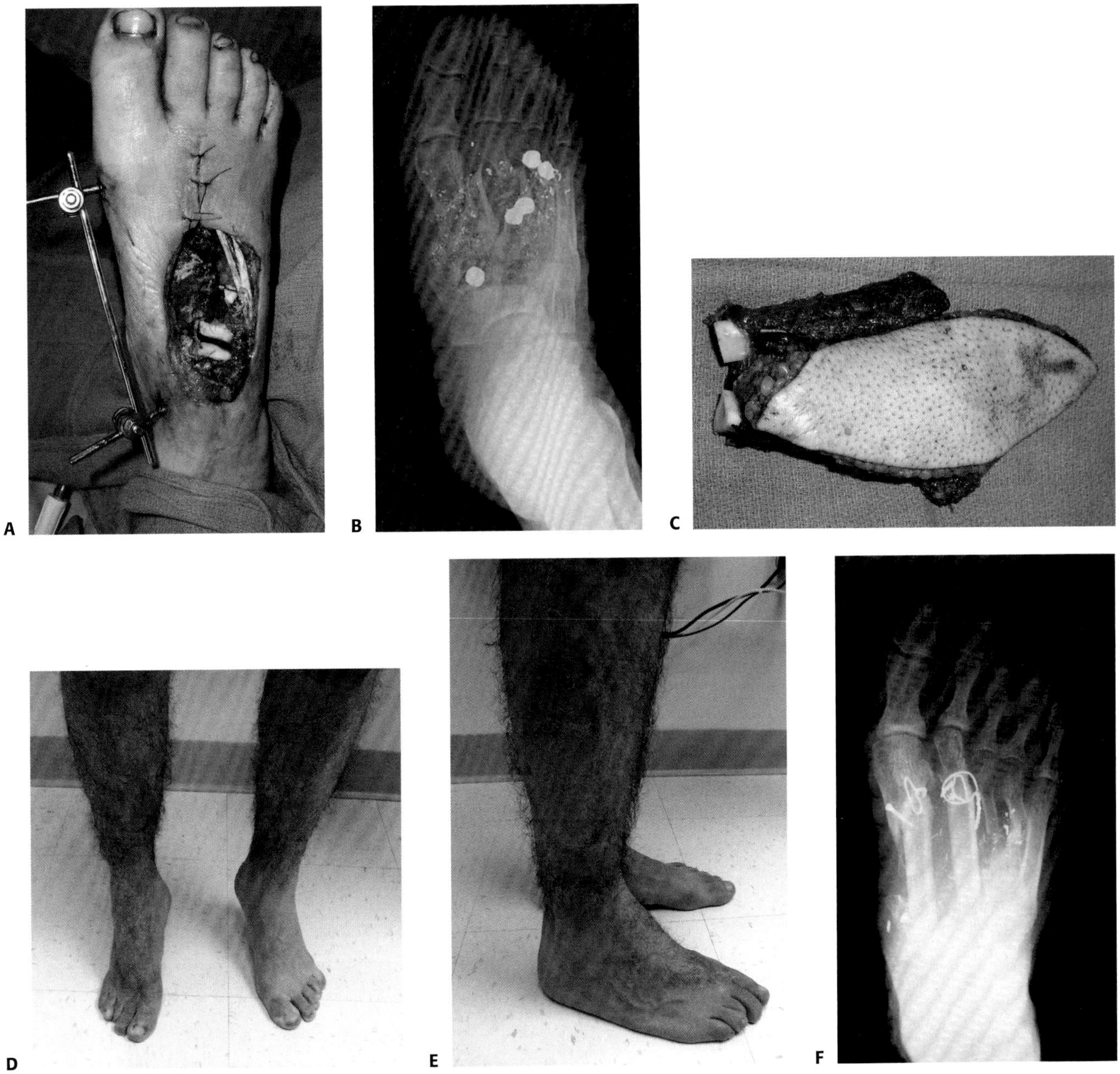

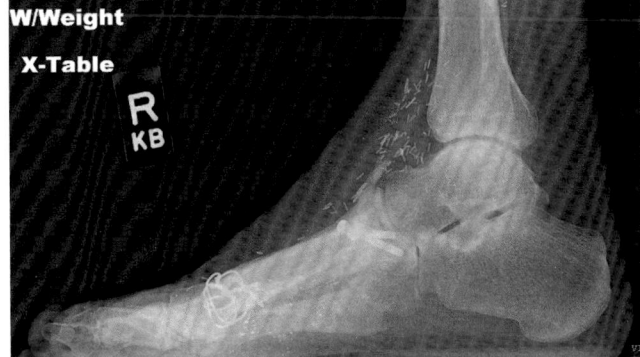

FIGURE 15-3 A, B: Following a gunshot wound to the foot, there was loss of the first and second metatarsals and an extensive dorsal foot wound. **C:** Intraoperative view of the fibular osteocutaneous flap with a longitudinally split fibula. **D–G:** Clinical photographs and x-rays 16 months following the free fibular osteocutaneous flap for first and second metatarsal ray reconstruction. The patient was able to ambulate without difficulty and play soccer.

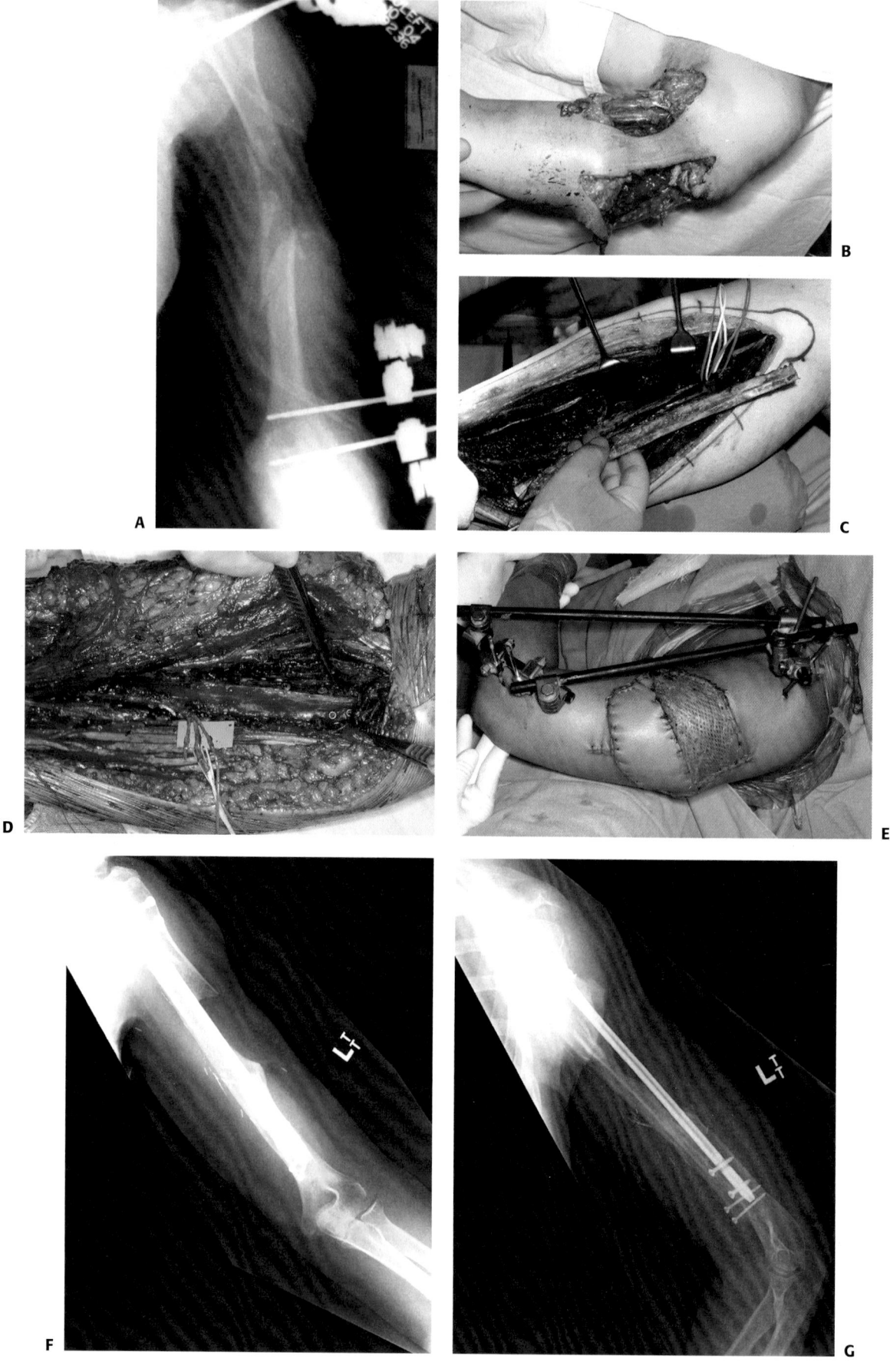

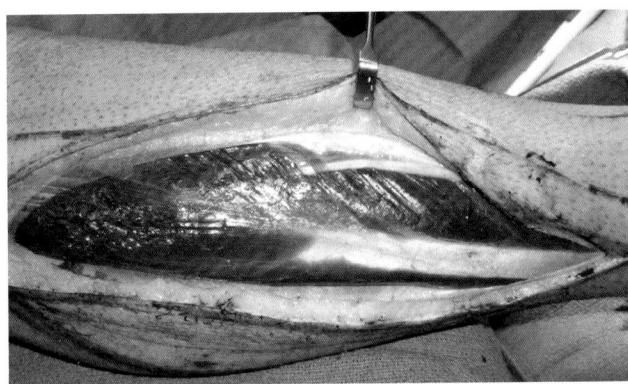

FIGURE 15-5 The superficial peroneal nerve is shown in the lateral compartment of the right leg during free fibula osteoseptocutaneous flap harvest.

posterior muscles. Minimizing dissection at the level of the fibular head will also help to avoid injury to the peroneal nerve.

Once the bone has been divided, the peroneal artery is identified distally deep to the tibialis posterior muscle and just dorsal to the FHL. The artery is divided and ligated distally. Dissection proceeds proximally to the peroneal-posterior tibial arterial bifurcation. Here the artery is ligated distal to the junction, preserving the posterior tibial artery. The surgeon should always verify the position of the tibial nerve and posterior tibial artery before ligation of the peroneal vessels.

If a skin paddle is taken with the fibular graft, a meshed skin graft is always used to cover the donor site; a tight primary closure can increase the risk of compartment syndrome within the donor leg and should be avoided. Meticulous closure of the donor site, with particular attention to the FHL muscle, is critical to decreasing donor limb morbidity. Patients are typically able to resume pain free weight-bearing ambulation 4 to 6 weeks after fibular harvest.

Bone fixation using a fibular graft needs to be performed with care as inadvertent screw placement can injure or avulse the pedicle or nutrient vessels. Plates applied to the surface of the fibula should use unicortical screws and ideally the plate and screws should be placed on the lateral surface of the fibula, away from the vascular pedicle. The periosteum at the bone/plate interface should not be stripped and only minimal periosteal stripping should be performed at the points of screw insertion. The bone-to-bone contact between the fibula and the recipient site can be maximized by creating step cuts, or the fibula can be telescoped into the recipient bone when the size is appropriate, such as the femur or humerus. Spanning plates are

ideal as they allow for firm fixation above and below the intercalated fibula, yet allow for unicortical purchase of the fibula for stabilization.[329]

Iliac Crest

The iliac crest receives a dual blood supply from the superficial circumflex iliac artery and deep circumflex iliac artery (DCIA).[315] Of the two, the DCIA system is most important.[296] Musculocutaneous perforators penetrating the abdominal wall 1 cm proximal to the iliac crest provide its nutrition. In the experience of several authors, the skin paddle has been less reliable than a standard groin flap, particularly if it is slightly rotated in relation to the underlying bone.[234,294] Its size, when based on the DCIA, is quite variable, ranging between 7 to 10 and 15 to 30 cm. The entire iliac bone, however, is well supplied by the DCIA via multiple perforating arteries at the points of muscle attachment.[260] It remains the pedicle of choice for osteocutaneous flaps, although double-pedicle flaps have been described using both the superficial and deep circumferential iliac vessels and may be desirable.[189]

Although the entire crest may be harvested, it has a practical limit of 10 cm in length as a vascularized graft because of its curved shape. It is relatively less suited for diaphyseal reconstruction than the fibula, as remodeling to tolerate weight bearing is prolonged. Further, osteosynthesis is difficult and weak.

Vascularized Periosteal Grafts

Periosteal grafts have been demonstrated experimentally to produce predictable new bone formation, provided they have adequate vascularity.[186,327] Bone formation after free vascularized transfer of periosteum may be enhanced by enclosing a cancellous bone graft in a periosteal wrap.[283] A variety of donor sites have been identified, including clavicle, fibula, ilium, humerus, tibia and femur, among others.[67,85,201,267] In the upper extremity, thin corticoperiosteal grafts and small periosteal bone grafts harvested from the supracondylar region of the femur have proved to be of great use, based on either the descending genicular or medial superior genicular artery and vein (Fig. 15-6). This graft is elastic and can be readily conformed to the shape of small tubular bones. It has been successfully used for clavicle, humerus, and forearm applications, including pathologic fractures from radiation necrosis and other recalcitrant nonunions.[85]

Vascularized Medial Femoral Condyle Structural Grafts

Vascularized bone grafts from the medial femoral condyle are particularly useful for treating fracture nonunion, which

FIGURE 15-4 **A, B:** A 44-year-old woman sustained a gunshot wound to the left humerus resulting in a large entrance and exit wound (greater than 15 cm each) with segmental bone loss of the humerus exceeding 10 cm in length. The fractures were temporarily stabilized with external fixation and the soft tissue defect addressed with an ipsilateral free latissimus dorsi flap. **C–E:** Once the soft tissues were stabilized, a free vascularized fibula was used to bridge the bony defect after an intramedullary nail had been placed. **F, G:** The fibula had incorporated into the proximal and distal ends of the humerus by 3 months, resulting in a salvaged and very functional upper extremity.

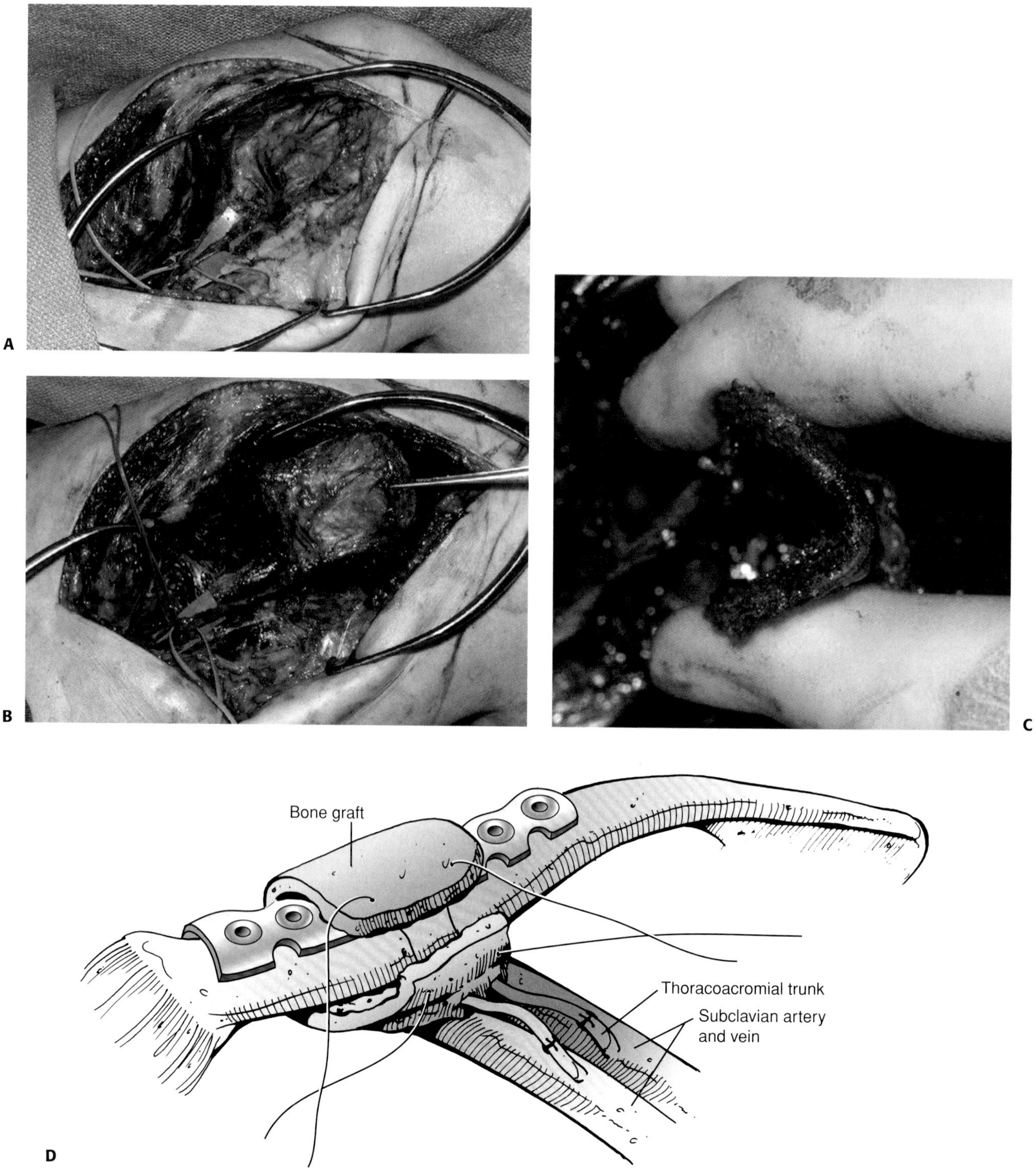

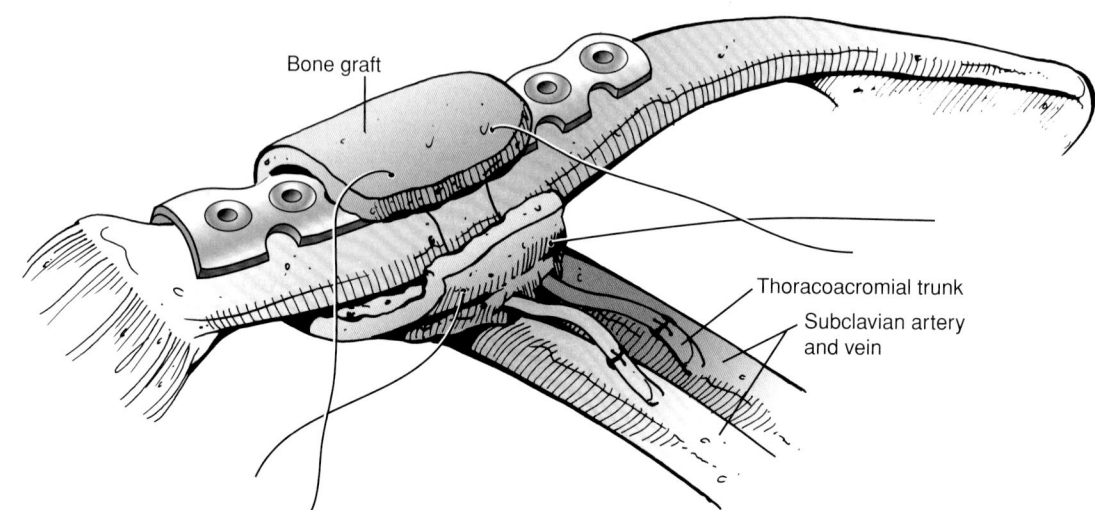

FIGURE 15-6 Medial femoral condyle corticoperiosteal grafts can be used to span shorter defects or be used to wrap around difficult fractures to provide a vascularized bone graft option. After elevating the vastus medialis, the medial femoral condyle is exposed to demonstrate a ring of periosteal vessels based on the descending genicular or medial superior genicular artery and vein **(A)**, a corticocancellous graft is elevated **(B)**. The graft is quite flexible and can be molded around the bones at the recipient site **(C, D)**.

often occurs in areas that are poorly vascularized. The medial femoral condyle has become a popular donor site as it provides a large quantity of cancellous bone graft of excellent quality and density with a robust blood supply, and it is technically straightforward to harvest.[169] The periosteum of the medial femoral condyle is supplied by the descending genicular artery (DGA) and the superomedial genicular artery (SGA).

The graft is harvested with the patient in the supine position and the leg externally rotated and flexed at hip and knee. A longitudinal incision is made along the posterior border of the vastus medialis extending proximally to the adductor hiatus. The vastus medialis is retracted anteriorly to expose the underlying descending genicular vessels, which emerge from the adductor hiatus proximally. Either the DGA or the SGA is used as the pedicle for the bone graft, depending on which is larger.[17] A bone graft up to 8 cm long and 6 cm wide can be harvested, with care taken to preserve the attachment of the periosteum to underlying bone. The size of the corticoperiosteal flap that can be harvested is limited anteriorly by the medial patellar facet, posteriorly by the posterior border of the femur, distally by the origin of the medial collateral ligament, and proximally by the flare of the medial femoral condyle.[108] Caution should be taken in harvesting larger bone grafts as this may result in fracture of the femur.

Vascularized medial femoral condyle bone grafts have been used successfully for the treatment of scaphoid,[169] clavicle,[108] metacarpal,[295] humerus, radius, femur, and tibial[17,54] nonunions, and have been found to result in faster bony union compared to distal radial pedicle grafts when used to treat scaphoid waist nonunions.[168]

Rib Plus Serratus and Latissimus Dorsi

The rib, although used in early reports,[139] is generally not suitable for upper extremity reconstruction because of its membranous, weak structure and curved shape. When based on its anterior internal mammary or supracostal arterial blood supply, only periosteal vessels are supplied.[139] The posterior rib graft, which includes its nutrient artery, requires ligation of the dorsal branch of the posterior intercostal artery. Because this vessel supplies the spinal cord, the potential for causing paraplegia exists. Further, dissection is difficult and usually requires a thoracotomy.

Composite vascularized bone grafts including a muscle flap with vascularized bone graft on a single pedicle have multiple advantages, including the ability to have a vascularized bone graft and then cover it with healthy muscle. One such vascularized bone graft and muscle flap composite graft is the rib, serratus anterior, and latissimus dorsi flap.[182,212,254,266,328,375] Based on the thoracodorsal vessel and its branches to the serratus and latissimus, up to two nonadjacent ribs can be harvested with the overlying serratus muscle which provides the vascularity to the bone. A significant length of rib can be harvested and by making a corticotomy on its concave side, the curved rib can be straightened to be applied to a long bone or long bone defect (Fig. 15-7). Hypertrophy of the ribs, in comparison to a fibular graft, does occur with time.

SOFT TISSUE RECONSTRUCTION
Classification of Soft Tissue Injury

Soft tissue injury may be of several varieties: Lacerations, abrasions, contusions, degloving injuries, and burns. In addition, soft tissue damage can occur in the absence of frank skin lacerations and can result in tissue damage that is even more extensive than that seen in open fractures.[336,337] Closed injuries that are associated with skin contusions, deep abrasions, burns, or frank separation of the dermal layer from the subcutaneous tissues have been classified by Tscherne et al. (Table 15-2).[336,337] Although not critically validated, this classification system has heightened our awareness of the importance of soft tissue injuries associated with closed fractures.

The mechanism of injury will also provide clues as to the severity of the underlying soft tissue injury. Penetrating injury will cause local and immediate surrounding tissue trauma; therefore, the surgical debridement required will typically be limited to the surrounding region of penetration. Blunt force resulting from motor vehicle crashes or falls will lead to more extensive soft tissue trauma and possible associated neurovascular injury with increased muscle contusion, devascularization, and necrosis. A ringer injury or press injury typically carries a poorer prognosis because of the amount of associated tissue damage. Electrical injuries associated with fractures may

(text continues on page 486)

TABLE 15-2	Classification of Soft Tissue Injury Associated with Closed Fractures
Grade 0	Minimal soft tissue injury, indirect injury causing simple fracture. A typical example is a spiral fracture of the tibia in a skiing injury.
Grade 1	Injury from within, superficial abrasion/contusion, resulting in simple or medium to severe fracture types. A typical example is a pronation–external rotation fracture-dislocation of the ankle joint, with soft tissue damage occurring from fragment pressure at the medial malleolus.
Grade 2	Direct injury with localized skin or muscle contusions, more extensive soft tissue injury or deep contaminated abrasions. Injury results in transverse or complex fracture patterns. A typical example is a segmental fracture of the tibia from a direct blow by a car fender. Imminent compartment syndrome also falls in this group.
Grade 3	Severe degloving with destruction of subcutaneous muscle and/or subcutaneous tissue, extensive skin contusions. Fracture patterns are complex. This grade includes manifest compartment syndrome and vascular injuries.

Adapted from: Tscherne H, Gotzen L. *Fractures with Soft Tissue Injuries*. Berlin: Springer-Verlag; 1984 and Tscherne H, Oestern HJ. Die Klassifizierung des Weichteilschadens bei offenen und geschlossenen Frakturen. *Unfallheilkunde*. 1982;85:111–115.

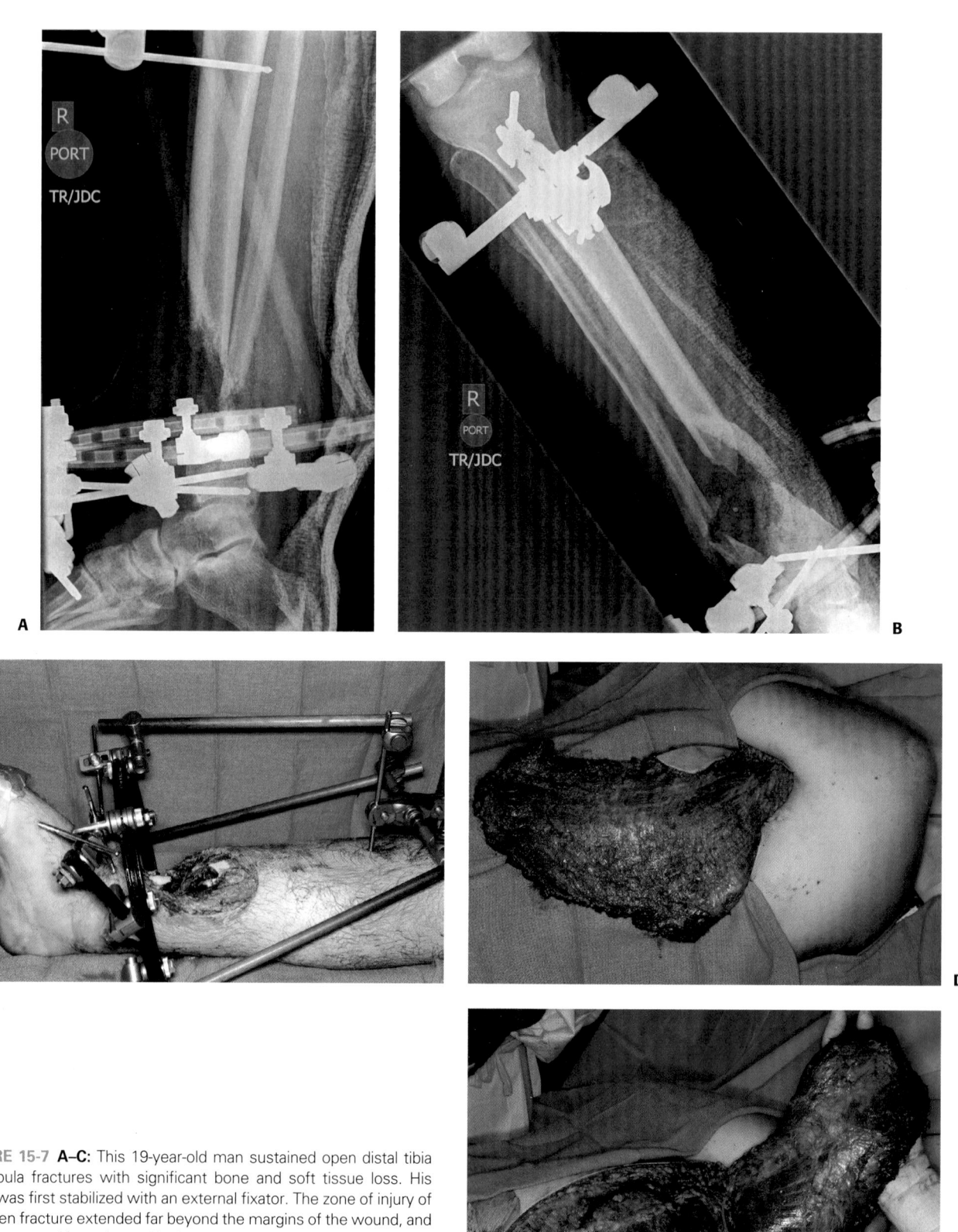

FIGURE 15-7 **A–C:** This 19-year-old man sustained open distal tibia and fibula fractures with significant bone and soft tissue loss. His injury was first stabilized with an external fixator. The zone of injury of the open fracture extended far beyond the margins of the wound, and with segmental bone loss, skin loss, and extensive soft tissue injury, the decision for a composite rib, serratus, and latissimus flap was made. The latissimus was raised with a cutaneous paddle **(D)** and after elevation, the serratus and its branch of the thoracodorsal artery and vein were identified over the fourth and sixth ribs **(E).**

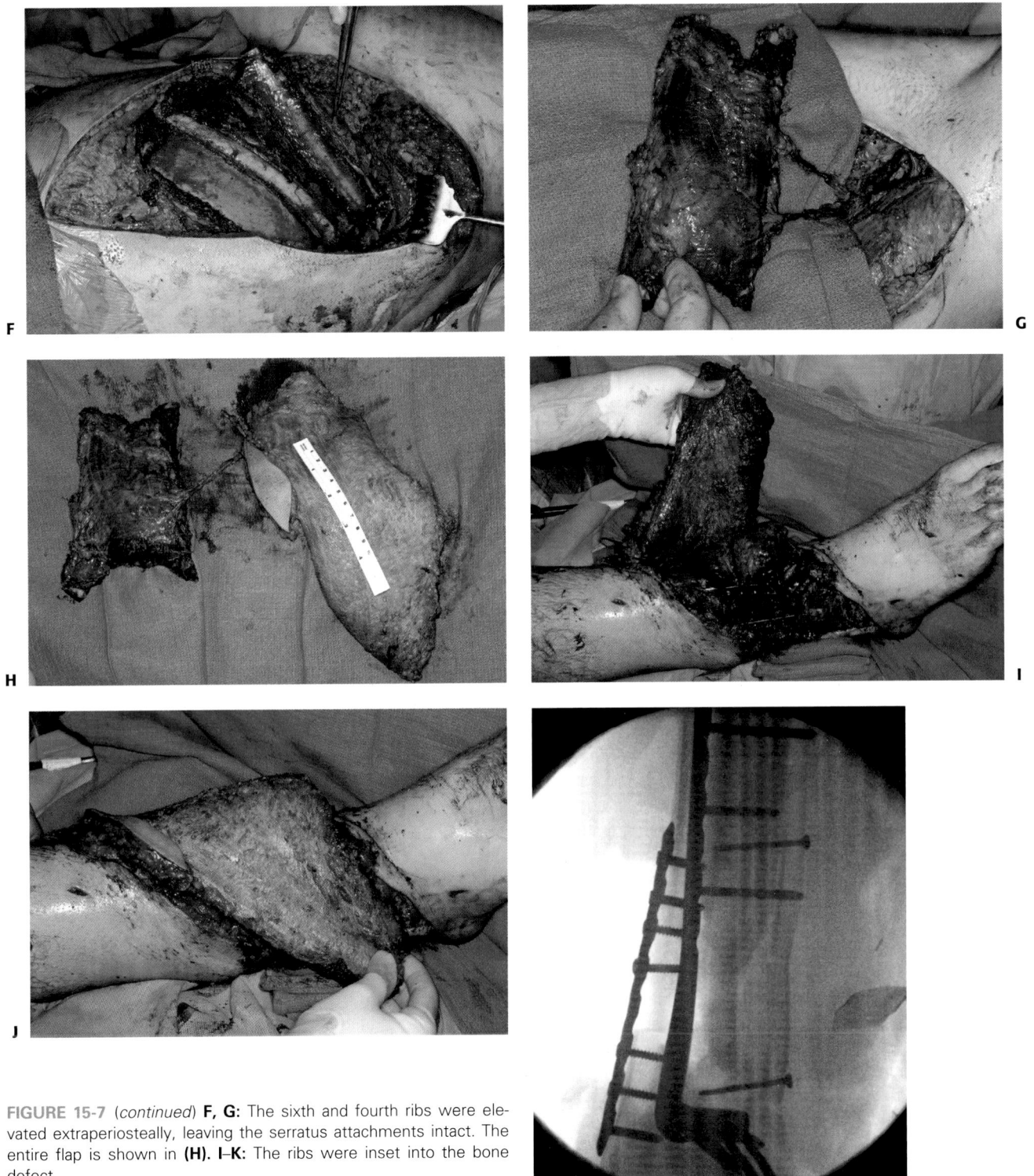

FIGURE 15-7 (*continued*) **F, G:** The sixth and fourth ribs were elevated extraperiosteally, leaving the serratus attachments intact. The entire flap is shown in **(H). I–K:** The ribs were inset into the bone defect.

(*continues*)

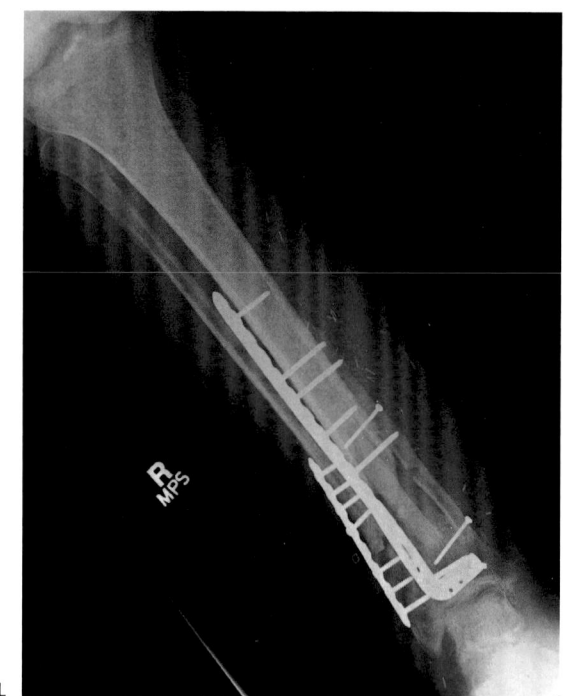
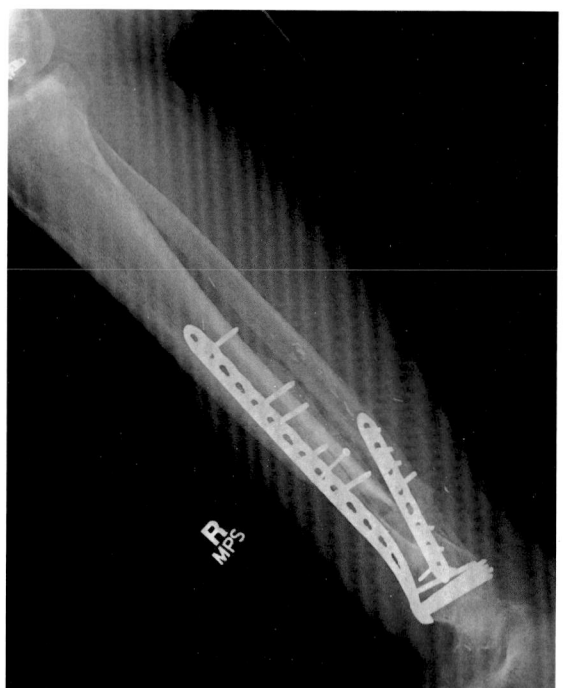
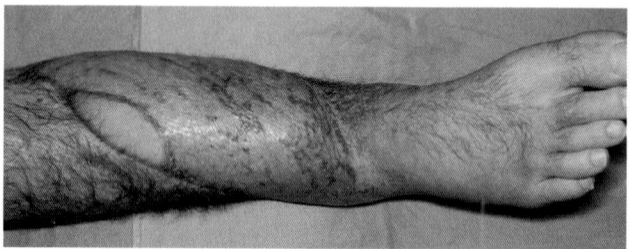

FIGURE 15-7 (continued) **L–N:** Seven months after reconstruction, the flap has contoured nicely and there was consolidation of the ribs to the tibia.

appear innocuous but will always be associated with significant underlying soft tissue damage.

Wound Healing

To fully appreciate the nature of the soft tissue injury the surgeon must have some understanding of the normal wound healing process. Surgically induced wounds heal in several stages. The wound passes through phases of coagulation, inflammation, matrix synthesis and deposition, angiogenesis, fibroplasia, epithelialization, contraction, and remodeling. These processes have been divided into three main stages: Inflammation, fibroplasia, and maturation. Interruption in any of these stages can lead to wound healing complications.[165]

The inflammatory phase of wound healing involves cellular responses to clear the wound of debris and devitalized tissue. Increased capillary permeability and leukocyte infiltration occur secondary to inflammatory mediators and vasoactive substances. Inflammatory cells clean the wound of harmful bacteria and devitalized tissue. Fibronectin and hyaluronate deposition from fibroblasts in the first 24 to 48 hours provides scaffolding for further fibroblast migration.[96,318]

The fibroblast proliferation phase starts within the first 2 to 3 days as large populations of fibroblasts migrate to the wound.

Secretion of a variety of substances is necessary for wound healing and includes large quantities of glycosaminoglycans and collagen. Collagen levels rise for approximately 3 weeks corresponding to increasing wound tensile strength. After 3 weeks the rate of degradation of collagen equals the rate of deposition. Angiogenesis is an important aspect of the fibroblast proliferation phase, as it helps to support new cells in the healing wound.

The maturation phase starts at around 3 weeks lasting up to 2 years. It is characterized by collagen remodeling and wound strengthening. Collagen is the principal building block of connective tissue and is found in at least 13 different types. Early wounds are composed of a majority of type III collagen. As the wound matures, type III collagen is replaced by type I collagen. Collagen cross-linking improves tensile strength. There is a rapid increase in the strength of the wound by 6 weeks as the wound reaches 70% of the strength of normal tissue. The wound then gradually plateaus to 80% of normal strength, but never returns to preinjury levels.[165]

Wound re-epithelialization occurs as adjacent cells migrate through a sequence of mobilization, migration, mitosis, and cellular differentiation of epithelial cells. Wound contraction starts at about 1 week. It is facilitated by the transformation of certain fibroblasts into myofibroblasts. These cells adhere to the wound margins as well as to each other and effect contraction of the wound. These stages are imperative for proper wound healing, as interruption of these processes results in chronic wound complications.[96,318]

Large wounds, or wounds incapable of primary healing, heal through a process of "secondary wound healing," which is dominated by wound contraction and re-epithelialization. If infection, ischemia, or ongoing trauma inhibit the wound from completing the re-epithelialization process, it will then enter into a protracted inflammatory state.[266] In these chronic wounds the environment is predominated by neutrophils with the increased production of proteolytic enzymes.[81] In most situations a chronic wound must be converted to a clean acute wound through the process of surgical debridement for healing to occur. Surgical debridement re-establishes a normal healing environment, allowing the wound to heal through primary or secondary intention.

Debridement

Debridement is the cornerstone of success for the management of any traumatic wound. Adequate debridement requires the complete removal of foreign material and devitalized tissue. Inadequate debridement can promote wound infection, delay surgical healing, and attenuate the inflammatory response.

Careful wound evaluation and wound debridement should take place as soon as possible after the injury, under general anesthesia in the operating room. Debridement performed in the emergency room or on the ward is often inadequate, as it is limited by poor lighting and inadequate patient analgesia. Debridement in the operating room also allows the surgeon to have on hand the appropriate surgical tools for the removal of devitalized bone and soft tissue and to obtain hemostasis.

For all trauma patients, the surgeon must determine the "zone of injury," which refers to the area throughout which trauma has occurred. The extent of the zone of injury is not always apparent on initial assessment, particularly in degloving, crush, and electrical injuries. If one cannot assure complete excision of all necrotic tissue, soft tissue and bony reconstruction should be postponed and a second debridement planned within 24 hours. The need for fasciotomy should be considered at the first debridement. Injuries sustained in an agricultural setting or in industrial machinery are subject to heavier and deeper contamination. Mechanical roller injuries involving crushing, avulsion, or degloving will also result in more severe tissue damage and have a worse prognosis than blunt trauma or guillotine-type injuries.[33,125,126,179] Such injuries should routinely undergo serial debridements over the course of 48 hours to ensure that all devitalized tissue is removed before soft tissue reconstruction begins.

After sharp debridement, all wounds should be irrigated to remove additional loose debris and decrease bacterial contamination. Several different solutions are available for irrigation. Antibiotic solutions (bacitracin, neomycin, and polymyxin) and detergents (Castile soap, benzalkonium chloride) are used by many surgeons in an attempt to minimize infection rates. Although wound irrigation with antibiotic solutions has been effective in some experimental studies,[82,284] there is still a lack of convincing clinical data that it provides a benefit over soap lavage alone.

High pressure flow, although beneficial for decreasing bacterial counts, should be used prudently. When using high pressure irrigation, one should avoid driving foreign material further into the wound bed, hydrodissection of uninjured areas, and tissue insufflation.[113,232] High pressure irrigation should be utilized judiciously in the hand, as the water jet can injure or avulse nerves or digital vessels. In such cases, copious amounts of gravity fed irrigation in conjunction with careful debridement will suffice.

Newer debridement devices have been designed to exert variable pressure throughout the debridement process. Devices such as the Versajet Hydrosurgery System (Smith and Nephew, USA) use a controlled fluid jet that allows for precise debridement over tendons in addition to gross debridement of acute and chronic wounds.[39,187,303] In a prospective trial, this device has been shown to decrease operative times and allow for increased precision during the debridement process.[122]

Inadequate debridement can often result from the surgeon's concerns over wound closure. If the surgeon is at all concerned about wound closure, early consultation with a plastic surgeon or other wound management specialist should be carried out to allow for a multidisciplinary approach to wound management. Such collaborations will allay concerns and allow for an aggressive initial debridement minimizing late wound complications.

Debridement of Acute Wounds

The first step in any major reconstructive effort is an adequate debridement. With each debridement the surgeon's goal should be to remove all foreign and necrotic tissues. Wound debridement and careful wound evaluation should take place as soon as possible after the injury, under general anesthesia in the operating room. The debridement process starts with a careful wound scrub using a surgical brush and sterile soap or iodine solution, followed by irrigation with 4 to 8 L of sterile saline, ideally heated to 37°C to avoid excessive cooling of the patient. If there is excessive bleeding, a tourniquet may be inflated before the irrigation process.

Important structures including nerves and vessels should be identified, marked, and protected before sharp debridement of the nonviable soft tissues. Major motor nerves should never be debrided, but rather dissected from necrotic tissue and preserved. Free bony fragments that are completely denuded of soft tissue attachments, and therefore avascular, should be removed from the wound. Avulsed parts can often be used as a source of "spare-parts" for wounds requiring skin grafting or flap closure, and this option should always be considered before discarding them.[32] After debridement, the final assessment of tissue viability must be made with the tourniquet deflated.

Skin that is insensate, and does not blanch or bleed at the wound edges should be removed. Clotted venules are a sign of skin devitalization and they should be debrided with the surrounding skin and soft tissue. Healthy muscle is bright red and shiny and will contract when grasped with the forceps. If there is any question regarding muscle viability it may be stimulated with the electrocautery; if there is no evidence of contraction, it should be debrided.

If the surgeon has removed all foreign material and devitalized tissue, immediate reconstruction can be considered. Clean surgical instruments, ideally on a separate operating tray, should be used for any immediate reconstructive procedure, as it has been shown that instruments used for debridement can carry a bacterial concentration in excess of 10^3 organisms.[14] If one cannot assure complete excision of all necrotic tissue, reconstruction should be postponed and a second debridement planned within 24 hours. Debridement should continue at 24- to 48-hour intervals until the wound is clean and ready for reconstruction.

Debridement of Chronic Wounds

As discussed, a chronic wound is a wound that has failed to progress through the normal stages of healing and remains arrested in the inflammatory stage.[14,165] In traumatic cases, such wounds exist because of an infection associated with a retained sequestrum, hardware, or other foreign material. To allow these wounds to heal, all necrotic and infected materials must be removed before any attempt at soft tissue reconstruction. Thus, one must turn the chronic wound into an acute wound through the process of thorough debridement. The one caveat to this recommendation is the removal of hardware that is providing critical and stable fracture fixation. If the application of an external fixator is not possible, hardware can be maintained within an infected field until more definitive fixation is possible or bony healing has occurred, providing systemic antibiotics have been administered and the hardware is covered with well-vascularized tissue.[38,279]

Chronic wounds present a greater challenge, as vital structures are often hidden within scar and granulation tissue. Debridement must be extended beyond the zone of injury, into normal tissue, to ensure complete resection of all contaminated tissue. Use of a tourniquet early in the case is important to best visualize and avoid injury to vital structures such as nerves and blood vessels. The tourniquet should be released before closure or dressing application to confirm the removal of all devascularized tissue.

A centripetal approach should be used working from superficial tissues to deep, from the margins to the center of the wound. Every effort is made to preserve nerves and blood vessels crossing the zone of injury. If nerves must be transected, they should be tagged with dyed monofilament suture and documented in the operative records so that they may be more easily identified during later wound debridements or reconstructive efforts. Tissue from the wound should always be sent for bacterial cultures as well as pathologic analysis to rule out the possibility of osteomyelitis or vasculitis.[14]

Adjuvants to Debridement

Management of the wound between debridements is an issue of some debate. Normal saline wet to dry dressings have been the most common form of wound dressing after surgical debridement. They help to prevent soft tissue desiccation and obliterate dead space, and the dressing changes provide an opportunity for continuous surveillance of the wound, in addition to providing excellent mechanical wound debridement. One disadvantage is patient discomfort with dressing changes, which may be alleviated by moistening the gauze before removal. For contaminated wounds immediately after injury, Dakin solution or Betadine solution may be used judiciously. Dakin solution is bacteriostatic and Betadine is bactericidal. Their use is controversial, especially if used for more than 3 days, because of soft tissue toxicity and their negative effects on wound healing.[18,190] In cases of established infection, the application of topical antibiotics such as silver sulfadiazine, Sulfamylon (mafenide acetate), and silver nitrate has been shown to reduce bacterial counts.[103,194] For *Pseudomonas* infections, 0.25% acetic acid may be used to reduce surface bacterial counts. Consultation with an infectious disease specialist is recommended in such cases.

The advantage of all these forms of dressing changes is that they ensure consistent monitoring of the wound site. This is in contrast specifically to the use of a VAC device, in which the sponge is commonly not changed for 2 to 4 days, thus preventing wound surveillance by the surgeon who will be performing the reconstruction.

Emollient-type soft tissue coverage with various wound gels, semipermeable films, or even antibiotic impregnated ointments may be used in cases in which there has been avulsion of the dermal surface but without damage to the underlying muscle. The dressings may take the form of a hydrogel, antibiotic impregnated gauze, or a simple semipermeable film. Semipermeable films and semiocclusive hydrogels are impermeable to water and bacteria but permeable to oxygen and water vapor. Occlusive hydrocolloids are impermeable to even water vapor and oxygen. Thus these dressings are not as useful in wounds that require mechanical debridement or wounds that are exudative because of accumulation of fluid under them.

Vessels and nerves that are exposed in the wound should always be covered with a nonadherent gauze or hydrogel dressing to protect them until soft tissue coverage can be obtained. Nerve repairs and blood vessel repairs should be covered with local soft tissue, immediately after repair, to allow for a moist healing environment, as opposed to gauze dressings.

Vacuum-Assisted Closure

If the wound is clean and wound reconstruction is not going to be performed immediately, whether because of concomitant life-threatening injuries or other medical issues, a negative pressure dressing can be used until definitive closure. A wound VAC can help to remove surrounding edema, decrease local metalloproteinases and other inhibitors of wound healing while promoting angiogenesis.[11,253]

The VAC consists of an open polyurethane ether foam sponge, in some cases impregnated with silver for more contaminated cases, sealed by an adhesive drape and attached to suction. All pores in the sponge communicate so that negative pressure applied to the sponge by the suction is applied equally and completely to the entire wound surface. The effects of the

VAC on the wound are multiple. The application of negative pressure causes the sponge to collapse toward its center. Traction forces are thus applied to the wound perimeter pulling the wound edges together progressively making the wound smaller. The VAC sponge should be cut to fit inside the wound to maximize these traction forces on the wound edges. The sponge should not overlap intact skin, as skin maceration may occur. In addition, the VAC removes wound edema fluids, and it appears to increase circulation and decrease bacterial counts (see Fig. 15-2).[253]

The use of the VAC in traumatic lower extremity wounds has been associated with a decreased requirement for skin grafting, free tissue transfers, and flap coverage.[74,99] Herscovici et al. reported on 21 patients, 16 of whom had lower extremity wounds because of high-energy trauma. At the time of initial presentation, all wounds "would have required flap coverage"; however, after an average of 19 days of VAC treatment, 12 of the wounds no longer required flap procedures to achieve wound coverage.[143]

Vacuum-assisted therapy must be used with caution over tendons and nerves, as continuous suction can produce desiccation and injury to these structures. When neurovascular structures are exposed, local tissue or flap coverage should be performed in an urgent or emergent manner to prevent desiccation. If wounds remain contaminated despite surgical debridement, wet to dry dressing changes can be performed every 8 hours until the next scheduled surgical debridement or until the wound is clean enough to accept a VAC device.

Hyperbaric Oxygen Therapy

Hyperbaric oxygen therapy (HBOT) involves the intermittent inhalation of 100% oxygen in specialized chambers at pressures greater than that at sea level (>1 atmosphere absolute, ATA). Typical protocols recommended by the Undersea and Hyperbaric Medical Society (UHMS) for treating wounds expose the patient to pressures of 2 to 2.5 ATA lasting 90 to 120 minutes per session for approximately 40 treatments. Oxygen tensions can approach 500 mm Hg in soft tissue and 200 mm Hg in bone.[178]

Traumatized and osteomyelitic limbs and bones have been shown to be hypoxic, with a partial pressure of 20 to 25 mm Hg in animal models, and thus oxygen content can be dramatically raised under hyperbaric conditions.[219] The hypoxic conditions in the diseased bone reduce the ability of neutrophils to generate the reactive oxygen species necessary to kill bacteria. Hyperbaric oxygen (HBO), therefore, enhances bactericidal activity by increasing oxygen tension in tissues.[21] The processes of collagen synthesis and osteogenesis are also inhibited in a hypoxic state, and studies have suggested that improved oxygen tension can normalize, if not enhance, these functions.[188] A review of 57 studies examining HBOT[350] concluded that it had potential beneficial adjunctive effects for conditions such as chronic non-healing diabetic wounds, compromised skin grafts, osteoradionecrosis, soft tissue radionecrosis, gas gangrene, and chronic osteomyelitis. However, the definitive value of HBOT remains to be determined through prospective randomized trials.

TIMING OF SOFT TISSUE RECONSTRUCTION

The timing of soft tissue reconstruction in the trauma setting is often debated, and different authors have advocated different time scales including immediate (emergency) closure,[214] early closure (before 5 days), and delayed closure (6 to 21 days).[80] In our opinion, the requirements for wound closure should be no different when dealing with primary closure, pedicled flaps, or free tissue transfer; wounds must be free of necrotic tissue and infection. There is experimental and clinical evidence that quantitative bacteriology obtained immediately before wound closure correlates with the likelihood of subsequent infection.[44,64] Breidenbach and Trager[31] evaluated 50 free tissue transfers carried out for complex wound closure in the extremities to determine predictors of subsequent infection, and found that quantitative cultures had the highest positive-predictive value (89%), negative-predictive value (95%), sensitivity, and specificity. Mechanism of injury, type and degree of contamination, wound location, and systemic factors such as diabetes, corticosteroid use, immunosuppression, advanced age, and malnutrition also affect the likelihood of clinical infection.

In 1986, Godina published the results of 532 free flaps used for extremity reconstruction. In that study, he was able to reduce the postoperative infection rate in patients with open fractures to 1.5% in a subset of patients undergoing reconstruction within 72 hours.[118] Many subsequent studies support these data, and when free tissue transfer is to be used, reconstruction within 5 days of the injury is a commonly adopted guideline. This approach has been extrapolated into the general practice of trauma reconstruction. "Emergency" free flap reconstruction in the upper limb (within 24 hours of injury) potentially can allow for earlier rehabilitation and a quicker resolution of the inflammatory response after trauma. Several authors have reported successful series of emergency free flaps in the upper extremity.[48,214,256] Nevertheless, no prospective comparative studies have examined the benefits of very early versus later coverage with regard to outcome or functionality. In contrast, studies have shown that flap reconstruction performed beyond the frequently quoted critical interval of 72 hours with or without temporary VAC coverage yields results similar to those of immediate reconstruction within the first 3 days.[176,319]

Yaremchuk[373] proposed that treatment of the severely injured lower extremity be done in four distinct phases: (i) emergency evaluation, orthopedic stabilization, and debridement of obviously devitalized structures and tissues; (ii) wound management with serial debridement; (iii) soft tissue coverage; and (iv) delayed bone reconstruction. Soft tissue coverage and bone reconstruction may be performed simultaneously using osteocutaneous flaps. In summation, a wound should be closed when it is clean. The quicker the wound is made clean, the sooner reconstruction may occur. When the surgeon is sure all necrotic material has been removed from the wound, then reconstruction should proceed.

WOUND COVERAGE OPTIONS

Once the wound is clean and the decision for limb salvage has been made, definitive bony fixation and wound coverage may proceed. Wound coverage may be obtained by multiple means, including primary closure, local flaps, and free tissue transfer. As experience and success with free tissue transfer has increased, surgeons have moved away from the classic reconstructive ladder and now opt to reconstruct defects with more complex procedures if they can provide a more rapid and complete reconstructive solution.[225] The most common reconstructive techniques will now be discussed in detail.

Skin Grafting

Skin grafting involves the transfer of the most superficial epidermal and dermal elements of the skin to a new location where the graft is capable of re-establishing blood flow. Skin grafts may be taken as split thickness (including only part of the dermis) or full thickness (including all of the dermis).[231] Full-thickness grafts have greater *primary* contracture rates (the amount the graft rolls or shrinks initially once it is harvested) because of a higher percentage of elastin retained within the graft; however, full-thickness grafts are less likely to contract *secondarily* (after healing has occurred) because of greater preservation of the deep dermal architecture when compared with split-thickness grafts.[300,347] Return of sensation is also superior when compared with split-thickness grafts.[4]

Split-thickness grafts have fewer dermal components and thus undergo less primary contracture but have greater secondary contracture rates. Because of high secondary contracture rates, split-thickness grafts should be avoided over joints (Fig. 15-8). Split-thickness grafts are more likely to take over compromised beds as compared with full thickness grafts.[65] The split-thickness graft donor site heals through a process of re-epithelialization and contraction as keratinocytes migrate out of retained hair follicles within the donor site.[19,298] In contrast, the full graft donor site heals by primary intention.

Skin grafts require a well-nourished tissue bed to survive and will not do well in an area of frank infection or when placed on tendon devoid of paratenon, bone, or cartilage. In wounds in which these structures predominate, local, regional, or free tissue transfers are required for successful wound closure. In addition, skin grafting should be avoided in areas that may require secondary surgery for bone or nerve grafting. The greatest risks for graft failure include infection, shearing, motion at the graft site, seroma or hematoma accumulation beneath the graft, and finally poor wound bed vascularity.[231]

Skin grafts survive for the first several days through a process called serum imbibition. During this stage of healing, the graft obtains nutrients from the underlying wound bed through a diffusion process. This commonly occurs in the first 24 to 48 hours. After this point the skin graft undergoes revascularization through an ingrowth of capillary buds primarily from the wound bed.[22,62,63] Clinically most grafts are adherent to the wound bed by the fourth to fifth postoperative day.

The wound bed or recipient site must be debrided and clean before attempts at skin grafting. Infection is one of the leading

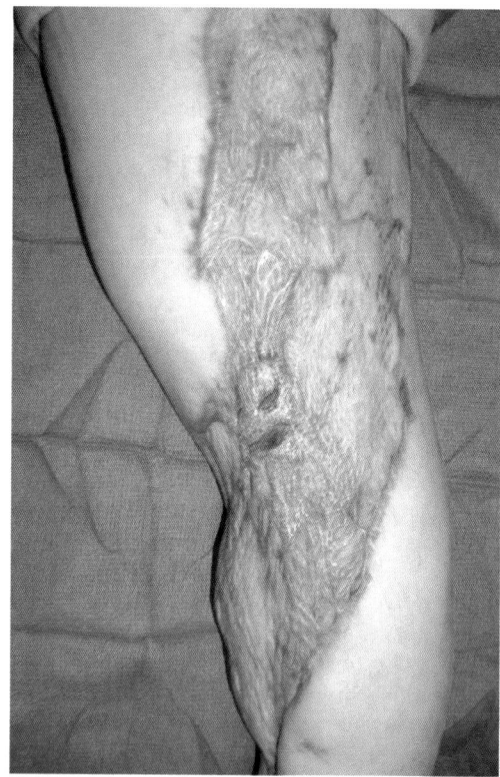

FIGURE 15-8 Late effects of skin grafting over the popliteal fossa. Although the wound is healed, the split-thickness skin graft has not provided durable coverage and is subject to chronic breakdown with knee extension.

causes of skin graft failure. Because skin grafts are completely dependent on the wound bed they are transplanted to for nutrition, they possess no intrinsic ability to resolve infection.[192]

Tissue expansion may have a role in resurfacing healed skin grafted wounds subsequently to optimize the aesthetic result but it has no role in acute coverage of wounds.

Flaps

Classification of Flaps

A flap consists of tissue transferred from one anatomic location to another. The flap may be based on a random or axial pattern blood supply. Random flaps have no named or defined blood supply. They are raised in a subdermal or subfascial plane and rely on the subdermal vascular plexus of the skin for circulation. To ensure adequate circulation, random flaps should be limited to a length no greater than 2.5 times the width of their base, which is the uncut border of the flap. This ratio may be even more limited in poorly perfused extremities. Varied random pattern flaps include z-plasty, four flap z-plasty, rhomboid flap, banner flap, V-Y advancement flaps, and rotational flaps.

Axial pattern flaps can be raised pedicled regional flaps or used as a free tissue transfer. The flaps can contain more than one type of tissue. Fasciocutaneous flaps contain skin and the underlying fascia, musculocutaneous flaps contain skin, fascia, and muscle, and osteocutaneous flaps contain bone, fascia, and skin.

Muscle flaps are classified on the basis of five patterns of muscle circulation.[227] A muscle for free tissue transfer must be able to survive on one vascular pedicle that is dominant and that will support the entire muscle mass. The classification (with examples) is as follows.

Type I: One vascular pedicle (extensor digitorum brevis or tensor fascia latae)

Type II: One dominant pedicle and minor pedicles (gracilis muscle)

Type III: Two dominant pedicles (rectus abdominis muscle)

Type IV: Segmental vascular pedicles (sternocleidomastoid)

Type V: One dominant pedicle and secondary vascular pedicles (latissimus dorsi, pectoralis major)

Animal studies have shown that muscle flaps are able to control a 10-fold higher bacterial count than fasciocutaneous flaps, and improve antibiotic delivery to the wound site.[37] Although the potential antimicrobial advantages of muscle flaps have also been demonstrated clinically, a recent study by Yazar et al.[374] comparing lower limb wounds reconstructed with free fasciocutaneous or free muscle flaps in a total of 177 cases showed no difference in outcomes or infection rates. This highlights the important role of adequate debridement, regardless of the type of flap used.

Free Flaps

The coverage of traumatic wounds of the extremities has historically been accomplished with the use of pedicled, local, or distant rotational flaps. However, when defects are very large or encompass multiple structures including nerve, bone, or muscle, the use of composite free tissue transfer provides a reliable and single stage means of reconstruction.

The benefits of free tissue transfer within the extremity include the transfer of additional vascularized tissue to the injured area, the ability to carry vascularized nerve, bone, skin, and muscle to the injured area in one procedure, and the avoidance of any additional functional deficits to the injured limb that may be incurred with the use of a local or pedicled flap. Free flaps are not tethered at one end, as is the case for pedicled laps, and this allows for more freedom in flap positioning and insetting. More recently developed fasciocutaneous and perforator flaps also allow for primary closure of donor sites with minimal sacrifice of donor site muscle. With current microsurgical techniques free flap loss rates range between 1% and 4% for elective free tissue reconstruction.[16,180] The upper extremity is particularly suited for free tissue transfer as the majority of recipient blood vessels utilized for anastomosis are located close to the skin, and are of relatively large caliber.

Major indications for free tissue transfer include: (i) the primary coverage of large traumatic wounds with exposed bone, joint, tendons, or hardware; (ii) the coverage of complex composite defects requiring bone and soft tissue replacement; (iii) the coverage of soft tissue deficits resulting from the release of contractures or scarring from previous trauma; and (iv) the coverage of extensive burns or electrical injuries.[191,205,206,286,297]

There are few absolute contraindications for free flap transfer within the upper and lower extremities, and in many cases free tissue transfer may be the only option for limb salvage after severe soft tissue loss. Despite this, *relative contraindications to free tissue transfer* include a history of a hypercoagulable state, a history of a recent upper extremity deep venous thrombosis, and evidence of ongoing infection within the traumatic defect. Other contraindications would include an inadequate recipient vessel for flap anastomosis. Disregarding technical error, the status of the recipient vessel used for flap anastomosis may play the greatest role in flap failure; recipient vessels within the zone of injury are prone to postoperative and intraoperative thrombosis. Recipient vessels for microvascular transfer ideally should be located out of the zone of injury, radiation, or infection. Petechial staining of the adventitia, a ribbon-like appearance of the recipient vessels, and poor flow at the time of arteriotomy are all suggestive of vessel injury, and alternative vessels should be chosen as recipient vessels for microvascular anastomosis. In rare cases, arterial-venous fistulas may be created proximally within the upper extremity or axilla using the cephalic or saphenous vein. These fistulas can be brought into the zone of injury and divided to provide adequate inflow and outflow for a free tissue transfer.[210] Commonly used recipient vessels in the upper extremity are the thoracodorsal, thoracoacromial, circumflex scapular, transverse cervical, brachial, circumflex humeral, superior ulnar collateral, radial collateral, ulnar, radial, and digital vessels.[359] Common recipient vessels in the lower extremity are the superficial femoral, the popliteal, the posterior tibial, and the anterior tibial arteries.[207]

The choice of flap should take into account both functional requirements and the surgeon's experience. Muscle flaps are useful for large three-dimensional defects when soft tissue bulk is necessary; however, direct coverage of tendons with muscle flaps encourages dense adhesions limiting postoperative tendon excursion. In general, fascial or fasciocutaneous flaps are more useful for coverage of exposed tendons and areas in which a gliding tissue plane needs to be preserved.

SOFT TISSUE RECONSTRUCTIVE ALGORITHMS BY REGION

Lower Extremity Reconstructive Options

Lower extremity reconstruction has historically followed an algorithm that is based on the location of the defect (Table 15-3). The gastrocnemius muscle flap has been used to cover defects around the knee and proximal tibia; the soleus muscle flap has been used to cover defects within the middle third of the tibia, and free flaps have been reserved to cover defects overlying the lower third of the tibia and ankle. Nonetheless, with continuing advancements in microsurgery, there are now several reliable fasciocutaneous flaps and free flaps that may be used for proximal and distal defects in addition to the standard options. An overview of the standard options will be provided with a subsequent explanation of newer approaches for soft tissue coverage.

TABLE 15-3	Reconstructive Options for the Lower Extremity
Pelvis/groin	Rectus abdominis muscle Rectus femoris muscle Transverse rectus abdominis myocutaneous flap Tensor fascia lata Free flap
Thigh	Pedicled anterolateral thigh flap Rectus abdominis muscle Rectus femoris muscle Tensor facia lata Vastus lateralis Gracilis Sartorius Free flap
Knee/proximal third of tibia	Gastrocnemius muscle Reversed anterolateral thigh flap Anterior tibial perforator flap Free flap
Middle third of tibia	Soleus Free flap
Lower third of tibia/ankle	Free flap Sural artery island flap Posterior tibial perforator flap Posterior tibial flap Reverse soleus muscle flap
Foot/dorsum	Free flap Sural artery island flap
Foot/plantar	STSG/FTSG Free flaps Medial plantar island flap Abductor hallucis muscle

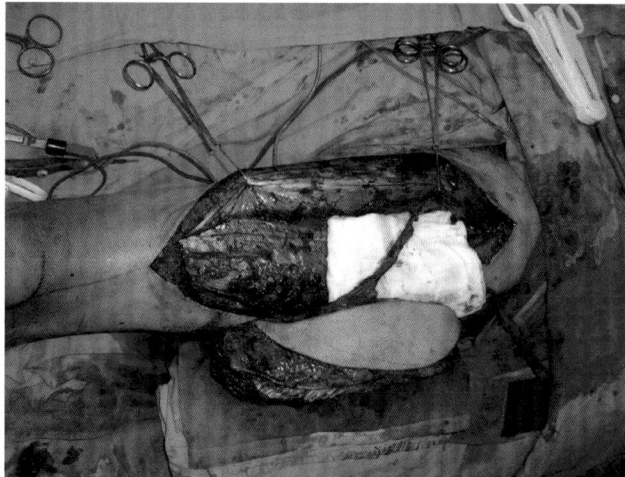

FIGURE 15-9 Anterolateral thigh flap with a vastus lateralis muscle component prior to pedicle division.

Upper Thigh, Groin, and Pelvis

Wounds within the pelvis and upper thigh rarely require flap coverage. The bone in this area is covered with enough soft tissue that most defects can be covered with skin grafts. Should the size of the defect prohibit primary closure or skin grafting, the rectus abdominis or the rectus femoris muscle flap may be used in a pedicled fashion to cover most defects in this region. The anterolateral thigh (ALT) flap and tensor fascia lata muscle can also be used to cover wounds surrounding the femur and the greater trochanter.

Anterolateral Thigh Flap

The ALT flap is a versatile flap harvested from the anterolateral region of the thigh. It is most often used as a free flap for lower third injuries in the leg or for reconstruction in the upper extremities, but it may also be pedicled to cover defects in the groin and thigh. Its blood supply is through the descending branch of the lateral femoral circumflex artery. Several branches of this vessel supply the overlying skin. These skin vessels are either septocutaneous or they take a course through the vastus lateralis muscle before supplying the skin.[196] Inclusion of the lateral femoral cutaneous nerve allows for the flap to become

sensate. The length of the pedicle is approximately 8 cm, but it can have a longer effective length when the skin paddle is designed so that the perforator is eccentrically located. The flap is easy to design and can be as large as 40×20 cm (Fig. 15-9). The skin is relatively pliable and the flap can be thinned to a great degree without compromising the blood supply. This flap can also be used as a flow-through flap that maintains distal blood supply in the extremity,[9] which is particularly useful in extremities that have compromise of one or more vessels.[110,224]

The ALT flap can be dissected to include a variety of tissue components such as muscle (vastus lateralis or rectus femoris), fascia, and skin in a variety of combinations.[52] It has disadvantages such as a color mismatch (when reconstructing defects in distant locations) and the presence of hair in some patients. When large defects are reconstructed, skin grafts are required at the donor site. Donor site morbidity is minimal when the donor site is closed primarily, and some residual functional deficit is sometimes noted when a large skin graft is required.[195] If necessary the flap can be thinned down to a 5-mm thickness. This allows for an aesthetically appealing reconstruction while providing a tendon gliding surface when necessary.

The ALT flap can also be harvested as an adipofascial flap for areas with adequate skin but a lack of soft tissue. This type of flap can then be buried or skin grafted. When reconstructing lower extremity defects, the flap is designed with a variation in tissue types tailored to the recipient site requirement. Certain areas such as the foot and ankle will require thin cutaneous flaps, whereas other areas will require more tissue bulk. For defects closer to the thigh such as the groin or knee, a pedicled flap can be elevated with the pedicle based proximally or distally. A distally based pedicled ALT flap is based on retrograde blood flow from the descending branch of the lateral femoral circumflex artery with the pivot point greater than 2 cm above the knee. Longer pedicle length can be achieved by designing the flap more proximally on the upper thigh.

This flap is also extremely useful in lower extremity reconstruction.[261,262,376] Areas such as the foot and ankle, which require a pliable thin flap for defect coverage, can be covered with a cutaneous flap. Harvested as a myocutaneous flap, it can be used to cover amputation stump defects. A strip of fascia lata can be incorporated with the flap and used for tendon reconstruction.[46] For areas with exposed bone or extensive soft tissue loss, the cutaneous portion is often adequate for reconstruction[147]; however, if necessary, a myocutaneous flap can be used.

Knee and Proximal Third of Tibia

Proximal third tibial injuries and injuries around the knee may be covered with the medial or lateral gastrocnemius muscle flap. These flaps may be used in conjunction with each other for large defects. The medial head of the gastrocnemius will cover the *inferior thigh, knee, and proximal tibia* and is more frequently used than the lateral head as it is larger in size. The lateral head may also be used alone or in combination with the medial head for coverage of *lateral knee defects and lateral distal thigh* wounds. The tendinous inferior margin of the gastrocnemius muscle may be used to augment the repair of an injured quadriceps tendon. For coverage of extremely large defects, or in situations in which compromise of the gastrocnemius muscles will hinder ambulation, a free flap can be used for proximal third coverage. Other nonmicrosurgical options for proximal third coverage include the reverse ALT flap.

Gastrocnemius

The gastrocnemius muscle is located in the superficial posterior compartment and its function is to flex the knee and plantar flex the foot. It has two heads, which lie superficial to the soleus. It is dispensable only if the soleus muscle is intact. Its blood supply is via the medial and lateral sural arteries, which are branches from the popliteal artery. This is a type I muscle and the pedicle length is 6 cm. Ideally, only one head of the gastrocnemius is needed for a reconstruction around the knee; however, both heads may be used, depending on the reconstructive requirements. Each head is considered a separate unit for the purpose of flap design. The medial head is longer and its muscular fibers extend more inferiorly. The distal soleus tendon unites with the gastrocnemius to form the Achilles tendon. For defects at the level of the midportion of the tibia, the gastrocnemius may not provide adequate coverage and the soleus muscle is preferred for coverage.

Contraindications to the use of the gastrocnemius muscle flap include active infection and/or significant disruption of the soft tissue and/or vascular pedicle. Additional contraindications for the flap include any procedure or injury that may have traumatized or injured the sural artery, such as a previous repair of a popliteal arterial laceration or repair of a popliteal aneurysm. Occasionally, severe compartment syndromes may render the muscle fibrotic and unusable for transfer.

Although the medial and lateral heads of the gastrocnemius can support a skin paddle, a paddle is not commonly used because of its unreliability and the limitation in size of the skin. The medial gastrocnemius is dissected through a posterior midline incision. The sural nerve and lesser saphenous vein are two key landmarks that are seen superficial to the muscle belly and preserved. The muscle fascia is split, and the junction

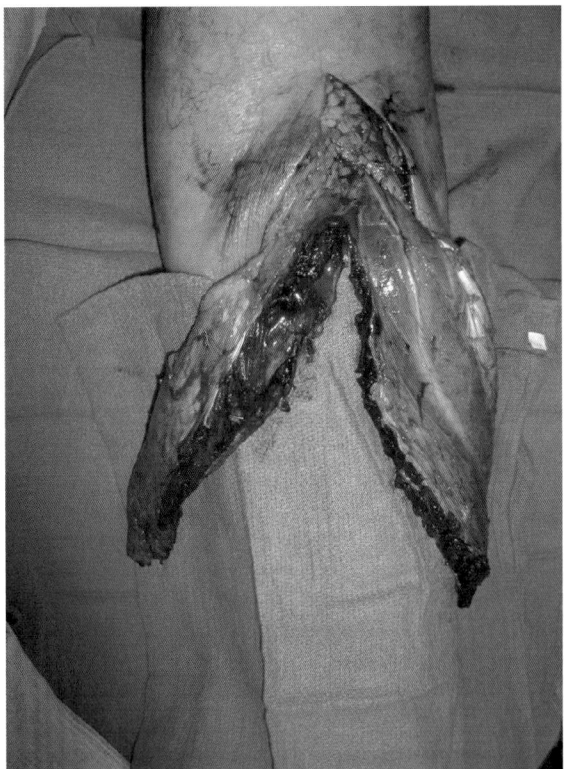

FIGURE 15-10 Gastrocnemius muscle flap after separation of the medial and lateral heads along the raphe.

between the two heads is incised (Fig. 15-10). Blunt dissection in the plane between the gastrocnemius and the soleus is gently done with the finger. The superficial dissection is then performed, and the muscle is transected distally with a cuff of tendon attached for use in fixation to the wound edge. The tunnel through which the muscle is passed should be of adequate size so as to not constrict the blood supply of the flap. To expand the muscle area, the fascia may be incised, with careful attention being paid to not injure the underlying muscle. The flap may be used as an advancement flap to cover part of an amputation stump or upper tibial defects, or as a cross leg flap.

Middle Third of Tibia

Historically the soleus has been the muscle of choice for reconstruction of middle third tibia defects; however, we use this flap sparingly, and often opt for free tissue coverage in this area, especially if there is comminution of the bone.[53] There are several factors that may prohibit the successful transfer of the soleus muscle: (i) the size of the defect, (ii) the status of the muscle, and (iii) the status of the surrounding tissue and bone.[200] The standard soleus flap can cover most defects under 75 cm². Large defects occupying the majority of the middle third and lower third of the leg are best covered with a free tissue transfer. The soleus can be used in conjunction with the medial or lateral gastrocnemius muscles for larger defects spanning the upper aspect of the leg, but doing so will compromise active plantar flexion.

Because the soleus muscle is closely adherent to the deep posterior surface of the interosseous membrane, tibia, and fibula, it can often be traumatized with comminuted fractures of the tibia and fibula. Often, during initial wound evaluation and debridement, the muscle can be inspected through the soft tissue defect. If the muscle is extensively lacerated by fracture fragments or contains a significant amount of intramuscular hematoma, one should use another flap for soft tissue coverage. In addition, any associated injury to the popliteal, peroneal, or posterior tibial arteries can adversely affect the survival of the soleus muscle.[200]

Soleus

The soleus muscle is a type II muscle, with dominant pedicles from the posterior tibial, popliteal, and peroneal arteries and minor segmental pedicles from the posterior tibial artery. The muscle originates from the posterior surface of the tibia, the interosseous membrane, and the proximal fibula. It lies in the superficial posterior compartment deep to the plantaris muscle and distally joins the gastrocnemius muscle as the conjoined, Achilles tendon. It is a bipennate muscle with the medial and lateral muscle bellies each receiving an independent neurovascular supply; this allows the lateral and medial portions to be mobilized independently while preserving some function of the remaining soleus muscle. The medial head originates from the tibia and receives the majority of its blood supply from the posterior tibial artery. The lateral head originates from the fibula and receives the majority of its blood supply from the peroneal artery. Typically the soleus muscle is used as a proximally based flap (Fig. 15-11). Dividing the muscle longitudinally at the level of the septum allows for the elevation of medial and lateral hemisoleus flaps; however, the proximal dissection is typically more tedious because the distinction between the two heads is often not clear.

In the distal one-third of the muscle, the soleus receives segmental arterial perforators from the posterior tibial artery. These distal perforators may be absent in up to 26% of patients; in these cases distal perfusion to the muscle is provided by axial blood flow from more proximal perforators. The diameter and position of these distal perforators is variable but, if present and of large enough caliber, they can allow for a portion of the muscle to be harvested in a reverse fashion (Fig. 15-12).

Knee and ankle motion may begin once the skin graft is adherent to the underlying muscle bed. Weight-bearing status is determined by the stability of the underlying fractures. In a study by Hallock of 29 soleus flaps, 24 were used for coverage of high-energy impact defects. All of the flaps in this study were based on a proximal pedicle. The complication rate was low (13.8%) and there were no cases of total flap loss.[131] Similar results were found by both Pu and Tobin,[217,332] when using a proximally based flap.

Distal Third of Tibia/Ankle

Free tissue transfer has historically been recommended for lower third tibia coverage; however, other nonmicrosurgical options for soft tissue closure of ankle defects include the reversed soleus flap (described above) and the sural artery flap.

Sural Artery Flap

The distally based sural artery flap is perfused by reverse flow through the anastomosis between the superficial sural artery and the lowermost perforator of the peroneal artery. This flap has

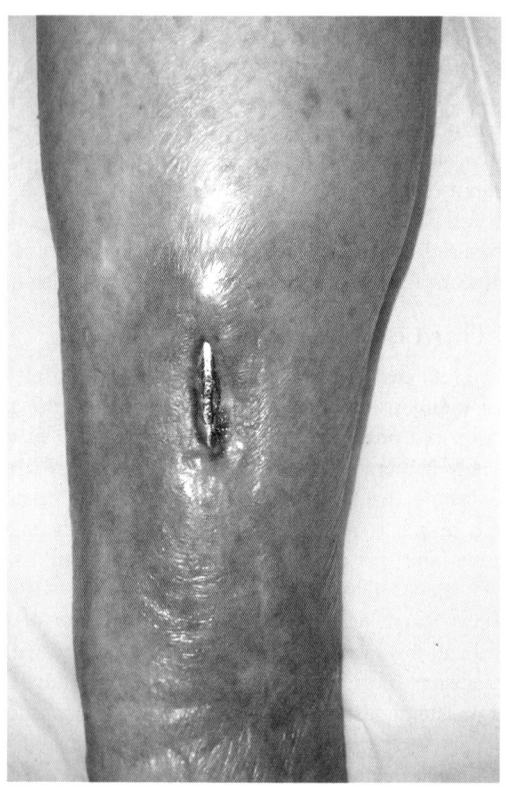
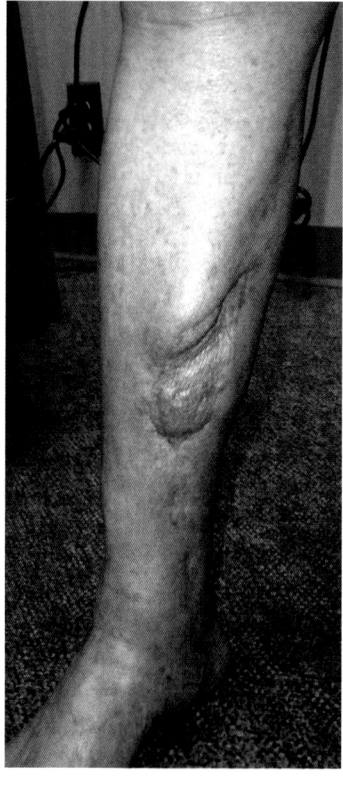

FIGURE 15-11 A medial hemisoleus flap was used to cover this healed infected tibia fracture in a 75-year-old diabetic woman after the hardware was removed. **A:** Preoperative image. **B:** Postoperative view at 6 months. The infection is resolved, and the patient is ambulating without difficulty.

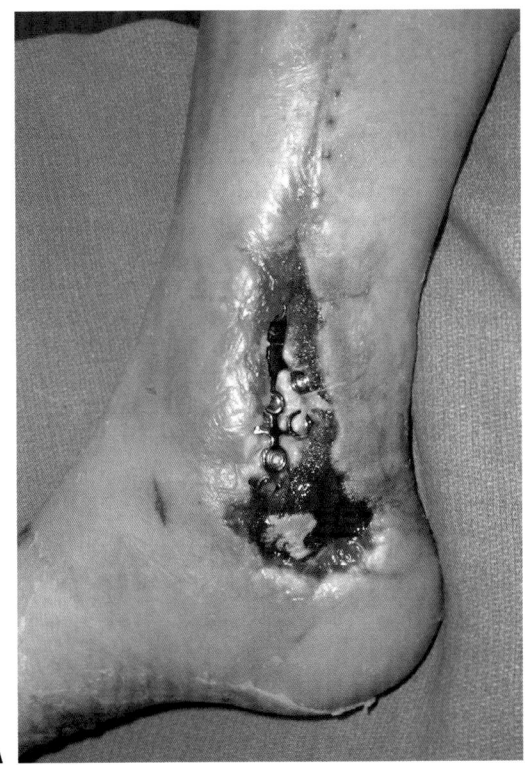

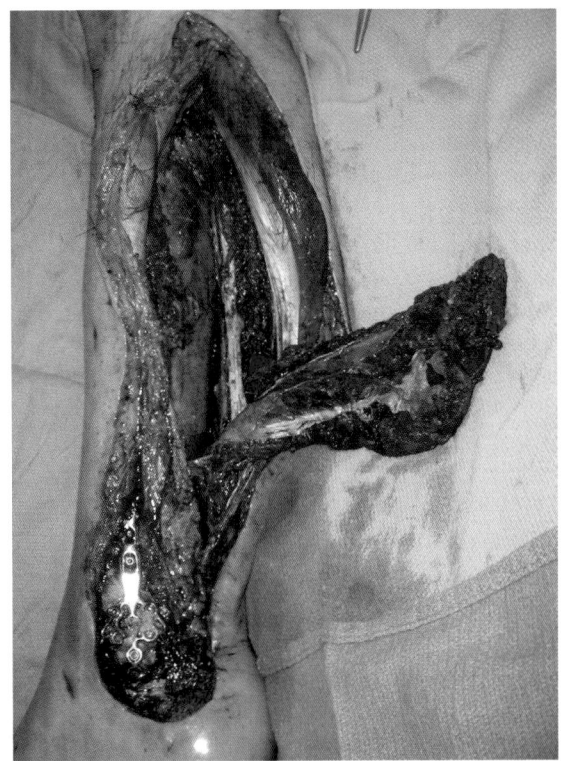

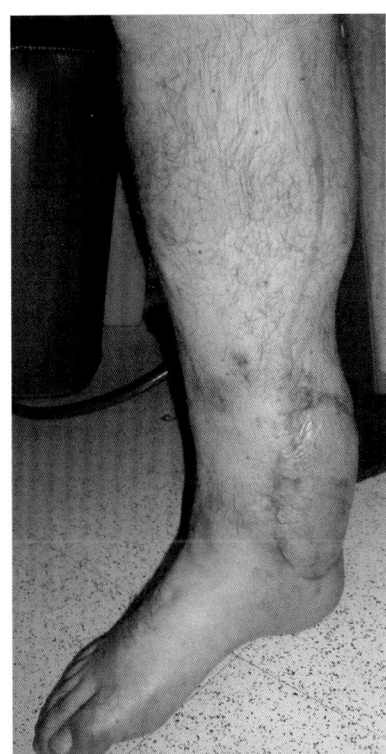

FIGURE 15-12 **A:** An infected Gustilo IIIB distal tibia-fibular fracture after open reduction and internal fixation. **B:** Intraoperative view shows the raised, distally based right hemisoleus flap. Blue markers indicate the distally based perforating vessels from the posterior tibial artery. **C:** One year after surgery, the wound is healed.

been used for the successful coverage of defects of the posterior and inferior surface of the heel, the Achilles tendon, the middle and distal one-third of the leg, the dorsum of the foot, and the medial and lateral malleoli. The flap is contraindicated in patients with destruction of the vascular pedicle or the lowermost perfo-

rator of the peroneal artery. Sacrifice of the sural nerve results in hyposensitivity of the lateral border of the foot and a higher rate of complications may be anticipated in patients with comorbid conditions such as peripheral vascular disease, diabetes mellitus, and venous insufficiency. In this patient population, a delay procedure (wherein the flap is incised along its boundary but not elevated until a subsequent second surgery 2 to 3 weeks later, to optimize blood supply through its pedicle) may be performed to increase its survival rate.

Many different methods have been described for flap harvest all in an effort to decrease its main problem of vascular congestion. Our technique is as follows.

- The patient is placed in the prone position

- An axial line is drawn from the superior aspect of the lateral malleolus to the midpoint of the popliteal flexion crease. The skin island, at least 2 to 3 cm distal to the popliteal flexion crease, is centered on this axis and planned according to defect size.

- The pivot point of the subcutaneous pedicle is at least three finger breadths (4 to 6 cm) superiorly from the superiormost aspect of the lateral malleolus.

- The subcutaneous pedicle should be at least 3 to 4 cm wide and the skin raised over the subcutaneous pedicle must be very thin so as to not injure the pedicle.

- Dissection is performed in a plane deep to the fascia with an incision isolating the skin paddle and dividing the proximal blood supply if a delay is not planned (Fig. 15-13).

- The distally based sural flap is then transferred to the recipient site usually with the division of the intervening skin bridge to alleviate any possible compression of the subcutaneous pedicle.

- Skin grafts are used liberally over the flap pedicle and at the donor site of the flap.

Postoperatively, the most important issue is prevention of congestion or compression of the vascular pedicle. This can be achieved either by an adequately elevated position of the leg and/or by the use of conventional splints with a gap over the flap; however, some authors prefer the use of external fixation devices that serve to not only immobilize the limb, but also obviate the need for tight compressive dressings. External fixation also allows the treatment of concomitant fractures and prevents the development of an equinus deformity as well as facilitating elevation of the limb.

Surveillance of flap perfusion in terms of arterial as well as venous flow must be performed regularly during the first several postoperative days. Capillary refill should be tested every several hours in the postoperative period so that interventions may be made to prevent flap loss. A revision procedure should be performed if any signs of poor arterial perfusion or venous congestion are identified. The administration of anticoagulants in the postoperative period after pedicled flap reconstruction remains controversial; however, we commonly will use anticoagulation therapy such as heparin and/or aspirin in mildly congested flaps reserving leech therapy for those with more significant congestion.[50,241] If serious compromise of the flap is evident, the flap may be laid back in the donor site bed as a last resort, in essence creating a delayed flap.

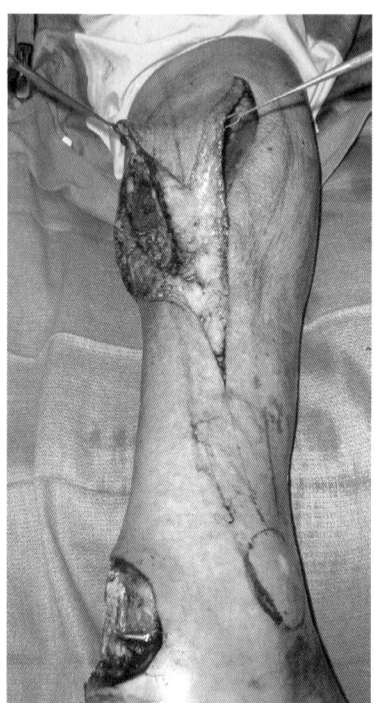
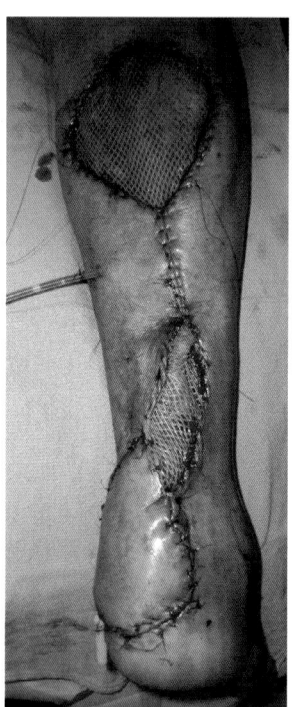
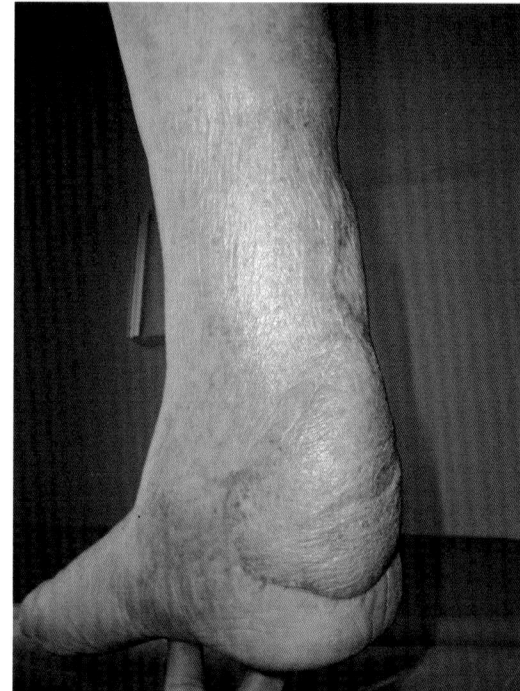

A   **B**   **C**

FIGURE 15-13 **A:** Intraoperative view of a distally based sural flap being raised for coverage of a calcaneal wound. Note the superior skin bridge has not been divided. **B:** Intraoperative view of the distally based sural flap at the time of flap inset with division of the skin bridge over the pedicle and liberal use of skin grafts over the pedicle of the flap and the donor site. **C:** View of the healed distally based sural flap 16 months postoperatively.

The patient should be at complete bed rest for approximately 4 to 5 days after the procedure with a gradual dangling protocol of the limb to assess tissue tolerance. If signs of significant edema or venous compromise are evident in the flap tissue after 10 to 15 minutes of dangling the extremity, bed rest with elevation should be prolonged for several more days until the flap can tolerate the dependent position. Donor site morbidity is generally low, with the most common finding being sural nerve neuroma and scarring. Neuromas that are painful and significantly distressing to the patient may be resected and the nerve stump buried in the gastrocnemius muscle.

Foot/Dorsum

Most dorsal foot wounds may be treated with a split-thickness skin graft if there is no exposed tendon or bone. Local toe fillet flaps are capable of covering smaller distal defects. Transmetatarsal amputation may be considered if there is extensive concomitant injury to the toes. In such cases, the plantar surface can be advanced to cover the remaining dorsal defect. When tendon or bone is exposed, free tissue transfer provides the most reliable means of durable coverage and preserves the remaining foot function. Smaller defects can be treated with the sural artery flap.

Foot/Plantar

Free flaps are good options for heel wounds as well as defects covering the majority of the plantar surface of the foot. Another option for heel coverage is the medial plantar artery flap, which provides sensate coverage of heel defects without the need for microsurgery. This flap is based on the medial plantar artery. The sural artery flap can also be extended to cover moderate-sized heel defects (Fig. 15-14).

Free Flaps for Lower Extremity Coverage

We have found the latissimus dorsi muscle, gracilis muscle, ALT, and scapular flaps to be the most versatile for lower extremity coverage. For osteocutaneous defects, we most frequently use a free fibular flap or a fibular flap in combination with a latissimus dorsi muscle flap. For moderate-sized ankle defects the gracilis

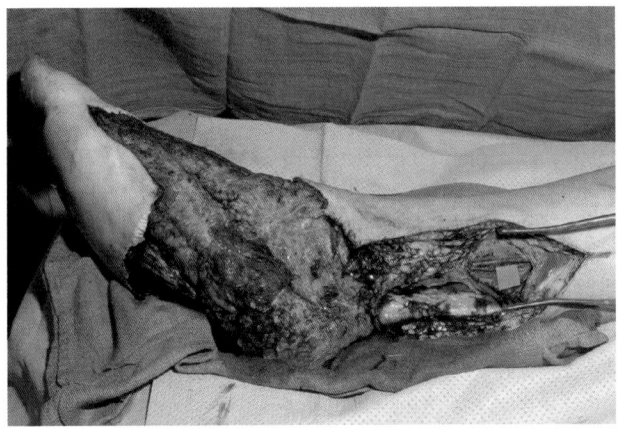
A

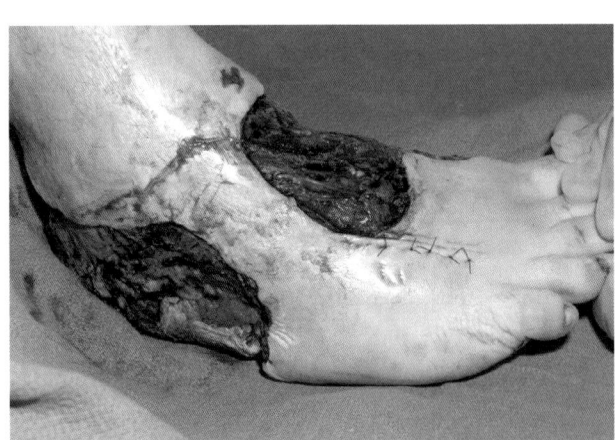
B

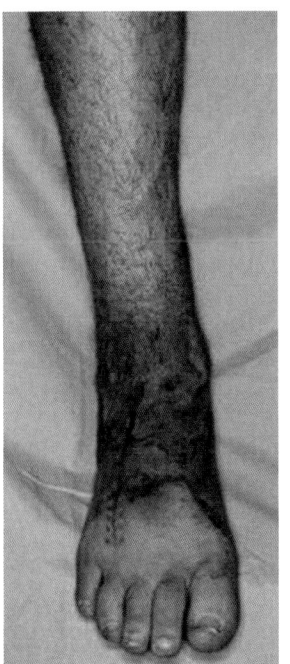
C

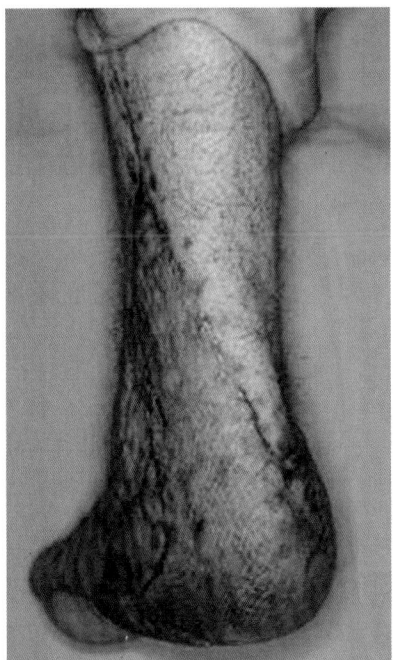
D

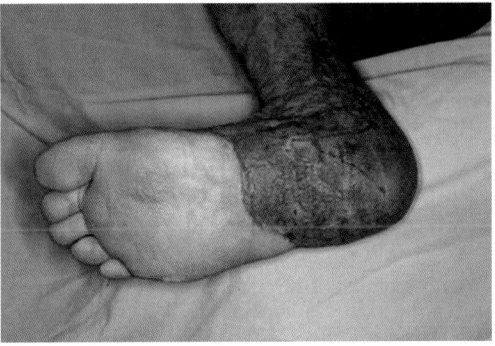
E

FIGURE 15-14 Small- to moderate-sized foot and ankle defects can be covered with the sural artery flap. **A:** This 55-year-old man has developed wound breakdown following ankle fracture fixation. **B:** The sural artery flap is harvested and pedicled to cover the defect. **C:** The donor site is skin grafted. **D, E:** The flap allows for thin pliable coverage of the area and will eventually allow for normal shoe wear.

muscle is our flap of choice as it produces minimal donor site morbidity and can be contoured nicely to the malleolar region and will not interfere with normal shoewear.

Latissimus Dorsi

The latissimus dorsi has proved to be a very reliable muscle for coverage of soft tissue defects for the chest, shoulder, and elbow. The muscle provides a workhorse flap for extremity coverage and is based on the thoracodorsal artery as the major pedicle and on branches of the intercostals and lumbar arteries as secondary segmental vessels. It is a type IV muscle and has a pedicle length of 8 to 12 cm, which can be obtained by dissecting the thoracodorsal vessels proximally toward the axillary artery and vein. Its innervation is the thoracodorsal nerve, which is a direct branch of the brachial plexus, and it enters the muscle 10 cm from the apex of the axilla. It is important to identify the anterior border of the muscle preoperatively by having the patient contract the muscle with the hand supported on the hip in a standing position. Preoperative marking of the skin over the posterior–superior iliac spine and the scapular tip is helpful also.

The indication for the use of this flap is to cover a large skin and soft tissue defect that cannot be managed with local flaps. Contraindications for flap use include previous injury, or in some cases, axillary lymphadenectomy. Breast cancer surgery, in particular, axillary node dissection, may injure the nerve or arterial supply, rendering the muscle fibrotic and inadequate for transfer.

The latissimus dorsi flap may be harvested as not only a muscle flap but also a musculocutaneous flap. A muscle flap covered with a split-thickness skin graft is often less bulky and can seal deep defects (Fig. 15-15), whereas musculocutaneous flaps give better aesthetic reconstruction because the skin paddle can conform to the skin texture of the surrounding tissues, particularly when it is used as a pedicled flap.

Technique

The patient under general anesthesia is placed in a lateral decubitus position with an axillary roll. Dissection is most easily accomplished beginning from the anterior border of the muscle, and this method allows early pedicle identification. If a skin paddle is chosen, then it may be oriented along the muscle fibers with care being taken to center the paddle on the muscle belly. If no skin paddle is selected, the skin flaps are elevated commonly parallel to the muscle fibers to expose the muscle origins and insertions. The muscle is released from the lumbosacral fascia and iliac crest. The pedicle is identified and the serratus branch is then divided so that the muscle may be reflected toward the axilla. Pedicle dissection should be performed with loupe magnification (2.5× or greater). If performing a functional muscle transfer, marking sutures should be placed along the long axis of the muscle to allow adequate tension adjustment at the recipient site. The muscle can be split longitudinally into halves based on the medial and lateral branches of the thoracodorsal artery, which bifurcate upon entering the muscle.

Upon dissection of the neurovascular pedicle, the insertion of the muscle at the humerus is divided. Additional distal cov-

erage, if it is being used as a pedicled flap for extremity reconstruction, can be obtained by releasing its insertion from the intertubercular groove of the humerus as well. When the latissimus dorsi flap is transferred as a free flap, the vascular pedicle is divided at the juncture with the axillary artery and vein to obtain the maximum pedicle length. Large suction drains should be left beneath the skin flaps and in the axilla to avoid postoperative hematoma or seroma problems. Frequently there is difficulty elevating the flap simultaneously with donor site preparation, particularly when it is used for upper extremity reconstruction. In addition, if used as a musculocutaneous flap it may be excessively thick in obese patients.

Donor site seroma is the most common complication after harvest of a latissimus dorsi flap. Seromas can be relieved with frequent aspiration and compressive garments. Scarring over the donor site is inevitable, and endoscopic harvest can be entertained to minimize subsequent scarring.[366] Total flap necrosis is rare when used as a pedicled flap; however, partial flap necrosis because of an inconsistent blood supply to the lower third of the muscle is not uncommon. Bleeding at the distal edge of the flap should be checked when it is elevated. Kinking and tension on the pedicle can cause a disturbance of flap circulation and must be recognized immediately.

Rectus Abdominis

The rectus abdominis muscle may be harvested with the patient in the supine position. This vertically oriented, type III muscle (two dominant vascular pedicles), extends between the costal margin and the pubic region and is enclosed by the anterior and posterior rectus sheaths. The superior blood supply is from the superior epigastric artery, which is a continuation of the internal mammary artery. Distally the blood supply is from the inferior epigastric artery, which is a branch of the external iliac artery. The pedicle length is 5 to 7 cm superiorly and 8 to 10 cm inferiorly. Because of the larger size of the inferior epigastric artery and the venae comitantes, it is more commonly used as a free tissue transfer. Large defects of the thigh, where local soft tissues are either not sufficient in area or unusable because of radiation, for example, may be covered with pedicled rectus muscle only or myocutaneous flaps (Fig. 15-16).

The motor innervation is supplied by the seventh through twelfth intercostal nerves that enter the deep surface of the muscle at its middle to lateral aspects. The size of the muscle is up to 25×6 cm^2. The skin territory that can be harvested is 21×14 cm^2 and its blood supply is based on musculocutaneous perforators. The donor site created via the fascial incision in the anterior rectus sheath to access a muscle-only flap may be closed primarily with a running or interrupted absorbable or nonabsorbable suture on a tapered needle. When harvesting a myocutaneous flap, a portion of the anterior rectus sheath is taken with the flap and a mesh or biologic implant may be used to reinforce the closure of the abdominal wall fascia to prevent hernia or bulge. Drains are commonly used under the raised skin flaps after muscle harvest. An abdominal wall binder may be used to aid in postoperative recovery in cases of a free tissue transfer. Although the rectus abdominis muscle is considered a workhorse flap, its popularity has decreased slightly because

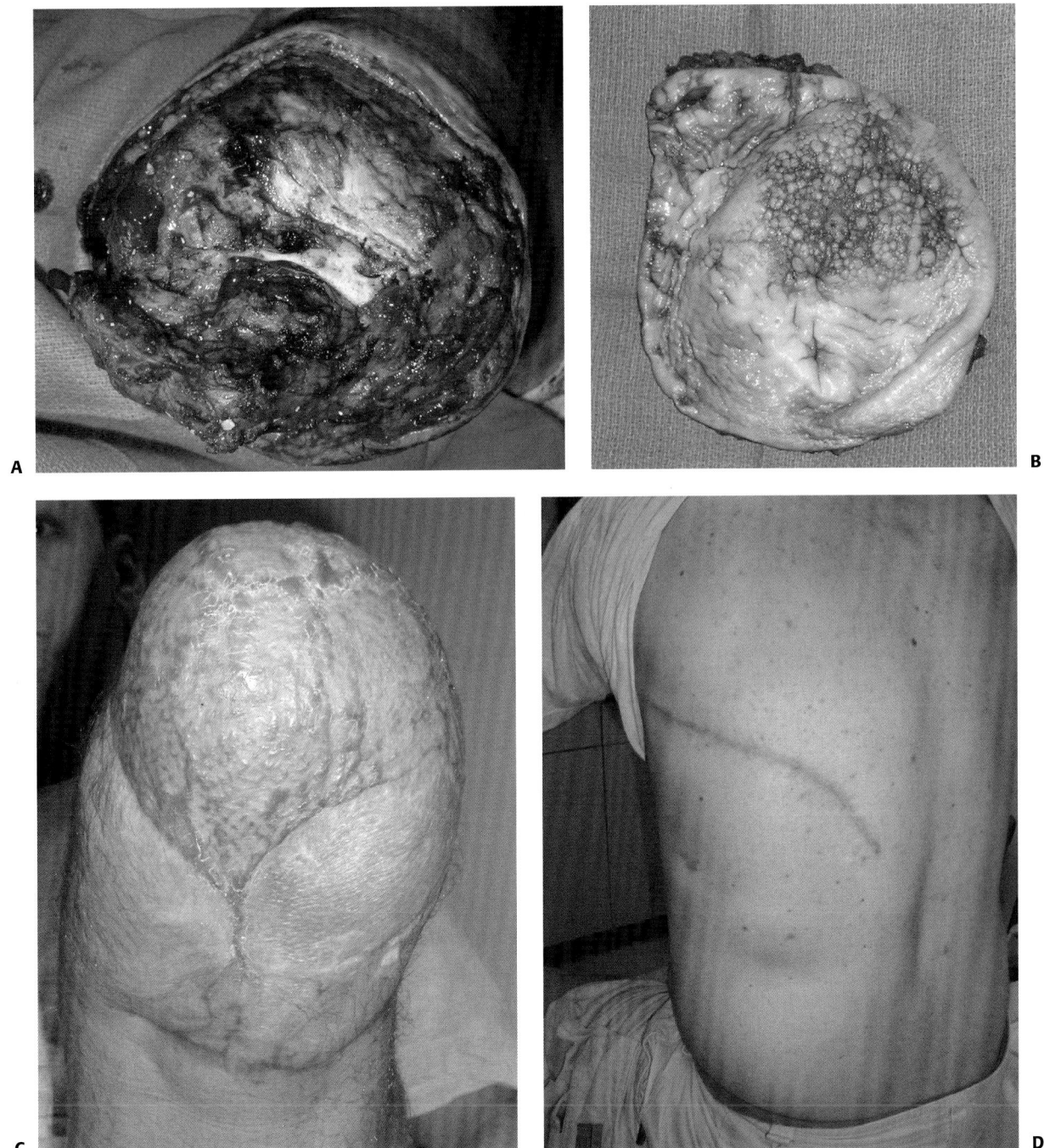

FIGURE 15-15 A: A below-knee amputation stump following resection of poor quality skin. **B:** Following thorough debridement of osteomyelitis of the distal tibia, the stump was covered with a latissimus dorsi muscle flap and split-thickness skin graft. **C:** At 6 months postoperatively, the stump has been resurfaced nicely. **D:** The latissimus dorsi flap donor site at 6 months.

of the lower donor site morbidity that other muscle and non-muscle flaps have to offer.

Gracilis

The gracilis muscle is a very commonly chosen donor site for free tissue transfer to cover foot and ankle soft tissue defects.[277] Typically, the ipsilateral limb is chosen so that only one limb is immobilized. The blood supply to the muscle is from the medial femoral circumflex artery, which originates from the profunda femoris artery. The major pedicle can be identified 8 to 10 cm inferior to the pubic tubercle. The flap also has a minor arterial pedicle, which enters the muscle at the level of the midthigh. This artery originates from the superficial femoral artery. The muscle receives its innervation from the anterior branch of the

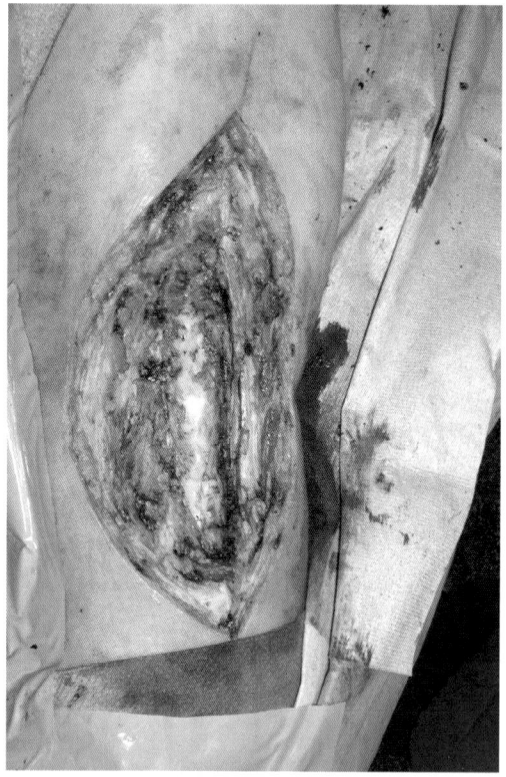
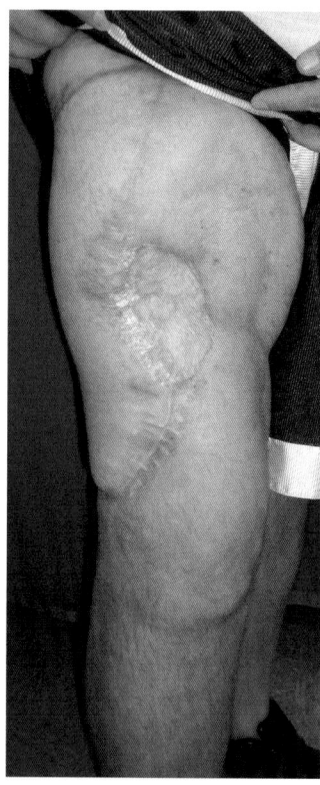

FIGURE 15-16 A: After resection of a recurrent liposarcoma in a radiated field in the thigh, there is extensive exposure of the femur and the scarred wound bed. **B:** Six months after a pedicled vertical rectus abdominis myocutaneous flap for soft tissue coverage. Anteriorly, a skin graft was used over a portion of the flap to minimize the size of the skin paddle and facilitate abdominal wall closure.

obturator nerve. This branch can be harvested with the muscle if there are requirements for a functional muscle transfer.

The muscle is exposed through a medial thigh incision as it lies between the adductor longus medially and the semitendinous muscle inferiorly. It lies superficial to the adductor magnus. The gracilis may be confused with the sartorius and is differentiated from the sartorius and semimembranous by identification of its musculotendinous portion. At the level of the medial femoral condyle the gracilis consists of muscle and tendon, whereas the semimembranous is entirely composed of tendon and the sartorius is entirely muscular.

Once the major pedicle has been identified with loupe magnification and determined to be adequate for a microvascular anastomosis, the secondary pedicle is divided. The origin of the muscle and the branch of the obturator nerve are then divided. The muscle is left to perfuse on its major pedicle until the recipient vessels have been prepared for microvascular anastomosis. Before muscle transfer, a final definitive debridement of the defect site is performed and the flap transfer is performed (Fig. 15-17).

Upper Extremity Reconstructive Options

Advances in microsurgery have expanded our reconstructive armamentarium over the last three decades, and the options for most soft tissue defects are now extensive (Table 15-4). As innovations in flap design continue to develop, reconstructive algorithms move away from the traditional reconstructive ladder toward delivering composite flaps to provide the best possible reconstructive solution.[45] Although free flaps are often the preferred method of reconstruction, all surgeons should be familiar with other options for upper limb reconstruction. The

major factors determining flap choice are location, size, and tissue involvement.[144]

Skin Grafting

As discussed previously, wounds with exposed muscle and subcutaneous tissue will accept skin grafts; however, exposure of

TABLE 15-4	**Reconstructive Options for the Upper Extremity**
Palm	Radial forearm flap
	Ulnar forearm flap
	Free flap
	Groin flap
Dorsal hand	Radial forearm flap
	Posterior interosseous flap
	Free flap
	Groin flap
Forearm	Radial forearm flap
	Posterior interosseous flap
	Free flap
Elbow	Radial forearm flap
	Posterior interosseous flap
	Pedicled latissimus dorsi flap
	Anconeus muscle flap
	Reverse lateral arm flap
	Free flap
Humerus	Pedicled latissimus dorsi flap
	Scapular flap
	Parascapular flap

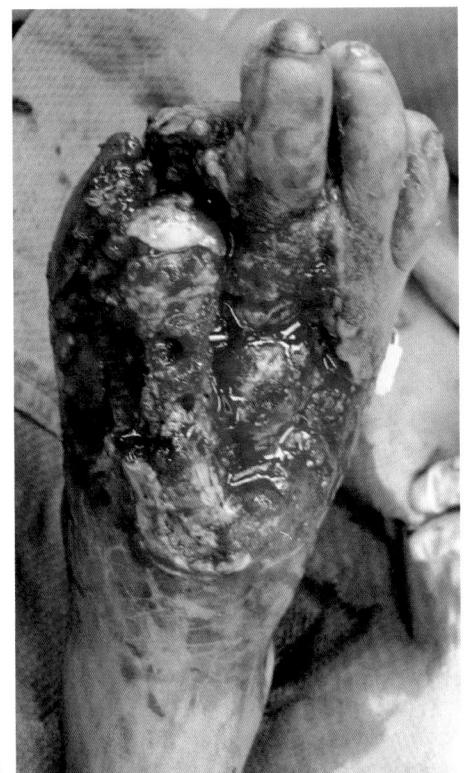

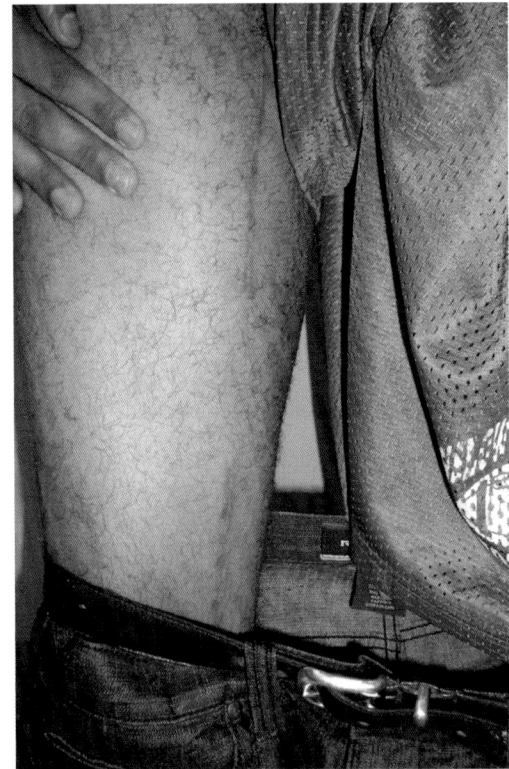

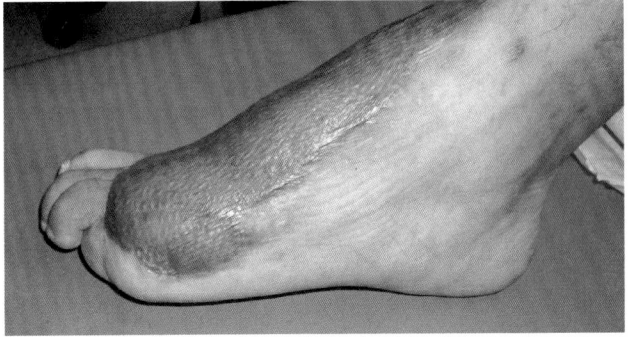

FIGURE 15-17 **A:** A gunshot wound to the dorsum of the foot with severe comminution of the metatarsals and loss of the hallux and second toe. **B:** The donor site after gracilis muscle harvest using two incisions and preserving a central skin bridge. **C:** One and a half years after gracilis muscle transfer for coverage of the dorsal foot wound.

vital structures such as tendons devoid of paratenon, nerves, vessels, bone, and hardware requires flap coverage. Although a split skin graft (Fig. 15-18) *will* typically survive when grafted onto major nerves, vessels, periosteum, and paratenon large areas of exposed bone need durable coverage, nerves and vessels need robust protection, and the preservation of tendon excursion requires that the overlying tissue is not firmly adherent to the paratenon. Flap coverage is also indicated in situations in which there is a need for the restoration of sensation.

Fasciocutaneous Flaps

Within the upper extremities, fasciocutaneous flaps can be either pedicled or free. The two most common pedicled fasciocutaneous flaps used in the upper extremity are the radial forearm flap and the posterior interosseous flap. Both can be used in an anterograde or retrograde fashion and can provide thin pliable coverage for most defects involving the *dorsum of the hand, the palm, the forearm, and the elbow.*

Radial Forearm Flap

This can be used as a local pedicled flap, or as a free flap from the contralateral limb (Fig. 15-19). The radial artery gives off fasciocutaneous perforators along its length, to supply the radial two-thirds of the forearm skin, and it also gives branches to the distal half of the radius. A flap measuring up to 15 × 35 cm can be raised as a fascial flap, a fasciocutaneous flap, or an osteocutaneous flap, in an antegrade or retrograde manner.[177] Palmaris longus, flexor carpi radialis, and the lateral and medial antebrachial nerves can also be included.[102,367] The pivot point can be as proximal as the origin of the radial artery, approximately 1 to 4 cm distal to the intercondylar line of the humerus, or as distal as the wrist crease, allowing it to be used for defects anywhere from the elbow to the dorsum of the hand. The versatility of this flap and the relative ease in flap elevation have made it a workhorse flap for forearm and hand reconstruction.

An adequate collateral circulation to the hand *must* be confirmed before the flap is elevated. The patient should have a

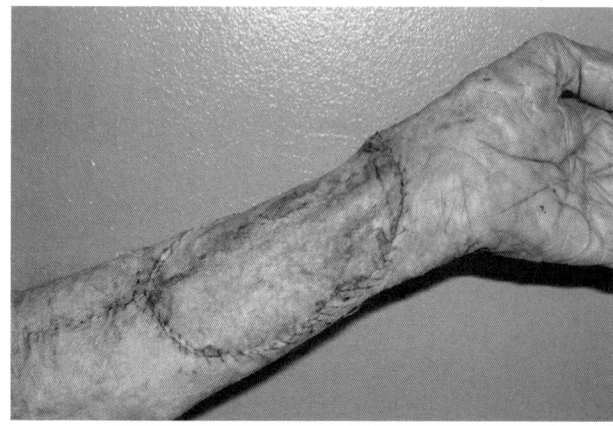

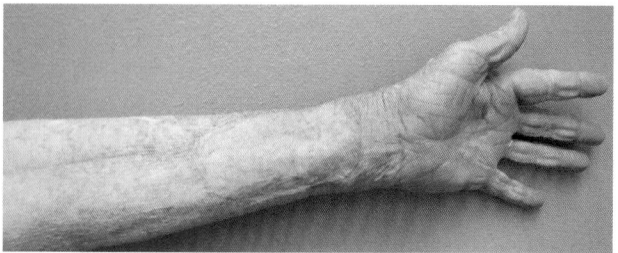

FIGURE 15-18 A split-thickness skin graft on the patient's forearm shown **(A)** 1 week and **(B)** 8 months after surgery.

normal Allen test to ensure safe flap harvest. If there is concern about the patency of the ulnar artery during the surgical procedure, the radial artery can be temporarily clamped, before flap division, and perfusion to the hand can be examined. The importance of checking collateral circulation to the hand when raising the flap from the already traumatized forearm cannot be overemphasized.

Posterior Interosseous Flap

The posterior interosseous flap was designed in an attempt to find alternatives to the radial forearm flap. The posterior interosseous artery, which this flap is based on, arises from the common interosseous artery in the antecubital fossa and passes dorsally through the interosseous membrane. The descending branch runs in the septum between the extensor carpi ulnaris and extensor digiti minimi, giving rise to several fasciocutaneous perforators to the skin. A fasciocutaneous flap up to 8 cm in width and 12 cm in length can be raised centered over a line drawn from the lateral epicondyle to the distal radioulnar joint.

The posterior interosseous branch of the radial nerve, which also runs in this septum, gives off its branches to the extensor digitorum communis and extensor carpi ulnaris at this level, and these branches are prone to injury when dissecting the flap. The posterior interosseous flap can also be used in a

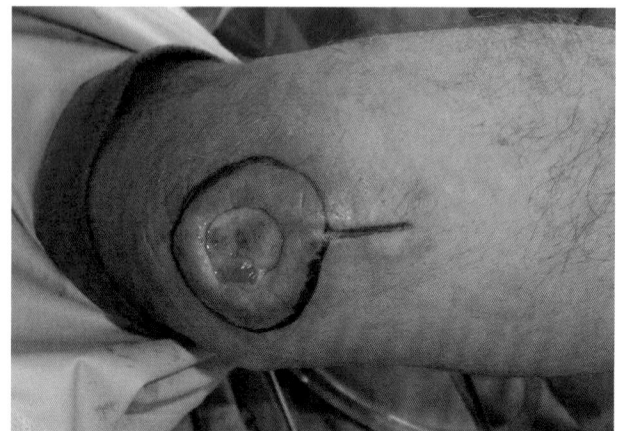

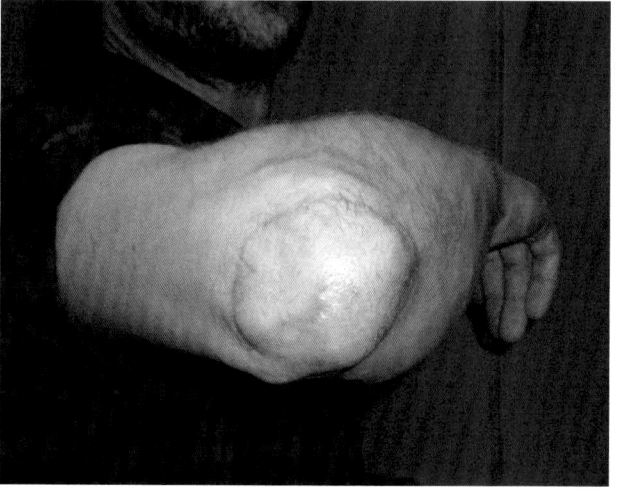

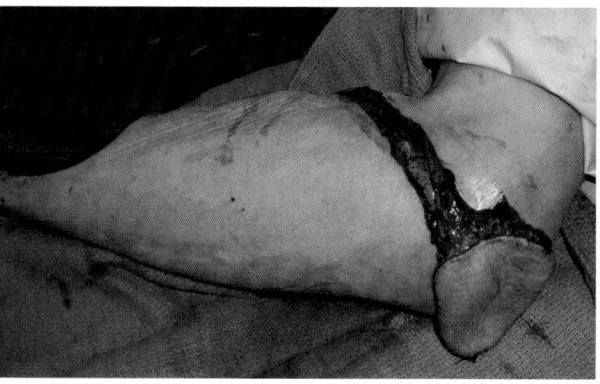

FIGURE 15-19 **A:** A 34-year-old man with chronic wound of the elbow with osteomyelitis of the olecranon, after a fall from a bike. **B:** Intraoperative view of radial forearm pedicled flap for elbow reconstruction. **C:** Appearance at 6 months postoperatively.

retrograde manner, making use of the collateral flow to the posterior interosseous artery through its distal anastomosis with the anterior interosseous artery. The principal advantages of this flap are as an alternative when the radial or ulnar artery has already been damaged or sacrificed, and when a thin pliable skin flap is needed.[7,230]

Free Fasciocutaneous Flaps

These flaps can be used anywhere throughout the upper extremity. If joints are to be crossed, fasciocutaneous flaps are much preferred as muscle flaps can undergo atrophy and restrict flexion and extension across joints. Some fasciocutaneous free flaps, such as the lateral arm flap and scapular flap, have limitations in size and overall thickness. If a larger skin island is needed, tissue expansion can be performed before flap transfer.

Scapular Flap

The scapular flap provides a large area of fasciocutaneous tissue based on the circumflex scapular branch of the subscapular artery.[322] This is an excellent choice for coverage of large wounds of the forearm. The dissection is relatively easy, and a flap of up to 10 × 25 cm (scapular flap) or 15 × 30 cm (parascapular flap) can be raised and used to reconstruct large defects of the forearm. For defects involving the radius or ulna, the scapular flap can be harvested as an osteocutaneous flap by incorporating the lateral part of the scapula, with very little extra morbidity.[342] Coverage can be extended even further by combining this flap with the latissimus dorsi or serratus anterior muscle flaps on one pedicle.[366] Donor sites of up to 7 to 8 cm in width can usually be closed directly.

Parascapular Flap

This flap has similar characteristics to the scapular flap but is based on the descending branch of the circumflex scapular artery. Similarly, it provides a large area of pliable and relatively thin tissue for forearm coverage, but the donor site usually requires skin grafting.

Anterolateral Thigh Flap

This flap has been previously discussed. It has recently seen a huge gain in popularity as a free flap, with some authors proclaiming it as the ideal soft tissue flap. Its vascular pedicle is reliably at least 8 cm long and can be lengthened up to 20 cm, the flap is easy to design and can be made up to 40 × 20 cm in size. It can be thinned to 3 to 5 mm without compromising its vascularity.[185,274] Some subcutaneous fat can be included to minimize tendon adhesion in the forearm and hand. Wei et al.[353] reviewed a series of 672 flaps with a success rate of over 98%. Its many advantages make it a versatile flap that has been reliably used in upper limb reconstructions including defects of the forearm and elbow (Fig. 15-20).[164,351]

Lateral Arm and Reverse Lateral Arm Flaps

The lateral arm flap is a fasciocutaneous flap perfused by the septal perforators of the posterior radial collateral artery, the terminal branch of the profunda brachii. An area of thin, pliable skin can be harvested up to 20 × 14 cm in size; however, only donor sites 6 cm in width or less can be closed primarily. This flap has a very short vascular leash, and its use as a pedicle flap is therefore limited, with most surgeons preferring to use it as a free flap. The radial recurrent artery provides the retrograde flow when this flap is used as a reversed flap. The reverse lateral arm flap has been used successfully for olecranon and antecubital coverage. As a free flap, the lateral arm flap is extremely versatile, capable of carrying bone (the humerus) and nerve (the posterior antebrachial nerve). Historically this has been a workhorse flap for upper extremity reconstruction.[21,257,339]

Muscle Flaps

The muscle flaps most commonly used to reconstruct the forearm, elbow, and humerus are the latissimus dorsi, rectus abdominis, serratus anterior, and gracilis muscles. The choice of muscle flap depends on the size of the defect, donor site availability, and donor site morbidity.

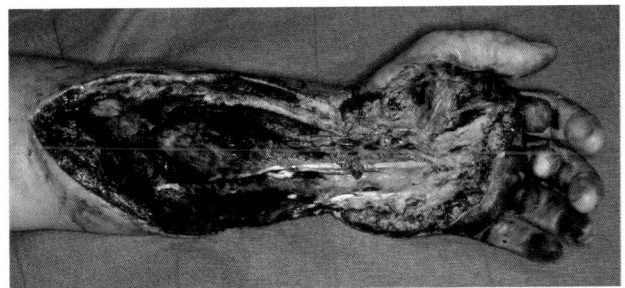

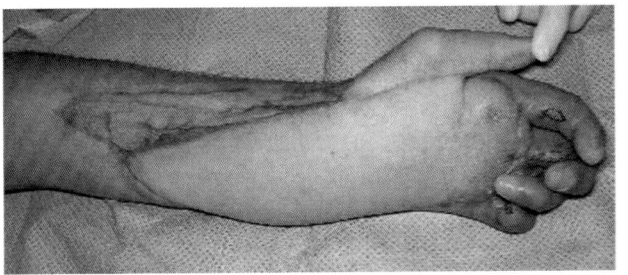

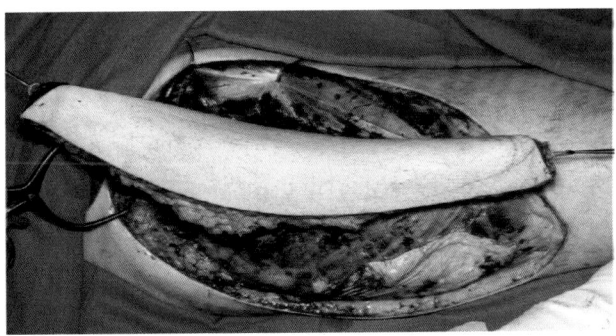

FIGURE 15-20 A: A 48-year-old man had a roller press injury resulting in loss of most of the palmar and forearm skin. **B:** Coverage was obtained with use of an anterolateral thigh flap. **C:** The flap appearance at 3 months, at the time of secondary flexor tendon tenolysis surgery.

Latissimus Dorsi. This is the largest single muscle flap and has a long pedicle (8 to 11 cm), making it one of the most versatile flaps for reconstructing large defects in the upper extremity. In addition, in the majority of patients, the thoracodorsal trunk has two major divisions, allowing the surgeon to harvest only a portion of the muscle if a narrower flap is needed. Conversely, if a broader flap is required, the serratus muscle (± a vascularized rib) can be raised with the flap, taking care to preserve its arterial supply, which arises as a branch from the thoracodorsal artery.

As a pedicle flap, the latissimus dorsi can be transferred as a functional muscle to re-establish lost biceps or triceps function. It can be used in a pedicled fashion for coverage of the elbow, but should not be used for elbow defects extending distal to the olecranon. For such defects the radial forearm flap has been found to provide more reliable coverage.[55,164] Functional morbidity of the donor site is variable, with conflicting reports in the literature. If it is anticipated that a resulting degree of shoulder weakness (adduction, as in patients who walk with crutches and those with paraplegia) would have a major impact on the patient, then an alternative flap should be considered.

Serratus Anterior. The lower three slips of the serratus can be harvested with or without the underlying ribs, based on the thoracodorsal pedicle. This flap is a relatively thin, broad sheet of muscle but can be very versatile when combined with components of rib or the latissimus dorsi muscle.

Rectus Abdominis. This muscle has a consistent vascular pedicle (5 to 7 cm) arising from the deep inferior epigastric vessels, and can be used for coverage in most situations encountered in forearm trauma. Its main disadvantage is an abdominal wall hernia, which can sometimes occur at the donor site, especially if the fascia is harvested.

Gracilis. This muscle is well suited for small defects requiring muscle coverage. The dominant pedicle is the medial femoral circumflex artery arising from the profunda femoris; it is usually approximately 6 to 7 cm in length. The muscle is unipennate, and has an excursion of approximately 10 cm. The main advantage of this muscle flap in the forearm is its use as a functional motor unit as discussed previously.

Distant Pedicled Flaps

Groin Flap

The workhorse flap before the advent of microsurgery was the groin flap. This flap is based on the superficial femoral circumflex artery, which arises from the femoral artery along with the superficial inferior epigastric artery in the femoral triangle.[249,312] The flap has shown great versatility. It may include the lateral cutaneous branch of the femoral nerve if a sensate flap is required.[172] The flap may be combined with the abdominohypogastric flap for large defects or it may be expanded before transfer. If bone is required, a portion of the iliac crest may be harvested.[98] The flap may also be split longitudinally to cover defects on both aspects of the hand.[313]

The flap can often be divided safely at 3 weeks, especially if the wound is well healed at the flap's distal margin. Any compromise to the arm's vascularity, such as preoperative radiation

or electrical injury may prolong the period of revascularization. If there is doubt about the vascularity of the flap prior to division, the pedicle may be occluded with a tourniquet and the vascular flow assessed.[365] The disadvantage of the groin flap is the mandatory period of hand immobilization before pedicle division. This can result in hand, elbow, and shoulder stiffness. Despite this the groin flap still remains a reliable means of providing soft tissue coverage for large hand wounds without the need for microvascular experience (Fig. 15-21).[249]

Upper Extremity Reconstructive Pearls

For free flap options, our preferred flaps for soft tissue reconstructions of the forearm are the ALT flap and the scapular flap. If bone is required, the fibular osteocutaneous flap is a good match for the radius or ulna. Flaps based on the subscapular or thoracodorsal system and taken with rib are also very versatile for the reconstruction of smaller bony defects.[112,153,174,222,321]

Musculocutaneous flaps such as the latissimus dorsi and rectus abdominis flaps result in functional loss and donor site morbidity including, particularly in the abdomen, the potential for hernia formation. In addition, in the coverage of joint surfaces, muscle flaps tend to undergo fibrosis and atrophy over time, which may limit joint excursion, particularly when they are placed over the elbow or the dorsum of the hand. Muscle is still indicated for those circumstances involving osteomyelitis or soft tissue contamination.

POSTOPERATIVE CARE AND MONITORING OF PATIENTS AFTER FLAP TRANSFER

Free flap success is not always guaranteed at the completion of the case, as 5% to 25% of transferred flaps require re-exploration for microcirculatory compromise, which can be caused by arterial or venous thrombosis.[34,46,180] Free flap salvage rates after thrombosis range from 42% to 85%.[46,193] Early recognition of vascular compromise has been shown to provide the best chance of successful flap salvage.[46,145,302]

Methods for monitoring free tissue transfers have advanced from clinical observation to implantable Doppler probes. The best method for monitoring has yet to be established. Clinical observation of the nonburied free flap remains the gold standard to which monitoring systems are generally compared.[83] Monitoring devices should ideally be sensitive enough to supersede clinical evidence of vascular thrombosis but specific enough to avoid unnecessary re-exploration. Here we review the current literature regarding monitoring methods and protocols.

Conventional Flap Monitoring Methods

Clinical Observation

In clinical observation, the flap is observed by assessing capillary refill, temperature, swelling, and flap color. Its use is confined to monitoring surface skin flaps and is less reliable in the monitoring of muscle flaps and buried flaps.[83] Capillary refill can be assessed by simply applying deep pressure to the transferred tissue using one's finger or the flat end of a surgical instrument and then releasing the pressure and evaluating capillary refill time, which is commonly 2 to 3 seconds. With increasing disturbance

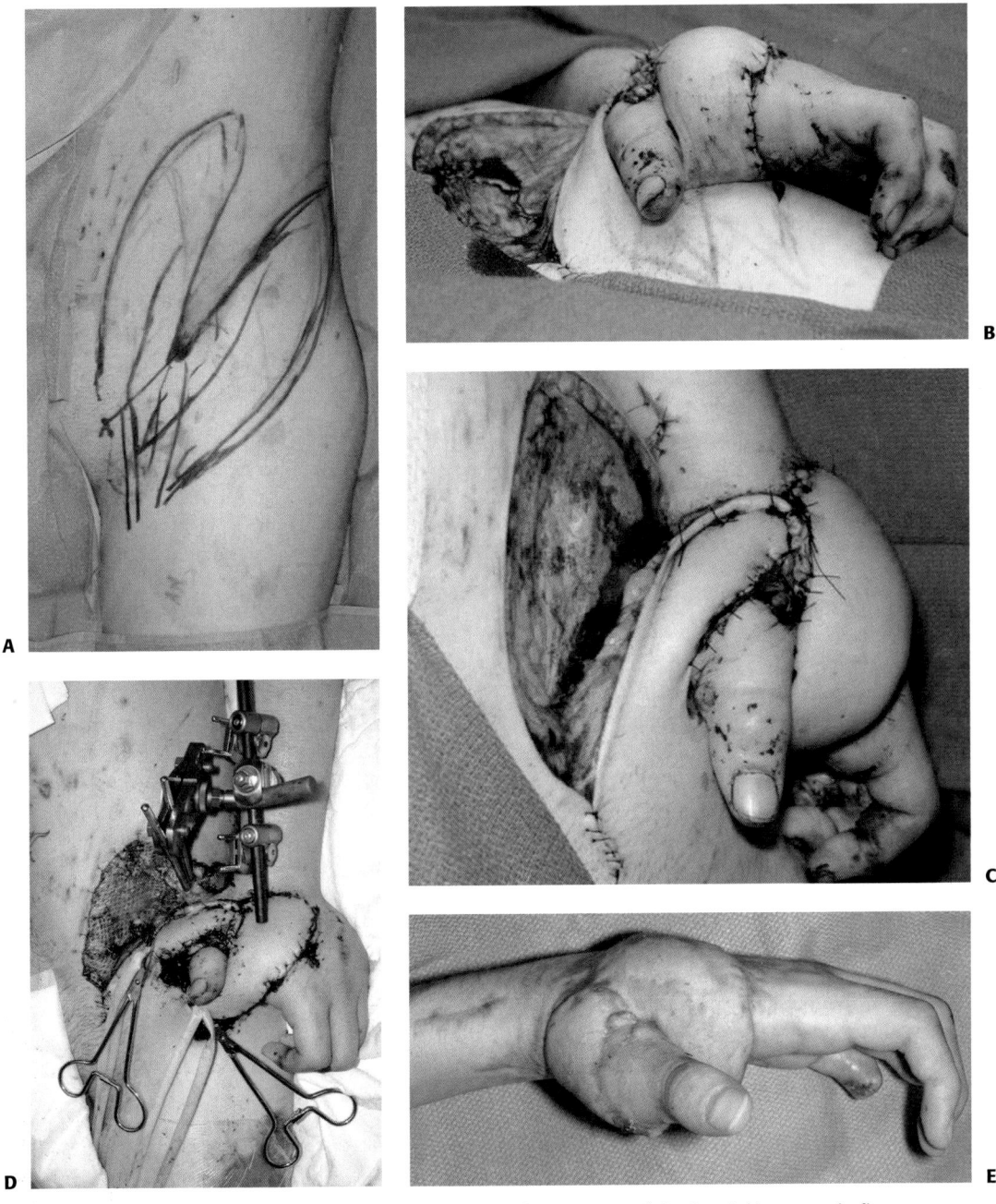

FIGURE 15-21 A: The groin flap can provide versatile coverage of the hand. Here a groin flap was designed with two separate skin paddles to cover both the palmar **(B)** and dorsal **(C)** surfaces of the hand. **D:** The hand was temporarily stabilized to the groin with the use of an external fixator. **E:** The appearance of the hand following flap division and insetting.

of the blood supply, a livid bluish discoloration (shortened capillary refill of less than 2 seconds) or paleness of the flap (delayed capillary refill of greater than 3 seconds) appears in a venous congested or ischemic flap, respectively. When these criteria cannot be reliably assessed or for confirmation, one may then use the pin prick test.

It is important to remember that for clinical observation to be effective, the person performing flap evaluation needs to be educated with regard to the signs of flap failure. Nursing units and new house staff members require annual in-service education to improve their diagnostic acumen, as these two groups are in constant flux in most medical centers.

Pin Prick Testing

The pin prick test is commonly used on flaps with a cutaneous component. The test is performed by puncturing the cutaneous paddle of the flap with a 24- or 25-gauge needle. The puncture should not be too deep into the tissue, and it should be in a portion of the flap that is not in close proximity to the vascular pedicle and microanastomosis. An indicator of flap viability is a stream of continuous bright red blood upon puncture. A congested flap will produce a continuous stream of dark venous blood. Care should be taken not to perform this test too frequently, particularly in patients on anticoagulants, because repeated puncture trauma may lead to a bruised flap, which may hinder further evaluation of the tissue. This test is certainly the least expensive of the various methods of flap monitoring.

Surface Temperature Monitoring

A difference of greater than 3°C between the surface temperature of the flap and the adjacent skin is associated with arterial compromise and a difference of between 1°C and 2°C is more indicative of venous compromise. A simple liquid crystal temperature probe may be placed on the flap tissue with a second probe placed on the adjacent normal skin. Temperature changes in flaps such as toe flaps placed on an extremity will be more accurate than flaps placed on the trunk, where the flap temperature may be a direct reflection of the body part on which it is placed.

Hand-Held Doppler Ultrasonography

Currently, there is no single adjunctive monitoring technique widely accepted as the method of choice, but ultrasonography with a hand-held Doppler (5 to 8 MHz) device is the most common technique in use.[290,314,345] Its most important limitation is differentiating between the recipient vessels and the flap's vascular pedicle because of their potential close proximity. A clinician may detect the Doppler signal of the recipient vessels instead of the signal from the flap's vascular pedicle, which may mislead the observer into believing that the flap's pedicle is patent when in reality a thrombosis has occurred. This limitation may be overcome by performing a Doppler ultrasound examination of an arterial signal within the flap tissue intraoperatively and then simultaneously compressing the donor (flap) artery to ensure that this is a true artery within the flap. Upon compression of the donor (flap) artery there should be loss of the arterial ultrasonic signal within the flap.

Hand-held Doppler ultrasonography is also an effective method of determining the status of the vein of a flap. The Doppler signal of a vein is detected intraoperatively after flap revascularization and a suture may be placed to mark it. The venous sound is at times difficult to detect but, when heard, it is a clear indication that the vein is patent. When a venous signal is detected, the flap can be compressed and a "venous augment" sound should be heard.

Implantable Doppler Ultrasonography

The implantable Doppler device can measure blood flow across a microvascular anastomosis and is an effective tool to monitor flap perfusion and improve salvage rates, especially in buried flaps.[72] Initial research demonstrated a 3% false-positive rate, which led to unnecessary re-explorations, and a 5% false-negative rate when the probe was placed on the artery.[326] Further, up to a 5-hour delay was found between a venous obstruction and the loss of the arterial signal in large muscle flaps. Best results occur if an implantable probe is placed on the vein instead of the artery

allowing the detection of venous obstruction immediately followed by the detection of arterial thrombosis.

Pulse Oximetry

The pulse oximeter consists of two light-emitting diodes that transmit two separate wavelengths of visible red (660 nm) and infrared (940 nm) light and a photodiode receiver. It can distinguish the difference in light absorption between oxyhemoglobin and reduced hemoglobin and thereby measure oxygen saturation. By the way of photoplethysmography, the oximeter can identify pulsatile flow and will therefore provide a continuous display of both the pulse rate and arterial saturation. This is an excellent monitor for replanted and revascularized digits and toe-to-hand transfers.[121]

Laser Doppler

Light from a helium neon laser of uniform wavelength will penetrate 1.5 mm below the surface of the flap, and this light is reflected by the red blood cells moving within the capillaries enclosed within a 1-mm^3 volume of tissue. The frequency shift between the transmitted and reflected light is directly proportional to the velocity of capillary blood flow. This flow value provides an objective measurement of flap perfusion. Laser Doppler interpretation requires experience, as values differ depending on tissue type and patient. Furthermore, perfusion readings may fluctuate for any given patient because of physiologic microcirculation variation or artifacts. Therefore, the observer must monitor the trend rather than the absolute values. This method is limited to monitoring cutaneous circulatory phenomena, as the probe only penetrates 1.5 mm into the flap. Estimated sensitivity and specificity values have been reported at 93% and 94%, respectively, and this technique has been found to be superior to thermometry when used alone for the evaluation of replantations.[148]

AUTHORS' PREFERRED METHOD

How often and for how long flap monitoring should be performed has been debated, but most series recommend a minimum of hourly monitoring for the first 24 to 48 hours after surgery.[146,193] The majority (greater than 80%) of vascular complications occur within the first 48 to 72 hours postoperatively. Postoperative venous thrombosis is the most common vascular complication.[193] With these factors in mind our current recommendations for flap monitoring include the following.

1. Placement of an implantable venous Doppler probe when feasible.
2. Flap inspection every hour by experienced nursing staff for first 48 hours, moving to every 2 hours for the next 24 hours.
3. Discontinuation of flap monitoring after day 4, unless there are extenuating circumstances.

Anticoagulation Considerations in Free Flap Surgery

Ninety-six percent of reconstructive surgeons use some type of anticoagulation regimen after free tissue transfer, and in pedicled flap reconstruction the frequency of use is dependent on its vascular supply.[70,117] Unfortunately, there is no consensus on anticoagulation therapy after free tissue transfer, and a full discussion of all pertinent studies pertaining to postoperative anticoagulation is beyond the scope of this chapter. It is sufficient to say that scientific findings are often clouded by anecdotal experience. The three most common anticoagulants in use are aspirin, heparin, and dextran.

Aspirin, through its activity on the cyclooxygenase pathway, decreases the production of thromboxane and prostacyclin, both of which are powerful platelet aggregators. Aspirin's effectiveness in decreasing macrovascular graft occlusion has been clearly demonstrated in several studies.[15,60] The effective dose of aspirin to inhibit thromboxane while preserving some of the provasodilatory effects of prostacyclin function is relatively low, within the range of 50 to 100 mg per day.[58,61,358] Despite its use postoperatively to prevent thrombosis, aspirin's most beneficial effect may be when it is given several hours before surgery. The administration of aspirin 10 hours before surgery has been shown to result in a significant increase in vessel patency and a decrease in platelet aggregation.[288]

Heparin has been shown to provide a beneficial effect on anastomotic patency in animal models.[124] Large prospective randomized human trials are not yet in existence. Hematoma formation with the potential for flap loss has been linked to full systemic postoperative anticoagulation. In Pugh's retrospective study, the incidence of hematoma formation after lower-leg reconstruction and systemic anticoagulation with heparin was 66%.[272] The use of subcutaneous heparin or low-molecular-weight heparin (LMWH) is warranted for prevention of deep venous thrombosis, while also providing a benefit with regard to vessel patency. Khouri et al.[180] found, in the largest multicenter prospective free flap tissue study, that only postoperatively administered subcutaneous heparin had a statistically significant effect on the prevention of postoperative free flap thrombosis.

The combination of subcutaneous heparin and low-dose aspirin has been shown to produce no increase in the rate of postoperative hematoma formation. In our opinion, this combination of drugs provides a safe and economical means of providing thrombosis prophylaxis for routine free flap procedures. This combination therapy also provides the benefits of coronary protection and deep venous thrombosis prophylaxis.[57] Subcutaneous heparin does not require monitoring of coagulation factors, and both medications may be given without intravenous access. LMWH also provides the benefits of higher bioavailability, a longer plasma half-life, and a steady dose-response curve and it causes fewer cases of hematoma formation and thrombocytopenia when compared with unfractionated heparin.[13]

Finally, dextran, like heparin, has shown benefit in improving patency rates in the immediate postoperative period when given as a single preoperative bolus[289,381]; however, the effectiveness of prolonged administration is debatable.[270,285,287] An increasing number of reports have noted significant morbidity associated with the use of dextran and have questioned its use in routine microsurgical cases.[135,137] Complications from dextran administration can include renal failure, congestive heart failure, myocardial infarction, pulmonary edema, pleural effusion, and pneumonia.

Because flap failure rates are so low, large prospective randomized multicenter trials will be necessary to definitively decide which anticoagulation therapy is the most effective in preventing postoperative flap thrombosis. *Until that time we feel that a combination of low-dose aspirin and subcutaneous or low-molecular-weight heparin provides adequate flap protection with minimal associated morbidity and little additional cost.*

Hemodynamic Management

Effective medical management of all patients with flaps will improve flap survival and prevent morbidity and mortality. From a cardiac standpoint, surgical patients with coronary artery disease or risk factors for coronary artery disease who undergo tissue transfer surgery should undergo an appropriate evaluation by their cardiologist or internist before surgical intervention. The administration of beta-blockade with Atenolol has been shown to have reduced cardiovascular complications and mortality for up to 2 years in this patient population.[223] Hyperglycemia associated with relative insulin resistance or diabetes has been reported to increase the incidence of complications in the surgical patient.[97,247] For this patient population, intensive insulin therapy to maintain blood sugar levels between 80 and 110 mg/dL has been shown to substantially reduce morbidity and mortality from 8% to 4.6%.[346]

Patients must also have adequate intravenous fluid hydration in the perioperative period, and commonly a Foley catheter will be used to record and maintain a urine output of at least 50 cm^3/hour. In our institution, patients commonly are given nothing by mouth until the morning after surgery in the event reoperation is necessary. Hematocrit levels are kept at greater than 30% in patients with coronary artery disease and greater than 25% in those without it.

Flap Failures and Management

Despite our greatest efforts in reconstructive microsurgery, flap failure will occur. The failure can be partial or complete. It is important to recognize the cause of flap failure so it may be reversed or prevented in the next reconstructive attempt. Arterial insufficiency leading to flap complications can be recognized by decreased capillary refill, pallor, reduced temperature, and the absence of bleeding on pin prick testing. This complication can result from arterial spasm, vessel plaque, torsion of the pedicle, pressure on the flap, technical error with injury to the pedicle, a flap harvested that is too large for its blood supply, or small vessel disease secondary to diabetes or smoking. If pharmacologic agents do not relieve spasm at the level of arterial inflow, the vessel anastomosis should be redone.

Venous outflow obstruction can be suspected when the flap has a violaceous color and brisk capillary refill, and dark blood is seen after pin prick. Venous obstruction can occur as a result of flap edema, hematoma, tight closure over the pedicle, or pedicle torsion. Venous compromise will lead to microvascular thrombi, which will then compromise arterial flow if not promptly addressed.[239] Conservative treatment in the acute phase, besides pharmacologic therapy as discussed, may include drainage of an underlying hematoma with suture release to decrease the pressure. Leeches may also be helpful if sufficient venous outflow cannot be established despite a patent venous anastomosis. The leeches work by biting the venous congested tissue and extracting blood via direct suction and injecting *hirudin,* a potent anticoagulant present in their saliva. *Aeromonas hydrophila* is an important microbe present in the leech, and prophylactic antibiotics (usually a second- or third-generation cephalosporin or an aminoglycoside or fluoroquinolone) must be given when patients are undergoing leech therapy.[71,236] Because of blood loss from the therapy, it is also important to check serial hemoglobin levels and have the patient typed and cross-matched for blood transfusion at all times.

Nonviable flaps should be debrided promptly as they may serve as a source of infection in an already compromised limb. The timing of removal is dependent on the recipient bed on which it was inset. Scarred, radiated, or dysvascular wound beds only provide minimal blood supply to the overlying flap tissue; therefore, upon flap compromise more flap tissue is lost.[293,357] If a second free flap is considered, obvious errors that led to the original flap compromise need to be recognized and avoided.

Nerve Reconstruction

Nerve Injuries Associated with Fractures

Much of our modern understanding of the treatment of acute nerve injuries comes from the works of Seddon,[301] which stemmed from the treatment of World War II patients. Seddon introduced a simple classification of traumatic nerve injuries: Neurapraxia, which was minimal injury with localized ischemic demyelination of the nerve; axonotmesis, characterized by interruption of the axons and their myelin sheath with the endoneurial tubes remaining intact; and neurotmesis, which is a completely severed nerve or one that is so seriously disorganized that spontaneous regeneration is impossible. Sunderland[325] in 1951 proposed a five-level classification that related to the internal structure of the nerve; however, it relied on pathologic examination of the nerve, which is quite impractical in the trauma setting.

The treatment of the injured nerve is dependent on the type of injury to it (neurapraxic, axonotmetic, and neurotmetic), the time from the injury, the soft tissue bed quality, the defect size if the nerve is transected, and associated nerve/muscle injuries. In acute fractures with nerve injury, there is tremendous debate on whether to explore or observe. Depending on the energy of the trauma, the decisions may vary. In particular, debate continues regarding treatment of radial nerve injury associated with distal humeral fractures (see Chapter 36).[73,88,89,90,101,136,152,160,181,198,215, 275,281,305,310,311] Generally in acute closed fractures, observation of the nerve injury with serial examination for 3 to 6 months should be undertaken. If no recovery is seen, electrodiagnostic testing should be considered as early as 6 weeks after injury. If no improvement is observed by 4 to 6 months, exploration with interposition nerve grafting or alternatively nerve transfers should be considered.

In injuries where the nerve is obviously sectioned with a high degree of trauma (i.e., not a sharp laceration) with associated soft tissue injuries, the nerve ends should be tagged and the soft tissue and bone injury addressed. The greatest challenge is the

determination of the zone of injury of the nerve.[76,77,94,218,333,348] If acute nerve grafting is to be performed, resecting the injured portion is imperative. Unfortunately, intraoperative assessment by histologic section, touch, or visualization of the injured nerve cannot inform us of the zone of injury. Delay of a few weeks allows the development of intraneural fibrosis, and allows tactile and pathologic visualization of the zone of injury; however, the scarred tissues make the surgical reconstruction more difficult. If acute soft tissue reconstruction is performed, and a delayed nerve reconstruction is planned, the surgeon should consider placing the nerve to be reconstructed in a location where it can be easily accessed. Finally, if more than 6 to 12 months pass between injury and reconstruction, tendon transfers or free functioning muscle transfers should be considered as there is a time dependent, irreversible degradation of the motor endplate that occurs after motor nerve injury.[309]

Brachial Plexus Injuries

Treatment recommendations for complete nerve root avulsions have varied widely over the past 50 years, and the results of treatment have ranged from fair to dismal. After World War II, the standard approach was surgical reconstruction by shoulder fusion, elbow bone block, and finger tenodesis.[140] In the 1960s, transhumeral (above elbow) amputation combined with shoulder fusion in slight abduction and flexion was advocated.[100] Yeoman and Seddon noted the tendency for injured patients to become "one-handed" within 2 years of injury, which led to a dramatic reduction in successful outcomes regardless of the treatment approach. Their retrospective study revealed no good results from the primitive surgical reconstruction of that era, but predominantly good and fair outcomes when amputation plus shoulder fusion were performed within 24 months of injury. They also noted that the loss of glenohumeral motion caused by brachial plexus injuries limited the effectiveness of body-powered prostheses and that manual laborers seemed to accept hook prostheses much more readily than did office workers with similar injuries. Although these observations remain valid today, there have been advances in brachial plexus reconstruction that have yielded outcomes superior to the historical results. A better understanding of the pathophysiology of nerve injury and repair, as well as the recent advances in microsurgical techniques, have allowed reliable restoration of elbow flexion and shoulder abduction in addition to useful prehension of the hand in some cases. The specific treatment of these injuries is beyond the scope of this chapter; however, there are multiple modalities, including nerve grafting, nerve repair, nerve transfers, tendon transfers, and free tissue transfers that can be used to improve function and outcome.[20,40,252]

Recent Advances in Reconstructive Surgery of the Extremities

Aesthetic Improvements in Reconstructive Surgery of the Extremities

As with any reconstructive surgical procedure, the goal is to restore form and function. In some areas of the body, the priority of improving the aesthetic outcome of the procedure is higher than others. Clearly, when reconstructing a facial defect, this becomes a high focus of the reconstruction. With advancements in the understanding of flap anatomy, major advancements have been seen in the aesthetic refinements that can be achieved when reconstructing defects in the extremities as well.[273] Improvements in aesthetic outcomes come at two stages in the reconstruction. The first is during the initial reconstructive procedure, when a flap is chosen to meet the functional needs at the recipient site and to achieve a reasonable aesthetic outcome. Choosing a flap that has qualities that match the recipient site, such as color, thickness, and pliability is important. Primary flap thinning can be performed in the operating room to achieve the best aesthetic outcome in the initial setting. The second stage is carried out with the use of additional surgical procedures to refine flap shape; several months after the initial procedure, secondary procedures may be performed, such as flap debulking through direct excision or liposuction[364] or even using the arthroscopic shaver device,[330] flap advancement, and serial excision of the flap.[306] Workhorse flaps in reconstructive surgery that are thin include the radial forearm flap, the lateral arm flap, and many of the discussed perforator flaps. In addition, depending on the needs at the recipient site, fascia flaps covered with skin grafts often produce aesthetically and functionally good results. These flaps include the temporoparietal fascia flap,[282] the posterior rectus sheath flap,[292] the lateral arm fascia flap,[323] as well as the ALT fascia flap.[150]

Another important concept in improving aesthetics in reconstructive surgery is tissue expansion. This tool has been used in both upper and lower extremity reconstructions.[129,130] The flap is expanded before harvest and transfer to the defect site.[133,334] Alternatively tissue expanders can be used to expand the tissue surrounding a defect to provide additional tissue to help in reconstruction, minimizing flap requirements. After acute reconstruction, if the patient is unhappy with the shape or color of the flap, tissue expanders can be placed around the flap, under the normal skin of the extremity, and once expansion is complete the flap can be excised, with the native expanded local skin used to cover the resultant defect. Tissue expansion is associated with complications including infection and implant extrusion, and is usually not recommended in cases of acute reconstruction of contaminated wounds.

Endoscopic harvest and minimally invasive dissection of flaps provide another refinement in reconstructive surgery,[291] the benefit of which has not been fully used at this point. Endoscopic technique now allows for the successful harvest of flaps such as the latissimus dorsi,[240] the rectus abdominis,[213] the gracilis, the temporoparietal fascia flap,[56] and others. It is also used in harvesting vein grafts and nerve grafts which are often used in reconstructive surgery.[209] Comparative studies between open and endoscopically assisted muscle harvest have found patients to have less donor site pain and shorter scar lengths after endoscopic harvest.[211]

Perforator Flaps and Free Style Flaps

One of the most significant advancements in limiting donor site morbidity has been the advent of perforator flap surgery. Whereas the muscle was always thought to be a necessary car-

rier of the blood supply in musculocutaneous flaps, perforator flaps are performed by harvesting the skin and subcutaneous tissue, with a variety of tissue components, while preserving the muscle at the donor site. The skin and subcutaneous tissue are elevated and a large perforator is found. This perforator is then dissected from the surrounding muscle and traced to the origin vessel. The flap is harvested while the muscle is left intact. The remaining muscle is supplied through its secondary blood supply, and innervation of the muscle is maintained by preserving the nerves in the region. Functionally, the patient experiences minimal donor site morbidity. The blood supply to the flap is through a perforator that is clearly visualized intraoperatively, with its anatomic basis as has been studied through anatomic dissections.[344] Hence the flap can be thinned during the initial reconstructive procedure, preserving the perforator, to provide a nicely contoured flap without the need for a second surgery to thin the flap.[75] Preoperative planning with the aid of CT and ultrasound to identify perforating blood vessels can improve surgical success.[28,42,116,128] Once the surgeon's skill in microsurgical techniques and flap dissection has reached a high level, one can perform microdissection of a perforator, which allows a detailed visualization of the arterial anatomy of the flap, eventually allowing for aggressive and accurate thinning of that flap.[92,183,184,369]

Commonly used perforator flaps include the deep inferior epigastric perforator (DIEP) flap based on the deep inferior epigastric artery (DIEA), the ALT flap, the thoracodorsal artery perforator (TAP) flap,[8] and the gastrocnemius perforator flap.[127] As previously discussed, the most commonly used perforator flap is the ALT perforator flap because of its versatility and the ability to include a variety of structures as well as the ability to thin and tailor the flap to fit the defect.[376] Harvest of the ALT flap has previously been described in this chapter in the section entitled "Lower Extremity Reconstructive Options."

Deep Inferior Epigastric Perforator Flap

The DIEP flap is an abdominal flap based on a single or multiple transmuscular perforators originating from the DIEA. The DIEA originates from the external femoral artery and then travels superomedially in the extraperitoneal tissue and subsequently pierces the transversalis fascia. The DIEA then enters the rectus sheath and usually divides into a lateral and medial branch which gives off perforators which pierce the rectus muscle to supply the overlying skin and subcutaneous tissue. The DIEP flap is used extensively for breast reconstruction. However, it can also be used for extremity reconstruction as it allows a large skin paddle measuring on average 34×13 cm to be harvested. The flap is harvested with the patient supine, and is usually designed as an ellipse extending over the infraumbilical region of abdomen from one anterior superior iliac spine to the other. Preoperative identification and marking of major perforators using a Doppler probe, CT, or MRI angiography are useful adjuncts to aid perforator dissection.

Lateral Thoracic Perforator Flaps

Perforator flaps in the lateral thoracic region were developed as an attempt to utilize the skin over the lateral thoracic region without the requirement for harvesting the underlying latissimus dorsi muscle, therefore reducing the bulk of the flap and obviating sacrifice of the latissimus dorsi muscle. Three distinct rows of perforators supply the skin of the lateral thoracic region. The most anterior row usually consists of direct cutaneous perforators, and originates from the lateral thoracic vessels, usually found on the serratus anterior muscle at the lateral border of the pectoralis major muscle. The middle row consists of septocutaneous perforators from the thoracodorsal system and the posterior row consists of musculocutaneous perforators through the latissimus dorsi muscle. When harvested off perforators from the lateral thoracic vessels, the flap is termed a lateral thoracic perforator flap; when harvested off the middle row it is called a TAP flap; and when harvested off the posterior row it is called a latissimus dorsi perforator flap. Flaps in this region have the advantage of reduced donor site morbidity, with flap harvest leaving a small linear scar. In addition, the flap is thin, providing supple tissue for limb resurfacing. Furthermore, composite flaps consisting of muscle and/or bone can be harvested with skin and subcutaneous tissue off the subscapular artery system. Disadvantages are an inconsistent perforator anatomy, which can make the learning curve for flap harvest steep. In addition, for female patients, harvest of a large flap may cause deviation and deformity of the breast.

Free Style Flaps

Free style flaps have been proposed by Wei and Mardini,[354] and greatly increase the repertoire of the reconstructive surgeon. Instead of harvesting a flap off a named axial vessel, the flap is based on a perforator in any area of the body, which is usually detected with the aid of the Doppler probe. Retrograde dissection until a pedicle of sufficient length is obtained allows utilization as a local or free flap. Typically these flaps are harvested as skin and subcutaneous only flaps in the suprafascial or subfascial plane. The donor site is matched to the recipient site such that tissue which most closely approximates the recipient site in terms of thickness, color, and texture is harvested. In the extremities, these flaps have particular application as local flaps utilized in a propeller flap fashion, or as small free flaps used for resurfacing of areas such as the digits of the hand.

New Modalities for Soft Tissue Coverage

Artificial Skin

The role of artificial skin has advanced significantly over the past 15 years; materials are now available which can provide a scaffold for the ingrowth of fibroblasts and blood vessels over avascular or minimally vascularized structures such as tendon and bone. Integra dermal regeneration template (Integra Life Sciences, Plainsboro, NJ) was initially developed in the late 1980s as a means of facilitating burn wound management.[36,371] More recently, the indications for this material have been extended to include the treatment of acute and chronic traumatic wounds (Fig. 15-22).[138,243,349]

The material is bilayered, consisting of a deep layer of a collagen glycosaminoglycan biodegradable matrix and a superficial semipermeable silicone layer. The deep layer allows for the ingrowth of native fibroblasts. Fibroblasts can form a "neodermis" upon the collagen scaffold, which is similar in appearance

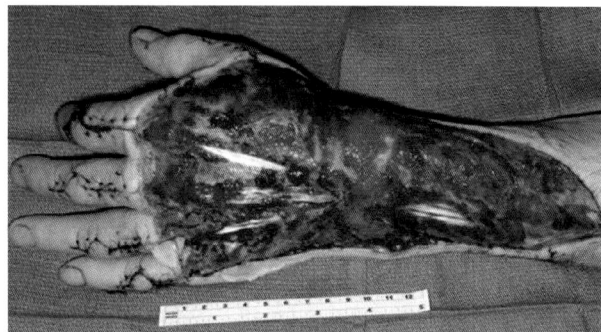

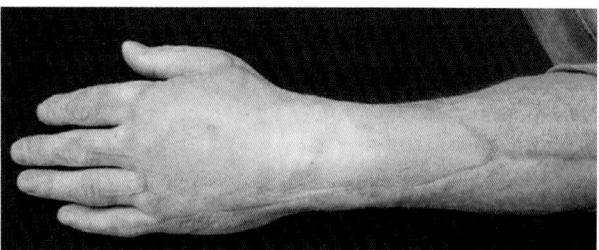

FIGURE 15-22 The application of Integra can allow for skin grafting to be performed over wounds previously requiring flap coverage. **A:** This 32-year-old man sustained an extensive degloving injury to the dorsum of his hand. Integra was applied over the exposed tendons and then VAC therapy was instituted for 14 days. **B:** After the establishment of a neodermis, the Integra was covered with a split-thickness skin graft providing stable and functional coverage of the hand.

to normal dermis.[242,320] This neodermis can then support a thin split-thickness skin graft. The silicone layer prevents desiccation during the ingrowth period and it is removed before the application of a skin graft. Major contraindications to the use of this material include ongoing infection and open fractures exposed within the wound.

Helgeson described the use of Integra in conjunction with skin grafting in 16 combat-related soft tissue wounds. The average wound size was 87 cm². Eleven wounds contained exposed tendon and five wounds had exposed bone devoid of overlying periosteum. Integra application was combined with overlying VAC therapy for an average of 19 days before the application of a split-thickness skin graft to the wounds. Treatment was successful in 83% cases. Failure was associated with the application over cortical bone.[138]

Acceleration of fibroblast ingrowth can be accomplished with the use of fibrin glue for fixation of the Integra and subsequent VAC therapy. In a retrospective review, Jeschke et al. found the use of fibrin glue and VAC therapy improved the "take rate" of split-thickness skin grafts from 78% to 98% and shortened the time to skin grafting. The overall hospital stay was also decreased.[166]

The use of the VAC and Integra has led to a decrease in the need for flap coverage for many traumatic wounds.[263] Despite this trend, the surgeon should exercise restraint in trying to apply these technologies to exposed bone, tendon, and large defects. Pedicled flaps and free tissue transfer provide reliable solutions to even the largest soft tissue defects, and should be considered the standard of care until formal comparative outcome studies are available to assess functional outcome and long-term consequences of these newer reconstructive technologies.

REFERENCES

1. Aberg M, Rydholm A, HolmbergJ, et al. Reconstruction with a free vascularized fibular graft for malignant bone tumor. *Acta Orthop Scand.* 1988;59(4):430–437.
2. Adani R, Delcroix L, Innocenti M, et al. Free fibula flap for humerus segmental reconstruction: Report on 13 cases. *Chir Organi Mov.* 2008;91(1):21–26.
3. Adani R, Delcroix L, Innocenti M, et al. Reconstruction of large posttraumatic skeletal defects of the forearm by vascularized free fibular graft. *Microsurgery.* 2004;24:423–429.
4. Adeymo O, Wyburn GM. Innervation of skin grafts. *Transplant Bull.* 1957;4:152–153.
5. Advanced Trauma Life Support. American College of Surgeons. 2012.
6. Allieu Y, Gomis R. Congenital pseudarthrosis of the forearm treated by the fibular graft. *J Hand Surg Am.* 1981;6:475–481.
7. Angrigiani C, Grilli D, Dominikow D, et al. Posterior interosseous reverse forearm flap: Experience with 80 consecutive cases. *Plast Reconstr Surg.* 1993;92:285–293.
8. Angrigiani C, Grilli D, Siebert J. Latissimus dorsi musculocutaneous flap without muscle. *Plast Reconstr Surg.* 1995;96(7):1608–1614.
9. Ao M, Nagase Y, Mae O, et al. Reconstruction of posttraumatic defects of the foot by flow-through anterolateral or anteromedial thigh flaps with preservation of posterior tibial vessels. *Ann Plast Surg.* 1997;38(6):598–603.
10. Arata M, Wood M, Cooney WR. Revascularized segmental diaphyseal bone transfers in the canine. An analysis of viability. *J Reconstr Microsurg.* 1984;1(1):11–19.
11. Argenta LC, Morykwas MJ. Vacuum-assisted closure: A new method for wound control and treatment: Clinical experience. *Ann Plast Surg.* 1997;38:563.
12. Arnez ZM, Kersnic M, Smith RW, et al. Free lateral arm osteocutaneous neurosensory flap for thumb reconstruction. *J Hand Surg Br.* 1991;16:395–399.
13. Askari M, Fisher BS, Weniger FG, et al. Anticoagulation therapy in microsurgery: A review. *J Hand Surg Am.* 2006;31:836.
14. Attinger CE, Janis JE, Steinberg J, et al. Clinical approach to wounds: Debridement and wound bed preparation including the use of dressings and wound-healing adjuvants. *Plast Reconstr Surg.* 2006;117:72S–109S.
15. Awtry EH, Loscalzo J. Aspirin. *Circulation.* 2000;101:1206.
16. Bakri K, Moran SL. Initial assessment and management of complex forearm defects. *Hand Clin.* 2007;23:255–268.
17. Bakri K, Shin AY, Moran SL. The vascularized medial femoral corticoperiosteal flap for reconstruction of bony defects within the upper and lower extremities. *Semin Plast Surg.* 2008; 22:228–233.
18. Balin AK. Dilute povidone-iodine solutions inhibit human skin fibroblast growth. *Dermatol Surg.* 2002;28(3):210–214.
19. Barnett AB, Ott R, Laub DR. Failure of healing of split skin donor sites in anhidrotic ectodermal dysplasia. *Plast Reconstr Surg.* 1979;64:97–100.
20. Barrie KA, Steinmann SP, Shin AY, et al. Gracilis free muscle transfer for restoration of function after complete brachial plexus avulsion. *Neurosurg Focus.* 2004;16(5):E8.
21. Barth E, Sullivan T, Berg E. Animal model for evaluating bone repair with and without adjunctive hyperbaric oxygen therapy (HBO): Comparing dose schedules. *J Invest Surg.* 1990;3(4):387–392.
22. Bellman S, Velander E, Frank HA, et al. Survival of arteries in experimental full thickness skin autografts. *Transplantation.* 1964;2:167–174.
23. Berggren A, Weiland AJ, Dorfman A. The effect of prolonged ischemia time on osteocyte and osteoblast survival in composite bone grafts revascularized by microvascular anastomoses. *Plast Reconstr Surg.* 1982;69(2):290–298.
24. Berggren A, Weiland AJ, Dorfman H. Free vascularized bone grafts: Factors affecting their survival and ability to heal to recipient bone defects. *Plastic Reconstr Surg.* 1982; 69(1):19–29.
25. Beris AE, Lykissas MG, Korompilias AV, et al. Vascularized fibula transfer for lower limb reconstruction. *Microsurgery.* 2011;31(3):205–211.
26. Bieber EJ, Wood MB. Bone reconstruction. *Clin Plast Surg.* 1986;13(4):645–655.
27. Bishop AT, Wood MB, Sheetz KK. Arthrodesis of the ankle with a free vascularized autogenous bone graft. Reconstruction of segmental loss of bone secondary to osteomyelitis, tumor, or trauma. *J Bone Joint Surg Am.* 1995;77(12):1867–1875.
28. Blondeel PN, Ali SR. Planning of perforator flaps. In: Bolondeel PN, Morris SF, Hallock GG, Neligan PC, eds. *Perforator Flaps: Anatomy, Technique, and Clinical Application.* 1st ed. St. Louis, MO: QMP; 2006:109–114.
29. Bosse MJ, MacKenzie EJ, Kellam JF, et al. An analysis of outcomes of reconstruction or amputation of leg threatening injuries. *N Engl J Med.* 2002;347:1924–1931.
30. Bosse MJ, McCarthy ML, Jones AJ, et al. The insensate foot following severe lower extremity trauma: An indication for amputation. *J Bone Joint Surg Am.* 2005; 87(12): 2601–2608.
31. Breidenbach WC, Trager S. Quantitative culture technique and infection in complex wounds of the extremities closed with free flaps. *Plast Reconstr Surg.* 1995;95(5): 860–865.
32. Brown RE, Wu TY. Use of "spare parts" in mutilated upper extremity injuries. *Hand Clin.* 2003;19(1):73–87, vi.
33. Bueno RA Jr, Neumeister MW. Outcomes after mutilating hand injuries: Review of the literature and recommendations for assessment. *Hand Clin.* 2003;19(1):193–204.
34. Bui DT, Cordeiro PG, Hu QY, et al. Free flap re-exploration: Indications treatment and outcomes in 1193 free flaps. *Plast Reconstr Surg.* 2007;119:2092–2100.
35. Burchardt H. The biology of bone graft repair. *Clin Orthop Relat Res.* 1983;(174):28–42.
36. Burke JF, Yannas IV, Quinby WC, et al. Successful use of a physiologically acceptable artificial skin in the treatment of extensive burn injury. *Ann Surg.* 1981;194:413–427.
37. Calderon W, Chang N, Mathes SJ. Comparison of the effect of bacterial inoculation in musculocutaneous and fasciocutaneous flaps. *Plast Reconstr Surg.* 1986;77(5): 785–794.
38. Calvert JW, Kohanzadeh S, Tynan M, et al. Free flap reconstruction for infection of ankle fracture hardware: Case report and review of the literature. *Surg Infect (Larchmt).* 2006;7:315–322.
39. Caputo WJ, Beggs DJ, DeFede JL, et al. A prospective randomised controlled clinical trial comparing hydrosurgery debridement with conventional surgical debridement in lower extremity ulcers. *Int Wound J.* 2008;5:288–294.
40. Carlsen BT, Bishop AT, Shin AY. Late reconstruction for brachial plexus injury. *Neurosurg Clin North Am.* 2009;20(1):51–64, vi.
41. Carpenter EB. Management of fractures of the shaft of the tibia and fibula. *J Bone Joint Surg Am.* 1966;48(8):1640–1646.
42. Celik N, Wei FC. Technical tips in perforator flap harvest. *Clin Plast Surg.* 2003;30: 469–472.
43. Chacha PB. Vascularised pedicular bone grafts. *Int Orthop.* 1984;8(2):117–138.
44. Chang N, Mathes SJ. Comparison of the effect of bacterial inoculation in musculocutaneous and random-pattern flaps. *Plast Reconstr Surg.* 1982;70(1):1–10.
45. Chen HC, Tang YB, Mardini S, et al. Reconstruction of the hand and upper limb with free flaps based on musculocutaneous perforators. *Microsurgery.* 2004;24(4):270–280.
46. Chen KT, Mardini S, Chuang DC, et al. Timing of presentation of the first signs of vascular compromise dictates the salvage outcome of free flap transfers. *Plast Reconstr Surg.* 2007;120(1):187–195.
47. Chen MC, Chang MC, Chen CM, et al. Double-strut free vascularized fibular grafting for reconstruction of the lower extremities. *Injury.* 2003;34:763–769.
48. Chen SH, Wei FC, Chen HC, et al. Emergency free-flap transfer for reconstruction of acute complex extremity wounds. *Plast Reconstr Surg.* 1992;89(5):882–888; discussion 9–90.
49. Chen ZW, Yan W. The study and clinical application of the osteocutaneous flap of fibula. *Microsurgery.* 1983;4(1):11–16.
50. Chien W, Varvares MA, Hadlock T, et al. Effects of aspirin and low-dose heparin in head and neck reconstruction using microvascular free flaps. *Laryngoscope.* 2005; 115(6):973–976.
51. Chim H, Sontich JK, Kaufman BR. Free tissue transfer with distraction osteogenesis is effective for limb salvage of the infected traumatized lower extremity. *Plast Reconstr Surg.* 2011;127(6):2364–2372.
52. Chou EK, Ulusal B, Ulusal A, et al. Using the descending branch of the lateral femoral circumflex vessel as a source of two independent flaps. *Plast Reconstr Surg.* 2006; 117(6):2059–2063.
53. Choudry U, Moran S, KaracorZ. Soft tissue coverage and outcome of Gustilo grade IIIB midshaft tibia fractures: A 15-year experience. *Plast Reconstr Surg.* 2008;122:479–485.
54. Choudry UH, Bakri K, Moran SL, et al. The vascularized medial femoral condyle periosteal bone flap for the treatment of recalcitrant bony nonunions. *Ann Plast Surg.* 2008;60:174–180.
55. Choudry UH, Moran SL, Li S, et al. Soft tissue coverage of the elbow: An outcome analysis and reconstructive algorithm. *Plast Reconstr Surg.* 2007;11:1852–1857.
56. Chung KC, Cederna PS. Endoscopic harvest of temporoparietal fascial free flaps for coverage of hand wounds. *J Hand Surg Am.* 2002;27A(3):525–533.
57. Clagett GP, Reisch JS. Prevention of venous thromboembolism in general surgical patients: Results of meta-analysis. *Ann Surg.* 1998;208:227.
58. Clarke RJ, Mayo G, Price P, et al. Suppression of thromboxane A2 but not of systemic prostacyclin by controlled-release aspirin. *N Engl J Med.* 1991;325:1137.
59. Clemens MW, Chang EI, Selber JC, et al. Composite extremity and trunk reconstruction with vascularized fibula flap in postoncologic bone defects: A 10-year experience. *Plast Reconstr Surg.* 2012;129(1):170–178.
60. Collaborative overview of randomised trials of antiplatelet therapy-III. Reduction in venous thrombosis and pulmonary embolism by antiplatelet prophylaxis among surgical and medical patients. Antiplatelet Trialists' Collaboration. *BMJ.* 1994:308(6923):235–246.
61. Conrad MH, Adams WP. Pharmacologic optimization of microsurgery in the new millennium. *Plast Reconstr Surg.* 2001;108:2088.
62. Converse JM, Rapaport FT. The vascularization of skin autografts and homografts: An experimental study in man. *Ann Surg.* 1956;143:306–315.
63. Converse JM, Smahel J, Ballantyne DL, et al. Inosculation of vessels of skin graft and host bed: A fortuitous encounter. *Br J Plast Surg.* 1975;28(4):274–282.
64. Cooney WP 3rd, Fitzgerald RH Jr, Dobyns JH, et al. Quantitative wound cultures in upper extremity trauma. *J Trauma.* 1982;22(2):112–117.
65. Corps BVM. The effect of graft thickness, donor site and graft bed on graft shrinkage in the hooded rat. *Br J Plast Surg.* 1969;22:125–133.
66. Court-Brown CM, Rimmer S, Prakash U, et al. The epidemiology of open long bone fractures. *Injury.* 1998;29(7):529–534.
67. Crock JG, Morrison WA. A vascularised periosteal flap: Anatomical study. *Br J Plast Surg.* 1992;45(6):474–478.
68. Cutting CB, McCarthy JG. Comparison of residual osseous mass between vascularized and nonvascularized onlay bone transfers. *Plast Reconstr Surg.* 1983;72(5):672–675.
69. Dagum AB, Best AK, Schemitsch EH, et al. Salvage after severe lower-extremity trauma: Are the outcomes worth the means? *Plast Reconstr Surg.* 1999;103(4):1212–1220.
70. Davies DM. A world survey of anticoagulation practice in clinical microvascular surgery. *Br J Plast Surg.* 1982;35:96.
71. de Chalain TMB. Exploring the use of the medicinal leech: A clinical risk-benefit analysis. *J Reconstr Microsurg.* 1996;12:165–172.
72. de la Torre J, Hedden W, Grant JH 3rd, et al. Retrospective review of the internal Doppler probe for intra- and postoperative microvascular surveillance. *J Reconstr Microsurg.* 2003;19(5):287–290.
73. DeFranco MJ, Lawton JN. Radial nerve injuries associated with humeral fractures. *J Hand Surg Am.* 2006;31(4):655–663.
74. DeFranzo AJ, Argenta LC, Marks MW, et al. The use of the vacuum-assisted closure therapy for treatment of lower-extremity wound with exposed bone. *Plast Reconstr Surg.* 2001;108:1184.
75. del Piñal F, Garda-Bemal FJ, Studer A, et al. Super-thinned iliac flap for major defects on the elbow and wrist flexion creases. *J Hand Surg Am.* 2008;33(10):1899–1904.

76. Dellon AL. "Think nerve" in upper extremity reconstruction. *Clin Plast Surg.* 1989; 16(3):617–627.
77. Dellon AL. Management of peripheral nerve problems in the upper and lower extremity using quantitative sensory testing. *Hand Clin.* 1999;15(4):697–715, x.
78. Dendrinos GK, Kontos S, Katsenis D, et al. Treatment of high-energy tibial plateau fractures by the Ilizarov circular fixator. *J Bone Joint Surg Br.* 1996;78(5):710–717.
79. Dendrinos GK, Kontos S, Lyritis E. Use of the Ilizarov technique for treatment of non-union of the tibia associated with infection. *J Bone Joint Surg Am.* 1995;77(6):835–846.
80. Derderian CA, Olivier WA, Baux G, et al. Microvascular free-tissue transfer for traumatic defects of the upper extremity: A 25-year experience. *J Reconstr Microsurg.* 2003; 19(7):455–462.
81. Diegelmann RF, Evans MC. Wound healing: An overview of acute, fibrotic, and delayed healing. *Front Biosci.* 2004;1:283–289.
82. Dirschl DR, Wilson FC. Topical antibiotic irrigation in the prophylaxis of operative wound infections in orthopedic surgery. *Orthop Clin North Am.* 1991;22(3):419–426.
83. Disa JJ, Cordeiro PG, Hidalgo DA. Efficacy of conventional monitoring techniques in free tissue transfer: An 11 year experience in 750 consecutive cases. *Plast Reconstr Surg.* 1999;104:97–101.
84. Disa JJ, Cordeiro PG. The current role of preoperative arteriography in free fibula flaps. *Plast Reconstr Surg.* 1998;102:1083–1088.
85. Doi K, Sakai K. Vascularized periosteal bone graft from the supracondylar region of the femur. *Microsurgery.* 1994;15(5):305–315.
86. Doi K, Tominaga S, Shibata T. Bone grafts with microvascular anastomoses of vascular pedicles: An experimental study in dogs. *J Bone Joint Surg Am.* 1977;59(6):809–815.
87. Dunham WK, Meyer RD. Vascularized bone grafts for reconstruction after tumor surgery. *Ala J Med Sci.* 1984;21(4):407–411.
88. Ekholm R, Ponzer S, Tornkvist H, et al. Primary radial nerve palsy in patients with acute humeral shaft fractures. *J Orthop Trauma.* 2008;22(6):408–414.
89. Ekholm R, Ponzer S, Tornkvist H, et al. The Holstein-Lewis humeral shaft fracture: Aspects of radial nerve injury, primary treatment, and outcome. *J Orthop Trauma.* 2008;22(10):693–697.
90. Elton SG, Rizzo M. Management of radial nerve injury associated with humeral shaft fractures: An evidence-based approach. *J Reconstr Microsurg.* 2008;24(8):569–573.
91. Enneking WF, Eady JL, Burchardt H. Autogenous cortical bone grafts in the reconstruction of segmental skeletal defects. *J Bone Joint Surg Am.* 1980;62(7):1039–1058.
92. Eo S, Kim D, Jones NF. Microdissection thinning of a pedicled deep inferior epigastric perforator flap for burn scar contracture of the groin case report. *J Reconstr Microsurg.* 2005;21(7):447–450; discussion 51–52.
93. Eren S, Klein W, Paar O. [Free, vascularized, folded fibula transplantation]. *Handchir Mikrochir Plast Chir.* 1993;25(1):33–38.
94. Faibisoff B, Daniel RK. Management of severe forearm injuries. *Surg Clin North Am.* 1981;61(2):287–301.
95. Fairhurst MJ. The function of below-knee amputee versus the patient with salvaged grade III tibial fracture. *Clin Orthop.* 1994;301:227–232.
96. Falanga V. Wound healing and its impairment in the diabetic foot. *Lancet.* 2005; 366(9498):1736–1743.
97. Fietsam R Jr, Bassett J, Glover JL, et al. Complications of coronary artery surgery in diabetic patients. *Am Surg.* 1992;57:551–557.
98. Finseth F, May JW, Smith RJ. Composite groin flap with iliac bone for primary thumb reconstruction. Case report. *J Bone Joint Surg Am.* 1976;58:130–132.
99. Fleischman W, Lang E, Klinzl L. Vacuum-assisted wound closure after dermatofasciotomy of the lower extremity. *Unfallchirurg.* 1996;99:283 (in German).
100. Fletcher I. Traction lesions of the brachial plexus. *Hand.* 1969;1:129–136.
101. Foster RJ, Swiontkowski MF, Bach AW, et al. Radial nerve palsy caused by open humeral shaft fractures. *J Hand Surg Am.* 1993;18(1):121–124.
102. Foucher G, van Genechten F, Merle N, et al. A compound radial artery forearm flap in hand surgery: An original modification of the Chinese forearm flap. *Br J Plast Surg.* 1984;37(2):139–148.
103. Fox CL. Silver sulfadiazine, a new topical therapy for Pseudomonas in burns. *Arch Surg.* 1968;96:184.
104. Francel TJ. Improving re-employment rates after limb salvage of acute severe tibial fractures by microvascular soft-tissue reconstruction. *Plast Reconstr Surg.* 1994;93:1028–1034.
105. Friedrich JB, Moran SL, Bishop AT, et al. Free vascularized fibular graft salvage of complications of long-bone allograft after tumor reconstruction. *J Bone Joint Surg Am.* 2008;90(1):93–100.
106. Friedrich JB, Moran SL, Bishop AT, et al. Vascularized fibula flap onlay for salvage of pathologic fracture of the long bones. *Plast Reconstr Surg.* 2008;121(6):2001–2009.
107. Friedrich JB, Shin AY. Management of forearm compartment syndrome. *Hand Clin.* 2007;23(2):245–254, vii.
108. Fuchs B, Steinmann P, Bishop AT. Free vascularized corticoperiosteal bone graft for the treatment of persistent nonunion of the clavicle. *J Shoulder Elbow Surg.* 2005;14: 264–268.
109. Fujimaki A, Suda H. Experimental study and clinical observations on hypertrophy of vascularized bone grafts. *Microsurgery.* 1994;15(10):726–732.
110. Gedebou TM, Wei FC, Lin CH. Clinical experience of 1284 free anterolateral thigh flaps. *Handchir Mikrochir Plast Chir.* 2002;34(4):239–244.
111. Geiger S, McCormick F, Chou R, et al. War wounds: Lessons learned from Operation Iraqi Freedom. *Plast Reconstr Surg.* 2008;122(1):146–153.
112. Georgescu AV, Ivan O. Serratus anterior-rib free flap in limb bone reconstruction. *Microsurgery.* 2003;23(3):217–225.
113. German G, Sherman R, Levin LS. *Decision Making in Reconstructive Surgery of the Upper Extremity.* New York, NY: Springer-Verlag; 1999.
114. Gerwin M, Weiland AJ. Vascularized bone grafts to the upper extremity. Indications and technique. *Hand Clin.* 1992;8(3):509–523.
115. Gidumal R, Wood MB, Sim FH, et al. Vascularized bone transfer for limb salvage and reconstruction after resection of aggressive bone lesions. *J Reconstr Microsurg.* 1987;3(3):183–188.
116. Giunta RE, Geisweid A, Feller AM. The value of preoperative Doppler sonography for planning free perforator flaps. *Plast Reconstr Surg.* 2000;105:2381–2386.
117. Glicksman A, Gerder M, Casale P, et al. Fourteen hundred fifty-seven years of microsurgical experience. *Plast Reconstr Surg.* 1997;100(2):355–363.
118. Godina M. Early microsurgical reconstruction of complex trauma of the extremities. *Plast Reconstr Surg.* 1986;78(3):285–292.
119. Goldberg VM, Shaffer JW, Field G, et al. Biology of vascularized bone grafts. *Orthop Clin North Am.* 1987;18(2):197–205.
120. Gornet MF, Randolph MA, Schofield BH, et al. Immunologic and ultrastructural changes during early rejection of vascularized bone allografts. *Plast Reconstr Surg.* 1991; 88(5):860–868.
121. Graham B, Paulus DA, Caffee HH. Pulse oximetry for vascular monitoring in upper extremity replacement surgery. *J Hand Surg Am.* 1986;11A:687.
122. Gravante G, Delogu D, Esposito G, et al. Versajet hydrosurgery versus classic escharectomy for burn debridement: A prospective randomized trial. *J Burn Care Res.* 2007; 28:720–724.
123. Green SA. Ilizarov method. *Clin Orthop Relat Res.* 1992;(280):2–6.
124. Greenberg BM, Masem M, May JW. Therapeutic value of intravenous heparin in microvascular surgery: An experimental vascular thrombosis study. *Plast Reconstr Surg.* 1988;82:463.
125. Gustilo RB, Anderson JT. Prevention of infection in the treatment of 1025 open fractures of long bones: Retrospective and prospective analyses. *J Bone Joint Surg Am.* 1976; 58(4):453–458.
126. Gustilo RB, Simpson L, Nixon R, et al. Analysis of 511 open fractures. *Clin Orthop Relat Res.* 1969;66:148–154.
127. Hallock GG. Anatomic basis of the gastrocnemius perforator based flap. *Ann Plast Surg.* 2001;47(5):517–522.
128. Hallock GG. Doppler sonography and color duplex imaging for planning a perforator flap. *Clin Plast Surg.* 2003;30(3):347–357.
129. Hallock GG. Extremity tissue expansion. *Orthop Rev.* 1987;16(9):606–611.
130. Hallock GG. Free flap donor site refinement using tissue expansion. *Ann Plast Surg.* 1988;20(6):566–572.
131. Hallock GG. Getting the most from the soleus muscle. *Ann Plast Surg.* 1996;36: 139–146.
132. Hallock GG. Severe lower-extremity injury. The rationale for microsurgical reconstruction. *Orthop Rev.* 1986;15(7):465–470.
133. Hallock GG. The pre-expanded anterolateral thigh free flap. *Ann Plast Surg.* 2004;53(2): 170–173.
134. Han CS, Wood MB, Bishop AT, et al. Vascularized bone transfer. *J Bone Joint Surg Am.* 1992;74(10):1441–1449.
135. Hardin CK, Kirk WC, Pederson WC. Osmotic complications of low-molecular-weight dextran therapy in free flap surgery. *Microsurgery.* 1992;13:36.
136. Heckler MW, Bamberger HB. Humeral shaft fractures and radial nerve palsy: To explore or not to explore…that is the question. *Am J Orthop.* 2008;37(8):415–419.
137. Hein KD, Wechsler ME, Schwartzstein RM, et al. The adult respiratory distress syndrome after dextran infusion as an antithrombotic agent in free TRAM flap breast reconstruction. *Plast Reconstr Surg.* 1999;103:1706.
138. Helgeson MD, Potter BK, Evans KN, et al. Bioartificial dermal substitute: A preliminary report on its use for the management of complex combat-related soft tissue wounds. *J Orthop Trauma.* 2007;21:394–399.
139. Hendel PM, Hattner RS, Rodrigo J, et al. The functional vascular anatomy of rib. *Plast Reconstr Surg.* 1982;70(5):578–587.
140. Hendry HAM. The treatment of residual paralysis after brachial plexus lesions. *J Bone Joint Surg.* 1949;31B:42.
141. Hentz VR, Pearl RM. The irreplaceable free flap: Part I. Skeletal reconstruction by microvascular free bone transfer. *Ann Plast Surg.* 1983;10(1):36–42.
142. Hentz VR, Pearl RM. The irreplaceable free flap: Part II. Skeletal reconstruction by microvascular free bone transfer. *Ann Plast Surg.* 1983;10(1):43–54.
143. Herscovici D, Sanders RW, Scaduto JM, et al. Vacuum-assisted wound closure (VAC therapy) for management of patients with high-energy soft tissue injuries. *J Orthop Trauma.* 2003;17:683–688.
144. Herter F, Ninkovic M, Ninkovic M. Rational flap selection and timing for coverage of complex upper extremity trauma. *J Plast Reconstr Aesthet Surg.* 2006;60:760–768.
145. Hidalgo DA, Jones CS. The role of emergent exploration in free tissue transfer: A review of 150 consecutive cases. *Plast Reconstr Surg.* 1990;86:492–498.
146. Hirigoyen MB, Urken ML, Weinberg H. Free flap monitoring: A review of current practice. *Microsurgery.* 1995;16:723.
147. Hong JP, Shin HW, Kim JJ, et al. The use of anterolateral thigh perforator flaps in chronic osteomyelitis of the lower extremity. *Plast Reconstr Surg.* 2005;115(1): 142–147.
148. Hovius SER, van Adrichem LNA, Mulder HD, et al. Comparison of laser Doppler flowmetry and thermometry in the postoperative monitoring of replantations. *J Hand Surg Am.* 1995;20:88–93.
149. Howe H, Poole GV, Hansen, KJ, et al. Salvage of lower extremities following combined orthopaedic and vascular trauma: A predictive salvage index. *Clin Am.* 1987;53: 205–208.
150. Hsieh CH, Yang CC, Kuo YR, et al. Free anterolateral thigh adipofascial perforator flap. *Plast Reconstr Surg.* 2003;112(4):976–982.
151. Huang WC, Lin JY, Wallace CG, et al. Vascularized bone grafts within composite tissue allotransplants can autocreate tolerance through mixed chimerism with partial myeloablative conditioning: An experimental study in rats. *Plast Reconstr Surg.* 2010;125(4): 1095–1103.
152. Hugon S, Daubresse F, Depierreux L. Radial nerve entrapment in a humeral fracture callus. *Acta Orthop Belg.* 2008;74(1):118–121.
153. Hui KC, Zhang F, Lineaweaver WC, et al. Serratus anterior-rib composite flap: Anatomic studies and clinical application to hand reconstruction. *Ann Plast Surg.* 1999;42(2): 132–136.

154. Hussl H, Sailer R, Daniaux H, et al. Revascularization of a partially necrotic talus with a vascularized bone graft from the iliac crest. *Arch Orthop Trauma Surg.* 1989;108(1):27–29.

155. Ikeda K, Tomita K, Hashimoto F, et al. Long-term follow-up of vascularized bone grafts for the reconstruction of tibial nonunion: Evaluation with computed tomographic scanning. *J Trauma.* 1992;32(6):693–697.

156. Ilizarov GA, Ledyaev VI. The replacement of long tubular bone defects by lengthening distraction osteotomy of one of the fragments. 1969. *Clin Orthop Relat Res.* 1992;(280):7–10.

157. Ilizarov GA. Clinical application of the tension-stress effect for limb lengthening. *Clin Orthop Relat Res.* 1990;(250):8–26.

158. Ilizarov GA. The tension-stress effect on the genesis and growth of tissues. Part I. The influence of stability of fixation and soft-tissue preservation. *Clin Orthop Relat Res.* 1989;(238):249–281.

159. Ilizarov GA. The tension-stress effect on the genesis and growth of tissues: Part II. The influence of the rate and frequency of distraction. *Clin Orthop Relat Res.* 1989;(239):263–285.

160. Ilyas AM, Jupiter JB. Treatment of distal humerus fractures. *Acta Chir Orthop Traumatol Cech.* 2008;75(1):6–15.

161. Innis PC, Randolph MA, Paskert JP, et al. Vascularized bone allografts: In vitro assessment of cell-mediated and humoral responses. *Plast Reconstr Surg.* 1991;87(2):315–325.

162. Ippolito E, Peretti G, Bellocci M, et al. Histology and ultrastructure of arteries, veins, and peripheral nerves during limb lengthening. *Clin Orthop Relat Res.* 1994;(308):54–62.

163. Janis JE, Kwon RK, Attinger CE. The new reconstructive ladder: Modifications to the traditional model. *Plast Reconstr Surg.* 2011;127(suppl 1):205S–212S.

164. Jensen M, Moran SL. Soft tissue coverage of the elbow: A reconstructive algorithm. *Orthop Clin North Am.* 2008;39:251–264.

165. Jensen MH, Moran SL. Why wounds fail to heal. In: Moran SL, Cooney WP, eds. *Soft Tissue Surgery.* Baltimore, MD: Lippincott Williams & Wilkins; 2008:1–10.

166. Jeschke MG, Rose C, Angele P, et al. Development of new reconstructive techniques: Use of Integra in combination with fibrin glue and negative-pressure therapy for reconstruction of acute and chronic wounds. *Plast Reconstr Surg.* 2004;113:525–530.

167. Johansen K, Daines M, Hower T, et al. Objective criteria accurately predict amputation following lower extremity trauma. *J Trauma.* 1990;30:568–573.

168. Jones DB Jr, Bürger H, Bishop AT, et al. Treatment of scaphoid waist nonunions with an avascular proximal pole and carpal collapse. Surgical technique. *J Bone Joint Surg Am.* 2009;91(suppl 2):169–183.

169. Jones DB Jr, Moran SL, Bishop AT, et al. Free-vascularized medial femoral condyle bone transfer in treatment of scaphoid nonunions. *Plast Reconstr Surg.* 2010;125:1176–1184.

170. Jones DB Jr, Rhee PC, Bishop AT, et al. Free vascularized medial femoral condyle autograft for challenging upper extremity nonunions. *Hand Clin.* 2012;28(4):493–501.

171. Jones NF, Swartz WM, Mears DC, et al. The "double barrel" free vascularized fibular bone graft. *Plast Reconstr Surg.* 1988;81(3):378–385.

172. Joshi BB. Neural repair for sensory restoration in a groin flap. *Hand.* 1977;9:221–225.

173. Jupiter JB, Bour CJ, May JW Jr. The reconstruction of defects in the femoral shaft with vascularized transfers of fibular bone. *J Bone Joint Surg Am.* 1987;69(3):365–374.

174. Jupiter JB, Gerhard HJ, Guerrero J, et al. Treatment of segmental defects of the radius with use of the vascularized osteoseptocutaneous fibular autogenous graft. *J Bone Joint Surg Am.* 1997;79(4):542–550.

175. Jupiter JB, Tsai TM, Kleinert HE. Salvage replantation of lower limb amputations. *Plast Reconstr Surg.* 1982;69:1–8.

176. Karanas YL, Nigriny J, Chang J. The timing of microsurgical reconstruction in lower extremity trauma. *Microsurgery.* 2008;28(8):632–634.

177. Kaufman MR, Jones NF. The reverse radial forearm flap for soft tissue reconstruction of the wrist and hand. *Tech Hand Up Extrem Surg.* 2005;9(1):47–51.

178. Kawashima M, Tamura H, Nagayoshi I, et al. Hyperbaric oxygen therapy in orthopedic conditions. *Undersea Hyperb Med.* 2004;31(1):155–162.

179. Khatod M, Botte MJ, Hoyt DB, et al. Outcomes in open tibial fractures: Relationship in delay in treatment and infection. *J Trauma.* 2003;55:951.

180. Khouri RK, Cooley BC, Kunselman AR, et al. A prospective study of microvascular free-flap surgery and outcome. *Plast Reconstr Surg.* 1998;102(3):711–721.

181. Kim DH, Kam AC, Chandika P, et al. Surgical management and outcome in patients with radial nerve lesions. *J Neurosurg.* 2001;95(4):573–583.

182. Kim PD, Blackwell KE. Latissimus-serratus-rib free flap for oromandibular and maxillary reconstruction. *Arch Otolaryngol Head Neck Surg.* 2007;133(8):791–795.

183. Kimura N, Saito M, Sumiya Y, et al. Reconstruction of hand skin defects by microdissected mini anterolateral thigh perforator flaps. *J Plast Reconstr Aesthet Surg.* 2008;61(9):1073–1077.

184. Kimura N, Saitoh M, Okamura T, et al. Concept and anatomical basis of microdissected tailoring method for free flap transfer. *Plast Reconstr Surg.* 2009;123(1):152–162.

185. Kimura N, Satoh K. Consideration of a thin flap as an entity and clinical applications of the thin anterolateral thigh flap. *Plast Reconstr Surg.* 1996;97(5):985–992.

186. King KF. Periosteal pedicle grafting in dogs. *J Bone Joint Surg Br.* 1976;58(1):117–121.

187. Klein MB, Hunter S, Heimbach DM, et al. The Versajet water dissector: A new tool for tangential excision. *J Burn Care Rehabil.* 2005;26:483–487.

188. Knighton DR, Silver IA, Hunt TK. Regulation of wound-healing angiogenesis: Effect of oxygen gradients and inspired oxygen concentration. *Surgery.* 1981;90(2):262–270.

189. Koshima I, Higaki H, Soeda S. Combined vascularized fibula and peroneal composite-flap transfer for severe heat-press injury of the forearm. *Plast Reconstr Surg.* 1991;88(2):338–341.

190. Kozol RA, Gilles C. Effects of sodium hypochlorite (Dakin's solution) on cells of the wound module. *Arch Surg.* 1988;123(4):420–423.

191. Kremer T, Bickert B, Germann G, et al. Outcome assessment after reconstruction of complex defects of the forearm and hand with osteocutaneous free flaps. *Plast Reconstr Surg.* 2006;118(2):443–454; discussion 55–56.

192. Krizek TJ, Robson MC, Kho E. Bacterial growth and skin graft survival. *Surg Forum.* 1967;18:518–519.

193. Kroll S, Schusterman MA, Reece GP, et al. Timing of pedicle thrombosis and flap loss after free-tissue transfer. *Plast Reconstr Surg.* 1996;98(7):1230–1233.

194. Kucan JO, Robson MC, Heggers JP, et al. Comparison of silver sulfadiazine, povidone-iodine, and physiological saline in the treatment of chronic pressure ulcers. *J Am Geriatr Soc.* 1981;29:232.

195. Kuo YR, Jeng SF, Kuo MH, et al. Free anterolateral thigh flap for extremity reconstruction: Clinical experience and functional assessment of donor site. *Plast Reconstr Surg.* 2001;107(7):1766–1771.

196. Kuo YR, Seng-Feng J, Kuo FM, et al. Versatility of the free anterolateral thigh flap for reconstruction of soft-tissue defects: Review of 140 cases. *Ann Plast Surg.* 2002;48(2):161–166.

197. Lange RH. Limb reconstruction versus amputation decision making in massive lower extremity trauma. *Clin Orthop.* 1989;243:92–99.

198. Larsen LB, Barfred T. Radial nerve palsy after simple fracture of the humerus. *Scand J Plast Reconstr Surg Hand Surg.* 2000;34(4):363–366.

199. Lee J, Oh SJ, Jung SW, et al. Ilizarov distraction and vascularized fibular osteocutaneous graft for postosteomyelitis skeletal deformity of the forearm. *J Reconstr Microsurg.* 2012;28(9):627–630.

200. Lettieri SC, Moran SL. The pedicled soleus muscle flap for coverage of the middle and distal third of the tibia. In: Moran SL, Cooney WPI, eds. *Soft Tissue Surgery.* Philadelphia, PA: Lippincott Williams & Wilkins; 2008:345–360.

201. Letts M, Pang E, Yang J, et al. Periosteal augmentation of the acetabulum. *Clin Orthop Relat Res.* 1998;(354):216–223.

202. Leung PC, Hung LK. Bone reconstruction after giant-cell tumor resection at the proximal end of the humerus with vascularized iliac crest graft. A report of three cases. *Clin Orthop Relat Res.* 1989;(247):101–105.

203. Leung PC. Femoral head reconstruction and revascularization. Treatment for ischemic necrosis. *Clin Orthop Relat Res.* 1996;(323):139–145.

204. Levin LS, Condit DP. Combined injuries—soft tissue management. *Clin Orthop Relat Res.* 1996;(327):172–181.

205. Levin LS, Erdmann D. Primary and secondary microvascular reconstruction of the upper extremity. *Hand Clin.* 2001;17(3):447–455, ix.

206. Levin LS, Goldner RD, Urbaniak JR, et al. Management of severe musculoskeletal injuries of the upper extremity. *J Orthop Trauma.* 1990;4:432–440.

207. Levin SL, Baumeister S. Lower extremity. In: Wei FC, Mardini S, eds. *Flaps and Reconstructive Surgery.* London: Elsevier; 2009:63–70.

208. Liang K, Cen S, Xiang Z, et al. Massive juxta-articular defects of the distal femur reconstructed by series connected double-strut free-vascularized fibular grafts. *J Trauma Acute Care Surg.* 2012;72(2):E71–E76.

209. Lin CH, Mardini S, Levin SL, et al. Endoscopically assisted sural nerve harvest for upper extremity posttraumatic nerve defects an evaluation of functional outcomes. *Plast Reconstr Surg.* 2007;119(2):616–626.

210. Lin CH, Mardini S, Lin YT, et al. Sixty-five clinical cases of free tissue transfer using long arteriovenous fistulas or vein grafts. *J Trauma.* 2004;56:1107–1117.

211. Lin CH, Wei FC, Levin LS, et al. Donor-site morbidity comparison between endoscopically assisted and traditional harvest of free latissimus dorsi muscle flap. *Plast Reconstr Surg.* 1999;104:1070–1078.

212. Lin CH, Wei FC, Levin LS, et al. Free composite serratus anterior and rib flaps for tibial composite bone and soft-tissue defect. *Plast Reconstr Surg.* 1997;99(6):1656–1665.

213. Lin CH, Wei FC, Lin YT, et al. Endoscopically assisted fascia-saving harvest of rectus abdominis. *Plast Reconstr Surg.* 2001;108(3):713–718.

214. Lister G, Scheker L. Emergency free flaps to the upper extremity. *J Hand Surg Am.* 1988;13(1):22–28.

215. Livani B, Belangero WD, Castro de Medeiros R. Fractures of the distal third of the humerus with palsy of the radial nerve: Management using minimally-invasive percutaneous plate osteosynthesis. *J Bone Joint Surg Br.* 2006;88(12):1625–1628.

216. Lutz BS, Wei FC, Ng SH, et al. Routine donor leg angiography before vascularized free fibula transplantation is not necessary: A prospective study of 120 clinical cases. *Plast Reconstr Surg.* 1999;103:121–127.

217. MacKenzie EJ, Bosse MJ. Factors influencing outcome following limb threatening lower limb trauma: Lessons learned from the Lower Extremity Assessment Project (LEAP). *J Am Acad Orthop Surg.* 2006;14:S205–S210.

218. Mackinnon SE, Novak CB. Nerve transfers. New options for reconstruction following nerve injury. *Hand Clin.* 1999;15(4):643–666, ix.

219. Mader JT, Brown GL, Wells CH, et al. A mechanism for the amelioration by hyperbaric oxygen of experimental staphylococcal osteomyelitis in rabbits. *J Infect Dis.* 1980;142(6):915–922.

220. Malizos KN, Dailiana ZH, Innocenti M, et al. Vascularized bone grafts for upper limb reconstruction: Defects at the distal radius, wrist, and hand. *J Hand Surg Am.* 2010;35(10):1710–1718.

221. Malizos KN, Quarles LD, Seaber AV, et al. An experimental canine model of osteonecrosis: Characterization of the repair process. *J Orthop Res.* 1993;11(3):350–357.

222. Malizos KN, Zalavras CG, Soucacos PN, et al. Free vascularized fibular grafts for reconstruction of skeletal defects. *J Am Acad Orthop Surg.* 2004;12(5):360–369.

223. Mangano DT, Layug EL, Wallace A, et al. Effect of atenolol on mortality and cardiovascular morbidity after noncardiac surgery. *N Engl J Med.* 1996;335(23):1713–1720.

224. Mardini S, Lin LC, Moran SL, et al. Anterolateral thigh flap. In: Wei FC, ed. *Flaps and Reconstructive Surgery.* London: Elsevier; 2009:93–101.

225. Mardini S, Wei FC, Salgado CJ, et al. Reconstruction of the reconstructive ladder. *Plast Reconstr Surg.* 2005;115(7):2174.

226. Mast BA, Schultz GS. Interaction of cytokines, proteases and growth factors in acute and chronic wounds. *Wound Repair Regen.* 1996;4:411–420.

227. Mathes SJ, Nahai F. Classification of the vascular anatomy of muscles: Experimental and clinical correlation. *Plast Reconstr Surg.* 1981;67:177–187.

228. Mathoulin C. Comment on "Scaphoid nonunion: Treatment with a pedicled vascularized bone graft based on the 1,2 intercompartmental supraretinacular branch of the radial artery". *J Hand Surg Br.* 2003;28(3):281–282; author reply 2.

229. Mazur KU, Bishop AT, Berger RA. *Vascularized bone grafting for Kienbock's disease: Method and results of retrograde-flow metaphyseal grafts and comparison with cortical graft sites (SS-03).* Presented at: 51st Annual Meeting of the American Society for Surgery of the Hand, August 4–7. Nashville, TN; 1996.

230. Mazzer N, Barbieri CH, Cortez M. The posterior interosseous forearm island flap for skin defects in the hand and elbow. A prospective study of 51 cases. *J Hand Surg Br.* 1996;21B:237–243.

231. McGregor IA, McGregor AD. *Fundamental Techniques of Plastic Surgery.* 9th ed. Edinburgh, SA: Churchill-Livingstone; 1995.

232. McKay PL, Nanos G. Initial evaluation and management of complex traumatic wounds. In: Moran SL, Cooney WP, eds. *Soft Tissue Surgery.* Philadelphia, PA: Lippincott Williams & Wilkins; 2009:11–37.

233. McNamara MG, Heckman JD, Corley FG. Severe open fractures of the lower extremity: A retrospective evaluation of the Mangled Extremity Severity Score (MESS). *J Orthop Trauma.* 1994;8:81–87.

234. Medalie DA, Llull R, Heckler F. The iliacus muscle flap: An anatomical and clinical evaluation. *Plast Reconstr Surg.* 2011;127(4):1553–1560.

235. Medrykowski F, Barbary S, Gibert N, et al. Vascularized proximal fibular epiphyseal transfer: Two cases. *Orthop Traumatol Surg Res.* 2012;98(6):728–732.

236. Mercer N, Beere D, Bornemisza A, et al. Medicinal leeches as sources of wound infection. *BMJ.* 1987;294:937.

237. Metaizeau JP, Olive D. [Conservative treatment of malignant bone tumors by vascularized bone grafts]. *Presse Med.* 1983;12(15):960–961.

238. Minami A, Kaneda K, Itoga H. Treatment of infected segmental defect of long bone with vascularized bone transfer. *J Reconstr Microsurg.* 1992;8(2):75–82.

239. Mirzabeigi MN, Wang T, Kovach SJ, et al. Free flap take-back following postoperative microvascular compromise: Predicting salvage versus failure. *Plast Reconstr Surg.* 2012;130:579–589.

240. Missana MC, Pomel C. Endoscopic latissimus dorsi flap harvesting. *Am J Surg.* 2007;194(2):164–169.

241. Miyawaki T, Jackson IT, Elmazar H, et al. The effect of low-molecular-weight heparin in the survival of a rabbit congested skin flap. *Plast Reconstr Surg.* 2002;109(6):1994–1999.

242. Moiemen NS, Staiano JJ, Ojeh NO, et al. Reconstructive surgery with a dermal regeneration template: Clinical and histologic study. *Plast Reconstr Surg.* 2001;108:93–103.

243. Molnar JA, Defranzo AJ, Hadaegh A, et al. Acceleration of Integra incorporation in complex tissue defects with subatmospheric pressure. *Plast Reconstr Surg.* 2004;113:1339–1346.

244. Mommsen P, Zeckey C, Hildebrand F, et al. Traumatic extremity arterial injury in children: Epidemiology, diagnostics, treatment and prognostic value of Mangled Extremity Severity Score. *J Orthop Surg Res.* 2010;5:25.

245. Moore JR, Weiland AJ, Daniel RK. Use of free vascularized bone grafts in the treatment of bone tumors. *Clin Orthop Relat Res.* 1983;(175):37–44.

246. Moore JR, Weiland AJ. Free vascularized bone and muscle flaps for osteomyelitis. *Orthopedics.* 1986;9(6):819–824.

247. Moran CG, Wood MB. Vascularized bone autografts. *Orthop Rev.* 1993;22(2):187–197.

248. Moran SL, Bakri K, Mardini S, et al. The use of vascularized fibular grafts for the reconstruction of spinal and sacral defects. *Microsurgery.* 2009;29:393–400.

249. Moran SL, Johnson CH. Skin and soft tissue: Pedicled flaps. In: Berger RA, Weiss AP, eds. *Hand Surgery.* Philadelphia, PA: Lippincott Williams & Wilkins; 2004:1131–1160.

250. Moran SL, Salgado CJ. Free tissue transfer in patients with renal disease. *Plast Reconstruct Surg.* 2004;113(7):2006–2011.

251. Moran SL, Shin AY, Bishop AT. The use of massive bone allograft with intramedullary free fibular flap for limb salvage in a pediatric and adolescent population. *Plast Reconstr Surg.* 2006;118:413–419.

252. Moran SL, Steinmann SP, Shin AY. Adult brachial plexus injuries: Mechanism, patterns of injury, and physical diagnosis. *Hand Clin.* 2005;21(1):13–24.

253. Morykwas, MJ, Argenta, LC, Shelton-Brown EL, et al. Vacuum-assisted closure: A new method for wound control and treatment: Animal studies and basic foundation. *Ann Plast.* 1997;38(6):553–562.

254. Netscher D, Alford EL, Wigoda P, et al. Free composite myo-osseous flap with serratus anterior and rib: Indications in head and neck reconstruction. *Head Neck.* 1998;20(2):106–112.

255. Newington DP, Sykes PJ. The versatility of the free fibula flap in the management of traumatic long bone defects. *Injury.* 1991;22(4):275–281.

256. Ninkovic M, Deetjen H, Ohler K, et al. Emergency free tissue transfer for severe upper extremity injuries. *J Hand Surg Br.* 1995;20(1):53–58.

257. Ninkovic M, Harpf C, Schwabegger AH, et al. The lateral arm flap. *Clin Plast Surg.* 2001;28:367–374.

258. Nusbickel FR, Dell PC, McAndrew MP, et al. Vascularized autografts for reconstruction of skeletal defects following lower extremity trauma. A review. *Clin Orthop Relat Res.* 1989;(243):65–70.

259. Ostrowski DM, Eilert RE, Waldstein G. Congenital pseudarthrosis of the ulna: A report of two cases and a review of the literature. *J Pediatr Orthop.* 1985;5(4):463–467.

260. Ostrup LT. Free bone transfers. Some theoretical aspects. *Scand J Plast Reconstr Surg Suppl.* 1982;19:103–104.

261. Ozkan O, Coskunfirat OK, Ozgentas HE. The use of free anterolateral thigh flap for reconstructing soft tissue defects of the lower extremities. *Ann Plast Surg.* 2004;53(5):455–461.

262. Park JE, Rodriguez ED, Bludbond-Langer R, et al. The anterolateral thigh flap is highly effective for reconstruction of complex lower extremity trauma. *J Trauma.* 2007;62(1):162–165.

263. Parrett BM, Maros E, Pribaz JJ, et al. Lower extremity trauma: Trends in the management of soft-tissue reconstruction of open tibia-fibula fractures. *Plast Reconstr Surg.* 2006;117:1315–1322.

264. Paskert JP, Yaremchuk MJ, Randolph MA, et al. Prolonging survival in vascularized bone allograft transplantation: Developing specific immune unresponsiveness. *J Reconstr Microsurg.* 1987;3(3):253–263.

265. Paskert JP, Yaremchuk MJ, Randolph MA, et al. The role of cyclosporin in prolonging survival in vascularized bone allografts. *Plast Reconstr Surg.* 1987;80(2):240–247.

266. Penfold CN, Davies HT, Cole RP, et al. Combined latissimus dorsi-serratus anterior/rib composite free flap in mandibular reconstruction. *Int J Oral Maxillofac Surg.* 1992;21(2):92–96.

267. Penteado CV, Masquelet AC, Romana MC, et al. Periosteal flaps: Anatomical bases of sites of elevation. *Surg Radiol Anat.* 1990;12(1):3–7.

268. Pho RW, Levack B, Satku K, et al. Free vascularised fibular graft in the treatment of congenital pseudarthrosis of the tibia. *J Bone Joint Surg Br.* 1985;67(1):64–70.

269. Pirela-Cruz MA, DeCoster TA. Vascularized bone grafts. *Orthopedics.* 1994;17(5):407–412.

270. Pomerance J, Truppa K, Bilos ZJ, et al. Replantation and revascularization of the digits in a community microsurgical practice. *J Reconstr Microsurg.* 1997;13:163.

271. Pu LLQ. Medial hemisoleus muscle flap: A reliable flap for soft tissue reconstruction of the middle third tibial wound. *Int Surg.* 2006;91:194–200.

272. Pugh CM, Dennis RHI, Massac EA. Evaluation of intraoperative anticoagulants in microvascular free-flap surgery. *J Natl Med Assoc.* 1996;88:655.

273. Rainer C, Schwabegger AH, Gardetto A, et al. Aesthetic refinements in reconstructive microsurgery of the lower leg. *J Reconstr Microsurg.* 2004;20(2):123–131.

274. Rajacic N, Gang RK, Krishnan J, et al. Thin anterolateral thigh free flap. *Ann Plast Surg.* 2002;48(3):252–257.

275. Ramachandran M, Birch R, Eastwood DM. Clinical outcome of nerve injuries associated with supracondylar fractures of the humerus in children: The experience of a specialist referral centre. *J Bone Joint Surg Br.* 2006;88(1):90–94.

276. Rasmussen MR, Bishop AT, Wood MB. Arthrodesis of the knee with a vascularized fibular rotatory graft. *J Bone Joint Surg Am.* 1995;77(5):751–759.

277. Redett RJ, Robertson BC, Chang B. Limb salvage in the lower extremity using free gracilis muscle reconstruction. *Plast Reconstr Surg.* 2000;106:1507–1513.

278. Reinisch JF, Winters R, Puckett CL. The use of the osteocutaneous groin flap in gunshot wounds of the hand. *J Hand Surg Am.* 1984;9:12–17.

279. Rightmire E, Zurakowski D, Vrahas M. Acute infections after fracture repair: Management with hardware in place. *Clin Orthop Relat Res.* 2008;466:466–472.

280. Rindell K, Solonen KA, Lindholm TS. Results of treatment of aseptic necrosis of the femoral head with vascularized bone graft. *Ital J Orthop Traumatol.* 1989;15(2):145–153.

281. Ring D, Chin K, Jupiter JB. Radial nerve palsy associated with high-energy humeral shaft fractures. *J Hand Surg Am.* 2004;29(1):144–147.

282. Rogachefsky RA, Quellette EA, Mendietta CG, et al. Free temporoparietal fascial flap for coverage of a large palmar forearm wound after hand replantation. *J Reconstr Microsurg.* 2001;17(6):421–423.

283. Romana MC, Masquelet AC. Vascularized periosteum associated with cancellous bone graft: An experimental study. *Plast Reconstr Surg.* 1990;85(4):587–592.

284. Rosenstein BD, Wilson FC, Funderburk CH. The use of bacitracin irrigation to prevent infection in postoperative skeletal wounds. An experimental study. *J Bone Joint Surg Am.* 1989;71(3):427–430.

285. Rothkopf DM, Chu B, Bern S, et al. The effect of dextran on microvascular thrombosis in an experimental rabbit model. *Plast Reconstr Surg.* 1993;92:511.

286. Saint-Cyr M, Daigle JP. Early free tissue transfer for extremity reconstruction following high-voltage electrical burn injuries. *J Reconstr Microsurg.* 2008;24:259–266.

287. Salemark L, Knudsen F, Dougan P. The effect of dextran 40 on patency following severe trauma in small arteries and veins. *Br J Plast Surg.* 1995;48:121.

288. Salemark L, Wiesland JB, Dougan P, et al. Effects of low and ultralow oral doses of acetylsalicylic acid in microvascular surgery. An experimental study in rabbits. *Scand J Plast Reconstr Surg Hand Surg.* 1991;25:203.

289. Salemark L, Wieslander JB, Dougan P, et al. Studies of the antithrombotic effects of dextran 40 following microarterial trauma. *Br J Plast Surg.* 1991;44:15.

290. Salgado CJ, Chim H, Schoenoff S, et al. Postoperative care and monitoring of the reconstructed head and neck patient. *Semin Plast Surg.* 2010;24(3):281–287.

291. Salgado CJ, Orlando GS, Herceg S, et al. Pfannenstiel incision as an alternative approach for harvesting the rectus abdominis muscle for free-tissue transfer. *Plast Reconstr Surg.* 2000;105(4):1330–1333.

292. Salgado CJ, Orlando GS, Serletti JM. Clinical applications of the posterior rectus sheath-peritoneal free flap. *Plast Reconstr Surg.* 2000;106(2):321–326.

293. Salgado CJ, Smith A, Kim S, et al. Effects of late loss of arterial inflow on free flap survival. *J Reconstr Microsurg.* 2002;18(7):579–584.

294. Salibian AH, Anzel SH, Salyer WA. Transfer of vascularized grafts of iliac bone to the extremities. *J Bone Joint Surg Am.* 1987;69(9):1319–1327.

295. Sammer DM, Bishop AT, Shin AY. Vascularized medial femoral condyle graft for thumb metacarpal reconstruction: Case report. *J Hand Surg Am.* 2009;34:715–718.

296. Sanders R, Mayou BJ. A new vascularized bone graft transferred by microvascular anastomosis as a free flap. *Br J Surg.* 1979;66(11):787–788.

297. Sauerbier M, Ofer N, Germann G, et al. Microvascular reconstruction in burn and electrical burn injuries of the severely traumatized upper extremity. *Plast Reconstr Surg.* 2007;119:605–615.

298. Sawhney CP, Subbaraju GV, Chakravarti RN. Healing of donor sites of split skin graft. *Br J Plast Surg.* 1969;22:359–364.

299. Schneeberger S, Morelon E, Landin L. ESOT CTA Committee. Vascularized composite allotransplantation: A member of the transplant family? *Transplantation.* 2012;93(11):1088–1091.

300. Schwanholt C, Greenhalgh DG, Warden GD. A comparison of full-thickness versus split-thickness autografts for the coverage of deep palm burns in the very young pediatric patient. *J Burn Care Rehabil.* 1993;14:20–33.

301. Seddon HJ. Three types of nerve injury. *Brain.* 1943;66:237–238.

302. Serletti JM, Moran SL, Orlando GS, et al. Urokinase protocol for free-flap salvage following prolonged venous thrombosis. *Plast Reconstr Surg.* 1998;102:1947–1953.

303. Shafer DM, Sherman CE, Moran SL. Hydrosurgical tangential excision of partial thickness hand burns. *Plast Reconstr Surg.* 2008;122:96e–97e.

304. Shaffer JW, Field GA, Wilber RG, et al. Experimental vascularized bone grafts: Histopathologic correlations with postoperative bone scan: The risk of false-positive results. *J Orthop Res.* 1987;5(3):311–319.
305. Shao YC, Harwood P, Grotz MR, et al. Radial nerve palsy associated with fractures of the shaft of the humerus: A systematic review. *J Bone Joint Surg Br.* 2005;87(12):1647–1652.
306. Shaw W. Aesthetic reconstructions of the leg after trauma. *Clin Plast Surg.* 1986;13(4):723–733.
307. Sheetz KK, Bishop AT, Berger RA. The arterial blood supply of the distal radius and its potential use in vascularized pedicled bone grafts. *J Hand Surg Am.* 1995;20A:902–914.
308. Shigetomi M, Doi K, Kuwata N, et al. Experimental study on vascularized bone allografts for reconstruction of massive bone defects. *Microsurgery.* 1994;15(9):663–670.
309. Shin AY, Spinner RJ, Steinmann SP, et al. Adult traumatic brachial plexus injuries. *J Am Acad Orthop Surg.* 2005;13(6):382–396.
310. Shin R, Ring D. The ulnar nerve in elbow trauma. *J Bone Joint Surg Am.* 2007;89(5):1108–1116.
311. Shivarathre DG, Dheerendra SK, Bari A, et al. Management of clinical radial nerve palsy with closed fracture shaft of humerus—a postal questionnaire survey. *Surgeon.* 2008;6(2):76–78.
312. Smith PJ FB, McGregor IA, Jackson IT. The anatomical basis of the groin flap. *Plast Reconstr Surg.* 1972;49:41–47.
313. Smith PJ. The Y-shaped hypogastric-groin flap. *Hand.* 1982;14:263–270.
314. Solomon GA, Yaremchuk MJ, Manson PN. Doppler ultrasound surface monitoring of both arterial and venous flow in clinical free tissue transfers. *J Reconstr Microsurg.* 1986;3:39.
315. Solonen KA, Rindell K, Paavilainen T. Vascularized pedicled bone graft into the femoral head—treatment of aseptic necrosis of the femoral head. *Arch Orthop Trauma Surg.* 1990;109(3):160–163.
316. Soni A, Tzafetta K, Knight S, et al. Gustilo IIIC fractures in the lower limb: Our 15-year experience. *J Bone Joint Surg Br.* 2012;94(5):698–703.
317. Sowa DT, Weiland AJ. Clinical applications of vascularized bone autografts. *Orthop Clin North Am.* 1987;18(2):257–273.
318. Stadelmann WK, Digenis AG, Tobin GR. Impediments to wound healing. *Am J Surg.* 1998;176(2 suppl 1):39S–47S.
319. Steirt AE, Gohritz A. Delayed flap coverage of open extremity fractures after previous vacuum-assisted closure (VAC) therapy—worse or worth? *J Plast Reconstr Aesthet Surg.* 2008;62(5):675–683.
320. Stern R, McPherson M, Longaker MT. Histologic study of artificial skin used in the treatment of full-thickness thermal injury. *J Burn Care Rehabil.* 1990;11:7–13.
321. Stevanovic M, Gutow AP, Sharpe F. The management of bone defects of the forearm after trauma. *Hand Clin.* 1999;15(2):299–318.
322. Strauch B, Yu H-L. Atlas of Microvascular Surgery. *Anatomy and Operative Approach.* 2nd ed. New York, NY: Thieme; 2006.
323. Summers AN, Sanger JR, Matloub HS. Lateral arm fascial flap microarterial anatomy and potential. *J Reconstr Microsurg.* 2000;16(4):279–286.
324. Sunagawa T, Bishop AT, Muramatsu K. Role of conventional and vascularized bone grafts in scaphoid nonunion with avascular necrosis: A canine experimental study [in proc cit]. *J Hand Surg Am.* 2000;25A(5):849–859.
325. Sunderland S. A classification of peripheral nerve injuries producing loss of function. *Brain.* 1951;74:491–516.
326. Swartz WM, Izquierdo R, Miller MJ. Implantable venous Doppler microvascular monitoring. *Plast Reconstr Surg.* 1994;93:152–163.
327. Takato T, Harii K, Nakatsuka T, et al. Vascularized periosteal grafts: An experimental study using two different forms of tibial periosteum in rabbits. *Plast Reconstr Surg.* 1986;78(4):489–497.
328. Takayanagi S, Ohtsuka M, TsukieT. Use of the latissimus dorsi and the serratus anterior muscles as a combined flap. *Ann Plast Surg.* 1988;20(4):333–339.
329. Tan CH. Reconstruction of the bones and joints of the upper extremity by vascularized free fibular graft: Report of 46 cases. *J Reconstr Microsurg.* 1992;8:285–292.
330. Tan NC, Cigna E, Varkey P, et al. Debulking of free myocutaneous flaps for head and neck reconstruction using an arthroscopic shaver. *Int J Oral Maxillofac Surg.* 2007;36(5):450–452.
331. Tanaka K, Maehara H, Kanaya F. Vascularized fibular graft for bone defects after wide resection of musculoskeletal tumors. *J Orthop Sci.* 2012;17(2):156–162.
332. Tobin GR. Hemisoleus and reversed hemisoleus flaps. *Plast Reconstr Surg.* 1985;76:87–96.
333. Trumble TE, McCallister WV. Repair of peripheral nerve defects in the upper extremity. *Hand Clin.* 2000;16(1):37–52.
334. Tsai FC. A new method: Perforator-based tissue expansion for a preexpanded free cutaneous perforator flap. *Burns.* 2003;29(8):845–848.
335. Tsai TM, Ludwig L, Tonkin M. Vascularized fibular epiphyseal transfer. A clinical study. *Clin Orthop Relat Res.* 1986;(210):228–234.
336. Tscherne H, Gotzen L. *Fractures with Soft Tissue Injuries.* Berlin: Springer-Verlag; 1984.
337. Tscherne H, Oestern HJ. Die Klassifizierung des Weichteilschadens bei offenen und geschlossenen Frakturen. *Unfallheilkunde.* 1982;85:111–115.
338. Tscherne H. The management of open fractures. In: Tscherne H, Gotzen L, eds. *Fractures with Soft Tissue Injuries.* New York, NY: Springer Verlag; 1984:10–32.
339. Tung TC, Wang KC, Fang CM, et al. Reverse pedicle lateral arm flap for reconstruction of posterior soft-tissue defects of the elbow. *Ann Plast Surg.* 1997;38:635–641.
340. Uchida Y, Sugioka Y. Effects of vascularized bone graft on surrounding necrotic bone: An experimental study. *J Reconstr Microsurg.* 1990;6(2):101–107; discussion 9, 11.
341. Urbaniak JR, Coogan PG, Gunneson EB, et al. Treatment of osteonecrosis of the femoral head with free vascularized fibular grafting. A long-term follow-up study of one hundred and three hips. *J Bone Joint Surg Am.* 1995;77(5):681–694.
342. Urken ML, Bridger AG, Zur KB, et al. The scapular osteofasciocutaneous flap: A 12-year experience. *Arch Otolaryngol Head Neck Surg.* 2001;127(7):862–869.
343. Usami F, Iketani M, Hirukawa M, et al. Treatment of congenital pseudoarthrosis of the tibia by a free vascularized fibular graft: Case report. *J Microsurg.* 1981;3(1):40–47.
344. Uysal AC, Lu F, Mizuno H, et al. Defining vascular supply and territory of thinned perforator flaps: Part I. Anterolateral thigh perforator flap. *Plast Reconstr Surg.* 2006;118(1):288–289.
345. Van Beek AL, Link WJ, Bennet JE, et al. Ultrasound evaluation of microanastomosis. *Arch Surg.* 1975;110:945.
346. Van Den Berghe G, Wouers P, Weekers F, et al. Intensive insulin therapy in critically ill patients. *N Engl J Med.* 2001;345(19):1359–1366.
347. Vande Berg JS, Rudolph R. Immunohistochemistry of fibronectin and actin in ungrafted wound and wounds covered with full-thickness and split-thickness skin grafts. *Plast Reconstr Surg.* 1993;91:684–692.
348. Varitimidis SE, Sotereanos DG. Partial nerve injuries in the upper extremity. *Hand Clin.* 2000;16(1):141–149.
349. Violas P, Abid A, Darodes P, et al. Integra artificial skin in the management of severe tissue defects, including bone exposure, in injured children. *J Pediatr Orthop.* 2005;14:381–384.
350. Wang C, Schwaitzberg S, Berliner E, et al. Hyperbaric oxygen for treating wounds: A systematic review of the literature. *Arch Surg.* 2003;138:272–279.
351. Wang HT, Erdmann D, Fletcher JW, et al. Anterolateral thigh flap technique in hand and upper extremity reconstruction. *Tech Hand Up Extrem Surg.* 2004;8(4):257–261.
352. Wei FC, El-Gammal TA, Lin CH, et al. Free fibular osteoseptocutaneous graft for reconstruction of segmental femoral shaft defects. *J Trauma.* 1997;43:784–792.
353. Wei FC, Jain V, Celik N, et al. Have we found an ideal soft-tissue flap? An experience with 672 anterolateral thigh flaps. *Plast Reconstr Surg.* 2002;109(7):2219–2226; discussion 27–30.
354. Wei FC, Mardini S. Free-style free flaps. *Plast Reconstr Surg.* 2004;114:910–916.
355. Weiland AJ, Moore JR, Daniel RK. Vascularized bone autografts. Experience with 41 cases. *Clin Orthop Relat Res.* 1983;(174):87–95.
356. Weiland AJ. Vascularized bone transfers. *Instr Course Lect.* 1984;33:446–460.
357. Weinzweig N, Gonzalez M. Free tissue failure is not an all-or-none phenomenon. *Plast Reconstr Surg.* 1995;96(3):648–660.
358. Weksler BB, Pett SB, Alonso D, et al. Differential inhibition by aspirin of vascular and platelet prostaglandin synthesis in atherosclerotic patients. *N Engl J Med.* 1983;308(14):800–805.
359. Winograd JM, Guo L. Upper extremity. In: Wei FC, Mardini S, eds. *Flaps and Reconstructive Surgery.* London: Elsevier; 2009:51–61.
360. Wong CH, Ong YS, Chew KY, et al. The fibula osteoseptocutaneous flap incorporating the hemisoleus muscle for complex head and neck defects: Anatomical study and clinical applications. *Plast Reconstr Surg.* 2009;124(6):1956–1964.
361. Wong CH, Tan BK, Wei FC, et al. Use of the soleus musculocutaneous perforator for skin paddle salvage of the fibula osteoseptocutaneous flap: Anatomical study and clinical confirmation. *Plast Reconstr Surg.* 2007;120(6):1576–1584.
362. Wood MB. Femoral reconstruction by vascularized bone transfer. *Microsurgery.* 1990;11(1):74–79.
363. Wood MB. Free vascularized bone transfers for nonunions, segmental gaps, and following tumor resection. *Orthopedics.* 1986;9(6):810–816.
364. Wooden WA, Shestak KC, Newton ED, et al. Liposuction-assisted revision and recontouring of free microvascular tissue transfers. *Aesthetic Plast Surg.* 1993;17(2):103–107.
365. Wray RC, Wise DM, Young VL, et al. The groin flap in severe hand injuries. *Ann Plast Surg.* 1982;9:459–462.
366. Wu WC, Chang YP, So YC, et al. The combined use of flaps based on the subscapular vascular system for limb reconstruction. *Br J Plast Surg.* 1997;50(2):73–80.
367. Yajima H, Inada Y, Shono M, et al. Radical forearm flap with vascularized tendons for hand reconstruction. *Plast Reconstr Surg.* 1996;98(2):328–333.
368. Yajima H, Tamai S, Ono H, et al. Free vascularized fibular grafts in surgery of the upper limb. *J Reconstr Microsurg.* 1999;15:515–521.
369. Yang WG, Chiang YC, Wei FC, et al. Thin anterolateral thigh perforator flap using a modified perforator microdissection technique and its clinical application for foot resurfacing. *Plast Reconstr Surg.* 2006;117(3):1004–1008.
370. Yannas IV, Burke JF, Gordon PL, et al. Design of an artificial skin. II. Control of chemical composition. *J Biomed Mater Res.* 1980;14:107–131.
371. Yannas IV, Orgill DP, Burke JF. Template for skin regeneration. *Plast Reconstr Surg.* 2011;127(suppl 1):60S–70S.
372. Yaremchuk MJ, Nettelblad H, Randolph MA, et al. Vascularized bone allograft transplantation in a genetically defined rat model. *Plast Reconstr Surg.* 1985;75(3):355–362.
373. Yaremchuk MJ. Acute management of severe soft-tissue damage accompanying open fractures of the lower extremity. *Clin Plast Surg.* 1986;13:621–629.
374. Yazar S, Lin CH, Lin YT, et al. Outcome comparison between free muscle and free fasciocutaneous flaps for reconstruction of distal third and ankle traumatic open tibial fractures. *Plast Reconstr Surg.* 2006;117(7):2468–2475; discussion 76–77.
375. Yazar S, Lin CH, Wei FC. One-stage reconstruction of composite bone and soft-tissue defects in traumatic lower extremities. *Plast Reconstr Surg.* 2004;114(6):1457–1466.
376. Yildirim S, Giderolu K, Akoz T. Anterolateral thigh flap: Ideal free flap choice for lower extremity soft-tissue reconstruction. *J Reconstr Microsurg.* 2003;19(4):225–233.
377. Yoshimura M, Shimamura K, Iwai Y, et al. Free vascularized fibular transplant. A new method for monitoring circulation of the grafted fibula. *J Bone Joint Surg Am.* 1983;65(9):1295–1301.
378. Yoshizaki K. [Experimental study of vascularized fibular grafting including the epiphyseal growth plate—autogenous orthotopic grafting]. *Nihon Seikeigeka Gakkai Zasshi.* 1984;58(8):813–828.
379. Zaidemberg C, Siebert JW, Angrigiani C. A new vascularized bone graft for scaphoid nonunion. *J Hand Surg Am.* 1991;16A(3):474–478.
380. Zeng BF, Chen YF, Zhang ZR, et al. Emergency rotationplasty of ankle to knee. *Plast Reconstr Surg.* 1998;101:1608–1615.
381. Zhang BM, Wieslander JB. Dextrin's antithrombotic properties in small arteries are not altered by low-molecular-weight heparin or the fibrinolytic inhibitor tranexamic acid: An experimental study. *Microsurgery.* 1993;14:289.
382. Zinberg EM, Wood MB, Brown ML. Vascularized bone transfer: Evaluation of viability by postoperative bone scan. *J Reconstr Microsurg.* 1985;2(1):13–19.

16

OUTCOME STUDIES IN TRAUMA

Mohit Bhandari

INTRODUCTION

The "outcomes" movement in orthopedic surgery involves careful attention to the design, statistical analysis, and critical appraisal of clinical research. The delineation between "outcomes" research and "evidence-based medicine (EBM)" is vague.

Orthopedic surgeons and researchers have adopted their own style of critical appraisal, often coined as "evidence-based orthopedics" (EBO). EBO entails using a clear delineation of relevant clinical questions, a thorough search of the literature relating to the questions, a critical appraisal of available evidence and its applicability to the clinical situation, and a balanced application of the conclusions to the clinical problem.[29,50,51]

The balanced application of the evidence (the clinical decision-making) is the central point of practicing EBO and involves, according to EBM principles, integration of our clinical expertise and judgment, patients' perceptions and societal values, and the best available research evidence.[2,22]

EBO involves a hierarchy of evidence, from meta-analyses of high-quality randomized trials showing definitive results directly applicable to an individual patient, to relying on physiologic rationale or previous experience with a small number of similar patients. The hallmark of the evidence-based surgeon is that, for particular clinical decisions, he or she knows the strength of the evidence, and therefore the degree of uncertainty.

In the process of adopting EBO strategies, surgeons must avoid common misconceptions about EBO. Critics have mistakenly suggested that evidence can be derived only from the results of randomized trials or that statistical significance automatically means clinical relevance. These things are not true. That being said, new methods for measurement of fracture healing and function and quality of life outcomes will likely see their value demonstrated in the conduct of high-quality clinical trials that test new innovative approaches to trauma care.[5]

This chapter provides an evaluation of all study designs with recommendations to their appropriate use in orthopedic clinical research.

HIERARCHY OF EVIDENCE

Among various study designs, there exists a hierarchy of evidence with randomized controlled trials (RCTs) at the top, controlled observational studies in the middle, and uncontrolled studies and opinion at the bottom (Fig. 16-1).[19,22,23,50] Understanding the association between study design and level of evidence is important. The *Journal of Bone and Joint Surgery* (JBJS), as of January 2003, has published the level of evidence associated with each published scientific article to provide readers with a gauge of the validity of the study results. Based upon a review of several existing evidence ratings, the JBJS uses five levels for each of the four different study types (therapeutic, prognostic, diagnostic, and economic or decision-modeling studies)

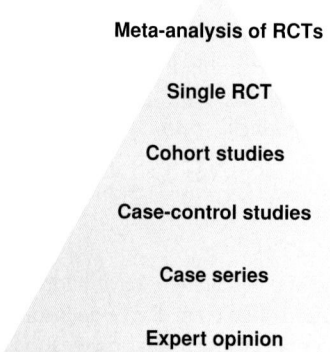

Meta-analysis of RCTs

Single RCT

Cohort studies

Case-control studies

Case series

Expert opinion

FIGURE 16-1 The hierarchy of evidence with high-quality randomized trials at the top and expert opinion at the bottom.

(Table 16-1).[60] Level I studies may be deemed appropriate for the application to patient care, whereas level IV studies should be interpreted with caution. For example, readers should be more confident about the results of a high-quality multicenter randomized trial of arthroplasty versus internal fixation on revision rates and mortality (level I study) than two separate case series evaluating either arthroplasty or internal fixation on the same outcomes (level IV studies).

Bhandari and Tornetta[18] have evaluated the interobserver agreement among reviewers with varying levels of epidemiology training in categorizing clinical studies published in the JBJS into levels of evidence. Among 51 included articles, the majority were studies of therapy (68.6%) constituting level IV evidence (56.9%). Overall, the agreement among reviewers for the study type, level of evidence, and subcategory within each level was substantial (range: 0.61 to 0.75). Epidemiology-trained reviewers demonstrated greater agreement (range: 0.99 to 1) across all aspects of the classification system when compared with nonepidemiology-trained reviewers (range: 0.6 to 0.75). The findings suggested that epidemiology- and nonepidemiology-trained reviewers can apply the levels of evidence guide to published studies with acceptable interobserver agreement. Although reliable, it remains unknown whether this system is valid.[18]

The hierarchy of evidence bases its classification on the validity of the study design. Thus, those designs that limit bias to the greatest extent find themselves at the top of the pyramid and those inherently biased designs are at the bottom (Fig. 16-1). Application of the levels of evidence also requires a fundamental understanding of various study designs.

Sackett et al.[50] proposed a grading system that categorizes the hierarchy of research designs as levels of evidence. Each level (from 1 to 5) is associated with a corresponding grade of recommendation: (i) grade A—consistent level I studies, (ii) grade B—consistent level II or level III studies, (iii) grade C—level IV studies, and (iv) grade D—level V studies.[19,22,23,50]

More recently, the grading of recommendations assessment, development and evaluation (GRADE) working group suggested that, when making a recommendation for treatment, four areas should be considered (Table 16-2)[3,4,6]: (i) what are the benefits versus the harms? Are there clear benefits to an intervention or are there more harms than good?; (ii) what is the quality of the evidence?; (iii) are there modifying factors affecting the clinical setting such as the proximity of qualified persons able to carry out the intervention?; and (iv) what is the baseline risk for the potential population being treated?

STUDY DESIGNS

The types of study designs used in clinical research can be classified broadly according to whether the study focuses on describing the distributions or characteristics of a disease or on elucidating its determinants (Fig. 16-2).[23] *Descriptive studies* describe the distribution of a disease, particularly what type of people have the disease, in what locations, and when. Cross-sectional studies, case reports, and case series represent the types of descriptive studies. *Analytic studies* focus on determinants of a disease by testing a hypothesis with the ultimate goal

TABLE 16-1	Level of Evidence			
	Types of Studies			
	Therapeutic Studies— Investigating the Results of Treatment	**Prognostic Studies Investigating the Outcome of Disease**	**Diagnostic Studies— Investigating a Diagnostic Test**	**Economic and Decision Analyses—Developing an Economic or Decision Model**

Level I	1. Randomized trial
	  a. Statistically significant difference
	  b. No statistically significant difference but narrow CIs
	2. Systematic review[a] of level I RCTs (and studies were homogenous)
		1. Prospective study[b]
		2. Systematic review[a] of level I studies
			1. Testing of previously developed diagnostic criteria on consecutive patients (with universally applied reference criterion standard)
			2. Systematic review[a] of level I studies
				1. Clinically sensible costs and alternatives; values obtained from many studies; with multiway sensitivity analyses
				2. Systematic review[a] of level I studies

Level II	1. Prospective cohort study[c]
	2. Poor-quality RCT (e.g., <80% follow-up)
	3. Systematic review[a]
	  a. Level II studies
	  b. Nonhomogeneous level I studies
		1. Retrospective[d] study
		2. Untreated controls from an RCT
		3. Systematic review[a] of level II studies
			1. Development of diagnostic criteria on consecutive patients (with universally applied reference criterion standard)
			2. Systematic review[a] of level II studies
				1. Clinically sensible costs and alternatives; values obtained from limited studies; with multiway sensitivity analyses
				2. Systematic review[a] of level II studies

Level III	1. Case-control study[e] 2. Retrospective[d] cohort study 3. Systematic review[a] of level III studies		1. Study of nonconsecutive patients; without consistently applied reference criterion standard 2. Systematic review[a] of level III studies	1. Analyses based on limited alternatives and costs and poor estimates 2. Systematic review[a] of level III studies
Level IV	Case series (no, or historical, control group)	Case series	1. Case-control study 2. Poor reference standard	Analyses with no sensitivity analyses
Level V	Expert opinion	Expert opinion	Expert opinion	Expert opinion

[a]Patients treated one way (e.g., with cemented hip arthroplasty) compared with patients treated another way (e.g., with cementless hip arthroplasty) at the same institution.
[b]Study was started before the first patient enrolled.
[b]A combination of results from two or more prior studies.
[d]Study was started after the first patient enrolled.
[e]Patients identified for the study on the basis of their outcome (e.g., failed total hip arthroplasty), called "cases," are compared with those who did not have the outcome (e.g., had a successful total hip arthroplasty), called "controls."
Adapted from JBJS Guidelines. Available online at http://www2.ejbs.org/misc/instrux.dtl#levels.

of judging whether a particular exposure causes or prevents disease. Analytic design strategies are broken into two types: Observational studies, such as case-control and cohort studies, and experimental studies, also called clinical trials. The difference between the two types of analytic studies is the role that the investigator plays in each of the studies. In the observational study, the investigator simply observes the natural course of events. In the trial, the investigator assigns the intervention or treatment.

Bhandari et al.[17] reviewed each type of study to highlight methodologic issues inherent in their design (Table 16-3).

Meta-Analysis (Level I Evidence; Grade A Recommendation)

Although not considered to be a primary study design, meta-analysis deserves mention because it is frequently utilized in the surgical literature. A meta-analysis is a systematic review

that combines the results of multiple studies (of small sample size) to answer a focused clinical question. Meta-analyses are retrospective in nature. The main advantage of meta-analysis is the ability to increase the "total sample size" of the study by combining the results of many smaller studies. When well-designed studies are available on a particular question of interest, a meta-analysis can provide important information to guide clinical practice. Consider the following example. Several small randomized trials have attempted to resolve the issue of whether operative repair of acute Achilles tendon ruptures in younger patients reduces the risk of rerupture compared with conservative treatment. Of five randomized trials (ranging in sample size from 27 to 111 patients), four found nonsignificant differences in rerupture rates. These studies were underpowered. Using meta-analytic techniques, the results of these small studies were combined ($n = 336$ patients) to produce a summary estimate of 3.6% surgery versus 10.6% conservative

TABLE 16-2	Criteria for Assessing Grade of Evidence

Type of Evidence
Randomized trial = high quality
Quasi-randomized = moderate quality
Observational study = low quality
Any other evidence = very low quality

Decrease Grade(s) If
Serious (–1) or very serious (–2) limitation to study quality
Important inconsistency (–1)
Some (–1) or major (–2) uncertainty about directness
Imprecise or sparse data (–1)
High probability of reporting bias (–1)

Increase Grade(s) If
Strong evidence of association—significant relative risk greater than 2 (<0.5) based on consistent evidence from two or more observational studies, with no plausible confounders (+1)
Very strong evidence of association—significant relative risk greater than 5 (<0.2) based on direct evidence with no major threats to validity (+2)
Evidence of a dose response gradient (+1)
All plausible confounders would have reduced the effect (+1)

(relative risk = 0.41; 95% confidence interval [CI], 0.17% to 0.99%; p = 0.05) of adequate study power (>80%) to help guide patient care.[10]

Another benefit of meta-analysis is the increased impact over traditional reviews (i.e., narrative or nonsystematic reviews). Rigorous systematic reviews received over twice the number of mean citations compared with other systematic or narrative reviews (13.8 vs. 6; p = 0.008).[13]

Authors of meta-analyses can be limited to summarizing the outcomes available and not necessarily the outcomes of interest. There is often a trade-off between pooling data from many studies on common and sometimes less relevant outcomes (i.e., nonunion) versus fewer studies reporting less common outcomes of interest (i.e., avascular necrosis). Thus, the definition eligibility criteria for the studies to be included is an important step in the conduct of a meta-analysis.

Meta-analysis of high-quality randomized trials represents the current standard in the translation of evidence to practice. Although meta-analysis can be a powerful tool, its value is diminished when poor quality studies (i.e., case series) are included in the pooling. Pooled analyses of nonrandomized studies are prone to bias and have limited validity. Surgeons should be aware of these limitations when extrapolating such data to their particular clinical settings.

Randomized Trial (Level I Evidence; Grade A Recommendation)

When considering a single study, the randomized trial is the single most important design to limit bias in clinical research.[12] Randomized trials are by no means easy to conduct even when the fracture is a common one. In a systematic review of hip fracture trials around the world, Yeung and Bhandari[20] identified 199 randomized trials.[61] Sweden ranked highest with 50 trials (8,941 patients). The United Kingdom followed with 40 trials (7,589 patients). The United States and Canada together contributed only a tenth of the total number of trials contributed by European countries.

Although it may seem elementary to explain the term "randomization," most surgeons are unfamiliar with the rationale for random allocation of patients in a trial. Orthopedic treatment studies attempt to determine the impact of an intervention on events such as nonunions, infections, or death—occurrences that we call the trial's target outcomes or target events. Patients' age, the underlying severity of fracture, the presence of comorbid conditions, health habits, and a host of other factors typically determine the frequency with which a trial's target outcome occurs (prognostic factors). Randomization gives a patient entering a clinical trial an equal probability (or chance) of being allocated to alternative treatments. Patients can be randomized to alternative treatments by random number tables or computerized randomization systems. Randomization is the only method for controlling for known and unknown prognostic factors between two comparison groups. For instance, in a study comparing plates and intramedullary nails for the treatment of tibial shaft fractures in patients with concomitant head injury, investigators reported imbalance in acetabular fractures between treatment groups. Readers will agree that differences in patient function or mortality may not be attributed to treatment groups, but rather, differences in the proportion of patients with acetabular fractures. Realizing this imbalance because of lack of randomization, the investigators employed a less attractive strategy to deal with the imbalance—statistical adjustment for differences between groups. By controlling for the difference in the number of acetabular fractures between groups, the effect of plates versus nails in patients was determined.

Equally important is the concept of "concealment" (not to be confused with blinding).[12] Concealed randomization ensures

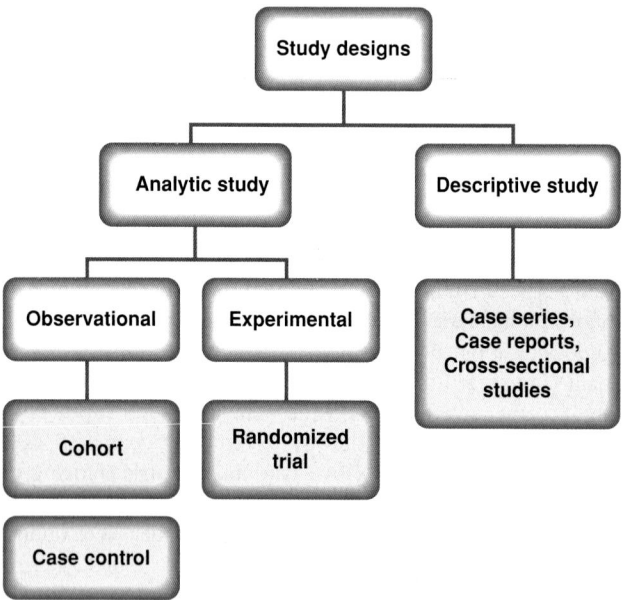

FIGURE 16-2 Categorization of study designs.

TABLE 16-3	**Study Designs and Common Errors**	
Study Design	**Summary**	**Common Errors**
Meta-analysis	High-quality studies addressing a focused clinical question are critically reviewed and their results statistically combined	Major differences between pooled studies (heterogeneity) Poor-quality studies pooled = less valid results
Randomized trial	Patients are randomized to receive alternative treatments (i.e., cast vs. intramedullary nail for tibial shaft fracture) Outcomes (i.e., infection rates) are measured prospectively	Type II (β) errors: Insufficient sample size Type I (α) error: Overuse of statistical tests and multiple outcomes Lack of blinding Lack of concealed randomization
Prospective cohort (with comparison group)	Patients who receive two different treatments are followed forward in time. Choice of treatment is not randomly assigned (i.e., surgeon preference, patient preference) Comparison group is identified and followed at the same time as the treatment group (i.e., concurrent comparison group) Outcomes (i.e., infection rates) are measured prospectively	Type II (β) errors: Insufficient sample size Type I (α) error: Overuse of statistical tests and multiple outcomes Lack of adjustment for differences in characteristics between treatment and comparison groups
Prospective case series (without comparison group)	Patients who receive a particular treatment are followed forward in time (i.e., intramedullary nailing of tibial fractures) No concurrent comparison group is utilized	Lack of independent or blinded assessment of outcomes Lack of follow-up
Case-control study	Patients with an outcome of interest (i.e., infection) are compared backward in time (retrospective) to similar patients without the outcome of interest (i.e., no infection) Risk factors for a particular outcome can be determined between cases and controls	Type II (β) errors: Insufficient sample size Type I (α) error: Overuse of statistical tests and multiple outcomes Problems in ascertainment of cases and controls
Retrospective case series (with comparison group)	Patients with a particular treatment are identified backward in time (i.e., retrospectively) Comparison patients are also identified retrospectively	Type II (β) errors: Insufficient sample size Type I (α) error: Overuse of statistical tests and multiple outcomes Incomplete reporting in patient charts

that surgeons are unable to predict the treatment to which their next patient will be allocated. The safest manner in which to limit this occurrence is a remote 24-hour telephone randomization service. Historically, treatment allocations in surgical trials have been placed within envelopes; although seemingly concealed, envelopes are prone to tampering.

Whereas it is believed that surgical trials cannot be double-blinded because of the relative impossibility of blinding surgeons, Devereaux et al.[26] have recently challenged the "classic" definition of double-blinding. In a survey of 91 internists and researchers, 17 unique definitions of "double-blinding" were obtained. Moreover, randomized trials in five high-profile medical journals (*The New England Journal of Medicine, The Lancet, British Medical Journal, Annals of Internal Medicine,* and *Journal of the American Medical Association*) revealed considerable variability in the reporting of blinding terminology. Common sources of blinding in a randomized trial include physicians, patients, outcome assessors, and data analysts. Current recommendations for reporting randomized trials include explicit statements about who was blinded in the study rather than using the term "double-blinded." Surgical trials can always blind the data analyst, almost always blind the outcome assessor, occasionally blind the patient, and never blind the surgeon. In a review of orthopedic trials, outcome assessors were blinded only 44% of the time and data analysts were never blinded. However, at least two-thirds of surgical trials could have achieved double-blinding by blinding the outcome assessors, patients, or data analysts.[14]

The principle of attributing all patients to the group to which they were randomized results is an *intention-to-treat* (ITT) principle (Fig. 16-3).[12] This strategy preserves the value of randomization: Prognostic factors that we know about and those we do not know about will be, on average, equally distributed in the two groups, and the effect we see will be just that because of the treatment assigned. When reviewing a report of a randomized trial, one should look for evidence that the investigators analyzed all patients in the groups to which they were randomized. Some suggest that an ITT approach is too conservative and more susceptible to type II error because of increased biologic variability. Their argument is that an ITT analysis is less likely to show a positive treatment effect, especially for those studies that randomized patients who had little or no chance of benefiting from the intervention.

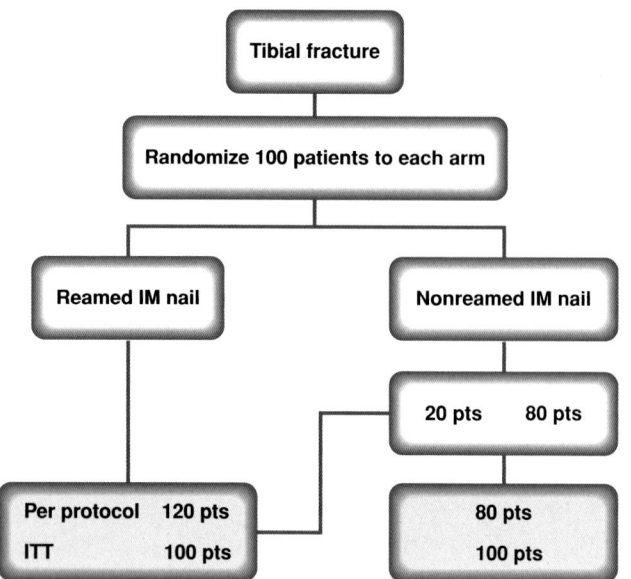

FIGURE 16-3 The intention to treat principle: A per protocol analysis analyzes patient outcomes to the treatment they "actually received" whereas intention to treat analysis evaluates outcomes based upon the treatment to which patients were originally randomized.

An alternative approach, referred to as a *per protocol* analysis, reports outcomes on the treatments patients actually received regardless of the number of crossovers from one treatment to another. This approach is often utilized to determine whether imbalances in baseline factors actually affect the final result. It may be particularly important when patients who are randomized

to one treatment (i.e., reamed or unreamed tibial nail) but never receive either treatment. For example, in a trial of reamed versus unreamed tibial nailing, a patient randomized to a reamed tibial nail who ultimately receives an external fixator because of an intraoperative surgical decision will be excluded from in per protocol analysis; however, recall that this same patient would be included in the reamed tibial nail group in an ITT analysis.

The overall quality of a randomized trial can be evaluated with a simple checklist (Table 16-4). This checklist provides guides to the assessment of the methodologic rigor of a trial.

Randomized Trial (Expertise-Based Design)

In conventional surgical hip fracture trials, all surgeons involved in the trial have performed both total hip arthroplasties (THAs) and hemiarthroplasties. Surgeons performing arthroplasty are frequently less experienced (or expert) in one or both surgical alternatives. This trial aims to limit this differential expertise across treatment alternatives. In our proposed expertise-based design, we will randomize patients to receive THA (by surgeons who are experienced and committed to performing only THA) or to hemiarthroplasty (by surgeons with expertise in hemiarthroplasty who are committed to performing only hemiarthroplasty). Devereaux et al.[26] have outlined the advantages of this trial design, which include the following: (i) elimination of differential expertise bias where, in conventional designs, a larger proportion of surgeons are expert in one procedure under investigation than the other; (ii) differential performance, cointervention, data collection, and outcome assessment are less likely than in conventional RCTs; (iii) procedural crossovers are less likely because surgeons are committed and experienced in

TABLE 16-4 Checklist for Assessing Quality of Reporting			
Randomization	1 Yes	1 Partly	0 No
Were the patients assigned randomly?	2 Yes		0 No
Randomization adequately described?	1 Yes		0 No
Was treatment group concealed to investigator?			
Total/4			
Description of outcome measurement adequate?	1 Yes	1 Partly	0 No
Outcome measurements objective?	2 Yes		0 No
Were the assessors blind to treatment?	1 Yes		0 No
Total/4			
Were inclusion/exclusion criteria well defined?	2 Yes	1 Partly	0 No
Number of patients excluded and reason?	2 Yes	1 Partly	0 No
Total/4			
Was the therapy fully described for the treatment group?	2 Yes	1 Partly	0 No
Was the therapy fully described for the controls?	2 Yes	1 Partly	0 No
Total/4			
Statistics	1 Yes	1 Partial	0 No
Was the test stated and was there a p value?	2 Yes		0 No
Was the statistical analysis appropriate?	1 Yes		0 No
Was the trial negative, were confidence intervals of post hoc power calculations performed?	1 Yes		0 No
Sample size calculation before the study?			
Total/4 (if positive trial); total/5 (negative trial)			
Total score: 20 points (if positive trial); 21 points (if negative trial)			

their procedures; and (iv) ethical concerns are reduced because all surgeries are conducted by surgeons with expertise and conviction concerning the procedure.[26]

Observational Study (Cohort, Case Series)

Studies in which randomization is not employed can be referred to as nonrandomized, or *observational,* study designs. The role of observational comparative studies in evaluating treatments is an area of continued debate: Deliberate choice of the treatment for each patient implies that observed outcomes may be caused by differences among people being given the two treatments, rather than the treatments alone.[11] Unrecognized confounding factors can interfere with the attempts to correct for identified differences between groups. There has been considerable debate about whether the results of nonrandomized studies are consistent with the results of RCTs.[8,25,32,36] Nonrandomized studies have been reported to overestimate or underestimate the treatment effects.[32,36]

One example of the pitfalls of nonrandomized studies was reported in a study comparing study designs that addressed the general topic of comparison of arthroplasty and internal fixation for hip fracture.[19] Mortality data was available in 13 nonrandomized studies (n = 3,108 patients) and in 12 randomized studies (n = 1,767 patients). Nonrandomized studies overestimated the risk of mortality by 40% when compared with the results of randomized trials (relative risk: 1.44 vs. 1.04, respectively) (Fig. 16-4). If we believe the data from the nonrandomized trials, then no surgeon would offer a patient a hemiarthroplasty for a displaced hip fracture, given the significant risk of mortality. However, in practice, arthroplasty is generally favored over internal fixation in the treatment of displaced femoral neck fractures. Thus, surgeons believe the

randomized trials that report no significant differences in mortality and significant reductions in revisions with arthroplasty.

Important contradictory examples of observational and RCT results can be found in the surgical literature. An observational study of extracranial-to-intracranial bypass surgery suggested a "dramatic improvement in the symptomatology of virtually all patients" undergoing the procedure.[31] However, a subsequent large RCT demonstrated a 14% relative increase in the risk of fatal and nonfatal stroke in patients undergoing this procedure compared with medical management.[1] These considerations have supported a hierarchy of evidence, with RCTs at the top, controlled observational studies in the middle, and uncontrolled studies and opinion at the bottom. However, these findings have not been supported in two publications in the *New England Journal of Medicine* that identified nonsignificant differences in results between RCTs and observational studies.[8,25]

Although randomized trials, when available, represent the most valid evidence, information from nonrandomized studies can provide invaluable data to generate hypotheses for future studies.

Prospective Observational Study (Level II Evidence; Grade B Recommendation)

A prospective observational study identifies a group of patients at a similar point in time and follows them forward in time. Outcomes are determined prior to the start of the study and evaluated at regular time intervals until the conclusion of the study. A comparison group (controls) may also be identified concurrently and followed for the same time period.

Whereas comparison groups are helpful when comparing the outcomes of two surgical alternatives, a prospective evaluation of a single group of patients with complex injuries can

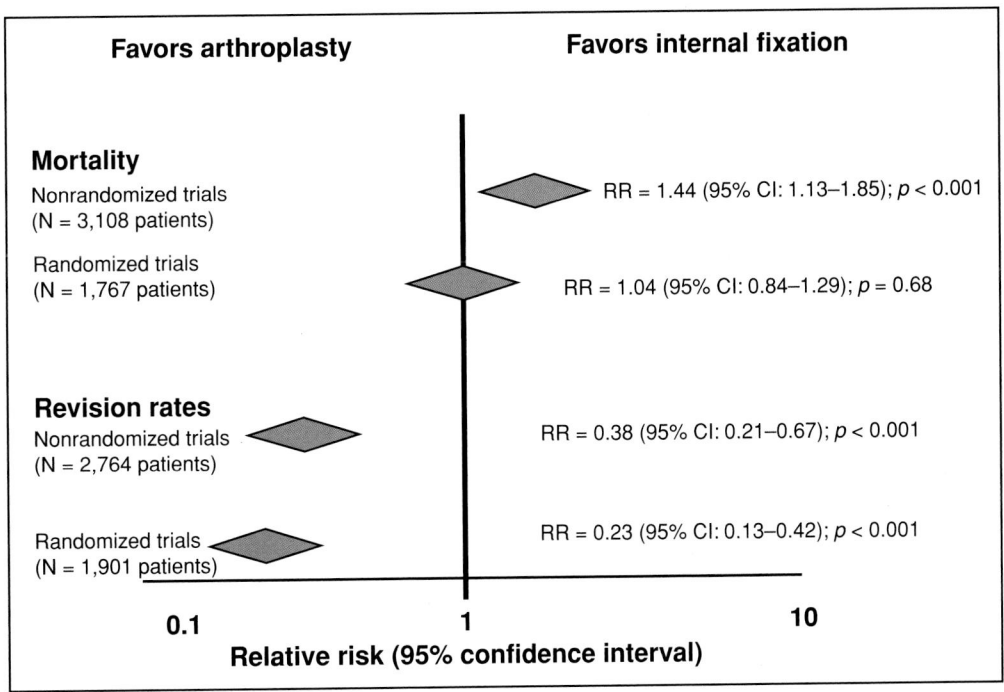

FIGURE 16-4 Estimates from randomized trials tend to provide a more conservative estimate of a treatment effect when compared with nonrandomized studies. Nonrandomized studies overestimate the benefit of internal fixation regarding mortality by 40%.

Favors arthroplasty   Favors internal fixation

Mortality
Nonrandomized trials
(N = 3,108 patients)   RR = 1.44 (95% CI: 1.13–1.85); *p* < 0.001

Randomized trials
(N = 1,767 patients)   RR = 1.04 (95% CI: 0.84–1.29); *p* = 0.68

Revision rates
Nonrandomized trials
(N = 2,764 patients)   RR = 0.38 (95% CI: 0.21–0.67); *p* < 0.001

Randomized trials
(N = 1,901 patients)   RR = 0.23 (95% CI: 0.13–0.42); *p* < 0.001

0.1   1   10
Relative risk (95% confidence interval)

provide information on the frequency of success (radiographic and functional outcomes) and expected complications. This information is most useful when the data collected remains consistent over time, the data collected includes important baseline patient characteristics and patient outcomes, and efforts are made to ensure patients are followed over time. Professor Joel Matta's acetabular fracture database is one striking example of a carefully designed single-surgeon, prospective database that has consistently collected data on patients for more than 20 years (personal communication). With over 1,000 patients with acetabular fractures included in this database, the current limits of technique, results, and complications can be reported to serve as a benchmark for future studies. In addition, these types of studies can assist surgeons in discussing the expected risk and outcomes of surgery with their patients during the informed consent process.

Case-Control Study (Level III Evidence; Grade B Recommendation)

If the outcome of interest is rare (i.e., mortality or infection), conducting a prospective cohort study may be cost-prohibitive. A case-control study is a useful strategy in such circumstances.[23] Cases with the outcome of interest are identified retrospectively from a group of patients (i.e., databases) and matched (i.e., by age, gender, severity of injury) with control patients who do not have the outcome of interest. Both groups can be compared for differences in "risk" factors.[11] One control may be matched for each case that is identified (1:1 matching). Alternatively, multiple controls may be matched to each case (i.e., 3:1 or 4:1 matching). The validity of results from case-control studies depends upon the accuracy of the reporting of the outcomes of interest. For example, investigators conducted a study to determine risk factors for hip fracture among elderly women.[30] To accomplish this, they identified 159 women with their first hip fracture and 159 controls (1:1 matching) matched for gender, age, and residence. Risk factors included perceived safety of the residence, psychotropic drug use, and tendency to fall. Comparison of these factors between the hip fracture and control groups revealed an increased risk of perceived safety (odds ratio = 5.8), psychotropic drug use (odds ratio = 2.6), and tendency to fall (odds ratio = 2.3) among patients who sustained a fracture compared with those who did not.

Retrospective Case Series (Level IV Evidence; Grade C Recommendation)

The retrospective study design, although less costly and less time consuming, is often limited by bias in the ascertainment of cases and the evaluation of outcomes. Comparison groups can be identified during the same time period as the treatment group (concurrent controls). However, controls from a different period of time can also be utilized (historical controls). Patient follow-up may be conducted passively (via patient records) or actively (patient follow-up appointment and examination). When patient charts have formed the basis for the outcome evaluation, readers should be convinced that the outcomes were objective measures accurately obtained from patient records. For example, in-hospital mortality data is an objective outcome that is likely to have been well documented in patient charts; however, patient satisfaction or functional outcome is subjective and far less likely to have been recorded with any standardization or consistency.

A case series can provide initial useful information about the safety and complication profile of a new surgical technique or implant. This information is most valid when eligibility criteria for patient inclusion are clearly defined, consecutive patients are screened for eligibility, surgery and perioperative care are consistent, outcomes are objective and independently assessed, and follow-up is complete. Unfortunately, the validity of the results can be compromised by inadequate and incomplete reporting of patient characteristics and outcomes in patient charts.

Case Study: The Study to Prospectively Evaluate Reamed Intramedullary Nails in Tibial Fractures Trial (Level I Study)

The debate of reamed versus nonreamed insertion of tibial intramedullary nails was largely fueled decades ago by case series (level IV evidence). Case series eventually led to prospective cohort comparison of reamed and unreamed nailing techniques (level II). Realizing the biases inherent in nonrandomized designs, a number of investigators conducted randomized trials ranging in sample size from 50 to 136 patients.[55] Despite a strong design, these trials were limited by small sample sizes, imprecise treatment effects, lack of outcome assessment blinding, and unconcealed allocation of patients to treatment groups.

The Study to Prospectively evaluate Reamed Intramedullary Nails in Tibial fractures (SPRINT) trial was designed to compare the effects of reamed and nonreamed intramedullary nailing approaches.[56] To overcome the limitations of previous studies, the design involved concealed central randomization, blind adjudication of outcomes, and disallowing reoperation before 6 months.

SPRINT enrolled 1,339 patients from July 2000 to September 2005 across 29 clinical sites in Canada, the United States, and the Netherlands. The final follow-up occurred in September 2006 and final outcomes adjudication was completed in January 2007. Participating investigators randomized patients by accessing a 24-hour toll-free remote telephone randomization system that ensured concealment. Randomization was stratified by center and severity of soft tissue injury (open, closed, or both open and closed) in randomly permuted blocks of two and four. Patients and clinicians were unaware of block sizes. Patients were allocated to fracture fixation with an intramedullary nail following reaming of the intramedullary canal (reamed group) or with an intramedullary nail without prior reaming (nonreamed group).

All patients received postoperative care according to the same protocol. SPRINT investigators hypothesized that the benefits of reamed nails suggested by previous literature may have been because of a lower threshold for early reoperation in patients with nonreamed nails. Therefore, reoperations were disallowed within the first 6 months following surgery. Exceptions to the 6-month rule included reoperations for infections, fracture gaps, nail breakage, bone loss, or malalignment. Patients, outcome assessors, and data analysts were blinded to treatment allocation. Reoperation rates were monitored at hospital discharge; 2 weeks post discharge; 6 weeks post surgery; and 3, 6, 9, and 12 months post surgery.

The SPRINT trial set a number of important benchmarks in study methodology including: (i) a sample size 10-fold greater than the largest previous tibial fracture trial; (ii) a modern trial organization including an independent blinded adjudication and data safety monitoring committee; (iii) use of innovative trial infrastructure for randomization and data management; and (iv) large-scale multimillion collaborative funding from the National Institutes of Health and the Canadian Institutes of Health proving that orthopedic surgical trials belong in the same arena as the large cardiovascular and osteoporosis trials.

UNDERSTANDING STATISTICS IN TRAUMA OUTCOME STUDIES

Hypothesis Testing

The essential paradigm for statistical inference in the medical literature has been that of hypothesis testing. The investigator starts with what is called a *null hypothesis* that the statistical test is designed to consider and possibly disprove. Typically, the null hypothesis is that there is no difference between treatments being compared. In a randomized trial in which investigators compare an experimental treatment with a placebo control, one can state the null hypothesis as follows: The true difference in effect on the outcome of interest between the experimental and control treatments is zero. We start with the assumption that the treatments are equally effective, and we adhere to this position unless data make it untenable.

In this hypothesis-testing framework, the statistical analysis addresses the question of whether the observed data are consistent with the null hypothesis. The logic of the approach is as follows: Even if the treatment truly has no positive or negative impact on the outcome (i.e., the effect size is zero), the results observed will seldom show exact equivalence; that is, no difference at all will be observed between the experimental and control groups. As the results diverge further from the finding of "no difference," the null hypothesis that there is no difference between treatment effects becomes less and less credible. If the difference between results of the treatment and control groups becomes large enough, clinicians must abandon belief in the null hypothesis. We will further develop the underlying logic by describing the role of chance in clinical research.

Let us conduct a hypothetical experiment in which the suspected coin is tossed 10 times and, on all 10 occasions, the result is heads.[2] How likely is this to have occurred if the coin was indeed unbiased? Most people would conclude that it is highly unlikely that chance could explain this extreme result. We would therefore be ready to reject the hypothesis that the coin is unbiased (the null hypothesis) and conclude that the coin is biased. Statistical methods allow us to be more precise by ascertaining just how unlikely the result is to have occurred simply as a result of chance if the null hypothesis is true. The law of multiplicative probabilities for independent events

(where one event in no way influences the other) tells us that the probability of 10 consecutive heads can be found by multiplying the probability of a single head (1/2) 10 times over; that is, $1/2 \times 1/2 \times 1/2$, and so on.[2] The probability of getting 10 consecutive heads is slightly less than 1 in 1,000. In a journal article, one would likely see this probability expressed as a p value, such as $p < 0.001$.

What is the *p* Value?

What is the precise meaning of this p value? Statistical convention calls results that fall beyond this boundary (i.e., p value <0.05) *statistically significant*. The meaning of statistically significant, therefore, is that it is "sufficiently unlikely to be due to chance alone that we are ready to reject the null hypothesis." In other words, the p value is defined as the probability, under the assumption of no difference (null hypothesis), of obtaining a result equal to or more extreme than what was actually observed. Let us use the example of a study that reports the following: Patient function scores following tibial intramedullary nailing were significantly greater than those patients treated with plates (75 points vs. 60 points, $p < 0.05$). This may be interpreted as the probability that the difference of 15 points observed in the study was because the chance is less than 5% (or 1 in 20).

The 95% Confidence Interval

Investigators usually (though arbitrarily) use the 95% CI when reporting the precision around a proportion. One can consider the 95% CI as defining the range that includes the true difference 95% of the time.[12] In other words, if the investigators repeated their study 100 times, it would be expected that the point estimate of their result would lie within the CI 95 of those 100 times. The true point estimate will lie beyond these extremes only 5% of the time, a property of the CI that relates closely to the conventional level of statistical significance of $p < 0.05$. For example, if a study reports that nails reduced the risk of infection by 50% compared with plates in patients with tibial shaft fractures (95% CI: 25% to 75%), one may interpret the results consistent with as little as a 25% risk reduction or as much as a 75% risk reduction. In other words, the true risk reduction of infection with nails lies somewhere between 25% and 75% (95% of the time).

Measures of Central Tendency and Spread

Investigators will often provide a general summary of data from a clinical or experimental study. A number of measures can be utilized. These include measures of central tendency (mean, median, and mode) and measures of spread (standard deviation, range). The sample mean is equal to the sum of the measurements divided by the number of observations. The median of a set of measurements is the number that falls in the middle. The mode, however, is the most frequently occurring number in a set of measurements. Continuous variables (such as blood pressure or body weight) can be summarized with a mean if the data is normally distributed. If the data is not normally distributed, then the median may be a better summary statistic. Categorical variables (pain grade: 0, 1, 2, 3, 4, or 5) can be summarized with a median.

Along with measures of central tendency, investigators will often include a measure of spread. The standard deviation is derived from the square root of the sample variance. One standard deviation away from the mean accounts for somewhere around 68% of the observations. Two standard deviations away from the mean account for roughly 95% of the observations and three standard deviations account for about 99% of the observations.

The variance is calculated as the average of the squares of the deviations of the measurements about their mean. The range of a dataset reflects the smallest value and the largest value.

Measures of Treatment Effect (Dichotomous Variables)

Information comparing the outcomes (dichotomous: Mortality, reoperation) of two procedures can be presented to patients as an odds ratio, a relative risk, a relative risk reduction (RRR), an absolute risk reduction, and the number needed to treat. Both reduction in relative risk and reduction in absolute risk have been reported to have the strongest influences on patient decision-making.[15]

Common Statistical Tests

Common statistical tests include those that examine differences between two or more means, differences between proportions, and associations between two or more variables (Table 16-5).[28]

Comparing Two Independent Means

When we wish to test the null hypothesis that the means of two independent samples of normally distributed continuous data are the same, the appropriate test statistic is called t, hence the t-test. The author of the original article describing the distribution of the t-statistic used the pseudonym *Student* leading to the common attribution Student's t-test.[21] When the data is nonnormally distributed, a nonparametric test such as the Mann–Whitney U or Wilcoxon rank-sum test can be utilized. If the means are paired, such as left and right knees, a paired t-test is most appropriate. The nonparametric correlate of this test is the Wilcoxon signed-rank test.

Comparing Multiple Independent Means

When three or more different means have to be compared (i.e., hospital stay among three tibial fracture treatment groups: Plate fixation, intramedullary nail, and external fixation), single factor analysis of variance is a test of choice. If the test yields statistical significance, investigators can conduct post hoc comparison tests (usually a series of pairwise comparisons using t-tests) to determine where the differences lie. It should be recalled that the p value (α-level) should be adjusted for multiple post hoc tests. One rather conservative method is the Bonferroni correction factor that simply divides the α-level ($p = 0.05$) by the number of tests performed.

Comparing Two Proportions

A common situation in the orthopedic literature is that two proportions are compared. For example, these may be the proportion of patients in each of two treatment groups who experience an infection. The chi-squared (χ^2) test is a simple method of determining whether the proportions are really different. When samples are small, the χ^2 test becomes rather approximate because the data is discrete but the χ^2 distribution from which the p value is calculated is continuous. A "Yates' correction" is a device that is sometimes used to account for this, but when cell counts in the contingency table become very low (say, less than five), the χ^2 test becomes unreliable and a Fisher's exact test is the test of choice.

TABLE 16-5 **Common Statistical Tests**[a]

Samples		Categorical	Ordered Categorical or Continuous and Nonnormal	Continuous and Normal
Two samples	Different individuals	χ^2 test Fisher's exact test	Mann–Whitney U test Wilcoxon rank-sum test	Unpaired t-test
	Related or matched samples	McNemar's test	Wilcoxon signed-rank test	Paired t-test
Three or more samples	Different individuals	χ^2 test Fisher's exact test	Kruskal–Wallis statistic	ANOVA
	Related samples	Cochran Q test	Friedman statistic	Repeated measures ANOVA

Column group header: Data Type and Distribution

[a]Consult a statistician when planning an analysis or planning a study.

Adapted from Griffin D, Audige L. Common statistical methods in orthopaedic clinical studies. *Clin Orthop Relat Res.* 2003;413:70–79.

Determining Association Between One or More Variables Against One Continuous Variable

When two variables have been shown to be associated, it may be logical to try to use one variable to predict the other. The variable to be predicted is called the dependent variable and the one to be used for prediction is the independent variable. For such a linear relationship, the equation $y = a + bx$ is defined as the regression equation. a is a constant and b the regression coefficient. Fitting the regression equation, generally using a software package, is the process of calculating values for a and b, which allows the regression line represented by this equation to best fit the observed data. The p value reflects the result of a hypothesis test that x and y are in fact unrelated, or in this case that b is equal to zero.

Correlation

The strength of the relationship between two variables (i.e., age vs. hospital stay in patients with ankle fractures) can be summarized in a single number: The *correlation coefficient*. The correlation coefficient, which is denoted by the letter r, can range from -1 (representing the strongest possible negative relationship in which the person who scores the highest on one variable scores the lowest on the other variable) to 1 (representing the strongest possible positive relationship in which the person who is older also has the longest hospital stay). A correlation coefficient of 0 denotes no relationship between the two variables.

COMMON ERRORS IN THE DESIGN OF ORTHOPEDIC STUDIES

Any study that compares two or more treatments (i.e., comparative study: Randomized trial, observational study with control group, case-control) can be subject to errors in hypothesis testing. For example, when investigators conduct studies to determine whether two treatments have different outcomes, there are four potential outcomes (Fig. 16-5)[50]: (i) a true positive result (i.e., the study correctly identifies a true difference between treatments); (ii) a true negative result (i.e., the study

		Difference	No difference
Results of the study	Difference	Correct conclusion (1-β)	False positive (α error or type I error)
	No difference	False negative (β error or type II error)	Correct conclusion (1-α)

FIGURE 16-5 Errors in hypothesis testing: Type I and type II errors are presented along with the power of a study (1–p).

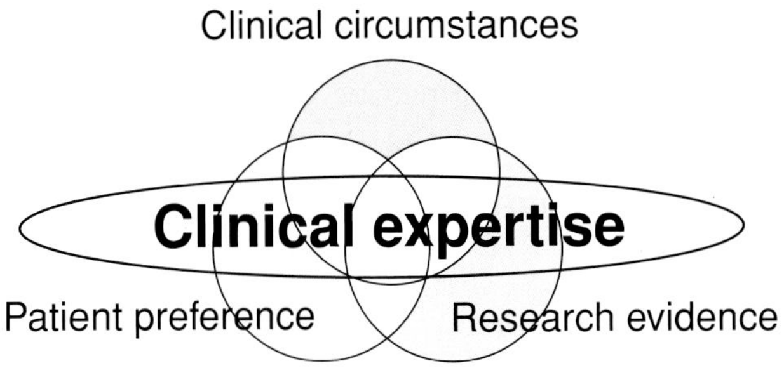

Clinical circumstances

Clinical expertise

Patient preference   Research evidence

FIGURE 16-6 The current conceptual framework for evidence-based practice encompassing research findings, patients' values and preferences, clinical circumstances, and expertise.

correctly identifies no difference between treatments); (iii) a false negative result—type II (β) error (i.e., the study incorrectly concludes no difference between treatments when a difference really exists); and (iv) a false positive result—type I (α) error (i.e., the study incorrectly concludes a difference between treatments when no difference exists).

Type II Errors (β-Error)

It is perceived that trials of surgical therapies may be sufficiently undersized to have a meaningful impact on clinical practice. Such trials of small sample size are subject to β-errors (type II errors): The probability of concluding that no difference between treatment groups exists when, in fact, there is a difference (Fig. 16-6). Typically, investigators will accept a β-error rate of 20% (β = 0.2), which corresponds with a study power of 80%. Most investigators agree that β-error rates greater than 20% (study power less than 80%) are subject to unacceptably high risks of false negative results.

In an effort to quantify the extent to which orthopedic trauma trials were underpowered, Lochner et al.[37] reviewed 117 randomized trials in trauma for type II error rates. The mean overall study power was 24.65% (range 2% to 99%). The potential type II error rate for primary outcomes was 91%. For example, one study demonstrated "no difference" between reamed and non-reamed tibial intramedullary nailing; however, this study was underpowered for this conclusion (study power = 32%). Thus, these conclusions should be interpreted with caution.

Case Study—The Risk of Small Sample Sizes

The SPRINT trial evaluated reamed versus unreamed nailing of the tibia in 1,226 patients, as well as in open and closed fracture subgroups ($N = 400$ and $N = 826$, respectively).[16] To evaluate the impact of smaller sample sizes on the results, the SPRINT investigators analyzed the reoperation rates and relative risk comparing treatment groups at 50, 100, and then increments of 100 patients up to the final sample size. Results at various enrollments were compared with the final SPRINT findings. In the final analysis, there was a statistically significant decreased risk of reoperation with reamed nails for closed fractures (RRR 35%). Results for the first 35 patients enrolled suggested reamed nails increased the risk of reoperation in closed fractures by 165%. Only after 543 patients with closed fractures were enrolled did the results reflect the final advantage for reamed nails in this subgroup. Had the SPRINT trial stopped at few than 100 patients, the findings may have represented a misleading estimate of the true effect of reamed nailing.

Type I Error (α-Error)

Most surgeons are less familiar with the concept of concluding that the results of a particular study are true, when, in fact, they are really because of chance (or random sampling error). This erroneous false positive conclusion is designated as a type I or α-error (Fig. 16-6).[20] By convention, most studies in orthopedics adopt an α-error rate of 0.05. Thus, investigators can expect a false positive error about 5% of the time. Ideally, a type I error rate is based on one comparison between alternative treatment groups usually designated as the primary outcome measure. In situations where no primary outcome variable has been determined, there is a risk of conducting multiple tests of significance on multiple outcomes measures. This form of data dredging by investigators risks spurious false positive findings. Several techniques are available to adjust for multiple comparisons, such as the Bonferroni correction.

Most readers are intuitively skeptical when 1 in a list of 20 outcomes measured by an investigator is significant ($p < 0.05$) between two treatment groups. This situation typically occurs when investigators are not sure what they are looking for and therefore test several hypotheses hoping that one may be true. Statistical aspects of the multiple testing issues are straightforward. If n independent associations are examined for statistical significance, the probability that at least one of them will be found statistically significant is $1-(1-\alpha)^n$ if all n of the individual null hypotheses are true. Therefore, it is argued that studies that generate a large number of measures of association have markedly greater probability of generating some false positive results because of random error than does the stated α-level for individual comparisons.

Bhandari et al.[20] conducted a review of recently published randomized trials (within the last 2 years) to determine the risk of type I errors among surgical trials that did not explicitly state a primary outcome. One study examining outcomes in two different uncemented total knee arthroplasty designs evaluated 21 different outcome measures and found 13 outcomes that were significantly different between groups. As there was no clear statement about a designated primary outcome measure, the risk of a false positive result was 66%.[20]

The Misuse of Subgroup Analyses in Orthopedic Outcome Studies

Subgroup analyses can be defined as treatment outcome comparisons for patients subdivided by baseline characteristics.[46,62] For instance, in a study of operative versus nonoperative management of calcaneal fractures, investigators may report no difference in the overall outcome (patient function), but subsequently conduct a series of comparisons across different patient subgroups (gender, disability status, or comorbidities). Subgroup analyses are frequently post hoc analyses that risk false positive results (type I error) in which ineffective (or even harmful) treatments may be deemed beneficial in a subgroup. Conducting multiple statistical tests risks spurious false positive

findings. Alternatively, false negative results may occur because negative subgroup analyses are often underpowered.

Bhandari et al.[9] identified important errors in surgical RCTs related to subgroup analyses. The majority of authors did not report whether subgroup analyses were planned a priori, and these analyses often formed the basis of the RCT conclusions. Inferences from such RCTs may be misleading and their application to clinical practice unwarranted.[46,62]

In a review of 72 RCTs published in orthopedics and other surgical subspecialties, 27 (38%) RCTs reported a total of 54 subgroup analyses with a minimum of 1 and a maximum of 32 subgroup analyses per study.[9] The majority of subgroup analyses, 49 (91%), were performed post hoc and not stated to be preplanned at the outset of the study nor included in the hypothesis. The majority of investigators inappropriately used tests of significance when comparing outcomes between subgroups of patients (41 subgroup analyses, 76%); however, only three of the analyses were performed using statistical tests for interaction. Investigators reported differences between subgroups in 31 (57%) of the analyses, all of which were featured in the summary or conclusion of the published paper.

Subgroup analyses should be undertaken and interpreted with caution. The validity of a subgroup analysis can be improved by defining a few important (and biologically plausible) subgroups before conducting a study and conducting statistical tests of interaction. When faced with a subgroup analysis in a published scientific paper, readers should ask the following questions: Is the subgroup difference suggested by comparisons within rather than between studies? Did the hypothesis precede rather than follow the analysis? Was the subgroup effect one of a small number of hypothesized effects tested? Is the magnitude of the effect large? Was the effect statistically significant? Is the effect consistent across studies? Is there indirect evidence that supports the hypothesized subgroup effect?

Statistical Versus Clinical Significance

Statistically significant differences between two treatments may not necessarily reflect a clinically important difference. Although it is well known that orthopedic studies with small sample sizes risk underpowered false negative conclusions (β-errors), statistically significant findings in small trials can occur at the consequence of very large differences between treatments (treatment effect). It is not uncommon for randomized trials to report RRRs larger than 50% when comparing one treatment with another.

Sung et al.[57] conducted a comprehensive search for all RCTs between January 1, 1995 and December 31, 2004. Eligible studies included those that focused upon orthopedic trauma. Baseline characteristics and treatment effects were abstracted by two reviewers. Briefly, for continuous outcome measures (i.e., functional scores), effect sizes (mean difference / standard deviation) were calculated. Dichotomous variables (i.e., infection, nonunion) were summarized as absolute risk differences and RRRs. Effect sizes >0.8 and RRRs greater than 50% were defined as large effects.

These investigators identified 433 RCTs, of which 76 RCTs had statistically significant findings on 184 outcomes

(122 continuous / 62 dichotomous outcomes). The average study reported large reductions (>50% RRR) in the risk of an adverse outcome event versus a comparative treatment; however, almost 1 in 2 study outcomes (47%) had RRRs less than 50%, and over 1 in 5 (23%) had RRRs less than 20%.

Study Power and Sample Size Calculation

The power of a study is the probability of concluding a difference between two treatments when one actually exists. Power $(1-\beta)$ is simply the complement of the type II error (β). Thus, if we accept a 20% chance of an incorrect study conclusion $(\beta = 0.2)$, we are also accepting that we will come to the correct conclusion 80% of the time. Study power can be used before the start of a clinical trial to assist with sample size determination, or following the completion of study to determine if the negative findings were true (or because of chance).

The power of a statistical test is typically a function of the magnitude of the treatment effect, the designated type I error rate (α), and the sample size (n). When designing a trial, investigators can decide upon the desired study power $(1-\beta)$ and calculate the necessary sample to achieve this goal.[28] Numerous free sample size calculators are available on the internet and use the same principles and formulae estimating sample size in clinical trials.

Comparing Two Continuous Variables

A continuous variable is one with a scale (i.e., blood pressure, functional outcome score, time to healing). For example, in planning a trial of alternative strategies for the treatment of humeral shaft fractures, an investigator may identify a systematic review of the literature that reports that the time to fracture healing with treatment A is 110 ± 45 days, whereas time to healing with treatment B (control group) can be expected to be up to 130 ± 40 days. The expected treatment difference is 20 days and the effect size (mean difference/standard deviation) is 0.5 (20/40). Effect sizes can be categorized as small (0.1), medium (0.3), and large (0.5). The anticipated sample size for this continuous outcome measure is determined by a standard equation.

A particular study will require approximately 63 patients in total to have sufficient power to identify a difference of 20 days between treatments, if it occurs. An investigator may then audit his or her center's previous year and decide if enough patients will present to the center to meet the sample size requirements. Table 16-6 provides additional scenarios and the sample size requirements for varying differences in healing times between treatment and control groups. As the difference between treatments diminishes, the sample size requirements increase (Table 16-6).

Let us consider another study that aims to compare functional outcome scores in patients with ankle fractures treated operatively versus nonoperatively. Previous studies using the functional outcome score have reported standard deviations for operative and nonoperative cases of 12 points, respectively. Based upon previous studies, we want to be able to detect a difference of 5 points on this functional outcome score between treatments. From the equation in the Appendix at the end of this chapter, our proposed study will require 90 patients per treatment arm to have adequate study power.

TABLE 16-6	Sample Size Requirements for Continuous Outcome (Time to Fracture Healing)		
Time to Healing (Control Group)	Time to Healing (Treatment Group)	% Reduction in Time to Healing	Number of Patients Needed per Group
150 days	120	20%	16
150 days	135	10%	63
150 days	143	5%	289

Reworking the above equation, the study power can be calculated for any given sample size by transforming the above formula and calculating the z-score:

$$z_{1-\beta} = (n_1(\Delta^2) / 2(\sigma^2))^{1/2} - z_{1-\alpha/2}$$

The actual study power that corresponds to the calculated z-score can be looked up in readily available statistical literature[19] or on the internet (keyword: "z-table").[23,60] From the above example, the z-score will be 0.84 for a sample size of 90 patients. The corresponding study power for a z-score of 0.84 is 80%.

When the Outcome Measure is Dichotomous (Proportion)

A dichotomous variable is typically one that has one of two options (i.e., infection or not, nonunion or not, alive or dead). Let us assume that this same investigator chooses nonunion as the primary outcome instead of time to union. Based upon the previous literature, he or she believes that treatment A will result in a 95% union rate and treatment B (control group) will result in a 90% union rate. Eight-hundred-and-sixty-nine patients are required for the study to identify a 5% difference in nonunion rates between treatments. An investigator may realize that this number is sufficiently large enough to prohibit the trial being conducted at one center and may elect to gain support at multiple sites for this trial. For example, in a proposed trial using pulmonary embolus risk as the primary outcome, the number of patients required may be prohibitive (Table 16-7).

TABLE 16-7	Sample Size Requirements for Difference Baseline Risks of Pulmonary Embolus		
Pulmonary Embolus Rate Control Group	Pulmonary Embolus Rate Treatment Group	% Reduction in Pulmonary Embolus Risk	Number of Patients Needed Per Group
10%	8%	20%	3,213
1%	0.8%	20%	35,001
0.10%	0.08%	20%	352,881

Returning to our example of ankle fractures, let us now assume that we wish to change our outcome measure to differences in secondary surgical procedures between operatively and nonoperatively treated ankle fractures. A clinically important difference is considered to be 5%. Based upon the previous literature, it is estimated that the secondary surgical rates in operative and nonoperative treated ankles will be 5% and 10%, respectively. The number of patients required for our study can now be calculated from the equation presented in the Appendix.

Thus, we need 433 patients per treatment arm to have adequate study power for our proposed trial.

Reworking the above equation, the study power can be calculated for any given sample size by transforming the above formula and calculating the z-score:

$$z_{1-\beta} = ((n(\Delta^2))^{1/2} - (2p_m q_m)^{1/2} z_{1-\alpha/2}) / (p_1 q_1 + p_2 q_2)^{1/2}$$

From the above example, the z-score will be 0.84 for a sample size of 433 patients. The corresponding study power for a z-score of 0.84 is 80%.

MEASURING PATIENT HEALTH AND FUNCTION

The basis of the "outcomes movement" in trauma is the move toward identifying patient-relevant and clinically important measures to evaluate the success (or failure) of surgical interventions. Common to any outcome measure that gains widespread use should be its reliability and validity. Reliability refers to the extent to which an instrument yields the same results in repeated applications in a population with stable health. In other words, reliability represents the extent to which the instrument is free of random error. Validity is an estimation of the extent to which an instrument measures what it was intended to measure. The process of validating an instrument involves accumulating evidence that indicates the degree to which the measure represents what it was intended to represent. Some of these methods include face, content, and construct validity.[7,33]

What is Health-Related Quality of Life?

The World Health Organization defines health as "a state of complete physical, mental, and social well-being." Thus, when measuring health in a clinical or research setting, questioning a patient's well-being within each of these domains is necessary to comprehensively represent the concept of health. Instruments that measure aspects of this broad concept of health are often referred to as health-related quality of life (HRQOL) measures. These measures encompass a broad spectrum of items including those associated with activities of daily life such as work, recreation, household management, and relationships with family, friends, and social groups. HRQOL considers not only the ability to function within these roles, but also the degree of satisfaction derived from performing them.

A generic instrument is one that measures general health status inclusive of physical symptoms, function, and emotional dimensions of health. A disadvantage of generic instruments, however, is that they may not be sensitive enough to be able to detect small but important changes.[28]

Disease-specific measures, on the other hand, are tailored to inquire about the specific physical, mental, and social aspects of health affected by the disease in question, allowing them to detect small, important changes.[33] Therefore, to provide the most comprehensive evaluation of treatment effects, no matter the disease or intervention, investigators often include both a disease-specific and a generic health measure. In fact, many granting agencies and ethics boards insist that a generic instrument be included in the design of proposed clinical studies.

Often, the combination of objective endpoints in a surgical study (i.e., quality of fracture reduction) and validated measures of patient function and quality of life is an ideal combination. Whereas an intra-articular step-off in a tibial plafond fracture may be viewed as a less-than-satisfactory radiograph outcome, there may be no detectable effect on patient function or quality of life.[38]

Another factor to consider is the ability of the outcome measure to discriminate between patients across a spectrum of the injury in question. Questionnaires may sometimes exhibit ceiling and floor effects. Ceiling effects occur when the instrument is too easy and all respondents score the highest possible score. Alternatively, floor effects can occur if the instrument is very difficult or tapping into rare issues associated with the disease. Most patients will score the lowest possible score. Miranda et al.,[42] in a study of 80 patients with pelvic fractures, found that the severity of pelvic fracture did not alter Short Form-36 (SF-36) and Iowa pelvic scores.

Despite increasing severity of the pelvic injury, functional outcomes remained equally poor. This was likely related to the associated soft tissue injuries that created a "floor effect" limiting the ability to discriminate between the orthopedic injuries.

Common Outcome Instruments Used in Trauma

Beaton and Schemitsch[6] have reported commonly used measures of outcome in orthopedics (Table 16-8). These include both generic and disease-specific instruments. Properties of these instruments follow.

EQ-5D/EuroQOL

The EQ-5D, formally described as the EuroQOL, is a five-item scale that is designed to allow people to describe their health state across five dimensions.[19] There are three response categories that combine for a total of 243 possible health states. The preference weight allows a single numeric score from slightly less than zero (theoretically worse than death) to one (best health state). EQ-5D scores are used in economic appraisals (such as cost utility analyses) in the construction of quality-adjusted life years for the calculation of cost per quality of life year gained and its comparison across interventions.

Short Form-36

The SF-36 is a generic measure of health status. It is probably one of the most widely used measures. The SF-36 has 35 items that fit into one of 8 subscales. One additional item is not used in the scores. In 1994, the developers, led by Ware,[59] produced two summary scores for the SF-36: The physical component score (more heavily weights dimensions of pain,

TABLE 16-8 Commonly Used Outcome Measures

Type	Measure	Domains/Scales	Number of Items	Response Categories	Target Population	Internal Consistency	Test-Retest Reliability	Construct Validity	Responsiveness	Comments
										Measurement Properties
Utility	EQ-5D	Mobility Self care Usual activities Anxiety/depression Pain	1 1 1 1 1 Total: 5	3	All	NA	Y	YY	Y	Describes health state that is transcribed into utility using UK data. Indirect measure of utility.
Generic	SF-36 version 2	Physical function bodily pain Role function—physical Role function—emotional Mental health vitality Social functioning General health	10 2 4 3 5 4 2 5 Total = 35 + 1 item	3–6	All	YY	Y	YY	YY	Version 2 now in use. Uses improved scaling for role functioning, and clearer wording. Reliability is lower than desired for individual level of interpretation, fine for group.
Region	SMFA	Daily activities Emotional status Arm/hand function Mobility Above combined for functional index Bothersome index	10 7 **8** **9** **34** **12**	5 points	Musculoskeletal	YY	YY	YY	YY	Normative data now available Only measure designed for any musculoskeletal problem.
	DASH	Physical function, symptoms (one scale)	30	5	All upper limb musculoskeletal disorders	YY	YY	Y	YY	Normative data now available. Manual available. Developed in oncology; used in hip fractures.
	Toronto extremity salvage score (TESS)	Physical function in surgical oncology	30	5	Lower limb sarcoma	YY	YY	Y	YY	
Specific	WOMAC	Physical function Pain Stiffness	17 5 2	5 or VAS	Osteoarthritis of knee, hip	YY	YY	YY	YY	Adopted as key outcome for evaluating knee arthroplasty.

(continues)

TABLE 16-8 Commonly Used Outcome Measures (continued)

Type	Measure	Domains/Scales	Number of Items	Response Categories	Target Population	Measurement Properties Internal Consistency	Test–Retest Reliability	Construct Validity	Responsiveness	Comments
	Roland and Morris	Physical function because of low back pain	24	2 (Yes/No)	Low back pain	Y	YY	YY	YY	Excellent review and comparison with Oswestry in Roland and Fairbanks.[48]
	Oswestry	Pain Personal care Lifting Walking Sitting Standing Sleeping Sex life Social life Traveling	1 each	6 points	Low back pain	YY	YY	YY	YY	Excellent review and comparison with Roland in Roland and Fairbanks.[48]
	Simple Shoulder Test (SST)	Function-8 Pain Sleep position	8 1 1 2	2 (Yes difficult Yes/No)	Shoulder disorders	Y	YY	YY	YY	Developers suggest reporting % with difficulty in each item, not a summative score. Some psychometrics done using sum of items.
	Neck disability index	Pain Personal care Lifting Reading Headaches Concentration Work Driving Sleeping Recreation	1 each	6 points	Whiplash disorders	Y	Y	Y	Y	Neck pain has few instruments that have been evaluated for psychometrics. This is most tested.
Patient-specific	—	—	—	—	—	—	—	—	—	No patient-specific measure found in literature reviewed.

NA, not available; Y, one or two articles found in support of this attribute; YY, multiple articles supporting this attribute.

From Beaton DE, Schemitsch E. Measures of health-related quality of life and physical function. *Clin Orthop Relat Res.* 2003;413:90–105.

physical function, and role function physical) and the mental component score (more weight given to mental health, vitality, etc.). The two physical component scores are standardized, so the general population (based on a US sample) will score 50 on average, with a standard deviation of 10. The subscale scores, often presented as a profile graph, are scored on a scale of 0 to 100 where 100 is a good health state.

Short Musculoskeletal Function Assessment Form

The short musculoskeletal function assessment (SMFA) form is a 46-item questionnaire that is a shortened version of Swionkowski's full musculoskeletal functional assessment.[53] The SMFA has two main scores: The function index (items 1 to 34) and the bothersome index (items 35 to 46). The functional index is subdivided into 4 subscales (daily activities, emotional status, arm and hand function, and mobility). The SMFA has been tested in patients with musculoskeletal disorders, as this is the target population. The psychometric properties are high, suggesting that it can be used for monitoring individual patients. The SMFA was designed to describe the various levels of function in people with musculoskeletal disorders, as well as monitor change over time. The SMFA correlates highly with the SF-36 and use of both instruments in the same patient population is likely redundant.

Disabilities of the Arm, Shoulder, and Hand Form

The Disabilities of the Arm, Shoulder, and Hand (DASH) form is a 30-item questionnaire designed to measure physical function and disability in any or all disorders of the upper limb. It is therefore designed to be sensitive to disability and change in disability in the hand as well as in the shoulder. In one study, it was directly compared to a shoulder and a wrist measure, and had similar levels of construct validity, responsiveness, and reliability. Another study showed slightly lower properties in the DASH as compared with a wrist-specific measure in patients with wrist fracture. Like the SMFA, the measurement properties of the DASH are quite high (internal consistency 0.96, test–retest 0.95, good validity and responsiveness) suggesting it could also be used in individual patients in a clinical setting.

Western Ontario and McMaster Universities Osteoarthritis Index

The Western Ontario and McMaster Universities Osteoarthritis Index (WOMAC) is a 24-item scale divided into three dimensions: Function, pain, and stiffness. The most commonly used response scale is a five-point Likert; however, there is a visual analogue scale version. It has been widely used and tested in the field of osteoarthritis and rheumatoid arthritis and a review of its psychometric properties was summarized by McConnell et al.[40] in 2001. The WOMAC is the most commonly used and endorsed patient-based outcome after hip or knee arthroplasty.

Hip Rating Questionnaire

The Hip Rating Questionnaire (HRQ) is a patient-administered, 14-item questionnaire that uses a 100-point summated rating scale. A higher score suggests better health status. Equal weight is given to the domains of the overall impact of arthritis, pain,

walking, and function. This questionnaire is designed to assess outcomes after total hip replacement surgery. According to Johanson et al.,[35] 2-week test–retest administrations produced a weighted κ-score of 0.7, and the sensitivity to change was deemed to be excellent.

Harris Hip Score

The Harris Hip Score (HHS) is a patient- and clinician-administered questionnaire designed to assess patients with traumatic arthritis of the hip.[47] It is a 10-item questionnaire that uses a 100-point summated rating scale and takes approximately 15 to 30 minutes to administer. There are four domains: The pain domain contributes 44 points; function, 47; range of motion, 5; and absence of deformity, 4. The function domain is divided into gait and activities, whereas deformity considers hip flexion, adduction, internal rotation, and limb-length discrepancy and range-of-motion measures.[47] A higher score suggests better health status. The HHS is the most commonly used scoring system for evaluating hip arthroplasty. Its responsiveness has been found to be comparable to, and in some cases, better than the WOMAC pain and function subscales.[47]

The Hospital for Joint Diseases Hip Fracture Recovery Score (Functional Recovery Score)

The Hospital for Joint Diseases Hip Fracture Recovery Score (FRS) is an interviewer-administered questionnaire with 11 items comprising three main components: Basic activities of daily living assessed by four items and contributing 44 points, instrumental activities of daily living assessed by six items and contributing 33 points, and mobility assessed by one item and contributing 33 points. Therefore, complete independence in basic and instrumental activities of daily living and mobility will give a score of 100 points.[63,64] It is a patient-oriented outcomes measure that is designed to assess functional recovery for ambulatory hip fracture patients.[63,64] Use of the FRS can provide the means of assessing the recovery of prefracture function.[63,64] The FRS has been found to be responsive to change, reliable, and has predictive validity as well as discriminant validity.[64]

Get-Up and Go Test

The Get-Up and Go (GUG) test was developed as a clinical measure of balance in elderly people and is an in-person assessment. The GUG test measures the time a person takes to get up from a chair and walk 15.2 m (50 ft) as fast as possible along a level and unobstructed corridor. Thus, this performance-based measure of physical function requires the patient to be able to rise from a seated position, walk, and maintain his or her balance.[45] The scoring of this instrument is based on balance function, which is scored on a 5-point scale, with 1 indicating normal and 5 indicating severely abnormal. A patient with a score of 3 or more is at risk for falling. Mathias et al.[39] found that when patients underwent laboratory tests of balance and gait, there was good correlation between the laboratory tests and the objective assessment.

Merle d'Aubigne-Postel Score

The Merle d'Aubigné-Postel (MDP) score contains three domains: Pain, mobility, and walking ability. These three domains have the same impact. The scores for pain and walking ability can be added and subsequently classified into the grades very good, good, medium, fair, and poor. These grades are then adjusted down by one to two grades to account for the mobility score, which results in the final clinical grade. The modified MDP is slightly different from the original in terms of language and grading, as the modified version is calculated on a scale of 0 to 6 (as opposed to 1 to 6) and does not combine the scores to obtain a total score.[44]

Knee Injury and Osteoarthritis Outcome Score

The Knee injury and Osteoarthritis Outcome Score (KOOS) is designed to assess short- and long-term patient-relevant outcomes after knee injury.[49] The KOOS was designed based on the WOMAC, literature review, and an expert panel and has been statistically validated for content validity, construct validity, reliability, and responsiveness. The questionnaire is composed of 42 items that are scored on a Likert scale. A higher score indicates better health status. Subscales include pain, symptoms, activities of daily living, sport and recreation, and knee-related quality of life.[49]

Lower Extremity Measure

The Lower Extremity Measure is a patient-administered instrument designed to assess physical function.[34] This questionnaire is a modification of the Toronto Extremity Salvage Score and has been statistically confirmed for reliability, validity, and responsiveness. The Lower Extremity Measure is composed of 29 items on a Likert scale and administration takes approximately 5 minutes. This questionnaire has been designed for an elderly population, with 10 points indicating significant clinical change.[34]

Olerud and Molander Scoring System

The Olerud and Molander Scoring System is a patient-administered questionnaire designed to assess the symptoms after ankle fracture.[43] It is composed of nine items on a summated rating scale and has been compared with the visual analog scale (VAS), range of motion, osteoarthritis, and dislocation for statistical validation. A higher score indicates better health status.[43]

American Shoulder and Elbow Surgeons Assessment Form

The American Shoulder and Elbow Surgeons (ASES) Assessment Form is designed to assess the shoulder and elbow and is patient- and clinician-administered.[41] There is no cost to obtain this instrument. Subscales include shoulder score index pain, instability, activities of daily living, range of motion, signs, and strength. A higher score indicates better health status. The instrument is a combination of VAS and Yes/No scaled questions. Administration by the patient takes approximately 3 minutes.[41]

American Orthopedic Foot and Ankle Scale

The American Orthopedic Foot and Ankle Scale was designed for use among patients with foot or ankle dysfunction. It contains four region-specific scales, including ankle–hindfoot, midfoot, hallux metatarsophalangeal, and lesser metatarsophalangeal–

interphalangeal scales. Patients self-report information about pain and function in each region. This scale also incorporates physical examination results recorded by the clinician. Although the American Orthopedic Foot and Ankle Scale has been widely used in studies of foot and ankle surgical outcomes, limitations have also been reported.[52,54]

UTILIZING OUTCOME STUDIES IN DECISION-MAKING (EVIDENCE-BASED ORTHOPEDICS)

What is Evidence-Based Orthopedics?

The term EBM first appeared in the fall of 1990 in a document for applicants to the Internal Medicine Residency Program at McMaster University in Ontario, Canada, which described EBM as an attitude of enlightened skepticism toward the application of diagnostic, therapeutic, and prognostic technologies. As outlined in the text *Clinical Epidemiology* and first described in the literature in the *ACP Journal Club* in 1991, the EBM approach to practicing medicine relies on an awareness of the evidence upon which a clinician's practice is based and the strength of inference permitted by that evidence.[29] The most sophisticated practice of EBM requires, in turn, a clear delineation of relevant clinical questions, a thorough search of the literature relating to the questions, a critical appraisal of available evidence and its applicability to the clinical situation, and a balanced application of the conclusions to the clinical problem. The balanced application of the evidence (i.e., the clinical decision-making) is the central point of practicing EBM and involves, according to EBM principles, integration of our clinical expertise and judgment with patients' preferences and societal values and with the best available research evidence (Fig. 16-6). The EBM working group at McMaster University has proposed a working model for evidence-based clinical practice that encompasses current research evidence, patient preferences, clinical circumstances, and clinical expertise. EBM is commonly misunderstood as removing clinical expertise as a factor in patient decision-making. This is not so. The common thread that weaves the relationships between patients, circumstances, and research is the experience and skill of the surgeon.

Finding Current Evidence in Trauma

To be effective EBM practitioners, surgeons must acquire the necessary skills to find the "best" evidence available to answer clinically important questions. Reading a few articles published in common orthopedic journals each month is insufficient preparation for answering the questions that emerge in daily practice. There are at least 100 orthopedic journals indexed by MEDLINE.[2] For surgeons whose principal interest is orthopedic traumatology, the list is even larger. Given their large clinical demands, surgeons' evidence searches must be time-efficient. Evidence summaries (such as those published in the *Journal of Orthopaedic Trauma*) and systematic reviews (comprehensive literature reviews) are useful resources for surgeons (Table 16-9). The most efficient way to find them is by electronic searching of databases and/or the internet. With time at a premium, it is

TABLE 16-9	Finding Current Evidence: Resources

Publications

EBM

Using the Medical Literature

Journal of American Medical Association User's Guides

Canadian Medical Association Journal User's Guides

Journal of Bone and Joint Surgery User's Guides

Canadian Journal of Surgery User's Guides

Databases

Best Evidence

Cochrane Library and Cochrane Randomized Trials Register (www.update-software.com/cochrane/)

OrthoEvidence (www.myorthoevidence.com)

Database of Abstracts and Reviews of effectiveness (DARE)

Internet Database of Evidence-based Abstracts and Articles (IDEA)

Medline/PubMED (www.ncbi.nlm.nih.gov/entrez/query.fcgi)

EMBASE (European equivalent of Medline)

Clinical Evidence (www.clinicalevidence.org/)

SUMSearch (www.sumsearch.uthscsa.edu)

TRIP database (www.tripdatabase.com/)

Electronic Publications

ACP Journal Club (American College of Physicians) (www.acpjc.org/)

Bandolier: Evidence-based healthcare

EBM

National Guideline Clearinghouse (Agency of Health Care Policy and Research [AHCPR]; www.guidelines.gov)

Internet Resources

HealthWeb: Evidence-based Health Care (www.healthweb.org)

EBM from McMaster University (www.hiru.hirunet.mcmaster.ca)

Center for Evidence-based Medicine (www.cebm.net)

Critically Appraised Topics (CAT) databank (www.cebm.net/toolbox.asp)

New York Academy of Medicine EBM resource center (www.ebmny.org)

University of Alberta EBM (cebm.med.ualberta.ca/ebm/ebm.htm)

Trauma Links—Edinburgh Orthopaedic Trauma Unit (http://www.trauma.co.uk/traumalinks.htm)

OrthoEvidence: (www.myorthoevidence.com)

important to know where to look and how to develop a search strategy, or filter, to identify the evidence most efficiently and effectively. Recently, we have developed a point of care resource in orthopedics that provides timely and regularly updated evidence reports in trauma. The site, known as OrthoEvidence (www.myorthoevidence.com) searches journals each month and identifies high-quality evidence (namely randomized clinical trials or meta-analyses). Data from these trials are abstracted and a careful risk of bias assessment is conducted. The end result, termed an "Advanced Clinical Evidence (ACE) report," is posted on the site.

User's Guide to Evaluate an Orthopedic Intervention

Most surgical interventions have inherent benefits and associated risks. Before implementing a new therapy, one should ascertain the benefits and risks of the therapy, and be assured that the resources consumed in the intervention will not be exorbitant. A simple three-step approach can be used when reading an article from the orthopedic literature (Table 16-10). It is prudent to ask whether the study can provide valid results (internal validity), to review the results, and to consider how the results can be applied to patient care (generalizability). Lack of randomization, no concealment of treatment allocation, lack of blinding, and incomplete follow-up are serious threats to the validity of a published randomized trial. The user's guide focuses the assessment on assuring that investiga-

tors have considered these issues in the conduct of their study. Understanding the language of EBM is also important. Table 16-11 provides a summary of common terms used when considering the results of a clinical paper. Although randomized trials sit atop the hierarchy of an intervention, not all orthopedic research questions are suitable for randomized trials. For example, observational studies (prospective cohorts) are more suitable designs when evaluating prognosis (or risk factors) for outcome following a surgical procedure. However, common problems with alternative (and accepted) surgical treatments argue strongly in favor of randomized trials. Complex problems with nonconsensus in surgical technique or lack of acceptance of one approach argue in favor of observational studies to further elucidate the technique as well as understand the indications for alternative approaches before embarking on a randomized trial.

Incorporating Evidence-Based Orthopedics into Daily Trauma Practice

EBM is becoming an accepted educational paradigm in medical education at a variety of levels. An analysis of the literature related to journal clubs in residency programs in specialties other than orthopedic surgery reveals that the three most common goals were to teach critical appraisal skills (67%), to have an impact on clinical practice (59%), and to keep up with the current literature (56%).[58] The implementation of the structured article review checklist has been found to increase

---

TABLE 16-10 User's Guide to Orthopedic Randomized Trials

Validity
Did experimental and control groups begin the study with a similar prognosis?
Were patients randomized?
Was randomization concealed?
Were patients analyzed in the groups to which they were randomized?
Were patients in the treatment and control groups similar with respect to known prognostic factors?
Did experimental and control groups retain a similar prognosis after the study started?

Blinding
Did investigators avoid effects of patient awareness of allocation—were patients blinded?
Were aspects of care that affect prognosis similar in the two groups—were clinicians blinded?
Was outcome assessed in a uniform way in experimental and control groups—were those assessing the outcome blinded?
Was follow-up complete?

Results
How large was the treatment effect?
How precise was the estimate of the treatment effect?

Applicability
Can the results be applied to my patient?
Were all patient-important outcomes considered?
Are the likely treatment benefits worth the potential harms and costs?

---

resident satisfaction and improve the perceived educational value of the journal club without increasing resident workload or decreasing attendance at the conference.

Structured review instruments have been applied in a number of orthopedic training programs; assessments of the outcomes and effectiveness of this format for journal club are ongoing. One example of one structured review instrument for use in orthopedic training programs is provided in Figure 16-7.

THE FUTURE OF OUTCOME STUDIES IN ORTHOPEDIC TRAUMA

Over the past 50 years, there has been a vast proliferation of randomized trials. Although the strength of evidence is most persuasive in large, randomized trials with small CIs around their treatment effect, this is not always feasible for many clinical problems in orthopedics. Indeed, only 3% (72 of 2,498 studies) of studies published in orthopedics reflect randomized trial methodology.[14] The design, conduct, and analysis of orthopedic research has gained widespread appreciation in surgery, particularly in orthopedic surgery. Still, only 14% of the original contributions in JBJS represent level I evidence.[18] When randomization is either not feasible or unethical, prospective observational studies represent the best evidence. Approximately, one in five scientific articles published in JBJS represent this level II evidence.[18] In a more recent review of the literature, Chan and Bhandari[23] identified 87 randomized trials in orthopedic surgical procedures, representing 14% of the published studies. JBJS contributed 4.1% of the published randomized trials in this report.

Future studies can provide high-quality data on which to base practice if we conduct RCTs whenever feasible, ensure adequate sample size, involve biostatisticians and methodologists, collect data meticulously, and accurately report our results using sensible outcomes and measures of treatment effect. Limiting type II errors (β-errors) will need multicenter initiatives. These larger trials have the advantage of increased

---

TABLE 16-11 Presentation of Results

	Infection	No Infection
Treatment Group	**10** A	90 B
Control Group	50 C	50 D

Treatment event rate (TER): A / (A + B) = 10/100 = 10%
The incidence of infection in the treatment group

Control event rate (CER): C / (C + D) = 50/100 = 50%
The incidence of infection in the control group

Relative risk: TER / CER = 10/50 = 0.2 or 20%
The relative risk of infection in the treatment group relative to the control group

RRR: 1–RR = 1 – 0.2 = 0.8 or 80%
Treatment reduces the risk of infection by 80% compared with controls

Absolute risk reduction (ARR): CER – TER = 50% – 10% = 40%
The actual numerical difference in infection rates between treatment and controls

Number needed to treat: 1 / ARR = 1 / 0.4 = 2.5
For every 2.5 patients who received the treatment, 1 infection can be prevented

Odds ratio: AD / BC = (10)(50) / (90)(50) = 500 / 4500 = 0.11
The odds of infection in treatment compared with controls is 0.11

1. Study design

Randomized trial or Meta-analysis (MA) of randomized trial	12
Prospective observational study with a comparison group or MA	10
Retrospective observational study with a comparison group or MA	8
Prospective observational study with no comparison group or MA	6
Retrospective observational study with no comparison group or MA	4
Cross-sectional (single point in time)/survey	2
Not reported/unable to discern	0

/12

2. Eligibility criteria

Eligibility criteria defined	3
Eligibility criteria partially defined	2
Eligibility criteria not reported	0

/3

Ineligible or excluded patients reported	3
Ineligible or excluded patients partially reported	2
Ineligible patients or excluded not reported	0

/3

3. Similarity of comparison groups at beginning of study

Groups similar due to randomization	8
Groups similar by matching cases to controls or p values shown	6
Groups not similar but statistical tests utilized to correct for imbalances	4
Authors report groups similar but with no supporting information	2
Groups not similar, single group only or not reported	0

/8

4. Similarity of comparison groups at completion of study (omit, if MA)

Groups remained similar (no crossovers occurred)	4
Groups dissimilar (crossovers occurred)	2
Single group only or unsure/not reported/not applicable	0

/4

5. Outcomes assessment

Main outcomes are objective (i.e., do not require major judgement-mortality)	3
Main outcomes are not objective	1

/3

Outcome assessors independent or blinded	3
Outcome assessors not independent or not blinded	0
Unsure	0

/3

6. Follow-up

90% or greater follow-up achieved (prospective, active)	6
80–89% follow-up (prospective, active)	4
70–79% follow-up (prospective, active)	2
Less than 70% follow-up achieved	1
Not reported or unsure or not applicable or passive follow-up	0

/6

7. Sample size

Prestudy sample size or power calculation reported	4
Poststudy power calculation reported	2
Prestudy sample size or power calculation not reported	0

/4

8. Statistical tests

p value and confidence interval(s) reported	4
p value or confidence interval(s) reported	2
No statistics reported	0

/4

Total score   /50

If meta-analysis   /46

FIGURE 16-7 A checklist to assess the quality of surgical therapies.

generalizability of the results and the potential for large-scale and efficient recruitment (1,000 patients or more). Single-center trials that may have taken a decade to recruit enough patients can now be completed in a few years with collaborative research trials. The obvious drawback with multicenter initiatives is the relative complexity of the design and the cost. It is reasonable to expect that a trial of over 1,000 patients will cost more than $3 to 4 million to conduct.

CONCLUSION

The purpose of the "outcomes movement" and EBM is to provide healthcare practitioners and decision-makers (physicians, nurses, administrators, regulators) with tools that allow them to gather, access, interpret, and summarize the evidence required to inform their decisions and to explicitly integrate this evidence with the values of patients. In this sense, EBM is not an end in itself, but rather a set of principles and tools that help clinicians distinguish ignorance of evidence from real scientific uncertainty, distinguish evidence from unsubstantiated opinions, and ultimately provide better patient care.

APPENDIX: SAMPLE SIZE CALCULATIONS

1. Continuous Variables

The number of patients required per treatment arm to obtain 80% study power ($\beta = 0.2$) at a 0.05 α-level of significance is as follows:

$$n_1 = n_2 = 2(\sigma^2)(z_{1-\alpha/2} + z_{1-\beta})^2 / \Delta^2$$

where

n_1 = sample size of group one
n_2 = sample size of group two
Δ = difference of outcome parameter between groups (5 points)
σ = sample standard deviations (12)
$z_{1-\alpha/2} = z_{0.975} = 1.96$ (for $\alpha = 0.05$)
$z_{1-\beta} = z_{0.8} = 0.84$ (for $\beta = 0.2$)

2. Dichotomous Variables

The number of patients required per treatment arm to obtain 80% study power ($\beta = 0.2$) at a 0.05 α-level of significance is as follows:

$$n_1 = n_2 = [(2p_m q_m)^{1/2} z_{1-\alpha/2} + p_1 q_1 + p_2 q_2)^{1/2} z_{1-\beta}]^2 / \Delta^2$$

where

n_1 = sample size of group one
n_2 = sample size of group two
p_1, p_2 = sample probabilities (5% and 10%)
$q_1, q_2 = 1 - p_1, 1 - p_2$ (95% and 90%)
$p_m = (p_1 + p_2)/2$ (7.5%)
$q_m = 1 - p_m$ (92.5%)
Δ = difference = $p_2 - p_1$ (5%)
$z_{1-\alpha/2} = z_{0.975} = 1.96$ (for $\alpha = 0.05$)
$z_{1-\beta} = z_{0.8} = 0.84$ (for $\beta = 0.2$)

REFERENCES

1. American Medical Association. *User's guides to the medical literature: a manual for evidence-based clinical practice.* In Guyatt GH, Rennie D, eds. 2nd ed. Chicago, IL: American Medical Association Press; 2001.
2. Atkins D, Best D, Briss PA, et al. Grading quality of evidence and strength of recommendations. *BMJ.* 2004;328(7454):1490.
3. Atkins D, Briss PA, Eccles M, et al. Systems for grading the quality of evidence and the strength of recommendations II: pilot study of a new system. *BMC Health Serv Res.* 2005;5(1):25.
4. Atkins D, Eccles M, Flottorp S, et al. Systems for grading the quality of evidence and the strength of recommendations I: critical appraisal of existing approaches. The GRADE Working Group. *BMC Health Serv Res.* 2004;4:38.
5. Balogh ZJ, Reumann MK, Gruen RL, et al. Advances and future directions for management of trauma patients. *Lancet.* 2012;380(9847):1109–1119.
6. Beaton DE, Schemitsch E. Measures of health-related quality of life and physical function. *Clin Orthop Relat Res.* 2003;413:90–105.
7. Benson K, Hartz AJ. A comparison of observational studies and randomized, controlled trials. *N Engl J Med.* 2000;342:1878–1886.
8. Bhandari M, Devereaux PJ, Li P, et al. The misuse of baseline comparison tests and subgroup analyses in surgical randomized controlled trials. *Clin Orthop Relat Res.* 2006;447:247–251.
9. Bhandari M, Guyatt GH, Siddiqui F, et al. Operative versus nonoperative treatment of achilles tendon rupture—a systematic overview and meta-analysis. *Clin Orthop Relat Res* 2002:400:190–200.
10. Bhandari M, Guyatt GH, Swiontkowski MF. User's guide to the orthopaedic literature: how to use an article about a prognosis. *J Bone Joint Surg.* 2001;83A:1555–1564.
11. Bhandari M, Guyatt GH, Swiontkowski MF. User's guide to the orthopaedic literature: how to use an article about a surgical therapy. *J Bone Joint Surg.* 2001;83A:916–926.
12. Bhandari M, Montori VM, Devereaux PJ, et al. Doubling the impact: publication of systematic review articles in orthopaedic journals. *J Bone Joint Surg Am.* 2004;86:1012–1016.
13. Bhandari M, Richards R, Schemitsch EH. The quality of randomized trials in Journal of Bone and Joint Surgery from 1988–2000. *J Bone Joint Surg Am.* 2002;84A:388–396.
14. Bhandari M, Swiontkowski MF, Einhorn TA, et al. Interobserver agreement in the application of levels of evidence to scientific papers in the American volume of the Journal of Bone and Joint Surgery. *J Bone Joint Surg Am.* 2004;86A:1717–1720.
15. Bhandari M, Tornetta P III. Issues in the hierarchy of study design, hypothesis testing, and presentation of results. *Tech Orthop.* 2004;19:57–65.
16. Bhandari M, Tornetta P 3rd, Rampersad SA, et al. (Sample) Size Matters! An Examination of Sample Size from the SPRINT trial study to prospectively evaluate reamed intramedullary nails in patients with tibial fractures. *J Orthop Trauma.* 2013;27:183–188.
17. Bhandari M, Tornetta P III, Ellis T, et al. Hierarchy of evidence: differences in results between nonrandomized studies and randomized trials in patients with femoral neck fractures. *Arch Orthop Trauma Surg.* 2004;124(1):10–16.
18. Bhandari M, Tornetta P III. Communicating the risks of surgery to patients. *European J Trauma.* 2004;30:177–180.
19. Bhandari M, Whang W, Kuo JC, et al. The risk of false-positive results in orthopaedic surgical trials. *Clin Orthop Relat Res.* 2003;413:63–69.
20. Bhandari M, Zlowodzki M, Cole PA. From eminence-based practice to evidence-based practice: a paradigm shift. *Minn Med.* 2004;4:51–54.
21. Box JF. Guinness, Gosset, Fisher, and small samples. *Statistical Science.* 1987;2:45–52.
22. Brighton B, Bhandari M, Tornetta P III, et al. Hierarchy of evidence: from case reports to randomized controlled trials. *Clin Orthop Relat Res.* 2003;413:19–24.
23. Chan S, Bhandari M. The quality of reporting of orthopaedic randomized trials with use of a checklist for nonpharmacological therapies. *J Bone Joint Surg Am.* 2007;89:1970–1978.
24. Concato J, Shah N, Horwitz RI. Randomized, controlled trials, observational studies, and the hierarchy of research designs. *N Engl J Med.* 2000;342:1887–1894.
25. Devereaux PJ, Bhandari M, Clarke M, et al. Need for expertise-based randomized controlled trials. *BMJ.* 2005;330(7482):88.
26. Devereaux PJ, Manns BJ, Ghali W, et al. In the dark: physician interpretations and textbook definitions of blinding terminology in randomized controlled trials. *JAMA.* 2001;285:2000–2003.
27. Dirschl DR, Tornetta P III, Bhandari M. Designing, conducting, and evaluating journal clubs in orthopaedic surgery. *Clin Orthop Relat Res.* 2003;413:146–157.
28. Griffin D, Audige L. Common statistical methods in orthopaedic clinical studies. *Clin Orthop Relat Res.* 2003;413:70–79.
29. Guyatt GH. Evidence-based medicine. *ACP J Club.* 1991;114:A16.
30. Haentjens P, Autier P, Boonen S. Clinical risk factors for hip fracture in elderly women: a case-control study. *J Orthop Trauma.* 2002;6:379–385.
31. Haynes RB, Mukherjee J, Sackett D, et al. Functional status changes following medical or surgical treatment for cerebral ischemia: results in the EC/IC, Bypass Study. *JAMA.* 1987;257:2043–2046.
32. Ioannidis JP, Haidich AB, Pappa M, et al. Comparison of evidence of treatment effects in randomized and nonrandomized studies. *JAMA.* 2001;286:821–830.
33. Jackowski D, Guyatt G. A guide to health measurement. *Clin Orthop Relat Res.* 2003; 413:80–89.
34. Jaglal S, Lakhani Z, Schatzker J. Reliability, validity, and responsiveness of the lower extremity measure for patients with a hip fracture. *J Bone Joint Surg Am.* 2000;82-A:955–962.
35. Johanson NA, Charlson ME, Szatrowske TP, et al. A self-administered hip-rating questionnaire for the assessment of outcome after total hip replacement. *J Bone Joint Surg Am.* 1992;74:587–597.
36. Kunz R, Oxman AD. The unpredictability paradox: review of empirical comparisons of randomized and nonrandomized clinical trials. *BMJ.* 1998;317:1185–1190.

37. Lochner H, Bhandari M, Tornetta P III. Type II error rates (beta errors) in randomized trials in orthopaedic trauma. *J Bone Joint Surg.* 2002;83A:1650–1655.
38. Marsh JL, Weigel DP, Dirschl DR. Tibial plafond fractures. How do these ankles function over time? *J Bone Joint Surg Am.* 2003;85A:287–295.
39. Mathias S, Nayak USL, Isaacs B. Balance in the elderly patients: the "get-up-and-go" test. *Arch Phys Med Rehab.* 1986;67:387–389.
40. McConnell S, Kolopack P, Davis AM. The Western Ontario and McMaster Universities Osteoarthritis Index (WOMAC): a review of its utility and measurement properties. *Arthritis Rheum.* 2001;45:453–461.
41. Michener LA, McClure PW, Sennett BJ. American Shoulder and Elbow Surgeons Standardized Shoulder Assessment Form patient self-report section: reliability, validity, and responsiveness. *J Shoulder Elbow Surg.* 2002;11:587–594.
42. Miranda MA, Riemer BL, Butterfield SL, et al. Pelvic ring injuries. Along-term functional outcome study. *Clin Orthop Relat Res.* 1996;329:152–159.
43. Olerud C, Molander H. A scoring scale for symptom evaluation after ankle fracture. *Arch Orthop Trauma Surg.* 1984;103:190–194.
44. Ovre S, Sandvik L, Madsen JE, et al. Comparison of distribution, agreement, and correlation between the original and modified Merle d'Aubigne-Postel Score and the Harris Hip Score after acetabular fracture treatment: moderate-agreement, high-ceiling effect and excellent correlation in 450 patients. *Acta Orthop Scand.* 2005;76:796–802.
45. Piva SR, Fitzgerald GK, Irrgang JJ, et al. Get-up-and-go test in patients with knee osteoarthritis. *Arch Phys Med Rehabil.* 2004;85:284–289.
46. Pocock S, Assman S, Enos L, et al. Subgroup analysis, covariate adjustment, and baseline comparisons in clinical trial reporting: current practice and problems. *Stats Med.* 2002;21:2917–2930.
47. Rogers JC, IrrgangJJ. Measures of adult lower extremity function. *Arthitis Rheum.* 2003;49:S67–S84.
48. Roland M, Fairbank J. The Roland-Morris disability questionnaire and the Oswestry disability questionnaire. *Spine.* 2000;25:3115–3124.
49. Roos EM, Toksvig-Larsen S. Knee injury and Osteoarthritis Outcome Score (KOOS)—validation and comparison to the WOMAC in total knee replacement. *Health Qual Life Outcomes.* 2003;1:17.
50. Sackett DL, Haynes RB, Guyatt GH, et al. *Clinical Epidemiology: A Basic Science for Clinical Medicine.* Boston, MA: Little Brown; 1991.
51. Sackett DL, Richardson WS, Rosenberg WM, et al. *Evidence-based Medicine: How to Practice and Teach EBM.* New York, NY: Churchill Livingstone; 1997.
52. Saltzman CL, Domsic RT, Baumhauer JF. Foot and ankle research priority: report from the Research Council of the American Orthopaedic Foot and Ankle Society. *Foot Ankle Int.* 1997;18:447–448.
53. SMFA Swionkowski. Available online at http://www.med.umn.edu/ortho/research.html. Accessed September 10, 2009.
54. SooHoo NF, Shuler M, Fleming LL. Evaluation of the validity of the AOFAS Clinical Rating Systems by correlation to the SF-36. *Foot Ankle Int.* 2003;24:50–55.
55. SPRINT Investigators, Bhandari M, Guyatt G, et al. Randomized trial of reamed and unreamed intramedullary nailing of tibial shaft fractures. *J Bone Joint Surg Am.* 2008;90:2567–2578.
56. SPRINT Investigators, Bhandari M, Guyatt G, et al. Study to prospectively evaluate reamed intramedullary nails in patients with tibial fractures (SPRINT): study rationale and design. *BMC Musculoskeletal Discord.* 2008;9:91.
57. Sung J, Siegel J, Tornetta P III, et al. The orthopaedic trauma literature: an evaluation of statistically significant findings in orthopaedic trauma randomized trials. *BMC Musculoskelet Disord.* 2008;29(9):14.
58. The EC/IC Bypass Study Group. Failure of extracranial-intracranial arterial bypass to reduce the risk of ischemic stroke: results of an international randomized trial. *N Engl J Med.* 1985;313:1191–1200.
59. Ware J. Available online at http://www.qualitymetric.com. Accessed September 10, 2009.
60. Wright JG, Swiontkowski MF, Heckman JD. Introducing levels of evidence to the journal. *J Bone Joint Surg Am.* 2003;85A:1–3.
61. Yeung M, Bhandari M. Uneven global distribution of randomized trials in hip fracture surgery. *Acta Orthop.* 2012;83(4):328–333.
62. Yusuf S, Wittes J, Probstfield J, et al. Analysis and interpretation of treatment effects in subgroups of patients in randomized clinical trials. *JAMA.* 1991;266:93–98.
63. Zuckerman JD, Koval KJ, Aharonoff GB, et al. A functional recovery score for elderly hip patients: I. Development. *J Orthop Trauma.* 2000;14:20–25.
64. Zuckerman JD, Koval KJ, Aharonoff GB, et al. A functional recovery score for elderly hip patients: II. Validity and reliability. *J Orthop Trauma.* 2000;14:26–30.

17
IMAGING CONSIDERATIONS IN ORTHOPEDIC TRAUMA

Andrew H. Schmidt and Kerry M. Kallas

GENERAL CONSIDERATIONS

Medical imaging in the setting of acute musculoskeletal trauma contributes greatly to the initial diagnosis and subsequent management of orthopedic injuries. In many instances, patients are able to provide details of the injury, and imaging studies often confirm or exclude diagnoses already suggested by the clinical history, mechanism of injury, and physical examination findings. Imaging plays a critical role in the management of multitrauma patients who arrive obtunded or unconscious or are intubated and therefore unable to localize symptoms or cooperate during the physical examination. Multitrauma patients may also have coexisting neurologic and visceral injury, and in this setting orthopedic imaging is often deferred for other imaging studies and surgical triage for life-threatening injuries. However, plain radiographs must be made of all potential musculoskeletal injuries as soon as possible so that appropriate early treatment decisions are made.

A wide variety of imaging examinations are available in clinical practice today, and use of a particular modality may be influenced by multiple factors, such as availability, image resolution, invasiveness, cost-effectiveness, patient risk, and requirements for special handling of the trauma patient. Many imaging studies are routinely ordered for specific indications and need no justification; for example, conventional radiographs are used to evaluate acute bony trauma of the extremities. Particularly with regard to more advanced imaging techniques; however, clinicians must often consider these tradeoffs in deciding whether to pursue additional imaging. Clinicians also need to be aware of the limitations of imaging in selected patients. For example, in elderly female patients with trauma to the proximal femur and/or pelvis, plain radiographs are not nearly as accurate for the diagnosis of fractures as MR imaging.[103]

Availability

Although there is widespread availability of conventional radiography in both clinical and hospital settings, there is more variable access to advanced imaging modalities, particularly in rural communities and after hours.[76] In a random survey of 5% of US emergency departments (n = 262), CT scanners were present in 96% of institutions and were available 24 hours a day in 94%. Scanner resolution was variable; 39% had access to 16-slice or greater scanners. On-site MRI was available in two-thirds of the institutions, with another 20% having mobile MRI available. Smaller and rural hospitals had less access to CT and MRI, and when available, CT tended to be lower resolution.[76] Although data are lacking, access to other imaging modalities, such as ultrasound (US) and nuclear medicine (NM) is also

---

TABLE 17-1 | **The Limiting Spatial Resolutions of Various Medical Imaging Modalities: The Resolution Levels Achieved in Typical Clinical Usage of the Modality**

| Modality | Resolution | | Comments |
	lp/mm	mm	
Screen film radiography	6	0.08	Limited by focal spot and detector resolution
Digital radiography	3	0.17	Limited by size of detector elements
Fluoroscopy	4	0.125	Limited by detector and focal spot
CT	1	0.4	About V_2-mm pixels
NM: Planar imaging	<0.1	7	Spatial resolution degrades substantially with distance from detector
SPECT	<0.1	7	Spatial resolution worst toward the center of cross-sectional image slice
PET	0.1	5	Better spatial resolution than other nuclear medicine imaging modalities
MRI	0.5	1.0	Resolution can be improved at higher magnetic fields
US	1.7	0.3 (5 MHz)	Limited by wavelength of sound

CT, computed tomography; NM, nuclear medicine; SPECT, single-photon emission computed tomography; PET, positron emission tomography; MRI, magnetic resonance imaging; US, ultrasound.

Modified and reprinted with permission from: Brushberg JT, Seibert JA, Leidholt EM Jr, et al. The essential physics of medical imaging. 2nd ed. Philadelphia, PA: Lippincott Williams & Wilkins; 2002.

---

likely to be similarly variable, and may be available only on an "on-call" basis or not available at all after hours.

Fortunately, all that is needed to evaluate the orthopedic trauma patient in the immediate setting are plain radiographs, which provide information sufficient to diagnose any fracture or dislocation. The primary exception to this is in the evaluation of the spine, especially in the comatose patient and in the setting of specific injury patterns, where both CT and MRI have well-defined roles.[59,79,82] However, controversy continues over the relative merits of CT versus MRI in the evaluation of spine trauma, with one group considering that MRI is the new standard for the evaluation of blunt cervical spine trauma.[141] Although MRI has the added benefit of more clearly demonstrating soft tissue injuries in general, and disc herniation in the spine in particular, the inconsistent after-hours availability of MRI, as well as the obvious logistic problems of transporting and monitoring a trauma patient within an MRI unit, means that CT will remain the most common method of imaging the spine in the early evaluation of the trauma patient.[189]

The recent introduction of digital radiography (DR) and teleradiology provides a means to obtain after-hours interpretation of images by trained radiologists.[57,135,167,194] Although this is most often done in the management of acute neurologic emergencies and in the assessment of cross-sectional imaging of the abdomen and chest, such technology will no doubt benefit musculoskeletal trauma patients as well. In a recent report describing the benefits of a nighttime teleradiology service for emergencies, 43 of 75 studies were musculoskeletal.[57]

Image Resolution

The choice of a particular imaging examination may, in part, be influenced by spatial resolution and contrast resolution. The ability of an imaging modality to resolve small objects of high

subject contrast (e.g., bone–muscle interface) as distinct entities is referred to as spatial resolution, which is typically measured in line pairs per millimeter (lp/mm); higher values of lp/mm indicate greater resolution. For comparison, the limiting spatial resolution of the human eye is approximately 30 lp/mm. Resolution may also be expressed in millimeters, whereby smaller values represent greater spatial resolution. Table 17-1 lists representative values of limiting spatial resolution for common imaging modalities. Conventional radiographs have considerably better spatial resolution than cross-sectional imaging techniques, although overlapping bony structures often complicate evaluation of osseous anatomy. CT has better spatial resolution than MRI and is more commonly performed for evaluating finer bony abnormalities, such as avulsion fractures and calcification within tumor matrix.

Contrast resolution refers to the ability to resolve two tissues of similar subject contrast. Conventional radiographs typically have poor soft tissue contrast resolution, whereas CT and MRI, in particular, have much better contrast resolution, in part related to their tomographic nature. For example, on conventional radiographs, subcutaneous fat may be discerned from the underlying muscle groups, although the intermuscular fascial planes cannot be visualized. CT and MRI better demonstrate the subcutaneous fat and intermuscular fascial planes, although MRI shows superior soft tissue contrast resolution compared with CT.

Invasiveness

Most medical imaging procedures are noninvasive, or may require minimally invasive procedures, such as placement of intravenous access for contrast administration. Some imaging techniques are more invasive; however, such as peripheral angiography for vascular assessment in the trauma patient, and not only carry more inherent risk to the patient but also require greater resources and coordination on an emergent basis. When used appropriately, the diagnostic and therapeutic advantages of these procedures can contribute substantially to the patient's management.

Cost-Effectiveness

With increasing pressures on cost containment, studies have been performed to address the cost-effectiveness of algorithms incorporating conventional radiography in the diagnosis and follow-up of musculoskeletal trauma.[6] Significant costs may be incurred at receiving hospitals as a result of repeating radiographic workups for patients who have been transferred from referring facilities along with their original radiographs.[187] Several recent studies have shown the benefits of "rules" in deciding when to order radiographs for knee and ankle trauma, resulting in fewer radiographs ordered and reduced cost without increased incidence of missed fractures.[6] Additional studies have also shown the ability to reduce postoperative and follow-up radiographs in treatment of ankle fractures.[86] Similar studies have addressed the cost-effectiveness of routine pelvic radiography in the setting of blunt trauma, although with mixed results.[52,97] Study of pediatric torus fractures has shown that postcasting radiographs are unnecessary and follow-up radiographs do not change fracture management, with the implication of significant cost savings as a result of decreased radiography.[62]

Given the increases in health care costs each year in the United States, an area of particular concern is the perceived expense of advanced musculoskeletal imaging techniques such as MRI. According to one estimate, the use of musculoskeletal MRI has grown nearly 14 times faster than overall musculoskeletal imaging during the period 1996 to 2005 (353% increase vs. 26% increase).[153] Parker et al.[153] explored the possible cost savings that could be realized if ultrasound was used instead of MRI for the diagnosis of musculoskeletal disorders. According to their review of 3,621 musculoskeletal MRI reports, 45.4% of primary diagnoses and 30.6% of all diagnoses could have been made with US instead.[153] By extrapolating these data into the future, Parker et al.[153] predict that the substitution of musculoskeletal US for MRI in appropriate cases could save more than $6.9 billion in the period 2006 to 2020 and lead to large cost savings for Medicare.[153]

Other studies have shown that advanced imaging can be very cost-effective to the degree that such imaging improves initial diagnostic accuracy and avoids delays in treatment that can contribute to increased morbidity to the patient or delay to return to work. For example, several studies have shown that early MRI in cases of wrist trauma can be cost-effective by providing accurate diagnosis of scaphoid fractures in cases where initial conventional radiography was normal.[27,49,127] MRI also proved superior to follow-up radiography for diagnosis of occult fractures, resulting in a change in management in up to 89% of cases.[165] Cost was found to be similar or reduced in all studies comparing early MRI with more traditional algorithms of casting and radiographic follow-up.[27,49,173] Two studies showed cost benefits associated with earlier rather than later MRI scanning.[27,165] Similar studies have shown the cost-effectiveness of early limited MRI in the diagnosis and management of occult hip fractures.[118]

Patient Risk

As a rule, imaging procedures used in evaluating orthopedic trauma contribute very little increased risk to the patient. The exception is CT, for which there is increasing concern about the risks of radiation exposure, especially in children.[26,145,162,177,178] In addition to the risk of ionizing radiation with CT, other potential risks include patient handling, contrast reactions, and potential risk with MRI in patients with implanted devices containing metal.

Handling trauma patients requires special attention and care, especially when transferring patients from gurneys onto imaging equipment. Many trauma patients have potential spine injuries, necessitating the use of spinal precautions and special radiographic views during imaging procedures. Likewise, fractured limbs may be very painful when moved, and there may be changes in fracture reduction or redislocation of an injured joint during manipulation of an extremity for radiographs. Because of pain and disorientation, patients may be unable to lie still during imaging examinations and may require analgesia and sedation. Sometimes, mechanical ventilation and multiple lines as well as catheters must be managed. Life support equipment and external fixation devices may also be incompatible with or limit the usefulness of certain examinations, such as conventional radiography and MRI.

The risk of cancer associated with medical imaging has been the subject of recent reports.[66,145,162,177,178] Cancer risks associated with ionizing radiation vary with modality; CT generates considerably higher-radiation doses compared to conventional radiography, while US and MRI do not involve ionizing radiation. Radiation doses vary considerably among CT protocols and between manufacturers.[168] One study showed a 61% to 71% decrease in radiation dose between standard-dose and low-dose multidetector CT (MDCT) in cervical spine trauma.[142] The National Council of Radiation Protection and Measurements reported in 2009 that the average radiation dose in the United States has risen from 3.6 mSv in the early 1980s to a value of 6.2 mSv in 2006, with most of the increase attributed to CT and nuclear imaging.[145] Another report documented an increase between 1996 and 2012 in the use of advanced imaging and the per capita radiation dose, as well as the proportion of patients receiving high and very high doses of radiation.[178] It has been estimated that as many as 1.5% to 2% of all cancers in US patients may be attributable to radiation from CT studies.[26] CT is often used to evaluate to evaluate the multiply-injured and unconscious patient. These patients typically undergo head and body CT for evaluation of intracranial and body trauma, and the use of CT to clear the cervical spine, in lieu of conventional radiography, may be increasing. Body CT generates the greatest radiation dose. In the cervical region, the greatest risk of ionizing radiation is induction of thyroid malignancy. One study suggests that use of CT to clear the cervical spine in unconscious major trauma patients is justified given the relatively minor concern for inducing thyroid malignancy. However, in those patients who are conscious or with a Glasgow Coma Scale score between 9 and 12, clinical evaluation is more likely to be helpful, and the risk of thyroid malignancy in a young cohort does not justify the use of CT to clear the entire cervical spine.[168] A recent study reported radiation doses in common CT studies done at four hospitals in San Francisco, noting a mean 13-fold difference between the highest and lowest dose for each type of study.[177] Prasarn et al.[162] reported total radiation exposure in a cohort of 1,357 orthopedic trauma patients. The average effective radiation dose for all patients was 31.6 mSv. For patients with an Injury Severity Score of greater than 16, the average exposure was 48.6 mSv.[162] To put these findings in perspective, the International Commission on Radiological Protection recommends a permissible annual radiation dose of 20 mSv.[162] This suggests that more should be done to limit radiation exposure during routine medical imaging, and clinicians as well as radiologists should keep radiation exposure in mind when ordering and performing imaging studies, especially CT. Because of concerns regarding ionizing radiation, CT manufacturers are developing noise-reduction software tools that allow high-quality images to be provided at much lower-radiation doses.

Intravenous administration of iodinated contrast medium carries a small risk of adverse events, which may be categorized as mild, moderate, severe, and end organ.[4] With traditional high-osmolality ionic contrast media, most adverse reactions are mild to moderate and occur in 5% to 12% of all patients. This incidence is significantly decreased with use of the newer low-osmolality nonionic contrast agents. The occurrence of severe contrast reactions is approximately 1 to 2 per 1,000 patients receiving high-osmolality contrast agents, whereas this number decreases to approximately 1 to 2 per 10,000 patients receiving low-osmolality contrast media.[3] Examples of end-organ adverse events include thrombophlebitis related to the injection site, nephrotoxicity, pulseless electrical activity, seizures, and pulmonary edema.[4] Peripheral angiography carries a low risk of complications, including bleeding and further vascular injury, although these problems may be minimized with experience and careful technique.

MRI has unique risks in patients with implanted devices.[85] Ferromagnetic metals can experience strong forces, especially near the magnet when forces can be enough to cause motion of the implant. Secondly, some metals may experience heating, although the effects of this are negligible in orthopedic implants. Finally, metal implants always cause some degradation of the image, although this can often be mitigated using new signal processing techniques, as discussed later in this chapter.

SPECIFIC IMAGING MODALITIES

Radiography

Technical Considerations

Conventional Radiography. Conventional radiography (screen film radiography, plain film radiography) involves the use of x-rays, which are high-energy electromagnetic radiation with wavelengths smaller than ultraviolet light but longer than gamma rays. X-rays are produced using an x-ray tube, whereby electrons are emitted from a heated tungsten filament and accelerated across a voltage potential to strike an opposing tungsten target. The flow of electrons from filament to the target results in a tube current, and its interaction with the tungsten target generates a spectrum of x-rays and heat. Before leaving the x-ray tube, the x-rays are filtered and collimated into a useable beam. Factors that are set by the technologist to vary the quality and/or quantity of the x-ray beam include the voltage potential (measured in peak kilovoltage [kVp]), tube current (milliamperes [mA]), and exposure time (seconds). The output of the x-ray tube is expressed in mAs, calculated by multiplying the tube current (mA) by the exposure time (s). These factors are routinely recorded on digital radiographs, whereas they may be handwritten on portable radiographs for use with future examinations.

After leaving the x-ray tube, the x-ray beam is directed through the patient and onto a screen/film cassette. The x-ray beam is attenuated as it passes through the patient, primarily via two processes: The photoelectric effect and the Compton scatter. After passing through the patient and before reaching the screen/film cassette, the transmitted radiation may be further collimated using a lead grid to remove the scatted radiation. Scatter increases with increasing patient thickness and larger fields of view and is a significant source of image degradation. Scatter may be negligible with extremities, in part related to their smaller size and greater proximity to the cassette; hence, grids may not be required.

Screen/film cassettes are used to capture the transmitted radiation and create the latent image. Intensifying screens absorb x-ray photons and subsequently emit a greater number of light photons, which are then absorbed by the film. The film consists of a base, which is covered on one or both sides by an emulsion containing silver grains. Absorbed light photons result in liberation of free electrons within the emulsion, which subsequently reduce the silver atoms. When the film is developed, the reduced silver atoms are amplified and appear black on the film. Most screen/film cassettes use a dual-screen and dual-emulsion film combination, which is enclosed in a light-tight cassette and ensures good contact between the screens and film. To improve bone detail, a single-screen, single emulsion system may be used.

Portable Radiography. Portable radiography is frequently used to evaluate acute trauma patients, and its use may be complicated by several factors not encountered in the radiology department's controlled environment. Trauma patients frequently are immobile and require special handling precautions, which may make it difficult to obtain routine anteroposterior (AP) and lateral projections. Appropriate placement and alignment of the screen/film cassette may be especially challenging, and if placed behind a backboard or beneath the patient's cart, it may introduce artifacts into the radiograph and obscure anatomy of interest. Objects outside of the patient's body related to his or her resuscitation, including endotracheal tubes, nasogastric tubes, chest tubes, and intravenous access, frequently project onto the radiograph. Casts, splints, and other external fixation devices may also project onto extremity radiographs and limit visualization of underlying bony detail.

Technical factors, such as levels of kilovoltage peak (kVp) and mA, also need modification with portable radiography. Portable examinations are often performed with higher kVp settings, which provide for a wider margin of error in selecting other technical factors. Higher kVp values will result in greater scattered radiation; however, and may necessitate the use of a grid with the screen/film cassette. Precise alignment of the grid and cassette to the central beam of the portable x-ray tube is also more difficult because each of the components are not fixed in space, and malalignment results in significant obscuration of the image and degradation in image quality.

Digital Radiography. Several digital technologies for acquiring radiographs are in use and continue to be refined. In all DR systems, the creation of x-rays and attenuation of the x-ray beam as it passes through the patient are similar to conventional radiography systems. What differentiates DR systems is the type of image receptor that interacts with the attenuated x-ray beam to create a medical image.

Computed radiography (CR) was first introduced in the late 1970s and has gained wide popularity in radiology departments within the last decade. With CR, the screen/film cassette is replaced by a cassette containing a photostimulatable phosphor deposited onto a substrate. When this type of phosphor interacts with x-rays, electrons are elevated to and trapped at higher-energy levels within the phosphor. The amount of electron trapping is proportional to the incident x-rays and results in the creation of a latent image, which can later be read using a specialized CR cassette reader. The reader scans the phosphor plate using a laser, which releases the electrons from their higher-energy states, and results in emission of light as they drop down to lower-energy states. The emitted light is captured by a photomultiplier tube, which converts the light into an electrical signal, which is subsequently digitized and stored. This process is done on a point-by-point basis throughout the entire phosphor plate to create a digital image.

Relatively recent advances in flat panel detectors have led to a new digital imaging technology that has been referred to as direct capture radiography, or alternatively, indirect and direct DR. Each of these systems uses flat panel detectors that incorporate a large array of individual detector elements; each one corresponds to a pixel in the final image. In indirect DR, the detector elements are sensitive to light; hence, an x-ray intensifying screen is used to convert the incident x-rays into light, which is then captured by the individual detector elements and stored as a net negative charge. In direct DR, the individual detector elements are coated with a photoconductive material (selenium is commonly used). On exposure to x-rays, electrons are liberated from the photoconductor and are captured by the underlying detector elements, resulting in a net negative charge within each detector element. With both systems, the negative charges within the array of detector elements are read out electronically, digitized, and stored to create the final image.

Currently, the spatial resolution of conventional radiography is greater than for DR systems (Table 17-1). CR and DR; however, offer significant advantages over conventional radiography, including the ability to manipulate digital images and alter image contrast, decreased radiation dose to the patient and radiologic personnel, and greater ease of storage and transmission of radiographs both within and beyond the imaging department. New portable DR systems that incorporate wireless flat panel displays are much quicker and have improved workflow compared to conventional DR.[114] Unfortunately, DR systems are expensive to implement, as they require replacement of the entire radiography suite. CR systems are much more economical to implement, as they only require replacement of the screen/film cassettes and purchase of a CR reader. Both digital systems, though, offer ongoing cost savings as a result of decreased numbers of retakes and reduction in film costs.

Applications

Conventional radiography remains the primary diagnostic modality for assessing fractures and dislocations. Orthogonal views, occasionally supplemented by additional specific projections, are sufficient to identify and manage most fractures. Orthopedic surgeons' immediate interpretation of conventional radiographs of simple fractures has been shown to be timely, accurate, and inexpensive and contributes to patient care, whereas formal interpretation of the same studies by a radiologist typically occurs after care is rendered, may be inaccurate, adds expense, and does not contribute to patient management.[23]

For many injuries, including those in the spine, specific measurements have been reported that may characterize a given injury.[19] In addition to delineating the fracture pattern, conventional radiographs are useful for assessing limb length and alignment and are the primary means by which fracture healing is monitored. Numerous examples of the use of conventional radiographs are found throughout this text. In many cases, more subtle indications of injury apparent on conventional radiographs can suggest the need for further diagnostic imaging or intervention. Examples of such cases would be the identification of a posterior fat pad sign in a pediatric elbow, indicating an occult elbow injury, a joint effusion, or the finding of a fat-fluid level in the knee joint capsule indicating osteochondral fracture. Surrounding soft tissues may also be evaluated for and show additional evidence of trauma, including swelling, foreign bodies, and gas. Although conventional radiographs are universally used for assessing fracture healing, one recent report noted that there is very poor interobserver agreement regarding the determination of fracture healing after internal fixation.[43]

DR has largely replaced conventional radiography and has provided a platform on which to develop new methods of musculoskeletal imaging. Digital imaging facilitates computer processing of images, which may improve their diagnostic value. Botser et al.[24] studied a series of nondisplaced proximal femoral fractures and found that digital enhancement with the use of specific filter techniques improved fracture diagnosis. One recent advance is a full body scanner that can take rapid digital images of the entire body in one or multiple planes (StatScan Critical Imaging System; Lodox Systems Ltd., South Africa). The use of StatScan in the evaluation of multiple trauma patients and pediatric patients has been reported.[60,143,158] The primary advantages are the rapid detection of injuries and less time needed for resuscitation. In one study, 96% of fractures were identified on the initial StatScan.[158] In another study focusing on 37 consecutive pelvic injuries, findings on StatScan images were compared to those seen with CR and CT.[143] Of 73 abnormalities noted in these patients, 18 were not identifiable on the StatScan, although only one of the missed findings was considered significant for the initial management of the patient.[143] Although many patients initially evaluated with StatScan still need formal CT, such studies can be more limited and result in less overall radiation exposure to the patient than conventional imaging algorithms.[60]

Fluoroscopy

Technical Considerations

Conventional Fluoroscopy. Fluoroscopy involves the use of low-dose x-rays to image patient anatomy at high temporal resolutions—that is, in real time. Typical components of a fluoroscopy system include an x-ray tube, filters, and a collimator, similar to that used in conventional radiography. The x-ray tube is energized continuously using a low exposure rate, and the x-ray beam is directed through the patient onto an image intensifier. The image intensifier is responsible for converting the attenuated x-ray beam into a visible light image, which is frequently coupled to a closed-circuit television camera to produce a "live" image on a video monitor. An optical coupling system, using high-resolution lenses and mirrors, may also be used to direct the light image to recording devices, such as video recorders and photospot cameras.

The components of the image intensifier are housed in a glass vacuum tube and include a large input phosphor, a photo cathode, a series of electrostatic lenses, an anode, and a smaller output phosphor. Incident x-rays are directed onto the input phosphor and are converted into light photons, similar to a radiographic intensifying screen. The light photons are channeled by the phosphor to the adjacent photocathode as a result of the linear crystalline structure of the phosphor matrix. The photocathode is composed of a thin metal layer, containing cesium and antimony, applied to the posterior surface of the input phosphor, which interacts with the light photons and results in emission of electrons. The electrons are then accelerated from the photocathode to the anode by an applied voltage approximating 25,000 V. During the acceleration process, the electrons emitted across the entire cross-sectional area of the photocathode are kept in relative alignment by a series of electrostatic lenses, such that the spatial information they contain is preserved. The electrons are subsequently focused onto the output phosphor, which results in light emission and creation of an image.

Fluoroscopy systems vary in configuration, from permanently installed biplane angiography suites to mobile C-arm designs. Mini C-arm units have become increasingly popular for outpatient clinics. Image intensifiers are produced in different sizes, and measurements refer to the size of the input phosphor. Typical diameters range from 10 to 40 cm (4 to 16 in), and various sizes may be better suited or standardized to specific applications. Many fluoroscopy systems offer additional magnification modes, which use a smaller area of the input phosphor to create the magnified image. The theoretical resolution of an image intensifier is approximately 4 to 5 lp/mm, with somewhat better resolution obtained in magnification modes (Table 17-1). This is achievable only when the images are output to film. The image intensifier output is usually coupled to a video monitor for real-time viewing, which results in degradation of the resolution achievable by the image intensifier. Resolution of such closed-circuit television systems is typically 1 to 2 lp/mm.

Digital Fluoroscopy. Advances in digital technology have led to the development of digital fluoroscopy systems, which are now common in clinical practice. The output of the image intensifier may be coupled to a high-resolution video camera with subsequently digitized output, or directed onto a charge-coupled device (CCD). A CCD is a small plate containing a large array of photosensitive elements, each of which corresponds to a single pixel in the final digital image. Each element stores charge in proportion to the amount of absorbed light, which is then read out electronically and digitized to produce a pixel value. The matrix of pixel values is then used to create the final digital image. The resolution of a CCD depends on the size of each of its array elements; CCDs with a 1024×1024 matrix may achieve a resolution of 10 lp/mm. The digital nature of the image lends itself to computer postprocessing, including digital subtraction techniques, which improves image contrast. More recent advances in flat panel detector technology using thin-film transistor (TFT) arrays may allow replacement of the image intensifier and video camera by TFT panels, resulting in even greater improvement in image contrast.

Two- and Three-Dimensional Fluoroscopy. New fluoroscopic devices obtain fluoroscopic images in an arc around the patient, and contain imaging processing software that provides an immediate two-dimensional (2D) or three-dimensional (3D) reconstruction of the target. Several 3D-fluoroscopic imaging systems are available. C-arms that are adapted for this purpose incorporate a motor that rotates the x-ray tube and image intensifier around the patient while taking hundreds of images. Immediate computer processing generates a reconstructed cross-sectional image that is similar to an axial CT image. Different manufacturers' devices vary in the arc of rotation required to obtain an image, with newer devices capable of creating the reconstructed images with 136 degrees of arc compared to the 180 degrees required by first-generation scanners.[183] Although the devices that obtain images through a full 180-degree arc produce quality images, the devices that image through the smaller arc can provide images in anatomic regions like the shoulder that cannot be imaged with the 180-degree devices.[183]

Applications

Intraoperative Imaging. Intraoperative radiography and fluoroscopy are almost universally used during the operative

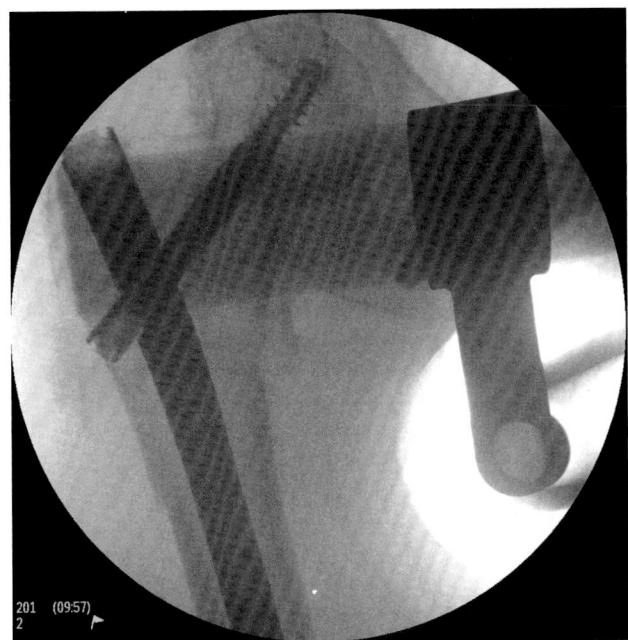
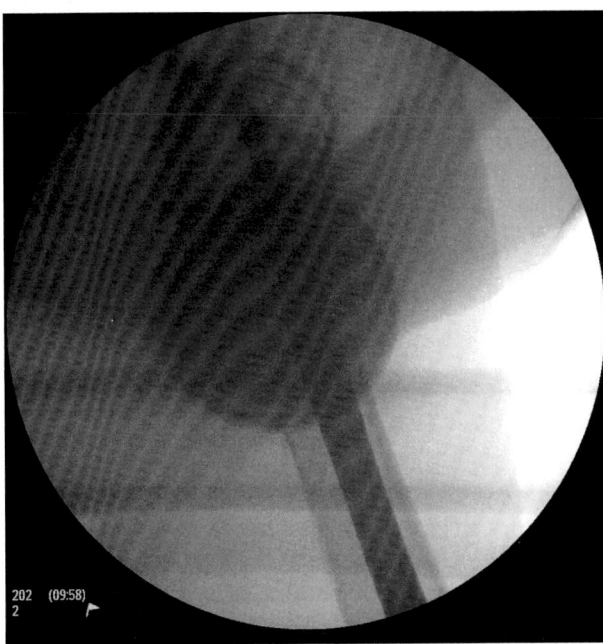

FIGURE 17-1 Intraoperative fluoroscopic views of the proximal femur used to evaluate fracture reduction and position of the femoral head screw during cephalomedullary nailing of an unstable reverse obliquity fracture. Here, intraoperative fluoroscopy is used to target drilling of a guide pin in the center of the femoral head, using both **(A)** anteroposterior and **(B)** lateral images. Information available on these images includes coronal and sagittal plane fracture alignment, position of the intramedullary nail itself, and finally, position of the screw in the femoral head.

care of fractures. Imaging techniques are needed during surgery to verify the reduction of fractures, identify the starting portals for intramedullary nails, target cannulated or interlocking screws, and verify implant position (Fig. 17-1). Fluoroscopic assessment of tibial plateau fracture reduction leads to results as good as or better than those obtained with arthroscopy-assisted reduction.[119] Norris et al.[147] used intraoperative fluoroscopy during the repair of acetabular fractures and found it as effective as postoperative radiographs to assess fracture reduction and comparable to postoperative CT to evaluate for intra-articular extension of hardware. Recent advances in "minimally invasive" fracture fixation rely even more on the interpretation of fluoroscopic images.[108]

Despite the benefits of intraoperative fluoroscopy, most surgeons insist on obtaining conventional radiographs at the completion of surgery. Although this practice requires further radiation exposure and adds time and expense, it is important for both clinical and medicolegal documentation. Fluoroscopic images have limited field-of-view and may not demonstrate the full extent of hardware fixation (as in the case of an intramedullary nail) or overall limb alignment as well as conventional radiographs. Finally, it may be difficult to compare intraoperative fluoroscopic images to later conventional radiographs, so the immediate postoperative radiograph represents an important baseline reference for future comparisons.

Several studies have examined the amount of ionizing radiation that operating room personnel are exposed to during the care of fractures when fluoroscopy is used.[16,95,186] Fortunately,

with modern fluoroscopic systems, measurable radiation exposure is limited to the surgeon's hands,[16,95] although he or she needs to limit excessive use of the fluoroscope during surgical procedures. Recently, Matthews et al.[132] showed that during surgery, repetitive fluoroscopic scout imaging is performed to reproduce a specific desired image. In a simulated test-rig, an average of seven scout images were required to reproduce a given C-arm position.[132] In contrast, these investigators showed that the use of navigation-assisted repositioning using a standard, commercially available image-guided surgical navigation system did not require a single additional scout image, with comparable positioning times.[132]

A recent advance in intraoperative fluoroscopy is the ability to generate cross-sectional, multiplanar 2D and 3D computer-reconstructed images in real-time.[9,11,31,98,99,192] The ability to obtain immediate cross-sectional images during surgery can help the surgeon assess reduction during the repair of certain intra-articular fractures when direct visualization of the articular surface is not possible.[31] Cross-sectional intraoperative imaging may also be of benefit in situations when hardware placement requires precision, such the insertion of pedicle screws or iliosacral screws.[11] In cadaver models of calcaneal fracture[98] and acetabular fracture,[99] 3D fluoroscopy was superior to standard 2D fluoroscopy and comparable to CT for the detection of intra-articular hardware and intermediate between the other modalities in demonstrating articular impaction of acetabular fracture[99] or the articular reduction or medial screw protrusion in calcaneal fractures.[98] In a clinical series of articular fractures, information obtained via intraoperative 3D fluoroscopy led to a decision to revise the fracture and/or fixation in 11% of cases.[9] In another series of patients undergoing surgery for foot and ankle trauma, 39% of cases with adequate conventional C-arm images were revised intraoperatively after 3D fluoroscopy was performed.[169] However, it is important to note that no one has documented that the use of 3D fluoroscopy improves outcomes, so for now this technology remains mostly investigational.

Surgical Navigation. Although computer-assisted surgical navigation techniques may be performed with cross-sectional imaging data obtained from preoperative CT, fluoroscopy is commonly used for surgical navigation because of its flexibility, convenience, low radiation exposure, and low cost. Although the field of surgical navigation is in its infancy, computer-assisted surgical navigation has already been applied to cervical and thoracic spine fracture fixation,[7] placement of percutaneous iliosacral and anterior column screws in the pelvis,[40,115,140] femoral neck fracture fixation,[115] and intramedullary nailing.[96,101,115,185]

Fluoroscopic surgical navigation requires a specialized computer-based system, which tracks the position of a hand-held tool in space. It is necessary to "register" the patient's bone within the computer based on preoperative CT data or the use of a generic dataset. Fluoroscopic views need be taken only once; thereafter, all movements of the tool are recorded against the registered bone image and may be displayed in different planes simultaneously, superimposed on the static images by the computer system. This dramatically reduces the need for repeated intraoperative imaging, decreasing the time of surgery and the radiation exposure of the patient and surgical team. However, intraoperative changes in the patient's position or in the dimensions of the registered bone (such as might occur during fracture reduction) decrease the accuracy of image registration. Surgical navigation has been used for hip fractures[35,117] and placement of iliosacral screws.[140] During intramedullary nailing of the femur, surgical navigation facilitates accurate entry-point location, fracture reduction, and insertion of interlocking and blocking screws and assists with determination of nail and screw length.[74,101,196] Weil et al.[196] used a cadaveric femur model to demonstrate that computerized navigation may increase the precision of fracture reduction, while at the same time lessening requirements for intraoperative fluoroscopy. In another cadaveric model, navigated distal interlocking was found to lead to less rotational deformity (2 degrees) compared with freehand distal interlocking (7 degrees).[74]

Although this technology has been proved to be feasible, the clinical importance and cost-effectiveness of surgical navigation remain undetermined. Collinge et al.[38] compared the safety and efficiency of standard multiplanar fluoroscopy with those of virtual fluoroscopy for use in the percutaneous insertion of iliosacral screws in 29 cadaver specimens. Interestingly, both methods were equally accurate; one screw was incorrectly inserted in each group, and both groups contained examples of screws with minor deviations in trajectory. Although the actual time for screw insertion was less with virtual fluoroscopy (3.5 minutes vs. 7.1 minutes), this was offset by the increased time needed to set up and calibrate the image-guided system.[38]

Liebergall et al.[117] showed improved screw parallelism and screw spread when navigation was used during repair of femoral neck fractures, and this correlated with fewer reoperations and overall complications in the navigated group.

Computed Tomography
Technical Considerations

CT has had the greatest clinical impact of any of the radiographic imaging modalities; its inventors (Godfrey Hounsfield and Allan Cormack) received the Nobel Prize for Medicine in 1979. Since its inception in the early 1970s, advances in technology and computer science have guided the development of several new generations of CT scanners, each capable of greater throughput and improved resolution. Although a more detailed review of the history of CT scanners is beyond the scope of this section, a brief description of current concepts in CT scanner technology is presented.

Helical (spiral) CT scanners were developed in the late 1980s and are so named because of the helical path the x-ray beam takes through the patient. The development of "slip ring" technology allowed the gantry (x-ray tube and detectors) to rotate continuously around the patient, whereas with previous-generation scanners, gantry rotation was constrained by electrical cables, which needed to be unwound in between slice acquisitions. With nonhelical scanners, table position was incrementally advanced in between slice acquisitions; with slip ring technology, the table position is advanced continuously while the gantry rotates, resulting in a helical x-ray beam path.

The first dual-slice helical scanner was demonstrated in 1992, with 4- and 16-slice models appearing in 1998 and 2001. On the whole, multislice (multidetector) scanners are similar to single-slice helical scanners in many respects. Instead of a single row of detectors; however, multiple rows of detectors are present within the gantry and are designed to allow acquisition of multiple slices at the same time.

With these new technologies, scanning algorithms needed to be modified, which resulted in new terminology and imaging parameters to adjust. For single-slice helical scanners (and older-generation scanners as well), slice thickness is determined by x-ray beam collimation, whereas, for multislice scanners, it is determined by detector width. For single-slice scanners, pitch is defined as the ratio of table movement (mm) per 360-degree rotation to slice thickness (mm). A pitch of 1 is comparable to older-generation scanners where the table movement increment was the same as the slice thickness. A pitch of less than 1 results in overlapping of the x-ray beam and higher patient radiation dose; a pitch greater than 1 results in increased coverage through the patient and decreased radiation dose. In practice, pitch is generally limited to 1.5 to 2, although protocols vary. For multislice scanners, the definition of pitch changes to incorporate the detector array width rather than the single slice width and is referred to as *detector pitch*.

The data sets from single-slice and multislice scanners are both helical in nature, and individual slices must be interpolated from the data set. Minimum slice thickness is set by the original x-ray beam collimation (single-slice scanners) or detector width (multislice scanners). Any number of slices may be reconstructed at any position along the long axis of the patient, and in any thickness equal to or greater than the minimal slice thickness. This allows reconstruction of overcontiguous slices (with typically 50% overlap), which increases the sensitivity for detecting small lesions that may otherwise be averaged between adjacent slices. This also results in twice as many images, although with no increase in scan time or additional radiation dose to the patient.

Multiplanar reconstructions (MPRs) and 3D reconstructions are also routinely performed with both single-slice and multislice helical scanners. This, in part, is related to the fact that today's CT examinations routinely produce hundreds of images, and MPR and 3D reformatting assist in interpreting these data. Advances in detector technology have allowed slice thickness to decrease such that slice thicknesses of 0.5 mm are routinely achieved clinically and allow acquisition of isotropic voxels. A voxel is the 3D equivalent of a pixel and represents the volume of tissue represented by a single pixel; isotropic voxels have uniform thickness in all directions (e.g., $0.5 \times 0.5 \times 0.5$ mm). Acquisition of images with isotropic voxels results in multiplanar (nonaxial) reconstructions that have in-plane resolutions equal to those of the original axial image. In addition, the use of overcontiguous images is useful in 3D reconstructions to eliminate stair-step artifact.

Developments in rapid-prototyping technology now readily allow Digital Imaging and Communications in Medicine (DICOM)-based CT data to be used to develop physical models of the imaging target. Such models have been extensively used in maxillofacial reconstruction, but are beginning to be utilized for complex fractures of the scapula and pelvis.[58]

Orthopedic hardware results in metallic streak artifact on standard CT images, which frequently obscures surrounding bone and soft tissue detail.[65] Standard CT protocols can be modified to reduce metal artifact by using a lower pitch setting, a higher tube current (250 to 350 mAs), and higher peak kilovoltage (140 kVp) during acquisition.[65] In addition, soft-tissue filters rather than edge-enhancing algorithms can be used to further reduce metal artifacts, and use of wide window settings at image display (width, 3,000 to 4,000 HU; level, 800 HU) is advocated.[65] Metal streak artifact is propagated on multiplanar reformatted images as well. Fortunately, volume rendering of an MDCT axial database can dramatically reduce streak artifact associated with hardware.[64] Fayad et al.[65] recently reviewed the use of 3D-CT images obtained using 64-MDCT in assessing postoperative complications in patients with orthopedic hardware, including nonunion, infection, new fracture, or hardware malposition. Postoperative MDCT after surgical repair of tibial plateau fractures has been shown to accurately image the articular surface in the early postoperative period and to be useful for assessing fracture healing later, despite the adjacent metal implant.[144]

Overall, the advantages of multislice helical scanners include faster scan times and patient throughput, reduced motion artifacts, reduced intravenous contrast requirements, improved lesion detection, and improved MPRs and 3D reconstructions. Disadvantages include the potential for decreased resolution along the long axis of the patient (related to increased pitch)

and a large number of images, resulting in increased reconstruction time and storage requirements. Another disadvantage of CT in general is the high radiation dose associated with this modality. However, radiation doses can be reduced by using low-dose, rather than standard-dose, scanning algorithms without differences in subjective image quality evaluation.[142] Furthermore, use of MDCT with volume visualization and postprocessing (3D CT) limits exposure to radiation by using single-plane acquisitions with isotropic data sets.

Advances are being made in not only the processing of images, but in image analysis. Although currently not in clinical use, automatic detection of fractures using a computer algorithm has been shown to be very fast and effective.[203]

Applications

Complex Fractures. CT remains the imaging modality of choice for evaluating complex fractures as well as ruling out injury to the spine. Axial (cross-sectional) CT cuts provide important information regarding 3D relationships that may not be evident on plain films (Fig. 17-2). In addition to high-resolution axial images, MPRs are commonly performed (Fig. 17-3). Such information provides critical data about the displacement of fracture fragments, including assessment of intra-articular displacement, articular surface depression, and bone loss.[8] Three-dimensional reconstructions using surface rendering techniques are often less helpful in fracture management compared with MPRs. With 3D imaging techniques, fracture planes are frequently obscured by overlying fracture fragments and underestimate the true degree of comminution; however, they may be helpful in evaluating angulation and displacement of fracture fragments, in addition to depression of articular surfaces. With previous-generation CT scanners, evaluation of fracture planes parallel to the scan plane was suboptimal because of volume averaging of the fracture plane with adjacent intact bone. With multislice scanners, image data are obtained as a volume rather than as individual slices, and MPRs typically have resolution equal to the axial images (due to isotropic voxels). For this reason, detection of transversely oriented fracture planes is significantly enhanced. Typical indications for CT include fractures of the spine, scapula, proximal humerus, distal radius, pelvis and acetabulum, tibial plateau, tibial plafond, calcaneus, and midfoot.

In the spine, helical CT has become the imaging modality of choice. The latest American College of Radiologists' appropriateness criteria recommend axial MDCT with sagittal and coronal reconstructions as the primary imaging modality of choice for suspected spine trauma.[41] In addition to its high diagnostic sensitivity, MDCT is more time effective, reducing imaging time by as much as 50% compared to radiography; time that may be critical to a trauma patient.[42] A variety of measurements that incorporate CT data have been described that are useful in the assessment of the cervical spine following injury, including cervical translation and vertebral body height loss, canal compromise, spinal cord compression, and facet fracture and/or subluxation.[19] Despite its greater initial expense, CT has been shown to have sensitivity and specificity of 96%, both greater than for conventional plain radiography.[82]

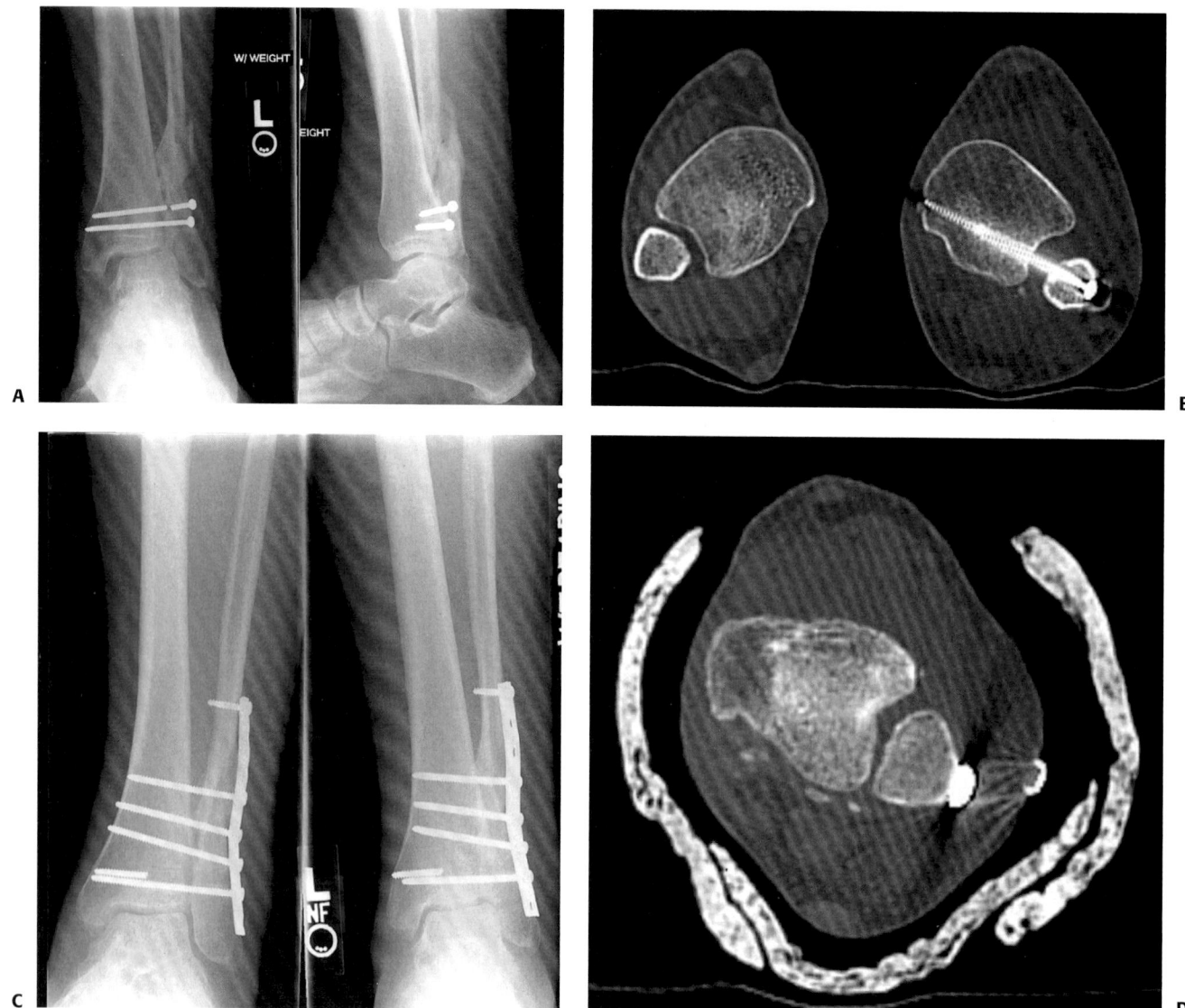

FIGURE 17-2 A: Anteroposterior and lateral plain images of an ankle with recurrent syndesmotic widening following previous screw fixation. Once cannot tell from the plain films alone whether the fibula is malpositioned anteriorly or posteriorly as well. **B:** Axial CT of both ankles demonstrates that the primary deformity is widening. **C:** Plain views after revision fixation. **D:** Postoperative CT showing that the syndesmosis has been reduced.

Grogan et al.[82] present a decision analysis emphasizing cost minimization and conclude that helical CT is the preferred initial screening test for detecting cervical spine injury in moderate- to high-risk trauma patients. However, clinicians depending on MDCT of the spine for the imaging of trauma should be aware of potential diagnostic pitfalls, including accessory ossification centers, developmental disk abnormalities, vascular channels, and image artifacts.[100] Finally, one recent study suggested that CT of the cervical spine in trauma is overutilized, and that strict adherence to NEXUS guidelines for imaging could reduce the need for CT of the neck by 20%.[80]

In the upper extremity, CT is commonly performed to evaluate fractures of the scapula, proximal humerus, and distal radius.[8,83,134,206] MPRs of these fractures assist in surgical planning.

For proximal humeral fractures, simple axial images provide important information about the glenohumeral relationship, demonstrate glenoid rim fractures, and reveal whether the tuberosities of the humerus are fractured. Occult fractures of the coracoid process and lesser tuberosity are readily seen.[83] Despite the valuable information that CT provides (with or without MPRs), several studies have shown that the interobserver assessment of proximal humeral and scapular neck fractures was not improved with the addition of CT.[134] For distal radial fractures that mandate surgical reconstruction, CT is more accurate than conventional radiography in demonstrating involvement of the distal radioulnar joint, the extent of articular surface depression, and the amount of comminution.[8,37,163,206] Three-dimensional CT was found to further

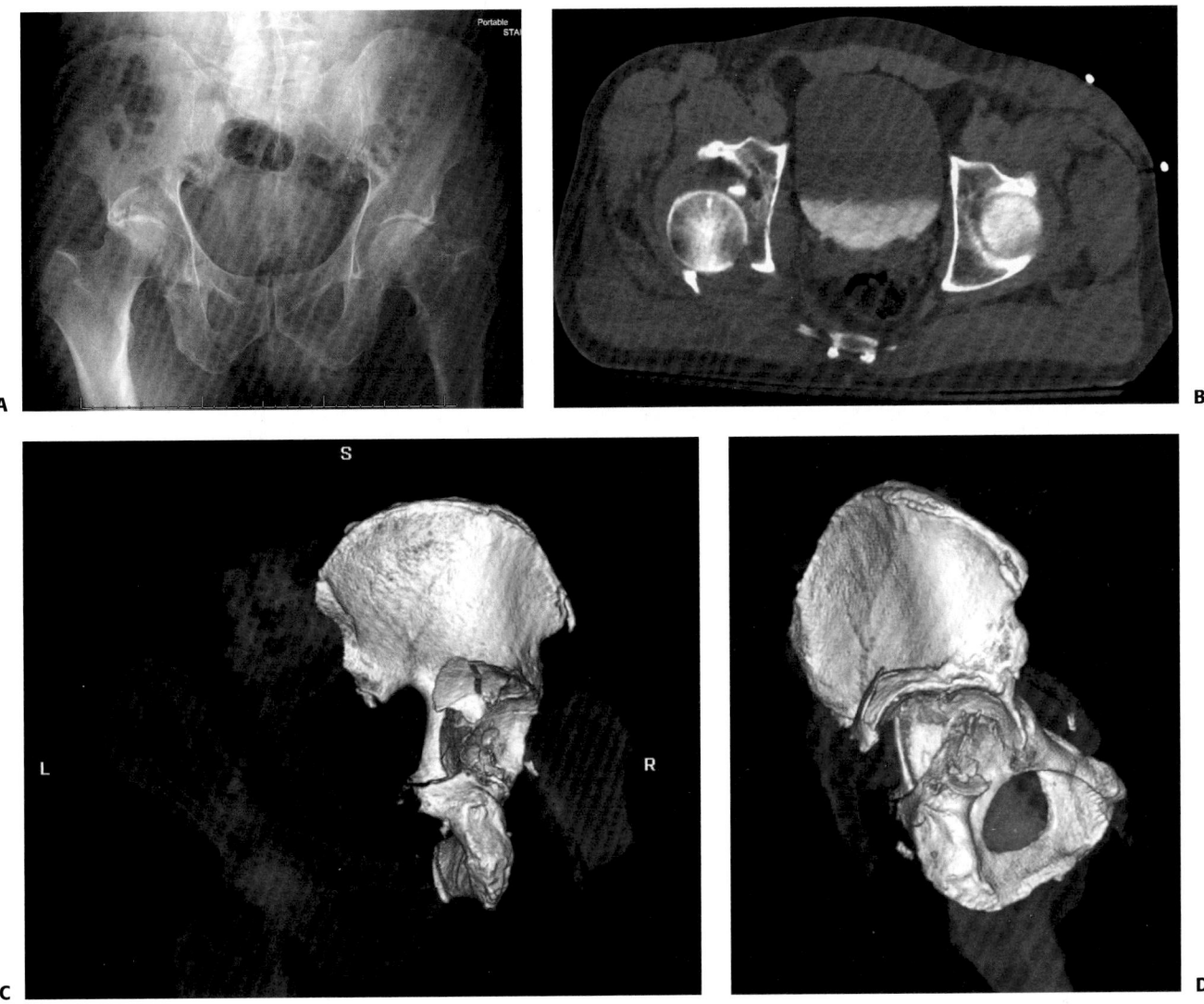

FIGURE 17-3 A: Anteroposterior view of a right acetabular fracture-dislocation. Axial computed tomography (CT) **(B)** better reveals the extent of comminution of the posterior wall, as well as demonstrating the persistent posterior dislocation of the hip. **C and D:** With high-resolution 3D reconstructions, a more "anatomic" appreciation of the fracture pattern is possible, similar to what the surgeon would view at surgery. Note the "ghosting" technique used to remove the other bones, most notably the femoral head, that would otherwise obscure the view. For complex fractures such as this, advanced CT scanning is unparalleled.

improve the accuracy of fracture classification and to influence treatment decisions compared to standard 2D CT in a series of 30 intra-articular distal radius fractures.[87] In another study, MDCT was compared to conventional radiography in a series of 120 distal radius fractures.[8] In this study, MDCT was dramatically better at demonstrating central articular impaction than plain, and 26 radiographically occult injuries to the carpus were identified. Furthermore, the recommended treatment plan changed in 23% of the cases based on information provided by the CT evaluation.[8]

CT is routinely used in evaluating pelvic fractures. CT with sagittal reconstruction is the best way to diagnose the so-called "U" fracture of the sacrum.[160] A CT-based classification of acetabular fractures has been proposed.[88] For the assessment of

acetabular fractures, classification according to the system of Letournel is more accurate when CT is used compared to plain radiographs alone.[148] CT is also better than conventional plain radiography at identifying intra-articular step-offs and gaps and is considered an essential part of the preoperative evaluation.[20] Reformatted images can be obtained in oblique planes to simulate standard Judet radiographs (Fig. 17-4).[75,148] Use of CT-reformatting avoids the pain and risk of fracture displacement or hip redislocation that might occur while repositioning the patient 45 degrees on each side for Judet views. A potential disadvantage is the slight loss of information resulting from volume averaging and computer reconstruction that could affect interpretation of the images. In one study, 5 orthopedic trauma surgeons with varying trauma experience compared 77 images

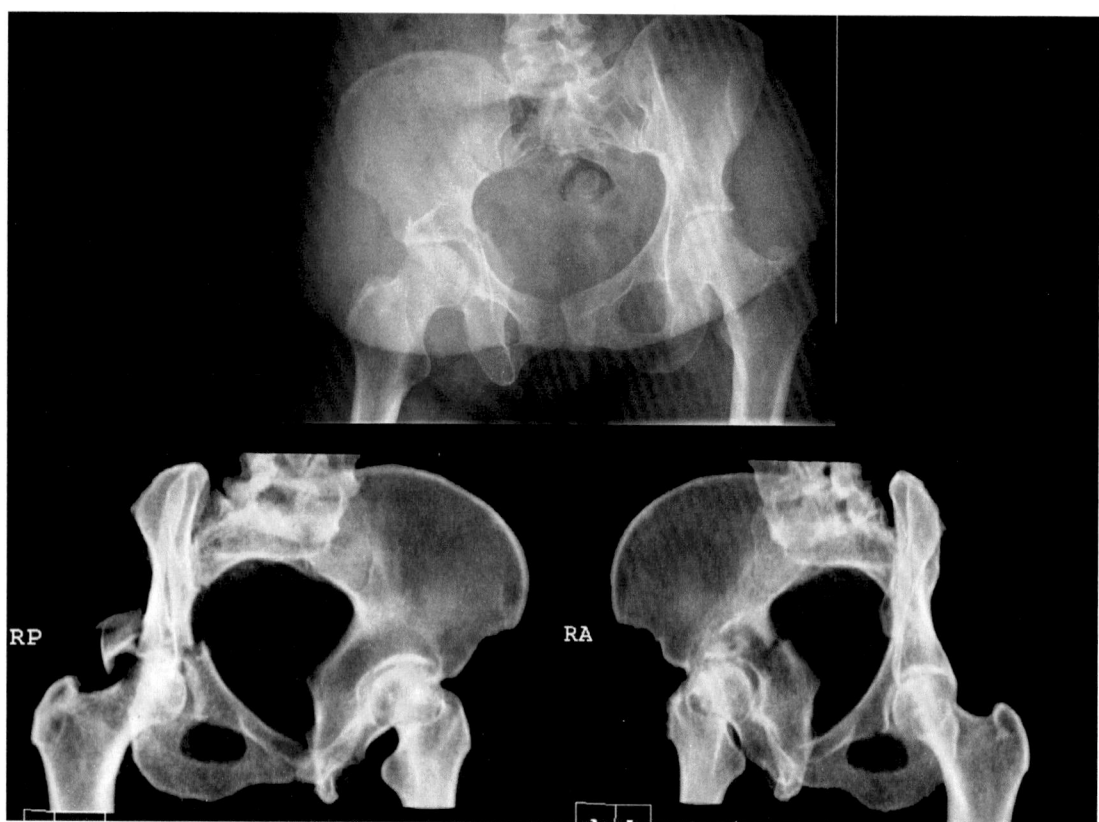

FIGURE 17-4 Computed tomography of the pelvis reformatted in 45-degree right and left oblique planes (*bottom*) to simulate the traditional plain film Judet views of the pelvis. The corresponding anteroposterior view is shown above. (Courtesy of Dr Rena Stewart.)

from 11 different patients with acetabular fractures.[22] The reviewers were asked to identify primary fracture lines and to classify each fracture according to the Judet-Letournel system; each patient had two sets of three images (one with traditional Judet radiographs and one with reformatted CT scans). When compared to the surgical findings, both sets of images performed equally well, and reviewers reported equivalent confidence in their ability to recognize fracture characteristics with each type of imaging.[22] Postoperative CT after acetabular fracture repair identifies residual articular defects or incongruities better than plain radiographs.[21] CT demonstrates intra-articular debris in a significant number of patients after hip dislocation,[92] and CT should be performed in any patient whose conventional plain radiographs show an incongruent reduction. Because small intra-articular bodies may not be visible on radiographs, one should consider obtaining CT images in all patients who sustain a hip dislocation, even when conventional plain radiographs appear to be normal.

The impact of CT on tibial plateau fracture management is well described.[33] In one study, when using just conventional radiographs for formulating a treatment plan, the mean interobserver kappa coefficient was 0.58, which increased to 0.71 after adding CT. The mean intraobserver kappa coefficient for fracture classification using radiographs was 0.70, which increased to 0.80 with addition of CT. The mean intraobserver kappa coefficient for treatment plan based on radiographs

alone was 0.62, which increased to 0.82 after adding CT. With the addition of CT, the fracture classification was changed in 12% of cases, whereas the treatment plan was altered 26% of the time.[33] In another study, Wicky et al.[199] compared helical CT with 3D reconstructions to conventional radiography in patients with tibial plateau fractures and found that, for the purpose of classification, fractures were underestimated in 43% of cases by radiographs. Among a smaller subset of patients in whom operative plans were formulated with and without CT, the same investigators found that the addition of helical CT 3D reconstructions led to modifications in the surgical plan in more than half the cases.[199]

Tornetta and Gorup[190] evaluated the use of preoperative CT in the management of tibial pilon fractures. Twenty-two patients were studied with both conventional radiographs and CT. The fracture pattern, number of fragments, degree of comminution, presence of articular impaction, and location of the major fracture line were recorded. CT revealed more fragments in 12 patients, increased impaction in 6 patients, and more severe comminution in 11 patients. The operative plan was changed in 14 (64%) patients, and additional information was gained in 18 (82%) patients.[190]

CT is valuable for assessing fractures of the hindfoot. CT reveals bone debris in the subtalar joint of patients with lateral process fractures of the talus.[56] In children with Tillaux fractures of the anterolateral distal tibia, CT is better than

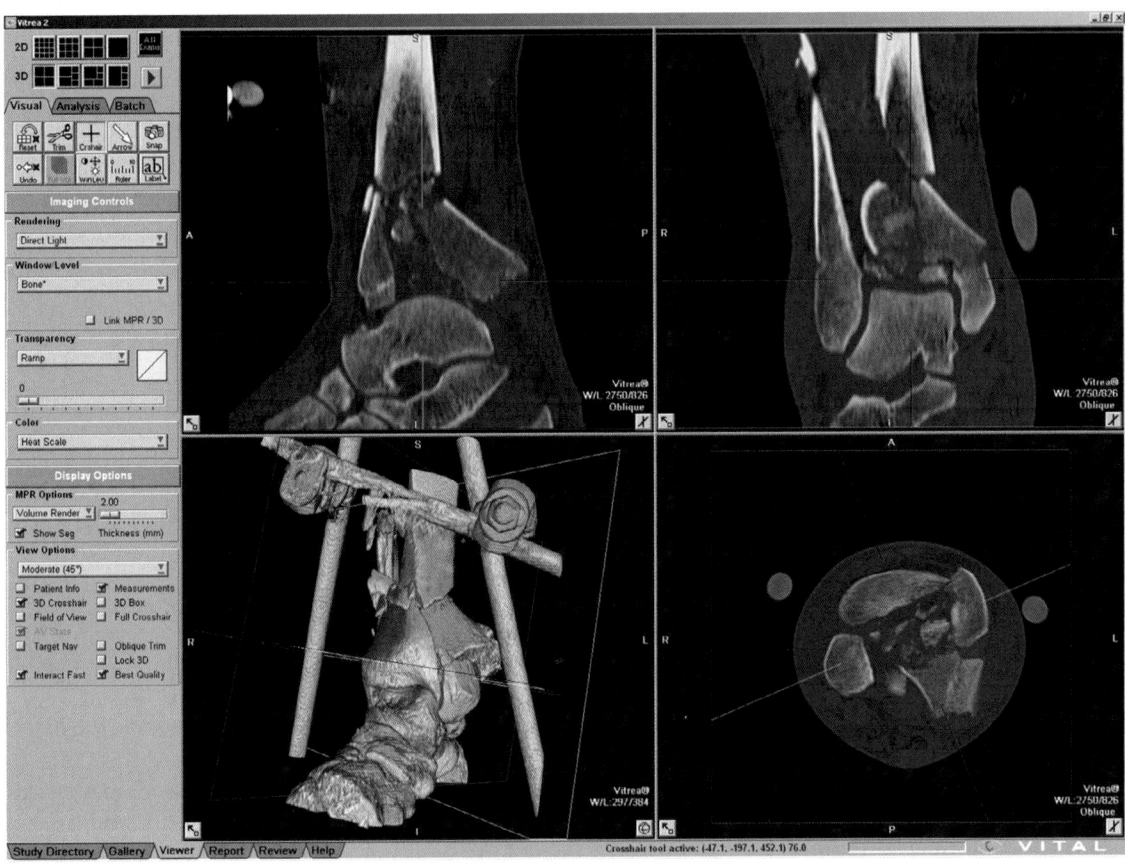

FIGURE 17-5 Computed tomography of a triplane fracture as viewed on a digital workstation. Users can visualize axial and reconstructed coronal and sagittal images simultaneously.

conventional radiography in detecting displacement of more than 2 mm, which is considered an indication for surgery (Fig. 17-5).[91] Helical CT is valuable for the preoperative planning of calcaneal fractures.[68] Axial images of the calcaneus best show hindfoot deformity, whereas MPRs (including 3D imaging with dislocation of the joint) best reveal intra-articular involvement.[68]

Postoperative Evaluation of Fracture Reduction. CT is also useful for postoperative assessment of complex fractures. Moed et al.[136] compared the functional outcome of 67 patients with posterior wall acetabular fractures with the findings on postoperative CT. In this study, postoperative CT more accurately revealed the degree of residual fracture displacement compared with conventional radiographs, and the accuracy of surgical reduction seen on postoperative CT was highly predictive of the clinical outcome.[136] In a series of operatively treated tibial plateau fractures, clinically relevant information regarding articular depression or fracture healing that were not apparent on plain radiographs was found in 81% of cases imaged with MDCT.[144] Vasarhelyi et al.[191] found side-to-side torsional differences of greater than 10 degrees in one-quarter of 61 patients undergoing fixation of distal fibula fractures.[191] Kurozumi et al.[111] correlated postoperative radiographs and CT with functional outcomes in 67 patients with intra-articular calcaneal fractures and found that better reduction of the cal-

caneocuboid joint and posterior facet of the subtalar joint correlated with improved outcome.

Healing of Fractures. Conventional radiographs are often limited in demonstrating persistent fracture lines, while such nonunions are more readily demonstrated on CT (Fig. 17-6).[14] CT has replaced conventional tomography in most centers for the identification of fracture nonunions. Multiplanar CT reconstructions may be needed if the fracture pattern is complex. Assessing partially united fractures can also be difficult, even with CT. The accuracy of CT in detecting tibial nonunion was evaluated. Bhattacharyya et al.[14] studied 35 patients with suspected tibial nonunion and equivocal plain radiograph findings. In this series, the sensitivity of CT for detecting nonunion was 100%, but its accuracy was limited by a low specificity of 62%, because three patients who were diagnosed as having tibial nonunion by CT were found to have a healed fracture at surgery.[14]

A more interesting role for CT is evaluation of early fracture healing. CT reveals external callus formation earlier than conventional radiography and allows for more complete and detailed visualization of fracture healing, which may be obscured by overlying casts and/or fixation hardware on radiographs.[81] Lynch et al.[126] developed a means of measuring changes in CT density at fracture sites by quantifying the formation of mineralized tissue within fracture gaps, while

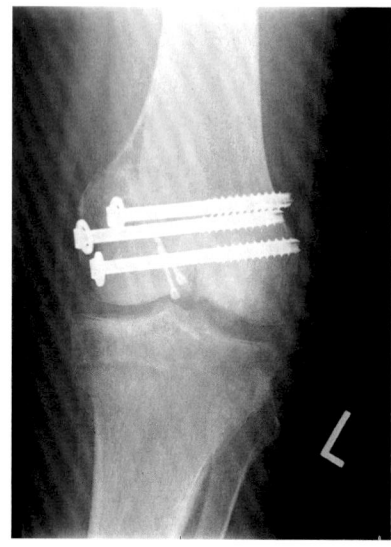 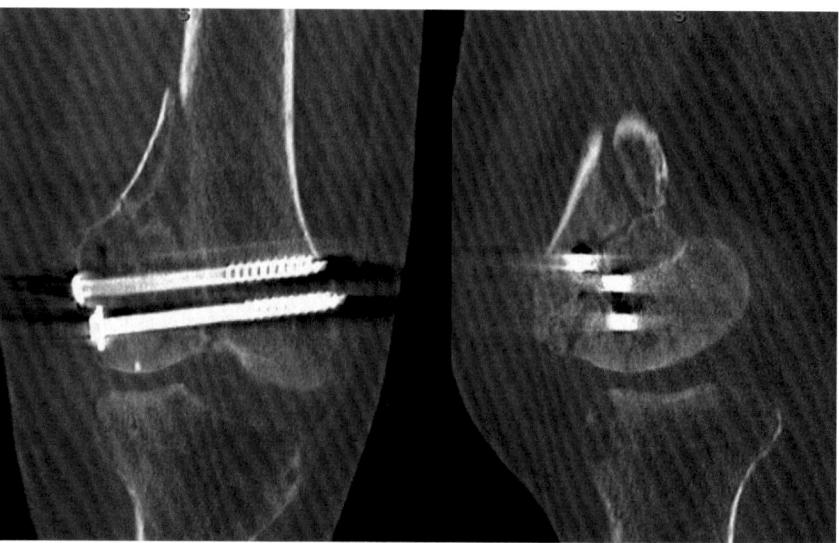

A

B

FIGURE 17-6 **A:** Anteroposterior radiograph of a patient who had persistent knee pain after surgical repair of a medial femoral condyle fracture. **B:** Computed tomography of the distal femur clearly with 2D reconstructions in the coronal and sagittal planes provides unambiguous evidence of fracture nonunion.

ignoring loss of bone mineral caused by disuse osteoporosis. In a preliminary study of seven patients with distal radial fractures, this technique demonstrated increased CT density 2 weeks postfracture that correlated with the visual appearance of sclerosis and blurring of the fracture line on conventional radiographs.[126] It is not yet known whether such information will be predictive of fracture healing complications. The use of new multidetector 3D-CT techniques can reduce metal artifact to further improve the visualization of nonunion adjacent to metal hardware.[65]

Evaluation of Combat Injuries. Combat injuries are now frequently caused by multiple ballistic fragments causing multiple penetrating injuries. State-of-the-art MDCT is available at all US deployed combat hospitals.[67] Use of 3D CT at the point of initial patient triage allows radiologists to identify retained fragments and depict wound paths, providing trauma surgeons with vitally important information regarding potential injury to vital organs and neurovascular structures. Such information assists in the initial stabilization of injured soldiers in the combat hospital without delaying emergent life-preserving intervention.[67] In a simulated mass casualty incident, use of 64-MDCT increases throughput and facilitates imaging of patients more rapidly.[107]

Magnetic Resonance Imaging
Technical Considerations

MRI does not use ionizing radiation. Rather, MRI uses radiofrequency (RF) waves, in the presence of a strong magnetic field, to interact with the patient's hydrogen atoms (protons) to create images of superb soft tissue contrast. Although the physics of MRI is complex and too detailed to review in this section, the more practical aspects of MRI relevant to the evaluation of orthopedic imaging will be discussed.

Present-day MRI scanners may be classified according to field strength. The basic unit of measurement of magnetic field strength is the Gauss (G); the earth's magnetic field measures approximately 0.5 G. Field strengths for MRI are much greater and are measured in Tesla (T), which is defined as 10,000 G. Low-field-strength scanners are typically 0.2 to 0.3 T and are commonly used in outpatient settings as "extremity" or "open" scanners. High-field-strength scanners are generally those greater than 1 T, with 1.5-T scanners dominating the market and representing more than 90% of installed scanners worldwide. The 3-T scanners have also become clinically available, although their acceptance has been limited because of the higher cost of these systems and relatively limited selection of receiver coils. Advantages to higher-field-strength scanners include increased capability, increased resolution and image quality, and decreased scan time.

The RF coils are an important element of any MRI system. RF coils are used to transmit RF waves into the patient, as well as receive RF signals ("echoes") from the patient during the course of the examination. A standard "body" coil is incorporated into scanners as a default coil from which to both send and receive RF signals. The body coil is located within the housing of the magnet and, as a result, is located some distance from the patient. This distance factor decreases the strength of the RF signal received from the patient, although this is not a problem for imaging larger body parts such as the abdomen and pelvis. For smaller body parts, such as extremities in orthopedic imaging, specialized RF coils are available and are widely used to increase the quality of MRI studies. These coils are usually "receive only" coils, meaning the body coil transmits the RF pulse; some specialty coils; however, incorporate both transmit and receive functions. These smaller coils are placed around or over the body part to be scanned, which decreases the distance from the patient's anatomy to the coil and results in greater signal return from the underlying tissue. This increases the signal-to-noise ratio (SNR) of the resulting images and produces images of greater contrast resolution and higher image quality, which may be used to improve image quality, increase spatial resolution, or decrease scan time.

Advances in RF coil technology have led to a wide variety of RF coil designs available today. Volume coils encircle the anatomy of interest and provide increased signal homogeneity. Surface coils are placed over the anatomy of interest and significantly improve near-field signal strength returning from the underlying anatomy. Quadrature and phased-array coil designs incorporate multiple coil elements with electronic coupling to increase signal strength and SNR. Specialized coils are available for orthopedic imaging and include dedicated phased-array coils, as well as various sizes of flexible surface coils.

MR images are generated using a series of pulse sequences. The term *pulse sequence* refers to sequence of RF pulses that are applied in concert with a series of magnetic gradients. These pulses are applied in a particular order and with a particular timing scheme, with the RF coils listening for the resulting "echoes" at specific time intervals. Pulse sequences determine the type of image contrast produced. During each pulse sequence, magnetic gradients are applied to the main magnetic field to achieve spatial localization. A magnetic gradient along the long axis of the bore of the magnet (and patient) is used for slice selection, whereas gradients along the transverse plane are responsible for frequency and phase encoding, which result in localization within the transverse plane. Most MRI examinations are particularly loud as a result of rapidly switching the gradients on and off, which necessitates use of earplugs or headphones during the test study. Inherent in all pulse sequences are specifications for parameters such as geometry (imaging plane, field of view, number of slices), resolution (number of frequency and phase encoding steps, slice thickness), and image contrast (repetition time [TR], echo delay time [TE]). A collection of multiple pulse sequences used for a particular examination is often referred to as a *protocol*.

Common sequences used in orthopedic imaging include spin-echo (SE) and gradient-echo (gradient recalled echo [GRE]) imaging. SE sequences are most frequently used in conjunction with a fast imaging technique, termed *fast* spin-echo (FSE) or *turbo* spin-echo (TSE) imaging, depending on the manufacturer. SE sequences provide T1-weighted (T1W), proton density (PD), and T2-weighted (T2W) image contrast based on selection of the parameters TR and TE. T1W images tend to depict anatomy well and are sensitive, but not specific, for pathology. T2W images are fluid-sensitive images and tend to depict pathology well. PD images are neither T1W nor T2W, and contrast is derived from differences in PD within the tissues. PD images are commonly used in orthopedic imaging, as they result in high SNR images and depict anatomy and pathology well. PD images are often acquired in conjunction with T2W images during the same pulse sequence; in this case, the PD image is referred to as the *first echo,* and the T2W image is called the *second echo.* This combination may also be referred to as a *double echo* (DE, 2E) sequence.

One consequence of FSE/TSE techniques is that fat, like fluid, is relatively bright on PD and T2W sequences. Fat suppression (FS) techniques are necessary to evaluate for edema or fluid with fat-containing tissues, such as bone marrow. Two techniques are commonly used: Short T1 inversion recovery (STIR) and chemical saturation ("fat-sat," spectral saturation, frequency-selective presaturation). STIR is a distinctive spin echo pulse sequence that results in suppression of a particular tissue based on the choice of an additional parameter, TI. A relatively short TI value of 150 ms results in suppression of fat-containing tissues. This sequence tends to be relatively low in SNR and, as a consequence, is often performed at lower resolution. The sequence is less affected by variations in magnetic field homogeneity; however, and results in fairly uniform FS throughout the image. Chemical saturation is a frequency-selective RF pulse, which is applied before the normal RF pulse, and effectively eliminates the signal from fat-containing tissues. This may be applied to any of the SE sequences (T1W, PD, T2W); T1W FS sequences are typically used after contrast (gadolinium) enhancement, whereas PD FS and T2W FS sequences are used in evaluating a variety of tissues, including bone marrow and articular cartilage. Chemical saturation is often used in conjunction with lower-resolution FSE sequences, as the technique decreases SNR as a result of eliminating fat signal, resulting in "grainier" images at higher resolutions. Chemical saturation is also sensitive to inhomogeneities in the external magnetic field, which may result in nonuniform FS across the field of view. This is particularly a problem with extremities positioned off-center with the bore of the magnet, such as the elbow, where the magnetic field is not as uniform compared with isocenter. When uniformity of FS is a problem, STIR images may be substituted. STIR images are not sensitive to gadolinium and cannot be used to evaluate gadolinium-contrast enhancement, and hence are less useful for MR arthrography or intravenous contrast studies.

Developing orthopedic imaging protocols is a challenging task that involves balancing tradeoffs in signal (SNR), spatial resolution, contrast resolution, and image acquisition time. Low SNR images tend to be "noisy" or "grainy" and unpleasant to view. Higher-resolution techniques result in both lower SNR and longer acquisition times and may not be practical for all patients; for this reason, lower-resolution techniques may be required. Many patients are unable to tolerate long scan times because of pain and limitations on movement during the examination, and, motion artifact may become a problem. MR artifacts (wrap around, motion artifact, pulsation artifact, metallic artifact) represent additional sources of image degradation and can be difficult at times to eliminate. Metal artifact is a particular problem in orthopedic imaging applications,[85] but fortunately the amount of artifact can be reduced with certain MR imaging techniques on high-field (1.5 to 3 T) MRI. These include the use of TSE sequences with smaller interecho spacing, with the frequency-encoding direction oriented away from the site of interest and the readout bandwidth increased.[63,85] When difficulties arise during an MRI examination, pulse sequences often need to be modified to obtain the information needed from the examination.

Applications

MRI is frequently performed in evaluating both osseous and soft tissue injuries after trauma. It is capable of defining fractures that are radiographically occult, pediatric articular fractures, and associated soft tissue injuries that may not be suspected or evaluable after physical examination and plain radiography.[34] Although MR angiography is a well-established technique for noninvasive evaluation of the arterial system, it may be impractical for evaluating the multitrauma patient. Evaluation of vascular trauma is accomplished much more rapidly with CT angiography (CTA) or conventional angiography, which also allows for interventional procedures (e.g., embolization of arterial bleeding). A more controversial application is MR venography (MRV) to detect deep venous thrombosis (DVT) of the proximal thigh and pelvic veins. In a recent review of the imaging of DVT, Orbell et al.[149] note that MRV has many advantages, including lack of exposure to ionizing radiation and avoidance of any need for vein cannulation and injection of contrast (for nonenhanced studies). MRV is as sensitive and specific for proximal leg DVT as ultrasonography (US) or venography[30] and is reported to be more accurate in the detection of isolated pelvic thrombi.[138] Unfortunately, the cost and logistical problems of MRI have limited its usefulness in the imaging of DVT.

MRI has been advocated to be the gold standard for imaging of the cervical spine following trauma,[141] and faster imaging protocols certainly make the use of MRI much more feasible in the acutely injured patient.[59] However, the practicality of using MRI in trauma patients may be limited by difficulties associated with transporting patients to the MRI suite, as well as MRI incompatibilities with various life-support equipment and patient implants. MRI scan times are also much longer than with CT and other imaging modalities and may not be tolerated by potentially unstable patients or those in considerable pain. Thus, for practical reasons, MRI continues to have only a limited role in the immediate management of the trauma patient.

Osseous Injury. Recent advances in MRI have made it possible to quantitatively assess bone structure and function, so that MRI may someday supplant bone densitometry as a tool to assess fracture risk caused by osteoporosis as well as the response to treatment.[195] It is now well known that bone marrow edema (bone bruise, bone marrow contusion) is frequently identified on MRI after extremity trauma. Histologically, these imaging findings correlate with cancellous bone microfractures as well as edema and hemorrhage within the fatty marrow.[166] The long-term sequelae of these radiographically occult lesions have not been well defined. Roemer and Bohndorf[172] evaluated 176 consecutive patients with acute knee injuries and found that nearly three-fourths had bone marrow abnormalities. The majority of lesions (69%) involved the lateral compartment of the knee; 29% were medial, and 2% were patellofemoral. Many of the lesions resembled edema of the subchondral bone, without other osseous or cartilage injury, while nearly one-fourth represented subchondral impaction fractures and one-third comprised osteochondral or chondral lesions. Forty-nine of these patients had repeat MR studies conducted at least 2 years after their injury. In these patients, only 7 of 49 (14%) had persistent signal changes within the marrow space. The extent of signal abnormality was less than originally seen, and none of the patients developed degenerative changes, regardless of the injury type that was initially present. No cases of posttraumatic osteonecrosis were found. Therefore, one must be careful to avoid interpreting marrow signal abnormalities alone on MRI as evidence of a true fracture, as this may lead to overtreatment. This distinction is especially problematic in the assessment of hip pain after a fall, where trochanteric bone marrow edema might be interpreted as a fracture, leading to a decision to perform internal fixation.

MRI is very useful in the evaluation of radiographically occult fractures. Fracture lines are distinctly visualized on PD or T2W images as linear, lower-signal intensity abnormalities silhouetted by higher-signal intensity marrow fat. Fracture lines can also be seen on STIR and PD/T2W FS images, which also show the degree of surrounding reactive marrow edema. Care is needed in interpreting T1W images; however, images as fracture lines may be obscured by surrounding marrow edema, both of which are hypointense in signal intensity on T1W images.[77]

MRI has become the imaging modality of choice for identifying occult fractures for which correct early diagnosis is essential, such as femoral neck fractures (Fig. 17-7),[118,124] scaphoid fractures,[49,109,165,173] and pediatric elbow injuries.[164] In elderly patients with hip pain after a fall, early MRI when radiographs are normal can avoid delays in diagnosis and treatment of hip fractures. In one study, 25 patients with hip pain were evaluated for occult fracture with conventional radiographs, scintigraphy, CT, or a combination of studies.[159] A final diagnosis was ultimately determined from repeat radiographs in 10 patients and by scintigraphy in 15 patients. The time to final diagnosis averaged 9.6 days when the diagnosis was made by serial radiographs and averaged 5.3 days when the diagnosis was made by scintigraphy. Given the delay in diagnosis associated with using more conventional methods of imaging, the authors point out that use of immediate MRI instead can dramatically decrease the number of imaging examinations performed and the time to diagnosis, resulting in decreased costs of care and possibly reduced complications.[159] In a more recent study, six elderly patients with hip pain after a fall had both MRI and CT, while seven others had MRI alone.[124] In the first group, four of the six CT studies were inaccurate, while all MRI studies were correctly defined the pathology.[124] In cases of occult hip fracture, the fracture pattern can be delineated using MRI, which may be of therapeutic importance. Occult fractures of the femoral neck that frequently are treated with screw fixation may be distinguished on MRI from occult intertrochanteric fractures, greater trochanter fractures, or pubic rami fractures that do not require surgical stabilization. Finally, if the MRI does not demonstrate fracture, it often does indicate another finding that explains a given patient's symptoms.[69] Clinicians may be more apt to rely on MRI alone than on NM studies; in one report, clinicians always requested additional imaging for cases in which the bone scan was positive.[46] MRI may also identify additional comorbid conditions such as pre-existing osteonecrosis or metastatic disease.[84]

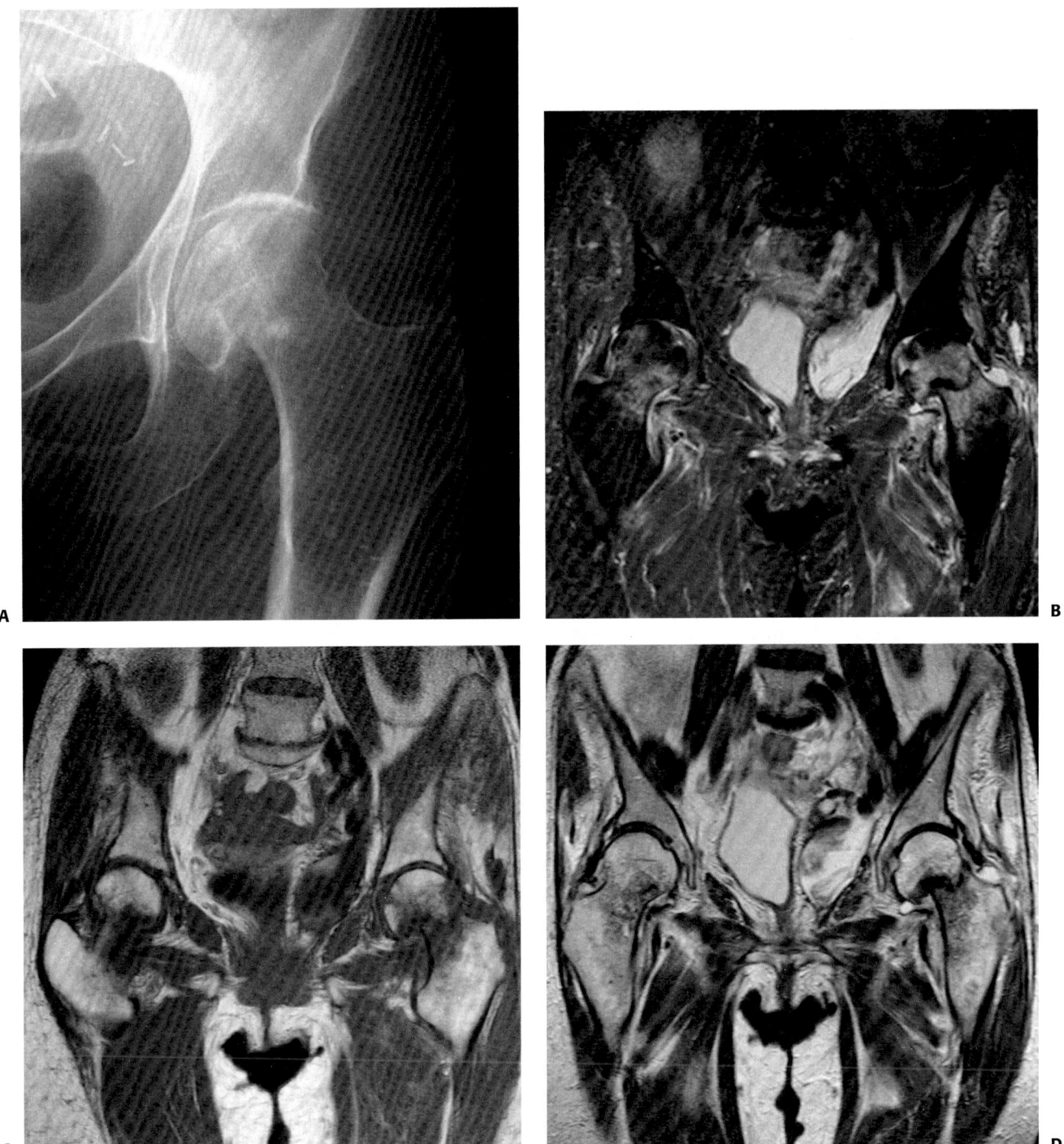

FIGURE 17-7 A: Conventional plain anteroposterior radiograph of a patient's hip demonstrates a femoral neck fracture. Although the fracture can be seen on routine radiographs, the patient was at risk for osteonecrosis because of corticosteroid use related to a kidney transplant. Some apparent changes are seen in the bone density of the femoral head. Magnetic resonance imaging of the pelvis confirms the presence of an acute left hip fracture and demonstrates that there was no osteonecrosis. Incidentally noted is a small developing fracture with surrounding stress reaction in the right femoral neck medially: **(B)** STIR, **(C)** T1-weighted, and **(D)** T2-weighted images. Higher-resolution images of the left hip fracture demonstrating mild impaction at the fracture site without significant angulation.

(continues)

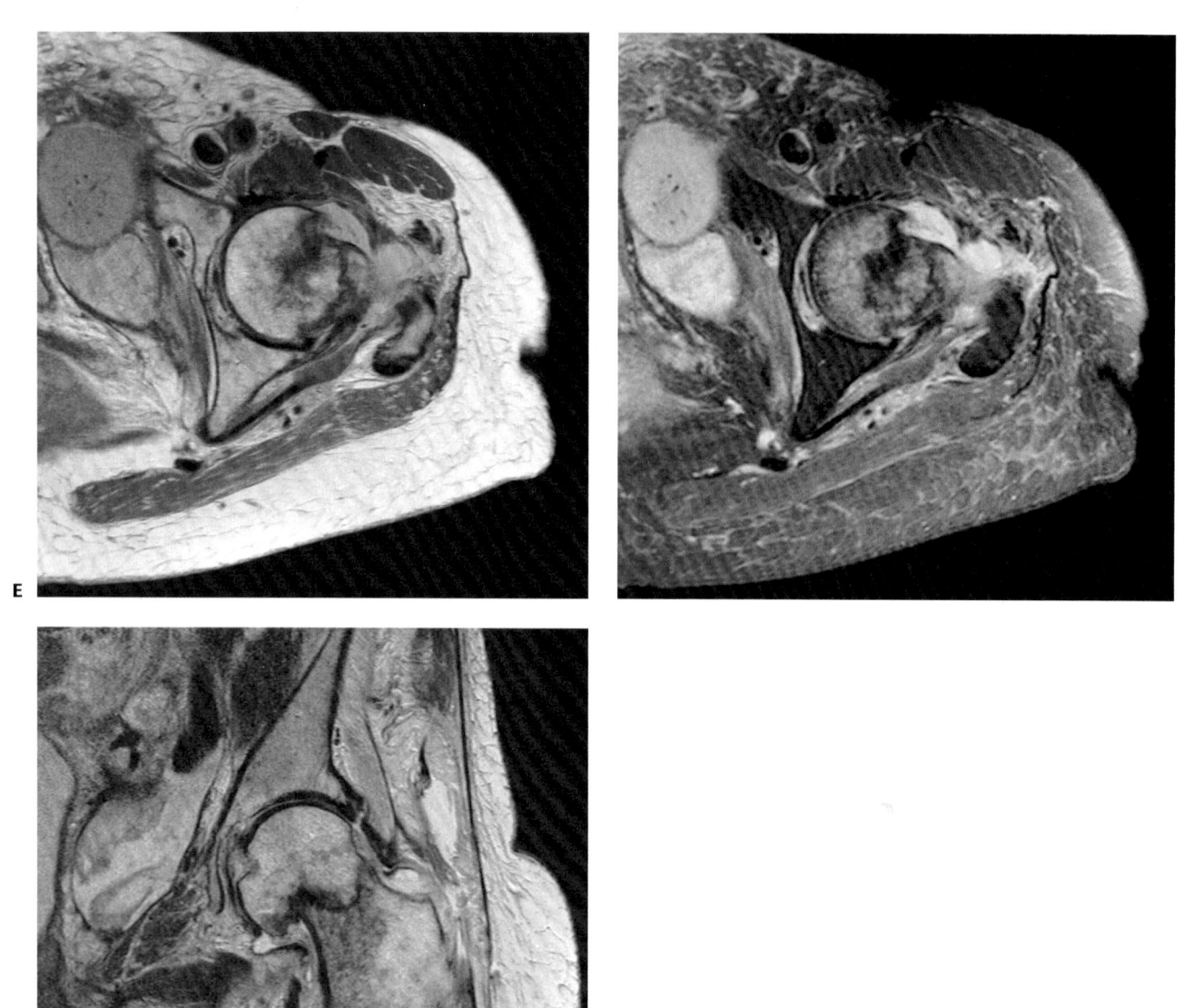

FIGURE 17-7 (*continued*) Axial proton density **(E)**, axial fat-suppressed proton density **(F)**, and coronal T2-weighted **(G)** images. Note inferior pole of kidney transplant in the lower left pelvis with surrounding complex fluid collection.

MRI is similarly advantageous in the assessment of pediatric elbow injuries. In one series, seven of nine pediatric patients with an elbow effusion after injury were found to have a radiographically occult fracture.[164] In the same series, MRI provided further useful diagnostic information in 16 other patients despite the presence of a visible fracture and/or dislocation of the elbow on plain radiographs.[164]

Although CT with multiplanar reformatting remains the modality of choice for imaging complex fractures, recent studies indicate that MRI may be valuable in assessing such injuries as well. In one such study, the impact of MRI on the treatment of tibial plateau fractures was assessed.[204] Patients presenting with tibial plateau fracture were assessed with conventional

radiography, CT, and MRI. Three sets of images were prepared for each injury: Radiographs alone, radiographs with CT, and radiographs with MRI. Three surgeons were asked to determine the fracture classification and suggest a treatment plan based on each set of images. The investigators found that the best interobserver variability for both fracture classification and fracture management was seen with the combination of conventional radiographs and MRI. The Schatzker classification of tibial plateau fractures based on conventional radiographs changed an average of 6% with the addition of CT and 21% with the addition of MRI. MRI changed the treatment plan in 23% of cases. Holt et al.[90] studied 21 consecutive patients with tibial plateau fractures who were evaluated with both conventional radiography and MRI before treatment. MRI was more accurate in determining fracture classification, in revealing occult fracture lines, and in measuring the displacement and depression of fragments. The MRI findings resulted in a change in the classification of 10 fractures (48%) and a change in the management of four patients (19%). MRI also allowed diagnosis of associated intra-articular and periarticular soft tissue injuries preoperatively.

The role of CT is well recognized in the assessment of spinal trauma, but MRI is increasingly being used to evaluate for associated injuries such as herniated discs with cervical spine injuries and possible spinal cord injury associated with thoracolumbar spine fracture/dislocations. Green and Saifuddin[79] have shown that 77% of patients with spine injury have a secondary injury level identified by whole spine MRI. Most commonly, these secondary injuries were bone marrow contusions, but 34% of patients had noncontiguous compression or burst fractures diagnosed by MRI.

Soft Tissue Injury. Because of its superb soft tissue contrast resolution and good spatial resolution, MRI provides an accurate means to assess soft tissue injury. MRI of the shoulder and knee is commonly ordered for evaluation of tendons, ligaments, and cartilage after trauma, frequently related to athletic injuries. Common indications for shoulder MRI following trauma include evaluation of the rotator cuff tendons for tearing, the superior glenoid labrum for superior labral anterior-posterior (SLAP) tears, and the anteroinferior labral-ligamentous complex after glenohumeral joint dislocation.[12,39,188] Standard indications for knee MRI following trauma include evaluation of the cruciate and posterolateral corner ligaments for sprain or disruption, the menisci for tears, and the articular cartilage for osteochondral injury.[53,70,198,200] Lonner et al.[120] compared MRI findings to examination under anesthesia in 10 patients with acute knee dislocations who had later surgical intervention, at which time the pathology was defined. Although the investigators considered MRI to be useful for defining the presence of ligamentous injuries in knee dislocations, the clinical examination under anesthesia was more accurate in this series when correlated with findings at surgery.[120] MRI has recently been shown to be useful at defining the nature of associated ligamentous injuries to the deltoid and tibiofibular syndesmosis in cases of distal fibular fracture, which may affect surgical decision making.[34]

MR arthrography is a potentially valuable technique for assessing intra-articular derangement in many joints. Common indications include distinguishing partial- from full-thickness rotator cuff tears and evaluating labral-ligamentous pathology in the shoulder, evaluating the collateral ligaments in the elbow and intercarpal ligaments in the wrist, demonstrating labral tears in the hip, evaluating postoperative menisci in the knee, assessing stability of osteochondral lesions, and delineating intra-articular bodies.[182] Direct MR arthrography is performed by intra-articular injection of a dilute gadolinium solution, resulting in distention of the joint capsule and improved delineation of intra-articular structures. Indirect MR arthrography is performed using intravenous injection of gadolinium, with a delay before scanning during which mild exercise may be performed. The indirect technique is based on recognition that the intravenous gadolinium diffuses from the highly vascular synovium into the joint space. The indirect technique does not produce controlled joint distention; however, and is best applied in smaller joints such as the elbow, wrist, ankle, and shoulder.[13]

Orthopedic Hardware. Orthopedic hardware presents a challenge in MRI because metal distorts the magnetic field and results in large areas of signal void, which frequently obscures adjacent anatomy.[63] Modifications of traditional MR pulse sequences have been developed on high-field MR scanners to reduce artifact associated with orthopedic implants. FSE (turbo) sequences are used, which inherently decrease metallic artifact compared with routine SE and GRE sequences. Modifications to FSE sequences include increasing receiver readout bandwidths, decreasing interecho spacing and reducing effective echo times to maintain SNRs.[63,179] These protocols are now commonly found in the sequence libraries of many newer MR scanners. Protocols based on modification of receiver bandwidth have been shown to reduce metallic artifact by an average of 60%, whereas additional experimental protocols (not commercially available) using a combination of several susceptibility artifact reduction techniques further reduce metallic artifact by an average of 79%.[106] The degree of artifact is also dependent on the metallic composition of the orthopedic hardware, with titanium generally exhibiting the least amount of artifact. Applications for these sequences include evaluation of painful joint replacements, particularly knee and hip prostheses,[161,179,180] and osteonecrosis of the femoral head after pinning femoral neck fractures (Fig. 17-8).

Ferromagnetic material placed within a magnetic field may experience linear force, torque, and heating. In general, most contemporary orthopedic implants are not ferromagnetic and are MRI compatible in terms of heating and migration. Most fracture implants are made of 316L stainless steel, titanium, or titanium alloy; none of these materials contain delta ferrite, so they are not magnetic.[47] MRI can be safely performed about plates, screws, and total joint implants, although artifacts may degrade the image as described earlier. In contrast, some external fixator components, especially clamps, contain strongly ferromagnetic materials and can be potentially unsafe in an MRI scanner.[44,110] Davison et al.[44] studied 10 sets of commercially available tibial external fixators that they applied to sawbone tibia. The external fixators were tested for magnetic attraction using a hand-held magnet while positioned 30 cm outside the entry portal of a 1.5-T scanner, at the level of the entry portal, and 30 cm inside the MRI tube. The EBI Dynafix with Ankle Clamp, EBI Dynafix, and EBI Dynafix Hybrid, along with the Hoffman II, Hoffman II Hybrid, Ilizarov with stainless steel rings, and Synthes Hybrid, all had more than 1 kg of magnetic attraction at all three locations, which is a significant enough force to cause potential movement of implant and pain. These devices were not scanned. Three devices—the Ilizarov fixator with carbon fiber rings, Richards Hex-Fix, and Large Synthes External Fixator—had less than 1 kg of magnetic attraction at all three locations and were scanned for 30 minutes while temperature measurements were obtained with a digital

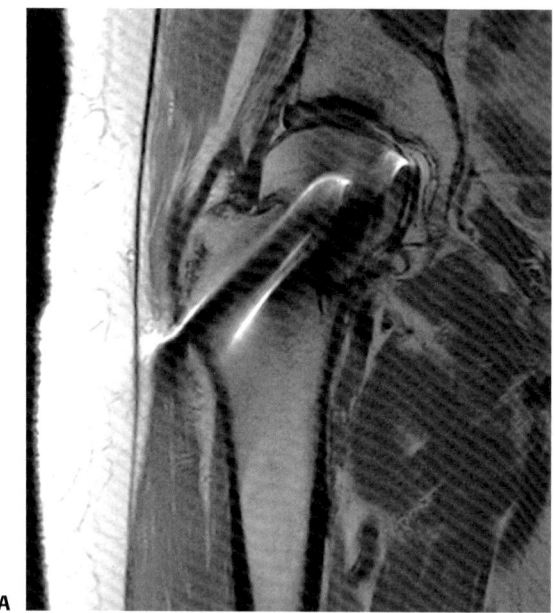
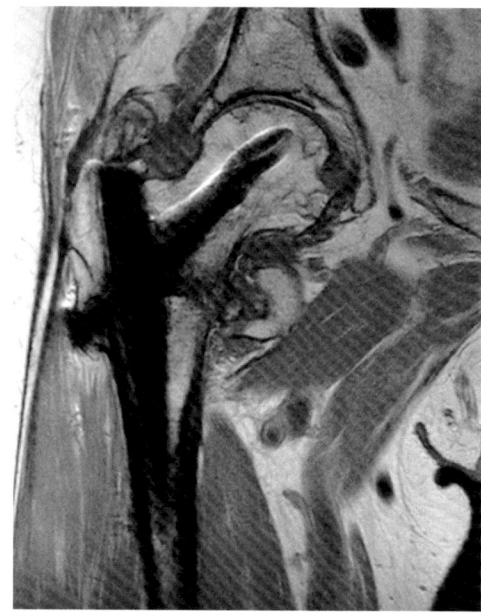

A   **B**

FIGURE 17-8 Metal artifact reduction sequences. **A:** A femoral neck fracture after pinning with four screws demonstrates nonunion. Magnetic resonance imaging using metal artifact reduction sequences shows no evidence of avascular necrosis of the femoral head. **B:** An additional case of nonunion of an intertrochanteric fracture that demonstrates avascular necrosis of the femoral head without subchondral fracture or collapse. The intramedullary rod and screw are titanium, which results in fewer artifacts than stainless steel or other alloys.

thermometer and thermocouple. No component of these three fixators experienced more than −16.67°C (2°F) of temperature elevation during a 30-minute MRI scan. Davison et al.[44] conclude that many commercially available external fixators have components that have significant magnetic attraction to the MRI scanner. Fixators that have less than 1 kg of attraction do not experience significant heating during MRI.

The American Society for Testing and Materials (ASTM) has established standards for MRI compatibility of implants.[202] Many orthopedic manufacturers have redesigned their implants to make them MRI compatible. Luechinger et al.[125] recently studied new MRI-compatible large external fixator clamps made by Synthes and found dramatic reductions in forces experienced in a 3-T field compared with older devices. All orthopedic surgeons should check with the manufacturer and be aware of the MRI compatibility of their particular external fixator inventory.

Arthrography

Technical Considerations

Conventional Arthrography. Arthrography involves distention of a joint capsule using positive or negative contrast agents. Water-soluble, iodinated contrast media is typically used to provide positive contrast, whereas air has been historically used to produce negative contrast. Double-contrast examinations may also be performed using both agents simultaneously, although these techniques are largely of historical interest, as advances in cross-sectional imaging have supplanted double-contrast arthrography techniques.

Injection technique involves placement of a needle into the joint capsule, usually under fluoroscopic or CT guidance. Typically, a 22-gauge needle is used for larger joints, including the shoulder, hip, and knee, and a 25-gauge needle is used for smaller joints, such as the elbow, wrist, ankle, and smaller joints of the hands and feet. The anatomic approach varies according to each joint; for example, a lateral approach into the radiocapitellar joint space is frequently used for the elbow, and anterior approaches are typically used for the shoulder, hip, and tibiotalar joint. Table 17-2 lists technical considerations for arthrography of selected joints. After needle placement, small amounts of contrast are injected until the intra-articular location of the needle tip is confirmed. Contrast is then injected with subsequent distention of the joint capsule; the amount also varies by joint.

Frequently, the injection is performed under fluoroscopy, and sequential spot films are obtained before and during the injection to evaluate the flow of contrast. Pathology is inferred by abnormal communication of contrast with extracapsular structures. Passive and active range of motion are often required to demonstrate pathology, as abnormalities may only be shown after contrast is allowed to work its way through defects in the capsule and into the surrounding soft tissues. Contrast extravasation through capsular abnormalities can be fairly rapid and may occur during passive or active range of motion. Extravasation may also occur during periods when the fluoroscope is not energized. In addition, the fluoroscope only provides 2D views of bony anatomy, and it is extremely limited in its evaluation of surrounding soft tissues. Consequently, localizing the site of

TABLE 17-2	**Arthrographic Techniques of Selected Joints**		
Joint	Injection Approach	Needle Size	Volume of Contrast (mL)[182]
Shoulder	Anterior glenohumeral joint space	22-gauge 3 V_2-inch spinal needle	15
Elbow	Lateral radiocapitellar joint space	25-gauge 1 V_2-inch needle	10
Wrist	Dorsal radioscaphoid joint space	25-gauge 1 V_2-inch needle	4
Hip	Anterior femoral head/neck junction	22-gauge 3 V_2-inch needle	15
Knee	Medial or lateral patellofemoral joint space	22-gauge 1 V_2-inch needle	40
Ankle	Anterior tibiotalar joint space	22-gauge 3 V_2-inch spinal needle	10–12

extravasation during conventional arthrography can be quite challenging. Care is also needed to avoid overdistention of the joint capsule, as extravasation through the capsule can occur, leading to subsequent decompression of intra-articular contrast and possible false-positive interpretations.

Complications of arthrography are uncommon but may include bleeding and infection at the injection site, in addition to allergic reactions related to iodinated contrast media. A small number of patients experience postprocedural pain, possibly related to a mild synovial inflammatory response to the contrast media. Although patients are generally apprehensive about the procedure, they generally tolerate the procedure with less discomfort than expected.[170]

Digital Subtraction Arthrography. With the advent of digital imaging, digital subtraction techniques have been developed for fluoroscopy. Typically, a preliminary scout film serves as a "mask," which is subsequently subtracted from images following contrast injection. This significantly improves contrast resolution of the fluoroscopic spot films and enables visualization of contrast that would otherwise not be apparent when adjacent to similar high-density objects, such as joint prostheses. Digital subtraction arthrography (DSA) also allows sequential injection and evaluation of adjacent joint compartments, as a new mask is obtained after injection of the first compartment, which is subsequently subtracted from images acquired during injection of the second compartment. DSA techniques are sensitive to patient motion; however, which produces misregistration artifact as a result of misalignment of the mask and subsequent images. DSA also requires specialized equipment, which may not be available outside of radiology departments.

CT and MR Arthrography. Cross-sectional techniques, such as CT and MRI, have largely replaced conventional arthrography for evaluating internal derangement, but these imaging modalities may be combined with arthrography using appropriate contrast agents for each modality.[61,182] For CTA, an arthrogram is first obtained using a contrast solution containing saline and water-soluble, iodinated contrast media, typically in a 1:1 dilution. Thin-section CT is then performed through the joint, and images in orthogonal planes are reconstructed. For MR arthrography, a very dilute gadolinium solution (typically 1:200 dilution) is injected into the joint, and MRI is subsequently performed. In addition to routine sequences, fat-suppressed T1W images are used to visualize the injected contrast. With both

imaging modalities, evaluation is aided not only by silhouetting intra-articular structures by relatively bright contrast but also by distention of the joint capsule. This results in separation of intra-articular ligaments and capsular structures and allows more precise evaluation of complex anatomy (Fig. 17-9). Bony and soft tissue abnormalities are directly visualized with these cross-sectional techniques, compared to conventional arthrography, whereby pathology is inferred based on the appearance of the contrast collection in relation to the bony landmarks.

Applications

Before advanced cross-sectional imaging techniques, arthrography was traditionally used for assessing periarticular soft tissue injuries associated with trauma. Today, there are more limited indications for arthrography, although it is frequently performed in combination with CT and MRI to increase the sensitivity and specificity for internal derangement.

Arthrography may be substituted in patients with contraindications to MRI, such as pacemakers or intracranial aneurysm clips. CTA is preferred; however, as advances in CT scanner technology have led to marked improvements in resolution and scan time, resulting in high spatial resolution images and MPRs of intra-articular structures.

Upper Extremity. In the upper extremity, shoulder arthrography may be performed to evaluate for full-thickness rotator cuff tears. Extravasation of contrast into the subacromial/subdeltoid bursa is diagnostic of a full-thickness tear. Even with careful fluoroscopic observation during the injection process, it is frequently impossible to delineate the site or extent of the tear, as contrast medium may accumulate in the bursa without visualization of an obvious tract through the torn tendon. Occasionally, no extravasation is seen after completing the injection; however, after passively and/or actively exercising the shoulder, subsequent fluoroscopy reveals contrast flooding the bursa as a result of the medium working itself through a full-thickness tear. Special care is needed in interpreting arthrography of the postoperative rotator cuff, because intact cuff repairs may continue to leak contrast into the bursa.

The value of three-compartment arthrography has been documented in the setting of acute wrist trauma,[78] as has the value of digital subtraction techniques in wrist arthrography.[45,205] Arthrography has historically been applied to the evaluation of ulnar collateral ligament injuries of the thumb ("gamekeeper's

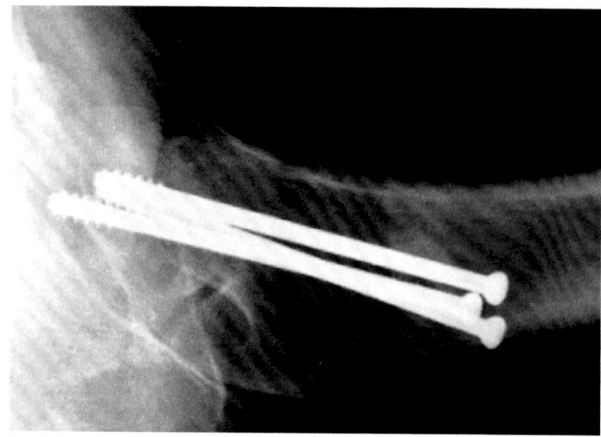

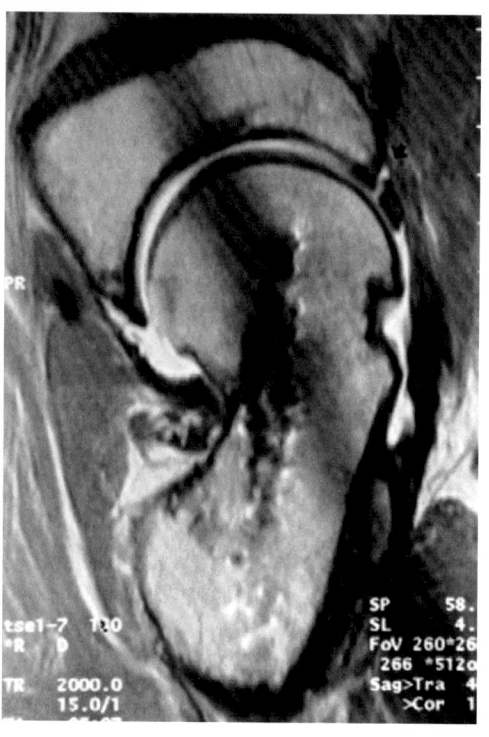

FIGURE 17-9 **A:** Lateral radiograph of the proximal femur after fixation of a femoral neck fracture, showing malunion with retroversion of the femoral neck. **B:** The patient had persistent hip pain, and magnetic resonance arthrography revealed a tear of the anterior acetabular labrum. Note angular deformity at the site of fracture malunion and residual micrometallic artifact related to insertion of prior screws. (Reprinted with permission from: Eijer H, Myers SR, Ganz R. Anterior femoroacetabular impingement after femoral neck fractures. *J Orthop Trauma.* 2001;15:475–481.)

thumb"). Recent literature has shown MR arthrography to be more accurate in detecting ulnar collateral ligament injuries and in evaluating displacement of the torn ligament[1] as well for evaluation of triangular fibrocartilage complex injury.[176]

Lower Extremity. In the lower extremity, arthrography alone is rarely performed for trauma but may be combined with CT or MRI for evaluating osteochondral abnormalities (Fig. 17-9).[121] A recent study comparing CTA with MR arthrography suggests that CTA may be more accurate in evaluating cartilage lesions of the ankle joint.[174]

Arthrography may also be useful in the evaluation of pain after treating calcaneal fractures with intra-articular extension. Matsui et al.[131] performed posterior subtalar joint arthrography at a mean of 6 months postinjury in 22 patients; 15 had undergone surgical repair and 7 had been treated nonoperatively. The patients were separated into four groups based on arthrographic findings: Normal, narrow, irregular, and ankylosis. Clinical follow-up performed at a mean of 23 months postinjury correlated very well with the earlier arthrographic findings, suggesting that subtalar arthrosis is responsible for much of the symptoms that develop after calcaneal fracture.

Pediatric Injuries. Arthrography is valuable in assessing pediatric physeal injuries (especially the elbow)[2,15,51,113,129] that are not visible on conventional radiographs. It is also used intraoperatively to assist with the reduction of pediatric radial head fractures.[94] The use of arthrography to assess pediatric injuries has been largely supplanted by MRI (when available), although in the pediatric population both procedures may require sedation.

Dynamic Imaging. Arthrography remains the investigation of choice when dynamic imaging is necessary. Using arthroscopy as the diagnostic standard, Kim et al.[102] compared dynamic arthrography with MRI arthrography for the diagnosis of wrist pain in 38 patients, finding both modalities had similar sensitivity and specificity for the diagnosis of scapholunate ligament, lunotriquetral ligament, and triangular fibrocartilage complex tears.

Ultrasonography

Technical Considerations

Conventional Ultrasonography. US refers to the spectrum of sound waves with frequencies greater than 20 kHz (20,000 Hz), which are beyond the audible range of the human ear. Typical frequencies used in medical diagnostic US range from 2 to 12 MHz, although frequencies of 20 MHz and higher are in clinical use for more specialized applications involving very small regions of anatomy. Lower frequencies within this range (2 to 5 MHz) allow deeper penetration of the US beam for evaluation of thicker body parts, although at lower spatial resolutions. Higher-frequency US beams (10 to 12 MHz) provide greater spatial resolution and are frequently used in evaluating superficial anatomy, such as tendons.

US beams are generated by transducers, which make use of piezoelectric materials to convert electrical energy into mechanical energy (sound waves). Today's transducer designs are complex and may incorporate hundreds of individual piezoelectric elements, each of which is energized in turn or in combination, such that the individual sound waves combine into a US beam. The US beam propagates into the underlying tissues and is partially reflected back at tissue boundaries because of differences in acoustic impedance between tissues. Acoustic impedance is defined as the product of tissue density and the speed of sound, both of which vary among tissues. Small differences in acoustic impedance will produce smaller reflections of sound waves, whereas large differences in acoustic impedances will result in larger reflections. The reflected echoes travel back to the transducer, where the transducer elements convert the sound waves into electrical signals, which are then used to create the US image.

A US image is composed of an array of pixels, each corresponding to a tissue element at a particular depth and location. Echoes returning from underlying soft tissue elements are generated from reflections of the US beam at tissue interfaces of different acoustic impedance. In addition, smaller cellular elements within tissues can also act as individual "scatterers." Each of these scatterers reflects a small portion of the US beam in all directions. A portion of these scattered echoes are reflected back toward the transducer and are displayed in the image as background "echogenicity" that is characteristic for that tissue. Echoes returning from superficial soft tissues have shorter round trip distances to travel back to the transducer and are detected earlier than those for deeper soft tissues. For this reason, the depth of a tissue element can be calculated using the return time of its corresponding echo. The amplitude of the returning echo determines the brightness, or echogenicity, of a tissue element. As the US beam travels deeper within the soft tissues, it progressively loses energy and subsequent echoes from deeper tissue elements are smaller in amplitude. A correction factor, termed *time gain compensation,* is applied to deeper soft tissues to account for this drop off in echo amplitude. Thus, differences in echogenicity in the resulting US image will be less dependent on tissue depth and more related to differences in acoustic impedance and scattering.

During a single cycle, the transducer sends a short burst of US waves (the US pulse) into the underlying tissues, and then listens for the returning echoes. The time spent sending out the US pulse is a tiny fraction of the listening time, typically about 0.5% of the total cycle time. The pulse repetition frequency determines how many pulses are sent into the underlying tissue over time, and typically ranges between 2000 and 4000 cycles/s (2 to 4 kHz). During routine scanning, the transducer is constantly steering and refocusing the US beam within the underlying tissue to generate echoes that will correspond to each pixel in the US image. The 2D US image that is generated is typically referred to as *B-mode* ("brightness" mode) *imaging.* The designs of current transducers are quite complex and rely on advanced electronics and scanning algorithms, but have resulted in greater spatial resolution and more advanced feature sets, including 3D, four-dimensional, and Doppler imaging.

Echogenicity is a term used to describe the relative brightness of echoes returning from tissues or tissue interfaces. Tissues may be described as *hypoechoic* or *hyperechoic* with regard to a reference tissue, in addition to *isoechoic* if two distinct soft tissues share the same level of echogenicity. The descriptor *anechoic* refers to a tissue or medium that produces no reflected echoes and is black on the corresponding US image. Water is the best example of an anechoic medium, because all of the sound waves are transmitted through the medium without any reflections. In such situations, the energy within the US beam will be greater as it reaches the tissues on the far side of the medium and the distal tissues will appear brighter; this is referred to as *increased through transmission.* Conversely, any tissue or medium that blocks transmission of all sound waves will appear highly echogenic at its proximal interface with the US beam and will exhibit "distal acoustic shadowing," whereby the more distal tissues appear black, resembling a shadow. Cortical bone and air are examples where the large differences in acoustic impedance result in marked attenuation of the US beam, producing distal acoustic shadowing.

US examinations are highly operator dependent, and the quality of the examination can be influenced by the sonographer's training, experience performing certain examinations, and understanding of normal anatomy and disease states. US is a real-time examination, and although images that represent the underlying anatomy are saved, these 2D images cannot provide the depth of understanding that real-time visualization provides. For this reason, it may be necessary for the interpreting physician to be present or to image the patient to interpret complex examinations.

Doppler US. Doppler US is used to evaluate moving tissues, such as blood flow within vessels. Velocity measurements and directions of flow may be ascertained on the basis of frequency shifts of the returning echoes. When the US beam is reflected from a tissue moving toward the transducer, the returning echoes undergo a slight increase in frequency. Similarly, when interacting with a tissue moving away from the transducer, the US beam will be reflected such that the returning echoes will incur a slight decrease in their frequency. These frequency shifts are used to calculate the speed of the moving tissue, whereas the direction of frequency shift (positive vs. negative) is used to determine the direction of motion relative to the transducer.

Various modes of Doppler operation are available on today's scanners and are frequently used for vascular evaluation. Duplex Doppler imaging combines 2D B-mode imaging with pulsed Doppler imaging; the 2D B-mode image provides an anatomical map to identify vessels for subsequent Doppler interrogation. Color Doppler combines B-mode grayscale imaging with color flow superimposed over vessels, as determined by Doppler imaging. Shades of red and blue are assigned to the vessels based on their velocities and directions and represent flow toward and away from the transducer, respectively. Power Doppler imaging is a signal processing algorithm that uses the total amplitude of the Doppler signal to generate maps of flow, which are then superimposed on B-mode grayscale images. The corresponding images demonstrate greater sensitivity to slow flow, although no directional information is available.

Applications

US is a simple, noninvasive, relatively inexpensive imaging modality that is now widely available in most hospitals and in many clinics. Diagnostic US has an established role in the immediate diagnosis of trauma patients according to the ATLS protocol, where it is used in the "Focused Abdominal Sonography for Trauma" (FAST) examination for intra-abdominal injury. US also has applications in evaluation of fractures, fracture healing, soft tissue trauma including ligamentous injury, and venous thromboembolism.

Fractures. US has potential in the assessment of fractures, and may be underused in this regard.[153] US compares favorably to conventional radiography in the assessment of occult scaphoid fracture in patients with wrist pain.[89] Durston and Swartzentruber[55] used US to assess the reduction of pediatric forearm fractures in the emergency department, thereby avoiding multiple trips to the radiology suite while gaining much more rapid assessment of the quality of fracture reduction. Assessing pediatric elbow injuries is notoriously difficult because of the complex joint anatomy and the multiplicity of its ossification centers, many of which are relatively unossified in childhood. US has proved to be valuable in evaluating lateral condylar fractures, in that it is able to assess the extent of the fracture line through the unossified capitellum and trochlea, to distinguish unstable intra-articular fractures from their stable extra-articular counter parts.[193]

US may also be clinically useful in evaluating fractures in settings where conventional radiography may not be readily available, such as in military or aerospace settings.[104] Dulchavsky et al.[54] prospectively evaluated 158 injured extremities by US. Nonphysician cast technicians, who had received limited training and were blinded to the patient's radiographic diagnoses, performed the US evaluations. Examinations only required an average of 4 minutes and accurately diagnosed injury in 94% of patients with no false-positive results. Injuries that were diagnosed by US included fractures in the upper arm, forearm, femur, tibia/fibula, hand, and foot.

Fracture Healing. US is a useful method to monitor fracture healing. Moed et al.[137] performed sonographic evaluation of patients 6 and 12 weeks after unreamed tibial nailing and found that persistent nail visualization indicated poor callus formation and predicted later healing complications. Color Doppler sonography has been shown to demonstrate progressive vascularization of fracture callus and predict delayed callus formation in another study of patients with tibial fractures.[32]

Soft Tissue Trauma. US is also well suited for diagnosing musculoskeletal soft tissue injuries and is of proven value in the assessment of many tendon injuries, such as those of the tendo Achillis, rotator cuff, and ankle.[17,29,36,171] US has been used to assess muscle injury, depicted as a tear or hematoma and subsequent complications such as fibrosis, cystic lesions, or heterotopic ossification.[154] US is valuable in localizing foreign bodies within soft tissues; an advantage over conventional radiography is that foreign objects do not need to be radiopaque to visualize them.[116]

Venous Thromboembolism. US has come to play a very important role in managing venous thromboembolism in trauma patients.[207] All trauma patients are at risk for developing DVT, and venous US has become the most widely used imaging modality for DVT diagnosis. Venous scanning performed by skilled operators is the most practical and cost-effective method for assessing DVT of the proximal and distal lower-extremity veins. Several US modalities are used to evaluate DVT, including B-mode for real-time visualization of compression of larger veins.

Duplex Doppler for evaluating waveforms and velocities and color Doppler for depicting patency of veins are particularly useful in the calf and iliac veins.[207] The diagnostic accuracy of US is well documented, and the sensitivity and specificity of venous US (including all types) for the diagnosis of symptomatic proximal DVT is 97% and 94%, respectively.[207] The high specificity of venous US is sufficient to initiate treatment of DVT without further confirmation, and the high sensitivity for proximal DVT makes it possible to withhold treatment if the examination is negative.[207] When US examinations cannot be performed (e.g., uncooperative patient, presence of bandages, casts), an alternative diagnostic procedure, such as contrast venography, may be needed. More advanced imaging modalities, such as CT or MRV are also available. US is less accurate in the diagnosis of proximal DVT involving the pelvis; MRV has been suggested as a more accurate modality for detecting intrapelvic DVT.[138]

Nuclear Medicine Imaging
Technical Considerations

Nuclear scintigraphy involves intravenous injection of a radiopharmaceutical with subsequent imaging using a gamma scintillation camera. The radiopharmaceutical is typically composed of two moieties: A radionuclide and a pharmaceutical compound. The pharmaceutical is responsible for localization of the molecule in the body, and the radionuclide allows imaging of the pharmaceutical distribution.

Radionuclides are radioactive isotopes that undergo spontaneous decay, which results in the emission of photons. Photons that are generated in the nucleus of the atom are gamma rays, whereas photons generated by electron transitions within their orbital shells are x-rays. Either may be used for imaging, although the particular choice of a radionuclide predetermines the types and energies of photons that are emitted. In many NM imaging applications, technetium (^{99m}Tc) is commonly used as the radionuclide because of its favorable imaging properties (140-keV gamma energy), clinically suitable half-life (6 hours), availability (^{99}Mo/^{99m}Tc generator) and ease in labeling of pharmaceuticals. Other radionuclides used in orthopedic imaging include gallium (^{67}Ga) and indium (^{111}In) and are discussed later in this section.

Pharmaceuticals are metabolically active molecules that are designed to localize to target tissues once injected intravenously. There are many different mechanisms of localization, but for orthopedic imaging, regional blood flow is important for all administered radiopharmaceuticals. Specific radiopharmaceuticals for orthopedic imaging and their method of localization are discussed later in this section.

Gamma scintillation cameras are specialized detectors that capture photons within a large flat crystal, commonly made of sodium iodide activated with thallium. Photons interact with the scintillation crystal and are converted to visible light, which is then captured by photomultiplier tubes (PMTs) coupled to the crystal. The PMT converts the light photon into an electrical signal, which is subsequently amplified and electronically processed. This process results in a single "count" in the final NM image corresponding to a single radioactive decay in the patient.

NM images are formed by placing the gamma scintillation camera over the anatomy of interest and accumulating counts for a specific amount of time or for a minimum number of counts, typically on the order of hundreds of thousands of counts. Imaging is often performed after a delay to allow localization and/or uptake of the radiopharmaceutical within the target tissues. Delayed imaging demonstrates characteristic patterns of distribution throughout the body for a particular radiopharmaceutical, in addition to abnormal accumulation or absence of activity corresponding to disease states. Consequently, nuclear imaging studies are based on visualization of metabolic function, rather than anatomy. Anatomic features are frequently visualized on NM images, although spatial resolution is typically quite poor compared with other imaging modalities (Table 17-1).

During routine acquisition of NM images, the gamma scintillation camera is left stationary in a single projection, resulting in a planar image. Single-photon emission computed tomography (SPECT) is an extension of planar imaging, whereby the gamma camera rotates around the patient, stopping at predefined intervals, to acquire multiple static planar images. Using techniques similar to those in CT, these planar data sets are then processed by computers. Images are typically created in orthogonal tomographic planes (axial, coronal, sagittal), in addition to 3D volumes. Although the main advantage of SPECT over planar images is the improved image contrast resolution as a result of eliminating radioactivity from overlapping anatomy, spatial resolution is similar or slightly decreased compared to planar imaging (Table 17-1).

Indwelling orthopedic hardware may affect image quality by introducing artifacts into the diagnostic image. Hardware can shield the gamma camera from photons arising behind the hardware, resulting in a photopenic defect. Knowledge of indwelling hardware and their characteristic photopenic appearances alleviates misinterpretation of these defects. Multiple projections are also frequently performed during a single examination, which allows evaluation of the activity on multiple sides of the hardware.

NM techniques relevant to trauma and orthopedics are described in the sections to follow.

Skeletal Scintigraphy.
Skeletal scintigraphy, commonly referred to as a *bone scan,* is the most commonly performed NM study with respect to the skeletal system. The radiopharmaceutical used is typically a ^{99m}Tc-labeled diphosphonate, which localizes to bone based on chemiadsorption of the phosphorus compound to the mineral phase of bone, particularly at sites of increased osteoblastic activity. Regional blood flow is also important for tracer distribution, as areas of increased regional blood flow deliver greater tracer to the adjacent skeleton, and result in greater uptake. The term *bone scan* typically refers to images obtained after a 2- to 4-hour delay, to allow localization of the diphosphonate compound. *Three-phase bone scans* incorporate additional dynamic and immediate imaging phases. A radionuclide angiogram (first phase) is

obtained during transit of radiopharmaceutical through the arterial system. Immediate static images are then obtained for an additional 5 minutes (second phase) and represent "blood pool" or "tissue phase" images. Both of these earlier imaging phases are used to evaluate for regional hyperemia, as evidenced by both increased blood flow and increased surrounding soft tissue uptake.

Normal bone scan images show a characteristic appearance of the skeleton, with slightly greater uptake in the axial skeleton (spine, pelvis) than the extremities. In skeletally immature individuals, there is normal avid uptake in the growth plates, resulting in symmetrically increased bands of activity occurring adjacent to joints and apophyses. Many diseases are characterized by both increased osteoblastic and osteoclastic activity within the bone, in addition to regional hyperemia, and result in greater tracer uptake ("hot" lesions) than normal bone. These abnormalities may be solitary or multiple, and focal or diffuse in nature. Some pathologic processes, particularly permeative processes (small round cell tumors) or those that elicit little surrounding bone reaction, result in regions of decreased tracer uptake, or "cold" lesions. These lesions may be difficult to detect on routine bone scans. Bone scans are highly sensitive for disease processes, although specificity is poor. A normal bone scan may rule out underlying skeletal abnormality, but a positive bone scan necessitates further workup of the underlying abnormality.

Marrow Imaging.
Marrow imaging is performed using ^{99m}Tc-labeled sulfur colloid. The sulfur colloid is composed of particles measuring between 0.1 and 2 micron, which are taken up by the reticuloendothelial cells within the liver (85%), spleen (10%), and bone marrow (5%). Uptake is rapid (half-life is 2 to 3 minutes), and imaging is performed after a 20-minute delay. Current indications for marrow imaging are limited but include evaluation of osteomyelitis in conjunction with ^{111}In-labeled white blood cell (WBC) imaging.

Gallium Imaging.
Gallium-67 citrate is a radiopharmaceutical that was originally developed as a bone-imaging agent but was later found to be useful in imaging infection and inflammation. After intravenous injection, gallium binds to transferrin and circulates in the bloodstream. At sites of inflammation or infection, increased regional blood flow and increased vascular permeability result in greater accumulation of gallium. In addition, neutrophils release large amounts of lactoferrin as a part of their inflammatory response; gallium has a higher binding affinity for lactoferrin than transferrin and localizes at the site of inflammation. Gallium is a relatively poor imaging agent, as its photons are not optimum for imaging with present-day gamma cameras, and total body clearance is slow with considerable background activity. Imaging is typically performed at 48 hours, which contributes to delays in diagnosis.

Gallium scans are often interpreted with bone scans for evaluation of osteomyelitis. Gallium activity that is greater than, or in different distribution than, corresponding activity on the bone scan is diagnostic for osteomyelitis.

White Blood Cell Imaging.
There are several approaches for using labeled WBCs for diagnosing infection and/or

inflammatory processes. Of these, ^{111}In oxine– and ^{99m}Tc-labeled hexamethylpropyleneamine oxime (HMPAO)–labeled WBCs are discussed briefly.

Indium-111 is complexed with oxine, which results in a lipid-soluble complex that readily crosses the cell membranes. Approximately 50 mL of blood must be withdrawn and the leukocytes need to be separated from the plasma and red cells. Labeling is accomplished by incubating the leukocytes with the ^{111}In oxine complex for 30 minutes. The leukocytes are then resuspended in plasma and reinjected into the patient within a total of 2 to 4 hours. Imaging is typically performed at 24 hours to allow for leukocyte localization and clearance from the blood pool.

[99m]Tc HMPAO is a cerebral perfusion agent that also crosses cell membranes and may be used to label WBCs, preferentially granulocytes. Approximately 50 to 75 mL of blood is withdrawn and incubated with the radiopharmaceutical; however, the labeling process is performed in plasma, and cell separation is not needed. The labeled cells are then reinjected, and imaging is performed at 4 hours for the peripheral skeleton.

Labeled WBC studies should be interpreted in combination with sulfur colloid marrow studies for evaluation of osteomyelitis and infected joint replacements. When used alone, labeled white cell studies may result in false-positive results, because labeled WBCs normally distribute to the bone marrow, in addition to the liver and spleen, after reinjection. The sulfur colloid marrow study is used to map out areas of normal residual marrow activity. Congruent activity is seen within the bone marrow on both examinations. Osteomyelitis results in replacement of marrow activity on the sulfur colloid study, resulting in a photopenic defect, whereas there is significantly increased activity on the corresponding labeled WBC study.

Applications

NM imaging is frequently used for further evaluation when conventional radiographs are normal or to evaluate the significance of abnormalities seen on radiographs. Although typically highly sensitive for disease processes, its poor specificity makes it necessary to correlate the findings with additional clinical history, laboratory evaluation, or imaging examinations. Applications of NM to orthopedic trauma include evaluation of fractures, osteomyelitis, and osteonecrosis.

Fractures. Bone scans are highly sensitive for acute fractures. Matin[130] demonstrated positive scans in 80% of fractures at 24 hours, and in 95% by 72 hours. Advanced age and debilitation contributed to nonvisualization of fractures beyond this time frame. The minimum time to return to normal was 5 months, and 90% of fractures returned to normal by 2 years. Because of its poor specificity, scintigraphy can lead to false-positive diagnoses of fracture. Garcia-Morales et al.[73] reported five cases of false-positive scans for hip fracture because of collar osteophytes; subsequent MRI in these patients was negative.

Radiographically negative stress fractures and insufficiency fractures are also well delineated on bone scintigraphy as focal areas of increased radiotracer uptake. Characteristic sites of stress fractures depend on the activity that produced them, although there is considerable overlap. Some fracture patterns show characteristic appearances on scintigraphy. For example, in elderly patients with chronic low back or hip pain, sacral insufficiency fractures reveal a classic "H" pattern of uptake, known as the "Honda" sign.[71,155] Not uncommonly, several focal areas of increased tracer uptake are seen in the skeleton, which presumably represent a combination of acute and more chronic findings. In these cases, three-phase scintigraphy can provide additional information regarding hyperemia and may help to differentiate acute from chronic injuries. Typically, hyperemia resolves within 4 to 8 weeks after initial injury, with the blood flow, then the blood pool, images normalizing.

Scintigraphy may be useful in the early identification of fracture healing complications. Barros et al.[10] performed scintigraphy at 6, 12, and 24 weeks with 25 mCi of MDP-^{99m}Tc in 40 patients with tibial shaft fractures that were treated nonsurgically. Using the normal leg as a control, an activity index (the ratio of the uptake counts of the injured leg to the normal leg) was calculated. All fractures in this series healed within 20 weeks and the activity ratio index progressively decreased at the three evaluations.[10] The investigators speculate that a persistently increased activity index would indicate future development of healing complications, such as delayed union or nonunion, although they did not have any such healing complications in their series.[10]

Bone scintigraphy may also be used in evaluating a child with nonaccidental trauma. In a study from Australia, studies of 30 children who were the victims of suspected child abuse and who had both skeletal surveys and bone scintigraphy were retrospectively reviewed.[128] Excluding rib fractures, there were 64 bony injuries, of which 33% were seen on both imaging modalities, 44% were seen on skeletal survey only, and 25% of the injuries were seen on bone scans alone. Metaphyseal lesions typical of child abuse were found in 20 cases (31%) on skeletal survey; only 35% of these were identified on bone scan. The investigators believed that both skeletal survey and bone scintigraphy should be performed in cases of suspected child abuse.

Infection. Osteomyelitis may result from hematogenous spread of microorganisms to bone, from direct extension from areas of adjacent soft tissue infection, or as a result of open fractures and/or surgery. Persistent pain or delayed healing after surgery can be difficult to evaluate with regard to infection, as conventional radiographs may show only more advanced destructive changes and MRI may be very difficult to interpret in light of recent surgery.

Radionuclide imaging has evolved over time with respect to imaging orthopedic infections. In addition to three-phase bone scans, dual gallium/bone scintigraphy and labeled WBC studies, including combination leukocyte/bone and leukocyte/marrow studies, are valuable in diagnosing both acute and chronic osteomyelitis as well as infected joint replacements. However, no one study is equally applicable to all clinical situations.[151]

Although three-phase bone scans have excellent accuracy for detecting osteomyelitis in normal underlying bone, the specificity of this test is markedly reduced in the presence of underlying bone disease.

Dual gallium (^{67}Ga)/bone scintigraphy has been used to evaluate osteomyelitis. Gallium scintigraphy demonstrates greater accuracy (86%) in diagnosing spinal osteomyelitis compared with ^{111}In-labeled WBCs (66%).[152] A recent evaluation of imaging techniques in spinal osteomyelitis and surrounding soft tissue infections has recommended SPECT ^{67}Ga as the radionuclide study of choice when MRI is unavailable or as an adjunct in patients with possible spinal infection in whom the diagnosis remains uncertain.[122] Gallium is also better suited for imaging of chronic osteomyelitis compared with ^{99m}Tc HMPAO–labeled WBCs, which are better for imaging acute infections.[157]

^{99m}Tc HMPAO–labeled WBC scintigraphy exhibits high sensitivity (97.7%) and specificity (96.8%) for acute osteomyelitis, although its sensitivity for chronic osteomyelitis is slightly decreased.[201] ^{99m}Tc HMPAO–labeled WBC scintigraphy is preferred for evaluating children because the radiation dose to the spleen is smaller and less blood is needed for labeling.[175] ^{99m}Tc HMPAO–labeled WBC scintigraphy is superior to ^{99m}Tc bone scintigraphy for children younger than 6 months because of the poor sensitivity of bone scintigraphy at this age.[157] ^{111}In-labeled WBC scintigraphy is preferred in evaluating chronic osteomyelitis, as dual ^{111}In WBC/^{99m}Tc sulfur colloid studies result in improved accuracy for diagnosis of osteomyelitis in regions containing active bone marrow.[157,175] In more complex regions with overlapping bone and soft tissues, such as the skull and hips, simultaneous ^{111}In WBC/^{99m}Tc bone SPECT imaging has been recommended.[175]

Dual ^{111}In WBC/^{99m}Tc bone scans have been used to evaluate for osteomyelitis at sites of delayed union or nonunion.[146] The sensitivity, specificity, positive and negative predictive values, and accuracy of this approach were 86%, 84%, 69%, 94%, and 82%, respectively.

Recently, a meta-analysis of ^{99m}Tc-radiolabeled antigranulocyte monoclonal antibodies has shown a sensitivity of 81% and specificity of 77% in the diagnosis of osteomyelitis. The authors conclude that antigranulocyte scintigraphy can be used as a major diagnostic method in patients with suspected osteomyelitis but cannot replace traditional methods such as

histologic examination and cell culture.[150] Similarly, Stucken et al.[184] reported the results of a prospective protocol designed to identify the presence of occult infection in patients with a nonunion of an open or previously operated fracture. The protocol included labeled leukocyte/sulfur colloid imaging, as well as measurement of inflammatory markers (C-reactive protein [CRP] and erythrocyte sedimentation rate [ESR]), serum WBC count, and histopathology. In this study of ununited fractures, the labeled leukocyte/sulfur colloid scan had a sensitivity of just 19%, and did not add anything to the positive predictive value of the combination of serum WBC, ESR, CRP and histopathologic examination alone.[184] The authors concluded that the addition of labeled WBC/sulfur colloid imaging had no clinical benefit and was not cost effective when trying to assess occult infection when fracture nonunion is present.[184]

Osteonecrosis. Because scintigraphy is able to demonstrate the vascularity of bone, it is often used to try to assess the risk of osteonecrosis after an injury. Although largely supplanted by MRI, bone scanning can be used to identify osteonecrosis of the femoral head before it is apparent on conventional radiographs (Fig. 17-10).[18] Studies by Drane and Rudd[50] and Mortensson et al.[139] have shown that bone scintigraphy cannot predict the risk of osteonecrosis after femoral neck fracture. Subsequent work has suggested that SPECT imaging may be more accurate in assessing vascularity of the femoral head in fractures of the femoral neck.[28]

Angiography
Technical Considerations

Conventional Angiography. Techniques in conventional angiography are well established and involve cannulation of a vessel, commonly a major artery, for subsequent diagnostic and therapeutic interventions. Typically, the right common femoral artery is accessed, although less common access sites include the left common femoral artery, the axillary and brachial arteries, and translumbar aortic approaches, the selection of which depend on the clinical situation and goal of angiography. The

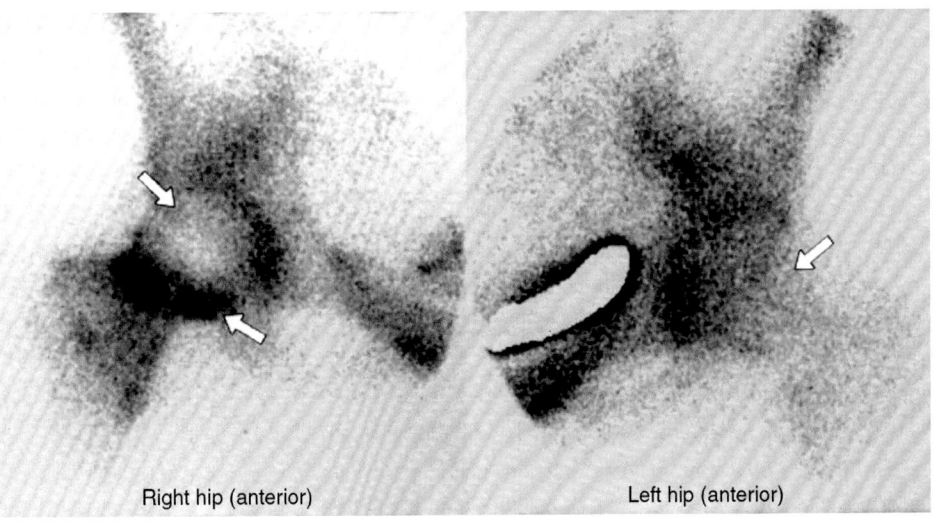

FIGURE 17-10 Pinhole bone scintigraphy (anteroposterior views) showing a photon-deficient area centrally in the right femoral head and increased uptake in the femoral neck and subcapital area compared with normal left hip findings. (Reprinted with permission from: Yoon TR, Rowe SM, Song EK, et al. Unusual osteonecrosis of the femoral head misdiagnosed as a stress fracture. *J Orthop Trauma.* 2004;18:43–47.)

Right hip (anterior)   Left hip (anterior)

Seldinger technique, the standard procedure for cannulating the common femoral artery, involves placing an 18-gauge needle into the artery at the level of the midfemoral head under fluoroscopic guidance. A double wall puncture is preferred, whereby the needle is advanced through both the anterior and posterior arterial walls until contact is made with the femoral head. The needle tip is pulled back slowly until it is within the arterial lumen and pulsatile flow is observed from the needle hub. A guidewire is then passed through the needle and into the vessel lumen, and the needle is then exchanged over the guidewire for a catheter or sheath. Selective catheterization of individual vessels involves advancing the guidewire into the arterial tree, with subsequent advancement of the catheter over the guidewire.

Diagnostic angiography is performed by positioning the catheter tip proximal within the artery of interest and rapidly injecting nonionic iodinated contrast medium, the rate and volume of which are proportional to the size of and flow within the vessel lumen. Rapid fluoroscopic spot filming is timed to coincide with contrast opacification of the arterial tree and documents progressive filling and washout of the vessels. Venous return may also be demonstrated with appropriate delays in filming. Abnormal findings associated with vascular trauma include transection, laceration, dissection, arteriovenous fistula, pseudoaneurysm, mural hematoma, intimal tears, and vasospasm.

Digital subtraction angiography (DSA) is a commonly used technique, whereby a preliminary fluoroscopic spot film (the "mask") is taken before contrast injection and is subsequently subtracted from dynamic images obtained during contrast injection. The background tissues (bones, soft tissues) are removed from the dynamic arterial images, resulting in greater image contrast resolution. The concentration of iodinated contrast may be reduced using this technique, resulting in a lower total volume of injected contrast medium. Disadvantages of this technique include lower-spatial resolution and misregistration artifact, which occurs as a result of patient motion after the mask image has been performed and results in misalignment of the mask during subtraction.

Therapeutic interventions may be performed during angiography and, for trauma patients, most commonly include embolization of bleeding arterial vessels in association with both visceral and bony fractures. Superselective catheterization of the bleeding vessel is first performed, with subsequent occlusion of the vessel using agents administered through the catheter. Temporary and permanent embolic agents are available, and their use is directed by the clinical situation and therapeutic goal. Temporary agents include autologous blood clots and Gelfoam pledgets, whereas permanent agents include microcoils and macrocoils, detachable balloons, polyvinyl alcohol, as well as various tissue adhesives and glues. Pre-embolization and postembolization angiograms are performed not only to document occlusion of the bleeding vessel but also to evaluate for collateral flow around the occluded vessel.

Complications of angiography include puncture site complications (e.g., groin hematoma, arteriovenous fistula, pseudoaneurysm), contrast complications (e.g., anaphylactoid reactions, renal failure), catheter-related complications (e.g., vessel wall dissection, thromboembolism), and therapy-related complications (e.g., tissue necrosis distal to embolization). Complications may be reduced with experience and careful technique by the angiographer.

Computed Tomography Angiography. CTA has become an established application of multislice helical CT technology. Intravenous nonionic iodinated contrast medium is injected, usually through an antecubital vein, using a volume of 120 to 150 mL at a rate of approximately 3 to 4 mL/s. Scanning is performed after an appropriate delay to ensure passage of contrast through the lungs and heart and into the arterial tree, so that imaging occurs during peak intravascular enhancement throughout the arterial segment of interest. Images are typically reconstructed from the helical dataset at 1-mm slice thicknesses with a 50% overlap. Because a typical CTA study generates hundreds to thousands of images, evaluation of the data is performed using 3D workstations, whereby the images may be viewed using cine modes, MPRs, and interactive real-time volume-rendering techniques. In addition to arterial injury, concomitant complex fractures are well evaluated on the same study. Factors that can limit accurate interpretation of CTA images include vasospasm, anatomic variants, atherosclerosis, displaced fracture fragments, metal hardware artifacts, foreign bodies, and patient motion or positioning problems.

Applications

Vascular Trauma. CTA using MDCT has become the imaging method of choice for the initial evaluation of vascular injury. CTA can be an important diagnostic and therapeutic modality in trauma patients with hemodynamic instability because of severe abdominal and pelvic trauma or extremity injuries with vascular damage (Fig. 17-11). Although management of a hemodynamically unstable patient with a pelvic fracture remains controversial, many experts suggest emergent angiography in these situations.[48] The yield in terms of identifiable arterial injury is low; however, when vascular injury is present, embolization using interventional techniques can be life saving. If necessary, pelvic angiography can be performed concomitantly with external fixation of the pelvis in patients with severe "open-book" injuries of the pelvic ring (Fig. 17-11).

More recently, CTA has emerged as a simple and effective means of assessing possible vascular injury of the pelvis and extremities. It is as accurate, less invasive, more time-efficient, and less expensive than standard angiography. CTA of the pelvis can be easily and successfully incorporated into standard CT evaluation protocols in patients with blunt trauma and is capable of differentiating active arterial and venous bleeding that can be useful information in guiding further care.[5] In a study of 48 trauma patients, contrast-enhanced CT was compared to formal angiography in detecting pelvic bleeding; CT had 94.1% sensitivity and 97.6% negative predictive value for the detection of active hemorrhage, and 92.6% sensitivity and 91.2% negative predictive value for predicting need for surgical or endovascular intervention.[133]

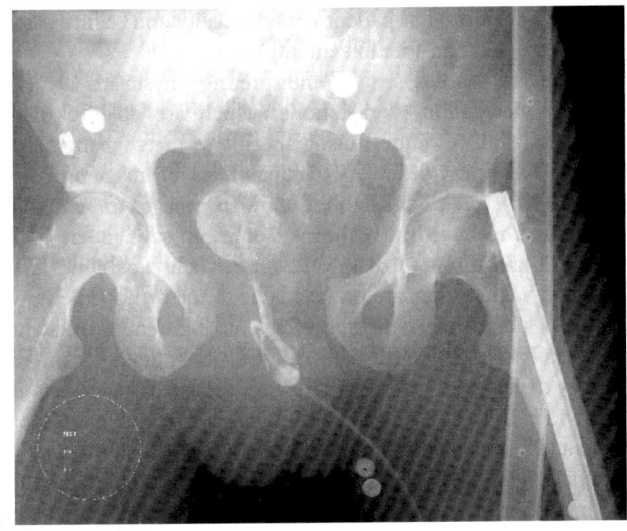

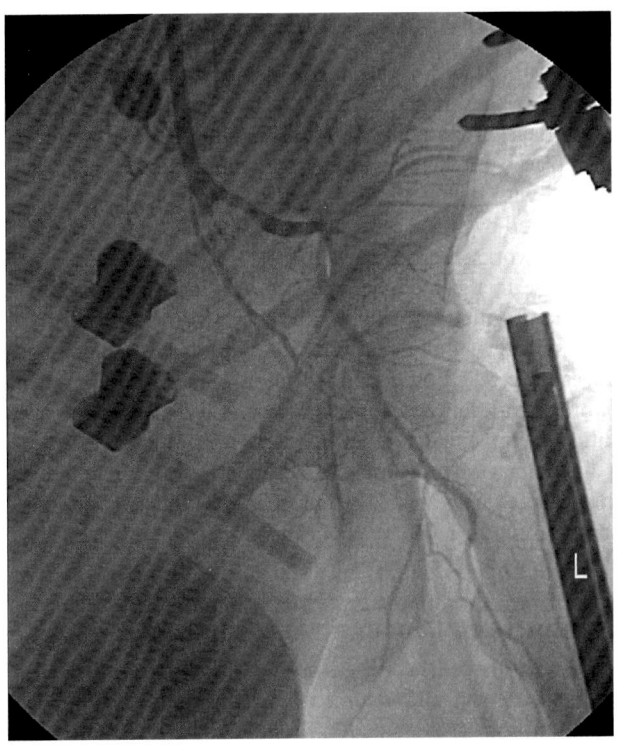

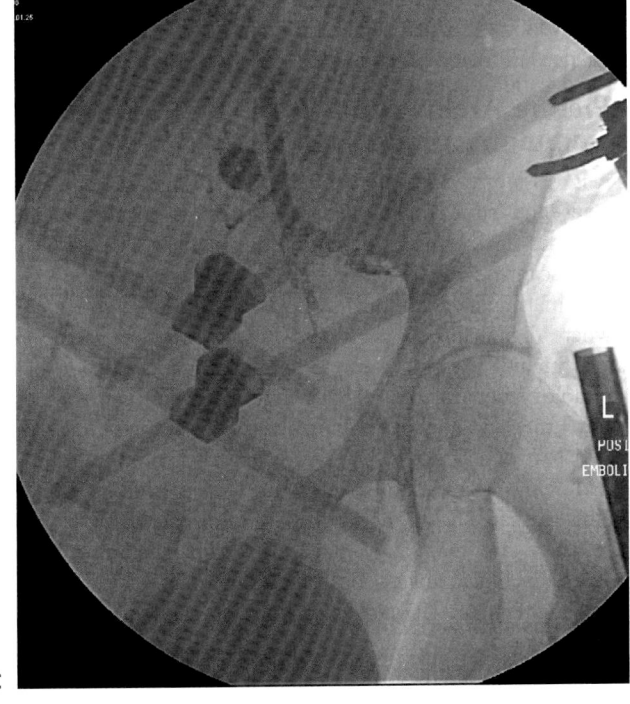

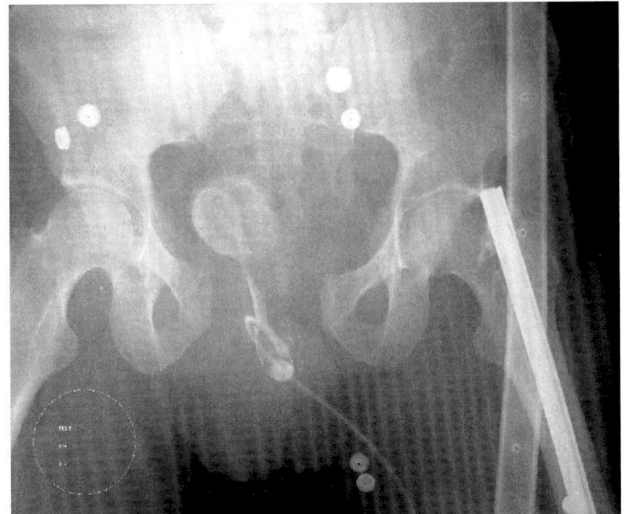

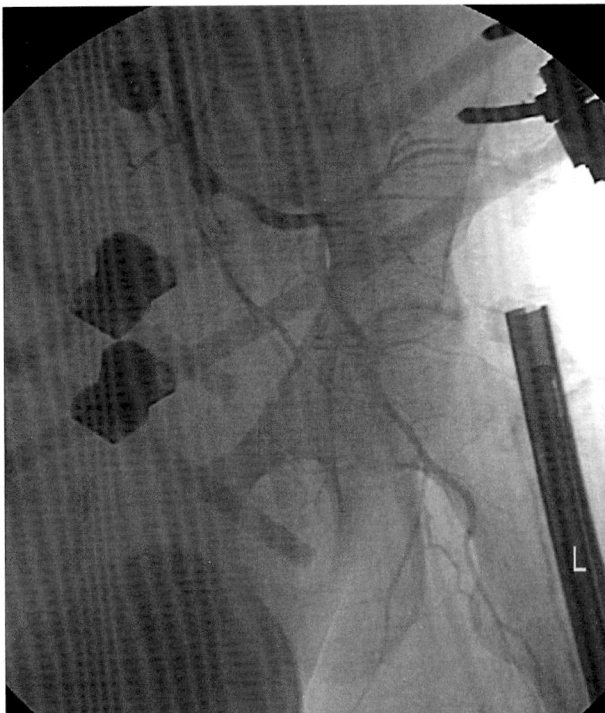

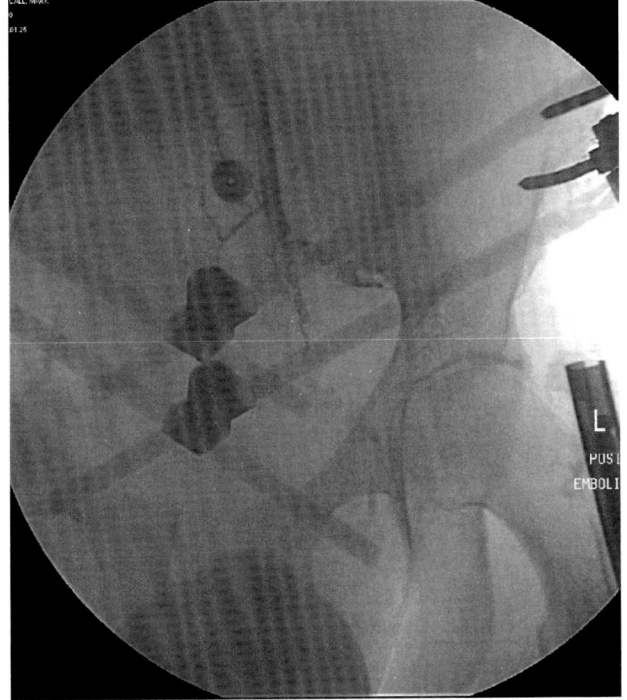

FIGURE 17-11 Pelvic angiography in a hemodynamically unstable trauma patient with a pelvic ring injury. **A:** The anteroposterior pelvic radiograph shows wide diastasis of the pubic symphysis. After emergent application of an anterior pelvic external fixator, the patient underwent selective embolization of both right and left internal iliac arteries. **B:** Spot film of the left internal iliac artery demonstrates dissection and nonfilling of multiple medial branches. Contrast fills the left internal iliac artery and its branches before embolization. **C:** Postembolization spot film demonstrates no flow of contrast distal to the embolization coils.

One traditional indication for angiography has been in the assessment of popliteal artery injury in the patient with definite or suspected knee dislocation. Recently, several studies have clarified the role of angiography in such patients, showing that urgent angiography is not needed unless there are deficits in distal pulses, ideally quantified by determination of the ankle-brachial index.[105,181]

CTA has significant advantages for the assessment of potential vascular injury in the lower extremity because of its noninvasiveness and immediate availability. CTA has supplanted arteriography as the imaging method of choice for the initial radiographic evaluation of peripheral vascular injuries.[72,156] Inaba et al.[93] used multislice CTA in 59 patients who underwent a total of 63 studies. In their

series, multislice CTA was both 100% sensitive and 100% specific for detecting clinically significant arterial injury.[93] A recent study by LeBus and Collinge[112] suggests that routine use of CTA in the evaluation of patients with high-energy tibial plafond injuries may be beneficial. Twenty-five consecutive patients were treated with a standard protocol that included preoperative CT (and CTA). In 13 of the patients (52%), notable arterial injury was identified, most involving the anterior tibial artery. The authors thought that information about associated vascular injury allowed them to make better decisions about surgical tactics to be used for a given procedure, including whether to use traditional open or minimally invasive approaches, as well as in choices about placement of incisions.[112]

MANAGEMENT OF IMAGING DATA

Advances in digital imaging modalities have necessarily been paralleled by advances in distributing, viewing, and storing imaging data. In many instances, the traditional light box has been replaced by digital workstations, the file room has been upgraded with digital archives, and the transport of films has been replaced by digital transmission of images across networks to remote workstations. Many of these changes have evolved in response to the increasing size of digital imaging studies, in addition to the need to use and distribute this information more efficiently within the health care environment. All of these changes have relied on continued improvements in computer networks, workstations, storage devices, and display media, in addition to implementation of standards, to support the evolving digital imaging infrastructure. Although a thorough discussion of digital image management is beyond the scope of this section, a brief review of some of the more common concepts and standards will be presented.

Distribution of Imaging Information

Distribution of medical images is influenced by several factors, including size and volume of imaging studies, computer network infrastructure, and clinical needs by interpreting and referring physicians. Current trends in digital imaging technology have resulted in greater image resolution and greater numbers of images, both of which substantially contribute to increasing sizes of imaging studies. For example, a typical 256×256 matrix image, using 2 bytes of storage for each pixel, requires approximately 125 KB of storage per image, whereas a 512×512 matrix image requires approximately 500 KB, or four times as much as its lower-resolution counterpart. CT and MRI studies routinely contain 100 to 200 images, resulting in storage requirements of 12 to 100 MB per study. Newer 64-slice and 256-slice CT scanners may result in data files of up to 2.5 and 10 GB, respectively, per study.

Media for distribution include printed films, CD-ROMs, and networks for remote viewing or processing on workstations (Fig. 17-5). When trauma patients are transported from one institution to another, import of images taken at the referring institution to a picture archive and communications system (PACS) at the receiving hospital, thereby reducing the need for repeat imaging at the receiving hospital.[123]

Many imaging devices are connected to networks for transmitting image data to remote locations for image viewing and storage, to which the term *teleradiology* applies. There is a wide variety of network configurations, with descriptors such as local or wide area networks (LAN, WAN), intranets, and the internet. Speed of transmission across networks depends on the various types of communication links within the network (modem, ISDN, DSL, cable modem, T1, T3, fiberoptic cable), as well as the level of network traffic. Data compression is used to decrease the size of imaging studies before electronic transmission, and compression schemes are categorized as "lossless" (no loss of original data, typically 3:1 compression) or "lossy" (some loss of data in original image, typically 15:1 or greater compression). Use of the internet to transmit imaging studies

is growing, although patient confidentiality and security issues have received considerable attention.

Imaging studies sent to interpreting physicians are commonly viewed on workstations, which are able to display images at full resolution using specific formats ("hanging protocols") and provide advanced capabilities for image processing (Fig. 17-5). Such workstations allow 3D images to be manipulated and reviewed in real-time; some can save movie files of the 3D image onto a disk. Of course, such capabilities are of limited value if they are not available to the orthopedic trauma surgeon in a timely manner. Current, high-end workstations are expensive and are usually not available outside of the radiology department; normally, less-sophisticated viewing stations provide basic access to images outside of the imaging department. In certain environments, use of hardcopy images will remain necessary. Examples of this situation include the operating room, where multiple images of different imaging modalities need to be viewed together by a surgeon in sterile operating garb, and in the clinic, where the viewing of multiple studies in chronologic order is necessary to observe fracture healing or changes in fracture alignment.

Picture Archive and Communications Systems

A PACS represents a network of mechanisms used to acquire, view, and store digital images and at its most basic level includes devices used to acquire digital images (e.g., CT and MRI scanners), workstations whereby images may be viewed and manipulated for diagnostic interpretations, and archives where digital images are stored for later retrieval. PACS may also include viewing stations for departments outside of the radiology department (e.g., emergency department, intensive care unit), and may be contained within their own LAN or exist as a part of a larger WAN. PACS may also communicate with Radiology Information Systems and Hospital Information Systems to share and/or modify patient information.

There are many advantages of PACS, including prompt access to clinical images, postprocessing of image data (window levels, MPRs and 3D reconstructions, measurement and annotations tools), the ability of more than one user to simultaneously view the same images, and reduced filming costs and lost films. On the other hand, significant disadvantages include initial and recurring expenses related to installing and maintaining PACS, massive storage requirements for image archival, and the necessity of support personnel to maintain the network and its components. One study showed that LCD personal computer monitors and PACS workstations did not differ significantly in the diagnostic quality of cervical spine fracture radiographs, suggesting that LCD personal computer monitors are sufficient for fast, accurate diagnosis in the emergency department for evaluation of cervical spine injuries at considerably reduced cost.[25]

Digital Imaging and Communications in Medicine Standards

In 1983, the American College of Radiology (ACR) and the National Electrical Manufacturers Association (NEMA) formed a joint committee to develop a standard by which users could retrieve images and associated information from digital imaging equipment in a form that would be compatible across all manufacturers. Two years later, the first version of the ACR-NEMA standard was published, and in 1988, an updated second version was published, which corrected errors and inconsistencies and added new data elements. The first two versions relied on point-to-point connections between equipment, and by 1988, the growing implementation of networks and PACS necessitated a complete rewriting of the standard, which is currently known as DICOM version 3.0.

The DICOM standard sets forth a uniform set of rules for communication of medical images and associated information, which are complex but practical and adaptable. The standard is flexible enough to accommodate a variety of images and image information across a broad range of medical imaging platforms. Conformance with the standard is voluntary, and manufacturers of medical imaging equipment or software who support the standard must provide conformance statements describing their particular implementation of the standard. This does not guarantee that two DICOM-compliant devices will communicate properly with one another; rather, the conformance statement serves as a guide to rule out obvious incompatibilities between equipment.

Digital Imaging and Teleradiology in Orthopedics

Digital Imaging

Digital imaging is the future of radiology and has definite advantages and disadvantages in the management of musculoskeletal injuries. In a recent review, Wade et al.[194] noted the many potential advantages of digital imaging: Reduction of foot traffic between clinics, wards, and the radiology department; increased availability of investigations; increase in the speed of availability; the virtual elimination of missing studies; less radiation exposure; fewer wasted films; and reduction in retrieval times. However, there are logistical problems associated with the adoption and use of filmless systems in an emergency department setting that must be overcome.[197] In addition, DR remains inferior to conventional radiography in terms of image spatial resolution (Table 17-1). Work is progressing in digital detector technology that may eventually provide spatial resolution equal to or exceeding that of conventional radiography. Miller et al.[135] describe the medical application of total-body DR for screening trauma patients, using a C-arm–based system initially developed in South Africa to detect theft by diamond miners. Full implementation of DR and PACS can be expensive and subject to the nuisances of technologic failure and requires technical support skills that may not be universally available. Traditional printed images will continue to have a role in the operating room, in the clinic, and in other venues where access to the PACS system is not available or appropriate.

Teleradiology

Teleradiology can affect the practice of fracture management in many ways. Teleradiology allows emergency physicians and/or house staff to send digital images of radiographs or clinical photographs to off-site attending orthopedic staff. There is potential application for community-based orthopedists to obtain second opinions about fracture management from specialists at tertiary care centers. Traditionally, such consultation required the referring orthopedic surgeon to obtain, duplicate, and mail hardcopies of radiographs to the consulting surgeon, who has then had to communicate his or her opinion to the referring surgeon by telephone. Using teleradiology, the transmission of patient information, imaging studies, and the consultant's evaluation can all be accomplished with greater convenience and less cost.

Ricci and Borrelli[167] demonstrated that teleradiology improved clinical decision making in the management of acute fractures. A series of 123 consecutive fractures was studied; in all cases, a junior orthopedic resident performed the initial orthopedic evaluation. All radiographs were digitized and electronically sent to the attending orthopedist. Treatment plans were formulated and documented at three different times: After verbal communication of the patient's history and injuries, after the digitized radiographs were viewed, and after the original hardcopy radiographs were viewed. The investigators recognized two different types of changes that were made to the initial plan of management: Acute treatment changes and changes in the definitive management of the fracture. Overall, the viewing of digitized radiographs resulted in a change of management in 21% of the fractures. No further changes in management were decided on after review of the original radiographs. The investigators concluded that the routine use of digitized radiographs improves fracture management.[167]

REFERENCES

1. Ahn JM, Sartoris DJ, Kang HS, et al. Gamekeeper thumb: Comparison of MR arthrography with conventional arthrography and MR imaging in cadavers. *Radiology.* 1998;206:737–744.
2. Akbarnia BA, Silberstein MJ, Rende RJ, et al. Arthrography in the diagnosis of fractures of the distal end of the humerus in infants. *J Bone Joint Surg Am.* 1986;68-A:599–602.
3. American College of Radiology Committee on Drugs and Contrast Media. Manual on contrast media, Version 5.0. 2004;13.
4. American College of Radiology Committee on Drugs and Contrast Media. Manual on contrast media, Version 5.0. 2004;7–10.
5. Anderson SW, Soto JA, Lucey BC, et al. Blunt trauma: Feasibility and clinical utility of pelvic CT angiography performed with 64-detector row CT. *Radiology.* 2008;246:410–419.
6. Anis AH, Stiell IG, Stewart DG, et al. Cost-effectiveness analysis of the Ottawa Ankle Rules. *Ann Emerg Med.* 1995;26:422–428.
7. Arand M, Hartwig E, Kinzl L, et al. Spinal navigation in cervical fractures: A preliminary clinical study on Judet-osteosynthesis of the axis. *Comput Aided Surg.* 2001;6:170–175.
8. Arora S, Grover SB, Batra S, et al. Comparative evaluation of postreduction intra-articular distal radial fractures by radiographs and multidetector computed tomography. *J Bone Joint Surg Am.* 2010;92-A:2523–2532.
9. Atesok K, Finkelstein J, Khoury A, et al. The use of intraoperative three-dimensional imaging (ISO-C-3D) in fixation of intraarticular fractures. *Injury.* 2007;38:1163–1169.
10. Barros JW, Barbieri CH, Fernandes CD. Scintigraphic evaluation of tibial shaft fracture healing. *Injury.* 2000;31:51–54.
11. Beck M, Kröber M, Mittlmeier T. Intraoperative three-dimensional fluoroscopy assessment of iliosacral screws and lumbopelvic implants stabilizing fractures of the os sacrum. *Arch Orthop Trauma Surg.* 2010;130:1363–1369.
12. Bencardino JT, Garcia AI, Palmer WE. Magnetic resonance imaging of the shoulder: Rotator cuff. *Top Magn Reson Imag.* 2003;14:51–67.
13. Bergin D, Schweitzer ME. Indirect magnetic resonance arthrography. *Skeletal Radiol.* 2003;32:551–558.
14. Bhattacharyya T, Bouchard KA, Phadke A, et al. The accuracy of computed tomography for the diagnosis of tibial nonunion. *J Bone Joint Surg Am.* 2006;88-A:692–697.
15. Blane CE, Kling TF, Andrews JC, et al. Arthrography in the posttraumatic elbow in children. *Am J Roentgenol.* 1984;143:17–21.
16. Blattert TR, Fill UA, Kunz E, et al. Skill dependence of radiation exposure for the orthopaedic surgeon during interlocking nailing of long-bone shaft fractures: A clinical study. *Arch Orthop Trauma Surg.* 2004;124:659–664.

17. Bleakney RR, Tallon C, Wong JK, et al. Long-term ultrasonographic features of the Achilles tendon after rupture. *Clin J Sports Med.* 2002;12:273–278.
18. Bonnarens F, Hernandez A, D'Ambrosia R. Bone scintigraphic changes in osteonecrosis of the femoral head. *Orthop Clin N Am.* 1985;16:697–703.
19. Bono CM, Vaccaro AR, Fehlings M, et al. Measurement techniques for lower cervical spine injuries: Consensus statement of the Spine Trauma Study Group. *Spine.* 2006;31:603–609.
20. Borrelli J Jr, Goldfarb C, Catalano L, et al. Assessment of articular fragment displacement in acetabular fractures: A comparison of computerized tomography and plain radiographs. *J Orthop Trauma.* 2002;16:449–456.
21. Borrelli J Jr, Ricci WM, Steger-May K, et al. Postoperative radiographic assessment of acetabular fractures: A comparison of plain radiographs and CT scans. *J Orthop Trauma.* 2005;19:299–304.
22. Borrelli J, Peelle M, McFarland E, et al. Computer-reconstructed radiographs are as good as plain radiographs for assessment of acetabular fractures. *Am J Orthop.* 2008;37:455–460.
23. Bosse MJ, Brumback RJ, Hash C. Medical cost containment: Analysis of dual orthopedic/radiology interpretation of X-rays in the trauma patient. *J Trauma.* 1995;38:220–222.
24. Botser IB, Herman A, Nathaniel R, et al. Digital image enhancement improves diagnosis of nondisplaced proximal femur fractures. *Clin Orthop Relat Res.* 2009;467:246–253.
25. Brem MH, Böhner C, Brenning A, et al. Evaluation of low-cost computer monitors for the detection of cervical spine injuries in the emergency room: An observer confidence based study. *Emerg Med.* 2006;23:850–853.
26. Bremer DJ, Hall EJ. Computed tomography: An increasing source of radiation exposure. *N Engl J Med.* 2007;357:2277–2284.
27. Brooks S, Cicuttini FM, Lim S, et al. Cost effectiveness of adding magnetic resonance imaging to the usual management of suspected scaphoid fractures. *Br J Sports Med.* 2005;39:75–79.
28. Calder SJ, McCaskie AW, Belton IP, et al. Single-photon-emission computerised tomography compared with planar bone scan to assess femoral head vascularity. *J Bone Joint Surg Br.* 1995;77-B:637–639.
29. Campbell DG, Menz A, Isaacs J. Dynamic ankle ultrasonography: A new imaging technique for acute ankle ligament injuries. *Am J Sports Med.* 1994;22:855–858.
30. Cantwell CP, Cradock A, Bruzzi J, et al. MR venography with true fast imaging with steady-state precession for suspected lower-limb deep vein thrombosis. *J Vasc Interv Radiol.* 2006;17:1763–1770.
31. Carelsen B, Haverlag R, Ubbink DTh, et al. Does intraoperative fluoroscopic 3D imaging provide extra information for fracture surgery? *Arch Orthop Trauma Surg.* 2008;128:1419–1424.
32. Caruso G, Lagalla R, Derchi L, et al. Monitoring of fracture calluses with color Doppler sonography. *J Clin Ultrasound.* 2000;28:20–27.
33. Chan PS, Klimkiewicz JJ, Luchetti WT, et al. Impact of CT scan on treatment plan and fracture classification of tibial plateau fractures. *J Orthop Trauma.* 1997;11:484–489.
34. Cheung Y, Perrich KD, Gui J, et al. MRI of isolated distal fibular fractures with widened medial clear space on stressed radiographs: Which ligaments are interrupted? *Am J Roentgenol.* 2009;192:W7–W12.
35. Chong KW, Wong MK, Rikhraj IS, et al. The use of computer navigation in performing minimally invasive surgery for intertrochanteric hip fractures—The experience in Singapore. *Injury.* 2006;37:755–762.
36. Churchill RS, Fehringer EV, Dubinsky TJ, et al. Rotator cuff ultrasonography: Diagnostic capabilities. *J Am Acad Orthop Surg.* 2004;12:6–11.
37. Cole RJ, Bindra RR, Evanoff BA, et al. Radiographic evaluation of osseous displacement following intra-articular fractures of the distal radius: Reliability of plain radiography versus computed tomography. *J Hand Surg Am.* 1997;22:792–800.
38. Collinge CA, Coons D, Tornetta P, et al. Standard multiplanar fluoroscopy versus a fluoroscopically based navigation system for the percutaneous insertion of iliosacral screws: A cadaver model. *J Orthop Trauma.* 2005;19:254–258.
39. Connell DA, Potter HG. Magnetic resonance evaluation of the labral capsular ligamentous complex: A pictorial review. *Australas Radiol.* 1999;43:419–426.
40. Crowl AC, Kahler DM. Closed reduction and percutaneous fixation of anterior column acetabular fractures. *Comput Aided Surg.* 2002;7:169–178.
41. Daffner RH, Wippold FJ III, Bennett DL, et al. ACR appropriateness criteria suspected spine trauma. 2009;2012. Available at: http://www.acr.org/~/media/ACR/Documents/AppCriteria/Diagnostic/SuspectedSpineTrauma.pdf. Accessed December 22, 2013.
42. Daffner RH. Helical CT of the cervical spine for trauma patients: A time study. *Am J Roentgenol.* 2001;177:677–679.
43. Davis BJ, Roberts PJ, Moorcroft CI, et al. Reliability of radiographs in defining union of internally fixed fractures. *Injury.* 2004;35:557–561.
44. Davison BL, Cantu R, Van Woerkom S. The magnetic attraction of lower extremity external fixators in an MRI suite. *J Orthop Trauma.* 2004;18:24–27.
45. Delcoigne L, Durant H, Kunnen M, et al. Digital subtraction in multicompartment arthrography of the wrist. *J Belge Radiol.* 1993;76:7–10.
46. Deutsch AL, Mink JH, Waxman AD. Occult fractures of the proximal femur: MR imaging. *Radiology.* 1989;170:113–116.
47. Disegi JA. Magnetic resonance imaging of AO/ASIF stainless steel and titanium implants. *Injury.* 1992;23:1–4.
48. Dondelinger RF, Trotteur G, Ghaye B, et al. Traumatic injuries: Radiological hemostatic intervention at admission. *Eur Radiol.* 2002;12:979–993.
49. Dorsay TA, Major NM, Helms CA. Cost-effectiveness of immediate MR imaging versus traditional follow-up for revealing radiographically occult scaphoid fractures. *Am J Roentgenol.* 2001;177:1257–1263.
50. Drane WE, Rudd TG. Femoral head viability following hip fracture. Prognostic role of radionuclide bone imaging. *Clin Nucl Med.* 1985;10:141–146.
51. Drvaric DM, Rooks MD. Anterior sleeve fracture of the capitellum. *J Orthop Trauma.* 1990;4(2):188–192.
52. Duane TM, Cole FJ Jr, Weireter LJ Jr, et al. Blunt trauma and the role of routine pelvic radiographs. *Am Surg.* 2001;67:849–852.
53. Duc SR, Pfirrmann CW, Schmid MR, et al. Articular cartilage defects detected with 3D water excitation true FISP: Prospective comparison with sequences commonly used for knee imaging. *Radiology.* 2007;245:216–223.
54. Dulchavsky SA, Henry SE, Moed BR, et al. Advanced ultrasonic diagnosis of extremity trauma: The FASTER examination. *J Trauma.* 2002;53:28–32.
55. Durston W, Swartzentruber R. Ultrasound-guided reduction of pediatric forearm fractures in the ED. *Am J Emerg Med.* 2000;18:72–77.
56. Ebraheim N, Skie MC, Podeszwa DA, et al. Evaluation of process fractures of the talus using computed tomography. *J Orthop Trauma.* 1994;8:332–337.
57. Eklof H, Radecka E, Liss P. Teleradiology Uppsala-Sydney for nighttime emergencies: Preliminary experience. *Acta Radiol.* 2007;48:851–853.
58. Esses SJ, Berman P, Bloom AI, et al. Clinical applications of physical 3D models derived from MDCT data and created by rapid prototyping. *Am J Roentgenol.* 2011;196:W683–W688.
59. Eustace S, Adams J, Assaf A. Emergency MR imaging of orthopaedic trauma. Current and future directions. *Radiol Clin North Am.* 1999;37:975–994.
60. Exadaktylos AK, Benneker LM, Jeger V, et al. Total-body digital X-ray in trauma. An experience report on the first operational full body scanner in Europe and its possible role in ATLS. *Injury.* 2008;39:525–529.
61. Farber JM. CT arthrography and postoperative musculoskeletal imaging with multichannel computed tomography. *Semin Musculoskelet Radiol.* 2004;8:157–166.
62. Farbman KS, Vinci RJ, Cranley WR, et al. The role of serial radiographs in the management of pediatric torus fractures. *Arch Pediatr Adolesc Med.* 1999;153:923–925.
63. Farrelly C, Davarpanah A, Brennan S, et al. Imaging of soft tissues adjacent to orthopedic hardware: Comparison of 3-T and 1.5-T MRI. *Am J Roentgenol.* 2010;194:W60–W64.
64. Fayad LM, Bluemke DA, Fishman EK. Musculoskeletal imaging with computed tomography and magnetic resonance imaging: When is computed tomography the study of choice? *Curr Probl Diagn Radiol.* 2005;34:220–237.
65. Fayad LM, Patra A, Fishman EK. Value of 3D CT in defining skeletal complications of orthopedic hardware in the postoperative patient. *Am J Roentgenol.* 2009;193:1155–1163.
66. Fazel R, Krumholz HM, Wang Y, et al. Exposure to low-dose ionizing radiation from medical imaging procedures. *N Engl J Med.* 2009;361:849–857.
67. Folio LR, Fischer T, Shogan P, et al. Blast and ballistic trajectories in combat casualties: A preliminary analysis using a Cartesian positioning system with MDCT. *Am J Roentgenol.* 2011;197:W233–W240.
68. Freund M, Thomsen M, Hohendorf B, et al. Optimized preoperative planning of calcaneal fractures using spiral computed tomography. *Eur Radiol.* 1999;9:901–906.
69. Frihagen F, Nordsletten L, Tariq R, et al. MRI diagnosis of occult hip fractures. *Acta Orthop.* 2005;76:524–530.
70. Fritz RC. MR imaging of meniscal and cruciate ligament injuries. *Magn Reson Imaging Clin N Am.* 2003;11:283–293.
71. Fujii M, Abe K, Hayashi K, et al. Honda sign and variants in patients suspected of having a sacral insufficiency fracture. *Clin Nucl Med.* 2005;30:165–169.
72. Gakhal MS, Sartip KA. CT angiography signs of lower extremity vascular trauma. *Am J Roentgenol.* 2009;193:W49–W57.
73. Garcia-Morales F, Seo GS, Chengazi V, et al. Collar osteophytes: A cause of false-positive findings in bone scans for hip fractures. *Am J Roentgenol.* 2003;181:191–194.
74. Gardner MJ, Citak M, Kendoff D, et al. Femoral fracture malrotation caused by free-hand versus navigated distal interlocking. *Injury.* 2008;39:17–180.
75. Geijer M, El-Khoury GY. Imaging of the acetabulum in the era of multidetector computed tomography. *Emerg Radiol.* 2007;14:271–287.
76. Ginde AA, Foianini A, Renner DM, et al. Availability and quality of computed tomography and magnetic resonance imaging equipment in U.S. emergency departments. *Acad Emerg Med.* 2008;15:780–783.
77. Grangier C, Garcia J, Howarth NR, et al. Role of MRI in the diagnosis of insufficiency fractures of the sacrum and acetabular roof. *Skeletal Radiol.* 1997;26:517–524.
78. Grechenig W, Peicha G, Fellinger M, et al. Wrist arthrography after acute trauma to the distal radius: Diagnostic accuracy, technique, and sources of diagnostic errors. *Invest Radiol.* 1998;33:273–278.
79. Green RA, Saifuddin A. Whole spine MRI in the assessment of acute vertebral body trauma. *Skeletal Radiol.* 2004;33:129–135.
80. Griffith B, Bolton C, Goyal N, et al. Screening cervical spine CT in a level I trauma center: Overutilization? *Am J Roentgenol.* 2011;197:463–467.
81. Grigoryan M, Lynch JA, Fierlinger AL, et al. Quantitative and qualitative assessment of closed fracture healing using computed tomography and conventional radiography. *Acad Radiol.* 2003;10:1267–1273.
82. Grogan EL, Morris JA Jr, Dittus RS, et al. Cervical spine evaluation in urban trauma centers: Lowering institutional costs and complications through helical CT scan. *J Am Coll Surg.* 2005;200:160–165.
83. Haapamaki VV, Kiuru MJ, Koskinen SK. Multidetector CT in shoulder fractures. *Emerg Radiol.* 2004;11:89–94.
84. Haramati N, Staron RB, Barax C, et al. Magnetic resonance imaging of occult fractures of the proximal femur. *Skeletal Radiol.* 1994;23:19–22.
85. Hargreaves Brian A., Worters PW, Pauly KB, et al. Metal-induced artifacts in MRI. *Am J Roentgenol.* 2011;197:547–555.
86. Harish S, Vince AS, Patel AD. Routine radiography following ankle fracture fixation: A case for limiting its use. *Injury.* 1990;30:231–235.
87. Harness NG, Ring D, Zurakowski D, et al. The influence of three-dimensional computed tomography reconstructions on the characterization and treatment of distal radial fractures. *J Bone Joint Surg Am.* 2006;88-A:1315–1323.
88. Harris JH, Coupe KJ, Lee JS, et al. Acetabular fractures revisited: Part 2, A new CT-based classification. *Am J Roentgenol.* 2004;182:1367–1375.
89. Herneth AM, Siegmeth A, Bader TR, et al. Scaphoid fractures: Evaluation with high-spatial-resolution US – initial results. *Radiology.* 2001;220:231–235.

90. Holt MD, Williams LA, Dent CM. MRI in the management of tibial plateau fractures. *Injury*. 1995;26:595–599.
91. Horn BD, Crisci K, Krug M, et al. Radiologic evaluation of juvenile Tillaux fractures of the distal tibia. *J Ped Orthop*. 2001;21:162–164.
92. Hougaard K, Lindequist S, Nielsen LB. Computerised tomography after posterior dislocation of the hip. *J Bone Joint Surg Br*. 1987;69-B:556–557.
93. Inaba K, Potzman J, Munera F, et al. Multi-slice CT angiography for arterial evaluation in the injured lower extremity. *J Trauma*. 2006;60:502–507.
94. Javed A, Guichet JM. Arthrography for reduction of a fracture of the radial neck in a child with a nonossified radial epiphysis. *J Bone Joint Surg Br*. 2001;83-B:542–543.
95. Jones DG, Stoddart J. Radiation use in the orthopaedic theatre: A prospective audit. *Aust NZ J Surg*. 1998;68:782–784.
96. Kahler DM. Virtual fluoroscopy: A tool for decreasing radiation exposure during femoral intramedullary nailing. *Stud Health Technol Inform*. 2001;81:225–228.
97. Kaneriya PP, Schweitzer ME, Spettell C, et al. The cost-effectiveness of routine pelvic radiography in the evaluation of blunt trauma patients. *Skeletal Radiol*. 1999;28:271–273.
98. Kendoff D, Citak M, Gardner M, et al. Three-dimensional fluoroscopy for evaluation of articular reduction and screw placement in calcaneal fractures. *Foot Ankle Int*. 2007;28:1165–1171.
99. Kendoff D, Gardner MJ, Citak M, et al. Value of 3D fluoroscopic imaging of acetabular fractures. Comparison to 2D fluoroscopy and CT imaging. *Arch Orthop Trauma Surg*. 2008;128:599–605.
100. Khoo JN, Chong LR, Chan EH-Y, et al. Pitfalls in multidetector computed tomography imaging of traumatic spinal injuries. *Emerg Radiol*. 2011;18:551–562.
101. Khoury A, Liebergall M, Weil Y, et al. Computerized fluoroscopic-based navigation-assisted intramedullary nailing. *Am J Orthop*. 2007;36:582–585.
102. Kim T-Y, Lee GY, Kim BH, et al. The usefulness of dynamic cine-arthrography for wrist instability as correlated with arthroscopic palmer classification. *J Korean Soc Radiol*. 2011;64:265–271.
103. Kirby MW, Spritzer C. Radiographic detection of hip and pelvic fractures in the emergency department. *Am J Roentgenol*. 2010;194:1054–1060.
104. Kirkpatrick AW, Brown R, Diebel LN, et al. Rapid diagnosis of an ulnar fracture with portable hand-held ultrasound. *Mil Med*. 2003;168:312–313.
105. Klineberg EO, Crites BM, Flinn WR, et al. The role of arteriography in assessing popliteal artery injury in knee dislocations. *J Trauma*. 2004;56:786–790.
106. Kolind SH, MacKay AL, Munk PL, et al. Quantitative evaluation of metal artifact reduction techniques. *J Magn Reson Imaging*. 2004;20:487–495.
107. Körner M, Geyer LL, Wirth S, et al. 64-MDCT in mass casualty incidents: Volume image reading boosts radiological workflow. *Am J Roentgenol*. 2011;197:W399–W404.
108. Krettek C, Miclau T, Grün O, et al. Intraoperative control of axes, rotation, and length in femoral and tibial fractures. Technical Note *Injury*. 1998;29:C29–C39.
109. Kukla C, Gaebler C, Breitenseher MJ, et al. Occult fractures of the scaphoid. The diagnostic usefulness and indirect economic repercussions of radiography versus magnetic resonance scanning. *J Hand Surg Br*. 1997;22:810–813.
110. Kumar R, Lerski RA, Gandy S, et al. Safety of orthopedic implants in magnetic resonance imaging: An experimental verification. *J Orthop Res*. 2006;24:1799–1802.
111. Kurozumi T, Jinno Y, Sato T, et al. Open reduction for intra-articular calcaneal fractures: Evaluation using computed tomography. *Foot Ankle Int*. 2003;24:942–948.
112. LeBus GF, Collinge C. Vascular abnormalities as assessed with CT angiography in high-energy tibial plafond fractures. *J Orthop Trauma*. 2008;22:16–22.
113. Leet AI, Young C, Hoffer MM. Medial condyle fractures of the humerus in children. *J Pediatr Orthop*. 2002;22:2–7.
114. Lehnert T., Naguib NN, Ackermann H, et al. Novel, portable, cassette-sized, and wireless flat-panel digital radiography system: Initial workflow results versus computed radiography. *Am J Roentgenol*. 2011;196:1368–1371.
115. Leung KS, Tang N, Cheung LWH, et al. Image-guided navigation in orthopaedic trauma. *J Bone Joint Surg Br*. 2010;92-B:1332–1337.
116. Levy AD, Harcke HT. Handheld ultrasound device for detection of nonopaque and semi-opaque foreign bodies in soft tissues. *J Clin Ultrasound*. 2003;31:183–188.
117. Liebergall M, Ben-David D, Weil Y, et al. Computerized navigation for the internal fixation of femoral neck fractures. *J Bone Joint Surg Am*. 2006;88-A:1748–1754.
118. Lim KB, Eng AK, Chng SM, et al. Limited magnetic resonance imaging (MRI) and the occult hip fracture. *Ann Acad Med Singapore*. 2002;31:607–610.
119. Lobenhoffer P, Schulze M, Gerich T, et al. Closed reduction/percutaneous fixation of tibial plateau fractures: Arthroscopic versus fluoroscopic control of reduction. *J Orthop Trauma*. 1999;13:426–431.
120. Lonner JH, Dupuy DE, Siliski JM. Comparison of magnetic resonance imaging with operative findings in acute traumatic dislocations of the adult knee. *J Orthop Trauma*. 2000;14:183–186.
121. Loredo R, Sanders TG. Imaging of osteochondral injuries. *Clin Sports Med*. 2001;20:249–278.
122. Love C, Patel M, Lonner BS, et al. Diagnosing spinal osteomyelitis: A comparison of bone and Ga-67 scintigraphy and magnetic resonance imaging. *Clinical Nucl Med*. 2000;25:963–977.
123. Lu MT, Tellis WM, Fidelman N, et al. Reducing the rate of repeat imaging: Import of outside images to PACS. *Am J Roentgenol*. 2012;198:628–634.
124. Lubovsky O, Liebergall M, Mattan Y, et al. Early diagnosis of occult hip fractures MRI versus CT scan. *Injury*. 2005;36:788–792.
125. Luechinger R, Boesiger P, Disegi JA. Safety evaluation of large external fixation clamps and frames in a magnetic resonance environment. *J Biomed Mater Res B*. 2007;82:17–22.
126. Lynch JA, Grigoryan M, Fierlinger A, et al. Measurement of changes in trabecular bone at fracture sites using X-ray CT and automated image registration and processing. *J Orthop Res*. 2004;22:362–367.
127. Mack MG, Keim S, Balzer JO, et al. Clinical impact of MRI in acute wrist fractures. *Eur Radiol*. 2003;13:612–617.
128. Mandelstam S, Cook D, Fitzgerald M, et al. Complementary use of radiological skeletal survey and bone scintigraphy in detection of bony injuries in suspected child abuse. *Arch Dis Child*. 2003;88:387–390.
129. Marzo JM, d'Amato C, Strong M, et al. Usefulness and accuracy of arthrography in management of lateral humeral condyle fractures in children. *J Pediatr Orthop*. 1990;10:317–321.
130. Matin P. The appearance of bone scans following fractures, including immediate and long-term studies. *J Nucl Med*. 1979;20:1227–1231.
131. Matsui Y, Myoui A, Nakahara H, et al. Prognostic significance of posterior subtalar joint arthrography following fractures of the calcaneus. *Arch Orthop Trauma Surg*. 1995;114:257–259.
132. Matthews F, Hoigne DJ, Weiser M, et al. Navigating the fluoroscope's C-arm back into position: An accurate and practicable solution to cut radiation and optimize intraoperative workflow. *J Orthop Trauma*. 2007;21:687–692.
133. Maturen KE, Adusumilli S, Blane CE, et al. Contrast-enhanced CT accurately detects hemorrhage in torso trauma: Direct comparison with angiography. *J Trauma*. 2007;62:740–745.
134. McAdams TR, Blevins FT, Martin TP, et al. The role of plain films and computed tomography in the evaluation of scapular neck fractures. *J Orthop Trauma*. 2002;16:7–11.
135. Miller LA, Mirvis SE, Harris L, et al. Total-body digital radiography for trauma screening: Initial experience. *Appl Radiol*. 2004;33:8–14.
136. Moed BR, Carr SEW, Gruson KI, et al. Computed tomographic assessment of fractures of the posterior wall of the acetabulum after operative treatment. *J Bone Joint Surg Am*. 2003;85-A:512–522.
137. Moed BR, Subramanian S, van Holsbeeck M, et al. Ultrasound for the early diagnosis of tibial fracture healing after static interlocked nailing without reaming: Clinical results. *J Orthop Trauma*. 1998;12:206–213.
138. Montgomery KD, Potter HG, Helfet DL. Magnetic resonance venography to evaluate the deep venous system of the pelvis in patients who have an acetabular fracture. *J Bone Joint Surg Am*. 1995;77-A:1639–1649.
139. Mortensson W, Rosenborg M, Gretzer H. The role of bone scintigraphy in predicting femoral head collapse following cervical fractures in children. *Acta Radiol*. 1990;31:291–292.
140. Mosheiff R, Khoury A, Weil Y, et al. First generation computerized fluoroscopic navigation in percutaneous pelvic surgery. *J Orthop Trauma*. 2004;18:106–111.
141. Muchow RD, Resnick DK, Abdel MP, et al. Magnetic resonance imaging (MRI) in the clearance of the cervical spine in blunt trauma: A meta-analysis. *J Trauma*. 2008;64:179–189.
142. Mulkens TH, Marchal P, Daineffe S, et al. Comparison of low-dose with standard-dose multidetector CT in cervical spine trauma. *Am J Neuroradiol*. 2007;28:1444–1450.
143. Mulligan ME, Flye CW. Initial experience with Lodox Statscan imaging system for detecting injuries of the pelvis and appendicular skeleton. *Emerg Radiol*. 2006;13:129–133.
144. Mustonen AOT, Koivikko MP, Kiuru MJ, et al. Postoperative MDCT of tibial plateau fractures. *Am J Roentgenol*. 2009;193(5):1354–1360.
145. NCRP. Report No. 160: Ionizing Radiation Exposure to the Population of the United States; 2009.
146. Nepola JV, Seabold JE, Marsh JL, et al. Diagnosis of infection in ununited fractures. Combined imaging with indium-111-labeled leukocytes and technetium-99m methylene diphosphonate. *J Bone Joint Surg Am*. 1993;75-A:1816–1822.
147. Norris BL, Hahn DH, Bosse MJ, et al. Intraoperative fluoroscopy to evaluate fracture reduction and hardware placement during acetabular surgery. *J Orthop Trauma*. 1999;13:414–417.
148. O'Toole RV, Cox G, Shanmuganathan K, et al. Evaluation of computed tomography for determining the diagnosis of acetabular fractures. *J Orthop Trauma*. 2010;24:284–290.
149. Orbell JH, Smith A, Burnand KG, et al. Imaging of deep vein thrombosis. *Br J Surg*. 2008;95:137–146.
150. Pakos EE, Koumoulis HD, Fotopoulos AD, et al. Osteomyelitis: Antigranulocyte scintigraphy with 99mTc radiolabeled monoclonal antibodies for diagnosis: Meta-analysis. *Radiology*. 2007;245:732–741.
151. Palestro CJ, Torres MA. Radionuclide imaging in orthopedic infections. *Semin Nucl Med*. 1997;27:334–345.
152. Palestro CJ. The current role of gallium imaging in infection. *Semin Nucl Med*. 1994;24:128–141.
153. Parker L, Nazarian LN, Carrino JA, et al. Musculoskeletal imaging: Medicare use, costs, and potential for cost substitution. *J Am Coll Radiol*. 2008;5:182–188.
154. Peetrons P. Ultrasound of muscles. *Eur Radiol*. 2002;12:35–43.
155. Peh WCG, Khong P-L, Yin Y, et al. Imaging of pelvic insufficiency fractures. *Radiographics*. 1996;16:335–348.
156. Peng PD, Spain DA, Tataria M, et al. CT angiography effectively evaluates extremity vascular trauma. *Am Surg*. 2008;74:103–107.
157. Peters AM. The utility of [99mTc]HMPAO-leukocytes for imaging infection. *Semin Nucl Med*. 1994;24:110–127.
158. Pitcher RD, van As AB, Sanders V, et al. A pilot study evaluating the "STATSCAN" digital X-ray machine in paediatric polytrauma. *Emerg Radiol*. 2008;15:35–42.
159. Pool FJ, Crabbe JP. Occult femoral neck fractures in the elderly: Optimisation of investigation. *N Z Med J*. 1996;109:235–237.
160. Porrino JA Jr, Kohl CA, Holden D, et al. The Importance of sagittal 2D reconstruction in pelvic and sacral trauma: Avoiding oversight of U-shaped fractures of the sacrum. *Am J Roentgenol*. 2010;194:1065–1071.
161. Potter HG, Nestor BJ, Sofka CM, et al. Magnetic resonance imaging after total hip arthroplasty: Evaluation of periprosthetic soft tissue. *J Bone Joint Surg Am*. 2004;86-A:1947–1954.
162. Prasarn ML, Martin E, Schreck M, et al. Analysis of radiation exposure to the orthopaedic trauma patient during their inpatient hospitalisation. *Injury*. 2012;43:757–761.
163. Pruitt DL, Gilula LA, Manske PR, et al. Computed tomography scanning with image reconstruction in evaluation of distal radius fractures. *J Hand Surg Am*. 1994;19:720–727.

164. Pudas T, Hurme T, Mattila K, et al. Magnetic resonance imaging in pediatric elbow fractures. *Acta Radiol.* 2005;46:636–644.
165. Raby N. Magnetic resonance imaging of suspected scaphoid fractures using a low field dedicated extremity MR system. *Clin Radiol.* 2001;56:316–320.
166. Rangger C, Kathrein A, Freund MC, et al. Bone bruise of the knee: Histology and cryosections in 5 cases. *Acta Orthop.* 1998;69:291–294.
167. Ricci WM, Borrelli J. Teleradiology in orthopaedic surgery: Impact on clinical decision making for acute fracture management. *J Orthop Trauma.* 2002;16:1–6.
168. Richards PJ, Summerfield R, George J, et al. Major trauma and cervical clearance radiation doses and cancer induction. *Injury.* 2008;39:347–356.
169. Richter M, Geerling J, Zech S, et al. Intraoperative three-dimensional imaging with a motorized mobile C-arm (SIREMOBIL ISO-C-3D) in foot and ankle trauma care: A preliminary report. *J Orthop Trauma.* 2005;19:259–266.
170. Robbins MI, Anzilotti KF, Katz LD, et al. Patient perception of magnetic resonance arthrography. *Skeletal Radiol.* 2000;29:265–269.
171. Roberts CS, Beck DJ Jr, Heinsen J, et al. Diagnostic ultrasonography: Applications in orthopaedic surgery. *Clin Orthop Rel Res.* 2002;401:248–264.
172. Roemer FW, Bohndorf K. Long-term osseous sequelae after acute trauma of the knee joint evaluated by MRI. *Skeletal Radiol.* 2002;31:615–623.
173. Saxena P, McDonald R, Gull S, et al. Diagnostic scanning for suspected scaphoid fractures: An economic evaluation based on cost-minimisation models. *Injury.* 2003;34:503–511.
174. Schmid MR, Pfirrmann CW, Hodler J, et al. Cartilage lesions in the ankle joint: Comparison of MR arthrography and CT arthrography. *Skeletal Radiol.* 2003;32:259–265.
175. Seabold JE, Nepola JV. Imaging techniques for evaluation of postoperative orthopaedic infections. *Q J Nucl Med.* 1999;43:21–28.
176. Smith TO, Drew B, Toms AP, et al. Diagnostic accuracy of magnetic resonance imaging and magnetic resonance arthrography for triangular fibrocartilaginous complex injury: A systematic review and meta-analysis. *J Bone Joint Surg Am.* 2012;94-A:824–832.
177. Smith-Bindman R, Lipson J, Marcus R, et al. Radiation dose associated with common computed tomography examinations and the associated lifetime attributable risk of cancer. *Arch Int Med.* 2009;169:2078–2086.
178. Smith-Bindman R, Miglioretti DL, Johnson E, et al. Use of diagnostic imaging studies and associated radiation exposure for patients enrolled in large integrated health care systems, 1996–2010. *JAMA.* 2012;307:2400–2409.
179. Sofka C, Potter HG, Figgie M, et al. Magnetic resonance imaging of total knee arthroplasty. *Clin Orthop Rel Res.* 2003;406:129–135.
180. Sofka CM, Potter HG. MR imaging of joint arthroplasty. *Semin Musculoskelet Radiol.* 2002;6:79–85.
181. Stannard JP, Sheils TM, Lopez-Ben RR, et al. Vascular injuries in knee dislocations: The role of physical examination in determining the need for arteriography. *J Bone Joint Surg Am.* 2004;86-A:910–915.
182. Steinbach LS, Palmer WE, Schweitzer ME. Special focus session. MR arthrography. *Radiographics.* 2002;22:1223–1246.
183. Stübig T, Kendoff D, Citak M, et al. Comparative Study of Different Intraoperative 3-D Image Intensifiers in Orthopedic Trauma Care. *J Trauma.* 2009;66:821–830.
184. Stucken C, Olszewski DC, Creevy WR, et al. The preoperative diagnosis of infection in nonunions. *J Bone Joint Surg Am.* 2013;95(15):1409–1412.
185. Suhm N, Jacob AL, Nolte LP, et al. Surgical navigation based on fluoroscopy: Clinical application for computer-assisted distal locking of intramedullary implants. *Comput Aided Surg.* 2000;5:391–400.
186. Theocharopoulos N, Damilakis J, Perisinakis K, et al. Image-guided reconstruction of femoral fractures: Is the staff progeny safe? *Clin Orthop.* 2005;430:182–188.
187. Thomas SH, Orf J, Peterson C, et al. Frequency and costs of laboratory and radiograph repetition in trauma patients undergoing interfacility transfer. *Am J Emerg Med.* 2000;18:156–158.
188. Tirman PFJ, Smith ED, Stoller DW, et al. Shoulder imaging in athletes. *Semin Musculoskelet Radiol.* 2004;8:29–40.
189. Tomycz ND, Chew BG, Chang YF, et al. MRI is unnecessary to clear the cervical spine in obtunded/comatose trauma patients: The four-year experience of a level I trauma center. *J Trauma.* 2008;64:1258–1263.
190. Tornetta P, Gorup J. Axial computed tomography of pilon fractures. *Clin Orthop.* 1996;323:273–276.
191. Vasarhelyi A, Lubitz J, Gierer P, et al. Detection of fibular torsional deformities after surgery for ankle fractures with a novel CT method. *Foot Ankle Int.* 2006;27:1115–1121.
192. Verlaan JJ, van de Kraats EB, Dhert WJ, et al. The role of 3-D rotational x-ray imaging in spinal trauma. *Injury.* 2005;36:B98–B103.
193. Vocke-Hell AK, Schmid A. Sonographic differentiation of stable and unstable lateral condyle fractures of the humerus in children. *J Pediatr Orthop B.* 2001;10:138–141.
194. Wade FA, Oliver CW, McBride K. Digital imaging in trauma and orthopaedic surgery: Is it worth it? *J Bone Joint Surg Br.* 2000;82-B:791–794.
195. Wehrli FW, Song HK, Saha PK, et al. Quantitative MRI for the assessment of bone structure and function. *NMR Biomed.* 2006;19:731–764.
196. Weil YA, Gardner MJ, Helfet DL, et al. Computer navigation allows for accurate reduction of femoral fractures. *Clin Orthop Rel Res.* 2007;460:185–191.
197. White FA, Zwemer FL Jr, Beach C, et al. Emergency department digital radiology: Moving from photos to pixels. *Acad Emerg Med.* 2004;11:1213–1222.
198. White LM, Miniaci A. Cruciate and posterolateral corner injuries in the athlete: Clinical and magnetic resonance imaging features. *Semin Musculoskelet Radiol.* 2004;8:111–131.
199. Wicky S, Blaser PF, Blanc CH, et al. Comparison between standard radiography and spiral CT with 3D reconstruction in the evaluation, classification, and management of tibial plateau fractures. *Eur Radiol.* 2000;10:1227–1232.
200. Winalski CS, Gupta KB. Magnetic resonance imaging of focal articular cartilage lesions. *Top Magn Reson Imag.* 2003;14:131–144.
201. Wolf G, Aigner RM, Schwarz T. Diagnosis of bone infection using 99m Tc-HMPAO labelled leukocytes. *Nucl Med Commun.* 2001;22:1201–1206.
202. Wood TO. MRI safety and compatibility of implants and medical devices. In: G.L. Winters and M.J. Nutt, eds. *Stainless Steels for Medical and Surgical Applications, ASTM STP 1438.* West Conshohocken, PA: ASTM International; 2003:187.
203. Wu J, Davuluri P, Ward KR, et al. Fracture detection in traumatic pelvic CT images. *Int J Biomed Imaging.* 2012;2012:327198.
204. Yacoubian SV, Nevins RT, Sallis JG, et al. Impact of MRI on treatment plan and fracture classification of tibial plateau fractures. *J Orthop Trauma.* 2002;16:632–637.
205. Yin Y, Wilson AJ, Gilula LA. Three-compartment wrist arthrography: Direct comparison of digital subtraction with nonsubtraction images. *Radiology.* 1995;197:287–290.
206. Youn MH, Roh J-Y, Kim S-B, et al. Evaluation of the sigmoid notch involvement in the intra-articular distal radius fractures: The efficacy of computed tomography compared with plain x-ray. *Clin Orthop Surg.* 2012;4:83–90.
207. Zierler BK. Ultrasonography and diagnosis of venous thromboembolism. *Circulation.* 2004;109:I9–I14.

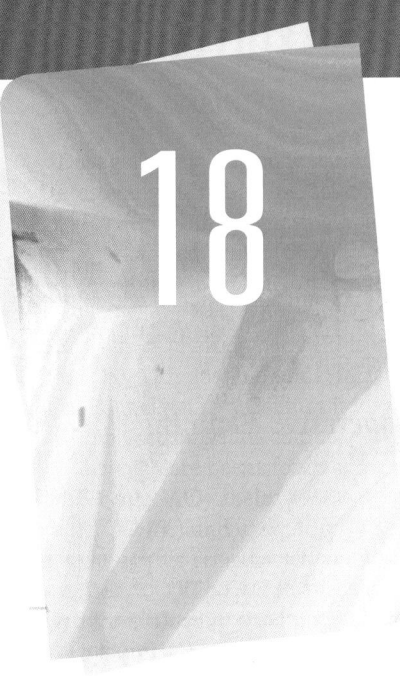

18 COMPUTER-AIDED ORTHOPEDIC SURGERY IN SKELETAL TRAUMA

Meir Liebergall, Rami Mosheiff, and Leo Joskowicz

INTRODUCTION

Computers are becoming pervasive in all fields of human endeavor, and medicine is no exception. Starting with the advent of computed tomography (CT) in the 1970s, computer-based systems have become the standard of care in many clinical fields, most notably in radiology, radiation therapy, neurosurgery, and orthopedics. These systems assist the surgeon in planning, executing, and evaluating the surgery, often improving existing procedures and at times enabling new procedures that could not have been realized without them.

The first computer-based systems for surgery were developed in the mid-1980s for neurosurgery. The key characteristic of these systems was an integration of preoperative information with intraoperative execution. Traditionally, preoperative radiographs, CT scans, and magnetic resonance images (MRIs) showing the patient's condition and the planned approach are brought into the operating room to guide the surgeon. However, when performing surgical actions, it is not possible to determine exactly where the surgical tools and implants are with respect to these images, especially when direct line of sight is limited, such as in keyhole, minimally invasive, and percutaneous surgery. Often, intraoperative images, such as fluoroscopic radiographs, are acquired to monitor the location of tools, implants, and anatomy. The surgeon must then mentally recreate the spatiotemporal situation from these images and decide on a course of action. This mental integration is qualitative and imprecise, as is the surgeon's hand–eye coordination, which requires significant skill, experience, and judgment and varies from surgeon to surgeon.

Computer-aided surgery (CAS) systems perform this integration automatically and accurately, thereby providing the surgeon with a precise, more complete, and up-to-date view of the intraoperative situation.[55] By incorporating real-time tracking of the location of instruments and anatomy, and their precise relation to preoperative and intraoperative images, the systems create a new modality akin to continuous imaging. In this sense, CAS systems are like navigators based on global positioning systems (GPSs), currently found in cars that help drivers find their way to a desired destination. During driving, the system shows the exact location of the car at all times on a computerized map and provides turn-by-turn directions ahead of time.

In orthopedics, the first CT-based navigation commercial systems were introduced in the mid-1990s for spinal surgery.[30] Several years later, fluoroscopic radiography-based systems were developed for total hip and total knee replacement.[39] Today, a variety of image-free and image-based systems exist for planning and executing a variety of orthopedic procedures, including primary and revision total hip and total knee replacement; anterior cruciate ligament reconstruction; spinal pedicle screw insertion; and trauma.[9,10,16,18,31,39,43]

CAS has already become an integral part of the orthopedic trauma surgery setup. The rapid advancement in the use of computers in this field provides many feasible options at all stages of treatment of the orthopedic trauma patient, from preoperative planning to postoperative evaluation. The role of computerization in the treatment of trauma patients is not only to enhance the surgical options in the preplanning stage but also to shorten surgery, an advantage that could be crucial for patient morbidity in a trauma setup. Although computerized imaging equipment can be moved into the admitting area and/or the trauma unit of the emergency department, this may involve adaptation of an existing setup, requiring administrative changes and incurring high costs. Another option is the use of comprehensive imaging provided by the improvement of conventional image intensifiers in achieving accurate three-dimensional (3D) information in a minimal period of time inside the operating room, such as can be achieved with isocentric fluoroscopy and mobile CT-like machines.

Computerized navigation has thus been a key factor in expanding the use of CAS from the preplanning to the intraoperative stage. This expansion integrates well with the current tendency toward minimal invasive surgery. CAS technology brings important digitized information into the operating room, enabling the accomplishment of three main goals: Minimal invasive surgery, maximal accuracy, and robustness. Moreover, both surgeon and patient benefit from a significant reduction in the amount of radiation exposure usually associated with orthopedic trauma surgery. The main modality, which is currently in various stages of application and has been adapted to trauma surgery, is fluoroscopy-based navigation including modern mobile 3D image intensifiers. While this technology might be viewed by some as only improved fluoroscopy, it is undoubtedly this modality that has allowed computer-based navigation systems to become a pioneer in the process of CAS integration into the orthopedic trauma operating room.

TECHNICAL ELEMENTS

Computer-aided orthopedic surgery in skeletal trauma (CAOS–ST) systems consist mainly of preoperative planning, when available and feasible, and intraoperative navigation. Robotic and verification technologies are still experimental and at present are seldom used.[9] We will describe the technical principles of each and the existing types of navigation systems.

Computerized Preoperative Planning and Model Construction

Preoperative planning for skeletal trauma surgery has traditionally been accomplished using radiographic and CT films. The drawbacks of this traditional practice are that anatomic measurements are either approximate or cannot be obtained; that fixation plates and implant templates are usually not available; that the size, position, and orientation of the implants can only be approximately determined; and that spatial views are unavailable. Consequently, only a few surgical alternatives can be explored.

Digital radiographic and CT data have significantly improved and allow for better planning. Digital radiographic images can be correlated and anatomic measurements, such as anteversion angle and leg length, can be performed on them. Digital templates of fixation and implant devices can be superimposed onto the radiographic images to explore a variety of alternatives. Computer-aided planning packages allow surgeons to select digital templates of fixation devices, position them, and take appropriate measurements. This computerized support allows for greater accuracy, versatility, and simplicity as compared with traditional analog templating and measuring techniques.[4,38] Figure 18-1A shows a screenshot of a preoperative planning session for internal fixation of a fractured tibia.

For CT data, preoperative planning allows for 3D measurements and spatial visualization of complex structures and fractures. It allows for the construction of computer *models,* such as bone *surface mesh,* anatomic axes, and osteotomy planes. Bone fragment models and implants can be visualized in three dimensions and manipulated to analyze several possible scenarios. The resulting fixation can be evaluated in three dimensions and with a simulated postoperative radiograph, known as a digitally reconstructed radiograph, obtained from the preoperative CT in cooperation with templates of fixation hardware. In certain situations the healthy side can be inverted ("mirror image") and can be used for templating of the fractured side. Figures 18-1B(1 to 4) illustrate the concepts of preoperative planning in reduction and fixation, as well as applying virtual forces using finite element analysis of a humeral fracture.

An increasing number of computer programs have been developed enabling visualization of virtually all steps of the real surgical procedure; however, clinically it is mainly two-dimensional (2D) technology that is available.[3,6] This ability to exercise a virtual surgical procedure marking out safe zones allows for precise planning of screw dimensions and pathways and enables prechecking of the percutaneous option as an alternative to the open approach.

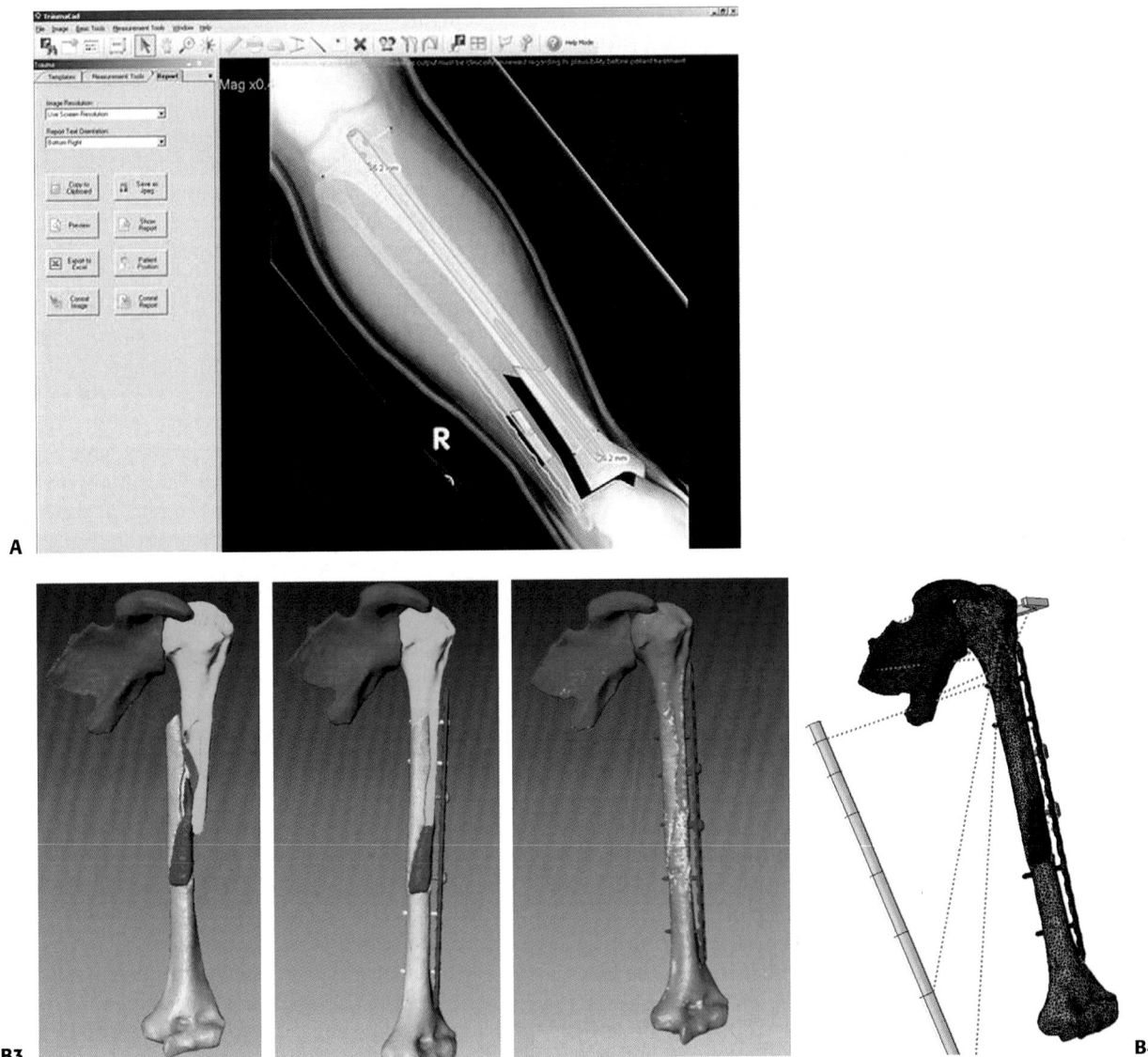

FIGURE 18-1 Preoperative planning. **A:** Preplanning for internal fixation of a distal tibia and fibula fracture using an intramedullary nail and fibular plate. Interlocking screw sizes are estimated using a ruler tool. **B:** Preplanning for reduction and fixation of a humeral fracture: Three-dimensional visualization of the humerus and fragment (each fragment is indicated in a different color). *B1:* The bone fragments of the fractured humerus were segmented enabling the creation of a 3D surface model. *B2:* The fragments were reduced to construct the best anatomical model. The side plate and screws were positioned and then a Boolean cut was carried out between implants and bone. *B3:* Material properties were applied to all elements of the bone according to a density-based empirical relationship. *B4:* A finite element model of a plated humerus. The muscles attach the proximal humerus to the scapula element, the artificial clavicle, and an additional artificial element (Image courtesy of Dr. E. Peleg).

There is consensus among most orthopedic surgeons that preplanning is mandatory and that it helps to improve performance.

Principles of Navigation and Guidance

The goal of *navigation* is to provide precise, real-time visual feedback of the spatial location of surgical instruments and anatomic structures that cannot be directly observed. In current practice, this information is obtained by repeated use of fluoro-scopic radiography, which produces a time-frozen 2D view; is not updated in real time; and results in cumulative radiation to the surgeon, staff, and patient. The goal of *guidance* is to indicate to the surgeon in real time, via images, graphics, or sound, the best course of action during surgery.

Navigation systems show the current location of surgical instruments with respect to images of the anatomy using either preoperative CT or intraoperative fluoroscopic radiography images and continuously update the image as the instruments and bone structures move. The resulting display, called *navigation images,* is equivalent to continuous intraoperative imaging without radiation.

Navigation requires *tracking, registration, visualization,* and *validation.* Tracking determines in real time the location of moving objects in space. Registration establishes a common reference frame between the moving objects and the images. Visualization creates navigation images showing the location of moving objects with respect to the anatomy. Validation ensures that the updated images match the clinical intraoperative situation.

The key advantage of navigation is that it obviates the need for repeated fluoroscopic radiography. However, it requires additional procedures, including setting up the navigation system and attaching trackers to both instruments and bone structures of interest, as well as additional surgical training.

System Components and Mode of Operation

A navigation system consists of a computer unit, a tracking unit, and tracker mounted hardware. Figure 18-2 shows the equipment setup in the operating room. A rolling cart usually holds the computer unit and the *tracking base unit.* The cart is placed next to the patient, so that the surgeon can conveniently see the display. Tracking requires a *position sensor* and one or more *trackers.* The position sensor determines the spatial location of the trackers at any given moment in time. By attaching trackers to surgical tools and bones, their relative spatial position can continuously be followed and updated in the computer display. Trackers are rigidly mounted on tools and bones with *tracker mounting jigs,* which are mechanical jigs similar to screws and clamps. Because the trackers and their mounting jigs come in contact with the patient, they must be sterilized. The position sensor is either mounted on the cart, part of a separate unit, or attached to the ceiling or to a wall. It is aimed at the surgical field so that the expected tracker motions are within its working area throughout surgery. The position sensor's location can be changed during surgery as needed. When fluoroscopic radiography images are used for navigation, the computer unit is also connected to a C-arm

and imports images acquired with it. The C-arm is usually fitted with its own tracker to determine its relative location with respect to the tracked objects and imaged anatomy.

The tracking base unit receives and integrates the signals from the position sensor and the trackers. The computer integrates the signals from the base unit with fluoroscopic radiography or CT images and instrument models (registration), and creates one or more views for display (visualization). The navigated images are updated in real time by the computer as the instruments and anatomy move. The *tool calibration unit* is used to obtain geometric data of surgical tools fitted with trackers, such as the tool tip's offset. These geometric data are used to create the instrument model for display.

Tracking

A tracking system obtains the position and orientation of trackers by measuring spatially dependent physical properties, which can be optical, magnetic, acoustic, or mechanical. Currently, two types of tracking technologies are available for medical applications: optical and magnetic, with optical being by far the most commonly used (Fig. 18-3).

Optical Tracking

In optical tracking, the position sensor consists of two or more *optical cameras* that detect the light emitted or reflected by *markers.* Each camera measures the distance of the markers from the camera. Because the base distance between the optical cameras is known, the position of the marker with respect to the camera's base line can be computed by a method known as triangulation. A *tracker* consists of three or more markers mounted on a rigid base (Fig. 18-3A). The tracker's position and orientation are determined by the markers' positions relative to each other and by their sensed position with respect to the position sensor. A key requirement is the maintenance of an unobstructed *line of sight* between the position sensor and the trackers. Optical tracking systems can be *active, passive,* or *hybrid.*

Active Tracking

Active tracking uses active markers, which are light-emitting diodes (LEDs) that are strobbed (turned on and off) in tandem

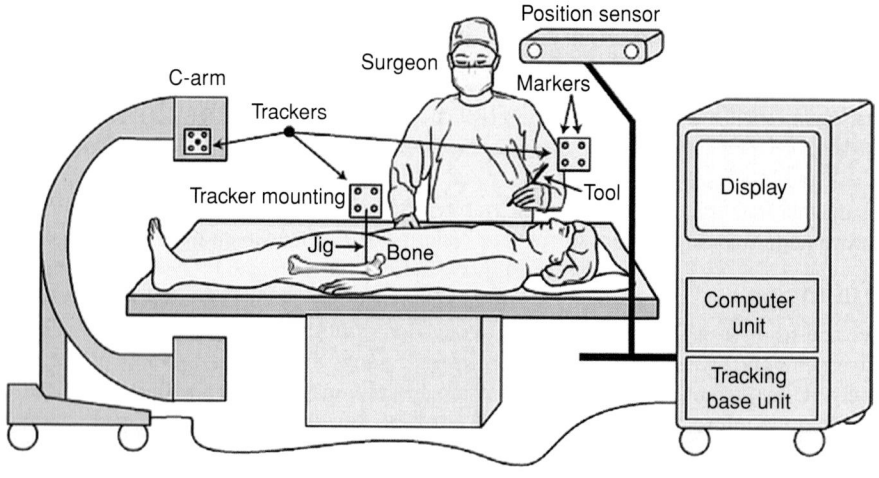

FIGURE 18-2 Equipment setup in the operating room. A navigation system consists of a computer unit, tracker unit, and tracker mounting hardware. The computer unit consists of a computer, keyboard, mouse, and display monitor or touch screen. The tracking unit consists of a tracking base unit, position sensor, one or more trackers, and a tool calibration unit (optional). (Image property of authors.)

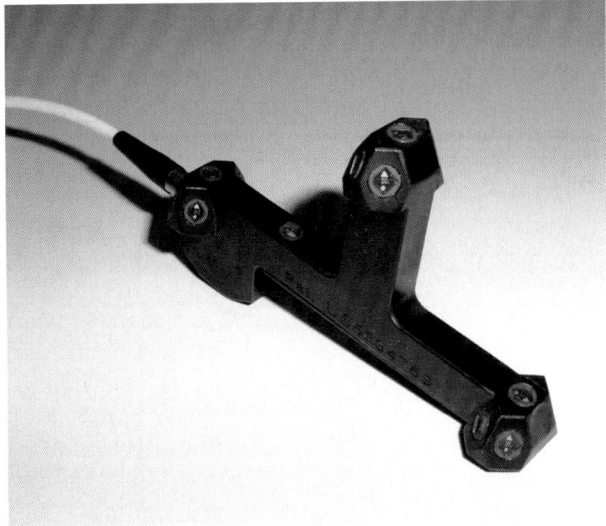

A

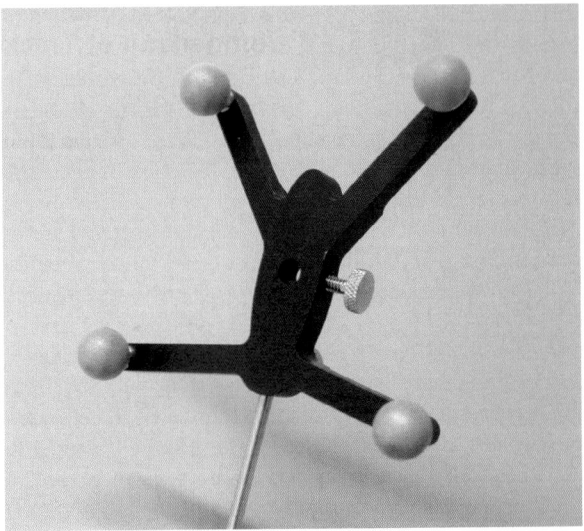

B

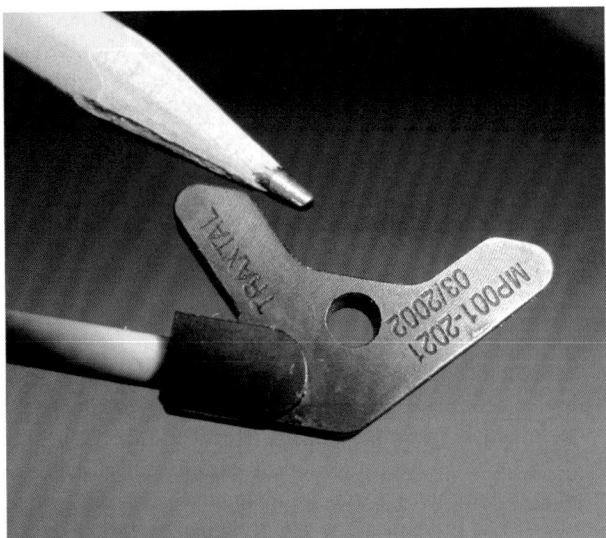

C

FIGURE 18-3 Trackers. **A:** Active optical tracker. **B:** Passive optical tracker. **C:** Magnetic tracker. (Courtesy of Traxtal Technologies, Toronto, Canada)

by the base unit. LEDs emit infrared light that is detected by the cameras. The cameras' capture is synchronized with the LED strobbing so that the identity of the lighting marker is known. Active trackers consist of three or more wired LEDs mounted onto a rigid base and connected by a cable or by a wireless link (tetherless communication) to the tracking base unit. Each active tracker has a unique identifier. Active trackers are built so that they can be sterilized many times over.

Passive Tracking

Passive tracking uses passive markers, which can be reflective spheres or printed patterns (Fig. 18-3B). Reflective spheres reflect the infrared light generated by the position sensor, which is then detected by the cameras. Unlike the active markers, passive markers are not controlled by the tracking base unit and are "seen" simultaneously by the cameras. Passive trackers consist of three or more passive markers. The identity of the passive tracker is determined by the configuration of the markers on the rigid mounting base. Consequently, no two passive

trackers can have the same marker configuration. The tracking base unit must know the tracker configuration. Because the markers lose their reflectance with sterilization and touch, they must be replaced after several uses.

Hybrid Tracking

Hybrid tracking incorporates both active and passive tracking. Hybrid tracking systems simultaneously track both passive and active trackers, thus providing the advantages of both technologies. Table 18-1 summarizes the advantages and disadvantages of active (wired and tetherless) and passive trackers. Because neither technology is always superior to the other in all categories, the anatomy, the surgical instruments, and the clinical situation determine the best choice of trackers.

In terms of physical characteristics, passive trackers are lightest, while tetherless active trackers are heaviest because of the battery required to activate the circuitry and the LEDs. Passive trackers are more rugged than active ones because they have no electronics. Tetherless trackers are more convenient because there

TABLE 18-1	**Comparison of Tracking Technologies**			
		Optical		
Characteristic	Active Wired	Active Tetherless	Passive	Magnetic
Physical				
Size	0	0	0	+
Weight	0	–	+	+
Ruggedness	0	–	+	+
Ergonomics	–	0	+	–
Functional				
Activation indicator	+	+	NA	+
Integrated switch	+	+	NA	+
Tool recognition	+	+	NA	+
Reliability	0	–	+	0
Performance				
Orientation dependency	–	–	+	–
Accuracy	+	+	0	–
Cost				
Upfront cost	0	–	+	+
Running cost	+	–	0	+
Amortized cost	0	–	+	+

Scores (+, 0, –) are relative: + indicates most favorable; 0, neutral; and –, least favorable. NA, feature is not available.

are no cables to get in the way. In terms of functionality, active trackers have the advantage that they indicate, on the tracker itself (via a light indicator), when the line of sight is maintained, while passive tracker obstruction can only be shown on the display. Active trackers are automatically recognized as soon as they are plugged in. Passive trackers are the most reliable, because there are no electric connections; tetherless active trackers are the least reliable because of possible communication interferences and their short battery life (LEDs require substantial power for illumination). In terms of performance, active trackers are somewhat more accurate than passive trackers but they are also more sensitive to their orientation with respect to the cameras. In terms of cost, it is the highest for active tetherless tracking because of the additional electronics and lowest for passive trackers, which have no electronics at all. The running cost of active wired tracking is lowest, because there are no batteries or reflective spheres to replace. The amortized cost over time of the wired active trackers represents significant savings.

Magnetic Tracking

Magnetic tracking works by measuring variations of generated magnetic fields. The position sensor consists of a magnet that generates a uniform magnetic field and a sensor that measures its phase and intensity variations. Trackers consist of one or more miniature coils mounted on a rigid base that generate a local magnetic field from an electric current, either alternating or pulsed direct (Fig. 18-3C). Both the position sensor and the

trackers are connected to the tracking base unit. The tracker magnetic field modifies the sensor's magnetic field characteristics according to its position in space. The location of the tracker is computed from the relative variations of the sensor's intensity and its phase magnetic field. A key requirement is the maintenance of a uniform magnetic field, which is altered by the vicinity of magnetic fields from other electronic devices and by nearby ferromagnetic objects.

Magnetic trackers are usually much smaller, lighter, and cheaper than optical trackers and their functionality is similar to that of active optical trackers (Table 18-1). However, the accuracy of existing magnetic tracking systems is less than that of optical tracking systems. Their main advantages are that they are small and do not require a direct line of sight, and therefore they are useful in percutaneous procedures. However, they do require careful control of the environment in which they operate, because the nearby presence of ferrous objects and electrical instruments in the operating room can influence their measurements.

Tracking: Technical Issues

The best way to visualize a tracking system is as a 3D measurement instrument, also known as a *coordinate measuring machine*. A 3D measurement instrument provides a stream of spatial location measurements in a given range, accuracy, and rate (frequency). It measures the *location* of an object (a tracker) with respect to a fixed coordinate frame centered at the position sensor's origin.

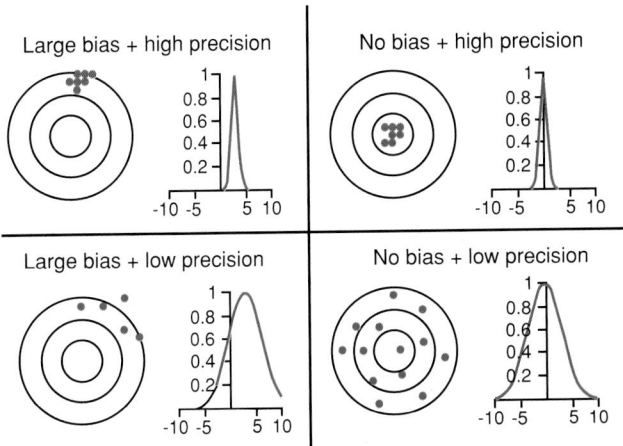

FIGURE 18-4 Accuracy and bias. Accuracy is a combination of precision and bias. High accuracy requires no bias and high precision (top right). The concentric circles represent the distance from the true value (the common center of the circles); dots represent actual measurements. (Image property of authors.)

The location of an object in space, its position and orientation, is uniquely determined by six parameters: Three translational (vertical, horizontal, and depth) and three rotational (roll, yaw, and pitch).

Tracking systems measure the position of markers in a predefined volume in space, called the *tracking work volume*. Its shape is usually simple, such as a sphere, pyramid, or cube, depending on the type of position sensor technology used. The distance between the position sensor and the tracking work volume center is fixed.

Accuracy is defined as the measure of an instrument's capability to approach a true or absolute value. Accuracy is a function of both *bias* and *precision* (Fig. 18-4). Bias is a measure of how closely the mean value in a series of replicated measurements approaches the true value. Precision is a measure of how closely the values within a series of replicated measurements agree with each other. It has no units and indicates the relative degree of repeatability. *Repeatability* is a measure of *resolution*

and *stability*. Resolution is the smallest discernible difference between two measurements. Stability refers to making identical measurements at a steady state and over a sufficiently long period. *Frequency* is the number of overall measurements per second. Static accuracy refers to measurements obtained when the trackers are at rest, while dynamic accuracy refers to measurements obtained as the trackers move.

The factors influencing tracking accuracy are as follows:

Position sensor accuracy: For optical tracking, the number of cameras, the distance between them, and their resolution. For magnetic tracking, the intensity of the magnetic field and the resolution of the magnetic sensor.

Marker accuracy: For optical tracking, the type of LEDs, sphere size, and reflectance. For magnetic tracking, the strength of the coil magnetic field.

Tracker accuracy: Depends on marker accuracy, number of markers, their configuration, and the distance between them.

Tracking system accuracy: Depends on all of the above, and on the relative position and orientation of the position sensor with respect to the trackers.

It should be noted that accuracy is not uniform within the tracking work volume. It is usually highest at the center, with decay toward the boundaries of the tracking work volume. Therefore, the position sensor should always be placed as close as possible to the center of the expected operating volume. It is often useful to distinguish between position and orientation accuracy. Statistics on accuracy include average, minimum, maximum, and root-mean-square (RMS) error. Table 18-2 summarizes the typical characteristics of current tracking systems.

Tool and Bone Tracking

Tool and bone tracking are achieved by rigidly attaching trackers to them with mounting hardware (Fig. 18-5). To track a surgical tool, a tracker can be added to it or the tool can be custom designed, with markers integrated within the tool. To track the C-arm, a ring with several dozen markers is attached to its image intensifier. It is very important that the trackers do not move with respect to the tracked body during surgery,

TABLE 18-2 **Typical Characteristics of Commercial Tracking Systems**

Characteristic	Optical		Magnetic
	Active	**Passive**	
Work volume	Sphere 1 m³ diameter	Sphere 1 m³ diameter	Cube 0.5 × 0.5 × 0.5 m³
Distance from center	2.25 m	1 m	0.55 m
Accuracy (root-mean-square)	0.1–0.35 mm	0.35 mm	1–2 mm 0.8–1.7 degrees
Frequency	60–450 Hz	60–250 Hz	20–45 Hz
Interferences	Line of sight	Line of sight	Ferrous objects Magnetic fields
Number of tools	3	6	3

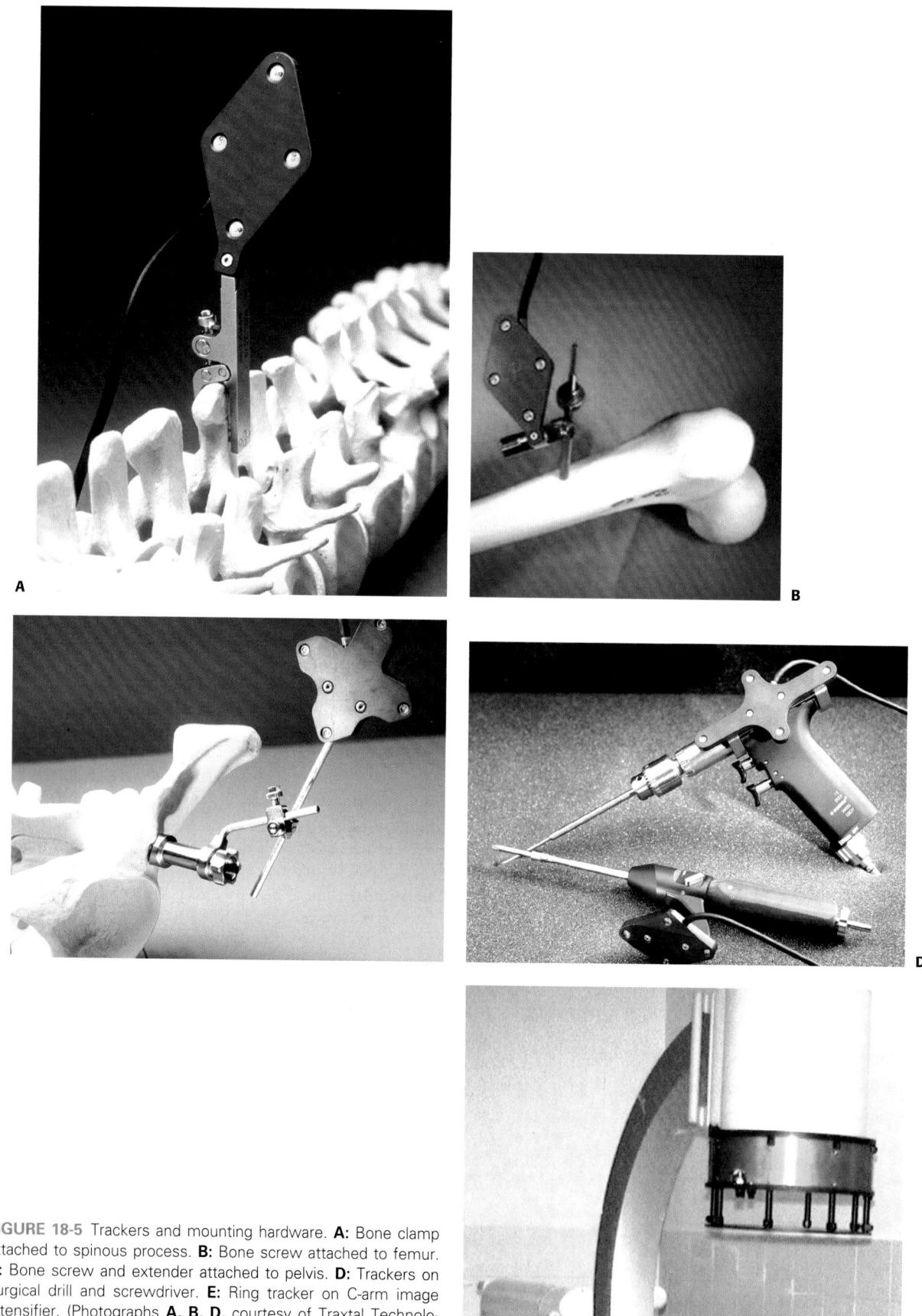

FIGURE 18-5 Trackers and mounting hardware. **A:** Bone clamp attached to spinous process. **B:** Bone screw attached to femur. **C:** Bone screw and extender attached to pelvis. **D:** Trackers on surgical drill and screwdriver. **E:** Ring tracker on C-arm image intensifier. (Photographs **A, B, D,** courtesy of Traxtal Technologies, Toronto, Canada; **C,** courtesy of MedVision, Unna, Germany; **E,** property of authors.)

because relative movement cannot be detected and measured and will increase system error.

Registration

Registration is the process of establishing a common reference frame between objects and images. It is a prerequisite for creating a reliable image of the intraoperative situation, accurately showing the relative locations of the anatomy and the surgical tools of interest with respect to the preoperative and/or intraoperative images.[14] Registration is achieved by *transformations* between the objects' *coordinate frames* at all times.

A coordinate frame serves as a reference within which the spatial locations (position and orientation) of objects can be described. Each object of interest has its own coordinate frame. The relative location of objects is described by a transformation T_B^A, describing the location of B's coordinate frame with respect to A. A transformation is a matrix describing the relationship between the three rotational and three translational parameters of the objects. The transformation is *static* (constant) when the relative locations of A and B do not change or *dynamic* $T_B^A(t)$ (a function of time t) when one or both of the objects move. The relative locations of objects are obtained by *chaining* (composing) transformations. Thus, the location of C with respect to A is obtained from the location of B with respect to A and the location of C with respect to B.

$$T_C^A = T_B^A \bullet T_C^B$$

The goal is to compute the location of the surgical tools with respect to the displayed images $T_{tool}^{display}(t)$, as illustrated in Figure 18-6. This registration involves four types of transformations: (1) tracker transformations; (2) tool transformations; (3) image transformations; and (4) display transformations.

1. *Tracking transformations:* Tracking transformations $T_{tracker}^{sensor}(t)$ indicate the location of each tracker with respect to the position sensor coordinate system. They are provided in real time by the tracking system and can be static or dynamic, depending on whether the objects attached to the tracker move or do not move. The relative location of one tracker with respect to the other is obtained by chaining their transformations:

$$T_{tracker^1}^{tracker^2}(t) = T_{sensor}^{tracker^1}(t) \bullet T_{tracker^2}^{sensor}(t)$$

where $T_{sensor}^{tracker^1}(t) = [T_{tracker^1}^{sensor}(t)]^{-1}$ is the inverse transformation.

2. *Tool transformations:* Tool transformations $T_{tool}^{t\_tracker}$ indicate the location of the tool coordinate frame with respect to the tracker. Because the tracker is rigidly attached to the tool, the transformations are static. They are provided at shipping time when the tracker and the tool come from the same manufacturer (i.e., precalibrated tools). Alternatively, they are computed shortly before surgery with a *tool calibration* procedure, which typically consists of attaching the tool to a tracked calibration object and computing with custom calibration software the transformation and the tool's geometric features, such as its main axis and tip position.

3. *Image transformations:* Image transformations T_{images}^{sensor} indicate the location of the images with respect to the position sensor. There are two types of transformations, T_{CT}^{sensor} and $(T_{x-ray}^{sensor})_i$, depending on the type of images used: either one preoperative CT or several intraoperative fluoroscopic radiography images. The transformation between the position sensor and the CT image T_{CT}^{sensor} is static and unknown and must be computed with a *CT registration procedure*. The transformation between the position sensor and fluoroscopic radiography images $(T_{x-ray}^{sensor})_i$, where i indicates each C-arm viewpoint, is computed from the transformation $(T_{i\_tracker}^{sensor})_i$ of the ring tracker attached to the C-arm image intensifier transformation and $(T_{x-ray}^{i\_tracker})_i$ the C-arm internal imaging transformation:

$$(T_{x-ray}^{sensor})_i = (T_{i\_tracker}^{sensor}) \bullet (T_{x-ray}^{i\_tracker})$$

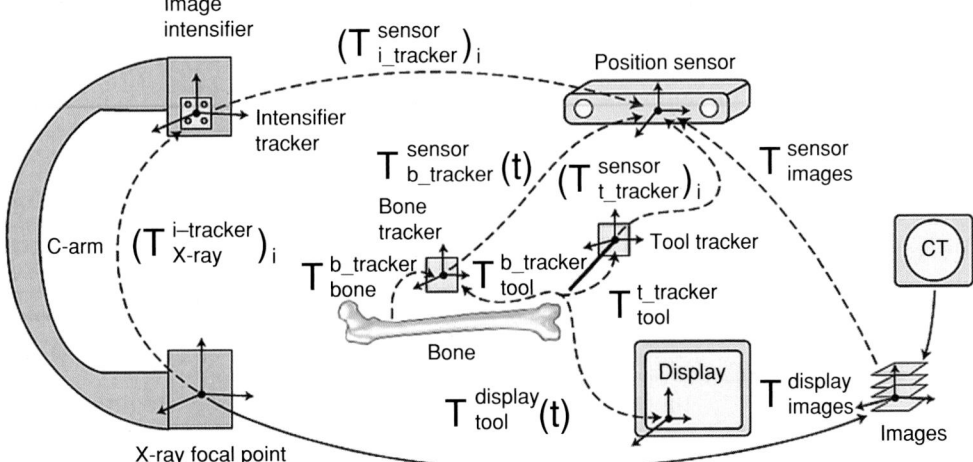

FIGURE 18-6 Coordinate frames and transformations between objects. The goal is to compute the location of the surgical tools with respect to the displayed images $T_{tool}^{display}$. (Image property of authors.)

In older fluoroscopic units, this internal transformation is orientation-dependent and thus must be computed for each C-arm viewpoint i.[32]

4. *Display transformations:* Display transformations $T_{CT}^{display}$ and $(T_{x\text{-}ray}^{display})_i$ indicate the location of the CT and fluoroscopic radiography images with respect to the display shown to the surgeon, respectively. The transformations are determined by the viewpoint shown to the surgeon. Note that the transformation between the bone and the tracker $T_{bone}^{b\_tracker}$ is unknown and cannot be computed, because the exact location of the tracker mounting jig with respect to the bone is not known. Instead, the relative location of the tool with respect to the tracker is used:

$$T_{tool}^{b\_tracker}(t) = T_{sensor}^{b\_tracker}(t) \bullet T_{t\_tracker}^{sensor}(t) \bullet T_{tool}^{t\_tracker}$$

In effect, the bone tracker becomes the reference coordinate frame and therefore is also called the *dynamic reference frame.*

The registration between the tool coordinate frame and the display coordinate frame $T_{tool}^{display}(t)$ is computed by chaining the transformations:

$$T_{tool}^{display}(t) = T_{image}^{display} \bullet T_{sensor}^{image} \bullet T_{t\_tracker}^{sensor} \bullet T_{tool}^{t\_tracker}$$

For fluoroscopic radiography images, there is one transformation $(T_{x\text{-}ray}^{sensor})_i$ and $(T_{tool}^{display})_i(t)$ for every C-arm viewpoint i.

Registration Accuracy

The accuracy of the registration depends on the accuracy of each transformation and on the cumulative effect of transformation chaining. Because the transformation includes rotation, the translational error is amplified as the distance from the reference frame increases (Fig. 18-7).

Tracking transformation accuracy depends on the accuracy of the tracking system and on the location of the tracker with respect to the center of the position sensor working volume. Tool transformation accuracy depends on the accuracy of the tool calibration procedure and on the relative location

of the tracker with respect to the tool tip. Image transformation accuracy depends on the accuracy of the imaging modality used and on the tracking system's accuracy. For CT images, it depends on the resolution (slice spacing and pixel size) of the CT scan and on the accuracy of the CT registration procedure. For fluoroscopic radiography images, it depends on the C-arm calibration and on distortion correction procedures. Display transformation accuracy is very high, as it only involves numerical computations.

Note that any accidental shift in the location of the bone tracker with respect to the bone will introduce an error in the registration. It is therefore essential that the bone tracker remain rigidly secured to the bone at all times during navigation.

Visualization

Visualization creates updated images that show the location of moving objects with respect to the anatomy. The navigation images are created by merging the preoperative and intraoperative images with the tools and bone location information. The navigation images can be augmented with relevant procedure-dependent data, such as anteversion angle and distance from a predefined safe zone.

The type of navigation images created depends on the preoperative and intraoperative images that are used, on the surgical tools, and on the surgical procedure. In fluoroscopic-based navigation systems, the navigation images consist of fluoroscopic radiography images from the C-arm typically used in conventional surgical procedure poses (anterior–posterior, lateral, oblique), with the surgical tool silhouette at its present location superimposed on them. For example, when the tool is a long cylinder (e.g., drill, pointer, or screwdriver), the tool's location and its prolongation are displayed in two different colors to indicate what would be the tool's location if the current directions were followed. The number of images, tool silhouette, and additional navigation information are procedure-dependent.

In CT-based navigation systems, the navigation images typically consist of sagittal, coronal, and transverse CT cross sections, and a spatial view with the preoperative plan (e.g., fixation screws, fixation plate at their desired location); with the

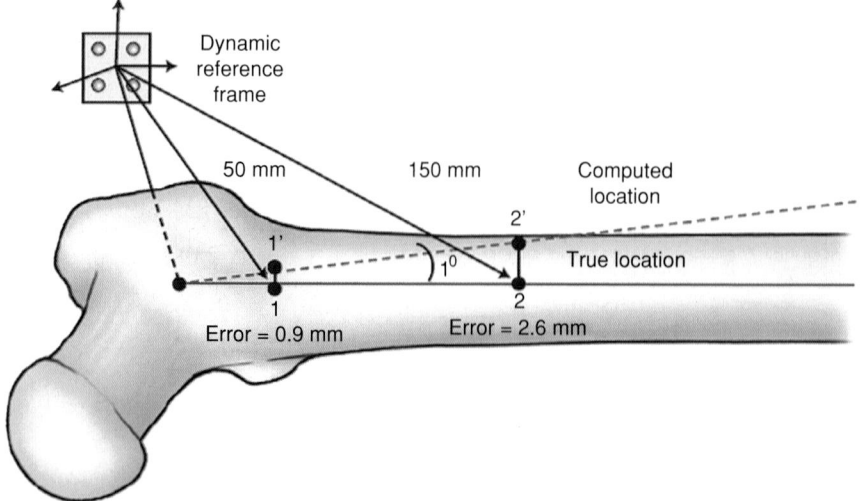

FIGURE 18-7 Influence of the angular error on the translational offset. A dynamic reference frame is attached to the proximal femur. With an angular transformation error of only 1 degree, a nearby target **(1)** 50 mm from the origin of the bone coordinate frame will be offset by 0.9 mm (*1'*), which is acceptable in most situations. However, a farther target **(2)** 150 mm away will be offset by 2.6 mm (*2'*), which may not be acceptable. (Image property of authors.)

surgical tool's silhouette at its current location superimposed on them. Typically, the tool tip corresponds to the crosshair location in the CT cross sections.

Visualization software usually provides the surgeon with various image processing, viewpoint selection, and information display features such as contrast enhancement, viewpoint rotation and translation, window selection, and tool silhouette thickness and color control.

Validation

Validation is the task of verifying that the images and data used for intraoperative navigation closely correspond to the clinical situation. It is essential to verify and quantify the correlation; otherwise the data can mislead the surgeon and yield unwanted results. Validation is an integral part of the navigation surgical protocol. It is performed both before the surgery starts and at key points during the surgery.

There are three main types of verification.

1. *Tool calibration verification:* Verifies that the tool's geometric information is accurate. Sources of inaccuracy include deformations in the tool as a result of high-temperature sterilization; bending; wear and tear; tracker relative motion; and marker drift.

2. *Dynamic reference frame verification:* Verifies that the bone tracker has not moved with respect to the bone to which it is attached.

3. *Registration accuracy verification:* Verifies that the tool, implant, and bone fragment locations are indeed where they are shown in the navigation images. Over time, registration accuracy depends on variations in the tool's calibration accuracy; on the dynamic reference frame's relative location with respect to the bone to which it is attached; on the tracking system's drift over time; and on the accumulation of small computational numerical errors.

The validation procedure depends on the type of surgery, the navigated surgical tools, and the images used. Tool calibration verification usually consists of verifying with a calibration jig that the tool tip is at its computed location. Dynamic reference frame and registration accuracy verification usually consist of verifying that the tracked bones and tools are indeed where the navigated images indicate. This is done by acquiring one or more fluoroscopic radiography images and comparing them with the navigation images. Alternatively, it is done by touching with the tip of a surgical tool the known anatomic landmarks and verifying that the tool tip appears close to the landmark in the navigated image. Registration accuracy is quantified by measuring the drift between the actual and the computed location of tools and anatomic landmarks. When registration accuracy is inadequate, the surgeon must repeat the registration process.

NAVIGATION SYSTEMS

There are currently two types of navigation systems for CAS in skeletal trauma: Fluoroscopy-based and CT-based navigation systems.

Fluoroscopy-Based Systems

Fluoroscopy-based systems create navigation images by superimposing the surgical tool silhouette onto conventional fluoroscopic images and updating its location in real time, thereby creating the impression of continuous fluoroscopy without the ensuing radiation. The resulting effect is called *virtual fluoroscopy*. Fluoroscopy-based systems are thus closest to the current practice of conventional fluoroscopy because the navigation images are in close proximity to the familiar fluoroscopic images, with the advantage being that only a dozen fluoroscopic radiography images are used, instead of tens or even hundreds.

There are two types of fluoroscopy-based navigation systems: Systems that use conventional C-arm fluoroscopy and those that use new 3D fluoroscopy, such as the Siemens Iso-C 3D C-arm. Virtually any C-arm can be used, provided that the images are corrected for geometric distortion and the C-arm imaging properties are calibrated. The correction is usually done with an online C-arm calibration procedure that relies on imaged patterns of metallic spheres mounted on the C-arm ring tracker (the spheres appear as a grid of black circles in the images). Newer conventional and 3D C-arms do not require calibration.

Conventional C-Arm Fluoroscopy

The surgical protocol is as follows: Shortly before surgery, the rolling cart with the display, computer unit, and tracking base unit is positioned in the operating room so that the display can be easily seen by the surgeon. The position sensor is positioned so that it does not get in the way and its working volume is roughly at the center of where the surgical actions will take place. Next, the ring tracker is mounted on the C-arm's image intensifier and covered with a transparent plastic for sterility. The patient is then brought into the operating room and surgical preparations proceed as usual. Next, the surgeon validates the tool calibration and installs the dynamic reference frame with tracker mounting hardware. Touching known anatomic landmarks with the tip of a surgical tool and verifying that the tool tip appears close to the landmark in the navigated image validates the registration. Once registration validation is successful, the navigated surgery begins. At key points during surgery, such as before drilling a pilot hole or inserting a fixation screw, one or more validation fluoroscopic radiography images can be taken to verify that the navigated images correspond to the actual situation. The navigation procedure can be repeated with other tools and implants. At any time during the procedure, the navigation system can be stopped and the procedure can continue in a conventional manner.

Three-Dimensional Fluoroscopy

3D fluoroscopy is a new imaging modality that allows for the acquisition of CT-like images during surgery by taking about 100 fluoroscopic radiography images at one-degree intervals with a motorized isocentric C-arm. This fluoroscopic machine can also be used as a conventional C-arm, with the added advantage that CT and fluoroscopic radiography images acquired with it are already registered. Although these images are not of as high a quality as those obtained with a preoperative CT, and can only be used to image limbs, the radiation dose is

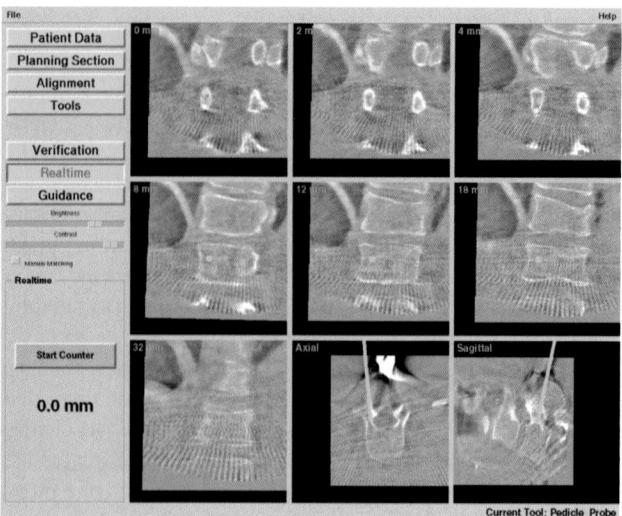

FIGURE 18-8 Pedicle screw insertion with three-dimensional fluoroscopy. Screen view of three-dimensional fluoroscopy navigation during pedicle screw insertion in a fractured thoracic vertebra with the SireMobil Iso-C 3D (Siemens Medical Solutions, Erlangen, Germany). (Image courtesy of Prof. F. Gebhard.)

about half of the dose of a regular CT and accurately reflects the actual intraoperative situation. The navigation images consist of both CT images and fluoroscopic radiography images. The advantages are that complex fractures can be better visualized and that CT images can be taken before and after reduction. In addition, CT images present an entree for better intraoperative planning and thus might advantageously blur the distinction between preoperative and intraoperative planning. The surgical protocol is very similar to that of conventional fluoroscopy, with the additional step of acquiring, when necessary, the intraoperative CT images during surgery.[8,12] Figure 18-8 shows an example of navigation with 3D fluoroscopy. Recently, mobile CT-like imaging technology using an O-arm (Medtronic) has been introduced. This technology has potential but has not as yet been proven to be efficient in trauma applications.

Computed Tomography-Based Systems

CT-based systems create navigation images by superimposing the surgical tool silhouette onto preoperative CT cross-sectional and spatial images and updating its location in real time. This type of navigation is only feasible when a CT data set is available.

The surgical protocol is as follows: Any time between a few hours and a day before surgery, a CT scan is acquired and transferred to the computer, within which the planning will be performed by the surgeon. With the help of preoperative planning and model construction software, the surgeon visualizes the clinical situation, takes measurements, and plans the target location of implants and fixation screws for navigation. The plan is then saved for use during surgery. Shortly before surgery, the rolling cart with the display, computer unit, and tracking base unit is positioned in the operating room so that the surgeon can easily see the display. The position sensor is positioned so that it does not get in the way and its working area is roughly placed at the center of where the surgical actions will take place. The

preoperative plan is loaded into the computer unit. The patient is then brought into the operating room and surgical preparations proceed as usual. Next, the surgeon validates the tool calibration and installs the dynamic reference frame with tracker mounted hardware. Before the beginning of surgery, the preoperative CT is registered to the actual intraoperative anatomic site with a *CT registration procedure*. Touching known anatomic landmarks with the tip of a surgical tool and verifying that the tool tip appears close to the landmark in the navigated image validates the registration. Once registration validation is successful, the navigated surgery begins. At key points during surgery, such as before drilling a pilot hole or inserting a fixation screw, one or more validation fluoroscopic radiography images are taken to verify that the navigated images correspond to the actual situation. The navigation procedure can be repeated with other tools and implants. At any time during the procedure, the navigation system can be stopped and the procedure can continue in a conventional manner. Figure 18-9 shows images of a typical CT-based navigation system.[21,22]

A key step in the protocol is the CT registration procedure. The relationship between the CT and the intraoperative situation is established by matching a set of points on the surface of the bone region to the corresponding points on the CT surface model. The intraoperative point set is obtained by touching the surface of the bone region of interest with a precalibrated tracked pointer and recording the location of a few dozen of these points by pressing on a foot pedal. The point set is then matched to a corresponding point set, automatically extracted from the CT surface model of the same bone region. The points must be a representative sample of the bone surface; that is, they must be as far apart as is possible and cover the entire region of interest.

Comparison of Fluoroscopy- and Computed Tomography-Based Systems

Table 18-3 summarizes the advantages and disadvantages of navigation systems. Only CT-based systems allow for preoperative planning. Spatial visualization is only available with a CT data set and thus is only available in CT-based and 3D fluoroscopy-based systems. No additional registration procedure is necessary for intraoperative imaging, as the position sensor provides a common reference frame for trackers and images. All navigation systems require additional setup procedures, which is a drawback as compared with conventional practice. CT-based systems are not suitable for fracture reduction, as there is no way to determine bone fragment locations during and after reduction. The 3D fluoroscopy-based systems can be used before and after, but not during, reduction, provided that both before and after, images are acquired. In fluoroscopy-based systems, reduction navigation is feasible when the bone fragments have trackers attached to them and new images are acquired at key points during reduction. Currently, CT-based navigation requires the surgeon to touch the surface of the bone; therefore, it cannot be used for percutaneous procedures. In terms of radiation, the best option for the patient and the surgeon is fluoroscopy-based navigation. The indications for fluoroscopy-based systems present the most options, while 3D fluoroscopy-based and CT-based systems are

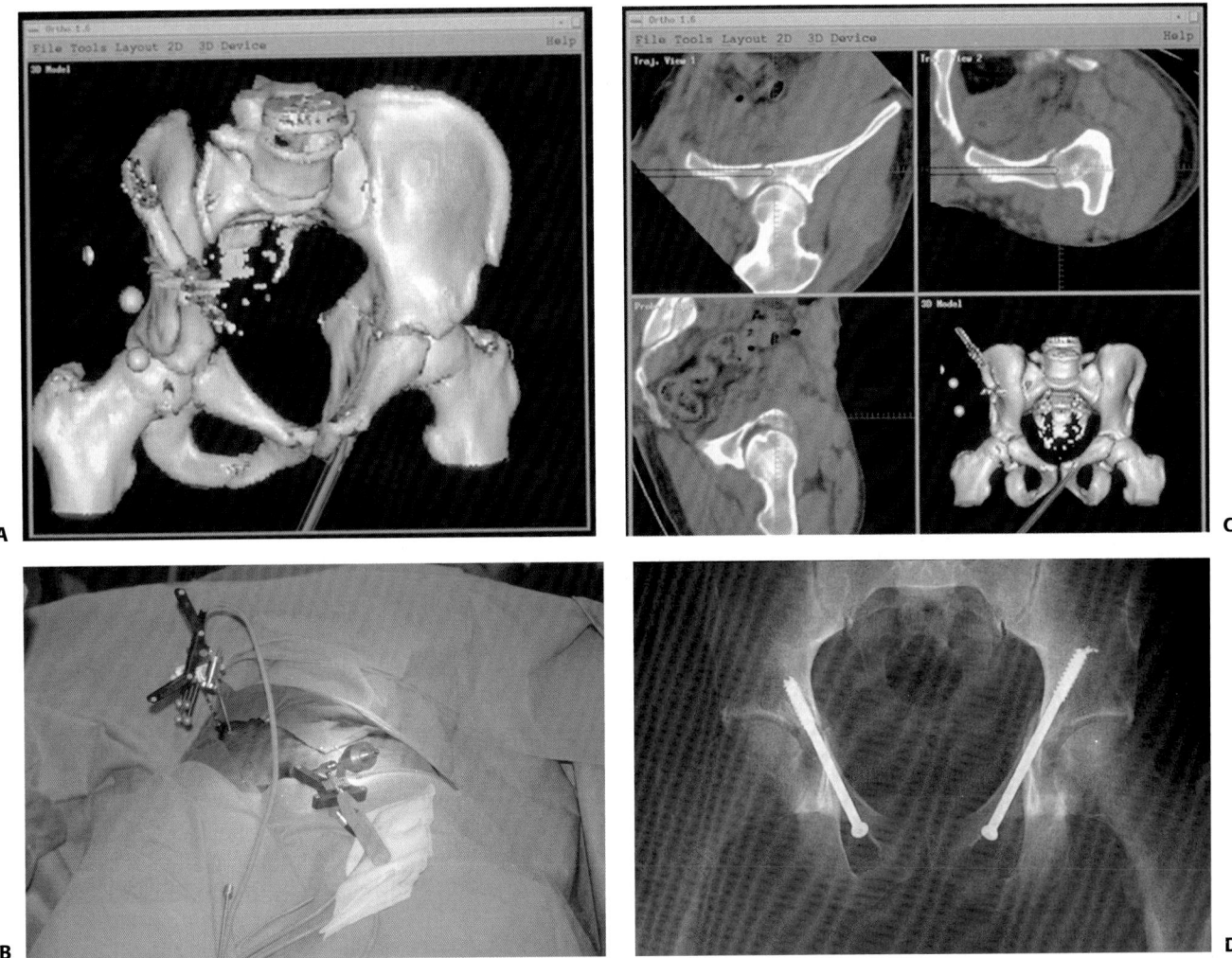

FIGURE 18-9 Retrograde anterior column screw. **A:** Three-dimensional model of the patient's pelvis built on the computer-guided surgery workstation (StealthStation; Sofamor-Danek, Memphis, TN). The position of a virtual drill guide for placement of a retrograde anterior column screw has been added to the virtual image. **B:** Intraoperative photograph taken during placement of the right retrograde anterior column screw (view from the foot of the bed). The reference frame attached to the external fixator is visible at the top left. Also visible are the navigated drill guide, chuck, and guidewire. **C:** The two top images show a preoperative plan for placement of the left-sided retrograde anterior column screw. Two customized orthogonal planes relative to the drilling path are depicted, with a planned trajectory diameter of 7 mm. There is a small safe zone available between the planned position of the implant and the pelvic brim, as well as the articular surface of the acetabulum. The implant path is perpendicular to the fracture line, allowing lag screw reduction and fracture fixation. **D:** Anteroposterior pelvis image at 6 weeks post fixation shows accurate implant placement and early fracture healing without displacement. (Images courtesy of Dr. D. Kahler.)

best used with complex situations requiring spatial visualization. Currently, CT-based systems are mostly used for pelvic fracture fixation, while fluoroscopy-based systems are used for intramedullary nailing and fixation screw insertion.

SURGICAL TECHNIQUES

Clinical Considerations

The concept of combining computer-aided procedures in the treatment of trauma patients should take into account available

innovative technologies together with the clinical situation, as part of the decision-making process. The main goals of CAS are less invasiveness and maximal accuracy in surgical procedures. It has been shown that, if used appropriately, this combination has added value. While the first generation of CAS uses computerized technology for current surgical concepts, it is clear that in the future the surgeon will be able to develop new ways of approaching surgical conditions.

There is no doubt that the timing and duration of procedures are of major concern in trauma management. Damage

TABLE 18-3 **Comparison Between the Conventional Technique and Fluoroscopy-Based and Computed Tomography (CT)-Based Navigation Systems**

Characteristics	No Computerized Navigation	Conventional Technique	Fluoroscopy-Based Three-Dimensional Fluoroscopy	CT-Based
Preoperative planning	No (−)	No (−)	No (−)	Yes (+)
Three-dimensional views	No (−)	No (−)	Yes (+)	Yes (+)
Registration	No (+)	No (+)	No (+)	Yes (−)
Additional operating room setup	None (+)	Yes (−)	Yes (−)	Yes (−)
Reduction	Yes (+)	Yes (+)	Limited (−)	No (−)
Percutaneous procedures	Yes (+)	Yes (+)	Yes (+)	No (−)
Radiation to surgeon	Yes (−)	Very limited (+)	Very limited (+)	None (+)
Radiation to patient	Yes (−)	Very limited (+)	Yes (−)	Yes (−)
Indications	Current practice	Wide range of procedures	Complex anatomy	CT available; partially open
Current use	All of trauma	Intramedullary nailing; screw fixation	Just beginning	Pedicle screw insertion

+, an advantage; −, a disadvantage.

control principles are considered the leading guidelines in the treatment of the severely injured patient. Alternatively, isolated skeletal trauma may be treated in a semielective fashion. Adding computer-assisted procedures to the trauma armamentarium is definitely influenced by, and affects, time-related factors. This is relevant to all stages of the trauma patients' treatment, beginning with the preplanning stage and up to the end of the surgery itself.

Currently, most surgeons believe that CAS is a time-consuming, expensive, and cumbersome procedure. The system's setup time and registration process prolong the preparation phase and might not suit acute trauma management considerations. Moreover, experienced surgeons believe that most surgical tasks can be easily, sufficiently, and accurately carried out, without the use of computer-related technologies. This conservative approach is well known in medical history, whenever a new technology emerges. For example, many years elapsed from the introduction of laparoscopic procedures until surgeons were ready to routinely use them.

Although computer-aided technology has been available for several years, it appears that we are still in the learning phase for CAS systems, and therefore, indications for their use are still being selected. Further assimilation of these promising technologies requires them to become easier to use (i.e., more user friendly). The setup time for the computerized system will definitely be reduced in the modern surgical suite when it is built directly into the operating theatre environment, as presently available in several pioneering institutions. Furthermore, the execution of some surgical tasks is faster and more accurate with CAS equipment and will, in the future, allow for procedures that are presently considered almost unfeasible. For example, the placement of a sacroiliac screw in the fixation of pelvic and

acetabular fractures becomes a fast and accurate procedure with minimal radiation by using a navigation system.[7,8,21]

Retrograde percutaneous posterior column screw placement is an example of a procedure that previously had been considered an almost impossible task to perform and is now an available option with computer assistance.[33,48] Robotic surgery may also play a role in this developing field. Robots are usually useful for several tasks; they offer precision and reproducibility, and are suitable for intensive labor and tedious and monotonous activities. Robots in the OR free the surgeon from such activities allowing him to concentrate on the surgery. Medical robots were introduced into the OR in the late 80s, followed by Robodoc (1992), an active robot for total hip arthroplasty. More recently, the da Vinci Surgical System (2003) was introduced for use in elective abdominal surgery and prostatectomy. Two modern commercial robots in orthopedics are the MAKO (2009) robot for hip and knee arthroplasty and Mazor Surgical Technology's SpineAssist (2004) surgical robot, now called the Renaissance (2011), for spinal surgery, mainly pedicular localization for screw insertion and vertebral augmentation. Robotic technology has been used in spinal trauma and may, in the future, be useful in selected pelvic surgery. Several advantages were reported in spine surgery including a 50–70% reduction in radiation exposure to the patient and reduced radiation to the OR staff[25] in 1815 implants used in 120 scoliotic adolescents.[9] There was increased safety in 593 cases with a 0.7% transient nerve deficit[10] as well as a short learning curve and simple integration into the OR flow.

The different CAS solutions including navigation, robotics, etc. may be categorized into "enablers" and "improvers." While enablers refer to procedures that are not possible without CAS (i.e., the introduction of a new concept or ability rather than a translation of a current technique into CAS), improvers mainly yield improved accuracy and not a new concept. A simple but extremely important example of improvement is the significant reduction in radiation exposure that can be achieved with CAS.[25] As more orthopedic procedures are found to be suitable for CAS applications and as younger surgeons, born into the era of information technologies, enter the operating theatre, the adoption of CAS will become more natural and routine in the operating room.

Currently the simple indications for using CAOS–ST systems in trauma care are percutaneous surgical procedures in which added imaging can provide essential information that will contribute to reducing invasiveness and increasing accuracy.[23,30] Clearly, the fixation of nondisplaced fractures is most suitably carried out with navigation systems, although often the indication for internal fixation is questionable. Alternatively, because available systems can only follow one or two tracked bony fragments, they are not suitable for treating displaced multiple fragment fractures such as comminuted articular fractures, where careful anatomic reduction is required.

In general, navigation systems function better in static or stable situations. For example, using a fracture reduction table or an external fixator eliminates movement between fragments and creates a temporary situation in which there is little or no movement at the fracture site. Moreover, it has been shown that in such "stable" situations, the reference frame can be attached to the fracture table, avoiding additional harm to the patient, while maintaining acceptable accuracy.[19] Following fracture reduction, a guidewire or fixation tool can be inserted using the navigation system according to specific clinical guidelines.

Required accuracy is a key factor for deciding whether to use a CAOS–ST system. For example, the accuracy needed for pedicular screw insertion is by far greater than that needed for hip fracture fixation with cannulated screws. Required accuracy is directly influenced by the cost of inaccuracy (e.g., the cost of inaccuracy in spinal surgery is much greater than in intramedullary nailing).

Computerized navigation has been shown to increase placement accuracy and reduce variability as compared with manual placement. The accuracy of computerized navigation in cannulated screw placement in hip fracture fixation was evaluated.[30] After verifying stable reduction on a fracture table, the reference tracker was attached to the anterior superior iliac crest. The reference frame was not attached to the affected bone so as to improve working convenience during the procedure and minimize morbidity. It was found that the accuracy of the procedure was much better than that of conventional manual procedures. The navigation system enabled the surgeon to place screws with optimal alignment including configuration, parallelism, and scattering. This experience demonstrates that stable reduction creates an acceptable situation for navigational systems and that the reference-tracked frame may be fixed, on such occasions, to an adjacent bone as well as to an external fixator or to the operating table, as mentioned earlier.[18]

Preparation for Surgery

Before surgery, the decision as to whether the procedure is suitable for CAOS–ST is determined by the surgeon's knowledge and capabilities. In most trauma cases, fluoroscopy-based navigation (2D or 3D) is the method of choice.

It is very important to plan and prepare the operating room to create a surgeon-friendly environment and to enable proper tracking without interference (Fig. 18-10). Adding CAOS–ST equipment (computer, monitor, position sensor, and trackers) to an already crowded room requires careful planning. The computer screen should be positioned so that the surgeon can see it without any effort, because, as in arthroscopic procedures, most of the time the surgeon will watch the screen rather than the operative site. Easy access to the computer's control panel is also important and is usually realized with a sterile touch screen. When using optical tracking, maintaining an unobstructed line of sight between the position sensor and the trackers is very important. Thus, the location of the position sensor with respect to the surgeon, nurses, and patient must be carefully examined. These ergonometric issues will definitely be easier in newly designed operating rooms in which computer screens and modern remote controls will be built-in.

Inherent to the implementation of a new technique is the learning curve. In CAS, the learning curve affects all members of the surgical team. It affects surgeons performing the operation, nurses having to cope with new tools, anesthetists who need to adjust the anesthesia time to the expected operation time, and x-ray technicians who sometimes need to operate fluoroscopy-based navigation. The entire team should be aware that there is a "new partner" in the operating theater (i.e., the computer), and sometimes a computer technician will also need to be part of the surgical team.

During the initial phase, the minimal required free field of vision is determined by the location of the C-arm and the calibrating targeting device, the reference frame tracker attached to the patient's anatomy, and by the optical camera. The calibrating targeting device is typically a ring tracker attached to the fluoroscope or the newly designed hands-free trackers that overcome the obstacle of attachment of the cumbersome targeting device to the C-arm. During the navigation phase, tracked surgical instruments replace the ring tracker and the tracking space changes accordingly. Continuous tracking of the patient's anatomy and of the surgical instrument is required. Verification and validation are extremely important at every stage in order to achieve optimal accuracy. Tracking the surgical instrument is more simple and precise, whereas tracking the anatomy, especially in trauma surgery, is more problematic, particularly in those cases where two fragments are simultaneously tracked, as in the fracture reduction process.

Registration and tracking of the patient's anatomy are usually the main cause of inaccuracy. The first obstacle is attaching the rigid frame to the patient. The problem of inserting a stable screw into the bone fragment is well known from the use of external fixation. Screw or pin grip depends on their design and on bone quality. For each procedure, the location needs to be selected according to local morbidity (soft tissue access and crucial anatomic structures); convenience during the procedure (line of sight and free surgical site); and stability of anatomic frame fixation. The stability of the screw holding

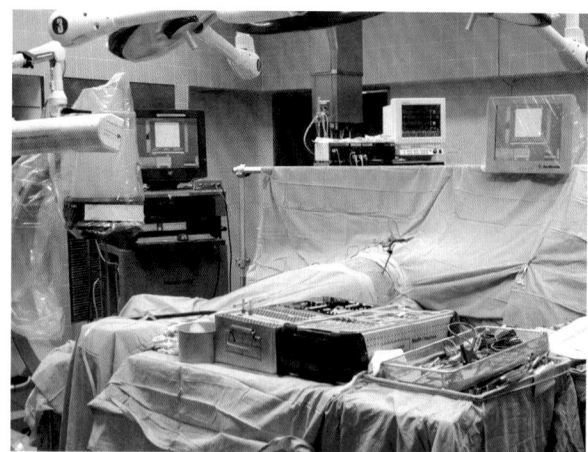

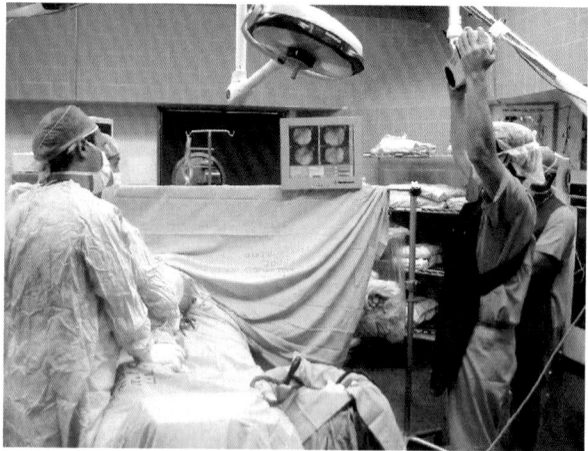

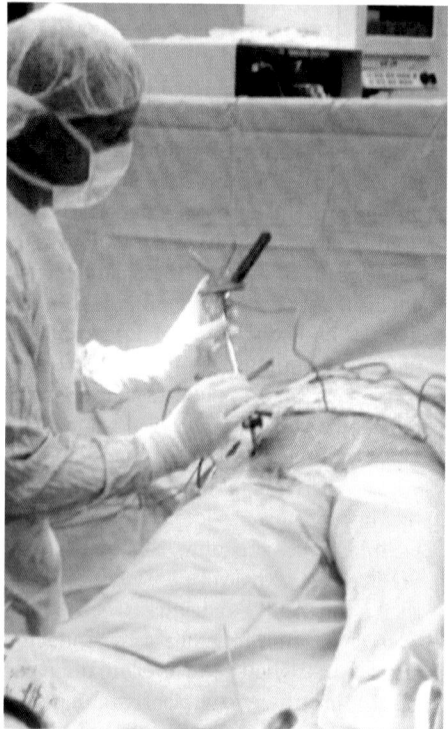

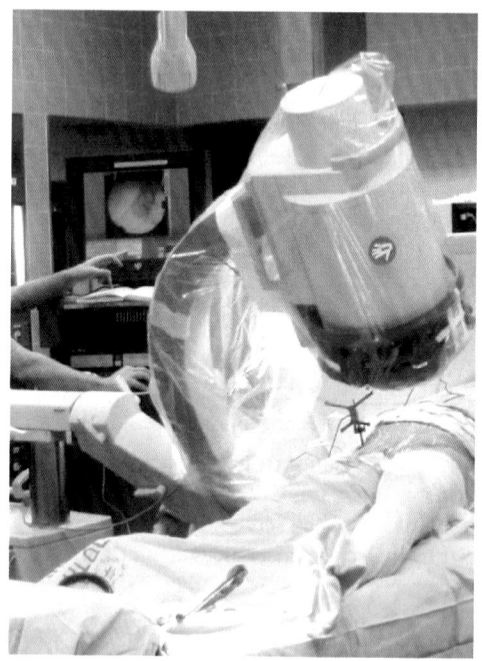

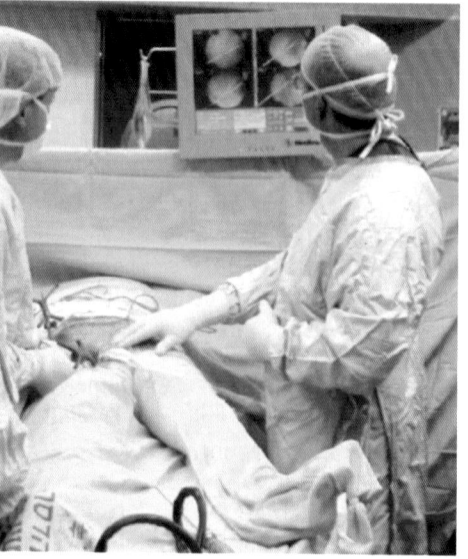

FIGURE 18-10 Operating room setup. **A:** View of the operating room showing locations of the computer unit, position sensor, and bone-mounted reference frame. **B:** Reorientation of the position sensor during surgery. **C:** Surgical tool calibration. **D:** Acquisition of fluoroscopic images. **E:** Navigation with fluoroscopy-based system. (Images property of authors.)

the anatomically referenced tracked frames depends on bone quality and soft tissue interference. Subcutaneous locations such as the iliac crest or the medial aspect of the tibia are preferable. The site of frame fixation should also take into account the surgical task (e.g., avoiding the medullary canal in intramedullary long bone fracture reduction).

Newly designed frames contain more than one screw as well as several soft tissue adaptors and are able to detach from the frame during the non-navigational steps of the procedure. Improvements in bone tracking technology, as well as the ability to track more than one or two large bone fragments, significantly enhance the surgeon's surgical performance in the treatment of fractures.

Basic Procedures Under Navigation

The clinical situations in which computerized navigation is recommended will be presented. For each clinical application, both the rationale and the contribution of these systems will be discussed. The aim of this section is to expose the reader to the first generation of computerized navigation systems. The specific indication for each surgical procedure is beyond the scope of this discussion. All the surgical navigation procedures discussed are based on optical infrared tracking.

When using fluoroscopy-based navigation, the first step is to mount the ring tracker on the C-arm and drape it for sterility or to use a portable calibration device that requires a special attachment to the C-arm. Next, a reference frame (either one or two) is attached to the patient's anatomy and several base fluoroscopic images are acquired—typically, between one and four for 2D navigation or computerized controlled imaging for 3D navigation using an isocentric C-arm or mobile CT technology. The optimal images are stored in the computer and activated during the navigation process. It should be noted that, for all of the clinical examples to be discussed, the preliminary fluoroscopic views can be taken while the operating team stands at a distance of 2 m or more from the radiation source, thus almost eliminating the team's radiation exposure.

The next stage relates to the activation of the designated surgical tool (i.e., wires, awls, drill bits, etc.) or the actual implant, which is to be attached to a tracker, commonly referred to as the *instrument tracker*. The contour of the instrument in its current location is displayed on the previously activated fluoroscopic images thereby creating the effect of virtual fluoroscopy. Similar concepts may be used for tracking fracture reduction—in this case, instead of following the relationship between the tracked instrument and the tracked bone, we track the relationship between the two tracked bone fragments (Fig. 18-11).

Currently available procedures are as follows.

- Trajectory navigation—drill guide applications (hip and pelvic fractures)

- Fracture reduction

- Intra-articular fracture fixation

- Novel uses of navigation: Localization of bone lesions or removal of surgical hardware and shrapnel

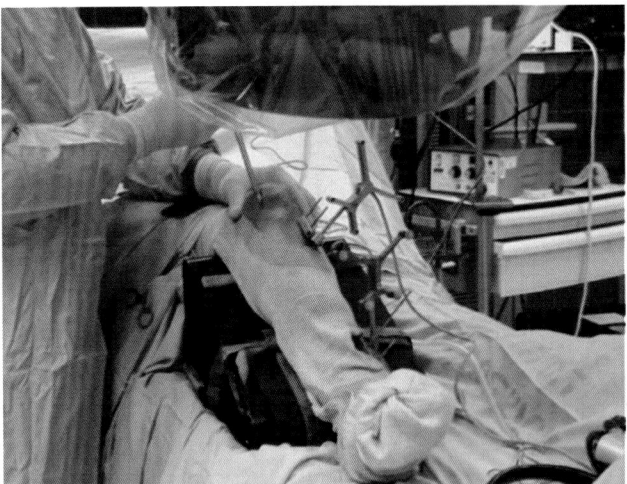

FIGURE 18-11 Tibial intramedullary nailing using fracture reduction software with two frames attached to the two bone fragments. (Image property of authors.)

Trajectory Navigation—Drill Guide Applications (Hip and Pelvic Fractures)

Insertion of straight surgical fixation implants such as nails and screws is a common task in orthopedic traumatology. This procedure can often be performed percutaneously and thereby fit the CAS philosophy of minimal invasiveness with high accuracy. Navigated 2D fluoroscopy provides a natural computerized enhancement for this surgical application. Thus, the most common current indication for the use of CAOS–ST systems is the insertion of cannulated screws. This surgical procedure requires high accuracy and unusually large radiation exposure for the surgeon and for the patient. Both issues can be successfully addressed with fluoroscopy-based navigation.

The percutaneous treatment of pelvic and acetabular fractures and internal fixation of slipped capital femoral epiphyses are procedures that can greatly benefit from computerized navigation. The use of computerized navigation turns the procedure into a simple task to perform, while using minimal radiation.[23] Internal fixation of intracapsular fractures of the femoral neck is considered straightforward, although accurate performance requires high proficiency on the one hand and large exposure to radiation on the other. A prospective comparison between patients who underwent internal fixation of intracapsular fracture of the femoral neck by means of cannulated screws, with and without the assistance of a navigation system, was performed.[30] This study revealed that computerized navigation increased the accuracy of screw placements in all measured parameters. Having acquired proficiency with the computerized system, the surgeon is ready to move on to the next level, which includes percutaneous fixation of pelvic and acetabular fractures.

Internal pelvic fracture fixation is a challenging task for the orthopedic trauma surgeon. The pelvis is a complex 3D structure that contains important anatomic structures in a confined environment. Therefore, surgical fixation of displaced fractures

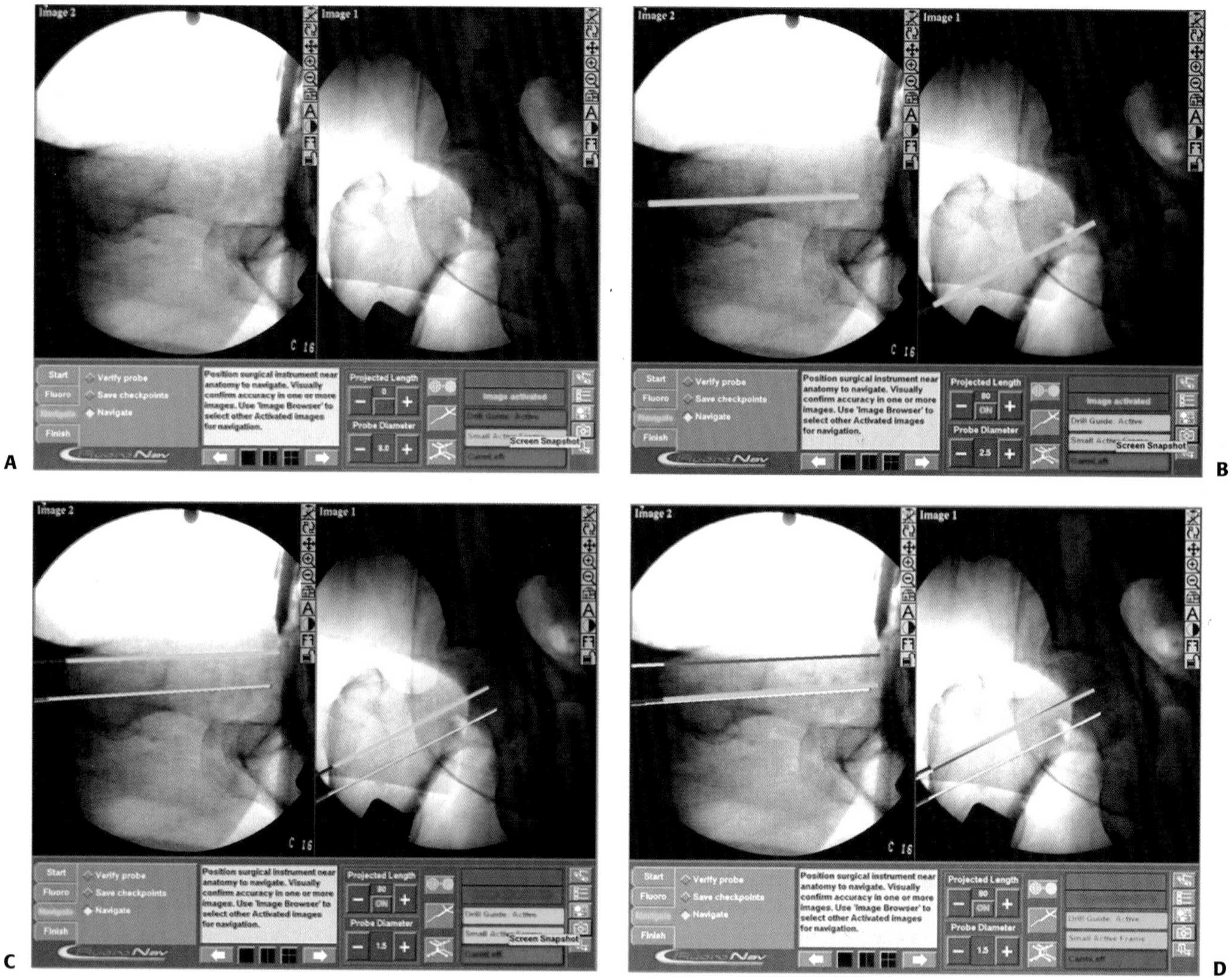

A

B

C

D

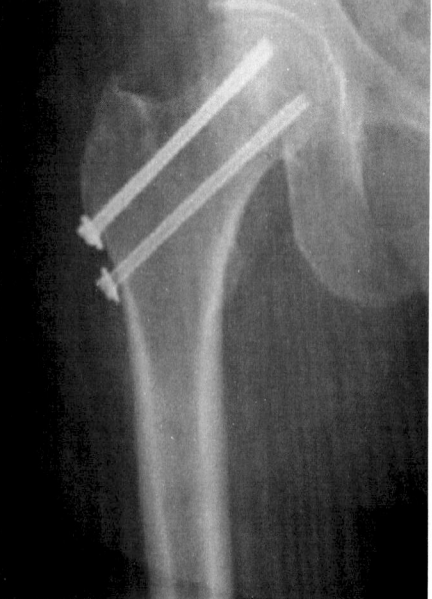

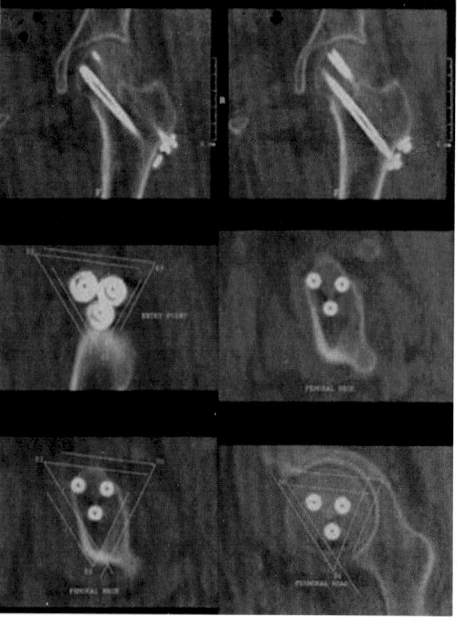

FIGURE 18-12 Cannulated screws. **A:** Anteroposterior and lateral views of a reduced intracapsular fracture of the femoral neck displayed on the computer's screen. **B–D:** Insertion of the three guidewires without additional radiation. **E, F:** Radiograph and CT scan showing the precise scattering of the three screws in a spatial configuration of an inverted triangle. (Images property of authors.)

E

F

should be meticulously performed under strict visual control, because the "safe zones" are narrow. With CAS technologies, it is possible to define several "safe corridors" for the insertion of different screws around the pelvis including the acetabulum. It has been shown that navigation is advantageous for these challenging procedures.[13,49,50]

In many cases, closed reduction and percutaneous fixation is feasible and provides enough stability to allow for immediate patient mobilization. A conventional image intensifier is most frequently used in percutaneous pelvic fixation. However, it provides only a 2D image and requires multiple images in different projections to determine the correct point of entry and the direction of the screw. Furthermore, the use of conventional fluoroscopy makes the procedure long and tedious and exposes both the patient and the medical team to prolonged radiation.[8,21,22] Fluoroscopy-based navigation systems (2D and 3D) have the potential to significantly reduce radiation exposure and operative time, while allowing the surgeon to achieve maximum accuracy.[8,13,27,36,44]

The indications for percutaneous pelvic and acetabular surgery are controversial and are not discussed here. A selected population with traumatic pelvic and acetabular fractures can be treated percutaneously under three conditions: (i) cases with minimally displaced pelvic and acetabular fractures; (ii) displaced fractures where closed reduction is feasible; and (iii) in cases of open pelvic surgery when the insertion of several screws is very challenging and demands the assistance of guiding systems such as fluoroscopy or navigated fluoroscopy following appropriate open reduction.

It is important to note that the percutaneous approach to fracture fixation of the pelvis continues to evolve and undergo many improvements and developments in which computerized technology may be of great assistance. For example, in preplanning, the use of standard axial CT data to create computer-reconstructed 3D images and/or models may replace the standard radiographic assessment of pelvic and acetabular fractures.[5,11,15,36,40] Similarly, 3D fluoroscopy technology allows the surgeon to obtain immediate and accurate 3D reconstructions in the operating room. By integrating these images into navigation systems, preplanning becomes easier and more accurate and allows for direct, truly spatial surgical navigation. It also enables the precise evaluation of closed reduction (using a fracture table, external fixator, and/or other fixation instruments) before insertion of the navigated screws.

Surgical Technique

For both acetabular and pelvic surgery, the dynamic reference frame can be rigidly attached to the patient's iliac crest. Several appropriate fluoroscopic images of the pelvis are acquired and saved in the system's computer. No further fluoroscopic imaging is necessary, except for verification fluoroscopy prior to the insertion of the cannulated screw, or in the case of reduced fracture, the crossing of the fracture site.

During surgery, following the activation of the fluoroscopic images, the surgeon can accurately determine the entry point and direction of each screw. At the same time, by means of a virtual trajectory line, the correct length and diameter of the screw can be calculated (Fig. 18-12). After satisfactory virtual alignment and length have been achieved, the conventional guidewire pertaining to the cannulated screw system is driven through the drill guide. Before insertion of a self-drilled cannulated screw, the position of the guidewire should be verified by fluoroscopy. When the insertion of several screws in the same area is required, such as in the fixation of fractures or dislocations in the sacroiliac zone, the acquired fluoroscopic views can be used for the insertion of more than one screw (Figs. 18-13 and 18-14).

In pelvic surgery, serious complications can arise from the surgical procedure and intervention, rather than from the initial injury. Therefore, it is only natural that percutaneous minimal surgical approaches are sought to overcome the difficulties that arise in relation to fractures in the complex anatomy of the pelvis and acetabulum. Figure 18-9 illustrates the placement of a retrograde anterior column screw using a CT-based navigation system.

Fracture Reduction

Intramedullary nailing is the preferred surgical option in many long bone fractures Although it is a routine procedure, performed by most trauma surgeons, it is not devoid of technical pitfalls and complications. Achieving accurate and successful results with conventional techniques involves exposure to significant amounts of radiation for both patients and the surgical team.

Fluoroscopy-based navigation can be helpful in closed intramedullary nailing by increasing precision, minimizing soft tissue damage, and significantly decreasing radiation exposure.[14,20,24] Several surgical goals can be achieved by using computerized navigation systems. The insertion of instruments based on real-time information becomes possible and significantly increases the accuracy of nail placement. Determining the exact point of entry of the nail is critical because it is one of the main sources of morbidity in intramedullary nailing as well as a cause of misalignment. As previously discussed, computerized navigation systems help to precisely locate the nail entry point by means of trajectory navigation, thus minimizing soft tissue dissection. This is particularly helpful in special cases such as in obese patients where anatomic landmarks are obscured. Working with several images simultaneously can also decrease unnecessary drill holes, tissue damage, and cartilage perforation, because all targeting is done virtually, prior to the introduction of the actual instrument. The insertion of locking screws into certain nails can be a potential hazard for neurovascular structures.[24,47,48] Additional improvement in nailing techniques is achieved by the facilitation of Poller screw insertion. When precisely placed, better angular correction of metaphyseal fractures is achieved. Another important future contribution of the new generation of navigation technology will be to allow for the tracking and aligning of two fragments, thus enabling fracture reduction without radiation and reduction wire insertion, and perhaps most critically, its ability to provide the surgeon with accurate information to restore alignment, including length and rotation.[17,24,38] The precision of length measurement may also decrease the rate of complications associated with nailing such as protrusion of the nail or screw ends.[26,52,62]

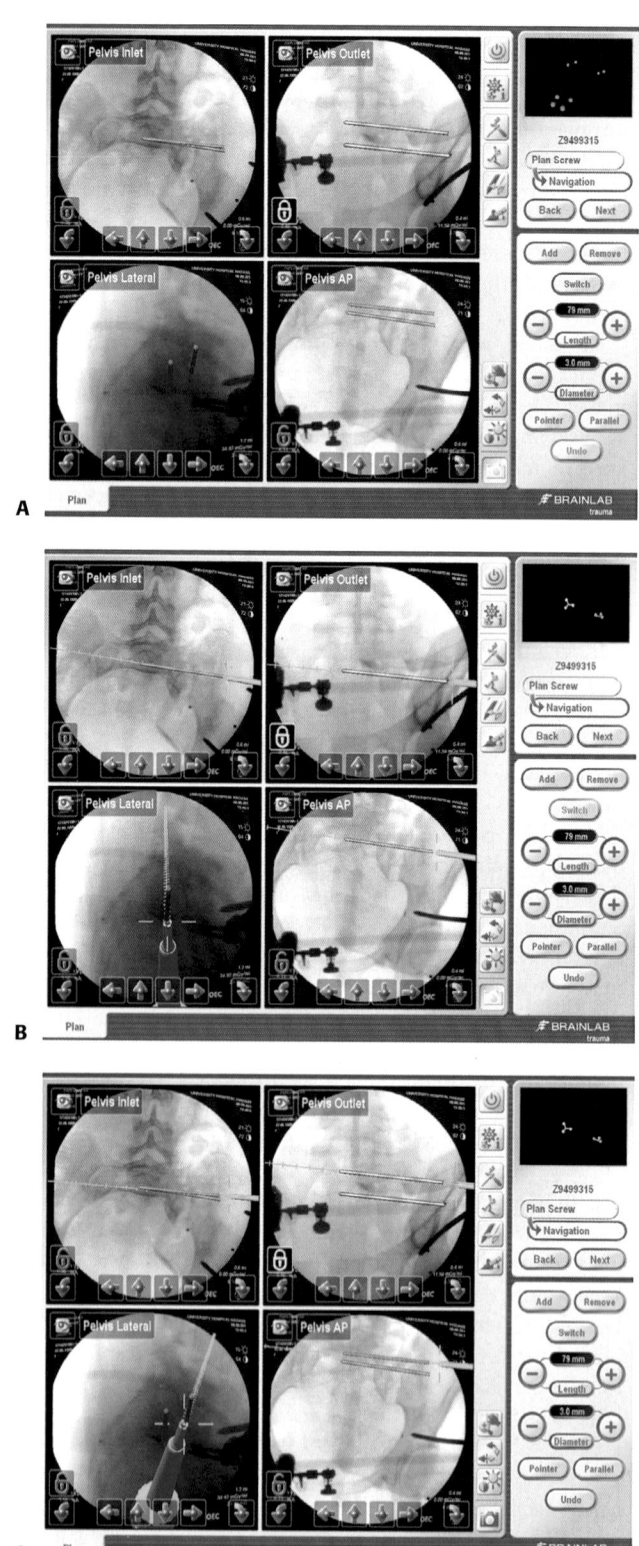

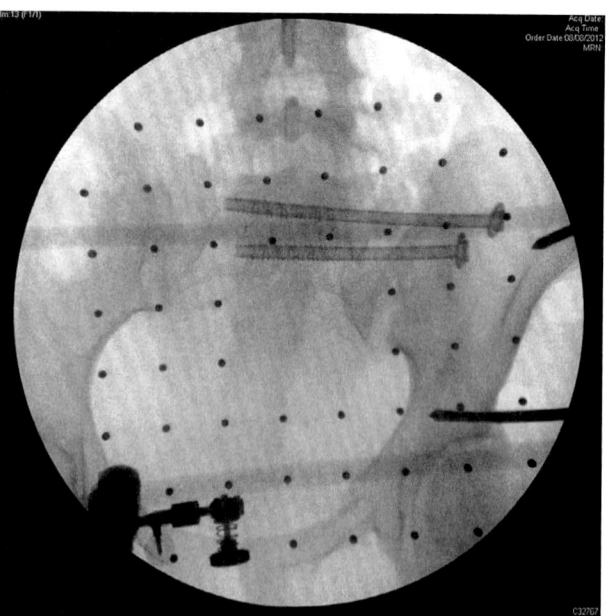

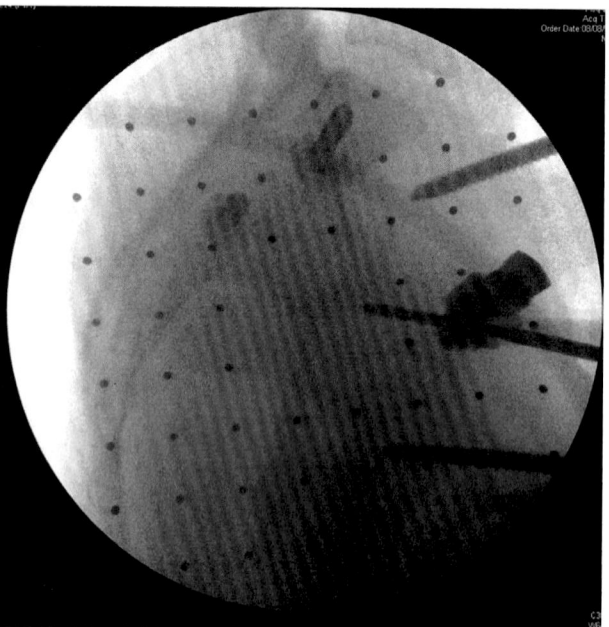

FIGURE 18-13 Sacroiliac screws. **A:** The optimal screw position is planned on the screw and later by the virtual drill guide **B, C:** Typical intraoperative display of computer screen during insertion of two sacroiliac screws. The live spatial position of the drill guide is simultaneously presented on four views (inlet and outlet AP and lateral) with a virtual continuation representing the track of the guide. **D, E:** Postoperative verification fluoroscopic images showing the accurate real position of the two sacroiliac screws after the navigation process. (Brainlab Trauma Package [Ver 3], images property of authors.)

Surgical Technique

A fluoroscopy-based surgical navigation system can be used, either for the entire operation, or for different stages of intramedullary nailing. These include the nail's entry point, nail and screw measurements, freehand locking, placement of auxiliary screws, as well as fracture reduction and the assessment of length and rotation. Navigation of the entrance point and the locking procedure are performed by using straight line trajectory. The reference frame should be attached to the tracked bone fragment, either proximal or distal, depending on the specific task.

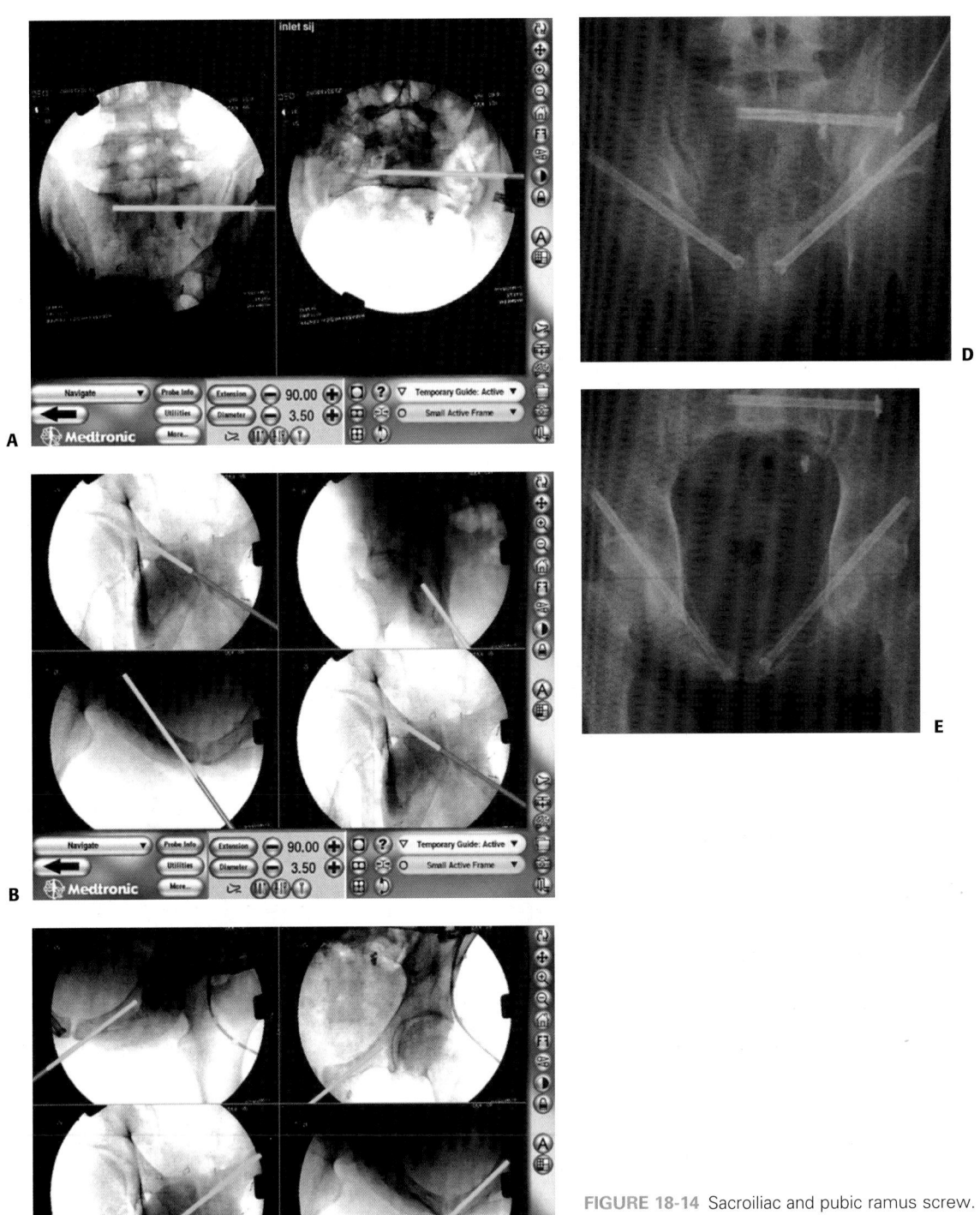

FIGURE 18-14 Sacroiliac and pubic ramus screw. **A–C:** An intraoperative display of the computer screen during insertion of a sacroiliac screw and two intramedullary pubic ramus screws. **D, E:** Inlet and outlet postoperative verification radiographs showing the accurate real placement of the three screws. (Images property of authors.)

1. *Nail entry point:* The actual point of entry is determined by the use of simultaneous virtual fluoroscopic views, usually anteroposterior (AP) and lateral views. Before incision, the tracked drill guide is drawn next to the skin. Its position is adjusted by viewing its virtual trajectory superimposed on the activated fluoroscopic images so as to minimize the surgical exposure. The entry point location is established while moving the tracked drill guide to an optimal position (Fig. 18-15A). No further fluoroscopy is required and a verification fluoroscopic image is taken only after insertion of the guidewire. After this task is performed a cannulated awl or a larger cannulated drill is inserted, according to the manufacturer's instructions, through this guide to open the medullary canal.[24]

2. *Freehand locking:* This technique is relatively easy to perform and involves minimal radiation exposure. The bone tracker is fixed close to the location of the locking screws. Using the "perfect circle" technique, an AP or lateral view of the locking hole, in which the holes almost resemble circles, is obtained. An additional AP or lateral view may be taken to determine the screw length. The tracked drill guide is then drawn toward the locking screw area and is navigated until a circle appears within the hole on the computer screen (Figs. 18-15B, C). This is followed by drilling through the tracked drill guide and inserting the locking screw. Sometimes, such as with tibial nailing, the same AP and lateral views can be used for insertion of two or even three adjacent locking screws. New advanced technologies are designed to facilitate easy locking with less radiation than conventional navigation.[63]

3. *Placement of other screws:* Poller screws are important tools for correcting bone alignment when nailing metaphyseal fractures. Precise placement of these screws can now be performed using a technique similar to that of locking screws. Virtual fluoroscopy based on AP and lateral images enables easy and precise positioning of Poller screws. For "miss-a-nail" screws, additional AP and lateral images of the proximal femur are obtained following the insertion of the intramedullary nail. The goal is to insert the cross-neck screw without interfering with the intramedullary nail. The navigation system enables the surgeon to determine the precise position of the "miss-a-nail" cross-neck screws and to safely navigate through the narrow safe zone[24,38,61] (Fig. 18-16).

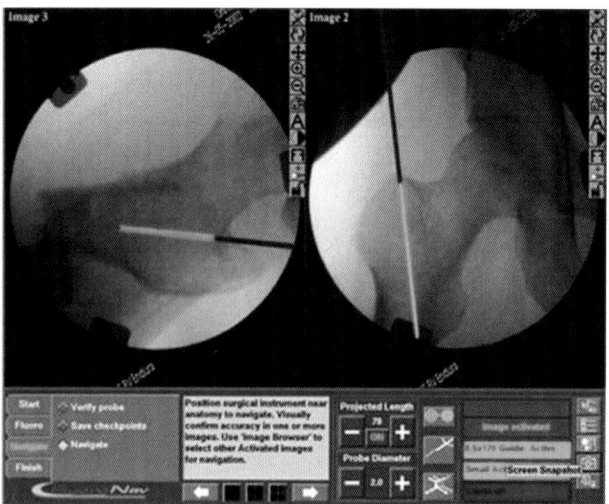

A

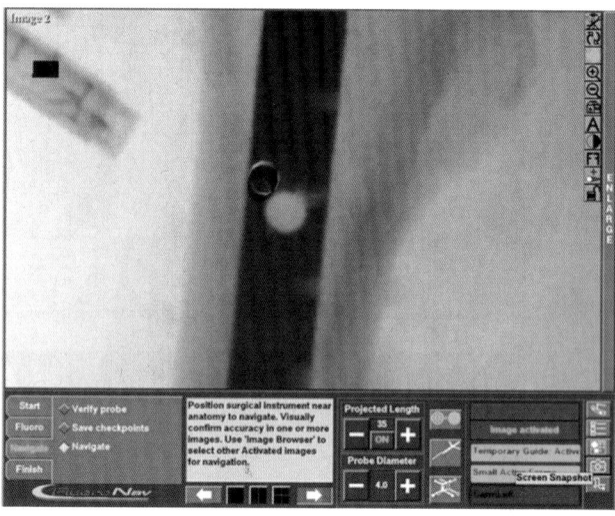

B

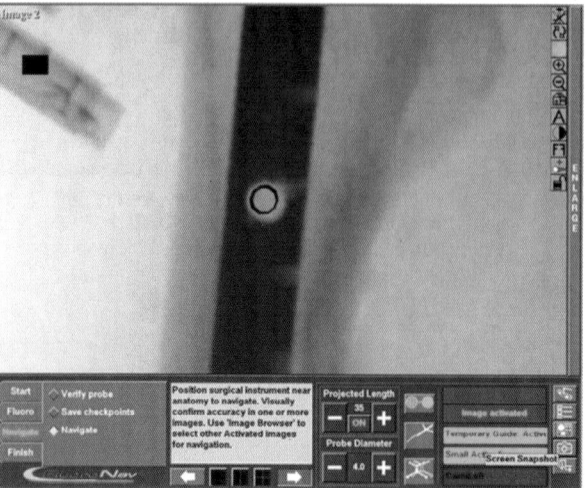

C

FIGURE 18-15 Intramedullary nailing. **A:** Typical computer display used during antegrade femoral intramedullary nailing consisting of simultaneous anteroposterior and lateral views, where the pink line represents the guide's insertion point at the precise entry point in the piriformis fossa and the green line represents the nail's direction. **B, C:** Proximal locking hole in the retrograde femoral nail. Note the hole as a perfect circle enabling precise aiming of the locking screw. (Images property of authors.)

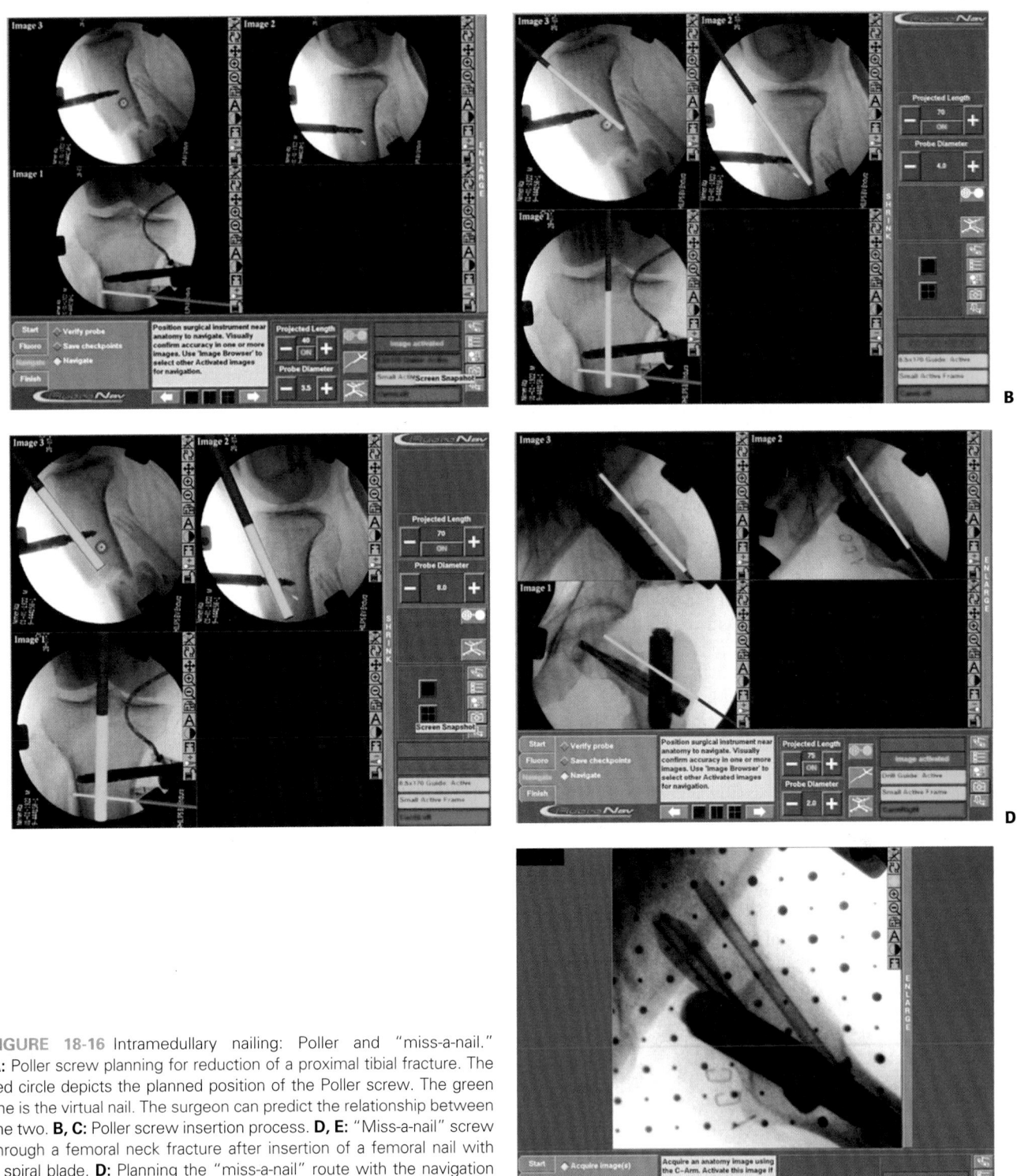

FIGURE 18-16 Intramedullary nailing: Poller and "miss-a-nail." **A:** Poller screw planning for reduction of a proximal tibial fracture. The red circle depicts the planned position of the Poller screw. The green line is the virtual nail. The surgeon can predict the relationship between the two. **B, C:** Poller screw insertion process. **D, E:** "Miss-a-nail" screw through a femoral neck fracture after insertion of a femoral nail with a spiral blade. **D:** Planning the "miss-a-nail" route with the navigation system displayed as a green line. **E:** Fluoroscopic image after nail insertion. Note the parallelism between the planned and real route of the nail. (Images property of authors.)

4. *Fracture reduction:* New software is available for the entire fracture reduction procedure. This became possible because of the ability to simultaneously track two reference frames. The frames are attached to the distal and proximal long bone fragments. Several AP and lateral views are acquired, enabling visualization of the entire bone. Usually, six views (three AP and three lateral) are needed to visualize the proximal fragment, the fracture site, and the distal fragment in two planes. It is possible to virtually define each segment on the computer display and to track each fragment by navigation as already described. The special location of each fragment in relationship to the other enables actual fracture reduction and insertion of the reduction wire. The procedure resembles the fluoroscopic process of fracture reduction surgery with two major advantages: No radiation and simultaneous two-plane tracking. The ability to track and visualize the entire bone enables the taking of several measurements including length and rotation. Newly computerized navigation software provides accurate measurements of length and rotation (Brainlab navigation, Brainlab Trauma 3.0). It enables access to biomechanical data of the nonfractured side for reproduction on the fractured side. A noninvasive optical tracker is placed on the noninjured thigh at the beginning of the case, using a Velcro strap. Tracked AP and lateral images of the proximal and distal femur are obtained. A handheld tracker placed in the vicinity of a C-arm fluoroscope (X-Spot™) is used to track and register the images along with the noninvasive tracking. The resultant images are marked by the surgeon on four landmarks: the center of the femoral head; the tip of the greater trochanter; the most posterior part of the femoral condyles; and in the center of the knee. The software automatically calculates the axial rotation angle between the proximal and distal femoral landmarks as well as the femoral length and stores the values for later reproduction. The injured extremity is then prepped and the femoral nailing procedure commences in a standard surgical fashion according to the surgeon's preference. Following nail insertion and prior to any nail interlocking, trackers are placed both proximally and distally to the injured femur and an identical process of imaging acquisition and landmarking, as described above for the uninjured extremity, is repeated. At this point, the tracking camera of the navigation system records the length and rotation of the injured nailed extremity. The rotation and length is corrected, followed by interlocking screw placement to secure the alignment. Preliminary data indicate that this technology is feasible in the clinical setup and may significantly contribute to the clinical outcome of long bone fracture reduction (Fig. 18-17). Recently, several software packages have been developed that also enable the tracking of implants, particularly plates. Thus, it is possible to track the position of the implant in relationship to the bone. This technique overcomes some of the drawbacks of the first generation of computer navigation systems. In the future, customized tracked instruments based on these principles will further improve and facilitate computer-aided intramedullary nailing.[9,15,24,38,40,52,58]

Intra-Articular Fracture Fixation

Intra-articular fracture fixation presents unique technical difficulties. In many cases, the fracture is comminuted and has complex geometry that is difficult to evaluate on conventional CT slices or fluoroscopic radiography images. Recently introduced 3D intraoperative imaging, such as Iso C-arm imaging, is a useful tool for this visualization. However, it too has limitations. It can be used only once or twice during surgery because of radiation exposure and it is a static view. Other difficulties include tracking of small bone fragments and possible fragment motion during fixation.

Intraoperative Control

Intraoperative, rather than postoperative, confirmation of the reduction and fixation of intra-articular fractures can save patients and surgeons from uncertainty relating to the quality of the reduction. Recent developments have yielded new options for intraoperative 3D imaging. The SireMobil Iso-C 3D (Siemens Medical Solutions), for example, combines the capabilities of routine intraoperative C-arm fluoroscopy with resultant 3D images. The 3D imaging equipment has the ability to automatically revolve around a fixed surgical target (isocentric) acquiring up to 100 images. Of these images, axial cuts and 2D and 3D reformations can be generated which are comparable to CT images. Using this unique imaging modality can help the surgeon to intraoperatively assess not only the fracture anatomy,[1,2] but also the position and configuration of the implants in correlation to the area of surgery,[57] including those in the vicinity of the acetabulum and the posterior pelvic ring.[41] The performance of the Iso-C 3D has already been described in several studies for intraoperative demonstration of high-contrast skeletal objects, with encouraging results.[1,2] The persisting disadvantages of 3D fluoroscopes are their limited image size of 12.5 cm³, which is sufficient for the sacroiliac joint but not for the entire posterior pelvic ring, and their relatively inferior image quality. Modifications of the isocentric C-arm have recently been introduced, offering superior image quality, increased field of view, higher spatial resolution, and soft tissue visibility, as well as the elimination of the need to rotate around a fixed point (isocentricity).[45] In addition, newly developed patented software modules have recently been developed which allow for intraoperative 3D assessment, with decreased cost and less radiation, using conventional fluoroscope techniques.[35,41,51,60]

Fracture Fixation

An improved method for image guidance in intra-articular fracture fixation is 3D fluoroscopy-based navigation. Of the intraoperative axial cuts, 2D and 3D reformations can be generated and the data can be transferred to the navigation system. With inherent registration, the navigation procedure can be performed, similar to CT navigation, but without any registration procedure.[49]

New developments integrating a second-generation 3D fluoroscope (e.g., the ARCADIS Orbic; Siemens AG, Erlangen, Germany; O-arm Surgical Imaging System; Metronic, Minneapolis, MN, USA)[28,41,42,53] and a multifunctional navigation system onto one common trolley markedly improve data transfer and

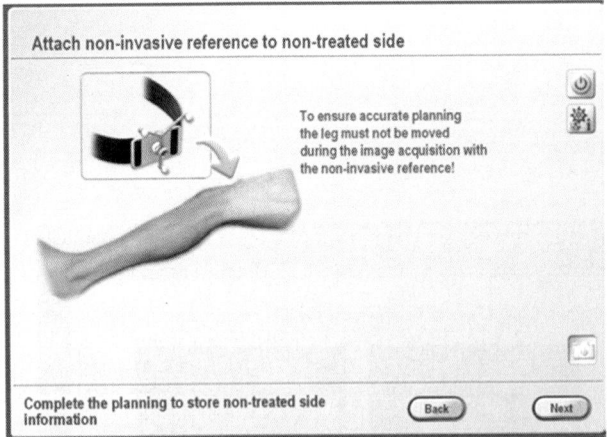

A1

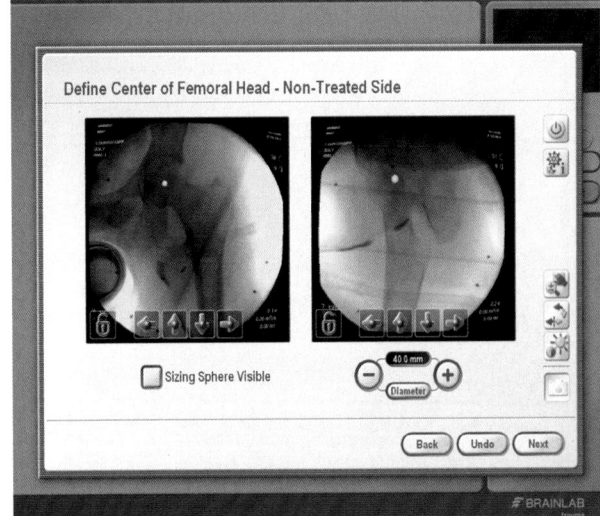

B1

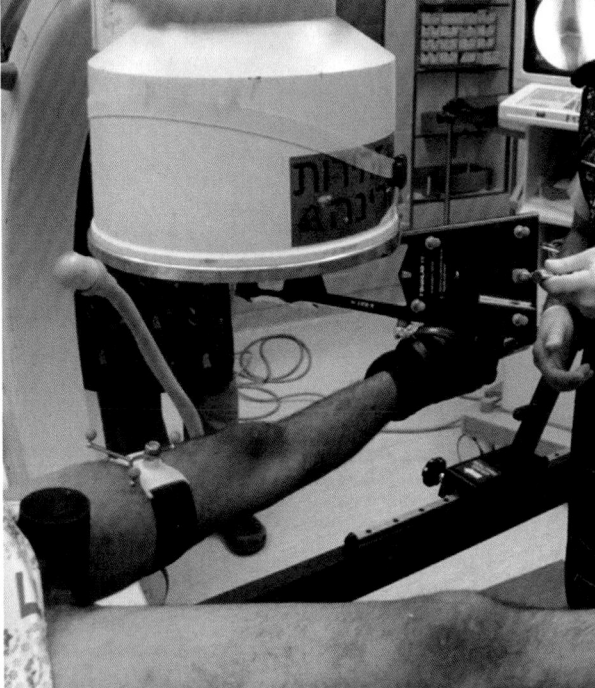

A2

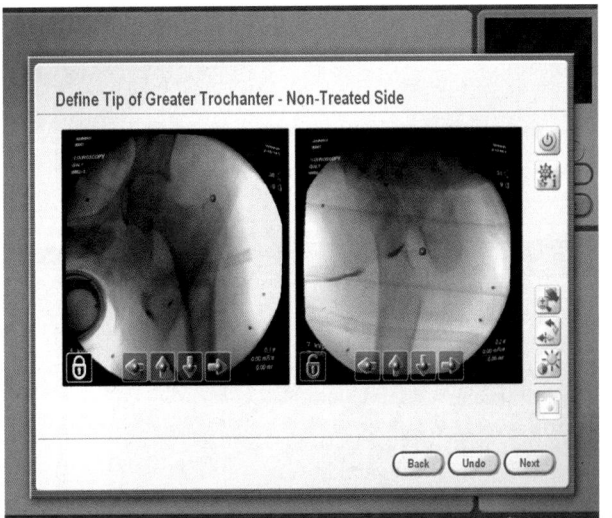

B2

B3

FIGURE 18-17 Femoral fracture reduction procedure including length & rotation control. **A:** Attachment of noninvasive strap to the noninjured side. *A1*: Instruction on display. *A2*: Clinical picture. **B:** Measurements of length and rotation of the nontreated side as a reference for the treated side. *B1*: Definition of femoral head center. *B2*: Definition of greater trochanter. *B3*: Distal femur and posterior condyle reference.

(*continues*)

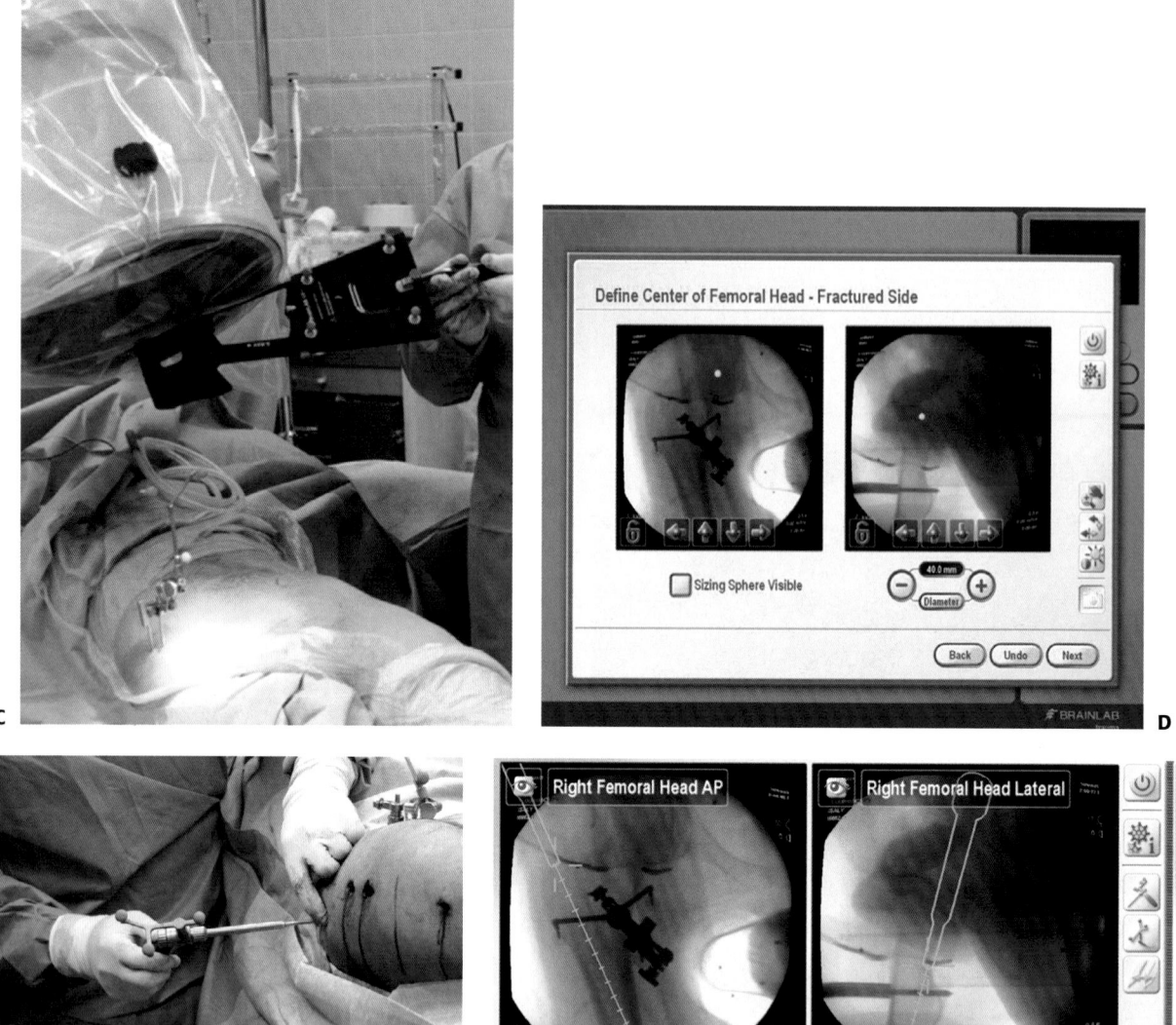

FIGURE 18-17 (*continued*) **C:** Acquisition of fluoroscopic images of the treated side with two reference frames attached to the distal and proximal fragments using a new image registration method that has been introduced consisting of a portable device "Expot" that is not connected to the fluoroscope and includes trackers and markers that allow for an easy registration process. **D:** Definition of the same anatomical landmarks on the treated side, not the rigidity attached reference frame. **E:** Navigation of entry point. *E1:* Clinical. *E2:* Display image.

system handling. Thus, the indications for image guidance in intra-articular fractures, including pelvic surgery, have expanded in order to reduce open procedures (Fig. 18-18). The increasing use of these new technologies provides intraoperative control, thus facilitating their use in trauma surgery of the spine.[50,54,64]

Novel Uses of Navigation: Localization of Bone Lesions or Removal of Surgical Hardware and Shrapnel

The simplest indication for using CAOS–ST systems is a situation in which a foreign body is retained in bone or soft tissue,

such as surgical hardware or penetrating injuries with retained metals (e.g., shrapnel, nuts, and bolts), that need to be removed. It is not necessary to track foreign bodies, as they usually remain in place and do not drift. They can be reached with a navigated tool by following the tool's location with respect to the foreign body in the activated fluoroscopic images (Fig. 18-19). Given the simplicity of the procedure, we recommend that this be the first surgical procedure using computerized navigation systems to be performed by inexperienced surgeons.[30,37,59]

The main indication for metal/hardware removal is local discomfort, although other indications include infection or risk of

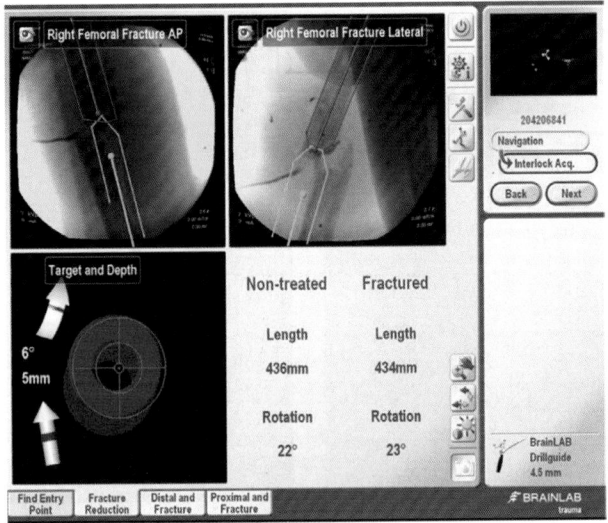

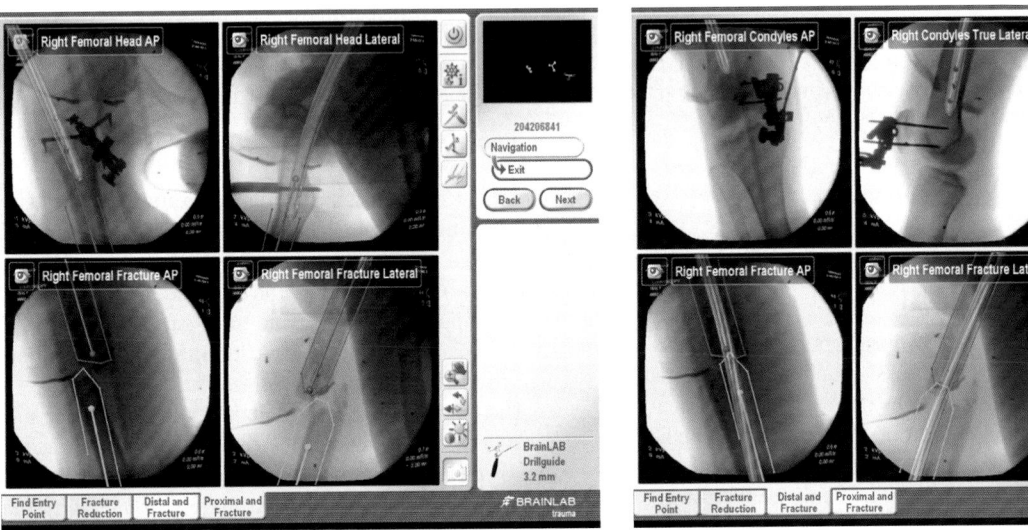

FIGURE 18-17 (*continued*) **F:** Fracture reduction—the navigation process of two fragments. The software enables simultaneous tracking of the two fragments, with information regarding length, angulation, and rotation. **G:** Implant navigation: Navigation of intramedullary nail. *G1:* Navigation of intramedullary nail into the entrance point and (*G2*) into the distal fragment. (Images property of authors.)

toxicity. The removal of missiles retained in an inaccessible location poses a major problem for the trauma surgeon because they can be hazardous to the integrity of adjacent internal structures.

Fluoroscopy-based navigation is the method of choice for these situations. Unlike CT-based systems, it requires very short preoperative preparation, making it appropriate in emergency situations as well, where its effectiveness has already been proven even during the urgent stages of treatment. Thanks to the high accuracy of fluoroscopy-based navigation, its use in complex and dangerous situations where a foreign body is located in the proximity of structures such as blood vessels and/or nerves is promising. In comparison to other conventional techniques, the use of fluoroscopy-based navigation has allowed orthopedic surgeons to minimize soft tissue dissection. The same principle can be used for guided bone biopsy.

Surgical Technique

Tracked reference frames are rigidly attached to the patient's adjacent bone and to a calibrated pointer. Several fluoroscopic images of the required anatomic site are acquired and stored in the computer, or 3D information using Iso-C technology is acquired. The accurate spatial location of the foreign object can be seen in the images displayed on the computer's screen (Fig. 18-19). The surgeon then plans the most accurate and safest minimal surgical approach for the foreign body that needs to be removed. Once the stored fluoroscopic images have been activated, the location of the guided probe with respect to the patient's anatomy is continuously displayed and updated on all of the fluoroscopic images. This enables accurate determination of the entry point and spatial advancement of the probe toward the foreign body.[29]

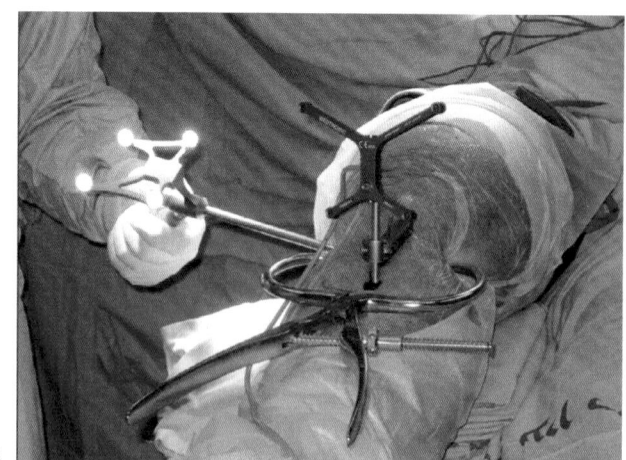
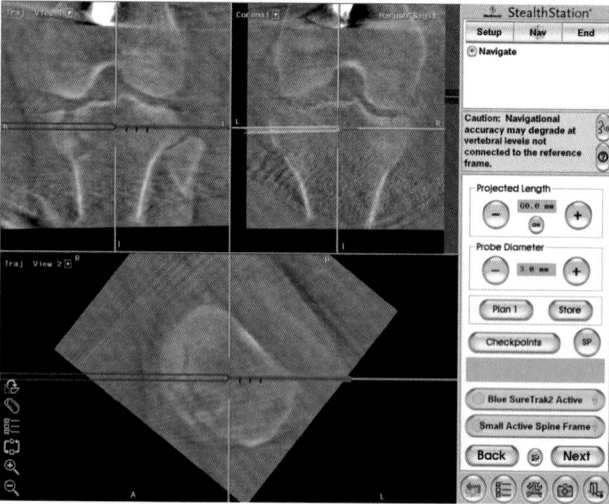

FIGURE 18-18 Using SireMobil Iso-C 3D (Siemens Medical Solutions, Erlangen, Germany) for fracture reduction. **A:** Percutaneous reduction of a tibial plateau fracture using reduction instruments with application of a reference frame. **B:** Three images displayed on the system's screen (coronal and sagittal), showing the location of the surgical tool (*blue*) and allowing for real-time tracking with the virtual green line, which assists in determining the direction of the surgical tool in a three-dimensional environment. (Images property of authors.)

COMPLICATIONS AND CONTROVERSIES

The most frequent clinical and technical complications that lead to navigation errors and failure are listed below.

1. *Loss of line of sight*

    An unobstructed view between the optical camera and the trackers at all times is the basic requirement of optical navigation. Loss of line of sight occurs when the view between the optical camera and one or more of the trackers is obstructed by the surgeon or another member of the surgical team, the patient's body, the fluoroscopy C-arm, the overhead lamps, or any other object in the vicinity of the surgical field. When there is no line of sight, the tracker, which is not seen, either disappears from the display or the entire display freezes. Navigation resumes as soon as the obstruction disappears.

    Loss of line of sight can be remedied by moving the object causing the interference, by repositioning the optical camera, or by changing the surgical team's location around the patient. In some situations, because of the surgical approach, it is not possible to see all of the trackers at once. In this case, partial navigation is possible with the visible trackers. In some surgical situations, maintenance of the line of sight is not possible and therefore navigation should be avoided. As previously discussed, the surgeon can control some of the obstacles by appropriate placement of the trackers and the camera. In practical terms the availability of line of sight should be considered as an integral part of the preplanning stage of CAOS–ST.

2. *Shift of the dynamic reference frame rigid bone mounting*

    Maintaining a rigid attachment between the bone tracker and the bone throughout surgery is essential in order to guarantee registration accuracy. Shifting is usually the result of bone fixation loosening, poor jig fixation, or unintentionally pushing or hitting the tracker and its mounting jig. An undetected shift will result in inaccurate navigation images that might mislead the surgeon and lead to undesired results and complications. To avoid this situation, the surgeon should ensure that the tracker mounting jig is securely fixated to the bone structure.

    The only way to detect dynamic reference frame motion is by validation. Validation is performed either by acquiring one or more fluoroscopic radiography images and comparing them with the navigation images, or by using the tip of a surgical tool to touch known anatomic landmarks and verifying that the tool tip appears close to the landmark in the navigated image. Validation should be performed at key points during surgery and always when in doubt.

3. *Tool decalibration*

    Tool decalibration occurs when the geometric data of the tracked tool does not match its actual geometry. Tool decalibration is caused by tool wear and tear (e.g., tip bending, frame deformation because of repeated sterilization or tool tracker shift). To avoid these situations, the surgeon should verify tool calibration before surgery, at key points during the surgery, and always when in doubt. Tool decalibration cannot be detected automatically. The surgeon must perform a tool calibration verification procedure, which usually involves the use of custom calibration software and hardware.

4. *Navigation image inaccuracy*

    Inaccuracy of navigation images is the mismatch between the displayed images and the intraoperative situation. Inaccuracy is the result of errors in the registration chain. The main causes of the errors include the shift of the dynamic reference frame, tool decalibration, and the shift of the

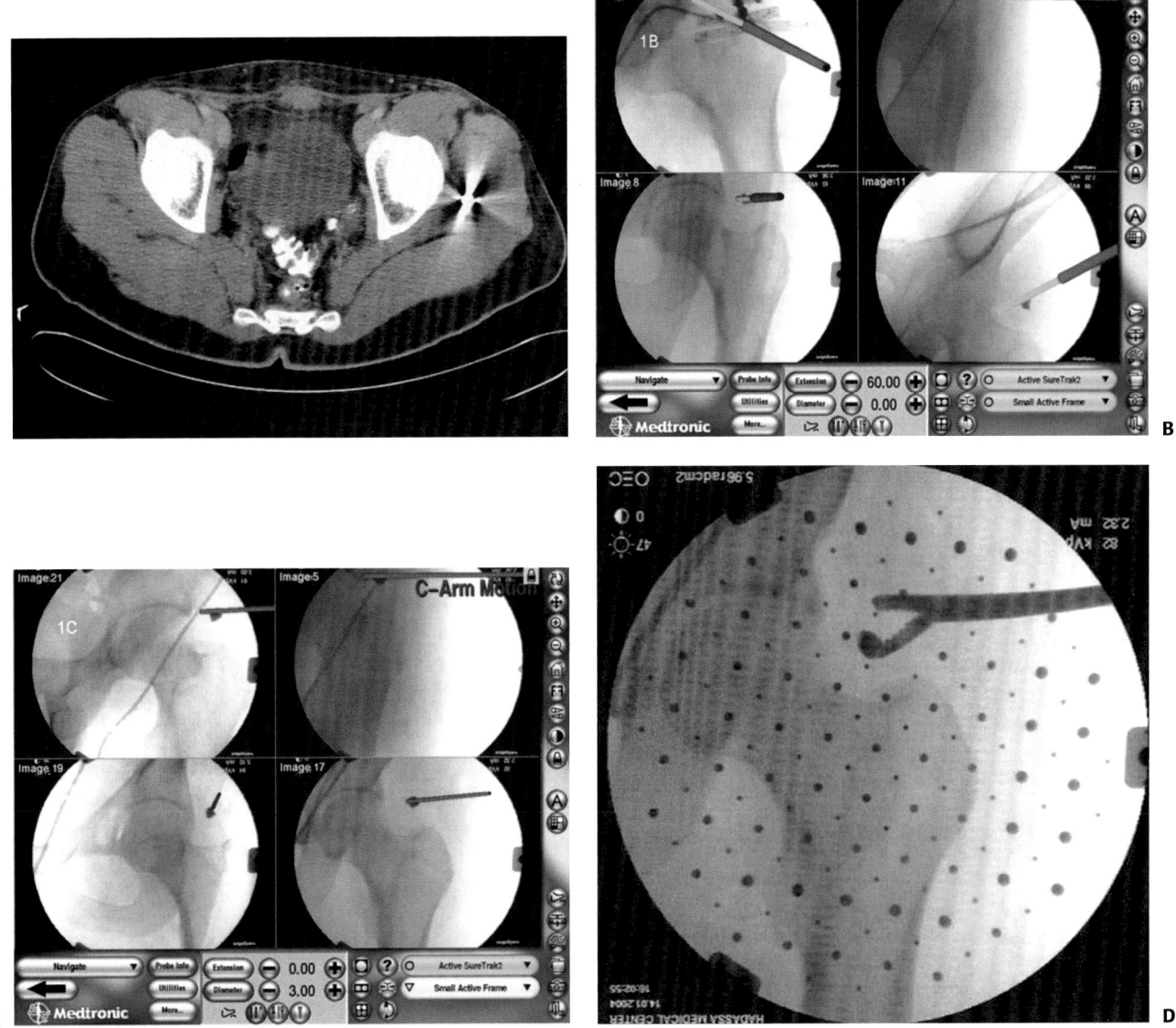

FIGURE 18-19 Shrapnel removal. **A:** Preoperative computed tomography scan showing shrapnel that needs to be removed because of its proximity to the left hip joint. **B:** Four acquired images displayed on the system's screen, showing the location of the missile and allowing for immediate presurgical planning of the percutaneous surgical approach. The pink line represents the surgical tool and the virtual green line assists in determining the point of entry and direction of the surgical tool. **C:** The surgical tool, represented by the pink line, arrives at the missile. **D:** Verification fluoroscopy followed by removal of the missile. (Images property of authors.)

C-arm tracker ring. Secondary causes include tracking system drift over time and navigation at the edge of the position sensor working volume. Other causes are related to the images themselves. In CT images, they include poor contrast, low slice resolution, insufficient radiation dose, large spacing between slices, patient motion during the CT scan, and blooming artifacts as a result of the presence of metallic objects. In fluoroscopic radiography images, they include poor image resolution, poor contrast because of insufficient or excessive radiation, inappropriate viewpoints, and patient motion during image acquisition.

The surgeon must realize that the acquired images serve as the basis for the entire navigated surgical procedure.[17,19,46] Therefore, optimization of these images (contrast, field, viewing angle, etc.) is crucial and should be done during the image acquisition stage, before surgery begins. Note that navigation image inaccuracy can be observed by the surgeon but cannot automatically be detected. It requires performing validation tests for C-arm ring and dynamic reference frame shift, tool decalibration, restarting of the tracking system, repositioning of the position sensor, and the acquisition of new images.[27]

5. *System robustness issues*

Robustness is the ability of a system to perform its intended tasks with a minimum number of failures over time. The more robust the system, the more acceptable it will be to the surgeon. Robustness depends on both software and hardware components. Software failures include flaws in the computer operating system, in the custom-designed software, and in the tracking base unit controller. At best, software flaws can be temporarily overcome by restarting the system. At worst, they require pre-empting navigation and reporting the flaw to the company. Hardware failures include failure of the computer unit, poor cable connections, and failure of the tracking unit.

6. *Verification of surgical tool and implant spatial position*

The surgeon should always remember to make a distinction between the virtual and nonvirtual situations displayed on the computer screen. This is of great importance in trauma surgery because the surgeon is used to working under fluoroscopic guidance that provides a true view of the surgical site as opposed to the virtual display in CAOS–ST procedures. For example, a perfect virtual position of a guidewire may be a false presentation of the real situation, because during insertion of the real guidewire, it may slip or bend and point to a wrong position, without being detected or shown on the augmented image. There are several ways to tackle this critical obstacle. The best is to use rigid guidewires to prevent bending so as to penetrate the cortical bone in the right location. Experience and/or the use of rigid drills can usually overcome this problem. In addition, it is also very important to perform real-time fluoroscopic verification at critical or questionable time points during the surgical procedure.

7. *Adaptation to different surgical techniques*

The main addition to computer-assisted navigation compared with conventional fluoroscopic trauma surgery is the bone-mounted reference frame. The significant ramifications of the loosening of the reference frame have been previously described. The actual location of the frame can interfere with the surgical procedure. For example, while inserting the reference frame screw into the bone diaphysis during intramedullary nailing, it should not obstruct nail passage within the medullary canal. In addition, during the insertion of a locking screw, the reference frame might be in the way and prevent either an accurate line of sight or the proper positioning of certain surgical instruments (e.g., drills). The surgeon must choose between placing the frame close to the operative site, to increase the accuracy of the procedure and to improve triangulation, and placing the frame where it establishes a convenient working distance.

PERSPECTIVES

Technical and Economic Perspectives

Navigation systems are limited by technical elements. Currently, their main limitations, in decreasing order of importance, and perspectives for improvements are as follows.

1. *Support for implants and instrumentation*

Navigation systems are designed to be used with specific tools, implants, and hardware from specific manufacturers. The choice of supported instruments and implants depends on decisions made by the navigation and instrument companies, which are primarily dictated by commercial interests. Often, the software module only accepts models from one manufacturer. In some cases, tools from other manufacturers can be incorporated following a tool calibration procedure. Currently, only a handful of instruments and implants are supported.

2. *Support for surgical procedures*

Navigation systems require software modules (software surgical protocols) that implement the surgical protocol for navigation for specific procedures. Without the custom software module for the surgical procedure, the navigation system cannot be used, although in principle it is technically feasible in procedures other than those for which they were designed. Currently, only a handful of procedures are supported.

3. *Improvements in tracking technology*

Current optical tracking technology has several drawbacks, including line of sight, size of trackers, cables, number of trackers, accuracy, and cost. Magnetic tracking offers a variety of potential advantages, including no line of sight requirement, reduced tracker size, and reduced cost. Although the technology is not as yet ready for routine clinical use, it is likely that some of the obstacles will be overcome in the near future, offering the possibility of tracking bone fragments and easing tracker fixation to the bone, thus significantly reducing or eliminating dynamic reference frame shift and opening the door for navigation during reduction.

4. *Image-based CT registration*

Current CT-based navigation systems require the surgeon to acquire points on the surface of the anatomy of interest to perform the registration between the CT data set and the intraoperative situation. This precludes its use in percutaneous procedures because it is time consuming and error prone and produces suboptimal registration results. An alternative is to use fluoroscopic radiography images instead of points harvested from the bone surface. This type of registration, called anatomy-based CT to fluoroscopic radiography registration, has been demonstrated in the laboratory and will soon be available in navigation systems.

5. *Planning*

Current intraoperative planning is either nonexistent or limited at best. Intraoperative definition of goals, such as screw path safety zone and insertion axis, can greatly help the surgeon perform the surgery. The blurring of the distinction between preoperative and intraoperative planning opens the door for better, more adaptive planning and consequently better and more consistent results.

6. *Spatial visualization without CT*

A drawback of fluoroscopy-based navigation systems is that they do not show spatial views of the intraoperative situation, which can only be produced when CT data are available. Isometric fluoroscopic technology (Iso-C) overcomes this obstacle; however, it provides a relatively small visual field. Newly designed technology is now available with better quality and a larger view. Another way to overcome this limitation has been proposed—to acquire several fluoroscopic radiography images and adapt a closely related CT or generic anatomic model so as to match the patient-specific fluoroscopic radiography images. This approach, called *atlas-based matching,* is currently under investigation.

7. *Ergonometric factors*

Most operating rooms were not designed with new technology in mind in terms of size; placement of the computer, computer screen, and cables; etc. A surgeon experienced with CAS can appreciate the advanced ease of use in newer generations of navigation systems. However, the insertion of a navigation system into the operating room still warrants special consideration. The machine occupies space. Its positioning is dictated by line of sight between the tracker sensor and the markers.

These obvious technical and economic factors need to be taken into account along with the human factors.

Clinical Perspectives

The use of computerized navigation systems in orthopedic trauma surgery is rather new. The four main contributions to trauma surgery are as follows:

1. They facilitate less invasive surgery by reducing soft tissue damage, thus shortening the postoperative rehabilitation process.

2. They improve the accuracy of fracture reduction and implant placement compared with that obtained with conventional methods and reduce the outcome variability.

3. They significantly reduce radiation exposure to both the patient and the surgeon.

4. They create a powerful educational and quality control tool.

Most of the contributions achieved to date are in the preplanning stage. For example, if we look at the imaging field, it is clear that computerized imaging supplies a better 3D understanding that may influence the planning of the surgical procedure. Undoubtedly, this technology can, and should, change our way of thinking in relation to other stages of surgical treatment.

It is quite obvious that computerized navigation systems are continuously advancing and offer additional possibilities. Although these systems are still in their infancy, it appears that they have already managed to change the setting in several trauma centers. The CT suite can be transformed into an operating room or, alternatively, the modern hi-tech fluoroscope can now be altered to produce 3D images. These technologies together with surgeons' preferences and compliance will in the future determine the setup of the operating room. Future generations of computerized navigation systems will be characterized not only by improved accuracy but also by improvements to robustness and improving working convenience in the computerized environment. When these changes finally take place, it is expected that computerized technology will be of assistance not only in navigation but also in the execution of the surgical procedure by means of robots.[56] If the trauma surgeon can overcome the difficulties entailed in integrating the new technology, we may experience a revolution in surgical approaches and education.

GLOSSARY

General

CAOS (computer-aided orthopedic surgery). Planning and execution of orthopedic surgery with the help of a computer system.

CAOS–ST (computer-aided orthopedic surgery in skeletal trauma). Planning and execution of orthopedic trauma surgery with the help of a computer system.

CAS (computer-aided surgery). Planning and execution of orthopedic surgery with the help of a computer system. Synonyms: Computer-assisted surgery, computer-integrated surgery (CIS), image-guided surgery (IGS), surgical navigation.

Planning

Model. Computer representation of the relevant characteristics (e.g., shape, location, main axis) of an object of interest (e.g., a bone, bone fragment, surgical instrument, implant, fixation plate, cutting plane). Synonym: *Digital template.*

Preoperative planning. Process of creating a computerized plan for the purposes of surgery.

Surface mesh. Geometric description of a bone surface consisting of a collection of interconnected points, usually extracted from CT data. Synonym: *Surface model.*

Navigation

CT-based navigation. Navigation with images created by superimposing onto a preoperative CT cross section and spatial images the surgical tool silhouette and updating its location in real time.

Fluoroscopy-based navigation. Navigation using images created by superimposing onto conventional fluoroscopic images the surgical tool silhouette and updating its location in real time, thereby creating the impression of continuous fluoroscopy without the ensuing radiation. Synonyms: *Virtual fluoroscopy, augmented fluoroscopy.*

Guidance. Process of indicating in real time to the surgeon, via images, graphics, or sound, the best course of action during surgery.

Navigation. Process of determining the spatial location of surgical instruments and anatomic structures in real time for the purposes of guiding surgical gestures during surgery.

Navigation images. Images created by a navigation system for the purposes of navigation. Synonyms: *Active display, navigation display, real-time visualization.*

Navigation system. System that shows the current location of surgical instruments with respect to images of the anatomy and continuously updates this image as the instruments and bone structures move. It requires tracking, registration, visualization, and validation. Synonyms: *Surgical navigator, guidance system.*

Tracking

Line of sight. Basic requirement of optical tracking systems in which there must be no occluding objects between the position sensor and the trackers.

Marker. Basic element recognized by the position sensor; can be an LED or a reflective sphere. Synonyms: *Infrared light-emitting diode (IRED)*

Position sensor. System that determines the spatial location of the trackers at any moment in time. It is an **optical camera** for optical systems and a **magnetic field generator** for magnetic systems. Synonym: *Localizer.*

Tracked pointer. Pointer with a tracker used for pointing and probing during navigation. Synonym: *Digitizing probe.*

Tracker. Rigid body with markers that are recognized by the position sensor. Synonyms: *Optical localizer, 3D localizer, sensor, marker carrier.*

Tracker mounting jigs. Mechanical jigs, such as screws and clamps, used to rigidly attach trackers to surgical instrumentssand bone structures and whose purpose is to mechanically fix their positional relationship. Synonym: *Attachment.*

Tracking. Process of determining in real time the spatial location of moving objects. Synonym: *Localization.*

Tracking base unit. Unit that controls and processes the information from the position sensor and the trackers. Synonym: *Tracking data acquisition unit.*

Tracking system. System that obtains the position and orientation of trackers by measuring spatially dependent physical properties, such as optical and magnetic properties. Synonym: *Localization system.*

Tracking technology. Physical means by which the location of trackers is measured. Tracking technology is optical or magnetic. Optical tracking is active (light-emitting diodes), passive (reflective spheres), or hybrid (both active and passive), and is called semi-active. Synonym: *Localization technology.*

Tracking work volume. Volume of space covered by the position sensor in which measurements can be made. Synonym: *Measurement volume.*

Accuracy

Accuracy. Measure of an instrument's capability to approach a true or absolute value. Static accuracy refers to measurements that do not change over time, while dynamic accuracy refers to time-varying measurements. Accuracy is a function of both bias and precision.

Bias. Measure of how closely the mean value in a series of replicate measurements approaches the true value.

Frequency. Number of overall measurements per second. Static accuracy refers to measurements obtained when the trackers are at rest, while dynamic accuracy refers to measurements obtained as the trackers move. Synonyms: *Rate, frame rate, display rate.*

Precision. Measure of how closely the values within a series of replicate measurements agree with each other.

Repeatability. Measure of resolution and stability. Resolution is the smallest discernible difference between two measurements. Stability refers to measurements made at steady state and over a sufficiently long period of time.

Registration

Coordinate frame. Fixed reference within which the spatial locations of objects can be described. Each object of interest has its own coordinate frame. Synonym: *Coordinate system (COS).*

CT registration. Process of establishing a common reference frame between the preoperative CT images and the intraoperative situation. Synonyms: *Point registration, surface registration, contact registration.*

Dynamic reference frame. Tracker attached to the bone used to track the bone motions to determine the relative location of the bone with respect to the tool. Synonyms: *Reference, reference base, dynamic reference base (DRB), dynamic referencing.*

Location. Six parameters determining the position and orientation of an object in space. Synonyms: *Placement, degrees of freedom (DOF).*

Registration. Process of establishing a common reference frame between objects and images. Synonym: *Alignment.*

Registration chain. Series of transformations that relate the locations of objects in space.

Tool calibration. Process of computing the transformation and the tool's geometric features, such as its main axis and its tip position. Tool calibration verification is the process of comparing the actual and computed calibration. The tool calibration unit is the device used for calibrating tools.

Transformation. Mathematical description of the relationship between the locations of two objects. Transformations are static (constant) when the relative locations of the objects do not change, dynamic otherwise. There are four types of transformations: Tracking transformations, tools transformations, image transformations, and display transformations.

Visualization

Silhouette. Projection of the contours of a 3D object onto a plane.

Viewpoint. Location from which navigation images are created.

Visualization. Process of creating, manipulating, and displaying images showing the location of objects in space.

Validation

Validation. Process of verifying that the navigation images match the clinical intraoperative situation. There are three types of validation: tool calibration validation, dynamic reference frame validation, and registration accuracy validation. Synonym: *Verification.*

REFERENCES

1. Atesok K, Finkelstein J, Khoury A, et al. CT (ISO-C-3D) image-based computer-assisted navigation in trauma surgery: a preliminary report. *Injury.* 2008;39:39–43.
2. Atesok K, Finkelstein J, Khoury A, et al. The use of intraoperative three-dimensional imaging (ISO-C-3D) in fixation of intraarticular fractures. *Injury.* 2007;38:1163–1169.
3. Attias N, Lindsey RW, Starr AJ, et al. The use of a virtual three-dimensional model to evaluate the intraosseous space available for percutaneous screw fixation of acetabular fractures. *J Bone Joint Surg Br.* 2005;87B:1520–1523.
4. Bono JV. Digital templating in total hip arthroplasty. *J Bone Joint Surg Am.* 2004; 86A:118–122.
5. Borrelli J, Peele M, Ricci WM, et al. Validation of CT-reconstructed images for the evaluation of acetabular fractures. Proceedings of the American Academy of Orthopedic Surgery, 2004, San Francisco: 610.
6. Cimerman M, Kristan A. Preoperative planning in pelvic and acetabular surgery: the value of advanced computerized planning modules. *Injury.* 2007;38:442–449.
7. Citak M, Hufner T, Geerling J, et al. Navigated percutaneous pelvic sacroiliac screw fixation: experimental comparison of accuracy between fluoroscopy and Iso-C 3D navigation. *Comput Aided Surg.* 2006;11:209–213.
8. Crowl AC, Kahler DM. Closed reduction and percutaneous fixation of anterior column acetabular fractures. *Comput Aided Surg.* 2002;7:169–178.
9. Devito DP, Gaskill T, Erikson M, et al. Robotic Assisted Image-based guidance for pedicle screw instrumentation of the scoliotic spine. Presented at Pediatric Society of North America (POSNA); May 2011; Montreal, Canada.
10. Devito DP, Kaplan L, Dietl R, et al. Clinical acceptance and accuracy assessment of spinal implants guided with SpineAssist surgical robot: retrospective study. *Spine.* 2010;35(24):2109–2115.
11. Gardner MJ, Citak M, Kendoff D, et al. Femoral fracture malrotation caused by free-hand versus navigated distal interlocking. *Injury.* 2008;39:176–180.
12. Gautier E, Bachler R, Heini PF, et al. Accuracy of computer-guided screw fixation of the sacroiliac joint. *ClinOrthop.* 2001;393:310–317.
13. Gras F, Marintschev I, Klos K, et al. Screw placement for acetabular fractures: Which navigation modality (2-Dimensional vs. 3-Dimensional) should be used? An experimental study. *J Orthop Trauma.* 2012;8:466–473.
14. Hajnal J, Hill D, Hawkes D. *Medical Image Registration.* Boca Raton: CRC Press; 2001.
15. Hazan E, Joskowicz L. Computer-assisted image-guided intramedullary nailing of femoral shaft fractures. *Techn Orthop.* 2003;18:191–201.
16. Hazan E. Computer aided orthopaedic surgery: special issue. *TechnOrthop.* 2003;18.
17. Hofstetter R, Slomczykowski M, Krettek C, et al. Computer-assisted fluoroscopy-based reduction of femoral fractures and anteversion correction. *Comput Aided Surg.* 2000;5:311–325.
18. Hufner T, Pohlemann T, Tarte S, et al. Computer-assisted fracture reduction of pelvic ring fractures: an in vitro study. *Clin Orthop.* 2002;399:231–239.
19. Ilsar I, Weil YA, Joskowicz L, et al. Fracture-table-mounted versus bone-mounted dynamic reference frame tracking accuracy using computer-assisted orthopaedic surgery: a comparative study. *Comput Aided Surg.* 2007;12:125–130.
20. Jaramaz B, Eckman K. Virtual reality simulation of fluoroscopic navigation. *Clin Orthop Relat Res.* 2006;442:30–34.
21. Joskowicz L, Milgrom C, Simkin A, et al. FRACAS: a system for computer-aided image-guided long bone fracture surgery. *Comput Aided Surg.* 1999;3:271–288.
22. Kahler DM. Computer-assisted closed techniques of reduction and fixation. In: Tile M, Helfet D, Kellam J, eds. *Surgery of the Pelvis and Acetabulum.* Philadelphia, PA: Lippincott Williams & Wilkins; 2003:604–615.
23. Kahler DM. Computer-assisted fixation of acetabular fractures and pelvic ring disruptions. *Techn Orthop.* 2000;10:20–24.
24. Kahler DM. Virtual fluoroscopy: a tool for decreasing radiation exposure during femoral intramedullary nailing. *Stud Health Technol Inform.* 2001;81:225–228.
25. Kaplan L. Robotic assisted vertebral cement augmentation: a Major radiation reduction tool. Aging Spine Symposium, March 2011. Jerusalem, Israel.
26. Keast-Butler O, Lutz MJ, Angelini M, et al. Computer navigation in the reduction and fixation of femoral shaft fractures: A randomized control study. *Injury* (Netherlands). 2012;43(6):749–756.
27. Khoury A, Liebergall M, Weil Y, et al. Computerized fluoroscopic-based navigation-assisted intramedullary nailing. *Am J Orthop.* 2007;36:582–585.
28. Kluba T, Rühle T, Schulze-Bövingloh A, et al. [Reproducibility of readings of ISO C 3D and CT lumbar pedicle screw scans]. *Rofo.* 2009;181(5):477–482. [German]
29. Langlotz F. Potential pitfalls of computer aided orthopaedic surgery. *Injury.* 2004;35(suppl 1):17–23.
30. Lavallee S, Sautot P, Troccaz J, et al. Computer-assisted spine surgery: a technique for accurate transpedicular screw fixation using CT data and a 3D optical localizer. *Comput Aided Surg* (formerly *J Image Guid Surg*). 1995;1:65–73.
31. Liebergall M, Ben-David D, Weil Y, et al. Computerized navigation for the internal fixation of femoral neck fractures. *J Bone Joint Surg Am.* 2006;88A:1748–1754.
32. Liebergall M, Mosheiff R, Segal D. Navigation in orthopaedic trauma. *Oper Techn Orthop.* 2003;13:64–72.
33. Livyatan H, Yaniv Z, Joskowicz L. Robust automatic C-arm calibration for fluoroscopy-based navigation: a practical approach. Proceedings of the Fifth International Conference on Medical Computing and Computer-Aided Intervention. Lecture Notes in Computer Science 2488. *Springer Verlag.* 2002;2:60–68.
34. Martirosyan NL, Kalb S, Cavalcanti DD, et al. Comparative analysis of isocentric 3-dimensional C-arm fluoroscopy and biplanar fluoroscopy for anterior screw fixation in odontoid fractures. *J Spinal Disord Tech.* 2013;26(4):189–193.
35. Meier R, Geerling J, Hüfner T, et al. [The isocentric C-arm. Visualization of fracture reduction and screw position in the radius]. *Unfallchirurg.* 2011;114(7):587–590. [German]
36. Mosheiff R, Khoury A, Weil Y, et al. First generation of fluoroscopic navigation in percutaneous pelvic surgery. *J Orthop Trauma.* 2004;18:106–111.
37. Mosheiff R, Weil Y, Khoury A, et al. The use of computerized navigation in the treatment of gunshot and shrapnel injury. *Comput Aided Surg.* 2004;9:39–43.
38. Mosheiff R, Weil Y, Peleg E, et al. Computerized navigation for closed reduction during femoral intramedullary nailing. *Injury.* 2005;36:866–870.
39. Nolte L, Beutler T. Basic principles of CAOS. *Injury.* 2004;35(suppl 1):6–16.
40. Nolte LP, Ganz R. *Computer-Assisted Orthopaedic Surgery.* Bern: Hogrefe and Huber Publishers; 1999.
41. Ochs BG, Gonser C, Shiozawa T, et al. Computer-assisted periacetabular screw placement: Comparison of different fluoroscopy-based navigation procedures with conventional technique. *Injury.* 2010;41(12):1297–1305.
42. Park MS, Lee KM, Lee B, et al. Comparison of operator radiation exposure between C-arm and O-arm fluoroscopy for orthopaedic surgery. *Radiat Prot Dosimetry.* 2012;148(4):431–438.
43. Reddix RN, Webb LX. Computed-assisted preoperative planning in the surgical treatment of acetabular fractures. *J Surg Orthop Adv.* 2007;16:138–143.
44. Ruan Z, Luo CF, Zeng BF, et al. Percutaneous screw fixation for the acetabular fracture with quadrilateral plate involved by three-dimensional fluoroscopy navigation: surgical technique. *Injury.* 2012;43(4):517–521.
45. Schafer S, Nithiananthan S, Mirota DJ, et al. Mobile C-arm cone-beam CT for guidance of spine surgery: image quality, radiation dose, and integration with interventional guidance. *Med Phys.* 2011;38(8):4563–4574.
46. Schep NW, Haverlag R, van Vugt AB. Computer-assisted versus conventional surgery for insertion of 96 cannulated iliosacral screws in patients with postpartum pelvic pain. *J Trauma.* 2004;57:1299–1302.
47. Schmucki D, Gebhard F, Grutzner P, et al. Computer-aided reduction and imaging. *Injury.* 2004;35(suppl 1):96–104.
48. Slomczykowski MA, Hofstetter R, Sati M, et al. Novel computer-assisted fluoroscopy system for intraoperative guidance: feasibility study for distal locking of femoral nails. *J Orthop Trauma.* 2001;15:122–131.
49. Stockle U, Krettek C, Pohlemann T, et al. Clinical applications: pelvis. *Injury.* 2004; 35(suppl 1):46–56.
50. Stockle U, Schaser K, Konig B. Image guidance in pelvic and acetabular surgery: expectations, success, and limitations. *Injury.* 2007;38:450–462.
51. Stübig T, Kendoff D, Citak M, et al. Comparative study of different intraoperative 3-D image intensifiers in orthopedic trauma care. *J Trauma.* 2009;66(3):821–830.
52. Stübig T, Min W, Arvani M, et al. Accuracy of measurement of femoral anteversion in femoral shaft fractures using a computer imaging software: a cadaveric study. *Arch Orthop Trauma Surg.* 2012;132(5):613–616.
53. Stuby F, Seethaler AC, Shiozawa T, et al. [Evaluation of image quality of two different three-dimensional cone-beam-scanners for orthopedic surgery in the bony structures of the pelvis in comparison with standard CT scans]. *Z Orthop Unfall.* 2011;149(6):659–667. [German]
54. Sugimoto Y, Ito Y, Tomioka M, et al. Clinical accuracy of three-dimensional fluoroscopy (IsoC-3D)-assisted upper thoracic pedicle screw insertion. *Acta Med Okayama.* 2010;64(3):209–212.
55. Taylor R, Lavallee S, Burdea C, et al. *Computer-Integrated Surgery: Technology and Clinical Applications.* Boston, MA: The MIT Press; 1995.
56. Taylor RH. Medical robotics. IEEE Trans Robot Automat 2003;Special Issue:19.
57. von Recum J, Wendl K, Vock B, et al. [Intraoperative 3D C-arm imaging. State of the art]. *Unfallchirurg.* 2012;115(3):196–201. [German]
58. Weil YA, Gardner MJ, Helfet DL, et al. Computer navigation allows for accurate reduction of femoral fractures. *Clin Orthop Relat Res.* 2007;460:185–191.
59. Weil YA, Liebergall M, Khoury A, et al. The use of computerized fluoroscopic navigation for removal of pelvic screws. *Am J Orthop.* 2004;33:384–385.
60. Weil YA, Liebergall M, Mosheiff R, et al. Assessment of two 3-D fluoroscopic systems for articular fracture reduction: a cadaver study. *Int J Comput Assist Radiol Surg.* 2011;6(5):685–692.
61. Weil YA, Liebergall M, Mosheiff R, et al. Long bone fracture reduction using a fluoroscopy-based navigation system: a feasibility and accuracy study. *Comput Aided Surg.* 2007;12:295–302.
62. Wilharm A, Gras F, Rausch S, et al. Navigation in femoral-shaft fractures—from lab tests to clinical routine. *Injury* (Netherlands). 2011;42(11):1346–1352.
63. Windolf M, Schroeder J, Fliri L, et al. Reinforcing the role of the conventional C-arm - a novel method for simplified distal interlocking. *BMC Musculoskelet Disord.* 2012;13:18.
64. Yang YL, Zhou DS, He JL. Comparison of isocentric C-Arm 3-dimensional navigation and conventional fluoroscopy for C1 lateral mass and C2 pedicle screw placement for atlantoaxial instability. *J Spinal Disord Tech.* 2013;26:127–134.

19

OSTEOPOROSIS

Stuart H. Ralston

INTRODUCTION

Osteoporosis is a common metabolic bone disease characterized by reduced bone mass, microarchitectural deterioration of bone tissue, and an increased risk of fragility fracture.[36] The diagnosis is made by measurements of bone mineral density (BMD) using dual energy x-ray absorptiometry (DEXA). Individuals with BMD values more than 2.5 standard deviations below the average in young healthy subjects (T-score <−2.5) are classified as having osteoporosis. People with lesser reductions in BMD (T-score between −1 and −2.5) are classified as having osteopenia whereas people with T-score values between −1 and +2.5 are said to have normal bone mass. Patients with T-score values above +2.5 in the absence of a known cause such as osteoarthritis of the spine considered to have abnormally high bone mass.

Bone mass increases through growth and adolescence to reach a peak in the early 20s (Fig. 19-1). It remains relatively stable in healthy individuals thereafter until the age of about 45 years when bone loss starts to occur. Although bone is lost with age in both genders, there is an accelerated phase of bone loss after the menopause in women as the result of estrogen deficiency. By the age of 80 years it has been estimated that about 50% of white women and about 20% of men will have osteoporosis as defined on the basis of a T-score of −2.5 or below.

The clinical importance of osteoporosis lies in the fact that it is a risk factor for fractures and the risk of fracture increases by a factor of 1.5- to 3-fold for each standard deviation reduction in BMD.[45] Osteoporosis is classically associated with an increased risk of low-trauma fractures (fragility fractures), but recent studies indicate that perhaps not surprisingly, low levels

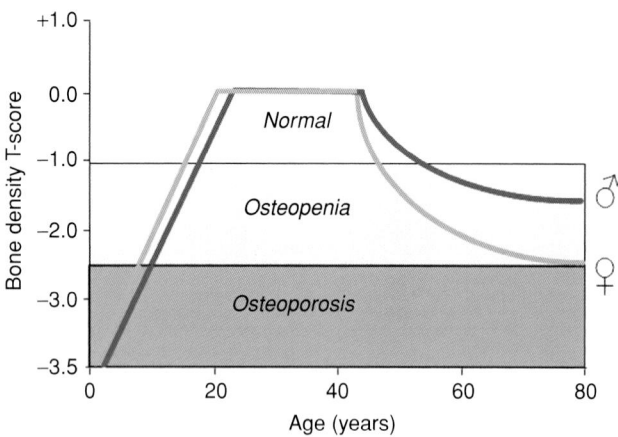

FIGURE 19-1 Changes in bone mass with age. Bone mass gradually increases during childhood and adolescence to reach a peak by the age of about 20. Thereafter bone mass is stable until the age of 45 when bone loss starts to occur, particularly in women. By the age of 80 it is estimated that BMD values will have fallen to within the osteoporotic range (T-score < –2.5) in about 50% of all women.

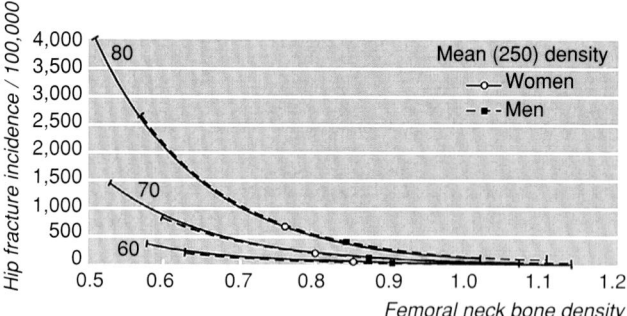

FIGURE 19-2 Relation between BMD, age, and fractures. The incidence of hip fracture increases with age in both genders but is about five times greater in those aged 80 as compared with those aged 60 as BMD values fall below 0.8. (From: De Laet CE, van Hout BA, Burger H, et al. Bone density and risk of hip fracture in men and women: Cross sectional analysis. *BMJ.* 1997;315:221–225, with permission.)

of BMD are associated with the risk of all types of fractures including high energy fractures.[44]

Fractures are a major public health problem in developed countries. For example, it has been estimated that in North America, white women aged 50 have a remaining lifetime risk of 17.5% for hip fracture, 15.6% for clinical vertebral fracture, and 16% for wrist fracture. For men corresponding risks are 6%, 5%, and 2.5%. In the United Kingdom the lifetime risk of any fracture at the age of 50 has been estimated as about 53% for women and 21% for men.[34] Although the risk of fracture is significantly increased in patients with osteoporosis as defined by DEXA, most fractures occur in patients who do not have osteoporosis.[73] This is because the occurrence of fracture is not only determined by bone strength (which is strongly correlated with BMD) but also other factors such as risk of falling, the type of fall, bone geometry, and bone quality. In keeping with this, it has been shown that reduced BMD values only account for a small proportion of the exponential increase in fracture risk that occurs with increasing age (Fig. 19-2).

PATHOPHYSIOLOGY

Bone Structure

Bone is a composite material comprising matrix and mineral phases. The main component of bone matrix is type I collagen which is a fibrillar protein comprising two alpha 1 and one alpha 2 chains wound together in a triple helix. Bone matrix also contains small amounts of other collagens, growth factors, and other noncollagenous proteins and glycoproteins. The mineral phase of bone consists of calcium and phosphate in the form of hydroxyapatite crystals $(Ca_{10}(PO_4)_6(OH)_2)$ which are deposited in the spaces between collagen fibrils. Mineralization confers upon bone the property of mechanical rigidity, which complements the tensile strength and elasticity derived from bone collagen. Anatomically bone is divided into cortical

and trabecular subtypes. Most of the skeleton consists of cortical bone which forms the shafts of the long bones such as the femur, tibia, humerus, and radius and forms a thin envelope around the trabecular bone which is abundant at the metaphyses of long bones and in the vertebral bodies. Both types of bone undergo a process of renewal and repair throughout life as a result of bone remodeling (Fig. 19-3). During bone remodeling old and damaged bone is removed by multinucleated osteoclasts which dissolve bone mineral through secretion of acid and degrade bone matrix through secretion of proteases. Following completion of bone resorption, bone marrow stromal cells are attracted to the resorption lacuna and differentiate into osteoblasts. The osteoblasts lay down new bone matrix which is initially unmineralized (osteoid) and subsequently becomes mineralized to form mature calcified bone. During the process of bone formation some osteoblasts become trapped in the bone matrix and differentiate into osteocytes. Osteocytes are the most abundant cells in bone. They communicate with each other and with cells on the bone surface through long cytoplasmic processes which run through channels in the bone matrix termed canaliculi. Osteocytes play a critical role in the regulation of bone remodeling at a local level. They sense and respond to mechanical stimuli by producing regulatory molecules including receptor activator of nuclear factor kappa B (RANK) which regulates bone resorption and sclerostin (SOST) which regulates bone formation. Osteocytes also have an important endocrine function by producing a circulating hormone called fibroblast growth factor 23 (FGF23) which acts on the renal tubule to regulate serum phosphate levels.

Bone Resorption

Bone resorption is carried out by osteoclasts which are multinucleated cells derived from the monocytes/macrophage lineage. The RANK signaling pathway plays a critical role in regulating osteoclast differentiation and bone resorption.[39] The RANK receptor is a member of the tumor necrosis factor (TNF) receptor superfamily which is expressed on osteoclast precursors and mature osteoclasts. It is activated by a molecule called RANK ligand (RANKL) which is a member of the TNF superfamily

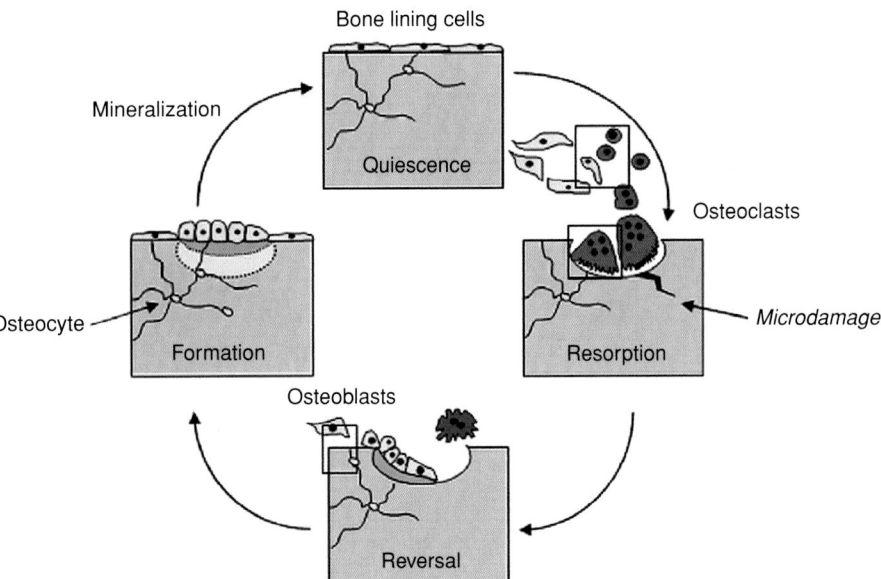

FIGURE 19-3 The bone remodeling cycle. The bone remodeling cycle is responsible for renewal and repair of bone throughout life. Bone is removed by multinucleated osteoclasts which are thought to be able to detect and remove areas of microdamage. After about 10 to 12 days osteoclasts undergo programmed cell death (apoptosis) and are replaced by osteoblasts which lay down new bone in the resorption lacuna. Some osteoblasts become trapped in bone matrix and differentiate into osteocytes which are responsible for detecting and responding to mechanical strain. When bone formation is complete the matrix mineralizes and the bone surface becomes quiescent and covered with flat lining cells.

(Fig. 19-4). When RANKL binds to RANK several intracellular signaling pathways are activated which cause osteoclast differentiation and bone resorption. Osteoprotegerin (OPG) has homology to RANK, but lacks a signaling domain and acts as a decoy receptor for RANKL. In the presence of OPG, the stimulatory effects of RANKL on osteoclasts are blocked causing osteoclast inhibition. The importance of this system is underscored by the fact that loss of function mutations in RANK and RANKL result in osteoclast poor osteopetrosis due to the failure of osteoclast differentiation,[79] whereas loss of function mutations in OPG result in juvenile Paget's disease, a condition associated with markedly elevated bone turnover, fractures, and bone deformity.[42] Rarely, neutralizing autoantibodies to OPG may develop in patients with autoimmune disease and this causes a severe form of osteoporosis with high bone turnover.[64] Mature osteoclasts form a tight seal over the bone surface and resorb bone by secreting hydrochloric acid and proteolytic enzymes onto the bone surface. The acid dissolves hydroxyapatite, allowing the proteolytic enzymes to degrade collagen and other bone matrix proteins. Osteoclast-rich osteopetrosis is caused by mutations in the genes that encode molecules which are involved in acid secretion and matrix degradation.[79] These include the *CA2* gene which encodes carbonic anhydrase type II, which is necessary for acid generation in osteoclasts; the *TCIRG1* gene that encodes a 117 kD subunit of the osteoclast proton pump which is necessary for acid secretion; the *CLCN7* gene which encodes the osteoclast chloride channel; and the *CATK* gene which encodes cathepsin K, a protease that is necessary for collagen degradation.

Bone Formation

Bone is formed by osteoblasts which are mononuclear cells derived from mesenchymal stem cells. Several molecules are involved in regulating osteoblast differentiation. They include core-binding factor alpha 1 (Cbfa1) and osterix which are transcription factors that promote differentiation of mesenchymal stem cells to osteoblasts; bone morphogenic proteins which

are members of the transforming growth factor beta superfamily that upregulate Cbfa1 expression in osteoblast precursors; and members of the *Wnt* superfamily which affect osteoblast differentiation and function by regulating the transcription factor beta-catenin.[82] The *Wnt* molecules are a series of glycoproteins that are highly conserved throughout evolution. They bind to a receptor complex which comprises a member of the frizzled family in a heterodimer with either Lipoprotein receptor-related protein 5 (LRP5) or LRP6 (Fig. 19-4). Binding of *Wnt* to the frizzled/LRP receptor complex is antagonized by various proteins including Dickkopf 1 (DKK1), secreted frizzled-related proteins (sFRPs) and sclerostin (SOST) (Fig. 19-4). Accordingly, regulation of bone formation by this pathway depends on a fine balance between the stimulatory effects of *Wnt* and the inhibitory effects of DKK1, sFRP, and SOST on LRP5/LRP6 signaling.

There are 19 different *Wnt* genes in mammals and it is currently unclear how many of these interact with frizzled/LRP to regulate bone mass. Experimental evidence has been gained to suggest that at the very least, *Wnt3A*[6] and *Wnt10B*[75] play a role.

Emerging evidence suggests that production of SOST by osteocytes plays a critical role in regulating bone mass and bone turnover in response to mechanical loading. Mechanical loading of bone inhibits production of SOST by osteocytes and this increases bone formation and reduces bone resorption by increasing levels of OPG.[65] The importance of SOST in regulating bone mass is reflected by the fact that recessive (loss of function) mutations in SOST result in bone overgrowth and high bone mass in the syndromes of sclerosteosis and van Buchem disease.[35] Similarly, heterozygous mutations in the LRP5 receptor also result in high bone mass by preventing SOST–LRP5 binding, allowing *Wnt* to activated LRP5 signaling.[3]

Systemic Factors That Regulate Bone Remodeling

In addition to the local mediators mentioned above, several systemic hormones regulate bone remodeling. Parathyroid hormone

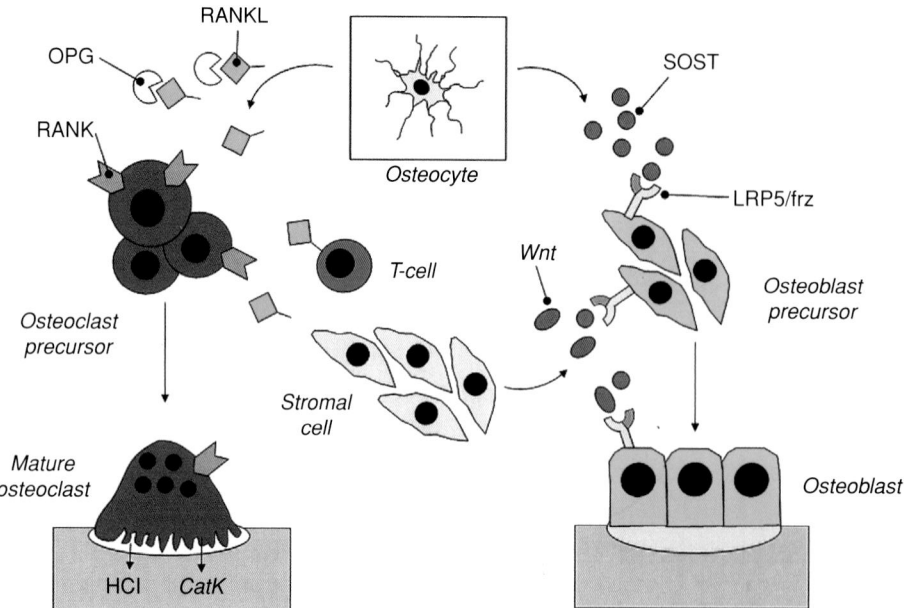

FIGURE 19-4 Molecular regulation of bone turnover. Osteocytes play a central role in regulating bone resorption and formation. They regulate bone resorption (*left side*) by releasing RANKL which binds to RANK on osteoclast precursors triggering osteoclast differentiation and bone resorption, which is mediated by secretion of hydrochloric acid (HCl) and cathepsin K (*CatK*) onto the bone surface. Osteoprotegerin (OPG) inhibits bone resorption by binding to RANKL and preventing it activating RANK. Other sources of RANKL include T-cells and stromal cells. Osteocytes regulate bone formation by secreting sclerostin (SOST) which binds to the LRP5/frizzled (LRP5/frz) coreceptor, preventing its activation by *Wnt* family members, thereby suppressing bone formation.

(PTH) and 1,25-dihydroxyvitamin D act together to increase bone remodeling allowing skeletal calcium to be mobilized for maintenance of plasma calcium homeostasis. Bone remodeling is also increased by thyroid hormone and growth hormone, but suppressed by estrogen and androgens. These factors are thought to work in part by modulating production of locally produced factors such as RANKL, OPG, and SOST as well as by exerting direct effects on osteoblast and osteoclast activity.

In addition to suppressing bone turnover, estrogen is also involved in regulating coupling between bone resorption and bone formation such that in states of estrogen deficiency, bone formation fails to keep pace with bone resorption, resulting in bone loss. This is thought to account for the phase of accelerated bone loss that occurs after the menopause in women.

RISK FACTORS FOR OSTEOPOROSIS

Osteoporosis is a complex disease with both environmental and genetic components and several risk factors have been identified as summarized in Table 19-1.

Genetics

Twin and family studies have shown that genetic factors account for between 70% to 85% of the variance in bone mass[2] although the heritability of fracture is considerably lower than this especially in the elderly.[49] Although the genetic influences on fracture risk are partly mediated by the effects on BMD, other determinants of fracture risk such as bone turnover and bone geometry also have a heritable component.[59] Current evidence indicates that BMD is influenced by a large number of genetic variants which individually have a small effect size.[59] The same applies to fracture, although fewer variants have been identified.[27] It is of interest that many of the genetic variants that are associated with BMD or fractures lie close to genes in the RANK and *Wnt* signaling pathways.[27]

Diet

Most research in this area has focused on calcium intake. Several studies have shown a positive relationship between calcium intake during youth and peak bone mass although there is no convincing evidence linking dietary calcium intake with fracture risk in adults.[8]

Mechanical Loading

There is evidence to suggest that mechanical loading increases bone mass whereas immobility causes bone loss.[50,74] Population-based studies have also shown an association between increased levels of physical exercise and reduced fracture risk,[15] although

TABLE 19-1	Risk Factors for Osteoporosis and Fractures

- Smoking
- Excessive alcohol intake (>3 units/day)
- Low body weight (BMI <19)
- Early menopause
- Genetic factors
  - Race
  - Family history hip fracture

- Diseases
  - Thyrotoxicosis
  - Rheumatoid arthritis
  - Primary hyperparathyroidism
  - Cushing syndrome
  - Hypogonadism
  - Anorexia nervosa
  - Cancer
  - Chronic liver disease
  - Celiac disease
  - Cystic fibrosis
  - Epilepsy
- Drugs
  - Corticosteroids
  - Thyroxine
  - Gonadotrophin releasing hormone agonists
  - Sedatives
  - Anticonvulsants

this is probably due to increased muscle strength and a reduced risk of falling rather than the effects on BMD.

Smoking

Cigarette smokers are at increased risk of fractures.[33,41] The mechanisms are likely to be multifactorial including the fact that female smokers have an earlier menopause, accelerated metabolism of exogenous estrogens, and impaired peripheral conversion of adrenal androgens to estrogen due to reduced body weight.

Alcohol

Moderate alcohol intake does not seem to affect fracture risk significantly, but there is strong evidence that the risk of fracture increases significantly in those who drink more than 3 units of alcohol per day and is increased substantially in those who drink more than 6 units per day.[33] The association between excessive alcohol intake and fracture risk is likely to be multifactorial in nature and probably involves effects on BMD as well as nonskeletal factors such as an increased risk of falling.

Social Deprivation

Social deprivation is strongly associated with fracture risk.[17] The mechanisms are unclear but likely to be multifactorial involving differences in lifestyle factors such as diet, smoking, alcohol, and physical activity.

Diseases

Diseases that are associated with an increased risk of osteoporosis or fractures are summarized in Table 19-1. The mechanisms underlying these associations are discussed in more detail below. Hypogonadism is an important cause of osteoporosis in both genders. This may be physiologic as in the case of postmenopausal osteoporosis or pathologic as in patients with pituitary disease, Klinefelter syndrome, and Turner syndrome. Hypogonadism during growth predisposes to osteoporosis by reducing peak bone mass whereas hypogonadism in adults predisposes to osteoporosis by causing increased bone loss with uncoupling between bone resorption and bone formation. Although testosterone protects against osteoporosis in men, current evidence suggests that it does so through peripheral conversion to estrogen through aromatization.[38] Chronic inflammatory rheumatic diseases such as rheumatoid arthritis and ankylosing spondylitis are associated with an increased risk of osteoporosis and fractures. Several mechanisms are likely to contribute including relative immobility, increased production of proinflammatory cytokines such as interleukin-1 and TNF, and corticosteroid treatment. Similar mechanisms are likely to be responsible for osteoporosis in gastrointestinal (GI) diseases such as Crohn disease and ulcerative colitis. Celiac disease is associated with an increased risk of osteoporosis and fractures presumably due to impaired intestinal absorption of calcium, vitamin D, and other nutrients. Osteoporosis may coexist with osteomalacia in patients with celiac disease and malabsorption or in patients with inflammatory bowel disease. Thyrotoxicosis is associated with osteoporosis due to increased bone turnover as is over-replacement with thyroxine.

Primary hyperparathyroidism is associated with osteoporosis due to increased bone turnover with relative uncoupling of bone resorption from bone formation.

Corticosteroids

Corticosteroids are a strong risk factor for osteoporosis and fractures.[78] The risk of fracture is directly related to the dose and duration of therapy. Several mechanisms have been implicated including reduced intestinal calcium absorption, increased renal calcium losses by an effect of glucocorticoids on renal tubular calcium absorption, and reduced bone formation and inhibition of bone formation by apoptosis of osteoblasts and osteocytes. Inhaled corticosteroids are generally considered to be safe with respect to the risk of osteoporosis but high-dose inhaled steroids have been associated with reduced bone mass.

Thyroxine

Over-replacement with thyroxine in patients with hypothyroidism is associated with reduced bone mass, presumed to be due to a direct stimulatory effect on bone turnover.[4]

Other Drugs

Several other drugs including benzodiazepines, selective serotonin reuptake inhibitors (SSRIs), and anticonvulsants have been associated with an increased risk of fragility fractures.[33] The mechanisms are incompletely understood but are likely multifactorial due to adverse effects on balance and cognitive function and/or direct effects on bone cells.

CLINICAL PRESENTATION OF OSTEOPOROSIS

The most common clinical presentation of osteoporosis is with fractures of various types, details of which are reviewed elsewhere in these volumes. Vertebral fractures deserve special mention since their presence is easily missed. Some patients with vertebral fractures present with acute back pain which can be localized to the affected site or can radiate to the anterior chest wall or abdomen, mimicking intrathoracic pathology or an acute abdomen. In some cases there is a predisposing factor such as bending, coughing, or lifting whereas other fractures occur spontaneously. Many patients with vertebral fractures present insidiously with height loss or kyphosis and chronic back pain. In addition to pain and height loss, patients with multiple vertebral fractures may experience abdominal discomfort and distension due to compression of abdominal organs by severe kyphosis.

CLINICAL ASSESSMENT

Bone Density

Assessment of BMD by DEXA has a pivotal role in the diagnosis of osteoporosis, in fracture risk assessment, and in selecting patients for treatment. Measurements of BMD are usually made at the femoral neck and lumbar spine in routine practice, but it is also possible to obtain measurements at the wrist and the whole body. Reduced levels of BMD are significantly associated with an increased risk of fracture such that fracture risk increases by a factor of 1.5 to 3-fold for each standard deviation reduction in BMD.[45] It is important to emphasize that BMD measurements do not accurately predict fractures occurring since many people with BMD values in the osteoporotic range do not suffer fractures and many people with fractures do not have osteoporosis as defined by BMD measurements. It has been estimated that the sensitivity and specificity of BMD in predicting fractures is similar to that of high blood pressure in predicting stroke, or raised cholesterol in predicting myocardial infarction.

Osteoporosis is diagnosed if T-score values at either the lumbar spine (typically the average of lumbar vertebrae L1 to L4), femoral neck, or total hip sites lie below −2.5. Although BMD values at these sites are moderately correlated with one another ($r = 0.6$), it is not uncommon to encounter patients who have low BMD at one site and normal BMD at another. Several factors are thought to contribute to these differences. Trabecular bone has a greater surface than cortical bone and therefore is remodeled more rapidly under states of increased bone turnover such as occurs after the menopause. Accordingly, women with postmenopausal osteoporosis in the 5th and 6th decades often have a greater reduction in spine BMD than hip BMD. There is also evidence that genetic factors may have site-specific effects on BMD depending on the content of cortical and trabecular bone.[27] Indications for bone densitometry differ in different countries, depending on the availability of DEXA and economic factors. In the United Kingdom, DEXA is indicated in patients aged 50 years and over who suffer low-trauma fractures and in those with strong clinical risk factors for osteoporosis. In the USA, DEXA is indicated in all women above the age of 65 years and in younger women and men with an equivalent fracture risk.

Fracture Risk Assessment

Clinical risk factors can be used in the assessment of fracture risk, with or without BMD measurements. Several risk factor tools have been developed, but the ones that are used most commonly are the FRAX tool (www.shef.ac.uk/frax/) and the QFracture score (http://www.qfracture.org/).[33] Both provide estimates of 10-year fracture risk by combining information on weight, height, age, and gender with other clinical risk factors such as corticosteroid use, smoking, alcohol intake, and other diseases. In the United Kingdom, the National Institute for Health and Care Excellence (NICE) guidance recommends that fracture risk should be assessed by one of these tools before proceeding to DEXA. It has been suggested that people who have a high absolute fracture risk should be treated for osteoporosis without recourse to a BMD measurement but the evidence base for this is lacking. In one study it was estimated that only 50% of patients over the age of 75 with a history of fragility fractures actually had osteoporosis on a DEXA scan.[57]

Radiography

Standard radiographs have poor sensitivity for the detection and monitoring of osteoporosis, since large amounts of bone mineral (up to 30%) must be lost or gained from the skeleton before it can be reliably detected on plain radiographs. The lack of sensitivity of radiographs in detecting early osteoporosis is offset by a relatively high specificity, since most patients who are found to have osteopenia on X-ray do indeed have reduced bone mass on DEXA. The principal application of radiographic examination in the assessment of patients with osteoporosis is in the diagnosis of fractures. The diagnosis of long bone fracture is based on the subjective opinion of a clinician looking for characteristic features such as deformity, displacement, and cortical discontinuity. For vertebral fractures morphometric criteria are increasingly being used for diagnosis and classification.[29]

Biochemical Markers

Bone turnover can be assessed biochemically by analysis of bone cell-specific proteins or products of matrix formation and degradation, which are released during bone remodeling. Biochemical markers have been investigated clinically in three main areas: Predicting rates of bone loss, predicting the response to treatment, and assessing compliance with medication. The biochemical markers that are used most commonly in current clinical practice are summarized in Table 19-2. Several investigators have reported a positive correlation between changes in biochemical markers of bone turnover and changes in bone mass in patients who are being treated with antiresorptive agents, but there is limited evidence as yet to show that changes in bone markers are associated with fracture risk reduction. Other studies have investigated the possibility that feedback to patients of biochemical markers might improve adherence but the results have been inconclusive.

Other Investigations

Several other investigations may be helpful in the assessment of patients with osteoporosis, particularly to exclude secondary causes of the disease such as hypogonadism, primary hyperparathyroidism, thyrotoxicosis, celiac disease, and chronic renal and liver disease. Rarely, transiliac bone biopsy may be required

TABLE 19-2	Biochemical Markers of Bone Turnover	
Marker Type	**Correlates With**
Bone Resorption	
• Deoxypyridinoline	Bone collagen degradation
• Collagen telopeptides (CTX, NTX)	Bone collagen degradation
• Tartrate-resistant acid phosphatase	Osteoclast numbers
Bone Formation	
• Total alkaline phosphatase	Osteoblast numbers, liver, and kidney disease
• Bone-specific alkaline phosphatase	Osteoblast numbers
• Osteocalcin	Osteoblast numbers
• Collagen propeptides (PINP, PICP)	Type I collagen synthesis

CTX, C-terminal crosslinking telopeptide of type I collagen; NTX, N-terminal crosslinking telopeptide of type I collagen; PINP, N-terminal propeptide of type I procollagen; PICP, C-terminal propeptide of type I procollagen.

in unusual cases of osteoporosis or in patients where an infiltrative disorder is suspected.

SYSTEMS OF CARE

Increasing interest has focused over recent years on improving systems of care for patients with osteoporosis and fragility fractures, based on the observation that relatively few patients with fractures related to osteoporosis are appropriately treated.

Fracture Liaison Service

The fracture liaison service (FLS) was developed in the United Kingdom to try and increase the proportion of individuals with fragility fractures who are investigated for possible osteoporosis and to ensure that they are treated appropriately.[46] The FLS system involves offering DEXA examination as a routine to patients above a certain age who suffer low-trauma fractures (typically age >50) and treating those that have osteoporosis with an appropriate therapy. In one study, implementation of an FLS increased the proportion of patients being investigated for osteoporosis from about 10% to over 90%.[46] Recent modeling studies indicate that the FLS approach is probably cost effective in reducing overall fracture burden.[47]

Population-Based DEXA Screening

No controlled studies have evaluated the effect of screening for osteoporosis on rates of fractures or fracture-related morbidity or mortality. In some healthcare systems such as the United States, it is recommended that DEXA should be performed in all women aged 65 and above and in younger women and men who have similar estimates of fracture risk, although the cost effectiveness of this approach has not been tested.[52]

MANAGEMENT

Effective management of osteoporosis depends on correcting modifiable risk factors for the disease, treating secondary causes of osteoporosis where possible, addressing falls risk, and commencing drug therapy where appropriate.

Lifestyle Modifications and Other Measures

Lifestyle modifications and other measures aimed at reducing the risk of falls or addressing predisposing disease are frequently employed in the management of patients with osteoporosis.

Diet

Patients with osteoporosis should be advised to take a balanced diet with an adequate protein and energy intake. Adequate amounts of dietary calcium are considered to be important for optimal bone health but the evidence base is poor. In the United Kingdom, the current recommended daily intake for calcium is 700 mg per day, whereas in the United States it has been suggested that premenopausal women and men should take 1,000 mg daily and postmenopausal women 1,500 mg daily.[1] Vitamin D is required for optimal absorption of calcium and there is evidence (summarized later) that calcium and vitamin D supplements reduce the risk of fractures. Only a few

foods contain substantial amounts of vitamin D, however, and in northern latitudes the amount of vitamin D synthesized by the skin is very limited. The Scientific Advisory Committee on Nutrition in the United Kingdom (www.sacn.gov.uk) recommends a daily intake of 400 International Units of vitamin D to maintain serum 25(OH)D levels above 50 nmol/L which is considered optimal for bone health, but acknowledges that this cannot be achieved easily by dietary means alone. Recent USA-based guidelines recommend 600 International Units of vitamin D up to the age of 70 and 800 International Units of vitamin D thereafter.[66]

Exercise

There is no direct evidence that exercise can reduce the risk of osteoporotic fractures, but exercise programs have been shown to reduce falls risk and have potential benefits in terms of improving muscle strength, morale, and general well-being.[72] Patients with osteoporosis and a history of fragility fractures should therefore be encouraged to take exercise if possible. Exercise programs have also been shown to be beneficial in improving pain and quality of life after vertebral fractures.[7]

Smoking and Alcohol

It is customary to advise patients who have osteoporosis or a history of fragility fractures to reduce cigarette intake or stop smoking, although there is no direct evidence that this affects fracture risk. Similarly patients who consume more than three units of alcohol daily should be advised to reduce intake although it is unclear if this reduces the risk of fractures.

Falls Reduction

The increased risk of fracture with increasing age is thought to be due in large part to an increase in risk of falling. It is possible to reduce the number of falls significantly by structured multidisciplinary assessment and interventions.[14] On this basis, interventions such as correction of cardiovascular or circulatory disorders or poor visual acuity and elimination of environmental hazards should be considered in patients with a history of fragility fracture who have a history of falls. Reduced visual acuity is a risk factor for falls and surgery for cataract has been reported to reduce fracture rates significantly.[77] Accordingly, patients with poor vision should be referred to the appropriate specialists for advice and treatment, as appropriate.

TREATMENT OF UNDERLYING DISEASE

Patients with osteoporosis should be screened for the presence of predisposing diseases and these should be treated where possible, since in some cases this can avoid the need for drug treatment. Examples include a gluten-free diet and calcium and vitamin D supplements in celiac disease and parathyroidectomy in primary hyperparathyroidism.

Drug Treatments

Several drug treatments are available for the treatment of osteoporosis (Table 19-3). They can broadly be divided into

TABLE 19-3 **Drug Treatments for Osteoporosis**

Antiresorptive agents	Anabolic agents
Bisphosphonates	Parathyroid hormone 1-34
Etidronate	Parathyroid hormone 1-84
Alendronic acid	**Other agents**
Risedronate	Strontium ranelate
Ibandronate	Nutritional supplements
Zoledronic acid	Calcium and vitamin D
Denosumab	Vitamin D
Hormone replacement therapy	Active vitamin D metabolites
Raloxifene	
Tibolone	

those that suppress bone resorption (antiresorptive agents) and those that increase bone turnover, but stimulate bone formation more than resorption (anabolic agents). Some agents, such as strontium ranelate, combine a weak antiresorptive effect with a weak stimulatory effect on biochemical markers of bone formation.

Bisphosphonates

Bisphosphonates are stable analogues of pyrophosphate, a naturally occurring inhibitor of mineralization and ectopic calcification. They share in common a central core structure of phosphorus–carbon–phosphorus atoms to which are attached various side chains at the R_1 and R_2 positions (Fig. 19-5). Bisphosphonates bind strongly to calcium ions causing the drugs to preferentially target bone and become incorporated within hydroxyapatite. The binding affinity for hydroxyapatite varies widely between drugs, but is particularly high for zoledronic acid. The potency with which bisphosphonates inhibit bone resorption is highly variable, and mainly determined by the chemical structure of the side chains. Specifically, incorporation of nitrogen into the side chain markedly increases potency. After oral or intravenous administration, the bisphosphonate is targeted to bone surfaces at sites of increased bone turnover. When bone containing the bisphosphonate undergoes resorption, the drug is released at high concentration within the osteoclast, causing osteoclast inhibition and inhibition of bone resorption.

Etidronate

Etidronate is now seldom used in the treatment of osteoporosis due to the fact that it has not been shown to prevent nonvertebral fractures.[18] It is given in a dose of 400 mg daily for 2 weeks followed by calcium supplementation of 500 mg daily for 11 weeks (Didronel PMO). The etidronate component should be given on an empty stomach at least 2 hours before eating, with a glass of water.

Alendronic Acid

Alendronic acid is one of the most widely used treatments for osteoporosis. It has been shown to reduce vertebral fractures by about 50%, nonvertebral fractures by about 17%, and hip fractures by 40% in women with postmenopausal osteoporosis when given in a dose of 10 mg daily in combination with calcium and vitamin D supplements (NICE, systematic review 2008). Alendronic acid has also been shown to increase BMD in corticosteroid induced osteoporosis[68] and men with osteoporosis,[53] but evidence for antifracture efficacy in these indications is lacking.

Alendronic acid in a dose of 70 mg once weekly has been found to give an equivalent increase in BMD as 10 mg daily[71] and on this basis, the once-weekly dosing regimen is now used virtually in all patients. Alendronic acid is poorly absorbed from the GI tract and should be taken at least 30 minutes before food or other medication with a large glass of water and the patient instructed to remain upright during this time. The most common adverse effect of alendronic acid is upper GI upset which resolves when the treatment is stopped. Less commonly severe esophagitis and esophageal ulcers may occur especially in patients with swallowing difficulty and those who fail to take the drug correctly. Rare adverse effects include osteonecrosis of the jaw,[37] and atypical subtrochanteric femoral fractures.[70]

Risedronate

Risedronate has similar antifracture efficacy to alendronic acid in patients with postmenopausal osteoporosis when given in a dose of 5 mg daily in combination with calcium and vitamin D supplements.[19] Efficacy has also been demonstrated in the prevention of vertebral fractures in corticosteroid-induced osteoporosis.[80] Risedronate increases BMD in male

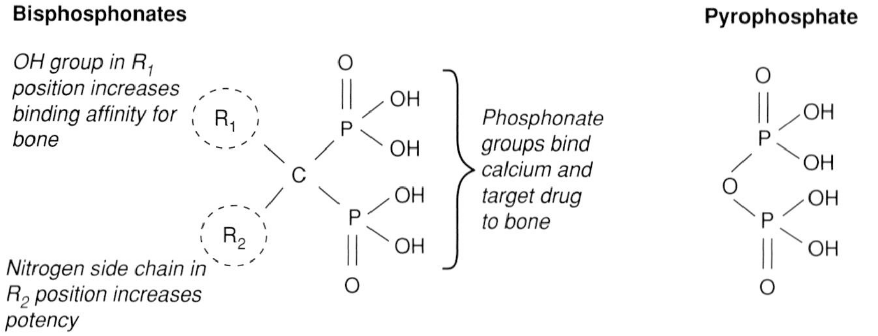

Bisphosphonates

OH group in R_1 position increases binding affinity for bone

Nitrogen side chain in R_2 position increases potency

Phosphonate groups bind calcium and target drug to bone

Pyrophosphate

FIGURE 19-5 Structure of bisphosphonates. Bisphosphonates are based on the structure of pyrophosphate, an endogenously produced inhibitor of mineralization. The carbon atom in bisphosphonates renders the drugs resistant to hydrolysis.

osteoporosis but there are no data on fracture prevention. Risedronate in a dose of 35 mg weekly has been found to give an equivalent increase in BMD as 5 mg daily and once-weekly dosing is used most commonly in routine clinical practice. Adverse effects are as described for alendronic acid although there is weak evidence from observational studies that risedronate may have a slightly better upper GI tolerability than alendronic acid.[58]

Zoledronic Acid

Zoledronic acid is an effective treatment for osteoporosis. When given intravenously at a dose of 5 mg once a year, along with calcium and vitamin D supplements, it has been shown to reduce the risk of vertebral, nonvertebral, and hip fractures in patients with postmenopausal osteoporosis.[10] Zoledronic acid is the only agent that has been shown to reduce mortality in osteoporosis. When administered to men and postmenopausal women who had suffered hip fractures, treatment reduced overall mortality by 28% and reduced the risk of recurrent fracture by about 35%.[43] It has also been shown to be effective in the prevention and treatment of glucocorticoid-induced osteoporosis with effects on BMD that are superior to those of risedronate.[62] The most common adverse effect is a transient influenza-like illness for 2 to 3 days after the first infusion which is self limiting. This reaction can occur after subsequent infusions but is milder and usually asymptomatic. Other less common adverse effects include hypocalcemia, atrial fibrillation, and renal impairment. Rare side effects include osteonecrosis of the jaw and uveitis. Prior to administration of zoledronic acid renal function should be checked and the drug administered only if the estimated GFR is greater than 35 mL/min. Vitamin D deficiency should also be corrected to reduce the risk of hypocalcemia.

Ibandronate

Ibandronate can be given orally or intravenously in the management of osteoporosis. A randomized controlled trial in patients with postmenopausal osteoporosis showed that it reduced the risk of vertebral fractures by about 50% when given orally in a dose of 2.5 mg daily.[23] However no overall reduction in the risk of nonvertebral or hip fractures was found in this study. As with other bisphosphonates, bridging studies have shown that 150 mg monthly gives an equivalent or greater increase in BMD as 2.5 mg daily[60] and this is the dose that is used in routine clinical practice. Intravenous ibandronate is given in a dose of 3 mg every 3 months in osteoporosis. The antifracture efficacy of the 3-mg/3-month regimen has not specifically been investigated but a post hoc analysis of data from patients treated with oral ibandronate 150 mg monthly and various doses of intravenous ibandronate showed evidence of efficacy at preventing vertebral and nonvertebral fractures with higher cumulative doses of the drug.[32] Adverse effects and dosing instructions for administration of oral ibandronate are as described for alendronate. Patients who receive intravenous ibandronate may experience a transient "flu-like illness" as described for zoledronic acid.

Denosumab

Denosumab is a fully humanized monoclonal antibody directed against RANKL, a key stimulator of bone resorption (see above). It has powerful inhibitory effects on bone resorption and is given subcutaneously in a dose of 60 mg every 6 months in the treatment of osteoporosis. Large-scale clinical trials have shown that denosumab reduces the risk of vertebral fractures by about 68%, hip fractures by 40%, and nonvertebral fractures by 20% in patients with postmenopausal osteoporosis.[22] Although adverse effects are uncommon, it is important to ensure that patients are vitamin D replete at the time of therapy to reduce the risk of hypocalcemia. Osteonecrosis of the jaw has been reported in patients receiving long-term treatment with denosumab, but this is rare.[55] Denosumab is not subject to clearance by the kidney and because of this can be used in osteoporotic patients with renal impairment, although care should be exercised in such patients to ensure they do not have renal osteodystrophy since this is predicted to increase the risk of hypocalcemia considerably. Unlike bisphosphonates, the effect of denosumab on bone resorption is relatively short lived and when treatment is stopped there is a rebound increase in bone turnover with significant bone loss. Accordingly, treatment must be given on a continuing basis for a sustained therapeutic effect.

Strontium Ranelate

Strontium ranelate has weak inhibitory effects on bone resorption and weak stimulatory effects on biochemical markers of bone formation. It is also incorporated into bone, substituting for calcium in hydroxyapatite crystals. Randomized trials have shown that strontium ranelate 2 g daily reduces the risk of vertebral fractures by about 50% and nonvertebral fractures by about 16% in women with postmenopausal osteoporosis.[48,56] The pivotal trials of strontium ranelate showed no overall efficacy at preventing hip fractures but a positive effect was identified in a post hoc subgroup analysis of patients with hip BMD values less than −3. Absorption of strontium is inhibited by food and it is usually given as a single dose at night at least 2 hours after eating. The most common side effect is diarrhea and other GI side effects, but other less common adverse effects include skin rashes and venous thrombosis. Strontium ranelate has recently been found to increase the risk of myocardial infarction and is contraindicated in patients with known cardiovascular disease and those with strong risk factors for cardiovascular disease such as diabetes. Patients who are treated with strontium often have large increases in BMD as assessed by DEXA. This however is mainly due to the fact that strontium ions (atomic mass, 87.6) substitute for calcium ions (atomic mass, 40.1) in hydroxyapatite. In view of this it is difficult to truly assess bone mass in patients who have been receiving strontium. The effects of strontium on bone density persist for about 12 months after stopping treatment and there is evidence that antifracture efficacy is also sustained during this time.

Parathyroid Hormone

PTH differs from the other drugs mentioned above in that it is an anabolic agent which works by stimulating bone remodeling and producing new bone.[61] Although bone resorption and bone formation are both increased by PTH, the cyclical mode of administration causes bone formation to increase more than bone resorption, resulting in a net gain of bone. This differs from the situation in primary hyperparathyroidism where the sustained elevation in PTH levels causes bone resorption to increase more than bone formation resulting in bone loss, especially in cortical bone. Two types of PTH are currently licensed, the 1-34 fragment and the full length molecule (1-84). PTH 1-34 20 mcg daily given by subcutaneous injection has been shown to be effective in reducing the risk of vertebral fractures by 65% and nonvertebral fractures by 50% in women with postmenopausal osteoporosis.[51] The 1-34 fragment has also been shown to be effective in male osteoporosis with regard to the effects on BMD, although there are no fracture studies in males.[54] PTH 1-34 is effective in the treatment of corticosteroid-induced osteoporosis and has been shown to be superior to alendronic acid at reducing the risk of vertebral fractures in this situation.[69] The 1-84 fragment of PTH has been shown to reduce the risk of vertebral fractures by about 60% but there are no data on efficacy for nonvertebral fractures.[31] Adverse effects of PTH include headache, muscle cramps, and mild hypercalcemia which is usually asymptomatic and does not require therapy to be stopped. The recommended duration of therapy is 2 years at which point patients should be given an antiresorptive agent to prevent loss of the bone that has been newly formed. Raloxifene, alendronic acid, and zoledronic acid have all been reported to be effective at maintaining the increases in bone mass and preventing bone loss in patients previously treated with PTH.[9,26,40,63] There is evidence to suggest that concurrent administration of alendronic acid blunts the anabolic effect of PTH by inhibiting bone formation[30] and that previous treatment with oral bisphosphonates results in a slightly blunted anabolic response.[11] Interestingly, concomitant administration of intravenous zoledronic acid with PTH does not appear to blunt the anabolic response.[16]

Calcium and Vitamin D

There is evidence to suggest that combined calcium and vitamin D supplements can reduce the risk of nonvertebral fractures with effects that are most pronounced in elderly institutionalized patients who are at risk of vitamin D deficiency.[13] Calcium and vitamin D supplements are seldom used as stand-alone therapy for younger patients with osteoporosis but are frequently used as an adjunct to other osteoporosis treatments including bisphosphonates, strontium ranelate, denosumab, and PTH.

Calcitonin

Intranasal calcitonin (200 units/day) has been shown to reduce the risk of vertebral fractures by about 30% in postmenopausal women with osteoporosis but it does not appear to be effective at preventing nonvertebral fractures.[12] Calcitonin has a number of side effects including flushing and nausea, and recently long-term use of calcitonin was reported to be associated with an increased risk of cancer resulting in withdrawal

of authorization for its use in the treatment of osteoporosis in Europe.

Hormone Replacement Therapy

Hormone replacement therapy (HRT) is effective at preventing postmenopausal bone loss and has been shown to be effective in preventing vertebral fractures, nonvertebral fractures, and hip fractures in postmenopausal women,[76] even if they have not been diagnosed with osteoporosis on the basis of DEXA.[67] Although HRT is clearly effective at preventing fractures, it is seldom used clinically in the treatment of osteoporosis because long-term use in older women has been associated with an increased risk of cardiovascular disease, venous thrombosis, and breast cancer. It remains an option in younger women (age <60) with osteoporosis and is the treatment of choice for preventing bone loss in women with an early menopause.

Raloxifene

Raloxifene belongs to a class of compounds termed selective estrogen receptor modulators (SERM). It acts an estrogen receptor agonist in bone and as an antagonist in other tissues, most notably the breast. Raloxifene, given orally at a dose of 60 mg/day, has been shown to reduce the risk of vertebral fractures in postmenopausal women with osteoporosis by about 30%.[28] No efficacy has been demonstrated for nonvertebral and hip fractures and because of this it is used infrequently. Adverse effects include hot flushes, muscle cramps, and an increased risk of venous thrombosis.

Tibolone

Tibolone is a steroid hormone which acts as a partial agonist at estrogen, progesterone, and androgen receptors. It alleviates vasomotor symptoms and enhances libido in postmenopausal women with similar efficacy to HRT. Tibolone has been shown to reduce the risk of vertebral fractures by about 45% and nonvertebral fractures by about 26% in a randomized trial of older (age >65) postmenopausal women with osteoporosis.[20] In this study tibolone treatment was associated with a reduced risk of breast cancer (68% reduction) but an increased risk of stroke (119% increase), although the number of events were small. Currently tibolone is mainly used as an alternative to HRT in postmenopausal women with low BMD and menopausal symptoms.

Testosterone

Testosterone replacement therapy is often used in the treatment of osteoporosis in men who have hypogonadism where it has added benefits of increasing muscle strength and general well-being. Treatment can either be given by injection every 4 to 6 weeks or by transdermal patches. Testosterone has no clear role in the treatment of male osteoporosis in the absence of hypogonadism.

Combination Therapy

There is no clear indication for using combination therapy in the treatment of osteoporosis. Although several clinical trials have been performed using combination therapy these have not been powered to look at fractures and so the clinical value of this approach remains uncertain.

MONITORING RESPONSE TO TREATMENT

It remains uncertain whether patients on treatment for osteoporosis should be monitored or how this should best be achieved. Although most drug treatments for osteoporosis have stimulatory effects on BMD, the role of BMD monitoring remains controversial since changes in BMD are poorly associated with fracture risk reduction.[21,81] This may be partly because of limitations in the precision of BMD measurements and the fact that fracture risk is only partly explained by BMD. Biochemical markers of bone turnover have also been explored as a means of predicting good and poor responders to treatment in terms of fracture risk reduction. Although pretreatment levels of bone turnover as assessed by biochemical markers have been associated with subsequent risk of fracture on alendronate therapy,[5] clinical trials designed to investigate the effectiveness of feeding back the results of biochemical markers to patients on therapy showed no significant benefit in terms of fracture risk reduction.[24] In clinical practice, repeat DEXA measurements are often performed in patients on treatment to assess response. Such measurements should not normally be repeated within 2 years of starting antiresorptive therapy since the precision of the measurement is such that significant changes are unlikely to be detected before this time.

TREATMENT FAILURE

Treatment failure has recently been defined as the occurrence of two or more fragility fractures in a patient who has been established on therapy or the occurrence of one fragility fracture in a patient who has experienced bone loss or failed to respond in terms of biochemical markers of bone turnover.[25] It is unclear how patients with treatment failure should best be managed. There are several potential options including switching from one oral agent to another, switching from an oral agent to a parenteral agent, or switching from an antiresorptive to an anabolic agent. In the absence of an evidence base the author's personal approach is to first ensure that the patient is taking oral medication correctly. This is especially important with oral bisphosphonates and strontium ranelate. If the treatment is being taken properly then I recommend a switch to a parenteral therapy, except in patients with severe osteoporosis (T-score −4 or below) where I would offer treatment with PTH.

REFERENCES

1. Anonymous. Optimal calcium intake. Sponsored by National Institutes of Health Continuing Medical Education. *Nutrition.* 1995;11:409–417.
2. Arden NK, Spector TD. Genetic influences on muscle strength, lean body mass, and bone mineral density: A twin study. *J Bone Miner Res.* 1997;12:2076–2081.
3. Balemans W, Piters E, Cleiren E, et al. The binding between sclerostin and LRP5 is altered by DKK1 and by high-bone mass LRP5 mutations. *Calcif Tissue Int.* 2008;82: 445–453.
4. Bassett JH, O'Shea PJ, Sriskantharajah S, et al. Thyroid hormone excess rather than thyrotropin deficiency induces osteoporosis in hyperthyroidism. *Mol Endocrinol.* 2007; 21:1095–1107.
5. Bauer DC, Garnero P, Hochberg MC, et al. Pretreatment levels of bone turnover and the antifracture efficacy of alendronate: The fracture intervention trial. *J Bone Miner Res.* 2006;21:292–299.
6. Berendsen AD, Fisher LW, Kilts TM, et al. Modulation of canonical Wnt signaling by the extracellular matrix component biglycan. *Proc Natl Acad Sci USA.* 2011;108: 17022–17027.
7. Bergland A, Thorsen H, Karesen R. Effect of exercise on mobility, balance, and health-related quality of life in osteoporotic women with a history of vertebral fracture: A randomized, controlled trial. *Osteoporos Int.* 2011;22:1863–1871.
8. Bischoff-Ferrari HA, wson-Hughes B, Baron JA, et al. Calcium intake and hip fracture risk in men and women: A meta-analysis of prospective cohort studies and randomized controlled trials. *Am J Clin Nutr.* 2007;86:1780–1790.
9. Black DM, Bilezikian JP, Ensrud KE, et al. One year of alendronate after one year of parathyroid hormone (1-84) for osteoporosis. *N Engl J Med.* 2005;353:555–565.
10. Black DM, Delmas PD, Eastell R, et al. Once-yearly zoledronic acid for treatment of postmenopausal osteoporosis. *N Engl J Med.* 2007;356:1809–1822.
11. Boonen S, Marin F, Obermayer-Pietsch B, et al. Effects of previous antiresorptive therapy on the bone mineral density response to two years of teriparatide treatment in postmenopausal women with osteoporosis. *J Clin Endocrinol Metab.* 2008;93:852–860.
12. Chesnut CH, Silverman S, Andriano K, et al. A randomized trial of nasal spray salmon calcitonin in postmenopausal women with established osteoporosis: the prevent recurrence of osteoporotic fractures study. PROOF Study Group. *Am J Med.* 2000;109:267–276.
13. Chung M, Lee J, Terasawa T, et al. Vitamin D with or without calcium supplementation for prevention of cancer and fractures: an updated meta-analysis for the U.S. Preventive Services Task Force. *Ann Intern Med.* 2011;155:827–838.
14. Close J, Ellis M, Hooper R, et al. Prevention of falls in the elderly trial (PROFET): A randomised controlled trial. *Lancet.* 1999;353:93–97.
15. Cooper C, Barker DJP, Wickham C. Physical activity, muscle strength, and calcium intake in fracture of the proximal femur in Britain. *Br Med J.* 1988;297:1443–1446.
16. Cosman F, Eriksen EF, Recknor C, et al. Effects of intravenous zoledronic acid plus subcutaneous teriparatide [rhPTH(1-34)] in postmenopausal osteoporosis. *J Bone Miner Res.* 2011;26:503–511.
17. Court-Brown CM, Aitken SA, Ralston SH, et al. The relationship of fall-related fractures to social deprivation. *Osteoporos Int.* 2011;22:1211–1218.
18. Cranney A, Guyatt G, Griffith L, et al. Meta-analyses of therapies for postmenopausal osteoporosis. IX: Summary of meta-analyses of therapies for postmenopausal osteoporosis. *Endocr Rev.* 2002;23:570–578.
19. Cranney A, Tugwell P, Adachi J, et al. Meta-analyses of therapies for postmenopausal osteoporosis. III. Meta-analysis of risedronate for the treatment of postmenopausal osteoporosis. *Endocr Rev.* 2002;23:517–523.
20. Cummings SR, Ettinger B, Delmas PD, et al. The effects of tibolone in older postmenopausal women. *N Engl J Med.* 2008;359:697–708.
21. Cummings SR, Karpf DB, Harris F, et al. Improvement in spine bone density and reduction in risk of vertebral fractures during treatment with antiresorptive drugs. *Am J Med.* 2002;112:281–289.
22. Cummings SR, San MJ, McClung MR, et al. Denosumab for prevention of fractures in postmenopausal women with osteoporosis. *N Engl J Med.* 2009;361:756–765.
23. Delmas PD, Recker RR, Chesnut CH III, et al. Daily and intermittent oral ibandronate normalize bone turnover and provide significant reduction in vertebral fracture risk: Results from the BONE study. *Osteoporos Int.* 2004;15:792–798.
24. Delmas PD, Vrijens B, Eastell R, et al. Effect of monitoring bone turnover markers on persistence with risedronate treatment of postmenopausal osteoporosis. *J Clin Endocrinol Metab.* 2007;92:1296–1304.
25. Diez-Perez A, Adachi JD, Agnusdei D, et al. Treatment failure in osteoporosis. *Osteoporos Int.* 2012;23:2769–2774.
26. Eastell R, Nickelsen T, Marin F, et al. Sequential treatment of severe postmenopausal osteoporosis after teriparatide: Final results of the randomized, controlled European Study of Forsteo (EUROFORS). *J Bone Miner Res.* 2009;24:726–736.
27. Estrada K, Styrkarsdottir U, Evangelou E, et al. Genome-wide meta-analysis identifies 56 bone mineral density loci and reveals 14 loci associated with risk of fracture. *Nat Genet.* 2012;44:491–501.
28. Ettinger B, Black DM, Mitlak BH, et al. Reduction of vertebral fracture risk in postmenopausal women with osteoporosis treated with raloxifene. *JAMA.* 1999;282:637–645.
29. Ferrar L, Jiang G, Schousboe JT, et al. Algorithm-based qualitative and semiquantitative identification of prevalent vertebral fracture: Agreement between different readers, imaging modalities, and diagnostic approaches. *J Bone Miner Res.* 2008;23: 417–424.
30. Finkelstein JS, Hayes A, Hunzelman JL, et al. The effects of parathyroid hormone, alendronate, or both in men with osteoporosis. *N Engl J Med.* 2003;349:1216–1226.
31. Greenspan SL, Bone HG, Ettinger MP, et al. Effect of recombinant human parathyroid hormone (1-84) on vertebral fracture and bone mineral density in postmenopausal women with osteoporosis: A randomized trial. *Ann Intern Med.* 2007;146:326–339.
32. Harris ST, Blumentals WA, Miller PD. Ibandronate and the risk of non-vertebral and clinical fractures in women with postmenopausal osteoporosis: Results of a meta-analysis of phase III studies. *Curr Med Res Opin.* 2008;24:237–245.
33. Hippisley-Cox J, Coupland C. Derivation and validation of updated QFracture algorithm to predict risk of osteoporotic fracture in primary care in the United Kingdom: prospective open cohort study. *Br Med J.* 2012;344:e3427.
34. Holroyd C, Cooper C, Dennison E. Epidemiology of osteoporosis. *Best Pract Res Clin Endocrinol Metab.* 2008;22:671–685.
35. Johnson ML, Harnish K, Nusse R, et al. LRP5 and Wnt signaling: A union made for bone. *J Bone Miner Res.* 2004;19:1749–1757.
36. Kanis JA, Melton LJ III, Christiansen C, et al. The diagnosis of osteoporosis. *J Bone Miner Res.* 1994;9:1137–1141.
37. Khosla S, Burr D, Cauley J, et al. Bisphosphonate-associated osteonecrosis of the jaw: Report of a task force of the American Society for Bone and Mineral Research. *J Bone Miner Res.* 2007;22:1479–1491.

38. Khosla S, Melton LJ III, Riggs BL. Estrogens and bone health in men. *Calcif Tissue Int.* 2001;69:189–192.

39. Khosla S. Minireview: The OPG/RANKL/RANK system. *Endocrinology.* 2001;142:5050–5055.

40. Kurland ES, Heller SL, Diamond B, et al. The importance of bisphosphonate therapy in maintaining bone mass in men after therapy with teriparatide [human parathyroid hormone(1-34)]. *Osteoporos Int.* 2004;15:992–997.

41. Law MR, Hackshaw AK. A meta-analysis of cigarette smoking, bone mineral density and risk of hip fracture: recognition of a major effect. *Br Med J.* 1997;315:841–846.

42. Lucas GJ, Daroszewska A, Ralston SH. Contribution of genetic factors to the pathogenesis of Paget's disease of bone and related disorders. *J Bone Miner Res.* 2006;21(suppl 2):31–37.

43. Lyles KW, Colon-Emeric CS, Magaziner JS, et al. Zoledronic acid and clinical fractures and mortality after hip fracture. *N Engl J Med.* 2007;357:1799–1809.

44. Mackey DC, Lui LY, Cawthon PM, et al. High-trauma fractures and low bone mineral density in older women and men. *JAMA.* 2007;298:2381–2388.

45. Marshall D, Johnell O, Wedel H. Meta-analysis of how well measures of bone mineral density predict occurrence of osteoporotic fractures. *Br Med J.* 1996;312:1254–1259.

46. McLellan AR, Gallacher SJ, Fraser M, et al. The fracture liaison service: Success of a program for the evaluation and management of patients with osteoporotic fracture. *Osteoporos Int.* 2003;14:1028–1034.

47. McLellan AR, Wolowacz SE, Zimovetz EA, et al. Fracture liaison services for the evaluation and management of patients with osteoporotic fracture: A cost-effectiveness evaluation based on data collected over 8 years of service provision. *Osteoporos Int.* 2011;22:2083–2098.

48. Meunier PJ, Roux C, Seeman E, et al. The effects of strontium ranelate on the risk of vertebral fracture in women with postmenopausal osteoporosis. *N Engl J Med.* 2004;350:459–468.

49. Michaelsson K, Melhus H, Ferm H, et al. Genetic liability to fractures in the elderly. *Arch Intern Med.* 2005;165:1825–1830.

50. Minaire P, Meuniere P, Edouard C, et al. Quantitative histological data on disuse osteoporosis: Comparison with biological data. *Calcif Tiss Res.* 1974;17:57–73.

51. Neer RM, Arnaud CD, Zanchetta JR, et al. Effect of parathyroid hormone (1-34) on fractures and bone mineral density in postmenopausal women with osteoporosis. *N Engl J Med.* 2001;344:1434–1441.

52. Nelson HD, Haney EM, Dana T, et al. Screening for osteoporosis: An update for the U.S. Preventive Services Task Force. *Ann Intern Med.* 2010;153:99–111.

53. Orwoll E, Ettinger M, Weiss S, et al. Alendronate for the treatment of osteoporosis in men. *N Engl J Med.* 2000;343:604–610.

54. Orwoll ES, Scheele WH, Paul S, et al. The effect of teriparatide [human parathyroid hormone (1-34)] therapy on bone density in men with osteoporosis. *J Bone Miner Res.* 2003;18:9–17.

55. Papapoulos S, Chapurlat R, Libanati C, et al. Five years of denosumab exposure in women with postmenopausal osteoporosis: Results from the first two years of the FREEDOM extension. *J Bone Miner Res.* 2012;27:694–701.

56. Pleiner-Duxneuner J, Zwettler E, Paschalis E, et al. Treatment of osteoporosis with parathyroid hormone and teriparatide. *Calcif Tissue Int.* 2009;84:159–170.

57. Ralston SH, de'Lara G, Farquhar DJ, et al. NICE on osteoporosis. Women over 75 with fragility fractures should have DEXA. *Br Med J.* 2009;338:b2340.

58. Ralston SH, Kou TD, Wick-Urban B, et al. Risk of upper gastrointestinal tract events in risedronate users switched to alendronate. *Calcif Tissue Int.* 2010;87:298–304.

59. Ralston SH, Uitterlinden AG. Genetics of osteoporosis. *Endocr Rev.* 2010;31:629–662.

60. Reginster JY, Adami S, Lakatos P, et al. Efficacy and tolerability of once-monthly oral ibandronate in postmenopausal osteoporosis: 2-year results from the MOBILE study. *Ann Rheum Dis.* 2006;65:654–661.

61. Reginster JY, Seeman E, de Vernejoul MC, et al. Strontium ranelate reduces the risk of nonvertebral fractures in postmenopausal women with osteoporosis: TROPOS study. *J Clin Endocrinol Metab.* 2005;90:2816–2822.

62. Reid DM, Devogelaer JP, Saag K, et al. Zoledronic acid and risedronate in the prevention and treatment of glucocorticoid-induced osteoporosis (HORIZON): A multicentre, double-blind, double-dummy, randomised controlled trial. *Lancet.* 2009;373:1253–1263.

63. Rhee Y, Won YY, Baek MH, et al. Maintenance of increased bone mass after recombinant human parathyroid hormone (1-84) with sequential zoledronate treatment in ovariectomized rats. *J Bone Miner Res.* 2004;19:931–937.

64. Riches PL, McRorie E, Fraser WD, et al. Osteoporosis associated with neutralizing autoantibodies against osteoprotegerin. *N Engl J Med.* 2009;361:1459–1465.

65. Robling AG, Niziolek PJ, Baldridge LA, et al. Mechanical stimulation of bone in vivo reduces osteocyte expression of Sost/sclerostin. *J Biol Chem.* 2008;283:5866–5875.

66. Rosen CJ, Abrams SA, Aloia JF, et al. IOM committee members respond to Endocrine Society vitamin D guideline. *J Clin Endocrinol Metab.* 2012;97:1146–1152.

67. Rossouw JE, Anderson GL, Prentice RL, et al. Risks and benefits of estrogen plus progestin in healthy postmenopausal women: Principal results from the Women's Health Initiative randomized controlled trial. *JAMA.* 2002;288:321–333.

68. Saag KG, Emkey R, Schnitzer TJ, et al. Alendronate for the prevention and treatment of glucocorticoid-induced osteoporosis. Glucocorticoid-Induced Osteoporosis Intervention Study Group. *N Engl J Med.* 1998;339:292–299.

69. Saag KG, Zanchetta JR, Devogelaer JP, et al. Effects of teriparatide versus alendronate for treating glucocorticoid-induced osteoporosis: Thirty-six-month results of a randomized, double-blind, controlled trial. *Arthritis Rheum.* 2009;60:3346–3355.

70. Schilcher J, Michaelsson K, Aspenberg P. Bisphosphonate use and atypical fractures of the femoral shaft. *N Engl J Med.* 2011;364:1728–1737.

71. Schnitzer T, Bone HG, Crepaldi G, et al. Therapeutic equivalence of alendronate 70 mg once-weekly and alendronate 10 mg daily in the treatment of osteoporosis. Alendronate Once-Weekly Study Group. *Aging (Milano).* 2000;12:1–12.

72. Sherrington C, Tiedemann A, Fairhall N, et al. Exercise to prevent falls in older adults: An updated meta-analysis and best practice recommendations. *N S W Public Health Bull.* 2011;22:78–83.

73. Siris ES, Miller PD, Barrett-Connor E, et al. Identification and fracture outcomes of undiagnosed low bone mineral density in postmenopausal women: Results from the National Osteoporosis Risk Assessment. *JAMA.* 2001;286:2815–2822.

74. Skerry TM. Mechanical loading and bone: What sort of exercise is beneficial to the skeleton? *Bone.* 1997;20:179–181.

75. Stevens JR, Miranda-Carboni GA, Singer MA, et al. Wnt10b deficiency results in age-dependent loss of bone mass and progressive reduction of mesenchymal progenitor cells. *J Bone Miner Res.* 2010;25:2138–2147.

76. Torgerson DJ, Bell-Syer SE. Hormone replacement therapy and prevention of nonvertebral fractures. A meta-analysis of randomized trials. *JAMA.* 2001;285:2891–2897.

77. Tseng VL, Yu F, Lum F, et al. Risk of fractures following cataract surgery in Medicare beneficiaries. *JAMA.* 2012;308:493–501.

78. van Staa TP. The pathogenesis, epidemiology and management of glucocorticoid-induced osteoporosis. *Calcif Tissue Int.* 2006;79:129–137.

79. Villa A, Guerrini MM, Cassani B, et al. Infantile malignant, autosomal recessive osteopetrosis: The rich and the poor. *Calcif Tissue Int.* 2009;84:1–12.

80. Wallach S, Cohen S, Reid DM, et al. Effects of risedronate treatment on bone density and vertebral fracture in patients on corticosteroid therapy. *Calcif Tissue Int.* 2000;67:277–285.

81. Watts NB, Geusens P, Barton IP, et al. Relationship between changes in BMD and nonvertebral fracture incidence associated with risedronate: Reduction in risk of nonvertebral fracture is not related to change in BMD. *J Bone Miner Res.* 2005;20:2097–2104.

82. Williams BO, Insogna KL. Where Wnts went: The exploding field of Lrp5 and Lrp6 signaling in bone. *J Bone Miner Res.* 2009;24:171–178.

20 FRACTURES IN THE ELDERLY PATIENT

Nicholas D. Clement and Leela C. Biant

INTRODUCTION

An "elderly" person is generally defined by age, with those aged 65 years and older being assigned "elderly" status. This chronologic definition is related to policies and social norms related to retirement and legislation.[152] In contrast, a physiologic definition of aging is more complex, and would vary depending on individual well-being, relative to the society in which the person lives.

In the United States of America the retirement age was introduced in the 1930s as a way of encouraging people to leave the labor force to be replaced by younger people, thereby lowering the unemployment rate. Such legislation made it "customary" to "finish working," thus giving people an expectation of retirement at 65 years. A survey in Manitoba, Canada revealed that nearly 80% of people aged 65 and over, who considered themselves retired, stated that they had done so voluntarily, although health also entered into the equation for about a third of the patients.[159]

The elderly population is commonly subdivided into three groups that show marked physiologic variation. Thus, young–old (65 to 69), middle–old (70 to 74), and old–old (over 75) cohorts are often identified. Sometimes the age divisions vary and being over 80 or over 85 years may define the "oldest–old" category. The terminology also changes with oldest–old and super-elderly being used to define the oldest patients. The term "super-elderly" has been used in orthopedics for both elective and trauma patients. The definition, however, varies from those patients greater than 80 years old to those greater than 90 years old.[18,37] For the purpose of this chapter, we will define the super-elderly population as those patients 80 years old or more. This group of patients is thought to be more vulnerable to the physical and social challenges that we associate with old age, such as widowhood, worsening health, and an increasing difficulty completing the activities of daily life without assistance.[159]

INCIDENCE AND EPIDEMIOLOGY OF FRACTURES IN THE ELDERLY

Aging Population

The elderly population is on the threshold of a boom. According to the United States Census Bureau[75] projections, a substantial increase in the number of older people will occur during the 2010 to 2030 period, after the first "baby boomers" have turned 65. The older population in 2030 is projected to be twice as large as it was in 2000, growing from 35 million to 72 million, which will represent nearly 20% of the total United States population. The median age rose from 22.9 years in 1900 to 35.3 years in 2000 and is projected to increase to 39 years by 2030. In 2000, the oldest–old, defined as those 85 years and older, was 34 times greater than that recorded in 1900, whereas the elderly population aged between 65 and 84 years was only 10 times as large. In 2000, 420 million people in the world were at least 65 years of age, this constituting 7% of the world's population. However, this number is projected to more than double by 2030, reaching 974 million. This changing population demographic is affecting developing countries at a rapid rate; in the year 2000, 60% of the world's elderly population lived in developing countries. This is projected to increase to 70% by 2030.

People in developed countries are not only living longer but they are enjoying increasingly healthier lifestyles than ever before. The effect of the obesity epidemic on longevity is yet to peak. The average life expectancy in the United States at birth rose from 47.3 years in 1900 to 76.9 years in 2000. Furthermore, disability among the older population is declining, with studies over the past two decades demonstrating a substantial decline in the rate of disability and functional limitation. The growth of this more active and physically fitter elderly population is challenging policy makers, families, businesses, and health-care providers to meet the needs of aging individuals. This will have major repercussions upon the type and severity of fragility fractures presenting to orthopedic surgeons. Fracture management in the elderly and super-elderly patients will consume a greater proportion of the trauma workload and expense in the future with an ever-increasing population being at risk.

Life Expectancy of the Super-Elderly

There is evidence that increases in the population of centenarians over the 20th century were largely a result of increases in survival between 80 and 100 years and at birth, as well as increases in the size of the birth cohorts available to survive.[141] The increases in survival from birth to 80 years, combined with the increases in survival from 80 to 100 years seen over the second half of the 20th century, are expected to continue. This suggests that considerable extension to the length of life has been, and will continue to be, achieved in very old age. Table 20-1 presents the life expectancy at age 80 for cohorts born between 1901 and 1961 in England and Wales and the estimated and projected population aged 80 between 1981 and 2041. Life expectancy at age 80 for females born in England and Wales at the beginning of the 20th century was about 8 years. The estimated mid-year population of females aged 80 years in 1981 was 152,000. The cohort of females born in England and Wales in 1961 is expected to live, on an average, for a further 13 years after their 80th birthday in 2041. The population of females aged 80 in 2041 is projected to be twice the size of that of the same age in 1901. The remaining life expectancy, at age 80, for men born during the 20th century has increased and is expected to increase at a greater pace than that of women. Life expectancy at age 80 for the cohort of men born in 1901 was 6 years but will be 12 years for those born in 1961. The population of men aged 80 in 1901 was 74,000, half that of women of the same age. The population of men aged 80 years projected to be alive in 2041 is 3.5 times larger than that in 1901. The super-elderly population is growing and is projected to continue to grow. In addition, expectation of life at older ages is expected to continue to increase.

| TABLE 20-1 | The Life Expectancy at 80 Years and the Estimated Mid-Year Population for Males and Females Aged ≥80 Years Born Between 1901 and 1961 |

Birth Cohort	Year Aged 80	Life Expectancy at 80 (yrs)		Population ≥80 yrs (1000s)	
		Male	Female	Male	Female
1901	1981	6	8	74	152
1911	1991	7	8	96	172
1921	2001	8	9	127	202
1931	2011	9	11	136	180
1941	2021	11	12	157	187
1951	2031	12	13	207	244
1961	2041	12	13	252	295

Trends in Fracture Incidence

A simple fall from standing height is the commonest cause of injury in the elderly population.[99,167] Out of all fall-related injuries needing medical attention in older people, every second injury is reported to be a fracture.[90] In 2000, the worldwide occurrence of fragility fractures in adults aged 50 years or older was estimated to be approximately 9 million.[91] In Finland, the annual number of hip fractures has remained static at approximately 7,000 fractures per year in patients aged 50 years or older between 1997 and 2004.[95] However, due to increasing longevity and a growing elderly population the number of fractures presenting to orthopedic surgeons is estimated to double[150] and the number of hip fractures to double or even triple by the year 2030.[95]

The cost of fracture care in the elderly is relatively high compared with younger patients.[22,140] In Finland, the average total cost of a patient with a hip fracture during the first postoperative year was $17,750 in 2003.[140] More recently, Nikitovic et al.[139] demonstrated the costs to be far greater reaching nearly $40,000 in the first year. This continued into the second postoperative year with a further $10,000 of costs being recorded. This was mainly due to the cost of institutional care after injury, with 24% of females and 19% of males who were living independently in the community before their fracture needing long-term postoperative care. In the United States, medical expenditure has been reported to be two to three times greater for women compared with men.[167] It is predicted, however, that in the future the number and the costs of fall-related injuries will rise more rapidly in older men relative to women.[150,151] The insult of the fracture upon the functional status of elderly patients can be serious[91] and can lead to excess morbidity and mortality and foreshorten the frailty trajectory.[21] In addition to altering physical performance and the management of activities of daily living tasks, hip fractures may seriously affect health-related quality of life.[22,180] Thus, fracture prevention is an important public health issue.

Falls and fractures can be prevented.[68,101] There is inconsistency regarding the role of fall-related factors and bone fragility in predicting whether a person will sustain a fracture.[100] Factors associated with an increased risk of falls differ according to gender.[26] Thus, more detailed information about the gender-specific predictors of fractures are needed to make prevention of fractures more effective.

Fragility Fracture Burden

Elderly Fractures over the Last Decade

Three analyses of fracture epidemiology have been undertaken in Edinburgh since 2000 with the third analysis, undertaken over a period of 1 year in 2010/11, being analyzed in Chapter 3. The previous two studies were undertaken in 2000[48] and 2007/08.[46] Each study has analyzed all adult fractures from a defined population in a developed country. This data from Scotland has been used to assess the change in fracture epidemiology during the last decade with regard to the elderly and super-elderly population, and in relation to common fragility fractures. Spinal fractures were excluded because of the fact that not all spinal fractures in the elderly are admitted to the hospital and analysis would underestimate the exact incidence.

The overall incidence of all adult fractures during the last decade has significantly increased from $1,113/10^5$/year in 2000 to $1,352/10^5$/year in 2010/11 (odds ratio 1.2, $p < 0.0001$). The age group in which fracture incidence has increased most rapidly during this time period is the elderly, and more specifically, the super-elderly (Tables 20-2 and 20-3). The incidence of fractures in the elderly increased from $2,028/10^5$/year in the year 2000 to $2,318/10^5$/year in 2010/11 (odds ratio 1.2, $p < 0.001$). A similar rate of increase was also observed for the super-elderly group which increased from $3,733/10^5$/year in the year 2000 to $4,045/10^5$/year in 2010/11 (odds ratio 1.1, $p < 0.001$). This was the greatest increase in any age group. Hence, elderly patients are the fastest-growing age group that are currently presenting with fractures. This will have significant repercussions upon the provision of future trauma

TABLE 20-2 **Epidemiology of Fractures Treated in a 1-Year Period. The Numbers, Prevalence, Incidence, and Gender Ratios are Shown Together with the Average Ages and Percentages of Patients ≥65 Years and ≥80 Years of Age**

All Fractures	n	%	n/10⁵/yr	Average Age (yrs)	≥65 yrs (%)	≥80 yrs (%)	Male/Female
Distal radius/ulna	1,221	17.5	235.9	58.4	41.8	18.1	28/72
Metacarpus	781	11.2	150.9	33.6	8.2	3.1	80/20
Proximal femur	753	10.8	145.5	80.7	90.6	63.7	27/73
Ankle	720	10.3	139.1	48.8	23.6	6	47/53
Finger phalanges	696	9.9	134.5	41.6	13.6	5.8	60/40
Proximal humerus	478	6.8	92.4	66.3	55.6	23	31/69
Metatarsus	465	6.6	89.8	44.6	17	5.2	37/63
Proximal forearm	378	5.4	73	45.6	17.2	5.8	46/54
Clavicle	257	3.7	49.7	44.5	21	9.7	70/30
Toe phalanges	248	3.5	47.9	35.7	3.9	1	59/41
Carpus	194	2.8	37.5	38	7.7	1.5	64/36
Pelvis	119	1.7	23	75.6	74.8	58.8	30/70
Femoral diaphysis	82	1.2	15.8	70.2	67.1	39	48/52
Tibial diaphysis	69	1	13.3	42.3	8.7	0	71/29
Calcaneus	65	0.9	12.6	41	9.2	3.1	74/26
Humeral diaphysis	62	0.9	12	59.5	46.8	22.6	47/53
Proximal tibia	59	0.8	11.4	54.5	30.5	11.9	52/48
Distal humerus	56	0.8	10.8	56.4	50	25	43/57
Forearm diaphysis	55	0.8	10.6	48	27.3	16.4	69/31
Patella	49	0.7	9.5	64.8	55.1	28.6	41/59
Scapula	37	0.5	7.1	54.8	32.4	16.2	76/24
Fibula	41	0.5	7.9	46.8	14.6	2.4	46/54
Distal femur	36	0.5	7	67.3	52.8	38.9	17/83
Distal tibia	35	0.5	6.8	44.6	22.9	5.7	63/27
Mid-foot	28	0.4	5,4	39.4	7.1	0	61/39
Talus	12	0.2	2.3	30.1	0	0	83/17
All fractures	6,996	100	1,351.7	53.2	34	17.3	47/53

| TABLE 20-3 | The Numbers of Fractures in Younger Patients and in the Elderly. The Odds Ratios for Each Fracture are Given |||||

Fracture	All	15–64	65+	Odds Ratio
Proximal femur	753	70	683	45.36
Pelvis	119	30	89	13.71
Femoral diaphysis	82	27	55	9.41
Proximal humerus	478	211	267	5.86
Patella	49	22	27	5.67
Distal femur	36	17	19	5.16
Distal humerus	56	28	28	4.62
Humeral diaphysis	62	33	29	4.06
Distal radius/ulna	1,221	711	510	3.32
Scapula	37	25	12	2.22
Proximal tibia	59	41	18	2.03
Forearm diaphysis	55	40	15	1.73
Ankle	720	550	170	1.43
Distal tibia	35	27	8	1.37
Clavicle	257	203	54	1.23
Proximal forearm	378	313	65	0.96
Metatarsus	465	386	79	0.95
Fibula	41	35	6	0.79
Finger phalanges	696	602	94	0.72
Calcaneus	65	59	6	0.47
Tibial diaphysis	69	63	6	0.44
Metacarpus	781	717	64	0.41
Carpus	194	179	15	0.39
Mid-foot	28	26	2	0.36
Toe phalanges	248	238	10	0.19
Talus	12	12	0	0
All fractures	6,996	4,665	2,331	2.34

services. Not only are the absolute numbers in the elderly age group increasing but also it would seem that the fracture incidence is also increasing. If the incidence of fractures continues to increase at the same rate, by 2050, the incidence of fractures in the elderly will be $4,079/10^5$/year which is double that observed in the year 2000. This, combined with the increasing elderly population at risk, will result in a considerable change in the delivery of orthopedic trauma services, where the majority of the workload will involve fragility fractures in frail patients.

Fracture epidemiology varies widely according to the demographics, socioeconomic status, and health and safety standards in a particular country. However, data from Scotland should be representative of the fracture incidence of the Western world.[93] Figures from both Europe and America affirm the increasing rate of fragility fractures.

In developed and developing countries the incidence of osteoporosis is increasing at a rate faster than would be predicted simply by the increasing longevity of the population.[109] The increasing rate of osteoporosis may be one aspect of the increasing rate of fragility fractures we have observed in Scotland. Osteoporosis is a metabolic bone disease leading to microarchitectural deterioration, which results in bone fragility and increased fracture risk.[42] The estimated prevalence of osteoporosis in Europe varies; in Denmark approximately 20% of men and 40% of women aged 50 years or more have osteoporosis,[175] whereas in southern European countries such as Spain, the prevalence is lower but still significant, the condition affecting one in four Spanish women who are at least 50 years of age.[55] Over two million people are affected by osteoporosis in Australia,[160] with 1 in 10 men and 1 in 4 women aged over 60 years being diagnosed with osteoporosis.[138] In China, osteoporosis affects almost 70 million people over the age of 50 years, whereas, in India, bone mineral density at all the skeletal sites showed a high prevalence of osteopenia (52%) and osteoporosis (29%).[162] The prevalence of osteoporosis in the Japanese female population aged 50 to 79 years has been estimated to be about 35% in the spine and 9.5% in the hip.[86] This considerable global rate of osteoporosis, which seems to be accelerating, may explain the increasing incidence of fractures we have observed in our elderly population over the last decade. This makes elderly fractures one of the most important groups to understand as this growing group of patients will constitute more of the orthopedic trauma workload of the future.

Epidemiology of Elderly Fractures

More than a third of all fractures presenting to orthopedic trauma services are sustained by elderly patients, of which half occur in the super-elderly age group. It is not surprising that more than half of proximal femoral and proximal humeral fractures occur in elderly patients (Table 20-2), as these are generally accepted as fragility fractures of the elderly. However, it is interesting to note that Table 20-2 shows that more than half of pelvic, distal femoral, and femoral diaphyseal fractures occur in this elderly group. These fractures may not be as readily accepted as fragility fractures by all surgeons. Each of these fractures, except femoral diaphyseal fractures, are associated with an approximate 70/30 female to male ratio, which is likely to be caused by the effect of osteoporosis in this elderly population. In contrast, femoral diaphyseal fractures demonstrate a 50/50 female to male ratio. This difference may be due to the fracture distribution curve which formerly demonstrated a type A curve, this being a unimodal distribution in younger males and older females. However it is likely that the distribution curve is now a type G curve (see Chapter 3).

The definition of what constitutes a fragility fracture lies in the pattern of presentation and relates to age and the low-energy mechanism of injury. It is discussed further in Chapters 3 and 19. However, if we accept that these are fractures that are more likely to occur in the elderly population, then more than half of all fractures are fragility fractures (Table 20-3). Overall, the elderly population is more likely to sustain a fracture relative to the population aged between 15 and 64 years of age (odds ratio 2.3). Fractures of the femur, humerus, pelvis, patella, and distal radius were all at least three times more likely to occur in the elderly age group (Table 20-3). Interestingly, fractures affecting the scapula, proximal tibia, forearm diaphysis, ankle, distal tibia, and clavicle were also more likely to occur in the elderly age group; however, the risk was not as great as the fractures mentioned above. In contrast, fractures less likely to occur in the elderly were those involving the foot and the hand. This difference probably relates to the mechanism by which these fractures are sustained. Younger patients are more likely to sustain their fracture by a fall from height, a direct blow, sport, or a motor vehicle accident which are the typical mechanisms by which foot and hand fractures occur. These fractures are less likely, even in the presence of osteoporosis, to occur after a simple fall from standing height.

The incidence of proximal femoral fractures in the elderly (≥65 years) is 679/10^5/year (Table 20-4). If the elderly population of the United States continues to increase as predicted and reach an estimated 71 million in 2030 this would double the number of proximal femoral fractures presenting to orthopedic trauma services resulting in half a million hip fractures per year.[129] Similar figures would also be observed for fractures of the distal radius and proximal humerus, with 360,000 and 190,000 presenting to orthopedic services in the United States alone. This will have considerable repercussions upon trauma services and the management of these frail patients. Currently proximal humeral fractures are the sixth most common fracture in the population. However, the overall incidence will increase because of the growing elderly population who are more likely to sustain a proximal humerus fracture.

Table 20-5 shows the modes of injury that caused fractures in the 2010/11 study. The commonest mode of injury for all ages is falls from a standing height and almost 40% of fractures

TABLE 20-4	The Prevalence and Incidence of Each Fracture Type in the Younger-Elderly and the Super-Elderly Groups					
	≥65 yrs			≥80 yrs		
	Number	%	Incidence (x/10⁵/year)	Number	%	Incidence (x/10⁵/year)
Ankle	170	7.3	169	43	3.7	147.8
Calcaneus	6	0.3	6	2	0.2	6.9
Carpus	15	0.6	14.9	3	0.3	10.3
Clavicle	54	2.3	53.7	25	2.1	85.9
Distal femur	19	0.8	18.9	14	1.2	48.1
Distal humerus	28	1.2	27.8	14	1.2	48.1
Distal radius/ulna	510	21.9	507.1	221	18.8	759.6
Distal tibia	8	0.3	8	2	0.2	6.9
Femoral diaphysis	55	2.4	54.7	32	2.7	110
Fibula	6	0.3	6	1	0.1	3.4
Finger phalanges	94	4	93.5	39	3.3	134
Forearm diaphysis	15	0.6	14.9	9	0.8	30.9
Humeral diaphysis	29	1.2	28.8	14	1.2	48.1
Metacarpus	64	2.7	63.6	24	2	82.5
Metatarsus	79	3.4	78.6	24	2	82.5
Mid-foot	2	0.1	2	0	0	0
Patella	27	1.2	26.8	14	1.2	48.1
Pelvis	89	3.8	88.5	70	5.9	240.6
Proximal femur	683	29.3	679.2	479	40.7	1,646.3
Proximal forearm	65	2.8	64.6	22	1.9	75.6
Proximal humerus	267	11.5	265.5	111	9.4	381.5
Proximal tibia	18	0.8	17.9	7	0.6	24.1
Scapula	12	0.5	11.9	6	0.5	20.6
Talus	0	0	0	0	0	0
Tibial diaphysis	6	0.3	6	0	0	0
Toe phalanges	10	0.4	9.9	1	0.1	3.4
Total	2,331	100	2,318	1,177	100	4,045.2

TABLE 20-5 Epidemiology of the Different Modes of Injury

| | % | Average Age (yrs) | | | ≥65 yrs | ≥80 yrs | Male/Female |
		All	Males	Females			
Falls (standing height)	62.5	62.3	54.3	65.7	38.9	20.6	30/70
Falls (stairs/low height)	4.2	51.7	48.2	55.2	27.1	10.8	51/49
Falls (height)	2.3	36	37.5	30	8.1	2.5	88/12
Direct blow/assault/crush	13.6	33.3	31.1	40.1	3.6	1	75/25
Sport	11.1	31.3	30.4	35.5	3	0.3	82/18
Motor vehicle accident	5.2	42.6	41.7	45.8	10.2	3	78/22
Pathologic	0.4	67.3	63.5	70.3	60	24	44/56
Stress/Spontaneous	0.3	49.9	44.5	54	21.4	21.4	43/57

The prevalence and gender ratios are shown. The average ages and prevalence of patients ≥65 years and ≥80 years are also shown. Low falls include falls down stairs and slopes. Direct blows/assaults include crush injuries.

TABLE 20-6 Epidemiology of Fractures in Males Aged ≥65 Years

Males ≥65 yrs	Number	%	Multiple Fractures (%)	Open (%)	Causes
Proximal femur	180	32.7	3.9	0	92.2% falls, 3.9% low fall
Proximal humerus	59	10.7	13.6	0	94.9% falls, 1.7% low fall
Distal radius/ulna	54	9.8	9.3	0	94.4% falls, 3.7% MVA
Ankle	47	8.5	4.3	0	83% falls, 6.4% sport
Finger phalanges	35	6.4	13.8	3.1	59.4% falls, 18.7% db/assault
Metacarpus	25	4.5	41.2	0	72% falls, 12% sport
Pelvis	20	3.6	10	0	90% falls, 10% MVA
Femoral diaphysis	20	3.6	5	0	80% falls, 15% pathologic
Clavicle	19	3.5	10.5	0	63.2% falls, 10.5% MVA
Proximal forearm	15	2.7	20	0	80% falls, 6.6% MVA
Metatarsus	11	2	18.2	0	63.6% falls, 18.2% db/assault
Humeral diaphysis	9	1.6	11.1	0	100% falls
Proximal tibia	8	1.5	37.5	12.5	50% falls, 12.5% fall height
Distal humerus	7	1.3	28.6	0	71.4% falls, 14.3% fall height
Carpus	6	1.1	0	0	100% falls
Patella	6	1.1	0	0	83.3% falls, 16.6% low fall
Scapula	5	0.9	20	0	40% falls, 20% fall height
Toe phalanges	5	0.9	0	0	80% db/assault, 20% falls
Tibial diaphysis	5	0.9	20	40	60% falls, 40% MVA
Forearm diaphysis	4	0.7	0	0	75% falls, 25% sport
Fibula	3	0.5	0	0	33.3% fall, 33.3% db/assault
Distal femur	3	0.5	0	0	100% falls
Calcaneus	2	0.4	50	0	50% fall height, 50% low fall
Distal tibia	2	0.4	0	0	100% falls
Mid-foot	0	0	0	0	
Talus	0	0	0	0	
	550	100	5.7	0.7	83.8% falls, 4% MVA

The numbers and prevalence of the different fractures are shown as are the prevalence of open fractures and patients with multiple fractures. The two commonest causes of each fracture are shown. (db = direct blow).

that followed a standing fall occurred in patients ≥65 years. If one simply examines the elderly age group between 65 and 79 years, 91.2% of all fractures followed a standing fall. Falls from a standing height were more common in females, whereas all other modes of injury were equally distributed between the genders or were male-predominant. There is marked difference in the fracture incidence between males and females in the elderly. The incidence of fractures in elderly males is 1,301/10^5/year, and in females is 3,055/10^5/year. Hence, female gender is associated with an increased risk of fracture in this elderly age group (odds ratio 2.4, $p < 0.001$).

Despite the marked difference in fracture incidence between elderly males and females, the prevalence of each fracture according to anatomical location is similar. Tables 20-6 and 20-7 show the incidence of fractures in males (Table 20-6) and females (Table 20-7) aged ≥65 years. Approximately 30% of

fractures in both males and females involve the proximal femur and 10% of fractures involve the proximal humerus. However, fractures involving the distal radius were less prevalent in males, accounting for 10% of fractures, compared with about 25% in females. The reason for this difference is not clear. The rate of multiple fractures varied with the anatomical site of the fracture but the overall incidence was about 5%. Fractures of the proximal humerus were associated with other fractures in about 10% of patients. The rate of open fractures was low, but was greater in elderly females (Tables 20-6 and 20-7).

Epidemiology of Super-Elderly Fractures

Knowledge and understanding of the fracture epidemiology of the super-elderly age group forms an important aspect of what the future may hold for orthopedic trauma services. The super-elderly population, comprising patients over the age of

TABLE 20-7 Epidemiology of Fractures in Females Aged ≥65 Years

Females ≥65 yrs	Number	%	Multiple Fractures (%)	Open (%)	Causes
Proximal femur	503	28.2	6.2	0	96.8% falls, 1.8% low fall
Distal radius/ulna	456	25.6	7.1	1.5	95.6% falls, 2.9% low fall
Proximal humerus	208	11.7	9.2	0	93.8% falls, 5.3% low fall
Ankle	123	6.9	5.7	2.4	95.1% falls, 2.4% low fall
Pelvis	69	3.9	8.7	0	97.1% falls, 2.9% low fall
Metatarsus	68	3.8	20	0	91.2% falls, 4.4% low fall
Finger phalanges	59	3.3	18	3.6	72.9% falls, 15.3% db/assault
Proximal forearm	50	2.8	16	4	94% falls, 4% MVA
Metacarpus	39	2.2	17.6	2.6	92.3% falls, 2.4% low fall
Clavicle	35	2	5.7	0	91.4% falls, 5.7% MVA
Femoral diaphysis	35	2	2.9	0	88.6% falls, 5.7% pathologic
Distal humerus	21	1.2	14.3	0	100% falls
Patella	21	1.2	0	4.8	95.2% falls, 4.8% db/assault
Humeral diaphysis	20	1.1	0	5	85% falls, 10% pathologic
Distal femur	16	0.9	12.5	6.2	81.2% falls, 12.5% low fall
Forearm diaphysis	11	0.6	9.1	0	90.9% falls, 9.1% pathologic
Proximal tibia	10	0.6	20	0	70% falls, 20% low fall
Carpus	9	0.5	11.1	0	88.9% falls, 11.1% db/assault
Scapula	7	0.4	14.3	0	100% falls
Distal tibia	6	0.3	0	0	83.3% falls, 16.6% low fall
Toe phalanges	5	0.3	0	0	80% falls, 20% db/assault
Calcaneus	4	0.2	25	0	100% falls
Fibula	3	0.2	63.3	0	66.6% falls, 33.3% MVA
Mid-foot	2	0.1	0	0	50% fall height, 50% sport
Tibial Diaphysis	1	0.06	0	100	100% falls
Talus	0	0	0	0	
	1,781	100	5	1.2	94.3% falls, 2.9% low fall

The numbers and prevalence of the different fractures are shown as are the prevalence of open fractures and patients with multiple fractures. The two commonest causes of each fracture are shown. (db = direct blow).

80 years, has doubled during the last 25 years and will probably double again in the next 25 years.[181] Approximately half of all fragility fractures occur in this super-elderly subgroup although they constitute only 29% of the elderly population. More than half of all proximal femur and pelvic fractures, and approximately a quarter of all humeral fractures, occur in the super-elderly age group (Table 20-2). Interestingly, 40% of femoral diaphyseal and distal femoral fractures occur in this age group, these being fractures that are traditionally associated with high-energy trauma.

The fracture risk is significantly increased for elderly patients relative to those aged between 15 and 64 years of age (Table 20-3). However, the risk of a super-elderly patient sustaining a fracture is also greater relative to the younger-elderly population. A comparison of the numbers of the different fractures presenting in the younger-elderly and the super-elderly populations is shown in Table 20-8 which shows that fractures of the pelvis, distal femur, proximal femur, forearm diaphysis, and femoral diaphysis are at least three times more common in the super-elderly group. It also shows that hand and foot fractures are less common in the super-elderly. Super-elderly patients are nearly three times more likely to sustain a fracture compared with younger-elderly patients (odds ratio 2.6, $p < 0.001$). Table 20-4 gives the prevalences and incidences of each fracture in the younger-elderly and super-elderly groups in 2010/11. The overall incidence of fractures in the super-elderly was 4,045/10⁵/year, which is nearly double that observed for the younger-elderly patients which was 2,318/10⁵/year. Fractures involving the proximal femur, distal radius, and proximal humerus have the greatest incidence in the super-elderly population (Table 20-4). This is also true of the younger-elderly population. However, the incidence for these fractures is significantly greater with increasing age. This is particularly obvious in proximal femoral fractures where the overall incidence is 145/10⁵/year. This increases to 679/10⁵/year in the younger-elderly population and increases further to 1,646/10⁵/year in the super-elderly population. Fractures of the femur, humerus, pelvis, patella, distal radius, scapula, proximal tibia, forearm diaphysis, and clavicle are all more likely to occur in the super-elderly age group relative to the younger-elderly group (Table 20-4). This confirms that a number of these fractures should be regarded as fragility fractures (see Table 3-19) and also suggests that other fractures, which are not currently regarded as fragility fractures, may be so regarded in the future. However, the increased risk of ankle and distal tibial fractures in the elderly group, was not demonstrated in the super-elderly group. The reason for this is not clear but it may be related to the mechanism of the fall in older patients.

The commonest mode of injury for all ages is falls from standing height (Table 20-5). The prevalence of simple fall-related fractures in the elderly age group was 91.2%; however, this increased to 94.3% in the super-elderly. The super-elderly age group was significantly more likely to sustain fractures from a fall compared with both the adult population, aged between 15 and 64 years of age (odds ratio 2.4, $p < 0.001$), and the younger-elderly population, aged between 65 and 79 years of age (odds ratio 1.2, $p = 0.02$).

TABLE 20-8 The Numbers of Fractures in Younger-Elderly Patients and in the Super-Elderly. The Odds Ratios for Each Fracture are Given

Fracture	65+ yrs	65–79 yrs	80+ yrs	Odds Ratio
Pelvis	89	19	70	9.07
Distal femur	19	5	14	6.88
Proximal femur	683	204	479	5.85
Forearm diaphysis	15	6	9	3.69
Femoral diaphysis	55	23	32	3.42
Patella	27	13	14	2.65
Distal humerus	28	14	14	2.46
Scapula	12	6	6	2.46
Humeral diaphysis	29	15	14	2.29
Clavicle	54	29	25	2.12
Distal radius/ulna	510	289	221	1.89
Proximal humerus	267	156	111	1.75
Finger phalanges	94	55	39	1.74
Proximal tibia	18	11	7	1.56
Metacarpus	64	40	24	1.47
Proximal forearm	65	43	22	1.26
Calcaneus	6	4	2	1.23
Metatarsus	79	55	24	1.07
Ankle	170	127	43	0.83
Distal tibia	8	6	2	0.82
Carpus	15	12	3	0.61
Fibula	6	5	1	0.49
Toe phalanges	10	9	1	0.27
Talus	0	0	0	0
Mid-foot	2	2	0	0
Tibial diaphysis	6	6	0	0
Total	2,331	1,154	1,177	2.57

There is a marked difference in the fracture incidence between males and females in the super-elderly group. The incidence of fractures in super-elderly males is 2,880/10⁵/year, and in females is 4,870/10⁵/year (odds ratio 1.7, $p < 0.001$). This would imply that super-elderly females, like their elderly counterparts, are twice as likely to sustain a fracture after a fall from standing height when compared with males if we assume the rate of falls is equal.

Tables 20-9 and 20-10 show the epidemiology of fractures in super-elderly males and females in 2010/11. Despite the gender difference in fracture incidence, the prevalence of a number of fractures is very similar. For example, approximately 40% of fractures involve the proximal femur and 10% involve the proximal humerus. However, fractures involving the distal radius

TABLE 20-9 Epidemiology of Fractures in Males Aged ≥80 Years

Males 80+ yrs	Number	%	Multiple Fractures (%)	Open (%)	Causes
Proximal femur	112	44.4	4.5	0	92.8% falls, 4.5% fall height
Proximal humerus	25	9.9	24	0	100% falls
Distal radius/ulna	18	7.1	16.7	0	94.4% falls, 5.6% MVA
Pelvis	13	5.2	0	0	100% falls
Finger phalanges	13	5.2	30	0	84.6% falls, 15.4% MVA
Femoral diaphysis	12	4.8	0	0	91.7% falls, 8.3% pathologic
Metacarpus	11	4.4	25	0	72.7% falls, 18.2% fall height
Ankle	10	4	0	0	90% falls, 10% MVA
Clavicle	6	2.4	0	0	83.3% falls, 16.6% low fall
Humeral diaphysis	6	2.4	16.6	0	100% falls
Proximal forearm	5	2	40	0	100% falls
Distal humerus	4	1.6	25	0	50% falls, 25% fall height
Metatarsus	3	1.2	0	0	77.7% falls, 18.2% fall height
Patella	3	1.2	0	0	100% falls
Distal femur	3	1.2	0	0	100% falls
Forearm diaphysis	3	1.2	0	0	66.6% falls, 33.3% sport
Proximal tibia	3	1.2	33.3	0	66.6% falls, 33.3% fall height
Carpus	1	0.4	0	0	100% falls
Toe phalanges	1	0.4	0	0	100% db/assault
Scapula	0	0	0	0	
Distal tibia	0	0	0	0	
Calcaneus	0	0	0	0	
Fibula	0	0	0	0	
Mid-foot	0	0	0	0	
Tibial diaphysis	0	0	0	0	
Talus	0	0	0	0	
	252	100	5.8	0	90.5% falls, 2.4% low fall

The numbers and prevalence of the different fractures are shown as are the prevalence of open fractures and patients with multiple fractures. The two commonest causes of each fracture are shown. (db = direct blow).

demonstrated a similar pattern to that observed in the elderly group (Tables 20-6 and 20-7). They only accounted for 7% of fractures in super-elderly males compared with 22% of fractures in super-elderly females. The prevalences of pelvic fractures were very similar but it is interesting to observe that there was a higher prevalence of femoral diaphyseal fractures in super-elderly males. The rate of multiple fractures varied according to the fracture site for both genders. The overall rate of multiple fractures was 5%, but this varied between fracture types. One in ten patients who sustained a proximal humerus or distal radius fracture had an associated fracture.

Pattern of Changing Fracture Incidence in the Elderly

We have already documented that the overall incidence of all adult fractures increased during the last decade, from 1,113/10^5/year in 2000 to 1,352/10^5/year in 2010/11 (odds ratio 1.2, $p < 0.0001$). This is shown diagrammatically in Figure 20-1 with the comparative figures for 2000 and 2010/11 being shown in Table 20-11. Table 20-11 shows that this was because of a significant increase in elderly fractures. Fractures affecting the proximal femur, distal radius, proximal humerus, ankle, and pelvis are the most common fractures of the elderly and their changing incidence will be examined in more detail.

The changing incidence of proximal femoral fractures between 2000 and 2010/11 is shown in Table 20-12. The overall incidence of proximal femoral fractures in the year 2000 was 129/10^5/year. This increased to 146/10^5/year in the 2010/11 study (odds ratio 1.1, $p = 0.33$). This increase in the incidence of proximal femoral fractures was not observed across all age groups There was an increase from 77/10^5/year in 2000 to 101/10^5/year in 2010/11 for

TABLE 20-10 Epidemiology of Fractures in Females Aged ≥80 Years

Females 80+ yrs	Number	%	Multiple Fractures (%)	Open (%)	Causes
Proximal femur	367	39.7	5.4	0	97% falls, 1.9% low fall
Distal radius/ulna	203	21.9	10.5	1	98.5% falls, 1.5% low fall
Proximal humerus	86	9.3	12.8	0	96.5% falls, 3.5% low falls
Pelvis	57	6.2	8.8	0	96.5% falls, 3.5% low falls
Ankle	33	3.6	12.1	6.1	93.9% falls, 3% low falls
Finger phalanges	26	2.8	25	7.7	88.5% falls, 7.7% db/assaults
Metatarsus	21	2.3	36.4	0	76.2% falls, 14.3% MVA
Femoral diaphysis	20	2.2	5	0	95% falls, 5% low fall
Clavicle	19	2.1	5.3	0	94.7% falls, 5.3% MVA
Proximal forearm	17	1.8	11.8	5.9	100% falls
Metacarpus	13	1.4	36.4	0	92.3% falls, 7.7% db/assaults
Patella	11	1.2	0	0	100% falls
Distal femur	11	1.2	9.1	0	90.9% falls, 9.1% low falls
Distal humerus	10	1.1	0	0	100% falls
Humeral diaphysis	8	0.9	0	0	87.5% falls, 12.5% pathologic
Forearm diaphysis	6	0.6	0	0	100% falls
Scapula	6	0.6	16.6	0	100% falls
Proximal tibia	4	0.4	25	0	75% falls, 25% MVA
Carpus	2	0.2	0	0	100% falls
Distal tibia	2	0.2	0	50	100% falls
Calcaneus	2	0.2	0	0	100% falls
Fibula	1	0.1	100	0	100% falls
Toe phalanges	0	0	0	0	
Mid-foot	0	0	0	0	
Tibial diaphysis	0	0	0	0	
Talus	0	0	0	0	
	925	100	5.4	0.9	96.1% falls, 2.1% low fall

The numbers and prevalence of the different fractures are shown as are the prevalence of open fractures and patients with multiple fractures. The two commonest causes of each fracture are shown. (db = direct blow).

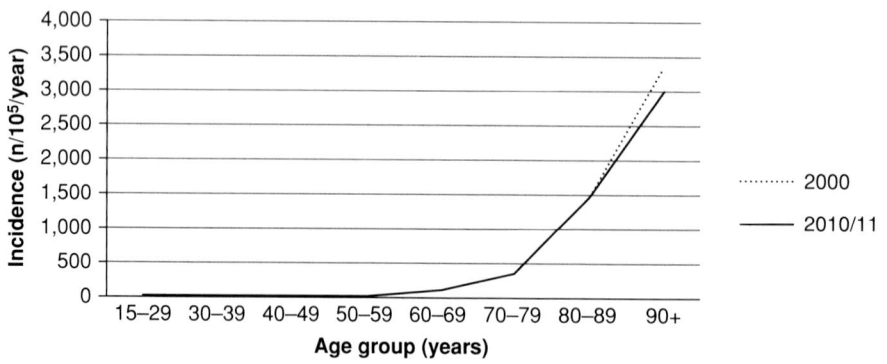

FIGURE 20-1 Fracture incidence, according to age, comparing the year 2000 with 2010/11.

TABLE 20-11 **The Patient Numbers and Fracture Incidences in 2000 and 2010/11. The Odds Ratios and *p* Values are Shown**

	2000		2010/11			
Patients	Number	Incidence	Number	Incidence	Odds Ratio	*p* Value
All	6,562	1,267.9	6,996	1,238.4	0.98	0.55
15–64 yrs	4,606	1,094.7	4,665	1,004.6	0.92	0.051
≥65 yrs	1,963	2,028.2	2,331	2,318	1.15	<0.0001
≥80 yrs	930	3,733.4	1,177	4,045.2	1.09	0.0003

Incidence, x/10⁵/yr.

patients aged between 60 and 69 years (Table 20-12). Otherwise the general trend was similar between these two time points. This is shown diagrammatically in Figure 20-2. However, there was a significant decrease in the incidence of proximal femoral fractures in those patients aged 90 years and older, although the absolute number increased from 132 patients in 2000 to 142 patients in 2010/11. The population in this age group increased in number, hence the decreased incidence.

The changing incidence of distal radial fractures between 2000 and 2010/11 is shown in Table 20-13. The overall incidence of distal radial fractures significantly increased from $195/10^5$/year in the year 2000 to $236/10^5$/year in 2010/11 (odds ratio 1.2, $p = 0.048$). Overall, the general trend was toward an increase in incidence for all age categories. This is shown diagrammatically in Figure 20-3. This increase, however, was more marked, and only became significant, from the age of 40 years (Table 20-13). The greatest increase in incidence was observed in the 40- to 60-year age group which suggests that younger patients are sustaining distal radial fractures. If this is the case and the predominant mode of injury remains a fall

from standing height, then it is possible that the bone quality of the population at risk may be worsening.

The changing incidence of proximal humeral fractures between 2000 and 2010/11 is shown in Table 20-14. The overall incidence of proximal humeral fractures in the year 2000 was $63/10^5$/year. This increased to $92/10^5$/year in 2010/11 (odds ratio 1.5, $p = 0.02$). There was no difference in the incidence in patients below the age of 50 years. After the age of 50 years, there was a significant increased risk of sustaining a fracture of the proximal humerus (Table 20-14). This is shown diagrammatically in Figure 20-4. Excluding those patients over 90 years, the risk seems to accelerate with increasing age.

The changing incidence of ankle fractures between 2000 and 2010/11 is shown in Table 20-15. The overall incidence of ankle fractures has significantly increased over the last decade from $101/10^5$/year in 2000 to $139/10^5$/year in 2010/11 (odds ratio 1.4, $p = 0.02$). A similar pattern to that of distal radial and proximal femoral fractures was observed for the change in incidence of ankle fractures with a trend from increased incidence in younger patients to a significant increase in older

TABLE 20-12 **The Incidence of Proximal Femoral Fractures in Different Age Groups in 2000 and 2010/11. The Odds Ratios, 95% Confidence Limits, and *p* Values are Shown**

Proximal Femoral Fractures

Age Group	Incidence (x/10⁵/year)		Odds Ratio	95% CI	*p* Value
	2000	2010			
15–29	4.5	1.3	0.2	0.02–1.7	0.9
30–39	3	3.1	1	0.2–5	0.9
40–49	10.6	4.2	0.4	0.1–1.1	0.12
50–59	38.5	35.2	0.9	0.6–1.5	0.82
60–69	76.9	100.5	1.3	0.9–1.8	0.08
70–79	380	349.4	0.9	0.8–1.1	0.26
80–89	1,439.9	1,445.3	1	0.9–1.1	0.9
90+	3,353.7	2,994.5	0.9	0.8–0.9	<0.001

TABLE 20-13 **The Incidence of Distal Radial Fractures in Different Age Groups in 2000 and 2010/11. The Odds Ratios, 95% Confidence Limits, and *p* Values are Shown**

Distal Radial Fractures

Age Group	Incidence (x/10⁵/year)		Odds Ratio	95% CI	*p* Value
	2000	2010			
15–29	144.2	155.8	1.1	0.9–1.4	0.49
30–39	85.3	109.9	1.3	0.97–1.7	0.07
40–49	76.8	125.5	1.6	1.2–2.2	0.0006
50–59	149.8	231.5	1.5	1.3–1.9	<0.001
60–69	273.6	339.1	1.2	1.1–1.5	0.009
70–79	500.7	430.6	0.9	0.7–0.97	0.02
80–89	677	788.4	1.2	1.1–1.3	0.003
90+	813	970.1	1.2	1.1–1.3	0.0002

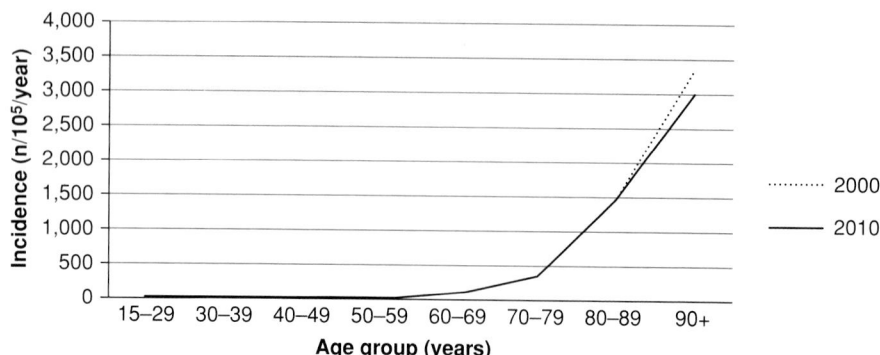

FIGURE 20-2 Incidence of proximal femoral fractures for the year 2000 and 2010/11, according to patient age.

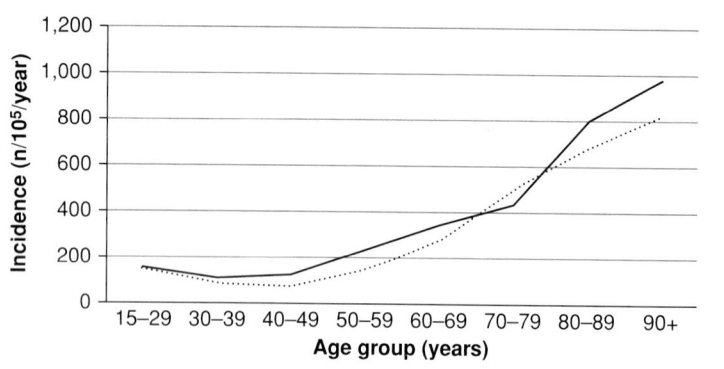

FIGURE 20-3 Incidence of distal radial fractures for the year 2000 and 2010/11, according to patient age.

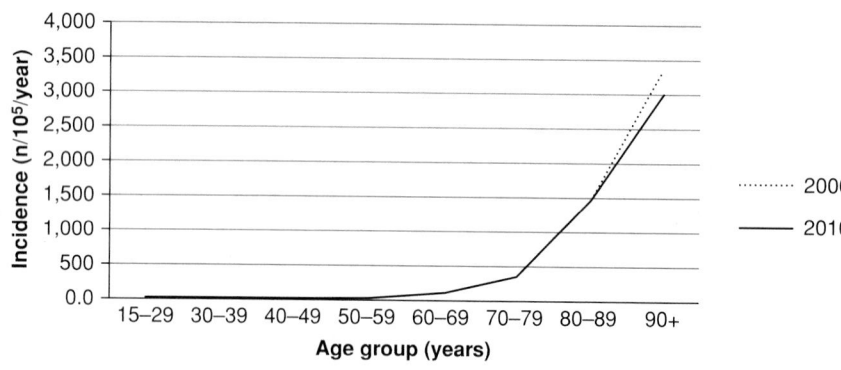

FIGURE 20-4 Incidence of proximal humeral fractures for the year 2000 and 2010/11, according to patient age.

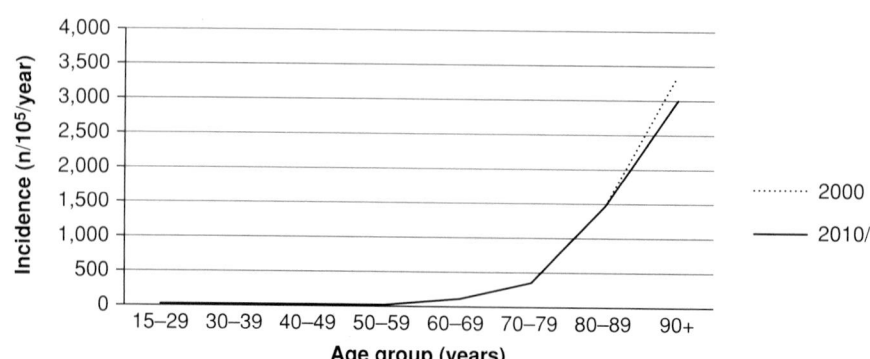

FIGURE 20-5 Incidence of ankle fractures for the year 2000 and 2010/11, according to patient age.

TABLE 20-14 The Incidence of Proximal Humeral Fractures in Different Age Groups in 2000 and 2010/11. The Odds Ratios, 95% Confidence Limits and *p* Values are Shown

Proximal Humeral Fractures

Age Group	Incidence (x/10^5/year) 2000	2010	Odds Ratio	95% CI	*p* Value
15–29	9.7	5.8	0.6	0.2–1.7	0.45
30–39	23.8	21.6	0.9	0.5–1.6	0.76
40–49	37.8	47.1	1.2	0.8–1.9	0.33
50–59	66	93.1	1.4	1.02–1.9	0.03
60–69	118	169.6	1.4	1.1–1.8	0.002
70–79	172.1	225.4	1.3	1.1–1.6	0.008
80–89	271.8	398.3	1.5	1.3–1.7	<0.001
90+	482.7	442.9	0.9	0.8–1.04	0.19

TABLE 20-16 The Incidence of Pelvic Fractures for the Different Age Groups in 2000 and 2010/11. The Odds Ratios, 95% Confidence Limits, and *p* Values are Shown

Pelvic Fractures

Age Group	Incidence (x/10^5/year) 2000	2010	Odds Ratio	95% CI	*p* Value
15–29	3	4.5	1	0.5–1.7	0.9
30–39	4	2.1	0.5	0.1–2.7	0.9
40–49	3.5	4.2	1	0.3–4	0.9
50–59	4.1	10.1	2.5	0.8–8	0.18
60–69	17.9	25.1	1.4	0.8–2.5	0.35
70–79	40.2	24.8	0.6	0.4–1.03	0.08
80–89	157.3	180.7	1.2	0.9–1.4	0.21
90+	228.7	611.6	2.7	2.3–3.1	<0.001

patients (Table 20-15). This is shown diagrammatically in Figure 20-5. The greatest increased incidence of ankle fractures was observed in patients aged 90 years or more.

The changing incidence of pelvic fractures between 2000 and 2010/11 is shown in Table 20-16. The overall incidence of pelvic fractures in 2000 was 17/10^5/year, compared with 23/10^5/year in 2010/11 (odds ratio 1.4, *p* = 0.42). The increase in incidence was only significant in very elderly patients, aged 90 years or older (Table 20-16). This is shown diagrammatically in Figure 20-6. This increase in the incidence in the very elderly suggests that fragility fractures of the pelvis are fractures

of extreme old age, and may explain the decrease in proximal femoral fractures observed for this age group. A simple fall in this age group may cause a pelvic fracture instead of a proximal femoral fracture.

Open Fractures in the Elderly and Super-Elderly

Table 20-17 shows the incidence of open fractures in the different age groups. The data comes from a 15-year study of open fractures and the overall data from the study is shown in Table 3-17 which gives the prevalences of different open fractures in the elderly and super-elderly groups. The overall incidence of open fractures is 30/10^5/year, and the most common fractures involved are the hand, tibia, distal radius, toes, and ankle (Table 20-17). The incidence in younger patients and elderly patients is similar but it rises to 46/10^5/year in the super-elderly aged 80 years or more. The incidence of open fractures associated with finger, metacarpal, and tibial fractures remains relatively constant across all age groups (Table 20-17). However, the reason for the increasing incidence of open fractures with age is because of a significant increase in the incidence of open distal radius and ankle fractures with age. The incidence of open distal radius fractures increases from 1/10^5/year for adults aged between 15 and 64 years of age to 6/10^5/year for elderly patients (odds ratio 4.5, *p* = 0.03), and increases further still to 15/10^5/year for super-elderly patients (odds ratio 7.5, *p* = 0.002). This is also true for open ankle fractures where the incidence increases from 1/10^5/year for adults aged between 15 and 64 years of age to 3/10^5/year for elderly patients, and again increases further still to 5/10^5/year for super-elderly patients (Table 20-17).

Although as a group the incidence of open fractures increases with age, analysis by gender demonstrates that the incidence of open fractures in male patients actually decreases with age whereas the incidence of open fractures in females

TABLE 20-15 The Incidence of Ankle Fractures in Different Age Groups in 2000 and 2010/11. The Odds Ratios, 95% Confidence Limits, and *p* Values are Shown

Ankle Fractures

Age Group	Incidence (x/10^5/year) 2000	2010	Odds Ratio	95% CI	*p* Value
15–29	97.9	113.3	1.2	0.9–1.5	0.33
30–39	79.4	92.4	1.2	0.9–1.6	0.35
40–49	92.2	118.2	1.3	0.97–1.7	0.08
50–59	103.1	159.8	1.6	1.2–2	0.0005
60–69	144.8	186.8	1.3	1.03–1.6	0.02
70–79	105.1	151	1.4	1.1–1.8	0.005
80–89	138.3	176.6	1.3	1.02–1.6	0.02
90+	76.2	147.6	2	1.5–2.7	<0.001

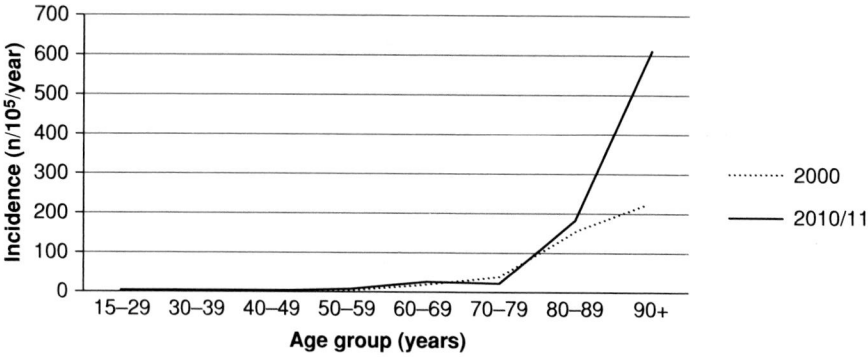

FIGURE 20-6 Incidence of pelvic fractures for the year 2000 and 2010/11, according to patient age.

TABLE 20-17	**The Number and Incidence of Open Fractures in Younger Patients, the Elderly, and the Super-Elderly**					
	15–64 yrs		**65–79 yrs**		**80+ yrs**	
	Number	**Incidence**	**Number**	**Incidence**	**Number**	**Incidence**
Finger phalanges	944	14.9	100	9.3	46	12.2
Tibial diaphysis	219	3.5	30	2.8	18	4.8
Distal radius	60	0.9	68	6.3	56	14.9
Toe phalanges	150	2.4	17	1.6	3	0.8
Ankle	72	1.1	36	3.3	18	4.8
Metacarpus	96	1.5	3	0.3	5	1.3
Proximal ulna	36	0.6	11	1	4	1.1
Metatarsus	42	0.7	5	0.5	2	0.5
Patella	41	0.6	3	0.3	2	0.5
Radius and ulna	35	0.6	6	0.6	3	0.8
Femoral diaphysis	40	0.6	1	0.1	1	0.3
Distal tibia	24	0.4	6	0.6	1	0.3
Proximal tibia	22	0.3	4	0.4	3	0.8
Distal femur	21	0.3	2	0.2	3	0.8
Ulna diaphysis	21	0.3	4	0.4	—	—
Calcaneus	14	0.2	4	0.4	—	—
Distal humerus	12	0.2	4	0.4	2	0.5
Humeral diaphysis	10	0.2	4	0.4	2	0.5
Proximal humerus	9	0.1	2	0.2	—	—
Clavicle	8	0.1	—	—	1	0.3
Pelvis	6	0.1	1	0.1	—	—
Talus	6	0.1	—	—	—	—
Radial diaphysis	4	0.06	1	0.1	—	—
Mid-foot	5	0.08	—	—	—	—
Scapula	2	0.03	—	—	—	—
Proximal radius/ulna	1	0.02	—	—	1	0.3
Proximal femur	1	0.02	—	—	—	—
Carpus	1	0.02	—	—	—	—
Total	1,902	30.1	312	28.9	172	45.7

Incidence, x/10⁵/yr.

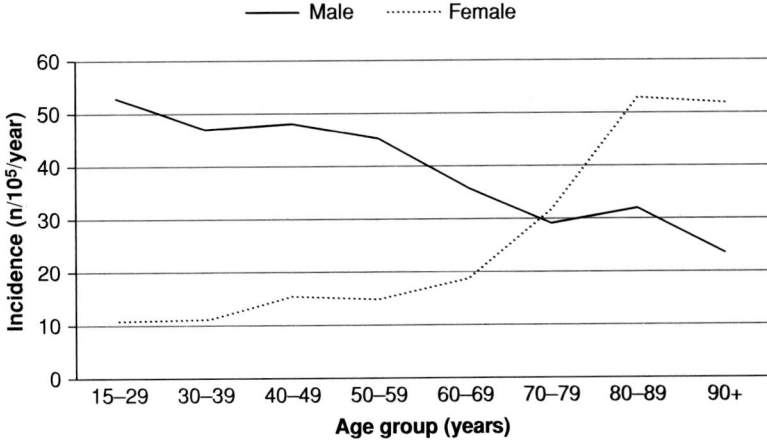

FIGURE 20-7 Incidence of open fractures, according to patient age and gender.

increases with age (Fig. 20-7). The incidence in males peaks in the 15- to 29-year age group and then gradually decreases with age to $24/10^5$/year in patients aged more than 90 years. However, the incidence of open fractures in females is relatively low from 15 to 60 years, at which point the incidence doubles to reach a peak of $52/10^5$/year in the super-elderly patients. This significant difference in the incidence of open fractures by age and gender is related to the increase in open distal radius and ankle fractures (Table 20-17), which are more common in super-elderly females (Tables 20-9 and 20-10). The reason why super-elderly females have a significantly increased risk of sustaining an open fracture (odds ratio 1.7, $p = 0.03$) relative to males is not clear. Assuming the mechanism of these open fractures is similar, with the majority occurring after a fall from standing height, then this suggests that the soft tissues in females may be more vulnerable to trauma.

THE FUTURE EFFECT ON TRAUMA SERVICES

There are few studies analyzing the outcome of all fractures in super-elderly patients.[49] The majority of the literature focuses upon proximal femoral fractures in this age group, as they are acknowledged to have major repercussions for the patient, their family, social services, and health-care services. These patients have an increased age- and gender-adjusted mortality rate when compared with the general population.[80] The outcome deteriorates with increasing age, mortality increases, and the patient is less likely to return to independent living and mobility after the fracture.[84]

The super-elderly account for 17% of all fractures presenting to orthopedic surgeons. However they account for 34% of all acute orthopedic trauma admissions. There are significant case-mix and comorbidity considerations in admissions of the super-elderly. Table 20-18 shows a comparison of the case-mix variables in the elderly and super-elderly patients admitted to the Royal Infirmary of Edinburgh.[36] These patients are less likely (odds ratio 3) to live in their own home and are less likely (odds ratio 4.5) to be independently mobile. Dementia is also significantly more common in the super-elderly group. Excluding hip fractures, the oldest patients are more likely to be admitted to hospital after injury even after upper limb

fractures where the patient may otherwise be ambulant. This reflects their frailty and failure to cope unaided.

Increasing age is associated with a higher rate of mortality after hip fracture.[80] However, a recent study also affirmed that in elderly patients this increased risk extends across all common

TABLE 20-18	Case-Mix Variables in Elderly and Super-Elderly Patients. See Text for Details	
	Age Group	
Case-mix Variables	**Elderly**	**Super-elderly**
Gender		
Male	18% (189)	18.2% (58)
Female	82% (808)	81.8% (260)
Prefracture Residence of Inpatients		
Own home[a]	82.6%	68.8%
Residential care[a]	5.9%	8.6%
Nursing home[a]	11.2%	22.3%
Hospital	0.4%	0.4%
Prefracture Mobility		
No aids[a]	49%	17.6%
One stick	33.7%	38.5%
Two sticks[a]	11.1%	14.6%
Zimmer frame[a]	4.4%	23.9%
Unable to walk[a]	1.8%	5.4%
Comorbidities		
Nil	6.1%	4.1%
One	23%	20.6%
Two	39.5%	40.2%
Three	22.3%	23.7%
Four or more	10.1%	11.4%
Dementia[a]	5.1%	11.6%

[a]This relates to a chi square test – demonstrating significant differences between the groups ($p < 0.01$).

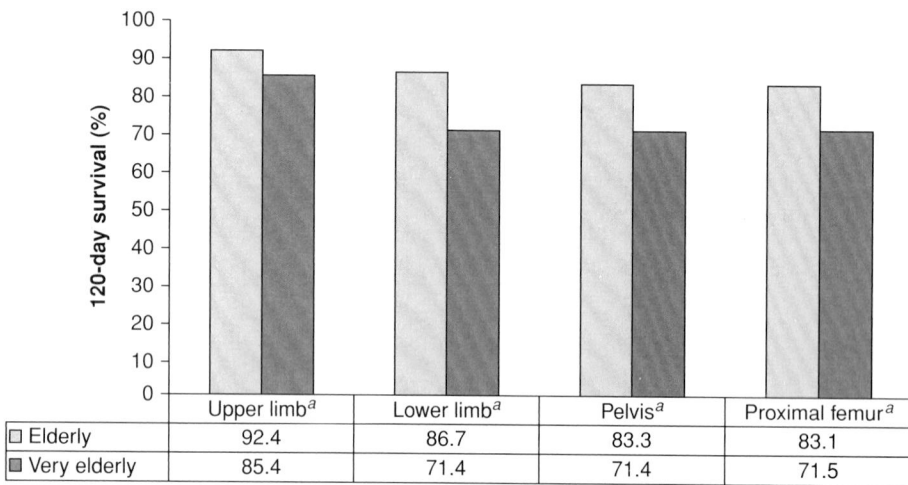

FIGURE 20-8 120-day patient survival for upper and lower limbs, pelvis and proximal femoral fractures for the elderly (80 to 90 years) and very elderly (90 years and older).

[a]Significant difference between the two groups ($p < 0.02$).

fractures. When survival outcome was analyzed, patients in the super-elderly group were less likely to survive 120 days in all fracture subgroups (Fig. 20-8).[36]

Several studies have demonstrated that advancing age is associated with increased length of hospital stay after surgery for the treatment of hip fractures.[88,89] The median length of hospital stay is significantly longer for the super-elderly group when compared with the elderly group.[36] Assuming that the cost of stay per day in an acute ward is similar to that of a fractured hip ($664[119]), then this would result in an increased cost of $6,640 per patient. This will have major implications for future resource allocation and service provision in the face of an aging population.

Those patients admitted from their own home form an important group. The aim of treatment should be to return the patient to independent living. Only 58.4% of the super-elderly patients documented in Table 20-18, who were living independently, returned to their original domicile (Table 20-19). Failure to discharge these patients directly to their domicile may reflect their worsening mobility when compared with elderly patients (Table 20-18), with their fracture finally initiating the need for increased care. It is difficult to analyze the cost implications of future care packages in all fractures in the super-elderly, but this financial burden is well recognized in hip fracture studies.[95,99]

The super-elderly patients are more likely to sustain a proximal femoral or pelvic fracture than a distal radius fracture.[36] This may be because of decreasing cognition with age and diminished protective reflexes.[6,153]

Table 20-20 presents an analysis of the management of elderly and super-elderly patients in Edinburgh, Scotland.[36] It shows that super-elderly patients are more likely to be managed nonoperatively for upper limb fractures. This is particularly true if they had more than two comorbidities or a diagnosis of dementia. This is because of their diminished functional demand, with nearly a third of patients residing in care homes. For those living at home at the time of admission, the rate of operative intervention increased.

Evidence demonstrates that operating on proximal femoral fractures within 48 hours of admission improves patient outcome, with decreased perioperative complication rates and shorter length of stay.[32] It would seem logical to apply this principle to all lower limb fractures requiring surgery in the elderly to aid early rehabilitation. A single study has demonstrated a significantly increased mortality risk for super-elderly patients with lower limb fractures who had delayed surgery (>48 hours).[36] However, this delay may also be because of optimization of the most physically unwell patients who may carry an increased mortality risk.

Due to the complex issues surrounding the inclusive care of these very-elderly patients, a multidisciplinary team approach has been shown to improve 1-year survival in hip fracture patients,[2] and may benefit all elderly patients with a fragility fracture.[72] The acute orthopedic trauma ward may also be a

TABLE 20-19	The Outcome of Elderly and Super-Elderly Patients Admitted to Hospital with a Fracture	
	Age Group	
Outcome	Elderly	Very-elderly
30-day survival for all inpatients		
Alive	94.6%	91.1%
Dead	5.4%	8.9%
120-day survival for all inpatients		
Alive	85.5%	74%
Dead	14.4%	26%
Residence at 120 days if patient lived at home prior to fracture		
Own home	81.3%	58.4%
Residential care	9.3%	15.7%
Nursing home	6.6%	18.9%
Rehabilitation ward	3%	6.5%
Hospital	0%	1.1%

TABLE 20-20 An Analysis of the Requirement for Surgery for Various Upper and Lower Limb Fractures and Pelvic Fractures in the Elderly and Super-Elderly

Fracture Group	Elderly		Super-elderly			
	Patients Number (%)	Surgery (%)	Patients Number (%)	Surgery (%)	Risk of Surgery	p Value
Lower Limb						
Ankle	30 (3)	8 (26.7)	10 (3.1)	3 (30)	OR 1.1	p = 0.6
Distal femur	8 (0.8)	6 (75)	6 (1.9)	5 (83.3)	OR 1.7	p = 0.6
Femoral diaphysis	29 (2.9)	27 (93.1)	12 (3.8)	11 (91.7)	OR 1.2	p = 0.7
Proximal tibia	10 (1)	7 (70)	6 (1.9)	4 (66.7)	OR 1.2	p = 0.7
Total	77	48 (62.3)	34	23 (67.6)	OR 1.3	p = 0.4
Upper Limb						
Distal radius	180 (18.2)	41 (22.8)	35 (11.1)	2 (5.7)	OR 4	p = 0.04
Proximal humerus	110 (11)	11 (10)	34 (10.8)	1 (2.9)	OR 3.4	p = 0.2
Total	290	52	69	3	OR 4.1	p = 0.006
Pelvis	43 (4.3)	0	23 (7.3)	0	OR 1.9	p = 0.6
Proximal femur	421 (42.5)	409 (97.1)	160 (50.6)	149 (93.1)	OR 2.4	p = 0.03

OR, Odds ratio.

suboptimal location to manage such patients who may need an environment that will address their multifaceted needs.

SPECIFIC COMMON FRACTURES IN THE ELDERLY

The management of specific fractures is comprehensively covered within the appropriate chapters of Rockwood and Green. This section offers a review of specific issues relating to super-elderly patients presenting with fragility fractures.

Proximal Femur

Hip fractures account for 12% of all adult fractures presenting to orthopedic trauma surgeons,[48] and are a major cause of morbidity and mortality for elderly patients.[82] Although the reported annual incidence of hip fractures during the last decade has declined,[81,95] the population at risk continues to increase.[147] Hence, these elderly patients will form an increasing proportion of the orthopedic trauma workload in the future. The mean age of patients with proximal femoral fractures is 80 years. The management of proximal femoral fractures is covered in Chapters 49 and 50. However, a question that particularly pertains to the super-elderly patient group is whether undisplaced intracapsular hip fractures should be managed with internal fixation or with an arthroplasty?

Approximately 50% of hip fractures are intracapsular,[83] of which 32% to 38% are undisplaced.[69,70] The conventional management of an undisplaced intracapsular hip fracture is by internal fixation. However, there is a reported revision rate of 12% to 30% at 1 year.[41,117] Recently, Gjertsen et al.[70] demonstrated that the outcome of displaced intracapsular hip fractures managed with a hemiarthroplasty was better than in patients with an undisplaced intracapsular hip fracture managed with

internal fixation. If patients with a high risk of revision surgery could be identified prior to fixation of their undisplaced intracapsular hip fracture, they might benefit from a primary hemiarthroplasty or potentially a total hip replacement.[104] Conn and Parker[41] identified age, mobility, and the lateral Garden angle to be risk factors for nonunion after fixation of undisplaced intracapsular hip fractures.

The 1-year mortality after a hip fracture is approximately 30%.[179] Independent patients surviving beyond this time may benefit from a total hip replacement when compared with a hemiarthroplasty.[12,27,104] Isolated independent predictors of survival have been identified for both intra- and extracapsular fractures hip fractures.[169,179] Holt et al.[82] specifically identified intracapsular fractures to be associated with a decreased early mortality rate relative to other hip fracture patterns.

Varying survival rates [52,117] have been reported for cannulated screw fixation of undisplaced intracapsular fractured neck of femur, with the largest series in the literature reporting 88% survival.[41] Increasing age has been associated with nonunion of femoral neck fractures,[14,33,41] and hence would result in a lower survivorship rate in the super-elderly cohort. Posterior tilt (anterior angulation) on the lateral radiograph of the hip is an independent predictor of fixation failure (Fig. 20-9). This was identified to be a risk factor by Conn and Parker.[41] The presence of posterior tilt probably relates to comminution of the posterior aspect of the femoral neck. This is associated with an inferior biomechanical construction when using cannulated screws.[53] Those patients with posterior tilt may benefit from the biomechanical advantage of either four screws or a fixed angle device, such as an extramedullary sliding hip screw, which could potentially improve their survival rate.[53,103] Recent evidence, however,

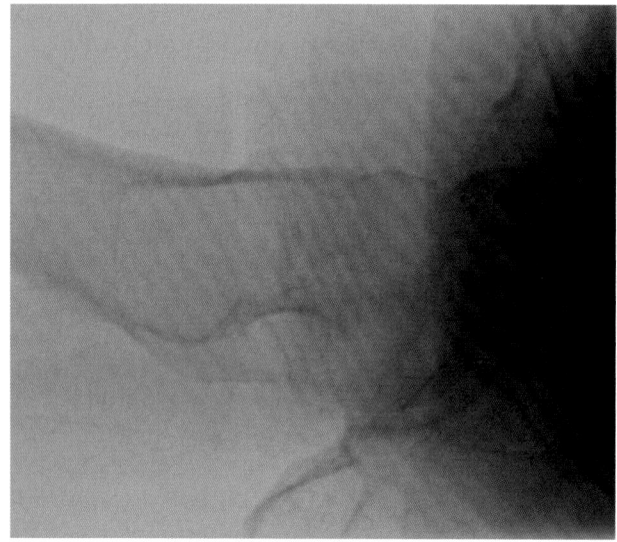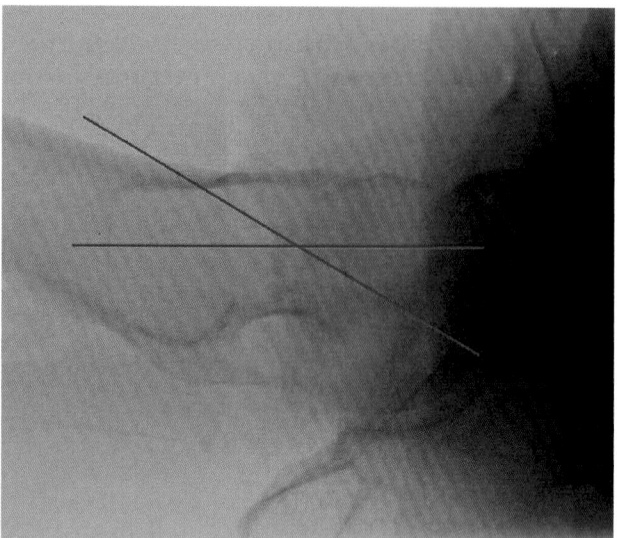

A

B

FIGURE 20-9 Lateral radiograph of the hip demonstrating posterior tilt **(A)** with a Garden lateral angle of 145 degrees **(B)**.

from the Norwegian hip fracture register found patients with displaced intracapsular hip fractures managed with hemiarthroplasty experienced greater patient satisfaction and pain relief and better functional results when compared with patients who had sustained undisplaced intracapsular hip fractures managed with internal fixation.[70] Gjertsen et al.[70] hypothesize that this difference in outcome may relate to the higher re-operation rate associated with internal fixation compared to hemiarthroplasty.

The 1-year unadjusted mortality rate reported after undisplaced femoral neck fractures is approximately 20%,[41] which is about 10% less than other hip fracture patterns.[179] The patient's age and gender have previously been shown to be independent predictors of mortality for hip fracture patients.[82,169] The American Society of Anesthesiologists (ASA) grade was designed to predict perioperative mortality,[11] and has been shown to be an independent predictor of early mortality for hip fracture patients.[82] Patients with a lower ASA grade, predicting longevity, but with risk factors for failure of internal fixation, may benefit from a primary total hip replacement if we apply the rationale that has already been discussed.[104]

The management of super-elderly patients with an undisplaced fractured neck of femur with a high risk of fixation failure is difficult, and randomized controlled trials are required to compare the outcome of the alternative methods of internal fixation and arthroplasty for these patients.

Distal Radius

Fractures of the distal radius account for 16% of all fractures, making it the commonest fracture that presents to orthopedic surgeons.[43] Undisplaced stable fractures can be managed conservatively with the expectation of a good functional outcome.[45,126] However the management of unstable fractures of the distal radius remains controversial.[73] The functional outcome of displaced fractures is generally accepted to correlate with the anatomical reduction of the fracture,[126] although some

authors suggest that this may not be the case.[10] This disparity may be because of the size of the reported cohorts, lack of standardized reporting, and the combination of both intra- and extra-articular fractures within a series. In addition, multiple studies have reported cohorts with a wide age range with one series including patients 18 to 86 years old.[168] Because age has been demonstrated to influence the outcome of distal radial fractures,[164] this may have influenced the outcome of these studies hence the differing functional results observed with and without anatomical restoration.

The effect of a distal radial malunion upon functional outcome has been demonstrated to diminish with increasing age.[56] Most studies reporting the outcome of distal radial fractures in the elderly, being defined as greater than 60 or 65 years of age, include low-demand patients only. The question remains whether malunion results in an inferior outcome in super-elderly patients who have a lower physical demand, because of their advanced age. Furthermore, manipulation and reduction of distal radial fractures has been shown to be of minimal benefit in frail elderly patients.[19]

Colles,[39] some 200 years ago, when describing his fracture, stated that "one consolation only remains, that the limb at some remote period will again enjoy perfect freedom in all its motions, and be completely exempt from pain: the deformity, however, will remain undiminished through life." This statement may not be applicable to all patients, but as functional demand decreases with age it may display a degree of insight into the problem. Even if there is a malunion in the elderly population the associated diminished grip strength and range of movement may not hinder limb function.

There is no association of malunion with poor functional outcome for low-demand patients. Beumer and McQueen[19] questioned whether attempted reduction of displaced distal radial fractures should be attempted in very elderly, frail, dependent, or demented patients after finding that 88.3% lost reduction and went on to malunion. Young and Rayan[182] and Chang et al.[30] showed that malunion did not correlate with poor functional outcome. These studies only included elderly patients with low physical demands. More recently, Grewal and MacDermid[71] included all patients, with no exclusions according to physical demands, and found no difference in the outcome of extra-articular fractures of the distal radius after malunion in patients greater than 65 years old. They did however demonstrate an increased risk of a poor functional outcome in younger patients. They assessed the outcome using the Disabilities of the Arm, Shoulder and Hand (DASH) score. The DASH score is not validated for patients at the extremes of age. To state that a DASH score of 20 points or more is a poor outcome for very elderly patients is difficult to support, as this score may be normal for them. In fact, one study found the mean DASH score to be 22 points for a group of patients with a mean age of 78 years after sustaining a distal radial fracture.[8]

The management of distal radial fractures, the most prevalent fracture of the super-elderly,[36] will form the greatest proportion of the emergency room and orthopedic trauma workload. If a conservative protocol was followed for all distal radial fractures in the super-elderly group in view of the limited disability incurred, a potential risk would be the development of a symptomatic malunion in some patients. A distal radial osteotomy is indicated in fit patients with a symptomatic malunion which interferes with function irrespective of age. Patients generally achieve a good functional outcome, but the rate of metalwork removal varies from 25% to 54% when plates are used to stabilize the osteotomy. However, more recently, the use of a nonbridging external fixator has been described to stabilize the osteotomy, offering a minimally invasive technique and good functional results without the subsequent need to remove internal metalwork.[127]

Proximal Humerus

Fractures of the proximal humerus account for about 7% of all adult fractures presenting to orthopedic surgeons, the prevalence being recorded as 7.3% in the seventh edition of Rockwood and Green[18] and 6.8% in this edition (Table 20-2). It is the third commonest fracture sustained by elderly patients. Proximal humeral fractures have a type F fracture distribution, being unimodal for both older males and females (Table 3-13). Table 20-2 shows that the average age of patients with proximal humeral fractures is about 66 years, hence more than half of these injuries occur in the elderly, and it is regarded as an osteoporotic fracture.[48] Proximal humeral fractures, like those of the proximal femur, are associated with an increased mortality, relative to a standardized population.[163] Modification in the management of proximal humeral fractures may address this excess mortality, as previously demonstrated for proximal femoral fractures.[72]

The incidence of proximal humeral fractures is increasing although the reason for this is not clear.[144] In Sweden, the incidence of proximal humeral fractures in females doubled between 1950 and 1980.[17] Kannus et al.[97] and Palvanen et al.,[144] reporting the epidemiology of proximal humeral fractures from Finland, demonstrated that the incidence in elderly patients tripled from 32/10⁵/year in 1970 to 105/10⁵/year in 2002. The most recent update of this study from Finland, reporting the incidence of proximal humeral fractures in super-elderly female patients, shows results that are nearly identical to the incidence and the rate of change observed in the Scottish super-elderly population. If the incidence of proximal humeral fractures in the super-elderly population continues to increase at the rate predicted by our results and those of Kannus et al.,[97] it will reach 1,000 to 1,600/10⁵/year by 2030. In addition, if this same population also doubles, as it is predicted to do,[141] then we will be managing four times as many proximal humeral fractures in the super-elderly than orthopedic trauma surgeons manage currently.

Proximal humeral fractures are regarded as fragility fractures.[48] The incidence of all fragility fractures in the elderly is increasing, with most occurring as the result of low-energy falls, which usually occurs in the patients' place of domicile.[46,98] Approximately one-third of the elderly population who live at home fall each year. This increases to two-thirds in those who live in residential homes.[125] One in ten of these falls results in a serious injury[172] and a recent Swedish study has suggested that 7% of falls in the elderly result in fracture.[178] It is likely that the incidence of fall-related fractures, including those affecting the proximal humerus, will increase in the future resulting in considerable expense for all healthcare systems. The Center for Disease Control and Protection in the United States has suggested that the cost of falls in 2020 may reach $35 billion.[28]

Fragility fractures are more likely to occur in patients with poor gait, festinant gait or who fall sideways, or are unable to break their fall with an outstretched arm.[105] Allum et al.[6] studied age-dependent balance correction and arm movements for falls in different age groups, and showed that compensatory movements to facilitate protection from falls were less effective with increasing age. Frailer patients are more likely to incur proximal limb girdle fractures because of diminished protective reflexes.[6,153]

The level of social deprivation of patients sustaining proximal humeral fractures has increased. A greater proportion of elderly patients sustaining such fractures suffer an increased level of comorbidity, which is associated with social deprivation,[38,47] and in turn is an independent risk factor for sustaining a proximal humeral fracture.[105] We have observed increasing fracture severity in the last 20 years and this may be, at least partially, due to increasing social deprivation (Table 3-12). Diminishing bone mineral density has been demonstrated to result in more severe fractures of the distal radius[34] and the same may be true for the proximal humerus. The increasing proportion of elderly patients sustaining proximal humeral fractures, in addition to their increased deprivation, with its associated comorbidities, may also have reduced bone mineral density[149] and hence more severe fractures.

The overall unadjusted mortality rate at 1 year is approximately 10%. Shortt and Robinson[163] demonstrated a significantly increased mortality associated with these fractures relative to the standard population in all age groups older than 45 years. The highest 1-year mortality rate that they observed was approximately 30% for patients 85 years or more, this being the same as the unadjusted mortality rate we observed for our super-elderly patients. They did not analyze the standardized mortality by gender, but they did identify male gender as an independent predictor of outcome. Morin et al.[131] more recently demonstrated that both female and male genders suffered a significantly increased standardized mortality rate at 1 year after a "nontraumatic" fracture of the proximal humerus.

It is not clear whether super-elderly patients benefit from operative intervention. Again, the functional demands of this patient population need to be acknowledged. Most studies reporting the outcome of operative intervention, open reduction and internal fixation, and hemiarthroplasty consist of cohorts of a younger mean age than that of the average for proximal humeral fractures. Hence, outcomes reported by these authors may not reflect that of the older low-demand patient. It can be expected that a good functional result will be obtained by nonoperative management for minimally displaced and two-part proximal humeral fractures, which is acknowledged for all age groups. However, for three- and four-part fractures of the proximal humerus the evidence is not as clear for elderly patients.

During the course of the last decade there has been over 60 studies published describing the outcome of proximal humeral fractures fixed using the proximal humeral internal locking system (PHILOS) plate. There has been an exponential rise in the published literature during this time period, from a single study in 2004[20] to 13 in 2012. The claimed advantages of the PHILOS plate are improved screw fixation in osteoporotic bone which facilitates fixation with minimal soft tissue dissection. The plate is precontoured for the proximal humerus, and direct compression of the plate against the bone is not required, which is thought to preserve the blood supply to the bone. The locking screws offer angular as well as axial stability and may reduce the risk of loss of reduction.[66]

Despite the escalation in the use of the PHILOS plate and in publications regarding its outcome the evidence as to whether this device is beneficial to the patients it was designed for remains difficult to decipher. It is not clear in which patients these plates should be used and whether they offer a functional advantage over nonoperative management.

There have been 29 studies, of the 63 cited on PubMed, that have used the Constant score as their outcome assessment tool (Table 20-21). There is, however, marked heterogeneity between these studies, with the mean age ranging from 42 to 78 years old, and the size of the reported cohorts varying from 9 to 294 fractures. The mean age of the patients in those studies reporting the outcome of the PHILOS plate is 62 years old but it should be remembered that while the average age of patients with proximal humeral fractures is 66 years,[97] the average age of patients who present with three- and four-part proximal humeral fractures is 72 years.[98] This suggests that there is an inclusion bias in some studies, which may reserve such an intervention for younger patients. However, this does seem to be at odds with the design and intention of the PHILOS plate.

Furthermore, it is interesting to note the outcome of these studies according to the Constant score. The Constant score has been demonstrated to diminish with age in a normal population.[43] The variation in the reported Constant score after PHILOS plating varies from 58 to 95 (Table 20-21). In part this may reflect the differing mean age between study cohorts. However, even if these scores are adjusted for age, the variation in score ranges from 24 points less than predicted to 21 points greater than predicted (Fig. 20-10). This variation may also be because of the inclusion criteria of the studies, which may reflect that only higher functioning patients were offered surgery. However, it is hard to believe that most patients will regain their prior functional status or even improve relative to their predicted score.

The only randomized controlled trial comparing the outcome of the PHILOS plate ($n = 30$) with conservative management ($n = 29$) for proximal humeral fractures in elderly patients concluded in favor of the PHILOS plate.[142] However, there was no statistical difference in any of the outcome measures assessed, and the three-point difference they found in the Constant score at 2 years (61 vs. 58) is not clinically significant.[43] The authors also demonstrated a re-operation rate of 17% for those plated. The cost and complication risk of operative intervention with a PHILOS plate would seem, with current

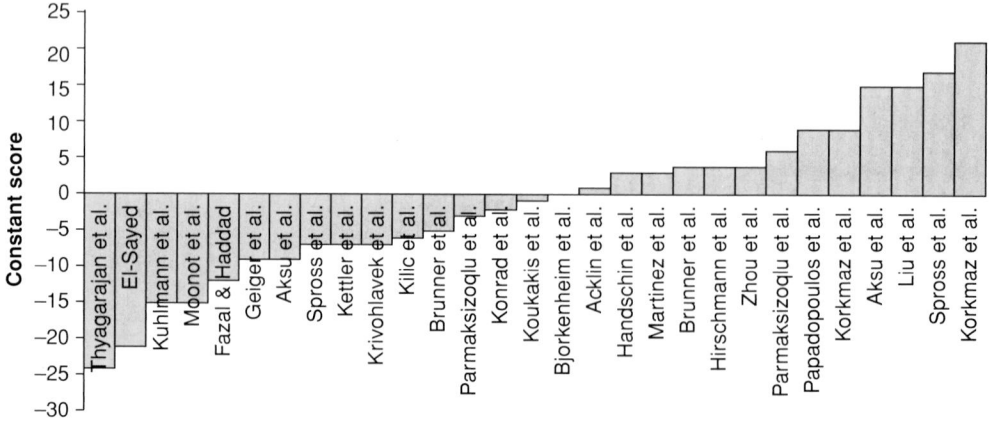

FIGURE 20-10 Difference in the reported Constant score relative to the age-matched score for the 29 identified studies reporting the outcome of the PHILOS plate for proximal humeral fractures (Table 20-21).

| TABLE 20-21 | Studies Reporting the Outcome of Proximal Humeral Fractures Treated with the Philos Plate | | | | | |

Author	Year	Number	Age (yrs)	Constant Score Reported	Constant Score Predicted*	Constant Score Difference
Brunner et al.[24]	2012	16	61	81	77	4
Zhao et al.[183]	2012	74	57	86	82	4
Aksu et al.[5]	2012	9	75	87	72	15
Spross et al.[166]	2012	294	73	89	72	17
Acklin and Sommer[1]	2012	29	64	78	77	1
Kuhlmann et al.[116]	2012	30	69	62	77	−15
Spross et al.[165]	2012	44	75	65	72	−7
Konrad et al.[110]	2012	153	65	75	77	−2
El-Sayed[61]	2010	59	42	65	86	−21
Hirschmann et al.[78]	2011	57	65	81	77	4
Parmaksizoğlu et al.[148]	2010	12	56	88	82	6
Parmaksizoğlu et al.[148]	2010	19	67	74	77	−3
Aksu et al.[4]	2010	103	62	68	77	−9
Thyagarajan et al.[171]	2009	30	58	58	82	−24
Geiger et al.[67]	2010	28	61	68	77	−9
Liu et al.[121]	2010	17	71	87	72	15
Papadopoulos et al.[145]	2009	29	62	86	77	9
Brunner et al.[25]	2009	158	65	72	77	−5
Fazal and Haddad[63]	2009	27	56	70	82	−12
Martinez et al.[124]	2009	58	61	80	77	3
Kilic et al.[107]	2008	22	57	76	82	−6
Krivohlavek et al.[115]	2008	49	57	75	82	−7
Korkmaz et al.[111]	2008	24	47	95	86	9
Korkmaz et al.[111]	2008	17	78	93	72	21
Handschin et al.[74]	2008	31	62	80	77	3
Moonot et al.[130]	2007	32	60	67	82	−15
Kettler et al.[106]	2006	225	66	70	77	−7
Koukakis et al.[112]	2006	20	62	76	77	−1
Bjorkenheim et al.[20]	2004	72	67	77	77	0

aPredicted Constant score according to the age of the reported cohort.
From Constant CR, Gerber C, Emery RJ, et al. A review of the Constant score: Modifications and guidelines for its use. *J Shoulder Elbow Surg.* 2008;17:355–361.

evidence, to be of no significant benefit to the elderly patients for whom this plate was designed.

In contrast to the fixation versus conservative management randomized control trial described above, the same study group performed another randomized controlled trial comparing non-operative with hemiarthroplasty for four-part proximal humeral fractures in the elderly (>57 years with a mean of 77 years). They demonstrated a significant functional improvement according to the EQ-5D questionnaire in the operative group but no difference in the DASH score, Constant score, pain, or range of movement. Whether these results translates to the super-elderly

remains unknown, but future studies should acknowledge this age group and analyze whether there is a diminishing improvement offered by operative intervention for proximal humeral fractures in these low-demand patients.

Pelvic Fractures

Although the predominant fracture of the super-elderly involves the proximal femur, 73% of all pelvic fractures occur in this age group.[48] Currently pelvic fractures are three times less common than proximal femoral fractures.[128] However, a recent epidemiologic study from Europe demonstrated a three-fold increase of pelvic fractures in the elderly from 1970 to 1997.[96] The predominant pelvic fracture in the elderly is that of the pubic rami,[46] which is associated with considerable morbidity and mortality.[23,77,113,132,173] The changing epidemiology of the elderly may have major repercussions on the trauma workload in the future, placing a major burden on medical resources both acutely and for the ongoing care of these frail patients after discharge.[92,113,132,154] The majority of what modest literature exists, regarding pelvic injuries in the elderly, focuses on pubic rami fractures.[23,77,113,114,173]

The average length of stay on an acute trauma ward for an elderly hip fracture patient is 23 days,[119] which is the same as elderly patients sustaining pelvic fractures other than those of the pubic rami. The length of stay of patients with pubic rami fractures ranges from 9 to 14 days, although the studies reporting these figures included all ages in their analysis.[77,113] Super-elderly patients have a significantly longer length of hospital stay relative to their elderly counterparts and the same can be assumed for pubic rami fractures.[36] Furthermore, a recent study demonstrated that the average length of stay was 45 days for elderly patients sustaining either combined pubic rami fractures or a sacral fracture,[7] which is a considerably longer length of stay than observed for isolated pubic rami fractures.

Koval et al.[113] demonstrated that three or more comorbidities increased the length of stay, and Hill et al.[77] found younger age to be a predictor of discharge to the patient's original domicile. In addition, the place of residence, level of mobility, and socioeconomic status are also isolated independent predictors of length of stay and discharge destination for patients sustaining a pubic rami fracture. These predictors could be used to identify patients who may have a longer-than-average stay or need an increased care package on discharge.

The 1-year mortality rate of super-elderly patients sustaining a pubic rami fracture is 22%,[36] which is greater than previous studies have observed.[77,113] This is clearly due to the exclusion of patients younger than 80 years of age, who have an improved 1-year survival. However, despite the absolute mortality rate being higher in the super-elderly, the standardized mortality ratio (SMR) at 1 year is actually lowest in the super-elderly group.[35] These frail patients may benefit from input from a geriatrician and multidisciplinary therapy team to medically optimize their comorbidities and rehabilitation as has been demonstrated for hip fractures.[120] Alternatively, in frail patients, a palliative care approach may be preferred to facilitate end-of-life management.[133] Although the standard treatment of pubic rami fractures is nonoperative, Krappinger et al.[114] and Beall et al.[15] suggested that "ramoplasty," percutaneous injection of polymethyl methacrylate into acute pubic rami fractures, may relieve pain and facilitate early mobilization, but this is not widespread practice nor is there any level 1 evidence to support this management intervention.

Tibia

Not all fractures show the same trend as fractures of the proximal femur, proximal humerus, and distal radius with an increasing prevalence in older males and females. A good example of this

is the tibial diaphyseal fracture. The epidemiology of tibial fractures has changed significantly during the last 20 years mainly because of improved road safety.[46] The overall incidence of tibial diaphyseal fractures is declining, nearly halving in number from $27/10^5$/year in 1990[50] to $13/10^5$/year in 2010/11 (Table 20-2). The gender distribution is predominately male (Table 20-2) but the literature suggests that there was a change in the distribution in the latter half of the last century with an increased incidence of female patients, including elderly patients.[16,62] The mean age of the patients, particularly females, increased during this period and Table 3-14 shows that in 1991, in Edinburgh, the average age of males and females who presented with tibial fractures was 33 years and 61 years, respectively. The mechanism of injury has also changed. In 1990 most tibial diaphyseal fractures occurred after a motor vehicle accident (37.5%) or a sports injury (30.9%),[50] whereas in 2008 two-thirds occurred after a low-energy fall from standing height.[46]

Table 3-14 shows that since 1991 there has been further changes in the epidemiology of tibial fractures. The average age of males has risen from 33 to 41 years whereas the average age of females has fallen from 61 to 44 years. However, in both males and females, the prevalence of tibial fractures caused by standing falls has risen from 16% to 37% in males and from 53% to 65% in females. The number of tibial diaphyseal fractures caused by road traffic accidents has fallen considerably and many fewer elderly female pedestrians are now being hit by automobiles. As tibial diaphyseal fractures are not osteoporotic fractures (Table 20-3) this means that although the relative number of fractures caused by standing falls will rise, the average age will fall. A review of the data from 2010/11 (Table 20-2) shows that 8.7% of open tibial diaphyseal fractures occurred in the elderly and there were no open fractures in the super-elderly population. The gender distribution of open fractures in the elderly population was 83/17.

There is a wealth of literature regarding the management and outcome of tibial diaphyseal fractures in young patients.[58,161] However, there is a very limited literature regarding the outcome in elderly patients after tibial diaphyseal fractures, with only a small cohorts reported.[51,156] The demographics and outcome of these fractures is different in the elderly patients relative to their younger counterparts and therefore a different management approach may be required.

Age has been shown to correlate with injury severity, as elderly patients are more likely to suffer an open fracture after a relatively minor injury.[50] In the 2010/11 study (Table 20-2) 50% of the tibial fractures in the elderly group were open compared with 17.4% of fractures in patients aged less than 65 years. These open fractures are more likely to occur as a result of minor injury, with falls being responsible for 66% of all elderly tibial fractures and 66% of open fractures. In the elderly population, whose bone and soft tissues are becoming increasingly fragile,[44] an increased injury severity for less severe modes of injury might be expected.

The 10% nonunion rate of elderly tibial fractures is greater than that expected relative to the general population.[143] Chatziyiannakis et al.[31] theorized that increased soft tissue injury and fracture comminution, combined with soft tissue stripping during surgery, may increase the rate of nonunion. There is another factor in open fractures which significantly increases the risk of nonunion in the elderly. Fracture fixation with an intramedullary nail significantly reduces the nonunion rate after adjusting for other confounding variables. Hence, the increased rate of nonunion in our elderly cohort may be explained by the greater rate of open fractures and increased rate of fixation by methods other than an intramedullary nail. There are, however, other factors which may contribute to this increased nonunion rate which are more prevalent within the elderly population. Examples are medications such as statins, nonsteroidal anti-inflammatory drugs and steroids, and diseases such as hypothyroidism, diabetes, and vascular insufficiency, which have all been associated with nonunion.[65]

Cox et al.[51] published the only other study to examine both closed and open elderly tibial diaphyseal fractures and compare the mortality of these injuries. They found no difference between the 6-month mortality rates. A lower mortality rate, compared to our elderly patients,[160] was demonstrated, with an 8% and 11% mortality rate at 6 months for closed and open fractures, respectively. Although our mortality rate at 6 months for closed fractures of 13% is similar to their 8%, the mortality associated with an open fracture in our group was significantly different with a 33% mortality rate at 6 months. The reason for this difference may reflect a type II statistical error because of their small number of patients ($n = 54$), which Cox et al. acknowledge in their discussion. In addition, their study centre is a tertiary referral unit for trauma, and did not exclude patients' resident out with their own catch area. This may have skewed the results, with the most unwell or frail patients not being referred, and hence the improved survivorship of their open elderly fractures.

The unadjusted mortality rate is 17% at 120 days and 27% at 1 year for elderly tibial fractures, with age and whether the fracture was open or closed predicting mortality. These unadjusted rates are similar to the 18%[82] 120 day and 29%[179] 1-year mortality rates observed after a fractured neck of femur. The unadjusted rate peaks at 33% for elderly patients with open tibial diaphyseal fractures at 120 days post injury. Clement et al.[36] demonstrated that unadjusted mortality rates of lower limb fractures in the elderly are similar to that of a fractured hip. They also suggested that if targets are set for operating on hip fractures within 48 hours of admission, which is associated with a decreased number of post-operative complications and shorter hospital stays,[32] then it would seem appropriate to apply this principle to all lower limb fractures requiring surgery in the elderly. For tibial diaphyseal fractures in the elderly, with a mortality rate similar to that of a hip fracture, outcome may also improve by adopting the fast-track care that now benefits hip fracture patients.[118]

The SMR we observed for elderly patients with tibial fractures is greater than that observed after an isolated hip fracture. The SMR for a hip fracture in the elderly is 3.4,[35] whereas the SMR we observed for elderly tibial diaphyseal fractures was 4.2, which increased to 8.1 in elderly females. This excess adjusted mortality associated with elderly tibial fractures confirms that they should

receive the same priority as those patients with a hip fracture in an effort to improve their morbidity and mortality.[157]

Olecranon

Undisplaced fractures of the olecranon are routinely managed nonoperatively[137,155] with tension band wiring and plate fixation being frequently employed for displaced fractures.[9,13,29,85,102,158,177] However, there is conflicting literature regarding the outcome and complications of operative fixation in elderly patients due to poor fixation in osteoporotic bone and wound breakdown.[76,79,108,123] Fracture excision with advancement of the triceps has been suggested as an alternative option for osteoporotic patients,[64,87] although some authors have also demonstrated triceps weakness with this technique.[40,57] There is a paucity of data on the outcome following nonoperative management for displaced fractures of the olecranon, particularly in elderly patients with multiple comorbidities, low functional demand, and poor bone quality.

There is an increasing incidence of olecranon fractures in the elderly,[59] and it is now acknowledged that further work is needed to determine whether the surgical treatment for displaced olecranon fractures in these patients provides any significant long-term benefit over nonoperative management.[60] There are two small case series reporting favorable short-term results following the nonoperative management of displaced olecranon fractures in both young and elderly patients.[146,174]

The use of operative fixation for a displaced olecranon fracture in elderly patients can be associated with an increased anesthetic risk, poor fixation in osteoporotic bone, problems with wound breakdown, and an inferior outcome.[76,79,108,123] However, it is necessary for nonoperative treatment to adequately manage pain, allow early movement, provide active extension power at the elbow, and meet the long-term demands of the patient.[40,57,174] Parker et al.[146] documented the short-term outcome of 23 patients with a mean age of 48 years (range, 13 to 91) who were managed conservatively using early active motion within the first 2 weeks following injury for a displaced fracture of the olecranon. In their study they included young patients, comminuted fractures, concomitant fractures to the ipsilateral elbow, and also open fractures. At a mean follow-up of 2 years the outcome was reported as good or fair in 21 (91%) patients, with comparable findings in patients over the age of 50 years. Only three patients noted a loss of power at the elbow and radiologic union was achieved in 30% of patients, with fibrous union achieved in the rest. The other series in the literature reports the short-term outcome of 12 elderly low-demand patients, who presented with a displaced fracture of the olecranon, with a mean age of 82 years managed in a 90-degree above elbow cast for a mean of 4 weeks.[149] They reported patient satisfaction was excellent in 11 (92%) cases at a mean of 15 months after injury. In their series, eight (67%) patients were pain-free and nine patients had radiologic evidence of a pseudoarthrosis.

The current evidence would suggest that nonoperative management of displaced olecranon fractures in low-demand patients with multiple comorbidities results in a satisfactory outcome in the majority of patients. However, further work is required to directly compare operative and nonoperative management in this low-demand patient group.

MULTIPLE FRACTURES IN THE ELDERLY

The majority of the literature concerning fractures in the elderly has focused on isolated fractures, particularly those of the proximal femur, proximal humerus, and distal radius. However elderly patients frequently present with more than one fracture.[48] The epidemiology of multiple fractures in the elderly was studied by Clement et al.[35] This study showed that the majority of multiple fractures in the elderly occur after low-energy trauma in females. Distal radius, proximal humerus, and pelvic fractures are associated with an increased risk of sustaining multiple fractures (Table 20-22). The commonest combination of multiple fractures is that of combined fractures involving the upper and lower limbs (Table 20-23). Most elderly patients sustaining multiple fractures required hospital admission, despite the fact that 42% did not require surgical treatment. However, 54% needed an increased level of social care at discharge (Table 20-24). There is a significantly increased SMR associated with multiple fractures that include a proximal humerus, pelvic, or proximal femur fracture (Table 20-25). However, this increased mortality risk diminished with increasing age, with very elderly patients actually having a lower risk. Combined fractures of the proximal humerus and femur are associated with the highest mortality risk at 1 year.

Surgeons may assume multiple fractures are the result of high-energy injuries and this is frequently the case in younger patients. High-energy modes of injury were associated with the highest incidence of multiple fractures in the elderly. However, these modes of injury are uncommon in the elderly and the majority of multiple fractures actually occur after low-energy trauma (88.1%).[35]

There is no significant difference in the average age or gender ratios in elderly patients who present with single or multiple fractures (Table 20-22). Patients who have multiple fractures are more likely to present with a distal radius, proximal humerus, or pelvic fracture. There is, however, no consistency in the distribution of fractures in the patients who presented with three or four fractures, or for fractures that had been sustained by high-energy modes of injury in the elderly.[35] This is probably because of the relative infrequency of these fractures. However, double fracture combinations that occur as a result of a fall demonstrate definite fracture patterns.

In the study 86.7% of the fractures in fall-related double fracture combinations were in the proximal femur, proximal humerus, and distal radius. Patients who presented with upper limb fracture combinations were significantly younger than those in the other groups, with the majority of patients sustaining a distal radial fracture. However, the highest frequency of double fractures following a fall was observed in patients with combined upper and lower limb fractures. The combination of a proximal femur fracture with either a proximal humerus or distal radius fracture accounted for 31% of all fall-related double fracture combinations with a mean age of 82.2 years.

There is a considerable difference between the double fractures caused by low-energy and high-energy modes of injury.

TABLE 20-22	The Demographic Characteristics of Elderly Patients Who Present with Single or Multiple Fractures from All Modes of Injury. The Prevalence and Risk of Sustaining One of the Most Common Six Fractures are Shown			
	Single Fractures	Multiple Fractures	Odds Ratio	p Value
Patients (%)	2,216 (94.9)	119 (5.1)	—	—
Average Age (yrs)				
All	78.9	78.7	—	0.78[a]
Male	77.7	76.5	—	0.61[a]
Female	79.2	79.4	—	0.54[a]
Male/Female (%)	23/77	22/78	1	0.9[b]
Fracture Prevalence (%)				
Proximal femur	30.6	32.8	1.1	0.34[b]
Distal radius	21.1	37	2.2	<0.0001[b]
Proximal humerus	9.9	35.3	5.1	<0.0001[b]
Ankle	6.7	9.2	1.4	0.19[b]
Finger phalanx	3.8	7.6	2.1	0.05[b]
Pelvis	3.1	12.6	4.9	<0.0001[b]

[a]Mann Whitney U test.
[b]Chi Squared.

| TABLE 20-23 | A Comparison of the Demographic Characteristics of Double Fractures in Elderly Patients Caused by a Fall with those Caused by Other Modes of Injury |

	Falls	Other Modes of Injury	Odds Ratio	p Value
Number of patients	90	19	—	—
Fractures	180	38	—	—
Average age (yrs)	79.1	77.9	—	0.4[a]
Male/female (%)	16/84	42/58	3.8	0.03[b]
Fracture combinations				
Upper limb fractures (%)	32.2	47.4	1.8	0.29[b]
Lower limb fractures (%)	12.2	31.6	3.4	0.04[b]
Combined fractures (%)	55.5	21	4.6	0.007[b]
Fracture types				
Proximal femur (%)	21.7	5.3	5	0.01[b]
Distal radius (%)	21.1	18.4	1	0.59[b]
Proximal humerus (%)	18.8	10.5	2	0.16[b]
Pelvis (%)	8.9	10.5	1.2	0.47[b]

[a]Mann Whitney U test.
[b]Fisher's Exact test.

Despite a similar mean age, high-energy trauma is significantly more common in males, with a higher prevalence of combined upper limb fractures, and less likelihood of proximal femoral fractures. This suggests that the patients who sustain double fractures, especially those of the lower limb, following a low-energy injury may be frailer than those who present with high-energy related double fractures, regardless of the fact that the mean ages are similar.

The frailty of patients who present with double fractures is confirmed by the associated increased standardized mortality rate at 1 year. This is supported by subgroup analysis. Elderly patients, relative to super-elderly patients, were demonstrated to have an increased mortality risk, which may reflect the frailty of this younger-elderly age group after sustaining low-energy multiple fractures. The mortality risk is significantly increased for multiple fractures that included pelvic or proximal humeral fractures in all elderly patients, or proximal femoral fractures in those aged 65 to 79 years old, relative to fractures sustained in isolation. Patients sustaining these multiple fracture combinations should be identified, and both the medical and surgical management should be prioritized in an effort to improve their outcome.

| TABLE 20-24 | Rate of Admission, Operative Intervention, Fixation of Both Fractures, Length of Stay, and Rate of Discharge to Original Domicile for those Patients Admitted to Hospital, for Each Double Fracture Group |

Outcome	Upper Limb	Lower Limb	Combined	p Value
Admission (%)	24/29 (82.8)	11/11 (100)	46/50 (92)	0.14[a]
Operative intervention (%)	7/29 (24.1)	5/11 (45.5)	40/50 (80)	<0.001[a]
Both fractures fixed (%)	2/29 (6.9)	1/11 (9.1)	6/50 (12)	0.75[a]
Length of stay (days)	8.3	32.8	29.3	0.002[b]
Return to original place of domicile (%)	21/24 (87.5)	2/11 (18.2)	21/46 (45.6)	<0.001[a]

[a]Chi Squared.
[b]Analysis of variance.

TABLE 20-25 The 1-Year Standardized Mortality Ratios and *p* Values for Single and Multiple Fractures of the Ankle, Distal Radius, Pubic Rami, Proximal Femur, and Proximal Humerus According to Age Group

| Fractures | Single Fracture (95% CI) | *p* Value[a] | Multiple Fractures (95% CI) | | | | | |
			All Ages	*p* Value[a]	65–79 yrs	*p* Value[a]	≥80 yrs	*p* Value[a]
Ankle	1.85 (1.03–3.10)	0.02	1.95 (0.34–6.61)	0.32	2.66 (0.33–6.61)	0.31	No deaths	—
Distal radius	0.75 (0.50–1.08)	0.13	1.43 (0.64–4.82)	0.15	2.18 (0.33–6.61)	0.31	1.07 (0.16–3.30)	1
Pelvis	2.28 (1.35–3.63)	<0.001	10.50 (2.43–13.05)	<0.001	11.64 (5.38–19.22)	0.03	3.45 (1.27–9.65)	0.003
Proximal femur	3.41 (2.99–3.87)	<0.001	4.66 (2.66–7.64)	<0.001	8.39 (1.83–11.08)	<0.001	3.53 (1.46–5.51)	<0.001
Proximal humerus	2.06 (1.47–2.80)	<0.001	4.95 (2.66–7.64)	<0.001	6.64 (1.83–11.08)	<0.001	4.34 (2.19–8.25)	<0.001

[a]Chi Squared.

1-year mortality approached 50% for the most common double fracture combination of a proximal femoral and proximal humeral fracture. However, in contrast, the combination of a proximal femoral fracture and a distal radial fracture is associated with a decreased mortality of 18%. Allum et al.[6] studied age-dependent balance correction and arm movements for falls in different age groups, and showed that compensatory movements to facilitate protection from falls were less effective with increasing age. Frailer patients were more likely to incur proximal limb girdle fractures because of diminished protective reflexes and hence sustain proximal humeral and femoral fractures.[6,153] Patients who retain their protective reflexes are more likely to sustain a distal radial fracture, which may reflect a superior physiologic status. This may account for the observed improved survival rate of proximal femoral fractures associated with distal radial fracture.

There is evidence that there is an increased incidence of fractures in socially deprived patients after falls[47] and one might therefore hypothesize that there is an association between multiple fractures and deprivation. In Scotland, the population can be divided into quintiles based on social deprivation with quintile 1 being the most affluent and quintile 5 the least affluent. Figure 20-11 illustrates the incidence of multiple fractures in the five social quintiles. It shows a significant increase in the incidence of multiple fractures in the most deprived social quintile (odds ratio 2.5, 95% confidence interval (CI) 1.8 to 3.9, *p* = 0.001). However, a similar pattern is observed for single fractures and there is no significant difference in the relationship between single and multiple fractures and social deprivation.[135]

END-OF-LIFE CARE

Multiple studies have demonstrated that one in five people sustaining a hip fracture will die within 4 months of injury.[82] This figure increases with increasing age, with a one in three mortality rate for super-elderly patients at 4 months.[36] This is not unique to hip fractures. The same mortality rate has been demonstrated for pelvic fracture and other lower limb fractures in super-elderly patients.[36] This unadjusted mortality rate is greater than for some malignant diseases.[94] A palliative care approach is therefore appropriate for patients with advanced nonmalignant as well as malignant diseases.[135] Thus a fragility fracture in

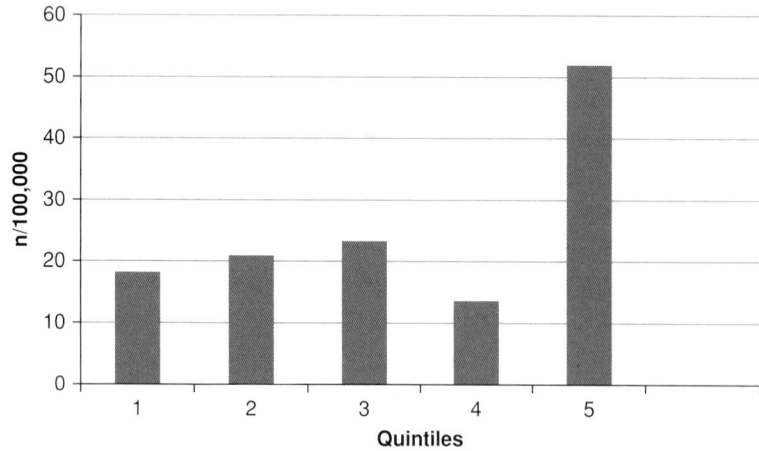

FIGURE 20-11 A histogram showing the relationship between social deprivation and the incidence of fractures.

a frail super-elderly person may reasonably trigger a palliative care approach: Anticipating and planning for physical, social, psychological and spiritual needs, and end-of-life care.[133]

1-year mortality following hip fracture (26% to 37%) is greater than the equivalent mortality of many solid tumors.[94] The mortality is even higher in specific groups, such as those graded preoperatively as ASA III or ASA IV, with 38% of patients dying within 4 months of surgery.[82] However, predicting those individuals who will die is very difficult. Many such patients have multiple comorbidities, including dementia, and the fracture may precipitate a rapid physical and social decline. Even in patients who may have only days or weeks to live, surgery may be indicated to achieve pain control and avoid prolonged immobility and opiate therapy with its associated side effects. Death in the year after their fracture may be because of acute cardiovascular, respiratory, or neurologic events, but a typical pattern of decline in the final months or years has not been described. Even trivial physical events in the frail older person can cause major decompensation.[136] A hip fracture is a major physical insult which can foreshorten the frailty trajectory where gradual physical or cognitive deterioration may last for many years.[134]

The question "Would I be surprised if this patient were to die in the next year?" is being increasingly used to identify non-malignant patients for a palliative care approach.[135] Orthopedic surgeons, orthogeriatric clinicians, and family physicians considering individual hip fracture patients might not be surprised in many cases. Relatives frequently underestimate the 1-year mortality associated with a hip fracture. In patients with a real risk of dying, even when the prognosis is uncertain, it is appropriate to make a care plan, together with the patient and relatives where appropriate, just in case this does happen. It is then possible to anticipate problems and possibly prevent unnecessary interventions and admissions. For the majority of such patients, postoperative care planning includes nutritional, cognitive, social, physiotherapy, and occupational therapy assessments.[122] In some trauma units a geriatrician is responsible for ensuring appropriate medical treatments are undertaken and is often involved in discussions with the patient and family over a poor prognosis. Comprehensive geriatric intervention may reduce short- and long-term mortality, but overall mortality remains high.[176] A recent controlled trial of advance care planning in geriatric inpatients was shown to improve end-of-life care and family anxiety.[54]

Active supportive care following their fracture is useful to help patients live and die well. It is currently good practice for a hip fracture in a frail, older person to trigger an orthogeriatric review to prevent and treat medical complications.[3] Some authors have suggested that for such patients, the orthopedic surgeons, orthogeriatricians, patient, and family should be involved in discussions about anticipatory care to optimize the quality of life, and in due course, death.[133] These care plans could then be reviewed and taken forward by family physicians, nurses, and social carers in the community. A fracture, especially those of the lower limb and pelvis, in the frail super-elderly patient may act as a stimulus to consider holistic planning and care typical of a palliative care approach. Specialist palliative care in people with lung cancer has been shown to be associated with improved quality of life and even longevity.[170] It may also be beneficial if clinicians adopt a palliative care approach in selected super-elderly patients with fractures.

REFERENCES

1. Acklin YP, Sommer C. Plate fixation of proximal humerus fractures using the minimally invasive anterolateral delta split approach. *Oper Orthop Traumatol.* 2012;24:61–73.
2. Adams AL, Schiff MA, Koepsell TD, et al. Physician consultation, multidisciplinary care, and 1-year mortality in Medicare recipients hospitalized with hip and lower extremity injuries. *J Am Geriatr Soc.* 2010;58:1835–1842.
3. Adunsky A, Lerner-Geva L, Blumstein T, et al. Improved survival of hip fracture patients treated within a comprehensive geriatric hip fracture unit, compared with standard of care treatment. *J Am Med Dir Assoc.* 2011;12:439–444.
4. Aksu N, Gogus A, Kara AN, et al. Complications encountered in proximal humerus fractures treated with locking plate fixation. *Acta Orthop Traumatol Turc.* 2010;44:89–96.
5. Aksu N, Karaca S, Kara AN, et al. Minimally invasive plate osteosynthesis (MIPO) in diaphyseal humerus and proximal humerus fractures. *Acta Orthop Traumatol Turc.* 2012;46:154–160.
6. Allum JH, Carpenter MG, Honegger F, et al. Age-dependant variations in the directional sensitivity of balance corrections and compensatory arm movements in man. *J Physiol.* 2002;542:643–663.
7. Alnaib M, Waters S, Shanshal Y, et al. Combined pubic rami and sacral osteoporotic fractures: A prospective study. *J Orthop Traumatol.* 2012;13:97–103.
8. Amorosa LF, Vitale MA, Brown S, et al. A functional outcomes survey of elderly patients who sustained distal radius fractures. *Hand (N Y).* 2011;6:260–267.
9. Anderson ML, Larson AN, Merten SM, et al. Congruent elbow plate fixation of olecranon fractures. *J Orthop Trauma.* 2007;21:386–393.
10. Anzarut A, Johnson JA, Rowe BH, et al. Radiologic and patient-reported functional outcomes in an elderly cohort with conservatively treated distal radius fractures. *J Hand Surg Am.* 2004;29:1121–1127.
11. ASA Physical Status Classification System. American Society of Anesthesiologists http://www.asahq.org/clinical/physicalstatus.htm (last accessed 10th October 2012).
12. Avery PP, Baker RP, Walton MJ, et al. Total hip replacement and hemiarthroplasty in mobile, independent patients with a displaced intracapsular fracture of the femoral neck: A seven- to ten-year follow-up report of a prospective randomised controlled trial. *J Bone Joint Surg Br.* 2011;93:1045–1048.
13. Bailey CS, MacDermid J, Patterson SD, et al. Outcome of plate fixation of olecranon fractures. *J Orthop Trauma.* 2001;15:542–548.
14. Barnes R, Brown JT, Garden RS, et al. Subcapital fractures of the femur. A prospective review. *J Bone Joint Surg Br.* 1976;58:2–24.
15. Beall DP, D'souza SL, Costello RF. Percutaneous augmentation of the superior pubic ramus with polymethylmethacrylate: Treatment of acute and chronic insufficiency fractures. *Skeletal Radiol.* 2007;36:979–983.
16. Bengner U, Ekbom T, Johnell O, et al. Incidence of femoral and tibial shaft fractures. Epidemiology 1950–1983 in Malmo, Sweden. *Acta Orthop Scand.* 1990;61:251–254.
17. Bengner U, Johnell O, Redlund-Johnell I. Changes in the incidence of fracture of the upper end of the humerus during a 30-year period: A study 2125 fracture. *Clin Orthop Relat Res.* 1988;231:179–182.
18. Bennett KM, Scarborough JE, Vaslef S. Outcome and health care resource utilization in super-elderly trauma patients. *J Surg Res.* 2010;163:127–131.
19. Beumer A, McQueen MM. Fractures of the distal radius in low-demand elderly patients: Closed reduction of no value in 53 of 60 wrists. *Acta Orthop Scand.* 2003;74:98–100.
20. Bjorkenheim JM, Pajarinen J, Savolainen V. Internal fixation of proximal humeral fractures with a locking compression plate: A retrospective evaluation of 72 patients followed for a minimum of 1 year. *Acta Orthop Scand.* 2004;75:741–745.
21. Bliuc D, Nguyen ND, Milch VE, et al. Mortality risk associated with low-trauma osteoporotic fracture and subsequent fracture in men and women. *JAMA.* 2009;301:513–521.
22. Borgstrom F, Zethraeus N, Johnell O, et al. Costs and quality of life associated with osteoporosis-related fractures in Sweden. *Osteoporos Int.* 2006;17:637–650.
23. Breuil V, Roux CH, Testa J, et al. Outcome of osteoporotic pelvic fractures: An underestimated severity. Survey of 60 cases. *Joint Bone Spine.* 2008;75:585–588.
24. Brunner A, Thormann S, Babst R. Minimally invasive plating osteosynthesis of proximal humeral shaft fractures with long PHILOS plates. *Oper Orthop Traumatol.* 2012;24:302–311.
25. Brunner F, Sommer C, Bahrs C, et al. Open reduction and internal fixation of proximal humerus fractures using a proximal humeral locked plate: A prospective multicenter analysis. *J Orthop Trauma.* 2009;23:163–172.
26. Campbell AJ, Borrie MJ, Spears GF. Risk factors for falls in a community-based prospective study of people 70 years and older. *J Gerontol.* 1989;44:M112–M117.
27. Carroll C, Stevenson M, Scope A, et al. Hemiarthroplasty and total hip arthroplasty for treating primary intracapsular fracture of the hip: A systematic review and cost-effectiveness analysis. *Health Technol Assess.* 2011;15:1–74.
28. Centre of Disease Control and Prevention. Cost of falls among older adults. Available online at: http//www.cdc.gov.homeand recreationalsafety/falls/fallscost (last accessed 10th October 2012).
29. Chalidis BE, Sachinis NC, Samoladas EP, et al. Is tension band wiring technique the "gold standard" for the treatment of olecranon fractures? A long term functional outcome study. *J Orthop Surg Res.* 2008;3:9.

30. Chang HC, Tay SC, Chan BK, et al. Conservative treatment of redisplaced Colles' fractures in elderly patients older than 60 years old - anatomical and functional outcome. *Hand Surg.* 2001;6:137–144.
31. Chatziyiannakis AA, Verettas DA, Raptis VK, et al. Nonunion of tibial fractures treated with external fixation. Contributing factors studied in 71 fractures. *Acta Orthop Scand Suppl.* 1997;275:77–79.
32. Chilov MN, Cameron ID, March LM. Evidence-based guidelines for fixing broken hips: An update. *Med J Aust.* 2003;179:489–493.
33. Chiu FY, Lo WH, Yu CT, et al. Percutaneous pinning in undisplaced subcapital femoral neck fractures. *Injury.* 1996;27:53–55.
34. Clayton RA, Gaston MS, Ralston SH, et al. Association between decreased bone mineral density and severity of distal radial fractures. *J Bone Joint Surg Am.* 2009;91:613–619.
35. Clement ND, Aitken S, Duckworth AD, et al. Multiple fractures in the elderly. *J Bone Joint Surg Br.* 2012;94:231–236.
36. Clement ND, Aitken SA, Duckworth AD, et al. The outcome of fractures in very elderly patients. *J Bone Joint Surg Br.* 2011;93:806–810.
37. Clement ND, Court-Brown CM. Four-score years and ten: The fracture epidemiology of the super-elderly [abstract]. *Injury Extra.* 2009;40:235.
38. Clement ND, Muzammil A, MacDonald D, et al. Socioeconomic status affects the early outcome of total hip replacement. *J Bone Joint Surg Br.* 2011;93B:464–469.
39. Colles A. On the fracture of the carpal extremity of the radius. *Edinb Med Surg J.* 1814;10:182–186.
40. Colton CL. Fractures of the olecranon in adults: Classification and management. *Injury.* 1973;5:121–129.
41. Conn KS, Parker MJ. Undisplaced intracapsular hip fractures: Results of internal fixation in 375 patients. *Clin Orthop Relat Res.* 2004;421:249–254.
42. Consensus development conference: Prophylaxis and treatment of osteoporosis. *Am J Med.* 1991;90:107–110.
43. Constant CR, Gerber C, Emery RJ, et al. A review of the Constant score: Modifications and guidelines for its use. *J Shoulder Elbow Surg.* 2008;17:355–361.
44. Cook JL, Dzubow LM. Aging of the skin: Implications for cutaneous surgery. *Arch Dermatol.* 1997;133:1273–1277.
45. Cooney WP. Management of Colles' fractures. *J Hand Surg Br.* 1989;14:137–139.
46. Court-Brown CM, Aitken SA, Forward D, et al. The epidemiology of fractures. In: Bucholz RW, Heckman JD, Court-Brown CM, et al., eds. *Rockwood and Greens Fractures in Adults.* 7th ed. Philadelphia, PA: Lippincott, Williams & Wilkins; 2010:53–77.
47. Court-Brown CM, Aitken SA, Ralston SH, et al. The relationship of fall-related fractures to social deprivation. *Osteoporos Int.* 2011;22:1211–1218.
48. Court-Brown CM, Caesar B. Epidemiology of adult fractures: A review. *Injury.* 2006;37:691–697.
49. Court-Brown CM, Clement N. Four score years and ten: An analysis of the epidemiology of fractures in the very elderly. *Injury.* 2009;40:1111–1114.
50. Court-Brown CM, McBirnie J. The epidemiology of tibial fractures. *J Bone Joint Surg Br.* 1995;77:417–421.
51. Cox G, Jones S, Nikolaou VS, et al. Elderly tibial shaft fractures: Open fractures are not associated with increased mortality rates. *Injury.* 2010;41:620–623.
52. Cserhati P, Kazar G, Manninger J, et al. Non-operative or operative treatment for undisplaced femoral neck fractures: A comparative study of 122 non-operative and 125 operatively treated cases. *Injury.* 1996;27:583–588.
53. Deneka DA, Simonian PT, Stankewich CJ, et al. Biomechanical comparison of internal fixation techniques for the treatment of unstable basicervical femoral neck fractures. *J Orthop Trauma.* 1997;11:337–343.
54. Detering KM, Hancock AD, Reade MC, et al. The impact of advance care planning on end of life care in elderly patients: Randomised controlled trial. *BMJ.* 2010;340:c1345.
55. Diaz CM, Garcia JJ, Carrasco JL, et al. Prevalence of osteoporosis assessed by densitometry in the Spanish female population. *Med Clin (Barc).* 2001;116:86–88.
56. Diaz-Garcia RJ, Oda T, Shauver MJ, et al. A systematic review of outcomes and complications of treating unstable distal radius fractures in the elderly. *J Hand Surg Am.* 2011;36:824–835.
57. Didonna ML, Fernandez JJ, Lim TH, et al. Partial olecranon excision: The relationship between triceps insertion site and extension strength of the elbow. *J Hand Surg Am.* 2003;28:117–122.
58. Duan X, Al-Qwbani M, Zeng Y, et al. Intramedullary nailing for tibial shaft fractures in adults. *Cochrane Database Syst Rev.* 2012;1:CD008241.
59. Duckworth AD, Clement ND, Aitken SA, et al. The epidemiology of fractures of the proximal ulna. *Injury.* 2012;43:343–346.
60. Duckworth AD, Court-Brown CM, McQueen MM. Isolated displaced olecranon fracture. *J Hand Surg Am.* 2012;37:341–345.
61. El-Sayed MM. Surgical management of complex humerus head fractures. *Orthop Rev (Pavia).* 2010;2:e14.
62. Emami A, Mjoberg B, Ragnarsson B, et al. Changing epidemiology of tibial shaft fractures. 513 cases compared between 1971–1975 and 1986–1990. *Acta Orthop Scand.* 1996;67:557–561.
63. Fazal MA, Haddad FS. Philos plate fixation for displaced proximal humeral fractures. *J Orthop Surg (Hong Kong).* 2009;17:15–18.
64. Gartsman GM, Sculco TP, Otis JC. Operative treatment of olecranon fractures. Excision or open reduction with internal fixation. *J Bone Joint Surg Am.* 1981;63:718–721.
65. Gaston MS, Simpson AH. Inhibition of fracture healing. *J Bone Joint Surg Br.* 2007; 89:1553–1560.
66. Gautier E, Sommer C. Guidelines for the clinical application of the LCP. *Injury.* 2003;34(suppl 2):B63–B76.
67. Geiger EV, Maier M, Kelm A, et al. Functional outcome and complications following PHILOS plate fixation in proximal humeral fractures. *Acta Orthop Traumatol Turc.* 2010;44:1–6.
68. Gillespie WJ. Extracts from "clinical evidence": Hip fracture. *BMJ.* 2001;322:968–975.
69. Gjertsen JE, Engesaeter LB, Furnes O, et al. The Norwegian Hip Fracture Register: Experiences after the first 2 years and 15,576 reported operations. *Acta Orthop.* 2008;79:583–593.
70. Gjertsen JE, Fevang JM, Matre K, et al. Clinical outcome after undisplaced femoral neck fractures. *Acta Orthop.* 2011;82:268–274.
71. Grewal R, MacDermid JC. The risk of adverse outcomes in extra-articular distal radius fractures is increased with malalignment in patients of all ages but mitigated in older patients. *J Hand Surg Am.* 2007;32:962–970.
72. Handoll HH, Cameron ID, Mak JC, et al. Multidisciplinary rehabilitation for older people with hip fractures. *Cochrane Database Syst Rev.* 2009:CD007125.
73. Handoll HH, Madhok R. Surgical interventions for treating distal radial fractures in adults. *Cochranse Database Syst Rev.* 2009:CD003209.
74. Handschin AE, Cardell M, Contaldo C, et al. Functional results of angular-stable plate fixation in displaced proximal humeral fractures. *Injury.* 2008;39:306–313.
75. He W, Sengupta M, Velkoff VA, et al. 65+ *in the United States: 2005*, Current Population Reports. *U.S. Census Bureau and National Institute on Aging.* 2005;23–209.
76. Helm RH, Hornby R, Miller SW. The complications of surgical treatment of displaced fractures of the olecranon. *Injury.* 1987;18:48–50.
77. Hill RM, Robinson CM, Keating JF. Fractures of the pubic rami. Epidemiology and five-year survival. *J Bone Joint Surg Br.* 2001;83:1141–1144.
78. Hirschmann MT, Fallegger B, Amsler F, et al. Clinical longer-term results after internal fixation of proximal humerus fractures with a locking compression plate (PHILOS). *J Orthop Trauma.* 2011;25:286–293.
79. Holdsworth BJ, Mossad MM. Elbow function following tension band fixation of displaced fractures of the olecranon. *Injury.* 1984;16:182–187.
80. Holt G, Macdonald D, Fraser M, et al. The outcome after hip surgery for fracture of the hip in patients aged over 95 years. *J Bone Joint Surg Br.* 2006;88:1060–1064.
81. Holt G, Smith R, Duncan K, et al. Changes in population demographics and the future incidence of hip fracture. *Injury.* 2009;40:722–726.
82. Holt G, Smith R, Duncan K, et al. Early mortality after surgical fixation of hip fractures in the elderly: An analysis of data from the Scottish hip fracture audit. *J Bone Joint Surg Br.* 2008;90:1357–1363.
83. Holt G, Smith R, Duncan K, et al. Gender differences in epidemiology and outcome after hip fracture: Evidence from the Scottish Hip Fracture Audit. *J Bone Joint Surg Br.* 2008;90:480–483.
84. Holt G, Smith R, Duncan K, et al. Outcome after surgery for the treatment of hip fracture in the extremely elderly. *J Bone Joint Surg Am.* 2008;90:1899–1905.
85. Hume MC, Wiss DA. Olecranon fractures. A clinical and radiographic comparison of tension band wiring and plate fixation. *Clin Orthop Relat Res.* 1992:229–235.
86. Iki M, Kagamimori S, Kagawa Y, et al. Bone mineral density of the spine, hip and distal forearm in representative samples of the Japanese female population: Japanese Population-Based Osteoporosis (JPOS) Study. *Osteoporos Int.* 2001;12:529–537.
87. Inhofe PD, Howard TC. The treatment of olecranon fractures by excision or fragments and repair of the extensor mechanism: Historical review and report of 12 fractures. *Orthopedics.* 1993;16:1313–1317.
88. Jensen JS, Bagger J. Long-term social prognosis after hip fractures. *Acta Orthop Scand.* 1982;53:97–101.
89. Jette AM, Harris BA, Cleary PD, et al. Functional recovery after hip fracture. *Arch Phys Med Rehabil.* 1987;68:735–740.
90. Johansson B. Fall injuries among elderly persons living at home. *Scand J Caring Sci.* 1998;12:67–72.
91. Johnell O, Kanis JA. An estimate of the worldwide prevalence and disability associated with osteoporotic fractures. *Osteoporos Int.* 2006;17:1726–1733.
92. Johnell O. The socioeconomic burden of fractures: Today and in the 21st century. *Am J Med.*1997;103:20S–26S.
93. Kanis JA, Oden A, McCloskey EV, et al. A systematic review of hip fracture incidence and probability of fracture worldwide. *Osteoporos Int.* 2012;23:2239–2256.
94. Kannegaard PN, van der Mark S, Eiken P, et al. Excess mortality in men compared with women following a hip fracture. National analysis of comedications, comorbidity and survival. *Age Ageing.* 2010;39:203–209.
95. Kannus P, Niemi S, Parkkari J, et al. Nationwide decline in incidence of hip fracture. *J Bone Miner Res.* 2006;21:1836–1838.
96. Kannus P, Palvanen M, Niemi S, et al. Epidemiology of osteoporotic pelvic fractures in elderly people in Finland: Sharp increase in 1970–1997 and alarming projections for the new millennium. *Osteoporos Int.* 2000;11:443–448.
97. Kannus P, Palvanen M, Niemi S, et al. Rate of proximal humeral fractures in older Finnish women between 1970 and 2007. *Bone.* 2009;44:656–659.
98. Kannus P, Parkkari J, Koskinen S, et al. Fall-induced injuries and deaths among older adults. *JAMA.* 1999;281:1895–1899.
99. Kannus P, Sievanen H, Palvanen M, et al. Prevention of falls and consequent injuries in elderly people. *Lancet.* 2005;366:1885–1893.
100. Kannus P, Uusi-Rasi K, Palvanen M, et al. Non-pharmacological means to prevent fractures among older adults. *Ann Med.* 2005;37:303–310.
101. Karinkanta S, Piirtola M, Sievanen H, et al. Physical therapy approaches to reduce fall and fracture risk among older adults. *Nat Rev Endocrinol.* 2010;6:396–407.
102. Karlsson MK, Hasserius R, Karlsson C, et al. Fractures of the olecranon: A 15- to 25-year followup of 73 patients. *Clin Orthop Relat Res.* 2002;403:205–212.
103. Kauffman JI, Simon JA, Kummer FJ, et al. Internal fixation of femoral neck fractures with posterior comminution: A biomechanical study. *J Orthop Trauma.* 1999;13: 155–159.
104. Keating JF, Grant A, Masson M, et al. Randomized comparison of reduction and fixation, bipolar hemiarthroplasty, and total hip arthroplasty. Treatment of displaced intracapsular hip fractures in healthy older patients. *J Bone Joint Surg Am.* 2006;88:249–260.
105. Kelsey JL, Browner WS, Seeley DG, et al. Risk factors for fractures of the distal forearm and proximal humerus. The Study of Osteoporotic Fractures Research Group. *Am J Epidemiol.* 1992;135:477–489.

106. Kettler M, Biberthaler P, Braunstein V, et al. Treatment of proximal humeral fractures with the PHILOS angular stable plate. Presentation of 225 cases of dislocated fractures. *Unfallchirurg.* 2006;109:1032–1040.
107. Kilic B, Uysal M, Cinar BM, et al. Early results of treatment of proximal humerus fractures with the PHILOS locking plate. *Acta Orthop Traumatol Turc.* 2008;42:149–153.
108. Kiviluoto O, Santavirta S. Fractures of the olecranon. Analysis of 37 consecutive cases. *Acta Orthop Scand.* 1978;49:28–31.
109. Kohrt WM, Bloomfield SA, Little KD, et al. American College of Sports Medicine Position Stand: Physical activity and bone health. *Med Sci Sports Exerc.* 2004;36:1985–1996.
110. Konrad G, Audige L, Lambert S, et al. Similar outcomes for nail versus plate fixation of three-part proximal humeral fractures. *Clin Orthop Relat Res.* 2012;470:602–609.
111. Korkmaz MF, Aksu N, Gogus A, et al. The results of internal fixation of proximal humeral fractures with the PHILOS locking plate. *Acta Orthop Traumatol Turc.* 2008;42: 97–105.
112. Koukakis A, Apostolou CD, Taneja T, et al. Fixation of proximal humerus fractures using the PHILOS plate: Early experience. *Clin Orthop Relat Res.* 2006;442:115–120.
113. Koval KJ, Aharonoff GB, Schwartz MC, et al. Pubic rami fracture: A benign pelvic injury? *J Orthop Trauma.* 1997;11:7–9.
114. Krappinger D, Struve P, Schmid R, et al. Fractures of the pubic rami: A retrospective review of 534 cases. *Arch Orthop Trauma Surg.* 2009;129:1685–1690.
115. Krivohlavek M, Lukas R, Taller S, et al. Use of angle-stable implants for proximal humeral fractures: Prospective study. *Acta Chir Orthop Traumatol Cech.* 2008;75:212–220.
116. Kuhlmann T, Hofmann T, Seibert O, et al. Operative treatment of proximal humeral four-part fractures in elderly patients: Comparison of two angular-stable implant systems. *Z Orthop Unfall.* 2012;150:149–155.
117. Lagerby M, Asplund S, Ringqvist I. Cannulated screws for fixation of femoral neck fractures. No difference between Uppsala screws and Richards screws in a randomized prospective study of 268 cases. *Acta Orthop Scand.* 1998;69:387–391.
118. Larsson G, Holgers KM. Fast-track care for patients with suspected hip fracture. *Injury.* 2011;42:1257–1261.
119. Lawrence TM, White CT, Wenn R, et al. The current hospital costs of treating hip fractures. *Injury.* 2005;36:88–91.
120. Leung AH, Lam TP, Cheung WH, et al. An orthogeriatric collaborative intervention program for fragility fractures: A retrospective cohort study. *J Trauma.* 2011;71: 1390–1394.
121. Liu XW, Fu QG, Xu SG, et al. Application of PHILOS plate with injectable artificial bone for the treatment of proximal humeral fractures in elderly patients. *Zhongguo Gu Shang.* 2010;23:180–182.
122. Lynn J. Palliative Care Beyond Cancer: Reliable comfort and meaningfulness. *BMJ.* 2008;336:958–959.
123. Macko D, Szabo RM. Complications of tension-band wiring of olecranon fractures. *J Bone Joint Surg Am.* 1985;67:1396–1401.
124. Martinez AA, Cuenca J, Herrera A. Philos plate fixation for proximal humeral fractures. *J Orthop Surg (Hong Kong).* 2009;17:10–14.
125. Masud T, Morris RO. Epidemiology of falls. *Age Ageing.* 2001;30(suppl 4):3–7.
126. McQueen M, Caspers J. Colles fracture: Does the anatomical result affect the final function? *J Bone Joint Surg Br.* 1988;70:649–651.
127. McQueen MM, Wakefield A. Distal radial osteotomy for malunion using non-bridging external fixation: Good results in 23 patients. *Acta Orthop.* 2008;79:390–395.
128. Melton LJ III, Sampson JM, Morrey BF, et al. Epidemiologic features of pelvic fractures. *Clin Orthop Relat Res.* 1981;155:43–47.
129. Midyear population, by age and sex. U.S. Census Bureau, 2012. (last accessed 10th October 2012).
130. Moonot P, Ashwood N, Hamlet M. Early results for treatment of three- and four-part fractures of the proximal humerus using the PHILOS plate system. *J Bone Joint Surg Br.* 2007;89:1206–1209.
131. Morin S, Lix LM, Azimaee M, et al. Mortality rates after incident non-traumatic fractures in older men and women. *Osteoporos Int.* 2011;22:2439–2448.
132. Morris RO, Sonibare A, Green DJ, et al. Closed pelvic fractures: Characteristics and outcomes in older patients admitted to medical and geriatric wards. *Postgrad Med J.* 2000;76:646–650.
133. Murray IR, Biant LC, Clement ND, et al. Should a hip fracture in a frail older person be a trigger for assessment of palliative care needs? *BMJ Support Palliat Care.* 2011;1:3–4.
134. Murray SA, Kendall M, Boyd K, et al. Illness trajectories and palliative care. *BMJ.* 2005;330:1007–1011.
135. Murray SA, Sheikh A. Palliative Care Beyond Cancer: Care for all at the end of life. *BMJ.* 2008;336:958–959.
136. Newall E, Dewar B, Balaam M, et al. Cumulative trivia: A holistic conceptualization of the minor problems of ageing. *Prim Health Care Res Dev.* 2006;7:331–340.
137. Newman SD, Mauffrey C, Krikler S. Olecranon fractures. *Injury.* 2009;40:575–581.
138. Nguyen TV, Eisman JA, Kelly PJ, et al. Risk factors for osteoporotic fractures in elderly men. *Am J Epidemiol.* 1996;144:255–263.
139. Nikitovic M, Wodchis WP, Krahn MD, et al. Direct health-care costs attributed to hip fractures among seniors: A matched cohort study. *Osteoporos Int.* 2013;24:659–669.
140. Nurmi I, Narinen A, Luthje P, et al. Cost analysis of hip fracture treatment among the elderly for the public health services: A 1-year prospective study in 106 consecutive patients. *Arch Orthop Trauma Surg.* 2003;123:551–554.
141. Office of National Statistics. Available online at: http://www.statistics.gov.uk (last accessed 10th October 2012).
142. Olerud P, Ahrengart L, Ponzer S, et al. Internal fixation versus nonoperative treatment of displaced 3-part proximal humeral fractures in elderly patients: A randomized controlled trial. *J Shoulder Elbow Surg.* 2011;20:747–755.
143. Oni OO, Hui A, Gregg PJ. The healing of closed tibial shaft fractures. The natural history of union with closed treatment. *J Bone Joint Surg Br.* 1988;70:787–790.
144. Palvanen M, Kannus P, Niemi S, et al. Update in the epidemiology of proximal humeral fractures. *Clin Orthop Relat Res.* 2006;442:87–92.
145. Papadopoulos P, Karataglis D, Stavridis SI, et al. Mid-term results of internal fixation of proximal humeral fractures with the Philos plate. *Injury.* 2009;40:1292–1296.
146. Parker MJ, Richmond PW, Andrew TA, et al. A review of displaced olecranon fractures treated conservatively. *J R Coll Surg Edinb.* 1990;35:392–394.
147. Parliament UK. Available online at: http://www.parliament.uk/documents/commons/lib/research/key_issues/Key Issues The ageing population2007.pdf (last accessed 10th October 2012).
148. Parmaksizoğlu AS, Sokucu S, Ozkaya U, et al. Locking plate fixation of three- and four-part proximal humeral fractures. *Acta Orthop Traumatol Turc.* 2010;44:97–104.
149. Pearson D, Taylor R, Masud T. The relationship between social deprivation, osteoporosis, and falls. *Osteoporos Int.* 2004;15:132–138.
150. Piirtola M, Hartikainen S, Akkanen J, et al. Injurious fall needing medical care in older population. *Suom Laakaril.* 2001;57:4903–4907.
151. Piirtola M, Sintonen H, Akkanen J, et al. The cost of acute care of fall injuries in older population. *Suom Laakaril.* 2002;57:4841–4848.
152. Pratt HJ. *Gray Agendas: Interest Groups and Public Pensions in Canada, Britain and the United States.* Ann Arbor, MI: University of Michigan Press; 1994.
153. Rankin JK, Woollacott MH, Shumway-Cook A, et al. Cognitive influence on postural stability: A neuromuscular analysis in young and older adults. *J Gerontol A Biol Sci Med Sci.* 2000;55:M112–M119.
154. Ray NF, Chan JK, Thamer M, et al. Medical expenditures for the treatment of osteoporotic fractures in the United States in 1995: Report from the National Osteoporosis Foundation. *J Bone Miner Res.* 1997;12:24–35.
155. Ring D. Elbow fractures and dislocations. In: Bucholz RW, Court-Brown CM, Heckman JD, et al., eds. *Rockwood and Green's Fractures in Adults,* 7th ed. Philadelphia, PA: Lippincott Williams & Wilkins; 2010:905–944.
156. Ritchie AJ, Small JO, Hart NB, et al. Type III tibial fractures in the elderly: Results of 23 fractures in 20 patients. *Injury.* 1991;22:267–270.
157. Rogers FB, Shackford SR, Keller MS. Early fixation reduces morbidity and mortality in elderly patients with hip fractures from low-impact falls. *J Trauma.* 1995;39:261–265.
158. Rommens PM, Kuchle R, Schneider RU, et al. Olecranon fractures in adults: Factors influencing outcome. *Injury.* 2004;35:1149–1157.
159. Rosenberg M, Everitt J. Planning for aging populations: Inside or outside the walls. *Progress in Planning.* 2001;56:119–168.
160. Sambrook PN, Seeman E, Phillips SR, et al. Preventing osteoporosis: Outcomes of the Australian Fracture Prevention Summit. *Med J Aust.* 2002;176(suppl):S1–S16.
161. Schmidt AH, Finkemeier CG, Tornetta P III. Treatment of closed tibial fractures. *Instr Course Lect.* 2003;52:607–622.
162. Shatrugna V, Kulkarni B, Kumar PA, et al. Bone status of Indian women from a low-income group and its relationship to the nutritional status. *Osteoporos Int.* 2005;16:1827–1835.
163. Shortt NL, Robinson CM. Mortality after low-energy fractures in patients aged at least 45 years old. *J Orthop Trauma.* 2005;19:396–403.
164. Slutsky DJ. Predicting the outcome of distal radius fractures. *Hand Clin.* 2005;21: 289–294.
165. Spross C, Platz A, Erschbamer M, et al. Surgical treatment of Neer Group VI proximal humeral fractures: Retrospective comparison of PHILOS(R) and hemiarthroplasty. *Clin Orthop Relat Res.* 2012;470:2035–2042.
166. Spross C, Platz A, Rufibach K, et al. The PHILOS plate for proximal humeral fractures–risk factors for complications at one year. *J Trauma Acute Care Surg.* 2012;72:783–792.
167. Stevens JA, Corso PS, Finkelstein EA, et al. The costs of fatal and non-fatal falls among older adults. *Inj Prev.* 2006;12:290–295.
168. Stewart HD, Innes AR, Burke FD. Functional cast-bracing for Colles' fractures. A comparison between cast-bracing and conventional plaster casts. *J Bone Joint Surg Br.* 1984;66:749–753.
169. Stewart NA, Chantrey J, Blankley SJ, et al. Predictors of 5 year survival following hip fracture. *Injury.* 2011;42:1253–1256.
170. Temel JS, Greer JA, Muzikansky A, et al. Early palliative care for patients with metastatic non-small-cell lung cancer. *N Engl J Med.* 2010;363:733–742.
171. Thyagarajan DS, Haridas SJ, Jones D, et al. Functional outcome following proximal humeral interlocking system plating for displaced proximal humeral fractures. *Int J Shoulder Surg.* 2009;3:57–62.
172. Tinetti ME, Speechley M, Ginter SF. Risk factors for falls among elderly persons living in the community. *N Engl J Med.* 1988;319:1701–1707.
173. van Dijk WA, Poeze M, van Helden SH, et al. Ten-year mortality among hospitalised patients with fractures of the pubic rami. *Injury.* 2010;41:411–414.
174. Veras Del Monte L, Sirera Vercher M, Busquets Net R, et al. Conservative treatment of displaced fractures of the olecranon in the elderly. *Injury.* 1999;30:105–110.
175. Vestergaard P, Rejnmark L, Mosekilde L. Osteoporosis is markedly underdiagnosed: A nationwide study from Denmark. *Osteoporos Int.* 2005;16:134–141.
176. Vidan M, Serra JA, Moreno C, et al. Efficacy of a comprehensive geriatric intervention in older patients hospitalized for hip fracture: A randomized, controlled trial. *J Am Geriatr Soc.* 2005;53:1476–1482.
177. Villanueva P, Osorio F, Commessatti M, et al. Tension-band wiring for olecranon fractures: Analysis of risk factors for failure. *J Shoulder Elbow Surg.* 2006;15:351–356.
178. Von Heideken P, Gustafson Y, Kallin K, et al. Falls in the very old people: The population based Umea 85+ study in Sweden. *Arch Gerontol Geriatr.*2009;49:390–396.
179. Wiles MD, Moran CG, Sahota O, et al. Nottingham Hip Fracture Score as a predictor of one year mortality in patients undergoing surgical repair of fractured neck of femur. *Br J Anaesth.* 2011;106:501–504.
180. Willig R, Keinanen-Kiukaaniemi S, Jalovaara P. Mortality and quality of life after trochanteric hip fracture. *Public Health.* 2001;115:323–327.
181. Wise J. Number of "oldest old" has doubled in the past 25 years. *BMJ.* 2010;340:c3057.
182. Young BT, Rayan GM. Outcome following nonoperative treatment of displaced distal radius fractures in low-demand patients older than 60 years. *J Hand Surg Am.* 2000;25:19–28.
183. Zhao JP, Hu WK, Zhang QL, et al. Application of PHILOS plate through mini-open deltoid-splitting approach for the treatment of proximal humeral fractures. *Zhongguo Gu Shang.* 2012;25:155–157.

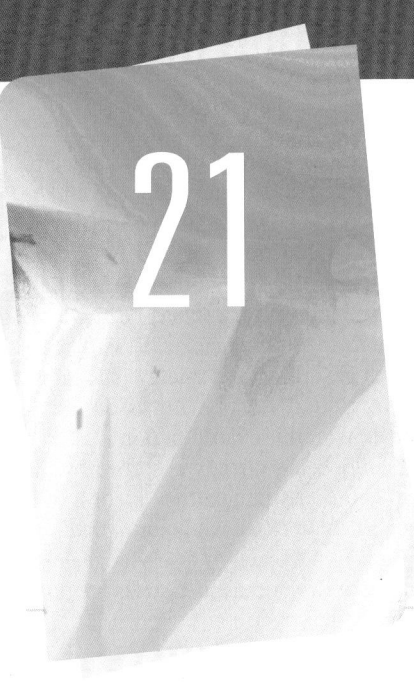

21

STRESS FRACTURES

Timothy L. Miller and Christopher C. Kaeding

HISTORICAL PERSPECTIVE

Stress fractures of bone, also known as fatigue fractures or march fractures, are common and troublesome injuries in athletes and nonathletes alike. Originally described by Breithaupt[21] in unconditioned Prussian military recruits in 1855, they typically occur in individuals who perform repetitive tasks and, therefore, result from an overuse mechanism.[32,84] Stress fractures are not a single consistent entity. They occur along a spectrum of severity which can impact treatment and prognosis.[64,65,67] Not only does the extent of these injuries vary, but the clinical behavior of these injuries varies by location and causative activity.[18,19]

Traditionally, stress fractures have been predominantly regarded as occurring in the weight-bearing bones of the lower extremities. Here the repeated stresses of running and jumping are the typical precipitating activity.[3,57,85] However, as awareness of potential overuse injuries of the upper extremity has increased, so has the diagnosis of stress fractures in the upper extremity.[6,11,12,24] This chapter is meant to provide general guidance on the causes, risks, classification, and treatment of stress fractures. It should be borne in mind that no two stress fractures behave exactly alike. Treatment protocols should be individualized to the patient, the causative activity, the anatomical site, and the severity of the fracture. A treatment algorithm employed by the authors is presented later in this chapter.

PATHOPHYSIOLOGY

Stress fractures are a material fatigue failure of bone.[10,62,68] These stress injuries result from an overuse mechanism. Repeated episodes of bone strain can result in the accumulation of enough microdamage to become a clinically symptomatic stress fracture.[62,75] Fatigue failure of bone has three stages: Crack initiation, crack propagation, and complete fracture. Crack initiation typically occurs at sites of stress concentration during bone loading.[74] Stress concentration occurs at sites of differential bone consistency such as lacunae or canaliculi.[74] Initiation of the microcrack alone is not sufficient to cause a symptomatic fracture. In fact, crack initiation is likely important for bone health because, when coupled with the reparative response, it is the first step in bone remodeling. It may serve to increase bone density and strength. Crack propagation occurs if loading continues at a frequency or intensity above the level at which new bone can be laid down and microcracks are repaired. Propagation, or extension of a microcrack, typically occurs along the cement lines of the bone. When propagating parallel to the cement lines, microcracks expand more rapidly than when propagating perpendicular to cement lines.[65] Continued loading and crack propagation allows for the coalescence of multiple cracks to the point of becoming a clinically symptomatic stress fracture.[68,74] If the loading episodes are not modified or the reparative response increased, crack propagation can continue until structural failure or complete fracture occurs.[15,65]

Any stress or load causes some strain of or deformation to bone, and any strain of bone results in some microdamage.[62,92] Since in vitro bone appears to have no endurance limit (a strain level below which a material may be loaded an infinite number of times without failure), with continued loading, microdamage will continue to occur and accumulate until complete fracture occurs.[10,132] Fortunately, in vivo bone has a reparative healing response to microcracks. Bone metabolic units (BMUs) traditionally known as "cutting cones" respond to repair microcracks.[74,119] Healthy bone is in homeostasis between microcrack creation and repair. If the healing response cannot stop crack propagation, a fatigue failure results. Propagation of a microcrack to a size of 1 to 3 mm is believed to be large enough to become symptomatic.[68,137] Through the adaptive process of remodeling, bone is able to respond to crack initiation and propagation such that the loaded bone is strengthened in preparation for future loading.[82] This positive adaptive response is known as Wolff's law and is an essential part of bone health.[62,68]

Risk Factors

A variety of biologic and mechanical factors are thought to influence the body's ability to remodel bone and therefore impact an individual's risk for developing a stress fracture. These include, but are not limited to sex, age, race, hormonal status, nutrition, neuromuscular function, and genetic factors. Other predisposing factors to consider include abnormal bony alignment, improper technique/biomechanics, poor running form, poor blood supply to specific bones, improper or worn-out footwear, and hard training surfaces.[13,38,75]

The key modifiable risk factors in the development of overuse injuries of bone relate to the preparticipation condition of the bone and the frequency, duration, and intensity of the causative activity. Without preconditioning and acclimation to a particular activity, athletes are at significantly increased risk for the development of overuse and fatigue-related injuries of bone.[53,89,117]

The Neuromuscular Hypothesis

Muscle contraction can have both provocative and protective effects on fatigue failure of bone.[62,68] Muscle contraction results in internally generated compressive, tensile, and/or rotational stresses on bone. In this way muscle contraction creates microdamage. An example of this "internal" loading of bone would be the rotational strain placed on the humerus during the throwing motion. Yet neuromuscular function can also be protective of the skeleton by facilitating the distribution of externally applied loads. Since the late 20th century, it has been widely accepted that neuromuscular conditioning plays a significant role in enhancing the shock absorbing and energy dissipating function of muscles to the ground reaction forces occurring during impact loading. This neuromuscular function is able to decrease the amount of energy being directly absorbed by the bones and joints.[62] Thus, as muscles fatigue they are less able to dissipate the applied external forces, allowing for more rapid accumulation of microtrauma to the bone.[65] Muscle fatigue may be a collaborative culprit in the development of stress fractures in overtrained athletes and military recruits.

General Treatment Principles

Stress fractures are the result of the loss of the normal balance between the creation and repair of microcracks in bone. Treatment principles include an evaluation of both sides of this equation. In order to decrease the creation of microcracks one must evaluate the patient's training regimen, biomechanics, and equipment. In order to maximize the patient's biologic capacity to repair microcracks, one must evaluate the general health of the patient, including nutritional status, hormonal status, and medication use. The clinician should be aware of the female athletic triad which is the interaction and frequent coexistence of disordered eating, amenorrhea, and stress fractures in female endurance athletes.[13,37,38,55]

Stress Fracture Versus Insufficiency Fracture

There is a subtle difference between stress fractures and insufficiency fractures. Both are the result of the loss of balance between the creation and repair of microdamage in bone. A stress fracture is generally felt to be the result of high loads placed on relatively normal bone, whereas an insufficiency fracture is the result of normal loads placed on bone with impaired healing capacity.[74] Insufficiency fractures are typically seen in elderly females. An example would be a metatarsal fatigue fracture in a household ambulator.

DIAGNOSIS

Clinical Presentation

Pain that is initially present only during activity is common in patients presenting with a stress fracture. Symptom onset is usually insidious, and typically patients cannot recall a specific injury or trauma to the affected area. If activity level is not decreased or modified, symptoms persist or worsen. Those who continue to train without modification of their activities may develop pain with normal daily activity and potentially sustain a complete fracture.[37] Physical examination reveals reproducible point tenderness with direct palpation of the affected bone

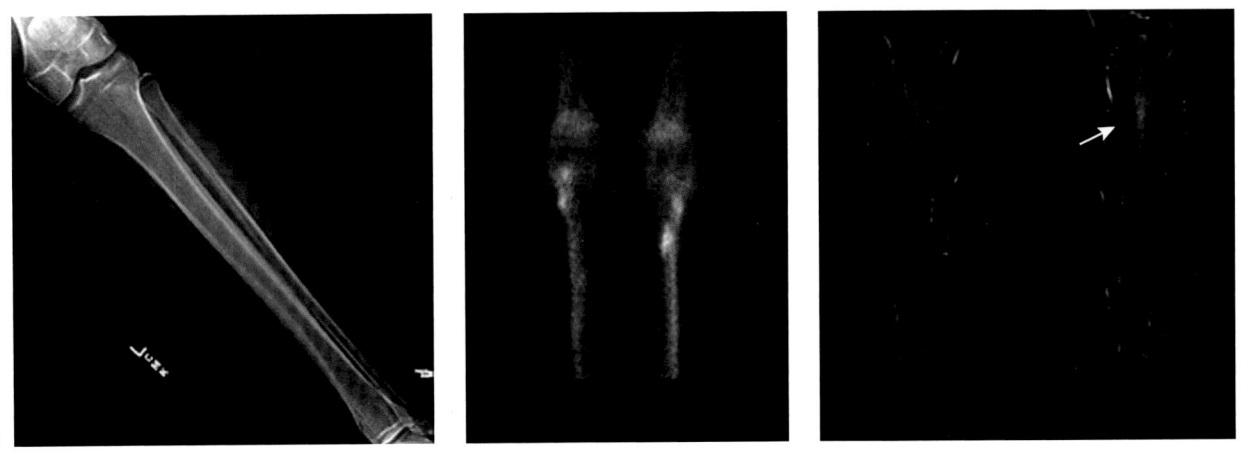

A, B   **C**

FIGURE 21-1 X-ray **(A)**, bone scan **(B)**, and T2-weighted MRI **(C)** images of a 23-year-old distance runner with left proximal tibia pain. *Arrow* indicates area of increased T2 signal on MRI. This correlated with the area of the patient's pain. All images were obtained within a 5-day period.

site. There may or may not be swelling or a palpable soft tissue or bone reaction.

Imaging

Plain x-rays are usually negative early on in the course of a stress fracture, especially in the first 2 to 3 weeks.[5,31,134] Two-thirds of initial x-rays are negative, but half ultimately prove positive once healing begins to occur making standard radiographs specific but not sensitive.[23]

Even after healing has begun to occur, radiographic findings can be subtle and may be easily overlooked if the images are not thoroughly scrutinized.[47,135] Likewise, diagnostic ultrasound imaging has not been shown to be reliable for diagnosing stress injuries of bone.[107]

Bone scintigraphy has been shown to be nearly 100% sensitive for stress injuries of bone, but with lower specificity than magnetic resonance imaging (MRI).[59,115] Bone scan-negative, but MRI-positive stress fractures have been reported.[73] Especially useful for tarsal, femoral, pelvic, and tibial plateau stress fractures, bone scans are usually positive in all phases of a triple-phase technetium scan (angiogram, blood pool, delayed). This allows for easier differentiation of stress fractures from periostitis, or medial tibial stress syndrome (shin splints), as periostitis is often negative in the angiogram and blood pool phases and positive in the delayed image phase. Periostitis has also been shown to have a more diffuse distribution along the medial border of the tibia as opposed to a focal "hotspot" indicating a stress fracture.[28,138]

In the clinical setting, the greatest value of bone scintigraphy is to allow early diagnosis of stress injuries.[39,133] Bone scans will often demonstrate increased uptake in the affected bone 1 to 2 weeks before radiographic changes occur (Fig. 21-1). Given that uptake on bone scan requires 12 to 18 months to normalize, often lagging behind the resolution of clinical symptoms, bone scans are less helpful for guiding return to activity and/or sports participation.[69,102,108] This, then, makes them less useful in the clinical setting for determining prognosis or assessing clinical union of the fracture.

Single photon emission computed tomography (SPECT) scan is a more specific nuclear medicine scanning technique than planar bone scan. Using analysis of the metabolic rate of cells, it is especially helpful in detecting stress fractures of the vertebral pars interarticularis (Fig. 21-2), pelvis, and femoral neck.[26]

Computed tomography (CT) delineates bone well and is useful when the diagnosis of a stress injury is difficult, particularly

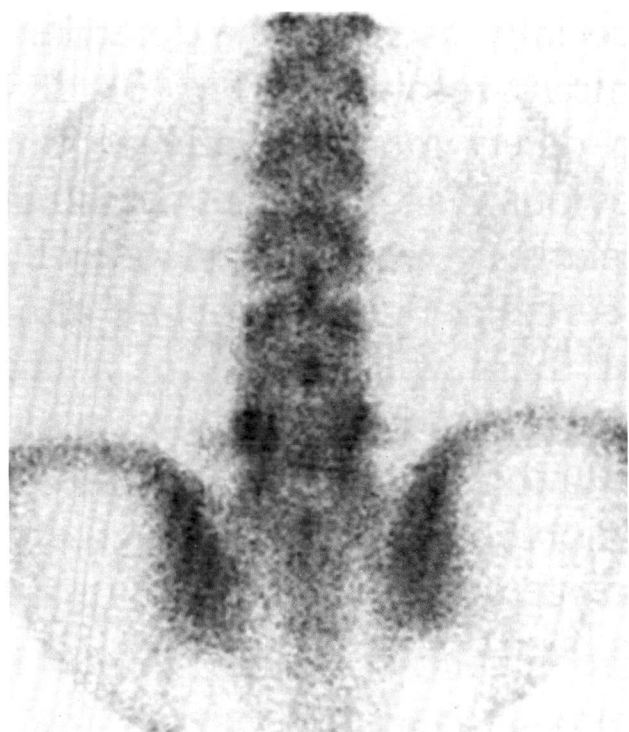

FIGURE 21-2 Single-photon emission computed tomography bone scan demonstrating increased contrast uptake at the site of bilateral L4 pars interarticularis stress fractures in a 15-year-old female gymnast.

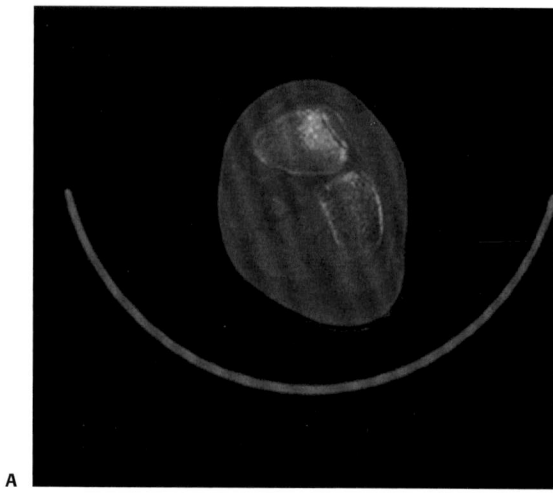
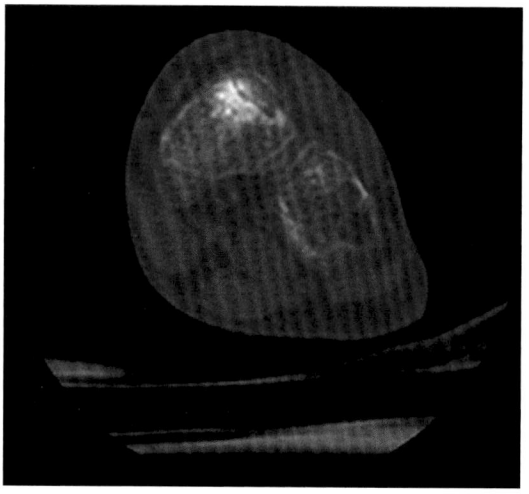

FIGURE 21-3 High-Risk stress fracture. **A:** CT example of a high-risk tarsal navicular stress fracture in a competitive dancer. **B:** After 3 months of nonoperative treatment, the fracture shows minimal signs of interval healing and has developed a nonunion.

in the case of tarsal navicular stress fractures (Fig. 21-3) as well as those of the vertebral pars interarticularis or linear stress fractures. CT scanning is useful for demonstrating evidence of healing by clearly showing the periosteal reaction and the absence of a discrete lucency or sclerotic fracture line.[20,26,31,50] It is also helpful in determining if the fracture is complete or incomplete.[98,126]

MRI is the most sensitive and specific imaging study available to evaluate stress injuries of bone.[59,73,118] This imaging modality has demonstrated superior sensitivity and specificity over bone scan and CT for associated soft tissue abnormalities and edema and may delineate injury earlier than bone scan.[59,115] MRI has been used more frequently recently as the primary diagnostic tool for stress fractures. Its sensitivity is similar to that of a bone scan; however, it is much more precise in delineating the anatomic location and extent of injury.[7,73,77]

Typical MRI findings on T2 sequences include a band of low signal corresponding to the fracture line, surrounded by diffuse high signal intensity representing marrow edema.[4] Though expensive, it has the additional benefit of identifying soft tissue injuries. In summary, MRI is highly useful clinically for the diagnosis of many stress fractures, especially if used by musculoskeletal radiologists familiar with specific imaging protocols.[7,118]

Classification/Grading

Stress fractures are classified in multiple ways but most commonly by the size of the fracture line seen on imaging, the severity of pain or disability, the biologic healing potential of the particular injury or location, the natural history of the particular fracture, or some combination of these parameters.[7,39,66,67,109] The classification of stress fractures as either "high risk" or "low risk," has been suggested by multiple authors.[18,19,22] High-risk stress fractures have at least one of the following characteristics: Risk of delayed union or nonunion, risk of refracture, and significant long-term consequences if they progress to complete fracture.[19,65] Table 21-1 shows a list of anatomic locations

considered high risk for stress fractures. This distinction allows clinicians to quickly determine if they can be aggressive or conservative with the decision to return an athlete to training or competition.

In addition to knowing the classification of whether a stress fracture is high risk or low risk as determined by its anatomic site, the extent of the fatigue failure or "grade" of the stress fracture is also needed to completely describe the injury and make appropriate treatment plans.[37,65–67] As described above, stress injuries to bone occur on a continuum from simple bone marrow edema (stress reaction) to a small microcrack with minor cortical disruption to a complete fracture with or without nonunion. The management of bony stress injuries should be based on the location and grade of the injury. These two details give us the amount of damage that has accumulated and whether it is a high- or low-risk injury. A combined clinical and radiographic classification system developed by the authors of this chapter is shown in Table 21-2. This system has shown high inter- and intra-observer reliability among sports medicine and orthopedic clinicians.[66] This chapter will later present a recommended treatment algorithm based on this classification system. Figures 21-4–21-7 show examples of the grades of stress fracture severity based on this classification system.[66]

TABLE 21-1 **Anatomic Sites for High-Risk Stress Fractures**[65]

- Femoral Neck (Tension Side)
- Patella (Tension Side)
- Anterior Tibial Cortex
- Medial Malleolus
- Talar Neck
- Dorsal Tarsal Navicular Cortex
- Fifth Metatarsal Proximal Metaphysis
- Sesamoids of the Great Toe

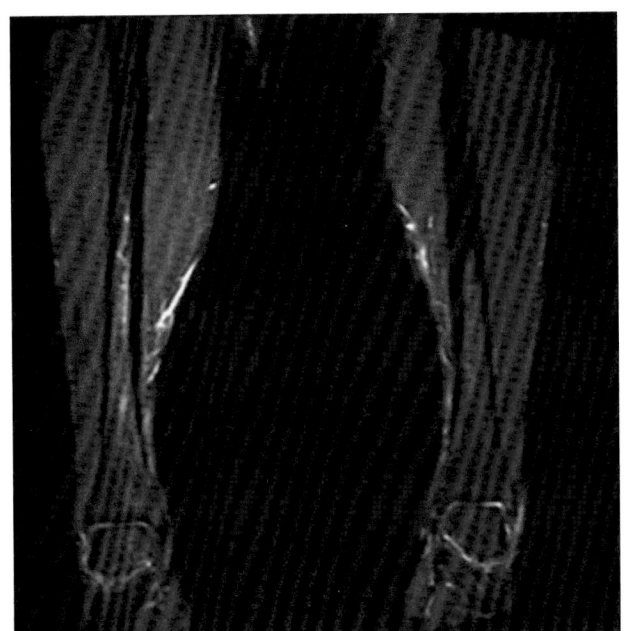
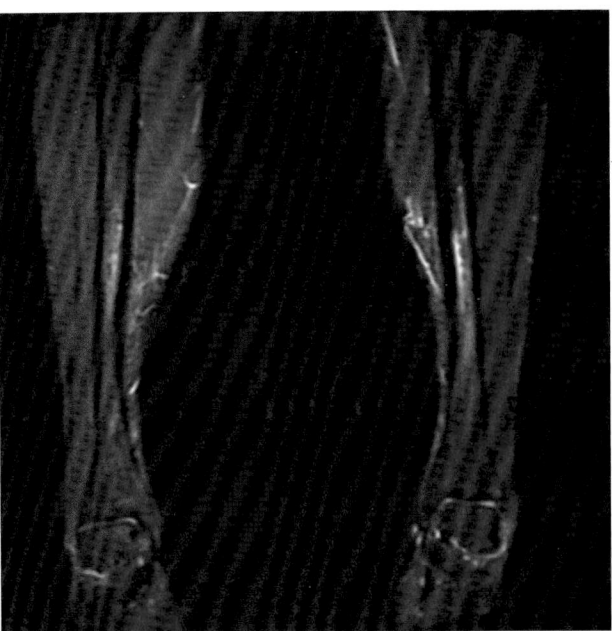

FIGURE 21-4 (A, B): T2 MRI examples of Kaeding–Miller Type I and Type II stress fractures of the tibia in a collegiate lacrosse player. The right tibial stress reaction was symptomatic with pain in this patient (Type II). The increased signal intensity in the left tibia representing a stress reaction was asymptomatic at the time of presentation (Type I).

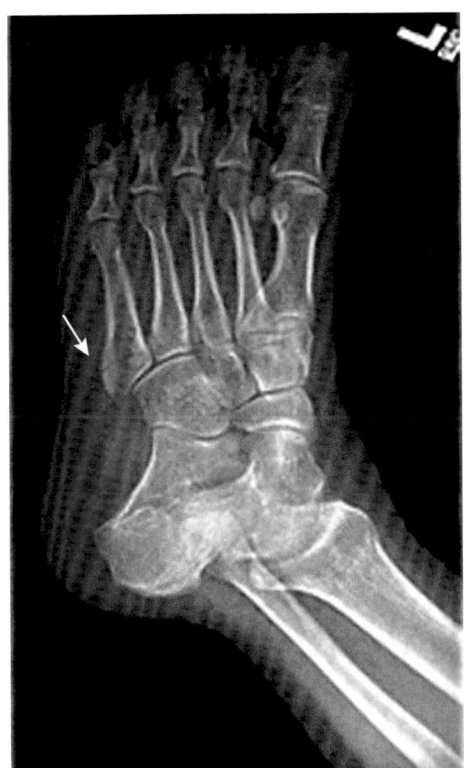

FIGURE 21-5 Kaeding–Miller Type III stress fracture of the fifth metatarsal in a 28-year-old male marathon runner.

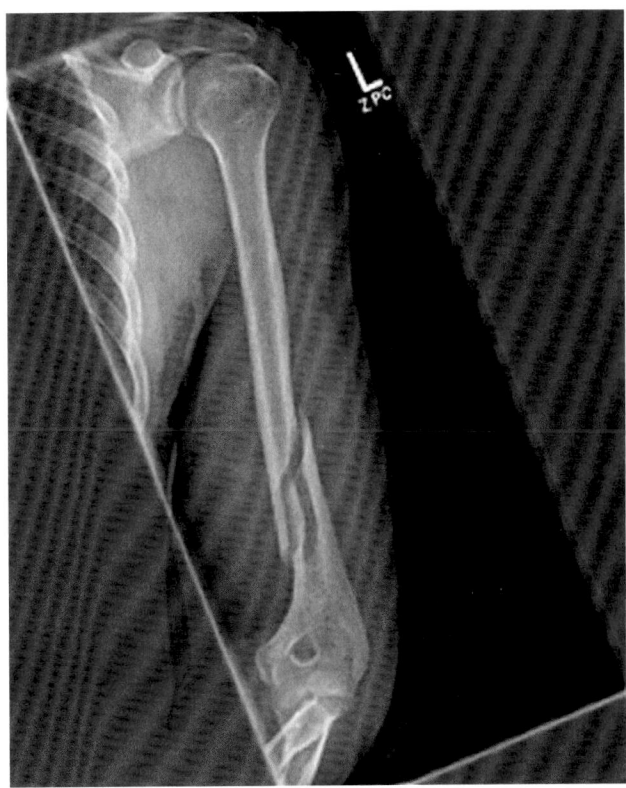

FIGURE 21-6 Kaeding–Miller Type IV stress fracture of the humeral shaft in baseball pitcher/football quarterback.

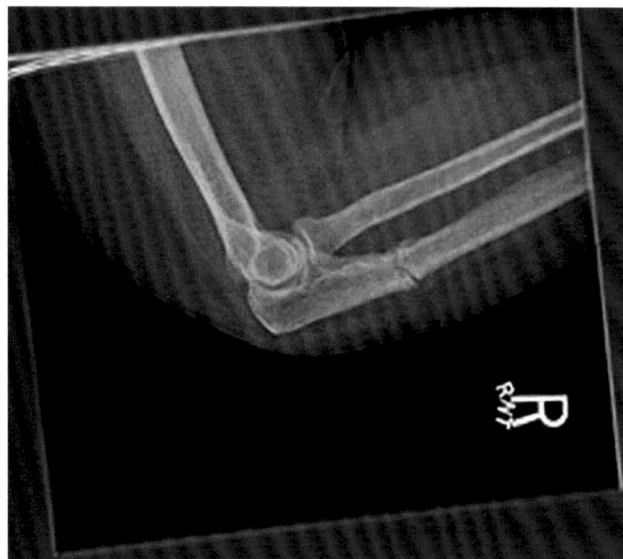

FIGURE 21-7 Kaeding–Miller Type V stress fracture of the ulnar shaft in a 35-year-old female who used crutches for 6 weeks following an ankle fracture.

HIGH-RISK STRESS FRACTURES VERSUS LOW-RISK STRESS FRACTURES

Low-risk stress fractures include the femoral shaft, medial tibia, ribs, ulnar shaft, and first through fourth metatarsals, all of which have a favorable natural history. These sites tend to be on the compressive side of the bone, and respond well to activity modification. A low-risk stress fracture is less likely to reoccur, develop nonunion, or have a significant complication should it progress to complete fracture.[18]

High-risk stress fracture locations are noted in Table 21-1. Not only do fractures at these anatomical sites have a predilection to progress to complete fracture, delayed union, or nonunion, have a refracture, or have significant long-term consequences

should they progress to a complete fracture, but they also often have worsening prognosis if they have a delay in diagnosis. A delay in treatment may prolong the patient's period of complete rest of the fracture site and potentially alter the treatment strategy to include surgical fixation with or without bone grafting. Due to their location on the tension side of the respective bones, these fractures possess common biomechanical properties regarding propagation of the fracture line. In comparison to low-risk stress fractures, high-risk stress fractures do not have an overall favorable natural history. With delay in diagnosis or with less aggressive treatment, high-risk stress fractures tend to progress to nonunion or complete fracture, require operative management, and recur in the same location.[19,94]

Management of High-Risk Stress Fractures

Treatment decision making for high-risk stress fractures should be based on radiographic findings with less consideration given to symptom severity. The immediate goal of treatment of a high-risk stress fracture is to avoid progression and get the fracture to heal. Typically this requires either complete elimination of loading of the site or surgical stabilization. Ideally while the fracture is healing, one works to avoid deconditioning of the athlete while minimizing the risk of a significant complication of fracture healing.[37,64] While overtreatment of a low-risk stress fracture may result in unnecessary deconditioning and loss of playing time, undertreatment of a high-risk injury puts the athlete and indeed all patients at risk of significant complications. Understanding the classification and grade of stress fractures and their implications is the key to providing optimal care to all patients with a high-risk injury.

The presence of a visible fracture line on a plain radiograph in a high-risk stress fracture should prompt serious consideration of operative management. Depending on injury classification, patients with stress injuries in high-risk locations may require immediate immobilization and/or restriction from weight-bearing activities with close monitoring. If an incomplete fracture is present on plain films with evidence of fracture on MRI or CT in a high-risk location, immobilization and strict nonweight bearing is indicated. Worsening symptoms or radiographic evidence of fracture progression despite nonoperative treatment is an indication for surgical fixation. All complete fractures at high-risk sites should receive serious consideration for surgical treatment. In summary, surgical fixation should be considered for high-risk stress fractures for several reasons. These include expediting healing of the fracture to allow earlier return to full activity as well as to minimize the risk of nonunion, delayed union, and refracture. Finally, surgical intervention may be necessary to prevent catastrophic fracture progression such as in the case of a tension-sided femoral neck fracture.[17,19]

Return to Sports Participation

Generally in athletes, return to play should only be recommended after proper treatment and complete healing of the injury. As previously mentioned, high-risk stress fractures have a significantly poorer prognosis when they progress to complete fracture as well as having more frequent complications. Because of the significant complications associated with progression to

TABLE 21-2	Kaeding–Miller Stress Fracture Classification System	
Grade	Pain	Radiographic Findings (CT, MRI, Bone Scan, or x-ray)
I	–	Imaging evidence of stress fracture No fracture line
II	+	Imaging evidence of stress fracture No fracture line
III	+	Nondisplaced fracture line
IV	+	Displaced fracture (>2 mm)
V	+	Nonunion

Note: Shown is a combined clinical and radiographic classification system for stress fractures that has shown high intra- and inter-observer reliability.
Kaeding, C, Miller T. The comprehensive description of stress fractures: A new classification system. *J Bone Joint Surg Am.* 2013;95:1214–1220.

complete fracture, it is not recommended that an individual be allowed to continue to participate in their activity with evidence of a high-risk stress fracture.[64] Complete rest, including weight-bearing restrictions, with or without immobilization or operative management is commonly required.[37]

The majority of early stress reactions at high-risk sites heal with nonoperative management.[19] A period of absolute rest to eliminate the individual's symptoms and gradual return to training with activity modification is suggested for early stress reactions at high-risk sites.[9] Return to play decision making for a low-grade injury at a high-risk location should be predicated on the patient's compliance level, healing potential, and risk of worsening of the injury. A key difference between a low-grade stress fracture at a high-risk location versus a low-risk location is that with the low-risk site the athlete or patient can be allowed to continue to train or otherwise be active, whereas the high-risk site needs to heal prior to full return to activity.

Regardless of the grade and location, the risk of continued participation should be discussed with each athlete, and the management of each fracture should be individualized. Cross-training while resting from the inciting activity allows maintenance of cardiovascular fitness while decreasing stresses at the healing fracture site.[37,60] Return to participation should be a joint decision between the physician, athletic trainer, coach, and athlete.

Management of Low-Risk Stress Fractures

Low-risk stress fractures may be treated nonoperatively with relative rest and activity modification. Decision making should be based in part on symptom severity. Those who experience enough pain to limit function should be treated with relative, if not complete, rest.[37] As the treatment algorithm in Figure 21-8 suggests, if the fracture does not heal or if symptoms persist beyond 4 to 6 weeks, the options for treatment are immobilization with restriction from weight-bearing or operative intervention. Those patients with a low-risk stress fracture who present with pain but have no functional limitation may continue their activities as tolerated using symptoms as a guide. The decision to continue activity despite the presence of a low-risk stress fracture and titrate the volume of activity to a low pain level can be made after a discussion with the patient of the possible progression to complete fracture with this approach. This approach is acceptable, if the risk and consequence of progression to complete fracture are acceptable to the patient due to the importance of their continuing their activity. If the goal is not to continue activity, but to heal the low-risk stress fracture, then rest to a pain-free level is required. The acceptable level of activity will differ among patients and may include discontinuation of only the aggravating activity, discontinuing all training activities, or placing the patient on a non–weight-bearing status. Unless otherwise contraindicated, a patient may be permitted to cross-train during this time with cycling, swimming, or aqua-running to maintain fitness as long it does not cause pain at the stress fracture site. As with high-risk stress fractures, close follow-up of these patients is necessary to assure compliance with activity restrictions and prevent fracture progression to a higher-grade injury.

Low-grade stress injuries at a low-risk site have a better prognosis for time to recovery than a higher-grade injury at the same low-risk site.[7,18] The difference in treatment of these two levels of severity, then, has to do with the expected time of treatment, the required degree of activity modification, and the need for immobilization. The goal of treating injuries with this level of severity is to decrease the repetitive stress at the fracture site enough to allow the body to restore the dynamic balance between damage and repair. This may include decreasing the volume and intensity of activity, equipment changes, technique changes, or cross-training. One benefit to such a strategy is that the individual typically does not suffer a substantial loss of conditioning while still allowing his or her body to repair the bone injury. If pain intensifies and activity modification alone is inadequate for healing, treatment should be intensified to include complete rest, immobilization, or surgical intervention (Fig. 21-8).

Return to Sports Participation

Despite advances in imaging and our understanding of stress fracture behavior, return to activity decisions continue to challenge sports medicine practitioners. Many factors need to be discussed with the athlete or patient. None of these considerations is more important than assessing and explaining the risks of continued participation, particularly in the setting of an ongoing injury. All patients should understand the risk of noncompliance with the treatment plan; this is especially true for high-risk stress fractures. A treatment plan should be tailored to the individual's athletic and personal goals with a thorough discussion of the risks and benefits of continued participation.[8,60,64,91]

In the treatment of low-risk stress fractures, the point in the competitive season at which the injury is diagnosed is often a major consideration for return to play. Athletes at the end of a competitive season or in their off season, often desire to be healed from their stress fracture before resumption of competition or preseason training.[64] For these individuals, the treatment plan should include relative rest and activity modification to a pain-free level. In contrast, athletes in mid-season with low-risk stress fractures often desire to finish the season and pursue treatment for a cure at a later time.[37] Low-risk stress fractures will usually heal by limiting the athlete to a pain-free level of activity for 4 to 8 weeks.[24] Gradual increase in activity can begin once the athlete is pain free with activities of daily living and when the site is nontender.[24]

UPPER-EXTREMITY STRESS FRACTURES

Stress fractures most commonly occur in the lower extremity as a result of the impact loading of walking, running, or jumping.[84] However, individuals performing repetitive tasks with the upper extremity and those who require upper extremity weight bearing may develop stress injuries of bone (Figs. 21-6 and 21-7). Upper-extremity stress fractures account for less than 10% of all stress fractures, and are commonly found in throwing athletes and rowers.[63,129] In recent years, there has been increased attention focused on upper-extremity stress fractures, and case

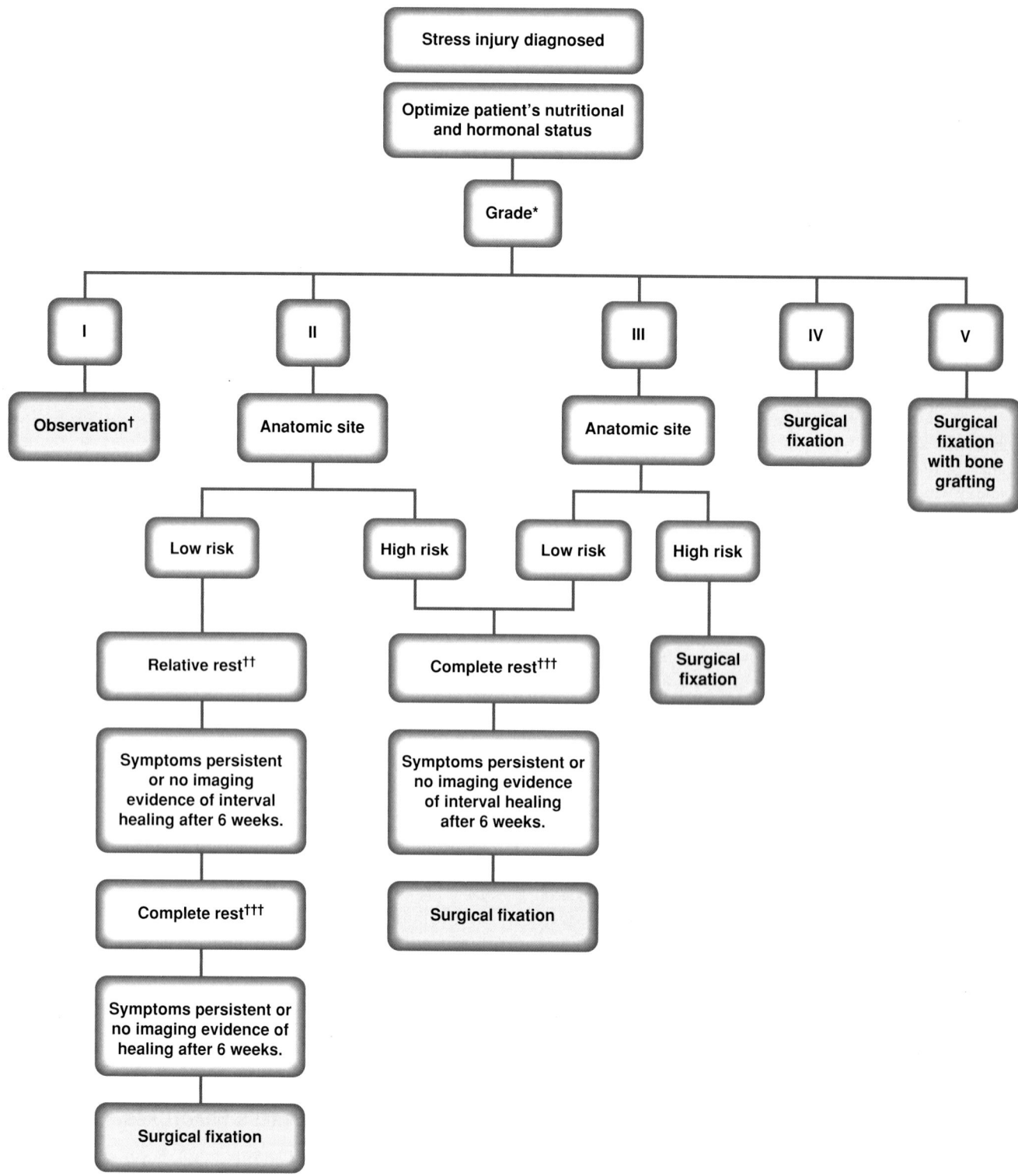

*Grade: Based on the Kaeding-Miller classification system presented in Table 21-2.
†Observation: Return to activity with close follow-up. Consider relative rest and cross-training.
††Relative rest: Decrease frequency or intensity of inciting activity. May cross-train gradual return to full pain-free activity.
†††Complete rest: Discontinuation of any activity that places stress at fracture site. May include immobilization.

FIGURE 21-8 Recommended treatment algorithm for stress injuries of bone.

reports of these injuries have increased. The great majority of these stress injuries are considered low risk and usually require only activity modification to heal. Repetitive torsion, weight bearing, and muscle contraction overload of bone must be considered when evaluating these injuries. Any repetitive overhead athlete or laborer complaining of the nontraumatic onset of pain in the upper extremity, with a normal examination and the presence of pain only with the repetitive activity should be considered as having a possible stress fracture.[63]

In the shoulder girdle, arm, forearm, and wrist, strain is generated by the rotational torque of swinging or throwing, as well as by the tension or compression generated by muscle contraction.[130] A third mechanism of creating bone stress in the upper extremity is repetitive axial loading. Sinha et al.[116] reviewed 40 stress fractures of the ribs and upper extremity. They noted that individuals performing weight-bearing activities of the upper extremity (gymnastics, cheerleading) developed all their stress fractures distal to the elbow, indicating that with such activities significant bony overload occurs in the distal upper extremity as opposed to the proximal portion.

As mentioned previously, the majority of upper-extremity stress injuries respond well to nonoperative treatment with rest and activity modification. One of the few stress fractures of the upper extremity that may require surgical intervention is the olecranon stress fracture in a competitive thrower. Though this injury has the potential to heal with conservative management, when a stress fracture line (Grade 3 injury) is discovered in a throwing athlete's olecranon process, internal fixation is the ideal treatment.[2,41,112]

Vertebral, Pelvic, and Sacral Stress Fractures

Spondylolysis, or a stress fracture of the pars interarticularis region of the posterior elements of the vertebrae, occurs most commonly in patients performing repetitive hyperextension of the spine (gymnasts, cheerleaders, divers, weight lifters), and is a common cause of pediatric low back pain.[77] The L4 and L5 levels are most commonly affected. Patients present with the insidious onset of low back pain ultimately with complaints of significant back spasms. This injury is often misdiagnosed as lumbar strain. Short periods of rest may temporarily relieve pain, but return to activity typically results in immediate exacerbation of symptoms.[25,77]

On examination, affected individuals may have clinical hyperlordosis in addition to pain with palpation over affected vertebral levels, and exquisite pain and muscle guarding with one- and two-leg standing trunk extension.[25] Pain may also be elicited by trunk rotation and extension, prone hip extension, and prone trunk extension. Neurologic evaluation is usually normal but occasionally the patient may have associated radiculopathy.[77]

On radiographic evaluation, x-rays have low sensitivity for stress fracture of the pars interarticularis.[25] Anteroposterior, lateral, and bilateral oblique views should be obtained. If positive, the classic defect of a "collar" on the neck (pars interarticularis) of the "Scotty dog" is seen on oblique views. X-ray imaging however has fallen out of favor in recent years because of low sensitivity and high radiation exposure. A SPECT scan has a greater sensitivity and is becoming the gold-standard test for diagnosis of a pars interarticularis stress fractures[77] (Fig. 21-2). A thin-cut CT scan (1.5- to 2-mm cuts) may additionally aid in determining the extent and age of a stress fracture in this area. Furthermore, a combination of SPECT and CT findings may help determine the likelihood of healing and may help define the treatment protocol.[77]

The treatment protocol for stress fractures of the pars interarticularis is somewhat controversial. Initially, activity modification and avoidance of lumbar hyperextension is recommended. If symptoms persist, a nonrigid brace such as a corset may be applied. After 2 to 4 weeks of rest and bracing, patients should begin a regimen of physical therapy which includes trunk stabilization, core strengthening, and lumbar spine flexibility exercises.[77] If pain is still present by 4 weeks, a thoracolumbosacral orthosis (TLSO) or low-profile rigid antilordotic Boston brace should be considered to unload posterior elements and prevent hyperextension. Treatment should be continued until the patient is symptom-free. Complete healing, however, may take as long as 3 to 6 months, and a repeat axial-cut CT scan may be considered to assess the amount of healing.[25]

Return to play may be as early as 8 weeks if the patient remains pain free at rest, in hyperextension, and while performing aggravating activities.[25] Surgical fixation may be considered if the patient continues to experience persistent pain despite rigid bracing, especially if neurologic symptoms are present or progressive.[77]

Pelvis and Sacrum

Stress fractures of the pelvis and sacrum are uncommon and typically involve the pubic rami. These injuries occur most often in women, military recruits, long-distance runners, or joggers after increases in duration, frequency, or intensity of impact-loading exercise.[55] Patients with stress fractures of the pubic rami present with insidious pain in the inguinal, perineal, or adductor regions that is relieved by rest. Sacral stress fractures present with vague, poorly localized pain in the gluteal or groin area.[42] Therefore, a high index of suspicion must be maintained.

On physical examination, patients may demonstrate an antalgic gait, tenderness over the pubic rami, or an inability to stand unsupported on the affected side. Patients with a sacral stress fracture may also demonstrate pain with hip flexion, abduction, and external rotation in addition to increased pain when asked to hop. These patients usually will have normal hip and spine range of motion but complain of deep groin pain at the extremes of hip motion.

X-rays are initially negative in most cases of both pelvic and sacral stress fractures.[25,42] Later in the healing process callus may be present on plain films. Bone scan or MRI is usually necessary for early diagnosis. Treatment requires cessation of running and jumping activities, protected weight bearing, and relative rest lasting from 6 weeks to 8 months. An initial brief period of nonweight bearing may be necessary based on the patient's pain level. Surgery is not typically necessary if the fracture is diagnosed in a timely manner.

LOWER-EXTREMITY STRESS FRACTURES

Femur

Stress injuries and fatigue fractures may occur at a variety of sites in the femur. The most commonly involved areas are the shaft, the intertrochanteric region, and the neck. As mentioned previously, the tension or superior side of the femoral neck is a high-risk site for fracture propagation. Here, a missed or delayed diagnosis significantly increases the patient's risk for a potentially catastrophic complete fracture.

Femoral Neck

Seen most frequently in runners, dancers, and military recruits, the diagnosis of a femoral neck stress fracture is often delayed for 5 to 13 weeks.[43,61,89] Unlike femoral shaft stress fractures, which are low risk and therefore heal with activity modification, femoral neck fractures are high-risk injuries.[19,36] Tension-sided femoral neck stress fractures possess the greatest risk for fracture progression.[19,36] The diagnosis requires a high degree of suspicion and usually occurs in runners with vague hip or groin pain. Examination will likely reveal an antalgic gait, pain with palpation in the groin, hip, or anterior thigh as well as pain at the extremes of hip range of motion.[40,42,48,49] Subtle limitation of flexion and internal rotation may also be present with or without a positive log roll test.[87]

Confirmation of the diagnosis usually requires bone scan and/or MRI. The radiographic appearance lags behind symptoms and may not be evident until some healing has occurred.[61] X-rays have a high false-negative rate. Bone scan or SPECT scans have proven useful for early diagnosis, but false negatives have been reported up to 12 days after symptom onset.[26] MRI is becoming more popular and is a sensitive study identifying early marrow edema, which typically resolves in 8 to 12 weeks.[59,115]

Femoral neck stress fractures require aggressive management with inferior cortex fractures requiring restricted weight bearing for 6 weeks or longer.[40,42,48,49] Weekly radiographs should be obtained until the patient can walk pain free with a cane. Return to play or other vigorous activity may be delayed up to 2 years.[114] We believe tension-sided stress fracture is an indication for surgical fixation with parallel screws or a sliding hip screw device.[131] If no displacement is present, some authors have advocated bed rest as the first-line treatment without immediate surgery.[9] Regardless, recognition of the tension-sided femoral neck stress fracture and immediate appropriate treatment is of utmost importance to prevent complete fracture, nonunion, and the potential development of femoral head osteonecrosis.[40,42,48,49]

Femoral Shaft Stress Fractures

Stress fractures of the femoral shaft are diagnosed most commonly in runners, in particular female runners, with the most common location being the junction of the proximal and middle thirds of femoral shaft.[55,101,123] As with most stress injuries of bone, the history often reveals a recent increase in frequency, intensity, or duration of a repetitive activity. Pain with running then progresses to pain with activities of daily living and functional limitation. Examination is positive for an antalgic gait

with normal knee and hip range of motion. Pain with palpation may be present at the anterior thigh with hopping on the affected leg reproducing the pain. The fulcrum or "hanging leg" test involves having the patient seated on an examination table with the leg hanging freely. A three-point bending force is then applied to the thigh with the edge of the table being used as a fulcrum. Pain elicited is indicative of a stress fracture. As with most stress injuries plain x-rays are typically negative early in the course of the injury. Fracture callus and a radiolucent fracture line usually appear 2 to 6 weeks after symptom onset. Bone scan or MRI may be necessary for an early diagnosis.

Nonoperative treatment of femoral shaft stress fractures is usually successful. First-line interventions include protected weight bearing with crutches for 1 to 4 weeks depending on symptom severity and radiologic grade of the injury. Activity modification with cross-training during this time period allows maintenance of aerobic fitness, skill, and strength. If the patient is pain free with day-to-day activities at 2 weeks, a rehabilitation program with low-impact exercise may be initiated. Time to full recovery varies, but has been reported as 5 to 10 weeks from diagnosis with return to full athletic participation at 8 to 16 weeks.

Knee and Lower Leg Stress Fractures
Patella

Patellar stress fractures are rare but troublesome injuries occurring most often in basketball players, soccer players, and high jumpers.[65,122] Risk factors for a tension-sided (anterior cortex) stress fracture of the patella are flexion contracture and/or harvest of a patellar tendon graft for ACL reconstruction.[122] The patient's history reveals anterior knee pain, worse with jumping. The key diagnostic features are point tenderness to palpation of the anterior patella and increased pain with resisted knee extension.[65] Radiographic studies may show fracture lines in longitudinal or transverse directions, but these must be differentiated from a bipartite or tripartite patella.[122] A bone or MRI scan identifying bone edema can clarify the diagnosis.

Due to the distractive forces of the extensor mechanism, transverse fractures are prone to displacement. Nondisplaced fractures are treated in a hinged knee brace with the knee in full extension for 4 to 6 weeks, followed by progressive range of motion and quadriceps rehabilitation.

Displaced fractures should be treated with open reduction and surgical fixation.[65] Fractures in a longitudinal direction occur most often at the lateral patellar facet, and if displaced, the lateral fragment may be excised. Case series have reported that acute nondisplaced fractures can heal with immobilization and relative rest, but open reduction and internal fixation is recommended for chronic or displaced fractures.

Tibial Shaft Stress Fractures

Stress fractures of the tibia represent 20% to 75% of all stress fractures in athletes.[8,16] To effectively treat stress injuries at this anatomical site, a distinction must be made between medial tibial stress syndrome (shin splints), a compression-sided stress fracture, and a tension-sided stress fracture. The most predominant

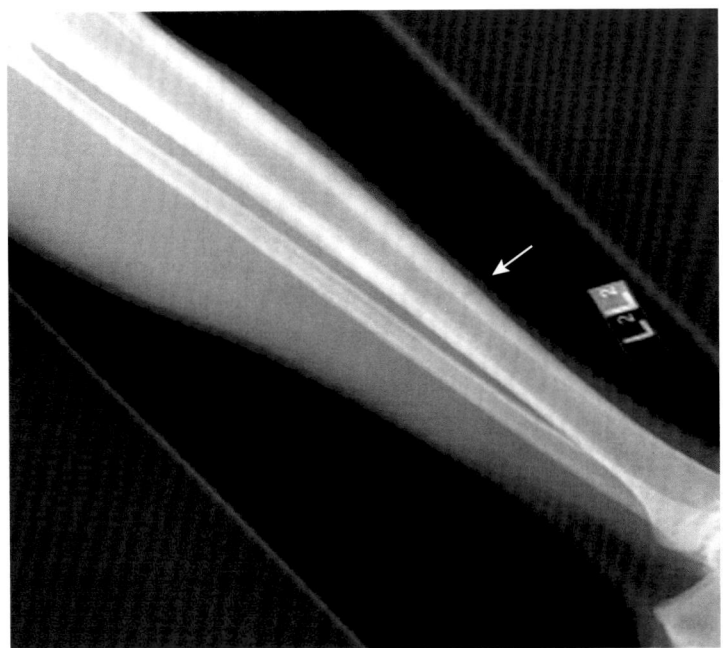
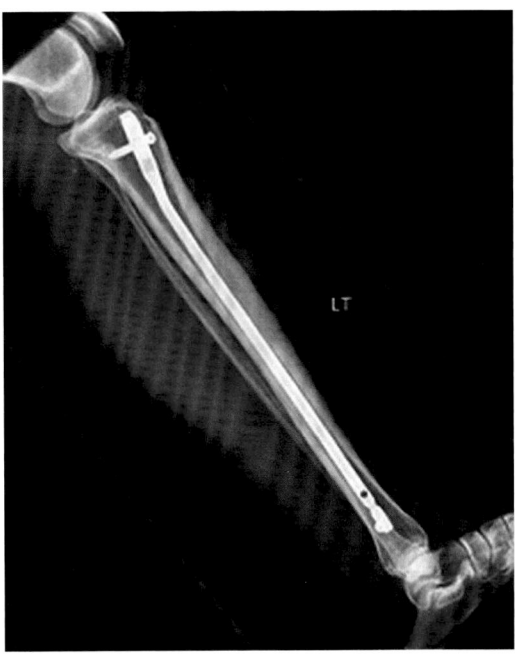

FIGURE 21-9 A: Case example of a 23-year-old female college soccer player with chronic anterior tibial pain and stress fracture of the anterior tibial cortex *(arrow)*. **B:** Final treatment required operative fixation with a statically locked intramedullary rod. Cortical thickening remains evident 6 months post surgery.

type is a low-risk posteromedial cortex (compression side) stress fracture with the much less common type being the high-risk "dreaded black line" of the anterolateral cortex of the central shaft (Fig. 21-9A).[54,128] Most commonly occurring in running sports such as soccer, track, and field, basketball or ballet, the pain occurs initially after activity. Pain later develops during running and progresses to eventually affect activities of daily living. On examination, there is localized pain with point tenderness at the anterior or medial tibia. Edema, palpable periosteal thickening, and pain with percussion may also be present. A "tuning fork test" may be performed to elicit pain if a high pretest probability is present but is generally not performed due to a high false-negative rate and limited availability of the proper equipment.[81]

X-rays may be positive if symptoms have persisted for 4 to 6 weeks. Bone scan often demonstrates focal fusiform uptake, which differs from the linear uptake seen with medial tibial stress syndrome.[28,39] MRI is more useful for grading and providing a prognosis for return to play (Figs. 21-1 and 21-4A,B).[46]

Treatment should initially involve steps to control pain and limit, if not completely discontinue, running or jumping activities. The use of crutches, immobilization, and limited weight bearing may be necessary depending on symptom severity and fracture classification.[83,134] If the fracture is diagnosed early, it frequently may be treated by limiting practice activities but still participate in competitions. Once pain free, cross-training with low-impact or nonimpact aerobic training may begin and be used to supplement training during a gradual return to running. Compression-sided injuries may take 2 to12 weeks to heal. Tension-sided injuries achieve faster return to play with intramedullary (IM) rod fixation (Fig. 21-9B).[27,128] The options for treatment of

injuries in this location include 4 to 6 months of rest, bone grafting, electrical stimulation, or IM nailing.[65] If a patient or athlete desires to resume training for sports at the same or increased intensity, IM nailing is usually recommended.[105]

Medial Malleolus

Stress fractures of the medial malleolus are relatively rare and are usually associated with running and jumping sports.[95,113] They are inherently unstable and prone to nonunion.[104] A high index of suspicion is the key to their early recognition as patients typically present with the insidious onset of medial ankle pain that is increased with exercise and relieved by rest. Physical examination reveals medial malleolar tenderness to palpation and an effusion of the ankle joint. It is important to also evaluate the patients for any predisposing factors that may contribute to stress overloading in the area such as foot or lower limb alignment.[95,113] Varus alignment in particular, can cause medial overload.[93] On x-ray, the fracture line extends vertically or horizontally from the medial articular surface of the tibial plafond.

Treatment of an incomplete fracture requires no weight bearing and immobilization with gradual rehabilitation in low-demand individuals. In high-demand athletes and those who wish early return to sports participation, a more aggressive approach may be warranted. Complete fractures require treatment with open reduction and malleolar screw fixation. As with traumatic ankle fractures, most patients return to full activity by 6 to 8 weeks postoperatively. Nonunion of a medial malleolar stress fracture requires bone grafting and screw fixation.[104]

Fibula

Stress fractures of the fibula are also rare given the limited amount of weight-bearing stress borne by this bone. The most common location is in the distal third of the diaphysis just proximal to the distal tibiofibular syndesmosis. It may be associated with overpronation and a valgus hind foot.[88] Patients typically present with lateral leg and ankle pain with mild swelling and may have a notable limp. Point tenderness can be elicited by palpation of the bone or by performing a syndesmosis squeeze test. Recommended initial treatment is weight bearing as tolerated in a protective fracture brace, followed by gradual return to activity once pain and swelling have resolved. With early diagnosis, athletes may return to participation after 3 to 6 weeks of rest.[18] Complete healing occurs within approximately 8 to 12 weeks.

Stress Fractures of the Foot

Calcaneus

Calcaneal stress fractures occur most commonly in long-distance runners and military recruits from repetitive loading of the heel with weight-bearing activities. Patients present with the insidious onset of diffuse heel pain with running that may be increased by toe walking or during the toe-off phase of running. Examination reveals edema and a positive "heel squeeze" test. This is performed by compressing the body of the calcaneus between the palms of both hands. Increased pain with hop testing may also be present.

Plain x-rays become positive after 2 to 4 weeks. At that time a sclerotic line with callus perpendicular to the trabecular lines of the calcaneal tuberosity may be visualized. Bone scan and MRI usually demonstrate increased reactive bone in this region as well, confirming the diagnosis. Initial treatment is to decrease activity and use cushioned heel inserts until symptoms have improved and healing is evident radiographically. The use of a cast or brace and a brief period of nonweight bearing may be necessary if ambulation is painful. The estimated time to return to sports participation is 3 to 8 weeks.

Tarsal Navicular

Previously thought to be uncommon, navicular stress fractures are now frequently recognized in jumping and running athletes.[14,29,30,58,79] This is a high-risk stress fracture.[19,65,78] Patients present with vague midfoot and medial arch symptoms of insidious onset often leading to delayed diagnosis[110,125,126] and the final diagnosis may be delayed from 2 to 7 months.[71,126] On examination, patients report tenderness at the "N spot" (the dorsal aspect of the navicular), but pain may be diffuse rather than localized. Continued weight-bearing activity may delay the healing process, resulting in progression to a complete fracture or nonunion. Therefore, midfoot pain in a running or jumping athlete requires a high index of suspicion and early aggressive management.

Since most fractures occur in the sagittal plane and in the central third of the dorsal navicular cortex, x-rays are usually negative.[86] It has been proposed that this site has a poor blood supply predisposing the bone to stress-related injury.[56,96] This region has also been correlated with the plane of maxi-

mum shear stress during a combination of plantar flexion and pronation.[34,52,72] Associated foot anomalies that may predispose a patient to this type of fracture include a short first metatarsal, a long second metatarsal or a calcaneonavicular coalition.[98,125,126]

Bone scan can confirm the diagnosis, but CT (Fig. 21-3) or MRI may be necessary to determine the exact location and extent of the fracture and the amount of healing or to diagnose a nonunion.[86] The key to a successful outcome in treating this injury is early diagnosis with aggressive treatment.[111] Current literature supports nonsurgical treatment of incomplete fractures and no weight bearing is recommended in a cast for 6 to 8 weeks followed by gradual rehabilitation.[97,100,125] Upon return to play the use of orthotics should be considered if a bony abnormality or poor biomechanics are present.[72]

The decision to surgically treat a navicular fracture has typically been ascribed to fractures that are complete and/or show evidence of sclerosis at the margins.[86] Surgical fixation with or without bone grafting is suggested for those in whom nonsurgical management has failed.[45,70,71,100] Because of the poor blood supply to the region where the fracture occurs, it is crucial to immobilize the fracture site after surgery and until radiographic healing has occurred.[98]

Metatarsal Stress Fractures

First Through Fourth Metatarsals

Stress fractures of the first through fourth metatarsals are generally considered low-risk injuries. Excluding the fifth metatarsal, first metatarsal stress fractures make up 10% of all metatarsal stress injuries and are associated with overpronation during running. The remaining 90% are distributed between the second, third, and fourth metatarsals.[44] Stress injuries to these bones are associated with running over 20 miles/week. Pes planus deformity increases the impact stress to the medial four metatarsals. In runners, most injuries occur in the distal shaft. However, in ballet dancers, fractures may occur proximally and often involve the medial border of the second metatarsal due to weight bearing in the *en pointe* position. Patients present with localized pain and swelling in the absence of trauma and report symptom onset after an increase in training intensity. Close inspection of the foot may reveal low arches, overpronation while running, and point tenderness over the involved metatarsal. Pain is often exacerbated with inversion of the foot.[44]

Weight-bearing AP, lateral, and oblique radiographs should be obtained. In dancers with second metatarsal pain, internal and external oblique radiographs of the foot may be necessary to fully evaluate the involved bone. Treatment involves rest and the use of a stiff-soled shoe or fracture boot to decrease bending stresses across the midfoot.[44] Gradual reconditioning with progression of repetitive loading such as pool running progressing to cycling, then land running is recommended in athletes to maintain cardiovascular fitness and prevent progression of the injury. Once the fracture has healed, orthotic devices should be prescribed if abnormal bony alignment or foot biomechanics are present. In dancers, proximal second metatarsal stress fractures may progress to nonunion and must be aggressively

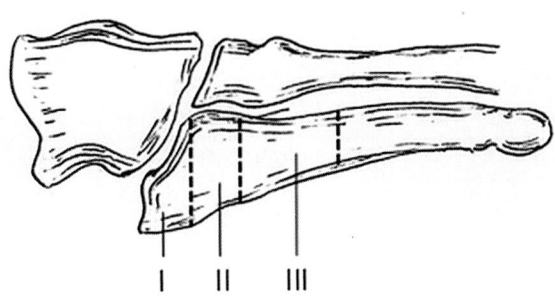

FIGURE 21-10 Illustration demonstrating the three zones of the proximal fifth metatarsal. Zone I, tuberosity; Zone II, watershed (avascular) zone at the metaphyseal–diaphyseal junction; Zone III, proximal diaphysis.[124]

managed with casting or fracture bracing until radiographic healing is present (usually 6 to 8 weeks).

Fifth Metatarsal

The proximal fifth metatarsal is considered a high-risk site for stress fracture. Because of the poor blood supply to the affected area, both stress injuries and traumatic injuries are prone to nonunion.[1,120,121] Figure 21-10 demonstrates the three zones of the proximal fifth metatarsal. Zone I represents the tuberosity; zone II the watershed or avascular area at the metaphyseal–diaphyseal junction.[116] Zone III represents the proximal diaphysis. Fractures occurring in zone II have the greatest risk for delayed healing due to the limited vascularity of this site.[1,120,124] Occurring commonly in basketball players and runners, these injuries present with the insidious onset of lateral foot pain that is worse during and after running or jumping activity.[120] Pain steadily worsens if the causative activity is continued. Not uncommonly an acute fracture occurs following days to weeks of antecedent pain. On clinical evaluation, point tenderness is present directly over the fracture.[124] Plain x-rays usually show sclerotic change around the fracture site (Fig. 21-5). Bone scans are only occasionally necessary for diagnosis, but bone scan or MRI may be employed if an occult fracture is suspected.

Treatment for stress fractures of the proximal fifth metatarsal, as with all high-risk anatomical sites, should be aggressive.[33,35] In nonathletes, a short-leg non–weight-bearing cast or fracture brace for 6 to 8 weeks is recommended. Longer immobilization may be required if no radiographic evidence of healing has occurred during that time period.[33] Because of the potentially prolonged healing time and risk of refracture or nonunion following conservative treatment, there is now a greater tendency to use surgical fixation as the primary treatment.[51,76,80,90] This tendency is shared by the authors of this chapter.

In high-demand athletes, IM screw fixation with a 4- or 4.5-mm cannulated screw permits faster return to play since casting alone in this population has been shown to have a high failure rate.[99,103] If nonunion is not present, bone grafting usually is not necessary at the time of IM fixation. Weight bearing should be initiated 7 to 14 days postoperatively, with training progressing to full unrestricted activity over 9 weeks. Return

to sports activities is expected at approximately 3 to 9 weeks postoperatively in patients with zone II or III fractures.[126] A risk, however, remains for fracture nonunion and fatigue failure of the screw.[136]

Sesamoids

Sesamoid stress fracture is a rare and difficult diagnosis to make. This injury must be differentiated from sesamoiditis, bipartite, and tripartite sesamoids, hallux rigidus and a painful soft tissue callous.[127] The medial sesamoid is most frequently involved. Because most of the body's weight is transferred through the medial aspect of the first metatarsal during the toe-off phase of activity, the medial sesamoid receives both tensile and compressive stresses.[65] Patients with this injury typically present with pain localized to the plantar surface of the first metatarsal head which is worse upon weight bearing and during the toe-off phase of the gait cycle. Pain on palpation, pain with resisted active great toe plantarflexion, and pain over the sesamoids with stretch into full dorsiflexion of the first metatarsophalangeal joint are positive indicators on physical examination.[127] Diagnosis of sesamoid stress fracture by x-ray is challenging, if not impossible, when the fracture is nondisplaced. Additional imaging, including bone scan or MRI, is often required to identify marrow edema and differentiate stress fracture from a bipartite sesamoid.

Conservative treatment with 6 weeks of non–weight-bearing cast immobilization to prevent dorsiflexion of first ray is the recommended initial treatment.[65] Unloading of the first metatarsal head is the primary goal. Consideration should also be given to the use of orthotic devices in the shoe after casting. Complete resolution of this fracture and its symptoms may take as long as 4 to 6 months.[88] Surgical excision is recommended for delayed union or chronic pain.[106] Removal of the entire medial sesamoid may, however, result in weakening of the flexor hallucis brevis insertion on the proximal phalanx, resulting in the great toe drifting into valgus. Partial sesamoidectomy has been suggested as an alternative to complete sesamoidectomy to effectively resolve symptoms and maintain normal mechanics of the great toe.[65] Surgery is considered to be a last resort and generally should be avoided in athletes.

PREVENTION OF STRESS INJURIES

Prevention is the ideal treatment of stress injuries of bone. An assessment of the athlete's risk should be made at preparticipation evaluations, especially in those with a history of previous stress fractures.[37,64] Correction of amenorrhea in females and calcium and Vitamin D supplementation is recommended in addition to general nutritional optimization. If biomechanical abnormalities are encountered, the use of appropriately designed orthotic devices should be considered as an initial corrective measure. However, gait analysis, appropriate running form, and technique changes may be necessary to prevent future injuries.

SUMMARY

The diagnosis of a stress fracture is usually straightforward if a high index of suspicion is maintained and the proper imaging studies are obtained. They are common injuries particularly in endurance athletes and military recruits. The authors' classification system for stress fractures characterizes these injuries based on the patient's symptoms as well as their position on a radiographic continuum of severity. Our recommended treatment algorithm further stratifies these injuries as either high risk or low risk based upon the biomechanical environment in which they are located. High-risk stress fractures are primarily loaded in tension, have a poor natural history, and commonly require surgical intervention. Low-risk fractures are most often those loaded in compression, have a better prognosis, and are unlikely to progress to complete fracture. The goal of this algorithm is to provide clinicians with general guidelines for the management of stress fractures based on recent literature findings and the authors' clinical experience. It should not be interpreted as a set of rigid rules for treatment. Stress fracture management should be individualized to the patient taking into consideration injury site (low risk vs. high risk), grade (extent of microdamage accumulation), the individual's activity level, competitive situation, and risk tolerance.

REFERENCES

1. Agarwal A. Jones' fracture. *Tex Med.* 1993;89(6):60–61.
2. Ahmad C, ElAttrache NS. Valgus extension overload syndrome and stress injury of the olecranon. *Clin Sports Med.* 2004;23(4):665–676.
3. Albe E, Youngber R. Occult fractures of the femoral neck. *Am J Sports Med.* 1994;17:65–76.
4. Amendola A, Sitler D. *MRI of the Foot and Ankle: The Orthopaedic Surgeon's Perspective in Practical MR Imaging of the Foot and Ankle.* Boca Raton, FL: CRC Press LLC; 2000.
5. Anderson M, Greenspan A. Stress fractures. *Radiology.* 1966;199:1–12.
6. Anderson M. Imaging of upper extremity stress fractures in the athlete. *Clin Sports Med.* 2006;25(3):489–504.
7. Arendt EA, Griffiths HJ. The use of MR imaging in the assessment and clinical management of stress reactions of bone in high-performance athletes. *Clin Sports Med.* 1997;16:291–306.
8. Arendt EA, Agel J, Heikes C, et al. Stress injuries to bone in college athletes. *Am J Sports Med.* 2003;31(6):959–968.
9. Aro H, Dahlstrom S. Conservative management of distraction-type stress fractures of the femoral neck. *J Bone Joint Surg Br.* 1986;68:65–67.
10. Baker J, Frankel VH, Burstein A. Fatigue fractures: Biomechanical considerations. *J Bone Joint Surg Am.* 1972;54:1345–1346.
11. Balius R, Pedret C, Estruch A, et al. Stress fractures of the metacarpal bones in adolescent tennis players. *Am J Sports Med.* 2010; 38(6):1215–1220.
12. Banks K, Ly JQ, Beall DP, et al. Overuse injuries of the upper extremity in the competitive athlete. *Curr Probl Diagn Radiol.* 2005;34(4):127–142.
13. Barrow GW, Saha S. Menstrual irregularity and stress fractures in collegiate female distance runners. *Am J Sports Med.* 1988;16:209–216.
14. Bartz RL, Marymont JV. Tarsal navicular fractures in major league baseball players at bat. *Foot and Ankle International.* 2001;22(11):908–910.
15. Bennell K, Brukner P. Epidemiology and site specificity of stress fractures. *Clin Sports Med.* 1997;16:179–196.
16. Bennell KL, Malcolm SA, Thomas SA, et al. The incidence and distribution of stress fractures in competitive track and field athletes. A twelve-month prospective study. *Am J Sports Med.* 1996;24(2):211.
17. Blickenstaff LD, Morris JM. Fatigue fractures of the femoral neck. *J Bone Joint Surg Am.* 1966;48:1031–1047.
18. Boden B, Osbahr DC, Jimenez C. Low-risk stress fractures. *Am J Sports Med.* 2001;29(1):100–111.
19. Boden B. High-risk stress fractures: Evaluation and treatment. *J Am Acad Orthop Surg.* 2000;8:344–353.
20. Bradshaw C, Khan K, Brukner P. Stress fracture of the body of the talus in athletes demonstrated with computer tomography. *Clin J Sport Med.* 1996;6:48–51.
21. Breithaupt MD. Zur pathologie des menschlichen fusses. *Med Zeitung.* 1855;36:169–171,37:175–177.
22. Brukner P, Bradshaw C, Bennell K. Management of common stress fractures: Let risk level guide treatment. *Phys Sportsmed.* 1998;26(8):39–47.
23. Brukner P, Bradshaw C, Khan KM, et al. Stress fractures: A review of 180 cases. *Clin J Sport Med.* 1996;6(2):85–89.
24. Brukner P. Stress fractures of the upper limb. *Sports Med.* 1998;26:415–424.
25. Brukner P, Bennell K, Matheson G. Stress fractures of the trunk. In: Brukner P, ed. *Stress Fractures.* Victoria: Blackwell Science; 1999:119–138.
26. Bryant L, Song WS, Banks KP, et al. Comparison of planar scintigraphy alone with SPECT for the initial evaluation of femoral neck stress fractures. *Am J Roentgenol.* 2008;191:1010–1015.
27. Chang PS, Harris RM. Intramedullary nailing for chronic tibial stress fractures: A review of five cases. *Am J Sports Med.* 1996;24:688–692.
28. Chisin R, Milgrom C, Giladi M, et al. Clinical significance of nonfocal scintigraphic findings in suspected tibial stress fractures. *Clin Orthop Relat Res.* 1987;220:200–205.
29. Coris EE, Lombardo JA. Tarsal navicular stress fractures. *Am Fam Physician.* 2003;67(1):85–90.
30. Coughlin M. Tarsal navicular stress fractures. *Tech Foot Ankle Surg.* 2002;1(2):112–122.
31. Coughlin MJ, Grimes JS, Traughber PD, et al. Comparison of radiographs and CT scans in the prospective evaluation of the fusion of hindfoot arthrodesis. *Foot Ankle Int.* 2006;27(10):780–787.
32. Daffner RH, Pavlov H. Stress fractures: Current concepts. *Am J Roentgenol.* 1992;159:245–252.
33. Dameron TB Jr. Fractures of the proximal fifth metatarsal: Selecting the best treatment option. *J Am Acad Orthop Surg.* 1995;3:110–114.
34. Daniels T, DiGiovanni C, Lau JTC, et al. Prospective clinical pilot trial in a single cohort group of rhPDGF in foot arthrodesis. *Foot Ankle Int.* 2010;31(6):473–479.
35. DeLee JC, Evans JP, Julian J. Stress fracture of the fifth metatarsal. *Am J Sports Med.* 1983;11:349–353.
36. Devas MB. Stress fractures of the femoral neck. *J Bone Joint Surg Br.* 1965;47:728–738.
37. Diehl J, Best TM, Kaeding CC. Classification and return-to-play consideration for stress fractures. *Clin Sports Med.* 2006;25(1):17–28.
38. Drinkwater BL, Nilson K, Chesnut CH III, et al. Bone mineral content of amenorrheic and eumenorrheic athletes. *N Engl J Med.* 1984;311:277–281.
39. Dutton J. Clinical value of grading the scintigraphic appearances of tibial stress fractures in military recruits. *Clin Nucl Med.* 2002;27(1):18–21.
40. Egol K. Stress fractures of the femoral neck. *Clin Orthop Relat Res.* 1998;348:72–78.
41. El Attrache NS, Ahmed CS. Valgus extension overload syndrome and olecranon stress fractures. *Sports Med Arthrosc Rev.* 2003;11:25–29.
42. Eller DJ, Katz DS, Bergman AG, et al. Sacral stress fractures in long-distance runners. *Clin J Sport Med.* 1997;7:222–225.
43. Ernst J, et al. Stress fracture of the neck of the femur. *J Trauma.* 1964;4:71–83.
44. Fetzer G, Wright RW. Metatarsal shaft fractures and fractures of the proximal fifth metatarsal. *Clin Sports Med.* 2006;25:139–150.
45. Fitch KD, Blackwell JB, Gilmour WN. Operation for the non-union of stress fracture of the tarsal navicular. *J Bone Joint Surg Br.* 1989;71:105–110.
46. Fredericson M, Bergman AG, Hoffman KL, et al. Tibial stress reaction in runners: Correlation of clinical symptoms and scintigraphy with a new magnetic resonance imaging grading system. *Am J Sports Med.* 1995;23:472–481.
47. Fredericson M, Jennings F, Beaulieu C, et al. Stress fractures in athletes. *Top Magn Reson Imaging* 2006;17(5):309–325.
48. Fullerton LR Jr, Snowdy HA. Femoral neck stress fractures. *Am J Sports Med.* 1988;16:365–377.
49. Fullerton L. Femoral neck stress fractures. *Sports Med.* 1990;9(3):192–197.
50. Gaeta M, Minutoli F, Vinci S, et al. High-resolution CT grading of tibial stress reactions in distance runners. *Am J Roentgenol.* 2006;187:789–793.
51. Glasgow MT, Naranja RJ Jr, Glasgow SG, et al. Analysis of failed surgical management of fractures of the base of the fifth metatarsal distal to the tuberosity: The Jones fracture. *Foot Ankle Int.* 1996;17:449–457.
52. Goergen TG, Venn-Watson EA, Rossman DJ, et al. Tarsal navicular stress fractures in runners. *Am J Roentgenol.* 1981;136(1):201–203.
53. Greaney RB, Gerber FH, Laughlin RL, et al. Distribution and natural history of stress fractures in U.S. Marine recruits. *Radiology.* 1983;146:339–346.
54. Green NE, Rogers RA, Lipscomb AB. Nonunions of stress fractures of the tibia. *Am J Sports Med.* 1985;13:171–176.
55. Hod N, Ashkenazi I, Levi Y, et al. Characteristics of skeletal stress fractures in female military recruits of the Israel Defense Forces on bone scintigraphy. *Clin Nucl Med.* 2006;31:742–749.
56. Hulkko A, Orava S, Peltokallio P, et al. Stress fracture of the navicular bone: Nine cases in athletes. *Acta Orthop Scand.* 1985;56(6):503–505.
57. Hulkko A, Orava S Stress fractures in athletes. *Int J Sports Med.* 1987;8:221–226.
58. Hunter LY. Stress fracture of the tarsal navicular: More frequent than we realize? *Am J Sports Med.* 1981;9(4):217–219.
59. Ishibashi Y, Okamura Y, Otsuka H, et al. Comparison of scintigraphy and MRI for stress injuries of bone. *Clin J Sport Med.* 2002;12(2):79–84.
60. Jensen S. Stress fracture in the world class athlete: A case study. *Med Sci Sports Exerc.* 1998;30:783–787.
61. Johansson C, Ekenman I, Törnkvist H, et al. Stress fractures of the femoral neck in athletes. The consequence of a delay in diagnosis. *Am J Sports Med.* 1990;18:524–528.
62. Jones BH, Harris JM, Vinh TN, et al. Exercise-induced stress fractures and stress reactions of bone: Epidemiology, etiology, and classification. *Exerc Sport Sci Rev.* 1989;17:379–422.
63. Jones G. Upper extremity stress fractures. *Clin J Sport Med.* 2006;25(1):159–174.
64. Kaeding CC, Yu JR, Wright R, et al. Management and return to play of stress fractures. *Clin J Sport Med.* 2005;15(6):442–447.
65. Kaeding CC, Spindler KP, Amendola A. Management of troublesome stress fractures. *Instr Course Lect.* 2004;53:455–469.
66. Kaeding, C, Miller T. The comprehensive description of stress fractures: A new classification system. *J Bone Joint Surg Am.* 2013;95:1214–1220.
67. Kaeding CC, Najarian RG. Stress fractures: Classification and management. *Phys Sportsmed.* 2010;38(3):45–54.
68. Keaveny TM, Hayes WC. Mechanical properties of cortical and trabecular bone. In: Hall BK, ed. *Bone.* Vol 7. Boca Raton, FL: CRC Press; 1993:285–344.
69. Kempfer G, et al. Stress fracture and nuclear medicine. *Rev Bras Med Esporte.* 2004;10(6):532–534.
70. Khan KM, Brukner PD, Kearney C, et al. Tarsal navicular stress fracture in athletes. *Sports Med.* 1994;17(1):65–76.

71. Khan KM, Fuller PJ, Brukner PD, et al. Outcome of conservative and surgical management of navicular stress fracture in athletes: Eighty-six cases proven with computerized tomography. *Am J Sports Med.* 1992;20(6):657–666.

72. Kitaoka H, Luo Z, An K. Contact features of the talonavicular joint of the foot. *Clin Orthop Relat Res.* 1996;325:290–295.

73. Kiuru MJ, Pihlajamäki HK, Perkiö JP et al. Dynamic contrast-enhanced MRI in symptomatic bone stress of the pelvis and the lower extremity. *Acta Radiol.* 2001;42(3):277–285.

74. Koch JC. The laws of bone architecture. *Am J Anat.* 1917;21:177–298.

75. Korpelainen R, Orava S, Karpakka J, et al. Risk factors for recurrent stress fractures in athletes. *Am J Sports Med.* 2001;29:304–310.

76. Larson CM, Almekinders LC, Taft CN, et al. Intramedullary screw fixation of Jones fractures: Analysis of failure. *Am J Sports Med.* 2002;30:55–60.

77. Lawrence JP, Greene HS, Grauer JN. Back pain in athletes. *J Am Acad Orthop Surg.* 2006;14(13):726–735.

78. Lee JK, Yao L. Stress fractures: MR imaging. *Radiology.* 1988;169:217–220.

79. Lee S, Anderson RB. Stress fractures of the tarsal navicular. *Foot Ankle Clin.* 2004;9(1):85–104.

80. Lehman RC, Torg JS, Pavlov H, et al. Fractures of the base of the fifth metatarsal distal to the tuberosity: A review. *Foot Ankle.* 1987;7:245–252.

81. Lesho EP. Can tuning forks replace bone scans for identification of tibial stress fractures? *Mil Med.* 1997;162(12):802–803.

82. Li GP, Zhang SD, Chen G, et al. Radiographic and histologic analyses of stress fracture in rabbit tibias. *Am J Sports Med.* 1985;13:285–294.

83. Matheson G, Bruckner P. Pneumatic leg brace after tibial stress fracture for faster return to play. *Clin J Sport Med.* 1998;8:66.

84. Matheson GO, Clement DB, McKenzie DC, et al. Stress fractures in athletes: A study of 320 cases. *Am J Sports Med.* 1987;15:46–58.

85. McBryde AM Jr. Stress fractures in athletes. *J Sports Med.* 1975;3(5):212–217.

86. McCormick JJ, Bray CC, Davis WH et al. Clinical and computed tomography evaluation of surgical outcomes in tarsal navicular stress fractures. *Am J Sports Med.* 2011; 39(8):1741–1748

87. McKeag D, Moeller J. *Primary Care Sports Medicine.* Philadelphia, PA: The American College of Sports Medicine; 2007:449.

88. Meyer SA, Saltzman CL, Albright JP. Stress fractures of the foot and leg. *Clin Sports Med.* 1993;12:395–413.

89. Milgrom C, Giladi M, Stein M, et al. Stress fractures in military recruits: A prospective study showing an unusually high incidence. *J Bone Joint Surg Br.* 1985;67:732–735.

90. Mindrebo NK, Shelbourne D, Van Meter CD, et al. Outpatient percutaneous screw fixation of the acute Jones fracture. *Am J Sports Med.* 1993;21:720–723.

91. Monteleone GP Jr. Stress fractures in the athlete. *Orthop Clin North Am.* 1995;2:423–432.

92. Morris JM, Blickenstaff LD. *Fatigue Fractures: A Clinical Study.* Springfield, IL: Charles C. Thomas; 1967:3–6.

93. Niva MH, Sormaala MJ, Kiuru MJ et al. Bone stress injuries of the ankle and foot: An 86-month magnetic resonance imaging-based study of physically active young adults. *Am J Sports Med* 2007;35(4):643–649.

94. Noakes TD, Smith JA, Lindenberg G, et al. Pelvic stress fractures in long distance runners. *Am J Sports Med.* 1985;13:120–123.

95. Orava S, Hulkko A. Delayed unions and nonunions of stress fractures in athletes. *Am J Sports Med.* 1988;16:378–382.

96. Orava S, Karpakka J, Taimela S, et al. Stress fracture of the medial malleolus. *J Bone Joint Surg Am.* 1995;77-A:362.

97. Ostlie DK, Simons SM. Tarsal navicular stress fracture in a young athlete: Case report with clinical, radiologic, and pathophysiologic correlations. *J Am Board Fam Pract.* 2001;14(5):381–385.

98. Pavlov H, Torg J, Freiberger R. Tarsal navicular stress fractures: radiographic evaluation. *Radiology.* 1983;148(3):641–645.

99. Porter DA, Duncan M, Meyer SJF. Fifth metatarsal Jones fracture fixation with a 4.5 mm cannulated stainless steel screw in the competitive and recreational athlete: A clinical and radiographic evaluation. *Am J Sports Med.* 2005;33:726–733.

100. Potter NJ, Brukner PD, Makdissi M, et al. Navicular stress fractures: Outcomes of surgical and conservative management. *Br J Sports Med.* 2006;40(8):692–695.

101. Pouilles JM, Bernard J, Tremollières F, et al. Femoral bone density in young male adults with stress fractures. *Bone.* 1989;10:105–108.

102. Prather JL, Nusynowitz ML, Snowdy HA, et al. Scintigraphic findings in stress fractures. *J Bone Joint Surg Am.* 1977;59:869–874.

103. Reese K, Litsky A, Kaeding C, et al. Cannulated screw fixation of Jones fractures: A clinical and biomechanical study. *Am J Sports Med.* 2004;32:1736–1742.

104. Reider B, Falconiero R, Yurkofsky J. Nonunion of a medial malleolus stress fracture: A case report. *Am J Sports Med.* 1993;21:478–481.

105. Rettig AC, Shelbourne KD, McCarroll JR, et al. The natural history and treatment of delayed union stress fractures of the anterior cortex of the tibia. *Am J Sports Med.* 1988; 16(3):250–255.

106. Richardson EG. Injuries to the hallucal sesamoids in the athlete. *Foot Ankle.* 1987; 7:229–244.

107. Romani W, Perrin DH, Dussault RG, et al. Identification of tibial stress fractures using therapeutic continuous ultrasound. *J Orthop Sports Phys Ther.* 2000;30(8):444–452.

108. Roub L, Gumerman LW, Hanley EN Jr, et al. Bone stress: A radionuclide imaging perspective. *Radiology.* 1979;132:431–483.

109. Savoca CJ. Stress fractures. A classification of the earliest radiographic signs. *Radiology.* 1971;100(3):519–524.

110. Saxena A, Fullem B, Hannaford D, et al. Results of treatment of 22 navicular stress fractures and a new proposed radiographic classification system. *J Foot Ankle Surg.* 2000;39(2):96–103.

111. Saxena A, Fullem B. Navicular stress fractures: A prospective study on athletes. *Foot Ankle Int.* 2006;27(11):917–921.

112. Schickendantz M, Ho C, Koh J. Stress injury of the proximal ulna in professional baseball players. *Am J Sports Med.* 2002;30:737–741.

113. Shelbourne KD, Fisher DA, Rettig AC, et al. Stress fractures of the medial malleolus. *Am J Sports Med.* 1988;16:60–63.

114. Shin AY, Gillingham BL. Fatigue fractures of the femoral neck in athletes. *J Am Acad Orthop Surg.* 1997;5:293–302.

115. Shin AY, Morin WD, Gorman JD, et al. The superiority of magnetic resonance imaging in differentiating the cause of hip pain in endurance athletes. *Am J Sports Med.* 1996;24:168–176.

116. Sinha A, Kaeding CC, Wadley GM. Upper extremity stress fractures in athletes: Clinical features of 44 cases. *Clin J Sport Med.* 1999;9(4):199–202.

117. Sormaala M, Niva MH, Kiuru MJ , et al. Bone stress injuries of the talus in military recruits. *Bone.* 2006;39(1):199–204.

118. Stafford SA, Rosenthal DI, Gebhardt MC, et al. MRI in stress fracture. *Am J Roentgenol.* 1986;147:553–556.

119. Stanitski CL, McMaster JH, Scranton PE. On the nature of stress fractures. *Am J Sports Med.* 1978;6:391–396.

120. Strayer S, Reece SG, Petrizzi MJ. Fractures of the proxima fifth metatarsal. *Am Fam Physician.* 1999;59(9):2516–2522.

121. Swenson E, DeHaven K, Sebastianelli W, et al. The effect of a pneumatic leg brace on return to play in athletes with tibial stress fractures. *Am J Sports Med.* 1997;25: 322–328.

122. Teitz CC, Harrington RM. Patellar stress fracture. *Am J Sports Med.* 1992;20:761–765.

123. Toren A, Goshen E, Katz M, et al. Bilateral femoral stress fractures in a child due to in-line (roller) skating. *Acta Paediatr.* 1997;86:332–333.

124. Torg JS, Balduini FC, Zelco RR. Fractures of the base of the fifth metatarsal distal to the tuberosity: Classification and guidelines for non-surgical and surgical management. *J Bone Joint Surg Am.* 1984;66:209–214.

125. Torg JS, Moyer J, Gaughan JP, et al. Management of tarsal navicular stress fractures: Conservative versus surgical treatment. *Am J Sports Med.* 2010;38(5):1048–1053.

126. Torg JS, Pavlov H, Cooley LH, et al. Stress fractures of the tarsal navicular: A retrospective review of twenty-one cases. *J Bone Joint Surg Am.* 1982;64:700–712.

127. Van Hal ME, Keene JS, Lange TA, et al. Stress fractures of the great toe sesamoids. *Am J Sports Med.* 1982,10(2):122–128.

128. Varner K, Younas S, Lintner D, et al. Chronic anterior midtibial stress fractures in athletes treated with reamed intramedullary nailing. *Am J Sports Med.* 2005;33:1071–1076.

129. Verma R., Sherman O. Athletic stress fractures: Part III. The upper body. *Am J Orthop.* 2001;20(12):848–860.

130. Vinther A, Kanstrup IL, Christiansen E et al. Exercise-induced rib stress fractures: Potential risk factors related to thoracic muscle co-contraction and movement pattern. *Scand J Med Sci Sports.* 2006;16(3):188–196.

131. Visuri T, Vara A, Meurman KOM. Displaced stress fractures of the femoral neck in young male adults: A report of twelve operative cases. *J Trauma.* 1988;28:1562–1569.

132. Voss LA, Fadale PD, Hulstyn MJ. Exercise-induced loss of bone density in athletes. *J Am Acad Orthop Surg.* 1998;6:349–357.

133. Wall J, Feller JF. Imaging of stress fractures in runners. *Clin Sports Med.* 2006;25(4): 781–802.

134. Whitelaw G, Wetzler M, Levy A, et al. A pneumatic leg brace for the treatment of tibial stress fractures. *Clin Orthop Relat Res.* 1991;270:301–305.

135. Wilson E, Katz FN . Stress fractures: Analysis of 250 consecutive cases. *Radiology.* 1969;92:481–486.

136. Wright RW, Fisher DA, Shively HA, et al. Refracture of proximal fifth metatarsal (Jones) fractures after intramedullary screw fixation in athletes. *Am J Sports Med.* 2000;28: 732–736.

137. Yao L, Johnson C, Gentili A, et al. Stress injuries of bone. *Acad Radiol.* 1998;5:34–40.

138. Zwas S. Interpretation and classification of bone scintigraphic findings in stress fractures. *J Nucl Med.* 1987;28:452–457.

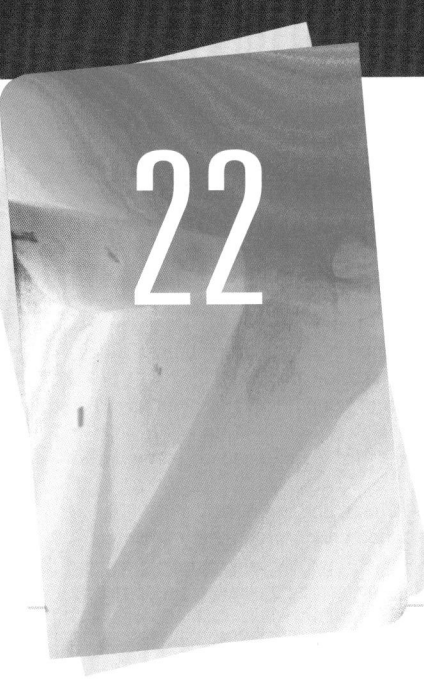

22

PATHOLOGIC FRACTURES

Rajiv Rajani and Robert T. Quinn

INTRODUCTION

Pathologic fractures occur in abnormal bone. Weakened bone predisposes the patient for failure during normal activity or after minor trauma. Failure (pathologic fracture) of bone under these circumstances should alert the orthopedic surgeon to the presence of an underlying condition. Successful management of the patient requires recognition, diagnosis, and treatment of the condition affecting the bone. The management of the fracture may be dramatically altered by the associated pathologic condition, and failure to recognize a condition such as osteoporosis or metastatic bone disease may be detrimental to the patient's life or limb.

When planning the management of patients with a pathologic fracture and systemic, non-neoplastic skeletal disease, it is best to separate the underlying problem into correctable and uncorrectable conditions. Correctable conditions include renal osteodystrophy, hyperparathyroidism, osteomalacia, and disuse osteoporosis. Uncorrectable conditions include osteogenesis imperfecta, polyostotic fibrous dysplasia, postmenopausal osteoporosis, Paget disease, and osteopetrosis. All of these disorders involve weak bones that are predisposed to fracture or

plastic deformation. Fracture callus may not form normally, and healing often occurs slowly. Many of these patients have an increased incidence of additional fractures, delayed union, and nonunion.

If the underlying process is correctable, appropriate medical treatment should be initiated. If the underlying process cannot be corrected, the condition of the remainder of the skeleton must be considered when planning treatment of the fracture. In the management of patients with systemic skeletal disease, it is important to prevent disuse osteoporosis, which may lead to additional pathologic fractures.

Osteoporosis is the most common condition associated with pathologic fractures, and the management of patients with this condition may only require minor modifications of typical fracture care. In contrast, the treatment of patients with metastatic bone disease who have actual or impending pathologic fractures necessitates a multidisciplinary approach with different principles applied to fracture fixation.

This chapter will primarily focus on the evaluation and treatment of patients with metastatic bone disease and actual or impending pathologic fractures. It will briefly cover the management of pathologic fractures in patients with primary benign or malignant bone tumors. Treatment of patients with metabolic abnormalities and decreased bone density unrelated to malignancy will be addressed in a less comprehensive fashion. The majority of patients with pathologic fractures are treated by general orthopedic surgeons. It is important that all orthopedic surgeons have a basic understanding of the principles involved in the care of these patients so that pathologic fractures are recognized and appropriate treatment is initiated.

Demographics

Currently, an estimated 10 million Americans have osteoporosis, while another 34 million have osteomalacia and are at risk for developing osteoporosis.[34] It is a major public health concern for 55% of people who are 50 years or older. Eighty percent of those affected by osteoporosis are women, and approximately 2 million people sustain a pathologic fracture related to osteoporosis each year.[34] Of patients older than 50 years of age, 24% who sustain a hip fracture die within 1 year.[34] One of every two women will have an osteoporosis-related fracture in her lifetime.[17] Spine, proximal femur, distal femur, and distal radius fractures are the most common locations for pathologic fractures in this population. Other skeletal conditions such as Paget disease affect an estimated 1 million people in the United States, while approximately 20,000 to 50,000 Americans have osteogenesis imperfecta while worldwide approximately 300,000 are affected.[34]

The American Cancer Society predicts almost 1.6 million new cancer cases will be diagnosed in 2011, and nearly 50% of these tumors can metastasize to the skeleton.[50] With improved medical treatment of many cancers, especially those originating in the breast and prostate, patients are living longer. There is an increased prevalence of bone metastasis in this population, which increases the chances that these patients will develop a pathologic fracture. The vast majority of bone metastasis originate from cancers of the breast, lung, prostate, thyroid, and kidney.[87] The most common sites of metastasis in the skeleton include the spine, pelvis, ribs, skull, proximal femur, and proximal humerus.[99]

EVALUATION OF THE PATIENT WITH AN IMPENDING OR ACTUAL PATHOLOGIC FRACTURE

Clinical

History

A comprehensive evaluation of a patient with a lytic bone lesion or pathologic fracture is essential (Table 22-1).[81,99] A thorough history must be obtained to understand the circumstances surrounding the current injury. Certain symptoms should alert the orthopedic surgeon to the possibility of an associated pathologic process (Table 22-2). The degree of trauma required to cause the fracture and presence of prodromal pain before the injury may provide information about the underlying bone strength. Pain is the most common presenting symptom before fracture, ranging from a dull constant ache to an intense pain

---

TABLE 22-1	Comprehensive Evaluation of a Patient with a Lytic Bone Lesion

1. *History:* Thyroid, breast, or prostate nodule
2. *Review of systems:* Gastrointestinal symptoms, weight loss, flank pain, hematuria
3. *Physical examination:* Lymph nodes, thyroid, breast, lungs, abdomen, prostate, testicles, rectum
4. *Plain x-rays:* Chest, affected bone (additional sites as directed by bone scan findings)
5. *^{99m}Tc total body bone scan* (FDG-PET scan in selected cases such as lymphoma)
6. *CT scan with contrast:* Chest, abdomen, pelvis
7. *Laboratory:* Complete blood count, erythrocyte sedimentation rate, calcium, phosphate, urinalysis, prostate specific antigen, immunoelectrophoresis, and alkaline phosphatase
8. *Biopsy:* Needle vs. open

FDG, fluorine-18-deoxyglucose; PET, positron emission tomography; CT, computed tomography.

---

exacerbated by weight bearing. Patients must be asked specifically about previously diagnosed or treated cancer; otherwise, they may consider themselves cured and not volunteer this information. Specifically, breast cancer can have a long latent period until bony metastases present. A history of radiation is important. Standard review of systems questions about constitutional symptoms such as recent weight loss, fevers, night sweats, and fatigue are important. Questions about relevant risk factors such as smoking, dietary habits, and toxic exposures should be asked.

Physical Examination

The physical examination should include a thorough evaluation of the affected skeletal region. Palpation of a mass, identification of an obvious deformity, and a detailed neurovascular examination of the extremities are essential. All extremities and the entire spine should be evaluated for additional lesions or lymphadenopathy, as patients can have multiple sites of involvement with bone metastasis, lymphoma, multiple myeloma, or osteoporosis. A physical examination should include careful

---

TABLE 22-2	Factors Suggesting a Pathologic Fracture

- Spontaneous fracture
- Fracture after minor trauma
- Pain at the site before the fracture
- Multiple recent fractures
- Unusual fracture pattern ("banana fracture")[a]
- Patient older than 45 years
- History of primary malignancy

[a]A "banana fracture" is a transverse fracture after minimal trauma through an abnormal area of bone. It is a frequent pattern in pathologic situations and has the appearance of breaking a segment off of a banana.

evaluation of all possible primary sites (breast, prostate, lung, thyroid) and a stool test for occult blood.[99]

Laboratory Studies

Laboratory tests will not often make the diagnosis, especially in cases of cancer, but they are supporting data relevant to the overall patient evaluation. A baseline laboratory profile should include a complete blood count with manual differential, erythrocyte sedimentation rate (ESR), serum chemistries, blood urea nitrogen (BUN), serum glucose, liver function tests, protein, albumin, calcium, phosphorus, and alkaline phosphatase. Patients with widespread bone metastasis may exhibit anemia of chronic disease, hypercalcemia, and increased alkaline phosphatase. The hemoglobin is also often low in patients with multiple myeloma. A standard urinalysis is necessary to look for microscopic hematuria, which suggests renal cell carcinoma (RCC), and a 24-hour urine collection is necessary for a complete metabolic evaluation. Serum and urine protein electrophoreses are important to exclude multiple myeloma. Thyroid function tests, carcinoembryonic antigen (CEA), CA125, and prostate specific antigen (PSA) are serum markers for specific tumors that can be useful for particular individuals. N-telopeptide and C-telopeptide are new biomechanical markers of bone collagen breakdown that can be measured in the serum and urine. These markers are used to confirm increased destruction caused by bone metastasis, measure the overall extent of bone involvement, and assess the response of the bone to bisphosphonate treatment.[22]

Patients with osteoporosis have normal values for the aforementioned laboratory tests, whereas patients with osteomalacia have low serum calcium and phosphorus, high serum alkaline phosphatase, high urinary phosphorus, and high urinary hydroxyproline values (Table 22-3). Patients with primary hyperparathyroidism have high serum calcium, alkaline phosphatase, and parathyroid hormone levels with low serum phosphorus. They also have high urinary calcium, phosphorus, and hydroxyproline levels. Patients with renal osteodystrophy have low serum calcium with high serum phosphorus, alkaline phosphatase, and BUN levels. When secondary hyperparathyroidism

develops in these patients, the serum calcium increases to normal or elevated values with elevated parathyroid hormone levels. Urine values are difficult to assess in patients with secondary hyperparathyroidism caused by abnormal glomerular filtration. Patients with Paget disease have normal values for serum calcium and phosphorus, but markedly elevated levels of alkaline phosphatase and urinary hydroxyproline. PSA is a sensitive measurement of prostate cancer. A value less than 10 ng/mL essentially excludes the presence of bone metastasis. Serum calcium is a measurement of unbound calcium in the serum and, therefore, determination of serum protein is necessary to interpret the calcium level. If the serum protein is lower than normal, the normal range of serum calcium is lowered.

Associated Medical Problems

The clinical problems encountered by patients with metastatic bone disease are substantial. Patients often have marked pain or pathologic fractures that leave them unable to ambulate or perform their activities of daily living (ADLs). Patients with spinal fractures may develop neurologic deficits that lead to paralysis. Patients with impending or actual extremity fractures may be forced to remain in bed for prolonged periods of time, predisposing them to hypercalcemia. Anemia is a common hematologic abnormality in these patients. The most encompassing and tragic concern of patients with pathologic fractures from metastatic disease is the general loss in their quality of life.

Approximately 40% of the 75,000 cases of hypercalcemia diagnosed in the United States each year are related to hypercalcemia of malignancy, most commonly associated with cancers of the lung, breast, kidney, genitourinary tract, and multiple myeloma.[78] Much of the remainder is caused by primary hyperparathyroidism. Rarely, the two causes occur simultaneously. The orthopedic surgeon managing a patient with metastatic carcinoma to bone must be aware of the risks, symptoms, and management of hypercalcemia as it can be lethal if untreated (Table 22-4).

Hypercalcemia is not usually the presenting sign of malignancy, but it portends a poor prognosis for the patient. As

TABLE 22-3	Disorders Producing Osteopenia			
	Laboratory Value			
Disorder	Serum Calcium	Serum Phosphorus	Serum Alkaline Phosphatase	Urine
Osteoporosis	Normal	Normal	Normal	Normal calcium
Osteomalacia	Normal	Normal	Normal	Low calcium
Hyperparathyroidism	Normal to high	Normal to low	Normal	High calcium
Renal osteodystrophy	Low	High	High	
Paget disease	Normal	Normal	Very high	Hydroxyproline
Myeloma[a]	Normal	Normal	Normal	Protein

[a]Abnormal serum or urine immunoelectrophoresis.

Signs and Symptoms of Hypercalcemia

- *Neurologic:* Headache, confusion, irritability, blurred vision
- *Gastrointestinal:* Anorexia, nausea, vomiting, abdominal pain, constipation, weight loss
- *Musculoskeletal:* Fatigue, weakness, joint and bone pain, unsteady gait
- *Urinary:* Nocturia, polydipsia, polyuria, urinary tract infections

many as 60% of patients with hypercalcemia will survive less than 3 months, and only 20% will be alive at 1 year. Often the symptoms are nonspecific, so it is easiest to diagnose the problem by measuring the serum calcium. There is not a reliable correlation between the severity of the hypercalcemia and the degree of metastatic bone disease. Patients with lung cancer may develop hypercalcemia without obvious bone metastases due to PTH-like proteins made by the tumor, whereas hypercalcemia in multiple myeloma or breast carcinoma correlates with the extent of bone metastases.[78] Diffuse osteoclastic activity associated with clinical hypercalcemia can be seen histologically without the presence of metastasis in the bone.

A treatment plan for the patient with hypercalcemia often requires inpatient care. Vigorous volume repletion is a temporizing measure, so treatment must focus on reducing the degree of bone resorption. This can be accomplished by treating the primary tumor directly or by using bisphosphonates to reduce osteoclastic activity.[67] Correction of any electrolyte imbalance or hypercalcemia should be done before surgery.

Radiographic Investigations

Plain Radiographs

The first and most important imaging study used to evaluate a patient with a destructive bone lesion or pathologic fracture is a plain radiograph in two orthogonal planes.[99] The radiographs should be carefully reviewed with attention to specific lesions and overall bone quality. Specifically they should be examined for diagnostic clues such as generalized osteopenia, periosteal reaction, cortical thinning, Looser lines, and abnormal soft tissue shadows. A series of questions to assist in determining the underlying process was popularized by W. Enneking, MD, and can be reviewed in Table 22-5. The entire affected bone should be imaged to identify all possible lesions, and it must be remembered that pain referred to distal sites may be caused by a more proximal lesion.

Osteopenia is the radiographic term used to indicate inadequate bone (osteoporosis) or inadequately mineralized bone (osteomalacia). These two disorders cannot be definitively distinguished on plain radiographs, but there are some suggestive differential clues. Looser lines (compression-side radiolucent lines), calcification of small vessels, and phalangeal periosteal reaction are features of osteomalacia or hyperparathyroidism. Thin cortices and loss of the normal trabecular pattern without other abnormalities are more suggestive of osteoporosis.

When an osteolytic or osteoblastic lesion is noted in otherwise normal bone, the process is most likely neoplastic. It is important to determine whether the lesion is inactive, active, or aggressive. Small osteolytic lesions surrounded by a rim of reactive bone without endosteal or periosteal reaction are usually inactive or minimally active benign bone tumors. Lesions that erode the cortex but are contained by periosteum are usually active benign or low-grade malignant bone tumors. Large lesions that destroy the cortex are usually aggressive, malignant lesions that can be primary or metastatic. A permeative or "moth-eaten" pattern of cortical destruction is highly suggestive of malignancy. Most destructive bone lesions in patients older than 40 years of age are caused by metastatic carcinoma followed in order of incidence by multiple myeloma and lymphoma; however, a solitary bone lesion should be fully evaluated to rule out a primary bone tumor such as a chondrosarcoma, malignant fibrous histiocytoma, or osteosarcoma.[99]

TABLE 22-5 **Evaluation of Plain Radiographs**

Question	Option	Interpretation
1. Where is the lesion?	Epiphysis vs. metaphysis vs. diaphysis Cortex vs. medullary canal Long bone (femur, humerus) vs. flat bone (pelvis, scapula)	
2. What is the lesion doing to the bone?	Bone destruction (osteolysis) • Total • Diffuse • Minimal	
3. What is the bone doing to the lesion?	Well-defined reactive rim Intact but abundant periosteal reaction Periosteal reaction that cannot keep up with tumor (Codman triangle)	Benign or slow growing Aggressive Highly malignant
4. What are the clues to the tissue type within the lesion?	Calcification Ossification Ground-glass appearance	Bone infarct/cartilage tumor Osteosarcoma/osteoblastoma Fibrous dysplasia

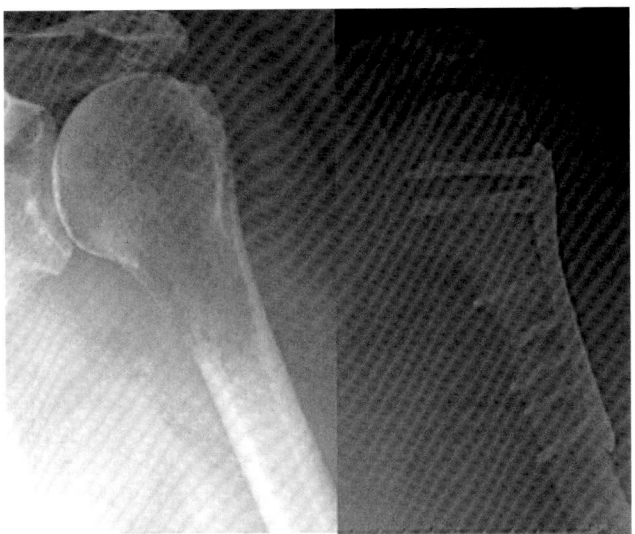

FIGURE 22-1 Anteroposterior (AP) radiograph of a 55-year-old man with metastatic renal cell carcinoma. He had pain for approximately 3 months prior to presentation. The impending pathologic fracture was treated with plate fixation and cement augmentation after embolization and curettage.

The radiographic appearance of bone metastasis can be osteolytic, osteoblastic, or mixed. Osteolytic destruction is most common and occurs in metastases from cancers of the lung, thyroid, kidney, and colon (Fig. 22-1). An osteoblastic appearance with sclerosis of the bone is common in metastatic prostate cancer. Metastatic breast cancer often has a mixed osteolytic and osteoblastic appearance in the bone (Fig. 22-2). The radiographic

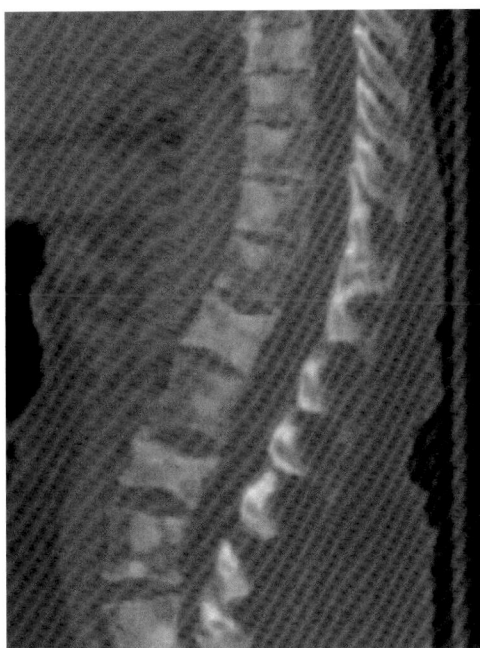

FIGURE 22-2 Multiple lytic and blastic lesions are noted throughout the thoracolumbar spine, consistent with breast cancer. Note the collapse of vertebrae even in blastic metastases.

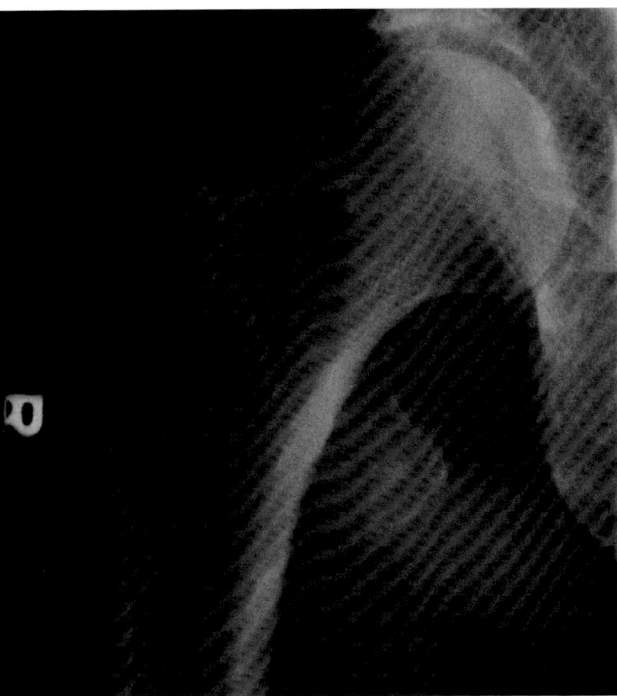

FIGURE 22-3 AP radiograph of an isolated lesser trochanter fracture. This is highly suggestive of an impending fracture of the inter-trochanteric region or femoral neck.

appearance is determined by the balance of bone destruction by osteoclasts and bone production by osteoblasts. Tumor cells secrete factors that interact with host cells in the bone microenvironment and affect the cycle of normal bone turnover.[23,79,95,98] An isolated avulsion of the lesser trochanter is almost always pathologic, and this specific injury should arouse suspicion of occult metastatic disease or lymphoma and an imminent femoral neck fracture (Fig. 22-3).[9] A cortical lesion in an adult is usually a metastasis, most commonly from lung cancer.[37]

Nuclear Medicine Studies

When a bone metastasis is diagnosed or suspected, the remainder of the skeleton should be evaluated for additional bony sites of disease. Technetium bone scintigraphy is helpful in determining the extent of metastatic disease to the skeleton, as it detects osteoblastic activity and is quite sensitive. Multiple myeloma is falsely negative on a bone scan as are occasional cases of metastatic RCC because of the decreased osteoblastic response to the tumor. More recently, positron emission tomography (PET) scanning has been available but the indications for staging patients with metastatic bone disease are not clear at present.[74] For lung cancer, fluorine-18-deoxyglucose (FDG)-PET with correlated CT images is superior to standard CT images for detecting metastatic disease in small lesions.[94] It has also been useful in staging patients with lymphoma and monitoring response to lymphoma treatment.[56] In a recent study, PET/computed tomography (CT) scanning had higher sensitivity and specificity than PET scanning alone for detection of malignant bone lesions.[28]

Additional Staging and Three-Dimensional Studies

Further imaging studies are necessary to search for a primary lesion when metastatic carcinoma to the skeleton is suspected.[81] The recommended radiographic staging study is a CT scan of the chest, abdomen, and pelvis with oral and intravenous contrast. A mammogram should also be done if breast cancer is suspected; however, MRI can also be used for early detection. If multiple myeloma is considered, a skeletal survey including skull films is recommended.

Magnetic resonance imaging (MRI) is not generally used to evaluate metastatic lesions in the extremity, but it is useful in the evaluation of patients with spinal metastasis to define the relationship of tumor to the underlying neurologic structures. A standard angiogram is still useful when embolizing feeding tumor vessels in vascular lesions such as metastatic RCC or multiple myeloma as definitive treatment or before surgery.

When and How to Perform a Biopsy

A thorough history and physical examination with appropriate imaging studies often leads to the correct diagnosis, particularly in the case of widespread metastatic bone disease. However, a solitary bone lesion in a patient with or without a history of cancer should be biopsied to obtain an accurate diagnosis. Presuming a solitary lesion is a bone metastasis in an older patient may lead to the wrong operation, cause extensive contamination, and potentially compromise the life or limb of the patient if the lesion is actually a primary sarcoma of bone.

If a tissue diagnosis is necessary, a biopsy must be performed. Either a needle or open incisional biopsy is reasonable depending on the availability of expert musculoskeletal radiologists and pathologists.[96] A needle biopsy is usually definitive when differentiating a carcinoma from a sarcoma. Specific immunohistochemical staining may allow determination of the primary site of origin of a carcinoma, most commonly from the lung, breast, thyroid, or prostate. When there is a pathologic fracture through a lytic lesion, the biopsy can be complicated due to bleeding and early fracture callus. The fracture should be stabilized initially with traction or a cast to allow preliminary staging studies to be completed, which may allow the diagnosis to be made on imaging alone, or there may be a different lesion more amenable to biopsy.

If a needle biopsy is nondiagnostic or unable to be done, a careful incisional biopsy should be performed using oncologic principles so as not to preclude subsequent definitive surgical treatment.[68] When possible, the tissue should be obtained from a site near but unaffected by the fracture. The biopsy should be as small as possible, in a longitudinal fashion in line with the extremity, and performed with excellent hemostasis. Tissues contaminated by a postbiopsy hematoma must be considered contaminated by tumor cells. Cultures should always be sent at the time of biopsy to rule out infection, which can be confused radiographically with a tumor. If a definitive diagnosis of metastatic disease can be made on an intraoperative frozen section, surgical treatment of the pathologic fracture can be performed at the same operative setting. If the frozen section is not diagnostic, it is best to wait for the permanent sections before definitively treating the tumor and fracture.

IMPENDING PATHOLOGIC FRACTURES

Bone metastases are painful even without an associated fracture. Treatment options for known skeletal metastasis include (a) prophylactic surgical stabilization before radiation therapy or (b) radiation and/or chemotherapy without prophylactic fixation.[49,99] The term *impending fracture* is used throughout the literature on metastatic disease, but there are no clear guidelines supported by prospective clinical studies to define this term. Retrospective studies have formed the basis to guide the indications for prophylactic fixation, but they are often limited by the use of plain radiographs, subjective patient information, and an inadequate understanding of the biomechanical factors involved in the bone affected by a neoplastic process.[31,72,86] Although experienced orthopedic oncologists may have an intuitive sense for which lesions are at high risk for fracture, there is considerable controversy about what constitutes an impending fracture and little reliable data to guide treatment.

Classification Systems

Factors necessary for the assessment of fracture risk include the radiographic appearance of the lesion and the patient's symptoms. Fidler[31] assessed preoperative and postoperative pain in patients with impending fractures and found that among patients with 50% to 75% cortical involvement, all had moderate to severe pain preoperatively and none or minimal pain after prophylactic internal fixation. Commonly, a lesion is considered to be at risk for fracture if it is painful, larger than 2.5 cm, and involves over 50% of the cortex.[86] In an attempt to quantify this risk, Mirels[70] developed a scoring system based on the presence or absence of pain and the size, location, and radiographic appearance of the lesion. Each of the four variables is assigned from 1 to 3 points (Table 22-6). Mirels analyzed 78 lesions previously irradiated without prophylactic surgical fixation. Over a 6-month period, 27 lesions (35%) fractured and 51 remained stable. A mean score of 7 in the nonfracture group and 10 in the fracture group was calculated. The author concluded that lesions scoring 7 or lower can be safely irradiated, while lesions scoring 8 or higher require prophylactic internal fixation before radiation.[70] However, this is a general treatment guide and each individual patient's medical comorbidities should also be considered.

Subsequently, investigators have attempted to quantify the risk of pathologic fracture in patients with metastatic bone disease. *Fracture risk* is defined as the load-bearing requirement of the bone divided by its load-bearing capacity. The load-bearing requirement depends on the patient's age, weight, activity level, and ability to protect the site. The load-bearing capacity depends on the amount of bone loss, modulus of the remaining bone, and location of the defect with respect to the type of load applied.[72] A biomechanical study of simulated lytic defects in whale vertebral bodies demonstrated that relative fracture risk in vivo could be predicted by a structural rigidity analysis using cross-sectional imaging data.[47] Although this system provides a comprehensive method to determine the risk of pathologic fracture, it is not yet routinely used in the clinical setting. Quantitative CT structural analysis has also been proposed as a method for predicting fracture risk, but it also is not routinely used in the clinical setting.[61]

TABLE 22-6	Mirels Criteria for Risk of Fracture		
	Number Assigned		
Variable	**1**	**2**	**3**
Site	Upper extremity	Lower extremity	Peritrochanteric
Pain	Mild	Moderate	Severe
Lesion[a]	Blastic	Mixed	Lytic
Size	$<1/3$ diameter of the bone	$1/3$–$2/3$ diameter of the bone	$>2/3$ diameter of the bone

Each patient's situation is assessed by assigning a number (1, 2, or 3) to each aspect of his or her presentation (site, pain, lesion, and size) and then adding the numbers to obtain a total number to indicate the patient's risk for fracture. Mirels's data suggest that those patients whose total number is 7 or less can be observed, but those with a number of 8 or more should have prophylactic internal fixation.

[a]By radiography.

Patients treated by prophylactic stabilization of an impending fracture versus those treated after an actual fracture have the following outcomes: Shorter hospitalization (average 2 days), discharge to home more likely (40%), more immediate pain relief, faster and less complicated surgery, less blood loss, quicker return to premorbid function, improved survival, and fewer hardware complications.[13,53] Elective stabilization also allows the medical oncologist and surgeon to coordinate operative treatment and systemic chemotherapy. One critical caveat when treating patients with impending pathologic fractures is that fracture risk is greatest during the surgical positioning, preparation, and draping. When patients are anesthetized, they cannot protect the affected extremity and must rely on the surgical team to proceed carefully. Low-energy fractures will occur after very minor trauma or a twisting movement. If a pathologic fracture occurs, damage to the surrounding soft tissues is minimal compared to traumatic fractures in healthy bone.

The goals of surgical treatment in a patient with an impending pathologic fracture are to alleviate pain, reduce narcotic utilization, restore skeletal stability, and regain functional independence.[49,99] However, the decision to proceed with operative intervention is multifactorial and must be individualized. Factors included in the decision making are (a) life expectancy of the patient, (b) patient comorbidities, (c) extent of the disease, (d) tumor histology, (e) anticipated future oncologic treatments, and (f) degree of pain. Patients with a life expectancy of less than 6 weeks may not gain significant benefit from major reconstructive surgery. However, an accurate prognosis is not always possible, and the decision of whether to proceed with surgery should be discussed with the multidisciplinary team, the patient, and the patient's family.

TREATMENT OPTIONS FOR PATIENTS WITH METASTATIC OR SYSTEMIC DISEASE

General Considerations

As stated earlier in this chapter, the most common pathologic fracture is caused by osteoporosis. In most situations, these fractures should be managed in a standard fashion as recommended in the accompanying chapters of this text. Modifica-tions such as the addition of methyl methacrylate or locking plate fixation may be necessary because of the weakened bone.[6] Pathologic fractures caused by metastatic bone disease demand special considerations, which will be discussed in further detail.

Patients with cancer are living longer. More patients are living with bone metastasis. Because of the advances in systemic treatment, pain control, and local modalities including radiation and surgery, the philosophy has changed from one of palliation for immediate demise to aggressive care to improve the quality of remaining life. The local bone lesion can be treated with nonsurgical management (radiation, functional bracing, and bisphosphonates) or surgical stabilization with or without resection. Medical treatment with bisphosphonates has decreased the incidence of pathologic fractures because of inhibition of osteoclast-mediated bone destruction.[43,64,65] Patients with small bone lesions, especially in nonweight-bearing bones, are often candidates for radiation therapy rather than surgical stabilization. Surgical intervention is usually employed for large lytic lesions at risk for fracture or for existing pathologic fractures. Postoperatively, external beam radiation is used as an adjuvant local treatment for the entire operative field and implant unless the metastatic lesion is completely resected.[92,99]

Patients who present with a pathologic fracture are often medically debilitated and require multidisciplinary care. In addition to an orthopedic surgeon, the comprehensive team includes medical oncologists, radiation oncologists, endocrinologists, radiologists, pathologists, pain specialists, nutritionists, physical therapists, and psychologist/psychiatrists. Nutrition is of particular concern; serum prealbumin should be measured and improved if it is low. This may require the addition of enteral or parenteral hyperalimentation perioperatively. Patients may have relative bone marrow suppression and will require adequate replacement of blood products. Perioperative antibiotic coverage, prophylaxis for embolic events, aggressive postoperative pulmonary toilet, and early mobilization are all instituted as standard treatment.

Nonoperative Treatment

Bracing an impending or actual pathologic fracture is indicated if the patient is not a surgical candidate. Nonsurgical candidates are those with limited life expectancies, severe comorbidities, small lesions, or radiosensitive tumors.[99] The use of a fracture brace works well for lesions in the upper extremity. Patients should limit weight bearing on the affected extremity. A braced lesion may heal with or without radiation therapy. Lesions most amenable to bracing are those in the humeral diaphysis, forearm, and occasionally the tibia. Patients with proximal humeral lesions can be treated with a sling, and those with distal humeral lesions can be immobilized in a posterior elbow splint with or without a hinge. If a patient has multiple lesions requiring the use of all extremities to ambulate, surgical stabilization will provide better support than a brace.

After treatment for a pathologic fracture, the bone may or may not heal. The factors that influence whether healing will occur include location of the lesion, extent of bony destruction, tumor histology, type of treatment, and length of patient survival. Gainor and Buchert[33] determined the most important factor affecting union was length of patient survival. Of 129 pathologic long bone fractures, the overall rate of fracture healing was 34%; however, it was 74% in the group of patients who survived greater than 6 months. Among different tumor histologies, fractures secondary to multiple myeloma were most likely to heal.[33]

Operative Treatment

Surgical treatment of metastatic bone disease uses the most current internal fixation devices and prosthetic replacements. The ideal reconstruction allows immediate weight bearing and is durable enough to last for the increased total life span of patients with metastatic bone disease.[49,99] It should be assumed that the fixation device used will be load bearing, as only 30% to 40% of pathologic fractures unite even after radiation treatment.[12,33]

Depending on the external forces, bone quality, and likelihood of tumor progression, standard internal fixation may be contraindicated. An intramedullary device or modular prosthesis provides more definitive stability. Polymethyl methacrylate (PMMA) is often used to increase the strength of the fixation, but it should not be used alone to replace a segment of bone. PMMA improves the bending strength of a fixation construct and the outcome of fixation in both animal and human studies.[42,85] It does not affect the use of therapeutic radiation, nor are the properties of the PMMA affected adversely by the radiation.[27] Autogenous bone graft is not generally used in the treatment of extremity fractures from metastatic bone disease. Segmental allografts are also rarely indicated, as they have extremely poor rates of healing after radiation.

The most expedient reconstruction with the least risk of complication or failure should be used for patients with metastatic bone disease. In the vast majority of cases, this requires metal and PMMA. When a prosthesis is used to replace a joint affected by a metastatic lesion or a pathologic fracture, it should be cemented into the host bone. The goal is to have the patient weight bearing as tolerated after the surgical procedure. Another guideline when treating patients with metastatic disease is to prophylactically stabilize as much of the affected bone as possible. When an intramedullary device is indicated, the entire femur, humerus, or tibia should be treated with a statically locked nail.[101,107] For femoral lesions, a reconstruction nail is used to stabilize the femoral neck even if no lesion is present there at the time of surgery. Patients with metastatic disease often develop subsequent lesions and the reconstruction nail is helpful in preventing a future pathologic femoral neck fracture.

Some carcinomas are relatively resistant to chemotherapy and radiation therapy when they spread to the skeleton. RCC is a notable example. Surgical treatment is often indicated for even small RCC lesions, as they tend to progress despite standard medical treatment and external beam radiation.[51,88] Depending on the patient's expected life span and location of the lesion, open treatment with thorough curettage of metastatic RCC followed by intramedullary fixation and PMMA will decrease the tumor burden.[63] Postoperative radiation is often used to prevent growth of the residual microscopic disease.[92] When complete resection and joint replacement is performed for metastatic disease, the chances of progressive bone destruction from recurrent tumor are decreased.[51,88]

Hypervascular metastases put the patient at risk for life-threatening intraoperative hemorrhage when adequate preoperative precautions are not taken. Metastatic RCC is the most likely lesion to cause excessive blood loss, but metastatic thyroid cancer and multiple myeloma are also hypervascular. When possible, a tourniquet should be used during surgery. However, most metastases occur in the proximal extremities, precluding use of a tourniquet. Excessive blood loss can often be avoided if preoperative embolization is performed by an interventional radiologist within 36 hours of the surgical procedure.[15] Patients with metastatic RCC may have only one functioning kidney, so a careful evaluation of their renal status should be performed before injecting nephrotoxic dye for angiography.

Upper-Extremity Fractures

Twenty percent of osseous metastases occur in the upper extremity with approximately 50% occurring in the humerus. Upper-extremity metastases can result in substantial functional impairment by hindering personal hygiene, independent ambulation, meal management, ability to use external aids, and general ADLs.[99] When making decisions about treatment of upper-extremity metastasis, the benefits to quality of life should outweigh the risks of potential surgery. Contractures of the shoulder and elbow are common with or without surgical treatment, and these joints should be kept moving. Gentle pendulum exercises can maintain motion in the shoulder and, with appropriate precautions against using torsion, are safe for most proximal and midhumeral impending fractures. Gravity-assisted elbow flexion and extension exercises can also be performed safely by most patients.

Scapula/Clavicle

Metastatic lesions to the clavicle and scapula are generally treated nonoperatively with shoulder immobilization, radiation, and/or medical management. Occasionally a large, destructive metastasis will occur in the inferior body or articular portion (glenoid) of the scapula. As pain dictates, these areas of the scapula can be resected.

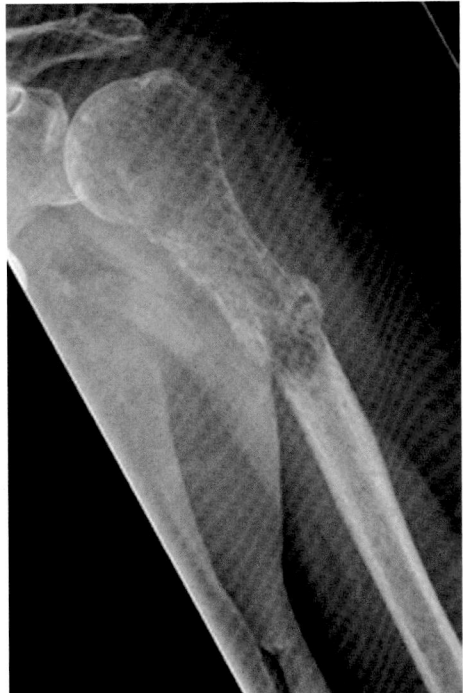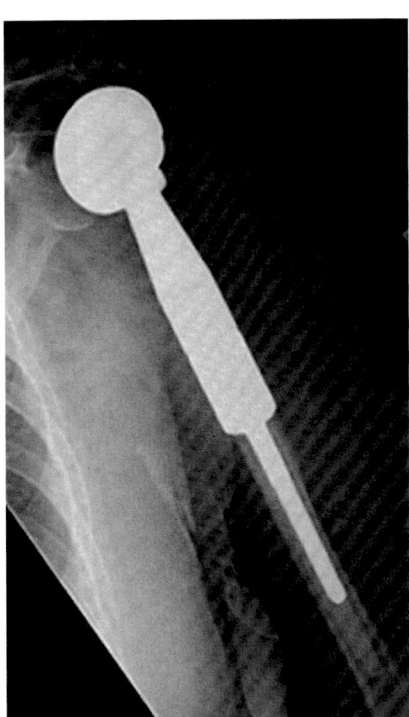

FIGURE 22-4 A: A destructive lesion with pathologic fracture through the proximal humerus due to myeloma. **B:** After proximal humerus megaprosthetic reconstruction, the patient has reasonable function but limitations in abduction and forward flexion.   **A**   **B**

Proximal Humerus

Pathologic fractures involving the humeral head or neck are treated with a proximal humeral replacement or intramedullary fixation. If enough bone is available in the proximal humerus, an intramedullary locked device with multiple proximal screws is acceptable and maintains shoulder range of motion.[107] PMMA may be required to supplement the fixation. When there is extensive destruction of the proximal humerus or a fracture leaving minimal bone for adequate fixation, resection of the lesion and reconstruction with a cemented proximal humeral endoprosthesis are indicated.[54] This modular construct replaces a variable amount of proximal humerus and has a long cemented stem to protect the remainder of the bone (Fig. 22-4). In the face of distal disease progression, it can be modified to a total humeral prosthesis. Involvement of the glenoid is rare, so replacement of this articular surface is generally not necessary. The goal of a proximal humeral replacement is pain relief and local control of the tumor: Shoulder range of motion and stability are often compromised because of poor soft tissue attachments (especially the rotator cuff) to the metal construct. A synthetic vascular graft or mesh sutured to the glenoid labrum and around the prosthetic humeral head can offer some stability. Postoperative radiation therapy is used for patients when intralesional treatment is performed.

Humeral Diaphysis

Humeral diaphyseal lesions of fractures can be surgically treated with locked intramedullary fixation or an intercalary metal spacer.[19,20,107] Locked intramedullary humeral nails span the entire humerus and provide mechanical and rotational stability (Fig. 22-5). In addition, when inserted in a closed fashion, this type of fixation allows unrestricted radiation to the shaft without

fear of incisional breakdown. As previously mentioned, PMMA improves implant stability and supplements poor bone quality when used with surgical stabilization.[42] Intercalary spacers offer a modular reconstructive option after resection of large diaphyseal lesions.[20] They are used in segmental defects and cases of failed fixation caused by progressive disease. Intercalary spacers can be used for reconstruction after complete resection of a metastatic lesion in the humeral diaphysis, minimizing blood loss in hypervascular lesions and often alleviating the need for postoperative radiation. Damron et al. reported that intercalary spacers provide immediate stable fixation, excellent pain relief, and early return of function.[20,45] Plate fixation produces good to excellent functional results in nonpathologic humeral fractures; however, drawbacks for their use in metastatic disease include the need for extensive exposure of the humerus and the inability to protect the entire bone. With disease progression, there is risk of hardware failure when plate fixation is used (Fig. 22-6).

Distal Humerus

Distal humeral lesions or fractures are treated with flexible intramedullary nails, bicondylar plate fixation, or resection with modular distal humeral reconstruction. Flexible nails, inserted in a retrograde manner through small medial and lateral incisions, offer ease of insertion, the ability to span the entire humerus, excellent functional recovery, and preservation of the native elbow joint. Curettage of the distal humeral lesion allows an open reduction in the case of a fracture and the opportunity to use PMMA in the lesion to gain rotational stability (Fig. 22-7). Orthogonal plate fixation is similar to nonpathologic fracture care but, when combined with PMMA, it can provide a stable construct about the elbow. This method of fixation does not protect the proximal humerus against a

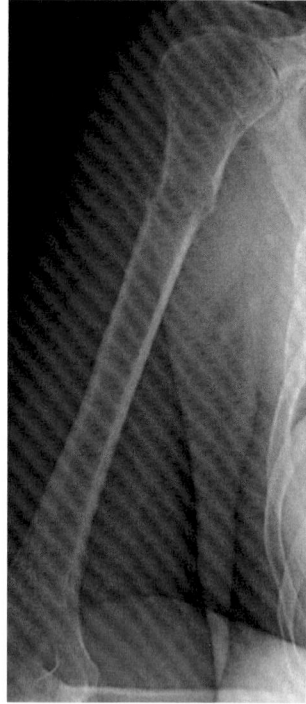
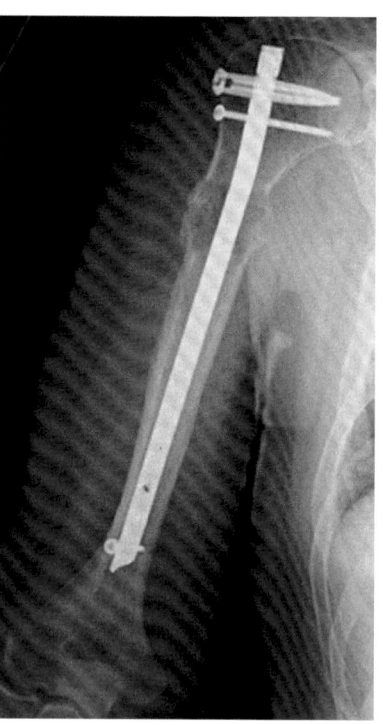

A

B

FIGURE 22-5 **A:** AP radiograph of a right proximal humerus fracture in a 63-year-old male with metastatic lung cancer. Multiple other metastatic lesions were identified on his surveillance examinations and therefore a decision was made not to proceed with resection. **B:** A biopsy and curettage was performed with intramedullary nailing of the right humerus. At 1 year, the patient has no pain and full range of motion of the shoulder and elbow.

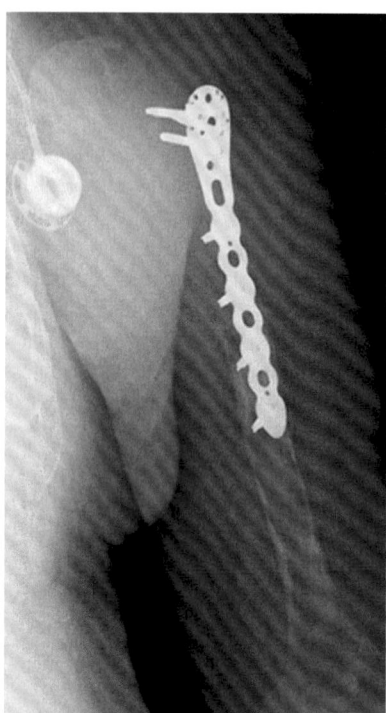

FIGURE 22-6 AP radiograph of the left humerus in a 57-year-old man with multiple myeloma. Initial radiographs showed a small lesion and minimally displaced fracture. Plate fixation was performed but was inadequate as the tumor progressed, resulting in massive bone loss. Ultimately, the patient was treated with a shoulder disarticulation.

future metastatic lesion or fracture. A distal humeral resection and modular endoprosthetic reconstruction of the elbow is the best option for massive bone loss involving the condyles.[100]

Forearm/Hand

Metastases distal to the elbow are unusual, and the most common are from the lung, breast, and kidney.[59] Metastatic lesions to the radius and ulna can be treated with flexible rods or rigid plate fixation. Pathologic fractures of the radial head can be treated with resection. Intralesional surgery is preferred for hand metastasis with curettage, internal fixation, and cementation. If the lesion is distal or extensive, amputation may be the best option.

Pelvic/Acetabular Fractures

Many bone metastasis or pathologic fractures in the bony pelvis do not affect weight-bearing functions; consequently, they do not require surgical intervention. Lesions of the iliac wing, superior/inferior pubic rami, or sacroiliac region fit into this category. Insufficiency fractures caused by osteoporosis frequently occur in these locations and are managed with protected weight bearing until the pain diminishes followed by assessment of bone density and appropriate medical treatment.[11,73]

Periacetabular lesions or fractures; however, affect ambulatory status and often present a difficult surgical problem.[41,55,69,89] The situation is magnified if there is protrusion of the femoral head through a pathologic acetabular fracture or defect (Fig. 22-8). All pathologic fractures or defects in this location should be assessed with CT scans with three-dimensional reconstruction. There are several classification systems for acetabular

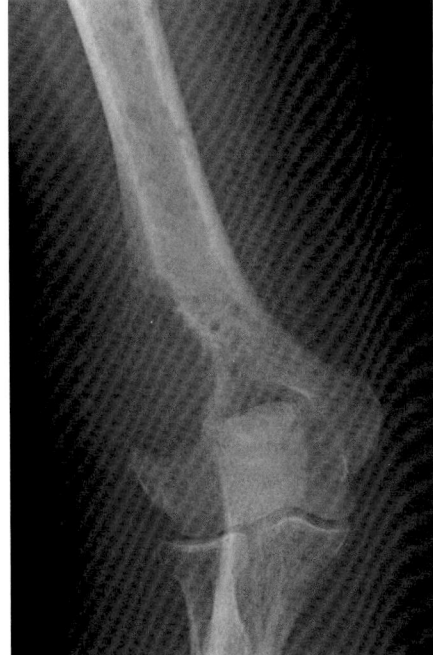
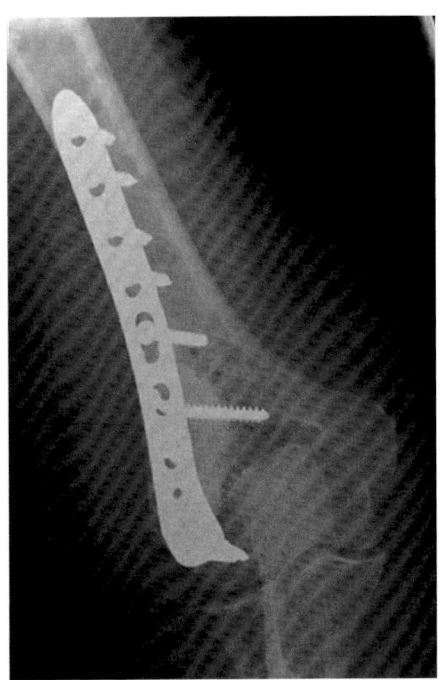

FIGURE 22-7 **A:** AP radiograph of a right distal humerus in a 74-year-old male with metastatic renal cell carcinoma. **B:** Due to a relatively poor prognosis, the patient underwent curettage, cementation, and plating of the lesion. Numerous nonstructural metastases remain untreated.

defects, but various modifications of the Harrington classification are considered to be most useful for assessing metastatic disease. This system classifies the location and extent of the defect and guides the technical considerations of fixation.[41] The modification often used describes Class I lesions as minor acetabular defects with maintenance of the lateral cortices, superior walls, and medial walls. A conventional cemented acetabular component provides sufficient support. Class II lesions are major acetabular defects with a deficient medial wall and superior dome. An antiprotrusion device and/or medial mesh is necessary (Fig. 22-9). Class III lesions are massive defects with deficient lateral cortices and superior dome. There is no substantial peripheral rim for fixation of a metal component; therefore, weight-bearing stresses must be transmitted from the acetabular component into bone unaffected by the tumor, usually near the sacroiliac joint. An acetabular cage should be used

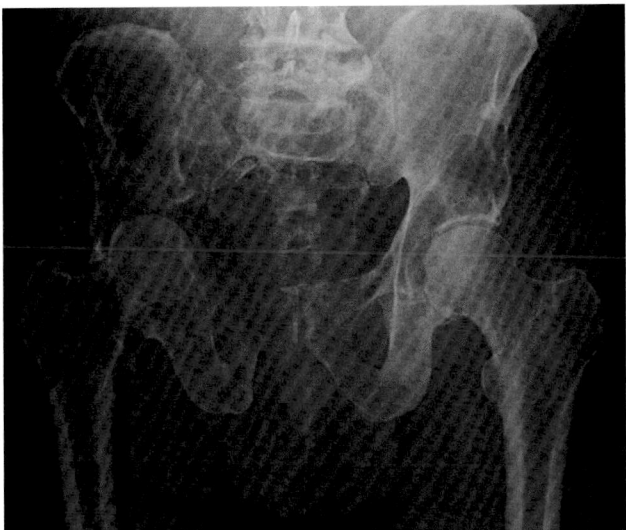
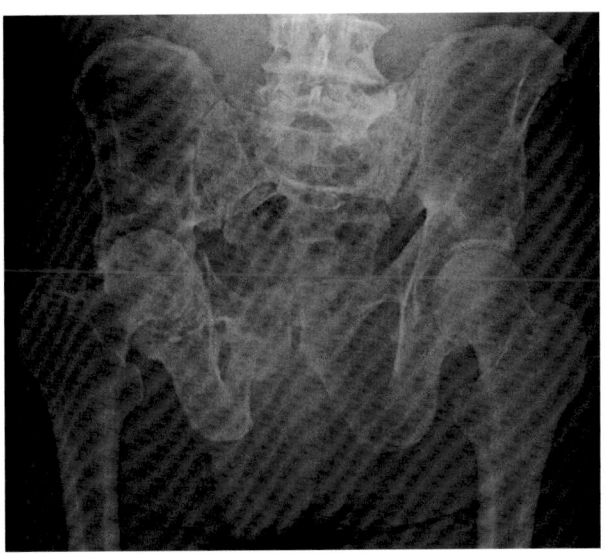

FIGURE 22-8 **A:** An AP pelvis of a 53-year-old male with multiple myeloma. He sustained a fracture of the pelvis at the time of his diagnosis. Due to the severe lack of bone stock and advanced stage, he was treated with intravenous bisphosphonates, radiation, and limited weight bearing. **B:** At 1 year postinitiation of treatment, he ambulates with a cane, no pain. Radiographs show that the acetabulum, ischium, and proximal femur have increased bone stock. The patient does not desire any surgery.

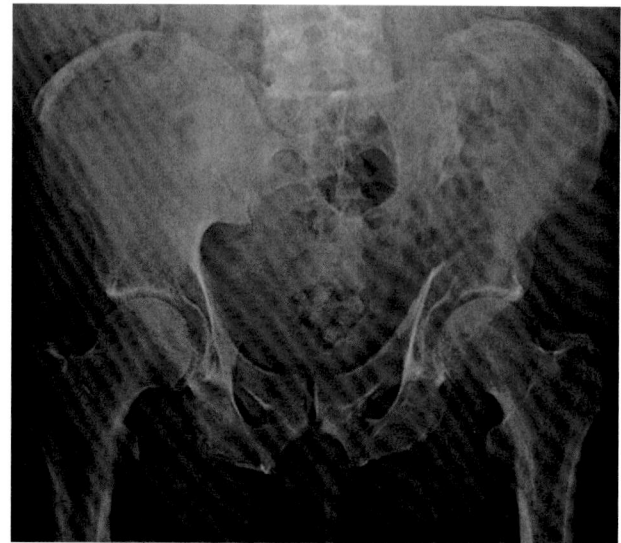
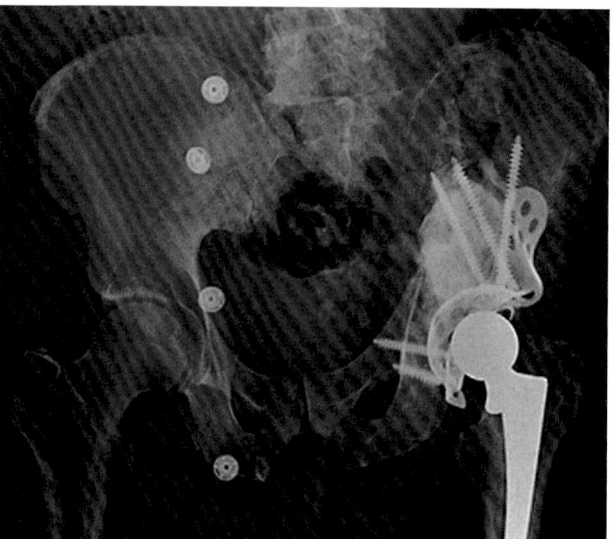

A

B

FIGURE 22-9 **A:** AP radiograph of the pelvis in a 68-year-old-male with multiple myeloma. There is a fracture through a lytic lesion on the left acetabulum and ilium. **B:** Cement is placed in the location of the lesion with a pelvic cage and long screws in the ilium for stabilization. A cemented total hip replacement is placed to manage the lesions in the femur.

with long screw fixation into any remaining pubis, ischium, and ilium. The massive bony defect is filled with PMMA to provide immediate stability after long screws and threaded $^5/_{16}$-inch Steinmann pins anchor the construct. A polyethylene cup is then cemented into the acetabular cage in the correct orientation Class IV lesions involve pelvic discontinuity and can be treated expediently with resection and reconstruction using a saddle prosthesis or a resection arthroplasty depending on patient factors and expected life span.[1] With these techniques, satisfactory pain relief and function can be achieved in 70% to 75% of patients. Complications are common and occur in 20% to 30% of cases.[1,2,41,55,69,89] Extensive blood loss can be anticipated with massive lytic defects. This demanding surgery is best done by surgeons with extensive experience treating this type of lesion. The trabecular metal tantalum provides new options for acetabular fixation by allowing early bone ingrowth. It can be used in combination with a cemented acetabular cage.[80]

Lower-Extremity Fractures

The femur is the most common long bone to be affected by metastasis.[101] The proximal third is involved in 50% of cases, with the intertrochanteric region accounting for 20% of cases. Metastatic disease to the femur is the most painful of the bone metastasis, likely because of the high weight-bearing stresses through the proximal region. Pathologic fractures of the femur severely impact the quality of a patient's life and threaten an individual's level of independence. Without proper surgical attention, the patient with a pathologic fracture of the femur will be confined to bed, a situation that is medically and psychologically devastating.

Painful destructive lesions in the proximal femur should be prophylactically stabilized whenever possible because of the high incidence of subsequent fracture and the comparative

ease of the operation. The development of bone metastasis is a continuous process, so it is important to stabilize as much of the femur as possible to avoid future peri-implant failure.[101] At a minimum, it is recommended that the tip of the chosen fixation device should bypass a given lesion by at least twice the diameter of the femur.

Femoral Neck. Pathologic fractures of the femoral head and neck rarely heal, and the neoplastic process tends to progress.[58] Accordingly, there is a high incidence of failure if traditional fracture fixation devices are used. The procedure of choice for patients with metastatic disease to the femoral head or neck is a cemented replacement prosthesis (Fig. 22-10).[58,75] The decision to use a hemiarthroplasty versus a total hip replacement depends on the presence of acetabular involvement. This must be carefully scrutinized as acetabular disease may go unrecognized and may be present microscopically in a surprisingly high percentage of cases. All tumor tissue should be curetted from the femoral canal before implanting the prosthesis. When there are adjacent lesions in the subtrochanteric region or proximal diaphysis, a long-stemmed cemented femoral component should be used for prophylactic fixation distally, avoiding a future pathologic fracture through a distal lesion and allowing full weight bearing postoperatively. When there are no additional lesions in the femur, the length of the cemented femoral stem is controversial. The risk of cardiopulmonary complications from cement monomer/marrow content embolization after pressurizing the extra cement and long stem within the canal must be weighed against the potential risk of future metastasis distal to the tip of the prosthesis if a shorter stem is used.[99] If long-stemmed femoral components are used, it is important to inject the cement into the canal while still in a fairly liquid state after thorough canal preparation.[7,16]

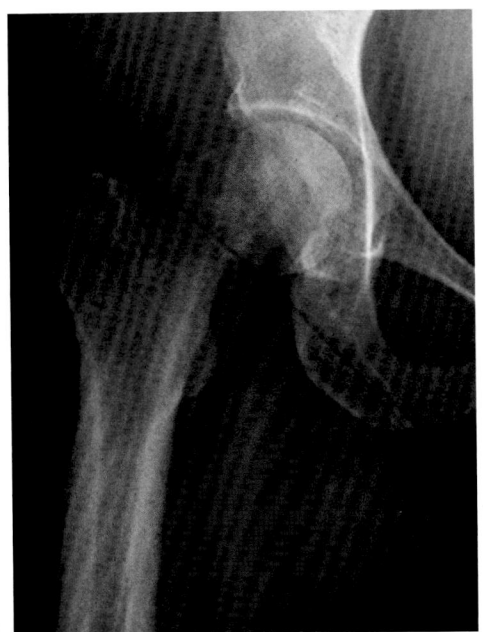
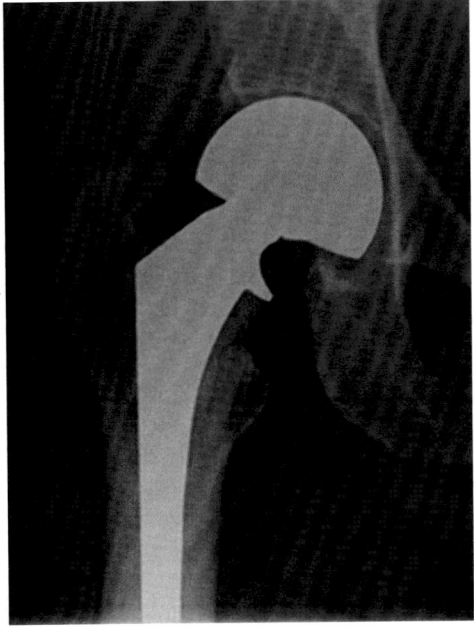

A **B**

FIGURE 22-10 A: AP radiograph of a right hip in a 49-year-old female with metastatic breast cancer. The femoral neck is displaced and due to the presence of tumor, has little biologic ability to heal. **B:** AP radiograph of a right hip after a cemented long-stem bipolar arthroplasty. The patient has no limitations in activities, no pain, and performs all activities at 2 years postop.

Intertrochanteric Region. Traditional fixation of an intertrochanteric fracture with screw and side-plate fixation has a high rate of failure when used in the setting of metastatic bone disease, even when supplemented with adjuvant PMMA and postoperative radiation. The standard of care is intramedullary fixation or prosthetic replacement.[101] The choice of fixation in this region of the femur depends on the extent of the lesion and whether it is radiosensitive. If bone with sufficient strength remains in the femoral head and neck and local control is likely to be achieved with postoperative external beam radiation, an intramedullary reconstruction device is recommended, which will allow the highest level of function. A cephalomedullary nail protects the femoral neck and is used for all metastatic lesions or pathologic fractures of the femur when an intramedullary device is indicated. If the destruction is more extensive, a cemented calcar-replacing prosthesis is required (Fig. 22-9). The same issues arise related to the length of the femoral stem as discussed in the previous section.

Subtrochanteric Region. Using plate and screw internal fixation for subtrochanteric fractures in patients with metastatic bone disease will usually end in failure. This region of the femur is subjected to forces of up to four to six times body weight. Statically locked intramedullary fixation with or without PMMA will stabilize the area and provide weight-bearing support.[102] Even impending fractures should be statically locked as the lesion can fracture later causing shortening of the femur. A modular proximal femoral prosthesis is reserved for cases with extensive bone destruction or used as a salvage device for failed internal fixation (Fig. 22-11).[75] It can also be used when a wide resection is necessary for a pathologic fracture through a

primary bone sarcoma. There is an increased risk of dislocation and abductor mechanism weakness with a megaprosthesis, but this should not prevent its use in patients with radioresistant or locally aggressive tumors. A bipolar head is used to provide more stability if the acetabulum is not involved with metastatic disease. Excellent pain relief and local tumor control can be obtained after tumor resection and prosthetic reconstruction.

Femoral Diaphysis. Pathologic fractures of the femoral diaphysis are treated most effectively with a statically locked cephalomedullary nail, with or without PMMA (Fig. 22-12).[101,107] Plate fixation, although more rigid, will not protect a large enough segment of bone and is prone to failure with disease progression. Cephalomedullary nail fixation protects the entire bone and is technically simple, especially when performed prophylactically. A trochanteric or piriformis entry point can be used, and the canal is slowly overreamed 1 to 1.5 mm to avoid high impaction forces during rod placement.[7] Because the device will be load bearing if the fracture does not unite, a nail with the largest possible diameter should be used. The fields for postoperative radiation should encompass the entire implant.

Supracondylar Femur. The choice of fixation for pathologic supracondylar femur fractures depends on the extent of local bone destruction and the presence of additional lesions in the proximal femur. The distal lesions can be a treatment challenge caused by frequent comminution and poor bone stock, especially in older patients. Options include lateral locking plate fixation supplemented with PMMA or a modular distal femoral prosthesis.[98] A retrograde nail has the drawback of potentially seeding the knee joint with tumor while failing to

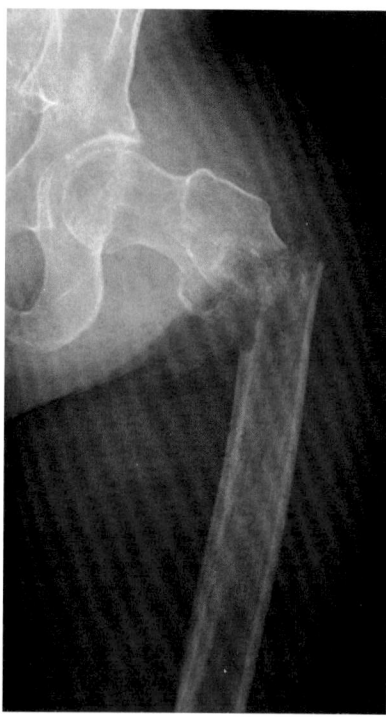
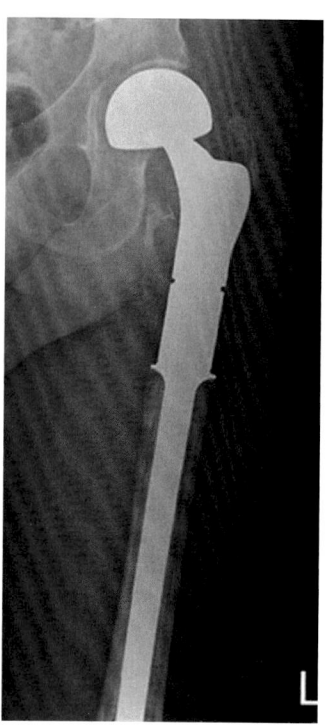

FIGURE 22-11 A: AP radiograph of the left proximal femur in a 37-year-old male with metastatic hepato-cellular carcinoma. The patient had received radiation therapy and had a long period of hip pain prior to fracture. **B:** AP radiograph of the left proximal femur shows a cemented long-stem bipolar arthroplasty performed. The greater trochanter is reattached to the prosthesis while still attached to the vastus late-ralis and gluteus medius tendons.

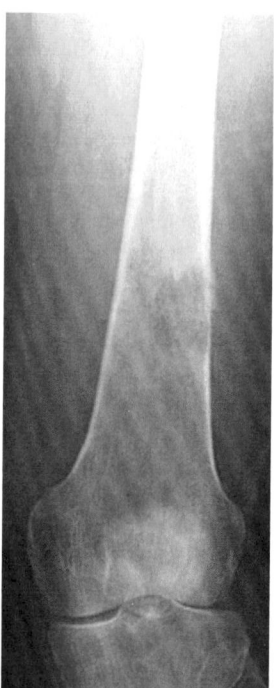
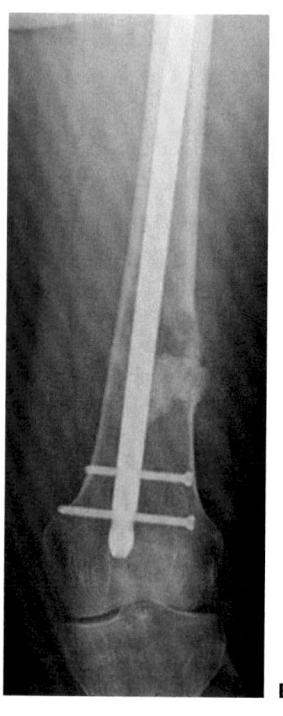

FIGURE 22-12 A: AP radiograph of the left distal femur in a 61-year-old male with multiple myeloma. The patient has a nondisplaced fracture through the lateral cortex of the femur with pain. **B:** AP radiograph shows a cephalomedullary intramedullary nail coursing the distal femoral lesion with cement augmentation to assist with early stability. A cephalomedullary device is chosen to prophylacti-cally stabilize the femoral neck.

provide fixation to the femoral neck region. The locking plate provides stable fixation after curettage and cementation of the metastatic lesion. The modular endoprosthesis is the optimal choice for local control when there is massive destruction of the femoral condyles, as it allows the lesion to be resected en bloc.[26]

Tibia. Metastases distal to the knee are uncommon but, for proximal tibial lesions, similar principles should be used as for lesions in the supracondylar femoral area. A locking plate with PMMA after thorough curettage of the lesion is generally sufficient. Extensive lesions may require a modular proximal tibial prosthesis. Tibial diaphyseal lesions and fractures should be managed with a locked intramedullary device. Various techniques can be employed for pathologic fractures of the distal tibia, but standard internal fixation methods are generally advised with generous use of PMMA to augment the construct.[21,59] The treatment of foot and ankle lesions must be individualized to maintain maximal function.[44]

Spinal Fractures

Between 5% and 10% of patients who die of metastatic carcinoma will have microscopic disease in their spine. The metastases most commonly involve the vertebral body rather than the posterior elements. The majority of these patients will not have clinically significant spine disease during their lifetime and will not need treatment specific to this location. The lesions are often discovered incidentally on a bone scan during a routine metastatic workup in a patient with known cancer. However, if the disease progresses, it can cause moderate to severe pain persisting for months before the onset of focal neurologic deficits.

Occasionally, the onset of pain is sudden following a pathologic compression fracture.

When the patient does not have a history of cancer, it must be decided whether a compression fracture is secondary to osteoporosis or a bone metastasis. If the patient has a history of cancer or if the patient's current symptoms, physical examination, laboratory studies, or imaging suggests a primary carcinoma or myeloma, the patient should be evaluated for a compression fracture caused by metastatic disease. It is imperative to consider spinal metastasis in any cancer patient with back pain. A delay in diagnosis can allow progression and possible neurologic compromise, leading to permanent functional deficits. Patients with a suspected malignancy should have a biopsy, but others should be treated symptomatically. If a patient treated for an osteoporotic compression fracture does not respond to the treatment or if there is progressive destruction of bone, a biopsy should be performed. Percutaneous CT-guided needle biopsy of vertebral lesions can be performed with local anesthesia and intravenous sedation.

The classic plain radiographic finding in metastatic involvement of the spine is loss of a pedicle on an anteroposterior view. MRI can be used to differentiate an osteoporotic compression fracture from one caused by a malignant lesion.[108] When there is complete replacement of the vertebral segment, multiple vertebral body lesions, pedicle involvement, and an intact intervertebral disk, metastatic disease is most likely (Fig. 22-13). Some patients with myeloma, lymphoma, or leukemia may present with osteopenia of the vertebra. To determine if the patient has a hematologic malignancy, a bone marrow aspirate should be considered. Most of these patients will have systemic findings (e.g., weight loss, fatigue, fever). If a metastatic lesion in the spine is identified, the patient is at risk of having additional skeletal lesions.

Treatment options for patients with symptomatic metastatic disease to the spine include nonoperative management with radiation, corticosteroids, and/or bracing; minimally invasive techniques such as kyphoplasty and vertebroplasty; and surgical treatment with adjuvant radiation.[29,38,40,66,84] Scoring systems for the evaluation of patients with vertebral metastasis have been reported, but no system has been universally adopted to guide treatment.[60,90] Quality of life must be considered as these are painful lesions, but surgical treatment is often a major undertaking that has significant morbidity and may require a prolonged recovery.[48]

Generally, symptoms from a vertebral compression fracture caused by osteoporosis are minor and can be successfully controlled with temporarily decreased activity or bracing. If the patient has asymptomatic vertebral metastases that are not at risk for pathologic fracture, systemic treatment can be used to address the primary and metastatic disease. Regular imaging of the spine should be performed to ensure that any disease progression is identified quickly. Often, early recognition of a spinal metastasis allows pain relief with nonoperative management. If the patient has pain but no neurologic compromise or risk of impending fracture, radiation treatment is indicated. Radiation is also used for radiation-sensitive tumors such as lymphoma or myeloma even when they present with neurologic compromise. The tumor response is usually sufficiently rapid such that the risk of permanent neurologic loss is no higher than that seen after surgical decompression. When there is minimal or no bone destruction but cord compression is caused by tumor extension, emergent radiation is recommended.[77] The patient should also be treated with a short course of high-dose corticosteroids to reduce edema surrounding the tumor that contributes to compression and neurologic damage. Other indications for radiation of vertebral metastasis include patients with medical comorbidities precluding surgery, patients with 6 weeks or less to live, and those with multilevel disease. Radiation should be added preoperatively or postoperatively to improve local disease control when patients are treated with surgery.[92] More recently, cyberknife radiosurgery has provided effective pain relief in patients with spinal metastases. It can be used in patients who have had prior external beam radiation as it focuses small beams of radiation into the tumor from many different directions via a robotic arm. This minimizes radiation exposure to the surrounding tissues. Cyberknife is a computer-assisted, minimally invasive procedure that can be performed as an outpatient in only one to three sessions and serves as another alternative to major surgery.[35]

Indications for surgical treatment of vertebral metastasis include progression of disease after radiation, neurologic compromise caused by bony impingement or radioresistant tumor within the spinal canal, an impending fracture, or spinal instability caused by a pathologic fracture or progressive deformity. The goals of surgery are to maintain or restore neurologic function and spinal stability.

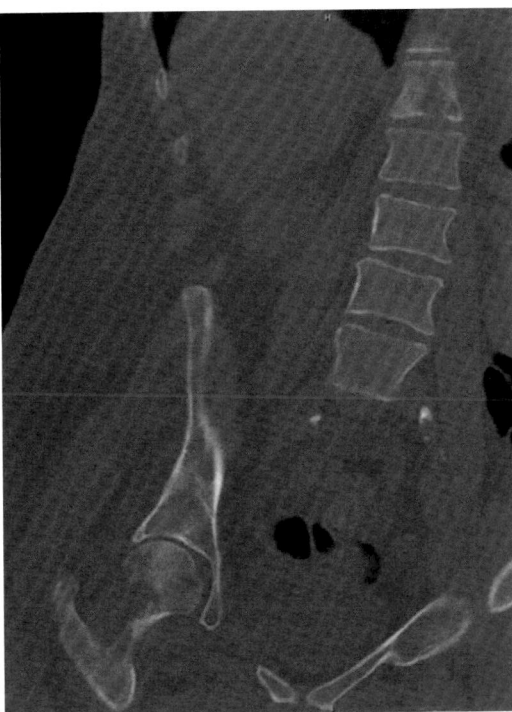

FIGURE 22-13 Multiple lytic lesions in a 55-year-old female including the body of L1 and the right femoral neck suggest a malignant process. A biopsy and treatment of the femoral neck lesion revealed a squamous lesion consistent with lung cancer.

When surgical treatment is necessary to relieve compression of the spinal cord, decompression and stabilization are required. Before surgery, MRI is used to verify the level of the lesion and rule out the possibility of compression at additional levels. A preoperative angiogram with embolization of feeder vessels should be considered in patients with highly vascular metastasis, such as RCC, to reduce intraoperative blood loss.[15] Relief of symptoms can often be accomplished via a posterior decompression and fusion using instrumentation.[3] When there is anterior collapse of the vertebrae and anterior compression of the spinal cord resulting in kyphosis, the patient is also treated with an anterior decompression and stabilization.[29,40,52,66] When the posterior elements are involved with tumor and the cord is compressed anteriorly, the patient should have an anterior decompression with posterior stabilization and fusion (Fig. 22-14).[90] Internal fixation is indicated to provide immediate stability for all but the most limited decompressions. In recent years, there has been considerable improvement in the available implants to manage structural deficiency of the spine, including pedicle screws, cages, and more sophisticated plates and rods. Specific techniques for anterior and posterior decompression and stabilization, including the use of modern instrumentation systems, are described in the literature.[29,90] Surgical implants made of titanium allow easier assessment of recurrent disease on MRI. As patients live longer with their metastatic disease, aggressive surgical treatment of spinal lesions can enhance quality of life. However, the magnitude of the operative procedure should not exceed the patient's chance of surviving the surgery or the surgeon's level of competence.

Kyphoplasty/Vertebroplasty. Minimally invasive treatments for metastatic disease to the spine have been used to control pain in patients who have developed compression fractures.[24,84] Vertebroplasty or kyphoplasty can be used for pathologic vertebral body fractures caused by osteoporosis, metastatic carcinoma, or multiple myeloma. The literature suggests that the results are similar in patients with malignancy versus osteoporosis, although these procedures have not been directly compared. Indications include patients with stable compression fractures who have normal neurologic function but persistent pain. One technique, vertebroplasty, involves percutaneous direct injection of PMMA through the pedicle to maintain vertebral height. Kyphoplasty is a way of regaining vertebral body height by expanding the compression fracture with a balloon before injecting the PMMA (Fig. 22-15). Reported complications include extrusion of cement around the neurologic structures, so this procedure should only be performed after careful consideration of the risks.

Complications

Because patients with pathologic fractures are often older with multiple associated medical problems, the chance of them developing a perioperative complication is increased. These patients have the same risks as those with nonpathologic fractures when

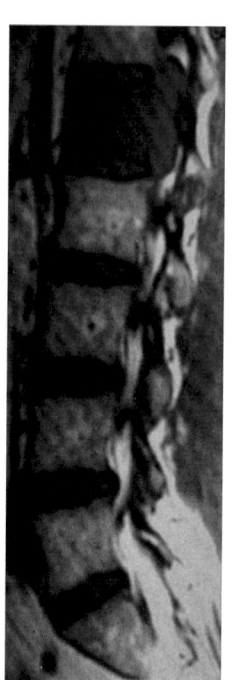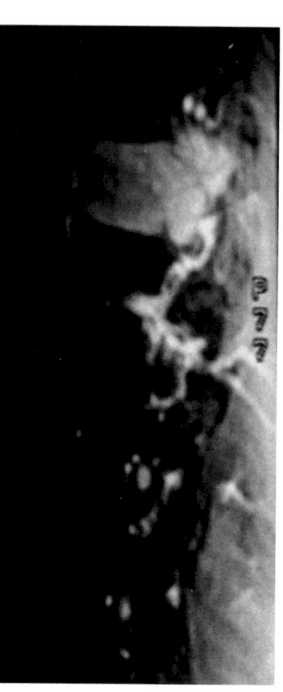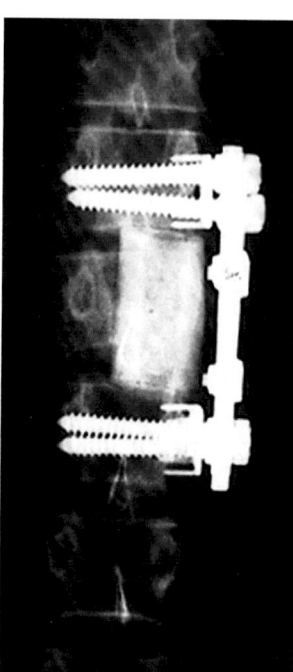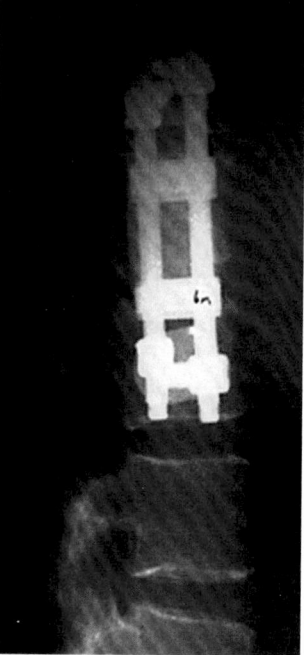

A, B

C, D

FIGURE 22-14 A: Sagittal T1-weighted image of the lumbar spine in a 53-year-old male with lung cancer shows an infiltrative lesion throughout L1 with complete marrow involvement and an extraosseous soft tissue mass abutting the anterior cord. The patient had significant leg weakness and inability to ambulate at presentation. **B:** A T2-weighted image with infiltration along the left epidural space at L1. **C:** AP radiograph of the lumbar spine after anterior decompression of the lumbar spine with screw fixation from T12 to L2 and allograft strut. **D:** Lateral radiograph of the thoracolumbar junction showing appropriate screw and hardware position. The patient had resolution of leg pain and weakness.

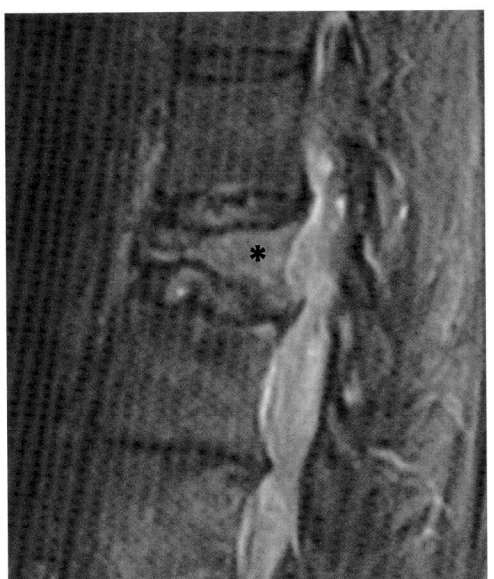 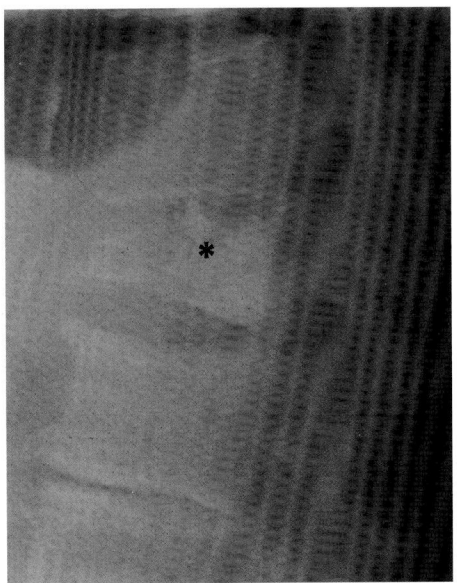

FIGURE 22-15 A: Sagittal T2 fat-suppressed image of the L1 vertebra in a patient with metastatic squamous cell carcinoma of the lungs (* = L1 vertebrae). The patient had significant pain associated with this lesion. **B:** Postvertebroplasty lateral x-ray of the lumbar spine shows cement filling the tumor void. Although restoration of vertebral height was not obtained, pain control was adequate and the deformity was corrected.

they consent to surgical treatment, but some complications are more likely in patients with widespread cancer. Two of the most concerning problems are tumor progression with resultant hardware failure and cardiopulmonary compromise.

Bone metastases that are unresponsive to chemotherapy and radiation will continue to destroy bone so that the existing hardware or prosthesis is load bearing rather than load sharing. Using the principles of surgical treatment outlined in this chapter will minimize the risk of hardware failure, but inevitably some constructs will fail, especially with increasing patient longevity. The salvage of failed reconstructions must be individualized, but modular endoprostheses can frequently be used to salvage failed intramedullary fixation.[49] Again, the patient's life span and general health must be favorable before they are indicated for a prolonged procedure.

Cardiopulmonary compromise is a noted risk in patients with bone metastasis. First, many of these patients have pulmonary metastasis or primary lung tumors that compromise lung function. Some patients will have a surgical procedure to stabilize a pathologic fracture and fail postoperative attempts at extubation, remaining in an intensive care setting for a prolonged time. Second, the placement of long-stemmed cemented femoral prostheses or prophylactic femoral or humeral nails must be done carefully to avoid embolic events. The orthopedic literature details how thorough canal preparation (brushing, irrigation, and careful suction of the canal in addition to slow reaming and possibly "venting" distally) are all tips to decrease this complication.[7,16] It is unclear from the available literature whether the actual incidence of fat emboli is increased during placement of intramedullary rods or long cemented femoral stems in patients with malignancy compared to those without cancer. However, patients with cancer are

hypercoagulable and are less likely to be able to compensate for fat emboli to the lung due to significantly reduced cardiopulmonary reserve, than are patients without cancer, especially if they have primary or metastatic pulmonary disease.

Role of Adjuvant Radiation and Medical Treatment

External Beam Radiation

External beam radiation is used to treat pain secondary to bone metastases, halt the progression of bony destruction, and allow healing of an impending pathologic fracture. It is a reasonable alternative to surgical treatment for certain lesions. When the endpoint is pain relief, local radiation therapy typically results in partial relief in over 80% of patients with bone metastasis and complete pain relief in 50% to 60% of cases.[99] Variability in response rates depends on multiple factors including the histology and location of the lesion.[104] The onset of symptomatic relief usually occurs in the first 1 to 2 weeks, but maximal relief may take several months. Radiation is used in the postoperative setting to increase local tumor control after surgical stabilization. Retrospective data have shown that postoperative radiation improves limb function and decreases the rates of second orthopedic procedures.[92] The majority of patients in this study had the entire prosthesis or internal fixation device included in the treatment field. Radiation can usually begin 2 weeks after the surgical procedure if there are no wound complications.

Systemic Radionucleotides

Systemic therapy for bone metastasis using radioactive bone-seeking agents provides palliation of bone pain. It may be appropriate for widespread bone metastases when more traditional forms of radiation have reached their limit or when standard radiation techniques are not feasible because of surrounding normal tissue tolerances. Strontium-89 is used clinically and preferentially taken up at sites of active bone mineral turnover, similar to bisphosphonates. There is a greater uptake of the radionucleotides in metastatic lesions than in normal bone. A systematic review of the published literature on palliation of painful bone metastasis with radiopharmaceuticals revealed better pain relief with fewer sites of disease using strontium-89 compared to placebo or local radiation therapy.[8]

Bisphosphonates

Bisphosphonates bind preferentially to the bone matrix and inhibit osteoclastic bone resorption. Receptor activator of nuclear factor kappa-B ligand (RANKL) on osteoblasts acts as an activator of osteoclast function. Bisphosphonates act as a competitive inhibitor of RANKL and thus decrease the depth of resorption cavities at osteoclastic binding sites, inhibit osteoclastic function, alter the morphology of the osteoclast ruffled border, and inhibit maturation and recruitment of osteoclasts from the monocyte/macrophage cell line. They promote osteoclast apoptosis, and there are some data to suggest direct effects on tumor cells. Intravenous bisphosphonates have been used with success to treat bone pain and hypercalcemia in breast cancer, and they are most commonly used as an adjunct to other systemic therapies.[65]

There have been multiple, well-organized studies that document a decrease in the time to skeletal-related events as well as a decrease in the rate of these events in patients with bone metastasis treated with various bisphosphonates.[43,64,65] Acutely, these medications are not used to prevent large lesions from fracture as their ability to provide structural rigidity requires many months of treatment.

Controversies and Future Directions

Two of the main controversies in the management of patients with metastatic bone disease are (a) the ideal length of a cemented femoral stem in patients with metastatic disease about the hip and (b) the specific characteristics that define an impending fracture. These topics were discussed previously.

There is also continued debate as to the surgical treatment of patients with a solitary metastasis. There is literature to suggest that wide resection of a solitary RCC metastasis leads to increased survival.[51,88] However, it has not been shown that these data are applicable to metastatic disease from other primary sites. The study recommending resection of solitary RCC metastasis was conducted before widespread use of PET scanning, which allows discovery of smaller foci of active disease. It is likely that many patients presumed to have solitary metastasis would have additional sites of disease if screened with PET imaging. However, a patient with a solitary metastasis from any origin who has been tumor free for several years should be theoretically considered a candidate for a resection. RCC and follicular thyroid carcinoma are the two tumor types most likely to produce isolated bone metastasis years after treatment of the primary tumor.

Future directions in the surgical treatment of patients with metastatic bone disease of the spine and extremities will likely include continued use and new applications for trabecular metal.[62] The tantalum acetabular components allow excellent bone ingrowth and are being used more routinely in revision joint arthroplasty to reconstruct large acetabular defects.[49,80] Thus, surgical experience with this material in the field of revision joint arthroplasty is rapidly increasing, expanding its use in other situations. Further advances in this type of metal fixation may allow improvement in the attachment of soft tissues to megaprostheses after tumor resection. Endoprostheses made of porous tantalum have been used in limb-sparing surgery in patients with lower-extremity sarcomas with short-term follow-up.[46]

Interventional radiologists are working more closely with orthopedic surgeons to manage patients with bone metastasis. Radiofrequency ablation (RFA) and cryotherapy are now being used routinely for palliative treatment of painful metastatic lesions. These techniques provide an alternative to external beam radiation or surgery.[36] A recent study of patients with pelvic and sacral metastasis treated with RFA showed a clinical benefit with significant pain relief in 95% of patients.[36] Most of these patients had failed to respond to prior treatment or were considered to be poor candidates for narcotic medication or radiation. Another new procedure termed acetabuloplasty is similar to vertebroplasty in that PMMA is injected percutaneously into an acetabular defect to provide pain relief and possibly avoid a major surgical reconstruction.[49,103]

TREATMENT OPTIONS FOR PATIENTS WITH PATHOLOGIC FRACTURES THROUGH PRIMARY BONE TUMORS

Benign Bone Tumors

Benign bone tumors occur most commonly in children and young adults. Most tumors gradually enlarge until the patient reaches skeletal maturity and then resolve or become inactive. Inactive lesions do not require surgical treatment. Active or aggressive benign lesions often require intralesional curettage with or without bone grafting to remove the tumor and allow healing of the underlying bone. A pathologic fracture through a benign bone tumor may change the course of treatment. Due to the younger age and higher activity level of patients who have benign bone tumors, pathologic fractures are not uncommon.

In general, the treatment of a pathologic fracture through a benign bone lesion depends on the activity of the underlying lesion. Most can be treated nonoperatively in a cast until the fracture heals. At that time, treatment of the benign tumor can be addressed. Indications for surgical treatment of the fracture include unacceptable deformity in a cast, open fracture, fracture nonunion, or an association with active or aggressive lesions such as giant cell tumor (GCT) or aneurysmal bone cyst (ABC). The treatment of pathologic fractures in the context of specific benign bone tumors is discussed next. The reader is referred to comprehensive musculoskeletal oncology textbooks to learn more about the diagnosis and treatment of individual tumors.

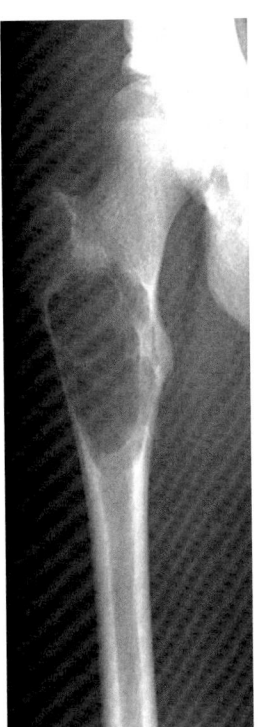 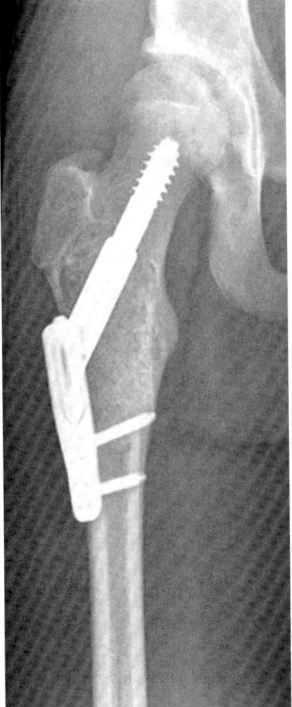

A   B

FIGURE 22-16 A: AP radiograph of a right proximal femur in an 11-year-old male shows a unicameral bone cyst with a medial non-displaced fracture. **B:** Treatment with a biopsy, curettage, bone grafting, and side plate allows for full weight bearing, mobilization, and treatment of the cyst.

Unicameral Bone Cyst

A pathologic fracture is the presenting complaint in two-thirds of patients with a unicameral bone cyst (UBC).[14] The majority of these lytic lesions are located in the proximal humerus or proximal femur (Fig. 22-16). A humeral fracture should be allowed to heal in a satisfactory position as the fracture occasionally stimulates healing of the cyst. If the cyst does not heal spontaneously after the fracture callus remodels, corticosteroid injection with bone graft or bone marrow aspirate into the cyst is recommended. A displaced fracture through a proximal femoral UBC in a child usually requires open reduction, bone grafting of the cyst, and internal fixation due to weight-bearing requirements.

Aneurysmal Bone Cyst

An ABC is an active benign lesion that can grow rapidly in the metaphysis of a young patient, simulating a malignancy.[14] Care should be taken in performing a biopsy for a presumed ABC as telangiectatic osteosarcomas can appear radiographically similar. Despite its occasional aggressive growth pattern, pathologic fractures are uncommon. Approximately 15% to 20% of lesions occur in the posterior elements of the spine and can cause neurologic compromise. The standard treatment of an ABC with or without a fracture is intralesional curettage and bone grafting. Depending on the age of the patient and location of the ABC, a pathologic fracture might require internal fixation at the time of curettage.

Eosinophilic Granuloma

An eosinophilic granuloma is a solitary lesion in the spectrum of disease known as Langerhans cell histiocytosis. It is a benign bone tumor, and affected patients present with pain. This tumor can cause collapse of a vertebral body (vertebra plana) and neurologic symptoms. Patients with symptomatic vertebra plana are braced, and eventually the vertebral height is restored without surgery (Fig. 22-17).[76] For extremity lesions that do not spontaneously resolve, the standard of care is an intralesional corticosteroid injection. Open curettage is reserved for selected lesions that fail to respond or are unsuitable for steroid injection because of the size, location, or aggressiveness of the lesion.[106] A pathologic fracture should be allowed to heal before performing a needle biopsy and injection, so the fracture callus does not confuse the histologic picture.

Nonossifying Fibroma

Nonossifying fibromas are extremely common lytic lesions in young patients. They spontaneously resolve after skeletal maturity. They are asymptomatic, but large lesions can fracture. Common pathologic fracture locations include the distal tibia, distal femur, and proximal tibia. Patients with multiple lesions have a higher risk of fracture. Pathologic fractures can be treated successfully in the majority of cases with closed reduction and cast immobilization.[25] If the lesion persists after fracture consolidation, curettage and bone grafting can be performed if necessary. If a fracture is unstable and cannot be reduced in a closed

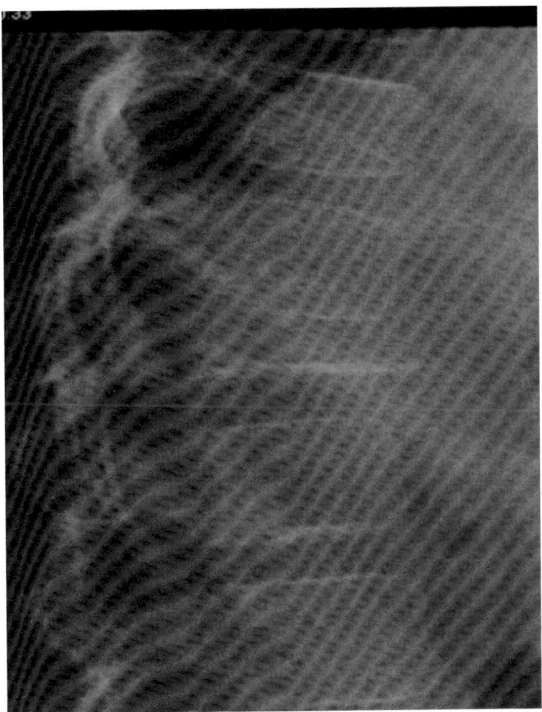

FIGURE 22-17 Lateral radiograph of the thoracolumbar spine of an 8-year-old female shows a compression of the vertebral body. This is a classic radiographic appearance of eosinophilic granuloma. Over time, the vertebral body will reconstitute in height.

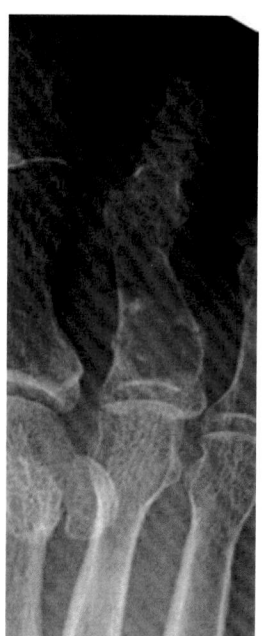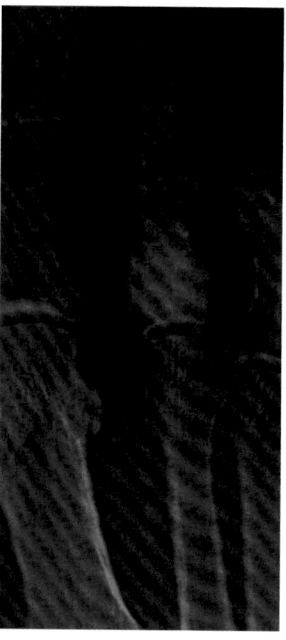

A **B**

FIGURE 22-18 A: AP radiograph of a second toe that shows a non-displaced fracture through the second toe, midshaft proximal phalanx lesion. **B:** The fracture was allowed to heal and subsequently, a biopsy, curettage, and bone grafting was performed which revealed a low-grade chondroid lesion consistent with enchondroma.

fashion, curettage and bone grafting is combined with internal fixation.

Enchondroma

Enchondromas are benign cartilage tumors that are asymptomatic unless associated with a pathologic fracture.[82] These lesions, when they occur in long bones, rarely fracture. Those most prone to pathologic fractures and pain occur in the small bones of the hand and foot (Fig. 22-18). Some advocate nonsurgical treatment of these lesions, as the fracture occasionally stimulates resolution of the enchondroma. Most agree that surgical intervention, if performed, should be delayed until the fracture has healed.[91] Occasionally, other factors (such as a tendon avulsion fracture through a phalangeal enchondroma) may prompt urgent surgery. Surgical treatment of the enchondroma eliminates the future risk of pathologic fracture and avoids progressive deformity. Whether to perform a bone graft to the defect after curettage remains controversial. Multiple enchondromas with frequent hand fractures and deformities occur in Ollier disease and Maffucci syndrome. Both of these conditions are associated with malignant transformation of the lesion. Although the actual rate of malignant transformation is unknown, Ollier's is estimated to be 25% lifetime risk, while Maffucci's is near 100% lifetime risk.

Fibrous Dysplasia

Fibrous dysplasia is defined as a developmental abnormality rather than a true neoplasm and occurs in both monostotic and polyostotic forms.[39] Most solitary lesions of fibrous dysplasia are asymptomatic, but patients can present with a painful patho-

logic fracture or a bowed extremity. In the polyostotic form, lesions involve multiple areas of a single bone or multiple bones in one extremity, and fractures occur in 85% of these patients. The structural bone strength is decreased in fibrous dysplasia, and sequential fractures can result in progressive deformity producing the classic shepherd's crook varus appearance of the proximal femur. The fractures are rarely displaced and heal well.

Pathologic fractures or symptomatic lesions in the upper extremity and spine can be treated nonoperatively, whereas lower-extremity fractures usually require internal fixation.[39] Extensive areas of fibrous dysplasia in high-stress weight-bearing areas are treated with prophylactic internal fixation. The lesion should be biopsied at the time of surgery to confirm the diagnosis before proceeding with intramedullary fixation to stabilize long bones. The goal is to strengthen and straighten the bone, not to resect the lesion. If bone graft is used, it should be allograft, as autograft has the same genetic abnormality as the dysplastic bone and may not heal properly. Internal fixation does not alter the disease process but provides mechanical support and pain relief. Another option is medical treatment with bisphosphonates alone or in combination with surgery.[57]

Giant Cell Tumor

GCT is an aggressive benign bone tumor that occurs in young adults. Ten percent of patients present with a pathologic fracture. In patients whose adjacent joint can be preserved, the GCT should be treated with thorough curettage and bone grafting or cementation.[93] Internal fixation is often necessary after a pathologic fracture as there is usually extensive bone loss and deformity. Adjuvant treatment with phenol or cryosurgery should be used with caution in patients when a pathologic fracture exposes adjacent soft tissues. Adjuvant treatments such as high-speed burr, argon beam, phenolization, cryosurgery, and cementation have been shown to lower local recurrence rates. Primary wide resection and reconstruction is only necessary when the associated joint is beyond salvage.

Malignant Bone Tumors

Primary malignant bone tumors are treated with a combination of surgery, chemotherapy, and/or radiation. Multiple myeloma is a primary malignant bone tumor with a systemic presentation that occurs in older patients. Pathologic fractures in patients with myeloma, lymphoma, and metastatic carcinoma can be treated with fixation through the tumor as they are systemic diseases treated primarily with chemotherapy and radiation. The overall survival of these patients is not compromised by palliative surgical stabilization.

Primary malignant bone tumors such as osteosarcoma, Ewing sarcoma, and chondrosarcoma are treated much differently than systemic neoplastic disease.[97] These tumors grow initially in the bone and can metastasize to the lungs. Local control of the primary lesion is achieved by complete surgical resection. A pathologic fracture through the lesion theoretically decreases the chance of local control, because tumor cells spread throughout the hematoma. Amputation should be discussed as a potential surgical option for patients with a pathologic fracture through a primary malignant bone tumor. The traditional literature has suggested that amputation is the treatment of choice for pathologic fractures through a primary malignant bone tumor, but with improved adjuvant care and surgery, there are recent studies that describe good rates of limb salvage with local disease control.[30,83,105] Ferguson in 2010 showed that in 31 patients with pathologic fractures associated with an osteosarcoma, the rate of limb salvage and local control was equal to 201 patients without a pathologic fracture with osteosarcoma. However, the overall survival was also shown to be worse in patients with pathologic fracture. To some degree this depends on the amount of fracture displacement, histology of the tumor, and response to chemotherapy.

Before initiating treatment for a patient with a pathologic fracture through a presumed primary bone sarcoma, the patient should be staged and a biopsy performed. An appropriate staging workup includes a CT scan of the chest for all patients, and a bone marrow biopsy when Ewing sarcoma is suspected. The biopsy of a presumed bone sarcoma is especially difficult in the setting of an associated pathologic fracture. The fracture hematoma and healing process alters the histology and may make the pathology difficult to properly interpret. Whenever possible, the biopsy should be performed away from the fracture. When there is an extraosseous soft tissue mass associated with the tumor, an image-guided needle biopsy is usually adequate. When the lesion is intraosseous and fracture callus is present, an open biopsy may be necessary. The surgeon who will eventually perform the definitive surgical treatment of the lesion should be the one who orders or performs the diagnostic biopsy.

Internal fixation of a pathologic fracture through a primary sarcoma may compromise the limb and life of the patient. If the patient will be treated with preoperative chemotherapy, cast immobilization or limited internal fixation of the fracture is preferred. The fracture usually heals during systemic treatment, and a cast avoids potential pin tract infections in neutropenic patients stabilized with an external fixator.

Patients with a pathologic fracture through a primary malignancy of bone require a coordinated multidisciplinary team that includes a medical oncologist, radiation oncologist, musculoskeletal pathologist, radiologist, physical therapist, and orthopedic oncologist; only with the full complement of care can these patients achieve the best quality of life and maximum overall survival.

Osteosarcoma/Ewing Sarcoma

These are the two most common primary malignant bone tumors in children. Approximately 10% of patients present with a pathologic fracture. Closed treatment of the fracture in a cast is indicated after a needle or open biopsy is performed. When staging is complete, preoperative chemotherapy is used for patients with osteosarcoma or Ewing sarcoma. After 3 to 4 months of systemic therapy, a decision is made about local control of the primary tumor. For patients with osteosarcoma, surgical resection is indicated. If patients have a clinical and radiographic response to chemotherapy, a limb salvage procedure is generally preferred. Articles have shown no difference in local control for patients with osteosarcoma and a pathologic fracture that are treated with limb salvage compared to ampu-

tation.[5,83] However, if the sarcoma shows a poor response to chemotherapy or neurovascular invasion has progressed since treatment, limb salvage is potentially contraindicated. Close follow-up is necessary to identify a possible local recurrence or the presence of metastatic disease.

Local control in Ewing sarcoma can be achieved with surgical resection, radiation, or both. In reconstructable sites, most patients are treated with limb salvage surgery to remove all chemotherapy-resistant clones and avoid the risks of radiation in a growing child. However, in patients with a pathologic fracture treated with surgical resection, consideration should be given to adding radiation as a postoperative adjuvant to improve the chance of local control and avoid amputation.[32]

Chondrosarcoma

Chondrosarcoma occurs in middle-aged and older adults.[10] The pelvis is a common site, but displaced pathologic fractures are rare in this location. The most common location of a pathologic fracture through a chondrosarcoma is in the proximal femur (Fig. 22-19). A serious mistake is to assume the fracture is secondary to metastatic carcinoma and place an intramedullary rod through the lesion. This act contaminates multiple tissue planes (such as the glutei) with malignant cells and generally precludes any safe limb salvage option for the patient. Although no data has shown that reaming directly results in systemic spread of disease, the implication is that tumor cells may be forced into the blood stream or lymphatics and this could lead to seeding distant sites. An older patient with a solitary lytic lesion should be staged appropriately with a biopsy to confirm the diagnosis before any surgical treatment.

The treatment of a patient with a pathologic fracture through a chondrosarcoma is wide resection by an orthopedic oncologist. Chemotherapy and radiation are generally not effective for this tumor. Recent studies have shown that proton beam radiation to be useful in some patients with chondrosarcoma.[4,18] This is reserved for specific cases that include skull base tumors or recurrent, unresectable tumors. A pathologic fracture greatly compromises the local area, as any stray tumor cells not resected will likely grow into a locally recurrent lesion. A displaced fracture through a chondrosarcoma is a reason to consider amputation, especially if wide resection cannot be achieved with a limb salvage procedure.

SUMMARY AND KEY POINTS

- Any process that reduces bone strength predisposes a patient to a pathologic fracture during normal activity or after minimal trauma. It must be recognized as a pathologic fracture if the patient is to be treated properly.

- The most common cause for a pathologic fracture is osteoporosis or osteomalacia.

- Patients with osteoporosis or osteomalacia require evaluation and management of the underlying disorder.

- Patients older than 40 years of age with a pathologic fracture through a discrete bone lesion are much more likely to have metastatic bone disease than a primary bone tumor.

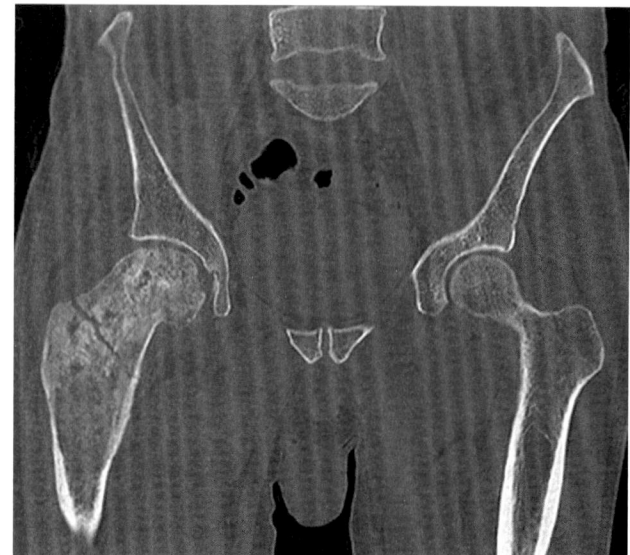 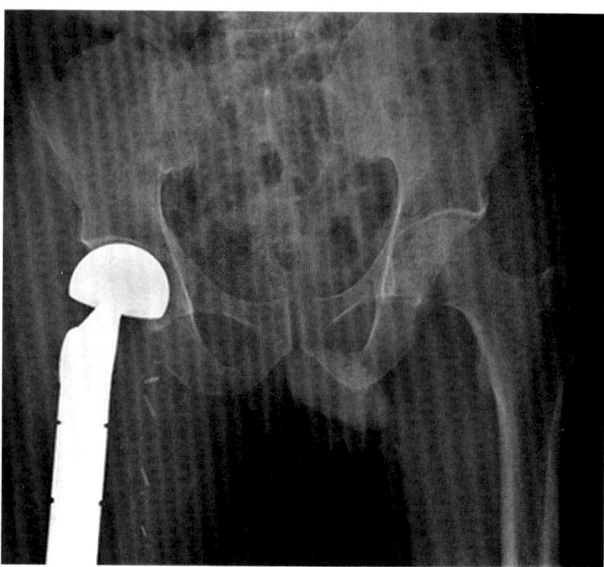

FIGURE 22-19 A: Coronal CT of the pelvis in a 48-year-old male with right hip pain. Note the pathologic fracture through a lesion that was diagnosed as clear cell chondrosarcoma. Initially, a plate was used to stabilize the bone until his pathology was determined. **B:** After a final diagnosis, he underwent resection of the right proximal femur followed by megaprosthetic reconstruction and bipolar hemiarthroplasty.

- The prognosis for patients with metastatic bone disease is improving because of early recognition and better adjuvant treatment; therefore, many patients will live longer than 2 years.

- Do not immediately assume that a lytic lesion or pathologic fracture is from metastatic disease. A thorough workup and possible biopsy are required.

- Prophylactic fixation for impending (vs. actual) fractures from metastatic disease is technically easier for the surgeon and allows a quicker patient recovery.

- The Mirels's scoring system is available to guide the treatment of an impending fracture from metastatic bone disease.

- Femoral neck fractures caused by metastatic bone disease require a cemented hip prosthesis, as internal fixation has a high rate of failure with disease progression.

- An isolated fracture of the lesser trochanter is usually a sign of a metastatic femoral neck lesion with impending fracture.

- When surgery is required for metastatic disease to the spine, decompression and stabilization with internal fixation are generally necessary.

- Surgical reconstruction for pathologic fractures should be durable enough to allow immediate weight bearing and last the patient's expected life span.

- A pathologic fracture through a primary malignant bone tumor is treated much differently than a fracture through a metastatic lesion. The treating surgeon should keep in mind with proper surgery there is a chance for long-term cure.

- Treatment of patients with pathologic fractures requires the presence of a multidisciplinary team comprises orthopedic surgeons, medical oncologists, radiation oncologists, endocrinologists, radiologists, pathologists, pain specialists, nutritionists, physical therapists, and psychologists/psychiatrists.

REFERENCES

1. Aboulafia AJ, Buch R, Mathews J, et al. Reconstruction using the saddle prosthesis following excision of primary and metastatic periacetabular tumors. *Clin Orthop Relat Res.* 1995;(314):203–213.
2. Abudu A, Grimer RJ, Cannon SR, et al. Reconstruction of the hemipelvis after the excision of malignant tumors. Complications and functional outcome of prostheses. *J Bone Joint Surg Br.* 1997;79:773–779.
3. Akeyson EW, McCutcheon IE. Single-stage posterior vertebrectomy and replacement combined with posterior instrumentation for spinal metastasis. *J Neurosurg.* 1996;85:211–220.
4. Amichetti M, Amelio D, Cianchetti M, et al. A systematic review of proton therapy in the treatment of chondrosarcoma of the skull base. *Neurosurg Rev.* 2010;33(2):155–165.
5. Bacci G, Ferrari S, Longhi A, et al. Nonmetastatic osteosarcoma of the extremity with pathologic fracture at presentation: Local and systemic control by amputation or limb salvage after preoperative chemotherapy. *Acta Orthop Scand.* 2003;74:449–454.
6. Bartucci EJ, Gonzalez MH, Cooperman DR, et al. The effect of adjunctive methylmethacrylate on failures of fixation and function in patients with intertrochanteric fractures and osteoporosis. *J Bone Joint Surg Am.* 1985;67:1094–1107.
7. Barwood SA, Wilson JL, Molnar RR, et al. The incidence of acute cardiorespiratory and vascular dysfunction following intramedullary nail fixation of femoral metastasis. *Acta Orthop Scand.* 2000;71:147–152.
8. Bauman G, Charette M, Reid R, et al. Radiopharmaceuticals for the palliation of painful bone metastasis: A systemic review. *Radiother Oncol.* 2005;75:258–270.
9. Bertin KC, Horstman J, Coleman SS. Isolated fractures of the lesser trochanter in adults: An initial manifestation of metastatic malignant disease. *J Bone Joint Surg Am.* 1984;66:770–773.
10. Bjornsson J, McLeod RA, Unni KK, et al. Primary chondrosarcoma of long bones and limb girdles. *Cancer.* 1998;83:2105–2119.
11. Brahme SK, Cervilla V, Vinct V, et al. Magnetic resonance appearance of sacral insufficiency fractures. *Skeletal Radiol.* 1990;19:489–493.
12. Brown RK, Pelker RR, Friedlaender GE, et al. Postfracture radiation effects on the biomechanical and histologic parameters of fracture healing. *J Orthop Res.* 1991;9:876–882.
13. Bunting RW, Boublik M, Blevins FT, et al. Functional outcome of pathologic fracture secondary to malignant diseases in a rehabilitation hospital. *Cancer.* 1992;69:98–102.
14. Campanacci M, Capanna R, Picci P. Unicameral and aneurysmal bone cysts. *Clin Orthop Relat Res.* 1986;(204):25–36.
15. Chatziioannou AN, Johnson ME, Penumaticos SG, et al. Preoperative embolization of bone metastases from renal cell carcinoma. *Eur J Radiol.* 2000;10:593–596.

16. Churchill DL, Incavo SJ, Uroskie JA, et al. Femoral stem insertion generates high bone cement pressurization. *Clin Orthop Relat Res.* 2001;(393):335–344.
17. Cummings SR, Melton LJ. Epidemiology and outcomes of osteoporotic fractures. *Lancet.* 2002;359:1761–1767.
18. Dallas J, Imanirad I, Rajani R, et al. Response to sunitinib in combination with proton beam radiation in a patient with chondrosarcoma: A case report. *J Med Case Rep.* 2012;6:41.
19. Damron TA, Rock MG, Choudhury SN, et al. Biomechanical analysis of prophylactic fixation for middle third humeral impending pathologic fractures. *Clin Orthop Relat Res.* 1999;363:240–248.
20. Damron TA, Sim FH, Shives TC, et al. Intercalary spacers in the treatment of segmentally destructive diaphyseal humeral lesions in disseminated malignancies. *Clin Orthop Relat Res.* 1996;(324):233–243.
21. De Geeter K, Reynders P, Samson I, et al. Metastatic fractures of the tibia. *Acta Orthop Belg.* 2001;67:54–59.
22. Demers LM, Costa L, Lipton A. Biochemical markers and skeletal metastases. *Clin Orthop Relat Res.* 2003;(415):S138–S147.
23. Dougall WC, Chaisson M. The RANK/RANKL/OPG triad in cancer-induced bone disease. *Cancer Metastasis Rev.* 2006;25:541–549.
24. Dudeney S, Lieberman IH, Reinhardt MK, et al. Kyphoplasty in the treatment of osteolytic vertebral compression fractures as a result of multiple myeloma. *J Clin Oncol.* 2002;20:2382–2387.
25. Easley ME, Kneisl JS. Pathologic fractures through nonossifying fibromas: Is prophylactic treatment warranted? *J Pediatr Orthop.* 1997;17:808–813.
26. Eckardt JJ, Kabo M, Kelly CM, et al. Endoprosthetic reconstructions for bone metastases. *Clin Orthop Relat Res.* 2003;(415 suppl):S254–S262.
27. Eftekhar NS, Thurston CW. Effect of radiation on acrylic cement with special reference to fixation of pathological fractures. *J Biomech.* 1975;8:53–56.
28. Even-Sapir E, Metser U, Flusser G, et al. Assessment of malignant skeletal disease: Initial experience with 18 F-fluoride PET/CT and comparison between 18 F-Fluoride PET and 18 F-fluoride PET/CT. *J Nucl Med.* 2004;45:272–278.
29. Feiz-Erfan I, Rhines LD, Weinberg JS. The role of surgery in the management of metastatic spinal tumors. *Semin Oncol.* 2008;35:108–117.
30. Ferguson PC, McLaughlin CE, Griffin AM, et al. Clinical and functional outcomes of patients with a pathologic fracture in high-grade osteosarcoma. *J Surg Oncol.* 2010;102(2):120–124.
31. Fidler M. Prophylactic internal fixation of secondary neoplastic deposits in long bones. *BMJ.* 1973;1:341–343.
32. Fuchs B, Valenzuela RG, Sim FH. Pathologic fracture as a complication in the treatment of Ewing's sarcoma. *Clin Orthop Relat Res.* 2003:25–30.
33. Gainor BJ, Buchert P. Fracture healing in metastatic bone disease. *Clin Orthop Relat Res.* 1983;(178):297–302.
34. Gass M, Dawson-Hughes B. Preventing osteoporosis-related fractures: An overview. *Am J Med.* 2006;119(4 suppl 1):S3–S11.
35. Gerszten PC, Welch WC. Cyberknife radiosurgery for metastatic spine tumors. *Neurosurg Clin N Am.* 2004;15:491–501.
36. Goetz MP, Callstrom MR, Charboneau JW, et al. Percutaneous image-guided radiofrequency ablation of painful metastases involving bone: A multicenter study. *J Clin Oncol.* 2004;22:300–306.
37. Greenspan A, Norman A. Osteolytic cortical destruction: An unusual pattern of skeletal metastases. *Skeletal Radiol.* 1988;17:402–406.
38. Gronemeyer DH, Schirp S, Gevargez A. Image-guided radiofrequency ablation of spinal tumors: Preliminary experience with an expandable array electrode. *Cancer J.* 2002;8:33–39.
39. Guille JT, Jumar SJ, MacEwin GD. Fibrous dysplasia of the proximal part of the femur. Long-term results of curettage and bone-grafting and mechanical realignment. *J Bone Joint Surg Am.* 1998;80:648–658.
40. Harrington KD. Anterior decompression and stabilization of the spine as a treatment for vertebral collapse and spinal cord compression from metastatic malignancy. *Clin Orthop Relat Res.* 1988;233:177–197.
41. Harrington KD. The management of acetabular insufficiency secondary to metastatic malignant disease. *J Bone Joint Surg Am.* 1981;63:653–664.
42. Harrington KD, Sim FH, Enis JE, et al. Methylmethacrylate as an adjunct in internal fixation of pathologic fractures. *J Bone Joint Surg Am.* 1976;58:1047–1055.
43. Hatoum HT, Lin SJ, Smith MR, et al. Zoledronic acid and skeletal complications in patients with solid tumors and bone metastases: Analysis of a national medical claims database. *Cancer.* 2008;113:1438–1445.
44. Hattrup SJ, Amadio PC, Sim FH, et al. Metastatic tumors of the foot and ankle. *Foot Ankle.* 1988;8:243–247.
45. Henry JC, Damron TA, Weiner MM, et al. Biomechanical analysis of humeral diaphyseal segmental defect fixation. *Clin Orthop Relat Res.* 2002:231–239.
46. Holt GE, Christie MJ, Schwartz HS. Trabecular metal endoprosthetic limb salvage reconstruction of the lower limb. *J Arthroplasty.* 2009;24(7):1079–1085.
47. Hong J, Cabe GD, Tedrow JR, et al. Failure of trabecular bone with simulated lytic defects can be predicted noninvasively by structural analysis. *J Orthop Res.* 2004;22:479–486.
48. Ibrahim A, Crockard A, Antonietti P, et al. Does spinal surgery improve the quality of life for those with extradural (spinal) osseous metastases? An international multicenter prospective observational study of 223 patients. Invited submission from the Joint Section Meeting on Disorders of the Spine and Peripheral Nerves, March 2007. *J Neurosurg Spine.* 2008;8:271–278.
49. Jacofsky DJ, Papagelopoulos PJ, Sim FH. Advances and challenges in the surgical treatment of metastatic bone disease. *Clin Orthop Relat Res.* 2003;(415 suppl):S14–S18.
50. Jemal A, Siegel R, Ward E, et al. Cancer statistics, 2008. *CA Cancer J Clin.* 2008;58:71–96.
51. Jung ST, Ghert MA, Harrelson JM, et al. Treatment of osseous metastases in patients with renal cell carcinoma. *Clin Orthop Relat Res.* 2003;223–231.
52. Kanayama M, Ng JT, Cunningham BW, et al. Biomechanical analysis of anterior versus circumferential spinal reconstruction for various anatomic stages of tumor lesions. *Spine.* 1999;24:445–450.
53. Katzer A, Meenen NM, Grabbe F, et al. Surgery of skeletal metastases. *Arch Orthop Trauma Surg.* 2002;122:251–258.
54. Kumar D, Grimer RJ, Abudu A, et al. Endoprosthetic replacement of the proximal humerus. Long-term results. *J Bone Joint Surg Br.* 2003;85:717–722.
55. Kunisada T, Choong PF. Major reconstruction for periacetabular metastasis: Early complications and outcome following surgical treatment in 40 hips. *Acta Orthop Scand.* 2000;71:585–590.
56. Kwee TC, Kwee RM, Nievelstein RA: Imaging in staging of malignant lymphoma: A systematic review. *Blood.* 2008;111:504–516.
57. Lane JM, Khan SN, O'Connor WJ, et al. Bisphosphonate therapy in fibrous dysplasia. *Clin Orthop Relat Res.* 2001;382:6–12.
58. Lane JM, Sculco TP, Zolan S. Treatment of pathological fractures of the hip by endoprosthetic replacement. *J Bone Joint Surg Am.* 1980;62:954–959.
59. Leeson MC, Makley JT, Carter JR. Metastatic skeletal disease distal to the elbow and knee. *Clin Orthop Relat Res.* 1986;(206):94–99.
60. Leithner A, Radl R, Gruber G, et al. Predictive value of seven preoperative prognostic scoring systems for spinal metastases. *Eur Spine J.* 2008;17:1488–1495.
61. Leong NL, Anderson ME, Gebhardt MC, et al. Computed tomography-based structural analysis for predicting fracture risk in children with benign skeletal neoplasms: Comparison of specificity with that of plain radiographs. *J Bone Joint Surg Am.* 2010;92(9):1827–1833.
62. Levine BR, Sporer S, Poggie RA, et al. Experimental and clinical performance of porous tantalum in orthopaedic surgery. *Biomaterials.* 2006;27:4671–4681.
63. Lin PP, Mirza AN, Lewis VO, et al. Patient survival after surgery for osseous metastases from renal cell carcinoma. *J Bone Joint Surg Am.* 2007;89:1794–1801.
64. Lipton A. Efficacy and safety of intravenous bisphosphonates in patients with bone metastases caused by metastatic breast cancer. *Clin Breast Cancer.* 2007;7(suppl 1):S14–S20.
65. Lipton A. Treatment of bone metastasis and bone pain with bisphosphonates. *Support Cancer Ther.* 2007;4:92–100.
66. Liu JK, Apfelbau RI, Chiles BW III, et al. Cervical spinal metastasis: Anterior reconstruction and stabilization techniques after tumor resection. *Neurosurg Focus.* 2003;15:E2.
67. Major P, Lortholary A, Hon J, et al. Zoledronic acid is superior to pamidronate in the treatment of hypercalcemia of malignancy: A pooled analysis of two randomized, controlled clinical trials. *J Clin Oncol.* 2001;19:558–567.
68. Mankin HJ, Mankin CJ, Simon MA. The hazards of the biopsy, revisited. Members of the Musculoskeletal Tumor Society. *J Bone Joint Surg Am.* 1996;78:656–663.
69. Marco RA, Sheth DS, Boland PJ, et al. Functional and oncological outcome of acetabular reconstruction for the treatment of metastatic disease. *J Bone Joint Surg Am.* 2000;82:642–651.
70. Mirels H. Metastatic disease in long bones. A proposed scoring system for diagnosing impending pathologic fractures. *Clin Orthop Relat Res.* 1989;249:256–265.
71. Morrow M, Waters J, Morris E. MRI for breast cancer screening, diagnosis, and treatment. *Lancet.* 2011;378(9805):1804–1811.
72. Nazarian A, von Stechow D, Zurakowski D, et al. Bone volume fraction explains the variation in strength and stiffness of cancellous bone affected by metastatic cancer and osteoporosis. *Calcif Tissue Int.* 2008;83(6):368–379.
73. Newhouse KE, El-Khoury GY, Buckwalter JA. Occult sacral fractures in osteopenic patients. *J Bone Joint Surg Am.* 1992;74:1472–1477.
74. Ohta M, Tokuda Y, Suzuki Y, et al. Whole body PET for the evaluation for bony metastases in patients with breast cancer: Comparison with 99Tcm-MDP bone scintigraphy. *Nucl Med Commun.* 2001;22:875–879.
75. Papagelopoulos PJ, Galanis EC, Greipp PR, et al. Prosthetic hip replacement for pathologic or impending pathologic fractures in myeloma. *Clin Orthop Relat Res.* 1997:192–205.
76. Raab P, Hohmann F, Kuhl J, et al. Vertebral remodeling in eosinophilic granuloma of the spine. A long-term follow-up. *Spine.* 1998;23:1351–1354.
77. Rades D, Blach M, Nerreter V, et al. Metastatic spinal cord compression. Influence of time between onset of motoric deficits and start of radiation on therapeutic effect. *Strahlenther Onkol.* 1999;175:378–381.
78. Ralston S, Fogelman I, Gardner MD, et al. Hypercalcemia and metastatic bone disease: Is there a causal link? *Lancet.* 1982;2:903–905.
79. Roodman GD. Biology of osteoclast activation in cancer. *J Clin Oncol.* 2001;19:3562–3571.
80. Rose PS, Halasy M, Trousdale RT, et al. Preliminary results of tantalum acetabular components for THA after pelvic radiation. *Clin Orthop Relat Res.* 2006;453:195–198.
81. Rougraff BT. Evaluation of the patient with carcinoma of unknown primary origin metastatic to bone. *Clin Orthop Relat Res.* 2003;415:S105–S109.
82. Scarborough M, Moreau G. Benign cartilage tumors. *Orthop Clin North Am.* 1996;27:583–589.
83. Scully SP, Ghert MA, Zurakowski D, et al. Pathologic fracture in osteosarcoma: Prognostic importance and treatment implications. *J Bone Joint Surg Am.* 2002;84A:49–57.
84. Siemionow K, Lieberman IH. Vertebral augmentation in osteoporosis and bone metastasis. *Curr Opin Support Palliat Care.* 2007;1:323–327.
85. Sim FH, Daugherty TW, Ivins JC. The adjunctive use of methylmethacrylate in fixation of pathological fractures. *J Bone Joint Surg Am.* 1974;56:40–48.
86. Snell W, Beals RL. Femoral metastases and fractures from breast carcinoma. *Surg Gynecol Obstet.* 1964;119:22–24.
87. Sugiura H, Yamada K, Sugiura T, et al. Predictors of survival in patients with bone metastasis of lung cancer. *Clin Orthop Relat Res.* 2008;466:729–736.
88. Swanson DA. Surgery for metastases of renal cell carcinoma. *Scand J Surg.* 2004;93:150–155.
89. Tillman RM, Myers GJ, Abudu AT, et al. The three-pin modified "Harrington" procedure for advanced metastatic destruction of the acetabulum. *J Bone Joint Surg Br.* 2008;90B:84–87.

90. Tomita K, Kawahara N, Kobayashi T, et al. Surgical strategy for spinal metastasis. *Spine*. 2001;26:298.

91. Tordai P, Lugnegard H. Is the treatment of enchondroma in the hand by simple curettage a rewarding method? *J Hand Surg*. 1990;15B:331–334.

92. Townsend P, Smalley S, Cozad S. Role of postoperative radiation therapy after stabilization of fractures caused by metastatic disease. *Int J Radiat Oncol Biol Phys*. 1995;31:43.

93. Turcotte RE, Wunder JS, Isler MH, et al. Giant cell tumor of long bone: A Canadian Sarcoma Group study. *Clin Orthop Relat Res*. 2002:248–258.

94. Vansteenkiste JF, Stroobants SS. PET scan in lung cancer: Current recommendations and innovation. *J Thorac Oncol*. 2006;1(1):71–73.

95. Virk MS, Petrigliano FA, Liu NQ, et al. Influence of simultaneous targeting of the bone morphogenetic protein pathway and RANK/RANKL axis in osteolytic prostate cancer lesion in bone. *Bone*. 2009;44(1):160–167.

96. Weber KL. Specialty update: What's new in musculoskeletal oncology. *J Bone Joint Surg*. 2004;86:1104–1109.

97. Weber K, Damron TA, Frassica FJ, et al. Malignant bone tumors. *Instr Course Lect*. 2008;57:673–688.

98. Weber KL, Gebhardt MC. Specialty update: What's new in musculoskeletal oncology. *J Bone Joint Surg*. 2003;85:761–767.

99. Weber KL, Lewis VO, Randall L, et al. An approach to the management of the patient with metastatic bone disease. *Instr Course Lect*. 2004;53:663–676.

100. Weber KL, Lin PP, Yasko AW. Complex segmental elbow reconstruction after tumor resection. *Clin Orthop*. 2003;415:31–44.

101. Weber KL, O'Connor MI. Operative treatment of long bone metastases: Focus on the femur. *Clin Orthop Relat Res*. 2003;S276–S278.

102. Weikert DR, Schwartz HS. Intramedullary nailing for impending pathological subtrochanteric fractures. *J Bone Joint Surg Br*. 1991;73B:668–670.

103. Weill A, Kobaiter H, Chiras J. Acetabulum malignancies: Technique and impact on pain of percutaneous injection of acrylic surgical cement. *Eur Radiol*. 1998;8:123–129.

104. Wu J, Wong R, Johnston M, et al. Meta-analysis of dose-fractionation radiotherapy trials for the palliation of painful bone metastases. *Int J Radiat Oncol Biol Phys*. 2003;55:594.

105. Xie L, Guo W, Li Y, et al. Pathologic fracture does not influence local recurrence and survival in high-grade extremity osteosarcoma with adequate surgical margins. *J Surg Oncol*. 2012;106(7):820–825.

106. Yasko AW, Fanning CV, Ayala AG, et al. Percutaneous techniques for the diagnosis and treatment of localized Langerhans-cell histiocytosis (eosinophilic granuloma of bone). *J Bone Joint Surg Am*. 1998;80:219–228.

107. Yazawa Y, Frassica FJ, Chao EY, et al. Metastatic bone disease: A study of the surgical treatment of 166 pathologic humeral and femoral fractures. *Clin Orthop Relat Res*. 1990;(251):213–219.

108. Yuh WTC, Zacharck CK, Barloon TJ, et al. Vertebral compression fractures: Distinction between benign and malignant causes with MR imaging. *Radiology*. 1989;172:215–218.

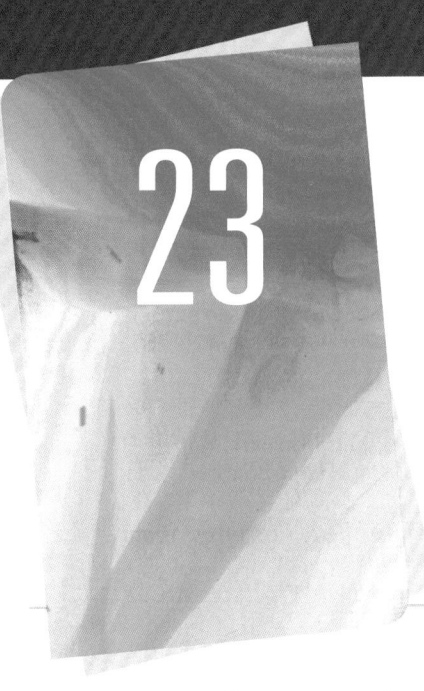

23

PERIPROSTHETIC FRACTURES

William M. Ricci

INTRODUCTION TO PERIPROSTHETIC FRACTURES

Periprosthetic fractures continue to increase in frequency. This is due, in part, to the increasing number of primary and revision arthroplasties performed annually and also to the increasing age and fragility of patients with such implants. All types of periprosthetic fractures can present unique and substantial treatment challenges. In each situation, the presence of an arthroplasty component either obviates the use of, or increases the difficulty of, standard fixation techniques. In addition, these fractures often occur in elderly patients with osteoporotic bone making stable fixation with traditional techniques even more problematic.

The difficulty in management of periprosthetic fractures regardless of location is evidenced by the array of treatment options described in the literature without a clear consensus emerging on the most appropriate method.[140,160,228,229,230] Treatment of the most common periprosthetic fractures, those of the femoral shaft and those of the femoral supracondylar region, has focused on open reduction and internal fixation (ORIF) or revision arthroplasty procedures with or without supplementary autologous or allogeneic bone grafting.[39,99,222] Most recently, treatment strategies to accelerate weight bearing have suggested benefits with regard to mortality.[149,151,210] Successful application of these strategies can be extrapolated to periprosthetic fractures in other anatomic locations but must also consider the fracture location relative to the arthroplasty component, the implant stability, the quality of the surrounding bone, and the patient's medical and functional status.[64]

ASSESSMENT OF PERIPROSTHETIC FRACTURES

Injury Mechanisms for Periprosthetic Fracture

Low-energy falls account for the mechanism of injury in most patients with periprosthetic fractures of both the upper and lower extremity.[81,147,165,229] Lower extremity fractures tend to occur postoperatively rather than intraoperatively whereas a relatively larger proportion of upper extremity periprosthetic fractures, especially those about humeral shoulder arthroplasty stems, occur intraoperatively. Postoperative low-energy falls account for greater than 75% of all periprosthetic femur fractures from the Swedish registry database,[165] whereas a majority, up to 76% of humeral fractures, have been reported to occur intraoperatively.[32,261] Periprosthetic fractures are noted to be more common after revision arthroplasty than after primary arthroplasty. This is likely because of the reduced bone stock often present after revision.[165] High-energy trauma accounts for only a small percentage of periprosthetic fractures and these are usually associated with a more comminuted fracture pattern than seen with low-energy fractures.[13] Intraoperative fractures of both the upper and lower extremities occur more commonly during revision procedures and with implantation of large noncemented stems.[188,236] The risk increases when there is mismatch between the shape of long prosthetic stems and the shape of the bone.[305] Specific to periprosthetic fractures about a total knee arthroplasty (TKA), another mechanism is related to forced manipulation of a stiff knee.

Injuries Associated with Periprosthetic Fractures

Given the predominance of low-energy injury mechanisms associated with periprosthetic fractures, associated injuries are relatively uncommon. Of course, vigilance is required to avoid missing the occasional associated injury. On the occasion when high-energy mechanism is the cause of a periprosthetic fracture, that patient should be evaluated just as any other patient with a high-energy injury mechanism.

Signs and Symptoms of Periprosthetic Fractures

When evaluating patients with obvious or even suspected periprosthetic fractures, the history should include a detailed account of the status of the arthroplasty including as much detail as possible on the date of implantation, the specific prosthesis used, the index diagnosis for implantation, and the relevant history related to the associated arthroplasty. Additional secondary procedures should be carefully cataloged as well as other complications such as prior infection. Occult infection may be associated with and potentially contributing to periprosthetic fracture.[42] Laboratory markers such as ESR and C-reactive protein, in the setting of fracture, are likely to be elevated regardless of infection status and are therefore of limited value for the diagnosis of infection in this setting.[42]

The baseline functional status specific to the involved joint as well as to the patient as a whole, such as handedness, occupation, ambulatory status, and any need for assist devices, are a standard part of the history. The time course of any recent change in status or symptoms related to the arthroplasty can heighten suspicion of a subtle periprosthetic fracture or prefracture implant loosening. A history of mechanical symptoms such as start-up pain, increasing difficulty with ambulation, progressive limb shortening, and deformity of the extremity are all associated with prosthetic loosening prior to the fracture and will impact the treatment.

The standard comprehensive orthopedic examination is warranted with specific attention to prior surgical wounds about the joint in question, the presence or absence of associated lesions such as venous stasis or diabetic ulcers of the ipsilateral or contralateral limbs, limb length evaluation, as well as strength and neurologic evaluation. Status of the abductors for the hip and the extensor mechanism for the knee are essential parts of the evaluation. Obviously, in cases of displaced fracture, many of these parameters will be abnormal and not represent the patient's baseline status. However, it is still important to obtain a comprehensive history, as clues to potential etiologic factors to the acute fracture such as implant loosening,

osteolysis, and infection may need to be addressed during the course of fracture repair.

Direct observation of periprosthetic fractures occurs when the fracture happens intraoperatively. A pitch change during insertion of the trial or final prosthesis alerts the surgeon to the possibility of fracture and should prompt an appropriate investigation starting with direct observation. Similarly, an abrupt easing of insertion resistance can be a subtle sign of fracture or perforation.

Imaging and Other Diagnostic Studies for Periprosthetic Fractures

The diagnosis of a postoperative periprosthetic fracture is usually obvious. The patient typically has an abrupt onset of pain and deformity associated with trauma. However, more subtle fractures can occur especially when associated with significant osteopenia or osteolysis. In cases of fracture related to severe osteolysis, the trauma is usually trivial or absent. The extent of bone loss is usually significant and makes treatment more difficult. Although challenging, it is important to recognize these cases. Clinical suspicion is necessary to instigate a specific radiographic evaluation to rule out fracture.

The standard radiographic evaluation of periprosthetic fractures should include plain AP and lateral views to include the joint in question and full length radiographs of the bones above and below the joint. Attention should be paid not only to fracture specifics but also to an evaluation of the prosthesis relative to the fracture as well as the prosthesis relative to the native bone to which it is secured. It is useful to assess for prosthetic loosening, presence of bone loss and osteolysis, and prosthetic and limb alignment. Prefracture radiographs, when available, can provide insight to the time course of any existing or impending prosthetic failure, specifically osteolysis, progression of cortical erosions, and presence of any cortical penetrations or notching. In addition, in more subtle cases, prefracture radiographs can help to identify subtle changes in implant position which may be the only clue to a loose implant associated with a fracture. Radiographic features of a loose stem include progressive change in stem position (e.g., subsidence), global radiolucency around the stem, distal pedestal formation, and cement mantle fracture (for cemented stems). Despite radiographic appearance of implant stability, components may be loose based on intraoperative findings.[49] Therefore, surgical planning should account for this contingency.

Identifying a well-fixed stem is also important. Radiographic features of this include bony "spot welding" to the implant, proximal stress shielding or remodeling above a distally well-fixed stem, and distal bone condensation or remodeling around a proximally fixed stem.

Diagnosis of intraoperative fracture can be from direct observation or indirectly based on suspicion from auditory changes in the pitch of sounds coming from mallet blows of a broach or implant. In such circumstances, intraoperative radiographs should be obtained to define the extent of the fracture which can be more extensive than seen under direct vision. Immediate postoperative radiographs are done in many institutions and should be checked meticulously to ensure the imaged area is adequate to diagnose subtle fractures.

Cross-sectional imaging is not routinely required to evaluate periprosthetic fractures. However, significant advances have been made to reduce metal artifact of both CT scans and MRI scans which may help in evaluating subtle fractures or in the evaluation of available bone stock for fracture repair.[199,204,290]

Outcome Goals and Outcome Measures for Periprosthetic Fractures

In the most general sense, the goals of periprosthetic fracture care are no different than the goals of treatment of any other periarticular fracture. These goals include timely and uncomplicated fracture union, restoration of alignment, and return to preinjury level of pain and function. By definition, periprosthetic fractures are not associated with normal joints. Therefore, neither baseline painless normal joint function and normal anatomic alignment cannot be assumed nor can return to normal function be the *de facto* goal. Instead, an accurate history of prefracture function should be elicited to help guide goals and prognosis. In the setting of a poorly functioning loose prosthesis, return to a better functional level after fracture fixation and revision arthroplasty may be a reasonable goal. If prefracture malalignment existed, a careful determination must be made whether restoring baseline alignment or normal alignment should be the goal. This decision is often predicated on the alignment of the prosthesis relative to the bone on the nonfractured side of the joint which may provide an inherent compensatory alignment. A unique consideration when treating periprosthetic, rather than native, periarticular fractures is consideration of prosthesis stability and the potential need for future revision arthroplasty. The additional goal therefore is to assure stability of the prosthesis and restoration of adequate bone stock to maximize the potential success of any subsequent procedures.

PERIPROSTHETIC ACETABULAR FRACTURES

Incidence, Risk Factors, and Prevention of Periprosthetic Acetabular Fractures

Periprosthetic acetabular fractures are very uncommon. They may occur intraoperatively or postoperatively. Intraoperative fractures are most commonly associated with insertion of noncemented components.[101,252] Identification of intraoperative fractures can be difficult. It has been suggested that published results of intraoperative fractures that use only AP radiographs for diagnosis may underestimate the true incidence as oblique views were found to be required to accurately identify the presence of an occult fracture.[135]

The incidence of intraoperative fracture was found to be 0.3% in a series of 7,121 primary total hip arthroplasties (THAs) performed at the Mayo Clinic between 1990 and 2000.[101] All 21 fractures occurred during insertion of a noncemented component resulting in a fracture incidence of 0.4% for noncemented components and 0% for cemented components. The fracture occurrence was most common during impaction of the final component (16/21) but fracture was also noted to occur during reaming (3/21) and during initial dislocation (2/21). This study also demonstrated that elliptical designs had a significantly

higher rate of fracture (0.7%) compared to hemispherical designs (0.09%). This increased risk of fracture with elliptical designs was largely related to the association with a monoblock design, one with the liner bound to the shell such that visualization of implant seating through screw holes is not possible. Monoblock elliptical components had a 3.5% incidence of fracture whereas modular elliptical components had a 0.3% incidence. There was no statistical difference in fracture between the modular elliptical and hemispherical designs supporting the theory that the reduced feedback from the monoblock design may be a greater contributing factor than the elliptical shape. The size of the component relative to the reamed acetabulum also affects risk of fracture. In a cadaveric study, there were more fractures with components oversized by 4 mm than with components oversized by 2 mm.[135] This study also showed that more force was required to seat the 4-mm oversized components (3,000 N) than the 2-mm oversized components (2,000 N).

Postoperative periprosthetic acetabular fractures have an exceedingly low rate of occurrence. In another largely cohort study from the Mayo Clinic (23,850 patients), the incidence of postoperative acetabular fracture was 0.07%.[216] A number of factors have been implicated to be associated with periprosthetic acetabular fracture. Although low-energy trauma, most notably falls from a standing height, is the most common mechanism,[216] fractures may also be seen without antecedent trauma or on occasion from high-energy trauma.[89,107] In some occult cases, especially those diagnosed soon after arthroplasty, a missed intraoperative fracture may be causative. *De novo* fractures in the postoperative period that are not associated with trauma are normally associated with reduced bone quality or quantity or both. Osteolytic lesions clearly reduce bone stock and not surprisingly fractures through such lesions have been reported.[243] An apparent acetabular fracture years removed from surgery with minimal trauma is likely related to progressive particle disease. Based on indirect evidence, usually in the form of a disproportionately high ratio of females, many authors have implicated osteoporosis as a risk factor.[101,252,260] Weakening of the pelvic bone stock associated with reaming required to obtain a secure fit of a large-diameter hemispherical component for revision resulted in a 1.2% incidence of transverse acetabular fracture without associated trauma.[260] Stress fracture has also been reported in association with primary cemented and revision arthroplasty and should be considered with acute pain onset especially when associated with abrupt increased activity level.[8,189] Infection may be an etiologic factor predisposing to stress fracture[189] and therefore concomitant infection should be considered anytime a stress fracture is identified. The prudent clinician should also consider periprosthetic acetabular fracture whenever there is acute onset of pain associated with total hip arthroplasty especially in situations with compromised bone stock.

Avoidance of fracture may be the first step. To this end, the degree of reaming is of paramount importance. Too much reaming, especially in the revision setting where bone stock is already compromised or in the presence of serve osteoporosis, should be avoided. Careful reaming without violation of the acetabular walls including the medial wall will reduce risk for fracture and also provide the necessary foundation for component stability.[58] The degree of reaming relative to the size of an uncemented implant is also critical. Under reaming of the acetabulum more than 2 mm is ill advised as the more oversized the component is, the higher is the risk of fracture.[135] Trialing is helpful to identify areas of impingement and the aggressiveness of the bony press fit. Care must also be exercised during insertion of the component. Excessive force should be avoided and failure of the component to seat properly with successive mallet blows should be an indication for increased caution and possibly additional reaming.

Classification of Periprosthetic Acetabular Fractures

Peterson and Lewallen distinguished two types of periprosthetic acetabular fractures based on the stability of the acetabular component.[216] Type I fractures are associated with a radiographically stable component, one where there was no change in the position of the component compared with that seen on radiographs made before the fracture (if available) and where gentle passive range of motion (ROM) of the hip caused little or no pain. Fractures were considered type II if the acetabular component was obviously displaced or radiographically loose and there was notable pain with any motion of the hip. This classification scheme neither does account for the morphology of the fracture nor does it include the relative location of the fracture. A modification of the acetabular fracture classification system of Letournel (see Chapter 47 Acetabulum Fractures) that includes a category for fractures of the medial wall of the acetabulum, a location that is common when these fractures occur postoperatively, provides more insight into the fracture pattern and location. In Peterson's series of postoperative periprosthetic acetabular fractures occurring at an average of 6.2 years after the index arthroplasty procedure, there were eight type I fractures and three type II fractures.[216] Medial wall fracture was the most common pattern (5 of the 11 cases) followed by posterior column in three, transverse in two, and anterior column in one patient. Given the need to consider both the stability of the component and the fracture location and pattern to determine a treatment plan, it seems that neither classification system is sufficient without consideration of the other.

Management Principles for Periprosthetic Acetabular Fractures

Treatment of periprosthetic acetabular fractures requires consideration of many factors. In addition to the obvious consideration of patient factors such as medical condition and functional demands, the timing of the fracture (intraoperative or postoperative), the displacement, the location, and the stability of the component should be accounted for in the decision algorithm, the overall goals being union of the fracture and return of the patient to their prefracture functional level with a stable acetabular component.

Nonoperative treatment of a periprosthetic acetabular fracture is not usually indicated when associated with a loose or unstable component. For early fractures, those identified on radiographs shortly after surgery, nonoperative treatment may be an option assuming that the component had good stabil-

ity intraoperatively and did not migrate on serial x-rays, and that there is no pelvic discontinuity or major interruption of the columns. For late fractures associated with osteolysis (and usually with trivial trauma) there are only rare indications for nonoperative treatment. For those late fractures associated with a significant high speed mechanism in a well-functioning hip without osteolysis, nonoperative treatment has a role if the pelvic fracture does not destabilize the socket or predispose to migration (similar criteria as in the immediate postoperative period).

Operative management of periprosthetic acetabular fractures can take many forms. The strategy is determined by a number of factors: the timing of the diagnosis (intraoperative or postoperative), the stability of the acetabular component, the fracture location, and the fracture displacement. Fixation of minimally displaced fractures identified intraoperatively can be achieved with screws through a multihole acetabular component. More widely displaced fractures may require formal ORIF with plate fixation with revision of the acetabular component.[89] Percutaneous screw fixation utilizing computer navigation has also been reported.[94]

Management Principles for Intraoperative Periprosthetic Acetabular Fractures

Treatment of intraoperative acetabular fractures begins with the evaluation of the acetabular component stability and definition of the fracture location and displacement. Any change in pitch upon implantation of the component or sudden loosening of a component should alert the surgeon to the possible presence of a periprosthetic fracture. The acetabular shell should be removed and the pelvis visually inspected systematically with particular attention to the posterior column, dome, and anterior column. Intraoperative radiographs may help define the location and degree of displacement. Anterior–posterior radiographs alone may not be sufficient to identify such fractures, therefore obturator and iliac oblique views should also be included.[135] Small fractures of either the anterior, medial, or posterior walls may not affect the stability of the implant and can be treated without any further surgery. If the component is relegated unstable by a large wall fracture or a fracture that traverses one of the acetabular columns, then additional steps are required to insure component stability that may involve adjunctive fracture fixation. When the fracture is nondisplaced, screw fixation through holes in the acetabular component may be sufficient to provide component stability. However, if a column is involved there should be a low threshold for independent reduction and plate and screw fixation of the acetabular fracture, especially if it is displaced. Bone grafting of the fracture site with reamings or morselized femoral head may be beneficial to speed fracture healing.[252] After plate and screw fixation of the acetabulum, the acetabulum should be reamed line-to-line for a new multihole component which is carefully impacted and then stabilized with multiple screws. When possible, screws on either side of the fracture are preferred. Weight bearing is typically restricted for at least 6 weeks based on radiographic and clinical evidence of fracture healing unless the fracture is of the acetabular wall and is very small.

Management Principles for Postoperative Periprosthetic Acetabular Fractures

Postoperative periprosthetic acetabular fractures are very different than those occurring intraoperatively. Intraoperative fractures are usually minimally displaced, most commonly involve the acetabular walls rather than columns, generally require minimally additional surgical management, and are generally associated with good results. Postoperative fractures, on the other hand, are usually more complex, require a greater degree of surgical intervention, and in general have poorer results. Before treatment can be instituted, etiologic factors should be considered, the stability of the cup determined, and the available bone stock quantified.

Fractures about stable components (type I fractures) with good bone stock can be expected to have a high union rate with nonoperative management consisting of protected weight bearing for 6 to 12 weeks. Despite union and in distinction from similar intraoperative fractures, the fate of the component is dubious. These components have a high likelihood of loosening and therefore have results inferior to those seen for type I fractures occurring intraoperatively. Immediate surgical treatment for fractures with stable components in the absence of osteolysis may be indicated for widely displaced fractures. Component revision should be considered to accompany reduction and fixation of the fracture in such instances; however, there is little in the way of published results to guide this decision making.

Fractures that are associated with a loose acetabular component, type II fractures, generally require revision of the acetabular component and supplemental fracture fixation with plates and screws. The type of component revision is highly dependent upon the available bone stock. CT scan is useful to identify the type of reconstruction option needed. If there is an intact posterior column and dome, bone grafting and use of a hemispherical revision socket with screws is feasible though backup options should always be available. In cases with severe osteolysis or pelvic discontinuity, reconstruction typically requires bone grafting, augments, a reconstruction cage, or some combination of these methods. After removal of the acetabular component, the fracture is fixed with plates and screws based on the fracture pattern to restore, to the extent possible, the integrity of the acetabular columns. Bone grafts, either morselized or structural depending upon the size and location of the defect, are used to re-establish any residual structural deficiencies. A large multihole cup with screws or a cage is used to complete the reconstruction. There is little published data to guide subtle variations in treatment or to establish prognosis.

Periprosthetic acetabular fractures in association with osteolysis have been the subject of case reports.[40,243] Regardless of the healing potential of the fracture, which in most cases is nondisplaced, surgical management is indicated for the underlying osteolytic process as well to deal with the loose component that in most instances accompanies these fractures. Treatment is primarily directed to management of the osteolytic lesions with bone graft. Revision of the acetabular component is usually required even if stable so that adequate access to the lesions for bone grafting can be accomplished.

TABLE 23-1 **Surgical Treatment of Periprosthetic Acetabular Fractures**

Preoperative Planning Checklist

- OR table: Radiolucent table that allows imaging of hip and pelvis
- Position: Lateral
- Fluoroscopy location: From front of patient (opposite from operating surgeon)
- Equipment:
  Reduction clamps specific to ORIF of acetabular fractures
  Retractors specific to ORIF of acetabular fractures
  Bone mill or other method to morselize allograft
- Implants:
  3.5-mm pelvic reconstruction plates and associated screws
  Array of acetabular components including:
  Cups with multiholes
  Jumbo-sized cups
  Acetabular cages
  Allograft

Preoperative Planning for Management of Periprosthetic Acetabular Fractures

Component revision, ORIF, and bone grafting should be prepared for, even if one or more of these options is considered unlikely based on preoperative assessment (Table 23-1). Intraoperative findings can be different than expected based on preoperative evaluations. An array of acetabular components may be required, including multiholed cups, jumbo sizes, as well as cages. ORIF of periprosthetic acetabular fractures requires standard 3.5-mm pelvic reconstruction plates and 3.5-mm cortical screws. 4.5-mm cortical screws may also be required, either to serve as anchor points for reduction clamps or as a lag screw across a column fracture. Specialized clamps (see Chapter 47 Acetabular Fractures) are often required for the reduction maneuvers. Allograft, usually in the form of morselized femoral head or cancellous croutons or chips, is typically used for osteolytic lesions.

Positioning and Surgical Approach for Management of Periprosthetic Acetabular Fractures

The patient is generally positioned laterally on a radiolucent operating table with a beanbag used for support. Peg boards and other positioners often used for positioning during hip arthroplasty are typically not radiolucent, so they should be avoided when fracture fixation will require fluoroscopy. Although other approaches can be successfully utilized for hip arthroplasty, simultaneous fixation of the acetabular fracture and management of the acetabular component generally necessitate the posterior Kocher–Langenbeck approach. The C-arm for intraoperative fluoroscopic imaging is placed from the front of the patient, on the side opposite to the operating surgeon. The knee should remain flexed throughout the procedure to reduce tension and risk of injury to the sciatic nerve.[22]

TABLE 23-2	**Surgical Treatment of Periprosthetic Acetabular Fractures with a Stable Cup**

Surgical Steps

- Expose the acetabulum including the posterior wall and column
  - Protect sciatic nerve with retractors, hip extension, and knee flexion
- Identify and debride fracture lines and fragments
- Confirm cup stability
- Fill osteolytic lesions through fracture or via separate window
  - Be careful to avoid blocking fracture reduction
  - If window is used, this step can come after reduction and fixation
- Apply reduction maneuvers and clamp fracture
- Insert a lag screw, if possible, across the fracture for provisional fixation
- Definitively stabilize fracture with a contoured 3.5-mm reconstruction plate
- Standard closure

TABLE 23-3	**Surgical Treatment of Periprosthetic Acetabular Fractures with an Unstable Cup**

Surgical Steps

- Expose the acetabulum including the posterior wall and column
- Protect sciatic nerve with retractors, hip extension, and knee flexion
- Perform hip arthrotomy
- Identify and debride fracture lines and fragments
- Dislocate femoral head and retract it anteriorly to expose acetabular component
- Remove loose cup
- Apply reduction maneuvers and clamp fracture
- Insert a lag screw, if possible, across the fracture for provisional fixation
- Definitively stabilize fracture with a contoured 3.5-mm reconstruction plate
- Fill osteolytic lesions and bone defects through exposed acetabular surface
- Implant new acetabular component
- Reduce hip
- Reconstruct posterior pseudocapsule
- Standard wound closure

Surgical Technique for Management of Periprosthetic Acetabular Fractures

Details for the surgical technique for ORIF of acetabular fractures as presented in Chapter 47 Acetabular Fractures generally apply to ORIF of periprosthetic acetabular fractures. The differences come with regard to management of the acetabular cup and any associated osteolytic lesions. When the cup is stable, steps for ORIF of the periprosthetic acetabular fracture (Table 23-2) are little different from ORIF of a native fracture. Exposure is followed by identification and debridement of the primary fracture lines. Cup stability should be confirmed and osteolytic lesions bone grafted through the fracture if easily accessible. Care must be taken not to overpack the lesion so as to prevent fracture reduction. An alternative to filling osteolytic lesions through the fracture is to fill them through separate cortical windows which can be done after reduction of the fracture. A basic tenet of acetabular fracture surgery is anatomic reduction of the articular surface. In the presence of an acetabular cup, such precision is not required, but anatomic reduction should still be strived for to maximize healing potential. Fixation of reduced fractures is with standard pelvic reconstruction plates and screws.

When the acetabular component is loose, surgical treatment includes component revision (Table 23-3). The loose component can be removed either before or after provisional fracture reduction. Sometimes the presence of the loose cup can provide a template for fracture reduction. More often, the component is removed after exposure and prior to fracture reduction. The femoral head is dislocated from the component and retracted anteriorly to allow unencumbered exposure to the acetabulum. This can require wide exposure and extensive release of the soft tissues about both the acetabulum as well as the proximal femur. Fracture reduction and fixation as described previously is followed by grafting of any bone defects and implantation of a new acetabular component. When massive bone loss is present, reconstruction with an acetabular cage is indicated.

Potential Pitfalls and Preventative Measures for Management of Periprosthetic Acetabular Fractures

It is often difficult to determine the status of the acetabular cup stability after periprosthetic acetabular fracture (Table 23-4). A careful history of signs of cup loosening prior to fracture as well as careful scrutinization of prefracture radiographs, if available, and postfracture radiographs with particular attention to cup stability should be performed on a routine basis. Even when preoperative evaluation points to a stable cup, careful intraoperative evaluation of component stability should be performed. Because unexpected cup instability can occur, the surgeon should be prepared for cup revision in all operative cases for periprosthetic acetabular fracture.

Because there is no articular surface remaining, it is tempting to settle for an imperfect fracture reduction. Poor reduction with remaining fracture gaps can lead to nonunion and therefore efforts should be made to obtain an anatomic reduction. To obtain a satisfactory reduction, careful preoperative evaluation of the fracture morphology and a comprehensive plan for reduction and fixation, just as is performed for native acetabular fractures, should be performed. Occasionally, an intraoperative acetabular fracture is identified postoperatively. Although usually these are minimally displaced and can be treated nonoperatively with good results, occasionally these fractures require revision surgery. To avoid missing intraoperative fractures, a low threshold for intraoperative imaging should coincide with any suspicion for intraoperative fracture.

TABLE 23-4	Surgical Treatment of Periprosthetic Acetabular Fractures

Potential Pitfalls and Preventions

Pitfalls	Preventions
1. Cup instability	Obtain accurate history of potential symptoms of prefracture implant instability Careful evaluation of prefracture and postfracture imaging Careful intraoperative assessment of cup stability even when history and radiographs indicate cup stability
2. Fracture malreduction and/or nonunion	Careful preoperative evaluation of fracture morphology with Judet radiographs and CT scanning Comprehensive plan for reduction and fixation based on principles of acetabular fracture management Avoid temptation to accept imperfect reduction because of lack of need for reduction of articular surface
3. Missed intraoperative fracture	Low threshold for intraoperative radiographs with any suspicion for intraoperative fracture

Outcomes for Periprosthetic Acetabular Fractures

Sharkey et al.[252] identified nine intraoperative fractures. Two were small posterior wall fractures that did not compromise component stability and therefore had no additional treatment and were allowed immediate weight bearing. One similar fracture had no additional intraoperative treatment but had restricted postoperative weight bearing. The other six were managed with screws either through the component or placed peripherally outside the cup and in four of these autograft was packed into the fracture site. Other than one patient who required resection arthroplasty because of infection, all fractures healed and no patient required revision at an average follow-up of 42 months. Haidukewych et al.[101] identified 21 intraoperative fractures occurring during primary arthroplasty. Seventeen were judged not to compromise component stability and received no additional intraoperative treatment. In 4 of their 21 patients, the component was found to be unstable necessitating a change in component to one that provided supplemental screw fixation. No adjunctive plates or screws outside the component were used. All patients were treated with protected weight bearing. All fractures healed and no patient required revision for loosening at an average follow-up of 44 months.

In the series of Peterson and Lewallen,[216] 75% of patients treated nonoperatively for a type I fracture (stable component) eventually required revision of their acetabular component. Of the eight fractures, six healed but four eventually required revision of the acetabular component for loosening. The other two patients developed delayed union or nonunion and both eventually required revision. The fractures in the two patients without revision healed and they had no requirement for subsequent revision. All eight patients had a stable prosthesis at a mean of 36 months after their latest revision procedure.

Springer et al.[260] reported seven displaced transverse periprosthetic acetabular fractures after uncemented acetabular revision about well-fixed components. Two were identified on routine radiographs, were asymptomatic, and were treated nonoperatively with a period of protective weight bearing and healed. Of the five symptomatic patients all were treated operatively. Four patients with the component well fixed to the superior portion of the ilium were treated with ORIF of the posterior column of the acetabulum without revision of the acetabular component. In one case where the cup was fixed to the inferior, ischial segment treatment was with a reconstruction cage. Of the five operatively treated fractures, one went on to nonunion and the other four healed and at the latest follow-up had a stable, well-fixed cup.

Two patients in the series of Peterson and Lewallen with type II fractures had immediate revision of the acetabular component without adjuvant plate and screw fixation of the fracture.[216] In one a cemented component was utilized and the fracture healed. The other was revised with a noncemented component with screw fixation through the shell. This patient went on to nonunion and required repeat revision with a cemented acetabular component and plate and screw fixation of the acetabular nonunion. Desai and Ries[61] reported on two cases of likely missed intraoperative pelvic fractures associated with pelvic discontinuity in octogenarian patients with poor bone quality. This report emphasizes the importance of meticulous attention to bone preparation, appropriate underreaming for the socket, careful insertion, and awareness of potential fractures because the salvage for these fractures consists of extensive pelvic reconstruction.

AUTHOR'S PREFERRED TREATMENT OF PERIPROSTHETIC ACETABULAR FRACTURES

The optimal treatment of periprosthetic acetabular fractures is primarily dictated by component stability and fracture pattern stability (Fig. 23-1). In the setting of a stable component, stable fracture patterns are generally treated nonoperatively with protected weight bearing. Fracture patterns of

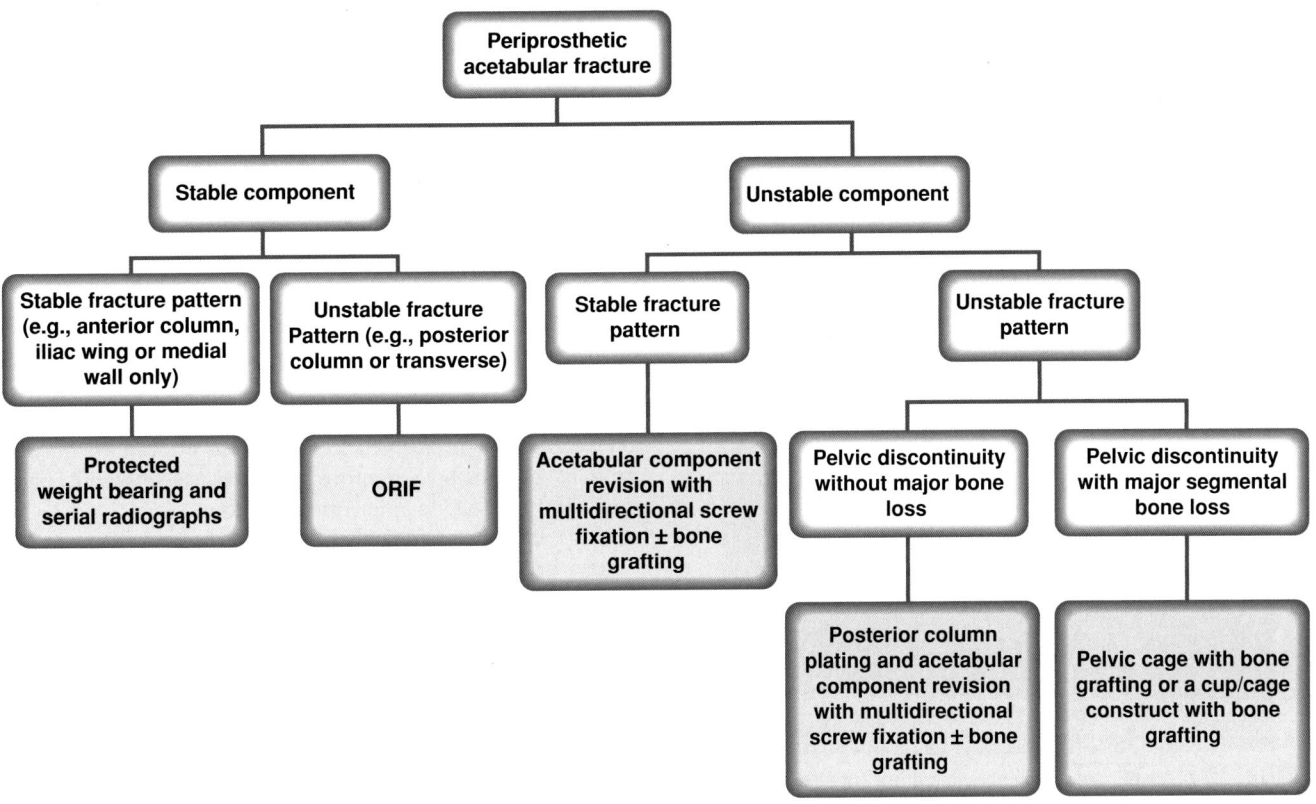

FIGURE 23-1 Algorithm depicting the author's preferred method of treatment for periprosthetic acetabular fractures.

this type include non- or minimally displaced anterior column fractures, fractures of the iliac wing, or medial wall fractures. Close follow-up, with weekly or biweekly radiographs are used to confirm progressive healing without secondary loss of reduction. Weight bearing is increased at about 6 weeks based on clinical and radiographic evidence of fracture healing.

Surgical treatment with ORIF is preferred for management of unstable fractures about a stable acetabular component. Typical patterns of bony injury encountered in this scenario are displaced posterior column or transverse fractures. The fixation strategy, surgical approach, and implants are dictated by the details of the fracture pattern and generally follow those utilized for treatment of native acetabular fractures. Adjuvant bone grafts in these situations are generally not indicated.

In the setting of an unstable acetabular component, treatment requirements become much more complex. In such cases when there is a stable fracture pattern, revision of the acetabular component may be all that is required. In such cases, revision of the acetabular component with a press-fit shell utilizing multiple screw fixation on either side of the fracture may serve to provide a stable component as well as help stabilize the fracture. When the periprosthetic fracture involves both an unstable component and an unstable fracture pattern, the degree of bone loss should also be considered in the treatment algorithm. When there is no substantial bone loss, fixation of the unstable acetabular fracture as well as revision of the loose acetabular

component is recommended. This usually takes the form of plating of the posterior column of the acetabulum. Revision also includes use of multiple screws preferably on either side of the major fracture line. In the setting of a pelvic discontinuity, reconstruction of the columns of the acetabulum may require substantial structural bone grafting with the possibility of the use of an acetabular cage. These cases represent some of the most challenging acetabular revisions and should be undertaken by an experienced surgical team with a substantial amount of necessary resources available.

PERIPROSTHETIC FEMUR FRACTURES ABOUT HIP ARTHROPLASTY PROSTHESES

Incidence, Risk Factors, Prevention, and Mortality for Periprosthetic Femur Fractures About Hip Arthroplasty Prostheses

Vancouver A Periprosthetic Femur Fractures

Trochanteric fractures about hip arthroplasty stems, Vancouver type A fractures, can occur intraoperatively or postoperatively with similar frequency. They were found to occur intraoperatively in 21 of 373 (5.6%) patients operated on using a lateral approach with the patient in the supine position.[112] All of these fractures occurred in women. Broach-only metaphyseal medial–lateral fit stems have a fracture rate that is

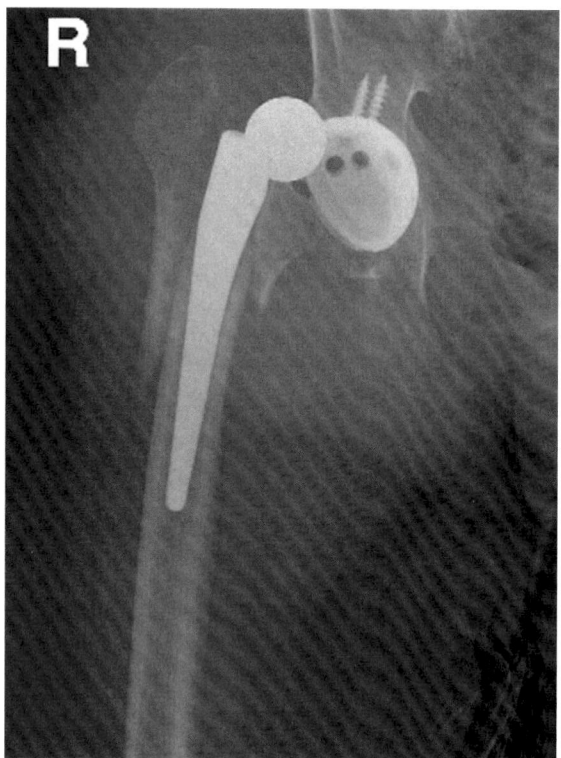

FIGURE 23-2 An AP radiograph showing stem subsidence and hip dislocation after trochanteric periprosthetic fracture. (Courtesy of Hari Parvataneni, MD.)

technique dependent. Associated fractures usually involve the metaphyseal area and can be visualized within the surgical field along the medial aspect of the neck osteotomy. If there is an unrecognized intraoperative metaphyseal fracture, there is usually propagation and subsidence early in the postoperative period (Fig. 23-2). Postoperative fracture occurred in 2.6% of 887 cases treated with a single type of uncemented prosthesis.[120] These fractures occurred through osteolytic cysts between 4 and 11 years after THA.

Vancouver B and C Periprosthetic Femur Fractures

Periprosthetic femoral shaft fractures are increasing in frequency because of the increasing number of patients with hip arthroplasties. The incidence of periprosthetic femur fracture after primary hip arthroplasty has been considered to be less than 1%,[130,160,184] but has been reported to be as high as 2.3%.[16,82,86,160] A recent survivorship analysis on 6,458 primary cemented femoral hip prostheses revealed a fracture incidence of 0.8% at 5 years and 3.5% at 10 years.[46] Another series of 354 hips in 326 patients all treated with the same uncemented, straight, collarless tapered titanium stem and followed for a mean of 17 years showed a cumulative incidence of periprosthetic fracture of 1.6% at 10 years that increased to 4.5% at 17 years.[263] The rate of fracture was low in the first 8 years after THA then increased into the second decade. In a comparison to the rate of aseptic loosening, the cumulative occurrence of periprosthetic fracture became equivalent to aseptic loosening

at 17 years indicating the relative importance of periprosthetic fracture in the long term.

After revision arthroplasty, the incidence of periprosthetic femoral shaft fractures climbs to between 1.5% and 7.8%.[16,130,160,184,193] The risk further increases after an increasing number of revision surgeries.[81] The lapsed time period from an index primary hip arthroplasty to periprosthetic femur fracture averages 6.3 to 7.4 years[46,165] and is reduced to an interval of 2.3 years after a third revision procedure.[165]

Risk factors for periprosthetic femoral shaft fractures about hip arthroplasty femoral stems are related to the age of the patient, gender, index diagnosis, presence or absence of osteolysis, presence or absence of aseptic loosening, primary or revision status, the specific type of implant utilized, and whether cemented or noncemented technique was utilized. Identifying risk factors can both improve patient counseling and potentially improve efforts at fracture prevention.

Age, although commonly cited as a risk factor for periprosthetic femur fracture, is not clearly an independent risk factor.[263] Coexisting medical comorbidities,[255,256] osteoporosis,[298] increased activity level,[245] and fall risk also contribute. A recent report revealed a doubled risk of fracture in patients with higher medical comorbidities.[255] Furthermore, the number of years after arthroplasty must be considered as each year after arthroplasty has been associated with a 1.01 additional risk ratio per year.[81]

Although a higher proportion of periprosthetic femur fractures among female patients (52% to 70%) has been reported in many series,[13,17,125,255,291] associated osteoporosis and a higher percentage of procedures being performed in female patients makes gender less clear as an independent risk factor. Accordingly, reports that account for such biases indicate no[164,246,263] or even reduced risk for females.[81]

The index diagnosis leading to arthroplasty may also be a risk factor with rheumatoid arthritis (RA) and arthroplasty for hip fracture each being identified as having increased risk ratios for fracture: RA having an increased ratio of 1.56 to 2.1[81,246] and hip fracture having a reported risk ratio of 4.4.[246]

Osteolysis, especially near the tip of a loose femoral stem represents an impending pathologic fracture, a growing problem in arthroplasty, and a complex reconstructive challenge. Fracture, deficient bone stock, a loose implant, and an inciting particle generator may each need to be addressed during fracture repair and reconstruction. Osteolytic reaction associated with the use of a biodegradable cement restrictor has also been implicated as a potential etiologic factor.[62]

Reports vary as to whether periprosthetic femur fracture is most often associated with a loose prosthesis. Some clinical data indicate that the presence of a loose stem represents a risk factor for subsequent fracture[121,279] and other data show no such association.[165,276] A cadaveric biomechanical comparison showed a 58% reduction in torsion to failure in specimens with loose as compared to those with well-fixed prostheses.[106]

In the setting of revision hip arthroplasty, univariate and multivariate analyses of a large population of patients with postoperative periprosthetic fractures (n = 330) showed female gender, younger age, higher comorbidity index, and operative diagnosis associated with risk/hazard ratio of periprosthetic fracture.[256] Women had a 66% higher risk than men, patients of age 61 to 80 had a 40% lower risk than those younger than 60, those with a Deyo–Charlston comorbidity index of 2 had 50% higher risk and those with an index of 3 or more had 100% higher risk than those with an index of 0. Operative diagnosis of nonunion and fracture was associated with a five-time higher risk of subsequent periprosthetic fracture.

Intraoperative fracture has a unique subset of associated risk factors. During primary total hip or hemiarthroplasty, implantation of a cementless femoral component presents a reported 3% to 5.4% risk of intraoperative fracture compared to 0% to 1.2% for a cemented stem.[16,79,102,250,271] The force utilized during insertion, the relative geometry of the stem and the femur, and the strength of the bone all may influence the risk of fracture during insertion of noncemented stems. Surgical experience helps dictate the required force for insertion. The "feel" and pitch of the sound made during each successive mallet blow are used to guide the experienced surgeon. Novel research has investigated the pitch and vibratory changes that occur as a potential means to minimize intraoperative fractures.[185,241] Stem design also influences fracture rate and the surgeon must be aware of the unique aspects of each stem design and each patient's femoral morphology which may predispose to fracture.[37] Stems with a combination of metaphyseal and diaphyseal fit with a cylindrical diaphyseal design can predispose to diaphyseal fractures if the distal press fit is too aggressive or the reamers are not advanced to the full length of the stem (Fig. 23-3). Certain bone morphology patterns have been correlated with fracture during noncemented fixation[47] because of a metaphysis–diaphysis mismatch. Cemented stems may also protect against postoperative fracture in patients with poor bone quality by virtue of internal stiffening of the femoral canal.[275]

Impaction grafting for revision of a femoral hip component carries up to a 22.4% perioperative risk for fracture.[73,188,236] Most of these fractures, many incidental perforations, have been found to occur with cement removal rather than the reconstructive procedure.[73] Revision with large porous-coated diaphyseal stems have been reported to be associated with a nearly 30% risk,[183] and long straight revision stems have an intermediate reported fracture occurrence of 18% with an additional 55% of cases thought to be at increased potential subsequent risk because of impingement of the distal stem tip on the anterior femoral cortex.[305]

Patients with periprosthetic femur fractures have increased mortality.[81] In multiple recent series, 7% to 18% of patients with periprosthetic fractures died within 1 year following surgical treatment.[6,18,302] In one study, this mortality rate approached that of hip fracture patients (16.5%) treated during the same time period and was significantly higher than the mortality of patients undergoing primary joint replacement (2.9%).[18] Data from the New Zealand National Registry indicated the 6-month mortality after revision THA associated with periprosthetic fracture (7.3%) was significantly higher than in a matched cohort undergoing revision for aseptic loosening (0.9%).[302]

Fractures About Femoral Resurfacing Prostheses

Hip resurfacing arthroplasty is currently considered as a reasonable alternative to THA in a select patient population. Periprosthetic fracture during or after femoral resurfacing is a potentially devastating complication that requires abandonment of this arthroplasty technique and conversion to THA. The prevalence of periprosthetic fracture about hip resurfacing components has been identified as being approximately 1% in most studies but as high as 2.5%. Multiple large cohort studies have produced similar low short-term fracture rates. Fifty fractures were identified from 3,497 Birmingham hips inserted by 89 different surgeons (1.46%),[254] five fractures were found in a series of 600 metal-on-metal surface arthroplasties (0.8%),[5] and one fracture occurred in another series of 230 Birmingham hip resurfacings (0.4%).[12] Another study of 550 cases revealed an overall fracture rate of 2.5%, but 12 of 14 fractures occurred in the first 69 resurfacing procedures performed by a single surgeon.[173] After the first 69 cases, the incidence of fracture dropped to 0.4% demonstrating the importance of surgeon experience. It should be noted that long-term fracture rates remain largely unknown. Extrapolation of data for periprosthetic femoral shaft fractures about traditional femoral stems would indicate that these low rates of fracture about resurfacing implants may rise substantially at longer follow-up. However, the younger age of patients undergoing resurfacing may be protective against such a late rise in periprosthetic fracture rates.

The risk of periprosthetic fracture has been tied to subtle aspects of surgical technique, bone quality, and patient selection. Notching of the superior aspect of the femoral neck, a varus position of the femoral component, and inadequate coverage of the reamed portion of the femoral head have each been implicated

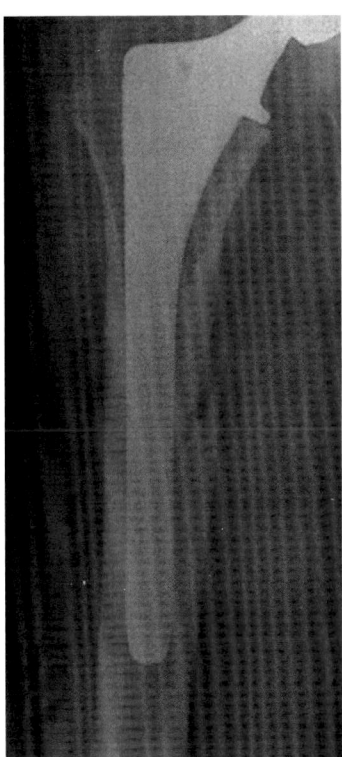

FIGURE 23-3 Cylindrical press-fit stems, especially when under reamed, pose a risk for fracture at the tip of the stem upon insertion as shown in this AP radiograph. (Courtesy of Hari Parvataneni, MD.)

as surgeon-controlled risk factors for periprosthetic fracture[5,254] that may be present in up to 85% of these fractures.[254] Biomechanical analyses support the clinical findings that a valgus orientation decreases the risk of femoral neck fracture[169,231] and suggested that maximum valgus, while avoiding notching, may provide maximum protection from periprosthetic fracture.[231] Poor bone quality has been subjectively described as a risk factor for periprosthetic fracture.[191] This theory is supported by biomechanical investigation, but bone quality was found to be less important than varus–valgus orientation of the component.[9] A change in indications was one factor attributed to a reduction in femoral neck fracture rate from 7.2% to 0.8% although the specific changes were not detailed and technique modifications occurred simultaneously. The technical aspects may have been largely responsible for the reduced fracture rate seen.[191] Another study suggested that female gender and obesity may be patient-related risk factors for fracture.[173]

Classification of Periprosthetic Femur Fractures About Hip Arthroplasty Prostheses

Classification of Postoperative Periprosthetic Femur Fractures

The Vancouver classification is most useful to direct communication about and treatment of periprosthetic femoral shaft fractures about hip arthroplasty stems.[64] Its reliability and validity

have been confirmed and therefore it represents the current standard for assessing and reporting these fractures.[25,64,88,198,225] It considers the location of the fracture relative to the stem, the stability of the implant, and associated bone loss (Fig. 23-4). Type A fractures are in the trochanteric region, type B fractures involve the area of the stem, and type C fractures are distal to the tip of the stem such that their treatment is considered independent of the hip prosthesis (except relating to overlap of the fixation device and the prosthesis). Type A fractures are subdivided into fractures of the greater trochanter, A_G (Fig. 23-5), and the much less common fractures about the lesser trochanter, A_L. Type B fractures are also further subdivided: B1 fractures are associated with a stable implant, B2 fractures are associated with a loose implant, and B3 fractures are associated with bone loss and usually a loose implant (Table 23-5). The ability to distinguish a well fixed from a loose implant in the setting of periprosthetic fracture may be difficult; therefore intraoperative testing of implant stability and preparation for dealing with a loose stem are prudent.[225]

Classification of Intraoperative Periprosthetic Femur Fractures

The original Vancouver classification was developed to describe postoperative fractures but has been expanded to address intraoperative periprosthetic femur fractures.[177] Similarly to the original, the intraoperative Vancouver

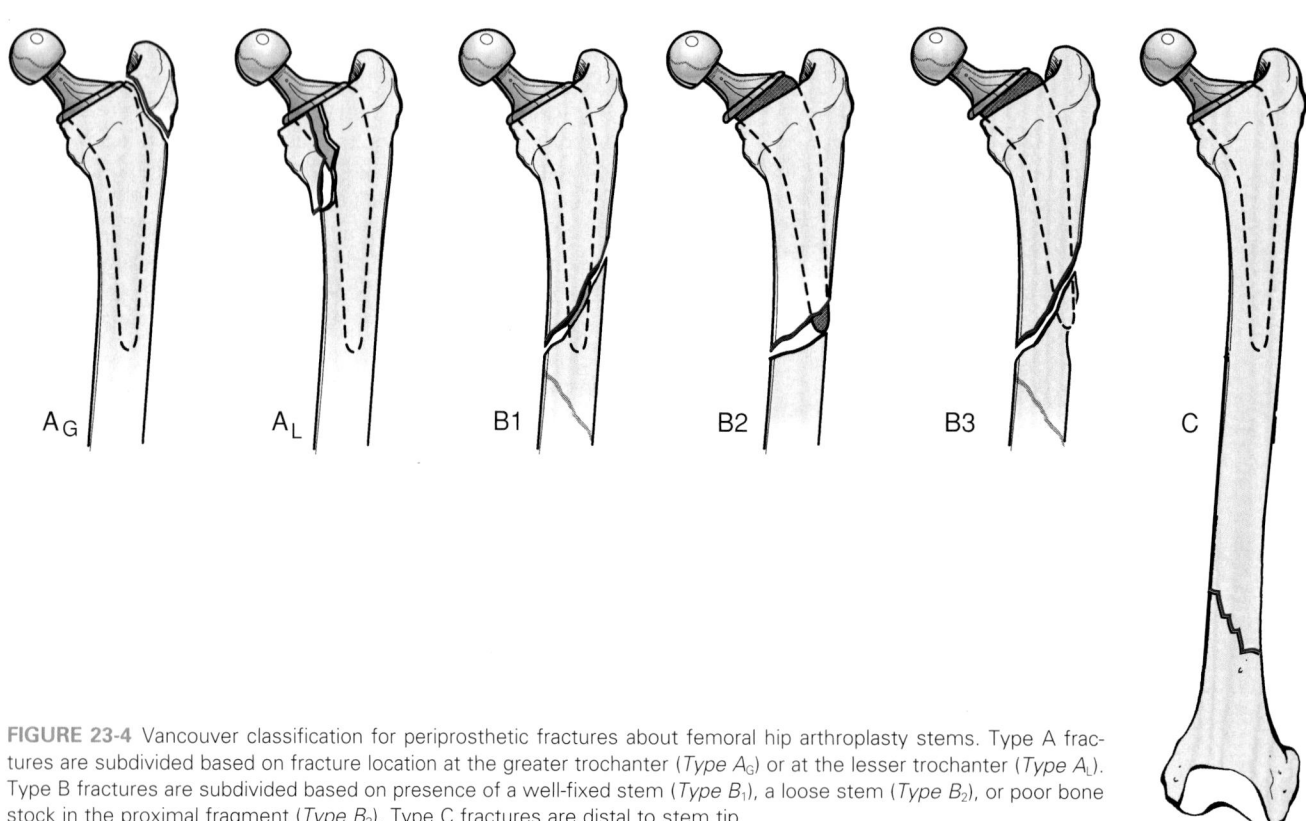

FIGURE 23-4 Vancouver classification for periprosthetic fractures about femoral hip arthroplasty stems. Type A fractures are subdivided based on fracture location at the greater trochanter (*Type A_G*) or at the lesser trochanter (*Type A_L*). Type B fractures are subdivided based on presence of a well-fixed stem (*Type B_1*), a loose stem (*Type B_2*), or poor bone stock in the proximal fragment (*Type B_3*). Type C fractures are distal to stem tip.

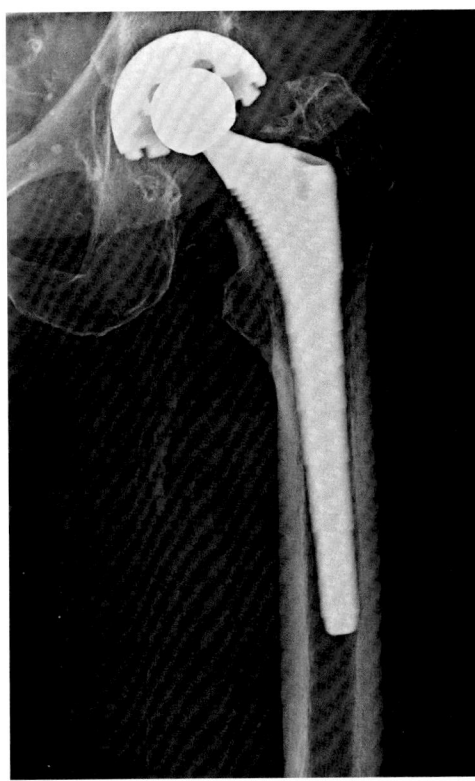

FIGURE 23-5 A minimally displaced fracture of the greater trochanter (Vancouver type A$_G$) that occurred postoperatively.

classification divides fractures into three zones: Type A being of the proximal metaphysis without extension to the diaphysis, type B are diaphyseal about the tip of the stem, and type C fractures extend beyond the longest revision stem and include fractures of the distal metaphysis. The subclassification of each type distinguishes the intraoperative from the postoperative classification and reflects fracture stability: Subtype I represents a simple cortical perforation; subtype II is a nondisplaced linear cortical crack; and subtype III is a displaced or otherwise unstable fracture (Table 23-6). The treatment options for fractures occurring intraoperatively vary somewhat based on when the fracture was detected. Intraoperative identification, in general, leads to more surgical interventions than identification in the recovery room or later (Table 23-6).

Classification of Periprosthetic Femur Fractures After Hip Resurfacing

No universally accepted or tested classification of periprosthetic femoral fractures associated with hip resurfacing currently exists. A systematic analysis of 107 specimens retrieved at the time of revision hip arthroplasty because of periprosthetic fracture revealed three distinct fracture patterns.[309] Type A were described as biomechanical fractures, type B as acute postnecrotic fractures, and type C chronic biomechanical fractures. Type A fractures occurred at an average of 41 days postoperatively. They were characterized by changes consistent with acute fracture without signs of osteonecrosis, regenerative fibrosis, or vascular proliferation. Type B fractures occurred at an average of 149 days postoperatively and all of these fractures were associated with osteonecrosis. Type C fractures were seen at an average of 179 days postoperatively. These were characterized by evidence of refracture or pseudoarthrosis through a previous fracture. Fractures were also categorized based on the location of the fracture, inside or outside the bounds of the edge of the femoral head component. The majority occurred inside the femoral component (59%). All acute biomechanical fractures were located exclusively outside of the component and were located in the neck.

Management Principles for Periprosthetic Femur Fractures

Management Principles for Vancouver Type A Periprosthetic Femur Fractures

The majority of periprosthetic fractures of the greater trochanter, Type A$_G$, are stable. They are usually nondisplaced or minimally displaced and are stabilized by the opposite pull and continuity of the soft tissue sleeve connecting the abductors and the vastus lateralis.[281] Such stable fractures when occurring postoperatively can be managed nonoperatively with symptomatic treatment. Weight bearing to tolerance is generally allowed. Intraoperative stable fractures of the greater trochanter can be managed similarly especially when recognized after wound closure. When recognized intraoperatively internal fixation may be considered. Nonoperative treatment is contraindicated if there is a complete fracture of the greater trochanter including the abductor attachment without a stabilizing soft tissue sleeve as the chance of migration, nonunion, and hip instability is high. In addition, if stability of the implant is compromised, or if the patient is unable to comply with abductor restrictions during the healing process, nonoperative treatment is not recommended.

Protected weight bearing may be used for nondisplaced or incomplete fractures about hip stems or resurfacing implants that are recognized after surgery. Typically, partial or toe-touch weight bearing is recommended with a walker or crutches. Abductor precautions can be added to protect nondisplaced greater trochanter fractures. The use of a walking device to unload the abductors during gait as well as avoidance of abductor strengthening or active abduction exercises is recommended while these fractures heal. It is important to obtain regular imaging using similar radiographic projections with increased frequency in the early post-op period. This will monitor displacement and allow decisions for continued observation or operative intervention if there is fracture displacement or loss of implant stability.

Widely displaced, or otherwise unstable fractures of the greater trochanter (Vancouver Type A$_G$), especially when associated with substantial pain, weakness, or limp, are generally treated operatively with ORIF typically with a claw plate that engages the soft tissue attachment of the gluteus medius as well as the bone of the greater trochanter

TABLE 23-5 Vancouver Classification Scheme and Treatment Options for Postoperative Fractures

Classification	Trochanteric		Diaphyseal			Distal to Stem
	A$_L$	A$_G$	B1	B2	B3	C
Bone Stock	Good	Good	Good	Good	Poor	Good
Stem Fixation	Well fixed	Well fixed	Well fixed	Loose	Loose	Well fixed
Author's Preferred Treatment Options	Symptomatic treatment unless substantial medial cortex is involved	Symptomatic treatment or ORIF with claw plate to treat pain, weakness, limp, or instability	Lateral plate applied with biologic fracture reduction techniques. Consider extending plate to include lateral femoral condyle	Uncemented revision long stem with or without lateral plate	Long stem revision with allograft with or without a lateral plate or revision to a tumor prosthesis	Distal femoral locking plate extending proximal to overlap the femoral stem

(Fig. 23-6). Results with these modern plates represent an improvement over other techniques.[165,166] Fractures of the lesser trochanter, Vancouver type A$_L$, are typically avulsion fractures that can be managed nonoperatively. However, larger fractures that involve a segment of the proximal medial femoral cortex are typically associated with tapered press-fit stem designs and are usually treated operatively with cerclage cables or wires with or without revision of the stem to one that provides fixation distal to the fracture.[282] Nondisplaced fractures of this nature noted intraoperatively can be managed with cerclage cables with retention of the femoral stem if stable. Displaced medial fractures noted intraoperatively or postoperatively are managed with cables and revision to a stem with distal fixation.

TABLE 23-6 Vancouver Classification Scheme and Treatment Options for Intraoperative Fractures

Classification	Metaphyseal			Diaphyseal			Distal to Stem		
	A1	A2	A3	B1	B2	B3	C1	C2	C3
Fracture Morphology	Cortical perforation	Undisplaced crack	Displaced or unstable	Cortical perforation	Undisplaced crack	Displaced or unstable	Cortical perforation	Undisplaced crack	Displaced or unstable
Author's Preferred Treatment Options									
Recognized Fractures	Protected weight bearing or bone graft	Protected weight bearing or cerclage cables	ORIF with claw plate with conversion to long stem if implant unstable	Cortical strut with or without conversion to long stem implant	Lateral plate with conversion to long stem if implant unstable	Lateral plate with conversion to long stem if implant unstable	Cortical strut	Lateral plate	Lateral plate
Unrecognized Fractures	Protected weight bearing	Protected weight bearing	ORIF with claw plate with revision to long stem if implant unstable	Cortical strut	Lateral plate with revision to long stem if implant unstable	Lateral plate with revision to long stem if implant unstable	Cortical strut	Protected weight bearing or lateral plate	Lateral plate

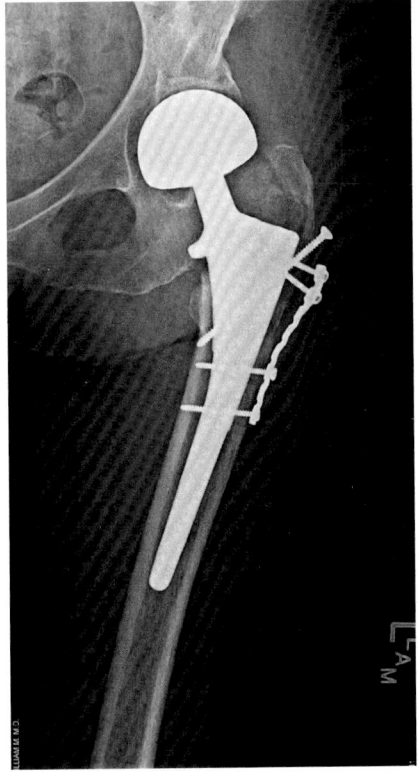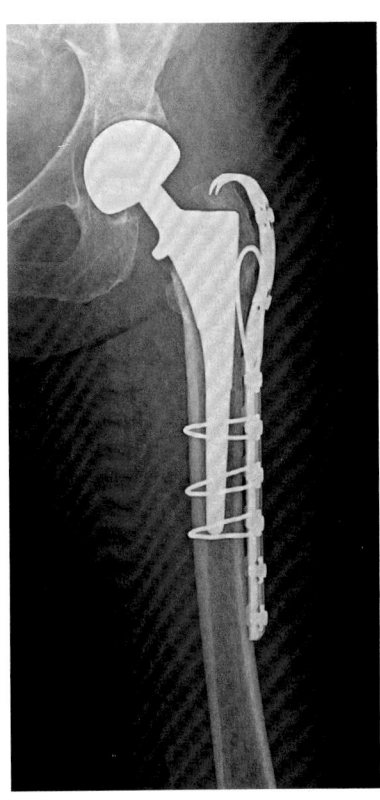

FIGURE 23-6 A fracture of the greater trochanter (Vancouver A_G) treated with a small buttress plate and lag screws that resulted in nonunion **(A)** is successfully treated with a claw plate **(B)**.

Management Principles for Vancouver Type B Periprosthetic Femur Fractures

Vancouver type B fractures identified during surgery are rarely treated nonoperatively. Those recognized postoperatively can be treated nonsurgically in certain cases (Table 23-7). If there is excellent implant stability and the fracture is incomplete or a nondisplaced diaphyseal crack, these can be observed with protected weight bearing and close follow-up. In addition, if there

TABLE 23-7	Periprosthetic Femur Fractures About Hip Arthroplasty Prostheses

Nonoperative Treatment

Indications	Relative Contraindications
Stable femoral stem and non-displaced diaphyseal fracture	Loose implant
Proximal fracture related to osteolysis with adequate distal stem fixation	Proximal metaphyseal fracture with a proximal fit stem
Nondisplaced neck fracture associated with hip resurfacing	Displaced diaphyseal or distal fracture
Minimally displaced trochanteric fracture	Widely displaced greater trochanteric fracture with altered abduct or function

is adequate distal stem fixation and a strictly proximal fracture, this can be observed. If there is a high predicted chance of stem subsidence or fracture displacement, operative management should be pursued early. This is typically the case with proximal (metaphyseal) fit stems with an intraoperative metaphyseal fracture where the risk of fracture propagation and stem subsidence is high.

The difficulty in operative management of periprosthetic femoral shaft fractures that involve the tip of hip arthroplasty stems, Vancouver type B fractures, is evidenced by the array of treatment options described without a clear consensus emerging on the most appropriate method.[140,160] Operative treatment of these femur fractures is indicated in most circumstances, except for those fractures that are truly nondisplaced or when the patient's condition prohibits operation. ORIF with plates and revision arthroplasty with or without supplementary autologous or allogeneic bone grafting are the most common methods for operative stabilization.[39,99,222] Stabilization using ORIF techniques with plates and screws or cortical onlay allografts or a combination of both is indicated for femoral shaft fractures about well-fixed implants (Vancouver type B1 fractures).[24,98,276,294] Historically, there has been little role for revision arthroplasty for B1 fractures given the stable prosthesis. However, revision of an associated well-fixed stem to a long stem modular prosthesis nail that spans the fracture has recently been advocated by multiple authors for Vancouver B fractures regardless of stem stability.[149,151,210] The earlier weight bearing and improved mobilization associated with revision arthroplasty with implants that span the fracture may provide

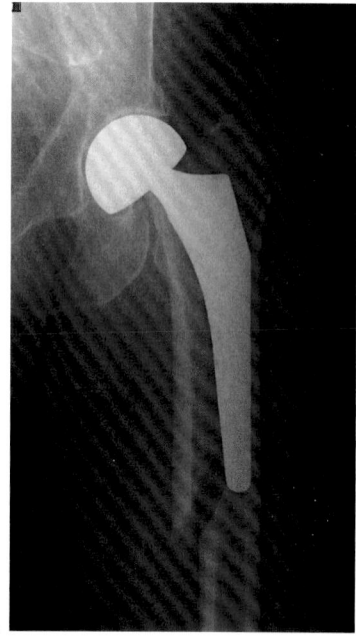
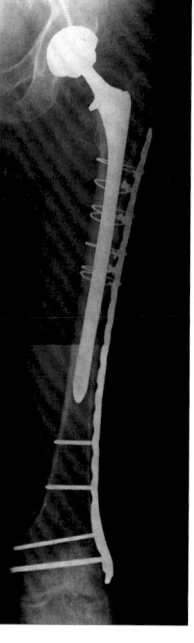

A   **B**

FIGURE 23-7 Fracture about a loose hemiarthroplasty stem with good bone stock (Vancouver B$_2$) **(A)** is treated with a long porous-coated revision stem and lateral plating **(B)** that protects the entire length of the femur.

for improved mortality rates if patients who can withstand the magnitude of such surgery are properly selected. Femoral component revision with or without adjuvant plate and/or allograft strut fixation is indicated for Vancouver types B2 and B3 fractures where the femoral stem is loose. The indication for including allograft struts in the operative strategy is most clear when there is associated bone loss from long standing component motion, type B3 fractures.

For femoral shaft fractures around a loose implant, Vancouver types B2 and B3 fractures, revision of the femoral component is typically recommended (Fig. 23-7). This strategy addresses both the loose component and the fracture and provides intramedullary stability by virtue of longer femoral stems used for revision. Fracture fixation with a lateral plate or reconstitution of bone stock with allograft strut or sometimes a combination of both plates and struts are utilized in addition to femoral component revision. In more severe cases of bone loss, an allograft prosthesis composite, impaction bone grafting technique, or proximal femoral replacement may be considered.[153,194] Knowledge of specific revision techniques is necessary to effectively handle these challenging cases. In addition to the above mentioned radiographic evaluation of the fracture and femoral stem stability, quality orthogonal radiographs are also mandatory to evaluate the fixation status of the acetabular component and remaining acetabular and femoral bone stock. If possible, the operative note from the original arthroplasty should be obtained to determine the manufacturer of the components, so that new acetabular liners, if needed, can be available. The presence of prefracture hip symptoms, such as mechanical thigh or groin pain, can alert the surgeon to potential component loosening, if the radiographs are equivocal. Serologies such as sedimentation

rate and C-reactive protein are of unknown benefit in the presence of an acute fracture. If there is any concern for infection, a preoperative hip aspiration should be considered.

Management Principles for Vancouver Type C Periprosthetic Femur Fractures

In the initial description of the Vancouver classification type C fractures were described as those "well distal" to the stem.[64] It has been inferred that treatment indications and fixation techniques for these fractures are independent of the femoral prosthesis. This, however, is an oversimplification of the typical situation. Distal femoral shaft fractures in the absence of a hip prosthesis are typically treated with intramedullary nails (either antegrade or retrograde) and supracondylar or intercondylar fractures are treated with either a lateral plate or retrograde nail. Vancouver type C periprosthetic fractures, by virtue of the femoral stem, obviate standard techniques and implants utilized for nailing of native femoral shaft fractures. Attempts to insert standard retrograde nails in this short segment are ill advised because of inadequate fixation within the proximal fragment and propensity for nonunion[187] and malunion (Fig. 23-8). A unique retrograde nail designed to slide over the tip of the femoral stem has shown reasonable results as described in a small clinical series and has been studied in a biomechanical analysis that supports immediate weight bearing with this device.[310,311] ORIF remains the most applicable method of internal fixation. Ending a plate at or just distal to the femoral stem should also be avoided to minimize the stress rise effect (Fig. 23-9). Instead, the plate should span the fracture and overlap the zone of the stem (Fig. 23-10). The indications and contraindications for surgical management follow closely those for Vancouver type B Fractures. Additional principles and results of treating these distal femoral shaft fractures and metaphyseal fractures are presented in Chapter 52 Femoral Shaft Fractures and Chapter 53 Distal Femoral Fractures.

Management Principles for Fractures About Femoral Resurfacing Prostheses

Nonoperative management is often cited as a viable treatment option for nondisplaced femoral neck fractures associated with hip resurfacing.[50,54,123] Fractures that are completely displaced or those with components that have shifted are generally treated with revision arthroplasty.

Although nonoperative management has been described for nondisplaced fractures of the femoral neck associated with hip resurfacing,[50] revision to a conventional THA is typically performed.[5,173,309] There is little role for internal fixation of these femoral neck fractures after resurfacing, although successful plate and screw fixation and intramedullary nailing (IMN) has been reported for management of intertrochanteric and subtrochanteric fractures in the setting of hip resurfacing.[33,212]

ORIF of Periprosthetic Femur Fractures

Indirect fracture reduction techniques have favorable biologic features that minimize soft tissue disruption, preserve the vascular supply to bone, enhance healing, and decrease the incidence of nonunion for many fractures including periprosthetic femur

FIGURE 23-8 **A:** Ill-advised treatment of a Vancouver Type C femur fracture distal to a hip arthroplasty stem. **B:** The nail eroded through the anterior cortex and a nonunion developed. This was treated with nail removal, ORIF with a lateral plate, autologous bone graft to stimulate nonunion healing, and an anterior strut graft to restore bone stock.

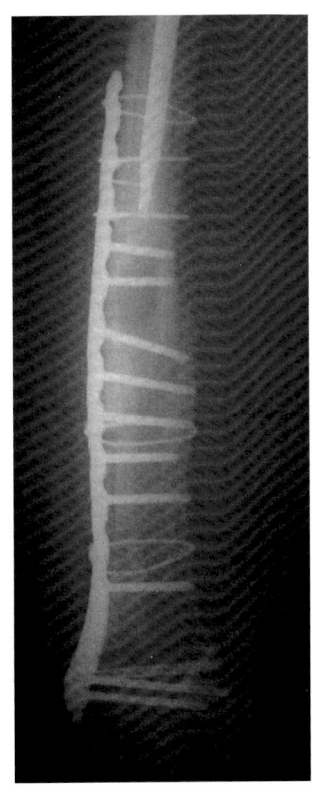

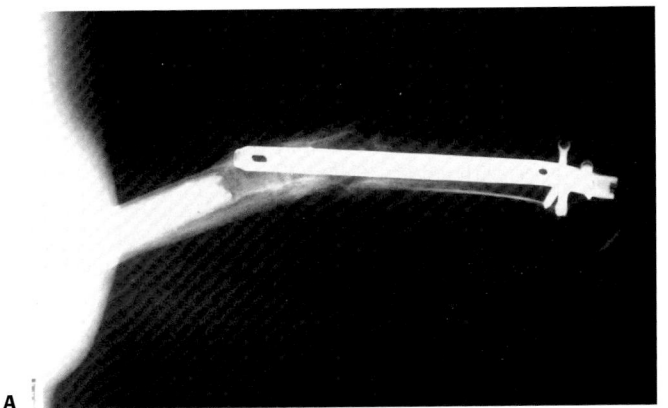

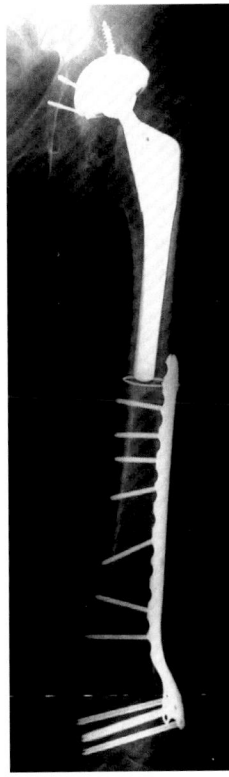

FIGURE 23-9 Ill-advised treatment of a Vancouver Type C fracture with a plate that is too short because it creates an unnecessary additional stress riser at the tip of the arthroplasty stem.

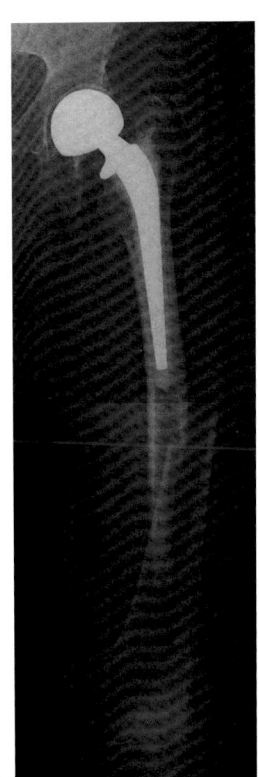
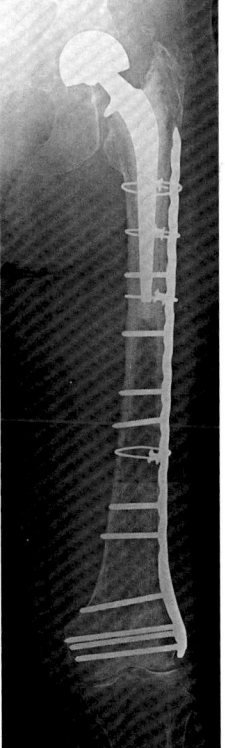

FIGURE 23-10 A Vancouver C fracture **(A)** treated with an optimal plate construct **(B)** that spans the fracture, the zone of the femoral stem, and the entire unprotected femur distally.

fractures,[116] often obviating the need for supplemental bone grafting.[227] Successful application of these techniques to periprosthetic fractures must consider the fracture location relative to the femoral component, the implant stability, the quality of the surrounding bone, and the medical and functional status of the patient.[64] The following are principles for ORIF of periprosthetic femoral shaft fractures about hip arthroplasty stems, Vancouver type B. These general principles also apply for Vancouver types A and C fractures. Subtleties in technique and differences in implant choices distinguish techniques for Vancouver types A and C fractures.

Preoperative Planning for ORIF of Periprosthetic Femoral Fractures

When ORIF of periprosthetic femur fractures is planned, the surgeon should be prepared for encountering an unexpected intraoperative finding of a loose femoral component (Table 23-8). Radiographically stable implants may be loose in up to 20% of cases of B1- and C-type fractures.[49] Therefore, all aspects of the preoperative plan should allow for the contingency that revision arthroplasty may be required. A radiolucent OR table is required and although ORIF can be performed with the patient in the supine or lateral position, the lateral position is preferred to accommodate the possibility of revision arthroplasty via a posterior approach. A radiolucent positioner,

---

TABLE 23-8	**ORIF of Periprosthetic Femoral Fractures About Hip Arthroplasty Stems**

Preoperative Planning Checklist

- **OR table:** Radiolucent table that allows fluoroscopic imaging of the entire involved femur and hip
- **Position/positioning aids:** Lateral decubitus using a radiolucent positioner such as a beanbag (peg boards are typically not radiolucent) or supine
- **Fluoroscopy location:** Opposite side from the primary surgeon's position with the monitor at the foot
- **Equipment:**
  An array of reduction forceps
  Burr
  Sagittal saw
  Cable set
  Equipment required for revision arthroplasty should be immediately available
- **Implants:**
  Large fragment set
  Straight or bowed plates (or specialty plates) long enough to span the entire femur
  At least six cables (approximately 1.7-mm diameter)
  Femoral allograft strut
  Implants required for revision arthroplasty should be immediately available
  For Vancouver Type A fractures, specialized trochanteric "claw" plates are typically needed rather than long plates that span the entire femur
- **Tourniquet (sterile/nonsterile):** None required
- **Blood:** PRBCs typed and crossmatched

---

such as a beanbag, is required. It should be noted that positioners, such as peg boards, used for hip arthroplasty may not be radiolucent. Fluoroscopic access to the entire limb and hip should be planned for. The equipment needed for ORIF of periprosthetic femur fractures can be extensive to accommodate all contingencies: ORIF, revision of the femoral stem, revision of the acetabular component, strut grafting, and autologous bone grafting (Table 23-8). Similarly, the implants required for these contingencies should be confirmed to be readily available.

Surgical Approach for ORIF of Periprosthetic Femur Fractures

For ORIF of periprosthetic femoral shaft fractures, a straight lateral thigh incision is used for exposure of the lateral aspect of the femur. Posterior incisions from prior hip arthroplasty are incorporated. Dissection is carried down to the iliotibial fascia with care to minimize stripping of the subcutaneous fat from the fascia. Self-retaining retractors are not utilized until they can be placed at a fascial level. The iliotibial fascia is incised parallel to its fibers and the fascia of the vastus lateralis is also incised parallel to its fibers approximately 3 cm from its attachment to the intermuscular septum. The vastus lateralis muscle is carefully elevated off the posterior fascial flap and retracted anteriorly. This is done in a distal to proximal motion based on the orientation of the muscle fibers attachment to the fascia. Dissection done in this manner takes advantage of the axilla created between the muscle fibers and the fascia and allows the muscle to be elevated cleanly off the fascia. Perforating vessels are identified and ligated as needed. Meticulous deep soft tissue dissection is used to minimize devascularization of bone. Exposure is limited to the lateral surface of the femur spanning the region needed to apply and secure a plate proximal and distal to the fracture. Whenever possible, the muscle is left undisturbed in the region of the fracture and the plate slid in an extraperiosteal plane deep to the muscle in this region. When direct access to the fracture is required, to remove entrapped soft tissue for instance, great care is taken to work through the fracture site rather than to strip muscle from around the bone.

Reduction Strategy for ORIF of Periprosthetic Femur Fractures

Once adequate exposure is obtained, and hemostasis assured, attention is turned to fracture reduction and fixation. The reduction technique is distinct based on the fracture pattern. Either an anatomic reduction and rigid fixation (lag screws or compression plating or both) (Table 23-9) or a bridge plating technique is chosen (Table 23-10). The simple patterns typically seen with these fractures are amenable to the anatomic reduction and rigid fixation strategy. This strategy can easily lead to inadvertent excessive soft tissue stripping more so than a bridge plating technique. Therefore, great care and patience during reduction maneuvers is required. Although cerclage cables have a reputation of being associated with excessive soft tissue stripping, this is not absolute. Properly and carefully placed cables can ease the effort of reduction, especially with the long oblique or spiral fractures that are commonly encountered. The afforded ease of reduction that cables

TABLE 23-9 ORIF of Simple Periprosthetic Femoral Shaft Fractures About Hip Arthroplasty Stems (Vancouver Types B and C)

Surgical Steps

- Expose the lateral femur
- Debride displaced fractures without causing unnecessary soft tissue stripping
  - For comminuted fractures, this step is neither required nor advised
- Reduce the fracture incrementally with manual traction and gentle manipulation
  - Provisional cable fixation of spiral oblique fractures to help obtain and maintain reduction
  - Goal is an anatomic reduction
- Apply precontoured lateral plate
  - Consider spanning entire length of the femur to protect from subsequent peri-implant fractures
  - Plate should be contoured to match the lateral femur
- Provisionally secure plate to the proximal fragment with cables
- Provisionally secure plate to distal fragment with nonlocked screws
- Apply lag screw across fracture through plate, if possible
- Loosen provisional fixation and lag screw enough to remove initial reduction cable from beneath plate
  - This step is optional, as reduction cable can be left beneath plate
- Finally tighten distal screws
- Finally tighten lag screw
- Sequentially tighten proximal cables
  - Finally secure cables once all cables are sufficiently and equally tightened
- Add additional screws into greater trochanter and distal fragment as necessary
  - Consider locked screws

TABLE 23-10 ORIF of Comminuted Periprosthetic Femoral Shaft Fractures About Hip Arthroplasty Stems (Vancouver Types B and C)

Surgical Steps

- Expose the lateral femur
- Avoid disruption of the comminuted fracture zone. Formal debridement of fracture fragments is unnecessary.
- Apply precontoured lateral plate
  - Consider spanning entire length of the femur to protect from subsequent peri-implant fractures
  - Plate should be contoured to match the lateral femur
  - Fracture reduction is not required at this step
- Provisionally secure plate to the proximal fragment with cables
- Re-establish length and rotation
- Finally secure plate to distal fragment with nonlocked screws
  - Coronal plane alignment is restored by using the plate contour as a reduction aid
  - Sagittal plane alignment is restored by having the plate centered on the proximal and distal fragments on a lateral x-ray view
- Sequentially tighten proximal cables
  - Finally secure cables once all cables are sufficiently and equally tightened
- Add screws into greater trochanter and distal fragment as necessary
  - Consider locked screws

provide can actually reduce soft tissue disruption associated with prolonged and repeated reduction attempts without cables. The cables and any adjunctive clamps are placed through muscle rather than underneath muscle. This strategy sacrifices very few muscle fibers and minimizes subperiosteal stripping and has been employed successfully in clinical series.[227,300] When a bridge plating construct is utilized, when there is fracture comminution, a properly contoured plate is used as a reduction template for alignment in the coronal and sagittal planes. The surgeon then only needs to assure proper length. Because, with this strategy, individual fracture fragments do not require anatomic reduction, the risk of excessive iatrogenic stripping should be minimal.

For typical spiral fractures, the first step is to restore gross alignment and length. The latter requires complete muscle relaxation. With complete paralysis, manual longitudinal traction by an assistant can usually restore length, at least to within 2 to 3 cm upon the first attempt. The fracture is provisionally stabilized with pointed reduction clamps. Anatomic reduction need not be accomplished all at once prior to initial clamping of the reduction. Rather, reduction is accomplished with stepwise improvements. Residual deformity at each step is identified via direct vision, palpation, and/or fluoroscopy and requirements for successive reduction maneuvers determined. During these maneuvers, great care is taken not to inadvertently strip soft tissue. The orientation of clamps is critical. To hold an established reduction, clamps placed perpendicular to the fracture work well. However, clamps used to help obtain a reduction are not necessarily placed perpendicular to the fracture plane. They are placed in an orientation such that squeezing the clamps will provide a force vector that serves to better reduce the fracture. Once the reduction is close, within about 1 cm in length, one or two cables are passed around the fracture and provisionally tightened. Two cables are used for longer oblique fractures. The cable tension can be relaxed to afford final reduction maneuvers, typically rotation and additional traction via appropriately placed clamps or via manual traction of an assistant. Once the fracture has "keyed in" and the reduction is confirmed with fluoroscopy, the cables are definitively retensioned.

Fixation Technique for ORIF of Periprosthetic Femur Fractures

ORIF Technique for Vancouver A Fractures. Claw plates are typically used for fixation of greater trochanteric fractures. The tines of the claw are placed through the tendinous insertion of the gluteus medius and impacted into the tip of the trochanter thereby gaining soft tissue and bony purchase proximally. A plate is selected to bypass the apex of the fracture by enough distance to apply two to three well-spaced (approximately 2 cm apart) cables around the zone of the femoral stem. A vertically applied cable is recommended to augment the claw fixation proximally. There is usually no requirement to extend the plate beyond the tip of the femoral prosthesis. However, very short plates have been associated with fixation failure.[166] Of course, the stability of the arthroplasty components is considered, and when loose they are revised. When these fractures are associated with substantial osteolysis, bone grafting is indicated with care to maintain the soft tissue stabilizers.[281]

ORIF Technique for Vancouver B and C Fractures. The preferred plate construct for Vancouver type B1 fractures includes a lateral plate contoured proximally to accommodate the trochanteric flare. Distally, the plate should have a minimum of six to eight holes covering the native femur distal to the fracture or extend to the condylar region (where a distal femoral plate design may be utilized). A bowed plate to accommodate the sagittal bow of the femur is preferred. When the strategy for fracture reduction includes provisional fracture fixation with cables, plate fixation of the reduced fracture is very simple; however, several principles should be adhered to. A well-contoured plate can be secured to either the proximal and distal fragment with cables or nonlocked screws without affecting the reduction. However, when the plate contour deviates from the bone contour, nonlocked screws and cables can potentially disrupt an anatomic reduction. In such circumstances, additional efforts to contour the plate anatomically are advised, especially with regard to the proximal fragment where nonlocked means, primarily cables, are the primary method of fixation. Deviations between the distal fragment and distal plate contour can be accommodated with the use of locked screws without disrupting a pre-established anatomic reduction. When the fracture pattern allows, a lag screw distal to the stem and across the fracture is utilized (Table 23-9). Screws through an existing cement mantle, either in the proximal or distal fragment, provide excellent points of fixation. If such

a screw can be placed in the proximal fragment, this screw is tightened prior to definitive tensioning of cables. Three or more equally spaced cables are used proximally between the lesser trochanter and the tip of the stem. Devices to attach or hold cables to the plate are not required; the cables are simply passed around the plate with the crimping connection purposely positioned either just anterior or just posterior to the plate to minimize prominence and to allow easy access for locking the cable. The cables are individually tightened and provisionally secured, then retightened sequentially akin to the method of tightening lug nuts on a car wheel. This assures that tightening one cable does not result in loosening of an adjacent cable. A recent study indicates that cerclage wires and cables provide point contact fixation and are unlikely to strangulate blood supply.[154] Screws, typically locked screws, are placed in the trochanteric region after all cables are tensioned.

Proximal fragment screw fixation without the use of cables has been successfully employed.[28,66] With this strategy, multiple short locked screws are supplemented with bicortical locked screws into the trochanteric region or around the stem or both. To increase the screw density in the trochanteric region, reversed application of plates designed for the distal femur have been utilized.[66,70] Isolated use of unicortical locked screws is not recommended because of marginal rotational control.

Several considerations go into distal fixation details: the plate length covering the distal segment, the location of screws, the number of screws, and the type of screws. The minimum plate length to obtain satisfactory distal fixation usually corresponds to six plate holes but this minimum threshold is increased when poor quality bone is encountered. Longer plates that extend to the lateral femoral condyle have recently been advocated to protect the entire femur (Fig. 23-11) and reduce the risk of subsequent peri-implant fracture at the distal margin of the plate (Fig. 23-12).[229] This strategy is at the expense of an increased risk of plate-related pain over the subcutaneously located condylar extent of the plate. The holes nearest to the fracture and farthest from the fracture are the most important for maximizing construct stability. These holes and two in between are typically filled with screws. Locked or additional screws should be considered when osteoporotic bone is present. When nonlocked screws could cause a malreduction because of plate and bone contour mismatch, locked screws should be utilized. In general, locked screws should be placed after nonlocked screws and appear to be most advantageous near to the fracture. The initially placed reduction cables can either be left under the plate or removed from beneath the plate after two points of provisional fixation are established in both the proximal and distal fragments. These provision points of fixation, cables and screws, must be loosened slightly to allow cable removal from beneath the plate.

Strut allografts are reserved for situations with associated bone loss (Vancouver B3 fractures). The strut is secured anteriorly with cables placed proximal and distal to the fracture. These are a combination of cables independent of an associated plate (cables over the strut and under the plate) and with cables around both the plate and strut.

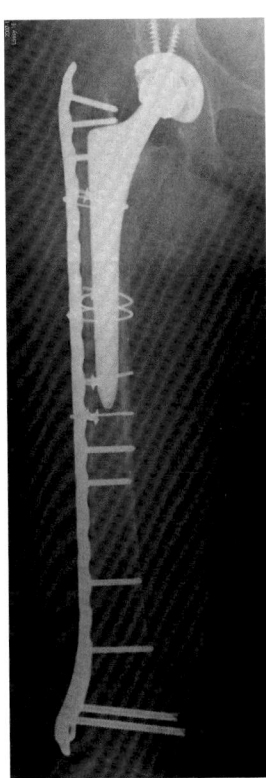

FIGURE 23-11 AP view of a modern modification of the Ogden construct with a long distal femoral plate to protect the entire femur and with locked screws to augment fixation.

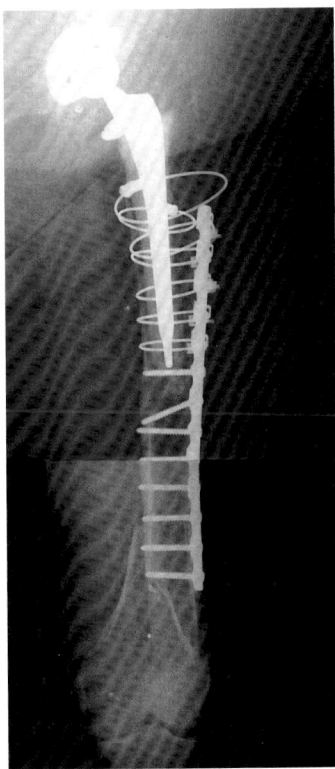

FIGURE 23-12 A Vancouver Type B femur fracture treated successfully with a lateral plate until fracture occurred at the distal tip of the plate. Constructs that span the entire femur avoid such complications.

When fractures of the medial calcar are noted intraoperatively, x-rays are obtained to delineate the extent of fracture, as occasionally these splits can spiral down toward the stem tip. Limited, nondisplaced medial cracks noted intraoperatively are treated with one or two cerclage cables. When propagation is present, a lateral plate is used to bypass the distal extent of the fracture. Displaced fractures of either the lesser or greater trochanter are treated operatively with an anatomic ORIF. Limited sized lesser trochanteric fractures are treated with cables alone.

Vancouver type C fractures were originally defined as being "well distal" to the femoral stem. These are usually in the supracondylar femur region and are occasionally intercondylar. Although the fracture fixation is not entirely dictated by the presence of the femoral stem, the femoral stem must be considered. There is almost always not enough proximal shaft bone to allow stable fixation of a retrograde nail. The mainstay of treatment of distal femur fractures in the presence of a femoral stem is ORIF with lateral plates. The principles for lateral plating (LP) for Vancouver C fractures are similar to those for Vancouver B fractures. Locked plates are used to provide fixed-angle stability of the end segment and improved fixation in an osteoporotic shaft segment. The main deviation from standard fixation of these fractures because of the presence of the hip arthroplasty stem comes with fixation proximally. It is rare that a lateral plate used to provide stable fixation of the distal femur fracture is short enough to avoid creating a stress riser effect between the top of the plate and the hip arthroplasty femoral stem. Therefore, we recommend that plates utilized for Vancouver type C fractures be long enough to overlap the femoral stem. Fixation in the proximal fragment is with multiple screws distal to the stem into the native shaft fragment and supplemented with two cables around the plate in the zone of the femoral prosthesis. This construct provides satisfactory stability for fixation of the distal femur fracture and protects the entire femur from future fracture.

Postoperative Care for ORIF of Periprosthetic Femur Fractures

Postoperatively, early rehabilitation is concentrated on mobilization and knee ROM. Weight bearing is protected to some degree for approximately 6 to 8 weeks. Initial weight-bearing restrictions are typically toe-touch for balance or up to 50% weight bearing if the bone quality and fixation were both optimal. Immediate weight bearing has been advocated after minimally invasive plate application;[68,69] however, little clinical results to support such an aggressive protocol are available. Therapy for knee ROM, transfer training, and use of assist devices are initiated immediately postoperatively. Based on progressive clinical and radiographic signs of fracture healing, weight bearing is gradually advanced. Full weight bearing is typically accomplished by 6 to 8 weeks and at this time formal strengthening and gait training therapy are useful.

Potential Pitfalls and Preventative Measures for ORIF of Periprosthetic Femur Fractures

ORIF of periprosthetic femoral shaft fractures are demanding procedures (Table 23-11). These fractures are most commonly simple spiral oblique fracture patterns. They are therefore,

TABLE 23-11   **ORIF of Periprosthetic Femoral Shaft Fractures**

Potential Pitfalls and Preventions

Pitfalls	Preventions
Extensive soft tissue stripping during reduction	Adherence to biologic fracture fixation techniques Comminuted fractures are bridge plated Simple fractures are anatomically reduced and compression plated. Simple patterns are at greatest risk for excessive stripping
Extensive soft tissue stripping during cable application	Cables should be passed through muscle rather than circumferentially under muscle
Mismatch between plate contour and bone causes malreduction	Fine adjustments to precontoured plates especially in the zone of greater trochanter and distal metaphyseal flare are often required Locked screws placed after reduction should not alter reduction
Inadequate proximal fragment fixation	Standard fixation around the zone of femoral implant with cables can be supplemented with locked screws into trochanteric region Screws can be placed into cement mantle just distal to stem Cables are sequentially tightened and retightened akin to tightening lug nuts Exclusive use of unicortical locked screws in the proximal fragment provides poor rotational control and should be avoided
Femoral stem is unexpectedly found to be loose	Even when stems appear radiographically stable, revision of a loose stem should be considered a contingency

typically amenable to anatomic reduction with compression techniques. To obtain anatomic reduction it is often possible to inadvertently strip substantial amounts of soft tissues. The surgeon must be continually aware of this potential problem and should adhere to biologic fracture fixation techniques. The use of cables to provisionally obtain and hold a reduction of long spiral fractures can actually make the reduction process easier and may limit soft tissue stripping if properly applied (Fig. 23-10B). Cables should be passed through muscle rather than circumferentially under the muscle.

When spanning the entire length of the femur with a lateral plate, it is difficult to contour these thick plates to accommodate for both the trochanteric and distal femoral flares. However, when the reduction is obtained prior to plate application, this contour is critical if nonlocked screws or cables are going to be applied. A mismatch between plate contour and bone contour can be accommodated with the placement of locked screws.

One of the challenges for ORIF of periprosthetic femoral shaft fractures is obtaining adequate fixation in the proximal fragment around the zone of the hip stem. Cables are typically supplemented with screws into the trochanteric region or with unicortical locked screws in the zone of the stem. Relying on unicortical locked screws without cables should be avoided as these constructs have inadequate rotational control.

Unexpectedly finding a loose femoral stem can be avoided with a careful history and careful observation of prefracture and postfracture radiographs. Even when a careful preoperative evaluation indicates that the stem is stable, intraoperative

evaluation of the stem should be performed for confirmation. Access to the distal aspect of the stem is via the fracture. Some authors have advocated performing a hip arthrotomy in all cases to confirm stem stability.

Revision Arthroplasty of Periprosthetic Femur Fractures

Preoperative Planning for Revision Arthroplasty of Periprosthetic Femoral Fractures

When planning for revision arthroplasty, adequate preoperative imaging is essential for preoperative planning (Table 23-12). These images should be used to determine the type and extent of implants needed. Even for femoral fractures, the status and

TABLE 23-12   **Revision Hip Arthroplasty for Periprosthetic Femur Fractures**

Preoperative Planning Checklist

- OR table: Radiolucent table with pelvic positioner that allows fluoroscopy
- Intraoperative fluoroscopy or plain radiograph capability
- Good quality and templated x-rays
- Cell saver and blood products
- Equipment: Bone graft based on preoperative plan, cerclage wires, large fragment plate, and screw system
- Implants: Revision acetabular and femoral options as outlined above

type of socket is important. Even if the socket appears well fixed, it is reasonable to have revision options. For liners, modular liners can be very helpful and time saving. Increasing head size and using lipped, lateralized, or constrained liners are often necessary for hip stability. The size of the socket will determine the liners that can be cemented in if this becomes necessary. Bone defects on the femur or socket evident on x-rays will dictate the need for particulate bone graft or structural bone graft such as cortical strut. Cerclage wires should always be available. Trochanteric fixation options including plates, heavy suture, or wires should be available based on the particular radiographic features. The extent of the fracture and the quality of the bone can be determined on x-ray and this will guide the femoral fixation options. A proximal fracture can be solved with many standard nonmodular stems but distal fractures or complex femoral problems often require modular titanium stems, and having bowed options is essential for long-stemmed implants or very bowed femurs. Some very osteoporotic femurs require very wide stems that are best prepared using hand reamers. Fluoroscopy will be useful for reaming close to a bowed femur. If there is only a very short segment available for fixation before the distal femoral metaphyseal flare, there should be options for a megaprosthesis or allograft–prosthesis composite. If the femur has a very severe bow or varus remodeling, preoperatively, there should be plans for a femoral osteotomy and this would require fixation options (often cerclage wires) and may require cortical strut grafts or plates for supplemental fixation. Many cases require a "plan A" and a "plan B" and the implants for either plan should be arranged preoperatively. Imaging should be readily accessible in the operating suite and templating will allow implant suppliers to provide outlier sizes and nonroutine bone graft.

Positioning for Revision Arthroplasty of Periprosthetic Femoral Fractures

The patient position for ORIF of periprosthetic femoral shaft fractures can be either lateral decubitus or supine and must take into consideration positioning requirements of the preferred approach for fracture fixation (usually the lateral approach) and revision arthroplasty if needed. Vancouver type A fractures are typically treated in the lateral decubitus position to facilitate access to the trochanteric region. The OR table must provide for unencumbered fluoroscopy of the entire femur and hip. In general, lateral positioning is preferred as it provides greater ease for the surgeon. In this position, the soft tissues require less retraction and the surgeons' view is in the preferred vertical plane rather than the horizontal as compared to operating with the patient supine. Positioning aids used to hold the patient lateral must be radiolucent. Typically, beanbags meet this requirement but peg boards do not. The torso and contralateral pelvis should be stabilized and the ipsilateral hip should be free to flex, extend, abduct, and adduct with minimal interference from the positioning aids. The contralateral hip is flexed to minimize interference with lateral fluoroscopic radiographs. Consistent with lateral positioning for any procedure, an axillary roll is used and the down leg is padded to protect the bony prominences, namely the proximal fibular head and lateral malleolus, and protect the peroneal nerve from compression. The

torso and down leg are secured to the OR table in standard fashion. When supine positioning is utilized, the ipsilateral limb is brought to the edge of the OR table and a small bump can be placed beneath the ipsilateral hip to place the limb in neutral rotation at rest.

Standard surgical prep and draping is performed with care to allow access to the limb from the top of the ilium to at least the midcalf. The affected extremity is draped free and typically a tourniquet is not used. However, for distal exposure and reduction of Vancouver type C fractures, a sterile tourniquet may be utilized and then removed.

Fluoroscopy is generally required. The C-arm is positioned on the opposite side from the operating surgeon toward the patient's front when positioned lateral, and on the contralateral side when supine. The monitor is placed on the contralateral side near the table foot to allow easy visualization by the primary surgeon. The contralateral lower extremity has the propensity to block lateral views, whether lateral or supine positioning is used. This is one reason why, when positioned lateral, hip motion should be unencumbered. By flexing or extending the hip, overlap of the contralateral leg can be avoided. With the patient supine, 10 to 20 degrees of external rotation of the limb and a matching amount of C-arm rotation allows a lateral x-ray without overlap of the contralateral leg.

For revision hip arthroplasty, the patient should be positioned to allow the most extensile and flexible approaches to the pelvis, hip joint, and femur. Typically, the lateral position with the operative side up and a suitable pelvic positioner, one that allows for unencumbered fluoroscopic radiographs, is the most versatile option. Supine positions allow easier access by fluoroscopy but little extensile options. With the lateral position, orthogonal plain radiographic views can be obtained easily though fluoroscopy is challenging.

Surgical Approach(es) for Revision Arthroplasty of Periprosthetic Femoral Fractures

For revision arthroplasty, the most extensile approach to the femur, hip, and pelvis is the posterior-lateral approach. This approach can be extended down the femur, as described previously in this chapter for ORIF, to the knee as needed. The muscular (and vascular) attachments to the femur and fracture fragments can be preserved.

Revision Arthroplasty Technique of Periprosthetic Femoral Fractures

The specific revision strategy chosen depends on the quality of the remaining bone stock, the diameter of the femoral canal distal to the fracture, and patient factors such as age and baseline functional status (Table 23-13). Through the fracture site, cement and cement restrictors can be removed. If necessary, an extended trochanteric osteotomy of the proximal fracture fragment can allow excellent access for stem removal and direct visualization of the distal canal to allow accurate reaming.[158,262] The acetabular component is typically exposed more easily after the femoral component is removed. The liner is removed if modular and the acetabular component is manually tested for stability. If it is loose, acetabular revision is performed. If it

> **TABLE 23-13** **Revision Arthroplasty for Periprosthetic Femoral Shaft Fractures**
>
> **Surgical Steps**
>
> - Appropriate patient position with a suitable pelvic positioner that provides excellent stability to limb manipulation but does not encroach on the surgical field or block limb flexion
> - Drape and prep widely (up to the iliac wing and below the knee)
> - Allow free movement of the operative extremity in all planes. Allow access to the contralateral limb for referencing femoral length and knee position
> - During exposure, recreate plane between gluteus maximus and abductors
> - Maintain abductor–greater trochanter–vastus lateralis sleeve, especially if the greater trochanter is mobile
> - Extend incision along femur distally. Deep to the fascia, follow intermuscular plane posterior to vastus lateralis proximally and along intermuscular septum distally. Identify and coagulate perforator vessels. The sciatic nerve can be palpated and can be detensioned by releasing the gluteus maximus sling off the linea aspera. Preserve soft tissue attachments to femur as much as possible. Dissect down to the intact femoral shaft
> - The femoral component can be removed through the fracture if feasible or a coronal split of the proximal involved femur can be utilized if it will not be used for fixation later
> - Acetabular work is easier after the femoral component is removed. If the acetabular component is well fixed, a modular exchange of the polyethylene can be done, increasing the head size if possible. Cementing a liner is a good option if modular options are not available
> - The distal intact femur is prepared for the appropriate stem. A cerclage wire is recommended at the mouth of the distal femoral bone to prevent fracture here. This is especially important at the distal diaphysis
> - The trial femur is assembled. Length can be referenced via the other limb and tension of the abductor/vastus sleeve if the usual soft tissue tension measures are absent. Stability of the hip joint is an important part of the evaluation with the trials. Special attention should be made to anteversion of the trials so this can be recreated with the implant. Combined anteversion can be optimized through the stem if the existing socket does not have adequate anteversion
> - If there is adequate distal fixation, soft tissue tension, and hip stability, the final stem can be assembled and inserted in a meticulous manner to avoid distal fracture and to recreate the anteversion and length of the trials
> - Closure is done in a standard manner with attention to hemostasis and repair of the posterior pseudocapsule or abductor tendon depending on the approach. If the trochanter is mobile, this can be repaired with a trochanteric plate, cerclage wires, or heavy suture depending on the specific procedure.

is well fixed, the liner is typically exchanged, and the head size increased, if possible, to allow improved hip stability.

Often, the greater trochanter with its abductor attachments is compromised by the fracture or surgical treatment. In addition to repairing it as described previously, maintenance of the abductor/vastus lateralis soft tissue sleeve attachments is highly recommended as this will prevent trochanteric escape and proximal migration from the pull of the abductors. In many cases, stable trochanteric bony union is not feasible or likely and maintaining this soft tissue sleeve will help to achieve a stable fibrous union.

Several strategies can be used for the femur, but all rely on obtaining secure distal fixation. Only rarely is cemented long stem revision considered. This can be useful in very osteopenic bone with a capacious canal[129] or in elderly patients with limited life expectancy and who are unable to undergo prolonged protected weight bearing or extensive procedures.[48] If the fracture is anatomically reduced and fixed with cerclage cables and if the cement not vigorously pressurized, cement extravasation will not typically occur. After cementation, intraoperative radiographs are recommended to determine if any problematic cement extravasation has occurred. Cement extrusion into the fracture site will impair fracture healing. It should be emphasized that cemented reconstructions are rarely useful in the setting of periprosthetic fractures. The most effective strategies include noncemented distal fixation techniques.

Preoperative radiographic findings can help guide the selection of the appropriate uncemented reconstruction. These include the endosteal diameter and morphology of the distal fragment. If the distal fragment demonstrates parallel endosteal cortices with 5 cm or more of tubular diaphysis (usually with a diameter of less than 18 mm), then an extensively coated uncemented long stem prosthesis with or without lateral plate augmentation is appropriate (Fig. 23-7B). The distal canal is reamed and a trial stem is potted into the distal fragment. The proximal fragments can then be reduced using the trial implant as a template. Cerclage cables are applied and a trial reduction is performed. Once leg length and stability are acceptable, the trial is removed and the femoral component is impacted. The cerclage cables are then retensioned, crimped, and cut. The appropriate femoral head length is selected and the reconstruction completed. These types of stems have demonstrated

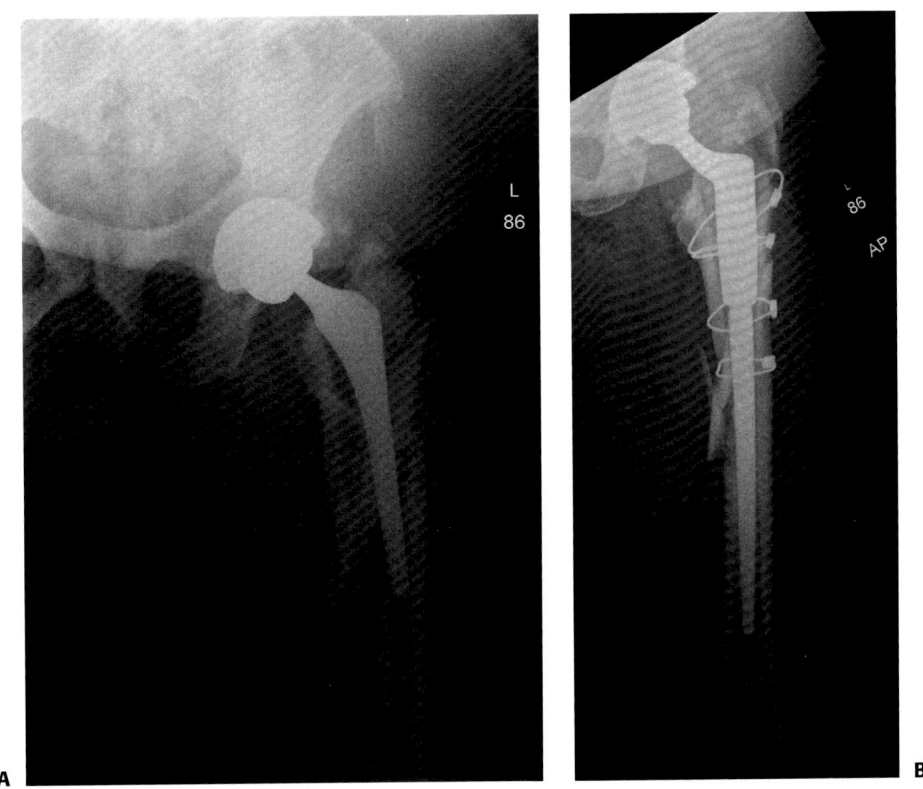

A   B

FIGURE 23-13 A highly comminuted fracture about a loose femoral stem (Vancouver Type B2) **(A)** is managed with a long stem modular prosthesis **(B)**. (Courtesy of Hari Parvataneni, MD.)

excellent long-term survivorship in the revision setting and for periprosthetic fracture situations.[140,160,195,206] Union occurs reliably and functional outcome is, as expected for complex revision arthroplasty, modest. At a mean follow-up of 10.8 years, 17 of 22 patients treated with an extensively porous-coated implant had a satisfactory functional result with delayed union occurring in only one.[206] Concomitant acetabular revision was required in 19 patients. Another similarly treated group of 24 patients had an average Harris Hip Score of 69 with 91% of fractures uniting uneventfully.[195]

If the distal diaphysis demonstrates divergent endosteal morphology, or large diameters (typically over 18 mm), fluted titanium-tapered modular stems can be used effectively. These stems are commercially available in diameters up to 30 mm and can be useful in capacious canals. Reaming under fluoroscopic control and "by hand," especially in osteopenic bone, can help to avoid anterior femoral cortical perforation. When axial stability is obtained by diaphyseal reaming, the implant is impacted into place. It is wise to place a prophylactic cable at the mouth of the distal fragment prior to stem impaction. The proximal bodies of the modular implants are then chosen to restore appropriate leg length, offset, and hip stability. In addition, these stems allow flexibility with femoral anteversion which can be useful in enhancing hip stability. After trialing, the components are assembled and the hip reduced. The proximal fragments are then reduced and cerclaged around the body of the implant (Fig. 23-13). The author finds this strategy effective for Vancouver type B2 and even some B3 fractures;

however, concerns remain about the durability of the modular junction of such stems without proximal bony support. Modular, tapered titanium stems have gained popularity in any revision setting but the issue of modular junction failures has not clearly been solved. There have been numerous clinical series in the last few years verifying the utility and clinical success of noncemented fixation especially with modular diaphyseal engaging titanium stem.[77,200,226]

Rarely, the proximal bone is so deficient that either a modular proximal femoral replacement (so called "tumor prosthesis") (Fig. 23-14),[137,303] proximal femoral allograft,[133,178] or impaction grafting with plate fixation[278,280] is appropriate. The former two methods are typically used in very osteopenic bone; therefore, cemented distal fixation is recommended. Preserving a sleeve of remaining proximal bone, albeit deficient, provides some soft tissue attachment and assists in maintaining a stable hip. In addition, maintaining the abductor/vastus sleeve attached to the greater trochanter bone fragment helps to prevent trochanteric escape (Fig. 23-14C). A coronal split (Wagner type) of the proximal bone can facilitate stem removal. The new implant is cemented into the distal fragment, and then the proximal sleeve of remaining bone and soft tissue can be cerclaged around the body of the proximal femoral replacing prosthesis or the proximal femoral allograft/revision stem composite (Fig. 23-15) with cable or heavy braided suture. Results of these extreme revision scenarios are not as good as seen with the less complex revisions associated with type B1 fractures. Patients should be counseled that neither bone

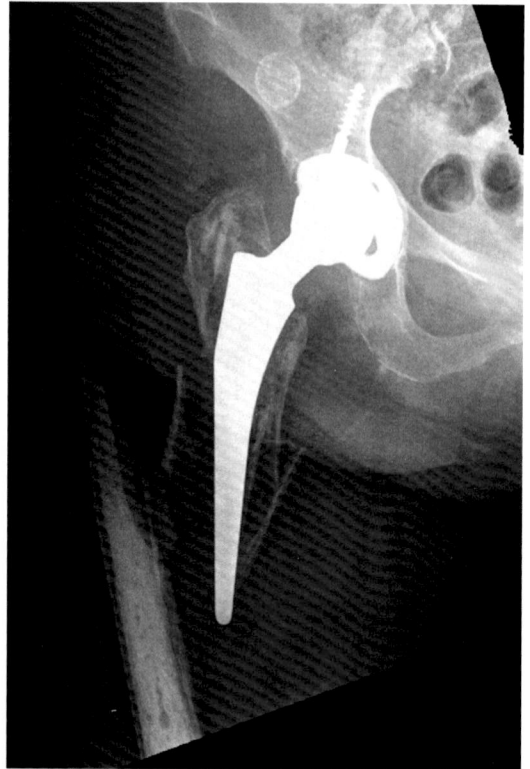

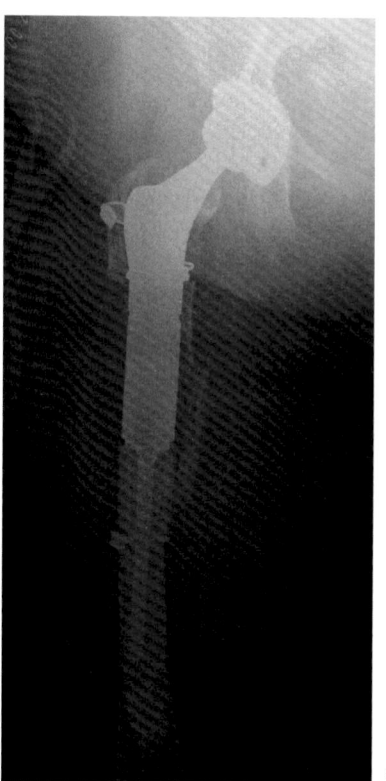

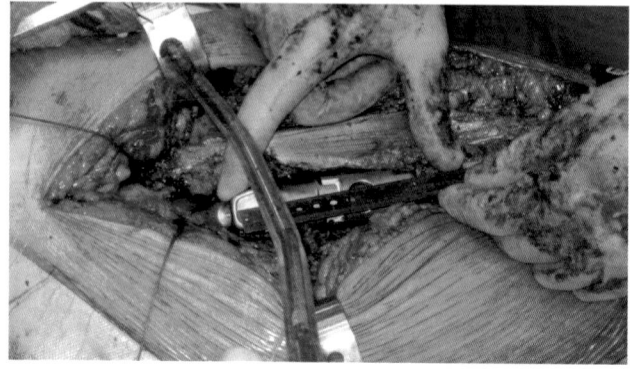

A

C

B

FIGURE 23-14 A fracture associated with a loose prosthesis and bone loss from osteolysis (Vancouver Type B3) **(A)** is treated with a proximal femoral replacement. An intraoperative photograph **(B)** shows sizing of the stem and postoperative radiographs show reattachment of the abductor/vastus lateralis sleeve **(C)**. (Courtesy of Hari Parvataneni, MD).

healing nor function are predictably good, but that both can be satisfactory. Twenty-three of 24 patients treated with such an allograft/implant composite for Vancouver type B3 fractures were able to walk but 15 required a walker.[133,178] Osseous union of the allograft to host femur occurred in 80% and union of the greater trochanter occurred in 68%. At a mean follow-up of 5.1 years, 16% had required a repeat revision. In a series of 21 similar fractures treated with a proximal femoral replacement and followed for 3.2 years, all but one was able to walk.[137] Despite a relatively high complication rate (two wound drainage, two dislocations, one refracture distal to the femoral stem, one acetabular cage failure) the authors concluded this was a viable option for patients with a severe problem. A more recent review of 20 patients undergoing megaprosthesis reconstruction for periprosthetic fracture confirms acceptable results in terms of function and satisfaction at a mean of 48 months but with a high complication rate (six major complications in

20 patients).[182] When impaction grafting technique is chosen, better results have been demonstrated with the use of a long-stem femoral component that bypasses the fracture then with a short stem.[280] It is important to note that if the abductors are deficient then any of these constructs should include a constrained acetabular liner to minimize the risk of postoperative dislocation. If the acetabular component is of sufficient diameter and a compatible constrained liner is not available, some surgeons have recommended cementing a constrained liner into a well-fixed acetabular component. Good containment of the locked liner by the acetabular component is required, and cup position should be acceptable. Contouring the backside of the liner to be cemented is recommended (if it is smooth) to allow cement interdigitation.

When postoperative fractures occur around loose implants, revision strategies should rely on diaphyseal, not proximal fixation. The diameter, geometry, and bone quality of the

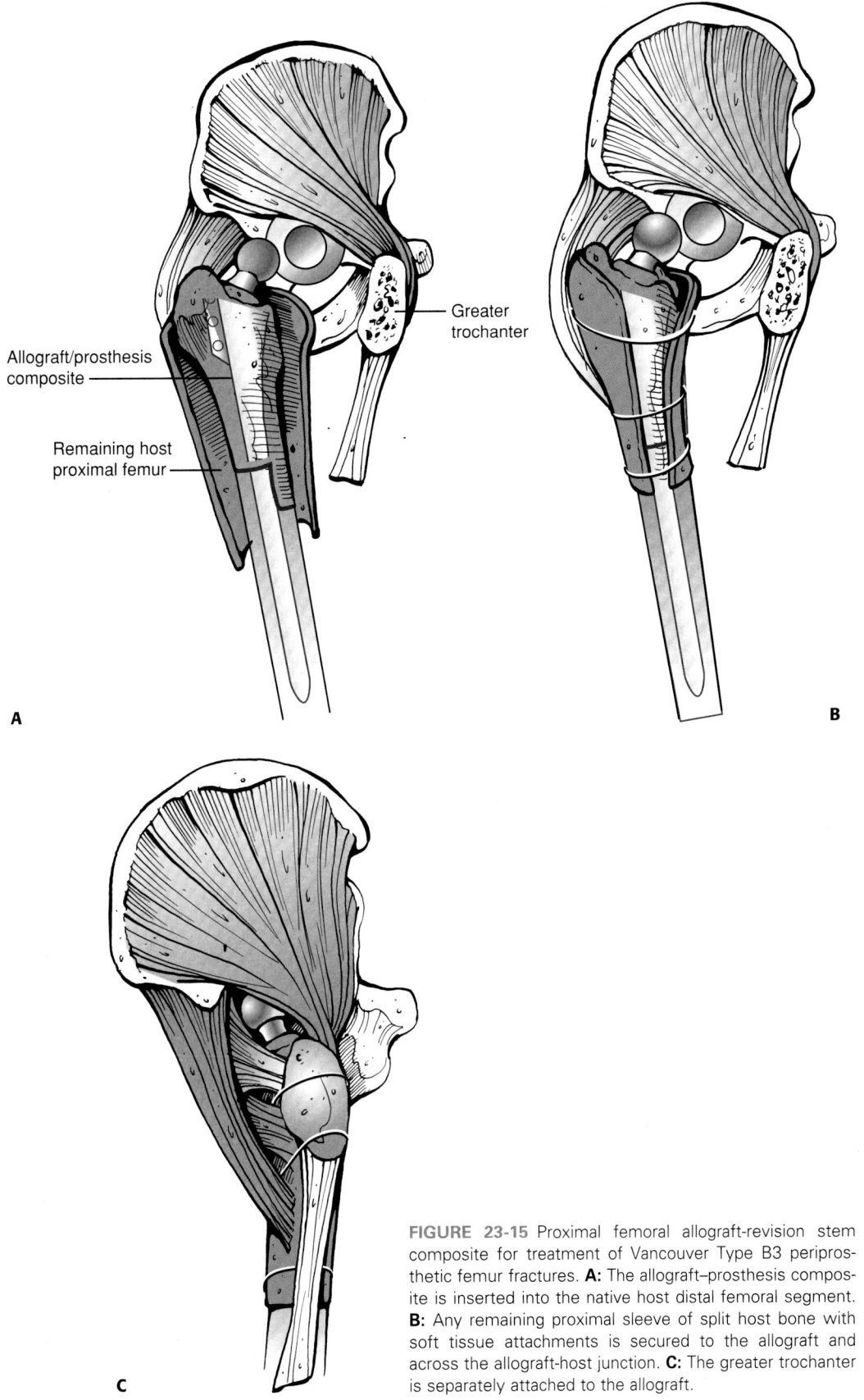

Allograft/prosthesis
composite

Greater
trochanter

Remaining host
proximal femur

A

B

C

FIGURE 23-15 Proximal femoral allograft-revision stem composite for treatment of Vancouver Type B3 periprosthetic femur fractures. **A:** The allograft–prosthesis composite is inserted into the native host distal femoral segment. **B:** Any remaining proximal sleeve of split host bone with soft tissue attachments is secured to the allograft and across the allograft-host junction. **C:** The greater trochanter is separately attached to the allograft.

diaphyseal bone will determine whether an extensively coated cylindrical stem or a tapered modular stem is appropriate. Extensively coated cylindrical stems are appropriate in smaller canals (<18 mm), simple fracture patterns, and in situations where 5 cm of parallel diaphyseal endosteum is available for fixation. This situation is rare, therefore we generally prefer to osteotomize the proximal femur, utilizing existing fracture lines, if possible, for direct access to the diaphysis, and then obtain distal fixation with a tapered modular stem. Modular trials are used to restore leg length and hip stability. After the assembly of the implant, the proximal fragments are stabilized with cerclage, typically utilizing cables, using the intramedullary stem as an "endoskeleton." Rarely, the proximal bone is so deficient that proximal femoral replacement with a modular megaprosthesis is necessary. An effort should be made to preserve the proximal femoral muscular attachments. We prefer to "wrap" any residual bony fragments around the megaprosthesis with cerclage in an attempt to improve construct stability. Obviously, if there are any acetabular component issues, they can be addressed simultaneously, either with modular liner exchange or cup revision as indicated.

Postoperative Care for Revision Arthroplasty of Periprosthetic Femoral Fractures

Weight-bearing status will depend on the quality of the bone and fixation. Typically, protected weight bearing is recommended for 6 weeks to 3 months to allow early bony incorporation of the implants. Special precautions should be emphasized for dislocation which is much more likely with complex revision surgery and if the greater trochanter is repaired. Trochanteric precautions (protected weight bearing and minimal active abduction) may be indicated if there is a high chance of trochanteric escape. Close attention should be given to wound issues or persistent drainage. Regularly scheduled radiographs will guide activity advancement and need for further intervention.

Potential Pitfalls and Preventative Measures for Revision Arthroplasty of Periprosthetic Femoral Fractures

Revision hip arthroplasty in the setting of periprosthetic femur fracture requires wide surgical exposure (Table 23-14). Wide draping as well as care that positioners do not inhibit extensile exposure should be taken. A wide array if revision implants may be required and should be confirmed as being available, including multiple lengths and sizes. Occasionally, a worn or cracked acetabular liner or a loose acetabular component is unexpectedly encountered. Therefore, implants and equipment for acetabular revision should also be confirmed as available.

Implantation of a long femoral stem across a femoral shaft fracture can generate substantial stress on the bone. This establishes a risk of fracture propagation. Preparation of the canal with flexible reamers can accommodate for the normal femoral bow. With meticulous preparation of the canal, careful selection of the appropriate size prosthesis, and with meticulous insertion technique, iatrogenic fracture risk can be minimized. As with any revision hip arthroplasty, stability of the hip joint is a potential issue. Proper anteversion, adequate soft tissue tension, larger head size, and an elevated liner each can improve stability. A constrained liner should be available if hip stability cannot be accomplished with standard means.

TABLE 23-14 | **Revision Arthroplasty for Periprosthetic Femoral Shaft Fractures**

Potential Pitfalls and Preventions

Pitfalls	Preventions
Inadequate surgical field	Drape and prep widely (above iliac crest to below knee)
	Ensure pelvic positioner does not encroach on the field anteriorly or posteriorly
	Use an extensile incision that allows access to the entire femur and much of the pelvis
Limited implant options	Preoperative planning for selection of acetabular socket, liner, femoral fixation, and bone graft options
	Pay special attention to large femurs requiring outlier sizes, bowed femurs, small sockets that will not allow many options for hip stability, constrained liners if the abductors are dysfunctional, trochanteric fixation options, and "backup implants" such as a megaprosthesis
Propagation of the fracture distally	Meticulous bone preparation with trialing prior to stem insertion. If the stem is not advancing, reprepare the femur. Cerclage wire (s) at the mouth of the diaphysis just distal to the fracture
	For bowed stems, flexible reamers are needed and often require variable over reaming
Inadequate hip stability	Pay attention to combined anteversion, status of abductors, and soft tissue tension. Increase head size if possible. Have lipped and lateralized liners available. Constrained liners must be available if there are deficient abductors or instability that cannot be solved with other options

Outcomes of Periprosthetic Femur Fractures

Outcomes of Vancouver A Periprosthetic Femur Fractures

Among Vancouver types A, B, and C periprosthetic fractures, only type A fractures are treated nonoperatively with any regularity. In a series of 30 Vancouver type A fractures treated nonoperatively, 90% had displacement of 2.5 cm or less.[221] A combination of superior and medial displacement was typically observed and only three patients (10%) had a secondary increase in displacement. Functional outcomes were marginal with 12 patients (40%) experiencing pain or limp. However, only three had symptoms persistent and severe enough to warrant operative repair. Two of these three experienced improvement. No dislocations occurred in this series; however, in another small series of six patients treated nonoperatively for a Vancouver type A fracture, two had subsequent dislocation within 2 months.[112] Minimally displaced postoperative fractures occurring through osteolytic lesions 4 to 11 years after THA treated nonoperatively yielded union in 15 of 17 patients.[120] At a mean follow-up of 3 years after fracture 16 had revision THA, the majority for excessive wear and component loosening.

There is very little in the way of published modern series of acute Vancouver type A_G fractures to guide treatment and establish expected outcomes. Much of the available information includes or is exclusively related to treatment of greater trochanteric osteotomies or nonunions.[96,163,165,166] In a recent series of 31 cases of claw plate fixation of the greater trochanter, only eight were for acute fracture.[166] Results for these patients were not distinguished. Overall, union occurred in 28 of 31 patients with three having fibrous union of the trochanter. Other complications included painful bursitis requiring plate removal in three patients and deep infection in one. In the setting of greater trochanteric nonunion, adjunctive vertically oriented wires have resulted in better osseous contact and union.[290]

Outcomes of Internal Fixation of Vancouver Types B and C Periprosthetic Femur Fractures

The results of traditional nonlocked plate and screw fixation for periprosthetic femoral shaft fractures using now outdated direct reduction techniques have been varied.[30,53,76,87,186,190,192,268,276,285,308,312] Failure of traditional cable-plate constructs with cable fixation in zone of intramedullary implant and nonlocked screws distally is likely related, at least in part, to older direct reduction techniques and not necessarily to an inappropriate construct (Fig. 23-16). Soft tissue stripping associated with direct reduction can delay healing which eventually manifests as implant failure. The addition of strut grafts 90 degrees to a lateral plate offers increased immediate as well as prolonged construct stability (Fig. 23-17) and has been associated with good results.[98,286] In a report on 40 patients, Haddad et al.[98] concluded that cortical allografts should be used routinely to augment fixation and healing of periprosthetic femoral fracture around well-fixed implants. Treatment methods varied in this study and included cortical onlay strut allograft alone, a plate and one cortical strut, or a plate and two struts. The nonstandardized use of other adjuvant bone grafting materials in this study further increased the heterogeneity of the treatment methods: eight patients received autograft, 29 received

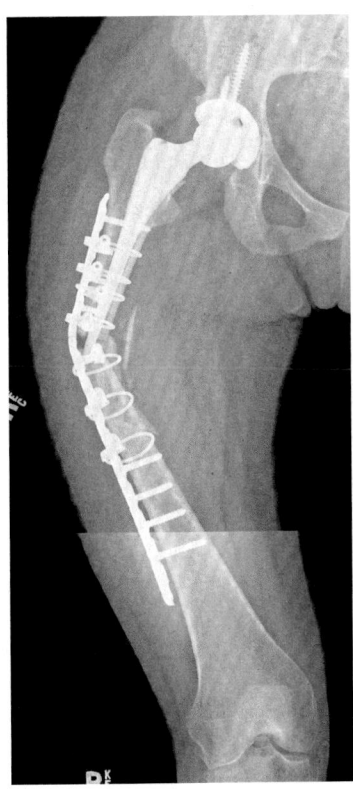
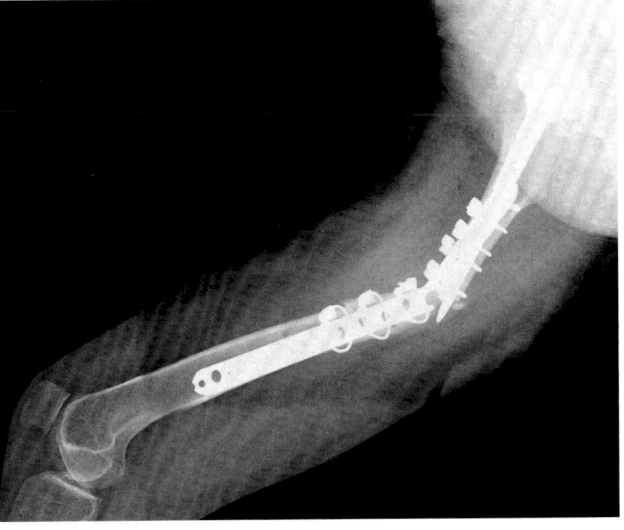

FIGURE 23-16 High failure rates have been associated with lateral plate fixation when older, direct, nonbiologically friendly reduction techniques are utilized **(A, B)**.

A

B

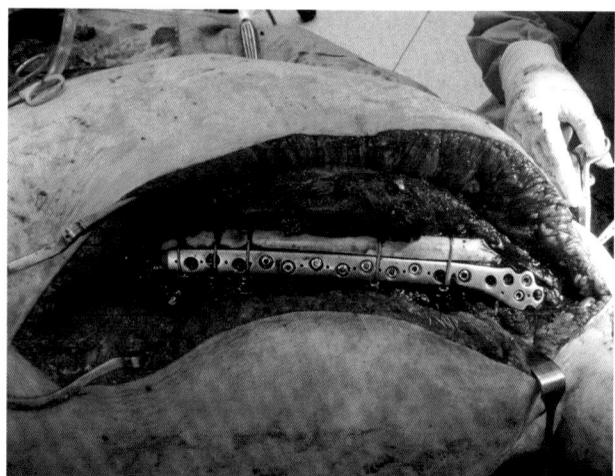

FIGURE 23-17 An intraoperative clinical photograph showing lateral plate fixation augmented with an anterior femoral strut allograft.

morselized allograft, and 15 received demineralized bone matrix. Based on 100% healing, it is logical to conclude that the use of strut allografts plus adjuvant bone graft and/or lateral plate fixation can achieve good results. However, it may be overstated to conclude that allograft is a requirement for treatment of Vancouver B1 fractures.

Newer biologic plating techniques that maximally preserve the soft tissue attachments about a fracture have been shown to be successful without adjuvant bone grafting for fractures in other anatomic areas that traditionally were treated with adjuvant bone grafts. Abhaykumar and Elliott[2] and Ricci et al.[227] were among the first to apply biologic plating techniques to periprosthetic femoral shaft fractures. Neither indirect fracture reduction and a single, laterally applied, plate without the use of structural allograft nor any other substitute was uniformly utilized in the series of Ricci et al.[227] Union occurred after the index procedure in all of the 41 patients who lived beyond the perioperative period. The average time required for healing was relatively short, 11 weeks, and was very homogenous with the standard deviation being only ±4 weeks. All patients healed in satisfactory alignment (less than 5 degrees of malalignment). Although minor implant-related complications such as cable fracture occurred in three patients, this did not appear to complicate the healing process. Each of these three fractures healed at between 10 and 12 weeks in satisfactory alignment and without the need for further operation. The consistent healing was attributed to care in preserving the soft tissue envelope around the fracture. Xue et al.[300] and Anakwe et al.[6] had very similar results in smaller series, 12 and 11 cases, respectively treated in nearly the identical manner: single lateral plate, screw fixation distally, screw and cerclage fixation proximally, and without the use of adjuvant bone grafts. All patients from both studies healed after the index procedure, with one patient having a delayed union and one with proximal screw loosening in Xue's series. These results compare favorably to treatment of similar fractures using cortical onlay grafts alone,[38,39,98,294] where nonunion requiring revision surgery has been reported in 8% to 10% of cases[38,39,294] and where angular malunion has been reported to occur in 5% to 10% of cases.[38,98]

The reason for the higher malunion rate seen when allograft strut fixation is used alone may be because these struts cannot be bent or contoured as can plates. Fracture alignment, therefore, cannot be adjusted with struts as precisely as with the use of plates. Good clinical results of isolated locked compression plating technique, without the use of cables, has been reported in small series of patients (10 to 13), all who accomplished union after the index procedure.[28,66] It is important to recognize that in these series all patients had bicortical fixation in the proximal fragment including bicortical locking screws anterior or posterior to the prosthesis, bicortical fixation into the lesser trochanter, or bicortical fixation into the greater trochanter, or some combination of these methods. Constructs relying on unicortical fixation, without any bicortical fixation, have poor rotational control and are not recommended. Other recent series of ORIF for Vancouver types B and C fractures utilizing plates have not shown universally good results. Plating with the less invasive stabilization system (LISS) for 19 patients yielded two delayed unions and four implant-related complications each requiring revision ORIF.[196] Another small study of 10 patients treated with ORIF reported surgery-related complication in 62.5% of cases.[151]

A host of biomechanical studies exist to define the characteristics of various plate constructs used for Vancouver type B fractures.[29,59,60,84,269,306] The so-called Ogden-type construct (Fig. 23-18), cables proximally and standard nonlocked screws distally, is the typical control construct in these biomechanical studies. Prior to the advent of locking plates, cortical allograft struts either in place of or in addition to the Ogden concept were the focus of testing.[60,59] More recently, the use of proximal

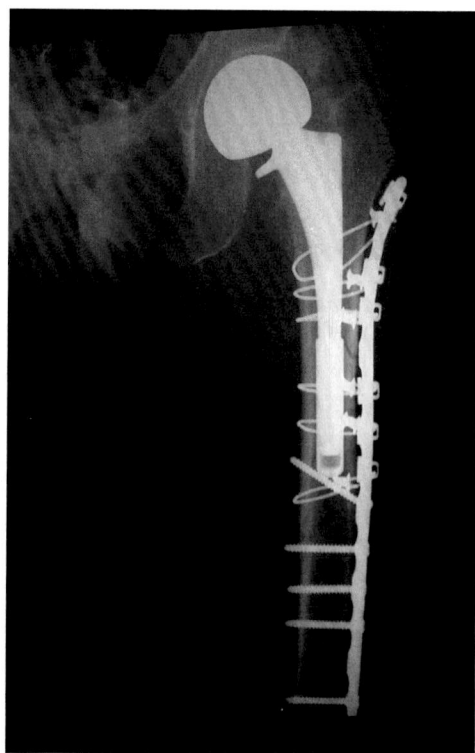

FIGURE 23-18 AP view of the traditional Ogden type construct with cable fixation proximally and nonlocked screw fixation distally.

unicortical locking screws either in lieu of or in addition to cables has been investigated.[84,269,306] In each of these studies, the stiffness of various experimental constructs was greater than the Ogden construct but fatigue characteristics were not investigated in the majority of studies, limiting the clinical applicability of these investigations.[59,60,84,306] The recent clinical series utilizing modern biologic plating techniques have shown good results with slight modification of the Ogden construct. Addition of locked screws in the proximal segment to augment (but not replace) cables and bicortical locked screws in the distal segment to augment nonlocked screws in the presence of osteoporotic bone has been reported with good results (Figs 23-18 and 23-19).[2,227] Unicortical locked screws alone, without cables or bicortical screws around the prosthesis, have not been shown to provide adequate fixation for these fractures. This is primarily because of the poor rotational stability of such short unicortical screws. Therefore, locked screws should be used as an adjunct to, but not as a substitute for, cable fixation in the zone of the hip prosthesis. A biomechanical study attempting to evaluate the effect of unicortical and bicortical screws on the cement mantle provided mixed results: unicortical screws induced few cracks but had less holding power than bicortical screws.[128] Any clinical long-term detrimental effect of unicortical or bicortical screws inserted into a cement mantle remains unknown.

The specific type of plate utilized for fixation of periprosthetic femoral shaft fractures is probably less important than the technique utilized for its implantation. A number of designs that employ various mechanisms for attachment of cables through or around the plate are available. However, good results have been achieved with standard plates.[2,98,227,228] A plate that is bowed in the sagittal plane to match the anterior femoral bow makes sense to assist in obtaining an anatomic reduction in this plane (Fig. 23-19).

The subsidence of stems after wiring of minimally displaced intraoperative fractures was evaluated in a series of 38 patients all with the same short-stemmed prosthesis and compared to a control group without a fracture.[307] There was no significant migration at an average 5.7 years of the stems in the study group compared to the control group. Also, the frequency of radiolucent lines was not different between the study and control groups.

Outcomes of Revision Arthroplasty for Vancouver Types B and C Periprosthetic Femur Fractures

The overall functional outcome based on the Oxford Hip Score (OHS) for revision arthroplasty in the setting of periprosthetic fracture has been found, in a large comparative analysis (n = 232 revisions for fracture), to be worse than when revision is

for aseptic loosening.[302] Further, this study demonstrated an eightfold higher mortality rate (7.3%) seen in the periprosthetic fracture patients. These data are consistent with the high mortality rates (11%) seen in patients treated with ORIF for periprosthetic femur fractures[269] and together paint a sobering picture of the seriousness of these injuries. Langenhan et al.,[149] because of high mortality rates after ORIF, altered their treatment protocol in 2001 and began performing stem replacement with a distally locked modular prosthesis nail for the majority of periprosthetic femur fractures, Vancouver B and C, regardless of stem stability. This strategy permitted immediate full weight bearing and therefore improved mobility compared to patients treated with ORIF and protected weight bearing. The authors attribute the decrease in mortality to the improved mobility seen in their group of 29 patients who underwent revision arthroplasty (10 died at final follow-up and three died early) compared to the 23 patients treated with ORIF (21 died at final follow-up and seven died early). Subgroup analysis of patients with Vancouver B1 fractures showed no significant difference in 6-month mortality between groups, but this analysis was likely underpowered. Another retrospective study comparing ORIF to revision arthroplasty for Vancouver B and C fractures failed to show differences in systemic complications between groups.[151] This study did, however, reveal more surgery-related complications in the ORIF group (62.5% vs. 18.8%).

Results after revision THA associated with periprosthetic femur fractures appear to be inferior to those for revision for aseptic loosening. Data from the New Zealand National Registry showed functional outcomes based on the Oxford Hip Score (OHS) to be worse following revision THA for periprosthetic fracture than in reference patients (mean OHS: 29 vs. 24).[302] Also, there was a higher likelihood of revision (7.3% vs. 2.6%) and higher 6-month mortality (7.3% vs. 0.9%).Reoperation in 7 of 25 patients with Vancouver B2 and B3 fractures treated with revision alone or revision + ORIF was reported.[312]

Outcomes of Fractures About Femoral Resurfacing Prostheses

Cossey et al.[50] reported on seven patients with nondisplaced femoral neck fractures associated with the Birmingham hip resurfacing procedure that were treated nonoperatively. All fractures occurred within 4 months of surgery and all were treated with non–weight-bearing. At a minimum of 16 months post fracture, all fractures were united and all patients were without impaired function. One patient was noted to have marked femoral neck narrowing that appeared asymptomatic. Jacobs et al.[123] described 13 patients treated nonoperatively for

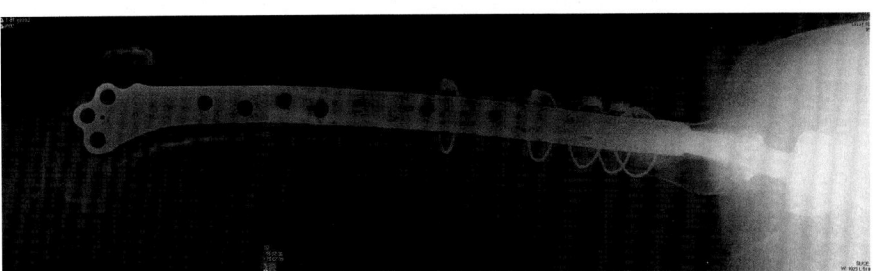

FIGURE 23-19 Fixation of midshaft femur fractures with a bowed plate helps preserve anatomic alignment in the sagittal plane.

femoral neck fracture after hip resurfacing. All healed with nonoperative management; however, four healed in varus. No follow-up beyond fracture healing was presented, so the consequence of varus union in this population remains unknown. Nonoperative management for nondisplaced fractures and revision to THA for displaced fractures was advocated.

AUTHOR'S PREFERRED TREATMENT OF PERIPROSTHETIC FEMUR FRACTURES ABOUT HIP ARTHROPLASTY STEMS

We find the Vancouver classification very useful in determining treatment for periprosthetic femoral shaft fractures (Fig. 23-20). Nondisplaced Vancouver A fractures are generally treated nonoperatively with protected weight bearing based on comfort unless the fracture is noticed intraoperatively. In such cases, we have a lower threshold for cable or claw plate fixation. Widely displaced Vancouver A fractures are generally treated with ORIF with a claw plate and cables.

Vancouver B1 fractures are usually treated with ORIF via a lateral approach. These fractures are typically simple spiral patterns and we prefer to use cables to help obtain and maintain a provisional reduction. Fixation is with a lateral locked plate which is secured proximately with cables and then with locked screws into the trochanteric region. Distal fixation is with a combination of nonlocked and locked screws depending upon the bone quality. Lag screws are placed across the fracture through the plate whenever feasible. We prefer to protect the entire length of the femur and therefore select a plate that extends at

least to the distal metaphyseal flare and we usually utilize a distal femoral locking plate. Comminuted fractures are treated similarly except a bridge plating technique is utilized. We neither generally utilize any bone grafts for Vancouver B1 fractures nor do we perform revision arthroplasty for well-fixed stems.

By definition, Vancouver B2 fractures have a loose stem and therefore our treatment incorporates revision of the femoral component. However, in select cases when the patient's functional demands are severely limited, and when the patient had no preoperative symptoms associated with the loose prosthesis, we may forgo revision arthroplasty especially if the patient has substantial cardiopulmonary comorbid disease that increases the risk of intraoperative or postoperative medical complications. In most cases, we perform revision arthroplasty with bowed noncemented stems across the fracture. We also generally supplements revision arthroplasty with a long lateral plate that protects the entire femur from future fracture. If there are bone defects, these are managed with structural allograft in addition to the lateral plate.

Vancouver B3 fractures present substantial technical challenges. We highly recommend these fractures be placed in the hands of a surgeon that is well versed with revision hip arthroplasty technique as well as proximal femoral replacement technique. As with other types of periprosthetic femur fractures, we typically protect the entire femur with a lateral plate after revision arthroplasty.

We treat Vancouver C fractures according to the techniques outlined for plate and screw treatment of distal femur fractures. Typically, a lateral lock plate is utilized. We are careful to use plates long enough to overlap the femoral stem such that two cables can be placed that are spaced apart by 3 to 4 cm.

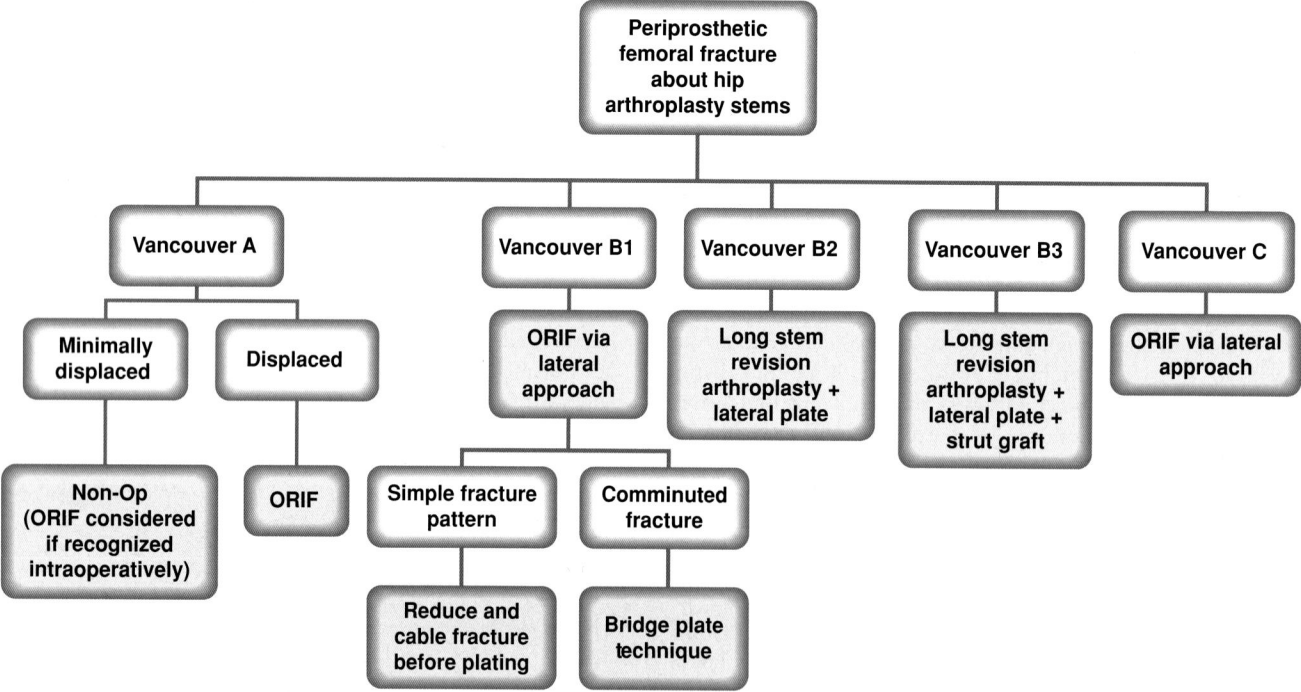

FIGURE 23-20 Algorithm depicting the author's preferred method of treatment for periprosthetic femur fractures about hip arthroplasty stems.

PERIPROSTHETIC DISTAL FEMUR FRACTURES ABOUT TOTAL KNEE ARTHROPLASTY

Incidence, Risk Factors, Prevention, and Mortality for Periprosthetic Distal Femur Fractures

Approximately 300,000 primary knee arthroplasties are performed annually in the United States, and this number continues to increase. It is estimated that 0.3% to 2.5% of patients will sustain a periprosthetic fracture as a complication of primary TKA.[11,56,184,190] The prevalence of these fractures is substantially higher (1.7% to 38%) after revision TKA.[184,209] Patient-specific risk factors such as RA, osteolysis, osteopenic bone, use of steroid medications, frequent falls common in the elderly population, and technique-specific risk factors such as anterior femoral cortical notching have all been implicated as potential causes of periprosthetic fractures. In a large population-based study from Scotland that included 44,511 primary and 3,222 revision TKAs, female gender, age >70, and revision arthroplasty were associated with risk of fracture.[184] Although tibia fractures about unicompartmental knee arthroplasty has been identified in a number of reports, fractures about the femur in association with unicompartmental knee arthroplasty has rarely been reported.[136]

Intraoperative fracture of the femur during TKA is much less common than femur fracture during THA. It has been reported to occur in 49 cases out of 17,389 primary TKAs.[3] Of the 49 fractures identified in this series, 20 were of the medial condyle, 11 of the lateral condyle, 8 were complete supracondylar fractures, 7 involved the medial epicondyle, 2 the lateral epicondyle, and 1 the posterior cortex. The majority of fractures occurred in females and most occurred during exposure, bone preparation, and component trialing.

Osteopenia, from a multitude of potential causes, is a major contributing factor to periprosthetic fractures in TKA.[1,30,53,186] Bone mineral density (BMD) in the distal femur has been shown to decrease between 19% and 44% 1 year after TKA compared to initial values.[214] Progressive loss in BMD has been reported at 2 years after surgery, possibly from stress shielding in the anterior distal femur. Such reductions in BMD may be an important determinant of periprosthetic fracture.[215] Neurologic disorders have also been implicated as etiologic factors,[53,157] but this too may be primarily related to osteopenia from associated disuse or neuroleptic medications.

Stress fractures in the femur and tibia associated with a sudden increase in activity soon after TKA have been described and may be related to relative disuse osteopenia occurring with extended periods of inactivity prior to TKA.[71] In the femur these stress fractures may occur at any location and may present a diagnostic challenge in a patient that complains of sudden onset of pain without antecedent trauma and without signs of infection.[51,105,148,157,207,224] Repeat plain radiographs a period of weeks after the onset of symptoms may reveal the previously occult stress fracture or a bone scan may be diagnostic earlier. With an index of suspicion, protected weight bearing is prudent until stress fracture is ruled out. When ruled in, protected weight bearing for approximately 6 weeks followed by gradual advancements is usually a successful treatment plan.

With or without associated osteopenia, several local factors may further contribute to the occurrence of periprosthetic fractures above TKAs. Fractures through an osteolytic lesion about TKAs are much less common than their occurrence about femoral hip components, but these certainly may occur.[213] Anterior femoral notching has been implicated as another risk factor for subsequent periprosthetic supracondylar femur fracture. Biomechanical evaluations, including cadaveric studies and finite element models, implicate anterior notching as a risk factor for periprosthetic fracture.[156,304] When loaded in bending, notched femora failed with a short oblique fracture originating at the cortical defect whereas unnotched femora sustained a midshaft fracture. No difference in failure mode was noted with loading in torsion. The force to failure was significantly less for notched femora than unnotched, 18% less in bending and 39% less than torsion. Finite element analysis has also yielded results that indicate notching reduces the fracture threshold.[304] Larger notches, sharper notches, and proximity to the prosthesis each lead to increased local stresses. Despite common sense and laboratory investigations indicating notching as a risk factor for periprosthetic supracondylar femur fractures, clinical data remains unconvincing. The lack of statistical association between notching and fracture may be because of underpowered studies and extremely small numbers of observed fractures. Lesh et al.[156] reviewed 164 supracondylar periprosthetic femur fractures reported in the literature and noted more than 30% were associated with notching. Many of these patients, however, were noted to have other risk factors for fracture. Three separate large retrospective studies (>200 patients) failed to find an association between notching and fracture.[97,234,235] However, with very few fractures (three or less) in each of these cohorts, statistical power is lacking in each to rule out an association between notching and fracture. Other studies, however, suggest notching may predispose to subsequent fracture. Aaron and Scott[1] found that 42% of patients with excessive notching suffered fracture, whereas none of those without encroachment of the anterior cortex fractured. A study that included a cohort of patients with supracondylar fractures, but without a denominator indicating how many patients without fracture did and did not have notching, found a large proportion (up to 25%) of fractures associated with notching.[155] Further supporting the association of notching and fracture are the findings that the time from index arthroplasty to fracture was 37.5 months in patients with notching compared to 80.3 months in those without and that the distance from the anterior flange of the femoral component to the fracture was significantly shorter in patients with notching (3.6 mm) than in patients without notching (39 mm).[155] It has also been postulated that bone remodeling around notched areas may reduce risk of fracture[97] and that notching is of minimal concern beyond the early postoperative period.[235] However, the rate of periprosthetic distal femur fracture has been shown to increase with the number of years after both primary and revision TKA.[184]

Prosthetic designs with a posterior stabilized femoral component that removes bone from the intercondylar region has been noted to increase risk for intraoperative fracture.[238] Fracture, typically of the medial femoral condyle, is more likely to occur if the component is not centered between the condyles. A relatively new potential risk factor has been described in a case report of periprosthetic supracondylar femur fractures through a navigation pin hole.[162] With the increasing popularity of surgical navigation for TKA, this potential complication should be considered when choosing a location for navigation instruments. Another new technology, saline-cooled bipolar radiofrequency, used on the synovium overlying the femoral condyles for hemostasis has been implicated in periprosthetic femoral condyle fractures after TKA.[201] Four such fractures occurred shortly after increasing usage of this technology whereas the senior author had no fractures of this kind in 2,500 prior TKAs. It was hypothesized that thermal damage to the bone caused by saline-cooled bipolar radiofrequency reduced the mechanical integrity and predisposed to fracture.

It is well established that geriatric patients who sustain hip fractures have high mortality rates at any time point relative to their fracture. The combination of stress associated with fracture and treatment, and the comorbid medical conditions commonly present in this population are attributed to the high mortality rates seen. These conditions are also seen in patients with periprosthetic distal femur fractures. It is therefore not surprising that patients with distal femur fractures were found to have high mortality rates (6% at 30 days, 18% at 6 months, 25% at 1 year) that were similar to hip fracture patients.[265] Furthermore, in this study, TKA was found to be an independent risk factor for decreased survival.

Classification of Periprosthetic Distal Femur Fractures

The Lewis and Rorabeck classification scheme for periprosthetic femur fractures about TKAs accounts for fracture displacement and prosthesis stability (Fig. 23-21).[161,237] Type I are stable, essentially nondisplaced, fractures and the bone–prosthesis

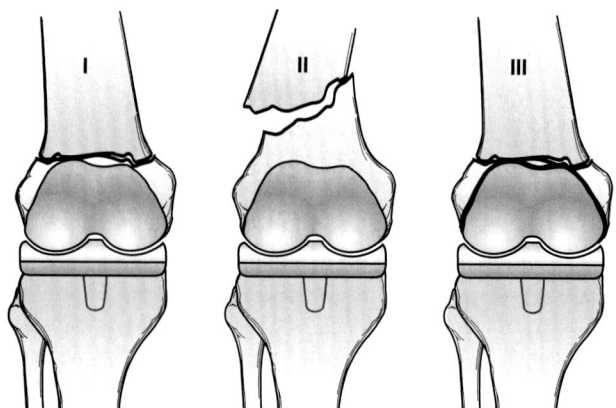

FIGURE 23-21 Classification scheme for periprosthetic fractures about the femoral component of the knee. Type I fractures are minimally displaced with an intact prosthesis–bone interface; Type II fractures are displaced but maintain an intact bone–prosthesis interface; and Type III fractures may be displaced or nondisplaced, but have a loose femoral component. (Modified from: Lewis PL, Rorabeck CH. Periprosthetic fractures. In: Engh GA, Roabeck CH, eds. *Revision Total Knee Arthroplasty.* Baltimore, MD: Williams & Wilkins; 1997: 275–295).

interface remains intact. Type II fractures are displaced with a well-fixed prosthesis. Type III fractures have a loose or failing prosthesis regardless of the fracture displacement.

This classification does not account for the fracture location relative to the prosthesis, a factor that has the potential to dictate treatment. The classification scheme of Su et al.[267] divides fractures into three types according to the fracture location relative to the proximal border of the femoral component: Type I fractures are proximal to the femoral component; type II originate at the proximal end of the component and extend proximally; and type III extend distal to the proximal border of the femoral component (Fig. 23-22).

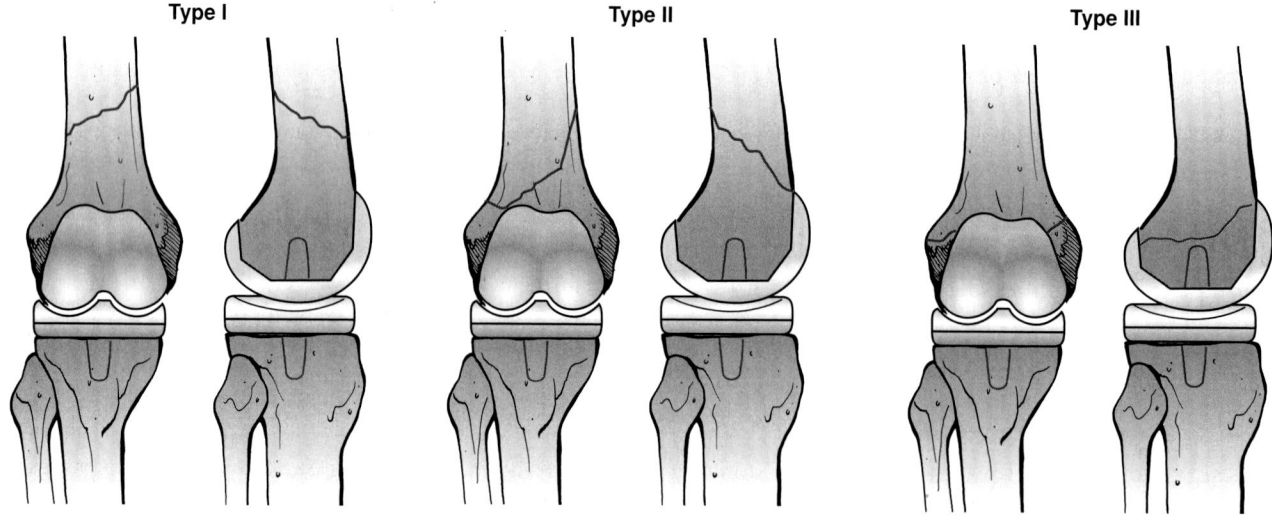

FIGURE 23-22 The Su classification of periprosthetic distal femur fractures accounts for location of the fracture relative to the femoral TKA component.

Nonoperative Management of Periprosthetic Distal Femur Fractures

Nonoperative treatment of periprosthetic supracondylar femur fractures is reserved for nondisplaced fractures or for displaced fractures where patient-based results of nonoperative treatment would be at least as good as operative treatment. For displaced fractures, nonoperative treatment is indicated for nonambulatory patients or those patients who are not likely to survive surgery because of medical comorbidities.

Nondisplaced fractures can be treated nonoperatively with skeletal traction, splints, casts, and braces or a combination of these methods. Initial treatment, especially if the limb is substantially swollen, is typically with a long leg splint. Once the soft tissue swelling has subsided and the patient has regained reasonable comfort, a long leg brace, such as a knee immobilizer or an unlocked hinged knee brace can be utilized. As with other nondisplaced fractures treated nonoperatively, it is prudent to monitor for secondary displacement with frequent, usually weekly or biweekly, radiographs. Any secondary displacement noted early in the treatment course (e.g., the first 2 weeks) is a relative indication for operative intervention as such early displacement is typically followed by progressive later displacement.

Outcomes of Nonoperative Treatment for Periprosthetic Distal Femur Fractures

Related to improvements in operative techniques and implants, the vast majority of these fractures are treated operatively, especially displaced fractures. Accordingly, very little attention has been paid to nonoperative management outcomes of periprosthetic supracondylar femur fractures over the last three decades. Only one case focusing on nonoperative treatment could be identified in the last 25 years.[258] The poor results, especially malalignment, associated with nonoperative treatment for displaced supracondylar femur fractures was one of the driving forces toward operative management.[30,53,76,87,186,192] For example, in the study of Moran et al.,[192] eight of nine displaced fractures treated closed resulted in malunion.

Principles for Operative Treatment of Periprosthetic Distal Femur Fractures

Most displaced periprosthetic distal femur fractures are treated operatively. Only in special circumstances are such displaced fractures treated nonoperatively. When comorbid medical issues make survival of operative treatment questionable, these risks must be weighed against the likely poor outcome of nonoperative management. Nonambulatory patients can be successfully treated nonoperatively; however, even in this circumstance there are potential benefits to operative management. Internal fixation improves patient comfort, facilitates mobilization, and improves ease of care.

Operative treatment of patients with supracondylar femur fractures associated with TKA prostheses presents unique challenges. The presence of a TKA prosthesis can complicate operative treatment of these fractures by interfering with or precluding the use of standard fixation methods. A TKA prosthesis with a narrow or closed intracondylar space either limits the diameter for a retrograde nail or completely obviates its use.[172] Traditional nonlocked plate fixation is prone to varus collapse.[56] Fixed-angle implants such as blade plates or condylar screws have limited applicability for very distal fractures or when associated with a TKA prosthesis that has a deep intracondylar box, but may be used successfully when adequate bone above the femoral prosthesis is available.[139] These challenges induce the application of alternative methods. Although varying degrees of success have been reported with such alternative methods including thin-wire external fixation,[15] the so-called "nailed cementoplasty,"[19] fibular allograft supplementation of plate fixation,[145] and upside down use of a proximal femoral nail,[219] locked plating has become the treatment method of choice for many surgeons as this device offers many theoretic advantages. The multiple locked distal screws provide both a fixed angle to prevent varus collapse and the ability to address distal fractures[264] even when associated with a deep intracondylar box. The provision for locked screw insertion into the diaphyseal fragment theoretically improves fixation in the often associated osteoporotic bone. These devices can also be inserted with relative ease and familiarity.

The results of locked plate fixation for treatment of periprosthetic supracondylar femur fractures above a TKA have been investigated by numerous authors with the initial enthusiasm being tempered by an inability to obtain consistently high union rates.[113,220,228,230,272] Intramedullary nailing represents another viable and efficacious option for these fractures.[4,91,113,292] Whereas locked plate fixation is applicable to nearly all periprosthetic supracondylar fractures, regardless of the prosthesis design and even for extreme distal fractures, IMN is reserved for a subset of these fractures. The associated femoral component must accommodate the diameter of the driving end of a retrograde nail, a diameter that may be larger than the diameter of the nail shaft, and sufficient distal bone is required. Published galleries of radiographic profiles and reference lists that include intercondylar dimensions of various prostheses are helpful to avoid unanticipated problems when documentation of the component type is unavailable.[270] Distal femoral replacement also has a role in certain subsets of patients with periprosthetic distal femur fractures.[142,192,240] This treatment method is gaining in popularity and indications are expanding from primarily those patients with loose TKA prostheses to also include patients with well-fixed and well-functioning prosthesis when the prolonged period of protected weight bearing associated with internal fixation methods is undesirable or impractical.

ORIF of Periprosthetic Distal Femur Fractures

The vast majority of periprosthetic supracondylar femur fractures about a TKA are in the presence of a stable femoral component. Therefore, ORIF can generally be performed in this scenario. Fractures that are distal to the diaphyseal/metaphyseal junction are treated with ORIF with locked plates, even when fracture extension is extremely distal. We have found that locked plating constructs offer satisfactory fixation distally even in these short segments (Fig. 23-23). The important principle

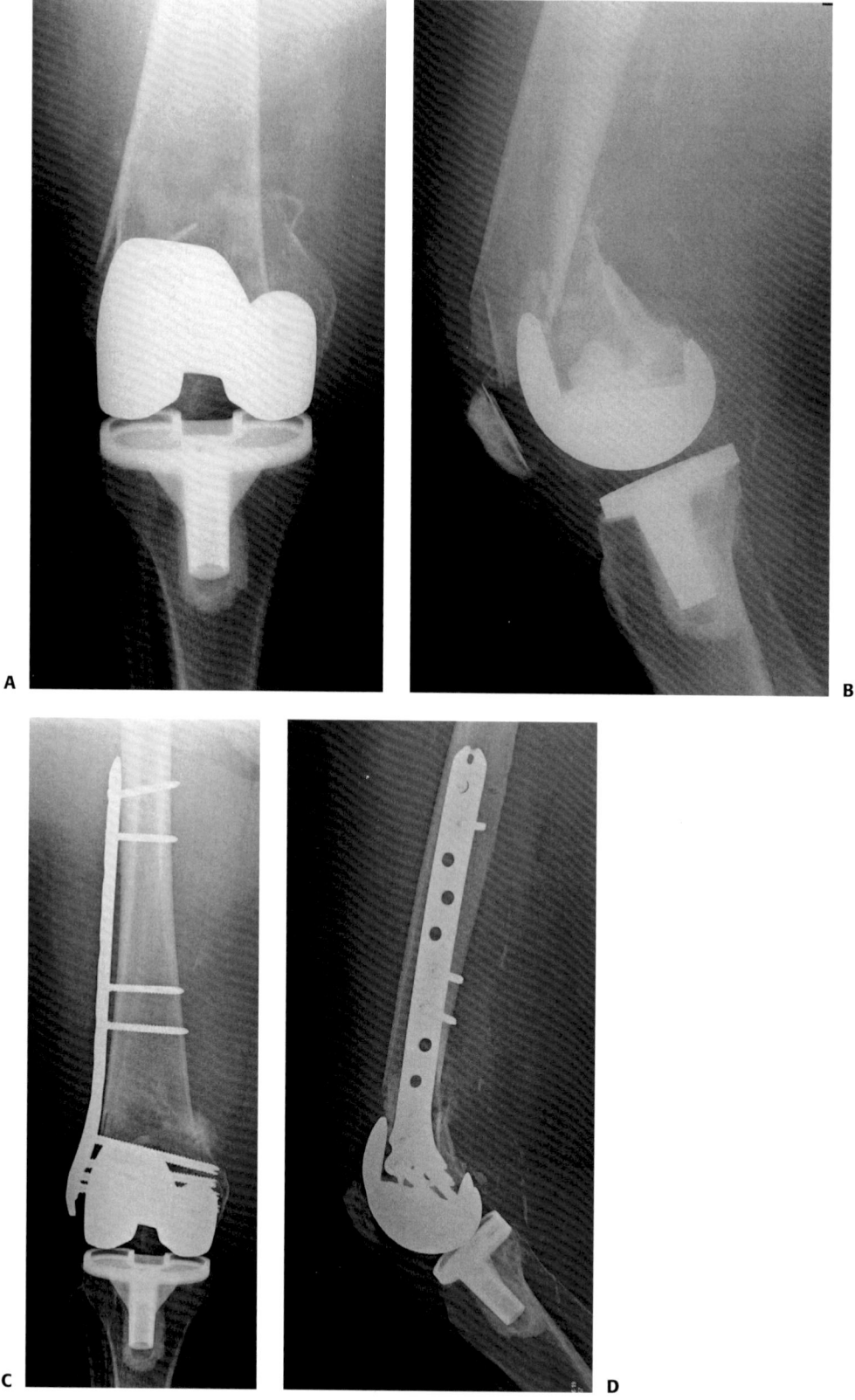

FIGURE 23-23 An extreme distal periprosthetic fracture above a TKA **(A, B)** treated successfully with a distal lateral femoral locking plate **(C, D)**.

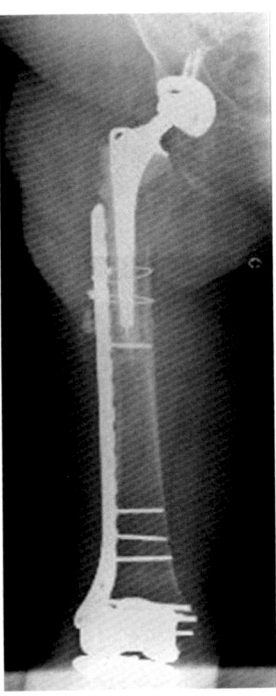

FIGURE 23-24 An interprosthetic fracture located in the distal femur is treated with a long distal lateral femoral locking plate that protects the entire femur by overlapping the hip arthroplasty stem.

for plate fixation of these fractures is the use of biologically friendly, indirect, fracture reduction techniques.

A unique situation that is becoming more and more common is periprosthetic fracture between a TKA and THA, the so-called interprosthetic fracture.[171] These fractures have been found to be in the supracondylar region above the TKA about two times more frequently than in the shaft about the THA stem. Treatment of these interprosthetic fractures should follow the principles of the individual type of fracture encountered and simultaneously protect against future fracture. This situation almost universally lends to plate fixation with a long distal femoral locking plate that spans from the distal femur to overlap with the region of the femoral stem (Fig. 23-24) as described for treatment of Vancouver type C fractures taking into account the issues of distal fixation in the presence of the TKA femoral component discussed in this section.

Preoperative Planning for ORIF of Periprosthetic Distal Femur Fractures

The strategy for ORIF of periprosthetic supracondylar femur fractures starts with consideration of the fracture details to determine the fixation method (Table 23-15). A simple fracture pattern amenable to compression plating techniques will require an anatomic reduction and rigid fixation whereas a comminuted fracture is treated with indirect reduction techniques and bridge plating. This has implications for the required exposure. Anatomic reduction typically requires exposure that spans the fracture site whereas indirect reduction requires only the exposure needed for plate insertion. Potential hindrances to standard screw placement, such as a deep intercondylar box of

TABLE 23-15 **ORIF of Periprosthetic Distal Femur Fractures**

Preoperative Planning Checklist

- OR table: Radiolucent table that allows fluoroscopic imaging of the entire involved femur and knee
- Position/positioning aids: Supine using a radiolucent leg ramp to support and elevate the injured extremity
- Fluoroscopy location: Opposite side from the injured extremity with the monitor at the foot
- Equipment: Large and small fragment sets; distal femoral locking plates long enough to span the proximal fragment with at least eight screw holes; an array of reduction forceps; for interprosthetic fractures, a cable set with two cables (approximately 1.7-mm diameter)
- Tourniquet: A sterile tourniquet may be utilized for distal exposure, reduction, and plate insertion. Proximal fixation may require removal of any tourniquet
- Blood: PRBCs typed and crossmatched

the femoral component or the existence of proximal implants such as a hip arthroplasty stem, a short trochanteric nail, or a plate device are identified and a strategy for overcoming such issues is made. Availability of additional needed equipment, such as cables to attach the plate in the zone of an existing hip arthroplasty stem, is confirmed. Other aspects of the plan are similar regardless of the plating strategy selected.

Positioning for ORIF of Periprosthetic Distal Femur Fractures

The patient is typically positioned supine with the injured extremity pulled over to the edge of the OR table. The selected OR table should allow fluoroscopic imaging of the entire femur, especially if there are any proximal implants to be dealt with. It is helpful, but not essential that the foot of the bed be free of any hindrance to access by surgical personnel. Fracture shortening may be treated with traction applied via an assistant pulling on the limb from the foot of the bed. A bump may be placed under the ipsilateral hip to position the limb in neutral rotation. A radiolucent leg ramp is helpful to elevate the limb such that lateral radiographs are unencumbered by the contralateral leg. The entire leg and hip are prepped and draped free. To keep the entire leg in the surgical field, a sterile rather than unsterile tourniquet is utilized. The C-arm is placed on the contralateral side with the monitor at the foot of the bed.

Surgical Approach(es) for ORIF of Periprosthetic Distal Femur Fractures

The surgical approach used for ORIF of periprosthetic distal femur fractures is essentially identical to that used for ORIF of native distal femur fractures as described in Chapter 53. Given the presence of the distal femoral prosthesis, there is obviously no need for access to the articular surface. Therefore, the standard lateral approach to the distal femur is utilized. In most cases, limited exposure to the lateral femoral condyle is supplemented with small incisions proximally to center and

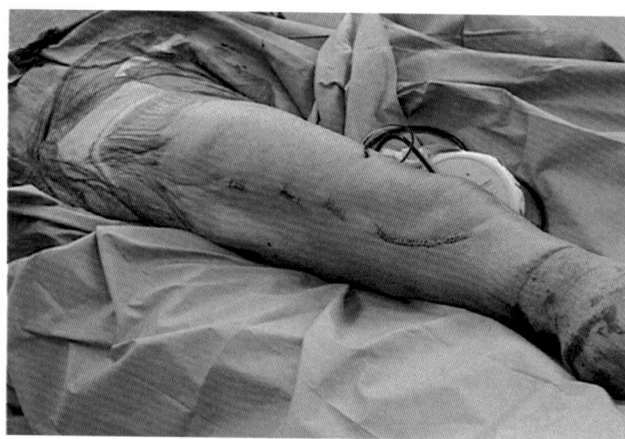

FIGURE 23-25 An intraoperative photograph **(A)** demonstrates limited incisions utilized for ORIF of a periprosthetic distal femur fracture. **B:** The lateral distal femur is exposed for plate insertion and small proximal incisions are used to place proximal screws.

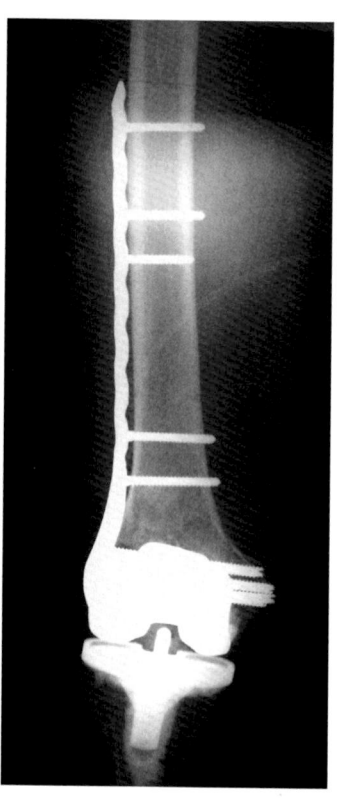

fix the proximal portion of the plate to the proximal fragment (Fig. 23-25). When there is a simple fracture pattern and an anatomic reduction and lag screw fixation to promote primary bone healing is the surgical tactic, a longer lateral incision and wider exposure is needed. In these cases, it is critical to avoid excessive soft tissue disruption during exposure and during reduction maneuvers.

Surgical Technique for ORIF of Periprosthetic Distal Femur Fractures

Details for the surgical technique for ORIF of periprosthetic distal femur fractures depend largely on whether a bridge plating technique will be utilized in the context of a comminuted fracture, or whether a compression or neutralization plating technique is utilized for a simple fracture anatomically reduced and secured with lag screws (Table 23-16).

With bridge plating, a limited surgical approach is utilized. The lateral femoral condyle is exposed and the plate is slid submuscularly across the fracture. Reduction is deferred until after provisional placement of the plate. Ultimately, the plate must be aligned properly with regard to the proximal fragment and aligned properly with regard to the distal fragment to obtain a satisfactory fracture reduction. Whether the plate is secured first to the proximal fragment or first to the distal fragment is largely a matter of personal preference. It is relatively easy to align and secure the plate with the shaft fragment. However, when there is a comminuted fracture it is often difficult to judge the proximal/distal position of the plate to assure proper length reduction of the fracture. Therefore, alignment and provisional fixation of the plate to the proximal fragment with a

single screw via percutaneous or limited incisions is preferred. A single nonlocked screw is usually sufficient to hold the plate well reduced to the proximal fragment. In severely osteoporotic bone, more than one screw may be required for this purpose. The distal fragment is then reduced to the plate which is already aligned and secured to the proximal fragment. The plate is used as a reduction aid. Sagittal plane alignment of the distal fragment can be adjusted using joysticks or a clamp placed from anterior to posterior on the distal fragment. Varus/valgus alignment is often difficult to establish. There is a tendency for valgus malalignment. Comparison to radiographs taken of the contralateral limb can be useful for properly recreating coronal plane alignment.

Once coronal and sagittal plane alignment is established, the distal fragment is provisionally fixed to the plate, usually with a nonlocked screw. Proper length and rotation are confirmed. If adjustments to length or rotation are required, the provisional fixation in the proximal fragment is temporarily removed to allow these adjustments. Once satisfactory length, alignment, and rotation are confirmed, the plate is definitively secured to both the proximal and distal fragments. Multiple locking screws are inserted across the distal femoral condyle. If the prosthesis blocks placement of screws across to the medial condyle, unicortical screws are utilized. In the proximal fragment, screws are placed near and far from the fracture. If the bone quality is poor, locked screws are utilized to supplement nonlocked screws. Plate length should allow at least eight holes to cover the proximal shaft fragment.

When dealing with a simple fracture pattern, an anatomic reduction and provisional fixation of the fracture is usually

TABLE 23-16 ORIF of Periprosthetic Distal Femur Fractures

Surgical Steps

- Expose the distal lateral femur
  - For bridge plating, exposure is limited to the lateral femoral condylar region. Exposure of the fracture is neither required nor desired.
  - For compression plating, exposure across the fracture zone is required to obtain an anatomic reduction of fracture fragments
- Fracture reduction
  - For bridge plating, reduction is deferred until after plate insertion. The plate is generally used as a reduction aid.
  - For compression plating, the fracture is reduced anatomically with care to avoid excessive soft tissue stripping
    - Small fragment lag screw(s) can be helpful to maintain reduction for unencumbered plate insertion
- Plate insertion for bridge plating
  - The plate is inserted submuscularly and used as a reduction aid
  - The plate is aligned and provisionally secured to the proximal fragment through percutaneous or limited proximal incisions
  - The distal fragment is reduced to the plate, with the plate acting as a reduction aid. Alignment relative to the distal fragment is confirmed on the AP and lateral views.
  - The plate is provisionally secured to the distal fragment
  - If needed, length and rotation are restored. This requires removal of the provisional proximal fixation
  - The plate is aligned and secured to the proximal fragment with nonlocked screws through separate limited or percutaneous exposure
  - Alignment is confirmed and adjustments made as needed prior to definitive fixation
- Plate insertion for compression plating
  - The plate is inserted submuscularly
  - Plate alignment relative to the proximal and distal fragments is confirmed
- Definitive plate fixation
  - Distal fixation
    - Multiple locked screws are inserted across the distal femoral condyle
  - Proximal fixation
    - Screws are inserted near and far from the fracture
- Closure
  - A drain in the knee joint can facilitate postoperative knee ROM
  - Standard wound closure

accomplished prior to plate fixation (Fig. 23-26). This generally requires a larger surgical exposure. Great care must be taken to avoid excessive stripping when attempting to anatomically reduce the fracture. Once the fracture is anatomically reduced, it can be held with reduction clamps or countersunk lag screws. Lag screws, in contrast to clamps, allow unencumbered plate insertion and fixation. The plate is applied to the lateral femur with the proximal portion of the plate slid along the lateral femur submuscularly. Fixation of the plate to the already reduced fracture must assure that the fracture reduction is not disturbed. If there is a mismatch between the contour of the plate and the

contour of the bone, nonlocked screw fixation runs the risk of disrupting the reduction. In this scenario, either the plate must be recontoured to match the bone, or fixation with locked screws can be utilized. In addition, it is often possible to get additional lag screw fixation across the fracture through the plate.

Postoperative Care for ORIF of Periprosthetic Distal Femur Fractures

There is generally no need for postoperative immobilization. Early rehabilitation is concentrated on patient mobilization and knee ROM. Weight bearing is protected to some degree for approximately 6 to 8 weeks. Initial weight-bearing restrictions are toe-touch for balance or up to 50% weight bearing if the bone quality and fixation were both optimal. Therapy for knee ROM, transfer training, and use of assist devices are initiated immediately postoperatively. It is important to know baseline knee ROM limits to determine postoperative goals. Continuous passive motion (CPM) for knee ROM is usually familiar to this patient population given their prior knee arthroplasty. The use of CPM after periprosthetic supracondylar femur fracture is of unknown long-term benefit but can be useful to obtain early functional ROM. CPM to 90 degrees of flexion can generally be obtained within 48 hours of surgery if any knee joint hemarthrosis is decompressed with a drain, the limits of flexion are advanced 10 degrees three times daily, and adequate postoperative analgesia is provided.

Based on progressive clinical and radiographic signs of fracture healing, weight bearing is gradually advanced. Full weight bearing is typically accomplished by 6 to 8 weeks postoperatively and at this time formal strengthening and gait training therapy are useful.

Potential Pitfalls and Preventative Measures for ORIF of Periprosthetic Distal Femur Fractures

One of the most common pitfalls during ORIF of distal femur fractures is reduction in valgus (Table 23-17). True AP radiographs and comparison to the contralateral limb should be used to assure proper alignment. Most locked plating systems have screw(s) that are designed to be 95 degrees from the long axis of the plate shaft. When these screws are parallel to the articular surface, 5 degrees of valgus results. In the sagittal plane, apex posterior malreduction is common. Joysticks or clamps in the distal fragment can be used to manipulate the articular segment into proper alignment. Loss of distal fixation, a concern when the femoral component blocks screw placement, is fortunately uncommon. Use of multiple locking screws and the largest diameter screws available will minimize this potential problem. Proximal fixation is optimized with the use of relatively long plates, eight or more holes covering the proximal fragment secured with at least four screws. Locked screws are utilized in the proximal fragment when bone stock is poor. The mechanics of the construct should be optimized to promote the desired method of fracture healing. Simple fractures are fixed with relatively rigid constructs with lag screws to promote primary bone healing. More comminuted fractures are managed with bridge plating constructs that provide relative stability and promote secondary bone healing.

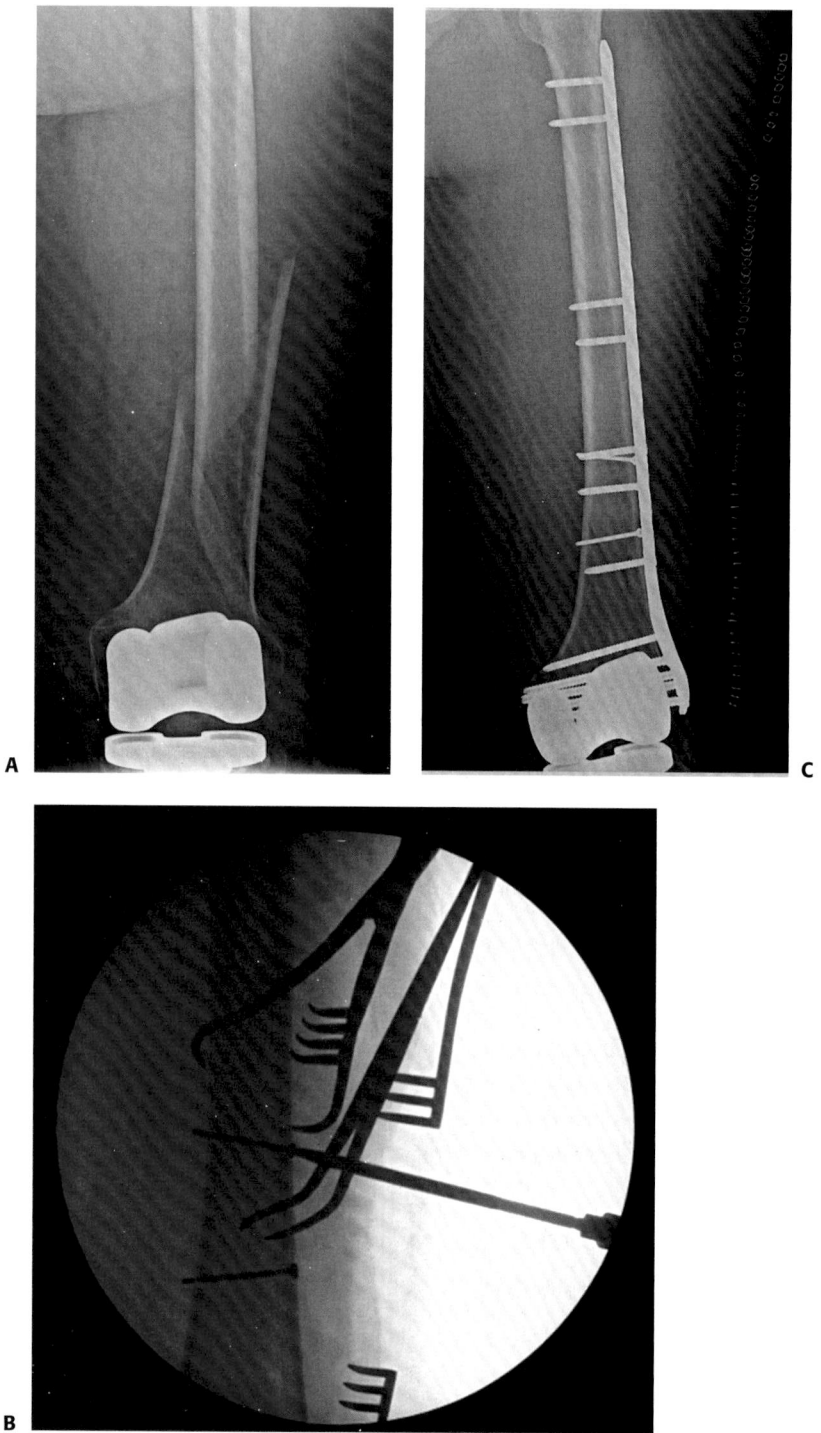

FIGURE 23-26 A relatively simple spiral periprosthetic fracture of the distal femur **(A)** is reduced anatomically and provisionally secured with small fragment lag screws **(B)** to allow unencumbered definitive plate fixation **(C)**.

Outcomes of ORIF for Periprosthetic Distal Femur Fractures

Older methods of plate fixation of supracondylar femur fractures that included traditional condylar buttress plates are prone to complications. These non–fixed-angle implants are especially prone to varus collapse when comminution is present.

Davison[56] reported more than 5 degrees of collapse to occur in 11 of 26 (42%) such comminuted distal femur fractures. These problems can be magnified in patients with fractures associated with a TKA as these patients are often elderly with osteoporotic bone making stable internal fixation even more unreliable. This is further confounded by a potentially reduced

TABLE 23-17	ORIF of Periprosthetic Distal Femur Fractures

Potential Pitfalls and Preventions

Pitfalls	Preventions
The femoral prosthesis is found intraoperatively to have a closed intercondylar box obviating retrograde nailing	Preoperative identification of femoral prosthesis geometry from past surgical records and x-rays Intraoperative notch view of the knee prior to initiation of retrograde nailing
Axial shortening of the fracture	Compare leg lengths preoperatively with a radiopaque ruler Muscle paralysis can aid in restoring length
Loss of reduction between reaming and nail placement	Recreate reduction maneuvers used to obtain reduction for guidewire placement for reaming and nail placement
Fracture malalignment	Starting point and starting trajectory are colinear with the long axis of the distal fracture fragment Blocking screws used to obtain and maintain colinearity of nail with long axis of distal fracture fragment
Secondary loss of fracture alignment	Use of blocking screws to help maintain fracture alignment, especially in osteoporotic bone Use of multiple fixed angle distal interlocking screws
Painful medial interlocking screws	Careful measurement of screw length without reliance on AP radiographs Confirm screw length with "roll-over" fluoroscopic view
Knee pain from intra-articular nail protrusion	Confirm countersinking of nail by direct vision, palpation, and true lateral knee radiograph Do not rely on AP radiograph of knee to judge nail position relative to articular surface

ability to gain bicondylar screw purchase because of interference of the TKA prosthesis. Figgie et al.[76] reported failure of internal fixation in 5 of 10 patients with periprosthetic femur fractures above a TKA treated with traditional plating methods and Merkel and Johnson[186] reported satisfactory results in only three of five such patients. Traditional fixed-angle plate constructs, such as 95-degree condylar plates and blade plates, reduce the risk for varus collapse of distal femur fractures when compared to traditional nonlocked plating, but have limited application for fractures about a TKA prosthesis because of potential interference of the femoral component. In the setting of relatively proximal supracondylar fractures, where there is sufficient bone for seating of a blade, 95-degree condylar blade plating using indirect reduction techniques has been shown to yield very good results. Kolb et al.[139] applied this technique in 21 cases, four of which were supplemented with bone graft and three were supplemented with bone cement. All but one fracture healed after the index procedure with only one case of varus malalignment.

Anatomically contoured locking plates for the distal lateral femur have potential advantages for the fixation of supracondylar femur fractures associated with TKA. In contrast to traditional 95-degree plate devices, locking plates offer multiple, rather than single, distal fixed-angle screw options. Ricci et al.[230] showed that at least two such locked screws were typically able to be placed across to the medial condyle despite the presence of a TKA femoral component. When bicondylar screw fixation was blocked by the TKA, unicondylar locked screws were utilized. This combination of bicondylar and unicondylar locked screw fixation provided excellent distal fixation. In

the series of Ricci et al.[230] no distal fixation failures occurred. Another study from the same group showed that extreme distal fractures, those that extended to the anterior flange of the TKA femoral component or beyond, treated with locked plates have similar results as more proximal fractures.[264] These results are consistent with those of other series of locked plate fixation of native distal femur fractures[247,249] indicating that the presence of the TKA femoral component has little effect of the outcome of supracondylar distal femur fractures treated with locked plates. The use of polyaxial locked screws has also shown promising results (90% union) for these fractures with a purported advantage of better ease of screw insertion to avoid interference of the TKA component.[72]

Although locked plate fixation has become the *de facto* standard method for ORIF at many centers, nonunion and implant failure rates for this method of fixation remain a concern. Hoffmann et al.,[115] in a series of 36 fractures in patients with mean age of 73.2 years treated with locked plates at two trauma centers, reported nonunion in 22.2% of cases and implant failure in 8.3%. They noted that surgical handling of the soft tissues affected the risk of nonunion. Patients treated with submuscular plating had a reduced risk of nonunion compared to those treated with an extensive lateral approach. Ricci et al.,[230] in a series of 22 patients treated with locked distal femoral plates, also showed a relatively high nonunion rate of 14%. The three patients with nonunion were insulin-dependent diabetics who were also obese. Fulkerson et al.[85] also had a high complication rate (33%) after treatment of 18 supracondylar femur fractures above a TKA with a first generation locking plate. These included plate failure (n = 1), delayed union (n = 2), nonunion (n = 2), and component loosening

($n = 1$). In contrast, Anakwe et al.[6] and Large et al.[150] had no non-unions among a total of 40 patients treated with locked plating and Kolb et al.[138] reported just one nonunion among 19 patients at midterm follow-up of 46 months.

Head-to-head comparisons of modern locked plating and retrograde nailing have shown similar results for the two methods of treatment. A systematic review of 415 cases showed locked plating and retrograde IMN to provide superior results compared to conventional nonlocked plating.[113] Overall, the nonunion rate was 9%, the fixation failure rate was 4%, the infection rate was 3%, and the revision surgery rate was 13%. Retrograde nailing was found to offer relative risk reductions for nonunion (87%) and revision surgery (70%) compared to traditional nonlocked plating. Locked plating showed non-significant trends toward similar risk reductions compared to traditional plating (57% for nonunions, 43% for revision surgery). Other retrospective comparative studies of LP or IMN of periprosthetic femur fractures above a TKA have showed varying results. Hou et al.[117] reported similar nonunion (9% for LP and 6% for IMN) and malunion (9% for LP and 11% for IMN) rates for the two methods, whereas Platzer et al.[217] found better union rates with IMN and better alignment after LP.[217]

Given the modest nonunion rates reported after locked plating of distal femur periprosthetic fractures, it is not surprising that there is a parallel reported occurrence of implant failure. As with all internally fixed fractures, there is a race between fracture healing and implant failure. For plate constructs implant failure may occur in one of three zones: the zone of distal fragment fixation, the zone of fracture (the so-called working length

of the plate), or the zone of the proximal fragment. The weak link of locked plate constructs has been shown to be the plate failure over the zone of fracture or screw failure in the proximal fragment in up to 33% of cases.[113,220,230,264] Of note, three of the four proximal screw failures in one series occurred when exclusively nonlocking screws were used in the shaft fragment.[230] This study was among the first to describe modern "hybrid" locked fixation, where nonlocked and locked screws were used in the same construct. Only one failure occurred among the 14 cases where locking screws supplemented nonlocked fixation in the shaft, this being a patient with diabetes and obesity who developed an aseptic nonunion.

Inserting nonlocked screws prior to locked screws in any given fragment during hybrid locked plating allows the plate to be used as a reduction aid where the contour of the plate helps dictate the reduction in the coronal plane. Malreductions using the hybrid locked-plating technique were present in only 2 of 22 cases (9%).[230] This compares favorably with the reduction (6% to 20% malreductions) reported with internal fixator systems (such as LISS) where exclusive use of locked screws makes reduction independent of plate contour.[143,150,174,247,249]

Biomechanical investigations suggest that locked screws in the diaphysis may protect from this type of screw failure, especially in osteoporotic bone.[67,211]

Intramedullary Nailing of Periprosthetic Distal Femur Fractures

Retrograde intramedullary nailing has evolved as a satisfactory treatment option for fixation of supracondylar femur fractures

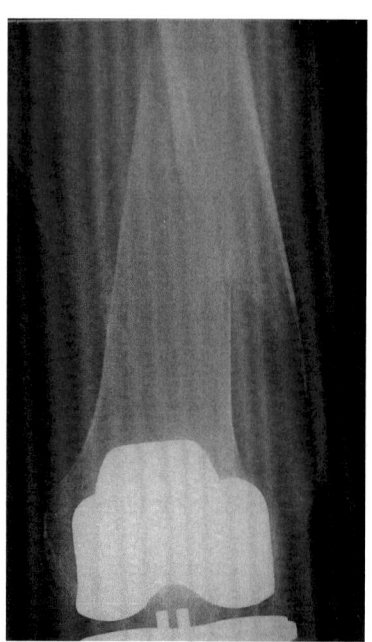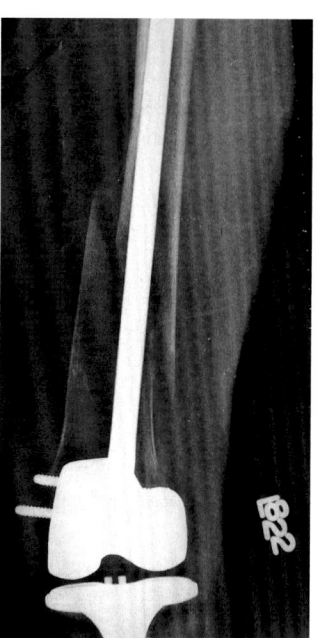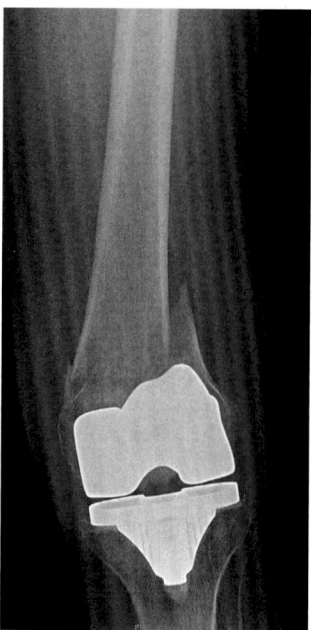

A, B   **C**

FIGURE 23-27 Retrograde nailing of distal femur fractures with wide metaphyseal regions **(A)** runs the risk of malalignment **(B)**. Proper technique requires the nail be aligned with the axis of both the proximal and distal fragments. The isthmus of the femur helps align long nails within the proximal fragment, but it is incumbent upon the surgeon to establish alignment in the distal fragment. With attention to detail, successful alignment can be accomplished even with distal fractures **(C)**.

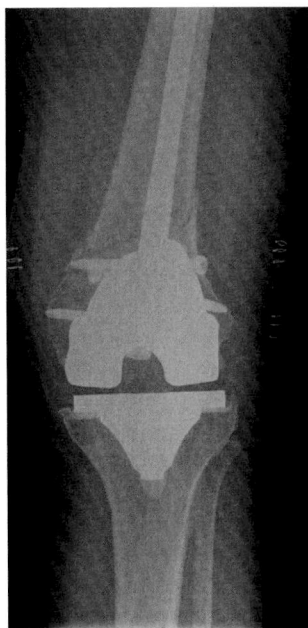

D

FIGURE 23-27 (*continued*) Nails with multiple distal locking options are recommended **(D)**. (C & D, courtesy of Paul Tornetta, III, MD).

that are not associated with TKA. This fixation method is advantageous because of the indirect nature of the fracture reduction and associated minimization of soft tissue disruption about the fracture. However, problems obtaining stable fixation with intramedullary nails in patients with wide metaphyseal areas, with osteopenia, or both can lead to loss of fixation and malalignment.[4] When a TKA is present, the potential difficulties of retrograde nailing of supracondylar femur fractures are also increased (Fig. 23-27). As previously described, some TKA designs, because of a closed or narrow intercondylar notch, preclude the use of retrograde nails or limit their maximum diameter, respectively. Furthermore, the specific prosthesis type may be unknown at the time of fracture fixation. In these cases, the choice of an anterior surgical approach used for retrograde nailing may need to be aborted in favor of a lateral approach for plate fixation if a nonaccommodating prosthesis is encountered. Despite these potential pitfalls, retrograde IMN can be successfully applied to periprosthetic supracondylar femur fractures that have adequate distal bone stock and is the preferred method of treatment by some authors (Figs. 23-27 C and D).[91]

Preoperative Planning for IM Nailing of Periprosthetic Distal Femur Fractures

In general, planning for retrograde nailing of periprosthetic distal femur fractures follows that described for standard retrograde nailing in Chapter 53 Femoral Shaft Fractures (Table 23-18). Ideally, the femoral component type and the intercondylar dimensions are identified from prior operative records to assure that retrograde nailing through the intercondylar notch of the femoral component is possible. If documentation is unobtainable, reference sources can help identify the component based on radiographic profiles and provide details

TABLE 23-18	**Intramedullary Nailing of Periprosthetic Distal Femur Fractures**

Preoperative Planning Checklist

- Assessment of the femoral prosthesis: Compatibility of the femoral prosthesis with retrograde nailing is confirmed
- OR table: Radiolucent table that allows fluoroscopic imaging of the entire involved femur and knee and allows unencumbered access to the foot of the table
- Position/positioning aids: Supine using a radiolucent triangle
- Fluoroscopy location: Opposite side from the injured extremity with the monitor at the head
- Equipment: Retrograde nailing set and associated implants. Femoral distractor available
- Tourniquet: A sterile tourniquet may be utilized for obtaining distal exposure, the starting point, and instrumentation of the distal fragment. Proximal fixation usually requires removal of any tourniquet
- Blood: PRBCs typed and crossmatched

of the intercondylar notch dimensions.[111] It is very unusual to unexpectedly encounter a loose femoral component. However, if there is clinical suspicion for component loosening, then the preoperative plan should consider the contingency for component revision or distal femoral replacement.

Positioning and Surgical Approach for IM Nailing of Periprosthetic Distal Femur Fractures

Patient positioning, typically supine, and the surgical approach for IMN of periprosthetic distal femur fractures is essentially identical to that for retrograde nailing of native femur fractures as discussed in Chapter 53 Femoral Shaft Fractures. Of course, consideration must be given to old incisions about the knee from the prior knee arthroplasty. The longitudinal midline incision typically used for TKA is usually well positioned for the standard approach for retrograde nailing.

Surgical Technique for IM Nailing of Periprosthetic Distal Femur Fractures

As with nailing any long bone, the first critical step for retrograde nailing of distal femur fractures is securing the location and trajectory of the starting point in the distal fragment (Table 23-19). The location of the starting point is in line with the long axis of the distal fragment, or slightly off this line based on the geometry of the selected nail. On the AP view, a starting point located on the center axis line is typically just medial to the center of the intercondylar notch. On the lateral view, a starting point on the center axis line corresponds to the apex of Blumensaat line or just anterior to it. Because most retrograde nails have an apex posterior bend at the driving end, the starting point can be just posterior to the center axis line on the lateral view. Unique to retrograde nailing of periprosthetic fractures are the constraints imposed by the location of the femoral component intercondylar space. The location of the prosthetic notch may force a starting location from the ideal points discussed above.

The starting trajectory should be collinear with the long axis of the femur in both the sagittal and coronal planes. Given the often coexistent osteopenic bone and wide metaphyseal areas in the patient population with periprosthetic fractures, an initial opening reamer passed in an ideal trajectory will not necessarily guarantee that subsequent reamers or the retrograde nail will follow the same path. Therefore, the surgeon must be prepared to utilize supplementary techniques to assure that the nail is aligned properly within the distal fragment. We prefer the use of blocking screws. These screws are placed anterior to posterior to control varus/valgus alignment and from lateral to medial to control flexion/extension alignment. The blocking screws should be placed relatively near the fracture to optimally affect alignment. Additional technical details of retrograde femoral nailing and blocking screw placement can be found in multiple chapters throughout this book including Chapter 7 – Principles of Internal Fixation, Chapter 54 – Distal Femur Fractures, and Chapter 57– Tibia and Fibula Fractures.

TABLE 23-19 **Intramedullary Nailing of Periprosthetic Distal Femur Fractures**

Surgical Steps

- Confirm open intercondylar box with notch view fluoroscopic radiograph
- Confirm muscle paralysis is complete
- Midline surgical incision and medial parapatellar arthrotomy
- Place starting guidewire colinear with the long axis of the distal femoral fracture fragment
- Insert stiff starting reamer over guidewire and adjust trajectory
- Reduce fracture with manual forces (e.g., longitudinal traction and gentle manipulation with the use of strategically placed bumps) and be prepared to use accessory means such as blocking screws, a femoral distractor, or Schanz pin joysticks.
- Pass guidewire across reduced fracture to a location above the lesser trochanter
- Depth gauge measurement to determine nail length with fracture out to proper length
- Ream over guidewire to a diameter 0.5 to 1.5 mm beyond the initiation of cortical chatter at the femoral isthmus
- Select appropriate size nail with determined diameter 1 to 1.5 mm smaller than largest reamer diameter
- Assemble nail to insertion handle and confirm alignment of drill sleeves for interlocking screws
  - Insert nail over guidewire
  - Confirm final location of nail with fluoroscopic radiographs proximally and distally
  - Confirmation of distal nail location, countersunk beyond the articular margin, is performed with direct vision, palpation, and/or true lateral radiographs of the knee
- Confirm satisfactory angular fracture reduction before interlocking. Be prepared to remove nail and place blocking screws if reduction is unsatisfactory
- Perform multiple distal interlocking and assure screws are of appropriate length so as to avoid medial prominence
- Confirm satisfactory rotational fracture reduction and satisfactory length
- Perform proximal interlocking

Postoperative Care for IM Nailing of Periprosthetic Distal Femur Fractures

Patients are mobilized as soon as possible postoperatively. Weight bearing is typically protected for 4 to 6 weeks after retrograde nailing of a comminuted distal femur fracture in osteoporotic patients, the typical scenario for periprosthetic distal femur fractures. Weight bearing can be initiated earlier when there is confidence in the distal fixation and bone quality is good. CPM is generally initiated in the recovery room and is usually better tolerated if the knee is decompressed with a suction drain. The goals of CPM must not assume full knee ROM was achievable at baseline. A careful history of prefracture knee function helps identify reasonable goals for postoperative ROM and function. Weight bearing is advanced based on clinical and radiographic evidence of progressive fracture healing.

Potential Pitfalls and Preventative Measures for IM Nailing of Periprosthetic Distal Femur Fractures

One of the most disheartening potential pitfalls of retrograde nailing of periprosthetic distal femur fractures is unexpectedly finding a closed or a narrow intercondylar box of the femoral component that prevents passage of the retrograde nail (Table 23-20). Prevention of this situation is certainly preferred to managing it intraoperatively. In the absence of accurate documentation of the knee arthroplasty design, an intraoperative notch view can be used to confirm an open intercondylar notch. In situations where there is such uncertainty, the preoperative

---

TABLE 23-20 **Intramedullary Nailing of Periprosthetic Distal Femur Fractures**

Potential Pitfalls and Preventions

Pitfalls	Preventions
Fracture malreduction, typically valgus	Intraoperative evaluation of fracture alignment with true AP and true lateral radiographs Comparison to contralateral limb radiographs Clinical comparison to the contralateral limb
Loss of distal fixation	Maximize the number and diameter of bicondylar locking screws in distal fragment Unicondylar locking screws may be required if bicondylar screws are blocked by the prosthesis
Loss of proximal fixation	Use of long plate, eight or more holes spanning proximal fragment Secure with at least two screws near the fracture and two screws far from fracture
Inadequate biomechanics of fixation construct	Identify the desired mode of fracture healing, primary or secondary, and design construct with appropriate mechanics

plan should include the contingency for alternative fixation methods than retrograde nailing, including immediate availability of all equipment and implants.

Obtaining and maintaining satisfactory fracture alignment is often difficult in the setting of a periprosthetic fracture. The patient population that sustains these injuries often has substantial osteoporosis, leaving the metaphyseal region of the distal fracture fragment relatively vacuous and often incapable of supporting a proper nail trajectory. Even when the starting guidewire and opening portal are perfectly aligned, the nail often migrates to a different trajectory leading to malalignment of the fracture. In such cases, placement of blocking screws helps obtain and maintain proper position of the nail, centered along the long axis of the distal fragment, and in turn results in a satisfactory fracture reduction. With the use of long retrograde nails that span the isthmus of the femur, alignment of the nail within the proximal fragment is infrequently an issue. The isthmus, located at the junction of the proximal and middle thirds of the femoral diaphysis, serves to center the nail in the proximal fragment. When the nail is colinear with the long axis of both the distal and proximal fragments, a proper reduction, with regard to varus/valgus and flexion/extension, will result. Secondary loss of reduction can occur as a result of poor fixation within the distal fragment, also owing to the presence of substantial osteoporotic bone. As described earlier, blocking screws can help maintain reduction as they stabilize the nail relative to the surrounding bone. When blocking screws are used for this purpose, screws on both sides of the nail, medial and lateral to control varus/valgus and anterior and posterior to control flexion/extension, are beneficial. Whereas blocking screws used purely to control alignment are placed only on one side of the nail, for example, lateral side to control valgus and anterior side to control extension deformities. It is recommended to place as many interlocking screws as possible (typically three or four depending upon the nailing system selected) in various planes to support distal fixation in osteoporotic bone. Interlocking screws should be bicortical to capture the strength of the cortical shell, but care should be taken to avoid excessively long screws. AP radiographs should not be relied upon to judge screw length because of the trapezoidal shape of the distal femur. A screw that is relatively anterior in the distal femur, which is the same width as the distal femoral condyles, will protrude through the medial distal femur by 1 cm or more and cause pain. Careful length measurement with a depth gauge and confirmation of screw length with roll-over fluoroscopic views can help avoid this potential problem. Just as proper views are necessary to judge interlocking screw length, proper views are needed to judge position of the distal end of the nail relative to the articular surface of the prosthesis. Again, AP views should not be relied upon for this purpose. A true lateral of the knee is necessary to judge nail position relative to the knee prosthesis. Even with a true lateral, confirmation of proper positioning of the nail can be obscured by the radio-opaque prosthesis. In such scenarios, direct vision and/or palpation should be used to assure the nail end is not too proud. A nail that protrudes into the knee can interfere with patellofemoral motion and even damage the patellar component.

Outcomes of IM Nailing for Periprosthetic Distal Femur Fractures

Most studies of periprosthetic supracondylar femur fractures treated with retrograde nailing are small retrospective series. Reported union rates are generally favorable, especially in comparison to locked plating. However, the risk of malunion after retrograde nailing is high.

Four small series (14 or less patients) of periprosthetic supracondylar femur fractures treated with retrograde nailing each reported 100% union.[41,91,104] Alignment at healing is variable as this is one of the main technical challenges of this treatment method: Han et al. had no malalignment greater than 10 degrees. They paid particular attention to alignment and used cerclage fixation to improve reduction in three of eight cases when closed reduction resulted in greater than or equal to 5 degrees of malalignment.[104] Malunion of 35-degree valgus requiring revision to a stemmed TKA occurred in 1 of 10 cases reported by Gliatis.[91] Another study of 14 patients reported valgus of 8 to 12 degrees in three cases, 15-degree extension in one, and 50% posterior translation in another.[41] The malalignment seen in these series may, in part, be related to the use of short nails, which, because they do not benefit from the stability and alignment control that comes from passing the nail across the femoral isthmus, are not currently recommended for treatment of distal femur fractures.

Wick et al.[292] found comparable results for retrograde nailing and locked plating of periprosthetic distal femur fractures in a small comparative series of nine fractures each. They noted that locked plates were preferred in cases with osteoporotic bone.

Recent advances in nail design that provide multiple interlocks at various angles may provide improved fixation of the distal segment and may therefore expand the indications for this technique.

Revision Total Knee Arthroplasty for Periprosthetic Distal Femur Fractures

For patients with loose implants associated with a supracondylar fracture, revision is typically considered. Bony defects, areas of osteolysis, osteopenia, and short periarticular fragments all pose challenges to a successful revision arthroplasty in this setting. In elderly patients, distal femoral replacement "megaprostheses" are often required to reconstruct massive bony defects. Attention to specific technical details is necessary for a successful result, and the surgeon undertaking such reconstructions should be experienced in both arthroplasty and fracture management techniques. In patients with a loose implant or a history of prefracture knee pain, the routine preoperative evaluation of these patients should include a complete blood count with manual differential, sedimentation rate, C-reactive protein serologies, and a knee aspiration to exclude occult infection.

If available, the operative note from the original arthroplasty should be obtained. This is especially important if isolated component revision is contemplated. Older implant designs may not offer varying degrees of constraint, augmentations, polyethylene insert sizes, etc., and thus compatibility issues may necessitate complete arthroplasty revision. Previous incisions and the status of the soft tissues should be circumferentially evaluated and the neurovascular status of the limb should be carefully documented. Wounds are especially important around the knee since the probability of flap necrosis and wound problems is much higher around the knee than the hip. Great care should be taken to prevent narrow, acutely angled skin bridges between connecting incisions and to develop full thickness flaps during dissection. As best as possible, prior incisions should be used. If a distinct incision is needed, appropriate separation of the incisions should be maintained to provide a suitable skin bridge. The status of the extensor mechanism is very important for treatment and prognosis and this should be determined during evaluation.

The need for revision TKA secondary to periprosthetic fracture has become less common in our practice with the advent of improved internal fixation devices such as locked plates. Typically, revision arthroplasty is reserved for fractures around a loose prosthesis, fractures with inadequate bone stock to allow for stable internal fixation, or for recalcitrant supracondylar nonunions which require resection and megaprosthesis implantation (Fig. 23-28). Surgeons who treat periprosthetic fractures around a TKA must have the expertise and technical support to be able to perform either long-stemmed revision TKA or revision to a megaprosthesis. Bony defects secondary to comminution, multiple previous procedures, the presence of broken hardware, and the presence of deformity all may present technical challenges to a successful outcome.

Revision TKA with intramedullary femoral stems that engage the diaphysis and simultaneously stabilize the fracture can be used. Cemented stems may be used, but care must be taken to prevent extrusion of cement into the fracture site. Allograft struts with cerclage wiring can be used to reinforce the stability provided by a long stem prosthesis. It is very unusual, however, to have distal femoral bone stock that is inadequate for internal fixation yet adequate for formal revision. The ideal indication for long stem revision TKA would be the presence of adequate bone stock in the face of a supracondylar fracture with a grossly loose femoral component.[11,71,217]

Revision arthroplasty is typically chosen for fractures around loose implants and fractures of the distal femur with distal fragments that offer no reasonable opportunity for internal fixation. Revision of femoral components typically requires metal augmentation because of the inevitable bone deficiency associated with component removal. Stems should be used routinely, and it is recommended that the stem engage the femoral diaphysis both for alignment and fixation reasons. Commercially available metaphyseal sleeves and trabecular metal cones can be useful for managing capacious metaphyseal defects. These implant types have limited published data on outcomes but do offer increased revision options including a combination of cemented and noncemented fixation and modular options allowing increased constraint and stemmed implants mated to the metaphyseal fixation. These hybrid constructs may offer improved longevity over cemented-only designs. It should be noted that implants with increased varus–valgus constraint and hinged implants should be available, since ligamentous insufficiency is common in this setting. More commonly, with a distal femoral fracture above a loose implant, there is simply not enough bone to support a traditional revision, even with the use of diaphyseal engaging stems. This situation is not

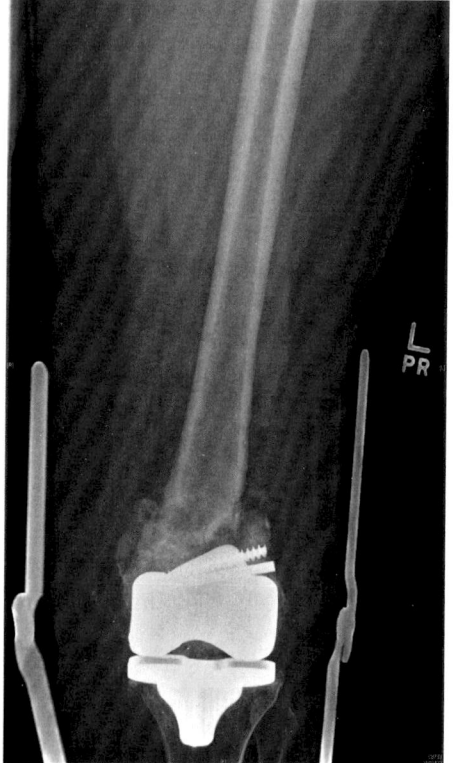

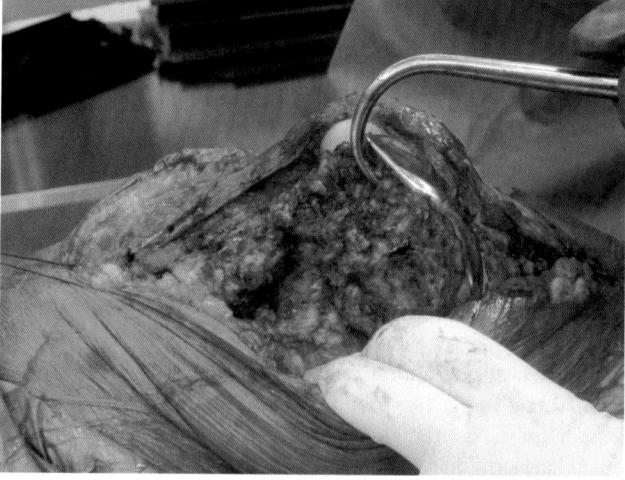

FIGURE 23-28 A: A radiograph of a periprosthetic distal femoral nonunion. **B:** An intraoperative photograph shows extensive bone loss.

FIGURE 23-28 *(continued)* **C, D:** This was treated with a distal femoral replacement. (Courtesy of Hari Parvataneni, MD).

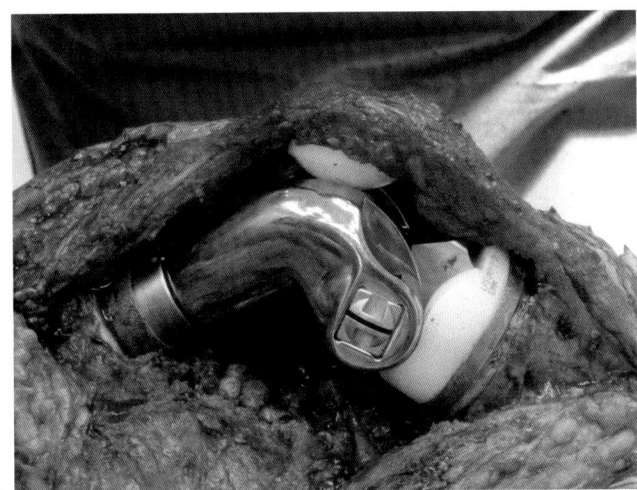

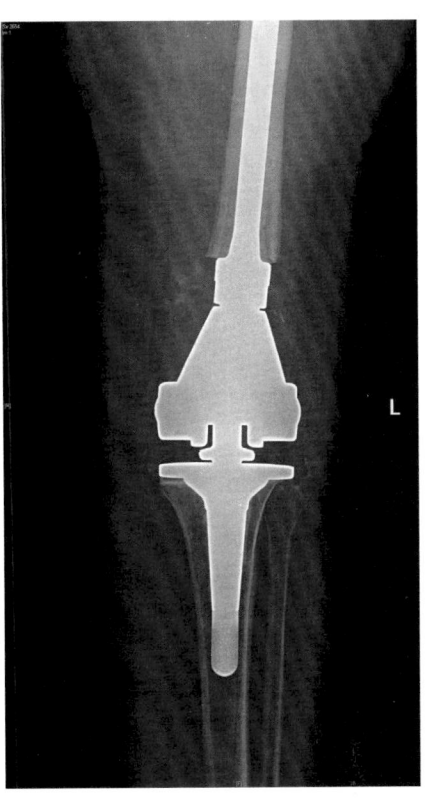

uncommon in the elderly, low-demand patient. In these cases, a modular megaprosthesis (distal femoral replacement) is performed. Careful dissection of the residual distal femoral bone is performed to avoid vascular injury. Various modular segments are available to manage metaphyseal bone loss because of fracture comminution, yet still allow restoration of appropriate leg length, limb alignment, and knee stability. Cement fixation is typically used in this setting.

Preoperative Planning, Positioning, Surgical Approaches, and Surgical Technique for Revision TKA for Periprosthetic Distal Femur Fractures

Incision planning is essential in preventing skin necrosis or wound issues (Table 23-21 and 23-22). The prior incision should be used if possible and if it allows extensile approaches. If a separate incision is needed, an adequate skin bridge should be maintained. If the surgical incision contacts or crosses another, the junctional area should not have too acute an angle. Skin flaps should be of full thickness. A full thickness anteromedial capsular flap should be maintained to reduce the risk of wound-healing problems in this area.

The extensor mechanism should be protected and continuously evaluated for risk of rupture. The medial and lateral gutters must be recreated. Peripatellar and infrapatellar scar must be excised to mobilize the extensor mechanism. A quadriceps snip or tibial tubercle osteotomy should be performed if there is undue tension on the extensor mechanism or inadequate exposure.

Once an adequate exposure is obtained, the status of the patellar component, tibial and femoral bone stock, and the sta-

tus of the collaterals are determined. At this point, decisions about metaphyseal/diaphyseal/combined fixation, length of the stems needed, augments, and need for metaphyseal sleeves or megaprosthesis are made.

Typically the patellar component should be retained unless loose or defective. If a megaprosthesis is required, subperiosteal dissection of the bone to be removed should be done for safety and to preserve a good soft tissue sleeve. The joint line level can be determined based on the position of the patella. The

TABLE 23-21 Revision Total Knee Arthroplasty for Periprosthetic Distal Femur Fractures

Preoperative Planning Checklist

- OR table: Radiolucent
- Position/positioning aids: Knee bumps for working in midflexion and full flexion
- Fluoroscopy: Usually needed for hardware removal or to confirm adequate bypass of stress risers
- Equipment: Hardware removal equipment, flexible osteotomes, high speed burr, curettes, and appropriate implant options including stem options, implant constraint, backup options
- Tourniquet (sterile/nonsterile): Sterile for distal femoral replacements or any procedure requiring exposure up to the proximal thigh. Nonsterile tourniquet otherwise
- Confirm incision and prior wound conflicts as well as infection workup

TABLE 23-22
| **TABLE 23-22** | **Revision Total Knee Arthroplasty for Periprosthetic Fractures About the Knee** |

Surgical Steps

- Incision planning and placement: Full thickness flaps
- Extensile approach: Quadriceps snip or tibial tubercle osteotomy if needed
- Assess collateral ligaments to determine level of constraint needed: A hinged prosthesis would be necessary with megaprosthesis that removes the collateral ligaments
- Evaluate bone stock to determine if metaphyseal, diaphyseal, or combined fixation is needed: Use augments, sleeves, stems, and/or megaprosthesis as needed
- Retain patellar component unless grossly loose
- Both femoral and tibial component revision may be needed if additional constraint is used
- Femoral rotation should be marked on the remaining femur before removal of the distal femur. The joint line can be restored by referencing the patella
- Trialing should be done carefully to evaluate soft tissue tension, joint line, stability of the flexion gap, patellar tracking, and the ability to close the soft tissue sleeve

| **TABLE 23-23** | **Revision Total Knee Arthroplasty for Periprosthetic Distal Femur Fractures** |

Potential Pitfalls and Preventions

Pitfalls	Preventions
Skin necrosis	Careful incision planning Full thickness skin flaps Restrict postoperative flexion if needed
Inadequate exposure	Recreate gutters, excise peripatellar and infrapatellar scar tissue Quadriceps snip or tibial tubercle osteotomy
Inadequate fixation options	Careful preoperative planning and implant selection Availability of metaphyseal sleeves, stems, augments, and/or megaprosthesis
Instability	Plan adequate constraint options including varus/valgus constraint options and hinged prosthesis. Pay special attention to flexion laxity

femoral and tibial rotation should be marked on the remaining diaphysis before removal of the metaphysis.

Trialing should be done to evaluate soft tissue tension, position of the joint line, patella tracking, stability of the gaps, and the tension on the soft tissue sleeve. If the trials are too bulky and closure is difficult, downsizing the implant and shortening the construct can help in closure.

If cemented implants are used, they can be cemented in separate phases to allow for better control of implant position. For cases where there is diaphyseal-only noncemented fixation, cerclage wires at the opening will help to prevent fracture propagation.

The tourniquet should be deflated and hemostasis should be obtained before closure to reduce hematomas in the large potential spaces.

After closure, the skin should be checked carefully in extension and flexion for vascularity.

Postoperative Care After Revision TKA for Distal Femur Fracture

Weight bearing is dictated by fixation quality and stability. ROM should be restricted until it is clear that the wound has adequate vascularity and is healing well. A hinged knee brace may provide additional external protection during the recovery period while the patient regains strength and improved gait.

Potential Pitfalls and Preventative Measures After Revision TKA for Distal Femur Fracture

Revision arthroplasty is a demanding procedure that has many potential issues at various stages (Table 23-23). In the setting of a periprosthetic fracture, the soft tissue envelope may be compromised more so than in the setting of a standard revision. Great care must be taken to avoid skin necrosis by carefully

planning incisions and using meticulous surgical technique. As with any TKA revision, adequate exposure and recreating of the normal medial and lateral gutter tissue planes facilitate component removal and implantation, maximizes ROM potential, and minimizes the need for excessive soft tissue retraction. Stable component fixation may require specialized devices such as metaphyseal sleeves, augments, long stems, and highly constrained or hinged components, and/or megaprostheses. A full complement of such fixation options should be available.

Outcomes of Revision Total Knee Arthroplasty for Periprosthetic Distal Femur Fractures

Most of the clinical data evaluating the outcomes of a simultaneous revision arthroplasty with intramedullary stem fixation of a supracondylar fracture have been gathered from the treatment of distal femoral nonunions in this situation. Kress et al.[144] reported a small series of nonunions about the knee treated successfully with revision and uncemented femoral stems with bone grafting. They achieved union in 6 months.

Distal femoral replacement "megaprostheses" have been used for salvage of failed internal fixation of supracondylar periprosthetic femur fractures. The long-term results of the kinematic rotating hinge prosthesis for oncologic resections about the knee have been good, with a 10-year survivorship of approximately 90%. As their success becomes more predictable, the indications for megaprostheses are expanding. Elderly patients with refractory periprosthetic supracondylar nonunions or those with acute fractures with bone stock inadequate for internal fixation are reasonable candidates for megaprostheses. Davila et al.[55] have reported a small series of supracondylar distal femoral nonunions treated with a megaprostheses in elderly patients. They have shown that a cemented megaprosthesis in this patient population permits early ambulation and return to activities of daily living. Freedman[83] performed distal femoral replacement in five elderly patients with acute fractures and reported four good results and one poor result secondary to infection. The four patients with good results regained ambulation in less than 1 month and had an average arc of motion of 99 degrees. All patients had some degree of extension lag.

For a younger, active patient, an allograft-prosthetic composite may be a better alternative. Distal femoral reconstruction with an allograft-prosthetic composite, providing a biologic interface, can help restore bone stock and potentially make future revision easier.[45,71] Kraay et al.[142] have reported a series of allograft-prosthetic reconstructions for the treatment of supracondylar fractures in patients with TKAs. At a minimum 2-year follow-up, the mean Knee Society Score was 71 and the mean arc of motion was 96 degrees. All femoral components were well fixed at follow-up. Results of this study indicate that large segmental distal femoral allograft-prosthetic composites can be a reasonable treatment method in this setting.

AUTHOR'S PREFERRED TREATMENT OF PERIPROSTHETIC DISTAL FEMUR FRACTURES

As with most periprosthetic fractures, the typical first branch of the decision tree is at the determination of the stability of the existing prosthesis (Fig. 23-29). When a distal femur fracture involves an associated loose prosthesis, revision arthroplasty is indicated. Because of the paucity of critical soft tissue attachments in this anatomic region, distal femoral replacement is our treatment of choice for these fractures. These prostheses provide adequate stability through their built-in constraint mechanisms and their insertion is technically straightforward for the surgeon practiced in this technique. They allow immediate weight bearing and therefore early rehabilitation, and they

have reasonable outcomes. The longevity and complication rates associated with distal femoral replacement, however, do not favorably compare with fracture fixation of distal femoral fractures about stable implants.

ORIF and IMN both are reasonable options for the management of distal femur fractures about stable and well-functioning femoral components. The decision for one or the other is based on fracture fragment size, the morphology of the femoral arthroplasty component, and surgeon's preference. When the distal fracture fragment is so small that control of it with a retrograde nail is suspect, ORIF is indicated. We reserve IMN for cases where the distal fragment extends into the diaphyseal region but we recognize that it is reasonable to consider this option anytime the distal fragment is at least long enough to allow placement of two to three distal interlocks. Another absolute requirement for IM nailing is the presence of a prosthesis with an open intercondylar notch. Lateral locked plate fixation is our preferred method for any fracture confined to the distal metaphyseal region, even fractures that extend beyond the confines of the anterior flange of the femoral component. Our results of ORIF of extreme distal fractures are similar to results for more proximal fractures with larger distal fragments. However, in certain individual cases, we consider distal femoral replacement for these extreme distal fractures.

PERIPROSTHETIC PATELLA FRACTURES

A number of factors guide treatment of periprosthetic patella fractures. The integrity and tracking of the extensor mechanism, locations and displacement of the fracture, stability of the implant, and the available remaining bone stock must all be considered. As with management of other periprosthetic fractures, the determination of the optimal method can be complex

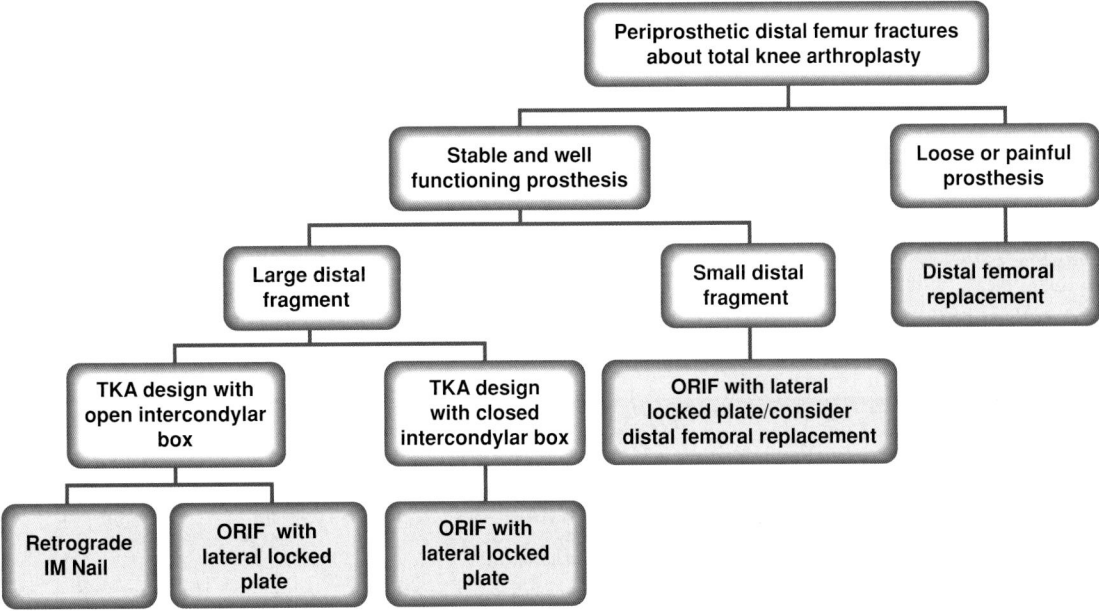

FIGURE 23-29 Algorithm depicting the author's preferred method of treatment for periprosthetic distal femur fractures.

and fracture management can be difficult. A clear vision of the ultimate management goals, typically restoration of the extensor mechanism and at least return to baseline function and pain levels, helps define the optimal individual management scheme. Treatment options include nonoperative management, ORIF, component resection, and patellectomy (partial or complete).

Incidence, Risk Factors, and Prevention of Periprosthetic Patella Fractures

Patellar fracture is the second most frequent periprosthetic fracture around the knee joint, and given the critical nature of the extensor mechanism for knee function, these fractures are significant to the ultimate arthroplasty success. Fractures of the patella generally occur postoperatively and may occur with either an unresurfaced or a resurfaced patella.[3,36,253] An analysis of fractures about TKAs from the Mayo Clinic joint registry published in 1999 indicated that postoperative fracture of the patella occurred in 0.7% of cases after primary TKA (n = 16,906) and 1.8% of cases after revision TKA (n = 2,904).[16] The only intraoperative patella fractures occurred during revision TKA in 8 of 2,904 cases. These data should be interpreted with caution since they do not include postoperative fractures treated at institutions other than the Mayo Clinic and the duration of follow-up was not presented. Several other published series indicate that the frequency of periprosthetic patella fractures is up to 21% with revision TKAs.[11,56,209,232,277]

Etiologic factors related to periprosthetic patella fractures may be either systemic or local. Systemic risk factors are not unique to these anatomic locations and are therefore similar to those for other types of periprosthetic fractures and primarily include osteopenia from a variety of causes. Patients with RA, especially those taking corticosteroids, are at a particularly high risk for fracture about a TKA.[20,30,114] Chalidis et al.,[36] in a literature review, found that only 11.68% of 539 reported fractures were directly associated with trauma. The remaining occurred spontaneously and most fractures occurred during the first 2 years after arthroplasty. Etiologic factors specific to the patella are component design, excessive resection of bone, limb and prosthesis alignment, and presence or absence of a lateral release.[26,31,75,92,110,232] Intraoperative fractures, although very uncommon, can occur with aggressive clamping of the patellar component, bone resection leaving less than 10 to 15 mm of bone, in the setting of revision arthroplasty, and in cases with poor remaining bone stock. Devascularization of the patella from lateral retinacular release may be a risk factor for subsequent fracture as well as for failure of subsequent fracture management.

Tria et al.[277] reported that all 18 patella fractures in a series of 504 primary TKAs were associated with a prior lateral release. In this series, 4% of those with lateral release (n = 413) had subsequent fracture of the patella compared to 0% of those without lateral release (n = 91). The association of lateral release and fracture was significant. However, opposite results were found in another study by Ritter and Campbell.[232] In this series, the vast majority of the 555 patients did not have a lateral release (n = 471). Fractures occurred in 1.2% of cases with and 3.6% of those without lateral release. These conflicting reports, both from large series, make it difficult to determine if lateral release should be considered an independent risk factor for patella fracture. Any prior bony defects, such as from bone-patellar tendon-bone donor sites used for ligament reconstructions are additional potential risk factors for fracture of the patella.

Classification of Periprosthetic Patella Fractures

There are many classification schemes utilized for periprosthetic patella fractures.[92,119,205] In an extensive literature review, Chalidis et al.,[36] found that the classification scheme of Ortiguera and Berry[205] was utilized most frequently in the available literature. This classification takes into account the integrity of the extensor mechanism, the status of the patellar component (well fixed or loose), and the amount of available bone stock (Table 23-24). Type I fractures have an intact extensor mechanism and a stable implant, type II have disruption of the extensor mechanism with or without a stable implant, and type III have an intact extensor mechanism and a loose implant. Type III subtype A has reasonable remaining bone stock, and subtype B has poor bone stock. Among 265 fractures in the literature classified using this system approximately 50% were type III with the rest almost equally divided between types I and II.[36]

Management of Periprosthetic Patella Fractures

Nonoperative management is usually appropriate in a majority of patients with periprosthetic patella fractures. When the extensor mechanism is intact and even sometimes when it is not, nonoperative management is recommended. Surgical management of periprosthetic patella fractures is usually reserved for disturbance of the extensor mechanism integrity, a loose patellar component, and patellar maltracking.

When there is adequate bone stock (more than 10 mm), revision of the patellar component is reasonable. Avulsion

TABLE 23-24	Ortiguera and Berry Classification for Periprosthetic Patella Fractures[205]			
Classification	Type I	Type II	Type IIIa	Type IIIb
Extensor Mechanism	Intact	Disrupted	Intact	Intact
Implant Fixation	Well fixed	Well fixed or Loose	Loose	Loose
Bone Stock	Unspecified	Unspecified	Reasonable	Poor

fractures of the proximal or distal pole are amenable to suture repair. Severe bone deficiency, however, usually mandates patellar resection arthroplasty with partial or complete patellectomy. A novel reconstructive technique for management of type IIIB fractures, those with bone loss and a loose component, has recently been reported.[7] Multiple Steinmann pins are used to reduce and stabilize the patella and act as a scaffold for bone grafting and a patellar button is cemented into the construct.

Outcomes for Periprosthetic Patella Fractures

The results of surgical management of periprosthetic patella fractures are marginal. ORIF with tension band technique or cerclage wiring results in nonunion (Fig. 23-30) in a very large proportion of patients in many reports, with an overall average nonunion rate of 92%.[26,36,43,93,119,132,205,251] Although fibrous union can, on occasion, restore painless extensor mechanism function, poor results in the face of nonunion can be expected. The relatively small and avascular fracture fragments have limited healing potential which can be negatively influenced by surgical dissection potentially leading to nonunion and infection. Therefore, nonoperative management is not an unreasonable consideration even in the face of a disrupted extensor mechanism. The presence of fracture and a loose implant is understandably associated with high complication rates regardless of treatment method. These situations usually lead to surgery for either removal or revision of the component.

Knee function among all patients treated for periprosthetic patella fracture reveals an extensor lag of no more than 10 degrees and a limitation of approximately 20 to 30 degrees of flexion in most patients.[36] However, function is highly variable and related to the ultimate status of the extensor mechanism.

Potential Pitfalls and Preventative Measures for Periprosthetic Patella Fractures

Too aggressive surgical indications of periprosthetic patella fractures are perhaps the greatest potential pitfall. These fractures have high complication rates associated with surgical management. Nonsurgical management should therefore at least be strongly considered for nearly all of these fractures.

AUTHOR'S PREFERRED TREATMENT OF PERIPROSTHETIC PATELLA FRACTURES

Patella fractures are among the most difficult periprosthetic fractures to manage (Fig. 23-31). Operative management is associated with relatively high nonunion and infection rates and nonoperative management may require prolonged immobilization and does not address loose components. We tend to lean toward nonoperative management for these fractures unless displacement is severe or the component is so loose that it may dislodge. A staged management protocol that treats a periprosthetic patella fracture associated with a loose component sequentially rather than simultaneously is sometimes prudent to avoid major complications. Nonoperative fracture management to healing followed by surgical management of a loose component, if symptomatic, is a

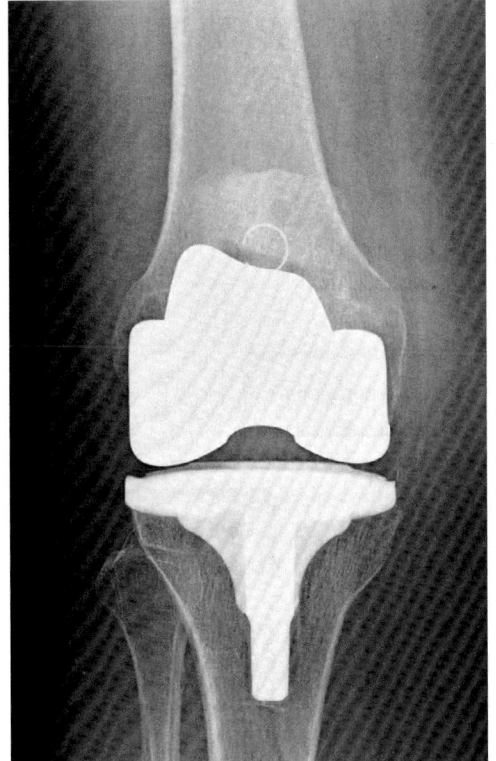

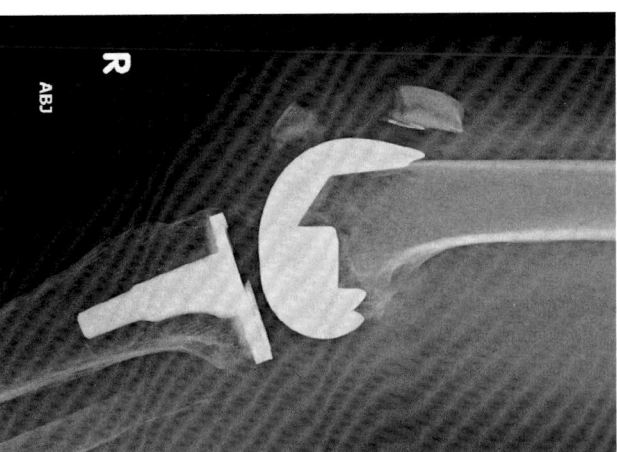

FIGURE 23-30 An acute periprosthetic patella fracture (**A, B**) treated with a K-wire and suture tension band results in secondary displacement and nonunion (**C, D**).

(*continues*)

A

B

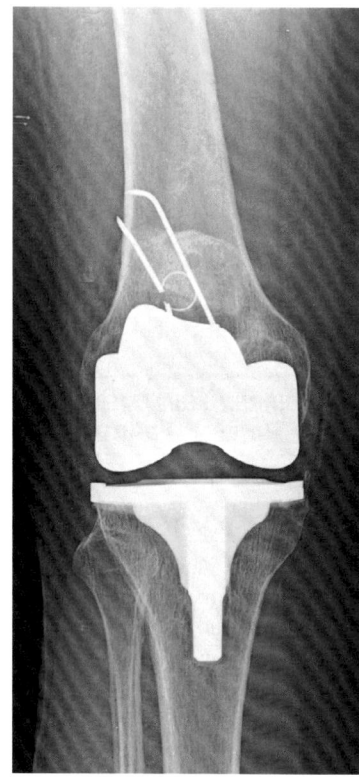

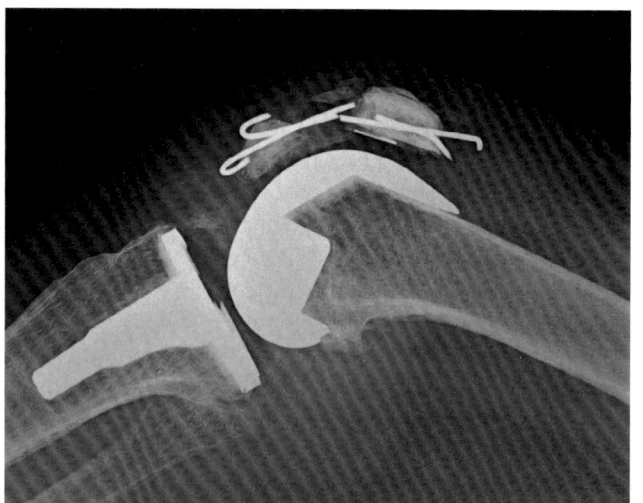

FIGURE 23-30 (*continued*)

C

D

strategy that takes longer to complete but may ultimately result in fewer complications. When acute operative management is undertaken in the face of a stable component, we have a low threshold for excision of small- to moderate-sized superior or inferior pole fragments with suture repair of the associated tendon to the remaining bone. Patellectomy is our operative treatment of choice for cases with a loose prosthesis and poor bone stock.

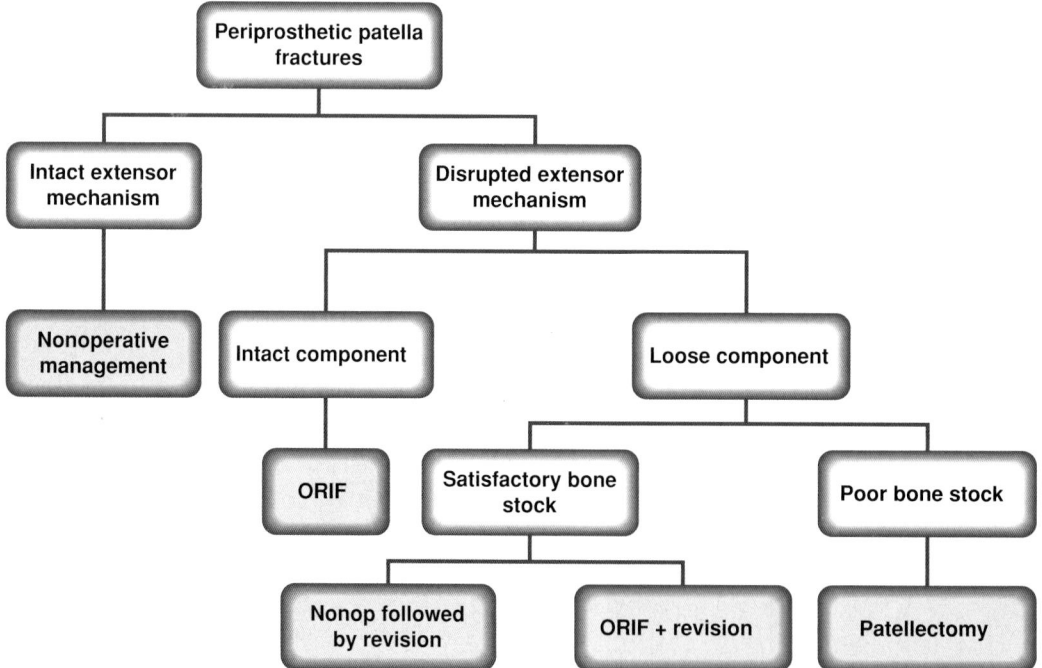

FIGURE 23-31 Algorithm depicting the author's preferred method of treatment for periprosthetic patella fractures.

PERIPROSTHETIC PROXIMAL TIBIA FRACTURES

Incidence, Risk Factors, and Prevention of Periprosthetic Proximal Tibia Fractures

Tibia Fractures About Total Knee Components

Periprosthetic tibia fractures about TKA are uncommon. An analysis of fractures about TKAs from the Mayo Clinic Joint Registry published in 1999 indicated that postoperative tibia fracture occurred in 0.4% of cases after primary TKA and 0.9% of cases after revision TKA.[16] Intraoperative fractures, in this series, were found to occur in 0.67% of primary and 0.8% of revision TKAs. These data should be interpreted with caution because they do not include postoperative fractures treated at institutions other than the Mayo Clinic and the duration of follow-up was not presented. In a more recent report of 17,389 primary TKAs performed between 1985 and 2005, intraoperative tibia fracture was found to be much less common than the Mayo experience: fracture occurred in 18 of the 17,389 cases (0.1%).[3]

Nonspecific etiologic factors related to periprosthetic tibia fractures are similar to those described in the prior section regarding periprosthetic patella fractures and include poor bone quality. BMD in the tibia below the tibial component has been shown to progressively decrease at 3 years follow-up after arthroplasty.[215,289]

Local risk factors for periprosthetic tibia fractures may be related to technique as well as to implant design. The largest series of periprosthetic tibial fractures around loose prostheses was reported by Rand and Coventry.[223] They reported that all 15 knees had varus axial malalignment when compared to a control group. Similar studies have confirmed that varus malalignment may be a potential risk factor for periprosthetic tibial fracture.[170,293] Osteotomy of the tibial tubercle facilitates exposure for the very stiff knee but it reduces the structural integrity of the proximal tibia. In a small series of nine TKAs with tibial tubercle osteotomy, Ritter et al.[233] reported two proximal tibia fractures. Both cases occurred soon after surgery (within 2 months) and each healed with nonoperative management. Any prior bony defects, such as from patellar tendon donor sites or tunnels associated with anterior cruciate ligament reconstructions, are additional risk factors for fracture of the tibia. Prior fracture malunion and holes from prior fixation devices for high tibial osteotomy or tibial plateau fracture fixation pose stress risers and are also potential sites for fracture.

Fracture associated with uncemented insertion of the low-contact stress (LCS) knee system tibial component has been reported.[274] The technique used for implantation of this prosthesis, reaming a conical hole for the tibial stem without impaction and absence of trialing, rather than the implant itself may have been causative.

Tibia Fractures About Unicompartmental Components

A small number of tibia fractures associated with unicompartmental knee arthroplasty have been reported including both intraoperative and postoperative fractures.[146,239,284] Suggested risk factors include broaching the posterior cortex during preparation of the tibia,[257] using multiple guide pinholes in the proximal tibia,[27] an extended vertical saw cut,[239] improper component positioning, malalignment, loosening,[74] and obesity.[239] A biomechanical study indicates that extending the vertical cut posteriorly by increasing the sagittal plane cut angle caudally by just 10 degrees reduces fracture load by 30%.[44]

Classification of Periprosthetic Proximal Tibia Fracture

Location of the fracture, stability of the implant, and timing of the fracture (intra- or postoperative) are incorporated into the classification of periprosthetic tibia fractures according to Felix et al.[74,266] Type I fractures occur in the tibial plateau. Postoperative fractures of this type were thought to be stress fractures related to loosening or malalignment of the component. These were a common fracture type prior to introduction of keeled components. Type II fractures are adjacent to the stem tip and are generally related to trauma in the setting of osteolysis. Type III fractures are distal to the prosthesis, and Type IV involve the tibial tubercle. Subtype A has a well-fixed implant, subtype B has a loose implant, and subtype C occur intraoperatively (Table 23-25) (Fig. 23-32).

Management of Periprosthetic Proximal Tibia Fractures

Management of Tibia Fractures About Total Knee Components

On the occasion where periprosthetic tibia fracture is associated with a well-fixed component, nonoperative management with a cast or brace is indicated for nondisplaced fractures. If cast management is chosen, great care should be taken to monitor for pressure sores especially in patients with RA and those with diabetes. Maintenance of limb alignment is important;

TABLE 23-25 **Classification for Periprosthetic Tibia Fractures**

Classification	Type I	Type II	Type III	Type IV
Fracture Location	Tibial plateau	Adjacent to stem	Distal to prosthesis	Tibial tubercle
Subtype				
A	Prosthesis well fixed	Prosthesis well fixed	Prosthesis well fixed	Prosthesis well fixed
B	Prosthesis loose	Prosthesis loose	Prosthesis loose	Prosthesis loose
C	Intraoperative	Intraoperative	Intraoperative	Intraoperative

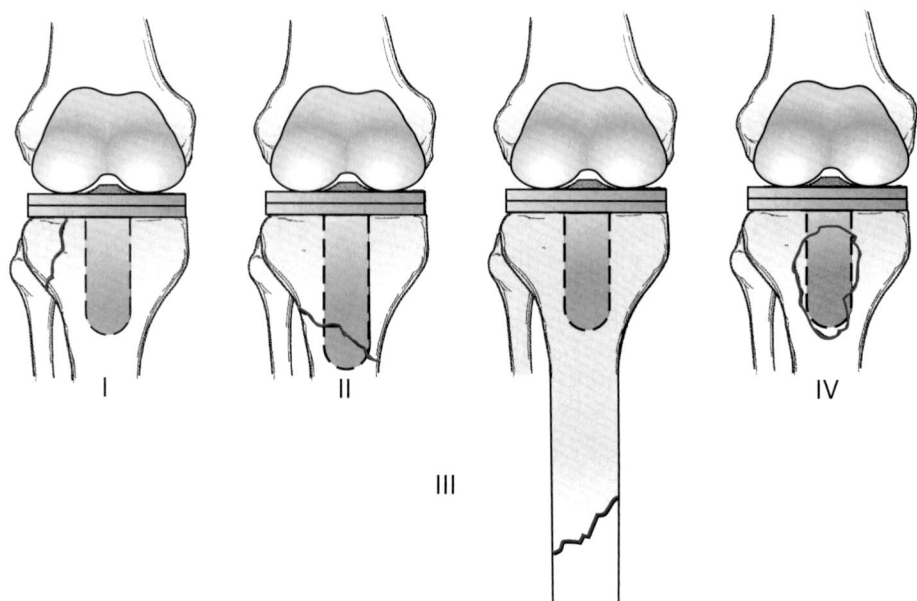

FIGURE 23-32 Classification scheme for periprosthetic tibia fractures about a TKA: Type I fractures involve only a small portion of the tibial plateau; type II fractures are about the stem; type III fractures are distal to the stem; and Type IV fractures are of the tibial tubercle. The subtypes are described in Table 25.

therefore, frequent, usually weekly, radiographic surveillance is advisable with conversion to ORIF for failure to maintain satisfactory alignment. As with any other immobilized joint, arthrofibrosis is a potential risk factor.

ORIF is indicated for displaced periprosthetic proximal tibia fractures associated with a well-fixed component. ORIF is advisable for displaced fractures involving the metaphyseal–diaphyseal junction (Fig. 23-33). Plate and screw constructs

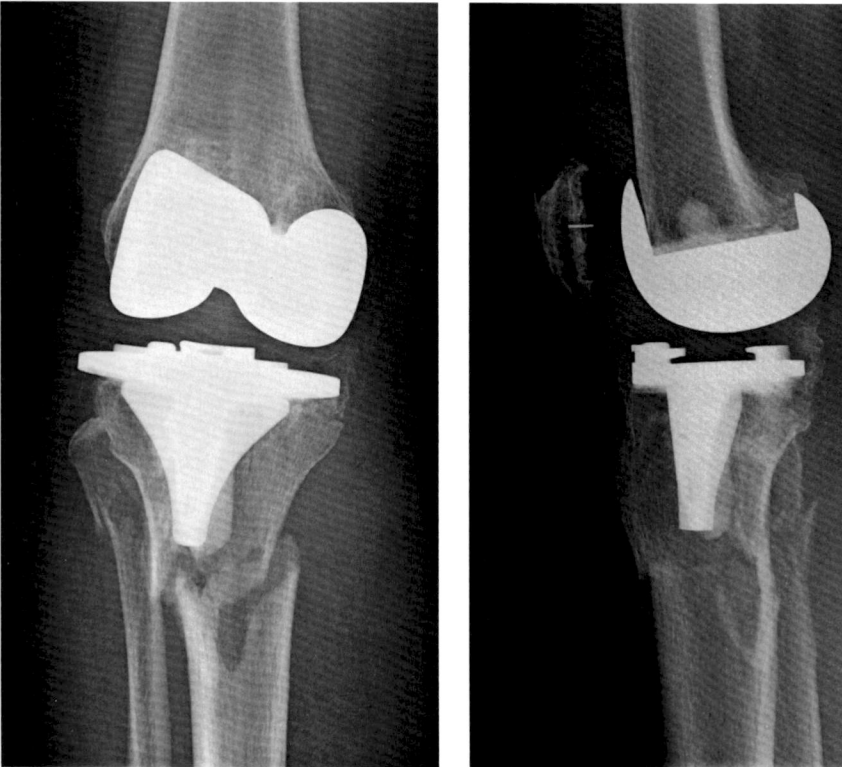

FIGURE 23-33 A periprosthetic proximal tibia fracture **(A, B)** treated with a lateral proximal tibia locking plate that is supplemented with a posterior lateral plate **(C, D)**.

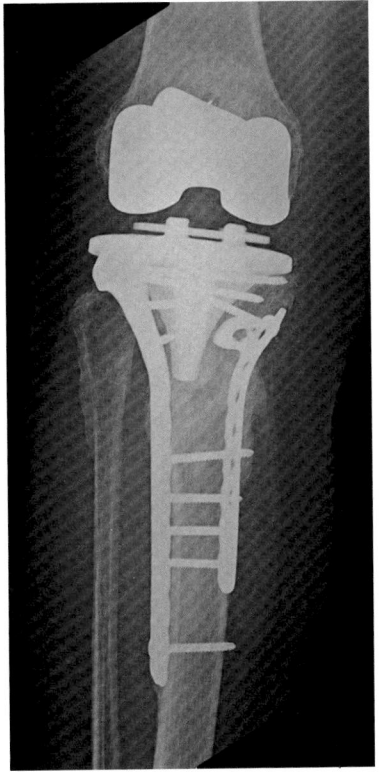
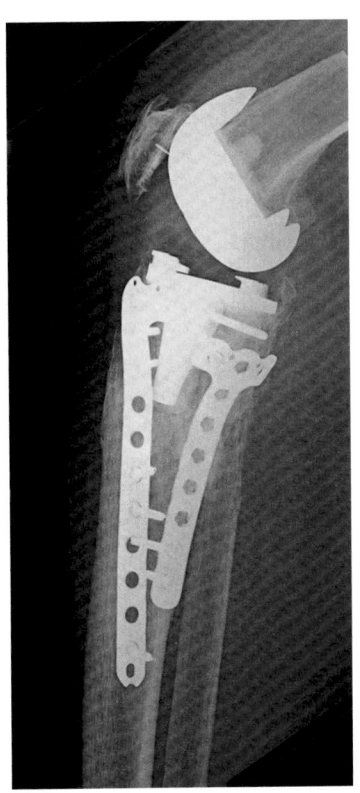

FIGURE 23-33 (*continued*)   **C**   **D**

are limited by the available bone proximally to pass bicortical screws. This is highly dependent upon the prosthesis design with regard to the degree of metaphyseal filling. The inability to pass multiple screws across the proximal fragment can lead to insufficient fixation and calls for adjunctive fixation with unicortical locked screws, cables, secondary posterior-medial plates, or some combination thereof (Fig. 23-34). This scenario

is common, so the surgeon should be prepared to deal with marginal fixation in the proximal fragment afforded by a lateral plate and screw construct. A medial plate usually adds sufficient stability even when a limited number of proximal fixation points are obtained.

Fractures in the midtibial shaft, distal to a tibial component, are typically treated with ORIF, especially when associated with

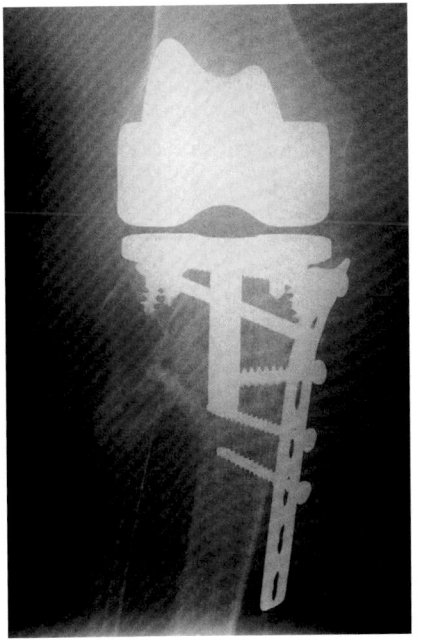
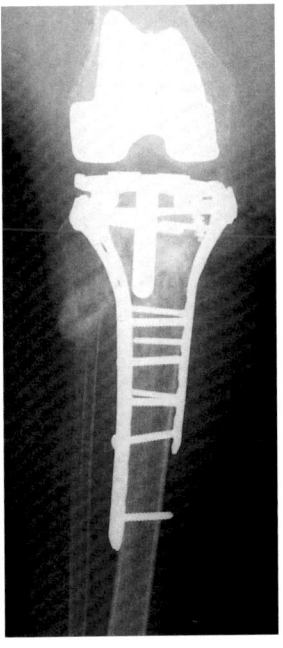

FIGURE 23-34 A periprosthetic proximal tibial fracture treated with a single medial plate that offered marginal fixation progresses to nonunion **(A)** that is treated successfully with a combination of lateral locked plating, posterior-medial locked plating, bone grafting, and adjuvant BMP **(B)**.   **A**   **B**

stemmed components (Fig. 23-35). When a nonstemmed THA component is present, IMN of tibial shaft fractures can be successfully performed (Fig. 23-36). Care must be taken to assure there is adequate space for the nail anterior to the tibial component so that the tibial tubercle is not disturbed (Fig. 23-36C).

Tibial fractures associated with loose components are best treated with revision arthroplasty, frequently utilizing a long stem to bypass the fracture.[11,71,74] It is wise to have an entire revision system available, because, often the femoral component will need to be revised as well for sizing, constraint, exposure, or gap balancing reasons. Often these fractures are associated with extensive osteolysis and therefore may require structural or morselized bone grafting, the use of metal wedges, or in the most severe cases proximal tibial megaprosthesis or allograft-prosthetic composites. Maximizing host bone support is critical for a good result. General principles for arthroplasty treatment of periprosthetic tibia fractures include the use of stem extensions with either metaphyseal cementation or longer, diaphyseal press-fit strategies. More contemporary techniques utilize metaphyseal-filling sleeves that provide rotational and axial stability, however, long-term data on such reconstructions is lacking.

Specific technical considerations include careful soft tissue dissection and retraction to minimize soft tissue trauma to the already compromised skin flaps. The anteromedial capsule is a major source of wound-healing problems or postoperative drainage. If there is a deficiency in this area that cannot be approximated well, a gastrocnemius flap may be indicated. The extensor mechanism and its insertion along the proximal tibia is a crucial consideration. The tibial tuberosity can be osteotomized and repaired for exposure or repaired directly to the

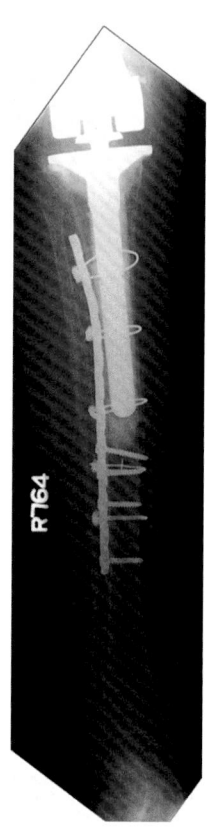

FIGURE 23-35 A fracture about a well-fixed stemmed tibial component of a TKA had a previously untreated perforation near the tip of the stem. This was managed with a lateral plate and an anterior medial strut allograft.

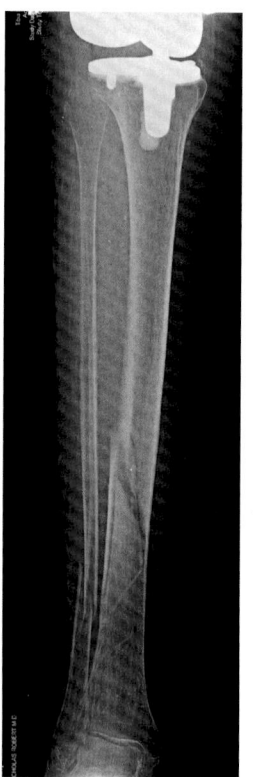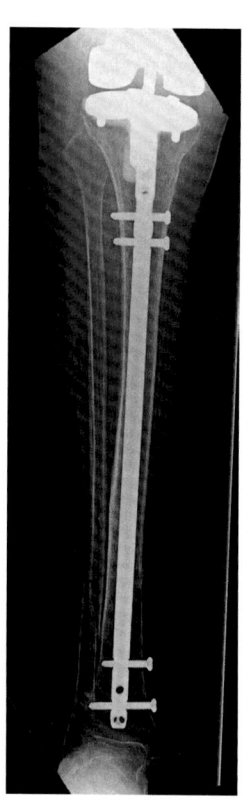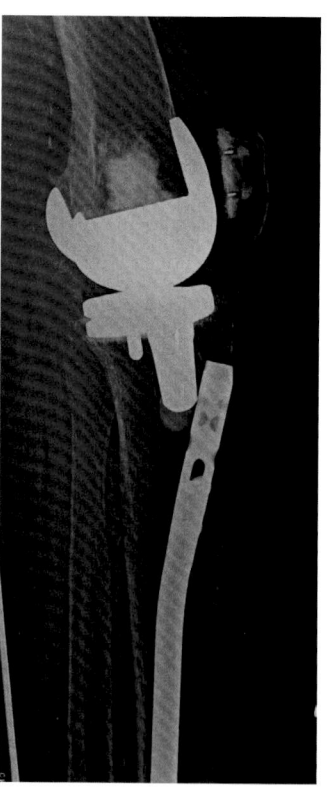

A, B

C

FIGURE 23-36 A tibial shaft fracture below a nonstemmed TKA **(A)** is treated with an IM nail **(B)**. Note that there must be sufficient space between the tibial component and the nail **(C)** to allow insertion without disturbing the tibial tubercle.

implant for proximal tibial replacement prosthesis. It is important that the surgeon undertaking these reconstructions be experienced in both revision arthroplasty techniques and fracture management techniques to achieve a successful outcome.

Management of Tibia Fractures About Unicompartmental Components

Tibia fractures about unicompartmental knee arthroplasties can be managed in a variety of ways including with nonoperative means,[14] ORIF,[239,257] and revision to TKA.[27,167,284] There is very little literature available at this point to guide decision making, therefore general principles of periprosthetic fracture management must be relied upon. Under usual circumstances, stable fractures with stable components can be managed nonoperatively,[14] unstable fractures with stable components can be managed with ORIF,[239,257] and any fracture associated with an unstable component would demand revision arthroplasty,[27,167,284] typically revision to a TKA. As with native medial tibial plateau fractures, nondisplaced periprosthetic fractures of the medial plateau about a unicompartmental component have a propensity to displace over time. Therefore careful observation is warranted and changes in fracture alignment should prompt consideration of operative management as progressive displacement of these fractures is common.

Outcomes for Periprosthetic Proximal Tibia Fractures

There is exceedingly little published literature regarding outcomes after periprosthetic proximal tibia fracture after TKA. Felix et al.,[74] in 1997, reported on a large series of 102 fractures. The majority of types I and II fractures were associated with loose prostheses and were treated successfully with revision arthroplasty. Fractures associated with well-fixed components were managed with the usual principles of tibia fracture management of that time period.

Several case reports demonstrate isolated results for various methods of treating tibia fractures about unicompartmental knee arthroplasties but few describe much detail or long-term outcomes. Berger et al.[14] presented results of 38 patients followed for 10 years after unicompartmental knee arthroplasty. Three patients had tibial plateau fractures, two noted intraoperatively and one that occurred intraoperatively, but was not recognized until the first postoperative visit. All were treated nonoperatively, healed, and had a good ultimate outcome. Rudol et al.[239] described a postoperative, and Sloper et al.[257] an intraoperative, vertical medial tibial plateau fracture, each treated successfully with buttress plating.[239] Pandit et al.[208] described eight fractures about a unicompartmental knee arthroplasty treated in a variety of ways resulting in a variety of outcomes. Two minimally displaced fractures were treated nonoperatively, healed, and had good outcomes with retained unicompartmental components at either 1 or 3 years. Three others failed nonoperative management and ultimately required conversion to TKA. Two of these three also failed intermediate surgical management of their nonunited fractures, but all three had good outcomes at between 1 and 4 years. Two others had occult fractures that upon initial diagnosis had already subsided and these two patients were managed with conversion to TKA and were with

TABLE 23-26 Periprosthetic Proximal Tibia Fractures

Potential Pitfalls and Preventions

Pitfalls	Preventions
Loss of proximal fixation after ORIF	Medial and lateral locked plates Maximize number of locked screws in proximal fragment
Skin necrosis	Maintain adequate skin bridge between incisions
Devitalization of bone	Minimize soft tissue stripping from bone Use multiple incisions

good results at 2 years. The eighth patient in the series was treated to union with a buttress plate and had a good result at 2 years. Van Loon et al.[284] reported three cases where revision to TKA was performed either immediately after intraoperative fracture ($n = 1$), after initial ORIF ($n = 1$), or after nonoperative management ($n = 1$). The precise indications for conversion to TKA were not identified in this report, but were related to pain and reduced mobility in the latter two cases. Follow-up was 2 years or less and results at this short follow-up were mixed.

Potential Pitfalls and Preventative Measures for Management of Periprosthetic Proximal Tibia Fractures

Obtaining adequate fixation during ORIF of periprosthetic proximal tibia fractures can be a challenge (Table 23-26). The tibial component often fills a substantial volume of the proximal tibial metaphysis, making placement of bicortical screws difficult or impossible. Dual plating of these fractures is often required to obtain adequate fracture stability. Care must be taken to maintain adequate skin bridges between medial and lateral incisions used for ORIF and any anterior incision pre-existing from the knee arthroplasty. The medial incision can be placed sufficiently posterior to minimize risk of skin necrosis while still allowing adequate exposure for posterior-medial plating. Despite the potential risk for skin necrosis, using multiple incisions is still preferred to extensive deep dissection through fewer incisions.

AUTHOR'S PREFERRED TREATMENT OF PERIPROSTHETIC TIBIA FRACTURES

Fortunately, periprosthetic tibia fractures around TKAs are relatively uncommon (Fig. 23-37). When they do occur, most often they are associated with a loose tibial component; therefore revision is preferred in these situations. Tibial revision for periprosthetic fracture requires the routine use of stems and augments and metaphyseal-filling metal implants can be useful for managing bone deficiencies. The tibial base trays have often subsided into varus, and anticipating medial and central defects is wise. The surgeon should be aware that isolated tibial

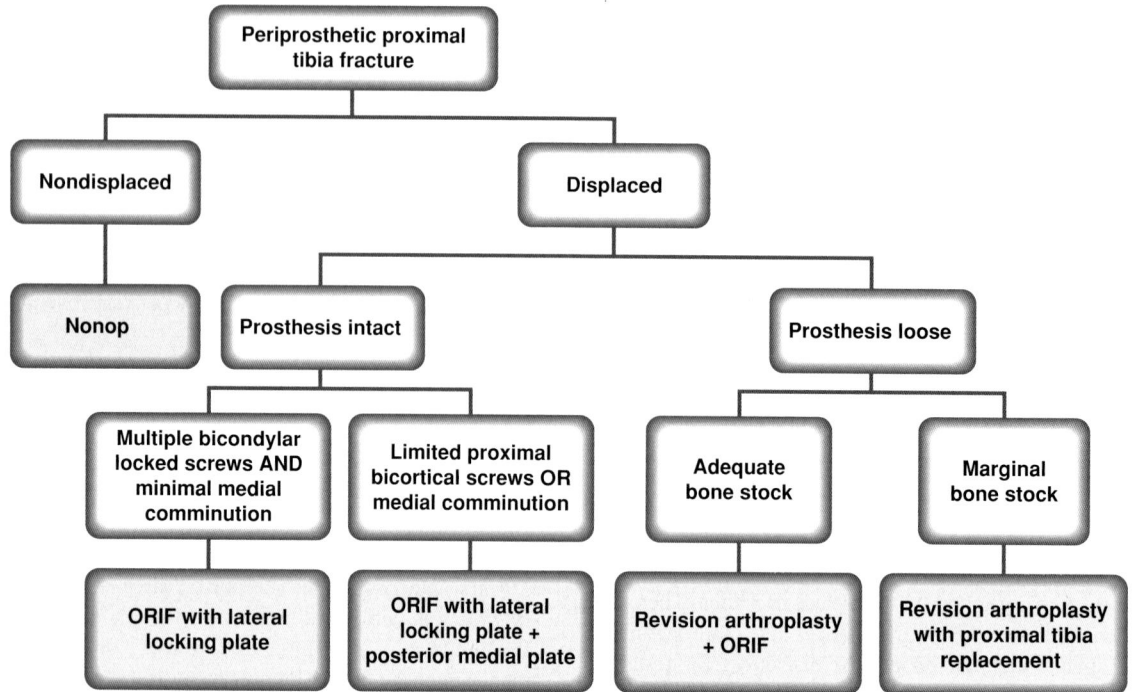

FIGURE 23-37 Algorithm depicting the author's preferred method of treatment for periprosthetic proximal tibia fractures.

component revision is rare, and commonly, one should be prepared to revise the entire arthroplasty.

When the tibial component is stable and the fracture displaced, our preferred method of treatment is with lateral locked plates. Although there is scant literature supporting this or any other practice for these fractures, it is our feeling that locked plates are invaluable for these fractures. The amount and quality of bone proximally is usually marginal and in these situations nonlocked screws rarely obtain adequate fixation. Locked screws proximally and either locked or nonlocked screws distally through a lateral plate may provide sufficient stability. We, however, have a low threshold to supplement a lateral plate with a posterior-medial locked plate (Figs. 23-33 and 23-34). Medial comminution and an inability to pass lateral screws across to the medial side are indications for dual plating. It is critical that these exposures be through separate incisions so as to maximally preserve the soft tissue envelope. Even in the presence of a midline incision from the TKA, separate lateral and medial incisions can provide an adequate skin bridge in all but the thinnest of patients.

PERIPROSTHETIC FRACTURES ABOUT ANKLE ARTHROPLASTY

Incidence, Risk Factors, and Prevention of Periprosthetic Fractures About Ankle Arthroplasty

There have been a number of reports of malleolar fractures complicating total ankle arthroplasty (TAA), but no large series have been published to date clearly elucidating specific etiologic factors or classification schemes.[108,152,181,197,242,248,295] One risk

factor, however, seems to be clear. Multiple studies have demonstrated that intraoperative fractures of the malleoli decrease with increasing surgeon experience with the procedure. Lee et al.[152] and Myerson and Mroczek[197] each compared results of their first 25 TAA cases to their next 25. Both showed substantial reduction in intraoperative malleolar fractures with experience: Lee had four fractures among the first 25 cases (16%) and one in the subsequent 25 (4%), and Myerson had five from the initial group (20%) and two from the second group (8%). These results are similar to those of several other authors. Haskell and Mann[108] found a reduction in intraoperative fracture from 12% in the initial 50 cases to 9% in the subsequent 137 cases, and Schuberth et al.[248] reported 19 intraoperative fractures from 50 cases (38%) and noted that this complication decreased with experience.

The medial malleolus is the most common site of intraoperative fracture, occurring approximately twice as frequently as lateral malleolus fracture.[63,108,181,242,295] In a series of 93 TAAs performed for inflammatory joint disease, there were 27 intraoperative fractures: 15 of the medial malleolus, 7 of the anterolateral distal tibia, and 5 of the lateral malleolus.[63]

Although the vast majority of periprosthetic fractures about TAAs occur intraoperatively (Fig. 23-38), postoperative malleolar fracture has been reported.[63,100,108,181,295] Wood and Deakin[295] had 10 postoperative fractures occurring between 3 days and 23 months postoperatively in their series of 200 TAAs. Two of the 10 were associated with implant loosening. Doets et al.[63] reported four fractures occurring between 4 and 6 months postoperatively in a series of 93 TAAs performed in patients with inflammatory joint disease. Severe osteopenia was noted in all four patients with postoperative fractures.

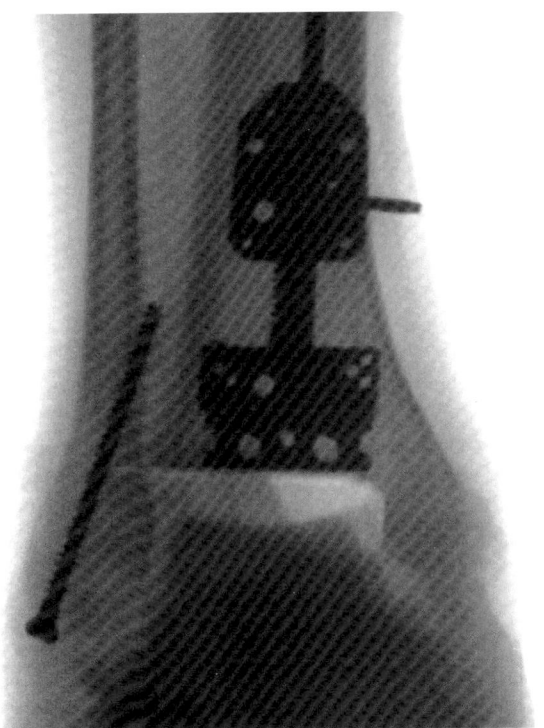
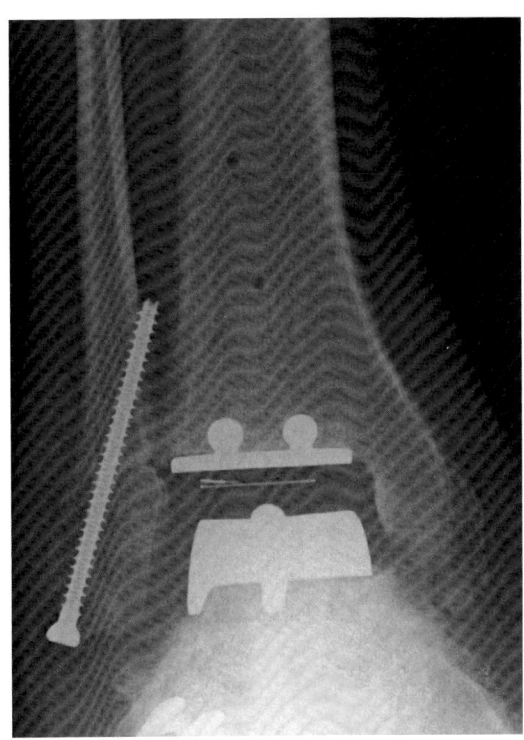

A   **B**

FIGURE 23-38 An intraoperative lateral malleolus fracture related to inadvertent saw cut of the lateral malleolus **(A)** heals with screw fixation **(B)**.

Management and Outcomes of Periprosthetic Fractures About Ankle Arthroplasty

There are no accepted standards for treatment of periprosthetic fractures about TAA. However, the general principles of management of other periprosthetic fractures can be applied. Fracture union, implant stability, and re-establishment of any associated loss of bone stock are general goals of management with the hope of restoring baseline function. Several authors describe internal fixation for intraoperative malleolar fractures that compromised implant stability[108,181] and yet others treated many of these fractures nonoperatively.[152,197,295] Nonunion occurred after intraoperative fracture in one of six nonoperatively treated from one study[108] and in one of five treated with ORIF from another.[181] Either screw fixation or cast immobilization was used for treatment of 27 intraoperative fractures in the series of Doets et al.[63] Six of 15 with medial malleolar fractures, one of seven with anterolateral distal tibia fractures, and two of five with lateral malleolar fractures were treated with screw fixation. Among these patients, two with medial malleolar fractures were ultimately considered failures.

Most postoperative fractures are also of the malleolus and are typically treated nonoperatively unless associated with implant loosening or osteolysis.[108,181,295] A very small number of displaced postoperative fractures of the distal tibia metaphysis associated with TAA, six to the best of our knowledge, have been reported.[63,100,301] Each was associated with a stemmed tibial component. Treatment with either an anterolateral or medial locked plate in two cases that were associated with trauma

mimicked standard treatment of a native extra-articular distal tibia fracture.[100,301]

Periprosthetic ankle fractures are uncommonly dealt with, except by those surgeons who perform a high volume of TAAs, especially since the majority of these fractures occur intraoperatively (Fig. 23-39). When an intraoperative fracture is encountered, ORIF is preferred, except for the most minimally displaced fracture, to maximize stability of the arthroplasty. Postoperative fractures about stable implants are treated operatively with ORIF when the fracture potentially affects joint stability or when displacement is great enough to risk nonunion with nonoperative treatment.

PERIPROSTHETIC FRACTURES ABOUT SHOULDER ARTHROPLASTY

Incidence, Risk Factors, and Prevention of Periprosthetic Fractures About Shoulder Arthroplasty

Humeral Shaft Fractures About Stemmed Shoulder Arthroplasty Components

Fractures of the humerus associated with total shoulder arthroplasty (TSA) or hemiarthroplasty occur with intermediate

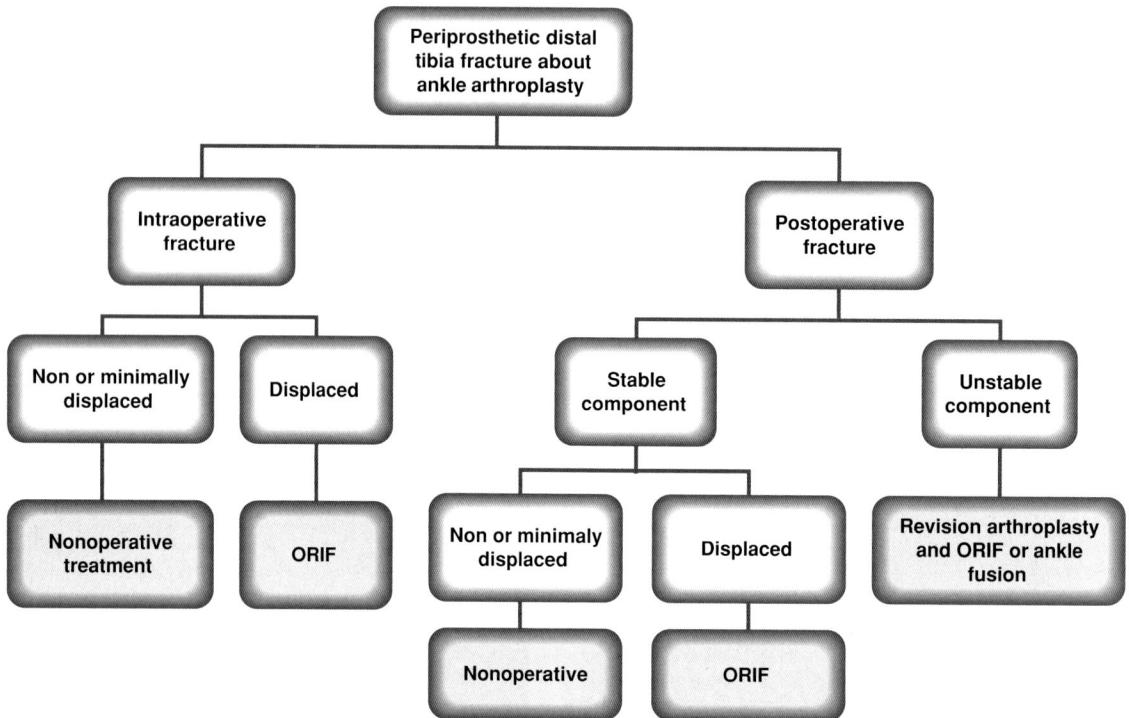

FIGURE 23-39 Algorithm depicting the author's preferred method of treatment for periprosthetic fractures about a total ankle arthroplasty.

frequency relative to other periprosthetic fractures. Among series that focus exclusively on fractures that occurred postoperatively, the incidence has been remarkably consistent at between 0.6% and 2.3%.[23,147,296,297] With only limited data to rely on, the incidence of intraoperative fracture may be substantially higher. Two studies that distinguish between intraoperative and postoperative fractures both found two times more fractures occurred intraoperatively.[32,95] A recent study focusing on intraoperative fractures found the rate of humeral fracture after primary shoulder arthroplasty to be 1.7% and the rate during revision arthroplasty to be 3.3%.[10] Of the 45 fractures in this report, 19 were of the greater tuberosity, 16 of the humeral shaft, 6 of the metaphysis, 3 of the greater tuberosity with shaft extension, and one that included the greater and lesser tuberosities.

Many risk factors for fracture have been postulated, but the limited number of fractures in most series, usually less than 10, makes scientific analysis impossible. It is logical, however, that conditions that further weaken a bone that already has a stress riser would put that patient at a particularly high risk of fracture after even minor trauma.

RA has been implicated as a significant risk factor. In Boyd's series of seven postoperative fractures, five patients had RA. The incidence of fracture among those treated with their initial arthroplasty because of RA (1.8%), however, was only slightly higher than for those treated for other diagnoses (1.5%). Studies from the Mayo Clinic, where a large proportion of patients had a primary diagnosis of RA have shown higher incidences of fracture among patients with RA. Wright and Cofield[297] reported on nine postoperative fractures from a cohort of 499, 144 of whom had RA. The incidence of fracture was 3.4% among those

with RA and 1.1% among the rest. A more recent study from the Mayo Clinic that included a larger cohort of patients found a relatively low overall incidence of postoperative fracture of 0.6%, 19 fractures among 3,091 patients.[147] The proportion of fractures that occurred in patients with RA was high (31%) but the relative numbers of patients in the entire cohort who had RA were not reported, so evaluation of RA as a risk factor is not possible.

Osteopenia or severe cortical thinning has been cited as a risk factor for periprosthetic humeral fracture, especially among patients with revision arthroplasty stems.[32,95,261] Is should be noted, however, that such statements have been made with indirect data regarding the degree of osteopenia in some series.[32,95] Campbell et al.[32] quantified the degree of osteopenia as the ratio of the combined width of the middiaphyseal cortices to the diameter of the diaphysis. Normal bone was considered to have a ratio of greater than 50%, mild osteopenia had a ratio of between 25% and 50%, and severe osteopenia less than 25%. Although the validity of these criteria and definitions is unsubstantiated, Campbell et al. found 25% of 20 patients with a fracture had normal bone, 45% mild osteopenia, and 30% severe osteopenia. It is useful to note that their 75% prevalence of osteopenia in this cohort is very high; however, without data on the bone quality of those without fracture, it is inaccurate to conclude that this truly represents a risk factor for fracture. Kumar et al.[147] also utilized this system to grade bone quality and found all of their patients with fracture had osteopenia (44% severe). The presence or degree of osteopenia has not been correlated with a particular injury mechanism or a particular treatment strategy. It seems intuitive, however, that any treatment algorithm in a patient with severely compromised bone stock should include consideration of minimizing the presence of stress risers in the final fracture treatment construct to avoid subsequent additional fractures.

Other implicated risk factors for postoperative fracture, advanced age and female gender,[180] are also limited by a lack of data for patients without fracture. When such data is available, age does not appear to be substantially different in those with and without fracture. The average age of all 3,091 patients who had undergone shoulder arthroplasty at the Mayo Clinic between 1976 and 2001 was 63 years and the age of those who sustained a fracture was also 63 years.[147] The female-to-male ratio was slightly higher in those with fracture (63%) compared to the entire group (56%).

A number of technical issues may relate to intraoperative fracture. Most of these relate to manipulations of the humerus during surgical exposure or to preparation of the canal with reamers or an oversized broach.[32,95] Excessive external rotation required to provide exposure in patients with large muscles or scars was causative for half of all intraoperative fractures in one series.[32] In half of the cases with fracture associated with external rotation, over reaming of the diaphysis caused notching of the endosteum resulting in a stress riser for spiral fracture formation during subsequent external rotation. Hoop stresses associated with an oversized broach or prosthesis can cause transverse or oblique fractures.[32,95] Fracture during revision shoulder arthroplasty may be intentional[32] as the least destructive method to remove a stem. Unintentional fracture may also occur during explantation of the prosthesis, removal of associated cement, or during implantation of the revision prosthesis.

Treatment of periprosthetic humeral shaft fractures, as much as any other periprosthetic fracture, starts with prevention of intraoperative fracture. Steps include detailed preoperative planning particularly with regard to templating stem diameter. This requires good quality preoperative radiographs taking into account magnification. Substantive soft tissue releases reduce risk of fracture by reducing stresses that accompany arm manipulations during arthroplasty. Capsular contractures as well as scar formations in the subacromial and subdeltoid spaces should be addressed to allow gentle delivery of the bone so stress-free preparation and implantation can occur. Proper sizing of the implant and meticulous care to be colinear with the long axis of the bone during canal preparation will help to avoid perforation. Small perforations that are diagnosed intraoperatively can easily be treated with a stem that bypasses the defect by two or more bone diameters. There should be a low threshold for intraoperative radiographs to assure a split that propagated distally did not accompany the perforation, as this might require additional treatment to stabilize the distal extent of such a fracture.

Humeral Fracture About Resurfacing Shoulder Arthroplasty Components

Periprosthetic fracture of the humerus after resurfacing has been reported infrequently.[126,273] One case occurred intraoperatively and was managed successfully without operation.[273] Another reported case occurred postoperatively secondary to a fall and resulted in a surgical neck fracture. Initial nonoperative management was abandoned in favor of ORIF with a locked

plate because of progressive displacement.[126] These authors point out that the specific design of the resurfacing implant may dictate treatment. The Epoca prosthesis involved in their case is a shell-like design that allowed screws to penetrate the head fragment. Other resurfacing designs would make screw placement more challenging and would therefore make revision to a stemmed humeral component more attractive. It is also unclear how the risk or consequence of avascular necrosis after ORIF of these fractures would affect outcome.

Fractures About Reverse Shoulder Arthroplasty

Acromial fracture after a reverse TSA has been reported in several series.[52,80,109,159] These fractures are generally atraumatic and are associated with stress on the deltoid origin and are therefore often nondisplaced or minimally displaced. They occur relatively commonly, with a prevalence of up to 10%,[52,80,159] but can be missed on plain radiographs[159] and therefore may be underreported. When suspected, based on pain or tenderness along the acromion or scapular spine, a CT scan is indicated when plain films are negative.

Classification of Periprosthetic Fractures About Shoulder Arthroplasty

Classification of Periprosthetic Humeral Fractures About Shoulder Arthroplasty

Several classification schemes have been reported for periprosthetic humeral shaft fractures about shoulder arthroplasty stems. Most distinguish fractures by their location relative to the tip of the stem,[32,95,297] and a smaller subset account for fractures of the tuberosities or the stability of the stem.[296] None are universally accepted. Wright and Cofield[297] described three fracture patterns occurring in their series of nine postoperative fractures, type A centered at the tip of the stem and extending proximally more than one-third the length of the stem, type B also centered at the tip of the stem but with less proximal extension, and type C involved the distal humeral diaphysis, distal to the tip of the stem, extending into the metaphysis. Campbell et al.[32] categorized fractures into one of four regions. Region 1 included the greater or lesser tuberosities, region 2 the proximal metaphysis, region 3 the proximal humeral diaphysis, and region 4 the mid- and distal diaphysis. They classified their 21 fractures based on the distal most fracture extent. Groh et al.,[95] like Wright and Cofield, classified fractures of the shaft into three types. Type I occur proximal to the tip of the prosthesis, type II fractures originate proximal to the tip and extend distal to it, and type III fractures originate below the tip. Worland et al.[296] considered each fracture location, fracture obliquity, and implant stability. They also made treatment recommendations based on the fracture classification. Types A, B, and C were designated by the location of the fracture: A about the tuberosities, B around the stem, and C well distal to the stem. Type B fractures were subdivided: B1 fractures were spiral with a stable stem; B2 were transverse or short oblique with a stable stem; and B3 were any fracture associated with a loose stem. Their recommended treatment was very general, with conservative management or ORIF recommended for all but B2 and B3 types where long stem revision was recommended.

Classification of Scapular Fracture About Shoulder Arthroplasty

Two classification systems have been reported for periprosthetic acromial fractures associated with reverse shoulder arthroplasty.[52,159] Levy et al.[159] described type I acromial fractures as distal and involving the anterior and middle deltoid origin, type II fractures as being of the central portion of the acromion and involving at least the entire middle deltoid origin, and type III fractures being of the base of the acromion and involving the entire middle and posterior deltoid origin. This classification scheme was based on evaluation of 16 fractures. Five of these fractures were not evident on plain radiographs and required CT for diagnosis. The interobserver reliability was found to be excellent.

Because of the relative rarity of periprosthetic fractures about glenoid components and an absence of large series dealing with them, no generally accepted fracture classification exists for these fractures.

Management of Periprosthetic Fractures About Shoulder Arthroplasty

Management of Intraoperative Periprosthetic Tuberosity Fractures

Nondisplaced or minimally displaced fractures of the lesser tuberosity can occur with some frequency during placement of the trial humeral component. Treatment of these is generally with suture repair using heavy nonabsorbable sutures placed through the subscapularis tendon and either through or around the lesser tuberosity then into the adjacent intact bone on the other side of the fracture. Similarly, cracks about the greater tuberosity are stabilized with sutures to assure displacement does not ensue.

Management of Periprosthetic Humeral Shaft Fractures

Humeral shaft fractures are treated with goals of uneventful fracture healing and implant stability (Table 23-27).[57,261] This can be accomplished by a variety of means. Intraoperative frac-

---

TABLE 23-27 **ORIF for Periprosthetic Humeral Shaft Fractures About Shoulder Arthroplasty**

Surgical Steps

- Develop plane between long and lateral heads of triceps
- Identify radial neurovascular bundle
- Split triceps distally
- Dissect plane between radial neurovascular bundle and posterior humerus
  - Debride fracture
- Reduce fracture and provisionally secure reduction with clamps, reduction plates, and/or cables
- Apply plate across fracture and beneath radial neurovascular bundle
  - Secure plate proximally with cables and distally with screws
- Confirm reduction and implant location with radiographs
- Close triceps fascia
- Close skin

---

tures of the shaft are carefully examined with intraoperative radiographs. A long-stemmed noncemented prosthesis with adjunctive cerclage cables is useful for spiral fractures. More transverse intraoperative fractures that are not amenable to cable stabilization are more appropriately treated with a long-stemmed prosthesis and either plate or strut stabilization. As with other diaphyseal periprosthetic fractures, when there is compromised bone stock, strut allografts are utilized.

Fractures that occur postoperatively can be treated nonoperatively if the implant is stable and the fracture is otherwise amenable to bracing (Fig. 23-40). This usually means the fracture is middiaphyseal, spiral, or short oblique (not transverse), and there is no drastic displacement, where interposed muscle may inhibit fracture healing. A lower threshold for surgical management of periprosthetic humerus fractures compared to similar fractures of the native humerus may be justified. Whether the presence of the humeral component stem inhibits fracture healing is unproven, but it is reasonable to assume that instrumentation of the humeral canal may negatively affect the endosteal blood supply. However, the degree and duration of such an effect as well as the clinical significance remains unclear. Nonetheless surgical management, especially for transverse or short oblique fractures (Fig. 23-41), is commonplace. The preferred exposure is through a posterior approach. This is extensile and allows visualization of the entire shaft of the humerus. Furthermore, this exposure allows clear identification and protection of the radial nerve during reduction and plating, and most importantly during cable fixation in the zone of the prosthesis. Applying cables through an anterior exposure is dangerous with regard to potential injury and entrapment of the radial nerve. Consideration is given to the timing of the fracture relative to the arthroplasty. When the fracture occurs shortly after joint replacement, surgical fixation offers better capability to perform shoulder rehabilitation and therefore a low threshold exists to treat these fractures operatively.

In the setting of a loose prosthesis with or without osteolysis, revision arthroplasty is indicated. A revision stem that crosses the fracture provides intramedullary stabilization and is usually accompanied by plate fixation in the absence of bone loss. Strut grafts (Fig. 23-42), with or without plates are used to restore any associated deficient bone stock. A noncemented technique is preferred whenever there is good quality bone to provide a reasonably tight fit. A low threshold for supplemental plate fixation is the norm. If either of the fragments has poor quality bone, a cemented technique can be utilized in that fragment (usually the distal fragment) and a noncemented technique in the other. When osteolysis is severe, either impaction bone grafting, an allograft–prosthesis composite, or a tumor prosthesis is utilized. These are extremely technically demanding cases that are individualized based on secondary factors and should be undertaken by surgeons and in centers familiar with and stocked with appropriate equipment, respectively.

Management of Periprosthetic Glenoid Fractures

Periprosthetic fractures of the glenoid most commonly occur intraoperatively and are related to retraction. A retractor that is placed on the posterior glenoid margin to retract the humerus

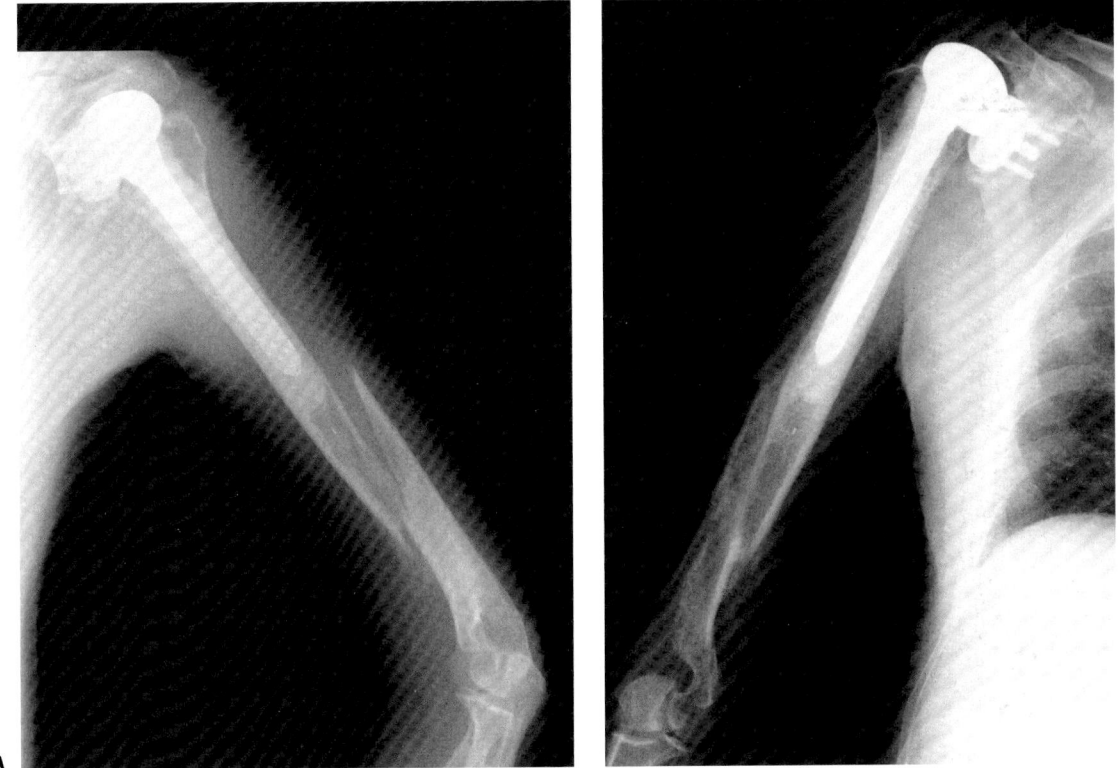

FIGURE 23-40 A humeral shaft fracture distal to a humeral prosthesis **(A)** treated nonoperatively to union **(B)**.

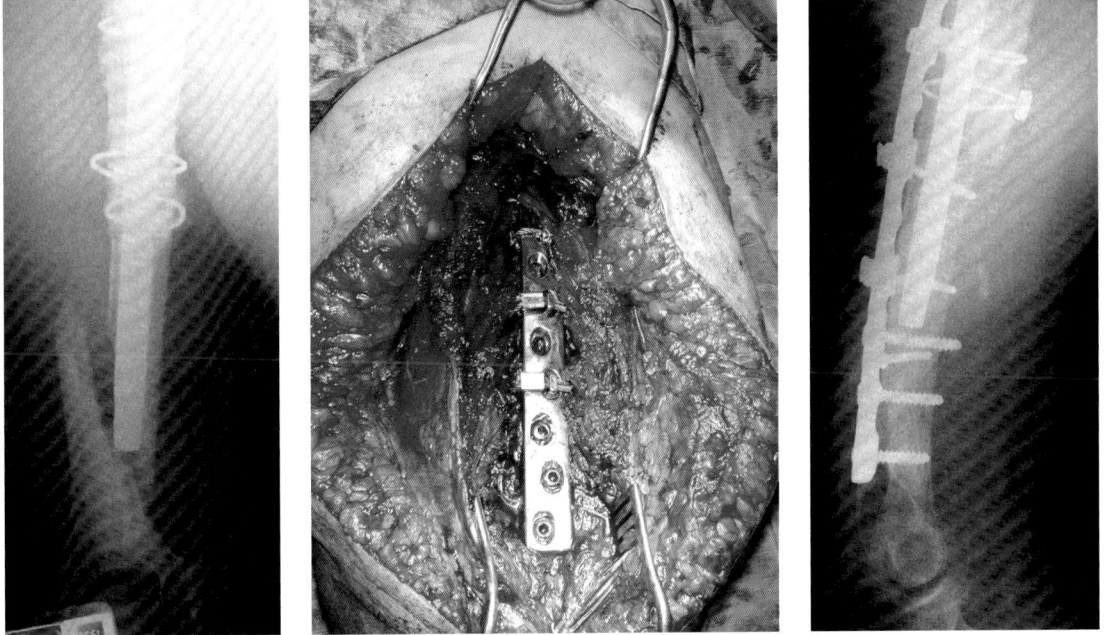

FIGURE 23-41 A periprosthetic humeral shaft fracture distal to a revision humeral component **(A)**. The proximal allograft was used previously during the revision arthroplasty. The acute periprosthetic fracture was treated via the posterior approach using biologic reduction techniques seen in an intra-operative photograph **(B)** that preserved the majority of the soft tissue attachments. A posterior plate with cables proximally and screws distally was used for fixation **(C)**.

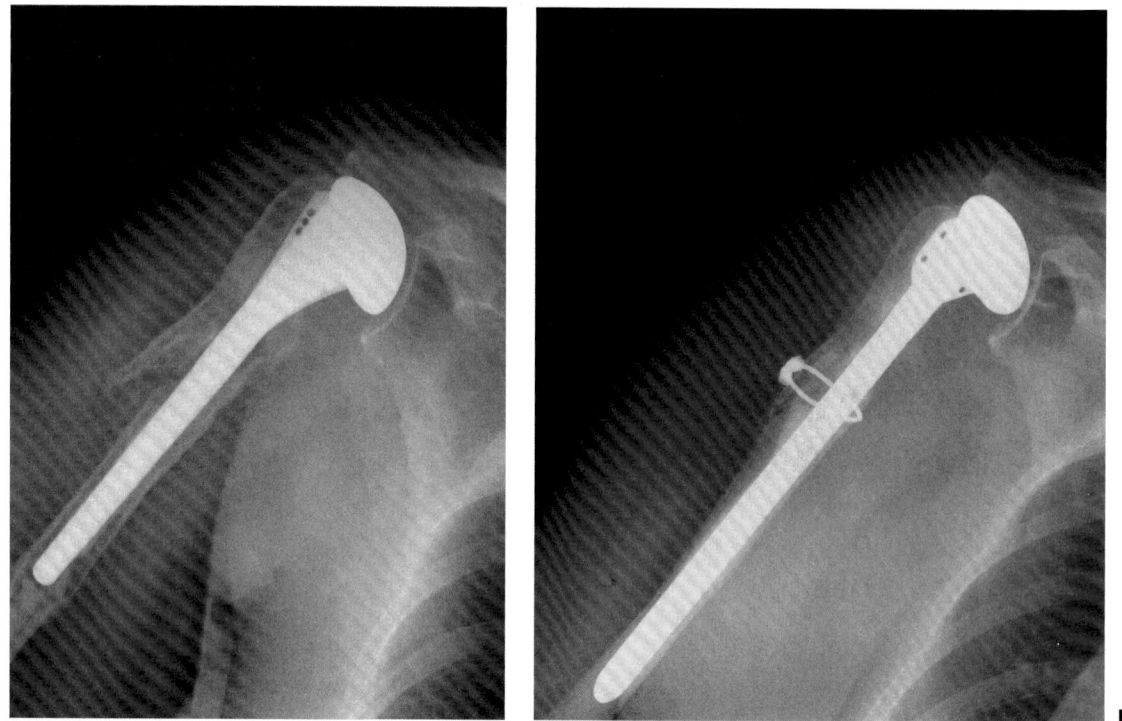

FIGURE 23-42 Treatment of a periprosthetic humeral shaft fracture associated with a loose prosthesis **(A)** with a long stem revision, allograft, and a cerclage cable **(B)**.

posteriorly during preparation of the glenoid articular surface can cause fracture. Patients undergoing revision surgery and those with severe osteopenia are at a particularly high risk. Large fragments may be treated with screws or plates. However, commonly, the fragments are small and comminuted and are not amenable to screw fixation. With inadequate bone support, glenoid resurfacing should be abandoned and the defect bone grafted. After fracture healing, conversion of the hemiarthroplasty to a TSA can be contemplated if symptoms require.

Management of Periprosthetic Acromial Fractures About Reverse Shoulder Arthroplasty

Many fractures of the acromion about reverse shoulder arthroplasties are stress fractures.[202] They are typically nondisplaced or minimally displaced and are usually amenable to nonoperative management with a sling or shoulder immobilizer and limited activity based on pain.[159] Fracture healing is usually reliable and full activities can be resumed in 6 to 12 weeks. On the occasion of a displaced fracture, ORIF may be indicated.[287]

Outcomes for Periprosthetic Fractures About Shoulder Arthroplasty

Outcomes of Periprosthetic Humeral Fractures About Shoulder Arthroplasty

The results of treating periprosthetic humeral shaft fractures about TSA nonoperatively are mixed in the literature and some advocate ORIF in this setting.[21,23,32,95,134,147,180,261,296,297] Kumar et al.[147] treated 11 postoperative periprosthetic humeral shaft fractures nonoperatively. Six healed uneventfully but five required

eventual operative intervention, three had ORIF with bone grafting, and two underwent revision arthroplasty with a long stem for associated loosening. Failure of nonoperative management in this series may be related to the presence of loose implants. Immediate ORIF was performed in only two patients with stable prostheses; both had uneventful union. Similarly marginal results were reported by Boyd et al.[23] in a small series where nonunion occurred in four of seven patients treated nonoperatively and radial nerve palsy occurred in another two. To the contrary, Groh et al. reported union in all five postoperative fractures treated nonoperatively.[95] Nonunion after nonoperative treatment is typically managed with a combination of bone grafting, ORIF, and revision to a long-stemmed arthroplasty.[147,297]

There are no large series demonstrating outcomes of operative management of periprosthetic humeral shaft fractures. Multiple small case series show relatively consistent results: high union rates with little effect on functional outcome in the absence of complications. Wutzler et al.[299] reported on six patients with periprosthetic humeral shaft fractures all with well-fixed stems and all treated with plate fixation. Screws were used distally and either cables or screws or a combination of both were used for proximal fixation. Five of the six fractures healed without complication. One developed a nonunion requiring multiple surgeries and eventual revision to a long-stemmed prosthesis, bone grafting, and bone morphogenic protein to achieve union. This patient also had a persistent radial nerve palsy related to the initial periprosthetic fracture and was the only patient with a poor functional result in this series. Martinez et al.,[176] based on union of six of six patients, advocated augmentation of a typical plate construct, screws distally and cables proximally, with strut allograft to improve stability. Just as in the femur, plate fixation for humeral periprosthetic fractures in the presence of a stable prosthesis with or without the addition of strut allografts is associated with good results. Therefore, the benefit of the adjuvant use of struts remains unclear.

In the setting of a nonunion, the complexity of treatment increases. Kumar et al.[147] treated five periprosthetic humeral fractures or nonunions after nonoperative treatment with revision arthroplasty (three with adjuvant allograft). One of the patients with nonunion had persistent nonunion after revision arthroplasty and ultimately required a free fibular transfer.

Outcomes of Periprosthetic Scapula Fractures About Shoulder Arthroplasty

Outcomes after periprosthetic glenoid fractures about traditional TSA have been scarcely reported.

Acromial fracture after reverse shoulder arthroplasty can have varying effects on outcome. Residual pain, even in the presence of a nonunion may be minimal, but function can be reduced.[103] Union of acromial fractures with nonoperative treatment has been variable. Hamid et al.[103] reported six nonunions out of eight fractures and Wahlquist et al.[287] reported one of three fractures treated nonoperatively eventually requiring surgery to promote union. Fractures at the base of the acromion have been associated with poorer outcomes than more lateral fractures.[109,159,287] In general, patients sustaining an acromial fracture can be expected to have minimal pain but poorer functional outcomes than those without fracture.[159,288]

Potential Pitfalls and Preventative Measures for Treatment of Periprosthetic Fractures About Shoulder Arthroplasty

Operative intervention should not be considered mandatory for all periprosthetic humeral shaft fractures. Strong consideration for nonoperative management should be given to nondisplaced and minimally displaced fractures. Patients with more widely displaced fractures and those with fractures occurring shortly after shoulder arthroplasty, who require aggressive shoulder motion to achieve a good functional outcome, are less ideal candidates for nonoperative management. Given the typical necessity for cable fixation and the immediate proximity of the radial nerve to the posterior humerus in the zone of injury, there is substantial potential for injury to the radial nerve. Passing cables from an anterior approach, without the benefit of direct visualization of instrumentation relative to the radial nerve, is risky. Clear and careful delineation of the proximal and distal margins of the radial neurovascular bundle, as it crosses the posterior humerus, followed by dissection of the plane between the bundle and the posterior cortex is a good first step to avoid potential injury to the nerve. This bundle is often very wide and is less distinct than most other neurovascular bundles. Careful dissection of the plane between the bundle and the posterior cortex allows for visualization of fracture margins in this zone and for safe passage of plates beneath the bundle. A longer plate that allows easy access proximal to the bundle is preferred to aggressive retraction of the nerve to allow access to a shorter plate. The radial nerve is also very sensitive to traction injury.

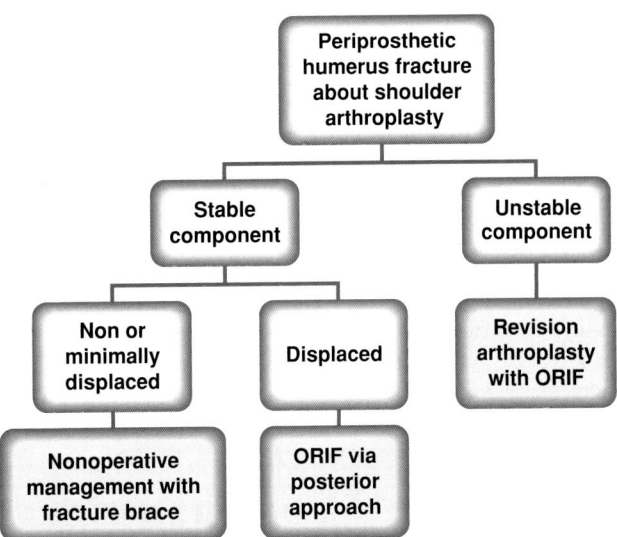

FIGURE 23-43 Algorithm depicting the author's preferred method of treatment for periprosthetic fractures about a total shoulder arthroplasty.

Retraction should avoid leverage (such as a Hohmann retractor placed between the bone and nerve) in favor of gentle controlled direct retraction such as with an army–navy retractor.

AUTHOR'S PREFERRED TREATMENT OF PERIPROSTHETIC FRACTURES ABOUT SHOULDER ARTHROPLASTY

Management of periprosthetic humeral fractures about shoulder arthroplasty stems is relatively straightforward and is based on the stability of the stem and the displacement of the fracture (Fig. 23-43). Most of these fractures occur about stable stems so revision arthroplasty is rarely required. Nondisplaced or minimally displaced fractures are managed nonoperatively with a fracture brace, similar to a native humeral shaft fracture, one that is not associated with a prosthesis. The indications for operative treatment are also similar to native humeral shaft fractures although the threshold for recommending operative treatment is somewhat lower. As opposed to native fractures that can be treated with either IMN or ORIF, operative treatment of periprosthetic fractures is limited to ORIF. A posterior approach is preferred to allow direct visualization and protection of the radial neurovascular bundle. A posterior large fragment plate is secured proximally with cables and distally with screws. Locked screws are utilized when osteoporotic bone is encountered.

PERIPROSTHETIC FRACTURES ELBOW ARTHROPLASTY

Incidence, Risk Factors, and Prevention of Periprosthetic Fractures About Elbow Arthroplasty

There are few large scale evaluations of periprosthetic fractures about total elbow prostheses. One notable exception is the

Mayo Clinic experience with 1,072 linked Coonrad–Morrey procedures performed between 1983 and 2003. Periprosthetic fractures occurred with 9% of primary and 23% of revision procedures. These were equally distributed between fractures of the humerus and those of the ulna. All ulna fractures, in a different series of 30 consecutive fractures about a total elbow arthroplasty (TEA) treated surgically, were associated with loose components at a mean of 8 years after the index arthroplasty.[78] Ulnar bone loss was considered moderate in 14 and severe in 6 of these cases.

Risk factors specific to fracture about TEA have not been clearly elucidated because of the relative paucity of published data related to this topic. However, it is probably safe to consider that systemic or local conditions that reduce or weaken the bone stock in proximity to TEAs would predispose to periprosthetic fracture.

Classification of Periprosthetic Fractures About Total Elbow Arthroplasty

O'Driscoll and Morrey[203] classified humeral and ulnar periprosthetic fractures about total elbow components according to fracture location, component fixation, and bone quality, (Fig. 23-44). Type I fractures are metaphyseal, type II are of the shaft and in the zone of the stem, and type III are beyond the stem. As popularized by the Vancouver classification of periprosthetic femur fractures, periprosthetic elbow fractures are further subdivided by the status of the stem fixation. Subtype A fractures are well fixed and subtype Bs are associated with a loose implant.

Management of Periprosthetic Fractures About Elbow Arthroplasty

Treatment of periprosthetic fractures about TEAs depends upon the location and displacement of the fracture, the time of occurrence (intra- or postoperative), the status of the implant (well fixed or loose), and the type of prosthesis (constrained or unconstrained). Type A fractures, those associated with a well-fixed component, are typically treated by either nonoperative means if nondisplaced or minimally displaced; otherwise, they are treated with ORIF. Type B fractures, those with a loose prosthesis, merit revision arthroplasty.

Management of Periprosthetic Metaphyseal Fractures of the Humerus

Type I periprosthetic fractures of the humerus represent condylar fractures and may occur intraoperatively or postoperatively. Intraoperative fractures are associated with implant preparation in the metaphyseal region. Avulsion fracture of either the medial or lateral condyle can occur with stressing the collateral ligaments especially if bone resection was generous. This weakened area may be subject to spontaneous postoperative fracture or occur with minor trauma. Treatment of Type IA fractures, condylar fractures associated with well-fixed components, depends upon the prosthesis being used. A linked prosthesis such as the Coonrad–Morrey device does not rely upon the collateral ligaments for stability; therefore, these fractures with

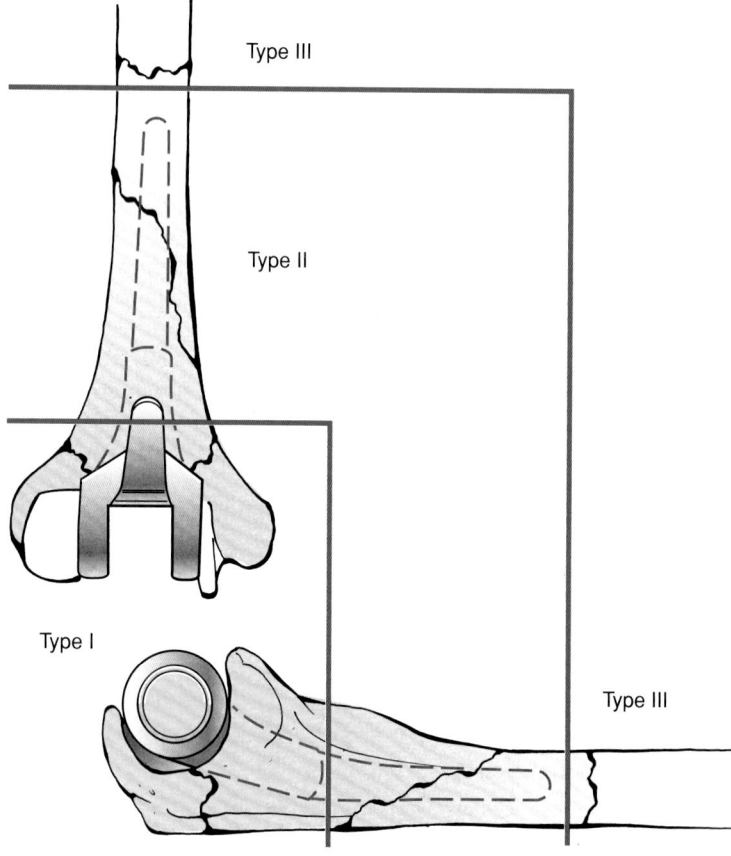

FIGURE 23-44 The Mayo classification of periprosthetic fractures about a total elbow arthroplasty. Type I fractures are metaphyseal, Type II involve bone occupied by the implant, and Type III fractures extend beyond the stem. The subdivisions of these fractures are presented in the text.

this implant type have little implications regarding prognosis. Therefore, nonoperative management is the mainstay so long as displacement is not so great as to compromise eventual union as nonunion may cause pain. In the setting of prostheses that rely upon the collateral ligaments for elbow stability, surgical fixation of these fractures is indicated. Peer-reviewed data to guide decision making for these fractures is lacking.

Management of Periprosthetic Metaphyseal Fractures of the Ulna

Type I periprosthetic ulna fractures are either of the olecranon or coronoid. Coronoid fractures are very uncommon and usually occur intraoperatively. If the fragment is large, extends toward the diaphysis, or compromises ulnar stem fixation, then cable or wire fixation is performed. Type I fractures involving the olecranon are more likely to affect function as these fractures may disrupt the extensor mechanism. Thinning of the olecranon either because of systemic disease such as from RA or from intraoperative bone resection predisposes to fracture, and in these instances extreme care must be taken to avoid critical stress on the olecranon, particularly during intraoperative ulnar component trialing and forearm manipulation. Postoperative fracture can, of course, be related to direct trauma but may also occur spontaneously because of the force generated by triceps muscle contraction when there is compromised bone. Treatment is generally with ORIF utilizing a tension band technique for intraoperative fractures. Postoperative fractures are typically treated nonoperatively unless displacement is greater than approximately 2 cm. Nonunion has been reported in up to 50% of these fractures, but fibrous union and lack of displacement of more than 1 cm has been attributed to the generally good results despite lack of healing.[175]

Management of Periprosthetic Diaphyseal Fractures of the Humerus and Ulna

Type IIA fractures of the humerus and of the ulna, diaphyseal fractures about well-fixed components, are very uncommon. They can theoretically occur at the time of implantation, especially if a long humeral component is inserted into an excessively bowed humerus. Fractures around the stem of the implant are more likely to occur postoperatively and be associated with osteolysis (Type IIB) or with relatively high-energy trauma. Treatment of these fractures should provide fracture stabilization, restoration of bone stock, and a stable prosthesis. The treatment principles follow that for the much more common and extensively studied Vancouver type B femoral fractures (Table 23-28). In the absence of a loose prosthesis, ORIF of a humeral shaft fracture with a strut allograft or plate can provide the required stability. ORIF with a plate and cable construct applied through a posterior approach is the most utilized means. Critical aspects of this procedure are identification and protection of the ulnar nerve distally and the radial nerve proximally. Formal exposure of the median nerve is generally not necessary as long as great care is taken to pass cables around the anterior aspect of the distal humerus adjacent to the anterior surface of the bone. Proximal fixation is with standard screws or, if the bone is osteoporotic, locked screws. A

TABLE 23-28 ORIF for Periprosthetic Fractures About Elbow Arthroplasty

Preoperative Planning Checklist

- OR table: Any table that allows fluoroscopy of the positioned arm
- Position/positioning aids:
  Humerus—lateral or prone with upper arm horizontal for posterior approach; supine for anterior approach
  Ulna—supine with arm over chest or lateral with forearm vertical
- Fluoroscopy location: Ipsilateral to fracture
- Equipment: Small and large fragment sets, cerclage cable system
- Tourniquet (sterile/nonsterile):
  Humerus—sterile
  Ulna—nonsterile

plate long enough to extend proximal to the radial neurovascular bundle allows ease of proximal screw fixation. The plate is gently slid beneath the bundle and fixed to the proximal fragment above and below the bundle. Historically, large fragment broad plates have been advocated for plating humeral fractures. However, with utilization of modern biologic fracture reduction techniques, the strength and associated bulk of these implants is somewhat excessive and narrow large fragment plates are now commonly utilized. Occasionally, fractures about the stem of the humeral component are nondisplaced or minimally displaced or the patient is otherwise not a candidate for surgery. In these cases, nonoperative treatment of the periprosthetic shaft fracture follows standard means with a fracture brace.

When the prosthesis is loose, implant revision with a long stem that bypasses the fracture provides intramedullary stability. Unlike the femur where canal-filling fully porous-coated stems are mainstream, long humeral stems do not reliably provide such stabilization. Therefore, plate or strut fixation is used. When bone deficiencies are present, strut allografts are indicated with or without an adjunctive plate.

Successful use of a novel IMN technique for the management of such a nonunited fracture with massive bone loss has been reported.[131] The fixation implant consisted of a custom IM nail and supplemental autologous bone graft. A commercially available cannulated nail was further hollowed at its distal end to form a sleeve that would nest over the stem of the humeral component.

For fracture of the ulna shaft, plates are preferred if there is a stable implant with no associated bone loss. However, if there is significantly diminished bone stock, a strut allograft with or without a supplemental plate is typically utilized. Revision arthroplasty is indicated when there is a loose prosthesis on either side of the joint, osteolysis, or both.

Fractures of the humerus and ulna distant to the stem tip are relatively uncommon and are usually associated with trauma and a loose stem. By definition, these fractures of the humerus are relatively proximal and may be difficult to control with splints or braces. Control of such fractures of the ulna is generally easier by closed means. Operative treatment is

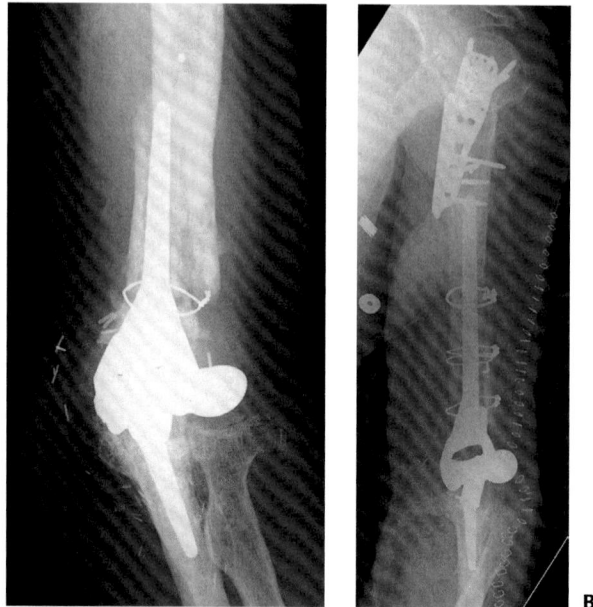

FIGURE 23-45 A periprosthetic humerus fracture about the humeral component of a TEA **(A)** treated with ORIF **(B).**

Outcomes for Periprosthetic Fractures About Total Elbow Arthroplasty

Foruria et al.[78] reported on a series of 30 periprosthetic ulna fractures, all were about loose components. Management included a variety of methods all including ulnar component revision. Strut allograft was utilized in 20 and impaction grafting techniques in eight. Three were revised with only impaction grafting and five were reconstructed with an allograft ulnar prosthetic composite. Twenty-one of these patients were ultimately available for follow-up at a mean of 4.9 years. Eighteen were with mild or no pain. The mean ROM of the elbow was 112 degrees and the mean Mayo Elbow Performance Score was 82. Fracture healing was achieved in all 21 of the followed patients. Complications included three deep infections, one case of ulnar component loosening, and one case of transient nerve palsy.

Results of strut fixation of 11 humeral and 22 ulnar fractures revealed approximately 99% success at 3 to 5 years of both anatomic sites.[127,244]

AUTHOR'S PREFERRED TREATMENT OF PERIPROSTHETIC FRACTURES ABOUT ELBOW ARTHROPLASTY

Decision making for treatment of periprosthetic fractures about an elbow arthroplasty is relatively straightforward (Fig. 23-46). Diaphyseal fractures, or either the humerus or ulna, associated

indicated for displaced fractures and those associated with a loose prosthesis (Fig. 23-45). The goals are to obtain stable fixation, adequate bone stock, and a stable prosthesis. When revision is indicated, a long stem is inserted across the fracture if practical. Regardless of stem position, ORIF with plates and struts are relied upon to provide fracture stability.

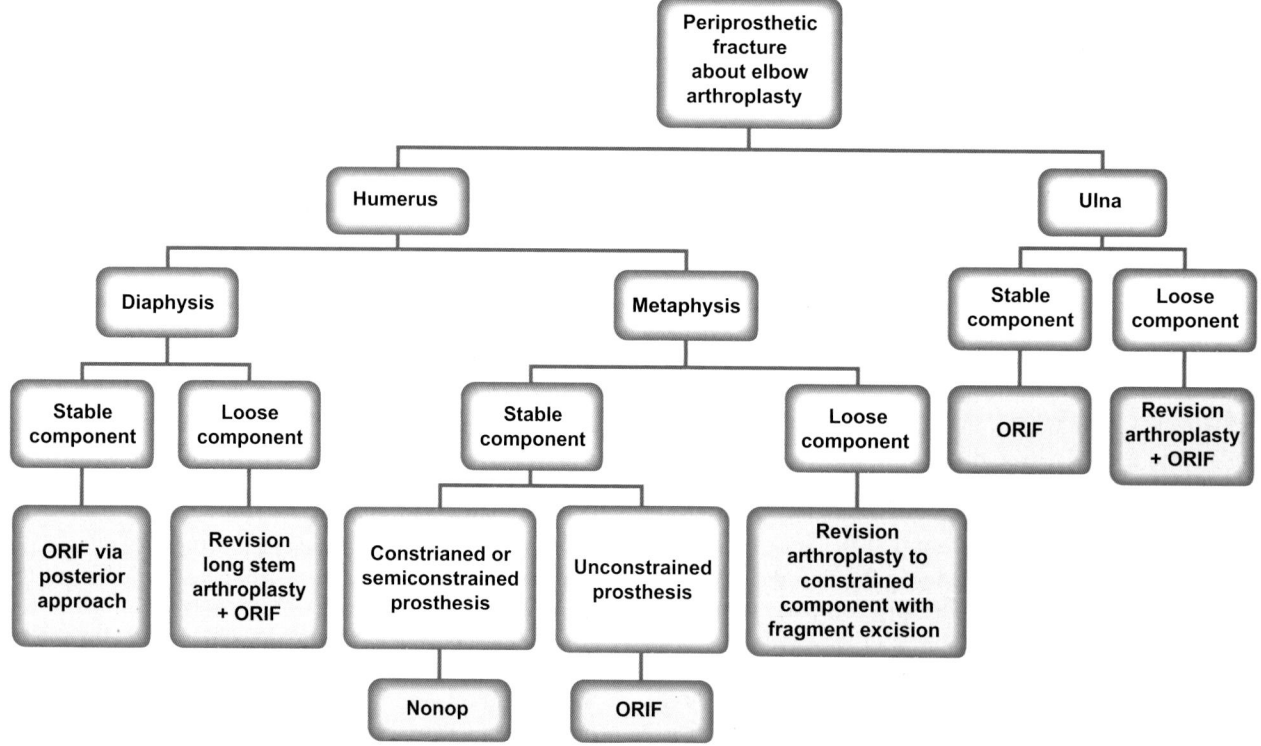

FIGURE 23-46 Algorithm depicting the author's preferred method of treatment for periprosthetic fractures about a total elbow arthroplasty.

with a stable prosthesis are managed with ORIF. The preferred approach to the humeral shaft is posterior so that the radial and ulnar nerves can be directly visualized and protected. Passing cables from an anterior approach puts the radial nerve at substantial risk for injury given its immediate proximity to the posterior humeral cortex. Passing cables from posterior does not put the median nerve at such high risk as the median nerve is not in such close approximation to the anterior bone. Even when the prosthesis stem crosses the fracture, adjunctive ORIF is recommended. This is because long-stemmed humeral components are not canal filling and therefore provide little stability to the fracture. Long-stemmed ulna components provide marginal stability because they are typically either very thin or barely cross the fracture. Bone loss is managed with strut allografting. When diaphyseal fractures of either the humerus or ulna are associated with a loose component, revision arthroplasty is indicated.

A special circumstance relates to periprosthetic metaphyseal fractures of the distal humerus. Management of these fractures considers the prosthesis type. Constrained or semiconstrained prostheses do not rely on ligamentous stability, so the epicondyles are not critical to prosthesis function. Therefore, metaphyseal fractures involving the epicondyles can often be treated nonoperatively, even if displaced. If displacement is so great that there is concern for nonunion, then ORIF is indicated. When these fractures occur around an unconstrained prosthesis, reduction and fixation is generally performed to restore ligamentous stability.

SPECIAL CIRCUMSTANCES, EXPECTED ADVERSE OUTCOMES, AND UNEXPECTED COMPLICATIONS FOR PERIPROSTHETIC FRACTURES

The complications encountered during treatment of periprosthetic fractures is a compilation of the typical complication scene after acute fracture through native bone and the complications associated with joint arthroplasty. These can occur in isolation or in combination. Clearly, treatment must consider both the implications relative to the fracture and the implications with regard to arthroplasty stability and function. It is sometimes useful to prioritize the goals of treatment and decide if the outcome for the fracture is paramount or if preservation of the arthroplasty function is the primary goal. These are sometimes conflicting goals.

Interprosthetic Fractures

Fractures between arthroplasties at opposite ends of a long bone have been termed interprosthetic fractures. As the number of patients with various joint arthroplasties increases, the likelihood of having a fracture that is between two existing arthroplasties similarly increases. Interprosthetic femur fractures between THA and TKA[6,118,171,187,218,259] appear to be most common, but interprosthetic fractures of the humerus between TSA and TEA[34,179] and of the tibia between TKA and TAA may also occur. As with any other femoral fractures, these interprosthetic fractures are typically treated operatively.

In the upper extremity, nonoperative[90,122] and operative[34,179] management of interprosthetic humeral fractures has been described.

Operative treatment of any interprosthetic fracture presents additional technical challenges relative to management of standard periprosthetic fractures. Extramedullary fixation, namely plate constructs, must account for interference by the associated arthroplasty in both the proximal and distal fracture fragments. Intramedullary devices, including nails and stemmed arthroplasty components that span the fracture, must be sized carefully so as to avoid interference from a stemmed component at the opposite end of the bone. For example, in the setting of an interprosthetic femoral shaft fracture between a stemmed THA component and a stemmed TKA component, a revision long stem THA femoral component must not be too long as to contact the stem of the TKA. When the final construct for management of an interprosthetic fracture leaves two stemmed components or a plate and an arthroplasty component in close proximity, the stress riser effect of each implant is potentially magnified. It is not surprising that in this patient population, who, by definition, have proven to be at risk for interprosthetic fracture, secondary interprosthetic fractures have been reported[35,65] Plate fixation long enough to avoid a stress riser effect or the addition of a plate or strut graft to span a zone between two stemmed implants may be prudent to avoid future fracture.

Nonunion

Nonunion is perhaps the most common complication associated with periprosthetic fractures. Nonunion rates for periprosthetic fracture fixation are generally higher than the rate for treatment of the same fracture in the absence of a prosthesis. It has been postulated that damage to the endosteal blood supply related to the intramedullary implant could alter the healing response to fracture, but this remains theory. A more influential cause of higher nonunion rates is the potentially compromised fixation caused by the prosthesis inhibiting optimal fixation. Cable fixation, the mainstay for plate or strut fixation around the zone of prostheses, has inferior strength compared to bicortical screws. However, advances in surgical technique and implant technologies have led to recent improvement in union rates. These advancements include biologic reduction techniques and the use of locked plates where locking screws can augment cable fixation in the zone of the implant and also augment fixation when osteopenic bone is encountered. Treatment of a periprosthetic nonunion can be extremely challenging. Results of nonunion repair of periprosthetic fracture are marginal. A multimodal approach is required.[124] Correction of any systemic process that could inhibit fracture healing is done prior to nonunion repair. This consists of smoking cessation, discontinuation of NSAIDs, strict control of diabetes, and discontinuation of any other dispensable medications that could alter bone metabolism. Operative strategies include utilization of long stem prostheses in conjunction with extramedullary strut and plate fixation. Generous use of osteogenic and osteoinductive grafts and graft substitutes is imperative. Autologous iliac crest bone graft remains the gold standard, but rhBMP is a growing part of the armamentarium for these difficult cases.

It goes without saying that restoration of anatomic limb alignment is another critical step.

Infection

Infection may predate a periprosthetic fracture or may occur as a complication related to the treatment of one. A study evaluating inflammatory markers at the time of periprosthetic fracture associated with THA found evidence of infection to be present in 11.6% of 204 patients.[42] The white blood cell count was elevated in 16.2%, the ESR increased in 33.3%, and the C-reactive protein level increased in 50.5%. The positive predictive value of these markers for infection were found to be poor, therefore clinical history is primarily relied upon to generate an index of suspicion for infection and operative findings are used for determining if infection should be considered during management.

Infection can complicate any surgical procedure but when infection occurs after periprosthetic fracture it can be particularly devastating. Not only is fracture healing compromised but also the survivorship of the associated arthroplasty. Two competing goals must be addressed simultaneously: fracture stability and eradication of infection. Relatively aggressive early surgical treatment with irrigation and debridement and parental organism-specific antibiotics followed by long-term oral suppression has a potential to spare the fracture fixation and arthroplasty implants. Failure to control infection can have serious results including resection arthroplasty or amputation at or above the involved joint. Therefore, removal of the fracture fixation device, or the arthroplasty component, or removal of both should be considered. Use of antibiotic cement spacers typically used in the setting of infected joint arthroplasty in the absence of fracture may not provide adequate fixation in the setting of an associated nonunited fracture. Accordingly, infection surrounding a nonunited fracture associated with a joint arthroplasty often requires creative treatment means. To provide stability in such cases, the use of an antibiotic-impregnated cement-coated plate[168] and the use of an interlocking prosthesis[141] during staged treatment of a Vancouver B periprosthetic femur fracture have been successfully reported.

There is little data specifically regarding infection after treatment of periprosthetic fractures. The majority of available data relates to periprosthetic femur fractures about hip stems. The rate of infection after modern treatment of Vancouver type B fractures with either ORIF or revision arthroplasty has been reported to be 5.94% in 202 cases[210] and as high as 10%.[141] Eleven of 17 patients with infected nonunited Vancouver type B periprosthetic femur fractures treated with debridement, removal of the hip stem, and replacement with an interlocking prosthesis eventually had definitive revision hip arthroplasty and were without residual evidence of infection.[141] Of the other six patients, two had elevated inflammatory markers and were managed with long-term oral antibiotics with retention of the interlocking prosthesis and four were without serologic evidence of infection but electively retained the interlocking prosthesis. All 17 patients were without clinical evidence of infection at the final follow-up. The success of this strategy was attributed to the lack of ingrowth potential with the utilized

locking prosthesis. This affords the opportunity for relatively easy revision to a definitive ingrowth prosthesis and also provides a reasonable long-term solution for low-demand patients unfit or unwilling to undergo such revision.

The use of structural allograft has been implicated to increase infection rates although it remains unclear if the use of allograft is an independent risk factor for infection.[283] Other factors commonly associated with the use of structural allograft such as length of operation, wound complications, inadequate soft tissue coverage, presence of nonunion, and multiple prior operations may influence the risk of infection. Management of an established infection associated with structural allograft usually involves complete removal of the allograft. Because the allograft is a nonvascular organic tissue, it serves as an optimal environment for bacterial growth. The lack of perfusion makes antibiotics and host immune responses ineffective and therefore making removal necessary.

Neurologic Injury

Neurologic injury associated with periprosthetic fracture is reported in a number of series especially with fixation of humeral fractures. One partial radial and two partial ulnar nerve palsies were reported in a series of 11 periprosthetic humeral shaft fractures.[244] The proximity of the radial and ulnar nerves to the fracture, the fixation devices, and securing cerclage cables put these structures at particular risk for injury. The best strategy for dealing with neurologic injury is one based on prevention. Appropriate choice of surgical approach is the first step. We prefer to directly expose any and all nerves that are potentially compromised. Therefore, the posterior approach is preferred for access to the humeral shaft. This way, the radial nerve is precisely located and can be protected throughout the procedure. Gentle soft tissue handling is also important with avoidance of forceful or prolonged retraction of nerves. Passing cerclage cables can be a harrowing experience. There is no substitute for direct knowledge of nerve location and direct protection during passage of cables.

Joint Stiffness

Treatment of any periarticular fracture can result in temporary or permanent stiffness of the involved joint because of contracture and scar of the surrounding soft tissues from the processes leading to and associated with the index joint arthroplasty as well as from the trauma of fracture and subsequent surgery. Immobilization of the joint as part of fracture care can compound the tendency for stiffness. These issues are also relevant to the treatment of periprosthetic fractures. Fortunately, by nature, most periprosthetic fractures are at some distance from the involved joint and by definition are not intra-articular. Nevertheless, every effort should be made to obtain stable enough fixation to minimize the requirement for joint immobilization and to allow as early as possible ROM exercises. Hoffmann et al.[115] reported that most patient in their series treated for a supracondylar periprosthetic femur fracture had loss of ROM with 13.5% having loss of extension of greater than 5 degrees. A shortcoming of this and similar reports is that any loss of motion related to the fracture is difficult to differentiate from baseline loss of motion related to the joint arthroplasty. This is an inherent problem with the evaluation of ROM related to any periprosthetic fracture. By definition, the affected joint is not normal by virtue of having been subjected to surgical joint replacement. This is unlike fractures about native joints, where a careful history producing no prior issues with joint mobility makes baseline ROM equal to the contralateral joint a reasonable assumption.

REFERENCES

1. Aaron RK, Scott R. Supracondylar fracture of the femur after total knee arthroplasty. *Clin Orthop Relat Res.* 1987;(219):136–139.
2. Abhaykumar S, Elliott DS. Percutaneous plate fixation for periprosthetic femoral fractures–a preliminary report. *Injury.* 2000;31(8):627–630.
3. Alden KJ, Duncan WH, Trousdale RT, et al. Intraoperative fracture during primary total knee arthroplasty. *Clin Orthop Relat Res.* 2010;468(1):90–95.
4. Althausen PL, Lee MA, Finkemeier CG, et al. Operative stabilization of supracondylar femur fractures above total knee arthroplasty: A comparison of four treatment methods. *J Arthroplasty.* 2003;18(7):834–839.
5. Amstutz HC, Campbell PA, Le Duff MJ. Fracture of the neck of the femur after surface arthroplasty of the hip. *J Bone Joint Surg Am.* 2004;86-A(9):1874–1877.
6. Anakwe RE, Aitken SA, Khan LA. Osteoporotic periprosthetic fractures of the femur in elderly patients: Outcome after fixation with the LISS plate. *Injury.* 2008;39(10):1191–1197.
7. Anderson AW, Polga DJ, Ryssman DB, et al. Case report: The nest technique for management of a periprosthetic patellar fracture with severe bone loss. *Knee.* 2009;16(4):295–298.
8. Andrews P, Barrack RL, Harris WH. Stress fracture of the medial wall of the acetabulum adjacent to a cementless acetabular component. *J Arthroplasty.* 2002;17(1):117–120.
9. Anglin C, Masri BA, Tonetti J, et al. Hip resurfacing femoral neck fracture influenced by valgus placement. *Clin Orthop Relat Res.* 2007;465:71–79.
10. Athwal GS, Sperling JW, Rispoli DM, et al. Periprosthetic humeral fractures during shoulder arthroplasty. *J Bone Joint Surg Am.* 2009;91(3):594–603.
11. Ayers DC. Supracondylar fracture of the distal femur proximal to a total knee replacement. *Instr Course Lect.* 1997;46:197–203.
12. Back DL, Dalziel R, et al. Early results of primary Birmingham hip resurfacings. An independent prospective study of the first 230 hips. *J Bone Joint Surg Br.* 2005;87(3):324–329.
13. Beals RK, Tower SS. Periprosthetic fractures of the femur. An analysis of 93 fractures. *Clin Orthop.* 1996;(327):238–246.
14. Berger RA, Meneghini RM, Jacobs JJ, et al. Results of unicompartmental knee arthroplasty at a minimum of ten years of follow-up. *J Bone Joint Surg Am.* 2005;87(5):999–1006.
15. Beris AE, Lykissas MG, Sioros V, et al. Femoral periprosthetic fracture in osteoporotic bone after a total knee replacement: Treatment with Ilizarov external fixation. *J Arthroplasty.* 2010;25(7):1168–1112.
16. Berry DJ. Epidemiology: Hip and knee. *Orthop Clin North Am.* 1999;30(2):183–190.
17. Bethea JS III, DeAndrade JR, Fleming LL, et al. Proximal femoral fractures following total hip arthroplasty. *Clin Orthop Relat Res.* 1982;(170):95–106.
18. Bhattacharyya T, Chang D, Meigs JB, et al. Mortality after periprosthetic fracture of the femur. *J Bone Joint Surg Am.* 2007;89(12):2658–2662.
19. Bobak P, Polyzois I, Graham S, et al. Nailed cementoplasty: A salvage technique for rorabeck type II periprosthetic fractures in octogenarians. *J Arthroplasty.* 2010;25(6):939–944.
20. Bogoch E, Hastings D, Gross A, et al. Supracondylar fractures of the femur adjacent to resurfacing and MacIntosh arthroplasties of the knee in patients with rheumatoid arthritis. *Clin Orthop Relat Res.* 1988;(229):213–220.
21. Bonutti PM, Hawkins RJ. Fracture of the humeral shaft associated with total replacement arthroplasty of the shoulder. A case report. *J Bone Joint Surg Am.* 1992;74(4):617–618.
22. Borrelli J Jr, Kantor J, Ungacta F, et al. Intraneural sciatic nerve pressures relative to the position of the hip and knee: A human cadaveric study. *J Orthop Trauma.* 2000;14(4):255–258.
23. Boyd AD Jr, Thornhill TS, Barnes CL. Fractures adjacent to humeral prostheses. *J Bone Joint Surg Am.* 1992;74(10):1498–1504.
24. Brady OH, Garbuz DS, Masri BA, et al. The treatment of periprosthetic fractures of the femur using cortical onlay allograft struts. *Orthop Clin North Am.* 1999;30(2):249–257.
25. Brady OH, Garbuz DS, Masri BA, et al. The reliability and validity of the Vancouver classification of femoral fractures after hip replacement. *J.Arthroplasty.* 2000;15(1):59–62.
26. Brick GW, Scott RD. The patellofemoral component of total knee arthroplasty. *Clin Orthop Relat Res.* 1988;(231):163–178.
27. Brumby SA, Carrington R, Zayontz S, et al. Tibial plateau stress fracture: A complication of unicompartmental knee arthroplasty using 4 guide pinholes. *J Arthroplasty.* 2003;18(6):809–812.
28. Bryant GK, Morshed S, Agel J, et al. Isolated locked compression plating for Vancouver Type B1 periprosthetic femoral fractures. *Injury.* 2009;40(11):1180–1186.
29. Buttaro MA, Farfalli G, Paredes NM, et al. Locking compression plate fixation of Vancouver type-B1 periprosthetic femoral fractures. *J Bone Joint Surg Am.* 2007;89(9):1964–1969.
30. Cain PR, Rubash HE, Wissinger HA, et al. Periprosthetic femoral fractures following total knee arthroplasty. *Clin Orthop Relat Res.* 1986;(208):205–214.
31. Cameron HU, Jung YB. Noncemented stem tibial component in total knee replacement: The 2- to 6-year results. *Can J Surg.* 1993;36(6):555–559.
32. Campbell JT, Moore RS, Iannotti JP, et al. Periprosthetic humeral fractures: Mechanisms of fracture and treatment options. *J Shoulder Elbow Surg.* 1998;7(4):406–413.
33. Carpentier K, Govaers K. Internal fixation of an intertrochanteric femoral fracture after Birmingham hip resurfacing arthroplasty. *Acta Orthop Belg.* 2012;78(2):275–278.
34. Carroll EA, Lorich DG, Helfet DL. Surgical management of a periprosthetic fracture between a total elbow and total shoulder prostheses: A case report. *J Shoulder Elbow Surg.* 2009;18(3):e9–e12.
35. Chakravarthy J, Bansal R, Cooper J. Locking plate osteosynthesis for Vancouver Type B1 and Type C periprosthetic fractures of femur: A report on 12 patients. *Injury.* 2007;38(6):725–733.
36. Chalidis BE, Tsiridis E, Tragas AA, et al. Management of periprosthetic patellar fractures. A systematic review of literature. *Injury.* 2007;38(6):714–724.
37. Chana R, Mansouri R, Jack C, et al. The suitability of an uncemented hydroxyapatite coated (HAC) hip hemiarthroplasty stem for intra-capsular femoral neck fractures in osteoporotic elderly patients: The Metaphyseal-Diaphyseal Index, a solution to preventing intra-operative periprosthetic fracture. *J Orthop Surg Res.* 2011;6:59.
38. Chandler HP, King D, Limbird R, et al. The use of cortical allograft struts for fixation of fractures associated with well-fixed total joint prostheses. *Semin Arthroplasty.* 1993;4(2):99–107.
39. Chandler HP, Tigges RG. The role of allografts in the treatment of periprosthetic femoral fractures. *Instr Course Lect.* 1998;47:257–264.
40. Chatoo M, Parfitt J, Pearse MF. Periprosthetic acetabular fracture associated with extensive osteolysis. *J Arthroplasty.* 1998;13(7):843–845.
41. Chettiar K, Jackson MP, Brewin J, et al. Supracondylar periprosthetic femoral fractures following total knee arthroplasty: Treatment with a retrograde intramedullary nail. *Int Orthop.* 2009;33(4):981–985.
42. Chevillotte CJ, Ali MH, Trousdale RT, et al. Inflammatory laboratory markers in periprosthetic hip fractures. *J Arthroplasty.* 2009;24(5):722–727.
43. Chun KA, Ohashi K, Bennett DL, et al. Patellar fractures after total knee replacement. *AJR Am J Roentgenol.* 2005;185(3):655–660.
44. Clarius M, Haas D, Aldinger PR, et al. Periprosthetic tibial fractures in unicompartmental knee arthroplasty as a function of extended sagittal saw cuts: An experimental study. *Knee.* 2010;17(1):57–60.
45. Clatworthy MG, Ballance J, Brick GW, et al. The use of structural allograft for uncontained defects in revision total knee arthroplasty. A minimum five-year review. *J Bone Joint Surg Am.* 2001;83-A(3):404–411.
46. Cook RE, Jenkins PJ, Walmsley PJ, et al. Risk factors for periprosthetic fractures of the hip: A survivorship analysis. *Clin Orthop Relat Res.* 2008;466(7):1652–1656.
47. Cooper HJ, Rodriguez JA. Early post-operative periprosthetic femur fracture in the presence of a non-cemented tapered wedge femoral stem. *HSS J.* 2010;6(2):150–154.
48. Corten K, Macdonald SJ, McCalden RW, et al. Results of cemented femoral revisions for periprosthetic femoral fractures in the elderly. *J Arthroplasty.* 2012;27(2):220–225.
49. Corten K, Vanrykel F, Bellemans J, et al. An algorithm for the surgical treatment of periprosthetic fractures of the femur around a well-fixed femoral component. *J Bone Joint Surg Br.* 2009;91(11):1424–1430.
50. Cossey AJ, Back DL, Shimmin A, et al. The nonoperative management of periprosthetic fractures associated with the Birmingham hip resurfacing procedure. *J Arthroplasty.* 2005;20(3):358–361.
51. Cracchiolo A. Stress fractures of the pelvis as a cause of hip pain following total hip and knee arthroplasty. *Arthritis Rheum.* 1981;24(5):740–742.
52. Crosby LA, Hamilton A, Twiss T. Scapula fractures after reverse total shoulder arthroplasty: Classification and treatment. *Clin Orthop Relat Res.* 2011;469(9):2544–2549.
53. Culp RW, Schmidt RG, Hanks G, et al. Supracondylar fracture of the femur following prosthetic knee arthroplasty. *Clin Orthop Relat Res.* 1987;(222):212–222.
54. Cumming D, Fordyce MJ. Non-operative management of a peri-prosthetic subcapital fracture after metal-on-metal Birmingham hip resurfacing. *J Bone Joint Surg Br.* 2003;85(7):1055–1056.
55. Davila J, Malkani A, Paiso JM. Supracondylar distal femoral nonunions treated with a megaprosthesis in elderly patients: A report of two cases. *J Orthop Trauma.* 2001;15(8):574–578.
56. Davison BL. Varus collapse of comminuted distal femur fractures after open reduction and internal fixation with a lateral condylar buttress plate. *Am J Orthop.* 2003;32(1):27–30.
57. Dehghan N, Chehade M, McKee MD. Current perspectives in the treatment of periprosthetic upper extremity fractures. *J Orthop Trauma.* 25(suppl 2):S71–S76.
58. Della Valle CJ, Momberger NG, Paprosky WG. Periprosthetic fractures of the acetabulum associated with a total hip arthroplasty. *Instr Course Lect.* 2003;52:281–290.
59. Dennis MG, Simon JA, Kummer FJ, et al. Fixation of periprosthetic femoral shaft fractures occurring at the tip of the stem: A biomechanical study of 5 techniques. *J Arthroplasty.* 2000;15(4):523–528.
60. Dennis MG, Simon JA, Kummer FJ, et al. Fixation of periprosthetic femoral shaft fractures: A biomechanical comparison of two techniques. *J Orthop Trauma.* 2001;15(3):177–180.
61. Desai G, Ries MD. Early postoperative acetabular discontinuity after total hip arthroplasty. *J Arthroplasty.* 2011;26(8):1570, e17–e19.
62. Dhawan RK, Mangham DC, Graham NM. Periprosthetic femoral fracture due to biodegradable cement restrictor. *J Arthroplasty.* 2012;27(8):1581, e13–15.
63. Doets HC, Brand R, Nelissen RG. Total ankle arthroplasty in inflammatory joint disease with use of two mobile-bearing designs. *J Bone Joint Surg Am.* 2006;88(6):1272–1284.
64. Duncan CP, Masri BA. Fractures of the femur after hip replacement. *Instr Course Lect.* 1995;44:293–304.
65. Duwelius PJ, Schmidt AH, Kyle RF, et al. A prospective, modernized treatment protocol for periprosthetic femur fractures. *Orthop Clin North Am.* 2004;35(4):485–492.
66. Ebraheim NA, Gomez C, Ramineni SK, et al. Fixation of periprosthetic femoral shaft fractures adjacent to a well-fixed femoral stem with reversed distal femoral locking plate. *J Trauma.* 2009;66(4):1152–1157.
67. Egol KA, Kubiak EN, Fulkerson E, et al. Biomechanics of locked plates and screws. *J Orthop Trauma.* 2004;18(8):488–493.
68. Ehlinger M, Adam P, Moser T, et al. Type C periprosthetic fractures treated with locking plate fixation with a mean follow up of 2.5 years. *Orthop Traumatol Surg Res.* 2010;96(1):44–48.

69. Ehlinger M, Bonnomet F, Adam P. Periprosthetic femoral fractures: the minimally invasive fixation option. *Orthop Traumatol Surg Res.* 2010;96(3):304–309.

70. Ehlinger M, Brinkert D, Besse J, et al. Reversed anatomic distal femur locking plate for periprosthetic hip fracture fixation. *Orthop Traumatol Surg Res.* 2011;97(5):560–564.

71. Engh GA, Ammeen DJ. Periprosthetic fractures adjacent to total knee implants: Treatment and clinical results. *Instr Course Lect.* 1998;47:437–448.

72. Erhardt JB, Grob K, Roderer G, et al. Treatment of periprosthetic femur fractures with the non-contact bridging plate: A new angular stable implant. *Arch Orthop Trauma Surg.* 2008;128(4):409–416.

73. Farfalli GL, Buttaro MA, Piccaluga F. Femoral fractures in revision hip surgeries with impacted bone allograft. *Clin Orthop Relat Res.* 2007;462:130–136.

74. Felix NA, Stuart MJ, Hanssen AD. Periprosthetic fractures of the tibia associated with total knee arthroplasty. *Clin Orthop Relat Res.* 1997;(345):113–124.

75. Figgie HE III, Goldberg VM, Figgie MP, et al. The effect of alignment of the implant on fractures of the patella after condylar total knee arthroplasty. *J Bone Joint Surg Am.* 1989;71(7):1031–1039.

76. Figgie MP, Goldberg VM, Figgie HE III, et al. The results of treatment of supracondylar fracture above total knee arthroplasty. *J Arthroplasty.* 1990;5(3):267–276.

77. Fink B, Grossmann A, Singer J. Hip revision arthroplasty in periprosthetic fractures of vancouver type B2 and B3. *J Orthop Trauma.* 2012;26(4):206–211.

78. Foruria AM, Sanchez-Sotelo J, Oh LS, et al. The surgical treatment of periprosthetic elbow fractures around the ulnar stem following semiconstrained total elbow arthroplasty. *J Bone Joint Surg Am.* 2011;93(15):1399–1407.

79. Foster AP, Thompson NW, Wong J, et al. Periprosthetic femoral fractures–a comparison between cemented and uncemented hemiarthroplasties. *Injury.* 2005;36(3):424–429.

80. Frankle M, Siegal S, Pupello D, et al. The reverse shoulder prosthesis for glenohumeral arthritis associated with severe rotator cuff deficiency. A minimum two-year follow-up study of sixty patients. *J Bone Joint Surg Am.* 2005;87(8):1697–1705.

81. Franklin J, Malchau H. Risk factors for periprosthetic femoral fracture. *Injury.* 2007;38(6):655–660.

82. Fredin HO, Lindberg H, Carlsson AS. Femoral fracture following hip arthroplasty. *Acta Orthop Scand.* 1987;58(1):20–22.

83. Freedman EL, Hak DJ, Johnson EE, et al. Total knee replacement including a modular distal femoral component in elderly patients with acute fracture or nonunion. *J Orthop Trauma.* 1995;9(3):231–237.

84. Fulkerson E, Koval K, Preston CF, et al. Fixation of periprosthetic femoral shaft fractures associated with cemented femoral stems: A biomechanical comparison of locked plating and conventional cable plates. *J Orthop Trauma.* 2006;20(2):89–93.

85. Fulkerson E, Tejwani N, Stuchin S, et al. Management of periprosthetic femur fractures with a first generation locking plate. *Injury.* 2007;38(8):965–972.

86. Garcia-Cimbrelo E, Munuera L, Gil-Garay E. Femoral shaft fractures after cemented total hip arthroplasty. *Int Orthop.* 1992;16(1):97–100.

87. Garnavos C, Rafiq M, Henry AP. Treatment of femoral fracture above a knee prosthesis. 18 cases followed 0.5–14 years. *Acta Orthop Scand.* 1994;65(6):610–614.

88. Gaski GE, Scully SP. In brief: Classifications in brief: Vancouver classification of postoperative periprosthetic femur fractures. *Clin Orthop Relat Res.* 2011;469(5):1507–1510.

89. Gelalis ID, Politis AN, Arnaoutoglou CM, et al. Traumatic periprosthetic acetabular fracture treated by acute one-stage revision arthroplasty. A case report and review of the literature. *Injury.* 2010;41(4):421–424.

90. Gill DR, Cofield RH, Morrey BF. Ipsilateral total shoulder and elbow arthroplasties in patients who have rheumatoid arthritis. *J Bone Joint Surg Am.* 1999;81(8):1128–1137.

91. Gliatis J, Megas P, Panagiotopoulos E, et al. Midterm results of treatment with a retrograde nail for supracondylar periprosthetic fractures of the femur following total knee arthroplasty. *J Orthop Trauma.* 2005;19(3):164–170.

92. Goldberg VM, Figgie HE III, Inglis AE, et al. Patellar fracture type and prognosis in condylar total knee arthroplasty. *Clin Orthop Relat Res.* 1988;(236):115–122.

93. Grace J N, Sim FH. Fracture of the patella after total knee arthroplasty. *Clin Orthop Relat Res.* 1988;(230):168–175.

94. Gras F, Marintschev I, Klos K, et al. Navigated percutaneous screw fixation of a periprosthetic acetabular fracture. *J Arthroplasty.* 2010;25(7):1169–1164.

95. Groh GI, Heckman MM, Wirth MA, et al. Treatment of fractures adjacent to humeral prostheses. *J Shoulder Elbow Surg.* 2008;17(1):85–89.

96. Guidera KJ, Borrelli J Jr, Raney E, et al. Orthopaedic manifestations of Rett syndrome. *J Pediatr Orthop.* 1991;11(2):204–208.

97. Gujarathi N, Putti AB, Abboud RJ, et al. Risk of periprosthetic fracture after anterior femoral notching. *Acta Orthop.* 2009;80(5):553–556.

98. Haddad FS, Duncan CP, Berry DJ, et al. Periprosthetic femoral fractures around well-fixed implants:Use of cortical onlay allografts with or without a plate. *J Bone Joint Surg Am.* 2002;84-A(6):945–950.

99. Haddad FS, Marston RA, Muirhead-Allwood SK. The Dall-Miles cable and plate system for periprosthetic femoral fractures. *Injury.* 1997;28(7):445–447.

100. Haendlmayer KT, Fazly FM, Harris NJ. Periprosthetic fracture after total ankle replacement: Surgical technique. *Foot Ankle Int.* 2009;30(12):1233–1234.

101. Haidukewych GJ, Jacofsky DJ, Hanssen AD, et al. Intraoperative fractures of the acetabulum during primary total hip arthroplasty. *J Bone Joint Surg Am.* 2006;88(9):1952–1956.

102. Hailer NP, Garellick G, Karrholm J. Uncemented and cemented primary total hip arthroplasty in the Swedish Hip Arthroplasty Register. *Acta Orthop.* 2010;81(1):34–41.

103. Hamid N, Connor PM, Fleischli JF, et al. Acromial fracture after reverse shoulder arthroplasty. *Am J Orthop (Belle Mead NJ).* 2011;40(7):E125–E129.

104. Han HS, Oh KW, Kang SB. Retrograde intramedullary nailing for periprosthetic supracondylar fractures of the femur after total knee arthroplasty. *Clin Orthop Surg.* 2009;1(4):201–206.

105. Hardy DC, Delince PE, Yasik E, et al. Stress fracture of the hip. An unusual complication of total knee arthroplasty. *Clin Orthop Relat Res.* 1992;(281):140–144.

106. Harris B, Owen JR, Wayne JS, et al. Does femoral component loosening predispose to femoral fracture?: An in vitro comparison of cemented hips. *Clin Orthop Relat Res.* 2010;468(2):497–503.

107. Harvie P, Gundle R, Willett K. Traumatic periprosthetic acetabular fracture: Life threatening haemorrhage and a novel method of acetabular reconstruction. *Injury.* 2004;35(8):819–822.

108. Haskell A, Mann RA. Perioperative complication rate of total ankle replacement is reduced by surgeon experience. *Foot Ankle Int.* 2004;25(5):283–289.

109. Hattrup SJ. The influence of postoperative acromial and scapular spine fractures on the results of reverse shoulder arthroplasty. *Orthopedics.* 2010;33(5).

110. Healy WL, Wasilewski SA, Takei R, et al. Patellofemoral complications following total knee arthroplasty. Correlation with implant design and patient risk factors. *J Arthroplasty.* 1995;10(2):197–201.

111. Heckler MW, Tennant GS, Williams DP, et al. Retrograde nailing of supracondylar periprosthetic femur fractures: A surgeon's guide to femoral component sizing. *Orthopedics.* 2007;30(5):345–348.

112. Hendel D, Yasin M, Garti A, et al. Fracture of the greater trochanter during hip replacement: A retrospective analysis of 21/372 cases. *Acta Orthop Scand.* 2002;73(3):295–297.

113. Herrera DA, Kregor PJ, Cole PA, et al. Treatment of acute distal femur fractures above a total knee arthroplasty: Systematic review of 415 cases (1981-2006). *Acta Orthop.* 2008;79(1):22–27.

114. Hirsh DM, Bhalla S, Roffman M. Supracondylar fracture of the femur following total knee replacement. Report of four cases. *J Bone Joint Surg Am.* 1981;63(1):162–163.

115. Hoffmann MF, Jones CB, Sietsema DL, et al. Outcome of periprosthetic distal femoral fractures following knee arthroplasty. *Injury.* 2012;43(7):1084–1089.

116. Holden CE. The role of blood supply to soft tissue in the healing of diaphyseal fractures. An experimental study. *J Bone Joint Surg Am.* 1972;54(5):993–1000.

117. Hou Z, Bowen TR, Irgit K, et al. Locked plating of periprosthetic femur fractures above total knee arthroplasty. *J Orthop Trauma.* 2012;26(7):427–432.

118. Hou Z, Moore B, Bowen TR, et al. Treatment of interprosthetic fractures of the femur. *J Trauma.* 2011;71(6):1715–1719.

119. Hozack WJ, Goll SR, Lotke PA, et al. The treatment of patellar fractures after total knee arthroplasty. *Clin Orthop Relat Res.* 1988;(236):123–127.

120. Hsieh PH, Chang YH, Lee PC, et al. Periprosthetic fractures of the greater trochanter through osteolytic cysts with uncemented Microstructured Omnifit prosthesis: Retrospective analyses pf 23 fractures in 887 hips after 5-14 years. *Acta Orthop.* 2005;76(4):538–543.

121. Incavo SJ, Beard DM, Pupparo F, et al. One-stage revision of periprosthetic fractures around loose cemented total hip arthroplasty. *Am J Orthop.* 1998;27(1):35–41.

122. Inglis AE, Inglis AE Jr. Ipsilateral total shoulder arthroplasty and total elbow replacement arthroplasty: A caveat. *J Arthroplasty.* 2000;15(1):123–125.

123. Jacobs MA, Kennedy WR, Bhargava T, et al. Postresurfacing periprosthetic femoral neck fractures: Nonoperative treatment. *Orthopedics.* 2012;35(5):e732–e736.

124. Jani MM, Ricci WM, Borrelli J, et al. A protocol for treatment of unstable ankle fractures using transarticular fixation in patients with diabetes mellitus and loss of protective sensibility. *Foot Ankle Int.* 2003;24(11):838–844.

125. Johansson JE, McBroom R, Barrington TW, et al. Fracture of the ipsilateral femur in patients wih total hip replacement. *J Bone Joint Surg Am.* 1981;63(9):1435–1442.

126. Jonas SC, Walton MJ, Sarangi PP. Management of a periprosthetic fracture after humeral head resurfacing total shoulder replacement: A case report. *J Shoulder Elbow Surg.* 2011;20(5):e18–e21.

127. Kamineni S, Morrey BF. Proximal ulnar reconstruction with strut allograft in revision total elbow arthroplasty. *J Bone Joint Surg Am.* 2004;86-A(6):1223–1229.

128. Kampshoff J, Stoffel KK, Yates PJ, et al. The treatment of periprosthetic fractures with locking plates: Effect of drill and screw type on cement mantles: A biomechanical analysis. *Arch Orthop Trauma Surg.* 2010;130(5):627–632.

129. Katzer A, Ince A, Wodtke J, et al. Component exchange in treatment of periprosthetic femoral fractures. *J Arthroplasty.* 2006;21(4):572–579.

130. Kavanagh BF. Femoral fractures associated with total hip arthroplasty. *Orthop Clin North Am.* 1992;23(2):249–257.

131. Kawano Y, Okazaki M, Ikegami H, et al. The "docking" method for periprosthetic humeral fracture after total elbow arthroplasty: A case report. *J Bone Joint Surg Am.* 2010;92(10):1988–1991.

132. Keating EM, Haas G, Meding JB. Patella fracture after post total knee replacements. *Clin Orthop Relat Res.* 2003;(416):93–97.

133. Kellett CF, Boscainos PJ, Maury AC, et al. Proximal femoral allograft treatment of Vancouver type-B3 periprosthetic femoral fractures after total hip arthroplasty. Surgical technique. *J Bone Joint Surg Am.* 2007;89(suppl 2 Pt.1):68–79.

134. Kim DH, Clavert P, Warner JJ. Displaced periprosthetic humeral fracture treated with functional bracing: A report of two cases. *J Shoulder Elbow Surg.* 2005;14(2):221–223.

135. Kim YS, Callaghan JJ, Ahn PB, et al. Fracture of the acetabulum during insertion of an oversized hemispherical component. *J Bone Joint Surg Am.* 1995;77(1):111–117.

136. Kim KT, Lee S, Cho KH, et al. Fracture of the medial femoral condyle after unicompartmental knee arthroplasty. *J Arthroplasty.* 2009;24(7):1143–1144.

137. Klein GR, Parvizi J, Rapuri V, et al. Proximal femoral replacement for the treatment of periprosthetic fractures. *J Bone Joint Surg Am.* 2005;87(8):1777–1781.

138. Kolb W, Guhlmann H, Windisch C, et al. Fixation of periprosthetic femur fractures above total knee arthroplasty with the less invasive stabilization system: A midterm follow-up study. *J Trauma.* 2010;69(3):670–676.

139. Kolb K, Koller H, Lorenz I, et al. Operative treatment of distal femoral fractures above total knee arthroplasty with the indirect reduction technique: A long-term follow-up study. *Injury.* 2009;40(4):433–439.

140. Kolstad K. Revision THR after periprosthetic femoral fractures. An analysis of 23 cases. *Acta Orthop Scand.* 1994;65(5):505–508.

141. Konan S, Rayan F, Manketelow AR, et al. The use of interlocking prostheses for both temporary and definitive management of infected periprosthetic femoral fractures. *J Arthroplasty.* 2011;26(8):1332–1337.

142. Kraay MJ, Goldberg VM, Figgie MP, et al. Distal femoral replacement with allograft/prosthetic reconstruction for treatment of supracondylar fractures in patients with total knee arthroplasty. *J Arthroplasty.* 1992;7(1):7–16.

143. Kregor PJ, Stannard JA, Zlowodzki M, et al. Treatment of distal femur fractures using the less invasive stabilization system: Surgical experience and early clinical results in 103 fractures. *J Orthop Trauma*. 2004;18(8):509–520.
144. Kress KJ, Scuderi GR, Windsor RE, et al. Treatment of nonunions about the knee utilizing custom total knee arthroplasty with press-fit intramedullary stems. *The Journal of Arthroplasty*. 1995;8(1):49–55.
145. Kumar A, Chambers I, Maistrelli G, et al. Management of periprosthetic fracture above total knee arthroplasty using intramedullary fibular allograft and plate fixation. *J Arthroplasty*. 2008;23(4):554–558.
146. Kumar A, Chambers I, Wong P. Periprosthetic fracture of the proximal tibia after lateral unicompartmental knee arthroplasty. *J Arthroplasty*. 2008;23(4):615–618.
147. Kumar S, Sperling JW, Haidukewych GH, et al. Periprosthetic humeral fractures after shoulder arthroplasty. *J Bone Joint Surg Am*. 2004;86-A(4):680–689.
148. Kumm DA, Rack C, et al. Subtrochanteric stress fracture of the femur following total knee arthroplasty. *J Arthroplasty*. 1997;12(5):580–583.
149. Langenhan R, Trobisch P, Ricart P, et al. Aggressive surgical treatment of periprosthetic femur fractures can reduce mortality: Comparison of open reduction and internal fixation versus a modular prosthesis nail. *J Orthop Trauma*. 2012;26(2):80–85.
150. Large TM, Kellam JF, Bosse MJ, et al. Locked plating of supracondylar periprosthetic femur fractures. *J Arthroplasty*. 2008;23(6 suppl 1):115–120.
151. Laurer HL, Wutzler S, Possner S, et al. Outcome after operative treatment of Vancouver type B1 and C periprosthetic femoral fractures: Open reduction and internal fixation versus revision arthroplasty. *Arch Orthop Trauma Surg*. 2011;131(7):983–989.
152. Lee KB, Cho SG, Hur CI, et al. Perioperative complications of HINTEGRA total ankle replacement: Our initial 50 cases. *Foot Ankle Int*. 2008;29(10):978–984.
153. Lee GC, Nelson CL, Virmani S, et al. Management of periprosthetic femur fractures with severe bone loss using impaction bone grafting technique. *J Arthroplasty*. 2010;25(3): 405–409.
154. Lenz M, Perren SM, Gueorguiev B, et al. Underneath the cerclage: An ex vivo study on the cerclage-bone interface mechanics. *Arch Orthop Trauma Surg*. 2012;132(10):1467–1472.
155. Lenz M, Windolf M, Muckley T, et al. The locking attachment plate for proximal fixation of periprosthetic femur fractures–a biomechanical comparison of two techniques. *Int Orthop*. 2012;36(9):1915–1921.
156. Lesh ML, Schneider DJ, Deol G, et al. The consequences of anterior femoral notching in total knee arthroplasty. A biomechanical study. *J Bone Joint Surg Am*. 2000;82-A(8): 1096–1101.
157. Lesniewski PJ, Testa NN. Stress fracture of the hip as a complication of total knee replacement. Case report. *J Bone Joint Surg Am*. 1982;64(2):304–306.
158. Levine BR, Della Valle CJ, Lewis P, et al. Extended trochanteric osteotomy for the treatment of vancouver B2/B3 periprosthetic fractures of the femur. *J Arthroplasty*. 2008;23(4):527–533.
159. Levy JC, Anderson C, Samson A. Classification of postoperative acromial fractures following reverse shoulder arthroplasty. *J Bone Joint Surg Am*. 2013;95(15):e104.
160. Lewallen DG, Berry DJ. Periprosthetic fracture of the femur after total hip arthroplasty: Treatment and results to date. *Instr Course Lect*. 1998;47:243–249.
161. Lewis PL, Rorabeck CH. Periprosthetic Fractures. In: Engh GA, Rorabeck CH, eds. *Revision Total Knee Arthroplasty*. Baltimore, MD: Williams & Wilkins; 1997: 275–295.
162. Li CH, Chen TH, Su YP, et al. Periprosthetic femoral supracondylar fracture after total knee arthroplasty with navigation system. *J Arthroplasty*. 2008;23(2):304–307.
163. Lindahl H. Epidemiology of periprosthetic femur fracture around a total hip arthroplasty. *Injury*. 2007;38(6):651–654.
164. Lindahl H, Garellick G, Regner H, et al. Three hundred and twenty-one periprosthetic femoral fractures. *J Bone Joint Surg Am*. 2006;88(6):1215–1222.
165. Lindahl H, Malchau H, Herberts P, et al. Periprosthetic femoral fractures classification and demographics of 1049 periprosthetic femoral fractures from the Swedish National Hip Arthroplasty Register. *J Arthroplasty*. 2005;20(7):857–865.
166. Lindahl H, Oden A, Garellick G, et al. The excess mortality due to periprosthetic femur fracture. A study from the Swedish National Hip Arthroplasty Register. *Bone*. 2007;40(5):1294–1298.
167. Lindstrand A, Stenstrom A, Ryd L, et al. The introduction period of unicompartmental knee arthroplasty is critical: A clinical, clinical multicentered, and radiostereometric study of 251 Duracon unicompartmental knee arthroplasties. *J Arthroplasty*. 2000;15(5):608–616.
168. Liporace FA, Yoon RS, Frank MA, et al. Use of an "antibiotic plate" for infected periprosthetic fracture in total hip arthroplasty. *J Orthop Trauma*. 2012;26(3):e18–e23.
169. Long JP, Bartel DL. Surgical variables affect the mechanics of a hip resurfacing system. *Clin Orthop Relat Res*. 2006;453:115–122.
170. Lotke PA, Ecker ML. Influence of positioning of prosthesis in total knee replacement. *J Bone Joint Surg Am*. 1977;59(1):77–79.
171. Mamczak CN, Gardner MJ, Bolhofner B, et al. Interprosthetic femoral fractures. *J Orthop Trauma*. 2010;24(12):740–744.
172. Maniar RN, Umlas ME, Rodriguez JA, et al. Supracondylar femoral fracture above a PFC posterior cruciate-substituting total knee arthroplasty treated with supracondylar nailing. A unique technical problem. *J Arthroplasty*. 1996;11(5):637–639.
173. Marker DR, Seyler TM, Jinnah RH, et al. Femoral neck fractures after metal-on-metal total hip resurfacing: A prospective cohort study. *J Arthroplasty*. 2007;22(7 suppl 3):66–71.
174. Markmiller M, Konrad G, Sudkamp N. Femur-LISS and distal femoral nail for fixation of distal femoral fractures: Are there differences in outcome and complications? *Clin Orthop Relat Res*. 2004;(426):252–257.
175. Marra G, Morrey BF, Gallay SH, et al. Fracture and nonunion of the olecranon in total elbow arthroplasty. *J Shoulder Elbow Surg*. 2006;15(4):486–494.
176. Martinez AA, Calvo A, Cuenca J, et al. Internal fixation and strut allograft augmentation for periprosthetic humeral fractures. *J Orthop Surg (Hong Kong)*. 2011;19(2):191–193.
177. Masri BA, Meek RM, Duncan CP. Periprosthetic fractures evaluation and treatment. *Clin Orthop Relat Res*. 2004;(420):80–95.
178. Maury AC, Pressman A, Cayen B, et al. Proximal femoral allograft treatment of Vancouver type-B3 periprosthetic femoral fractures after total hip arthroplasty. *J Bone Joint Surg Am*. 2006;88(5):953–958.
179. Mavrogenis AF, Angelini A, Guerra E, et al. Humeral fracture between a total elbow and total shoulder arthroplasty. *Orthopedics*. 2011;34(4).
180. McDonough EB, Crosby LA. Periprosthetic fractures of the humerus. *Am J Orthop*. 2005;34(12):586–591.
181. McGarvey WC, Clanton TO, Lunz D. Malleolar fracture after total ankle arthroplasty: A comparison of two designs. *Clin Orthop Relat Res*. 2004;(424):104–110.
182. McLean AL, Patton JT, Moran M. Femoral replacement for salvage of periprosthetic fracture around a total hip replacement. *Injury*. 2012;43(7):1166–1169.
183. Meek RM, Garbuz DS, Masri BA, et al. Intraoperative fracture of the femur in revision total hip arthroplasty with a diaphyseal fitting stem. *J Bone Joint Surg Am*. 2004;86-A(3): 480–485.
184. Meek RM, Norwood T, Smith R, et al. The risk of peri-prosthetic fracture after primary and revision total hip and knee replacement. *J Bone Joint Surg Br*. 2011;93(1):96–101.
185. Meneghini RM, Cornwell P, Guthrie M, et al. A novel method for prevention of intraoperative fracture in cementless hip arthroplasty: Vibration analysis during femoral component insertion. *Surg Technol Int*. 2010;20:334–339.
186. Merkel KD, Johnson EW Jr. Supracondylar fracture of the femur after total knee arthroplasty. *J Bone Joint Surg Am*. 1986;68(1):29–43.
187. Michla Y, Spalding L, Holland JP, et al. The complex problem of the interprosthetic femoral fracture in the elderly patient. *Acta Orthop Belg*. 2010;76(5):636–643.
188. Mikhail WE, Wretenberg PF, Weidenhielm LR, et al. Complex cemented revision using polished stem and morselized allograft. Minimum 5-years' follow-up. *Arch Orthop Trauma Surg*. 1999;119(5–6):288–291.
189. Miller AJ. Late fracture of the acetabulum after total hip replacement. *J Bone Joint Surg Br*. 1972;54(4):600–606.
190. Mont MA, Maar DC. Fractures of the ipsilateral femur after hip arthroplasty. A statistical analysis of outcome based on 487 patients. *J Arthroplasty*. 1994;9(5):511–519.
191. Mont MA, Seyler TM, Ulrich SD, et al. Effect of changing indications and techniques on total hip resurfacing. *Clin Orthop Relat Res*. 2007;465:63–70.
192. Moran MC, Brick GW, Sledge CB, et al. Supracondylar femoral fracture following total knee arthroplasty. *Clin Orthop*. 1996;(324):196–209.
193. Morrey BF, Kavanagh BF. Complications with revision of the femoral component of total hip arthroplasty. Comparison between cemented and uncemented techniques. *J Arthroplasty*. 1992;7:71–79.
194. Mukundan C, Rayan F, Kheir E, et al. Management of late periprosthetic femur fractures: A retrospective cohort of 72 patients. *Int Orthop*. 2010;34(4):485–489.
195. Mulay S, Hassan T, Birtwistle S, et al. Management of types B2 and B3 femoral periprosthetic fractures by a tapered, fluted, and distally fixed stem. *J Arthroplasty*. 2005;20(6): 751–756.
196. Muller M, Kaab M, Tohtz S, et al. Periprosthetic femoral fractures: Outcome after treatment with LISS internal fixation or stem replacement in 36 patients. *Acta Orthop Belg*. 2009;75(6):776–783.
197. Myerson MS, Mroczek K. Perioperative complications of total ankle arthroplasty. *Foot Ankle Int*. 2003;24(1):17–21.
198. Naqvi GA, Baig SA, Awan N. Interobserver and intraobserver reliability and validity of the Vancouver classification system of periprosthetic femoral fractures after hip arthroplasty. *J Arthroplasty*. 2012;27(6):1047–1050.
199. Naraghi AM, White LM. Magnetic resonance imaging of joint replacements. *Semin Musculoskelet Radiol*. 2006;10(1):98–106.
200. Neumann D, Thaler C, Dorn U. Management of Vancouver B2 and B3 femoral periprosthetic fractures using a modular cementless stem without allografting. *Int Orthop*. 2012;36(5):1045–1050.
201. Ng VY, Arnott L, McShane M. Periprosthetic femoral condyle fracture after total knee arthroplasty and saline-coupled bipolar sealing technology. *Orthopedics*. 2011;34(1):53.
202. Nicolay S, De Beuckeleer L, Stoffelen D, et al. Atraumatic bilateral scapular spine fracture several months after bilateral reverse total shoulder arthroplasty. *Skeletal Radiol*. 2013.
203. O'Driscoll SW, Morrey BF. Periprosthetic fractures about the elbow. *Orthop Clin North Am*. 1999;30(2):319–325.
204. Olsen RV, Munk PL, Lee MJ, et al. Metal artifact reduction sequence: Early clinical applications. *Radiographics*. 2000;20(3):699–712.
205. Ortiguera CJ, Berry DJ. Patellar fracture after total knee arthroplasty. *J Bone Joint Surg Am*. 2002;84-A(4):532–540.
206. O'Shea K, Quinlan JF, Kutty S, et al. The use of uncemented extensively porous-coated femoral components in the management of Vancouver B2 and B3 periprosthetic femoral fractures. *J Bone Joint Surg Br*. 2005;87(12):1617–1621.
207. Palance MD, Albareda J, Seral F. Subcapital stress fracture of the femoral neck after total knee arthroplasty. *Int Orthop*. 1994;18(5):308–309.
208. Pandit H, Murray DW, Dodd CA, et al. Medial tibial plateau fracture and the Oxford unicompartmental knee. *Orthopedics*. 2007;30(5 suppl):28–31.
209. Parvizi J, Jain N, Schmidt AH. Periprosthetic knee fractures. *J Orthop Trauma*. 2008;22(9):663–671.
210. Pavlou G, Panteliadis P, Macdonald D, et al. A review of 202 periprosthetic fractures–stem revision and allograft improves outcome for type B fractures. *Hip Int*. 2011;21(1):21–29.
211. Perren SM, Linke B, Schwieger K, et al. Aspects of internal fixation of fractures in porotic bone. Principles, technologies and procedures using locked plate screws. *Acta Chir Orthop Traumatol Cech*. 2005;72(2):89–97.
212. Peskun CJ, Townley JB, Schemitsch EH, et al. Treatment of periprosthetic fractures around hip resurfacings with cephalomedullary nails. *J Arthroplasty*. 2012;27(3):494, e1–e3.
213. Peters CL, Hennessey R, Barden RM, et al. Revision total knee arthroplasty with a cemented posterior-stabilized or constrained condylar prosthesis: A minimum 3-year and average 5-year follow-up study. *J Arthroplasty*. 1997;12(8):896–903.
214. Petersen MM, Lauritzen JB, Pedersen JG, et al. Decreased bone density of the distal femur after uncemented knee arthroplasty. A 1-year follow-up of 29 knees. *Acta Orthop Scand*. 1996;67(4):339–344.
215. Petersen MM, Olsen C, Lauritzen JB, et al. Changes in bone mineral density of the distal femur following uncemented total knee arthroplasty. *J Arthroplasty*. 1995;10(1):7–11.

216. Peterson CA, Lewallen DG. Periprosthetic fracture of the acetabulum after total hip arthroplasty. *J Bone Joint Surg Am.* 1996;78(8):1206–1213.
217. Platzer P, Schuster R, Aldrian S, et al. Management and outcome of periprosthetic fractures after total knee arthroplasty. *J Trauma.* 2010;68(6):1464–1470.
218. Platzer P, Schuster R, Luxl M, et al. Management and outcome of interprosthetic femoral fractures. *Injury.* 2011;42(11):1219–1225.
219. Pot JH, van Heerwaarden RJ, Patt TW. An unusual way of intramedullar fixation after a periprosthetic supracondylar femur fracture. *J Arthroplasty.* 2012;27(3):494–498.
220. Pressmar J, Macholz F, Merkert W, et al. [Results and complications in the treatment of periprosthetic femur fractures with a locked plate system.] *Unfallchirurg.* 2010;113(3):195–202.
221. Pritchett JW. Fracture of the greater trochanter after hip replacement. *Clin Orthop Relat Res.* 2001;(390):221–226.
222. Radcliffe SN, Smith DN. The Mennen plate in periprosthetic hip fractures. *Injury.* 1996;27(1):27–30.
223. Rand JA, Coventry MB. Stress fractures after total knee arthroplasty. *J Bone Joint Surg Am.* 1980;62(2):226–233.
224. Rawes ML, Patsalis T, Gregg PJ. Subcapital stress fractures of the hip complicating total knee replacement. *Injury.* 1995;26(6):421–423.
225. Rayan F, Dodd M, Haddad FS. European validation of the Vancouver classification of periprosthetic proximal femoral fractures. *J Bone Joint Surg Br.* 2008;90(12):1576–1579.
226. Rayan F, Konan S, Haddad FS. Uncemented revision hip arthroplasty in B2 and B3 periprosthetic femoral fractures - A prospective analysis. *Hip Int.* 2010;20(1):38–42.
227. Ricci WM, Bolhofner BR, Loftus T, et al. Indirect reduction and plate fixation, without grafting, for periprosthetic femoral shaft fractures about a stable intramedullary implant. *J Bone Joint Surg Am.* 2005;87(10):2240–2245.
228. Ricci WM, Borrelli J Jr. Operative management of periprosthetic femur fractures in the elderly using biological fracture reduction and fixation techniques. *Injury.* 2007;38(suppl 3):S53–S58.
229. Ricci WM, Haidukewych GJ. Periprosthetic femoral fractures. *Instr Course Lect.* 2009;58:105–115.
230. Ricci WM, Loftus T, Cox C, et al Locked plates combined with minimally invasive insertion technique for the treatment of periprosthetic supracondylar femur fractures above a total knee arthroplasty. *J Orthop Trauma.* 2006;20(3):190–196.
231. Richards CJ, Giannitsios D, Huk OL, et al. Risk of periprosthetic femoral neck fracture after hip resurfacing arthroplasty: Valgus compared with anatomic alignment. A biomechanical and clinical analysis. *J Bone Joint Surg Am.* 2008;90(suppl 3):96–101.
232. Ritter MA, Campbell ED. Postoperative patellar complications with or without lateral release during total knee arthroplasty. *Clin Orthop Relat Res.* 1987;(219):163–168.
233. Ritter MA, Carr K, Keating EM, et al. Tibial shaft fracture following tibial tubercle osteotomy. *J Arthroplasty.* 1996;11(1):117–119.
234. Ritter MA, Faris PM, Keating EM. Anterior femoral notching and ipsilateral supracondylar femur fracture in total knee arthroplasty. *J Arthroplasty.* 1988;3(2):185–187.
235. Ritter MA, Thong AE, Keating EM, et al. The effect of femoral notching during total knee arthroplasty on the prevalence of postoperative femoral fractures and on clinical outcome. *J Bone Joint Surg Am.* 2005;87(11):2411–2414.
236. Robinson DE, Lee MB, Smith EJ, et al. Femoral impaction grafting in revision hip arthroplasty with irradiated bone. *J.Arthroplasty.* 2002;17(7):834–840.
237. Rorabeck CH, Taylor JW. Classification of periprosthetic fractures complicating total knee arthroplasty. *Orthop Clin North Am.* 1999;30(2):209–214.
238. Rorabeck CH, Taylor JW. Periprosthetic fractures of the femur complicating total knee arthroplasty. *Orthop Clin North Am.* 1999;30(2):265–277.
239. Rudol G, Jackson MP, James SE. Medial tibial plateau fracture complicating unicompartmental knee arthroplasty. *J Arthroplasty.* 2007;22(1):148–150.
240. Saidi K, Ben-Lulu O, Tsuji M, et al. Supracondylar periprosthetic fractures of the knee in the elderly patients: A comparison of treatment using allograft-implant composites, standard revision components, distal femoral replacement prosthesis. *J Arthroplasty.* 2014;29(1):110–114.
241. Sakai R, Kikuchi A, Morita T, et al. Hammering sound frequency analysis and prevention of intraoperative periprosthetic fractures during total hip arthroplasty. *Hip Int.* 2011;21(6):718–723.
242. Saltzman CL, Amendola A, Anderson R, et al. Surgeon training and complications in total ankle arthroplasty. *Foot Ankle Int.* 2003;24(6):514–518.
243. Sanchez-Sotelo J, McGrory BJ, Berry DJ. Acute periprosthetic fracture of the acetabulum associated with osteolytic pelvic lesions: A report of 3 cases. *J Arthroplasty.* 2000;15(1):126–130.
244. Sanchez-Sotelo J, O'Driscoll S, Morrey BF. Periprosthetic humeral fractures after total elbow arthroplasty: Treatment with implant revision and strut allograft augmentation. *J Bone Joint Surg Am.* 2002;84-A(9):1642–1650.
245. Sarvilinna R, Huhtala H, Pajamaki J. Young age and wedge stem design are risk factors for periprosthetic fracture after arthroplasty due to hip fracture. A case-control study. *Acta Orthop.* 2005;76(1):56–60.
246. Sarvilinna R, Huhtala HS, Sovelius RT, et al. Factors predisposing to periprosthetic fracture after hip arthroplasty: A case (n = 31)-control study. *Acta Orthop Scand.* 2004;75(1):16–20.
247. Schandelmaier P, Partenheimer A, Koenemann B, et al. Distal femoral fractures and LISS stabilization. *Injury.* 2001;32(suppl 3):SC55–SC63.
248. Schuberth JM, Patel S, Zarutsky E. Perioperative complications of the Agility total ankle replacement in 50 initial, consecutive cases. *J Foot Ankle Surg.* 2006;45(3):139–146.
249. Schutz M, Muller M, Krettek C, et al. Minimally invasive fracture stabilization of distal femoral fractures with the LISS: A prospective multicenter study. Results of a clinical study with special emphasis on difficult cases. *Injury.* 2001;32(suppl 3):SC48–SC54.
250. Schwartz JT Jr, Mayer JG, Engh CA. Femoral fracture during non-cemented total hip arthroplasty. *J Bone Joint Surg Am.* 1989;71(8):1135–1142.
251. Scott RD, Turoff N, Ewald FC. Stress fracture of the patella following duopatellar total knee arthroplasty with patellar resurfacing. *Clin Orthop Relat Res.* 1982;(170):147–151.
252. Sharkey PF, Hozack WJ, Callaghan JJ, et al. Acetabular fracture associated with cementless acetabular component insertion: A report of 13 cases. *J Arthroplasty.* 1999;14(4):426–431.

253. Sheth NP, Pedowitz DI, Lonner JH. Periprosthetic patellar fractures. *J Bone Joint Surg Am.* 2007;89(10):2285–2296.
254. Shimmin AJ, Back D. Femoral neck fractures following Birmingham hip resurfacing: A national review of 50 cases. *J Bone Joint Surg Br.* 2005;87(4):463–464.
255. Singh JA, Jensen MR, Harmsen SW, et al. Are gender, comorbidity, and obesity risk factors for postoperative periprosthetic fractures after primary total hip arthroplasty? *J Arthroplasty.* 2013;28(1):126–131.
256. Singh JA, Jensen MR, Lewallen DG. Patient factors predict periprosthetic fractures after revision total hip arthroplasty. *J Arthroplasty.* 2012;27(8):1507–1512.
257. Sloper PJ, Hing CB, Donell ST, et al. Intra-operative tibial plateau fracture during unicompartmental knee replacement: A case report. *Knee.* 2003;10(4):367–369.
258. Sochart DH, Hardinge K. Nonsurgical management of supracondylar fracture above total knee arthroplasty. Still the nineties option. *J Arthroplasty.* 1997;12(7):830–834.
259. Soenen M, Migaud H, Bonnomet F, et al. Interprosthetic femoral fractures: Analysis of 14 cases. Proposal for an additional grade in the Vancouver and SoFCOT classifications. *Orthop Traumatol Surg Res.* 2011;97(7):693–698.
260. Springer BD, Berry DJ, Cabanela ME, et al. Early postoperative transverse pelvic fracture: A new complication related to revision arthroplasty with an uncemented cup. *J Bone Joint Surg Am.* 2005;87(12):2626–2631.
261. Steinmann SP, Cheung EV. Treatment of periprosthetic humerus fractures associated with shoulder arthroplasty. *J Am Acad Orthop Surg.* 2008;16(4):199–207.
262. Stiehl JB. Extended osteotomy for periprosthetic femoral fractures in total hip arthroplasty. *Am J Orthop.* 2006;35(1):20–23.
263. Streit MR, Merle C, Clarius M, et al. Late peri-prosthetic femoral fracture as a major mode of failure in uncemented primary hip replacement. *J Bone Joint Surg Br.* 2011;93(2):178–183.
264. Streubel PN, Gardner MJ, Morshed S, et al. Are extreme distal periprosthetic supracondylar fractures of the femur too distal to fix using a lateral locked plate? *J Bone Joint Surg Br.* 2010;92(4):527–534.
265. Streubel PN, Ricci WM, Wong A, et al. Mortality after distal femur fractures in elderly patients. *Clin Orthop Relat Res.* 2011;469(4):1188–1196.
266. Stuart MJ, Hanssen AD. Total knee arthroplasty: Periprosthetic tibial fractures. *Orthop Clin North Am.* 1999;30(2):279–286.
267. Su ET, DeWal H, Di Cesare PE. Periprosthetic femoral fractures above total knee replacements. *J Am Acad Orthop Surg.* 2004;12(1):12–20.
268. Tadross TS, Nanu AM, Buchanan MJ, et al. Dall-Miles plating for periprosthetic B1 fractures of the femur. *J. Arthroplasty.* 2000;15(1):47–51.
269. Talbot M, Zdero R, Schemitsch EH. Cyclic loading of periprosthetic fracture fixation constructs. *J Trauma.* 2008;64(5):1308–1312.
270. Taljanovic MS, Hunter TB, Miller MD, et al. Gallery of medical devices: Part 1: Orthopedic devices for the extremities and pelvis. *Radiographics.* 2005;25(3):859–870.
271. Taylor MM, Meyers MH, Harvey JP Jr. Intraoperative femur fractures during total hip replacement. *Clin Orthop Relat Res.* 1978;(137):96–103.
272. Tharani R, Nakasone C, Vince KG. Periprosthetic fractures after total knee arthroplasty. *J Arthroplasty.* 2005;20(4 suppl 2):27–32.
273. Thomas SR, Wilson AJ, Chambler A, et al. Outcome of Copeland surface replacement shoulder arthroplasty. *J Shoulder Elbow Surg.* 2005;14(5):485–491.
274. Thompson NW, McAlinden MG, Breslin E, et al. Periprosthetic tibial fractures after cementless low contact stress total knee arthroplasty. *J Arthroplasty.* 2001;16(8):984–990.
275. Thomsen MN, Jakubowitz E, Seeger JB, et al. Fracture load for periprosthetic femoral fractures in cemented versus uncemented hip stems: An experimental in vitro study. *Orthopedics.* 2008;31(7):653.
276. Tower SS, Beals RK. Fractures of the femur after hip replacement: The Oregon experience. *Orthop Clin North Am.* 1999;30(2):235–247.
277. Tria AJ Jr, Harwood DA, Alicea JA, et al. Patellar fractures in posterior stabilized knee arthroplasties. *Clin Orthop Relat Res.* 1994;(299):131–138.
278. Tsiridis E, Amin MS, Charity J, et al. Impaction allografting revision for B3 periprosthetic femoral fractures using a Mennen plate to contain the graft: A technical report. *Acta Orthop Belg.* 2007;73(3):332–338.
279. Tsiridis E, Haddad FS, Gie GA. The management of periprosthetic femoral fractures around hip replacements. *Injury.* 2003;34(2):95–105.
280. Tsiridis E, Narvani AA, Haddad FS, et al. Impaction femoral allografting and cemented revision for periprosthetic femoral fractures. *J Bone Joint Surg Br.* 2004;86(8):1124–1132.
281. Tsiridis E, Spence G, Gamie Z, et al. Grafting for periprosthetic femoral fractures: Strut, impaction or femoral replacement. *Injury.* 2007;38(6):688–697.
282. Van Houwelingen AP, Duncan CP. The pseudo A(LT) periprosthetic fracture: It's really a B2. *Orthopedics.* 2011;34(9):e479–e481.
283. Van Houwelingen AP, Schemitsch EH. Infection associated with cortical allograft strut fixation of a periprosthetic femoral shaft fracture: A case report and review of the literature. *J Trauma.* 2008;64(6):1630–1634.
284. Van Loon P, de Munnynck B, Bellemans J. Periprosthetic fracture of the tibial plateau after unicompartmental knee arthroplasty. *Acta Orthop Belg.* 2006;72(3):369–374.
285. Venu KM, Koka R, Garikipati, R, et al. Dall-Miles cable and plate fixation for the treatment of peri-prosthetic femoral fractures-analysis of results in 13 cases. *Injury.* 2001;32(5):395–400.
286. Virolainen P Mokka J, Seppanen M, et al. Up to 10 years follow up of the use of 71 cortical allografts (strut-grafts) for the treatment of periprosthetic fractures. *Scand J Surg.* 2010;99(4):240–243.
287. Wahlquist TC, Hunt AF, Braman JP. Acromial base fractures after reverse total shoulder arthroplasty: Report of five cases. *J Shoulder Elbow Surg.* 2011;20(7):1178–1183.
288. Walch G, Mottier F, Wall B, et al. Acromial insufficiency in reverse shoulder arthroplasties. *J Shoulder Elbow Surg.* 2009;18(3):495–502.
289. Wang CJ, Wang JW, Weng LH, et al. The effect of alendronate on bone mineral density in the distal part of the femur and proximal part of the tibia after total knee arthroplasty. *J Bone Joint Surg Am.* 2003;85-A(11):2121–2126.
290. White LM, Kim JK, Mehta M, et al. Complications of total hip arthroplasty: MR imaging-initial experience. *Radiology.* 2000;215(1):254–262.

291. Whittaker RP, Sotos LN, Ralston EL. Fractures of the femur about femoral endopros-theses. *J Trauma.* 1974;14(8):675–694.
292. Wick M, Muller EJ, Kutscha-Lissberg F, et al. [Periprosthetic supracondylar femoral fractures: LISS or retrograde intramedullary nailing? Problems with the use of mini-mally invasive technique]. *Unfallchirurg.* 2004;107(3):181–188.
293. Wilson FC, Venters GC. Results of knee replacement with the Walldius prosthesis: An interim report. *Clin Orthop Relat Res.* 1976;(120):39–46.
294. Wong P, Gross AE. The use of structural allografts for treating periprosthetic fractures about the hip and knee. *Orthop Clin North Am.* 1999;30(2):259–264.
295. Wood PL, Deakin S. Total ankle replacement. The results in 200 ankles. *J Bone Joint Surg Br.* 2003;85(3):334–341.
296. Worland RL, Kim DY, Arredondo J. Periprosthetic humeral fractures: Management and classification. *J Shoulder Elbow Surg.* 1999;8(6):590–594.
297. Wright TW, Cofield RH. Humeral fractures after shoulder arthroplasty. *J Bone Joint Surg Am.* 1995;77(9):1340–1346.
298. Wu CC, Au MK, Wu SS, et al. Risk factors for postoperative femoral fracture in cement-less hip arthroplasty. *J Formos Med Assoc.* 1999;98(3):190–194.
299. Wutzler S, Laurer HL, Huhnstock S, et al. Periprosthetic humeral fractures after shoul-der arthroplasty: Operative management and functional outcome. *Arch Orthop Trauma Surg.* 2009;129(2):237–243.
300. Xue H, Tu Y, Cai M, et al. Locking compression plate and cerclage band for type B1 periprosthetic femoral fractures preliminary results at average 30-month follow-up. *J Arthroplasty.* 2011;26(3):467–471.
301. Yang JH, Kim HJ, Yoon JR, et al. Minimally invasive plate osteosynthesis (MIPO) for periprosthetic fracture after total ankle arthroplasty: A case report. *Foot Ankle Int.* 2011;32(2):200–204.
302. Young SW, Walker CG, Pitto RP. Functional outcome of femoral peri prosthetic fracture and revision hip arthroplasty: A matched-pair study from the New Zealand Registry. *Acta Orthop.* 2008;79(4):483–488.
303. Zaki SH, Sadiq S, Purbach B, et al. Periprosthetic femoral fractures treated with a modular distally cemented stem. *J Orthop Surg (Hong Kong).* 2007;15(2):163–166.
304. Zalzal P, Backstein D, Gross AE, et al. Notching of the anterior femoral cortex during total knee arthroplasty characteristics that increase local stresses. *J Arthroplasty.* 2006;21(5):737–743.
305. Zalzal P, Gandhi R, Petruccelli D, et al. Fractures at the tip of long-stem prostheses used for revision hip arthroplasty. *J. Arthroplasty.* 2003;18(6):741–745.
306. Zdero R Walker R, Waddell JP, et al. Biomechanical evaluation of periprosthetic femo-ral fracture fixation. *J Bone Joint Surg Am.* 2008;90(5):1068–1077.
307. Zeh A, Radetzki F, Diers V, et al. Is there an increased stem migration or compromised osteointegration of the Mayo short-stemmed prosthesis following cerclage wiring of an intrasurgical periprosthetic fracture? *Arch Orthop Trauma Surg.* 2011;131(12):1717–1722.
308. Zenni EJ Jr, Pomeroy DL, Caudle RJ. Ogden plate and other fixations for fractures complicating femoral endoprostheses. *Clin Orthop.* 1988;(231): 83–90.
309. Zustin J, Krause M, Breer S, et al. Morphologic analysis of periprosthetic fractures after hip resurfacing arthroplasty. *J Bone Joint Surg Am.* 2010;92(2):404–410.
310. Zuurmond RG, Pilot P, Verburg AD. Retrograde bridging nailing of periprosthetic femoral fractures. *Injury.* 2007;38(8):958–964.
311. Zuurmond RG, Pilot P, Verburg AD, et al. Retrograde bridging nail in periprosthetic femoral fracture treatment which allows direct weight bearing. *Proc Inst Mech Eng H.* 2008;222(5):629–635.
312. Zuurmond RG, van Wijhe W, van Raay JJ, et al. High incidence of complications and poor clinical outcome in the operative treatment of periprosthetic femoral fractures: An analysis of 71 cases. *Injury.* 2010;41(6):629–633.

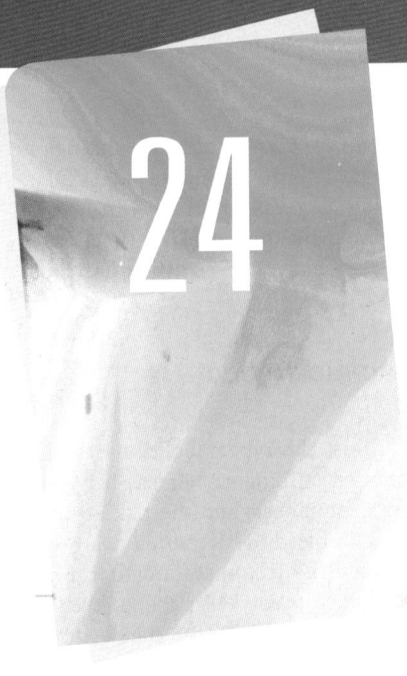

24

VENOUS THROMBOEMBOLIC DISEASE IN PATIENTS WITH SKELETAL TRAUMA

Robert Probe and David Ciceri

INTRODUCTION

Unbeknownst to Rudolph Virchow, when he described the classic triad of factors that lead to thrombotic disease in the nineteenth century, he was also providing an accurate depiction of the contemporary orthopedic trauma patient. To varying degrees, these individuals all have endothelial injury, stasis, and hypercoagulability as a part of their physiologic response to injury. Validating this triad as contributory to this potentially lethal disease, recent decades have produced reports suggesting that over half of polytraumatized patients without prophylaxis will develop thrombi within their legs.[21] This epiphany has led traumatologist to recognize that strategies to mitigate risks are an essential component of the comprehensive care of trauma patients. Unfortunately, despite universal recognition of risk, pulmonary embolism (PE) remains the third most common cause of death in patients surviving the first 24 hours following trauma.[2] It is becoming increasingly clear that PE and deep vein thrombosis (DVT), collectively referred to as venous thromboembolic disease (VTE) is a complex interplay of fluid dynamics, bioactive factors, and mechanics. This chapter will focus on the pathophysiology of the clotting pathways in the trauma patient, examine the sub-sets of trauma patients and their inherent risk of VTE, explore the pharmacologic and mechanical measures that can reduce the incidence, and conclude with a discussion of diagnostic and therapeutic strategies.

PATHOPHYSIOLOGY

Clot formation is a process involving the interaction of the endothelium, subendothelial matrix, platelets, and circulating proenzymes (zymogens). Traditionally, the coagulation cascade has been conceptualized as consisting of two intersecting arms, the extrinsic and intrinsic pathways. This construct, although recognized as a fairly drastic simplification, served adequately in many routine clinical settings when the major therapeutic options for anticoagulation were unfractionated heparin (UFH) and warfarin. In this schema, the extrinsic pathway was activated by the interaction of tissue factor and factor VII. Factor VIIa then activated factor X and the common coagulation pathway. The intrinsic pathway was felt to be initiated by exposure to a foreign surface (test tube) or damaged vessel surface causing activation of factor XII followed by factors XI, IX, and ultimately X and the common pathway (Fig. 24-1).

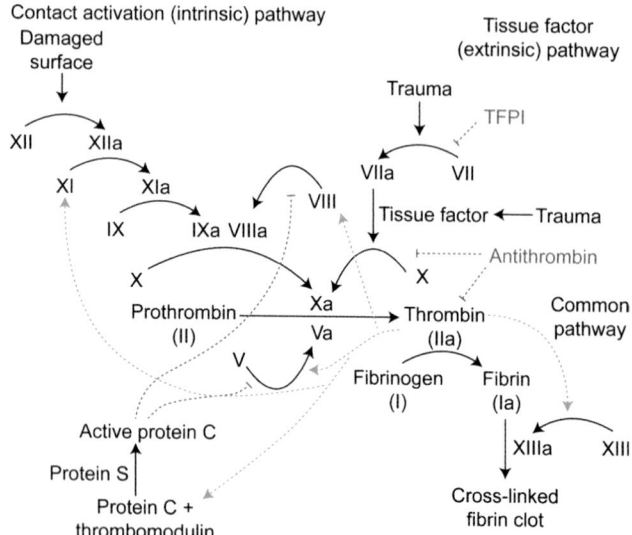

FIGURE 24-1 Intrinsic and extrinsic pathways leading to cross-linked thrombin clot.

It is now recognized that clot formation is a dynamic process in constant interplay with processes maintaining blood fluidity, retarding clot formation, and causing clot dissolution. These processes act in concert to rapidly achieve hemostasis even at the level of the myriad minor injuries which occur in the microvascular level every day. At the same time, these vital processes must limit clot formation to the actual site of vascular injury and restore patency of the micro- and macrovasculature. These systems are also closely interrelated to a host of other systems which mediate local and systemic inflammation.

Vessel injury triggers muscular contraction of the vessel wall and exposure of platelets to the subendothelial matrix. This is termed primary hemostasis. Platelets adhere to the exposed subendothelial tissue by a variety of mechanisms depending upon local shear stress conditions. This is followed by changes in platelet morphology, secretion of a host of products that enhance clot formation, aggregation, and surface expression of a negatively charged phosphatidylserine which serves as a catalytic surface for coagulation factors.[39]

The first stage of the coagulation cascade, initiation, is triggered by exposure of tissue factor to factor VII and small amounts of circulating activated factor VIIa. This leads to the formation of the extrinsic tenase complex which produces small amounts of FIXa, FXa, and thrombin. The amplification phase occurs at the platelet surface and the resulting intrinsic tenase complex (FIXa:VIIIa) and prothrombinase complex (FXa:FVA) leads to significant thrombin generation. The propagation phase is dependent upon an adequate number of platelets to support continued high levels of thrombin production that leads to the conversion of fibrinogen to fibrin and a stable fibrin clot.[3] The clinical consequences of venous thrombus formation are diverse. The majority of thrombi serve the purpose of hemostasis and ultimately undergo fibrinolysis with restoration of physiologic flow; however, there

are circumstances in which this process becomes pathologic. These include obstructive DVT, thromboembolism (VTE), and obstruction of the pulmonary vascular flow (PE). This review is intended to examine the prophylaxis, diagnosis, and treatment of these disease states in the setting of orthopedic trauma.

TRAUMA-RELATED THROMBOEMBOLIC RISK FACTORS

Appropriate prophylaxis against thromboembolic disease in the setting of trauma requires striking a balance between the risk of morbidity from a thrombosis and the risk of prophylaxis causing harm through bleeding.[14] Trauma has been identified as one of the strongest risk factors leading to thromboembolism. In a venographic study of 349 patients, Geerts et al.[21] identified a 58% rate of DVT and 18% incidence of proximal vein thrombosis in their population of patients with an Injury Severity Score (ISS) of >9 in the absence of any prophylactic measures. Natural history analysis of more contemporary studies is challenged by the fact that significant variation exists in the timing and method of prophylaxis, the screening tools utilized, and the definition of disease.[28] Despite these challenges, an understanding of relative risk between subsets of trauma patients is an important component of any risk benefit analysis.

Injury Severity Score

There are a multitude of reasons why the polytrauma patient is predisposed to thromboembolic disease. These patients are typically immobile, often ventilator-dependent, and subject to a hypercoagulable state.[51] In the era prior to prophylaxis, patients requiring transfusion, those with head injury, spinal cord injury, lower-extremity fracture, and those with pelvic fracture were found to be at increased relative risk of deep thrombosis.[21] While the dramatic increase in prophylactic measures has led to a substantial reduction in the incidence of VTE, the association of increasing injury severity with disease persists. In a review of the German National Trauma Data Bank, Paffrath et al.[49] noted an overall 1.8% incidence of "clinically significant" thromboembolic disease despite the vast majority of patients receiving prophylaxis. Within this group, multivariate analysis suggested ISS as a significant independent variable (Fig. 24-2). In a review of the American National Trauma Data Bank over the period 1994 through 2001, Knudson et al.[35] identified an overall rate of VTE of 0.36% in 450,375 patients. Independent risk factors in this review included an age ≥40 years, the presence of lower-extremity fracture (Abbreviated Injury Score [AIS] ≥ 3), the presence of a major head injury (AIS ≥3), days requiring mechanical ventilation greater than 3, the presence of a venous injury, and the need for at least one major operative procedure (Table 24-1).

Spinal Cord Injury

Several studies have noted large increase in relative risk of VTE with spinal cord injury.[53] The stasis that results from

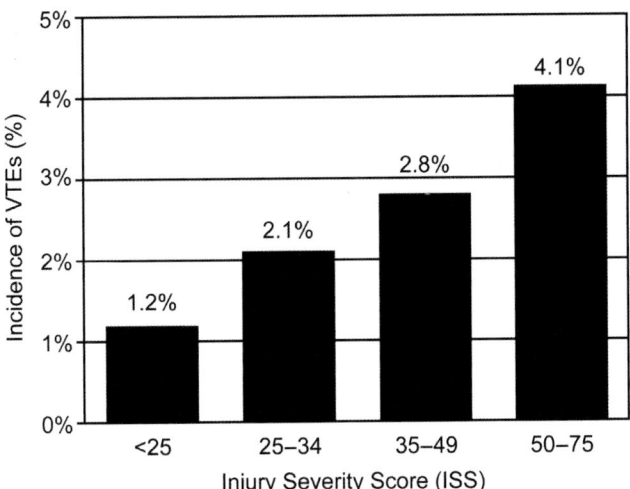

FIGURE 24-2 Rising incidence of VTE with increasing injury severity score. (Reproduced with permission from: Paffrath T, Wafaisade A, et al. Trauma Registry of DGU. Venous thromboembolism after severe trauma: Incidence, risk factors and outcome. *Injury.* 2010;41(1): 97–101.)

the absence of vascular tone combined with the attendant loss of muscle contractions are likely contributory factors to this heightened risk. In an analysis of the spinal cord injury patients within the National Trauma Data Bank, identified rates of VTE were 3.4% for high cervical (C1 to C4), 6.3% for high thoracic (T1 to T6), and 3.2% with lumbar injury. Additional independent risk factors from the Data Bank

TABLE 24-1 Risk Factors Associated with VTE (Univariate Analysis)

Risk Factor (Number with Risk)	Odds Ratio (95% CI)
Age ≥40 yrs. (n = 178,851)	2.29 (2.07–2.55)
Pelvic fracture (n = 2,707)	2.93 (2.01–4.27)
Lower-extremity fracture (n = 63,508)	3.16 (2.85–3.51)
Spinal cord injury with paralysis (n = 2,852)	3.39 (2.41–4.77)
Head injury (AIS ≥ 3) (n = 52,197)	2.59 (2.31–2.90)
Ventilator days >3 (n = 13,037)	10.62 (9.32–12.11)
Venous injury (n = 1,450)	7.93 (5.83–10.78)
Shock on admission (BP < 90 mm Hg) (n = 18,510)	1.95 (1.62–2.34)
Major surgical procedure (n = 73,974)	4.32 (3.91–4.77)

p <0.001 for all factors.

Risk factors associated with univariate analysis of venous thromboembolic disease from the National Trauma Data Bank.

Reproduced with permission from: Knudson MM, Ikossi DG, Khaw L, et al. Thromboembolism after trauma: An analysis of 1602 episodes from the American College of Surgeons National Trauma Data Bank. *Ann Surg.* 2004;240(3):490–496.

included increasing age, increasing ISS, male gender, traumatic brain injury, and chest trauma.[46]

Head Injury

Many of the same predisposing features of the spinal cord injured patient also apply to the head injured patient. In a review of 577 patients with head injury AIS > 3, a DVT incidence of 34% was identified when only mechanical prophylactic measures were utilized with weekly duplex ultrasound screening. In this series, the incremental risk of clinical VTE with other injuries was also noted. In patients with isolated head injury, the DVT rate was 26% compared to 35% in those patients with associated injury. In addition to head injury, advancing age, ISS > 15, and the presence of a lower-extremity injury were strong predictors for developing DVT in this study.[17]

Fracture Risks

Fractures of the lower extremity and pelvis have also been noted to increase the risk of VTE. The natural history of operatively treated fractures can be inferred from the work of Abelseth et al.[1] In an era prior to routine prophylaxis, a prospective study of 102 patients with lower-extremity fracture was conducted. Patients were examined with venography, an average of 9 days following injury, and followed clinically for 6 weeks. The overall incidence of clinically occult DVT was 28% and rose as the level of skeletal injury became more proximal. Other independent risk factors noted in this series included older age, longer operating times, and longer times before fracture fixation.[1]

Another fracture specific concern arises in those patients provisionally stabilized with damage control external fixation. The forced joint immobilization inherent to this technique and the limitations for the application of sequential pneumatic devices raises concern over the VTE risk. In a retrospective review, Sems et al.[59] evaluated 143 patients with bridging frames for an average of 18 days who received low-molecular-weight heparin (LMWH) as prophylaxis against VTE. In this group, there were only three cases of VTE and each was in a patient with multiple concomitant injuries. This review would suggest that under protection of appropriate prophylaxis, temporary bridging external fixation does not produce additive risk of DVT.

Geriatric hip fractures present another patient population at risk for VTE. The recognized effects of advancing age, immobility, and proximal femoral fracture are collectively causes for concern. Without prophylaxis, rates of 50% for DVT and 4% for PE are reported in systematic review.[27] This risk also increases with delay to surgery. In a review of 101 consecutive patients with >24-hour delay to surgery, Smith et al.[60] demonstrated a correlation between the length of delay and DVT identified by duplex ultrasound screening. Despite LMWH prophylaxis, the overall group demonstrated a DVT rate of 10% with those with a DVT averaging a 5.7-day delay and those without averaging a 3.2 day delay.

While the majority of available literature on VTE focuses on the incidence of DVT, the most feared complication is PE because of its potential for mortal consequences. Knudson et al. analyzed the National Trauma Data Bank and determined that in this large data set, the overall incidence of PE was 0.49% with an 11% mortality.[35] Head injury, more than three ventilator days, chest injury, pelvic fracture, lower-extremity injury, spine injury, and shock were all independent variables associated with this complication.

NONTRAUMATIC RISK FACTORS

In light of the fact that risk factors for VTE appear to be additive, individual patient risk factors unassociated with trauma must also be considered when determining composite risk. The use of estrogen-based oral contraceptives is common in the female trauma population and carries distinct additional risk. From pooled data, the estimated odds ratio for VTE from these drugs is 3.8. This additional risk is compounded in the obese and in those patients over the age of 40.[42]

In addition, genetically determined protein abnormalities predispose to VTE. The most common of these are protein C deficiency, protein S deficiency, antithrombin deficiency, factor V Leiden, and prothrombin mutations. In a review of patients presenting with VTE, one of these deficiencies was present in 35% compared to an incidence in the general population of 10%.[45] Relative risk for these genetic tendencies range from 2.2 to 8.5 times higher than the unaffected population.[44]

While testing for these deficiencies is complex and costly, a simple family history can be of significant value. A history of VTE in one or more first-degree relatives under age 50 should raise the question of a genetic predisposition. This was most conclusively shown in a population-based study of the incidence of VTE according to the presence or absence of VTE in a sibling. Standard incidence ratios for VTE were 2.27, 51.9, and 53.7 for patients with one, two, or three or more affected siblings, respectively.[6]

With the multitude of important individual risk factors and their variable weighting, it becomes a complex equation to incorporate all of these factors and their relative risk into a composite risk profile. Several scoring systems have been developed to assist the practitioner in calculating a cumulative risk. One such scoring system is the Caprini Index (Table 24-2).[10] This index coalesces multiple clinical parameters into a single

---

TABLE 24-2 **Caprini Index**

Each Risk Factor Represents 1 Point
- Age 41–60 yrs
- Minor surgery planned
- History of prior major surgery
- Varicose veins
- History of inflammatory bowel disease
- Swollen legs (current)
- Obesity (BMI > 30)
- Acute myocardial infarction (<1 mo)
- Congestive heart failure (<1 mo)
- Sepsis (<1 mo)
- Serious lung disease including pneumonia (<1 mo)
- Abnormal pulmonary function (COPD)
- Medical patient currently at bed rest
- Leg plaster cast or brace
- Other risk factors_____

Each Risk Factor Represents 3 Points
- Age over 75 yrs
- Major surgery lasting 2–3 hrs
- BMI > 50 (venous stasis syndrome)
- History of SVT, DVT/PE
- Family History of DVT/PE
- Present cancer of chemotherapy
- Positive factor V Leiden
- Positive prothrombin 20210A
- Elevated serum homocysteine
- Positive lupus anticoagulant
- Elevated anticardiolipin antibodies
- Heparin-induced thrombocytopenia (HIT)
- Other thrombophilia

Type_____

Each Risk Factor Represents 2 Points
- Age 60–74 yrs
- Minor surgery (>60 min)
- Arthroscopic surgery (>60 min)
- Laparoscopic surgery (>60 min)
- Previous malignancy
- Central venous access
- Morbid obesity (BMI > 40)

Each Risk Factor Represents 5 Points
- Elective major lower-extremity arthroplasty
- Hip, pelvis, or leg fracture (<1 mo)
- Stroke (<1 mo)
- Multiple trauma (<1 mo)
- Acute spinal cord injury (paralysis)(<1 mo)
- Major surgery lasting over 3 hrs

For Women Only (Each Represents 1 Point)
- Oral contraceptives or hormone replacement therapy
- Pregnancy or postpartum (<1 mo)
- History of unexplained stillborn infant, recurrent spontaneous abortion (≥3), premature birth with toxemia or growth-restricted infant

Total Risk Factor Score

The Caprini index can be used to sum the factors thought to be of additive risk in predisposition to venous thromboembolic disease. Patients with scores greater than 3 should have consideration given to prophylaxis.
BMI, Body mass index.
Reproduced with permission from: Caprini JA. Individual risk assessment is the best strategy for thromboembolic prophylaxis. *Dis Mon.* 2010;56(10):552–559.

sum that then stratifies patients into low, moderate, high, or highest risk. While no specific guidelines exist in the setting of fracture management, it would seem prudent to give consideration to some form of prophylaxis in patients with scores of 3 or greater (moderate risk) and the need for lower-extremity immobilization. In the setting of more significant trauma, it should be noted that major fracture of the lower extremity places patients in the highest-risk category by definition. The usefulness of this screen; therefore, applies only to those fractures that are low risk in isolation, but become high risk because of the cumulative effect of injury factors and idiosyncratic predisposition.

CHEMICAL PROPHYLACTIC OPTIONS

Aspirin

Several characteristics of acetylsalicylic acid make it an attractive agent for the prevention of DVT. It is inexpensive, easily administered, and produces a low rate of bleeding. The antiplatelet effect that results from the inhibition of thromboxane A2 disrupts an important component of clot initiation and formation.

In a group of 13,356 patients undergoing surgery for hip fracture or joint replacement, a relative risk reduction of 36% was noted by using low-dose aspirin.[54] Aspirin has also been shown to be effective in prospective trials in the reduction of risk for secondary DVT.[5] While these findings of benefit are attractive, it does not appear as though the treatment effect is as large as that offered by LMWH. To date, large prospective trials in the setting of trauma are lacking. Currently, aspirin's use for VTE prophylaxis should be restricted to patients in low-to-moderate risk categories as an alternative to no prophylaxis or to situations where extended prophylaxis is desired.

Heparin

The realization of the effectiveness of low-dose UFH led to its rapid adoption as one of the earliest forms of chemical prophylaxis against DVT. The anticoagulant effect of heparin is complex, but primarily involves the activation of antithrombin III through an increase in flexibility and activity of its reactive site.[7] Heparin also possesses a strong electrostatic attraction to thrombin and other cascade proteases (IX, Xa) creating a direct binding which limits their biologic effect.[25] One notable concern over the use of UFH is the potential for heparin-induced thrombocytopenia (HIT). While conflicting reports exist, UFH appears to have a much narrower therapeutic index when compared to LMWH. In a systematic review of prophylaxis in spinal cord injury patients, UFH had a 2.6 odds ratio for DVT and a 7.5 odds ratio for bleeding complications when compared to LMWH.[53] Given these factors, the best indication of UFH is in the short-term perioperative period of moderate-risk patients with advantages being restricted to its reduced cost.

Low-Molecular-Weight Heparin

In 1976, it was discovered that the direct factor Xa binding mechanism of heparin could be selected for by decreasing the size of the heparin molecule.[29] This preferential inactivation of factor Xa was found to be more effective than UFH in one of the earliest prospective trials of DVT prophylaxis. Geerts et al.[22] studied 360 trauma patients randomized to treatment with either UFH or LMWH. Their results showed a reduction in the rate of proximal DVT from 15% to 6% with the use of LMWH.[22] LMWH, including dalteparin, enoxaparin, and tinzaparin are cleared through renal mechanism and have a greater bioavailability and longer plasma half-life than heparin. Early recommendations for enoxaparin dosing called for twice daily administration. Several studies have suggested equivalent efficacy with once daily dosing.[56] Because of the short half-life, this provides windows without anticoagulation that allow for surgical procedures while simultaneously reducing administration cost. More recently, some have suggested variable dosing based on either weight or factor Xa inactivation.[43] To date, increased effectiveness with dose adjustment has not been shown and most continue with the standard dosages of enoxaparin of 30 mg bid or 40 mg daily. Because of its renal excretion, reduced dosing should be considered with calculated creatinine clearance below 30 mL/min. LMWH has emerged as the drug of choice in the majority of trauma patients for VTE prophylaxis. The probable improved effectiveness over UFH and the shorter half-life in comparison to fondaparinux, rivaroxaban, and dabigatran make it an ideal drug in the setting of trauma.

Fondaparinux

Fondaparinux is a synthetic pentasaccharide which closely mimics the active pentasaccharide of heparin. This molecule targets factor Xa exclusively with the aim of facilitating a more predictable regulation of coagulation and an improved therapeutic index.[66] In a prospective hip fracture trial of 1,711 patients, fondaparinux was found to have a greater incidence reduction than enoxaparin 8.3% versus 19.1% for VTE. Importantly, the improved risk reduction was not accompanied by an increased rate of bleeding.[19] While impressive in this phase III hip fracture trial, this decrease in VTE rate was not reproduced in a retrospective single center review for a larger population undergoing major orthopedic surgery. Donath et al.[16] noted similar rates of VTE and mortality in their comparison of LMWH to fondaparinux with an increased rate of distal DVT in the fondaparinux group. In trauma, Lu et al.[41] found fondaparinux prophylaxed group to have a DVT rate of 1.2% in high-risk patients. While this study had no controls, it does provide some indication that it may prove effective in trauma prophylaxis.

Rivaroxaban and apixaban are two other direct factor Xa inhibitors that have the advantage of predictable gut absorption allowing for oral administration. In a large prospective series of total hip and total knee patients, rivaroxaban has shown significant risk reduction for DVT without increase in bleeding complications. Dabigatran is another newly developed oral agent that is effective by virtue of its direct inhibition of thrombin. The drug has performed impressively in a comparative trial of stroke prevention in patients with atrial fibrillation. Despite their promise, to date, no large studies examining the performance of these drugs in the trauma setting have been performed. The lengthened half-life and irreversibility of these agents is cause for concern in the early days following trauma; however, because of their ease of administration, a role may evolve for their use in extended prophylaxis postdischarge.[15]

TIMING OF ADMINISTRATION

As the heightened risk of VTE can begin immediately after trauma, prophylactic measures are most effective when administered as soon as the immediate risk of bleeding has passed. This requires that the patient be warmed, volume resuscitated, and any consumptive coagulopathy reversed. Even after these milestones are achieved, some clinical situations continue to be controversial with regard to the advisability of chemical prophylaxis. These would include hemorrhagic intracranial injury and spinal cord injury. In the latter situation, recent systemic review suggests that chemical prophylaxis can be instituted within 72 hours of injury without additional risk of neurologic complication.[11] Similarly, in hemorrhagic head injury, large retrospective reviews are also demonstrating that closely monitored administration of chemical prophylaxis within 72 hours does not lead to an increased incidence of recurrent bleeding.[36] Taking advantage of the relatively short 4.5-hour half-life of enoxaparin, a pragmatic protocol is to discontinue dosing the evening prior to any invasive procedure. Following the procedure, dosing is resumed when clinical judgment suggests that primary hemostasis has occurred. This is typically 8 to 12 hours following most surgeries. Longer delays may be warranted when the consequences of bleeding carry high morbidity such as with intracranial or spinal procedures.

MECHANICAL DEVICES

While the body of evidence regarding safe chemical prophylaxis is increasing, there will always be situations in which bleeding concern exist with this strategy. These situations have led to interest in the effects of mechanical prophylaxis in the prevention of VTE. External mechanical devices can be broadly categorized as graduated compressive stockings and pneumatic pumps. The principle of the compressive stockings is to reduce the predisposition to venous stasis by reducing the resting volume of extremity veins. This theory has been validated through ultrasonic volume estimates with and without stockings and the clinical benefit documented in a systematic review.[58] Although the biologic and clinical evidence suggests that graduate compression stockings are an effective, relatively cheap, and more comfortable thromboprophylactic measure, they appear less effective overall than intermittent pneumatic compression (IPC).[40]

Intermittent Pneumatic Devices

IPC devices are postulated to be useful in VTE prevention by initiating return flow of blood pooled within the venous system. In circumstances where chemical prophylaxis is contraindicated, IPC has demonstrated a significant reduction in relative risk of VTE.[12] A few randomized trials comparing

mechanical methods to chemical alternatives have been performed. In a study of 442 trauma patients, Ginzburg et al.[23] demonstrated a DVT rate of 2.7% in the IPC group compared to 0.5% in the group prophylaxed with LMWH group. PE rates and bleeding rates were comparable.[23] In a population of 120 randomized patients with head and spinal trauma, Kurtoglu et al.[38] found no difference in the rate of DVT, PE, or mortality between treatment randomized groups treated with either LMWH or isolated IPC. Prospectively studying a population of 290 total hip patients, Warwick et al.[67] found no difference in rates of VTE between those randomized to foot pumps or those randomized to LMWH. They did note a significant increase in limb swelling and wound drainage in the LWMH group. While these comparatively small studies suggest effectiveness, combined systemic review concludes that their efficacy is not that of chemical prophylaxis.[26] The contemporary role of mechanical devices has evolved into four categories: (1) Patients at low risk, (2) patients with a bleeding diathesis, (3) transient use in trauma patients with concern for bleeding, and (4) as an adjunct in patients deemed at high risk. Relative to the third category, prospective study has shown safety in delay of 7 days prior to LMWH administration in high-risk trauma patients bridged with the use of foot pumps.[61] Relative to the fourth category, mechanical devices have been shown to be an effective addition to chemical prophylaxis. In a systematic review of 7,431 patients, Kakkos et al.[31] identified a risk reduction for DVT from 3% to 1% when chemical prophylaxis was added to mechanical. Similarly, combined therapy reduced PE rates from 4% to 1%. Given this demonstrated efficacy and the absence of risk, the addition of mechanical prophylaxis, should be given consideration in all high-risk patients.

INFERIOR VENA CAVA FILTERS

The use of inferior vena cava (IVC) filters in trauma patients, as in most other types of patients, is highly controversial. Accepted indications for IVC filter placement are patients at very high risk of VTE with an absolute contraindication to chemical thromboprophylaxis; bleeding on anticoagulation for a PE or DVT; and re-embolization despite therapeutic anticoagulation. IVC filters can be permanent or retrievable and may be placed using fluoroscopy or even at the bedside using intravascular ultrasound.

It is exceptionally difficult to prove an outcome benefit for an expensive intervention which is associated with infrequent short-term complications and uncertain long-term risks when the incidence of clinically significant PE even in the highest-risk patients is relatively low with other mechanical and chemical prophylactic measures. This benefit is so uncertain that the 2012 American College of Chest Physicians (ACCP) guidelines do not recommend the use of IVC filters as prophylactic measure for trauma patients.[26] Some recent literature may support questioning that recommendation. Angel et al.[4] published a review on the use of retrievable IVC filters for prophylaxis and treatment in 6,834 patients in 37 studies which met the authors' selection criteria. The individual studies were of intermediate quality, but the authors concluded that retrievable

IVC filters seemed to be effective in preventing PE (1.7% all indications). Long-term complications were infrequent, but could be severe: Filter migration (<1% except G2 filter), filter fracture, IVC thrombosis or stenosis (2.8%), and IVC perforation. One repeatedly reported problem which was highlighted in this review was the poor rate of device retrieval which occurred in only 34% of these 6,000 patients. Strategies to improve this retrieval rate have included removal prior to discharge and the creation of filter registries with retrieval protocols. These have proven moderately successful with improved retrieval rates of 59%.[57]

Kidane et al.[34] published a systematic review of the prophylactic use of IVC filters in trauma patients in 2012. The studies are all matched with historical control or case series limiting the conclusions which can be reached. The incidence of subsequent PE ranged from 0% to 9.1% and PE-associated mortality was 0% to 0.8%. The incidence of device-related complication was also very low although limited by the duration of patient follow-up in most studies. The most common complication was device migration/tilt. Device tilt was a radiologic determination and could be associated with a reduction in efficacy, but that clinical outcome was not observed in these studies. Given the existing uncertainty in the existing data, these authors do infrequently place an IVC filter in an occasional very high-risk patient when VTE chemoprophylaxis cannot be administered or must be significantly delayed beyond 3 or 4 days after injury (Fig. 24-3A–D). When they are placed, we coordinate our efforts with the trauma administrative support team to help ensure that they are removed prior to hospital discharge whenever possible.

SCREENING

Routine screening of patients with high risk of VTE has not proven to be an effective strategy. Borer et al.[9] compared the incidence of PE during a period in which no screenings were performed and a period when both ultrasound and magnetic resonance venography were performed in patients with pelvic or acetabular fractures. In this series of 973 patients, the rates of PE actually increased from 1.4% to 2%. The value of pelvic screening was also challenged by Stover[63] who identified a high rate of false-positive testing with both computed tomographic venography and magnetic resonance venography.

Despite its common use in practice, the use of routine screening with compression ultrasonography has not been recommended because of the low yield. One exception to this may be the high-risk patient who was not effectively prophylaxed following injury. The known high incidence of VTE in this setting makes consideration of ultrasound screening reasonable.

DIAGNOSIS

Despite recommendations to avoid routine screening, there are clinical signs which suggest the need to rule out VTE in the perioperative period. These would include inordinate limb swelling, tachycardia, hypoxia, hemoptysis, and unexplained fever. The clinical examination findings associated with DVT have long been acknowledged to have a poor predictive value.

TABLE 24-3 Wells Score (PE)	
Clinical signs and symptoms compatible with DVT	3
PE judged to be the most likely diagnosis	3
Surgery or bedridden for more than 3 d during past 4 wks	1.5
Previous DVT or PE	1.5
Heart rate >100 mins	1.5
Hemoptysis	1
Active cancer (treatment ongoing or within previous 6 mos or palliative treatment)	1

≤4, LOW (or "PE Unlikely") pretest probability; 4.5–6, MODERATE pretest probability; >6, HIGH pretest probability.
Adapted with permission from: Wells PS, Anderson DR, Rodger M, et al. Derivation of a simple clinical model to categorize patients probability of pulmonary embolism: Increasing the models utility with the SimpliRED D-dimer. *Thromb Haemost.* 2000;83(3):416–420.

In a systematic review that examined the effectiveness of differential calf diameter, limb swelling, erythema, Homan's sign, and tenderness, Goodacre et al.[24] found that none of these findings possessed the sensitivity or specificity to accurately predict disease. The single finding with the best predictive value was the presence of a differential of 2 cm or greater in calf diameter. This carried a likelihood ratio when positive of 1.8 and when negative of 0.57.[24] Time from injury also does little to affect the probability of VTE as there is relatively even distribution of events in the 4 weeks following injury.

Improving diagnostic probability with history and physical examination has been improved with the use of composite scoring. One of the more commonly used composite scores was described by Wells et al. (Table 24-3).[68] This scoring system has been through modifications with both the original and modified scores being of helpful predictive value in the outpatient setting. This score rapidly allows patients to be placed into categories of low, intermediate, or high risk of DVT with corresponding rates of DVT of 7%, 18%, and 37%.[18]

Knowing an individual's risk has bearing on testing sequence. In patients with a low risk of disease, a sensitive test for D-dimer is a reasonable screen. D-dimer is the final fragment of the plasmin-mediated degradation of cross-linked fibrin. Plasma D-dimer has proven to be a highly sensitive test for the presence of VTE with plasma levels being elevated eightfold. It also has advantage in that pelvic thrombi, often invisible to the ultrasonographer, can be detected in addition to being sensitive to PE, which may occur in the absence of DVT. The drawback with D-dimer as a diagnostic tool is its limited specificity. Conditions such as age, hospitalization, systemic inflammation, and surgery can all raise D-dimer level. With these characteristics, this tool then becomes effective in outpatient situations of low probability as a test of exclusion and insufficiently specific to initiate aggressive anticoagulant therapy.[55] In circumstances of intermediate or high risk, the more effective strategy is to directly investigate the entire lower limb with compression

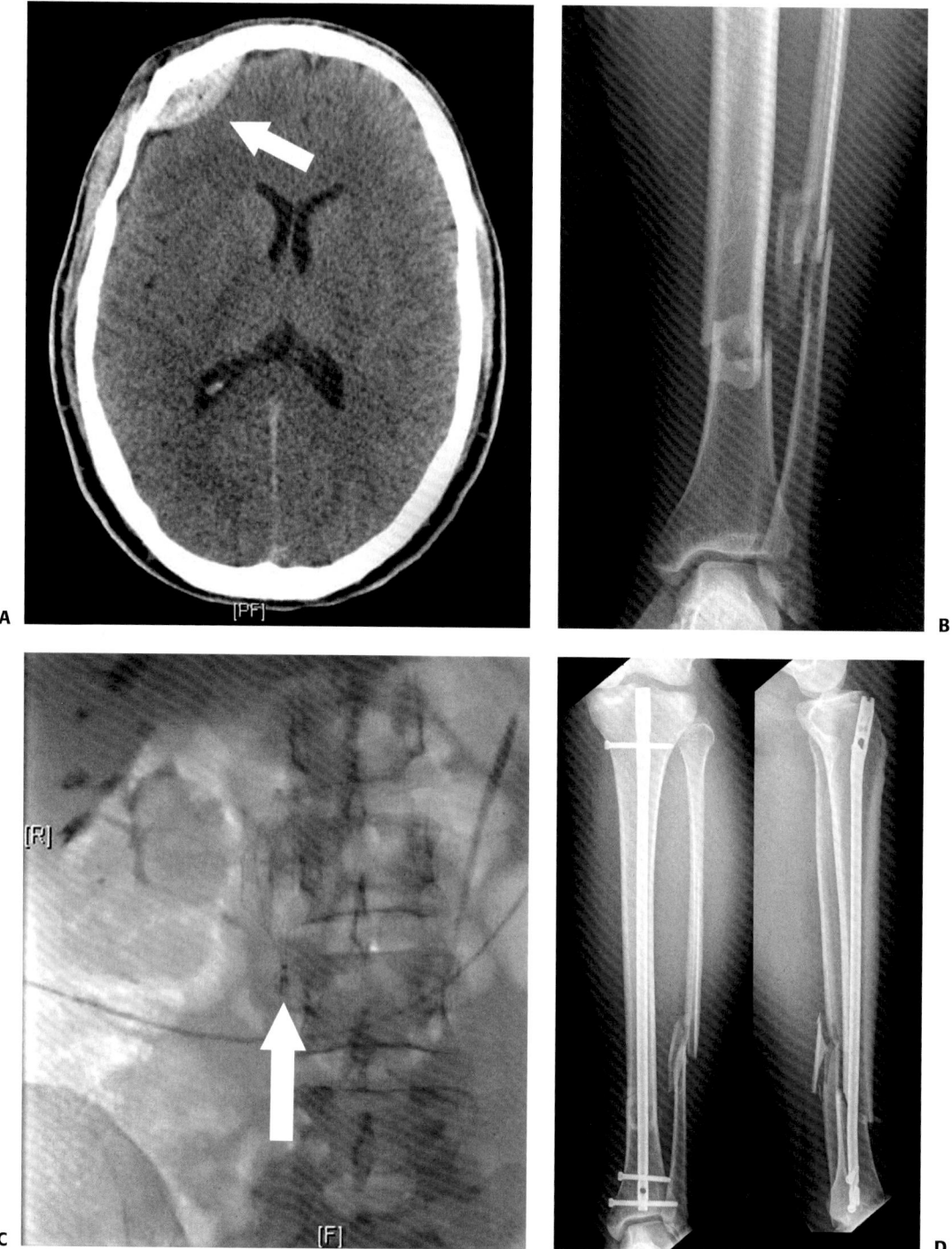

FIGURE 24-3 (A) Computed tomography of the head demonstrating right frontal epidural hematoma, **(B)** closed tibial shaft fracture, **(C)** retrievable filter placed because of concern over the safety of chemical prophylaxis and risk of VTE, and **(D)** intramedullary nail treatment of tibial shaft fracture following filter placement.

ultrasonography when DVT is suspected. This imaging technique has proven both 83% sensitive and 98% specific for both distal and proximal thrombotic disease.[33]

Just as disease Wells scores can predict DVT probability, a separate score exist for estimating probability of a PE. Risk stratification using this tool results in incidences of 75%, 17%,

and 3% found respectively in the high, intermediate, and low-risk groups.

Just as in DVT, low-risk patients may have disease excluded with a sensitive D-dimer test; however, high-risk patients are best evaluated with pulmonary imaging (Table 24-4). Classically, this has involved either a pulmonary angiogram or

TABLE 24-4 Wells Score (DVT)

Active cancer (treatment ongoing or within previous 6 mos, or palliative treatment)	1
Paralysis, paresis, or recent plaster immobilization of the lower extremities	1
Recently bedridden for 3 days or more, or major surgery within the previous 12 weeks requiring general or regional anesthesia	1
Localized tenderness along the distribution of the deep venous system	1
Entire leg swollen	1
Calf swelling >3 cm compared to asymptomatic leg (measuring 10 cm below tibial tuberosity)	1
Pitting edema confined to the symptomatic leg	1
Nonvaricose collateral superficial veins	1
Previously documented DVT	1
Alternative diagnosis at least as likely as DVT	−2

≤0, LOW pretest probability; 1 or 2, MODERATE pretest probability; ≥3, HIGH pretest probability.

ventilation perfusion scanning. More recently, these invasive and low-resolution tests have been supplanted with multidetector computed tomography pulmonary angiography with a reported sensitivity of 83% and specificity of 96%.[62] One consequence of this improved imaging resolution is that previously missed asymptomatic subsegmental emboli are now being diagnosed.[65]

TREATMENT

When prophylaxis fails and VTE is diagnosed, the reasons for treatment are fourfold: Prevention of clot extension, prevention of acute PE, prevention of recurrent thrombosis, and limiting late complications of DVT. When considering DVT, clots identified proximal to the calf are treated more aggressively as 90% of the DVT-related cases of acute PE stem from proximal DVT.[20] Because of the need for prompt anticoagulation, treatment is initiated with therapeutic doses of one of the fast-acting agents to include LMWH, fondaparinux, UFH intravenous heparin, or adjusted-dose subcutaneous heparin. Assuming patients are ambulatory and at low bleeding risk, outpatient management can be considered. Simultaneous with the initiation of one of these agents, vitamin K agonist (warfarin) is initiated for extended treatment. Heparin agents are continued for a minimum of 5 days with at least 2 days of overlap with warfarin at therapeutic levels.[26] As an alternative to dual agent therapy, oral rivaroxaban 15 mg twice daily has recently been shown to be effective for both the initial and extended treatment of DVT.[13] The treatment simplification and safety offered by this single oral medication is likely to make this an increasingly popular treatment strategy. Once the acute pain and swelling of the DVT improves, patients are encouraged to resume activity and rehabilitation appropriate to their orthopedic injury. When DVT is precipitated by a transient risk factor such as trauma, the recommended duration of anticoagulant treatment is 3 months.

Beyond the traditional anticoagulation treatment strategy just outlined, increasing attention is being paid to reduction of post-thrombotic symptoms with acute thrombolysis. While current evidence of effectiveness is not strong, consideration of thrombolysis should be given in cases of large iliofemoral clot and in the unusual cases of phlegmasia cerulea dolens.[47]

In contrast to proximal DVT, there is much less consensus on the appropriate treatment of clot restricted to the veins of the calf. Many authors recommend an aggressive approach with treatment similar to proximal DVT, while others recommend close observation. Small retrospective series report similar outcomes with ultrasound monitoring or therapeutic anticoagulation,[64] while others have demonstrated the effectiveness of short-course anticoagulant therapy.[50] At a minimum, these patients should be followed with clinical or ultrasound monitoring.

Aggressive treatment of clinically relevant PE is imperative as it reduces the mortality rate from 30% to 6%.[32] First-line therapy is directed at respiratory and circulatory support. Hypoxia is addressed with oxygen therapy and in extreme cases, mechanical ventilation for impending respiratory failure. Hypoperfusion is addressed with cautious fluid resuscitation and early introduction of vasopressors to guard against right heart overload.[37] Empiric anticoagulation should be utilized if there is no excessive risk for bleeding and a high clinical suspicion for PE exist. Once PE is confirmed, anticoagulation should be continued as the 25% risk of recurrent thromboembolism exceeds the 3% risk of significant hemorrhage. LMWH is preferred for hemodynamically stable patients with PE as evidence suggests lower mortality, less major bleeding, and fewer recurrences of thromboembolic events when compared to UFH.[32] In cases where contraindication to rapid anticoagulation exist, consideration of IVC filter should be given. In cases where hemodynamic stability is not rapidly restored with resuscitation, consideration of thrombolytic therapy or embolectomy is warranted. Just as in DVT, urgent anticoagulation is transitioned to oral warfarin and continued for 3 months in patients with transient risk factors.[32]

While this aggressive therapeutic intervention is warranted in documented pulmonary emboli that result in hypoxia, hypotension or tachycardia, the increasing ability of modern imaging to detect small clots, raises the question of appropriate treatment for physiologically irrelevant segmental and subsegmental pulmonary thrombi. In a retrospective review of 312 orthopedic trauma patients with documented PE treated with anticoagulants, 12% incurred surgical site bleeding complications.[8] As the natural history of these small pulmonary thrombi are unknown, judgment and shared decision making become necessary to balance the risks and benefits of traditional anticoagulation.

AUTHORS' TREATMENT RECOMMENDATIONS FOR PROPHYLAXIS

It is universally recognized that trauma in general and skeletal trauma in particular are strong risk factors for VTE. Regardless of ultimate prophylactic intervention, it is incumbent upon the treating physician to carefully consider the patient's risk of VTE morbidity and react to this risk with a commensurate prophylactic strategy.

Unfortunately, the multitude of patient and injury variables compounded by an incomplete body of scientific evidence makes dogmatic recommendations for VTE prophylaxis impossible. The quest for a set of routine universally accepted interventions is also challenged by the disparate views of clinicians. The ACCP has a long history of diligent review of existing evidence with regard to the prophylaxis of VTE. Their ninth edition of these guidelines was published in 2012 based on available evidence[26] and is felt to be a significant improvement over previous versions as increasing acceptance of mechanical measures and bleeding complications are now incorporated into their recommendations. Also incorporated into the latest guidelines are the practical issues of patient acceptance with latitude provided based on patient desires.

The value of these guidelines is that they provide the clinician ready access to evidence- based conclusions that lie within an enormous body of scientific work. The disadvantage of strictly adhering to evidence-based guidelines is that there are likely prophylactic algorithms that safely, conveniently, and inexpensively provide adequate protection that have not been rigorously studied. The following section of author's preferred guidelines will largely follow the recommendations of the ACCP and this is not the case, mention will be made.

ISOLATED FRACTURES

Regardless of fracture site, promoting mobilization to the extent permitted by the injury raises cardiac output, augments venous flow through muscle compression, and should be encouraged as a first-line prevention of VTE. In isolated fractures of the upper extremity and those of the ankle and foot, strong evidence does not suggest that routine prophylaxis is effective in lessening the risk of VTE and is therefore not recommended. In a review of 4,696 patients undergoing shoulder fracture repair within the English National Health Service Data Set, Jameson et al.[30] found no difference in VTE rates before or after institution of a national protocol to provide LMWH prophylaxis. Similarly, in a retrospective review of 1,540 operatively treated ankle fractures, Pelet et al.[52] found that the overall incidence of VTE of 2.99% was not affected by chemical prophylaxis. It should be recognized that in this group where prophylaxis is not routinely recommended, the risk presented by injury is additive to baseline patient risk. This makes assessment of an individual's predisposing factors advisable before making recommendations for no prophylaxis. In patients with 3 or greater on a Caprini score and presenting with these "low-risk" fractures, shared decisions with the patient regarding the need for prophylaxis should be strived for. While evidence is nonexistent in this population, an argument could be made for aspirin, LMWH, or oral factor X inhibitors for those patients concerned over the risk of VTE. The ACCP recommends no prophylaxis in injuries to the foot and ankle.

Isolated fractures of the pelvis, femur, and tibia are all known to place patients in the highest-risk categories of VTE. In this population, LMWH carries the greatest strength of evidence. In the preoperative period, the short half-life allows for surgical windows if single daily dosing is administered in the

evening. In a survey of the membership of the Orthopaedic Trauma Association (OTA), LMWH was the preferred principle agent of prophylaxis for approximately 75% of respondents. Of those utilizing LMWH, half utilized the single daily dose and half split dosing.[48] Because of the relatively low cost and additive effectiveness, a convenient form of mechanical prophylaxis could be justified in the early days following injury. In the OTA survey, mechanic methods of prophylaxis were added 40% of the time and most commonly involved graduated compressive stockings with or without pneumatic compression. While good data do not exist for length of treatment, it would seem beneficial to continue such dosing until patients are easily mobilized from bed. Once patients are mobile and discharged from the hospital, a common practice without supporting evidence is the recommendation for 81 mg of aspirin for 1 month. This practice is not recommended by the ACCP.

The geriatric hip fracture population likely represents a subgroup at heightened risk because of the cumulative effects of age, proximal fracture, and resultant immobility. In this setting, extending treatment with LMWH until 28 days is recommended because of their frequent delay in return of function.

In the setting of polytrauma with ISS > 10, there appears to be sufficient concern for VTE to routinely prophylax with LMWH. The controversies that persist in this population include the specific contraindications to chemical prophylaxis and the threshold for adding mechanical to chemical prophylaxis. With regard to the former question, there is a moderate amount of evidence that patients with traumatic brain injury can safely receive prophylaxis with LMWH, if they are clinically stable and computed tomography shows no evidence of progression. There are no similar outcome data regarding early initiation of chemical prophylaxis in patients who have suffered spinal cord injury. In those situations where the immediate risk is deemed unacceptably high, mechanical prophylaxis should be emphasized. The contraindication to chemical prophylaxis should be reevaluated and prophylaxis introduced when bleeding risk diminishes. Given the evidence of effectiveness with mechanical devices, these should always be utilized when chemical means are not employed and employed in combination with patients at high risk such as those with SCI, head injury, pelvic trauma, and prolonged ventilation.

In conclusion, it is imperative that those caring for skeletal trauma are cognizant of the heightened risk for VTE in their patients. It is equally important to have knowledge of the multitude of chemical and mechanical methods by which this risk may be mitigated. Recent decades have seen a rapidly morphing series of guidelines to help direct our preventative efforts. Given the significance of the disease, its potential for mortality and the plethora of newly released chemical prophylactic agents, it is likely that alternative strategies will continue to evolve.

REFERENCES

1. Abelseth G, Buckley RE, Pineo GE, et al. Incidence of deep-vein thrombosis in patients with fractures of the lower extremity distal to the hip. *J Orthop Trauma*. 1996;10:230–235.
2. Acosta JA, Yang JC, Winchell RJ, et al. Lethal injuries and time to death in a level I trauma center. *J Am Coll Surg*. 1998;186:528–533.
3. Adams RL, Bird RJ. Review article: Coagulation cascade and therapeutics update: Relevance to nephrology. Part 1: Overview of coagulation, thrombophilias and history of anticoagulants. *Nephrology (Carlton)*. 2009;14:462–470.

4. Angel LF, Tapson V, Galgon RE, et al. Systematic review of the use of retrievable inferior vena cava filters. *J Vasc Interv Radiol.* 2011;22:1522–1530.
5. Becattini C, Agnelli G, Schenone A, et al. Aspirin for preventing the recurrence of venous thromboembolism. *N Engl J Med.* 2012;366:1959–1967.
6. Bezemer ID, van der Meer FJ, Eikenboom JC, et al. The value of family history as a risk indicator for venous thrombosis. *Arch Intern Med.* 2009;169:610–615.
7. Bjork I, Lindahl U. Mechanism of the anticoagulant action of heparin. *Mol Cell Biochem.* 1982;48:161–182.
8. Bogdan Y, Tornetta P, Leighton R, et al. *Treatment and Complications in Orthopaedic Trauma Patients with Pulmonary Embolism.* Annual Meeting of the Orthopaedic Trauma Association, Minneapolis, MN; October 6, 2012.
9. Borer DS, Starr AJ, Reinert CM, et al. The effect of screening for deep vein thrombosis on the prevalence of pulmonary embolism in patients with fractures of the pelvis or acetabulum: A review of 973 patients. *J Orthop Trauma.* 2005;19:92–95.
10. Caprini JA. Individual risk assessment is the best strategy for thromboemboli prophylaxis. *Dis Mon.* 2010;56:552–559.
11. Christie S, Thibault-Halman G, Casha S. Acute pharmacological DVT prophylaxis after spinal cord injury. *J Neurotrauma.* 2011;28:1509–1514.
12. Chung SB, Lee SH, Kim ES, et al. Incidence of deep vein thrombosis after spinal cord injury: A prospective study in 37 consecutive patients with traumatic or nontraumatic spinal cord injury treated by mechanical prophylaxis. *J Trauma.* 2011;71:867–870; discussion 870–871.
13. Cohen AT, Dobromirski M. The use of rivaroxaban for short- and long-term treatment of venous thromboembolism. *Thromb Haemost.* 2012;107:1035–1043.
14. Datta I, Ball CG, Rudmik L, et al. Complications related to deep venous thrombosis prophylaxis in trauma: A systematic review of the literature. *J Trauma Manag Outcomes.* 2010;4:1.
15. Deftereos S, Hatzis G, Kossyvakis C, et al. Prevention and treatment of venous thromboembolism and pulmonary embolism: The role of novel oral anticoagulants. *Curr Clin Pharmacol.* 2012;7:175–194.
16. Donath L, Lützner J, Werth S, et al. Efficacy and safety of venous thromboembolism prophylaxis with fondaparinux or low-molecular weight heparin in a large cohort of consecutive patients undergoing major orthopaedic surgery—findings from the ORTHO-TEP registry. *Br J Clin Pharmacol.* 2012;74:947–958.
17. Ekeh AP, Dominguez KM, Markert RJ, et al. Incidence and risk factors for deep venous thrombosis after moderate and severe brain injury. *J Trauma.* 2010;68:912–915
18. Engelberger RP, Aujesky D, Calanca L, et al. Comparison of the diagnostic performance of the original and modified Wells score in inpatients and outpatients with suspected deep vein thrombosis. *Thromb Res.* 2011;127:535–539.
19. Eriksson BI, Bauer KA, Lassen MR, et al. Fondaparinux compared with enoxaparin for the prevention of venous thromboembolism after hip-fracture surgery. *N Engl J Med.* 2001;345:1298–1304.
20. Galanaud JP, Sevestre-Pietri MA, Bosson JL, et al. Comparative study on risk factors and early outcome of symptomatic distal versus proximal deep vein thrombosis: Results from the OPTIMEV study. *Thromb Haemost.* 2009;102:493–500.
21. Geerts WH, Code KI, Jay RM, et al. A prospective study of venous thromboembolism after major trauma. *N Engl J Med.* 1994;331:1601–1606.
22. Geerts WH, Jay RM, Code KI, et al. A comparison of low-dose heparin with lowmolecular-weight heparin as prophylaxis against venous thromboembolism after major trauma. *N Engl J Med.* 1996;335:701–707.
23. Ginzburg E, Cohn SM, Lopez J, et al. Miami deep vein thrombosis study group. Randomized clinical trial of intermittent pneumatic compression and low molecular weight heparin in trauma. *Br J Surg.* 2003;90:1338–1344.
24. Goodacre S, Sutton AJ, Sampson FC. Meta-analysis: The value of clinical assessment in the diagnosis of deep venous thrombosis. *Ann Intern Med.* 2005;143:129–139.
25. Gray E, Hogwood J, Mulloy B. The anticoagulant and antithrombotic mechanisms of heparin. *Handb Exp Pharmacol.* 2012;(207):43–61.
26. Guyatt GH, Akl EA, Crowther M, et al. Executive summary: Antithrombotic therapy and prevention of thrombosis, 9th ed: American College of Chest Physicians Evidence-Based Clinical Practice Guidelines. *Chest.* 2012;141(2 suppl):7S–47S.
27. Handoll HH, Farrar MJ, McBirnie J, et al. Heparin, low molecular weight heparin and physical methods for preventing deep vein thrombosis and pulmonary embolism following surgery for hip fractures. *Cochrane Database Syst Rev.* 2002;(4):CD000305.
28. Haut ER, Pronovost PJ. Surveillance bias in outcomes reporting. *JAMA.* 2011;305:2462–2463.
29. Hirsh J, Warkentin T, Shaughnessy S, et al. Heparin and low-molecular-weight heparin: Mechanisms of action, pharmacokinetics, dosing, monitoring, efficacy, and safety. *Chest.* 2001;119:64S–94S.
30. Jameson SS, James P, Howcroft DW, et al. Venous thromboembolic events are rare after shoulder surgery: Analysis of a national database. *J Shoulder Elbow Surg.* 2011;20:764–770.
31. Kakkos SK, Warwick D, Nicolaides AN, et al. Combined (mechanical and pharmacological) modalities for the prevention of venous thromboembolism in joint replacement surgery. *J Bone Joint Surg Br.* 2012;94:729–734.
32. Kearon C, Akl EA, Comerota AJ, et al. Antithrombotic therapy for VTE disease: Antithrombotic Therapy and Prevention of Thrombosis, 9th ed: American College of Chest Physicians Evidence-Based Clinical Practice Guidelines. *Chest.* 2012;141 (2 suppl):e419S–e494S.
33. Keller ME, Metzler MH, Phillips JO, et al. Evaluation of a disease management plan for prevention and diagnosis of thromboembolic disease in major trauma patients. *Curr Surg.* 2000;57:456–459.
34. Kidane B, Madani AM, Vogt K, et al. The use of prophylactic inferior vena cava filters in trauma patients: A systematic review. *Injury.* 2012;43:542–547.
35. Knudson MM, Ikossi DG, Khaw L, et al. Thromboembolism after trauma: An analysis of 1602 episodes from the American College of Surgeons National Trauma Data Bank. *Ann Surg.* 2004;240:490–498.
36. Koehler DM, Shipman J, Davidson MA, et al. Is early venous thromboembolism prophylaxis safe in trauma patients with intracranial hemorrhage. *J Trauma.* 2011;70:324–349.
37. Kucher N, Goldhaber SZ. Management of massive pulmonary embolism. *Circulation.* 2005;112:e28–e32.
38. Kurtoglu M, Yanar H, Bilsel Y, et al. Venous thromboembolism prophylaxis after head and spinal trauma: Intermittent pneumatic compression devices versus low molecular weight heparin. *World J Surg.* 2004;28:807–811.
39. Lasne D, Jude B, Susen S. From normal to pathological hemostasis. *Can J Anaesth.* 2006;53(6 suppl):S2–S11.
40. Lippi G, Favaloro EJ, Cervellin G. Prevention of venous thromboembolism: Focus on mechanical prophylaxis. *Semin Thromb Hemost.* 2011;37:237–251.
41. Lu JP, Knudson MM, Bir N, et al. Fondaparinux for prevention of venous thromboembolism in high-risk trauma patients: A pilot study. *J Am Coll Surg.* 2009;209:589–594.
42. Malinoski D, Jafari F, Ewing T, et al. Standard prophylactic enoxaparin dosing leads to inadequate anti-Xa levels and increased deep venous thrombosis rates in critically ill trauma and surgical patients. *J Trauma.* 2010;68:874–880.
43. Manzoli L, De Vito C, Marzuillo C, et al. Oral contraceptives and venous thromboembolism: A systematic review and meta-analysis. *Drug Saf.* 2012;35:191–205.
44. Martinelli I, Mannucci PM, De Stefano V, et al. Different risks of thrombosis in four coagulation defects associated with inherited thrombophilia: A study of 150 families. *Blood.* 1998;92:2353–2358.
45. Mateo J, Oliver A, Borrell M, et al. Laboratory evaluation and clinical characteristics of 2,132 consecutive unselected patients with venous thromboembolism–results of the Spanish Multicentric Study on Thrombophilia (EMET-Study). *Thromb Haemost.* 1997;77:444–451.
46. Maung AA, Schuster KM, Kaplan LJ, et al. Risk of venous thromboembolism after spinal cord injury: Not all levels are the same. *J Trauma.* 2011;71:1241–1245.
47. Meissner MH, Gloviczki P, Comerota AJ, et al. Early thrombus removal strategies for acute deep venous thrombosis: Clinical practice guidelines of the Society for Vascular Surgery and the American Venous Forum. *J Vasc Surg.* 2012;55:1449–1462.
48. Obremskey W, Sagi C, Molina C, et al. *OTA Current Practice Survey of IN-Patient DVT Prophylaxis in the Trauma Patient.* : Annual Meeting of the Orthopaedic Trauma Association, Minneapolis, MN; October 5, 2012.
49. Paffrath T, Wafaisade A, Lefering R, et al. Venous thromboembolism after severe trauma: Incidence, risk factors and outcome. *Injury.* 2010;41:97–101.
50. Parisi R, Visonà A, Camporese G, et al. Isolated distal deep vein thrombosis: Efficacy and safety of a protocol of treatment. Treatment of Isolated Calf Thrombosis (TICT) Study. *Int Angiol.* 2009;28:68–72.
51. Park MS, Owen BA, Ballinger BA, et al. Quantification of hypercoagulable state after blunt trauma: Microparticle and thrombin generation are increased relative to injury severity, while standard markers are not. *Surgery.* 2012;151:831–836.
52. Pelet S, Roger ME, Belzile EL, et al. The incidence of thromboembolic events in surgically treated ankle fracture. *J Bone Joint Surg Am.* 2012;94:502–506.
53. Ploumis A, Ponnappan RK, Maltenfort MG, et al. Thromboprophylaxis in patients with acute spinal injuries: An evidence-based analysis. *J Bone Joint Surg Am.* 2009;91:2568–2576.
54. [No authors listed]. Prevention of pulmonary embolism and deep vein thrombosis with low dose aspirin: Pulmonary Embolism Prevention (PEP) trial. *Lancet.* 2000;355:1295–1203.
55. Righini M, Perrier A, De Moerloose P, et al. D-Dimer for venous thromboembolism diagnosis: 20 years later. *J Thromb Haemost.* 2008;6:1059–1071.
56. Riha GM, Van PY, Differding JA, et al. Incidence of deep vein thrombosis is increased with 30 mg twice daily dosing of enoxaparin compared with 40 mg daily. *Am J Surg.* 2012;203:598–602.
57. Rogers FB, Shackford SR, Miller JA, et al. Improved recovery of prophylactic inferior vena cava filters in trauma patients: The results of a dedicated filter registry and critical pathway for filter removal. *J Trauma Acute Care Surg.* 2012;72:381–384.
58. Sachdeva A, Dalton M, Amaragiri SV, et al. Elastic compression stockings for prevention of deep vein thrombosis. *Cochrane Database Syst Rev.* 2010;(7):CD001484.
59. Sems SA, Levy BA, Dajani K, et al. Incidence of deep venous thrombosis after temporary joint spanning external fixation for complex lower extremity injuries. *J Trauma.* 2009;66:1164–1166.
60. Smith EB, Parvizi J, Purtill JJ. Delayed surgery for patients with femur and hip fractures-risk of deep venous thrombosis. *J Trauma.* 2011;70:E113–E116.
61. Stannard JP, Lopez-Ben RR, Volgas DA, et al. Prophylaxis against deep-vein thrombosis following trauma: A prospective, randomized comparison of mechanical and pharmacologic prophylaxis. *J Bone Joint Surg Am.* 2006;88:261–266.
62. Stein PD, Fowler SE, Goodman LR, et al. Multidetector computed tomography for acute pulmonary embolism. *N Engl J Med.* 2006;354:2317–2327.
63. Stover MD, Morgan SJ, Bosse MJ, et al. Prospective comparison of contrast-enhanced computed tomography versus magnetic resonance venography in the detection of occult deep pelvic vein thrombosis in patients with pelvic and acetabular fractures. *J Orthop Trauma.* 2002;16:613–621.
64. Sule AA, Chin TJ, Handa P, et al. Should symptomatic, isolated distal deep vein thrombosis be treated with anticoagulation? *Int J Angiol.* 2009;18:83–87.
65. Tornetta P, Bogdan Y. Pulmonary embolism in orthopaedic patients: Diagnosis and management. *J Am Acad Orthop Surg.* 2012;20:586–595.
66. Turpie AG, Eriksson BI, Bauer KA, et al. Fondaparinux. *J Am Acad Orthop Surg.* 2004;12:371–375.
67. Warwick D, Harrison J, Glew D, et al. Comparison of the use of a foot pump with the use of low-molecular-weight heparin for the prevention of deep-vein thrombosis after total hip replacement. A prospective, randomized trial. *J Bone Joint Surg Am.* 1998;80:1158–1166.
68. Wells PS, Anderson DR, Bomanis J, et al. Value of assessment of pretest probability of deep-vein thrombosis in clinical management. *Lancet.* 1997;350:1795–1798.

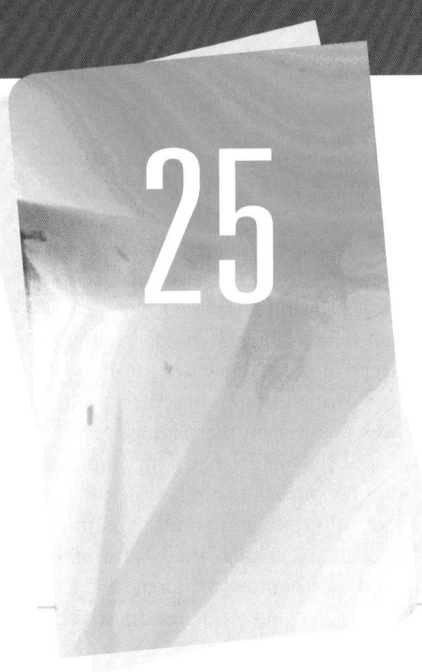

25

COMPLEX REGIONAL PAIN SYNDROME

Roger M. Atkins

INTRODUCTION

During the American Civil War, Silas Weir Mitchell et al.[137] described a syndrome which occurred in patients who had suffered gunshot injuries to major nerves. Noting that a leading feature was burning pain, he called the condition causalgia. At the beginning of the 20th century, Paul Sudeck,[170,171] a clinician in Hamburg, Germany, used the newly invented technique of roentgenology to investigate patients with severe pain after injury. He described a post-traumatic pain syndrome with edema, trophic changes, and osteoporosis. In 1979, the AO group advocated open reduction and rigid internal fixation to prevent fracture disease, which was defined as a combination of circulatory disturbance, inflammation, and pain as a result of dysfunction of joints and muscles.[138] In an intriguing vignette, Channon and Lloyd[35] noted that finger stiffness after Colles fracture could be either simple or associated with swelling and changes in hand temperature. In the latter case it did not respond well to physiotherapy. The modern term for the syndrome described in different circumstances by these researchers is complex regional pain syndrome, usually abbreviated to CRPS.

CRPS is characterized by abnormal pain, swelling, vasomotor and sudomotor dysfunction, contracture, and osteoporosis. It is used to be considered a rare, devastating complication of injury, caused by abnormalities in the sympathetic nervous system (SNS), and seen mainly in psychologically abnormal patients. Modern research is altering this view radically. This chapter will specifically examine CRPS within the context of orthopedic trauma surgery. For this reason, the emphasis, descriptions, and concepts differ slightly from those routinely found in publications from the International Association for the Study of Pain (IASP). It is important to appreciate that these apparent differences are merely counterpoints. The theme is identical.

SOME IMPORTANT DEFINITIONS

A cardinal feature of CRPS is abnormalities of pain perception which are mainly foreign to orthopedic surgeons. They have been codified by Merskey and Bogduk,[135] and since they will be used throughout this text, they are described here.

Allodynia (literally "other pain") is a painful perception of a stimulus which should not usually be painful. Thus, for example, a patient will find gentle stroking of the affected part painful. Allodynia differs from referred pain, but allodynic pain can occur in areas other than the one stimulated. There are several forms of allodynia:

Mechanical (or tactile) allodynia implies pain in response to touch. It may be subdivided into *static mechanical allodynia,* implying pain in response to light touch or pressure, and *dynamic mechanical allodynia,* where pain is due to brushing.[121]

In *thermal (hot or cold) allodynia,* the pain is caused by mild changes in skin temperature in the affected area.

Hyperalgesia is an increased sensitivity to pain, which may be caused by damage to nociceptors or peripheral nerves. Thus the patient finds gentle touching with a pin unbearably painful. Hyperalgesia is usually experienced in focal, discrete areas, typically associated with injury. Focal hyperalgesia may be divided into two subtypes:

- *Primary hyperalgesia* describes pain sensitivity that occurs directly in the damaged tissues.

- *Secondary hyperalgesia* describes pain sensitivity that occurs in the surrounding undamaged tissues.

Rarely, hyperalgesia is seen in a more diffuse, body-wide form.

Hyperpathia is a temporal and spatial summation of an allodynic or hyperalgesic response. The patient finds gentle touching painful, but repetitive touching either on the same spot or on another part of the affected limb becomes increasingly unbearable, and the pain continues for a prolonged period after the stimulus has been withdrawn. In severe cases the pain may be accentuated by unusual, extraneous things such as the sudden noise of a door shutting or a draft of cold air.

It is important for the orthopedic surgeon to realize that these patients are not malingering or mad. These are genuine perceptions of pain.

A HISTORIC VIEW OF TAXONOMY

A historic review of nomenclature will help to elucidate much confusion which surrounds this condition. In the past, CRPS was diagnosed using a variety of nonstandardized and idiosyncratic diagnostic systems derived solely from the authors' clinical experiences, none of which achieved wide acceptance. The condition was given a number of synonyms (Table 25-1) reflecting the site affected, cause, and clinical features. During the American Civil War, Mitchell[137] noted the burning nature of pain following

---

TABLE 25-1 **Synonyms for Complex Regional Pain Syndrome**

Complex regional pain syndrome
Reflex sympathetic dystrophy
Sudeck atrophy
Causalgia
Minor causalgia
Mimo-causalgia
Algodystrophy
Algoneurodystrophy
Post-traumatic pain syndrome
Painful post-traumatic dystrophy
Painful post-traumatic osteoporosis
Transient migratory osteoporosis

---

nerve trauma and described this as *causalgia* (from the Greek "burning pain"). In contrast, in the 1900s, Sudeck[170,171] investigated conditions characterized by severe osteoporosis, including some cases of CRPS. The condition was named *Sudeck atrophy* by Nonne[140] in 1901. Leriche[113,114] demonstrated that sympathectomy could alter the clinical features associated with *post-traumatic osteoporosis,* and De Takats[43] suggested *reflex dystrophy* in 1937. Evans[52] introduced the term *reflex sympathetic dystrophy* (RSD) based on the theory (following Leriche's observations) that sympathetic hyperactivity was involved in the pathophysiology, and this term was popularized by Bonica.[21] In 1940, Homans[95] proposed *minor causalgia* to imply a relationship between Mitchell's causalgia, renamed *major causalgia,* and similar conditions arising without direct nerve injury. *Causalgic state*[42] and *mimo-causalgia*[144] followed to add to the confusion. Today the term causalgia is reserved for the original Mitchell's use in which a major nerve injury produces burning pain.[166]

Steinbrocker[168] introduced the term *shoulder hand syndrome* for a condition which may be separate from true CRPS, and *algoneurodystrophy* was suggested by Glick and Helal.[75,76] *Algodystrophy,* from the Greek "painful disuse," was introduced by French rheumatologists in the late 1970s.[49]

Sympathetically maintained pain (SMP) is characterized by pain, hyperpathia, and allodynia which are relieved by selective sympathetic blockade. The relationship between CRPS and SMP is disputed.[166] In CRPS a proportion of the pain is usually sympathetically maintained and is therefore relieved by sympathetic blockade. However in CRPS a process is also taking place which leads to initial tissue edema followed by severe contracture. This is not an inevitable part of SMP.[102] SMP is not a particularly helpful concept for the orthopedic surgeon; however, it will be explored further when the etiology of CRPS is considered.

MODERN TAXONOMY AND DIAGNOSIS

Fortunately, all the above confusion is now of historic interest. The IASP has undertaken a major work in analyzing the features of CRPS and reclassifying the condition.[135] IASP changed the name of the condition to CRPS at a consensus workshop in Orlando, Florida, in 1994[19,166] and proposed new standardized diagnostic criteria (Table 25-2).[135] A broad description of CRPS is as follows[25,88]:

"CRPS describes an array of painful conditions that are characterized by a continuing (spontaneous and/or evoked) regional pain that is seemingly disproportionate in time or degree to the usual course of any known trauma or other lesion. The pain is regional (not in a specific nerve territory or dermatome) and usually has a distal predominance of abnormal sensory, motor, sudomotor, vasomotor, and/or trophic findings, including osteoporosis. The syndrome shows variable progression over time."

CRPS was divided into CRPS type 2 (CRPS-2), where the cause was direct nerve damage, and CRPS type 1 (CRPS-1), where it was not. These syndromes may have different clinical features,[24]; however, the distinction becomes blurred since post-surgery CRPS, where one might assume peripheral nerves to be damaged, is invariably classified as CRPS-1.[129] Furthermore,

TABLE 25-2	**The Original IASP Diagnostic Criteria for Complex Regional Pain Syndrome**

1. The presence of an initiating noxious event, or a cause of immobilization (Not required for diagnosis; 5–10% of patients will not have this).
2. Continuing pain, allodynia, or hyperalgesia in which the pain is disproportionate to any known inciting event.
3. Evidence at some time of edema, changes in skin blood flow, or abnormal sudomotor activity in the region of pain (can be sign or symptom).
4. This diagnosis is excluded by the existence of other conditions that would otherwise account for the degree of pain and dysfunction.

If the condition occurs in the absence of "major nerve damage," the diagnosis is CRPS-1.
If "major nerve damage" is present, the diagnosis is CRPS-2.

(Adapted from Merskey H, Bogduk N. *Classification of Chronic Pain: Descriptions of Chronic Pain Syndromes and Definitions of Pain Terms.* Seattle, WA: IASP Press; 1994.)

in amputation and biopsy specimens from CRPS-1 cases, small (C and Aδ) nerve fiber degeneration is seen.[1,141] From a surgeon's perspective, the most useful distinction would be a diagnosis of CRPS-2 where nerve damage susceptible to surgical intervention was causative, for example, sural nerve entrapment following a percutaneous tendo Achilles repair.

Clinical Features

Since the etiology of CRPS is obscure, the diagnosis must be clinical, and therefore, precise descriptions of symptoms and signs acquire great importance. Classical descriptions emphasize three sequential stages.[20,43,49,74,161,162,183] Modern evidence suggests that CRPS does not always follow this course[14,24,183,200,201] and supports the clinical impression that this evolution is seen in more severe cases (as might be expected from historic series). Since the classical descriptions provide the greatest information concerning clinical features, the following description will refer to the staging system where helpful.

CRPS is a biphasic condition with early swelling and vasomotor instability (VMI) giving way over a variable timescale to late contracture and joint stiffness.[49] The hand and foot are most frequently involved, although the knee is increasingly recognized.[38,39,104] The elbow is rarely affected, whereas shoulder disease is common and some cases of frozen shoulder are probably CRPS.[168] The hip is affected in transient osteoporosis of pregnancy.

CRPS usually begins up to a month after the precipitating trauma, although the delay may be greater. Antecedent trauma is not essential, but within an orthopedic context it is almost invariable.[49] As the direct effects of injury subside, a new diffuse, unpleasant, neuropathic pain arises.[194] Neuropathic pain is a pain which occurs without any precipitating noxious stimulus; and spontaneous or burning pain, mechanical or thermal hyperalgesia, allodynia, and hyperpathia are common but not

universal features.[51,125,135,163] Pain is unremitting (although sleep may be unaffected), worsening, and radiating with time and may be increased by limb dependency, physical contact, emotional upset, or even by extraneous factors such as sudden loud noise or a blast of cold air.

Early Phase of CRPS

VMI and edema dominate the early phase (Fig. 25-1), although this is less marked with more proximal CRPS. The classical description of the temporal evolution of the condition divides the early phase of CRPS into two stages depending on the type of the VMI.[49] In this description, initially the limb is dry, hot, and pink (vasodilated, stage 1), but after a variable period of days to weeks, it becomes blue, cold, and sweaty (vasoconstricted, stage 2). As noted above, this classical evolution is rarely seen. Most commonly, especially in more mild cases, the VMI is characterized by an increase in temperature sensitivity, with variable abnormality of sweating. Alternatively, some patients remain substantially vasodilated, while others are vasoconstricted with no history of vasodilatation.[14,24,183,199]

In the early phase of CRPS, edema is marked, particularly where the distal part of the limb is affected. Initially the edema is simple tissue swelling and may be overcome by physical therapy and elevation if the patient will permit. With time (in the classical description, passing from stage 1 to stage 2), the edema becomes more fixed and indurated with coalescence of tissue planes and structures.

Initially, in the early phase of CRPS, loss of joint mobility is due to swelling and pain combined with an apparent inability to

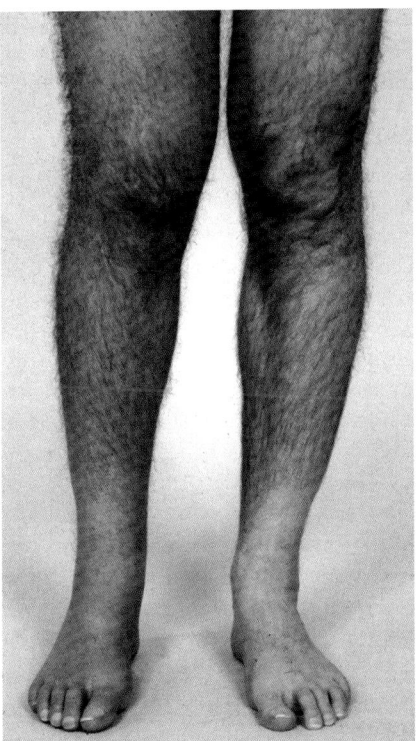

FIGURE 25-1 A patient with early CRPS-1 affecting the leg. Note the swelling of the leg and the discoloration of the shin.

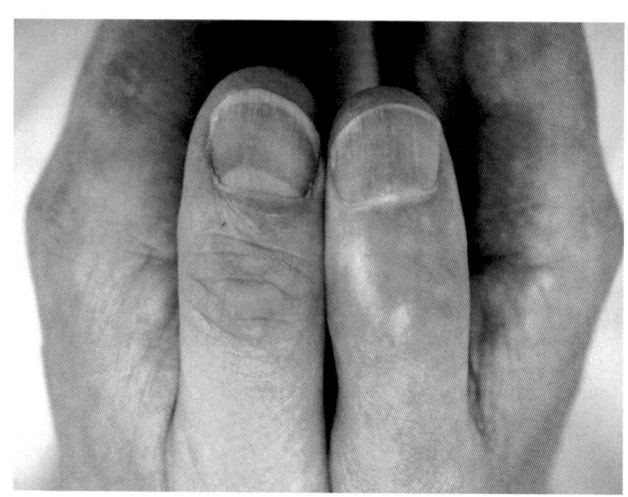
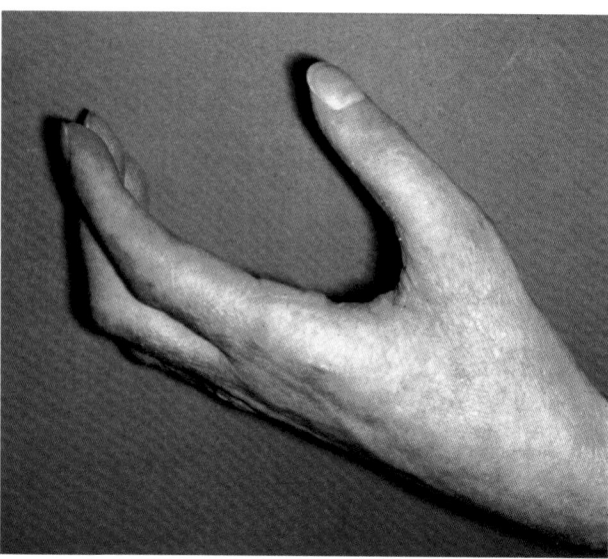

A   **B**

FIGURE 25-2 The late phase of CRPS. **A:** Detail of the thumbs of a patient with late CRPS-1 of the right hand. There is spindling of the digit particularly distally. The nail is excessively ridged and is discolored. **B:** The hand of a patient with late CRPS-1. The patient is trying to make a fist. Note the digital spindling and extension contractures with loss of joint creases.

initiate movement or state of neglect or denial with respect to the limb.[30–32,64,66–68,111,151] Weakness, dystonia, spasms, tremor, and myoclonus have also been reported[17,161,178,179]; however, these are not usually prominent within an orthopedic context. As the early phase progresses, loss of joint mobility is increasingly due to development of contracture. Only if the disease can be halted before fixed contracture has occurred can complete resolution occur.

Late Phase of CRPS

Passing into the late phase, VMI recedes, edema resolves, and atrophy of the limb occurs (Fig. 25-2), affecting every tissue. The skin is thinned, and joint creases and subcutaneous fat disappear. Hairs become fragile, uneven, and curled, while nails are pitted, ridged, brittle, and discolored brown. Palmar and plantar fascias thicken and contract simulating Dupuytren disease.[49,120] Tendon sheaths become constricted causing triggering and increased resistance to movement. Muscle contracture combined with tendon adherence leads to reduced tendon excursion. Joint capsules and collateral ligaments become shortened, thickened, and adherent, causing joint contracture.

It is important to restate that the progression of CRPS is very variable. Within orthopedic practice, the large majority of patients who demonstrate the features of the early phase of CRPS after trauma will not go on to develop severe late-phase contracture, although a significant proportion will show chronic subclinical contracture.[61]

Bone Changes

Bone involvement is universal with increased uptake on bone scanning in early CRPS (Fig. 25-3). This was originally thought

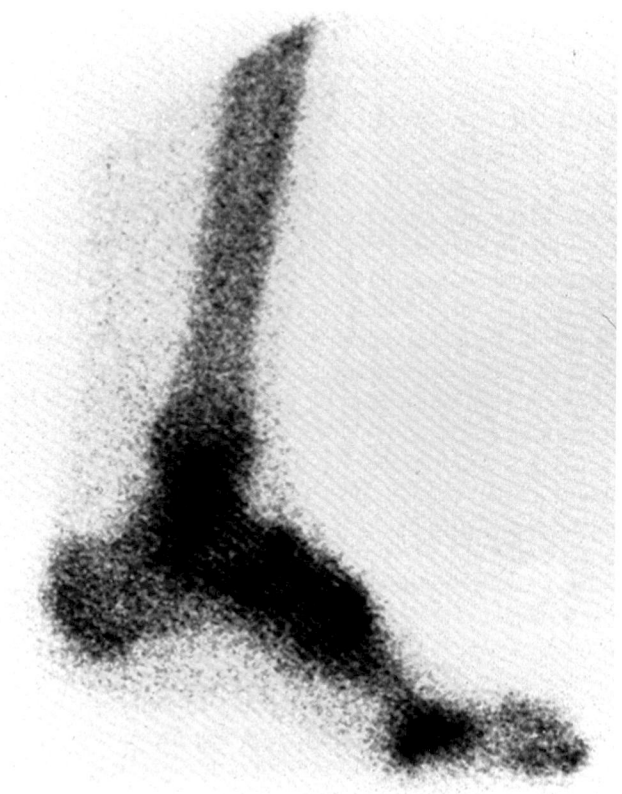

FIGURE 25-3 Bone scan changes in CRPS. The delayed phase of a bone scan of a patient with early CRPS-1 of the lower leg. There is increased uptake throughout the affected region. The bone scan will usually revert to normal after 6 months.

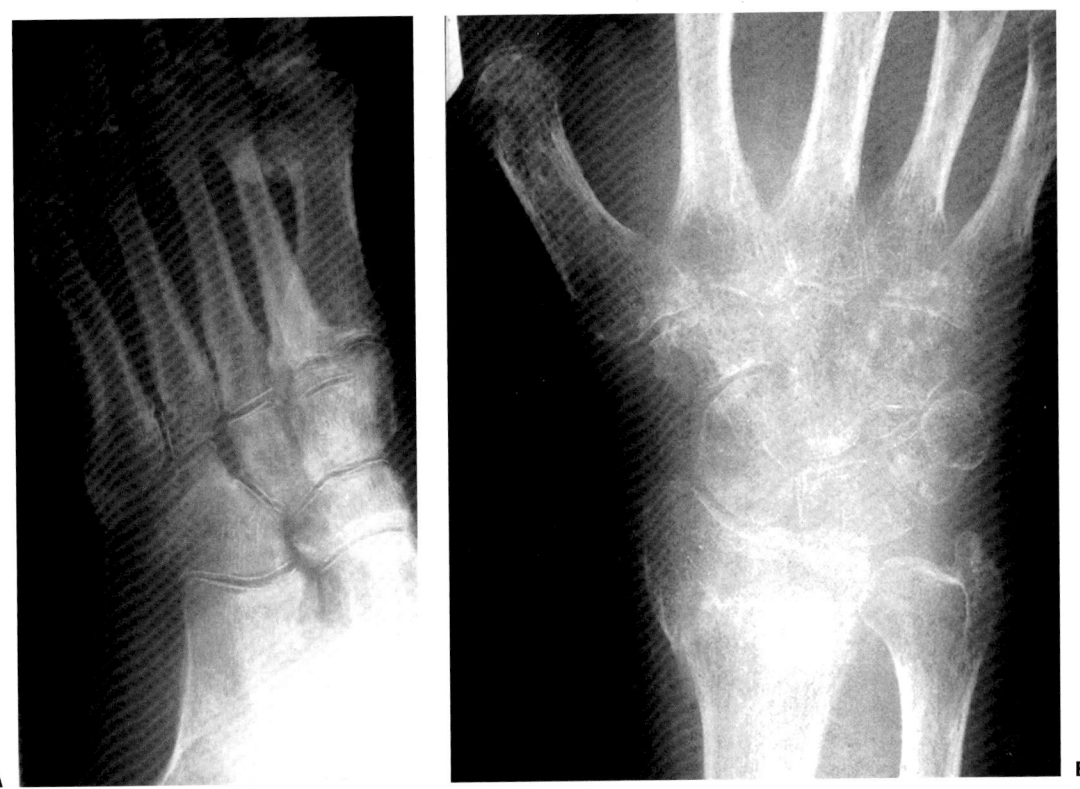

FIGURE 25-4 Radiographic features of CRPS. **A:** Oblique radiograph of a patient with CRPS-1 of the foot. There is patchy osteoporosis with accentuation of the osteoporosis beneath the joints. **B:** Profound osteoporosis in a patient with late severe CRPS-1 affecting the hand.

to be periarticular, suggesting arthralgia[94,109,124]; however, CRPS does not cause arthritis, and more recent studies have shown generalized hyperfixation,[6,37,45] confirming the view of Doury.[49] Increased uptake is not invariable in children.[192] Later, the bone scan returns to normal, and there are radiographic features of rapid bone loss: Visible demineralization with patchy, subchondral, or subperiosteal osteoporosis; metaphyseal banding; and profound bone loss (Fig. 25-4).[110] Despite the osteoporosis, fracture is uncommon, presumably because the patients protect the painful limb very effectively.

Incidence

It is the common experience of orthopedic surgeons that patients such as shown in Figure 25-2 are extremely rare. Thus severe, chronic CRPS associated with severe contracture is uncommon with a reported prevalence of less than 2% in historic retrospective series.[9,82,116,122,147] Two recent population-based studies have yielded contrasting results with 5.5 cases per 100,000 person-years in the United States[155] and 26.2 per 100,000 person-years in the Netherlands[41] In contrast, prospective studies designed to look specifically for the early features of CRPS show that they occur after up to 30% of fractures and surgical trauma (e.g., total knee replacement)[3,4,8,14,15,56,90,156,157,164] where the features of CRPS have been actively sought. Furthermore, statistically, the features tend to occur together.[4,156] These common early cases of CRPS are usually not specifically diagnosed,[164] and some would, contro-

versially, dispute the diagnosis.[16] They resolve substantially either spontaneously or with standard treatment by physical therapy and analgesia within a year.[14,15,119,164] Some features, particularly stiffness, may remain suggesting that CRPS may be responsible for significant long-term morbidity even when mild.[14,61] The truly intriguing question is, if CRPS is so common, why is it not a universal finding after trauma or orthopedic surgery?

Etiology

CRPS may occur after any particular trauma while an identical stimulus in a different limb does not cause it. The incidence is not changed by treatment method and open anatomic reduction, and rigid internal fixation does not abolish it.[157] It is unclear whether injury severity or quality of fracture reduction alters the incidence.[4,15] There is, however, an association with excessively tight casts,[60] and there may be a genetic predilection.[46,105,108,127,128] The following etiologies have been proposed.

Psychological Abnormalities

A psychological cause for chronic pain was first suggested by Breuer and Freud,[22] and historically, it has been suggested that CRPS may be purely a psychological problem.[36] Most orthopedic clinicians immediately recognize a "Sudecky" patient, that is, broadly speaking, a patient who appears to the clinician to be somebody who is likely to fare poorly after surgical intervention or trauma perhaps due to their inability to cooperate fully with physical therapy. In fact, the literature fails to identify this sort of patient and the evidence does not support the notion that CRPS is primarily psychological.[27] Studies of premorbid personality show no consistent abnormality.[139,198] Most patients are psychologically normal[184] although emotional lability, low pain threshold,[44] hysteria,[145] and depression[169] have been reported. There is an association with antecedent psychological stress[23,27,58,69–72,182] which probably exacerbates pain in CRPS, as in other diseases.[26] It seems likely that the severe chronic pain of CRPS causes depression and that a "Sudecky" type of patient who develops CRPS is at risk of a poor outcome because they will not mobilize in the face of pain.

Abnormal (Neuropathic) Pain

CRPS is characterized by excessive and abnormal pain. Pain is usually caused when an intense noxious stimulus activates high-threshold nociceptors, and it prevents tissue damage. Neuropathic pain in CRPS occurs without appropriate stimulus and has no protective function. However, injured peripheral nerve fibers undergo cellular changes which cause usually innocuous tactile inputs to stimulate the dorsal horn cells via A-β fibers from low-threshold mechanoreceptors, causing allodynia in CRPS-2.[103,195] Similar C-nociceptor dysfunction explains causalgia. Furthermore, axonal injury prevents nerve growth factor transport which is essential for normal nerve function.[118,194] In CRPS-1, covert nerve lesions with artificial synapses have been postulated.[48] These "ephases" have not been demonstrated and are unnecessary since inflammatory mediators released by the initial trauma (and possibly retained due to a failure of free radical clearance) can sensitize nociceptors to respond to normally innocuous stimuli.[137,138]

Sympathetic Nervous System (SNS) Abnormalities

That CRPS is associated with apparent abnormalities in the SNS is obvious. Hence the popularity of the eponym RSD. Furthermore, since Leriche's early studies,[113,114] generations of therapists have treated CRPS with sympathetic manipulation, noting an acute change in the clinical features,[34,77,84–87,97] although recent studies cast some doubt on whether sympathetic manipulation improves the long-term outcome of the condition.[98,119]

The features of CRPS which suggest SNS dysfunction include abnormalities in skin blood flow, temperature regulation and sweating, and edema. However, SNS activity is not usually painful.[99,100] In CRPS, however, some pain (termed SMP[166]) is SNS-dependent. This accounts for spontaneous pain and allodynia, which may therefore be relieved by stellate ganglion blockade[148] and then restored by noradrenalin injection.[2,173] Furthermore, there is an abnormal difference in cutaneous sensory threshold between the limbs, which is reversed by sympathetic blockade,[59,63,149,150] while increasing sympathetic activity worsens pain.[101]

What then is the cause of SMP in CRPS? It is due to the body's reaction to injury. After partial nerve division, injured and uninjured somatic axons express α-adrenergic receptors,[33] and sympathetic axons come to surround sensory neuron cell bodies in dorsal root ganglia.[134,186,194] These changes, which

may be temporary,[173,185,187] make the somatic sensory nervous system sensitive to circulating catecholamines and noradrenalin released from postganglionic sympathetic terminals.

Abnormal Inflammation

CRPS resembles an inflammatory state leading to gross scarring. Therefore, the orthopedic differential diagnoses are occult causes of inflammation such as soft tissue infection or stress fracture. CRPS is associated with inflammatory changes including macromolecule extravasation[143] and reduced oxygen consumption.[80,175] Serum concentrations of substance P, a neuropeptide associated with inflammatory processes and pain,[159] and calcitonin gene-related peptide (CGRP)[18] are higher in CRPS patients than controls, causing an augmented flare response[129] and excessive protein extravasation.[112] Substance P stimulates keratinocytes to express cytokines in vitro,[40] and keratinocytes in skin biopsies from CRPS-affected limbs show increased substance P receptors.[107,129] This suggests that excess neuropeptide activity causes extravasation, limb edema, and increased cytokine expression that characterize CRPS. However, how the immune and nervous systems interact in the bones, muscles, and connective tissue is not understood.

Cytokine levels are higher in CRPS-affected limbs than in the contralateral limb or control patients.[83,96,174] These changes do not correlate well with the clinical features except in mechanical hyperalgesia.[126]

In animals, infusion of free radical donors causes a CRPS-like state,[176] and amputated human specimens with CRPS show basement membrane thickening consistent with overexposure to free radicals.[177] This suggests that CRPS is an exaggerated local inflammatory response to injury[79,81] and that CRPS represents a local form of the systemic free radical disease that causes adult respiratory distress syndrome and multiple organ failure after severe trauma. This concept is supported by the preliminary evidence that the free radical scavenger vitamin C is an effective prophylaxis against post-traumatic CRPS.[196,197]

An alternative explanation for the inflammatory changes in early CRPS is a primary capillary imbalance causing stasis, extravasation, and consequent local tissue anoxia.[54,55,131,153]

The aberrant inflammatory response to tissue injury in CRPS does not seem to be caused by a cellular-mediated immune response since ESR, antigen titers, autoimmune antibody concentrations, and blood cell counts are all normal, and in histologic studies there is minimal inflammatory cell infiltrate.[154,160,183]

Immobilization and Failure to Use the Affected Limb

The popular French term for CRPS, algodystrophy, means painful disuse.[49] It is a common clinical observation that patients who appear to be at risk of developing CRPS are unable or unwilling to cooperate with physical therapy to mobilize their limb after trauma or orthopedic surgery. Indeed, undue immobilization has traditionally been believed to be at least an important contributory factor in the generation of CRPS or even the sole cause.[10,53,138,189]

CRPS obviously involves a significant abnormality of afferent sensory perception, but only recently has the possibility of abnormal efferent motor function been systematically explored. Classically, it was believed that the "immobile RSD limb" was guarded by the patient in order to prevent inadvertent painful movement or sensory contact.[49,67] In fact, CRPS is associated with an abnormality of motor function which is often overlooked partially due to patient embarrassment and partly because in the past it has been labeled as hysterical.[36,179] In 1990, Schwartzman and Kerrigan[161] reported a subgroup of CRPS patients with a variety of motor disorders, and a minority of patients with CRPS demonstrate obvious dystonia or spasms.[11,12,50,130] A prospective study of 829 CRPS patients showed that abnormalities of motor function were reported by 95%, varying from weakness to incoordination and tremor.[183] Objective testing in small numbers of patients shows that CRPS patients have impaired grip force coordination, target reaching, and grasping.[158,190]

Interviews with patients suggest further possible reasons for the lack of movement in CRPS. Patients demonstrate evidence of "neglect" of the affected limb, similar to that seen after parietal lobe stroke. When asked about moving the limb, statements are made such as "…my limb feels disconnected from my body…" and "…I need to focus all my mental attention and look at the limb in order for it to move the way I want…".[66] Another study revealed bizarre perceptions about a body part including a desperate desire for amputation. There was a mismatch between limb sensation and appearance with mental erasure of the affected part. These authors suggested the term "body perception disturbance" rather than "neglect" to describe this phenomenon.[115] There appears to be a central sensory confusion, in that when a non-noxious stimulus is provided, which the patient finds painful due to allodynia, the patient is unable to determine whether it is truly painful, and by impairing integration between sensory input and motor output, movement is impaired.[93,132]

Overall, in CRPS, patients tend to ignore their affected limb and find it difficult to initiate or accurately direct movement, and there is a mismatch between sensation, perception, and movement.[32,67,179] Failure to use the limb appears to relate to this rather than the traditional view of learned pain avoidance behavior in response to allodynia. Whatever the exact cause, failure of mobilization may be central to the etiology of CRPS since all the features of phase 1 CRPS, except pain, are produced in volunteers after a period of cast immobilization.[30–32] This may be explained by the fact that activity-dependent gene function is common in the nervous system,[194] and normal tactile and proprioceptive input are necessary for correct central nerve signal processing.[117,129]

A study of the treatment with mirror visual feedback (MVF) supports the central role of movement disorder in CRPS.[132] The rationale for MVF is restoration of the congruence between sensory and motor information, and it was originally used for the treatment of phantom limb pain.[152] Patients are instructed to exercise both the unaffected and the affected limb. However, a mirror is placed so that they cannot see the affected limb, and when they think they are looking at it, they are actually observing the mirror image of their normal limb. As might be expected, MVF resulted in improvement in range of movement; however, in addition, in early CRPS, MVF also abolished or substantially improved pain and VMI.[133]

MAKING A DIAGNOSIS

Considerable confusion has been generated by a failure to understand the recent work from the IASP. In 1994, when the IASP produced the new diagnostic entity of CRPS, it was descriptive and general and based on a consensus.[135] Deliberately, it did not imply any etiology or pathology (including any direct role for the SNS). The intention was to provide an officially endorsed set of standardized diagnostic criteria to improve clinical communication and facilitate research.[136] In other words, this was intended as a starting point from which individual researchers could move forward. It was not thought of as a mature clinical diagnostic device, and further validation has been carried out.[89]

Since their original publication, the diagnostic criteria have been validated, refined, and developed. The validation studies suggest that the original criteria are adequately sensitive *within the context of a pain clinic* (i.e., they rarely miss a case of actual CRPS); however, the criteria cause problems of over-diagnosis due to poor specificity.[65,88] Comparison of CRPS patients to other proven pain states such as chronic diabetic patients with ascending symmetrical pain, whose neuropathy is confirmed by nerve conduction studies, also shows that the criteria are very sensitive but have low specificity, so that a diagnosis of CRPS may be erroneous in up to 60% of cases.[25]

Other problems are evident. For example, the criteria assume that any sign or symptom of vasomotor, sudomotor, and edema-related change is sufficient to justify the diagnosis, and there is no possibility of providing greater diagnostic or prognostic accuracy by observing more than one of these features. An additional weakness is the failure to include motor or trophic signs and symptoms. Numerous studies have described various signs of motor dysfunction (e.g., dystonia, tremor) as important characteristics of this disorder, and trophic changes have frequently been mentioned in historical clinical descriptions.[161,162] These differentiate CRPS from other pain syndromes.[65,162] Finally, the wording of the criteria permits diagnosis based solely on patient-reported historical symptoms. This may be inappropriate in the context of litigation.

Factor analysis of 123 CRPS patients has indicated that the features cluster into four statistically distinct subgroups.[88]

1. A set of signs and symptoms indicating abnormalities in pain processing (e.g., allodynia, hyperalgesia, hyperpathia)
2. Skin color and temperature changes, indicating vasomotor dysfunction
3. Edema and abnormalities of sweating
4. Motor and trophic signs and symptoms

The statistical separation of edema and sudomotor dysfunction from VMI and the finding of motor and trophic abnormalities are at variance with the original IASP criteria which were therefore modified (Table 25-3[25,65,88]) The important changes are inclusion of clinical signs, their separation from symptoms, and the inclusion of features of motor abnormalities and trophic changes. Intriguingly these sub-groups are virtually identical to those suggested by our group a decade earlier.[4]

Statistical analysis has been undertaken to investigate sensitivity and specificity of decision rules for diagnosis of CRPS

TABLE 25-3 **The Modified IASP Diagnostic Criteria for CRPS**

General definition of the syndrome: CRPS describes an array of painful conditions that are characterized by a continuing (spontaneous and/or evoked) regional pain that is seemingly dispro-portionate in time or degree to the usual course of any known trauma or other lesion. The pain is regional (not in a specific nerve territory or dermatome) and usually has a distal predominance of abnormal sensory, motor, sudomotor, vasomotor, and/or trophic findings. The syndrome shows variable progression over time.

To make the *clinical* diagnosis, the following criteria must be met (sensitivity 0.85, specificity 0.69):
1. Continuing pain, which is disproportionate to any inciting event
2. Must report at least one symptom in *three of the four* following categories:
   Sensory: Reports of hyperesthesia and/or allodynia
   Vasomotor: Reports of temperature asymmetry and/or skin color changes and/or skin color asymmetry
   Sudomotor/edema: Reports of edema and/or sweating changes and/or sweating asymmetry
   Motor/trophic: Reports of decreased range of motion and/or motor dysfunction (weakness, tremor, dystonia) and/or trophic changes (hair, nail, skin)

3. Must display at least one sign *at the time of evaluation* in *two or more* of the following categories:
   Sensory: Evidence of hyperalgesia (to pinprick) and/or allodynia (to light touch and/or tempera-ture sensation and/or deep somatic pressure and/or joint movement)
   Vasomotor: Evidence of temperature asymmetry (>1°C) and/or skin color changes and/or asymmetry
   Sudomotor/edema: Evidence of edema and/or sweating changes and/or sweating asymmetry
   Motor/trophic: Evidence of decreased range of motion and/or motor dysfunction (weakness, tremor, dystonia)and/or trophic changes (hair, nail, skin)
4. There is no other diagnosis that better explains the signs and symptoms

For *research* purposes, the diagnostic decision rule should be at least one symptom *in all four* symptom categories and at least one sign (observed at evaluation) in two or more sign catego-ries (sensitivity 0.70, specificity 0.94).

(Data from Bruehl S, et al. External validation of IASP diagnostic criteria for complex regional pain syndrome and proposed research diagnostic criteria. International Association for the Study of Pain. *Pain.* 1999;81(1–2):147–154; Harden RN, et al. Complex regional pain syndrome: Are the IASP diagnostic criteria valid and sufficiently comprehensive? *Pain.* 1999;83(2):211–219.)

compared to neuropathic pain of a proven non-CRPS cause using these criteria (Table 25-4[25]). These propose different diag-nostic criteria depending on the clinical circumstances. Thus for purely clinical diagnosis, the criteria provide a sensitivity of 0.85 and a specificity of 0.69, whereas for research diagnosis, the criteria provide a sensitivity of 0.7 and a specificity of 0.94, since in the former circumstance, one wishes to avoid failing to offer treatment to a possible candidate, while in the latter situa-tion one is more concerned to be investigating a homogeneous group in whom the diagnosis cannot be in doubt.

It is critical to understand that the Bruehl modification of the original IASP criteria[25] given in Table 25-3 applies to the diagnosis of CRPS *within a pain clinic setting* and is therefore intended to differentiate CRPS from other causes of chronic pain within that setting. They do not apply directly to the diag-nosis of CRPS within the context of an orthopedic practice. The reason for this apparent conundrum is that the precise nature of CRPS remains unclear, and it is therefore a diagnosis of exclusion. Conditions from which CRPS must be distinguished in a pain clinic (e.g., neuropathic pain in association with dia-betic neuropathy) are different from those which apply in an

orthopedic or fracture clinic (e.g., soft tissue infection or stress fracture). Therefore, the diagnostic criteria must be slightly dif-ferent, just as slightly different criteria are required within a pain clinic for diagnosis of CRPS depending on whether the diagnosis is being made for clinical or research purposes.

Atkins et al.[3] proposed a set of diagnostic criteria for CRPS specifically in an orthopedic context (Table 25-5[3–5]). These were derived empirically in a manner similar to the IASP approach but critically in a fracture clinic rather than a pain clinic envi-ronment. The criteria were designed to be as far as possible objective but the patient's veracity was assumed, so no attempt was made to separate reports of vasomotor or sudomotor abnormalities from observation of them. A number of criteria are quantifiable,[3,4,62] which allows their powerful use to inves-tigate treatment.[57,59,119] The original criteria were developed in the context of CRPS of the hand following Colles fracture of the wrist, but they have subsequently been generalized for use in the diagnosis of CRPS in other orthopedic scenarios and in the lower limb.[14,157] Diagnosis by these criteria, when used after Colles fracture, maps virtually exactly with the Bruehl criteria suggesting their reliability.[172]

TABLE 25-4 Diagnostic Sensitivity and Specificity for the IASP Modified Criteria (Table 25-3) in Distinguishing CRPS from Patients with Neuropathic Pain from a Documented Non-CRPS Cause

Decision Rule	Sensitivity	Specificity
2+ sign categories & 2+ symptom categories	0.94	0.36
2+ sign categories & 3+ symptom categories	0.85	0.69
2+ sign categories & 4 symptom categories	0.70	0.94
3+ sign categories and 2+ symptom categories	0.76	0.81
3+ sign categories and 3+ symptom categories	0.70	0.83
3+ sign categories and 4 symptom categories	0.86	0.75

(From Bruehl S, et al. External validation of IASP diagnostic criteria for complex regional pain syndrome and proposed research diagnostic criteria. International Association for the Study of Pain. *Pain.* 1999;81(1–2):147–154.)

Clinical Diagnosis in an Orthopedic Setting

1. Pain

A history of excessive pain is elicited. Abnormalities of pain perception are examined in comparison with the opposite normal side. Excessive tenderness is found by squeezing digits in the affected part between thumb and fingers. This may be quantitated using dolorimetry, but this is usually a research tool.[5,7] Allodynia is demonstrated by fine touch and hyperalgesia using a pin. Hyperpathia is examined by serial fine touch or pin prick.

TABLE 25-5 Suggested Criteria for the Diagnosis of CRPS Within an Orthopedic Setting

The diagnosis is made clinically by the finding of the following associated sets of abnormalities:
1. Neuropathic pain. Nondermatomal, without cause, burning, with associated allodynia and hyperpathia.
2. Vasomotor instability and abnormalities of sweating. Warm red and dry, cool blue, and clammy or an increase in temperature sensitivity. Associated with an abnormal temperature difference between the limbs.
3. Swelling.
4. Loss of joint mobility with associated joint and soft tissue contracture, including skin thinning and hair and nail dystrophy.

These clinical findings are backed up by:
1. Increased uptake on delayed bone scintigraphy early in CRPS
2. Radiographic evidence of osteoporosis after 3 months

The diagnosis is excluded by the existence of conditions that would otherwise account for the degree of dysfunction.

Modified from Atkins RM, Duckworth T, Kanis JA. Algodystrophy following Colles' fracture. *J Hand Surg Br.* 1989;14(2):161–164; Atkins RM, Duckworth T, Kanis JA. Features of algodystrophy after Colles' fracture. *J Bone Joint Surg Br.* 1990;72(1):105–110.

2a. Vasomotor instability

VMI is often transitory, and so it may not be present at the time of examination. If the patient is reliable, then a history confirms its presence. Visual inspection is the usual means of diagnosis.

Thermography can be used to quantitate temperature difference between the limbs. This is greater in CRPS than other pain syndromes,[146,188] and this can be used to distinguish CRPS from other causes of neuropathic pain. However, thermography has not been validated within an orthopedic context and must therefore be employed with caution. It is not usually used in an orthopedic context.

2b. Abnormal sweating

Whether this feature should be considered with VMI as proposed by Atkins[4,7] or should be with edema as suggested recently by Harden[88] is as yet unclear. As for VMI, the feature is inconstant, and it may be necessary to rely on history. Excessive sweating is usually clinically obvious. In a doubtful case, the resistance to a biro or a pencil gently stroked across the limb is useful. The extent of sweating can be quantified by iontophoresis, but this is rarely undertaken.

3. Edema and swelling

This is usually obvious on inspection. In the hand it may be quantified by hand volume measurement. Similarly, skin-fold thickness and digital circumference may be measured.[4,7]

4. Loss of joint mobility and atrophy

Loss of joint mobility is usually diagnosed by standard clinical examination. The range of finger joint movement may be accurately quantified.[4,7,62] As outlined above, atrophy will affect every tissue within the limb.

5. Bone changes

X-ray appearances and bone scans are discussed above. CRPS does not cause arthritis, and joint space is preserved. Sudeck's technique of assessing bone density by radiographing two extremities on one plate[170,171] remains useful, but densitometry is not usually helpful.[13] A normal bone scan without radiographic osteoporosis virtually excludes adult CRPS.

Other Clinical Examinations

Making a diagnosis of "neglect"-like phenomena is relatively easy clinically but may not as yet be useful. Sensory neglect can be elucidated either by history or direct sensory examination with the patient watching or looking away from the affected limb. Motor neglect is examined by asking the patient to undertake a simple task initially while looking away and then while watching the limb. In the upper limb this can be repetitively opening the closing the fingers, or in the lower limb tapping the foot. If there is a significant improvement when the patient is watching the limb, a degree of motor neglect is present.[67]

Investigations

CRPS is a clinical diagnosis and there is no single diagnostic test. The classic case is obvious, and direct effects of trauma, fracture, cellulitis, arthritis, and malignancy are common alternative diagnoses. The patient is systemically well with normal general clinical examination, biochemical markers, and infection indices.

The MRI shows early bone and soft tissue edema with late atrophy and fibrosis but is not diagnostic. However in CRPS-2 an MRI scan may be useful to demonstrate nerve thinning with poststenotic dilatation due to compression and may even demonstrate a fibrous band causing the compression. It may also demonstrate neuroma formation; however, many neuromas are too small to be adequately shown.

CT scanning may also be useful in demonstrating a bony compressing lesion.

EMG and nerve conduction studies are normal in CRPS-1 but may demonstrate a nerve lesion in CRPS-2.

Differential Diagnosis

Pain, swelling, and VMI are common associations of trauma and orthopedic surgery. The following are common differential diagnoses.

1. Soft tissue infection. The clinical features are usually clear. The patient is systemically unwell with raised inflammatory markers.

2. "Mechanical" problems. Classical examples are incorrect sizing of a total knee replacement causing pain, swelling, and stiffness; overlong screws impinging on a joint; or malreduction of an intra-articular fracture (Fig. 25-5). In accordance with category 4 of the original IASP criteria for CRPS, all mechanical causes for the symptoms and signs must be excluded before making a diagnosis of CRPS. However, it must be borne in mind that the chronic pain of a mechanical problem can itself be the precipitating cause of CRPS.

3. Conscious exaggeration of symptoms. This is usually seen in the context of litigation, but the secondary gain from exaggeration may also relate to complex and pathologic interpersonal relationships. This problem has been accidentally made more acute and severe by the IASP criteria for CRPS diagnosis. The original criteria (Table 25-2) are readily mim-

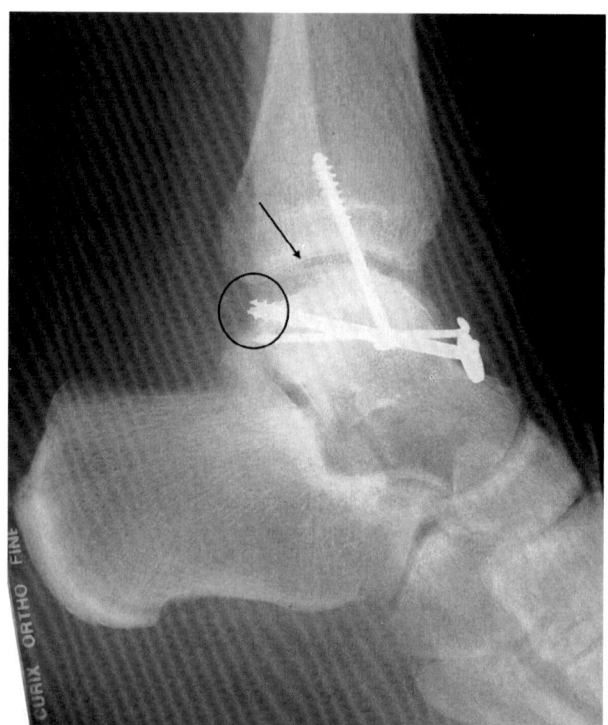

FIGURE 25-5 A patient referred with a diagnosis of CRPS. This patient with severe pain in his foot was referred some years after internal fixation of a talar body fracture. He has severe pain and dysfunction. The lateral radiograph shows no evidence of significant osteoporosis, which is inconsistent with the diagnosis. The talar body fracture is not reduced which renders the ankle and subtalar joints incongruous. Furthermore the screws are overlong and impinge on the ankle joint. This patient does not have CRPS; he has a mechanical cause for his severe pain, which was resolved by talar osteotomy, anatomic reduction, and refixation. It is important to exclude mechanical causes for pain before invoking the diagnosis of CRPS.

icked by a patient determined to deceive the examining clinician. Unfortunately, the modified criteria may also provide a diagnosis of CRPS in a deceitful patient. Categories 1 and 2 are simple. The patient merely has to report these problems. Category 3 refers to objective criteria. However, sensory abnormalities rely on the patient's subjective response to stimulus. Skin color change can be caused by deliberate dependency and immobility of the limb. Loss of joint range of movement can be caused by conscious resistant to movement; and dystonia, tremor, and weakness can likewise be produced artifactually. The rise of the internet means that any reasonably determined patient can have a very great knowledge of the features of CRPS and the diagnostic criteria. The solution to this problem is to remember that the IASP criteria are designed to differentiate CRPS from other chronically painful conditions; they are not intended to deal with a patient whose veracity is open to question. CRPS is a condition which inevitably leads to dystrophy,[24,49,65,162] and in a patient who has suffered from significant CRPS for any significant length of time, objective features of dystrophy such as nail or hair dystrophy, skin and subcutaneous tissue atrophy, fixed joint contracture, and radiographic features of significant osteoporosis with abnormalities of bone scanning should be present. If the patient's veracity is in doubt, the astute clinician will give only limited or no credence to those features which can be mimicked and look for incontrovertible physical signs.

4. Psychiatric disease. Separately from the conscious exaggeration described above, psychiatric disease may cause a patient subconsciously to exaggerate the level or impact of physical disease. Somatoform disorders describe conditions in which patients subconsciously exaggerate physical symptoms, and conversion disorders refer to subconscious exaggeration of physical signs. These patients are often psychologically fragile, they may have a history of an unusually severe reaction to multiple minor medical problems, and they may show a tendency to "catastrophize" life events. In addition to this direct influence on a diagnosis of CRPS, patients with CRPS may be depressed due to chronic pain, and psychiatric disease may play an indirect part in the condition. It is often very useful to obtain formal psychiatric or psychological opinion and treatment.[180–182]

5. Neuropathic pain. This has been defined and discussed. Neuropathic pain is part of CRPS, but a patient may have neuropathic pain without having CRPS. However, neuropathic pain may give rise to CRPS.

6. Chronic pain state. Patients with long-lasting and unremitting pain may become depressed, particularly when there is a neuropathic element. They learn to avoid activities which cause pain, and their relatives and carers act to protect them from perceived injury. This generates a complex psychosocial situation which may require psychological, psychiatric, pain therapeutic, and orthopedic combined management.

Management

A bewildering array of treatments have been proposed, but proper, scientifically constructed, prospectively randomized blinded studies are few,[106] and uncontrolled investigations are particularly unreliable in CRPS because of the variety of symptoms and the trend toward self-resolution in the majority of cases. This is well illustrated by a series of publications investigating the treatment of early CRPS after Colles fracture with intravenous regional guanethidine blockade (IVRGB). An initial investigation showed that IVRGB caused improvement in objective criteria of CRPS severity.[59] A subsequent pilot study appeared to confirm that the immediate improvement induced by IVRGB was associated with sustained symptomatic improvement.[57] However, a full prospectively randomized double-blind controlled study demonstrated that IVRGB actually seemed to worsen the condition.[119] The lesson is that these potentially fragile patients must be approached with caution.

This chapter has presented evidence that CRPS is very common in orthopedic trauma practice. Most sufferers are sensible people, concerned at the development of inexplicable pain, but the occasional "Sudecky" patient fares poorly and should be

treated vigorously. Early treatment, begun before contractures occur, gives optimal results, so a high index of clinical suspicion must be maintained. It is not reprehensible to have caused a case of CRPS through surgery or nonoperative management of injury. However, delay in diagnosis and treatment may contribute to a poor outcome.

Modern CRPS treatment emphasizes functional rehabilitation of the limb to break the vicious cycle of disuse,[91,92,165] rather than SNS manipulation.[29] Initial treatment from the orthopedic surgeon is by reassurance, excellent analgesia, and intensive, careful physical therapy avoiding exacerbation of pain.[73] Nonsteroidal anti-inflammatory drugs may give better pain relief than opiates, and a centrally acting analgesic such as amitriptyline is often useful even at this early stage. Immobilization and splintage should generally be avoided, but if used, joints must be placed in a safe position, and splintage is a temporary adjunct to mobilization. It seems sensible to give the patients vitamin C in view of the early evidence of its efficacy.[196,197]

Abnormalities of pain sensation will often respond to desensitization. The patient is asked to stroke the area of allodynia, where stroking is painful. They are reminded that simple stroking cannot by definition be painful, and they are instructed to stroke the affected part repetitively while looking at it and repeatedly saying "this does not hurt, it is merely a gentle touch." The earlier this is begun, the more effective it is. A similar attitude can be taken with early loss of joint mobility due to perceived pain rather than contracture.

The use of mirror virtual therapy is an exciting new concept which is as yet unproven in an orthopedic context.[133,152]

If the patient does not respond rapidly, a pain specialist should be involved and treatment continued on a shared basis. Psychological or psychiatric input may be important.[28] Second-line treatment is often unsuccessful, and many patients are left with pain and disability. Further treatments include centrally acting analgesic medications such as amitriptyline, gabapentin, or carbamazepine; regional anesthesia; calcitonin; the use of membrane-stabilizing drugs such as mexiletine; sympathetic blockade and manipulation; desensitization of peripheral nerve receptors with capsaicin; transcutaneous nerve stimulation; or an implanted dorsal column stimulator.[123,142,167] Behavioral therapy may be necessary in children.[191–193] Where the knee is affected, epidural anesthesia and continuous passive motion may be appropriate.[38,39]

It is important to ensure that a patient with CRPS within an orthopedic context under the management of a pain clinic is reviewed by an orthopedic surgeon with an interest in CRPS to ensure that there is no treatable orthopedic condition which better explains the symptoms (Tables 25-2, 25-3, 25-5[78]).

The role of surgery is limited and hazardous. These patients are very fragile and difficult. They respond abnormally to pain, and because of sensory and motor neglect, they rehabilitate poorly. Where the cause of CRPS is a surgically correctable nerve lesion, treatment should be cautiously directed at curing the nerve lesion. Occult nerve compression should be sought and dealt with. For example, decompression of a median nerve at the wrist which is causing CRPS of the hand may abort the CRPS and should be undertaken cautiously in the presence of active disease.

Surgery is rarely indicated to treat fixed contractures which usually involve all of the soft tissues. Surgical release must therefore be radical and expectations limited. Surgery for contracture should be delayed until the active phase of CRPS has completely passed, and ideally there should be a gap of at least a year since the patient last experienced pain and swelling.

Amputation of a limb affected by severe CRPS should be approached with great caution. Dielissen et al.[47] reported a series of 28 patients who underwent 34 amputations in 31 limbs. Surgery was usually performed for recurrent infection or to improve residual function. Pain relief was rare and unpredictable, and neither was infection always cured nor function universally improved. CRPS often recurred in the stump, especially if the amputation level was symptomatic at the time of surgery. For this reason only two patients wore a prosthesis.

Generally, surgery represents a painful stimulus which may exacerbate CRPS or precipitate a new attack. This risk must be balanced carefully against the proposed benefit. The risk of surgically precipitated recurrence is greatest when the same site is operated upon in a patient with abnormal psychology in the presence of active disease and lowest when these conditions do not apply. Surgery must be performed carefully with minimal trauma with excellent and complete postoperative analgesia. The surgery may be covered by gabapentin. Ideally the anesthetist will have a particular interest in the treatment of CRPS.

CONCLUSION

This chapter has presented the proposal that CRPS in a mild form, which is often not formally diagnosed, is very common but not universal in an orthopedic trauma practice. Although the majority of cases will resolve with simple management, CRPS is responsible for significant acute disability and may cause long-term problems.

REFERENCES

1. Albrecht PJ, Hines S, Eisenberg E, et al. Pathologic alterations of cutaneous innervation and vasculature in affected limbs from patients with complex regional pain syndrome. *Pain*. 2006;120(3):244–266.
2. Ali Z, Raja SN, Wesselmann U, et al. Intradermal injection of norepinephrine evokes pain in patients with sympathetically maintained pain. *Pain*. 2000;88(2):161–168.
3. Atkins RM, Duckworth T, Kanis JA. Algodystrophy following Colles' fracture. *J Hand Surg Br*. 1989;14(2):161–164.
4. Atkins RM, Duckworth T, Kanis JA. Features of algodystrophy after Colles' fracture. *J Bone Joint Surg Br*. 1990;72(1):105–110.
5. Atkins RM, Kanis JA. The use of dolorimetry in the assessment of post-traumatic algodystrophy of the hand. *Br J Rheumatol*. 1989;28(5):404–409.
6. Atkins RM, Tindale W, Bickerstaff D, et al. Quantitative bone scintigraphy in reflex sympathetic dystrophy. *Br J Rheumatol*. 1993;32(1):41–45.
7. Atkins RM. Algodystrophy. *Orthopaedic Surgery*. Oxford: University of Oxford, DM; 1989.
8. Aubert PG. *Etude sur le risque algodystrophique*. Paris: University of Paris, Val de Marne; 1980.
9. Bacorn R, Kurtz J. Colles' fracture: a study of 2000 cases from the New York State Workmen's Compensation Board. *J Bone Joint Surg Am*. 1953;35A:643–658.
10. Bernstein BH, Singsen BH, Kent JT, et al. Reflex neurovascular dystrophy in childhood. *J Pediatr*. 1978;93(2):211–215.
11. Bhatia KP, Marsden CD. Reflex sympathetic dystrophy. May be accompanied by involuntary movements. *BMJ*. 1995;311(7008):811–812.
12. Bhatia KP, Bhatt MH, Marsden CD. The causalgia-dystonia syndrome. *Brain*. 1993;116(Pt 4):843–851.
13. Bickerstaff DR, Charlesworth D, Kanis JA. Changes in cortical and trabecular bone in algodystrophy. *Br J Rheumatol*. 1993;32(1):46–51.
14. Bickerstaff DR, Kanis JA. Algodystrophy: an under-recognized complication of minor trauma. *Br J Rheumatol*. 1994;33(3):240–248.
15. Bickerstaff DR. The natural history of post traumatic algodystrophy. *Department of Human Metabolism and Clinical Biochemistry*. University of Sheffield; 1990.
16. Birklein F, Künzel W, Sieweke N. Despite clinical similarities there are significant differences between acute limb trauma and complex regional pain syndrome I (CRPS I). *Pain*. 2001;93(2):165–171.
17. Birklein F, Riedl B, Sieweke N, et al. Neurological findings in complex regional pain syndromes–analysis of 145 cases. *Acta Neurol Scand*. 2000;101(4):262–269.
18. Birklein F, Schmelz M, Schifter S, et al. The important role of neuropeptides in complex regional pain syndrome. *Neurology*. 2001;57(12):2179–2184.
19. Boas R. Complex regional pain syndromes: symptoms, signs and differential diagnosis. In: Janig W, Stanton-Hicks M, eds. *Reflex Sympathetic Dystrophy: A Reappraisal*. Seattle, WA: IASP Press; 1996;79–92.
20. Bonica JJ. Causalgia and other reflex sympathetic dystrophies. In: Bonica JJ, ed. *Management of Pain*. Philadelphia PA: Lea and Feibiger; 1990:220–243.
21. Bonica JJ. *The Management of Pain*. Philadelphia, PA: Lea and Febiger; 1953.
22. Breuer J, Freud S. *Studies in Hysteria*. Strachey J, Freud A, trans-eds. New York, NY: Basic Books; 1982.
23. Bruehl S, Carlson CR. Predisposing psychological factors in the development of reflex sympathetic dystrophy. A review of the empirical evidence. *Clin J Pain*. 1992;8(4):287–299.
24. Bruehl S, Harden RN, Galer BS, et al. Complex regional pain syndrome: are there distinct subtypes and sequential stages of the syndrome? *Pain*. 2002;95(1–2):119–124.
25. Bruehl S, Harden RN, Galer BS, et al. External validation of IASP diagnostic criteria for complex regional pain syndrome and proposed research diagnostic criteria. International Association for the Study of Pain. *Pain*. 1999;81(1-2):147–154.
26. Bruehl S, Husfeldt B, Lubenow TR, et al. Psychological differences between reflex sympathetic dystrophy and non-RSD chronic pain patients. *Pain*. 1996;67(1):107–114.
27. Bruehl S. Do psychological factors play a role in the onset and maintenance of CRPS-1? In: Harden RN, Baron R, Seattle JW, eds. *Complex Regional Pain Syndrome*. Vol. 22. Seattle, WA: IASP Press; 2001.
28. Bruehl S. Psychological interventions. In: Wilson P, Stanton-Hicks M, Harden RN, eds. *CRPS: Current Diagnosis and Therapy*. Vol. 32. Seattle, WA: IASP Press; 2005:201–216.
29. Burton AW, Lubenow TR, Raj PP. Traditional interventional therapies. In: Wilson P, Stanton-Hicks M, Harden RN, eds. *CRPS: Current Diagnosis and Treatment*. Seattle: IASP Press; 2005;32:217–233.
30. Butler SH, Galer BS, Benirsche S. Disuse as a cause of signs and symptoms of CRPS. *Abstracts: 8th World Congress on Pain*. Seattle, WA: IASP Press; 1996:401.
31. Butler SH, Nyman M, Gordh T. Immobility in volunteers produces signs and symptoms of CRPS and a neglect-like state. *Abstracts: 9th World Congress on Pain*. Seattle, WA: IASP Press; 1999.
32. Butler SH. Disuse and CRPS. In: Harden RN, Baron R, Janig W, eds. *Complex Regional Pain Syndrome*. Seattle, WA: IASP Press; 2001:141–150.
33. Campbell J, Raga S, Meyer R. Painful sequelae of nerve injury. In: Dubner R, Gebhart G, Bond M, eds. *Proceedings of the 5th World Congress on Pain*. Amsterdam: Elsevier Science Publishers; 1988:135–143.
34. Casale R, Glynn CJ, Buonocore M. Autonomic variations after stellate ganglion block: are they evidence of an autonomic afference?" *Funct Neurol*. 1990;5(3):245–246.
35. Channon GN, Lloyd GJ. The investigation of hand stiffness using Doppler ultrasound, radionuclide scanning and thermography. *J Bone Joint Surg Br*. 1979;61B:519.
36. Charcot JM. Two cases of hysterical contracture of traumatic origin (Lectures VII and VIII). *Lectures on Diseases of the Nervous System*. Nijmegen: Arts and Boeve; 1889:84–106.
37. Constantinesco A, Brunot B, Demangeat JL, et al. Three phase bone scanning as an aid to early diagnosis in reflex sympathetic dystrophy of the hand. A study of eighty-nine cases. *Ann Chir Main*. 1986;5(2):93–104.
38. Cooper DE, DeLee JC, Ramamurthy S. Reflex sympathetic dystrophy of the knee. Treatment using continuous epidural anesthesia. *J Bone Joint Surg Am*. 1989;71(3):365–369.
39. Cooper DE, DeLee JC. Reflex sympathetic dystrophy of the knee. *J Am Acad Orthop Surg*. 1994;2(2):79–86.
40. Dallos A, Kiss M, Polyánka H, et al. Effects of the neuropeptides substance P, calcitonin gene-related peptide, vasoactive intestinal polypeptide and galanin on the production of nerve growth factor and inflammatory cytokines in cultured human keratinocytes. *Neuropeptides*. 2006;40(4):251–263.
41. de Mos M, de Brujin AG, Huygen FJ, et al. The incidence of complex regional pain syndrome: a population-based study. *Pain*. 2007;129(1–2):12–20.
42. De Takats G. Causalgic states in peace and war. *JAMA*. 1945;128:699–704.
43. De Takats G. Reflex dystrophy of the extremities. *Arch Surg*. 1937;34:939–956.
44. De Takats G. The nature of painful vasodilatation in causalgic states. *Arch Neurol*. 1943;53:318–326.
45. Demangeat JL, Constantinesco A, Brunot B, et al. Three-phase bone scanning in reflex sympathetic dystrophy of the hand. *J Nucl Med*. 1988;29(1):26–32.
46. Devor M, Raber P. Heritability of symptoms in an experimental model of neuropathic pain. *Pain*. 1990;42(1):51–67.
47. Dielissen PW, Claassen AT, Veldman PH, et al. Amputation for reflex sympathetic dystrophy. *J Bone Joint Surg Br*. 1995;77(2):270–273.
48. Doupe J, Cullen CH, Chance GQ. Post traumatic pain and the causalgic syndrome. *J Neurol Psychiatry*. 1944;7:33–48.
49. Doury P, Dirheimer Y, Pattin S. *Algodystrophy: Diagnosis and Therapy of a Frequent Disease of the Locomotor Apparatus*. Berlin: Springer Verlag; 1981.
50. Dressler D, Thmpson PD, Gledhill RF, et al. The syndrome of painful legs and moving toes. *Mov Disord*. 1994;9(1):13–21.
51. Drummond PD. Sensory disturbances in complex regional pain syndrome: clinical observations, autonomic interactions, and possible mechanisms. *Pain Med*. 2010;11(8):1257–1266.
52. Evans JA. Reflex sympathetic dystrophy. *Surg Clin North Am*. 1946;26:780–790.

53. Fam AG , Stein J. Disappearance of chondrocalcinosis following reflex sympathetic dystrophy syndrome. *Arthritis Rheum.* 1981;24(5):747–749.
54. Ficat P, Arlet J, Lartique G, et al. [Post-injury reflex algo-dystrophies. Hemodynamic and anatomopathological study]. *Rev Chir Orthop Reparatrice Appar Mot.* 1973;59(5): 401–414.
55. Ficat P, Arlet J, Pujol M, et al. [Injury, reflex dystrophy and osteonecrosis of the femoral head]. *Ann Chir.* 1971;25(15):911–917.
56. Field J, Atkins RM. Algodystrophy is an early complication of Colles' fracture. What are the implications? *J Hand Surg Br.* 1997;22(2):178–182.
57. Field J, Atkins RM. Effect of guanethidine on the natural history of post-traumatic algodystrophy. *Ann Rheum Dis.* 1993;52(6):467–469.
58. Field J, Gardner FV. Psychological distress associated with algodystrophy. *J Hand Surg Br.* 1997;22(1):100–101.
59. Field J, Monk C, Atkins RM. Objective improvements in algodystrophy following regional intravenous guanethidine. *J Hand Surg Br.* 1993;18(3):339–342.
60. Field J, Protheroe DL, Atkins RM. Algodystrophy after Colles fractures is associated with secondary tightness of casts. *J Bone Joint Surg Br.* 1994;76(6):901–905.
61. Field J, Warwick D, Bannister GC. Features of algodystrophy ten years after Colles' fracture. *J Hand Surg Br.* 1992;17(3):318–320.
62. Field J. Measurement of finger stiffness in algodystrophy. *Hand Clin.* 2003;19(3): 511–515.
63. Francini F, Zoppi M, Maresca M, et al. Skin potential and EMG changes induced by electrical stimulation. 1. Normal man in arousing and non-arousing environment. *Appl Neurophysiol.* 1979;42:113–124.
64. Frettlöh J, Hüppe M, Maier C. Severity and specificity of neglect-like symptoms in patients with complex regional pain syndrome (CRPS) compared to chronic limb pain of other origins. *Pain.* 2006;124(1–2):184–189.
65. Galer BS, Bruehl S, Harden RN. IASP diagnostic criteria for complex regional pain syndrome: a preliminary empirical validation study. International Association for the Study of Pain. *Clin J Pain.* 1998;14(1):48–54.
66. Galer BS, Butler S, Jensen MP. Case reports and hypothesis: a neglect-like syndrome may be responsible for the motor disturbance in reflex sympathetic dystrophy (complex regional pain syndrome-1). *J Pain Symptom Manage.* 1995;10(5):385–391.
67. Galer BS, Harden N. Motor abnormalities in CRPS: A neglected but key component. In: Harden N, Baron R, Seattle JW, eds. *Complex Regional Pain Syndrome.* Seattle, WA: IASP Press; 2001:22.
68. Galer BS, Jensen M. Neglect-like symptoms in complex regional pain syndrome: results of a self-administered survey. *J Pain Symptom Manage.* 1999;18(3):213–217.
69. Geertzen JH, de Brujin H, de Brujin-Kofman AT, et al. Reflex sympathetic dystrophy: early treatment and psychological aspects. *Arch Phys Med Rehabil.* 1994;75(4):442–446.
70. Geertzen JH, de Brujin-Kofman AT, de Brujin HP, et al. Stressful life events and psychological dysfunction in Complex Regional Pain Syndrome type I. *Clin J Pain.* 1998; 14(2):143–147.
71. Geertzen JH, Dijkstra PU, Groothoff JW, et al. Reflex sympathetic dystrophy of the upper extremity—a 5.5-year follow-up. Part I. Impairments and perceived disability. *Acta Orthop Scand Suppl.* 1998;279:12–18.
72. Geertzen JH, Dijkstra PU, Groothoff JW, et al. Reflex sympathetic dystrophy of the upper extremity—a 5.5-year follow-up. Part II. Social life events, general health and changes in occupation. *Acta Orthop Scand Suppl.* 1998;279:19–23.
73. Geertzen JH, Harden RN. Physical and occupational therapies. In: Wilson P, Stanton-Hicks M, Harden RN. eds. *CRPS: Current Diagnosis and Therapy.* Vol. 32. Seattle, WA: IASP Press; 2005:173–179.
74. Gibbons JJ, Wilson PR. RSD score: criteria for the diagnosis of reflex sympathetic dystrophy and causalgia. *Clin J Pain.* 1992;8(3):260–263.
75. Glick EN, Helal B. Post-traumatic neurodystrophy. Treatment by corticosteroids. *Hand.* 1976;8(1):45–47.
76. Glick EN. Reflex dystrophy (algoneurodystrophy): results of treatment by corticosteroids. *Rheumatol Rehabil.* 1973;12(2):84–88.
77. Glynn CJ, Basedow RW, Walsh JA. Pain relief following post-ganglionic sympathetic blockade with I.V. guanethidine. *Br J Anaesth.* 1981;53(12):1297–1302.
78. Goebel A, Turner-Stokes L, Atkins RM, et al. *Complex Regional Pain Syndrome in Adults: UK Guidelines for Diagnosis, Referral and Management in Primary and Secondary Care.* London: Royal College of Physicians; 2012.
79. Goris RJ, Dongen LM, Winters HA. Are toxic oxygen radicals involved in the pathogenesis of reflex sympathetic dystrophy? *Free Radic Res Commun.* 1987;3(1–5):13–18.
80. Goris RJ. Conditions associated with impaired oxygen extraction. In: Gutierrez G, Vincent JL, eds. *Tissue Oxygen Utilisation.* Berlin: Springer Verlag; 1991:350–369.
81. Goris RJ. Treatment of reflex sympathetic dystrophy with hydroxyl radical scavengers. *Unfallchirurg.* 1985;88(7):330–332.
82. Green JT, Gay FH. Colles' fracture residual disability. *Am J Surg.* 1956;91:636–642.
83. Groeneweg JG, Huygen FJ, Heijmans-Antonissen C, et al. Increased endothelin-1 and diminished nitric oxide levels in blister fluids of patients with intermediate cold type complex regional pain syndrome type 1. *BMC Musculoskelet Disord.* 2006;7:91.
84. Hannington-Kiff JG. Hyperadrenergic-effected limb causalgia: relief by IV pharmacologic norepinephrine blockade. *Am Heart J.* 1982;103(1):152–153.
85. Hannington-Kiff JG. Pharmacological target blocks in hand surgery and rehabilitation. *J Hand Surg Br.* 1984;9(1):29–36.
86. Hannington-Kiff JG. Relief of causalgia in limbs by regional intravenous guanethidine. *Br Med J.* 1979;2(6186):367–368.
87. Hannington-Kiff JG. Relief of Sudeck's atrophy by regional intravenous guanethidine. *Lancet.* 1977;1(8022):1132–1133.
88. Harden RN, Bruehl S, Galer BS, et al. Complex regional pain syndrome: are the IASP diagnostic criteria valid and sufficiently comprehensive? *Pain.* 1999;83(2):211–219.
89. Harden RN, Bruehl S, Perez RS, et al. Validation of proposed diagnostic criteria (the "Budapest Criteria") for complex regional pain syndrome. *Pain.* 2010;150(2):268–274.
90. Harden RN, Bruehl S, Stanos S, et al. Prospective examination of pain-related and psychological predictors of CRPS-like phenomena following total knee arthroplasty: a preliminary study. *Pain.* 2003;106(3):393–400.
91. Harden RN, Swan M, King A, et al. Treatment of complex regional pain syndrome: functional restoration. *Clin J Pain.* 2006;22(5):420–424.
92. Harden RN. The rationale for integrated functional restoration. In: Wilson P, Stanton-Hicks M, Harden RN, eds. *CRPS: Current Diagnosis and Therapy.* Vol. 32. Seattle, WA: IASP Press; 2005:163–171.
93. Harris AJ. Cortical origin of pathological pain. *Lancet.* 1999;354:1464–1466.
94. Holder LE, Mackinnon SE. Reflex sympathetic dystrophy in the hands: clinical and scintigraphic criteria. *Radiology.* 1984;152(2):517–522.
95. Homans J. Minor causalgia. A hyperaesthetic neurovascular syndrome. *New Eng J Med.* 1940;222:870–874.
96. Huygen FJ, Ramdhani N, van Toorenenbergen A, et al. Mast cells are involved in inflammatory reactions during complex regional pain syndrome type 1. *Immunol Lett.* 2004;91(2–3):147–154.
97. Jacquemoud G, Chamay A. Treatment of algodystrophy using intravenous guanethidine regional block. *Ann Chir Main.* 1982;1(1):57–64.
98. Jadad AR, Carroll D, Glynn CJ. Intravenous regional sympathetic blockade for pain relief in reflex sympathetic dystrophy: a systematic review and a randomized, double-blind crossover study. *J Pain Symptom Manage.* 1995;10(1):13–20.
99. Janig W, Koltzenburg M. Possible ways of sympathetic afferent interaction. In: Janig W, Schmidt RF, eds. *Reflex Sympathetic Dystrophy: Pathophysiological Mechanisms and Clinical Implications.* New York, NY: VCH Verlagsgesellschaft; 1992:213–243.
100. Janig W, Koltzenburg M. What is the interaction between the sympathetic terminal and the primary afferent fibre? In: Basbaum AI BJ-M, ed. *Towards a New Pharmacology of Pain.* Chichester: John Wiley and Sons; 1991:331–352.
101. Janig W. CRPS 1 and CRPS 2: a strategic view. In: Harden RN, Baron R, Janig W, eds. *Complex Regional Pain Syndrome.* Vol. 22. Seattle, WA: IASP Press; 2001:3–15.
102. Janig W. The sympathetic nervous system in pain: physiology and pathophysiology. In: Stanton-Hicks M, ed. *Pain in the Sympathetic Nervous System.* Boston, MA: Kluwer Academic Publishers; 1990:17–89.
103. Jensen TS, Baron R. Translation of symptoms and signs into mechanisms in neuropathic pain. *Pain.* 2003;102(1):1–8.
104. Katz MM, Hungerford DS. Reflex sympathetic dystrophy affecting the knee. *J Bone Joint Surg Br.* 1987;69(5):797–803.
105. Kimura T, Komatsu T, Hosoda R, et al. Angiotensin-converting enzyme gene polymorphism in patients with neuropathic pain. In: Devor M, Rowbotham MC, Wiesenfeld-Hallin Z, eds. *Proceedings of the 9th World Conference on Pain.* Vol. 16. Seattle, WA: IASP Press; 2000:471–476.
106. Kingery WS. A critical review of controlled clinical trials for peripheral neuropathic pain and complex regional pain syndromes. *Pain.* 1997;73(2):123–139.
107. Kingery WS. Role of neuropeptide, cytokine, and growth factor signaling in complex regional pain syndrome. *Pain Med.* 2010;11(8):1239–1250.
108. Knepper R. [Pathogenic evaluation of pain]. *Med Welt.* 1967;35:1994–1996.
109. Kozin F, Genant HK, Bekerman C, et al. The reflex sympathetic dystrophy syndrome. II. Roentgenographic and scintigraphic evidence of bilaterality and of periarticular accentuation. *Am J Med.* 1976;60(3):332–338.
110. Kozin F, McCarty DJ, Sims J, et al. The reflex sympathetic dystrophy syndrome. I. Clinical and histologic studies: evidence for bilaterality, response to corticosteroids and articular involvement. *Am J Med.* 1976;60(3):321–331.
111. Legrain V, Bultitude JH, De Paepe AL, et al. Pain, body, and space: what do patients with complex regional pain syndrome really neglect? *Pain.* 2012;153(5): 948–951.
112. Leis S, Weber M, Isselmann A, et al. Substance-P-induced protein extravasation is bilaterally increased in complex regional pain syndrome. *Exp Neurol.* 2003;183(1): 197–204.
113. Leriche R. Oedeme dur aigu post-traumatique de la main avec impotence fonctionelle complete. Transformation soudaine cinq heures apres sympathectomie humerale. *Lyon Chir.* 1923;20:814–818.
114. Leriche R. Traitement par la sympathectomie periarterielle des osteoporoses traumatiques. *Bull Mem Soc Chir Paris.* 1926;52:247–251.
115. Lewis JS, Kersten P, McCabe CS, et al. Body perception disturbance: a contribution to pain in complex regional pain syndrome (CRPS). *Pain.* 2007;133(1–3):111–119.
116. Lidstrom A. Fractures of the distal end of the radius. A clinical and statistical study of end results. *Acta Orthop Scand Suppl.* 1959;41:1–118.
117. Liepert J, Tegenthoff M, Malin JP. Changes of cortical motor area size during immobilization. *Electroencephalogr Clin Neurophysiol.* 1995;97(6):382–386.
118. Lindsay RM, Harmar AJ. Nerve growth factor regulates expression of neuropeptide genes in adult sensory neurons. *Nature.* 1989;337:362–364.
119. Livingstone JA, Atkins RM. Intravenous regional guanethidine blockade in the treatment of post-traumatic complex regional pain syndrome type 1 (algodystrophy) of the hand. *J Bone Joint Surg Br.* 2002;84(3):380–386.
120. Livingstone JA, Field J. Algodystrophy and its association with Dupuytren's disease. *J Hand Surg Br.* 1999;24(2):199–202.
121. LoPinto C, Young WB, Ashkenazi A. Comparison of dynamic (brush) and static (pressure) mechanical allodynia in migraine. *Cephalalgia.* 2006;26(7): 852–856.
122. Louyot P, Gaucher A, Montet Y, et al. [Algodystrophy of the lower extremity]. *Rev Rhum Mal Osteoartic.* 1967;34(12):733–737.
123. Lubenow TR, Buvanendran A, Stanton-Hicks M. Implanted therapies. In: Wilson P, Stanton-Hicks M, Harden RN, eds. *CRPS: Current Diagnosis and Therapy.* Vol. 32. Seattle, WA: IASP Press; 2005:235–253.
124. Mackinnon SE, Holder LE. The use of three-phase radionuclide bone scanning in the diagnosis of reflex sympathetic dystrophy." *J Hand Surg Am.* 1984;9(4):556–563.
125. Maier C, Baron R, Tölle TR, et al. Quantitative sensory testing in the German Research Network on Neuropathic Pain (DFNS): somatosensory abnormalities in 1236 patients with different neuropathic pain syndromes. *Pain.* 2010;150(3):439–450.

126. Maihöfner C, Handwerker HO, Neundörfer B, et al. Mechanical hyperalgesia in complex regional pain syndrome: a role for TNF-alpha? *Neurology*. 2005;65(2):311–313.
127. Mailis A, Wade J. Profile of Caucasian women with possible genetic predisposition to reflex sympathetic dystrophy: a pilot study. *Clin J Pain*. 1994;10(3):210–217.
128. Mailis A, Wade JA. Genetic considerations in CRPS. In: Harden RN, Baron R, Janig W, eds. *Complex Regional Pain Syndrome*. Vol. 22. Seattle, WA: IASP Press; 2001:227–238.
129. Marinus J, Moseley GL, Birklein F, et al. Clinical features and pathophysiology of complex regional pain syndrome. *Lancet Neurol*. 2011;10(7):637–648.
130. Marsden CD, Obeso JA, Traub MM, et al. Muscle spasms associated with Sudeck's atrophy after injury. *Br Med J (Clin Res Ed)*. 1984;288(6412):173–176.
131. Matsumura H, Jimbo Y, Watanabe K. Haemodynamic changes in early phase reflex sympathetic dystrophy. *Scand J Plast Reconstr Surg Hand Surg*. 1996;30(2):133–138.
132. McCabe CS, Haigh RC, Halligan PW, et al. Referred sensations in patients with complex regional pain syndrome type 1. *Rheumatology (Oxford)*. 2003;42(9):1067–1073.
133. McCabe CS, Haigh RC, Ring EF, et al. A controlled pilot study of the utility of mirror visual feedback in the treatment of complex regional pain syndrome (type 1). *Rheumatology (Oxford)*. 2003;42(1):97–101.
134. McLachlan EM, Jänig W, Devor M, et al. Peripheral nerve injury triggers noradrenergic sprouting within dorsal root ganglia. *Nature*. 1993;363:543–546.
135. Merskey H, Bogduk N. *Classification of Chronic Pain: Descriptions of Chronic Pain Syndromes and Definitions of Pain Terms*. Seattle, WA: IASP Press; 1994.
136. Merskey H. Essence, investigation, and management of "neuropathic" pains: hopes from acknowledgment of chaos. *Muscle Nerve*. 1995;18(4):455–456; author reply 458–462.
137. Mitchell SW, Morehouse GR, Keen WW. *Gunshot Wounds and Other Injuries of Nerves*. Philadelphia, PA: JB Lippincott Co; 1864.
138. Muller ME, Allgower M, Schneider R, et al. *Manual of Internal Fixation. Techniques Recommended by the AO Group*. London/New York: Springer Verlag; 1979.
139. Nelson DV, Novy DM. Psychological characteristics of reflex sympathetic dystrophy versus myofascial pain syndromes. *Reg Anesth*. 1996;21(3):202–208.
140. Nonne N. Über die Radiolographische nachweisbare akute und kronische "Knochenatrophie" (Südeck bie Nerven-Erkrankungen). *Fortschr Geb Rontgenstr*. 1901;5:293–297.
141. Oaklander AL, Rissmiller JG, Gelman LB, et al. Evidence of focal small-fiber axonal degeneration in complex regional pain syndrome-I (reflex sympathetic dystrophy). *Pain*. 2006;120(3):235–243.
142. Oaklander AL. Evidence-based pharmacotherapy for CRPS and related conditions. In: Wilson P, Stanton-Hicks M, Harden RN, eds. *CRPS: Current Diagnosis and Therapy*. Vol. 32. Seattle, WA: IASP Press; 2005:181–200.
143. Oyen WJ, Arntz IE, Claessens RM, et al. Reflex sympathetic dystrophy of the hand: an excessive inflammatory response? *Pain*. 1993;55(2):151–157.
144. Patman RD, Thompson JE, Persson AV. Management of post-traumatic pain syndromes: report of 113 cases. *Ann Surg*. 1973;177(6):780–787.
145. Pelissier J, et al. La personnalite du sujet souvrant d'algodystrophie sympathique reflexe. Etudes Psychometrques par le test MMPI. *Rheumatologie*. 1981;23:351–354.
146. Perelman RB, Adler D, Humphreys M. Reflex sympathetic dystrophy: electronic thermography as an aid in diagnosis. *Orthop Rev*. 1987;16(8):561–566.
147. Plewes LW. Sudeck's atrophy in the hand. *J Bone Joint Surg Br*. 1956;38B:195–203.
148. Price DD, Long S, Wilsey B, et al. Analysis of peak magnitude and duration of analgesia produced by local anesthetics injected into sympathetic ganglia of complex regional pain syndrome patients. *Clin J Pain*. 1998;14(3):216–226.
149. Procacci P, Francini F, Maresca M, et al. Skin potential and EMG changes induced by cutaneous electrical stimulation. II. Subjects with reflex sympathetic dystrophies. *Appl Neurophysiol*. 1979;42(3):125–134.
150. Procacci P, Francini F, Zoppi M, et al. Cutaneous pain threshold changes after sympathetic block in reflex dystrophies. *Pain*. 1975;1(2):167–175.
151. Punt TD, Cooper L, Hey M, et al. Neglect-like symptoms in complex regional pain syndrome: learned nonuse by another name? *Pain*. 2013;154(2):200–203.
152. Ramachandran VS, Roger-Ramachandran D. Synaesthesia in phantom limbs induced with mirrors. *Proc R Soc Lond B Biol Sci*. 1996;263:377–386.
153. Renier JC, Moreau R, Bernat M, et al. [Contribution of dynamic isotopic tests in the study of algodystrophies]. *Rev Rhum Mal Osteoartic*. 1979;46(4):235–241.
154. Ribbers GM, Oosterhuis WP, van Limbeek J, et al. Reflex sympathetic dystrophy: is the immune system involved? *Arch Phys Med Rehabil*. 1998;79(12):1549–1552.
155. Sandroni P, Benrud-Larson LM, McClelland RL, et al. Complex regional pain syndrome type I: incidence and prevalence in Olmsted county, a population-based study. *Pain*. 2003;103(1–2): 199–207.
156. Sandroni P, Low PA, Ferrer T, et al. Complex regional pain syndrome I (CRPS I): prospective study and laboratory evaluation. *Clin J Pain*. 1998;14(4):282–289.
157. Sarangi PP, Ward AJ, Smith EJ, et al. Algodystrophy and osteoporosis after tibial fractures. *J Bone Joint Surg Br*. 1993;75(3):450–452.
158. Schattschneider J, Wenzelburger R, Deuschl G, et al. Kinematic analysis of the upper extremity in CRPS. In: Harden RN, Baron R, Janig W, eds. *Complex Regional Pain Syndrome*. Vol. 22. Seattle, WA: IASP Press; 2001:119–128.
159. Schinkel C, Gaertner A, Zaspel J, et al. Inflammatory mediators are altered in the acute phase of posttraumatic complex regional pain syndrome. *Clin J Pain*. 2006;22(3): 235–239.
160. Schinkel C, Scherens A, Köller M, et al. Systemic inflammatory mediators in post-traumatic complex regional pain syndrome (CRPS I)—longitudinal investigations and differences to control groups. *Eur J Med Res*. 2009;14(3):130–135.
161. Schwartzman RJ, Kerrigan J. The movement disorder of reflex sympathetic dystrophy. *Neurology*. 1990;40(1):57–61.
162. Schwartzman RJ, McLellan TL. Reflex sympathetic dystrophy. A review. *Arch Neurol*. 1987;44(5):555–561.
163. Sethna NF, Meier PM, Zurakowski D, et al. Cutaneous sensory abnormalities in children and adolescents with complex regional pain syndromes. *Pain*. 2007;131(1–2):153–161.
164. Stanos SP, Harden RN, Wagner-Raphael L, et al. A prospective clinical model for investigating the development of CRPS. In: Harden RN, Baron R, Janig W, eds. *Complex Regional Pain Syndrome*. Vol. 22. Seattle, WA: IASP Press; 2001:151–164.
165. Stanton-Hicks M, et al. Complex regional pain syndromes: guidelines for therapy. *Clin J Pain*. 1998;14(2):155–166.
166. Stanton-Hicks M, Jänig W, Hassenbusch S. Reflex sympathetic dystrophy: changing concepts and taxonomy. *Pain*. 1995;63(1):127–133.
167. Stanton-Hicks M, Rauck RL, Hendrickson M, et al. Miscellaneous and experimental therapies. In: Wilson P, Stanton-Hicks M, Harden RN, eds. *CRPS: Current Diagnosis and Therapy*. Vol. 32. Seattle, WA: IASP Press; 2005:255–274.
168. Steinbrocker O. The shoulder-hand syndrome: present perspective. *Arch Phys Med Rehabil*. 1968;49(7):388–395.
169. Subbarao J, Stillwell GK. Reflex sympathetic dystrophy syndrome of the upper extremity: analysis of total outcome of management of 125 cases. *Arch Phys Med Rehabil*. 1981;62(11):549–554.
170. Sudeck P. Über die akute (reflektorische) Knochenatrophie nach Entzündungen und Verletzungen in den Extremitäten und ihre klinischen Erscheinungen. *Fortschr Geb Rontgenstr*. 1901;5:227–293.
171. Sudeck P. Über die Akute (reflektorische) Knochenatrophie. *Arch Klin Chir*. 1900; 762:147–156.
172. Thomson McBride AR, Barnett AJ, Livingstone JA, et al. Complex regional pain syndrome (type 1): a comparison of 2 diagnostic criteria methods. *Clin J Pain*. 2008;24(7):637–640.
173. Torebjörk E, Wahren L, Wallin G, et al. Noradrenaline-evoked pain in neuralgia. *Pain*. 1995;63:11–20.
174. Uceyler N, Eberle T, Rolke R, et al. Differential expression patterns of cytokines in complex regional pain syndrome. *Pain*. 2007;132(1–2):195–205.
175. van der Laan L, Goris RJ. Reflex sympathetic dystrophy. An exaggerated regional inflammatory response? *Hand Clin*. 1997;13(3):373–385.
176. van der Laan L, Kapitein P, Verhofstad A, et al. Clinical signs and symptoms of acute reflex sympathetic dystrophy in one hindlimb of the rat, induced by infusion of a free-radical donor. *Acta Orthop Belg*. 1998;64(2):210–217.
177. van der Laan L, ter Laak HJ, Gabreëls-Festen A, et al. Complex regional pain syndrome type I (RSD): pathology of skeletal muscle and peripheral nerve. *Neurology*. 1998;51(1): 20–25.
178. van Hilten JJ, van de Beek WJ, Vein AA, et al. Clinical aspects of multifocal or generalized tonic dystonia in reflex sympathetic dystrophy. *Neurology*. 2001;56(12):1762–1765.
179. van Hilten, JJ, Blumberg H, Robert Schwartzman RJ. Factor IV: movement disorders and dystrophy. Pathophysiology and measurement. In: Wilson PR, Stanton-Hicks M, Harden RN, eds. *CRPS: Current Diagnosis and Therapy*. Seattle, WA: IASP Press; 2005;32:119–137.
180. Van Houdenhove B, Vasquez G, Onghena P, et al. Etiopathogenesis of reflex sympathetic dystrophy: a review and biopsychosocial hypothesis. *Clin J Pain*. 1992;8(4):300–306.
181. Van Houdenhove B, Vasquez G. Is there a relationship between reflex sympathetic dystrophy and helplessness? Case reports and a hypothesis. *Gen Hosp Psychiatry*. 1993; 15(5):325–329.
182. Van Houdenhove B. Neuro-algodystrophy: a psychiatrist's view. *Clin Rheumatol*. 1986;5(3):399–406.
183. Veldman PH, Reynen HM, Arntz IE, et al. Signs and symptoms of reflex sympathetic dystrophy: prospective study of 829 patients. *Lancet*. 1993;342(8878):1012–1016.
184. Vincent G, Ernst J, Henniaux M, et al. [Attempt at a psychological approach in algoneurodystrophy]. *Rev Rhum Mal Osteoartic*. 1982;49(11):767–769.
185. Wahren LK, Gordh T Jr., Torebjörk E. Effects of regional intravenous guanethidine in patients with neuralgia in the hand; a follow-up study over a decade. *Pain*. 1995;62(3):379–385.
186. Wall PD, Devor M. Sensory afferent impulses originate from dorsal root ganglia as well as from the periphery in normal and nerve injured rats. *Pain*. 1983;17(4):321–339.
187. Wall PD. Noradrenaline-evoked pain in neuralgia. *Pain*. 1995;63(1):1–2.
188. Wasner G, Schattschneider J, Baron R. Skin temperature side differences—a diagnostic tool for CRPS? *Pain*. 2002;98(1–2):19–26.
189. Watson Jones SR. *Fractures and Joint Injuries*. London: ES Livingstone Ltd; 1952.
190. Wenzelburger R, Schattschneider J, Wasner G, et al. Grip force coordination in CRPS. In: Harden RN, Baron R, Janig W, eds. *Complex Regional Pain Syndrome*. Vol. 22. Seattle, WA: IASP Press; 2001:129–134.
191. Wilder R, Olsson GL. Management of pediatric patients with CRPS. In: Wilson P, Stanton-Hicks M, Harden RN, eds. *CRPS: Current Diagnosis and Therapy*. Vol. 32. Seattle, WA: IASP Press; 2005:275–289.
192. Wilder RT, Berde CB, Wolohan M, et al. Reflex sympathetic dystrophy in children. Clinical characteristics and follow-up of seventy patients. *J Bone Joint Surg Am*. 1992;74(6): 910–919.
193. Wilder RT. Management of pediatric patients with complex regional pain syndrome. *Clin J Pain*. 2006;22(5):443–448.
194. Woolf CJ, Mannion RJ. Neuropathic pain: aetiology, symptoms, mechanisms, and management. *Lancet*. 1999;353:1959–1964.
195. Woolf CJ, Salter MW. Neuronal plasticity: increasing the gain in pain. *Science*. 2000;288:1765–1768.
196. Zollinger PE, Tuinebreijer WE, Breederveld RS, et al. Can vitamin C prevent complex regional pain syndrome in patients with wrist fractures? A randomized, controlled, multicenter dose-response study. *J Bone Joint Surg Am*. 2007;89(7):1424–1431.
197. Zollinger PE, Tuinebreijer WE, Kreis RW, et al. Effect of vitamin C on frequency of reflex sympathetic dystrophy in wrist fractures: a randomised trial. *Lancet*. 1999;354(9195): 2025–2028.
198. Zucchini M, Alberti G, Moretti MP. Algodystrophy and related psychological features. *Funct Neurol*. 1989;4(2):153–156.
199. Zyluk A. [The three-staged evolution of the post-traumatic algodystrophy]. *Chir Narzadow Ruchu Ortop Pol*. 1998;63(5):479–486.
200. Zyluk A. Results of the treatment of posttraumatic reflex sympathetic dystrophy of the upper extremity with regional intravenous blocks of methylprednisolone and lidocaine. *Acta Orthop Belg*. 1998;64(4):452–456.
201. Zyluk A. The natural history of post-traumatic reflex sympathetic dystrophy. *J Hand Surg Br*. 1998;23(1):20–23.

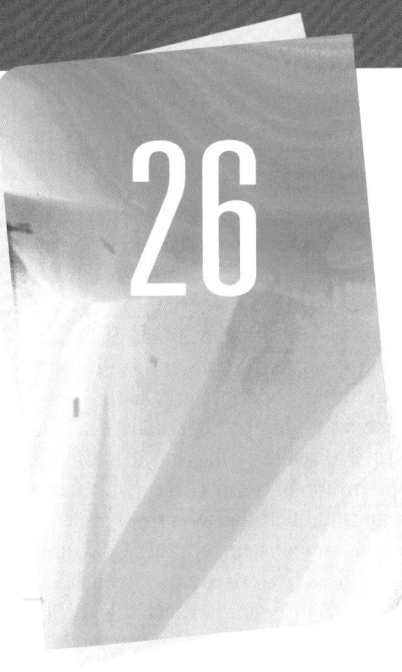

26

ORTHOPEDIC INFECTIONS AND OSTEOMYELITIS

Bruce H. Ziran, Wade R. Smith, and Nalini Rao

INTRODUCTION

The first descriptions of infections date back to the early Sumerian carvings, when the tenets of treatment were irrigation, immobilization, and bandaging.[83] In these early times, the practice of infection and wound care was essentially an art and there was very little science applied to it. Treatment included the use of honey, wine, and donkey feces, and there were a number of philosophies regarding the value of purulence. Dominant personalities had a significant influence over medical practice and the value of purulence persisted because of the writings of Galen of Pergamum (120 to 201 AD). It was not until the latter third of the second millennium that the concept of the value of purulence would be challenged.[83]

In the past three centuries, the treatment of infection has involved the use of local ointments or salves and the maintenance of an open wound that permitted purulence to exit the body. Some important terms were adopted into medical parlance. A *sequestrum* was defined as "a fragment of dead bone separated from the body." The word *sequestrum* is derived from the Latin words *sequester* meaning "depositary" and *sequestrate*

meaning "to give up for safe keeping." The word *sequestrum* is used to describe a detached piece of bone lying within a cavity formed by necrosis. The term *involucrum* derives from the Latin word *involucrum* meaning "enveloping sheath or envelope." This term describes the effects of the body's inflammatory response when trying to envelope and isolate the sequestrum from the host. The natural history of osteomyelitis was seen as the process of isolation of the infective material followed by a slow attempted resorption of the material by the immune system. However, the term *osteomyelitis* was not coined until the mid-1800s, when it was adopted by Nelaton.[99]

In his book *The Story of Orthopaedics*, Mercer Rang[99] describes the three pivotal discoveries that allowed orthopedic surgery to be successful: anesthesia, antisepsis, and radiography. The first two were important in all surgical specialties. Anesthesia made surgery tolerable, but there was still considerable morbidity secondary to infection. It was not until the mid-1800s that progress with antisepsis permitted infection control and more effective surgical intervention. As a result of this, infection issues became an integral part of medicine and were studied in a more formal basis. However, descriptions of the first sequestrectomies of the tibia had been illustrated as early as 1593 by Scultetus.[99]

Before anesthesia, most operative procedures were performed using forced immobility and inebriation. Operating rooms were created because procedures undertaken in the wards horrified patients who witnessed them and the screams of agony did nothing to encourage other patients to seek surgical treatment. Thus, the patients were isolated from the rest of the ward. In the same era, many modern drugs were developed, including morphine, heroin, nitrous oxide, and ether. Ether was in fact serendipitously identified as an anesthetic agent during one of the drug parties that were common at this time. However, it was first used for anesthesia in Massachusetts General Hospital in 1846 by William TG. Morton, and its use quickly caught on around the world. This increased the incentive to undertake surgical procedures. The ensuing increase in the number of surgical procedures, together with the lack of antisepsis, meant that the morbidity and mortality of surgery also increased.[99] Pasteur and Lister are most commonly credited as being the forerunners of antisepsis, but the most notable achievement in demonstrating the efficacy of bacterial transmission is the work of Semmelweis, who, in 1848, demonstrated that hand washing between obstetric deliveries reduced maternal mortality from 18% to about 1%. Lister read Pasteur's work on fermentation and likened tissue putrefaction to the same process. He subsequently developed carbolic acid, which reduced mortality from amputation from 43% in an untreated cohort of patients to 15% in a treated cohort. Despite this significant discovery, his findings were resisted for decades. Even when his concepts were adopted, the remaining pieces of the puzzle required for successful aseptic surgery did not come together for another 100 years.

The initial use of antibiotics was just as serendipitous as the use of anesthesia and antisepsis. Some antibacterial treatments were introduced, but it was not until the discovery of penicillin (PCN) by Alexander Fleming in 1928 that the proven usefulness of antibiotics became understood. Even Fleming did not vigorously pursue his discovery. However, when Florey and Chain read Fleming's initial report, they pursued and found the true impact of PCN, which was effective against streptococci. Since then, many antibiotics have been developed,[101] but the number of resistant bacteria has also increased. Hand washing, gloves, hats, enclosed rooms, aseptic techniques, and early antibiotics all slightly decreased the incidence of surgical infection. However, the operating theaters in the early 1900s still admitted observers who coughed, did not use masks, and wore street clothes. It was not until the mid-20th century that surgeons began to integrate all the controllable aspects of patient exposure to infectious agents by attempting to standardize the contributive effects of the environment, patient, surgeon, wound, antisepsis, antibiotics, and surgical techniques. It is likely, though, that many of the answers to the problem of infection remain undiscovered, and it seems likely that at the moment we do not fully understand the complex symbiosis between bacteria and humans.

This chapter will concentrate on the description, etiology, diagnosis, and management of orthopedic infections, but will have a specific focus on posttraumatic conditions. There will be an additional focus on institutional infection control and on infections in the geriatric orthopedic patient, this being a section of the population that is growing rapidly.

To treat orthopedic infection, one must first understand the basics of the interdependence of humans and bacteria. Bacteria are a necessary part of our existence and normal flora live in abundance on our bodies. It is worth considering that an individual's skin can contain up to 180 different types of bacteria at any given time.[46] There are up to 10 colony-forming units (CFUs) of bacteria in the mouth and perineum. Nearly 95% of bacteria found in the hands exist under the fingernails. The average human is composed of 100 trillion cells, but it is thought that we harbor over a 1,000 trillion bacteria in or on our bodies. Our blood is constantly infiltrated with bacteria from breaks in the skin, translocation across mucous membranes, and other roots. However, nearly all of these bacteria are quickly and efficiently eradicated by our host defense mechanisms. It is the disruption of our own homeostasis that provides an opportunity for either external contamination or opportunistic host bacteria to become pathogenic and cause infection. Although colonization necessarily precedes infection, the presence of bacteria by itself does not constitute infection. This is highlighted by the findings of one study of hardware removal in which 50% of cultures were positive in patients with no signs of symptoms or infection.[81] Thus, there is an important distinction between colonization and infection. Understanding the factors that have changed the local or systemic environment with resultant bacterial infection is the key to effective prophylaxis, treatment, and improved outcomes in orthopedic surgery.

Historically, the treatment of orthopedic infection was either ablative, when an amputation was performed, or temporizing with the treatment of a chronic wound or sinus. There was little chance of limb salvage as we know it today, and infections that were not adequately treated would occasionally become systemic and fatal.

Certainly, the high mortality of open gunshot wounds to the femur in the American Civil War and World War I was largely caused by sepsis. In every war, the science of surgery and medicine advances, and this is particularly true for trauma surgery and extremity injuries, which still account for approximately 65% of all war-related injuries.[84] Thus, many advances in infection treatment and extremity injuries have ironically come about as a result of war. The recent Middle East conflicts have been associated with a lower mortality than earlier wars with most orthopedic casualties being caused by blast injuries. This has mainly influenced infection control and prosthetics. Many soldiers presented with severe contamination from battlefield injuries that precluded acute definitive fixation. This prompted researchers to investigate the best methods of tissue reconstruction in the presence of significant contamination. The inevitable amputations that were required caused a renaissance in the prosthetics industry.

CLASSIFICATION

Historically, osteomyelitis was classified as either acute or chronic depending on the duration of symptoms. Kelly[61] documented a classification system based on the etiology of the osteomyelitis.

There were four types with type I being hematogenous osteomyelitis. Type II was osteomyelitis associated with fracture union, whereas type III was osteomyelitis without fracture union and type IV was postoperative or posttraumatic osteomyelitis without a fracture. Weiland et al.[127] in 1984 suggested another classification scheme based on the nature of the bony involvement. In this classification system, there were three types, with type I being characterized by open exposed bone without evidence of osseous infection, but with evidence of soft tissue infection. In type II fractures, there was circumferential cortical and endosteal infection, and in type III fractures, the cortical and endosteal infection was associated with a segmental defect.

In 1989, May et al.[71] proposed another classification scheme for osteomyelitis focusing on the tibia. This system was based on the nature of the bone following soft tissue and bony debridement. They proposed that there were five different categories.

Type I posttraumatic tibial osteomyelitis was defined as being present when the intact tibia and fibula were able to withstand functional loads and no reconstruction was required. In type II osteomyelitis, the intact tibia was unable to withstand functional loading and required bone grafting. In type III osteomyelitis, there was an intact fibula but a tibial defect that measured no more than 6 cm. The tibial defect required cancellous bone grafting, tibiofibular synostosis, or distraction histogenesis. Type IV osteomyelitis was characterized by an intact fibula but with a defect of more than 6 cm in length, which required distraction osteogenesis, tibiofibular synostosis, or a vascularized bone graft. Type V osteomyelitis was characterized by a tibial defect of more than 6 cm without an intact fibula, which often required amputation.

The Waldvogel classification[125] categorized osteomyelitis into three primary etiologies—hematogenous, contiguous (from an adjacent root such as an open fracture or a seeded implant), or chronic, this being a long-standing osteomyelitis with mature host reaction.

These various classification systems were predicated on the beliefs and treatment options of the times, and they have all become less relevant with current diagnostic and treatment modalities. However, each classification represented an important effort to categorize the pathophysiology of bone infection to facilitate the choice of an effective treatment.

The currently accepted classification remains the Cierny–Mader classification,[20] which not only describes the pathology in the bone, but more importantly, also classifies the host or patient (Tables 26-1 and 26-2). The usefulness of the Cierny–Mader system is its applicability to clinical practice and the wealth of experience and data gleaned from a single surgeon's practice with meticulous records. The hallmark of Cierny's and Mader's approach is the use of oncologic principles for treatment. In fact, osteomyelitis behaves very similarly to a benign bone tumor in that it is rarely lethal but has a tendency to return without complete eradiation. Interestingly, the outcome data reported by Cierny et al.[20] indicate that once appropriate surgical treatment is undertaken, the host may be the most important variable affecting treatment and outcome.

The hallmark of the Cierny–Mader classification is its analysis of the physiologic state of the patient or host. The host is classified by the number of systemic and local comorbidities. An A host has a healthy physiology and limb with little systemic or local compromise. The B host is further divided into one with local compromise (B local), systemic compromise (B systemic), or both (B systemic/local systemic compromise, which includes any immunocompromised condition, poor nutrition, diabetes, old age, multiple trauma, chronic hypoxia, vascular disease, malignancy, or organ failure such as renal insufficiency or liver failure). Local compromise includes conditions such as previous surgery or trauma, cellulitis, radiation fibrosis, scarring from burns or trauma, local manifestations of vascular disease, lymphedema, or zone-of-injury issues. We believe that a new variable of compromise can be identified in the trauma patient where systemic compromise is because of multiple organ damage, and the consequent systemic response to trauma and local compromise is defined by the zone-of-injury effects on local tissues.

The C host is a patient in whom the morbidity of treatment is greater than the morbidity of disease because of multiple and severe comorbid conditions that cannot be treated safely. In these patients, the risks of curative treatment such as extensive surgery, as might be used with free flaps, or prolonged reconstruction with bone transport would be greater than that caused by the infective condition itself. Type C hosts are often better treated with limited nonablative surgery and suppression or, if appropriate, by an amputation.

In the Cierny–Mader classification,[20] the bone lesion is classified by the extent of involvement and stability. Type I is a medullary or endosteal infection without penetration through cortex. This is the type of infection that occurs after intramedullary nailing. Type II is a superficial osteomyelitis that involves only the outer cortex and is frequently contiguous with a pressure ulcer or adjacent abscess. Type III is permeative in that there is involvement of both cortical and medullary bone, but importantly, there is no loss of axial stability of the bone. Type IV also involves cortical and medullary bone but in a segmental fashion such that axial stability is lost. Types III and IV would be typical infections related to open fractures. In type IV lesions, the segmental resection that is required necessitates reconstruction of the bone, whereas in type III lesions, additional stabilization may not be required (Tables 26-1 and 26-2).

The pairing of the four types of osteomyelitis with the three host classes allows for the development of practical treatment strategies. Cierny et al.[20] proposed a detailed treatment regimen defining optimal treatment modalities for each stage. They achieved an overall clinical 2-year success rate of 91% for all states. As one would expect, when their results were broken down by class of host and type of lesion, Class A hosts fared the best. In class A hosts, success rates of 98% were achieved even with type IV osteomyelitis. The compromised class B host's success rates were far lower, ranging from 79% to 92% depending on anatomic type. In his series, Cierny found that the host class seemed to be more important than the type of infection. A cumulative success rate of greater than 90% was achieved with most of the failures being in B hosts. C hosts were recommended for amputation or suppressive treatment.[19] The lessons that stem from their findings are that it is important not just to treat the disease but also the host and that the patient's physiologic

TABLE 26-1 Cierny–Mader Classification of Bone

Type I—Medullary
Infection is limited to the medullary canal. Typically seen after intramedullary nailing.

Type II—Superficial
Infection is limited to the exterior of the bone and does not penetrate the cortex. Typically seen from pressure ulcers.

Type III—Permeative/Stable
Infection penetrates cortex but bone is axially stable and generally will not require supplemental stabilization. Typically seen after internal fixation with plates.

Type IV—Permeative/Unstable
Infection is throughout the bone in segmental fashion and results in axial instability. Typically seen in extensive infections or after aggressive debridement of type III infections that results in loss of axial stability.

Osseous Location

Medullary

Superficial

Localized

Diffuse

Involvement

condition should be optimized. Thus, a B systemic-local host who has had a previous open fracture but also smokes and has uncontrolled diabetes, renal insufficiency, and malnutrition should have all of these problems treated together with the bone disease. Improving host status would appear to be a fruitful endeavor when one considers Cierny et al.'s[19,20] findings.

It should be noted that Cierny et al.'s[19,20] results used outcome criteria that were commonly used at that time. Current outcome studies focus more on subjective patient-based assessments than on surgeon-based assessments. We do not have much data on the functional outcomes in the scenarios described by Cierny et al., and it is possible that some of the

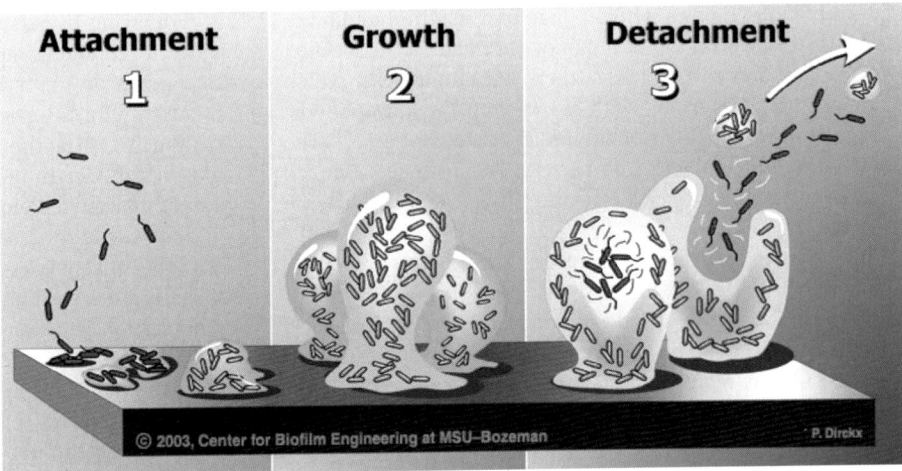

FIGURE 26-1 Illustration of the process of biofilm bacterial colonization. Firstly the bacteria need to find an inert surface such as an implant or dead tissue to attach to. Growth then occurs and the colonization process will continue until mature colonies are formed. Once mature, the colonies can detach depending on environmental signals or signals between colonies (from Center for Biofilm Engineering Montana State University—Bozeman, with permission).

patients whom they salvaged would have fared better with prosthetic replacement and vice versa.

PATHOGENESIS

Before a discussion of diagnosis and treatment, it is vital to understand the mechanisms by which infections occur. Most infections encountered in orthopedics are related to biofilm-forming bacteria. Much of our understanding of biofilm bacteria has come from the Centre for Biofilm Engineering in Bozeman, Montana. Biofilm bacteria are also important in the oil, food processing, naval, paper manufacturing, and water processing industries.

Biofilm bacteria exist in one of two states—the planktonic state or the colonized state (Fig. 26-1). Planktonic state bacteria are free floating in the blood stream and are isolated and relatively small in quantity. In this state, the body host defenses can easily eradicate the organism through the usual immunologic mechanisms. It is rare for planktonic bacteria to survive long in the blood stream despite numerous and repeated occurrences of entry. However, if the bacterial load is large and sustained, they can overwhelm the host defenses and escape the effects of antibiotics with the ensuing bacteremia leading to septicemia and death. Planktonic bacteria are also metabolically active and reproductive. This is an important consideration for antibiotic treatments that work by either interfering with cell wall or protein synthesis or with reproduction.

If planktonic bacteria encounter a suitable inert surface such as dead or necrotic tissue, foreign bodies, or any avascular body part by either direct contamination, contiguous spreading, or hematogenous seeding, they can attach and begin the process of colonization. Juxtaposition of the bacteria with a surface or biomaterial is accomplished by van der Waals forces, which allow bacteria to develop irreversible cross-links with the surface (adhesion–receptor interaction).[26] Adhesion is based on time-dependent specific protein adhesion–receptor interactions, as well as carbohydrate polymer synthesis in addition to charge and physical forces.[59] Following adhesion to a surface, bacteria begin to create a mucopolysaccharide layer called *biofilm* or *slime*. They then develop into colonies. These colonies exhibit remarkably resilient behavior. Figure 26-2 illustrates

TABLE 26-2	Cierny–Mader Classification of the Host
Host Class	**Description**
A host	Healthy physiology and limb
B host: Systemic	Diabetes, stable multiple organ disease, nicotine use, substance abuse, immunologic deficiency, malnutrition, malignancy, old age, vascular disease **Trauma context:** Multiple injuries
B host: Local	Previous trauma, burns, previous surgery, vascular disease, cellulitis, scarring, previous radiation treatment, lymphedema **Trauma context:** Zone of injury
B host: Systemic/local	Combinations of systemic and local conditions
C host	Multiple uncorrectable comorbidities. Unable to tolerate the extent of surgical reconstruction required. Treatment of the disease is worse than the disease itself

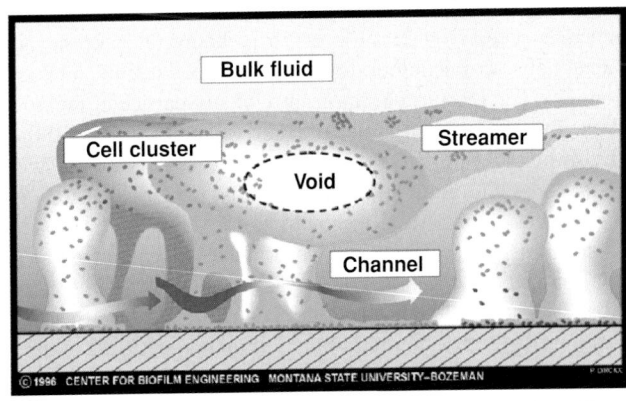

FIGURE 26-2 Illustration of biofilm colonies and interactions (from Center for Biofilm Engineering Montana State University—Bozeman, with permission).

mature biofilm colonies where pillars of a mature biofilm are visibly distributed on top of a monolayer of surface-associated cells. In addition to fixed cells, there are motile cells, which maintain their association with the biofilm for long periods, swimming between pillars of biofilm-associated bacteria.[126] The interaction of the colonies and bacteria demonstrates complex communication via proteins or markers that can alter bacterial behavior.

In the early stages of colonization, sessile bacteria can be killed or neutralized by the host defenses. However, some of these bacteria may escape destruction and potentially act as a nidus for future infection. Transition from colonization to infection usually requires other conditions to exist. This might occur if there was an inoculum that was larger than threshold levels, impaired host immune defense mechanisms, traumatized or necrotic tissues, a foreign body, or an acellular or inanimate surface such as dead bone, cartilage, or biomaterials. These complex mechanisms help explain why every open fracture or infected implant does not result in osteomyelitis.

As previously discussed, the first step in the transition from colonization to infection requires bacterial adhesion, which will usually not occur on viable tissue surfaces. Thus, when foreign material or dead tissue is found in the body, a "race for the surface" begins. Host cells will attempt to incorporate nonliving material or sequester nonviable tissue via encapsulation so that a well-incorporated biomaterial implant that has such a tissue-integrated neocapsule will be resistant to bacterial adhesion. Furthermore, the same tissue integration can often isolate bacteria that have become sessile on an implant surface by sequestering the bacteria from necessary nutrients until host mechanisms can act.

However, if bacteria encounter the surface and develop mature colonies, tissue integration by the host may be impaired and the process of infection may proceed. Damaged bone, necrotic tissues, and implants can act as a suitable surface for bacterial adhesion and colonization.[69] Devitalized bone devoid of normal periosteum presents a collagen matrix to which bacteria can bind. Moreover, it has been suggested that bone sialoprotein can act as a ligand for bacterial binding to bone.[69] Biomaterials and other foreign bodies are usually inert and susceptible to bacterial colonization because they are inanimate. Regardless of how inert a metal is, it may still modulate molecular events on its surfaces, these being receptor–ligand interactions, covalent bonding, and thermodynamic interactions.[44,50] The most important feature of any particular method is the interaction between its outer surface atomic layer and the glycoproteins of prokaryotic and eukaryotic cells. Stainless steel and cobalt–chromium and titanium alloys are resistant to corrosion because of several mechanisms including surface oxide passivations. These surface oxides form a reactive interface with bacteria that can promote colony formation. There is therefore a balance between implanting devices with surface structures that lower the corrosion rates but might increase the likelihood of surface binding by bacteria. Thus, a large surface area and bacterial inoculum, combined with local tissue damage and a compromised or insufficient host response, can collectively create the necessary conditions for infection.

Following bacterial adherence and colonization, the resistance to antibiotics appears to increase.[85,86] This resistance is dependent on the type of surface to which the organisms are attached. Organisms that adhere to hydrocarbon polymers are extremely resistant to antibiotics. These same organisms, when attached to metals, do not resist antibiotic therapy to the same extent. Bacterial colonies can undergo phenotypic changes and appear to hibernate. They can survive in a dormant state without causing infection, and this can explain the recovery of bacteria from asymptomatic hardware removal.[81] So, whereas colonization is a necessary antecedent for infection, colonization alone does not necessarily lead to infection.

Two characteristics of colonized bacteria may help understand and explain this pseudoresistance. Because the passage of antibiotics through tissues is based on a diffusion gradient, colonized bacteria are insulated with a natural barrier of glycocalyx, often referred to as *slime*, through which the circulating antibiotic must diffuse before arriving at the bacterial cell wall (Fig. 26-3). The antibiotic molecules must then diffuse into the bacterial cell or be transported by metabolically active bacterial cell membranes. Because it is theorized that bacteria within biofilms have a decreased metabolic rate and undergo phenotypic changes, active processes such as cell membrane formation, which are targeted by antibiotics, would be similarly decreased (Fig. 26-4).[117] Consequently, antibiotic concentrations of 1,500 times normal may be required to penetrate both the biofilm and the bacterial cell wall. Even then, most antimicrobials work via interference with cell wall synthesis or cellular reproduction, and they therefore require metabolically active bacteria to be effective. Thus, bacteria in the biofilm may be dormant and appear to be pseudoresistant. The more metabolically inactive the bacteria, the less bactericidal will be the antibiotic therapy, which is why mature or chronic infections can rarely be cured with antibiotics alone. Table 26-3 outlines the major antibiotic classes and their mechanisms of action, all of which may be limited by the bacterial state in biofilm.

Once colonization occurs, body defenses continue to identify bacteria as foreign. There may be chemotactic mechanisms

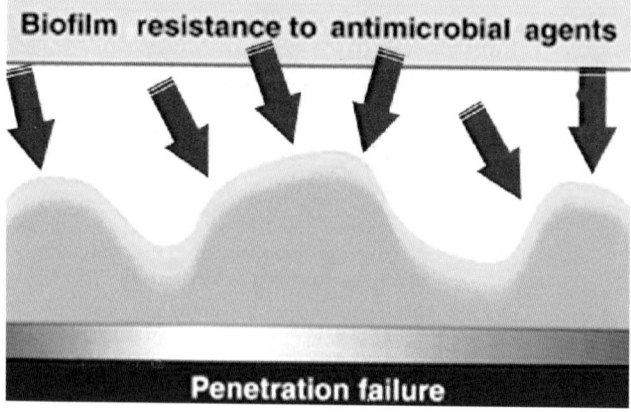

FIGURE 26-3 Illustration demonstrating the resistance to diffusion through biofilm for systemic antibiotics (from Center for Biofilm Engineering Montana State University—Bozeman, with permission).

TABLE 26-3	Major Antibiotic Classes and Their Mechanism of Action
Inhibition of cell wall synthesis/development	Penicillin, cephalosporins, vancomycin, bacitracin, chlorhexidine
Inhibition of protein synthesis	Chloramphenicol, macrolides, lincosamides, tetracyclines
Inhibition of RNA synthesis	Rifampin
Inhibition of DNA synthesis	Quinolones, macrolides
Inhibition of enzymatic/ metabolic activity	Trimethoprim/sulfamethoxazole (blocks folic acid production)

Data from www.sigmaaldrich.com/Area_of_Interest/Biochemicals/Antibiotic_Explorer/Mechanism_of_Action.html.

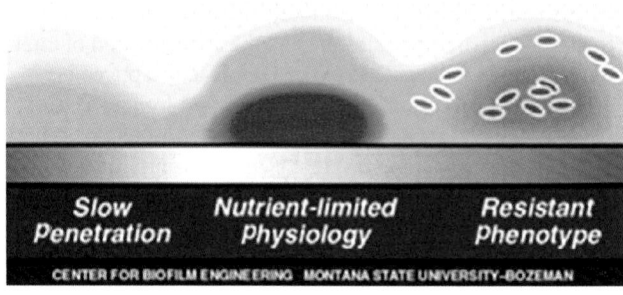

FIGURE 26-4 The phenomenon of "pseudoresistance." Biofilm bacteria can reduce their metabolic activity. Because many antibiotics interfere with such metabolic activity as their mechanism of action, any such attenuation may render antibiotics less effective. (From Center for Biofilm Engineering Montana State University—Bozeman, with permission.)

that keep immune cells active. The subsequent collection of inflammatory cells brought in to wall off the bacteria via chemotaxis manifests as *purulence*, which is a symptom of the host's attempt to isolate and destroy the infection. The acute inflammatory cells will also release a spectrum of oxidative and enzymatic products in an attempt to penetrate the glycocalyx. These mediators and enzymes are nonspecific and may be toxic to host tissue. Increased host tissue damage can lead

to more surface substrate for local bacteria, creating a cycle of tissue damage, host response, and exacerbation of infection (Fig. 26-5). The host tissues will eventually react to limit the spread of infection macroscopically as well as microscopically. The clinical manifestation of a sequestered infection is an

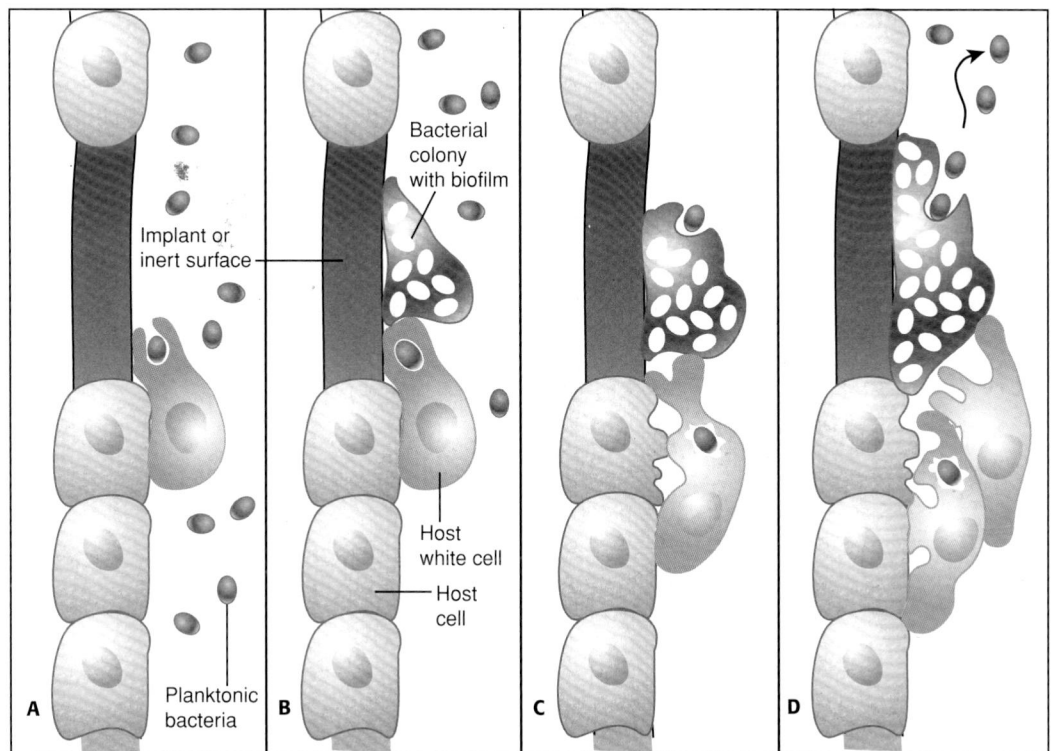

FIGURE 26-5 Autoinjury mechanism of host white cells in response to biofilm bacteria. **A:** Host white cells engulf planktonic bacteria and then **(B)** moves to engulf a bacterial colony that has developed but is unable to do so. **C:** Host white cells next response to engulfed bacteria is to release oxidative enzymes, but those enzymes also cause damage to local host cells. **D:** Unsuccessful eradication of bacteria and colony growth attracts more host white cells, resulting in increased damage to host tissue.

abscess or involucrum. Alternatively, if the infection grows and reaches the skin or an internal epithelial surface, a sinus tract forms as a route to dispel detritus. Although the appearance of a sinus tract is a manifestation of a locally devastating disease process and indicates severe underlying infection, it should be remembered that it may also prevent the accumulation of internal fixation, which can lead to bacteremia and septicemia.

Eventually, an equilibrium may exist in the form of a chronic infection, which is what many surgeons see in practice. There is usually a history of intermittent symptoms and drainage that has responded to some type of antibiotic regimen. What this probably represents is the inhibition of colony expansion at the borders of the infectious site. Clinically harmful manifestations of infection are generally caused by the release of bacteria into the bloodstream that are metabolically active and release toxins in addition to the release of oxidative enzymes by the host cell. Although the bacteria remain susceptible to the body's host defenses and to antibiotics, their numbers and continued release into the bloodstream represent a chronic debilitating disease. Any acute stress on the host environment from trauma, disease, or immunosuppression can allow the infection to strengthen and spread. Thus, long-standing infections that were tolerated by young healthy individuals may suddenly become limb- or life-threatening as the individuals age.

New developments stemming from the work of the Bozeman group provide novel opportunities to treat bacterial infection of orthopedic implants. These include surface coatings, agents that inhibit colonization or promote dissolution of colonies, small electric fields, and low pH and acidic and negatively charged surfaces that are resistant to biofilms. Surface proper-

ties of implants or local or systemic drugs may help decrease the risk to infection, particularly in the elderly population, who have decreased immune system activity.

INFECTION AFTER FRACTURE

Infection after fracture is most likely to be associated with open fractures or invasive surgical procedures. Few closed fractures treated nonoperatively develop osteomyelitis. To improve the diagnosis of posttraumatic bone infection, it is necessary to understand the mechanisms of infection, particularly for open fractures.

Approximately 60% to 70% of open fractures are contaminated by bacteria, but a much smaller percentage develops infection. The risk of infection correlates significantly with the degree of soft tissue injury.[121] If one remembers that merely the presence of bacteria in an open wound is not sufficient to cause infection, it is important to recognize that a severely contaminated fracture can rarely be debrided to the point of achieving a sterile or bacteria-free tissue bed. We believe that next to removing the majority of bacteria from the contaminated tissue bed, the second major goal of a wide and aggressive debridement is to leave behind a viable tissue bed with minimal necrotic or inert surfaces for the remaining bacteria to colonize. By minimizing the bacterial contamination by eliminating adhesions and nutrition, the host gains an opportunity to eradicate any remaining contaminants in the zone of injury. Figure 26-6 demonstrates the concept of open fracture debridement where a contaminated wound is debrided until the remaining wound looks as if it is created surgically, with residual tissue

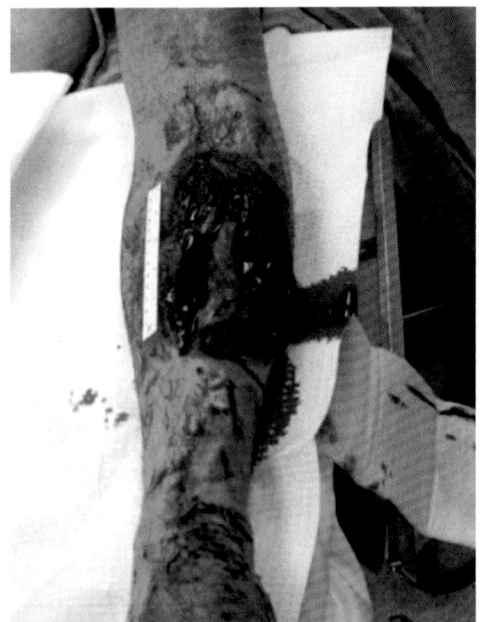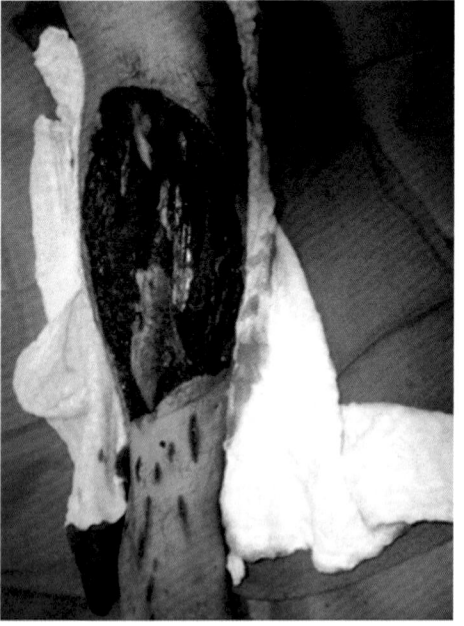

FIGURE 26-6 Operative photographs of a severe open tibial fracture. **A:** The appearance before surgical debridement. **B:** The appearance after surgical debridement. Note that after debridement the tissues and wound appear to have been made surgically. Although it is unlikely that all bacteria have been removed, a thorough exploration and debridement, leaving only viable tissues, will minimize the risk of subsequent infection.

being healthy with little evidence of contamination. It is important to remember that contamination can penetrate into tissue planes or locations that are not obvious in the initial wound. This may be a particular problem with blast injuries. The use of pulsatile irrigation before surgical exploration and debridement may in fact push the initial contaminants deeper into the tissues and result in contaminants being left behind in a locally compromised tissue bed. This will increase the likelihood of both acute and delayed infection.

An important fact that is often unrecognized is that the bacteria recovered from clinical infections are not necessarily the bacteria found acutely in the contaminated tissue bed. Several studies have found that routine cultures of open fractures are not useful because the predominant organism recovered from acute cultures is frequently not the organism recovered if and when an infection occurs. Antibiotic treatment based on the acute culture, whether before or after debridement, may be detrimental because the antibiotic that is chosen may not be specifically indicated and has the potential to promote changes and overgrowth in the bacterial flora. In the worst case scenario, routine antibiotic treatment based on initial wound cultures may promote the development of resistant bacterial strains.[64,92,122]

Many of the organisms responsible for eventual osteomyelitis are often hospital-acquired pathogens such as resistant *Staphylococcus aureus* or gram-negative bacilli, including *Pseudomonas aeruginosa*,[51,67] which are not initially present in a traumatic wound. This does not mean that other bacteria should not be considered and these may depend on the environment. *Clostridium perfringens* must be considered if there is soil contamination and *Pseudomonas*, and *Aeromonas hydrophila* may be present following a freshwater injury. *Vibrio* and *Erysipelothrix* may be present in saltwater injuries. One possible explanation for the lack of correlation between acute cultures and the eventual infection may be that the initial contaminants are of low virulence and easily neutralized by a combination of debridement and antibiotics, but that the locally and, in polytrauma, the systemically, compromised tissue bed is susceptible to the more aggressive nosocomial organisms.

ACUTE POSTTRAUMATIC OSTEOMYELITIS

Acute posttraumatic osteomyelitis is a bone infection that results in traumatic injury that allows pathogenic organisms to make contact with damaged bone and soft tissues, with a proliferation and expression of infection.[75] In a patient with traumatic injuries, additional factors that contribute to the subsequent development of osteomyelitis are the presence of hypotension, inadequate debridement of the fracture site, malnutrition, sustained intensive care unit hospitalization, alcoholism, and smoking.[41,118] Trauma may lead to interference with the host response to infection. Tissue injury or the presence of bacteria triggers activation of the complement cascade that leads to local vasodilatation, tissue edema, migration of polymorphonuclear leukocytes (PMNs) to the site of the injury, and enhanced ability of phagocytes to ingest bacteria.[56] Trauma has been reported to delay the inflammatory response to bacteria

as well as to depress cell-mediated immunity and to impair the functions of PMNs, including chemotaxis, superoxide production, and microbial killing.[56] The commonly used system of Cierny–Mader[20] has been shown to have a close correlation with the general condition of the patient rather than the specifics of bone involvement.

CHRONIC OSTEOMYELITIS

This condition is often the result of an acute osteomyelitis that is inadequately treated. General factors that may predispose to chronic osteomyelitis include the degree of bone necrosis, poor nutrition, the infecting organism, the age of the patient, the presence of comorbidities, and drug abuse.[25] The infecting organism generally varies with the cause of the chronic osteomyelitis. Chronic osteomyelitis results from acute osteomyelitis and is frequently caused by *S. aureus*, although chronic osteomyelitis that occurs after a fracture can be polymicrobial or gram negative. Intravenous drug users are commonly found to have *Pseudomonas* as well as *S. aureus* infections. Gram-negative organisms are now seen in up to 50% of all cases of chronic osteomyelitis, and this may be because of variables such as surgical intervention, chronic antibiotics, nosocomial causes, or changes in the bacterial flora of the tissue bed.[25] The fundamental problem in chronic osteomyelitis is a slow progressive revascularization of bone that leaves protected pockets of necrotic material to support bacterial growth that are relatively protected from systemic antibiotic therapy. This collection of necrotic tissue, bone, and bacteria is what becomes termed a *sequestrum,* and the body's attempt to wall off the offending material with reactive inflammatory tissue, whether this is bone or soft tissue, is termed the *involucrum.* The involucrum can be highly vascular and may be viable and structural, and this should be taken into consideration during surgical debridement.

FUNGAL OSTEOMYELITIS

Fungal osteoarticular infections are caused by two groups of fungi. The dimorphic fungi, which include *Blastomyces dermatitidis, Coccidioides* sp., *Histoplasma capsulatum,* and *Sporothrix schenckii,* typically cause infections in healthy hosts in endemic regions, whereas *Candida* sp., *Cryptococcus,* and *Aspergillus* cause infections in immunocompromised hosts. Infection is introduced by direct trauma or injury but may be associated with a penetrating foreign body or hematogenous spread.

Candida sp. is the most common fungus seen in osteomyelitis. It affects both native and prosthetic joints, vertebrae, and long bones. Risk factors include loss of skin integrity, diabetes, malnutrition, immunosuppressive therapy, intravenous drug use, hyperalimentation, the use of central venous catheters, intra-articular steroid injections, and the use of broad-spectrum antibiotics. A combined approach to therapy using medical and surgical modalities is necessary for optimal results. Azole antifungals and lipid preparations of amphotericin B have expanded the therapeutic options in fungal osteomyelitis as there is reduced toxicity associated with long-term therapy.[75]

CLINICAL AND LABORATORY DIAGNOSTIC TESTS

A history of infection or intercurrent illness as well as of remote surgery or trauma should raise the clinical suspicion of osteomyelitis. Normal signs of inflammation may be absent and thus the diagnosis of infection may be difficult. Patients may have a history of infection at another site, such as the lungs, bladder, or skin in conjunction with a history of trauma. They usually complain of pain in the affected area and feel generally unwell. Moreover, reduced activity, malaise, anorexia, fever, tachycardia, and listlessness may be present. Local findings include swelling and warmth, occasional erythema, tenderness to palpation, drainage, and restricted range of motion in adjacent joints.

Aspects of the clinical history that should alert the surgeon to look for infection include a history of open fracture, severe soft tissue injury, a history of substance abuse and smoking, inadequate previous treatment, or an immunocompromised state. These are all factors that contribute to a B host. Factors affecting treatment that need to be assessed include the time of onset of the infection, the status of the soft tissues, the viability of the bone, the status of fracture healing, implant stability, the condition of the host, and the neurovascular examination.

Routine blood cultures are of little help unless patients show manifestations of systemic disease, but they may be positive in up to 50% to 75% of cases where there is concomitant bacteremia or septicemia.[128] Blood cultures that yield coagulase-negative staphylococci, a common contaminant and pathogen, must be correlated with other clinical findings before attribution of clinical significance. Blood results that are suggestive of infection include an elevation of the white blood cell (WBC) count and elevations in the C-reactive protein (CRP) and erythrocyte sedimentation rate (ESR) levels. The ESR may be normal in the first 48 hours, but rises to levels about 100 mm/hr and may remain elevated for several weeks. It is, however, a nonspecific marker.[128] Combination of the ESR with the CRP improves specificity such that if both are negative, the specificity is 90% to 95% for acute osteomyelitis. In other words, a negative CRP and ESR make osteomyelitis unlikely. Their values are also age-dependent, and there is a steady increase in normal values with aging. In one recent study, the ESR and CRP were found to be useful diagnostic tools for the detection of an infected arthroplasty. Although they had low sensitivities and positive predictive values and therefore were of little value for screening, they had high specificity and negative predictive value and therefore were useful for treatment decisions.[49] These studies and other diagnostic studies may not be as useful in acute postoperative and chronic infections. In the acute setting, the ESR and CRP are expected to be elevated because of local and systemic inflammation from the surgical procedure. In chronic infections, the host has had time to adapt to the offending condition and thus may not mount the response required to trigger an elevation in these tests. Once osteomyelitis treatment is initiated, the CRP and ESR are useful in following the response to treatment. We use the ESR and CRP to establish a baseline value before debridement and initiation of antibiotic therapy and to monitor the subsequent response to treatment.

Radiographic Imaging

Radiologic findings in the initial presentation of acute osteomyelitis are often normal. The most common radiographic signs of bone infection are rarefaction, which represents diffuse demineralization secondary to inflammatory hyperemia; soft tissue swelling with obliteration of tissue planes; trabecular destruction; lysis; cortical permeation; periosteal reaction; and involucrum formation. Radiologically detectable demineralization may not be seen for at least 10 days after the onset of acute osteomyelitis.[128] When present, mineralization usually signifies trabecular bone destruction. If the infection spreads to the cortex, usually within 3 to 6 weeks, a periosteal reaction may be seen on radiographs. One study reported that in cases of proven osteomyelitis, 5% of radiographs were abnormal initially, 33% were abnormal by 1 week, and 90% were abnormal by 4 weeks.[6] In trauma and fracture treatment, the nature of callus formation and the obfuscation of bone by hardware may make radiologic changes difficult to recognize in the early or middle states of infection. Often it is not until there is a clear sequestrum, sinus, or involucrum that parallels the clinical findings that specific radiographic changes are recognized (Fig. 26-7).

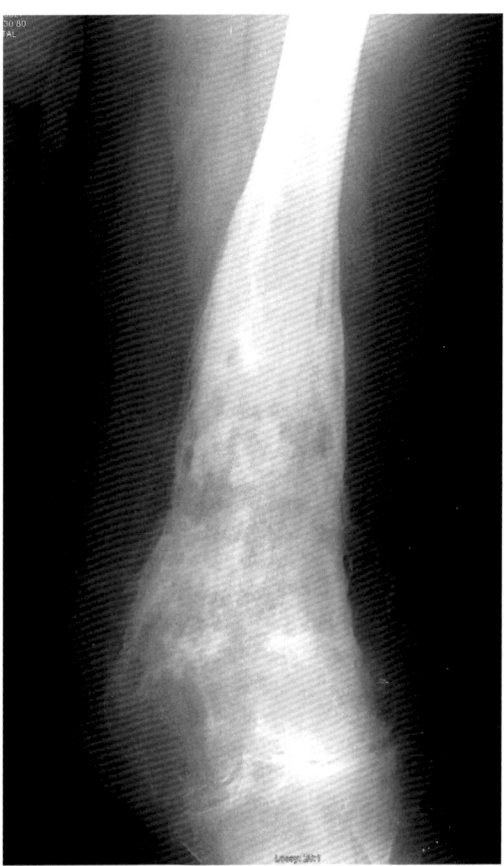

FIGURE 26-7 A radiograph showing the changes seen in bone with osteomyelitis. Note the periosteal reaction and the permeative changes in the bone.

Bone Scintigraphy

Scintigraphy has been widely used and remains a very useful diagnostic tool. However as noted below the usefulness of this test is governed by a number of variables such as technique and reader accuracy and the mainstay of diagnosis remains the clinical history together with the common screening examinations of CRP and ESR. There are numerous types of scintigraphy, but three scan types are commonly used to diagnose musculoskeletal infection. These are the bone scan, which uses tagged red cells; the leukocyte scan, which uses tagged white cells; and the bone marrow scan, which investigates marrow cell activity. Recently, positron emission tomography (PET) has shown promise and is undergoing increased investigation and use.

Technetium-99m is the principal radioisotope used in most whole-body red cell bone scans.[27,31,43] Technetium is formed as a metastable intermediate during the decay of molybdenum-99. It has a 6-hour half life and is relatively inexpensive and readily available.[27] After intravenous injection, there is a rapid distribution of this agent throughout the extracellular fluid. Within several hours, more than half the dose will accumulate in bone, whereas the remainder is excreted in the urine. Technetium phosphates bind to both the organic and inorganic matrix. However, the key characteristic that makes technetium scanning useful is that there is preferential incorporation into metabolically active bone. Bone images are usually acquired 2 to 4 hours following intravenous injection of the isotope. A triple-phase bone scan is one that is useful for examining general inflammation and related processes. Following the initial injection, dynamic images are captured over the specified region. These are followed by static images at later time points. The first phase represents the blood flow phase, the second phase immediately post injection represents the bone pooling phase, and the third phase is a delayed image made at 3 hours when there is decreased soft tissue activity. Classically, osteomyelitis presents as a region of increased blood flow, and it should appear "hot" in all phases with focal uptake in the third phase (Fig. 26-8). Other processes such as healing fractures, loose prostheses, and degenerative change do not appear hot in the early phase despite a hot appearance in the delayed phase. Reported sensitivities of bone scintigraphy for the detection of osteomyelitis vary considerably from 32% to 100%. Reported specificities have ranged from 0% to 100%.[106,124]

Gallium-67 citrate binds rapidly to serum proteins, particularly transferrin.[10,102] There is also uptake in the blood, especially by leukocytes. Gallium has been used in conjunction with technetium-99 to increase the specificity of the bone scanning.[39,52] Several mechanisms have been postulated to explain the increased activity at sites of inflammation. Enhanced blood flow and increased capillary permeability cause enhanced delivery. Bacteria have high iron requirements and thus take up gallium. Gallium is strongly bound to bacterial siderophores and leukocyte lactoferrins. In regions of inflammation, these proteins are available extracellularly and can avidly bind with gallium. Chemotaxis also acts to localize gallium-labeled WBCs at the sites of infection. In a typical study, gallium is injected intravenously and delayed images are acquired at 48 to 72 hours.

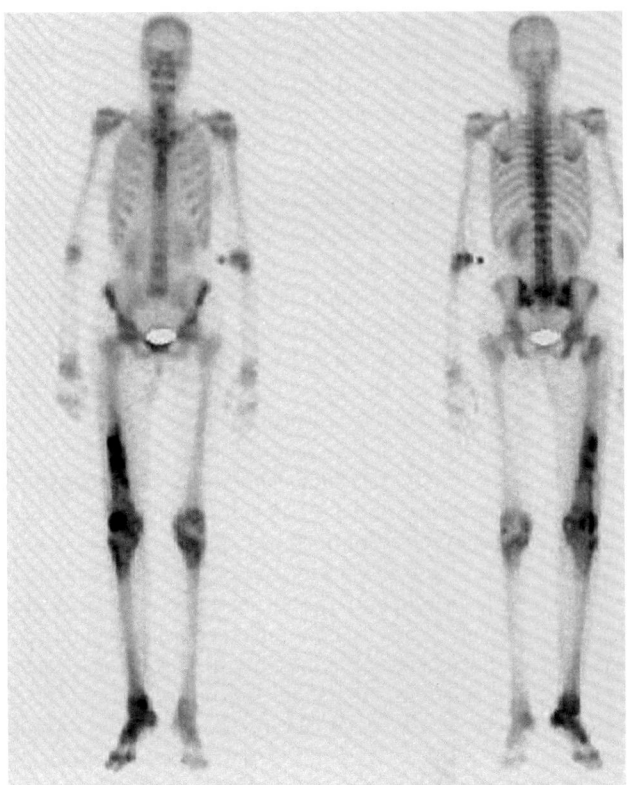

FIGURE 26-8 A standard bone scan demonstrating increased activity in the distal femur.

The hallmark of osteomyelitis is the focal increased uptake of gallium. Unfortunately, gallium's nonspecific bone uptake can be problematic because any processes causing reactive new bone formation will appear hot. In patients with fractures or a prosthesis, osteomyelitis cannot be easily diagnosed with gallium alone. Gallium images are usually interpreted in conjunction with a technetium bone scan. Gallium activity is interpreted as abnormal either if it is incongruous with the bone scan activity or if there is a matching pattern with gallium activity. Reported sensitivities and specificities for the diagnosis of osteomyelitis range from 22% to 100% and 0% to 100%, respectively.[27,52,77,106] Despite its lower-than-optimal diagnostic value, gallium still has some advantages. It is easily administered and it is the agent of choice in chronic soft tissue injection, although it is less effective in bone infections. It has also proved useful in following the resolution of an inflammatory process by showing a progressive decline in activity.

An indium-111 or 99mTc-hexamethylpropyleneamine oxime (99mTc-HMPAO) (Ceretec; GE Healthcare) labeled leukocyte scan is the most common scan used in conjunction with a standard bone scan. The labeled leukocytes migrate to the region of active infection resulting in a hot white cell scan over the area of active inflammation. The use of a combined red cell and white cell scan significantly increases both the sensitivity and specificity and now represents the gold standard of radionuclide testing for infection.[68] Because of the variable accuracy of both technetium and gallium scans most laboratories routinely use 111 In-labeled leukocytes.[102,105,109,123] Indium WBC preparations require the withdrawal of approximately 50 mL of autologous whole blood with a leukocyte count of at least 5,000 cells/mm³. The leukocytes are labeled with 1 mCi of indium oxine and then reinjected. They redistribute in the intravascular space. Immediate images show activity in the lungs, liver, spleen, and blood pool. The half life is about 7 hours. After 24 hours, only the liver, spleen, and bone marrow show activity. Wounds that heal normally and fully treated infections show no increase in uptake. Leukocytes that migrate to an area of active bone infection will show increased uptake (Fig. 26-9). Most results show improved sensitivity (80% to 100%) and specificity (50% to 100%) for the diagnosis of osteomyelitis.[28–30,54,58] Indium-labeled WBC scans are generally superior to bone scans and gallium scans in the detection of infection. McCarthy et al.[73] reported on the use of indium scans in 39 patients who had suspected osteomyelitis confirmed by bone biopsy. They found indium scans to be 97% sensitive and 82% specific for osteomyelitis. The few false-positive results occurred in patients who had overlying soft tissue infections. An accompanying bone scan can help to differentiate bone infection from soft tissue infection. In these situations, the indium scan should be performed before the bone scan to avoid false-positive results. With both tests, the sensitivities and specificities are in excess of 90%.

Until recently, a clinician investigating the site of infectious foci using nuclear medicine had a choice between 67Ga-citrate imaging and 111In-oxine leukocyte imaging.[28] Scientific advances, especially in nuclear medicine, have increased these choices considerably. Several techniques in nuclear medicine

have significantly aided the diagnosis of infection including imaging with 99mTc-HMPAO and 99mTc-stannous fluoride colloid-labeled leukocytes.[58] The principal clinical indications for 99mTc-HMPAO leukocytes include osteomyelitis and soft tissue sepsis. Chronic osteomyelitis, including infected joint prostheses, is better diagnosed with 111In-labeled leukocytes.[93] The use of 99mTc-HMPAO leukocyte scintigraphy in patients with symptomatic total hip or knee arthroplasty has shown improved diagnostic accuracy through the use of semiquantitative evaluation.[129]

Sulfur colloid bone scanning is a newer modality that is being increasingly used for the diagnosis of infection. The scan evaluates the bone marrow activity in an area where infection is suspected. The marrow may be reactive in several conditions that are not infected and is generally suppressed when infection is present. With the use of microcolloid bone marrow scans, more information is available to increase the specificity of diagnosis. There is the possibility of leukocyte accumulation with certain inflammatory conditions that could result in a false-positive indium scan. An infection will tend to suppress marrow activity and thus render the marrow scan cold, whereas the white cell scan may still be hot (Fig. 26-10). If the white cell scan is as hot as the marrow scan, it is possible that an infection may not be present. Segura et al.[112] examined technetium-labeled white cell scans (Tc-HMPAO) and technetium microcolloid marrow scans in total joint replacements. They found that in 77 patients, the white cell scans by themselves

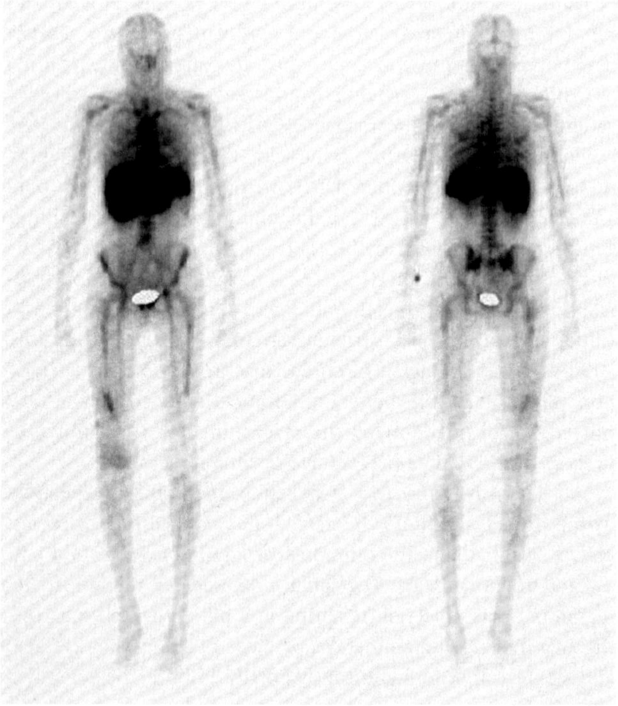

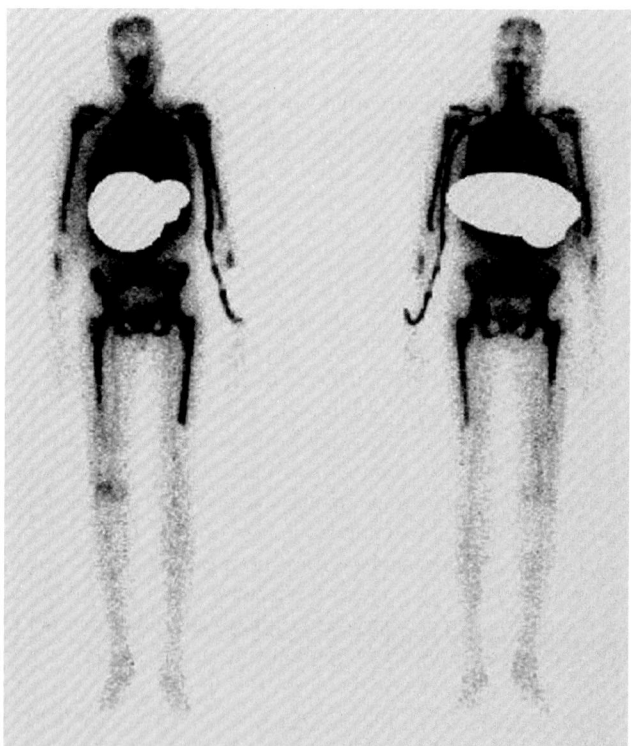

FIGURE 26-10 A marrow scan of the patient shown in Figure 26-8 demonstrating suppression of marrow in distal femur. Sulfur colloid scanning. Positive or "hot" scans indicate marrow activity and can be seen in inflammatory marrow conditions.

FIGURE 26-9 A white cell scan of the patient shown in Figure 26-8 demonstrating increased accumulation of tracer in the distal femur.

had a sensitivity of 96% and a specificity of 30%. When the colloid scan was added, the sensitivity decreased to 93% but the specificity increased to 98%. The addition of a regular red cell scan was not helpful.[109] In another study by Palestro et al.,[90] an indium-labeled white cell scan was compared with technetium sulfur colloid scans to differentiate infection from Charcot arthropathy. They found that white cell scans were positive in 4 of 20 cases, of which 3 were infected. In the 16 negative white cell scans, the marrow scan was also negative. However, in the four positive cases, the marrow scan was positive in two cases that were confirmed to be infected. They concluded that white cell scans can be positive in hematopoietically active bones, which can occur in the absence of infection, and that marrow scans should be used to confirm the diagnosis.

Classically, a combination of red cell bone scan and a labeled leukocyte scan has been used. Because standard bone scan agents and gallium are usually both positive at fracture sites; they have limited value in the detection of infection following a fracture. With no discernible uptake in reactive bone, indium-labeled WBC scans are superior in the detection of infection following fracture. In a prospective study of 20 patients with suspected osteomyelitis together with delayed union, Esterhai et al.[40] reported 100% accuracy of indium-labeled WBC scans. Seabold et al.[110] have shown that the use of indium-labeled WBC scans and bone scans, to differentiate between soft tissue infections, can be 97% specific for osteomyelitis. In chronic or recurrent osteomyelitis, bone scans by themselves are of less value because they show increased uptake for 2 years following the successful treatment and resolution of infection.[48] Although gallium scans have historically been shown to be successful in following the resolution of chronic osteomyelitis, indium-labeled WBC scans appear to be superior. Merkel et al.[76] compared indium-labeled WBC and gallium scans in a prospective study of 50 patients. They found that indium-labeled WBC scans had an accuracy of 83% compared with 57% for gallium scans in the detection of osteomyelitis. However, it is important to remember that all clinical data, including a detailed clinical history, a characterization of the host, appropriate laboratory studies, clinical examination, and radiographic studies, are important in determining the likelihood and extent of infection.

We have investigated the usefulness of these three scans read by a nuclear medicine specialist in a blinded fashion using receiver operating curves. We did not find any particular scan combinations that provided a reliable screening tool (sensitivity), but we did find that certain combinations provided good treatment decisions (specificity). Furthermore, the combination of white cell and marrow scans was equivalent to the combination of all three scans and better than the combination of red and white cell scans, which implies that the red cell scan may be of limited value. Whereas the sensitivities of all of these tests and combinations were low, the specificities remained at about 90% and the conclusion was that standard red cell scanning may not be necessary for the diagnosis of posttraumatic infection. Furthermore, we corroborated the findings of Segura et al.[112] and found that the red cell scan added little. Unfortunately, surgeons often continue to base their suspicion of infection on a simple

TABLE 26-4 Matrix of Scintigraphic Combinations and Potential for Infection

	Scan Results (Activity)			
Bone scan	Cold	Hot	Hot	Hot
White cell scan	Cold	Cold	Hot	Hot
Marrow scan	Cold	Cold	Cold	Hot
Infection present?	No	Unlikely	Probably	Maybe

bone scan. Table 26-4 illustrates the matrix as a guide to assist the interpretation of bone scan combinations.[22]

Other Scintigraphic Methods

In general, the accumulation of radiolabeled compounds and infectious conditions occurs via several routes. The labeled agents can bind to activate endothelium (anti-E-selectin). They can also enhance the influx of leukocytes or related byproducts (autologous leukocytes, antigranulocyte antibodies, or cytokines), and they can enhance glucose uptake by activated leukocytes (F-fluorodeoxyglucose [FDG]).[65] In addition, they bind directly to microorganisms (radiolabeled ciprofloxacin or antimicrobial peptides). Labeling of polyclonal immunoglobulin is a newer technique to investigate infection. It uses antigranulocyte antibodies, radiolabeled nonspecific human IgG, interleukins, and antimicrobial peptides.[9] The nonspecific polyclonal IgG prepared from human serum gamma globulin can be labeled with various agents, including indium, gallium, or technetium, and can be used for the detection of osteomyelitis.[9,95,102] Unlike labeled leukocyte scans, the IgG agent is easily prepared with short blood half lives of about 24 hours. The primary uptake occurs in the liver with less bone marrow uptake.[75] Indium IgG scintigraphy is useful for the detection of musculoskeletal infection in patients in whom sterile inflammatory events stimulate infectious processes.[79] However, despite its usefulness, this modality has not yet found its way into common clinical practice.

PET with 18F-FDG has been shown to delineate various infective and inflammatory disorders with a high sensitivity. The FDG–PET scan enables noninvasive detection and demonstration of the extent of chronic osteomyelitis with 97% accuracy.[32] PET scanning is especially accurate in the central skeleton within active bone marrow.[31] Although not yet in widespread use, it may well prove to be the single most useful test in specifically diagnosing bone infection. In one study, the overall accuracy of FDG–PET in evaluating infection involving orthopedic hardware was 96.2% for hip prostheses, 81% for knee prostheses, and 100% in 15 additional patients with other orthopedic implants. In patients with chronic osteomyelitis, the accuracy is 91%.[17] FDG–PET scanning appears to be a sensitive and specific method for the detection of infective foci because of metallic implants, which makes it useful in patients with trauma. Sensitivity, specificity, and accuracy were 100%, 93.3%, and 97%, respectively, for all PET data. The figures were 100%, 100%, and 100% for the central skeleton and 100%, 87.5%, and 95%, respectively, for the peripheral skeleton.[107] PET scanning may soon become the preferred diagnostic modality for the diagnosing and staging of skeletal infections.

Magnetic Resonance Imaging

MRI continues to play an important role in the evaluation of musculoskeletal infection.[78,98,114] The sensitivity and specificity of MRI scans for osteomyelitis ranges from 60% to 100% and from 50% to 90%, respectively. MRI has the spatial resolution necessary to accurately evaluate the extent of infection in preparation for surgical treatment and particularly to localize abscess cavities. T1- and T2-weighted imaging is usually sufficient; fat suppression and short tau inversion recovery (STIR) sequences may be added to improve the imaging of bone marrow and soft tissue abnormalities. MRI also has the ability to differentiate between infected bone and involved adjacent soft tissue structures. Images can be acquired in any orientation and there is no radiation exposure. Occasionally, a sinus tract can be identified (Fig. 26-11). Gadolinium enhancement should be obtained in the postoperative population to better differentiate postsurgical artifact from infection-related bone marrow edema patterns. Gadolinium may differentiate abscess formation from diffuse inflammatory changes and noninfectious fluid collections.

Active osteomyelitis characteristically displays a decreased signal in T1-weighted images and appears bright in T2-weighted images. The process presents the replacement of marrow fat with water from edema, exudates, hyperemia, and ischemia. However, the MRI signal characteristics that reflect osteomyelitis are intrinsically nonspecific, and tumors and fractures can also increase the marrow water content. In patients without prior complications, MRI has been found to be sensitive, but not specific, for osteomyelitis. When a fracture or prior surgery is evident, MRI is less specific in the diagnosis of infection. Furthermore, in the presence of metallic implants, artifacts make it difficult to comment on areas of interest that are near the implant. Certain external fixators are not compatible with MRI

and thus will preclude its use. We have found that the best use of MRI is helping to determine the extent of the infection for preoperative planning. Our experience has been that using MRI to plan the degree of bone resection or debridement is helpful, but that MRI may lead to an overestimation of the extent of the infection because of the detection of adjacent edema.

Computed Tomography

Computed tomography (CT) has assumed a lesser role in the evaluation of osteomyelitis with the widespread use of MRI.[31] However, CT remains unsurpassed in the imaging of cortical bone. It is especially useful in delineating the cortical details in chronic osteomyelitis, such as sequestra and foreign bodies.[115] CT is also useful in evaluating the adequacy of cortical debridement in the staged treatment of chronic osteomyelitis. Thus, it can help differentiate between type III and type IV infections. With modern equipment, CT scanning around fracture implants has improved and it can help evaluate both bone pathology and the extent of bone union. CT is also valuable in the treatment of extensive osteomyelitis in that it can determine the extent of bony involvement. In chronic cases, with some remodeling of both host and pathologic bone, it can often differentiate and identify sequestra or sclerosed diseased bone. It may often demonstrate useful pathologic findings (Fig. 26-12).

Cultures and Biopsy

Identification of an organism and determination of antibiotic resistance patterns are crucial to a successful outcome in the management of osteomyelitis. With regard to open fractures, the issue of culturing the predebridement or postdebridement tissue bed is often discussed among surgeons and infectious disease specialists. In civilian wounds, gram-positive bacteria usually predominate at the time of injury, but frequently change to gram-negative bacteria, which are often the cause of late infections. In one study, 119 of 225 open fractures had positive wound cultures with only 8% of predebridement cultures

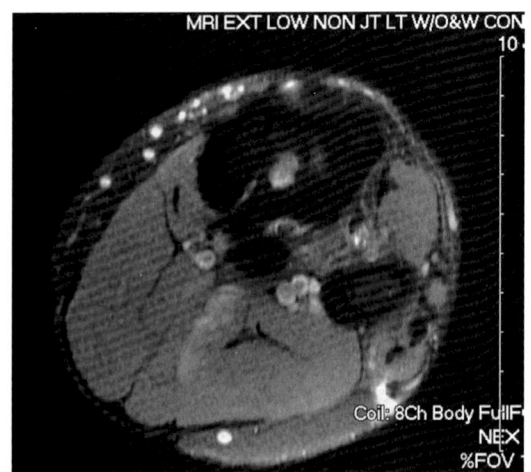
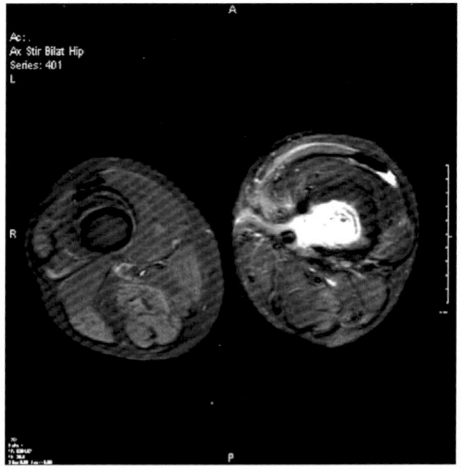

FIGURE 26-11 Magnetic resonance images of an infected tibia. In **(A)** the sinus tract can be seen leading to a central sequestrum (white area in the intramedullary canal). In **(B)** there is contrast entering into a bone abscess.

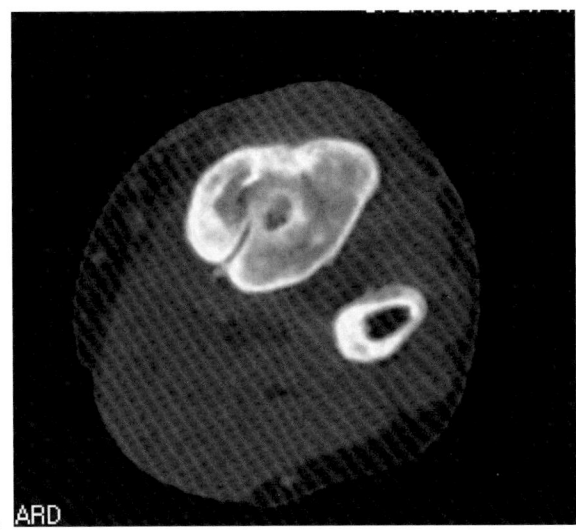
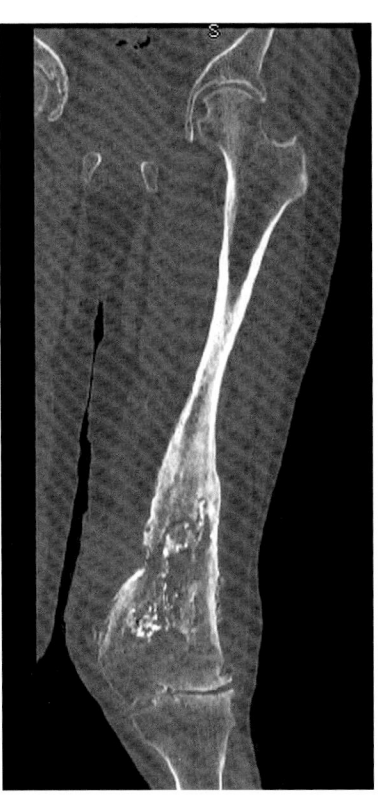

FIGURE 26-12 **A:** Computed tomography images of the sinus shown in Figure 26-11A. There is evidence of cortical changes suggestive of a sequestrum. In **(B)** there is clear evidence of a sequestrum which is avascular and infected bone that has not undergone resorption and remains a surface for colonized bacteria to proliferate. Systemic and even local antibiotics would not be sufficient to eradicate infection at this stage.

correctly identifying the infecting organism, whereas 7% of those with negative predebridement cultures also developed infection. In only 22% did the postdebridement cultures correlated with the ultimate infecting organism. These data are clinically relevant because treating the wrong bacteria can promote overgrowth of the true infecting bacteria or add to the development of resistant organisms. In recent war experience, military surgeons have noted different bacteria flora causing infection, but the same principles still apply to their treatment.[14,64,84,122] Although cultures of the sinus tract can be helpful, they should not be the sole guide for antibiotic treatment.[40] A study by Moussa et al.[82] found that 88.7% of sinus tract isolates were identical to operative specimens in 55 patients with chronic bone infection. However, other researchers have reported a concordance rate of between 25% and 45%.[66] The ability to obtain true deep cultures of the sinus improves concordance, but it is still not helpful. One study concluded that nonbone specimens had a worse concordance than bone specimens and were associated with 52% false negatives and 36% false positives. It is important to recognize that not only the superficial cultures of sinus tracts, open wounds, and fractures are unhelpful but also an error in bacterial identification may lead to inappropriate antibiotic selection and ultimately compromise patient outcome. Bone biopsy remains the preferred diagnostic procedure in chronic osteomyelitis. Multiple specimens should be obtained if possible, not only to minimize sampling error but also to increase specificity and sensitivity. Histologic and microbiologic evaluation of percutaneous biopsy samples should be combined in cases of suspected osteomyelitis. The sensitivity of culture in the diagnosis of osteomyelitis can be improved from 42% to 84% by the addition of histologic evaluation.

Molecular Diagnostics

Identification procedures based on molecular analysis and RNA or DNA typing are currently in development to facilitate diagnosis in osteomyelitis. These techniques offer a precise method of organism identification in cases in which standard techniques do not identify a pathogen despite the clinical presence of infection. This scenario is not uncommon in patients who have been treated with antibiotics shortly before sample collection. These methods target specific macromolecules unique to the infecting pathogens that are absent in the host cells.[38,119] They have the potential to provide rapid results with high accuracy.[57] The most commonly used method for the diagnosis of orthopedic infections is the polymerase chain reaction (PCR).[57] This has been used to identify microremnants of bacteria by identifying their nuclear contents. Sequences within bacterial 16S ribosomal RNA have served as targets for amplification and detection.[57] Unfortunately, PCR cannot easily delineate between nuclear materials from living or dead bacteria. This increases the likelihood of false-positive studies. Further investigations are required before these techniques can be widely used, as currently they lack sufficient sensitivity and specificity. However, their use remains promising. There have been recent reports of real-time testing that also appear more reliable and rapid, which could be very useful when deciding whether there is ongoing infection before undertaking a procedure requiring the implantation of orthopedic hardware.[116]

A new screening technique for methicillin-resistant *Staphylococcus aureus* (MRSA), recently evaluated at an urban trauma center, directly examines bacterial DNA. It identifies the organisms, as well as their antibiotic sensitivities, with a multiplex polymerase chain reaction. Diatherix Laboratories (Huntsville, AL) provides a screening system that not only might avoid infection complications in trauma patients but also provide documentation that infections during the hospital stay were because of prehospital MRSA colonization. A review of 332 patients showed a significant reduction of clinically documented MRSA infections, from 2.7% to 0.3% ($p < 0.05$), if their protocol was applied. In addition, the results from the polymerase chain reaction were available an average of 1.5 days before the final culture data. A much higher rate of MRSA colonization was screened on admission than has previously been reported. This may be because of a higher rate of colonization, as MRSA becomes more prevalent in the community or it may be because of more accurate detection of MRSA by polymerase chain reaction. Implementation of an MRSA screening, surveillance, and control policy may be one way of reducing the MRSA infection rate in trauma patients.[42]

MANAGEMENT AND TREATMENT

In orthopedic surgery and particularly in the treatment of fractures, postoperative infection is an unfortunate reality. The important questions to be posed are "Is there an infection?" and then "What do I do now?" The challenge is the difficulty in being certain whether an infection exists because we do not have an absolutely reliable method of determining the necessary elements of true postoperative or posttraumatic infection. As previously discussed, the establishment of colonization followed by an opportunistic bacteria, in a compromised host or environment, is necessary to allow an infection to occur. Furthermore, the accuracy and reliability of available diagnostic tests are not 100% and therefore, experience and clinical judgment are vital and could be considered more important than the tests that are currently available.

As has already been noted, treatment must not only follow basic principles but also must be tailored to the reality of the individual clinical scenario. It would be naive to assume that an inflamed and draining postoperative wound in a polytraumatized patient (B systemic) with significant fracture treatment (B local) that responds to a short course of antibiotics has no chance of recurrence. In such a case, sufficient treatment might have been provided so the balance would tip to favor the host defense mechanism. However, what probably occurred was that the threshold level for infection was exceeded and the body manifested a response in the form of inflammation and drainage. With the use of antibiotic treatment, the bacterial counts were reduced so that the host was able to take over and sequester the infection effectively. Thus, an initial positive response to antibiotic therapy does not necessarily mean that the infection was eradicated. It simply means that it was suppressed and possibly sequestered. Using an oncologic analogy, the infection may have been forced into remission, possibly for an indefinite period, but many of these patients present later with signs of infection in the

same limb. Unfortunately, by this time the patient may be older, in poorer health, and less able or willing to tolerate an aggressive ablative procedure, thus lowering the potential for cure. In the long run, early suppression may cause the patient more physical and psychological harm than early aggressive measures to achieve complete eradication. On the other hand, an overaggressive approach may require extensive reconstructive efforts that lead to other problems. Thus, in a world seeking clear black and white answers, osteomyelitis usually presents as a shade of gray!

The principles of osteomyelitis management rely on a multidisciplinary approach that begins with diagnosis and optimization in the form of medicine and radiology and then combines debridement, soft tissue coverage, antimicrobial therapy using orthopedic surgery, microvascular surgery, and infectious disease. This gives the best chance of a cure.[37,70] Initially, the infection needs to be diagnosed and the host optimized. This involves treating any comorbidities and optimizing the physiologic condition of the host. Interventions involving nutrition, the use of nicotine, diabetes, vascular disease, and improvement of tissue oxygenation will increase the chances of successful treatment. Secondly, the osteomyelitis needs to be classified and staged. It is then important to identify the organism to determine appropriate antimicrobial treatment. This can be done independently with a bone biopsy or deep culture or, more commonly, it is done at the time of surgery. Identification will also give an idea of the potential virulence of the causative organism, which may influence decisions regarding treatment. We recommend that if the risk of sepsis or amputation is low, then a period of time off all antibiotics may improve bacterial identification. This may be more important in long-standing cases where the usual organisms may have been replaced by other, more exotic species.

Once the extent of the disease, the nature of the host, and the infecting organism are understood, determination should be made regarding one of several general treatment algorithms. Available treatment options include attempted ablation and cure of the infection, or, in selective cases such as C hosts who are not suitable for surgery, some type of suppressive treatment may be undertaken. Attempted ablation and complete cure have numerous issues and decision-making steps and will often require the oncologic equivalent of a wide resection with clean margins. Although a surgically clean bed with extensive resection is desirable, all efforts should be made to maintain skeletal axial stability where possible. Thus, retention of a well-vascularized, but affected, involucrum or a viable segment of bone adjacent to infection may be preferable to a segmental resection that would add a level of complexity to the treatment regime. If an adequate resection would result in an overextensive reconstruction that is unsuitable for the host's function or desire, an amputation is the best option and it should not be considered a failure. In some cases of life- or limb-threatening infection, debulking of the infection may be a suitable first step followed by chronic suppression. In these circumstances, identification of the infecting bacteria is required to allow the use of a specific antibiotic. Otherwise, broad-spectrum antibiotics are required.

We have embraced a collaborative approach with our infectious disease colleagues. Modern antimicrobials have become so numerous and complex that their expert involvement is likely to increase the chances of successful treatment. Increasingly, in many hospitals bone infection mandates an infectious disease consult because of the risk of inadvertently creating resistant pathogens, the efficacy of combined antibiotic protocols, patient safety issues, and the cost of new treatment regimens. However, it is still important that the orthopedist has an understanding of antimicrobial treatment because it is the orthopedist who will initiate the treatment before consulting his or her infectious disease colleagues. We also recommend that orthopedic surgeons recognize that not all infectious disease practices are evidence based and not all specialists have a specific interest and training in bone infections. Therefore, it is vital that the orthopedist initiates an open and collegial partnership with the infectious disease specialists in his or her community to work on behalf of the patient. Both the orthopedic surgeon and the infectious disease physicians should work together to employ a consistent strategy of surgical and chemotherapeutic treatment predicated on the best evidence and logic available. Ziran et al.[131] showed that a dedicated team approach can enhance the outcomes of treatment, providing higher cure and successful suppression rates. The subsequent sections in this chapter will briefly review both systemic and local antimicrobial agents as well as discuss the techniques and implants used during treatment. Specific scenarios and algorithms will then be reviewed.

Antimicrobial Therapy

Prophylaxis

On the basis that prevention is always better than cure, prophylactic antibiotics have an important role in the treatment of closed fractures. The prophylactic use of appropriate antibiotics for closed fractures and elective cases will reduce the incidence of postoperative osteomyelitis. Antibiotic administration is not a substitute for proper aseptic technique, but it is a validated additional measure to reduce postoperative infection.

The use of prophylactic antibiotics was demonstrated in a Dutch trauma trial that found, in 2,195 cases of closed fracture surgery, a single preoperative dose of ceftriaxone resulted in an infection rate of 3.6% in comparison to a placebo group infection rate of 8.3% ($p < 0.001$).[12] Furthermore, the trial also found that there was a lower incidence of nosocomial urinary tract and respiratory tract infections in the first 30 postoperative days (2.3% vs. 10.2%, $p < 0.001$). In another retrospective study of 2,847 surgical cases, the timing of antibiotic administration was also found to be an important factor. If the antibiotics were given more than 2 hours before or 3 hours after the incision, there was a six-fold increase in the rate of surgical site infection.[21] The current recommendation is that antibiotics should be administered 30 to 60 minutes before the incision is made, except when using vancomycin, where a longer delay permits appropriate infusion rates.[12,47,108] For routine uncomplicated closed fracture surgery, prophylaxis should not be administered for greater than 24 hours, and many surgeons believe that only a single dose is necessary. Gillespie and Walenkamp performed a meta-analysis of 8,307 patients undergoing surgical treatment of hip and long bone fractures, to determine whether antibiotic prophylaxis reduced the incidence of wound infection. A total of 22 studies were analyzed. Single doses of antibiotic prophylaxis were found to significantly reduce the incidence of wound infection (relative risk, 0.4; 95% confidence interval, 0.24 to 0.67).[47] Controversy exists regarding the appropriate prophylaxis for orthopedic surgical patients in hospitals with high rates of MRSA. Traditional first-generation cephalosporins may not provide adequate coverage, and given the increasing prevalence of MRSA infections in Europe and North America, further studies are needed to understand the risk–benefit ratio of using routine vancomycin as a prophylaxis agent. The disadvantages of potential nephrotoxicity and an increase in the emergence of vancomycin-resistant *S. aureus* (VRSA) must be weighed against the risk of increased postoperative infection rates. Currently, neither vancomycin nor clindamycin is routinely used except in cases of known PCN or cephalosporin allergy. All institutions should have an infection control committee, including infectious disease specialists, to determine the bacterial spectrum of the institution. An "antibiogram" can then be provided to help determine the best agents to use for prophylactic and therapeutic treatments. In our institution the infection disease specialists recommend the use of vancomycin and rocephin based on our nosocomial bacterial flora. In cases of reported PCN allergy, patients can be given a small test dose of cephalosporin after anesthesia induction to determine if there is any cross-reactivity.

Open Fractures

Historically, the teaching in open fractures has been to use a first-generation cephalosporin followed by the addition of an aminoglycoside for more contaminated wounds using supplementary PCN if there is any soil contamination. It is perhaps surprising to realize that this recommendation is more than 30 years old and is not supported by any newer, high-level evidence-based studies. This practice was primarily an empirical and theoretical recommendation. Since the incidence of infection is so low that any treatment will also have a small statistical effect size, it may not be possible to undertake a sufficiently powered study to adequately test the success of this antibiotic regimen. A number of studies have examined the role of antibiotics, but the most recent review by the Surgical Infection Society found that current standard antibiotic prophylaxis is based on very limited data.[55]

Another question that remains unanswered concerns the true requirement for aminoglycosides at the time of injury. Given that the initial organism is often a *Staphylococcus* but that the eventual infective organism is a resistant gram-negative organism, it begs the question of whether early aminoglycoside administration, which is often given in adequate doses, will promote the development of a resistant organism. In two studies, a cephalosporin alone performed as well as the combination of a cephalosporin and PCN or the combination of a cephalosporin and an aminoglycoside.[92] Another study examining the use of broad-spectrum antibiotics proposed that their use could result in the development of resistant bacteria.

Analysis of the US military experience with high-energy open fractures has shown that there is sufficient level I data to support the use of a cephalosporin but that the use of amino-glycosides, even for grade III open fractures, may be deleterious. These recommendations are based on timely and adequate surgical debridement. If there is a delay to treatment whereby bacterial colonization may have begun and matured or if the wound is such that gram-negative bacteria or anaerobic conditions exist, then supplementation with appropriate antibiotics, in addition to a more aggressive initial debridement, may be useful. Because there is little scientific evidence about the subject, much current surgical practice is anecdotal. The authors believe that the initial debridement is the most important principle of open fracture treatment as well as in the management of acute or chronic infection. Minimalist approaches to the removal of devitalized tissue, in the hopes of preventing extensive later reconstructive surgery, are usually doomed to failure. By the surgeon taking less initially, the patient is often condemned to lose more later because of ongoing infection and diffuse tissue destruction.

The duration of antibiotic use in open fractures has also been poorly studied, but the current recommendation is to use antibiotics for 1 to 3 days following wound closure or coverage with ongoing treatment based on a reassessment of the injury zone. However, the current practice of continuing the use of antibiotics until definitive wound closure has occurred has no scientific basis. In fact, the literature suggests that the long duration of empirical or prophylactic antibiotic use may breed resistant organisms. The current recommendation is to use antibiotics for an extended period only if this is supported by the condition of the wound which will show signs of infection.[83] The author's institutions summarized the available literature and concluded that open fractures should be treated with antibiotics for 24 hours following definitive wound closure. These are also the recommendations being developed in new guidelines by the U.S. Centers for Disease Control and Prevention (CDC). Recently, a journal supplement focusing on military injuries has examined and summarized the current thinking on extremity infection in war time injury.[83,84] A recent study evaluated the timing of wound closure based on cultures. Antibiotics were continued based on ongoing positive cultures and wounds were only closed after negative culture results. Antibiotics were resumed, based on clinical evaluation, if cultures were positive after wound closure.

Established Infection

As the duration of antibiotic administration for chronic infections may be prolonged the antibiotics that are used to treat the infection should ideally be nontoxic, convenient to administer, affordable and based on the in vitro susceptibilities of the organisms. All antibiotics have potential adverse effects and complications and an infection disease specialist should be involved in the treatment regime. Table 26-5 lists treatment regimes for a number of different organisms that commonly cause osteomyelitis. Any antibiotic that is used should have reliable bone penetration, and the serum and bone concentrations for a number of antibiotics are shown in Table 26-6. There is no general consensus about the duration of antibiotic administration for osteomyelitis with some researchers suggesting 2 weeks and others considerably longer. Short-term therapy may be used in other-

wise healthy patients who have healthy tissue and have had a total debridement. Longer-term therapy will usually be used in patients with virulent or long-standing infections in whom the initial debridement will be followed at a later date by staged reconstruction. It is also used if there are retained implants.

If the patient requires grafting or reconstruction after a successful debridement, antibiotics will often be administered for 6 to 8 weeks followed by a period of antibiotics with monitoring of the CRP and ESR. A rebiopsy may also be undertaken. If there are no ongoing indicators of infection, reconstruction can usually be performed without additional long-term antibiotic treatment. There are a number of factors which should be considered when considering long-term antibiotics. There are reports of immunosuppression, allergic reaction, poor tolerance, poor compliance, and financial hardship that must also be considered when deciding on long-term antibiotic administration. To increase patient compliance the antibiotics that are used should be the least toxic and least expensive and preferably require administration once or twice daily. The oral antibiotics with excellent bioavailability are listed in Table 26-7. These antibiotics may be substituted for intravenous agents whenever possible, provided that the organism is susceptible and the bone penetration is adequate.

Because of increased incidences of vancomycin-resistant *Enterococcus,* especially in intensive care units, and VRSA, vancomycin should be used only if there is a high institutional incidence of MRSA or methicillin-resistant *Staphylococcus epidermidis* (MRSE). A single dose of vancomycin administered before surgery and followed by two or three doses postoperatively should provide adequate perioperative prophylaxis in high-risk cases. Vancomycin should only be used with type I hypersensitivity to cephalosporins that includes patients with urticaria, laryngeal edema, and bronchospasm, with or without cardiovascular shock. Clindamycin is considered the substitute of choice when cephalosporins are contraindicated.

There are also little data with regard to the use and duration of antibiotics in established infection. The most common practice is to begin with a 2- to 6-week course of a species-specific, bioavailable agent.[63] Such an agent may be used until adequate revascularization occurs. With the advent of many new and expensive oral agents, it may be possible to reduce the morbidity associated with intravenous use with an early step-down program converting to an oral agent. Obviously, this regimen may be less successful with resistant organisms. Thus, to date there have been few recommendations for the duration of antibiotics in established osteomyelitis.

A common clinical scenario is the partially treated infection. Patients who may have been suppressed but incompletely treated may present with an acutely inflamed, limb-threatening condition. Our approach has been to continue the use of antibiotics during the diagnostic and staging period when the necessary tests are undertaken and the host is optimized. However, we believe that as long as there are no signs of impending sepsis or limb loss, it is worthwhile stopping antibiotic treatment 1 to 2 weeks before surgical intervention so that more precise and reliable bacterial identification is possible. Begin an empirical course of antibiotics intraoperatively after all the cultures have been taken and continue until the culture results are available.

TABLE 26-5 Common Bacteria-Specific Antibiotic Regimens

Organism	First-Line Antibiotic(s)	Alternative Antibiotic(s)
Staphylococcus aureus or coagulase-negative staphylococci (methicillin-sensitive), MSSA	Oxacillin 2 g IV q6h Clindamycin 600 mg IV q8h	First-generation cephalosporin, vancomycin, daptomycin, tigecycline
S. aureus or coagulase-negative staphylococci (methicillin-resistant), MRSA	Vancomycin 1 g IV q12h ± Rifampin 300 mg PO BID	Linezolid, trimethoprim/sulfamethoxazole or minocycline + rifampin, daptomycin, tigecycline
Penicillin-sensitive *Streptococcus pneumoniae,* varied streptococci (groups A and B hemolytic organisms)	Penicillin G, 4 million units IV q6h Ceftriaxone 2 g IV QD Cefazolin 1 g IV q8h	Clindamycin, erythromycin, vancomycin
Intermediate penicillin-resistant *S. pneumoniae*	Ceftriaxone 2 g IV q24h	Erythromycin, clindamycin, or fluoroquinolone
Penicillin-resistant *S. pneumoniae*	Vancomycin 1 g IV q12h	Fluoroquinolone
Enterococcus spp.	Penicillin G, 4 million units IV q6h Ampicillin 2 g IV q6h + Gentamicin 3–5 mg/kg/day Vancomycin 1 g IV q12h	Ampicillin–sulbactam, linezolid, daptomycin, tigecycline + gentamicin
Pseudomonas spp., *Serratia* spp., or *Enterobacter* spp.	Cefepime 2 g IV q12h ± Fluoroquinolone (Table 26-7) Meropenem 1 g IV q8h	Fluoroquinolone, ertapenem
Enteric gram-negative rods	Ceftriaxone 2 g IV q24h Fluoroquinolone (see later)	Third-generation cephalosporin
Anaerobes	Clindamycin 600 mg IV q8h Metronidazole 500 mg PO q4h	For gram-negative anaerobes: amoxicillin–clavulanate or metronidazole
Mixed aerobic and anaerobic organisms	Amoxicillin–clavulanate 3 g IV q6h	Ertapenem

Fluoroquinolones: ciprofloxacin 750 mg PO BID, levofloxacin 500 mg PO QD, moxifloxacin 400 mg PO QD.
Note that use of fluoroquinolones has been associated with altered bone healing in animal models and increased risk of tendon rupture in humans.
Note that many antibiotics may result in development of severe colitis.

In chronic cases, we will cover both gram-negative and MRSA and collaborate with our infectious disease colleagues regarding final antibiotic selection and management.

Irrigation Solutions

The original use of pulsatile irrigation was based on early studies of infections, which recommended that colonized bacteria are adherent to tissue and needed to be moved from the surface.

Although such mechanical cleansing may work, mature colonies of bacteria are not easily eradicated with this method. Furthermore, there is evidence that the velocity of the fluid stream may be deleterious to both bone and soft tissue cells.[3,8,13,53,113] So

TABLE 26-6 Serum and Bone Concentrations After Antibiotic Administration

Antibiotic	Serum	Bone	% Serum
Clindamycin (7 mg/kg)	2.1 ± 0.6	1.9 ± 1.9	98.3
Vancomycin (30 mg/kg)	36.4 ± 4.6	5.3 ± 0.8	14.5
Nafcillin (40 mg/kg)	21.8 ± 4.6	2.1 ± 0.3	9.6
Moxalactam (40 mg/kg)	65.2 ± 5.2	6.2 ± 0.7	9.5
Tobramycin (5 mg/kg)	14.3 ± 1.3	1.3 ± 0.1	9.1
Cefazolin (15 mg/kg)	7.2 ± 2.6	4.1 ± 0.7	6.1
Cefazolin (5 mg/kg)	45.6 ± 3.2	2.6 ± 0.2	5.7
Cephalothin (40 mg/kg)	34.8 ± 2.8	1.3 ± 0.2	3.7

TABLE 26-7 Selected Oral Antimicrobial Agents with Excellent Oral Bioavailability Commonly Used to Treat Osteomyelitis

	Antimicrobial Agents
Fluoroquinolones	Ciprofloxacin 750 mg q12h Levofloxacin 500 mg q12h Moxifloxacin 400 mg q12h
Mixed	Metronidazole 500 mg q8h Linezolid 600 mg q12h Rifampin 300 mg q12h (not to be used alone) Trimethoprim/sulfamethoxazole 1 DS QD Minocycline–doxycycline 100 mg q12h
Azoles (antifungal)	Fluconazole 400 mg q24h Itraconazole 200 mg q12h

while high-pressure flow has been shown to damage bone or push bacteria even deeper into the wound, low-pressure lavage appears to be adequate without having the tissue-damaging effects.[8,13,53]

Irrigation with saline alone has been shown in animal studies to reduce colony counts by about 50% in contaminated wounds.[7] However, conflicting studies have shown no beneficial effect of the use of saline.[15,23] In one study, tap water was compared with sterile saline irrigation and no difference was found in infection rates.[80] The effect of adding bacteriocidal agents to irrigation solutions to aid with both bacterial removal and destruction has also been studied in an adherent staphylococci model.[8] These studies have shown that although solutions such as Betadine and hydrogen peroxide are effective in eliminating bacteria, they are also toxic to osteoblasts. Also, the addition of antibiotics to irrigation solutions has had mixed results, and overall it appears to have little benefit but there is a significant increase in cost. Their use as an adjunct to irrigation solutions is questionable at best.[4,34,94] One study, using a goat model, found that the use of certain bacteriocidal agents in irrigating solutions resulted in a rebound bacterial count 24 to 48 hours after irrigation.[89] Another study used gentamicin placed into the wound bed together with a systemic cephalosporin in an animal model. They found significantly lower bacterial counts.[16] Our institution has been using clorpactin (WCS-90, USA Guardian Laboratories, Hauppauge, NY) solution in their irrigation for decades. It is typically used as a topical agent for complicated burn wounds and is similar to sodium hypochlorite. We currently use a combination of clorpactin and gentamicin in our irrigating solutions because it is inexpensive and has low morbidity together with reasonable supportive evidence of efficacy.

Given the minimal effects of antibiotics in irrigation fluids, detergent-type compounds or surfactant solutions have been recently investigated as a way of disrupting the hydrophobic or electrostatic forces that drive the initial stages of bacterial surface adhesion. A sequential surfactant–irrigation protocol was developed and shown to be effective in polymicrobial wounds associated with an established infection.[5,35,82] Detergents, or soaps, have been shown to be the only irrigation solutions that remove additional bacteria beyond the effect of mechanical irrigation alone.[8] Moreover, soap solutions have been found to have minimal effects on bone formation and osteoblast numbers in vitro.[7] The proposed mechanism of their effect is based on the formation of micelles that overcome the strength of the interaction between the organisms and the bone. Castile soap has recently been reported to be useful in this situation.[5,82]

Antibiotic Depot Devices and Techniques

The concept of local antibiotic therapy in the form of antibiotics impregnated in bone cement to reduce infected arthroplasties was introduced in the 1970s. As a result of the success of this work, interest developed in using antibiotic-impregnated bone cement as treatment for osteomyelitis. Keating et al.[60] reported a 4% infection rate in 53 open tibial fractures with tobramycin-impregnated beads. Ostermann et al.[88] reported a significant difference in infection rates with grade IIIB fractures treated

with aminoglycoside beads together with parenteral antibiotics compared with patients who only received parenteral antibiotics. They reported a 6.9% infection rate in 112 patients with combined therapy compared with a 40.7% infection rate in 27 patients who only had parenteral antibiotics. The use of antibiotic depots allows for high local concentrations of antibiotic with little systemic absorption. Antibiotic release is biphasic with most occurring during the first few days to weeks after implantation. However, elution of the antibiotic persists for several weeks. Occasionally, antibiotics can be recovered after several years, but because the elution is based on a diffusion gradient, only the outer 1 cm or so of large-volume depots will elute antibiotic. The core of such large-volume depots will often contain antibiotic but it will not be useful.[62,111]

The key issue of the polymethyl methacrylate (PMMA) antibiotic depot is the need for a heat-stable antibiotic agent because during the cement hardening process, the exothermic reaction can render heat-labile antibiotics ineffective. Some of the antibiotics that have been tried with PMMA include clindamycin, which elutes well but is not available as a pharmaceutical grade power. Fluoroquinolones have been reported to have suitable elution, but clinical reports of their success are lacking.[33] Erythromycin was used in some earlier studies, but a subsequent study showed inadequate elution of erythromycin from Palacos cement. Macrolides and azalides are unavailable, and tetracycline and polymyxin E (Colistin) fail to elute from the Palacos cement in clinically useful quantities. Another issue with PMMA depot systems is that they require removal. If they are left for a prolonged period, the PMMA spaces can become encased in scar and may be difficult to remove. After antibiotics have eluted from the outer surface of the cement mass, the surface is rendered unprotected and may provide a suitable surface for secondary colonization. When used acutely for open fractures or for a short period, removal is not generally problematic and may even be undertaken percutaneously. There are entire issues of *Clinical Orthopaedics and Related Research* (numbers 295 and 420) dedicated to the use of PMMA antibiotic depot methods to which the reader is referred for more in-depth information.[1,2] The authors' formulation for PMMA antibiotic-laden beads uses vancomycin and tobramycin. Although up to 4 g of vancomycin and 4.8 g of tobramycin can be mixed per 40-g bag of cement, the cement may become difficult to manage. Other PMMA formulations such as Cranioplast do not tolerate even small amounts of antibiotic powder. For routine use, we place between 1 and 2 g of vancomycin and 1.2 to 2.4 g of tobramycin per bag. Depending on the clinical situation, we have developed a method to create three forms of antibiotic beads. We first cut a length of 18-gauge steel wire and loop one end. As the bowl becomes doughy, we roll multiple cement balls of about 1 to 2 cm in diameter. The wire is then moistened with water and the bead is allowed to slide and drop on the wire. The adherent cement is cleaned off the wire to allow subsequent beads to slide down. After the beads are placed, they can be left to cure as balls or they may be checked into oblong sausage-shaped beads by rolling them like dough. Alternatively, they can be shaped into discs by simply pressing each bead flat on the wire. We prefer the use of discs because

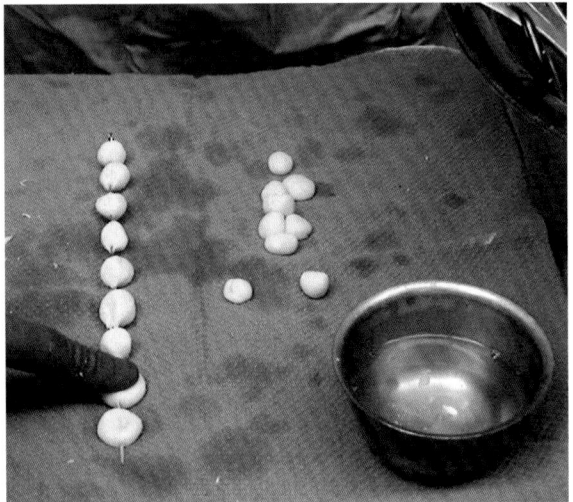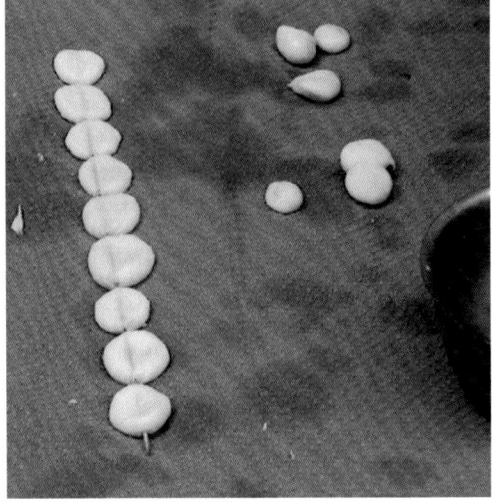

FIGURE 26-13 The manufacture of antibiotic bone cement beads and discs. **A:** Antibiotic balls placed on a stainless steel wire to form beads. One ball has been flattened to form a disc. **B:** The final appearance of antibiotic discs. They produce less local tissue pressure and ischemia than antibiotic balls.

they fit better between tissue planes and are less likely to have local compressive effects on the tissues (Fig. 26-13).

Recently, intramedullary antibiotic cement rods have been used. These are fashioned by using a large 36 French thoracotomy tube and placing an 18- to 20-gauge wire inside. After the tube has been cut to discard the ventholes, bone wax or a Kelly clamp can be used to obstruct the thin end. The antibiotic–cement mixture is then injected into the tube in a liquid state. Once the cement cures, the thoracostomy tube is cut off with a scalpel and the rod can then be used. It is important to ensure that both canal diameter and rod length have been measured (Fig. 26-14).

Most of the antibiotic cement used in the United States has been off-label use by the surgeon, and despite encouraging results from several studies, their approval by the U.S. Food and Drug Administration has been discouragingly slow. There are a number of commercial antibiotic-impregnated PMMA cements becoming available in the United States, and of course they have been available for some time in other parts of the world. We believe that the use of an aminoglycoside in antibiotic-impregnated cement does not provide the versatility that we need because vancomycin should be considered when there is a chance of resistant staphylococcal organisms. Thus, commercially produced antibiotic-laden cement may best be suited as prophylaxis during cemented arthroplasty.

There are also newer types of material available for local delivery of antibiotics that are resorbable and do not require removal. Surgical grade calcium sulfate has been used recently, and its use is reported in both open fractures and infections.[74] Although calcium sulfate products have been promoted as a bone graft substitute, there are little data in human fractures and infections demonstrating the efficacy of this dual function of depot and graft. Calcium sulfates and carbonate will absorb or dissolve independently of bone formation, whereas calcium phosphates tend to be replaced very slowly with bone. Furthermore, large volumes of calcium sulfate can cause an osmotic effect that results in fluid accumulation and the potential for

seroma formation and wound drainage. When mixed with fluid and blood, the calcium drainage looks like bloody pus and may prompt extra surgical treatments resulting in unacceptable complication rates.[11,132] In one study, the use of a calcium

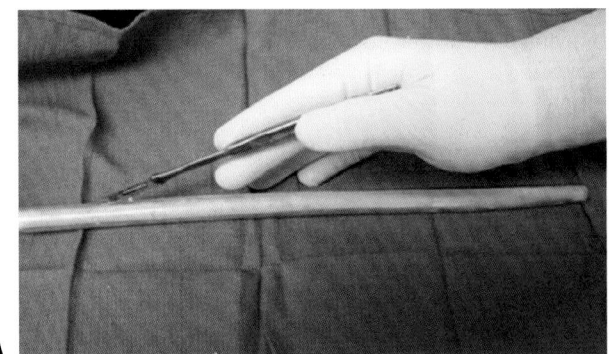

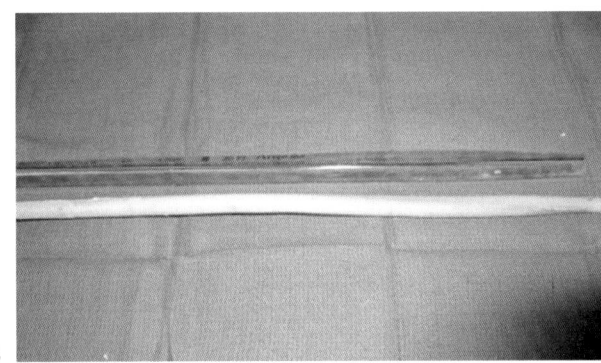

FIGURE 26-14 The manufacture of an antibiotic nail. Several methods have been advocated. **A:** In this example a stainless steel wire is placed within a thoracotomy tube and the tube is filled with antibiotic impregnated cement. It is then cut to allow removal of the rod. **B:** This shows the antibiotic-impregnated rod. An alternative is to use a threaded bone transport rod. This will enhance strength but may reduce the size and strength of the cement mantle.

sulfate-demineralized bone matrix (DBM) mixture (Allomatrix; Wright Medical, Memphis, TN) resulted in an unacceptably high rate of drainage, infection, and failure. We have heard of numerous anecdotal reports concerning the drainage problem of calcium sulfate and we do not recommend its use as a bone graft substitute. However, we have found it useful as an antibiotic depot. To minimize the drainage problem, we do not recommend placing a large amount of calcium sulfate beads into a cavity, but if this is unavoidable, a multiple-level watertight closure is essential. We have not found any problems with drainage when the beads are interspersed in small spaces and tissue planes. Another feature to note is that the addition of tobramycin to calcium sulfate greatly prolongs the setting time, which may be 30 to 45 minutes. Vancomycin greatly shortens the setting time, which may be as fast as 2 minutes, and for this reason the agent may be impractical. We routinely use both vancomycin and tobramycin for high-risk infections and find that the effect of tobramycin dominates the settling profile. Thus, despite a seemingly novel concept and marketing claims, such products should be used with caution and experience.

The use of impregnated hydroxyapatite ceramic beads may simulate a bone graft by serving as an osteoconductive matrix, but they are resorbed slowly, and after elution may behave as a foreign body with potential reinfection as may occur with PMMA beads. Gentamicin-impregnated polylactide–polyglycolide copolymer implants are biodegradable and may not need removal once they have been implanted. However, there is little clinical experience, and it is possible that they elicit an inflammatory response that may mimic acute infection.

Debridement Techniques

If surgical treatment is chosen, the hallmark of treatment is debridement. All nonviable and inert structures should be debrided to remove infected material and debris without destabilizing the bony structure. The goal is to convert a necrotic, hypoxic, infected wound to a viable wound. The critical judgment for the surgeon occurs when there is a potentially infected bone, which might be partially vascularized, which is needed to maintain the structural stability of the bone. Sinus tracts that are present for longer than 1 year should be excised and sent for pathologic examination to rule out an occult carcinoma.[104] Soft tissue retraction should be minimal and flaps should not be created. There is a balance between leaving behind infection, which may result in recurrence, and resection and subsequent destabilization, which might necessitate extensive surgical reconstruction with its associated risks. The risk–benefit ratio must be evaluated in each case and should form the basis of thorough informed consent.

Meticulous debridement is one of the most important initial steps in the treatment of infected bone and soft tissue. The limits of debridement have classically been determined by the "paprika sign," which is characterized by punctuate cortical or cancellous bleeding (Fig. 26-15). Efforts should be made to limit any periosteal stripping that may further devitalize the bone. Reactive new bone surrounding an area of chronic inflammation is living and sometimes does not require debridement.[18] Any sequestrated dead bone needs to be identified and removed,

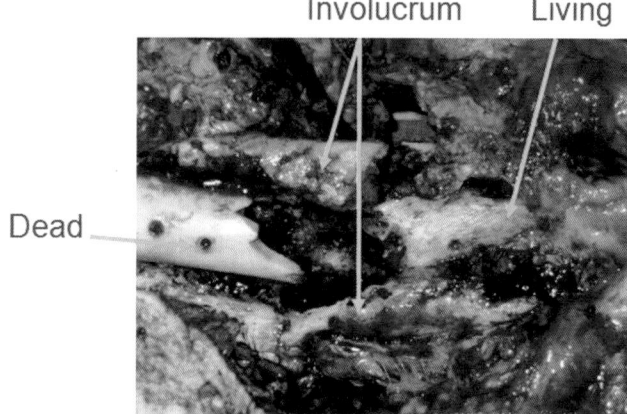

FIGURE 26-15 The appearance of bone at debridement. Note that the living bone has a pinkish hue and a petechial appearance indicating vascularity. The surrounding bone is involucrum and is also vascular. Resection of the involucrum should be at the judgment of the surgeon. The dead bone is clearly avascular and requires resection.

whereas live bone may be preserved. Rapid debridement can be achieved with a high-speed burr but used with continuous irrigation to limit thermal necrosis. Laser Doppler flowmetry may facilitate accurate assessment of the microvascular status of bone, thereby identifying it for removal.[36] However, we have found this technique to have little benefit compared with visual inspection. Laser Doppler flowmetry is the only nondestructive in vivo method of blood flow determination that provides instantaneous determination of perfusion.

When the medullary canal is infected, intramedullary reaming is an effective method of debridement that preserves cortical stability.[24] In general, one should overream the medullary canal by 2 mm. Excessive reaming may cause cortical necrosis and exacerbate infection by increasing the surface area of dead bone. Lavage can be performed from the reaming entry portal with the canal irrigator tips used in arthroplasty, with egress being provided through a vent or previous locking screw holes (Fig. 26-16). Dull reamers and the generation of heat should be avoided to prevent further cortical necrosis.

The recent use of the reamer–irrigator–aspirator (RIA) system[72,97] provides high-speed reaming debridement combined with continuous irrigation and aspiration of the medullary contents. Numerous centers have advocated its use in the debridement of infected long bones. We routinely use this technique in intramedullary canal debridement. Its advantages include vigorous cleaning of the canal and a decrease in embolization of marrow contents, and potentially bacteria, into the systemic circulation. Disadvantages include increased cost and a learning curve regarding matching the size of the reamer to the canal size. Choosing too small a reamer provides inadequate debridement and too large may cause a shaft fracture. Sizing should be performed preoperatively with digital radiography and then rechecked intraoperatively with fluoroscopy and an intraoperative measuring guide.

Intramedullary reaming of the medullary canal as a debridement technique has shown favorable results in the treatment

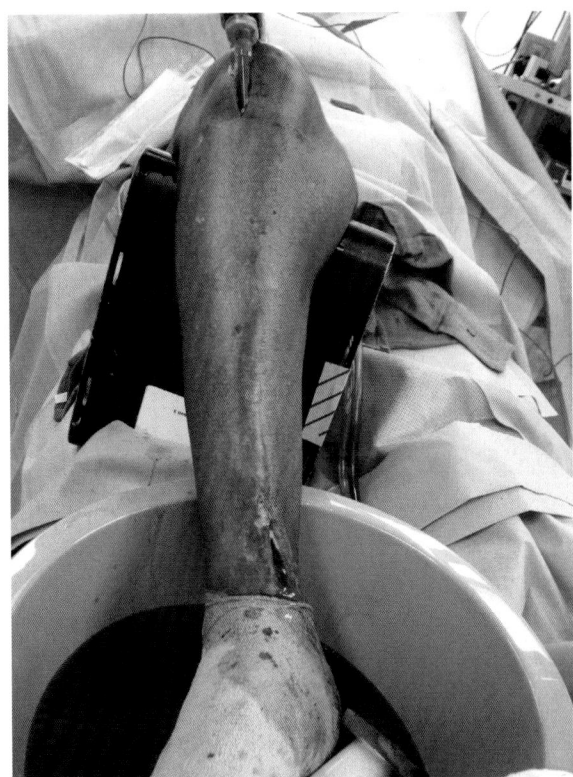

FIGURE 26-16 Intraoperative photograph of medullary canal lavage after removal of an intramedullary rod and the use of a medullary canal irrigator. The distal screw holes are connected and opened to create an efflux portal.

of medullary osteomyelitis. In a cohort of 32 patients who had had an average of 3.2 surgical operations for osteomyelitis, Pape et al.[91] found that reaming of the medullary canal was successful in that 84% of patients were able to return to their previous profession and 97% were pain-free. Evidence for the treatment of an infected intramedullary nail has been largely derived from observational data. Pommer et al.[96] found that reaming of an infected intramedullary canal resulted in eradication of infection in all patients when the infection occurred after primary intramedullary nailing compared with 62% of those with multiple operations before reaming and nailing. Ochsner et al. treated 25 patients with posttraumatic osteomyelitis, of whom 22, who were treated with intramedullary reaming, were followed for at least 6 months. Twenty-one of the twenty-two patients were free of any recurrent infection after an average period of 26 months. In a more recent study Ochsner et al. documented 40 patients with chronic osteomyelitis who were treated with intramedullary reaming. Only four patients had a recurrent infection.[87] If the medullary infection is too proximal or distal for a tight reamer fit, saucerization must be undertaken with the trough being created to debride the canal directly. Biomechanically, the most desirable shape for the trough is an oval, with this shape resulting in minimal diminution of the bone's torsional strength. If segmental resection is undertaken or there is more than 30% loss of circumferential cortical contact, stabilization is required.

Considerations in the Geriatric Patient

The geriatric patient population is not only increasing because of the increased birth rate after World War II, but also because advances in healthcare have resulted in increased longevity. Unfortunately, like most physical processes and materials, wear and tear and aging have irreversible consequences that can only mitigated or delayed. Thus the older patient will experience deterioration in bodily function that affects orthopedic treatment, whether it is for acute trauma, reconstruction, or infection.

The treatment principles are the same as for any age group, namely diagnosis, staging, and attempted eradication. In the geriatric population, several additional considerations must be taken into account. First is their physiologic ability to tolerate the extent of reconstruction that is necessary. Most of the elderly will, by definition, be B hosts, and many will be considered C hosts because of multiple comorbidities. Thus, a stage IV, B-systemic/local osteomyelitis of the distal tibia requiring a 6-cm resection and free tissue transfer, followed by bone transport, may not be feasible in such a patient. Instead, this patient should be considered for a limited resection and chronic suppressive therapy or an amputation, despite the cardiopulmonary drawbacks. The tenet that optimization of the host is needed is even more important in this age group. Not only should nutritional and local tissue conditions be optimized, but underlying physiologic disorders should be addressed to minimize the risk of perioperative complications.

Secondly, the expectations and demands of the patient must be considered. Most of these patients will be retired and have limited demands, and therefore may not require what a 30-year old-construction worker or mother of three requires. Once again, the consideration of limited nonablative treatment that allows a comfortable existence with a "treated" infection, with or without chronic suppressive therapy, becomes much more attractive in this population. In some patients, an appropriately done debridement with the use of depots and stabilization, along with suppressive antibiotics, may be sufficient for their lower demands, especially if they have concomitant comorbidities that make repeated surgical interventions risky (Fig. 26-17).

The option of arthroplasty must also be considered. While arthroplasty is contraindicated in active infection a staged treatment consisting of an aggressive debridement and antibiotic suppression (local and systemic) may be a reasonable option in such patients. The use of an antibiotic cement spacer and suppressive antibiotic therapy may be so successful that the patients may be happy and not want to undergo subsequent treatment (Figs. 26-18 and 26-19).

AUTHOR'S PREFERRED METHODS

Initial Evaluation

The authors assume that any patient with a history of surgical fracture treatment, subsequent drainage, wound dehiscence, antibiotic treatment, or unplanned surgery may potentially have osteomyelitis. Many of these patients present with a paucity of medical records and other details, and often their own

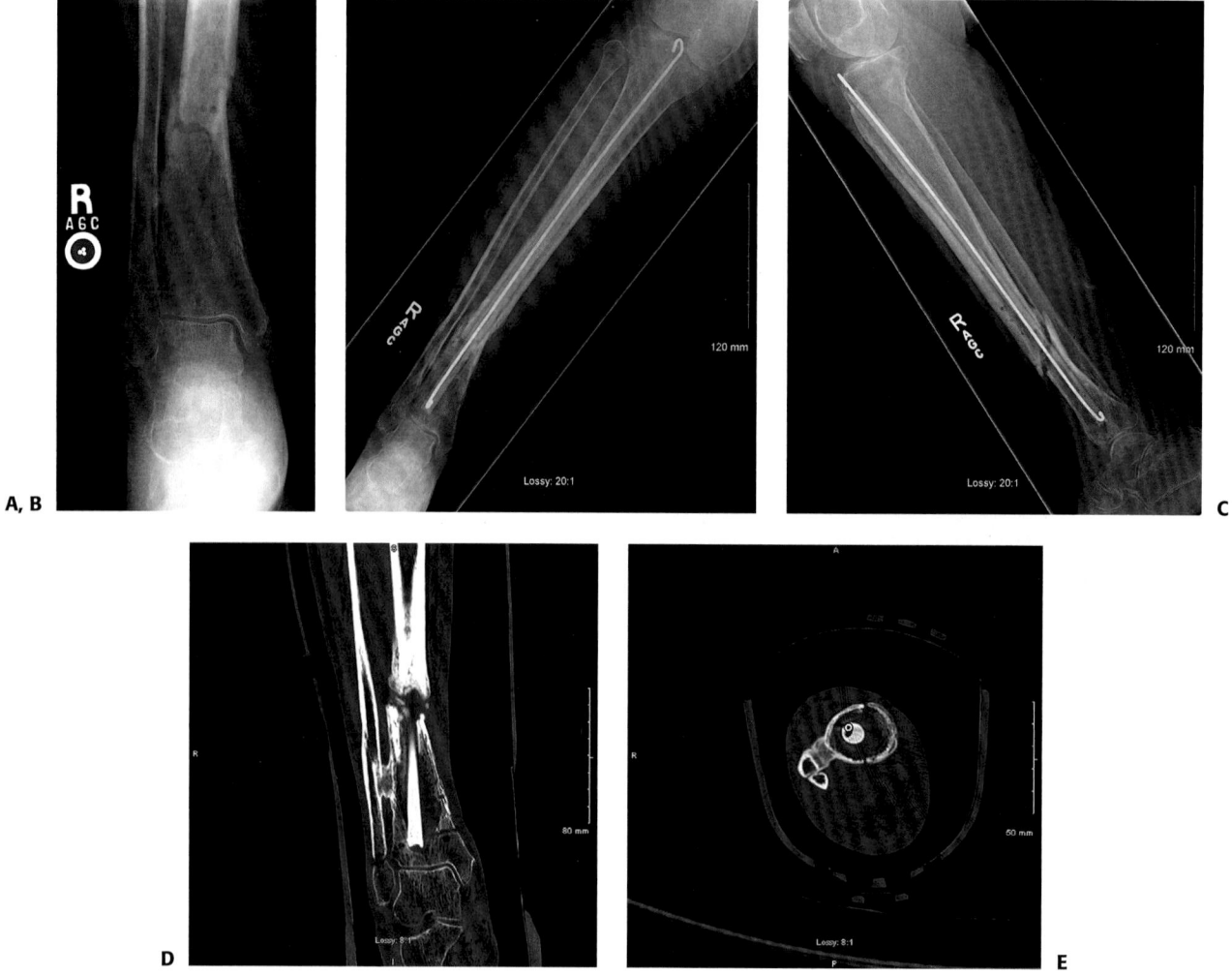

FIGURE 26-17 The case of a 75-year-old female with previous plating and intramedullary nailing. She had developed intramedullary infection and nonunion. **A:** Her nail was removed and intramedullary irrigation was performed using a reamer–irrigator–aspirator. **B:** She then had an antibiotic-impregnated PMMA rod, with a metal core, placed into the intramedullary canal. **C:** She developed a small area of posterior bridging, which may have been stimulated by the reaming and debridement, but she had not completely healed by 9 months. She had no evidence of infection after discontinuation of oral antibiotics. **D, E:** She had little or no pain despite a CT scan which showed no evidence of healing and was happy wearing a cam walker when outside. Further attempts to gain union would have put the patient through several surgical procedures including the need for soft tissue cover. In her case, her expectations and demands warranted a less aggressive approach.

recollection of events is poor. Therefore, we presume infection until we have strong evidence to the contrary, particularly if symptoms occur in conjunction with fracture nonunion.

The host is classified first and efforts are made to optimize the host status. Improving nutrition and tissue oxygenation is important before embarking on surgical treatment. Occasionally, hyperbaric oxygen is helpful if it is available and can be tolerated by the patient. Ideally, the patient should stop smoking, but this is generally difficult to accomplish. However, we encourage patients to limit nicotine use because it is thought that nicotine causes local microvascular effects. Therefore, nicotine patches and gum, although useful for smoking cessation programs, may not be useful for local tissue optimization. We

now routinely check vitamin D levels in all cases of delayed or failed osseous healing. Supplementation is usually 50,000 units per week for several weeks but underlying causes of the deficiency should be sought and corrected. Consultation with a primary care physician will help stabilize chronic medical conditions in many patients.

The limb is also evaluated for its ability to tolerate surgical intervention. Multiply operated limbs are B local by definition and heavily scarred and immobilized tissues may present risks for subsequent wound healing. Some patients may not be candidates or may not tolerate the extensive surgery that is required, and therefore compromises in treatment and patient expectations may be necessary. Many surgeons are now opting

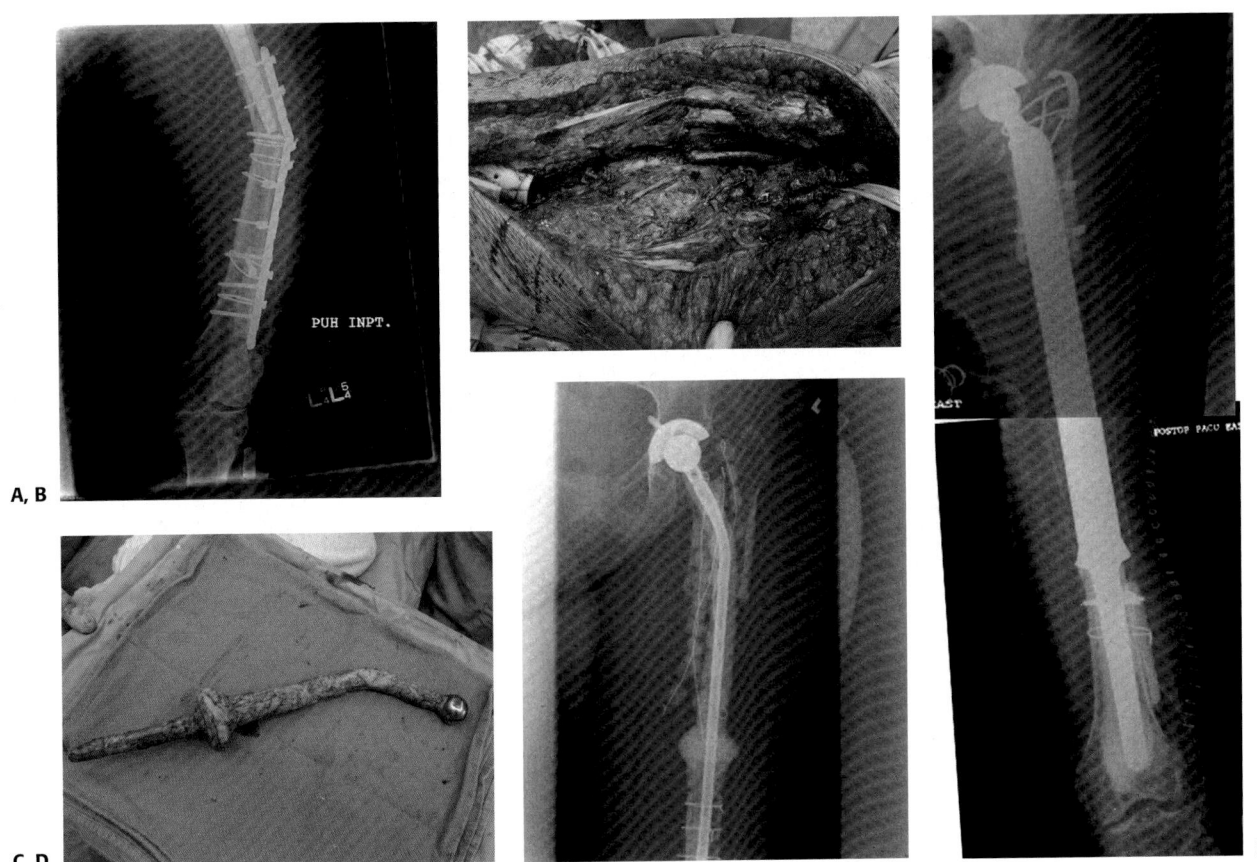

A, B

C, D

E

FIGURE 26-18 The case of an 80-year-old female who had undergone several attempts at reconstruction of a periprosthetic fracture. **A:** She presented with distally based infection that involved the plate, allograft, and distal aspect of the stem. She was a B-systemic/local host and extensive reconstruction efforts were not feasible. The plan was to perform a staged reconstruction using an arthroplasty. **B:** Intraoperatively, the infection was localized mostly to the middle part of the femur. The cup was well fixed and did not appear to have any involvement in the infection. **C, D:** A custom-made, weight-bearing antibiotic spacer was created using a coated tibial nail. **E:** After a 6-week course of IV antibiotics, during which time she was allowed to weight bear for transfers, she returned for reconstruction with a partial femoral replacement. Because of the proximity of the infection and potential for colonization, as well as her host status, she was maintained on suppressive oral antibiotics for an extended period of time as recommended by a musculoskeletal infectious disease specialist.

to treat exposed bone with a vacuum-assisted closure (VAC) device. Although this can often produce a healthy granulating tissue bed, it should be remembered that the underlying bone is compromised and has a higher risk of nonunion and infection. Another problem is that the soft tissue envelope tends to be an adherent layer of scar over the bone, which may not tolerate secondary surgery well. Secondary surgery under these circumstances may well result in further infection. For this reason, we still advocate the use of healthy muscle or fascial flaps that not only help being an external blood supply to the surface of the bone but can better tolerate subsequent surgical procedures.

Diagnostic Evaluation

Initially, laboratory testing including assessment of the WBC, ESR, and CRP is undertaken. If these tests are negative and there is no further reason to suspect infection, then we treat the patient as having an aseptic nonunion but we will pay

attention to our intraoperative findings. If there is any indication of infection despite normal laboratory findings, we obtain intraoperative cultures or undertake a biopsy and await results. One common scenario is a presumed aseptic case where routine cultures end up growing a few colonies of bacteria. The issue is whether the culture results represent a real infection or contamination. In these cases, we discuss the surgical findings with the infectious disease specialist who explains their assessment of the validity of the cultures. If we believe that the risk of infection is low, we may cover the patient with a short course of culture-specific oral antibiotics. However, if we believe that the risk is high, we use a longer course of antibiotic treatment. We have found that even when there is little diagnostic and operative evidence of infection, patients may still develop later infection. We have no way of knowing if the subsequent infection was a resurgence of an old occult infection or a secondary infection from the recent surgical intervention. A recent

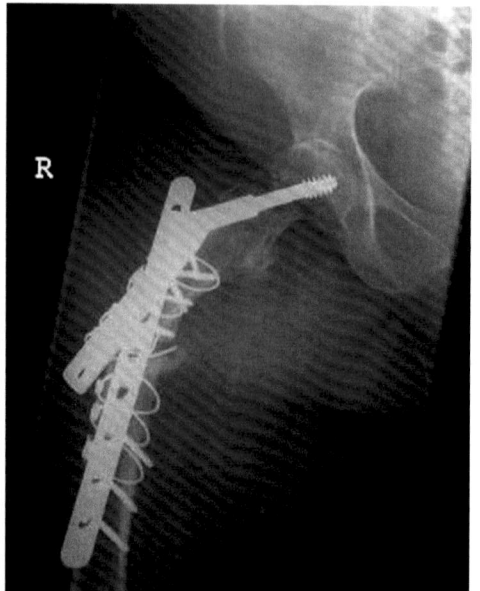 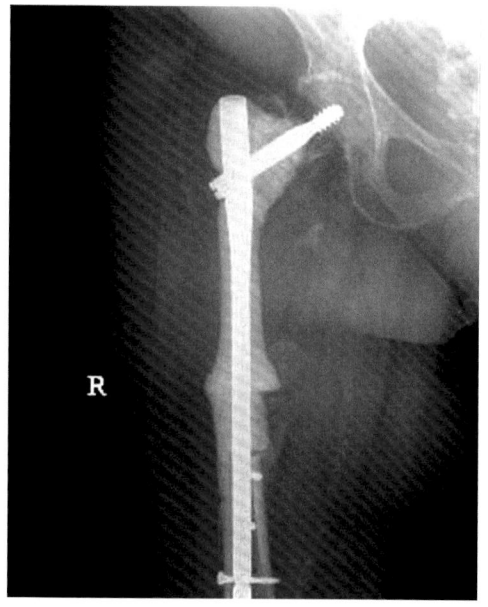

FIGURE 26-19 The case of a 78-year-old female who had multiple comorbidities and was nearly a C host. **A:** She had undergone an attempted reconstruction of a periprosthetic fracture in a rural community hospital. Her workup indicated a high likelihood of infection in the diaphyseal region without involvement of the hip area. **B:** She underwent a staged reconstruction that maintained the femoral head and neck using a custom-made antibiotic-coated prosthesis. After a 6-week course of antibiotics, during which she was ambulatory with assistance, she was scheduled for reconstruction with a total hip arthroplasty and partial femoral replacement. She felt "so good" that she refused any further treatment and she died prior to reconstruction.

study found that over 20% of nonunion cases, that had cultures taken intraoperatively, had positive cultures. These patients were given antibiotics and just over 2% developed infection from the same organism as was cultures preoperatively.[120]

In cases in which we suspect infection but do not know the organism, we will often remove the initial hardware and then take numerous cultures and biopsy samples of bone and soft tissue (often six or more). We will then temporarily stabilize the bone in the least invasive manner using a cast, brace, or monolateral external fixator. Sometimes it is helpful to obtain two different sets of cultures. One set of cultures is obtained from the most suspicious areas during the initial part of the surgical procedure. The second set of cultures is obtained after debridement from the margins of the tissue bed. If this methodology is used, one can assess whether the debridement was adequate, especially if the initial cultures were positive. If we remain uncertain about the extent of the infection, we will attempt to use MRI with contrast to determine the intramedullary and soft tissue extent of the infection and then plan our treatment accordingly. Unfortunately, in a majority of cases, there is implanted metal, which makes the use of MRI less applicable. When possible, we use scintigraphic studies preoperatively despite their limitations. We have anecdotally noted significant variations in the accuracy of the readings between various radiologists and encourage working with a few radiologists who are interested and experienced with musculoskeletal infection. Because of our own findings and those in the literature, we now depend less on scintigraphy than on other signs

and generally no longer use the red cell scan. The initial findings of PET scanning are encouraging.

Treatment

Once infection has been confirmed, an organism is identified, and the extent of the infection is delineated, we decide whether the goal is to cure the infection, suppress the infection, or recommend amputation. In compromised hosts, cure can usually be achieved only by complete excision of all the infected tissue, which often means that amputation is required. In healthier hosts, marginal resection leaving some bacteria behind or even intralesional resections when the infection is periarticular can lead to cure with appropriate antibiotic therapy. Generally speaking, our preference is to advise the patient that resection with a clean margin has the best chance of cure.

If bone resection and limb salvage are chosen, we follow the general principles that bone defects of 6 cm or greater require bone transport with distraction osteogenesis, whereas smaller defects can often undergo bone grafting. In the tibia, we prefer the posterolateral tibia-pro-fibula technique, but in some cases we will undertake central bone grafting. We try to avoid the exclusive use of demineralized bone matrix (DBM) and allograft because we have found a relatively low incidence of bone union. The low success rates using DBM products may be because of the poor vascularity found in such tissue beds and patients. Anecdotally, we have noted cases where patients present years after failed DBM grafting of the distal tibia, and during reoperation the original DBM material appears to be

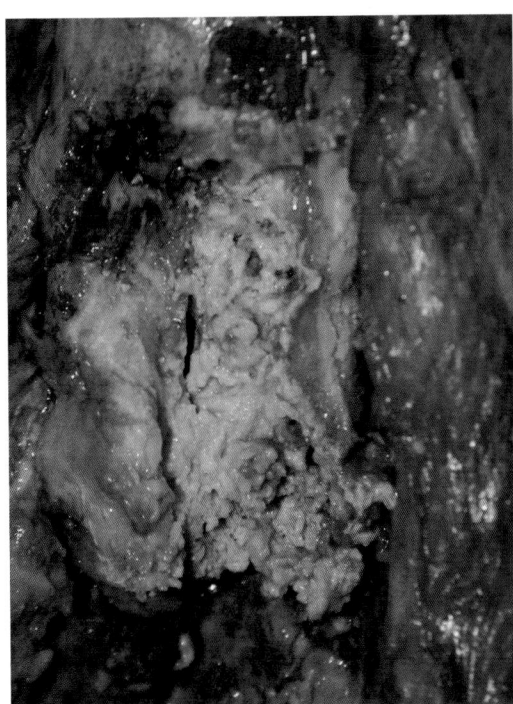

FIGURE 26-20 An intraoperative photograph of a distal tibial non-union. At the time of surgery the demineralized bone matrix (DBM) that was placed in situ over 5 years earlier appears to have changed little. Although DBM may be considered an inductive and conductive agent, its effects are weak to moderate at best, and without an improvement in bone vascularity, it may be of very limited value in those cases where it is needed the most.

unchanged. This indicates failure of angiogenesis (Fig. 26-20). DBM reports in the literature are limited but they do not support its general use as a bone graft substitute for nonunions, especially if there is bone loss. Ironically, cases in which bone graft is most needed, such as those where there is poor bone vascularity or a compromised host, are those in which DBM is of least value and the success of DBM may well be in those cases where bone graft is not needed.[132]

Bone morphogenetic proteins (BMPs) show significant promise and they are a much more powerful inductive agent than DBM. Currently surgeons still have to use them "off-label" as they have not been released for general use. There are numerous anecdotal cases of their successful use in nonunion and infection surgery, and their usefulness in limb salvage is unquestionable. However, there are some concerns about their potency and their use in females considering pregnancy within a year of its use.

The newer technique of graft harvest with the RIA has been shown to be successful for large defects and the graft harvested seems to have excellent osteogenic potential. Mixture with BMP may provide an even greater effect because the BMP is acellular and only an inductor, whereas the RIA aspirate supplies conductive elements and cellular components needed for healing. Experience with RIA has been positive.[72,97]

Another technique combining the use of RIA graft with an induced biomembrane has gained some popularity. The technique of Masquelet incorporates a cement spacer into the defect after bone resection. A biologic membrane grows over the spacer and the spacer is removed weeks to months later, once antibiotic elution has concluded. At the time of spacer removal, the membrane is maintained as best as possible to promote angiogenesis and a large-volume autograft, using iliac crest or RIA, is placed within the site.

If there is a sinus tract, we have found the technique of injecting diluted methylene blue dye into the sinus tract very helpful in localizing the path to any deep collection of fluid or sequestrum (Fig. 26-21). It helps minimize the amount of local tissue resection. The technique is relatively simple but does not always identify the whole lesion. Sinus tract resection is undertaken using a longitudinal elliptical skin incision to allow closure. The deep dissection follows the tract until the bone component is identified. Bone debridement is undertaken based on involvement. If the bone involvement is such that it is a Cierny III where there is axial stability, then all efforts are made to maintain axial stability, and avoid turning a type III lesion into a type IV, although sometimes this is not possible. Type IV lesions by definition require supplemental fixation and reconstruction. Some extensive type III lesions, although having some axial connection, are still unstable and may require additional treatment, thus essentially making them a type IV lesion. In salvageable type III lesions, we do not undertake a bulk resection and we often use a high-speed water-cooled burr to remove only as much bone as necessary.

In obvious type IV lesions, bone reconstruction is mandatory and it is a matter of how much reconstruction is required. We have found that bone transport is the most reliable method for reconstruction. This is discussed in Chapter 28. In certain areas, or in patients where transport may not be tolerated, the Masquelet technique or the use of bone cages with massive graft and BMP are the only other alternatives.

The use of antibiotic-coated nails for infected nonunions continues to evolve. Several reports have shown the efficacy of statically locked nails that are coated with a 2-mm cement mantle. We increasingly use this technique for infected long bone nonunions. The antibiotic cement must be mixed early in the procedure and the nail should be coated by the use of oversized cardiac pump tubing or other large bore tubing that is sterile and can be easily removed. We have not found chest tubes to be large enough. A 9-mm nail is selected for the tibia or femur. The nail and cement are prepared at the start of the case and the cement is allowed to cure on the nail for at least 45 minutes. The use of tubing insures a smooth, glass-like coating, which combined with the curing process, decreases the likelihood of debonding at insertion. The canal is overreamed by at least 5 mm to accommodate the nail and the cement. Once inserted, distal and proximal interlocking is undertaken using standard techniques. The nail permits early weight bearing. In cases of bone loss, we perform later grafting at 8 to 12 weeks, once the ESR and CRP tests are normal and the antibiotics have been stopped.[45,100,103]

In general, the mainstay of reconstruction for complex infection remains the bone transport techniques described by Ilizarov. These are described in detail in Chapter 28. Although this technique is not simple for either the patient or the surgeon, there are notable advantages compared with grafting

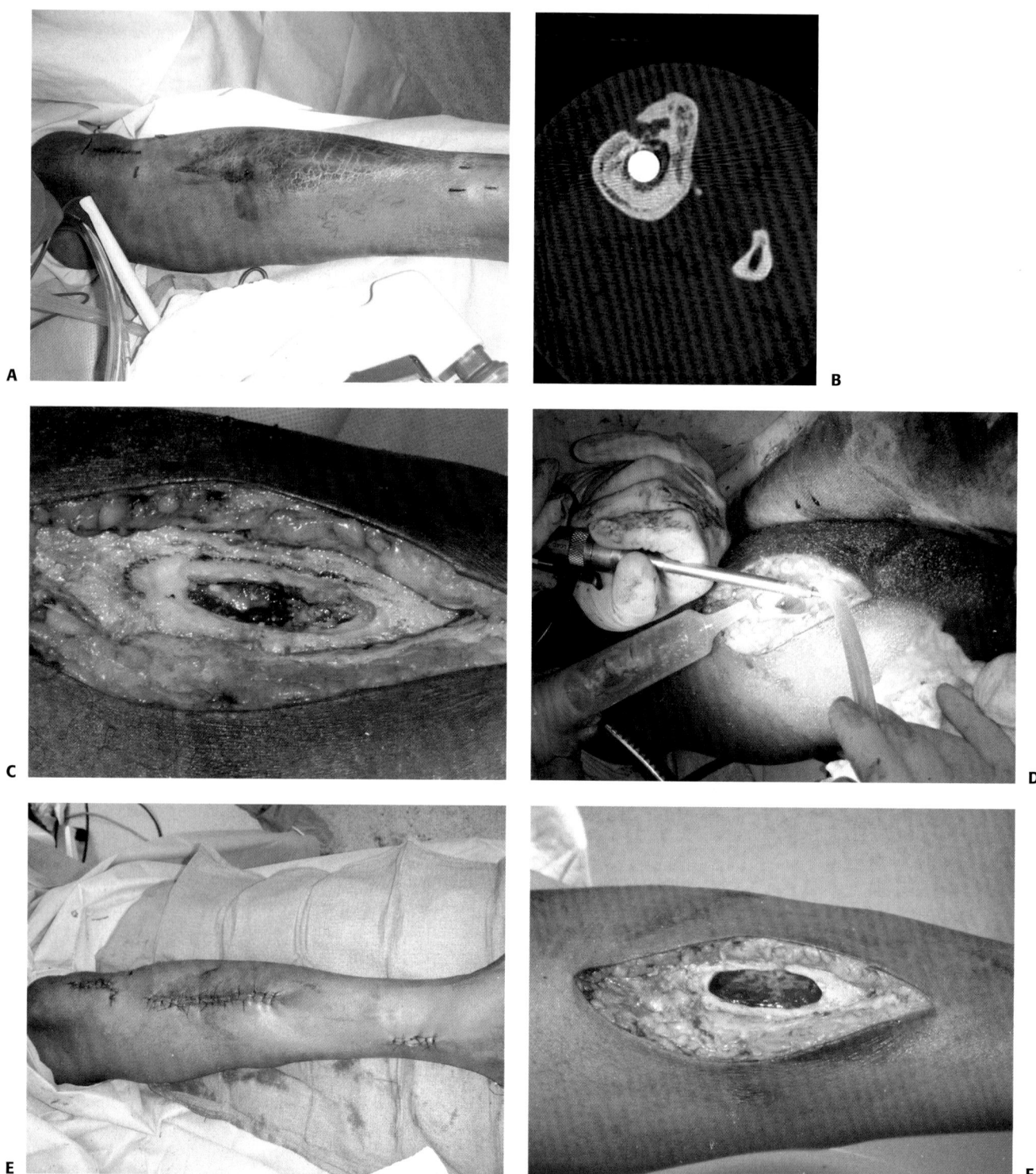

FIGURE 26-21 Images depicting the debridement technique in a case of type III osteomyelitis with a sinus tract. **A, B:** Methylene blue is injected into the sinus in the hope that it will find its way into the bone cavity and sequestrum. **C:** The skin resection is elliptical until the bone defect is identified. **D:** Because the lesion is type III and stable, we use a water-cooled high-speed burr to resect only as much bone as is required to remove the sequestrum and avascular tissue. **E:** This figure demonstrates the final resection and **(F)** demonstrates skin closure at follow-up.

techniques. These include the early development of regenerate bone soon after bone resection. If bone grafting is used, one must wait 8 weeks or longer as part of a staged reconstruction plan. Also, the effects of corticotomy include increasing blood flow in the limb for 4 to 6 weeks, and this may have a positive effect in infection cases. Most importantly, function is improved. The patient is encouraged to weight bear and to resume most activities of daily living. In many cases, patients can return to work, participate in recreational activities, and even swim. In cases where transport takes a considerable period or where transport has finished but one has to wait for maturation of regenerate bone, we have used long percutaneously inserted locked plates as an internal fixator that spans and protects maturing regenerate bone. This allows for early removal of the ring fixator (Fig. 26-22). Alternatively, some cases are amenable to transport over a nail (Fig. 26-23). We encourage

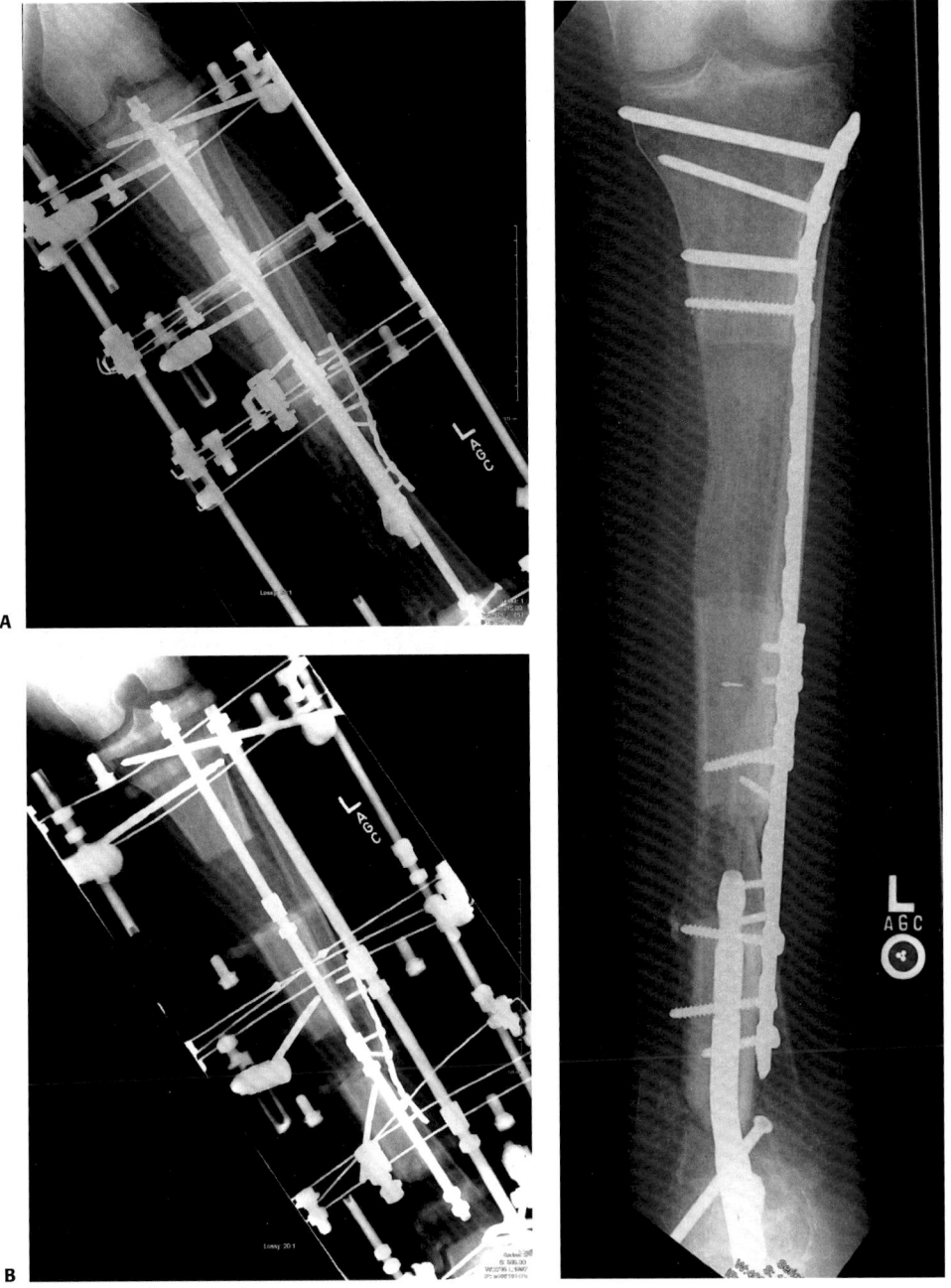

FIGURE 26-22 Radiographs of a long distal tibial transport. The patient had a very large (~16 cm) defect. **A, B:** To shorten transport time, bifocal transport was performed to an ankle fusion. **C:** At the time of docking, the subtalar joint was sacrificed and a retrograde hindfoot nail was inserted. This was overlapped with a long tibial locking plate. Screws were placed through the plate and nail. The regenerate was protected while simultaneously compressing the ankle docking site.

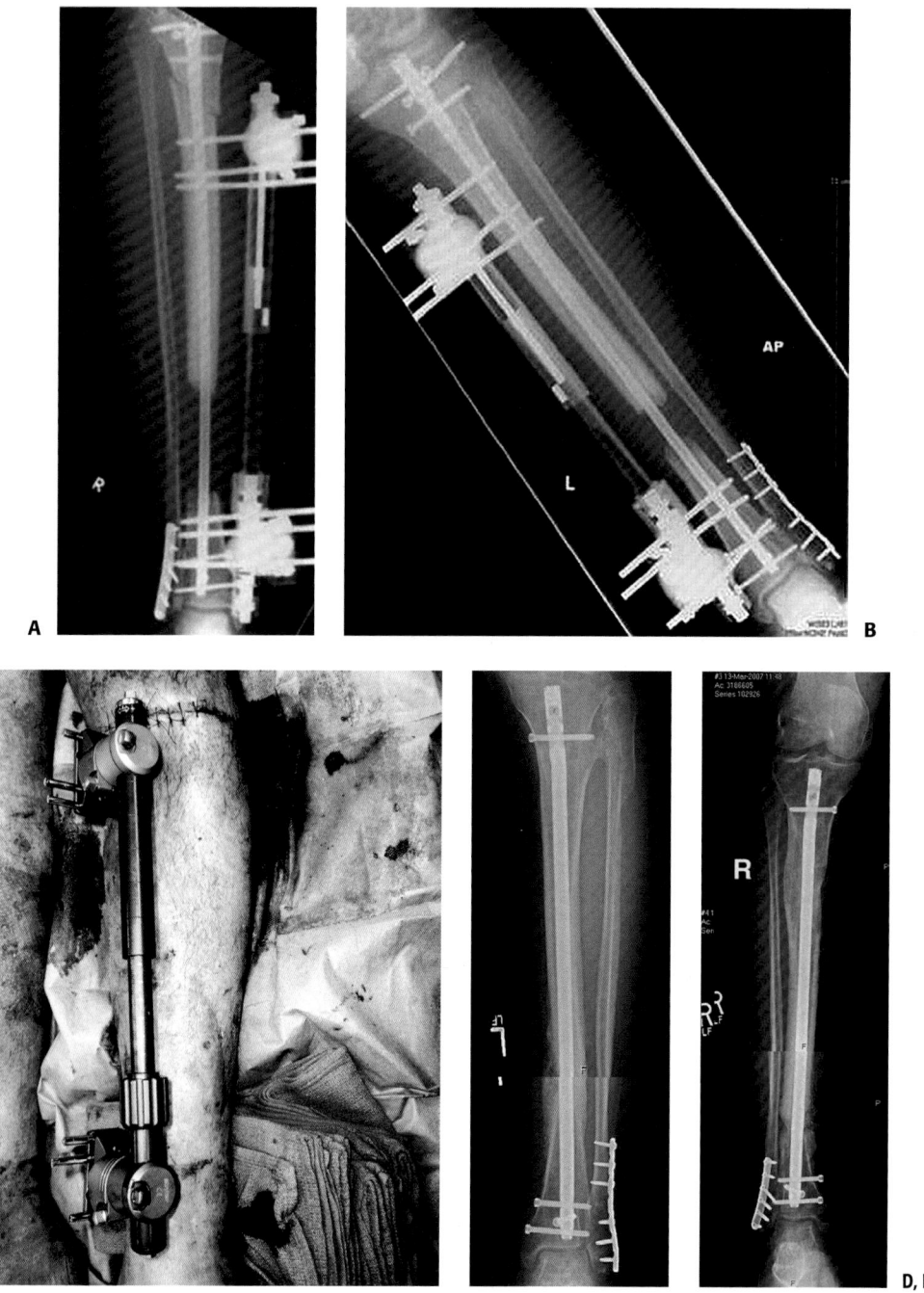

FIGURE 26-23 **A, B:** Images depicting length stable transport over a nail. In this case the patient had a sizeable bilateral defect. **C:** Functional treatment consisted of monolateral transport over a nail. **D, E:** At the time of docking, the bone ends were freshened and grafted, followed by a period of compression using the external fixator. Final healing occurred bilaterally.

surgeons who wish to treat bone infection to be familiar with Ilizarov method and to seek out appropriate training.

A key component in the management of infection is functional rehabilitation. Often, the patients are extremely debilitated from years of disability because of their condition. Treatments that permit early weight bearing and encourage range of motion in adjacent joints promote physical and psychological well-being.

It is unusual for treatment to fail because patients have been walking on their limb. Usually failure is caused by inadequate resection, inadequate stability, and inadequate biology.

It is very difficult for surgeons who operate infrequently on infection to achieve the results published by experts. Not only is bone transport labor intensive but successful treatment requires an integrated team who are trained and willing to meet the demands of the patients and to facilitate the work of the surgeon. It is also imperative to collaborate and enlist the expertise of colleagues in infectious disease, psychiatry, medicine, microvascular surgery, social work, physical therapy, and occupational therapy. All staff must also be aware of the special needs of these patients, many of whom have undergone multiple failed procedures. It is very common to find depression, anxiety, and other psychological issues in both patients and their families. In fact, the burdens of the caregiver have only recently been identified, with many caregivers reporting depression, financial loss, and other problems as they care for their family members.[130]

There is no doubt that, given the difficulties of treating bone infection, the best strategy is prevention. Surgeons have always been aware of this, but recently the medical community, patients, and bodies that fund medicine have become more aware of the problem. As a consequence of this, increased research is expanding our knowledge of surgical infection and this has significant implications for the prevention of osteomyelitis. There is more knowledge about the factors that increase the risk of infection. Controllable patient factors such as perioperative body temperature, glucose levels, and preoperative hygiene are being standardized. Improved surgical techniques and the optimization of the patient environment are also having an effect, and hopefully we will be able to minimize the incidence of osteomyelitis in the future.

TRIBUTE TO GEORGE C CIERNY III

Orthopedic surgeons, particularly those who treat osteomyelitis, were saddened by the loss of George C. Cierny III last year on June 24th, 2013. Dr. Cierny was pivotal in studying and understanding the treatment of bone infections. His incredible energy and drive resulted in the accumulation of data that transformed the diagnosis, classification, and treatment of osteomyelitis. With his partner Dr. J. Mader (infectious disease), they developed the widely quoted and utilized Cierny-Mader classification of osteomyelitis. Dr. Cierny and Mader recognized the importance of the host, and approached osteomyelitis in a systematic way, intuitively recognizing the utility of applying the principles of tumor surgery to bone infections. His surgical skills and patient care were difficult to match, and he was internationally sought as a surgeon and speaker. Dr. Cierny was a physician who worked for weeks on a specific plan for each patient, revisiting the plan daily and making changes until he felt it was perfect. Perfection is what he demanded of himself and everyone around him, including the patient. This was particularly true in the operating room. He was a founding member of the Musculoskeletal Infection Society (MSIS), and has left behind a legacy for his colleagues, students, and friends. Orthopaedic surgeons are indebted to him and will miss his veracity and wisdom.

REFERENCES

1. Zalavras CG, Patzakis MJ, Holtom P. Local antibiotic therapy in the treatment of open fractures and osteomyelitis. *Clin Orth Relat Res.* 2004;427:86–93.
2. Nelson CL. The current status of material used for depot delivery of drugs. *Clin Orthop Relat Res.* 2004;427:72–78.
3. Anglen JO. Wound irrigation in musculoskeletal injury. *J Am Acad Orthop Surg.* 2001;9(4):219–226.
4. Anglen JO. Comparison of soap and antibiotic solutions for irrigation of lower-limb open fracture wounds. A prospective, randomized study. *J Bone Joint Surg Am.* 2005;87(7):1415–1422.
5. Anglen JO, Apostoles S, Christensen G, et al. The efficacy of various irrigation solutions in removing slime-producing Staphylococcus. *J Orthop Trauma.* 1994;8(5):390–396.
6. Ash JM, Gilday DL. The futility of bone scanning in neonatal osteomyelitis: Concise communication. *J Nucl Med.* 1980;21(5):417–420.
7. Benjamin JB, Volz RG. Efficacy of a topical antibiotic irrigant in decreasing or eliminating bacterial contamination in surgical wounds. *Clin Orthop Relat Res.* 1984;(184):114–117.
8. Bhandari M, Schemitsch EH, Adili A, et al. High and low pressure pulsatile lavage of contaminated tibial fractures: An in vitro study of bacterial adherence and bone damage. *J Orthop Trauma.* 1999;13(8):526–533.
9. Boerman OC, Rennen H, Oyen WJ, et al. Radiopharmaceuticals to image infection and inflammation. *Semin Nucl Med.* 2001;31(4):286–295.
10. Borman TR, Johnson RA, Sherman FC. Gallium scintigraphy for diagnosis of septic arthritis and osteomyelitis in children. *J Pediatr Orthop.* 1986;6(3):317–325.
11. Borrelli JJ, Prickett WD, Ricci WM. Treatment of nonunions and osseous defects with bone graft and calcium sulfate. *Clin Orthop Relat Res.* 2003;411:245–254.
12. Boxma H, Broekhuizen T, Patka P, et al. Randomised controlled trial of single-dose antibiotic prophylaxis in surgical treatment of closed fractures: The Dutch Trauma Trial. *Lancet.* 1996;347(9009):1133–1137.
13. Boyd JI 3rd, Wongworawat MD. High-pressure pulsatile lavage causes soft tissue damage. *Clin Orthop Relat Res.* 2004;(427):13–17.
14. Carsenti-Etesse H, Doyon F, Desplaces N, et al. Epidemiology of bacterial infection during management of open leg fractures. *Eur J Clin Microbiol Infect Dis.* 1999;18(5):315–323.
15. Casten DF, Nach RJ, Spinzia J. An experimental and clinical study of the effectiveness of antibiotic wound irrigation in preventing infection. *Surg Gynecol Obstet.* 1964;118:783–787.
16. Cavanaugh DL, Berry J, Yarboro SR, et al. Better prophylaxis against surgical site infection with local as well as systemic antibiotics. An in vivo study. *J Bone Joint Surg Am.* 2009;91(8):1907–1912.
17. Chacko TK, Zhuang H, Nakhoda KZ, et al. Applications of fluorodeoxyglucose positron emission tomography in the diagnosis of infection. *Nucl Med Commun.* 2003;24(6):615–624.
18. Cierny G. Treating chronic osteomyelitis: evolving our antibiotic protocol. Paper presented at Musculoskeletal Infection Society, August, 2000.
19. Cierny G, Mader JT, Pennick JJ. A clinical staging system for adult osteomyelitis. *Contemp Orthop.* 1985;10:17–37.
20. Cierny G 3rd, Mader JT, Penninck JJ. A clinical staging system for adult osteomyelitis. *Clin Orthop Relat Res.* 2003;(414):7–24.
21. Classen DC, Evans RS, Pestotnik SL, et al. The timing of prophylactic administration of antibiotics and the risk of surgical-wound infection. *N Engl J Med.* 1992;326(5):281–286.
22. Collier BD. Scintigraphic diagnosis of acute bone infection: Is the red cell scan necessary? *Personal communication.*
23. Condie JD, Fergerson DJ. Experimental wound infections: Contamination versus surgical technique. *Surgery.* 1961;50:367.
24. Court-Brown CM, Keating JF, McQueen MM. Infection after intramedullary nailing of the tibia. Incidence and protocol for management. *J Bone Joint Surg Br.* 1992;74(5):770–774.
25. Cunha B, Klein N. Bone and joint infections. In: Dee R, Hurst LC, Gruber MA, Kottmeier SA, eds. *Principles of Orthopaedic Practice.* 2nd ed. New York, NY: McGraw-Hill; 1997:317–344.
26. Dankert J, Hogt AH, Feijen J. Biomedical polymers:Bacterial adhesion, colonization, and infection. *CRC Crit Rev Biocompat.* 1986;2:219–301.
27. Datz FL. *Minutes in Nuclear Medicine.* 2nd ed. New York, NY: Appleton Century Crofts; 1983:82–85.
28. Datz FL. Infection imaging. *Semin Nucl Med.* 1994;24(2):89–91.
29. Datz FL. Abdominal abscess detection: Gallium, 111In-, and 99mTc-labeled leukocytes, and polyclonal and monoclonal antibodies. *Semin Nucl Med.* 1996;26(1):51–64.
30. Datz FL, Seabold JE, Brown ML, et al. Procedure guideline for technetium-99m-HMPAO-labeled leukocyte scintigraphy for suspected infection/inflammation. Society of Nuclear Medicine. *J Nucl Med.* 1997;38(6):987–990.
31. David R, Barron BJ, Madewell JE. Osteomyelitis, acute and chronic. *Radiol Clin North Am.* 1987;25(6):1171–1201.
32. Dich VQ, Nelson JD, Haltalin KC. Osteomyelitis in infants and children. A review of 163 cases. *Am J Dis Child.* 1975;129(11):1273–1278.
33. DiMaio FR, O'Halloran JJ, Quale JM. In vitro elution of ciprofloxacin from polymethylmethacrylate cement beads. *J Orthop Res.* 1994;12(1):79–82.
34. Dirschl DR, Duff GP, Dahners LE, et al. High pressure pulsatile lavage irrigation of intraarticular fractures:Effects on fracture healing. *J Orthop Trauma.* 1998;12(7):460–463.
35. Dirschl DR, Wilson FC. Topical antibiotic irrigation in the prophylaxis of operative wound infections in orthopedic surgery. *Orthop Clin North Am.* 1991;22(3):419–426.
36. Duwelius PJ, Schmidt AH. Assessment of bone viability in patients with osteomyelitis:Ppreliminary clinical experience with laser Doppler flowmetry. *J Orthop Trauma.* 1992;6(3):327–332.
37. Eckardt JJ, Wirganowicz PZ, Mar T. An aggressive surgical approach to the management of chronic osteomyelitis. *Clin Orthop Relat Res.* 1994;(298):229–239.
38. Eisenstein BI. The polymerase chain reaction. A new method of using molecular genetics for medical diagnosis. *N Engl J Med.* 1990;322(3):178–183.
39. Esterhai J, Alavi A, Mandell GA, et al. Sequential technetium-99m/gallium-67 scintigraphic evaluation of subclinical osteomyelitis complicating fracture nonunion. *J Orthop Res.* 1985;3(2):219–225.
40. Esterhai JL Jr, Goll SR, McCarthy KE, et al. Indium-111 leukocyte scintigraphic detection of subclinical osteomyelitis complicating delayed and nonunion long bone fractures: A prospective study. *J Orthop Res.* 1987;5(1):1–6.
41. Evans RP, Nelson CL, Harrison BH. The effect of wound environment on the incidence of acute osteomyelitis. *Clin Orthop Relat Res.* 1993;(286):289–297.

42. Fennessy JM, Franzus M, Schlatterer D, et al. MRSA screening, surveillance, and control protocol in trauma patients. Poster. Annual Meeting of the AAOS, March 9–13, 2010.

43. Fink-Bennett D, Balon HR, Irwin R. Sequential technetium-99m sulfur colloid/indium-111 white blood cell imaging in macroglobulinemia of Waldenstrom. Clin Nucl Med. 1990;15(6):389–391.

44. Fischer B, Vaudaux P, Magnin M, et al. Novel animal model for studying the molecular mechanisms of bacterial adhesion to bone-implanted metallic devices: Role of fibronectin in Staphylococcus aureus adhesion. J Orthop Res. 1996;14(6):914–920.

45. Fuchs T, Stange R, Schmidmaier G, et al. The use of gentamicin-coated nails in the tibia: Preliminary results of a prospective study. Arch Orthop Trauma Surg. 2011; 131(10):1419–1425.

46. Gao Z, Tseng CH, Pei Z, et al. Molecular analysis of human forearm superficial skin bacterial biota. Proc Natl Acad Sci U S A. 2007;104(8):2927–2932.

47. Gillespie WJ, Walenkamp G. Antibiotic prophylaxis for surgery for proximal femoral and other closed long bone fractures. Cochrane Database Syst Rev. 2001;1:CD000244.

48. Graham GD, Lundy MM, Frederick RJ, et al. Predicting the cure of osteomyelitis under treatment: Concise communication. J Nucl Med. 1983;24(2):110–113.

49. Greidanus NV, Masri BA, Garbuz DS, et al. Use of erythrocyte sedimentation rate and C-reactive protein level to diagnose infection before revision total knee arthroplasty. A prospective evaluation. J Bone Joint Surg Am. 2007;89(7):1409–1416.

50. Gristina AG, Barth E, Webb LX. Microbial adhesion and the pathogenesis of biomaterial-centered infections. In: Gustilo RB, Tsukayama DT, eds. Orthopaedic Infection. Philadelphia, PA: WB Saunders; 1989:3–25.

51. Haas DW, McAndrew MP. Bacterial osteomyelitis in adults: Evolving considerations in diagnosis and treatment. Am J Med. 1996;101(5):550–561.

52. Hartshorne MF, Graham G, Lancaster J, et al. Gallium-67/technetium-99m methylene diphosphonate ratio imaging: Early rabbit osteomyelitis and fracture. J Nucl Med. 1985;26(3):272–277.

53. Hassinger SM, Harding G, Wongworawat MD. High-pressure pulsatile lavage propagates bacteria into soft tissue. Clin Orthop Relat Res. 2005;439:27–31.

54. Hauet JR, Barge ML, Fajon O, et al. Sternal infection and retrosternal abscess shown on Tc-99m HMPAO-labeled leukocyte scintigraphy. Clin Nucl Med. 2004;29(3): 194–195.

55. Hauser CJ, Adams CA Jr, Eachempati SR. Surgical Infection Society guideline: Prophylactic antibiotic use in open fractures: An evidence-based guideline. Surg Infect (Larchmt). 2006;7(4):379–405.

56. Hoch RC, Rodriguez R, Manning T, et al. Effects of accidental trauma on cytokine and endotoxin production. Crit Care Med. 1993;21(6):839–845.

57. Hoeffel DP, Hinrichs SH, Garvin KL. Molecular diagnostics for the detection of musculoskeletal infection. Clin Orthop Relat Res. 1999;(360):37–46.

58. Hughes DK. Nuclear medicine and infection detection: The relative effectiveness of imaging with 111In-oxine-, 99mTc-HMPAO-, and 99mTc-stannous fluoride colloid-labeled leukocytes and with 67Ga-citrate. J Nucl Med Technol. 2003;31(4):196–201; quiz 203–204.

59. Jefferson KK. What drives bacteria to produce a biofilm? FEMS Microbiol Lett. 2004; 236(2):163–173.

60. Keating JF, Blachut PA, O'Brien PJ, et al. Reamed nailing of open tibial fractures: Does the antibiotic bead pouch reduce the deep infection rate? J Orthop Trauma. 1996;10(5):298–303.

61. Kelly PJ. Infected nonunion of the femur and tibia. Orthop Clin North Am. 1984; 15(3):481–490.

62. Law HT, Flemming RH, Gilmore MF, et al. In vitro measurement and computer modelling of the diffusion of antibiotic in bone cement. J Biomed Eng. 1986;8(2):149–155.

63. Lazzarini L, Lipsky BA, Mader JT. Antibiotic treatment of osteomyelitis: What have we learned from 30 years of clinical trials? Int J Infect Dis. 2005;9(3):127–138.

64. Lee J. Efficacy of cultures in the management of open fractures. Clin Orthop Relat Res. 1997;(339):71–75.

65. Lenarz CJ, Watson JT, Moed BR, et al. Timing of wound closure based on cultures obtained after debridement. J Bone Joint Surg Am. 2010;92:1921–1926.

66. Mackowiak PA, Jones SR, Smith JW. Diagnostic value of sinus-tract cultures in chronic osteomyelitis. JAMA. 1978;239(26):2772–2775.

67. Mader JT, Calhoun J. Long-bone osteomyelitis diagnosis and management. Hosp Pract (Off Ed). 1994;29(10):71–76.

68. Magnuson JE, Brown ML, Hauser MF, et al. In-111-labeled leukocyte scintigraphy in suspected orthopedic prosthesis infection: Comparison with other imaging modalities. Radiology. 1988;168(1):235–239.

69. Mann S. Molecular recognition in biomineralization. Nature. 1988;332:119–124.

70. Marsh JL, Prokuski L, Biermann JS. Chronic infected tibial nonunions with bone loss. Conventional techniques versus bone transport. Clin Orthop Relat Res. 1994;(301): 139–146.

71. May JW Jr, Jupiter JB, Weiland AJ, et al. Clinical classification of post-traumatic tibial osteomyelitis. J Bone Joint Surg Am. 1989;71(9):1422–1428.

72. McCall TA, Brokaw DS, Jelen BA, et al. Treatment of large segmental bone defects with reamer-irrigator-aspirator bone graft. Technique and case series. Orthop Clin North Am. 2010;41(1):63–73.

73. McCarthy K, Velchik MG, Alavi A, et al. Indium-111-labeled white blood cells in the detection of osteomyelitis complicated by a pre-existing condition. J Nucl Med. 1988;29(6):1015–1021.

74. McKee MD, Wild LM, Schemitsch EH, et al. The use of an antibiotic-impregnated, osteoconductive, bioabsorbable bone substitute in the treatment of infected long bone defects: Early results of a prospective trial. J Orthop Trauma. 2002;16(9):622–627.

75. Meadows SE, Zuckerman JD, Koval KJ. Posttraumatic tibial osteomyelitis: Diagnosis, classification, and treatment. Bull Hosp Jt Dis. 1993;52(2):11–16.

76. Merkel KD, Brown ML, Dewanjee MK, et al. Comparison of indium-labeled-leukocyte imaging with sequential technetium-gallium scanning in the diagnosis of low-grade musculoskeletal sepsis. A prospective study. J Bone Joint Surg Am. 1985;67(3):465–476.

77. Merkel KD, Brown ML, Fitzgerald RH Jr. Sequential technetium-99m HMDP-gallium-67 citrate imaging for the evaluation of infection in the painful prosthesis. J Nucl Med. 1986;27(9):1413–1417.

78. Modic MT, Feiglin DH, Piraino DW, et al. Vertebral osteomyelitis: Assessment using MR. Radiology. 1985;157(1):157–166.

79. Molina-Murphy IL, Palmer EL, Scott JA, et al. Polyclonal, nonspecific 111In-IgG scintigraphy in the evaluation of complicated osteomyelitis and septic arthritis. Q J Nucl Med. 1999;43(1):29–37.

80. Moscati RM, Mayrose J, Reardon RF, et al. A multicenter comparison of tap water versus sterile saline for wound irrigation. Acad Emerg Med. 2007;14(5):404–409.

81. Moussa FW, Anglen JO, Gehrke JC, et al. The significance of positive cultures from orthopedic fixation devices in the absence of clinical infection. Am J Orthop. 1997;26(9):617–620.

82. Moussa FW, Gainor BJ, Anglen JO, et al. Disinfecting agents for removing adherent bacteria from orthopaedic hardware. Clin Orthop Relat Res. 1996;(329):255–262.

83. Murray CK, Hinkle MK, Yun HC. History of infections associated with combat-related injuries. J Trauma. 2008;64(3 suppl):S221–S231.

84. Murray CK, Hsu JR, Solomkin JS, et al. Prevention and management of infections associated with combat-related extremity injuries. J Trauma. 2008;64(3 suppl):S239–S251.

85. Naylor P, Jennings R, Myrvik Q. Antibiotic sensitivity of biomaterial-adherent Staphylococcus epidermidis. Orthop Trans. 1988;12:524–525.

86. Nichols WW, Dorrington SM, Slack MP, et al. Inhibition of tobramycin diffusion by binding to alginate. Antimicrob Agents Chemother. 1988;32(4):518–523.

87. Ochsner PE, Brunazzi MG. Intramedullary reaming and soft tissue procedures in treatment of chronic osteomyelitis of long bones. Orthopedics. 1994;17(5):433–440.

88. Ostermann PA, Henry SL, Seligson D. [Value of adjuvant local antibiotic administration in therapy of open fractures. A comparative analysis of 704 consecutive cases]. Langenbecks Arch Chir. 1993;378(1):32–36.

89. Owens BD, White DW, Wenke JC. Comparison of irrigation solutions and devices in a contaminated musculoskeletal wound survival model. JBJS (Am). 2009;91: 92–98.

90. Palestro CJ, Mehta HH, Patel M, et al. Marrow versus infection in the Charcot joint: Indium-111 leukocyte and technetium-99m sulfur colloid scintigraphy. J Nucl Med. 1998;39(2):346–350.

91. Pape HC, Zwipp H, Regel G, et al. [Chronic treatment refractory osteomyelitis of long tubular bones–possibilities and risks of intramedullary boring]. Unfallchirurg. 1995;98(3):139–144.

92. Patzakis MJ, Wilkins J. Factors influencing infection rate in open fracture wounds. Clin Orthop Relat Res. 1989;(243):36–40.

93. Peters AM. The utility of [99mTc]HMPAO-leukocytes for imaging infection. Semin Nucl Med. 1994;24(2):110–127.

94. Petrisor B, Jeray K, Schemitsch E, et al. Fluid lavage in patients with open fracture wounds (FLOW): An international survey of 984 surgeons. BMC Musculoskelet Disord. 2008;23(9):7.

95. Poirier JY, Garin E, Derrien C, et al. Diagnosis of osteomyelitis in the diabetic foot with a 99mTc-HMPAO leucocyte scintigraphy combined with a 99mTc-MDP bone scintigraphy. Diabetes Metab. 2002;28(6 Pt 1):485–490.

96. Pommer A, David A, Richter J, et al. [Intramedullary boring in infected intramedullary nail osteosyntheses of the tibia and femur]. Unfallchirurg. 1998;101(8):628–633.

97. Porter, RM, Fangjun L, Carmencita P, et al. Osteogenic potential of reamer irrigator aspirator from patients undergoing hip arthroplasty. J Orthop Res. 2009;27(1):42–49.

98. Quinn SF, Murray W, Clark RA, et al. MR imaging of chronic osteomyelitis. J Comput Assist Tomogr. 1988;12(1):113–117.

99. Rang M. The Story of Orthopaedics. Philadelphia, PA: WB Saunders; 2000.

100. Riel RU, Gladden PB. A simple method for fashioning an antibiotic cement-coated interlocking intramedullary nail. Am J Orthop (Belle Mead NJ). 2010;39(1):18–21.

101. Rosenstein BD, Wilson FC, Funderburk CH. The use of bacitracin irrigation to prevent infection in postoperative skeletal wounds. An experimental study. J Bone Joint Surg Am. 1989;71(3):427–430.

102. Rubin RH, Fischman AJ, Needleman M, et al. Radiolabeled, nonspecific, polyclonal human immunoglobulin in the detection of focal inflammation by scintigraphy: Comparison with gallium-67 citrate and technetium-99m-labeled albumin. J Nucl Med. 1989;30(3):385–389.

103. Sancineto CF, Barla JD. Treatment of long bone osteomyelitis with a mechanically stable intramedullar antibiotic dispenser: Nineteen consecutive cases with a minimum of 12 months follow-up. J Trauma. 2008;65(6):1416–1420.

104. Sankaran-Kutty M, Corea JR, Ali MS, et al. Squamous cell carcinoma in chronic osteomyelitis. Report of a case and review of the literature. Clin Orthop Relat Res. 1985;(198):264–267.

105. Schauwecker DS. Osteomyelitis: Diagnosis with In-111-labeled leukocytes. Radiology. 1989;171(1):141–146.

106. Schauwecker DS, Braunstein EM, Wheat LJ. Diagnostic imaging of osteomyelitis. Infect Dis Clin North Am. 1990;4(3):441–463.

107. Schiesser M, Stumpe KD, Trentz O, et al. Detection of metallic implant-associated infections with FDG PET in patients with trauma: Correlation with microbiologic results. Radiology. 2003;226(2):391–398.

108. Schmidt AH, Swiontkowski MF. Pathophysiology of infections after internal fixation of fractures. J Am Acad Ortho Surg. 2000;8(5):285–291.

109. Seabold JE, Flickinger FW, Kao SC, et al. Indium-111-leukocyte/technetium-99m-MDP bone and magnetic resonance imaging: Difficulty of diagnosing osteomyelitis in patients with neuropathic osteoarthropathy. J Nucl Med. 1990;31(5): 549–556.

110. Seabold JE, Nepola JV, Conrad GR, et al. Detection of osteomyelitis at fracture nonunion sites: Comparison of two scintigraphic methods. AJR Am J Roentgenol. 1989; 152(5):1021–1027.

111. Seeley SK, Seeley JV, Telehowski P, et al. Volume and surface area study of tobramycin-polymethylmethacrylate beads. Clin Orthop Relat Res. 2004;(420):298–303.

112. Segura AB, Munoz A, Brulles YR, et al. What is the role of bone scintigraphy in the diagnosis of infected joint prostheses? *Nucl Med Commun.* 2004;25(5):527–532.
113. Svoboda SJ, Bice TG, Gooden HA, et al. Comparison of bulb syringe and pulsed lavage irrigation with use of a bioluminescent musculoskletal wound model. *J Bone Joint Surg Am.* 2006;88(10):2167–2174.
114. Tang JS, Gold RH, Bassett LW, et al. Musculoskeletal infection of the extremities: Evaluation with MR imaging. *Radiology.* 1988;166(1 Pt 1):205–209.
115. Tehranzadeh J, Wang F, Mesgarzadeh M. Magnetic resonance imaging of osteomyelitis. *Crit Rev Diagn Imaging.* 1992;33(6):495–534.
116. Thomas LC, Gidding HF, Ginn AN, et al. Development of a real-time Staphylococcus aureus and MRSA (SAM-) PCR for routine blood culture. *J Microbiol Methods.* 2007;68(2):296–302.
117. Toguchi A, Siano M, Burkart M, et al. Genetics of swarming motility in Salmonella enterica serovar typhimurium: Critical role for lipopolysaccharide. *J Bacteriol.* 2000;182(22):6308–6321.
118. Toh CL, Jupiter JB. The infected nonunion of the tibia. *Clin Orthop Relat Res.* 1995;(315):176–191.
119. Tompkins LS. The use of molecular methods in infectious diseases. *N Engl J Med.* 1992;327(18):1290–1297.
120. Tornetta, P, Olszewski D, Jones, CB, et al. The fate of patients with a surprise positive culture after nonunion surgery. AAOS 2011, San Diego.
121. Tsukayama DT. Pathophysiology of posttraumatic osteomyelitis. *Clin Orthop Relat Res.* 1999;(360):22–29.
122. Valenziano CP, Chattar-Cora D, O'Neill A, et al. Efficacy of primary wound cultures in long bone open extremity fractures: Are they of any value? *Arch Orthop Trauma Surg.* 2002;122(5):259–261.
123. Van Nostrand D, Abreu SH, Callaghan JJ, et al. In-111-labeled white blood cell uptake in noninfected closed fracture in humans: Prospective study. *Radiology.* 1988;167(2):495–498.
124. Wald ER, Mirro R, Gartner JC. Pitfalls on the diagnosis of acute osteomyelitis by bone scan. *Clin Pediatr (Phila).* 1980;19(9):597–601.
125. Waldvogel FA, Medoff G, Swartz MN. Osteomyelitis: A review of clinical features, therapeutic considerations and unusual aspects. *N Engl J Med.* 1970;282(4):198–206.
126. Watnick P, Kolter R. Biofilm, city of microbes. *J Bacteriol.* 2000;182(10):2675–2679.
127. Weiland AJ, Moore JR, Daniel RK. The efficacy of free tissue transfer in the treatment of osteomyelitis. *J Bone Joint Surg Am.* 1984;66(2):181–193.
128. Wheat J. Diagnostic strategies in osteomyelitis. *Am J Med.* 1985;78(6B):218–224.
129. Wolf G, Aigner RM, Schwarz T. Diagnosis of bone infection using 99m Tc-HMPAO labelled leukocytes. *Nucl Med Commun.* 2001;22(11):1201–1206.
130. Ziran BH, Barrette-Grishow MK, Hull TF. Hidden burdens of orthopedic injury care: The lost providers. *J Trauma.* 2009;66(2):536–549.
131. Ziran BH, Rao N, Hall RA. A dedicated team approach enhances outcomes of osteomyelitis treatment. *Clin Orthop Relat Res.* 2003;414:31–36.
132. Ziran BH, Smith WR, Morgan SJ. Use of calcium-based demineralized bone matrix/allograft for nonunions and posttraumatic reconstruction of the appendicular skeleton: Preliminary results and complications. *J Trauma.* 2007;63(6):1324–1328.

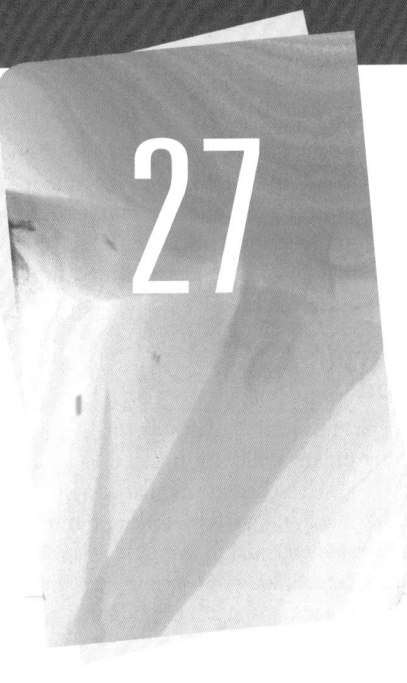

27

PRINCIPLES OF NONUNION TREATMENT

William M. Ricci and Brett Bolhofner

INTRODUCTION TO THE PRINCIPLES OF NONUNION TREATMENT AND DEFINITIONS

Bone healing is an elegant but complex biologic phenomenon. Most other tissues in the human body can only manage to heal with scar, but bone heals by forming new bone. Although fracture healing usually occurs unencumbered, it may be adversely affected or interrupted in many ways. The associated treatments, functional disability, prolonged pain, and lost wages can lead to substantial psychosocial impairment, economic burden to the patient, and stress on the health care system.[72]

Nonunion occurs when a fracture has failed to heal in the expected time and is not likely to heal without new intervention.[35,37,197] Delayed union occurs when a fracture has not completely healed in the time expected, but still has the potential to heal without further intervention. While these descriptions may seem simply put, defining the expected time for healing and identifying when healing has finally occurred can be elusive. Establishment of a nonunion can also be defined based on a lack of complete bone healing in a specified time frame, commonly 6 to 8 months, but this is arbitrary.[134]

In delayed union, clinical and radiographic evidence of healing lags behind what would ordinarily be present in a similar fracture in the same bone. This, of course, depends on the particular bone involved, the anatomic region of that bone, the fracture pattern, the energy of the original injury, the associated soft tissue damage, and the method of treatment. Comparison with healing times reported in the literature for similar fractures along with clinical experience is necessary to identify delayed union. The potential inaccuracies in this analysis are confounded by the fact that attempts to define a cellular process by reviewing radiographic data are inherently flawed. It has been suggested that cessation of the periosteal and not the endosteal healing response prior to fracture bridging may define delayed union at the cellular level.[199]

Nonunion, while often obvious in retrospect, is often difficult to define and diagnose in real time. For example, in the tibia the time for a metaphyseal fracture to be considered ununited will be different than for a fracture in the diaphysis. Both clinical and radiographic findings are necessary for the diagnosis of nonunion. However, such signs may be elusive as primary and secondary healing may be occurring simultaneously. On a cellular level, nonunion occurs when there is cessation of a reparative process antecedent to bony union.[115,318] Prior operative fracture treatment may alter the definition of nonunion and may also further complicate the ability to diagnose nonunion. While hardware failure may make the diagnosis obvious, with newer implants and techniques (locked nails and plates), a paucity of clinical symptoms and radiographic findings may persist long after progress in healing has ceased. This chapter will review the important aspects of nonunion pathophysiology including risk factors for the development of a nonunion, discuss the current methods for evaluating and diagnosing nonunions, present the common nonoperative and operative methods for treating nonunions including adjuncts to surgical treatments and their outcomes, and present and discuss the author's preferred treatments for nonunions.

PATHOPHYSIOLOGY AND ETIOLOGY OF NONUNION

Failure of an acute fracture to progress to timely union may be caused by a myriad of factors. Impaired fracture healing, delayed union and nonunion, is estimated with a combined prevalence of 6.9%.[248] A host of factors have been identified that may affect bone healing including patient age, gender, nutritional status, bone quality, endocrine disorders (most notably diabetes), smoking, fracture energy, location and pattern, associated injuries, exposure to radiation, and exposure to medications (most notably steroids, chemotherapy, and nonsteroidal anti-inflammatory drugs [NSAIDs]).[20,46] Some of these factors are and some are not within the surgeon's control.

The risk for nonunion increases with greater injury energy. Higher energy of injury is associated with greater damage to the bone and greater damage to the surrounding tissues. The damaged bone has a reduced inherent capacity to form new bone and the damaged soft tissues have a reduced ability to stimulate the reparative process. The incidence of nonunion in the presence of an open fracture and extensive soft tissue injury, not surprisingly, approaches 20%.[297] The characteristics of the original injury, the patient's ability

(or inability) to generate a normal healing response to the particular injury, the mechanical and biologic environment created by the chosen treatment method, and the presence or absence of associated infection are among the factors that can influence the rate and the likelihood of uncomplicated and timely fracture healing.

Fracture-Specific Factors Related to Nonunion

The involved bone and the specific location of the fracture within any given bone influence the innate ability for fracture healing. This is related, in large part, to the associated vascular supply to the fractured region. The talar neck, the proximal metaphyseal–diaphyseal junction of the fifth metatarsal, the femoral neck, and the waist of the scaphoid are examples of anatomic sites that have relatively limited or watershed vascular supplies that are potentially disrupted by fracture. Hence, fractures in these sites have a propensity for healing complications or the development of osteonecrosis. On the other hand, the metaphyseal regions of most other long bones as well as the pelvic bones and scapula have a robust vascular supply, and in the absence of other complicating factors, heal reliably. The diaphyseal regions of long bones, especially the tibia, fall between these extremes. The diaphyseal region of long bones has a relatively limited blood supply and therefore diaphyseal fractures usually require longer periods of time to achieve union than metaphyseal fractures and are more likely to proceed to nonunion.

Independent of the anatomic location of the fracture, the degree of bone and surrounding soft tissue injury influences the healing potential. The degree of soft tissue injury was recently identified in a survey of surgeons as one of the most important factors that contribute to the development of a nonunion.[22] High-energy fractures cause devascularization of the fractured bone in the form of periosteal stripping or disruption of the endosteal blood supply or both. This is clearly evident with open fractures (Fig. 27-1), but internal soft tissue stripping can occur equally in closed fractures. In addition, severe high-energy injuries can render the bone ends nonviable either from immediate cell death or via the process of apoptosis.[34] Bone loss, either traumatically associated with open fracture or the result of surgical debridement, is a potential precursor of nonunion. Nonunion is also closely related to the degree of open fracture by virtue of its providing a source of bacterial contamination and creating the potential for infection.

Host Factors Related to Nonunion

Host factors clearly play a major role in the potential for alterations in fracture healing. Specific conditions that are most notably considered to affect fracture healing are smoking, diabetes, and vascular disease.[22,109,208] Smoking was considered to be a major factor in the development of nonunion by 81% of polled orthopedic trauma surgeons, diabetes by 59%, and vasculopathy by 53%.[22] Other factors such as exposure to certain medications, the presence of osteoporosis, advanced age, and immunosuppression have also been implicated, with varying degrees of supportive data, as risk factors for nonunion.

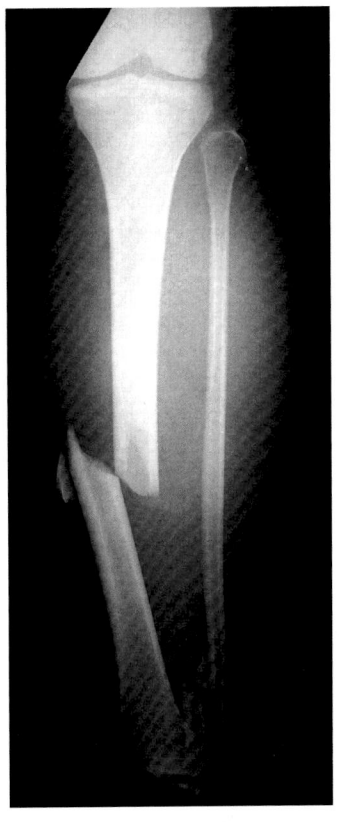

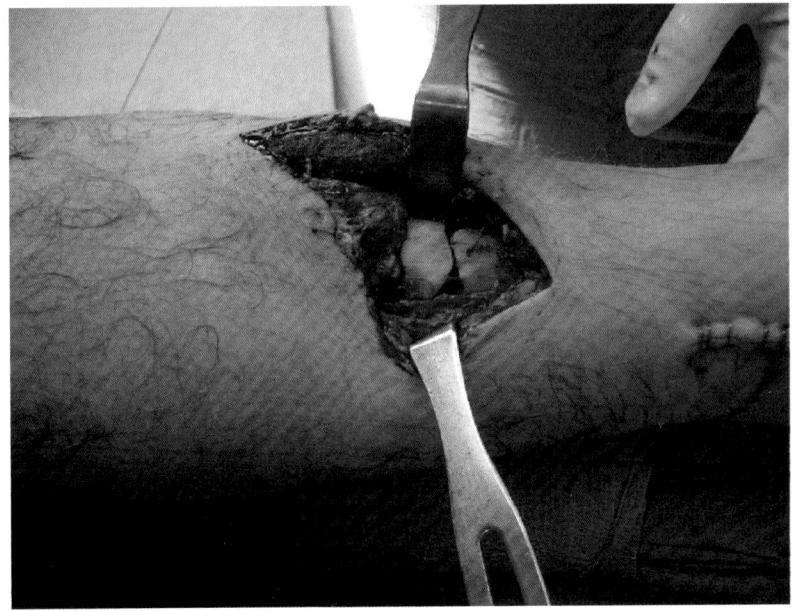

FIGURE 27-1 AP radiograph **(A)** of an open tibial shaft fracture with associated periosteal stripping seen in the clinical photograph **(B)**.

Diabetes

Laboratory evidence demonstrates that most phases of fracture healing are affected by diabetes mellitus. Decreased cellular proliferation is seen in the early phases of fracture healing[194] and decreased callus strength at the later phases.[14,107] The ultimate clinical effect of long-standing and especially uncontrolled diabetes is to increase the risk for delayed union and nonunion. It is postulated that the microvascular disease, and perhaps the reduced immunocompetence and the neuropathy associated with diabetes, leads to alterations in bone metabolism leading to delayed fracture healing.[249] Diabetes also poses greater risks for soft tissue healing complications as well as increased risk for infection after surgical fracture management.[158] The association of hyperglycemia with complications related to orthopedic surgery has been established.[122,263,301] However, it is unclear which, if any, diabetic-related comorbidities might also affect bone healing. A recent study suggested that peripheral neuropathy and hemoglobin A1c levels >7% were significantly associated with bone-healing complications in the foot and ankle.[301]

Smoking

Cigarette smoking is commonly identified by orthopedic trauma surgeons as one of the factors to cause delayed union and nonunion.[22] This perception is grounded by sound evidence linking smoking to delayed acute fracture healing,[49,148,193] and failure of nonunion treatment,[208] as well as failure of bone healing associated with spinal fusion and osteotomies.[177] Even a history of prior smoking and exposure to second-hand smoke

has been shown to delay bone healing.[49,177] Not only does smoking affect bone healing, it also increases the risk of other complications such as acute infection and osteomyelitis.[208]

Animal studies suggest that the vasoconstrictive properties of nicotine inhibit tissue differentiation and the normal angiogenic responses in the early stages of fracture healing, and that nicotine directly interferes with osteoblast function.[71,323,360] Recent human data, where samples of fractured and nonfractured bones from smokers and nonsmokers were assayed for BMP-2, -6, -4, and -7 using polymerase chain reaction, indicate that smoking reduces periosteal bone morphogenetic protein (BMP) gene expression.[53]

Smokers with open tibia fractures treated with intramedullary (IM) nails were found, in a prospective study by Castillo et al.,[49] to be 37% less likely to achieve union and 3.7 times more likely to develop osteomyelitis than nonsmokers. Smoking was also found to delay healing in a dose-dependent manner after closed management of tibial shaft fractures.[180,287] In the setting of Ilizarov limb reconstruction, McKee et al.[208] demonstrated that smoking was associated with multiple complications. The overall complication rate was over three times higher in the smokers compared with nonsmokers including higher rates of persistent infection, nonunion, and amputation.

Despite being one of the few risk factors that is potentially modifiable, smoking cessation in the face of the stresses associated with acute fracture is exceedingly difficult. Despite these challenges, it is prudent to advocate and support smoking cessation in all patients with fractures at risk for nonunion and in those facing nonunion repair. Given the direct adverse effects of nicotine on bone healing, nicotine supplementation (e.g., nicotine patch) as part of a smoking cessation program should be avoided. This concept is supported by animal data linking transdermal nicotine to nonunion and decreased mechanical strength of healing fractures.[84]

Nonsteroidal Anti-Inflammatory Drugs

Nonsteroidal anti-inflammatory medications, once used ubiquitously to control postfracture pain, have been implicated in inducing fracture nonunion.[215] These medications are now used much more sparingly in the setting of acute fracture or nonunion repair, especially in the initial weeks after injury, a time corresponding to the inflammatory phase of fracture healing. The initial biologic healing response to fracture is an inflammatory process. Therefore, it is logical that NSAIDs may be inhibitors of this process. Prostaglandins are inflammatory mediators present during the initial phases of fracture healing. Their synthesis from arachidonic acid is catalyzed by the cyclooxygenase (COX) enzymes. Both traditional NSAIDs and selective COX-2 inhibitors have been found to interfere with COX-2 up-regulation and therefore prostaglandin synthesis, including such synthesis in healing bone.[116,258]

Results of clinical studies on the effect of NSAIDs on fracture healing have yielded conflicting recommendations.[15,60,114,175,255,295] Adding to the controversy is alleged fraudulent research activity in this area that led to retraction of at least 20 articles and has cast doubt on some results.[83,341] A number of important clinical factors related to NSAID use in the face of fracture healing were investigated in a recent meta-analysis of over 10,000 patients.[83] Exposure was found to increase the risk of nonunion (odds ratio 3); however, lower study quality was found to be a confounding variable. Lower study quality was associated with higher risk of nonunion. Lower quality studies affected the association of NSAID use with spinal union rate, but not with long-bone fracture healing. When only moderate quality long-bone fracture studies were considered in isolation, NSAID exposure still was associated with an increased risk of nonunion (odds ratio 4.4). No association of factors, including dose or route (parenteral or oral) of administration or duration of treatment, was found to affect the risk of nonunion. Although these data provide no clear contraindication to NSAIDs in patients with healing bone, it appears reasonable to use alternative medications when possible.

Other Medications and Systemic Conditions

Other chronic health conditions, although not directly shown to negatively impact fracture healing, empirically can lead to altered healing responses. Any state leading to malnutrition or immunosuppression, including steroid use, rheumatoid disease, and malignancy, can negatively impact the body's healing response including fracture healing. Previously irradiated bone or bone actively infiltrated with tumor also are at high risk for delayed union or nonunion.[47] Although children clearly have higher healing potential than adults, whether advanced age, once physeal closure has occurred, is an independent risk factor for nonunion is unclear.[132] Advanced age was found to be an independent risk factor for nonunion in patients with an acute clavicle fracture,[269]

but other prognostic studies have failed to identify age as a risk factor for nonunion in other anatomic locations.[25,61] Although osteoporosis is clearly a risk factor for acute fracture, once fracture has occurred, osteoporosis does not appear to be a risk factor for the subsequent occurrence of nonunion.[329]

Bisphosphonates are a class of drugs that prevent bone loss by decreasing osteoclastic mediated bone turnover and have been used successfully in the treatment of osteoporosis, most commonly in the form of the drug alendronate. Recently, long-term use of bisphosphonates have been implicated in the development of atypical stress fractures,[124,186,220,298] and with impaired healing of these fractures. According to the task force of the American Society for Bone and Mineral Research, the major criteria for atypical femur fractures are location between the lesser trochanter and the supracondylar flare, association with minimal trauma, transverse or short oblique configuration, lack of comminution, and a medial spike in complete fractures.[298] The atypical fractures have characteristic radiographic findings including a simple transverse fracture, cortical thickening, and medial beaking at the fracture site. Additional minor features include prodromal symptoms, the use of bisphosphonates, and delayed healing. Cessation of bisphosphonates has been suggested to help promote union in the face of an atypical fracture.[76,227] However, given the long half-life of the drug and that physiologic effects are thought to continue for at least 5 years after discontinued use, it is unclear if cessation is of any clinical utility.

Treatment Factors Related to Nonunion

Appropriate mechanical stability is required to create an environment conducive to fracture healing. Unfortunately, appropriate stability is very difficult to define and even more difficult to quantify. In fact, the desired degree of stability depends, to a great extent, on the chosen method of stabilization. The natural process of bone healing, commonly referred to as secondary bone healing, through the formation of callus relies on micromotion at the fracture site. In nature, fractures can heal without stabilization, but stabilization can reduce the risk of nonunion. The use of external immobilization such as with a splint, as a method to effect fracture healing, evolved from an effort to control pain. Medical practice has similarly evolved to understand that fractures heal more reliably when immobilized. Indeed, most fractures heal with the relatively limited stability provided by splint or cast immobilization. Rigid internal fixation, as provided by the compression plating technique, represents the opposite end of the stability spectrum associated with fracture care. Rigidly stabilized fractures heal without callus via primary bone healing, a relatively unnatural, yet successful, strategy.

Regardless of whether the chosen treatment method relies on primary or secondary bone healing, improper technique can lead to an increased risk of nonunion. A poorly applied cast or one applied to a severely lipomatous extremity, for instance, may provide inadequate stability resulting in excessive fracture site motion and the development of nonunion. It is often difficult to predict the fracture healing response to excessive motion, as either abundant callus or a paucity of callus may result (Fig. 27-2). Relatively rigid internal fixation techniques that fail to accomplish bone-to-bone contact and compression

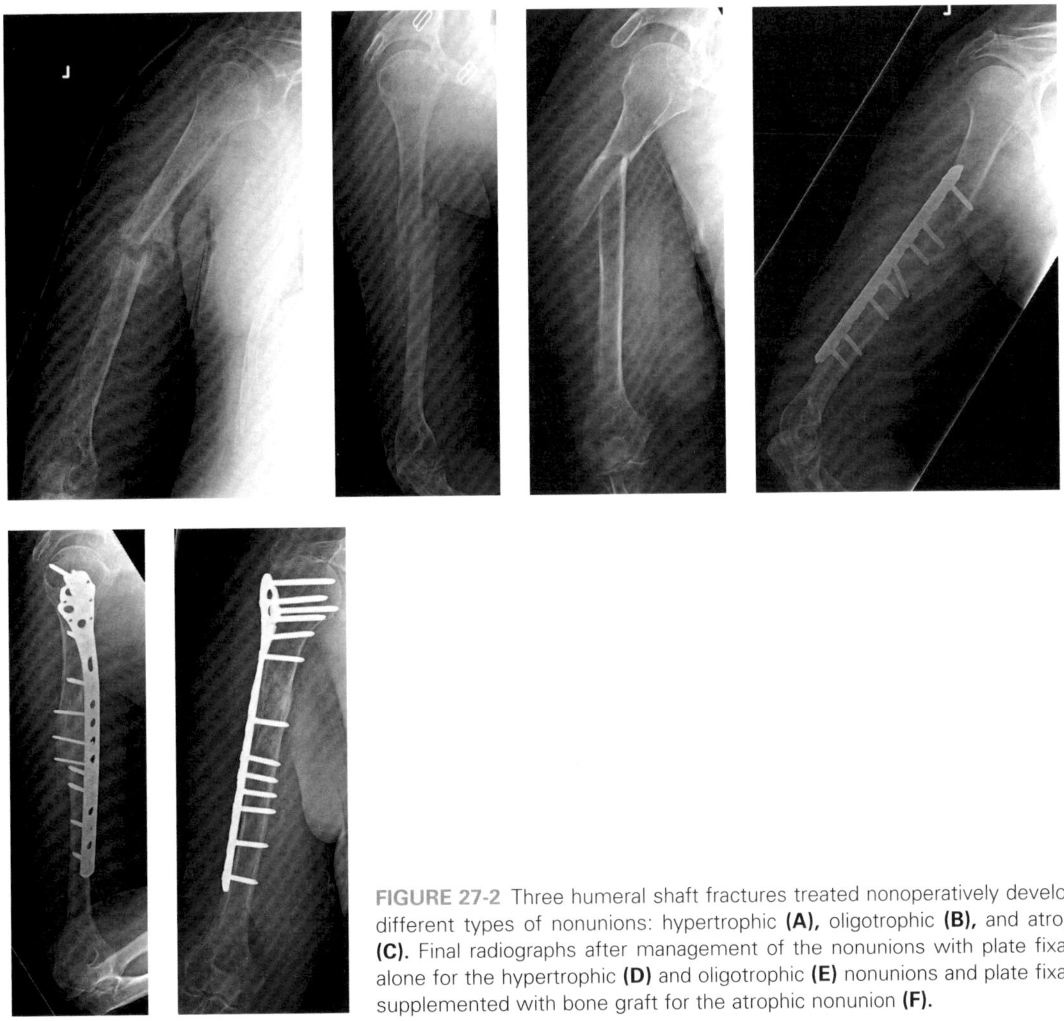

A, B

C, D

E, F

FIGURE 27-2 Three humeral shaft fractures treated nonoperatively developed different types of nonunions: hypertrophic **(A)**, oligotrophic **(B)**, and atrophic **(C)**. Final radiographs after management of the nonunions with plate fixation alone for the hypertrophic **(D)** and oligotrophic **(E)** nonunions and plate fixation supplemented with bone graft for the atrophic nonunion **(F)**.

(i.e., ones with gaps at the fracture site) do not support the primary bone healing process, which relies upon direct remodeling of bone via cutting cones that traverse the fracture, and can also lead to nonunion (Fig. 27-3). Whereas modern surgical techniques emphasize biologically friendly tissue handling, older techniques that included anatomic reduction of individual fracture fragments were at the expense of soft tissue stripping from the fracture fragments and led to a suboptimal environment for fracture healing. Whether fracture reduction is direct or indirect, or the fixation construct is relatively stable or rigid,

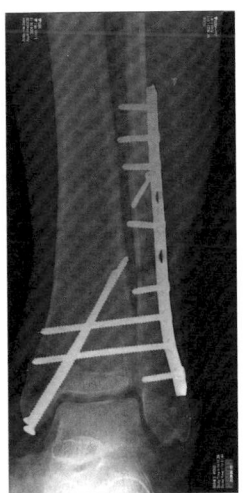
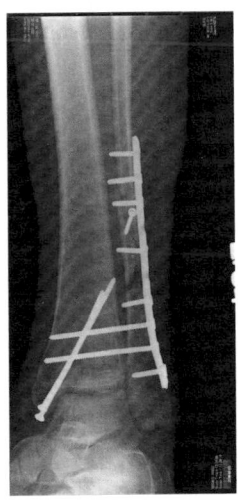
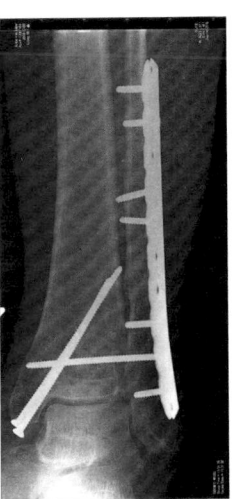

FIGURE 27-3 Postoperative radiograph showing fibular fracture gap **(A)**. At 3 months postoperatively, the gap persists **(B)**. Nonunion repair with bone grafting yields union **(C)**.

A, B

C

minimizing soft tissue disruption is paramount to maximizing the healing potential and minimizing other complications that relate to devitalization of bone, namely infection.

Infection as a Factor Related to Development of Nonunion

Fractures can heal in the face of infection; however, even a suppressed infection may substantially alter the healing process, and uncontrolled osteomyelitis can inhibit normal fracture healing altogether (Fig. 27-4). The inflammatory process in response to infection may inhibit fracture healing by causing excessive remodeling and osteolysis.[105] Tissue necrosis may be accelerated by infection, but histologic evidence indicates that soft tissue disruption caused by the initial trauma and surgical insult are the primary events leading to bone necrosis in cases of osteomyelitis associated with fracture.[226] Loose nonvital bone fragments and bone pieces demarcated by osteoclastic activity are eventually transformed into sequestra (Fig. 27-5).[226] Infection not only predisposes to nonunion, but makes nonunion repair substantially more complex, often requiring multistaged treatment protocols that are discussed later in this chapter.

CLASSIFICATION OF NONUNION

Nonunions may be classified based on the presence or absence of infection and the relative biologic activity of the fracture site. Septic nonunion implies that there is an infectious process at the site while aseptic nonunion is the absence of infection. Further

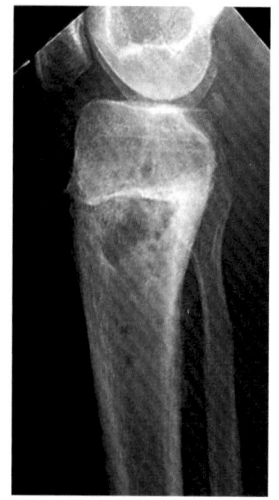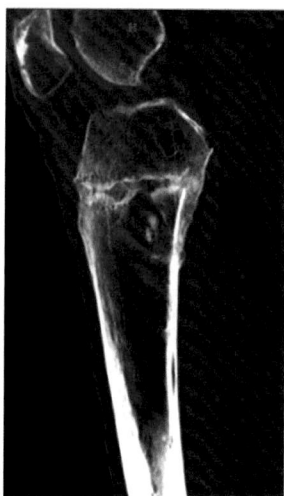

FIGURE 27-5 Lateral radiograph **(A)** and sagittal CT scan **(B)** showing a sequestrum.

classification of nonunion is an attempt at describing the biologic occurrences or lack thereof at the fracture site. Atrophic, oligotrophic, and hypertrophic nonunions represent increasing biologic potential for fracture healing. Radiographic analysis is the most common method used to distinguish among these classification types. Any inherent interpretation inaccuracies are confounded by attempting to identify a biologic phenomenon by radiographic analysis.

Atrophic Nonunion

Atrophic nonunion, also referred to as avascular, nonviable, or avital nonunion indicates poor healing response with little or no bone-forming cells active at the fracture site.[205,210] The blood supply to an atrophic nonunion is typically poor. This is typically manifested radiographically by the absence of any bone reaction (Figs. 27-2C and 27-3). This lack of healing response may be because of the injury (e.g., open fracture) or subsequent surgical treatment (e.g., surgical stripping of soft tissues about the fracture site) or because of host issues (e.g., diabetes or smoking).[285] Strategies for the treatment of atrophic nonunions generally include a method to provide a biologic stimulus to the fracture site, most commonly with autogenous bone graft or BMP. Debridement or excision of nonvital bone ends is another principle for the management of atrophic nonunion. The degree of bone resection can vary greatly depending upon the mode of treatment to be utilized and the presence or absence of infection. An aseptic atrophic nonunion treated with compression plating will require little bone resection, whereas a septic atrophic nonunion treated with Ilizarov methods including bone transport may benefit from a relatively large area of bone resection.

Hypertrophic Nonunion

At the other end of the spectrum from atrophic nonunion is hypertrophic nonunion, also referred to as hypervascular, viable, or vital nonunion. Associated is an adequate healing response with satisfactory vascularity.[206,211] These fractures lack adequate stability to progress to union. The viable healing fibrocartilage

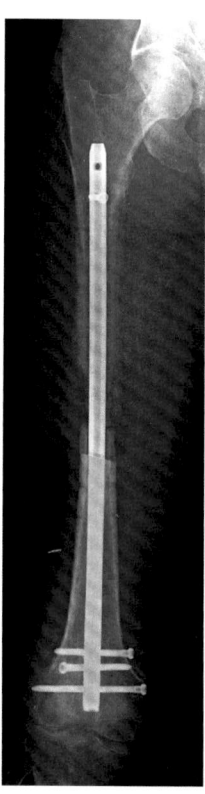

FIGURE 27-4 AP radiograph of an infected nonunion of the femur after IM nailing.

cannot mineralize because of unfavorable mechanical factors at the fracture site.[285] This is manifested radiographically by callus formation, usually abundant, with an interceding area of fibrocartilage-lacking mineral, and so appearing dark on standard radiographs. Hypertrophic nonunions can occur after initial nonoperative management (Fig. 27-2A) or after attempts at operative stabilization (Fig. 27-6A,B). Successful treatment of hypertrophic nonunions utilizes methods to provide the stability required to allow the adequate biologic response to complete (Figs. 27-2D and 27-6C–F). Rigid stabilization allows chondrocyte-mediated mineralization of the fibrocartilage at the hypertrophic nonunion site, usually by 8 weeks. Resection or debridement of the aseptic hypertrophic nonunion is neither required nor desired. Unlike atrophic nonunions, biologic stimulus, such as bone grafting, is not a treatment necessity for hypertrophic nonunions.

Oligotrophic Nonunion

Oligotrophic nonunions probably represent a condition somewhere between atrophic and hypertrophic nonunions. They are viable, but usually manifest minimal radiographic healing reaction (callus), often because of inadequate approximation of the fracture surfaces (Figs. 27-2B and 27-7). A bone scan may be necessary to distinguish this type of nonunion from a frankly atrophic one. The oligotrophic situation will be manifested by increased uptake where the atrophic situation would be relative cold on bone scan.[306] Management of oligotrophic nonunions usually involves addressing deficiencies in bone contact either by mechanical compression or bone grafting of associated defects or a combination of biologic and mechanical methods (Fig. 27-7B and C).

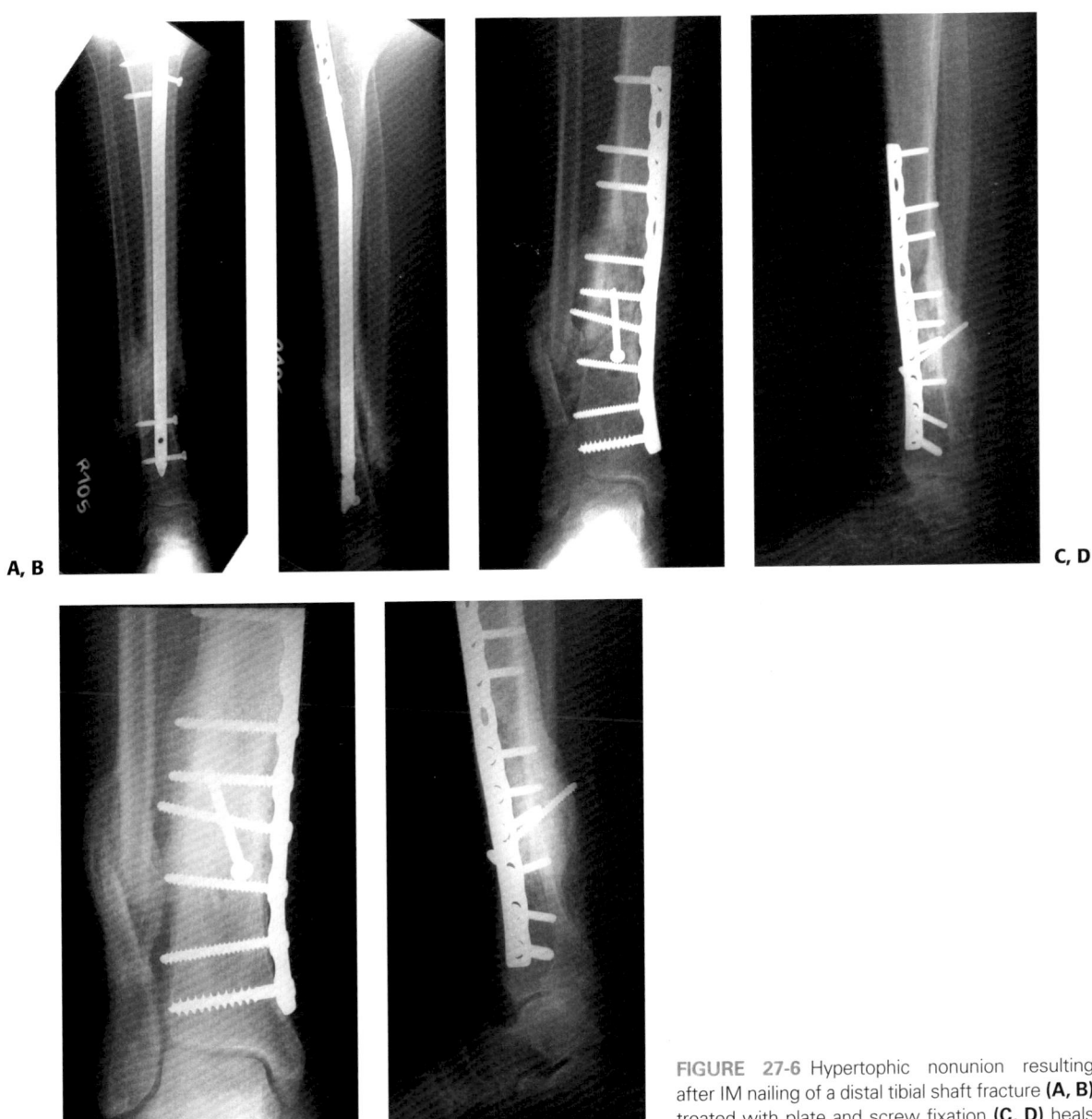

A, B

C, D

E, F

FIGURE 27-6 Hypertrophic nonunion resulting after IM nailing of a distal tibial shaft fracture **(A, B)** treated with plate and screw fixation **(C, D)** heals without adjuvant bone graft **(E, F)**.

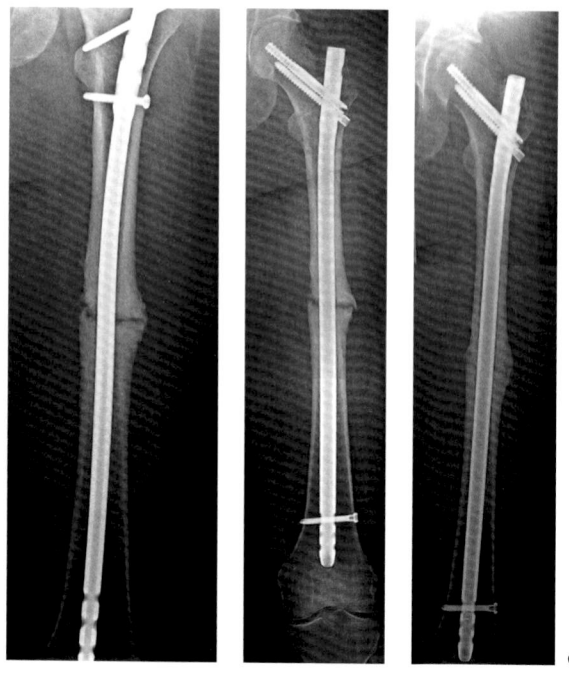

A, B   **C**

FIGURE 27-7 An oligotrophic femoral shaft nonunion after initial IM nailing **(A)** treated with exchange nailing **(B)** heals uneventfully **(C)** probably as the result of bone graft generated by reaming and improved stability.

Pseudoarthrosis

Pseudoarthrosis, a subclassification of nonunion, has properties of hypertrophic nonunion, but because of excessive and chronic motion, an actual synovial pseudocapsule is formed, containing fluid much like an actual synovial joint (Fig. 27-8).

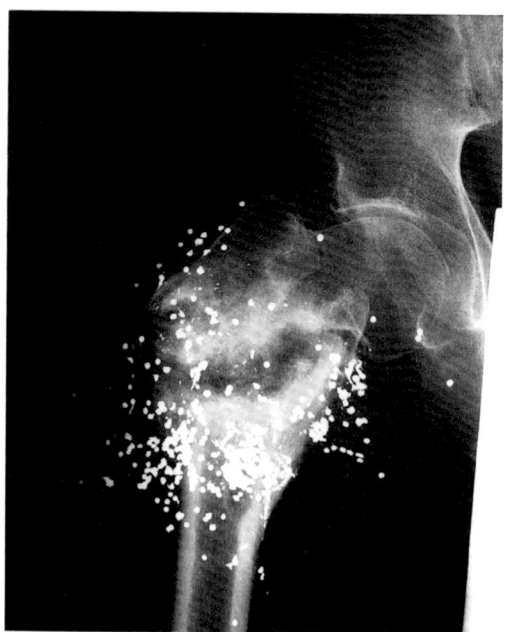

FIGURE 27-8 Pseudoarthrosis 20 years after shotgun injury and nonoperative treatment.

The medullary ends are usually sealed and an interceding cold cleft is noted on bone scan. Management of these nonunions usually requires debridement of the pseudoarthrosis, opening of the medullary canal, and enhancement of stability, typically with compression at the nonunion site. Although these nonunions are technically vital, biologic stimulation can be helpful to promote more rapid and reliable healing.

EVALUATION AND DIAGNOSIS OF NONUNION

The diagnosis of nonunion is an inexact science even when ignoring the temporal issues of defining when a fracture should or should not yet be considered a nonunion. At any given time point, determining if a fracture is united or not, is more straightforward than diagnosing a nonunion, but this is not a simple task either. Bone healing is a progressive process where the strength of the reparative process, under usual circumstances, gradually increases over a period of time. Clinical attempts to define union are hampered by utilizing indirect means to evaluate the strength of the healing process. Further, even if the strength of the healing bone could be accurately evaluated, neither the baseline strength of the uninjured bone nor the fraction of that value required to achieve union is known. However, technologic advances in microelectronics have made measurement of mechanical properties of healing bone possible. A recent preliminary report evaluated a telemetric system to measure bending load in a titanium internal fixator to determine if clinically relevant information could be drawn from its application.[294] Well before radiographic signs of healing could be detected, a substantial decrease in elasticity of the fixator was recorded. This and similar technologies have the potential to revolutionize the evaluation of fracture healing and also to change the management of healing fractures. It will be possible to identify progression towards union or nonunion and to accurately define a healed fracture without the use of ionizing radiation. Accelerated weight bearing could be allowed or reduction in activity recommended based on automated systems that evaluate real time data. Prior to the maturation of this exciting new technology, clinicians must continue to rely on indirect means in the evaluation of fracture healing and in determining if union has occurred.

Depending on the modality being used, the diagnosis of a nonunion may be one of inclusion or exclusion. That is, when evidence of union exists, then nonunion is ruled out. Some diagnostic modalities such as a bone scan may directly identify nonunion by a positive test result. In usual clinical practice, the information gathered from many modalities, such as history, physical examination, radiographs, and other special tests is used in concert to determine the presence or absence of fracture union. Since the majority of these evaluation tools are subjective, each clinician can interpret results differently and assign different relative importance to various measures. This leads to inherent difficulty in establishing uniform and agreed-upon definitions of delayed union and nonunion.[22,24,67,199] A recent survey of 335 orthopaedic trauma surgeons endorsed that currently there exists a lack of standardization in the definitions of delayed union and nonunion.[22] These surgeons did agree that these definitions should account for both radiographic and clinical criteria.

History and Physical Examination Related to Nonunion

History and physical examination are critically important to both the initial evaluation of the patient being scrutinized to determine the presence or absence of fracture union after acute fracture, as well as the patient suspected of having an established nonunion. The history of the events surrounding the index injury provides insight into any deviations from the normal course of fracture healing for the particular fracture being evaluated. This information may heighten the index of suspicion for not only nonunion but also for associated problems such as infection. The mechanism of injury, and perhaps more importantly, the energy associated with injury, have implications regarding fracture healing. Higher energy injuries, by virtue of the greater damage done to the bone and surrounding tissues, have a higher risk for healing complications. Similarly, the nature of the associated soft tissue injury may be prognostic for delayed bone healing. If the fracture was open, delayed fracture healing is expected and infection becomes more common.

The details of prior treatments and subsequent recovery complete the history of the problem at hand. It is important to uncover the type and timing of the initial treatments and any subsequent interventions. The indication for the specific details of, and the result of any additional procedures should be identified. Specifically, it is critical to distinguish if secondary debridement procedures were done as planned prophylactic procedures or for the treatment of a documented infection. Causative organisms, antibiotic susceptibilities, and details of antibiotic treatments should be elucidated. The clinical response to such treatments can provide valuable insight into future responses to similar treatment. The nature of prior surgical procedures aimed at augmenting fracture healing provides useful information regarding the diagnosis and helps direct future treatments. It is important to distinguish prior implant removal performed for pain from similar procedures done to promote fracture healing such as nail dynamization. With a history of prior bone grafting, it should be clarified if the graft was autologous or otherwise. If autologous, the prior harvest site is confirmed with physical examination such that if future graft harvest is contemplated a unique site can be prepared for. If there was treatment with bone growth stimulators, such devices may be incorporated in future treatments with little or no additional patient expense.

The typical signs and symptoms of nonunion are a combination of pain, tenderness, and detectible motion at the site of fracture. It should be noted that symptoms of nonunion can be masked in patients with relatively stable or rigid fixation such as is seen with locked plate constructs. It is not uncommon for such patients to present with the acute or subacute onset of pain and disability associated with implant fracture subsequent to a period of full weight bearing with no or a relative paucity of symptoms (Fig. 27-9). In these circumstances, the loss of stability accompanying implant failure incites the onset of symptoms. In a recent opinion poll of orthopedic trauma surgeons, the lack of ability to bear weight was felt to be the most important clinical factor in diagnosing a lower extremity nonunion followed by fracture pain, weight-bearing status, and tenderness on palpation.[22]

Radiographic Assessment of Nonunion
Plain Radiographs

Plain radiographs are used ubiquitously in the evaluation of fractures as they provide timely, accurate, and inexpensive

A, B 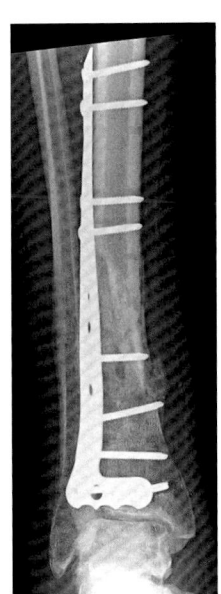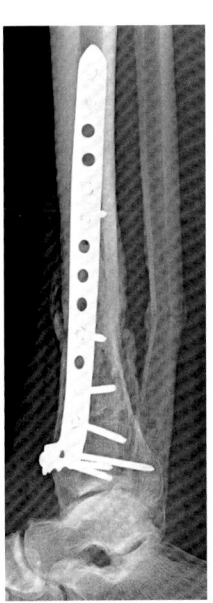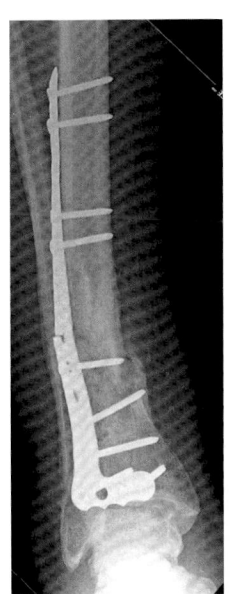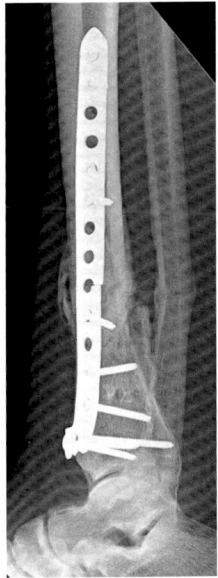 **C, D**

FIGURE 27-9 At 4 months after distal tibia nonunion repair, radiographs **(A, B)** and painless weight bearing suggest union. Two weeks later, the patient presents with increasing pain with weight bearing. Radiographs **(C, D)** show plate failure indicating a persistent nonunion.

means to diagnose an acute fracture. The utility of plain radiographs in evaluating fracture union is less clear. As the process of fracture healing is slow and progressive, when "union" occurs is often difficult to determine. Plain radiographs often help with the diagnosis of nonunion by excluding union.

The diagnosis of fracture union by plain radiographs is typically defined by the presence of bridging callus across the fracture. Whether circumferential bridging, as evidenced by bridging across four cortices on orthogonal x-rays, is required to accurately diagnose union is without consensus. The orthopedic literature is conflicted with regard to this requirement as different studies can define union as healing across only two or three, rather than four, cortices on orthogonal views.[22] Although identifying the number of healed cortices may seem straightforward, in practice this is a very subjective and imprecise exercise especially in the presence of implants that obscure visualization. Furthermore, it is often difficult to know if the radiograph and fracture are coplanar. When not, fracture gaps may be disguised by overlying bone. Minor variances in the angle of the x-ray beam can completely disguise a nonunion (Fig. 27-10). Scoring systems have been proposed to better quantify information gathered from plain radiographs to help predict healing, most notably the Radiographic Union Score for Tibia Fractures (RUST), but they have not yet gained widespread clinical use.[340]

The location and type of fracture and the relative stability of the fixation method creates great variations in the expected biologic healing response, and therefore, variations in the expected radiographic appearance of union. Simple diaphyseal fractures fixed anatomically with rigid compression plate techniques that promote primary bone healing without fracture callus may look nearly identical at healing as they did immediately after fixation (Fig. 27-11). Abundant fracture callus would be unexpected.

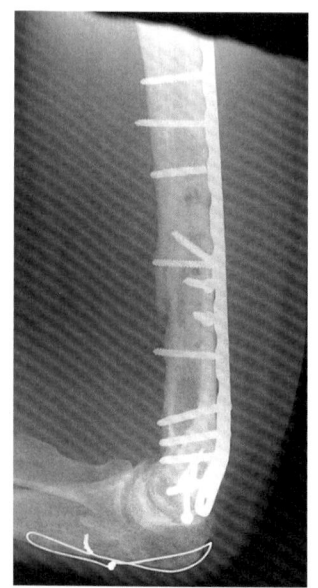
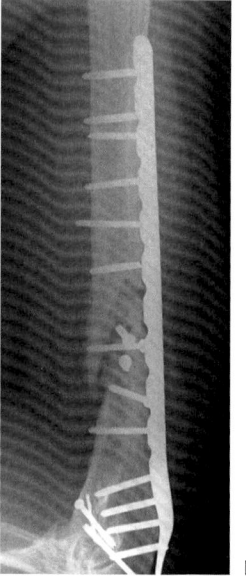

FIGURE 27-10 A lateral radiograph **(A)** fails to clearly identify a nonunion 8 months after ORIF of a distal humeral shaft fracture, whereas a slight oblique from the lateral projection **(B)** clearly shows the nonunion.

Under these circumstances, accurate diagnosis of union may be difficult, but lack of union may be directly or indirectly evident. Direct evidence is a fracture gap seen on a radiograph taken coplanar with the fracture (Fig. 27-10B). In the absence of direct evidence of nonunion, plain radiographs should be carefully scrutinized for indirect evidence for incomplete healing. Progressively loosened or broken implants indicate persistent motion at the fracture. More subtle findings are motion artifacts seen in bone at or around the margin of seemingly stable implants or fractured screws without complete loss of fixation (Fig. 27-12). Judicious utilization of other imaging methods helps to confirm the diagnosis of nonunions when only indirect evidence is present using plain radiographs. It should be noted that fracture healing can continue and sometimes is augmented by implant fracture. An example is "auto-dynamization" of an IM nail where interlocking screws fracture allowing dynamic compression at the fracture site. This phenomenon can also occur after plate fixation (Fig. 27-13), but is often associated with progressive malalignment which may or may not be problematic.

Computed Tomography

Computed tomography (CT) offers an opportunity to more accurately delineate bony anatomy at the site of a suspected nonunion than does plain radiography. Modern CT scans can be reformatted in high quality in any plane. This allows image orientation precisely optimized to evaluate potential absence of bridging bone, eliminating the major shortcoming of plain radiography. CT scans have been shown to be highly sensitive (100%) for detecting tibial nonunion.[26] The limitation of CT, however, is a relative lack of specificity (62%) that can lead to surgery in patients who have healed fractures (Fig. 27-14).[26]

In the future, CT may prove to provide a quantitative evaluation of not just union, but fracture stability. In one study, patients with less than 25% bridging of the circumference of bone were found to be at high risk (37.5%) for clinical failure of fracture union, whereas those with greater than 25% bridging had only a 9.7% failure rate.[68] Finally, an added benefit of CT is the ability to evaluate rotational deformities associated with nonunion.

Nuclear Imaging

The use of bone scintigraphy dates back to the 1920s. A multitude of radioactive materials have been applied to the diagnosis of musculoskeletal pathologies including Technetium-99m (^{99m}Tc), Indium-111 (^{111}In), Galliumcitrate-67 (^{67}Ga), and Fluorine-18 (^{18}F).[219,292] Technetium-99m methylene diphosphonate (Tc-99m) bone scintigraphy can be used to help diagnose nonunion. The major limitation of this technique is that a positive result can be relatively nonspecific. The vast majority of nonunions show an intense tracer uptake at the fracture site, as do fractures undergoing normal healing.[284] Various other types of scans used individually or in combination have been used in attempts to differentiate simple nonunion from those that are complicated by infection. Increased blood flow and blood pool as demonstrated during the first and second phases of a three-phase bone scan are consistent with the inflammatory reaction seen with infection, but are not pathognomonic

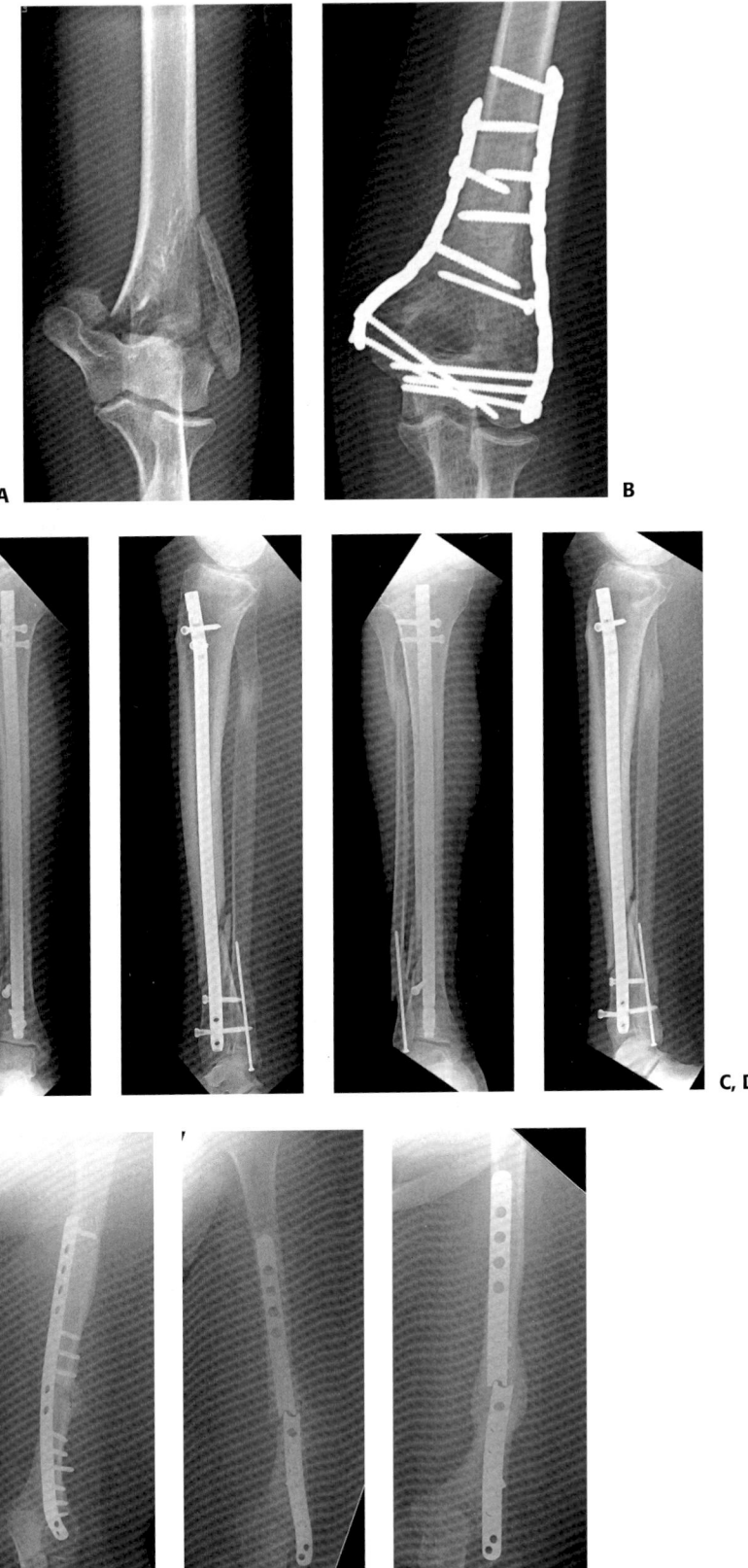

FIGURE 27-11 A distal humerus fracture. **A:** treated with rigid fixation. **B:** yields fracture healing without callus.

FIGURE 27-12 Radiographs showing a healing tibia fracture after IM nailing **(A, B).** One month later a fractured distal interlock confirms fracture nonunion **(C, D).**

FIGURE 27-13 A patient with an open distal humeral shaft fracture **(A)** was treated with irrigation and debridement and plate fixation **(B).** Despite having a nonunion at 6 months, she was functioning well and without pain because of the stability provided by the plate. An acute increase in pain resulted from failure of the plate **(C).** The fracture then healed in slight varus without further surgery **(D).**

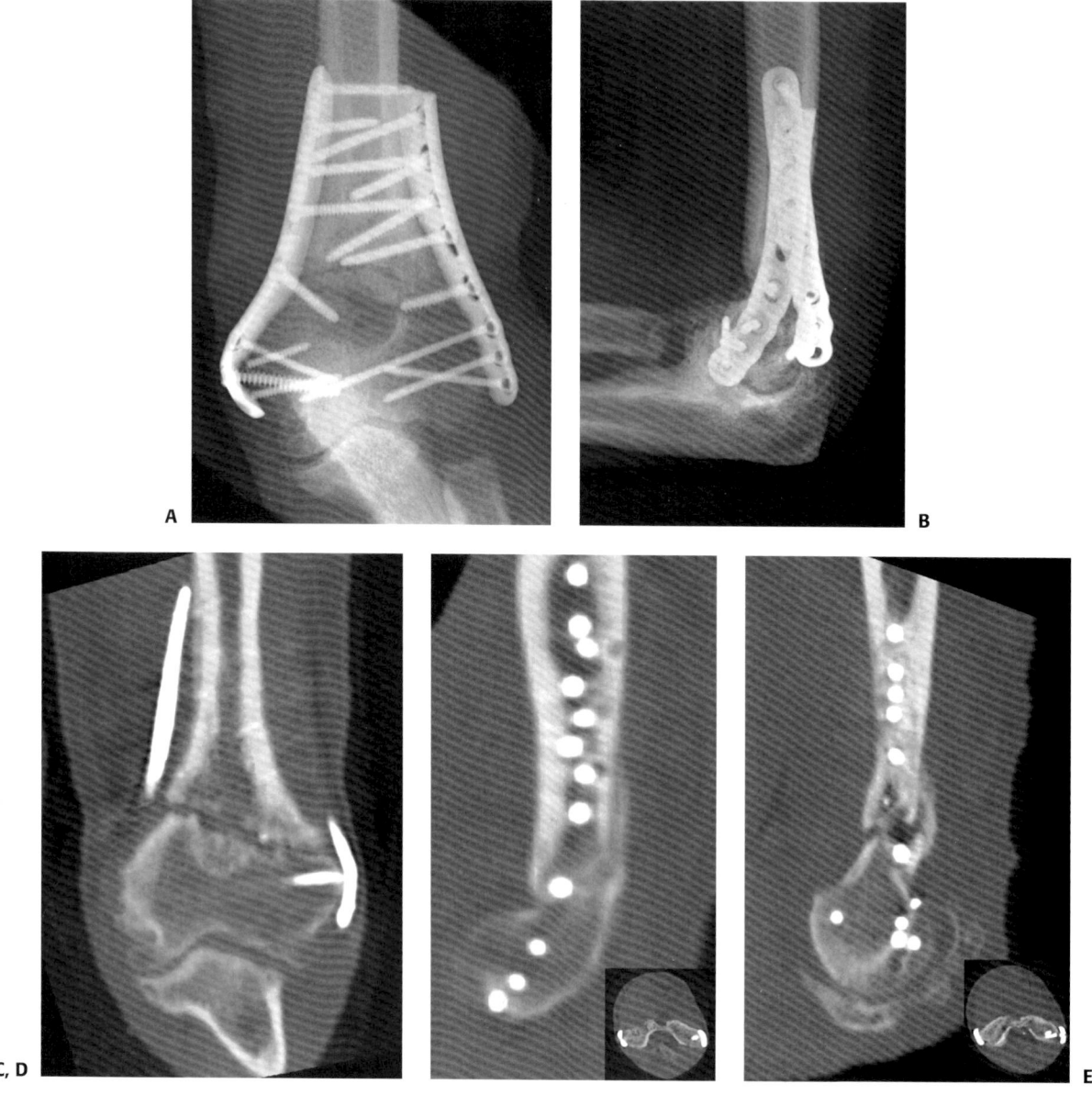

FIGURE 27-14 Lack of specificity of CT in the diagnosis of nonunion. AP and lateral radiographs **(A, B)** 6 months after repair of a distal humeral nonunion show equivocal healing. Coronal CT **(C)** demonstrates a lucent line consistent with nonunion prompting revision nonunion repair where solid healing, rather than nonunion, was encountered. Further scrutiny of the CT reveals healing of the posterior cortices of the medial **(D)** and lateral **(E)** columns.

for infection. Combined use of a Tc-99m and a Gallium-67 scan has produced inconsistent results for accurately detecting infection at the site of nonunion.[92,284] In contrast to other forms of nonunion, a synovial pseudoarthrosis correlates with the presence of a cold cleft between two intense areas of uptake on scintigraphy.[93] Newer technologies such as single-photon emission computed tomography (SPECT) have been investigated for use in differentiating infected from noninfected and vital from nonvital nonunions.[189] The technology appears to have high specificity but low sensitivity to confirm nonviability at a nonunion site.

Laboratory Studies for the Diagnosis of Nonunion

Given that clinical and radiographic evidence is unreliable for the early detection and prediction of eventual nonunion, repeated efforts have been made to identify reliable laboratory tests to evaluate bone healing. If reliable, early prediction of eventual nonunion would provide an opportunity for early intervention to prevent subsequent nonunion and thereby reduce associated time, pain, costs, and disability. Markers of bone metabolism are natural targets for such investigation but have not yet been proven to be clinically reliable.[69] The main application of laboratory tests in the setting of a nonunion is to help diagnose associated infection. This topic is discussed briefly in the later section of this chapter related to infected nonunions and in detail in the chapter dedicated to orthopedic infections and osteomyelitis, Chapter 26.

Nonunion Treatment

Objectives and General Principles of Nonunion Treatment

Regardless of the chosen method for operative nonunion repair, there are common principles that can be applied. As with most medical conditions, accurately identifying the diagnosis is a critical first step to designing a rational treatment plan. This is especially important when dealing with nonunions. Classifying the nonunion as either hypertrophic, oligotrophic, atrophic, or pseudoarthrosis, identifying whether it is septic or aseptic, and recognizing associated deformity are each critical to the formulation of a complete diagnosis and then the preferred treatment plan. The classification of the nonunion dictates whether a direct exposure and debridement is required and if adjuvant bone grafting is indicated. Hypertrophic nonunions, by definition, have inherent biologic capacity but lack sufficient mechanical stability required for completion of union. Treatment for this diagnosis is therefore focused upon increasing, and often maximizing, mechanical stability. More rigid forms of fixation such as plate fixation or a snug fitting nail in a diaphyseal region are generally preferred to less rigid means such as bridge plating techniques or loose fitting nails in metaphyseal regions. Because hypertrophic nonunions have the biologic potential to heal, debridement of the nonunion site and bone grafting is not an absolute requirement to accomplish union (Figs. 27-2A and 27-2D).[155]

Atrophic nonunions and pseudoarthroses have in common the need for debridement of the nonunion site despite atrophic nonunions being considered avital whereas pseudoarthroses are vital. Principles of atrophic nonunion management call for debridement of the nonviable bone ends back to healthy bleeding bone. Both of these classes of nonunions also typically require bone grafting. The relative paucity of healing potential of an atrophic nonunion calls for a graft with osteoinductive or osteogenic properties. A pseudoarthrosis, once debrided, has viable vascular ends, and technically speaking, may therefore not require a bone graft. However, in the absence of bone transport or purposeful shortening, graft material is usually used to fill the gap that is invariably left by debriding the synovial tissue central to the pseudoarthrosis. Oligotrophic nonunions are intermediate in their biologic capacity. Whether failure to unite was related to a primary problem of biology or a problem related to mechanics or a combination of both can be difficult to establish. It is therefore prudent to aim treatment of oligotrophic nonunions at improving both the biologic and mechanical environment.

Control, and preferably eradication, of any associated infection is another general principle of nonunion treatment. Even complex nonunions can be successfully treated in the absence of infection while simple nonunions can be recalcitrant in the presence of infection. If infection is diagnosed before initiating nonunion treatment, then treatment of the infection becomes a priority over treatment of the nonunion. Occasionally, infection and nonunion can be treated simultaneously with success. However, in most circumstances, it is prudent to optimize infection treatment first followed by optimal nonunion treatment. This strategy of serial, rather than parallel, treatments for infection and nonunion is at the expense of additional treatment duration. Optimal management of infection associated with nonunion begins with removal of associated implants. Serial debridement of necrotic soft tissues and bone follows until a stable healthy environment is accomplished. Skeletal stabilization by means that are conducive to eradication of infection calls for sparing the zone of infection from implants, typically with external fixation devices. Internal fixation is generally avoided with the notable exception of antibiotic-coated IM nails that have recently been shown to be successful in this scenario.[229,257,319] Also, certain anatomic areas, most notably the proximal femur, are not well suited for external fixation or antibiotic nails. In these circumstances, clinical judgment dictates whether plate/screw constructs or no internal fixation should be pursued. Infection treatment continues with organism-specific antibiotics, usually delivered parentally for 6 weeks. Once clinical and laboratory data indicate infection control, definitive treatment of the nonunion ensues. If conversion of external to internal fixation is planned, then a staged protocol consisting of removal of the external fixators and cast application (when it is reasonably appropriate) allows pin site healing prior to definitive nonunion surgery. On occasion, union can be accomplished concurrent with the antibiotic phase of nonunion treatment, but infection treatment should not be compromised toward this goal.

In the presence of a malaligned nonunion, correction of any associated deformity is paramount to a successful outcome. Correction of alignment not only restores normal anatomy and improves the potential for functional recovery, but it is also critical to establishing appropriate mechanics at the site of nonunion to maximally promote healing.

Finally, of critical importance to the choices made for treatment of a nonunion are the patient's individual response to prior treatment, their current level of disability, time constraints for future weight-bearing restrictions, and their occupational needs. With all other factors being equal, the patient with a progressive increase in pain and disability from an ununited fracture is more likely to benefit from surgical intervention than a patient with minimal or improving symptoms. Conversely, the patient with clear radiographic signs of nonunion but with limited pain and marginal functional disability may be more suited for less invasive treatment means such as external bone growth stimulation, especially if comorbid conditions made surgery risky or if restrictions after operative management would result in untimely loss of employment.

Soft Tissue Management Associated with Nonunion

In many cases, the soft tissues about nonunions are compromised by the original injury or subsequent surgeries. In situations where operative treatment is planned, it may be necessary to acquire soft tissue coverage with local, rotational, or free tissue flaps prior to successful nonunion repair. This is especially true if plate fixation is contemplated for stabilization of the nonunion. This requires forethought as a perfect osseous procedure may be planned and carried out only to have insufficient tissue for a tension-free closure to occur at the conclusion of the case. Preoperative consultation with a soft tissue reconstructive team to allow planning of any needed coverage and to coordinate logistic issues related to their availability is prudent. In the setting of an infected nonunion there is often the need for soft tissue reconstruction. This is usually performed after one or more debridements once control of infection has been obtained.

Of the myriad of flaps available, only tissue transfer brings something new to the local environment by way of vascularity and oxygen.[52,97,100,202] Particular attention should be paid to the soft tissue on the concave side of any associated deformity when angular correction of a malaligned nonunion is planned. When soft tissue coverage is lacking and flap coverage is not practical, deficient soft tissues can be dealt with using an external fixation technique or primary shortening by other means. Purposeful shortening and bone deformation to allow soft tissue closure without tension followed by gradual correction of alignment and distraction osteogenesis has been described utilizing the Taylor Spatial Frame device.[222] Another successful strategy is primary shortening during nonunion repair, followed by secondary lengthening after union has occurred.[196,235]

Indications and Contraindications for Nonoperative and Operative Treatment

Given the inherent inability to accurately evaluate the biologic potential of ununited fractures, nonoperative means can be considered for most. Additional time for the completion of fracture healing, without any other intervention, may be all that is required. When serial examinations show little or no progress to healing and the diagnosis of nonunion, defined as a fracture that is unlikely to heal without further intervention, is established, treatment interventions are indicated. On the surface there may appear to be little downside to nonoperative treatment other than the time required for successful treatment with nonoperative methods. These issues, however, should not be discounted. The socioeconomic and psychological aspects of prolonged periods of pain, functional loss, disability, and economic hardship can be profound. Also, there are some inherent associated risks with prolonged nonoperative management. Progressive fracture malalignment can occur, especially when implants fail. This represents one relative contraindication to nonoperative management of nonunions. Persistent and excessive motion at a nonunion site also can cause bone resorption, especially when an indolent infection is present. Known infection at the site of nonunion is another relative contraindication to nonoperative management. Therefore, the ideal situation for nonoperative management of a nonunion is when the limb has acceptable alignment and this method is thought to have a reasonable potential for success and the time anticipated for healing is associated with little morbidity. Most nonunions do not

meet these criteria; therefore, most nonunions are best suited for operative management.

Nonoperative Treatment of Nonunion

Nonoperative interventions for bone healing problems can accelerate the existing healing process or promote additional healing that would otherwise not have taken place. Such strategies may be most successful for promoting a delayed union to proceed to union, but healing of established nonunion can also be accomplished. The attractiveness of nonoperative treatment is the avoidance of surgical complications.

Nonoperative treatment can be divided into direct and indirect interventions. Direct intervention implies application of treatment directly to the ununited bone. Examples include electrical stimulation and ultrasound. Indirect intervention implies institution of treatment directed more toward the patient as a whole. Examples of indirect intervention would include nutritional augmentation or vitamin supplementation, alteration of certain medications, and smoking cessation (Table 27-1).

Indirect Nonoperative Treatment Interventions

Adequate nutrition is probably the most obvious and necessary ingredient for healing of all tissues including bone. Adequate caloric intake, vitamins, and protein are necessary to optimize the healing process.[133,135,307] Patient nutrition can be indirectly investigated by assessing total albumin levels. If low, nutritional supplementation and nutrition counseling can be helpful.

Smoking is probably the most commonly studied patient comorbidity that affects bone healing. Higher rates of delayed union and nonunion have been reported in smokers and the effect is probably proportional to the number of cigarettes smoked.[180,287] The mechanism, although not completely understood, likely relates to diminished osteoblast function and decreased local vascularity.[71,96] Therefore, cessation of smoking would logically be very important for any patient with a fracture or nonunion regardless of the treatment method. However, smoking cessation in the face of the stresses associated with an acute fracture is exceedingly difficult. Referral to a physician with expertise in smoking cessation or to a smoking cessation program can provide the support necessary for success. Given the direct adverse effects of nicotine on bone healing,

TABLE 27-1 Nonoperative Treatment of Nonunions

Indirect Intervention
- Smoking cessation
- Optimizing nutrition
- Correction of endocrine and metabolic disorders
- Elimination or reduction of certain medications

Direct Intervention
- Weight bearing
- External immobilization or support (e.g., cast or orthosis)
- Electromagnetic stimulation
- Ultrasound stimulation
- Parathyroid hormone

nicotine supplementation (e.g., nicotine patch) as part of a smoking cessation program should be avoided. This concept is supported by animal data linking transdermal nicotine to nonunion and decreased mechanical strength of healing fractures.[84]

Medical conditions such as diabetes also affect bone healing and increase the risk of nonunion. Diabetic patients with one or more comorbidities are at increased risk for the development of nonunion.[165] Diet modification and maintenance of well controlled blood sugar levels should be encouraged as they may minimize the negative effect of hyperglycemia on fracture and wound healing.[14]

Other metabolic and endocrine abnormalities may also play a role in nonunion in some patients. Conditions like calcium imbalance, hypogonadism, and thyroid and parathyroid disorders should be addressed medically by the appropriate specialist.[39] Patients with an established nonunion have a very high likelihood of having some endocrine dysfunction. The precise screening tests that should be obtained are not clearly defined. Serum vitamin D levels, at a minimum, are commonly obtained during the evaluation of the patient with a nonunion. This is an easy test to perform (as it is a relatively routine serologic test), is relatively inexpensive, may elucidate a potential confounding factor in fracture healing, and is relatively easily treated.[57] Nonunion repair surgery, if contemplated, is deferred until vitamin D levels are restored to normal whenever possible. Patients with low vitamin D levels are treated with 50,000 IU of vitamin D weekly in single doses for 4 to 6 weeks. If levels remain low, this regimen is repeated. Patients with low vitamin D levels, recalcitrant to such treatment, deserve a thorough evaluation by an endocrine or metabolic bone disease specialist.[39]

In addition to nicotine, other drugs and medications including steroids, dilantin, chemotherapeutic agents, NSAIDs, and some antibiotics (fluroquinolones) negatively affect bone healing.[40,120,244] Any adverse effects associated with cessation of such drugs must be balanced with benefits associated with nonunion treatment.

Adequate medical treatment of systemic infections, including HIV, is desirable in the face of fracture, and probably necessary in the treatment of an established nonunion, especially when CD4 counts are low.[143]

There appears to be no clinical evidence at this time to support the use of hyperbaric oxygen for the treatment of nonunion.[17]

Weight Bearing and External Stabilization

Probably the simplest and most long-standing direct intervention for a nonunion would be application of weight bearing in a functional brace. This, however, is only reasonably practical for the tibia. The mechanism for the success of this treatment is said to be stimulation of osteoblastic activity by mechanical loading.[252,282] The improved stability of a cast or brace can be most effective in the treatment of hypertrophic nonunions. Sarmiento et al.[282] managed 16 delayed unions and 57 nonunions of the tibia with below-the-knee functional braces. In 48 cases, a fibular osteotomy was performed to allow compression at the nonunion site with weight bearing and 10 patients had adjuvant bone grafting. Healing occurred in 91.3% of the

patients at a median of 4 months with an average of 5 mm of shortening for the nonunions. External supportive devices have little role in the management of atrophic nonunions, pseudoarthrosis, malaligned nonunions, and infected nonunions. These methods are generally considered to be less effective that modern operative means for almost all nonunions are associated with the potential for progressive deformity, and can result in skin breakdown.

Electrical Stimulation

Four forms of electrical stimulation including direct current (DC), capacitive coupling (CC), pulsed electromagnetic field stimulation (PEMF), and combined magnetic fields (CMFs) are currently used for the treatment of delayed unions and nonunions. It is estimated that more than 400,000 fracture nonunions and delayed unions have been treated with these physical forces.[218] DC electrical stimulation is unique in that it involves surgical implantation and potentially surgical removal of the stimulation device. The other methods are noninvasive and involve daily external application for various durations. PEMF is typically recommended for approximately 8 to 12 hours per day; CC must be worn for 24 hours a day; and CMFs are applied for 30 minutes a day. The substantial daily time requirements for PEMF and CC provide limitations with regard to patient compliance.

The mechanism of action with all of these devices is thought to be alteration of electrical potentials at the fracture site.[102,245,291] Electromagnetic fields have shown, in animal studies, to reduce osteoclastic-related bone resorption, increase osteoid formation, and stimulate angiogenesis.[232]

Although PEMF has been reported to be equally effective as compared to operative treatment of nonunions,[127] some degree of skepticism for these methods still exists because of the lack of well designed clinical trials of this technology. The only prospective double blind trial of CC, published in 1994, showed a 0% healing rate in the placebo group with no treatment, compared with 60% healing in the treated group. The series, however, was small with only 21 patients enrolled.[291] Four meta-analyses of electrical stimulation have recently been compared.[125] The most rigorous of these reported that the evidence available is insufficient to conclude a benefit of electromagnetic stimulation in improving fracture union rates or preventing nonunions.[212]

With regard to prevention of nonunion, Adie et al. reported on a large multicenter, prospective, randomized double-blind trial.[1] Two hundred and eighteen patients with acute tibial shaft fractures completed the 12-month trial. There was no difference in the need for secondary surgical intervention because of delayed union or nonunion in the group with active PEMF devices and the group with inactive devices (risk ratio 1.02). Because of moderate compliance with the recommended treatment protocol of 10 hours per day for 12 weeks (average daily use was 6.2 hours), a subanalysis between compliant patients with active units and patients with inactive units combined with noncompliant patients with active units also failed to demonstrate any benefit of pulsed electromagnetic field devices (risk ratio 0.97).

Requisite conditions for the successful application of electrical stimulation to nonunions include acceptable limb alignment, bone edge proximity, and the absence of pseudoarthrosis. Risk factors and relative contraindications for electrical stimulation are considered to be prolonged nonunion, prior bone graft surgery, prior electrical stimulation which failed, open fractures, active osteomyelitis, extensive comminution, and atrophic nonunion.[36] Electrical stimulation at this time can probably be considered to be a reasonable, acceptable nonoperative form of treatment for nonunion. Additional large double-blind trials offering level I evidence can probably not be expected because of the necessity of the control group having no treatment for nonunion for a prolonged time period.

Ultrasound Stimulation

Low-intensity pulsed ultrasound (LIPUS) is one of various noninvasive biophysical methods used to promote fracture and nonunion healing. LIPUS signals have a frequency of 1.5 MHz, a signal burst width of 200 μs, a repetition frequency of 1 kHz, an intensity of 300 mW/cm[37] (Fig. 27-15), and an administration time of approximately 20 minutes per day.[335] The LIPUS signal is of low energy, similar to that used for diagnostic ultrasound of vital organs and fetuses (10 to 50 mW/cm^2). Its side effect profile is therefore negligible as compared to high-energy shock wave therapy.

The mechanism is believed to be in part related to the actual mechanical phenomenon created by the ultrasound. LIPUS is a form of low mechanical energy which may be simulative to ossification.[344] It has been theorized that the acoustic waves of LIPUS can provide a surrogate for the forces involved in Wolff's law.[126] In addition, other investigations indicate that LIPUS affects cellular interactions, gene expression, signal transduction, and cellular level calcium regulation.[7,136,240,271,273,274] As a result of these complex cellular effects, multiple phases of fracture healing including inflammation, repair and remodeling, as well as angiogenesis, chondrogenesis and osteoblastic activity, are each thought to be influenced by LIPUS.[7,259,273,354]

LIPUS has been shown to accelerate fracture healing in both animal models[85,334,354,355] and in clinical trials.[145,178,187] Clinically, LIPUS has a role to speed fracture healing, to reduce healing complications in the high-risk population (diabetics, smokers, etc.), and to treat existing delayed unions and nonunions. In a study of closed or Gustilo type I open tibial shaft fractures treated with cast immobilization, significant improvements in time to healing were demonstrated for LIPUS with the proportion of fractures healed at 120 days being 88% in the LIPUS group and 44% in the controls.[145] The benefit of LIPUS appears to be greater for patients with risk factors for delayed healing such as smoking.[65,146] Laboratory data also indicates that LIPUS can increase the usually blunted fracture response associated with diabetes to nearly normal levels.[66]

High-quality, double-blind placebo-controlled clinical trials for the use of ultrasound in the treatment of nonunions does not exist and will probably not be done. Once again, there is an ethical consideration as the control group as a necessity would essentially need to have no treatment for their nonunions for a long period of time. There are, however, studies supporting its use (primarily self-pared controls for nonunion cases) with healing rates approaching 90% and healing times ranging from approximately 100 to 180 days.[101,113,204,224,271,335] The success rate for deeper bones seems to be lower than for subcutaneous bones.[335] Again, acceptable limb alignment, bone edge proximity, and the absence of a pseudoarthrosis are requisite conditions for ultrasound treatment.

Extracorporal Shock Wave Therapy

Extracorporal shock wave therapy (ESWT) is a higher energy treatment modality than LIPUS. It has been applied in the treatment of many musculoskeletal disorders including tendinopathy of the rotator cuff, lateral epicondylitis, and chronic plantar fasciopathy. Unlike LIPUS, which is patient self-administered on a daily basis, high-energy shock wave therapy typically requires general or regional anesthesia and investment in capital equipment by the treating institution. Studies have shown that the shock waves generated can elicit augmented osteogenic differentiation of mesenchymal stem cells, and can enhance biomechanical properties of bone and angiogenesis.[90] These properties make this technology potentially applicable to the treatment of nonunion. Early experiences have demonstrated a favorable response and side effect profile.[27,90,283,328,332] Side effects have included swelling, hematoma formation, and petechial hemorrhages. In a report of 115 patients with established nonunions or delayed unions treated with high-energy shock waves, 75.7% healed after one treatment[283] and in a follow-up report from the same group 80.2% healed after one to three treatments at an average of 4.8 ± 4 months.[90] A recent review of ESWT identified 10 studies (all level IV evidence) that included 924 patients.[358] The overall union rate was 76% and was significantly higher in hypertrophic nonunions. The majority of these studies were confounded by associated treatment with cast or external fixator immobilization, and, in the absence of a control group without shock wave treatment, it remains unproven how much effect this therapy has on nonunion healing.

Parathyroid Hormone

Parathyroid hormone (PTH) is a regulator of calcium metabolism and also assists in the regulation of bone turnover. Animal

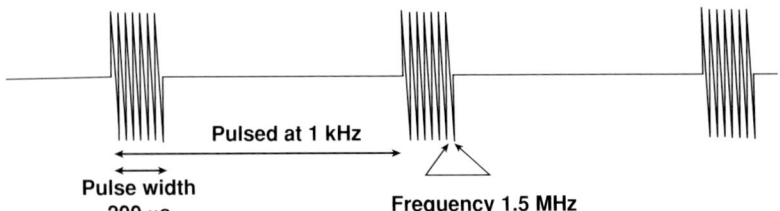

Pulsed at 1 kHz

Pulse width
200 μs

Frequency 1.5 MHz

FIGURE 27-15 A schematic diagram depicting characteristics of the low-intensity pulsed ultrasound signal.

research has established PTH as having an important role during fracture healing. PTH binds to osteoblasts stimulating release of mediators that in turn stimulate osteoclasts to resorb bone.[79] This oversimplification of the action of PTH in the complex interplay of osteoclasts and osteoblasts suggests a potential role for PTH in fracture healing. The utility of PTH to augment acute fracture healing and stimulate healing of nonunions has been the subject of several recent reports. Teriparatide is a synthetic hormone, containing the 1–34 amino acid fragment of recombinant human PTH, that has been used in such human investigations. Case reports have demonstrated healing of nonunions and atypical fractures related to bisphosphonate therapy after administration of teriparatide.[54,117,230] Whether bone healing would have occurred without the drug administration casts some doubt on the efficacy of PTH in these settings. Controlled clinical studies evaluating the effectiveness of PTH for the treatment of nonunions are anxiously awaited.[250]

Gene Therapy

A growing body of research indicates that gene therapies have the potential to augment fracture healing and to treat nonunions. Answers to critical questions such as what gene to transfer, where to transfer them, how to transfer them, does transfer work, and is transfer safe are beginning to unfold.[94] Genetically engineered stem cells have been successfully utilized in segmental defect and nonunion models.[73,214,230,247,299] Another approach that does not require stem cell isolation utilizes direct introduction of an osteogenic gene into a target tissue, some with viral vectors[21,108,188] and others without.[173,300] These direct methods rely on transient expression of the delivered gene. Such transient expression of members of the BMP family (BMP-2, -4, -6, and -9) has been shown to be sufficient for bone formation.[300] These targeted gene therapy techniques are promising in that they rely on relatively small quantities of inexpensive plasmid DNA in contrast to the mega doses of expensive recombinant proteins (e.g., rhBMP) used currently in clinical practice. Although the proof of concept has been demonstrated in small animal models, a few large animal studies have yielded encouraging results.[94] Progress toward developing clinically relevant gene therapies to augment bone healing is limited by substantial financial constraints and the ever changing regulatory environment.[217]

Operative Treatment of Nonunion

Although a common goal of surgical nonunion treatment is bone healing, there is large variation in the methods available for achieving this. Whereas a single treatment option is often clearly superior for an acute fracture such as IM nailing for a closed mid-diaphyseal tibia fracture, several options may be equally suited for the treatment of a nonunion of the same injury (e.g., exchange nailing, nail dynamization, plate osteosynthesis, circular external fixation, and external bone stimulation for a mid-diaphyseal tibial nonunion). The vast array of options can usually be refined with consideration of the integrity of the soft tissue envelope, the degree of bone loss, and coexisting conditions. For instance, nonunion in the face of associated infection makes repair with plates less, and external fixation more attrac-

tive. Malaligned nonunions are not well suited for interventions that do not address the deformity such as external stimulation or nail dynamization. Further refinement of the most desired treatment method considers surgeon experience and skill with, the relative risks and benefits of, as well as patient tolerance for, the remaining treatment methods.

Timing of Operative Intervention

Difficulty in establishing the optimal time to intervene surgically in the treatment of a nonunion parallels the difficulty in the diagnosis of a nonunion. Once the diagnosis of a nonunion is firmly established, operative intervention can reasonably be recommended at any time thereafter. However, if a future nonunion can be accurately predicted at an early stage, before meeting the criteria for the establishment of a nonunion, early operative intervention may be beneficial. This strategy could save patients from the prolonged adverse effect of living with an ununited facture and all the incumbent physical and psychological morbidities and socioeconomic hardships. However, if the prediction for eventual nonunion was inaccurate, patients could be subjected to unnecessary operations. Several recent studies have addressed these issues. A multicenter prospective study to evaluate reamed and unreamed IM nailing of tibia fractures suggested that delaying any surgical intervention for at least 6 months postoperatively may decrease the need for reoperation.[23] Other investigators suggest that nonunion repair be performed as early as 3 months.[38,51,98] In a survey of orthopedic trauma surgeons, >55% of them felt more confident about predicting nonunions at and past the 14th week after fracture for tibial and femoral shaft fractures and by the 12th week after humeral shaft, pubic rami, and scaphoid fractures.[22] The overall diagnostic accuracy of early (12 weeks) prediction of eventual nonunion was recently reported to be 74% with a sensitivity of 62% and specificity of 77%.[352] The diagnostic accuracy was higher in patients with less callus formation, high energy mechanisms, closed injuries, and diabetes. These authors concluded that a standardized protocol of waiting for 6 months before reoperation in all patients with nailed tibia fractures may subject a large proportion of the patients to unnecessary, prolonged disability and discomfort.

Plate and Screw Fixation for Nonunion Repair

Nonunion repair with plate and screw constructs is applicable to most anatomic locations (Fig. 27-16), and plates are applicable to repair of diaphyseal as well as end segment nonunions. Whereas IM nailing is almost universally considered the treatment of choice for acute mid-diaphyseal fractures of the femur and tibia, and by some the humerus, plate fixation is applicable and may be preferred for repair of ununited fractures in these locations. Additional relative advantages of plate and screw fixation of nonunions are the ability to address angular, rotational, and translational deformities, and with minor technical modifications the ability to manage periprosthetic nonunions. In the absence of soft tissue concerns, where the local soft tissues can accommodate the bulk of the implant and the dissection required for insertion, nonunion repair with plate constructs is a very powerful method that can be used successfully for any class of nonunion (i.e., atrophic or hypertrophic) by providing

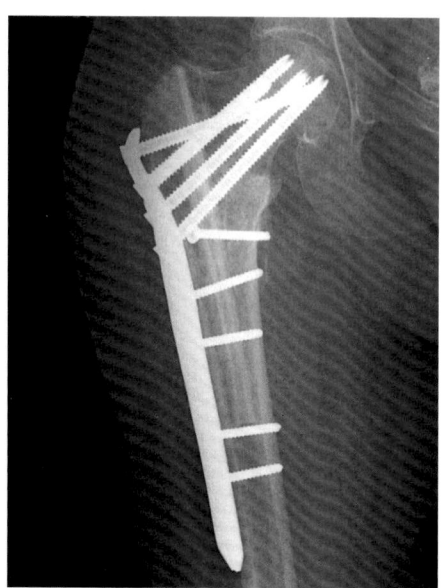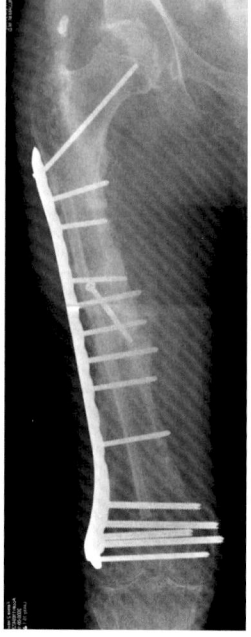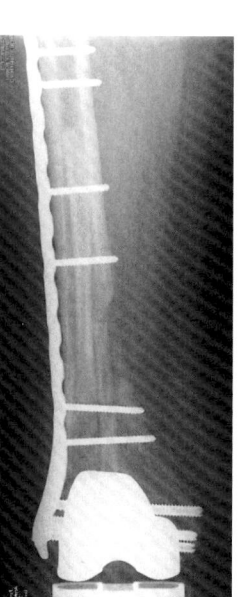

A, B   **C**

FIGURE 27-16 Plates can be used to treat nonunions at almost any part of any long bone. A proximal femur nonunion was repaired with a proximal femoral locking plate with adjuvant ICBG and an intra-medullary fibular strut **(A).** Nonunions of the midshaft **(B)** and distal **(C)** portions of the femur were repaired with distal femoral locking plates.

the stability, alignment control, and (when appropriate) the compression required for successful nonunion treatment.

Whether the tibia, femur, or humerus is involved, a pre-existing IM nail is, in most circumstances, removed at the time of nonunion repair with plates. However, successful locked and compression plate fixation of nonunions without nail removal has been reported.[216,356] Eccentric plate positioning allows bicortical screw fixation around the nail to augment unicortical locked screws.[216]

There are some inherent limitations of plate and screw techniques in the management of nonunions. Nonunion repair with plates is limited most by its relative invasiveness, most notably with regard to the potential compromise of any already marginal soft tissue envelope that is often encountered when dealing with nonunions. These constructs are generally load bearing and therefore, early postrepair weight bearing typically must be limited. The extreme stresses on plates spanning long segmental defects, because of their eccentric extramedullary location, may lead to premature implant failure (Fig. 27-17). Plate and screw constructs are also limited by an inability to correct limb shortening from bone loss.

Aftercare specific to plate-repaired nonunions must consider the soft tissue envelope. These procedures are often extensive and postoperative swelling can be substantial and lead to blistering, unforeseen wound issues, and even compartment syndrome. Therefore, efforts to minimize limb swelling are paramount. A well padded splint, one without proximal occlusiveness, is often used, even if not required, to protect the mechanical integrity of the repair. Elevation of the limb above the heart level and cold therapy are mainstays of the

initial postoperative regimen. Careful and timely observation of wounds is a practice that can identify and potentially help avoid impending problems. The results of nonunion repair with plate and screw constructs will be presented in each chapter that is specific to an anatomic location.

IM Nailing of Nonunions

IM nailing of nonunions and delayed unions can take three forms: primary nailing of a nonunion in the absence of a pre-existing nail, exchange nailing, and dynamization. Regardless of which situation is present, nail treatment is most applicable to diaphyseal nonunions. Nailing metaphyseal nonunions has been associated with mixed results and is dependent upon the specific region being treated with success most notably being reported for the distal femur and the distal tibia.[265,349]

Primary and Exchange Nailing. Primary IM nailing of a nonunion is less common than exchange nailing. This is because nonunions that are amenable to nailing would most likely have had IM nailing as an attractive initial method of treatment. Therefore primary nailing of mid-diaphyseal nonunions usually occurs after primary nonoperative management of tibia and humeral shaft fractures. Well aligned end segment nonunions initially treated with plate fixation are also potential candidates for primary nailing.

Exchange nailing, the practice of removing a pre-existing nail in favor of a new nail, is most applicable to situations where deficiencies of the pre-existing nail can be overcome with a new, larger reamed nail. Such deficiencies can include a lack of rotational control by absence or fracture of interlocking

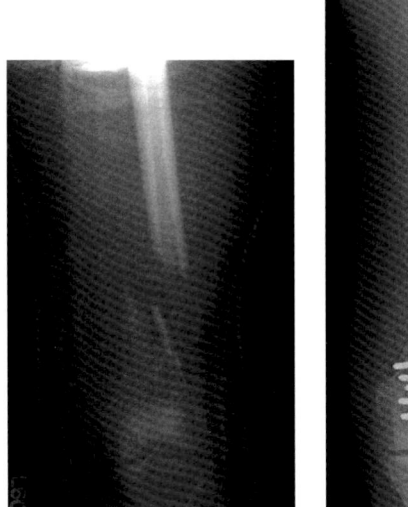
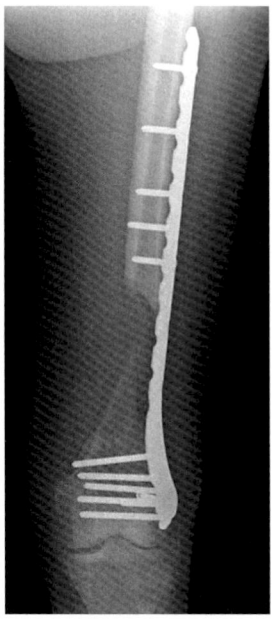
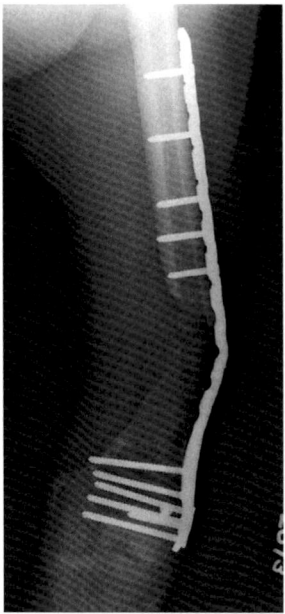
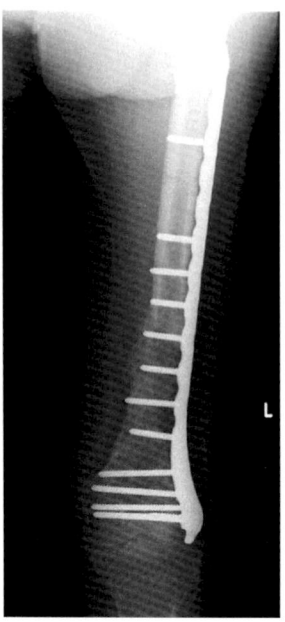

A, B

C, D

FIGURE 27-17 An open distal femur fracture treated with debridement and lateral plating resulted in a large segmental defect **(A)**. High varus stresses on the eccentrically placed plate **(B)** resulted in plate fracture prior to union despite bone grafting **(C)**. Nonunion repair with revision plating and additional autologous bone graft led to fracture union **(D)**.

screws and lack of adequate stability caused by an undersized nail. Even when there are no obvious mechanical deficiencies of the pre-existing nail, the reaming associated with an exchange nailing procedure can deposit small amounts of local bone graft and can stimulate an inflammatory response sufficient to promote healing.[62] It should be noted, however, that the local graft deposition provided by exchange nailing cannot be expected to fill defects of any substantial size. Therefore, exchange nailing is most applicable to situations without bone loss, unless adjuvant open bone grafting accompanies the procedure. Also, exchange nailing is best considered when angular alignment is satisfactory. The new nail will tend to follow the pre-existing IM path of the prior nail, and therefore, angular malalignments tend to persist after exchange nailing without specific efforts being taken to correct them (Fig. 27-18).

The technique for IM nailing of nonunions is generally similar to the technique used for nailing of acute fractures. The degree of overreaming required for effective application of exchange nailing is somewhat controversial. Newer evidence suggests that 1 mm of overreaming is sufficient rather than the historical recommendations for at least 2 mm of overreaming.[348] It should be clear that a minimum requirement for exchange nailing is the ability to insert a large enough nail to provide mechanical strength to the repair. When considering exchange nailing for the tibia, an associated fibular osteotomy to allow fracture compression during repair has been considered an integral part of the procedure, but recent evidence suggests this is not always essential.[154]

Alterations of angular alignment can be made during exchange nailing, but this adds substantial technical challenges to the procedure with any correction of malalignment needing to be made before reaming. This requires mobility of the non-

union, either at baseline or created by surgical means such as debridement of the nonunion and, for the tibia, osteotomy of the fibula. Externally applied devices, such as a femoral distractor, are invaluable tools to help obtain and maintain alignment during the procedure. When multiplanar deformities are present, simultaneous use of two distractors can be helpful, one in the sagittal plane and one in the coronal plane. Obviously, all distractor pins should be placed in locations that will not interfere with nailing.

Union rates for exchange nailing of femoral and tibial diaphyseal nonunions have ranged substantially, from less than 50% to over 90%.[38,139,228,338,346,348] With regard to the major long bones, success is most often reported for the tibia and femur, with exchange nailing of humeral nonunions being less consistent unless supplemental bone graft is utilized.[38,139,176,331,348] Results for exchange nailing of the femur were found to be better for isthmal fractures (87% union) compared with results for nonisthmal fractures (50% union).[353]

Dynamization. Dynamization, the practice of removing interlocking screws at one end of a nail to allow axial shortening with weight bearing, is a method advocated to promote healing of delayed unions or nonunions when small gaps are present at the fracture site. Such gaps may be present because of bone loss, osteoclastic bone resorption, or prior static nailing with distraction at the fracture site. Dynamization with modern nails that provide a dynamic interlocking slot can take two forms. Removal of static screws with retention or addition of a dynamic screw has the advantage of maintaining rotational control, but limits the amount of shortening to the amount of excursion of the dynamic screw within the oval dynamic

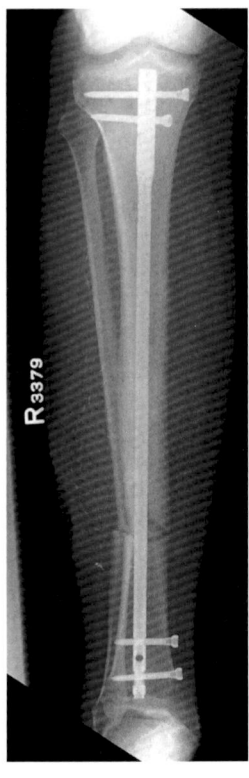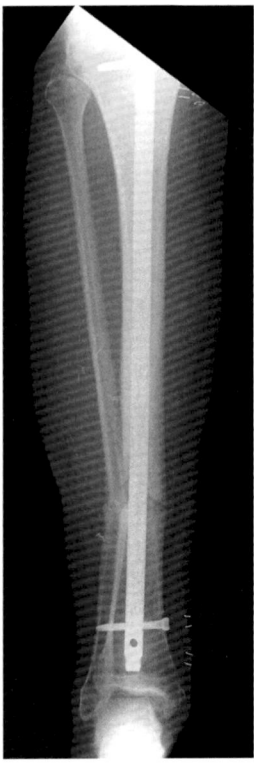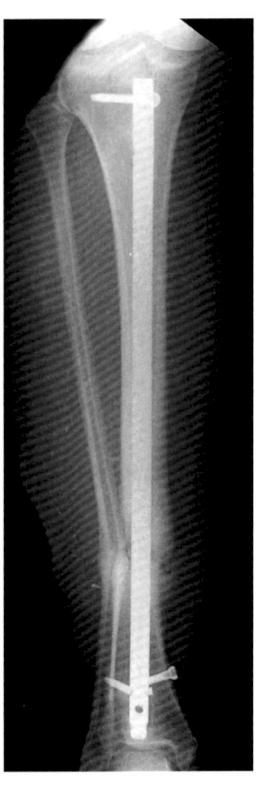

A, B   C

FIGURE 27-18 Exchange nailing of a malaligned tibia nonunion. An undersized nail was used to treat an open tibial shaft fracture leading to an atrophic nonunion in slight valgus alignment **(A)**. Exchange nailing was performed without specific consideration of the malalignment resulting in an almost identical amount of valgus **(B)**. A persistent nonunion, although now oligotrophic, with fractured interlocking screws has resulted **(C)**.

slot in the nail, usually just a few millimeters with most nail designs. This limit may on one hand be advantageous to avoid excessive shortening or, on the other hand, it may be detrimental by preventing sufficient compression at the fracture to accomplish union. The other form of dynamization is removal of all interlocking screws from one end of the nail. This allows more freedom for shortening at the expense of a lack of any axial or rotational control inherent in the nail construct, and therefore, creating the potential for complications of excessive shortening and malrotation.[41] The ideal situation for this form of dynamization is when the fracture pattern itself will result in limited shortening and when the existing healing response is thought to provide some inherent rotational stability. The compression allowed by dynamization will also provide increasing rotational stability. Several considerations should go into the decision regarding which end of a nail should be dynamized. Stability is maximized if screws near the fracture are retained and those on the opposite side of the isthmus relative to the nonunion site are removed. Another consideration relates to which end should be allowed to telescope over the nail. As the bone shortens, the nail will become more prominent on the end of the nail with removed screws. Therefore, screws should not be removed if this result (such as protrusion of the nail into the adjacent joint) is undesirable. One must also realize that predicting the degree of shortening can be imprecise. Removal of distal screws, those near the knee, in the case of a retrograde femoral nail is a notable example. In this scenario, the driving end of the nail, if devoid of interlocking screws, can theoretically back into the knee joint and potentially cause devastating damage to the patellar articulate cartilage.[261]

The practice of dynamization, given its relatively simplicity and minimal patient morbidity, was at one time commonplace, and even became a routine planned staged procedure after femoral nailing in some cases. This practice was utilized despite a lack of clinical evidence to support its use. Good results after routine dynamization of acute femur fractures was a justification for the practice.[170,171,320] Later evidence revealed that high union rates could be expected with static femoral nailing without secondary dynamization.[42] In the case of an established femoral delayed union or nonunion, dynamization has been shown to be successful in promoting union in only approximately 50% of cases.[239,251,345,347,351] Despite the marginal results of dynamization, it has a role in the management of femoral and tibial nonunions and should be considered in cases where shortening is unlikely. Its advantages are minimal morbidity and the potential for immediate full weight bearing.

External Fixation for Nonunion Treatment

Of the many different types of external fixation frames and techniques used to treat fractures, circular ring fixators utilizing thin wires and the concepts of Ilizarov are the mainstays for treatment of nonunions by external fixation. The general principles of these techniques are presented in Chapter 8 (Principles of External Fixation). The applicability of thin wire fixators in the treatment of nonunions extends to almost any location within any long bone as well as to the hand, foot, and even to the clavicle.[4,45,50,157,168,174,182,277,321] These techniques can even be applied in the setting of failed plate fixation.[13] Other advantages of Ilizarov techniques are the relative paucity of soft tissue trauma imparted by this nonunion repair method and the ability to slowly correct the associated deformities. The latter advantage also protects the soft tissues from the stretching that can accompany acute deformity correction with other methods. Other advantages of circular external fixation include the ability to fine tune correction and the potential for early weight bearing.

Computer-guided treatment with the Taylor Spatial Frame is a recent advance that has considerably simplified Ilizarov type correction of any malalignment, even complex multiplanar deformities.[89,270] The Taylor Spatial Frame differs from traditional Ilizarov fixators by utilizing adjustable struts that are oriented in a hexapod configuration. In conjunction with special web-based software programs, six axes of deformity can simultaneously and accurately be corrected (Fig. 27-19).

Decision making for nonunion treatment with ring fixators must consider if adjuvant open bone grafting is prudent either at the initial nonunion procedure or later in a staged manner. The nonunion characteristics dictate this aspect of the treatment strategy, with stiff nonunions being differentiated from mobile nonunions. Stiff nonunions rarely require bone grafting, whereas mobile nonunions often will benefit from the osteogenic stimulus of a graft. Radiographic evaluation of the stiff nonunion usually reveals hypertrophic callus formation and upon physical examination stress on the nonunion site is accompanied by pain with resistance to deformation. In contrast, mobile nonunions are characterized by either atrophic features on radiographic examination or by features of a synovial pseudoarthrosis. The mobile nonunion moves easily with stress, often without substantial pain. Stiff nonunions have inherent biologic activity and therefore usually do not require a bone graft and respond favorably to closed external fixation methods that utilize compression, distraction, or a combination of both.[50,157,168,174] According to the principles of distraction osteogenesis, gradual distraction of the hypertrophic nonunion can stimulate new bone formation and eventual union. Hypertrophic nonunions act similarly to the regenerate seen with limb lengthening or bone transport procedures. Modest lengthening,

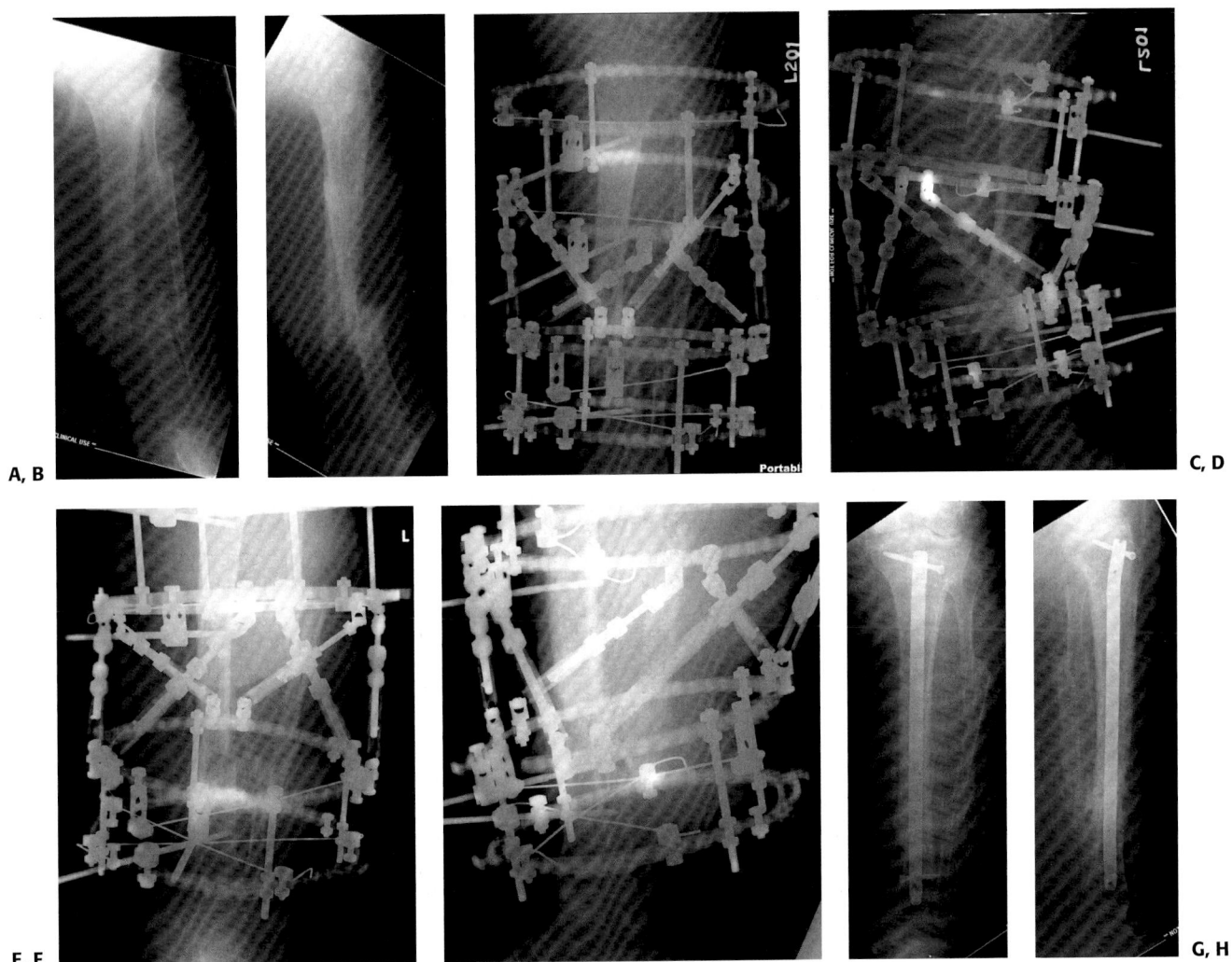

FIGURE 27-19 A malaligned tibial nonunion **(A, B)** is treated with a Taylor Spatial Frame (TSF) **(C, D)** which allows gradual correction of alignment **(E, F)**. The frame was removed after the correction and union was achieved with IM nailing **(G, H)**.

of up to approximately 1.5 cm, can typically be accomplished through a hypertrophic nonunion. If more length is required, lengthening can be performed separately through a distant osteotomy. Before distraction, a short period of compression, typically 7 to 14 days, may be helpful to "prime" the site for the osteogenic process. In certain circumstances, when there exists a transverse nonunion site where external compression will result in compression of the fracture fragments, union can be accomplished with pure compression. Clearly, an advantage of the gradual treatment afforded by thin wire external fixation, especially when associated with deformity correction, is the preservation of the often compromised soft tissue envelope.

Treatment of mobile nonunions with ring fixators usually requires opening the nonunion site to surgically convert the nonviable atrophic nonunion to fresh viable bone ends, or in the case of a pseudoarthrosis, to resect the synovium, pseudocapsule, and the fibrocartilage covering the bone ends. In either case, the medullary canal is opened and the site is typically bone grafted. Pure adherents to the Ilizarov techniques may, instead of bone grafting, perform a corticotomy of the involved bone at a site surrounded by healthy soft tissues followed by transport of the intercalary segment to eventually achieve healing by compression at the nonunion and regenerate formation at the corticotomy site, respectively. This technique is technically much more demanding, potentially more time consuming, relies on healing at two sites rather than one, and has the potential complications inherent with bone transport. But, despite this, it is a powerful strategy in experienced hands especially when lengthening of more than 2 cm is required.

Aftercare specific to nonunion treatment with circular frames obviously requires management of the pin sites. Pin site infection near a joint has the potential for joint sepsis, and in these cases careful pin site care and close observation can avoid disastrous consequences. The accepted strategies for pin site care are many, but at least one should be chosen and clearly outlined to the patient and caregivers. Signs and symptoms of infection should prompt more aggressive treatment such as initiation of antibiotic therapy or wire exchange. The potential for safe and early weight bearing is an advantage of nonunion treatment with ring fixators. Once any associated deformities are corrected and any soft tissue deficiencies are healed, some degree of weight bearing in the frame is generally permitted in all but the most extreme cases.

Ring fixators have limitations for the treatment of end segment nonunions related to the proximity of thin wires to the involved joint.[313] Wires that puncture joint capsule pose a risk for the development of joint sepsis if pin site infection develops.

Arthroplasty for Nonunion Treatment

There are limited circumstances that make total joint arthroplasty or hemiarthroplasty a viable option for the treatment of nonunion. However, when circumstances are appropriate, arthroplasty can result in rapid and profound symptomatic and functional improvement. Several factors determine the appropriateness for arthroplasty. A minimum requirement is nonunion in a periarticular location that has an associated arthroplasty option that can accommodate the bone resection required to eliminate the nonunion. Depending upon other factors, arthroplasty for nonunion can either be an excellent first choice, an option of last resort, or contraindicated. In the elderly, especially with associated joint arthrosis, which may be in the form of pre-existing arthritis, post-traumatic arthritis, joint destruction from prior implants, or osteonecrosis, arthroplasty is preferred to other methods of nonunion treatment. In contrast to the distal metaphyseal ends of the femur and humerus, metaphyseal nonunions of the proximal ends of these bones are somewhat less ideal for arthroplasty. The common reason is related to the tendon insertions onto the greater trochanter of the femur and the greater and lesser tuberosities of the humerus, respectively. These tendon attachments must be preserved to maintain normal function, and therefore, proximal replacing arthroplasty in these regions should only be considered in extreme circumstances where other options are of equal or greater disfavor.[262] When arthroplasty is selected it usually offers the advantages of immediate weight bearing and concomitant treatment of the associated arthrosis, two things that are not accomplished with nonunion repair.

In physiologically younger patients, arthroplasty becomes less advantageous because of limited longevity of the implants. In the absence of substantial and debilitating arthrosis in this patient population, periarticular nonunions are usually best treated with repair. Regardless of the patient's age, active infection at the site of nonunion is a contraindication to arthroplasty. Strategies for arthroplasty after eradication of infection, often accompanied with antibiotic spacer placement, are not unreasonable, but are associated with substantial risk of recurrent infection. Arthroplasty can be considered after aggressive treatment of an infected nonunion. This typically involves relatively radical debridement of involved bone, internal implantation of antibiotic-impregnated cement spacers, and prolonged administration of organism-specific parental antibiotics. Whether an infection-free period of time off antibiotics prior to arthroplasty, aimed to prove eradication of the infection, or whether arthroplasty should be accompanied by long-term oral suppression, are both unresolved issues and these decisions are typically individualized and made in concert with consultant infectious disease specialists. A more distant history of infection presents a similar quandary. Biopsy or joint aspiration prior to arthroplasty can be a useful guide to decision making.

One of the most suitable metaphyseal nonunion locations that is amenable to arthroplasty is the distal femur. Here, a knee arthroplasty that includes distal femoral replacement is relatively mainstream, technically of moderate, but not extreme, complexity, and, because of a lack of critical soft tissue attachments on the distal femur, is generally associated with good functional outcomes.[5,30,77,138,225,327] However, good results with this method are certainly not universal and complication rates, especially for infection, are potentially high.[142,153] Noninfectious complications occurred in 6 of 15 cases in one series[153] and a revision rate of 13% after a follow-up period of 24 months has been reported in another.[18] In the absence of complications, and even in some patients with treated complications, distal femoral replacement offers the potential for substantial improvement in function.[153,327]

Standard hip arthroplasty, either partial or total as dictated by other factors such as the condition of the hip joint and patient demand, are options for nonunions of the femoral neck and intertrochanteric region.[78,137,359]

Arthroplasty for nonunion of the proximal tibia, although reported,[153] is typically avoided in favor of staged knee arthroplasty after nonunion repair even in the presence of knee arthrosis because of the critical importance of the tibial tubercle for extensor function. In addition, infection was reported in 50% of proximal tibia replacements in one recent small series.[153]

Critical soft tissue attachments do not limit the applicability of total ankle replacement for nonunion of the distal tibia, but the lack of prostheses that can accommodate bone loss in this location does.

Nonunions of the distal humerus can often be treated with standard total elbow replacements rather than requiring distal humeral replacement.[8,213,281] This is because of a combination of the high frequency of fractures occurring within the articular block of the distal humerus, the potential problems with fixation of very distal fractures in this region, and the common association of osteoporosis with these factors. When nonunions are more proximal, a distal humeral replacing total elbow prosthesis can be used.[59]

Amputation for Nonunion Treatment

Amputation as definitive treatment for nonunions is often dictated by associated comorbid conditions and by patient preference rather than a technical inability to eventually achieve union.[195,231] Psychological and psychosocial factors specific to each individual patient are important to recognize, discuss, and consider before pursuing shared decision making for amputation in the setting of nonunion. The time and effort invested in prior treatments makes some patients reluctant to consider amputation and eager for fresh ideas and strategies for repair, whereas the same investments in prior failures may leave other patients frustrated, worn out, and ready to proceed with a definitive procedure such as amputation. Candid assessments for potential success with additional attempts at nonunion repair, the required investment of time and energy of the patient, and the relative functional, cosmetic, and neurologic (i.e., pain, neuralgia) outcomes of success versus failure of nonunion repair should be discussed and used to guide treatment decisions. Chronic pain from nonunion that will dissipate with bone healing needs to be differentiated from neurogenic pain which is likely to linger. If such neurogenic pain is chronically disabling, then efforts at nonunion repair may be misguided and amputation deserves serious consideration. Also, a contingency plan for what follows if a future nonunion repair fails is useful. A plan for amputation if failure occurs with the next intervention may make it much easier for some patients to reconcile amputation.

Arthrodesis for Nonunion Treatment

Arthrodesis is sometimes indicated for the management of periarticular nonunions.[12,44] The choice of arthrodesis is typically one of last resort when repair with standard techniques or arthroplasty is either contraindicated, unavailable, or not desired. Nonreconstructable periarticular nonunions without good arthroplasty options that can accommodate bone defects (e.g., ankle), nonreconstructable periarticular nonunions with good arthroplasty options, but in young patients who are likely to have poor long term success with arthroplasty, and infected periarticular nonunions, are typical indications for arthrodesis. Often, especially when dealing with infected nonunions of the lower extremity in a compromised host, the choice is between arthrodesis and amputation. It is useful to expose patients trying to make such a decision to other patients who have undergone either arthrodesis or amputation.

Fragment Excision and Resection Arthroplasty for Nonunion Treatment

Nonunions can be treated directly or indirectly with excision. Direct excision of one or more nonunited bone fragments is most applicable when the excision is designed to eliminate pain-associated contact of the fracture fragments with each other and when the excision minimally disrupts function. Ununited avulsion fracture fragments, where a portion of the ligamentous attachment to the intact bone remains in continuity, are prime candidates for excision. Anatomic examples include avulsion fractures of the base of the fifth metatarsal,[268] fractures of the medial malleolus, the inferior pole of the patella, the greater trochanter of the femur,[48] the ulnar styloid,[144] the olecranon,[238] and the greater tuberosity of the humerus. Although avulsed fragments represent a large category of ununited bone fragments amenable to excision, any ununited fragment is a potential candidate for excision. Excisions of an ununited radial head fragment,[86] the proximal pole of the scaphoid,[44,272] and the anterior process of the calcaneus[192] have been reported.

The utility of this method of nonunion treatment has recently been reported for excision of proximal fifth metatarsal avulsion fractures in six elite athletes.[268] All patients experienced relief of activity-related pain and all returned to competitive play at a mean of 11.7 weeks after surgery. The majority of the peroneus brevis tendon attachment to the fifth metatarsal was found to be preserved in all except one case. In the case with more than 50% of the tendon attached to the excised fragment, the tendon was repaired to the remaining fifth metatarsal base.

Nonunions may be treated indirectly with partial excision of an intact adjacent bone to facilitate healing of the ununited bone. A prime example is excision of a segment of fibula to allow compression of the tibia. As osteotomy and excision serve the same purpose; this type of excision will be discussed further in the next section on osteotomy.

Osteotomy for Nonunion Treatment

Osteotomy related to the treatment of nonunions usually serves the purpose to realign the nonunion directly or to allow secondary axial shortening of an adjacent bone (e.g., fibular osteotomy for tibial nonunion). In either case, the ultimate goal of osteotomy is to allow compression at the nonunion site to promote healing. The prototypical realignment osteotomy is the Pauwels osteotomy for a femoral neck nonunion described in 1935 and still used today.[9,200,242,309] In this case, a closing wedge osteotomy distal to a femoral neck nonunion serves to reorient a vertical nonunion to a more horizontal plane. Fixation across

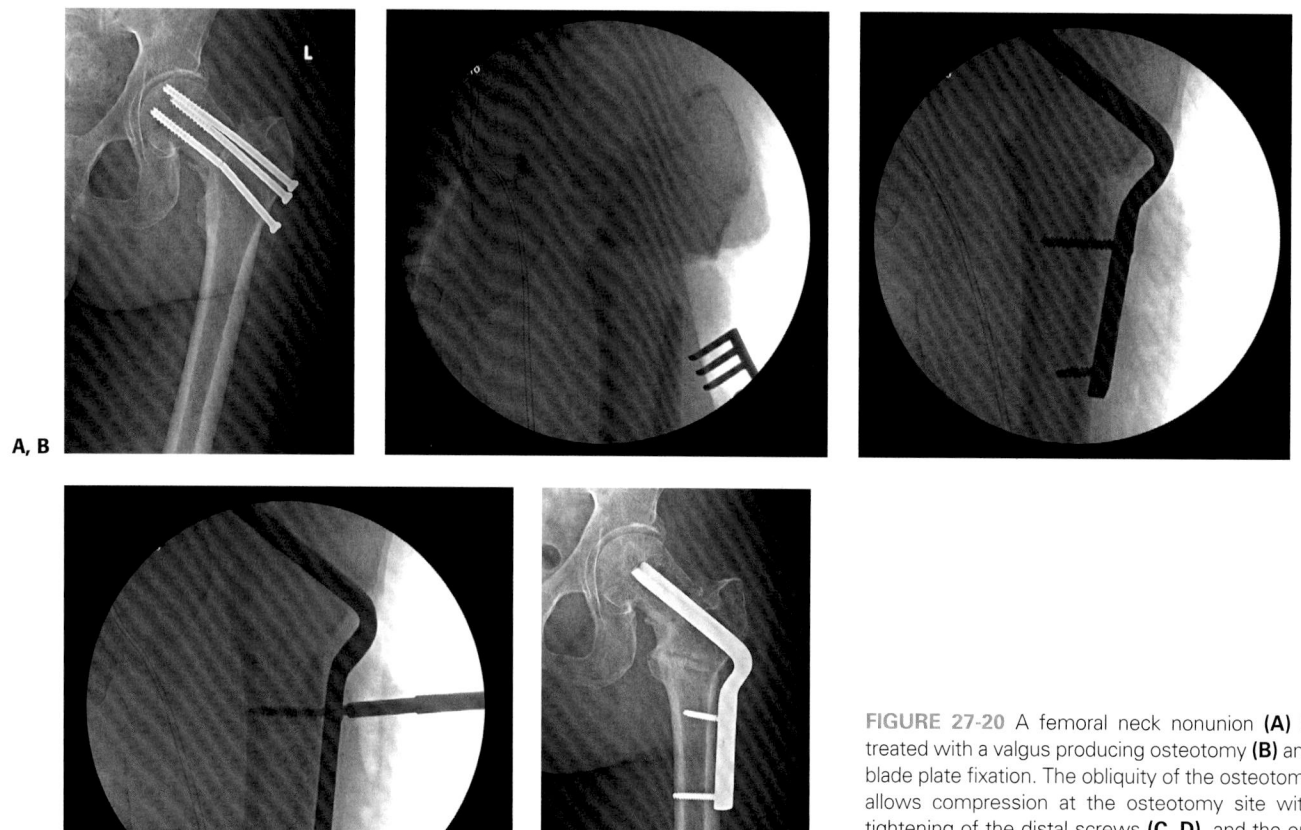

A, B

C

D

E

FIGURE 27-20 A femoral neck nonunion **(A)** is treated with a valgus producing osteotomy **(B)** and blade plate fixation. The obliquity of the osteotomy allows compression at the osteotomy site with tightening of the distal screws **(C, D)**, and the orientation of the nonunion relative to the blade plate allows compression of the nonunion with weight bearing. Union is achieved at both the nonunion and osteotomy sites **(E)**.

both the osteotomy and the femoral neck nonunion, typically with a blade plate, provides direct compression at the osteotomy and allows secondary dynamic compression across the nonunion (Fig. 27-20). This procedure has reported success rates of up to 90%.[200,309]

When manipulation of tibial length, either compression or distraction (associated with bifocal Ilizarov methods), is required during nonunion treatment and the fibula is intact, a fibular osteotomy or partial excision is performed. Osteotomy without excision allows compression for a relatively short period of time, until healing of the osteotomy occurs. When more time is needed to accomplish the desired compression of the tibia, an excision of a fibular segment large enough that healing is unlikely to occur is preferred over a simple osteotomy. The level of fibular excision has been suggested to be at a site other than that of the nonunion to avoid destabilization.[63] However, this recommendation is most applicable to nonunion treatment with cast immobilization without other fixation.[282] The level of fibular excision in the setting of adequate internal or external fixation is likely to be of less importance.

Synostosis for Nonunion Treatment

The lower leg and the forearm, by virtue of having paired bones, are amenable to synostosis techniques for treatment of nonunions of one of the bones. These techniques are most

applicable to tibial nonunions as synostosis between fibula and tibia is of little functional consequence.[181,305] This is in contrast to the forearm, where synostosis of the radius and ulna eliminates supination and pronation. Forearm synostosis may, however, be a reasonable option in situations where loss of forearm rotation is already a forgone conclusion, such as in the late management of a mangled extremity. Synostosis of the fibula and tibia may be identified by a number of terms: fibula transfer; fibula-pro-tibia; fibular transposition; fibulization; fibular medialization; posterolateral bone grafting, tibialization of the fibula, transtibio-fibular grafting; and synostosis. Synostosis techniques generally attempt to create continuity between the paired bones above and below the nonunion. Weight-bearing forces are transmitted, via the synostosis, around the nonunion through the adjacent bone. Healing of the nonunion is not a requisite for success of the synostosis procedure.

ADJUNCTS TO OPERATIVE NONUNION REPAIR

Approximately 500,000 bone graft procedures are performed annually in the United States.[129] Autologous bone grafts are the gold standard for use in fracture nonunions, but allografts and other bone graft substitutes are each part of the armamentarium for those treating nonunions. The optimal choice of graft material is determined by factors such as the required properties (e.g., osteogenic, osteoinductive, or osteoconductive), the required volume, the accessibility of the material, the cost, and known efficacy.

Autogenous Bone Graft

Autogenous bone graft remains the standard graft substance used in the repair of atrophic nonunions, some oligotrophic nonunions, and some pseudoarthroses. It has the best and longest documentation and experience and does not confer the risk of spreading infectious diseases. For instance, autograft from the iliac crest used in the treatment of tibial and femoral nonunion typically results in union rates exceeding 90%.[275] Cancellous autogenous bone graft supplies osteogenic and osteoconductive materials. Osteogenic cells, including stroma cells, are present in the graft material. It provides an excellent osteoconductive scaffold by way of cancellous bone spicules. It is estimated that 15% of the osteocytes and osteoblasts can survive the bone graft procedure.[88] Recent data also indicate that various growth factors and BMPs are present in autologous bone graft and that these levels seem to be independent of harvest site.[286,317]

The disadvantages of autogenous bone grafting relate to limited quantities that can be harvested, variable quality, and donor site morbidity. The volume required to fill a cylindrical defect in the femoral or tibial diaphysis has been estimated to be 11.3 cm^3/cm and 7.1 cm^3/cm, respectively.[311] Defects of several centimeters or more in length may therefore exceed the volume of autogenous graft that is available. It has been estimated that the limit of defect length that can be filled using iliac crest bone graft (ICBG) is 5 to 7 cm.[169] The quality of the autogenous graft is dependent on host health in general and perhaps to some degree on bone health, such as osteoporosis, as well. Donor site morbidity includes the potential for infection, pain (acute and chronic), neurovascular injury, secondary fracture, and hematoma.[6,316] Iliac crest is the most commonly used site for large volume grafts, but other sites such as the greater trochanter and the femoral and tibial condyles can be used for small amounts.

Iliac Crest Bone Graft (ICBG)

The anterior iliac crest is the most common site of autologous bone graft harvest for the treatment of nonunions. It is a relatively accessible location in all but the most obese patient, and it can provide relatively large quantities of graft, which can be either cancellous, cortical, or a combination of both. Furthermore, the efficacy of this graft is proven. The posterior iliac crest is a nearly identical alternative except for the obvious implications for patient positioning and surgical approach.

The disadvantages of using the anterior iliac crest are those described for autologous bone graft harvest in general.[2,11,80,303,316,339] The reported rates have varied from 2% to 26% for pain,[2,80,190,303,316,339] from 0% to 7.5% for infection,[2,16,80,339] and from 0% to 16% for persistent lateral femoral cutaneous nerve symptoms.[2,11,179,190,303,316] Less common, but severe complications related to ICBG harvest include arterial injury,[91] abdominal herniation,[260] pelvic instability,[70] and secondary fracture through the harvest site.[2,6,253] A recent prospective study of 92 patients who underwent anterior iliac crest bone grafting for delayed union or nonunion indicated that this was a well-tolerated procedure. Only two patients (2%) reported a pain value of >3 at 1 or more years postoperatively, there was no functional impairment compared to controls without ICBGs, there were no sensory deficits related to the lateral femoral cutaneous nerve, and deep infection was minimal (3%). These data are in contrast to those of one of the most cited articles in the history of the *Journal of Orthopaedic Trauma*[185] where an 8.6% major and a 20.6% minor complication rate were reported after autogenous bone grafting.[357] This report included harvest from different donor sites, a heterogeneous patient population, and multiple surgeons.

A number of techniques are available for harvesting anterior iliac crest graft. It can be harvested via a trap door in the crest, from the inner table, or from the outer table. Structural graft is available in the form of a tricortical wedge from the crest.[32] Cancellous graft may be harvested in isolation via the trap door approach or in combination with the thin cortical bone of the inner or outer table. Curettes, osteotomes, and gouges are useful tools for harvest. Alternatively, acetabular reamers can be used to shave the table and the underlying cancellous bone providing a homogeneous combination of cortical and cancellous bone (Fig. 27-21).[339]

Alternative Sites for Autologous Bone Graft Harvest

Although the iliac crest, anterior and posterior, are the most common sites for autologous bone graft harvest, other anatomic regions can provide cancellous graft for use in nonunion surgery, especially when small volumes of graft are required. The distal femur and proximal tibia can provide a modest volume of graft material as can the distal tibia, proximal humerus, and olecranon. Concerns regarding the efficacy of graft obtained from these alternative harvest sites have been one factor limiting their use. Recent data, however, suggests that sites other than the iliac crest have similar levels of endogenous BMP as crest graft[317] and grafts from such sites are associated with good clinical results.[184,233] However, another recent study suggested that the iliac crest may have a superior content of hematopoietic and osteogenic progenitor cells based on histologic differences.[55]

Reamer–Irrigator–Aspirator

Autogenous graft can also be harvested using the reamer–irrigator–aspirator (RIA) (Synthes, Paoli, PA) (Fig. 27-22).[221] This device was originally designed as a one-pass reamer for IM nailing to minimize embolic phenomenon.[74,75,162,163,290,315] Using this device, reamings are evacuated via suction and collected to be used as bone graft. In the relatively limited experiences reported so far, minimal complications have occurred, but potential certainly exists for mechanical malfunction, femur fracture, embolism, and excessive blood loss.[221,310] Reamings in general have been shown in in vitro analysis to contain pleuripotential stem cells with the possibility of dedifferentiation into osteoblasts.[337] Specifically quantitative assessment has

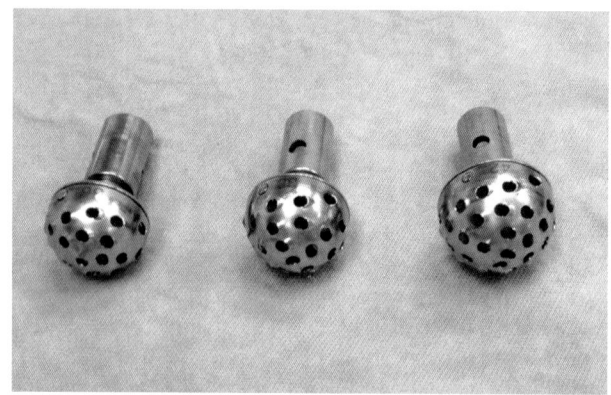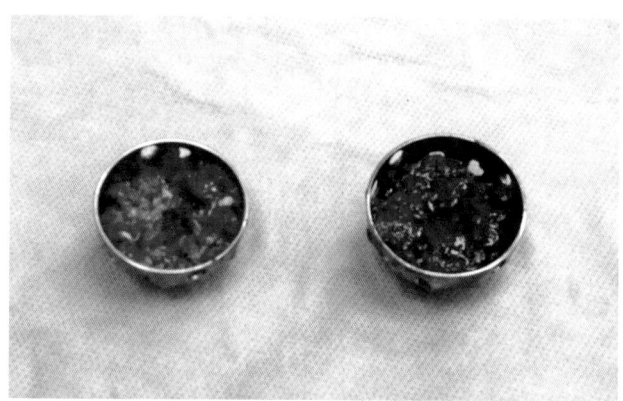

FIGURE 27-21 Acetabular reamers **(A)** can be used to harvest bone graft from the iliac crest **(B).**

demonstrated the presence of significant growth factors using the RIA technique[106,152,254,286,337] and also that the complement of osteogenic elements in the aspirate may be superior to those in ICBG.[342] In addition, an animal study has suggested that a superior quality of callus may result from implantation of graft material harvested in this way.[140]

Clinical results of RIA graft used for segmental defects and nonunions are generally favorable. Stafford and Norris[311] reported a 70% union rate at 6 months and 90% union rate after 12 months in 27 segmental long bone defect nonunions (average defect 5.8 cm, range 1 to 25 cm) managed with a femoral RIA bone graft. McCall et al.[205] reported on a similar group of 21 patients with defects averaging 6.6 cm. Seventeen of the twenty-one healed at 11 months; however, only ten of the twenty-one healed without a secondary intervention. The combined use of RIA graft plus rhBMP-2 in recalcitrant tibial nonunions resulted in union in a small case series of nine patients reported by Desai et al.[81]

Trials comparing RIA harvest with other standard methods of reaming and graft harvest are emerging. Streubel et al.[314] retrospectively compared conventional reaming with RIA during IM nailing of femoral shaft fractures. They found no benefit to RIA with regard to reducing pulmonary complications and found a trend toward increased healing complications in the RIA group. Belthur et al.[16] found the pain associated with graft harvest with RIA to be less than the pain after traditional ICBG.

Complications associated with RIA bone graft harvest have most notably included fracture and excessive blood loss. Lowe et al.[191] reported five postoperative fractures after RIA bone graft harvest and suggested that harvest in osteoporotic or osteopenic patients be avoided and that the degree of cortical reaming be carefully monitored.

A reamer is selected that is 1 to 4 mm greater than the narrowest part of the femoral canal as measured on preoperative or intraoperative images. The starting point is the same as for IM nailing and may be a piriformis or trochanteric entry site.

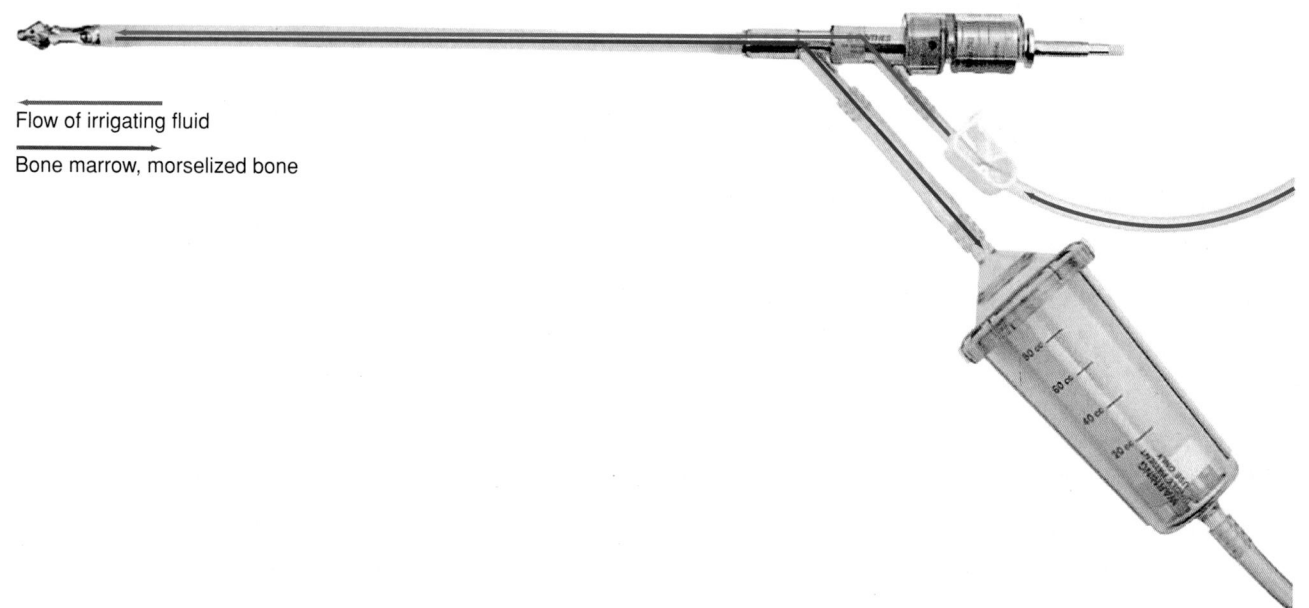

Flow of irrigating fluid

Bone marrow, morselized bone

FIGURE 27-22 The reamer–irrigator–aspirator (RIA).

Using standard IM nailing technique, a guidewire is inserted into the canal of the femur with image control and a one-time pass reamer is gently used to ream the femoral canal with an in and out motion so as not to advance too aggressively. A trap is used to collect the reamings. Typically 60 to 80 cm^{35} of graft can be harvested with experience without critically weakening the donor bone.[99,256]

Vascularized Grafts

Vascularized grafts are most commonly used to treat segmental defects and nonunions of the femoral neck.[167] They are advantageous in this situation as they provide a live bone graft that also has structural properties. These are properties not provided by standard iliac crest cancellous autograft. The fibula is the most commonly harvested bone although other sites such as the iliac crest[279] and rib[336] have been used. Vascularized grafts typically must undergo some degree of hypertrophy for ultimate success in addition to healing to the host tissue at each end.[156] Double vascularized grafts (fibula) combined with cancellous grafts have been proposed to gain additional and more rapid stability.[10] This is, however, a technically demanding procedure requiring mircovascular anastomosis. Complications include recurrent graft fractures and donor site morbidity.[141]

Bone Graft Substitutes and Other Modifiers of Bone Healing

Autologous bone graft has recently been challenged as the gold standard bone graft substance for nonunions.[297] Alternatives to autologous bone graft including demineralized bone matrix (DBM), bone marrow aspirate, platelet-rich plasma (PRP), allograft, and ceramics have been developed and utilized for nonunion treatment with varying degrees of success. New advances in bioengineering based on enhanced understanding of the cellular and molecular aspects of fracture healing have led to the development and clinical use of growth factors, such as BMPs, that are used to augment fracture healing. The details of the basic science and mechanism of action of these alternatives are presented in Chapter 5. The advantages of these substitutes, relative to autologous bone graft, in the treatment of nonunion include reduced or eliminated patient morbidity and increased or unlimited supply.

The ideal graft substitute for nonunion treatment would be inexpensive, of unlimited supply, easy to prepare and handle, easy to implant, without adverse reactions, and 100% efficacious. Each of the above mentioned graft substitutes has some of these ideal graft attributes but none have all. Effectiveness in the treatment of nonunion has been reported for each of these substitutes but there is little in the way of direct comparison to autologous bone grafting.[28,64,119,123,151,172,198,304] The utility of BMPs to enhance the effects of autogenous bone graft is controversial.[118] It seems logical that adding a bone growth stimulator such as BMP to autogenous bone graft would augment healing capacity. In a noninstrumented spinal fusion model, the combination of osteogenic protein-1 (OP-1) with autograft yielded a 55% fusion rate that was similar to historical controls.[325] In the setting of fracture nonunion, a similar lack of efficacy has been demonstrated recently.[264]

Recombinant Proteins

BMPs have been increasingly studied as potential substitutes for autologous bone graft.[288] Their production from recombinant gene technology makes them available in unlimited quantities. Furthermore, BMPs are available in exact concentrations therefore allowing accurate therapeutic dosing. Their major drawback nevertheless remains the high cost at which they are available. Recombinant human osteogenic protein-1 (rhOP-1), also known as BMP-7, has been studied in the setting of upper and lower extremity nonunions showing high healing rates when used either alone or in combination with autologous or allogeneic bone graft.[31,82,280,361] When used only in combination with a type I collagen carrier, BMP-7 has been shown to achieve healing rates similar to iliac crest autograft in tibial nonunions without the associated donor site morbidity.[103,104] BMP-7 has however only been approved in the United States under a humanitarian device exemption stipulating that its use is limited to situations where autologous graft is not available, thereby limiting its clinical applicability.[112] BMP-2 has been shown to improve healing rates and reduce the risk for infection and secondary procedures after IM nailing of acute open tibia fractures.[128] Similar healing rates to autologous ICBG have been reported for the combination of BMP-2 and freeze dried cancellous allograft in the management of diaphyseal tibial shaft fractures with segmental defects.[164] While approved by the US FDA only for the treatment of acute open tibia fractures, spinal fusions and oral facial bone augmentation, BMP-2 has been used off-label for the management of established nonunions alone or in combination with ICBG.[159,160,161,280,312,322,326]

rhOP-1 was directly compared to autograft in the treatment of 124 tibial nonunions in a prospective randomized study.[104] At 9 months after repair using an IM nail, 81% of the rhOP-1 and 85% of the autograft-treated nonunions had healed clinically. Radiographic healing in the rhOP-1 group was 75%, whereas it remained essentially unchanged from clinical healing in the autologous group (84%). The main advantage of rhOP-1 was elimination of the donor site pain which was present in 20% of the patients receiving autograft. Noncomparative data has shown good healing rates, 89% to 92%, with rhBMP-7 (rhOP-1) in the treatment of various upper and lower extremity nonunions.[82,206] One randomized controlled study exists comparing rhBMP-2 and allograft to autogenous bone graft for reconstruction of diaphyseal tibial fractures with cortical defects.[164] Thirteen patients in the rhBMP-2 group had comparable results to 10 patients in the autograft group. These fractures were not nonunions, but with an average 4-cm defect, they were certainly unlikely to heal without intervention. A recent retrospective comparison of BMP-2 plus cancellous allograft to autologous ICBG for the treatment of long bone nonunion revealed a moderate but not statistically significant difference in healing rates between the two groups of 68.4% and 85.1%, respectively.[322] The authors concluded that BMP-2 might provide a suitable alternative to ICBG, but acknowledged the potential for a β-error in their study. Although a disadvantage of recombinant BMPs is their cost, recent data suggests their use could actually reduce costs when treating complex or recalcitrant nonunions by reducing the number of procedures and the number of hospital days.[72]

Demineralized Bone Matrix

DBM is produced by extraction of proteins from allograft bone.[324] DBM contains type I collagen and noncollagenous proteins including osteoinductive growth factors. There is a requirement from the American Association of Tissue Banks and the US FDA that each batch of DBM be from a single donor. This requirement produces the potential for substantial differences in biologic activity between batches. Further heterogeneity between different formulations of DBM exists because of different manufacturing processes and different carriers used by various commercial producers.[246]

A number of studies report good results after nonunion treatment using DBM either alone or in combination with other graft materials.[266,343,362,363] These studies suffer from a lack of controls leaving definitive conclusions regarding the efficacy of DMB uncertain. DBM used as an adjunct to locked compression plating of osteoporotic humeral shaft nonunions resulted in union in 11 out of 13 patients.[366] Both failures united after secondary iliac crest bone grafting. By comparison in the same study, all 12 nonunions in patients treated with autograft healed without further intervention.

Bone Marrow Aspirate

Bone marrow aspirate, primarily from the iliac crest, has been shown to contain osteoprogenitor cells and has osteogenic and osteoinductive properties.[19] The generally low concentration of such cells ($612/cm^3$) and the variability between patients (12 to $1,224/cm^3$) has led to the development of improved aspiration techniques with specialized aspiration needles and cell concentration systems aimed at increasing both the number and density of the progenitor cells.[149] Without concentration, the evidence suggests that the number of cells in a marrow aspirate is suboptimal for nonunion treatment.[150] Furthermore, some controversy exists as to whether concentrated cells should be injected directly and percutaneously into nonunion sites or if applications with an osteoconductive carrier after open debridement of the nonunion are required for optimal results.[297] The actual efficiency of direct marrow injection is difficult to interpret in the face of associated interventions including cast immobilization and IM nailing that have accompanied the injection in series reporting union rates ranging from 75% to 90%.[64,111,123]

Platelet-Rich Plasma

PRP is harvested as the thin layer between clear plasma and red blood cells in centrifuged peripheral blood. This fluid contains concentrated platelets (300% to 600%) which are believed to promote osteoblast proliferation and differentiation.[330] However, to date no clinical evidence exists to support PRP in the treatment of nonunions.

Allograft and Ceramics

Other graft substitute materials such as ceramics (calcium sulfate, calcium phosphates, beta tricalcium phosphate, and hydroxyapatite) and allograft lack osteoinductive or osteogenic properties and have little role in promoting bone healing in the setting of nonunion. These ceramic materials are primarily osteoconductive and function best as graft extenders or carriers for other osteoinductive compounds.[33] The structural properties of allograft struts have been exploited most commonly for periprosthetic nonunions with bone loss[241] and in the management of proximal humeral nonunions.[110]

Graft Site Preparation

Successful application of a bone graft or a bone graft substitute requires preparation of the local recipient site.

The general principles are to expose healthy bone by removing local scar or other intervening materials, to increase surface area for graft adherence, and to stimulate blood flow to the affected area. These principles can be extended to the situation of a nonunion being repaired primarily with compression without the use of adjuvant graft. Debridement of a nonunion site is tedious and time consuming, but it is perhaps one of the most critical steps in nonunion management. Thorough debridement is at times at odds with preservation of local soft tissue attachments. Debridement of the space directly between the bone ends can be accomplished with exposure from one direction and therefore with limited circumferential soft tissue stripping. However, application, adherence, and consolidation of graft to the periphery of a long bone nonunion are biomechanically advantageous. Graft material placed at a further radius from the center axis provides substantially more strength than centrally placed material. This is based on calculations of cylinder strength: Torsional strength is proportional to the third power of the radius and bending strength is proportional to the fourth power of the radius. Therefore it is advantageous to circumferentially prepare either side of a diaphyseal nonunion while at the same time minimizing soft tissue stripping.

The technique of Judet and Patel,[166] which dates back over 40 years, remains a standard method to prepare the bone for grafting. This technique involves raising osteoperiosteal fragments from the periphery of the nonunion, either through cortex or callus. An osteotome is used to create small, 2- to 3-mm, fragments of cortex, each with an attached soft tissue sleeve. An area 3 to 4 centimeters in length on each side of the nonunion and covering approximately two-thirds of its circumference is so treated. This method increases surface area for bone graft healing and may stimulate the healing process. Various modifications have been proposed,[203,223] yet the original Judet principles remain steadfastly utilized. Petaling or fish scaling represents a less elegant and technically easier modification. An osteotome or a small gauge is used to simply raise flakes of bone that resemble flower petals or fish scales. This increases surface area and can promote bleeding into the area, but may have more limited biologic effects than the true Judet technique. These techniques should be applied with caution in osteoporotic bone, as iatrogenic fractures and weakening of the bone may hamper fixation.

SPECIAL CIRCUMSTANCES IN THE TREATMENT OF NONUNIONS

Managing Articular Nonunion

Articular nonunions are relatively uncommon. A potential causative factor is inadequate compression of the articular fracture gap leading to prolonged exposure of the fracture surfaces to synovial fluid. These nonunions are therefore commonly oligo-trophic and amenable to compression techniques.[293] Evaluation of and operative planning for articular nonunions should consider, in addition to standard factors evaluated for nonarticular nonunions, articular congruity, associated arthrosis, stability, and stiffness of the affected joint. The ideal situation for repair of an articular nonunion is one without associated joint arthrosis, without joint instability, and with minimal stiffness. Repair will not address or improve arthrosis and joint stability is often difficult to accomplish with nonunion repair alone. A stiff joint will put the nonunion repair under greater stress during postoperative rehabilitation than is seen with the repair of a nonunion involving a supple joint. Therefore, either the joint contracture should be released during nonunion repair or postoperative range of motion exercises should be modified to minimize the risk of implant failure before union can occur. As with any articular fracture, the goals of articular nonunion treatment include restoration of articular congruity, recreation of proper limb alignment, maximization of joint function, and minimization of pain. When these goals cannot be accomplished with nonunion repair, joint arthroplasty becomes a relatively attractive option.[18,30,78] Arthroplasty is particularly beneficial when patient age is advanced or baseline function is low. In the presence of active infection total joint arthroplasty is contraindicated and resection arthroplasty or arthrodesis become considerations. Both arthroplasty and arthrodesis as treatments for nonunion are discussed in further detail in prior sections of this chapter.

Managing Segmental Bone Loss

Segmental defects related to trauma may result from acute bone loss or be related to established nonunions. Regardless of the etiology, these are very challenging problems for the patient and the surgeon alike. Management of the chronic skeletal defect may be only part of the challenge, as infection and soft tissue compromise are often associated. Several surgical options are available to manage segmental defects including autogenous bone grafting, free vascularized fibular bone grafts, and bone transport. The relative rarity of these problems and the substantial variability between cases means that high-level evidence to guide treatment is difficult to come by. Therefore, treatment decisions are based on knowledge of the available low-level evidence, but more importantly, knowledge of contemporary principles of nonunion management, and consideration of personal experience and skill with the various methods.

A critical-sized defect is generally regarded as one that requires an intervention, most commonly some type of grafting or transport procedure, in addition to bony stabilization to achieve union. What constitutes a critical-sized defect varies based on a number of factors including the particular bone involved, the relative location within the bone, the state of the surrounding soft tissues, and the expected biologic response of the host (acute fracture vs. established nonunion, healthy patient vs. diabetic smoker, etc).

Autogenous Bone Grafting Using the Masquelet Technique

For segmental loss, the technique of Masquelet or primary shortening followed by lengthening is favored. In the technique of Masquelet, the area of segmental loss is filled with a PMMA cement. At 4 to 6 weeks, when an osteogenic membrane has been formed around the cement, the membrane is surgically reopened, the cement is removed, and generous cancellous grafting is carried out (Fig. 27-23). Recorticalization generally occurs slowly but usually by 3 to 6 months. This, of course, is done in conjunction with internal stabilization most frequently using a locked IM rod for diaphyseal defects or locked plates for metaphyseal defects.[201] The initial role of the spacer is to maintain the space for future grafting by avoidance of fibrous ingrowth. The secondary role of the spacer is the induction of membrane formation. This membrane is synovial-like with few

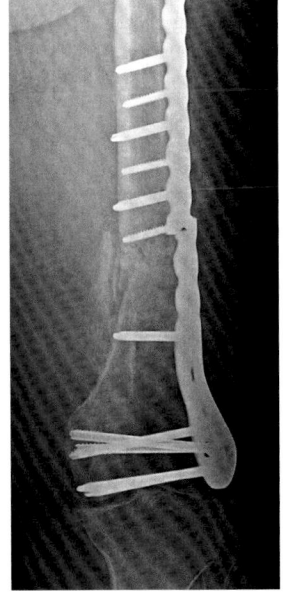 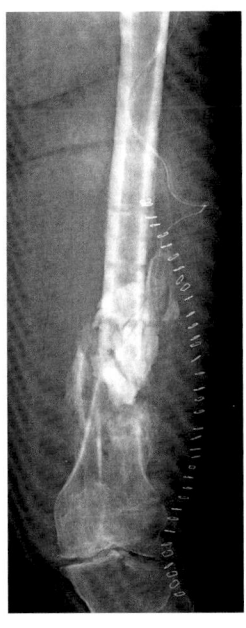 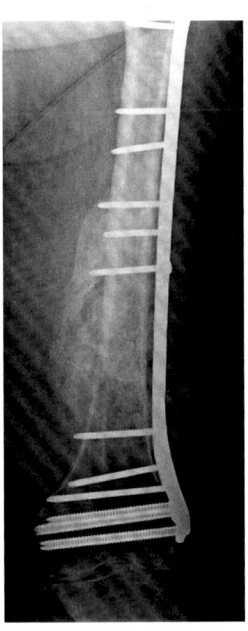

FIGURE 27-23 An infected nonunion of the distal femur **(A)** is treated with removal of failed implants, debridement, and implantation of an antibiotic-impregnated cement spacer according to the Masquelet technique **(B)**. Healing is accomplished after appropriate antibiotic therapy followed by nonunion repair with removal of the cement spacer, iliac crest bone grafting of the defect, and plate stabilization **(C)**.   A, B   C

inflammatory cells.[243] The membrane itself serves to contain the graft, prevent fibrous ingrowth, and provide growth factors.[3] Immunochemistry has shown that the membrane produces growth factors and inductive factors including BMP-2 which are probably maximal around 4 weeks.[243] In his original article, Masquelet reported successful use of this two-stage technique in 35 cases with defects ranging from 4 to 25 cm in length.[201] Other authors have had similar success with this staged membrane-induced technique.[267,289] The underlying mechanism of the membrane formation is not well understood but cases when the membrane itself has generated enough bone so that secondary grafting is not necessary have been observed in our practices. It is unclear whether this membrane can form with substances other than methyl methacrylate and this technique requires an excellent soft tissue envelope.[201]

Ilizarov Techniques for Bone Defects

Using Ilizarov techniques to treat nonunions without associated bone defects typically involves simple compression or distraction or some combination of compression and distraction at the nonunion site. This is considered a monofocal Ilizarov technique (Fig. 27-24). When bone defects are present, corticotomy at an adjacent site followed by distraction osteogenesis through the corticotomy (bone transport) and eventual compression at the nonunion site is a bifocal (distraction-compression) Ilizarov method for management of bone defects (Fig. 27-25). Two-level lengthening with compression at the nonunion site is considered trifocal bone transport. These methods have been applied with success for more than the last two decades in the management of tibial defects.[58,234,237,308]

Blum et al.,[29] in a retrospective series of 50 consecutive patients treated with distraction osteogenesis for an infected femoral nonunion, evaluated the associated complications. The infected nonunion sites were widely debrided creating segmental defects. In this exceedingly difficult group of patients who had an average of 3.8 prior surgical procedures, it is not unexpected that treatment was protracted, and a majority of patients experienced some complication. The duration of the distraction osteogenesis was 24.5 months; all patients sustained pin tract infections; knee range of motion was consistently reduced; 26% had persistent pain; and the residual leg length discrepancy was 1.9 cm on average. However, union was achieved in all but one patient.

The relative ease of use and the ability for simultaneous deformity correction have made the use of the Taylor Spatial Frame an attractive option for these cases.[270,278] Good results in a small (n = 12) retrospective series were recently reported by Sala et al.[278] for the management of postinfectious atrophic tibial nonunions using techniques of bifocal and trifocal bone transport. All patients were treated using Ilizarov principles but with the Taylor Spatial Frame apparatus. All patients achieved union and eradication of the infection.

Management of Infected Nonunions

The diagnosis of an infected nonunion can be obvious or very subtle. The diagnostic gold standard is a positive deep tissue or bone culture. However, the morbidity and expense of a separate surgical procedure to obtain deep cultures from a nonunion site is not warranted unless there is a sufficient index of suspicion. Establishing the correct threshold for what constitutes a "sufficient" index of suspicion is more art than science. An astute

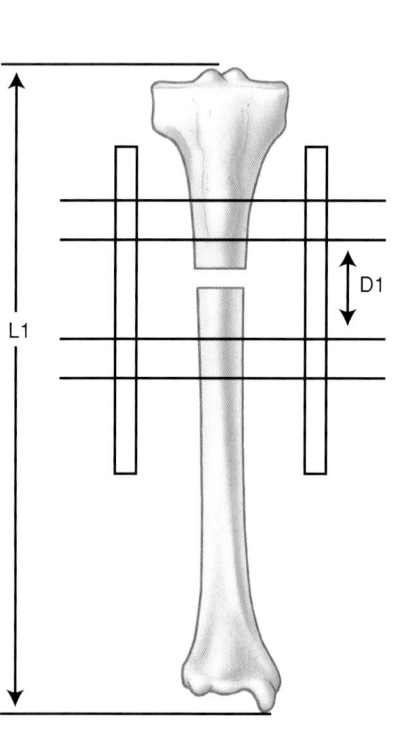
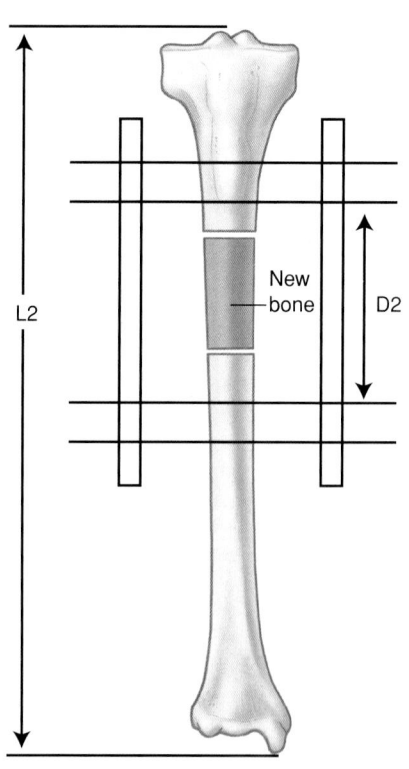

Before   **After**

FIGURE 27-24 Schematic diagram of monofocal Ilizarov lengthening technique. Increased length (L2–L1) is accomplished by increasing distance at one location (D2–D1).

Before   **After**

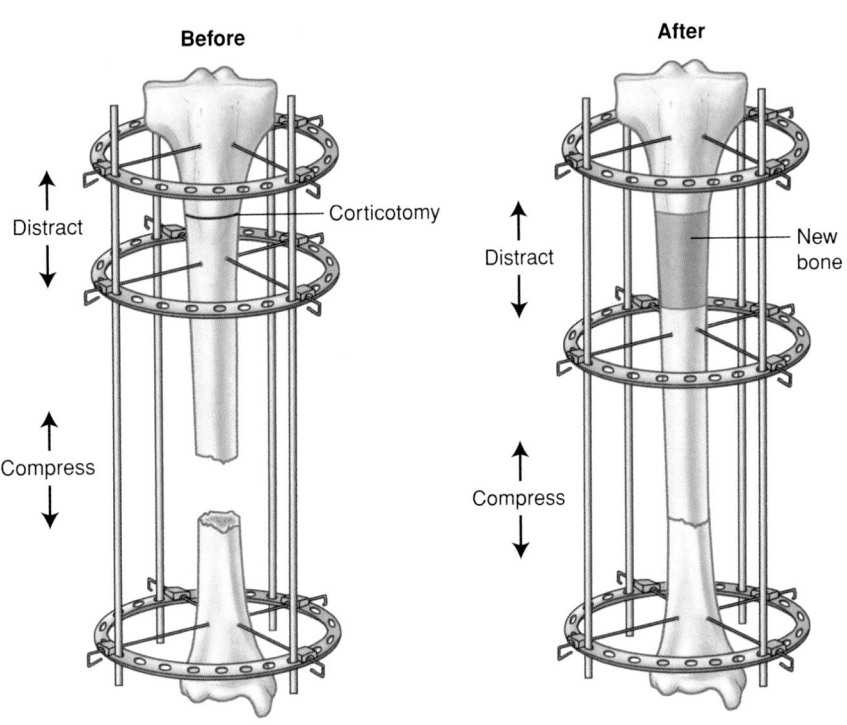

FIGURE 27-25 Schematic diagram of bifocal Ilizarov technique.

history and physical examination are of critical importance. A history of a previous open fracture or open fracture management raises the suspicion more than a prior closed fracture treated nonoperatively. Any history of a confirmed prior infection or of persistently draining traumatic or surgical wounds also substantially raises suspicion for infection. Pain at a nonunion site that is constant rather than activity-related may be another clue to an underlying infection. Any physical examination finding consistent with acute or chronic inflammation should also be considered a sign of potential deep infection in the setting of nonunion. Laboratory evaluation for the diagnosis of infection associated with nonunion typically includes a complete blood count (CBC), erythrocyte sedimentation rate (ESR), and C-reactive protein (CRP) level. The utility of these and other tests to diagnose bone infection are discussed further in Chapter 26.

After gathering diagnostic information regarding the potential for an infected nonunion, the clinician is often left contemplating the relative risk of infection and the appropriate course of action. It is useful to stratify risk as low, moderate or high. Again, as stated above, such stratification is largely based on experience rather than established guidelines. In a low risk setting, nonunion repair may proceed with the assumption that infection does not exist. Intra-operative cultures prior to the administration of antibiotics is a consideration but not mandatory in such cases. Surprise positive cultures in this scenario, when pre-operative clinical or laboratory evidence of infection was minimal or absent, are occasionally encountered. Internal fixation and bone grafts used in such a clinically non-infected but culture positive nonunion site can be successfully left in-situ with continuation of antibiotic therapy until union is achieved.[87]

When there is a moderate suspicion for infection it is prudent to plan for deep intraoperative cultures, intraoperative frozen section of the associated soft tissue (as frozen section of bone is usually not possible), careful inspection of the local environment for signs of infection, and a potentially staged treatment strategy. Patients should be advised of this possibility preoperatively. When intraoperative findings are benign, nonunion repair at this operative setting is reasonable. Suspicious findings usually trigger a staged protocol directed at infection control and eradication while awaiting definitive culture results. If final cultures are negative, nonunion repair can then commence.

When the suspicion for infection is high but not yet established, the initial management plan usually proceeds with the assumption that infection is present. The initial operative setting is therefore dedicated to confirming the diagnosis and preparing the nonunion for eventual repair as discussed in the following paragraphs. In the setting of an established infected nonunion, control, and when possible eradication, of infection normally takes precedence over efforts to achieve union. In the absence of infection, achieving union, even in the setting of a segmental defect, is usually achievable in all but the most challenging host. However, each case must be individualized and at times a reasonable strategy can be formulated to manage infection simultaneously with efforts to achieve bone healing or even to prioritize bone healing.

One consideration in the management of infected nonunions is whether to remove or retain existing implants. When evidence suggests that existing implants are providing no or marginal stability, removal is the usual course because retention provides little or no benefit. In the circumstance when the existing implants are providing sufficient stability and appear that they will continue to provide sufficient stability during the course of management of the infected nonunion, the decision to remove or retain implants is more controversial.[87,183] This

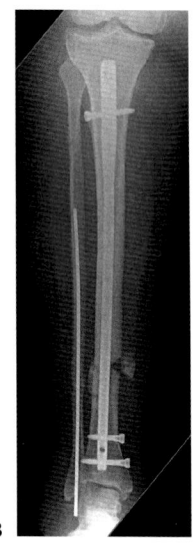
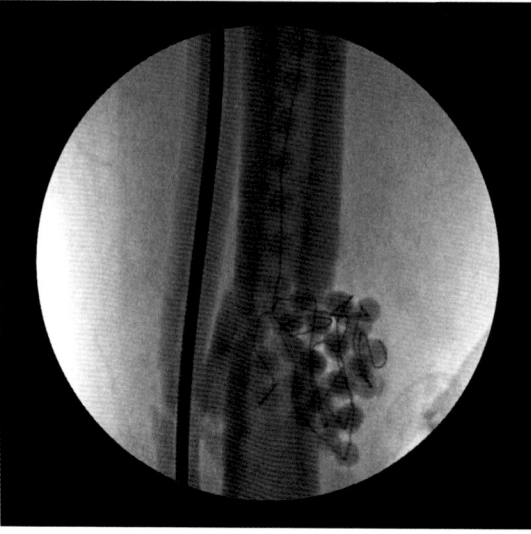
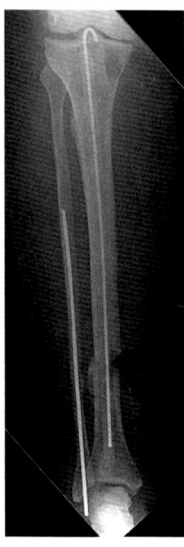

A, B   C

FIGURE 27-26 An infected tibial nonunion **(A)** is managed initially with removal of implants, debridement, and local antibiotic delivery (in addition to IV antibiotics) **(B)**, then repeat debridement and placement of an antibiotic impregnated IM "nail" **(C)**.

decision represents a conundrum. Internal implants may
increase the risk for persistent infection and impair the host's
ability to eradicate it, yet the stability imparted by the implants
may benefit the treatment of infection and may provide patient
comfort and retained function. Situations most amenable to
implant retention are those where union can be expected without the need for grafting procedures. The strategy relies on
suppression of infection while allowing the existing biologic
process, with the existing implants, to progress toward union.
Once union occurs, implant removal becomes part of the strategy to eradicate infection. The alternative strategy, removal of
implants, is most applicable when control of infection is particularly problematic or when bone grafting is thought to be
required. Metal implants are known to promote both adherence of microbes and biofilm formation and adversely affect
phagocytosis, thereby making control of infection more difficult, especially in a compromised host.[130,131] Bone graft,
whether autograft or allograft, is generally considered avascular upon initial implantation and therefore can provide fertile
ground for infection. In the situation when removal of internal
implants leaves the nonunion unstable, external fixation with
pins and wires placed outside the zone of infection, is normally
selected. In the long bones, a reinforced antibiotic bone cement
rod can serve to simultaneously provide local antibiotic administration and stability (Fig. 27-26).[229,236,296,319] This technique
is relatively simple and well tolerated. The cement nail is fashioned using an appropriately sized chest tube as a mold. Chest
tube sizing units, French (Fr), represent the outer circumference. The inner diameter depends on the wall thickness of the
chest tube, a parameter that varies based on the manufacturer.
The approximate outer and inner diameters of various-sized
chest tubes is presented in Table 27-2. Cement in a semi-liquid
state is injected into a chest tube of appropriate inner diameter,
usually about 1.5 mm smaller than the reamed canal to avoid
excessive stress on the nail during insertion. Length is based

upon intraoperative measurements. A thin rod, such as a guidewire used for IM reaming, is inserted as a reinforcing metal core
before curing of the cement. A hook can be fashioned at the
driving end of the nail to facilitate removal. Once the cement has
hardened and cooled down, the chest tube is cut off. The cement
nail is then inserted through the same portal as used for prior IM
nailing, is easily removed, and allows easy subsequent exchange
nailing. When additional strength is required, such as a very unstable femoral nonunion in a large patient, cement can be manually
placed around a standard small-diameter nail. One retrospective analysis revealed success in 14 of 16 patients with infected
nonunions of long bones treated with a protocol of culture-
specific IV and oral antibiotics, surgical debridement, and stabilization with an antibiotic-impregnated bone cement rod.[296]

Management of the infectious process in the setting of an
infected nonunion follows the general principles for the treatment of osteomyelitis as presented in Chapter 26. Surgical
debridement of the infected nonviable bone and surrounding
nonviable soft tissues, culture-specific parenteral antibiotics, and
bone stabilization are the primary goals. Local antibiotic delivery is often included, especially when a dead space results from
debridement, in the form of an antibiotic-impregnated synthetic
material. Polymethylmethacrylate (PMMA) as cement beads or

TABLE 27-2	Inner and Outer Diameters of Chest Tubes	
Chest Tube Size	Outer Diameter	Approximate Inner Diameter
38 Fr	12.1 mm	9.4 mm
40 Fr	12.7 mm	10 mm
42 Fr	13.3 mm	10.5 mm
44 Fr	14 mm	11.3 mm

as a cement spacer is the most common vehicle used for antibiotic delivery in this setting.[43,56,95] Beads have greater surface area than a spacer and therefore may provide higher initial antibiotic concentrations, but the effective duration for antibiotic elution may be shorter.[302] Creation of a bead pouch is an excellent method for local antibiotic delivery between serial debridement procedures. With regard to longer term implantation, beads can be substantially more difficult to remove after more than 4 weeks than a block of cement because of the ingrowth of scar tissue. Also, an antibiotic cement spacer prepares the defect for bone grafting according to the Masquelet technique previously described. An obvious shortfall of a nonabsorbable delivery system such as PMMA is the typical need for removal. Bioabsorbable bone substitutes that can be impregnated with antibiotics are osteoconductive, may promote bone healing, and do not necessarily require a second stage procedure for removal. Numerous animal, and more recently human, clinical trials support this approach.[121,210] McKee et al.[209] have recently reported promising results in a prospective randomized trial comparing an antibiotic-impregnated calcium sulfate bone substitute to standard antibiotic-impregnated PMMA beads in the treatment of chronic osteomyelitis and infected nonunion. Infection was eradicated in 86% of the patients from both groups; seven of the eight patients achieved healing of their nonunion in the bioabsorbable group compared to six of the eight in the PMMA group, and there were more operations in the PMMA group.

Infected nonunions are generally treated in a staged manner. However, Wu[350] reported success with one-stage surgical treatment of infected nonunion of the distal tibia. Twenty-two consecutive patients were successfully managed to union with a protocol of implant removal, intra- and extramedullary debridement, cancellous autograft with antibiotics (vancomycin and gentamycin), and stabilization with an Ilizarov fixator.

Management of Soft Tissue Compromise Associated with Nonunion

When soft tissues are poor or deficient and free tissue transfer is not possible, primary shortening with an IM rod followed by full weight bearing and an elevated shoe is preferred. Once healing has occurred, the limb can be relengthened if the patient desires with either an internal skeletal distraction nail (ISKD Orthofix Inc, McKinney, Texas) (Fig. 27-27) or the Ilizarov technique.[222,276,333] In some cases with less than 3 or 4 cm of shortening, patients are often satisfied with the result and do not desire secondary lengthening. The internal skeletal distraction nail seems to be better tolerated than the skinny

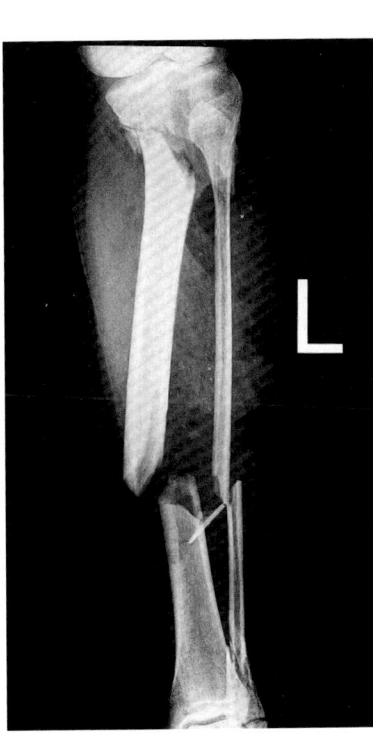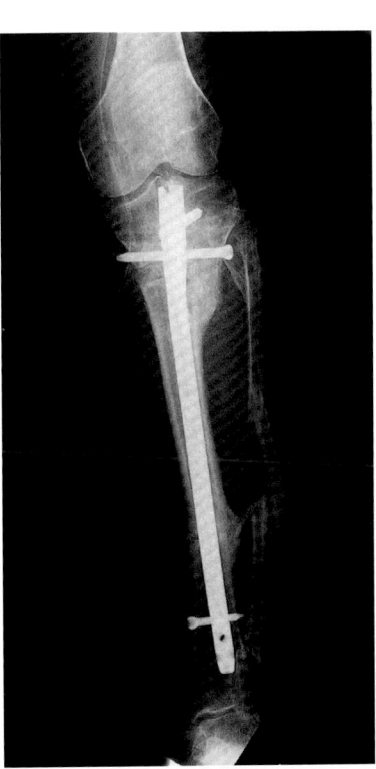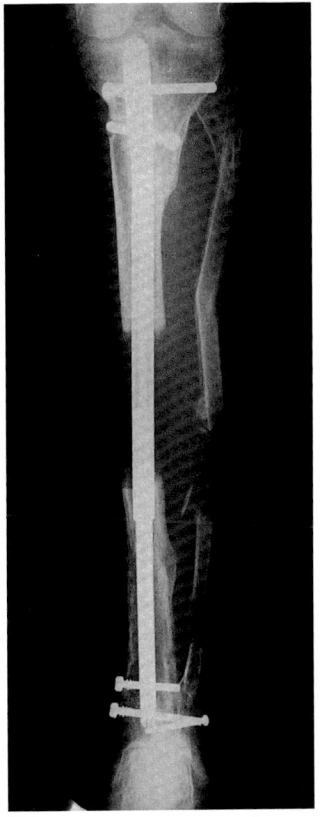

A, B   **C**

FIGURE 27-27 A 40-year-old female with a grade IIIB open tibia. The central fragment was completely stripped of soft tissue. She was not a candidate for free tissue transfer. **(B)** After resection of the devitalized bone, the leg was shortened and treated with a locked rod. The fracture healed with full weight-bearing ambulation in a built-up shoe. Note the overlapping fibula. Only local soft tissues, which were adequate in volume after shortening, were used for coverage. **(C)** Subsequent lengthening with the internal skeletal distraction nail.

(continues)

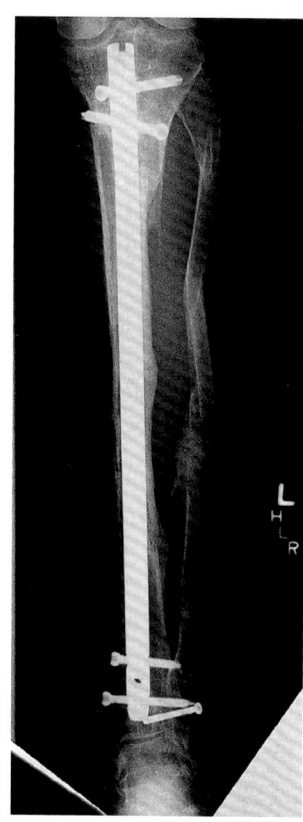

D

FIGURE 27-27 (*continued*) **(D)** After exchange nailing the regenerate was mature at about 6 months. (Case courtesy of Dr. Timothy Weber Orthoindy Indianapolis, IN.)

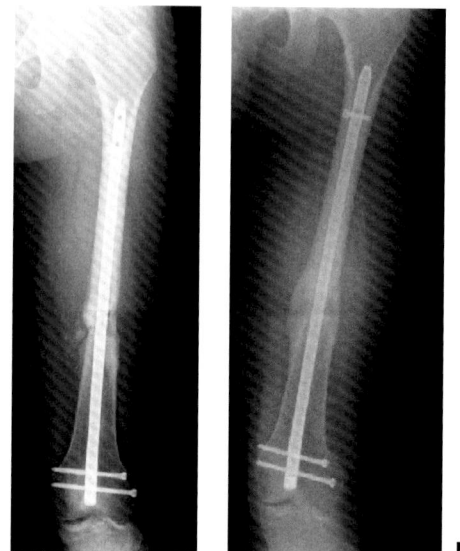

A **B**

FIGURE 27-28 AP radiograph **(A)** showing a nonunion in a 27-year-old man 6 months after intramedullary nailing of a mid-diaphyseal femur fracture. At this point, the patient was fully weight bearing with minimal pain and an ultrasound external bone stimulator was applied 20 minutes daily. Six months later and without further surgical intervention the nonunion is healed **(B)**.

wire external fixator techniques. It is, however, no faster. Complications similar to those with other distraction or transport techniques still exist including too fast or too slow distraction, failure or delay of regenerate bone formation, adjacent joint problems, a need for exchange nailing, and failure of the distraction device itself.

AUTHOR'S PREFERENCES IN THE TREATMENT OF NONUNIONS

Nonoperative Nonunion Treatment

External stimulation alone, typically ultrasound, is reserved for patients who are minimally symptomatic from their nonunion and who are not candidates for surgery or additional procedures (Fig. 27-28). Ultrasound stimulation is sometimes used in conjunction with operative treatment in high-risk patients such as smokers and diabetics.

Operative Treatment of Nonunion
Preferred Treatment of Septic Nonunions

Septic nonunions are one of the most challenging reconstructive procedures facing the orthopaedic traumatologist. These patients deserve the expertise of a team fluent in their management. Often, infected nonunions are limb-threatening condi-

tions. Given the seriousness of this condition, our approach is to maximize the treatment decisions toward eradicating infection. Therefore, hardware removal, wide debridement, soft tissue coverage as needed, culture-specific local and IV antibiotics, and bony stabilization are utilized in the initial phase of a multistage management protocol. Local antibiotic delivery is typically with antibiotic beads between serial debridements and with antibiotic PMMA spacers or antibiotic rods after definitive closure. Stabilization is with an antibiotic rod when applicable (e.g., diaphyseal tibia nonunion), otherwise with external fixation.

The second phase of management is dedicated to treatment with IV antibiotics and monitoring. We rely on an infectious disease team experienced in the management of osteomyelitis to direct the selection and duration of antibiotic therapy and manage any encountered side effects. The second phase ends when clinical, laboratory, and radiographic signs of infection are absent, usually after 6 weeks of therapy.

The third phase in the management of infected nonunions typically mimics the management of atrophic aseptic nonunions as discussed in the following section. One important decision at this juncture is whether to discontinue antibiotic therapy prior to nonunion repair or to continue therapy through and after nonunion repair. We generally lean toward continuation of oral therapy until union has occurred whenever there is any doubt regarding the success in eradication of infection.

Preferred Treatment of Aseptic Nonunions
Preferred Treatment of Atrophic and Oligotrophic Nonunions

The first consideration when dealing with nonviable or marginally vital nonunions is whether direct compression of the bone ends is possible without unacceptable shortening. When the answer is yes, then compression with a nail or plate is desired unless the soft tissues dictate the need for thin wire external fixation. If the nonunion is well aligned, then the choice of IM nailing or plating is largely based on the location of the nonunion. Well aligned nondiaphyseal nonunions, in the absence of bone loss, are preferably managed with compression plating. Diaphyseal nonunions without bone defects are preferably managed with primary IM nailing or exchange nailing (if a nail was previously used) if well aligned. If the nonunion is malaligned, compression plating is preferred regardless of location. When direct compression of atrophic nonunions can be accomplished without any remaining defects, we find it unnecessary to add bone graft. This is an unusual circumstance most commonly encountered when dealing with humeral and clavicle nonunions. When direct compression still leaves some

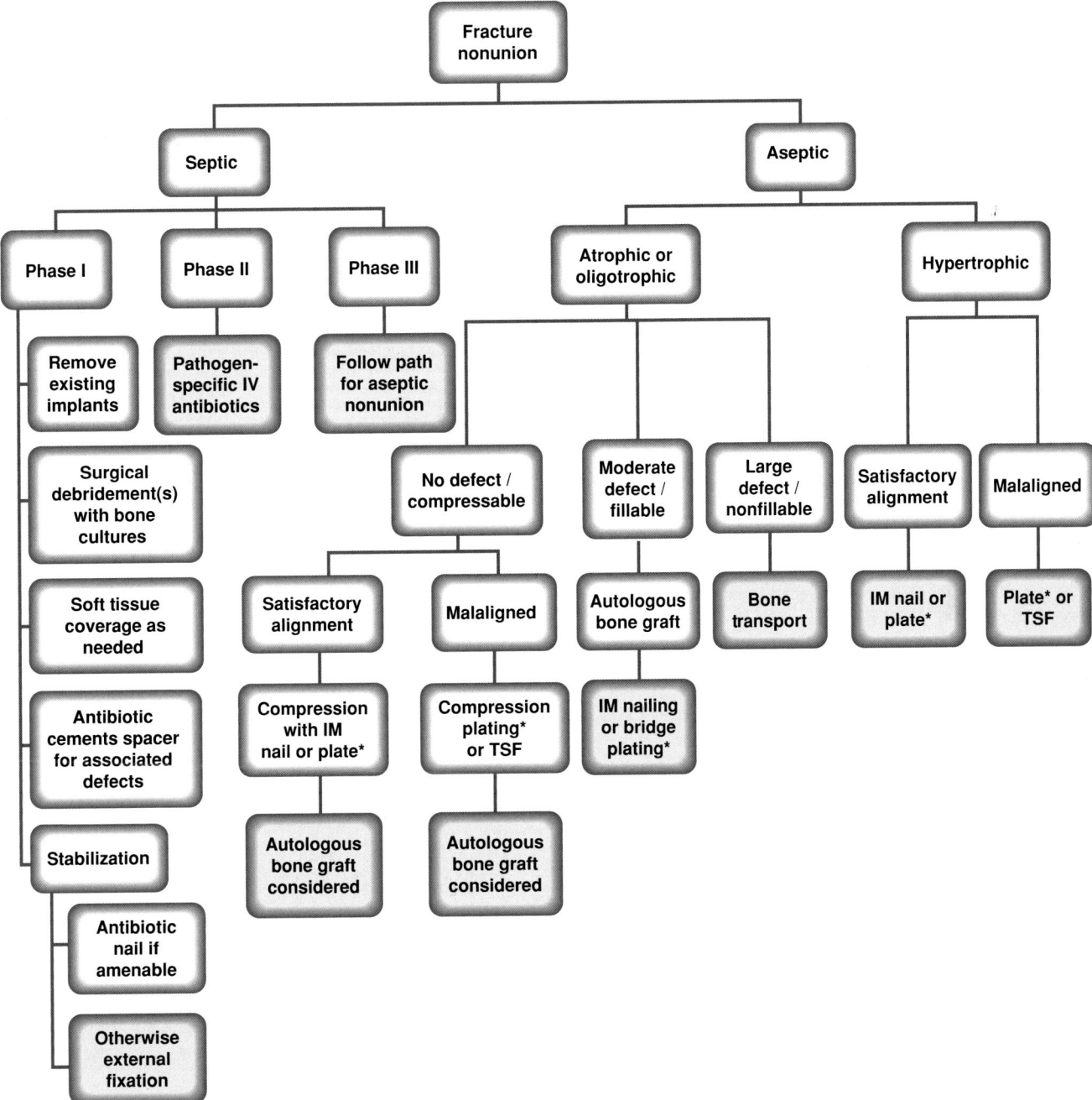

FIGURE 27-29 Author's preferred treatment algorithm for nonunions. *When soft tissues are compromised IM nailing is favored over plate fixation unless tissue transfer precedes nonunion treatment. For diaphyseal nonunions, IM nailing is preferred over plating and for metaphyseal or articular nonunions, plating is preferred over IM nailing (TSF = Taylor Spatial Frame).

bony defect, autologous cancellous bone is our primary choice of graft material. Cancellous allograft combined with BMP is a reasonable alternative. We find no utility in grafting atrophic nonunions with allograft alone.

When bone defects are present we prefer to fill the defect with autologous bone graft when available in sufficient quantities. Graft from the iliac crest harvested with an acetabular reamer and graft harvested from the femur using the RIA system have been found to be equally effective in our experience. When the volume of autologous graft is insufficient to fill the defect, we preferentially use cancellous allograft to expand the volume. As a rule of thumb, a ratio of autograft to allograft of up to 1:2 is acceptable. When greater relative quantities of allograft are expected to be required, bone transport methods rather than direct void filling is generally utilized. We prefer to think of the autologous and allograft mixture as being one of three grades. Grade A graft is pure autograft. This has the greatest potential for healing and is used in the most important regions of the nonunion, typically at the periphery. Grade B graft is a mixture of autograft and allograft. This has intermediate biologic potential for healing and is used centrally to fill the medullary canal of long bone nonunions. Grade C graft is pure allograft. It has the least potential for healing of the three grades and it is used sparingly and in locations that are the least important for rapid healing. Fixation in the presence of a filled defect is either with an IM nail or a bridge plate.

Preferred Treatment of Hypertrophic Nonunions

Hypertrophic nonunions are simply realigned if necessary, then stabilized and when possible, compressed (Fig. 27-2A and 27-2D). The choice of implant depends upon the location of the nonunion and limb alignment. Well aligned hypertrophic nonunions at the end segment of long bones or of flat bones are preferably managed with plating. Hypertrophic diaphyseal nonunions are preferably managed with primary IM nailing or exchange nailing (if a nail was previously used) when well aligned. If the nonunion is malaligned, plating is preferred regardless of location (Fig. 27-29).

REFERENCES

1. Adie S, Harris IA, Naylor JM, et al. Pulsed electromagnetic field stimulation for acute tibial shaft fractures: a multicenter, double-blind, randomized trial. *J Bone Joint Surg Am.* 2011;93(17):1569–1576.
2. Ahlmann E, Patzakis M, Roidis N, et al. Comparison of anterior and posterior iliac crest bone grafts in terms of harvest-site morbidity and functional outcomes. *J Bone Joint Surg Am.* 2002;84-A(5):716–720.
3. Aho OM, Lehenkari P, Ristiniemi J, et al. The mechanism of action of induced membranes in bone repair. *J Bone Joint Surg Am.* 2013;95(7):597–604.
4. Al-Sayyad MJ. Taylor spatial frame in the treatment of upper extremity conditions. *J Pediatr Orthop.* 2012;32(2):169–178.
5. Appleton P, Moran M, Houshian S, et al. Distal femoral fractures treated by hinged total knee replacement in elderly patients. *J Bone Joint Surg Br.* 2006;88(8):1065–1070.
6. Arrington ED, Smith WJ, Chambers HG, et al. Complications of iliac crest bone graft harvesting. *Clin Orthop Relat Res.* 1996;(329):300–309.
7. Azuma Y, Ito M, Harada Y, et al. Low-intensity pulsed ultrasound accelerates rat femoral fracture healing by acting on the various cellular reactions in the fracture callus. *J Bone Miner Res.* 2001;16(4):671–680.
8. Baksi DP, Pal AK, Baksi D. Prosthetic replacement of elbow for intercondylar fractures (recent or ununited) of humerus in the elderly. *Int Orthop.* 2011;35(8):1171–1177.
9. Ballmer FT, Ballmer PM, Baumgaertel F, et al. Pauwels osteotomy for nonunions of the femoral neck. *Orthop Clin North Am.* 1990;21(4):759–767.
10. Banic A, Hertel R. Double vascularized fibulas for reconstruction of large tibial defects. *J Reconstr Microsurg.* 1993;9(6):421–428.
11. Banwart JC, Asher MA, Hassanein RS. Iliac crest bone graft harvest donor site morbidity. A statistical evaluation. *Spine (Phila Pa 1976).* 1995;20(9):1055–1060.
12. Barwick TW, Montgomery RJ. Knee arthrodesis with lengthening: Experience of using Ilizarov techniques to salvage large asymmetric defects following infected peri-articular fractures. *Injury.* 2013;44:1043–1048.
13. Basbozkurt M, Kurklu M, Yurttas Y, et al. Ilizarov external fixation without removal of plate or screws: effect on hypertrophic and oligotrophic nonunion of the femoral shaft with plate failure. *J Orthop Trauma.* 2012;26(8):e123–e128.
14. Beam HA, Parsons JR, Lin SS. The effects of blood glucose control upon fracture healing in the BB Wistar rat with diabetes mellitus. *J.Orthop.Res.* 2002;20(6):1210–1216.
15. Beck A, Salem K, Krischak G, et al. Nonsteroidal anti-inflammatory drugs (NSAIDs) in the perioperative phase in traumatology and orthopedics effects on bone healing. *Oper Orthop Traumatol.* 2005;17(6):569–578.
16. Belthur MV, Conway JD, Jindal G, et al. Bone graft harvest using a new intramedullary system. *Clin Orthop Relat Res.* 2008;466(12):2973–2980.
17. Bennett MH, Stanford R, Turner R. Hyperbaric oxygen therapy for promoting fracture healing and treating fracture non-union. *Cochrane Database Syst Rev.* 2005;(1):CD004712.
18. Berend KR, Lombardi AV Jr. Distal femoral replacement in nontumor cases with severe bone loss and instability. *Clin Orthop Relat Res.* 2009;467(2):485–492.
19. Beresford JN. Osteogenic stem cells and the stromal system of bone and marrow. *Clin Orthop Relat Res.* 1989;(240):270–280.
20. Bergmann P, Schoutens A. Prostaglandins and bone. *Bone.* 1995;16(4):485–488.
21. Betz OB, Betz VM, Nazarian A, et al. Direct percutaneous gene delivery to enhance healing of segmental bone defects. *J Bone Joint Surg Am.* 2006;88(2):355–365.
22. Bhandari M, Fong K, Sprague S, et al. Variability in the definition and perceived causes of delayed unions and nonunions: a cross-sectional, multinational survey of orthopaedic surgeons. *J Bone Joint Surg Am.* 2012;94(15):e1091–1096.
23. Bhandari M, Guyatt G, Tornetta P 3rd, et al. Randomized trial of reamed and unreamed intramedullary nailing of tibial shaft fractures. *J Bone Joint Surg Am.* 2008;90(12):2567–2578.
24. Bhandari M, Guyatt GH, Swiontkowski MF, et al. A lack of consensus in the assessment of fracture healing among orthopaedic surgeons. *J.Orthop.Trauma.* 2002;16(8):562–566.
25. Bhandari M, Tornetta P III, Sprague S, et al. Predictors of reoperation following operative management of fractures of the tibial shaft. *J.Orthop.Trauma.* 2003;17(5):353–361.
26. Bhattacharyya T, Bouchard KA, Phadke A, et al. The accuracy of computed tomography for the diagnosis of tibial nonunion. *J.Bone Joint Surg.Am.* 2006;88(4):692–697.
27. Biedermann R, Martin A, Handle G, et al. Extracorporeal shock waves in the treatment of nonunions. *J Trauma.* 2003;54(5):936–942.
28. Bielecki T, Gazdzik TS, Szczepanski T. Benefit of percutaneous injection of autologous platelet-leukocyte-rich gel in patients with delayed union and nonunion. *Eur Surg Res.* 2008;40(3):289–296.
29. Blum AL, BongioVanni JC, Morgan SJ, et al. Complications associated with distraction osteogenesis for infected nonunion of the femoral shaft in the presence of a bone defect: a retrospective series. *J Bone Joint Surg Br.* 2010;92(4):565–570.
30. Boileau P, Trojani C, Walch G, et al. Shoulder arthroplasty for the treatment of the sequelae of fractures of the proximal humerus. *J Shoulder Elbow Surg.* 2001;10(4):299–308.
31. Bong MR, Capla EL, Egol KA, et al. Osteogenic protein-1 (bone morphogenic protein-7) combined with various adjuncts in the treatment of humeral diaphyseal nonunions. *Bull Hosp Jt Dis.* 2005;63(1–2):20–23.
32. Borrelli J Jr, Leduc S, Gregush R, et al. Tricortical bone grafts for treatment of malaligned tibias and fibulas. *Clin Orthop Relat Res.* 2009;467(4):1056–1063.
33. Borrelli J Jr, Prickett WD, Ricci WM. Treatment of nonunions and osseous defects with bone graft and calcium sulfate. *Clin Orthop Relat Res.* 2003;(411):245–254.
34. Borrelli J Jr, Tinsley K, Ricci WM, et al. Induction of chondrocyte apoptosis following impact load. *J.Orthop.Trauma.* 2003;17(9):635–641.
35. Brashear HR. Treatment of ununited fractures of the long bones; diagnosis and prevention of non-union. *J.Bone Joint Surg.Am.* 1965;47:174–178.
36. Brighton CT, Shaman P, Heppenstall RB, et al. Tibial nonunion treated with direct current, capacitive coupling, or bone graft. *Clin.Orthop.Relat Res.* 1995;(321):223–234.
37. Brinker MR. Nonunions: evaluation and treatment. In: Browner BD, Jupiter JB, Levine AM, Trafton PG, eds. *Skeletal Trauma Basic Science Management and Reconstruction.* Philadelphia, PA: WB Saunders; 2003:507–604.
38. Brinker MR, O'Connor DP. Exchange nailing of ununited fractures. *J.Bone Joint Surg. Am.* 2007;89(1):177–188.
39. Brinker MR, O'Connor DP, Monla YT, et al. Metabolic and endocrine abnormalities in patients with nonunions. *J.Orthop.Trauma.* 2007;21(8):557–570.
40. Brown KM, Saunders MM, Kirsch T, et al. Effect of COX-2-specific inhibition on fracture-healing in the rat femur. *J.Bone Joint Surg.Am.* 2004;86-A(1):116–123.
41. Brumback RJ, Reilly JP, Poka A, et al. Intramedullary nailing of femoral shaft fractures. Part I: Decision-making errors with interlocking fixation. *J Bone Joint Surg Am.* 1988;70(10):1441–1452.
42. Brumback RJ, Uwagie-Ero S, Lakatos RP, et al. Intramedullary nailing of femoral shaft fractures. Part II: Fracture-healing with static interlocking fixation. *J Bone Joint Surg Am.* 1988;70(10):1453–1462.
43. Buchholz HW, Elson RA, Heinert K. Antibiotic-loaded acrylic cement: current concepts. *Clin Orthop Relat Res.* 1984;(190):96–108.
44. Buijze GA, Ochtman L, Ring D. Management of scaphoid nonunion. *J Hand Surg Am.* 2012;37(5):1095–1100; quiz 1101.
45. Bumbasirevic M, Tomic S, Lesic A, et al. The treatment of scaphoid nonunion using the Ilizarov fixator without bone graft, a study of 18 cases. *J Orthop Surg Res.* 2011;6:57.
46. Calori GM, Albisetti W, Agus A, et al. Risk factors contributing to fracture non-unions. *Injury.* 2007;38(Suppl 2):S11–S18.
47. Cannon CP, Lin PP, Lewis VO, et al. Management of radiation-associated fractures. *J Am Acad Orthop Surg.* 2008;16(9):541–549.

48. Capello WN, Feinberg JR. Trochanteric excision following persistent nonunion of the greater trochanter. *Orthopedics.* 2008;31(7):711.
49. Castillo RC, Bosse MJ, MacKenzie EJ, et al. Impact of smoking on fracture healing and risk of complications in limb-threatening open tibia fractures. *J.Orthop.Trauma.* 2005;19(3):151–157.
50. Catagni MA, Guerreschi F, Holman JA, et al. Distraction osteogenesis in the treatment of stiff hypertrophic nonunions using the Ilizarov apparatus. *Clin Orthop Relat Res.* 1994;(301):159–163.
51. Chalidis BE, Petsatodis GE, Sachinis NC, et al. Reamed interlocking intramedullary nailing for the treatment of tibial diaphyseal fractures and aseptic nonunions. Can we expect an optimum result? *Strategies Trauma Limb Reconstr.* 2009;4(2):89–94.
52. Chang N, Mathes SJ. Comparison of the effect of bacterial inoculation in musculocutaneous and random-pattern flaps. *Plast.Reconstr.Surg.* 1982;70(1):1–10.
53. Chassanidis CG, Malizos KN, Varitimidis S, et al. Smoking affects mRNA expression of bone morphogenetic proteins in human periosteum. *J Bone Joint Surg Br.* 2012;94(10):1427–1432.
54. Chintamaneni S, Finzel K, Gruber BL. Successful treatment of sternal fracture nonunion with teriparatide. *Osteoporosis international: a journal established as result of cooperation between the European Foundation for Osteoporosis and the National Osteoporosis Foundation of the USA.* 2010;21(6):1059–1063.
55. Chiodo CP, Hahne J, Wilson MG, et al. Histological differences in iliac and tibial bone graft. *Foot Ankle Int.* 2010;31(5):418–422.
56. Cho SH, Song HR, Koo KH, et al. Antibiotic-impregnated cement beads in the treatment of chronic osteomyelitis. *Bull Hosp Jt Dis.* 1997;56(3):140–144.
57. Christodoulou S, Goula T, Ververidis A, et al. Vitamin D and bone disease. *BioMed research international.* 2013;2013:396–541.
58. Cierny G 3rd, Zorn KE. Segmental tibial defects. Comparing conventional and Ilizarov methodologies. *Clin Orthop Relat Res.* 1994;(301):118–123.
59. Cil A, Veillette CJ, Sanchez-Sotelo J, et al. Linked elbow replacement: a salvage procedure for distal humeral nonunion. *J Bone Joint Surg Am.* 2008;90(9):1939–1950.
60. Clarke S, Lecky F. Best evidence topic report. Do non-steroidal anti-inflammatory drugs cause a delay in fracture healing? *Emergency medicine journal: EMJ.* 2005;22(9):652–653.
61. CM C-B, McQueen MM. Nonunions of the proximal humerus: their prevalence and functional outcome. *J.Trauma.* 2008;64(6):1517–1521.
62. Cole JD. The vascular response of bone to internal fixation. In: BD B, ed. *The Science and Practice of Intramedullary Nailing.* 2nd ed. Baltimore: Williams & Wilkins; 1996:43–69.
63. Connolly JF. Common avoidable problems in nonunions. *Clin Orthop Relat Res.* 1985; (194):226–235.
64. Connolly JF, Guse R, Tiedeman J, et al. Autologous marrow injection as a substitute for operative grafting of tibial nonunions. *Clin Orthop Relat Res.* 1991;(266):259–270.
65. Cook SD, Ryaby JP, McCabe J, et al. Acceleration of tibia and distal radius fracture healing in patients who smoke. *Clin Orthop Relat Res.* 1997;(337):198–207.
66. Coords M, Breitbart E, Paglia D, et al. The effects of low-intensity pulsed ultrasound upon diabetic fracture healing. *J Orthop Res.* 2011;29(2):181–188.
67. Corrales LA, Morshed S, Bhandari M, et al. Variability in the assessment of fracture-healing in orthopaedic trauma studies. *J Bone Joint Surg Am.* 2008;90(9):1862–1868.
68. Costelloe CM, Dickson K, Cody DD, et al. Computed tomography reformation in evaluation of fracture healing with metallic fixation: correlation with clinical outcome. *J.Trauma.* 2008;65(6):1421–1424.
69. Coulibaly MO, Sietsema DL, Burgers TA, et al. Recent advances in the use of serological bone formation markers to monitor callus development and fracture healing. *Critical reviews in eukaryotic gene expression.* 2010;20(2):105–127.
70. Coventry MB, Tapper EM. Pelvic instability: a consequence of removing iliac bone for grafting. *J Bone Joint Surg Am.* 1972;54(1):83–101.
71. Daftari TK, Whitesides TE Jr, Heller JG, et al. Nicotine on the revascularization of bone graft. An experimental study in rabbits. *Spine.* 1994;19(8):904–911.
72. Dahabreh Z, Dimitriou R, Giannoudis PV. Health economics: a cost analysis of treatment of persistent fracture non-unions using bone morphogenetic protein-7. *Injury.* 2007;38(3):371–377.
73. Dai KR, Xu XL, Tang TT, et al. Repairing of goat tibial bone defects with BMP-2 gene-modified tissue-engineered bone. *Calcified tissue international.* 2005;77(1):55–61.
74. Danckwardt-Lilliestrom G, Lorenzi GL, Olerud S. Intramedullary nailing after reaming. An investigation on the healing process in osteotomized rabbit tibias. *Acta Orthop Scand Suppl.* 1970;134:1–78.
75. Danckwardt-Lilliestrom G, Lorenzi L, Olerud S. Intracortical circulation after intramedullary reaming with reduction of pressure in the medullary cavity. *J Bone Joint Surg Am.* 1970;52(7):1390–1394.
76. Das De S, Setiobudi T, Shen L, et al. A rational approach to management of alendronate-related subtrochanteric fractures. *J Bone Joint Surg Br.* 2010;92(5):679–686.
77. Davila J, Malkani A, Paiso JM. Supracondylar distal femoral nonunions treated with a megaprosthesis in elderly patients: a report of two cases. *J Orthop Trauma.* 2001;15(8):574–578.
78. Dean BJ, Matthews JJ, Price A, et al. Modular endoprosthetic replacement for failed internal fixation of the proximal femur following trauma. *Int Orthop.* 2012;36(4):731–734.
79. Della Rocca GJ, Crist BD, Murtha YM. Parathyroid hormone: is there a role in fracture healing? *J Orthop Trauma.* 2010;24(Suppl 1):S31–S35.
80. DeOrio JK, Farber DC. Morbidity associated with anterior iliac crest bone grafting in foot and ankle surgery. *Foot Ankle Int.* 2005;26(2):147–151.
81. Desai PP, Bell AJ, Suk M. Treatment of recalcitrant, multiply operated tibial nonunions with the RIA graft and rh-BMP2 using intramedullary nails. *Injury.* 2010;41(Suppl 2):S69–S71.
82. Dimitriou R, Dahabreh Z, Katsoulis E, et al. Application of recombinant BMP-7 on persistent upper and lower limb non-unions. *Injury.* 2005;36(Suppl 4):S51–S59.
83. Dodwell ER, Latorre JG, Parisini E, et al. NSAID exposure and risk of nonunion: a meta-analysis of case-control and cohort studies. *Calcif Tissue Int.* 2010;87(3):193–202.
84. Donigan JA, Fredericks DC, Nepola JV, et al. The effect of transdermal nicotine on fracture healing in a rabbit model. *J Orthop Trauma.* 2012;26(12):724–727.
85. Duarte LR. The stimulation of bone growth by ultrasound. *Arch Orthop Trauma Surg.* 1983;101(3):153–159.
86. Duckworth AD, McQueen MM, Ring D. Fractures of the radial head. *Bone Joint J.* 2013;95-B(2):151–159.
87. Dunbar RP Jr. Treatment of infection after fracture fixation. Opinion: retain stable implant and suppress infection until union. *J Orthop Trauma.* 2007;21(7):503–505.
88. Ebraheim NA, Elgafy H, Xu R. Bone-graft harvesting from iliac and fibular donor sites: techniques and complications. *J Am Acad Orthop Surg.* 2001;9(3):210–218.
89. Elbatrawy Y, Fayed M. Deformity correction with an external fixator: ease of use and accuracy? *Orthopedics.* 2009;32(2):82.
90. Elster EA, Stojadinovic A, Forsberg J, et al. Extracorporeal shock wave therapy for nonunion of the tibia. *J Orthop Trauma.* 2010;24(3):133–141.
91. Escalas F, DeWald RL. Combined traumatic arteriovenous fistula and ureteral injury: a complication of iliac bone-grafting. *J Bone Joint Surg Am.* 1977;59(2):270–271.
92. Esterhai J, Alavi A, Mandell GA, et al. Sequential technetium-99 m/gallium-67 scintigraphic evaluation of subclinical osteomyelitis complicating fracture nonunion. *J.Orthop.Res.* 1985;3(2):219–225.
93. Esterhai JL Jr, Brighton CT, Heppenstall RB, et al. Detection of synovial pseudarthrosis by 99mTc scintigraphy: application to treatment of traumatic nonunion with constant direct current. *Clin.Orthop.Relat Res.* 1981;(161):15–23.
94. Evans CH. Gene therapy for bone healing. *Expert Rev Mol Med.* 2010;12:e18.
95. Evans RP, Nelson CL. Gentamicin-impregnated polymethylmethacrylate beads compared with systemic antibiotic therapy in the treatment of chronic osteomyelitis. *Clin Orthop Relat Res.* 1993;(295):37–42.
96. Fang MA, Frost PJ, Iida-Klein A, et al. Effects of nicotine on cellular function in UMR 106–01 osteoblast-like cells. *Bone.* 1991;12(4):283–286.
97. Feng LJ, Price DC, Mathes SJ, et al. Dynamic properties of blood flow and leukocyte mobilization in infected flaps. *World J Surg.* 1990;14(6):796–803.
98. Finkemeier CG, Schmidt AH, Kyle RF, et al. A prospective, randomized study of intramedullary nails inserted with and without reaming for the treatment of open and closed fractures of the tibial shaft. *J Orthop Trauma.* 2000;14(3):187–193.
99. Finnan RP, Prayson MJ, Goswami T, et al. Use of the Reamer-Irrigator-Aspirator for bone graft harvest: A mechanical comparison of three starting points in cadaveric femurs. *J Orthop Trauma.* 2010;24(1):36–41.
100. Fisher J, Wood MB. Experimental comparison of bone revascularization by musculo-cutaneous and cutaneous flaps. *Plast Reconstr Surg.* 1987;79(1):81–90.
101. Frankel VH. Results of prescription use of pulse ultrasound therapy in fracture management. *Surg Technol Int.* 1998;VII:389–393.
102. Friedenberg ZB, Brighton CT. Bioelectric potentials in bone. *J Bone Joint Surg Am.* 1966;48(5):915–923.
103. Friedlaender GE. Osteogenic protein-1 in treatment of tibial nonunions: current status. *Surg Technol Int.* 2004;13:249–252.
104. Friedlaender GE, Perry CR, Cole JD, et al. Osteogenic protein-1 (bone morphogenetic protein-7) in the treatment of tibial nonunions. *J Bone Joint Surg Am.* 2001;83-A Suppl 1(Pt 2):S151–S158.
105. Friedrich B, Klaue P. Mechanical stability and post-traumatic osteitis: an experimental evaluation of the relation between infection of bone and internal fixation. *Injury.* 1977;9(1):23–29.
106. Frolke JP, Nulend JK, Semeins CM, et al. Viable osteoblastic potential of cortical reamings from intramedullary nailing. *J Orthop Res.* 2004;22(6):1271–1275.
107. Funk JR, Hale JE, Carmines D, et al. Biomechanical evaluation of early fracture healing in normal and diabetic rats. *J Orthop Res.* 2000;18(1):126–132.
108. Gafni Y, Pelled G, Zilberman Y, et al. Gene therapy platform for bone regeneration using an exogenously regulated, AAV-2-based gene expression system. *Mol Ther.* 2004;9(4):587–595.
109. Gandhi A, Liporace F, Azad V, et al. Diabetic fracture healing. *Foot Ankle Clin.* 2006;11(4):805–824.
110. Gao K, Gao W, Huang J, et al. Treatment of surgical neck nonunions of the humerus with locked plate and autologous fibular strut graft. *Med Princ Pract.* 2012;21(5):483–487.
111. Garg NK, Gaur S, Sharma S. Percutaneous autogenous bone marrow grafting in 20 cases of ununited fracture. *Acta Orthop Scand.* 1993;64(6):671–672.
112. Garrison KR, Donell S, Ryder J, et al. Clinical effectiveness and cost-effectiveness of bone morphogenetic proteins in the non-healing of fractures and spinal fusion: a systematic review. *Health Technol Assess.* 2007;11(30):1–150.
113. Gebauer D, Mayr E, Orthner E. Nonunions treated by pulsed low-intensity ultrasound. *J Orthop Trauma.* 2000;14(2):154–154.
114. Gerner P, O'Connor JP. Impact of analgesia on bone fracture healing. *Anesthesiology.* 2008;108(3):349–350.
115. Gerstenfeld LC, Cullinane DM, Barnes GL, et al. Fracture healing as a post-natal developmental process: molecular, spatial, and temporal aspects of its regulation. *J Cell Biochem.* 2003;88(5):873–884.
116. Gerstenfeld LC, Thiede M, Seibert K, et al. Differential inhibition of fracture healing by non-selective and cyclooxygenase-2 selective non-steroidal anti-inflammatory drugs. *J Orthop Res.* 2003;21(4):670–675.
117. Giannotti S, Bottai V, Dell'osso G, et al. Atrophic femoral nonunion successfully treated with teriparatide. *Eur J Orthop Surg Traumatol.* 2013;23(Suppl 2):S291–S294.
118. Giannoudis PV, Dinopoulos HT. Autologous bone graft: when shall we add growth factors? *Foot Ankle Clin.* 2010;15(4):597–609.
119. Giannoudis PV, Kanakaris NK, Dimitriou R, et al. The synergistic effect of autograft and BMP-7 in the treatment of atrophic nonunions. *Clin Orthop Relat Res.* 2009;467:3239–3248.
120. Giannoudis PV, MacDonald DA, Matthews SJ, et al. Nonunion of the femoral diaphysis. The influence of reaming and non-steroidal anti-inflammatory drugs. *J Bone Joint Surg Br.* 2000;82(5):655–658.
121. Gitelis S, Brebach GT. The treatment of chronic osteomyelitis with a biodegradable antibiotic-impregnated implant. *J Orthop Surg (Hong Kong).* 2002;10(1):53–60.
122. Glassman SD, Alegre G, Carreon L, et al. Perioperative complications of lumbar instrumentation and fusion in patients with diabetes mellitus. *Spine Jl.* 2003;3(6):496–501.

123. Goel A, Sangwan SS, Siwach RC, et al. Percutaneous bone marrow grafting for the treatment of tibial non-union. *Injury*. 2005;36(1):203–206.
124. Goh SK, Yang KY, Koh JS, et al. Subtrochanteric insufficiency fractures in patients on alendronate therapy: a caution. *J Bone Joint Surg Br*. 2007;89(3):349–353.
125. Goldstein C, Sprague S, Petrisor BA. Electrical stimulation for fracture healing: current evidence. *J Orthop Trauma*. 2010;24(Suppl 1):S62–S65.
126. Goodship AE, Cunningham JL, Kenwright J. Strain rate and timing of stimulation in mechanical modulation of fracture healing. *Clin Orthop Relat Res*. 1998;355(Suppl):S105–S115.
127. Gossling HR, Bernstein RA, Abbott J. Treatment of ununited tibial fractures: a comparison of surgery and pulsed electromagnetic fields (PEMF). *Orthopedics*. 1992;15(6):711–719.
128. Govender S, Csimma C, Genant HK, et al. Recombinant human bone morphogenetic protein-2 for treatment of open tibial fractures: a prospective, controlled, randomized study of four hundred and fifty patients. *J Bone Joint Surg Am*. 2002;84-A(12):2123–2134.
129. Greenwald AS, Boden SD, Goldberg VM, et al. Bone-graft substitutes: facts, fictions, and applications. *J Bone Joint Surg Am*. 2001;83-A(Suppl 2 Pt 2):98–103.
130. Gristina AG. Biomaterial-centered infection: microbial adhesion versus tissue integration. *Science*. 1987;237(4822):1588–1595.
131. Gristina AG, Naylor PT, Myrvik QN. Mechanisms of musculoskeletal sepsis. *Orthop Clin North Am*. 1991;22(3):363–371.
132. Gruber R, Koch H, Doll BA, et al. Fracture healing in the elderly patient. *Exp Gerontol*. 2006;41(11):1080–1093.
133. Guarniero R, Barros Filho TE, Tannuri U, et al. Study of fracture healing in protein malnutrition. *Rev Paul Med*. 1992;110(2):63–68.
134. Rosen H. Treatment of nonunion. In: Chapman WM, ed. *Operative Orthopaedics*. Philadelphia, PA: Lippincott-Raven; 1988:489–509.
135. Rosen H. Nonunion and malunion. In: Browner BD, Levine AM, Jupiter JB, eds. *Skeletal Trauma*. Philadelphia, PA: WB Saunders; 1998:501–541.
136. Hadjiargyrou M, McLeod K, Ryaby JP, et al. Enhancement of fracture healing by low intensity ultrasound. *Clin Orthop Relat Res*. 1998;355(Suppl):S216–S229.
137. Haidukewych GJ. Salvage of failed treatment of femoral neck fractures. *Instr Course Lect*. 2009;58:83–90.
138. Haidukewych GJ, Springer BD, Jacofsky DJ, et al. Total knee arthroplasty for salvage of failed internal fixation or nonunion of the distal femur. *J Arthroplasty*. 2005;20(3):344–349.
139. Hak DJ, Lee SS, Goulet JA. Success of exchange reamed intramedullary nailing for femoral shaft nonunion or delayed union. *J Orthop Trauma*. 2000;14(3):178–182.
140. Hammer TO, Wieling R, Green JM, et al. Effect of re-implanted particles from intramedullary reaming on mechanical properties and callus formation. A laboratory study. *J Bone Joint Surg Br*. 2007;89(11):1534–1538.
141. Han CS, Wood MB, Bishop AT, et al. Vascularized bone transfer. *J Bone Joint Surg Am*. 1992;74(10):1441–1449.
142. Hardes J, von Eiff C, Streitbuerger A, et al. Reduction of periprosthetic infection with silver-coated megaprostheses in patients with bone sarcoma. *J Surg Oncol*. 2010; 101(5):389–395.
143. Harrison WJ, Lewis CP, Lavy CB. Open fractures of the tibia in HIV positive patients: a prospective controlled single-blind study. *Injury*. 2004;35(9):852–856.
144. Hauck RM, Skahen J 3rd, Palmer AK. Classification and treatment of ulnar styloid nonunion. *J Hand Surg Am*. 1996;21(3):418–422.
145. Heckman JD, Ryaby JP, McCabe J, et al. Acceleration of tibial fracture-healing by non-invasive, low-intensity pulsed ultrasound. *J.Bone Joint Surg.Am*. 1994;76(1):26–34.
146. Heckman JD, Sarasohn-Kahn J. The economics of treating tibia fractures. The cost of delayed unions. *Bull Hosp Jt Dis*. 1997;56(1):63–72.
147. Hernandez RK, Do TP, Critchlow CW, et al. Patient-related risk factors for fracture-healing complications in the United Kingdom General Practice Research Database. *Acta Orthop*. 2012;83(6):653–660.
148. Hernigou J, Schuind F. Smoking as a predictor of negative outcome in diaphyseal fracture healing. *Int Orthop*. 2013;37(5):883–887.
149. Hernigou P, Mathieu G, Poignard A, et al. Percutaneous autologous bone-marrow grafting for nonunions. Surgical technique. *J Bone Joint Surg Am*. 2006;88(Suppl 1 Pt 2):322–327.
150. Hernigou P, Poignard A, Beaujean F, et al. Percutaneous autologous bone-marrow grafting for nonunions. Influence of the number and concentration of progenitor cells. *J Bone Joint Surg Am*. 2005;87(7):1430–1437.
151. Hierholzer C, Sama D, Toro JB, et al. Plate fixation of ununited humeral shaft fractures: effect of type of bone graft on healing. *J Bone Joint Surg Am*. 2006;88(7):1442–1447.
152. Hoegel F, Mueller CA, Peter R, et al. Bone debris: dead matter or vital osteoblasts. *J Trauma*. 2004;56(2):363–367.
153. Holl S, Schlomberg A, Gosheger G, et al. Distal femur and proximal tibia replacement with megaprosthesis in revision knee arthroplasty: a limb-saving procedure. *Knee Surg Sports Traumatol Arthrosc*. 2012;20:2513–2518.
154. Hsiao CW, Wu CC, Su CY, et al. Exchange nailing for aseptic tibial shaft nonunion: emphasis on the influence of a concomitant fibulotomy. *Chang Gung Med J*. 2006;29(3):283–290.
155. Huang HK, Chiang CC, Hung SH, et al. The role of autologous bone graft in surgical treatment of hypertrophic nonunion of midshaft clavicle fractures. *J Chin Med Assoc*. 2012;75(5):216–220.
156. Ikeda K, Tomita K, Hashimoto F, et al. Long-term follow-up of vascularized bone grafts for the reconstruction of tibial nonunion: evaluation with computed tomographic scanning. *J Trauma*. 1992;32(6):693–697.
157. Inan M, Karaoglu S, Cilli F, et al. Treatment of femoral nonunions by using cyclic compression and distraction. *Clin Orthop Relat Res*. 2005;(436):222–228.
158. Jani MM, Ricci WM, Borrelli J Jr, et al. A protocol for treatment of unstable ankle fractures using transarticular fixation in patients with diabetes mellitus and loss of protective sensibility. *Foot Ankle Int*. 2003;24(11):838–844.
159. Johnson EE, Urist MR, Finerman GA. Bone morphogenetic protein augmentation grafting of resistant femoral nonunions. *Clin Orthop*. 1988;230:257–265.
160. Johnson EE, Urist MR, Finerman GA. Repair of segmental defects of the tibia with cancellous bone grafts augmented with human bone morphogenetic protein. *Clin Orthop*. 1988;236:249–257.
161. Johnson EE, Urist MR, Finerman GA. Resistant nonunions and partial or complete segmental defects of long bones. *Clin Orthop*. 1992;277:229–237.
162. Joist A, Schult M, Frerichmann U, et al. [A new irrigation-suction boring system facilities low-pressure intramedullary boring of isolated swine femurs]. *Unfallchirurg*. 2003;106(10):874–880.
163. Joist A, Schult M, Ortmann C, et al. Rinsing-suction reamer attenuates intramedullary pressure increase and fat intravasation in a sheep model. *J Trauma*. 2004;57(1):146–151.
164. Jones AL, Bucholz RW, Bosse MJ, et al. Recombinant human BMP-2 and allograft compared with autogenous bone graft for reconstruction of diaphyseal tibial fractures with cortical defects. A randomized, controlled trial. *J Bone Joint Surg Am*. 2006;88(7):1431–1441.
165. Jones KB, Maiers-Yelden KA, Marsh JL, et al. Ankle fractures in patients with diabetes mellitus. *J.Bone Joint Surg.Br*. 2005;87(4):489–495.
166. Judet PR, Patel A. Muscle pedicle bone grafting of long bones by osteoperiosteal decortication. *Clin Orthop Relat Res*. 1972;87:74–80.
167. Jun X, Chang-Qing Z, Kai-Gang Z, et al. Modified free vascularized fibular grafting for the treatment of femoral neck nonunion. *J Orthop Trauma*. 2010;24(4):230–235.
168. Kabata T, Tsuchiya H, Sakurakichi K, et al. Reconstruction with distraction osteogenesis for juxta-articular nonunions with bone loss. *J Trauma*. 2005;58(6):1213–1222.
169. Keating JF, Simpson AH, Robinson CM. The management of fractures with bone loss. *J Bone Joint Surg Br*. 2005;87(2):142–150.
170. Kellam JF. Early results of the Sunnybrook experience with locked intramedullary nailing. *Orthopedics*. 1985;8(11):1387–1388.
171. Kempf I, Grosse A, Lafforgue D. [Combined Kuntscher nailing and screw fixation (author's transl)]. *Rev Chir Orthop Reparatrice Appar Mot*. 1978;64(8):635–651.
172. Kettunen J, Makela EA, Turunen V, et al. Percutaneous bone grafting in the treatment of the delayed union and non-union of tibial fractures. *Injury*. 2002;33(3):239–245.
173. Kishimoto KN, Watanabe Y, Nakamura H, et al. Ectopic bone formation by electroporatic transfer of bone morphogenetic protein-4 gene. *Bone*. 2002;31(2):340–347.
174. Kocaoglu M, Eralp L, Sen C, et al. Management of stiff hypertrophic nonunions by distraction osteogenesis: a report of 16 cases. *J Orthop Trauma*. 2003;17(8):543–548.
175. Koester MC, Spindler KP. NSAIDs and fracture healing: what's the evidence? *Curr Sports Med Rep*. 2005;4(6):289–290.
176. Kontakis GM, Papadokostakis GM, Alpantaki K, et al. Intramedullary nailing for non-union of the humeral diaphysis: a review. *Injury*. 2006;37(10):953–960.
177. Krannitz KW, Fong HW, Fallat LM, et al. The effect of cigarette smoking on radiographic bone healing after elective foot surgery. *J Foot Ankle Surg*. 2009;48(5):525–527.
178. Kristiansen TK, Ryaby JP, McCabe J, et al. Accelerated healing of distal radial fractures with the use of specific, low-intensity ultrasound. A multicenter, prospective, randomized, double-blind, placebo-controlled study. *J Bone Joint Surg Am*. 1997;79(7):961–973.
179. Kurz LT, Garfin SR, Booth RE Jr. Harvesting autogenous iliac bone grafts. A review of complications and techniques. *Spine (Phila Pa 1976)*. 1989;14(12):1324–1331.
180. Kyro A, Usenius JP, Aarnio M, et al. Are smokers a risk group for delayed healing of tibial shaft fractures? *Ann Chir Gynaecol*. 1993;82(4):254–262.
181. Lamb RH. Posterolateral bone graft for nonunion of the tibia. *Clin Orthop Relat Res*. 1969;64:114–120.
182. Lammens J, Bauduin G, Driesen R, et al. Treatment of nonunion of the humerus using the Ilizarov external fixator. *Clin Orthop Relat Res*. 1998;(353):223–230.
183. Leduc S, Ricci WM. Treatment of infection after fracture fixation. Opinion: two-stage protocol: treatment of nonunion after treatment of infection. *J Orthop Trauma*. 2007;21(7):505–506.
184. Lee M, Song HK, Yang KH. Clinical outcomes of autogenous cancellous bone grafts obtained through the portal for tibial nailing. *Injury*. 2012;43(7):1118–1123.
185. Lefaivre KA, Guy P, O'Brien PJ, et al. Leading 20 at 20: top cited articles and authors in the Journal of Orthopaedic Trauma, 1987–2007. *J Orthop Trauma*. 2010;24(1):53–58.
186. Lenart BA, Lorich DG, Lane JM. Atypical fractures of the femoral diaphysis in postmenopausal women taking alendronate. *N Engl J Med*. 2008;358(12):1304–1306.
187. Leung KS, Lee WS, Tsui HF, et al. Complex tibial fracture outcomes following treatment with low-intensity pulsed ultrasound. *Ultrasound Med Biol*. 2004;30(3):389–395.
188. Li JZ, Hankins GR, Kao C, et al. Osteogenesis in rats induced by a novel recombinant helper-dependent bone morphogenetic protein-9 (BMP-9) adenovirus. *J Gene Med*. 2003; 5(9):748–756.
189. Liodakis E, Liodaki E, Krettek C, et al. Can the viability of a nonunion be evaluated using SPECT/CT? A preliminary retrospective study. *Technol Health Care*. 2011;19(2):103–108.
190. Loeffler BJ, Kellam JF, Sims SH, et al. Prospective observational study of donor-site morbidity following anterior iliac crest bone-grafting in orthopaedic trauma reconstruction patients. *J Bone Joint Surg Am*. 2012;94:1649–1654.
191. Lowe JA, Della Rocca GJ, Murtha Y, et al. Complications associated with negative pressure reaming for harvesting autologous bone graft: a case series. *J Orthop Trauma*. 2009;24(1):46–52.
192. Lui TH. Endoscopic excision of symptomatic nonunion of anterior calcaneal process. *J Foot Ankle Surg*. 2011;50(4):476–479.
193. Lynch JR, Taitsman LA, Barei DP, et al. Femoral nonunion: risk factors and treatment options. *J Am Acad Orthop Surg*. 2008;16(2):88–97.
194. Macey LR, Kana SM, Jingushi S, et al. Defects of early fracture-healing in experimental diabetes. *J Bone Joint Surg Am*. 1989;71(5):722–733.
195. MacKenzie EJ, Bosse MJ, Kellam JF, et al. Factors influencing the decision to amputate or reconstruct after high-energy lower extremity trauma. *J Trauma*. 2002;52(4):641–649.
196. Mahaluxmivala J, Nadarajah R, Allen PW, et al. Ilizarov external fixator: acute shortening and lengthening versus bone transport in the management of tibial non-unions. *Injury*. 2005;36(5):662–668.
197. Mandt PR, Gershuni DH. Treatment of nonunion of fractures in the epiphyseal-metaphyseal region of long bones. *J Orthop Trauma*. 1987;1(2):141–151.
198. Mariconda M, Cozzolino F, Cozzolino A, et al. Platelet gel supplementation in long bone nonunions treated by external fixation. *J Orthop Trauma*. 2008;22(5): 342–345.
199. Marsh D. Concepts of fracture union, delayed union, and nonunion. *Clin Orthop Relat Res*. 1998;355(Suppl):S22–S30.

200. Marti RK, Schuller HM, Raaymakers ELF. Intertrochanteric osteotomy for Nonunion of the femoral neck. *J Bone Joint Surg [Br]*. 1989;71-B(5):782–787.
201. Masquelet AC, Fitoussi F, Begue T, et al. [Reconstruction of the long bones by the induced membrane and spongy autograft]. *Ann Chir Plast Esthet*. 2000;45(3):346–353.
202. Mathes SJ, Alpert BS, Chang N. Use of the muscle flap in chronic osteomyelitis: experimental and clinical correlation. *Plast Reconstr Surg*. 1982;69(5):815–829.
203. Matsushita T, Watanabe Y. Chipping and lengthening technique for delayed unions and nonunions with shortening or bone loss. *J Orthop Trauma*. 2007;21(6):404–406.
204. Mayr E, Frankel V, Ruter A. Ultrasound–an alternative healing method for nonunions? *Arch Orthop Trauma Surg*. 2000;120(1–2):1–8.
205. McCall TA, Brokaw DS, Jelen BA, et al. Treatment of large segmental bone defects with reamer-irrigator-aspirator bone graft: technique and case series. *Orthop Clin North Am*. 2009;41(1):63–73; table of contents.
206. McKee M. Aseptic nonunion. In: Ruedi TP, Murphy W, eds. *AO Principles of Fracture Management*. Stuttgart and New York: Georg Thieme Vercal; 2000:748–762.
207. McKee MD. Recombinant human bone morphogenic protein-7: applications for clinical trauma. *J Orthop Trauma*. 2005;19(10 Suppl):S26–S28.
208. McKee MD, DiPasquale DJ, Wild LM, et al. The effect of smoking on clinical outcome and complication rates following Ilizarov reconstruction. *J Orthop Trauma*. 2003;17(10):663–667.
209. McKee MD, Li-Bland EA, Wild LM, et al. A prospective, randomized clinical trial comparing an antibiotic-impregnated bioabsorbable bone substitute with standard antibiotic-impregnated cement beads in the treatment of chronic osteomyelitis and infected nonunion. *J Orthop Trauma*. 2010;24(8):483–490.
210. McKee MD, Wild LM, Schemitsch EH, et al. The use of an antibiotic-impregnated, osteoconductive, bioabsorbable bone substitute in the treatment of infected long bone defects: early results of a prospective trial. *J Orthop Trauma*. 2002;16(9):622–627.
211. Megas P. Classification of non-union. *Injury*. 2005;36(Suppl 4):S30–S37.
212. Mollon B, da Silva V, Busse JW, et al. Electrical stimulation for long-bone fracture-healing: a meta-analysis of randomized controlled trials. *J Bone Joint Surg Am*. 2008; 90(11):2322–2330.
213. Morrey BF, Adams RA. Semiconstrained elbow replacement for distal humeral nonunion. *J Bone Joint Surg Br*. 1995;77(1):67–72.
214. Moutsatsos IK, Turgeman G, Zhou S, et al. Exogenously regulated stem cell-mediated gene therapy for bone regeneration. *Mol Ther*. 2001;3(4):449–461.
215. Murnaghan M, Li G, Marsh DR. Nonsteroidal anti-inflammatory drug-induced fracture nonunion: an inhibition of angiogenesis? *J Bone Joint Surg Am*. 2006;88(Suppl 3):140–147.
216. Nadkarni B, Srivastav S, Mittal V, et al. Use of locking compression plates for long bone nonunions without removing existing intramedullary nail: review of literature and our experience. *J Trauma*. 2008;65(2):482–486.
217. Nauth A, Miclau T 3rd, Li R, et al. Gene therapy for fracture healing. *J Orthop Trauma*. 2010;24(Suppl 1):S17–S24.
218. Nelson FR, Brighton CT, Ryaby J, et al. Use of physical forces in bone healing. *J Am Acad Orthop Surg*. 2003;11(5):344–354.
219. Nepola JV, Seabold JE, Marsh JL, et al. Diagnosis of infection in ununited fractures. Combined imaging with indium-111-labeled leukocytes and technetium-99 m methylene diphosphonate. *J Bone Joint Surg Am*. 1993;75(12):1816–1822.
220. Neviaser AS, Lane JM, Lenart BA, et al. Low-energy femoral shaft fractures associated with alendronate use. *J Orthop Trauma*. 2008;22(5):346–350.
221. Newman JT, Stahel PF, Smith WR, et al. A new minimally invasive technique for large volume bone graft harvest for treatment of fracture nonunions. *Orthopedics*. 2008; 31(3):257–261.
222. Nho SJ, Helfet DL, Rozbruch SR. Temporary intentional leg shortening and deformation to facilitate wound closure using the Ilizarov/Taylor spatial frame. *J Orthop Trauma*. 2006;20(6):419–424.
223. Niikura T, Miwa M, Lee SY, et al. Technique to prepare the bed for autologous bone grafting in nonunion surgery. *Orthopedics*. 2012;35(6):491–495.
224. Nolte PA, van der KA, Patka P, et al. Low-intensity pulsed ultrasound in the treatment of nonunions. *J Trauma*. 2001;51(4):693–702.
225. Norris TR, Green A, McGuigan FX. Late prosthetic shoulder arthroplasty for displaced proximal humerus fractures. *J Shoulder Elbow Surg*. 1995;4(4):271–280.
226. Ochsner PE, Hailemariam S. Histology of osteosynthesis associated bone infection. *Injury*. 2006;37(Suppl 2):S49–S58.
227. Odvina CV, Zerwekh JE, Rao DS, et al. Severely suppressed bone turnover: a potential complication of alendronate therapy. *J Clin Endocrinol Metab*. 2005;90(3):1294–1301.
228. Oh JK, Bae JH, Oh CW, et al. Treatment of femoral and tibial diaphyseal nonunions using reamed intramedullary nailing without bone graft. *Injury*. 2008;39(8):952–959.
229. Ohtsuka H, Yokoyama K, Higashi K, et al. Use of antibiotic-impregnated bone cement nail to treat septic nonunion after open tibial fracture. *J Trauma*. 2002;52(2):364–366.
230. Oteo-Alvaro A, Moreno E. Atrophic humeral shaft nonunion treated with teriparatide (rh PTH 1–34): a case report. *J Shoulder Elbow Surg*. 2010;19(7):e22–e28.
231. O'Toole RV, Castillo RC, Pollak AN, et al. Determinants of patient satisfaction after severe lower-extremity injuries. *J Bone Joint Surg Am*. 2008;90(6):1206–1211.
232. Otter MW, McLeod KJ, Rubin CT. Effects of electromagnetic fields in experimental fracture repair. *Clin Orthop Relat Res*. 1998;355(Suppl):S90–S104.
233. Owoola AM, Odunubi OO, Yinusa Y, et al. Proximal tibial metaphysis: its reliability as a donor site for grafting. *West Afr J Med*. 2010;29(6):403–407.
234. Paley D. Treatment of tibial nonunion and bone loss with the Ilizarov technique. *Instr Course Lect*. 1990;39:185–197.
235. Paley D, Catagni MA, Argnani F, et al. Ilizarov treatment of tibial nonunions with bone loss. *Clin Orthop Relat Res*. 1989;(241):146–165.
236. Paley D, Herzenberg JE. Intramedullary infections treated with antibiotic cement rods: preliminary results in nine cases. *J Orthop Trauma*. 2002;16(10):723–729.
237. Paley D, Maar DC. Ilizarov bone transport treatment for tibial defects. *J Orthop Trauma*. 2000;14(2):76–85.
238. Papagelopoulos PJ, Morrey BF. Treatment of nonunion of olecranon fractures. *J Bone Joint Surg Br*. 1994;76(4):627–635.
239. Papakostidis C, Psyllakis I, Vardakas D, et al. Femoral-shaft fractures and nonunions treated with intramedullary nails: the role of dynamisation. *Injury*. 2011;42(11):1353–1361.
240. Parvizi J, Parpura V, Greenleaf JF, et al. Calcium signaling is required for ultrasound-stimulated aggrecan synthesis by rat chondrocytes. *J Orthop Res*. 2002;20(1): 51–57.
241. Patel AA, Ricci WM, McDonald DJ, et al. Treatment of periprosthetic femoral shaft nonunion. *J Arthroplasty*. 2006;21(3):435–442.
242. Pauwels F. *Der Schenkelhalsbruch: Ein mechanisches problem*. Stuttgart: Ferdinand Enke Verlag; 1935.
243. Pelissier P, Masquelet AC, Bareille R, et al. Induced membranes secrete growth factors including vascular and osteoinductive factors and could stimulate bone regeneration. *J Orthop Res*. 2004;22(1):73–79.
244. Perry AC, Prpa B, Rouse MS, et al. Levofloxacin and trovafloxacin inhibition of experimental fracture-healing. *Clin Orthop Relat Res*. 2003;(414):95–100.
245. Perry CR. Bone repair techniques, bone graft, and bone graft substitutes. *Clin Orthop Relat Res*. 1999;(360):71–86.
246. Peterson B, Whang PG, Iglesias R, et al. Osteoinductivity of commercially available demineralized bone matrix. Preparations in a spine fusion model. *J Bone Joint Surg Am*. 2004;86-A(10):2243–2250.
247. Peterson B, Zhang J, Iglesias R, et al. Healing of critically sized femoral defects, using genetically modified mesenchymal stem cells from human adipose tissue. *Tissue Eng*. 2005;11(1–2):120–129.
248. Phieffer LS, Goulet JA. Delayed unions of the tibia. *J Bone Joint Surg Am*. 2006;88(1):206–216.
249. Piepkorn B, Kann P, Forst T, et al. Bone mineral density and bone metabolism in diabetes mellitus. *Horm Metab Res*. 1997;29(11):584–591.
250. Pietrogrande L, Raimondo E. Teriparatide in the treatment of non-unions: Scientific and clinical evidences. *Injury*. 2013;44(Suppl 1):S54–S57.
251. Pihlajamaki HK, Salminen ST, Bostman OM. The treatment of nonunions following intramedullary nailing of femoral shaft fractures. *J Orthop Trauma*. 2002;16(6):394–402.
252. Polyzois VD, Papakostas I, Stamatis ED, et al. Current concepts in delayed bone union and non-union. *Clin Podiatr Med Surg*. 2006;23(2):445–453.
253. Porchet F, Jaques B. Unusual complications at iliac crest bone graft donor site: experience with two cases. *Neurosurgery*. 1996;39(4):856–859.
254. Porter RM, Liu F, Pilapil C, et al. Osteogenic potential of reamer irrigator aspirator (RIA) aspirate collected from patients undergoing hip arthroplasty. *J Orthop Res*. 2009; 27(1):42–49.
255. Pountos I, Georgouli T, Blokhuis TJ, et al. Pharmacological agents and impairment of fracture healing: what is the evidence? *Injury*. 2008;39(4):384–394.
256. Pratt DJ, Papagiannopoulos G, Rees PH, et al. The effects of medullary reaming on the torsional strength of the femur. *Injury*. 1987;18(3):177–179.
257. Qiang Z, Jun PZ, Jie XJ, et al. Use of antibiotic cement rod to treat intramedullary infection after nailing: preliminary study in 19 patients. *Arch Orthop Trauma Surg*. 2007;127(10):945–951.
258. Raisz LG. Prostaglandins and bone: physiology and pathophysiology. *Osteoarthritis Cartilage*. 1999;7(4):419–421.
259. Rawool NM, Goldberg BB, Forsberg F, et al. Power Doppler assessment of vascular changes during fracture treatment with low-intensity ultrasound. *J Ultrasound Med*. 2003;22(2):145–153.
260. Reid RL. Hernia through an iliac bone-graft donor site. A case report. *J Bone Joint Surg Am*. 1968;50(4):757–760.
261. Ricci WM, Bellabarba C, Evanoff B, et al. Retrograde versus antegrade nailing of femoral shaft fractures. *J Orthop Trauma*. 2001;15(3):161–169.
262. Ricci WM, Haidukewych GJ. Periprosthetic femoral fractures. *Instr Course Lect*. 2009; 58:105–115.
263. Ricci WM, Loftus T, Cox C, et al. Locked plates combined with minimally invasive insertion technique for the treatment of periprosthetic supracondylar femur fractures above a total knee arthroplasty. *J Orthop Trauma*. 2006;20(3):190–196.
264. Ricci WMS, P.N.;McAndrew CM;Gardner MJ. If Treatment of Nonunions With ICBG Works, Adding BMP-2 Must Work Better—Right or Wrong? *Orthopaedic Trauma Association Annual Meeting*. October 3–6, 2012, 2012; Minneapolis, MN.
265. Richmond J, Colleran K, Borens O, et al. Nonunions of the distal tibia treated by reamed intramedullary nailing. *J Orthop Trauma*. 2004;18(9):603–610.
266. Ring D, Kloen P, Kadzielski J, et al. Locking compression plates for osteoporotic nonunions of the diaphyseal humerus. *Clin Orthop Relat Res*. 2004;(425):50–54.
267. Ristiniemi J, Lakovaara M, Flinkkila T, et al. Staged method using antibiotic beads and subsequent autografting for large traumatic tibial bone loss: 22 of 23 fractures healed after 5–20 months. *Acta Orthop*. 2007;78(4):520–527.
268. Ritchie JD, Shaver JC, Anderson RB, et al. Excision of symptomatic nonunions of proximal fifth metatarsal avulsion fractures in elite athletes. *Am J Sports Med*. 2011; 39(11):2466–2469.
269. Robinson CM, Court-Brown CM, McQueen MM, et al. Estimating the risk of nonunion following nonoperative treatment of a clavicular fracture. *J Bone Joint Surg Am*. 2004;86-A(7):1359–1365.
270. Rozbruch SR, Pugsley JS, Fragomen AT, et al. Repair of tibial nonunions and bone defects with the Taylor Spatial Frame. *J Orthop Trauma*. 2008;22(2):88–95.
271. Rubin C, Bolander M, Ryaby JP, et al. The use of low-intensity ultrasound to accelerate the healing of fractures. *J Bone Joint Surg Am*. 2001;83-A(2):259–270.
272. Ruch DS, Papadonikolakis A. Resection of the scaphoid distal pole for symptomatic scaphoid nonunion after failed previous surgical treatment. *J Hand Surg Am*. 2006; 31(4):588–593.
273. Ryaby JJ, Bachner EJ, Bendo JA, et al. Low intensity pulsed ultrasound increases calcium incorporation in both differentiating cartilage and bone cell cultures. *Trans Orthop Res Soc*. 1989;14:15–15.
274. Ryaby JT, Matthew J, Duarte-Alves P. Low intensity pulsed ultrasound affects adenylate cyclase activity and TGF-b synthesising osteoblastic cells. *Orthop Res Soc Trans*. 1992; 17:590.

275. Ryzewicz M, Morgan SJ, Linford E, et al. Central bone grafting for nonunion of fractures of the tibia: a retrospective series. *J Bone Joint Surg Br.* 2009;91(4):522–529.

276. Sabharwal S, Rozbruch SR. What's new in limb lengthening and deformity correction. *J Bone Joint Surg Am.* 2011;93(24):2323–2332.

277. Safoury YA, Atteya MR. Treatment of post-infection nonunion of the supracondylar humerus with Ilizarov external fixator. *J Shoulder Elbow Surg.* 2011;20(6):873–879.

278. Sala F, Thabet AM, Castelli F, et al. Bone transport for postinfectious segmental tibial bone defects with a combined ilizarov/taylor spatial frame technique. *J Orthop Trauma.* 2011;25(3):162–168.

279. Salibian AH, Anzel SH, Salyer WA. Transfer of vascularized grafts of iliac bone to the extremities. *J Bone Joint Surg Am.* 1987;69(9):1319–1327.

280. Salkeld SL, Patron LP, Barrack RL, et al. The effect of osteogenic protein-1 on the healing of segmental bone defects treated with autograft or allograft bone. *J Bone Joint Surg Am.* 2001;83-A(6):803–816.

281. Sanchez-Sotelo J. Distal humeral nonunion. *Instr Course Lect.* 2009;58:541–548.

282. Sarmiento A, Burkhalter WE, Latta LL. Functional bracing in the treatment of delayed union and nonunion of the tibia. *Int Orthop.* 2003;27(1):26–29.

283. Schaden W, Fischer A, Sailler A. Extracorporeal shock wave therapy of nonunion or delayed osseous union. *Clin Orthop Relat Res.* 2001;(387):90–94.

284. Schelstraete K, Daneels F, Obrie E. Technetium-99m-diphosphonate, gallium-67 and labeled leukocyte scanning techniques in tibial nonunion. *Acta Orthop Belg.* 1992;58(Suppl 1):168–172.

285. Schenk R. Histology of Fracture Repair and Nonunion. *Bulletin of the Swiss Association for Study of Internal Fixation, Bern, Swiss Association for Study of Internal Fixation.* 1978.

286. Schmidmaier G, Herrmann S, Green J, et al. Quantitative assessment of growth factors in reaming aspirate, iliac crest, and platelet preparation. *Bone.* 2006;39(5):1156–1163.

287. Schmitz MA, Finnegan M, Natarajan R, et al. Effect of smoking on tibial shaft fracture healing. *Clin Orthop Relat Res.* 1999;(365):184–200.

288. Schmokel HG, Weber FE, Seiler G, et al. Treatment of nonunions with nonglycosylated recombinant human bone morphogenetic protein-2 delivered from a fibrin matrix. *Vet Surg.* 2004;33(2):112–118.

289. Schottle PB, Werner CM, Dumont CE. Two-stage reconstruction with free vascularized soft tissue transfer and conventional bone graft for infected nonunions of the tibia: 6 patients followed for 1.5 to 5 years. *Acta Orthop.* 2005;76(6):878–883.

290. Schult M, Kuchle R, Hofmann A, et al. Pathophysiological advantages of rinsing-suction-reaming (RSR) in a pig model for intramedullary nailing. *J Orthop Res.* 2006;24(6):1186–1192.

291. Scott G, King JB. A prospective, double-blind trial of electrical capacitive coupling in the treatment of non-union of long bones. *J Bone Joint Surg Am.* 1994;76(6):820–826.

292. Seabold JE, Nepola JV, Conrad GR, et al. Detection of osteomyelitis at fracture nonunion sites: comparison of two scintigraphic methods. *AJR Am J Roentgenol.* 1989;152(5):1021–1027.

293. Sears BW, Lazarus MD. Arthroscopically assisted percutaneous fixation and bone grafting of a glenoid fossa fracture nonunion. *Orthopedics.* 2012;35(8):e1279–e1282.

294. Seide K, Aljudaibi M, Weinrich N, et al. Telemetric assessment of bone healing with an instrumented internal fixator: a preliminary study. *J Bone Joint Surg Br.* 2012;94(3):398–404.

295. Seidenberg AB, An YH. Is there an inhibitory effect of COX-2 inhibitors on bone healing? *Pharmacol Res.* 2004;50(2):151–156.

296. Selhi HS, Mahindra P, Yamin M, et al. Outcome in patients with an infected nonunion of the long bones treated with a reinforced antibiotic bone cement rod. *J Orthop Trauma.* 2012;26(3):184–188.

297. Sen MK, Miclau T. Autologous iliac crest bone graft: should it still be the gold standard for treating nonunions? *Injury.* 2007;38(Suppl 1):S75–S80.

298. Shane E, Burr D, Ebeling PR, et al. Atypical subtrochanteric and diaphyseal femoral fractures: report of a task force of the American Society for Bone and Mineral Research. *J Bone Miner Res.* 2010;25(11):2267–2294.

299. Shen HC, Peng H, Usas A, et al. Structural and functional healing of critical-size segmental bone defects by transduced muscle-derived cells expressing BMP4. *J Gene Med.* 2004;6(9):984–991.

300. Sheyn D, Kimelman-Bleich N, Pelled G, et al. Ultrasound-based nonviral gene delivery induces bone formation in vivo. *Gene Ther.* 2008;15(4):257–266.

301. Shibuya N, Humphers JM, Fluhman BL, et al. Factors associated with nonunion, delayed union, and malunion in foot and ankle surgery in diabetic patients. *J Foot Ankle Surg.* 2013;52(2):207–211.

302. Shinsako K, Okui Y, Matsuda Y, et al. Effects of bead size and polymerization in PMMA bone cement on vancomycin release. *Biomed Mater Eng.* 2008;18(6):377–385.

303. Silber JS, Anderson DG, Daffner SD, et al. Donor site morbidity after anterior iliac crest bone harvest for single-level anterior cervical discectomy and fusion. *Spine (Phila Pa 1976).* 2003;28(2):134–139.

304. Sim R, Liang TS, Tay BK. Autologous marrow injection in the treatment of delayed and non-union in long bones. *Singapore Med J.* 1993;34(5):412–417.

305. Simpson JM, Ebraheim NA, An HS, et al. Posterolateral bone graft of the tibia. *Clin Orthop Relat Res.* 1990;(251):200–206.

306. Smith MA, Jones EA, Strachan RK, et al. Prediction of fracture healing in the tibia by quantitative radionuclide imaging. *J Bone Joint Surg Br.* 1987;69(3):441–447.

307. Smith TK. Prevention of complications in orthopedic surgery secondary to nutritional depletion. *Clin Orthop Relat Res.* 1987;(222):91–97.

308. Song HR, Cho SH, Koo KH, et al. Tibial bone defects treated by internal bone transport using the Ilizarov method. *Int Orthop.* 1998;22(5):293–297.

309. Sringari T, Jain UK, Sharma VD. Role of valgus osteotomy and fixation by double-angle blade plate in neglected displaced intracapsular fracture of neck of femur in younger patients. *Injury.* 2005;36(5):630–634.

310. Stafford P, Norris B. Reamer-irrigator-aspirator as a bone graft harvester. *Tech Foot Ankle Surg.* 2007;6(2):100–107.

311. Stafford PR, Norris BL. Reamer-irrigator-aspirator bone graft and bi Masquelet technique for segmental bone defect nonunions: a review of 25 cases. *Injury.* 2010;41(Suppl 2):S72–S77.

312. Starman JS, Bosse MJ, Cates CA, et al. Recombinant human bone morphogenetic protein-2 use in the off-label treatment of nonunions and acute fractures: a retrospective review. *J Trauma Acute Care Surg.* 2012;72(3):676–681.

313. Stavlas P, Polyzois D. Septic arthritis of the major joints of the lower limb after periarticular external fixation application: are conventional safe corridors enough to prevent it? *Injury.* 2005;36(2):239–247.

314. Streubel PN, Desai P, Suk M. Comparison of RIA and conventional reamed nailing for treatment of femur shaft fractures. *Injury.* 2010;41(Suppl 2):S51–S56.

315. Sturmer KM, Schuchardt W. [New aspects of closed intramedullary nailing and marrow cavity reaming in animal experiments. II. Intramedullary pressure in marrow cavity reaming (author's transl)]. *Unfallheilkunde.* 1980;83(7):346–352.

316. Summers BN, Eisenstein SM. Donor site pain from the ilium. A complication of lumbar spine fusion. *J Bone Joint Surg Br.* 1989;71(4):677–680.

317. Takemoto RC, Fajardo M, Kirsch T, et al. Quantitative assessment of the bone morphogenetic protein expression from alternate bone graft harvesting sites. *J Orthop Trauma.* 2010;24(9):564–566.

318. Taylor J. Delayed union and nonunion of fractures. In: Crenshaw A, ed. *Campbell's Operative Orthopedics.* St. Louis: Mosby; 1992:1287–1345.

319. Thonse R, Conway J. Antibiotic cement-coated interlocking nail for the treatment of infected nonunions and segmental bone defects. *J Orthop Trauma.* 2007;21(4):258–268.

320. Thoresen BO, Alho A, Ekeland A, et al. Interlocking intramedullary nailing in femoral shaft fractures. A report of forty-eight cases. *J Bone Joint Surg Am.* 1985;67(9):1313–1320.

321. Tomic S, Bumbasirevic M, Lesic A, et al. Modification of the Ilizarov external fixator for aseptic hypertrophic nonunion of the clavicle: an option for treatment. *J Orthop Trauma.* 2006;20(2):122–128.

322. Tressler MA, Richards JE, Sofianos D, et al. Bone morphogenetic protein-2 compared to autologous iliac crest bone graft in the treatment of long bone nonunion. *Orthopedics.* 2011;34(12):e877–e884.

323. Ueng SW, Lin SS, Wang CR, et al. Bone healing of tibial lengthening is delayed by cigarette smoking: study of bone mineral density and torsional strength on rabbits. *J Trauma.* 1999;46(1):110–115.

324. Urist MR, Silverman BF, Buring K, et al. The bone induction principle. *Clin Orthop Relat Res.* 1967;53:243–283.

325. Vaccaro AR, Patel T, Fischgrund J, et al. A pilot safety and efficacy study of OP-1 putty (rhBMP-7) as an adjunct to iliac crest autograft in posterolateral lumbar fusions. *Eur Spine J.* 2003;12(5):495–500.

326. Vaccaro AR, Patel T, Fischgrund J, et al. A 2-year follow-up pilot study evaluating the safety and efficacy of op-1 putty (rhbmp-7) as an adjunct to iliac crest autograft in posterolateral lumbar fusions. *Eur Spine J.* 2005;14(7):623–629.

327. Vaishya R, Singh AP, Hasija R, et al. Treatment of resistant nonunion of supracondylar fractures femur by megaprosthesis. *Knee Surg Sports Traumatol Arthrosc.* 2011;19(7):1137–1140.

328. Valchanou VD, Michailov P. High energy shock waves in the treatment of delayed and nonunion of fractures. *Int Orthop.* 1991;15(3):181–184.

329. van Wunnik BP, Weijers PH, van Helden SH, et al. Osteoporosis is not a risk factor for the development of nonunion: A cohort nested case-control study. *Injury.* 2011;42(12):1491–1494.

330. Veillette CJ, McKee MD. Growth factors–BMPs, DBMs, and buffy coat products: are there any proven differences amongst them? *Injury.* 2007;38(Suppl 1):S38–S48.

331. Verbruggen JP, Stapert JW. Failure of reamed nailing in humeral non-union: an analysis of 26 patients. *Injury.* 2005;36(3):430–438.

332. Vogel J, Hopf C, Eysel P, et al. Application of extracorporeal shock-waves in the treatment of pseudarthrosis of the lower extremity. Preliminary results. *Arch Orthop Trauma Surg.* 1997;116(8):480–483.

333. Wang K, Edwards E. Intramedullary skeletal kinetic distractor in the treatment of leg length discrepancy–a review of 16 cases and analysis of complications. *J Orthop Trauma.* 2012;26(9):e138–e144.

334. Wang SJ, Lewallen DG, Bolander ME, et al. Low intensity ultrasound treatment increases strength in a rat femoral fracture model. *J Orthop Res.* 1994;12(1):40–47.

335. Watanabe Y, Matsushita T, Bhandari M, et al. Ultrasound for fracture healing: current evidence. *J Orthop Trauma.* 2010;24(Suppl 1):S56–S61.

336. Weiland AJ. Current concepts review: vascularized free bone transplants. *J Bone Joint Surg Am.* 1981;63(1):166–169.

337. Wenisch S, Trinkaus K, Hild A, et al. Human reaming debris: a source of multipotent stem cells. *Bone.* 2005;36(1):74–83.

338. Weresh MJ, Hakanson R, Stover MD, et al. Failure of exchange reamed intramedullary nails for ununited femoral shaft fractures. *J Orthop Trauma.* 2000;14(5):335–338.

339. Westrich GH, Geller DS, O'Malley MJ, et al. Anterior iliac crest bone graft harvesting using the corticocancellous reamer system. *J Orthop Trauma.* 2001;15(7):500–506.

340. Whelan DB, Bhandari M, Stephen D, et al. Development of the radiographic union score for tibial fractures for the assessment of tibial fracture healing after intramedullary fixation. *J Trauma.* 2010;68(3):629–632.

341. White PF, Kehlet H, Liu S. Perioperative analgesia: what do we still know? *Anesth Analg.* 2009;108(5):1364–1367.

342. Wildemann B, Kadow-Romacker A, Haas NP, et al. Quantification of various growth factors in different demineralized bone matrix preparations. *J Biomed Mater Res A.* 2007;81(2):437–442.

343. Wilkins RM, Kelly CM. The effect of allomatrix injectable putty on the outcome of long bone applications. *Orthopedics.* 2003;26(5 Suppl):s567–s570.

344. Williams JL. Ultrasonic wave propagation in cancellous and cortical bone: prediction of some experimental results by Biot's theory. *J Acoust Soc Am.* 1992;91(2):1106–1112.

345. Wu CC, Chen WJ. Healing of 56 segmental femoral shaft fractures after locked nailing. Poor results of dynamization. *Acta Orthop Scand.* 1997;68(6):537–540.

346. Wu CC, Shih CH, Chen WJ, et al. High success rate with exchange nailing to treat a tibial shaft aseptic nonunion. *J Orthop Trauma.* 1999;13(1):33–38.

347. Wu CC, Shih CH. Effect of dynamization of a static interlocking nail on fracture healing. *Can J Surg.* 1993;36(4):302–306.

348. Wu CC. Exchange nailing for aseptic nonunion of femoral shaft: a retrospective cohort study for effect of reaming size. *J Trauma.* 2007;63(4):859–865.

349. Wu CC. Retrograde dynamic locked nailing for femoral supracondylar nonunions after plating. *J Trauma.* 2009;66(1):195–199.

350. Wu CC. Single-stage surgical treatment of infected nonunion of the distal tibia. *J Orthop Trauma.* 2011;25(3):156–161.

351. Wu CC. The effect of dynamization on slowing the healing of femur shaft fractures after interlocking nailing. *J Trauma.* 1997;43(2):263–267.

352. Yang JS, Otero J, McAndrew CM, et al. Can tibial nonunion be predicted at 3 months after intramedullary nailing? *J Orthop Trauma.* 2013;27:599–603.

353. Yang KH, Kim JR, Park J. Nonisthmal femoral shaft nonunion as a risk factor for exchange nailing failure. *J Trauma Acute Care Surg.* 2012;72(2):E60–E64.

354. Yang KH, Parvizi J, Wang SJ, et al. Exposure to low-intensity ultrasound increases aggrecan gene expression in a rat femur fracture model. *J Orthop Res.* 1996;14(5):802–809.

355. Yang RS, Lin WL, Chen YZ, et al. Regulation by ultrasound treatment on the integrin expression and differentiation of osteoblasts. *Bone.* 2005;36(2):276–283.

356. Ye J, Zheng Q. Augmentative locking compression plate fixation for the management of long bone nonunion after intramedullary nailing. *Arch Orthop Trauma Surg.* 2012;132(7):937–940.

357. Younger EM, Chapman MW. Morbidity at bone graft donor sites. *J Orthop Trauma.* 1989;3(3):192–195.

358. Zelle BA, Gollwitzer H, Zlowodzki M, et al. Extracorporeal shock wave therapy: current evidence. *J Orthop Trauma.* 2010;24(Suppl 1):S66–S70.

359. Zhang B, Chiu KY, Wang M. Hip arthroplasty for failed internal fixation of intertrochanteric fractures. *J Arthroplasty.* 2004;19(3):329–333.

360. Zheng LW, Ma L, Cheung LK. Changes in blood perfusion and bone healing induced by nicotine during distraction osteogenesis. *Bone.* 2008;43(2):355–361.

361. Zimmermann G, Moghaddam A, Wagner C, et al. [Clinical experience with bone morphogenetic protein 7 (BMP 7) in nonunions of long bones]. *Unfallchirurg.* 2006;109(7):528–537.

362. Ziran BH, Hendi P, Smith WR, et al. Osseous healing with a composite of allograft and demineralized bone matrix: adverse effects of smoking. *Am J Orthop (Belle Mead NJ).* 2007;36(4):207–209.

363. Ziran BH, Smith WR, Morgan SJ. Use of calcium-based demineralized bone matrix/allograft for nonunions and posttraumatic reconstruction of the appendicular skeleton: preliminary results and complications. *J Trauma.* 2007;63(6):1324–1328.

28 PRINCIPLES OF MALUNIONS

Mark R. Brinker and Daniel P. O'Connor

EVALUATION

Each malunited fracture presents a unique set of bony deformities that are described in terms of abnormalities of length, angulation, rotation, and translation. Also describing the location, magnitude, and direction of the deformity completes the characterization of the malunion. Proper evaluation allows the surgeon to determine an effective treatment plan for deformity correction.

Clinical

Evaluation begins with a medical history and a review of all available medical records. The history should include the date and mechanism of injury of the initial fracture and all subsequent operative and nonoperative interventions. The history should also include descriptions of prior wound and bone infections, and prior culture reports should be obtained. All pre-injury medical problems, disabilities, or associated injuries should be noted. The patient's current level of pain and functional limitations as well as medication use should be documented.

Following the history, a physical examination is performed. The skin and soft tissues in the injury zone should be inspected. The presence of active drainage or sinus formation should be noted.

The malunion site should be manually stressed to rule out motion and assess pain. In a solidly healed fracture with deformity, manual stressing of the malunion site should not elicit pain. If pain is elicited on manual stressing, the orthopedic surgeon should consider the possibility that the patient has an ununited fracture.

A neurovascular examination of the limb and evaluation of active and passive motion of the joints proximal and distal to the malunion site should be performed. Reduced motion in a joint adjacent to a malunion site may alter both the treatment plan and the expectations for the ultimate functional outcome. Patients who have a periarticular malunion may also have a compensatory fixed deformity at an adjacent joint, which must be recognized to include its correction in the treatment plan. Correction of the malunion without addressing a compensatory joint deformity results in a straight bone with a maloriented joint, thus producing a disabled limb. The limb may appear aligned in these cases, but radiographic evaluation will reveal the joint deformity. If the patient cannot place the joint into the position that parallels the deformity at the malunion site (e.g., evert the subtalar joint into valgus in the presence of a tibial valgus malunion) the joint deformity is fixed and requires correction (Fig. 28-1).

Radiographic

The plain radiographs from the original fracture show the type and severity of the initial bony injury. Subsequent plain radiographs show the status of orthopedic hardware (e.g., loose, broken, undersized) as well as document the timing of insertion or removal. The evolution of deformity—for example, gradual versus sudden—should be evaluated.

The current radiographs are evaluated next. Anteroposterior (AP) and lateral radiographs of the involved bone, including the proximal and distal joints, are used to evaluate the axes of the involved bone. Manual measurement of standard radiographs or computer-assisted measurement of digital radiographs may

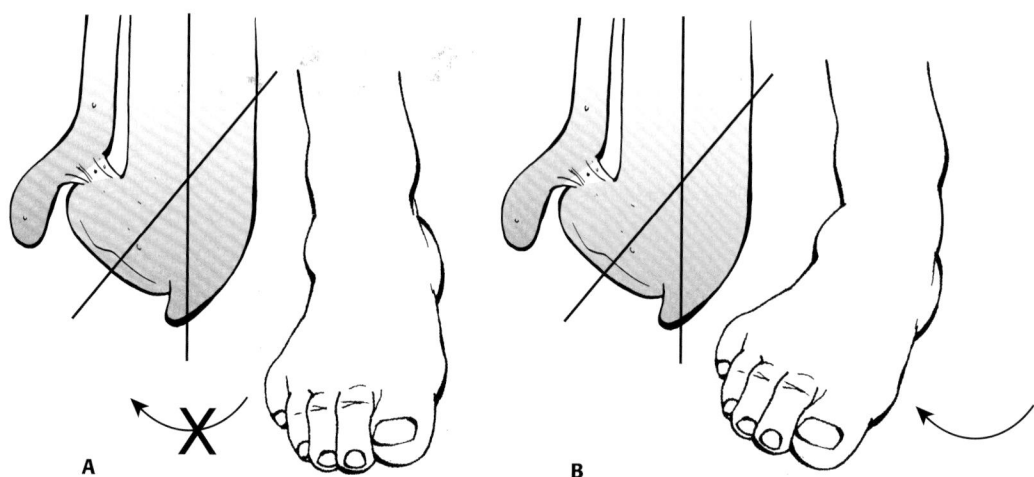

FIGURE 28-1 Angular deformity near a joint can result in a compensatory deformity through the joint. For example, frontal plane deformities of the distal tibia can result in a compensatory frontal plane deformity of the subtalar joint. The deformity of the subtalar joint is fixed **(A)** if the patient's foot cannot be positioned to parallel the deformity of the distal tibia or flexible **(B)** if the foot can be positioned parallel to the deformity of the distal tibia.

be used with equivalent accuracy.[88,92,99] Bilateral AP and lateral 51-inch radiographs are obtained for lower-extremity deformities to evaluate limb alignment (Fig. 28-2). Flexion/extension lateral radiographs may be useful to determine the arc of motion of the surrounding joints.

The current radiographs are used to document the following characteristics: Limb alignment, joint orientation, anatomic axes, mechanical axes, and center of rotation of angulation (CORA). Normative values for the relations among these various parameters[14,78] are used to assess deformities.

Limb Alignment

Evaluation of limb alignment involves assessment of the frontal plane mechanical axis of the entire limb rather than single bones.[35,45,47,76,77,91] In the lower extremity, the frontal plane mechanical axis of the entire limb is evaluated using the weight-bearing AP 51-inch alignment radiograph with the feet pointed forward (neutral rotation).[41,49,82]

Mechanical axis deviation (MAD) is measured as the distance from the knee joint center to the line connecting the joint centers of the hip and ankle. The hip joint center is located at the center of the femoral head. The knee joint center is half the distance from the nadir between the tibial spines to the apex of the intercondylar notch on the femur. The ankle joint center is the center of the tibial plafond.

Normally, the mechanical axis of the lower extremity lies 1 to 15 mm medial to the knee joint center (Fig. 28-3). If the lower-extremity mechanical axis is outside this range, the deformity is described as MAD (Fig. 28-3). MAD greater than 15 mm medial to the knee midpoint is varus malalignment; any MAD lateral to the knee midpoint is valgus malalignment.

Long Bone Anatomic Axes

The anatomic and mechanical axes of the long bones are assessed in both the frontal plane (AP radiographs) and sagittal

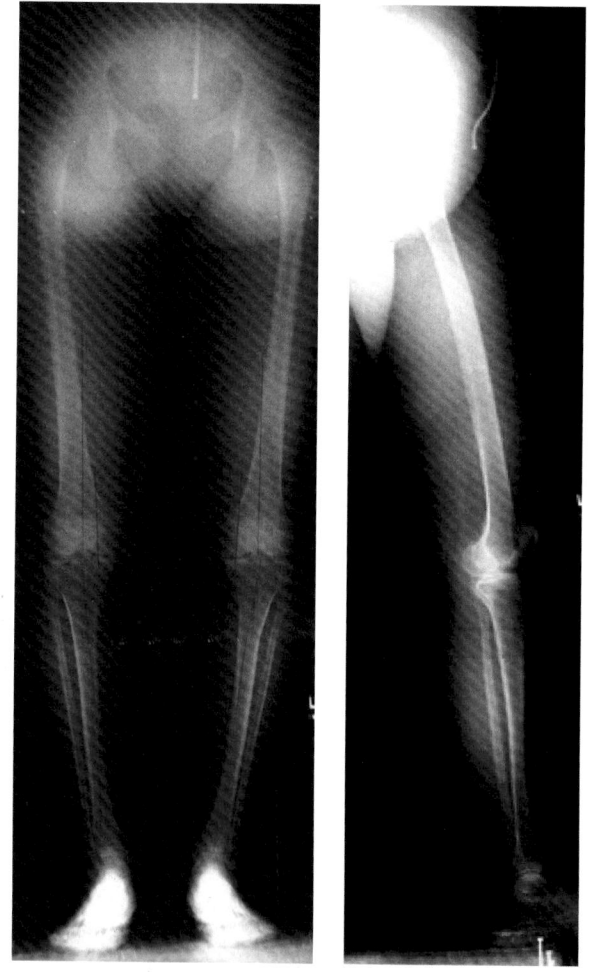

FIGURE 28-2 (A) Bilateral weight-bearing 51-inch AP alignment radiograph and **(B)** a 51-inch lateral alignment radiograph, which are used to evaluate lower-extremity limb alignment.

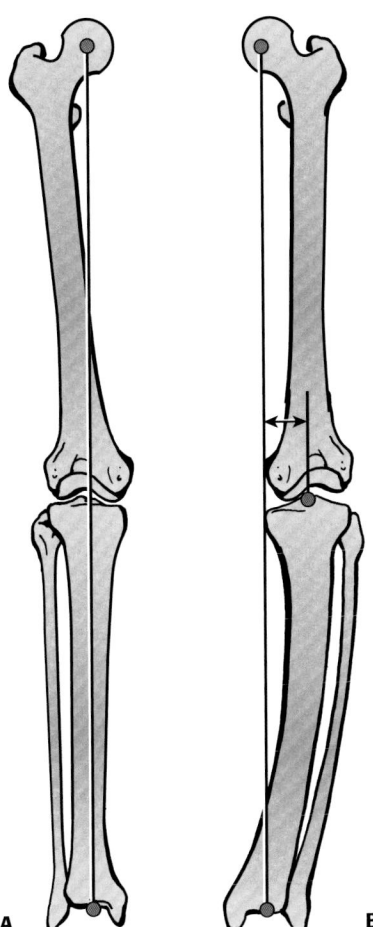

FIGURE 28-3 **A:** Mechanical axis of the lower extremity, which normally lies 1 to 15 mm medial to the knee joint center. **B:** Medial mechanical axis deviation, in which the mechanical axis of the lower extremity lies more than 15 mm medial to the knee joint center.

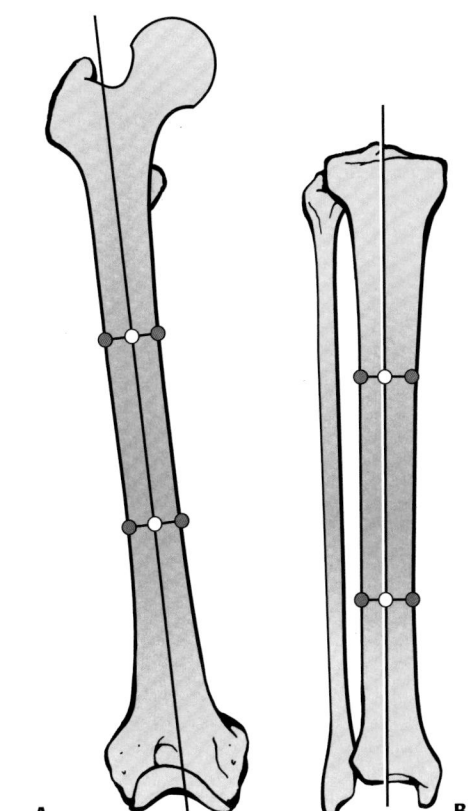

FIGURE 28-4 **A:** Anatomic axis of the femur. **B:** Anatomic axis of the tibia.

plane (lateral radiographs). The anatomic axes are defined by lines that pass through the center of the diaphysis along the length of the bone or bone segment. To identify the anatomic axis, the center of the transverse diameter of the diaphysis is identified at several points along the bone or bone segment. The line that passes through these points represents the anatomic axis (Fig. 28-4).

In a normal bone, the anatomic axis is a single straight line. In a malunited bone with angulation, each bony segment can be defined by its own anatomic axis with a line through the center of the diameter of the diaphysis of each bone segment representing the respective anatomic axis for that segment (Fig. 28-5). In bones with multiapical or combined deformities, there may be multiple anatomic axes in the same plane (Fig. 28-5).

Mechanical Axes

The mechanical axis of a long bone is defined as the line that passes through the joint centers of the proximal and distal joints. To identify the mechanical axis in a long bone, the joint centers are connected by a line (Fig. 28-6). The mechanical

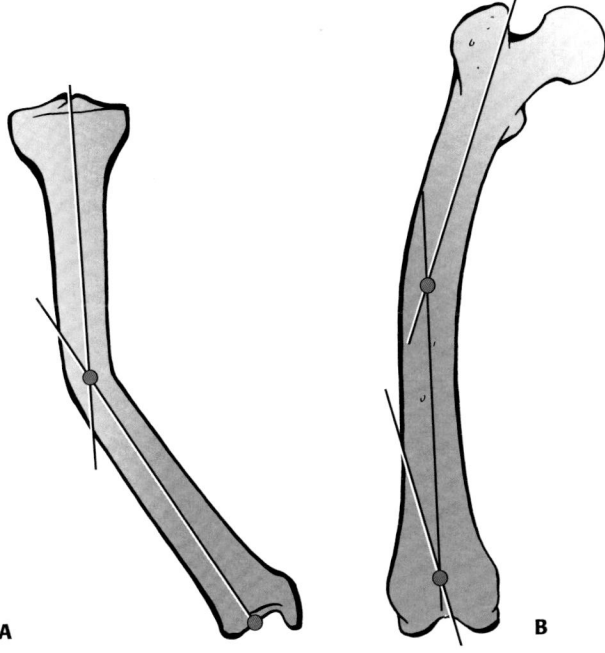

FIGURE 28-5 **A:** A malunited tibia fracture with angulation showing the anatomic axis for each bony segment as a line through the center of the diameter of the respective diaphyseal segments. **B:** A malunited femur fracture with a multiapical deformity, showing multiple anatomical axes in the same plane.

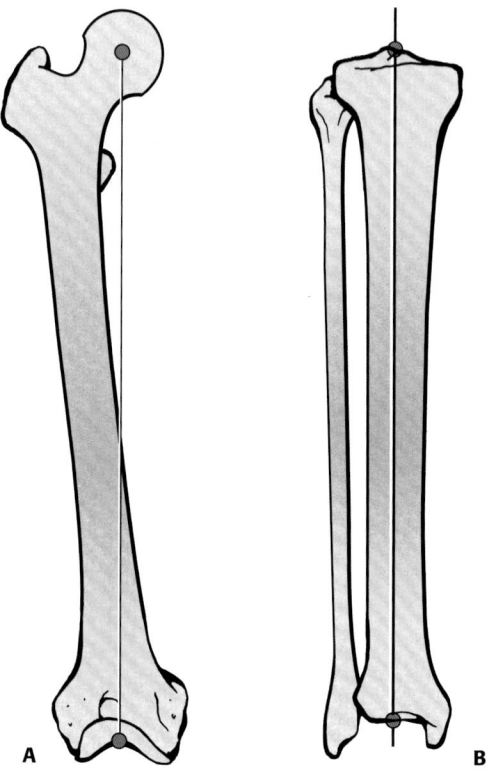

FIGURE 28-6 The mechanical axis of a long bone is defined as the line that passes through the joint centers of the proximal and distal joints. **A:** The mechanical axis of the femur. **B:** The mechanical axis of the tibia.

axis of the entire lower extremity was described above under limb alignment.

Joint Orientation Lines

Joint orientation describes the relation of a joint to the respective anatomic and mechanical axes of a long bone. Joint orientation lines are drawn on the AP and lateral radiographs in the frontal and sagittal planes, respectively.

Hip orientation may be assessed in two ways in the frontal plane. The trochanter-head joint orientation line connects the tip of the greater trochanter with center of the hip joint (the center of the femoral head). The femoral neck joint orientation line connects the hip joint center with a series of points which bisect the diameter of the femoral neck.

Knee orientation is represented in the frontal plane by joint orientation lines at the distal femur and the proximal tibia. The distal femur joint orientation line is drawn to connect the most distal points of the femoral condyles. The proximal tibial joint orientation line is drawn tangential to the subchondral lines of the medial and lateral tibial plateaus. The angle between the two knee joint orientation lines is called the joint line congruence angle (JLCA), which normally varies from 0 to 2 degrees medial JLCA (i.e., slight knee joint varus). A lateral JLCA of any degree represents valgus malorientation of the knee and a medial JLCA of 3 degrees or greater represents varus malorientation of the knee.

Knee orientation is represented in the sagittal plane by joint orientation lines at the distal femur and the proximal tibia. The sagittal distal femur joint orientation line is drawn through the anterior and posterior junctions of the femoral condyles with the metaphysis. The sagittal proximal tibial joint orientation line is drawn tangential to the subchondral lines of the tibial plateau.

Malorientation of the knee joint produces malalignment of the lower limb, but limb malalignment (MAD outside the normal range) is not necessarily due to knee joint malorientation.

Ankle orientation is represented in the frontal plane by a line drawn through the subchondral line of the tibial plafond. Ankle orientation is represented in the sagittal plane by a line drawn through the most distal points of the anterior and posterior distal tibia.

Joint Orientation Angles

The relation between the anatomic axes or the mechanical axes and the joint orientation lines can be referred to as joint orientation angles and are described using standard nomenclature (Table 28-1) (Fig. 28-7).

In order to draw a joint orientation angle in the lower extremity when a deformity is present, begin by drawing a joint orientation line. Next, identify the joint center, which will always lie on the joint orientation line and intersects the mechanical axis. The mechanical axis line of the bone segment immediately adjacent to the joint can then be drawn using one of the three methods: (1) using the population mean value for that particular joint orientation angle; (2) using the joint orientation angle of the contralateral extremity, assuming it is normal; or (3) by extending the mechanical axis of the neighboring bone.

For example, in order to draw the mechanical lateral distal femoral angle (mLDFA) in a femur with a frontal plane deformity, the steps would be as follows. Step 1: Draw the distal femoral joint orientation line. Step 2: Start at the joint center and draw an 88-degree mLDFA (population normal mean value), which will define the mechanical axis of the distal femoral segment. Alternately, draw the mLDFA which mimics the contralateral distal femur (if normal), or extend the mechanical axis of the tibia proximally (if the tibia is normal) to define the distal femoral mechanical axis.

Center of Rotation of Angulation

The intersection of the proximal axis and distal axis of a deformed bone is called the CORA (Fig. 28-8), which is the point about which a deformity may be rotated to achieve correction.[22,30,34,46,72,75–78,89] The angle formed by the two axes at the CORA is a measure of angular deformity in that plane. Either the anatomic or mechanical axes may be used to identify the CORA, but these axes cannot be mixed. For diaphyseal malunions, the anatomic axes are most convenient. For juxta-articular (metaphyseal, epiphyseal) deformities, the mechanical axis of the short segment is constructed using one of the three methods described above.

To define the CORA, the proximal axis and distal axis of the bone are identified, and then the orientations of the proximal

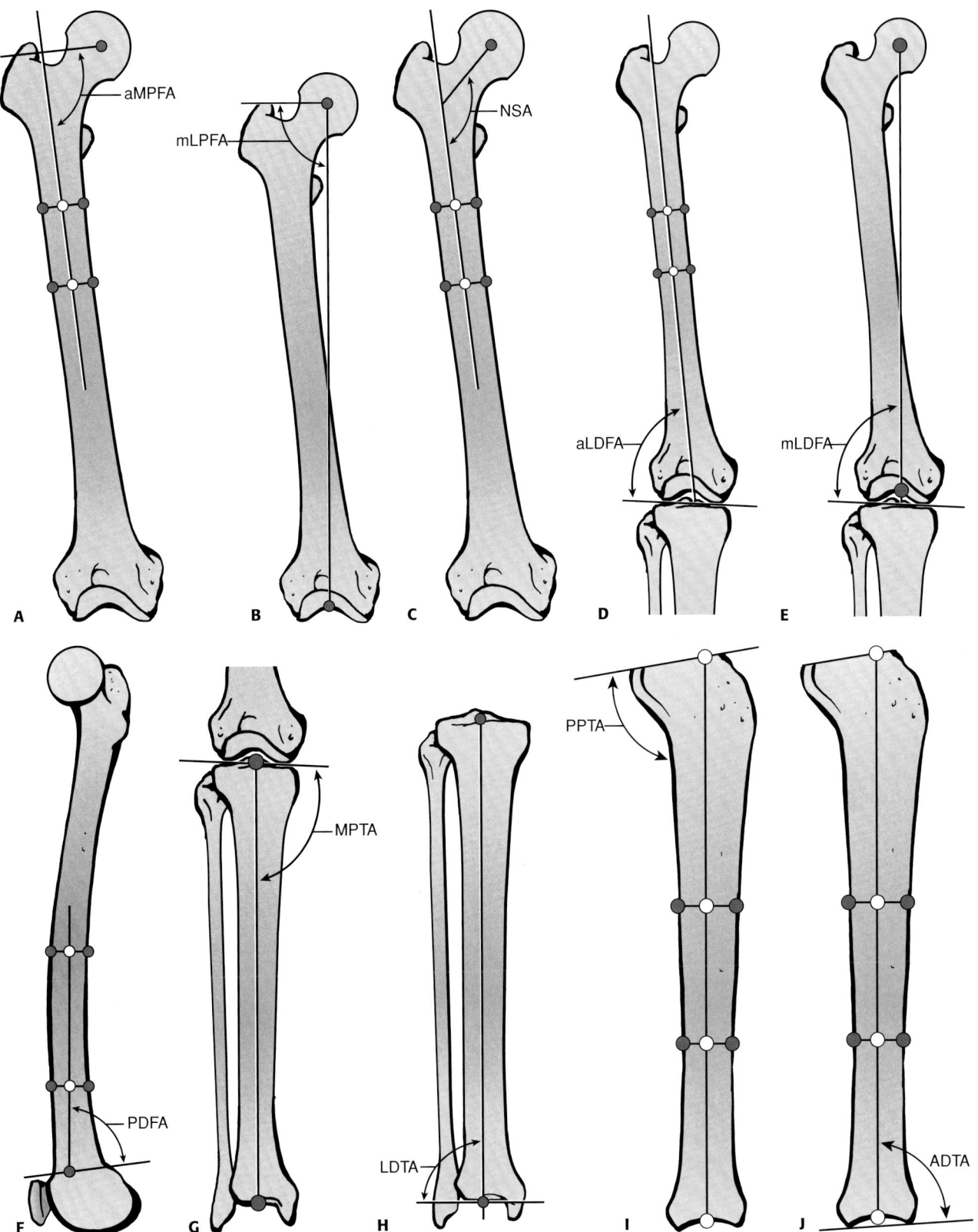

FIGURE 28-7 Joint orientation angles. **A:** Anatomic medial proximal femoral angle (aMPFA).
B: Mechanical lateral proximal femoral angle (mLPFA). **C:** Neck shaft angle (NSA). **D:** Anatomic lateral
distal femoral angle (aLDFA). **E:** Mechanical lateral distal femoral angle (mLDFA). **F:** Posterior distal
femoral angle (PDFA). **G:** Medial proximal tibial angle (MPTA). **H:** Lateral distal tibial angle (LDTA).
I: Posterior proximal tibial angle (PPTA). **J:** Anterior distal tibial angle (ADTA).

TABLE 28-1 | **Normal Values for Joint Orientation Angles in the Lower Extremity**

Bone–Plane	Components		Mean Value (degrees)	Normal Range (degrees)
Femur–Frontal				
Anatomic medial proximal femoral angle (aMPFA)	Anatomic axis	Trochanter-head line	84	80–89
Mechanical lateral proximal femoral angle (mLPFA)	Mechanical axis	Trochanter-head line	90	85–95
Neck shaft angle (NSA)	Anatomic axis	Femoral neck line	130	124–136
Anatomic lateral distal femoral angle (aLDFA)	Anatomic axis	Distal femoral joint orientation line	81	79–83
Mechanical lateral distal femoral angle (mLDFA)	Mechanical axis	Distal femoral joint orientation line	88	85–90
Femur–Sagittal				
Posterior distal femoral angle (PDFA)	Mid-diaphyseal line	Sagittal distal femoral joint orientation line	83	79–87
Tibial–Frontal				
Medial proximal tibial angle (MPTA)	Mechanical axis	Proximal tibial joint orientation line	87	85–90
Lateral distal tibial angle (LDTA)	Mechanical axis	Distal tibial joint orientation line	89	88–92
Tibial–Sagittal				
Posterior proximal tibial angle (PPTA)	Mid-diaphyseal line	Sagittal proximal tibial joint orientation line	81	77–84
Anterior distal tibial angle (ADTA)	Mid-diaphyseal line	Sagittal distal tibial joint orientation line	80	78–82

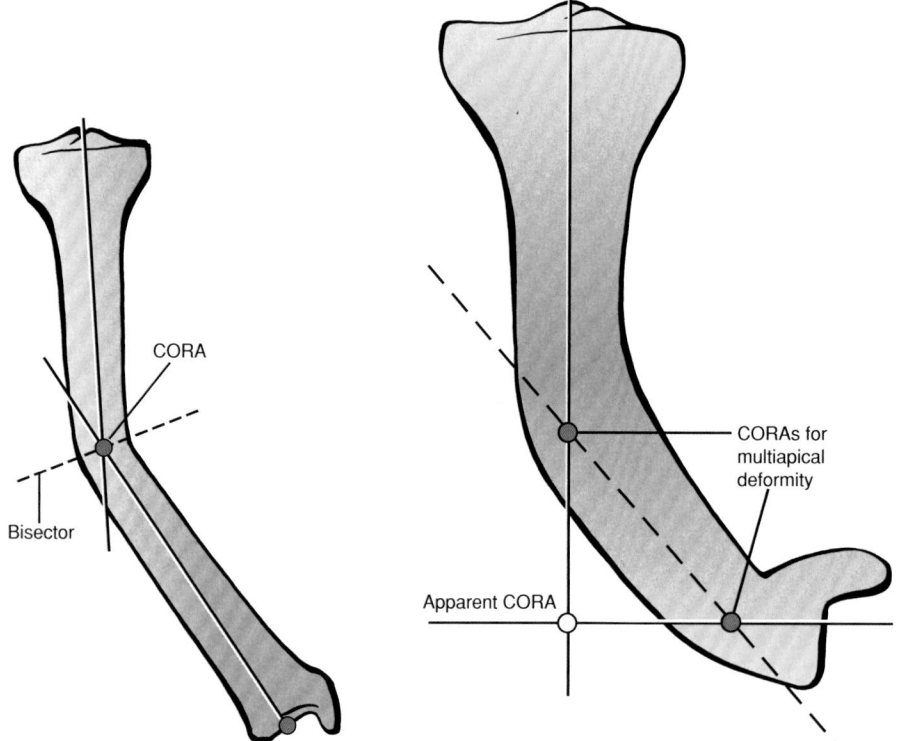

FIGURE 28-8 **A:** Center of rotation of angulation (CORA) and bisector for a varus angulation deformity of the tibia. **B:** Multiapical tibial deformity showing that the apparent CORA joining the proximal and distal anatomic axes (*solid lines*) lies outside of the bone. A third anatomic axis for the middle segment (*dashed line*) shows two CORAs for this multiapical deformity that both lie within the bone.

and distal joints are assessed. If the intersection of the proximal and distal axes lies at the point of obvious deformity in the bone and the joint orientations are normal, the intersection point is the CORA and the deformity is uniapical in the respective plane. If the intersection of the axes lies outside the point of obvious deformity or either joint orientation is abnormal, either a second CORA exists in that plane and the deformity is multiapical or a translational deformity exists in that plane, which is usually obvious on the radiograph.

The CORA is used to plan the operative correction of angular deformities. Correction of angulation by rotating the bone around a point on the line that bisects the angle of the CORA (the "bisector") ensures realignment of the anatomic and mechanical axes without introducing an iatrogenic translational deformity.[34] The bisector is a line that passes through the CORA and bisects the angle formed by the proximal and distal axes (Fig. 28-8).[78] Angular correction along the bisector results in complete deformity correction without the introduction of a translational deformity.[14,72,74,76,77] All points which lie on the bisector can be considered to be CORAs because angulation about these points will result in realignment of the deformed bone (see Treatment—Osteotomies below).

Note that the proximal half of the mechanical axis for the femur and a portion of the proximal humerus normally lie outside the bone, so the CORA that is identified using the mechanical axis of the femur may lie outside the bone as well although the deformity may be uniapical. By contrast, if the CORA identified using the anatomic axis of the femur or humerus, or either axis of the tibia, lies outside the bone, then a multiapical deformity exists (Fig. 28-8).

Evaluation of the Various Deformity Types
Length

Deformities involving length include shortening and overdistraction and are characterized by their direction and magnitude. They are measured from joint center to joint center in centimeters on plain radiographs and compared to the contralateral normal extremity, using an x-ray marker to correct for magnification (Fig. 28-9).[90] Shortening after an injury may result from bone loss (from the injury or debridement) or overriding of the healed fracture fragments. Overdistraction at the time of fracture fixation may result in a healed fracture with overlengthening of the bone.

Angulation

Deformities involving angulation are characterized by their magnitude and the direction of the apex of angulation. Angulation deformity of the diaphysis is often associated with limb malalignment (MAD), as described above. Angulation deformities of the metaphysis and epiphysis (juxta-articular deformities) can be difficult to characterize. The angle formed by the intersection of a joint orientation line and the anatomic or mechanical axis of the deformed bone should be measured. When the angle formed differs markedly from the contralateral normal limb (or normal values when the contralateral limb is abnormal), a juxta-articular deformity is present.[14,74,77] The identification of the CORA is key in characterizing angular deformities and planning their correction.

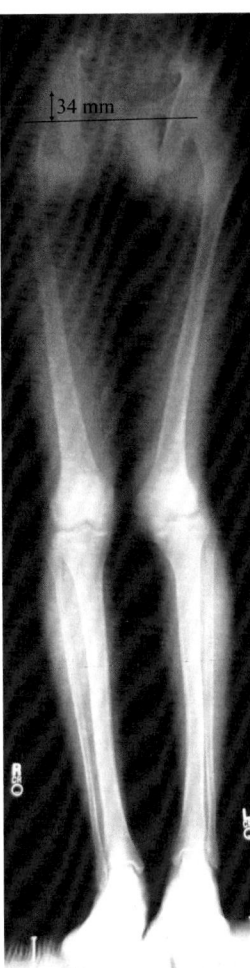

FIGURE 28-9 Bilateral standing 51-inch AP alignment radiograph reveals a 34-mm leg length inequality.

Pure frontal or sagittal plane angular deformities are simple to characterize. Since the deformity appears only on the AP or lateral radiograph, respectively. If, however, the AP and lateral radiographs both appear to have angulation with CORAs at the same level on both views, the orientation of the angulation deformity is in an oblique plane (Fig. 28-10). Characterization of the magnitude and direction of oblique plane deformities can be computed from the AP and lateral radiographic measures using either the trigonometric or graphic method.[18,36,78] Using the trigonometric method, the magnitude of an oblique plane angular deformity is

$$\text{oblique magnitude} = \tan^{-1}\sqrt{\tan^2(\text{frontal magnitude}) + \tan^2(\text{sagittal magnitude})}$$

and the orientation (relative to the frontal plane) of an oblique plane deformity is

$$\text{oblique orientation} = \tan^{-1}\left[\frac{\tan(\text{sagittal magnitude})}{\tan(\text{frontal magnitude})}\right]$$

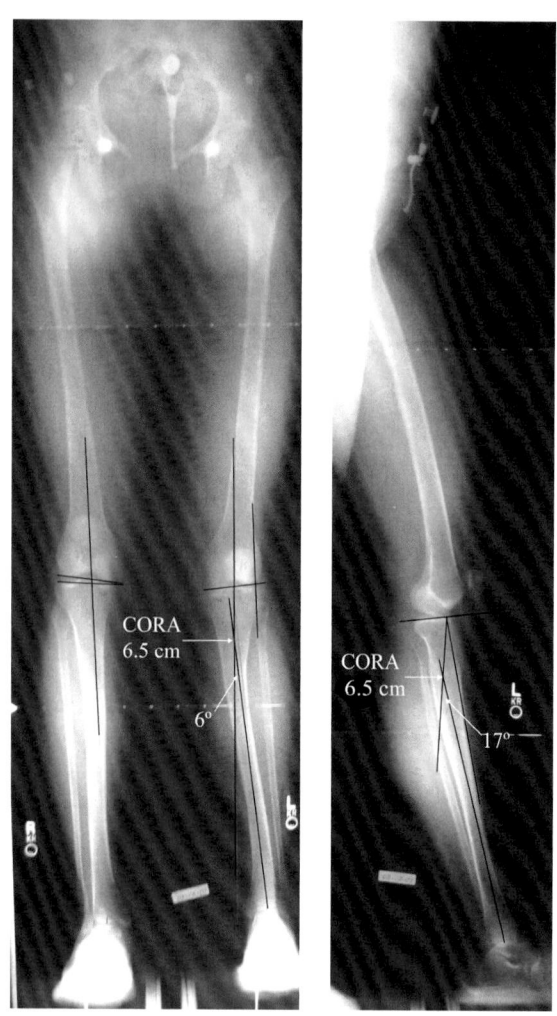

CORA
6.5 cm

6°

CORA
6.5 cm

17°

A

B

FIGURE 28-10 A 28-year-old woman presented with complaints of her leg "going out" and her knee hyperextending. **A:** 51-inch AP alignment radiograph reveals a 6-degree apex medial deformity with the CORA 6.5 cm distal to the proximal tibial joint orientation line, and **(B)** the lateral alignment radiograph shows a 17-degree apex posterior angulation with a CORA 6.5 cm distal to the proximal tibial joint orientation line. This patient has an oblique plane angular deformity without translation.

Using the graphic method, the magnitude of an oblique plane angular deformity is

$$\text{oblique magnitude} = \sqrt{(\text{frontal magnitude})^2 + (\text{sagittal magnitude})^2}$$

and the orientation (relative to the frontal plane) of an oblique plane deformity is

$$\text{oblique orientation} = \tan^{-1}\left(\frac{\text{sagittal magnitude}}{\text{frontal magnitude}}\right)$$

The graphic method, based on the pythagorean theorem, approximates the exact trigonometric method. The error of approximation for angular deformities using the graphic method is less than 4 degrees unless the frontal and sagittal plane magnitudes are both greater than 45 degrees.[14,46,72,74,76,77]

When the CORA is at a different level on the AP and lateral radiographs, a translational deformity is present in addition to an angulation deformity (Fig. 28-11).

A multiapical deformity is defined by the presence of more than one CORA on either the AP or lateral radiograph (or both). In a multiapical deformity without translation, one of the joints will appear maloriented relative to the anatomic axis of the respective segment. For multiapical deformity, the anatomic axis of the segment nearest the joint with malorientation provides a third line that intersects both of the existing lines within the bone. These intersections are the sites of the multiple CORAs (Fig. 28-12).

Rotation

A rotational deformity occurs about the longitudinal axis of the bone. Rotational deformities are described in terms of their magnitude and the position (internal or external rotation) of the distal segment relative to the proximal segment. Identification of a rotational deformity and quantification of the magnitude can be done using clinical measurements,[100] axial computed tomography (CT) (Fig. 28-13),[9] or AP and lateral radiographs with either trigonometric calculation or graphical approximation.[78] While axial CT and the radiographic methods allow for more precise measurement of rotational deformities, the more convenient clinical measurement method often results in measures of sufficient accuracy to allow for adequate correction.[100]

To measure tibial malrotation using clinical examination, the position of the foot axis, as indicated by a line running from the second toe through the center of the calcaneus, is compared

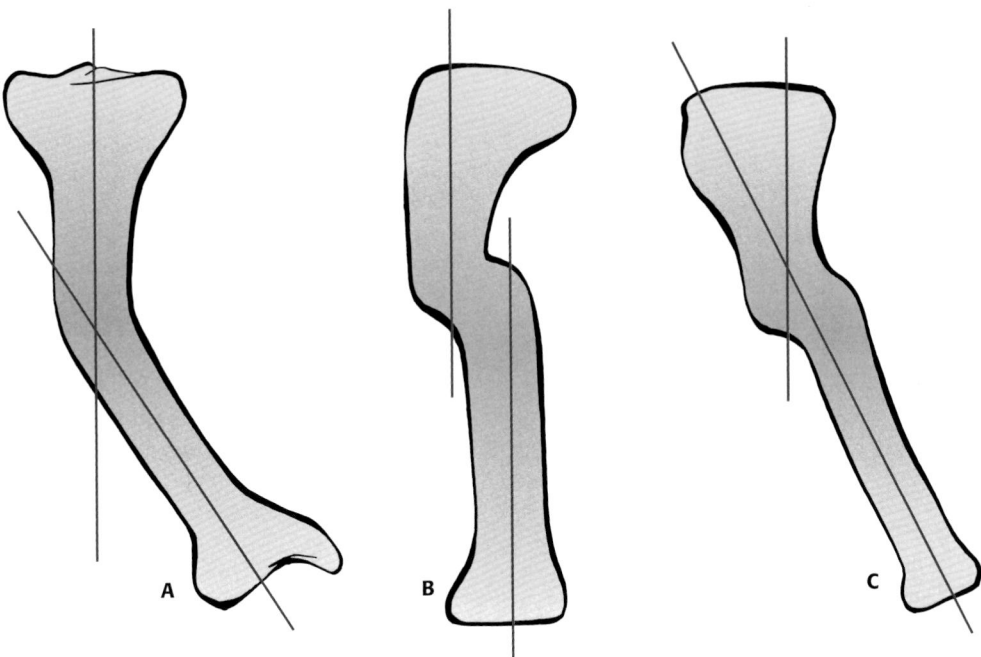

FIGURE 28-11 **A:** Frontal and **(B)** sagittal views of a tibia with an angulation–translational deformity. Note that the angulation deformity is evident only on the frontal view and the translational deformity is evident only on the sagittal view. **C:** The oblique view showing both deformities.

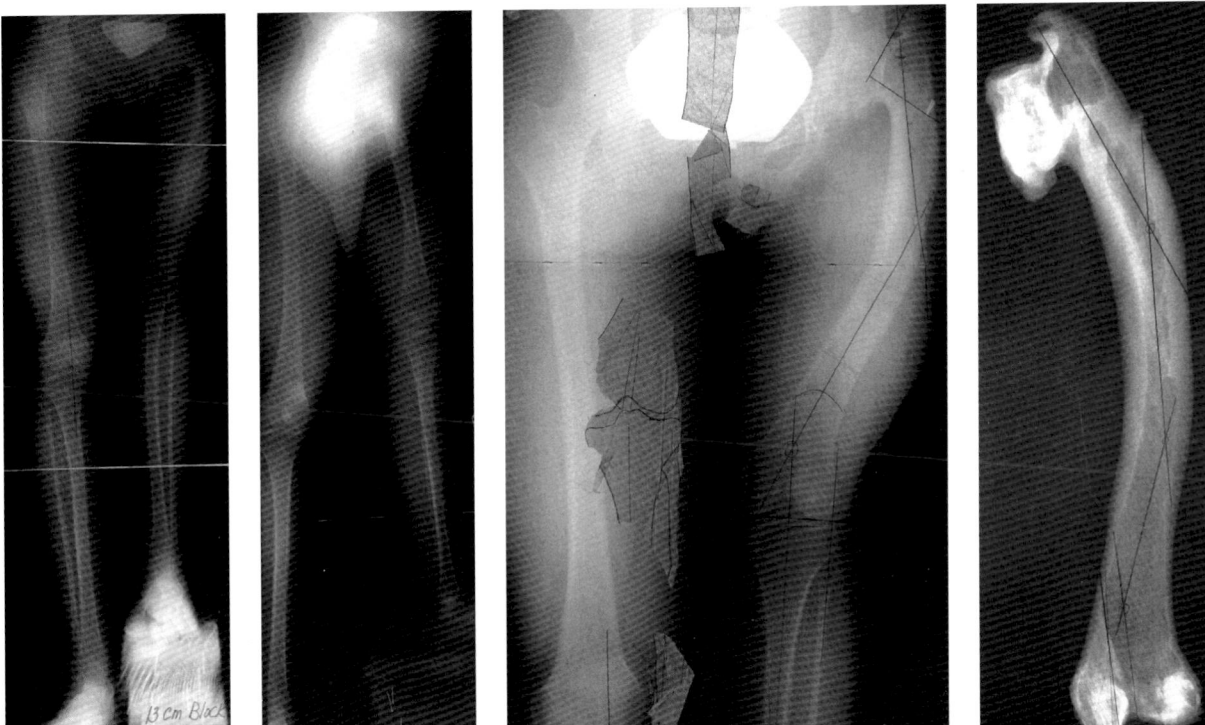

A, B

C, D

FIGURE 28-12 **(A)** AP and **(B)** lateral long-leg radiographs of a 27-year-old woman with a multiapical deformity of the femur, a large lateral mechanical axis deviation, a 13-cm leg length discrepancy, superior subluxation of the hip joint, degenerative hip joint disease, and a history of developmental dysplasia of the hip, proximal femoral focal deficiency, and Wagner osteotomy in childhood. The staged treatment plan included deformity correction, followed by femoral lengthening, and finally hip arthroplasty. **C:** Use of tracing paper and **(D)** three-dimensional CT reconstruction of the femur to facilitate treatment planning. The multiapical deformity and its three CORAs can be seen on these images.

(continues)

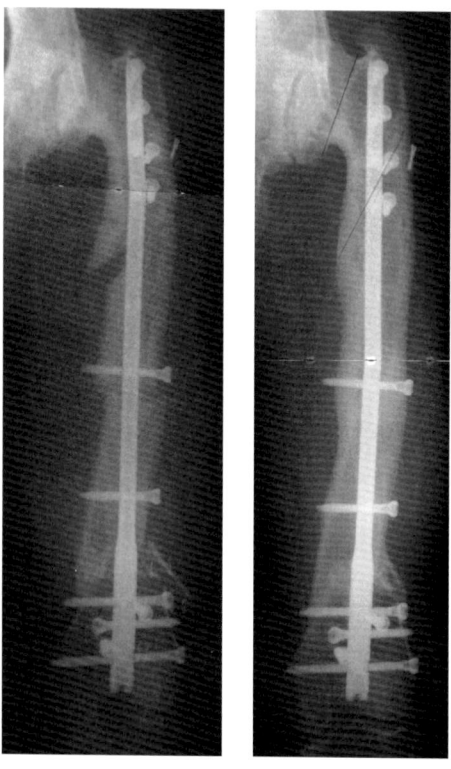

FIGURE 28-12 (*continued*) **E:** AP radiograph 1 month following multiapical deformity correction and intramedullary nailing showing the location and orientation of the three osteotomy sites. **F:** AP radiograph 7 months following deformity correction shows solid bony union at all three corticotomy sites.

to the projection of either the femoral or the tibial anatomic axis. To use the femoral axis, the patient is positioned prone or sits with the knee flexed to 90 degrees. The examiner measures the deviation of the foot axis from the line of the femoral axis;

any deviation is considered to represent tibial malrotation. To use the tibial axis, the patient stands with the patella facing anteriorly (i.e., aligned in the frontal plane). To measure tibial malrotation, the examiner measures the deviation of the foot axis from the anterior projection of the tibial anatomic axis in the sagittal plane; any deviation of the foot axis from the tibial anatomic axis is considered to represent tibial malrotation.

To measure a femoral rotational deformity using clinical examination, the patient is positioned prone with the knee flexed to 90 degrees and the femoral condyles parallel to the examination table. The femur is passively rotated internally and externally by the examiner, and the respective angular excursions of the tibia are measured. Asymmetry of rotation in comparison to the opposite side indicates a femoral rotational deformity. If the patient also has a tibial angulation deformity, the tibia will not be perpendicular to the examination table when the femoral condyles are so positioned; tibial angulation deformity will cause an apparent asymmetry in femoral rotation. In this case, the rotational excursions of the tibia must be adjusted for the magnitude of the tibial angular deformity to avoid an incorrect assessment of femoral rotation.

Translation

Translational deformities may result from malunion following either a fracture or an osteotomy. Translational deformities are characterized by their plane, direction, magnitude, and level. The direction of a translational deformity is described in terms of the position of the distal segment relative to the proximal segment (medial, lateral, anterior, posterior), except for the femoral and humeral heads in which case the description is the position of the head relative to the shaft. Translational deformities may occur in an oblique plane, and trigonometric or graphical methods similar to those described for characterizing angulation deformities may be used to identify the plane and direction of the deformity.[18,36,78] Magnitude of translation is

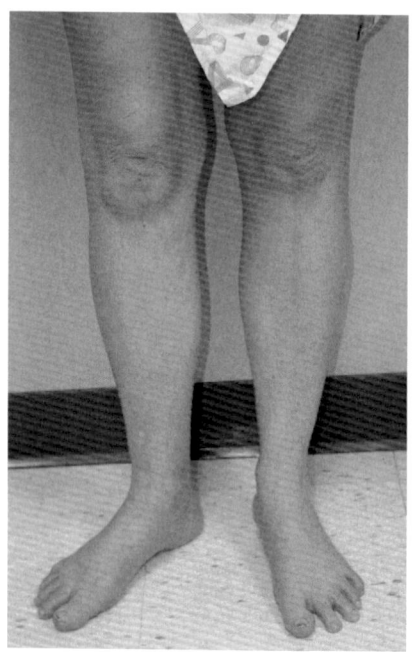

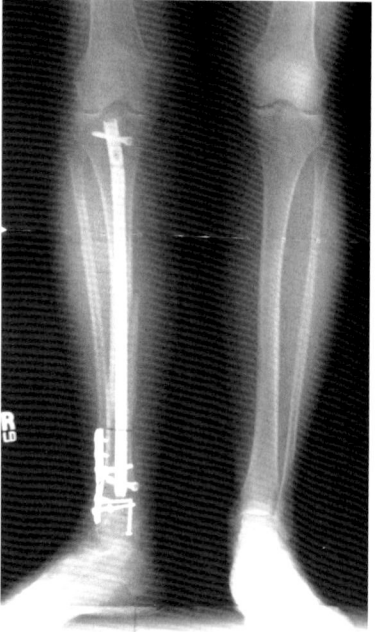

FIGURE 28-13 A: Clinical photograph of a 38-year-old woman who presented 9 months after nail fixation of a tibial fracture. She complained of her right foot "pointing outward." **B:** Plain radiographs show what appears to be a healed fracture following tibial nailing. Comparison of the proximal and distal tibias bilaterally was consistent with malrotation of the right distal tibia.

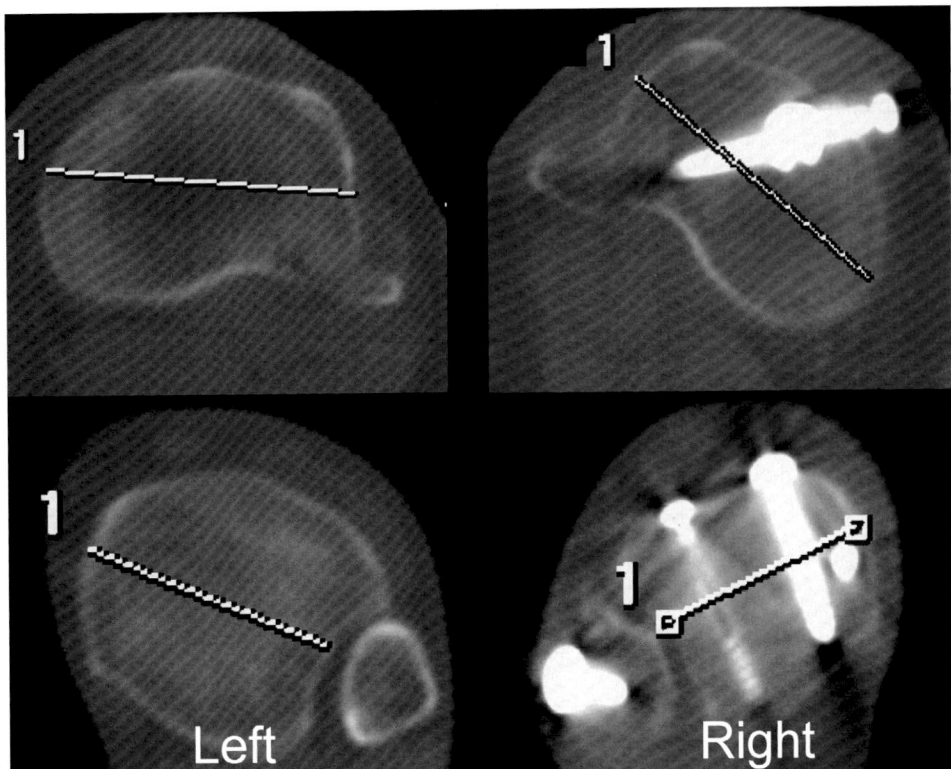

FIGURE 28-13 (*continued*) **C:** CT scans of both proximal and distal tibias show asymmetric external rotation of the right distal tibia which measures 42 degrees. The CT scan also confirmed solid bony union at the fracture site. **C**

measured as the horizontal distance from the proximal segment's anatomic axis to the distal segment's anatomic axis at the level of the proximal end of the distal segment (Fig. 28-14).

TREATMENT

The clinical and radiographic evaluation of the deformity provides the information needed to develop a treatment plan. Following evaluation, the deformity is characterized by its type (length, angulation, rotational, translational, or combined), the direction of the apex (anterior, lateral, posterolateral, etc.), its orientation plane, its magnitude, and the level of the CORA.

The status of the soft tissues may impact the surgical treatment of a bony deformity. Preoperative planning should include an evaluation of overlying soft tissue free flaps and skin grafts. In addition, scarring, tethering of neurovascular bundles, and infection may require modifications to the treatment plan in order to address these concomitant conditions in addition to correcting the malunion. Furthermore, if neurovascular structures lie on the concave side of an angular deformity, acute correction may lead to a traction injury and temporary or permanent complications. In such cases, gradual deformity correction may be preferable to allow for gradual accommodation of the nerves or vasculature to mitigate complications.

Osteotomies

An osteotomy is used to separate the deformed bone segments to allow realignment of the anatomic and mechanical axes. The ability of an osteotomy to restore alignment depends on

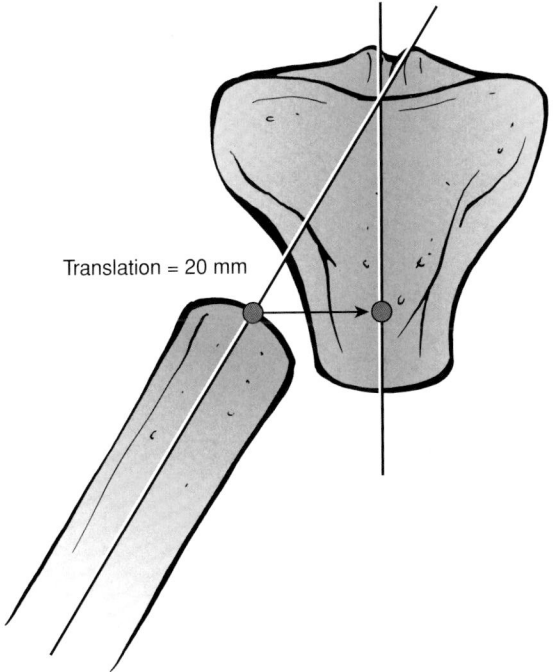

FIGURE 28-14 Method for measuring the magnitude of translational deformities. In this example, with both angulation and translation, the magnitude of the translational deformity is the horizontal distance from the proximal segment's anatomical axis to the distal segment's anatomical axis at the level of the proximal end of the distal segment.

the location of the CORA, the axis about which correction is performed (the correction axis), and the location of the osteotomy. While the CORA is defined by the type, direction, and magnitude of the deformity, the correction axis depends on the location and type of the osteotomy, the soft tissues, and the choice of fixation technique. The relation of these three factors to one another determines the final position of the bone segments. Reduction following osteotomy produces one of the three possible results: (1) realignment through angulation alone; (2) realignment through angulation and translation; and (3) realignment through angulation and translation with an iatrogenic residual translational abnormality.

When the CORA, correction axis, and osteotomy lie at the same location, the bone will realign through angulation alone, without translation (Fig. 28-15A). When the CORA and correction axis are at the same location but the osteotomy is made

proximal or distal to that location, the bone will realign through both angulation and translation (Fig. 28-15B). When the CORA is at a location different than the correction axis as well as different from the osteotomy, correction of angulation aligns the proximal and distal axes in parallel but excess translation occurs and results in an iatrogenic translational deformity (Fig. 28-15C).

Osteotomies can be classified by cut (straight or dome [actually not truly shaped like a dome, but cylindrical]) and type (opening, closing, neutral). A straight cut, such as a transverse or wedge osteotomy, is made such that the opposing bone ends have flat surfaces. A dome osteotomy is made such that the opposing bone ends have congruent convex and concave cylindrical surfaces. The type describes the rotation of the bone segments relative to one another at the osteotomy site.

Selection of the osteotomy type depends on the type, magnitude, and direction of deformity, the proximity of the deformity

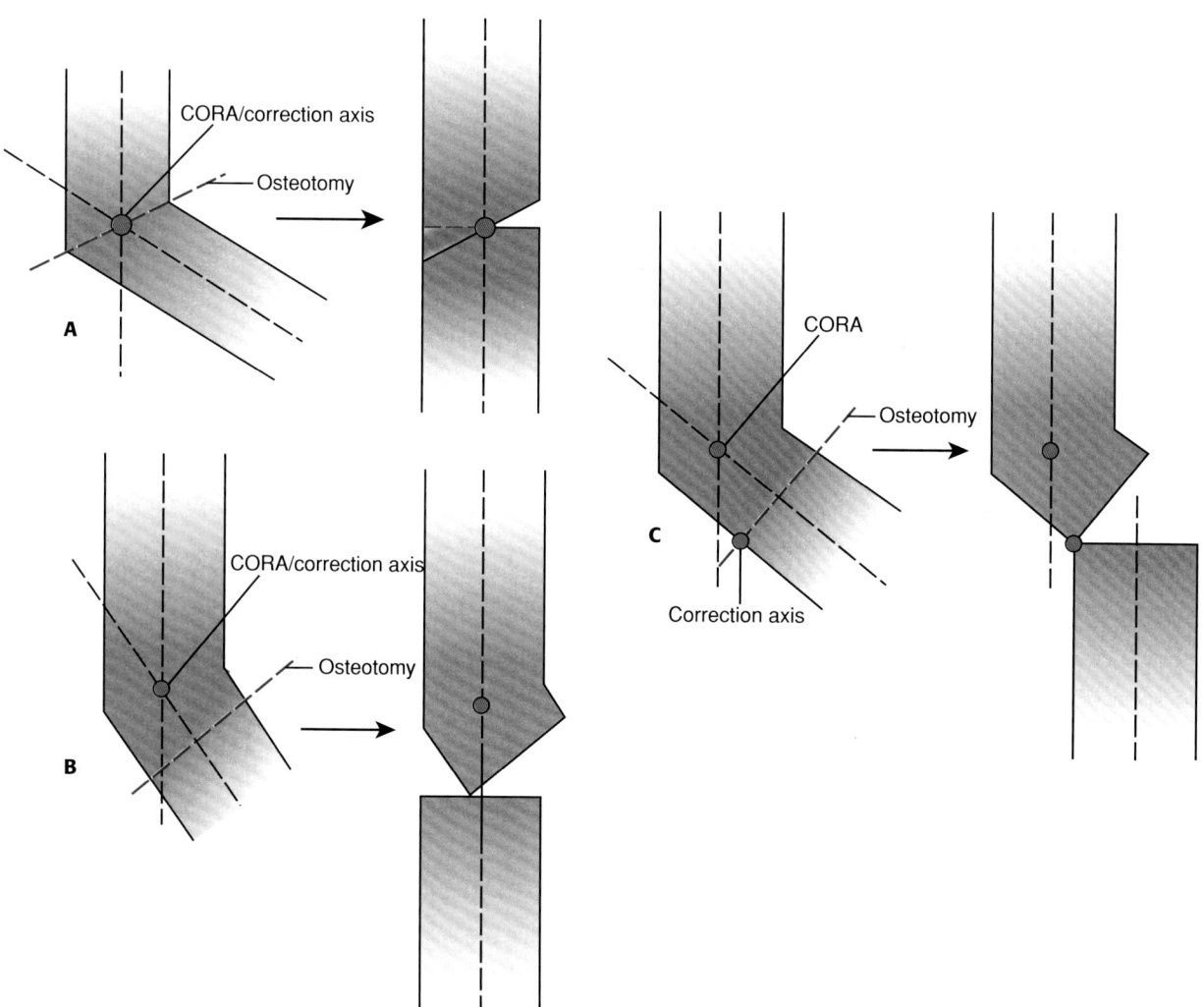

FIGURE 28-15 Possible results when using osteotomy for correction of deformity. **A:** The CORA, the correction axis, and the osteotomy all lie at the same location; the bone realigns through angulation alone, without translation. **B:** The CORA and the correction axis lie in the same location but the osteotomy is proximal or distal to that location; the bone realigns through both angulation and translation. **C:** The CORA lies at one location and the correction axis and the osteotomy lie in a different location; correction of angulation results in an iatrogenic translational deformity.

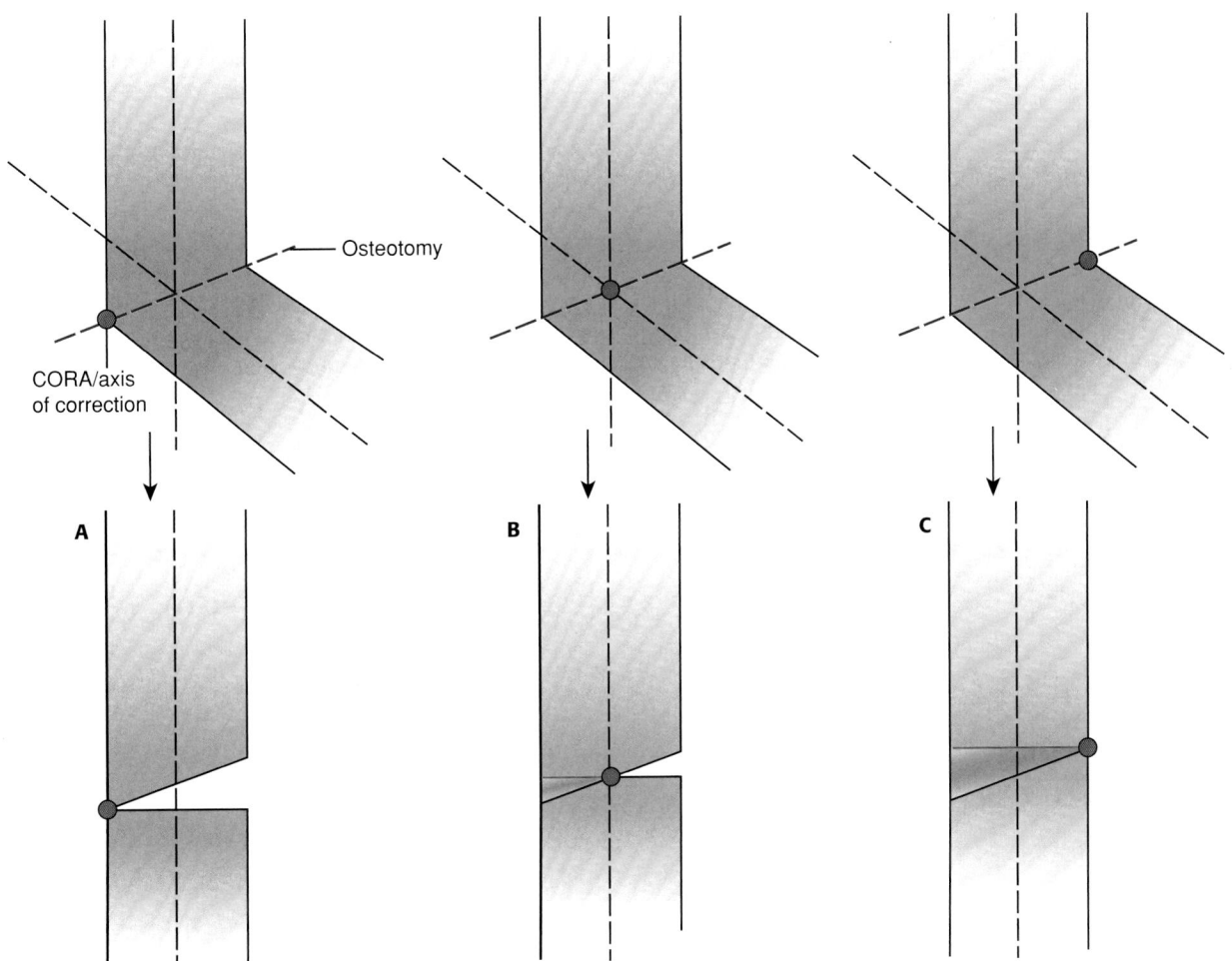

FIGURE 28-16 Wedge osteotomies; the osteotomy is made at the level of the CORA and the correction axis in all of these examples. **A:** Opening wedge osteotomy. The CORA and correction axis lie on the cortex on the convex side of the deformity. The cortex on the concave side of the deformity is distracted to restore alignment, opening an empty wedge that traverses the diameter of the bone. Opening wedge osteotomy increases final bone length. **B:** Neutral wedge osteotomy. The CORA and correction axis lie in the middle of the bone. The concave side cortex is distracted and the convex side cortex is compressed. A bone wedge is removed from the convex side. Neutral wedge osteotomy has no effect on final bone length. **C:** Closing wedge osteotomy. The CORA and correction axis lie on the concave cortex of the deformity. The cortex on the convex side of the deformity is compressed to restore alignment, requiring removal of a bone wedge across the entire bone diameter. A closing wedge osteotomy decreases final bone length.

to a joint, the location and its effect on the soft tissues, and the type of fixation selected. In certain cases, a small iatrogenic deformity may be acceptable if it is expected to have no effect on the patient's final functional outcome. This situation may be preferable to an osteotomy type that requires an unfamiliar fixation method or a fixation technique that the patient may tolerate poorly.

Wedge Osteotomy

The type of wedge osteotomy is determined by the location of the osteotomy relative to the locations of the CORA and the correction axis. When the CORA and correction axis are in the same location (to avoid translational deformity), they may lie on the cortex on the convex side of the deformity, on the cortex on the concave side of the deformity, or in the middle of the bone (Fig. 28-16).

When the CORA and correction axis lie on the convex cortex of the deformity, the correction will result in an opening wedge osteotomy (Fig. 28-16A). In an opening wedge osteotomy, the cortex on the concave side of the deformity is distracted to restore alignment, opening an empty, wedge-shaped space that traverses the diameter of the bone. An opening wedge osteotomy also increases bone length.

When the CORA and correction axis lie in the middle of the bone, the correction distracts the concave side cortex and compresses the convex side cortex. A bone wedge is removed from the convex, compression side to allow realignment. This neutral wedge osteotomy (Fig. 28-16B) has no effect on bone length.

When the CORA and correction axis lie on the concave cortex of the deformity, the correction will result in a closing wedge osteotomy (Fig. 28-16C). In a closing wedge osteotomy, the cortex on the convex side of the deformity is compressed to restore alignment; this requires removal of a bone wedge across the entire bone diameter. A closing wedge osteotomy decreases bone length (resulting in shortening).

These principles of osteotomy also hold true when the osteotomy is located proximal or distal to the mutual site of the CORA and correction axis, except that realignment in these cases occurs via angulation and translation. When the CORA and correction axis are not at the same point and the osteotomy is proximal or distal to the CORA, the correction maneuver results in excess translation and an iatrogenic translational deformity.

Dome Osteotomy

The type of dome osteotomy is also determined by the location of the CORA and the correction axis relative to the osteotomy. In contrast to a wedge osteotomy, however, the osteotomy site can never pass through the mutual CORA–correction axis (Fig. 28-17). Thus, translation will always occur with deformity correction using a dome osteotomy.

Ideally, the CORA and correction axis are mutually located such that the angulation and obligatory translation that occurs at

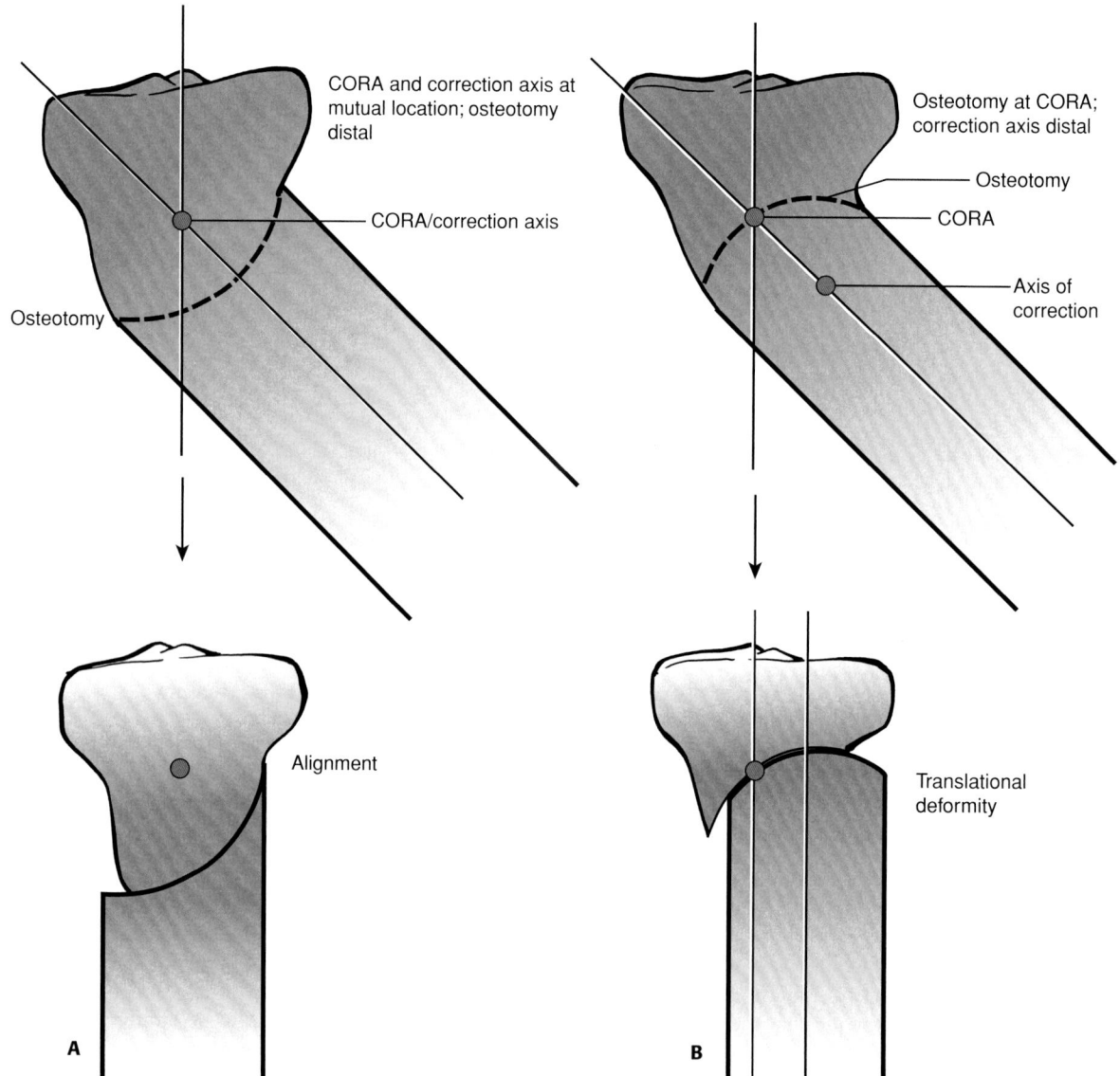

FIGURE 28-17 In a dome osteotomy, the osteotomy site cannot pass through both the CORA and the correction axis. Thus, translation will always occur when using a dome osteotomy. **A:** Ideally, the CORA and correction axis are mutually located with the osteotomy proximal or distal to that location such that the angulation and obligatory translation that occurs at the osteotomy site results in realignment of the bone axis. **B:** When the CORA and correction axis are not mutually located, a dome osteotomy through the CORA location results in a translational deformity.

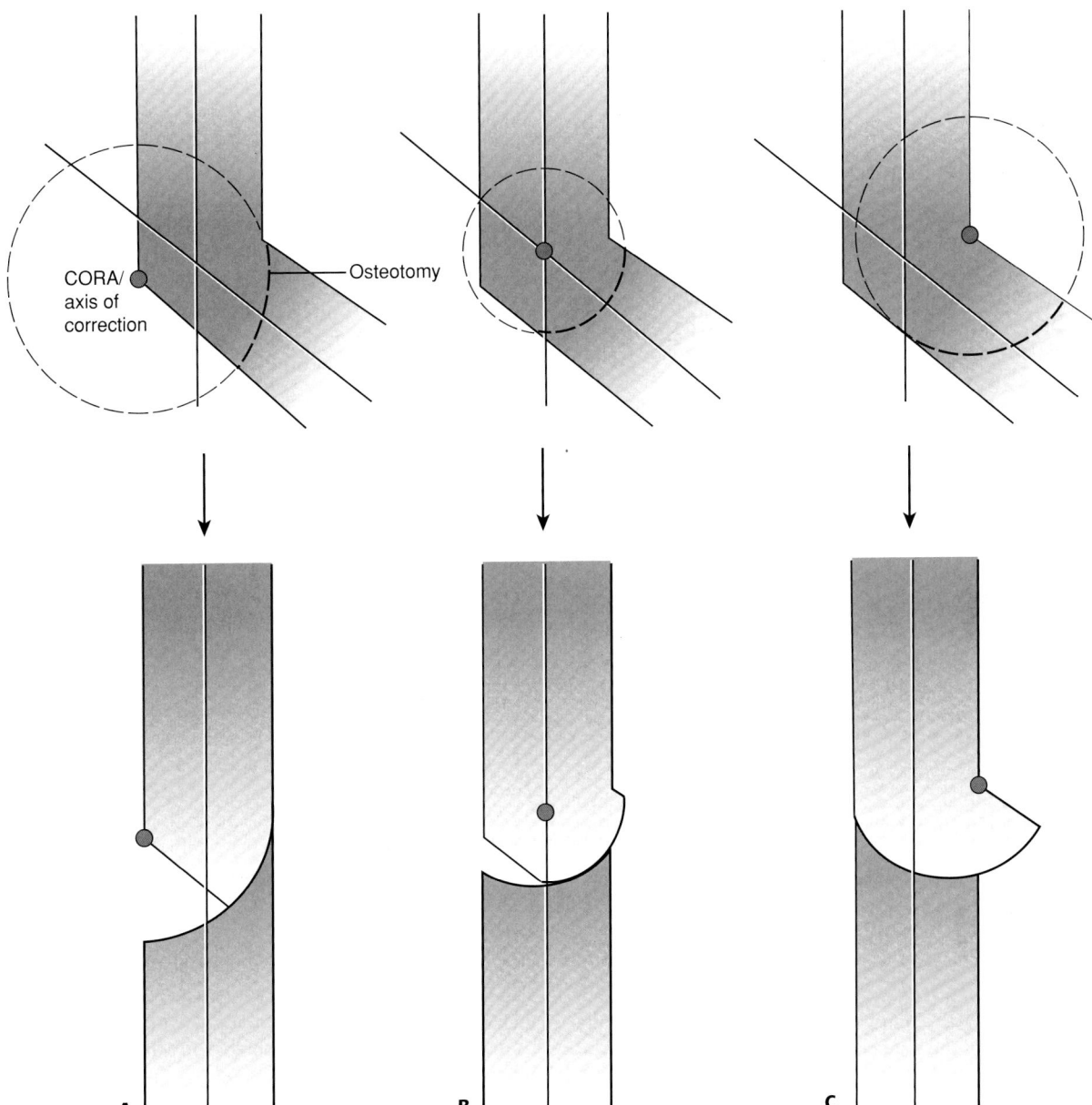

FIGURE 28-18 Dome osteotomies; the CORA and correction axis are mutually located with the osteotomy distal to that location in all of these examples. **A:** Opening dome osteotomy. The CORA and correction axis lie on the cortex on the convex side of the deformity. An opening dome osteotomy increases final bone length. **B:** Neutral dome osteotomy. The CORA and correction axis lie in the middle of the bone. A neutral dome osteotomy has no effect on final bone length. **C:** Closing dome osteotomy. The CORA and correction axis lie on the concave cortex of the deformity. A closing dome osteotomy decreases final bone length and can result in significant overhang of bone that may require resection.

the osteotomy site results in realignment. Attempts at realignment when the CORA and correction axis are not mutually located results in a translational deformity (Fig. 28-17B). Similar to wedge osteotomy, the CORA and correction axis may lie on the cortex on the convex side of the deformity, on the cortex on the concave side of the deformity, or in the middle of the bone.

The principles guiding wedge osteotomies hold true for dome osteotomies. When the CORA and correction axis lie on the convex cortex of the deformity, the correction will result

in an opening dome osteotomy (Fig. 28-18). The translation that occurs in an opening dome osteotomy increases final bone length. When the CORA and correction axis lie in the middle of the bone, the correction will result in a neutral dome osteotomy. A neutral dome osteotomy has no effect on bone length. When the CORA and correction axis lie on the concave cortex of the deformity, the correction will result in a closing dome osteotomy. The translation that occurs in a closing dome osteotomy decreases final bone length. Unlike wedge osteotomies, the movement of one bone segment on the other with a dome osteotomy is rarely impeded, so removal of bone is not typically required unless the final configuration results in significant overhang of the bone beyond the aligned bone column.

Treatment by Deformity Type

Length

Acute distraction or compression methods obtain immediate correction of limb length by acute lengthening with bone grafting or acute shortening, respectively. The extent of acute lengthening or shortening that is possible is limited by the soft tissues (soft tissue compliance, surgical and open wounds, and neurovascular structures).

Acute distraction treatment methods involve distracting the bone ends to the appropriate length, placing a bone graft in the resulting space between the bone segments, and stabilizing the construct to allow incorporation of the graft. Options for treating length deformities include the use of: (1) autogenous cancellous or cortical bone grafts; (2) vascularized autografts; (3) bulk or strut cortical allografts; (4) mesh cage-bone graft constructs; and (5) synostosis techniques. A variety of internal and external fixation treatment methods may be used to stabilize the construct during graft incorporation.[13]

The amount of shortening deformity that requires lengthening correction is uncertain.[38,65,102] In the upper extremity, up to 3 to 4 cm of shortening is generally well tolerated, and restoring length when shortening exceeds this value has been reported to improve function.[1,19,59,71,81,96,104,107] In the lower extremity, up to 2 cm of shortening may be treated with a shoe lift; tolerance for a 2- to 4-cm shoe lift is poor for most patients, and most patients with shortening of greater than 4 cm will benefit from restoration of bone length.[7,8,31,64,102,109]

Acute compression methods are used to correct overdistraction deformities by first resecting the appropriate length of bone, approximating the bone ends, and then stabilizing the approximated bone ends under compression. For the paired bones of the forearm and leg, the unaffected bone requires partial excision to allow shortening and compression of the affected bone. For example, partial excision of the intact fibula is necessary to allow shortening and compression of the tibia.

Gradual correction techniques for length deformities typically use tensioned-wire (Ilizarov) external fixation,[5,16,51,59,60,62,73,102,104,107] although gradual lengthening techniques using conventional monolateral external fixation or a special intramedullary nail that provides a continuous lengthening force have been described.[17,43,44,70,93,94] The most common form of gradual correction is gradual distraction to correct limb shortening. Gradual correction methods for length deformities can also be used to correct associated angular, translational, or rotational deformities simultaneously while restoring length.

Gradual distraction involves the creation of a corticotomy (usually metaphyseal) and distraction of the bone segments at a rate of 1 mm per day using a rhythm of 0.25 mm of distraction repeated four times per day. The bone formed at the distraction site is formed through the process of distraction osteogenesis, as discussed below in the Ilizarov Techniques section.

Angulation

Correction of angulation deformities involves making an osteotomy, obtaining realignment of the bone segments, and securing fixation during healing. The correction may be made acutely and then stabilized using a number of internal or external fixation methods.[28,39] Alternatively, the correction may be made gradually using external fixation to both restore alignment and stabilize the site during healing.[28,105]

Angulation deformities in the diaphysis are most amenable to correction using a wedge osteotomy at the same level as the correction axis and the CORA. For juxta-articular angulation deformities, however, the correction axis and the CORA may be located too close to the respective joint to permit a wedge osteotomy. Thus, juxta-articular angulation deformities may require a dome osteotomy with location of the osteotomy proximal or distal to the level of the correction axis and the CORA.

Rotation

Correction of a rotational deformity requires an osteotomy and rotational realignment followed by stabilization. Stabilization may be accomplished using internal or external fixation following acute correction, or external fixation may be used to gradually correct the deformity. The appropriate level for the osteotomy, however, can be difficult to determine. While the level of the deformity is obvious in the case of an angulated malunion, the level of deformity in rotational limb deformities is often difficult to determine. Consequently, other factors, including muscle and tendon line of pull, and the location of neurovascular structures and soft tissues, are usually considered to determine the level of deformity and level of osteotomy for correction of a rotational deformity.[32,56,57,78,80,101]

Translation

Translational deformities may be corrected in one of three ways. First, a single transverse osteotomy may be made to restore alignment through pure translation without angulation; the transverse osteotomy does not have to be made at the level of the deformity (Fig. 28-19). Second, a single oblique osteotomy may be made at the level of the deformity to restore alignment and gain length. Third, a translational deformity can be represented as two angulations with identical magnitudes but opposite directions. Therefore, two wedge osteotomies at the level of the respective CORAs and angular corrections of equal magnitudes in opposite directions may be used to correct a translational deformity. It should be noted that the osteotomy types used in this third method (opening, closing, or neutral) will affect final bone length. Internal or external fixation may be used to provide stabilization following acute correction of translational deformities, or gradual correction may be carried out using external fixation.

Combined Deformities

Combined deformities are characterized by the presence of two or more types of deformity in a single bone.[36,40] Treatment planning begins with identifying and characterizing each deformity independently from the other deformities. Once all deformities

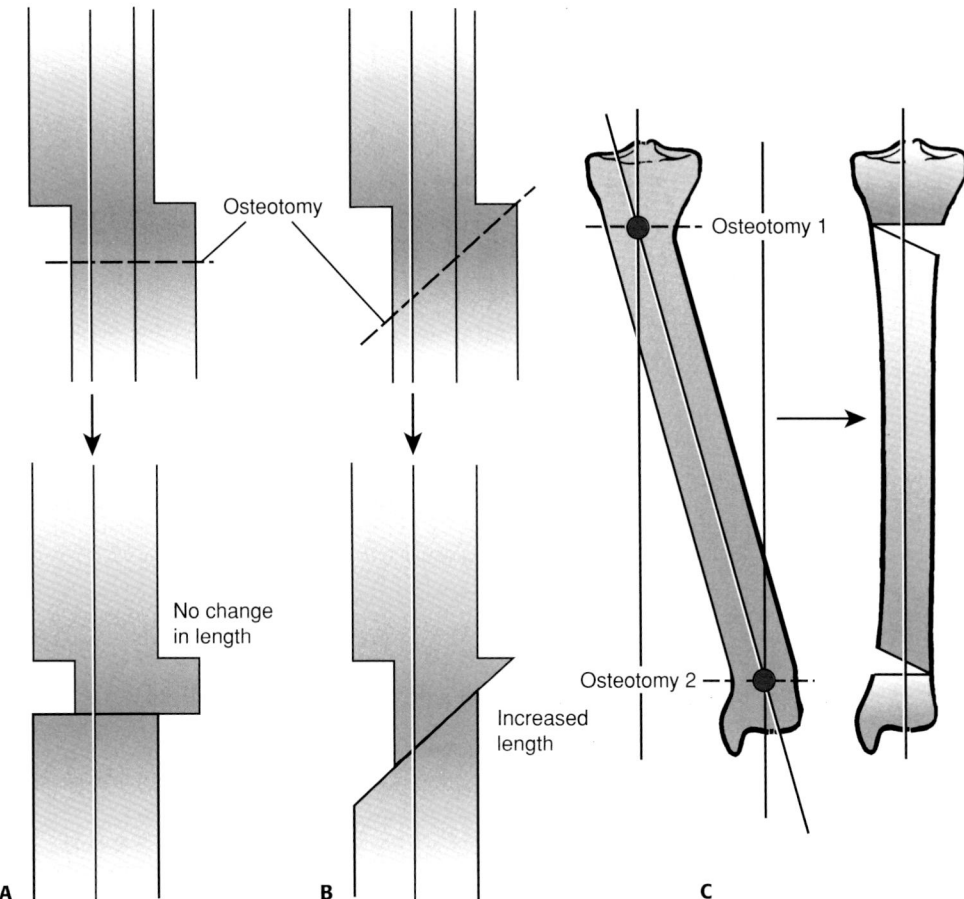

FIGURE 28-19 **A:** A single transverse osteotomy to restore alignment through pure translation without angulation. **B:** A single oblique osteotomy at the level of the deformity to restore alignment and gain length. **C:** A translational deformity represented as two angulations with identical magnitudes but opposite directions causing malalignment of the mechanical axis of the lower extremity. In this case, two wedge osteotomies of equal magnitudes in opposite directions at the levels of the respective CORAs may be used to correct a translational deformity and restore alignment of the mechanical axis of the lower extremity.

have been characterized, they are assessed as a group to determine which require correction to restore function. Correction of all of the deformities may be unnecessary. For example, small translational deformities or angulation deformities in the sagittal plane may not interfere with limb function and may remain untreated. Once those deformities requiring correction are identified, a treatment plan outlining the order and method of correction for each deformity can be developed.

In many instances, a single osteotomy can be used to correct two deformities. For example, a combined angulation–translational deformity can be corrected using a single osteotomy at the level of the apex of the angulation deformity. This method restores alignment and congruency of the medullary canals and cortices of the respective bone segments (Fig. 28-20). The deformities are then reduced one at a time—reducing translation and then angulation, for instance. Consequently, stabilization can be achieved using an intramedullary nail (Fig. 28-21) or other internal fixation and external fixation methods.

Combined angulation–translational deformities can also be treated as multiapical angulation deformities with an osteot-

omy through either or both CORAs in the frontal and sagittal planes. While this method restores alignment of the bone's mechanical axis, it can also result in incomplete bone-to-bone contact and incongruence of the medullary canals of the bone segments and cortices. As a result, stabilization cannot be achieved using an intramedullary nail and other internal fixation and external fixation methods are required to stabilize the bone segments.

A combined angulation–rotational deformity can be corrected by a single rotation of the distal segment around an oblique axis that represents the resolutions of both the component angulation axis and the rotation axis (Fig. 28-22).[66] The direction and magnitude of the combined angulation–rotational deformity are both characterized in this oblique axis. The angle of the oblique correction axis, which is perpendicular to the plane of the necessary osteotomy, can be approximated using trigonometry (axis angle = $\tan^{-1}$[rotation/angulation]; orientation of plane of osteotomy = 90 − axis angle).

This single osteotomy is made at a location such that it passes through the level of the CORA of the angulation deformity

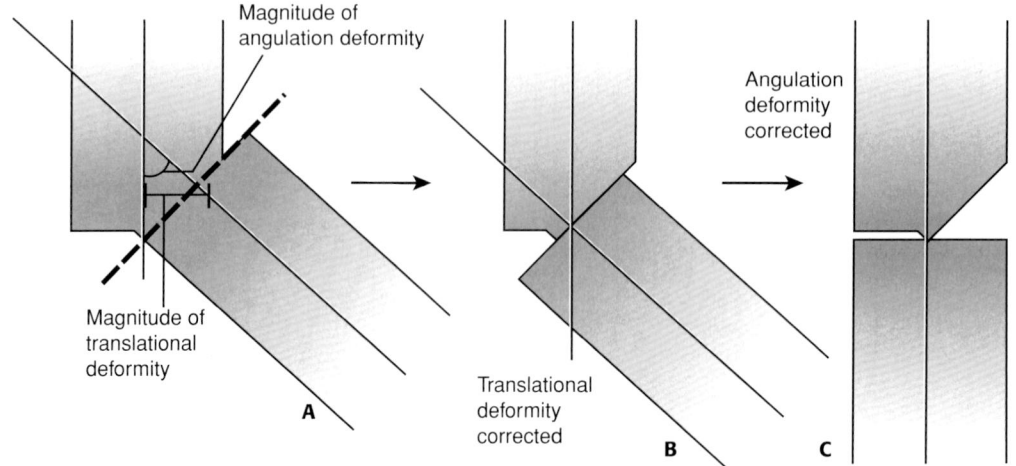

FIGURE 28-20 A single osteotomy to correct an angulation–translational deformity. **A:** A single osteotomy is made to allow correction of both deformities. **B:** Correction of the translational deformity, followed by **(C)** correction of the angulation deformity, resulting in realignment.

(i.e., the bisector of the axes of the proximal and distal segments). Rotation of the distal segment about this CORA in the plane of the osteotomy results in realignment; opening and closing wedge corrections can also be achieved by using the CORA located on the respective cortex. Rotation of the distal segment in the plane of the osteotomy but not about a CORA will lead to a secondary translational deformity. This secondary deformity can be corrected by reducing the translation after rotation is completed. Locating the level of the osteotomy distal to the level of the CORA and correcting the secondary translational deformity can be used to correct a combined deformity if locating the osteotomy at the level of the CORA is impractical, such as would occur if the osteotomy would violate a growth plate or place soft tissues or neurovascular structures at risk.

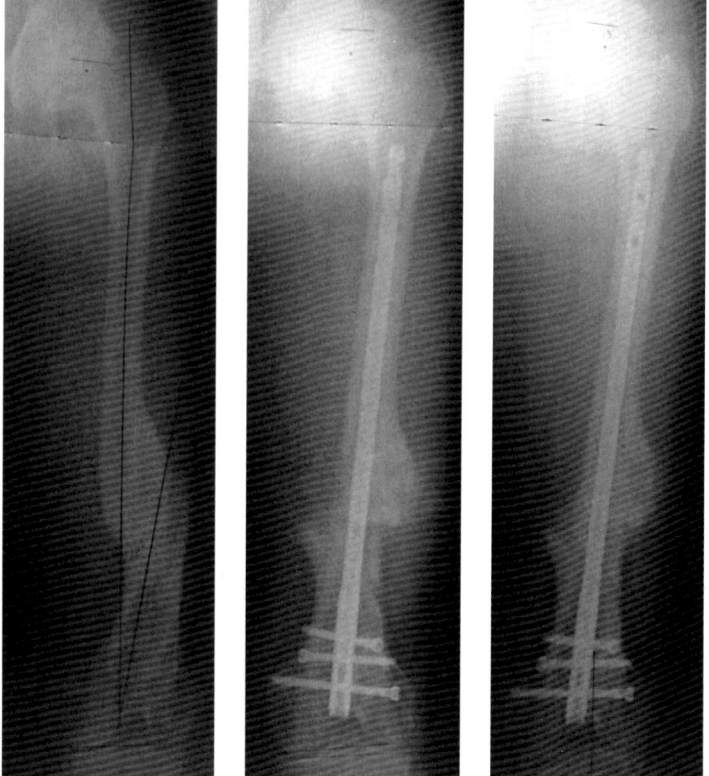

FIGURE 28-21 **A:** AP radiograph of a 50-year-old woman with a femur fracture sustained in a motor vehicle accident 28 years ago. The left femur has a 12-degree varus deformity with 23 mm of lateral translation. **B:** AP radiograph showing acute correction using a single osteotomy and statically locked intramedullary nail fixation. **C:** AP radiograph showing final deformity correction and solid union 8 months after surgery. Nail dynamization was performed 5 months after the corrective osteotomy.

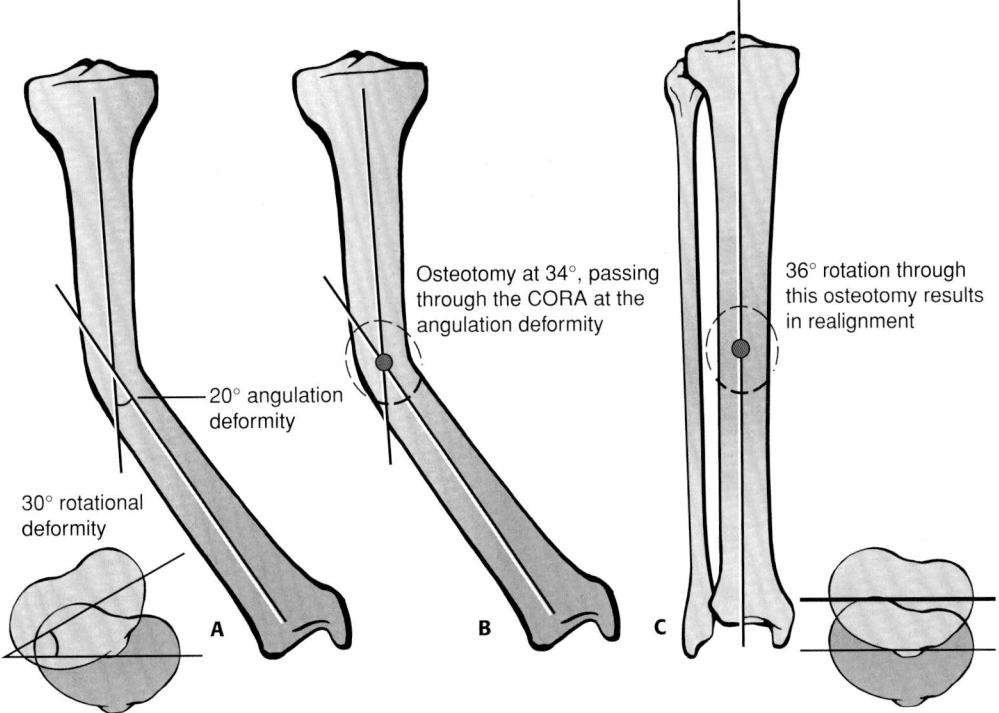

20° angulation
deformity

30° rotational
deformity

Osteotomy at 34°, passing
through the CORA at the
angulation deformity

36° rotation through
this osteotomy results
in realignment

A   **B**   **C**

FIGURE 28-22 A: Combined angulation-rotational deformity with a 20-degree angulation deformity and a 30-degree rotational deformity. Calculations of the correction axis show an inclination of 56 degrees, which corresponds to an osteotomy inclination of 34 degrees. **B:** The 34-degree osteotomy is made such that it passes through the CORA of the angulation deformity. **C:** Rotation of 36 degrees about the correction axis in the plane of the osteotomy results in realignment by simultaneous correction of both deformities.

Treatment by Deformity Location

The bone involved and the specific bone region or regions (e.g., epiphysis, metaphysis, diaphysis) define the anatomic location. While a bone-by-bone discussion is beyond the scope of this chapter, we will address the influence of the anatomic regions of long bones on the treatment of malunions in general terms.

Shaft

Diaphyseal deformities involve primarily cortical bone in the central section of long bones. Characterizing deformities is straightforward, as angulation and translational deformities are usually obvious on plain radiographs. In addition, the use of wedge osteotomies through the CORA for deformity correction is generally achievable, thus allowing reduction of the deformity without concerns about inducing secondary translational deformities. By virtue of their relatively homogeneous morphology, diaphyseal deformities are amenable to a wide array of fixation methods following correction. Intramedullary nail fixation is preferable when practical (Fig. 28-23).

Periarticular

Periarticular deformities located in the metaphysis and epiphysis are more difficult to identify, characterize, and treat. In addition to the juxta-articular deformities of length, angulation, rotation, and translation and the presence of joint malorientation,

there may also be malreduction of articular surfaces and compensatory joint deformities, such as soft tissue contractures and fixed joint subluxation or dislocation. Identification, characterization, and prioritization of each component are critical to forming a successful treatment plan.

Acute correction of periarticular deformities is most often accomplished using plate and screw fixation or external fixation. Gradual correction may also be accomplished using external fixation particularly for small periarticular bone segments (Fig. 28-24).

Treatment by Method
Plate and Screw Fixation

The advantages of plate and screw fixation include rigidity of fixation; versatility for various anatomic locations and situations (e.g., periarticular deformities); correction of deformities under direct visualization; and safety following failed or temporary external fixation. Disadvantages of the method include extensive soft tissue dissection; limitation of early weight-bearing and function; and inability to correct significant shortening deformity. A variety of plate types and techniques is available, and these are presented in the chapters covering specific fracture types. In cases of deformity correction with poor bone-to-bone contact following reduction; however, other methods of skeletal stabilization should be considered.

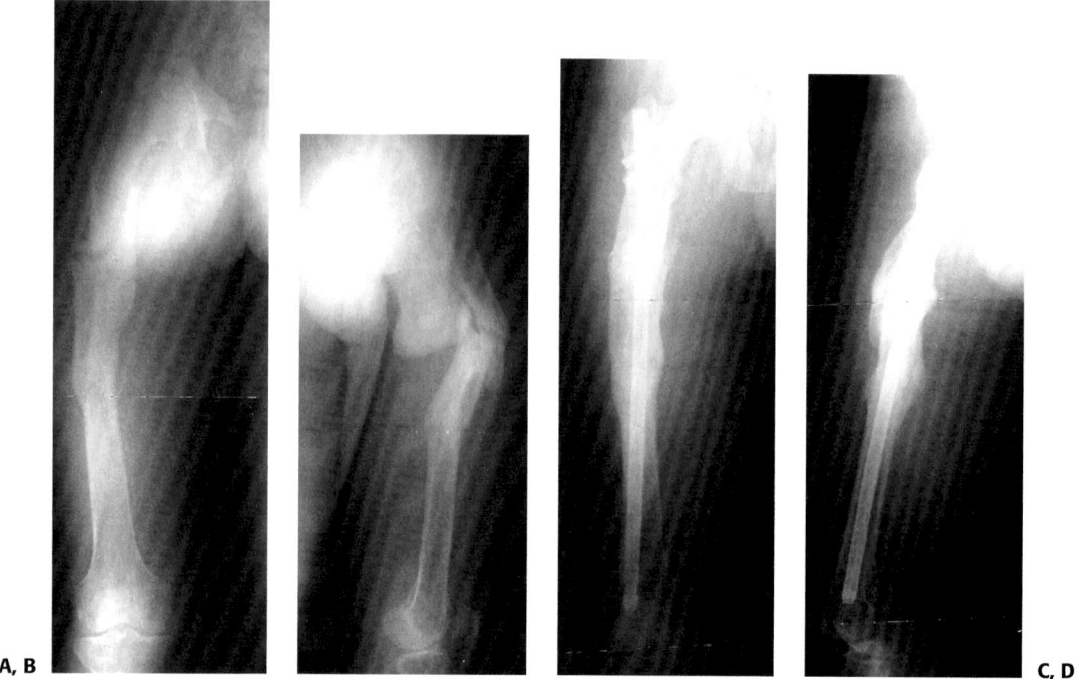

A, B

C, D

FIGURE 28-23 **A, B:** AP and lateral radiographs on presentation of a 37-year-old man initially definitively treated in traction in Africa for a femoral shaft fracture. **C, D:** AP and lateral radiographs following deformity correction with closed antegrade femoral nailing.

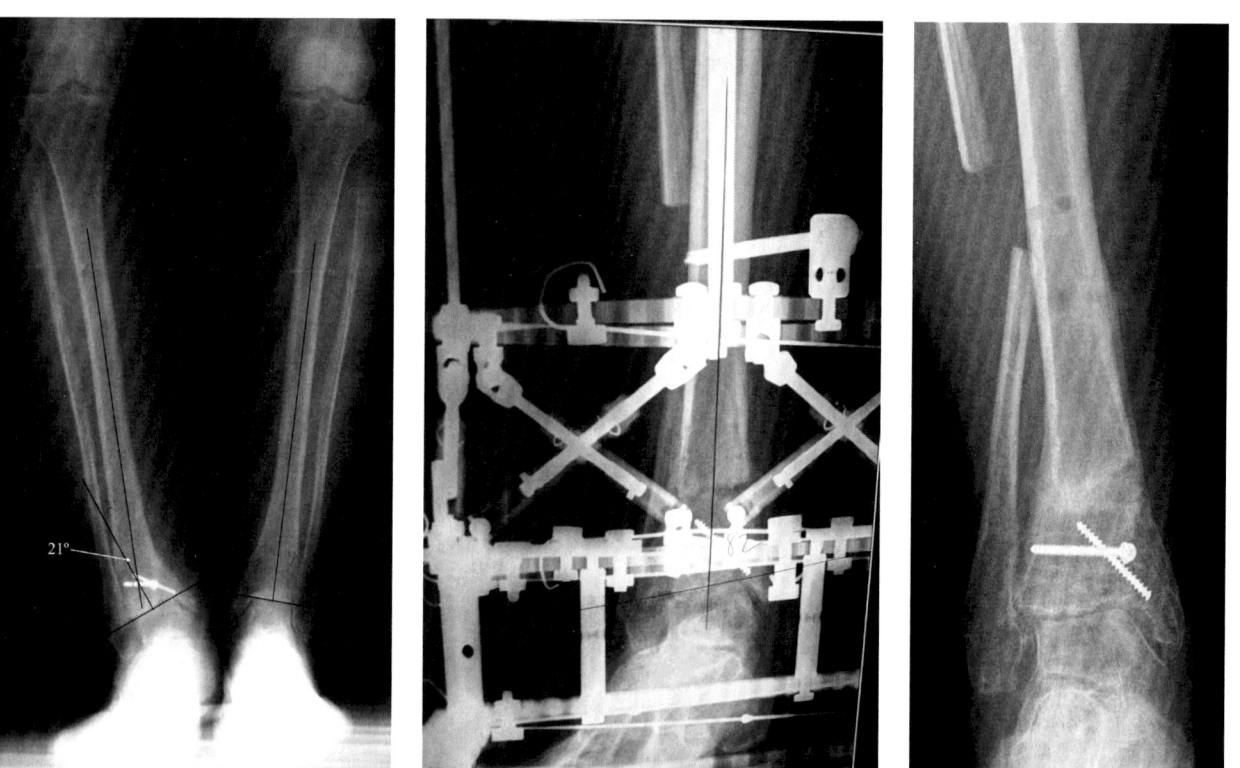

A, B

C

FIGURE 28-24 **A:** Presenting AP radiograph of a 45-year-old woman with a malunited distal tibial fracture. This pure frontal plane deformity measured 21 degrees of varus with a CORA located 21 mm proximal to the distal tibial joint orientation line. **B:** AP radiograph following transverse osteotomy and during gradual deformity correction (differential lengthening) using a Taylor Spatial Frame. **C:** Final AP radiograph following deformity correction and bony consolidation.

Locking plates have screws with threads that lock into threaded holes on the corresponding plate. This locking effect creates a fixed-angle device, or "single-beam" construct, because no motion occurs between the screws and the plate.[15,24,42] In contrast to traditional plate-and-screw constructs, the locked screws resist bending moments and the construct distributes axial load across all of the screw-bone interfaces.[24,42] As compared to compression plating where healing is by direct osteonal bridging, locked plating performed without compression results in healing via callus formation.[24,48,79,95,110] Due to the inherent axial and rotational stability with locked devices, obtaining contact between the plate and the bone is unnecessary; the construct can be thought of as functioning similarly to an external fixator but being located within the body. Consequently, periosteal damage and microvascular compromise are minimal. Locking plates are considerably more expensive than traditional plates and should be used primarily in deformity cases that are not amenable to traditional plate-and-screw fixation.[15]

Intramedullary Nail

Intramedullary nail fixation is particularly useful in the lower extremity because of the strength and load-sharing characteristics of intramedullary nails. This method of fixation is ideal for cases where diaphyseal deformities are being corrected (Fig. 28-25). The method may also be useful for deformities at the metaphyseal–diaphyseal junction. Intramedullary implants are excellent for osteopenic bone where screw purchase may be poor.

Ilizarov Techniques

Ilizarov techniques[3–6,9,10,12,21,23,26,33,37,39,46,51–55,61,72,73,81,84,85,104,105] have many advantages, including that they: (1) are primarily percutaneous, minimally invasive, and typically require only minimal soft tissue dissection; (2) can promote the generation of osseous tissue; (3) are versatile; (4) can be used in the presence of acute or chronic infection; (5) allow for stabilization of small intra-articular or periarticular bone fragments; (6) allow simultaneous deformity correction and enhancement of bone healing[3,5,6,11,13,37,50,55];

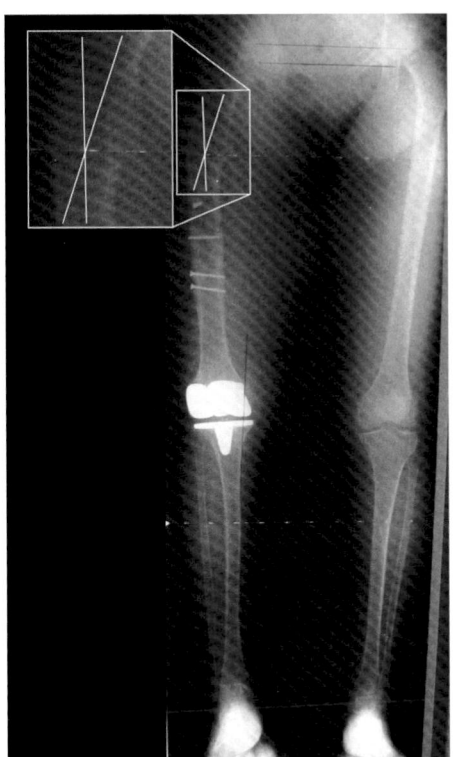
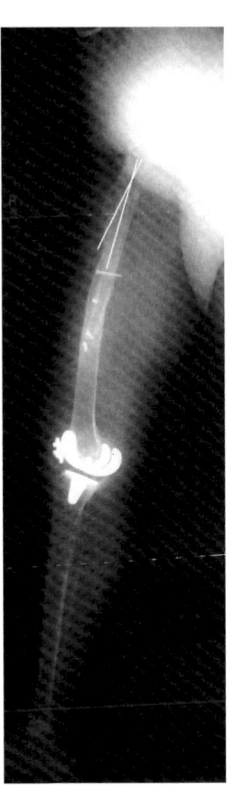
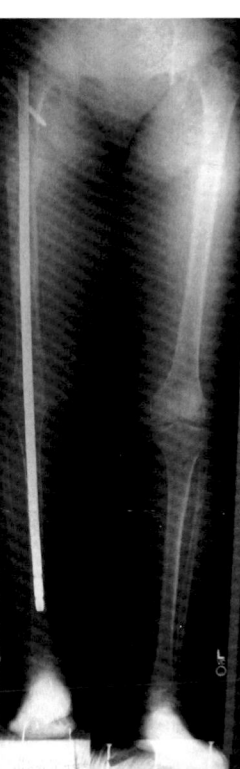
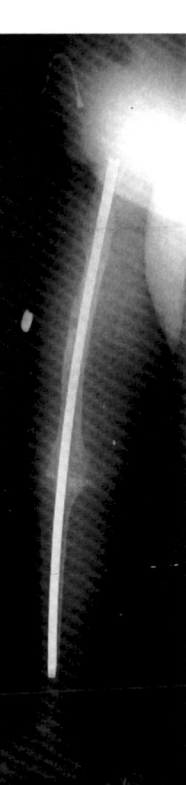

A, B   **C, D**

FIGURE 28-25 A, B: AP and lateral 51-inch alignment radiographs of a 52-year-old woman with a painful total knee arthroplasty. This patient had severe arthrofibrosis, severe pain, and had failed revision total knee arthroplasty. She was referred in for a knee fusion but was noted to have an oblique plane angular malunion of her proximal femur from a prior fracture, as indicated by the white lines superimposed on the femur. It was felt that without correction of this femoral malunion, passage of the knee fusion nail through the angled femoral diaphysis would have been difficult and the final clinical and functional results would likely have been suboptimal due to malalignment of the mechanical axis of the lower extremity. **C, D:** Follow-up radiographs 5 months after operative treatment with resection of her total knee arthroplasty, percutaneous corticotomy of her proximal femur to correct her deformity, and percutaneous antegrade femoral nailing to stabilize the corticotomy site and stabilize her knee fusion site.

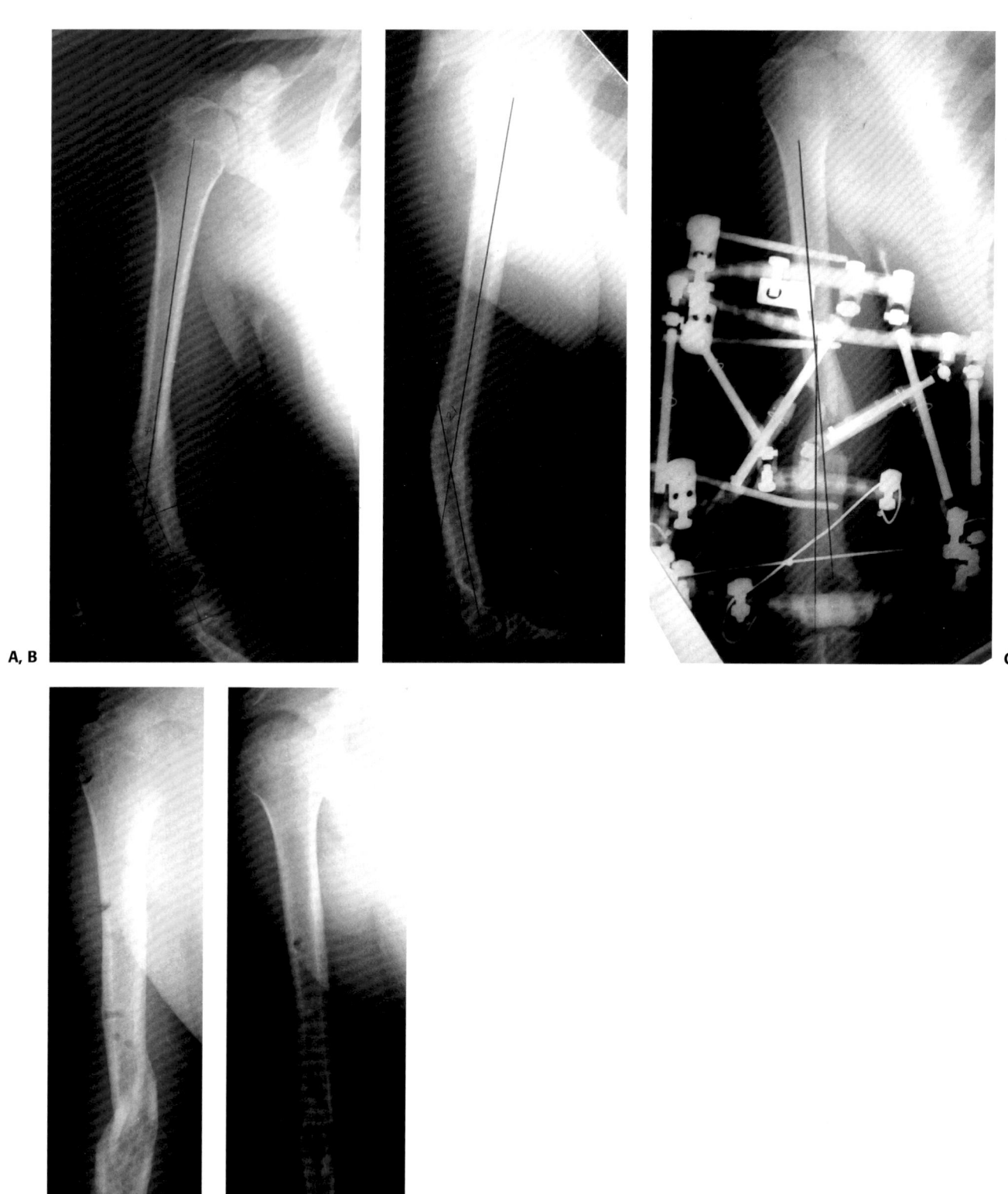

A, B

C

D, E

FIGURE 28-26 **(A)** AP and **(B)** lateral radiographs of a 25-year-old man 2 years after fracture of humerus while arm wrestling. This oblique plane deformity has 30 degrees AP varus, 21 degrees lateral posterior apex, and 5 mm of axial shortening, using the contralateral humerus as a reference. **C:** Ilizarov gradual deformity correction in progress. **(D)** AP and **(E)** lateral radiograph showing final deformity correction and solid bony union of the osteotomy site.

(7) allow immediate weight bearing and early joint function; (8) allow augmentation or modification of the treatment as needed through frame adjustment; and (9) resist shear and rotational forces while the tensioned wires allow the "trampoline effect" (axial loading–unloading) during weight-bearing activities.

The Ilizarov external fixator can be used to reduce and stabilize virtually any type of deformity, including complex combined deformities (Fig. 28-26), and restore limb length in cases of limb shortening. A variety of treatment modes can be employed using the Ilizarov external fixator, including distraction lengthening, and multiple sites in a single bone can be treated simultaneously. Monofocal lengthening involves a single site undergoing distraction. Bifocal lengthening denotes that two lengthening sites exist (Fig. 28-27).

Distraction Lengthening

The bone formed at the corticotomy site in distraction lengthening Ilizarov treatment occurs by distraction osteogenesis (Fig. 28-28).[3,4,20,51,67] Distraction produces a tension-stress effect that causes neovascularity and cellular proliferation in many tissues, including bone regeneration primarily through intramembranous bone formation. Corticotomy and distraction osteogenesis result in profound biologic stimulation. For example, Aronson[6] reported a nearly 10-fold increase in blood flow following corticotomy and lengthening at the proximal tibia distraction site relative to the control limb in dogs as well as increased blood flow in the distal tibia.

A variety of mechanical and biologic factors affect distraction osteogenesis. First, the corticotomy or osteotomy must be performed using a low-energy technique to minimize necrosis. Second, distraction of the metaphyseal or metaphyseal–

diaphyseal regions has superior potential for regenerate bone formation relative to diaphyseal sites. Third, the external fixator construct must be very stable. Fourth, a latency period of 7 to 14 days following the corticotomy and before beginning distraction is recommended. Fifth, since the formation of the bony regenerate is slower in some patients, the treating physician should monitor the progression of the regenerate on plain radiographs and adjust the rate and rhythm of distraction accordingly. Sixth, a consolidation phase in which external fixation continues in a static mode following restoration of length that generally lasts two to three times as long as the distraction phase is required to allow maturation and hypertrophy of the regenerate.

Complex Combined Deformities

All bone deformities can be characterized by describing the position of one bone segment relative to another in terms of angular rotations in each of three planes and linear displacements along each of three axes. Complex deformities can be characterized using magnitudes for each of these six parameters. Directions of the rotations or displacements are defined as positive and negative relative to the anatomic position. Positive rotations are defined by the right-hand rule: With the thumb pointed in the positive direction along the respective axis (defined identically to the displacement descriptions), the curled fingers indicate the direction of positive rotation (Fig. 28-29). For example, angulation in the frontal plane is rotation about an anterior–posterior axis. With anterior defined as the positive direction for this axis, counterclockwise rotation (to an examiner who is face to face with the patient) is positive and clockwise rotation is negative. Anterior, right, and superior displacements are defined as positive values.

Complex combined deformities often require gradual correction to allow adaptation of not only the bone but also the

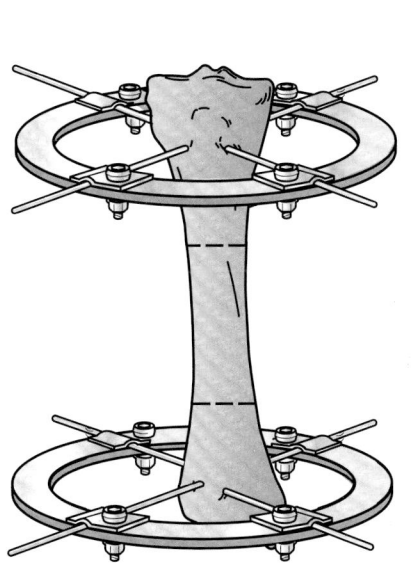
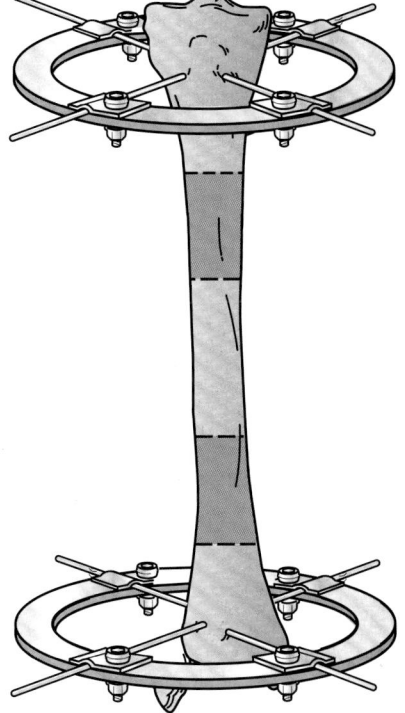

FIGURE 28-27 Bifocal lengthening. **A:** Tibia with length deformity showing two corticotomy sites. **B:** Tibia following distraction osteogenesis at both corticotomy sites showing restoration of length. **A**   **B**

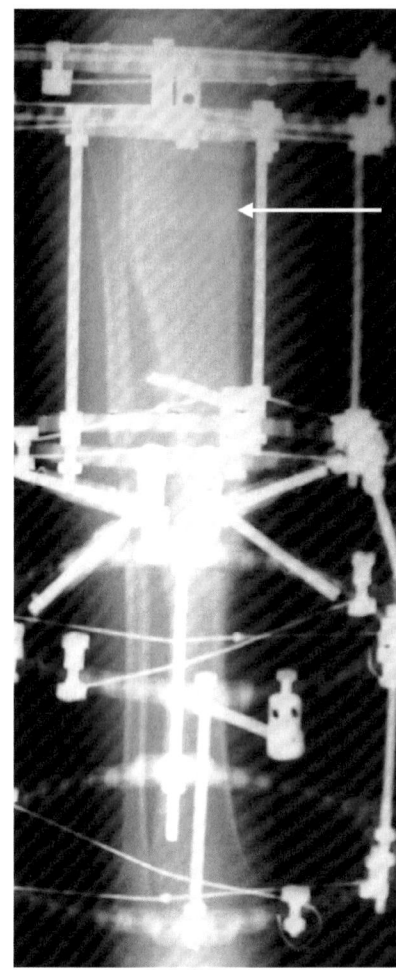
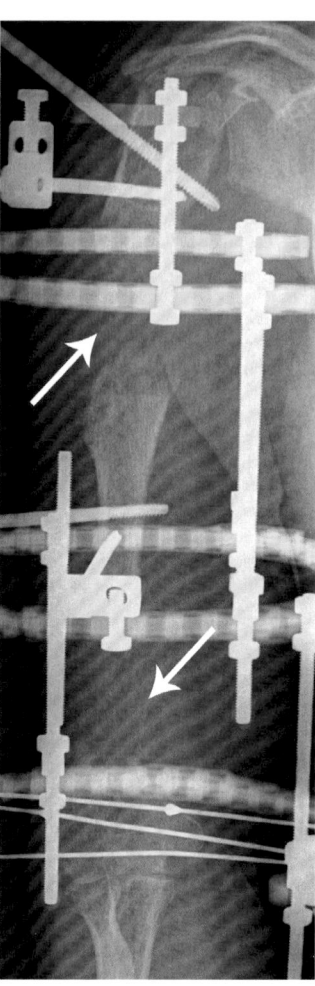

A

B

FIGURE 28-28 Regenerate bone (*arrows*) at the corticotomy site is formed via distraction osteogenesis. **A:** Monofocal lengthening of the tibia. **B:** Bifocal lengthening of the humerus.

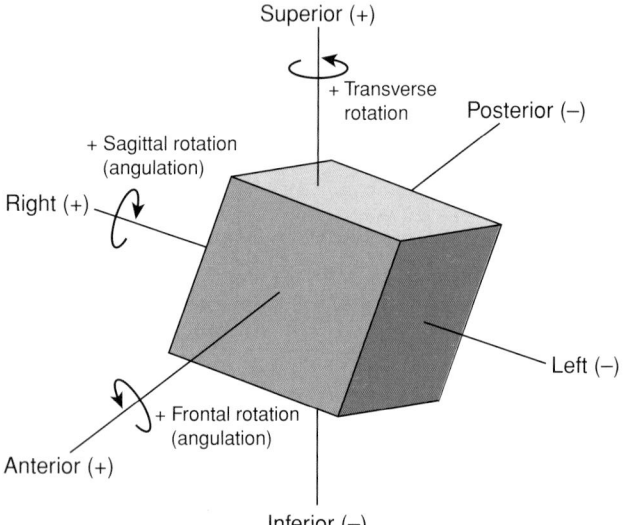

FIGURE 28-29 Definitions used to characterize complex deformities using three angular rotations and three linear displacements.

surrounding soft tissues and neurovascular structures. The modern Ilizarov hardware system uses different components (hinges, threaded rods, rotation–translation boxes) to achieve correction of multiple deformity types in a single bone. Alternatively, the Taylor Spatial Frame (Fig. 28-30), which uses six telescopic struts, can be used to correct complex combined deformities.[2,25–27,29,58,62,63,68,69,83–87,97,98,103,106,108,111,112] A computer program is used in treatment planning to determine strut lengths to connect the rings for the original frame construction around the deformity. The rings of the external fixator frame are attached perpendicular to the respective bone segments and the struts are gradually adjusted to attain neutral frame height (i.e., rings in parallel). Any residual deformity is then corrected by further adjusting the struts.

Correction can be simultaneous, in which all deformities are corrected at the same time, or sequential, in which some deformities (e.g., angulation–rotation) are corrected before others (e.g., translations). The rate at which correction occurs must be determined on a patient-by-patient basis and depends on the type and magnitude of deformity, the potential effects on the soft tissues, the health and healing potential of the patient, and the balance between premature consolidation and inadequate regenerate formation.

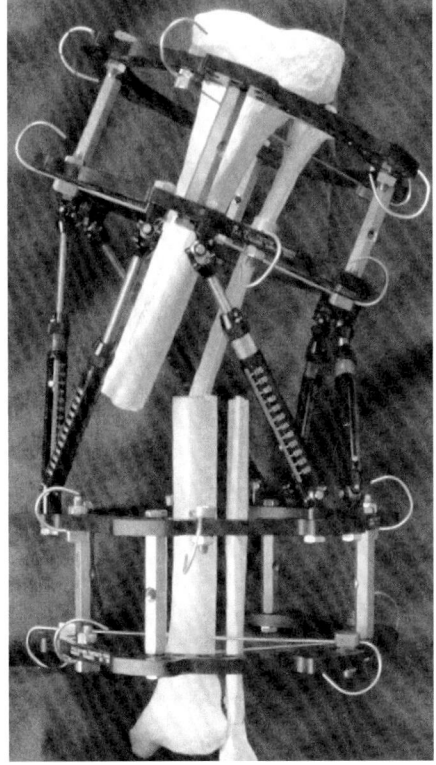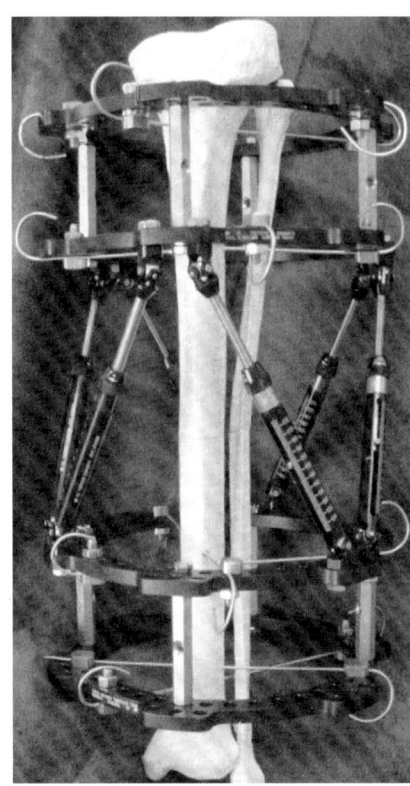

FIGURE 28-30 A: Taylor Spatial Frame with rings placed obliquely to one another and in parallel with the position of the tibial angular–translation deformity. **B:** Taylor Spatial Frame following correction of the deformity by adjusting the six struts to attain neutral frame height (i.e., rings in parallel).

A

B

REFERENCES

1. Abe M, Shirai H, Okamoto M, et al. Lengthening of the forearm by callus distraction. *J Hand Surg Br.* 1996;21:151–163.
2. Al-Sayyad MJ. Taylor Spatial Frame in the treatment of pediatric and adolescent tibial shaft fractures. *J Pediatr Orthop.* 2006;26:164–170.
3. Aronson J, Good B, Stewart C, et al. Preliminary studies of mineralization during distraction osteogenesis. *Clin Orthop Relat Res.* 1990;250:43–49.
4. Aronson J, Harrison B, Boyd CM, et al. Mechanical induction of osteogenesis: Preliminary studies. *Ann Clin Lab Sci.* 1988;18:195–203.
5. Aronson J. Limb-lengthening, skeletal reconstruction, and bone transport with the Ilizarov method. *J Bone Joint Surg Am.* 1997;79:1243–1258.
6. Aronson J. Temporal and spatial increases in blood flow during distraction osteogenesis. *Clin Orthop Relat Res.* 1994;301:124–131.
7. Bhave A, Paley D, Herzenberg JE. Improvement in gait parameters after lengthening for the treatment of limb-length discrepancy. *J Bone Joint Surg Am.* 1999;81:529–534.
8. Brady RJ, Dean JB, Skinner TM, et al. Limb length inequality: Clinical implications for assessment and intervention. *J Orthop Sports Phys Ther.* 2003;33:221–234.
9. Brinker MR, Gugenheim JJ, O'Connor DP, et al. Ilizarov correction of malrotated femoral shaft fracture initially treated with an intramedullary nail: A case report. *Am J Orthop.* 2004;33:489–493.
10. Brinker MR, Gugenheim JJ. The treatment of complex traumatic problems of the forearm using Ilizarov external fixation. *Atlas Hand Clin.* 2000;5:103–116.
11. Brinker MR, O'Connor DP. Basic sciences. In: Miller MD, ed. *Review of Orthopaedics.* Philadelphia, PA: W.B. Saunders; 2004:1–153.
12. Brinker MR, O'Connor DP. Ilizarov compression over a nail for aseptic femoral nonunions that have failed exchange nailing: A report of five cases. *J Orthop Trauma.* 2003; 17:668–676.
13. Brinker MR. Nonunions: Evaluation and treatment. In: Browner BD, Levine AM, Jupiter JB, Trafton PG, eds. *Skeletal Trauma: Basic Science, Management, and Reconstruction.* Philadelphia, PA: W.B. Saunders; 2003:507–604.
14. Brinker MR. Principles of fractures. In: Brinker MR, ed. *Review of Orthopaedic Trauma.* Philadelphia, PA: W.B. Saunders; 2001.
15. Cantu RV, Koval KJ. The use of locking plates in fracture care. *J Am Acad Orthop Surg.* 2006;14:183–190.
16. Cattaneo R, Catagni M, Johnson EE. The treatment of infected nonunions and segmental defects of the tibia by the methods of Ilizarov. *Clin Orthop Relat Res.* 1992;280: 143–152.
17. Cole JD, Justin D, Kasparis T, et al. The intramedullary skeletal kinetic distractor (ISKD): First clinical results of a new intramedullary nail for lengthening of the femur and tibia. *Injury.* 2001;32(suppl 4):SD129–SD139.
18. Dahl MT. Preoperative planning in deformity correction and limb lengthening surgery. *Instr Course Lect.* 2000;49:503–509.
19. Damsin JP, Ghanem I. Upper limb lengthening. *Hand Clin.* 2000;16:685–701.
20. Delloye C, Delefortrie G, Coutelier L, et al. Bone regenerate formation in cortical bone during distraction lengthening: An experimental study. *Clin Orthop Relat Res.* 1990;250:34–42.
21. DiPasquale D, Ochsner MG, Kelly AM, et al. The Ilizarov method for complex fracture nonunions. *J Trauma.* 1994;37:629–634.
22. Dismukes DI, Fox DB, Tomlinson JL, et al. Use of radiographic measures and three-dimensional computed tomographic imaging in surgical correction of an antebrachial deformity in a dog. *J Am Vet Med Assoc.* 2008;232:68–73.
23. Ebraheim NA, Skie MC, Jackson WT. The treatment of tibial nonunion with angular deformity using an Ilizarov device. *J Trauma.* 1995;38:111–117.
24. Egol KA, Kubiak EN, Fulkerson E, et al. Biomechanics of locked plates and screws. *J Orthop Trauma.* 2004;18:488–493.
25. Eidelman M, Bialik V, Katzman A. Correction of deformities in children using the Taylor spatial frame. *J Pediatr Orthop B.* 2006;15:387–395.
26. Fadel M, Hosny G. The Taylor spatial frame for deformity correction in the lower limbs. *Int Orthop.* 2005;29:125–129.
27. Feldman DS, Madan SS, Koval KJ, et al. Correction of tibia vara with six-axis deformity analysis and the Taylor Spatial Frame. *J Pediatr Orthop.* 2003;23:387–391.
28. Feldman DS, Madan SS, Ruchelsman DE, et al. Accuracy of correction of tibia vara: Acute versus gradual correction. *J Pediatr Orthop.* 2006;26:794–798.
29. Feldman DS, Shin SS, Madan S, et al. Correction of tibial malunion and nonunion with six-axis analysis deformity correction using the Taylor Spatial Frame. *J Orthop Trauma.* 2003;17:549–554.
30. Fox DB, Tomlinson JL, Cook JL, et al. Principles of uniapical and biapical radial deformity correction using dome osteotomies and the center of rotation of angulation methodology in dogs. *Vet Surg.* 2006;35:67–77.
31. Friend L, Widmann RF. Advances in management of limb length discrepancy and lower limb deformity. *Curr Opin Pediatr.* 2008;20:46–51.
32. Fujimoto M, Kato H, Minami A. Rotational osteotomy at the diaphysis of the radius in the treatment of congenital radioulnar synostosis. *J Pediatr Orthop.* 2005;25:676–679.
33. Gardner TN, Evans M, Simpson H, et al. Force-displacement behaviour of biological tissue during distraction osteogenesis. *Med Eng Phys.* 1998;20:708–715.
34. Gladbach B, Heijens E, Pfeil J, et al. Calculation and correction of secondary translation deformities and secondary length deformities. *Orthopedics.* 2004;27:760–766.
35. Goker B, Block JA. Improved precision in quantifying knee alignment angle. *Clin Orthop Relat Res.* 2007;458:145–149.
36. Green SA, Gibbs P. The relationship of angulation to translation in fracture deformities. *J Bone Joint Surg Am.* 1994;76:390–397.
37. Green SA. The Ilizarov method. In: Browner BD, Levine AM, Jupiter JB, eds. *Skeletal Trauma: Fractures, Dislocations, Ligamentous Injuries.* Philadelphia, PA: W.B. Saunders; 1998:661–701.
38. Gross RH. Leg length discrepancy: How much is too much? *Orthopedics.* 1978;1:307–310.
39. Gugenheim JJ Jr., Brinker MR. Bone realignment with use of temporary external fixation for distal femoral valgus and varus deformities. *J Bone Joint Surg Am.* 2003; 85-A:1229–1237.
40. Gugenheim JJ, Probe RA, Brinker MR. The effects of femoral shaft malrotation on lower extremity anatomy. *J Orthop Trauma.* 2004;18:658–664.

41. Guichet JM, Javed A, Russell J, et al. Effect of the foot on the mechanical alignment of the lower limbs. *Clin Orthop Relat Res.* 2003;415:193–201.
42. Haidukewych GJ. Innovations in locking plate technology. *J Am Acad Orthop Surg.* 2004;12:205–212.
43. Hankemeier S, Gosling T, Pape HC, et al. Limb lengthening with the Intramedullary Skeletal Kinetic Distractor (ISKD). *Oper Orthop Traumatol.* 2005;17:79–101.
44. Hankemeier S, Pape HC, Gosling T, et al. Improved comfort in lower limb lengthening with the intramedullary skeletal kinetic distractor. Principles and preliminary clinical experiences. *Arch Orthop Trauma Surg.* 2004;124:129–133.
45. Heijens E, Gladbach B, Pfeil J. Definition, quantification, and correction of translation deformities using long leg, frontal plane radiography. *J Pediatr Orthop B.* 1999;8:285–291.
46. Herzenberg JE, Smith JD, Paley D. Correcting tibial deformities with Ilizarov's apparatus. *Clin Orthop Relat Res.* 1994;302:36–41.
47. Hinman RS, May RL, Crossley KM. Is there an alternative to the full-leg radiograph for determining knee joint alignment in osteoarthritis? *Arthritis Rheum.* 2006;55:306–313.
48. Hofer HP, Wildburger R, Szyszkowitz R. Observations concerning different patterns of bone healing using the Point Contact Fixator (PC-Fix) as a new technique for fracture fixation. *Injury.* 2001;32(suppl 2):B15–B25.
49. Hunt MA, Fowler PJ, Birmingham TB, et al. Foot rotational effects on radiographic measures of lower limb alignment. *Can J Surg.* 2006;49:401–406.
50. Ilizarov GA, Kaplunov AG, Degtiarev VE, et al. Treatment of pseudarthroses and ununited fractures, complicated by purulent infection, by the method of compression-distraction osteosynthesis. *Ortop Travmatol Protez.* 1972;33:10–14.
51. Ilizarov GA. Clinical application of the tension-stress effect for limb lengthening. *Clin Orthop Relat Res.* 1990;250:8–26.
52. Ilizarov GA. The principles of the Ilizarov method. *Bull Hosp Jt Dis Orthop Inst.* 1988;48:1–11.
53. Ilizarov GA. The tension-stress effect on the genesis and growth of tissues: Part II. The influence of the rate and frequency of distraction. *Clin Orthop Relat Res.* 1989;239:263–285.
54. Ilizarov GA. The tension-stress effect on the genesis and growth of tissues. Part I. The influence of stability of fixation and soft-tissue preservation. *Clin Orthop Relat Res.* 1989;238:249–281.
55. Ilizarov GA. *Transosseous Osteosynthesis. Theoretical and Clinical Aspects of the Regeneration and Growth of Tissue.* Berlin: Springer-Verlag; 1992.
56. Inan M, Ferri-de Baros F, Chan G, et al. Correction of rotational deformity of the tibia in cerebral palsy by percutaneous supramalleolar osteotomy. *J Bone Joint Surg Br.* 2005;87:1411–1415.
57. Krengel WF 3rd, Staheli LT. Tibial rotational osteotomy for idiopathic torsion. A comparison of the proximal and distal osteotomy levels. *Clin Orthop Relat Res.* 1992;283:285–289.
58. Kristiansen LP, Steen H, Reikeras O. No difference in tibial lengthening index by use of Taylor spatial frame or Ilizarov external fixator. *Acta Orthop.* 2006;77:772–777.
59. Maffuli N, Fixsen JA. Distraction osteogenesis in congenital limb length discrepancy: A review. *J R Coll Surg Edinb.* 1996;41:258–264.
60. Mahaluxmivala J, Nadarajah R, Allen PW, et al. Ilizarov external fixator: Acute shortening and lengthening versus bone transport in the management of tibial non-unions. *Injury.* 2005;36:662–668.
61. Marsh DR, Shah S, Elliott J, et al. The Ilizarov method in nonunion, malunion and infection of fractures. *J Bone Joint Surg Br.* 1997;79:273–279.
62. Matsubara H, Tsuchiya H, Sakurakichi K, et al. Deformity correction and lengthening of lower legs with an external fixator. *Int Orthop.* 2006;30:550–554.
63. Matsubara H, Tsuchiya H, Takato K, et al. Correction of ankle ankylosis with deformity using the taylor spatial frame: A report of three cases. *Foot Ankle Int.* 2007;28:1290–1294.
64. McCarthy JJ, MacEwen GD. Management of leg length inequality. *J South Orthop Assoc.* 2001;10:73–85.
65. McCaw ST, Bates BT. Biomechanical implications of mild leg length inequality. *Br J Sports Med.* 1991;25:10–13.
66. Meyer DC, Siebenrock KA, Schiele B, et al. A new methodology for the planning of single-cut corrective osteotomies of mal-aligned long bones. *Clin Biomech (Bristol, Avon).* 2005;20:223–227.
67. Murray JH, Fitch RD. Distraction histiogenesis: Principles and indications. *J Am Acad Orthop Surg.* 1996;4:317–327.
68. Nakase T, Ohzono K, Shimizu N, et al. Correction of severe post-traumatic deformities in the distal femur by distraction osteogenesis using Taylor Spatial Frame: A case report. *Arch Orthop Trauma Surg.* 2006;126:66–69.
69. Nho SJ, Helfet DL, Rozbruch SR. Temporary intentional leg shortening and deformation to facilitate wound closure using the Ilizarov/Taylor spatial frame. *J Orthop Trauma.* 2006;20:419–424.
70. Noonan KJ, Leyes M, Forriol F, et al. Distraction osteogenesis of the lower extremity with use of monolateral external fixation. A study of two hundred and sixty-one femora and tibiae. *J Bone Joint Surg Am.* 1998;80:793–806.
71. Pajardi G, Campiglio GL, Candiani P. Bone lengthening in malformed upper limbs: A four year experience. *Acta Chir Plast.* 1994;36:3–6.
72. Paley D, Chaudray M, Pirone AM, et al. Treatment of malunions and mal-nonunions of the femur and tibia by detailed preoperative planning and the Ilizarov techniques. *Orthop Clin North Am.* 1990;21:667–691.
73. Paley D, Herzenberg JE, Paremain G, et al. Femoral lengthening over an intramedullary nail. A matched-case comparison with Ilizarov femoral lengthening. *J Bone Joint Surg Am.* 1997;79:1464–1480.
74. Paley D, Herzenberg JE, Tetsworth K, eds. *Program Manual: Annual Baltimore Limb Deformity Course.* Baltimore, MD: Maryland Center for Limb Lengthening; 2000.
75. Paley D, Herzenberg JE, Tetsworth K, et al. Deformity planning for frontal and sagittal plane corrective osteotomies. *Orthop Clin North Am.* 1994;25:425–465.
76. Paley D, Tetsworth K. Mechanical axis deviation of the lower limbs. Preoperative planning of multiapical frontal plane angular and bowing deformities of the femur and tibia. *Clin Orthop Relat Res.* 1992;280:65–71.
77. Paley D, Tetsworth K. Mechanical axis deviation of the lower limbs. Preoperative planning of uniapical angular deformities of the tibia or femur. *Clin Orthop Relat Res.* 1992;280:48–64.
78. Paley D. *Principles of Deformity Correction.* Berlin: Springer-Verlag; 2002.
79. Perren SM. Evolution of the internal fixation of long bone fractures. The scientific basis of biological internal fixation: Choosing a new balance between stability and biology. *J Bone Joint Surg Br.* 2002;84:1093–1110.
80. Pirpiris M, Trivett A, Baker R, et al. Femoral derotation osteotomy in spastic diplegia. Proximal or distal? *J Bone Joint Surg Br.* 2003;85:265–272.
81. Raimondo RA, Skaggs DL, Rosenwasser MP, et al. Lengthening of pediatric forearm deformities using the Ilizarov technique: Functional and cosmetic results. *J Hand Surg Am.* 1999;24:331–338.
82. Rauh MA, Boyle J, Mihalko WM, et al. Reliability of measuring long-standing lower extremity radiographs. *Orthopedics.* 2007;30:299–303.
83. Rogers MJ, McFadyen I, Livingstone JA, et al. Computer hexapod assisted orthopaedic surgery (CHAOS) in the correction of long bone fracture and deformity. *J Orthop Trauma.* 2007;21:337–342.
84. Rozbruch SR, Fragomen AT, Ilizarov S. Correction of tibial deformity with use of the Ilizarov-Taylor spatial frame. *J Bone Joint Surg Am.* 2006;88(suppl 4):156–174.
85. Rozbruch SR, Helfet DL, Blyakher A. Distraction of hypertrophic nonunion of tibia with deformity using Ilizarov/Taylor Spatial Frame. Report of two cases. *Arch Orthop Trauma Surg.* 2002;122:295–298.
86. Rozbruch SR, Pugsley JS, Fragomen AT, et al. Repair of tibial nonunions and bone defects with the Taylor Spatial Frame. *J Orthop Trauma.* 2008;22:88–95.
87. Rozbruch SR, Weitzman AM, Watson JT, et al. Simultaneous treatment of tibial bone and soft-tissue defects with the Ilizarov method. *J Orthop Trauma.* 2006;20:197–205.
88. Rozzanigo U, Pizzoli A, Minari C, et al. Alignment and articular orientation of lower limbs: Manual vs computer-aided measurements on digital radiograms. *Radiol Med (Torino).* 2005;109:234–238.
89. Sabharwal S, Lee J Jr., Zhao C. Multiplanar deformity analysis of untreated Blount disease. *J Pediatr Orthop.* 2007;27:260–265.
90. Sabharwal S, Zhao C, McKeon JJ, et al. Computed radiographic measurement of limb-length discrepancy. Full-length standing anteroposterior radiograph compared with scanogram. *J Bone Joint Surg Am.* 2006;88:2243–2251.
91. Sabharwal S, Zhao C. Assessment of lower limb alignment: Supine fluoroscopy compared with a standing full-length radiograph. *J Bone Joint Surg Am.* 2008;90:43–51.
92. Sailer J, Scharitzer M, Peloschek P, et al. Quantification of axial alignment of the lower extremity on conventional and digital total leg radiographs. *Eur Radiol.* 2005;15:170–173.
93. Sangkaew C. Distraction osteogenesis of the femur using conventional monolateral external fixator. *Arch Orthop Trauma Surg.* 2008;128:889–899.
94. Sangkaew C. Distraction osteogenesis with conventional external fixator for tibial bone loss. *Int Orthop.* 2004;28:171–175.
95. Schutz M, Sudkamp NP. Revolution in plate osteosynthesis: New internal fixator systems. *J Orthop Sci.* 2003;8:252–258.
96. Seitz WH Jr, Froimson AI. Callotasis lengthening in the upper extremity: Indications, techniques, and pitfalls. *J Hand Surg Am.* 1991;16:932–939.
97. Siapkara A, Nordin L, Hill RA. Spatial frame correction of anterior growth arrest of the proximal tibia: Report of three cases. *J Pediatr Orthop B.* 2008;17:61–64.
98. Sluga M, Pfeiffer M, Kotz R, et al. Lower limb deformities in children: Two-stage correction using the Taylor spatial frame. *J Pediatr Orthop B.* 2003;12:123–128.
99. Specogna AV, Birmingham TB, DaSilva JJ, et al. Reliability of lower limb frontal plane alignment measurements using plain radiographs and digitized images. *J Knee Surg.* 2004;17:203–210.
100. Staheli LT, Corbett M, Wyss C, et al. Lower-extremity rotational problems in children. Normal values to guide management. *J Bone Joint Surg Am.* 1985;67:39–47.
101. Staheli LT. Torsion–treatment indications. *Clin Orthop Relat Res.* 1989;61–66.
102. Stanitski DF. Limb-length inequality: Assessment and treatment options. *J Am Acad Orthop Surg.* 1999;7:143–153.
103. Taylor JC. Perioperative planning for two- and three-plane deformities. *Foot Ankle Clin.* 2008;13:69–121.
104. Tetsworth K, Krome J, Paley D. Lengthening and deformity correction of the upper extremity by the Ilizarov technique. *Orthop Clin North Am.* 1991;22:689–713.
105. Tetsworth KD, Paley D. Accuracy of correction of complex lower-extremity deformities by the Ilizarov method. *Clin Orthop Relat Res.* 1994;301:102–110.
106. Tsaridis E, Sarikloglou S, Papasoulis E, et al. Correction of tibial deformity in Paget's disease using the Taylor spatial frame. *J Bone Joint Surg Br.* 2008;90:243–244.
107. Villa A, Paley D, Catagni MA, et al. Lengthening of the forearm by the Ilizarov technique. *Clin Orthop Relat Res.* 1990;250:125–137.
108. Viskontas DG, MacLeod MD, Sanders DW. High tibial osteotomy with use of the Taylor Spatial Frame external fixator for osteoarthritis of the knee. *Can J Surg.* 2006;49:245–250.
109. Vitale MA, Choe JC, Sesko AM, et al. The effect of limb length discrepancy on health-related quality of life: Is the '2 cm rule' appropriate? *J Pediatr Orthop B.* 2006;15:1–5.
110. Wagner M, Frenk A, Frigg R. New concepts for bone fracture treatment and the Locking Compression Plate. *Surg Technol Int.* 2004;12:271–277.
111. Watanabe K, Tsuchiya H, Matsubara H, et al. Revision high tibial osteotomy with the Taylor spatial frame for failed opening-wedge high tibial osteotomy. *J Orthop Sci.* 2008;13:145–149.
112. Watanabe K, Tsuchiya H, Sakurakichi K, et al. Double-level correction with the Taylor Spatial Frame for shepherd's crook deformity in fibrous dysplasia. *J Orthop Sci.* 2007;12:390–394.

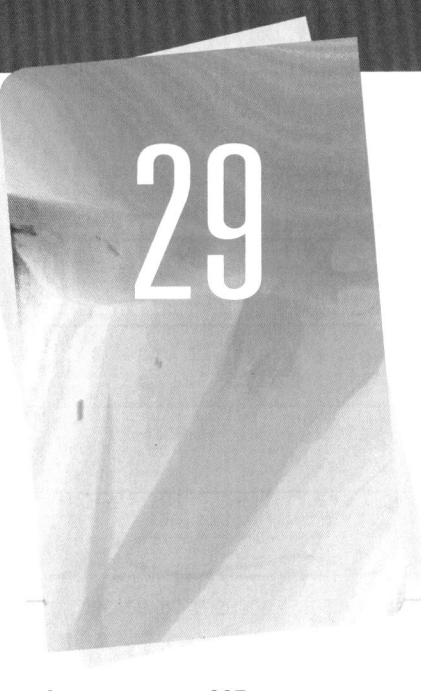

29

ACUTE COMPARTMENT SYNDROME

Margaret M. McQueen

INTRODUCTION TO ACUTE COMPARTMENT SYNDROME

Acute compartment syndrome occurs when pressure rises within a confined space in the body, resulting in a critical reduction of the blood flow to the tissues contained within the space. Without urgent decompression, tissue ischemia, necrosis, and functional impairment occur. The acute compartment syndrome should be differentiated from other related conditions, so awareness of the different definitions associated with a compartment syndrome is important.

Acute compartment syndrome is defined as the elevation of intracompartmental pressure (ICP) to a level and for a duration that without decompression will cause tissue ischemia and necrosis.

Exertional compartment syndrome is the elevation of intracompartmental pressure during exercise, causing ischemia, pain, and rarely neurologic symptoms and signs. It is characterized by resolution of symptoms with rest but may proceed to acute compartment syndrome if exercise continues.

Volkmann ischemic contracture is the end stage of neglected acute compartment syndrome with irreversible muscle necrosis leading to ischemic contractures.

The crush syndrome is the systemic result of muscle necrosis commonly caused by prolonged external compression of an extremity. In crush syndrome muscle necrosis is established by the time of presentation, but ICP may rise as a result of intracompartmental edema, causing a superimposed acute compartment syndrome.

HISTORY

Well over a century has passed since the first description of ischemic muscle contractures was published in the medical literature. The first report of the condition was attributed to Hamilton in 1850 by Hildebrand,[64] but Hamilton's original description has never been found. The credit for the first full description belongs to Richard Von Volkmann[155] who published a summary of his views in 1882. He stated that paralysis and

895

contractures appeared after too tight bandaging of the forearm and hand, were ischemic in nature, and were caused by prolonged blocking of arterial blood. He recognized that muscle cannot survive longer than 6 hours with complete interruption of its blood flow and that 12 hours or less of too tight bandaging were enough to result in "dismal permanent crippling." In 1888 Peterson[118] recognized that ischemic contracture could occur in the absence of bandaging but did not postulate a cause.

The first major reports appeared in the English speaking literature in the early twentieth century. At this time it was suggested that swelling after removal of tight bandaging might contribute to the contracture and that the contracture was caused by "fibrous tissue-forming elements" or a myositic process.[30,129,159] By the early part of the twentieth century published accounts of the sequence of events in acute compartment syndrome were remarkably similar to what is known today, with differentiation between acute ischemia caused by major vessel rupture, acute ischemia caused by "subfascial tension," the late stage of ischemic contracture, and the separate concept of nerve involvement.[9] This paper was the first description of fasciotomy to relieve the pressure. The importance of early fasciotomy was suggested at this time[9,110] and confirmed by prevention of the development of contractures in animal experiments.[70]

During the Second World War attention was directed away from these sound conclusions. A belief arose that ischemic contracture was caused by arterial injury and spasm with reflex collateral spasm. Successful results from excision of the damaged artery[36,47] were undoubtedly owing to the fasciotomy carried out as part of the exposure for the surgery. An unfortunate legacy of this belief persists today in the dangerously mistaken view that an acute compartment syndrome cannot exist in the presence of normal peripheral pulses.

The arterial injury theory was challenged by Seddon[132] in 1966. He noted that in all cases of ischemic contracture there was early and gross swelling requiring prompt fasciotomy, and that 50% of his cases had palpable peripheral pulses. He was unable to explain muscle infarcts at the same level as the injury on the basis of arterial damage. He recommended early fasciotomy.

In their classic paper McQuillan and Nolan[101] reported on 15 cases complicated by "local ischemia". They described the vicious circle of increasing tension in an enclosed compartment causing venous obstruction and subsequent reduction in arterial inflow. Their most important conclusion was that delay in performing a fasciotomy was the single cause of failure of treatment.

EPIDEMIOLOGY

Knowledge of the epidemiology of acute compartment syndrome is important in defining the patient at risk of developing acute compartment syndrome. The epidemiology of acute compartment syndrome has been described in a cohort of 164 patients drawn from a defined population in the United Kingdom.[100]

The incidence of acute compartment syndrome in a westernized population is 3.1 per 100,000 of the population per

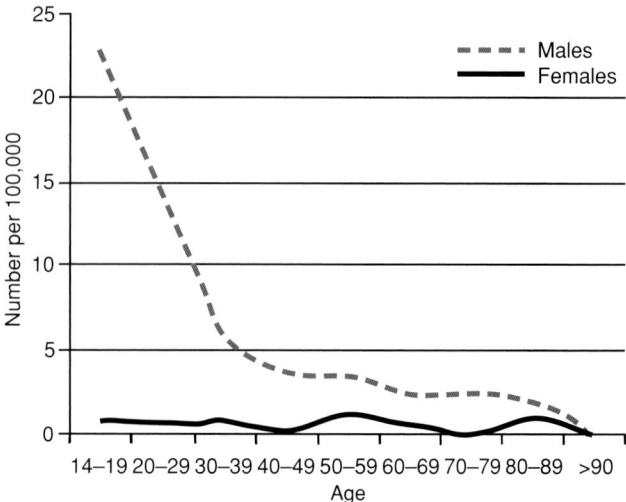

FIGURE 29-1 The annual age- and gender-specific incidence of acute compartment syndrome.

annum.[100] The annual incidence for males is 7.3 per 100,000 compared with 0.7 per 100,000 for females, a tenfold increase in risk for males. The age- and gender-specific incidences are illustrated in Figure 29-1, showing a type B pattern (see Chapter 3) or the L-shaped pattern described by Buhr and Cooke.[18] The mean age for the whole group was 32 years; the median age for males was 30 years and for females 44 years.

The underlying condition causing acute compartment syndrome was most commonly a fracture (69% of cases) (Table 29-1). Similar figures have been reported in children, with 76% of cases caused by fracture, predominantly tibial diaphyseal, distal radius, and forearm.[8] The most common

TABLE 29-1	Conditions Associated with Injury Causing Acute Compartment Syndrome Presenting to an Orthopaedic Trauma Unit	
Underlying Condition		**% of Cases**
Tibial diaphyseal fracture		36
Soft tissue injury		23.2
Distal radius fracture		9.8
Crush syndrome		7.9
Diaphyseal fracture forearm		7.9
Femoral diaphyseal fracture		3.0
Tibial plateau fracture		3.0
Hand fracture(s)		2.5
Tibial pilon fractures		2.5
Foot fracture(s)		1.8
Ankle fracture		0.6
Elbow fracture dislocation		0.6
Pelvic fracture		0.6
Humeral diaphyseal fracture		0.6

fracture associated with acute compartment syndrome in adults is tibial diaphyseal fracture. The prevalence of acute compartment syndrome in tibial diaphyseal fractures is reported as 2.7% to 15%,[3,16,24,34,98–100,109,141,163] with the differences in prevalences likely to be because of different diagnostic techniques and selection of patients.

The second most common cause of acute compartment syndrome is soft tissue injury, which when added to tibial diaphyseal fracture makes up almost two-thirds of the cases. The second most common fracture to be complicated by acute compartment syndrome is the distal radius fracture. It occurs in approximately 0.25% of cases. Forearm diaphyseal fractures are complicated by acute compartment syndrome in 3% of cases. The prevalence of acute compartment syndrome in other anatomic locations is rarely reported. Other less common causes of acute compartment syndrome are listed in Table 29-2.

From adolescence younger patients are at more risk of compartment syndrome. In tibial diaphyseal fracture the prevalence of acute compartment syndrome was reported as being three times greater in the under 35-year-old age group, and in distal radial fractures the prevalence is 35 times less in the older age group.[100] Adolescents have been recognized as having a high rate (8.3%) of compartment syndrome after tibial fracture.[24] More recently, in a cohort of 212 children with tibial diaphyseal fractures and a median age of 13 years a prevalence of 11.4% was reported. In the group older than 14 years who were injured in a motor vehicle accident the prevalence was 48%.[141] Analysis of 1,403 tibial diaphyseal fractures presenting to the Edinburgh Orthopaedic Trauma Unit over the period from 1995 to 2007 shows that there were 160 cases of acute compartment syndrome (11.4%). Using univariate analysis,

---

TABLE 29-2 **Causes of Acute Compartment Syndrome**

Conditions Increasing the Volume of Compartment Contents
Fracture
Soft tissue injury
Crush syndrome (including use of the lithotomy position)[84]
Revascularization
Exercise[94]
Bleeding diathesis/anticoagulants[66,125]
Fluid infusion (including arthroscopy)[10,133]
Arterial puncture[134]
Ruptured ganglia/cysts[31]
Osteotomy[45]
Snake bite[153]
Nephrotic syndrome[147]
Leukemic infiltration[152]
Viral myositis[78]
Acute hematogenous osteomyelitis[145]

Conditions Reducing Compartment Volume
Burns
Repair of muscle hernia[4]

Medical Comorbidity
Diabetes[21]
Hypothyroidism[67]

---

significant risk factors for the development of acute compartment syndrome were youth ($p < 0.001$) and male gender. Males were almost six times more likely to develop acute compartment syndrome if aged between 20 and 29 years compared with those aged over 40 years. Youth, regardless of gender, is therefore a significant risk factor for the development of acute compartment syndrome after tibial fracture. The only exception to youth being a risk factor in acute compartment syndrome is in cases with soft tissue injury only. These patients have an average age of 36 years and are significantly older than those with a fracture.[66]

High-energy injury is generally believed to increase the risks of developing an acute compartment syndrome. Nevertheless, in tibial diaphyseal fracture in adults complicated by acute compartment syndrome the proportion of high- and low-energy injury shows a slight preponderance of low-energy injury (59%).[100] In the same population there is an equal number of high-energy and low-energy injury in tibial diaphyseal fractures uncomplicated by acute compartment syndrome.[25] Adolescents may be an exception to this because of the high prevalence of 48% reported in teenagers after road accidents.[141] In the larger Edinburgh series there was an increased risk of acute compartment syndrome in closed compared with open fractures ($p < 0.05$). This suggests acute compartment syndrome may be more prevalent after low-energy injury, possibly because in low-energy injury the compartment boundaries are less likely to be disrupted and an "autodecompression" effect is avoided. The concept of patients with lower-energy injury being at higher risk is supported by the distribution of severe open fractures. In those complicated by acute compartment syndrome, 20% are Gustilo type III.[100] In the whole population of tibial fractures, 60% were type III.[25] It is important to note that open tibial diaphyseal fractures remain at risk of acute compartment syndrome, which occurs in approximately 3%,[100] but it appears that the lower Gustilo types are at more risk, again possibly because of the lack of disruption of the compartment boundaries.

Distal radial and forearm diaphyseal fractures associated with high-energy injury are more likely to be complicated by acute compartment syndrome, probably because of the high preponderance of young males who sustained these types of injury. This is illustrated by a comparison of the age- and gender-related incidence of distal radius fractures complicated by acute compartment syndrome (Fig. 29-2). The likely explanation for the preponderance of young patients with acute compartment syndrome is that the young have relatively large muscle volumes, whereas their compartment size does not change after growth is complete. Thus younger patients may have less space for swelling of the muscle after injury. Presumably the older person has smaller hypotrophic muscles allowing more space for swelling. There may also be a protective effect of hypertension in the older patient.

The second most common type of acute compartment syndrome is that arising in the absence of fractures. The majority of these arise subsequent to soft tissue injury, particularly a crushing type injury, but some arise with no preceding history of trauma.[66] In children 61% of cases of acute compartment

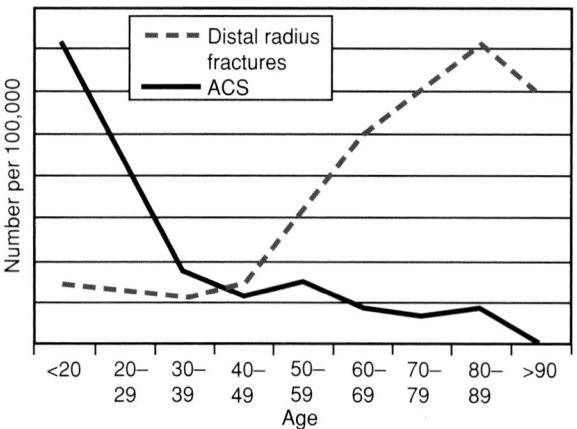

FIGURE 29-2 The annual age-specific incidence of all distal radius fractures compared with the annual age-specific incidence of acute compartment syndrome in distal radial fractures.

syndrome in the absence of fracture are reported as being iatrogenic.[120] Patients with acute compartment syndrome without fracture tend to be older and have more medical comorbidities than those with a fracture. They are more evenly distributed between the genders with a male to female ratio of five to one. The use of anticoagulants also seems to be a risk factor for the development of acute compartment syndrome.

Patients with polytrauma are at particular risk of delay in the diagnosis of their acute compartment syndrome, so identification of at-risk factors in this group is of particular importance.[37] Kosir et al.[75] examined risk factors for lower limb acute compartment syndrome in 45 critically ill trauma patients with the institution of an aggressive screening protocol. The prevalence of acute compartment syndrome was 20%. High base deficits, lactate levels, and transfusion requirements were significant risk factors in this group.

The possible risk factors for the development or late diagnosis of acute compartment syndrome are listed in Table 29-3. As well as demographic risk factors, altered pain perception can delay diagnosis. This can occur if the patient has an altered conscious state or with certain types of anesthesia or analgesia.[55,81,108]

TABLE 29-3 **Risk Factors for Development or Late Diagnosis of Acute Compartment Syndrome**

Demographic	Altered Pain Perception
Youth	Altered conscious level
Tibial fracture	Regional anesthesia
High-energy forearm fracture	Patient-controlled analgesia
High-energy femoral diaphyseal fracture	Children
Bleeding diathesis/anticoagulants	Associated nerve injury
Polytrauma with high base deficit, lactate levels, and transfusion requirement	

PATHOGENESIS

There remains uncertainty about the exact physiologic mechanism of the reduction in blood flow in the acute compartment syndrome, although it is generally accepted that the effect is at small vessel level, either arteriolar, capillary, or venous levels.

The critical closing pressure theory states that there is a critical closing pressure in the small vessels when the transmural pressure (TM) (the difference between intravascular pressure and tissue pressure) drops.[19] TM is balanced by a constricting force (TC) consisting of active and elastic tension derived from smooth muscle action in the vessel walls. The equilibrium between expanding and contracting forces is expressed in a derivation of Laplace law:

$$TM = TC \div r$$

where r is the radius of the vessel.

If, because of increasing tissue pressure, the TM drops to a level such that elastic fibers in the vessel wall are no longer stretched and therefore cannot contribute any elastic tension, then there will be no further automatic decrease in the radius. TC ÷ r then becomes greater than TM and active closure of the vessel will occur. This concept has been verified in both animal and human local vascular beds.[6,115,124,168] Ashton[7] was the first to relate these findings to acute compartment syndrome and concluded that whatever the cause of the raised tissue pressure, blood flow will be decreased and may temporarily cease altogether as a result of a combination of active arteriolar closure and passive capillary compression, depending on vasomotor tone and the height of the total tissue pressure. Critics of this theory doubt the possibility of maintaining arteriolar closure in the presence of ischemia, which is a strong local stimulus for vasodilatation.[85] Ashton[6] noted that flow resumes after 30 to 60 seconds of maintained tissue pressure and attributes this to vessel reopening possibly because of an accumulation of vasodilator metabolites.

A second theory is the arteriovenous (AV) gradient theory.[85,92] According to this theory the increases in local tissue pressure reduce the local AV pressure gradient and thus reduce the blood flow. When flow diminishes to less than the metabolic demands of the tissues (not necessarily to zero), then functional abnormalities result. The relationship between AV gradient and the local blood flow (LBF) is summarized in the equation:

$$LBF = (P_a - P_v) \div R$$

where P_a is the local arterial pressure, P_v is the local venous pressure, and R is the local vascular resistance. Veins are collapsible tubes and the pressure within them can never be less than the local tissue pressure. If tissue pressure rises as in the acute compartment syndrome, then the P_v must also rise, thus reducing the AV gradient ($P_a - P_v$) and therefore the local blood flow. At low AV gradients compensation from R is relatively ineffective[62] and local blood flow is primarily determined by the AV gradient. Matsen et al.[92] presented results on human subjects demonstrating reduction of the AV gradient with elevation of the limb in the presence of raised tissue pressure. This theory has been supported by work that demonstrated that with external pressure applied, simulating acute compartment syndrome, venous and capillary flow ceased, but arterioles were still capable of carrying flow.[156] This disproves the critical closing theory but supports the hypothesis of reduced AV gradient as the mechanism of reducing blood flow.

A third theory, the microvascular occlusion theory postulates that capillary occlusion is the main mechanism reducing blood flow in acute compartment syndrome.[52] Measurement of capillary pressure in dogs with normal tissue pressures revealed a mean level of 25 mm Hg. Hargens et al.[52] suggested that a tissue pressure of similar value is sufficient to reduce capillary blood flow. Resultant muscle ischemia leads to increased capillary membrane permeability to plasma proteins, increasing edema and obstruction of lymphatic by the raised tissue pressure. Nonetheless, the authors admitted that reactive hyperemia and vasodilatation both tend to raise the critical pressure level for microvascular occlusion. However, this work was done in the presence of normal tissue pressures and it has also been pointed out that capillaries are collapsible tubes[85] and their intravascular pressure ought to rise in the presence of raised tissue pressure. Hargens' theory[52] is supported by work demonstrating reduction of the number of perfused capillaries per unit area with raised tissue pressures.[57]

Effects of Raised Tissue Pressure on Muscle

Regardless of the mechanism of vessel closure, reduction in blood flow in the acute compartment syndrome has a profound effect on muscle tissue. Skeletal muscle is the tissue in the extremities most vulnerable to ischemia and is therefore the most important tissue to be considered in acute compartment syndrome. Both the magnitude and duration of pressure elevation have been shown experimentally to be important influences in the extent of muscle damage.

There is now universal agreement that rising tissue pressure leads to a reduction in muscle blood flow. A number of experimental studies have highlighted the importance of perfusion pressure as well as tissue pressure in the reduction of muscle blood flow. MR measurements of cellular metabolic derangement (pH, tissue oxygenation, and energy stores) and histologic studies, including electron microscopy and videomicroscopy studies of capillary blood flow, have shown that critical tissue pressure thresholds are 10 to 20 mm Hg below diastolic blood pressure or 25 to 30 mm Hg below mean arterial pressure.[57,60,63,83] Increased vulnerability in previously traumatized or ischemic muscle has been demonstrated when the critical threshold may occur at tissue pressures more than 30 mm Hg below mean arterial pressure.[12]

The ultimate result of reduced blood flow to skeletal muscle is ischemia followed by necrosis, with general agreement that increasing periods of complete ischemia produce increasing irreversible changes.[59,77,119] Evidence indicates that muscle necrosis is present in its greatest extent centrally in the muscle, and that external evaluation of the degree of muscle necrosis is unreliable. The duration of muscle ischemia dictates the amount of necrosis, although some muscle fibers are more vulnerable than others to ischemia. For example, the muscles of

the anterior compartment of the leg contain type I fibers or red slow twitch fibers, whereas the gastrocnemius contains mainly type II or white fast twitch fibers. Type I fibers depend on oxidative metabolism of triglycerides for their energy source and are more vulnerable to oxygen depletion than type II fibers whose metabolism is primarily anaerobic.[79] This may explain the particular vulnerability of the anterior compartment to raised ICP.

Effects of Raised Tissue Pressure on Nerve

There is little dispute about the effects of raised tissue pressure on neurologic function. All investigators note a loss of neuromuscular function with raised tissue pressures but at varying pressure thresholds and duration.[40,54,87,140] In a study on human neurologic function, Matsen et al.[89] found considerable variation of pressure tolerance that could not be attributed to differences in systemic pressure.

The mechanism of damage to nerve is as yet uncertain and could result from ischemia, ischemia plus compression, toxic effects, or the effects of acidosis.

Effects of Raised Tissue Pressure on Bone

Nonunion is now recognized as a complication of acute compartment syndrome.[23,27,71,98,103] It was first suggested by Nario in 1938 that "Volkmann's disease" caused obliteration of the "musculodiaphyseal" vessels and caused frequent pseudarthrosis.[113] McQueen[95] observed a reduction in bone blood flow and bone union in rabbit tibiae after an experimentally induced acute compartment syndrome. It is likely that muscle ischemia reduces the capacity for development of the extraosseous blood supply on which long bones depend for healing.

Reperfusion Injury

The reperfusion syndrome is a group of complications following re-establishment of blood flow to the ischemic tissues and can occur after fasciotomy and restoration of muscle blood flow in the acute compartment syndrome. Reperfusion is followed by an inflammatory response in the ischemic tissue that can cause further tissue damage. The trigger for the inflammatory response is probably the breakdown products of muscle.[15] Some breakdown products are procoagulants that activate the intrinsic clotting system. This results in increasing microvascular thrombosis, which in turn increases the extent of muscle damage.

If there is a large amount of muscle involved in the ischemic process, the inflammatory response may become systemic. In acute compartment syndrome this is most likely to occur in the crush syndrome. Procoagulants escape into the systemic circulation and produce systemic coagulopathy with parallel activation of inflammatory mediators. These then damage the vascular endothelium, leading to increased permeability, transcapillary fluid leakage and subsequent worsening of intracompartmental pressure,[46] and eventually multiple organ failure. Systemic clotting and the breakdown products of dead and dying cells also lead to activation of white blood cells, with the release of additional inflammatory mediators such as histamine, interleukin, oxygen free radicals, thromboxane, and many others.[15] This is the basis for the use of agents such as anti-oxidants, antithromboxanes, antileukotrienes, and antiplatelet-activating factors that modify the inflammatory process. Some of these agents have been shown in the laboratory to be capable of reducing muscle injury.[1,72,73,157]

DIAGNOSIS OF ACUTE COMPARTMENT SYNDROME

Prompt diagnosis of acute compartment syndrome is the key to a successful outcome. Delay in diagnosis has long been recognized as the single cause of failure of the treatment of acute compartment syndrome.[86,101,126,128] Delay in diagnosis may be because of inexperience and lack of awareness of the possibility of acute compartment syndrome, an indefinite and confusing clinical presentation,[102,151] or anesthetic or analgesic techniques that mask the clinical signs.[26,55,81,108]

Delay in treatment of the acute compartment syndrome can be catastrophic, leading to serious complications such as permanent sensory and motor deficits, contractures, infection, and at times, amputation of the limb.[109,120,128] In serious cases there may be systemic injury from the reperfusion syndrome. A clear understanding of the clinical techniques necessary to make an early diagnosis is therefore essential to any physician treating acute compartment syndrome to avoid such complications. As well as improving outcome, early recognition and treatment of acute compartment syndrome is associated with decreased indemnity risk in potential malpractice claims.[14]

Clinical Diagnosis

Pain is considered to be the first symptom of acute compartment syndrome. The pain experienced by the patient is by nature ischemic and usually severe and out of proportion to the clinical situation. Pain may, however, be an unreliable indication of the presence of acute compartment syndrome because it can be variable in its intensity.[32,88,162] Pain may be absent in acute compartment syndrome associated with nerve injury[65,167] or minimal in the deep posterior compartment syndrome.[86,88] Pain is present in most cases because of the index injury but cannot be elicited in the unconscious patient or where regional anesthesia is used.[26,55,108] Kosir at al.[75] abandoned clinical examination as part of their screening protocol for critically ill trauma patients because of the difficulty in eliciting reliable symptoms and signs in this group. Children may not be able to express the severity of their pain, so restlessness, agitation, and anxiety with increasing analgesic requirements should raise the suspicion of the presence of an acute compartment syndrome.[8] Both Shereff[139] and Myerson[112] state that clinical diagnosis of acute compartment syndrome in the foot is so unreliable that other methods should be used.

Pain has been shown to have a sensitivity of only 19% and a specificity of 97% in the diagnosis of acute compartment syndrome (i.e., a high proportion of false-negative or missed cases but a low proportion of false-positive cases).[151] There is general agreement, however, that pain, if present, is a relatively early symptom of acute compartment syndrome in the awake alert patient.[151] Increasing requirements for opiates should also be considered in assessing the severity of pain.

Pain with passive stretch of the muscles involved is recognized as a symptom of acute compartment syndrome. Thus pain is increased, for example, in an anterior compartment syndrome when the toes or foot are plantarflexed. This symptom is no more reliable than rest pain because the reasons for unreliability quoted above apply equally to pain on passive stretch. The sensitivity and specificity of pain on passive stretch are similar to those for rest pain.[151]

Paresthesia and hypoesthesia may occur in the territory of the nerves traversing the affected compartment and are usually the first signs of nerve ischemia, although sensory abnormality may be the result of concomitant nerve injury.[163,167] Ulmer[151] reports a sensitivity of 13% and specificity of 98% for the clinical finding of paresthesia in acute compartment syndrome, a false-negative rate that precludes this symptom from being a useful diagnostic tool.

Paralysis of muscle groups affected by the acute compartment syndrome is recognized as being a late sign.[151] This sign has equally low sensitivity as others in predicting the presence of acute compartment syndrome, probably because of the difficulty of interpreting the underlying cause of the weakness, which could be inhibition by pain, direct injury to muscle, or associated nerve injury. If a motor deficit develops, full recovery is unusual.[17,27,29,126,131,165] Bradley[17] reported full recovery in only 13% of patients with paralysis as a sign of their acute compartment syndrome.

Palpable swelling in the compartment affected may be a further sign of compartment syndrome, although the degree of swelling is difficult to assess accurately, making this sign very subjective. Casts or dressings often obscure compartments at risk and prevent assessment of swelling.[75] Some compartments such as the deep posterior compartment of the leg are completely buried under the muscle compartments, obscuring any swelling.

Peripheral pulses and capillary return are always intact in acute compartment syndrome unless there is major arterial injury or disease or in the very late stages of acute compartment syndrome when amputation is inevitable. If acute compartment syndrome is suspected and pulses are absent, then arteriography is indicated. Conversely, it is dangerous to exclude the diagnosis of acute compartment syndrome because distal pulses are present.

Using a combination of clinical symptoms and signs increases their sensitivity as diagnostic tools.[151] To achieve a probability of over 90% of acute compartment syndrome being present, however, three clinical findings must be noted. The third clinical finding is paresis; thus, to achieve an accurate clinical diagnosis of acute compartment syndrome the condition must be allowed to progress until a late stage. This is clearly unacceptable and has led to a search for earlier, more reliable methods of diagnosis.

Compartment Pressure Monitoring

Several techniques were developed to measure ICP once it was appreciated that acute compartment syndrome was caused by increased tissue pressure within the affected compartment. Because raised tissue pressure is the primary event in acute compartment syndrome, changes in ICP will precede the clinical symptoms and signs.[96]

There are a number of methods available to measure ICP. One of the first to be used was the needle manometer method, using a needle introduced into the compartment and connected to a column filled partly with saline and partly with air.[162] A syringe filled with air is attached to this column, as is a pressure manometer or transducer. The ICP is the pressure that is required to inject air into the tubing and flatten the meniscus between the saline and the air. This method was modified by Matsen et al. to allow infusion of saline into the compartment.[90,91] The ICP is the pressure resistance to infusion of saline. These methods, although simple and inexpensive, have some drawbacks. A danger exists of too large a volume being infused, possibly inducing acute compartment syndrome. It is probably the least accurate of the measurement techniques available, with falsely high values having been recorded in comparison with other techniques[104] and falsely low values in cases of very high ICP.[146] A needle with only one perforation at its tip also can become easily blocked.

The wick catheter was first described for use in acute compartment syndrome by Mubarak et al.[105] This is a modification of the needle technique, in which fibrils protrude from the bore of the catheter assembly. This allows a large surface area for measurement and prevents obstruction of the needle; it is ideal for continuous measurement. A disadvantage of this technique is the possibility of a blood clot blocking the tip or air in the column of fluid between the catheter and the transducer, which will dampen the response and give falsely low readings. There is a theoretical risk of retention of wick material in the tissues.

The slit catheter was first described by Rorabeck et al.[127] This operates on the same principle as the wick catheter in that it is designed to increase the surface area at the tip of the catheter by means of being cut axially at the end of the catheter (Fig. 29-3). The interstitial pressure is measured through a column of saline attached to a transducer. Patency can be confirmed by gentle pressure over the catheter tip; an immediate rise in the pressure should be seen. Care must be taken to avoid the presence of air bubbles in the system as this can, like the wick catheter, result in falsely low readings. The slit catheter is more accurate than the continuous infusion method[104] and is as accurate as the wick catheter.[138]

Attempts to improve the reliability of ICP measurement led to the placement of the pressure transducer directly into the compartment by siting it within the lumen of a catheter. The solid state transducer intracompartmental catheter (STIC) was described in 1984 and measurements were correlated with conventional pressure monitoring systems.[93] This device is now commercially available and widely used, although to retain patency of the catheter for continuous monitoring an infusion must be used with its attendant problems. The alternative is intermittent pressure measurements, which is likely to cause significant discomfort to patients and is more labor intensive. Newer systems with the transducer placed at the tip of the catheter do not depend on a column of fluid and therefore avoid the problems of patency.[166] These systems are more expensive, however, and are a potential problem for resterilization.

All the methods above measure ICP, which is an indirect way of measuring muscle blood flow and oxygenation. Near-infrared spectroscopy measures tissue oxygen saturation noninvasively by means of a probe placed on the skin. This has proved to correlate to tissue pressures experimentally[5] and in human volunteers.[42] In patients with acute compartment syndrome the reduction in oxygenation values compared to the opposite uninjured leg has been shown to correlate with reducing perfusion pressures but a critical level has not yet been established.[143] It has also been used to demonstrate the hyperemic response to injury in tibial fracture.[144] The technique has promise but requires further validation in humans subjected to injury.

ICP is usually monitored in the anterior compartment because this is most commonly involved in acute compartment syndrome and is easily accessible.[98] There is a risk of missing an acute compartment syndrome in the deep posterior compartments and some authors recommend measurement of both,[61] but measuring two compartments is much more cumbersome. If the anterior compartment alone is monitored, the surgeon must be aware of the small chance of deep posterior acute compartment syndrome and measure the deep posterior compartment pressures if there are unexplained symptoms in the presence of anterior compartment pressures with a safe difference between the diastolic pressure and the tissue pressure (ΔP). It is important to measure the peak pressure within the limb, which usually occurs within 5 cm of the level of the fracture.[61] Recommended catheter placement for each of the anatomic areas is summarized in Table 29-4.

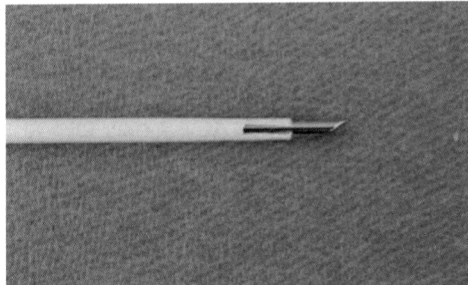

FIGURE 29-3 The tip of a slit catheter, which can be made easily from standard equipment by cutting two slits in the tip of the catheter.

TABLE 29-4	Recommended Catheter Placements for Compartmental Pressure Monitoring
Anatomic Area	**Catheter Placement**
Thigh	Anterior compartment
Leg	Anterior compartment Deep posterior if clinically suspected
Foot	Interosseous compartments Consider calcaneal compartment in hindfoot injuries
Forearm	Flexor compartment
Hand	Interosseous compartment

Threshold for Decompression in Acute Compartment Syndrome

Much debate has occurred about the critical pressure threshold, beyond which decompression of acute compartment syndrome is required. After appreciation of the nature of acute compartment syndrome being raised ICP, debate centered around the use of tissue pressure alone as indication of the need for decompression. One level believed to be critical was 30 mm Hg of ICP because this is a value close to capillary blood pressure.[53,107] Some authors felt that 40 mm Hg of tissue pressure should be the threshold for decompression,[50,90,93,131] although some recognized a significant variation between individuals in their tolerance of raised ICP.[50,92] In a series of patients with tibial fractures, a tissue pressure of 50 mm Hg was recommended as a pressure threshold for decompression in normotensive patients.[51]

It is now recognized that apparent variation between individuals in their tolerance of raised ICP is because of variations in systemic blood pressure. Whitesides et al.[162] were the first to suggest the importance of the difference between the diastolic blood pressure and tissue pressure, or ΔP. They stated that there is inadequate perfusion and relative ischemia when the tissue pressure rises to within 10 to 30 mm Hg of the diastolic pressure. There is now good evidence from experimental work to support this concept[60,83] or the similar concept that the difference between mean arterial pressure and tissue pressure should not be less than 30 mm Hg in normal muscle or 40 mm Hg in muscle subject to trauma[63] or antecedent ischemia.[12]

This concept was tested in a clinical study designed to test the hypothesis of the differential pressure as a threshold for decompression.[98] One hundred and sixteen patients with tibial diaphyseal fractures underwent continuous ICP monitoring both perioperatively and for at least 24 hours postoperatively. The differential pressure between the diastolic blood pressure and the ICP was recorded. Mean pressures over a 12-hour period were calculated to include the duration of elevated pressure in the analysis. Three patients had ΔP of less than 30 mm Hg for more than 2 hours and underwent fasciotomy. Of the remaining patients, all maintained a ΔP greater than 30 mm Hg despite a number of those having an ICP greater than 40 mm Hg. None of these patients underwent fasciotomy and none had any sequelae of acute compartment syndrome at final review. The authors concluded that a ΔP of 30 mm Hg is a safe threshold for decompression in acute compartment syndrome. This has been validated by the same group who examined the outcome in terms of muscle power and returned to function in two groups of patients with tibial fractures.[161] The first group of patients all had an ICP of greater than 30 mm Hg and the second all had an ICP less than 30 mm Hg. Both groups maintained a ΔP of greater than 30 mm Hg. There were no differences in the outcomes between the two groups. The concept of the use of ΔP is also supported by Ovre et al.,[117] who found an unacceptably high rate of fasciotomies (29%) using an ICP of 30 mm Hg as a threshold for decompression.

The sensitivity and specificity of continuous compartment pressure monitoring has recently been reported.[99] Using a pressure threshold of a ΔP of 30 mm Hg for more than 2 hours in 850 patients there were 11 false positives and 9 false negatives giving a sensitivity of 94% and a specificity of 98.4%. The positive predictive value was 92.8% and the negative predictive value was 98.7%. To achieve similar accuracy with clinical symptoms and signs three signs need to be present with the third being paralysis.[151] The authors stated that ideally there should be a 100% certainty of the diagnosis, but acknowledged that this is not possible in clinical practice when in most situations both the surgeon and the patient have to accept a small amount of risk. With acute compartment syndrome the risk should be weighted slightly toward false positives or so-called unnecessary fasciotomy which was felt to be preferable to false negatives or missing the acute compartment syndrome.[99]

To derive the full benefit of monitoring for acute compartment syndrome, the diagnosis should be made on the basis of sequential differential pressure measurements rather than awaiting the development of clinical symptoms and signs. It has been demonstrated that this approach reduces both the delay to fasciotomy and the development of sequelae[97] and that the appearance of clinical symptoms and signs lags behind the pressure changes.[98] This is well illustrated in a study in which the authors claimed to compare intracompartmental pressure monitoring with clinical findings in a randomized trial of[178] tibial fractures,[56] but their threshold for fasciotomy in both groups was the appearance of clinical signs regardless of the pressure measurement. Not surprisingly, the authors found no differences in the outcome of the two groups but had a total of 27 complications of neglected acute compartment syndrome excluding nonunions.

All of the work quoted above was performed in adults and with reference to leg compartment syndrome. The threshold may differ for children who have a low diastolic pressure and are therefore more likely to have a ΔP less than 30 mm Hg. Mars and Hadley[82] recommend the use of the mean arterial pressure rather than the diastolic pressure to obviate this problem. It has been assumed that these pressure thresholds apply equally to anatomic areas other than the leg, although this has not been formally examined.

Timing

Time factors are also important in making the decision to proceed to fasciotomy. It is well established experimentally and clinically that both the duration and severity of the pressure elevation influence the development of muscle necrosis and sequelae.[29,77,79,83,98,119,120,163] Continuous pressure monitoring allows a clear record of the trend of the tissue pressure measurements. In situations where the ΔP drops below 30 mm Hg if the ICP is dropping and the ΔP is rising, then it is safe to observe the patient in anticipation of the ΔP returning within a short time to safe levels. If the ICP is rising, the ΔP is dropping and less than 30 mm Hg, and this trend has been consistent for a period of 2 hours, then fasciotomy should be performed. Fasciotomy should not be performed based on a single pressure reading except in extreme cases. Using this protocol, delay to fasciotomy and the sequelae of acute compartment syndrome are reduced without unnecessary fasciotomies being performed.[98]

Overtreatment has been cited as a problem with continuous monitoring,[69] but this study did not consider the importance of the duration of raised ICP in the diagnosis of acute compartment syndrome. Some authors have found compartment pressure monitoring less useful but used clinical symptoms and signs as their indication for fasciotomy with pressure monitoring only as an adjunct.[3,56] For ICP monitoring to be most effective in reducing delay, it must be used as the primary indication for fasciotomy.

SURGICAL AND APPLIED ANATOMY

Thigh

The thigh is divided into three main compartments, both of which are bounded by the fascia lata and separated by the medial and lateral intermuscular septa (Fig. 29-4). Their contents and the clinical signs of compartment syndrome in each compartment are summarized in Table 29-5. Involvement of the adductor compartment is rare.

Leg

There are four compartments in the leg—anterior, lateral, superficial posterior, and deep posterior (Fig. 29-5).

The anterior compartment is enclosed anteriorly by skin and fascia, laterally by the intermuscular septum, posteriorly by the fibula and interosseous membrane, and medially by the tibia. Its contents and the clinical signs of acute compartment syndrome are listed in Table 29-6.

The lateral compartment is enclosed laterally by skin and fascia, posteriorly by the posterior intermuscular septum,

TABLE 29-5	Compartments of the Thigh, Their Contents, and Signs of Acute Compartment Syndrome	
Compartment	**Contents**	**Signs**
Anterior	Quadriceps muscles	Pain on passive knee flexion
	Sartorius	Numbness—medial leg/foot
	Femoral nerve	Weakness—knee extension
Posterior	Hamstring muscles	Pain on passive knee extension
		Sensory changes rare
	Sciatic nerve	Weakness—knee flexion
Adductor	Adductor muscles	Pain on passive hip abduction
	Obturator nerve	Sensory changes rare
		Weakness—hip adduction

medially by the fibula, and anteriorly by the anterior intermuscular septum. Its contents and the clinical signs of involvement in acute compartment syndrome are detailed in Table 29-6. The deep peroneal nerve may rarely be affected as it passes through the lateral compartment en route to the anterior compartment.

The superficial posterior compartment is bounded anteriorly by the intermuscular septum between the superficial and deep compartments and posteriorly by skin and fascia. Its

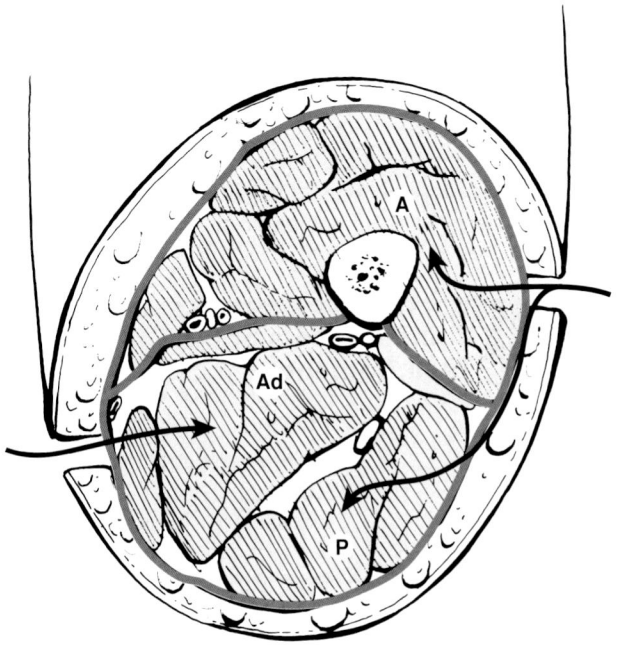

FIGURE 29-4 A cross section of the thigh demonstrating the three compartments and the access to them. A, anterior; Ad, adductor; P, posterior.

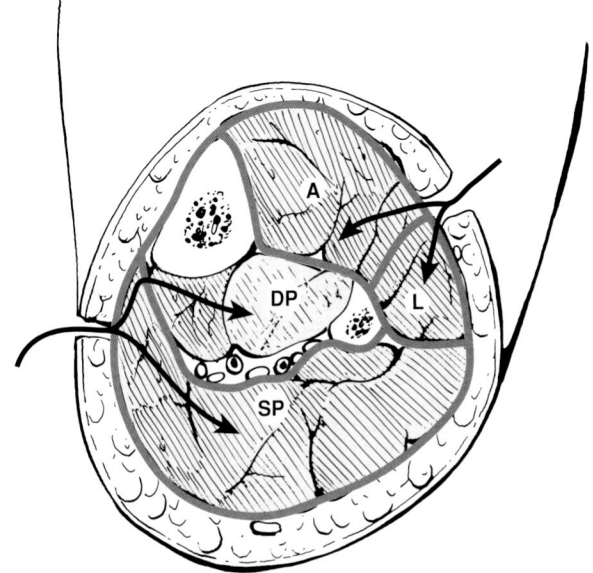

FIGURE 29-5 A cross section of the leg showing the four compartments. The arrows show the routes for double incision four-compartment fasciotomy. A, anterior compartment; DP, deep posterior compartment; L, lateral compartment; SP, superficial posterior compartment.

TABLE 29-6	**Compartments of the Leg, Their Contents, and Clinical Signs of Acute Compartment Syndrome**	
Compartment	**Contents**	**Signs**
Anterior	Tibialis anterior Extensor digitorum longus Extensor hallucis longus Peroneus tertius Deep peroneal (anterior tibial) nerve and vessels	Pain on passive flexion—ankle/toes Numbness—first web space Weakness—ankle/toe extension
Lateral	Peroneus longus Peroneus brevis Superficial peroneal nerve	Pain on passive foot inversion Numbness—dorsum of foot Weakness of eversion
Superficial posterior	Gastrocnemius Soleus Plantaris Sural nerve	Pain on passive ankle extension Numbness—dorsolateral foot Weakness—plantar flexion
Deep posterior	Tibialis posterior Flexor digitorum longus Flexor hallucis longus Posterior tibial nerve	Pain on passive ankle/toe extension/foot eversion Numbness—sole of foot Weakness—toe/ankle flexion, foot inversion

contents and the clinical signs of acute compartment syndrome are summarized in Table 29-6.

The deep posterior compartment is limited anteriorly by the tibia and interosseous membrane, laterally by the fibula, posteriorly by the intermuscular septum separating it from the superficial posterior compartment, and medially by skin and fascia in the distal part of the leg. Table 29-6 lists the contents of the deep posterior compartment and the likely clinical signs in acute compartment syndrome.

Foot

Until recently, most authorities believed that there were four compartments in the foot—medial, lateral, central, and interosseous (Fig. 29-6). The medial compartment lies on the plantar surface of the hallux, the lateral compartment is on the plantar surface of the fifth metatarsal, and the central compartment lies

on the plantar surface of the foot. The interosseous compartment lies dorsal to the others between the metatarsals. Their contents are shown in Table 29-7.

Manoli and Weber challenged the concept of four compartments using cadaver infusion techniques.[80] They believe that there are nine compartments in the foot, with two central compartments, one superficial containing flexor digitorum brevis, and one deep (the calcaneal compartment) (Fig. 29-7) containing quadratus plantae, which communicates with the deep posterior compartment of the leg. They demonstrated that each of the four interosseous muscles and adductor hallucis lie in separate compartments, thus increasing the number of compartments to nine. The clinical importance of these anatomic findings has been challenged after the finding that the barrier between the superficial and calcaneal compartments becomes incompetent at a pressure of 10 mm Hg, much lower than that required to produce an acute compartment syndrome.[49] The clinical diagnosis of acute compartment syndrome should be

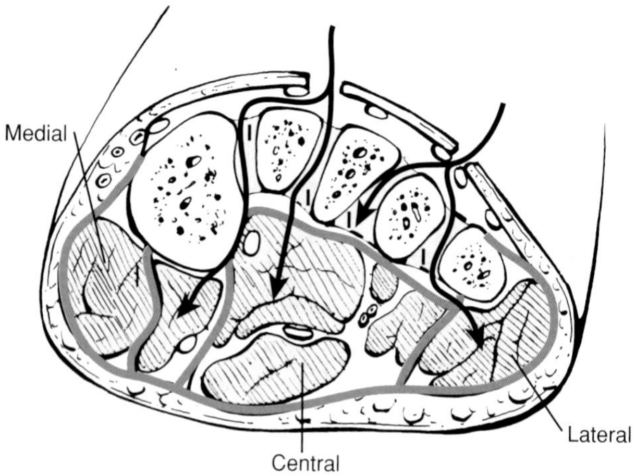

FIGURE 29-6 A cross section of the foot showing access from the dorsum of the foot to the compartments. I, interosseous.

TABLE 29-7	**Compartments of the Foot and Their Contents**
Compartment	**Contents**
Medial	Intrinsic muscles of the great toe
Lateral	Flexor digiti minimi Abductor digiti minimi
Central • Superficial • Deep (calcaneal)	Flexor digitorum brevis Quadratus plantae
Adductor hallucis	Adductor hallucis
Interosseous × 4	Interosseous muscles Digital nerves

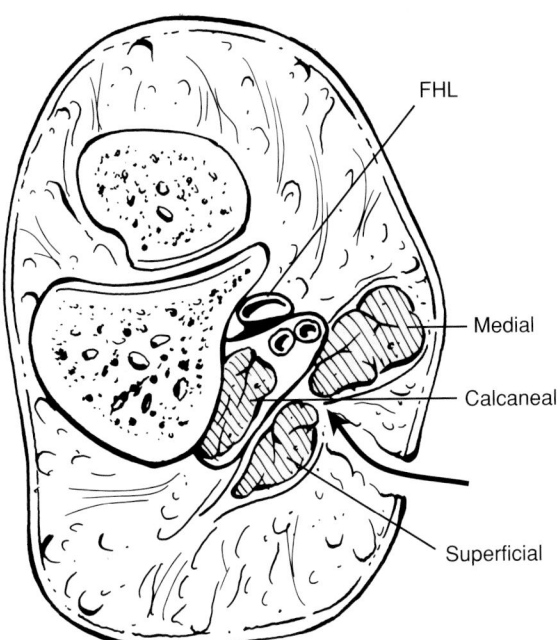

FIGURE 29-7 A section through the hindfoot showing the medial, superficial, and deep central (calcaneal) compartments. The medial approach for release of the calcaneal compartment is shown. FHL, flexor hallucis longus.

suspected in the presence of severe swelling, but differentiating the affected compartments is extremely difficult.

Arm

There are two compartments in the arm: anterior and posterior (Fig. 29-8). The anterior compartment is bounded by the humerus posteriorly, the lateral and medial intermuscular septa and the brachial fascia anteriorly. Its contents and the clinical signs of acute compartment syndrome are detailed in Table 29-8. In late cases paralysis of the muscles innervated by the median, ulna, and radial nerves is seen.

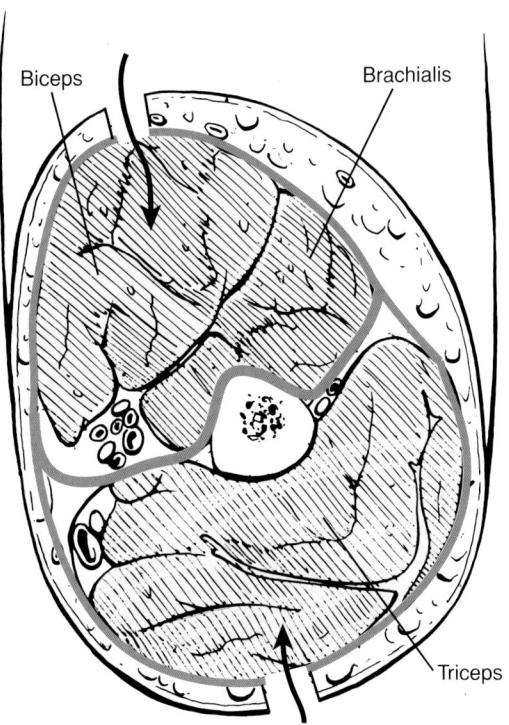

FIGURE 29-8 A cross section of the arm showing the anterior compartment containing biceps (B) and brachialis (Br), and the posterior compartment containing triceps (T).

The posterior compartment has the same boundaries as the anterior but lies posterior to the humerus. Its contents and the clinical signs of acute compartment syndrome are listed in Table 29-8.

Forearm

The forearm contains three compartments: volar, dorsal, and "the mobile wad" (Fig. 29-9). The volar compartment has the ulna, radius, and interosseous membrane as its posterior limit

TABLE 29-8	Compartments of the Arm, Their Contents, and Clinical Signs of Acute Compartment Syndrome	
Compartment	Contents	Signs
Anterior	Biceps Brachialis Coracobrachialis Median nerve Ulnar nerve Musculocutaneous nerve Lateral cutaneous nerve Antebrachial nerve Radial nerve (distal third)	Pain on passive elbow extension Numbness—median/ulnar distribution Numbness—volar/lateral distal forearm Weakness—elbow flexion Weakness—median/ulnar motor function
Posterior	Triceps Radial nerve Ulnar nerve (distally)	Pain on passive elbow flexion Numbness—ulnar/radial distribution Weakness—elbow extension Weakness—radial/ulnar motor function

The dorsal compartment of the forearm lies dorsal to the radius, ulna, and interosseous membrane and contains the finger and thumb extensors, abductor pollicis longus, and extensor carpi ulnaris. Its contents and the clinical signs of acute compartment syndrome are summarized in Table 29-9.

Hand

General agreement exists that the hand has ten muscle compartments: one thenar, one hypothenar, one adductor pollicis, four dorsal interosseous, and three volar interosseous compartments (Fig. 29-10). The thenar compartment is surrounded by the thenar fascia, the thenar septum, and the first metacarpal. The hypothenar compartment is contained by the hypothenar fascia and septum and the fifth metacarpal. The dorsal interosseous compartments lie between the metacarpals and are bounded by them laterally and the interosseous fascia anteriorly and posteriorly. The volar interosseous compartments lie on the volar aspect of the metacarpals, but it is unlikely that these are functionally separate from the dorsal interosseous compartments because the tissue barrier between the two cannot withstand pressures of more than 15 mm Hg.[48] The contents of the hand compartments are detailed in Table 29-10.

TREATMENT

The single most effective treatment for acute compartment syndrome is fasciotomy, which if delayed can cause devastating complications. Nevertheless, other preliminary measures should be taken in cases of impending acute compartment syndrome. The process may on occasion be aborted by release of external limiting envelopes such as dressings or plaster casts, including the padding under the cast. Splitting and spreading a cast has been shown to reduce ICP as has release of dressings.[38] The split and spread cast is the only method that can accommodate increasing limb swelling.[161] The limb should not be elevated above the height of the heart as this reduces the

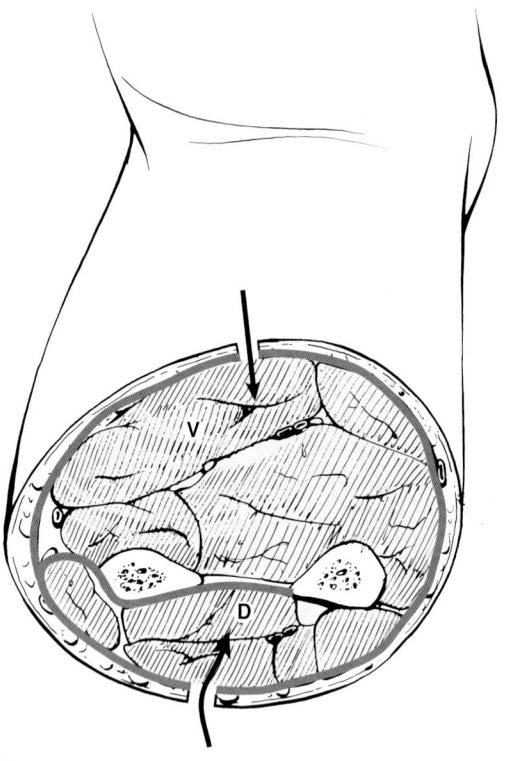

FIGURE 29-9 A cross section of the midforearm. The pronator quadratus compartment is not shown as it lies in the distal forearm. D, dorsal; V, volar.

and the antebrachial fascia as its anterior limit. Table 29-9 lists the contents and clinical signs of acute compartment syndrome in the volar compartment of the forearm. A suggestion has been made that the volar compartment of the forearm contains three spaces, the superficial volar, deep volar, and pronator quadratus spaces,[43] but in practice it is not usually necessary to distinguish between these at fasciotomy.[20]

TABLE 29-9	Compartments of the Forearm, Their Contents, and the Clinical Signs of Acute Compartment Syndrome
Compartment	**Contents**	**Signs**
Volar	Flexor carpi radialis longus and brevis Flexor digitorum superficialis and profundus Pronator teres Pronator quadratus Median nerve Ulnar nerve	Pain on passive wrist/finger extension Numbness—median/ulnar distribution Weakness—wrist/finger flexion Weakness—median/ulnar motor function in hand
Dorsal	Extensor digitorum Extensor pollicis longus Abductor pollicis longus Extensor carpi ulnaris	Pain—passive wrist/finger flexion Weakness—wrist/finger flexion
Mobile wad	Brachioradialis Extensor carpi radialis	Pain on passive wrist flexion/elbow extension Weakness—wrist extension/elbow flexion

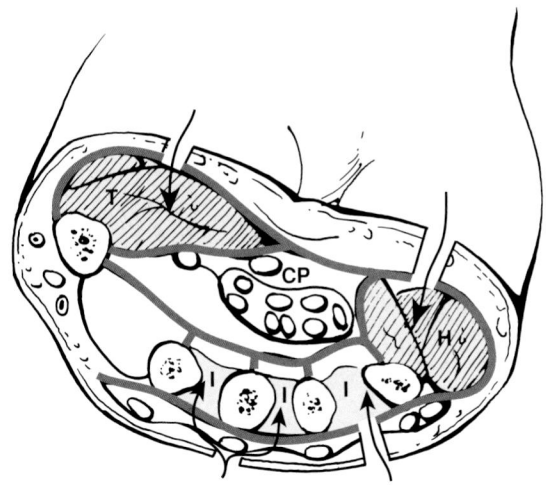

FIGURE 29-10 A cross section of the hand showing the muscle compartments. The adductor pollicis lies more distally. CP, central palmar; H, hypothenar; I, interosseous; T, thenar.

AV gradient.[92] Hypotension should be corrected because this will reduce perfusion pressure. Oxygen therapy should be instituted to ensure maximum oxygen saturation.

Fasciotomy

The basic principle of fasciotomy of any compartment is full and adequate decompression. Skin incisions must be made along the full length of the affected compartment. There is no place for limited or subcutaneous fasciotomy in acute compartment syndrome. It is essential to visualize all contained muscles in their entirety (Fig. 29-11) to assess their viability and any muscle necrosis must be thoroughly debrided to avoid infection. Subcutaneous fasciotomy is contraindicated for these reasons and also because the skin may act as a limiting boundary.[39]

In the leg, all four compartments should be released. One of the most commonly used techniques is the double incision four-compartment fasciotomy.[106] The anterior and lateral compartments are released through a lateral skin incision over the intermuscular septum between the compartments (Fig. 29-5). The skin may then be retracted to allow fascial incisions over

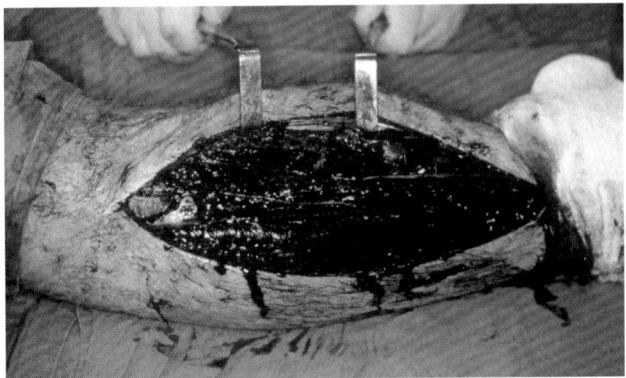

FIGURE 29-11 Fasciotomy of the anterior and lateral compartments of the leg. Note that the incision extends the whole length of the muscle compartment allowing inspection of all muscle groups.

both compartments. Care must be taken not to injure the superficial peroneal nerve that pierces the fascia and lies superficial to it in the distal third of the leg (Fig. 29-11). There is considerable variation in its course, with approximately three quarters of nerves remaining in the lateral compartment before its exit through the deep fascia and one quarter passing into the anterior compartment.[2]

The two posterior compartments are accessed through a skin incision 2 cm from the medial edge of the tibia (Fig. 29-5). This allows a generous skin bridge to the lateral incision but is anterior to the posterior tibial artery, especially in open fractures, to protect perforating vessels that supply local fasciocutaneous flaps. The superficial posterior compartment is easily exposed by skin retraction. The deep posterior compartment is exposed by posterior retraction of the superficial compartment and is most easily identified in the distal third of the leg (Fig. 29-12). It is sometimes necessary to elevate the superficial compartment muscles from the tibia for a short distance to allow release of the deep posterior compartment along its length. Care must be taken to protect the saphenous vein and nerve in this area and to protect the posterior tibial vessels and nerves.[121]

Single incision fasciotomy of all four compartments was first described using excision of the fibula,[74] but this is unnecessarily destructive and risks damage to the common peroneal

TABLE 29-10	The Compartments of the Hand and Their Contents
Compartment	Contents
Thenar	Abductor pollicis brevis Flexor pollicis brevis Opponens pollicis
Hypothenar	Abductor digiti minimi Flexor digiti minimi Opponens digiti minimi
Dorsal interosseous × 4	Dorsal interossei
Volar interossei × 3	Volar interossei
Adductor pollicis	Adductor pollicis

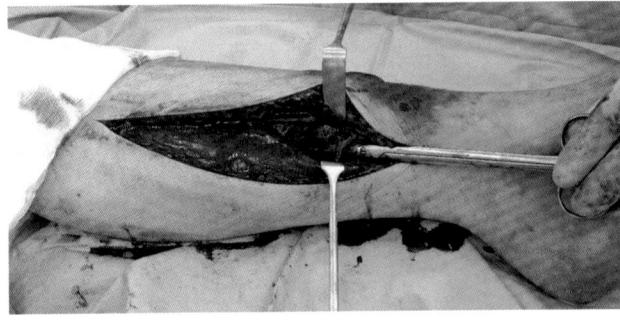

FIGURE 29-12 Decompression of the medial side of the leg. The superficial posterior compartment is being retracted to display the deep compartment. The scissors are deep to the fascia overlying the deep posterior compartment.

nerve. Single incision four-compartment fasciotomy without fibulectomy can be performed through a lateral incision that affords easy access to the anterior and lateral compartments.[22] Anterior retraction of the peroneal muscles allows exposure of the posterior intermuscular septum overlying the superficial posterior compartment. The deep posterior compartment is entered by an incision immediately posterior to the posterolateral border of the fibula.

Double incision fasciotomy is faster and probably safer than single incision methods because the fascial incisions are all superficial. Using the single incision method, it can be difficult to visualize the full extent of the deep posterior compartment. Both methods seem to be equally effective at reducing ICP.[106,154]

In the thigh and gluteal regions decompression is simple and the compartments are easily visualized. Both thigh compartments can be approached through a single lateral skin incision (Fig. 29-13),[148] although a medial incision can be used over the adductors if considered necessary (Fig. 29-4).

In the foot there are a number of compartments to decompress, and a sound knowledge of the anatomy is essential. Dorsal incisions overlying the second and fourth metacarpals allow sufficient access to the interosseous compartments and the central compartment that lies deep to the interosseous compartments (Fig. 29-6). The medial and lateral compartments can be accessed around the deep surfaces of the first and fifth metatarsal, respectively. Such a decompression is usually sufficient in cases of forefoot injury, but when a hindfoot injury, especially a calcaneal fracture, is present a separate medial incision may be required to decompress the calcaneal compartment (Fig. 29-7).[111,130]

Fasciotomy of the arm is performed through anterior and posterior incisions (Fig. 29-8) when the compartments are easily visualized. On rare occasions the deltoid muscle should also be decompressed.[28]

In the forearm both volar and dorsal fasciotomies may be performed. In most cases the volar compartment is approached first through an incision extending from the biceps tendon at the elbow to the palm of the hand to allow carpal tunnel decompression that is usually necessary (Fig. 29-14). Fascial incision then allows direct access to the compartment (Fig. 29-9). The deep flexors must be carefully inspected after fascial incision. Separate exposure and decompression of pronator

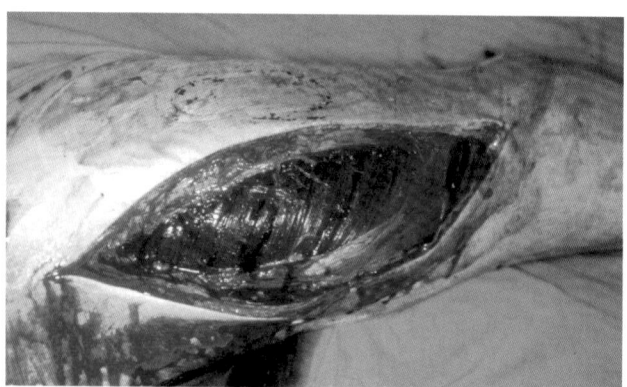

FIGURE 29-13 Fasciotomy of the thigh through a single lateral incision.

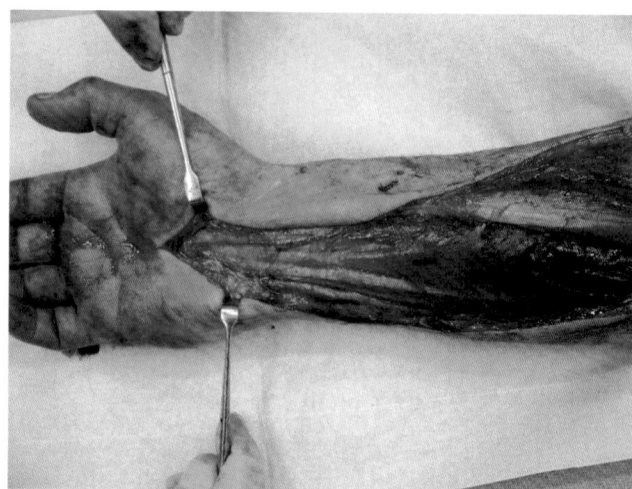

FIGURE 29-14 Fasciotomy of the forearm in a case of crush syndrome. There is necrosis of the forearm flexors proximally. The carpal tunnel has been decompressed.

quadratus may be necessary.[20] Usually volar fasciotomy is sufficient to decompress the forearm,[29] but if ICP remains elevated in the dorsal compartment perioperatively, then dorsal compression is easily performed through a straight dorsal incision (Fig. 29-9).

Decompression of the hand can usually be adequately achieved using two dorsal incisions that allow access to the interosseous compartments (Fig. 29-10). This may often be sufficient, but if there is clinical suspicion or raised ICP on measurement then incisions may be made over the thenar and hypothenar eminences, allowing fasciotomy of these compartments.

Management of Fasciotomy Wounds

Fasciotomy incisions must never be closed primarily because this may result in persistent elevation of ICP.[58] The wounds should be left open and dressed, and approximately 48 hours after fasciotomy a "second look" procedure should be undertaken to ensure viability of all muscle groups. Skin closure or cover should not be attempted unless all muscle groups are viable.

The type of closure or coverage required is predicted by age and type of injury with split skin grafting significantly more common in younger patients and crushing type injuries, presumably because of the increased muscle bulk in these groups.[29] The wounds may then be closed by delayed primary closure if possible, although this must be without tension on the skin edges. Commonly, in the leg this technique is possible in the medial but not the lateral wound. If delayed primary closure cannot be achieved, then the wound may be closed using either dermatotraction techniques or split skin grafting. Dermatotraction or gradual closure techniques have the advantage of avoiding the cosmetic problems of split skin grafting but may cause skin edge necrosis.[68] A further disadvantage is the prolonged time required to achieve closure, which may be up to 10 days.[11,68]

Split skin grafting, although offering immediate skin cover, has the disadvantage of a high rate of long-term morbidity.[35] The recent introduction of vacuum-assisted closure (VAC) systems is likely to be a significant advantage in this area and may reduce the need for split skin grafting with a low complication rate.[160]

Management of Associated Fractures

As is now generally accepted, fractures, especially of the long bones, should be stabilized in the presence of acute compartment syndrome treated by fasciotomy.[40,44,126,150] In reality the treatment of the fracture should not be altered by the presence of an acute compartment syndrome, although cast management of a tibial fracture is contraindicated in the presence of acute compartment syndrome. Fasciotomy should be performed prior to fracture stabilization to eliminate any unnecessary delay in decompression. Stabilization of the fracture allows easy access to the soft tissues and protects the soft tissues, allowing them to heal.

Reamed intramedullary nailing of the tibia confers excellent stabilization of a diaphyseal fracture and is now probably the treatment of choice in most centers for tibial diaphyseal fracture. Some authors, however, have implicated reaming as a possible cause of acute compartment syndrome.[76,103] This was refuted by other studies examining intercompartmental pressures during and after tibial nailing. McQueen et al.[97] studying reamed intramedullary nailing and Tornetta and French[149] studying unreamed intramedullary nailing agreed that the ICP increased perioperatively and dissipated postoperatively, and that nailing did not increase the likelihood of acute compartment syndrome. Nassif et al.[114] found no differences in ICP between reamed and unreamed nailing. In a group of 212 children and teenagers with tibial fractures treated with casting, external fixation, and locked and flexible nailing the fixation type was not predictive of acute compartment syndrome.[141]

Several factors may raise ICP during stabilization of tibial fractures. These include traction which raises pressure in the deep posterior compartment by approximately 6% per kilogram of weight applied.[137] .Countertraction using a thigh bar can cause external calf compression if the bar is wrongly positioned and can also decrease arterial flow and venous return, making the leg more vulnerable to ischemia. Elevation of the leg as in the 90-90 position decreases the tolerance of the limb to ischemia.[89] Thus excessive traction, poor positioning of the thigh bar, and high elevation of the leg should be avoided in patients at risk of acute compartment syndrome.

COMPLICATIONS OF ACUTE COMPARTMENT SYNDROME

Complications of acute compartment syndrome are unusual if the condition has been treated expeditiously. Delay in diagnosis has been cited as the single reason for failure in the management of acute compartment syndrome.[101] Delay to fasciotomy of more than 6 hours is likely to cause significant sequelae,[128] including muscle contractures, muscle weakness, sensory loss, infection, and nonunion of fractures.[23,27,41,54,59,71,79,87,89,98,103,123,140] In severe cases amputation may be necessary because of infection or lack of function.[33]

Late Diagnosis

There is some debate about the place of decompression when the diagnosis is made late and muscle necrosis is inevitable, whether because of a missed acute compartment syndrome or the crush syndrome. Little can be gained in exploring a closed crush syndrome when complete muscle necrosis is inevitable, except in circumstances where there are severe or potentially severe systemic effects when amputation may be necessary. Increased sepsis rates with potentially serious consequences have been reported when these cases have been explored.[122] Nonetheless, if partial muscle necrosis is suspected and compartment monitoring reveals pressures above the threshold for decompression, there may be an indication for fasciotomy to salvage remaining viable muscle. In these circumstances debridement of necrotic muscle must be thorough to reduce the chances of infection. In rare cases the ICP may be high enough to occlude major vessels. This is a further indication for fasciotomy to salvage the distal part of the limb.[122]

It is recommended that if there is no likelihood of any surviving muscle and compartment pressures are low, then fasciotomy should be withheld. If there is any possibility of any remaining viable muscle or if compartment pressures are above critical levels, fasciotomy should be performed to preserve any viable muscle. In any circumstances a thorough debridement of necrotic muscle is mandatory.

AUTHOR'S PREFERRED METHOD OF MANAGEMENT

Early diagnosis of acute compartment syndrome is essential, and it is important to be aware of the patients at risk of developing acute compartment syndrome. Good clinical examination techniques in the alert patient will help to identify the compartments at risk. Compartment monitoring should be used in all "at risk" patients as defined in Table 29-3. In practice this means that all tibial fractures should be monitored, but if resources to do so are limited, then younger patients should be selected for monitoring. The anterior compartment should be monitored, but in rare cases where symptoms are present that cannot be explained by the tissue pressures in the anterior compartment, the posterior compartment should also be monitored.

Fasciotomy is performed on the basis of a persistent differential pressure of less than 30 mm Hg (Fig. 29-15). If the ΔP is less than 30 mm Hg but the tissue pressure is dropping, as can happen for instance for a short time after tibial nailing, then the pressure may be observed for a short period in anticipation of the ΔP rising. On the other hand, if the ΔP remains less than 30 mm Hg or is reducing, then immediate fasciotomy is indicated. Delay and complications are minimized by making the decision to perform a fasciotomy primarily on the level of ΔP, with clinical symptoms and signs being used as an adjunct to diagnosis.

I prefer four-compartment fasciotomy in the leg because it is simpler and gives an excellent view of all compartments. If any muscle necrosis is present this should be thoroughly debrided. At this stage if a fracture is present, it should be stabilized if

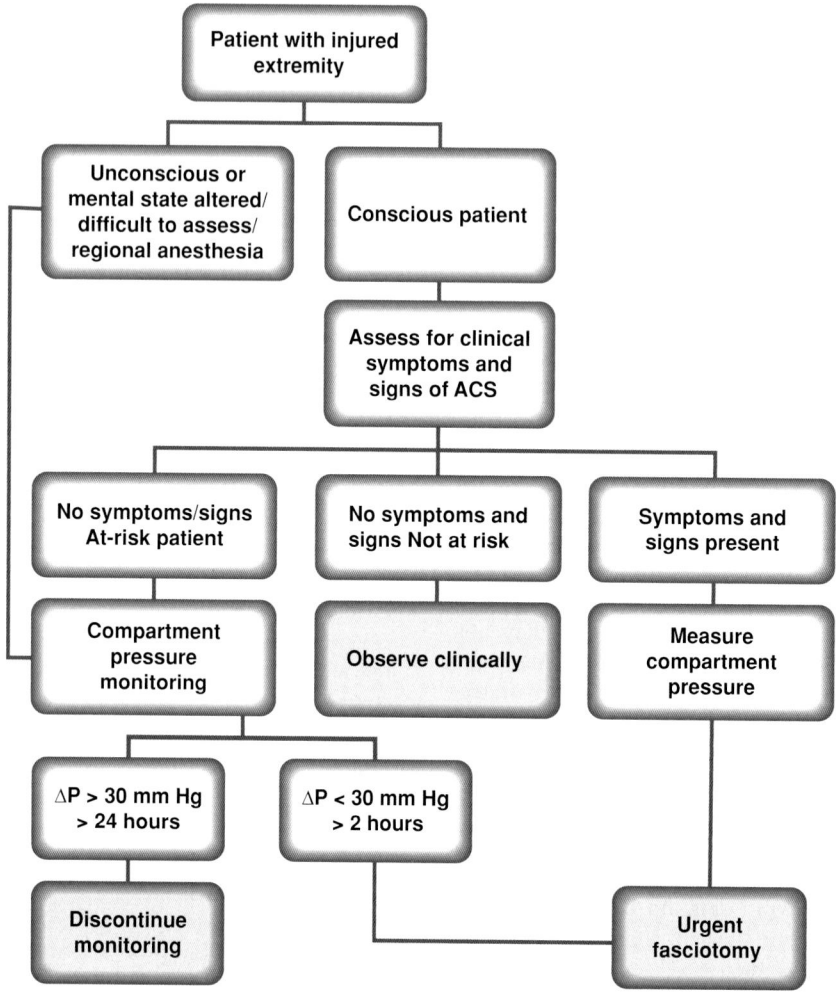

FIGURE 29-15 Compartment pressure monitoring.

this has not been done previously. Suction dressings if available should then be applied. A "re-look" procedure should be performed at 48 hours after fasciotomy with further debridement if necessary. If the wound is healthy closure should be undertaken at this stage with either direct closure or split skin grafting. I do not use gradual closure techniques because of the risk of wound edge necrosis and prolonged times to coverage. There is no indication to prolong closure beyond 48 hours unless there is residual muscle necrosis.

FUTURE DIRECTIONS

Acute compartment syndrome remains a potentially devastating complication of fracture that continues to be a significant cause of disability and successful litigation.[14,136] In a review of Canadian legal cases relating to ACS between 1998 and 2008 55% of cases had an unfavorable outcome for doctors or judgement for the plaintiff; 77% of plaintiffs had permanent disability. Orthopedic surgeons were assigned responsibility in the greatest numbers in both of these groups and the most frequent clinical issue was diagnostic failure or delay.[136] In a study from the United

States the most prominent risk factor for an indemnity payment was delay in diagnosis, and the number of hours delayed had a linear relationship to the value of the claim.[14] Delay to diagnosis was cited as the single cause of a poor outcome more than 40 years ago, yet there remains a remarkable lack of consistency in the methods used to diagnose the condition.[158,164] In light of the published high sensitivity and specificity of continuous ICP monitoring compared to that for the clinical diagnosis of ACS clinical diagnosis should no longer be the gold standard. Continuous ICP monitoring should be instituted in all patients at risk of ACS. Added to this, universally acceptable, clear, clinical guidelines are required to improve speed of diagnosis in all units managing trauma and would likely be the single biggest advance in the management of the condition.

Other future developments are likely to center on methods of measuring blood flow directly rather than indirectly by ICP measurement. Noninvasive methods of diagnosing acute compartment syndrome are being examined.[135] One such example is near-infrared spectroscopy, which measures the amount of oxygenated hemoglobin in muscle tissues transcutaneously.[5,42,64,142]

Methods of reducing the effects of acute compartment syndrome are also likely to play a part in the future. Some basic science research has already been published on the effects of antioxidants on the outcome of acute compartment syndrome with promising results.[72] This work should be extended to human studies in an attempt to reduce the effects of acute compartment syndrome in the clinical situation.

Prevention of acute compartment syndrome is the ultimate goal in its management. Attempts have been made to reduce ICP with the administration of hypertonic fluids intravenously,[13] but these have never been successful clinically. Nevertheless, an experiment on human subjects using tissue ultrafiltration to remove fluid from the compartment has been shown to reduce ICP.[116] Whether this technique can be useful clinically remains to be seen.

REFERENCES

1. Adams JG Jr, Dhar A, Shukla SD, et al. Effect of pentoxifylline on tissue injury and platelet-activating factor production during ischemia-reperfusion injury. J Vasc Surg. 1995;21:742–748.
2. Adkison DP, Bosse MJ, Gaccione DR, et al. Anatomical variations in the course of the superficial peroneal nerve. J Bone Joint Surg Am. 1991;73:112–114.
3. Al-Dadah OQ, Darrah C, Cooper A, et al. Continuous compartment pressure monitoring vs. clinical monitoring in tibial diaphyseal fractures. Injury. 2008;39:1204–1209.
4. Almdahl SM, Due J Jr, Samdal FA. Compartment syndrome with muscle necrosis following repair of hernia of tibialis anterior. Case report. Acta Chir Scand. 1987;153:695.
5. Arbabi S, Brundage SI, Gentilello LM. Near-infrared spectroscopy: a potential method for continuous, transcutaneous monitoring for compartmental syndrome in critically injured patients. J Trauma. 1999;47:829–833.
6. Ashton H. Critical closing pressure in human peripheral vascular beds. Clin Sci. 1962;22:79–87.
7. Ashton H. The effect of increased tissue pressure on blood flow. Clin Orthop Relat Res. 1975;15–26.
8. Bae DS, Kadiyala RK, Waters PM. Acute compartment syndrome in children: contemporary diagnosis, treatment, and outcome. J Pediatr Orthop. 2001;21:680–688.
9. Bardenheuer L. Die Anlang und Behandlung der ischaemische Muskellahmungen und Kontrakturen. Samml Klin Vortrage. 1911;122:437.
10. Belanger M, Fadale P. Compartment syndrome of the leg after arthroscopic examination of a tibial plateau fracture. Case report and review of the literature. Arthroscopy. 1997;13:646–651.
11. Berman SS, Schilling JD, McIntyre KE, et al. Shoelace technique for delayed primary closure of fasciotomies. Am J Surg. 1994;167:435–436.
12. Bernot M, Gupta R, Dobrasz J, et al. The effect of antecedent ischemia on the tolerance of skeletal muscle to increased interstitial pressure. J Orthop Trauma. 1996;10:555–559.
13. Better OS, Zinman C, Reis DN, et al. Hypertonic mannitol ameliorates intracompartmental tamponade in model compartment syndrome in the dog. Nephron. 1991;58:344–346.
14. Bhattacharyya T, Vrahas MS. The medical-legal aspects of compartment syndrome. J Bone Joint Surg Am. 2004;86-A:864–868.
15. Blaisdell FW. The pathophysiology of skeletal muscle ischemia and the reperfusion syndrome: a review. Cardiovasc Surg. 2002;10:620–630.
16. Blick SS, Brumback RJ, Poka A, et al. Compartment syndrome in open tibial fractures. J Bone Joint Surg Am. 1986;68:1348–1353.
17. Bradley EL III. The anterior tibial compartment syndrome. Surg Gynecol Obstet. 1973;136:289–297.
18. Buhr AJ, Cooke AM. Fracture patterns. Lancet. 1959;1:531–536.
19. Burton AC. On the physical equilibrium of small blood vessels. Am J Physiol. 1951;164:319–329.
20. Chan PS, Steinberg DR, Pepe MD, et al. The significance of the three volar spaces in forearm compartment syndrome: a clinical and cadaveric correlation. J Hand Surg Am. 1998;23:1077–1081.
21. Chautems RC, Irmay F, Magnin M, et al. Spontaneous anterior and lateral tibial compartment syndrome in a type I diabetic patient: case report. J Trauma. 1997;43:140–141.
22. Cooper GG. A method of single-incision, four compartment fasciotomy of the leg. Eur J Vasc Surg. 1992;6:659–661.
23. Court-Brown C, McQueen M. Compartment syndrome delays tibial union. Acta Orthop Scand. 1987;58:249–252.
24. Court-Brown CM, Byrnes T, McLaughlin G. Intramedullary nailing of tibial diaphyseal fractures in adolescents with open physes. Injury. 2003;34:781–785.
25. Court-Brown CM, McBirnie J. The epidemiology of tibial fractures. J Bone Joint Surg Br. 1995;77:417–421.
26. Davis ET, Harris A, Keene D, et al. The use of regional anaesthesia in patients at risk of acute compartment syndrome. Injury. 2006;37:128–133.
27. DeLee JC, Stiehl JB. Open tibia fracture with compartment syndrome. Clin Orthop Relat Res. 1981;160:175–184.
28. Diminick M, Shapiro G, Cornell C. Acute compartment syndrome of the triceps and deltoid. J Orthop Trauma. 1999;13:225–227.
29. Duckworth AD, Mitchell SE, Molyneux SG, et al. Acute compartment syndrome of the forearm. J Bone Joint Surg Am. 2012;94:e63.
30. Dudgeon LS. Volkmann's Contracture. Lancet. 1902;1:78–85.
31. Dunlop D, Parker PJ, Keating JF. Ruptured Baker's cyst causing posterior compartment syndrome. Injury. 1997;28:561–562.
32. Eaton RG, Green WT. Volkmann's ischemia. A volar compartment syndrome of the forearm. Clin Orthop Relat Res. 1975;113:58–64.
33. Finkelstein JA, Hunter GA, Hu RW. Lower limb compartment syndrome: course after delayed fasciotomy. J Trauma. 1996;40:342–344.
34. Finkemeier CG, Schmidt AH, Kyle RF, et al. A prospective, randomized study of intramedullary nails inserted with and without reaming for the treatment of open and closed fractures of the tibial shaft. J Orthop Trauma. 2000;14:187–193.
35. Fitzgerald AM, Gaston P, Wilson Y, et al. Long-term sequelae of fasciotomy wounds. Br J Plast Surg. 2000;53:690–693.
36. Foisie PS. Volkmann's Ischemic Contracture. N Engl J Med. 1942;226:679.
37. Frink M, Klaus AK, Kuther G, et al. Long term results of compartment syndrome of the lower limb in polytraumatised patients. Injury. 2007;38:607–613.
38. Garfin SR, Mubarak SJ, Evans KL, et al. Quantification of intracompartmental pressure and volume under plaster casts. J Bone Joint Surg Am. 1981;63:449–453.
39. Gaspard DJ, Kohl RD Jr. Compartmental syndromes in which the skin is the limiting boundary. Clin Orthop Relat Res. 1975;115–68.
40. Gelberman RH. Upper extremity compartment syndromes. In: Mubarak SJ, Hargens AR, eds. 1st ed. Philadelphia, PA: Saunders WB.; 1981.
41. Gelberman RH, Szabo RM, Williamson RV, et al. Tissue pressure threshold for peripheral nerve viability. Clin Orthop Relat Res. 1983;178:285–291.
42. Gentilello LM, Sanzone A, Wang L, et al. Near-infrared spectroscopy versus compartment pressure for the diagnosis of lower extremity compartmental syndrome using electromyography-determined measurements of neuromuscular function. J Trauma. 2001;51:1–8, discussion.
43. Gerber A, Masquelet AC. Anatomy and intracompartmental pressure measurement technique of the pronator quadratus compartment. J Hand Surg Am. 2001;26:1129–1134.
44. Gershuni DH, Mubarak SJ, Yaru NC, et al. Fracture of the tibia complicated by acute compartment syndrome. Clin Orthop Relat Res. 1987;217:221–227.
45. Gibson MJ, Barnes MR, Allen MJ, et al. Weakness of foot dorsiflexion and changes in compartment pressures after tibial osteotomy. J Bone Joint Surg Br. 1986;68:471–475.
46. Gillani S, Cao J, Suzuki T, et al. The effect of ischemia reperfusion injury on skeletal muscle. Injury. 2012;43:670–675.
47. Griffiths DL. Volkmann's ischemic contracture. Br J Surg. 1940;28:239–260.
48. Guyton GP, Shearman CM, Saltzman CL. Compartmental divisions of the hand revisited. Rethinking the validity of cadaver infusion experiments. J Bone Joint Surg Br. 2001A;83:241–244.
49. Guyton GP, Shearman CM, Saltzman CL. The compartments of the foot revisited. Rethinking the validity of cadaver infusion experiments. J Bone Joint Surg Br. 2001B;83:245–249.
50. Halpern AA, Nagel DA. Compartment syndromes of the forearm: early recognition using tissue pressure measurements. J Hand Surg Am. 1979;4:258–263.
51. Halpern AA, Nagel DA. Anterior compartment pressures in patients with tibial fractures. J Trauma. 1980;20:786–790.
52. Hargens AR, Akeson WH, Mubarak SJ, et al. Fluid balance within the canine anterolateral compartment and its relationship to compartment syndromes. J Bone Joint Surg Am. 1978;60:499–505.
53. Hargens AR, Akeson WH, Mubarak SJ, et al. Kappa Delta Award paper. Tissue fluid pressures: from basic research tools to clinical applications. J Orthop Res. 1989;7:902–909.
54. Hargens AR, Romine JS, Sipe JC, et al. Peripheral nerve-conduction block by high muscle-compartment pressure. J Bone Joint Surg Am. 1979;61:192–200.
55. Harrington P, Bunola J, Jennings AJ, et al. Acute compartment syndrome masked by intravenous morphine from a patient-controlled analgesia pump. Injury. 2000;31:387–389.
56. Harris IA, Kadir A, Donald G. Continuous compartment pressure monitoring for tibia fractures: does it influence outcome? J Trauma. 2006;60:1330–1335.
57. Hartsock LA, O'Farrell D, Seaber AV, et al. Effect of increased compartment pressure on the microcirculation of skeletal muscle. Microsurgery. 1998;18:67–71.
58. Havig MT, Leversedge FJ, Seiler JG III. Forearm compartment pressures: an in vitro analysis of open and endoscopic assisted fasciotomy. J Hand Surg Am. 1999;24:1289–1297.
59. Hayes C, Liauw S, Romaschin AD. Separation of reperfusion injury from ischemia induced necrosis. Surg Forum. 1988;39:306–308.
60. Heckman MM, Whitesides TE Jr, Grewe SR, et al. Histologic determination of the ischemic threshold of muscle in the canine compartment syndrome model. J Orthop Trauma. 1993;7:199–210.
61. Heckman MM, Whitesides TE Jr, Grewe SR, et al. Compartment pressure in association with closed tibial fractures. The relationship between tissue pressure, compartment, and the distance from the site of the fracture. J Bone Joint Surg Am. 1994;76:1285–1292.
62. Henriksen O. Orthostatic changes of blood flow in subcutaneous tissue in patients with arterial insufficiency of the legs. Scand J Clin Lab Invest. 1974;34:103–109.
63. Heppenstall RB, Sapega AA, Scott R, et al. The compartment syndrome. An experimental and clinical study of muscular energy metabolism using phosphorus nuclear magnetic resonance spectroscopy. Clin Orthop Relat Res. 1988;226:138–155.
64. Hildebrand O. Die Lehre von den ischamischen Muskellahmungen und Kontrakturen. Zeitschrift fur Chirurgie. 1906;108:44–201.
65. Holden CE. The pathology and prevention of Volkmann's ischaemic contracture. J Bone Joint Surg Br. 1979;61-B:296–300.
66. Hope MJ, McQueen MM. Acute compartment syndrome in the absence of fracture. J Orthop Trauma. 2004;18:220–224.
67. Hsu SI, Thadhani RI, Daniels GH. Acute compartment syndrome in a hypothyroid patient. Thyroid. 1995;5:305–308.
68. Janzing HM, Broos PL. Dermatotraction: an effective technique for the closure of fasciotomy wounds: a preliminary report of fifteen patients. J Orthop Trauma. 2001A;15:438–441.
69. Janzing HM, Broos PL. Routine monitoring of compartment pressure in patients with tibial fractures: Beware of overtreatment! Injury. 2001B;32:415–421.
70. Jepson PN. Ischaemic contracture: experimental study. Ann Surg. 1926;84:785–795.

71. Karlstrom G, Lonnerholm T, Olerud S. Cavus deformity of the foot after fracture of the tibial shaft. *J Bone Joint Surg Am.* 1975;57:893–900.

72. Kearns SR, Daly AF, Sheehan K, et al. Oral vitamin C reduces the injury to skeletal muscle caused by compartment syndrome. *J Bone Joint Surg Br.* 2004;86:906–911.

73. Kearns SR, Moneley D, Murray P, et al. Oral vitamin C attenuates acute ischaemia-reperfusion injury in skeletal muscle. *J Bone Joint Surg Br.* 2001;83:1202–1206.

74. Kelly RP, Whitesides TE. Transfibular route for fasciotomy of the leg. *J Bone Joint Surg Am.* 1967;49:1022–1023.

75. Kosir R, Moore FA, Selby JH, et al. Acute lower extremity compartment syndrome (ALECS) screening protocol in critically ill trauma patients. *J Trauma.* 2007;63:268–275.

76. Koval KJ, Clapper MF, Brumback RJ, et al. Complications of reamed intramedullary nailing of the tibia. *J Orthop Trauma.* 1991;5:184–189.

77. Labbe R, Lindsay T, Walker PM. The extent and distribution of skeletal muscle necrosis after graded periods of complete ischemia. *J Vasc Surg.* 1987;6:152–157.

78. Lam R, Lin PH, Alankar S, et al. Acute limb ischemia secondary to myositis-induced compartment syndrome in a patient with human immunodeficiency virus infection. *J Vasc Surg.* 2003;37:1103–1105.

79. Lindsay TF, Liauw S, Romaschin AD, et al. The effect of ischemia/reperfusion on adenine nucleotide metabolism and xanthine oxidase production in skeletal muscle. *J Vasc Surg.* 1990;12:8–15.

80. Manoli A, Weber TG. Fasciotomy of the foot: an anatomical study with special reference to release of the calcaneal compartment. *Foot Ankle.* 1990;10:267–275.

81. Mar GJ, Barrington MJ, McGuirk BR. Acute compartment syndrome of the lower limb and the effect of postoperative analgesia on diagnosis. *Br J Anaesth.* 2009;102:3–11.

82. Mars M, Hadley GP. Raised compartmental pressure in children: a basis for management. *Injury.* 1998;29:183–185.

83. Matava MJ, Whitesides TE Jr, Seiler JG III, et al. Determination of the compartment pressure threshold of muscle ischemia in a canine model. *J Trauma.* 1994;37:50–58.

84. Mathews PV, Perry JJ, Murray PC. Compartment syndrome of the well leg as a result of the hemilithotomy position: a report of two cases and review of literature. *J Orthop Trauma.* 2001;15:580–583.

85. Matsen FA III. *Compartmental Syndromes.* 1st ed. New York, NY: Grune and Stratton; 1980.

86. Matsen FA III, Clawson DK. The deep posterior compartmental syndrome of the leg. *J Bone Joint Surg Am.* 1975;57:34–39.

87. Matsen FA III, King RV, Krugmire RB Jr, et al. Physiological effects of increased tissue pressure. *Int Orthop.* 1979;3:237–244.

88. Matsen FA III, Krugmire RB Jr. Compartmental syndromes. *Surg Gynecol Obstet.* 1978;147:943–949.

89. Matsen FA III, Mayo KA, Krugmire RB Jr, et al. A model compartmental syndrome in man with particular reference to the quantification of nerve function. *J Bone Joint Surg Am.* 1977;59:648–653.

90. Matsen FA III, Mayo KA, Sheridan GW, et al. Monitoring of intramuscular pressure. *Surgery.* 1976;79:702–709.

91. Matsen FA III, Winquist RA, Krugmire RB Jr. Diagnosis and management of compartmental syndromes. *J Bone Joint Surg Am.* 1980;62:286–291.

92. Matsen FA III, Wyss CR, Krugmire RB Jr, et al. The effects of limb elevation and dependency on local arteriovenous gradients in normal human limbs with particular reference to limbs with increased tissue pressure. *Clin Orthop Relat Res.* 1980;187–195.

93. McDermott AG, Marble AE, Yabsley RH. Monitoring acute compartment pressures with the S.T.I.C. catheter. *Clin Orthop Relat Res.* 1984;190:192–198.

94. McKee MD, Jupiter JB. Acute exercise-induced bilateral anterolateral leg compartment syndrome in a healthy young man. *Am J Orthop (Belle Mead NJ).* 1995;24:862–864.

95. McQueen MM. The effect of acute compartment syndrome on bone blood flow and bone union [Thesis] University of Edinburgh; 1995.

96. McQueen MM, Christie J, Court-Brown CM. Compartment pressures after intramedullary nailing of the tibia. *J Bone Joint Surg Br.* 1990;72:395–397.

97. McQueen MM, Christie J, Court-Brown CM. Acute compartment syndrome in tibial diaphyseal fractures. *J Bone Joint Surg Br.* 1996;78:95–98.

98. McQueen MM, Court-Brown CM. Compartment monitoring in tibial fractures. The pressure threshold for decompression. *J Bone Joint Surg Br.* 1996;78:99–104.

99. McQueen MM, Duckworth AD, Aitken SA, et al. The estimated sensitivity and specificity of compartment pressure monitoring for acute compartment syndrome. *J Bone Joint Surg Am.* 2013;95:673–677.

100. McQueen MM, Gaston P, Court-Brown CM. Acute compartment syndrome. Who is at risk? *J Bone Joint Surg Br.* 2000;82:200–203.

101. McQuillan WM, Nolan B. Ischaemia complicating injury. A report of thirty-seven cases. *J Bone Joint Surg Br.* 1968;50:482–492.

102. Mithoefer K, Lhowe DW, Vrahas MS, et al. Functional outcome after acute compartment syndrome of the thigh. *J Bone Joint Surg Am.* 2006;88:729–737.

103. Moed BR, Strom DE. Compartment syndrome after closed intramedullary nailing of the tibia: a canine model and report of two cases. *J Orthop Trauma.* 1991;5:71–77.

104. Moed BR, Thorderson PK. Measurement of intracompartmental pressure: a comparison of the slit catheter, side-ported needle, and simple needle. *J Bone Joint Surg Am.* 1993;75:231–235.

105. Mubarak SJ, Hargens AR, Owen CA, et al. The wick catheter technique for measurement of intramuscular pressure. A new research and clinical tool. *J Bone Joint Surg Am.* 1976;58:1016–1020.

106. Mubarak SJ, Owen CA. Double-incision fasciotomy of the leg for decompression in compartment syndromes. *J Bone Joint Surg Am.* 1977;59:184–187.

107. Mubarak SJ, Owen CA, Hargens AR, et al. Acute compartment syndromes: diagnosis and treatment with the aid of the wick catheter. *J Bone Joint Surg Am.* 1978;60:1091–1095.

108. Mubarak SJ, Wilton NC. Compartment syndromes and epidural analgesia. *J Pediatr Orthop.* 1997;17:282–284.

109. Mullett H, Al-Abed K, Prasad CV, et al. Outcome of compartment syndrome following intramedullary nailing of tibial diaphyseal fractures. *Injury.* 2001;32:411–413.

110. Murphy JB. Myositis. *JAMA.* 1914;63:1249–1255.

111. Myerson M, Manoli A. Compartment syndromes of the foot after calcaneal fractures. *Clin Orthop Relat Res.* 1993;290:142–150.

112. Myerson MS. Management of compartment syndromes of the foot. *Clin Orthop Relat Res.* 1991;271:239–248.

113. Nario CV. La enfermedad de Volkman experimental. *Ann Fac Med Montivideo.* 1938;10:87–128.

114. Nassif JM, Gorczyca JT, Cole JK, et al. Effect of acute reamed versus unreamed intramedullary nailing on compartment pressure when treating closed tibial shaft fractures: a randomized prospective study. *J Orthop Trauma.* 2000;14:554–558.

115. Nichol J, Girling F, Jerrard W, et al. Fundamental instability of the small blood vessels and critical closing pressures in vascular beds. *Am J Physiol.* 1951;164:330–344.

116. Odland R, Schmidt AH, Hunter B, et al. Use of tissue ultrafiltration for treatment of compartment syndrome: a pilot study using porcine hindlimbs. *J Orthop Trauma.* 2005;19:267–275.

117. Ovre S, Hvaal K, Holm I, et al. Compartment pressure in nailed tibial fractures. A threshold of 30 mmHg for decompression gives 29% fasciotomies. *Arch Orthop Trauma Surg.* 1998;118:29–31.

118. Peterson F. Uber ischamische Muskellahmung. *Arch Klin Chir.* 1888;37:675–677.

119. Petrasek PF, Homer-Vanniasinkam S, Walker PM. Determinants of ischemic injury to skeletal muscle. *J Vasc Surg.* 1994;19:623–631.

120. Prasarn ML, Ouellette EA, Livingstone A, et al. Acute pediatric upper extremity compartment syndrome in the absence of fracture. *J Pediatr Orthop.* 2009;29:263–268.

121. Pyne D, Jawad AS, Padhiar N. Saphenous nerve injury after fasciotomy for compartment syndrome. *Br J Sports Med.* 2003;37:541–542.

122. Reis ND, Michaelson M. Crush injury to the lower limbs. Treatment of the local injury. *J Bone Joint Surg Am.* 1986;68:414–418.

123. Reverte MM, Dimitriou R, Kanakaris NK, et al. What is the effect of compartment syndrome and fasciotomies on fracture healing in tibial fractures? *Injury.* 2011;42:1402–1407.

124. Roddie IC, Shepherd JT. Evidence for critical closure of digital resistance vessels with reduced transmural pressure and passive dilatation with increased venous pressure. *J Physiol.* 1957;136:498–506.

125. Rodriguez-Merchan EC. Acute compartment syndrome in haemophilia. *Blood Coagul Fibrinolysis.* 2013;24:677–682.

126. Rorabeck CH. The treatment of compartment syndromes of the leg. *J Bone Joint Surg Br.* 1984;66:93–97.

127. Rorabeck CH, Castle GS, Hardie R, et al. Compartmental pressure measurements: an experimental investigation using the slit catheter. *J Trauma.* 1981;21:446–449.

128. Rorabeck CH, Macnab L. Anterior tibial-compartment syndrome complicating fractures of the shaft of the tibia. *J Bone Joint Surg Am.* 1976;58:549–550.

129. Rowlands RP. A case of Volkmann's contracture treated by shortening the radius and ulna. *Lancet.* 1905;2:1168–1171.

130. Sanders R. Displaced intra-articular fractures of the calcaneus. *J Bone Joint Surg Am.* 2000;82:225–250.

131. Schwartz JT Jr, Brumback RJ, Lakatos R, et al. Acute compartment syndrome of the thigh. A spectrum of injury. *J Bone Joint Surg Am.* 1989;71:392–400.

132. Seddon HJ. Volkmann's ischaemia in the lower limb. *J Bone Joint Surg Br.* 1966;48:627–636.

133. Seiler JG III, Valadie AL III, Drvaric DM, et al. Perioperative compartment syndrome. A report of four cases. *J Bone Joint Surg Am.* 1996;78:600–602.

134. Shabat S, Carmel A, Cohen Y, et al. Iatrogenic forearm compartment syndrome in a cardiac intensive care unit induced by brachial artery puncture and acute anticoagulation. *J Interv Cardiol.* 2002;15:107–109.

135. Shadgan B, Menon M, O'Brien PJ, et al. Diagnostic techniques in acute compartment syndrome of the leg. *J Orthop Trauma.* 2008;22:581–587.

136. Shadgan B, Menon M, Sanders D, et al. Current thinking about acute compartment syndrome of the lower extremity. *Can J Surg.* 2010;53:329–334.

137. Shakespeare DT, Henderson NJ. Compartmental pressure changes during calcaneal traction in tibial fractures. *J Bone Joint Surg Br.* 1982;64:498–499.

138. Shakespeare DT, Henderson NJ, Clough G. The slit catheter: a comparison with the wick catheter in the measurement of compartment pressure. *Injury.* 1982;13:404–408.

139. Shereff MJ. Compartment syndromes of the foot. *Instr Course Lect.* 1990;39:127–132.

140. Sheridan GW, Matsen FA III, Krugmire RB Jr. Further investigations on the pathophysiology of the compartmental syndrome. *Clin Orthop Relat Res.* 1977;123:266–270.

141. Shore BJ, Glotzbecker MP, Zurakowski D, et al. Acute compartment syndrome in children and teenagers with tibial shaft fractures: incidence and multivariable risk factors. *J Orthop Trauma.* 2013;27:616–621.

142. Shuler MS, Reisman WM, Cole AL, et al. Near-infrared spectroscopy in acute compartment syndrome: Case report. *Injury.* 2011;42:1506–1508.

143. Shuler MS, Reisman WM, Kinsey TL, et al. Correlation between muscle oxygenation and compartment pressures in acute compartment syndrome of the leg. *J Bone Joint Surg Am.* 2010;92:863–870.

144. Shuler MS, Reisman WM, Whitesides TE Jr, et al. Near-infrared spectroscopy in lower extremity trauma. *J Bone Joint Surg Am.* 2009;91:1360–1368.

145. Stott NS, Zionts LE, Holtom PD, et al. Acute hematogenous osteomyelitis. An unusual cause of compartment syndrome in a child. *Clin Orthop Relat Res.* 1995;317:219–222.

146. Styf JR, Crenshaw A, Hargens AR. Intramuscular pressures during exercise. Comparison of measurements with and without infusion. *Acta Orthop Scand.* 1989;60:593–596.

147. Sweeney HE, O'Brien GF. Bilateral anterior tibial syndrome in association with the nephrotic syndrome. Report of a case. *Arch Intern Med.* 1965;116:487–490.

148. Tarlow SD, Achterman CA, Hayhurst J, et al. Acute compartment syndrome in the thigh complicating fracture of the femur. A report of three cases. *J Bone Joint Surg Am.* 1986;68:1439–1443.

149. Tornetta P III, French BG. Compartment pressures during nonreamed tibial nailing without traction. *J Orthop Trauma.* 1997;11:24–27.

150. Turen CH, Burgess AR, Vanco B. Skeletal stabilization for tibial fractures associated with acute compartment syndrome. *Clin Orthop Relat Res.* 1995;315:163–168.

151. Ulmer T. The clinical diagnosis of compartment syndrome of the lower leg: are clinical findings predictive of the disorder? *J Orthop Trauma.* 2002;16:572–577.
152. Veeragandham RS, Paz IB, Nadeemanee A. Compartment syndrome of the leg secondary to leukemic infiltration: a case report and review of the literature. *J Surg Oncol.* 1994;55:198–200.
153. Vigasio A, Battiston B, De FG, et al. Compartmental syndrome due to viper bite. *Arch Orthop Trauma Surg.* 1991;110:175–177.
154. Vitale GC, Richardson JD, George SM Jr, et al. Fasciotomy for severe, blunt and penetrating trauma of the extremity. *Surg Gynecol Obstet.* 1988;166:397–401.
155. Volkmann RV. Die ischaemischen Muskellahmungen und Kontrakturen. *Zentrabl Chir.* 1882;8:801–803.
156. Vollmar B, Westermann S, Menger MD. Microvascular response to compartment syndrome-like external pressure elevation: an in vivo fluorescence microscopic study in the hamster striated muscle. *J Trauma.* 1999;46:91–96.
157. Walker PM, Lindsay TF, Labbe R, et al. Salvage of skeletal muscle with free radical scavengers. *J Vasc Surg.* 1987;5:68–75.
158. Wall CJ, Richardson MD, Lowe AJ, et al. Survey of management of acute, traumatic compartment syndrome of the leg in Australia. *ANZ J Surg.* 2007;77:733–737.
159. Wallis FC. Treatment of paralysis and muscular atrophy after the prolonged use of splints or of an Esmarch's cord. *The Practitioner.* 1907;67:429–436.
160. Webb LX. New techniques in wound management: vacuum-assisted wound closure. *J Am Acad Orthop Surg.* 2002;10:303–311.
161. White TO, Howell GE, Will EM, et al. Elevated intramuscular compartment pressures do not influence outcome after tibial fracture. *J Trauma.* 2003;55:1133–1138.
162. Whitesides TE, Haney TC, Morimoto K, et al. Tissue pressure measurements as a determinant for the need of fasciotomy. *Clin Orthop Relat Res.* 1975;113:43–51.
163. Williams J, Gibbons M, Trundle H, et al. Complications of nailing in closed tibial fractures. *J Orthop Trauma.* 1995;9:476–481.
164. Williams PR, Russell ID, Mintowt-Czyz WJ. Compartment pressure monitoring–current UK orthopaedic practice. *Injury.* 1998;29:229–232.
165. Willis RB, Rorabeck CH. Treatment of compartment syndrome in children. *Orthop Clin North Am.* 1990;21:401–412.
166. Willy C, Gerngross H, Sterk J. Measurement of intracompartmental pressure with use of a new electronic transducer-tipped catheter system. *J Bone Joint Surg Am.* 1999;81:158–168.
167. Wright JG, Bogoch ER, Hastings DE. The 'occult' compartment syndrome. *J Trauma.* 1989;29:133–134.
168. Yamada S. Effects of positive tissue pressure on blood flow of the finger. *J Appl Physiol.* 1954;6:495–500.

Upper Extremity

30

HAND FRACTURES AND DISLOCATIONS

Mark H. Henry

INTRODUCTION TO HAND FRACTURES AND DISLOCATIONS

Fractures and dislocations of the hand are some of the most frequently encountered musculoskeletal injuries. In Canada, the annual incidence was found to be 29 per 10,000 in people older than 20 years of age, and 61 per 10,000 in people younger than 20 years of age.[55] Males had 2.08 times greater risk until after age 65 when females become at greater risk.[55,153] Another study reported 3.7 hand fractures per year per 1,000 men compared with 1.3 hand fractures per year per 1,000 women.[8] The 1998

United States National Hospital Ambulatory Medical Care Survey found phalangeal (23%) and metacarpal (18%) fractures to be the second and third most common fractures below the elbow, peaking in the third decade for men and the second decade for women.[29] Another series of 1,358 fractures reported the distribution as 57.4% for proximal phalanx, 30.4% for middle phalanx, and 12.2% for metacarpal.[90] Of 502 phalangeal fractures, 192 were at the proximal phalanx (P1), 195 at the middle phalanx (P2), and 115 at the distal phalanx (P3).[175] The small finger axis is the most commonly injured, constituting as high as 37% of total hand fractures.[153]

ASSESSMENT OF HAND FRACTURES AND DISLOCATIONS

Hand Fractures and Dislocations Injury Mechanisms

The mechanism of injury description should include the magnitude, direction, point of contact, and type of force that caused the trauma. The high degree of variation with respect to mechanism of injury accounts for the broad spectrum of patterns seen in hand trauma. Axial load or "jamming" injuries are frequently sustained during ball sports or sudden reaches made during everyday activities such as in catching a falling object. Patterns frequently resulting from this mechanism are shearing articular fractures or metaphyseal compression fractures. Axial loading along the upper extremity must also raise suspicion of associated injuries to the carpus, forearm, elbow, and shoulder girdle. Diaphyseal fractures and joint dislocations usually require a bending component in the mechanism of injury, which can occur during ball-handling sports or when the hand is trapped by an object and unable to move with the rest of the arm. Individual digits can easily be caught in clothing, furniture, or workplace equipment to sustain torsional mechanisms of injury, resulting in spiral fractures or more complex dislocation patterns. Industrial settings or other environments with heavy objects and high forces lead to crushing mechanisms that combine bending, shearing, and torsion to produce unique patterns of skeletal injury and significant associated soft tissue damage.

Injuries Associated with Hand Fractures and Dislocations

Open Injuries

The integument is easily damaged, and open fractures are common. Open wounds should not be probed in the emergency department; doing so may only drive surface contaminants deeper and rarely yields useful information. The need for prophylactic antibiotics in open hand fractures is controversial. The previous standard administration of Ancef no longer appears applicable with methicillin-resistant *Staphylococcus aureus* (MRSA) dominating most community-acquired infection profiles. Clindamycin, vancomycin, Bactrim, and the quinolones are useful agents against MRSA. Aminoglycosides are added for contaminated wounds and penicillin for soil or farm environments. No hard evidence exists to support continuation of antibiotics beyond the initial 24 hours. The exception to this may be bite wounds whose potential for osteomyelitis is significant if the tooth directly penetrates the cortex, allowing the saliva into the cancellous structure. Aggressive and early surgical debridement is needed for all bite wounds.

The distal phalanx directly supports the nail matrix. With substantial displacement of the dorsal cortex, nail matrix disruption should be expected and direct repair planned. Reconstruction of residual open wounds overlying skeletal injury sites requires the use of flaps. Frequently, transposition flaps will suffice. Less frequently, pedicle or free flaps will prove necessary.[80,76] The greatest challenge in the hand, and particularly the digit, is to achieve both thin and supple tissue coverage. A fascial flap covered with a split thickness skin graft provides this combination of features except at the volar pulp where a directly innervated glabrous cutaneous flap is needed (Fig. 30-1).

Tendons

Closed extensor tendon ruptures near insertion points may accompany dislocations. Prime examples are terminal tendon ruptures sustained in association with distal interphalangeal (DIP) joint injuries and central slip ruptures sustained in association with proximal interphalangeal (PIP) joint injuries. Initial examination of the traumatized hand must include a survey that documents each potential tendon injury. Apart from these, tendon damage usually only occurs with an associated laceration or in open combined injuries.

Nerves and Vessels

Apart from open combined injuries, these tissues are rarely injured as part of simple fractures and dislocations of the hand. In major open hand trauma, there is usually a significant zone of injury. Appropriate treatment includes excision of the devitalized tissues in the zone of injury including nerve and vessel tissues followed by reconstruction with autogenous grafts or adjacent transfers.

Combined Injuries

The term combined refers to the association of a hand fracture with injury to at least one of the soft tissues listed above. These are most often open injuries with the soft tissue component of greatest significance being the injury to flexor tendons, extensor tendons, or both. The occurrence of this combined pattern of injury directly impacts the treatment strategy for the fracture itself. Many fracture patterns presenting as an isolated injury would be best cared for nonoperatively or with closed reduction and internal fixation (CRIF) using smooth stainless steel Kirschner wires (K-wires). The open wound leading to the fracture site automatically changes the surgical approach to open reduction, usually with open reduction and internal fixation (ORIF). The presence of an adjacent tendon repair site necessitates achieving skeletal stability sufficient to withstand the forces of an immediate tendon glide rehabilitation program. This often means the use of rigid internal fixation (Fig. 30-2). In a study limited to ORIF of intra-articular fractures, comminution and an initial open injury were identified as independent variables leading to a worse prognosis.[164] Only 6 of 16 patients in another study of comminuted phalangeal fractures and associated soft tissue injuries achieved greater than 180 degrees of total active motion (TAM).[34] The remainder of this chapter describes the most appropriate techniques for managing fractures and dislocations of the hand as isolated injuries.

Massive Hand Trauma

The comprehensive planning required for treatment of massive hand trauma merits a textbook in its own right and is beyond

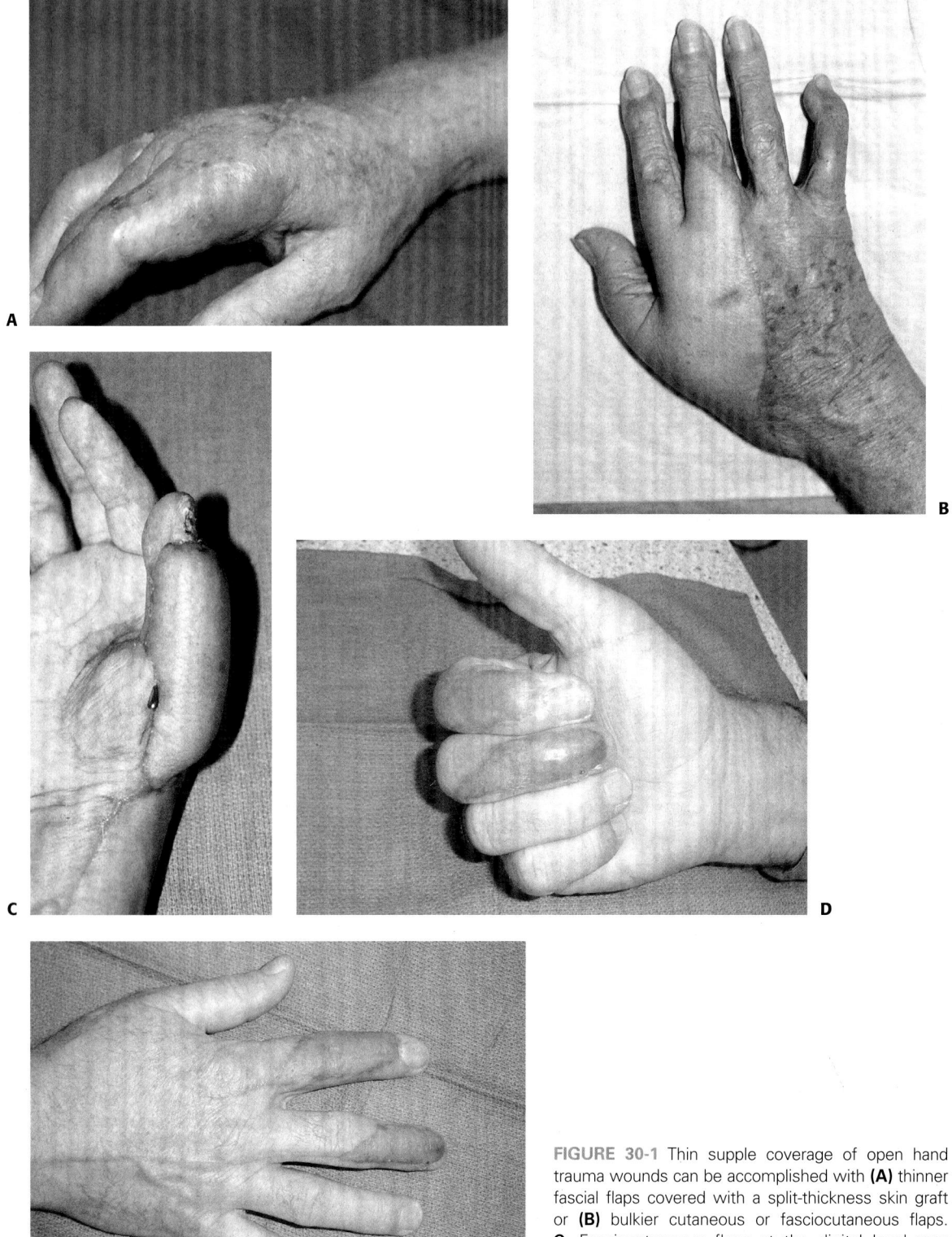

FIGURE 30-1 Thin supple coverage of open hand trauma wounds can be accomplished with **(A)** thinner fascial flaps covered with a split-thickness skin graft or **(B)** bulkier cutaneous or fasciocutaneous flaps. **C:** Fasciocutaneous flaps at the digital level may demonstrate an even more substantial difference when compared with the thinness and flexibility of a grafted fascial flap **(D, E).**

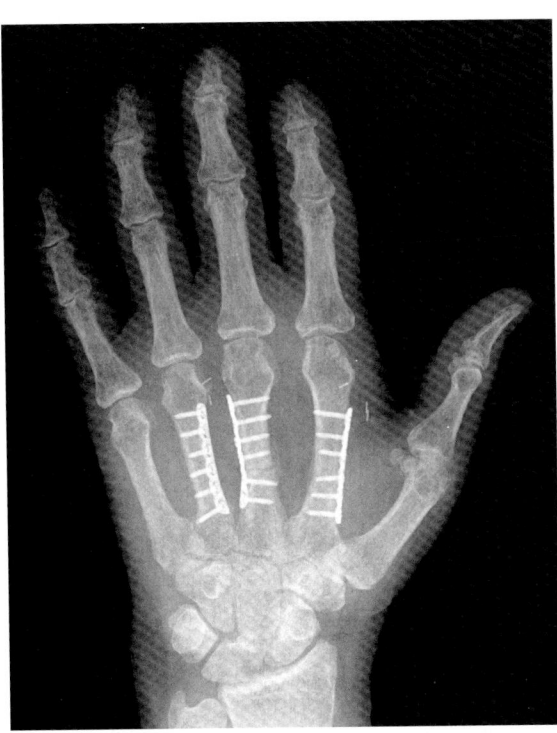

FIGURE 30-2 Major open hand trauma frequently requires the most stable forms of fixation to facilitate an aggressive early motion rehabilitation program focusing on tendon gliding.

the scope of this chapter. The majority of the complex decision-making in these injuries occurs with respect to the strategy chosen for the soft tissues (Fig. 30-3). With true degloving injuries and exposed bone and tendon, either pedicle or free flaps are required for coverage. Pedicle flaps are simpler and faster, but are limited in size and reach and are associated with a higher complication rate than thin fascial free flaps that can cover a defect of any size and shape.[80,76] Clinical evaluation of these injuries is quite difficult because the patient is often unable or unwilling to do very much with respect to an interactive examination. Much of the determination regarding the extent of injury is made intraoperatively. Good quality radiographs are rarely obtained initially and usually consist of semi-oblique views of the hand with a high degree of bone overlap. Every effort should be made within the scope of total patient management to obtain additional radiographic views that can be set up properly so that associated injuries are not missed. More often than not the opportunity for these views first presents itself in the operating room. A very easy pitfall is to draw attention to the most obvious radiographic findings without taking the time to search for more subtle injuries. Radiographic evidence of foreign matter embedded in the hand should be sought as well as its absence at the conclusion of the debridement.

The Gustilo classification of open fractures has been modified for the hand by reducing the 10-cm wound length threshold to 2 cm. The validity of the classification is supported by 62.5% normal hand function found after type I injuries compared with 21% following type III fractures.[116] Another series found 92% poor results associated with grade IIIB and III C

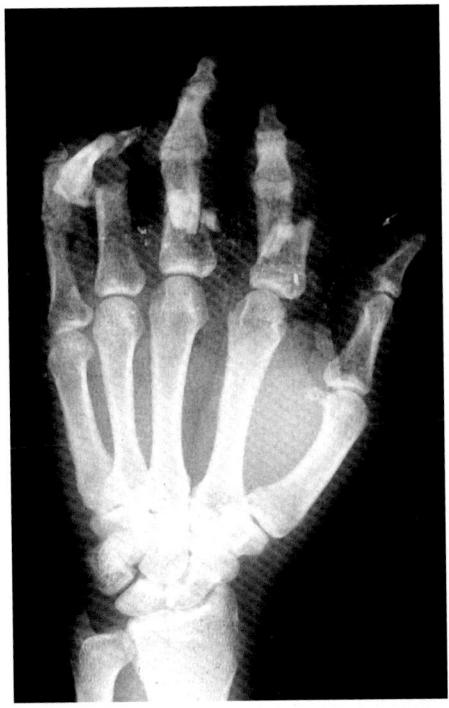

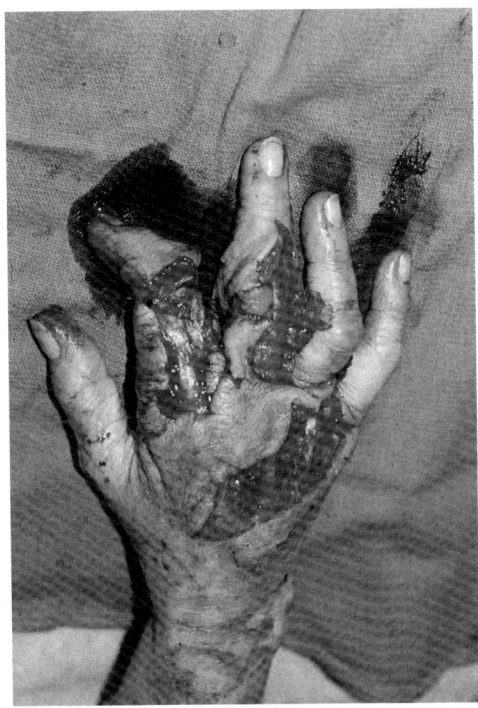

FIGURE 30-3 Massive crushing trauma to the hand usually causes its most devastating effects, not to **(A)** the skeletal elements themselves, but rather diffusely through devitalization of **(B)** the soft tissues covering the bone.

injuries.[46] From a series of 200 open hand fractures, Swanson et al.[159] differentiated type II wounds from type I wounds by three criteria: contamination at initial presentation, open for more than 24 hours before treatment, or in patients with systemic illness. Primary closure is not recommended for type II wounds.

Both internal and external fixation may be appropriate in massive hand injuries. Standard indications for external fixation include gross contamination of the original wound, segmental bone loss or comminution, or the lack of availability of good soft tissue coverage.[35] The biomechanics of external fixation in the hand are the same as elsewhere in the body with pin diameter constituting the chief determinant of fixator stiffness. Four pins, two proximally and two distally, are sufficient for most hand applications. A given hand injury may best be fixed by all internal, all external, or a combination of the two methods of fixation. An improved understanding and a wider array of elegant soft tissue coverage techniques have overcome previous concerns regarding exposure of hardware with internal fixation.[80,76]

Whenever the injury involves the first web space (especially with crush injuries) the thumb and index metacarpals should be pinned into abduction to prevent a first web space contracture. No matter how the injury is managed, the strategy should plan for rehabilitation to begin, unobstructed by bulky external dressings, by 72 hours after surgery. In one series, 72 metacarpal and phalangeal fractures with severe associated soft tissue injury were treated with plates and screws yielding 46% good, 32% fair, and 22% poor results by the American Society for Surgery of the Hand (ASSH) criteria of TAM.[24] The overall results for treatment of these severe injuries are most closely related to the soft tissue component rather than the status of the skeletal injury.[67] In 245 open injuries studied prospectively, extensor tendon injury alone had 50% poor results, but flexor tendon or multiple soft tissue injuries produced 80% poor results.[28] A series of 140 open fractures demonstrated better results at the metacarpal compared with the phalangeal level with the worst outcomes occurring for injuries at the proximal phalanx (P1) and PIP level, especially when associated with an overlying tendon injury.[46]

Bone Loss

Segmental bone loss is a frequent finding in massive hand injuries. Once the wound has been rendered clean through either a single or multiple debridements, bone grafting is appropriate using corticocancellous bone or just cancellous bone, shaped and sized to match the curvature and volume of the missing segment. Stable fixation is achieved with either internal plate or external fixator application (Fig. 30-4). With proper debridement, immediate primary bone grafting is safe. A series of 12 patients with type III open fractures and another 20 patients with low-velocity gunshot phalangeal fractures both demonstrated 0% infection rates with the use of immediate autograft.[66,139] If delayed bone grafting is planned, a temporary spacer may be used to preserve the volume that will later be occupied by the graft (Fig. 30-5). Bone loss that includes the articular surface represents an entirely different and much more complex problem. Strategies that have been advocated include autografts of metatarsal head, second, and third carpometacarpal (CMC) joints; immediate Silastic prosthetic replacement;

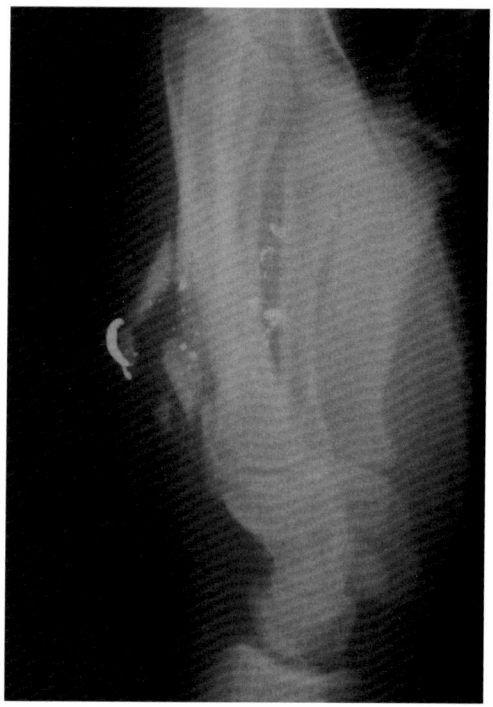
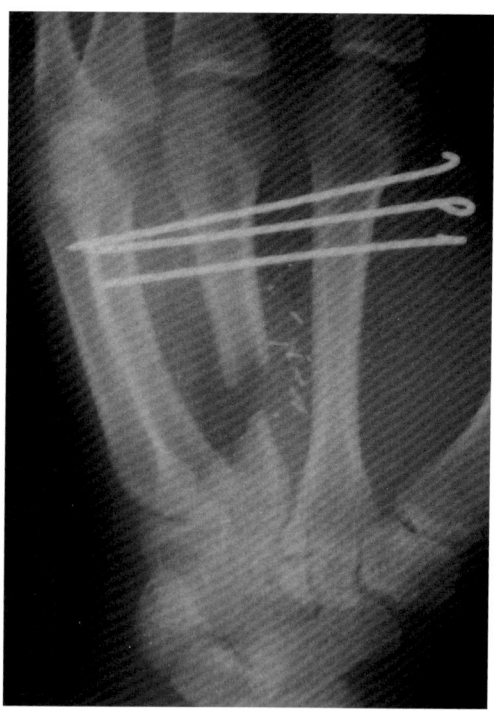

FIGURE 30-4 When segmental bone loss occurs **(A)**, shortening may be prevented by temporary stabilization **(B)**.

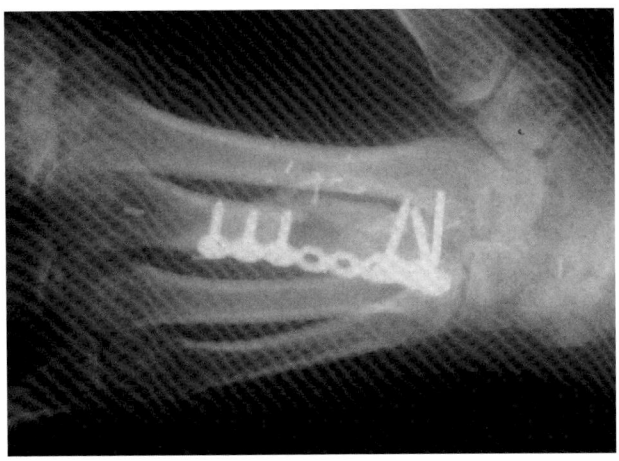

C

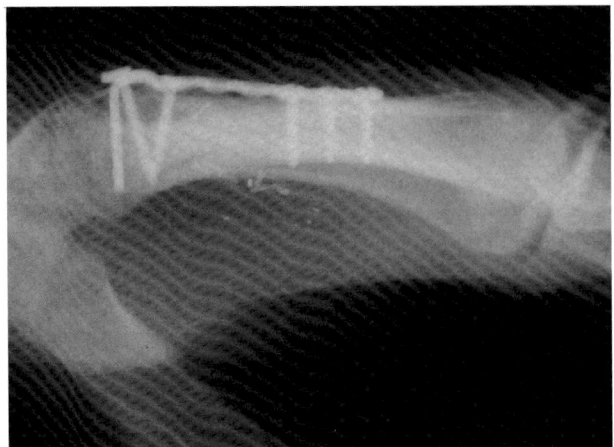

D

FIGURE 30-4 (*continued*) Subsequent internal fixation **(C, D)** and bone grafting can restore the original anatomic parameters of the skeletal unit.

osteoarticular allografts; primary arthrodesis; and free vascularized composite whole toe joint transfer.[91]

Signs and Symptoms of Hand Fractures and Dislocations

Symptoms associated with a fracture or dislocation of the hand include pain, swelling, stiffness, weakness, deformity, and loss of coordination. Numbness and tingling signify associated nerve involvement (either direct injury to the nerve or as a secondary effect of swelling). Signs include tenderness, swelling, ecchymosis, deformity, crepitus, and instability. A better skeletal examination can often be obtained with the aid of anesthesia applied directly at the injury site or regionally. Isolated metacarpophalangeal (MP) joint dislocations and metacarpal fractures can be treated with direct injection of anesthetic into the injury site. More distal injuries are easily anesthetized with a digital block. More global pain relief can be obtained through nerve blocks performed at the wrist to include the median nerve, ulnar nerve, and dorsal cutaneous branches of the radial and ulnar nerves. The time following administration of the anesthetic can be used to cleanse any superficial wounds and to prepare splinting supplies. Pain-free demonstration of tendon excursion and fracture and ligament stability can then be performed. At the conclusion of the anesthetized skeletal examination, the injury can be promptly reduced and splinted.

An important factor in many treatment algorithms is the presence of rotational deformity. The examiner must understand the appropriate method of assessment. The bones of the hand are short tubular structures. Malrotation at one bone segment is best represented by the alignment of the next more distal segment. This alignment is best demonstrated when the intervening joint is flexed to 90 degrees (Fig. 30-6). Comparing nail plate alignment is an inadequate method of evaluating

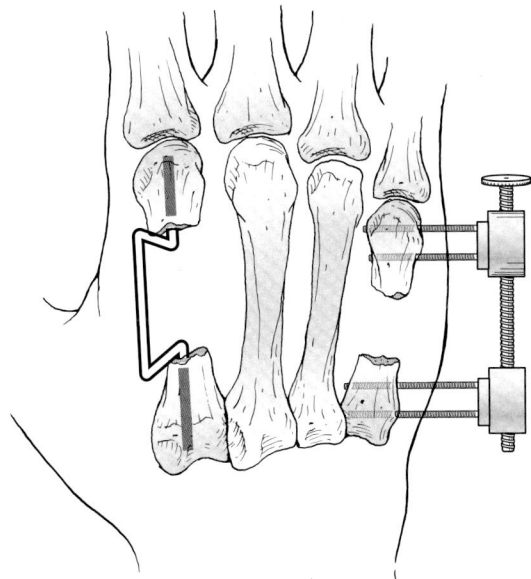

FIGURE 30-5 When extensive contamination precludes the use of internal fixation or when bone reconstruction is to be done at a later date, the use of spacer wires or the application of an external fixator with distraction and compression capabilities can be useful.

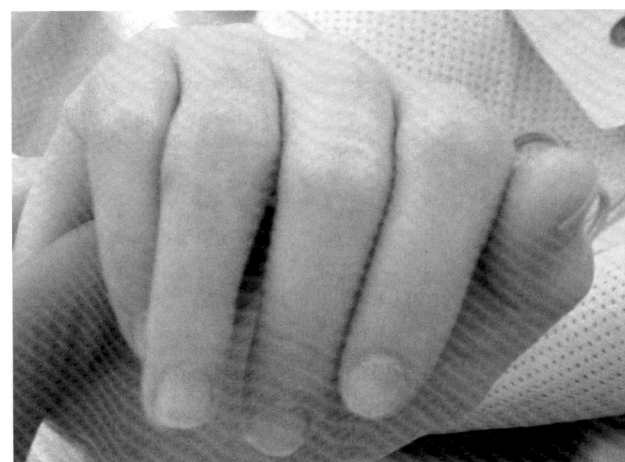

FIGURE 30-6 Pronation of the ring finger proximal phalanx is easily demonstrated by the angular discrepancy of the middle phalanges viewed with the PIP joints flexed 90 degrees.

rotation. Other unique physical examination findings will be discussed in association with specific injuries.

Hand Fracture and Dislocation Imaging and Other Diagnostic Studies

Plain radiographic evaluation includes at least two projections with the beam centered at the level of interest. A third oblique view is often quite instructive, revealing displacement not evident on the standard posterior–anterior (PA) or lateral. Rarely are other imaging studies necessary in evaluating fractures and dislocations of the hand. In complex periarticular fractures, such as "pilon" fractures at the base of P2, computed tomography (CT) scans assist some surgeons with operative planning. Foreign bodies may not always be detected by standard radiographic projections. Glass or gravel is best seen with soft tissue technique. CT scans may detect plastic, glass, and wood. Ultrasound can detect objects that lack radiopacity. Magnetic resonance imaging (MRI) remains a more expensive backup for all types of foreign materials.

Hand Fracture and Dislocation Classification

Unfortunately, the literature regarding these injuries has not been written in accordance with any defined classification scheme, and true comparisons are difficult to make. The AO comprehensive classification system proved to have poor interobserver (κ-coefficient of 0.44) and intraobserver (κ-coefficient of 0.62) agreement.[161] Descriptions of fractures have been based largely on the location within the bone (head, neck, shaft, base) and further modified by the direction of the fracture plane (transverse, spiral, oblique, comminuted) and the measurable degree of displacement. Dislocations have been described by the direction the distal segment travels (dorsal, volar, rotatory) and further modified by the capacity (simple) or incapacity (complex) for closed reduction. In the sections that follow regarding each injury, it will be assumed that the above stated designations are in effect unless specific exceptions are noted.

Hand Fracture and Dislocation Outcomes

In the modern era of hand surgery, outcomes research has become ever more refined with concepts such as the minimal clinically important difference, cost–utility analysis, Cochrane reviews, and a better understanding of how patient psychological status plays into reported symptoms.[30,95,122,142,143,168,177] Functional loss is often underappreciated and difficult to measure. No statistically significant correlation could be drawn in a study comparing the American Medical Association impairment rating with the Disability of the Arm, Shoulder, and Hand (DASH) questionnaire.[176] In a series of 924 hand fractures, overall results were excellent or good in 90% of thumbs but only 59% to 76% of fingers, citing comminution and open or multiple fractures as poor prognostic indicators.[90] Intra-articular extension appears to confer a worse prognosis with TAM of 169 degrees compared to TAM of 213 degrees in fractures without intra-articular extension.[66] Only a few patterns of

dislocation lead to residual instability. Fractures, however, can easily result in malunion. Some practitioners perceive a direct trade-off between stiffness and either residual instability or malunion. This is not necessarily the case. As the understanding of these difficult injuries improves along with new surgical techniques, it is becoming increasingly possible to achieve good hand function while avoiding complications for most isolated fractures and dislocations. Major hand trauma is another matter.

HAND FRACTURE AND DISLOCATION TREATMENT OPTIONS

One of the most fundamental principles of management is that the negative effects of surgery on the tissues should not exceed the negative effects of the original injury. Accordingly, nonoperative treatment plays a significant role in the management of fractures and dislocations of the hand. A corollary to this principle is that even though fractures and dislocations are fundamentally skeletal injuries, most of the difficult decision-making centers on management of the soft tissues. The injured part must not be considered in isolation. The multiple joints of the hand are maintained in a delicate balance by the intrinsic and extrinsic tendon systems such that a disturbance in one set of tissues will often significantly affect others.

The fundamental rationale for treatment in fractures and dislocations of the hand is to achieve sufficient stability of the bone or joint injury to permit early motion rehabilitation without resulting in malunion for fractures or residual instability for dislocations. The preferred treatment option is the least invasive technique that can accomplish these goals.[77] There are essentially five major treatment alternatives: immediate motion, temporary splinting, CRIF, ORIF, and immediate reconstruction.[164,99,105,154,166] External fixation is a variation that has been, surprisingly enough, applied to even initially closed fractures.[115] The general advantages of entirely nonoperative treatment are assumed to be lower cost and avoidance of the risks and complications associated with surgery and anesthesia. The generally presumed disadvantage is that stability is less assured than with some form of operative fixation. CRIF is expected to prevent overt deformity but not to achieve an anatomically perfect reduction. Pin tract infection is the prime complication that should be discussed with patients preparing for CRIF. Open fixation is considered to add the morbidity of surgical tissue trauma, titrated against the presumed advantage of achieving the most anatomic and stable reduction.

Nonoperative Treatment of Hand Fractures and Dislocations

Critical elements in selecting between nonoperative and operative treatment are the assessments of rotational malalignment and stability.[147] To define stability, some authors have used what seems to be the very reasonable criterion of maintenance of fracture reduction when the adjacent joints are taken through at least 30% of their normal motion.[28] Contraction of soft tissues begins approximately 72 hours following injury. Motion should be instituted by this time for all joints stable enough to tolerate rehabilitation. Elevation and elastic compression promote edema control. The more aggressive the surgeon's management of the injury has been, the more aggressive must be the rehabilitation. Low-energy isolated injuries have far less risk of stiffness than those created by high-energy trauma with large zones of injury.

Reduction maneuvers should not cause added tissue trauma. If the injury is reducible at all, gentle manipulation will accomplish the reduction far more successfully than forceful longitudinal traction. The principle is relaxation of deforming forces through proximal joint positioning such as MP joint flexion to relax the intrinsics or wrist flexion to relax the digital flexor tendons. Often, a gentle back-and-forth rotatory maneuver is necessary to free a bony prominence from soft tissue entrapment. The mobile distal part is then reduced to the stable proximal part.

Splints should immobilize the minimum number of joints possible and allow unrestricted motion of all other joints. One controversial point concerns the need to immobilize the wrist. Setting appropriate length–tension relationships in the extrinsic motors (in cases where they are deforming forces) is most easily accomplished through immobilization of the wrist in 25 to 35 degrees of extension. Wrist splinting in extension is extremely helpful in patients with low pain tolerance who tend to place the hand in a characteristic dysfunctional posture of wrist flexion–MP joint extension–interphalangeal (IP) joint flexion (the "wounded paw" position). Other patients who are capable of avoiding this position on their own often do not need wrist immobilization. A simple splint that is useful for injuries ranging from the CMC joints proximally to P1 fractures distally consists of a single slab of plaster or fiberglass applied dorsally. With a foundation at the forearm, the splint runs out to the level of the PIP joints distally with the wrist extended and the MP joints fully flexed. Full motion of the IP joints should be encouraged throughout the healing process. The total duration of immobilization should rarely exceed 3 to 4 weeks. Hand fractures are stable enough by this time to tolerate active range of motion (AROM) with further remodeling by 8 to 10 weeks.

From this point forward, nonoperative treatment is considered alongside potential operative treatments for each segment of the ray, working from distal to proximal (Table 30-1).

INTRODUCTION TO DISTAL PHALANX (P3) FRACTURES

As the terminal point of contact with the environment, the distal phalanx experiences stress loading with nearly every use of the hand. The soft tissue coverage is limited, and local signs of fracture can usually be detected at the surface. When fractures accompany a nail bed injury, hematoma can be seen beneath the nail plate. When the seal between the nail plate and the hyponychium is also broken, the fracture is open and should be treated as such. The mechanism of injury often involves crushing, and the soft tissue injury is frequently of greater significance for long-term prognosis than the fracture. When one is suspicious of a distal phalanx fracture, radiographs should be taken as isolated views of the injured digit.

PATHOANATOMY AND APPLIED ANATOMY RELATING TO DISTAL PHALANX FRACTURES

Unique features of the distal phalanx include the ligaments that pass from the distal margin of the widened lateral base to the expanded proximal margins of the tuft. Small branches of the proper digital artery that supply the dorsal arcade just proximal to the nail fold pass under these ligaments very close to the base of the shaft of the distal phalanx. The tuft is an anchoring point for the specialized architecture of the digital pulp, a honeycomb structure of fibrous septae that contains pockets of fat in each compartment. The proximal part of the pulp is thicker and more mobile than the distal pulp. The proximal portion of a tuft fracture may become entrapped in the septae of the pulp and prove irreducible.[5] The dorsal surface of the distal phalanx is the direct support for the germinal matrix and sterile matrix of the nail. The bone volarly and the nail plate dorsally create a three-layered sandwich with the matrix in the middle (Fig. 30-7).

Fractures in the distal phalanx can be conceived of as occurring in three primary regions: the tuft, the shaft, and the base (Fig. 30-8). The two mechanisms of injury experienced most frequently are a sudden axial load (as in ball sports) or crush

TABLE 30-1	Nonoperative Treatment	
Indications	**Contraindications**
Nondisplaced fracture	Open fracture or dislocation
Reduced fracture stable to motion stress	Irreducible fracture or dislocation
Reduced dislocation stable to motion stress	Associated soft tissue injuries requiring repair
Excessive patient comorbidity	Multiple musculoskeletal injuries in same limb
Medically unstable	Polytrauma patient, medically stable

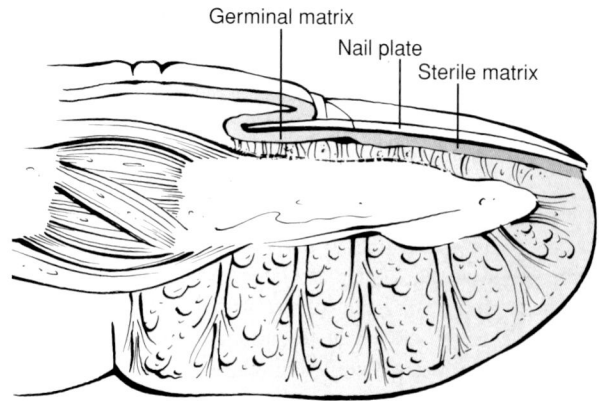

FIGURE 30-7 An intimate relationship exists between the three layers of the dorsal cortex of the distal phalanx, the nail matrix (both germinal and sterile), and the nail plate.

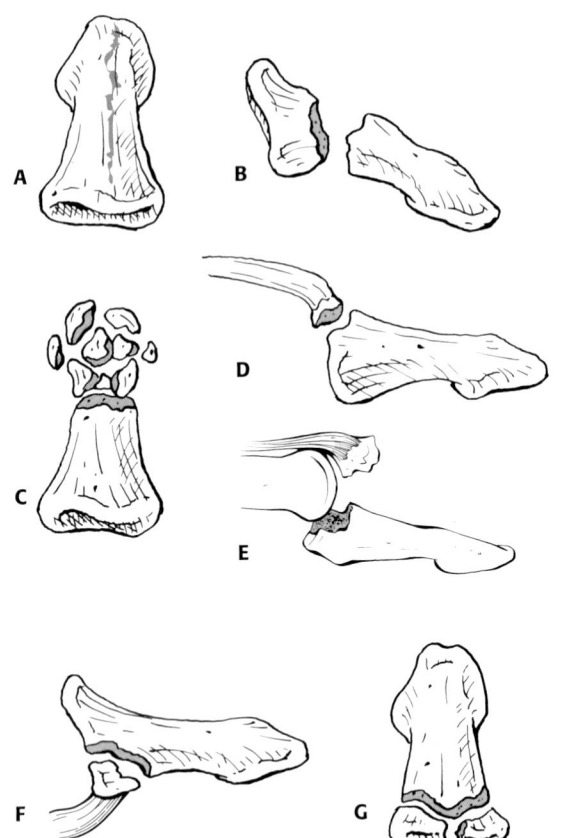

FIGURE 30-8 Fracture patterns seen in the distal phalanx include **(A)** longitudinal shaft, **(B)** transverse shaft, **(C)** tuft, **(D)** dorsal base avulsion, **(E)** dorsal base shear, **(F)** volar base, and **(G)** complete articular.

injuries. Crush fractures of the tuft are often stable injuries held in place by the fibrous network of the pulp volarly and the splinting effect of the nail plate dorsally. Proximally, the digital flexor and terminal extensor tendons insert on the volar and dorsal bases of the distal phalanx. Since these are the last tendon attachments in the digit, all fracture planes occurring distal to these tendon insertions have been separated from any internal deforming forces. In contrast, volar and dorsal base fractures are unstable, with the entire force of a tendon pulling the small base fragment away from the remainder of the bone. Controlling rotation in these small pieces may be particularly difficult. Dorsal base intra-articular fractures due to the shearing component of an axial load injury should be distinguished from avulsion fractures occurring under tension from the terminal tendon. The latter are smaller fragments with the fracture line perpendicular to the line of tensile force in the tendon, whereas the former are larger fragments comprising a significant (>20%) portion of the articular surface with the fracture line perpendicular to the articular surface. These are very different injuries with different treatment requirements. In a similar fashion, the majority of bone flakes at the volar base of P3 are really flexor digitorum profundus (FDP) tendon ruptures occurring through bone. A small percentage of volar base fractures, especially when large in size, are not FDP avulsions

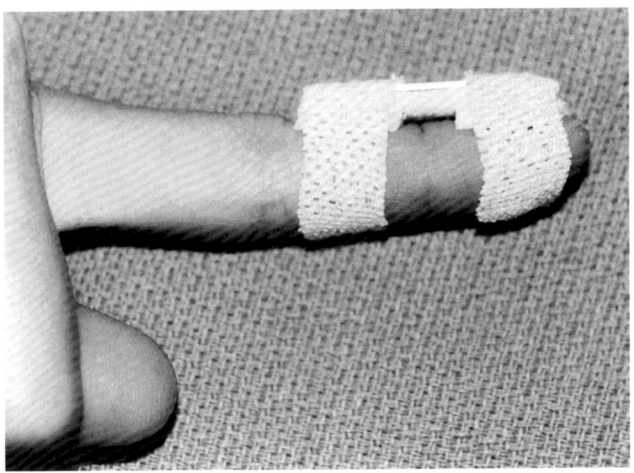

FIGURE 30-9 Dorsal splinting of the distal phalanx and the DIP joint is easily accomplished with an aluminum and foam splint. Cutting out the foam over the dorsal nail fold skin relieves direct pressure where the skin is at greatest risk for ischemic necrosis.

but rather shearing fractures that are amenable to extension block splinting or fixation.

DISTAL PHALANX FRACTURE TREATMENT OPTIONS

Many distal phalanx fractures can be treated with digital splints (Fig. 30-9). The splint should leave the PIP joint free but usually needs to cross the DIP joint simply to gain enough foundation to provide adequate stability. The splint may be removed daily to perform active DIP joint-blocking exercises. Aluminum and foam splints or plaster of Paris are common materials chosen. When surgery is contemplated the surgeon should consult a preoperative planning checklist (Table 30-2).

TABLE 30-2 Preoperative Planning Checklist

Hand table mounted to OR table rail with additional support by extendable leg

Nonsterile brachial level tourniquet

Single hole extremity drape specific to hand table coverage

Mini-fluoroscopy unit with C-arm horizontal, located at the end of hand table on surgeon's side

Technician's instrument table located at the end of hand table to assistant's side

Hand surgery instruments needed for fracture care: gauze packer, small elevators, microcurette

Power driver with both pistol grip (K-wires) and pencil grip (small drill bits) attachments

Kirschner wires of appropriate size to injured region (0.028- to 0.062-inch)

Modular plate and screw set ranging from 1- to 2.5-mm size

Tuft Fractures

If the dorsal surface of the distal portion of the phalanx that supports the nail matrix has a significant step-off, especially with a concomitant nail plate avulsion, the fracture should be restored to a level surface and pinned to render support to the surgical repair of the nail matrix. Conversely, if the nail plate has maintained its seal at the hyponychium, and the dorsal surface of the distal phalanx is level, formal removal of the plate to perform a nail matrix repair is not necessary despite any measured percentage of hematoma occupying the area under the nail. Matrix defects should be split-thickness grafted from the adjacent nail bed. Following repair, the dorsal nail fold should be stented to prevent adherence to the matrix but still allow fluid drainage. The patient should be warned of the potential for nail deformity and the time required (4 to 5 months) for regrowth.

Shaft Fractures

Most shaft fractures have sufficiently limited displacement that nonoperative management is appropriate. Active motion of the DIP joint can be pursued from the outset since the forces of the FDP and the terminal extensor tendon are not acting across the fracture. Only externally applied forces such as pinch will deform the fracture. Shaft fractures with wide displacement may not unite without closer approximation of the fragments. CRIF is usually sufficient for these fractures unless there is interposed tissue blocking the reduction (Fig. 30-10). K-wire fixation may also be preferable (0/5 malunions) compared with splinting (3/18 flexion malunions) when the fracture is transverse, extra-articular, and located at the base of the distal phalanx.[6] In extreme cases where the fragments continue to separate longitudinally along the smooth-sided wires, axial compression can be achieved with a micro-sized headless screw (Fig. 30-11).

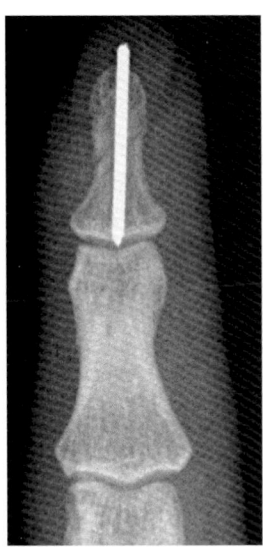 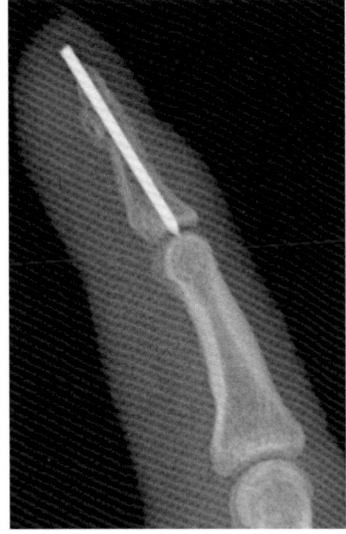

FIGURE 30-10 Shaft fractures should first be axially compressed, then stabilized with a longitudinal K-wire that is drilled just short of the subchondral bone plate, and then axially tapped into the subchondral bone without spinning the wire.

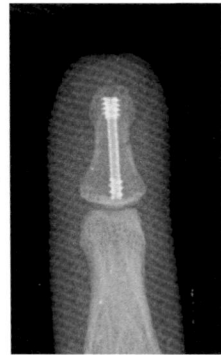 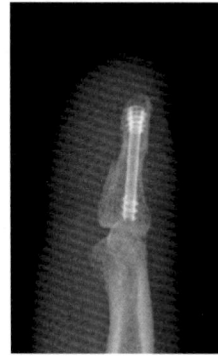

FIGURE 30-11 Shaft fractures can be axially compressed to avoid nonunion resulting from distraction by using a variable pitch headless compression microsized screw placed over a guidewire.

Dorsal Base Fractures—CRIF

Closed reduction and pin fixation is the treatment of choice for shearing dorsal base fractures comprising over 25% of the articular surface (Fig. 30-12). A variety of fixation techniques have been described, but the mainstay is extension block pinning (Figs 30-13 and 30-14).[84,93,112,133,186] Twenty-three patients treated with extension block pinning for fragments comprising an average of 40% of the joint surface had a mean flexion of 77 degrees with a 4-degree extensor lag with two losses of reduction.[84] The difficulty in comparing the published outcomes for these injuries is that the literature has usually failed to distinguish between dorsal fractures that are merely bony variants of terminal tendon injuries and those that are the more significant intra-articular fractures discussed in this section.

Dorsal Base Fractures—ORIF

Dorsal base fractures may rarely require ORIF. Although subluxation has been cited as a reason to perform ORIF, a biomechanical study showed that subluxation was not seen whenever the smaller fragment carried less than 43% of the articular surface.[88] Thirty-three patients treated with ORIF using K-wires had a mean arc of 4 to 67 degrees of final motion.[162] As an alternative method of ORIF, nine patients were treated with a custom "hook plate" formed by cutting a 1.3-mm modular straight

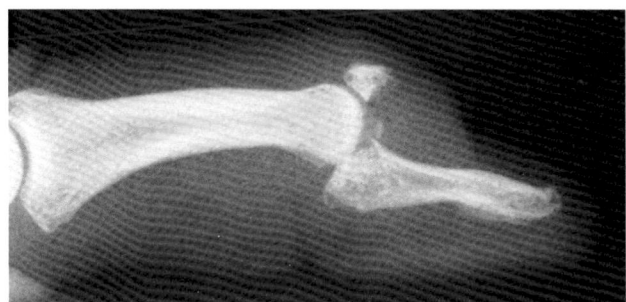

FIGURE 30-12 Dorsal base fractures from axial impaction with shearing rather than a traction avulsion injury may demonstrate subluxation of the volar fragment with rotation into extension of the smaller dorsal fragment. These features indicate the need for operative management of the injury.

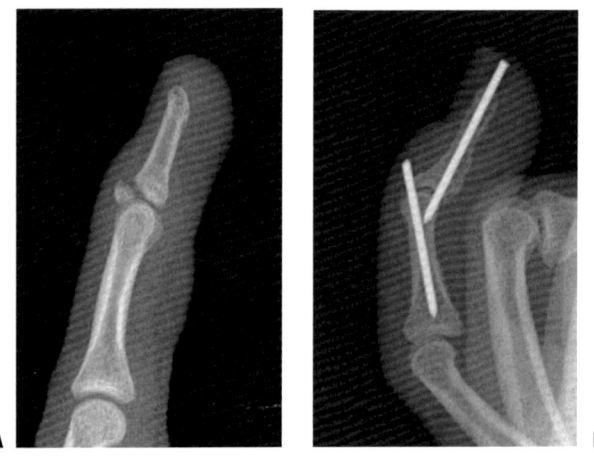

FIGURE 30-13 Dorsal base shearing articular fractures **(A)** can be stabilized by the extension block pinning technique **(B)** using two 0.045-inch K-wires.

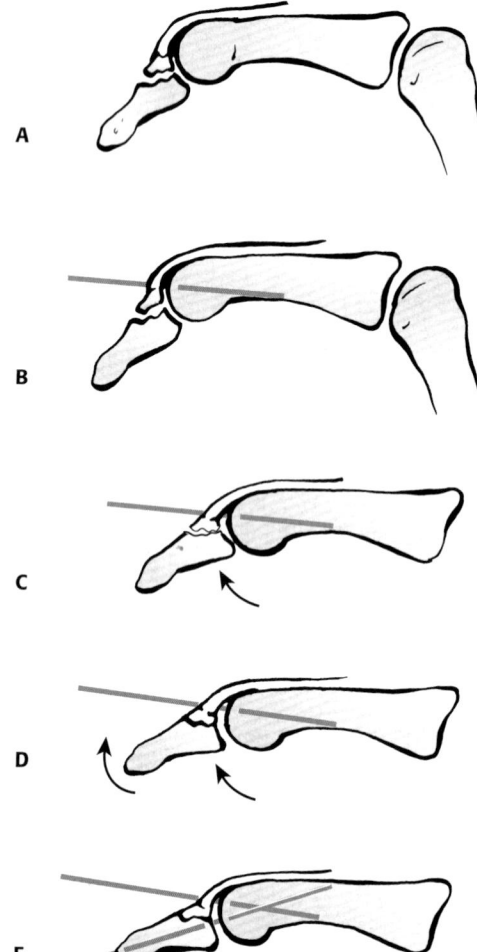

FIGURE 30-14 The steps of the extension block pinning method begin with **(A)** hyperflexion of the DIP joint to draw the smaller dorsal fragment volarly where it is **(B)** blocked from returning into further extension by the first 0.045-inch K-wire. The larger volar fragment is then reduced **(C)** first at the articular surface to meet the dorsal fragment followed by **(D)** extension of the shaft to approximate the metaphysis, and maintained by the second K-wire **(E)**.

plate and achieved an average of 64 degrees range of motion (ROM) of the DIP joint with no extensor lag.[165] One method of avoiding the complications potentially associated with open DIP joint surgery (0/19) might be the 5 weeks of external fixation employed in 19 patients resulting in 70 degrees of flexion with a 2-degree average extensor lag.[94]

Volar Base Fractures

ORIF is the treatment of choice for highly displaced volar base fractures that have a large intra-articular fragment and loss of FDP functional integrity. If the volar FDP fragment is large enough, it may be fixed with a compression screw. Extension block pinning is another rarely employed alternative. The remainder of small bone flakes located at the volar base of the distal phalanx are tendon avulsions and should be treated in accordance with modern principles of flexor tendon reinsertion.

Postoperative Care

Healing at this level of the digit is often prolonged. Transverse shaft fractures may take 3 to 4 months before being able to resist maximum pinch force. For stable tuft and longitudinal fractures, splints may be removed and functional use of the hand instituted as soon as tolerated. Dorsal base fractures usually have the K-wires removed by 4 weeks with continued external protection for 2 to 3 more weeks when using traditional pinning techniques. The dorsal base extension block method works through the institution of passive extension exercises beginning at 4 weeks and coinciding with wire removal. The more distal the injury is in the digit, the more hypersensitivity to surface contact the patient is likely to have. Desensitization through progressively more stimulating contact is the earliest component of the rehabilitation program, with the goal of reincorporating the fingertip into as many activities of daily living as possible.

Potential Pitfalls and Preventative Measures

The volar pulp space adjacent to distal phalanx fractures represents a tense three-dimensional hydrodynamic unit that will tend to expand when injured and forcibly distract fracture fragments from each other, resulting in the nonunions frequently seen at this level. The most common direction of displacement is in distraction. Smooth-sided K-wires are the most common devices used for P3 fracture fixation, but they can allow the fracture fragments to slide along the surface of the wires. The best way to defeat this is to place the wires as obliquely as possible and to use converging and diverging patterns (Fig. 30-15). To prevent K-wires from migrating into the DIP joint, tap, rather than drill them, into the subchondral bone at the base of the phalanx. To prevent pin tract infection, cut wires below skin level, but not too short resulting in an irretrievable pin. When performing the extension block pinning technique for dorsal base fractures, achieving a truly congruent joint is difficult. There are two typical problems: rotation of the smaller fragment into extension under the influence of the terminal extensor tendon and cantilevering of the volar articular-shaft fragment. A method to overcome the first problem is to use another K-wire percutaneously to hold pressure on the dorsal cortex of the small fragment while placing the extension block

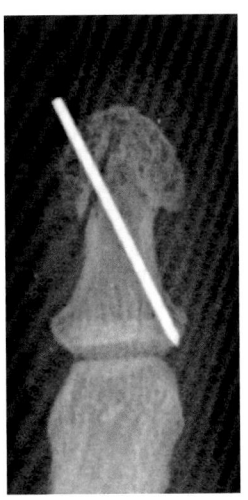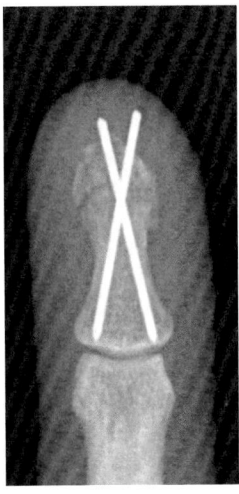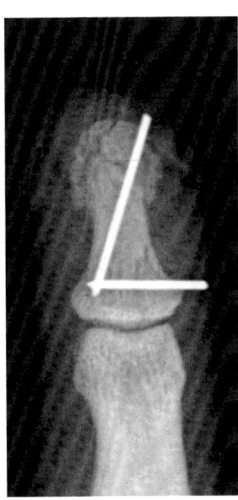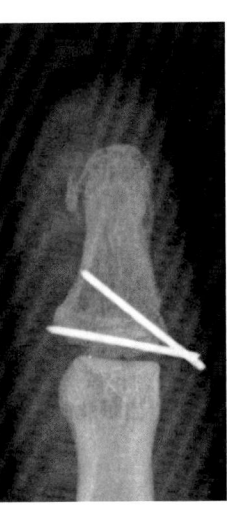

A, B   C, D

FIGURE 30-15 Fracture fragment sliding along the smooth shaft of the K-wire is prevented by **(A)** maximum oblique placement from one lateral edge of the tuft to the opposite far lateral corner of the base, **(B)** two wires targeting the lateral corners of the base, **(C)** converging wire patterns, and **(D)** diverging wire patterns.

wire. The flat side of the wire rather than the sharp tip should be used for this reduction maneuver. The second problem is created by the surgeon holding the distal phalanx shaft fragment manually and applying the extension force for reduction. Instead of achieving a congruent joint reduction, the larger fragment cantilevers and reduces at the metaphyseal level but leaves an incongruent articular gap. Placing an instrument handle, such as a Freer elevator, transversely across the volar base just distal to the flexion crease and using the instrument to apply the extension force directly at the level of the joint can overcome this second problem. The reduction will first occur congruently at the joint and then secondarily at the metaphysis.

Matrix tissue may fold into any dorsal opening of a fracture site, particularly at the base of the germinal matrix. If reduction of a distal phalanx fracture proves incomplete with a visible dorsal cortical gap on the lateral radiograph, this possibility must be considered and extrication performed to prevent both nonunion and nail deformity. Suturing the nail matrix can be difficult. Friable nail matrix tissue is easily torn as the needle is pushed rather than rolled along its axis during repair, a problem that is compounded by the needle tip's tendency to catch on the dorsal cortex during the bottom of the stroke. These problems are overcome by using a special 6–0 chromic suture with a spatula-tipped needle that can be passed with a rolling motion of the fingers when loaded on a Castroviejo needle driver (Table 30-3).

TABLE 30-3 Potential Pitfalls and Preventative Measures—P3 Fractures

Pitfall	Prevention
Hydrostatic distraction of fragments	Multiple wires converging/diverging
Pin migration into DIP joint	Tap pin into subchondral bone rather than drilling
Pin infection	Cut pins below skin level
Irretrievable pin	Do not cut pins too short
Extended dorsal base fragment	Direct nonpenetrating wire pressure held on fragment during reduction and fixation
Incongruent volar base fragment	Reduce at articular surface first with instrument pressure, then extend and close metaphysis
Nail matrix incarceration	Check lateral radiograph for contiguous dorsal cortex reduction
Tearing nail matrix during repair	Special small spatula needle with rolling technique, no pushing

AUTHOR'S PREFERRED TREATMENT (FIG. 30-16)

Tuft Fractures

Many tuft fractures can be splinted in a simple aluminum and foam splint for a duration determined by the patient's symptoms alone. The time course for healing of the associated soft tissue injury may well determine the total duration of disability far more than that of the fracture itself. When the seal of the nail plate with the hyponychium has been broken and the tuft fracture is displaced, this represents an open fracture that should be treated on the day of injury with debridement followed by direct nail matrix repair. If the distal fragment is of substantial size, the dorsal cortex of the distal phalanx that supports the nail matrix will provide a more level surface if pinned with one or more 0.028-inch K-wires for 4 to 6 weeks.

Shaft Fractures

Longitudinal sagittal plane shaft fractures of the distal phalanx can be treated entirely nonoperatively if minimally displaced

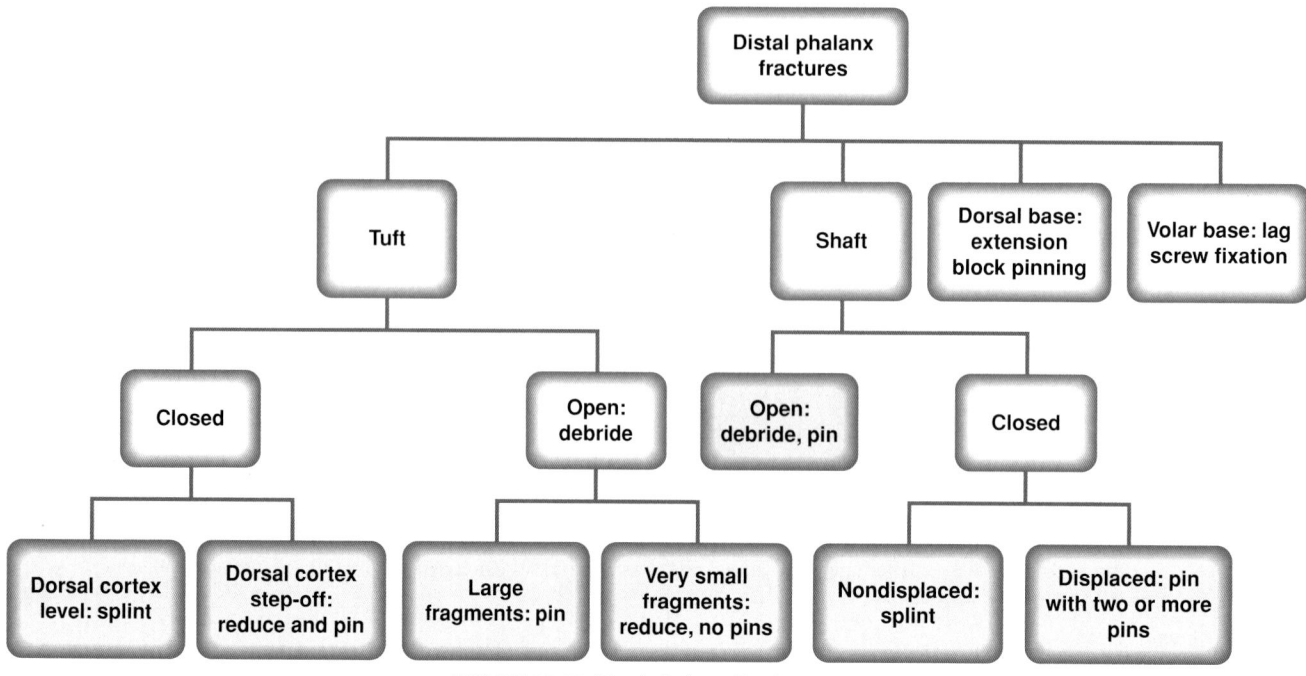

FIGURE 30-16 Distal phalanx (P3) fractures.

or with CRIF using oblique 0.028- to 0.035-inch K-wires for the rare displaced fracture. Two or more wires should be used to prevent sliding of the fracture along the smooth surface of a single wire. Care should be taken to avoid penetration of the nail matrix with the wire. If the fracture is at midshaft level or more distal, the wire will provide enough stability if driven to the subchondral base of the distal phalanx only. Fractures occurring at the metadiaphyseal junction may need to have the wire passed across the DIP joint to achieve sufficient stability.

Dorsal Base Fractures

Dorsal base intra-articular shear fractures produce a triangular dorsal fragment that is extended and translated by the pull of the terminal tendon. With proper collateral ligament damage, the larger articular fragment that is in continuity with the remainder of the phalanx may sublux volarly. ORIF adds excessive surgical trauma to this delicate set of tissues and the dorsal fragment is usually too small to accommodate fixation devices passing directly through it without experiencing comminution. The injury is best addressed by extension block pinning. The DIP joint is hyperflexed, drawing the dorsal fragment volarly to reach its natural position in relation to the head of P2. A 0.045-inch K-wire is then inserted at the dorsal margin of the fragment (but not through the fragment) to block it from returning to the retracted position under the influence of the terminal extensor tendon (Fig. 30-14). The remainder of the distal phalanx (consisting of the volar articular fragment and shaft) is then extended to meet the blocked smaller fragment and restore articular congruity. A second 0.045-inch K-wire is passed from the larger P3 fragment across the DIP joint into P2. The wires are retained for 4 weeks. Upon removal, passive

extension exercises further compress the two fragments and assist in the final stages of cancellous bone healing. The treatment can still be executed up to 4 to 5 weeks after the initial injury, but the early callus that has formed between the two fragments must be dispersed or satisfactory approximation will not be achieved (Table 30-4).

TABLE 30-4	Surgical Steps—Extension Block Pinning of Dorsal Base P3 Fractures

Flex DIP joint to draw all fragments volarly relative to the head of P2

Place nonpenetrating wire pressure against the small dorsal base fragment to prevent it from rotating into extension under the influence of the terminal tendon

Place the extension blocking wire dorsal to the small fragment into the intercondylar notch of the head of P2

Pre-position the axial transarticular wire in the shaft of P3 but not entering the fracture site yet

Check the placement of both wires and fragment relationships on lateral fluoroscopy

Reduce the articular surface using instrument pressure at the volar base of the shaft fragment

Extend the shaft fragment resulting in closure of the metaphysis while maintaining the instrument pressure

Advance the axial wire across the DIP joint

Check the final fixation on fluoroscopy, adjust if needed, cut off pins, dress, and splint

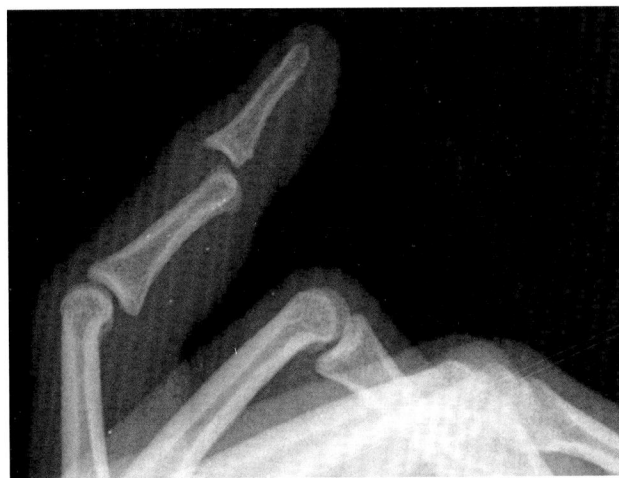

FIGURE 30-17 Dislocations of the DIP joint are nearly always dorsal.

INTRODUCTION TO DISTAL INTERPHALANGEAL (DIP) AND THUMB INTERPHALANGEAL (IP) JOINT DISLOCATIONS

Dislocations at the DIP/IP joint suffer from underappreciation and late presentation. Injuries are considered chronic after 3 weeks. Pure dislocations without tendon rupture are rare, usually result from ball-catching sports, are primarily dorsal in direction, and may occur in association with PIP joint dislocations (Fig. 30-17). Transverse open wounds in the volar skin crease are frequent (Fig. 30-18). Injury to a single collateral ligament or to the volar plate alone at the DIP joint is rare.

PATHOANATOMY AND APPLIED ANATOMY OF DISTAL INTERPHALANGEAL AND THUMB JOINT DISLOCATIONS

The DIP/IP joint is a bicondylar ginglymus joint stabilized on each side by proper and accessory collateral ligaments and the volar plate. The proper collateral ligaments insert on the lateral

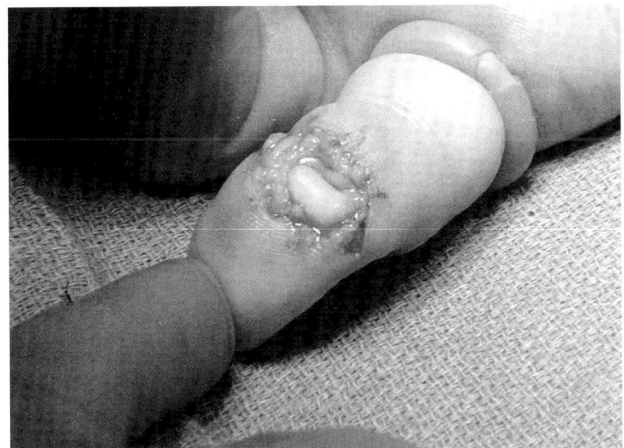

FIGURE 30-18 Dorsal DIP dislocations are often open injuries, with a transverse rent in the flexion crease resulting from tearing rather than from direct laceration. The wound should be debrided prior to reduction if possible.

tubercles at the base of P3, which also serve as the origin for the lateral ligaments to the tuft. The accessory collateral ligaments attach distally to the lateral margins of the volar plate. The volar plate of the DIP joint has a proximal attachment weakly confluent with the distal extent of the flexor digitorum superficialis (FDS) tendon but has no strong check-rein ligaments like those at the PIP joint. This is in keeping with the clinical observation that the volar plate detaches proximally when the DIP/IP joint dislocates dorsally. The joint is inherently stable owing to articular congruity and the dynamic balance of flexor and extensor tendons. However, the DIP/IP joint is not as intrinsically stable as the PIP joint and depends to a greater degree on its ligaments.

The DIP/IP joints have complex motion patterns involving axial rotation that are different for each digit and designed to ensure conformity when the hand surrounds an object. The capacity for passive DIP/IP hyperextension is unique to modern humans, but the role this plays in the etiology of dislocation is unclear. Irreducible dorsal dislocations are thought to occur through a variety of different anatomic circumstances. Reasons include a trapped volar plate, the FDP trapped behind a single condyle of P2 (marked lateral displacement), P2 buttonholed through the volar plate or through a rent in the FDP, and thumb sesamoids. Volar dislocations may also be irreducible with the extensor tendon displaced around the head of P2.

DISTAL INTERPHALANGEAL AND THUMB JOINT DISLOCATIONS TREATMENT OPTIONS

Nonoperative Management of Distal Interphalangeal and Thumb Joint Dislocations

Reduced dislocations that are stable may begin immediate AROM. The rare unstable dorsal dislocation should be immobilized in 20 degrees of flexion for up to 3 weeks before instituting AROM. The duration of the immobilization should be in direct proportion to the surgeon's assessment of joint stability following reduction. Complete collateral ligament injuries should be protected from lateral stress for at least 4 weeks. When splinting at the level of the DIP/IP joint, extreme caution must be exercised with regard to the vascularity of the dorsal skin between the extension skin crease and the dorsal nail fold. It is not only direct pressure but merely the angle of hyperextension that can "wash out" the blood supply to this skin, potentially resulting in full-thickness necrosis. This complication is thought to occur at an angle representing 50% of the available passive hyperextension of the DIP joint and can be identified by blanching of the skin.

Closed Reduction and Internal Fixation

It is possible that the degree of postreduction instability is great enough to require a brief period (3 to 4 weeks) of 0.045-inch K-wire stabilization across the joint (Fig. 30-19). The need for added stabilization occurs primarily when aggressive rehabilitation is required for adjacent hand injuries.

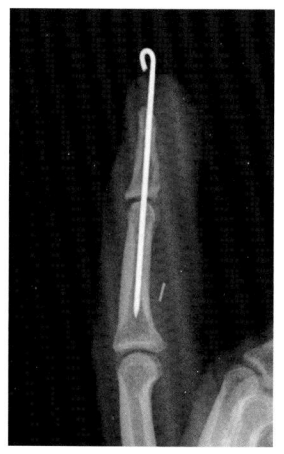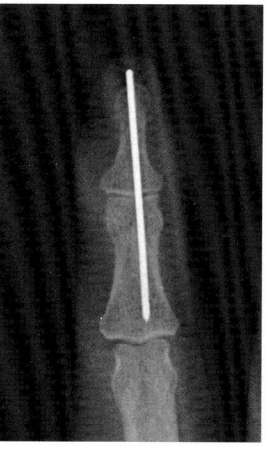

A   **B**

FIGURE 30-19 Closed reduction and internal fixation of the DIP joint should assure **(A)** a congruent articulation in neutral on the lateral view, and **(B)** neutral pin placement on the AP view.

Open Reduction

Delayed presentation (over 3 weeks) of a subluxed joint may require open reduction to resect scar tissue and permit a congruent reduction, but can result in additional postoperative stiffness. In one study, 10 patients with chronic dorsal fracture dislocations of the DIP and IP joints (average 8 weeks) underwent a volar plate arthroplasty with 4 weeks of K-wire fixation yielding a 42-degree average arc of motion for finger DIP joints and 51 degrees for thumb IP joints with an average flexion contracture of 12 degrees.[134] Open dislocations require thorough debridement to prevent infection. The need for fixation with a K-wire should be based on the assessment of stability and is not necessarily required for all open dislocations. The wire may be placed either longitudinally or on an oblique path. The duration of pinning should not be longer than 4 weeks. The advantage of longitudinal pinning is the absence of any lateral wire protrusion to contact adjacent digits. The advantage of oblique pinning is the ability to remove both sections of the wire should breakage across the joint occur. When open reduction of the joint is required, a transverse dorsal incision at

TABLE 30-5	Potential Pitfalls and Preventative Measures—DIP Dislocations
Pitfall	**Prevention**
Poor wound healing	Gentle technique, preserve dorsal veins
Hypersensitivity	Gentle technique, preserve small nerve branches

the distal joint crease from midaxial line to midaxial line provides ample exposure. Should additional exposure be required midaxial proximal extensions can be made.

Potential Pitfalls and Preventative Measures. Two primary complications of open surgery in this region are impaired wound healing and hypersensitivity. Dissecting and preserving longitudinal venous channels during the surgery facilitates venous drainage of the narrow skin flap between the wound and the dorsal nail fold. There is usually one major group of veins directly in the midline overlying the extensor tendon and one major group at each dorsolateral corner. The lateral venous groups are accompanied by the distal branches of the dorsal digital nerves. Transection of these small nerve branches with the subsequent formation of small neuromas adherent to the wound may be one reason for the high incidence of hypersensitivity in this region. The initial surgical incision should be just through dermis only, followed by careful longitudinal dissection of these neurovascular structures under magnification before proceeding with the remainder of the surgery (Table 30-5).

AUTHOR'S PREFERRED TREATMENT (FIG. 30-20)

Closed reduction and splinting is the preferred treatment for most injuries (Fig. 30-20). Should added pin stabilization prove necessary because of recurrent instability, a single longitudinal 0.045-inch K-wire is sufficient. Closed reduction may seem to be impossible. Interposed tissue is usually the cause and may include volar plate, collateral ligament, or tendon. Longitudinal

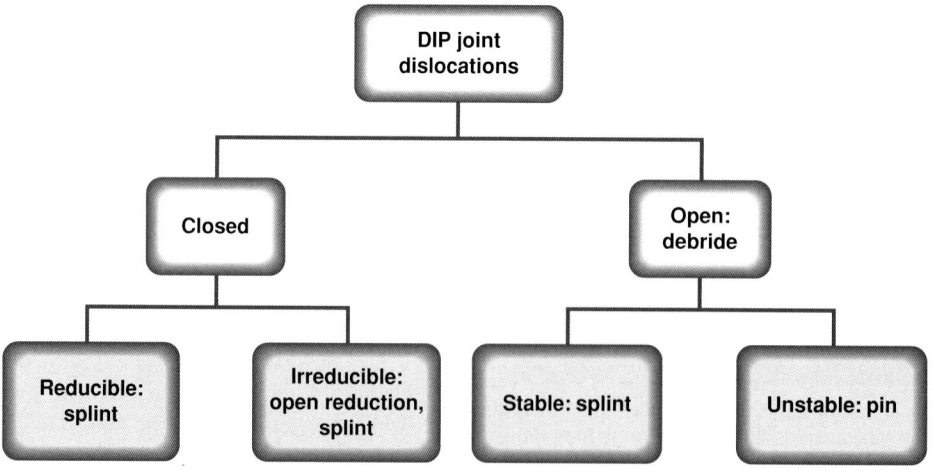

FIGURE 30-20 DIP joint dislocations.

traction rarely is successful in overcoming the blockade. Instead, proximal joint positioning to relax the involved tendons and gentle rotation may allow the interposed tissue to slip out of the joint.

Should open reduction prove necessary, my preferred incision for the DIP/IP joint is dorsal and transverse. The most distal of the major extensor creases corresponds to the joint level. Proximal extensions of 5 mm made in the midaxial lines create a small trapdoor effect that gives ample exposure for any procedure. The terminal extensor tendon or extensor pollicis longus (EPL) should be protected. Using a single prong skin hook is a gentle method to control the tendon without grasping and crushing its fibers with forceps while working to achieve reduction. One must search for small chondral or osteochondral injuries primarily for the purpose of removing the fragments from the joint to prevent subsequent third body wear.

INTRODUCTION TO MIDDLE PHALANX (P2) FRACTURES

This section is intentionally biased to concentrate on the intra-articular fractures that occur at the base of the middle phalanx. These are perhaps the most functionally devastating of all fractures and dislocations of the hand and the most technically difficult to treat. Many other fracture patterns that occur in the middle phalanx are the same as those patterns seen in the proximal phalanx. The literature rarely distinguishes between P1 and P2 when reporting on phalangeal fractures, and the majority of the published data on this subject is covered in the section on proximal phalanx fractures later in the chapter.

PATHOANATOMY AND APPLIED ANATOMY RELATING TO MIDDLE PHALANX FRACTURES

Fractures of the middle phalanx can be grouped by the anatomic regions of head, neck, shaft, and base (Fig. 30-21). Tendon insertions that play a role in fracture deformation include the central slip at the dorsal base and the terminal tendon acting through the DIP joint. The FDS has a long insertion along the volar lateral margins of the shaft of P2 from the proximal one-fourth to the distal one-fourth. Fractures at the neck of P2 will usually angulate apex volar as the proximal fragment is flexed by the FDS and the distal fragment is extended by the terminal

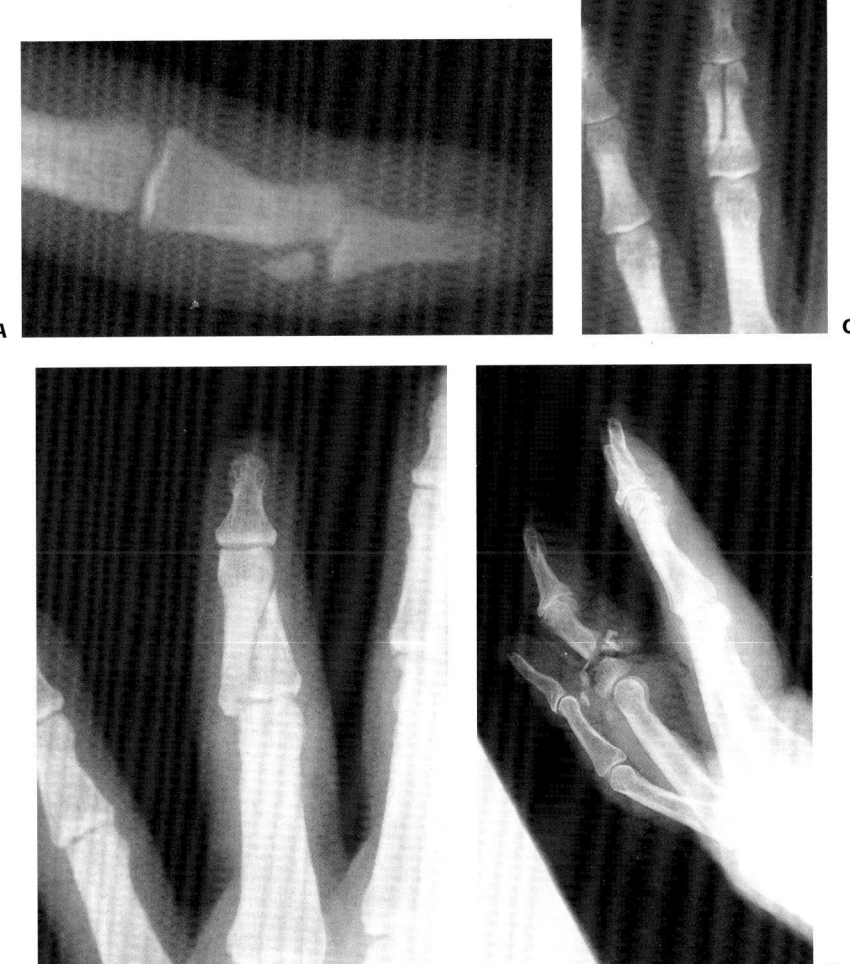

FIGURE 30-21 Fracture patterns of P2 other than the specific base patterns discussed later include **(A)** intra-articular fractures of the head, **(B)** oblique shaft fractures, **(C)** longitudinal shaft fractures, and **(D)** transverse shaft fractures.

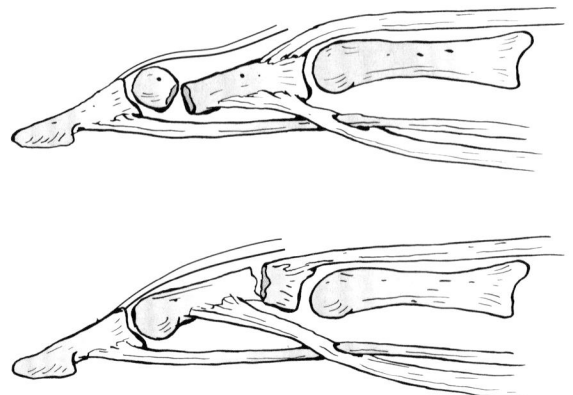

FIGURE 30-22 The insertions of the flexor digitorum superficialis, the flexor digitorum profundus, and the components of the extensor apparatus typically cause fractures in the distal one-fourth of P2 to angulate apex volarly and these in the proximal one-fourth of P2 to angulate apex dorsally.

tendon (Fig. 30-22). Those at the base will usually angulate apex dorsal as the distal fragment is flexed by the FDS and the proximal fragment is extended by the central slip. Despite the theoretical resolution of these force vectors, actual P2 fractures are less predictable and subject to any variety of displacement patterns. Axial loading patterns of injury may produce unicondylar or bicondylar fractures of the head or intra-articular fractures of the base. Base fractures can be divided into partial articular fractures of the dorsal base, volar base, and lateral base or complete articular fractures that are usually comminuted and often referred to as "pilon" fractures. "Pilon" fractures are unstable in every direction including axially.

Although the complete articular fractures are the most challenging ones in which to restore function, the force vectors of volar base fractures are perhaps more interesting. Fractures at the volar base of P2 can be particularly unstable in relation to the percentage of articular surface involved. When the volar fragment constitutes greater than around 40% of the articular surface, this fragment carries the majority of the proper collateral ligament insertion in addition to the accessory ligament and volar plate insertions (Fig. 30-23). The dorsal fragment and remainder of P2 will thus sublux proximally and dorsally

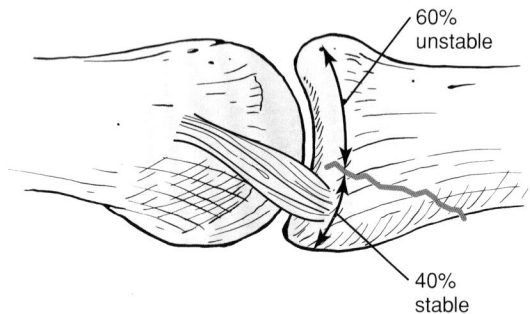

FIGURE 30-23 When the volar fragment of the base of P2 comprises more than 40% of the joint surface, the collateral ligaments attach to the volar, rather than the dorsal, fragment rendering the dorsal fragment with the shaft unstable in extension.

with displacement being driven by the pull of the FDS and the central slip. The joint then hinges rather than glides, pivoting on the fracture margin of the dorsal fragment and abrading the articular cartilage on the head of P1.

MIDDLE PHALANX FRACTURE TREATMENT OPTIONS

Static Splinting

Many P2 fractures can be effectively managed entirely nonoperatively. The presence of comminution alone does not necessitate surgery. When crushing is the mechanism of injury, the periosteal envelope may remain relatively intact as long as fracture displacement is not significant. The inherent stability of the fracture is more related to the degree of displacement than the direction or number of fracture planes. Nevertheless, certain patterns are more stable than others. Transverse fractures are more stable than long oblique or spiral fractures, both of which tend to shorten and either laterally deviate or rotate to cause interference patterns with neighboring digits. Splinting is confined to the digit alone with dorsally applied aluminum and foam or custom orthoplast splints. Motion rehabilitation should be initiated by 3 weeks post injury with interim splinting until clinical signs of healing are present (but not longer than 6 weeks).[22] Side strapping to an adjacent digit usually provides sufficient protection from external forces after the first 3 weeks.

Dynamic Extension Block Splinting

A nonoperative technique used specifically for volar base fractures is extension block splinting. Fractures at the volar base of P2 that involve less than 40% of the articular surface can usually be managed effectively with extension block splinting. The key to success with this treatment is absolute maintenance of a congruent reduction, avoiding the hinge motion that occurs with dorsal and proximal subluxation of the major fragment. Correct application of a dorsal extension block splint requires maintenance of contact between the dorsum of the proximal phalangeal segment and the splint. If the digit is allowed to "pull away" from the splint volarly, the PIP joint can extend beyond the safe range, sublux, and negate the desired effect of the splint. Once the splint is in place, weekly follow-up with a true lateral radiograph of the PIP joint is mandatory to monitor the advancement of extension at a rate of around 10 degrees per week (see below for details of extension block splinting).

Condylar Fractures of the Head

Displaced unicondylar or bicondylar fractures of the head of P2 require a transverse wire to be placed across the condyles to maintain a level distal articular surface at the DIP joint. A second wire passed obliquely to the diaphysis of the opposite cortex will prevent lateral migration of the condylar fragment along the smooth shaft of the first wire which would create an articular gap (Fig. 30-24). This second wire also controls the rotation of the fragment in the sagittal plane that can occur with single wire fixation alone. If the patient presents late or soft tissue lies interposed in the fracture plane between condyles, achieving an accurate closed reduction is unlikely and open reduction may be

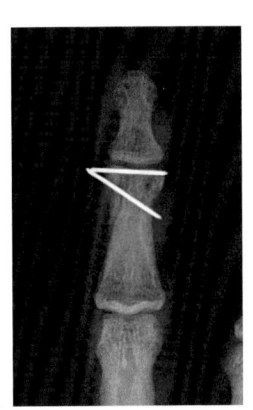
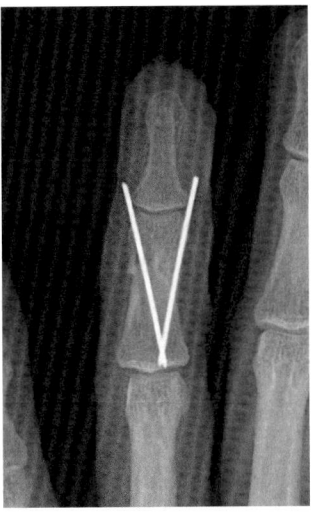

FIGURE 30-24 Condylar fractures at the head of P2 tend to slide along the pin interface producing an articular gap and/or step-off. **A:** Unicondylar fractures require diverging wires to prevent fragment separation. **B:** In bicondylar fractures, converging wires are used to prevent fragment separation.

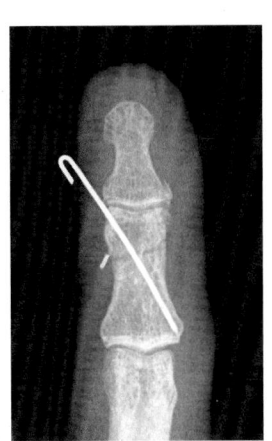
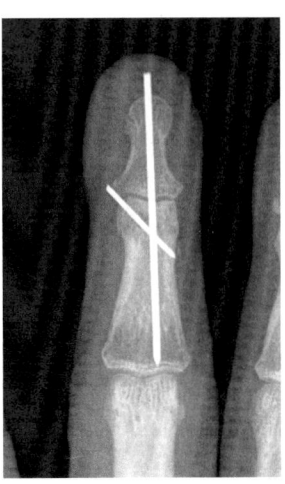

FIGURE 30-26 Fractures of the neck of P2 can be pinned with **(A)** a single oblique pin only when local soft tissues and the geometry of the fracture itself add some inherent stability. Correct placement is from the collateral recess distally to the opposite corner of the metaphyseal base. **B:** If there is a concomitant zone II extensor tendon repair needing protection, pinning can include the DIP joint with an oblique wire in P2 to prevent axial rotation.

required. Once opened, the opportunity for threaded lag screw fixation exists as opposed to smooth K-wire fixation. If the condylar fragment does not have a diaphyseal extension, then the location for lag screw placement is directly through the collateral ligament, which may negate the screw's theoretical advantage over two diverging K-wires in terms of early motion. More complex bicondylar fractures that extend into the shaft require individualized strategies for stabilization, including fixation as definitive as laterally placed plates (Fig. 30-25).

Unstable Shaft Fractures

CRIF is usually accomplished with 0.035-inch K-wires depending on patient size (Fig. 30-26). K-wires that cross in the middle of the shaft produce a less stable pattern of fixation, particularly

if the fracture is located at the level where the wires cross. For transverse or short oblique patterns, K-wire placement other than the crossing pattern may be difficult to achieve without violating either the DIP or PIP joint or directly penetrating a tendon (Fig. 30-27). Long oblique or spiral shaft fractures are amenable to relatively transverse placement of K-wires without joint or tendon penetration. When rotational alignment cannot be effectively restored by closed means, interfragmentary lag screw fixation is usually quite effective for spiral fractures. When comminution or axial instability is present, a limited number of P2 fractures may actually be most appropriately treated with plate and screw fixation (Fig. 30-28).

Temporary Transarticular Pinning for Partial Articular Base Fractures

Extension block pinning is an effective strategy for dorsal and volar base fractures (Fig. 30-29). An average PIP joint ROM of 91 degrees was achieved following CRIF of dorsal base fractures despite an extensor lag of over 10 degrees in five of nine patients.[135] Ten patients with transarticular pinning of volar base fractures for 3 weeks with 2 additional weeks of extension block splinting achieved an average 85-degree arc of motion with an 8-degree flexion contracture and no severe degenerative changes at 16 year follow-up.[120] Another study compared transarticular fixation (eight patients) to ORIF with lag screws (six patients) or ORIF with cerclage wires (five patients). At 7-year mean follow-up, cerclage wires produced the smallest arc of motion (median 48 degrees) compared to pinning (median 75 degrees). Eleven of the nineteen total patients healed with some degree of incongruence or frank subluxation.[3]

Volar Base Fractures

A closed fixation strategy uniquely designed for volar base fractures is a force couple device that works to dynamically

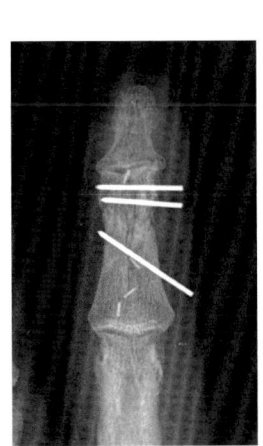
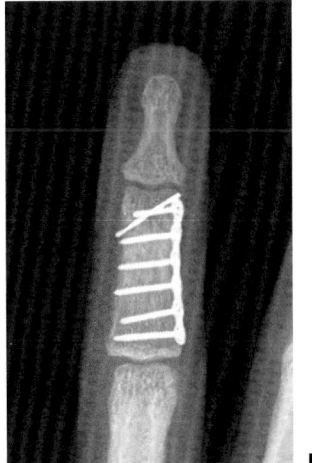

FIGURE 30-25 More complex bicondylar fractures can be stabilized by either **(A)** multiple wires in different planes or **(B)** a lateral plate and screws.

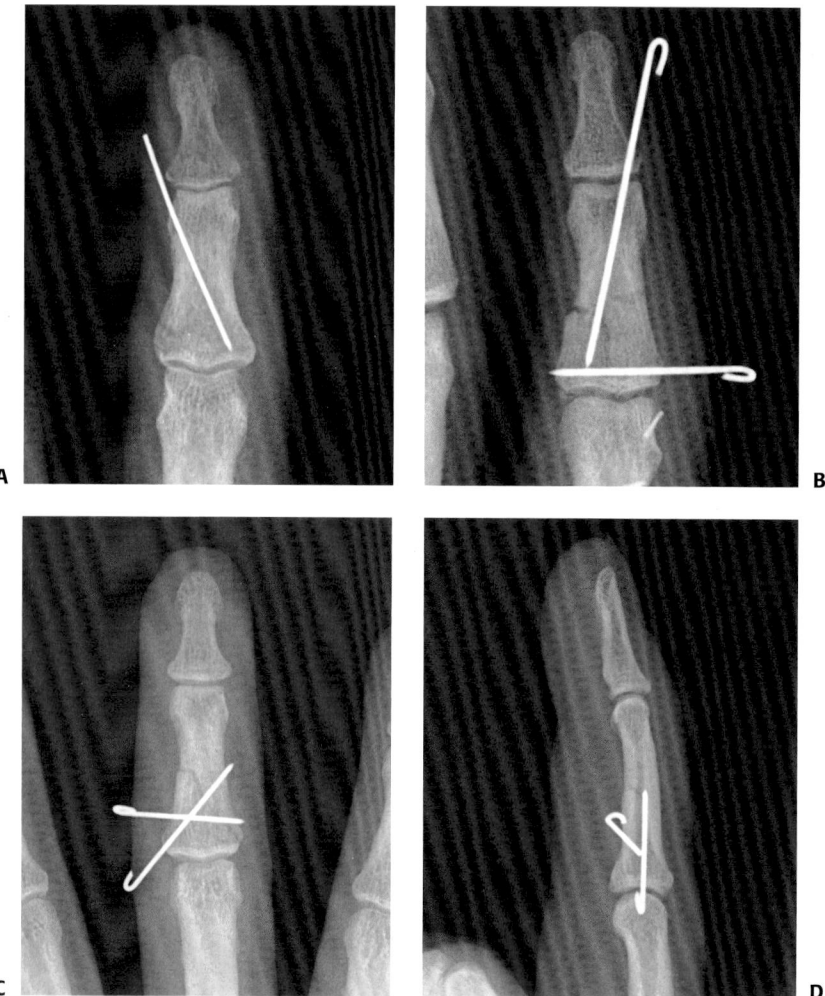

FIGURE 30-27 Shaft fractures of P2 can be stabilized with **(A)** a single oblique pin from the collateral recess to the opposite base if relatively stable upon reduction, **(B)** converging wires in different planes when added stability is needed, or **(C, D)** diverging wires.

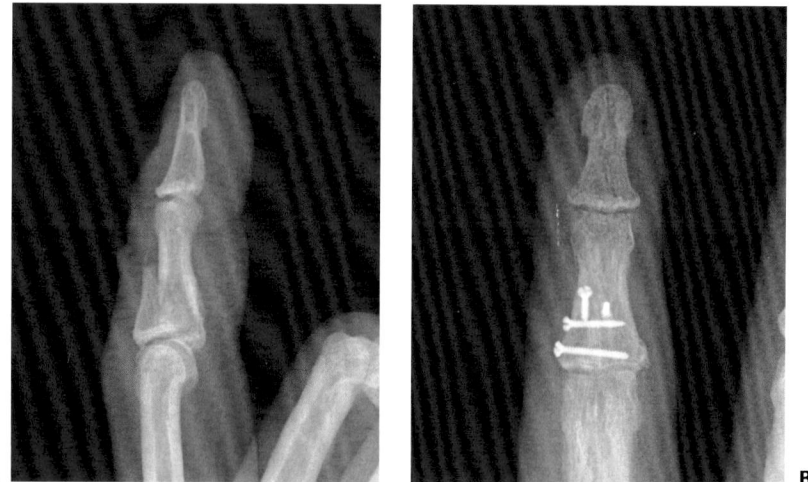

FIGURE 30-28 More complex shaft fractures **(A)** can be stabilized by **(B, C)** multiple lag screws or **(D)** a lateral plate and screws.

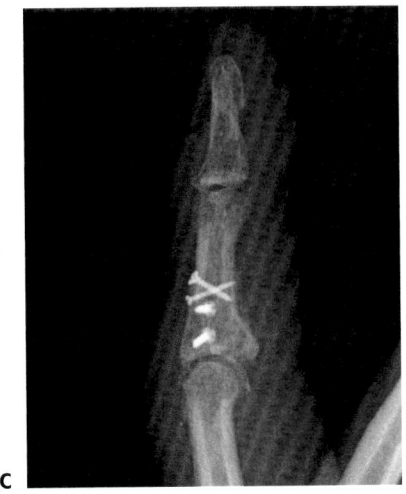
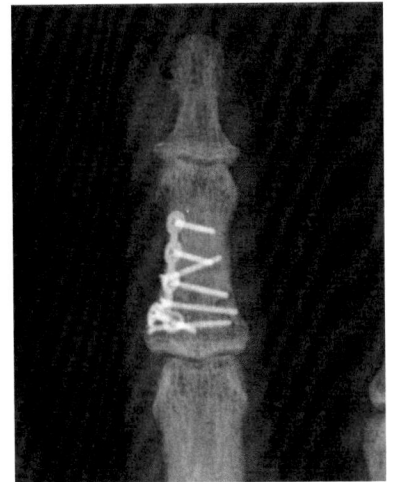

FIGURE 30-28 (continued)

reduce the tendency for dorsal subluxation of P2.[18] Acute volar base fractures involving more than 40% of the joint surface and those with sub-acute or chronic residual subluxation can be treated with volar plate arthroplasty. Seventeen patients followed at 11.5 years demonstrated a TAM of 85 degrees when operated on within 4 weeks of injury and 61 degrees when operated on later than 4 weeks from injury.[43] A series of 56 patients with volar base fracture-dislocations treated by either volar plate arthroplasty (23/56) or ORIF (33/56) had minimal pain in 83%, but radiographic evidence of degenerative changes in 96% at 46-month follow-up.[41]

Lag screw fixation is an excellent option for large volar fragments without comminution (Fig. 30-30). Seven patients undergoing lag screw fixation within 2 weeks of injury achieved an average PIP joint ROM of 100 degrees with a similar group of seven patients operated after 2 weeks achieving an average

of 86 degrees.[68] Another 12 digits followed for an average of 8.7 months after lag screw ORIF demonstrated combined PIP and DIP motion arcs that averaged 132 degrees.[104] When followed up at an average of 42 months from surgery, nine similar patients demonstrated an average PIP range of 70 degrees with a 14-degree flexion contracture.[70] Even displaced fractures more than 5 weeks from injury can be carefully corrected at the articular surface and supported by bone graft using the volar "shotgun" exposure.[38] When comminution is excessive, restoration of the volar buttress with true hyaline cartilage is possible using a hemi-hamate osteochondral autograft. Thirteen patients treated with this strategy at an average of 45 days post injury for comminution of the volar 60% of the P2 base had an average PIP arc of motion of 85 degrees at 16-month follow-up.[182] Another group of 33 patients achieved an average of a 70-degree arc of motion with a 20-degree flexion contracture

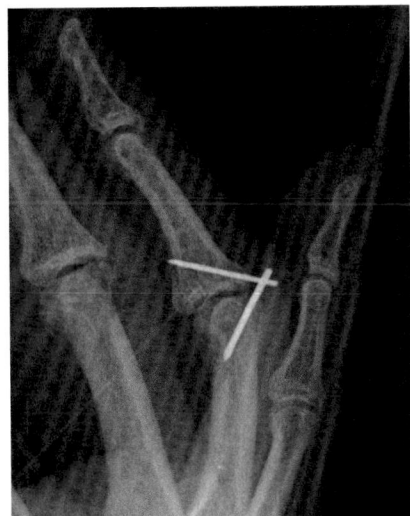

FIGURE 30-29 Extension block pinning includes at least one K-wire placed into the intercondylar notch of P1 to prevent dorsal displacement of the base of P2. A second interfragmentary wire may be added in the base of P2 itself.

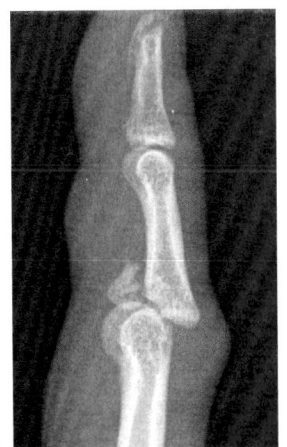
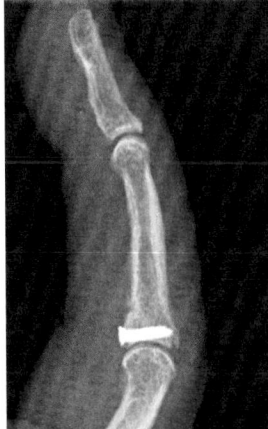

FIGURE 30-30 Volar base fractures of P2 allow the shaft and dorsal base fragment to (A) sublux dorsally and proximally resulting in hinge, rather than gliding, motion. Fixation of the volar base fragment must (B) restore the volar lip buttress against subluxation and re-create a congruent articulation.

and DASH score of 5.[21] Minimum 4-year follow-up of eight hemi-hamate osteochondral graft patients yielded an average arc of PIP motion of 67 degrees, mild arthritis in two patients, and severe arthritis in two patients (Table 30-6).[2]

"Pilon" Fractures

The most functionally devastating injuries to the PIP joint are "pilon" fractures that involve the complete articular surface combined with metaphyseal compaction. These are highly unstable injuries refractory to standard surgical techniques. Although other adverse events such as pin tract infection may intercede, the primary complication is stiffness. Unique forms of treatment have been devised for these injury patterns involving "dynamic traction."[11,37,49,98,114,137,140,160,167] An alternative design uses a dorsal spring mechanism.[53] The general principle is to establish a foundation at the center of rotation in the head of P1. From this foundation, traction (adjustable or elastic) is applied along the axis of P2 to hold the metaphyseal component of the fracture out to length while allowing early motion to remodel the articular surface. Dynamic traction with pins and rubber bands in 14 patients followed for 2.5 years produced average PIP motion of 74 degrees and a TAM of 196 degrees.[114] Dynamic fixation with wires but not elasticity in eight patients yielded a final average motion of 12 to 88 degrees following wire removal at 6 weeks.[89] Ideally, the patient should begin treatment acutely compared to delayed application of the device.[27] Many types of device constructs are possible (Fig. 30-31). The

TABLE 30-6	Surgical Steps—Osteochondral Reconstruction of Volar Base of P2 Fractures
	Bruner incision from DIP to palmodigital flexion crease, reflect, and tack back skin flap
	Mobilize neurovascular bundles to avoid traction during "shotgun" inversion of wound
	Open rectangular flap in flexor sheath from A2 to A4 pulleys
	Incise collateral ligaments tangentially from head of P1
	Excise volar plate
	Invert wound using "shotgun" maneuver, sweeping flexor tendons to side
	Evaluate fracture and prepare recipient defect using flat straight saw cuts to form right angle
	Harvest osteochondral graft from hamate larger than measurements at recipient defect
	Trim graft to orient sagittal ridge to match defect and to restore volar lip flexion posture
	Fix graft into defect with 2–3 lag screws (1.2–1.3 mm) and check orientation and fit
	Reduce joint and test stability, must not sublux or dislocate even in full extension
	Close flexor sheath and skin flaps, dress, and splint

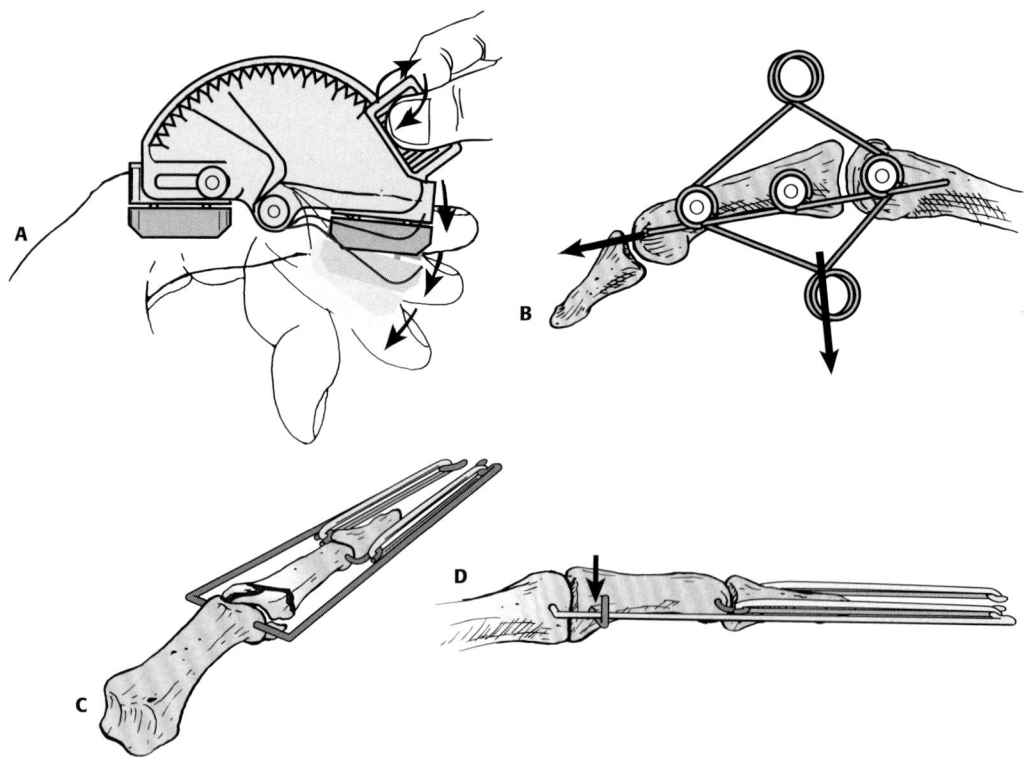

FIGURE 30-31 Strategies for managing "pilon" fractures at the base of P2 include **(A)** an adjustable unilateral hinged external fixator with distraction capabilities, **(B)** a wire spring construct, **(C)** the original configuration of pins and rubber bands, and **(D)** the same foundation augmented with an additional transverse wire across the metaphyseal base of P2 to resist dorsal subluxation.

TABLE 30-7	Potential Pitfalls and Preventative Measures—P2 Fractures	
Pitfall	**Prevention**	
Initially missing an incongruent PIP joint	Precise true lateral imaging to detect subtleties such as the dorsal V-sign	
Subsequent dorsal subluxation of P2 base	Using appropriately matched technique to resist subluxation: dorsal blocking splint, dorsal blocking wire, restored volar articular lip supported by internal fixation	
Axial collapse of pilon fracture	Sufficient external or internal fixation devices to resist the forces of tendon contraction	
Avascular necrosis of small articular fragments	Limit open dissection and preserve collateral ligament attachments to small fragments	
Inadequate restoration of volar articular lip in osteochondral reconstruction	Rotate graft correctly by cutting the cancellous surfaces to fit the recipient bed so that articular surface of graft is not perpendicular to neutral axis of P2	
Inadequate flexion after osteochondral reconstruction	Size graft correctly without overstuffing and excise volar plate	

simplest constructs involve only K-wires and rubber bands. Thirty-four patients from the armed services achieved a final average arc of motion at the PIP joint of 88 degrees and the DIP joint of 60 degrees using such a device with eight pin tract infections.[137] Another group of nonmilitary personnel achieved average PIP arcs of 64 degrees and DIP arcs of 52 degrees.[167] With the traction left in place for only 3.5 weeks on average, an average PIP arc of 94 degrees and thumb IP arc of 62.5 degrees were achieved in a total of six patients.[140] Another six patients having the device removed between 3 and 4 weeks achieved average PIP range from 5 degrees to 89 degrees with two pin tract infections.[11] Early removal of the device may be important as one group noted that their patients achieved minimal motion prior to removal of the device at a mean of 38 days with discomfort while in the device rated at 5.5/10.[57] By an average of 26 months postoperatively, five out of eight patients already demonstrated step-off deformities or arthritis.[49]

Potential Pitfalls and Preventative Measures. Successful management of P2 base fractures is predicated on a congruent joint. Thus, true lateral radiographs of the PIP joint are of paramount importance. A dorsal joint space shaped like the letter "V" is a subtle clue to an incongruent joint. With a volar base fracture dislocation of P2, the shaft fragment subluxes relative to the head of P1. To prevent subluxation, the shaft of P2 must be forcibly constrained by the appropriately matched technique to the degree and nature of the subluxation. By the same token, the axial collapse and splaying of fragments that occurs in a pilon fracture must be resisted by an adequate method of fixation, internal or external. When dealing with open procedures involving small articular fragments, dissection must be very precise and gentle, limiting the degree of soft tissue stripping to avoid avascular necrosis of the small fragments.

There are two critical steps in performing volar base osteochondral graft reconstructions. The first is to establish sharp and flat borders in the metaphyseal defect to receive and inset the graft in a stable fashion with broad cancellous surfaces for rapid bone healing. The second critical step is trimming the graft to fit this bed. The common pitfall is to set the graft's articular surface perpendicular to the neutral axis of the bone. This fails to re-establish the volar buttress and a truly congruent joint surface. If the graft is cut correctly, once inset, it should replicate the buttressing function of the native volar base and prevent dorsal dislocation. Another pitfall is simply overstuffing the space with too large a graft which will limit PIP joint flexion, partially remediable by volar plate excision (Table 30-7).

AUTHOR'S PREFERRED TREATMENT (FIG. 30-32)

Stable fractures are preferably treated by limited digital splints for 3 weeks or less and protected early motion thereafter with side strapping to an adjacent digit until clinically healed. Unstable but not comminuted fractures of the shaft can be treated well by temporary (3 weeks) closed pinning (Fig. 30-33). There are a few spiral fractures for which closed reduction will not achieve satisfactory control of rotation such that lag screw fixation with 1.2-mm screws is preferable to closed pinning techniques. These treatment strategies are also used in proximal phalanx fractures and more details may be found in that subsequent section of this chapter.

Dorsal Base Fractures

When a dorsal base fracture presents early, extension block pinning is an excellent treatment. The principles are all the same as described above for extension block pinning of dorsal base fractures in the distal phalanx. At the base of P2, the larger dorsal fragment (compared with the base of P3) is easier to work with and manipulate, but the PIP joint (compared with the DIP joint) imposes greater demands for a perfectly congruent joint reduction because of its more important role in overall digital function. The volar articular and shaft fragment is almost always subluxed proximally and volarly. When more

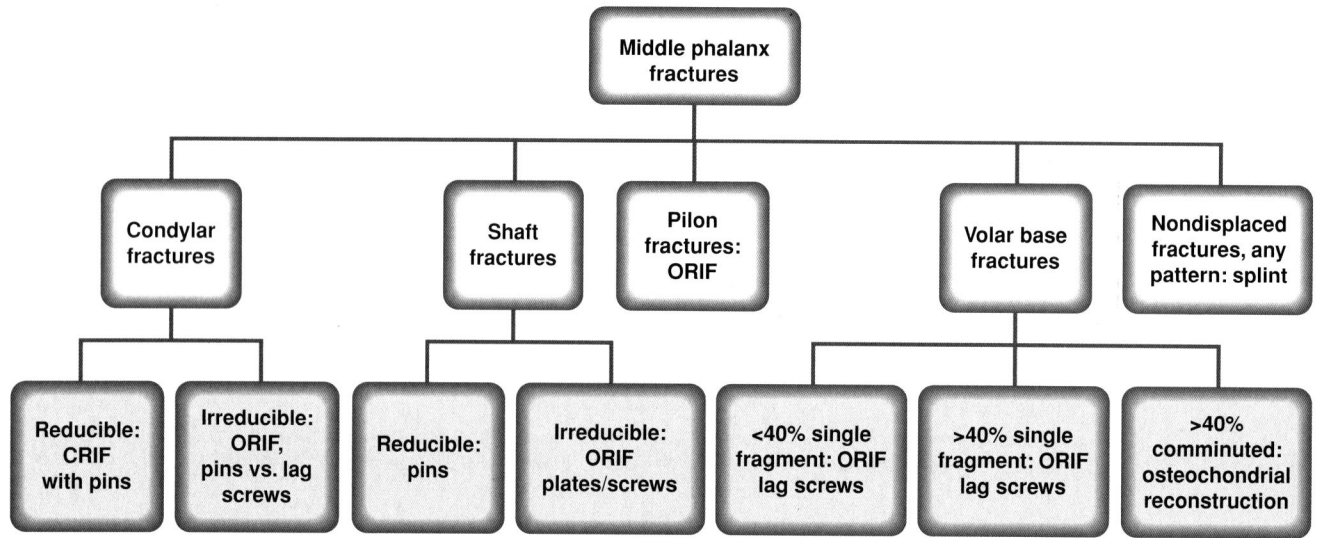

FIGURE 30-32 Middle phalanx (P2) fractures.

than 10 to 14 days have passed since injury, it can be quite difficult (because of early soft tissue contracture) to achieve a closed reduction of this fragment relative to the head of P1. It is for these reasons that late-presenting dorsal base fractures are often better managed with ORIF to ensure the clearance of consolidating hematoma from between the fragments and exact approximation of the articular reduction (Fig. 30-34). In this setting, fixation with two 1.2-mm lag screws usually affords enough stability to pursue early motion. Use of the countersink tap is important to minimize dorsal prominence of the screw heads and to avoid pressure concentration that might comminute the still relatively small dorsal fragment. Even though the surgical procedure occurs distal to extensor zone IV, a priority still must be placed on active extensor tendon excursion during rehabilitation to avoid a long-term extensor lag. In select cases, additional support may be needed in the form of a buttress plate (Fig. 30-34). Intraoperative assessment of the stability of the fixation will guide the progression of rehabilitation to ensure against fixation failure, recognizing the small size of the thread purchase in cancellous rather than cortical bone at the metaphyseal base of P2.

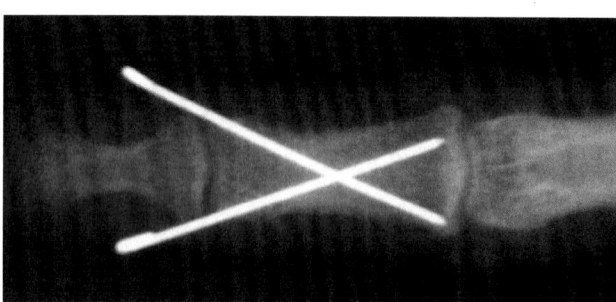

FIGURE 30-33 The relative biomechanical inferiority of K-wires crossing at the midshaft of the phalanx is offset by the lesser demands placed on P2 during rehabilitation than on P1 and the advantage of avoiding articular penetration to achieve a closed pinning.

Volar Base Fractures—Closed Treatment

Volar base fractures constituting less than 25% to 30% of the joint surface rarely require surgery unless presenting late with an incongruent joint. When seen acutely, these fractures are well managed with extension block splinting that begins at around 40 degrees and advances 10 to 15 degrees per week for the first 3 weeks. If the extension block splint cannot be eliminated in 3 weeks' time, this treatment strategy may not be appropriate. Fractures constituting more than 25% but less than 40% of the joint surface pose a difficulty in treatment planning as they are an intermediate group where the disadvantages of the two primary options are relatively well matched. It is difficult to predict in advance how the disadvantages will play out over the course of treatment for an individual patient. The disadvantage of extension block splinting or pinning is that with a greater amount of joint surface involved, the blocking must begin at a higher angle and it will take longer to achieve full extension. A permanent fixed flexion contracture is the consequence to be avoided. This must be compared with the overall tendency for loss of joint motion associated with ORIF or open reconstruction.

Volar Base Fractures—ORIF

When the volar fragment(s) constitute greater than 40% of the joint surface, an open procedure offers the greatest assurance of achieving a congruent joint as a final result. The distinction between the need for ORIF for one or two relatively large fragments or open reconstruction for highly comminuted multiple fragments often cannot be made until the time of surgery. One should always be prepared for both possibilities in the preoperative planning discussions with the patient. Dorsal base fractures usually provide a single fragment of reasonable size for direct lag screw fixation. Volar base fractures are not so easy. One or two large fragments that facilitate lag screw fixation are the exception rather than the rule. In this case, two 1.2-mm

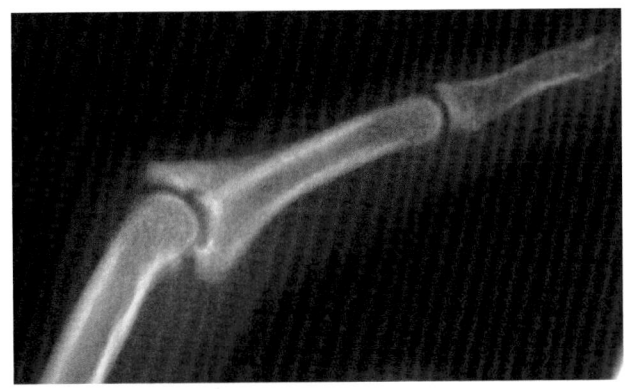
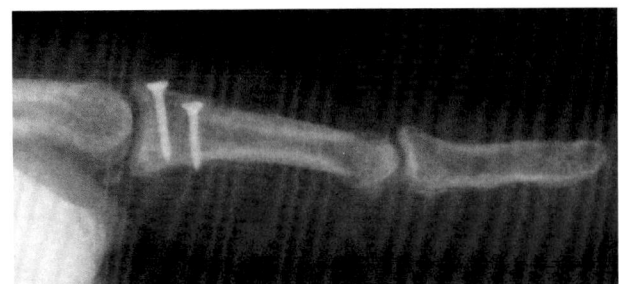

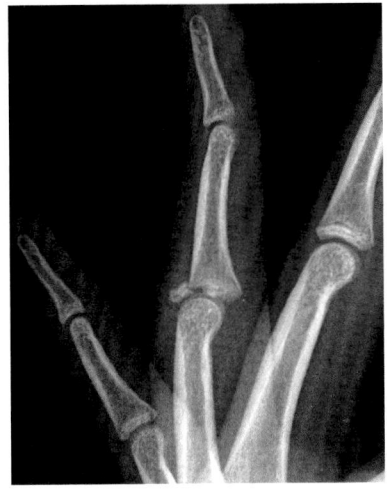
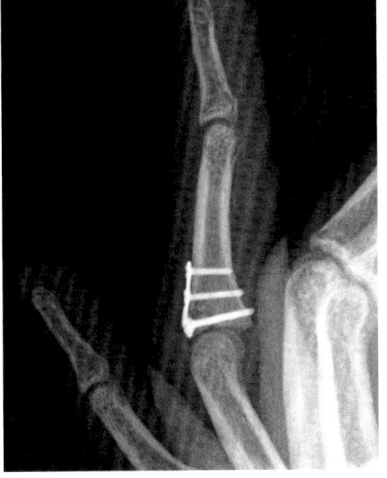

FIGURE 30-34 Dorsal base fractures allow **(A)** the volar articular fragment and the attached shaft of P2 to sublux volarly and proximally. **B:** A congruent joint is restored with sufficient stability to initiate early rehabilitation by lag screw fixation. An alternative fixation strategy is **(C, D)** a small custom-cut hook plate.

lag screws are appropriate. Placement is side by side with one screw in the radial half of the base fragment and the other in the ulnar half. If two separate radial and ulnar volar base fragments are found, this strategy is still acceptable provided that the fragment diameter is at least three times the screw diameter and compression can be achieved without causing fragment comminution. The countersink tap is useful in this regard. With increasing comminution and loss of metaphyseal support for the articular fragments, the original bone may still be salvaged by a volar buttress plate to avoid progressing to the next rung of the reconstructive ladder, osteochondral reconstruction.[23]

Volar Base Fractures—Osteochondral Reconstruction

A Bruner incision is made using one limb over P1 and a second over P2. The flexor tendon sheath is reflected as a single rectangular flap hinging on its lateral margin between the distal margin of the A2 pulley and the proximal margin of the A4 pulley. The FDS and FDP are retracted laterally, one to either side, and the collateral ligament origins are dissected as a sleeve from the lateral surfaces of the head of P1. Release of the volar plate allows complete hyperextension of the PIP joint and presentation of both joint surfaces toward the surgeon. This is the so-called "shotgun" approach, and its variations center on the management of the volar plate. This approach is also used for

volar plate arthroplasty and ORIF. In the former procedure, the volar plate is released distally so that it may be advanced to replace the defect in the volar articular surface. In the latter, it should remain attached to the fragments as an important source of blood supply. When performing a reconstruction of irreparable comminution, the volar plate no longer has an anatomic connection to the volar base of P2, and complete excision will facilitate restoration of PIP flexion after graft reconstruction. The defect in the volar articular surface may range anywhere from 40% up to almost 90%, often with irregular margins. A small saw or burr should be used to straighten the irregular margins into sharp orthogonal cuts that define a clear bed of cancellous bone in the metaphysis that can be accurately measured for reconstruction. The articular surface at the base of P2 has a sagittally oriented ridge that interdigitates with the groove between the two condyles at the head of P1. This relationship is important not only for preserving joint congruence but also for maintaining stability in the setting of collateral ligament releases. An excellent geometric match has been found in the distal articular surface of the hamate at the ridge that separates the ring from the small finger CMC joints. The measurements taken from the defect at the base of P2 are transposed to the hamate and a small saw and osteotomes are used to remove the osteochondral graft from its donor site. The graft is then exactly trimmed to match the defect and secured with two 1.2-mm lag

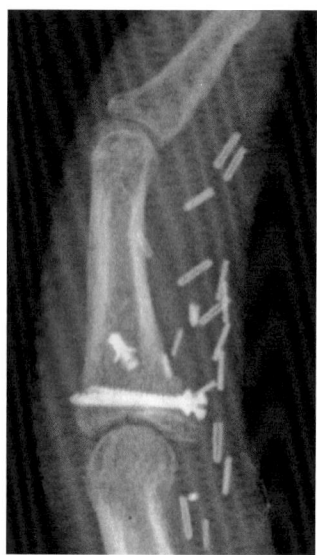

FIGURE 30-35 Volar base fractures with comminution of a substantial portion of the articular surface and subluxation can be reconstructed with an osteochondral graft from the hamate with particular emphasis placed on re-creating the volar lip buttress and a truly congruent reproduction of the radius of curvature.

screws (Fig. 30-35). The joint is checked clinically and radiographically for maintenance of congruence through a full ROM. The flexor sheath is reapproximated with 6–0 monofilament sutures and the PIP joint splinted for protection. Immediate active motion rehabilitation is begun within days of surgery. These same techniques can be extrapolated for use in alternative sites such as the thumb IP joint with the use of a partial FDP-reflecting approach (Fig. 30-36).

"Pilon" Fractures—ORIF

Complete articular fractures of the base of P2 may be treated by entirely closed reduction and stabilization. If significant metaphyseal bone loss is present or if the articular fragments

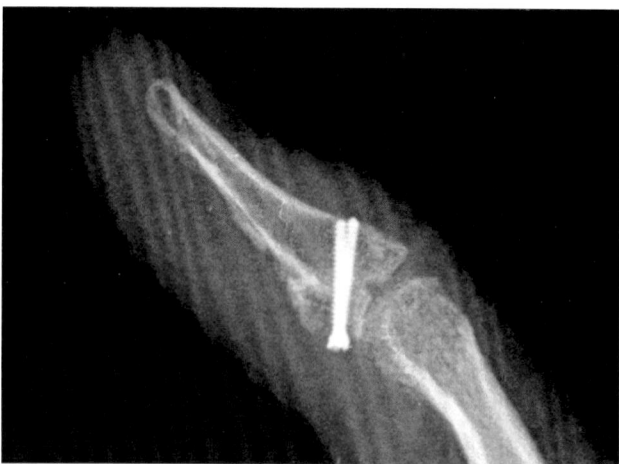

FIGURE 30-36 A congruent osteochondral reconstruction of a chronic volar base fracture dislocation can also be performed in the thumb with a partial FPL-reflecting approach.

at the base of P2 do not reduce sufficiently with traction alone, a small incision can be made through which cancellous bone graft can be added to fill the metaphyseal void and to assist in supporting a reduction of the articular fragments. Transverse 0.035-inch K-wires may be placed at the subchondral level to maintain the articular relationships. The fracture must then be reduced at the metaphyseal level and undergo stabilization sufficient to withstand the rigors of early motion that must accompany the rehabilitation of articular fractures. It is at this point that the significant variations in technique arise along with different devices available for stabilization. My previous preference was for an off-the-shelf unilateral hinged external fixator. The device, which is no longer available, allowed free AROM with a gear disengaged or passive range of motion (PROM) with the gear engaged and the ability to hold and stretch the end points of motion (Fig. 30-37). External fixators for "pilon" fractures are not well received by patients who tend to refuse to move the PIP joint much while the device is in place. For these reasons, my current preference is to treat "pilon" fractures with ORIF, a transition that has been aided by the increasing availability of small locking plates. This is a well-received option by patients, provided that stable fixation is achieved and the result maintained during the stress of therapy (Fig. 30-38).

INTRODUCTION TO PROXIMAL INTERPHALANGEAL (PIP) JOINT DISLOCATIONS

Dislocations of the PIP joint have a high rate of missed diagnoses that are passed off as "sprains." Although a large number of incomplete injuries occur (especially in ball-handling sports), complete disruptions of the collateral ligaments and the volar plate are also frequent. Since dramatic swelling is often present even with minor injuries to the PIP joint, this sign may often be dismissed by initial examiners of the patient. Careful palpation for localized tenderness may direct attention to one of the collateral ligaments, the volar plate, or the insertion of the central slip. The capacity for active PIP extension against resistance from a starting position of PIP flexion confirms the integrity of the central slip. Limitation of passive DIP flexion while the PIP joint is held in extension may appear several weeks following the initial injury and signifies a developing boutonnière deformity. Congruence on the lateral radiograph is the key to detecting residual subluxation. Correct axial rotational alignment is demonstrated when both P1 and P2 are seen in a true lateral projection on the same film.

Residual instability is quite rare in pure dislocations as opposed to fracture-dislocations where it is the chief issue at stake. It manifests as hyperextension laxity following volar plate injuries managed with an inadequate initial degree of extension blocking. Correction of hyperextension instability can be performed with either delayed reattachment of the volar plate or a capsulotenodesis reconstruction. In pure dislocations, stiffness is the primary concern. Stiffness can occur following any injury pattern and responds best at the late stage to complete collateral ligament excision.[108] Chronic missed dislocations require open reduction with a predictable amount of subsequent stiffness. Patients should be counseled to expect permanent residual

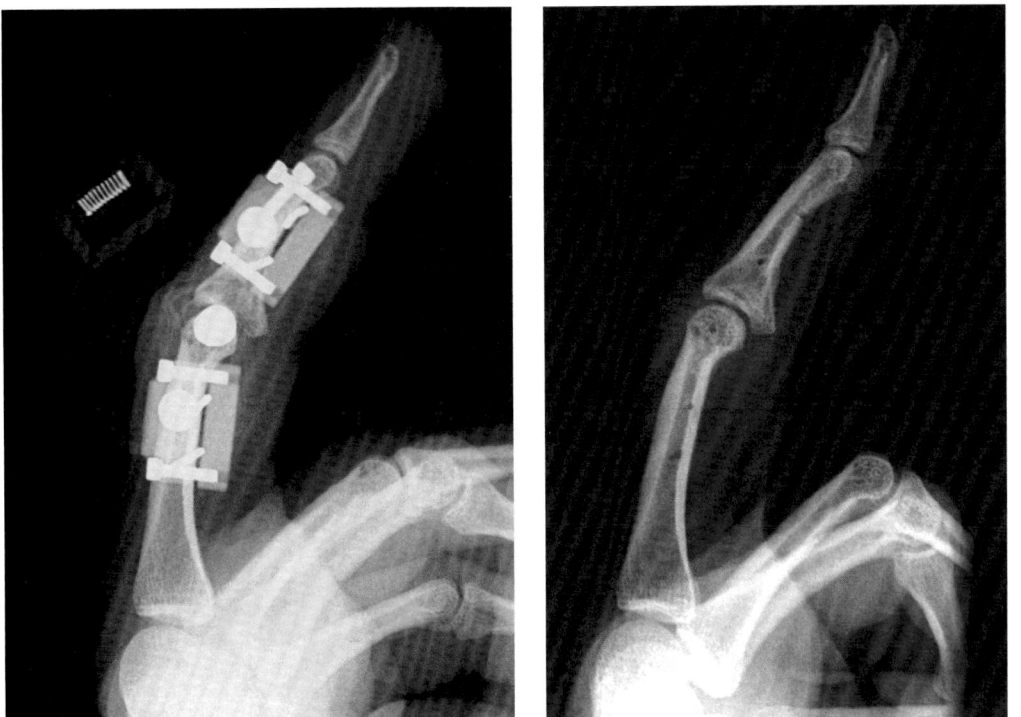

FIGURE 30-37 A hinged external fixator can be used to control "pilon" fractures beginning with **(A)** the placement of a transverse K-wire through the center of PIP rotation in the head of P1 followed by assembly of the device around that foundation wire. If performed correctly the result will be **(B)** a congruent joint when healed.

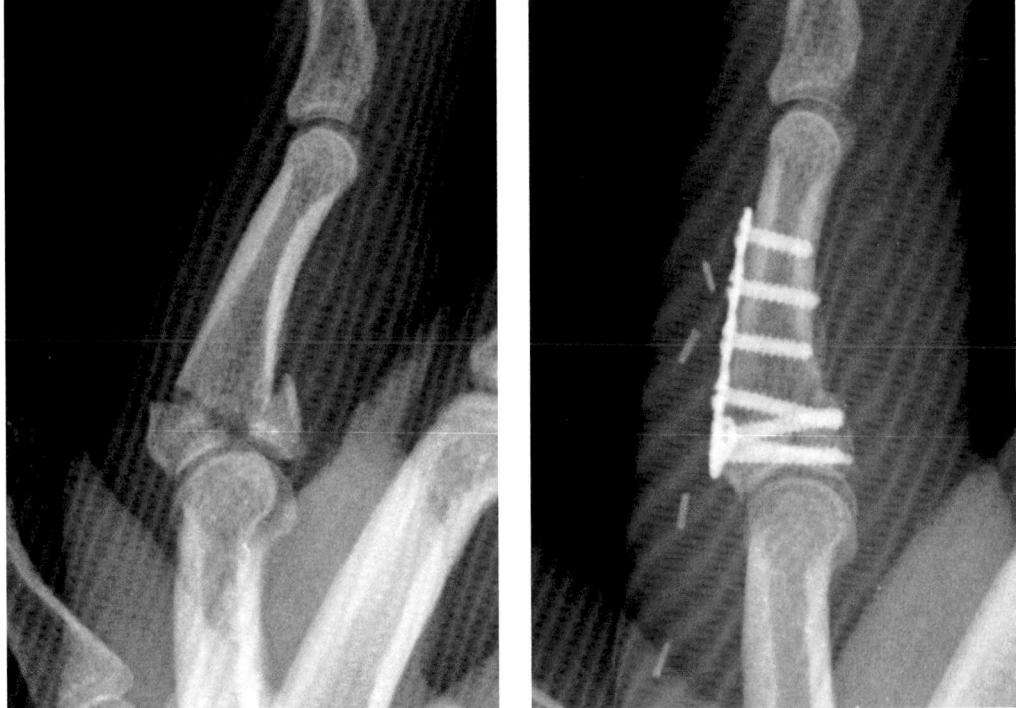

FIGURE 30-38 Some "pilon" fractures are amenable to ORIF which then avoids the complications of pin tract infection associated with the dynamic traction strategies.

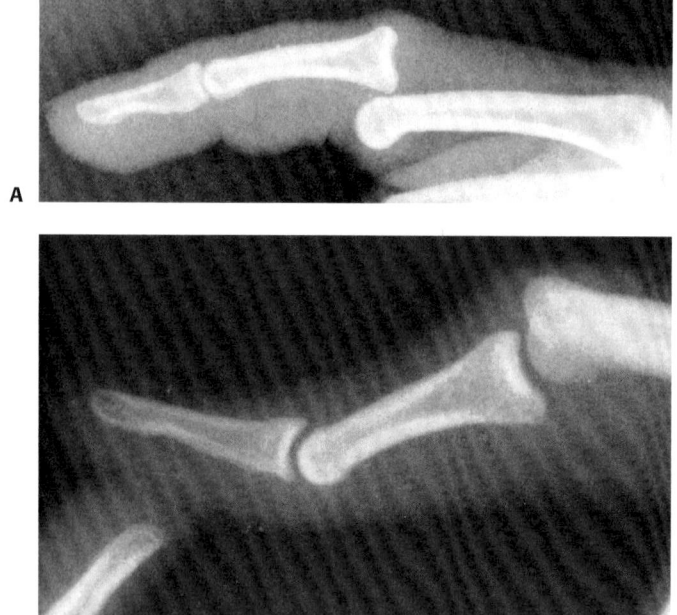

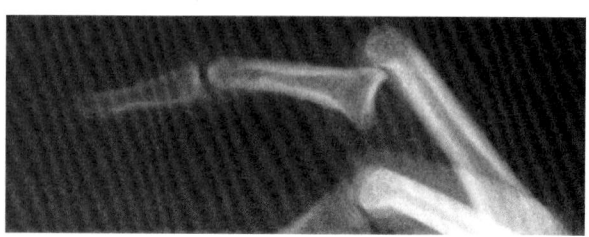

FIGURE 30-39 Three variants of PIP dislocation are seen. **A:** The most common, dorsal, **(B)** pure volar with central slip disruption, and **(C)** volar rotatory (note that P2 is seen as a true lateral whereas P1 is seen in oblique profile).

enlargement of the joint and for the final resolution of stiffness and aching to take as long as 12 to 18 months.

PATHOANATOMY AND APPLIED ANATOMY RELATING TO PROXIMAL INTERPHALANGEAL (PIP) JOINT DISLOCATIONS

The head of P1 is quite different from that of the metacarpal. There is no cam effect. The head is bicondylar, and the collateral ligaments originate from the center axis of joint rotation. Nevertheless, the accessory collateral ligaments and volar plate are lax in flexion and will become contracted if immobilized in that position. At the volar base of P2, there are tubercles for the confluence of the proper and accessory collateral ligaments with the volar plate. This junction is referred to as the "critical corner." This three-sided box design provides excellent inherent joint stability. The volar plate anatomy is unique at the PIP joint with the presence of strong check-rein ligaments that originate inside the margins of the A2 pulley, confluent with the C1 pulley fibers and the oblique retinacular ligament. The distal insertion of the volar plate is strong only at its lateral margins. The undersurface of the central slip has an articulating fibrocartilage that may aid in stabilization, prevent central slip attenuation, and increase the extensor moment arm. Although primarily a hinge, the PIP joint accommodates 7 to 10 degrees of lateral deviation and slight axial rotation. The normal ROM may be up to 120 degrees of flexion. In contrast to the other small joints of the hand, PIP joint volar plate disruptions usually occur distally. The proper collateral ligaments are the primary stabilizers to lateral stress, and a greater than 20-degree opening signifies complete disruption. Collateral ligament disruption is usually proximal, but the fibers traditionally stay positioned over their anatomic origin for subsequent healing.

Recognized patterns of dislocation are dorsal dislocation, pure volar dislocation, and rotatory volar dislocation (Fig. 30-39). Dorsal dislocations involve volar plate injury (usually distally, with or without a small flake of bone). To sustain a pure volar dislocation, the patient must rupture the volar plate, at least one collateral ligament, and the central slip. Rotatory volar dislocation occurs as the head of P1 passes between the central slip and the lateral bands, which can form a noose effect and prevent reduction (Fig. 30-40). Irreducible dislocations obstructed by the volar plate or flexor tendons are uncommon injuries.

PROXIMAL INTERPHALANGEAL (PIP) JOINT DISLOCATIONS TREATMENT OPTIONS

Dorsal Dislocations—Nonoperative Management

Isolated volar plate injuries can be managed with immediate AROM while strapped to an adjacent digit. Fortunately, the majority of hyperextension injuries remain congruent even at full extension and do not require extension block splinting.

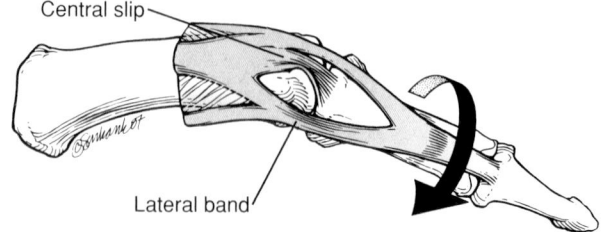

Central slip

Lateral band

FIGURE 30-40 In volar rotatory dislocations, the head of P1 protrudes between the intact central slip and one lateral band, which create a noose effect preventing reduction especially if longitudinal traction is applied.

However, one must consider that the distal volar plate is poorly vascularized, and a lack of early healing may lead to chronic hyperextension laxity. Swelling and pain serve to limit patients from full extension, and side strapping to an adjacent digit further inhibits maximum extension enough that extension block splinting is rarely necessary. When formal extension block splinting is chosen (usually only in the situation of fracture subluxation), the rate of progression each week is determined by the severity of the initial injury but should reach full extension no later than 3 weeks from injury.

Pure Volar Dislocations—Nonoperative Management

With pure volar dislocations, central slip disruption occurs and will result in a boutonnière deformity if not treated properly. Careful examination consisting of PIP extension against resistance from a starting position of full flexion will prevent missing the diagnosis of a central slip disruption. Limitation of passive DIP flexion is an early sign of a developing boutonnière deformity. Even when identified late, the treatment of choice is extension splinting at the PIP joint with immediate active DIP blocking exercises. Active DIP flexion pulls the whole extensor mechanism (including the ruptured central slip) distally through the intact lateral bands. The duration of PIP extension splinting is 6 weeks. Short arc of motion exercises can begin at 4 weeks, returning to the extension splint between sessions.

Rotatory Volar Dislocations—Nonoperative Management

Rotatory volar dislocations where the head of P1 is trapped between the central slip and lateral band may be difficult to reduce owing to the noose effect exerted by these two soft tissue structures. The key to closed reduction (if it is possible at all) is to relax both structures. Wrist extension relaxes the extrinsic component, and full MP joint flexion relaxes the intrinsic component. A gentle rotating maneuver that avoids excessive longitudinal traction stands the highest chance of success. A few of these dislocations remain irreducible even in the most skilled hands. When a reduction can be achieved, early mobilization is then instituted with adjacent digit strapping (usually the more radial) in an attempt to prevent stiffness.

Open Reduction

There are two indications for open treatment of PIP joint injuries: an open injury or an irreducible dislocation.[126] Lateral dislocations may also be irreducible because of interposition of a torn collateral ligament (Fig. 30-41). A midaxial (or dual midaxial) incision allows for management of both dorsal and volar dislocations. Controversy remains as to the need for direct repair of complete collateral ligament ruptures and volar plate injuries. Direct repair is probably only functionally necessary in the long term for the radial collateral ligament (RCL) of the index finger. Chronic reconstruction of collateral ligament deficiency is rarely necessary and is an even more technically demanding procedure with a high propensity for generating stiffness but may be accomplished by a variety of techniques.

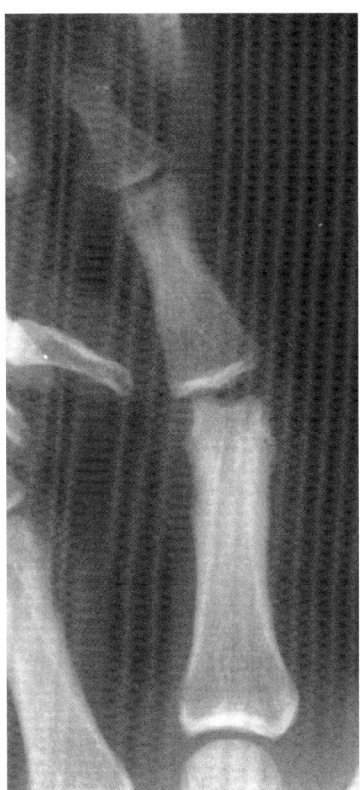

FIGURE 30-41 Entrapment of a collateral ligament can prevent reduction of the PIP joint; lateral stress examination demonstrates the high degree of instability in this situation.

Potential Pitfalls and Preventative Measures

Straight longitudinal traction is almost never the answer to accomplishing a reduction and certainly is the surest way to fail at the PIP joint. Relaxation of the most powerful tendon forces acting across the joint is the key to facilitating a smooth reduction that does not cause additional hyaline cartilage damage. Postreduction clinical and radiographic assessment is crucial with an emphasis on the lateral radiograph in full extension to assess congruence. The patient should be able to move the finger through a near full ROM under the influence of the digital block used to accomplish the reduction. Open dislocations should be taken seriously for their potentially high rate of complications and debrided prior to reduction (Table 30-8).

TABLE 30-8	Potential Pitfalls and Preventative Measures—PIP Joint Dislocations
Pitfall	**Prevention**
Attempting to use longitudinal traction to reduce the dislocation	Gentle rotatory maneuvers and strategic proximal joint positioning to relax tendons
Failing to achieve a congruent reduction	True lateral radiograph in flexion and extension or lateral fluoroscopy with motion
Infection following open dislocations	Definitive surgical debridement in operating room prior to reduction

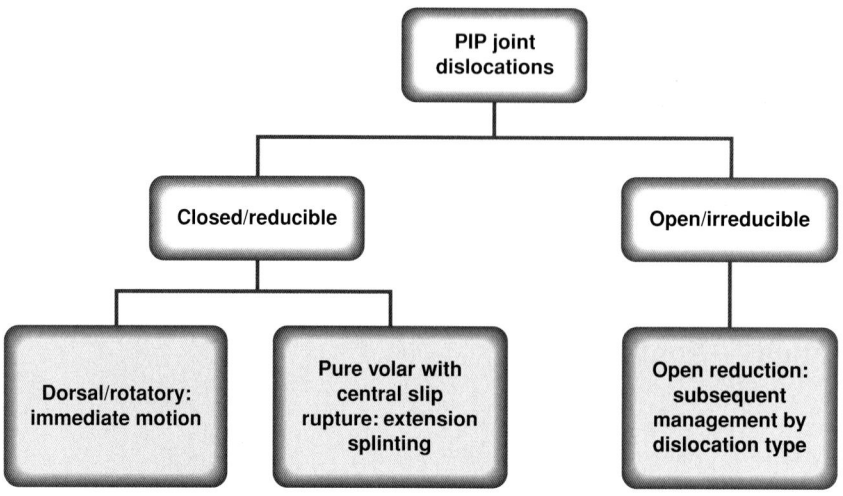

FIGURE 30-42 PIP joint dislocations.

AUTHOR'S PREFERRED TREATMENT (FIG. 30-42)

Once reduced, rotatory volar dislocations, isolated collateral ligament ruptures, and dorsal dislocations congruent in full extension on the lateral radiograph can all begin immediate AROM with adjacent digit strapping. Dorsal dislocations that are subluxed on the extension lateral radiograph require a few weeks of extension block splinting before progressing (however, this is an almost unheard of situation with pure dislocation and no fracture component). Volar dislocations with central slip disruptions require 6 weeks of PIP extension splinting followed by nighttime static extension splinting for 2 additional weeks. The DIP joint should be unsplinted and actively flexed throughout the entire recovery period. Short arc motion of the PIP joint can begin at 4 weeks.

Open dorsal dislocations usually have a transverse rent in the skin at the flexion crease. Debridement of this wound should precede reduction of the dislocation. Any joint debris should be cleared out to prevent third body wear. The "critical corner" warrants particular attention. For closed irreducible joints, unilateral or bilateral midaxial incisions allow excellent access to both volar and dorsal structures without violating the extensor mechanism. Postoperative management follows the same time courses stated above for nonoperative management based on the injury pattern and severity.

INTRODUCTION TO PROXIMAL PHALANX (P1) FRACTURES

Recognized proximal phalanx fracture patterns include intra-articular fractures of the head, extra-articular fractures of the neck and shaft, and both extra-articular and intra-articular fractures of the base (Fig. 30-43). Further describing the pattern

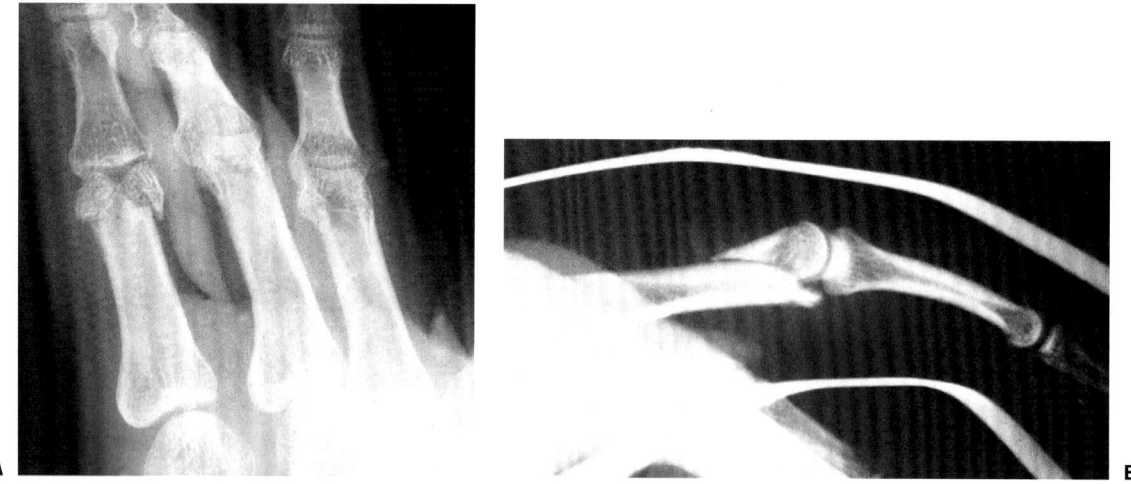

FIGURE 30-43 Fracture patterns appearing in P1 include **(A)** complete articular fractures of the head, **(B)** subcapital fractures with impingement in the volar plate recess, **(C)** transverse fractures of the shaft or base, **(D)** oblique fractures of the shaft, and **(E)** articular fractures of the base.

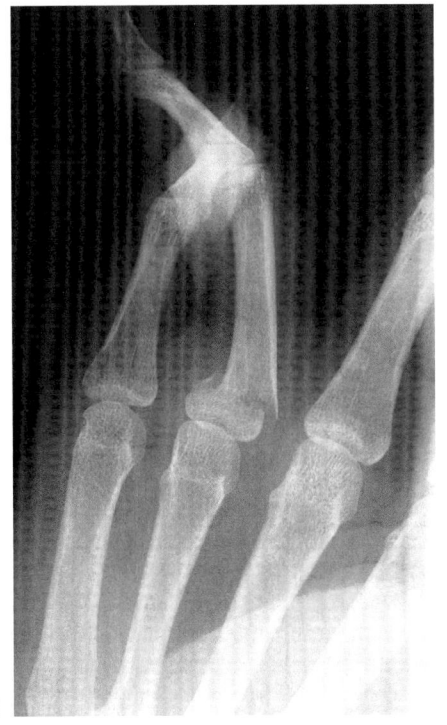
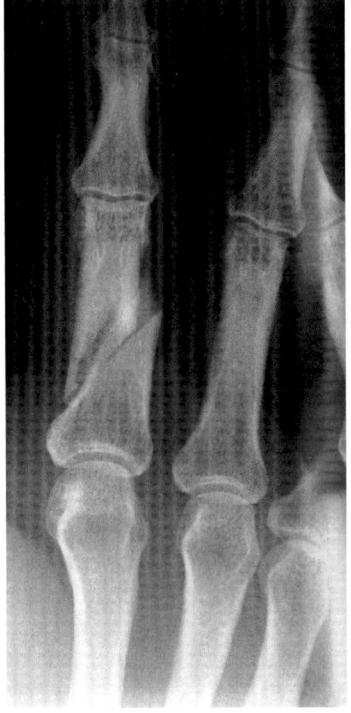
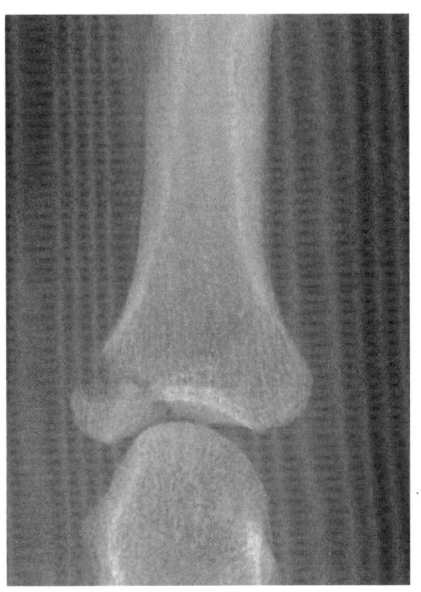

C, D

E

FIGURE 30-43 (*continued*)

of the fracture as transverse, short oblique, long oblique, or spiral for shaft fractures and partial or complete articular for intra-articular fractures (along with the degree and direction of displacement) provides the necessary information to support treatment decisions. A specific fracture pattern that risks extreme PIP limitation is that of the neck of the proximal phalanx, where a volar spike of bone from the proximal fracture fragment impinges into the subcapital recess volar to the neck of P1 (Fig. 30-43B). If the fracture heals in this position, full PIP flexion is prevented by obstruction of the space for volar plate in-folding. This pattern is best identified on an individual digital lateral radiograph and warrants operative treatment to prevent a functionally disabling malunion.

PATHOANATOMY AND APPLIED ANATOMY RELATING TO PROXIMAL PHALANX (P1) FRACTURES

Local Soft Tissue Relationships

Fracture of the proximal phalanx may well be one of the more frustrating hand injuries to manage owing to the local soft tissue anatomy.[99,105] Whereas the metacarpal has only a cord-like extensor tendon running well dorsal to it, the proximal phalanx is closely invested by a sheet-like extensor mechanism with a complex array of decussating collagen fibers (Fig. 30-44). Surgical disturbance of the fine balance between these fibers can permanently alter the long-term function of the digit. The operative approach to P1 can be either dorsal or lateral. The dorsal approach may be technically simpler but transgresses the extensor mechanism and should not be used unless an open trauma has already disrupted the tendon. The lateral midaxial

approach allows the fracture to be fully exposed and hardware placed in its proper lateral position (if hardware is indicated) without directly violating the extensor mechanism.[79] If prominent hardware is to be placed, the intrinsic tendon on that side (usually ulnar) may be resected. The proximal phalanx is not a cylinder, but rather highly elliptical (in fact, tunnel-shaped) in cross section, with a thicker dorsal cortex.

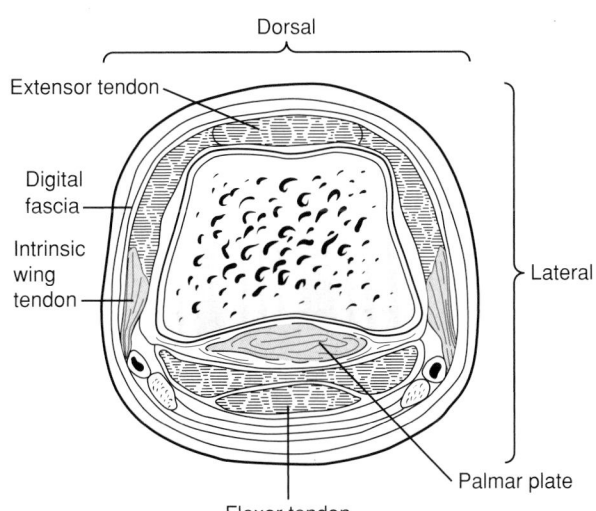

FIGURE 30-44 The proximal phalanx is closely invested by the sheet of the zone IV extensor tendon dorsally, the blending of the intrinsic wing tendons laterally and volarly, and the flexor tendons and flexor sheath directly volarly.

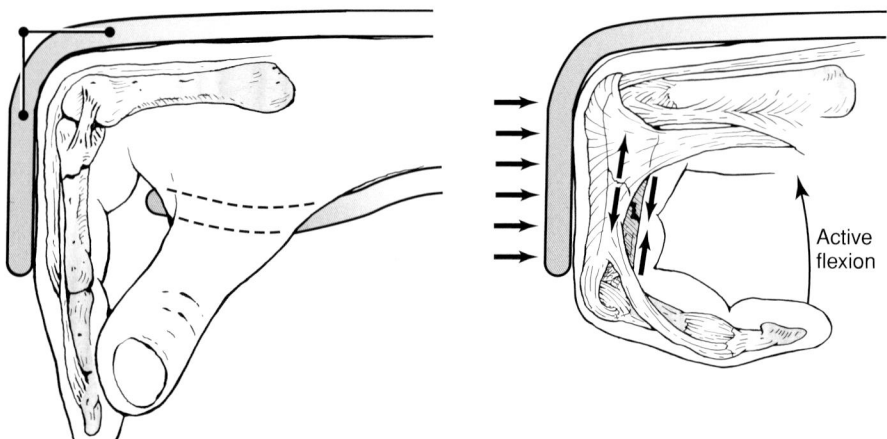

FIGURE 30-45 Flexing the MP joints fully causes the extensor apparatus to function as a tension band to a transverse fracture in the P1 shaft, helping to reduce the deformity and stabilize the fracture when the PIP joint is actively flexed.

Deforming Forces

At the proximal phalangeal level, both intrinsic and extrinsic tendon forces deform the fracture. They result in a predictable apex volar deformity for transverse and short oblique fractures. These forces can be used with benefit during rehabilitation. If the MP joints are maximally flexed (the intrinsic plus position), the intrinsic muscle forces acting through the extensor mechanism overlying P1 create a tension band effect that helps to maintain fracture reduction (Fig. 30-45). Active PIP joint motion will heighten this effect and forms the basis for nonoperative fracture management.[56] Spiral and long oblique fractures tend to shorten and rotate rather than angulate. These fractures also have more complex patterns of deformity that are not so easily controlled through the joint positioning just described. One can expect 12 degrees of extensor lag at the PIP joint for each millimeter of shortening and 1.5 degrees of extensor lag for each degree of apex palmar fracture angulation.[173]

Biomechanics of Fixation

Transverse and short oblique proximal phalanx shaft fractures deform through apex volar bending. Laboratory investigation has shown the biomechanical inefficiency of dorsally applied plates in an apex volar bending model that correlated with the clinical forces experienced at the P1 level.[111] Even with plate fixation, the soft tissue envelope has been shown to add stability under load application.[127] This is particularly true in the most proximal 6 to 9 millimeters at the base of P1.[181] The most valuable foundation in a fixation paradigm is a well-placed lag screw across a noncomminuted fracture interface, although some surgeons have bypassed the step of lagging the screw in favor of less labor-intensive bicortical screws.[136] Long oblique and spiral proximal phalanx fractures demonstrate less angular deformity than transverse fractures, instead shortening and rotating axially.

PROXIMAL PHALANX (P1) FRACTURE TREATMENT OPTIONS

Nonoperative Management

This is the preferred treatment for many phalangeal fractures that are either minimally displaced or easily rendered stable by reduc-

tion. Compared with oblique, spiral, or comminuted fractures, transverse fractures will generally prove to be stable after reduction. Stable proximal phalangeal fractures are ideal candidates for dorsal splinting with the MP joint in flexion. Only 4 of the 45 patients treated with intrinsic plus splinting failed to achieve full motion by 6 weeks.[48] Another 65 patients treated with intrinsic plus splinting achieved 86% of normal motion.[56] The splint should be discontinued at 3 weeks, followed by AROM exercises without resistance. Stable, nondisplaced fractures may even be treated by a program of immediate AROM, protected only with adjacent digit strapping. The key message for nonoperative management is that a carefully formed splint and/or adjacent digit strapping can effectively maintain an existing and reasonably stable reduction butt splints and strapping cannot accomplish a reduction in their own right. All patients undergoing nonoperative management should be reviewed at a week to verify maintenance of reduction both clinically and radiographically.

Operative Management
Closed Reduction and Internal Fixation

This is the treatment of choice for the category of reducible but unstable isolated fractures, both extra-articular and some intra-articular.[77] A higher degree of care must be exercised when pursuing CRIF in the phalanges compared with the metacarpals because of the close investment by the broad extensor mechanism. Pin entry sites should be chosen carefully to minimize tethering of the extensor mechanism. In the proximal two-thirds of P1, this is virtually impossible. As one approaches the distal one-third, a direct lateral approach can be made volar to the interosseous tendon. For long oblique and spiral fractures, three K-wires (0.045- or 0.035-inch) are placed perpendicular to the fracture plane (Fig. 30-46). For neck fractures, retrograde pinning may be necessary (Fig. 30-47). For short oblique and transverse fractures, longitudinal K-wires (0.045-inch) are placed through the MP joint (Fig. 30-48). Twelve patients achieved an average TAM of 265 degrees with two longitudinal pins placed across the MP joint and down the shaft of the proximal phalanx.[85] Trocar-tipped K-wires rather than diamond-tipped or surgeon-cut wires should be used. The wire should be passed through the soft tissues and down to bone before activating the wire driver. Pins should be

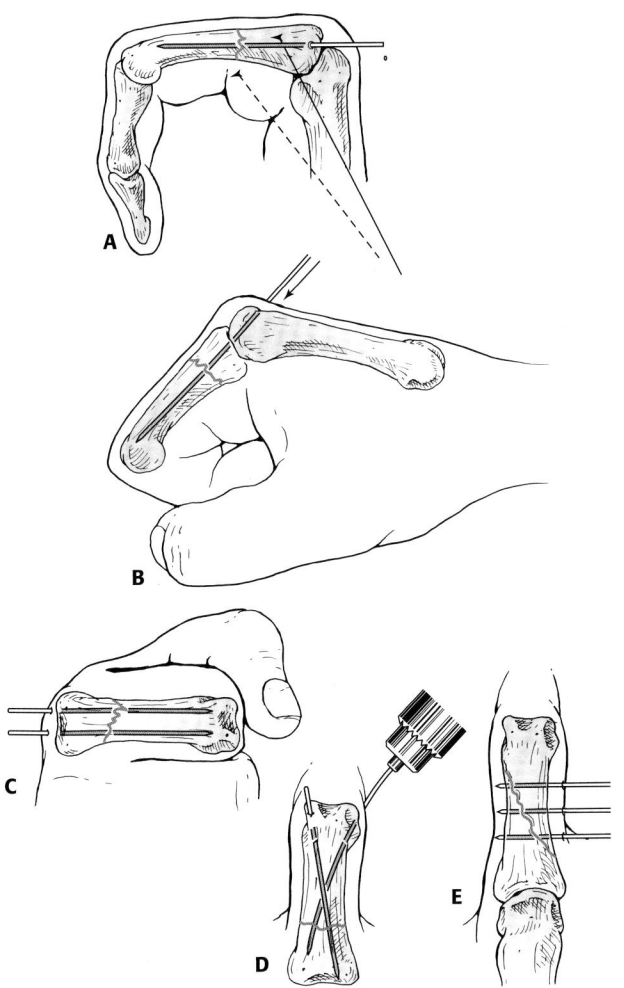

FIGURE 30-46 Closed reduction and internal fixation of P1 shaft fractures can be accomplished **(A)** longitudinally through the MP joint but not the metacarpal head, **(B)** or through the metacarpal head, **(C)** with the wires for either of these options running parallel in the phalanx, or **(D)** entering at the collateral recess and crossing, or **(E)** passing transversely.

cut just below the skin surface to prevent pin tract infection or left protruding for ease of removal at the surgeon's discretion. Absolute parallelism of the K-wires for oblique fractures risks the fracture displacing as it slides along the wires. Some degree of convergence or divergence of the wires will help to prevent this consequence of using smooth wires. The procedure of CRIF is made more difficult than it may initially appear by the challenge of obtaining a truly accurate reduction by closed means. Commercially available devices have been specially designed for closed intramedullary rodding of the phalanx (Fig. 30-49). Routinely, pins should be removed by 3 weeks. When this is done, any final limitations of motion are most likely due to the injury itself rather than the pins. In 35 fractures of the proximal phalanx treated by percutaneous pinning, 32% developed a PIP flexion contracture averaging 18 degrees.[50] A slight variation on the theme is "intrafocal" pinning used in five patients to achieve an average PIP range of 90 degrees.[32]

Open Reduction and Internal Fixation

ORIF is the technique of choice for severe open fractures with multiple associated soft tissue injuries and for patients with multiple fractures (within the same hand or polytrauma patients). It is also the technique of choice for intra-articular fractures with displacement in P1. In a series of 38 distal unicondylar fractures of P1, 5 of 7 initially nondisplaced and unfixed fractures and 4 of 10 fixed with a single K-wire went on to displace.[180] Displaced fractures at the intra-articular base of P1 with more than 20% articular involvement should be internally fixed. Using a volar A1 pulley approach, 10 patients had fixation of lateral base fractures with full motion recovery, good stability, and over 90% contralateral grip strength.[100] The role of ORIF for an isolated, noncomminuted, extra-articular fracture of the phalanx is clearly defined only for the rare irreducible fracture. Spiral fractures may benefit from ORIF with lag screws to achieve precise control over rotation, provided that surgeons experienced in this specific technique can minimize soft tissue disruption.[77,79] Most surgeons will be more comfortable with CRIF for those fractures that can be reduced. The 40-month follow-up of 32 patients prospectively randomized to percutaneous pinning versus lag screw fixation for long oblique and

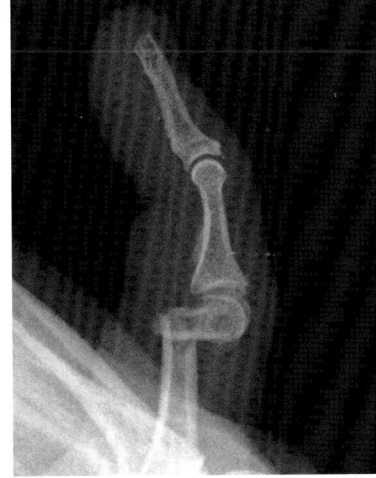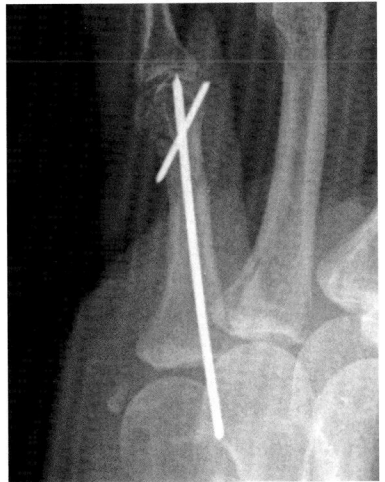

FIGURE 30-47 Fractures of the proximal phalangeal neck angulated apex volarly **(A)**, can be stabilized by **(B)** antegrade pinning with a rotational control crosswire if the fracture is sufficiently proximal, but very distal fractures **(C, D)** usually require retrograde pinning.

(*continues*)

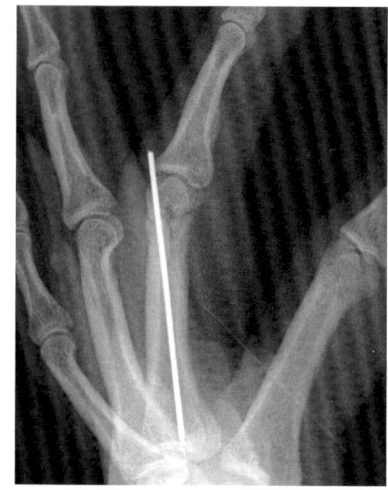
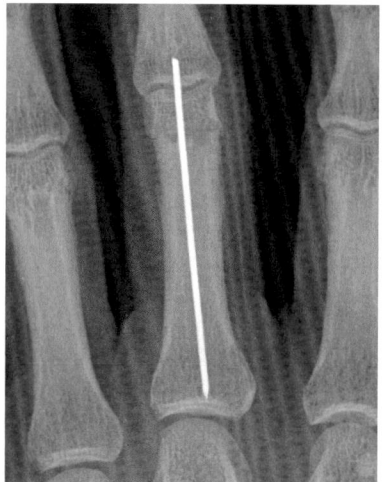

C

D   FIGURE 30-47 (continued)

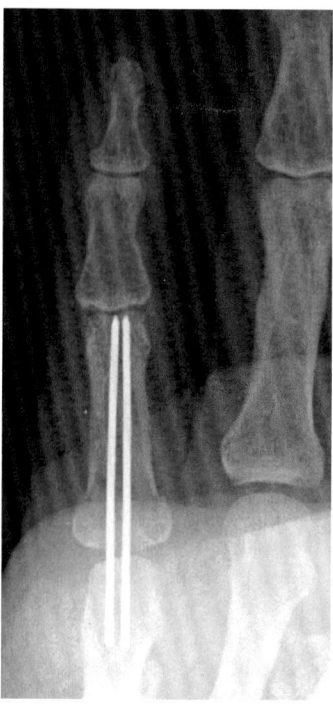
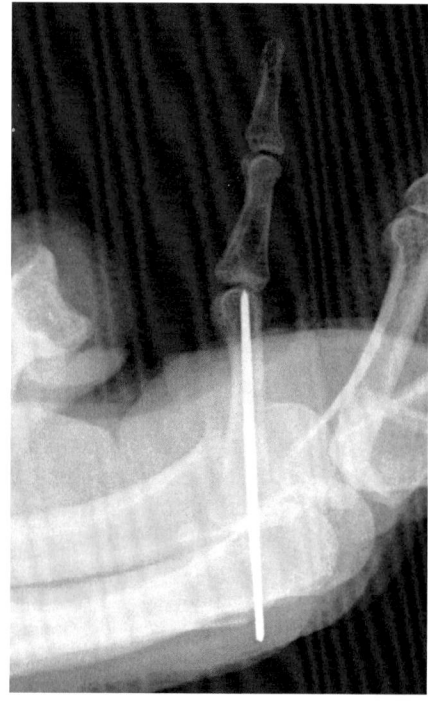

FIGURE 30-48 Transverse shaft fractures of P1 are best stabilized by 0.045-inch K-wires passed longitudinally through the metacarpal head and removed at 3 weeks.

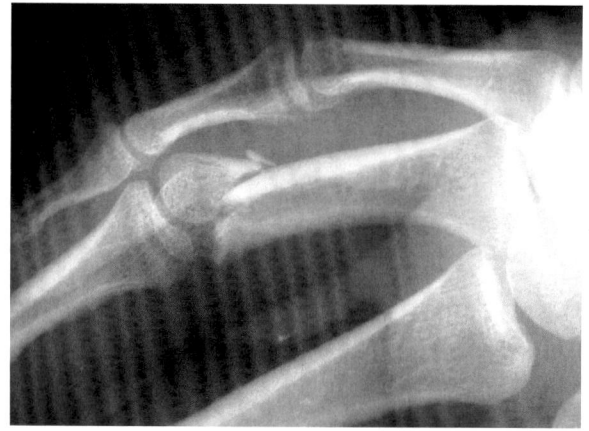
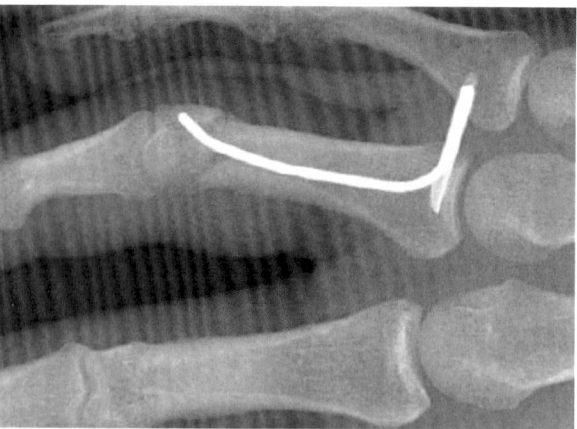

A

B

FIGURE 30-49 A: Proximal phalanx fractures can be stabilized by closed placement of a specially designed device that achieves (B) three-point fixation with a rotational locking sleeve proximally.

spiral shaft fractures found no differences in function, pain scores, ROM, or grip strength, but with a mean loss of active extension of 8 degrees in the pinning group and 27 degrees in the screw fixation group.[86] Surgical technique was such that there were 8 malunions out of the 15 lag screw patients using screws as large as 2 mm. Three of the seventeen K-wire patients required subsequent formal extensor tenolysis for tethering but none of the lag screw patients did.[86] ORIF with screws and/or plates is considerably more technically demanding than in the metacarpal for a number of reasons including the proximity of the extensor mechanism, the origins of the fibro-osseous flexor tendon sheath, and the size and consistency of the bone. More than just the technical complexity of ORIF is the problem of the postoperative response of the surrounding soft tissues to the surgical dissection and the presence of hardware (Table 30-9).

Options for ORIF include intra-osseous wiring, composite wiring, screw-only fixation, or screw and plate fixation.[34,66,139,77,79,26,74,138,158] The familiarity of the surgeon with the specific technique is probably the most important factor in the selection of a method. Of 30 patients followed for 2.3 years after tension band wiring, 17 had a TAM of over 195 degrees and 13 had a TAM of between 130 and 195 degrees.[138] More recently, attention has increasingly turned to the use of screw and plate technology (Figs 30-50 and 30-51). The relative

TABLE 30-9 Surgical Steps—Lag Screw Fixation of Spiral Proximal Phalanx Fractures

Midaxial incision, mobilizing dorsal branch of proper digital nerve dorsally

Single layer sleeve approach volar to zone IV extensor, through periosteum to bone

Elevate as one tissue flap from subperiosteal with no dissection between layers

Curette out clot and debris from fracture site to precisely define fracture edges

Reduce fracture with Adson-Brown forceps, precise interdigitation of fracture edges

Convert to bone-holding clamp to maintain reduction vs. continue holding with forceps

Carefully check rotation clinically using hands-free tenodesis testing

Core drill, overdrill, countersink, depth gauge, and place 2–3 lag screws, 1.2–1.7 mm

Return soft tissue sleeve into position, close wound with 5–0 monofilament, dress, and splint

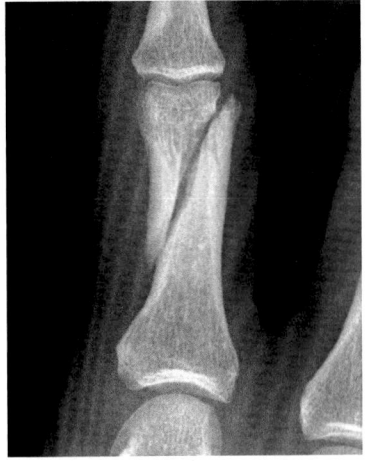 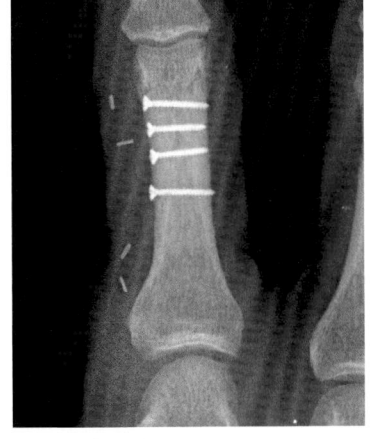 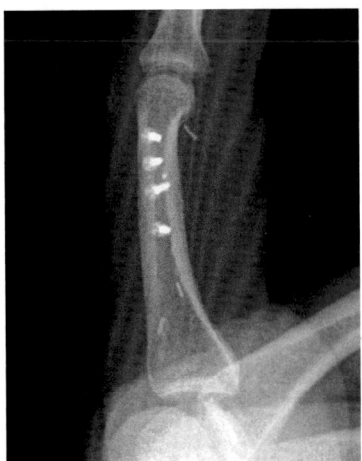 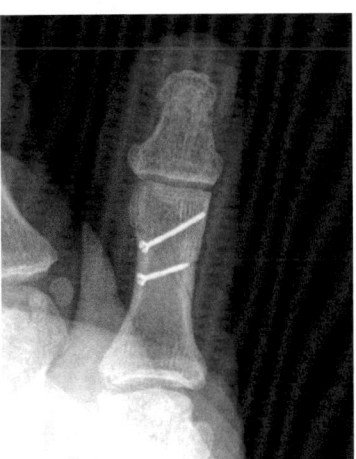

FIGURE 30-50 In long oblique fractures of the shaft with shortening an exact reduction and stability sufficient to withstand early motion can be achieved through lag screw fixation only.

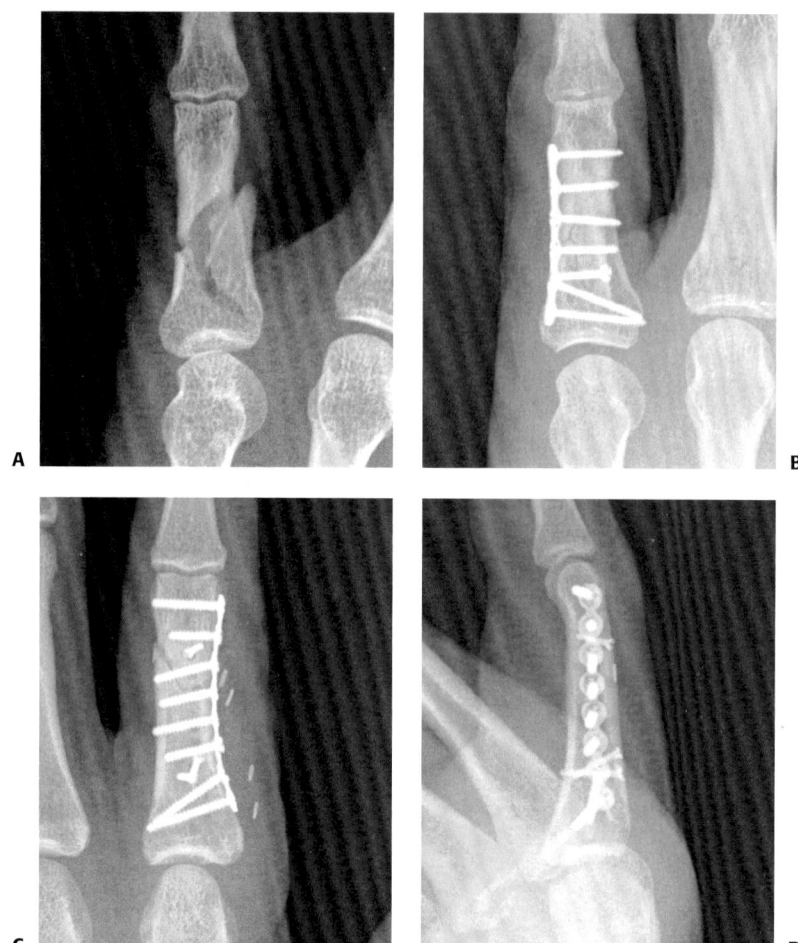

FIGURE 30-51 More complex fractures of the shaft **(A)** can be well stabilized by **(B)** lateral plating. Specific care should be taken to **(C)** contour the plate meticulously to fit the cortex and to place the hardware in **(D)** the true midlateral position.

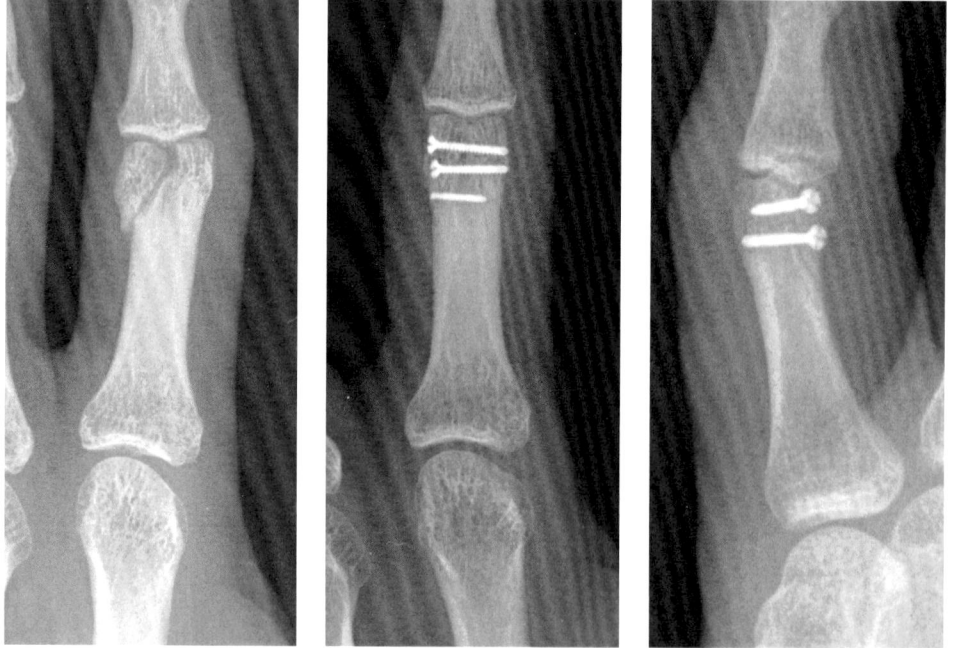

FIGURE 30-52 **A:** Unicondylar fractures of the head of P1 benefit from compression between the articular fragments through **(B, C)** lag screw fixation.

bulkiness of plates at the phalangeal level compared with the metacarpals can result in the need for their removal even with initially excellent results. The results of internal fixation are intimately related to the associated injuries present. The gravest danger, however, occurs when the surgeon elects ORIF but is then unable to secure rigid fixation of the fracture. In this situation, the patient has been subjected to the "worst of both worlds," and a poor outcome can be reliably predicted.

Intra-Articular Fractures

Two intra-articular patterns are seen distally at the phalangeal head, unicondylar (partial articular fracture), or bicondylar (complete articular fracture). The condylar fragments are usually extremely small, can be fragile, and receive their blood supply from the attached collateral ligaments. Fixation of a single condyle is most rigid when accomplished with a compression screw placed transversely, entering near the collateral ligament origin (Fig. 30-52). This can be quite challenging technically, and the bone stock may only tolerate K-wire or composite wiring techniques (Fig. 30-53). Tri-plane fractures of the head of the proximal phalanx are well managed with 1.2-mm lag screws (Fig. 30-54).[26] Complete articular fractures can be fixed with screws alone if one of the two condyles has an extended spike. If not, mini-condylar or locking plate fixation may be necessary to achieve excellent rigidity. Again, the bone stock may not tolerate the application of this device, and wiring techniques remain an alternative strategy.

The final group of articular fractures is that seen at the lateral corner of the phalangeal base. The most direct fixation uses a volar approach and a single lag screw for fixation to achieve full motion by 3 weeks.[144] Comminuted intra-articular fractures of the proximal phalangeal base can be stabilized by a small volar plate placed through the A1 pulley approach (Fig. 30-55).[74] A specific subset of proximal phalangeal base fractures that are purely impactions by nature may be treated by supporting

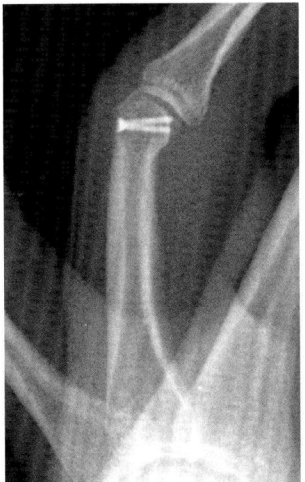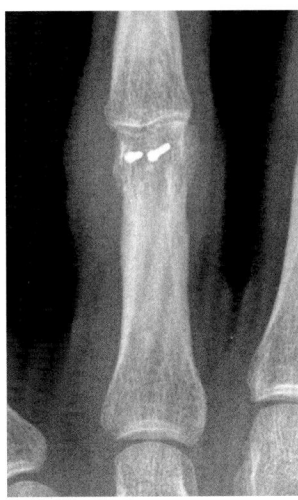

FIGURE 30-54 Tri-plane fractures of the proximal phalangeal head can be well stabilized by two small lag screws (1.2 to 1.5 mm).

the impacted fragments with packed cancellous bone only; in one series of 10 patients followed for 32 months there was no secondary displacement and an average MP joint flexion of 88 degrees, and a PIP joint flexion of 95 degrees was achieved.[158]

Postoperative Care. Nonoperative management should restrict splinting to 3 weeks followed by AROM that can include adjacent digit strapping if necessary. Similarly, CRIF should allow for pin removal at 3 weeks, with AROM beginning no later than this time. If ORIF is chosen, AROM should begin within 72 hours of surgery and edema control should be foremost in the treatment plan using cohesive elastic bandages.[58] AROM alone may be insufficient to counteract extensor lag at the joint distal to the site of fixation. Rapidly accelerating the extensor tendon concentrically without resistance best limits local adhesion formation (Fig. 30-56).[75] These exercises can

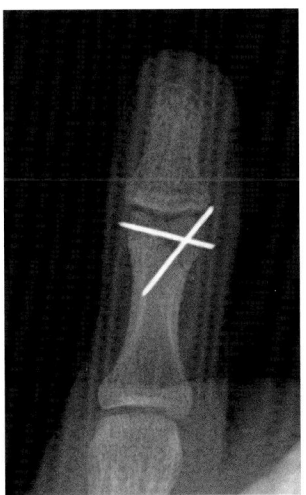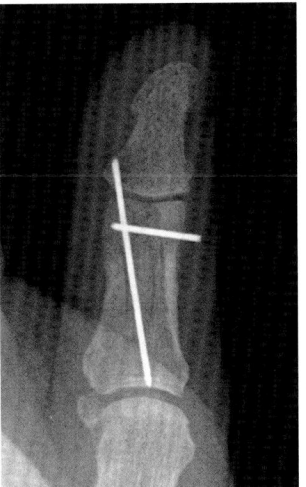

FIGURE 30-53 When a unicondylar fracture of the head of P1 has a proximal shaft extension on the smaller fragment, K-wire fixation in a diverging pattern can prevent migration of the fragment that would otherwise occur with a single smooth K-wire as the only fixation.

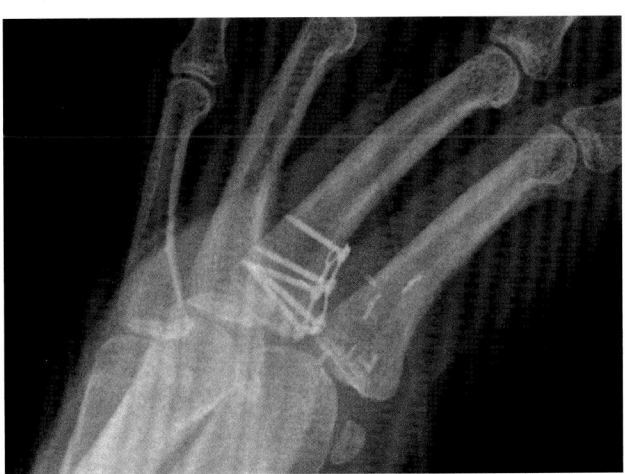

FIGURE 30-55 Comminuted volar shearing fractures of the base of P1 may require volar buttress plating for adequate stability to permit early rehabilitation.

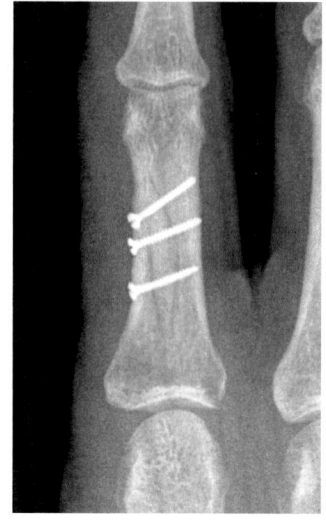

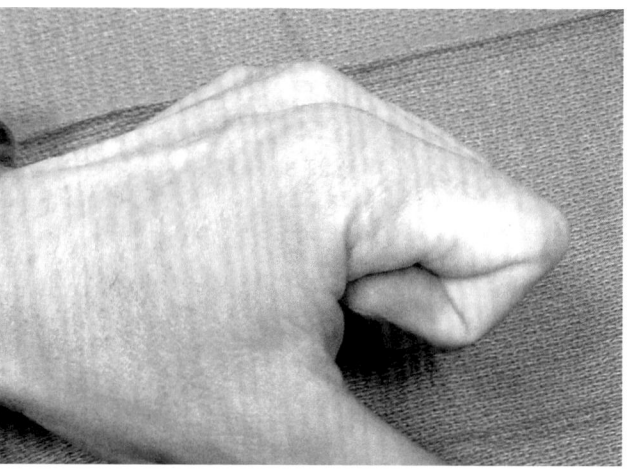

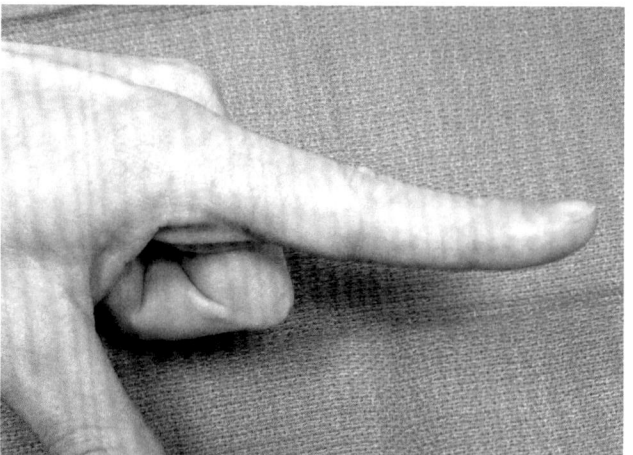

FIGURE 30-56 Following **(A)** lag screw fixation of a shaft fracture in P1, **(B)** complete PIP joint flexion and **(C)** PIP joint hyperextension are achievable with an aggressive special therapy program of resisted zone IV extensor tendon preload followed by sudden release with follow-through.

be supplemented with the use of electrical muscle stimulation during outpatient therapy sessions. Night splinting with the PIP joint in extension can be helpful but will not by itself overcome an extensor lag.

Potential Pitfalls and Preventative Measures. Longitudinal wires drilled past the head of P1 into the PIP joint and then later withdrawn may migrate back into the PIP joint during rehabilitation and cause hyaline cartilage damage to the base of P2. During initial placement, the wire should be drilled up to but not into the subchondral bone and then impacted. Pins should not be placed through tendons. All cases, closed or open, should be carefully checked clinically for angulation and rotation using a no-touch technique that does not distort the judgment of alignment. Open surgery should be performed strictly laterally with no dorsal incisions, no zone IV extensor splitting, and especially no dorsal plates. When approaching laterally, be careful not to transect the dorsal nerve branch that passes obliquely from the proper digital nerve. Drilling at too high a speed will create a larger hole than the diameter of the bit because of "whip" and the screw will lose purchase. Overtightening small titanium screws can shear off the heads, but rarely if a fingertip hold is used on the screwdriver. If the plate is not contoured correctly, as it is tightened down, the plate will induce a malunion (Table 30-10).

AUTHOR'S PREFERRED TREATMENT (FIG. 30-57)

Closed Reduction and Internal Fixation

CRIF is my preferred treatment for all isolated, closed transverse, and short oblique fractures of the proximal phalanx (Fig. 30-58). Longitudinal pinning with two K-wires passing through the metacarpal head with the MP joint flexed 80 to 90 degrees has yielded reliable results.[77] In larger patients, two 0.045-inch K-wires can be fitted into the medullary canal. In smaller patients, one 0.045-inch and one 0.035-inch wire may be more compatible. When rotational interlock is felt between the fragments, one wire can be used. The wires are placed one each on either side of the thick central extensor tendon dorsal to the MP joint, and may be placed just proximal to the sagittal band fibers. The wires are then passed through the base fragment, across the fracture site, and down the distal shaft of the phalanx to the head. Closed pinning is also a valuable technique for nondisplaced fractures at the head of P1. Both a transverse pin connecting the two condyles as well as an oblique pin from the condyle to the opposite diaphyseal cortex should be used for a unicondylar fracture. For bicondylar fractures, two oblique pins are needed. The oblique pins are best cut for

TABLE 30-10 Potential Pitfalls and Preventative Measures—P1 Fractures

Pitfall	Prevention
Distal pin migration into PIP joint	Tap rather than drill up to subchondral plate in head of P1 without penetrating
Tendon tethering by pins	Only place pins from entry points adjacent to but not through tendons; remove by 3 weeks, 4 weeks at the absolute latest
Malrotation leading to malunion	Careful clinical check of rotation; two axial pins for transverse fractures distal to metaphysis
Zone IV extensor adhesions	Midaxial surgery only, no dorsal incisions, no incisions through the zone IV extensor, no dorsally placed plates
Neuroma of dorsal digital nerve branch	Mobilize dorsal oblique branch out of operative field
Overdrilling the far hole on lag screws leading to poor fixation	Use low speed to avoid distal "whipping" of the small drill bit; larger size "rescue" screws
Shearing the head off small titanium screws	Use only fingertip tightening, no key pinch hold on the screwdriver
Inducing malunion with the plate	Take off and recontour the plate as many times as needed so that, when tightened down fully, it does not force the bone into malalignment or malrotation

retrieval proximally rather than distally as their passage through the periarticular soft tissues will interfere with PIP joint motion. Closed pinning also represents a reasonable treatment option for nondisplaced long oblique or spiral fractures that are suspected of subsequent displacement when subjected to the stress of motion rehabilitation. However, practically I have not found this fracture pattern to exist. I see either truly nondisplaced fractures that I expect to remain stable and treat nonoperatively or displaced long oblique and spiral fractures that I prefer to treat with open reduction.

Open Reduction and Internal Fixation with Lag Screws

This is my preferred treatment for long oblique and spiral fractures of the shaft and displaced partial articular fractures (Fig. 30-59). I have found it difficult to correct all the shortening and rotation of long oblique and spiral fractures by closed means alone. There is a natural trade-off between the undeniable added surgical trauma of an open approach and the benefits of an anatomically precise reduction. When lag screws alone are

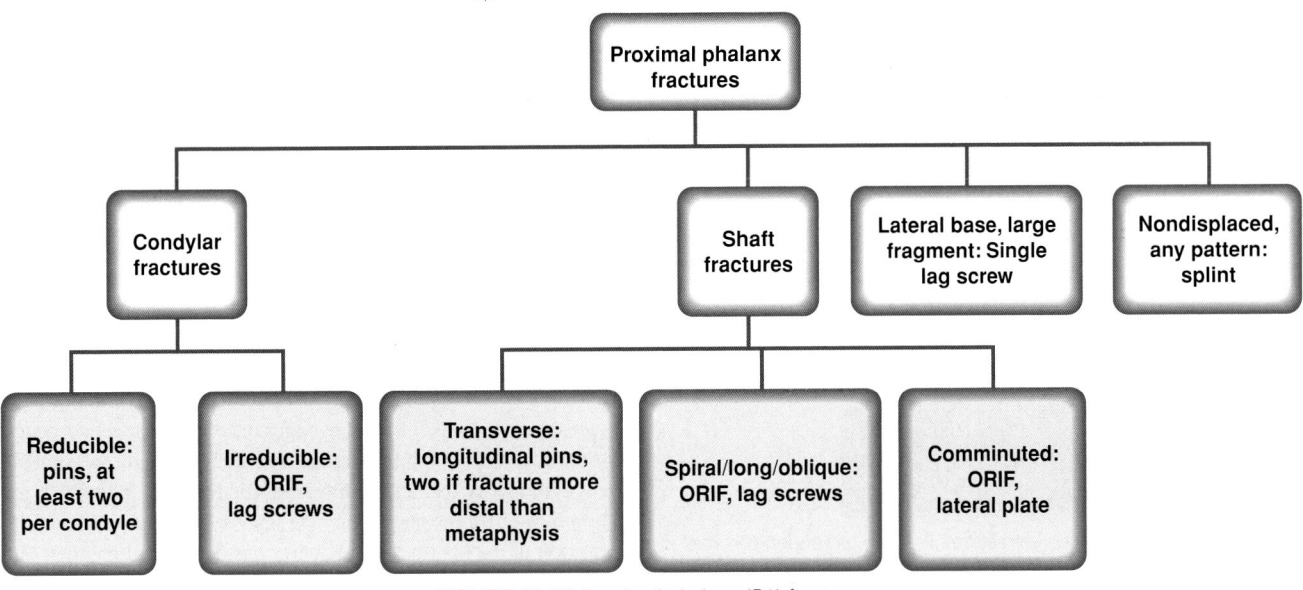

FIGURE 30-57 Proximal phalanx (P1) fractures.

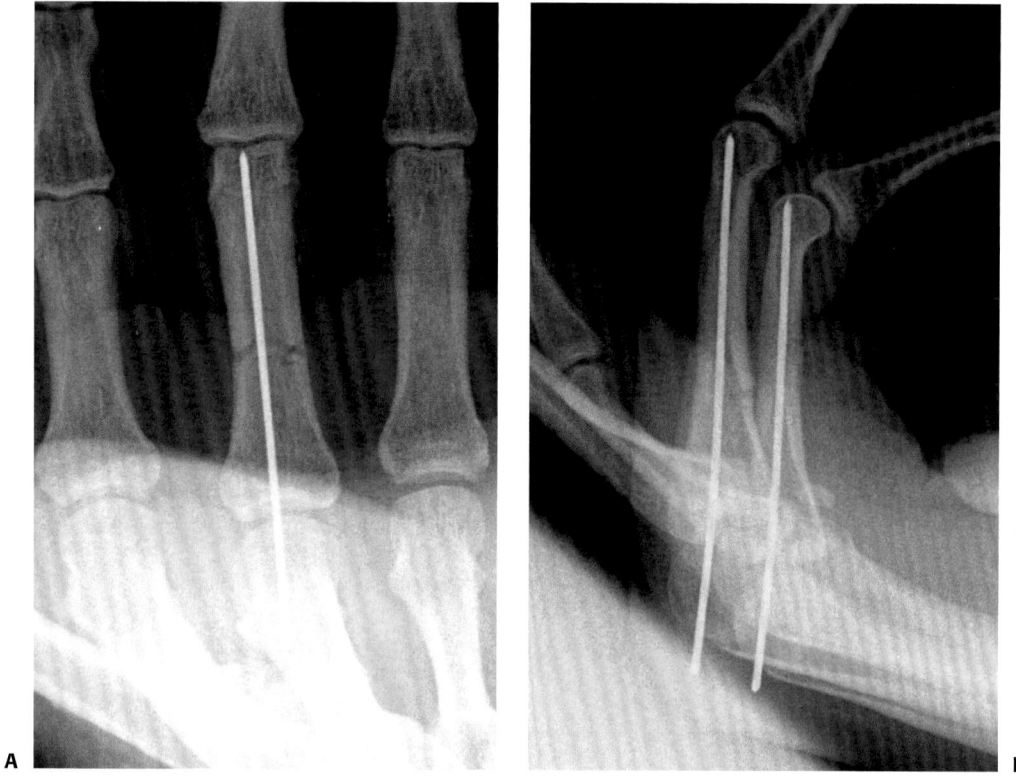

A   **B**

FIGURE 30-58 Transverse P1 fractures without comminution should achieve sufficient interfragmentary stability to have axial rotational control with a single wire alone that targets the **(A)** intercondylar notch and going **(B)** all the way to the subchondral bone.

used for fixation, full motion rehabilitation can begin immediately.[79,75] This is not the case with K-wires that tether soft tissues, limiting motion, and risking pin tract infection. Performing the open fixation gently and precisely to minimize soft tissue trauma is more easily described than executed. I prefer to

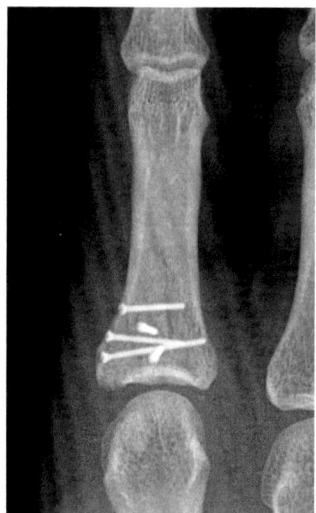

FIGURE 30-59 Partial articular fractures that can be rendered stable by interfragmentary compression are excellent candidates for lag screw fixation.

operate on closed fractures around postinjury day 3 to 5 when even adult periosteum will thicken dramatically in response to injury and can be surgically manipulated as a tissue flap. A true midaxial incision is in the neutral tension lines of the skin and brings the approach down to the volar leading edge of the intrinsic wing tendon. One of the most important principles in open fixation of a P1 fracture is not to create planes of surgical dissection either superficial or deep to the zone IV extensor tendon. The only dissection that should occur at the subcutaneous level is to identify dorsal cutaneous nerve branches passing obliquely from the proper digital nerves and to mobilize them effectively to avoid neuromas. Other than this, the approach should create a single tissue flap from skin through periosteum to bone.[79] A sharp blade is needed to carefully preserve the periosteum for later repair using fine monofilament resorbable sutures. This creates an additional gliding layer of protection for the extensor mechanism. A fine-tipped curette must be used to clear the fracture interface of all clot and soft tissue or a truly anatomic interdigitated reduction will not be possible. In a simple two-fragment diaphyseal fracture, there will be inherent stability between the bone edges once the fracture has been reduced. The role of internal fixation is then to exploit this inherent stability by further compressing the fracture line, which is optimized by interfragmentary lag screws. Although provisional fixation of the fracture with K-wires has been recommended by others, I have found that an absolutely perfect reduction is not well maintained by smooth wires, which invariably allow the reduction to slip a little. This ensures that the drill path will not be exactly in the desired location and that final placement of the screw or plate will thus be imperfect. I prefer to hold the reduction manually with either a bone clamp specialized for the short tubular bones of the hand or with Brown-Adson forceps. After reduction and provisional stabilization, the steps are core drilling followed by countersinking the near bone surface. Countersinking not only recesses the screw head but also distributes the force of compression, lessening the chance of propagating a new fracture line. Measuring for screw length is done next, and the time for the scrub technician to procure the correct screw can be used to drill the gliding hole. Self-tapping screws are a little difficult to start into bone as some axial load is necessary to get them to bite, but application of this load off the true axis will toggle the screw. A fine touch must be learned over the course of many cases using these implants. Screws are tightened with a "chuck" pinch on the screwdriver using three fingers, not with the more forceful key pinch that may shear the head off the shaft of the screw. The rules for selecting screw-only fixation include fracture length that is at least two times the bone diameter, and fragment width that is at least three times the screw diameter. Adherence to strict principles is mandatory; multiple drill bit passes are not well tolerated by the phalanx. Screws of 1.2- to 1.5-mm diameters are appropriate for P1. Biomechanically, it is desirable to have at least one screw placed perpendicular to the neutral axis of the bone. The remaining screws should be perpendicular to the fracture plane. In a spiral fracture, one screw can satisfy both of these requirements simultaneously and is termed the "ideal" screw. In an oblique fracture this will not be the case.

Plates at the Phalangeal Level

Plates at the phalangeal level are not desirable because of their bulk and propensity for tendon adherence, and I avoid using them whenever possible. This is my treatment of choice for fractures with comminution and bone loss and complete articular fractures of the phalangeal head that are unstable. Since the biomechanics of P1 fractures create an apex palmar sagittal plane deformity, the plate would (impossibly so) have to be applied to the volar surface of the bone to have its optimum tension band effect. Lateral placement is then the next most desirable option, and this corresponds well to the surgical access that is least harmful to the soft tissues.[79] A midaxial incision is carried volar to the margin of the extensor mechanism, straight through periosteum, and the entire soft tissue sleeve is elevated as a single unit, avoiding any dissection of planes surrounding the extensor tendon. When plates are used, one should attempt to place screws as perpendicular to the surface of the plate as possible (Fig. 30-60). The heads of obliquely placed screws have a prominent edge. Plates should also be painstakingly contoured to ensure both the lowest profile as well as proper biomechanical function (preload, dynamic compression, buttress effect). One must not hesitate to remove a plate and recontour it after the first two screws have been placed if it is clear that the shape is not correct. Application of an incorrectly contoured

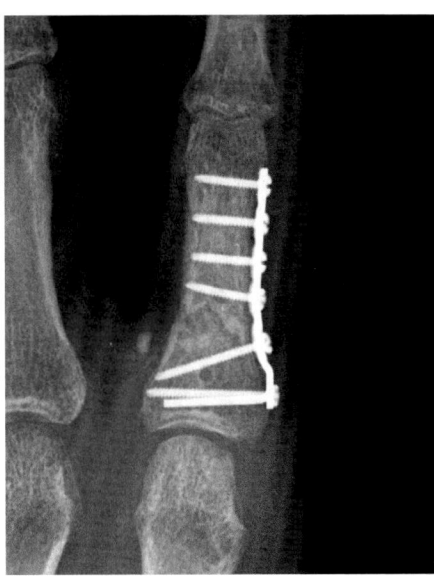

FIGURE 30-60 Plate fixation in P1 must be contoured meticulously to restore the normal anatomic shape of the bone. The condylar blade plate can also be used at the metaphyseal base of a proximal phalanx. An oblique screw is often advantageous to achieve an extra point of compression in the metaphyseal fragment.

plate guarantees an imperfect fracture reduction. A common error is with plates ending near the metaphyseal flare that must have a small bend at the last hole to accommodate the curvature of the bone at this level. Small-size locking plates represent a tremendous advantage over the only previously available implant that offered fixed angle stability, the minicondylar plate (Fig. 30-61). The minicondylar plate could not be fully contoured to the bone surface before placing the blade; a locking plate can. If more than 50% cross-sectional area of the bone is comminuted or lost, bone graft may be required.

INTRODUCTION TO METACARPOPHALANGEAL (MP) JOINT DISLOCATIONS

Dorsal MP joint dislocations are the most common. Simple dislocations are reducible and present with a hyperextension posture. They are really subluxations, as some contact remains between the base of P1 and the metacarpal head. The volar plate stays volar or distal to the metacarpal head. Reduction should be achieved with simple flexion of the joint; excessive longitudinal traction on the finger should be avoided. Longitudinal traction can convert a simple into a complex dislocation. A complex MP dislocation is, by definition, irreducible, most often because of volar plate interposition (Fig. 30-62). Complex dislocations occur most frequently in the index finger. A pathognomonic radiographic sign of complex dislocation is the appearance of a sesamoid in the joint space (Fig. 30-63). Concomitant injuries include small chip fractures on the dorsum of the metacarpal head that have been sheared off in complex dislocations by the volar base of P1.[69,83] Other difficult fractures to detect are bony collateral ligament avulsions.

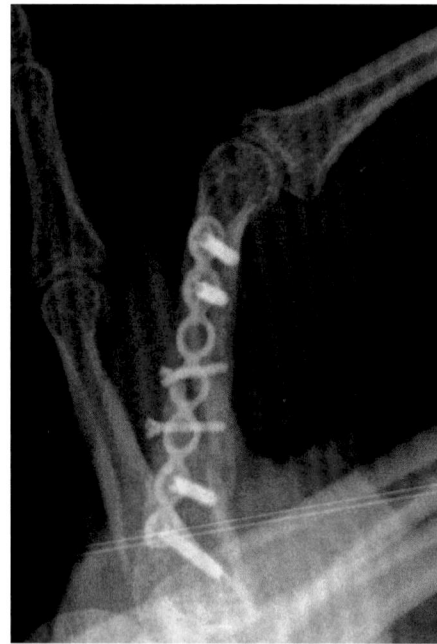
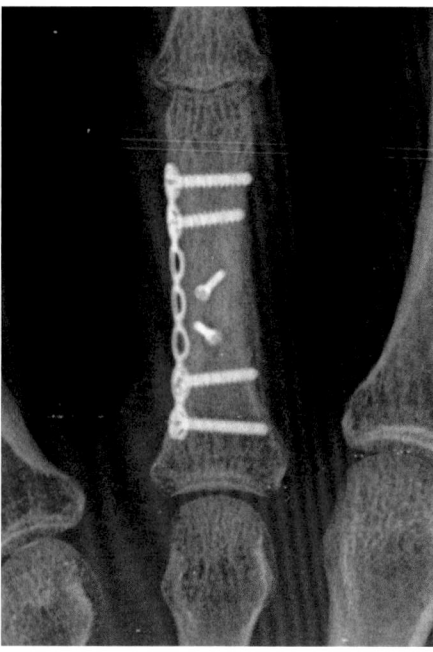

FIGURE 30-61 Small locking plates can span zones of comminution and obviate the need to use the fixed angle blade plate.

Most dorsal dislocations will be stable following reduction and do not need surgical repair of the ligaments or volar plate. Volar dislocations are rare but particularly unstable. Volar dislocations risk late instability and should have the ligaments repaired.[118] Obstructions to reducing volar dislocations include the volar plate, collateral ligament, and dorsal capsule. Irreducible thumb volar dislocations have been reported to involve the EPL, extensor pollicis brevis (EPB), flexor pollicis longus, and trapping of the radial condyle of the metacarpal in a rent dorsal to the accessory collateral–volar plate complex.[83]

Small fracture fragments at the collateral insertions (base of P1 or metacarpal head) need special consideration as such injuries share the features of ligament instability and the consequences of an intra-articular fracture.[144,141,145] Isolated collateral ligament injuries are more common on the radial aspect of the small finger followed by the index finger. A differential diagnosis to consider with posttraumatic swelling at the MP joint level is rupture of the sagittal bands (confirmed by visible

or palpable ulnar subluxation of the zone V extensor tendon), which requires protection in extension for 4 weeks. A rare variant injury to the MP joint is a dorsal capsular tear (Boxer's knuckle) that can prove persistently symptomatic. In a series of 16 patients that included extensor tendon dislocation in 7, surgical closure of the rent found in the dorsal capsule or extensor hood was reported to be successful in all cases.[9]

Complete rupture of the ulnar collateral ligament (UCL) of the thumb MP joint is a common injury that less frequently

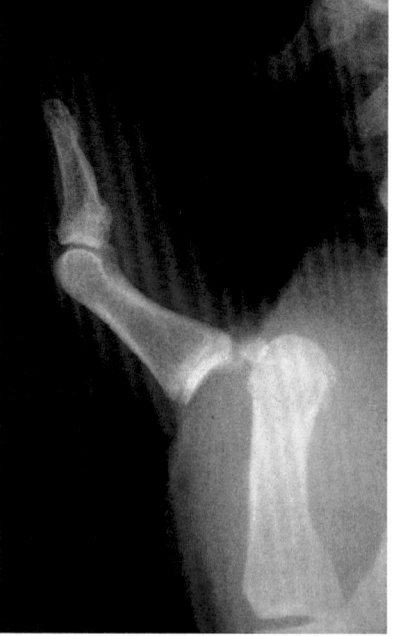

FIGURE 30-63 Metacarpophalangeal joint dislocation in the thumb, like the fingers, is typically dorsal. Note the sesamoid interposed in the joint space.

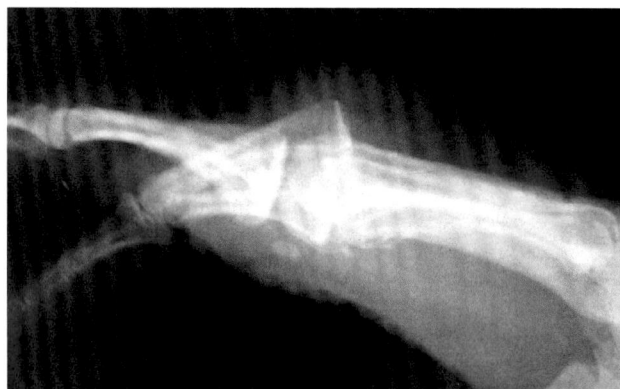

FIGURE 30-62 The typical complex dorsal dislocation of the MP joint presents with complete overriding of the phalanx on the metacarpal.

may accompany a full MP joint dislocation (Fig. 30-63). Circumferential palpation of the MP joint can often localize pain to the UCL, RCL, volar plate, or combinations of these. Following joint injection with local anesthetic, any instability can be revealed by stress testing in full extension and 30 degrees of flexion. Flexing the joint relaxes the volar plate so that only the collateral ligament resists examination force applied in the coronal plane. In full extension, an intact volar plate may mask a ruptured proper collateral ligament, yielding a false negative conclusion of stability. (Fig. 30-64A). If clinical uncertainty remains, stress radiographs may also be performed (Fig. 30-64B). A consistent role has not yet been found for MRI in the diagnosis of the Stener lesion (a distally ruptured UCL blocked from healing by the interposed adductor aponeurosis).[82] In a series of 24 patients, a palpable tender mass on the ulnar side of the MP joint was used as the sole diagnostic criterion for the Stener lesion. Operative treatment was performed for those felt to have the lesion and nonoperative management for those who did not, resulting in only a single case of long-term instability.[1]

PATHOANATOMY AND APPLIED ANATOMY RELATING TO METACARPOPHALANGEAL (MP) JOINT DISLOCATIONS

The anatomy of the MP joint is like the same three-sided box previously presented for the PIP joint, composed of the proper collateral ligaments, the accessory collateral ligaments, and the volar plate. The radial and ulnar proper collateral ligaments are the primary stabilizers to motion in all planes including distraction, dorsopalmar translation, abduction-adduction, and supination-pronation. The accessory collateral ligaments supplement adduction-abduction stability. The volar plates are connected to each other by the deep transverse intermetacarpal ligament. The MP collateral ligaments have an origin dorsal to the center axis of joint rotation. This feature combines with two others (a greater width of the metacarpal head volarly and a greater distance from the center of rotation to the volar articular surface than the distal articular surface) to maximize tension in the true collateral portion of the ligament when the joint is in full flexion. Consequently, stress testing to determine the presence of instability must be performed in full flexion.

Access for open reduction of complex dislocations is a topic of great controversy. Central MP joints can be approached either dorsally or volarly. Although the volar plate is the most commonly noted structure in the prevention of reduction, the flexor tendons, lumbricals, deep transverse intermetacarpal ligaments, juncturae tendinae, and dorsal capsule have all been implicated.[132] In a series of 10 operatively treated ligament ruptures, most were distal with the ligament occasionally trapped between the intrinsic tendon and the sagittal band, including 2 associated dorsal interosseous ruptures at the phalangeal insertion.[39]

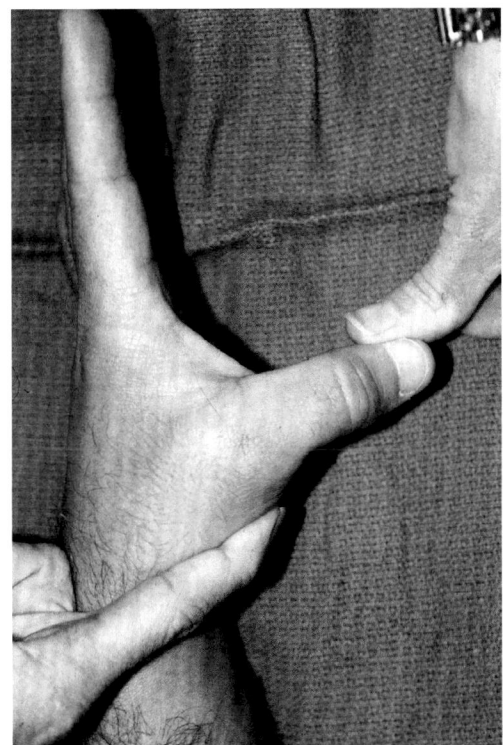
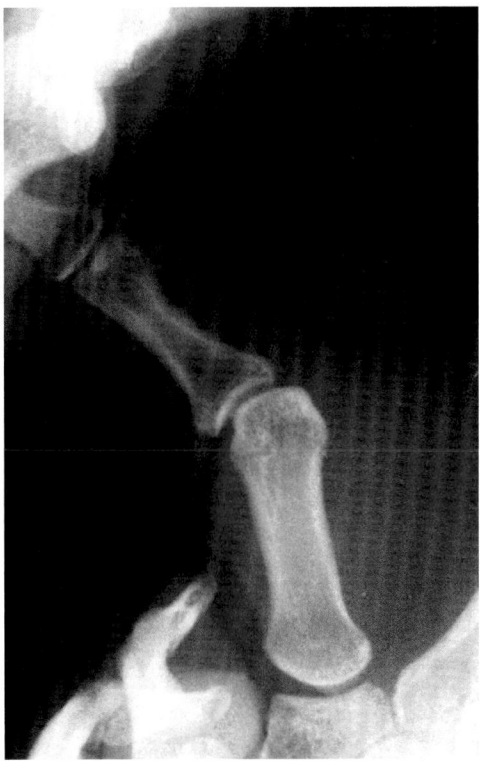

A   **B**

FIGURE 30-64 **A:** Clinical stress testing of the ulnar collateral ligament in 30 degrees of flexion prevents reaching a false negative conclusion when an intact volar plate obscures the instability of a complete proper ulnar collateral ligament rupture. **B:** Radiographic stress testing is also useful when there is clinical uncertainty.

The thumb MP joint, in addition to its primary plane of flexion and extension, allows abduction-adduction and a slight amount of rotation (pronation with flexion). The range of flexion and extension has a wide natural variation that may be related to the flatness of the metacarpal head and may also play a role in predisposition to injury for those with less motion. With a one-sided collateral ligament injury, the phalanx tends to subluxate volarly in a rotatory fashion, pivoting around the opposite intact collateral ligament. The UCL may have a two-level injury consisting of a fracture of the ulnar base of P1 with the ligament also rupturing off the fracture fragment.[63] Of particular importance is the proximal edge of the adductor aponeurosis that forms the anatomic basis of the Stener lesion. The torn UCL stump comes to lie dorsal to the aponeurosis and is thus prevented from healing to its anatomic insertion on the volar, ulnar base of the proximal phalanx. The true incidence of the Stener lesion remains unknown because of widely disparate reports. The abductor pollicis brevis also sends fibers to the extensor mechanism and the RCL can be obstructed from reaching the base of P1 to heal correctly even though the precise pattern that constitutes a classic Stener lesion does not exist on the radial side. RCL injuries have been found to occur at the phalangeal insertion in 13 of 38 cases and at the metacarpal origin in 25 of 38.[31]

METACARPOPHALANGEAL (MP) JOINT DISLOCATIONS TREATMENT OPTIONS

Nonoperative Management—Fingers

For reducible dorsal dislocations and collateral ligament injuries, nonoperative management is the treatment of choice. Collateral ligament injuries should be immobilized in incomplete flexion (50 degrees) for 3 weeks followed by AROM while the digit is strapped to an adjacent digit to resist lateral deviation stress. Even with fracture fragments constituting up to 25% of the width of the phalangeal base, early active mobilization using side strap protection led to normal motion and grip strength in six of seven patients with a mean DASH score of 3.1.[141] Dorsal dislocations will normally prove stable during early AROM. Only in an exceptional case would the use of extension block splinting of 20 degrees or so for 2 to 3 weeks be required. In a high-demand patient, the RCL of the index MP joint should be considered for operative repair.

Nonoperative Management—Thumb

Nonoperative management is the mainstay of treatment for thumb MP joint injuries. Only the complete UCL injury with a Stener lesion and volar dislocations require more aggressive treatment. The standard treatment consists of 4 weeks of static MP joint immobilization with the IP joint left free. Management in the presence of a fracture at the ulnar base of P1 is more controversial. Nine patients with less than 2-mm displacement of such a fragment treated nonoperatively all had chronic pain with pinch strength rated at 36% of normal. Following operative treatment, pinch improved to 89% of normal with symptom resolution.[42] Conversely, 28 patients with ulnar base fractures but with a joint clinically assessed as stable to stress testing

were managed nonoperatively resulting in equivalent grip and pinch strengths to the contralateral side, and 93% were pain-free despite a 60% rate of fibrous union.[149] RCL disruptions and pure dorsal dislocations can be successfully managed by a 4-week period of MP joint immobilization.

Open Reduction—Fingers

Volar dislocations, complex dorsal dislocations, and collateral ligament disruptions associated with large bone fragments should be treated with open reduction and repair (Fig. 30-65). RCL injuries repaired late risk a higher incidence of pinch weakness and should be attended to promptly. Open repair or reconstruction with a free tendon graft may also be required in chronic cases with persistent symptoms following initial nonoperative management. Of 33 patients with MP collateral ligament avulsion fractures from the base of the proximal phalanx, the 8 that were treated nonoperatively initially all went on to symptomatic nonunion requiring subsequent surgery.[144] In a similar series of 19 patients with the avulsion occurring at the metacarpal head, successful results occurred in the 11 displaced fragments internally fixed through a dorsal approach, but three of seven initially nondisplaced fragments went on to symptomatic nonunion requiring surgery.[145] Volar MP dislocations should have repair of the collateral ligaments and volar plate to prevent late instability. Either a dorsal or a volar approach is acceptable, and the one that provides access to the major pathology should be chosen based on the individual patient's preoperative findings. Dorsally, a midline longitudinal incision provides good access to manage any associated osteochondral fractures. One may have to split the volar plate longitudinally and draw it around the sides of the metacarpal head to accomplish a reduction. The volar approach avoids splitting the volar plate but risks injury to digital nerves which are tented over the deformity and lying directly under the dermis. With a volar approach, the volar plate can be pulled back out of the joint and reduced without splitting it.

The duration of immobilization should be in direct proportion to the surgeon's assessment of instability following reduction. Whereas most patients may begin AROM immediately, those injuries that demonstrate an extra degree of instability during the postreduction assessment should be immobilized in partial flexion for 3 weeks. Whether simple or complex, the dislocations should be immobilized in only partial (50-degree) flexion to allow ligament healing under appropriate tension. After 3 weeks, AROM is progressed until 6 weeks, when full passive motion including hyperextension is allowed.

Open Reduction—Thumb

Surgical management of thumb MP joint injuries is largely limited to UCL disruptions with a Stener lesion and volar or irreducible MP dislocations. Determining the presence of a Stener lesion on the ulnar side of the joint remains an inexact science; therefore, open management can be argued to be the treatment of choice for all widely unstable ulnar-sided disruptions. Pure ligamentous midsubstance ruptures can be repaired by direct suture. The usual site of disruption is distally at the phalangeal insertion where bone anchors can be used for ligament

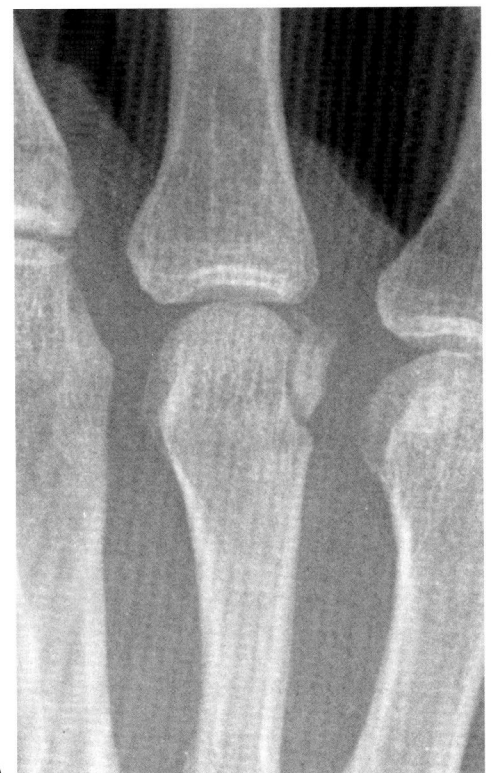
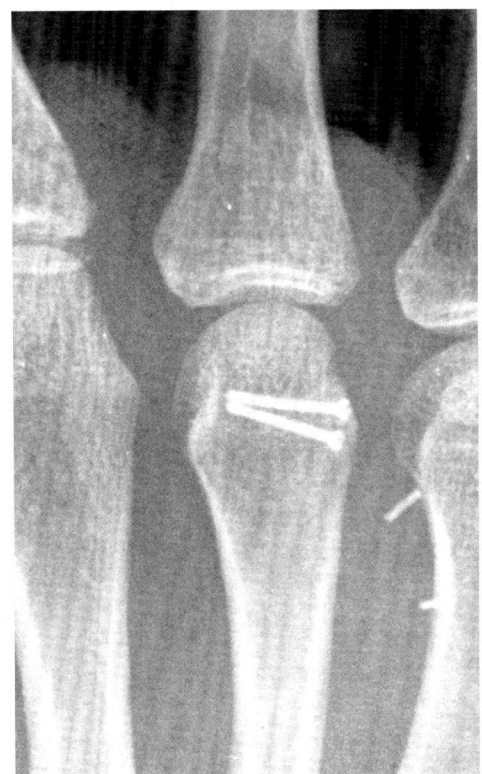

A   B

FIGURE 30-65 Collateral ligament injuries that **(A)** avulse a large bone fragment at the metacarpal head can be stabilized by direct bone fixation **(B)**.

reinsertion. Over-tensioning should be avoided as insertion sites malpositioned volarly or distally on the proximal phalanx will cause loss of motion.[12] With bony avulsion fragments, screw fixation, tension band wiring, intraosseous wiring, or fragment excision with ligament anchorage may all be used at the surgeon's discretion.

Ligament Reconstruction

Cases presenting late with residual instability (after degeneration of the ligament substance has occurred) may require reconstructive methods.[54] Twenty-six patients with tendon reconstruction for the thumb UCL followed for 4.5 years had 85% normal ROM and key pinch strength equal to the opposite side at 9.07 kg (20 lbs).[64] High-grade RCL tears that are widely unstable may benefit from direct soft tissue advancement and repair with 38 patients at 10-month follow-up achieving 92% of normal pinch; 87% were symptom free.[31]

Associated Osteochondral Injuries to the Metacarpal Head or a Base of P1 Fracture

Careful inspection of the dorsal aspect of the metacarpal head should identify any chondral or osteochondral fractures. There are three strategies to manage these fractures. If the fragment is small and extremely unstable, it should be excised. If the fragment has a large subchondral bone base, it can be fixed with a countersunk screw. If fixation is not possible but the fragment can be stably trapped in its bed by the congruent opposing joint surface, it can be further restrained with fine resorbable sutures. For collateral ligament injuries associated with bone fragments, there are two options. If the bone fragment is both large and solid enough to receive definitive fixation, ORIF may be performed with a tension band wire or lag screw. Twenty-five patients with base of P1 ligament avulsion injuries were reported to have recovered full motion by 3 weeks following volar approach single lag screw fixation.[144] If the bone fragment is too small or too comminuted, the bone can be excised and the end of the ligament reinserted to the cancellous bed of either the metacarpal head or the base of the proximal phalanx. This can be accomplished with a mini-bone anchor or by transosseous suture. Surgery may not always be necessary to achieve grip and key pinch strength in avulsion fractures of the lateral base of P1. For example, 27 of 30 nonoperatively treated patients achieved clinical stability despite a 25% incidence of radiographic nonunion, but with only 19 of 30 reporting no pain.[103]

Potential Pitfalls and Preventative Measures. Hypersensitivity and small cutaneous neuroma formation are often considered the banes of hand surgery. Although never totally avoidable, these unwanted complications can be minimized by a thorough knowledge of the branching patterns of the cutaneous nerves and meticulous attention to detail at the time of surgery. The dorsal digital nerve along the ulnar side of the thumb MP joint is at high risk of injury. It should be mobilized dorsally for the procedure and checked each time before drilling.

TABLE 30-11 **Potential Pitfalls and Preventative Measures—MP Joint Dislocations**

Pitfall	Prevention
Converting a simple MP dorsal finger dislocation to complex	No longitudinal traction, reduce by accentuating angular deformity, and sliding the base of the proximal phalanx back into place over the contour of the metacarpal head
Injury to proper digital nerve during open reduction of finger complex dislocation, particularly radial digital nerve to index	Once through dermis, must find and protect nerve, realizing pathoanatomy displaces the nerve from its normal position
Injury to dorsal digital nerve during closure of adductor aponeurosis after treating Stener lesion of thumb ulnar collateral	Must visualize dorsal digital nerve branch during each pass of the needle to close the aponeurosis
First web space contracture after ulnar collateral repair or reconstruction of thumb	Pin MP joint to support the radially directed force on proximal phalanx necessary to prevent first web contracture
Permanent loss of motion in thumb MP joint	Ensure anatomic targeting of anchor for repair and insertion points for graft. Typical error is too dorsal a placement on the proximal phalanx

Perhaps the greatest risk is during closure of the adductor aponeurosis along the margin of the EPL tendon. It is quite easy to simply capture the nerve branch with one of these sutures if it is not visualized to be clear with each suture pass.

First web space contracture can easily occur following immobilization of any hand injury and especially when the injury is located in the first web space. Since the first web is located at the level of the MP joint, all positioning forces designed to prevent contracture act on the proximal phalanx and across the MP joint. The value of pinning the thumb MP joint with a 0.045-inch K-wire during the 4-week period of immobilization in a thumb spica splint is that the splint may be appropriately molded to abduct the thumb and avoid web space contracture (Table 30-11).

AUTHOR'S PREFERRED TREATMENT (FIG. 30-66)

Careful review of the published literature regarding both finger and thumb MP joint ligament injuries indicates that the clinical assessment of instability is paramount in planning subsequent treatment. Local anesthetic injection into the MP joint allows vigorous stress testing of the ligament to be performed without fighting the patient or causing undue pain. Testing in both extension and flexion reveals the absolute value of deviation as well as the discrepancy compared with the uninjured side. The feel at the end point is also a significant piece of information. A greater than 15-degree difference side to side and a soft end point are stronger indicators of complete ligament disruption

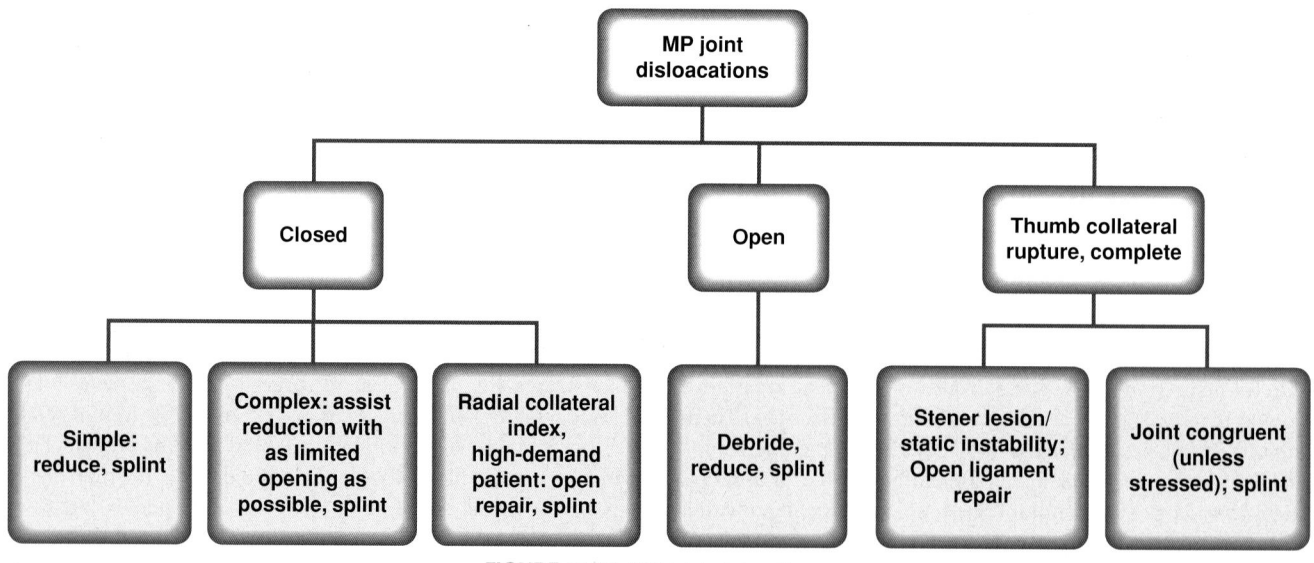

FIGURE 30-66 MP joint dislocations.

than the absolute value of the joint angle when stressed. The integrity of the volar plate should be assessed along with the appearance of rotatory subluxation. I use a combination of the clinical degree of instability and the presence of a palpable Stener lesion to choose direct repair of the thumb UCL, the index RCL, and large bony avulsion injuries. The management of complete RCL ruptures is currently in a state of transition in the field of hand surgery. Subluxation into pronation by the proximal phalanx pivoting on the intact UCL has led to increasing interest in early direct repairs. When I can appreciate rotatory subluxation on the examination, I now prefer RCL repair. Volar dislocations risk late instability if not surgically repaired. When the patient presents late following a complete ligament rupture, direct repair is rarely possible. The simplest reconstruction is then to create a proximally based flap of retracted ligament and advance it back to the anatomic insertion at the volar base of the proximal phalanx. This tissue is not always of sufficient quality. When that is the case, a free tendon graft (plantaris or palmaris longus) can be placed through drill holes to reconstruct the ligament. With appropriate rehabilitation, these patients can still achieve near-normal motion.

Open Reduction of Finger MP Dislocations

The border digits, the index and small fingers, can easily be approached with a midaxial incision that offers all the advantages that are proposed for both volar and dorsal approaches. Cartilage injuries on the metacarpal head can be well visualized, the digital nerves are easily protected, and the volar plate can be guided back into its correct position. For the long and ring fingers I prefer a dorsal transverse incision made at the level of the distal portion of the metacarpal head. This level can reliably be found at the dorsal apex of the sloping V shape of the web commissure. The sagittal bands do not need to be divided but rather they can be retracted distally to access the joint. The volar plate can be reduced without dividing it through a combination of wrist flexion to relax the extrinsic flexor tendons and MP hyperextension. A Freer elevator then guides the volar plate to the distal surface of the metacarpal head before attempting to reduce the joint itself. For the RCL of the index, an absorbable 1.3-mm bone anchor can be used for repair of insertional ruptures and a 4–0 absorbable monofilament suture for midsubstance ruptures. Pinning of the joint is not necessary in fingers as adjacent digit strapping provides enough restraint to excessive coronal plane deviation to protect the healing repair. The exception to this is the rare high-energy volar dislocation that is so unstable as to require 3 weeks of transarticular pin fixation.

Thumb MP Collateral Ligament Repair

The operative technique consists of a chevron incision over the ulnar aspect of the MP joint ensuring adequate volar exposure at the base of the proximal phalanx. Care must be taken with the superficial branches of the radial nerve to avoid neuroma formation. There is usually one large branch passing through the surgical field that is best mobilized dorsally. An incision in the adductor aponeurosis is made just ulnar to the EPL tendon with a cuff being left for repair. Reflection of this layer reveals the joint capsule and torn collateral ligament. Whereas all patterns of disruption have been reported, the most frequent is that of distal avulsion from the base of the proximal phalanx. Often there is a transverse rent in the dorsal capsule and evidence of volar plate injury as well. Direct repair is easiest with an absorbable 1.3-mm bone anchor placed at the true insertion site on the volar lateral tubercle to restore normal anatomy and reduce the rotatory subluxation of the joint. The repair may include a suture through the volar plate margin to re-create the "critical corner." The joint is pinned with a 0.045-inch K-wire before tying the anchor sutures to prevent inadvertent radial deviation and early rupture of the repair during the first 4 weeks postoperatively. A large bone fragment carrying the point of ligament insertion can be stabilized with one or two lag screws (Fig. 30-67). The IP joint should be left free for motion at all

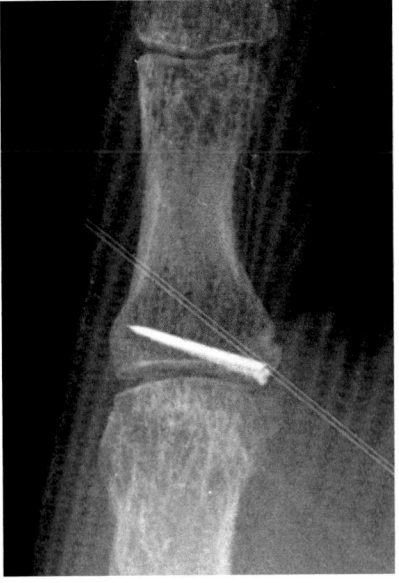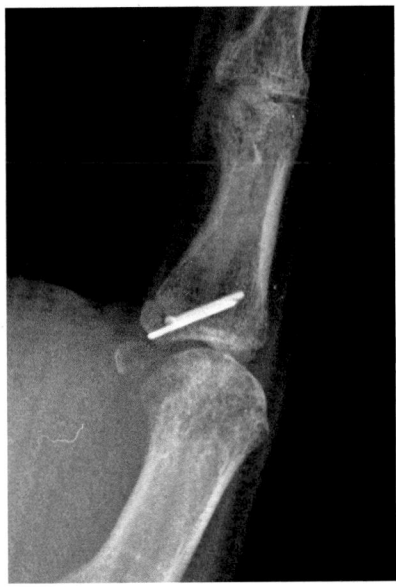

FIGURE 30-67 When a substantial bone fragment accompanies an ulnar collateral ligament injury to the MP joint, lag screw compression provides excellent stability through direct bone healing, provided that there is not a multilevel injury of the ligament separating it from the bone fragment as well.

times. Motion at the MP joint can begin in a protected fashion at 4 weeks following pin removal and then in an unprotected fashion by 6 weeks. Power pinch activities that stress the ligament in the coronal plane of the thumb should be avoided for up to 3 months after repair.

Free Tendon Graft Reconstruction of the Thumb UCL

The approach to the ulnar base of the thumb is the same as for simple repair. The correct anatomic sites of ligament origin at the metacarpal head and insertion at the phalangeal base should be easily discernable, having remnants of the original ligament fibers. Drill tunnels are made from each of these points obliquely directed away from the joint with a 3-mm bit. Free tendon graft may be harvested by conventional methods from either the palmaris longus (within the operative field) or the plantaris (a more appropriate size match). The tendon is passed through each of the drill holes, tensioned, and secured with 3-mm interference screws (Table 30-12).

INTRODUCTION TO METACARPAL FRACTURES

Fracture patterns may be broken down into those of the metacarpal head, neck, and shaft. Intra-articular fractures of the metacarpal base are covered in the next section on CMC joint fracture dislocations. Metacarpal head fractures present in a variety of patterns requiring different treatment strategies aimed at restoring a smooth congruent joint surface. Transverse metacarpal neck and shaft fractures will typically demonstrate apex dorsal angulation. The normal anatomic neck to shaft angle of 15 degrees should be recalled when assessing the amount of angulation in subcapital fractures. Radiographic assessment of apex dorsal angulation has a high interobserver

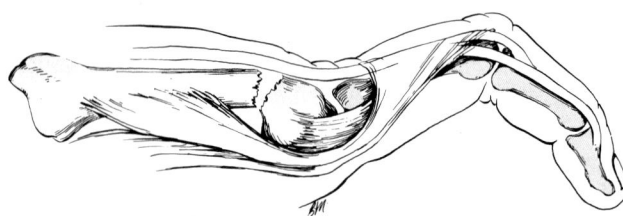

FIGURE 30-68 Pseudoclawing is an imbalance of compensatory MP joint hyperextension and PIP joint flexion that occurs on attempted digital extension in proportion to the degree of apex dorsal angulation at the metacarpal fracture site and represents one indication for surgery.

and intraobserver variability.[107] Pseudoclawing is a term used to describe a dynamic imbalance manifested as a hyperextension deformity of the MP joint and a flexion deformity of the PIP joint (Fig. 30-68). This occurs as a compensatory response to the apex dorsal angulation of the metacarpal fracture (usually at the neck) and represents a clinical indication for correcting the fracture angulation. Oblique and spiral fractures tend to shorten and rotate more than angulate (Fig. 30-69). As with all hand fractures, evaluation of rotation remains one of the most critical assessments to avoid a functionally disabling malunion. Ten degrees of malrotation (which risks as much as 2 cm of overlap at the digital tip) should represent the upper tolerable limit. The problem of overlapping bone shadows has led to the development of a number of specialized radiographic

TABLE 30-12	**Surgical Steps—Free Tendon Graft Reconstruction of Thumb UCL**

Midaxial ulnar approach, staying out of web space, and protecting dorsal digital nerve

Clear old scar and ruptured ligament fibers from anatomic points of UCL attachment

Drill oblique 3-mm tunnels from point of attachment out to radial cortex

Draw free tendon graft (palmaris or other) into tunnel by traction suture on straight Keith needle

Fix graft into place with 3-mm interference screw, pull back to test fixation

Repeat insertion of free graft into other tunnel, tension graft, and fix with interference screw

Check tension on graft and adjust fixation if needed, check range of motion

Check dorsal nerve branch, close wound with absorbable monofilament, dress, and splint

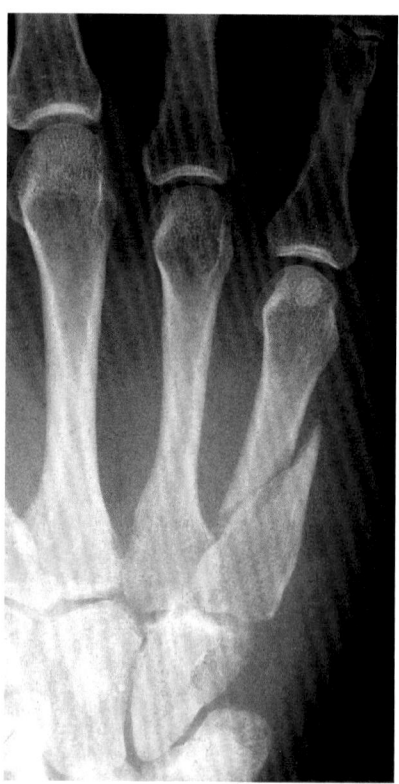

FIGURE 30-69 Long oblique and spiral fractures of the metacarpal shaft tend to shorten and rotate more than angulate.

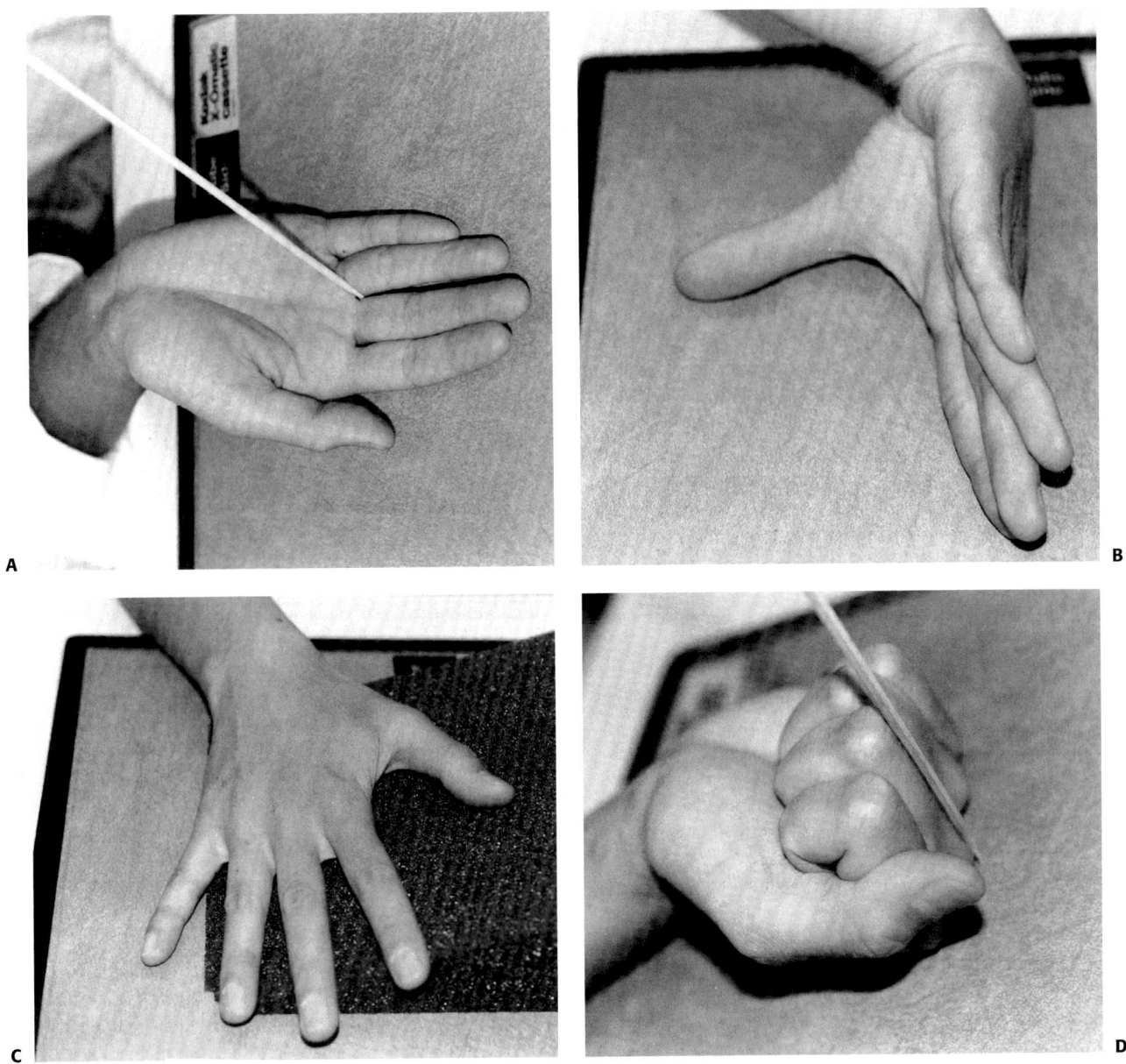

FIGURE 30-70 Specialized radiographic views may help to define injury patterns in the metacarpal including **(A)** the Brewerton view for the metacarpal bases, **(B)** the Mehara view for the index CMC relationships, **(C)** the reverse oblique view for angulation in the index metacarpal neck, and **(D)** the skyline view for vertical impaction fractures of the metacarpal head.

views (Fig. 30-70). The Brewerton and Mehara views may show otherwise occult fractures at the metacarpal bases. The reverse oblique projection allows a more accurate estimation of angulation at the second metacarpal neck. The skyline view may show vertical impaction fractures of the metacarpal head not appreciable on any other projection.

PATHOANATOMY AND APPLIED ANATOMY RELATING TO METACARPAL FRACTURES

The metacarpals are the key skeletal elements participating in the formation of the three arches of the hand. There are two transverse arches that exist at the CMC and MP joint levels. The metacarpals themselves are longitudinally arched with a fairly broad convex dorsal surface. Intramedullary geometry is highly variable but with a consistently 20% thicker volar cortex. Surgical access to the metacarpals is easily achieved through incisions placed over the intermetacarpal valleys and curved distally to avoid entering the digital web commissures.

The metacarpals are held tightly bound to each other by strong interosseous ligaments at their bases and by the deep transverse intermetacarpal ligaments distally. These connections help to maintain the transverse arches of the hand, but flattening can occur with multiple metacarpal fractures or crushing injuries. Shortening of individual metacarpal fractures is limited by these same ligaments (more effectively for the central metacarpals than for the border metacarpals). For each 2 mm of metacarpal shortening, 7 degrees of extensor lag can be expected.[157] One of the weakest points in the metacarpal is the volar aspect of the neck, where comminution is often present. In the sagittal plane, the primary deforming forces are the intrinsic muscles, which can be counteracted through MP joint flexion, an important component of the reduction maneuver for metacarpal fractures. Correction of apex dorsal angulation and rotational control is achieved indirectly by grasping the finger to exert control over the distal metacarpal fragment. Flexion of the PIP joint for reduction, as has been long recommended, is an unnecessary maneuver that actually encumbers the reduction process by tensioning the intrinsics.

METACARPAL FRACTURE TREATMENT OPTIONS

Nonoperative Management

Many metacarpal neck and shaft fractures can be treated nonoperatively. Twenty-seven small finger metacarpal fractures with initial angulation of 40 degrees were reduced and treated in a short hand cast for 4 weeks with only three patients losing reduction beyond 15 degrees.[36] Intra-articular fractures of the head and base may also be treated nonoperatively, provided the fracture plane is both stable and minimally displaced. Metacarpal fractures with significant rotation or shortening cannot be effectively controlled through entirely nonoperative means. However, initial shortening and extensor lag has been shown to improve over time where 42 such patients eventually achieved 94% of contralateral grip strength by 1 year.[7] An externally applied splint exerts indirect (but not direct) control over fracture position through positioning and reduction of myotendinous deforming forces. A splint is able to preserve a fracture position that is inherently stable but is not capable of reducing and maintaining an unstable position. The stability of a metacarpal fracture is determined primarily by the adjacent structures (periosteum, adjacent metacarpals, deep transverse

intermetacarpal, and proximal interosseous ligaments) as well as the degrees of initial displacement and comminution. Splinting should be directed at pain control and neutralization of deforming forces. Surface contact should be as broad as possible with an appropriate amount of padding. The splint may be discontinued as soon as the patient can comfortably perform ROM with the hand and not later than 3 weeks. IP joint motion should begin immediately following injury. A dorsal splint in full MP joint flexion meets the patient's needs well but may be more than is required. Some have advocated functional mobilization for metacarpal fractures without splinting at all.[16] Compared with simple adjacent digit strapping in 73 patients, a molded metacarpal brace for less than 40-degree angulated fractures of the small finger metacarpal neck yielded similar clinical results with less pain.[72] Defining the acceptable limits of deformity for each injury location is the subject of much controversy. Functionally, pseudoclawing is unacceptable. Also, the patient may be troubled by the appearance of a dorsal prominence at the fracture site or a shift in the metacarpal head from its dorsally visible position toward the palm. Only rarely will the shift toward the palm create a functional problem. Each patient may have different degrees of deformity that he or she is willing to tolerate. A correlation between deformity and symptoms has not been clearly established. Greater degrees of angulation are tolerable in neck fractures than in shaft fractures. Greater angulation is tolerable in the ring and small metacarpals than in the index and long metacarpals because of the increased mobility of the ulnar-sided CMC joints. Biomechanically significant decay in flexor tendon efficiency because of slack in the flexor digiti minimi and third volar interosseous occurs with angulations over 30 degrees in the fifth metacarpal neck, the site of greatest allowable angulation.[4,14]

Operative Management
Closed Reduction and Internal Fixation

CRIF is the mainstay of treatment for isolated metacarpal fractures not meeting the criteria for nonoperative treatment (Fig. 30-71). Twenty-five patients with small finger metacarpal fractures achieved excellent functional results following

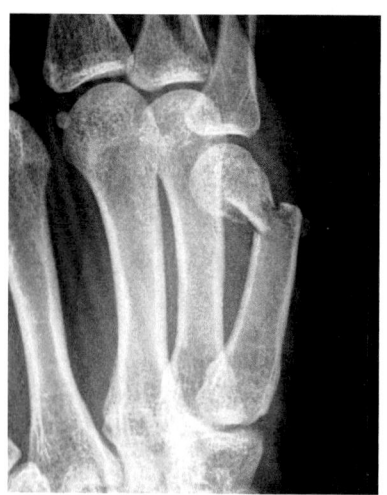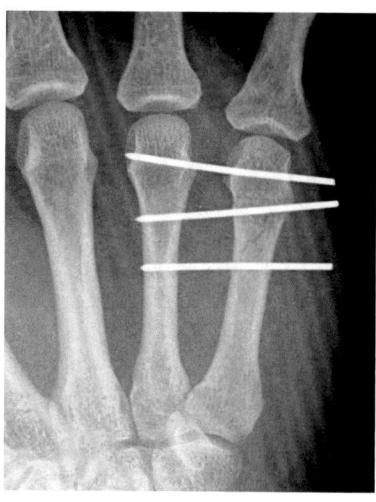

FIGURE 30-71 Closed reduction and internal fixation is effective for metacarpal neck fractures despite the smaller size of the head fragment and the need to achieve separation of the two wires that pass through it for control of fragment rotation in the sagittal plane.

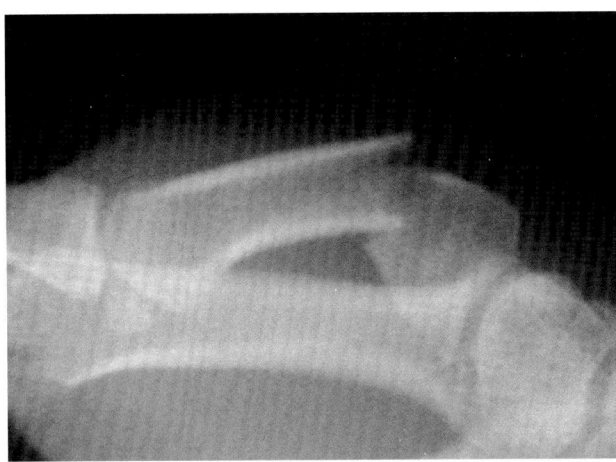
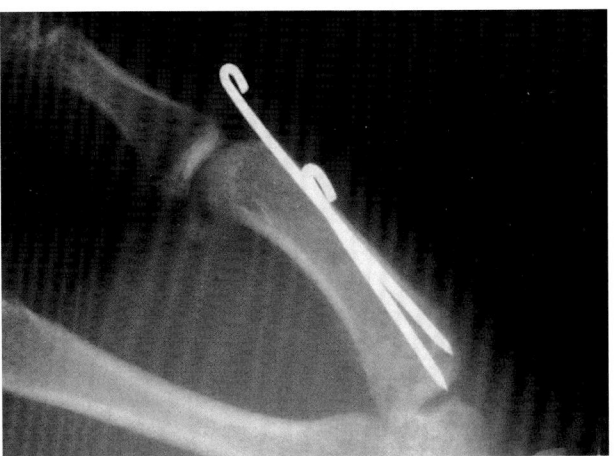

FIGURE 30-72 Extra-articular fractures of the thumb metacarpal **(A)** can be effective managed by **(B)** retrograde longitudinal pinning across the fracture into the base fragment.

stabilization with three transverse K-wires and demonstrated no shortening, appreciable angulation, or complications.[61] A comparison between transverse and intramedullary K-wires in 59 patients failed to show any differences in outcome with no complications in either group.[183] CRIF may be used for both extra-articular and intra-articular fractures provided that the fracture is anatomically reducible and stable to the stress of motion with only K-wire fixation. CRIF is the minimum treatment necessary for metacarpal base fractures that cannot be held reduced by nonoperative means (Fig. 30-72). Another closed reduction combined with stabilization option that has been reported is external fixation.[115]

Intramedullary Fixation

Intramedullary fixation strategies are best matched with transverse and short oblique fracture patterns and include a single large diameter rod such as a Steinmann pin, an expandable intramedullary device, multiple prebent K-wires, or specially manu-factured devices inserted at the metacarpal base designed to achieve three-point intramedullary fixation (Fig. 30-73).[10,10,125] A single Steinmann pin may be inserted open through the fracture site with the two fragments then impacted over it. Rotational control is achieved by fracture fragment interlock, and motion can be started immediately. The strategy of multiple, stacked prebent wires has received broader acceptance than the other two strategies, perhaps owing to the closed technique used for introduction.[110] The wires are prebent such that three point-contact is obtained dorsally at the proximal and distal ends of the metacarpal and volarly at the mid-diaphysis. This bow opposes the natural dorsal convexity of the metacarpal and is the basis for the apparently secure fixation achieved with this technique. The pins are stacked into the canal, filling it and imparting improved rotational control; as many as three to five 0.045-inch K-wires may be required. Locking intramedullary nails can also be used in special cases such as gunshot wounds.[10]

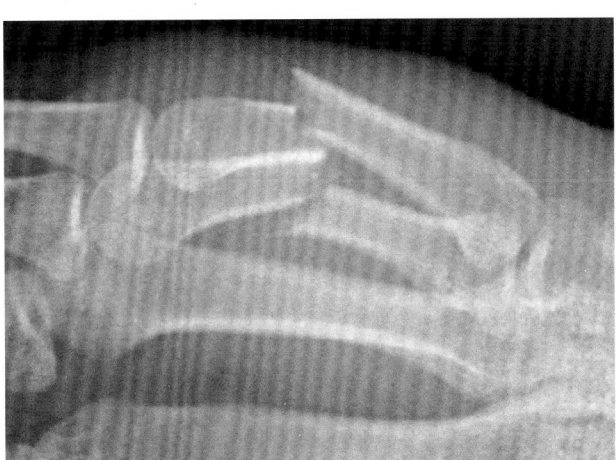
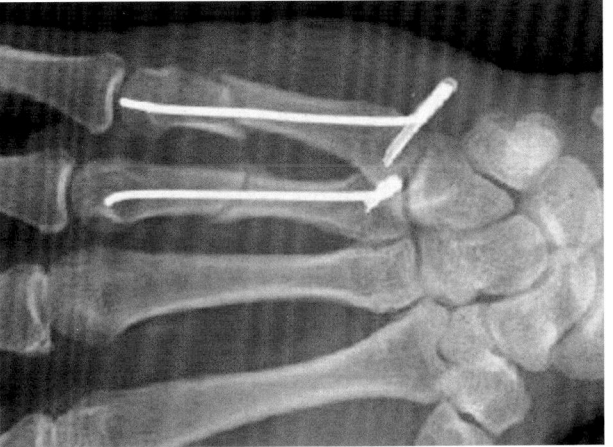

FIGURE 30-73 Fractures of the metacarpal at the same level that cannot be treated by transverse pinning **(A)** can be stabilized by **(B)** a specially manufactured device shaped for three-point fixation and closed intramedullary application with a rotational locking sleeve used proximally. This device is also effective **(C)** in oblique fracture patterns and **(D)** fractures near the base.

(continues)

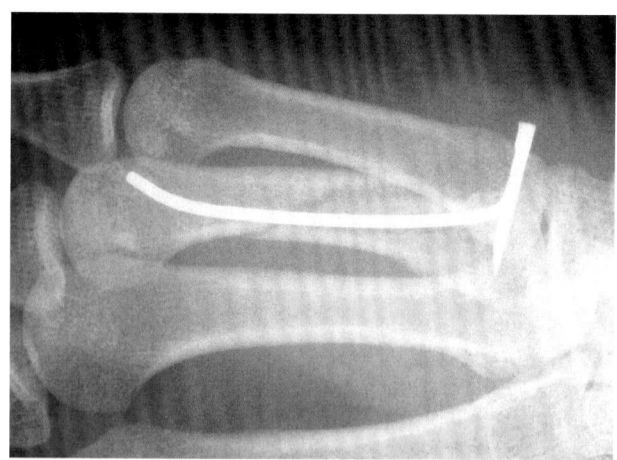

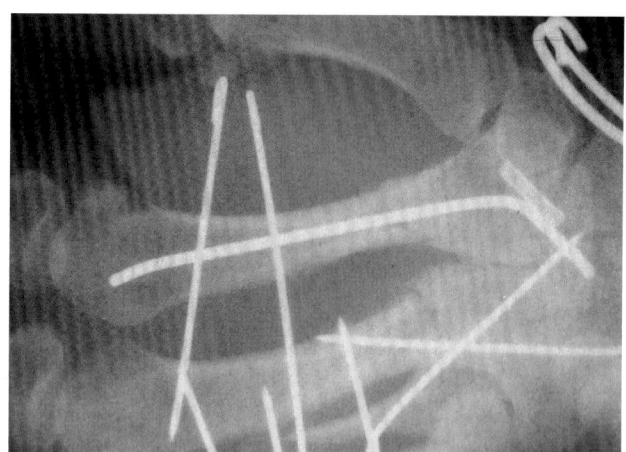

FIGURE 30-73 (continued)

Open Reduction and Internal Fixation

ORIF is the treatment of choice for intra-articular fractures that cannot be reduced and held by closed means. Internal fixation is also required for multiple fractures without inherent stability and for open fractures especially when associated with tendon disruptions.[59,150] Internal fixation can be accomplished with intraosseous wiring, composite wiring, screws only, or screws and plates (Fig. 30-74). Wiring techniques have traditionally held the advantage over plate and screw application in terms of technical ease and availability of materials. However, with the modular plating systems now available specifically for use in hand surgery, lower profile fixation can be achieved with greater rigidity (Fig. 30-75).[121] The most important consideration is that the surgeon should choose the method of internal fixation with which he or she is the most comfortable, keeping in mind that even plate fixation can fail.[40] A nonrandomized study of 52 patients found no statistically significant differences in functional outcome between intramedullary nailing and plate–screw fixation of extra-articular metacarpal fractures.[130]

Unlike the plate–screw patients, 5/38 intramedullary patients lost reduction, had intramedullary penetration into the MP joint, and had more secondary surgeries for hardware removal.

Metacarpal Head Fractures

For partial articular metacarpal head fractures, screw-only fixation is the treatment of choice with up to 79 degrees of ROM achieved.[163] If sufficient interlock of bone spicules occurs, a single 1.2- to1.5-mm countersunk screw can control rotation

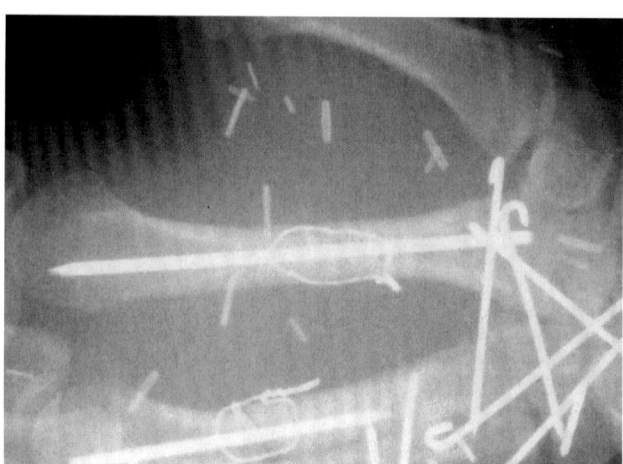

FIGURE 30-74 When rotational control is not sufficient with intramedullary fixation alone, composite wiring is useful and also adds a compressive force across the fracture site.

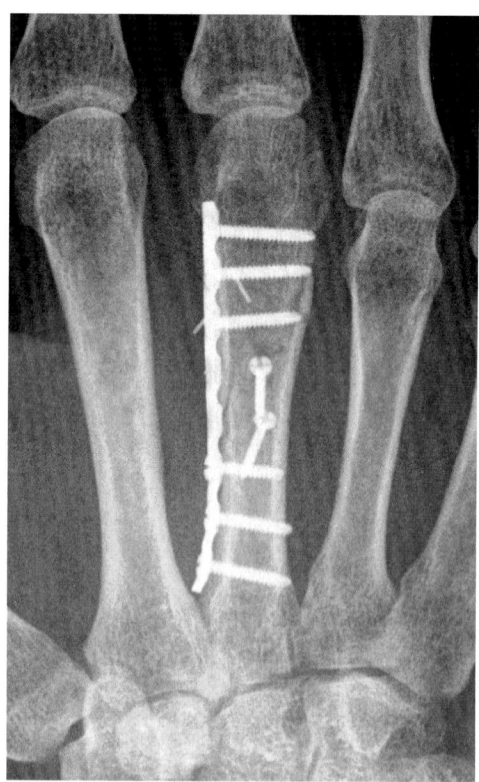

FIGURE 30-75 Plates are indicated for use with comminuted fractures lacking inherent stability and open fractures with associated soft tissue injury requiring immediate aggressive rehabilitation.

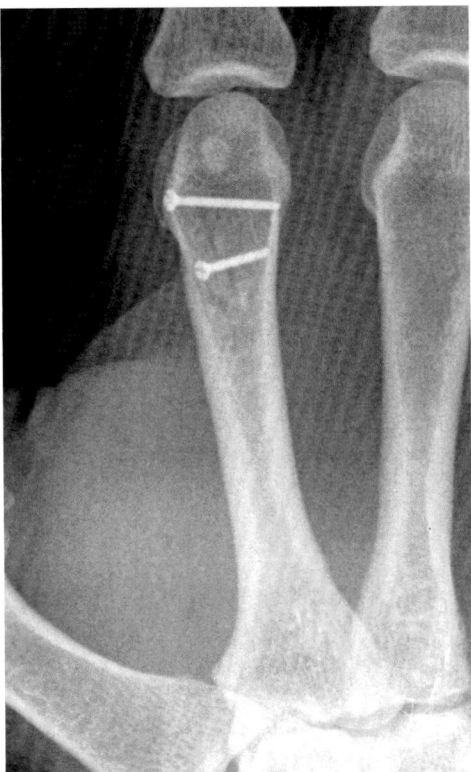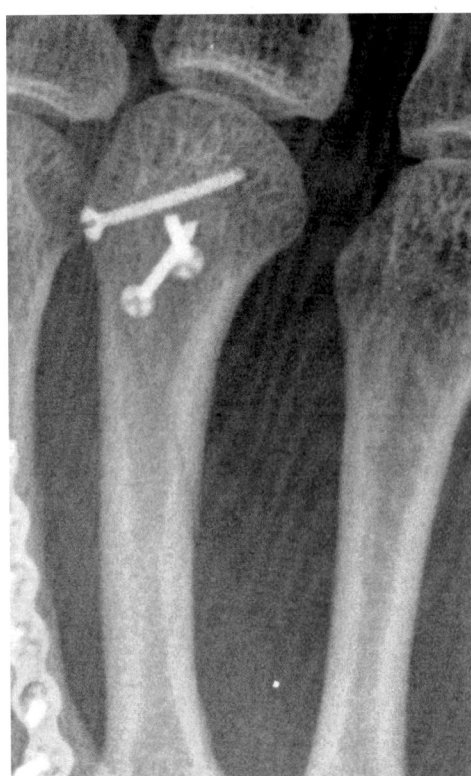

FIGURE 30-76 Metacarpal head fractures consisting of only a few fragments are best stabilized by countersunk small lag screws.

of the fragment. If interlock is not effective, two screws are preferred even if this means downsizing the screw diameter to accommodate both of them in the fragment without causing comminution (Fig. 30-76). For complete articular head fractures, the condylar blade plate used to be required. The currently available small size hand modular locking plates allow fixed angle support of comminuted periarticular fractures with the ability to contour the plate first and avoid the complexity associated with inserting the blade plate (Fig. 30-77).

Postoperative Care. The importance of early motion must be considered in direct proportion to the magnitude of the injury or the surgical procedure performed.[117] Modern plating systems tolerate applied loads in cadaver specimens sufficient for immediate full active motion rehabilitation.[148] The more tissue damage that is present, the more aggressive must be the motion program. One frequently overlooked factor that greatly confounds progress in therapy is edema control. External compression wraps to the zone of injury with cohesive elastic bandages work to minimize the presence of edema from the outset. When internal fixation has been required, one must anticipate the development of an extensor lag at the MP joint. Specific attention should be given to extensor tendon gliding in zone VI to overcome a developing lag. Rapid tendon activation has been successful in breaking free developing adhesions between the peritendinous tissues and their surroundings. (Fig. 30-78).[75] Patients should be allowed to use the hand for light activities throughout the healing period. Light resistance

activities can begin at 6 weeks. Extremely forceful use patterns should be deferred until 3 months.

Potential Pitfalls and Preventative Measures. The metacarpal is the most proximal bone in the ray. Rotational malunions here will be the most obvious and functionally disabling. In large part, the management of metacarpal fractures is all about ensuring that rotation is correct. Length and angulation are, of course, not to be forgotten. The assessment of rotation both preoperatively and intraoperatively merits discussion. In both cases, the examiner should not touch the digit during the assessment. The awake, preoperative patient may require an anesthetic block to relieve enough pain so that he or she is capable of flexing sufficiently to demonstrate the rotational status of the digit. In the anesthetized patient, tenodesis driven by full range wrist motion produces sufficient flexion and extension of the digit that rotational alignment can be accurately judged.

When performing transverse pinning of metacarpals, intraoperative imaging will effectively demonstrate depth of pin penetration and coronal plane fracture orientation. Metacarpal overlap obscures any individual metacarpal lateral view. Ensuring that the pins have penetrated both cortices of both metacarpals cannot be judged radiographically and must be determined by feel at the time of placement. If the reduction is difficult to obtain closed or tends to slip as the pins are driven, the case does not have to be converted to a full open reduction. A small instrument such as a dental pick or microelevator can be placed percutaneously at the fracture site to directly control reduction

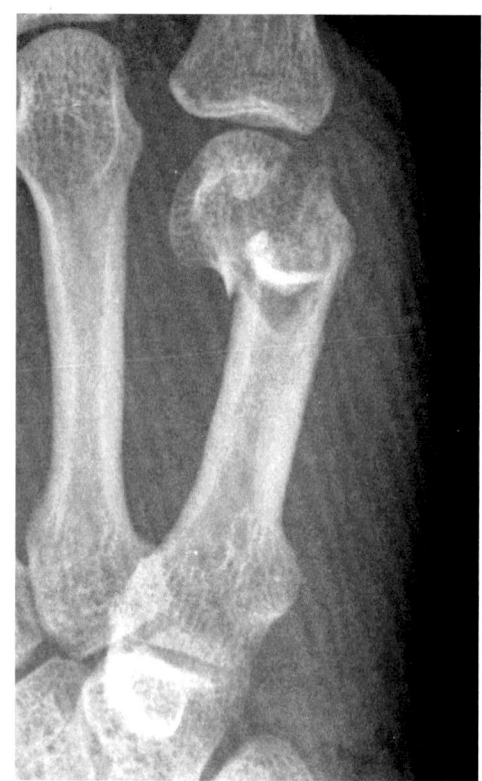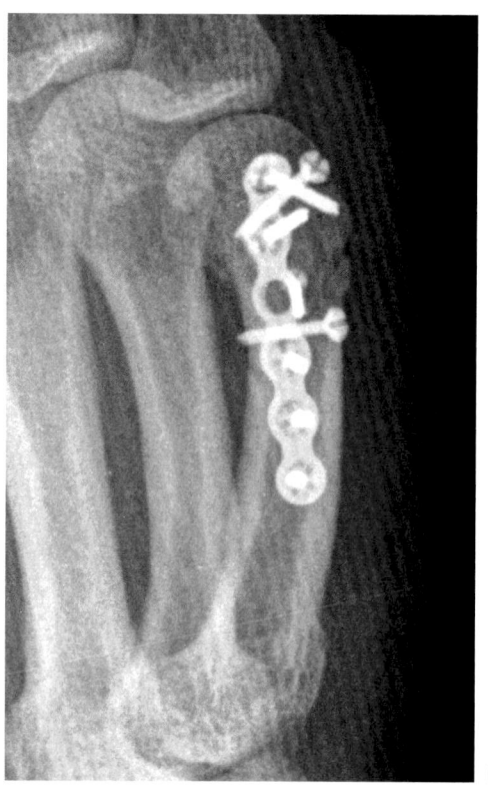

FIGURE 30-77 Metacarpal head fractures with **(A)** high degrees of comminution and inherent instability may require **(B)** plate stabilization to avoid collapse.

whereas the surgeon proceeds with the otherwise entirely closed pinning. Compared to plating of phalangeal fractures, there is even greater risk of inducing an iatrogenic rotational malunion when tightening down the screws. If a metacarpal plate has not been axially contoured correctly, when the screws are tightened, the plate will actually rotate the distal fragment out of an otherwise previously correct reduction. For this reason, no matter how many times the reduction has already been clinically evaluated, it must be evaluated at least one more time upon final placement of all fixations (Table 30-13).

AUTHOR'S PREFERRED TREATMENT (FIG. 30-79)

Nonoperative Management

Many extra-articular and some intra-articular fractures, which are categorized as stable by virtue of having over 30% normal ROM without motion at the fracture site, can be managed with entirely nonoperative means using temporary splinting. Patients with entirely nondisplaced fractures that have excellent inherent

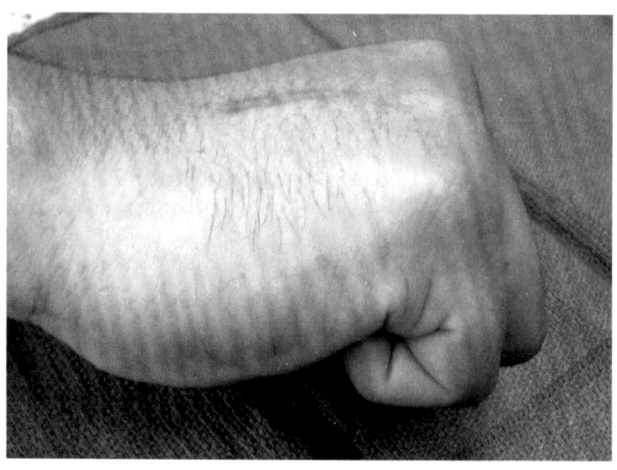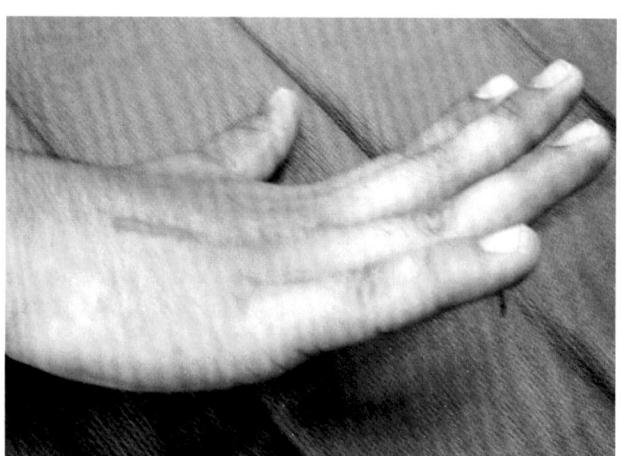

FIGURE 30-78 Even following ORIF, when a properly designed rehabilitation program is administered, **(A)** complete flexion and **(B)** hyperextension is possible.

TABLE 30-13 Potential Pitfalls and Preventative Measures— Metacarpal Fractures

Pitfall	Prevention
Tendon tethering by pins	Only place pins in the coronal plane and remain proximal to the sagittal bands; remove by 3 weeks, 4 weeks at the absolute latest
Malrotation leading to malunion	Careful clinical check of rotation
Failing to achieve purchase through all four cortices during transverse pinning	Judgment that the pin has passed all four cortices is by feel, not by radiographic image
Pin placement creates translation malposition of fragment	Resist translation with percutaneous placement of small bone elevator
Overdrilling the far hole on lag screws leading to poor fixation	Use low speed to avoid distal "whipping" of the small drill bit; larger size "rescue" screws
Shearing the head off small titanium screws	Use only fingertip tightening, no key pinch hold on the screwdriver
Inducing malunion with the plate	Take off and recontour the plate as many times as needed so that, when tightened down fully, it does not force the bone into malalignment or malrotation

stability do not require any external immobilization at all and can begin immediate AROM, usually with the added protection of adjacent digit strapping. Patients with stable metacarpal shaft fractures can be returned to nearly all light activities in a hand-based splint that is continued for a maximum of 3 weeks. Stable neck and intra-articular head fractures are more effectively protected by support that covers from the PIP level to the forearm with the MP joints in full flexion. At least one adjacent digit is included with the affected ray. IP joint motion should begin immediately with all strategies.

Closed Reduction and Internal Fixation

Transverse pinning to adjacent metacarpals is my treatment of choice for all unstable closed metacarpal fractures except multiple adjacent fractures at the same level that include a border

digit. The biomechanics of the transverse pinning strategy is that of external fixation. Four points of control are needed. The two points closest to the fracture site on either side should be as close together as possible. The two farthest from the fracture site should be as far apart as possible. The proximal intermetacarpal and CMC ligaments are stout enough to qualify as the most proximal point of fixation such that only one 0.045-inch K-wire is required proximal to the fracture site. The distalmost pin should avoid transgression of the sagittal bands. This must be titrated clinically against the goal of placing the point of fixation as far from the fracture site as possible. The transverse pinning strategy works equally well for central (long and ring) and border (index and small) metacarpals (Fig. 30-80). If the four finger metacarpals are thought of as occurring in two columns (a radial column for index and long and an ulnar column for

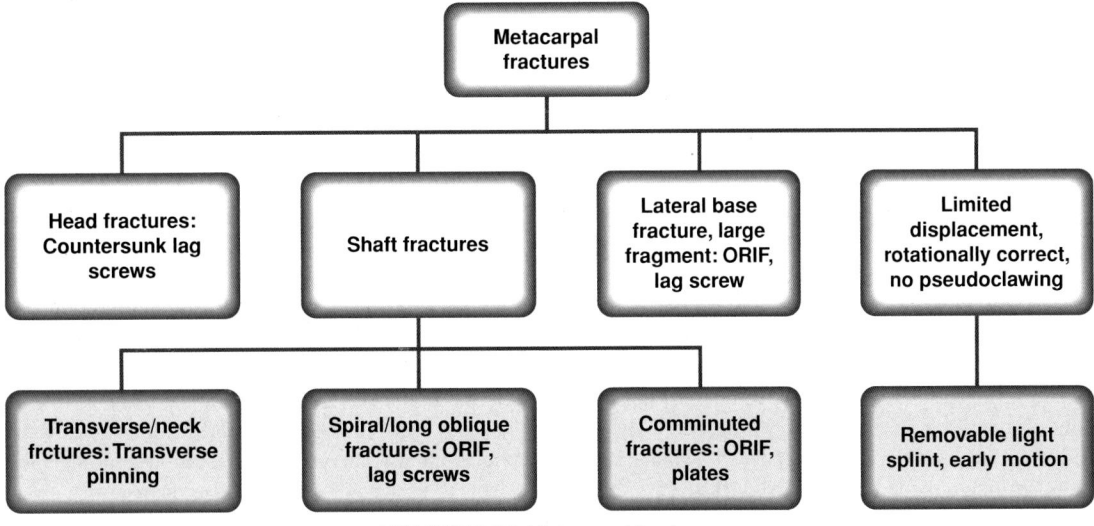

FIGURE 30-79 Metacarpal fractures.

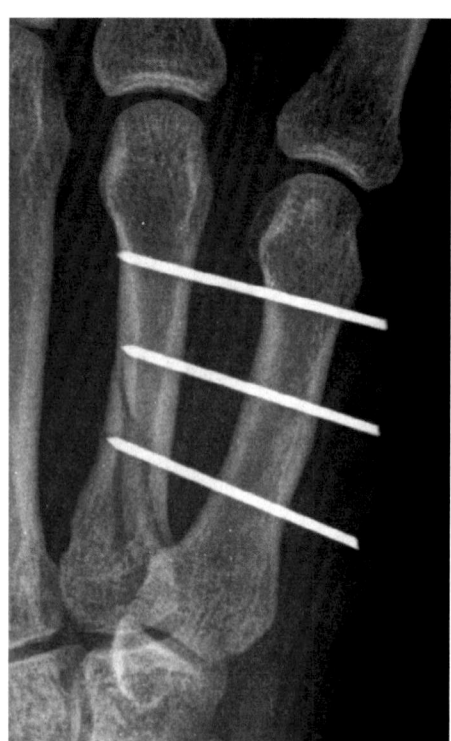

FIGURE 30-80 Transverse closed reduction and internal fixation functions under the same biomechanical principles as external fixation. Note the distal wire is placed just proximal to the collateral recess of both bones and has also avoided tethering the sagittal bands.

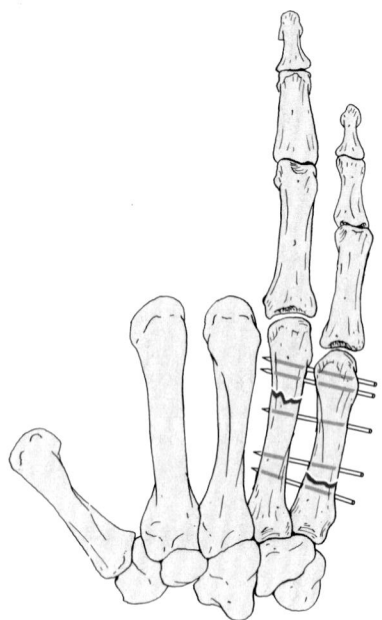

FIGURE 30-81 Reciprocal transverse stabilization of adjacent metacarpal fractures is possible when the levels of the two fractures are separated enough to be able to place two pins that fall distal to the first fracture and proximal to the second such that the first metacarpal is sufficiently stabilized in turn to provide stability to the other metacarpal.

ring and small) then most combinations of multiple metacarpal fractures can still be fixed with this strategy, and it can always be used if there is only one fracture per column. If both metacarpals in the column are fractured, but at different levels, they can be used to stabilize each other reciprocally (Fig. 30-81). The specific requirement for reciprocal stabilization to be effective is that there is a zone in the diaphysis of both bones where two pins can be placed with adequate spacing from each other (distal to one fracture site and proximal to the other). At the conclusion of the procedure, one has the choice of leaving the pins protruding through the skin or cutting them off beneath the skin. In previous editions of this chapter I had advocated allowing pins of less than 4 weeks' duration to be left outside the skin for ease of removal, but I now cut nearly all pins below the skin level given the prevalence of MRSA in the community. The hand is initially splinted in full MP flexion to resist the development of contractures. Early motion can proceed while the pins are still in place.

Open Reduction and Internal Fixation

ORIF is my treatment of choice for open fractures and multiple fractures not meeting the criteria for reciprocal transverse stabilization. When fracture plane interlock between bone spicules is present, intraosseous wiring, composite wiring, screw-only, or screw and plate fixation may all be considered. I prefer lag screw fixation for long-oblique or spiral fractures since CRIF cannot control the reduction of these patterns nearly as well as

transverse fractures (Fig. 30-82). To select screw-only fixation, the ratio of the length of the oblique or spiral fracture plane to the bone diameter must be at least 2:1. Furthermore, to avoid comminution, the screws must pass through an area in the bone spike where the screw's outer diameter is less than one-third the width of the spike. The screw sizes most appropriate for a metacarpal are 1.5 and 1.7 mm. Multiple open transverse or short oblique fractures of the mid-diaphysis from open crushing injuries are nicely managed with intramedullary pins. Rotational control can be supplemented with a composite wire loop. When interfragmentary compression cannot be achieved owing to the presence of comminution or bone loss, plates and screws are indicated.

As with all techniques of internal fixation, it is essential to cover the hardware with periosteal closure to provide a separate gliding layer. I prefer to operate 3 to 5 days following injury so that the periosteum will have thickened in response to injury and can be both dissected as a discrete tissue flap and closed with solid suture purchase. Unlike over the proximal phalanx, the extensor tendons at this level are discrete cords, and placement of the hardware away from them should be possible in most cases. Placement of the plate dorsally puts it on the tension cortex of the bone, but in this position it interferes most directly with the extensor tendons. Placement of the plate in a true lateral position allows sagittal plane forces to be resisted by the width of the plate rather than its thickness, and doing so is almost always possible, just technically more difficult. This is my choice for plate placement unless extenuating circumstances dictate dorsal placement. One such circumstance is

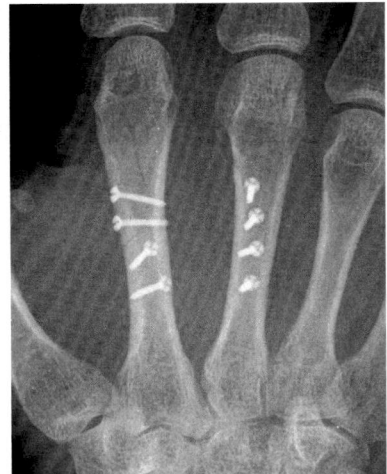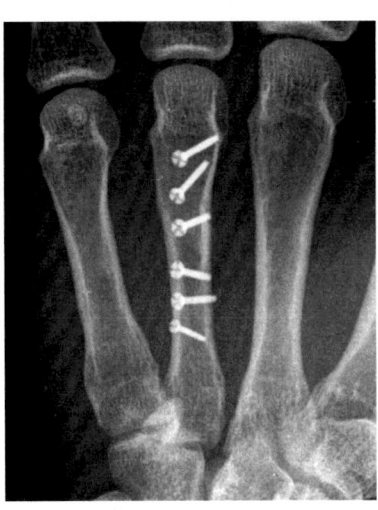

FIGURE 30-82 Interfragmentary lag screws allow stable fixation of **(A)** adjacent metacarpals and **(B)** three fragment fractures with an intermediate butterfly fragment sufficient to permit full immediate motion rehabilitation.

fracture comminution extending all the way to the base of the metacarpal. All the technical comments made in the section on proximal phalangeal fractures apply equally here (Table 30-14).

INTRODUCTION TO CARPOMETACARPAL (CMC) JOINT DISLOCATIONS AND FRACTURE DISLOCATIONS

Dislocations and fracture-dislocations at the finger CMC joints are usually high-energy injuries with involvement of associated structures, often neurovascular (Fig. 30-83). Particular care must be given to the examination of ulnar nerve function, especially motor, because of its close proximity to the fifth CMC joint. Frequently, the pattern is one of fracture-dislocation involving the metacarpal bases, the distal carpal bones, or both.[101] Overlap on the lateral x-ray obscures accurate depiction of the injury

pattern, and most authors recommend at least one variant of an oblique view.[185] The Brewerton view may be helpful in this respect, profiling individual metacarpal bases. When fracture dislocations include the dorsal cortex of the hamate, CT may be necessary to fully evaluate the pathoanatomy. Another pattern to recognize is dislocation of one CMC joint with fracture of an adjacent metacarpal base. Shortening can be evaluated by noting a disruption in the normal cascade seen distally at the MP joints. Volar CMC dislocations are rare.

Most thumb CMC dislocations are dorsal and are thought to occur through axial loading of a partially flexed thumb (Fig. 30-84). Motorcyclists may be uniquely prone to sustaining this rare injury and to having the injury missed on initial evaluation. The injury will often be reduced before being seen by the surgeon. Clinical diagnosis is then based on identifying the residual instability. Differentiating complete from

TABLE 30-14 **Surgical Steps—Plating of Comminuted Metacarpal Fractures**

Longitudinal incision not overlying path of extensor digitorum communis tendon

Avoid tendon and create single layer of musculoperiosteal envelope down to fracture, minimizing periosteal stripping from fracture to only the location where plate will be placed

Prepare fracture site with curettage of clot and debris to permit accurate reduction

Provisional reduction using Adson-Brown forceps and small elevators

Select plate length and type, including decision for locking vs. nonlocking (at least four diaphyseal cortices beyond zone of comminution)

Provisionally contour plate, check, recontour, check, repeat...

Fix plate to bone with one proximal and one distal screw near ends of plate, nonlocking screws

Check clinically and radiographically length, alignment, and rotation; redo earlier steps if not correct

Add second proximal and distal screws (if locking screws to be used, now is the time)

Recheck all parameters, but especially rotation at this key stage; redo earlier steps if not correct

Complete fixation by placing remaining midzone screws

Final check of all parameters clinically and radiographically, close wound with absorbable monofilament, dress, and splint intrinsic plus position

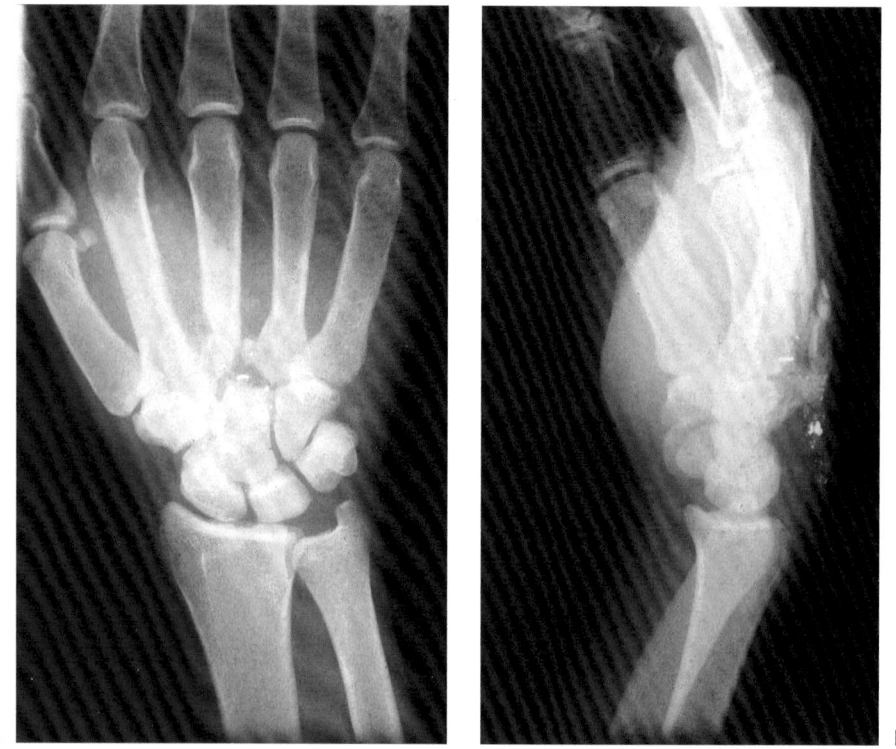

FIGURE 30-83 Fractures of CMC joints **(A)** are typically high-energy injuries with **(B)** comminution of both the metacarpal base and the distal carpal row.

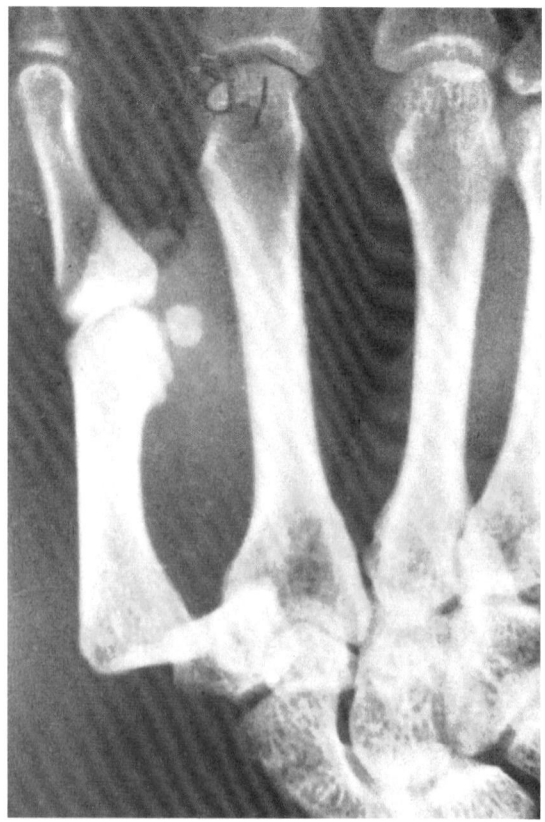

FIGURE 30-84 Pure dislocations of the thumb CMC joint are rare injuries and typically occur dorsoradially.

incomplete ligament rupture is essential, as initial operative treatment is appropriate only for complete disruptions. Instillation of local anesthetic into the joint may be required to allow an unimpeded examination. Manual stress testing compared to the contralateral side should allow for diagnosis in most cases.

The majority of thumb metacarpal base fractures are intra-articular (Fig. 30-85). The majority of thumb CMC joint injuries are fracture-dislocations rather than pure dislocations. The smaller fracture fragment at the thumb metacarpal volar base is deeply placed and not palpable. Eponyms associated with these fracture-dislocations are Bennett's (partial articular) and Rolando's (complete articular). Specific x-rays must be obtained in the true AP and lateral planes of the thumb (not a series of hand x-rays) if injuries along this axis are to be correctly identified (Fig. 30-86).

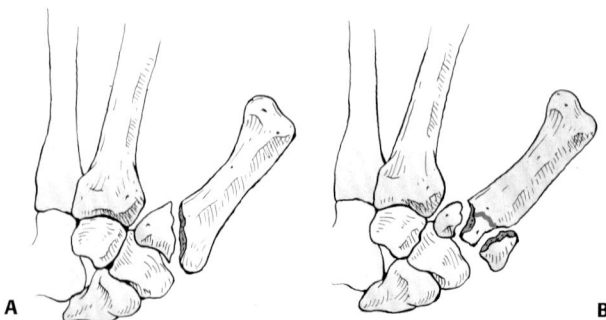

FIGURE 30-85 The most recognized patterns of thumb metacarpal base intra-articular fractures are **(A)** the partial articular Bennett fracture and **(B)** the complete articular Rolando fracture.

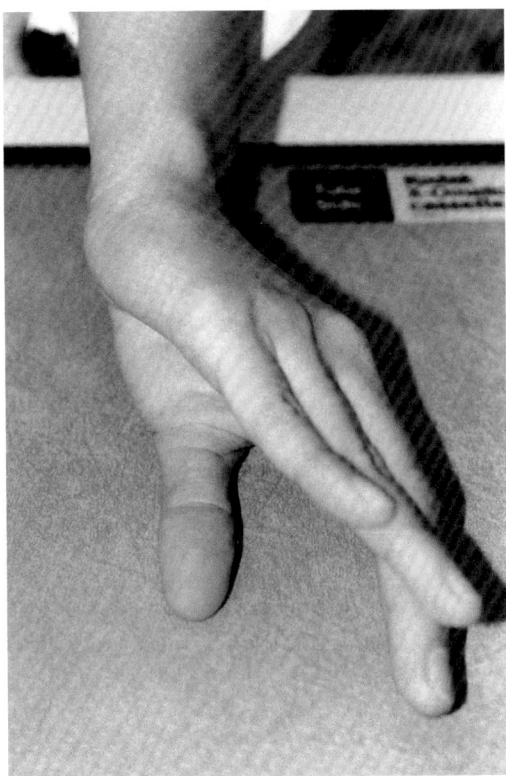

FIGURE 30-86 The thumb does not reside in the same plane as the rest of the hand. A true AP of the thumb can be obtained with the Robert's view.

PATHOANATOMY AND APPLIED ANATOMY RELATING TO CARPOMETACARPAL (CMC) JOINT DISLOCATIONS AND FRACTURE DISLOCATIONS

Finger CMC Joints

Stability at the finger CMC joints is provided by a system of four ligaments. There is a high degree of variation with dorsal, multiple palmar, and two sets of interosseous ligaments (only one between the long and ring metacarpals).[47,119] The interosseous ligaments are the strongest and have a V configuration with the base of the V oriented toward the fourth metacarpal. ROM of the index and long CMC joints is limited to less than 5 degrees, with 15 degrees at the ring, and up to 25 to 30 degrees at the small finger. Small finger CMC motion is reduced 28% to 40% when the ring finger is immobilized.[52] The axis of motion is located near the base of the metacarpal. The index metacarpal has a particularly stable configuration through its wedge-shaped articulation with the trapezoid. The small finger CMC joint is the only joint not having a gliding configuration but instead is a modified saddle-shaped joint. The increased mobility on the ulnar side of the hand may predispose to its greater frequency of injury. Critical soft tissue relationships to appreciate during treatment of injuries to the CMC joints are the positions of the motor branch of the ulnar nerve directly in front of the fifth CMC joint and the deep palmar arch in front of the third CMC joint. Of all hand fractures and dislocations, injury at the CMC level requires the highest degree of vigilance

regarding associated neurologic injury. The high-energy mechanism of these injuries and profound degrees of swelling may lead to worsened outcomes through residual long-term nerve compression.

Thumb CMC Joint

Branches of both the lateral antebrachial cutaneous and superficial radial nerve ramify throughout the region of the thumb base on the radial side. Three tendons pass through this region: The abductor pollicis longus (APL), extensor pollicis brevis (EPB), and EPL. The radial artery passes beneath the APL and EPB on its course to the first web space and lies just proximal to the CMC joint. The joint anatomy includes reciprocal saddle-shaped surfaces of the distal trapezium and proximal metacarpal. The axis of this concavoconvex joint is then itself curved in a third plane with the convexity lateral. The normal ROM at the thumb CMC joint is around 50 degrees of flexion-extension, 40 degrees of abduction-adduction, and 15 degrees of pronation-supination. There is consensus as to which ligaments are anatomically present at the trapeziometacarpal joint (Fig. 30-87). They are the superficial anterior oblique, deep anterior oblique (beak), ulnar collateral, intermetacarpal, posterior oblique, and dorsoradial ligaments.[13] A point of confluence exists at the palmar ulnar tubercle of the first metacarpal base. There was a period of disagreement regarding the primary stabilizing ligament in preventing dislocation between the deep anterior oblique and the dorsoradial ligament. Although the deep anterior oblique was previously considered the primary stabilizer, more recent research has effectively demonstrated that the dorsoradial ligament is the prime restraint to dislocation. The dorsoradial ligament is the shortest ligament in the group and the first to become taut with dorsal or dorsoradial subluxation.[13] Selective ligament sectioning showed that deficiency of the dorsoradial ligament led to the greatest degree of subluxation.[174] Dorsal dislocation usually occurs through rupture of the dorsal ligaments with a sleeve-type avulsion of the anterior oblique ligament as it peels off the volar surface of the first metacarpal.[156] Supination may also play a significant role in the mechanism of this injury. Deformation of fractures at the base of the thumb metacarpal occurs with a complex motion (Fig. 30-88). The distal metacarpal is adducted and supinated by the adductor pollicis. At the same time, the APL pulls the metacarpal radially and proximally. Reduction maneuvers must attempt to counteract each of these forces. Probably the most difficult aspect of the reduction to maintain through splinting is the radial displacement of the base.

CARPOMETACARPAL (CMC) JOINT DISLOCATIONS AND FRACTURE DISLOCATIONS TREATMENT OPTIONS

Nonoperative Management

Closed reduction is usually possible early but may be difficult later following injury. Dorsal finger CMC fracture-dislocations usually cannot be held effectively by external means alone. Although usually acceptable as the least invasive method of treatment for most injuries, entirely nonoperative management of pure thumb CMC dislocations does not provide sufficient

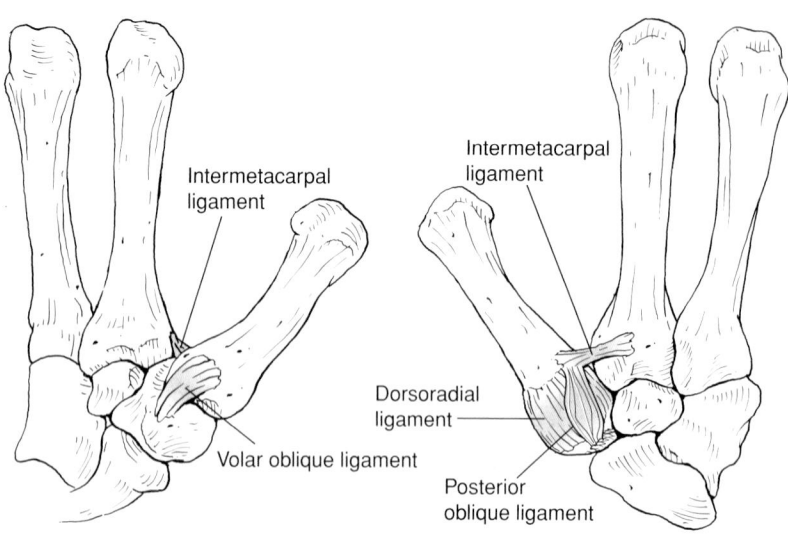

Intermetacarpal ligament

Intermetacarpal ligament

Dorsoradial ligament

Volar oblique ligament

Posterior oblique ligament

FIGURE 30-87 The primary stabilizing ligaments of the thumb CMC joint include the deep anterior oblique, dorsoradial, posterior oblique, and intermetacarpal ligaments. The superficial anterior oblique and ulnar collateral ligaments are not primary stabilizers.

stability for accurate healing of the ligaments. It is not possible through external means to maintain complete control over the reduction of a widely displaced intra-articular fracture-dislocation at the base of the thumb throughout the entire period of healing. However, the need to achieve anatomic union in these fractures has been questioned. Although no one study is definitive, the risk of significant malunion when managing an initially widely displaced intra-articular fracture is too great to warrant entirely nonoperative management.

Operative Management

Finger CMC Dislocations and Fracture Dislocations

For those injuries that can be accurately reduced, CRIF is the treatment of choice. The technique involves restoration of anatomic length to the shortened and dislocated metacarpals through the combined application of traction and direct pres-

sure at the metacarpal bases. Manual reduction is then followed by placement of 0.045-inch K-wires from the metacarpal bases into either the carpal bones or into adjacent stable metacarpals (Fig. 30-89). Adequacy of reduction as well as stability should be evaluated both radiographically and clinically. Pins should remain for 6 weeks. Unlike most other hand fractures, residual instability, rather than stiffness, is the risk with this injury. Initially open fractures and those with tissue interposition

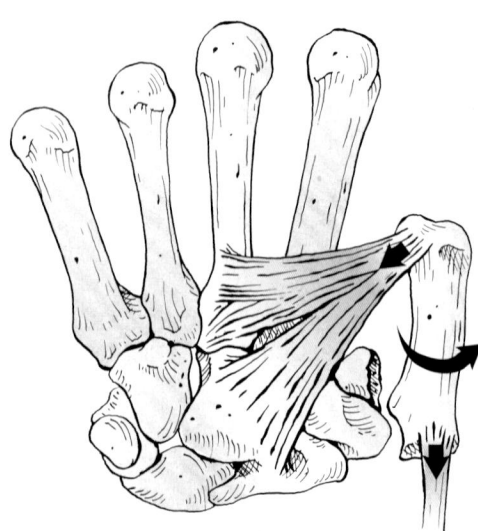

FIGURE 30-88 Displacement of Bennett fractures is driven primarily by the abductor pollicis longus (proximal migration) and the adductor pollicis (adduction and supination).

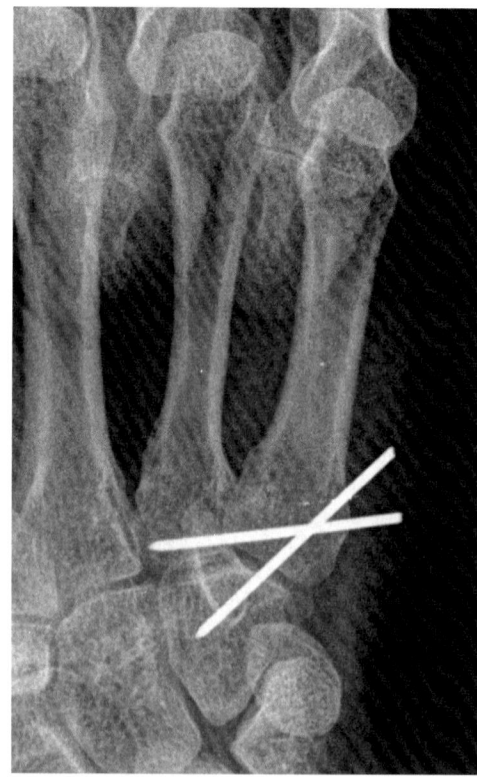

FIGURE 30-89 Isolated CMC fracture dislocations can be reduced and pinned closed to a stable adjacent metacarpal and to the distal carpal row.

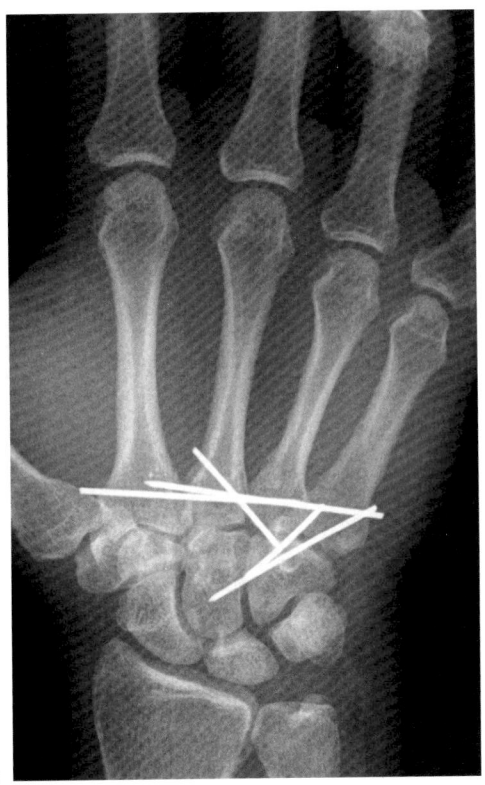 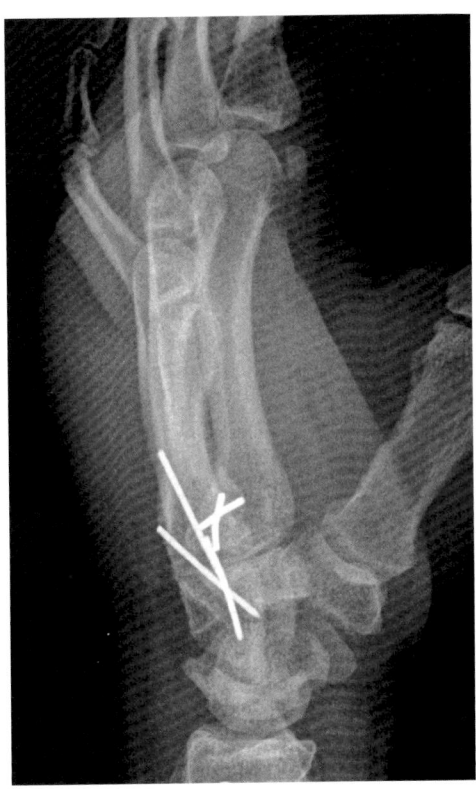

A **B**

FIGURE 30-90 Multiple highly unstable CMC dislocations are at high risk of incomplete reduction and require **(A)** multiple points of fixation and **(B)** a careful check on the lateral radiograph to identify any residual dorsal subluxation.

preventing reduction will require ORIF. Open reduction is much more likely to be required in cases presenting late and may be accomplished as long as 3 months after the initial injury (Fig. 30-90). The stabilization strategy is the same as for CRIF with the open part of the procedure being used strictly for reduction purposes. Excellent long-term stability without pain is achieved in the majority of cases. In more severe cases, immediate arthrodesis of the CMC joints may be required.[71]

Thumb CMC Pure Dislocations

Surprisingly, even the results of CRIF have not been sufficient to consistently prevent long-term symptoms of instability and arthritis in pure thumb CMC dislocations. In a series of eight dislocations pinned for 6 weeks and immobilized for a total of 7.4 weeks, four required ligament reconstruction (three for symptomatic instability and one for progression of early post-traumatic arthritis).[146] Based on these poor results, the same authors subsequently treated the next nine patients with early ligament reconstruction, resulting in no late symptoms, full motion, and normal grip strength (Fig. 30-91).

Thumb CMC Fracture Dislocations

Closed reduction and internal K-wire (0.045-inch) stabilization is the treatment of choice for nearly all Bennett fractures and most Rolando fractures (Fig. 30-92). Arthroscopy may be added to guide the reduction.[33] In a series of 32 patients followed for 7 years with intra-articular step-offs of less than 1 mm, no

difference was found between closed pinning and ORIF for Bennett fractures, with the exception of a higher incidence of adduction contracture in the pinning group.[113] Advocates of internal fixation may choose to manage less comminuted Rolando fractures and some Bennett fractures with ORIF.[109] When there are reasonably large fragments that will support purchase of at least one solid screw per fragment, one may consider plate and screw stabilization of a Rolando fracture (Fig. 30-93). However, ORIF of a Rolando fracture is not for the occasional hand surgeon. Comminution is the rule rather than the exception, and restoration of normal anatomy is quite difficult. The combination of limited internal fixation and external fixation to support the length and unload the articular reduction may be helpful in complex Rolando fractures.[51] A series of 10 patients managed this way and followed at 35 months showed 88% key pinch strength compared to the contralateral side with 9 of 10 patients having good or fair overall satisfaction.[20] Whereas some series have de-emphasized the role of anatomic reduction in improving long-term results, others have stressed its role. Eighteen patients followed to 10.7 years showed a clear correlation between the quality of reduction and posttraumatic arthritis.[170] A similar series with over 7-year follow-up demonstrated a clear correlation between radiographic posttraumatic arthritis and greater than 1-mm articular step-off in the final reduction.[169] Twenty-one patients achieved 80% of normal grip strength despite radiographic signs of degeneration in sixteen that did not correlate to clinical outcome.[17] Thirty-one patients

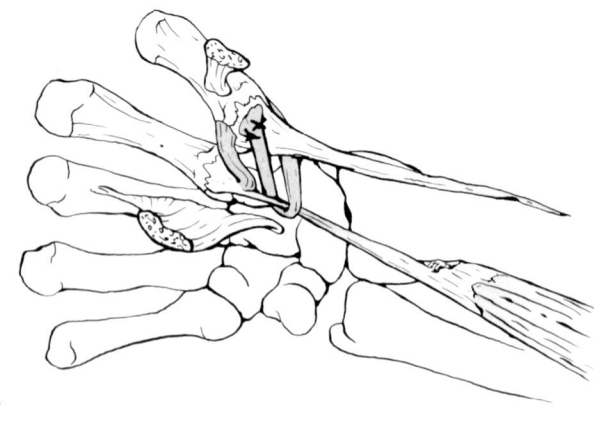

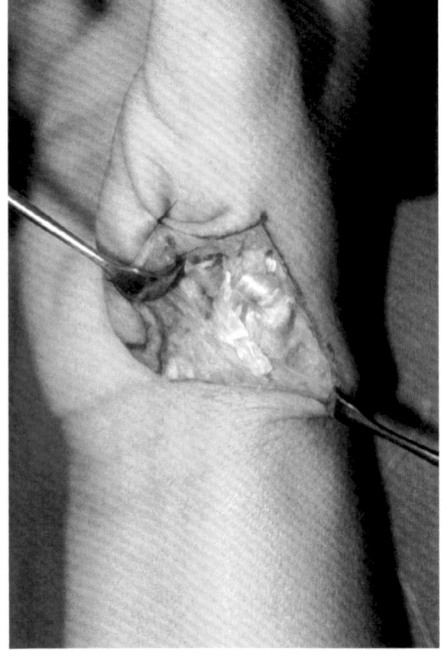

FIGURE 30-91 Reconstruction of the thumb CMC ligaments can be performed with **(A)** a split flexor carpi radialis graft woven through a bone tunnel in the thumb metacarpal base, exiting the dorsal cortex, passing deep to the abductor pollicis longus, around the intact remaining flexor carpi radialis, and back to the volar radial aspect of the metacarpal base. **B:** This procedure is accomplished through a traditional Wagner approach.

followed at 7.3 years demonstrated a correlation of both radiographic signs of osteoarthritis and (more importantly) symptoms of pain with the final residual displacement when healing occurred with more than a 2-mm articular step-off.[97]

Postoperative Care. Immobilization should last from 6 to 8 weeks in an orthoplast splint. The primary problem with finger CMC joint injuries is residual instability, not joint stiffness. The MP joints should be left free throughout the aftercare period with attention paid to excursion of the common digital extensor tendons. For thumb CMC joint injuries, immobilization is continued for 6 weeks in a thumb spica splint. The IP joint should be left free throughout the postoperative period. Following cast removal the patient undergoes a standard progression of ROM exercises that graduates as tolerated into functional use by 8 to 10 weeks. Forceful pinch loading is avoided for 3 months after surgery.

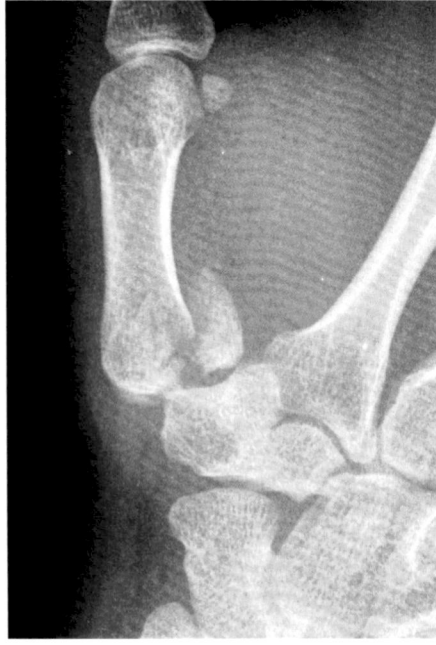

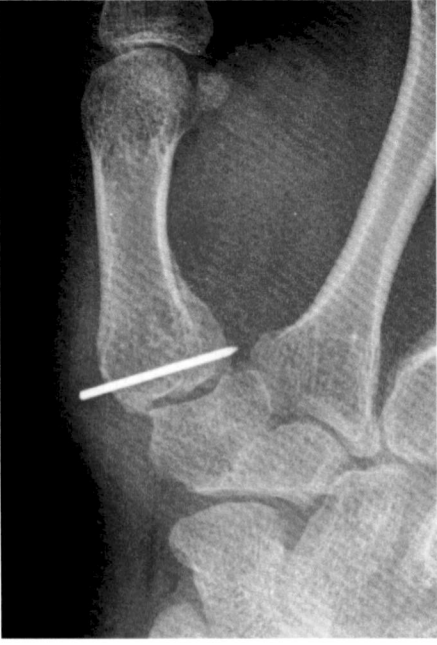

FIGURE 30-92 Bennett fractures can be stabilized by closed pinning of the articular reduction, with or without additional stabilization of the thumb metacarpal shaft to the trapezium.

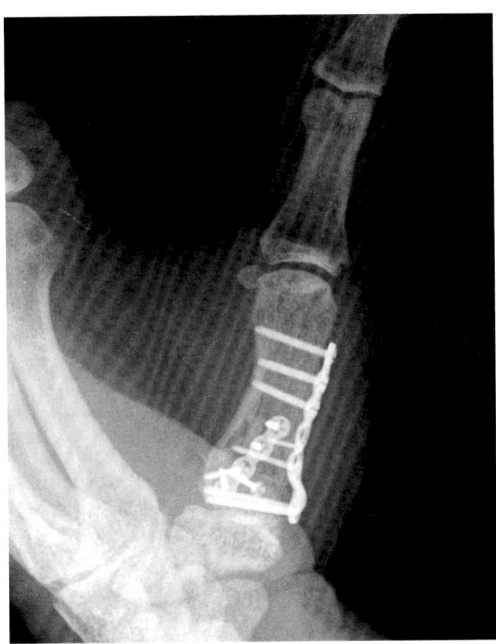

FIGURE 30-93 Rolando fractures are highly unstable and require techniques such as fixed angle plates adjacent to the subchondral bone to resist collapse and sometimes even a smaller second plate placed at 90 degrees to the primary plate.

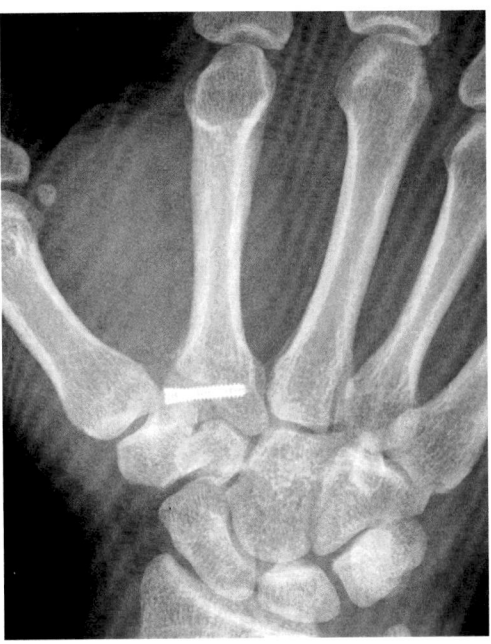

FIGURE 30-94 An isolated index metacarpal CMC fracture-dislocation can be percutaneously reduced and stably fixed with a headless variable pitch compression screw.

Potential Pitfalls and Preventative Measures. Treatment of both finger and thumb CMC joint injuries provides ample opportunity for the occurrence of two complications frequent in hand surgery: injury to cutaneous nerves and pin tract infections. The injury to cutaneous nerves is likely to occur by a pin rather than during dissection and particularly when approaching the radial side of the thumb base. Pins are retained longer here (6 weeks) than for stabilization of metacarpal (removed by 4 weeks) or phalangeal (removed by 3 weeks) fractures. There is thus more time for a pin tract infection to develop. The most important points for finger CMC joint fracture-dislocations are to be sure the joints are fully reduced, and not to miss associated carpal bone fractures. Although most isolated single ray CMC fracture-dislocations occur in the small

finger axis, there is a reproducible pattern that will occasionally be seen for the index ray where the articular base is split into two good-quality fragments very amenable to a percutaneous headless compression screw fixation (Fig. 30-94).

Comminuted fractures of the thumb CMC joint are indeed difficult injuries to treat but are made much simpler by approaching their management as follows: visualize where the shaft of the thumb metacarpal lies in a correct functional position relative to the rest of the hand and pin it there (to the index metacarpal) with two 0.062-inch K-wires. Then make the articular surface of the metacarpal base congruent with supportive bone graft and/or small subchondral wires through a limited opening. What originally appeared as an impossible undertaking now becomes a relatively simple two-step process (Table 30-15).

TABLE 30-15 Potential Pitfalls and Preventative Measures—CMC Dislocations and Fracture-Dislocations

Pitfall	Prevention
Cutaneous nerve injury by K-wire	Know the anatomy, place the wire tip all the way to bone by hand, do not spin the wire unless the tip has bone contact, do not make advance incisions and spread the tract around the wire
Pin tract infection	Cut the pins below the skin surface by enough distance that swelling reduction and external splint pressure cannot induce a protrusion
Incongruent joint	Imaging with beam oriented to accurately pass through CMC joint; when in doubt—open
Residual dorsal subluxation	Tangential profile views; when in doubt—open
Missed hamate/capitate fractures	Careful palpation; tangential profile views; when in doubt—open

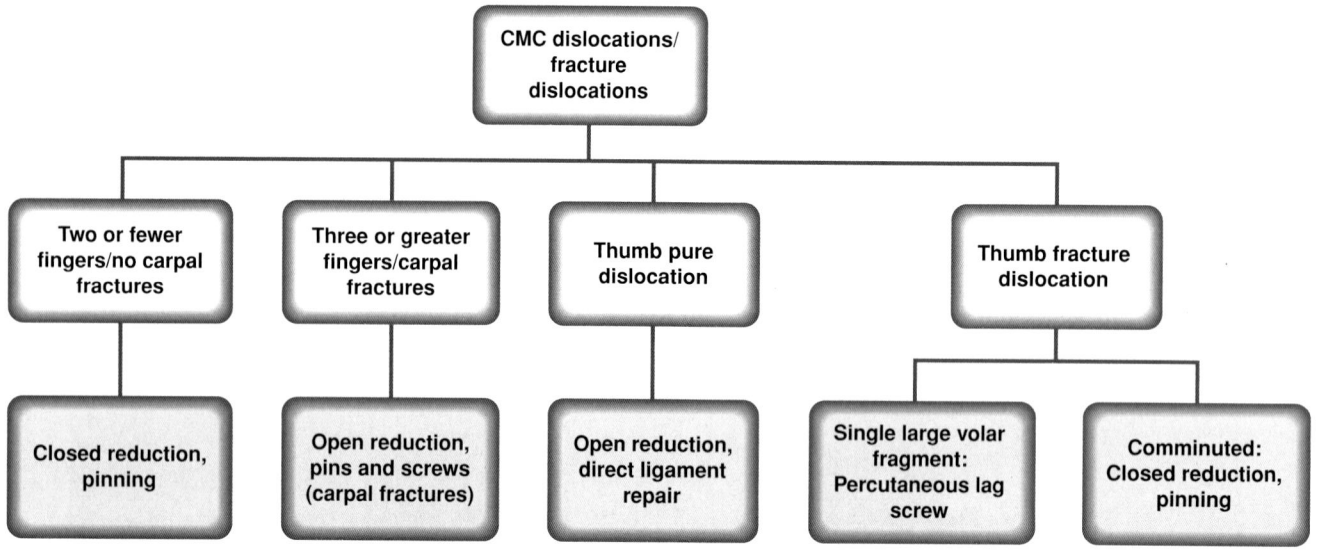

FIGURE 30-95 CMC joint dislocations and fracture dislocations.

AUTHOR'S PREFERRED TREATMENT (FIG. 30-95)

Finger CMC Joint Pure Dislocations

Pure dislocations rarely occur without fracture of either the metacarpal bases or carpal bones of the distal row. However, the absence of such fractures creates an opportunity for successful management by CRIF. The metacarpal bases must be felt to engage their articulations fully and demonstrate complete congruence on radiographs. Only when the x-ray beam passes tangentially through the joint can an accurate assessment be made. K-wires are retained for 6 weeks with an additional 2 weeks of splint protection before initiating wrist and CMC rehabilitation. All other joints remain mobile throughout the postoperative period.

Finger CMC Joint Fracture-Dislocations

If an accurate closed reduction can be achieved, CRIF is an excellent choice. Cases seen weeks after injury or those with tissue interposition will likely require ORIF to achieve accurate reduction. The approach may be dictated by the presence of an open traumatic wound. Branches of the superficial radial nerve and dorsal cutaneous branch of the ulnar nerve must be identified and protected not only from the surgical approach but also during pin placement. The common extensor tendons overlie the central metacarpal bases, and the wrist extensor tendons insert on the border metacarpals. Incision of the extensor retinaculum increases the lateral mobility of these tendons, allowing the surgeon to work around them. Bone and cartilage fragments too small for fixation but large enough to create third body wear in the joint should be removed. Fixation is founded upon 0.045-inch K-wire passage from the metacarpal bases across the CMC joints into the distal carpal row. If adjacent metacarpals are stable without CMC joint injury, transverse stabilization between metacarpal bases is an excellent addition. Evaluation of the dorsal cortices of the hamate

and capitate should be performed on each case as these are also often fractured. Large bone fragments should be restored to their cancellous beds and fixed with countersunk compression screws. Small bone fragments should be excised.

Thumb CMC Joint Pure Dislocations

The literature simply does not support CRIF as a valid treatment for this injury despite basic principles that should allow this method to produce satisfactory results. Although some articles suggest that one needs to perform immediate free tendon graft reconstruction of complete thumb CMC dislocations, this has not been my experience. I have consistently found open ligament repair to produce stable and pain-free motion. The reproducible surgical findings are a sleeve-like avulsion of the deep anterior oblique ligament from the volar surface of the metacarpal and a rupture of the dorsoradial and posterior oblique ligaments. The rupture has usually been distal from the metacarpal insertion. The procedure is easily accomplished by inserting a series of 1.3-mm bone anchors around the margin of the metacarpal base and using the sutures for anatomic repair of the dorsal ligaments. The joint should be pinned in a reduced position before tying down the dorsal ligaments. The deep anterior oblique ligament comes to lie flush with the metacarpal surface when the joint is reduced and stabilized. Pins are retained for 6 weeks with the thumb CMC joint motion instituted at that time. Light pinch is also allowed with progression to power pinch by 3 months postoperatively.

Thumb CMC Joint Fracture-Dislocations

The majority of these can be treated with CRIF, most of the remainder augmented with small openings to control small articular fragments or pack bone graft into the metaphysis, and the final minority with full ORIF. The soft tissue anatomy of this region should be taken into account when placing pins. The drill should not be activated until the pin is solidly placed down to bone. Pins may be placed from the main thumb metacarpal fragment into the small volar fragment, the trapezium, and the index metacarpal in variable combinations based on the unique fracture characteristics of each patient.

The goals of treatment in a Rolando fracture are different. The primary aim is to provide distraction to allow healing through the often-comminuted metaphyseal zone. This is best accomplished by pinning the thumb metacarpal (two 0.062-inch K-wires) to the index metacarpal rather than to the trapezium. It is in these cases of complete articular comminution that making a small opening to place an elevator into the metaphysis may prove useful. The articular fragments can be molded against the distal surface of the trapezium and kept there by either packing bone graft in behind them or with additional smaller caliber (0.035-inch) pins placed transversely at the subchondral level to maintain articular congruity. The advantage of plate and screw stabilization of an intra-articular fracture in general is usually to allow early motion of the joint for the sake of cartilage nutrition and preservation of long-term ROM. The small fragments at the base of the thumb metacarpal are more at risk of devascularization with a widely open procedure that includes periosteal stripping to place a small titanium plate. I have not experienced that long-term loss of motion is a problem at the trapeziometacarpal joint following 6 weeks of pin immobilization for these fractures but I have observed that the presence of the plate results in adherence of the EPL and EPB tendons and can cause long-term loss of motion of both the MP and IP joint, which is a clinically relevant problem.

If ORIF is chosen for a select case, a Wagner incision along the glabrous/nonglabrous border of the thumb base may be curved in a volar and transverse direction to expose the thenar muscle group. Reflection of these muscles reveals the joint capsule volar to the insertion of the APL. Arthrotomy reveals the intra-articular fracture, and subperiosteal dissection along the shaft allows for placement of a plate. Stable internal fixation of Rolando fractures is only possible when the fragments are large enough to accept the purchase of individual screws. My current fixation of choice in this situation is a titanium locking condylar plate (either 1.7 mm or 2.3 mm depending on the size of the patient). Eccentric drilling of the condylar holes can add transverse compression between the articular base fragments. If ORIF is chosen for a Bennett fracture, a smaller version of the same approach is used to allow sufficient access to compress the reduction and place an interfragmentary lag screw from dorsal to volar. Micro-sized variable pitch headless screws are also well suited to the fragment sizes seen in a Bennett fracture (Table 30-16).

MANAGEMENT OF EXPECTED ADVERSE OUTCOMES AND UNEXPECTED COMPLICATIONS

Published complication rates associated with rigid internal fixation are high and often attributable to the complex nature of the injuries for which this treatment method is selected. In a series of 41 metacarpal and 27 phalangeal fractures, complications of hardware (45%), extensor lag (19%), and infection (12%) were seen.[128] Another series of 37 phalangeal fractures

TABLE 30-16 Surgical Steps—Multiple CMC Fracture Dislocations

Approach short longitudinal at ulnar border of common digital extensors

Small arthrotomy at the junction of long metacarpal to capitate and ring metacarpal to hamate so both CMC joints can be visualized for true congruence

Curette and reduce all fracture and dislocation components to the injury, focusing on residual dorsal subluxation and shortening as the two most common reduction errors

Hold dorsal fragments of capitate/hamate approximated to volar counterparts with small bone instruments, and permanently fix with small lag screws in sagittal plane

Identify the most stable metacarpal and begin there as foundation (usually radial) and then link other metacarpals to this anchor point and to distal row

Progressively rebuild the transverse arch of the hand by pinning in coronal/oblique plane successive metacarpals to each other and to distal carpal row

Cut pins below skin level and away from extensor tendons

Check congruence by direct visualization through original arthrotomy and radiographically with tangential views; check for residual dorsal subluxation

Check clinical rotational alignment of each metacarpal axis; close wound with absorbable monofilament, dress, and splint

reported a 92% complication rate including 60% extensor lag and 38% fixed flexion contracture.[131] Increased complication rates were associated with intra-articular/periarticular locations, with extension to the shaft, open injuries, associated soft tissue injury, and the need for bone graft. As long as 18 months may be required for soreness and stiffness to abate following small joint dislocations. In 490 severe phalangeal fractures there were 31(6%) nonunions, 44(9%) malunions, and 8(2%) infections.[176]

In 200 open hand fractures there were 9 deep infections, 18 malunions, 17 delayed unions or nonunions, 23 fixation-related complications, and 2 late amputations.[159] These complications were usually associated with Swanson type II wounds (14% compared with 1.4% in type I wounds), but not with the use of internal fixation, high-energy injury, large wound size, or associated soft tissue injury.

Infection

Despite the excellent vascularity of the hand, infection still occurs with open fractures. In current practice, MRSA is the most commonly isolated species. The role of antibiotics in reducing the infection rate in noncontaminated open wounds with intact vessels has not been supported. When 198 patients were randomized in a double-blind placebo-controlled study with flucloxacillin for open distal phalangeal fractures, there were seven superficial and no deep infections (three with antibiotic, four without).[155] In 408 K-wire hand fracture fixation cases there was a 14% complication rate that was unaffected by the use of empiric antibiotics.[87]

Stiffness

Perhaps the most feared complication and certainly one of the most common following a fracture or dislocation in the hand is stiffness. Twenty-two of 54 patients failed to achieve TAM over 180 degrees following plate fixation of phalangeal fractures.[102] Stiffness is a product of the magnitude of the original trauma, the age and genetic composition of the patient, the duration of immobilization, the position of immobilization, and the invasiveness of any surgical intervention. The primary factors influencing stiffness are the associated soft tissue injury and the age of the patient.[28,180] Too often, the position of immobilization violates the fundamental principles of splinting ligaments at full length and balancing tendon forces that act across the fracture site.[58] First web space contractures are common and can be minimized by pinning or splinting the thumb metacarpal in maximum abduction. Active versus passive motion discrepancies most commonly appear in the form of an extensor lag. The overlying extensor tendon becomes adherent to the fracture site and its subsequent failure of excursion produces an extensor lag at the next most distal joint. This is most common at the PIP joint following fractures of P1 with adherence of the flat and broad extensor tendon in zone IV. Only 11% of phalangeal fractures fixed with plates had a TAM of >220 degrees.[131] A focused rehabilitation technique that uses the differential viscoelastic properties of tendon and scar tissue can be used to maximize extensor excursion over both phalangeal and metacarpal fractures.[75] Once a fixed contracture has been established by the time of tissue homeostasis following the initial trauma, tenocapsulolysis is required if the patient desires to improve motion.[108] One of the chief concerns with operative management of thumb MP ligament disruptions has been the loss of motion. Loss of motion may be more significant in patients undergoing late reconstructions as occurred in 21 patients from a series of 70 free tendon grafts.[103]

Hypersensitivity

The size and structure of the hand provides for very little padding between the surface and a complex array of small caliber nerve branches. There are very few locations for either surgical incisions or percutaneous pins where small nerve branches are more than a centimeter away. Hypersensitivity is a frequently seen consequence of the mechanism of injury itself. Crush injuries are almost invariably accompanied by some degree of hypersensitivity. When surgical management is performed soon after the injury, the procedure itself is often erroneously blamed for causing the hypersensitivity. Hypersensitivity may be further heightened by cold intolerance.[123] Some areas are at higher risk than others. Neuroma formation through direct injury or nerve encasement in postoperative scar should be guarded against when one is operating along the ulnar side of the thumb MP joint with its high concentration of small dorsal digital nerve branches and at the radial side of the wrist near the superficial radial nerve. Treatment is based on a combination of specific medications designed to reduce nerve pain such as gabapentin, amitriptyline, or pregabalin and a progressive contact desensitization therapy program. Gentle surface contact essentially trains the sensitive nerve fibers to tolerate that level of stimulation before then progressing to more intense stimulation. Eventually, the patient works his or her way up to normal use of the hand over a period of weeks. In the meantime, overstimulation of the nerve pain by traction and motion must be avoided even if this means slower progress in the motion program. Failure to heed this principle will result in progression from straightforward hypersensitivity to complex regional pain syndromes and a downward spiral of worsening pain and function that far exceeds the simple early reduction in motion.

Malunion and Deformity

Malunion is a frequently encountered complication in hand fractures owing to a lack of understanding regarding hand biomechanics, to an unfounded belief that all hand fractures do well with nonoperative treatment, or to a noncompliant patient. Malunions are managed with corrective osteotomy. Each aspect of the deformity must be well understood from angular to rotational to length considerations. The main decision is whether to place the osteotomy at the site of original deformity or to make a compensatory osteotomy that produces reciprocal deformities. Fundamentally, it is best to make the correction at the site of the original deformity. The problem is hardware interference with soft tissues. The plate and screws usually necessary to stabilize the correction may not fit well at the site of original deformity. Another consideration is the healing potential of metaphyseal as compared with diaphyseal regions, particularly if the diaphyseal bone has been stripped of its blood supply during prior procedures. A popular location for rotational corrections in particular is the metacarpal base for the above reasons.

Sagittal plane malunion of the proximal phalanx with apex volar usually occurs because of failure to splint the hand in the position of full MP flexion that will correct the dynamic imbalance across the fracture site. Rotational malunion typically stems from the improper choice of nonoperative treatment when direct fixation was needed to control rotation. Spiral fractures are difficult to correctly reduce closed, and rotational malunions can easily result from CRIF especially at the level of the proximal phalanx. Nail plate alignment is an inadequate method of assessing rotation, which should be judged by parallelism of the short tubular bone segment distal to the injured one with the intervening joint flexed to 90 degrees. Corrective osteotomy is more successful at the metacarpal level than the phalangeal level.[65] Correction of a sagittal plane or multidirectional malunion is best accomplished at the site of the original fracture (Fig. 30-96).[106,172] Significant stiffness often accompanies the malunion. A concomitant tenocapsulolysis can be performed if rigid fixation of the osteotomy is achieved. The alternative is to break the solution down into two parts: Stage one achieves correction of the skeletal deformity through osteotomy and stage two improves motion through tenocapsulolysis. These patients achieve the greatest gains in motion even though the

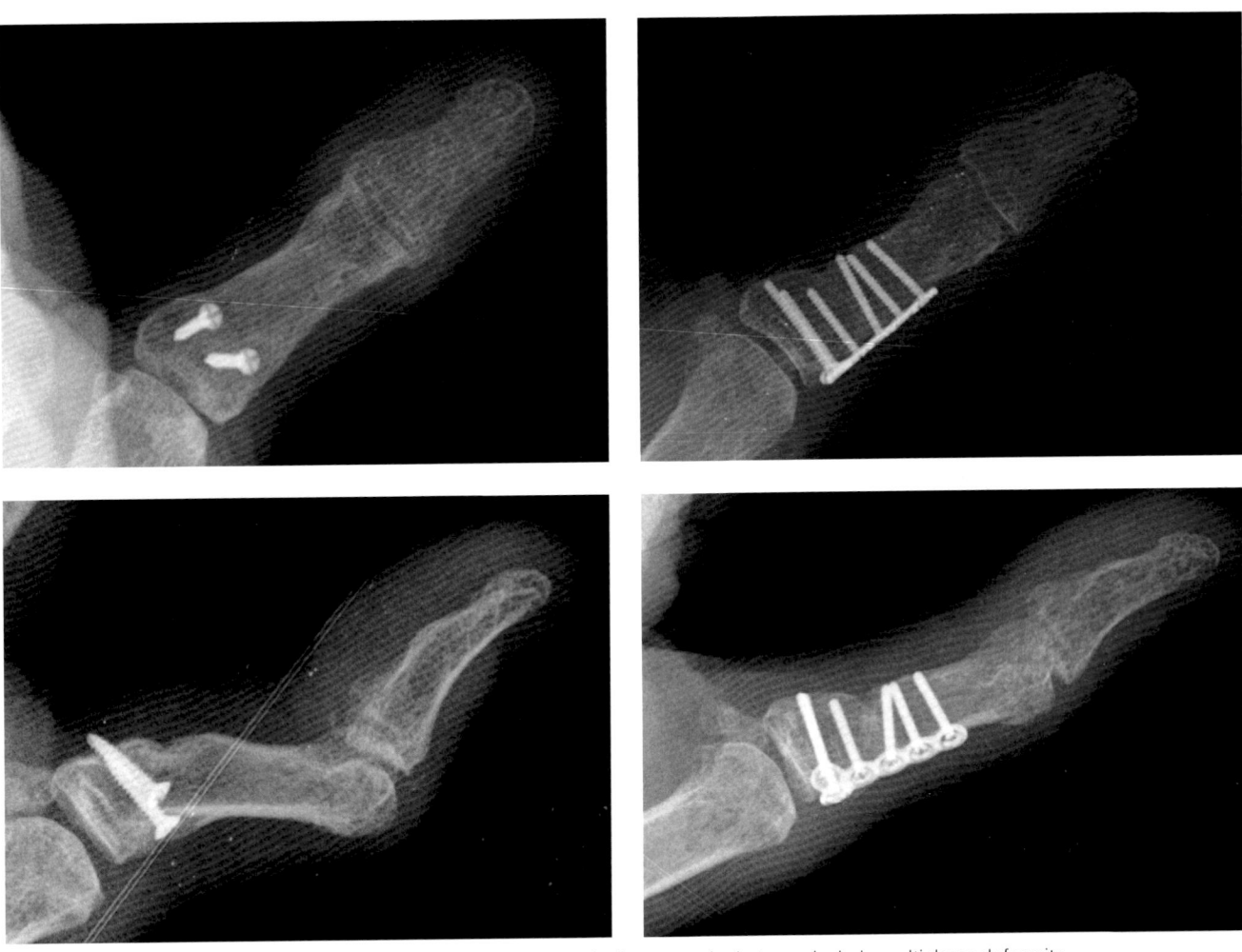

FIGURE 30-96 Malunion of P1 fractures is typically apex volar but may include multiplanar deformity, best corrected at the level of original trauma.

measured final range may be less than that of other patients with less severe injuries.[170,19] For mild to moderate malunions, a realistic assessment regarding the expected improvement in function must be weighed carefully against the predicted degree of digital stiffness created by the osteotomy procedure itself and the hardware utilized.[173,184] Intra-articular osteotomy is an extremely demanding undertaking and should be restricted to carefully selected patients (Fig. 30-97). Five patients undergoing extra-articular osteotomy for malunited unicondylar fractures of the proximal phalanx saw an increase in average PIP motion from 40 degrees preoperatively to 86 degrees postoperatively.[73] Surgery may be performed as late as several months after the initial injury through the original fracture plane.

Malunion of a metacarpal fracture usually presents as an apex dorsal sagittal plane deformity. Patients may complain of the cosmetic deformity, pain at the dorsal prominence, or grip discomfort with a prominent metacarpal head in the palm. Patients should be counseled to evaluate their defor-

mity and decide if their dissatisfaction is sufficient to warrant undergoing corrective osteotomy. The osteotomy should be delayed until tissue homeostasis has been achieved unless an opportunity for early intervention (less than 6 weeks) exists (Fig. 30-98). Correction is best achieved through the site of the original fracture with rigid internal fixation followed by immediate motion. In choosing between opening wedge, closing wedge, pivot osteotomy, or oblique osteotomy, the exact pattern of deformity needs to be assessed and the osteotomy designed to most closely restore normal anatomy. This will demand a different cut for each patient, but the simpler the intended osteotomy, the more likely the surgeon can achieve a good result. Shortening must be considered if a closing wedge is planned. An extensor lag at the MP joint of 7 degrees can be predicted for every 2 mm of shortening.[156] Rotational malunion in a metacarpal may also occur, causing digital overlap. Osteotomy can be performed at the site of original injury or at the metacarpal base. Rotational osteotomy performed at the base of the

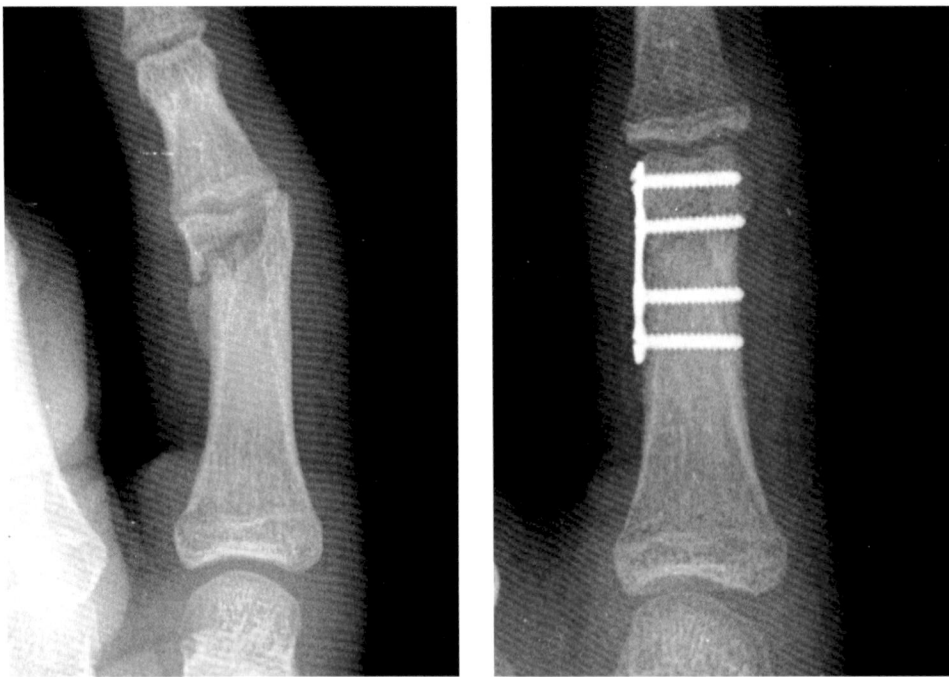

FIGURE 30-97 Intra-articular corrective osteotomy is a demanding undertaking but can produce excellent results when precise attention is given to restoring articular congruence.

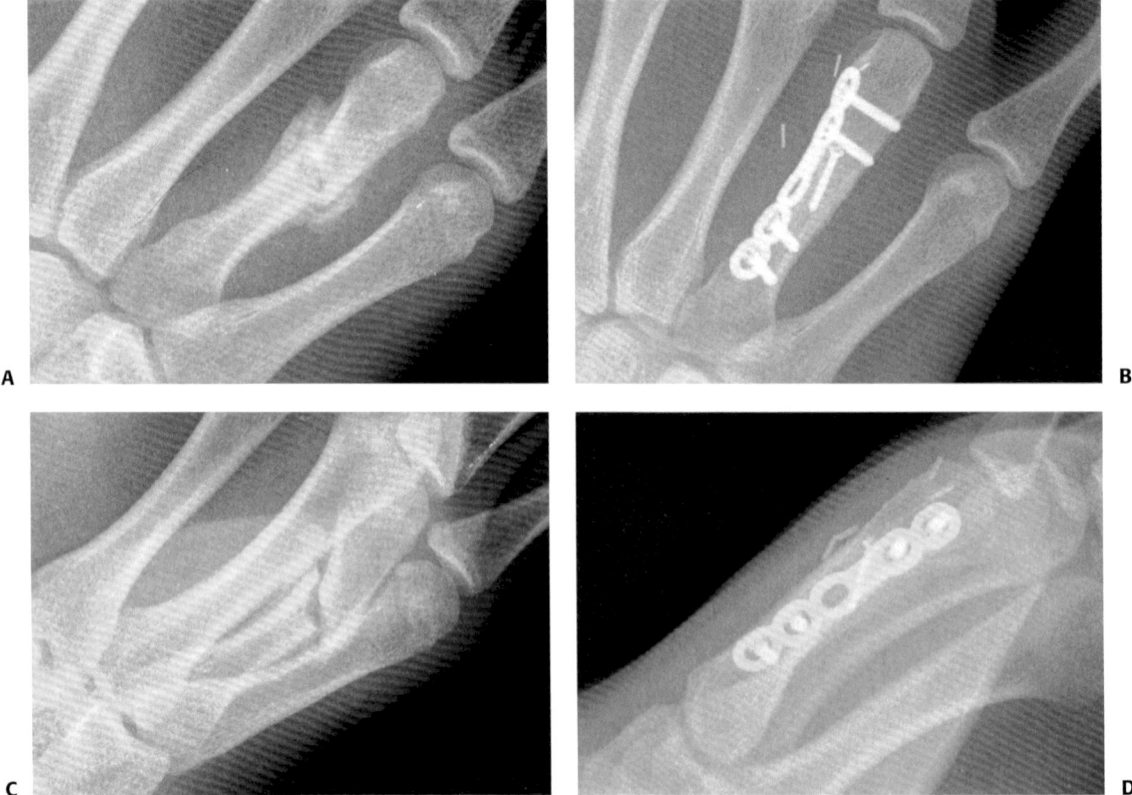

FIGURE 30-98 Nascent malunions that have healed by callus but where the original fracture plane can be cut with an osteotome by hand rather than a saw **(A, C)** are excellent opportunities to achieve a true anatomic restoration **(B, D)** as opposed to a close approximation.

metacarpal offers broader cancellous surfaces for healing and can correct up to 25 to 30 degrees of rotation.[92] If the plane of deformity is more complex than pure rotation, it may be wiser to attempt multiplanar correction through the original fracture site.

Intra-articular osteotomy at the metacarpal head has infrequent indications, as correction of an intra-articular malunion is extremely difficult. In long-term follow-up, intra-articular malunion at the metacarpal base leads to osteoarthritis (65%), decreased grip (49%), and pain (38%).[96] Arthrodesis is the preferred solution for these problems, even for the fifth metacarpal. It reliably improves grip strength with the elimination of pain. Compensatory triquetrohamate motion may alleviate the effect of arthrodesis on the mobility of the ulnar side of the hand. An alternative is a resection arthroplasty at the small CMC with the small metacarpal fused laterally to the ring metacarpal to prevent subsidence.[44]

Nonunion

Nonunion is a rare complication in hand fractures with the exception of distal phalanx fractures, when CRIF has caused distraction, or in fractures treated with ORIF where excessive periosteal stripping has occurred. Nonunions are treated no differently than anywhere else in the body. Hypertrophic nonunions may be addressed by compression alone using a dynamic compression plate. Nonunions with bone loss or inadequate vascular supply require supplementary bone grafting in addition to stable fixation. Tuft fractures of the distal phalanx frequently result in fibrous union but are rarely symptomatic long term. Transverse shaft fractures of the distal phalanx left without support too early may result in an apex volar malunion or nonunion after being repeatedly subjected to pinch forces. Micro-sized headless variable pitch screws can be used for percutaneous compression of P3 shaft nonunions, but caution is still required in assessing the relationship of the screw to the sagittal plane dimension of P3, risking both fracture extension and damage to the overlying nail apparatus (Fig. 30-99).[81] Other distal phalanx nonunions may have sufficient bone loss as to require supplementary bone graft (Fig. 30-100).[25,129] If no bone loss is present, simple compression across a tubular bone hypertrophic nonunion with a short plate should be sufficient to achieve healing. If bone loss is present, a longer plate and corticocancellous or cancellous bone graft may be required.

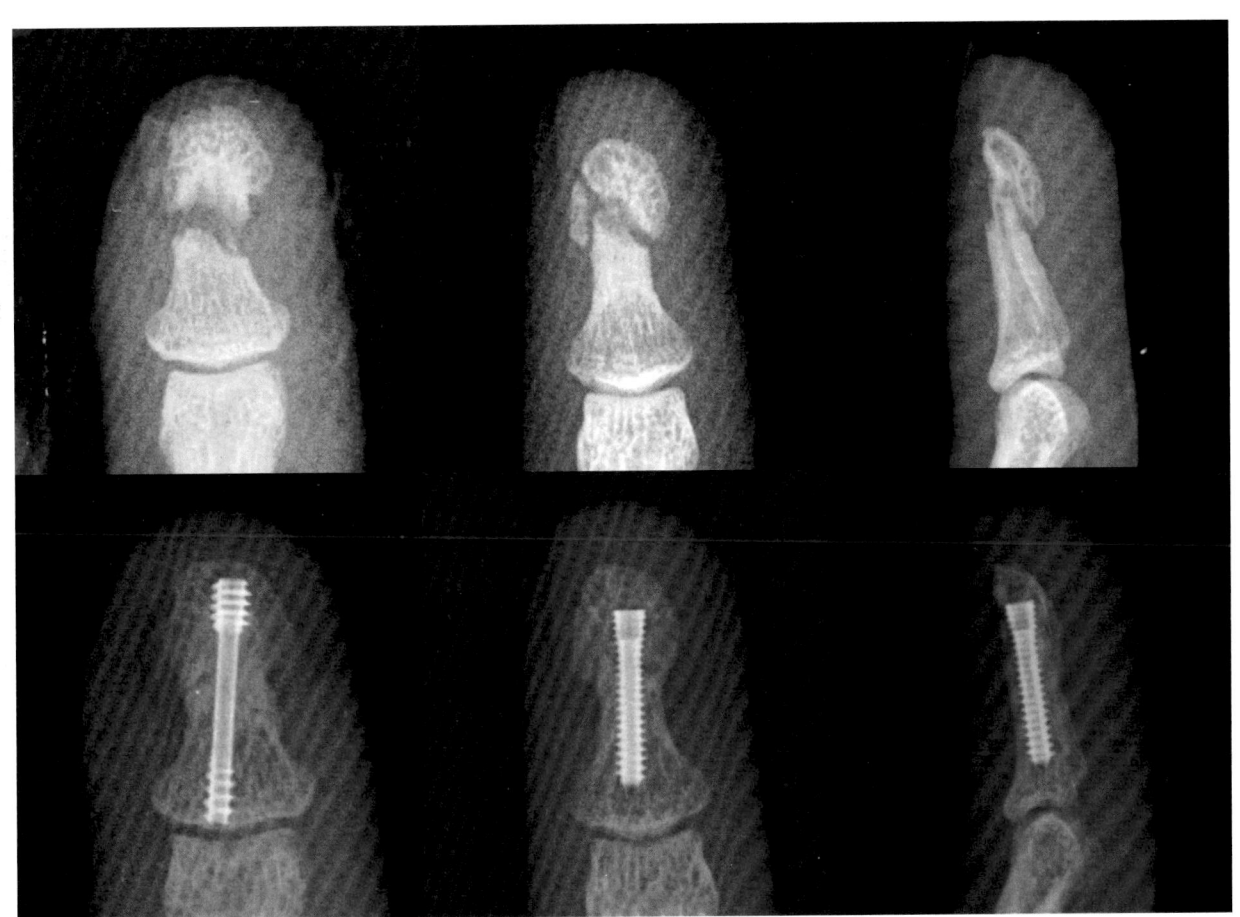

FIGURE 30-99 Nonunions of the distal phalanx shaft can be managed by adding compression across the nonunion site with a headless, variable pitch, cannulated micro screw; healing is prolonged.

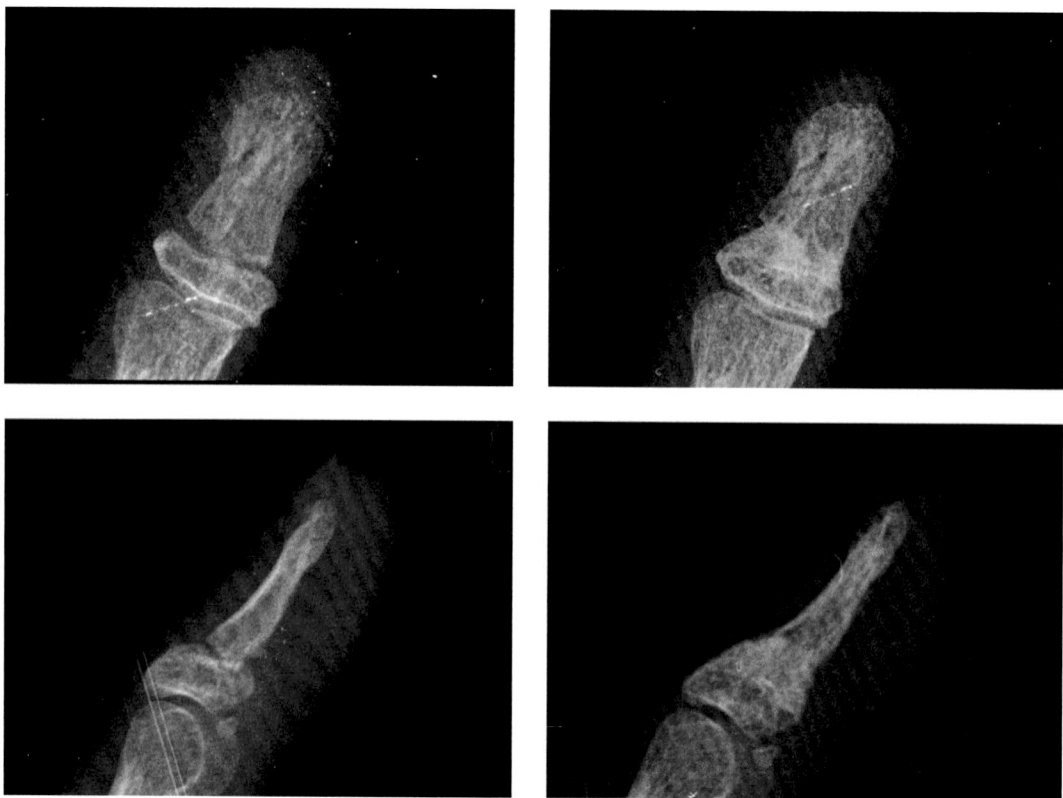

FIGURE 30-100 Some nonunions are primarily characterized by the lack of adequate bone stock and mostly require the dense packing of high-quality cancellous graft.

Residual Instability

Residual instability following dislocation is rare distally, but more common proximally. All five CMC joints are quite subject to recurrent instability particularly with pure dislocation patterns rather than fracture-dislocations. The reason is that in pure dislocation, all the ligaments are ruptured and require ligament-to-bone or ligament-to-ligament healing. Fracture-dislocations usually occur with one or more stabilizing ligaments remaining attached to key bone fragments so that bone-to-bone healing restores joint stability. In one series, re-dislocation occurred in 6 of 56 dorsal fracture-dislocations of the PIP joint.[29] Chronic instability following closed treatment of a complete MP joint RCL injury may need to be treated surgically. A small population of patients exists with chronic hyperextension laxity at the thumb MP joint that may be either passive (volar plate only) or active (involving the intrinsics) and may require surgical advancement of the volar plate for reconstruction and restoration of stability. Late symptomatic instability after finger CMC fracture-dislocation can be evaluated with lidocaine injection into the joint. If relief is provided, arthrodesis is a reliable way to eliminate the pain. The fifth CMC joint may be fused in 20 to 30 degrees of flexion with little long-term loss of hand motion, apparently through increased compensatory triquetrohamate motion. Thumb CMC painful residual instability is treated by ligament reconstruction rather than arthrodesis.

Posttraumatic Arthritis

As in other locations throughout the body, intra-articular fractures and residual joint instability may cause accelerated hyaline cartilage wear and lead to posttraumatic arthritis. A poor correlation exists between the radiographic appearance of posttraumatic arthritis and clinical loss of function and pain. Patients should be managed for the arthritis on the basis of clinical deficits and not based on radiographic abnormality. Posttraumatic arthritis of the thumb MP joint can be successfully managed by arthrodesis with excellent overall hand function. Few other joints in the hand can be fused with so little impact on function (index and long finger CMC joints) (Fig. 30-101). Finger MP and PIP joint fusions result in tremendous loss of function.

Hardware Complications

K-wires are appropriate tools for performing internal fixation of hand fractures and occasionally for stabilizing dislocations but they can demonstrate complication rates as high as 15%.[152] Pin tract infections are the most common complication seen. Infections used to be rare when pins were left in for less than 4 weeks and usually responded well to removal of the pin and administration of oral antibiotics. With the increasing prevalence of MRSA in the community, exposed pins pose a greater risk than in the past and may be more safely cut below the skin level. Another hardware complication is simply irritation of adjacent

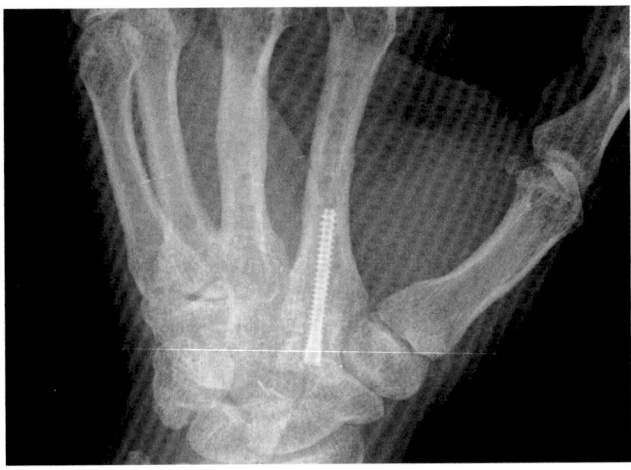

FIGURE 30-101 Index and long CMC joints tolerate fusion well without functional loss, especially when accomplished with low-profile fixation that avoids interference with the digital extensor tendons.

tissues such as overlying tendons by the presence of prominent hardware. Given the delicate and thin tissues of the hand, even implants measuring a few millimeters thick are enough to produce persistent symptoms for many patients. In one series, 7 of 57 patients required plate removal.[124] Another series reported a complication rate of 82% following plate fixation for phalangeal fractures compared with 31% for metacarpal plates.[171] A unique concern with plates, however, is the potential for delayed or nonunion in transverse metacarpal fractures (30%) as opposed to fracture sites with a broader interface (7%).[60]

Tendon Rupture

Tendon ruptures can occur in association with dislocations of the joint adjacent to the site of tendon insertion. Failure to recognize this associated injury may occur with an inadequate examination. The consequence is usually a deformity posture such as mallet finger at the DIP joint or a boutonnière deformity at the PIP joint. Open reconstructions of chronic terminal tendon ruptures with either local tissues or free tendon grafts have not proven particularly successful. For disabling terminal tendon deficiencies in a high angle of flexion, arthrodesis of the DIP joint is a permanent and durable solution to the problem. The loss of motion associated with arthrodesis is not as well tolerated at the PIP joint where every effort should be made to restore active extension. Mild deformities especially when identified reasonably early may respond to a program of PIP extension splinting and DIP joint flexion exercises. Success is dependent on the natural tendency of collagen-based scar to contract. For more substantial deficiencies, surgical reconstruction with local tissues or a free tendon graft may be required once passive motion has first been regained through either rehabilitation or a previously staged surgical capsulectomy.

Nail Matrix

Nail deformities can occur when a crush mechanism of injury includes the zone of the nail or when fixation hardware damages the delicate matrix tissues. Temporary or permanent passage

of fixation devices through the region of the germinal matrix should be avoided, and sterile matrix penetration should be either temporary or by suture material. A rare but troublesome complication is entrapment of the germinal matrix in a transverse fracture gap (which can occur with a reasonably normal external appearance of the digit) that both prevents fracture healing and results in permanent nail deformity (Table 30-17).

TABLE 30-17	Common Adverse Outcomes and Complications
Infection	
Stiffness	
Hypersensitivity	
Malunion and deformity	
Nonunion	
Residual instability	
Posttraumatic arthritis	
Hardware complications	
Tendon rupture	
Nail matrix abnormalities	

SUMMARY, CONTROVERSIES, AND FUTURE DIRECTIONS

Decision-Making

There is not a great deal of controversy surrounding the technical methods of reduction and fixation for fractures and dislocations of the hand. Controversy is much greater when it comes to deciding how specific fractures and dislocations should be managed. Most surgeons understand and accept the basic principle that the least invasive method should be employed that will result in stable, anatomically correct healing and still permit enough motion rehabilitation to achieve a useful and functional final result. The problem lies in the fact that the data simply do not exist anywhere in the published literature to definitively link specific treatment strategies to the many different fracture patterns that exist. Each of the various small bones in the hand (P3, P2, P1, metacarpal) responds to treatment differently. There are numerous varieties of the fracture pattern alone in each of these bones, not to mention the associated soft tissue injuries that impact final outcome substantially. No study has used sufficiently rigorous statistics to separate all the groups and stratify the results. The same holds true for dislocations.

The area where decision-making becomes particularly difficult is that of coordinating more complex reconstructions involving multiple tissues. When the original management of skeletal trauma to the hand yields unsatisfactory results, secondary surgery may be required. The timing and order of events is very much a matter of individual surgeon experience and preference. The foundation for good hand function is a stable inner skeletal structure and a well-vascularized and supple outer envelope of integument. These are the first steps to be accomplished in any reconstruction. The next step is to ensure passively supple joints that are also stable. This infrastructure is then powered by three groups of tendons responsible for active motion in the hand: the extrinsic extensors, the extrinsic flexors, and the intrinsics. Good motion facilitates interaction with the environment, a function that also requires sensibility. Reconstructive surgery of nerves is well timed to coincide with tendon procedures. Three stages have been outlined here, but this does not necessarily mean that three distinct surgical procedures are required. Judging, which combinations of procedures will yield the best results, is the province of an experienced revision hand surgeon. In general, procedures that require the same type of rehabilitation may be combined whereas those that have disparate therapy goals should be separated as distinct surgical events. When a series of surgical procedures is staged, tissue homeostasis after the former procedure should be achieved before executing the subsequent procedure.

Posttraumatic Arthritis

The only alternative to arthrodesis apart from microvascular whole joint transfer was previously the implantation of a Swanson-type one piece silicone prosthesis with the attendant high rates of prosthetic fracture and generation of silicone debris leading to osteolysis. Since earlier editions of this text, new prosthetic implants have become available for total joint replacement of the MP and PIP joints. There are models with metal on polyethylene-bearing surfaces as well as pyrolytic carbon-bearing surfaces. Rates of loosening, osteolysis from debris, and prosthetic breakage will determine if these models offer a new opportunity for improved hand motion and function to those with posttraumatic arthritis in the MP and PIP joints. Prosthetic hemiarthroplasty for unreconstructable intraarticular fractures with cartilage loss is being explored, but long-term wear tolerance has yet to be proven.[78]

Managing Skeletal Loss

Skeletal loss can occur at either periarticular locations or in the diaphysis. Diaphyseal loss is by far the more straightforward issue. Current controversies relate to the choice of purely cancellous graft with bridge plating as opposed to corticocancellous grafts. Additional controversy exists regarding the timing of bone grafting for open fractures. The traditions have been corticocancellous grafts with delay. New trends are for immediate grafting after extensive debridement and using purely cancellous graft.[151] Osteoarticular defects can be replaced with nonvascularized osteoarticular autografts as long as the defect only involves at most one-half of a joint.[91] Partial toe joint osteochondral grafts to the PIP joint of the hand resulted in significant motion loss in three of five cases and resorption in one.[62] The most common sites requiring partial osteoarticular grafts are single condyles at the head of P1 and the volar base of P2. Toe PIP joints provide well-matched condyle donor sites. The dorsal portion of the hamate provides an excellent donor site for the volar base of P2. Nonvascularized whole joint transfers have been unsuccessful. If an entire joint requires autogenous replacement, a vascularized whole joint transfer from the foot is required. Unique cases offer the opportunity to create a

pedicled, vascularized whole joint transfer from one unsalvageable digit to an adjacent digit.

Associated Wounds

Achieving stable wound coverage is a prerequisite to any other reconstruction. It is often performed at the same time as skeletal reconstruction and should be performed prior to most other reconstructions except first-stage tendon grafting. Methods of wound reconstruction include primary closure, secondary closure, split- or full-thickness skin grafts, transposition flaps, pedicle flaps, and free flaps. The simplest strategy that provides for optimum gliding of subjacent structures without contracture formation should be chosen. The challenge for more complex wounds that require flap reconstruction in the hand is finding tissue that is both supple and thin. Current trends are for earlier applications (within 72 hours) of increasingly thinner flaps. A useful strategy involves fascial flaps that are covered with split-thickness skin grafts. The lateral arm flap inverted to orient the muscular surface to receive the skin graft has performed particularly well in this respect.[76] The fascia overlying the serratus anterior is thin with a reliable, large, and long pedicle. One criticism of skin-grafted fascial flaps is that they are slightly more difficult to operate through at the time of further revision compared with cutaneous flaps. The current trend in microsurgery for perforator flaps has spawned a number of cutaneous flaps thin enough for use around the hand, wrist, and forearm but not the digits.

Bioabsorbable Implants

A polylactic acid plate and screw system tested in vitro showed maintenance of strength for 8 weeks comparable to titanium but then degraded with loss of strength over 12 weeks under four-point bending stress.[15] Testing in 112 fresh-frozen cadavers of 2-mm poly-L/DL-lactide plates demonstrated an overall stability comparable to that of 1.7-mm titanium plates.[178,179] Studies such as these appear in the literature, but the regular use of bioabsorbable implants in the hand simply has not caught on clinically. One concern may be reports of sterile abscess formation around implants of the same materials used in other orthopedic applications. In a small series of 12 cases, 2 lost reduction and 3 demonstrated a sustained excessive soft tissue reaction to the implant of copolymer L-lactide and glycolic acid with keloid formation.[45] Since the last edition of this text there has been no apparent advance toward greater use of bioabsorbable implants for hand fractures.

SUMMARY

Fractures and dislocations of the hand represent a diverse group of injuries that share a common theme in management. The hand is a delicate organ that requires both stability and flexibility; function follows form. Although rough guidelines can be drawn from the published literature, it remains the responsibility of individual surgeons to judge which fractures and dislocations can be managed by each of the various methods discussed in this chapter.

There are three basic treatment options for most fractures and dislocations of the hand: splinting, CRIF, and ORIF.

Many fractures and the majority of dislocations in the hand have enough inherent stability to be managed nonoperatively. Testing for inherent stability in the office setting using active motion under the protection of injectable anesthetics should demonstrate those fractures and dislocations that can safely be managed without surgery. Malrotated, multiple, high-energy, and open fractures are usually treated operatively. CMC dislocations and fracture dislocations (unlike MP and PIP joint injuries) are usually treated operatively. The majority of operatively treated hand fractures and dislocations are closed and isolated injuries for which CRIF is usually an appropriate method. The exceptions to this are noted throughout the chapter. A few select injury patterns such as intra-articular P2 base fractures have specific and unique treatments that must be remembered and used according to the indications described. Once underway with treatment, one should stay focused on edema control and promoting early motion. The final steps to a successful outcome lie in avoiding complications such as nerve hypersensitivity and pin tract infections. When complications do occur, the key is in planning a well-thought-out correction in terms of risk benefit analysis and staging. Finally, patients should be counseled regarding expectations, which are that fractures and dislocations of the hand produce swelling, stiffness, and aching that frequently takes more than a year to overcome.

REFERENCES

1. Abrahamsson SO, Sollerman C, Lundborg G, et al. Diagnosis of displaced ulnar collateral ligament of the metacarpophalangeal joint of the thumb. *J Hand Surg.* 1990;15A:457–460.
2. Afendras G, Abramo A, Mrkonjic A, et al. Hemi-hamate osteochondral transplantation in proximal interphalangeal dorsal fracture dislocations: a minimum 4 year follow-up in eight patients. *J Hand Surg.* 2010;35E:627–631.
3. Aladin A, Davis TRC. Dorsal fracture-dislocation of the proximal interphalangeal joint: a comparative study of percutaneous Kirschner wire fixation versus open reduction and internal fixation. *J Hand Surg.* 2005;30B:120–128.
4. Ali A, Hamman J, Mass DP. The biomechanical effects of angulated boxer's fractures. *J Hand Surg.* 1999;24:835–844.
5. Al-Qattan MM, Hashem F, Helmi A. Irreducible tuft fractures of the distal phalanx. *J Hand Surg.* 2003;28B:18–20.
6. Al-Qattan MM. Extra-articular transverse fractures of the base of the distal phalanx (Seymour's fracture) in children and adults. *J Hand Surg.* 2001;26B:201–206.
7. Al-Qattan MM. Outcome of conservative management of spiral/long oblique fractures of the metacarpal shaft of the fingers using a palmar wrist splint and immediate mobilisation of the fingers. *J Hand Surg.* 2008;33E:723–727.
8. Anakwe RE, Aitken SA, Cowie JG, et al. The epidemiology of fractures of the hand and the influence of social deprivation. *J Hand Surg.* 2011;36E:62–65.
9. Arai K, Toh S, Nakahara K, et al. Treatment of soft tissue injuries to the dorsum of the metacarpophalangeal joint (Boxer's knuckle). *J Hand Surg.* 2002;27B:90–95.
10. Bach HG, Gonzales MH, Hall Jr RF. Locked intramedullary nailing of metacarpal fractures secondary to gunshot wounds. *J Hand Surg.* 2006;31A:1083–1087.
11. Badia A, Riano F, Ravikoff J, et al. Dynamic intradigital external fixation for proximal interphalangeal joint fracture dislocations. *J Hand Surg.* 2005;30A:154–160.
12. Bean CHG, Tencer AF, Trumble TE. The effect of thumb metacarpophalangeal ulnar collateral ligament attachment site on joint range of motion: an in vitro study. *J Hand Surg.* 1999;24:283–287.
13. Bettinger PC, Linscheid RL, Berger RA, et al. An anatomic study of the stabilizing ligaments of the trapezium and trapeziometacarpal joint. *J Hand Surg.* 1999;24:786–798.
14. Birndorf MS, Daley R, Greenwald DP. Metacarpal fracture angulation decreases flexor mechanical efficiency in human hands. *Plast Reconstr Surg.* 1997;99:1079–1083.
15. Bozic KJ, Perez LE, Wilson DR, et al. Mechanical testing of bioresorbable implants for use in metacarpal fracture fixation. *J Hand Surg.* 2001;26:755–761.
16. Braakman M. Functional taping of fractures of the fifth metacarpal results in a quicker recovery. *Injury.* 1998;29:5–9.
17. Bruske J, Bednarski M, Niedzwiedz Z, et al. The results of operative treatment of fractures of the thumb metacarpal base. *Acta Orthop Belg.* 2001;67:368–373.
18. Buchanan RT. Mechanical requirements for application and modification of the dynamic force couple method. *Hand Clin.* 1994;10:221–228.
19. Buchler U, Gupta A, Ruf S. Corrective osteotomy for posttraumatic malunion of the phalanges of the hand. *J Hand Surg.* 1996;21B:33–42.
20. Buchler U, McCollam SM, Oppikofer C. Comminuted fractures of the basilar joint of the thumb: combined treatment by external fixation, limited internal fixation, and bone grafting. *J Hand Surg.* 1991;16A:556–560.
21. Calfee RP, Kiefhaber TR, Sommerkamp TG, et al. Hemi-hamate arthroplasty provides functional reconstruction of acute and chronic proximal interphalangeal fracture-dislocations. *J Hand Surg.* 2009;34:1232–1241.
22. Cannon NM. Rehabilitation approaches for distal and middle phalanx fractures of the hand. *J Hand Ther.* 2003;16:105–116.
23. Cheah AE, Tan DM, Chong AK, et al. Volar plating for unstable proximal interphalangeal joint dorsal fracture-dislocations. *J Hand Surg Am.* 2012;37:28–33.
24. Chen SH, Wei FC, Chen HC, et al. Miniature plates and screws in acute complex hand injury. *J Trauma.* 1994;37:237–242.
25. Chim H, Teoh LC, Yong FC. Open reduction and interfragmentary screw fixation for symptomatic nonunion of distal phalangeal fractures. *J Hand Surg.* 2008;33E:71–76.
26. Chin KR, Jupiter JB. Treatment of triplane fractures of the head of the proximal phalanx. *J Hand Surg.* 1999;24:1263–1268.
27. Chinchalkar SJ, Gan BS. Management of proximal interphalangeal joint fractures and dislocations. *J Hand Ther.* 2003;16:117–128.
28. Chow SP, Pun WK, So YC, et al. A prospective study of 245 open digital fractures of the hand. *J Hand Surg.* 1991;16B:137–140.
29. Chung KC, Spilson SV. The frequency and epidemiology of hand and forearm fractures in the United States. *J Hand Surg.* 2001;26:908–915.
30. Chung KC. Clinical research in hand surgery. *J Hand Surg.* 2010;35:109–120.
31. Coyle MP. Grade III radial collateral ligament injuries of the thumb metacarpophalangeal joint: treatment by soft tissue advancement and bony reattachment. *J Hand Surg.* 2003;28:14–20.
32. Crofoot CD, Saing M, Raphael J. Intrafocal pinning for juxta-articular phalanx fractures. *Tech Hand Up Extrem Surg.* 2005;9:169–171.
33. Culp RW, Johnson JW. Arthroscopically assisted percutaneous fixation of Bennett Fractures. *J Hand Surg.* 2010;35:137–140.
34. Curtin CM, Chung KC. Use of eight-hole titanium miniplates for unstable phalangeal fractures. *Ann Plast Surg.* 2002;49:580–586.
35. Dailiana Z, Agorastakis D, Varitimidis S, et al. Use of a mini-external fixator for the treatment of hand fractures. *J Hand Surg.* 2009;34:630–636.
36. Debnath UK, Nassab RS, Oni JA, et al. A prospective study of the treatment of fractures of the little finger metacarpal shaft with a short hand cast. *J Hand Surg.* 2004;29B:214–217.
37. Debus G, Courvoisier A, Wimsey S, et al. Pins and rubber traction system for intra-articular proximal interphalangeal joint fractures revisited. *J Hand Surg.* 2010;35E:396–401.
38. Del Pinal F, Garcia-Bernal FJ, Delgado J, et al. Results of osteotomy, open reduction, and internal fixation for late-presenting malunited intra-articular fractures of the base of the middle phalanx. *J Hand Surg.* 2005;30A:1039e1–e14.
39. Delaere OP, Suttor PM, Degolla R, et al. Early surgical treatment for collateral ligament rupture of metacarpophalangeal joints of the fingers. *J Hand Surg.* 2003;28:309–315.
40. Diaconu M, Facca S, Gouzou S, et al. Locking plates for fixation of extra-articular fractures of the first metacarpal base: a series of 15 cases. *Chir Main.* 2011;30:26–30.
41. Dietch MA, Kiefhaber TR, Comisar R, et al. Dorsal fracture dislocations of the proximal interphalangeal joint: surgical complications and long-term results. *J Hand Surg.* 1999;24:914–923.
42. Dinowitz M, Trumble T, Hanel D, et al. Failure of cast immobilization for thumb ulnar collateral ligament avulsion fractures. *J Hand Surg.* 1997;22A:1057–1063.
43. Dionysian E, Eaton RG. The long-term outcome of volar plate arthroplasty of the proximal interphalangeal joint. *J Hand Surg.* 2000;25:429–437.
44. Dubert TP, Khalifa H. "Stabilized arthroplasty" for old fracture dislocations of the fifth carpometacarpal joint. *Tech Hand Up Extrem Surg.* 2009;13:134–136.
45. Dumont C, Fuchs M, Burchhardt H, et al. Clinical results of absorbable plates for displaced metacarpal fractures. *J Hand Surg.* 2007;32A:491–496.
46. Duncan RW, Freeland AE, Jabaley ME, et al. Open hand fractures: an analysis of the recovery of active motion and of complications. *J Hand Surg.* 1993;18A:387–394.
47. Dzwierzynski WW, Matloub HS, Yan JG, et al. Anatomy of the intermetacarpal ligaments of the carpometacarpal joints of the fingers. *J Hand Surg.* 1997;22:931–934.
48. Ebinger T, Erhard N, Kinzl L, et al. Dynamic treatment of displaced proximal phalangeal fractures. *J Hand Surg.* 1999;24:1254–1262.
49. Ellis SJ, Cheng R, Prokopis P, et al. Treatment of proximal interphalangeal dorsal fracture-dislocation injuries with dynamic external fixation: a pins and rubber band system. *J Hand Surg.* 2007;32A:1242–1250.
50. Elmaraghy MW, Elmaraghy AW, Richards RS, et al. Transmetacarpal intramedullary K-wire fixation of proximal phalangeal fractures. *Ann Plast Surg.* 1998;41:125–130.
51. El-Sharkawy AA, El-Mofty AO, Moharram AN, et al. Management of Rolando fracture by modified dynamic external fixation: a new technique. *Tech Hand Up Extrem Surg.* 2009;13:11–15.
52. El-Shennawy M, Nakamura K, Patterson RM, et al. Three-dimensional kinematic analysis of the second through fifth carpometacarpal joints. *J Hand Surg.* 2001;26:1030–1035.
53. Fahmy N, Khan W. The S-Quattro in the management of acute intra-articular phalangeal fractures of the hand. *J Hand Surg.* 2006;31:79–92.
54. Fairhurst M, Hansen L. Treatment of "gamekeeper's thumb" by reconstruction of the ulnar collateral ligament. *J Hand Surg.* 2003;27B:542–545.
55. Feehan LM, Sheps SB. Incidence and demographics of hand fractures in British Columbia, Canada: a population-based study. *J Hand Surg.* 2006;31A:1068–1074.
56. Figl M, Weninger P, Hofbauer M, et al. Results of dynamic treatment of fractures of the proximal phalanx of the hand. *J Trauma.* 2011;70:852–856.
57. Finsen V. Suzuki's pins and rubber traction for fractures of the base of the middle phalanx. *J Plast Surg Hand Surg.* 2010;44:209–213.
58. Freeland AE, Hardy MA, Singletary S. Rehabilitation for proximal phalangeal fractures. *J Hand Ther.* 2003;16:129–142.
59. Freeland AE, Lineaweaver WC, Lindley SG. Fracture fixation in the mutilated hand. *Hand Clin.* 2003;19:51–61.
60. Fusetti C, Della Santa DR. Influence of fracture pattern on consolidation after metacarpal plate fixation. *Chir Main.* 2004;23:32–36.

61. Galanakis I, Aliquizakis A, Katonis P, et al. Treatment of closed unstable metacarpal fractures using percutaneous transverse fixation with Kirschner wires. *J Trauma*. 2003;55: 509–513.
62. Gaul JS. Articular fractures of the proximal interphalangeal joint with missing elements: repair with partial toe joint osteochondral autografts. *J Hand Surg*. 1999;24: 78–85.
63. Giele H, Martin J. The two-level ulnar collateral ligament injury of the metacarpophalangeal joint of the thumb. *J Hand Surg*. 2003;28B:92–93.
64. Glickel SZ, Malerich M, Pearce SM, et al. Ligament replacement for chronic instability of the ulnar collateral ligament of the metacarpophalangeal joint of the thumb. *J Hand Surg*. 1993;18A:930–941.
65. Gollamudi S, Jones WA. Corrective osteotomy of malunited fractures of phalanges and metacarpals. *J Hand Surg*. 2000;25B:439–441.
66. Gonzales MH, Hall M, Hall RF Jr. Low-velocity gunshot wounds of the proximal phalanx: treatment by early stable fixation. *J Hand Surg*. 1998;23A:142–149.
67. Graham TJ. The exploded hand syndrome: logical evaluation and comprehensive treatment of the severely crushed hand. *J Hand Surg*. 2006;31A:1012–1023.
68. Grant I, Berger AC, Tham SK. Internal fixation of unstable fracture dislocations of the proximal interphalangeal joint. *J Hand Surg*. 2005;30:492–498.
69. Hamada Y, Sairyo K, Tonogai I, et al. Irreducible fracture dislocation of a finger metacarpophalangeal joint: A case report. *Hand*. 2008;3:76–78.
70. Hamilton SC, Stern PJ, Fassler PR, et al. Miniscrew fixation for the treatment of proximal interphalangeal joint dorsal fracture-dislocations. *J Hand Surg*. 2006;31A:1349–1354.
71. Hanel DP. Primary fusion of fracture dislocations of central carpometacarpal joints. *Clin Orthop*. 1996;327:85–93.
72. Harding IJ, Parry D, Barrington RL. The use of a moulded metacarpal brace versus neighbour strapping for fractures of the finger metacarpal neck. *J Hand Surg*. 2001; 26B:261–263.
73. Harness NG, Chen A, Jupiter JB. Extra-articular osteotomy for malunited unicondylar fractures of the proximal phalanx. *J Hand Surg*. 2005;30A: 566–572.
74. Hattori Y, Doi K, Sakamoto S, et al. Volar plating for intra-articular fracture of the base of the proximal phalanx. *J Hand Surg*. 2007;32A:1299–1303.
75. Henry MH, Stutz C, Brown H. Technique for extensor tendon acceleration. *J Hand Ther*. 2006;19:421–424.
76. Henry MH. Degloving combined with structural trauma at the digital level: functional coverage with fascial free flaps. *J Reconstr Microsurg*. 2007;23:59–62.
77. Henry MH. Fractures of the proximal phalanx and metacarpals in the hand: preferred methods of stabilization. *J Am Acad Orthop Surg*. 2008;16:320–329.
78. Henry MH. Prosthetic hemi-arthroplasty for post-traumatic articular cartilage loss in the proximal interphalangeal joint. *HAND*. 2011;6:93–97.
79. Henry MH. Soft tissue sleeve approach to open reduction and internal fixation of proximal phalangeal fractures. *Tech Hand Up Extr Surg*. 2008;12:161–165.
80. Henry MH. Specific complications associated with different types of intrinsic pedicle flaps of the hand. *J Reconstr Microsurg*. 2008;24:221–225.
81. Henry MH. Variable pitch headless compression screw treatment of distal phalangeal nonunions. *Tech Hand Up Extrem Surg*. 2010;14:230–233.
82. Hinke DH, Erickson SJ, Chamoy L, et al. Ulnar collateral ligament of the thumb: MR findings in cadavers, volunteers, and patients with ligamentous injury (gamekeeper's thumb). *Am J Roentgenol*. 1994;163:1431–1434.
83. Hirata H, Tsujii M, Nakao E. Locking of the metacarpophalangeal joint of the thumb caused by a fracture fragment of the radial condyle of the metacarpal head after dorsal dislocation. *J Hand Surg*. 2006;31B:635–636.
84. Hofmeister EP, Mazurek MT, Shin AY, et al. Extension block pinning for large mallet fractures. *J Hand Surg*. 2003;28:453–459.
85. Hornbach EE, Cohen MS. Closed reduction and percutaneous pinning of fractures of the proximal phalanx. *J Hand Surg*. 2003;26B:45–49.
86. Horton TC, Hatton M, Davis TRC. A prospective randomized controlled study of fixation of long oblique and spiral shaft fractures of the proximal phalanx: closed reduction and percutaneous Kirschner wiring versus open reduction and lag screw fixation. *J Hand Surg*. 2003;28B:5–9.
87. Hsu LP, Schwartz EG, Kalainov DM, et al. Complications of K-wire fixation in procedures involving the hand and wrist. *J Hand Surg*. 2011;36:610–616.
88. Husain SN, Dietz JF, Kalainov DM, et al. A biomechanical study of distal interphalangeal joint subluxation after mallet fracture injury. *J Hand Surg*. 2008;33:26–30.
89. Hynes MC, Giddins GEB. Dynamic external fixation for pilon fractures of the interphalangeal joints. *J Hand Surg*. 2001;26B:122–124.
90. Ip WY, Ng KH, Chow SP. A prospective study of 924 digital fractures of the hand. *Injury*. 1996;27:279–285.
91. Ishida O, Ikuta Y, Kuroki H. Ipsilateral osteochondral grafting for finger joint repair. *J Hand Surg*. 1994;19:372–377.
92. Jawa A, Zucchini M, Lauri G, et al. Modified step-cut osteotomy for metacarpal and phalangeal rotational deformity. *J Hand Surg*. 2009;34:335–340.
93. Jorgsholm P, Bjorkman A, Emmeluth A, et al. Extension block pinning of mallet fractures. *Scand J Plast Reconstr Surg Hand Surg*. 2010;44:54–58.
94. Kaleli T, Ozturk C, Ersozlu S. External fixation for surgical treatment of a mallet finger. *J Hand Surg*. 2003;28B:228–230.
95. Keogh E, Book K, Thomas J, et al. Predicting pain and disability in patients with hand fractures: comparing pain anxiety, anxiety sensitivity and pain catastrophizing. *Eur J Pain*. 2010;14:446–451.
96. Kjaer-Peterson K, Jurik AG, Peterson LK. Intraarticular fractures at the base of the fifth metacarpal. A clinical and radiographic study of 64 cases. *J Hand Surg*. 1992;17B:144–147.
97. Kjaer-Peterson K, Langoff O, Andersen K. Bennett fracture. *J Hand Surg*. 1990;15B:58–61.
98. Korting O, Facca S, Diaconu M, et al. Treatment of complex proximal interphalangeal joint fractures using a new dynamic external fixator: 15 cases. *Chir Main*. 2009;28: 153–157.
99. Kozin SH, Thoder JJ, Lieberman G. Operative treatment of metacarpal and phalangeal shaft fractures. *J Am Acad Orthop Surg*. 2000;8:111–121.
100. Kuhn KM, Khiem DD, Shin AY. Volar A1 pulley approach for the fixation of avulsion fractures of the base of the proximal phalanx. *J Hand Surg*. 2001;26:762–771.
101. Kumar R, Malhotra R. Divergent fracture-dislocation of the second carpometacarpal joint and the three ulnar carpometacarpal joints. *J Hand Surg*. 2001;26:123–129.
102. Kurzen P, Fusetti C, Bonaccio M, et al. Complications after plate fixation of phalangeal fractures. *J Trauma*. 2006;60:841–384.
103. Kuz JE, Husband JB, Tokar N, et al. Outcome of avulsion fractures of the ulnar base of the proximal phalanx of the thumb treated nonsurgically. *J Hand Surg*. 1999;24:275–282.
104. Lee JYL, Teoh LC. Dorsal fracture dislocations of the proximal interphalangeal joint treated by open reduction and interfragmentary screw fixation: indications, approaches, and results. *J Hand Surg*. 2006;31B:138–146.
105. Lee SG, Jupiter JB. Phalangeal and metacarpal fractures of the hand. *Hand Clin*. 2000;16: 323–332.
106. Lester B, Mallik A. Impending malunions of the hand. Treatment of subacute, malaligned fractures. *Clin Orthop*. 1996;327:55–62.
107. Leung YL, Beredjiklian PK, Monaghan BA, et al. Radiographic assessment of small finger metacarpal neck fractures. *J Hand Surg*. 2002;27:443–448.
108. Levaro F, Henry MH. Management of the stiff proximal interphalangeal joint. *J Am Soc Surg Hand*. 2003;3:78–87.
109. Liebovic SJ. Treatment of Bennett and Rolando fractures. *Tech Hand Upper Ext Surg*. 1998;2:36–46.
110. Liew KH, Chan BK, Low CO. Metacarpal and proximal phalangeal fractures-fixation with multiple intramedullary Kirschner wires. *Hand Surg*. 2000;5:125–130.
111. Lins RE. A comparative mechanical analysis of plate fixation in a proximal phalanx fracture model. *J Hand Surg*. 1996;21A:1059–1064.
112. Lucchina S, Badia A, Dornean V, et al. Unstable mallet fractures: a comparison between three different techniques in a multicenter study. *Chin J Traumatol*. 2010;13:195–200.
113. Lutz M, Sailer R, Zimmerman R, et al. Closed reduction transarticular Kirshner wire fixation versus open reduction internal fixation in the treatment of Bennett fracture dislocation. *J Hand Surg*. 2003;28B:142–147.
114. Majumder S, Peck F, Watson JS, et al. Lessons learned from the management of complex intra-articular fractures at the base of the middle phalanges of fingers. *J Hand Surg*. 2003; 28B:559–565.
115. Margic K. External fixation of closed metacarpal and phalangeal fractures of digits. A prospective study of 100 consecutive patients. *J Hand Surg*. 2006;31B:30–40.
116. McLain RF, Steyers C, Stoddard M. Infections in open fractures of the hand. *J Hand Surg*. 1991;16A:108–112.
117. McNemar TB, Howell JW, Chang E. Management of metacarpal fractures. *J Hand Ther*. 2003;16:143–151.
118. Murase T, Morimoto H, Yoshikawa H. Palmar dislocation of the metacarpophalangeal joint of the finger. *J Hand Surg*. 2004;29B:90–93.
119. Nakamura K, Patterson RM, Viegas SF. The ligament and skeletal anatomy of the second through fifth carpometacarpal joints and adjacent structures. *J Hand Surg*. 2001;26: 1016–1029.
120. Newington DP, Davis TRC, Barton NJ. The treatment of dorsal fracture-dislocation of the proximal interphalangeal joint by closed reduction and Kirschner wire fixation: a 16-year follow-up. *J Hand Surg*. 2002;27B:537–540.
121. Nicklin S, Ingram S, Gianoutsos MP, et al. In vitro comparison of lagged and nonlagged screw fixation of metacarpal fractures in cadavers. *J Hand Surg*. 2008;33:1732–1736.
122. Niekel MC, Lindenhovius AL, Watson JB, et al. Correlation of DASH and QuickDASH with measures of psychological distress. *J Hand Surg*. 2009;34:1499–1505.
123. Nijhuis TH, Smits ES, Jaquet JB, et al. Prevalence and severity of cold intolerance in patients after hand fracture. *J Hand Surg*. 2010;35:306–311.
124. O'Sullivan ST, Limantzakis G, Kay SP. The role of low-profile titanium miniplates in emergency and elective hand surgery. *J Hand Surg*. 1999;24B:347–349.
125. Orbay JL, Indriago I, Gonzales E, et al. Percutaneous fixation of metacarpal fractures. *Oper Tech Plast Reconstr Surg*. 2002;9:138–142.
126. Otani K, Fukuda K, Hamanishi C. An unusual dorsal fracture-dislocation of the proximal interphalangeal joint. *J Hand Surg*. 2007;32E:193–194.
127. Ouellette EA, Dennis JJ, Latta LL, et al. The role of soft tissues in plate fixation of proximal phalanx fractures. *Clin Orthop*. 2004;418:213–218.
128. Ouellette EA. Use of the minicondylar plate in metacarpal and phalangeal fractures. *Clin Orthop*. 1996;327:38–46.
129. Ozcelik IB, Kabakas F, Mersa B, et al. Treatment of nonunions of the distal phalanx with olecranon bone graft. *J Hand Surg*. 2009;34:638–642.
130. Ozer K, Gillani S, Williams A, et al. Comparison of intramedullary nailing versus plate-screw fixation of extra-articular metacarpal fractures. *J Hand Surg*. 2008;33:1724–1731.
131. Page SM, Stern PJ. Complications and range of motion following plate fixation of metacarpal and phalangeal fractures. *J Hand Surg*. 1998;23A:827–832.
132. Patel MR, Bassini L. Irreducible palmar metacarpophalangeal joint dislocation due to juncture tendinum interposition: a case report and review of the literature. *J Hand Surg*. 2000;25:166–172.
133. Pegoli L, Toh S, Arai K, et al. The Ishiguro extension block technique for the treatment of mallet finger fracture: indications and clinical results. *J Hand Surg*. 2003;28B:15–17.
134. Rettig ME, Dassa G, Raskin KB. Volar plate arthroplasty of the distal interphalanageal joint. *J Hand Surg*. 2001;26A:940–944.
135. Rosenstadt BE, Glickel SZ, Lane LB, et al. Palmar fracture dislocation of the proximal interphalangeal joint. *J Hand Surg*. 1998;23A:811–820.
136. Roth JJ, Auerbach DM. Fixation of hand fractures with bicortical screws. *J Hand Surg*. 2005;30:151–153.
137. Ruland RT, Hogan CJ, Cannon DL, et al. Use of dynamic distraction external fixation for unstable fracture-dislocations of the proximal interphalangeal joint. *J Hand Surg*. 2008;33: 19–25.
138. Safoury Y. Treatment of phalangeal fractures by tension band wiring. *J Hand Surg*. 2001;26B:50–52.
139. Saint-Cyr M, Miranda D, Gonzalez R, et al. Immediate corticocancellous bone autografting in segmental bone defects of the hand. *J Hand Surg*. 2006;31B:168–177.

140. Sams I, Goitz RJ, Sotereanos DG. Dynamic traction and minimal internal fixation for thumb and digital pilon fractures. *J Hand Surg.* 2004;29A:39–43.

141. Sawant N, Kulikov Y, Giddins GEB. Outcome following conservative treatment of metacarpophalangeal collateral ligament avulsion fractures of the finger. *J Hand Surg.* 2007;32B:102–104.

142. Schadel-Hopfner M, Windolf J, Antes G, et al. Evidence-based hand surgery: the role of Cochrane reviews. *J Hand Surg.* 2008;33E:110–117.

143. Shauver MJ, Chung KC. The minimal clinically important difference of the Michigan hand outcomes questionnaire. *J Hand Surg.* 2009;34:509–514.

144. Shewring DJ, Thomas RH. Avulsion fractures from the base of the proximal phalanges of the fingers. *J Hand Surg.* 2003;28B:10–14.

145. Shewring DJ, Thomas RH. Collateral ligament avulsion fractures from the heads of the metacarpals of the fingers. *J Hand Surg.* 2006;31B:537–541.

146. Simonian PT, Trumble TE. Traumatic dislocation of the thumb carpometacarpal joint: early ligamentous reconstruction versus closed reduction and pinning. *J Hand Surg.* 1996;21A:802–806.

147. Smith NC, Moncrieff NJ, Hartnell N, et al. Pseudorotation of the little finger metacarpal. *J Hand Surg.* 2003;28B:395–398.

148. Sohn RC, Jahng KH, Curtiss SB, et al. Comparison of metacarpal plating methods. *J Hand Surg.* 2008;33A:316–321.

149. Sorene ED, Goodwin DR. Nonoperative treatment of displaced avulsion fractures of the ulnar base of the proximal phalanx of the thumb. *Scand J Plast Reconstr Surg Hand Surg.* 2003;37:225–227.

150. Souer JS, Mudgal CS. Plate fixation in closed ipsilateral multiple metacarpal fractures. *J Hand Surg.* 2008;33E:740–744.

151. Stahl S, Lerner A, Kaufman T. Immediate autografting of bone in open fractures with bone loss of the hand: a preliminary report. Case reports. *Scand J Plast Reconstr Surg Hand Surg.* 1999;33:117–122.

152. Stahl S, Schwartz O. Complications of K-wire fixation of fractures and dislocations in the hand and wrist. *Arch Orthop Trauma Surg.* 2001;121:527–530.

153. Stanton JS, Dias JJ, Burke FD. Fractures of the tubular bones of the hand. *J Hand Surg.* 2007;32E:626–636.

154. Stern PJ. Management of fractures of the hand over the last 25 years. *J Hand Surg.* 2000:25A:817–823.

155. Stevenson J, McNaughton G, Riley J. The use of prophylactic flucloxacillin in treatment of open fractures of the distal phalanx within an accident and emergency department: a double-blind randomized placebo-controlled trial. *J Hand Surg.* 2003;28B:388–394.

156. Strauch RJ, Behrman MJ, Rosenwasser MP. Acute dislocation of the carpometacarpal joint of the thumb: an anatomic and cadaver study. *J Hand Surg.* 1994;19:93–98.

157. Strauch RJ, Rosenwasser MP, Lunt JG. Metacarpal shaft fractures: the effect of shortening on the extensor tendon mechanism. *J Hand Surg.* 1998;23:519–523.

158. Strickler M, Nagy L, Buchler U. Rigid internal fixation of basilar fractures of the proximal phalanges by cancellous bone grafting only. *J Hand Surg.* 2001;26B:455–458.

159. Swanson TV, Szabo RM, Anderson DD. Open hand fractures: prognosis and classification. *J Hand Surg.* 1991;16A:101–107.

160. Syed AA, Agarwal M, Boome R. Dynamic external fixation for pilon fractures of the proximal interphalangeal joints: a simple fixator for a complex fracture. *J Hand Surg.* 2003; 28B:137–141.

161. Szwebel JD, Ehlinger V, Pinsolle V, et al. Reliability of a classification of fractures of the hand based on the AO comprehensive classification system. *J Hand Surg.* 2010;35E: 392–395.

162. Takami H, Takahashi S, Ando M. Operative treatment of mallet finger due to intra-articular fracture of the distal phalanx. *Arch Orthop Trauma Surg.* 2000;120:9–13.

163. Tan JS, Foo AT, Chew WC, et al. Articularly placed interfragmentary screw fixation of difficult condylar fractures of the hand. *J Hand Surg.* 2011;36:604–609.

164. Tan V, Beredjiklian PK, Weiland AJ. Intra-articular fractures of the hand: treatment by open reduction and internal fixation. *J Orthop Trauma.* 2005;19:518–523.

165. Teoh LC, Lee JYL. Mallet fractures: a novel approach to internal fixation using a hook plate. *J Hand Surg.* 2007;32B:24–30.

166. Teoh LC, Tan PL, Tan SH, et al. Cerclage wiring-assisted fixation of difficult hand fractures. *J Hand Surg.* 2006;31B:637–642.

167. Theivendran K, Pollock J, Rajaratnam V. Proximal interphalangeal joint fractures of the hand: treatment with an external dynamic traction device. *Ann Plast Surg.* 2007;58:625–629.

168. Thoma A, McKnight L, Knight C. The use of economic evaluation in hand surgery. *Hand Clin.* 2009;25:113–123.

169. Thurston AJ, Dempsey SM. Bennett fracture: a medium- to long-term review. *Aust NZ J Surg.* 1993;63:120–123.

170. Timmenga EJF, Blokhuis TJ, Maas M, et al. Long-term evaluation of Bennett fractures. A comparison between open and closed reduction. *J Hand Surg.* 1994;19B:373–377.

171. Trevisan C, Morganti A, Casiraghi A, et al. Low-severity metacarpal and phalangeal fractures treated with miniature plates and screws. *Arch Orthop Trauma Surg.* 2004;124:675–680.

172. Trumble T, Gilbert M. In situ osteotomy for extra-articular malunion of the proximal phalanx. *J Hand Surg.* 1998;23A:821–826.

173. Vahey JW, Wegner DA, Hastings H II. Effect of proximal phalangeal fracture deformity on extensor tendon function. *J Hand Surg.* 1998;23A:673–681.

174. Van Brenk B, Richards RR, Mackay MB, et al. A biomechanical assessment of ligaments preventing dorsoradial subluxation of the trapeziometacarpal joint. *J Hand Surg.* 1998;23:607–611.

175. Van Onselen EBH, Karim RB, Hage JJ, et al. Prevalence and distribution of hand fractures. *J Hand Surg.* 2003;28B:491–495.

176. Van Oosterom FJT, Brete GJV, Ozdemir C. Treatment of phalangeal fractures in severely injured hands. *J Hand Surg.* 2001;26B:108–111.

177. Waljee JF, Kim HM, Burns PB, et al. Development of a brief, 12-item version of the Michigan Hand Questionnaire. *Plast Reconstr Surg.* 2011;128:208–220.

178. Waris E, Ashammakhi N, Happonen H, et al. Bioabsorbable miniplating versus metallic fixation for metacarpal fractures. *Clin Orthop.* 2003;410:310–319.

179. Waris E, Ashammakhi N, Raatikainen T, et al. Self-reinforced bioabsorbable versus metallic fixation systems for metacarpal and phalangeal fractures: a biomechanical study. *J Hand Surg.* 2002;27:902–909.

180. Weiss APC, Hastings H II. Distal unicondylar fractures of the proximal phalanx. *J Hand Surg.* 1993;18A:594–599.

181. Widgerow AD, Ladas CS. Anatomical attachments to the proximal phalangeal base: a case for stability. *Scand J Plast Reconstr Surg Hand Surg.* 2001;35:85–90.

182. Williams RMM, Kiefhaber TR, Sommerkamp TG, et al. Treatment of unstable dorsal proximal interphalangeal fracture/dislocations using a hemi-hamate autograft. *J Hand Surg.* 2003;28:856–865.

183. Wong T-C, Ip FK, Yeung SH. Comparison between percutaneous transverse fixation and intramedullary K-wires in treating closed fractures of the metacarpal neck of the little finger. *J Hand Surg.* 2006;31B:61–65.

184. Yong FC, Tan SH, Tow BPB, et al. Trapezoid rotational bone graft osteotomy for metacarpal and phalangeal fracture malunion. *J Hand Surg.* 2007;32B:282–288.

185. Yoshida R, Shah MA, Patterson RM, et al. Anatomy and pathomechanics of ring and small finger carpometacarpal joint injuries. *J Hand Surg.* 2003;28:1035–1043.

186. Zhang X, Meng H, Shao X, et al. Pull-out wire fixation for acute mallet finger fractures with K-wire stabilization of the distal interphalangeal joint. *J Hand Surg.* 2010;35:1864–1869.

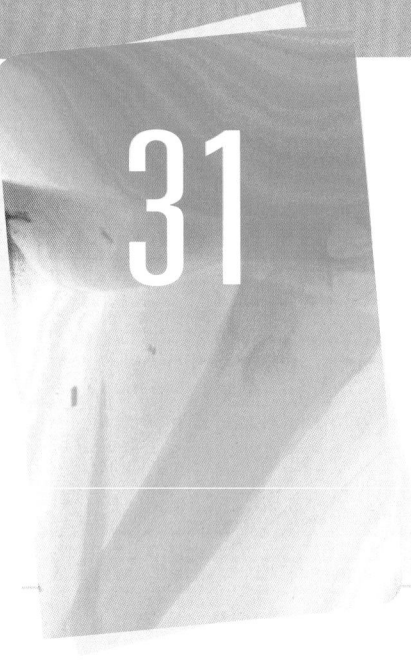

31

CARPUS FRACTURES AND DISLOCATIONS

Andrew D. Duckworth and David Ring

INTRODUCTION TO CARPAL FRACTURES AND DISLOCATIONS

Carpal injuries most frequently occur in young active patients and are not very common overall. We talk about them and study them disproportionately to their frequency because they can be difficult to manage. For instance, fractures of the scaphoid are notorious for nonunion and sometimes the fracture is initially not visible on radiographs. The diagnosis of true fractures among suspected scaphoid fractures remains a dilemma in spite of advances in imaging because even the most sophisticated imaging has false positives and false negatives, because true fractures are uncommon, and because there is no consensus reference standard for true fractures. The use of clinical predictions rules and latent class analysis, accepting that the best we can do is to define and refine the probability of a fracture, may help.

Nondisplaced scaphoid waist fractures have traditionally been treated in below-elbow casts including the thumb for nearly 3 months and issues with union persist. Screw fixation is an appealing option, but research suggests that with an accurate diagnosis of displacement, shorter less cumbersome methods of immobilization may suffice. Proximal pole fractures and displaced waist fractures are more routinely operated on, while distal pole fractures are treated symptomatically. Perilunate dislocations and fracture-dislocations are serious injuries, but effective treatment can maintain a mobile, useful wrist. Intercarpal ligament injuries and carpal malalignment remain confusing and debatable with many options for patients and surgeons to consider, and many questions worthy of study.

ANATOMY AND KINEMATICS OF CARPAL FRACTURES AND DISLOCATIONS

An understanding of the anatomy and kinematics of the eight carpal bones is essential for the diagnosis and management of carpal injuries. Advanced imaging techniques have increased our knowledge of the three-dimensional (3D) movements of the carpus, including their individual and combined contributions to wrist motion and stability.

Osseous and Ligamentous Anatomy of Carpal Fractures and Dislocations

The carpus encompasses two rows of eight bones (Fig. 31-1) that serve as a bridge between the forearm and the hand, providing movement at the wrist joint, while also retaining a notable degree of stability.[44,246,247,283,300,516] The proximal carpal row from radial to ulnar includes the scaphoid, lunate, and triquetrum. It is referred to as the key intercalated segment between the forearm and the distal row of the carpus, which is relatively fixed to the metacarpals distally, and movement results from the shape of the bones, their interaction with other bones, and the various ligamentous attachments.[247,277,283,502,530] Through these articulations the proximal carpal row provides wrist joint movement and congruency, as well as force transmission between the forearm and the hand.[43,46,300] To enable this to occur, the position and orientation of the scaphoid, lunate, and triquetrum is dynamic through their ligamentous attachments, as the proxi-

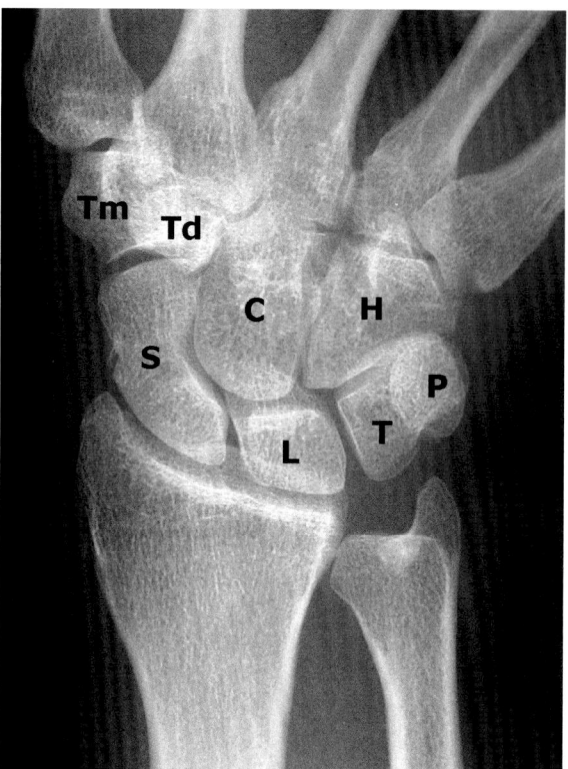

FIGURE 31-1 The wrist is composed of two rows of bones that provide motion and transfer forces. C, capitate; H, hamate; L, lunate; S, scaphoid; T, triquetrum; P, pisiform; Td, trapezoid; Tm, trapezium.

mal row has no direct tendinous attachments.[246,247,283] Although the pisiform bone may provide stability to the proximal carpal row through the pisotriquetral joint, it should not theoretically be considered to be within the proximal carpal row as it is a sesamoid bone enclosed within the sheath of the flexor carpi ulnaris tendon.[43,299]

The distal carpal row from radial to ulnar includes the trapezium, trapezoid, capitate, and hamate.[44,246,283,300,516] The distal row articulates with the proximal carpal row, and distally with the five metacarpals of the hand by forming a transverse arch on which they are supported. The trapezium articulates with the first metacarpal, the trapezoid with the second, the capitate with the third, and the hamate articulates with the fourth and fifth. The capitate and trapezoid are tightly connected to the metacarpals, whereas there is 30 to 40 degrees of flexion–extension and rotation at the metacarpotrapezial joint. Motion at the distal carpal row is controlled by the extrinsic wrist flexors and extensors.

Ligaments of the Carpus

The ligaments of the wrist are predominantly contained within the joint capsule. The inherent stability of the carpal rows, combined with the degree of movement achieved at the wrist joint, is predominantly due to the support of the extrinsic (Table 31-1) and intrinsic (Table 31-2) ligaments that reinforce the capsule of the carpus.[43,46,102,283,300,476,516] Buijze et al.[71] reviewed 58 anatomical studies and found that apart from the scaphocapite ligament, the carpal ligaments are not described consistently.

TABLE 31-1	The Extrinsic Ligaments of the Carpus		
Ligament	**Origin**	**Insertion(s)**	**Comments**
Transverse carpal[43,48,71,92,344,352,363,457]	Volar scaphoid tuberosity and trapezial ridge	Hook of hamate and pisiform	Extra-articular ligament Supports proximal carpal arch Contains flexor tendons Midportion of flexor retinaculum
Radioscaphocapitate[43,44,46,251,425,430,431,432,449,479]	Radial styloid at the level of the scaphoid fossa	Volar capitate	No scaphoid attachment Crosses scaphoid (part of arcuate ligament) allowing rotation Secondary stabilizer of scapholunate joint Separate radioscaphoid ligament debated Reinforces radial joint capsule
Radioscapholunate[39,41,43,46,221,300,340,476]	Distal radius ridge between scaphoid and lunate fossae	Proximal scaphoid and lunate	Pedicle derived from anterior interosseous artery, radial artery, and anterior interosseous nerve Neurovascular supply to scapholunate IOM Weak ligament, some consider not a true extrinsic ligament
Long/short radiolunate[42,43,46,300,345,476]	Radial styloid volar rim	Lunate (palmar horn) and triquetrum	Lies parallel to the radioscaphocapitate ligament Passes anterior to proximal pole of scaphoid
Radial collateral[42,43,46,251,319,476]	Radial styloid dorsal/volar rim	Scaphoid waist	Many question existence of collateral ligaments Some consider it part of the RSC ligament
Dorsal radiocarpal[42,43,46,319,433,434,447,476,513,514]	Distal radius, Lister tubercle	Lunate, lunotriquetral ligament, triquetrum (dorsal tubercle)	Origin debated Possible insertion scaphoid (dorsal radioscaphoid ligament) Role in scapholunate stability
Dorsal intercarpal[42,43,46,319,340,414,424,447,476,513,514]	Dorsoradial triquetrum	Dorsoradial groove of scaphoid	Multiple other insertions suggested (trapezium, trapezoid, lunate, capitate)
Ulnotriquetral[43,46,300,476]	Palmar edge TFCC	Proximal/ulnar surfaces of the triquetrum	Proximally, minimal distinction with ulnolunate ligament May have fibers attached to ulnar styloid Orifice provides communication between radiocarpal and pisotriquetral joint
Ulnolunate[43,46,300,476]	Palmar edge TFCC	Palmar cortex of the lunate	Continuous with short radiolunate ligament
Ulnocapitate[43,46,300,476]	Ulnar head, fovea region	Capitate	May act as ulnar anchor for the carpus 10% insertion on capitate, remainder arcuate ligament Reinforces palmar region of the LT interosseous ligament

Extrinsic Ligaments. The extrinsic ligaments of the carpus (Fig. 31-2) connect the carpal bones to the forearm bones (proximally) and the metacarpals (distally) (Table 31-1). They are often difficult to distinguish from the fibrous capsule of the wrist on dissection; however, they are out with the articulations of the joint.

The extrinsic palmar radiocarpal ligaments (Fig. 31-2A) include the transverse carpal, radioscaphocapitate (RSC), radioscapholunate (ligament of Testut; RSL), radial collateral, long radiolunate (radiolunotriquetral; RLT), and the short radiolunate ligaments.[5,43,46,63,286,300,355,426,476] The extrinsic ulnocarpal ligaments include the ulnotriquetral (dorsal and palmar), ulnolunate, and ulnocapitate ligaments.[5,43,46,63,286,300,355,426,476] These palmar ligaments predominantly originate from a lateral

position on the radial-palmar facet of the radial styloid and head in a distal ulnar direction, where they assemble with the palmar ulnocarpal ligaments originating medially from the distal ulna and triangular fibrocartilage complex (TFCC). The strong oblique extrinsic palmar radial ligaments prevent the carpus from translating medially on the angulated slope of the distal radius through two V-shaped ligamentous bands.[38,42,512,565] One is proximal (long radiolunate, RSC, ulnolunate, ulnotriquetral) and connects the forearm to the proximal carpal row and one is distal (RSC, ulnocapitate) and connects the forearm to the distal carpal row. Between the radial (RSC) and ulnar palmar ligaments (long radiolunate) there is a V-shaped interligamentous sulcus over the capitolunate articulation, which is an interval of capsular weakness known as the space of Poirier. Maximal space

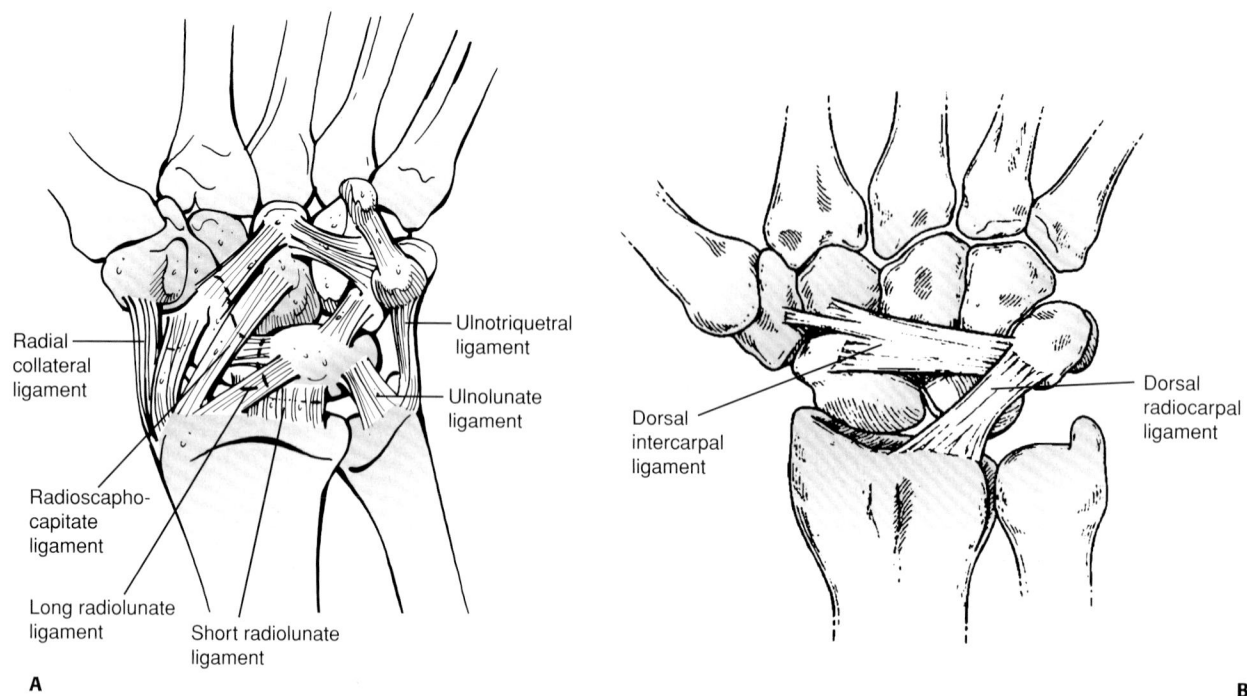

FIGURE 31-2 **A:** The extrinsic palmar ligaments of the carpus. **B:** The extrinsic dorsal ligaments of the carpus. (Part B redrawn from Duckworth AD, Buijze GA, Moran M, et al. Predictors of fracture following suspected injury to the scaphoid. *J Bone Joint Surg Br.* 2012;94-B(7):961–968.)

is seen when the wrist is dorsiflexed, with the space almost disappearing in palmar flexion. This is of clinical relevance during dorsal dislocations as it is through this area of weakness that the lunate displaces into the carpal canal. The arcuate ligament is found in the central third of the palmar joint capsule and is thought to be formed from the interdigitation of transverse fibers of the RSC, ulnocapitate, triquetrocapitate, and volar scaphotriquetral ligaments.[43,46,71,300,476] This ligament forms a support sling for the midcarpal region, in particular the head of the capitate, which is thought to improve midcarpal movement while also delivering carpal stability. Alternate names for the arcuate ligament include the deltoid ligament, palmar distal V ligament, or Weitbrecht oblique ligament.[46,71] Controversy exists regarding the existence of individual forms of some of the ligaments that make up the arcuate ligament, in particular the volar scaphotriquetral ligament.[46,425,449]

The extrinsic dorsal carpal ligaments (Fig. 31-2B) include the dorsal radiocarpal (DRC) ligament, which may also be known as the dorsal radioulnotriquetral ligament or the dorsal radiotriquetral ligament, and the dorsal intercarpal ligament, which form a V-shaped configuration. The ulnodorsal capsule of the wrist is reinforced by the ulnolunate and ulnotriquetral ligaments and the floors of the fifth and sixth extensor compartments.[5,43,46,63,286,300,355,426,444,513] Some studies have suggested an essential role of the dorsal carpal ligaments in scapholunate stability.[147,317,433,434]

Intrinsic Ligaments. The intrinsic ligaments connect the individual carpal bones to one another (Fig. 31-3 and Table 31-2). The ligaments are intra-articular short fibers that connect and hold the carpal bones of both the proximal and distal rows

to each other. There is a contiguous merging of the interosseous ligaments with the joint articular cartilage. The intrinsic ligaments include the palmar midcarpal ligaments (scaphotrapeziotrapezoid, scaphocapitate, triquetrocapitate, triquetrohamate), the proximal interosseous ligaments (scapholunate, lunotriquetral), and the distal interosseous ligaments (trapeziotrapezoid, trapeziocapitate, capitohamate).[43,46,63,286,300,355] Ligaments associated with the pisiform include the pisotriquetral ligament that bridges the pisotriquetral joint, and the pisohamate ligament, which is an extension of flexor carpi ulnaris.[43,46]

On the radial side of the wrist the V-shaped scaphotrapezium-trapezoid ligament is found, providing stability to the scaphoid-trapezium-trapezoid articulation as well as the scaphoid itself.[43,44,46,48,134,329,345,476] The V-shape is from the scaphotrapezial component of the ligament. Although insertion on the trapezoid bone is contested, recent studies have suggested the existence of two distinct ligaments: the scaphotrapezoid and scaphotrapezium ligaments, with the former thinner and less robust.[43,44,46,251,345] However, some have suggested that the soft tissue present is capsule.[134] Adjacent to the scaphotrapezium-trapezoid ligament is the scaphocapitate, which is a large robust ligament that provides midcarpal stability with fibers running in parallel to the RSC ligament.[43,46,134,344,345] One recent study analyzed eight fresh-frozen cadavers using 3D CT and cryomicrotome imaging to better define the osseous and ligamentous anatomy of the scaphoid.[67] They concluded that the scaphocapitate ligament was the thickest ligament of all those that attached to the scaphoid, with a mean thickness of 2.2 mm. On the ulnar side of the wrist, the remaining palmar midcarpal ligaments are the triquetrocapitate and triquetrohamate ligaments.[43,46,477]

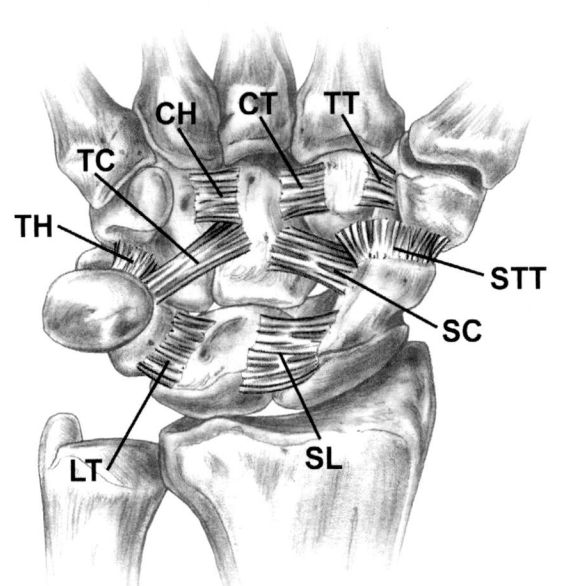
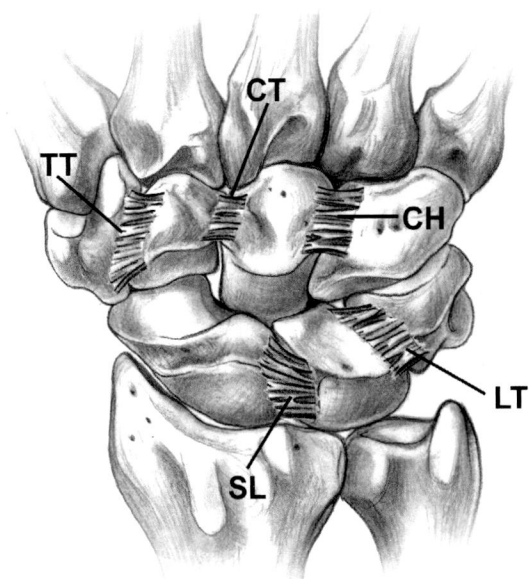

A   **B**

FIGURE 31-3 A: The palmar intrinsic ligaments—scaphotrapeziotrapezoid ligament (STT), scaphocapitate ligament (SC), triquetrocapitate ligament (TC), and triquetrohamate ligament (TH). **B:** The
dorsal intrinsic ligaments—capitohamate ligament (CH), capitotrapezoid ligament (CT), lunotriquetral
ligament (LT), scapholunate ligament (SL), trapeziotrapezoid ligament (TT). The dorsal intercarpal ligament is not shown. (From: Berger RA, Weiss APC. *Hand Surgery*. 1st ed. Philadelphia, PA: Lippincott
Williams & Wilkins; 2003.)

TABLE 31-2	The Intrinsic Ligaments of the Carpus, Excluding the Distal Interosseous Ligaments		
Ligament	**Origin**	**Insertion(s)**	**Comments**
Scaphotrapezium-trapezoid[43,44,46,48,134,329,345,430,431,432,476]	Distal pole of scaphoid	Proximal palmar aspect of trapezium/trapezoid	Insertion on trapezoid is controversial Secondary stabilizer scapholunate joint Prevents extreme scaphoid flexion
Scaphocapitate[43,46,134,344,345]	Distal pole of scaphoid	Radial volar body of the capitate	Origin large surface area distal scaphoid
Triquetrocapitate[43,46,477]	Distal/radial corner of triquetrum	Ulnar body of the capitate	Continuation of ulnotriquetral ligament
Triquetrohamate[43,46,477]	Distal palmar cortex of the triquetrum	Palmar aspect body of the hamate	Continuation of ulnotriquetral ligament
Scapholunate[37,40,43,45,46,67,340,428,448,453,476,497]			
Dorsal	Dorsal lateral horn Lunate	Ulnar-dorsal aspect proximal pole scaphoid	Transverse strong thick (2–4 mm) fibers Merges with dorsal intercarpal distally
Palmar	Dorsal lateral horn Lunate	Ulnar-dorsal aspect proximal pole scaphoid	Histologically comparable to dorsal portion but oblique fibers, thinner (1–2 mm) and less stiff
Proximal	Dorsal lateral horn lunate	Ulnar-dorsal aspect proximal pole scaphoid	Fibrocartilaginous membrane Merges with adjacent articular cartilage Widest, thinnest (1 mm), weakest section
Lunotriquetral[43,46,340,398,476]			
Dorsal	Lunate	Triquetrum	Transverse fibers but thinner and less stiff than palmar bundle
Palmar	Lunate	Triquetrum	Transverse strong thick bundle of fibers Interdigitates with ulnocapitate ligament
Proximal	Lunate	Triquetrum	Fibrocartilaginous membrane similar to scapholunate proximal portion

Data from Duckworth AD, Ring D, McQueen MM. Assessment of the suspected fracture of the scaphoid. *J Bone Joint Surg Br.* 2011;93:713–719, reprinted with permission.

The proximal interosseous scapholunate and lunotriquetral ligaments are found deep within the carpus and are considered the two most important intrinsic ligaments as they are critical to carpal stability.[183] The scapholunate interosseous ligament is a strong stiff C-shaped ligament that plays a vital role in carpal stability, with the thick and strong dorsal portion containing transversely oriented collagen fascicles key to the stability of the scapholunate joint.[37,40,43,45,46,67,340,428,448,453,476,497] The palmar/volar and proximal/central portions act as secondary stabilizers, contributing primarily to rotational stability of the joint.[40] Recent studies have demonstrated that the scapholunate interosseous ligament is the primary stabilizer of the scapholunate joint, with the scaphotrapezium-trapezoid ligament and the RSC ligament secondary stabilizers,[430–432] and the dorsal carpal ligaments likely having a tertiary role.[147,317,433,434] The lunotriquetral ligament interdigitates with three extrinsic ligaments: the ulnotriquetral, ulnolunate, and radiolunate ligaments.[43,46,340,398,476] The thickest and strongest zone of the lunotriquetral ligament is found palmarly.[43,340,398] A stronger kinematic relationship than the scapholunate ligament is seen due to the tight association of its fibers.[43,300,398,476] The scaphotriquetral ligament is a distal extension of the scapholunate and lunotriquetral ligaments.[43]

The distal interosseous ligaments have a comparable structure to the proximal interosseous ligaments, with both palmar and dorsal fibers.[43,46,396,397,476] The trapeziotrapezoid and trapeziocapitate ligaments similarly span their respective articulations, but with the latter having a deep ligament that bridges the joint. The capitohamate ligament spans only the distal part of the capitohamate joint articulation and again is reinforced by a large deep ligament that has extensions to the middle and ring finger metacarpals.

Neurovascular Anatomy of Carpal Fractures and Dislocations

The neurovascular supply to the carpus is through the regional vasculature and nerves.[47,164,185,186,298,366,474] Innervation is via the anterior interosseous and posterior interosseous nerves. Circulation to the carpus is composed of an extraosseous and intraosseous vasculature via both dorsal and palmar vascular systems, which are branches of the radial, ulnar, anterior interosseous, and deep palmar arch arteries (Fig. 31-4).[57,164,185,186,366] The extraosseous arterial supply is formed by an anastomotic network of dorsal and palmar transverse arches connected longitudinally from their medial and lateral borders by the radial, ulnar, and anterior interosseous arteries.[164,185,186,366,474] The three dorsal transverse arches of the carpus include the radiocarpal, the intercarpal, and the basal metacarpal arches.[164] The three palmar transverse arches of the carpus include the radiocarpal, the intercarpal, and the deep palmar arches.[164] For all of these arches, their presence in cadaveric specimens is inconsistent.[164]

The incidence of avascular necrosis (AVN) following injury to the carpal bones is related to their complex intraosseous blood supply.[57,164,185,186,366] Original work documented that the vascular supply of most carpal bones enters the distal half, leaving the proximal half at risk of AVN. The vascular supply of each carpal bone is shown in Table 31-3. From this, three general patterns of

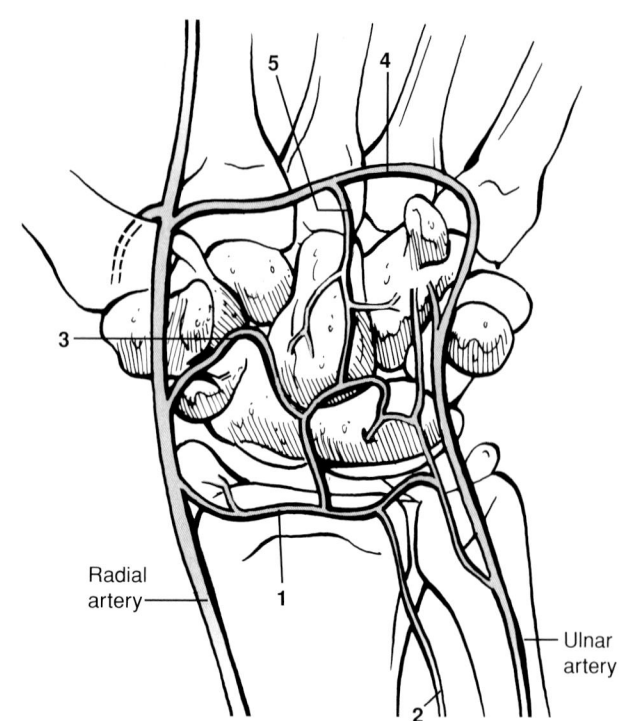

FIGURE 31-4 Schematic drawing of the arterial supply of the palmar aspect of the carpus. Circulation of the wrist is obtained through the radial, ulnar, and anterior interosseous arteries and the deep palmar arch. 1, palmar radiocarpal arch; 2, palmar branch of anterior interosseous artery; 3, palmar intercarpal arch; 4, deep palmar arch; 5, recurrent artery.

intraosseous vascularization have been described and help with identifying the carpal bones at risk of osteonecrosis.[57,164,184–186,366]

1. The scaphoid, capitate, and about 20% of all lunates are supplied by a single vessel increasing their risk to AVN.

2. The trapezium, triquetrum, pisiform, and 80% of lunates receive nutrient arteries through two nonarticular surfaces and have consistent intraosseous anastomoses; therefore, reducing the risk of AVN.

3. The trapezoid and 50% of hamates lack an intraosseous anastomosis and are at risk of avascular fragments.

Kinematics of Carpal Fractures and Dislocations

The study of carpal kinematics began in the late 1800s using plain radiographs, and knowledge has advanced through in vitro cadaveric work, as well as employing advanced imaging techniques such as 3D CT.

The biomechanics of the wrist joint need to allow for load transmission from the hand to the forearm and a wide range of motion, while also achieving stability throughout. Two predominant articulations are found at the wrist joint and include the proximal carpal bones (scaphoid, lunate, triquetrum) with the distal radius and ulna, which is considered as the key intercalated segment and provides principally extension and ulnar deviation at the wrist.[246,247,502,530] The second articulation is between the proximal and distal carpal rows and provides

TABLE 31-3	The Vascular Supply to All the Carpal Bones		
Carpal Bone	**Vascular Supply**	**Comments**
Scaphoid[57,164,185,186,366]	Scaphoid branches of the radial artery: • Dorsal branch supplies 70–80% proximally • Volar branch supplies 20–30% distally	No perforators at waist, cartilage, or SL ligament All surgical approaches potentially endanger some of the arterial branches
Lunate[57,164,182,186,366,542]	~80% receive vessels from palmar and dorsal surfaces • Dorsal originate from radiocarpal arch, intercarpal arch, and rarely dorsal branch of anterior interosseous ~20% receive vessels from palmar surface only • Palmar originate from radiocarpal arch, intercarpal arch, branches of anterior interosseous and ulnar recurrent arteries	Large articulating surface with nonperforators Proximal pole has marginally less vascularity Three intraosseous patterns: • Y (59%; dorsal or palmar) • I (30%; one dorsal, one palmar) • X (10%, two dorsal, two palmar)
Triquetrum[164,366]	Branches of ulnar artery, dorsal intercarpal arch, palmar intercarpal arch • Dorsal vessels supply 60% • Palmar vessels supply 40%	Vessels enter through two (dorsal ridge/palmar oval facet) nonarticulating surfaces Dorsal–palmar anastomoses found in 86%
Pisiform[164,366]	Branches of ulnar artery	Two entry points for vessels: • Proximal pole inferior to triquetral facet • Distal pole inferior to articular facets Proximal–distal anastomoses found
Trapezium[164,366]	Branches of radial artery • Dorsal supply predominates	Vessels enter through three (dorsal/lateral/palmar tubercle) nonarticulating surfaces Dorsal–lateral–palmar anastomoses found
Trapezoid[164,366]	Branches from the dorsal arch, the intercarpal arch, the basal metacarpal arch, and the radial recurrent artery • Dorsal vessels supply 70% • Palmar vessels supply 30%	Vessels enter through two (dorsal/palmar) nonarticulating surfaces
Capitate[164,366]	Branches of the dorsal intercarpal arch, dorsal basal metacarpal arch, palmar intercarpal arch, and ulnar recurrent artery	Vessels enter through two (dorsal/palmar) nonarticulating surfaces In 1/3 the supply to the capitate head is solely from the palmar side Dorsal–palmar anastomoses found in 30%
Hamate[164,366]	Branches of the dorsal intercarpal arch, the ulnar recurrent artery, and the ulnar artery • Dorsal vessels supply dorsal 30–40%	Vessels enter through three (dorsal/palmar/medial) nonarticulating surfaces Dorsal–palmar anastomoses found in 50%, but no anastomoses with medial vessels

Data from Duckworth AD, Ring D, McQueen MM. Assessment of the suspected fracture of the scaphoid. *J Bone Joint Surg Br.* 2011;93:713–719, reprinted with permission.

predominantly flexion and radial deviation. Motion predominantly occurs in two planes, with flexion–extension at approximately 70 degrees in both directions, and radioulnar deviation at approximately 20 and 40 degrees respectively.[246,247,283,516] The adjacent radioulnar joint provides a substantial rotatory arc of approximately 140 degrees around the longitudinal axis of the forearm.[282,364,365]

Although many theories have been described, there are two predominant theories used to explain carpal kinematics, which are known as the columnar and the oval-ring or row theories.[179,183] The columnar theory is the oldest, described by Navarro (Fig. 31-5).[349] He observed motion between the proximal carpal row bones, predominantly from data on birds, and put forward the theory of three longitudinal columns:

1. A *mobile lateral (radial) column* consisting of the scaphoid, trapezium, and trapezoid
2. A *central flexion–extension column* consisting of the lunate, capitate, and hamate

3. A *rotational medial (ulnar) column* consisting of the triquetrum and pisiform

This theory goes some way to explaining the load transmission of the wrist but not synchronous motion. Taleisnik[476] put forward a modification of this theory by including the trapezium and trapezoid (i.e., lunate + distal carpal row) to the central column, as well as removing the pisiform from the medial column. With this theory flexion and extension occur through the central column, but he suggested that the scaphoid was an essential stabilizer for the midcarpal joint (radial column), the triquetrum (triquetrohamate joint) was the pivot point for rotation of the carpus, and that radial and ulnar deviation was facilitated through rotation of the scaphoid laterally and the triquetrum medially.

The alternative oval-ring theory combines the theories of the carpal row and oval-ring concept (Fig. 31-6).[275,276,283] The key concepts for this theory include the proximal intercalated segment, variable geometry, as well as the synchronous and

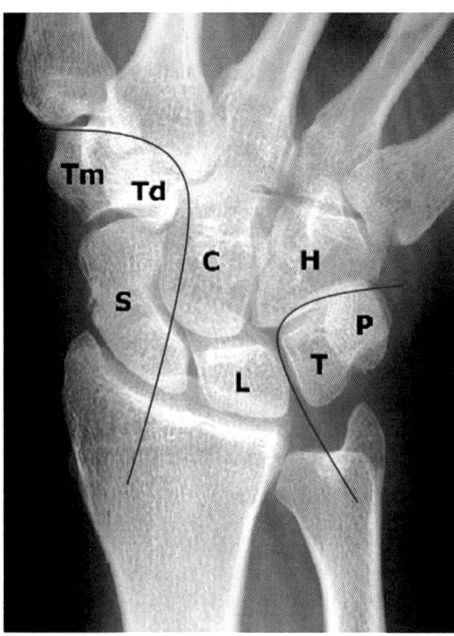

FIGURE 31-5 The columnar theory of carpal kinematics.

reciprocating motion of the carpal rows. What is key to providing versatility to the wrist joint, combined with the ability to remain stable throughout, is the proximal intercalated segment (proximal carpal row).[179,246,247,266,502,530] The primary axis for the combined motion of the carpus has been found to be within the head/neck of the capitate, which is not a singular point, but rather an oblique screw axis.[246,247,283,516,563] The scaphoid is found on an axis 45 degrees to the longitudinal axis that passes through the lunate and capitate, and provides stability to the midcarpal joint while also stabilizing the central column. By virtue of its

obliquity, the scaphoid will flex when under compression and exerts a similar force on the lunate. The lunate; however, is also under the influence of the triquetrum, which inherently prefers to extend. For this reason, the lunate may be thought of being in a state of dynamic balance between two antagonists, tending to lie in the position of least mechanical potential energy.

The movement of the individual components of the proximal carpal row allows the length and contour of the proximal carpal row to be dynamic, providing extreme movements at the wrist while also maintaining stability around the longitudinal axis.[246,247,283,502,516,530] This concept is known as the variable geometry of the proximal carpal row. To provide such a degree of motion, the individual carpal bones are multirotational moving not only up and down and back and forth, but also spinning and rolling about their own axes.[246,247,283,516]

During flexion and extension of the wrist, each carpal row bone angulates in the same direction with nearly equal amplitude and in a synchronous fashion, a concept known as synchronous angulation (Fig. 31-7).[64,246–249,283,306,325,413,516,549,563] However, the amplitude of movement is different for the bones of each column.[79] Recent studies using 3D noninvasive imaging have re-examined previous work analyzing the radiocarpal and midcarpal contributions to wrist flexion and extension.[64,248,249,306,325,413,549,563] Sarrafian et al.[413] documented that for flexion ~40% is at the radiocarpal joint with ~60% at the midcarpal joint, and that in extension ~66.5% is at the radiocarpal joint with ~33.5% at the midcarpal joint. More recent studies have documented that in flexion 62% to 75% of wrist motion occurred at the radioscaphoid joint, with 31% to 50% at the radiolunate joint.[249,325,549] In extension, 87% to 99% of wrist motion has been shown to occur at the radioscaphoid joint, with 52% to 68% at the radiolunate joint.

During radioulnar deviation, the proximal row exhibits a secondary out-of-plane angulation (sagittal plane) in conjunction

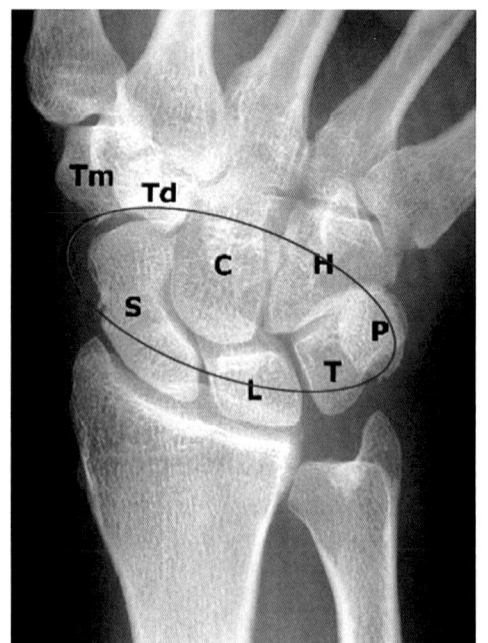

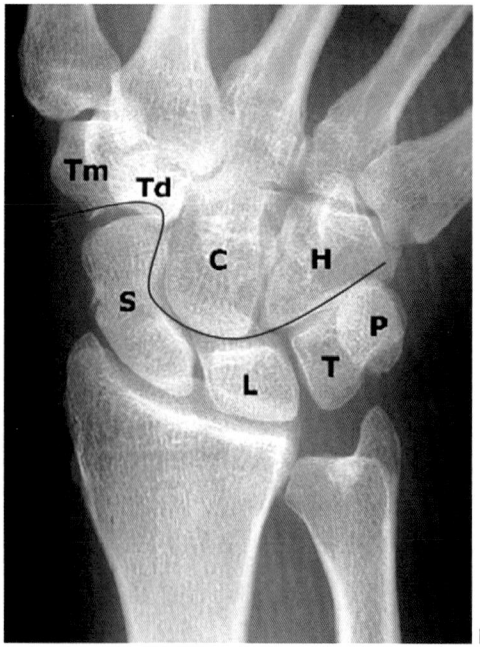

FIGURE 31-6 The oval **(A)** and row **(B)** theories of carpal kinematics.

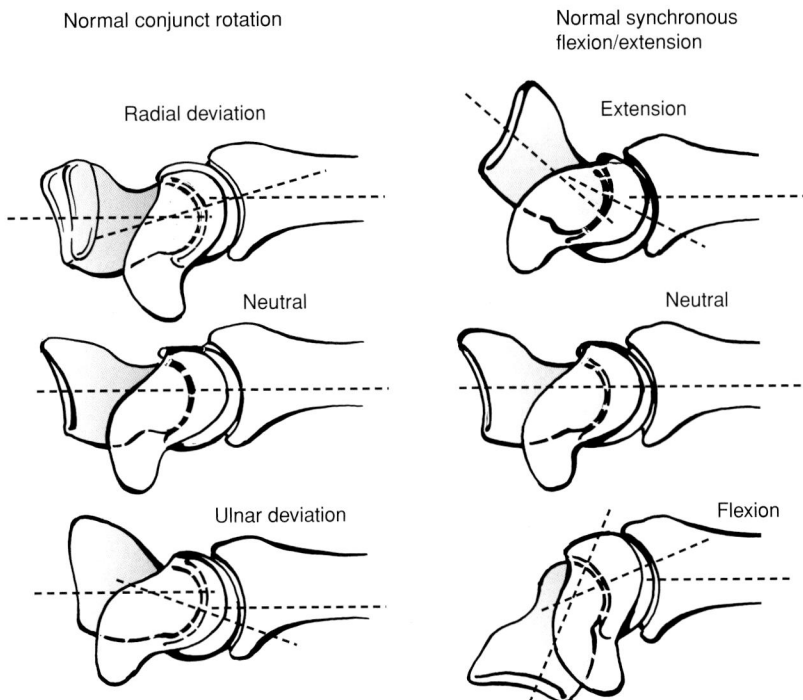

Normal conjunct rotation

Radial deviation

Neutral

Ulnar deviation

Normal synchronous
flexion/extension

Extension

Neutral

Flexion

FIGURE 31-7 Conjunct rotation of the entire proximal intercalated row occurs in flexion during radial deviation **(upper left).** The axes of the radius and carpal rows are collinear in neutral **(middle left),** and the proximal row extends with ulnar deviation **(lower left).** Angulatory excursions of the proximal and distal rows are essentially equal in amplitude and direction during extension **(upper right)** and flexion **(lower right).** This has been described as synchronous angulation.

to the synchronous motion occurring in the coronal plane.[64,248,306,325,563] In radial deviation the proximal carpal row flexes and the capitate extends (reciprocal motion). Flexion of the obliquely orientated scaphoid, as the trapezium and trapezoid approach the radius, is transmitted through the dorsal scapholunate ligament and onto the lunate and triquetrum, when flexion is at 10 to 20 degrees. In ulnar deviation the proximal carpal row extends and the capitate flexes, along with the proximal migration of the hamate, forcing the triquetrum to displace palmarly and extend, bringing the lunate with it. Recent studies have demonstrated that associated pronation (radial deviation) and supination (ulnar deviation) of the proximal carpal row is minimal.[248,325] These studies have also demonstrated that radial and ulnar deviation occurred primarily at the midcarpal joint, accounting for ~60% and ~85% of the movement respectively.

One study has suggested that as the wrist moves into ulnar deviation, the unique helicoidal shape of the triquetrohamate joint forces the distal carpal row to translate dorsally and the triquetrum to tilt into extension, leading to extension of the proximal carpal row.[530] The converse occurs during radial deviation.

Pathoanatomy of Carpal Fractures and Dislocations

An injury to the carpus commonly occurs following a mechanism in which an axial compression force is applied to the wrist, commonly leading to hyperextension where the palmar ligaments undergo tension and the dorsal articulations are subject to shear stresses.[255,279,302,529] It has been demonstrated that both the degree of force applied to the wrist and the degree of wrist radial or ulnar deviation will determine whether a ligament injury, a fracture, or both, occur. Minor injuries, such as ligamentous sprains, frequently result from a low-energy injury.

However, one study has demonstrated a relationship between a low-energy simple fall in women and sustaining a scaphoid fracture.[136] Higher-energy injuries that involve a more considerable force result in either a fracture to one or more of the carpal bones and/or a ligamentous disruption, with both intrinsic and extrinsic ligaments potentially involved.[255,279,302,529] Variations in bone quality, the direction and magnitude of the deforming force and the position of the wrist at the time of injury explain the variety of injuries that can occur.

Carpal Fractures

Fracture of the Scaphoid. Any shear strain that travels across the midcarpal joint is transferred through the scaphoid and may cause a fracture and/or dislocation. Fracture of the scaphoid has been shown to occur when the wrist is dorsiflexed to ≥95 degrees and radially deviated to ≥10 degrees.[255,279,302,529] In this position the proximal pole of the scaphoid is held firmly between the radius, capitate, RSC ligament, and the palmar capsule (Fig. 31-8).[302,529] With the wrist radially deviated the RSC ligament is relaxed and unable to relieve the increasing force being applied to the radiopalmar aspect of the scaphoid.[302,529] When axial loading and/or dorsal compression of the scaphoid occurs in this position, the scaphoid will fracture, most frequently through the waist as it is subject to the maximal bending movement.[173,529]

The degree of force and position of the wrist at the time of injury are the likely determinants for the type and severity of scaphoid fracture. Herbert[213] suggested that wrist deviation may predict the location of the fracture as the line of the midcarpal joint crosses the proximal pole in radial deviation and the distal pole in ulnar deviation. Fractures of the waist are usually the result of shear forces across the scaphoid, while tubercle fractures appear to be caused by either compression or

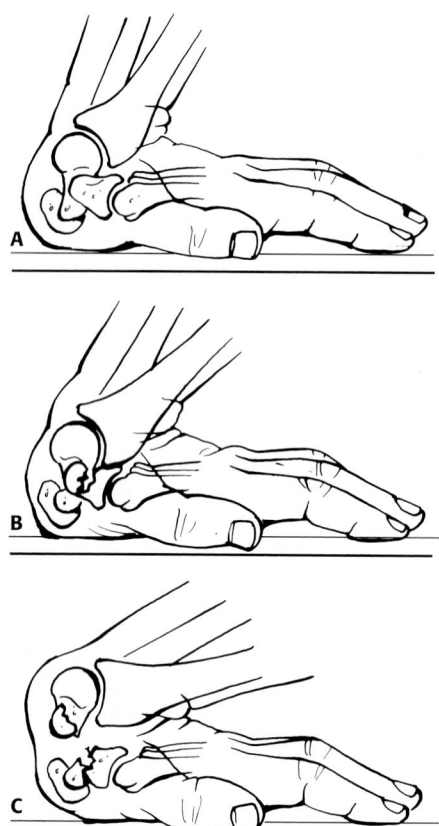

FIGURE 31-8 The schematic above demonstrates the progression to fracture of the scaphoid during a hyperextension injury to the wrist. The proximal pole of the scaphoid is trapped between the radius and tense palmar extrinsic ligaments, with the force concentrated at the scaphoid waist leading to fracture.

avulsion.[156,377] Compson[96] suggested that the size of a proximal pole fracture was dependent on the level of the proximal extent of the joint facet with the capitate, which is the most variable aspect of scaphoid anatomy. Smaller proximal pole fractures can also be caused by an avulsion of the attachment of the scapholunate ligament.

With an unstable displaced scaphoid fracture, the kinematics of the wrist are altered. Joint compressive forces, trapezium-scaphoid shear stress and capitolunate rotation moments all act upon the scaphoid, leading to a dissociation of the proximal and distal carpal rows that permits the natural tendency of the two carpal rows to fail by collapsing, assuming a lunate-extended posture. The scaphoid will assume an anteverted position, the lunate and triquetrum sublux forward and rotate dorsally, and the capitate and hamate sublux dorsally and proximally, producing the dorsal intercalated segment instability (DISI) deformity (see Carpal Ligament Injuries section below). This is demonstrated clinically by the collapse pattern seen with chronic scaphoid nonunion, a condition known as scaphoid nonunion advanced collapse (SNAC) appearing as a DISI deformity.[109,411,446] The proximal and distal fracture fragments can collapse giving a characteristic flexed or "humpback" position on radiographs with an intrascaphoid angle of greater than approximately 30 degrees.[411]

Fracture of the Capitate. It has been suggested that fracture of the capitate occurs through one of three potential mechanisms:

1. Scaphocapitate syndrome[154,296,314]: Occurs with a violent blow directed to the radial styloid which first fractures the scaphoid and then the capitate but produces no dislocation. The capitate fragment can be rotated 90 to 180 degrees, with the articular surface displaced anteriorly or facing the fracture surface of the capitate neck.[510] Some have questioned the nomenclature with reports suggesting a scaphoid fracture does not always occur.[24]

2. Anvil mechanism: An axial load with the wrist in dorsiflexion, forcing the capitate onto the dorsal rim of the radius. The dorsal border of the radius will impinge on the capitate and cause a fracture through its waist.

3. Direct blow or crush injury.

Fracture of the Lunate. Fracture of the lunate commonly occurs following a hyperextension injury to the wrist. In extension, the lunate is displaced onto the palmar aspect of the lunate fossa and rotated dorsally.[429,549] The capitate pushes against the palmar aspect of the lunate, and at the same time moves it into an ulnar direction, which is countered by the RSL ligament. When the forearm is pronated and there is an ulnar minus variant, the support offered by the TFCC and ulnar head will be reduced and the compressive stresses across the proximal convexity of the lunate are altered between the TFCC and the radial articular surface.[204,534] The reduced ulnar support may also allow proximal displacement of the triquetrum placing further tensile stress on the lunate surface through the lunotriquetral ligament. This chain of events can eventually result in a transverse fracture of the lunate in the sagittal plane.[204,534]

Avulsions of the dorsal pole of the lunate are often associated with scapholunate dissociation (SLD) and are thus likely secondary to tension placed on the scapholunate ligament. Avulsion fractures of the ulnar aspect of the palmar pole of the lunate are frequently associated with a perilunate dislocation and are thus likely secondary to tension placed on the lunotriquetral ligament (see below).

In the above scenarios, stress may be placed on the vasculature of the lunate (Table 31-3) prior to a fracture occurring, leading to the development of Kienböck disease. There is considerable evidence that the mechanisms of fracture are also associated with the development of Kienböck disease, with Kienböck disease known to be secondary to trauma, ulnar variance, and impaired vascularity.[33,182,265]

Carpal Ligament Injuries

Carpal instability usually follows a high-energy injury leading to the wrist undergoing a force associated with hyperextension, ulnar deviation, and intercarpal supination.[301–304] This can lead to an interruption of the oval ring, commonly in the proximal carpal row, leading to instability. The most common pattern of injury is associated with a perilunate dislocation or fracture dislocation (see below).

Although several systems exist, three interrelated classification systems are commonly used for defining carpal instability

TABLE 31-4 Classifications of Carpal Instability

Classification	Description	Examples
Dorsal intercalated segment instability (DISI)	Lunate extends, dorsal displacement of the capitate Scapholunate angle >60 degrees Capitolunate angle >15 degrees Radiolunate angle >10–15 degrees in dorsal direction	Scapholunate dissociation Displaced scaphoid fracture Scaphoid pseudarthrosis
Volar intercalated segment instability (VISI)	Lunate flexes, volar displacement of the capitate Scapholunate angle <30 degrees Capitolunate angle >30 degrees Radiolunate angle >10–15 degrees in volar direction	Lunotriquetral dissociation Multiple complex carpal instability
Dissociative	Instability due to injury within carpal row (intrinsic ligament injury)	Scaphoid fracture Scapholunate dissociation Perilunate dislocation
Nondissociative	Instability due to injury between the carpal rows (extrinsic ligament injury)	Radiocarpal instability Midcarpal instability Barton fracture-dislocations Die-punch fracture dislocations
Combined	Combination of dissociative and nondissociative	
Static instability	Standard (PA and lateral) nonstress views demonstrate carpal malalignment/instability	
Dynamic instability	Standard nonstress views demonstrate no carpal malalignment/instability, but positive stress views	

and are useful in understanding the pathoanatomy of the injury. The three classifications include intercalated segment instability,[277,278] static versus dynamic instability,[476] and dissociative versus nondissociative instability (Table 31-4). Linscheid described instability in relation to the appearance of the lunate and the intercalated segment on standard lateral radiographs (Fig. 31-9).[277] When the dynamic kinematic relationship between the scaphoid, lunate, and triquetrum is disrupted by either a fracture and/or a ligamentous injury, instability of the wrist ensues with loss of synchronous motion and intercarpal contact patterns. The lunate will flex with loss of ulnar support from the triquetrum and when in a fixed position of flexion of greater than 15 degrees, *volar intercalated segment instability (VISI)* has occurred. When the opposite occurs and

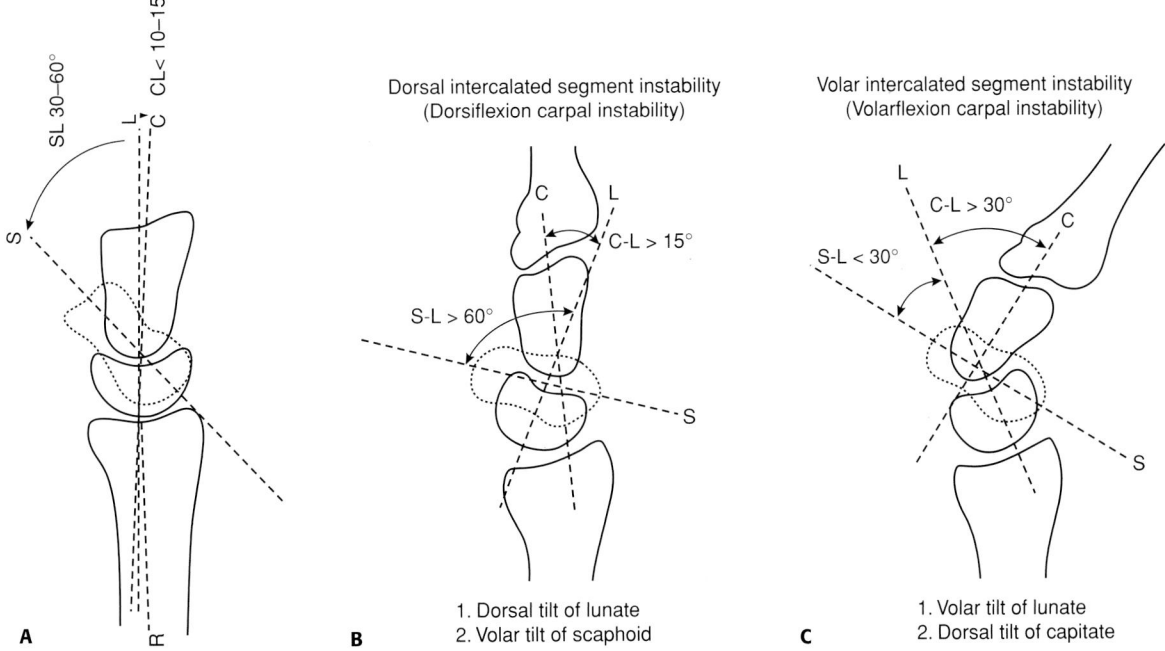

FIGURE 31-9 Schematic drawing of carpal instability. **A:** Normal longitudinal alignment of the carpal bones with the scaphoid axis at an approximately 45-degree angle to the axes of the capitate, lunate, and radius. **B:** DISI deformity (scapholunate angle >60 degrees). **C:** VISI deformity (scapholunate angle <30 degrees).

the lunate falls into fixed extension of more than 10 degrees, *DISI* has occurred. The fixed malpositioning of the lunate, even in radial and ulnar deviation of the wrist, affects the functioning of the proximal intercalated segment and thus the kinematics of the wrist. With persistent instability, degenerative changes will ensue as a consequence of increased shear forces and abnormal contact between the individual carpal bones.[15,267,524,527]

Dissociative instabilities of the carpus involve an isolated ligament disruption between two connected carpal bones (injury to major intrinsic ligament), with or without an associated bony disruption; for example, SLD ± a fracture of the scaphoid.[102,183,553] Nondissociative instabilities of the carpus include subluxations or incomplete dislocations of the entire carpus (radiocarpal subluxation or dislocation) that may be purely ligamentous (injury to major extrinsic ligament), but more commonly include a fragment of the distal radius.[183] These dislocations are frequently a palmar or dorsal Barton fracture-dislocation, or a radial styloid fracture-dislocation; for example, a chauffeur's fracture. DISI and VISI instabilities may be either dissociative or nondissociative depending on the degree of damage to the ligamentous connections of the proximal carpal row.

Static instability occurs when carpal malalignment and instability is found on standard PA and lateral radiographs of the wrist. With dynamic instability, carpal malalignment and instability is only apparent using specified clinical physical provocation tests and when stress radiographs are positive (normal standard radiographs). The term adaptive carpal instability relates to the development of carpal instability due a cause unrelated to the carpus; for example, carpal malalignment following a severe malunion of a distal radius fracture.

Perilunate Dislocation and Fracture-Dislocation

Perilunate dislocations and fracture-dislocation predominantly follow a high-energy mechanism of hyperextension, ulnar deviation, and intercarpal supination injury to the wrist.[301–304] There are rare cases of reversed perilunate instability, when the wrist is pronated at the time of impact thus adding an external force to the hypothenar region, forcing the wrist into extension and radial deviation. For these cases the lunotriquetral ligament injury occurs first and the scapholunate ligament may remain intact.[274,384]

Perilunate dislocations can be subdivided into two subgroups:[239,324]

1. *Lesser-arc perilunate dislocations:* Pure ligamentous injuries around the lunate
2. *Greater-arc perilunate dislocations:* Ligamentous injuries associated with a fracture of one or more of the bones around the lunate

Mayfield suggested that carpal instability predominantly occurs in relation to the lunate, which is the carpal keystone.[301–304] He put forward a pathoanatomic classification associated with progressive perilunate instability from a radial to ulnar direction (Fig. 31-10).

- Stage I: Scaphoid fracture, SLD, or both
  - As the distal carpal row is violently extended, supinated, and ulnarly deviated, the scaphotrapezium-trapezoid and scaphocapitate ligaments are tightened causing the

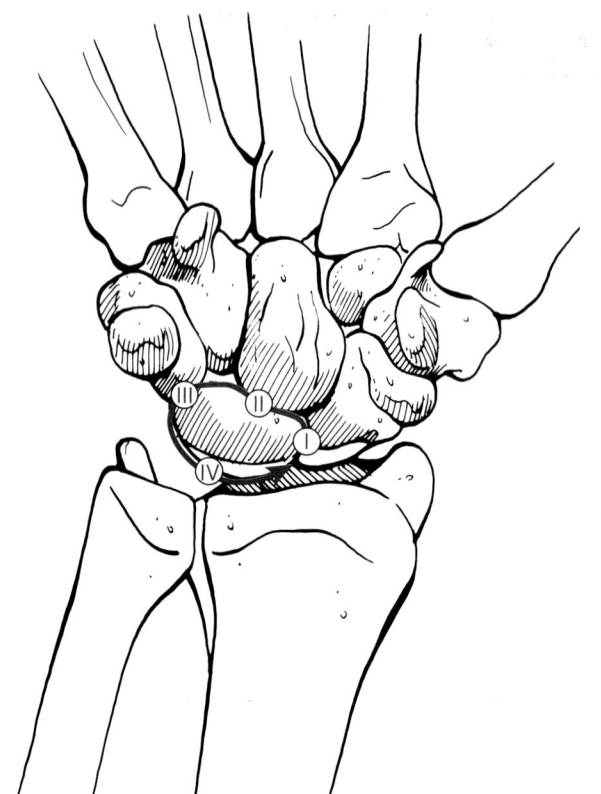

FIGURE 31-10 The Mayfield stages of progressive perilunate instability. Stage I results in SL instability. Stages II to IV result in progressively worse perilunate instability.

scaphoid to extend. As the scaphoid extends, the scapholunate ligament transmits the force to the lunate, which cannot rotate as much as the scaphoid because it is constrained by the palmarly located radiolunate and ulnolunate ligaments. As a consequence, a scaphoid fracture or a progressive elongation and tearing of the scapholunate and palmar RSC ligaments may occur, potentially leading to complete SLD.

- Stage II: Lunocapitate disruption
  - If the extension-supination force on the wrist persists once the proximal carpal row has been dislocated, transmission of the force distally to the capitate may lead to displacement and eventual dislocation dorsally through the space of Poirier. It is followed by the rest of the distal carpal row and the radial-most portion of the dislocated proximal carpal row. This may be the complete scaphoid or just its distal fragment.

- Stage III: Lunotriquetral disruption
  - If the extension-supination force to the wrist persists, once the capitate is displaced dorsally lunotriquetral (most common), ulnotriquetral, and/or triquetrum-hamate-capitate ligament disruptions may occur. Stage III is complete when the palmar lunotriquetral ligament, including the medial expansions of the long radiolunate ligament, is completely disrupted and the joint has displaced.

- Stage IV: Perilunate dislocation
    - If the extension-supination force to the wrist persists and the dorsally displaced capitate is pulled proximally, pressure is applied onto the dorsal aspect of the lunate, forcing it to dislocate in a palmar direction due to injury to the DRC ligament. As the palmar ligaments are much stronger than the dorsal capsule such a dislocation seldom involves a pure palmar displacement of the lunate, but rather a variable degree of palmar rotation of the bone into the carpal tunnel using the intact palmar ligaments as a hinge.

Lunate dislocation is the end stage of progressive perilunate dislocation. Along with ligamentous disruptions, fractures of the radial styloid, scaphoid, capitate, and the ulnar styloid can occur.

EPIDEMIOLOGY OF CARPAL FRACTURES AND DISLOCATIONS

When compared to fractures of the distal radius and hand, fractures of the carpus are uncommon, particularly those injuries not involving the scaphoid. There are minimal data documenting the global epidemiology of these injuries. The majority of literature is in relation to the epidemiology of scaphoid fractures, which is discussed later. An issue with many of the epidemiological studies in this area is that the majority of the data is collected retrospectively leading to inaccuracies in diagnosis and classification. Furthermore, many studies are performed within specific patient populations; for example, military, leading to wide ranging results regarding incidence, age, gender, and modes of injury.

Carpal Fractures

Using data that is presented in Chapter 3 on fracture epidemiology from the Edinburgh 2010 to 2011 database, carpal fractures are relatively frequent accounting for 2.8% of all fractures with an annual incidence of $37.5/10^5$ population per year. From the early 1900s Stimson[462] quoted a prevalence for carpal fractures of 0.2% of all fractures, although he acknowledged that the number of carpal fractures, particularly those of the scaphoid, was probably higher. Data from the past 60 years is consistent, with a prevalence ranging from 2% to 3% of all fractures.[107,148]

The mean age at the time of injury for all carpal fractures ranges from 35 to 40 years and a male predominance is seen.[218,227,507] Overall, fractures of the carpus have a type A fracture curve (Chapter 3) with a bimodal distribution involving younger males and older females. A fall from standing height accounts for almost two-thirds of all injuries, with other modes of injury including sports, direct blow, assault, and motor vehicle collision (MVC).[218,227,507]

It is consistently documented that scaphoid fractures and fractures of the triquetrum account for over 90% of all carpal fractures, with injuries to the hamate, pisiform, lunate, capitate, trapezium, and trapezoid being rare.[218,227,507] Fractures of the scaphoid, hamate, pisiform, and trapezium appear to occur predominantly in younger males, with the mean age ranging from 29 to 43 years and a male predominance ranging from 66% to 100%. These data are consistent with a type B fracture distribu-

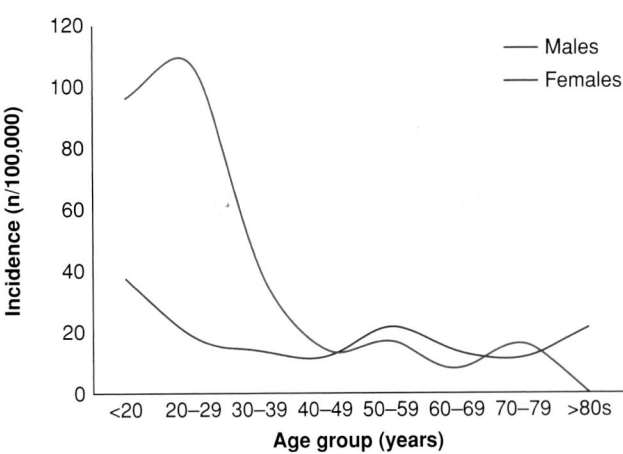

FIGURE 31-11 A type B fracture distribution curve for fractures of the scaphoid as seen in Edinburgh from 2007 to 2008. (Reprinted with permission from: *J Trauma Acute Care Surg.* 2012;72(2): E41–E45.)

tion curve (Fig. 31-11). Triquetral fractures appear to be a different fracture to other fractures of the carpus, occurring at a mean age of 51 years with an approximately equal gender distribution, thus most closely fitting a type A fracture distribution curve. One study analyzed the epidemiology of scaphoid fractures against that of the other carpal fractures and found youth and male gender to be associated with a fracture of the scaphoid.[218]

Injuries Associated with Carpal Fractures and Dislocations

Associated injuries are seen in approximately 7% of cases, with a fracture of the proximal or distal radius accounting for over 90% of all associated fractures. One study has demonstrated that of all patients with a carpal fracture only 7% sustain multiple carpal fractures, with almost half of these perilunate fracture-dislocations and over 90% involving a fracture to the scaphoid.[218] Work from Edinburgh on dislocations has demonstrated that perilunate dislocations have an incidence of $0.5/10^5$ population per year, occurring at a mean age of 26 years, and are frequently seen in males. Two studies have demonstrated that high-energy mechanisms are a risk factor for sustaining an associated injury following a fracture of the carpus.[136,218] Open carpal fractures are noted to be rare,[106,218] with only one documented in a 15-year study of 2,386 open fractures.[106]

DIAGNOSIS OF CARPAL INJURIES

Mechanism of Injury of Carpal Fractures and Dislocations

An injury to the carpus commonly occurs following a mechanism in which an axial compression force is applied to the wrist, commonly leading to hyperextension where the palmar ligaments undergo tension and the dorsal articulations are subject to shear stresses.[255,279,302,529] Given this, the most common mode of injury is a fall on the outstretched hand when an individual straightens the arm for protection and the body mass and external forces are placed across the wrist joint. Less common mechanisms occur when a forced is applied across the wrist when it is in palmar flexion. Most carpal instabilities, in particular perilunate dislocations, occur as a consequence of a high-energy injury; for example, a fall from a height on the outstretched hand or a motor vehicle accident.

Clinical Assessment and Diagnosis of Carpal Injuries

Patients with an injury to the carpus will commonly have wrist pain as their primary presenting complaint. Clinical examination uses a combination of clinical signs along with special tests to help determine the diagnosis; however, pain, swelling, and ecchymosis around the region of the carpus may be present in the acute phase. A full examination of the contralateral wrist can often be helpful, particularly when assessing for instability. The most constant and dependable sign of carpal injury is well-localized tenderness.[56,173]

- Anatomical snuffbox (ASB): Scaphoid injury

- Distal to Lister tubercle: Scapholunate and lunate injuries

- Dorsal margin, fingerbreadth distal to the ulnar head: Triquetral, lunotriquetral ligament and triquetrohamate ligament injuries

Changes in alignment of the hand, wrist, and forearm may be clinically evident on inspection of the extremity. Swelling over the proximal carpal row is suggestive of a ligament avulsion with or without an associated fracture. With carpal instability and/or dislocation a gross deformity may be apparent; for example, a marked prominence of the entire carpus dorsally is suggestive of a perilunate dislocation. Compressive stresses applied actively or passively may produce pain at the site of damage and cause a palpable and audible snap, click, shift, catch, or clunk, which may also be appreciated on movement of the wrist. Stress loading the wrist with compression and motion from radial to ulnar deviation may simulate midcarpal instability (MCI) and produce a "catch-up clunk" as the proximal row of carpal bones snap from flexion to extension. It should be noted that tendon displacements with audible snaps are easily produced in some patients but are seldom symptomatic. Despite poor diagnostic performance characteristics due to the rarity of these injuries, the following special tests are proposed as aids to the diagnosis of carpal ligament injury.

- Scaphoid shift test (Fig. 31-12)[370,523,528,547,548]
  - Pressure applied over scaphoid tubercle, wrist moving from radial to ulnar deviation
  - Positive if there is a "clunk" as the scaphoid subluxes dorsally out of the scaphoid fossa (up to 30% of normal wrists have positive test)[140]
  - Diagnostic of scapholunate disruption
- Midcarpal shift test[153,276]
  - Pressure applied over dorsum of the capitate, wrist moving from radial to ulnar deviation
  - Positive if there is a "clunk" as the lunate reduces from the palmar-flexed position
  - Diagnostic of MCI

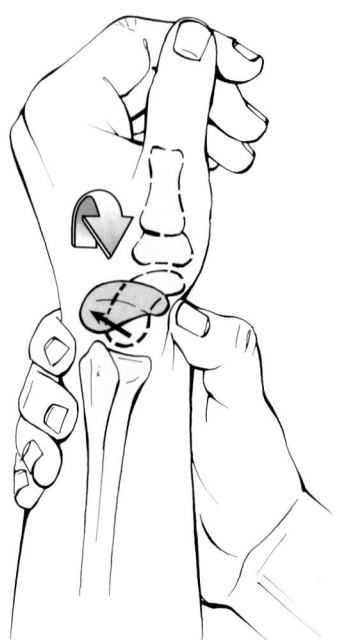

FIGURE 31-12 The scaphoid shift test: Pressure is applied to the palmar aspect of the scaphoid tubercle while moving the wrist from an ulnar to radial deviation.

- Lunotriquetral ballottement[384]
  - Lunate fixed with the thumb and index finger of one hand while the triquetrum is displaced palmarly and dorsally with the thumb of the other hand
  - Positive if painful
  - Diagnostic of lunotriquetral instability or arthritis
- Lunotriquetral shear test
  - Dorsally directed pressure to the pisiform (directly palmar to the triquetrum) and a palmarly directed pressure to the lunate (just distal to the palpable dorsoulnar corner of the distal radius)
  - Positive if results in reproducing patients pain along with palpable crepitation or clicking
  - Diagnostic of lunotriquetral instability

Imaging for Carpal Fractures and Dislocations
Radiographs

The four standard views commonly employed in the assessment of scaphoid fractures can be used to detect most injuries to the carpus.[85,170] These include neutral posteroanterior (PA) and lateral radiographs, along with a 45-degree radial oblique and a 45-degree ulnar oblique views (Fig. 31-13). Additional extension and flexion views are advocated for detecting intercarpal ligament injury, along with a clenched fist and stress views.[183] Some authors also advocate contralateral wrist views because of the wide range of normal alignment. The standard neutral PA and lateral radiographs are useful for determining the presence of clear fractures and assessing carpal alignment, but are often poor for scaphoid fracture detection due to the tubercle overhang on the PA and the overlap on the lateral.[96]

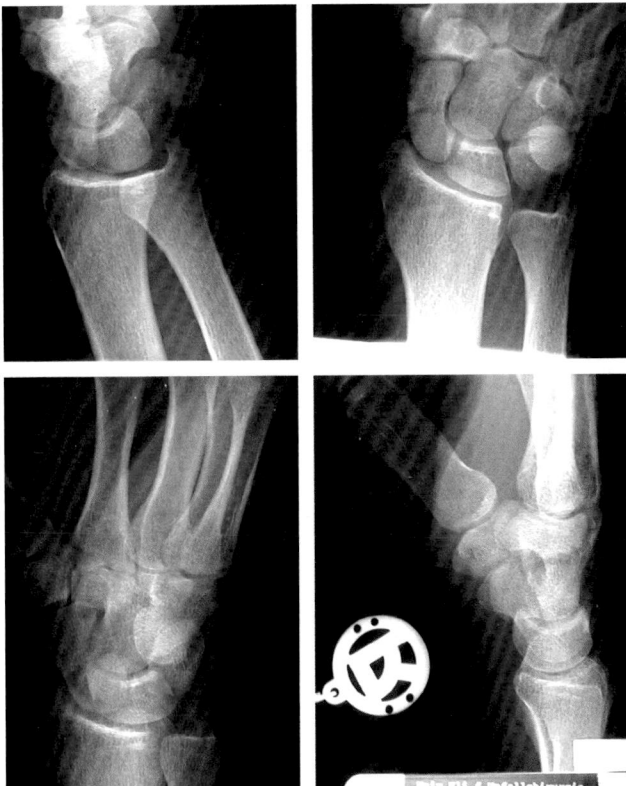

FIGURE 31-13 The four scaphoid views (PA, true lateral, radial oblique, ulnar oblique) detect most carpal fractures.

The 45-degree radial oblique, 45-degree ulnar oblique, ulnar deviated PA, Ziter (Fig. 31-14), and carpal box or tunnel views are purported to improve the ability to diagnose a fracture, particularly of the scaphoid, and are discussed later.[96,170,399,400,401,566] The VISI and DISI patterns of carpal malalignment are commonly detected using standard neutral lateral radiographs, with additional views in maximal radial and ulnar deviation if the diagnosis is in doubt.

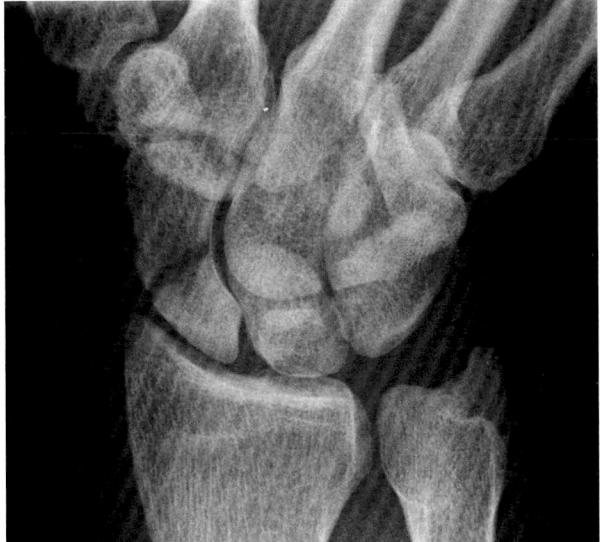

FIGURE 31-14 Ziter view is an additional image that can aid in the diagnosis of scaphoid fractures.

For the normal carpus with the wrist and hand in a neutral position, in the coronal (PA) plane a line drawn through the axis of rotation parallel with the anatomic axis of the forearm will pass through the head and base of the third metacarpal, the capitate, the radial aspect of the lunate, and the center of the lunate fossa of the radius.[306,563] In the sagittal (lateral) plane with the wrist and hand in a neutral position, a line will pass through the longitudinal axis of the index finger metacarpal, capitate, lunate, and the radius, with the scaphoid lying on an axis at a 45-degree angle to this line.[306,563] Standard radiographs should demonstrate a constant space between the scaphoid, lunate, and triquetrum throughout the range of wrist motion. Knowledge of these facts can aid in the diagnosis of carpal fracture displacement, instability, and collapse:

- Intercarpal, carpometacarpal, and radiocarpal joint spaces (neutral PA view)
  - Assessment of joint space between the individual carpal bones, the carpal bones and the metacarpals, and the carpal bones and radius
  - Space is normally ≤2 mm, with ligament disruption suspected at >3 mm and often diagnostic at >5 mm
  - Clenched fist views can accentuate the gap if equivocal
- Gilula lines (Fig. 31-15) (neutral PA view)[193]
  - Arc 1 runs along the proximal articular surface of the proximal carpal row
  - Arc 2 runs along the distal articular surface of the proximal carpal row
  - Arc 3 runs along the proximal cortical margins of the capitate and hamate
  - Three carpal arcs that produce smooth curves when drawn, with a broken arc diagnostic of a fracture and/or instability, particularly perilunate fracture dislocations
  - With lunotriquetral dissociation, an intercarpal gap may not be seen but a break in the normal carpal arc of the proximal carpal row is evident
- Carpal-height ratio = carpal height/length of third metacarpal (neutral PA view) (Fig. 31-16)
  - One method of measuring carpal height is to measure the distance between the base of the third metacarpal to the subchondral sclerotic line of the articular surface of the distal radius. The line should bisect the middle of the radius and metacarpal.
  - Used to quantify carpal collapse with the normal ratio 50% (45% to 60%) and less than 45% indicative of carpal collapse
  - One study has suggested gender specific normal values[520]
  - Limited diagnostic value for carpal instability
  - Alternate method uses height of the capitate instead of the third metacarpal[348]
- Inter- and intracarpal angles (neutral lateral view) (Table 31-4)
  - Scapholunate angle (normal 45 degrees, range 30 to 60)
    - Angle created by the longitudinal axes of the scaphoid and the lunate (Fig. 31-17)

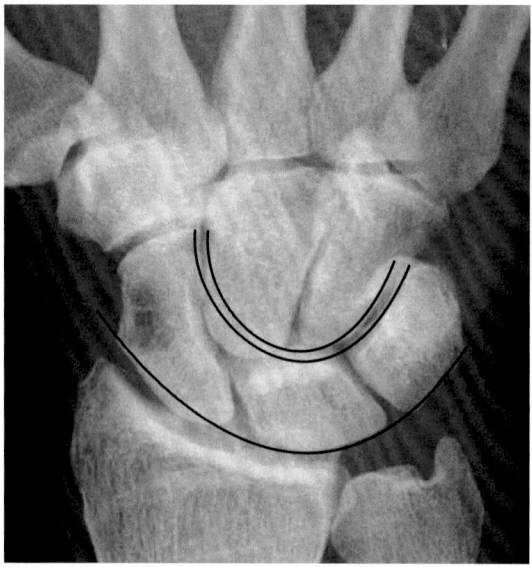 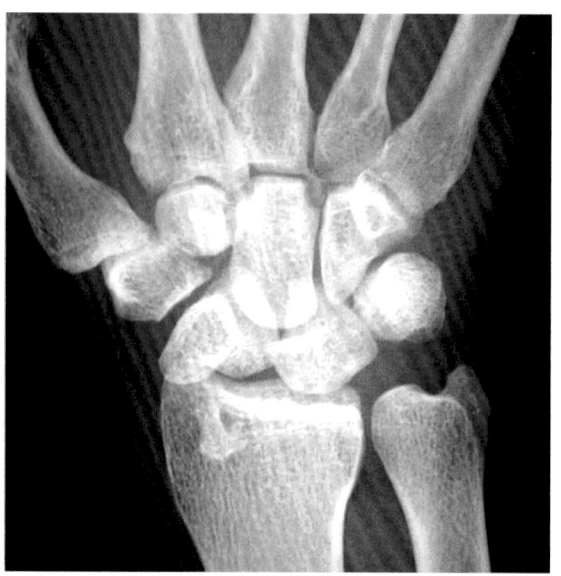

FIGURE 31-15 Gilula lines. **A:** AP views show three smooth Gilula arcs in a normal wrist. These arcs outline proximal and distal surfaces of the proximal carpal row and the proximal cortical margins of capitate and hamate. **B:** Arc I is broken, which indicates an abnormal lunotriquetral joint due to a peri-lunate dislocation. Additional findings are the cortical ring sign produced by the cortical outline of the distal pole of the scaphoid and a trapezoidal shape of the lunate.

- Long axis of the scaphoid is a line tangential to the palmar convex surfaces of the proximal and distal poles of the scaphoid
- Long axis of the lunate is a line perpendicular to the line connecting the dorsal and palmar lips of the lunate
- DISI pattern greater than 60 degrees, VISI pattern when less than 30 degrees; greater than 80 degrees is diagnostic of carpal (scapholunate) instability[183,277]

- Capitolunate angle (normal <15 degrees): Greater than 15 to 20 degrees is suggestive of carpal instability (Fig. 31-9)
- Radiolunate angle (normal <15 degrees): Greater than 15 to 20 degrees is suggestive of carpal instability

Secondary Imaging Modalities

Secondary imaging modalities are predominantly used in the assessment of scaphoid fractures and the diagnosis of

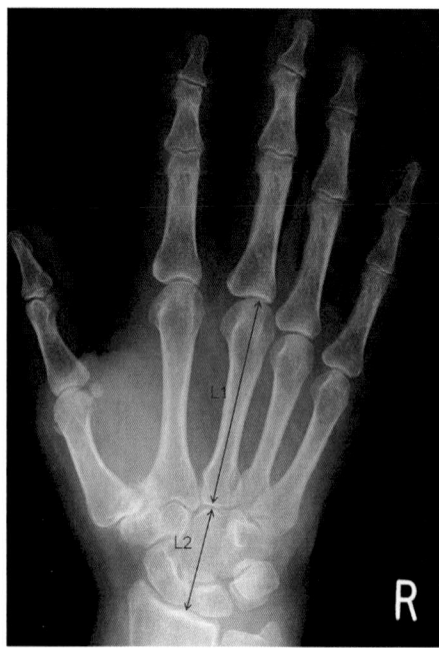

FIGURE 31-16 Carpal-height ratio, which is calculated by L2/L1.

TABLE 31-5	**Secondary Imaging Modalities for Carpal Injuries**
Modality	**Use(s)**
USS	Suspected carpal fractures, ligament injuries
CT (2D/3D)	Suspected carpal fractures, fracture displacement, malunion, nonunion, and bone loss
	3D imaging is useful in reconstructive procedures for malunions and nonunions
	Dynamic CT is used by some for ligament injuries
Bone scintigraphy	Suspected carpal fractures, avulsion injuries
Arthrography ± videofluoroscopy	Ligament injuries
MR imaging (MRI)	Suspected carpal fractures, AVN of carpal bones, ligament injuries
Wrist arthroscopy	Suspected carpal fractures, fracture displacement, ligament injuries

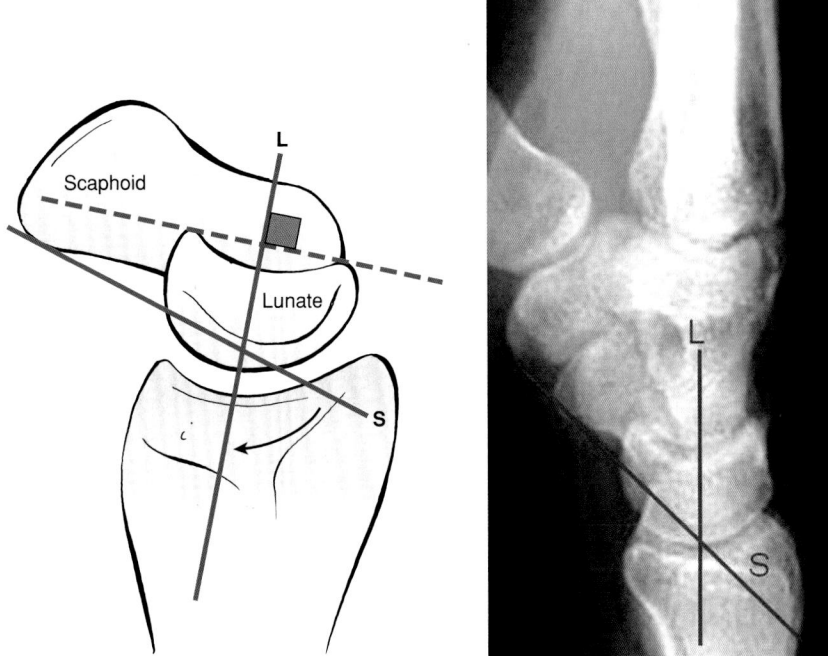

FIGURE 31-17 The scapholunate angle is created by the long axis of the scaphoid and a line perpendicular to the capitolunate joint.

intercarpal ligament injury and any associated instability (Table 31-5). For carpal fractures, further imaging is used for diagnosis, determining displacement, or in the assessment and management of malunions, nonunions, or bone loss. Detailed discussion of the use of secondary imaging modalities for fractures of the scaphoid is discussed in the scaphoid fracture section.

The following are measures of scaphoid fracture displacement, primarily assessed on CT and/or MR imaging:[18,30]

- Lateral intrascaphoid angle (normal 30 degrees ± 5 degrees; sagittal view)
  - Angle created by lines drawn perpendicular to the proximal and distal articular surfaces/poles of the scaphoid (Fig. 31-18A)

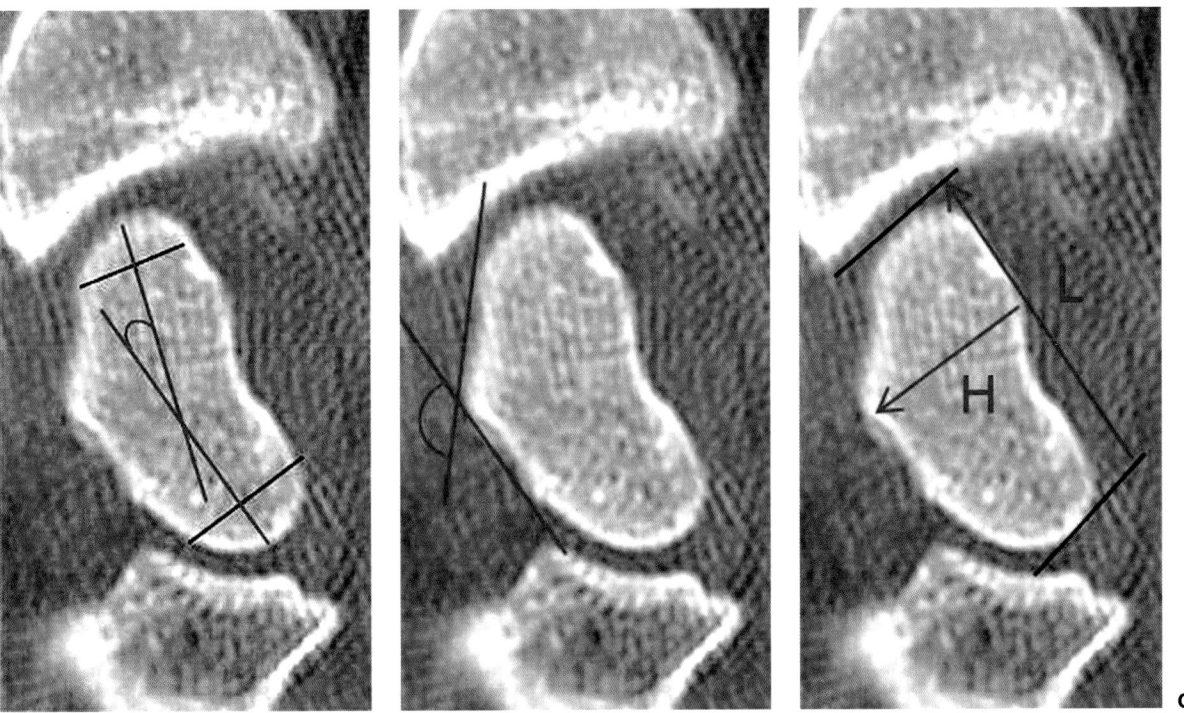

FIGURE 31-18 **A:** Lateral intrascaphoid angle measurement. **B:** Dorsal cortical angle measurement. **C:** Scaphoid height-to-length ratio measurement.

- An angle greater than 35 degrees is used as a cut-off for displacement[18]
- AP intrascaphoid angle (normal 40 degrees ± 5 degrees; coronal views)
  - Angle created by lines drawn perpendicular to the proximal and distal articular surfaces
- Dorsal cortical angle (normal 140 degrees, abnormal >160 degrees; sagittal view)
  - Angle created by tangential lines drawn along the dorsal cortices of the proximal and distal scaphoid fragments (Fig. 31-18B)
- Scaphoid height-to-length ratio (normal 0.60, abnormal >0.65; sagittal view)
  - Ratio of the lines measuring the height and length of the scaphoid
  - The length is determined by a palmar line drawn from the most proximal to the most distal edge of the scaphoid (Fig. 31-18C)
  - The height is the maximal point with a line perpendicular to the length line

Bain et al.[30] determined the intra- and interobserver reliability of the lateral intrascaphoid angle to be poor and poor to moderate respectively, the dorsal cortical angle to be moderate to excellent for both, and the height-to-length ratio was excellent and moderate to excellent respectively.

Diagnosis of Carpal Injuries: Pearls and Pitfalls

- Standard scaphoid radiographic views detect most carpal injuries
- DISI pattern is most commonly associated with displaced scaphoid fractures and SLD
- Perilunate dislocations can be missed
- Assessment of Gilula's line can aid in the diagnosis of perilunate dislocations
- CT is useful in the diagnosis of suspected carpal fractures and assessment of union
- MRI is useful in detecting suspected fractures and AVN of the carpus
- Wrist arthroscopy can be used as an aid to the diagnosis of ligament injuries and fracture displacement

SCAPHOID FRACTURES

The name scaphoid comes from the Greek word *"skaphos"* meaning boat, a reference to the shape of the bone.[173] Acute scaphoid fractures were first described by Cousin and Destot in 1889, with subsequent descriptions by Mouchet and Jeanne in 1919.[173] The position of the scaphoid on the radial side of the wrist, as the proximal extension of the thumb ray, makes it vulnerable to injury.

Some nondisplaced fractures of the scaphoid are not visible on radiographs taken at the time of injury (occult scaphoid fracture). Patients with radial-sided wrist pain and tenderness after a fall are often suspected of having an occult scaphoid fracture. The suspected scaphoid fracture remains a problematic clinical scenario despite advances in both knowledge and radiologic imaging. The mind-set and thrust of research in recent years has been aimed to find the optimal radiological test so that no fractures are missed, and to establish an early definitive diagnosis thus limiting immobilization, restrictions, and the number of further clinical assessments.[132,168,194,209,235,307,490,506] However, despite advocates for the various secondary imaging modalities, a clear answer to the problem has not emerged.

Displaced, comminuted, and unstable fractures of the scaphoid are routinely managed with surgical intervention. Much of the current controversy surrounds the undisplaced or minimally displaced acute fractures. Current opinion is that patients with undisplaced fractures of the scaphoid need protection and cast immobilization for 6 to 12 weeks, accounting for a considerable loss of time and productivity in a predominantly young and active population.[31,171,307,404,405] Advocates for early operative intervention claim that screw fixation not only limits the need for a cast, but may also allow earlier return to sports and work.[66,307,368,560]

Clinical Anatomy of Scaphoid Fractures

The scaphoid bone is located in the proximal carpal row on the radial aspect of the wrist and is a small irregular S-shaped tubular bone.[44,67,71] It lies entirely within the wrist joint and is located at a 45-degree plane to the longitudinal and horizontal axes of the wrist. It has a reduced capacity for periosteal healing and an increased tendency for delayed union and nonunion because just over 80% of its surface is articular cartilage.

The scaphoid is ridged across its nonarticular dorsoradial surface, along which the critical dorsal ridge vessels traverse. The ridge is the insertion point for both the dorsal component of the scapholunate ligament (Table 31-2) and the intercarpal ligament (Table 31-1). The distal pole is pronated, flexed, and ulnarly angulated with respect to the proximal pole. Articulations are with the trapezium/trapezoid (distal surface), radius (proximal/lateral surface), capitate (medial surface), and lunate (medial surface).[44,67,71]

The ligamentous attachments of the scaphoid are predominantly found on the nonarticular dorsoradial surface. The short intrinsic ligaments provide stability to the scaphoid through attachments to the other carpal bones, in particular the lunate, and merge with the extrinsic ligaments and capsule of the wrist.[43,44,46,53,67,71,300,476] The RSC ligament does not attach to the bone itself but crosses the waist, acting as a sling across it and allowing it to rotate.[43,44,46,251,425,430–432,449,476] There are no tendon attachments to the scaphoid.[283] Through these articulations and soft tissue attachments the scaphoid acts as a midcarpal joint "bridge" linking and synchronizing the motions of the proximal and distal carpal rows as part of the key intercalated segment.[44,246,247,434,530] Motion of the scaphoid includes rotation proximally and gliding distally, while providing stability to the midcarpal joint.

Vascular Supply

The potential for nonunion of the scaphoid is often ascribed to the meager, largely retrograde blood supply

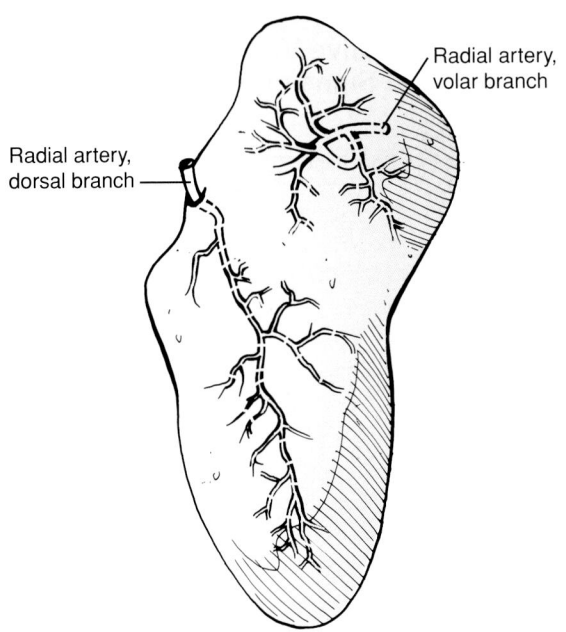

FIGURE 31-19 The vascular supply of the scaphoid is provided by two vascular pedicles.

(Table 31-3),[57,164,185,186,366,474] through soft tissue attachments via two vascular pedicles originating from the scaphoid branches of the radial artery (Fig. 31-19).[44,185,186,366]

- Dorsal branch: Enters via the small foramina along the spiral groove and dorsal ridge of the scaphoid and supplies 70% to 80% of the scaphoid proximally, including the proximal pole.

- Volar branch: Enters via the scaphoid tubercle and supplies the remaining 20% to 30% of distal scaphoid.

It should be noted that the waist of the scaphoid has been shown to have minimal or no perforating vasculature.[185] Furthermore, no vessels perforate the proximal dorsal cartilaginous area or through the scapholunate ligament.[164] For the detailed pathoanatomy of injury please see Page 999.

Epidemiology and Etiology of Scaphoid Fractures

Acute scaphoid fractures account for 2% to 3% of all fractures, approximately 10% of all hand fractures and between 60% and 80% of all carpal fractures.[173,226,270] The incidence of scaphoid fractures quoted in the literature is inconsistent with a range from 1.5 to 121 fractures per 100,000 persons per year.[136,226,242,270,506,509,546,558] It is most probable that the wide variation documented is due to the use of predominantly retrospective data, analysis of specific patient populations; for example, military, as well as the limitation of many large datasets to distinguish between a true and suspected fracture.[226,242,270,506,509,546,558] The lower quoted incidences appear to be more in keeping given that the average incidence of fractures of the distal radius is 195 per 100,000 population per year.[107,509] A recent study from Edinburgh documented the epidemiology of true radiographically confirmed acute fractures of the scaphoid in a defined adult population using a prospective dataset and found an annual incidence of 29 per 100,000 per year,[136] which is consistent with previous studies from Scandinavia quoting an annual incidence of 26 to 39 per 100,000 per year.[242,270] The mean age in the literature ranges from 25 to 35 years, with males significantly younger at the time of injury compared to females suggesting scaphoid fractures most closely fit a type B fracture distribution curve (Fig. 31-11). A male predominance is seen with a male-to-female ratio of approximately 2.5:1.[136,226,242,270,506,509,546,558] Two studies have documented male sex as a risk factor associated with a true fracture.[135,235]

Scaphoid fractures usually occur after a fall on to the outstretched hand or during sports,[136,235,270,509] with two studies reporting that sports injuries are associated with a true fracture.[135,235] One study has documented that a low-energy fall from standing height has been shown to occur more frequently in females, with males more likely to sustain their fracture after a high-energy injury such as sports or a motor vehicle collision.[136] This is in keeping with the younger age at which fracture occurs in males. Sports noted to cause increased risk include football, basketball, cycling, and skateboarding depending on the study origin.[136,509] Fractures of the scaphoid are being increasingly documented after punching or assault-related injuries.[224,468]

An exact understanding of the epidemiology and etiology of fractures of the scaphoid is essential when considering the diagnosis of the suspected scaphoid fracture, in particular the use of further imaging modalities such as CT or MRI. Given the increasing evidence for earlier return to function following fixation of the scaphoid,[66,307] it is important to consider that the population affected is predominantly young and active, with these patients more frequently sustaining unstable injuries.

Scaphoid Fractures Clinical Assessment and Diagnosis

The diagnosis of a fracture to the scaphoid is made by a combination of clinical history, examination, and radiographic assessment. Patients classically present with wrist pain following a fall onto the outstretched hand, with almost 90% recalling a hyperextension injury. Clinical examination uses a combination of clinical signs (Table 31-6). Generally pain, swelling, ecchymosis, and tenderness around the region of the scaphoid may be present in the acute phase. Standard four-view radiographs are subsequently used to confirm the diagnosis.

However, up to 30% to 40% of scaphoid fractures are not identified on initial assessment and investigation with standard four-view radiographs and are thus classified as having a suspected fracture.[31,62,170,172,173,255,393,505,517] Patients who are subsequently found to have a fracture confirmed on repeated assessment and radiologic imaging, most frequently at 10 to 14 days post injury, are said to have had an occult fracture of the scaphoid.[23,60,168,170,261,311,393] In these cases, the treating surgeon must balance employing immobilization and restriction of activities in a predominantly young and active population against the risks of nonunion and arthrosis associated with an undiagnosed and untreated scaphoid fracture.[104,250,405]

Symptoms

Patients present with a history of hyperextension to the wrist, often following a fall, sports, or punch injury. It is important to determine a history of previous trauma to the scaphoid and not

TABLE 31-6 **The Sensitivity, Specificity, Positive Predictive Value and Negative Predictive Value of Clinical Signs of Scaphoid Fractures**

	Sensitivity (%)	PPV (%)	Specificity (%)	NPV (%)
ASB tenderness	100	30	19	100
Scaphoid tubercle tenderness	100	34	30	100
Longitudinal thumb compression	100	40	48	100
Reduced thumb movement	66	41	66	85
ASB swelling	61	50	52	58
ASB pain in ulnar deviation/pronation	83	44	17	56
ASB pain in radial deviation/pronation	70	45	31	56
Pain on thumb/index pinch	48	44	31	41
Scaphoid shift (Kirk-Watson) test	66	49	31	69

PPV, positive predictive value; NPV, negative predictive value; ASB, Anatomical snuffbox.

treat a nonunion as if it is an acute fracture. The main complaint is of radial-sided wrist pain, with localized tenderness over the scaphoid in the region of the ASB.

Signs

No single sign has been found to be adequately sensitive or specific (Table 31-6).[150,167,200,350,371,376,505,517] The first studies in this area analyzed the sensitivity and specificity of the classic individual clinical signs. ASB tenderness is over sensitive and has poor specificity. In a study of 246 patients with a suspected fracture of the scaphoid, ASB tenderness was found to have a sensitivity of 90% and a specificity of 40%, with scaphoid tubercle tenderness having a sensitivity of 87% and specificity of 57%.[167] From another study that performed a prospective analysis of 73 patients with a suspected scaphoid fracture, the sensitivity and specificity of ASB pain on ulnar deviation of the pronated wrist was calculated.[376] That individual sign had a negative predictive value (NPV) of 100% and the authors concluded that patients with a negative test could be safely discharged at presentation as they did not have a scaphoid fracture.

Further studies aimed to improve the diagnostic performance characteristics, in particular specificity of the clinical signs, by combining them. Parvizi et al.[371] performed a prospective study of 215 consecutive patients and demonstrated that the use of one clinical sign in isolation was insufficient for the diagnosis of a fracture, but that a combination of ASB tenderness, scaphoid tubercle tenderness, and ASB pain on longitudinal compression of the thumb generated a sensitivity of 100% and a specificity of 74%. However, these findings were only valid for the first 24 hours after injury.

Recent studies have examined alternative clinical signs as predictors of a fracture of the scaphoid. Unay et al. analyzed 10 clinical examination maneuvers on 41 patients with suspected scaphoid fractures and used MRI to determine the presence or absence of a fracture. They demonstrated that pain on thumb-index finger pinch and ASB pain on pronation of the forearm

were most suggestive of a true scaphoid fracture.[505] Duckworth et al.[135] determined that the best predictors of fracture within 72 hours of injury were the absence of pain on ulnar deviation of the wrist and pain on thumb-index finger pinch, with scaphoid tubercle tenderness most predictive at week two.

Radiographs

Neutral PA and lateral radiographic views are useful for ascertaining carpal alignment and the assessment of perilunate fracture-dislocations; however, they are poor at fracture detection, particularly with the tubercle overhang found on the neutral PA view.[85,96] Views suggested to improve the ability to diagnose a scaphoid fracture are demonstrated in Table 31-7.[85,96,170,566]

Ziter view, or the "banana view," uses a PA view of the wrist in ulnar deviation with 20-degree tube angulation to the elbow (Fig. 31-14).[566] This modified view can aid in the identification of scaphoid waist fractures, although fractures oblique to the beam are not well identified. Carpal box views have been shown to increase agreement in the interpretation of the

TABLE 31-7 **Additional Radiographic Views Used in the Assessment of Scaphoid Fractures**

Radiologic View	Advantages
Ulnar-deviated	Detection of proximal pole fractures
45-degree ulnar oblique (semipronated)	Detection of oblique sulcal, waist (in particular displacement), and tubercle fractures
45-degree radial oblique (semisupinated)	Detection of proximal pole fractures, humpback deformities, and avulsion fractures
Ziter view	Detection of waist fractures as beam at right angles to long axis

standard four-view scaphoid radiographs from 36% to 55%, although they are not routinely utilized.[400,401] Some authors also suggest comparative views of the contralateral uninjured wrist can aid in the diagnosis of the suspected fracture.[1]

Some studies have suggested that when clinical and radiographical assessment is carried out by experienced surgeons, all suspected scaphoid fractures can be detected within 6 weeks of injury.[31,170] However, the vast majority of the literature consistently indicates that up to 30% to 40% of scaphoid fractures are not identified on initial assessment and investigation with four-view radiographs.[31,62,170,172,173,255,393,505,517] Standard four-view scaphoid radiographs have been demonstrated to have low inter- and intraobserver reliability for the diagnosis of suspected scaphoid fractures.[491,492] Repeated radiologic assessment has been documented to have low sensitivity, with one study only detecting 50% of suspected scaphoid fractures.[172] Barton suggested three possible reasons why standard scaphoid radiographs are often misinterpreted.[31]

1. A dark line may be formed by the dorsal lip of the radius overlapping the scaphoid

2. The presence of a white line formed by the proximal end of the scaphoid tuberosity

3. The dorsal ridge of the scaphoid may appear bent on the semisupinated view

Soft tissue signs of a scaphoid fracture on plain radiographs include the scaphoid fat pad sign (distortion or loss of adjacent fat stripes over the radial aspect of the scaphoid on the PA view with the wrist in ulnar deviation) and the pronator fat pad/stripe sign (a prominent pronator quadrates fat pad over the volar aspect of the wrist on the lateral view). Although there are advocates for these soft tissue signs,[268] most have demonstrated them to be unreliable detectors for the presence of a suspected scaphoid fracture.[23,123] Given the difficulty with confidently diagnosing a scaphoid fracture on standard radiographs, when clinical suspicion is present but radiographs are negative, immobilization is recommended with repeat examination and radiographs performed within 10 to 14 days of injury. The delay may lessen both tenderness and anxiety leading to a better examination.

Ultrasound

Ultrasound is a noninvasive and relatively inexpensive technique for diagnosing scaphoid fractures; however, it is operator dependent and has been shown to be least effective in detecting true fractures with a sensitivity ranging from 37% to 93% and a specificity ranging from 61% to 91%.[88,110,235,337,423] There are advocates for the use of high–spatial-resolution sonography for detecting the suspected scaphoid fracture, with the sensitivity rising up to 100% and the specificity as high as 91%.[168,214] Others have suggested it to be a useful precursor to further imaging modalities when used in the emergency department.[373]

Bone Scintigraphy

There are strong advocates for bone scintigraphy[34,35,490,491]; however, most authors feel that the specificity is too low when compared to both CT and MRI.[59,162,391,394,559] Beeres et al.[35] analyzed 100 patients with a suspected fracture and found bone scintig-

raphy had a sensitivity of 100% and a specificity of 90%, concluding that there was no advantage to MRI over this modality. Further work from this group found similar results when comparing CT with bone scintigraphy.[391] However, Fowler et al.[162] found in 43 patients with suspected scaphoid fractures that bone scintigraphy was inferior to MRI for both sensitivity and specificity, using 1-year follow-up as the reference standard.

CT

Many authors advocate the use of CT for diagnosing true fractures among suspected scaphoid fractures,[59,108,292,504,562] although some have cautioned against its use for undisplaced fractures.[3] In an analysis of 47 patients with a suspected scaphoid fracture, using 2-week radiographs and/or MRI as the reference standard, CT was found to be 94.4% sensitive and 100% specific with an NPV of 96.8% and a positive predictive value (PPV) of 100%.[198] CT has also been shown to be useful in detecting other injuries around the wrist, particularly in the acute assessment of the suspected fracture.[461,504] In a study of 28 patients with a suspected scaphoid fracture who underwent CT, undisplaced fractures of the distal radius or carpus were demonstrated in 36% of patients.[504] Stevenson et al. performed a retrospective analysis of 84 patients with suspected scaphoid fractures who underwent CT within 14 days of injury. Fifty-four scans were normal. Of the 30 abnormal scans the authors found that 7% were occult scaphoid fractures, 18% were occult carpal fractures (triquetrum, capitate, lunate), and 5% were distal radius fractures.[461] Overall, approximately one-third of CT scans for suspected scaphoid fractures found other wrist injuries.

To determine the intraobserver and interobserver reliability of CT for the diagnosis of an undisplaced scaphoid fracture, one study used eight observers to evaluate CT scans from 30 patients.[3] Although they found substantial intraobserver and interobserver reliability, they also noted a high false-positive rate, possibly from the misinterpretation of vascular channels as a unicortical fracture (Fig. 31-20). A very recent study has reported a kappa value of only 0.51 (moderate agreement) for the interobserver reliability among radiologists when using CT for the diagnosis of scaphoid fractures.[116]

MRI

For the suspected scaphoid fracture, MRI is argued to be the best investigation, although some institutions have limited access and there are inconsistencies regarding cost efficiency.[65,132,171,194,209,235,261,379,559] In a prospective blind study in which MRI scans were performed within 72 hours of injury in 32 patients with a suspected scaphoid fracture, it was found that the sensitivity and specificity of MRI were 100%, with potential savings of $7,200 per 100,000 of the population through avoiding unnecessary immobilization and review.[171] This study used clinical and/or radiographic follow-up at 6 weeks as their reference standard. A more recent randomized controlled trial allocated 84 patients with a suspected scaphoid fracture to early MRI and discharge if no injury, or to standard reassessment in clinic 10 to 14 days after injury.[372] They found no difference between the two groups in terms of mean management costs, pain, patient satisfaction, and time off work or sports.

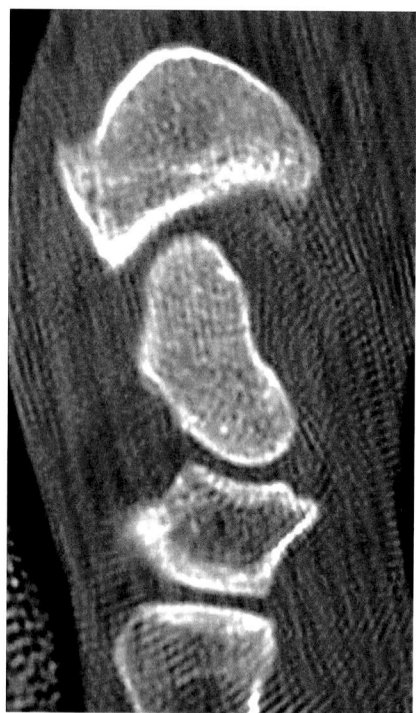

FIGURE 31-20 Sagittal CT slice demonstrating an undisplaced fracture of the scaphoid waist, although this could be mistaken for a vascular channel.

Although MRI is the most successful secondary imaging modality to date in terms of performance characteristics, in low prevalence situations the PPV has been found to be only 88% and recent work has documented the potential for false-positive MRI scans.[117] Ring and Lozano-Calderon[394] performed an analysis to determine the diagnostic performance characteristics of the various secondary imaging modalities utilized in the assessment of the suspected scaphoid fracture (Table 31-8). Using Bayesian formulae and an average published prevalence of scaphoid fractures among suspected fractures of 7%, the NPV for MRI was 88%, meaning that around 12% of patients with a suspected scaphoid fracture undergo an MRI that is interpreted as demonstrating a fracture when they may not actually have a fracture. A recent analysis of MRI scans in healthy individuals also highlighted the potential for false-positive MRI scans, with benign abnormalities diagnosed as fractures by numerous blinded radiologists.[117] This study concluded that MRI is not a suitable reference standard for true scaphoid fractures among patients with suspected fractures.

A prospective cohort study that again used 6-week radiographs as the reference standard demonstrated that CT and MRI had comparable diagnostic performance characteristics for detecting true fractures among suspected scaphoid fractures, with the PPV for CT being 76% compared to 54% for MRI.[292] This study also questioned whether or not bone edema on MRI and small unicortical lines on CT are diagnostic of a true scaphoid fracture. The rate of scaphoid bone bruising (Fig. 31-21) on MRI leading to occult fracture has been documented to be 2% in one study.[487]

Current Practice

Despite many advocates, the optimal imaging modality is not known. One paper has recently presented a meta-analysis of 26 studies to determine the prevalence adjusted diagnostic performance characteristics of bone scintigraphy, CT, and MRI for suspected scaphoid fractures.[559] Of the 26 studies, 9 used 6-week radiographic follow-up as their reference standard. Bone scintigraphy and MRI were shown to have comparable high sensitivity rates, though MRI was more specific (Table 31-9).

National guidelines of some professional associations, as well as advocates for MRI, suggest an overly optimistic assessment for its use. The Royal College of Radiologists (UK) recommends that on current evidence bone scintigraphy, CT, and MRI are comparable for triaging the suspected acute scaphoid fracture.[403] However, the American College of Radiology (ACR) concludes radiographs and MRI should be utilized.[19] An international survey of 105 hospitals worldwide was performed to determine their own imaging protocol for the suspected scaphoid fracture and reported a high rate of inconsistency among the hospitals with only 22% found to have a fixed protocol.[201]

TABLE 31-8 **The Sensitivity, Specificity, Accuracy as well as the Average Prevalence Adjusted PPV and NPV for Various Imaging Modalities as Determined by Ring et al. for Suspected Fractures of the Scaphoid**

Imaging Modality (Number of Studies Assessed)	Sensitivity (%)	Specificity (%)	Accuracy (%)	PPV	NPV
Ultrasound (n = 4)	93	89	92	0.38	0.99
Bone scintigraphy (n = 18)	96	89	93	0.39	0.99
CT (n = 8)	94	96	98	0.75	0.99
MRI (n = 22)	98	99	96	0.88	1.00

From Duckworth AD, Ring D, McQueen MM. Assessment of the suspected fracture of the scaphoid. *J Bone Joint Surg Br.* 2011;93-B(6):713–719.

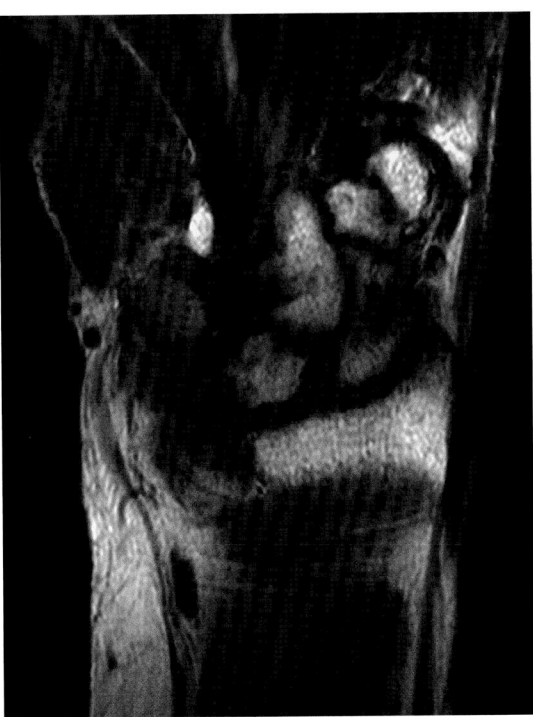

FIGURE 31-21 MRI demonstrating scaphoid bone bruising but no fracture.

Assessing Diagnostic Tests

Given the combination of oversensitive clinical signs and no consensus gold standard for diagnosing a scaphoid fracture, most patients with a suspected fracture of the scaphoid receive more protection and diagnostic testing than is required.[31,150,167,170,200,371,376] This can lead to issues with wrist stiffness and costs to both the healthcare system and the patient with time off work and sports in a predominantly young, healthy, and active patient group.[132,438,490,506]

It has been proposed that the assessment of the various diagnostic tests for the assessment of the suspected scaphoid

TABLE 31-9	The Sensitivity and Specificity as Determined by Yin et al. of Different Imaging Techniques in the Diagnosis of Occult Fractures of the Scaphoid		

Imaging Modality (Number of Studies Assessed)	Sensitivity (%)	Specificity (%)
Bone scintigraphy (n = 15)	97	89
CT (n = 6)	93	99
MRI (n = 10)	96	99

From Duckworth AD, Ring D, McQueen MM. Assessment of the suspected fracture of the scaphoid. *J Bone Joint Surg Br.* 2011;93-B(6):713–719; with data from Yin ZG, Zhang JB, Kan SL, et al. Diagnosing suspected scaphoid fractures: A systematic review and meta-analysis. *Clin Orthop Relat Res.* 2010;468:723–734.

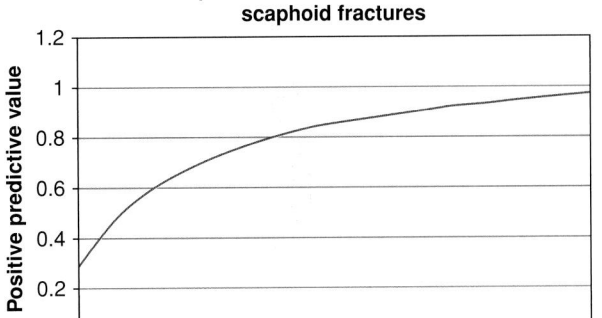

Positive predictive value of CT for suspected scaphoid fractures

FIGURE 31-22 The relationship between fracture prevalence and the positive predictive value of diagnostic tests, in this case, CT.

fracture must account for two important issues.[137,394] The first is the low prevalence of true fractures among suspected fractures, which greatly lowers the probability that a positive test will correspond with a true fracture as false positives are nearly as common as true positives.[3,137,226,235,255,270,390,394] Research has documented that between 5% and 20% of patients who attend the emergency department with a suspected scaphoid fracture are ultimately found to have a true fracture.[3,226,235,255,270,390,394] Given that false positives and false negatives are 5% to 10% for most diagnostic tests, this low prevalence of disease among assessed patients leads to low PPVs according to Bayes theorem even when the diagnostic test is both highly sensitive and specific (Fig. 31-22).[16,394]

The second issue relates to the fact that the calculation of the diagnostic performance characteristics (sensitivity, specificity, PPV and NPV, and accuracy) for the various imaging modalities using a traditional formula requires a consensus reference standard for the presence or absence of a fracture.[16,17] The most frequently used standard in the literature is the absence of a fracture on radiographs at 6 weeks post injury.[3,170,338,394,559] However, given the lack of consensus, an alternative method for calculating diagnostic performance characteristics based on a statistical method that identifies clinical factors that tend to associate (latent classes) in patients with a high probability of fracture is preferable.[3,338,394] This technique has been applied to the diagnosis of carpal tunnel syndrome,[263] as well as in two recently published studies on the assessment of the suspected scaphoid fracture.[72,135] These studies found small but potentially important differences between the results obtained using traditional formula and those obtained using latent class analysis.[72,135]

The upshot of the issues raised by the low prevalence and lack of consensus reference standard is that there will likely always be a small probability of missing a true fracture among suspected scaphoid fracture. If patients, doctors, and society can accept an approximate 1% chance of missing a true fracture, we may have adequate management strategies at the current time. It is not clear that imaging technology will improve these odds because better imaging has findings which are difficult to interpret. The best option might be to increase the pretest odds of a fracture before ordering advanced imaging, and this can be done by applying a clinical prediction rule to determine when to order further imaging.

Clinical Prediction Rules

The benefit of clinical prediction rules in medicine to guide, but not dictate, management of patients is well documented.[285,387] It has been suggested that an important step to improving the diagnostic performance characteristics of the various imaging modalities for the suspected scaphoid fracture would be to increase the prevalence of the true scaphoid fracture among suspected fractures through the development and promotion of clinical prediction rules.[137,394] These rules would incorporate a combination of demographic and clinical risk factors predictive of a true scaphoid fracture. Implementation of these rules could potentially increase the prevalence of true scaphoid fractures

among suspected fractures and subsequently allow the utilization of sophisticated secondary imaging in high risk patients, potentially leading to improved diagnostic performance characteristics of diagnostic imaging.

Two studies have demonstrated the potential of clinical prediction rules to improve the management of suspected scaphoid fractures. One study from Holland analyzed 78 patients with a suspected scaphoid fracture and determined using multivariate analysis that a reduction in extension of greater than 50%, supination strength of ≤10%, and the presence of a previous fracture were most predictive of a true fracture.[390] A recent prospective study from Edinburgh and Boston analyzed 223 patients with a clinically suspected or radiographically confirmed scaphoid fracture, using radiologic imaging at 6 weeks as their reference standard.[135] They demonstrated that risk factors for a true fracture were male gender, sports injury, ASB pain on ulnar

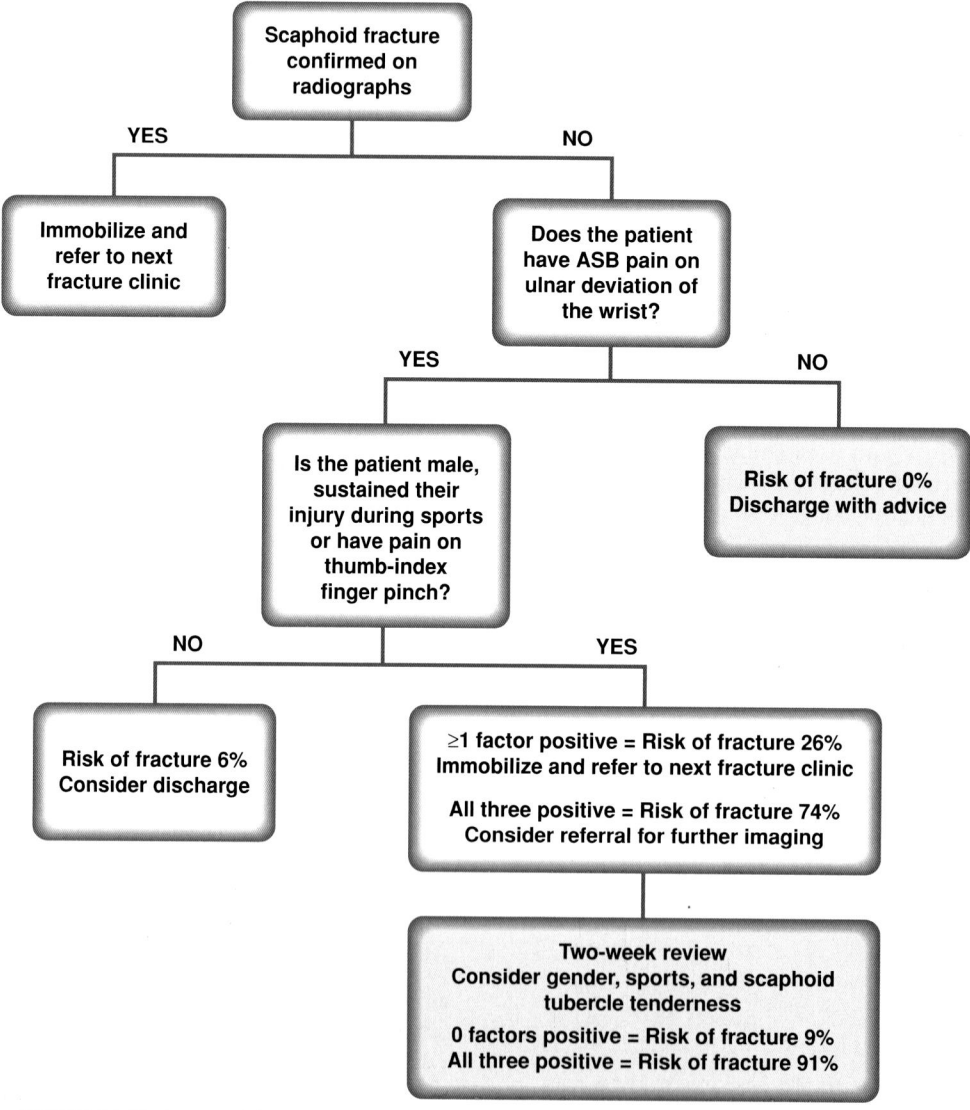

FIGURE 31-23 A potential management algorithm for suspected scaphoid fractures based on a clinical prediction rule developed by Duckworth et al. (Reprinted with permission from: *J Bone Joint Surg Br.* 2012;94(7):961–968, Figure 2.)

deviation of the wrist, and pain on thumb-index finger pinch at presentation, as well as persistent scaphoid tubercle tenderness at 2-week review. They incorporated these signs to develop clinical prediction rules that can guide assessment of these patients (Fig. 31-23). Ultimately, this study demonstrated that clinical prediction rules have a substantial and meaningful influence on the probability of a suspected scaphoid fracture.

Classification and Associated Injuries of Scaphoid Fractures

There are several classification systems available for fractures of the scaphoid. These include the following.

- Russe classification[407]
- AO classification
- Herbert and Fisher classification[211]
- Mayo classification[100]

The Russe classification predicts instability according to the inclination of the fracture line; for example, vertical oblique fractures. The AO classification breaks the fracture down into simple anatomic location (distal pole, waist, proximal pole) and comminution.

TABLE 31-10	The Prevalence of Different Herbert and Fisher Fracture Types of Acute Scaphoid Fractures	
Herbert Classification		**Prevalence (%)[136]**
Type A: Stable acute fractures		31.1
A1 (tuberosity)		14.6
A2 (unicortical waist)		16.5
Type B: Unstable acute fractures		68.9
B1 (distal oblique/pole)		21.2
B2 (complete waist)		36.4
B3 (proximal pole)		6
B4 (transscaphoid perilunate fracture dislocation)		2
B5 (comminuted)		3.3

Herbert and Fisher[211] proposed a classification intended to identify those fractures most applicable for operative fixation and is commonly used throughout the literature (Table 31-10 and Fig. 31-24). Type A fractures are stable fractures that often appear incomplete (unicortical), are associated with good union rates,

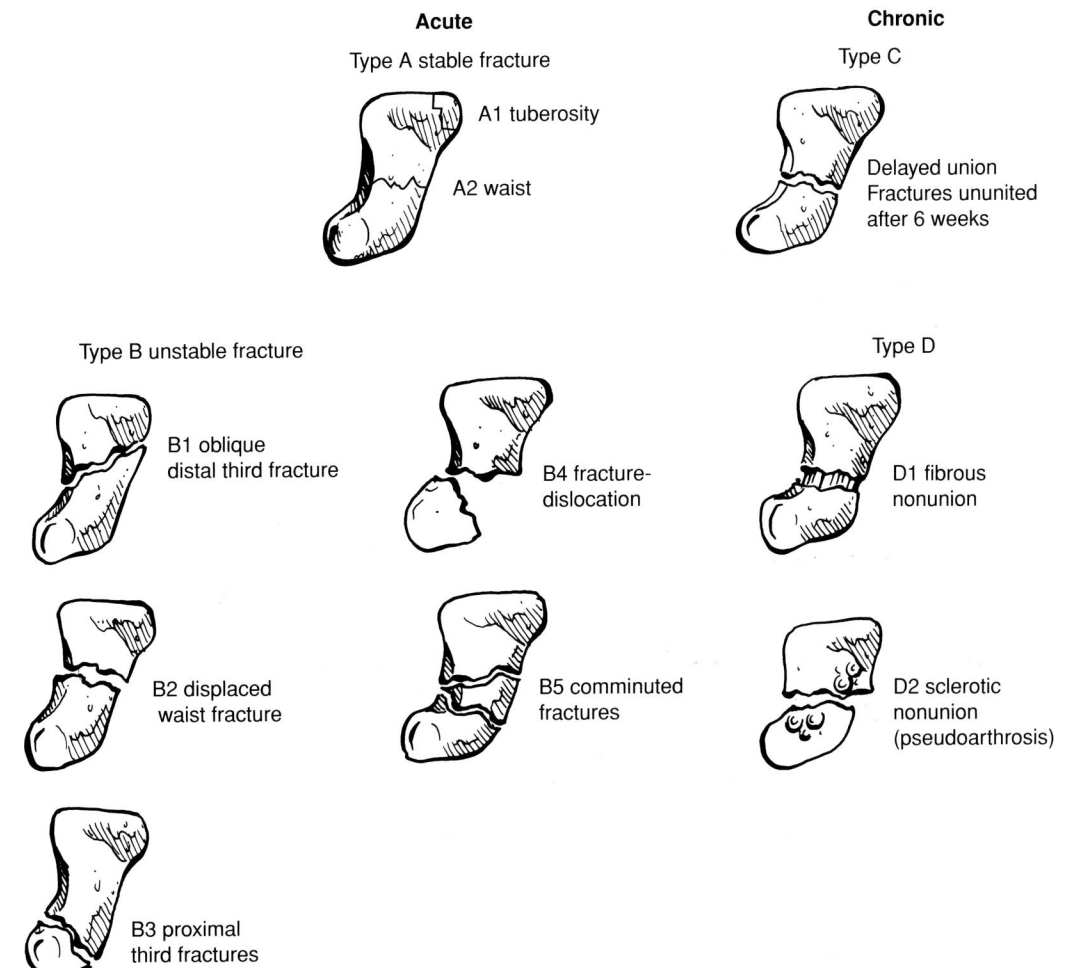

FIGURE 31-24 Schematic drawing of Herbert and Fisher classification of scaphoid fractures.

and minimal treatment is required. Type B fractures include any acute bicortical fracture and are defined as unstable and hence will most likely require surgery due to the potential for displacement in plaster and delayed union. There are now two studies that have demonstrated that displaced waist of scaphoid fractures (Herbert B2) account for over one-third of all fractures,[61,136] with one of these studies demonstrating that unstable Herbert type-B injuries were significantly more common in younger patients following a high-energy injury.[136] Type C and Type D fractures are associated with delayed and nonunion respectively. Characteristics of Type C delayed union are defined as widening of the fracture line, development of cysts adjacent to the fracture, and relative density of the proximal fragment.

Some argue the most useful classification for guiding treatment, particularly for displaced fractures, is the Mayo classification.[100,125] The criteria for instability they set out are as follows:

- >1 mm of fracture displacement[103,143]
- A lateral intrascaphoid angle of >35 degrees (see below)
- Bone loss or comminution
- Fracture malalignment
- Proximal pole fractures
- DISI deformity
- Perilunate fracture-dislocation

A criticism of all these classifications is that they do not clearly consider the extent of associated soft tissue injuries.

Diagnosis of Displacement and Instability

Assessment of scaphoid fracture displacement and instability is essential, given the higher rates of nonunion associated with nonoperative management.[143] All displaced fractures are unstable. A very small percentage of patients have a nondisplaced fracture (no radiologic signs of displacement) but are unstable (fracture fragments move easily with probing or external pressure on the distal pole of the scaphoid during wrist arthroscopy). There are various methods for determining scaphoid fracture displacement (Table 31-11). As with the assessment of the suspected scaphoid fracture, the various imaging modalities are hindered by the low prevalence of displaced scaphoid fractures among all fractures. This leads to all modalities being better at excluding displacement rather confirming it.

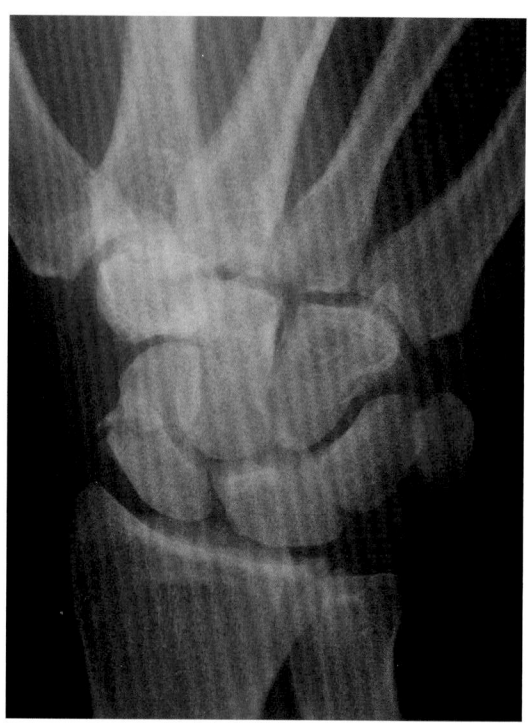

FIGURE 31-25 A displaced and comminuted fracture through the waist of the right scaphoid.

Standard scaphoid radiographs can be used to determine displacement in terms of translation, step-off, gap, rotation, and angulation (Fig. 31-25)[125]; however, some question the validity of its use with only moderate interobserver reliability being reported.[47,50,121] Some authorities advocate the use of wrist motion views to demonstrate displacement, with the length of the scaphoid determined by comparing ulnar and radial deviation views in both wrists. Assuming that the two views are identical, any difference in length is indicative of a scaphoid deformity as a consequence of either a fracture and/or a ligament injury. When displacement and instability is suspected, careful assessment of the lateral radiograph for the position of the lunate (Fig. 31-17) and intrascaphoid angulation (Fig. 31-18) is essential,[50,121] with repeat radiographs recommended as displacement may occur over time.

TABLE 31-11	The Sensitivity, Specificity, Accuracy as well as the PPV and NPV for Various Imaging Modalities Used in the Assessment of Scaphoid Fracture Displacement

Imaging Modality	Sensitivity (%)	Specificity (%)	Accuracy (%)	PPV	NPV
Radiographs	75	72	64	10	97
CT	72	80	80	13	98
Radiographs + CT	80	73	73	16	99

From: Dias JJ, Singh HP. Displaced fracture of the waist of the scaphoid. *J Bone Joint Surg Br.* 2011;93:1433–1439.

CT is more accurate and reliable than radiographs for the diagnosis of scaphoid fracture displacement,[287,343] but it is unclear whether routine CT scanning improves outcomes. One study determined that CT had a low sensitivity in the diagnosis of radial/ulnar scaphoid displacement, while radiographs had a low sensitivity in the diagnosis of volar/dorsal displacement.[486] Useful measurements include the following:

- Fracture displacement[103,143]
  - Step ≥1 mm at dorsal or radial cortices
  - Gap ≥1 mm (sagittal or coronal views)

Lozano-Calderon et al.[287] analyzed the diagnostic performance characteristic of radiographs and/or CT for detecting the displacement of acute scaphoid fractures. They concluded that CT improved the reliability of detecting scaphoid fracture displacement but with an accuracy still <80% with the utilization of CT limited by the low prevalence of displaced fractures. One study found that quantitative measurements of scaphoid fracture displacement using CT had limited intra- and interobserver reliability,[395] and others have suggested that measurement is influenced by the image plane and the thickness of the slices used.[388,446] However, one recent study has suggested that training can lead to a slight increase in reliability for detection of displacement using such methods.[68]

Alternate methods of determining fracture displacement include USS, MRI, or wrist arthroscopy.[50,70] One study has reported 100% specificity for determining scaphoid fracture instability when using USS; however, this is noted to be very user dependent.[124] A recent study analyzed 58 consecutive patients with a scaphoid fracture who underwent arthroscopy-assisted operative fracture fixation.[70] They found a significant correlation between radiographic comminution (>2 fragments) and arthroscopically determined displacement and instability. Using arthroscopy as the reference standard (Fig. 31-26), one study has found that radiographs and CT cannot be relied on to accurately diagnose scaphoid fracture displacement and/or instability.[69] This study was novel in making a clear distinction between displacement and instability, noting a few radiologically well-aligned fractures that were unstable on arthroscopic visualization. To our knowledge, there are no data regarding the prognosis of well-aligned unstable fractures.

Associated Injuries

Associated injuries occur in approximately 10% of all scaphoid fractures, commonly following a high-energy mode of injury, and proximal radial fractures are most frequently seen.[136,541] Fractures of the distal radius can occur, as can perilunate dislocations and transscaphoid perilunate fracture-dislocations.[136,218] A concomitant fracture of the distal radius can be indicative of more serious ligamentous disruption and carpal instability.[228] It is essential to consider that a radiograph never accurately exposes the true degree of joint and ligament damage.

Recent studies have aimed to document the incidence of associated ligamentous injuries given the increased use of wrist arthroscopy in the management of scaphoid fractures. Caloia

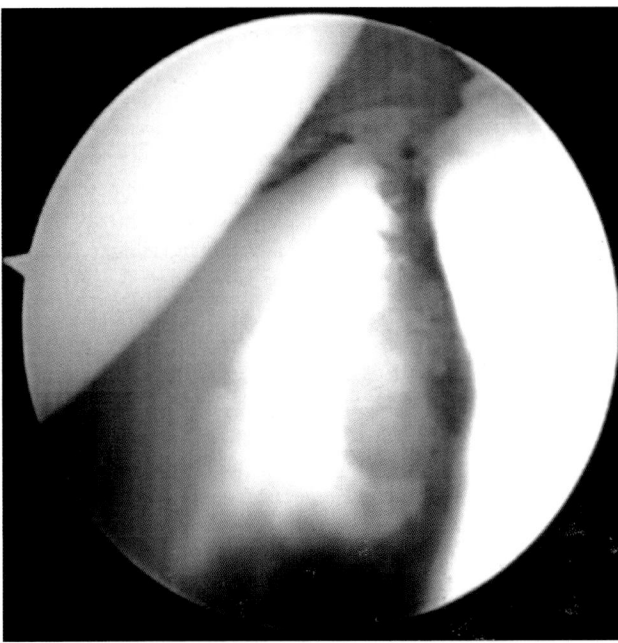

FIGURE 31-26 Arthroscopic diagnosis of scaphoid fracture displacement.

et al.[77] documented an associated ligamentous and/or bony injury in 63% of the 24 acute scaphoid fractures in their series. In a more recent study of 41 scaphoid waist fractures, fresh intrinsic ligament injuries were found in 34 cases, with 29 cases a scapholunate ligament injury (complete rupture in 10). Interestingly, there was no significant difference in the rate of ligament injury between nondisplaced and displaced scaphoid fractures.[243] The clinical relevance of these associated ligamentous injuries is yet to be determined.

Authors' Preferred Management— Imaging and Diagnosis of Displacement

Given the low prevalence of displacement and instability, we feel comfortable relying on radiographs that demonstrate no gapping or translation at the fracture, and no dorsal tilting of the lunate, if the patient agrees that a very small risk of healing problems is preferable to the radiation and other downsides of CT. If there is any uncertainty, we order CT in the planes defined by the long axis of the scaphoid.

Authors' Preferred Management—Acute Scaphoid Fractures

Suspected Scaphoid Fractures

Patients with a suspected occult scaphoid fracture are re-evaluated after 1 to 2 weeks of immobilization in a forearm cast or splint. An examination by a specialist after the injury has become less painful substantially decreases the probability of a scaphoid fracture in most circumstances. If the probability of a fracture remains unacceptable (a decision shared with the patient) and new scaphoid specific radiographs are also normal, the patient can either continue with immobilization (6 weeks of splint immobilization with normal scaphoid radiographs is likely sufficient) or advanced imaging (typically CT or MRI) can be used to attempt to exclude a fracture and avoid additional immobilization and activity restrictions. The higher the pretest odds of a fracture, the more likely an imaging diagnosis of a fracture will correlate with a true fracture. The lower the pretest odds; for example, "rule out" rather than "confirm," the less likely that a radiologic diagnosis of a fracture will correspond with a true fracture. Patients with more pressing needs to diagnose a fracture (some athletes and other occupations) can be considered for more sophisticated imaging early on, keeping in mind the limitations of this diagnostic strategy.

Scaphoid Tubercle Fractures

For tubercle fractures, we recommend 3 to 4 weeks in a splint followed by active mobilization.

Nondisplaced Scaphoid Fractures

We recommend as standard a below-elbow cast with the thumb free for nondisplaced stable scaphoid fractures. If there is any doubt about the presence of displacement, particularly if there is fragmentation at the fracture line, we would progress to a CT scan. Based more on tradition than data, the duration of immobilization is 8 to 10 weeks. Radiographs and clinical examination should not be used to determine duration of immobilization because they are unreliable for diagnosis of union. Return to sport and use of the hand with force is delayed until there is clear radiographic evidence of union or 4 to 6 months have passed. At this point it is reasonable to "put things to the test" no matter what the radiographs show since additional protection is unlikely to facilitate union.

We offer patients with nondisplaced or minimally displaced fractures the option of percutaneous screw fixation, including a balanced discussion on the risks and benefits of surgery based on the best available evidence. One of us prefers a volar approach to percutaneous fixation and the other uses either a dorsal or a volar approach. We feel the advantages of the volar approach are that the scaphoid tubercle is very superficial, the wrist can be maintained in neutral which makes imaging easier and decreases the chance of bending the guidewire, and there is no need to open the radiocarpal joint. On the other hand, care must be taken to ensure that an overhanging trapezium does not cause the surgeon to insert the screw too superficially (too volar) or too vertical. There may also be a risk of later scaphotrapezial arthrosis. Using this approach, the surgeon must be prepared to place the screw through the overhang of the trapezium which is usually extra-articular. If the screw is placed too vertically in the sagittal plane, the screw tip may penetrate the dorsal radial scaphoid cortex, which both endangers the

radioscaphoid cartilage and usually provides inadequate fixation of the proximal fragment.

We feel the advantages of a dorsal approach include easier central placement in the proximal pole and body of the scaphoid. Disadvantages include the need to keep the wrist in a flexed position, greater risk of bending the guidewire, risk to digital extensor tendons, and creation of a hole in the scaphoid articular surface. The starting point of the wire can be identified arthroscopically and a large bore needle used as a guidewire or this can be done entirely with the image intensifier. The hand is placed on top of a stack of towels on the image intensifier to maintain the wrist in flexion to provide access to the starting point and limit the potential for bending the wire. The wrist is kept flexed and the images are perpendicular to the carpus. After determining the length of the screw, the wire is placed into the trapezium to prevent unintended extraction if predrilling is used.

Some surgeons allow patients to return to sports and forceful activity sooner after screw fixation than they would after cast treatment (sometimes within a few weeks of screw placement), but we do not recommend that approach. Postoperatively, a bandage is applied and usually a cast is not required. Noncontact sports are allowed immediately. Contact sports, heavy lifting, or axial loading of the wrist can commence progressively 6 weeks after surgery.

Unstable and/or Displaced Scaphoid Fractures

Arthroscopic-assisted fixation or ORIF of the scaphoid is recommended if there is any gapping or angulation in the scaphoid, even if the fracture appears stable and impacted, because our impression is that displaced fractures are unstable and should be managed operatively.[543] If reduction can be achieved and monitored arthroscopically percutaneous fixation is possible, but we feel the standard treatment is open reduction and internal fixation. Reduction is facilitated by the use of K-wires used as joysticks in each fragment as well as other instruments used to push and guide the fragments into position. Bone grafting is considered in the face of comminution.

A splint is applied for comfort after operative fixation. In most cases the splint is maintained until suture removal about 2 weeks later. In unreliable patients or some very unstable or very proximal fractures a cast may be used for 4 to 8 weeks. Return to sports is risky until the fracture is healed (at least 2 to 3 months). Patients who wish to return sooner must agree to assume the associated risks.

Proximal Pole Scaphoid Fractures

For proximal pole fractures we recommend operative treatment using a small open dorsal approach to check alignment in case the fracture is unstable.[442] We prefer a straight 3-to 4-cm incision centered over the dorsal aspect of the wrist after checking the level of the scapholunate junction with the fluoroscope. The extensor pollicis longus tendon can usually be left in place. The dorsal capsule is then incised and the scaphoid exposed. Care is taken to avoid injury to the dorsal ridge vasculature during the approach. For unstable fractures, bone grafting might be considered to stimulate union. A compression screw is applied over a guidewire, using a second wire to control rotation if the fragment is unstable. Our postoperative protocol is as for unstable/displaced fractures.

Management of Scaphoid Fractures

Suspected Scaphoid Fractures

For suspected fractures, distal pole/tubercle fractures, and undisplaced waist fractures early diagnosis is important. If the diagnosis is confirmed at the time of injury following the use of secondary imaging; for example, CT or MRI, the patient is treated as an undisplaced scaphoid fracture. This is usually with a simple below-elbow forearm cast with or without thumb immobilization for 6 weeks, with check scaphoid radiograph views obtained at the time of cast removal. When there are persistent clinical and radiologic signs of a fracture, further immobilization in a cast for an additional 2 weeks is recommended. When secondary imaging is not used at presentation, repeat assessment and radiologic imaging, most frequently at 10 to 14 days post injury, is usually performed. In the interim, a below-elbow forearm cast with (scaphoid cast) or without (Colles cast) thumb immobilization should be applied until the diagnosis is confirmed or refuted.

Scaphoid Tubercle Fractures

Nonoperative management is routinely employed for scaphoid tubercle fractures (Herbert A1).[122,127,232] Scaphoid tubercle fractures are a generally benign avulsion injury. Although some authors suggest that splinting is adequate, others prefer cast immobilization for 4 weeks. Tubercle fractures managed with casting can have radiographs that show persistent displacement and fibrous union causing no disability, although these findings are more commonly seen in fractures treated without immobilization.[320]

Nondisplaced Scaphoid Fractures

Nonoperative Versus Operative Management. Controversy exists regarding the management techniques for nondisplaced or minimally displaced waist fractures (Herbert A2, B1, and B2). Studies in this area often include both nondisplaced and so-called minimally displaced fractures. Nondisplaced scaphoid fractures are usually stable, although there is no gold standard for confirming this, and achieve union rates between 95% and 99% when managed conservatively.[54] Some authors suggest that cast immobilization is the method of choice for the primary treatment of undisplaced or minimally displaced fractures of the scaphoid.[122,127,232] Variable rates (3% to 20%) of subsequent displacement in cast are reported,[91,272] due to a lack of consensus regarding the appropriate imaging modality to use and the criteria for displacement.

However, there is an increasing body of evidence to support early percutaneous screw fixation of these fractures, with advocates citing a minimally invasive technique associated with a low complication rate, a shorter time to union by over a month, a more rapid improvement in functional testing, as well as an earlier return to sports and work, all in a predominantly young and active population.[55,206,231,307,368,409,560] The shorter time to union is difficult to assess given radiographs are known to be unreliable.

Herbert and Fisher[211] reported an overall incidence of nonunion after conservative treatment at 50% and subsequently advocated the use of internal fixation for scaphoid fractures with a newly designed screw. More recently, there have been several studies advocating the use of early fixation for nondisplaced or minimally displaced fractures of the scaphoid,[206,231,368,560] with now several randomized controlled trials directly comparing the two treatment modalities (Table 31-12).[6,27,55,127,307,409,515]

McQueen et al. in their prospective randomized trial of 60 patients (30 percutaneous fixation, 30 casts) followed-up for 1 year reported a significantly decreased time to union with a more rapid return of function, sport, and full-time work when compared with those managed conservatively.[307] Low complication rates were also reported with the surgical technique. Arora et al.[27] found similar results in their prospective study of percutaneous fixation with comparable costs for both techniques; however, Davis et al.[112] reported cost savings of almost $6,000 in favor of surgical fixation.

Saeden et al. performed a long-term prospective randomized 12-year follow-up study comparing ORIF and nonoperative management and found an earlier return to function in the operative group, recommending surgery be offered to young and active patients.[409] This study did report an increased rate of radiologic signs of scaphotrapezial joint arthritis in the operative group, but this did not correlate with subjective clinical findings. Dias et al.[127] randomized 88 patients (44 ORIFs, 44 casts) and followed them for 1 year following injury. They reported superior earlier results in the operative group across many of the outcome measures. There were 10 (23%) patients in the conservative arm that developed nonunion compared to none in the operative group. There was a 30% complication rate in the operative group but all were minor, with the vast majority related to the scar due to the open technique. Despite these findings, the authors concluded that undisplaced or minimally displaced scaphoid waist fractures should be managed in a cast.

Three of four recent systematic reviews with meta-analysis have concluded that on current evidence neither method is clearly superior, not only with surgical management associated with improved functional outcome, a more rapid return to function/sports/work and superior union rates, but also with a significantly increased rate of complications.[13,66,232,470] However, these reviews included "minimally displaced" fractures and combined ORIF and percutaneous fixation under one umbrella for surgical management, with ORIF more commonly associated with complications.[127]

Technique—Nonoperative Management. For nondisplaced, minimally displaced or selected displaced fractures (see below), a below-elbow forearm cast with or without thumb

TABLE 31-12 **Details of Current PRCTs Comparing Operative and Nonoperative Management for Undisplaced or Minimally Displaced Fractures of the Scaphoid**

Study (Follow-up)	Mean Age (yr)	Male/ Female (%)	Treatment (n)		Fracture Type (Displaced)	Key Findings and Recommendations
			Conservative	Operative		
Adolfsson et al.[6] (Min 16 wks)	31	74/26	28	23	Herbert B1, B2 (none)	No significant difference for rate of union or time to union Operative group had a significantly better range of motion at 16 wks, grip strength no difference
Arora et al.[27] (Min 24 wks)	33	73/27	24	23	Herbert B2 (none)	No significant difference in the range of wrist motion or grip strength Operative group had a better mean DASH score, a faster time to union and a faster return to work
Bond et al.[55] (Mean 25 mos)	24	88/12	14	11	Herbert A2, B2 (none)	No significant difference in the range of wrist motion or grip strength Operative group had a significantly faster average time to union and average time to return to work Patient satisfaction high in both groups
Dias et al.[127] (Min 1 yr)	30	90/10	44	44	Herbert A2, B2, B5 (11 minimally displaced)	Operative group had significantly better range of motion, patient evaluation measure and grip strength at 8 wks, with significantly better grip strength at 12 wks No significant difference between groups with respect to any other outcome measure at any other time Return to work same in both groups Rate of nonunion was higher in conservative group, rate of complications (predominantly scar sensitivity) higher in operative group
McQueen et al.[307] (Min 1 yr)	29	83/17	30	30	Herbert B1, B2 (7 minimally displaced)	Operative group had significantly faster time to union Trend towards a higher rate of nonunion in the nonoperative group Operative group had a significantly more rapid return of function, sport and, work
Saeden et al.[409] (Min 12 yrs)	33	79/21	30	31	AO C2, C3 (none)	Return to work faster in operative group for blue-collar occupations No differences with respect to function, union, or carpal arthritis Operative group had a higher rate of scaphotrapezial joint arthritis but this did not correlate with subjective symptoms
Vinnars et al.[515] (Mean 10 yrs)	31	78/22	42	41	Herbert A2, B1, B2, B3 (none)	Operative group had a significant increase in rate of scaphotrapezial joint arthritis No differences in limb-specific outcome scores were found Range of motion and grip strength were greater (not significant) in the conservative group

Adapted from: Doornberg JN, Buijze GA, Ham SJ, et al. Nonoperative treatment for acute scaphoid fractures: A systematic review and meta-analysis of randomized controlled trials. *J Trauma.* 2011;71:1073–1081.

immobilization can be used for 2 weeks, and then clinical review is recommended with further scaphoid radiograph views mandatory as surgery may be necessary if the fracture has displaced. When in doubt, further imaging is recommended. If the fracture remains undisplaced, a cast can be reapplied until fracture union is confirmed clinically and radiographically. There is a general consensus that most stable scaphoid fractures unite in 6 to 8 weeks with cast immobilization; however, examination and radiographs are unreliable so duration of immobilization is based ultimately on surgeon preference.[126] However, bone consolidation can take 12 to 16 weeks and some fractures will not have healed even after this time.

One of the important questions regarding the nonoperative management of scaphoid fractures is the type of cast to be applied—an above-elbow cast, a Colles cast (below elbow without thumb immobilization), or a scaphoid cast. Three recent systematic reviews have concluded that on current evidence there is no advantage to any of these methods.[13,131,470] Although some authors still advocate the use of above-elbow casts, two randomized studies have demonstrated no significant advantage in the use of above-elbow casts.[10,188] In a further nonrandomized prospective study it was found that using an above-elbow cast may cause increased movement at the fracture site.[259]

The remaining debate is whether to use a scaphoid cast or a Colles cast. Prior to 1942, Bohler et al.[54] proposed the use of an unpadded dorsal backslab, but then changed the cast to include the proximal phalanx of the thumb—the scaphoid cast. Since then, there have been several studies demonstrating no difference between the two techniques. In one cadaveric study it was found that provided the wrist was not in ulnar deviation, the position of the thumb had no influence on the fracture gap.[557] Hambidge et al.[208] randomly allocated 121 acute scaphoid fractures for conservative treatment in a Colles cast with the wrist immobilized in either 20 degrees flexion (n = 58) or 20 degrees extension (n = 63). They found no difference between groups in terms of union rates, wrist flexion, or grip strength but did find that the wrists which had been immobilized in flexion had a greater reduction in wrist extension.

There are now two large prospective randomized trials (one published and one to be published) comparing the Colles cast and scaphoid cast for an acute fracture of the scaphoid, with both having demonstrated no advantage to either method.[91] For this reason, the use of Colles casts or forearm casts, rather than scaphoid casts, is advocated.

Technique—Percutaneous Fixation.
For undisplaced or minimally displaced fractures, percutaneous fixation is superior to ORIF providing superior union rates, faster functional recovery, and reduced surgical morbidity; for example, scar, complex regional pain syndrome (CRPS).[125,127,212,388] Percutaneous fixation is a simple technique and can be performed through either a volar or a dorsal approach, with neither reported to provide a superior outcome.[2,133,238,347]

Some feel it is easier to get the screw in the center of the scaphoid using the dorsal approach, particularly for fractures of the proximal pole.[205] The dorsal approach is often described utilizing a small open incision citing an increased risk to tendons or nerves, in particular the posterior interosseous nerve, extensor digitorum communis to the index finger, and extensor indicis proprius,[2] but the senior author and other advocates like Slade use a fully percutaneous approach.[442] Slade placed the wrist in a traction tower to facilitate arthroscopy and used a mini image intensifier placed lateral. The senior author of this chapter places the mini C-arm vertically, stacks towels on the collector to keep the wrist bent with the carpus perpendicular to the beam. Slade and Geissler found the starting point for the screw through the arthroscope and suggested marking the spot with a large gauge needle that could be used as a guide for wire insertion. The senior author finds the starting point under the image intensifier. Slade advanced the guidewires out the volar surface of the thumb to get the wire out of the wrist, facilitating a PA view of the wrist without risking bending the wire. The senior author keeps the wrist flexed to at least 45 degrees to avoid bending the wire and takes radiographs perpendicular to the scaphoid rather than the distal radius. Slade placed the scaphoid in the image intensifier with some wrist flexion and enough rotation so that the distal and proximal poles of the scaphoid overlap creating a near circular image in which the guidewire for the screw should be dead central. The senior author finds that view unpredictable and unreliable and uses real-time 360 imaging to judge the position of the screw, again, keeping the wrist flexed.

With the volar approach (Fig. 31-27), a potential disadvantage is an increased prevalence of later scaphotrapezial osteoarthrosis; however, this is commonly asymptomatic and has no impact on the final outcome.[515] For the volar approach, the hand is placed on a radiolucent table or with care directly on the collector of a small image intensifier with the shoulder abducted and the forearm in supination. The wrist is extended over a roll. The correct placement of the guidewire is crucial to the success of the procedure. It helps to remember that the scaphoid lies in a 45-degree plane to both the longitudinal and horizontal axes of the wrist. The incision point for the volar approach is found approximately 1 cm distal and radial to the scaphoid tubercle with entry point on the scaphoid tubercle. A 4- to 5-mm skin incision is made or the guidewire can be inserted percutaneously and an incision made around the wire just large enough for the screw to pass once the wire position is acceptable. In a few cases with an overhanging trapezium, it may be necessary to insert the guidewire through the trapezium, which does not seem to result in added morbidity.[190,191,308] The tip of the guidewire is placed on the scaphoid tubercle. The optimal entry point is one that will allow central placement of the screw in the proximal pole of the scaphoid. For the volar approach, this is often relatively radial on the distal pole. The guidewire is inserted at a 45-degree angle in both planes (roughly in line with the radially and palmarly abducted thumb metacarpal) aiming the tip at the apex of the proximal pole. The image intensifier is used to check wire placement utilizing anteroposterior, lateral and both supinated and pronated oblique views.[173]

When the wire is in a good position in the scaphoid (and the alignment of the scaphoid is confirmed for minimally displaced fractures), an attempt is made to measure the screw. The length of the screw should be measured carefully and several millimeters subtracted from the measured length to avoid prominence at either end. It is useful to estimate the length of the scaphoid based on preoperative measurement. Through a percutaneous insertion (incision just large enough to pass the screw) measurement can be difficult using the sleeve measure, but one can use a second wire of the same length and measure the difference. Some then drill the guidewire into the trapezium to anchor it. Predrilling is used depending on the type of screw. The drill is passed over the wire, stopping if there is any resistance as this may indicate a bend in the wire that will lead to drill or wire breakage. Even if the screw is self-drilling there is a

risk of distraction of the fracture and so if predrilling is not used the progress of the screw should be monitored using image intensification to ensure that no rotation or distraction occurs at the fracture site. If distraction occurs, the screw is removed and the track drilled. If there is a bend, the wire can usually be further advanced so that the drill passes over a nonbent part of the wire. After drilling, the screw is advanced under image intensification. It is important to judge screw length prior to fully seating the screw. The wire is then removed, and central positioning of the screw without joint penetration at the radiocarpal joint or prominence at the scaphotrapezial joint should be confirmed with AP, lateral, supinated, and pronated views of the wrist.[173]

There are a number of screws available that vary in size and pitch variation and can be partially, fully or tip threaded, and

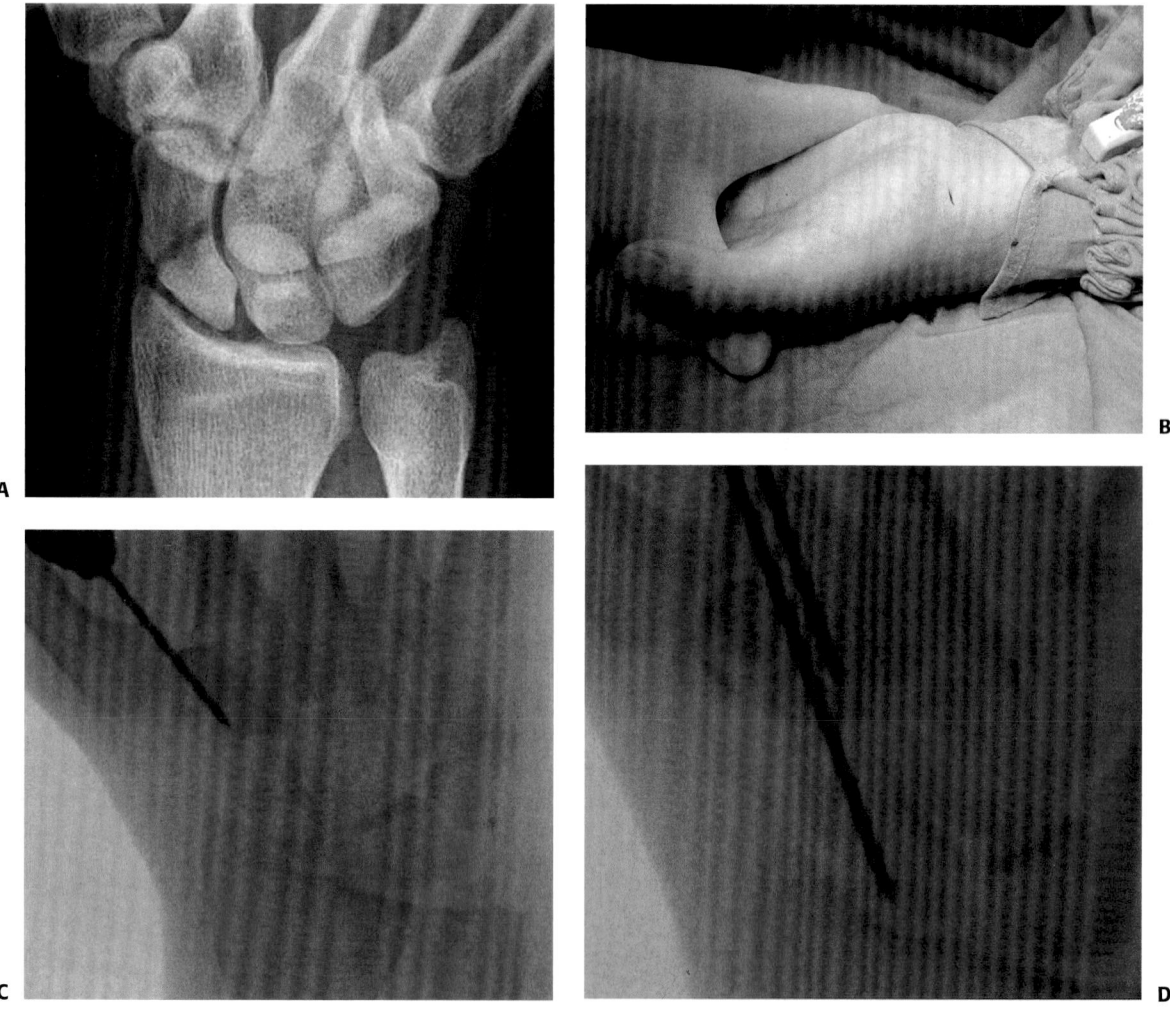

FIGURE 31-27 Percutaneous stabilization of scaphoid fracture. **A:** A fracture through the waist of the scaphoid. **B:** The wrist should be dorsiflexed prior to insertion of the K-wire and a 4-5 mm incision is made in the skin crease, sufficient for the insertion of the screw. **C:** The K-wire is inserted at a 45-degree angle in both planes and the position is checked using fluoroscopy. **D, E:** A second K-wire can be used if the position of the first wire is not quite adequate, or if there is concern regarding potential rotation of the fracture fragments.

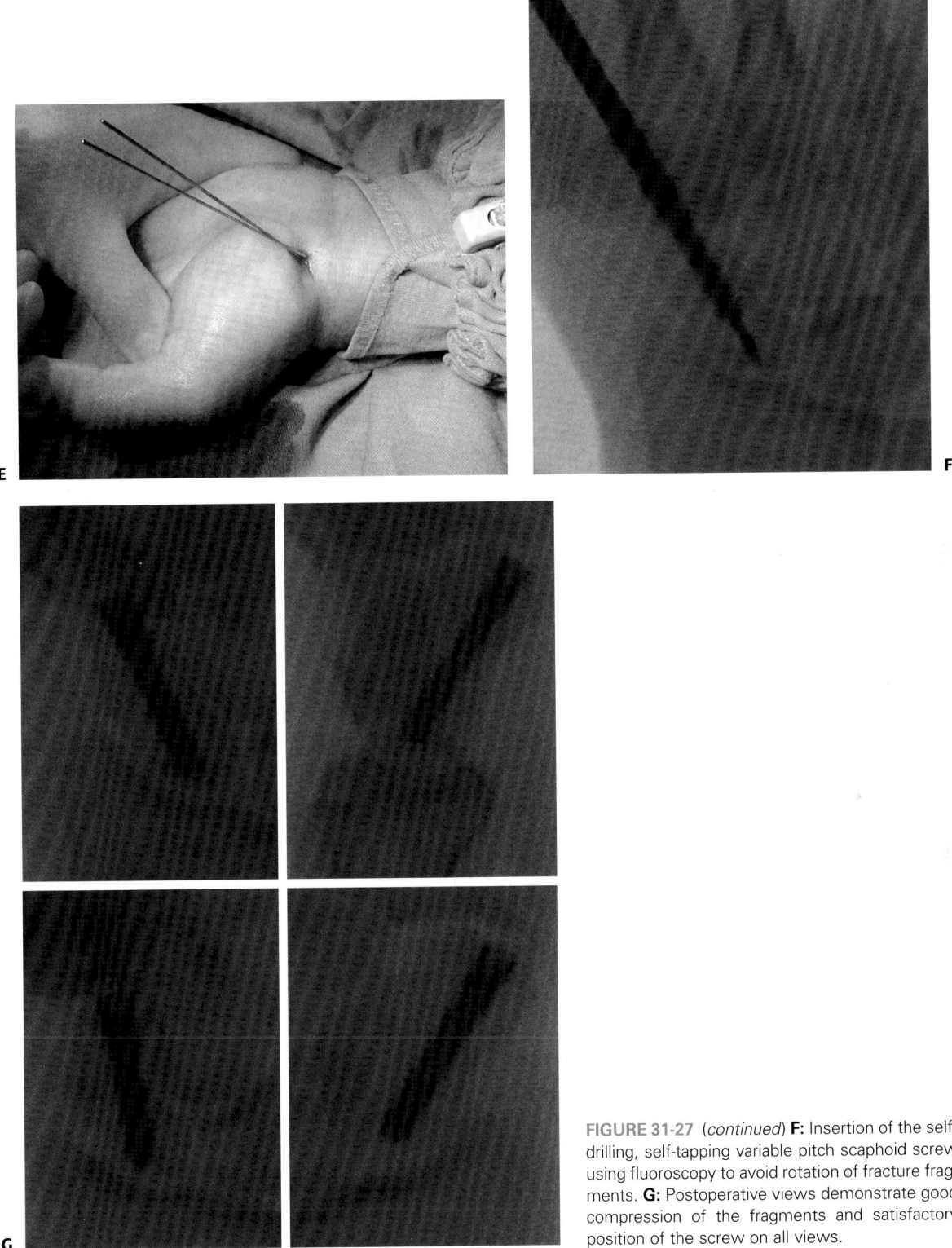

FIGURE 31-27 (*continued*) **F:** Insertion of the self-drilling, self-tapping variable pitch scaphoid screw using fluoroscopy to avoid rotation of fracture fragments. **G:** Postoperative views demonstrate good compression of the fragments and satisfactory position of the screw on all views.

with or without ancillary techniques for achieving compression (e.g., special screw drivers or even mobile parts of the screw). Biomechanical studies support the common sense view that larger screws are stronger[32,89,198,207,357,466]; however, there is no evidence that the type of screw affects the outcome with the exception that cannulated screws have been shown to improve central placement of the screw when compared with the Herbert screw.[503]

Unstable and/or Displaced Scaphoid Fractures

Surgical treatment is routinely employed for displaced scaphoid fractures (Herbert B1, B2), comminuted fractures (Herbert B5), and fractures associated with carpal instability and/or a dislocation (Herbert B4). Unstable or displaced fractures of the scaphoid, as well as proximal pole fractures, have an increased rate of redisplacement,[91] delayed union, and nonunion[143] when managed with cast immobilization alone.[73,367,551] A recent systematic review of displaced scaphoid fractures found a four times higher risk of nonunion when compared with undisplaced fractures following conservative management, with nonunion seventeen times more likely if a displaced fracture of the scaphoid is managed nonoperatively.[436]

It is debatable whether some displaced unstable scaphoid fractures can be treated in a cast.[73,367,551] Since displacement is the primary and only evidence-based risk factor for nonunion, displaced fractures should be strongly considered for either open or arthroscopic-assisted reduction plus internal fixation. Some patients may not be suitable for an operation; for example, noncompliant patients, elderly patients with or without significant medical comorbidities.[173] The consequence of managing these patients nonoperatively is not completely clear and it may be that in the elderly patient nonoperative management provides a comparable outcome to operative treatment, without the risks associated with surgery. Rates of redisplacement range from 12% to 22%,[10,91,103,143] union 50% to 90%,[10,103,125,409] and the development of osteoarthritis 16% to 31%.[122,409]

Technique—ORIF. McLaughlin[305] was the first to report the use of primary ORIF for fractures of the scaphoid, and subsequently positive results have been reported in many studies.[388] Displaced fractures are treated with either ORIF or arthroscopically assisted percutaneous fixation. There must be direct visualization of fracture reduction as the strange shape of the scaphoid and complex carpal anatomy makes image intensification inadequate. Some fractures reduce with radial deviation and extension, but many require direct manipulation which can be facilitated by the use of K-wires inserted into each fracture fragment. Both dorsal and volar approaches have been reported with success, with the palmar exposure limiting potential damage to the vascular supply, but the dorsal approach providing improved access to proximal fractures.[125,212,297] Once the fracture is reduced, screw placement is as described for percutaneous fixation.

For the volar approach, most use an incision across the transverse wrist creases in line with the flexor carpi radialis

(FCR) tendon. The incision starts distal to the distal pole of the scaphoid and is about 5 cm in length. The FCR tendon sheath is opened and the tendon is retracted in an ulnar direction. The superficial radial artery is either retracted distally or ligated. The wrist capsule is isolated and divided in line with the scaphoid, starting at the distal pole and ending as soon as the fracture is visualized, preserving as much of the RSC ligament as possible. The fracture is aligned and provisionally secured with a wire. Usually a volar screw is inserted as described above, but it is also possible to put in a dorsal screw percutaneously at this point.[173]

Technique—Arthroscopic-assisted Reduction and Fixation. Some authors advocate arthroscopic-assisted reduction and fixation, with high union rates reported and the added advantage of being able to assess for the presence of associated soft tissue injuries.[181,427,440,441,443,482] However, disadvantages are similar to that with the open technique and include a steep learning curve, extensor tendon damage, poor fracture reduction, nerve injury, and scaphotrapezial or radioscaphoid joint damage.[125,441] Ultimately, it is not clear that arthroscopic-assisted surgery has any advantages over open and might be more difficult and time consuming. Once the fracture is reduced, care must be taken not to flex, distract, translate, or rotate the fragments when inserting the screw and gaining compression.

For this technique, the fracture is best seen through a midcarpal portal, usually employing the 4/5 midcarpal portal. Angulation, translation, and gapping can be seen on the capitate articular surface of the scaphoid, but on the radial side is not seen. A reduction maneuver of extension and radial deviation with volar wire stabilization of the scaphoid often restores alignment. If a manipulative reduction is insufficient the K-wire is withdrawn to the volar side of the fracture and retained for later advancement across the reduced fracture. Additional K-wires in one or both fragments, as well as percutaneously inserted snaps or elevators, can help restore alignment. The volar wire is then advanced to stabilize the fracture. A screw is then placed percutaneously as described above.

Proximal Pole Scaphoid Fractures

A meta-analysis has demonstrated that the relative risk of nonunion for proximal pole fractures (Herbert B3) was 7.5 times more when compared with more distal fractures when all were managed nonoperatively (Fig. 31-28).[141] Temporary interruption of the blood supply to the proximal fragment is virtually certain with proximal pole fractures but, if stabilized, the proximal pole has the capacity to revascularize and heal.[187,290] Proximal pole fractures are uncommon and the use of operative management is based on intuition more than data.

Technique—ORIF. For proximal pole fractures, most authors recommend operative treatment using a small open dorsal approach to ensure alignment and to allow access to the proximal fragment.[442] Commonly, a straight 3- to 4-cm incision is centered over the dorsal aspect of the wrist after checking

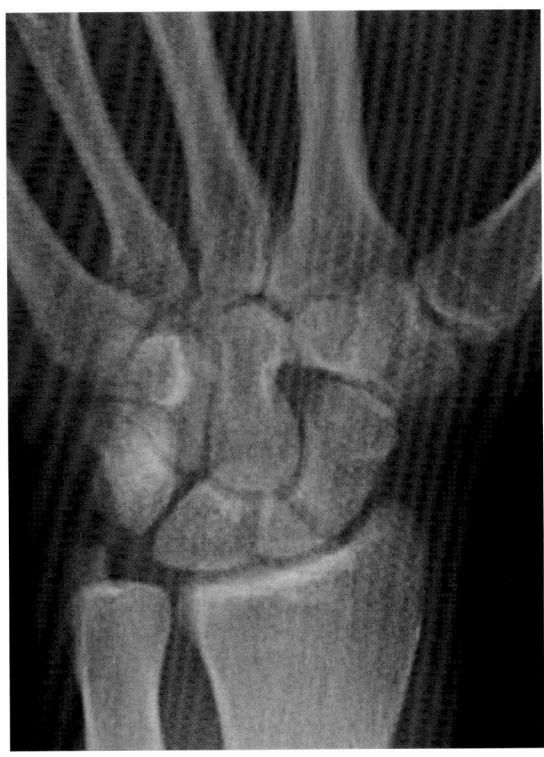

FIGURE 31-28 A fracture through the proximal pole of the scaphoid.

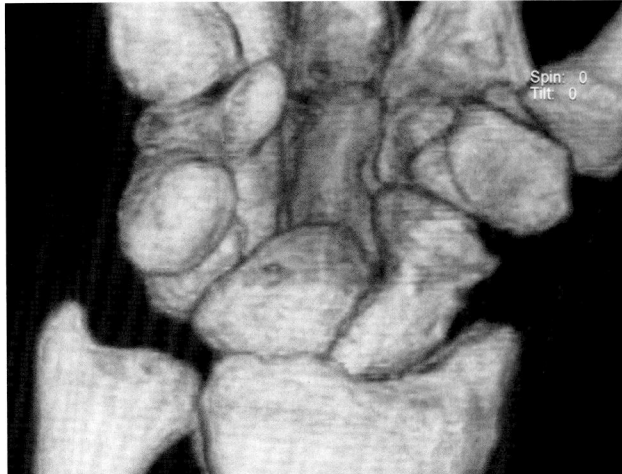

FIGURE 31-29 CT scan of a scaphoid fracture that has healed with a humpback deformity. The intrascaphoid angle measures 67 degrees.

the level of the scapholunate junction with the fluoroscope. The extensor pollicis longus tendon is routinely unmoved. The dorsal capsule is then incised and the scaphoid exposed. Care is taken throughout this approach to avoid injury to the dorsal ridge vasculature. Otherwise, the technique for fixation is as for ORIF above.

Complications of Scaphoid Fractures: Scaphoid Malunion

Some displaced scaphoid fractures can malunite, usually with a humpback deformity (Fig. 31-29). Pronation or ulnar translation of the distal fragment is less commonly seen.[125] The effect of this malalignment on symptoms and wrist function is debatable.[18,342] One cadaveric study has suggested that scaphoid malunion results in a notable reduction in wrist motion,[74] and a few small series of osteotomy for scaphoid malunion have reported improved motion and function with decreased symptoms.[289] However, studies of nonunions treated with no attempt to correct alignment (e.g., with Russe grafts) found no correlation of function or arthrosis with scaphoid malalignment in both the short and long term.[160,383]

Clinical Assessment and Diagnosis

Patients with scaphoid malunion are believed to be at risk of wrist pain, reduced wrist extension and diminished grip strength.[74,342] One study has demonstrated that the loss of

wrist extension is proportional to the angular deformity,[74] while another has suggested that the degree of DISI deformity correlates with symptom severity.[342] Standard radiographs are the first line of investigation, with further imaging in the form of CT to better delineate the deformity. Useful measurements include the following:

- Lateral intrascaphoid angle (Fig. 31-18A): An angle greater than 35 degrees is used as a cut-off for displacement[18]; noted to have poor interobserver reproducibility on both CT and MRI.[30,395]
- Height-to-length ratio (Fig. 31-18C): Found to have the best reproducibility for assessing angulation.[30,395]

Alternate measurements found to be of limited use include the dorsal cortical angle (Fig. 31-18B) and the AP intrascaphoid angle.[18] It should be noted that both short- and longer-term retrospective studies have demonstrated no correlation between any outcome measure and the degree of radiologic deformity.[160,383]

Management

The clinical consequences of malunion are not completely clear. Forward et al.[160] reported on the clinical outcome at 1 year of 42 consecutive patients with a malunited scaphoid waist fracture that had all been managed nonoperatively and found no significant correlation between any outcome measures (range of motion, grip strength, PROMs) and any of the three measures of malunion (height-to-length ratio, dorsal cortical angle, lateral intrascaphoid angle). Similar results have been reported in the longer term.[383]

An osteotomy is considered when there is objective impairment (e.g., loss of extension) that seems directly related to the scaphoid malalignment.[146,155] Lynch et al. reported a technique of corrective osteotomy that corrects the intrascaphoid angles, restores palmar length to the scaphoid, and reduces DISI deformity of the carpus.[281,289] They claim that this method could potentially prevent or delay the onset of arthritis in young patients with high functional demands.

Complications of Scaphoid Fractures: Scaphoid Nonunion

Scaphoid nonunion leads to a specific type of post-traumatic wrist arthrosis labeled scaphoid nonunion advance collapse (SNAC) similar to the arthrosis that develops after scapholunate ligament injury.[290] The development of SNAC (Fig. 31-30) is extremely variable in terms of the rapidity of progression and the association with pain, stiffness, disability, or union. One rationale for operative treatment to gain union of the scaphoid is to delay or prevent arthritis, but it is unclear if union can achieve these goals, particularly if the nonunion is more than a year old.

Epidemiology and Etiology

The natural history of scaphoid fracture nonunion is unknown as the majority of patients represent due to new or on-going symptoms. The quoted rate of nonunion is variable due to a lack of agreement regarding the criteria for union and the imaging modality that should be used. Nonunion is said to occur in approximately 10% of all scaphoid waist fractures, but the rate is much lower for nondisplaced fractures and approaches zero when a nondisplaced fracture is adequately treated and protected.[50,73] Displaced fractures have a 50% nonunion rate, with an increased rate also seen with proximal pole fractures (Table 31-13 and Fig. 31-31).[31,99,121,143,471] Other proposed risk factors for nonunion of scaphoid waist fractures include delayed diagnosis or treatment.[104,141,269,367,405,551]

Pathoanatomy and Classification

Fisk[156] described the triplane angulation and subsequent humpback deformity of the scaphoid that results from estab-

TABLE 31-13	Rates of Scaphoid Fracture Nonunion Based on Fracture Type and Management Used	
	Management	
Fracture Type	Nonoperative	Operative
Undisplaced/minimally displaced	1–5%	0–2%
Displaced	10–50%	0–7%

lished nonunion where the proximal scaphoid rotates dorsally into extension and the distal part faces downward in flexion. Impingement between the palmar-flexed scaphoid distal pole and the radial styloid process leads to the development of radiocarpal osteoarthritis.[173] At the same time, the unsupported carpus collapses into a DISI deformity with increasing subluxation and secondary arthritis of the midcarpal joint (Fig. 31-32). The articulation of the proximal pole with the radius and the radiolunate joint are relatively spared.

Some scaphoid nonunions have minimal or no deformity, there seems to be a firm fibrous union between the fracture fragments, and the progression to symptoms and the necessity for treatment is unclear.[73,126,128,367] According to the Herbert and Fisher classification (Fig. 31-24), Type D1 fractures are scaphoid fibrous nonunions that commonly occur in stable fractures following cast immobilization.[211]

Type D2 fractures are an established sclerotic scaphoid nonunion. These injuries are usually unstable with a progressive deformity that leads to the development of wrist arthritis (SNAC).[73,126,128,367] Two patterns of nonunion displacement have been described, dorsal or volar, with the location of the fracture

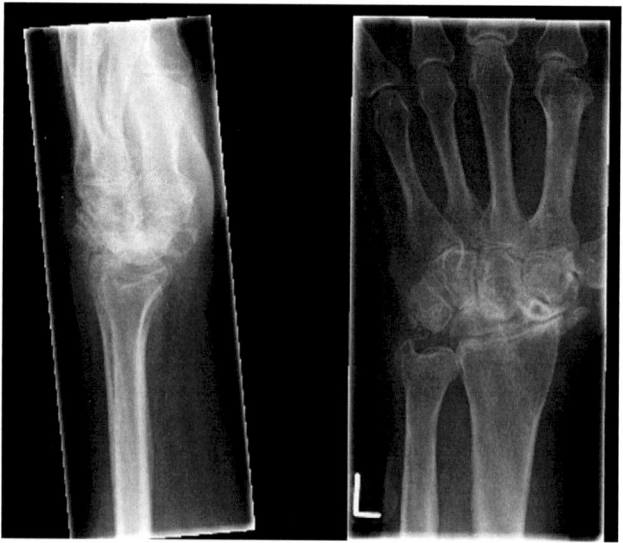

FIGURE 31-30 Scaphoid nonunion advanced collapse (SNAC) of the left wrist.

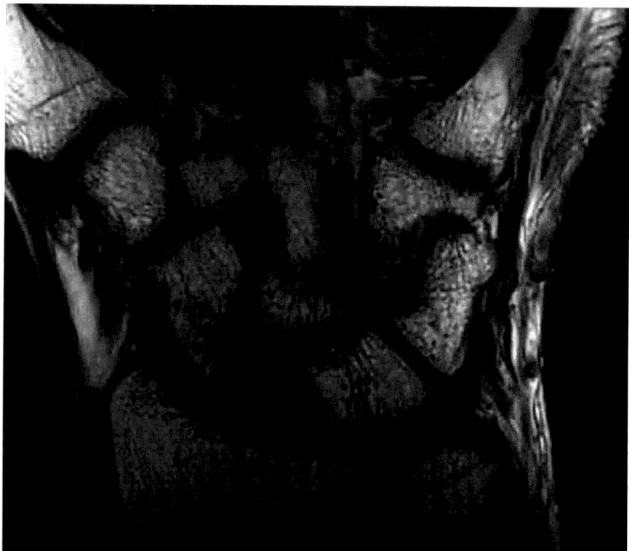

FIGURE 31-31 An established scaphoid proximal pole fracture nonunion found on MRI.

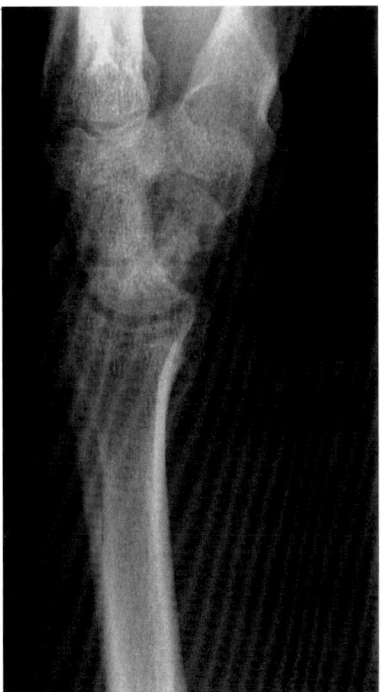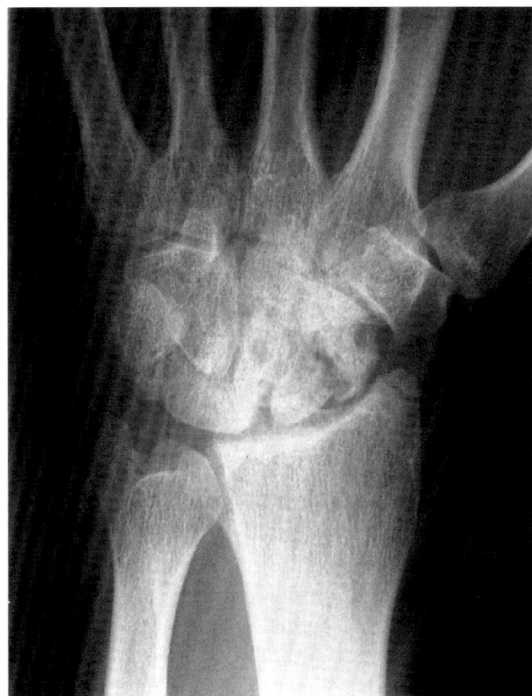

FIGURE 31-32 An established scaphoid nonunion with associated DISI deformity.

line relative to the dorsal apex of the scaphoid ridge predictive of the pattern.[328,358,359] Distal scaphoid waist fractures, with large triangular bone defects, are associated with the volar pattern, with the development of a humpback and/or DISI deformity. Proximal scaphoid waist fractures, with much smaller flat crescent-shaped bone defects, are associated with the dorsal pattern.[173] Similarly, one study has found that carpal instability after a scaphoid fracture nonunion is related to whether the fracture line passes distal or proximal to the scaphoid apex.[327]

Clinical Assessment and Diagnosis

Many scaphoid nonunions are unnoticed fractures that present with symptoms either gradually or after a later fall.[250] Missed diagnosis is not uncommon and often results in additional morbidity from secondary changes, including nonunion, collapse deformity, and degenerative arthritis.[290] Patients usually have radial-sided wrist pain, reduced wrist motion with pain at the limits of motion, and reduced grip strength.[73,74,250,367]

Imaging. A radiographic diagnosis of nonunion cannot be made confidently until 6 to 12 months after injury,[126,128] although some may argue that union can be confirmed if the patient is asymptomatic and the original fracture line is no longer visible.[121] Prior to that time radiographs may demonstrate the classic findings of nonunion, including widening of the fracture gap, cystic changes, and fracture line sclerosis even when the fracture is healing.[73,126,128] Radiographs can be compared with images of the opposite unaffected wrist, particularly for preoperative planning. Other options for diagnosing nonunion include USS, CT, or MRI. One study investigated the use of real-time linear USS in determining fracture site movement in 27

patients with a scaphoid nonunion, of which 24 had had surgical treatment, and found the technique to be 100% specific for visualization of movement at the fracture site although it was of no benefit in assessing proximal pole nonunion.[124]

Although MRI is utilized in the diagnosis of scaphoid AVN, it has not been found to be superior to CT for assessing fracture nonunion, alignment, and for comparison of findings before and after nonunion surgery.[21,309,326,420,435] Sagittal images from scans are considered to provide the best method of evaluating the location of the nonunion and the degree of collapse. The lateral intrascaphoid angle and the height-to-length ratio of the bone help determine angulation and collapse of the scaphoid, with an angle of more than 35 degrees associated with an increased incidence of arthrosis even in nonunions that eventually progress to union. One study has documented a good correlation between preoperative proximal pole sclerosis on CT with AVN and subsequent fracture union, with a specificity of 100%, but with a sensitivity of 60% and an accuracy of 74%.[450] CT is also cheaper and more readily available in many centers. The only definitive test for confirming AVN is the observation at surgery of the presence or absence of bleeding from bone.

Management

The quoted union rate following treatment for scaphoid fracture nonunion is wide ranging, with a recent systematic review concluding an 80% union rate for bone grafting without fixation and an 84% rate for grafting with internal fixation.[339]

The goals of management are to relieve symptoms, correct the carpal deformity, achieve union, and hopefully delay the onset of wrist arthrosis.[73,367] The major principles to follow are the following:[173]

1. Make an early diagnosis
2. Perform a complete resection of the nonunion
3. Correct the deformity secondary to carpal collapse and carpal instability
4. Preserve the blood supply throughout
5. Achieve bone apposition by an inlay graft
6. Achieve stability with screw fixation

Treatment options include bone grafting, fixation without bone grafting, fixation with either a vascularized or a nonvascularized graft, and finally wrist salvage procedures (Table 31-14). There is limited data on the ability of current techniques to either reduce symptoms or limit the onset of wrist arthrosis, as well as when salvage procedures should be utilized primarily.[73] Poor prognostic indicators are a prolonged nonunion time, prior failed surgery requiring revision, the more proximal the nonunion, and the absence of punctate bleeding at the proximal pole during surgery.[380,478,479] Generally, the number of punctuate bleeding points is a good indicator of bone vascularity. When the proximal pole is completely avascular, the likelihood of successful healing with a graft is virtually nil and an alternative salvage procedure should be considered.[197,380,478]

Stable Nonunions. The stable scaphoid nonunion is characterized by a firm fibrous nonunion that prevents deformity, with the risk of osteoarthritis being small. The indications to manage patients surgically with a stable nonunion are limited to improvement in symptoms, prevention of progression to an unstable nonunion, or delaying the development of degenerative changes. The earlier the surgery is performed, the lower the incidence of secondary osteoarthritis.[173]

For stable nonunions, structural graft support is not required, simply graft that will promote union; although some have suggested no graft at all is needed. Treating stable nonunions ordinarily gives good results using either an open or percutaneous technique.[291,386] One scientific exhibit presented data on stable scaphoid delayed unions or nonunions (defined by nonunions that were well aligned and without extensive sclerosis or bone resorption at the nonunion site) that were treated by percutaneous screw fixation with good results.[439] One study of 27 patients with established scaphoid nonunions (well-aligned fractures with extensive local bone resorption) managed with percutaneous screw fixation alone reported good results with all fractures uniting at an average of 3 months.[291] Additional study is needed to determine which nonunions are amenable to this approach.

Unstable Nonunions. The quoted success rates of achieving union with internal fixation and bone grafting for unstable nonunions range from 60% to 95%.[130,499] The differing rates may be explained by the heterogeneous nature of patient demographics, fracture nonunion characteristics, or the acknowledged difficulty in defining union.[173] Two studies have implicated smoking as a reason for failure of nonunion surgery.[130,284]

TABLE 31-14	Wrist Salvage Procedures for Scaphoid Nonunion
Fracture Type	**Comments**
Partial or complete scaphoidectomy	Excision of larger fragments (>8 mm) lead to wrist weakness and poor outcome[177]
Scaphoid replacement	Worth considering in selected patients
	Silicone implants abandoned due to progressive silicone arthritis in many cases and long-term results mixed[90,145,210,469]
	Unless the midcarpal joint is stable and painless, replacement should be combined with a fusion across the midcarpal joint to prevent carpal subluxation[173]
	Young and active patients are likely to complain of continued pain after this procedure and wrist arthrodesis is then often preferable
Wrist denervation	Good pain relief, but may be temporary[463]
Proximal row carpectomy (PRC)	Mixed results reported
	Recent systematic review compared PRC with four-corner fusion[335]
	Both procedures give improvements in pain and subjective outcome measures
	PRC gives marginally superior motion and reduced complications
	Risk of subsequent osteoarthritis is significantly higher in PRC
Wrist arthrodesis	Indicated for radiocarpal and midcarpal osteoarthritis associated with severe pain, weakness, and reduced wrist motion
	Good results, in particular pain relief and improved strength, reported in young patients with high functional demands[225]

Techniques and Bone Grafting. CT and radiographs of the opposite side can help determine the optimal size and shape of the bone graft required. The standard palmar approach (see above) with the advantage of avoiding damage to the blood supply can be used for most reconstructions of unstable scaphoid nonunions, except in fractures involving a small proximal pole fragment. Techniques of palmar and radiopalmar bone grafting have been developed to correct scaphoid malalignment and to restore normal scaphoid length. Failure to correct the humpback deformity results in intraoperative problems because the screw cannot be adequately placed and will cut out, leaving residual instability.[173] Even if the nonunion heals, the malunited scaphoid has a twofold increase in degenerative arthritis compared with a scaphoid

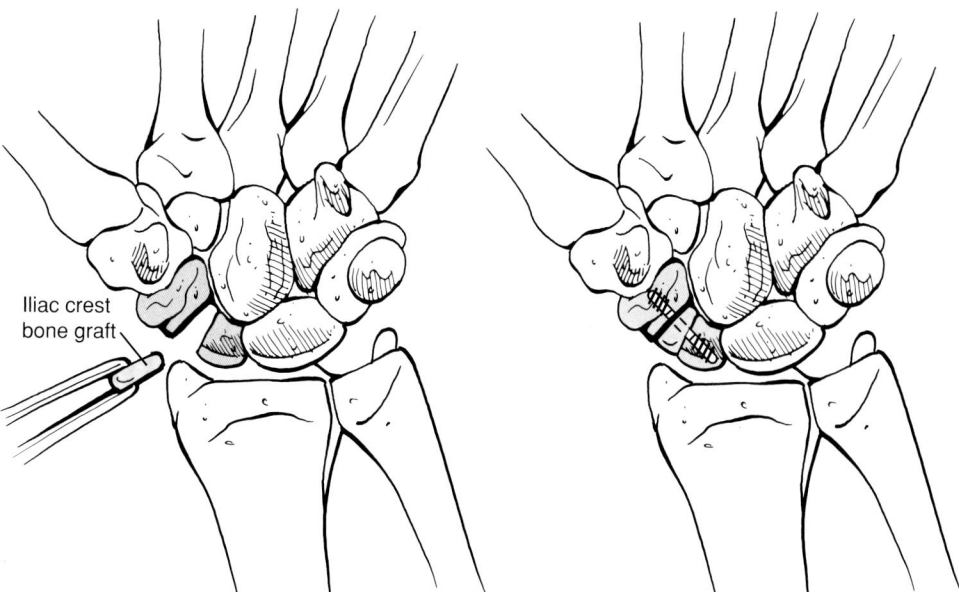

FIGURE 31-33 Standard Russe bone graft. His technique relied on packing a corticocancellous bone graft into a trough curetted through the volar cortex of both fragments. Because the volar cortex is often foreshortened by erosion of the fragments, loss of length is difficult to correct without introducing a cortical graft. Modified Russe winged graft can be impacted into a volar trough to lengthen the scaphoid.

that has healed with correct alignment.[500] Although AVN of the proximal fragment may potentially affect the healing potential of a scaphoid, diminished vascularity of the proximal scaphoid is not a contraindication to a palmar inlay bone graft.[173] If fracture union can be achieved, the relative avascularity will improve.

There are a number of methods of bone grafting in use but none has been found to be superior in terms of achieving union.[73,499] Prior to the introduction of modern fixation methods the Matti-Russe inlay graft was used in the treatment of scaphoid nonunion (Fig. 31-33), but this technique does not usually correct malalignment.[421] Anterior wedge grafting procedures, with initial reduction of the lunate and temporary pin fixation, are now in common use as humpback deformities can be corrected with this technique.[144,496] Screw fixation has generally been found to give superior union rates when compared to K-wire fixation when using nonvascularized graft.[73,313] No correlation between donor sites (iliac crest, distal radius) and union have been demonstrated.[478,479] Some authors advocate taking corticocancellous graft from the anterolateral corner of the radial metaphysis rather than the iliac crest, as it allows harvesting from one incision with reduced donor site morbidity and comparable union rates.[7,385] Cohen et al.[93] recently reported good clinical and radiologic results in 12 patients with established scaphoid waist nonunions using ORIF with only cancellous interposition graft from the ipsilateral distal radius. Potential disadvantages of nonvascularized grafts include increased nonunion rates in the presence of AVN and short-term donor site morbidity associated with graft taken from the iliac crest.[73]

Vascularized bone grafts from the distal radius (radial artery), distal ulna (ulnar artery), and based on the pronator quadratus (Fig. 31-34), have been described.[460] Union rates following distal radial pedicle grafts range from 27% to 100%, with poor rates seen when used for AVN.[73,459,464,564] New free vascularized grafts from the iliac crest and the medial femoral supracondylar

zone have been reported, with one study documenting superior union rates of the medial femoral supracondylar graft when compared to a vascularized graft from the distal radius.[240]

A recent randomized controlled trial compared vascularized (distal radius) with nonvascularized (iliac crest) bone grafting for scaphoid nonunion and found a 100% union rate in the nonvascularized group, with a rate of 85% in the vascularized group ($p > 0.05$).[58] No significant differences were found in time to union or function.

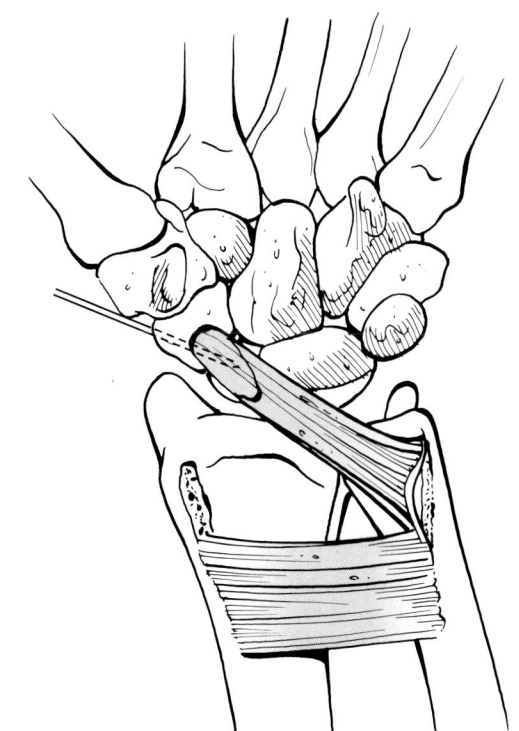

FIGURE 31-34 Pronator quadratus graft.

AUTHORS' PREFERRED MANAGEMENT — SCAPHOID FRACTURE NONUNION

For a stable scaphoid nonunion, we prefer an open palmar approach using a straight incision as opposed to the curved incision described by Russe.[173,407] The incision is based over or radial to the FCR from the scaphoid tubercle to the distal radius. The sheath of the FCR tendon is incised and the tendon retracted ulnarly. Directly beneath the tendon lies the palmar capsule of the wrist, just above the scaphoid. The capsule should be incised longitudinally. The superficial palmar branch of the radial artery is distal at the end of incision and needs to be ligated in cases of wider exposure of the distal scaphoid. Stable scaphoid nonunions might not be visible macroscopically and often need sharp division with the knife. It is useful to check the site of a nonunion as fusion of the proximal pole of the scaphoid with the lunate or the scaphoid distal pole and trapezium have been undertaken assuming that this joint was the site of nonunion. It is important to prepare the nonunion surfaces by removing any fibrous tissue and sclerotic bone. We usually leave the dorsal cartilage in place. This provides a hinge and facilitates assessment of scaphoid length. In most cases of stable nonunion, cancellous bone graft from the distal radius usually provides sufficient volume as structural support is not required, although iliac crest bone graft can be used if necessary. Screw fixation of the scaphoid is then used. Immobilization in a cast or splint is not required postoperatively except in occasional cases for pain relief.[173]

For an unstable nonunion, we feel a volar approach is necessary to correct the humpback deformity. The nonunion gap is exposed and debrided, and the fracture fragments are mobilized. It is best to leave a cartilage hinge posteriorly to provide a fulcrum around which the fragments may be hinged open although this is often not possible in older, unstable scaphoid fractures. If the hinge is released in an effort to regain all of the scaphoid length, the fracture fragments will become extremely unstable and difficult to align. Furthermore, the gap between the two fragments may be too great for the scaphoid to revascularize the proximal pole.[500] The wrist is extended and the two fragments gently distracted with small spreaders. This maneuver usually achieves adequate correction of the carpal deformity and a satisfactory improvement in wrist extension. Provided that reasonable correction is achieved and that the wrist extends to at least 45 degrees, most patients achieve satisfactory clinical results. The fracture surfaces are excised with a small osteotome, burr, or curette. We prefer a corticocancellous wedge graft from the iliac crest. This is an interposition graft, which is inserted on the palmar surface and serves to bridge the fracture gap and correct any displacement or angulation of the scaphoid that has occurred. Vascularized bone grafts from the distal radius (radial artery) or distal ulna (ulnar artery) have also been described, though we would prefer the pronator quadratus graft.[460] To correct angular deformity and restore normal scaphoid length, the amount of resection and size of the graft can be calculated preoperatively by CT scans. The indications

for interposition grafting include gross motion at the nonunion site, scaphoid resorption, and loss of carpal height. Most commonly, the operative procedure involves an anterior interposition bone graft, with the size based on comparative scaphoid views of the opposite wrist and intraoperative measurements. The width and depth of the defect is measured and a graft of the exact size is removed from the iliac crest with an osteotome. Oscillating saws should not be used, as thermal necrosis of the graft can occur. With the wedge graft in place and the scaphoid reduced and held with a K-wire, a compression screw is inserted. Internal fixation with K-wires alone is usually not successful as compression is required to achieve union. However, if the graft shows a tendency to rotate, additional fixation with a K-wire may be required. If there is a severe or longstanding DISI deformity with an RL angle greater than 20 degrees, additional pinning of the lunate to radius for 6 to 8 weeks is advised.[155] It may be difficult to completely correct carpal instability in long-standing cases, and these patients may be better served by various salvage procedures. Finally, a partial radial styloidectomy can be performed in patients with radiologic signs of stage I radioscaphoid arthritis, this being arthritis that is limited to the scaphoid and radial styloid. This is undertaken to relieve pain arising from arthritic joints or osteophyte impingement. If there are no radiologic signs of arthritis, a styloidectomy should not be undertaken at the same time as a scaphoid reconstruction often relieves symptoms.[173]

With stable fixation, postoperative immobilization is usually not required but a Colles cast can be used if there is doubt about stability or if pins have been used across the radiocarpal joint.

Complications of Scaphoid Fractures: Scaphoid AVN

AVN of the scaphoid can occur as a late complication of scaphoid fractures, especially those involving the proximal pole. Occasionally, AVN may occur without a fracture, either as a complication of SL ligament injury or as an idiopathic condition known as Preiser disease.

Clinical Assessment and Diagnosis

The typical symptoms of AVN are increasing pain and stiffness of the wrist. Standard radiographs demonstrate a small, deformed proximal pole fragment with cystic changes and areas of sclerosis. The value of MRI to diagnose AVN in the routine management of scaphoid nonunions is debated. Current best evidence has not demonstrated that MRI can reliably or accurately diagnose AVN, with MRI findings not prognostic.

Management

The natural history of scaphoid AVN is not known and it is not known if operative treatment can alter the natural course of the disease. One treatment option is a vascularized bone graft.[28,367,522] Arora et al.[28] reported the use of free vascularized iliac bone graft for the management of 21 patients with AVN and nonunion of the scaphoid for which conventional bone grafting had failed, achieving union and good symptom relief in 16 patients.

The bone graft can be harvested dorsally through the second dorsal compartment of the distal radius, anteriorly in the form of a pronator quadratus graft, or from the second metacarpal. It is important to adhere to the basic principles of nonunion treatment with meticulous preparation and stabilization of the nonunion site. There has been one report of using arthroscopic debridement in managing these patients.[312]

Directions for Future Research in Scaphoid Fractures

It is likely that we will never have a consensus reference standard for true fractures among suspected scaphoid fractures. More sophisticated imaging to date has simply identified more abnormalities that are difficult to interpret. Consequently, to move forward we may need to accept that we are ultimately dealing with probabilities rather than certainties in the diagnosis of fracture. Such an approach would no longer seek to diagnose the presence or absence of a fracture definitively. Rather, the goal would be optimal NPV and PPV with the ultimate aim of reaching certain accepted thresholds. Since the pretest odds of a fracture (or the prevalence of true fractures among suspected fractures) has a substantial effect on the PPV, future research should build on the attempts to develop clinical prediction rules that use demographic and clinical factors predictive of a true fracture to better identify patients in whom imaging will have an acceptable NPV and PPV. In addition, given the absence of an accepted reference standard, future research should use latent class analysis to estimate diagnostic performance characteristics.

Regarding the decision between operative or nonoperative treatment of nondisplaced fractures of the scaphoid waist, the following issues merit further investigation: The safety of a shorter duration of cast wear and the use of casts or even splints that are less cumbersome (e.g., thumb free); differences in quality of life, cost effectiveness, and the safety of earlier return to work or sport; the definition, diagnosis, and prevalence of "minimally displaced" fractures of the scaphoid waist; and a comparison of operative and nonoperative treatment for this subset of fractures.

Regarding scaphoid nonunion, more data is needed on the long-term outcome, including patient reported measures, following surgical intervention. There are also controversies regarding the use of vascularized bone grafts in reconstructive procedures, as well as when to progress to salvage procedures.

Scaphoid Fractures: Pearls and Pitfalls

- Male gender and sports injuries are risk factors for an acute fracture of the scaphoid
- Clinical prediction rules might aid in the assessment of the suspected fracture
- Displacement of scaphoid fractures may be difficult to diagnose and CT or arthroscopy can be helpful
- The criteria for displacement, in particular minimal displacement, needs to be further investigated and better defined

- Nonoperative management is routinely employed for suspected scaphoid fractures and tubercle fractures
- Percutaneous fixation for undisplaced or minimally displaced waist fractures may reduce time in cast, increase the rate of return to function and increase the rate of union
- Surgical management is recommended for displaced scaphoid fractures, proximal pole fractures, comminuted fractures, and fractures that are part of a greater perilunate injury

OTHER CARPAL FRACTURES

Triquetral Fractures

Triquetral fractures are the second most common fracture of the carpus,[218,227,507] with avulsion fractures (representing in essence a benign "wrist sprain") accounting for over 90% of all triquetral injuries.[114,218] Less common patterns of fracture include the following:

- Transverse fracture of the triquetrum as part of a perilunate dislocation, although more frequently dorsal displacement is seen[14,273,412,452,555]
- Impingement shear fracture type[178,489]
  - Ulnar impaction: Ulnar styloid against the dorsal triquetrum, which occurs with the wrist in extension and ulnar deviation, particularly when a long ulnar styloid is present.
  - Triquetrohamate impaction: Hamate against the posteroradial projection of the triquetrum, occurs through compression of the wrist in forced dorsal and ulnar extension while the forearm is pronated.

Clinical Assessment and Diagnosis

Patients present with pain and tenderness localized over the region of the triquetrum. Standard scaphoid views will detect most triquetral fractures, with dorsal avulsion fractures of the triquetrum often found on the oblique or lateral views.[114] PA radiographs of the wrist are useful in identifying transverse body fractures; however, they will often not detect avulsion fractures of the triquetrum due to the normal superimposition of the dorsal lip on the lunate. Additional views that can aid the diagnosis include an oblique pronated lateral radiograph that will project the triquetrum even more dorsal to the lunate.[114] Secondary imaging modalities are often not necessary, although CT for further delineation of body fractures is useful. Occult triquetral fractures can be identified when CT and MRI are used in the detection of occult scaphoid fractures.[171]

Management

Triquetral avulsions are managed with a splint for comfort only and active self-assisted stretches as comfort allows to limit stiffness.[114] Triquetral body fractures associated with carpal disruption often require internal fixation.[273,412,437,452]

Lunate Fractures

Lunate fractures account for less than 1% of all carpal fractures and most occur as part of a perilunate injury.[218,227,507]

Clinical Anatomy

The lunate is the middle bone of the proximal carpal row, acting as a keystone in the well-protected concavity of the lunate fossa of the radius, anchored on either side through interosseous ligaments that connect to the scaphoid and triquetrum.[247,277,283,502,530] Distally, the convex capitate head fits into the concavity of the lunate. The joint reaction forces from the capitate and radius move the lunate ulnarly. The proximal pole of the hamate has a variable articular facet on the distal ulnar surface of the lunate, and ulnar deviation increases the degree of contact between these two bones.

The vascular supply of the lunate is primarily through the proximal carpal arcade, with current literature suggesting that approximately 80% of lunates receive vessels from both the dorsal and palmar surfaces, with the remaining 20% from the palmar surface only (Table 31-3).[57,164,182,186,366,542] It is said that this limited blood supply renders the lunate vulnerable to AVN,[57,164,185,186,366] and yet AVN is almost unheard of after lunate or perilunate dislocations, presumably because the palmar radiocarpal arch usually remains intact as the dislocation is through the space of Poirier. The lunate blood supply is frequently endangered by common dorsal approaches to the wrist, but the blood supply from the palmar radiocarpal arch is usually sufficient.

Kienböck Disease. Kienböck disease is an eponym for idiopathic avascular osteonecrosis of the lunate.[75,116] It usually has an insidious onset without a history of injury; however, diagnosis is sometimes made after a simple fall that fractures the necrotic bone.[33,182] Osteonecrosis may be the result of interruption of the vascular supply to the lunate, which shows no radiographic evidence of injury until sclerosis and osteochondral collapse.[33,182,265] The condition is more common in patients with an ulnar minus variant.[173,204,534]

Some believe that unrecognized and untreated fractures of the lunate lead to Kienböck disease, predominantly due to the cadaveric work of Verdan who applied strong forces to cadaver bones and observed that the resulting fractures were not visible on standard radiographs but only on histology.[33,173,182] However, others have questioned these findings, with one study suggesting that early venous congestion, not fracture, of the lunate was responsible for the pathogenesis of Kienböck disease.[419] The lunate necrosis after perilunate dislocation is probably due to impairment of the arterial vasculature.[173]

Clinical Assessment and Diagnosis

Most patients with fractures of the lunate have a history of a hyperextension injury such as a fall on the outstretched hand.[81,229] Patients present with pain and tenderness localized over the region of the lunate and triquetrum.

Imaging. Standard scaphoid views are the primary investigation for suspected lunate fractures.[114] Some injuries may be difficult to visualize early, as an undisplaced fracture can be obscured by superimposed structures.[173]

- The palmar cortical line of the radial styloid is aligned with the division between the dorsal and palmar thirds of the lunate where a transverse fracture often occurs.

- The PA view of this is in a plane almost perpendicular to the fracture, which is overlapped by the rims of the distal radius and is therefore not apparent.

- The palmar horn of the lunate may also be hidden by the pisiform and scaphoid shadows.

Given this, there must be a low threshold for further imaging when the diagnosis is in doubt. Bone scan will be positive within 24 hours of injury. However, CT will provide the most precise detail regarding any fractures, as well as any osteonecrotic changes that may need to be differentiated from a primary fracture or secondary fracture associated with fragmentation. Arthroscopic examination permits a direct assessment, including of the articular surfaces and the intrinsic ligaments.[173]

Classification. Lunate fractures can be difficult to describe and part of the difficulty is that the fragmentation that occurs in Kienböck disease can be confused with fractures. However, acute fractures of the lunate were classified into five groups by Teisen and Hjarbaek.[484]

1. Frontal fractures of the palmar pole with involvement of the palmar nutrient arteries
2. Osteochondral fractures of the proximal articular surface without substantial damage to the nutrient vessels
3. Frontal fractures of the dorsal pole
4. Transverse fractures of the body
5. Transarticular frontal fractures of the body

Fresh fractures of the lunate include dorsal and palmar horn avulsion fractures that occur more often in the radial corner than in the ulnar corner. Fractures of the body are usually transverse in the coronal plane. The more common of these is between the middle and palmar thirds of the body.

Management

Nonoperative management in cast for approximately 4 weeks is suitable for most isolated lunate fractures,[81,229] with nonunion rarely reported. A transverse fracture of the body will heal if it remains nondisplaced, particularly in adolescents.

Indications for ORIF include displacement and/or associated carpal instability. If there is evidence of separation of the lunate fragments by the capitate, union will not occur and the risk of AVN is markedly increased.[78,258,323] Although the efficacy of internal fixation of the lunate is unproven and the obstacles to successful reduction and fixation are substantial, the consequences of inaction are as to be expected. Distraction with an external fixator may facilitate reduction of the lunate fragments, particularly in the chronic setting.[83]

Nonunion of a lunate body fracture is rare, as most will progress to Kienböck disease. If this does occur, the treatment includes radial shortening, radial wedge osteotomy, or ulnar lengthening in the early stages, with carpal arthodesis if the condition is advanced.[11,111,151,173,195,310,483,537]

Other Carpal Fractures

Carpal fractures other than those of the scaphoid, lunate and triquetrum are rare. The known facts about these are summarized in Table 31-15.

TABLE 31-15 Epidemiology, Etiology, Diagnosis and Management of Trapezium, Trapezoid, Capitate, Hamate, and Pisiform Fractures

Fracture	Epidemiology and Etiology	Clinical Assessment and Diagnosis	Management and Complications
Trapezium	Rare, <5% of all carpal fractures[218,467] Body (vertical), tuberosity or avulsion fracture types Ridge avulsion occur following forceful deviation, traction or rotation on capsular ligaments or flexor retinaculum[330] Tuberosity fractures associated with fractures of the hook of the hamate, or with dislocation of the hamate, due to the attachments of the flexor retinaculum[199,230,236,498] Articular surface fractures can be associated with dislocation or fracture-dislocation of the first CMCJ[176,230,330]	Localized pain and tenderness Standard scaphoid views primary investigation Carpal tunnel views for tuberosity fractures[230] Associated scaphoid fractures reported[222,508] Secondary imaging modalities for associated complex injuries	Undisplaced: Scaphoid cast Displaced/dislocation: CRIF[381] or ORIF[165,176,321,494] Recent report of the use of arthroscopy[540] 60% reported to have an unsatisfactory outcome[105] Nonunion (ridge fractures): Excision
Trapezoid	Least common carpal fracture (<1%)[218] Fracture patterns include sagittal, coronal, or crush[244] Vast majority undisplaced[244] Dislocations can occur in both directions[76,175,244,346,458] Associated fractures in one-third of cases[244] Strong ligamentous attachments mean high-energy injuries required for injury (e.g., RTA, crush, sports), with axial loading, forced flexion, forced extension, and direct blow all described[244,293,318]	Localized pain and tenderness (e.g., base of second metacarpal) Symptoms and signs can be minimal and imitate a scaphoid fracture[244] Standard scaphoid views primary investigation Oblique views can aid diagnosis Overlap of carpals can make diagnosis difficult[353] Coronal fractures rarely detected on radiographs[244] CT/MRI for diagnosis in over 80% of cases[244]	Undisplaced (<2 mm): Vast majority, scaphoid cast Excellent results often achieved even with delayed treatment[202,244,341] Displaced ± dislocation or delayed union: ORIF or excision[76,346,378,408,521]
Capitate	Controversy regarding frequency, <1% carpal fractures[75,218] Mechanism injury includes direct blow/crush, scaphocapitate syndrome[154,296,314] or the anvil mechanism theory of injury (see Pathoanatomy) Direct blow or crush injuries are often associated with injury to the other carpal bones and/or the metacarpals	Localized pain and tenderness Standard scaphoid views primary investigation Lateral views useful for determining displacement and rotation of the head Dynamic studies for displacement CT/MRI for occult fractures[8,115,356]	Undisplaced: Heals without immobilization, scaphoid cast Displaced ± dislocation: ORIF[166,382,392,488,510] Nonunion rare when undisplaced[98,561] AVN possible with displaced fractures[294,495]
Hamate	Rare, <5% of all carpal fractures, third most common[218] Hook (most common), body or dorsoulnar flake fracture types[161,354,536,567] Hook fracture is commonly a sports (racket sports and golf)-related injury[9,152,161,169,203,369,519] (Fig. 31-35) Body or coronal fractures are commonly seen in young men following a punch injury. Associated fracture or fracture-dislocation of metacarpals frequent[536] Flake or avulsion fractures usually occur following a low-energy fall or direct blow	Localized pain and tenderness, though often minimal Ulnar nerve lesion (deep branch of ulnar nerve passes around hook of hamate)[161,169,451] Tendon rupture with chronic presentations[315,485,556] Standard scaphoid views primary investigation Loss of bone contour is suspicious of dislocation One study suggested three signs indicative of a hook fracture[354]: 1. Absence of the hook 2. Sclerosis of the hook 3. Lack of cortical density Oblique and carpal tunnel views improving chance of diagnosing hook fractures[245,262] Important to distinguish from os hamulus proprium Alternate view with maximal radial deviation of the wrist and maximal abduction of the thumb[49] CT/MRI for suspected fractures[22,245,375]	Undisplaced: Cast with good results reported[519,535,536] Displaced ± dislocation ± nerve lesion: Excision or ORIF[9,220,417,451,519] ± decompression of Guyon canal With excision some authors advocate bone grafting to preserve the pulley effect on the flexor tendons[526] One study determined a concomitant soft tissue lesion was predictive of a poorer outcome[220] Nonunion (more common with hook fractures) can lead to chronic pain and little finger flexor tendon injury. Manage with excision or OIRF ± bone grafting[418,556]

(continues)

TABLE 31-15	Epidemiology, Etiology, Diagnosis and Management of Trapezium, Trapezoid, Capitate, Hamate, and Pisiform Fractures (continued)		
Fracture	Epidemiology and Etiology	Clinical Assessment and Diagnosis	Management and Complications
Pisiform	Rare, <5% of all carpal fractures[218] Predominantly body fractures[218] Dislocation is rare[119,336,415] Commonly sports-related fractures and often missed[262]	Localized pain and tenderness[336] Ulnar nerve lesion (terminal branch division at pisiform) Standard scaphoid views primary investigation Lateral in 20 to 45 degrees of supination and carpal tunnel views aid diagnosis[262] Subluxation of pisotriquetral joint diagnosed with ≥1 of 1. joint space <4 mm width 2. loss of parallelism >20 degrees 3. proximal or distal override of pisiform <15% width of joint surfaces	Cast treatment usually sufficient Excision through a volar approach for painful non-union (rare)[26,95,336] Complications of excision may include reduction of grip strength/wrist flexion, hammer syndrome, ulnar nerve neuropathy[26]; however, some studies have disputed the loss in wrist function[264]

AUTHORS' PREFERRED MANAGEMENT—OTHER CARPAL FRACTURES

For the vast majority of isolated, undisplaced or minimally displaced carpal fractures we prefer nonoperative management. We routinely use a standard Colles cast or wrist splint, depending on the requirements of the patient, for a period of approximately 4 weeks followed by routine mobilization. For simple avulsion fractures, immediate motion and a splint as required for discomfort is sufficient. For displaced fractures, which are routinely associated with other osseous or soft tissue injuries of the carpus, we prefer closed or open reduction, with internal fixation.

Directions for Future Research in Other Carpal Fractures

There is sparse literature on all the "other carpal fractures." Exact details regarding epidemiology, diagnosis using standard radiographs, as well as short-term and long-term outcomes following both conservative and operative management is not known.

Other Carpal Fractures: Pearls and Pitfalls

- Triquetral fractures are the second most common carpal fracture following a fracture of the scaphoid
- Routine scaphoid radiographs detect most carpal injuries
- A thorough assessment for other osseous and ligamentous injuries of the carpus is necessary

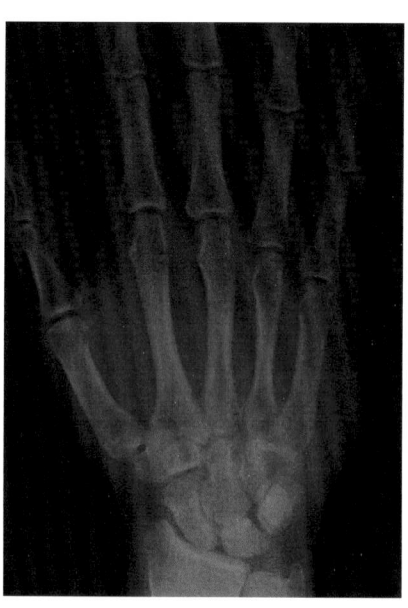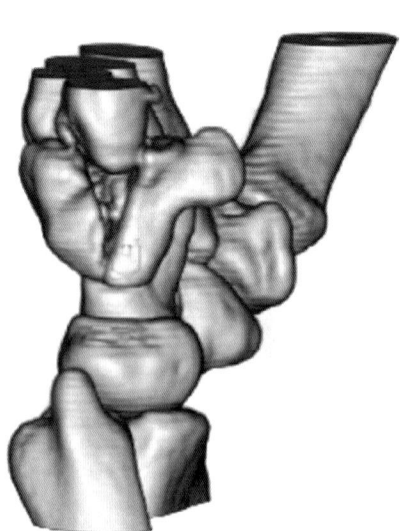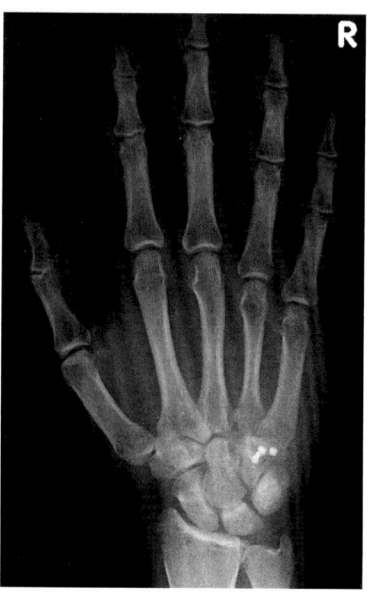

A, B   C

FIGURE 31-35 **A:** Radiograph of the right hand reveals a fracture through the hamate. **B:** 3D CT reconstruction confirms a fracture through the body of the hamate. **C:** Radiograph post ORIF.

- The vast majority of the other carpal fractures can be managed nonoperatively with good results

CARPAL LIGAMENT INJURIES

There are various classifications for carpal malalignment and carpal ligament injuries, which are discussed on Pages 1000–1002. A variety of imaging modalities are utilized when carpal ligament injury is suspected. Standard scaphoid radiographs with additional deviated views of the wrist, and possibly a clenched fist PA view form the primary investigation. MRI is imperfect for carpal ligament injuries and wrist arthroscopy is considered the reference standard, but it is not clear what to do with the so-called "partial" injuries and how these can be distinguished from normal variations or age-related changes.

Scapholunate Dissociation of Carpal Ligament Injuries

Etiology

SLD is the most common form of carpal ligament injury, with dynamic scapholunate instability the most common cause of instability in adolescents and young adults.[183,475,544] Instability can occur in isolation or in association with a fracture of the carpus or distal radius.[84,149,331,332,362,416,511] The most common mechanism of injury involves hyperextension of the wrist with associated ulnar deviation and intracarpal supination leading to injury of the scapholunate interosseous and palmar ligaments.[301–304] A previous injury, repetitive strain on the carpus, or the presence of acute or chronic synovitis appears to alter the magnitude of force required to cause ligamentous disruption, so much so that the presenting event may be following a trivial injury.[173]

SLD describes a spectrum of injuries ranging from ligamentous sprains through to dislocation of the scaphoid. A variety of ligament disruptions can occur including one or more of the scapholunate interosseous ligament, the RSL ligament, the RSC ligament, the scaphotrapezium-trapezoid ligament, the DRC ligament, and the dorsal intercarpal ligament.[173] Disruption of the scapholunate interosseous ligament leads to dyskinesia between the scaphoid and the lunate, ultimately resulting in progressive widening of the scapholunate joint with time.[480] The clinical consequences of the injury depend on the tightness or laxity of the capsuloligamentous system of the wrist, as well as the presence of any associated palmar radiocarpal or midcarpal ligament damage.[173]

Clinical Assessment and Diagnosis

Patients will often present with localized wrist pain and swelling following a fall onto an outstretched hand, with the wrist undergoing a forced hyperextension.[37,331,332,518] There will be tenderness in the region of the scaphoid and lunate. Movement of the wrist may be minimal, with pain on flexion–extension or radioulnar deviation and an audible clunk or click heard. A full assessment of the entire carpus and distal radius and ulna is necessary as there may be an associated fracture. A clinical deformity at the wrist may be apparent and a full neurovascular assessment is imperative, as acute carpal tunnel syndrome can occur with associated carpal fractures and dislocations.[331,332]

Clinical findings can be subtle, and the classic features of carpal instability may not be apparent without provocative stress testing. A simple general provocative maneuver is a vigorous grasp that induces pain, an audible clunk or click, a dorsal deformity in the region of the proximal scaphoid, and reduced power with repetitive grip strength testing. A positive Kirk-Watson (scaphoid shift) test is highly suggestive of scapholunate instability (Fig. 31-12), although not absolutely specific for SLD as it may reposition the entire proximal carpal row if the row, rather than the individual scaphoid, is unstable.[370,523,528,547,548] In addition, in individuals with lax ligaments there may be false-positive signs of dorsal subluxation of the scaphoid that are not pathologic. Generalized ligamentous laxity may be present in patients with true SLD as many wrists with an injury have some form of pre-existing ligamentous laxity.[303]

Imaging. The six standard views for carpal instability are mandatory in the assessment of suspected SL instability. Clenched fist views and contralateral wrist views can aid in the diagnosis. The following should be assessed (see Pages 1004–1008):

- A *scapholunate gap* of >3 mm is suggestive of instability, with a gap >5 mm diagnostic of SLD if there is a positive cortical ring sign (Fig. 31-36). The increased gap between the scaphoid and lunate has been named the Terry Thomas sign (Fig. 31-36) after the gap-toothed smile of the British comedian.[163] It is suggested that the gap should be compared to the uninjured opposite extremity,[80] particularly in the absence of a dorsiflexed lunate, which is most likely nontraumatic.[360]
- The appearance of the scaphoid.
  - A positive *cortical ring sign* is when the distal scaphoid tubercle is seen end-on with a PA view, suggestive that the scaphoid is flexed.[80]
- A *scapholunate angle* of >60 degrees is suggestive of instability, with an angle of >80 degrees diagnostic of SLD (Fig. 31-36).[183,277]
- The appearance of the lunate.
  - *DISI deformity* (Fig. 31-36) where the lunate is extended (dorsally angulated) is associated with a SLD (Table 31-4).
  - A normally positioned lunate projects as a quadrilateral shape on the neutral PA radiograph; however, the shape appears triangular when the lunate is malrotated and is often associated with a perilunate dislocation.
- A *capitolunate or radiolunate angle* of >15 degrees is suggestive of instability, with an angle >20 degrees diagnostic.
- *Gilula lines* for ligamentous instability (Fig. 31-15).
- Exclude associated fractures of the radius or carpus (Fig. 31-37), especially in younger patients.
  - An ulnar positive variance of >2 mm in nonosteoporotic patients with an intra-articular fracture of the distal radius has been found to be predictive of a severe scapholunate injury.[159]

When these findings are not found on initial radiographs, stress testing with the provocative maneuvers discussed can

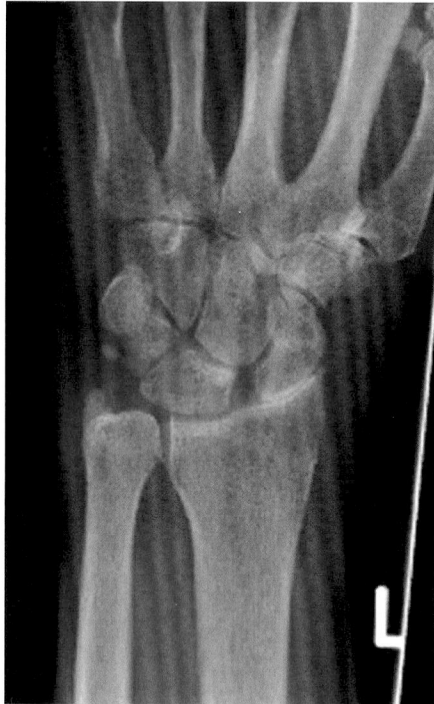
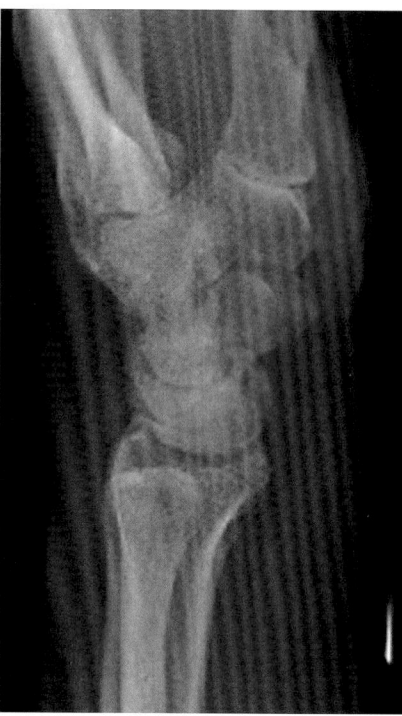

FIGURE 31-36 Scapholunate instability with an increased scapholunate gap (Terry Thomas sign) found on the AP view. A DISI deformity and an increased scapholunate angle are found on the lateral view.

be used with clenched-fist views or radioulnar stress views to determine the diagnosis and confirm dynamic SLD. Dynamic SLD is characterized by normal radiographs of the wrist, but with axial loading of the wrist a widening of the scapholunate gap is seen. Static instability is characterized by a widening of the scapholunate gap in an unloaded wrist and a scapholunate angle >60 degrees.[317]

Secondary imaging modalities include fluoroscopy or cineradiography using standard and provocative stress motions.[351,374] Arthrography has a high rate of false-positive and false-negative

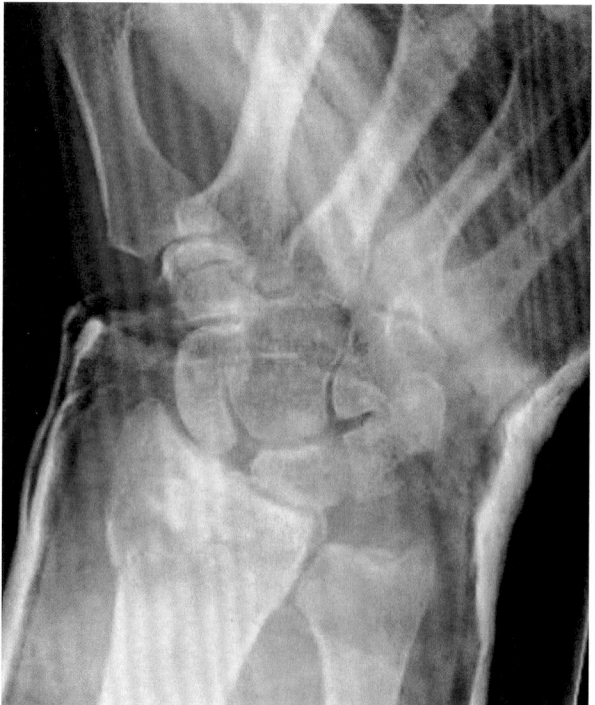
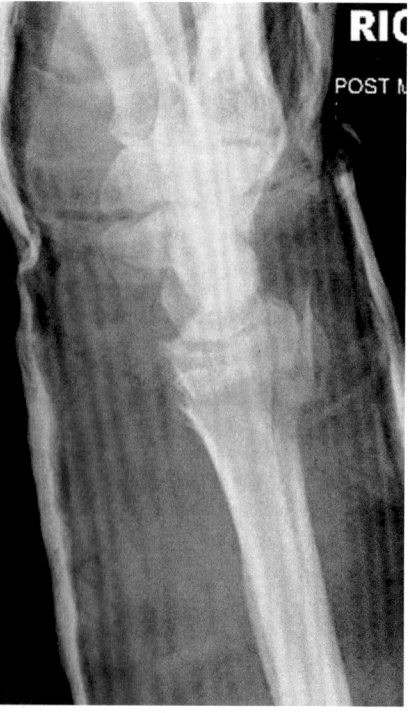

FIGURE 31-37 Radiographs of the wrist post manipulation for a fracture of the distal radius. An increased scapholunate gap indicative of SLD is seen, and was confirmed intraoperatively.

results and is therefore of limited use.[493,518] MRI is helpful in determining the extent of ligament injury. Wrist arthroscopy can be used to determine the extent of ligament disruption and the presence of radioscaphoid arthritis, as well as to classify and treat the injuries.[180,223,465,518] Arthroscopy has been shown to be effective in patients with suspected dynamic SLD (normal radiographs) for diagnosis and treatment in both acute and chronic cases, allowing assessment of both the ligaments, and midcarpal and radiocarpal joints.[223,532]

Classification. SLD encompasses a spectrum of injuries ranging from grade I ligament sprains, through all grades of ligament destabilization, to injuries of multiple ligaments, and finally dislocation.[173] A greater-arc injury encompasses SLD with a fracture of the radial styloid. The classification of scapholunate instability considers whether the injury is acute or chronic and whether it is static or dynamic, as this can be helpful for guiding management.

A static deformity does not occur with an isolated injury to the scapholunate ligament, is often only apparent on stress imaging; that is, dynamic instability.[45,317,331,332] Static instability occurs when the ligament is injured in conjunction with a multiple ligament disruption.

One study has described four grades of ligament injury according to arthroscopic findings.[180]

- Grade I: Attenuation or hemorrhage of the ligament is seen from the midcarpal space but the bones are congruent. Conservative treatment is usually sufficient.

- Grade II: Incongruency between the carpal bones when viewed from the midcarpal space. Arthroscopic reduction and fixation is normally required.

- Grade III: Carpal malalignment in both carpal spaces with a gap between the carpal bones allowing entry of a 1-mm probe. Arthroscopic ± open reduction with fixation is required.

- Grade IV: Carpal malalignment in both carpal spaces with gross instability and a gap between the carpal bones allowing entry of a 2.7-mm arthroscope. Open reduction and fixation is needed.

An alternative classification was put forward by Kuo and Wolfe,[260] which was subsequently used to define treatment (Table 31-16).[252]

Management

With appropriate treatment, it is possible to avoid potential complications of an SLD injury including advanced scapholunate collapse and progressive, painful arthritis of the wrist. Different treatment options need to be considered on the basis of the duration since the injury, the extent of ligamentous involvement, and the presence of associated carpal instabilities and/or fractures. The grade of ligament injury can guide treatment, as described above. However, a better guide is the duration since injury, which is best defined as follows:

- <4 weeks since injury = acute

- 4 to 24 weeks since injury = subacute

- >6 months = chronic

The primary goals of treatment are stabilization of the carpal bones in good alignment allowing restoration of wrist mobility. The earlier ligament repair takes place the easier it is to perform a direct repair.[173]

Acute SLD. Patients with a grade I ligament injury but with no evidence of carpal instability can be managed effectively with cast immobilization. In patients with partial ligament tears but with instability present arthroscopically, cast immobilization is unsuitable as the scaphoid requires wrist extension to maintain reduction and the lunate requires wrist flexion.[481] For these cases, percutaneous K-wire fixation in combination with cast immobilization for 8 weeks can be employed. One

---

TABLE 31-16 **An Alternate Classification for SLD, with an Aim to Guide Treatment, put Forward by Kuo and Wolfe**

	I. Occult	II. Dynamic	III. SL Dissociation	IV. DISI	V. SLAC
Ligaments	Partial SL ligament	Incompetent or complete SL ligament; partial volar extrinsics	Complete SLIL, volar or dorsal extrinsics	Complete SLIL, volar extrinsics, secondary changes in RL, STT, dorsal ligaments	As stage IV
Radiographs	Normal	Abnormal on stress testing	SL gap ≥3 mm, grossly abnormal on stress testing	SL angle ≥60 degrees, SL gap ≥3 mm, RL angle ≥15 degrees, CL angle ≥15 degrees	Progressive OA with pancarpal OA final stage
Management	Pinning or capsulodesis	Ligament repair with capsulodesis	Ligament repair with capsulodesis vs. triligament reconstruction	Reducible: Triligament reconstruction Irreducible: Fusion	Proximal row carpectomy or fusion

CL, capitolunate; RL, radiolunate; SL, scapholunate.
Adapted from: Kitay A, Wolfe SW. Scapholunate instability: Current concepts in diagnosis and management. *J Hand Surg Am.* 2012;37:2175–2196 and Kuo CE, Wolfe SW. Scapholunate instability: Current concepts in diagnosis and management. *J Hand Surg Am.* 2008;33:998–1013.

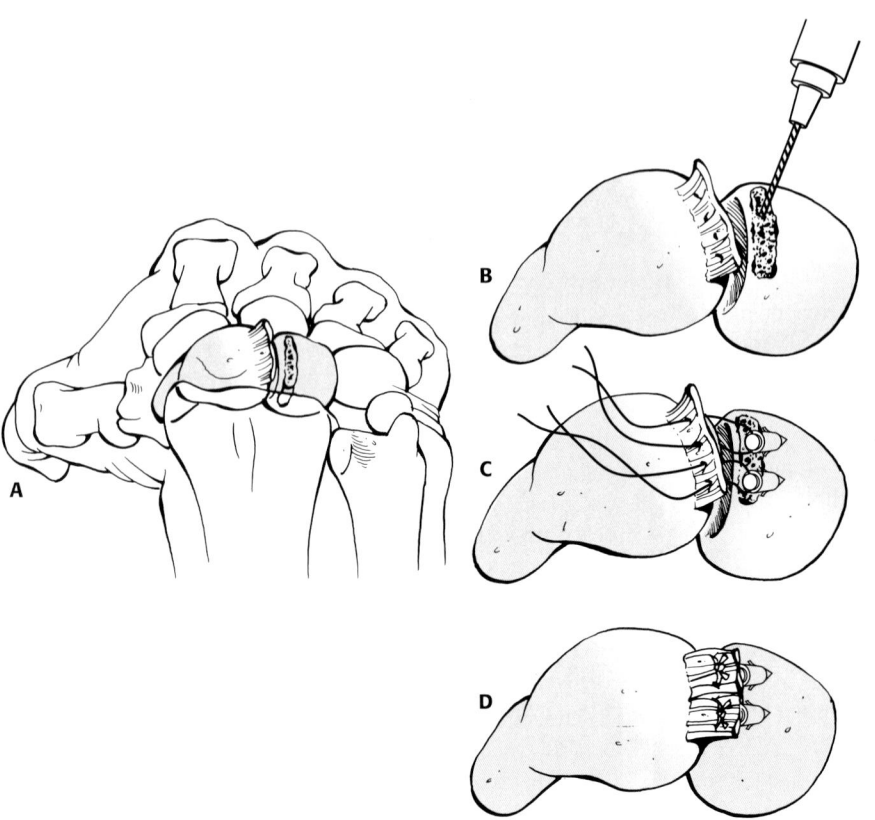

FIGURE 31-38 A–D: Ligament repair for scapholunate instability using anchors placed into the lunate (or scaphoid, depending on where the ligament has ruptured), and the ligament is sutured back into position.

K-wire is placed from the scaphoid to the lunate and another from the scaphoid to the capitate. Pins can be placed into the scaphoid and lunate and used as joysticks to reduce the scapholunate joint.[173] An 85% success rate in maintaining SL reduction has been reported in patients with a scapholunate interval that was greater than the unaffected wrist by 3 mm or less and in patients where the injury was less than 3 months old.[538,539] Such injuries, even if not initially associated with obvious instability, can progress to scapholunate collapse.[518]

When the carpus cannot be reduced by closed methods, open ligament repair and pin fixation is recommended in all cases of acute SLD. Cadaveric studies have demonstrated that reduction of the scapholunate articulation is essential to the recovery of normal wrist kinematics after SLD.[480] Soft tissue repair and reconstruction are popular because they attempt to restore the normal kinematics of the wrist, with current literature demonstrating superior results of direct ligament repair over ligament reconstruction.[36,94,316] The technique of repair has changed with the use of intraosseous suture retaining anchors allowing ligament attachment directly to the bone (Fig. 31-38).[29,51,402] Results of primary open ligament repair by a dorsal approach are conflicting.[51,271] Some authors advocate a combined dorsal and palmar approach suggesting improved reduction and outcome.[139,295]

Bickert et al.[51] reported on the short-term outcome of 12 patients following repair with a dorsal approach at a mean follow-up of 19 months and reported restoration of a normal scapholunate angle in 10 patients, with the mean range of motion at 78% of normal, the mean grip strength 81%, and 8 patients with an excellent or good result. However, no correlation was found between functional and radiologic results, although one of the two poor results was associated with lunate necrosis. Outcome in the long-term is unknown, although similar outcomes have been reported at 5 to 6 years following surgery.[258] Some authors are advocates of management using an arthroscopic technique that can aid in confirming the diagnosis, as well as determine the location and extent of ligamentous damage; for example, palmar extrinsic ligament attenuation.[257,538] However, whether this is superior remains unclear.

Subacute SLD. For subacute SLD, the addition of local tissue may be necessary if the ligament has retracted or is deficient.[173] Blatt's technique (Fig. 31-39) utilizes a proximally based dorsal capsular flap retracted onto the scapholunate

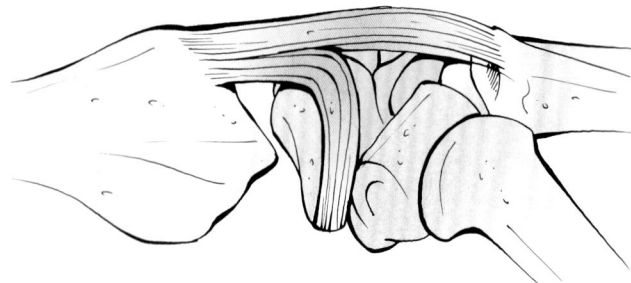

FIGURE 31-39 Blatt's technique of dorsal capsulodesis, with the scaphoid reduced a capsular flap is secured to the distal pole with an anchor.

articulation, and this is sutured as tightly as possible to the distal pole of the dorsal aspect of the scaphoid to act as a tether.[52,334] This flap can be added to the ligament repair process described earlier by placing nonabsorbable sutures from the lunate ligament remnant into the capsular tissue and then out through the scaphoid. An alternative method is to use a strip of tendon from the radial wrist extensors (extensor carpi radialis longus or extensor carpi radialis brevis), but tendon tissue is not an ideal ligament replacement with capsular tissue routinely preferred.[173]

Through a palmar approach, direct ligament repair using nonabsorbable sutures can be performed. If there is deficient tissue, a section of the FCR can be used to augment the repair process by placing drill holes through the proximal scaphoid and radial half of the lunate and passing one-half of the FCR tendon in a circular fashion to reinforce the dorsal and palmar ligaments. The RSC and RSL ligaments may be advanced into the gap. With a large, complete ligament tear associated with a gap of 5 mm or more, adjunct palmar ligament repair is usually needed.[173] A carpal tunnel incision extended slightly radially is performed, and the damaged area is identified with a probe inserted from a separate dorsal incision. The interval between the RSC ligament and the RSL ligament is developed. Sutures may then be placed with intraosseous anchors into the scaphoid proximal pole or remnants of the interosseous membrane, which are then used to pull the RSL ligament against the proximal pole to hold the over-reduction of the proximal scaphoid, which is stabilized by K-wires. The purpose of this palmar repair is to bring the dorsally subluxed and rotated proximal scaphoid in apposition with the palmar intracapsular ligaments.[173]

Whether the approach is dorsal, palmar, or combined, tight repair of the capsular structures is required. Internal fixation for a period of 12 weeks is preferred, supplemented with a below-elbow cast. After cast removal, a splint is worn as muscle strength and joint motion are restored with the aid of physiotherapy as required. Return to work or sports are best delayed for a minimum of 6 months, with continued protection being used during sports activities.

Chronic SLD. The major issues associated with chronic SLD and instability are whether the ligaments can be directly repaired, whether any residual carpal dislocation is reducible, and whether the joint has developed arthritis. When possible, restoration of normal carpal anatomy by repair and reconstruction of the support ligaments of the wrist remains the preferred treatment. This requires sufficient local tissue for a repair and a correctable carpal instability. Partial or complete fusion of the wrist may be required when:[173]

- there is a fixed carpal deformity; for example, the rotational subluxation of the scaphoid or DISI deformity cannot be reduced.
- the degree of ligament disruption and retraction precludes repair.
- there are local degenerative changes of the radiocarpal and midcarpal joints.
- the demands and expectations of the patient include heavy lifting or repetitive loading.

There are many techniques described to treat chronic scapholunate instability.[52,173,422,472] Current techniques for ligament reconstruction include repair with the dorsal capsular flap procedure, a palmar ligament reefing procedure, or combined dorsal and palmar procedures that add flexor or extensor tendon tissue to the repair site.[173] The goal of each of these repair techniques involves the addition of local tissue to provide a collagen framework for future stability.[52,173,422,472] Soft tissue reconstructions have several theoretical advantages that make them attractive alternatives to other procedures. In contrast to arthrodeses, soft tissue reconstructions provide a greater range of intercarpal motion.[472]

Tendon weave procedures and tenodeses (Fig. 31-40) have been attempted with variable success. Wrist extensor or flexor tendon augmentation procedures require placement of drill holes in bone. In this procedure, drill holes are carefully placed in a dorsal-to-palmar direction through the scaphoid and lunate. Tendon strips are then passed through these holes to attempt a reconstruction of the ligament. The large holes required to pass tendon grafts can lead to a fracture of the carpus.[173] An alternative technique is to take part of an extensor or flexor tendon and pass it through the capitate, scaphoid, lunate, and distal radius.[12] Another technique is the reconstruction of the dorsal part of the ligament using a bone-ligament-bone autograft; however, clinical results are not particularly convincing.[533]

The palmar approach for SL ligament repair (Conyers technique) is performed through a carpal tunnel incision.[97] A probe or needle passed dorsal to palmar is helpful in locating the ligament tear and palmar ligament intervals. Flaps of RSC and RSL ligaments are reflected laterally and medially. Palmar cortical bone is removed from the capitate, distal radius, scaphoid, and lunate on either side of the scapholunate interval and the cartilage surfaces of the scaphoid and lunate are denuded to subchondral bone to encourage a strong syndesmosis. The scaphoid and lunate are then reduced and pinned with threaded wires that are left in place for at least 8 weeks. The palmar ligaments are carefully repaired overlapping the edges over the denuded cortical bone to ensure sound healing to bone. Motion is delayed 10 to 12 weeks to encourage adequate strength of the syndesmosis.[173]

Several procedures have been designed to restrict rotatory subluxation of the scaphoid by creating a dorsal tether.[52,86,280,422] A commonly used method of dorsal capsulodesis is the Blatt type of capsular reconstruction.[52] Results of Blatt capsulodesis for chronic SLD are acceptable, although some clinical series have not reported favorable outcomes that could be a consequence of patient selection.[120] Both short- and longer-term series have reported promising results with the use of a dorsal intercarpal ligament capsulodesis, which is a soft tissue reconstruction procedure based on the dorsal intercarpal ligament of the wrist.[174,444,445,472] The theoretical advantage of this method is that it avoids a tether between the distal radius and the scaphoid, allowing the proximal carpal row to work as a functional unit. Wyrick et al.[554] assessed the use of ligament repair and dorsal capsulodesis for static SLD and found that no patients were free of pain at follow-up. Their experience, along with others, has suggested that dorsal capsulodesis is likely more suited to patients with dynamic instability than for those with static instability. Static instability requires an intercarpal fusion.[173]

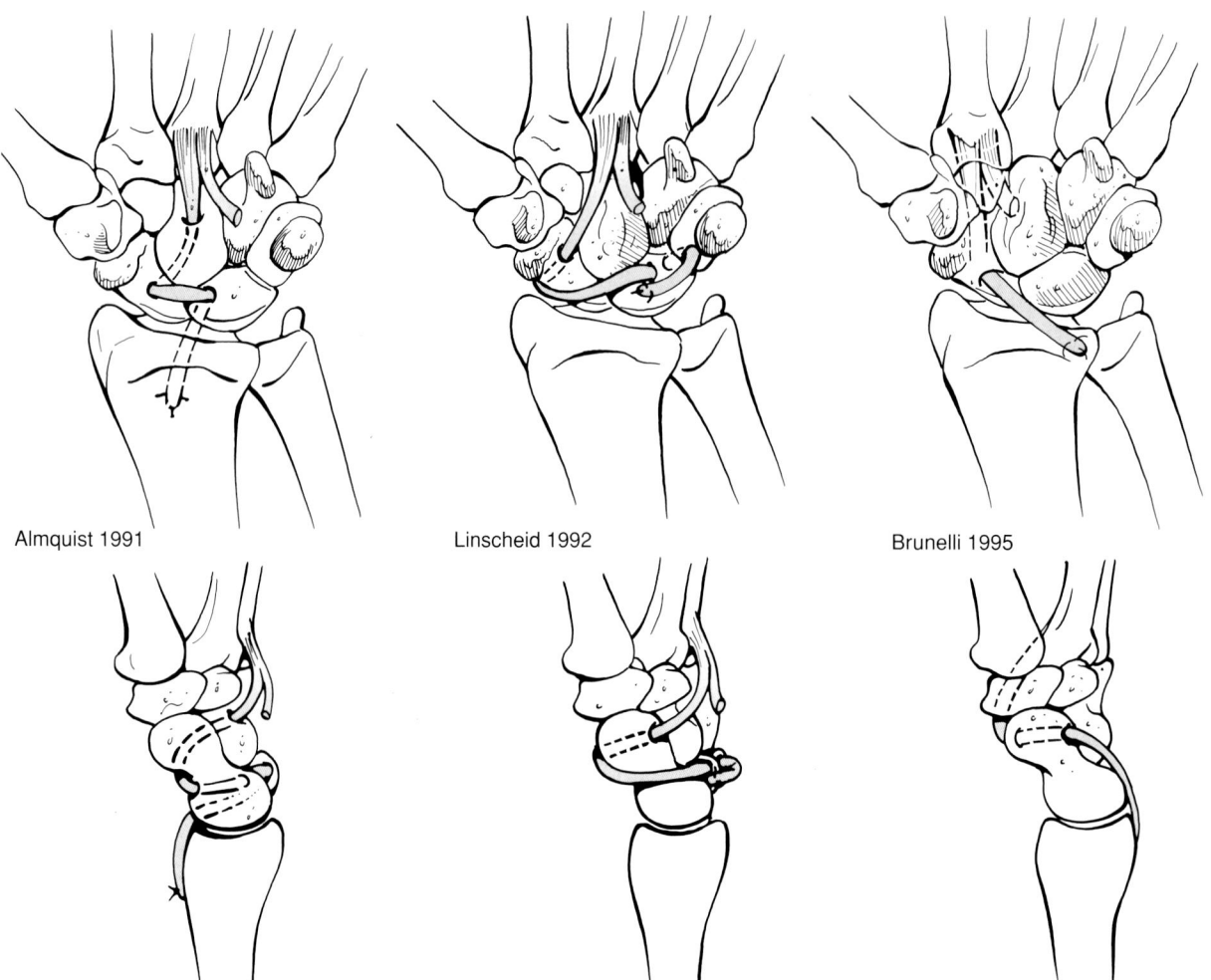

Almquist 1991   Linscheid 1992   Brunelli 1995

FIGURE 31-40 Tendon weaves and reconstructions proposed by various authors.

Wrist Fusion. Of the partial wrist fusions performed for wrist instability, the scaphotrapeziotrapezoidal (STT) fusion is frequently recommended in the literature.[142,173,525] The purpose of this procedure is to stabilize the distal scaphoid and thereby hold the proximal pole more securely within the scaphoid fossa of the distal radius.[173] Clinical studies have shown that STT fusion is reliable and effective, giving pain relief and reasonable functional results. Similar results have been recently reported for scaphocapitate fusion in the medium term.[118] However, in the longer term, degenerative changes in adjacent joints may be a problem.[158] Young active patients with chronic instability and severe arthritis can be treated with excision of the scaphoid and a four-corner fusion with arthrodesis of the capitate, lunate, hamate, and triquetrum.

STT fusion can be performed through a transverse incision centered over the STT joint or through the universal longitudinal incision. If either STT fusion or the equivalent scaphocapitate fusion is undertaken, it is important to reduce the palmar-flexed scaphoid, close the SL interval, and maintain carpal height.[118] The ideal flexion angle of the scaphoid is 45 degrees. Fixation of the STT or scaphocapitate joints is performed with K-wires,

screws, or staples. Bone graft from the distal radius or iliac crest is placed between the decorticated distal scaphoid and the proximal surfaces of the trapezium and trapezoid (STT fusion), or between the medial articular surface of the scaphoid and the lateral surface of the capitate (scaphocapitate fusion). Once scaphoid alignment is achieved, cancellous bone graft is inserted and K-wires are placed to support the fusion area. Prereduction placement of K-wires into the scaphoid facilitates correct orientation after reduction.[173] Immobilization after intercarpal fusion is usually for 8 weeks in a scaphoid cast, followed by a support splint for 4 to 6 weeks. CT scans of the wrist can help determine the degree of consolidation at the fusion site.

Authors' Preferred Management—SLD

We recommend primary repair and pin fixation for acute SLD using a dorsal approach.[173] The approach is centered over Lister tubercle, reflecting the dorsal wrist capsule to preserve the dorsal intercarpal and dorsal radiotriquetral ligaments, using a radial-based capsular flap. The radial capsule is reflected from the scaphoid to its waist. The open technique allows direct visualization of the injured ligament, reduction, and ligament repair. Most often, the SL ligament is torn off the scaphoid, but still attached to the lunate. In rare cases, avulsion from the lunate or an oblique tear will be seen. Reduction of the lunate and scaphoid is performed with K-wire joysticks inserted in a dorsal-to-palmar direction. The rim of the proximal scaphoid is freshened to subcortical bone with a fine rongeur to facilitate ligament healing. Ideally, high-speed burrs should be avoided as thermal necrosis may occur. When the ligament remains attached to the lunate, intraosseous anchors are inserted into the waist of the scaphoid. The anchors are placed in such a position that the suture lies in a slightly oblique direction in order to resist the rotational forces between scaphoid and lunate.[51] The sutures attached to the anchors are placed in the SL ligament in a palmar to dorsal direction. If anchors are not available, drill holes in the scaphoid are required to allow direct attachment of the ligament onto the scaphoid. When the sutures are positioned, the scaphoid and lunate are reduced with joysticks and held in the reduced position with K-wires. One K-wire is placed from the scaphoid to the lunate and another from the scaphoid to the capitate. The sutures are tied and the capsule repaired. A below-elbow cast is applied and retained for 12 weeks, when the K-wires are removed.

We prefer the Blatt's technique of capsule reconstruction, using dorsal capsulodesis for the treatment of chronic scapholunate instability.[52,120,173] For the Blatt type of capsule reconstruction, a long rectangular flap, about 1.5 cm wide, based on the dorsal aspect of the distal radius, is used. The distal edge of capsule is sutured to the distal pole of the scaphoid once the scaphoid is placed in a reduced position. A K-wire can be passed into the dorsum of the lunate to be used as a joystick to reduce any DISI. The scaphoid is reduced by pressure on the scaphoid tubercle and then transfixed to the capitate by another K-wire. The dorsal surface of the scaphoid is roughened with a fine rongeur just distal to the center of rotation. The dorsal flap of wrist capsule is sutured under tension with intraosseous anchors distal to the scaphoid center of rotation so that it tethers the proximal pole in the scaphoid fossa. The flap is sutured to reinforce the local tissue of the SL interval. For a distally based flap, one can raise a rectangular capsular flap, leaving the distal end of the flap attached to the scaphoid. After SL ligament reconstruction, immobilization in a below-elbow cast is recommended for 8 weeks. The K-wires are removed at 8 weeks. Splint immobilization for an additional 4 weeks is suggested to allow for tissue healing with gradual stress loading. Supporting splints are best worn intermittently for 6 months to prevent sudden stress to the wrist and to allow further collagen maturation.

Lunotriquetral Dissociation of Carpal Ligament Injuries

Lunotriquetral dissociation (LTD) includes sprains, partial or complete ligament tears, as well as part of the spectrum of

perilunate dislocation, or in association with ulnocarpal impingement and TFCC injuries.[173] Lunotriquetral ligament injuries are less common than scapholunate ligament injuries.[243] Although LTD is not associated with the development of degenerative changes in the carpus, it can lead to potentially devastating changes to carpal kinematics, especially if it advances to a stage of a VISI deformity. Even without this progression, the patient with chronic ulnar-sided pain experiences significant ongoing disability.[410]

The mechanism of an isolated LTD is relatively unknown when compared to LTD injury as part of a perilunate dislocation. The lunotriquetral joint is inherently stable, more so than the scapholunate joint, and it seems that associated ligament damage to the dorsal radiotriquetral ligament or palmar ulnocarpal ligaments must be present before severe fixed deformities occur.[274]

Clinical Assessment and Diagnosis

Patients present with a history of injury associated with ulnar-sided wrist pain, worse on activity.[384] Some patients describe a clunking sensation when the wrist moves from radial to ulnar deviation.[384] Clinical signs are often diffuse, although tenderness is often present directly over the lunotriquetral joint, and ballottement of the unstable triquetrum may be possible.[384] Stress provocation tests of the joint including compression, ballottement, or shear may be present, with the most sensitive test to diagnose LTD the LT shear test.[384]

Imaging. Primary assessment uses standard scaphoid radiographs; however, one of the major issues with diagnosing LTD is that many patients have a normal radiograph, with findings often subtle and dynamic, although stress-induced deformity is less frequent than with SLD.[384] The following may be found with an LTD:

- Disruption of Gilula lines on the PA view indicative of an altered intercarpal relationship
- A static VISI deformity on the lateral view (Fig. 31-41)
- Associated fractures; for example, a hamate fracture

Secondary imaging modalities may be required. Wrist arthrography is not a reliable diagnostic tool, but videofluoroscopy can be helpful.[173] Arthroscopy has become the most important diagnostic tool for confirming the presence and degree of LTD, with views of the radiocarpal and midcarpal joints allowing visualization of the scaphoid-trapezoid-trapezium joint, midcarpal extrinsic ligaments, the capitohamate joint, and the articular surfaces of the carpal bones.[180,223] Arthroscopic staging is applicable to all ligamentous dissociations.[180]

Management

Acute LTD with little deformity is routinely managed with a below elbow cast.[384] If conservative measures fail, surgical intervention should be considered. Closed reduction and percutaneous internal fixation of the lunate to the triquetrum is indicated when there is displacement.[173] Arthroscopy can be helpful in acute injuries to guide closed reduction and percutaneous pinning,[361,406] with some suggesting the arthroscope be

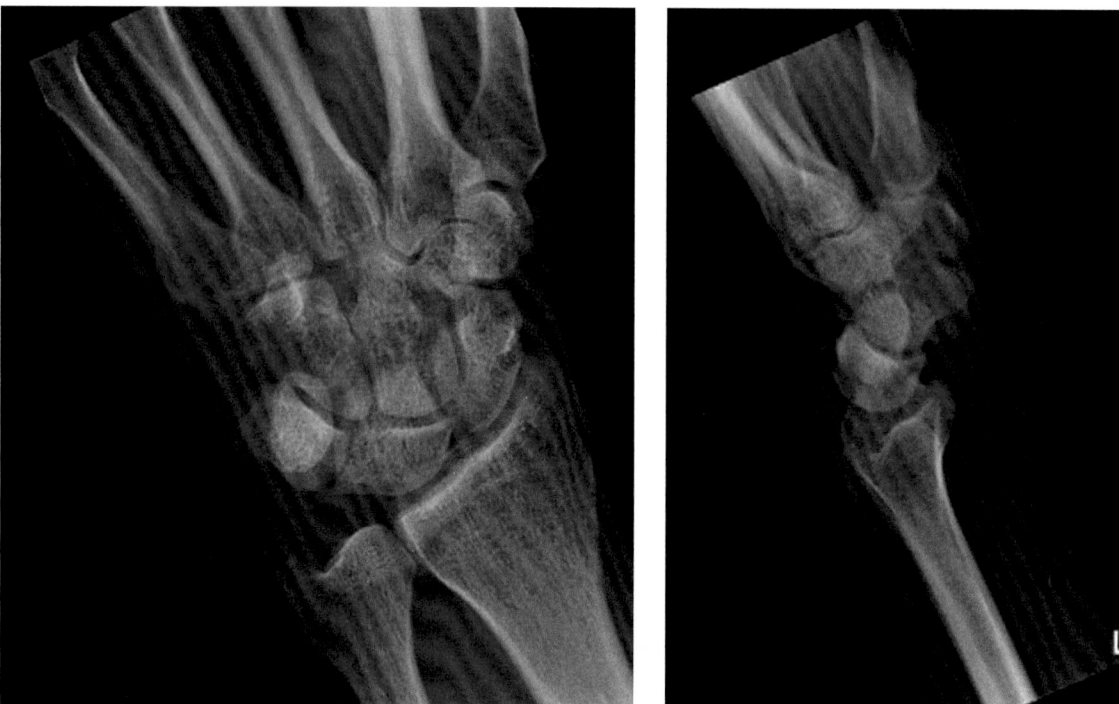

FIGURE 31-41 A VISI deformity of the left wrist. Subsequent MRI confirmed LTD.

placed in the radial midcarpal portal for this procedure because the alignment of the LT joint is much easier to evaluate.

Indications for open surgery include if closed reduction ± arthroscopy fails, when the LTD is associated with an angular deformity, or following unsatisfactory results from previous treatment. An open repair should be attempted only when there are sufficiently strong ligament remnants present, when the ligament remnants have a reasonable healing potential, and when the LT relationship is easily reduced.[173]

Open reduction, repair of lax or damaged ligaments, and temporary internal fixation with percutaneous wires across the triquetrum and lunate left in place for 6 to 8 weeks is recommended.[173] All ligaments that seem to be concerned with LT stability should be reattached and it is mandatory to correct any VISI deformity. The interosseous ligament repair is usually done through a dorsal approach. Care should be taken to avoid injury to the dorsal sensory branch of the ulnar nerve. The fifth extensor compartment is opened and an ulnar-based retinacular flap is elevated. The ligament is more likely to be stripped from the triquetrum. Intraosseous bone anchors with attached sutures are used for reconstruction. Capsular flaps are useful for reinforcing the dorsal portion of such a repair or augmenting the dorsal radiotriquetral and dorsal scaphotriquetral ligaments. For late presentations with complete ligament disruption and no tissue for repair, ligament reconstruction using part of the extensor carpi ulnaris tendon is recommended.[173,410]

In cases of recurrence and/or when soft tissue repair cannot control recurrent deformity, lunotriquetral joint fusion may be indicated, with or without accompanying denervation procedures. Concomitant ulnar shortening procedures should be considered (especially with ulnar plus variance) to tighten the palmar ulnocarpal ligaments in addition to fusion or ligament reconstruction. More aggressive treatments are proximal row carpectomy and total wrist arthrodesis in patients with radiologic signs of arthrosis.[173]

Perilunate Dislocation and Fracture-Dislocation

Etiology

A perilunate dislocation or fracture-dislocation is the most common form of wrist dislocation and encompasses a spectrum of injury, which can include both ligamentous and osseous disruption. In clinical practice, the prefix trans is commonly used to refer to associated fractures, whereas the prefix peri is used to describe a dislocation.[173] Perilunate fracture-dislocations (greater-arc injuries) are more frequently seen than perilunate dislocations (lesser-arc injuries) with the ratio reported to be two to one, with displacement in a dorsal direction in 97% of cases.[215] The injury is frequently seen in young males with strong bone as the distal radius and the scaphoid need to be strong enough to resist the amount of torque that results in a perilunate dislocation.[215]

Prompt management improves the chance of a good long-term outcome; however, all patients should be advised regarding the severity of these injuries and the guarded prognosis. Late diagnosis delays treatment, which is difficult and frequently less successful. Approximately 20% of patients are misdiagnosed at presentation and that delay between injury and treatment worsens the prognosis with neglected cases resulting in pain, weakness, stiffness, carpal tunnel syndrome, and post-traumatic osteoarthritis.[15,154,215,256]

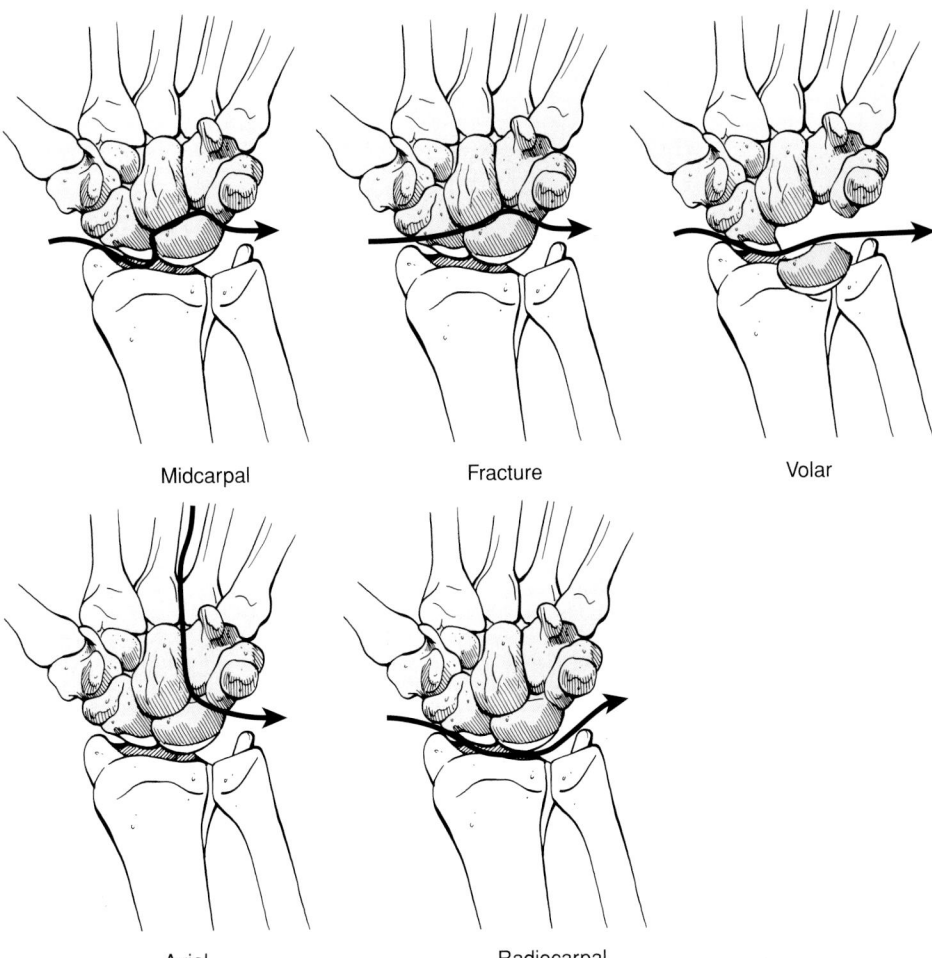

FIGURE 31-42 Different types of perilunate dislocations and fracture-dislocations.

Midcarpal

Fracture

Volar

Axial

Radiocarpal

Perilunate Dislocations. Perilunate dislocations (lesser-arc injury) are characterized by a progressive disruption of capsular and ligamentous connections of the lunate to the adjacent carpal bones and radius, without associated fractures to the carpus and distal radius. Ligament disruption typically begins radially and propagates around or through the lunate to the ulnar side of the carpus (Fig. 31-42). Classically, the distal row dislocates in a dorsal or dorsoradial direction followed by the entire scaphoid and triquetrum in pure perilunate dislocations or just by the distal portion of these bones in perilunate fracture-dislocations. SLD or LTD often persists even after relocation, with recurrence of instability common whether the injury involves one or both of the lesser or greater arc. It is important to define any associated ligamentous injuries such as LTD or SLD to prevent late carpal collapse.[173] For the detailed pathoanatomy of injury please see Page 1002.

Perilunate Fracture-dislocations. Perilunate fracture-dislocations (greater-arc injury) combine ligament ruptures, osseous avulsions and various types of fractures. The most common pattern of perilunate instability is the transscaphoid perilunate fracture-dislocation.[87,101,215] Fractures of the capitate, hamate, lunate, triquetrum, and radial styloid can also occur. In a series of 166 perilunate dislocations and fracture-dislocations, fracture-dislocations were twice as frequent as a dislocation alone, with 61% being dorsal transscaphoid perilunate fracture-dislocations.[215] Displaced transverse fractures of the neck of the capitate and sagittal fractures of the triquetrum are also quite frequent.[24,25,82,215,273] The capitate fragment is frequently rotated through 180 degrees so that its articular surface faces the raw cancellous surface of the major capitate fragment.[173] Both capitate and scaphoid fragments are devascularized by displacement and this is known as the scaphocapitate syndrome.[24,510]

Clinical Assessment and Diagnosis

Patients are often young males who present following a high-energy (e.g., fall from height, motor vehicle accident, sports) hyperextension injury, with persistent wrist pain, swelling, and deformity.[15,215,219] Approximately a quarter of presentations will be associated with a polytrauma, with one in ten sustaining an associated upper limb injury.[215] In around 16% of cases the clinical presentation includes median nerve symptoms and signs,[4] but an ulnar neuropathy, arterial injury, or tendon disruption may also be seen.[4,15,101,215,323]

Some perilunate dislocations may be seen several months or years after the initial injury.[473] The patient is more likely to present because of increasing nerve symptoms or tendon rupture than because of wrist deformity to which the patient has often become accustomed.

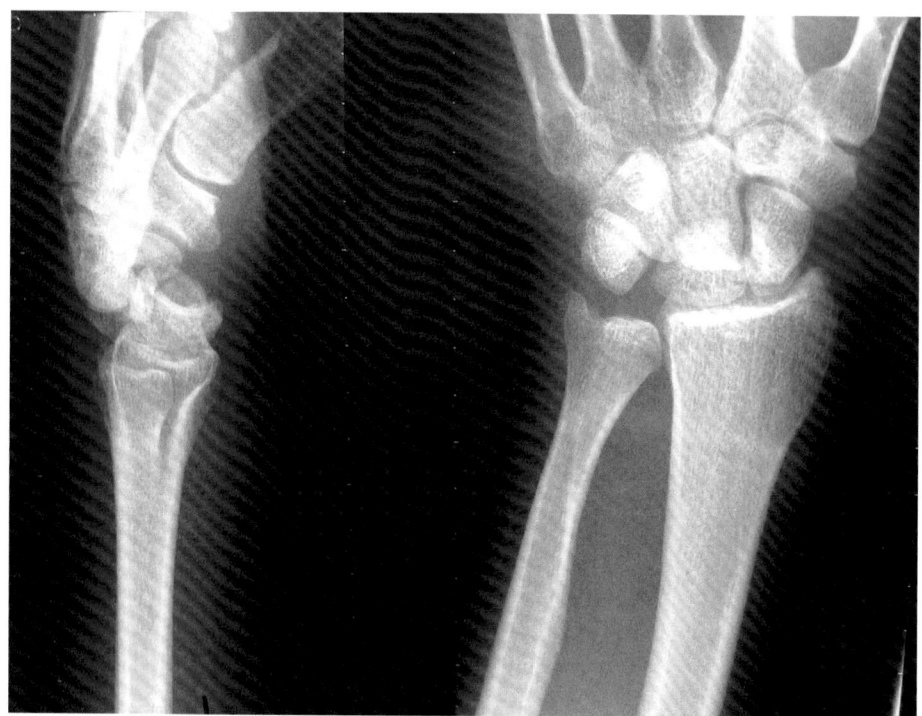

FIGURE 31-43 Wrist radiographs demonstrating typical radiologic signs of perilunate fracture-dislocation.

Imaging. Primary assessment uses standard scaphoid radiographs with the following appearances suggestive of a perilunate dislocation.[192,217]

- Disruption of Gilula lines on the PA view indicative of an altered intercarpal relationship (Fig. 31-43)

- "Spilled teapot sign" on the lateral view due to palmar rotation of the lunate and disruption of the lunate-capitate articulation

- Triangular appearance of lunate secondary to rotation

- Increased ulnocarpal translation[454,550]

  - Neutral PA and radial deviation radiographs recommended

  - Defined as >50% of lunate uncovering

  - Some suggest seen in 80% of perilunate injuries

Subtle signs of disruption may include loss of carpal height and increased intercarpal spaces. It is essential to assess for associated fractures of the carpus and distal radius. The literature suggests that 16% to 25% of perilunate dislocations are missed initially,[15,215,256] with lesser-arc injuries commonly missed because of the lack of an obvious osseous pathology and inexperience of the initial observer. Stress radiographs or an EUA may be necessary. Often secondary imaging modalities are necessary including CT and MRI, with arthrography and arthroscopy useful in determining the extent of the injury.[20,113]

Classification. The most frequent systems for describing perilunate injuries include the Mayfield classification (Fig. 31-10), and the greater- or lesser-arc injury patterns (Page 1002).[239,301–304] Injuries can also be classified as acute or chronic, and reducible or irreducible. The pattern of skeletal deformity is variable. The hand and distal carpal row usually remain intact, but the disruption pattern between distal and proximal carpal rows is quite variable. In the transscaphoid fracture-dislocation, the distal scaphoid dislocates with the distal row leaving the proximal scaphoid and lunate in near-normal relationship to the forearm. When the perilunate ligaments rupture, the lunate usually remains within the radiocarpal joint and the remainder of the carpus dislocates, usually dorsally but occasionally in a volar direction. Occasionally, the lunate is displaced and rotated palmarly and the remainder of the carpus settles into a seminormal alignment with the distal radius. Rarely, even the palmar attachment of lunate is torn, allowing extrusion into the forearm or through the skin.[173]

An alternate classification system was put forward by Witvoet and Allieu.[545]

- Grade I: Lunate appears normally aligned

- Grade II: Lunate rotated palmarly <90 degrees

- Grade III: Lunate rotated palmarly >90 degrees but still attached to the radius by its palmar ligaments

- Grade IV: Lunate totally enucleated without any connection to the radius

  Herzberg et al. suggested a three-stage classification.[531]

- Stage I: Dorsal dislocation of capitate, lunate remains in fossa

- Stage IIA: Dorsal dislocation of capitate, lunate dislocated from fossa, rotated <90 degrees

- Stage IIB: Dorsal dislocation of capitate, lunate dislocated from fossa, rotated >90 degrees

Management

Nonoperative management and delayed intervention of perilunate dislocations and fracture-dislocations has been shown to give poor results.[25,189,215,531] Early reduction and operative stabilization is now recommended for the vast majority of cases. However, patients need to be warned regarding the severity of this injury, and prognosis must always be guarded. Poor prognostic indicators have been found to be manual workers, a poor initial reduction, or those patients managed with a combined volar–dorsal surgical approach.[157,258]

Prompt reduction reduces swelling, as well as potential damage to the median nerve.[241] The earlier a reduction of a perilunate dislocation is performed, the easier it is. Ideally, reduction should be undertaken in the emergency room. Complete relaxation under general or regional anesthesia is required, with local anesthesia usually not sufficient. The most commonly used method of closed reduction is the Tavernier maneuver.[173] It consists of locking the capitate into the distal concavity of the lunate by combined axial traction and flexion of the distal row, followed by reduction of the capitate-lunate unit onto the radius by an extension movement, while externally applying a localized dorsally directed force to the lunate to help reposition it. When the injury cannot be reduced closed, urgent reduction in theatre

is required.[241] Post reduction radiographs are essential to assess the quality of the reduction and the presence of any concomitant fractures that may not have been apparent on initial radiographs.

Immediate closed reduction reduces any potential pressure on the median nerve, with the majority of patients experiencing resolution of their symptoms after closed reduction.[4,219] Immediate median nerve decompression is not usually required but should be performed where there is no resolution of symptoms or when late symptoms develop.[129] Severe or increasing median or ulnar neuropathy is always an indication for surgical exploration.

Surgery can be performed through either a dorsal or a volar approach, although a combined approach may be necessary especially if the dislocation is irreducible closed.[219,288,501] Some authors use a combined approach in all cases in order to repair the palmar capsule. The dorsal midline approach allows good exposure of the proximal carpal row and midcarpal joint (Fig. 31-44).[173] If there are neurovascular problems, an additional palmar approach allows access for median nerve decompression or repair, vascular repair if required, and repair of the damaged palmar carpal ligaments. This allows both intra-articular and

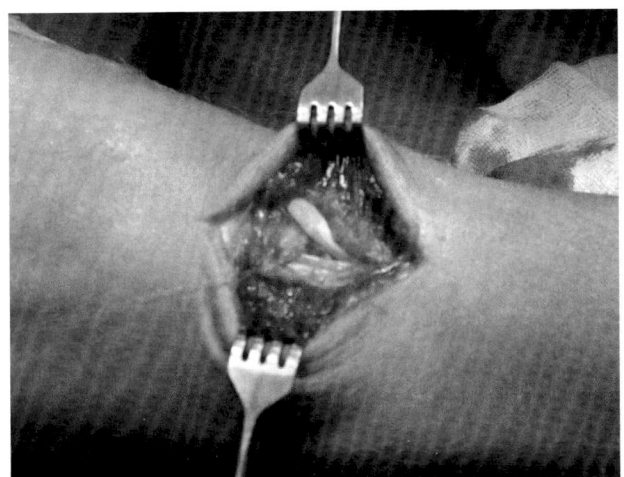

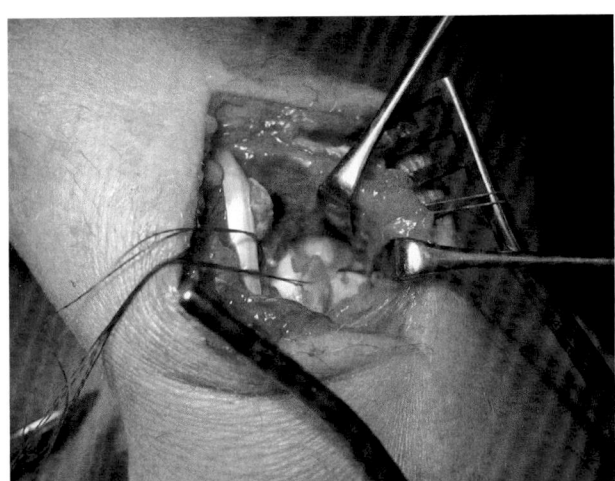

A

B

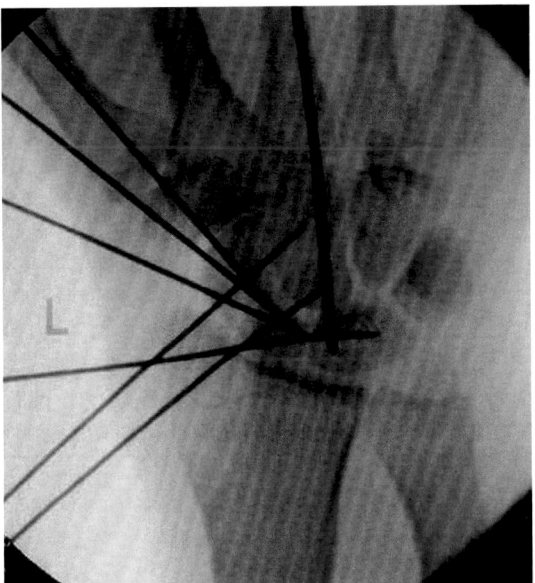

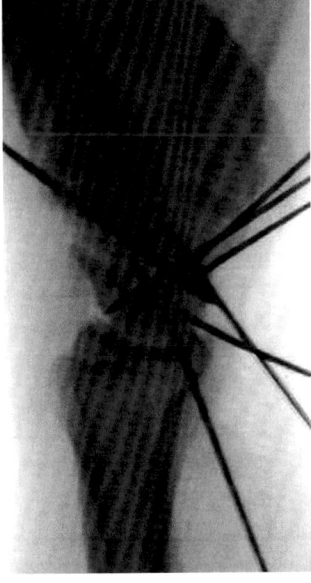

C

FIGURE 31-44 **A:** The dorsal capsule is exposed through a longitudinal incision that is centered on the Lister tubercle, dividing the extensor retinaculum between the second and third extensor compartments. The fourth compartment is opened by sectioning the septum between the third and fourth compartments. **B:** A ligament splitting capsulotomy is performed exposing the dorsal structures. **C:** Reduction and percutaneous pinning is performed under direct control. Additional K-wires can be inserted into scaphoid and lunate to help with the reduction. Ligaments are repaired using anchors and sutures.

extra-articular damage to be assessed and treated adequately. Some studies have suggested a combined approach can lead to complications (e.g., wound infection, flexor tendon adhesions) and inferior functional results; however, most authors acknowledge that a combined approach is routinely employed for more severe injuries that are associated with a difficult reduction and/or median nerve symptoms.[258,455] Minimally invasive and arthroscopic-assisted techniques of fixation and repair have also been used with satisfactory results.[237,531,552]

Lesser-Arc Injuries.

There are reductions that are so stable that it is difficult to determine whether a full perilunate-type dislocation took place, and there are others that reduce and can be maintained in near-normal alignment with cast immobilization. Successful closed reduction requires adequate imaging with good standardized AP and lateral radiographs of the wrist. Inadequate reduction leads to a poor prognosis. It is important to confirm any ligamentous stability with stress-test radiographs, MRI, arthroscopy, or open exploration. The very rare injury that reduces to normal alignment by closed reduction and appears stable can be treated with a scaphoid cast with the wrist in a neutral position. Many would advocate daily review in the first week to ensure there is no redisplacement. Review should then take place every week up until 12 weeks when the cast can be removed.[173]

However, the results of closed reduction and cast immobilization are unpredictable with loss of reduction common,[4,25] with one study finding that despite 17 weeks in cast carpal instability persisted.[101] It is now generally agreed that the risk of late deformity after successful reduction and cast management alone is unacceptably high and many advocate early operative intervention.[4,25,173] The use of percutaneous K-wire fixation to stabilize the carpus after closed reduction is now recommended. This reduces the incidence of late loss of reduction and enhances the healing capability of the intrinsic ligaments. If possible, pin fixation can be performed using arthroscopy.[237,531] Perilunate dislocations that are stable after reduction require only two pins for fixation. One transverse pin is placed from the scaphoid into the lunate (this can also be pinned through the radius into the lunate to neutralize the radiolunate alignment), and a second pin is placed from the scaphoid into the capitate. Pin stabilization of the lunotriquetral articulation is debated.[157,173,253] The pins can routinely be taken out at 8 weeks, but immobilization in a scaphoid cast should be continued for a total of 12 weeks post reduction.[173]

The vast majority of perilunate dislocations are irreducible or unstable. If reduction is not optimal or reduction cannot be achieved at all, then open exploration and repair is indicated.[25,78,196] Significantly superior results have been reported following open reduction, ligament repair, and K-wire stabilization when compared to closed reduction and percutaneous pinning.[25,216] Some authors advocate the use of temporary screw fixation as opposed to K-wires to facilitate early motion.[456]

The prognosis for these injuries is guarded even with successful reduction and maintenance of intercarpal stability, with longer-term studies reporting good patient satisfaction, but with high rates of loss of reduction and arthrosis although this does not correlate with outcome.[15,258] In a midterm study of 22 patients with perilunate dislocations treated with open reduction, cerclage wire fixation and ligament repair patient satisfaction was high for 15 patients, range of movement was 87% and grip strength 77% of the contralateral wrist, but only 10 patients returned to the same type of employment as before their injury.[501]

Greater-Arc Injuries.

Management is with closed reduction followed by ORIF, as it is the best method of achieving anatomic reduction of the fracture. This also allows repair of associated ligament injuries, as well as primary bone grafting when there is comminution of the scaphoid.[101] Cannulated screw fixation of the scaphoid is routinely recommended,[253,258,456] although there are some reports of K-wire fixation alone.[157,216] Again, stabilization of the lunotriquetral articulation is debated.[157,253]

Most series report satisfactory radiologic results, although the majority of cases have arthritis at longer-term review that does not seem to correlate with outcome.[157,215,216,253,258] Overall patient satisfaction is reported to be satisfactory with return to employment, although restoration of function is rarely complete with residual wrist stiffness and weakness of grip strength documented.[215,216,253,258]

Chronic Perilunate Dislocations.

Those injuries seen within 3 months are still potentially treatable by open reduction as long as no cartilage degeneration has already occurred, although treatment at this stage is often more difficult because of articular changes and capsular contracture, leading to inferior outcomes.[251,254] A good clue to the potential success of late reduction is gained by examining radiographs of the carpus under 25 to 30 pounds of traction.[173] An attempt at open reduction (by palmar and dorsal approaches), repair, and internal fixation should be offered if carpal bone realignment is feasible, because even in late cases results can be surprisingly good.[173,254,410,473] Late problems such as carpal bone ischemia and ligament contracture nearly always require some type of salvage operation; for example, a proximal row carpectomy or a total wrist arthrodesis.[219] Proximal row carpectomy usually provides satisfactory results when the capitate head and lunate fossa are preserved.[241,234,389]

Some patients undergo unsuccessful acute management. Depending on the time of presentation from injury and the extent and type of any surgery that has already been undertaken, the options for treatment are identical to those of acute treatment. When a bone or bone fragment has been removed such as a proximal scaphoid or capitate fragment, the alternatives are to rehabilitate the limb and assess the functional level or to consider a salvage procedure such as radiocarpal fusion or proximal row carpectomy.[173]

AUTHORS' PREFERRED MANAGEMENT—PERILUNATE DISLOCATION AND FRACTURE-DISLOCATIONS

All patients with an acute perilunate injury should undergo immediate closed reduction. For those patients with a *lesser-arc injury* that is reducible closed, we prefer K-wire fixation over conservative treatment in cast. The role of percutaneous reduction and fixation is unclear and still experimental.

We prefer a dorsal midline approach to expose and realign the bones (Fig. 31-44), with an additional palmar approach for neurovascular problems. The surgery is similar to that for treatment of SLD, except that an extended carpal tunnel release is performed when required. The palmar capsule should be examined either along its attachments to the radial rim or through the frequently damaged space of Poirier. The dorsal capsule is usually opened along its origin from the dorsal radial rim, as well as longitudinally in the space between the second and fourth extensor compartments, and the proximal carpal row is examined.[173]

If a scaphoid fracture is present (*greater-arc injury*), it can be reduced through the dorsal approach, temporarily stabilized with K-wires, and fixed with a cannulated screw. Autogenous cancellous bone graft from the distal radius is sometimes placed in comminuted scaphoid fractures. If there is not a scaphoid fracture, the scaphoid is aligned to the lunate and a screw is placed from radial to ulnar percutaneously. The dorsal scapholunate ligament is reattached with a small suture anchor. The screw is removed between 2 and 6 months after injury. Once the scaphoid is reduced, the lunotriquetral joint usually lines up. We sometimes stabilize it with K-wires or a temporary screw, but have left it unsecure more recently.

Reduction and K-wire fixation should be centered on the lunate. The lunate must be aligned and pinned first to the distal radius to neutralize the radiolunate alignment. The lunotriquetral joint is then reduced and fixed by a second K-wire. Ligaments are repaired as needed. The capitolunate joint alignment is then evaluated and correct colinear alignment is assessed. Lastly, the scapholunate joint is reduced and held with K-wires. Many of the patients have an associated radial styloid fracture, which should be reduced anatomically and stabilized with K-wires or a compression screw.[173]

Radiocarpal Instability
Etiology
The most common injuries at the radiocarpal joint are fracture-dislocations of the distal radius and carpus; for example, palmar and dorsal Barton fracture-dislocations, radial styloid fracture-dislocations, and die-punch fracture-dislocations. Less common are the pure ligamentous radiocarpal injuries that may result in a true ulnar, dorsal, or palmar dislocation of the wrist, with some missed as they may spontaneously reduce (Fig. 31-45). Ulnar translation is the most frequent radiocarpal instability. These injuries occur predominantly in young males and are often severe in nature.[173]

Clinical Assessment and Diagnosis
Radiocarpal instability may occur acutely, develop gradually, or be observed as a late sequela of a perilunate dislocation. In the acute phase, patients present with a history of high-energy trauma; for example, fall from height. They complain frequently of wrist swelling, deformity, and pain. Dorsal wrist

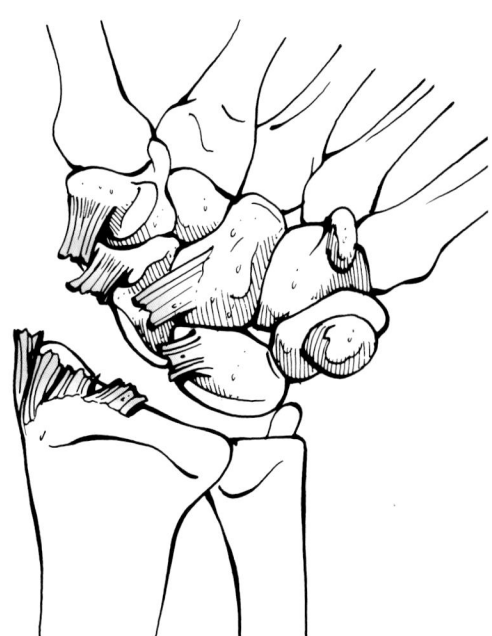

FIGURE 31-45 Radiocarpal dislocation with torn radiocarpal ligaments. This injury requires K-wire stabilization and direct repair of the radiocarpal ligaments.

swelling and tenderness are most noticeable at the radiocarpal level and are aggravated by wrist motion. Deformity may be due an ulnar, dorsal, or palmar translation of the carpus. With ulnar translation, the wrist and hand are offset in an ulnar direction. The majority of patients sustain an associated injury, with disruption to the ipsilateral distal radioulnar joint common, and thorough assessment is recommended.[138,333]

Imaging. Primary assessment uses standard scaphoid radiographs to detect displacement and associated fractures. Provocative stress tests may be required to demonstrate dynamic radiocarpal instability.[138,333] In those patients with an ulnar translation, the radiographic appearance is often dramatic with the lunate positioned just distal to the ulna and a large space between the radial styloid and the scaphoid. If a perilunate injury is also present the lunate and triquetrum slide ulnarly, opening a gap between scaphoid and lunate. In some cases, the ulnar shift is subtle, and a decrease in the ulnocarpal index may provide the only clue to diagnosis. Chronic causes for ulnar translation include rheumatoid arthritis and in developmental deformities; for example, Madelung deformity.[173]

To better define associated bony injuries, CT may be required. To determine the extent of ligamentous disruption, MRI can be used.

Classification. Radiocarpal dislocation has been classified into two groups by Dumontier et al.[138]

- Type I: Radiocarpal dislocation with no fracture, or a fracture of the tip of the radial styloid, when it is assumed that the radiocarpal ligaments are avulsed from the radius.

- Type II: Radiocarpal dislocation with a fracture of the radial styloid involving more than one-third of the scaphoid fossa, when it is assumed that the radiocarpal ligaments remain attached to the styloid process.

Moneim et al.[322] also classified these injuries into two groups, but his classification is dependent on the presence or absence of intercarpal ligament injury.

- Type I: Intact intercarpal ligaments
- Type II: A combination of radiocarpal and intercarpal dislocation

Dorsal translation of the carpus together with ulnar translation can be seen in two modes: one a true instability secondary to ligament damage, the other an apparent instability due to a carpal shift in response to a change in position of the distal radial articular surface. Pure dorsal translation usually occurs after a loss of the normal palmar slope of the distal radius from a flexion angle to an extension angle. The latter is a common problem after collapse of a distal radius fracture.[173]

Management

Dislocations of the radiocarpal joint require immediate reduction because the associated deformity may compromise adjacent neurovascular structures. Although reduction is usually possible, maintaining it is often difficult. Open treatment should be considered in most carpal dislocations.[173]

For type I injuries, the volar radiocarpal ligaments should be repaired using anchor sutures to prevent secondary ulnar or volar translation.[138] Where there is a substantial fracture fragment, the volar ligaments are likely to be attached to it; therefore, ORIF of the fragment is necessary. Added stabilization of the radiocarpal joint is recommended using percutaneous K-wires or external fixation to prevent late carpal translation, especially in type I injuries.[138,233] Concomitant intercarpal ligament injuries should also be repaired.[322] Limitation of wrist movement of 30% to 40% of normal should be expected following radiocarpal dislocation.[138,333]

For those with a delayed presentation or diagnosis, ligamentous repair does not usually provide a good result. The most certain method of controlling possible recurrence of deformity is to carry out a partial or total radiocarpal arthrodesis. Radiolunate fusion is an appropriate technique for this situation, although the variation of joint damage may indicate radioscaphoid fusion in some cases and RSL fusion in others. The latter is usually indicated in the combination of radiocarpal and perilunate instability.[173]

Directions for Future Research in Radiocarpal Instability

More short-term and long-term outcome data is needed in relation to all the carpal instabilities. Recently, substantial progress has been made in the understanding and detection of carpal ligament injuries, predominantly due to the ever-improving imaging modalities available. Hopefully, improved imaging and surgery will allow better prediction of the evolution of individual carpal instabilities and therefore determine the requirement for operative treatment at an earlier stage. It is likely that improved surgical methods will be devised to treat these problems. The use of closed fluoroscopically or arthroscopically

controlled techniques may increase and the results of treatment could improve.

It is interesting to speculate whether an increasingly aging society will affect the diagnosis and management of both carpal fractures and instabilities. Currently, they mainly occur in younger patients, but with altering patient demographics, this may not continue and a new set of challenges may emerge.

Carpal Ligament Injuries: Pearls and Pitfalls

- SLD is the most common pattern of carpal instability
- SLD without a dorsiflexed lunate is probably not traumatic
- For SLD the results of K-wire treatment are unpredictable and ligamentous repair should be undertaken if closed reduction is unsuccessful on serial radiographs
- For chronic scapholunate instability, partial or complete wrist fusion may be needed
- Perilunate dislocation patterns include a considerable spectrum of sprains, fracture-dislocations, and instabilities
- Up to a quarter of perilunate dislocations are initially missed
- Perilunate dislocation and fracture-dislocations routinely require immediate reduction and operative stabilization
- LTD may result in disruption of Gilula lines on radiograph
- Open repair of the lunotriquetral ligament is only possible in acute injury

REFERENCES

1. Abdel-Salam A, Eyres KS, Cleary J. Detecting fractures of the scaphoid: The value of comparative X-rays of the uninjured wrist. *J Hand Surg Br.* 1992;17:28–32.
2. Adamany DC, Mikola EA, Fraser BJ. Percutaneous fixation of the scaphoid through a dorsal approach: An anatomic study. *J Hand Surg Am.* 2008;33:327–331.
3. Adey L, Souer JS, Lozano-Calderon S, et al. Computed tomography of suspected scaphoid fractures. *J Hand Surg Am.* 2007;32:61–66.
4. Adkison JW, Chapman MW. Treatment of acute lunate and perilunate dislocations. *Clin Orthop Relat Res.* 1982;199–207.
5. Adler BD, Logan PM, Janzen DL, et al. Extrinsic radiocarpal ligaments: Magnetic resonance imaging of normal wrists and scapholunate dissociation. *Can Assoc Radiol J.* 1996;47:417–422.
6. Adolfsson L, Lindau T, Arner M. Acutrak screw fixation versus cast immobilisation for undisplaced scaphoid waist fractures. *J Hand Surg Br.* 2001;26:192–195.
7. Aguilella L, Garcia-Elias M. The anterolateral corner of the radial metaphysis as a source of bone graft for the treatment of scaphoid nonunion. *J Hand Surg Am.* 2012;37:1258–1262.
8. Albertsen J, Mencke S, Christensen L, et al. Isolated capitate fracture diagnosed by computed tomography. Case report. *Handchir Mikrochir Plast Chir.* 1999;31:79–81.
9. Aldridge JM III, Mallon WJ. Hook of the hamate fractures in competitive golfers: Results of treatment by excision of the fractured hook of the hamate. *Orthopedics.* 2003;26:717–719.
10. Alho A, Kankaanpää U. Management of fractured scaphoid bone. A prospective study of 100 fractures. *Acta Orthop Scand.* 1975;46:737–743.
11. Allan CH, Joshi A, Lichtman DM. Kienböck's disease: Diagnosis and treatment. *J Am Acad Orthop Surg.* 2001;9:128–136.
12. Almquist EE, Bach AW, Sack JT, et al. Four-bone ligament reconstruction for treatment of chronic complete scapholunate separation. *J Hand Surg Am.* 1991;16:322–327.
13. Alshryda S, Shah A, Odak S, et al. Acute fractures of the scaphoid bone: Systematic review and meta-analysis. *Surgeon.* 2012;10(4):218–229.
14. Alt V, Sicre G. Dorsal transscaphoid-transtriquetral perilunate dislocation in pseudarthrosis of the scaphoid. *Clin Orthop Relat Res.* 2004;135–137.
15. Altissimi M, Mancini GB, Azzara A. Perilunate dislocations of the carpus. A long-term review. *Ital J Orthop Traumatol.* 1987;13:491–500.
16. Altman DG, Bland JM. Diagnostic tests 2: Predictive values. *BMJ.* 1994;309:102.
17. Altman DG, Bland JM. Diagnostic tests. 1: Sensitivity and specificity. *BMJ.* 1994;308:1552.
18. Amadio PC, Berquist TH, Smith DK, et al. Scaphoid malunion. *J Hand Surg Am.* 1989;14:679–687.
19. American College of Radiology (ACR). Expert Panel on Musculoskeletal Imaging, ACR Appropriateness Criteria. In: Reston VA. ed. *Acute Hand and Wrist Trauma.* 1st ed. American College of Radiology; 2001:1–7.

20. Anderson ML, Skinner JA, Felmlee JP, et al. Diagnostic comparison of 1.5 Tesla and 3.0 Tesla preoperative MRI of the wrist in patients with ulnar-sided wrist pain. *J Hand Surg Am.* 2008;33:1153–1159.
21. Anderson SE, Steinbach LS, Tschering-Vogel D, et al. MR imaging of avascular scaphoid nonunion before and after vascularized bone grafting. *Skeletal Radiol.* 2005;34:314–320.
22. Andresen R, Radmer S, Sparmann M, et al. Imaging of hamate bone fractures in conventional X-rays and high-resolution computed tomography. An in vitro study. *Invest Radiol.* 1999;34:46–50.
23. Annamalai G, Raby N. Scaphoid and pronator fat stripes are unreliable soft tissue signs in the detection of radiographically occult fractures. *Clin Radiol.* 2003;58:798–800.
24. Apergis E, Darmanis S, Kastanis G, et al. Does the term scaphocapitate syndrome need to be revised? A report of 6 cases. *J Hand Surg Br.* 2001;26:441–445.
25. Apergis E, Maris J, Theodoratos G, et al. Perilunate dislocations and fracture-dislocations. Closed and early open reduction compared in 28 cases. *Acta Orthop Scand Suppl.* 1997;275:55–59.
26. Arner M, Hagberg L. Wrist flexion strength after excision of the pisiform bone. *Scand J Plast Reconstr Surg.* 1984;18:241–245.
27. Arora R, Gschwentner M, Krappinger D, et al. Fixation of nondisplaced scaphoid fractures: Making treatment cost effective. Prospective controlled trial. *Arch Orthop Trauma Surg.* 2007;127:39–46.
28. Arora R, Lutz M, Zimmermann R, et al. Free vascularised iliac bone graft for recalcitrant avascular nonunion of the scaphoid. *J Bone Joint Surg Br.* 2010;92:224–229.
29. Baczkowski B, Lorczynski A, Kabula J, et al. Scapholunate ligament repair using suture anchors. *Ortop Traumatol Rehabil.* 2006;8:129–133.
30. Bain GI, Bennett JD, MacDermid JC, et al. Measurement of the scaphoid humpback deformity using longitudinal computed tomography: Intra- and interobserver variability using various measurement techniques. *J Hand Surg Am.* 1998;23:76–81.
31. Barton NJ. Twenty questions about scaphoid fractures. *J Hand Surg Br.* 1992;17:289–310.
32. Beadel GP, Ferreira L, Johnson JA, et al. Interfragmentary compression across a simulated scaphoid fracture–analysis of 3 screws. *J Hand Surg Am.* 2004;29:273–278.
33. Beckenbaugh RD, Shives TC, Dobyns JH, et al. Kienböck's disease: The natural history of Kienböck's disease and consideration of lunate fractures. *Clin Orthop Relat Res.* 1980;98:106.
34. Beeres FJ, Hogervorst M, Rhemrev SJ, et al. A prospective comparison for suspected scaphoid fractures: Bone scintigraphy versus clinical outcome. *Injury.* 2007;38:769–774.
35. Beeres FJ, Rhemrev SJ, den HP, et al. Early magnetic resonance imaging compared with bone scintigraphy in suspected scaphoid fractures. *J Bone Joint Surg Br.* 2008;90:1205–1209.
36. Beredjiklian PK, Dugas J, Gerwin M. Primary repair of the scapholunate ligament. *Tech Hand Up Extrem Surg.* 1998;2:269–273.
37. Berger RA, Blair WF, Crowninshield RD, et al. The scapholunate ligament. *J Hand Surg Am.* 1982;7:87–91.
38. Berger RA, Blair WF, El-Khoury GY. Arthrotomography of the wrist. The palmar radiocarpal ligaments. *Clin Orthop Relat Res.* 1984;224–229.
39. Berger RA, Blair WF. The radioscapholunate ligament: A gross and histologic description. *Anat Rec.* 1984;210:393–405.
40. Berger RA, Imeada T, Berglund L, et al. Constraint and material properties of the subregions of the scapholunate interosseous ligament. *J Hand Surg Am.* 1999;24:953–962.
41. Berger RA, Kauer JM, Landsmeer JM. Radioscapholunate ligament: A gross anatomic and histologic study of fetal and adult wrists. *J Hand Surg Am.* 1991;16:350–355.
42. Berger RA, Landsmeer JM. The palmar radiocarpal ligaments: A study of adult and fetal human wrist joints. *J Hand Surg Am.* 1990;15:847-54.
43. Berger RA. The anatomy of the ligaments of the wrist and distal radioulnar joints. *Clin Orthop Relat Res.* 2001;32–40.
44. Berger RA. The anatomy of the scaphoid. *Hand Clin.* 2001;17:525–532.
45. Berger RA. The gross and histologic anatomy of the scapholunate interosseous ligament. *J Hand Surg Am.* 1996;21:170–178.
46. Berger RA. The ligaments of the wrist. A current overview of anatomy with considerations of their potential functions. *Hand Clin.* 1997;13:63–82.
47. Bernard SA, Murray PM, Heckman MG. Validity of conventional radiography in determining scaphoid waist fracture displacement. *J Orthop Trauma.* 2010;24:448–451.
48. Bettinger PC, Linscheid RL, Berger RA, et al. An anatomic study of the stabilizing ligaments of the trapezium and trapeziometacarpal joint. *J Hand Surg Am.* 1999;24:786–798.
49. Bhalla S, Higgs PE, Gilula LA. Utility of the radial-deviated, thumb-abducted lateral radiographic view for the diagnosis of hamate hook fractures: Case report. *Radiology.* 1998;209:203–207.
50. Bhat M, McCarthy M, Davis TR, et al. MRI and plain radiography in the assessment of displaced fractures of the waist of the carpal scaphoid. *J Bone Joint Surg Br.* 2004;86:705–713.
51. Bickert B, Sauerbier M, Germann G. Scapholunate ligament repair using the Mitek bone anchor. *J Hand Surg Br.* 2000;25:188–192.
52. Blatt G. Capsulodesis in reconstructive hand surgery. Dorsal capsulodesis for the unstable scaphoid and volar capsulodesis following excision of the distal ulna. *Hand Clin.* 1987;3:81–102.
53. Boabighi A, Kuhlmann JN, Kenesi C. The distal ligamentous complex of the scaphoid and the scapho-lunate ligament. An anatomic, histological and biomechanical study. *J Hand Surg Br.* 1993;18:65–69.
54. Bohler L, Trojan E, Jahna H. The results of treatment of 734 fresh, simple fractures of the scaphoid. *J Hand Surg Br.* 2003;28:319–331.
55. Bond CD, Shin AY, McBride MT, et al. Percutaneous screw fixation or cast immobilization for nondisplaced scaphoid fractures. *J Bone Joint Surg Am.* 2001;83-A:483–488.
56. Botte MJ, Gelberman RH. Fractures of the carpus, excluding the scaphoid. *Hand Clin.* 1987;3:149–161.
57. Botte MJ, Pacelli LL, Gelberman RH. Vascularity and osteonecrosis of the wrist. *Orthop Clin North Am.* 2004;35:405–421.
58. Braga-Silva J, Peruchi FM, Moschen GM, et al. A comparison of the use of distal radius vascularised bone graft and non-vascularised iliac crest bone graft in the treatment of non-union of scaphoid fractures. *J Hand Surg Eur Vol.* 2008;33:636–640.
59. Breederveld RS, Tuinebreijer WE. Investigation of computed tomographic scan concurrent criterion validity in doubtful scaphoid fracture of the wrist. *J Trauma.* 2004;57:851–854.
60. Breitenseher MJ, Metz VM, Gilula LA, et al. Radiographically occult scaphoid fractures: Value of MR imaging in detection. *Radiology.* 1997;203:245–250.
61. Brondum V, Larsen CF, Skov O. Fracture of the carpal scaphoid: Frequency and distribution in a well-defined population. *Eur J Radiol.* 1992;15:118–122.
62. Brooks S, Wluka AE, Stuckey S, et al. The management of scaphoid fractures. *J Sci Med Sport.* 2005;8:181–189.
63. Brown RR, Fliszar E, Cotten A, et al. Extrinsic and intrinsic ligaments of the wrist: Normal and pathologic anatomy at MR arthrography with three-compartment enhancement. *Radiographics.* 1998;18:667–674.
64. Brumbaugh RB, Crowninshield RD, Blair WF, et al. An in-vivo study of normal wrist kinematics. *J Biomech Eng.* 1982;104:176–181.
65. Brydie A, Raby N. Early MRI in the management of clinical scaphoid fracture. *Br J Radiol.* 2003;76:296–300.
66. Buijze GA, Doornberg JN, Ham JS, et al. Surgical compared with conservative treatment for acute nondisplaced or minimally displaced scaphoid fractures: A systematic review and meta-analysis of randomized controlled trials. *J Bone Joint Surg Am.* 2010;92:1534–1544.
67. Buijze GA, Dvinskikh NA, Strackee SD, et al. Osseous and ligamentous scaphoid anatomy: Part II. Evaluation of ligament morphology using three-dimensional anatomical imaging. *J Hand Surg Am.* 2011;36:1936–1943.
68. Buijze GA, Guitton TG, van Dijk CN, et al. Training improves interobserver reliability for the diagnosis of scaphoid fracture displacement. *Clin Orthop Relat Res.* 2012;470(7):2029–2034.
69. Buijze GA, Jorgsholm P, Thomsen NO, et al. Diagnostic performance of radiographs and computed tomography for displacement and instability of acute scaphoid waist fractures. *J Bone Joint Surg Am.* 2012;94(21):1967–1974.
70. Buijze GA, Jorgsholm P, Thomsen NO, et al. Factors associated with arthroscopically determined scaphoid fracture displacement and instability. *J Hand Surg Am.* 2012;37:1405–1410.
71. Buijze GA, Lozano-Calderon SA, Strackee SD, et al. Osseous and ligamentous scaphoid anatomy: Part I. A systematic literature review highlighting controversies. *J Hand Surg Am.* 2011;36:1926–1935.
72. Buijze GA, Mallee WH, Beeres FJ, et al. Diagnostic performance tests for suspected scaphoid fractures differ with conventional and latent class analysis. *Clin Orthop Relat Res.* 2011;469:3400–3407.
73. Buijze GA, Ochtman L, Ring D. Management of scaphoid nonunion. *J Hand Surg Am.* 2012;37:1095–1100.
74. Burgess RC. The effect of a simulated scaphoid malunion on wrist motion. *J Hand Surg Am.* 1987;12:774–776.
75. Calandruccio JH, Duncan SF. Isolated nondisplaced capitate waist fracture diagnosed by magnetic resonance imaging. *J Hand Surg Am.* 1999;24:856–859.
76. Calfee RP, White L, Patel A, et al. Palmar dislocation of the trapezoid with coronal shearing fracture: Case report. *J Hand Surg Am.* 2008;33:1482–1485.
77. Caloia MF, Gallino RN, Caloia H, et al. Incidence of ligamentous and other injuries associated with scaphoid fractures during arthroscopically assisted reduction and percutaneous fixation. *Arthroscopy.* 2008;24:754–759.
78. Campbell RD Jr, Thompson TC, Lance EM, et al. Indications for open reduction of lunate and perilunate dislocations of the carpal bones. *J Bone Joint Surg Am.* 1965;47:915–937.
79. Camus EJ, Millot F, Lariviere J, et al. [The double-cup carpus: A demonstration of the variable geometry of the carpus]. *Chir Main.* 2008;27:12–19.
80. Cautilli GP, Wehbe MA. Scapho-lunate distance and cortical ring sign. *J Hand Surg Am.* 1991;16:501–503.
81. Cetti R, Christensen SE, Reuther K. Fracture of the lunate bone. *Hand.* 1982;14:80–84.
82. Chantelot C, Peltier B, Demondion X, et al. A trans STT, trans capitate perilunate dislocation of the carpus. A case report. *Ann Chir Main Memb Super.* 1999;18:61–65.
83. Charalambous CP, Mills SP, Hayton MJ. Gradual distraction using an external fixator followed by open reduction in the treatment of chronic lunate dislocation. *Hand Surg.* 2010;15:27–29.
84. Cheng CY, Hsu KY, Tseng IC, et al. Concurrent scaphoid fracture with scapholunate ligament rupture. *Acta Orthop Belg.* 2004;70:485–491.
85. Cheung GC, Lever CJ, Morris AD. X-ray diagnosis of acute scaphoid fractures. *J Hand Surg Br.* 2006;31:104–109.
86. Choi J, Raskin KB. Rotatory subluxation of the scaphoid. *Bull Hosp Jt Dis.* 2000;59:197-200.
87. Chou YC, Hsu YH, Cheng CY, et al. Percutaneous screw and axial Kirschner wire fixation for acute transscaphoid perilunate fracture dislocation. *J Hand Surg Am.* 2012;37(4):715–720.
88. Christiansen TG, Rude C, Lauridsen KK, et al. Diagnostic value of ultrasound in scaphoid fractures. *Injury.* 1991;22:397–399.
89. Chung KC. A simplified approach for unstable scaphoid fracture fixation using the Acutrak screw. *Plast Reconstr Surg.* 2002;110:1697–1703.
90. Clark DW, Blackburn N. Treatment of periscaphoid osteoarthritis by Silastic scaphoid implant. *J R Soc Med.* 1989;82:464–465.
91. Clay NR, Dias JJ, Costigan PS, et al. Need the thumb be immobilised in scaphoid fractures? A randomised prospective trial. *J Bone Joint Surg Br.* 1991;73:828–832.
92. Cobb TK, Dalley BK, Posteraro RH, et al. Anatomy of the flexor retinaculum. *J Hand Surg Am.* 1993;18:91–99.
93. Cohen MS, Jupiter JB, Fallahi K, et al. Scaphoid waist nonunion with humpback deformity treated without structural bone graft. *J Hand Surg Am.* 2013;38(4):701–705.

94. Cohen MS, Taleisnik J. Direct ligamentous repair of scapholunate dissociation with capsulodesis augmentation. *Tech Hand Up Extrem Surg.* 1998;2:18–24.

95. Collins ED, Gharbaoui I. Imaging and anatomic study of the pisiform bone/ulnar nerve relationship-evaluation of the preferred surgical approach for the excision of the pisiform bone. *Tech Hand Up Extrem Surg.* 2010;14:150–154.

96. Compson JP. The anatomy of acute scaphoid fractures: A three-dimensional analysis of patterns. *J Bone Joint Surg Br.* 1998;80:218–224.

97. Conyers DJ. Scapholunate interosseous reconstruction and imbrication of palmar ligaments. *J Hand Surg Am.* 1990;15:690–700.

98. Cooney AD, Stuart PR. Symptomatic nonunion of an isolated capitate fracture in an adolescent. *J Hand Surg Eur Vol.* 2013;38(5):565–567.

99. Cooney WP III, Dobyns JH, Linscheid RL. Nonunion of the scaphoid: Analysis of the results from bone grafting. *J Hand Surg Am.* 1980;5:343–354.

100. Cooney WP III. Scaphoid fractures: Current treatments and techniques. *Instr Course Lect.* 2003;52:197–208.

101. Cooney WP, Bussey R, Dobyns JH, et al. Difficult wrist fractures. Perilunate fracture-dislocations of the wrist. *Clin Orthop Relat Res.* 1987;136–147.

102. Cooney WP, Dobyns JH, Linscheid RL. Arthroscopy of the wrist: Anatomy and classification of carpal instability. *Arthroscopy.* 1990;6:133–140.

103. Cooney WP, Dobyns JH, Linscheid RL. Fractures of the scaphoid: A rational approach to management. *Clin Orthop Relat Res.* 1980;90–97.

104. Cooney WP. Failure of treatment of ununited fractures of the carpal scaphoid. *J Bone Joint Surg Am.* 1984;66:1145–1146.

105. Cordrey LJ, Ferrer-Torells M. Management of fractures of the greater multangular. Report of five cases. *J Bone Joint Surg Am.* 1960;42-A:1111–1118.

106. Court-Brown CM, Bugler KE, Clement ND, et al. The epidemiology of open fractures in adults. A 15-year review. *Injury.* 2012;43:891–897.

107. Court-Brown CM, Caesar B. Epidemiology of adult fractures: A review. *Injury.* 2006; 37:691–697.

108. Cruickshank J, Meakin A, Breadmore R, et al. Early computerized tomography accurately determines the presence or absence of scaphoid and other fractures. *Emerg Med Australas.* 2007;19:223–228.

109. Dacho A, Grundel J, Holle G, et al. Long-term results of midcarpal arthrodesis in the treatment of scaphoid nonunion advanced collapse (SNAC-Wrist) and scapholunate advanced collapse (SLAC-Wrist). *Ann Plast Surg.* 2006;56:139–144.

110. DaCruz DJ, Taylor RH, Savage B, et al. Ultrasound assessment of the suspected scaphoid fracture. *Arch Emerg Med.* 1988;5:97–100.

111. Daecke W, Lorenz S, Wieloch P, et al. Lunate resection and vascularized Os pisiform transfer in Kienböck's disease: An average of 10 years of follow-up study after Saffar's procedure. *J Hand Surg Am.* 2005;30:677–684.

112. Davis EN, Chung KC, Kotsis SV, et al. A cost/utility analysis of open reduction and internal fixation versus cast immobilization for acute nondisplaced mid-waist scaphoid fractures. *Plast Reconstr Surg.* 2006;117:1223–1235.

113. Davis KW, Blankenbaker DG. Imaging the ligaments and tendons of the wrist. *Semin Roentgenol.* 2010;45:194–217.

114. de Beer JD, Hudson DA. Fractures of the triquetrum. *J Hand Surg Br.* 1987;12: 52–53.

115. De SF, De SL. Isolated fracture of the capitate: The value of MRI in diagnosis and follow up. *Acta Orthop Belg.* 2002;68:310–315.

116. de Zwart AD, Beeres FJ, Kingma LM, et al. Interobserver variability among radiologists for diagnosis of scaphoid fractures by computed tomography. *J Hand Surg Am.* 2012;37:2252–2256.

117. de Zwart AD, Beeres FJ, Ring D, et al. MRI as a reference standard for suspected scaphoid fractures. *Br J Radiol.* 2012;85:1098–1101.

118. Deletang F, Segret J, Dap F, et al. Chronic scapholunate instability treated by scaphocapitate fusion: A midterm outcome perspective. *Orthop Traumatol Surg Res.* 2011;97(2):164–171.

119. Demartin F, Quinto O. Isolated dislocation of the pisiform. A case report. *Chir Organi Mov.* 1993;78:121–123.

120. Deshmukh SC, Givissis P, Belloso D, et al. Blatt's capsulodesis for chronic scapholunate dissociation. *J Hand Surg Br.* 1999;24:215–220.

121. Dias JJ, Brenkel IJ, Finlay DB. Patterns of union in fractures of the waist of the scaphoid. *J Bone Joint Surg Br.* 1989;71:307–310.

122. Dias JJ, Dhukaram V, Abhinav A, et al. Clinical and radiological outcome of cast immobilisation versus surgical treatment of acute scaphoid fractures at a mean follow-up of 93 months. *J Bone Joint Surg Br.* 2008;90:899–905.

123. Dias JJ, Finlay DB, Brenkel IJ, et al. Radiographic assessment of soft tissue signs in clinically suspected scaphoid fractures: The incidence of false negative and false positive results. *J Orthop Trauma.* 1987;1:205–208.

124. Dias JJ, Hui AC, Lamont AC. Real time ultrasonography in the assessment of movement at the site of a scaphoid fracture non-union. *J Hand Surg Br.* 1994;19:498–504.

125. Dias JJ, Singh HP. Displaced fracture of the waist of the scaphoid. *J Bone Joint Surg Br.* 2011;93:1433–1439.

126. Dias JJ, Taylor M, Thompson J, et al. Radiographic signs of union of scaphoid fractures. An analysis of inter-observer agreement and reproducibility. *J Bone Joint Surg Br.* 1988;70:299–301.

127. Dias JJ, Wildin CJ, Bhowal B, et al. Should acute scaphoid fractures be fixed? A randomized controlled trial. *J Bone Joint Surg Am.* 2005;87:2160–2168.

128. Dias JJ. Definition of union after acute fracture and surgery for fracture nonunion of the scaphoid. *J Hand Surg Br.* 2001;26:321–325.

129. DiGiovanni B, Shaffer J. Treatment of perilunate and transscaphoid perilunate dislocations of the wrist. *Am J Orthop (Belle Mead NJ).* 1995;24:818–826.

130. Dinah AF, Vickers RH. Smoking increases failure rate of operation for established nonunion of the scaphoid bone. *Int Orthop.* 2007;31:503–505.

131. Doornberg JN, Buijze GA, Ham SJ, et al. Nonoperative treatment for acute scaphoid fractures: A systematic review and meta-analysis of randomized controlled trials. *J Trauma.* 2011;71:1073–1081.

132. Dorsay TA, Major NM, Helms CA. Cost-effectiveness of immediate MR imaging versus traditional follow-up for revealing radiographically occult scaphoid fractures. *AJR Am J Roentgenol.* 2001;177:1257–1263.

133. Drac P, Manak P, Cizmar I, et al. [A Palmar percutaneous volar versus a dorsal limited approach for the treatment of non- and minimally-displaced scaphoid waist fractures: An assessment of functional outcomes and complications]. *Acta Chir Orthop Traumatol Cech.* 2010;77:143–148.

134. Drewniany JJ, Palmer AK, Flatt AE. The scaphotrapezial ligament complex: An anatomic and biomechanical study. *J Hand Surg Am.* 1985;10:492–498.

135. Duckworth AD, Buijze GA, Moran M, et al. Predictors of fracture following suspected injury to the scaphoid. *J Bone Joint Surg Br.* 2012;94:961–968.

136. Duckworth AD, Jenkins PJ, Aitken SA, et al. Scaphoid fracture epidemiology. *J Trauma Acute Care Surg.* 2012;72:E41–E45.

137. Duckworth AD, Ring D, McQueen MM. Assessment of the suspected fracture of the scaphoid. *J Bone Joint Surg Br.* 2011;93:713–719.

138. Dumontier C, Meyer zu RG, Sautet A, et al. Radiocarpal dislocations: Classification and proposal for treatment. A review of twenty-seven cases. *J Bone Joint Surg Am.* 2001; 83-A:212–218.

139. Dunn MJ, Johnson C. Static scapholunate dissociation: A new reconstruction technique using a volar and dorsal approach in a cadaver model. *J Hand Surg Am.* 2001;26: 749–754.

140. Easterling KJ, Wolfe SW. Scaphoid shift in the uninjured wrist. *J Hand Surg Am.* 1994;19:604–606.

141. Eastley N, Singh H, Dias JJ, et al. Union rates after proximal scaphoid fractures; meta-analyses and review of available evidence. *J Hand Surg Eur Vol.* 2012.

142. Eckenrode JF, Louis DS, Greene TL. Scaphoid-trapezium-trapezoid fusion in the treatment of chronic scapholunate instability. *J Hand Surg Am.* 1986;11:497–502.

143. Eddeland A, Eiken O, Hellgren E, et al. Fractures of the scaphoid. *Scand J Plast Reconstr Surg.* 1975;9:234–239.

144. Eggli S, Fernandez DL, Beck T. Unstable scaphoid fracture nonunion: A medium-term study of anterior wedge grafting procedures. *J Hand Surg Br.* 2002;27:36–41.

145. Egloff DV, Varadi G, Narakas A, et al. Silastic implants of the scaphoid and lunate. A long-term clinical study with a mean follow-up of 13 years. *J Hand Surg Br.* 1993; 18:687–692.

146. El-Karef EA. Corrective osteotomy for symptomatic scaphoid malunion. *Injury.* 2005; 36:1440–1448.

147. Elsaidi GA, Ruch DS, Kuzma GR, et al. Dorsal wrist ligament insertions stabilize the scapholunate interval: Cadaver study. *Clin Orthop Relat Res.* 2004;152–157.

148. Emmett JE, Breck LW. A review and analysis of 11,000 fractures seen in a private practice of orthopaedic surgery, 1937–1956. *J Bone Joint Surg Am.* 1958;40-A:1169–1175.

149. Englseder WA. Scapholunate dissociation occurring with scaphoid fracture. *J Hand Surg Br.* 1993;18:272.

150. Esberger DA. What value the scaphoid compression test? *J Hand Surg Br.* 1994;19: 748–749.

151. Evans G, Burke FD, Barton NJ. A comparison of conservative treatment and silicone replacement arthroplasty in Kienböck's disease. *J Hand Surg Br.* 1986;11:98–102.

152. Evans MW Jr. Hamate hook fracture in a 17-year-old golfer: Importance of matching symptoms to clinical evidence. *J Manipulative Physiol Ther.* 2004;27:516–518.

153. Feinstein WK, Lichtman DM, Noble PC, et al. Quantitative assessment of the midcarpal shift test. *J Hand Surg Am.* 1999;24:977–983.

154. Fenton RL. The naviculo-capitate fracture syndrome. *J Bone Joint Surg Am.* 1956;38-A: 681–684.

155. Fernandez DL, Eggli S. Scaphoid nonunion and malunion. How to correct deformity. *Hand Clin.* 2001;17:631–646, ix.

156. Fisk GR. Carpal instability and the fractured scaphoid. *Ann R Coll Surg Engl.* 1970; 46:63–76.

157. Forli A, Courvoisier A, Wimsey S, et al. Perilunate dislocations and transscaphoid perilunate fracture-dislocations: A retrospective study with minimum ten-year follow-up. *J Hand Surg Am.* 2010;35:62–68.

158. Fortin PT, Louis DS. Long-term follow-up of scaphoid-trapezium-trapezoid arthrodesis. *J Hand Surg Am.* 1993;18:675–681.

159. Forward DP, Lindau TR, Melsom DS. Intercarpal ligament injuries associated with fractures of the distal part of the radius. *J Bone Joint Surg Am.* 2007;89:2334–2340.

160. Forward DP, Singh HP, Dawson S, et al. The clinical outcome of scaphoid fracture malunion at 1 year. *J Hand Surg Eur Vol.* 2009;34:40–46.

161. Foucher G, Schuind F, Merle M, et al. Fractures of the hook of the hamate. *J Hand Surg Br.* 1985;10:205–210.

162. Fowler C, Sullivan B, Williams LA, et al. A comparison of bone scintigraphy and MRI in the early diagnosis of the occult scaphoid waist fracture. *Skeletal Radiol.* 1998;27:683–687.

163. Frankel VH. The Terry-Thomas sign. *Clin Orthop Relat Res.* 1977;321–322.

164. Freedman DM, Botte MJ, Gelberman RH. Vascularity of the carpus. *Clin Orthop Relat Res.* 2001;47–59.

165. Freeland AE, Finley JS. Displaced vertical fracture of the trapezium treated with a small cancellous lag screw. *J Hand Surg Am.* 1984;9:843–845.

166. Freeland AE, Pesut TA. Oblique capitate fracture of the wrist. *Orthopedics.* 2004; 27:287–290.

167. Freeland P. Scaphoid tubercle tenderness: A better indicator of scaphoid fractures? *Arch Emerg Med.* 1989;6:46–50.

168. Fusetti C, Poletti PA, Pradel PH, et al. Diagnosis of occult scaphoid fracture with high-spatial-resolution sonography: A prospective blind study. *J Trauma.* 2005;59:677–681.

169. Futami T, Aoki H, Tsukamoto Y. Fractures of the hook of the hamate in athletes. 8 cases followed for 6 years. *Acta Orthop Scand.* 1993;64:469–471.

170. Gäbler C, Kukla C, Breitenseher MJ, et al. Diagnosis of occult scaphoid fractures and other wrist injuries. Are repeated clinical examinations and plain radiographs still state of the art? *Langenbecks Arch Surg.* 2001;386:150–154.

171. Gaebler C, Kukla C, Breitenseher M, et al. Magnetic resonance imaging of occult scaphoid fractures. *J Trauma.* 1996;41:73–76.
172. Gaebler C, Kukla C, Breitenseher MJ, et al. Limited diagnostic value of macroradiography in suspected scaphoid fractures. *Acta Orthop Scand.* 1998;69:401–403.
173. Gaebler C, McQueen MM. Carpus fractures and dislocations. In: Bucholz RW, Court-Brown CM, Heckman JD, Tornetta P, eds. *Rockwood and Green's Fractures in Adults.* 7th ed. Philadelphia, PA: Lippincott Williams & Wilkins; 2010:781–828.
174. Gajendran VK, Peterson B, Slater RR Jr, et al. Long-term outcomes of dorsal intercarpal ligament capsulodesis for chronic scapholunate dissociation. *J Hand Surg Am.* 2007;32:1323–1333.
175. Garcia-Elias M, Bishop AT, Dobyns JH, et al. Transcarpal carpometacarpal dislocations, excluding the thumb. *J Hand Surg Am.* 1990;15:531–540.
176. Garcia-Elias M, Henriquez-Lluch A, Rossignani P, et al. Bennett's fracture combined with fracture of the trapezium. A report of three cases. *J Hand Surg Br.* 1993;18:523–526.
177. Garcia-Elias M, Lluch A. Partial excision of scaphoid: Is it ever indicated? *Hand Clin.* 2001;17:687–695, x.
178. Garcia-Elias M. Dorsal fractures of the triquetrum-avulsion or compression fractures? *J Hand Surg Am.* 1987;12:266–268.
179. Gardner MJ, Crisco JJ, Wolfe SW. Carpal kinematics. *Hand Clin.* 2006;22:413–420.
180. Geissler WB, Freeland AE, Savoie FH, et al. Intracarpal soft-tissue lesions associated with an intra-articular fracture of the distal end of the radius. *J Bone Joint Surg Am.* 1996;78:357–365.
181. Geissler WB, Hammit MD. Arthroscopic aided fixation of scaphoid fractures. *Hand Clin.* 2001;17:575–588, viii.
182. Gelberman RH, Bauman TD, Menon J, et al. The vascularity of the lunate bone and Kienböck's disease. *J Hand Surg Am.* 1980;5:272–278.
183. Gelberman RH, Cooney WP III, Szabo RM. Carpal instability. *Instr Course Lect.* 2001;50:123–134.
184. Gelberman RH, Gross MS. The vascularity of the wrist. Identification of arterial patterns at risk. *Clin Orthop Relat Res.* 1986;40–49.
185. Gelberman RH, Menon J. The vascularity of the scaphoid bone. *J Hand Surg Am.* 1980;5:508–513.
186. Gelberman RH, Panagis JS, Taleisnik J, et al. The arterial anatomy of the human carpus. Part I: The extraosseous vascularity. *J Hand Surg Am.* 1983;8:367–375.
187. Gelberman RH, Wolock BS, Siegel DB. Fractures and non-unions of the carpal scaphoid. *J Bone Joint Surg Am.* 1989;71:1560–1565.
188. Gellman H, Caputo RJ, Carter V, et al. Comparison of short and long thumb-spica casts for non-displaced fractures of the carpal scaphoid. *J Bone Joint Surg Am.* 1989;71: 354–357.
189. Gellman H, Schwartz SD, Botte MJ, et al. Late treatment of a dorsal transscaphoid, transtriquetral perilunate wrist dislocation with avascular changes of the lunate. *Clin Orthop Relat Res.* 1988;196–203.
190. Geurts G, van RR, Meermans G, et al. Incidence of scaphotrapezial arthritis following volar percutaneous fixation of nondisplaced scaphoid waist fractures using a transtrapezial approach. *J Hand Surg Am.* 2011;36:1753–1758.
191. Geurts GF, van Riet RP, Meermans G, et al. Volar percutaneous transtrapezial fixation of scaphoid waist fractures: Surgical technique. *Acta Orthop Belg.* 2012;78:121–125.
192. Gilula LA, Destouet JM, Weeks PM, et al. Roentgenographic diagnosis of the painful wrist. *Clin Orthop Relat Res.* 1984;52–64.
193. Gilula LA, Weeks PM. Post-traumatic ligamentous instabilities of the wrist. *Radiology.* 1978;129:641–651.
194. Gooding A, Coates M, Rothwell A. Cost analysis of traditional follow-up protocol versus MRI for radiographically occult scaphoid fractures: A pilot study for the Accident Compensation Corporation. *N Z Med J.* 2004;117:U1049.
195. Graner O, Lopes EI, Carvalho BC, et al. Arthrodesis of the carpal bones in the treatment of Kienböck's disease, painful ununited fractures of the navicular and lunate bones with avascular necrosis, and old fracture-dislocations of carpal bones. *J Bone Joint Surg Am.* 1966;48:767–774.
196. Green DP, O'Brien ET. Classification and management of carpal dislocations. *Clin Orthop Relat Res.* 1980;55–72.
197. Green DP. The effect of avascular necrosis on Russe bone grafting for scaphoid non-union. *J Hand Surg Am.* 1985;10:597–605.
198. Gregory JJ, Mohil RS, Ng AB, et al. Comparison of Herbert and Acutrak screws in the treatment of scaphoid non-union and delayed union. *Acta Orthop Belg.* 2008;74: 761–765.
199. Griffin AC, Gilula LA, Young VL, et al. Fracture of the dorsoulnar tubercle of the trapezium. *J Hand Surg Am.* 1988;13:622–626.
200. Grover R. Clinical assessment of scaphoid injuries and the detection of fractures. *J Hand Surg Br.* 1996;21:341–343.
201. Groves AM, Kayani I, Syed R, et al. An international survey of hospital practice in the imaging of acute scaphoid trauma. *AJR Am J Roentgenol.* 2006;187:1453–1456.
202. Gruson KI, Kaplan KM, Paksima N. Isolated trapezoid fractures: A case report with compilation of the literature. *Bull NYU Hosp Jt Dis.* 2008;66:57–60.
203. Gupta A, Risitano G, Crawford R, et al. Fractures of the hook of the hamate. *Injury.* 1989;20:284–286.
204. Gupta R, Bingenheimer E, Fornalski S, et al. The effect of ulnar shortening on lunate and triquetrum motion–a cadaveric study. *Clin Biomech (Bristol. Avon).* 2005;20:839–845.
205. Gutow AP. Percutaneous fixation of scaphoid fractures. *J Am Acad Orthop Surg.* 2007;15:474–485.
206. Haddad FS, Goddard NJ. Acute percutaneous scaphoid fixation. A pilot study. *J Bone Joint Surg Br.* 1998;80:95–99.
207. Haddad FS, Goddard NJ. Acutrak percutaneous scaphoid fixation. *Tech Hand Up Extrem Surg.* 2000;4:78–80.
208. Hambidge JE, Desai VV, Schranz PJ, et al. Acute fractures of the scaphoid. Treatment by cast immobilisation with the wrist in flexion or extension? *J Bone Joint Surg Br.* 1999;81:91–92.
209. Hansen TB, Petersen RB, Barckman J, et al. Cost-effectiveness of MRI in managing suspected scaphoid fractures. *J Hand Surg Eur Vol.* 2009;34(5):627–630.
210. Haussman P. Long-term results after silicone prosthesis replacement of the proximal pole of the scaphoid bone in advanced scaphoid nonunion. *J Hand Surg Br.* 2002; 27:417–423.
211. Herbert TJ, Fisher WE. Management of the fractured scaphoid using a new bone screw. *J Bone Joint Surg Br.* 1984;66:114–123.
212. Herbert TJ. Open volar repair of acute scaphoid fractures. *Hand Clin.* 2001;17:589–599.
213. Herbert TJ. *The Fractured Scaphoid.* St. Louis, MO: Quality Medical Publishing; 1990.
214. Herneth AM, Siegmeth A, Bader TR, et al. Scaphoid fractures: Evaluation with high-spatial-resolution US initial results. *Radiology.* 2001;220:231–235.
215. Herzberg G, Comtet JJ, Linscheid RL, et al. Perilunate dislocations and fracture-dislocations: A multicenter study. *J Hand Surg Am.* 1993;18:768–779.
216. Herzberg G, Forissier D. Acute dorsal trans-scaphoid perilunate fracture-dislocations: Medium-term results. *J Hand Surg Br.* 2002;27:498–502.
217. Herzberg G. Perilunate and axial carpal dislocations and fracture-dislocations. *J Hand Surg Am.* 2008;33:1659–1668.
218. Hey HW, Chong AK, Murphy D. Prevalence of carpal fracture in Singapore. *J Hand Surg Am.* 2011;36:278–283.
219. Hildebrand KA, Ross DC, Patterson SD, et al. Dorsal perilunate dislocations and fracture-dislocations: Questionnaire, clinical, and radiographic evaluation. *J Hand Surg Am.* 2000;25:1069–1079.
220. Hirano K, Inoue G. Classification and treatment of hamate fractures. *Hand Surg.* 2005;10:151–157.
221. Hixson ML, Stewart C. Microvascular anatomy of the radioscapholunate ligament of the wrist. *J Hand Surg Am.* 1990;15:279–282.
222. Hodgkinson JP, Parkinson RW, Davies DR. Simultaneous fracture of the carpal scaphoid and trapezium–a very unusual combination of fractures. *J Hand Surg Br.* 1985;10:393–394.
223. Hofmeister EP, Dao KD, Glowacki KA, et al. The role of midcarpal arthroscopy in the diagnosis of disorders of the wrist. *J Hand Surg Am.* 2001;26:407–414.
224. Horii E, Nakamura R, Watanabe K, et al. Scaphoid fracture as a "puncher's fracture". *J Orthop Trauma.* 1994;8:107–110.
225. Houshian S, Schroder HA. Wrist arthrodesis with the AO titanium wrist fusion plate: A consecutive series of 42 cases. *J Hand Surg Br.* 2001;26:355–359.
226. Hove LM. Epidemiology of scaphoid fractures in Bergen, Norway. *Scand J Plast Reconstr Surg Hand Surg.* 1999;33:423–426.
227. Hove LM. Fractures of the hand. Distribution and relative incidence. *Scand J Plast Reconstr Surg Hand Surg.* 1993;27:317–319.
228. Hove LM. Simultaneous scaphoid and distal radial fractures. *J Hand Surg Br.* 1994; 19:384–388.
229. Hsu AR, Hsu PA. Unusual case of isolated lunate fracture without ligamentous injury. *Orthopedics.* 2011;34:e785–e789.
230. Hsu KY, Wu CC, Wang KC, et al. Simultaneous dislocation of the five carpometacarpal joints with concomitant fractures of the tuberosity of the trapezium and the hook of the hamate: Case report. *J Trauma.* 1993;35:479–483.
231. Iacobellis C, Baldan S, Aldegheri R. Percutaneous screw fixation for scaphoid fractures. *Musculoskelet Surg.* 2011;95:199–203.
232. Ibrahim T, Qureshi A, Sutton AJ, et al. Surgical versus nonsurgical treatment of acute minimally displaced and undisplaced scaphoid waist fractures: Pairwise and network meta-analyses of randomized controlled trials. *J Hand Surg Am.* 2011;36:1759–1768.
233. Ilyas AM, Mudgal CS. Radiocarpal fracture-dislocations. *J Am Acad Orthop Surg.* 2008;16:647–655.
234. Inoue G, Miura T. Proximal row carpectomy in perilunate dislocations and lunatomalacia. *Acta Orthop Scand.* 1990;61:449–452.
235. Jenkins PJ, Slade K, Huntley JS, et al. A comparative analysis of the accuracy, diagnostic uncertainty and cost of imaging modalities in suspected scaphoid fractures. *Injury.* 2008;39:768–774.
236. Jensen BV, Christensen C. An unusual combination of simultaneous fracture of the tuberosity of the trapezium and the hook of the hamate. *J Hand Surg Am.* 1990;15: 285–287.
237. Jeon IH, Kim HJ, Min WK, et al. Arthroscopically assisted percutaneous fixation for trans-scaphoid perilunate fracture dislocation. *J Hand Surg Eur Vol.* 2010;35:664–668.
238. Jeon IH, Micic ID, Oh CW, et al. Percutaneous screw fixation for scaphoid fracture: A comparison between the dorsal and the volar approaches. *J Hand Surg Am.* 2009;34:228–236.
239. Johnson RP. The acutely injured wrist and its residuals. *Clin Orthop Relat Res.* 1980; 33–44.
240. Jones DB Jr, Burger H, Bishop AT, et al. Treatment of scaphoid waist nonunions with an avascular proximal pole and carpal collapse. A comparison of two vascularized bone grafts. *J Bone Joint Surg Am.* 2008;90:2616–2625.
241. Jones DB Jr, Kakar S. Perilunate dislocations and fracture dislocations. *J Hand Surg Am.* 2012;37:2168–2173.
242. Jonsson BY, Siggeirsdottir K, Mogensen B, et al. Fracture rate in a population-based sample of men in Reykjavik. *Acta Orthop Scand.* 2004;75:195–200.
243. Jorgsholm P, Thomsen NO, Bjorkman A, et al. The incidence of intrinsic and extrinsic ligament injuries in scaphoid waist fractures. *J Hand Surg Am.* 2010;35:368–374.
244. Kain N, Heras-Palou C. Trapezoid fractures: Report of 11 cases. *J Hand Surg Am.* 2012;37:1159–1162.
245. Kato H, Nakamura R, Horii E, et al. Diagnostic imaging for fracture of the hook of the hamate. *Hand Surg.* 2000;5:19–24.
246. Kauer JM. Functional anatomy of the wrist. *Clin Orthop Relat Res.* 1980;(149):9–20.
247. Kauer JM. The mechanism of the carpal joint. *Clin Orthop Relat Res.* 1986;(202):16–26.
248. Kaufmann R, Pfaeffle J, Blankenhorn B, et al. Kinematics of the midcarpal and radiocarpal joints in radioulnar deviation: An in vitro study. *J Hand Surg Am.* 2005;30: 937–942.
249. Kaufmann RA, Pfaeffle HJ, Blankenhorn BD, et al. Kinematics of the midcarpal and radiocarpal joint in flexion and extension: An in vitro study. *J Hand Surg Am.* 2006;31:1142–1148.

250. Kawamura K, Chung KC. Treatment of scaphoid fractures and nonunions. *J Hand Surg Am.* 2008;33:988–997.

251. Kijima Y, Viegas SF. Wrist anatomy and biomechanics. *J Hand Surg Am.* 2009;34:1555–1563.

252. Kitay A, Wolfe SW. Scapholunate instability: Current concepts in diagnosis and management. *J Hand Surg Am.* 2012;37:2175–2196.

253. Knoll VD, Allan C, Trumble TE. Trans-scaphoid perilunate fracture dislocations: Results of screw fixation of the scaphoid and lunotriquetral repair with a dorsal approach. *J Hand Surg Am.* 2005;30:1145–1152.

254. Komurcu M, Kurklu M, Ozturan KE, et al. Early and delayed treatment of dorsal trans-scaphoid perilunate fracture-dislocations. *J Orthop Trauma.* 2008;22:535–540.

255. Kozin SH. Incidence, mechanism, and natural history of scaphoid fractures. *Hand Clin.* 2001;17:515–524.

256. Kozin SH. Perilunate injuries: Diagnosis and treatment. *J Am Acad Orthop Surg.* 1998;6:114–120.

257. Kozin SH. The role of arthroscopy in scapholunate instability. *Hand Clin.* 1999;15:435–444.

258. Kremer T, Wendt M, Riedel K, et al. Open reduction for perilunate injuries–clinical outcome and patient satisfaction. *J Hand Surg Am.* 2010;35:1599–1606.

259. Kuhlmann JN, Boabighi A, Kirsch JM, et al. [Experimental study on a plaster cast in fractures of the carpal scaphoid. Clinical deductions]. *Rev Chir Orthop Reparatrice Appar Mot.* 1987;73:49–56.

260. Kuo CE, Wolfe SW. Scapholunate instability: Current concepts in diagnosis and management. *J Hand Surg Am.* 2008;33:998–1013.

261. Kusano N, Churei Y, Shiraishi E, et al. Diagnosis of occult carpal scaphoid fracture: A comparison of magnetic resonance imaging and computed tomography techniques. *Tech Hand Up Extrem Surg.* 2002;6:119–123.

262. Lacey JD, Hodge JC. Pisiform and hamulus fractures: Easily missed wrist fractures diagnosed on a reverse oblique radiograph. *J Emerg Med.* 1998;16:445–452.

263. LaJoie AS, McCabe SJ, Thomas B, et al. Determining the sensitivity and specificity of common diagnostic tests for carpal tunnel syndrome using latent class analysis. *Plast Reconstr Surg.* 2005;116:502–507.

264. Lam KS, Woodbridge S, Burke FD. Wrist function after excision of the pisiform. *J Hand Surg Br.* 2003;28:69–72.

265. Lamas C, Carrera A, Proubasta I, et al. The anatomy and vascularity of the lunate: Considerations applied to Kienböck's disease. *Chir Main.* 2007;26:13–20.

266. Landsmeer JM. Studies in the anatomy of articulation. I. The equilibrium of the "intercalated" bone. *Acta Morphol Neerl Scand.* 1961;3:287–303.

267. Lane LB, Daher RJ, Leo AJ. Scapholunate dissociation with radiolunate arthritis without radioscaphoid arthritis. *J Hand Surg Am.* 2010;35:1075–1081.

268. Langer AJ, Gron P, Langhoff O. The scaphoid fat stripe in the diagnosis of carpal trauma. *Acta Radiol.* 1988;29:97–99.

269. Langhoff O, Andersen JL. Consequences of late immobilization of scaphoid fractures. *J Hand Surg Br.* 1988;13:77–79.

270. Larsen CF, Brondum V, Skov O. Epidemiology of scaphoid fractures in Odense, Denmark. *Acta Orthop Scand.* 1992;63:216–218.

271. Lavernia CJ, Cohen MS, Taleisnik J. Treatment of scapholunate dissociation by ligamentous repair and capsulodesis. *J Hand Surg Am.* 1992;17:354–359.

272. Leslie IJ, Dickson RA. The fractured carpal scaphoid. Natural history and factors influencing outcome. *J Bone Joint Surg Br.* 1981;63-B:225–230.

273. Leung YF, Ip SP, Wong A, et al. Transscaphoid transcapitate transtriquetral perilunate fracture-dislocation: A case report. *J Hand Surg Am.* 2006;31:608–610.

274. Li G, Rowen B, Tokunaga D, et al. Carpal kinematics of lunotriquetral dissociations. *Biomed Sci Instrum.* 1991;27:273–281.

275. Lichtman DM, Bruckner JD, Culp RW, et al. Palmar midcarpal instability: Results of surgical reconstruction. *J Hand Surg Am.* 1993;18:307–315.

276. Lichtman DM, Schneider JR, Swafford AR, et al. Ulnar midcarpal instability-clinical and laboratory analysis. *J Hand Surg Am.* 1981;6:515–523.

277. Linscheid RL, Dobyns JH, Beabout JW, et al. Traumatic instability of the wrist. Diagnosis, classification, and pathomechanics. *J Bone Joint Surg Am.* 1972;54:1612–1632.

278. Linscheid RL, Dobyns JH, Beckenbaugh RD, et al. Instability patterns of the wrist. *J Hand Surg Am.* 1983;8:682–686.

279. Linscheid RL, Dobyns JH. The unified concept of carpal injuries. *Ann Chir Main.* 1984;3:35–42.

280. Linscheid RL, Dobyns JH. Treatment of scapholunate dissociation. Rotatory subluxation of the scaphoid. *Hand Clin.* 1992;8:645–652.

281. Linscheid RL, Lynch NM. Scaphoid osteotomy for malunion. *Tech Hand Up Extrem Surg.* 1998;2:119–125.

282. Linscheid RL. Biomechanics of the distal radioulnar joint. *Clin Orthop Relat Res.* 1992;46–55.

283. Linscheid RL. Kinematic considerations of the wrist. *Clin Orthop Relat Res.* 1986;(202):27–39.

284. Little CP, Burston BJ, Hopkinson-Woolley J, et al. Failure of surgery for scaphoid nonunion is associated with smoking. *J Hand Surg Br.* 2006;31:252–255.

285. Llewelyn H. Assessing properly the usefulness of clinical prediction rules and tests. *BMJ.* 2012;344:e1238.

286. Logan SE, Nowak MD. Intrinsic and extrinsic wrist ligaments: Biomechanical and functional differences. *Biomed Sci Instrum.* 1987;23:9–13.

287. Lozano-Calderon S, Blazar P, Zurakowski D, et al. Diagnosis of scaphoid fracture displacement with radiography and computed tomography. *J Bone Joint Surg Am.* 2006;88:2695–2703.

288. Lutz M, Arora R, Kammerlander C, et al. [Stabilization of perilunate and transscaphoid perilunate fracture-dislocations via a combined palmar and dorsal approach]. *Oper Orthop Traumatol.* 2009;21:442–458.

289. Lynch NM, Linscheid RL. Corrective osteotomy for scaphoid malunion: Technique and long-term follow-up evaluation. *J Hand Surg Am.* 1997;22:35–43.

290. Mack GR, Bosse MJ, Gelberman RH, et al. The natural history of scaphoid non-union. *J Bone Joint Surg Am.* 1984;66:504–509.

291. Mahmoud M, Koptan W. Percutaneous screw fixation without bone grafting for established scaphoid nonunion with substantial bone loss. *J Bone Joint Surg Br.* 2011;93:932–936.

292. Mallee W, Doornberg JN, Ring D, et al. Comparison of CT and MRI for diagnosis of suspected scaphoid fractures. *J Bone Joint Surg Am.* 2011;93:20–28.

293. Malshikare V, Oswal A. Trapezoid fracture caused by assault. *Indian J Orthop.* 2007;41:175–176.

294. Mansberg R, Lewis G, Kirsh G. Avascular necrosis and fracture of the capitate bone: Unusual scintigraphic features. *Clin Nucl Med.* 2000;25:372–373.

295. Marcuzzi A, Leti AA, Caserta G, et al. Ligamentous reconstruction of scapholunate dislocation through a double dorsal and palmar approach. *J Hand Surg Br.* 2006;31:445–449.

296. Marsh AP, Lampros PJ. The naviculo-capitate fracture syndrome. *Am J Roentgenol Radium Ther Nucl Med.* 1959;82:255–256.

297. Martus JE, Bedi A, Jebson PJ. Cannulated variable pitch compression screw fixation of scaphoid fractures using a limited dorsal approach. *Tech Hand Up Extrem Surg.* 2005;9:202–206.

298. Mataliotakis G, Doukas M, Kostas I, et al. Sensory innervation of the subregions of the scapholunate interosseous ligament in relation to their structural composition. *J Hand Surg Am.* 2009;34:1413–1421.

299. May O. [The pisiform bone: Sesamoid or carpal bone?]. *Ann Chir Main Memb Super.* 1996;15:265–271.

300. Mayfield JK, Johnson RP, Kilcoyne RF. The ligaments of the human wrist and their functional significance. *Anat Rec.* 1976;186:417–428.

301. Mayfield JK, Johnson RP, Kilcoyne RK. Carpal dislocations: Pathomechanics and progressive perilunar instability. *J Hand Surg Am.* 1980;5:226–241.

302. Mayfield JK. Mechanism of carpal injuries. *Clin Orthop Relat Res.* 1980;45–54.

303. Mayfield JK. Patterns of injury to carpal ligaments. A spectrum. *Clin Orthop Relat Res.* 1984;36–42.

304. Mayfield JK. Wrist ligamentous anatomy and pathogenesis of carpal instability. *Orthop Clin North Am.* 1984;15:209–216.

305. McLaughlin HL. Fracture of the carpal navicular (scaphoid) bone; some observations based on treatment by open reduction and internal fixation. *J Bone Joint Surg Am.* 1954;36-A:765–774.

306. McMurtry RY, Youm Y, Flatt AE, et al. Kinematics of the wrist. II. Clinical applications. *J Bone Joint Surg Am.* 1978;60:955–961.

307. McQueen MM, Gelbke MK, Wakefield A, et al. Percutaneous screw fixation versus conservative treatment for fractures of the waist of the scaphoid: A prospective randomised study. *J Bone Joint Surg Br.* 2008;90:66–71.

308. Meermans G, Verstreken F. Percutaneous transtrapezial fixation of acute scaphoid fractures. *J Hand Surg Eur Vol.* 2008;33:791–796.

309. Megerle K, Worg H, Christopoulos G, et al. Gadolinium-enhanced preoperative MRI scans as a prognostic parameter in scaphoid nonunion. *J Hand Surg Eur Vol.* 2011;36:23–28.

310. Mehrpour SR, Kamrani RS, Aghamirsalim MR, et al. Treatment of Kienböck disease by lunate core decompression. *J Hand Surg Am.* 2011;36:1675–1677.

311. Memarsadeghi M, Breitenseher MJ, Schaefer-Prokop C, et al. Occult scaphoid fractures: Comparison of multidetector CT and MR imaging–initial experience. *Radiology.* 2006;240:169–176.

312. Menth-Chiari WA, Poehling GG. Preiser's disease: Arthroscopic treatment of avascular necrosis of the scaphoid. *Arthroscopy.* 2000;16:208–213.

313. Merrell GA, Wolfe SW, Slade JF III. Treatment of scaphoid nonunions: Quantitative meta-analysis of the literature. *J Hand Surg Am.* 2002;27:685–691.

314. Meyers MH, Wells R, Harvey JP Jr. Naviculo-capitate fracture syndrome. Review of the literature and a case report. *J Bone Joint Surg Am.* 1971;53:1383–1386.

315. Milek MA, Boulas HJ. Flexor tendon ruptures secondary to hamate hook fractures. *J Hand Surg Am.* 1990;15:740–744.

316. Minami A, Kato H, Iwasaki N. Treatment of scapholunate dissociation: Ligamentous repair associated with modified dorsal capsulodesis. *Hand Surg.* 2003;8:1–6.

317. Mitsuyasu H, Patterson RM, Shah MA, et al. The role of the dorsal intercarpal ligament in dynamic and static scapholunate instability. *J Hand Surg Am.* 2004;29:279–288.

318. Miyawaki T, Kobayashi M, Matsuura S, et al. Trapezoid bone fracture. *Ann Plast Surg.* 2000;44:444–446.

319. Mizuseki T, Ikuta Y. The dorsal carpal ligaments: Their anatomy and function. *J Hand Surg Br.* 1989;14:91–98.

320. Mody BS, Belliappa PP, Dias JJ, et al. Nonunion of fractures of the scaphoid tuberosity. *J Bone Joint Surg Br.* 1993;75:423–425.

321. Mody BS, Dias JJ. Carpometacarpal dislocation of the thumb associated with fracture of the trapezium. *J Hand Surg Br.* 1993;18:197–199.

322. Moneim MS, Bolger JT, Omer GE. Radiocarpal dislocation–classification and rationale for management. *Clin Orthop Relat Res.* 1985;199–209.

323. Moneim MS, Hofammann KE III, Omer GE. Transscaphoid perilunate fracture-dislocation. Result of open reduction and pin fixation. *Clin Orthop Relat Res.* 1984;227–235.

324. Moneim MS. Management of greater arc carpal fractures. *Hand Clin.* 1988;4:457–467.

325. Moojen TM, Snel JG, Ritt MJ, et al. In vivo analysis of carpal kinematics and comparative review of the literature. *J Hand Surg Am.* 2003;28:81–87.

326. Morgan WJ, Breen TF, Coumas JM, et al. Role of magnetic resonance imaging in assessing factors affecting healing in scaphoid nonunions. *Clin Orthop Relat Res.* 1997;240–246.

327. Moritomo H, Murase T, Oka K, et al. Relationship between the fracture location and the kinematic pattern in scaphoid nonunion. *J Hand Surg Am.* 2008;33:1459–1468.

328. Moritomo H, Viegas SF, Elder KW, et al. Scaphoid nonunions: A 3-dimensional analysis of patterns of deformity. *J Hand Surg Am.* 2000;25:520–528.

329. Moritomo H, Viegas SF, Nakamura K, et al. The scaphotrapezio-trapezoidal joint. Part 1: An anatomic and radiographic study. *J Hand Surg Am.* 2000;25:899–910.

330. Morizaki Y, Miura T. Unusual pattern of dislocation of the trapeziometacarpal joint with avulsion fracture of the trapezium: Case report. *Hand Surg.* 2009;14:149–152.

331. Mudgal C, Hastings H. Scapho-lunate diastasis in fractures of the distal radius. Pathomechanics and treatment options. *J Hand Surg Br.* 1993;18:725–729.

332. Mudgal CS, Jones WA. Scapho-lunate diastasis: A component of fractures of the distal radius. *J Hand Surg Br.* 1990;15:503–505.

333. Mudgal CS, Psenica J, Jupiter JB. Radiocarpal fracture-dislocation. *J Hand Surg Br.* 1999;24:92–98.

334. Muermans S, De SL, Van RH. Blatt dorsal capsulodesis for scapholunate instability. *Acta Orthop Belg.* 1999;65:434–439.

335. Mulford JS, Ceulemans LJ, Nam D, et al. Proximal row carpectomy vs four corner fusion for scapholunate (Slac) or scaphoid nonunion advanced collapse (Snac) wrists: A systematic review of outcomes. *J Hand Surg Eur Vol.* 2009;34:256–263.

336. Muniz AE. Unusual wrist pain: Pisiform dislocation and fracture. *Am J Emerg Med.* 1999;17:78–79.

337. Munk B, Bolvig L, Kroner K, et al. Ultrasound for diagnosis of scaphoid fractures. *J Hand Surg Br.* 2000;25:369–371.

338. Munk B, Frokjaer J, Larsen CF, et al. Diagnosis of scaphoid fractures. A prospective multicenter study of 1,052 patients with 160 fractures. *Acta Orthop Scand.* 1995; 66:359–360.

339. Munk B, Larsen CF. Bone grafting the scaphoid nonunion: A systematic review of 147 publications including 5,246 cases of scaphoid nonunion. *Acta Orthop Scand.* 2004;75:618–629.

340. Nagao S, Patterson RM, Buford WL Jr, et al. Three-dimensional description of ligamentous attachments around the lunate. *J Hand Surg Am.* 2005;30:685–692.

341. Nagumo A, Toh S, Tsubo K, et al. An occult fracture of the trapezoid bone. A case report. *J Bone Joint Surg Am.* 2002;84-A:1025–1027.

342. Nakamura P, Imaeda T, Miura T. Scaphoid malunion. *J Bone Joint Surg Br.* 1991;73: 134–137.

343. Nakamura R, Imaeda T, Horii E, et al. Analysis of scaphoid fracture displacement by three-dimensional computed tomography. *J Hand Surg Am.* 1991;16:485–492.

344. Nanno M, Buford WL Jr, Patterson RM, et al. Three-dimensional analysis of the ligamentous attachments of the second through fifth carpometacarpal joints. *Clin Anat.* 2007;20:530–544.

345. Nanno M, Patterson RM, Viegas SF. Three-dimensional imaging of the carpal ligaments. *Hand Clin.* 2006;22:399–412.

346. Nanno M, Sawaizumi T, Ito H. Dorsal fracture dislocations of the second and third carpometacarpal joints. *J Hand Surg Eur Vol.* 2007;32:597–598.

347. Naranje S, Kotwal PP, Shamshery P, et al. Percutaneous fixation of selected scaphoid fractures by dorsal approach. *Int Orthop.* 2010;34:997–1003.

348. Nattrass GR, King GJ, McMurtry RY, et al. An alternative method for determination of the carpal height ratio. *J Bone Joint Surg Am.* 1994;76:88–94.

349. Navarro A. Luxaciones del carpo. *An Fac Med (Lima).* 1921;6:113–141.

350. Nguyen Q, Chaudhry S, Sloan R, et al. The clinical scaphoid fracture: Early computed tomography as a practical approach. *Ann R Coll Surg Engl.* 2008;90:488–491.

351. Nielsen PT, Hedeboe J. Posttraumatic scapholunate dissociation detected by wrist cineradiography. *J Hand Surg Am.* 1984;9A:135–138.

352. Nigro RO. Anatomy of the flexor retinaculum of the wrist and the flexor carpi radialis tunnel. *Hand Clin.* 2001;17:61–64.

353. Nijs S, Mulier T, Broos P. Occult fracture of the trapezoid bone: A report on two cases. *Acta Orthop Belg.* 2004;70:177–179.

354. Norman A, Nelson J, Green S. Fractures of the hook of hamate: Radiographic signs. *Radiology.* 1985;154:49–53.

355. Nowalk MD, Logan SE. Distinguishing biomechanical properties of intrinsic and extrinsic human wrist ligaments. *J Biomech Eng.* 1991;113:85–93.

356. Obdeijn MC, van der Vlies CH, van Rijn RR. Capitate and hamate fracture in a child: The value of MRI imaging. *Emerg Radiol.* 2010;17:157–159.

357. Oduwole KO, Cichy B, Dillon JP, et al. Acutrak versus Herbert screw fixation for scaphoid non-union and delayed union. *J Orthop Surg (Hong Kong).* 2012;20:61–65.

358. Oka K, Moritomo H, Murase T, et al. Patterns of carpal deformity in scaphoid nonunion: A 3-dimensional and quantitative analysis. *J Hand Surg Am.* 2005;30:1136–1144.

359. Oka K, Murase T, Moritomo H, et al. Patterns of bone defect in scaphoid nonunion: A 3-dimensional and quantitative analysis. *J Hand Surg Am.* 2005;30:359–365.

360. Ono H, Gilula LA, Evanoff BA, et al. Midcarpal instability: Is capitolunate instability pattern a clinical condition? *J Hand Surg Br.* 1996;21:197–201.

361. Osterman AL, Seidman GD. The role of arthroscopy in the treatment of lunatotriquetral ligament injuries. *Hand Clin.* 1995;11:41–50.

362. Osti M, Zinnecker R, Benedetto KP. Scaphoid and capitate fracture with concurrent scapholunate dissociation. *J Hand Surg Br.* 2006;31:76–78.

363. Pacek CA, Chakan M, Goitz RJ, et al. Morphological analysis of the transverse carpal ligament. *Hand (N Y).* 2010;5(2):135–140.

364. Palmer AK, Werner FW. Biomechanics of the distal radioulnar joint. *Clin Orthop Relat Res.* 1984;26–35.

365. Palmer AK. The distal radioulnar joint. Anatomy, biomechanics, and triangular fibrocartilage complex abnormalities. *Hand Clin.* 1987;3:31–40.

366. Panagis JS, Gelberman RH, Taleisnik J, et al. The arterial anatomy of the human carpus. Part II: The intraosseous vascularity. *J Hand Surg Am.* 1983;8:375–382.

367. Pao VS, Chang J. Scaphoid nonunion: Diagnosis and treatment. *Plast Reconstr Surg.* 2003;112:1666–1676.

368. Papaloizos MY, Fusetti C, Christen T, et al. Minimally invasive fixation versus conservative treatment of undisplaced scaphoid fractures: A cost-effectiveness study. *J Hand Surg Br.* 2004;29:116–119.

369. Papilion JD, DuPuy TE, Aulicino PL, et al. Radiographic evaluation of the hook of the hamate: A new technique. *J Hand Surg Am.* 1988;13:437–439.

370. Park MJ. Radiographic observation of the scaphoid shift test. *J Bone Joint Surg Br.* 2003;85:358–362.

371. Parvizi J, Wayman J, Kelly P, et al. Combining the clinical signs improves diagnosis of scaphoid fractures. A prospective study with follow-up. *J Hand Surg Br.* 1998;23: 324–327.

372. Patel NK, Davies N, Mirza Z, et al. Cost and clinical effectiveness of MRI in occult scaphoid fractures: A randomised controlled trial. *Emerg Med J.* 2013;30(3): 202–207.

373. Platon A, Poletti PA, Van AJ, et al. Occult fractures of the scaphoid: The role of ultrasonography in the emergency department. *Skeletal Radiol.* 2011;40:869–875.

374. Pliefke J, Stengel D, Rademacher G, et al. Diagnostic accuracy of plain radiographs and cineradiography in diagnosing traumatic scapholunate dissociation. *Skeletal Radiol.* 2008;37:139–145.

375. Polivy KD, Millender LH, Newberg A, et al. Fractures of the hook of the hamate—a failure of clinical diagnosis. *J Hand Surg Am.* 1985;10:101–104.

376. Powell JM, Lloyd GJ, Rintoul RF. New clinical test for fracture of the scaphoid. *Can J Surg.* 1988;31:237–238.

377. Prosser AJ, Brenkel IJ, Irvine GB. Articular fractures of the distal scaphoid. *J Hand Surg Br.* 1988;13:87–91.

378. Pruzansky M, Arnold L. Delayed union of fractures of the trapezoid and body of the hamate. *Orthop Rev.* 1987;16:624–628.

379. Raby N. Magnetic resonance imaging of suspected scaphoid fractures using a low field dedicated extremity MR system. *Clin Radiol.* 2001;56:316–320.

380. Ramamurthy C, Cutler L, Nuttall D, et al. The factors affecting outcome after nonvascular bone grafting and internal fixation for nonunion of the scaphoid. *J Bone Joint Surg Br.* 2007;89:627–632.

381. Ramoutar DN, Katevu C, Titchener AG, et al. Trapezium fracture—a common technique to fix a rare injury: A case report. *Cases J.* 2009;2:8304.

382. Rand JA, Linscheid RL, Dobyns JH. Capitate fractures: A long-term follow-up. *Clin Orthop Relat Res.* 1982;209–216.

383. Raudasoja L, Rawlins M, Kallio P, et al. Conservative treatment of scaphoid fractures: A follow up study. *Ann Chir Gynaecol.* 1999;88:289–293.

384. Reagan DS, Linscheid RL, Dobyns JH. Lunotriquetral sprains. *J Hand Surg Am.* 1984;9:502–514.

385. Reed DN, Fulcher SM, Harrison SJ. Unstable scaphoid nonunion treatment technique: Use of a volar distal radius corticocancellous autograft. *Tech Hand Up Extrem Surg.* 2012;16:91–94.

386. Reigstad O, Grimsgaard C, Thorkildsen R, et al. Long-term results of scaphoid nonunion surgery: 50 patients reviewed after 8 to 18 years. *J Orthop Trauma.* 2012;26:241–245.

387. Reilly BM, Evans AT. Translating clinical research into clinical practice: Impact of using prediction rules to make decisions. *Ann Intern Med.* 2006;144:201–209.

388. Rettig ME, Kozin SH, Cooney WP. Open reduction and internal fixation of acute displaced scaphoid waist fractures. *J Hand Surg Am.* 2001;26:271–276.

389. Rettig ME, Raskin KB. Long-term assessment of proximal row carpectomy for chronic perilunate dislocations. *J Hand Surg Am.* 1999;24:1231–1236.

390. Rhemrev SJ, Beeres FJ, van Leerdam RH, et al. Clinical prediction rule for suspected scaphoid fractures A Prospective Cohort Study. *Injury.* 2010;41(10):1026–1030.

391. Rhemrev SJ, de Zwart AD, Kingma LM, et al. Early computed tomography compared with bone scintigraphy in suspected scaphoid fractures. *Clin Nucl Med.* 2010;35:931–934.

392. Richards RR, Paitich CB, Bell RS. Internal fixation of a capitate fracture with Herbert screws. *J Hand Surg Am.* 1990;15:885–887.

393. Ring D, Jupiter JB, Herndon JH. Acute fractures of the scaphoid. *J Am Acad Orthop Surg.* 2000;8:225–231.

394. Ring D, Lozano-Calderon S. Imaging for suspected scaphoid fracture. *J Hand Surg Am.* 2008;33:954–957.

395. Ring D, Patterson JD, Levitz S, et al. Both scanning plane and observer affect measurements of scaphoid deformity. *J Hand Surg Am.* 2005;30:696–701.

396. Ritt MJ, Berger RA, Bishop AT, et al. The capitohamate ligaments. A comparison of biomechanical properties. *J Hand Surg Br.* 1996;21:451–454.

397. Ritt MJ, Berger RA, Kauer JM. The gross and histologic anatomy of the ligaments of the capitohamate joint. *J Hand Surg Am.* 1996;21:1022–1028.

398. Ritt MJ, Bishop AT, Berger RA, et al. Lunotriquetral ligament properties: A comparison of three anatomic subregions. *J Hand Surg Am.* 1998;23:425–431.

399. Roolker L, Tiel-van Buul MM, Bossuyt PP, et al. The value of additional carpal box radiographs in suspected scaphoid fracture. *Invest Radiol.* 1997;32:149–153.

400. Roolker W, Tiel-van Buul MM, Bossuyt PM, et al. Carpal Box radiography in suspected scaphoid fracture. *J Bone Joint Surg Br.* 1996;78:535–539.

401. Roolker W, Tiel-van Buul MM, Ritt MJ, et al. Experimental evaluation of scaphoid X-series, carpal box radiographs, planar tomography, computed tomography, and magnetic resonance imaging in the diagnosis of scaphoid fracture. *J Trauma.* 1997;42:247–253.

402. Rosati M, Parchi P, Cacianti M, et al. Treatment of acute scapholunate ligament injuries with bone anchor. *Musculoskelet Surg.* 2010;94:25–32.

403. Royal College of Radiologists. *Making the Best Use of a Department of Clinical Radiology; Guidelines for Doctors.* 5th ed. London, UK: Royal College of Radiologists; 2003.

404. Ruby LK, Leslie BM. Wrist arthritis associated with scaphoid nonunion. *Hand Clin.* 1987;3:529–539.

405. Ruby LK, Stinson J, Belsky MR. The natural history of scaphoid non-union. A review of fifty-five cases. *J Bone Joint Surg Am.* 1985;67:428–432.

406. Ruch DS, Poehling GG. Arthroscopic management of partial scapholunate and lunotriquetral injuries of the wrist. *J Hand Surg Am.* 1996;21:412–417.

407. Russe O. Fracture of the carpal navicular. Diagnosis, non-operative treatment, and operative treatment. *J Bone Joint Surg Am.* 1960;42-A:759–768.

408. Sadowski RM, Montilla RD. Rare isolated trapezoid fracture: A case report. *Hand (N Y).* 2008;3:372–374.

409. Saeden B, Tornkvist H, Ponzer S, et al. Fracture of the carpal scaphoid. A prospective, randomised 12-year follow-up comparing operative and conservative treatment. *J Bone Joint Surg Br.* 2001;83:230–234.

410. Sammer DM, Shin AY. Wrist surgery: Management of chronic scapholunate and lunotriquetral ligament injuries. *Plast Reconstr Surg.* 2012;130:138e–156e.

411. Sanders WE. Evaluation of the humpback scaphoid by computed tomography in the longitudinal axial plane of the scaphoid. *J Hand Surg Am.* 1988;13:182–187.

412. Sandoval E, Cecilia D, Garcia-Paredero E. Surgical treatment of trans-scaphoid, trans-capitate, transtriquetral, perilunate fracture-dislocation with open reduction, internal fixation and lunotriquetral ligament repair. *J Hand Surg Eur Vol.* 2008;33:377–379.

413. Sarrafian SK, Melamed JL, Goshgarian GM. Study of wrist motion in flexion and extension. *Clin Orthop Relat Res.* 1977;153–159.

414. Savelberg HH, Kooloos JG, Huiskes R, et al. Stiffness of the ligaments of the human wrist joint. *J Biomech.* 1992;25:369–376.

415. Schadel-Hopfner M, Bohringer G, Junge A. Dislocation of the pisiform bone after severe crush injury to the hand. *Scand J Plast Reconstr Surg Hand Surg.* 2003;37: 252–255.

416. Schadel-Hopfner M, Junge A, Bohringer G. Scapholunate ligament injury occurring with scaphoid fracture—a rare coincidence? *J Hand Surg Br.* 2005;30:137–142.

417. Scheufler O, Andresen R, Radmer S, et al. Hook of hamate fractures: Critical evaluation of different therapeutic procedures. *Plast Reconstr Surg.* 2005;115:488–497.

418. Scheufler O, Radmer S, Erdmann D, et al. Therapeutic alternatives in nonunion of hamate hook fractures: Personal experience in 8 patients and review of literature. *Ann Plast Surg.* 2005;55:149–154.

419. Schiltenwolf M, Wrazidlo W, Brocai DR, et al. [A prospective study of early diagnosis of lunate necrosis by means of MRI]. *Rofo.* 1995;162:325–329.

420. Schmitt R, Christopoulos G, Wagner M, et al. Avascular necrosis (AVN) of the proximal fragment in scaphoid nonunion: Is intravenous contrast agent necessary in MRI? *Eur J Radiol.* 2011;77:222–227.

421. Schneider LH, Aulicino P. Nonunion of the carpal scaphoid: The Russe procedure. *J Trauma.* 1982;22:315–319.

422. Schweizer A, Steiger R. Long-term results after repair and augmentation ligamentoplasty of rotatory subluxation of the scaphoid. *J Hand Surg Am.* 2002;27:674–684.

423. Senall JA, Failla JM, Bouffard JA, et al. Ultrasound for the early diagnosis of clinically suspected scaphoid fracture. *J Hand Surg Am.* 2004;29:400–405.

424. Sennwald GR, Zdravkovic V, Kern HP, et al. Kinematics of the wrist and its ligaments. *J Hand Surg Am.* 1993;18:805–814.

425. Sennwald GR, Zdravkovic V, Oberlin C. The anatomy of the palmar scaphotriquetral ligament. *J Bone Joint Surg Br.* 1994;76:147–149.

426. Shahabpour M, De MM, Pouders C, et al. MR imaging of normal extrinsic wrist ligaments using thin slices with clinical and surgical correlation. *Eur J Radiol.* 2011;77:196–201.

427. Shih JT, Lee HM, Hou YT, et al. Results of arthroscopic reduction and percutaneous fixation for acute displaced scaphoid fractures. *Arthroscopy.* 2005;21:620–626.

428. Short WH, Werner FW, Fortino MD, et al. A dynamic biomechanical study of scapholunate ligament sectioning. *J Hand Surg Am.* 1995;20:986–999.

429. Short WH, Werner FW, Fortino MD, et al. Analysis of the kinematics of the scaphoid and lunate in the intact wrist joint. *Hand Clin.* 1997;13:93–108.

430. Short WH, Werner FW, Green JK, et al. Biomechanical evaluation of ligamentous stabilizers of the scaphoid and lunate. *J Hand Surg Am.* 2002;27:991–1002.

431. Short WH, Werner FW, Green JK, et al. Biomechanical evaluation of the ligamentous stabilizers of the scaphoid and lunate: Part II. *J Hand Surg Am.* 2005;30:24–34.

432. Short WH, Werner FW, Green JK, et al. Biomechanical evaluation of the ligamentous stabilizers of the scaphoid and lunate: Part III. *J Hand Surg Am.* 2007;32:297-309.

433. Short WH, Werner FW, Green JK, et al. The effect of sectioning the dorsal radiocarpal ligament and insertion of a pressure sensor into the radiocarpal joint on scaphoid and lunate kinematics. *J Hand Surg Am.* 2002;27:68–76.

434. Short WH, Werner FW, Sutton LG. Dynamic biomechanical evaluation of the dorsal intercarpal ligament repair for scapholunate instability. *J Hand Surg Am.* 2009;34:652–659.

435. Singh AK, Davis TR, Dawson JS, et al. Gadolinium enhanced MR assessment of proximal fragment vascularity in nonunions after scaphoid fracture: Does it predict the outcome of reconstructive surgery? *J Hand Surg Br.* 2004;29:444–448.

436. Singh HP, Taub N, Dias JJ. Management of displaced fractures of the waist of the scaphoid: Meta-analyses of comparative studies. *Injury.* 2012;43:933–939.

437. Skelly WJ, Nahigian SH, Hidvegi EB. Palmar lunate transtriquetral fracture dislocation. *J Hand Surg Am.* 1991;16:536–539.

438. Skirven T, Trope J. Complications of immobilization. *Hand Clin.* 1994;10:53–61.

439. Slade JF III, Geissler WB, Gutow AP, et al. Percutaneous internal fixation of selected scaphoid nonunions with an arthroscopically assisted dorsal approach. *J Bone Joint Surg Am.* 2003;85-A(suppl 4):20–32.

440. Slade JF III, Grauer JN, Mahoney JD. Arthroscopic reduction and percutaneous fixation of scaphoid fractures with a novel dorsal technique. *Orthop Clin North Am.* 2001;32:247–261.

441. Slade JF III, Gutow AP, Geissler WB. Percutaneous internal fixation of scaphoid fractures via an arthroscopically assisted dorsal approach. *J Bone Joint Surg Am.* 2002;84-A(suppl 2):21–36.

442. Slade JF III, Jaskwhich D. Percutaneous fixation of scaphoid fractures. *Hand Clin.* 2001;17:553–574.

443. Slade JF, Lozano-Calderon S, Merrell G, et al. Arthroscopic-assisted percutaneous reduction and screw fixation of displaced scaphoid fractures. *J Hand Surg Eur Vol.* 2008;33:350–354.

444. Slater RR Jr, Szabo RM, Bay BK, et al. Dorsal intercarpal ligament capsulodesis for scapholunate dissociation: Biomechanical analysis in a cadaver model. *J Hand Surg Am.* 1999;24:232–239.

445. Slater RR Jr, Szabo RM. Scapholunate dissociation: Treatment with the dorsal intercarpal ligament capsulodesis. *Tech Hand Up Extrem Surg.* 1999;3:222–228.

446. Smith DK, Gilula LA, Amadio PC. Dorsal lunate tilt (DISI configuration): Sign of scaphoid fracture displacement. *Radiology.* 1990;176:497–499.

447. Smith DK. Dorsal carpal ligaments of the wrist: Normal appearance on multiplanar reconstructions of three-dimensional Fourier transform MR imaging. *AJR Am J Roentgenol.* 1993;161:119–125.

448. Smith DK. Scapholunate interosseous ligament of the wrist: MR appearances in asymptomatic volunteers and arthrographically normal wrists. *Radiology.* 1994;192:217–221.

449. Smith DK. Volar carpal ligaments of the wrist: Normal appearance on multiplanar reconstructions of three-dimensional Fourier transform MR imaging. *AJR Am J Roentgenol.* 1993;161:353–357.

450. Smith ML, Bain GI, Chabrel N, et al. Using computed tomography to assist with diagnosis of avascular necrosis complicating chronic scaphoid nonunion. *J Hand Surg Am.* 2009;34:1037–1043.

451. Smith P III, Wright TW, Wallace PF, et al. Excision of the hook of the hamate: A retrospective survey and review of the literature. *J Hand Surg Am.* 1988;13: 612–615.

452. Soejima O, Iida H, Naito M. Transscaphoid-transtriquetral perilunate fracture dislocation: Report of a case and review of the literature. *Arch Orthop Trauma Surg.* 2003;123:305–357.

453. Sokolow C, Saffar P. Anatomy and histology of the scapholunate ligament. *Hand Clin.* 2001;17:77–81.

454. Song D, Goodman S, Gilula LA, et al. Ulnocarpal translation in perilunate dislocations. *J Hand Surg Eur Vol.* 2009;34:388–390.

455. Sotereanos DG, Mitsionis GJ, Giannakopoulos PN, et al. Perilunate dislocation and fracture dislocation: A critical analysis of the volar-dorsal approach. *J Hand Surg Am.* 1997; 22:49–56.

456. Souer JS, Rutgers M, Andermahr J, et al. Perilunate fracture-dislocations of the wrist: Comparison of temporary screw versus K-wire fixation. *J Hand Surg Am.* 2007;32: 318–325.

457. Stecco C, Macchi V, Lancerotto L, et al. Comparison of transverse carpal ligament and flexor retinaculum terminology for the wrist. *J Hand Surg Am.* 2010;35:746–753.

458. Stein AH Jr. Dorsal dislocation of the lesser multangular bone. *J Bone Joint Surg Am.* 1971;53:377–379.

459. Steinmann SP, Bishop AT, Berger RA. Use of the 1,2 intercompartmental supraretinacular artery as a vascularized pedicle bone graft for difficult scaphoid nonunion. *J Hand Surg Am.* 2002;27:391–401.

460. Steinmann SP, Bishop AT. A vascularized bone graft for repair of scaphoid nonunion. *Hand Clin.* 2001;17:647–653.

461. Stevenson JD, Morley D, Srivastava S, et al. Early CT for suspected occult scaphoid fractures. *J Hand Surg Eur Vol.* 2012;37:447–451.

462. Stimson LA. *A Practical Treatise on Fractures and Dislocations.* 4th ed. New York, NY, Philadelphia, PA; Lea Brothers & Co.; 1905.

463. Strauch RJ. Scapholunate advanced collapse and scaphoid nonunion advanced collapse arthritis–update on evaluation and treatment. *J Hand Surg Am.* 2011;36:729–735.

464. Straw RG, Davis TR, Dias JJ. Scaphoid nonunion: Treatment with a pedicled vascularized bone graft based on the 1,2 intercompartmental supraretinacular branch of the radial artery. *J Hand Surg Br.* 2002;27:413.

465. Stuffmann ES, McAdams TR, Shah RP, et al. Arthroscopic repair of the scapholunate interosseous ligament. *Tech Hand Up Extrem Surg.* 2010;14:204–208.

466. Sugathan HK, Kilpatrick M, Joyce TJ, et al. A biomechanical study on variation of compressive force along the Acutrak 2 screw. *Injury.* 2012;43:205–208.

467. Suresh S. Isolated coronal split fracture of the trapezium. *Indian J Orthop.* 2012;46: 99–101.

468. Sutton PA, Clifford O, Davis TR. A new mechanism of injury for scaphoid fractures: 'Test your strength' punch-bag machines. *J Hand Surg Eur Vol.* 2010;35:419–420.

469. Swanson AB. Silicone rubber implants for the replacement of the carpal scaphoid and lunate bones. *Orthop Clin North Am.* 1970;1:299–309.

470. Symes TH, Stothard J. A systematic review of the treatment of acute fractures of the scaphoid. *J Hand Surg Eur Vol.* 2011;36:802–810.

471. Szabo RM, Manske D. Displaced fractures of the scaphoid. *Clin Orthop Relat Res.* 1988;30–38.

472. Szabo RM, Slater RR Jr, Palumbo CF, et al. Dorsal intercarpal ligament capsulodesis for chronic, static scapholunate dissociation: Clinical results. *J Hand Surg Am.* 2002;27:978–984.

473. Takami H, Takahashi S, Ando M, et al. Open reduction of chronic lunate and perilunate dislocations. *Arch Orthop Trauma Surg.* 1996;115:104–107.

474. Taleisnik J, Kelly PJ. The extraosseous and intraosseous blood supply of the scaphoid bone. *J Bone Joint Surg Am.* 1966;48:1125–1137.

475. Taleisnik J. Classification of carpal instability. *Bull Hosp Jt Dis Orthop Inst.* 1984;44: 511–531.

476. Taleisnik J. The ligaments of the wrist. *J Hand Surg Am.* 1976;1:110–118.

477. Taleisnik J. Triquetrohamate and triquetrolunate instabilities (medial carpal instability). *Ann Chir Main.* 1984;3:331–343.

478. Tambe AD, Cutler L, Murali SR, et al. In scaphoid non-union, does the source of graft affect outcome? Iliac crest versus distal end of radius bone graft. *J Hand Surg Br.* 2006;31:47–51.

479. Tambe AD, Cutler L, Stilwell J, et al. Scaphoid non-union: The role of vascularized grafting in recalcitrant non-unions of the scaphoid. *J Hand Surg Br.* 2006;31:185–190.

480. Tang JB, Ryu J, Omokawa S, et al. Wrist kinetics after scapholunate dissociation: The effect of scapholunate interosseous ligament injury and persistent scapholunate gaps. *J Orthop Res.* 2002;20:215–221.

481. Tang JB, Shi D, Gu YQ, et al. Can cast immobilization successfully treat scapholunate dissociation associated with distal radius fractures? *J Hand Surg Am.* 1996;21: 583–590.

482. Taras JS, Sweet S, Shum W, et al. Percutaneous and arthroscopic screw fixation of scaphoid fractures in the athlete. *Hand Clin.* 1999;15:467–473.

483. Tatebe M, Hirata H, Iwata Y, et al. Limited wrist arthrodesis versus radial osteotomy for advanced Kienböck's disease–for a fragmented lunate. *Hand Surg.* 2006;11:9–14.

484. Teisen H, Hjarbaek J. Classification of fresh fractures of the lunate. *J Hand Surg Br.* 1988;13:458–462.

485. Teissier J, Escare P, Asencio G, et al. Rupture of the flexor tendons of the little finger in fractures of the hook of the hamate bone. Report of two cases. *Ann Chir Main.* 1983;2:319–327.

486. Temple CL, Ross DC, Bennett JD, et al. Comparison of sagittal computed tomography and plain film radiography in a scaphoid fracture model. *J Hand Surg Am.* 2005;30:534–542.

487. Thavarajah D, Syed T, Shah Y, et al. Does scaphoid bone bruising lead to occult fracture? A prospective study of 50 patients. *Injury.* 2011;42:1303–1306.

488. Thompson NW, O'Donnell M, Thompson NS, et al. Internal fixation of an isolated fracture of the capitate using the Herbert-Whipple screw. *Injury.* 2004;35:541–542.

489. Thomsen NO. A dorsally displaced capitate neck fracture combined with a transverse shear fracture of the triquetrum. *J Hand Surg Eur Vol.* 2012;38(2):210–211.

490. Tiel-van Buul MM, Broekhuizen TH, van Beek EJ, et al. Choosing a strategy for the diagnostic management of suspected scaphoid fracture: A cost-effectiveness analysis. *J Nucl Med.* 1995;36:45–48.

491. Tiel-van Buul MM, van Beek EJ, Borm JJ, et al. The value of radiographs and bone scintigraphy in suspected scaphoid fracture. A statistical analysis. *J Hand Surg Br.* 1993; 18:403–406.

492. Tiel-van Buul MM, van Beek EJ, Broekhuizen AH, et al. Radiography and scintigraphy of suspected scaphoid fracture. A long-term study in 160 patients. *J Bone Joint Surg Br.* 1993;75:61–65.

493. Tirman RM, Weber ER, Snyder LL, et al. Midcarpal wrist arthrography for detection of tears of the scapholunate and lunotriquetral ligaments. *AJR Am J Roentgenol.* 1985;144:107–108.

494. Tohyama M, Miya S, Honda Y. Trapezium fracture associated with occult fracture of the proximal pole of the scaphoid. *Arch Orthop Trauma Surg.* 2006;126:70–72.

495. Toker S, Ozer K. Avascular necrosis of the capitate. *Orthopedics.* 2010;33:850.

496. Tomaino MM, King J, Pizillo M. Correction of lunate malalignment when bone grafting scaphoid nonunion with humpback deformity: Rationale and results of a technique revisited. *J Hand Surg Am.* 2000;25:322–329.

497. Totterman SM, Miller RJ. Scapholunate ligament: Normal MR appearance on three-dimensional gradient-recalled-echo images. *Radiology.* 1996;200:237–241.

498. Tracy CA. Transverse carpal ligament disruption associated with simultaneous fractures of the trapezium, trapezial ridge, and hook of hamate: A case report. *J Hand Surg Am.* 1999;24:152–155.

499. Trezies AJ, Davis TR, Barton NJ. Factors influencing the outcome of bone grafting surgery for scaphoid fracture non-union. *Injury.* 2000;31:605–607.

500. Trumble T, Nyland W. Scaphoid nonunions. Pitfalls and pearls. *Hand Clin.* 2001; 17:611–624.

501. Trumble T, Verheyden J. Treatment of isolated perilunate and lunate dislocations with combined dorsal and volar approach and intraosseous cerclage wire. *J Hand Surg Am.* 2004;29:412–417.

502. Trumble TE, Bour CJ, Smith RJ, et al. Kinematics of the ulnar carpus related to the volar intercalated segment instability pattern. *J Hand Surg Am.* 1990;15:384–392.

503. Trumble TE, Clarke T, Kreder HJ. Non-union of the scaphoid. Treatment with cannulated screws compared with treatment with Herbert screws. *J Bone Joint Surg Am.* 1996;78:1829–1837.

504. Ty JM, Lozano-Calderon S, Ring D. Computed tomography for triage of suspected scaphoid fractures. *Hand (N Y).* 2008;3:155–158.

505. Unay K, Gokcen B, Ozkan K, et al. Examination tests predictive of bone injury in patients with clinically suspected occult scaphoid fracture. *Injury.* 2009;40:1265–1268.

506. van der Molen AB, Groothoff JW, Visser GJ, et al. Time off work due to scaphoid fractures and other carpal injuries in The Netherlands in the period 1990 to 1993. *J Hand Surg Br.* 1999;24:193–198.

507. van Onselen EB, Karim RB, Hage JJ, et al. Prevalence and distribution of hand fractures. *J Hand Surg Br.* 2003;28:491–495.

508. Van SP, De SC. Simultaneous fracture of carpal scaphoid and trapezium. *J Hand Surg Br.* 1986;11:112–114.

509. Van Tassel DC, Owens BD, Wolf JM. Incidence estimates and demographics of scaphoid fracture in the U.S. population. *J Hand Surg Am.* 2010;35:1242–1245.

510. Vance RM, Gelberman RH, Evans EF. Scaphocapitate fractures. Patterns of dislocation, mechanisms of injury, and preliminary results of treatment. *J Bone Joint Surg Am.* 1980;62:271–276.

511. Vender MI, Watson HK, Black DM, et al. Acute scaphoid fracture with scapholunate gap. *J Hand Surg Am.* 1989;14:1004–1007.

512. Viegas SF, Patterson RM, Ward K. Extrinsic wrist ligaments in the pathomechanics of ulnar translation instability. *J Hand Surg Am.* 1995;20:312–318.

513. Viegas SF, Yamaguchi S, Boyd NL, et al. The dorsal ligaments of the wrist: Anatomy, mechanical properties, and function. *J Hand Surg Am.* 1999;24:456–468.

514. Viegas SF. The dorsal ligaments of the wrist. *Hand Clin.* 2001;17:65–75.

515. Vinnars B, Pietreanu M, Bodestedt A, et al. Nonoperative compared with operative treatment of acute scaphoid fractures. A randomized clinical trial. *J Bone Joint Surg Am.* 2008;90:1176–1185.

516. Volz RG, Lieb M, Benjamin J. Biomechanics of the wrist. *Clin Orthop Relat Res.* 1980; 112–117.

517. Waizenegger M, Barton NJ, Davis TR, et al. Clinical signs in scaphoid fractures. *J Hand Surg Br.* 1994;19:743–747.

518. Walsh JJ, Berger RA, Cooney WP. Current status of scapholunate interosseous ligament injuries. *J Am Acad Orthop Surg.* 2002;10:32–42.

519. Walsh JJ, Bishop AT. Diagnosis and management of hamate hook fractures. *Hand Clin.* 2000;16:397–403, viii.

520. Wang YC, Tseng YC, Chang HY, et al. Gender differences in carpal height ratio in a Taiwanese population. *J Hand Surg Am.* 2010;35:252–255.

521. Watanabe H, Hamada Y, Yamamoto Y. A case of old trapezoid fracture. *Arch Orthop Trauma Surg.* 1999;119:356–357.

522. Waters PM, Stewart SL. Surgical treatment of nonunion and avascular necrosis of the proximal part of the scaphoid in adolescents. *J Bone Joint Surg Am.* 2002;84-A: 915–920.

523. Watson HK, Ashmead D, Makhlouf MV. Examination of the scaphoid. *J Hand Surg Am.* 1988;13:657–660.

524. Watson HK, Ballet FL. The SLAC wrist: Scapholunate advanced collapse pattern of degenerative arthritis. *J Hand Surg Am.* 1984;9:358–365.

525. Watson HK, Belniak R, Garcia-Elias M. Treatment of scapholunate dissociation: Preferred treatment–STT fusion vs other methods. *Orthopedics.* 1991;14:365–368.

526. Watson HK, Rogers WD. Nonunion of the hook of the hamate: An argument for bone grafting the nonunion. *J Hand Surg Am.* 1989;14:486–490.

527. Watson HK, Weinzweig J, Zeppieri J. The natural progression of scaphoid instability. *Hand Clin.* 1997;13:39–49.

528. Watson HK, Weinzweig J. Physical examination of the wrist. *Hand Clin.* 1997;13: 17–34.

529. Weber ER, Chao EY. An experimental approach to the mechanism of scaphoid waist fractures. *J Hand Surg Am.* 1978;3:142–148.

530. Weber ER. Concepts governing the rotational shift of the intercalated segment of the carpus. *Orthop Clin North Am.* 1984;15:193–207.

531. Weil WM, Slade JF III, Trumble TE. Open and arthroscopic treatment of perilunate injuries. *Clin Orthop Relat Res.* 2006;445:120–132.

532. Weiss AP, Sachar K, Glowacki KA. Arthroscopic debridement alone for intercarpal ligament tears. *J Hand Surg Am.* 1997;22:344–349.

533. Weiss AP. Scapholunate ligament reconstruction using a bone-retinaculum-bone autograft. *J Hand Surg Am.* 1998;23:205–215.

534. Werner FW, Palmer AK, Fortino MD, et al. Force transmission through the distal ulna: Effect of ulnar variance, lunate fossa angulation, and radial and palmar tilt of the distal radius. *J Hand Surg Am.* 1992;17:423–428.

535. Whalen JL, Bishop AT, Linscheid RL. Nonoperative treatment of acute hamate hook fractures. *J Hand Surg Am.* 1992;17:507–511.

536. Wharton DM, Casaletto JA, Choa R, et al. Outcome following coronal fractures of the hamate. *J Hand Surg Eur Vol.* 2010;35:146–149.

537. Wheatley MJ, Finical SJ. A 32-year follow-up of lunate excision for Kienböck's disease: A case report and a review of results from excision and other treatment methods. *Ann Plast Surg.* 1996;37:322–325.

538. Whipple TL. The role of arthroscopy in the treatment of scapholunate instability. *Hand Clin.* 1995;11:37–40.

539. Whipple TL. The role of arthroscopy in the treatment of wrist injuries in the athlete. *Clin Sports Med.* 1992;11:227–238.

540. Wiesler ER, Chloros GD, Kuzma GR. Arthroscopy in the treatment of fracture of the trapezium. *Arthroscopy.* 2007;23:1248–1244.

541. Wildin CJ, Bhowal B, Dias JJ. The incidence of simultaneous fractures of the scaphoid and radial head. *J Hand Surg Br.* 2001;26:25–27.

542. Williams CS, Gelberman RH. Vascularity of the lunate. Anatomic studies and implications for the development of osteonecrosis. *Hand Clin.* 1993;9:391–398.

543. Wilton TJ. Soft-tissue interposition as a possible cause of scaphoid non-union. *J Hand Surg Br.* 1987;12:50–51.

544. Wintman BI, Gelberman RH, Katz JN. Dynamic scapholunate instability: Results of operative treatment with dorsal capsulodesis. *J Hand Surg Am.* 1995;20:971–979.

545. Witvoet J, Allieu Y. [Recent traumatic lesions of the semilunar bone]. *Rev Chir Orthop Reparatrice Appar Mot.* 1973;59(suppl 1):98–125.

546. Wolf JM, Dawson L, Mountcastle SB, et al. The incidence of scaphoid fracture in a military population. *Injury.* 2009;40:1316–1319.

547. Wolfe SW, Crisco JJ. Mechanical evaluation of the scaphoid shift test. *J Hand Surg Am.* 1994;19:762–768.

548. Wolfe SW, Gupta A, Crisco JJ III. Kinematics of the scaphoid shift test. *J Hand Surg Am.* 1997;22:801–806.

549. Wolfe SW, Neu C, Crisco JJ. In vivo scaphoid, lunate, and capitate kinematics in flexion and in extension. *J Hand Surg Am.* 2000;25:860–869.

550. Wollstein R, Wei C, Bilonick RA, et al. The radiographic measurement of ulnar translation. *J Hand Surg Eur Vol.* 2009;34:384–387.

551. Wong K, von Schroeder HP. Delays and poor management of scaphoid fractures: Factors contributing to nonunion. *J Hand Surg Am.* 2011;36:1471–1474.

552. Wong TC, Ip FK. Minimally invasive management of trans-scaphoid perilunate fracture-dislocations. *Hand Surg.* 2008;13:159–165.

553. Wright TW, Dobyns JH, Linscheid RL, et al. Carpal instability non-dissociative. *J Hand Surg Br.* 1994;19:763–773.

554. Wyrick JD, Youse BD, Kiefhaber TR. Scapholunate ligament repair and capsulodesis for the treatment of static scapholunate dissociation. *J Hand Surg Br.* 1998;23:776–780.

555. Yamaguchi H, Takahara M. Transradial styloid, transtriquetral perilunate dislocation of the carpus with an associated fracture of the ulnar border of the distal radius. *J Orthop Trauma.* 1994;8:434–436.

556. Yamazaki H, Kato H, Nakatsuchi Y, et al. Closed rupture of the flexor tendons of the little finger secondary to non-union of fractures of the hook of the hamate. *J Hand Surg Br.* 2006;31:337–341.

557. Yanni D, Lieppins P, Laurence M. Fractures of the carpal scaphoid. A critical study of the standard splint. *J Bone Joint Surg Br.* 1991;73:600–602.

558. Yardley MH. Upper limb fractures: Contrasting patterns in Transkei and England. *Injury.* 1984;15:322–323.

559. Yin ZG, Zhang JB, Kan SL, et al. Diagnosing suspected scaphoid fractures: A systematic review and meta-analysis. *Clin Orthop Relat Res.* 2010;468:723–734.

560. Yip HS, Wu WC, Chang RY, et al. Percutaneous cannulated screw fixation of acute scaphoid waist fracture. *J Hand Surg Br.* 2002;27:42–46.

561. Yoshihara M, Sakai A, Toba N, et al. Nonunion of the isolated capitate waist fracture. *J Orthop Sci.* 2002;7:578–580.

562. You JS, Chung SP, Chung HS, et al. The usefulness of CT for patients with carpal bone fractures in the emergency department. *Emerg Med J.* 2007;24:248–250.

563. Youm Y, McMurthy RY, Flatt AE, et al. Kinematics of the wrist. I. An experimental study of radial-ulnar deviation and flexion-extension. *J Bone Joint Surg Am.* 1978;60:423–431.

564. Zaidemberg C, Siebert JW, Angrigiani C. A new vascularized bone graft for scaphoid nonunion. *J Hand Surg Am.* 1991;16:474–478.

565. Zdravkovic V, Sennwald GR, Fischer M, et al. The palmar wrist ligaments revisited, clinical relevance. *Ann Chir Main Memb Super.* 1994;13:378–382.

566. Ziter FM. A modified view of the carpal navicular. *Radiology.* 1973;108:706–707.

567. Zoltie N. Fractures of the body of the hamate. *Injury.* 1991;22:459–462.

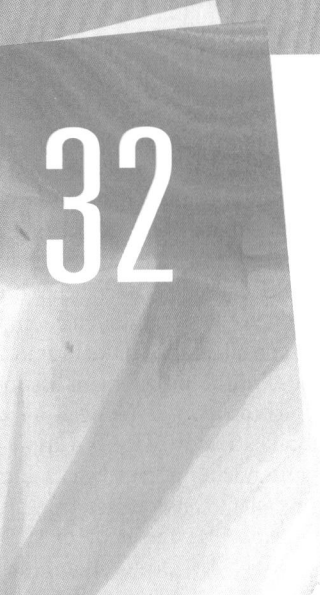

32

FRACTURES OF THE DISTAL RADIUS AND ULNA

Margaret M. McQueen

INTRODUCTION TO FRACTURES OF THE DISTAL RADIUS AND ULNA

Fracture of the distal radius and ulna is the most common fracture encountered by orthopedic trauma surgeons with around 120,000 fractures per year in the United Kingdom and 607,000 annually in the United States.[60,73]

The history of fractures of the distal radius reflects the evolution of the understanding of many conditions in orthopedic trauma. The credit for recognition of the true nature of the injury is shared between Petit, Pouteau, and Colles, prior to whose writings it was believed that the injury was a carpal or distal radioulnar joint dislocation. Petit first suggested in the early 18th century that these injuries might be fractures rather than dislocations but it was Pouteau[291] who first recognized that injuries to the wrist from a fall on to the outstretched hand were usually fractures of the distal radius with "outward" or dorsal displacement. He recognized "inward" or volar displacement but attributed it to ulnar fracture. His meticulous observations demonstrate the knowledge that can be accrued from clinical examination. Pouteau could not defend his opinion from the scepticism of his colleagues as this article was published post-

humously. Added to this little attention was paid to his views outside France.

Fractures of the distal radius were brought to the attention of the English speaking literature in 1814 when Abraham Colles published his views "On the fracture of the carpal extremity of the radius" in 1814. Colles was the Professor of surgery at the Royal College of Surgeons in Ireland from 1804 to 1836. He was renowned for his truthfulness and honesty having on one occasion informed his students: "Gentleman, it is no use mincing the matter; I caused the patient's death." Colles wrote: "This fracture takes place about an inch and a half above the carpal extremity of the radius ..... the posterior surface of the limb presents a considerable deformity; for a depression is seen in the forearm, about an inch and a half above the end of this bone, while a considerable swelling occupies the wrist and metacarpus. Indeed, the carpus and base of metacarpus appear to be thrown backward so much as on first view to excite a suspicion that the carpus has been dislocated forward. On viewing the anterior surface of the limb we observe a considerable fullness, as if caused by the flexor tendons being thrown forwards....On the posterior surface (the surgeon) will discover, by the touch, that the swelling on the wrist and metacarpus is not caused entirely by an effusion among the softer parts; he will perceive that the ends of the metacarpal and second row of the carpal bones form no small part of it......If the surgeon lock his hand in that of the patient and makes extension...he restores the limb to its natural form, but the distortion of the limb instantly returns on the extension being removed....Or, should he mistake the case for a dislocation of the wrist and attempt to retain the parts in situ by tight bandages and splints, the pain caused by the pressure on the back of the wrist will force him to unbind them in a few hours; and if they be applied more loosely, he will find, at the expiration of a few weeks, that the deformity still exists in its fullest extent. ...By such mistakes the patient is doomed to endure for many months considerable lameness and stiffness of the limb, accompanied by severe pains on attempting to bend the hand and fingers....The hard swelling which appears on the back of the hand is caused by the carpal surface of the radius being directed slightly backwards instead of looking directly downwards. The carpus and metacarpus, retaining their connections with this bone, must follow it in its derangement, and cause the convexity above alluded to. The broken extremity of the radius being thus drawn backwards causes the ulna to appear prominent toward the palmar surface......"[66] These observations were made more extraordinary by the fact that they were made without the benefit of anatomical dissection or x-rays.

With the publication of his "Leçons Orales," in 1841, Guillaume Dupuytren, the chief surgeon of L'Hôtel Dieu in Paris, brought the subject to the attention of a wider audience. Dupuytren was renowned not only for being an absolute perfectionist combined with intelligence, drive, and boundless energy but also for a complete disregard for the sensibilities of his colleagues about whom he is quoted as saying "nothing should be feared as much for a man as mediocrity." Most of his vast knowledge was imparted by lectures attended by hundreds from near and far and eventually published by his students as Leçons Orales de Clinique Chirurgicale. On fracture of the distal radius he acknowledged Petit and Pouteau's contributions and went on to state "one would have thought...that the observations of these writers would have raised some doubts in the minds of modern surgeons on this obscure point of doctrine: but not so;.........I have for a long time publicly taught that fractures of the carpal end of the radius are extremely common; that I had always found that these supposed dislocations turn out to be fractures; and that, in spite of all which has been said on the subject, I have never met with or heard of one single well authenticated and convincing case of the dislocation in question."[86]

In 1847 Malgaigne[237] defined the injury further and stated that most fractures of the distal radius were caused by a fall on the palm of the hand and fewer by a fall on the back of the hand. He identified extra- and intra-articular fractures, including undisplaced fractures. He recognized the sequelae of untreated fracture: deformity, reduction of pronation, supination and flexion, weakness of the hand, long-term swelling and pain, and permanent finger stiffness. He recorded that the prognosis is favorable if there is only dorsal displacement and the fracture is recognized early but with radial shortening and radial deviation it is "almost impossible to overcome it entirely." He also recognized the poorer prognosis for articular fractures.

The concept of a variety of types of distal radius fractures was developed by John Rhea Barton[24] from Philadelphia, who in 1838 described "a subluxation of the wrist consequent to a fracture through the articular surface of the carpal extremity of the radius." He described dorsal displacement of the wrist and the partial articular fracture. He also recognized the morbidity of distal radius fracture: "I do not know any subject on which I have been more frequently consulted than on deformities, rigid joints, inflexible fingers, loss of the pronating and supinating motions and on neuralgic complaints resulting from injuries of the wrist and of the carpal extremity of the forearm—one or more of these evils having been left, not merely as a temporary inconvenience but as a permanent consequence."

Robert William Smith, who was Professor of surgery in Dublin (and also performed Colles' postmortem) described "fracture of the lower extremity of the radius with displacement of the lower fragment forward" and stated that it was generally the result of a fall on the back of the hand.[337] This was the first description of volar displacement of distal radius fractures.

The next major step forward was the discovery of x-rays in 1895. Carl Beck,[26] a surgeon from New York City, concluded in 1901 that "in no fracture type were the Röntgen rays more urgently needed to realize how often we have erred in its true recognition" and he described eight different types of distal radius fracture.

Frederick Cotton[70,71] from Boston described his findings in distal radius fractures using a combination of postmortems and x-rays. He described comminution of the metaphysis, which he considered frequent and most common on the dorsum, and in two articles gives a clear and comprehensive review of the knowledge of the time.

During this time the main debate about treatment centered around the mechanics of reduction, the position of immobilization, and the types of splint used. Poor results and amputation were recorded because of tight bandages and splints. Lucas-Champonnière[227] described his new ideas in the management of fractures using massage and early mobilization, which were revolutionary in their time. He considered that distal radius fracture was best suited to this form of treatment.

Further contributions to the management of distal radius fractures were in the realms of fixation of the distal radius with the development of methods of stabilization, although the biggest influence was the advent of anesthesia and asepsis. External fixation of the distal radius was first reported by Ombredanne,[270] a Parisian surgeon in 1929. It is of interest that this was a nonbridging external fixator and was used in pediatric cases. Ombredanne concluded that "temporary osteosynthesis with external connections permits a mathematical adjustment of the surgical correction ..... and guarantees further retention with ample and sufficient precision."

Bridging external fixation was introduced by Roger Anderson and Gordon O'Neill from Seattle in 1944 because of the poor results of nonoperative management. They recognized the difficulty of maintaining a reduction particularly of radial length and attributed this to "crushing of the cancellous bone." The authors named the technique "castless fixation."[13] Meanwhile Raoul Hoffman of Geneva was designing his external fixator, which had universal clamps allowing reduction of the fracture by closed manipulation while the fixator was in place. Jacques Vidal et al.[380] introduced the concept of ligamentotaxis: "the device is placed beyond the involved joint in the unaffected bone, tension is applied and by means of distraction forces working through capsuloligamentous structures, reduction is obtained." The Hoffmann fixator, although modified, remains in use today.

Internal fixation of distal radius fractures has long been dominated by percutaneous pinning, which was first suggested for distal radius fracture treatment by Lambotte in 1907 with the use of one radial styloid pin.[295] This was followed by reports of many other techniques of multiple pinning in the middle to late 20th century.[295] Plating was first popularized by Ellis[93] in 1965. Since then, the development of initially dorsal plating and then volar locked plating has extended its indications.

EPIDEMIOLOGY OF FRACTURES OF THE DISTAL RADIUS AND ULNA

Fractures of the distal radius are the most frequent fractures encountered by orthopedic trauma surgeons accounting for 17.5% of all adult fractures.[73] A variety of incidences are reported (Table 32-1), but these are difficult to interpret because of varying ages of the populations and methods of recording the information. The most recent information comes from Edinburgh in 2010 to 2011(unpublished data) and Finland in 2008[105] with similar incidences being reported from each country (23.6 and 25.8 per 10,000 per year respectively) for adult distal radius fractures. In all studies the incidences in females are higher than males by a factor of two to three.

Men who sustain distal radius fractures are significantly younger than women. The average age of all distal radius fractures in adults has been reported to be between 57 and 66 years with females being on average in their 60s and men in their 40s. This is reflected in the age- and gender-specific distribution curves, which are type A (see Chapter 3). Low-energy injury is the cause of the majority of distal radius fractures with 66% to 77% of fractures being related to a fall from standing height[41,105,304,332] and increased numbers in winter conditions.[105] The Edinburgh data show that high-energy injury accounts for around 10% of all wrist fractures.

The majority (57% to 66%) of fractures are extra-articular (AO type A). Of the remainder between 9% and 16% are reported as partial articular (AO type B) and 25% to 35% as complete articular fractures (type C). From the Edinburgh data there were 51 type C3 or complex articular fractures (4.5%), whereas there were 543 fractures (48.3%) with metaphyseal comminution but without severe articular involvement. Thus a potentially unstable metaphyseal fracture is 10 times more common than a severe articular fracture. Using the Mackenney formula[234] the median risk of instability is 39.4%.

TABLE 32-1	**The Reported Incidences of Fracture of the Distal Radius**				
Area	Date	Incidence/ 10⁵/yr	Male Incidence/ 10⁵/yr	Female Incidence/ 10⁵/yr	Age Groups (yrs)
UK					
Dundee/Oxford[43]	1954–1958	20	7.2	29.9	≥15
Edinburgh[72]	1991–1993	17.2	7.7	25.7	
(see text and Chapter 3)	2000	19.3	11.7	26	
	2007–2008	20.6	12.9	27.8	
	2010–2011	23.6	13.9	32.2	
Dorset[368]	1996–1997	26.1	11.4	35.9	>25
Scotland/England[271]	1997–1998	23.6	9	36.8	>35
Denmark					
Frederiksborg[342]	1981	21.9	8.9	34.6	>20
Hvidovre[212]	1976–1984	19.7	N/A	39.7	≥20
Sweden					
Stockholm[324]	1981–1982	36.5	13.4	54.6	>15
Uppsala[238]	1989–1990	29	14.3	43.2	>15
Malmo[28]	1953–1957	17.6	9.6	24.8	≥10
	1980–1981	42.2	19.6	62.4	
	1991–1992	31.3	16.5	44.4	
SE Sweden[41]	2001	26	12	39	>18
Iceland[304,332]	1985	26	14	34	>15
	2004	27	17	37	
Finland					
Oulu[105]	2008	25.8	14.7	36.3	≥16
USA					
Rochester, MN[278]	1945–1974	17.6	7.8	25.7	≥50
All emergency rooms[272]	2001–2007	26.5	8.8	40.9	≥35

There is some evidence emerging from Scandinavia and the United Kingdom that the epidemiology of distal radius fractures is changing. In Iceland, between 1985 and 2004, the overall incidence of distal radius fractures did not change significantly, but there were changes within the age- and gender-specific incidences.[332] The incidence reduced in women aged 50 to 70 years over this time period, which the author speculated was because of the increased use of hormone replacement therapy (HRT). In men there was a trend showing an increase in incidence, which the author suggested was related to the increase in longevity of men whose mean age at fracture had risen by 8 years to 50 years over the 19-year period.

In contrast, data from Edinburgh shows an increase in the incidence of distal radius fractures over a 17-year period (Table 32-1), mainly attributable to an increase in incidence in both younger and older men (Fig. 32-1). In women there was a reduction in incidence in the 45- to 59-year-old age group, but an increase in the incidence in women over 75 years of age. It is of interest however that the percentage of patients who were independent for the activities of daily living increased significantly over the period confirming that although getting older, individuals were also getting fitter. In the fragility fractures there was an increase in extra-articular and partial articular fractures and a corresponding decrease in complete articular fractures. In the whole group there was no difference detected in the radiographic severity of the fractures. However, when fragility fractures (defined as those in patients aged 50 years or more) are examined, there are significant increases in the likelihood of metaphyseal instability in the extra-articular and complete articular fractures.

It would seem therefore that fractures of the distal radius are increasing in men and older women but remain most common in older women. Reducing numbers have been observed in middle-aged women, which may be the effect of successful programs to detect and treat osteoporosis. The Edinburgh data confirms that patients are becoming more independent for their activities of daily living but the fractures in the older age group are becoming more severe. If the population projections are accurate for westernized countries and the proportion of the elderly continues to rise, there will be an increasing burden on orthopedic trauma services for the treatment of more unstable distal radius fractures in older but more active patients. This increases the urgency of coming to a consensus on the recommended method of treatment for those fractures.

Risk Factors for Distal Radius Fractures

There are a number of methods of predicting the risk of an osteoporotic fracture and many published risk fractures. These are dealt with in more detail in Chapter 3. There are, however, some studies that consider the risk factors specific to distal radius fractures.

Reported lifetime risks of distal radius fractures from the age of 50 onward range from 12% to 52.7% for women and 2.4% to 6.2% for men (Table 32-2). These may be real differences in risk from country to country although it may be that the difficulties in fracture ascertainment account for some of the differences.

As is the case with all osteoporotic fractures, distal radius fractures occur because of a combination of a fall and low bone mineral density (BMD). Not surprisingly, low BMD is an important predictor of future fracture risk,[186,216,265,267] but there is also evidence that increasing falls, especially with aging, are a significant risk factor.[265,267] Some authors have found that the risk of distal radius fracture increases with a higher level

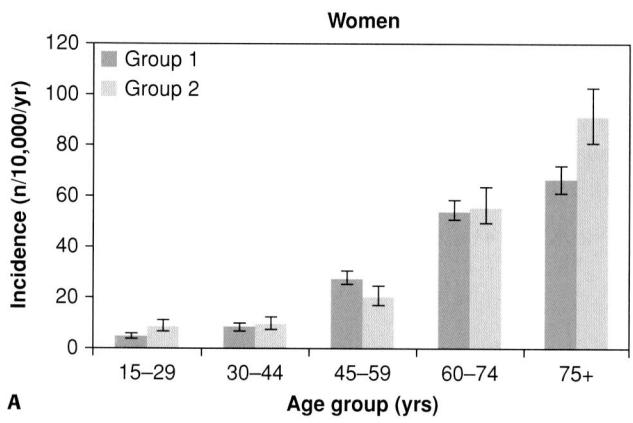

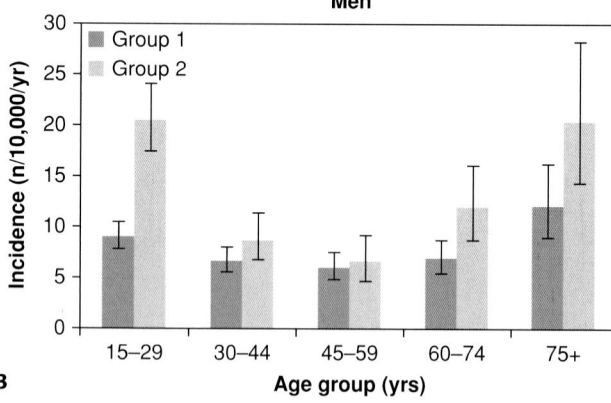

FIGURE 32-1 **A, B:** The incidence of distal radius fractures in men and women with 95% confidence intervals. Group 1 data were collected from 1991 to 1993 inclusive and group 2 data were collected in the year from 2007 to 2008. The increases in both younger and older men largely account for the overall increase in incidence of distal radius fractures.

TABLE 32-2	The Estimated Percentage Lifetime Risk of Sustaining a Distal Radius Fracture over the Age of 50 Years for Men and Women		
	Females	Males	Dates
Norway[7]	32.7	6.2	1994–2004
Sweden[181]	20.8	4.6	1987–1993
UK[376]	16.6	2.9	1988–1998
USA[74]	15	2.4	1979–1981
Tasmania[67]	12	5	1997–1999
S Korea[283]	21.7	4.9	2005–2008
Denmark[212]	18	N/A	1976–1984

of activity[127,168,333] implying that individuals who sustain distal radius fractures are in the fitter cohort of older people.

ASSESSMENT OF FRACTURES OF THE DISTAL RADIUS AND ULNA

Injury Mechanisms for Distal Radius and Ulna Fractures

The common injury mechanism that results in a fracture of the distal radius is a fall on to the outstretched hand from standing height, although a small proportion of patients will experience high-energy injury. Palvanen et al.[281] demonstrated that the typical osteoporotic upper extremity fractures in older adults have specific injury mechanisms with individuals with distal radius fractures significantly more frequently breaking their fall with an outstretched hand compared to those sustaining proximal humerus or elbow fractures. This suggests that patients with distal radius fractures have better preserved reflexes and are generally fitter than those with proximal humerus fractures.

The different characteristics of fractures of the distal radius are generally agreed to be influenced by the position of the hand at the time of impact, the type of surface with which it makes contact, and the velocity of the force. Added to this the quality and strength of the bone of the distal radius will influence the severity of the fracture.

Most attention has been focused on the position of the hand at the time of impact. In the late 19th century Lilienfeldt[220] used cadaver arms to show that both the position of the hand and the angle at which the forearm strikes the ground determine the type of fracture. Fracture of the distal radius resulted if the angle was between 60 and 90 degrees with a radial styloid fracture resulting from a hand in ulnar deviation and an ulnar styloid fracture from radial deviation. Lilienfeldt also reproduced a volar displaced fracture with the hand in flexion. Frykman[114] refined these experiments and concluded that clinical types of distal radius fractures occurred, provided dorsiflexion of the wrist was between 40 and 90 degrees. If less, a proximal forearm fracture resulted and if more, a carpal bone fracture. More force was required to produce a fracture with increasing dorsiflexion. He produced volar fractures when the hand was loaded in volar flexion. Frykman also noted that more force was required to fracture a male compared to a female specimen.

Fernandez and Jupiter[97] divided distal radius fractures into five types depending on the mechanism of the injury and this forms the basis for the Fernandez classification (see below). They believe that bending fractures occur because at impact the proximal carpal row transmits the force to the dorsal aspect of the radius and the volar cortex fails because of tensile stresses. As the radius bends dorsally, the dorsal cortex compresses producing dorsal comminution and a metaphyseal defect especially in an osteopenic patient. If the forearm is supinated and the elbow is extended, the force is applied with the wrist in flexion and the displacement is reversed producing compression of the volar lip and an extra-articular volar displaced bending fracture.

Partial articular or shearing fractures of the volar lip of the distal radius probably occur in the same way as extra-articular volar displaced fractures in younger patients. In these cases the compression of the volar lip results in an articular fracture with volar subluxation of the carpus. The fracture line is often vertical and usually unstable.

The severity of distal radius fractures is related to the quality of the bone. Clayton et al.[64] examined 37 distal radius fractures and showed that there was a linear correlation between dual energy x-ray absorptiometry T scores and early instability and malunion. Patients with osteoporosis had a 43% probability of having a metaphyseal unstable distal radius fracture and a 66% probability of malunion compared with patients with normal T-scores who had a 28% probability of instability and a 48% probability of malunion. Xie and Barenholdt[396] used multilayer peripheral quantitative CT scans and showed that cross-sectional volumetric density and geometric properties of cortical bone may be essential in determining the severity of a distal radius fracture.

Injures Associated with Distal Radius and Ulna Fractures

The main injuries associated with distal radius fractures are those to the interosseous ligaments of the carpus and to the triangular fibrocartilage complex (TFCC). Chondral lesions have also been reported in 32% of patients. Their significance is unknown although it has been suggested that they may be precursors of degenerative change.[222]

Interosseous Ligament Injury

Interosseous ligament injury associated with fractures of the distal radius is predominantly scapholunate and lunatotriquetral injury. The severity of these injuries has been graded arthroscopically by Geissler from grade 1 to grade 4. Grade 1 injuries are the least severe with attenuation or hemorrhage, grades 2 and 3 are increasing incongruity of the ligament, and grade 4 is gross instability with sufficient disruption to allow passage of an arthroscope from radiocarpal to midcarpal joints.

Scapholunate injury has been reported to occur in between 4.7% and 46% of distal radius fractures,[121,222,298,330,365] but it is difficult to estimate the true figure as most studies report highly selected series of young patients with predominantly intra-articular fractures which have been treated arthroscopically. The figure of 4.7% is derived from the least selective series of distal radius fractures and is likely to be closest to the true figure.[365] Lunatotriquetral injury is less common with prevalences between 12% and 34% being reported.[121,222,298,330]

The diagnosis of ligament injury can be made from static radiographs of the distal radius in the more severe cases (see Chapter 31). However, the diagnosis can be difficult when associated with a distal radius fracture. Arthroscopy is probably the best method but is expensive and may subject the patient to an unnecessary procedure. This can be minimized by the carpal stretch test when traction is applied to the wrist to emphasize disruption of Gilula's lines. This test has been reported to have a sensitivity of 78% and a specificity of 72% in cases with distal radius fracture. The authors concluded that it is a useful screening test to rule out the more severe grade 3 and 4 tears.[209] An increased risk of interosseous ligament injury has been demonstrated where there is more than 2 mm of positive ulnar variance and in intra-articular fractures.[109]

The significance of interosseous ligament tears to the outcome of distal radius fractures is unclear. It has been suggested that undetected lesions are a cause of ongoing pain, but in a series of 51 patients with displaced distal radius fractures reviewed at 11 to 27 months after injury there were no differences in patient-reported outcome measures (PROMs) between the grade 3 and 4 ligament injuries and those with grade 0 to 2 ligament injuries. There was increased pain in the more severe injuries but only when the Watson shift test was performed and not at rest or with use of the hand.[109] However, Tang et al.[365] reported worse function in 20 patients with radiographically obvious scapholunate instability compared to cases with normal carpal alignment.

Triangular Fibrocartilage Complex (TFCC) Injury

TFCC injury is commoner than interosseous ligament injury being reported in 39% to 82% of cases.[121,222,298,330] The majority are peripheral avulsions and may be associated with ulnar styloid fractures, the presence of which increases the risk of a TFCC tear by a factor of 5.1.[222] The natural history of these lesions remains unclear but in a long-term review at 13 to 15 years after injury there were no differences in any outcome measure including the Disabilities of Arm, Shoulder and Hand (DASH) score between patients with and without complete TFCC tears or between those with or without detectable laxity at the distal radioulnar joint (DRUJ) barring a reduction of grip strength to 83% in the patients with laxity.[260] It is debatable if this is clinically significant. Surgery to repair TFCC tears has good reported results although similar to nonoperatively managed patients with average grip strength of 78% and a DASH score of 13 at 2 years after surgery.[315] The indications for surgical treatment of these injuries have not yet been clearly defined.

Signs and Symptoms of Fractures of the Distal Radius and Ulna

Eliciting the symptoms of a fracture of the distal radius is usually straightforward with a history of a fall on to the outstretched hand or occasionally a higher-energy injury. Pain and swelling around the wrist are invariable features and where there is displacement the patient may also complain of a visible deformity. Specific questioning should include any paresthesia or numbness in the fingers to exclude any median or ulnar nerve injury. Evidence of pain elsewhere in the limb should be sought to diagnose an ipsilateral injury.

On examination swelling is usually evident around the wrist. In cases with displacement, the deformity can be seen. The classical dinner fork or silver fork deformity is caused by dorsal displacement of the carpus secondary to dorsal angulation of the distal radius (Fig. 32-2). The reverse deformity is seen in volar displaced fractures. The hand may be radially deviated and if there is shortening of the radius the ulna will be prominent. The skin should be inspected to rule out any open wounds, which most commonly occur on the ulnar side.

Palpation will elicit tenderness at the area of the fracture and is more useful in raising clinical suspicion where there is no obvious deformity. A thorough neurologic examination of

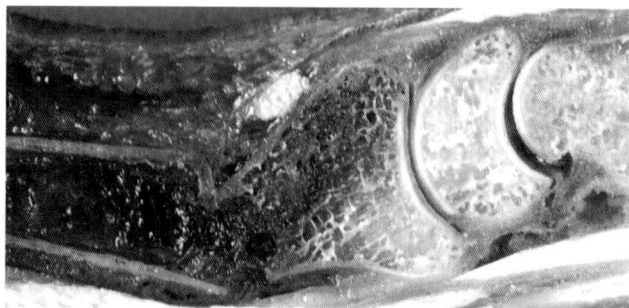

FIGURE 32-2 A sagittal section of a distal radius fracture. There is dorsal angulation with comminution of the metaphysis producing the classic dinner fork deformity which is caused by the malalignment of the carpus.

the hand should be performed as acute carpal tunnel syndrome (CTS) may require prompt treatment. It is also important to remember that distal radius fractures may be complicated by acute compartment syndrome and the symptoms and signs of this condition should also be sought (see Chapter 29).

Imaging and Other Diagnostic Studies for Fractures of the Distal Radius and Ulna

The standard series of posteroanterior (PA), lateral, and oblique x-ray views is useful to visualize a suspected fracture of the distal radius. Additional views may be obtained as needed to assess for displacement or additional injuries.

A number of radiologic measurements quantifying the orientation of the distal radius are in common use and it is important to understand these to reduce interobserver error. Significant discrepancy regarding intra- and interobserver reliability has been demonstrated in the measurement of standard radiographic criteria. For extra-articular fractures the mean standard deviation between surgeons was 3.2 degrees for radial angle, 3.6 degrees for conventional lateral palmar tilt, and 2.1 degrees for 15 degrees of lateral palmar tilt.[175]

Dorsal/palmar tilt: On a true lateral view a line is drawn connecting the most distal points of the volar and dorsal lips of the radius. The dorsal or palmar tilt is the angle created with a line drawn along the longitudinal axis of the radius (Fig. 32-3A).

Radial length: This is measured on the PA radiograph. It is the distance in millimeters between a line drawn perpendicular to the long axis of the radius and tangential to the most distal point of the ulnar head and a line drawn perpendicular to the long axis of the radius and at the level of the tip of the radial styloid (Fig. 32-3B).

Ulnar variance: This is a measure of radial shortening and should not be confused with the measurement of radial length. Ulnar variance is the vertical distance between a line parallel to the medial corner of the articular surface of the radius and a line parallel to the most distal point of the articular surface of the ulnar head, both of which are perpendicular to the long axis of the radius (Fig. 32-3B).

Radial inclination: On the PA view the radius inclines toward the ulna. This is measured by the angle between a line drawn from the tip of the radial styloid to the medial corner of the

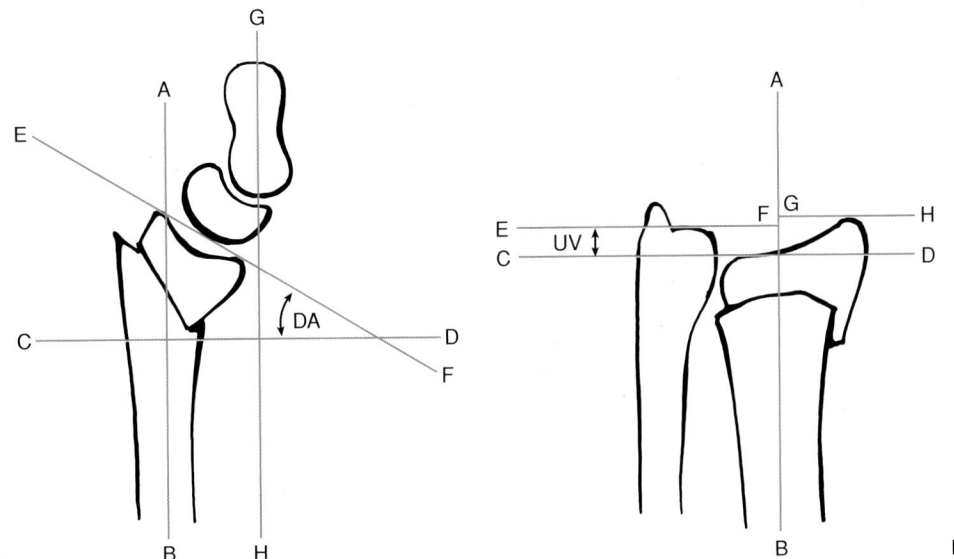

FIGURE 32-3 A: The dorsal angle *(DA)* is measured by finding the angle between a line (CD) perpendicular to the long axis of the radius (AB) and a line joining the dorsal and volar extremities of the radiocarpal joint (EF). Carpal alignment is assessed by the point of intersection of the line parallel to the long axis of the radius (AB) and a line parallel to the long axis of the capitate (GH). If these intersect outwith the carpus or do not intersect as in this illustration, then the carpus is malaligned. **B:** Ulnar variance *(UV)* is the distance between two lines perpendicular to the long axis of the radius (AB). The first is tangential to the ulnar corner of the radius (CD) and the second tangential to the ulnar head (EF). Radial length is the distance between line EF and a line tangential to the radial styloid (GH). (From Court-Brown C, McQueen M, Tornetta P. *Orthopaedic Surgery Essentials: Trauma.* Philadelphia, PA: Lippincott Williams & Wilkins; 2006, with permission.)

articular surface of the radius and a line drawn perpendicular to the long axis of the radius.

Carpal malalignment: There are two types of carpal malalignment associated with fracture of the distal radius. The commonest is malalignment which compensates for the tilt of the distal radius and is extrinsic to the carpus. On a lateral view one line is drawn along the long axis of the capitate and one down the long axis of the radius. If the carpus is aligned the lines will intersect within the carpus. If not they will intersect outwith the carpus (Fig. 32-3A). Carpal malalignment can also be caused by associated carpal ligament disruption. The radiologic diagnosis of this condition is detailed in Chapter 31.

Teardrop angle and anteroposterior (AP) distance: More recently, attention has been drawn to examination of the teardrop angle and AP distance, as measured on a lateral radiograph.[254] The teardrop of the distal radius articular surface refers to the U-shaped outline of the volar rim of the lunate facet. The teardrop angle refers to the angle between the central axis of the teardrop and the central axis of the radial shaft. Depression of the teardrop angle to less than 45 degrees indicates displacement of the lunate facet (Fig. 32-4). A depressed teardrop angle may be the only evidence that reduction is incomplete and articular incongruity remains. The AP distance is also a measure of articular incongruity and is defined by the distance between the apices of the dorsal and volar rims of the lunate facet. The normal AP distance averages 19 mm on a true lateral view,[254] but is probably best assessed by comparison with the contralateral normal wrist.

Specific features should be assessed on each view of the distal radius as follows.

PA View

For extra-articular fractures assess the following:

- Radial length/ulnar variance
- Extent of metaphyseal comminution
- Ulnar styloid fracture location (tip/waist/base)

In addition, for intra-articular fractures assess the following:

- Presence and orientation of articular fractures
- Depression of the lunate facet
- Gap between scaphoid and lunate facet
- Central impaction fragments
- Carpal bone assessment—Gilula's carpal arc 1 or evidence of a scaphoid fracture

Lateral View. For extra-articular fractures assess the following:

- Dorsal/palmar tilt
- Extent of metaphyseal comminution
- Carpal alignment
- Displacement of the volar cortex
- Position of the DRUJ

For intra-articular fractures assess the following:

- Depression of the palmar lunate facet
- Depression of the central fragment

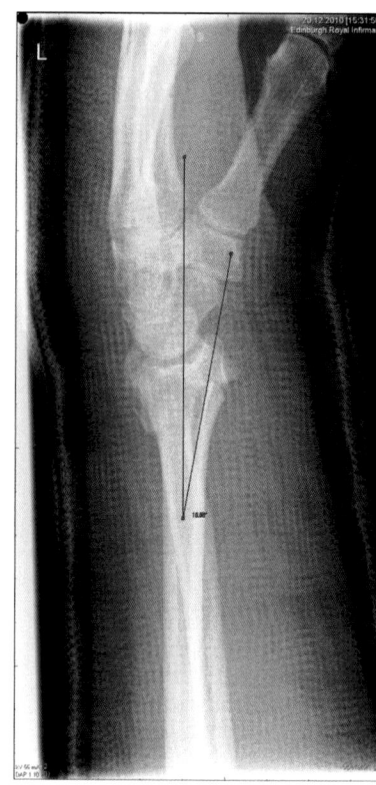

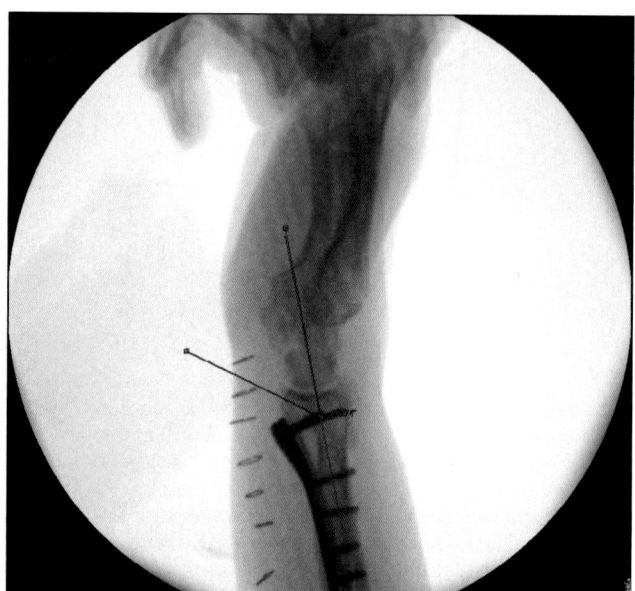

FIGURE 32-4 A: A lateral view of a displaced intra-articular distal radius fracture showing a depressed teardrop angle of just over 10 degrees. **B:** The fracture has been reduced and the teardrop angle is restored to just under 54 degrees.

- Gap between palmar and dorsal fragments
- Scapholunate angle for possible associated carpal injury
- Teardrop angle
- AP distance

Measurement of dorsal and volar tilt should be made on a true lateral view of the distal radius when the ulna is completely superimposed on the radius. Pronation of the forearm reduces the apparent volar tilt and supination increases it although it does not affect the measurement of radiolunate or carpal alignment.[46] Johnson and Szabo[175] found that a 5-degree rotational change produces a 1.6-degree change in palmar tilt on the conventional lateral view and a 1-degree change on the 15-degree lateral view.

Oblique Views. The pronated oblique view demonstrates the radial side of the distal radius and is particularly useful for assessing radial comminution, a split or depression of the radial styloid, and for confirming the position of screws on the radial side of the distal radius (Fig. 32-5A).[335]

The supinated oblique view demonstrates the ulnar side of the distal radius and is useful for assessing depression of the dorsal lunate facet and the position of ulnar-sided screws (Fig. 32-5B).

Tilted Lateral View. This is a lateral view taken with a pad under the hand to incline the radius 22 degrees toward the beam.[229] It provides a tangential view of the lunate facet and allows more accurate measurement of lunate facet depression and possible screw penetration into the radiocarpal joint (Fig. 32-5C, D).

Traction Views (AP and Lateral). These views are taken with manual traction or finger traps applied after reduction and under anesthetic. They are most useful in articular fractures and

allow the surgeon to plan whether closed techniques will be sufficient for treatment or whether open reduction will be necessary. A traction view also helps to identify fracture fragments that may be obscured by the displacement of the fracture and emphasizes any disruption of Gilula's arc in the proximal carpal row in associated interosseous ligament injury.

Contralateral Wrist (AP and Lateral). These x-rays may be indicated prior to surgery to assess the patient's normal ulnar variance, scapholunate angle, and AP distance, all of which vary between patients.

Computerized Tomography

Computerized tomography (CT) scanning is used to improve the visualization and accuracy of measurement of articular fractures in the distal radius. Clinical data suggest that CT demonstrates intra-articular fracture lines and measures intra-articular displacement more accurately than plain radiographs,[176] and in particular demonstrates the presence and displacement of sigmoid notch fractures more accurately than plain radiographs. In one study comparing plain radiographs to CT, the authors found that in 20 consecutive fractures plain x-rays documented sigmoid notch involvement in only 35% of the fractures compared with 65% found on CT.[312] A more recent study found that in 95 articular fractures there was 77% involvement of the sigmoid notch, 71% involvement of the dorsoulnar segment, 57% of the dorsoradial segment, and only 13% involvement of the volar ulnar segment.[364]

Three-dimensional CT scans are now commonly used in assessing intra-articular fractures of the distal radius. Their use has been shown to improve intraobserver but not interobserver

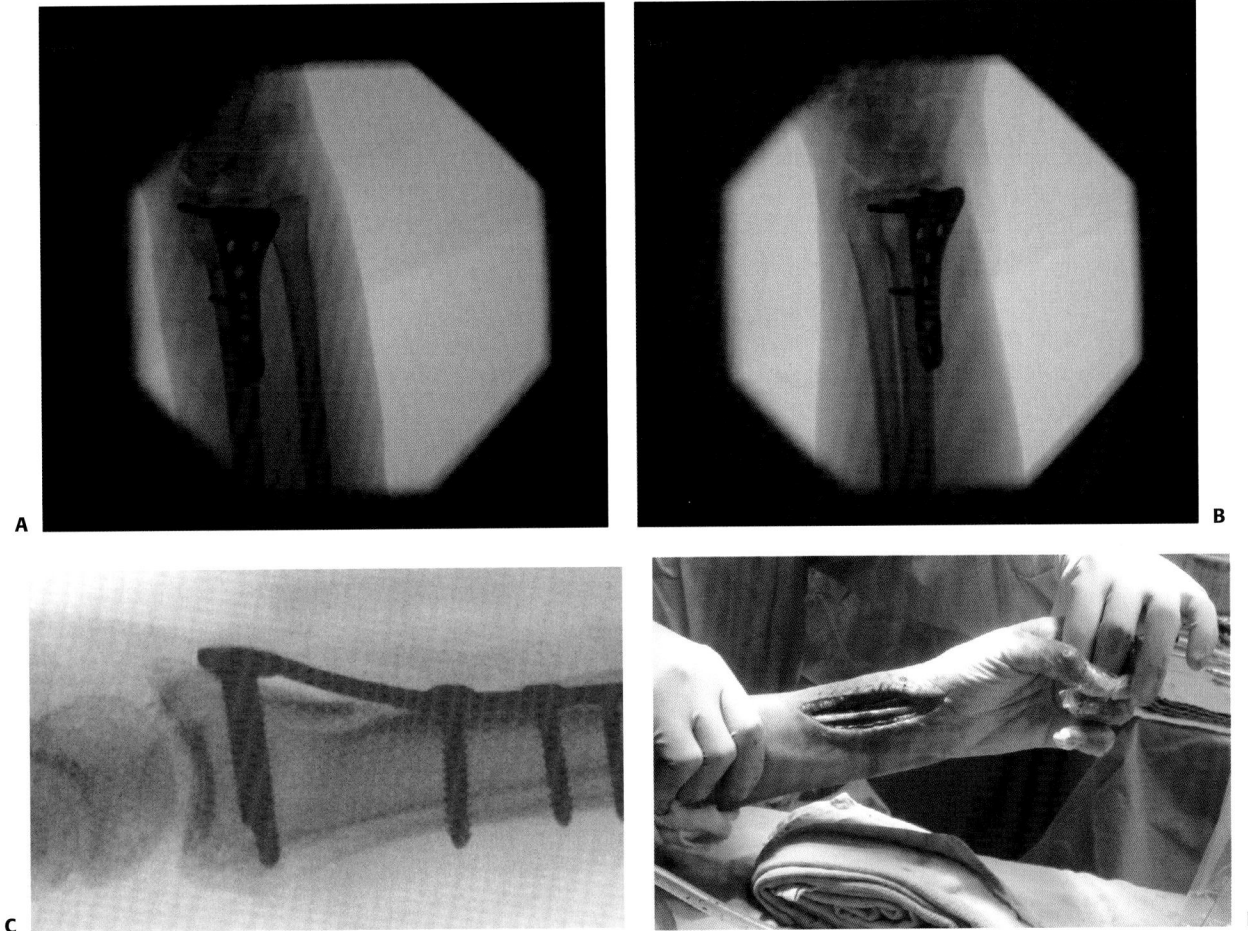

FIGURE 32-5 **A:** A pronated oblique view of the distal radius. This allows assessment of the radial side of the joint. In this case a volar plate is being inserted and it can be seen that the screws are outwith the radiocarpal joint. **B:** A supinated oblique view of the distal radius allowing assessment of the ulnar side of the joint. **C, D:** The forearm is elevated 20 degrees off the table to provide a tilted lateral view of the distal radius which captures a tangential view of the radiocarpal joint.

agreement and to allow a reliable determination of fracture characteristics which may influence treatment such as coronal fracture lines, central articular depression, and articular comminution. The use of this technique has been shown to increase the perceived need for open exposure of displaced articular segments when compared to conventional CT,[149] but the influence of this on functional outcome has yet to be determined.

Classification of Fractures of the Distal Radius and Ulna

Many classification systems have been proposed for fractures of the distal radius and ulna over the years, the majority of which are morphologic and consider in varying degrees the presence or absence of displacement, comminution, and articular involvement.

Previous Classifications

Of the older classification systems the most common still quoted are Gartland and Werley,[117] Older,[269] and the Frykman[114] classification, with the Melone classification for intra-articular fractures.[257] In 1951, Gartland and Werley described a classification system, which included articular involvement, comminution, and displacement. They described three groups:

Group 1—Simple Colles fracture with no involvement of the articular surface.

Group 2—Comminuted Colles fracture with fractures of the radial articular surface in which the fragments were not displaced.

Group 3—Comminuted Colles fracture with fractures of the radial articular surface in which the fragments were displaced.

Group 4—Gartland and Werley did not specify whether group 1 fractures were displaced but Solgaard[339] added a fourth group of extra-articular undisplaced fractures.

The Older classification was published in 1965 and aimed to assist the inexperienced resident in selecting treatment. It is based on severity of displacement and comminution. There are four types:

Type 1—Undisplaced:

1. Loss of some volar angulation up to 5 degrees dorsal angulation.

2. No significant radial shortening—2 mm or more above the distal ulna.

Type 2—Displaced with minimal comminution:

1. Loss of volar angulation or dorsal displacement of distal fragment.

2. Shortening—usually not below the distal ulna, occasionally up to 3 mm below it.

3. Minimal comminution of dorsal radius.

Type 3—Displaced with comminution of distal radius:

1. Comminution of dorsal radius.

2. Shortening—below distal ulna.

3. Comminution of distal radial fragment—usually not marked, often characterized by pieces.

Type 4—Displaced with severe comminution of distal radius:

1. Marked comminution of dorsal radius.

2. Comminution of distal radial fragment—shattered with fractures into the joint.

3. Shortening—usually 2 to 8 mm below the distal ulna.

4. Poor volar cortex in some cases.

Older et al. correlated their end results to the classification system and found that anatomical and functional results were worse with increasing severity of the fracture.

Frykman classified fractures of the distal radius concentrating on articular and ulnar (styloid or shaft) involvement. He specifically differentiated between radiocarpal and distal radioulnar joint involvement, as he believed that intra-articular involvement and ulnar involvement were the most prognostic factors:

Type I	Extra-articular, no ulnar fracture
Type II	Extra-articular, ulnar fracture
Type III	Radiocarpal articular, no ulnar fracture
Type IV	Radiocarpal articular, ulnar fracture
Type V	DRUJ articular, no ulnar fracture
Type VI	DRUJ articular, ulnar fracture
Type VII	Radiocarpal and DRUJ, no ulnar fracture
Type VIII	Radiocarpal and DRUJ, ulnar fracture

Melone classified intra-articular fractures of the distal radius by considering that each fracture consisted of four parts: radial styloid, dorsal medial fragment, volar medial fragment, and the radial shaft. He termed the two medial fragments, which make up the lunate fossa the medial complex and based his classification on the position of the medial complex (Fig. 32-6).

Type 1—Undisplaced or variable displacement of the medial complex as a unit. No comminution. Stable after closed reduction.

Type 2—Unstable, die punch. Moderate or severe displacement of the medial complex as a unit with comminution of dorsal and volar cortices.

    A—Irreducible, closed.

    B—Irreducible, closed because of impaction.

Type 3—As type 2 but with a spike of the radius on the volar side, which may compromise the median nerve.

Type 4—Split fracture, unstable. The medial complex fragments are severely comminuted with rotation of the fragments.

Type 5—Explosion injury. Severe displacement and comminution often with diaphyseal comminution.

Current Classifications

Probably the most widely used classification system in current use is the AO classification (Fig. 32-7), which has been adopted by the Orthopaedic Trauma Association and has been renamed

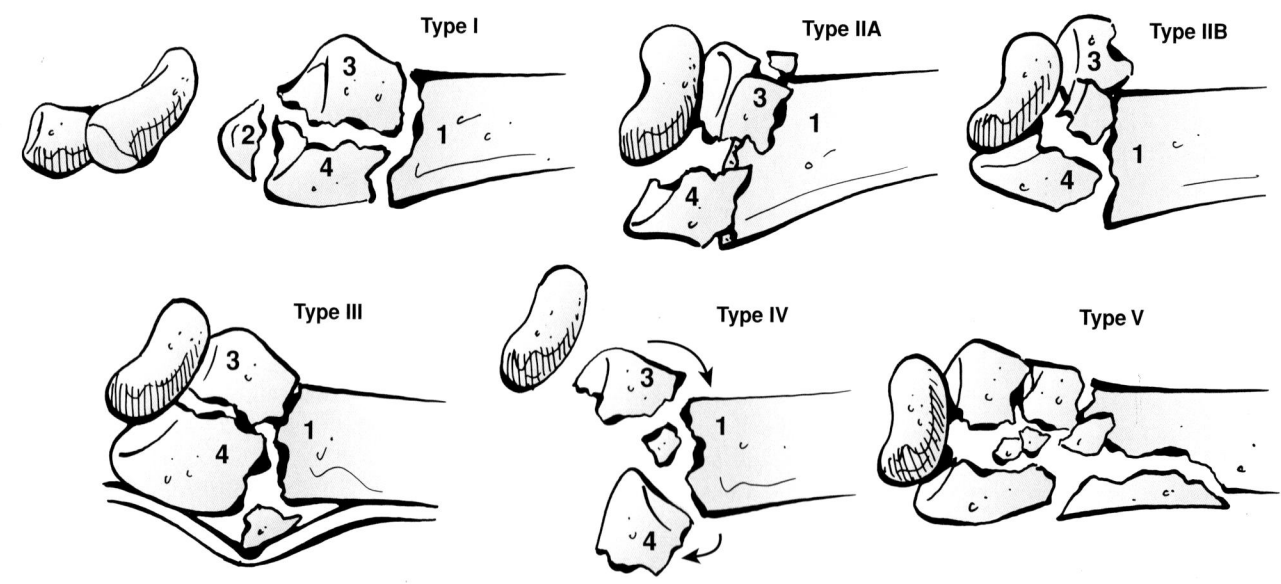

FIGURE 32-6 The Melone classification for intra-articular fractures of the distal radius. Four parts of the fractures are illustrated—the shaft, the radial styloid, the volar ulnar, and the volar dorsal components.

A. Extra-articular   B. Simple articular   C. Complex articular

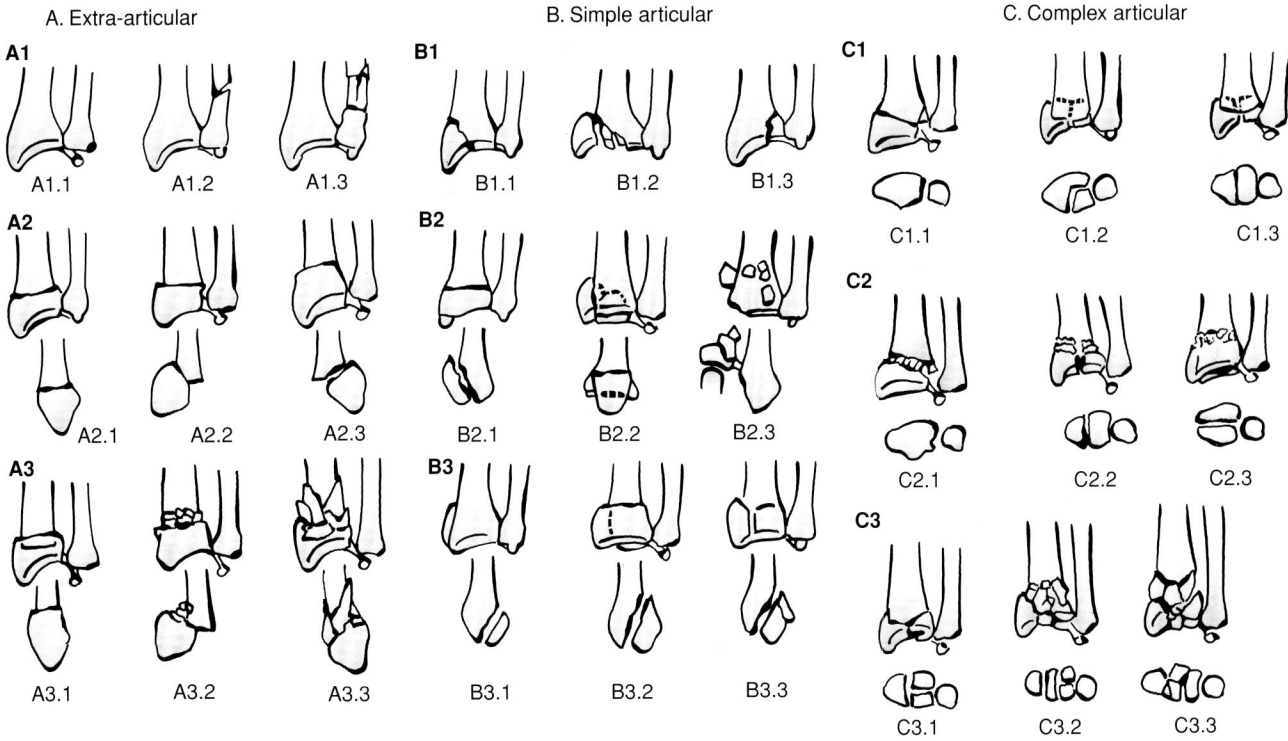

FIGURE 32-7 The AO/OTA classification.

the AO/OTA classification.[241] This is an inclusive, alphanumeric classification and has 27 different subgroups. Three different types (A—extra-articular, B—partial articular, and C—complete articular) are divided into 9 main groups and 27 different subtypes depending on comminution and direction of displacement.

In response to the AO classification, Fernandez and Jupiter[97] published a simplified classification intended to be more treatment-oriented and based on the mechanism of injury. There are five basic types—bending fracture of the metaphysis, shearing and compression fractures of the joint surface, avulsion fractures, and combined fractures from high-velocity injury (Fig. 32-8). The system is presented with the likely risk of instability and associated injuries and gives treatment recommendations. It has not as yet been validated in terms of the treatment recommendations.

Reliability of Classification Systems

Although classification systems are widely used for distal radius fractures, their reliability has not been established. A reliable classification system should be able to define and quantify the severity of a fracture and assist the surgeon in predicting the outcome of a fracture. The dilemma in constructing a classification system is that the more complex the system, the less reliable it becomes both within and between observers.

A number of studies have investigated the reliability of classification system for distal radius fractures. At best, inter- or intraobserver reliability has been demonstrated for the AO/OTA system[205,375] when only types A, B, or C are considered. Other studies considering both the AO/OTA and other clas-

sifications fail to demonstrate reliability[11,102,288] except for the Older classification in which Anderson et al. showed high inter- and intraobserver reproducibility. Solgaard[339] demonstrated the prognostic value of this system. However, undue reliance should not be placed on classification systems especially in considering treatment and prognosis. For research purposes it is preferable to classify distal radius fractures by consensus amongst authors.

Classification of Associated Ulnar Injury

Both the AO/OTA classification[241] and Fernandez classification[97] have constructed a system of classifying ulnar injury associated with distal radius fractures. The Fernandez classification concentrates on the residual stability of the DRUJ after the distal radius fracture has been reduced. There are three types.

Type 1—The distal radioulnar joint is clinically stable and congruous. The primary stabilizers of the joint are intact. Includes avulsion of the tip of the ulnar styloid and stable fractures of the ulnar neck.

Type 2—The distal radioulnar joint is subluxed or dislocated in association with a TFCC tear or fracture at the base of the ulnar styloid.

Type 3—Potentially unstable lesions. Displaced fracture involving sigmoid notch or ulnar head.

The AO/OTA classification system applies a qualification (Q) modifier to classify associated ulnar injuries as follows:

Q1—Distal radioulnar joint dislocation (base of styloid process fracture).

Q2—Simple neck fracture.

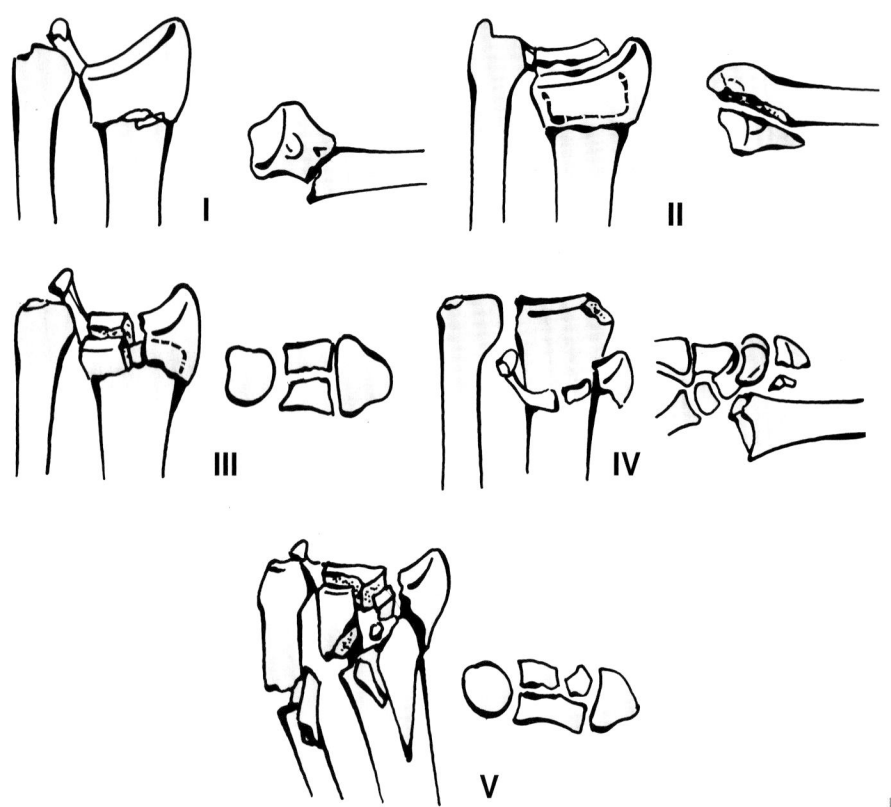

FIGURE 32-8 The Fernandez classification.

Q3—Multifragmentary neck fracture.
Q4—Ulnar head fracture.
Q5—Ulnar head and neck fracture.
Q6—Ulnar fracture proximal to neck.

Outcome Measures for Fractures of the Distal Radius and Ulna

Evaluation of the outcome of a fracture or its treatment is essential to the practice of modern surgery, but any system used for this purpose must be reliable, reproducible, and validated. The World Health Organization (WHO) developed a framework to measure health and disease, the International Classification of Impairments, Disabilities and Handicaps (ICIDH) which distinguishes between impairment, disability, and handicap. Impairment is abnormal physical function, for example, lack of forearm rotation following distal radius fracture, which is generally measured by clinical methods. Disability is the lack of ability to perform daily activities because of the impairment such as inability to open a tight jar because of the lack of forearm rotation. Disability is usually measured by patient reported outcome measures (PROMs). However the patient's perception of disability may be heavily influenced by psychosocial factors,[300] which surgical intervention will not influence. This suggests that those methods measured by clinicians (which treatment may influence) which can be correlated with PROMs may be the best method of measuring outcomes.

Initially, outcome measures for distal radius fracture concentrated on a combination of objective and subjective factors including pain, range of motion, grip strength, ability to undertake the activities of daily living, and radiologic measurements which mainly measure impairment. In recent years however, more emphasis has been placed on self-reported measures of symptoms and function after injury which measure perceived disability.

Clinician-Rated Outcome Measures

Clinician-measured outcomes depend on the measurement of grip strength, ranges of motion, and specialized grip strengths and may contain an element of assessment of the ability to undertake the normal activities of daily living. Although not patient related, it should be noted that although these measurements are theoretically objective the effort applied can be influenced by the patient's psychological state.[346]

The most frequently used physician-based scores for distal radius fractures are the Mayo wrist score,[68] the Gartland and Werley score,[117] and the Green and O'Brien[134] score. None have been examined to determine their reliability, responsiveness, or validity.

Mayo Wrist Score. This was developed for assessment of perilunate fracture dislocations[68] and includes four measures of outcome: pain intensity (25 points), functional status (25 points) based purely on work ability, range of motion (25 points), and grip strength (25 points). The resultant score (maximum 100) is then rated as excellent (90 to 100), good (80 to 90), satisfactory (60 to 80), and poor (below 60). It is based on the Green and O'Brien score, which was modified by Cooney et al.[68] in 1987 by removing any scoring for radiographic appearances.

Green and O'Brien Score. This was developed for assessment of carpal dislocations and includes assessment of pain (five categories, 25 points), occupation (five categories, 25 points), range of motion (five categories, 25 points), grip strength (three categories, 10 points), and radiology (five categories, 20 points).[135] The radiology can only be scored for carpal dislocation. The total score out of 100 was considered satisfactory if it was greater than 70.

Gartland and Werley Score. In 1951, Gartland and Werley[117] constructed an outcome score to evaluate the results of distal radius fractures. It is a demerit score with an excellent result being 0 to 2 points, good 3 to 8 points, fair 9 to 20 points, and poor greater than 20 points. Points are allocated for residual deformity, subjective (i.e., patient) evaluation of pain, disability and limitation of motion, objective (i.e., surgeon) evaluation of loss of movement and distal radioulnar joint pain, and complications of arthritic change, CTS, and stiff fingers. Radiologic results were reported separately.

Patient-Reported Outcome Measures

In recent years there have been a number of PROMs developed ranging from generic measures assessing the impact of injury on the patient's health and well-being (e.g., Short Form 36 [SF-36], sickness impact profile [SIP]) to more specific measures of outcome focused on anatomical regions or specific conditions.

There are two scoring systems in common usage which focus on the upper extremity or wrist.

The Disabilities of Hand, Arm and Shoulder (DASH) Score. The DASH score was first described in 1996[165] as a joint initiative of the American Academy of Orthopaedic Surgeons (AAOS), the Council of Musculoskeletal Research Societies, and the Institute for Work & Health in Toronto. The authors wished to produce a brief self-administered measure of symptoms and mainly physical functional status. The result was the DASH score, which is a 30-item disability/symptom score from 0 (no disability) to 100 (severe disability). Questions are asked about the degree of difficulty in performing tasks because of the upper extremity problem (21 items); the severity of pain; pain with use, tingling, weakness, or stiffness (five items); and the problems' effect on social activities, work, sleep, and self-image (four items). The normal DASH score is less than 15.[119]

Studies of the validity, reliability, and responsiveness of the use of the DASH score in upper limb disorders have demonstrated good validity, reliability, and responsiveness for upper extremity conditions[53,78,141] and specifically for distal radius fractures.[232] A 10-point difference in the mean DASH score is considered the minimal clinically important change.[141] A shorter form, the QuickDASH, is also available and consists of 11 items with similar results for validity and reliability for a variety of upper extremity conditions[141] although not specifically for distal radius fractures.

The Patient-Related Wrist Evaluation (PRWE) Score. The PRWE is a 15-item questionnaire, which examines the severity and frequency of pain in 5 questions and the ability to undertake activities of daily living in 10 questions.[233] It was developed and tested on patients with distal radius fractures and is therefore specific to the wrist rather than to the whole upper extremity. The developers reported excellent reliability and the ability to detect changes over time and concluded that the PRWE provides a brief, reliable, and valid measure of patient-related pain and disability. The responsiveness (or the ability to detect change) of the PRWE was rated highest in a comparison between SF-36, DASH, and PRWE.[232] Changulani et al.[53] summarized the validity, reliability, and responsiveness of four outcome measures, three of which (Gartland and Werley, DASH, and PRWE) are used for assessment of outcome in distal radius fractures and concluded that the PRWE validity was fair, but its reliability and responsiveness was good. The system has also been found to be reliable and valid when translated into different languages.[394]

PATHOANATOMY AND APPLIED ANATOMY OF FRACTURES OF THE DISTAL RADIUS AND ULNA

The distal end of the radius and ulna is an integral part of the wrist joint and preservation of its normal anatomy is essential for the mobility of the wrist and its ability to transmit axial load. The prime function of the wrist joint is to position the hand in space and allow full hand function. Fractures of the distal radius that malunite are therefore likely to have a significant effect on hand function.

The articular surface of the distal radius has two concavities, one for articulation with the scaphoid and one for the lunate. The two facets are divided by a ridge running from dorsal to volar. The surface is triangular in shape with the base formed by the sigmoid notch and the apex by the tip of the radial styloid. The articular surface is inclined both in a volar and an ulnar direction.

The palmar surface of the radius forms a curve concave from proximal to distal. It is relatively smooth, which allows easy contouring of plates in this area. It also allows attachment of stout radiocarpal ligaments, which act as restraints to the normal tendency of the carpus to slide in an ulnar and palmar direction. The curve is covered by the transverse fibers of pronator quadratus, which is attached to the radial side of the bone.

The dorsal surface is convex and much more irregular with Lister's tubercle, around which the extensor pollicis longus (EPL) tendon passes, being the most prominent area. There are grooves that form the floors of extensor compartments (Fig. 32-9). A knowledge of their anatomy is essential in approaching the dorsum of the distal radius surgically or in applying any form of fixation to the distal radius dorsally (Table 32-3).

As well as the radiocarpal articulation the distal radius forms one half of the distal radioulnar joint, the sigmoid notch, which is a uniform curve semicylindrical in shape allowing rotation of the radius around the ulnar head. As rotation occurs the ulnar head moves in a volar direction with supination and a dorsal direction with pronation. The ulnar head is largely covered in cartilage even on its inferior surface. However, it does not articulate with the carpus as the TFCC extends from the ulnar aspect of the radius to the base of the ulnar styloid and articulates with the triquetrum. The TFCC acts as a stabilizer of

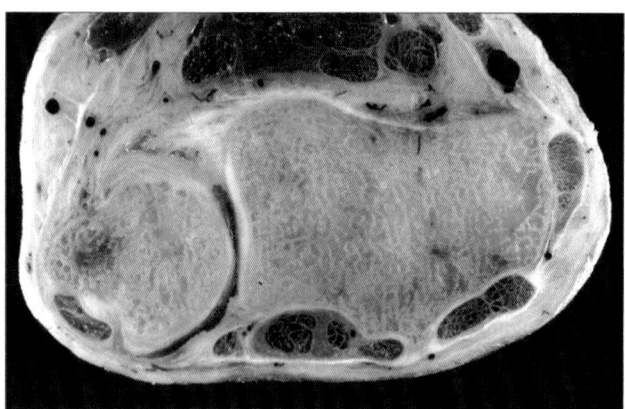

FIGURE 32-9 The cross-sectional anatomy of the radius immediately below the radiocarpal joint. The extensor tendons lie in their compartments in immediate contact with the bone whilst on the palmar surface the flexor tendons are protected by a layer of fat.

the distal radioulnar joint along with extensor carpi ulnaris and flexor carpi ulnaris, the pronator quadratus, and the interosseous membrane of the forearm.

TREATMENT OPTIONS

There are numerous treatment options for the management of distal radius fractures including nonoperative, external fixation, and internal fixation. The indications for each differ depending on the patient, their demands, and the type of fracture. As the main goal of treatment is to maximize function in the hand and wrist it is essential in planning treatment to consider the factors that may predict fracture instability or functional outcome.

Prediction of Instability

Several factors have been associated with re-displacement following closed manipulation of a distal radius fracture.

Age

Patients over 80 years of age with a displaced fracture of the distal radius are three times more likely to have instability than those under 30 years of age. This is even more striking in patients with minimally or undisplaced fractures when the risk of instability increases tenfold in older patients.[234] Fractures in elderly patients with osteopenic bones may also displace at a later stage.

Initial Fracture Displacement[340]

The greater the degree of initial displacement (particularly radial shortening), the more energy is imparted to the fracture resulting in a higher likelihood that closed treatment will be unsuccessful.

Metaphyseal Comminution

The presence of a metaphyseal defect as evidenced by either plain radiographs or computerized tomography increases the chance of instability.[340]

Displacement Following Closed Treatment

This is a predictor of instability as repeat manipulation is unlikely to result in a successful radiographic outcome.[104,250,251]

Mackenney and his co-authors[234] examined the natural history of over 3,500 distal radius fractures and detailed the independently significant predictors of early instability (redisplacement before two weeks), late instability (redisplacement between two weeks and fracture union) and malunion for both undisplaced and displaced fractures. Mathematical formulae were constructed to give a percentage chance of redisplacement or malunion for individual patients. The authors give an example of an independent 85 year old lady with a dorsally displaced fracture of the distal radius with metaphyseal comminution and a positive ulnar variance of 2 mm. The calculated probability of malunion is 82%. Clinical application of these formulae is likely to encourage early treatment in appropriate cases and reduce the prevalence of malunion.

Prediction of Function

Patient Factors

Age. The main consideration influencing a decision about the treatment of a patient with a distal radius fracture is the demand which an individual places on their wrist. The purpose

TABLE 32-3	The Extensor Compartments of the Wrist and Their Contents	
Extensor Compartment	Contents	Comments
1	Abductor pollicis longus Extensor pollicis brevis	Form the radial border of the anatomical snuff box
2	Extensor carpi radialis longus Extensor carpi radialis brevis	
3	Extensor pollicis longus	Ulnar to Lister's tubercle
4	Extensor digitorum Extensor indicis	
5	Extensor digiti minimi	Dorsal to the distal radioulnar joint
6	Extensor carpi ulnaris	Runs in groove between the ulnar head and styloid

of treatment is to maintain normal strength, mobility, and function in the hand and wrist. These factors are influenced by the age and psychological state, both of which may alter the demands placed on the wrist. Treatment methods usually serve to restore the normal anatomy, failing which malunion results. As demands upon the wrist become less, the symptoms from a malunion are likely to reduce and the importance of normal anatomy declines.

However, there is as yet no consensus on how patients should be treated as the definition of an elderly patient is not clear. Physiologic and actual age may vary greatly but the surgeon usually makes a judgment on a subjective impression. The use of more objective measures available in the geriatric and epidemiologic literature such as the Physical Activity Scale of the Elderly (PASE) score may be of value.[387] The PASE is a brief instrument designed to assess physical activity in older persons and includes assessment of participation in normal daily and leisure activities. It has been validated as a measure of physical activity, health, and physical function in older people.[327,386]

Lessening demands may account for reports of malunion of the distal radius in older people being compatible with good function. Jaremko et al.[170] reviewed 74 older patients with distal radius fractures treated nonoperatively. Seventy-one percent had at least one unacceptable radiographic deformity, but at review 6 months after fracture the authors reported that self-reported disability was low and patient satisfaction high despite a mean DASH score of 24 and a patient dissatisfaction rate of 28%. Mean DASH scores were higher if the radiologic deformity was outside the acceptable range but this was not statistically significant. The outcome scores could not be predicted by radiologic deformity possibly because the age range was wide from 50 years upward. Young and Rayan[399] studied 25 low-demand patients over 60 years of age. Thirty-two percent of patients had fair or poor radiographic results but only 12% had fair or poor functional outcomes. The most difficult task was jar opening. The authors concluded that nonoperative treatment yields satisfactory results in low-demand patients. No relationship between anatomy and function was found in a group of 74 older patients with conservatively managed distal radius fractures 6 months after injury, although only 59% of patients were satisfied with the outcome.[14] Grewal and MacDermid[136] found that the relative risk of a poor outcome with malalignment of the distal radius showed a decreasing trend with increasing age. In a comparison of operative versus nonoperative treatment in elderly patients despite better anatomical results in the operatively treated group there were no differences in DASH scores or pain scores between the groups up to a year after injury.[92]

In contrast to these studies Brogren et al.[40] examined 143 patients 1 year after distal radius fracture and classified them into three groups: No malunion, single malunion (either dorsal tilt of 10 degrees or positive ulnar variance) and combined malunion (both dorsal tilt of 10 degrees and positive ulnar variance). The average age was 65 years. The mean DASH score was 10.5 points worse than the no malunion group if there was single malunion (p = 0.015) and 8.7 points worse if there was a combined malunion (p = 0.034). With regression analysis the relative risk of higher disability was 2.5 with single malunion

and 3.7 with a combined malunion. There was no difference in these results when adjusted for age or gender. The authors concluded that malunion with a dorsal angle greater than 10 degrees or a positive ulnar variance leads to higher arm-related disability after distal radius fracture, regardless of age or gender.

Other Factors. A number of other factors have been linked to outcome after fractures of the distal radius. Work-related injury or compensation claims have been shown to have a negative influence on outcomes.[138,231] Poorer socioeconomic status,[58] lower education levels[138] and low bone density[158] have also been implicated in poorer outcomes.

Fracture Factors

There remains little consensus on what constitutes an "acceptable" radiologic result after distal radius fracture. This should be defined as a radiologic position which will predict satisfactory function in the substantial majority of cases. A number of authors have examined the influence of radiologic position on function, considering both metaphyseal and articular alignment.

Metaphyseal Alignment. All of the radiologic indices of anatomy detail earlier in this chapter have been examined in attempts to detect any correlation with function.

Radial Height. After retrospectively reviewing 269 distal radial fractures in adults, Solgaard[340] found that shortening had the most impact on the result and recommended restoration of the radial length to be the primary goal of surgery. Batra and Gupta,[25] in a retrospective review of 69 patients at 1 year after the injury that had been treated with various techniques, echoed the above findings by highlighting radial length as the most important determinant of functional outcome. Jenkins et al.[173] in a prospective study of 61 consecutive patients presenting with distal radial fractures treated by plaster immobilization showed that shortening of more than 4 mm was associated with wrist pain at a mean follow-up of 23 months. Trumble et al.[369] also concluded that the degree of surgical correction of the shortening was strongly associated with an improved outcome.

Ulnar Variance. Displacement and impaction of the distal fragment leads to relative shortening of the radius compared to the ulna (Fig. 32-10) or ulnar variance, which can be ascertained by comparison with the contralateral normal wrist. The ulna could appear longer (ulnar plus), shorter (ulnar minus), or level (ulnar neutral) with the radius in the normal population.[21] Hence the extent of radial shortening as a result of fracture cannot be determined by simply measuring the distance between the radius and ulna, without a preinjury or contralateral radiograph for comparison.

Adams[3] in a cadaveric experiment showed that positive ulnar variance caused the greatest alteration in the kinematics of the DRUJ and the most distortion of the triangular fibrocartilage, compared with loss of radial inclination and palmar tilt. In a prospective randomized trial involving 120 patients with redisplaced distal radial fractures, McQueen et al.[250] showed that radial shortening (more than 3 mm compared to the contralateral wrist) resulted in diminished grip strengths. More

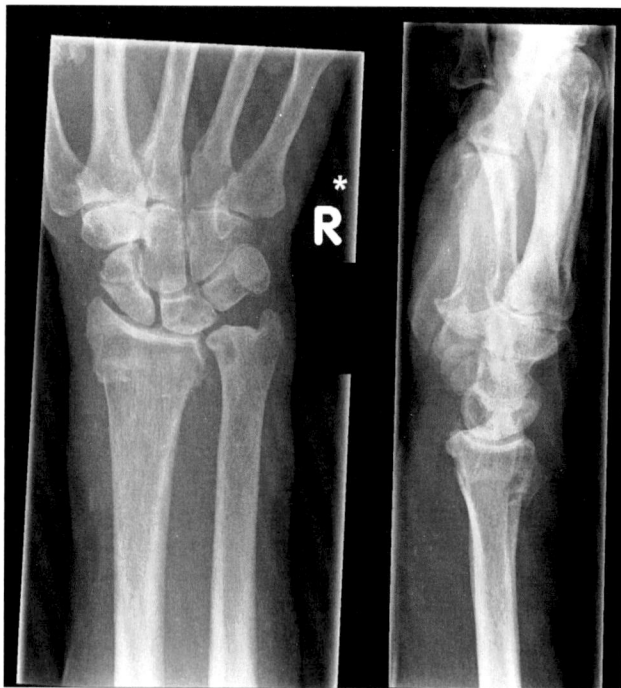

FIGURE 32-10 A fracture of the distal radius with an ulnar positive variance, dorsal angulation, and carpal malalignment.

recently in 118 patients with distal radius fractures treated with locked plating positive ulnar variance at presentation or at final review predicted ulnar-sided wrist pain at final review.[401] Brogren et al.[40] reported significantly worse DASH and SF-12 scores and weaker grip strength with positive ulnar variance 1 year after fracture.

Radial Inclination. Radial inclination is closely correlated with radial height and both are indications of axial compression.[374] At 1 to 3 years after a distal radial fracture, Jenkins and Mintowt-Czyz[173] showed a correlation between the loss of radial inclination and decreased grip strength. Axial compression predicted the presence of degenerative changes in the radiocarpal joint and the DRUJ in a study of 76 young patients after a mean of 30 years although no patient had altered his occupation or leisure activities as a result.[200] Wilcke et al.[392] highlighted the association between a loss of radial inclination of >10 degrees and a worse DASH score in a retrospective review of 78 healed distal radial fractures after a mean of 22 months.

Dorsal/Palmar Tilt. Cadaveric studies have provided some evidence of the mechanical effects of loss of palmar tilt. The pressure distribution on the ulnar and radial articular surfaces has been shown to change and become more concentrated as dorsal tilt increases.[331] In another study the effects of increasing dorsal tilt resulted in worsening incongruence of the distal radioulnar joint, increased tightness of the interosseous membrane, and limited rotation.[189] In addition, loss of the normal palmar tilt positions the carpus in a dorsal collapse alignment, leading to midcarpal instability, which may be corrected by a distal radial osteotomy.[362]

There has been conflicting evidence on the impact of loss of the normal palmar tilt on functional outcome, which may be because of different measurements and definitions of function or the difficulty in obtaining standard radiographs and a consequent wide margin of error in measurement. Some authors failed to find any relationship between radiology and function.[369] Forward et al.[108] observed that measurements of extra-articular malunion were not related to the Patient Evaluation Measure. However, in the same study, they noted that dorsal angulation was associated with worse narrowing of joint space and reduced grip strength when compared to the contralateral uninjured site.

In contrast, radiologic position has been shown to influence a number of individual surgeon-rated measures of function. Van der Linden and Ericson,[374] in a study of 250 consecutive cases of extra-articular distal radial fractures, noted that the better the reduction of the dorsal tilt, the better the range of movement, grip strength, and residual pain. In a study of 115 patients being followed up for 2 years post injury, Porter and Stockley[290] demonstrated that grip strength diminished significantly when the dorsal tilt exceeded 20 degrees. Gartland and Werley,[117] in a study of 60 cases after a mean follow-up of 18 months, showed that residual dorsal tilt of 11 degrees or more was associated with significant loss of wrist flexion. McQueen and Caspers[248] performed comprehensive functional assessment on 30 patients with extra-articular fractures after a mean of 5 years. They showed that malunion (dorsal tilt of 12 degrees or more and more than 2 mm of radial shift) was clearly associated with significant functional limitation.

A more recent study using DASH scores as the primary outcome demonstrated statistically and clinically significantly worse DASH scores with dorsal angle of 10 degrees or more 1 year after fracture.[40] The same effect was seen with SF-12 scores and grip strength.

Carpal Alignment. It is important to appreciate that most cases of carpal malalignment after distal radius fractures are caused by residual dorsal or volar tilt of the distal radius and not by intrinsic instability of the carpus. As the radius tilts, for example dorsally, the lunate tilts with it. The position of the hand is corrected at the midcarpal joint resulting in carpal malalignment (Fig. 32-10).

This was first appreciated by Linscheid et al.[223] in 1972. They described two cases of distal radius malunion and carpal malalignment and demonstrated correction of the malalignment and improvement in function with corrective osteotomy of the distal radius. Bickerstaff and Bell described carpal malalignment as the inevitable response of the carpus to the altered mechanics caused by dorsal tilt of the distal radius and believed that it explained the morbidity caused by the fracture. They examined 32 patients and concluded that the most significant indication of a poor result was the degree of carpal malalignment.[30] In a prospective randomized study of 120 patients with unstable fractures of the distal radius there was poorer recovery of grip strength and forearm rotation in those with carpal malalignment.[250] The authors concluded that carpal malalignment had the strongest negative influence on function. Gupta et al. differentiated between two types of carpal alignment, one where the lunate dorsiflexes with the distal radius displacement and one where the lunate remains colinear with the capitate. They believe that the latter is associated with radiocarpal ligament damage and carries a worse prognosis.[143]

Articular Alignment. The relationships between the initial insults to the cartilage, the effects of residual incongruity, and the subsequent development of degenerative changes remain debatable.[240] There are no robust data to guide the surgeon on the amount of residual articular displacement which can be accepted with a reasonable guarantee of a satisfactory outcome. This is likely to be caused by the many other factors which influence outcome and its measurement such as age, injury severity, inter- and intraobserver reliability, and difficulty in obtaining accurate measurements of the articular surface.[124]

Articular incongruity appears to adversely affect the biomechanics of the joint, and three separate cadaveric experiments using pressure-sensitive films have shown significant increases in contact stresses with articular step-offs varying between 1 and 3 mm.[23,383]

However, although radiologic degeneration can be demonstrated with articular displacement, it has been more difficult for investigators to show consistent relationships between articular incongruity, osteoarthrosis, and significant functional compromise. In 1986, Knirk and Jupiter correlated patient outcome with residual intra-articular incongruity. They found a 91% incidence of radiographically apparent arthrosis with any measurable intra-articular step-off and a 100% incidence with over 2 mm of articular step-off, of which 93% (26 of 28) were said to be symptomatic. However, only one patient with bilateral fractures had to stop working as a direct result of the injuries. Overall, 61% reported an excellent or good outcome.[196]

Subsequent authors also emphasized the relationship of as little as 1 mm or more of articular incongruity with a worse clinical outcome.[120,200] Although these studies indicate the importance of restoring articular congruity, other authors question the ability of plain radiographs to consistently demonstrate incongruity of less than 2 mm. Data on healed fractures indicate that clinicians measuring step and gap deformity on a random x-ray film will differ by more than 3 mm at least 10% of the time. Repeat step or gap measurements by the same observer are also expected to differ by more than 2 mm at least 10% of the time.[206]

In another retrospective review, 21 young patients were examined at a mean follow-up of 7.1 years following open reduction and internal fixation (ORIF) of a displaced intra-articular fracture. There was a 76% prevalence of radiocarpal arthritis, but no patient reported a poor functional outcome. Radiocarpal degenerative changes were noted to deteriorate over time, but the patients maintained a high level of function.[50]

More recently, Forward et al. reviewed 108 patients at a mean follow-up of 38 years after distal radial fracture. The majority was treated nonoperatively and only one patient underwent internal fixation. The mean age of the patients at the latest review was 64 years. Around two-thirds of the fractures were

malunited although none of the patients reported any limitation of activity as a result of the injuries, and none had required a salvage procedure. Intra-articular injury was found to be a strong predictor of radiologic degenerative changes and worse Patient Evaluation Measure and DASH scores.[108]

Can We Predict Outcome?

Prediction of outcome is made difficult by the numerous factors which have been shown to have an influence on the final result but would be useful in aiding the surgeon to make a management decision in individual patients. For example, one of the most difficult decisions is in treatment of the elderly patient where biologic and chronologic age may vary significantly and it is difficult to know whether age, level of comorbidity, and preinjury function, or combination of those are the most important factors in deciding whether there will be benefit in correcting the anatomical position.

In an attempt to predict the threshold above or below which correction of the anatomy should be undertaken, 642 patients treated for distal radius fractures in Edinburgh were examined. Poorer functional outcome was predicted by age, pain, residual dorsal angulation, positive ulnar variance, and carpal malalignment. Weighted equations are being developed which can be applied in individual cases to predict the outcome and assist the surgeon in making a treatment decision. Other authors have also examined the influence of multiple factors on functional outcome. In a prospective study of 96 patients with distal radius fractures treated nonoperatively, Wakefield and McQueen[384] found that malunion, the severity of the initial fracture displacement, and a high level of pain 6 weeks after fracture were independent predictors of a poor outcome. Finsen et al. found a highly statistically significant relationship between radiographic displacement and clinical outcome scores including the PRWE and DASH scores. With multiple regression analysis they found that complications, ulnar variance, dorsal angulation, and time since fracture significantly contributed to outcome scores, but that they only contributed 11% to 16% of the variability of the scores.[99]

In a recent study osteoporosis has been demonstrated to result in poorer outcomes after distal radius fracture.[101] In a cohort of 64 patients treated with ORIF, 20 were osteoporotic and 44 osteopenic on BMD scanning. At 1 year after injury the osteoporotic group had a mean DASH score 15 points higher than the osteopenic group. Using multivariate analysis the authors showed that osteoporosis was a strong independent predictor of a higher DASH score and a higher rate of major complications. This study used a comorbidity index to assess the patients' general state of health and also demonstrated that more comorbidity was a strong predictor of a poorer DASH score. A similar study published in the same year failed to demonstrate a relationship between osteoporosis and the DASH score, but showed a trend to more complications in the osteoporotic patients.[381]

As present knowledge stands we cannot predict the outcome of a distal radius fracture with any degree of confidence but can only recommend levels of displacement which can be accepted in the fit, active, and fully functioning patient.

TABLE 32-4	The Radiologic Limits Beyond Which Correction is Recommended	
Radiologic Measurement	Recommended Limits
Positive ulnar variance (mm)	2–3
Carpal malalignment	None
Dorsal tilt (degrees)	Neutral if carpus malaligned <10 degrees if carpus aligned
Palmar tilt (degrees)	No limit if carpus aligned
Gap or step in joint (mm)	2

These are detailed in Table 32-4. They are more stringent than those recommended by the AAOS, as the AAOS publication does not consider the effect of carpal malalignment. If the carpus is malaligned and the dorsal tilt is beyond neutral then correction should be undertaken. Some dorsal tilt can be accepted if the carpus is aligned.[264] Palmar tilt can be accepted provided the carpus is aligned.

Indications for Treatment

There are numerous treatment options for the management of distal radius fractures including nonoperative treatment, external fixation, and internal fixation. The indications for each differ depending on the patient, their demands, and the type of fracture.

The main factor influencing a decision about treatment of a distal radius fracture is the demand that an individual patient places on their wrist. The purpose of treatment of a distal radius fracture is to maintain normal strength, mobility, and function in the hand and wrist. These factors are influenced by the age and physiologic state of a patient, both of which may reduce the demands placed on the wrist. Treatment methods usually aim to restore normal anatomy and if this is not achieved malunion will result, which may cause difficulty with activities requiring strength in the hand and wrist. As demands on the wrist become less, the symptoms from a malunion become less thus reducing the need for treatment to maintain normal alignment.

Nonoperative Treatment of Fractures of the Distal Radius and Ulna

Nonoperative treatment remains the mainstay for fractures of the distal radius and consists of plaster or splint management with or without closed reduction. Rates of nonoperative treatment are probably around 70%,[72] with a range in the United States varying from 60% to 96% with geographic location.[60,96] Nonoperative treatment of distal radius fractures increases with increasing age and comorbidities[59,96] in males and in black patients.[60] It was postulated that this was the case because males and black patients were less likely to be osteoporotic and were therefore likely to have more stable fractures.[60] Nonoperative treatment is also less likely to be employed by hand surgeons compared to orthopedic trauma surgeons.[59,60]

Trends in the use of nonoperative treatment of distal radius fractures have changed over the years. In the early 1950s just over 95% were treated nonoperatively in an urban practice in

Southwest USA[94] in comparison to as few as 60% in some areas of the United States in this millennium.[96] Recent trends have shown an increase from 3% to 16% in the use of ORIF and an accompanying decrease from 82% to 70% in nonoperative management in the elderly since 2000.[60] The authors attribute the change to the introduction of volar locked plating systems around 2000. A striking shift has been recorded in fixation techniques amongst younger surgeons between 1999 and 2007 but not in response to improved surgeon-related outcomes.[201] This suggests vulnerability in the profession to marketing of new devices and emphasizes the importance of making management decisions based on scientific evidence.

Indications for Nonoperative Treatment

Nonoperative treatment is indicated for undisplaced stable fractures or displaced fractures which are stable after reduction (Fig. 32-11). Stability after reduction may be assessed by observation over time or by predictive algorithms.[234]

Manipulative reduction is indicated where the radiologic position falls outwith acceptable limits (Table 32-4) and nonoperative treatment is predicted to be successful, that is, if the fracture is likely to be stable (Fig. 32-12). It is also used when there is an impending complication which may be averted by early reduction even if further treatment may be necessary. In some situations manipulative treatment is not necessary. These include fracture with a high risk of instability where more definitive primary treatment should be used. Manipulative reduction should not be used where the fracture is displaced and unstable, but the patient is not considered suitable for surgical treatment, for example, in a low-demand patient.

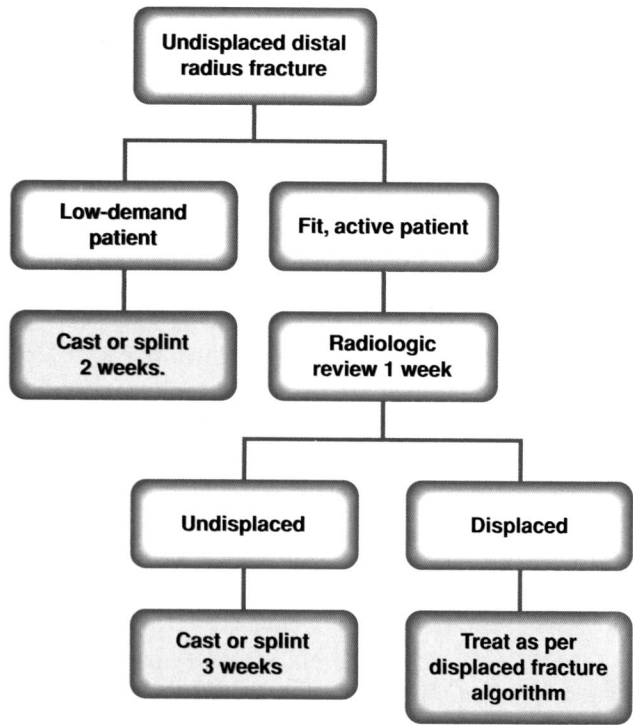

FIGURE 32-11 Management of the undisplaced distal radius fracture.

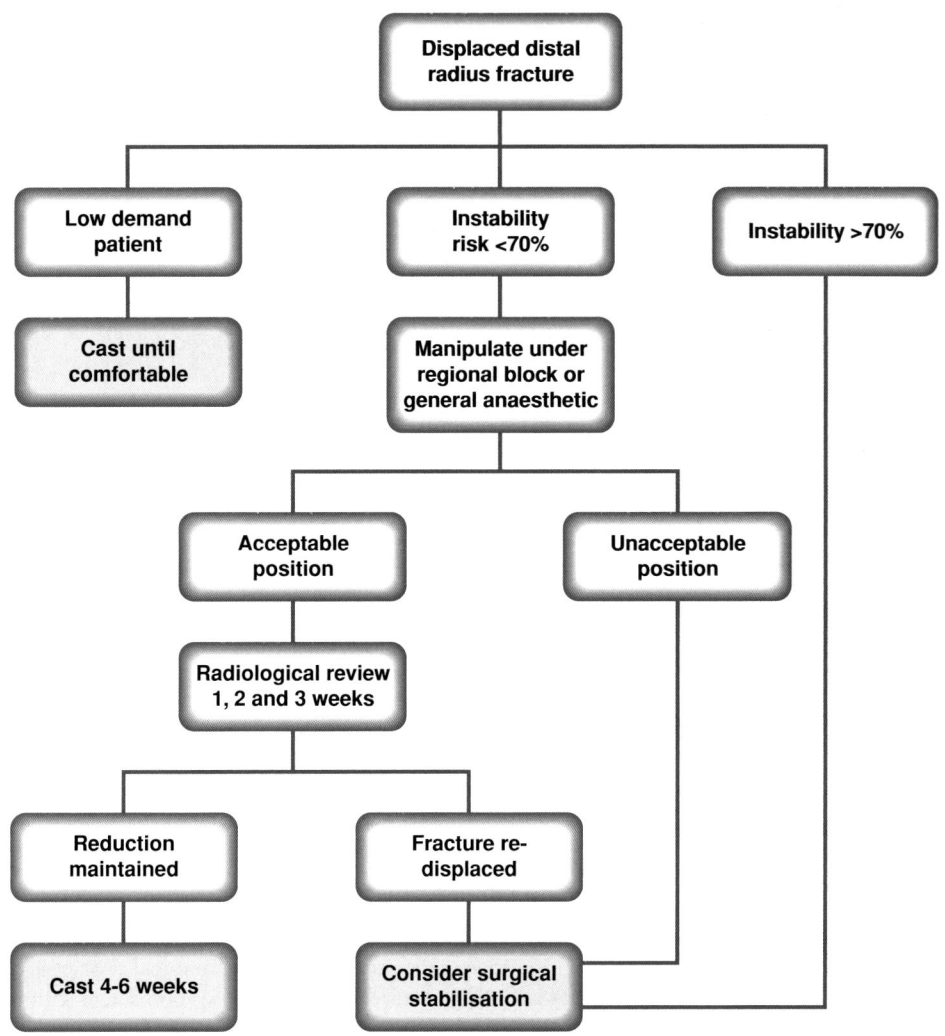

FIGURE 32-12 Nonoperative management of the displaced distal radius fracture.

In a series of 59 low-demand patients who had undergone manipulative reduction and who had a mean age of 82 years, 53 patients ultimately had a malunion. The authors concluded that primary reduction was ineffective in elderly frail patients and recommend that it should only be performed where there is a specific indication such as median nerve symptoms.[29]

Technique of Manipulative Reduction

Reduction of a displaced distal radius fracture requires adequate analgesia or pain relief, which can be achieved by hematoma block, regional or general anesthesia, or intravenous sedation. General anesthesia and intravenous sedation are used in smaller proportions[130,348] and the majority of patients are treated with either regional anesthesia or hematoma block. A number of randomized controlled trials (RCTs) have been published, all of which agree that regional anesthesia in the form of a Bier's block provides superior pain relief and reduction without a significant risk of complications. Hematoma block is cited as being more efficient because it requires only one doctor in attendance, although transit times in the emergency department are similar for both methods.[187] However, there is a consensus

that Bier's block is a safe, effective, and practical procedure and superior to hematoma block.[1,65,187,385] Despite this it is reported that hematoma block remains a common procedure[348] and is used in up to half of the cases.

Once adequate analgesia or anesthesia has been established, reduction of distal radius fractures is usually straightforward. The surgeon applies longitudinal traction to the forearm with an assistant providing countertraction above the elbow. This usually disengages the fracture and allows direct pressure to be applied to the distal radial fragment from dorsal to volar if dorsally displaced and volar to dorsal if volar displaced. Flexion of the wrist may assist in producing some restoration of volar tilt. However, dorsal ligaments only tighten with maximal wrist flexion.[4] This position cannot be maintained in a cast because excessive flexion, the Cotton-Loder position, increases carpal tunnel pressures[122,198] and therefore the risk of acute CTS. In recalcitrant cases with dorsal displacement, for example late reduction, Agee technique[4] of applying palmar translation of the hand in relation to the forearm is often successful (Fig. 32-13). Finger traps can also be used to apply longitudinal traction, which may be useful when no

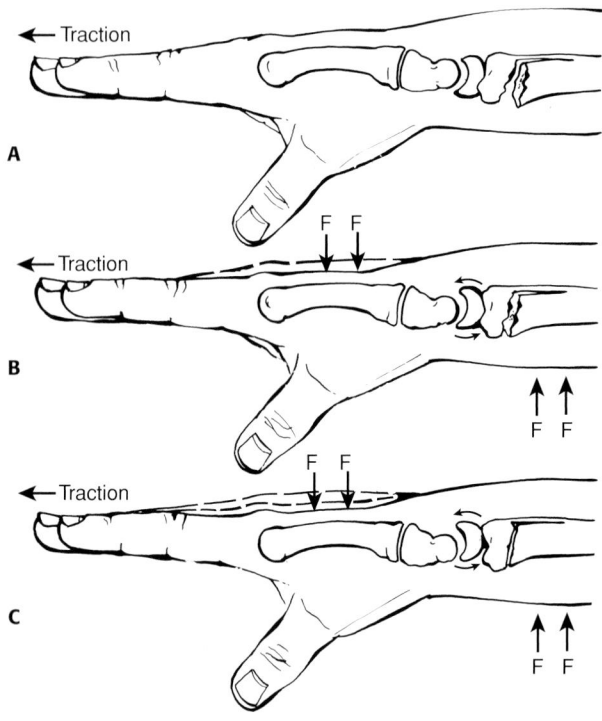

FIGURE 32-13 To apply the Agee maneuver, traction is first applied either manually or with fingertraps **(A)**. A volar translation force *(F)* is applied to the distal fragment of the radius **(B)**. The lunate translates on the distal radius, causing the distal fragment to tilt in a volar direction **(C)**. (From Court-Brown C, McQueen M, Tornetta P. *Orthopaedic Surgery Essentials: Trauma.* Philadelphia, PA: Lippincott Williams & Wilkins; 2006, with permission.)

assistant is available but have not been demonstrated to improve reduction.[88]

Cast Immobilization

Once the reduction maneuvers have been performed, a plaster cast is applied. There are a number of controversies around the use of plaster casts including the type of cast, the use of bracing, the position of immobilization, and the length of time required in cast.

Type of Cast. The initial cast is usually a back slab or sugar tong splint. These theoretically allow for swelling to occur in the cast but this has not been demonstrated by pressure measurements within casts which indicate that splitting a circumferential cast is the only method which allows for swelling after reduction.[400] The cast is then completed when swelling has reduced. It is important to allow free finger movement within a cast by ensuring that the cast ends proximal to the metacarpophalangeal joints.

Both forearm and above-elbow casts have been used for distal radius fractures. Above-elbow casts were used because it was believed that holding the forearm in supination prevented redisplacement from the deforming force of brachioradialis.[322] However, randomized studies have shown no benefit of above-elbow immobilization compared to forearm

casts in maintaining the fracture reduction,[36,129,289,352,374] with some showing a disadvantage because of long-term rotational contracture with above-elbow casts.[289] No advantage has been demonstrated by the use of braces rather than casts.[371]

Position of Immobilization. Extreme positions of the wrist such as the Cotton-Loder position of extreme flexion and ulnar deviation should be avoided because of their potential complications. Traditionally, slight flexion and ulnar deviation have been recommended but neutral or even dorsiflexed positions do not seem to affect the final radiologic position.[142,374] It is likely that fracture and patient factors rather than the wrist position determine the stability of a distal radius fracture.[234,374]

Length of Time in Cast. Undisplaced fractures need a very limited immobilization time with some evidence that no or minimal immobilization is required with functional recovery faster than when conventional cast immobilization is used.[76,80,355] If immobilization is used, removable wrist splints may be more acceptable to the patient than a cast.[268]

In displaced fractures, which have required manipulative reduction, the accepted length of time in a cast is 5 to 6 weeks. However, in an RCT, McAuliffe et al. found no significant anatomical differences but less pain in patients over 60 years of age whose casts were retained for 3 rather than 5 weeks. They recommended that casts be removed after 3 weeks and active mobilization encouraged.[244]

Radiologic and clinical review following fracture reduction should be undertaken at regular intervals. All fractures should be reviewed at 1 week as even minimally displaced fractures which have not required initial reduction may displace. Mackenney et al. reported that 10% of minimally displaced fractures and 43% of displaced fractures were unstable within 2 weeks and would have malunited without further treatment. Late instability, defined as loss of position after 2 weeks of injury, occurred in 22% of the remaining minimally displaced fractures and 47% of the remaining displaced fractures after the fractures with early instability were excluded.[234] These data indicate that fracture review should also be undertaken at 2 and 3 weeks after injury.

Outcome of Nonoperative Treatment

Cohort Studies. The majority of reports of outcomes after nonoperative treatment are in cohorts of older patients. One study has presented the results of nonoperative treatment at a review period of 9 to 13 years. The patients' ages ranged from 19 to 78 at the time of injury. There was a high rate of radiologic deformity with a mean dorsal angle of 13 degrees in patients less than 60 years of age and 18 degrees in the older patients. Fifty-two of sixty-six patients' outcomes were rated as excellent or good according to the modified Green and O'Brien score. The authors noted a slower recovery in the over 60 group and concluded that some patients with nonoperatively treated distal radius fractures still experience some impairment a decade after injury.[106]

Other reports concentrate on older patients and those who had access to radiographs after healing report a significant proportion of malunited fractures.[14,170,360,399] Mean DASH scores range from 15.7 to 24.[10,170,360] Patient satisfaction is rated from 59% to 92%.[14,170,399]

Randomized Controlled Trials. A number of RCTs have compared nonoperative treatment with percutaneous pinning. Most report no or minimal radiologic advantage with percutaneous pinning but no functional advantage.[20,357,395] The only study to report anatomical and functional advantages of percutaneous pinning compared to cast management was in patients under 65 years of age.[305]

There seems to be a consensus amongst authors of RCTs or pseudo-RCTs which compare nonoperative management with bridging external fixation that bridging external fixation results in a better anatomical position than nonoperative management,[8,57,160,164,203,250,308,341] but most reported no differences in the functional results.[160,203,250,308,341] The only series that reported DASH scores showed no differences,[8] whereas Christensen et al.[57] reported improvement in the Gartland and Werley scores for external fixation at 3 and 9 months after injury. Some authors reported either a trend toward poorer function[164,203] or worse results for nonoperative management in a small number of objective surgeon-orientated outcomes.[8] However, a lower rate of complications is reported for nonoperative management.[160,341] Only one study has reported on a randomized comparison of nonbridging external fixation and cast management. Jenkins et al. compared 26 cases treated in plaster with 30 cases treated with nonbridging external fixation. All of their patients were under 60 years of age. There was a mean loss of reduction of 10.5 degrees of dorsal angulation and 3.7 mm of radial length in the plaster group with the fixator group maintaining the reduced position. The authors concluded that a nonbridging external fixator was more effective in maintaining the reduced position of distal radial fractures.[171] The following year the same group published functional results in 106 patients under the age of 60 years with displaced distal radial fractures randomized between cast and nonbridging external fixation and confirmed the superiority of the external fixator in maintaining the reduced position. They reported better grip strength and a higher proportion of excellent results both subjectively and objectively in the external fixation group, although each group achieved similar proportions of satisfactory results.[172]

There is only one RCT comparing volar locked plating and nonoperative management. Arora et al. reported on 90 patients over 65 years with unstable distal radius fractures treated with a volar locked plate or manipulation under anesthetic and plaster management. Radiologic results were superior in the plated group, which was reflected by better grip strength in this group. The DASH and PRWE scores showed early advantages in the plated group but this was not sustained at later follow-up. The operative group had a higher complication rate (36% vs. 11%) with a 22 % tendon complication rate and a 31% secondary surgery rate.[16]

One study compared both external fixation and ORIF as a combined operative group with nonoperative management in patients over the age of 65 years with displaced distal radius fractures. Not surprisingly, the operative group not only had

better radiologic results but also had improved grip strength and supination. There were no significant differences in the mean DASH scores which were 12.1 for the nonoperative group and 10 for the operative group. The nonoperative group were significantly older which may have had an impact on the results.[92]

AUTHOR'S PREFERRED TREATMENT FOR NON-OPERATIVE MANAGEMENT OF FRACTURES OF THE DISTAL RADIUS AND ULNA

Undisplaced or minimally displaced fractures are treated without manipulative reduction. I define minimal displacement as fractures without carpal malalignment, less than 10 degrees of dorsal tilt and less than 3 mm of ulnar variance. Undisplaced or minimally displaced fractures are treated in either a forearm cast or removable splint with radiologic review at 1 week. If the fracture is undisplaced, the risk of metaphyseal instability is calculated at less than 70%, and the position has not changed, the patient is reviewed at 3 weeks and if x-rays are satisfactory the wrist is mobilized.

For minimally displaced fractures, the risk of instability is calculated and if this is less than 70%, review is undertaken at 1 week. I recommend further radiologic review at 2 weeks and immobilization in a forearm cast for a total of 4 weeks from injury. In a low-demand patient who is not considered suitable for fracture fixation, immobilization is required only for pain relief. Radiologic review is only required at cast or splint removal to confirm union.

Displaced distal radius fractures are carefully assessed for risk of instability and articular malalignment. If there is articular displacement of more than 2 mm gap or step or if the risk of metaphyseal instability is greater than 70%, I recommend early operative reduction and stabilization. Calculation of the instability risk[234] is easily performed online (www.trauma.co.uk/wristcalc).

If there is acceptable articular alignment and the risk of instability is less than 70%, manual manipulative reduction is performed under regional anesthesia. Agee's technique is used if necessary to restore volar tilt (Fig. 32-13). If an acceptable reduction (Table 32-4) is obtained then the wrist is immobilized in the neutral position in a forearm back slab. If the reduction maneuvers fail then surgery is planned. Reduced fractures are reviewed at 1, 2, and 3 weeks with the back slab being completed or replaced with a full forearm cast at 1 week. Cast immobilization is maintained for 4 to 6 weeks depending on the evidence of radiologic healing and the patient's symptoms.

Operative Treatment

There are a number of methods of operative treatment available for distal radius fractures including closed reduction and percutaneous pinning, ORIF, different types of external fixation, or combinations of each type of treatment. The indications for each are complex and relative and are to some extent guided by the type of fracture.

As indicated in this chapter on the section on epidemiology, around 60% of distal radius fractures are extra-articular and almost one-half of almost all distal radius fractures are likely to have metaphyseal instability. Of the total, one-third are articular fractures but fewer than 5% are complex articular fractures. A small proportion is volar displaced fractures including volar shearing fractures. For the purposes of making decisions about surgical treatment, three groups should be considered: metaphyseal unstable extra- or minimal articular fractures, displaced articular fractures, and partial articular fractures.

Metaphyseal Unstable, Extra- or Minimal Articular Fractures

These are the most common fractures requiring surgical treatment. Metaphyseal instability may be predicted or actual. A minimal articular fracture is one that has an articular component and that does not require articular reduction; most are undisplaced articular fractures (Fig. 32-14). In fit active patients with these fractures, reduction and stabilization is indicated to maximize the chance of good recovery. Metaphyseal unstable fractures can be stabilized by closed reduction and percutaneous pinning, ORIF, or external fixation. Closed remanipulation and plaster management was popular a number of years ago but has been shown to be ineffective by a number of authors.[250,251,324] This practice should be abandoned in favor of more stable fixation techniques.

Percutaneous Pinning. Percutaneous pinning of fractures of the distal radius was first suggested in the early 20th century and many different constructs of pins have been described.[295] The technique is appealing as it is minimally invasive and it has been widely used for the treatment of unstable extra-articular or minimal articular distal radius fractures as well as for intra-articular fractures.

Technique. Percutaneous pinning is performed under sterile conditions with the arm abducted on an arm board. The fracture should first be reduced and held either by an assistant or by finger traps. If intrafocal pinning is planned, complete reduction is not necessary as the pins are used as reduction tools. It can be of assistance to place the wrist in flexion over towels as this gives easier access for the dorsal ulnar pins.

There are three basic constructs for percutaneous pinning:

1. Distal radius pinning where pins are placed across the fracture in the distal radius. These may be only radial styloid

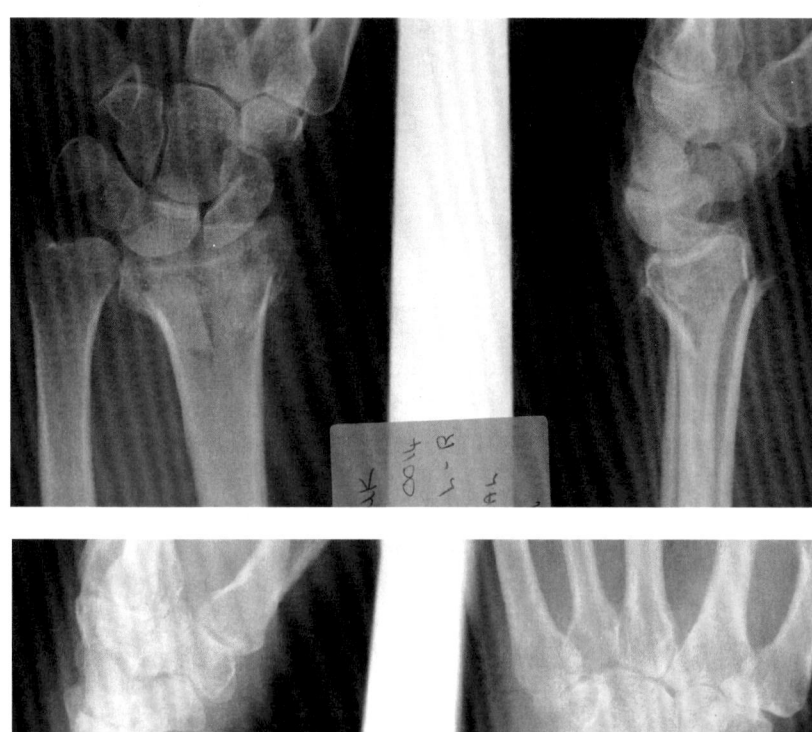

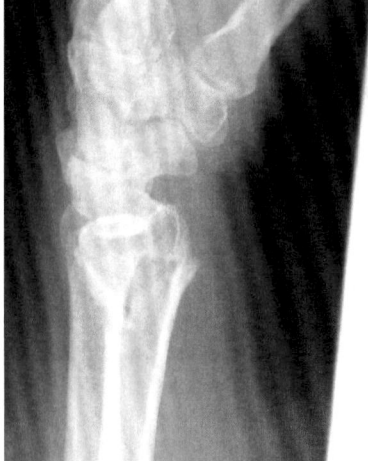

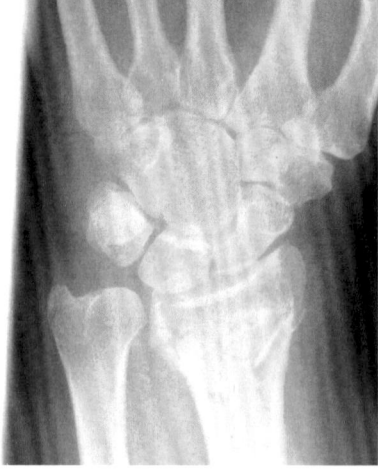

FIGURE 32-14 A: A minimal articular fracture of the distal radius. **B:** Despite initially successful manipulative reduction the fracture has lost position because of metaphyseal instability but the articular alignment is maintained.

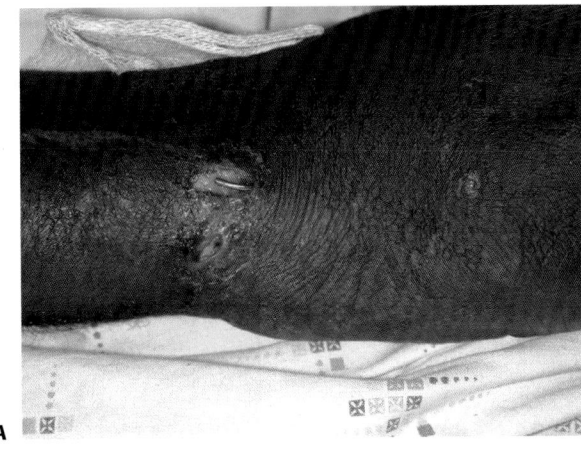

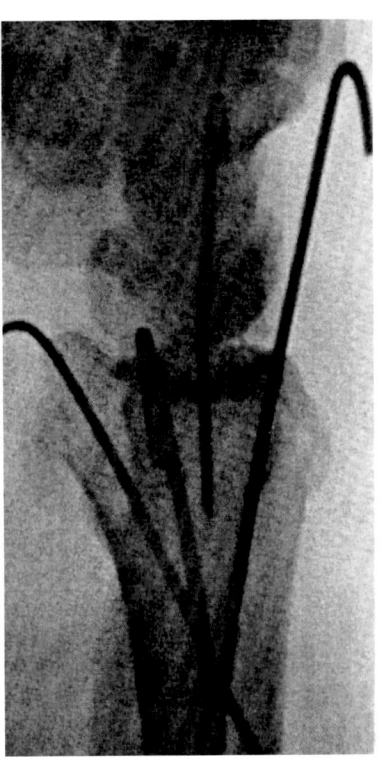

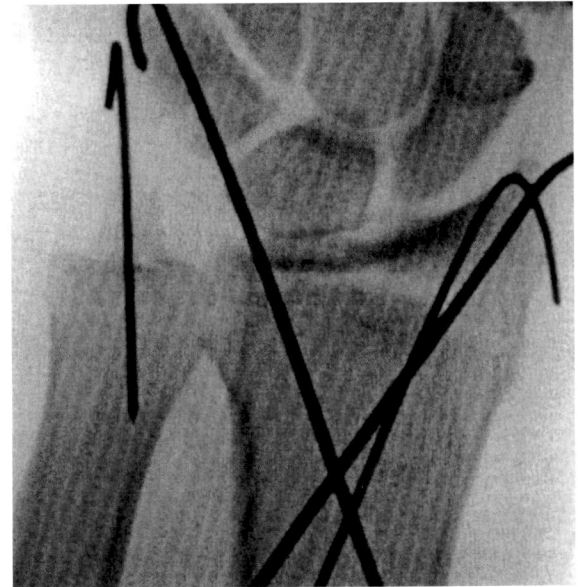

FIGURE 32-15 **A–C:** Comminuted radius fracture in a polytrauma patient treated with percutaneous pinning technique.

pins or may also include a pin from the dorsal ulnar aspect to the volar aspect of the radius.

2. Ulnar radial pinning where the pins are placed from the radius across the ulna.

3. Intrafocal pinning or the Kapandji technique where the pins are inserted into the fracture, used as reduction tools, and then driven into the proximal radius.

Whichever technique is used it is important to avoid damage to the dorsal sensory branch of the radial nerve or tendons which are close to the insertion points of both radial styloid and dorsal ulnar wires. A small incision should be made at the proposed point of pin entry with blunt dissection down to the bone to protect nerves and tendons.[56] Fluoroscopic control is used to confirm the correct placement of the K-wires. The styloid wire fixes the radial styloid to the radius and is usually placed first from a starting point on the lateral cortex of the radius either on or within 1 cm of the tip of the radial styloid.[55] The pin is then driven diagonally in an ulnar direction to engage the cortex proximal to the fracture on the ulnar side

of the radius (Fig. 32-15). The dorsal ulnar pin is placed from the dorsal ulnar corner of the radius and driven across the fracture to the volar radial cortex. Biomechanically, the use of two radial styloid and one dorsal ulnar pin is the most rigid construct.[262] These authors also recommend that at least a 0.062-in pin should be used.

For intrafocal pinning, pins are driven into the fracture site and used as levers to reduce the fracture (Fig. 32-16). Kapandji recommends three wires placed laterally, posterolaterally, and posteromedially. He describes making a small incision in the skin and using blunt dissection to avoid tendons and nerves.[182] A small vertical incision is made at the fracture site. On the radial side the pin is inserted in the plane between the tendons of extensor pollicis brevis (EPB) and abductor pollicis longus (APL) and the wrist extensors. The posterolateral incision is placed slightly lateral to and above Lister's tubercle and the pin is placed between the EPL and the tendons of EPB and APL. The posteromedial placement is in the fourth extensor compartment usually between the extensors of the ring and little fingers. The pins are introduced perpendicularly in the line of the

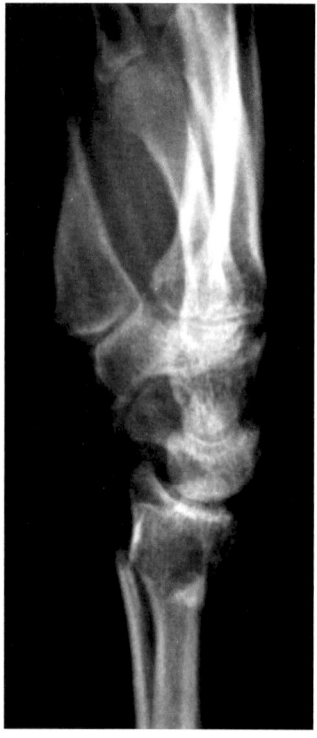
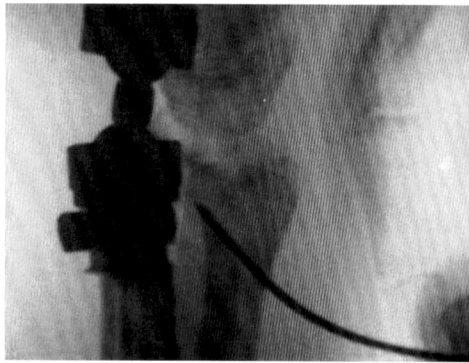
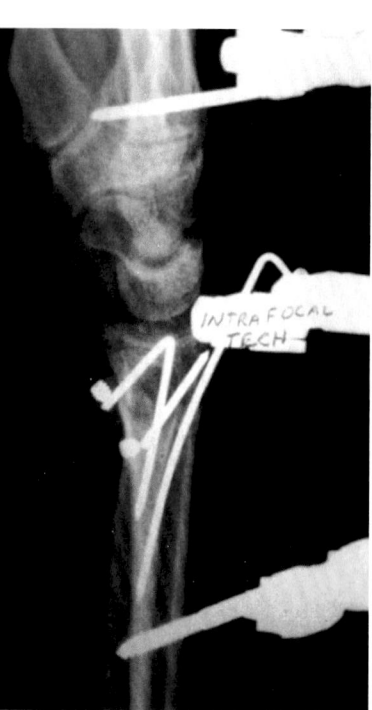

A, B

C

FIGURE 32-16 The Kapandji Technique: Metaphyseal fracture with redisplacement after reduction **(A)**. A pin is inserted into the fracture site, manipulated to elevate the fragment distally **(B)**, and then driven into the opposite cortex **(C)**. The fragments are thus trapped and prevented from dorsal displacement.

fracture and then inclined obliquely upward thus buttressing the cortex of the distal fragment. The pin is then driven into the opposite cortex of the radius.

Pins may be left protruding from the skin for ease of removal but a small RCT demonstrated lower pin track infection rates in wires buried below the skin.[147] This has the disadvantage of requiring a further minor procedure to remove the wires.

There are a number of controversies centered around percutaneous pinning for distal radius fractures. These include the best configuration of the pins, whether the pins should be buried, whether immobilization is required, and if so for how long.

Postoperative Immobilization. Although Kapandji stated, "plaster is strictly forbidden,"[182] most authors utilize a short arm cast for varying periods of up to 6 weeks after percutaneous pinning.[9,20,188,357] Allain performed an RCT of 60 patients using transstyloid pinning and compared 1 and 6 weeks in a cast. No difference was found between the groups, but only 24 patients had metaphyseal comminution, so the likelihood is that the majority were stable fractures. The author concluded that no plaster was required after percutaneous pinning but recognized that there was more loss of volar tilt in comminuted fractures.[9]

Type of Percutaneous Pinning. Neither intrafocal nor any type of extra-focal pinning has been shown to be superior. Lenoble[215] compared Kapandji fixation to transstyloid fixation with two pins in 96 patients with dorsally displaced distal radius fractures. No immobilization was used postoperatively for Kapandji pinning but a plaster was applied for over 6 weeks for the group treated with styloid pinning. Loss of reduction occurred in both groups with a worse loss of ulnar variance in the Kapandji group. There was better initial reduction in terms of volar tilt in the Kapandji group but some were overreduced in a volar direction. More complications occurred in the Kapandji group with sensory radial nerve symptoms and complex regional pain syndrome predominating. The Kapandji group had better movement at 6 weeks, which is not surprising as they were not immobilized, but they had more pain. Overall, there were disadvantages to Kapandji pinning but neither method performed particularly well considering that over half of the fractures had no comminution. A similar study was performed by Strohm et al.[358] comparing modified Kapandji pinning with two transstyloid pins. Radiologic results were not reported but 82% of the fractures had no comminution. The authors found better results in the Kapandji group but review times were not standardized and a significant number of patients were lost to follow-up leading to a recommendation that these results should not be considered as proven.[146] In a radiologic comparison of traditional Kapandji pinning versus modified Kapandji pinning with one transfocal radial styloid pin the latter gave better results.[131]

Outcome of Percutaneous Pinning

COHORT STUDIES. There have been a number of cohort studies examining the outcome of percutaneous pinning for distal radius fractures. Although some earlier papers were optimistic about the outcome of the technique[235,351] more recent papers have reported significant loss of position at final review.[38,188] This is particularly prevalent in older patients and patients with poor bone stock and comminuted fractures.[9,38,84,276]

RANDOMIZED CONTROLLED TRIALS. There have been a number of studies comparing percutaneous pinning with other methods. Stoffelen and Broos examined 98 patients with distal radius fractures randomized to Kapandji pinning and cast for 1 week or plaster cast for 6 weeks after closed reduction. The authors found no significant differences in the two groups for either functional or radiologic outcome.[357] Azzopardi et al.[20] found marginal radiographic advantage and no functional advantage in the use of percutaneous pinning. Wong et al. studied older patients and found small radiologic advantages in dorsal angulation but not in ulnar variance with the use of percutaneous pinning. They found no functional differences.[395] The only study to report anatomical and functional advantages of percutaneous pinning compared to cast management was in patients under 65 years of age.[305]

Three studies have compared the outcome of external fixation to percutaneous pinning. Ludvigsen[228] examined 60 patients with distal radius fractures with metaphyseal comminution randomized to bridging external fixation (average age 61 years) or percutaneous pinning (average age 58 years) reviewed at 6 months after injury. There were no significant differences in radiologic outcome, complication rates, or function as measured by the modified Gartland and Werley score. In a series of 50 younger patients aged less than 65 years and randomized to augmented bridging external fixation or percutaneous pinning, there were no differences in the radiologic outcome or DASH scores except for better articular surface reduction in the external fixation group.[148] Nonbridging external fixation allowed more rapid early rehabilitation than percutaneous pinning in a randomized study of 40 patients but no longer-term advantages.[111]

In the last few years there have been two retrospective comparisons and a number of prospective randomized comparisons of percutaneous pinning and ORIF with volar locking plates. The two retrospective studies found a greater loss of reduction with percutaneous pinning,[214,274] particularly ulnar variance, in patients with lower bone density measurements.[274] Locked plating demonstrated a faster recovery time and a better final grip strength in one study[274] but no significant differences in function in the other.[214] Two of the randomized studies showed no significant differences in the radiologic outcomes,[239,310] but one warned against overreduction with pinning in the presence of volar comminution.[239] All showed a consistent advantage in DASH scores for plating up to 6 months after injury.

There seems to be little advantage in the use of percutaneous pinning over plaster cast in older patients. Kapandji's published indications were primarily for younger patients with good bone stock and the use of this technique in older patients results in a significant secondary instability rate. This may be higher than is realized, as the definition of instability in most studies is vague. A number of studies use fractures without metaphyseal comminution, which suggest that many are stable fractures which would do well with minimal treatment. Comparison with external fixation or ORIF seems to show advantages in terms of earlier function in the external fixation and ORIF groups, but this may be because of earlier mobilization.

Complications of Percutaneous Pinning. The most common complication of this technique is damage to the superficial branch of the radial nerve which although poorly reported in some papers occurs in up to 15% of cases.[9,55,144,215] A number of authors note that it occurs after pin removal.[9,215] Placement of the pins should be done under direct visualization using small skin incisions and blunt dissection down to the bone. Care should be taken when removing pins that the incisions are large enough to ensure protection of the nerve.

Pin track infection is an often ignored complication of percutaneous pinning and is often poorly defined. Classification systems defining pin track infection are available[147] and should be used for research purposes, but in practice it is important to differentiate between minor and major pin track infections. Major pin track infection occurs when further surgery is required to eradicate the problem or the pins have to be removed early. The majority of pin track infections are minor after percutaneous pinning with rates recorded from 1.7% to 70%.[9,38,144,147,215,305] Major pin track infection occurs rarely with most authors reporting none. Burial of pins subcutaneously may contribute to avoidance of pin track infection, especially if the pins are in place for prolonged periods.[147]

External Fixation. External fixation for distal radius fractures was first used over 80 years ago and the first large series was reported by Anderson and O'Neill in 1944. The authors used K-wires into the metacarpal and the radius and described their technique as "castless fixation allowing full finger function."[13] The technique was not popularized until the late 1970s when Vidal et al.[380] described the principal of tension on the ligaments and capsule allowing reduction and coined the term "ligamentotaxis."

There are two different methods of utilizing external fixation, bridging or spanning fixation and nonbridging or nonspanning fixation (Fig. 32-17). Bridging external fixation employs pins in the second metacarpal and the radial shaft thus bridging the radiocarpal, intercarpal, and carpometacarpal joints and depends on ligamentotaxis. It may be static, dynamic, or augmented. Nonbridging external fixation employs pins in the distal fragment of the fracture and in the radial shaft and allows direct fixation of the fracture.

Bridging External Fixation

Indications. The most common indication for bridging external fixation is actual or predicted instability in the dorsally displaced extra-articular or minimal articular fracture of the distal radius, especially where the distal fragment is too small to allow nonbridging external fixation. It can also be used for severe articular fractures (see below) and open injuries.

Technique. The patient is placed supine on the operating table with the arm abducted to 90 degrees and placed on an arm table. A tourniquet is used on the upper arm. The surgeon sits in the axilla and the C-arm is brought in from the opposite side and diagonally to allow room for an assistant.

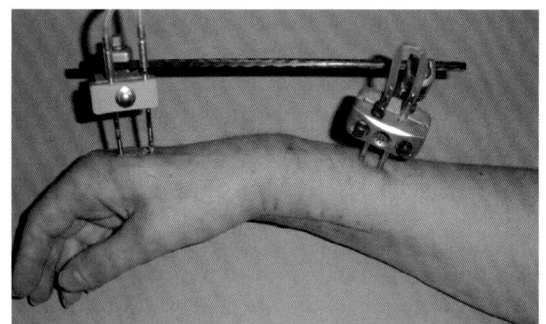

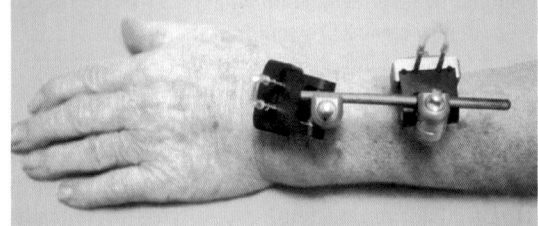

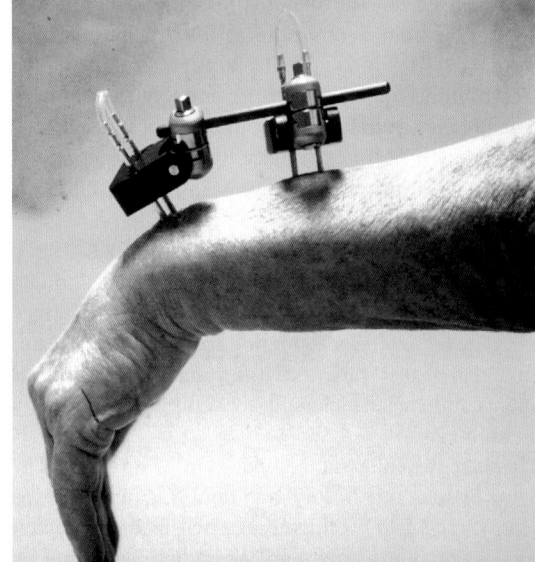

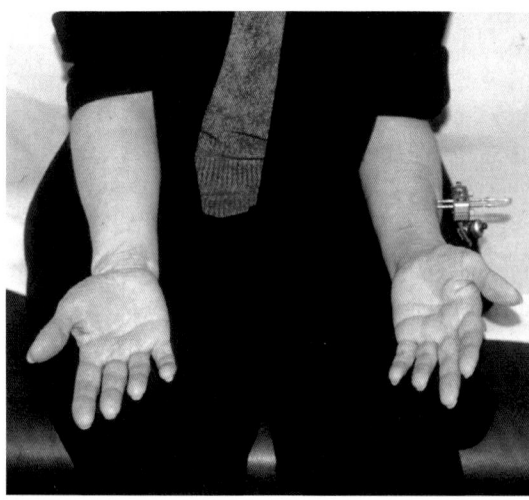

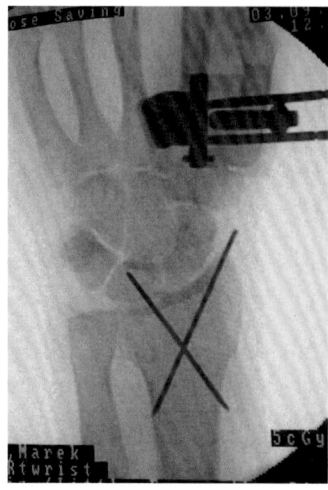

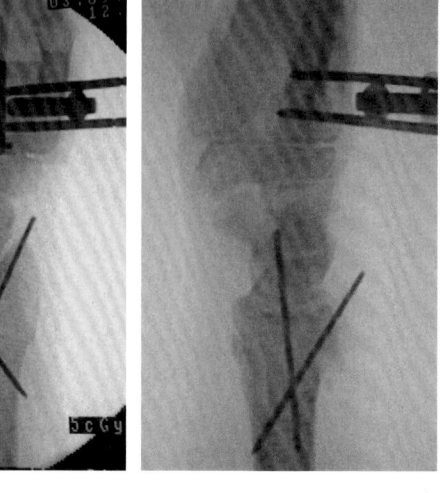

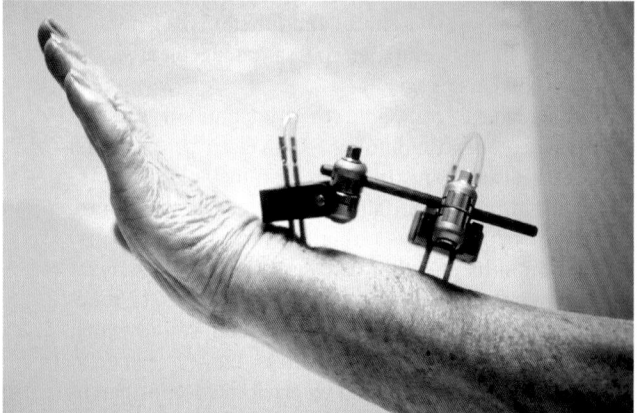

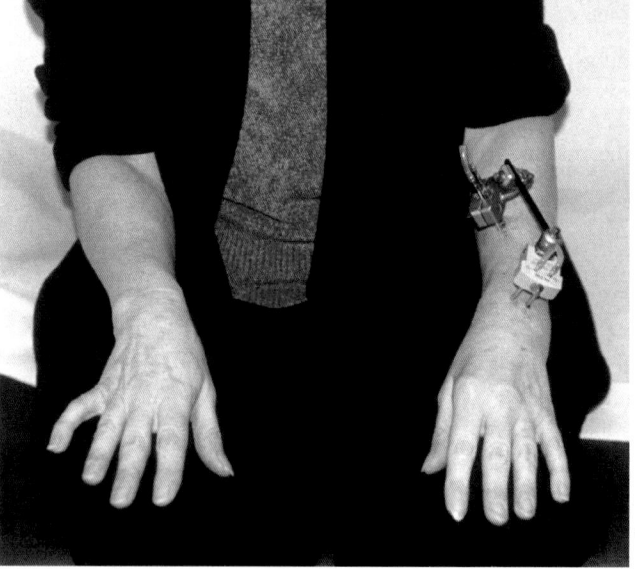

FIGURE 32-17 A: A bridging external fixator. The distal pins are fixed in the second metacarpal and the proximal pins in the radius immobilizing the radiocarpal, intercarpal, and carpometacarpal joints. **B:** Augmentation of a bridging external fixator with K-wires. **C:** A non-bridging external fixator with the distal pins proximal to the radiocarpal joint allowing early mobilization of the wrist **(D–G).**

The technique is similar regardless of whether the fixator is to be used as a static, dynamic, or augmented device. Two pins are first placed in the second metacarpal, the proximal of which should be close to the second carpometacarpal joint, which can be easily palpated. Either one or two incisions may be used depending on surgeon preference and are placed on the lateral side of the metacarpal in the gap between the extensor tendon and the first dorsal interosseous muscle. The incision is made down to bone and the pin track is first drilled using a drill diameter which is narrower than the thread diameter of the pin to be used. The drill should be placed at about 45 degrees to the frontal plane. A pin is then inserted by hand and should engage both cortices. A second pin is then placed more proximally in the same manner, using a template if necessary.

The proximal pins are placed in the radial diaphysis. A 2- to 3-cm longitudinal skin incision is made at the level of the junction of the middle and distal thirds of the radius. This is then deepened using blunt dissection to protect the superficial branch of the radial nerve. The radius is exposed by retraction of the brachioradialis muscle and superficial radial nerve allowing the proximal pins to be placed in the midlateral position. Clamps are then applied to the pins. There should be sufficient room to allow access for cleaning of the pin tracks. This can be ensured by placing a finger between the clamp and the skin as the clamp is tightened. A bar is then placed between the clamps.

The fracture is then reduced using the techniques described above and the fixator tightened. Care must be taken not to overdistract the wrist, which can be recognized by widening of the radiocarpal joint (Fig. 32-18) or by measuring the carpal height ratio. In cadaveric work it has been shown that wrist distraction of more than 5 mm increases the load required to generate metacarpophalangeal joint flexion,[282] although the results of clinical studies are conflicting, with some showing adverse effects of distraction[180] and others finding no disadvantage in distraction provided the distal radioulnar relationship is maintained[33] or provided the distraction is moderate.[48] At the end of the procedure the pin incisions should be examined to ensure that there is no tension on the skin edges and should be extended if necessary. Sutures are not required and may lead to skin tension around the pins.

Augmentation. Bridging external fixation can be augmented by percutaneous K-wires, limited ORIF with plates, bone graft, or bone substitute. The commonest method is with K-wires, which are inserted in a similar manner to percutaneous pinning (Fig. 32-17B). Bone graft or bone substitute may also be used where there is a large metaphyseal defect and are usually introduced through a small dorsal incision. Augmentation by using a fifth pin inserted dorsally into the distal fragment has been described[39,389] and is placed in a similar fashion to distal pins for nonbridging external fixation.

Postoperative Care. The presence of external fixation pins requires regular dressings to prevent pin track infection. A simple dry dressing is sufficient, changed twice weekly with cleansing of the pin sites with sterile saline if necessary. No benefit has been demonstrated by the use of hydrogen peroxide for cleaning or antiseptic dressings.[91]

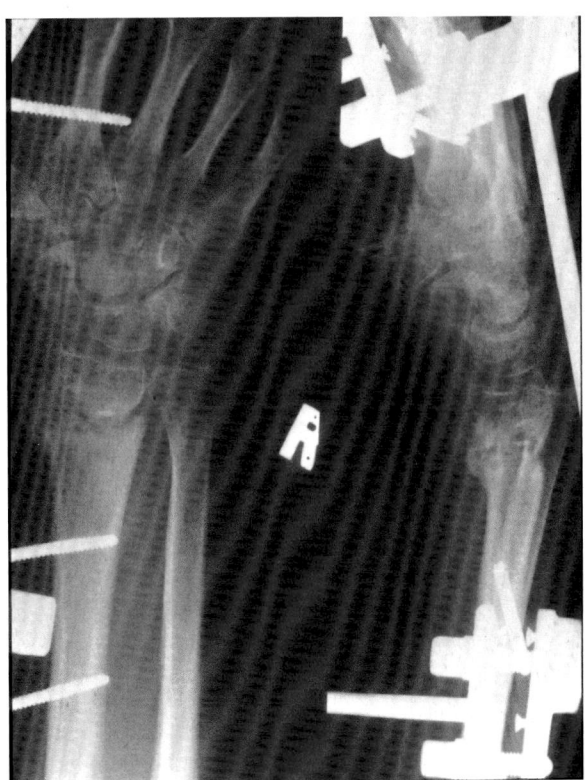

FIGURE 32-18 A bridging external fixation which has caused distraction of the wrist joint. There is regional osteoporosis raising the possibility of complex regional pain syndrome.

The patient should be instructed to mobilize the hand, elbow, and shoulder. Physiotherapy is required if any finger stiffness is detected. The fixator is usually removed at around 6 weeks. Removal does not usually require anesthetic.

Outcome

COHORT STUDIES. Most authors agree that with bridging external fixation alone unstable fractures of the distal radius will redisplace by varying degrees. Significant loss of reduction was reported by McQueen et al.[250] in 14 of 60 cases; furthermore, 10 of the 60 cases did not fully reduce with closed reduction. Twenty-four of sixty patients were considered to have malunion. At 1-year grip strength was around two-thirds of the opposite normal side, although recovery of movement was an average of 89% of the opposite wrist. Although the anatomical results were better with bridging external fixation than cast management, the functional results did not show clear benefit. The authors attributed this to the failure of either technique to restore volar tilt and therefore carpal alignment, which was significantly related to function.

In a series of 641 distal radius fractures treated with external fixation, 230 patients were treated in bridging fixators. Twenty-four percent had a malunion at final review despite successful initial reduction.[151] Similar findings of improved radiologic outcomes, but similar functional outcomes to those treated in a cast, have been reported by others.[8,203,250] Other authors have found that bridging external fixation fails to regain or maintain the volar tilt.[194,392] Wilcke et al. treated 30 patients with distal radius fractures with bridging external fixation but excluded those with severe comminution, which are the most likely to be unstable. Even so nine patients had residual dorsal angulation after healing.[392]

Augmentation of bridging external fixation has been suggested to reduce loss of reduction. Dicpinigaitis et al. reported that in a series of 70 cases treated with bridging external fixation augmented with percutaneous pins, half of the fractures lost more than 5 degrees of initially reduced volar tilt. However, no cases deteriorated sufficiently to be considered radiologically unacceptable.[82] Lin et al. reported a retrospective comparison of 20 cases treated with bridging external fixation without augmentation and 36 cases with augmentation of the bridging external fixator using percutaneous pins. They demonstrated that bridging external fixation alone did not regain volar tilt and that augmentation was better at retaining the initial reduction and provided a better range of movement and grip strength.[221]

Augmentation of bridging external fixation with a fifth pin inserted dorsally in the distal fragment and attached to the fixator was first described in 1994.[39] In 10 cases in which volar tilt could not be restored by closed reduction, volar tilt was regained and maintained by the addition of a fifth pin. Improvement in both radiographic and functional results using the five-pin technique was demonstrated in an RCT in 2003.[389] This technique combines the advantage of nonbridging external fixation with a disadvantage of bridging external fixation and probably does not have any advantages over the nonbridging technique.

Bone grafting or insertion of bone substitutes into the metaphyseal defect after reduction and bridging external fixation can assist in maintenance of the reduction[318,372] and may allow earlier removal of the fixator at 3 weeks without loss of reduction.[218] Bone substitutes seem to be equally effective to autograft[318,372] and are probably preferable to avoid graft donor site complications.

RANDOMIZED CONTROLLED TRIALS. Since the late 1980s, there have been a number of RCTs comparing bridging external fixation with other methods of treatment for distal radius fractures. Analysis of any RCT for the treatment of distal radius fractures is frequently hampered by varying definitions of instability, with widely varying inclusion and exclusion criteria, which makes comparisons difficult. Instability for these purposes should be defined as a fracture which has redisplaced in plaster or which can be predicted to have a chance of instability of more than 70%.[234]

Despite this, there largely seems to be a consensus amongst authors of RCTs or pseudo-RCTs, which compare bridging external fixation with cast management. All authors agree that bridging external fixation results in a better anatomical position than nonoperative management,[8,57,160,164,203,250,308,341] but most reported that improvement is not reflected in the functional results.[160,203,250,308,341] For patient-orientated measures the only series that reported DASH scores showed no differences,[8] whereas Christensen reported improvement in the Gartland and Werley scores for external fixation at 3 and 9 months after injury.[57] Some authors reported either a trend toward better function[164,203] or improvement in a small number of objective

surgeon-orientated outcomes.[8] However, these advantages in anatomy and function were usually accompanied by an increase in early complications,[160,341] usually because of minor pin track infection or radial nerve irritation.

Augmented bridging external fixation has not been compared in a prospective RCT with cast management. The only reported RCT on the subject is a comparison of standard nonaugmented bridging external fixation with bridging external fixation augmented by a fifth pin in the distal fragment.[389] Fifty patients with an unstable dorsally angulated distal radius fracture were randomized. Restoration and retention of reduction was better in the five-pin group as was the range of movement and grip strength. The authors concluded that their clinical findings supported the concept of augmentation of bridging external fixation of unstable distal radius fractures.

Dynamic bridging external fixation for unstable distal radius fractures was popular in the 1990s and was achieved by using bridging external fixators with a built-in hinge, which was released at 2 to 3 weeks after application of the fixator. No advantage has been identified with the use of this technique.[163,250,343]

Bridging external fixation has been compared with open reduction and plating for distal radius fractures in a number of randomized studies in the last 5 years.[2,90,137,174,211,388,393] Four of these studies showed no differences in the patient-orientated scores (DASH and PRWE) at any time period,[2,90,137,211] and three showed subjective improvement for the first few months after surgery, which was not sustained by 6 months.[174,388,393] Early improvement in the recovery of the range of movement with plates was reported by some authors,[2,90,388,393] but in all of these studies, the patients treated with plates were allowed to mobilize their wrist early in the postoperative period whereas the external fixation device immobilized the wrist until its removal. Landgren et al.[211] extended the outcome studies on a previously reported study[2] to 5 years and found no differences in function between external fixation and plating.

Radiologic results were equivalent between plating and augmented external fixation in most studies.[2,90,137,174,388] When poorer radiologic results were reported, the bridging external fixator was not augmented in all cases.[393] Only two studies reported malunion rates. Jeudy et al.[174] reported a 31% malunion rate for external fixation and 30% for ORIF, with both methods allowing loss of reduction after surgery. Loss of correction in both groups was also reported by Abramo et al.[2]

Complication rates were similar for the two methods of treatment in most studies.[2,90,137,388,393] Egol et al.[90] reported a higher reoperation rate for plates, with most reoperations being caused by hardware problems. Grewal et al. found more tendon complications in their ORIF group, a number of which would be deemed major complications. All but one complication (acute compartment syndrome) in the external fixation group were minor, mainly minor pin track infections.[137]

Esposito et al. undertook a meta-analysis of nine studies and concluded that overall there was very little clinical difference between the two methods of treatment. They cite lower DASH scores for plates but the difference did not reach the acknowledged clinically important difference of 10. They found that overall complication rates were similar but that external fixation had a higher rate of infection, although this was minor.[95]

Overall, therefore ORIF seems to allow earlier recovery than bridging external fixation in the first few months after fracture, probably because of the earlier mobilization the technique allows. Both Egol et al.[90] and Abramo et al.[2] allude to the better results for nonbridging external fixation compared with bridging external fixation because of direct fixation of the distal fragment, which may remove this advantage of plating. The rate of major complications or reoperation when plating is used is a disadvantage of the technique and may be a reason to use external fixation to limit the severity of complications when treating extra-articular or minimal articular unstable fractures of the distal radius.

Nonbridging External Fixation

Indications. The main indication for nonbridging external fixation is in fractures of the distal radius with actual or predicted instability, which are extra-articular or have an articular extension, which is undisplaced or reducible closed. There must be sufficient space in the distal fragment to site the pins. This usually requires 1 cm of intact volar cortex. The technique can also be used for displaced articular fractures if there is sufficient space for pins once the joint surface has been reduced and fixed. Nonbridging external fixation can also be used for distal radial osteotomy for dorsal malunion.

Technique. Positioning is similar to that for bridging external fixation except that the surgeon sits at the head end of the patient, as the distal pins are placed from dorsal to volar.

The distal pins are placed first usually from dorsal to volar, although some fixators use radial-sided pins. For dorsal to volar placement, a marker is placed on the skin at the estimated point of entry of the pin into the distal fragment. With the forearm in the lateral position, an image is obtained. The proximal end of the pin track incision should be level with the point of entry of the pin into the bone. The ulnar pin is placed first and should be on the ulnar side of Lister's tubercle in the ulnar corner of the radius (Fig. 32-19A); care should be taken not to penetrate the distal radioulnar joint. A 1-cm longitudinal incision is made in the skin at the appropriate point and deepened until the extensor retinaculum is visualized. A longitudinal incision is then made in the retinaculum taking care to avoid damage to any underlying extensor tendons. Using blunt dissection, the tendons are retracted until the bone is palpated. A pin is then placed on the bone, half way between the fracture and the radiocarpal joint on the lateral view (Fig. 32-19B) and its starting point is checked with the fluoroscope. The pin is adjusted until it is parallel to the radiocarpal joint on the lateral view and is then inserted by hand without predrilling into the distal fragment. The pin should penetrate the volar cortex (Fig. 32-19C). The forearm is then rotated to confirm free rotation and exclude penetration of the distal radioulnar joint. A second pin is then inserted in a similar manner on the radial side of Lister's tubercle using the clamp of the fixator as a template if necessary.

Two proximal pins are then placed in the radius proximal to the fracture in a similar fashion to that used for bridging exter-

nal fixation except that their position is usually more dorsal to volar than midlateral. Once the skin and subcutaneous tissues are opened, the interval between the flat tendons of extensor carpi radialis longus and extensor carpi radialis brevis can be seen. This interval is developed and the radius is exposed (Fig. 32-20). These pins are usually predrilled as it is more difficult to control their path in cortical bone.

The fixator is then assembled maintaining adequate space between the clamps and the skin to allow access for pin track dressings. The fracture is reduced by using the distal pins as a "joystick" to control the position of the distal fragment (Fig. 32-19D). Care should be taken to avoid overreduction where there is volar comminution (Fig. 32-19E). As the distal pins move with the reduction, they should move into the centre of correctly placed skin incisions, but each pin track should be released if there is any residual tension. Sutures should not be used on the pin tracks to avoid tension on the skin, which may lead to pin track infection.

Postoperative Care. Pin track care is carried out as for bridging external fixation. No other form of immobilization is necessary and the patient is encouraged to move the hand and wrist fully. Physiotherapy is not usually required unless finger stiffness develops. The fixator is usually removed after 5 to 6 weeks. Anesthesia is not required for removal.

Outcome of Nonbridging External Fixation

COHORT STUDIES. There are a number of cohort studies which report the outcome of nonbridging external fixator for extra- or minimal articular unstable fractures of the distal radius. The first study of the technique was published in 1981 in 22 cases of redisplaced distal radius fractures with an average age of 64 years. The authors reported 21 good or excellent results and concluded that the nonbridging external fixator maintained the reduced position and allowed rapid restoration of good function in the wrist and hand.[107]

Since then, a consensus has developed that nonbridging external fixation restores and maintains volar tilt[12,100,104,151,249,252,259] and carpal alignment[104,151,249,252] in patients of varying ages. Radial length is restored with a small increase in ulnar variance after removal of the fixator.[12,100,104,151,249,252] In a retrospective radiologic comparison of 588 bridging or nonbridging external fixators Hayes et al.[151] reported a 6.2 times increased chance of dorsal malunion in bridging external fixation compared with nonbridging external fixation and a 2.5 times increased chance of radial shortening in the bridging group.

Functional results in cohort studies are equally good. Andersen et al.[12] reported 88% excellent or good results with the Gartland and Werley score and concluded that nonbridging external fixation is a reliable method of maintaining radiologic reduction with a good functional outcome after 1 year. Flinkkila et al. reported 90% restoration of grip strength and up to 97% restoration of movement at a mean of 16 months after fracture and concluded that nonbridging external fixation is an easy, minimally invasive, and reliable method that restores the anatomy and function after unstable fracture of the distal forearm. The authors consider it their treatment of choice for these fractures.[104]

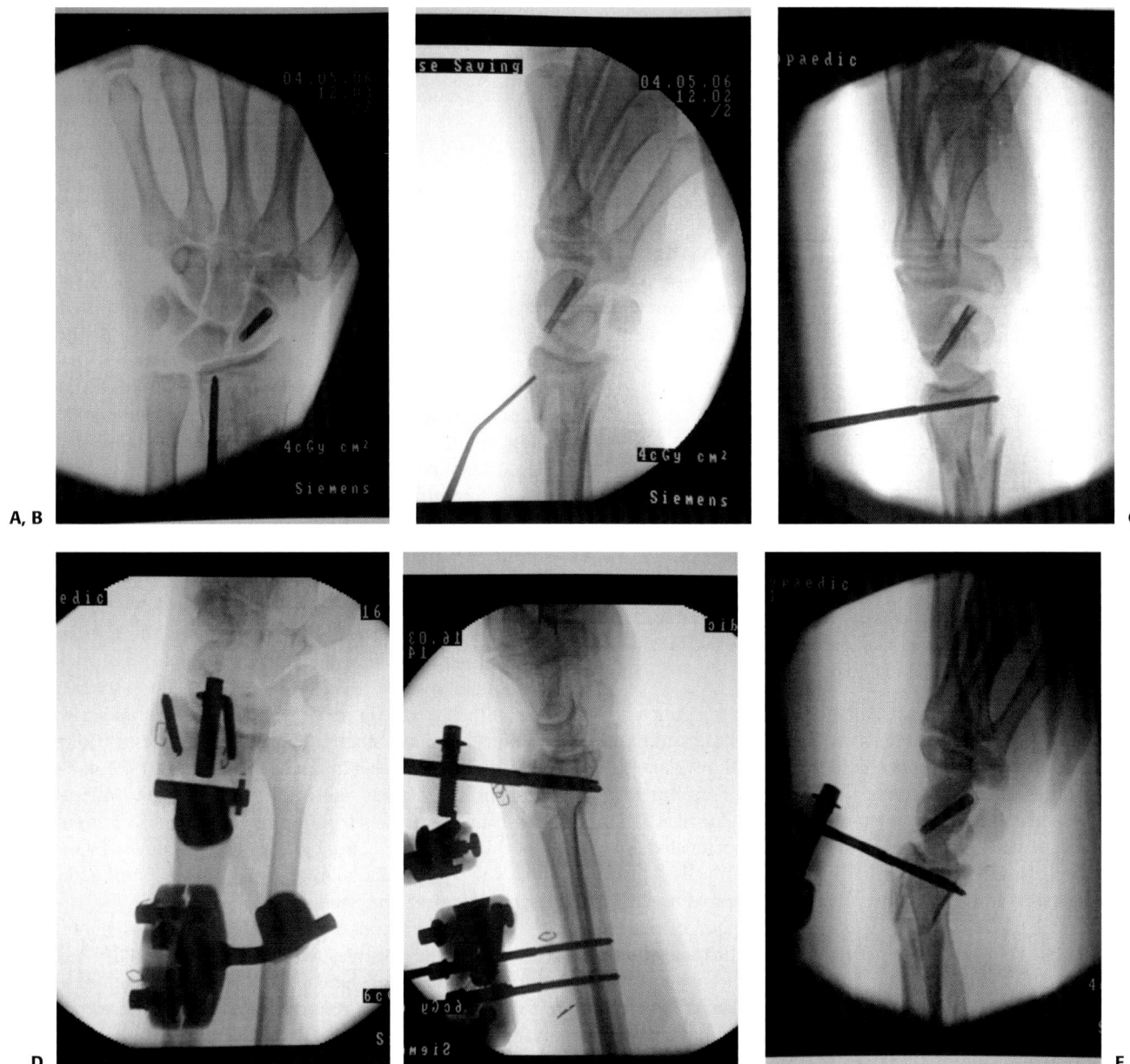

FIGURE 32-19 A: Placement of the distal pins for a nonbridging external fixator. On the AP view the ulnar pin starting point is shown. **B:** A marker on the starting point on the lateral view which should be halfway between the fracture and the joint. **C:** The pin is parallel to the radiocarpal joint and engages the volar cortex **D:** Reduction has been achieved by using the distal pins as a joystick **E:** Where there is volar comminution or bayoneting it is possible to overreduce the fracture in the volar direction.

The ease of the technique was demonstrated by Hayes et al.[151] who reported on the success of the technique in the hands of surgeons in training thus confirming its generalizability.

RANDOMIZED CONTROLLED TRIALS. The first randomized study to include nonbridging external fixation was reported in the late 1980s. Jenkins et al. initially reported radiologic results of external fixation versus cast management with their first two cases utilizing pins in the second metacarpal. The authors then concluded that "it seemed unnecessary to cross the wrist joint with a frame if a satisfactory hold could be obtained in the distal fracture fragments" and used nonbridging external fixation for their next 30 cases. They compared these with 26 cases treated in plaster. All of their patients were under 60 years of age. There was a mean loss of reduction of 10.5 degrees of dorsal angulation and 3.7 mm of radial length in the plaster group with the fixator group maintaining the reduced position. The authors concluded that a nonbridging external fixator was highly effective in maintaining the reduced position of distal radial fractures.[171] The following year the same group published functional results in 106 patients under the age of 60 years with

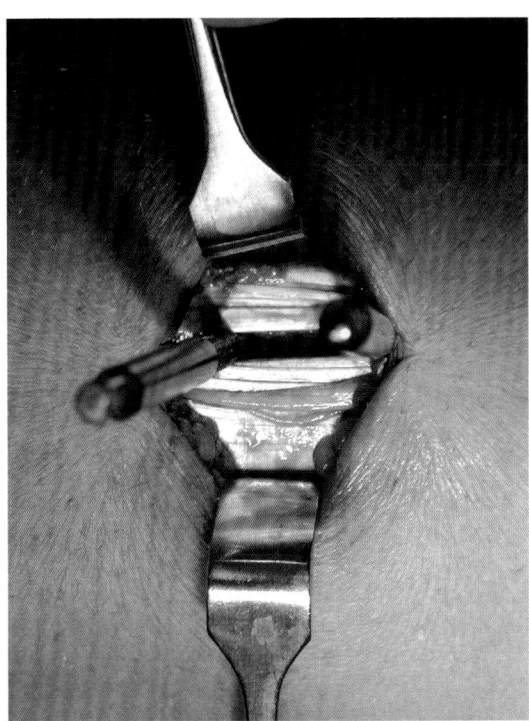

FIGURE 32-20 Pin position between the extensor carpi longus and brevis. Note the proximity of the dorsal sensory branch of the radial nerve. Iatrogenic injury to this nerve is a frequent cause of neurogenic pain after external fixation and may be minimized by open rather than percutaneous pin insertion.

displaced distal radial fractures randomized between cast and nonbridging external fixation and confirmed the superiority of the external fixator in maintaining the reduced position. They reported better grip strength and a higher proportion of excellent results both subjectively and objectively in the external fixation groups although each group achieved similar proportions of satisfactory results.[172]

McQueen reported on an RCT of nonbridging versus bridging external fixation in 60 patients with redisplaced fractures of the distal radius and an average age of 61 years. Because they had all redisplaced and all had metaphyseal comminution, there was little heterogeneity in the fractures. Both extra- and intra-articular fractures were randomized but displaced intra-articular fractures were excluded. Anatomical studies were statistically significantly better in the nonbridging group throughout the period of review. Nonbridging external fixation restored and maintained the volar tilt whereas bridging external fixation failed to restore volar tilt after reduction and had lost a mean of 8.6 degrees of tilt during and after the period of fixation. Nonbridging external fixation lost some radial length after removal of the fixator but at 1 year radial shortening was still only half that of the bridging group. Carpal alignment was restored in 28 of 30 patients in the nonbridging group but in only 13 of 30 patients in the bridging group at 1 year. There were 14 cases in the bridging group with malunion but none in the nonbridging group. It should be noted however that augmentation of the bridging group was not used in this study.[249] All ranges of movement were significantly

better in the early rehabilitation period in the nonbridging external fixation group, which was likely to be related to the freedom of wrist movement which the technique allows. Only the range of flexion showed sustained superiority with nonbridging external fixation possibly because volar tilt was retained. Pain scores were low at 1 year and the groups did not differ significantly in this respect. The author concluded that nonbridging external fixation was significantly better than bridging external fixation and should be the treatment of choice for unstable distal radius fractures where external fixation is contemplated and where there is space for pins in the distal fragment.[249]

Since then, three further RCTs comparing bridging and nonbridging external fixation in patients with extra-articular or minimal articular fractures of the distal radius have been reported.[19,208,373] All demonstrated better reduction in the nonbridging groups. The DASH score was used in two studies with no differences in one[19] and better DASH scores in the nonbridging group in the other.[208] The former study reported better early SF-12 physical health scores for the nonbridging group but no differences in pain scores.

There is only one RCT comparing nonbridging external fixation with percutaneous pinning. Similar ranges of movement and grip strength were found in each group but there was a higher proportion of excellent and good results with nonbridging external fixation. The study concluded that nonbridging external fixation had the advantages of early restoration of function, easy reduction, and free use of the hand during the treatment period.[111]

There has been one report of an RCT comparing nonbridging external fixation to volar locked plating.[128] One hundred and two patients with an average age of 63 years were recruited. Fractures were dorsally displaced by more than 20 degrees and 93 were either extra-articular (AO/OTA A3) or minimal articular (AO/OTA C2). The authors found that the surgery time was significantly less in the nonbridging external fixation group. Restoration of volar tilt was achieved in all cases in the nonbridging external fixation group but in none of the volar locked plating group. One year after surgery there were no differences in range of movement, grip strength, or pain. Although volar flexion was significantly better in the external fixation group at 6 months ($p < 0.03$) the difference of 7 degrees is unlikely to be clinically significant. The Garland and Werley, Castaing, and SF-36 scores were similar between the groups barring social functioning in the volar locked plate group at 8 weeks only. More differences are evident in the analysis of complications. There was a 10% prevalence of minor pin track infection in the external fixation group. There were two EPL ruptures in the external fixation group requiring reconstruction and four tendon problems in the volar locked plate group requiring further surgery. The overall complication rate was similar in each group (20% external fixation vs. 21% volar locked plate) but the more serious nature of the complications in the volar locked plate group is reflected in the reoperation rate of 36.5% in that group compared to 6% in the external fixation group.[128]

The main complication of nonbridging external fixation reported in cohort studies is minor pin track infection or irritation, defined as requiring antibiotic treatment and increased dressings but not compromising the final outcome. Rates range from 17% to 31% in cohort studies.[12,100,104,151] In a comparison between bridging and nonbridging fixation Hayes et al.[151] reported a three times increase of minor pin track infection with nonbridging compared with bridging external fixation, although this is not confirmed by RCTs despite some demonstrating a trend to more minor pin track infections in nonbridging external fixation.[19,249] No other complications occur more in either type of external fixation.

Complications of External Fixation

Pin Track Infection. The most common complication of external fixation is pin track infection. There are a number of classification systems for the assessment of the severity of pin track infections,[54,147,319] but practically it is important to differentiate between those which compromise the final outcome by early removal of the fixator or added surgical procedure (major pin track infections) and those which do not, merely requiring treatment with antibiotics and increased frequency of dressing changes (minor pin track infection).[151]

Rates of pin track infection reported in the literature vary from 0% to 39% for minor pin track infections.[2,6,12,19,91,104,163,208,249,259,390,393] Major pin track infections are rare in external fixation of the distal radius with none in most reports[12,19,91,104,163,208,390] and sporadic single cases in others.[100,249,250,393] In the biggest series of external fixation of distal radius fractures reported in the literature, minor pin track infection occurred in 126 of 588 cases (21%). Major pin track infection requiring early removal of the fixator or further surgery occurred in only 12 cases (2%).[151]

Other Pin Track Complications. Other pin track complications including pin track fracture, pin pull-out, and skin adherence are rare. The largest prevalence of pin track fracture was reported by Ahlborg with 11 pin track fractures in 314 cases of bridging external fixation, 5 in the radius, and 6 in the second metacarpal. Two of these were related to added trauma, one occurred during surgery, seven during the fixation period, and three after removal of the fixator. The authors found no relationship with pin track

infection.[6] In 588 cases, Hayes et al.[151] reported only three pin track fractures (0.5%), all in the second metacarpal. Pin track fractures that occur during treatment can be managed by resiting the pin; those occurring outwith this time should be treated by standard methods for the specific fracture.

Pin pull-out was originally cited as a potential problem for pins placed in the distal fragment with nonbridging external fixation but these fears have proven to be unfounded with only occasional cases occurring in both bridging and nonbridging external fixators.[151]

Tethering of the skin can occur after healing of the pin tracks but is poorly documented. Ahlborg and Josefsson[6] reported a 1% rate of surgery to correct skin tethering. This procedure is simple and can be done using local anesthetic.

Radial Nerve Damage. The superficial branch of the radial nerve runs deep to the brachial radialis muscle in the forearm and around 5 cm proximal to the radial styloid it emerges dorsally from beneath the brachioradialis tendon. At this point it is vulnerable to damage with insertion of the proximal pins of an external fixator. This is a preventable complication if care is taken to place pins using open incisions and the nerve is protected (Fig. 32-20).

The rate of damage to the radial nerve is reported to occur in between 0% and 13% of cases.[2,6,19,137,151,174,208,388,390,393] In one series there was a five-time increased prevalence with ORIF compared to bridging external fixation but this was with the use of a radial approach.[2] No study reports any difference in the rate of radial nerve injury between different types of external fixation with Hayes et al.[151] reporting a 1% rate in a large series of both bridging and nonbridging external fixations. Theoretically there may be an increased risk where percutaneous pins are used to augment a bridging external fixator but this has not been reported.

Joint Distraction. There is a risk that bridging external fixation will cause overdistraction of the radiocarpal and midcarpal joints with excessive force being applied in attempts to reduce a fracture (Fig. 32-18). This is usually measured by measuring the distance from the distal radius to the base of the third metacarpal and dividing that value by the length of the third metacarpal (carpal height ratio). The standard carpal height ratio is 0.54.[398]

Initial reports raised concerns that distraction of the wrist might lead to complex regional pain syndrome[180] or hand stiffness[180,282] and that outcome was compromised more with a longer duration of distraction. Biyani et al.[33] reported that distraction alone did not cause functional problems in seven patients with carpal distraction from 5 to 8 mm but if the distraction was sufficient to cause a negative ulnar variance then the result could be impaired. More recently, in a larger study of 42 patients with augmented external fixation for unstable distal radial fractures, Capo et al. found that the mean carpal height ratio in the group of patients with excellent results was 0.63 and of those with good or fair results was 0.58. The authors concluded that moderately increased distraction resulted in improved clinical outcome and did not cause subsequent joint stiffness but cautioned against extreme distraction, which

TABLE 32-5	Pitfalls and Prevention External Fixation	
Pitfall	**Prevention**
Bridging External Fixation	
Pin track infection	Ensure no skin tension
	Insert pins by hand, not power
Overdistraction	Examine fluoroscopic views for radiocarpal gap and carpal height ratio
Loss of reduction/ malunion	Always augment
	Use mini open reduction if closed reduction fails
Hand stiffness	Refer for physiotherapy at first signs
Radial nerve injury	Open pin placement
Nonbridging External Fixation	
Overreduction	Be wary if volar comminution, bayoneting volar cortex
Tendon injury	Open distal pin placement

could induce carpal malalignment, worsen intercarpal ligament injury, and induce finger stiffness.[48]

Plating. ORIF with plating is an alternative technique for stabilizing an extra-articular or minimal articular fracture of the distal radius. Plating was first popularized for volar displaced distal radial fractures by Ellis in 1965 with a plate which was placed on the volar surface of the radius and acted as a buttress to prevent volar displacement of the distal fragment.[93] Variations of the Ellis buttress plate were used for a number of years but only for volar displaced fractures.

The problem of maintaining the reduced position of a dorsally displaced distal radius fracture was first tackled with dorsal plating. This technique was designed to buttress the dorsally displaced fracture but had problems with soft tissue complications. Volar locking plates were then introduced to stabilize dorsally displaced fractures. As fixed angle devices, theoretically volar locked plates provide sufficient stability to the dorsally displaced distal fragments.

Volar Locked Plating

Indications. The main indication for volar locked plating in extra-articular or minimal articular displaced fractures is similar to that for nonbridging external fixation, namely for actual or predicted instability of a distal radius fracture, and there must be sufficient space for pins in the distal fragment. This technique is therefore contraindicated in cases with a very small distal fragment. Volar locked plating can be used for corrective osteotomy for malunion of the distal radius. It may also be used for volar displaced fractures, although in younger patients with good bone quality it is not necessary to use locking screws. It is advisable to use locking plates for volar displaced fractures in the older patient who is likely to be osteoporotic.

Technique

POSITIONING. Positioning of the patient is similar to that for other techniques with the patient supine and the arm abducted to 90 degrees, supinated, and placed on an arm table. A tourniquet is applied to the upper arm. The surgeon sits in the axilla and the C-arm is positioned diagonally from the opposite side of the arm table.

APPROACH. The approach used for the majority of distal radius fractures is the modified Henry's approach or trans-flexor carpi radialis (FCR) approach between the radial artery and FCR tendon. A longitudinal skin incision is used in line with the FCR tendon. The length of the incision depends on the plate size. The fascia is released to expose the FCR tendon, which is mobilized by incising the sheath. The tendon is then retracted in an ulnar direction and an incision made in the floor of the tendon sheath. This exposes the flexor pollicis longus (FPL) muscle belly, which is swept to the ulnar side by blunt dissection. The transverse muscle fibers of pronator quadratus are then evident and should be released from the radial side of the radius and elevated subperiosteally from the radius in a volar direction. A cuff of pronator quadratus should be left attached to the radius if repair is planned but there is no evidence that repair confers any advantage in range of rotation, pain levels, DASH scores, or prevention of FPL rupture.[155] The exposure should be as far radial

as the first dorsal compartment subperiosteally. The brachialis tendon may be released if necessary. This allows visualization of the dorsal surface of the radius, which is useful when fixation is late and early callus has formed dorsally. Further subperiosteal release dorsally allows the radius to be pronated away from the distal fragment. Articular displacement can then be seen and reduced and subarticular graft used.

The main limitation of this approach is visualization of the volar ulnar corner of the distal radius. The ideal position of a volar plate incorporates the volar ulnar corner with the ulnar side of the plate. Where there is an intra-articular fracture at the volar ulnar corner, it is mandatory to capture that fragment with the plate. In these circumstances, an approach between the flexor tendons and ulnar neurovascular bundle should be used. The incision for this approach is more ulnar over the ulnar border of palmaris longus. The flexor tendons are mobilized in a radial direction and the ulnar neurovascular bundle in an ulnar direction. The pronator quadratus is incised at its attachment to the ulna and elevated radially. This approach gives easy access to the carpal tunnel should the median nerve require release.

PLATE APPLICATION. The technique of volar plating for extra-articular or minimal articular fractures depends on whether the surgeon wishes to reduce the fracture manually or with the plate. Reduction with the plate allows easier restoration of the volar tilt. Screws are placed distally in the plate parallel to the joint surface in the lateral view, taking care not to penetrate the dorsal cortex (Fig. 32-21A). Pronated and supinated oblique views and a tilted lateral view are useful at this stage to ensure that the distal screws have not penetrated the radiocarpal or distal radioulnar joints (Fig. 32-5). The plate is then lying off the shaft of the radius. The proximal limb of the plate is then gently pushed on to the shaft, the so called lift technique[336] and fixed in place (Fig. 32-21B). This usually reduces the distal fragment in a similar manner to the joystick effect of nonbridging external fixation.

In volar displaced fractures the fracture must be reduced prior to application of the plate. The plate is then secured to the radial shaft using one screw, usually in an oval hole, which allows adjustment of the plate's position. The positioning of the plate is then confirmed on an image intensifier and adjusted distally or proximally as necessary to ensure correct placement of the distal screws. The plate should not be placed distal to the watershed line as this risks FPL rupture.[18] The distal screws are then inserted using oblique views or rotational fluoroscopy[344] to ensure that the radiocarpal or distal radioulnar joints are not penetrated. The length of the central two screws should be around 2 mm less than the measured length to avoid penetration of the dorsal cortex and to reduce the risk of tendon rupture. There is some evidence that inserting screws in all available holes in the distal fragment confers additional stability.[256]

In cases with a large metaphyseal defect there is a risk of subsidence of the fracture and migration of the screws into the radiocarpal joint. This may be prevented by augmentation by either bone substitute or grafting.[157,195]

Postoperative Care. Theoretically, after volar plating whether locked or not, there is no need for immobilization of the wrist

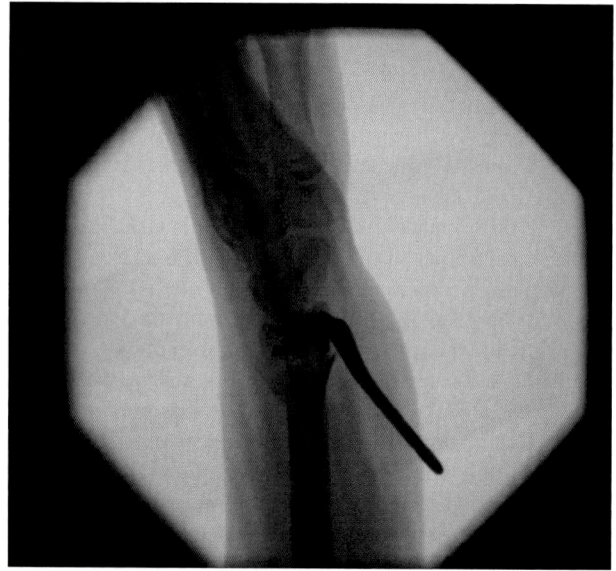

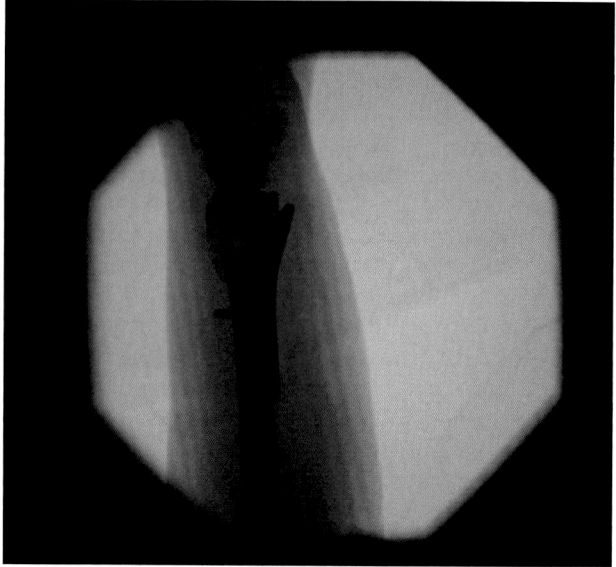

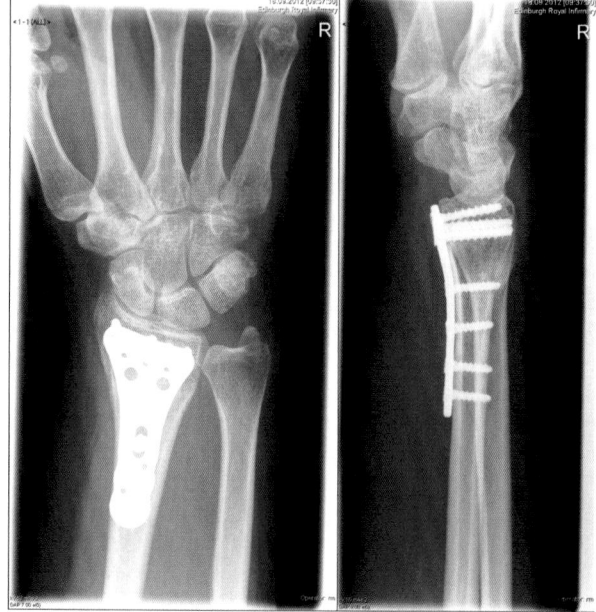

FIGURE 32-21 **A:** A volar plate has been fixed to the distal end of the radius in the unreduced position. The screws are parallel to the joint. **B:** The shaft of the plate has been reduced to the radial thereby reducing the fracture. **C:** AP and lateral views of the reduced fracture after healing.

as the fixation is very stable. However, in practice a plaster or splint is frequently used in the first few weeks.[62,98] Early finger motion is encouraged and wrist motion when comfort allows but certainly by 3 to 4 weeks after fracture.

Complications of Volar Locked Plating

Reported rates of complications after volar locked plating are high, ranging from 5.9% to 48%[16,90,128,195,366,393] with the majority of complications being hardware related. The main hardware-related complications are tendon rupture or irritation and screw penetration into the radiocarpal joint or DRUJ and frequently result in high reoperation rates.[16,90,128,195,317,393]

SCREW PENETRATION. Screw penetration into the radiocarpal joint or DRUJ is reported in a number of studies and ranges

from 3% to 57%.[16,85,195,311,317] Although screws may inadvertently be placed into a joint at the time of surgery this should largely be avoidable with the use of suitable imaging such as oblique and tilted lateral views. However, in patients with significant metaphyseal comminution, collapse around the plate is a concern with rates of collapse of up to 57% being reported.[17,145,195,311] As the plate is a fixed angle device the screws penetrate the radiocarpal joint as the fracture collapses (Fig. 32-22) which is more likely in a fracture with a small distal fragment as screws are of necessity close to the subchondral bone.[195] In intra-articular fractures there is also a danger of screws being placed in sagittal fracture lines allowing their migration into the joint.[317] Such penetration of the radiocarpal joint usually requires removal of the metalwork. It has been suggested that augmentation of the defect with bone substitutes

TABLE 32-6	Pitfalls and Prevention Volar Plating	
Pitfalls of Volar Plating	**Prevention**	
Fracture collapse/ malunion	Beware of overreduction of volar displaced fracture if dorsal comminution present	
	Ensure volar ulnar corner fragment captured by plate	
	Avoid screws in sagittal intra-articular fractures	
	Augment with bone substitute/ graft if large metaphyseal defect	
Tendon injury	Reduce measured size of distal screws by 2 mm	
	Ensure proximal screws not prominent dorsally	
	Ensure distal end of plate is proximal to watershed line	
	Look for signs of tendon irritation post-op and if present remove plate early	
Joint penetration by screws	Use oblique and tilted lateral views peroperatively	
	Examine flexion/extension and rotation at end of procedure	
	Prevent fracture collapse	

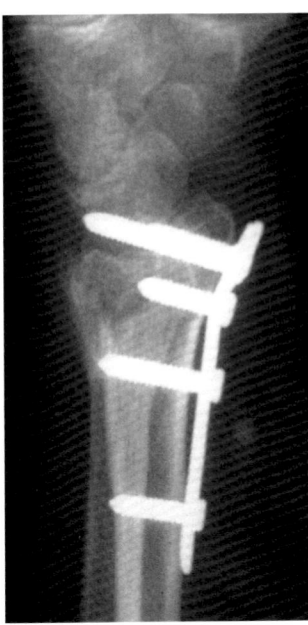

FIGURE 32-22 An unstable fracture of the distal radius fixed with a volar locked plate. The fracture has collapsed into dorsal angulation allowing the fixed angle screws to penetrate the radiocarpal joint. The leading edge of the plate is prominent risking flexor tendon rupture.

may prevent collapse.[195,317] This has been supported by cadaver experiments showing that subsidence of the distal fragment can be significantly decreased by augmentation.[157] However, in a recent RCT, no significant differences in radiologic or clinical measurements were found in elderly patients treated with volar locking plate with or without calcium phosphate bone cement augmentation.[191]

TENDON COMPLICATIONS. Hardware-related tendon problems are either tendon irritation or rupture and may involve flexor or extensor tendons with EPL and FPL being most commonly affected. A wide range of prevalences are reported from 0.8% to 19.6%.[16,85,195,311,359,366,391]

Extensor tendon pathology is likely to be related to screw prominence dorsally (Fig. 32-23) which can be difficult to visualize using radiographs because of the irregularity of the dorsal surface of the radius (Fig. 32-2) and the prominence of Lister's tubercle. Using ultrasound on 46 distal radius fractures treated with volar locking plates one study demonstrated that of 230 distal screws 59 were proud of the cortex distally and resulted in seven cases of tenosynovitis and two EPL ruptures.[359] Another study used CT and MR scanning to demonstrate that in a substantial number of cases the depth of the valley between Lister tubercle and the sigmoid notch was more than 2 mm.[284] Both sets of authors recommended that the measured length of the distal screws should be reduced by 2 mm and that symptoms of tenosynovitis should prompt hardware removal.

Flexor tendon irritation or rupture usually affects the FPL tendon although it has been reported in other flexor tendons.[183,391] It has been attributed to plate prominence, especially with placement distal to the watershed and was rarely reported as a complication of distal radius fractures before the advent of locked plating. A recent study analyzed the risk of flexor tendon rupture related to plate positioning and found that volar prominence of the distal end of the plate of more than 2 mm and plate positioning within 3 mm of the distal rim of the radius had high sensitivity and specificity for tendon rupture. Elective hardware removal after union was recommended in such cases.[193]

Outcome of Volar Plating

COHORT STUDIES. Despite initial enthusiasm, the radiologic and functional outcomes of volar locked plating for extra-articular and minimal articular distal radius fractures are similar to other techniques. Reported radiologic results indicate that volar locked plating is successful in restoring volar tilt and radial length[17,62,195,311] even in older patients.[61,98]

Functional outcome with volar locked plating is generally good with DASH scores ranging from 13 to 28.[17,98,195,311] Some of the differences are probably explained by the age of the patient with the oldest cohorts having the highest DASH scores.[98] Variations in the length of follow-up may also explain some of the differences. When other outcome measures are used, the percentages of good and excellent scores are usually high.

RANDOMIZED CONTROLLED TRIALS. There are now a number of RCTs comparing volar locked plates with other treatment methods, although they suffer from heterogeneity of inclusion criteria, especially in the definition of instability and the inclusion of both extra-articular and severe articular fractures.

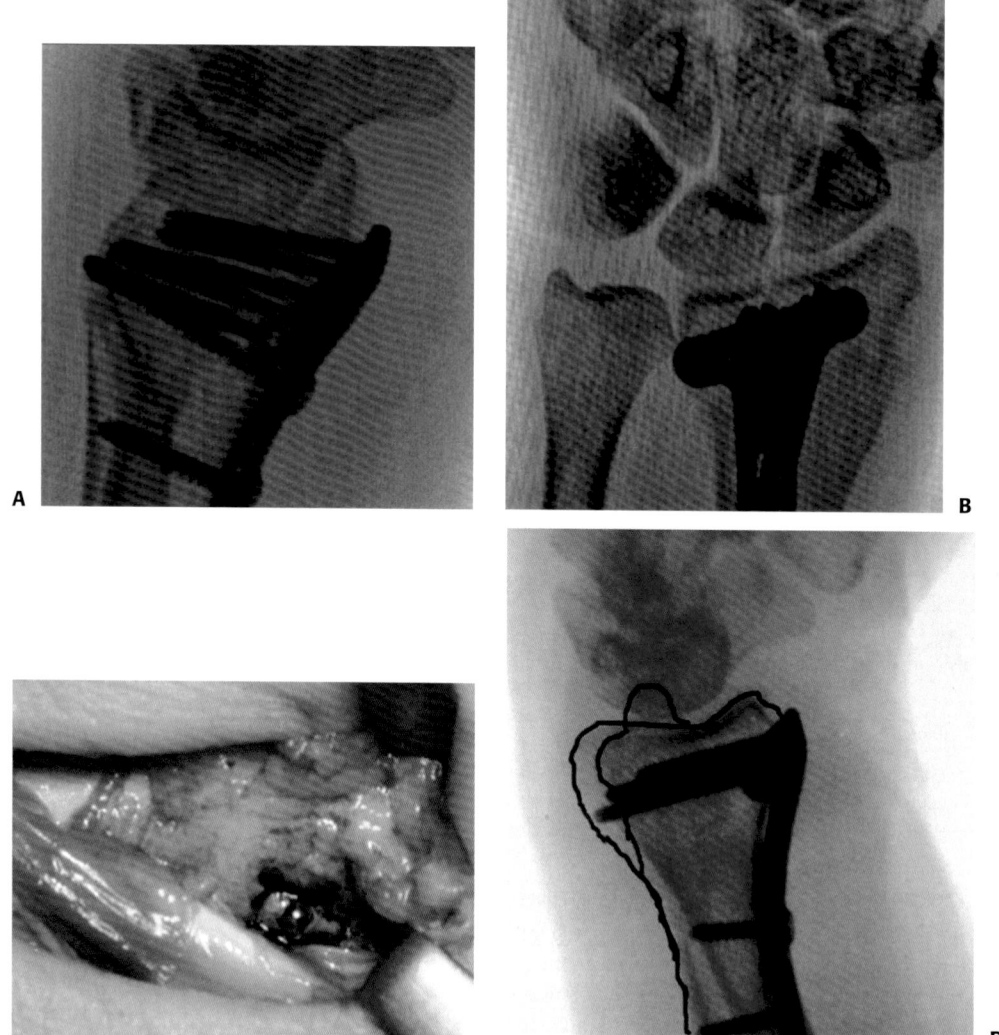

FIGURE 32-23 A, B: A patient with an extensor pollicis longus tendon rupture following palmar plate application. Note that on the initial lateral view from the OR **(A),** the screws appear to be well contained by the dorsal cortex. However, the Lister tubercle is the outline dorsally on the lateral view **(C, D)** and does not protect against dorsal cortical penetration either radially or ulnarly.

VOLAR LOCKED PLATING VERSUS NONOPERATIVE MANAGEMENT. There is only one RCT comparing volar locked plating and nonoperative management. Arora et al. reported on 90 patients over 65 years with unstable distal radius fractures treated with a volar locked plate or manipulation under anesthetic and plaster management. Radiologic results were superior in the plated group, which was reflected by better grip strength in this group. The DASH and PRWE scores showed early advantages in the plated group but this was not sustained at later follow-up. The operative group had a higher complication rate (36% vs. 11%) with a 22% tendon complication rate and a 31% secondary surgery rate.[16]

VOLAR LOCKED PLATING VERSUS EXTERNAL FIXATION. The largest number of RCTs compare volar locked plating and external fixation.[90,128,137,174,388,390,393] Six of the seven studies used bridging external fixation, five of which used augmentation with percutaneous pins.

Maintenance of reduction was achieved in both methods of treatment. Most studies found no differences in longer-term functional or patient-related outcomes, although some showed advantages to plating at the early stage of rehabilitation,[137,388,393] but this may reflect earlier immobilization in the plated group.

No studies found differences in the complication rates but when the types of complications are examined, some differences emerged. Westphal et al. reported that of 12 complications, 10 were minor in their external fixation group compared to 4 out of 4 major complications in their plated group. They recommended that all plates should be removed.[390] Grewal et al. reported that hardware-related tendon complications were significantly more frequent with their group treated with ORIF with a 23% rate of tendon complication. The external fixation group had a significantly increased infection rate but these were all minor pin track infections not requiring reoperation.[137]

There is only one study comparing nonbridging external fixation with volar locked plating.[128] The authors examined 102 patients randomized to either nonbridging external fixation or volar locked plating. They found that surgery time was significantly shorter in the external fixation group. Volar tilt was restored in all cases treated with external fixation but in none treated with ORIF. There were no significant differences in patient-related outcome scores. The complication rates were similar but the reoperation rate in the volar locked plate group was 36.5% compared to 6% in the external fixation group, reflecting the more major nature of complications encountered with volar locked plating.

VOLAR LOCKED PLATING VERSUS PERCUTANEOUS PINNING. Two RCTs have compared the use of volar locked plates versus closed reduction and percutaneous pinning.[245,311] Rozental et al. reported on 45 relatively young patients and found better early DASH and PRWE scores in the plated group but had mobilized this group earlier. There were no other significant differences barring an increased rate of minor complications in the form of minor pin track infection in the group treated with percutaneous pinning.[311]

In a later RCT the authors reported improved radiologic results, patient-related outcome scores, and fewer complications and reoperations in the plated group but this study suffers from a shorter review period of 6 months.[245]

DORSAL PLATING. Prior to the introduction of volar locked plates, dorsal plating was used for dorsally displaced extra-articular or minimally articular distal radius fractures. Theoretically, this technique should give improved stability as the plate is placed on the compression side of the fracture and acts as a buttress for dorsally displaced fractures. However, concerns about fracture collapse and tendon irritation or rupture have limited the use of this technique in extra-articular or minimal articular fractures although it is used in some displaced articular fractures.

Intramedullary Nailing.

In recent years there have been reports of the use of intramedullary nailing techniques for extra-articular or minimal articular fractures of the distal radius.[166,266,363,378] This technique requires closed reduction of the fracture and provisional fixation with percutaneous wires. The entry point for the nail is at the radial styloid between the first and second dorsal compartment. Reaming over a guidewire is necessary before introduction of the nail. Distal locking screws are placed subchondrally with a jig. Proximal locking is also used.

Two cohort studies have shown that the technique has good radiologic results although in common with most techniques allows slight shortening in terms of ulnar variance.[266] Good functional results have also been reported.[266,378] Reported complications are as yet few with some volar malunions and superficial radial nerve irritation. There is presumably also a risk of distal locking screw penetration into the radiocarpal joint and care must be taken to prevent this at surgery.

There are two comparative studies available, one an RCT comparing nonbridging external fixation and intramedullary nailing[326] and one retrospective comparison of cast management and intramedullary nailing.[363] The RCT showed better reduction of volar tilt in the external fixator group but better grip strength in the intramedullary nailing group, but only reviewed patients for 3 months after surgery. Patient-related outcome measures showed no significant differences between the two techniques.[326] In the retrospective comparison of intramedullary nailing and casting, it is not surprising that radiologic results were heavily in favor of the intramedullary nailing group. Restoration of function was better in the intramedullary nailing group.[363]

Clearly, the reported results of this technique are as yet limited and superficial radial nerve problems may be a concern, but intramedullary nailing may be an addition to the surgeon armamentarium.

AUTHOR'S PREFERRED METHOD OF TREATMENT FOR UNSTABLE EXTRA OR MINIMAL ARTICULAR FRACTURES OF THE DISTAL RADIUS AND ULNA (FIG. 32-24)

In low-demand patients with unstable extra- or minimal articular distal radius fractures, I do not recommend manipulative or operative treatment. The main effect of malunion of the distal radius is to reduce the individual's ability to undertake the activities of daily living which require strength in the hand and wrist. The frailer the patient, the less likely it is they will need such activities on a daily basis, which I believe explains the results of studies which show limited or no evidence of an advantage to frailer patients in restoration of normal anatomy by any means.[16,92,250] I therefore do not undertake any intervention in this patient group including manipulation. The deformity should be accepted with appropriate patient counseling and a plaster cast applied until the patient is comfortable mobilizing the wrist.

In the fitter, less dependent patients, my treatment of choice is nonbridging external fixation where there is space for pins in the distal fragment and when it can be predicted that the fracture is reducible by closed means. Augmentation with this technique is not required. I believe that the radiologic and functional outcomes of nonbridging external fixation and volar locked plating are similar in most cases but when complications are encountered, those associated with nonbridging external fixation are minor (usually minor pin track infection), do not result in reoperation, and do not affect the final outcome. In contrast, the complications associated with volar locked plating are usually major, result in a higher reoperation rate, and may affect the final outcome.

The external fixator is retained for 5 to 6 weeks and the patient is encouraged to mobilize the wrist and hand during this period. Removal is achieved in the outpatient setting and does not require a further anesthetic. Physiotherapy is rarely required.

Where the fracture is likely to be irreducible closed, usually because of marked bayoneting of the volar cortex or because there has been a delay in diagnosis and there is a nascent malunion, then I recommend open reduction and locked volar plating, provided there is room for screws in the distal fragment. It is important to counsel the patient about the risk of complications such as tendon rupture, fracture collapse, and the need for plate removal. If possible I use the lift technique

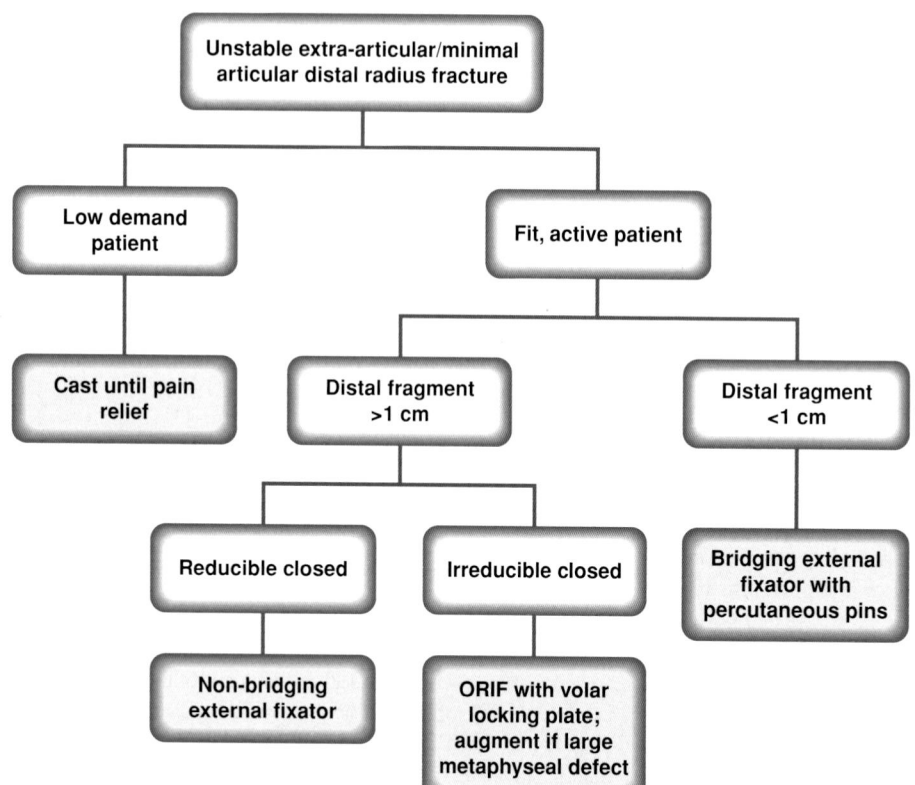

FIGURE 32-24 Management of the unstable extra-articular or minimal articular distal radius fracture.

(Fig. 32-21) to ensure restoration of the volar tilt. It is essential to ensure correct placement of the plate proximal to the watershed and to ensure that screws do not penetrate the dorsal cortex. If there is a large metaphyseal defect with a risk of fracture collapse, I augment the fixation with a bone substitute. Postoperatively, the wrist is placed in a removable splint for 10 days to 2 weeks after which the patient is advised to mobilize within limits of their comfort.

Where there is no space for pins or screws in the distal fragment, I use bridging external fixation augmented with percutaneous pins, one running diagonally from the radial styloid and extending through the cortex of the proximal radius and one from dorsal to volar in the midline. The fixator and pins are retained for 5 to 6 weeks when both are removed. I usually bury the percutaneous pins below the skin to reduce the possibility of pin track infection, so local anesthetic is required for their removal.

Displaced Intra-Articular Fractures

Although severe articular fractures account for less than 5% of distal radius fractures, they are the most challenging to treat. There remains debate about the effect of articular incongruity on the eventual outcome of these fractures but it is still recommended that intra-articular fractures with articular displacement of more than 2 mm in fit, active patients require surgical treatment (Table 32-4) (www.aaos.org/research/guidelines/drfguideline.pdf). However, as for extra-articular or minimal articular

fractures, nonoperative treatment with a cast for comfort is sufficient for the frail elderly patient. Articular fractures without articular displacement should be treated as extra- or minimal articular fractures.

Surgical treatment must address both the intra-articular displacement and any accompanying metaphyseal displacement and instability, so a combination of techniques may be required. Each fracture must be assessed to ascertain the fracture pattern and displacement of the fragments and a treatment strategy defined on this basis. A knowledge of the typical fracture patterns as described by Melone[257] is useful. He described four parts—radial styloid, dorsal and ulnar volar fragments, and the radial shaft (Fig 32-7). As the lunate impacts on to the articular surface, the lunate facet may be depressed as one or split into a volar and dorsal component with added central impaction. The impact of the scaphoid on the radial styloid typically causes a shearing fracture. An understanding of this mechanism is helpful to the surgeon in planning procedures.

Two techniques are used for the surgical treatment of displaced articular fractures: closed or percutaneous reduction of the articular surface with bridging external fixation to stabilize the metaphyseal comminution or ORIF. An RCT of the two techniques[204] demonstrated that if indirect reduction and percutaneous fixation was possible then better functional outcome was achieved compared to ORIF, provided the joint was reduced. If the closed method did not reduce the joint, the authors proceeded to ORIF. The authors recommended that open reduction be preceded by an attempt at a minimally invasive percutaneous reduction and if a good reduction is achieved then ORIF is unnecessary.

In practice, closed reduction and percutaneous fixation is generally possible in the less severe fractures, particularly when there is no volar ulnar fragment displacement. Traction radiographs are helpful to confirm the ability to reduce the metaphysis and the radial column. In general, residual compression is easier to correct percutaneously than residual rotatory displacement.

External Fixation with Percutaneous Reduction and Pinning

Technique. The positioning of the patient is identical to that for the application of a bridging external fixator. The first step is to reduce any metaphyseal malalignment and apply a bridging external fixator.

The articular surface is then assessed with a fluoroscope. If there is a radial styloid fragment, this is addressed first to reconstitute the radial column. The radial styloid may reduce with the longitudinal traction and slight ulnar deviation used to reduce the metaphysis, in which case two wires are driven from the tip of the styloid diagonally to engage in the ulnar cortex of the radius proximal to the fracture. If the styloid

remains displaced then percutaneous manipulation may be performed either by partially inserting a pin and using it as a lever or by inserting a small awl percutaneously and elevating the styloid.

Once the radial column is reduced, attention is turned to the lunate facet. If the lunate facet is reduced then pins are placed transversely from the styloid in the subchondral area as far as but not penetrating the DRUJ. Residual lunate facet displacement is either a depression or a sagittal gap when the facet itself is intact. The facet may be elevated with a small awl. Using a small 1-cm longitudinal incision on the dorsum of the wrist, an awl can be inserted into the radius through the dorsal comminution. Using image intensifier control, the tip of the awl is placed just proximal to the depressed fragment and the fragment is elevated (Fig. 32-25B). If a sagittal split remains, a large bone clamp can be placed percutaneously between the radial column and the dorsal ulnar corner. Transverse pins are then inserted.

If there is a four-part fracture with displacement of the volar and dorsal fragments of the volar facet then percutaneous

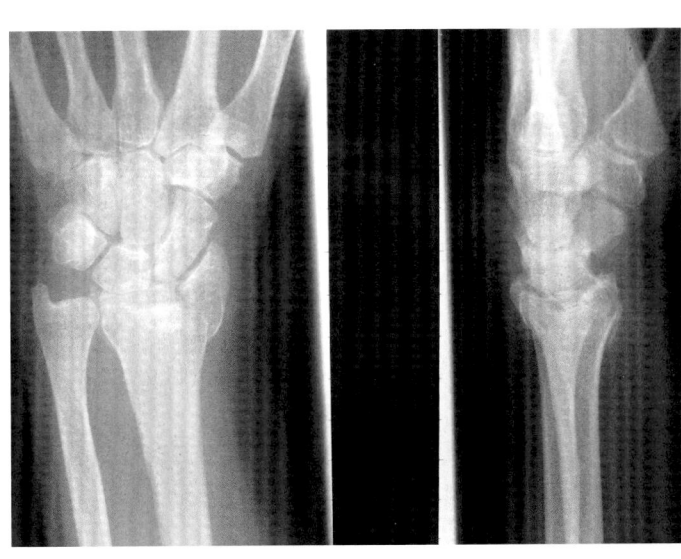

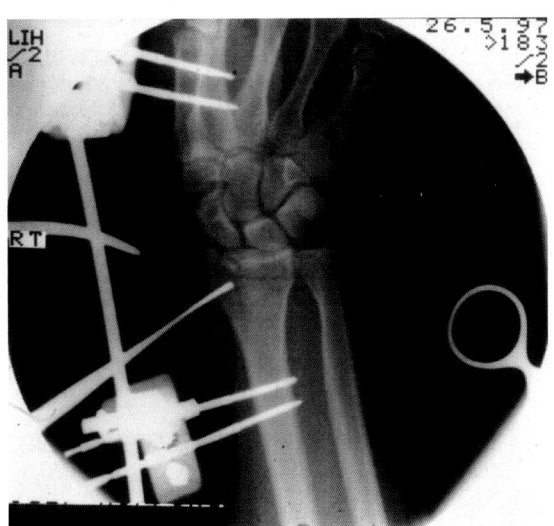

A

B

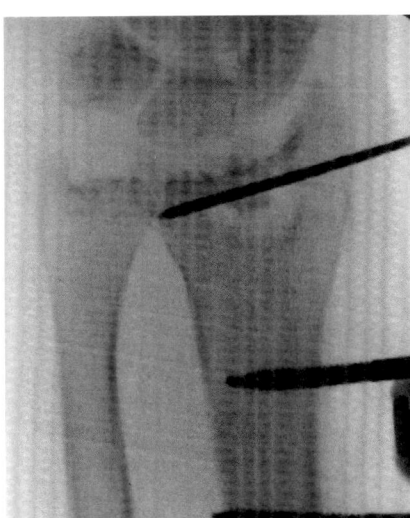

C

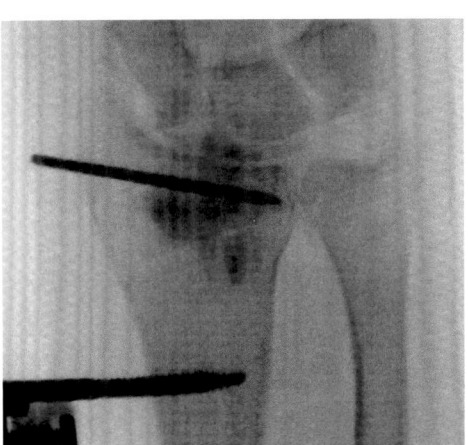

D

FIGURE 32-25 A: A complex intra-articular fracture of the distal radius with central impaction, a die punch lesion. **B:** A bridging external fixator has been applied. The central depression is reduced closed with a bone awl. **C:** The fragment is reduced and held with a transverse K-wire. There is a significant metaphyseal defect. **D:** The metaphyseal defect has been filled with bone substitute.

fixation is not usually possible. If the surgeon plans to retain the external fixator, the volar and dorsal fragments may be reduced and fixed through limited open approaches, using either K-wires or a buttress fixation with plate and screws on the dorsal or volar side or both as appropriate to the fracture and its reduction. It is usually best to reduce and fix the volar ulnar fragment first. This allows the use of the volar ulnar fragment as a fulcrum to reduce the dorsal ulnar fragment using palmar flexion and radial deviation followed by K-wire fixation from posterior to anterior.

If there are large metaphyseal defects after elevation of the fragment, then support from either cancellous bone grafting or bone substitute is recommended (Fig. 32-25C, D).[120,204,218,306]

Postoperative Care. Postoperatively, the external fixator and K-wires are removed at 6 weeks, provided radiographic control reveals fracture healing. Physiotherapy is started at this stage or earlier if there is any compromise of hand movement.

Open Reduction and Internal Fixation. ORIF of displaced articular fractures of the distal radius can be achieved using a single plate, usually a volar locked plate, or with a column- or fragment-specific approach with multiple plates. The choice of technique should be determined by the fracture configuration; if all the fragments can be captured by a single plate then this is used but if not, multiple plates are required.

Technique. The positioning for this technique is the same as plating for the extra-articular fracture. The approach to severe articular fractures is determined by the location and displacement of the intra-articular fragments and by the degree of metaphyseal comminution. If it is anticipated that a volar plate will capture all necessary fragments, then an open reduction using the modified Henry's approach as described above for extra- and minimal articular fractures is used. It is essential that the surgeon visualizes the volar ulnar corner of the radius

clearly to capture any volar ulnar corner fragments. Failure to do this may result in escape of the fragment from the plate and volar subluxation of the carpus (Fig. 32-26).

Where it is not possible to capture all fragments with a volar plate, for example, when there is a displaced dorsal ulnar fragment, then column-specific or fragment-specific fixation may be used. This was pioneered by Rikli and Regazzoni[299] who recognized intermediate and lateral columns in the distal radius corresponding to the lunate facet and radial styloid and used radial and dorsal ulnar plates (Fig. 32-27). However, the limitation of this technique was when a displaced volar ulnar column was present when a palmar plate was required. This technique therefore evolved into fragment-specific fixation where small implants are used depending on the configuration of the fracture.

Limited dorsal, radial, and volar approaches are used. For the radial approach, a longitudinal incision is made radial to the radial artery protecting the superficial branches of the radial nerve in the skin flaps. The first dorsal compartment is released proximally only and the tendons retracted. Brachioradialis is then released from the radius and the radial styloid exposed. If volar exposure of the radial styloid is required, pronator quadratus can be released from the distal radius and elevated to expose the volar aspect. The radial styloid is then reduced and held with a K-wire. In some cases, addition of a further K-wire is sufficient, but frequently a small (usually 2 mm) plate is required, which is contoured to fit the radial styloid on its lateral aspect.

Once the radial column is stabilized, attention is turned to the ulnar side of the radius. If dorsal fixation is required, a longitudinal incision is made between the third and fourth extensor compartments. If necessary the EPL tendon is released and the fourth compartment elevated subperiosteally which gives good exposure of the dorsal ulnar radius. The fracture is

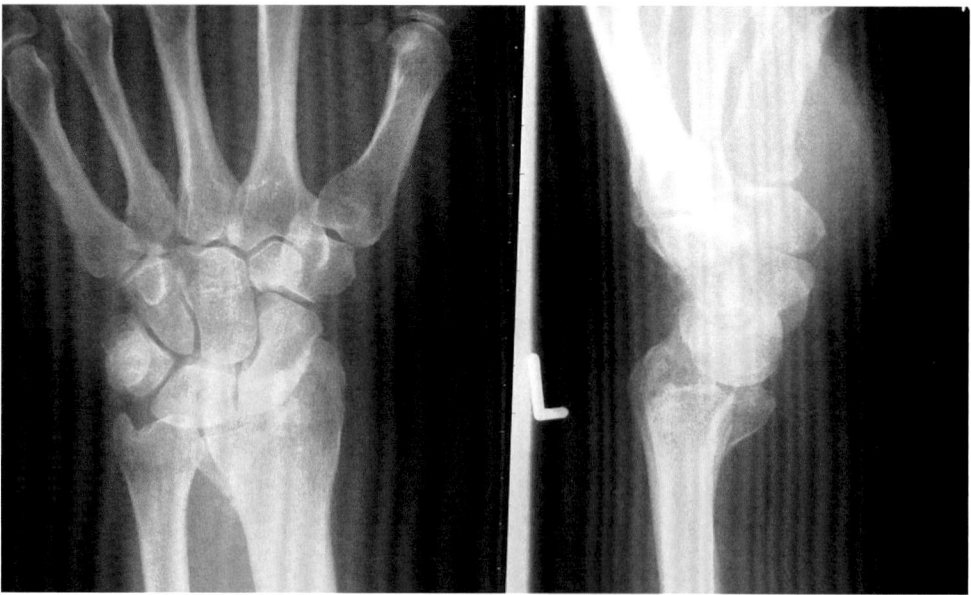

FIGURE 32-26 An intra-articular fracture of the distal radius with a volar ulnar corner fracture and subluxation of the carpus.

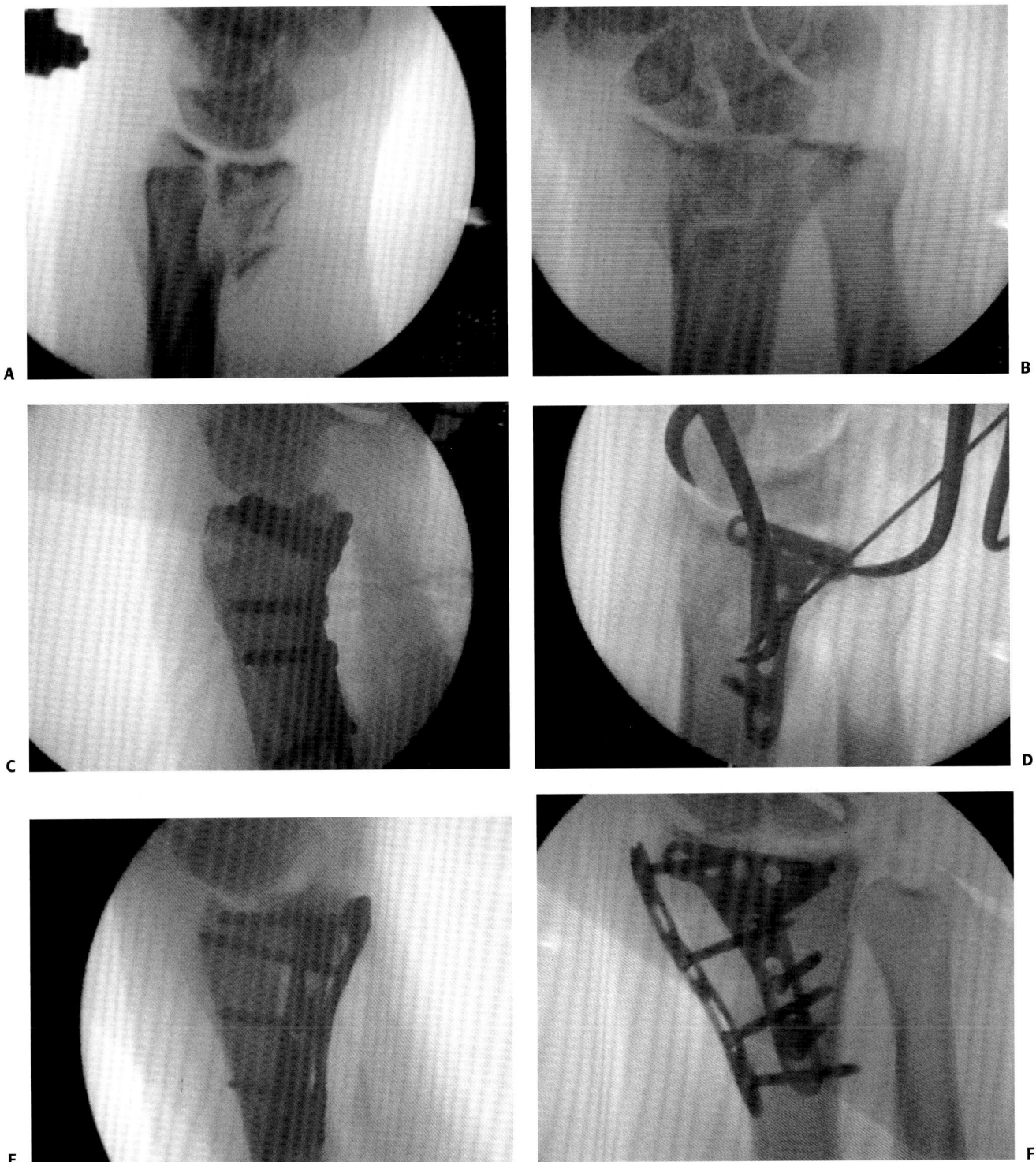

FIGURE 32-27 Lateral and PA fluoroscopy views **(A, B)** after reduction in traction of a highly comminuted intra-articular fracture. Note that the dorsal cortex comes out to length whereas the palmar cortex remains displaced. Following application of a palmar plate, there still remains some residual comminution of the radial styloid **(C, D)**. The radial styloid (particularly distally) may require adjunctive fixation with either a second plate or K-wires. For this case a separate radial column plate was used to create the final construct **(E, F)**.

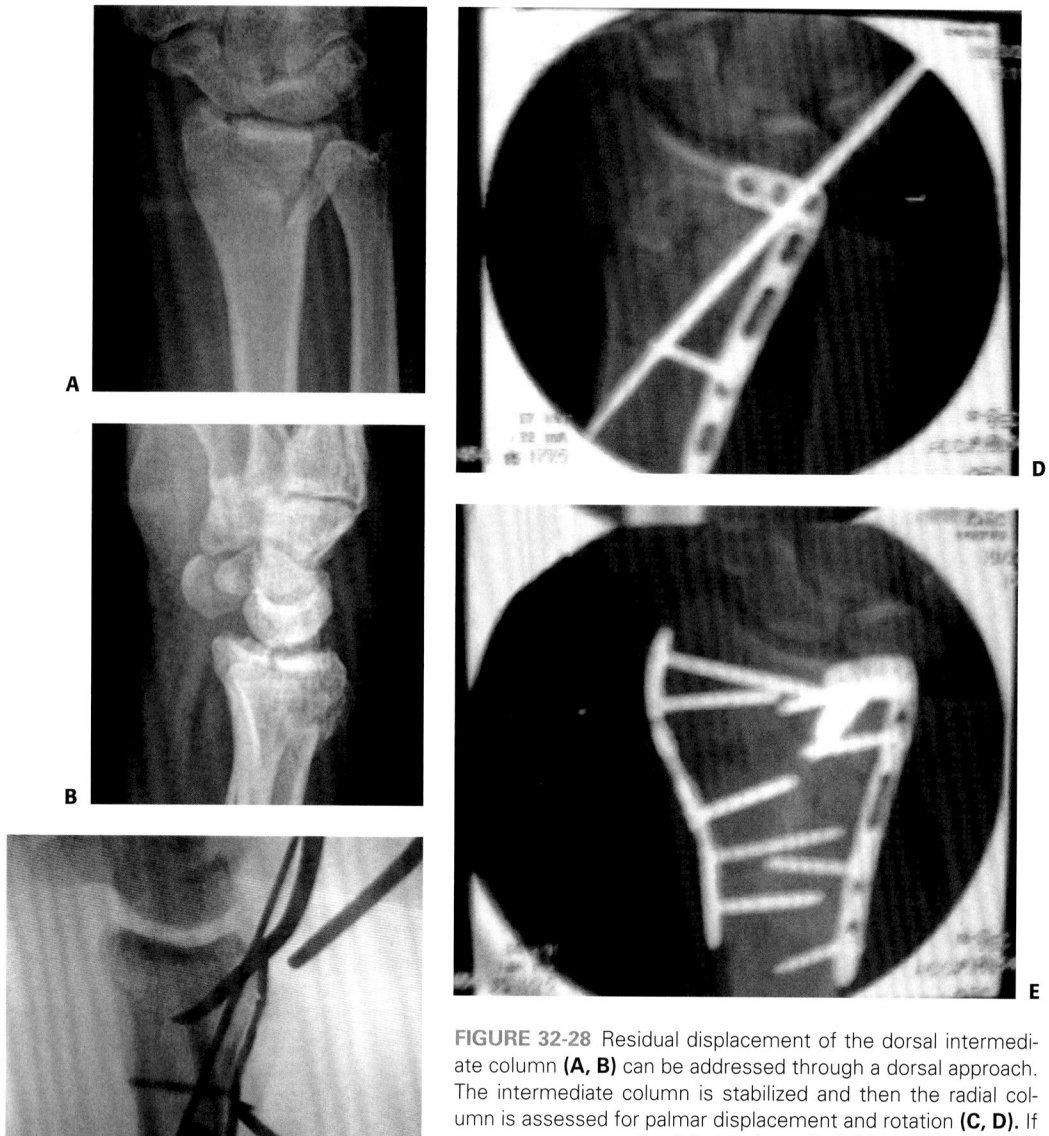

FIGURE 32-28 Residual displacement of the dorsal intermediate column **(A, B)** can be addressed through a dorsal approach. The intermediate column is stabilized and then the radial column is assessed for palmar displacement and rotation **(C, D)**. If necessary, a second radial plate is applied **(E)**.

reduced using bone graft, if necessary, to augment the elevated position. A T plate is usually necessary to maintain the reduction (Fig. 32-28).

On the volar side of the radius, a volar ulnar fracture is approached between the flexor tendons and the ulnar neurovascular bundle. The fracture is reduced, bone graft used as necessary, and a small T plate is applied (Fig. 32-29).

Postoperative Care. Postoperatively, if fixation is deemed satisfactory, a plaster is not required although a resting splint may be used for comfort. Active range of movement is started as soon as pain allows although patients should be cautioned to avoid weight bearing on the hand.

Outcomes

Combined External and Internal Fixation. There are a limited number of reports of the outcome of external fixation and limited open reduction. Limited open reduction without

external fixation has been reported but should be reserved for the treatment of fractures with articular displacement without metaphyseal comminution. In one study the authors reported on 40 patients with intra-articular fractures of the distal radius, of which 12 had AO type C3 fractures and 5 of the 12 had percutaneous reduction and fixation without external fixation. The authors found that there was loss of the metaphyseal reduction in patients with metaphyseal comminution. Articular reduction was achieved in half of the 40 patients but limited open reduction was required for displaced volar fractures or small impacted joint fragments. They cited the minimal soft tissue disruption as an advantage of the technique.[120]

A combination of external fixation and plating of the lunate facet was used in the treatment of 21 patients younger than 65 years of age by Ruch et al.[314] with good or excellent results in 18 patients. The most comprehensive cohort study of combined closed reduction and external fixation retrospectively

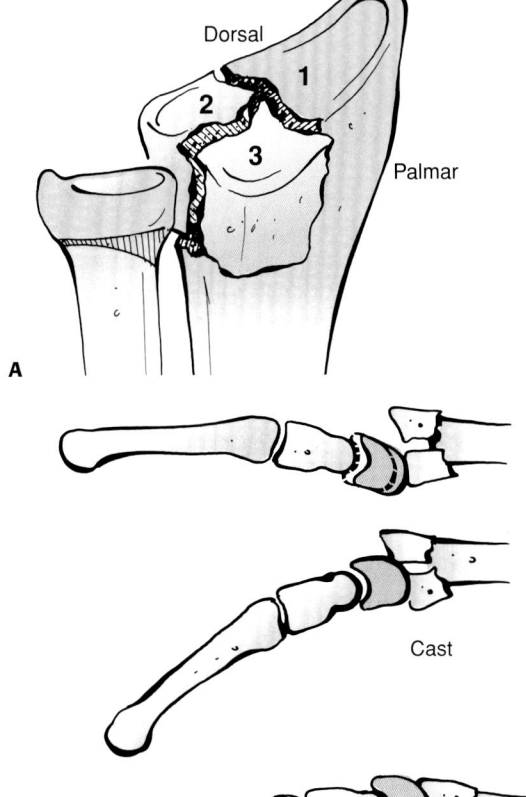

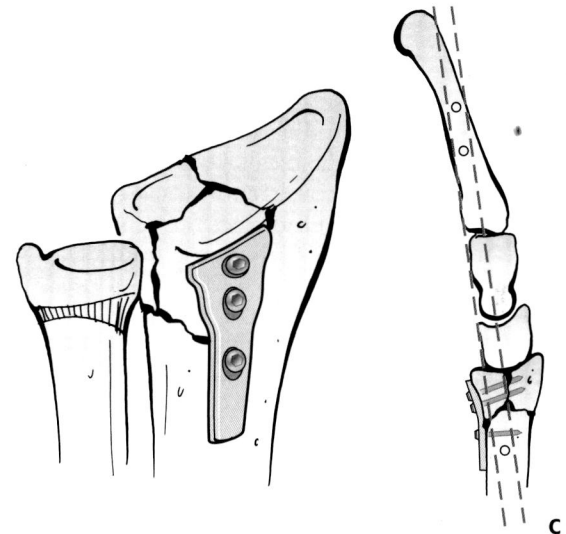

FIGURE 32-29 A: Typical three-part intra-articular fracture of the distal radius. **B:** Depression of the lunate facet palmarly is difficult to reduce by closed methods. **C:** A plate applied palmarly to the lunate facet reduces and mortars both the DRUJ and the radiocarpal joint.

examined 22 patients with 23 AO type C3 fractures at an average review time of 40 months. Excellent or good results using the Gartland and Werley scale were obtained in 17 cases with the average grip strength being 67.5% of the opposite sides. Five of twenty-three fractures healed with a step greater than 2 mm and two with a gap greater than 2 mm. There was statistical correlation between better results and patients aged less than 40 years and in those fractures which healed with a gap or step of less than 2 mm. The authors concluded that the technique led to a satisfactory outcome in most cases.[32] This study illustrates that closed reduction techniques are satisfactory, provided reduction of the joint is achieved.

Open Reduction and Internal Fixation. There are considerably more papers published on this subject than on limited reduction and external fixation. There are reports of the use of both single (usually volar locked) plates and of fragment-specific fixation. Caution should be used in comparing the results of these studies as a single plate will generally be used in less complex intra-articular fractures.[320] Even studies concentrating on one type of plating are difficult to interpret as the cohort usually contains a heterogeneous group of patients and fractures ranging from extra-articular to severely displaced intra-articular fractures.[62,85,90,95,388,393] Even if the studies are restricted to AO/OTA type C fractures, no attention is paid to whether the artic-

ular fragments are displaced requiring open reduction or not, which is likely to have a significant influence on their outcome.

The outcome of 54 patients with intra-articular fractures of the distal radius treated with volar locked plates was reported by Gruber et al. Forty-nine fractures were AO type C2 or C3 with the remaining five being type C1. The average age was 63 years with older women and younger men. The authors considered that a volar locked plate alone was not sufficient in "more difficult" fractures when K-wires were added. They reported good restoration of metaphyseal alignment and 89% of cases with articular incongruity of less than 1 mm. Radiologic arthritis was evident in 24% of cases at 2 years and 37% of cases at 6 years with the average severity increasing significantly over the time period.[140]

In the same year, Konstantinidis et al. reported the results of volar plating of 40 AO type C fractures, 60% of which were type C3. Metaphyseal alignment was well maintained but joint alignment was not reported. The mean DASH score was 18 at a minimum follow-up of 1 year. Ten percent required revision surgery which resulted in worse functional outcomes. As in other reports of the treatment of articular fractures, the complication rate was high. Ten cases required augmentation with external fixation or K-wires and the authors acknowledged that it may be difficult to treat both radial and ulnar column fractures with a single plate.[199]

Column- or fragment-specific internal fixation was reported by Jakob et al. in 2000. They included 77 patients, 40 of which were described as complex articular. One year after surgery 75% had no pain. Ninety-seven percent returned to work at a mean of 6 months after injury. There was no residual intra-articular incongruity and 7% had radiographic evidence of osteoarthritis. There was a 21.6% complication rate with nine patients experiencing tendon problems. Four fractures redisplaced and the reoperation rate was 23%. The authors concluded that the technique reliably restored joint congruency and extra-articular alignment but was technically demanding.[169]

The column-specific technique was extended to include fixation of any fragment with small implants, the fragment-specific technique. The largest series of intra-articular distal radius fractures reported using this technique contains 105 patients, all with AO type C fractures of which only 33 were type C3.[118] The remainder consisted of 41 C1 fractures and 31 C2 fractures. Six patients had additional bridging external fixators applied, demonstrating the need for a combination of techniques in the more complex cases. Thirty-one patients had nonanatomical joint reduction with the odds of achieving a good reduction being 0.25 for C2 fractures and 0.17 for C3 fractures compared to C1 fractures. Eleven patients had radiologic evidence of arthritis at 1 year, eight of whom had initial malreduction of the joint. The DASH and PRWE scores had not returned to baseline at 1 year but this was not affected by fracture subtype or quality of reduction. Five patients lost reduction because of unaddressed dorsal comminution or volar ulnar corner fractures and eight patients had tendon problems. The authors concluded that most articular fractures can be managed using a volar approach. Indications for an added dorsal approach were defined as a dorsal ulnar fragment, dorsal comminution, or joint impaction.

Other authors have reported similar outcomes with the fragment-specific type of technique. All studies report some residual articular incongruity.[52,178,323] In the more complex fractures, augmentation of the plates with external fixation, K-wires, bone graft, or bone substitute may be required.[52,178,323] Functional outcome scores rarely revert to baseline and complication rates are high, reflecting the complexity of the fractures treated.

Randomized Controlled Trials. Kreder et al.[204] performed a randomized controlled study on 179 patients with intra-articular distal radius fractures with 118 patients attending for review at 2 years. Eighty-eight patients were treated with indirect reduction, percutaneous fixation, and bridging external fixation, whereas 91 were treated with ORIF. The majority of fractures were AO type C. Bone graft was used in 13% of the closed group and 50% of the open group. Residual articular incongruity occurred in 12 in the closed group and 13 in the open group with radiologic osteoarthritis in 7 and 6 patients respectively. The closed reduction and external fixation group had superior upper limb Musculoskeletal Functional Assessment (MFA) scores, less pain and better grip strength, and specialized grip strength. Eight patients in this group had crossed over to the ORIF group because it proved impossible to reduce the fracture by closed means. The authors reported a more than 10-fold increase in the likelihood of osteoarthritis if there

was a residual step of more than 2 mm. They concluded that there was a more rapid return to function and superior overall function within 2 years in the closed reduction and external fixation group provided articular incongruity was minimized. They believe that neither the fixation nor the implant dictates outcome but rather the ability of the surgeon to obtain a satisfactory reduction with the least invasive procedure possible and recommended that ORIF of articular fractures of the distal radius be preceded by an attempted indirect reduction and percutaneous fixation supplemented by bridging external fixation.

Leung et al.[217] performed a similar RCT on 137 patients with 134 AO type C fractures with 113 patients followed for 2 years. The Gartland and Werley scores and radiologic osteoarthritis was less for C2 fractures treated with plating but no such difference could be demonstrated for the more complex C3 nor the simpler C1 fractures. The authors attributed the differences between theirs and Kreder's study to the use of fewer dorsal approaches in their study and the use of external fixation at the surgeon's discretion in the latter study.

An earlier comparison between dorsal plating and limited open reduction and external fixation was abandoned before completion of enrolment because of higher complication rates, more pain and worse grip strength in the dorsal plating group.[139]

Volar locked plating was compared retrospectively with external fixation for AO type C2 and C3 fractures in 115 patients.[297] Better grip strength, range of movement, and DASH scores, but higher complication rates were reported in the volar locked plating group but a trend toward the use of external fixation in open fractures and a higher proportion of C3 fractures in the external fixation group suggests that as this study was retrospective, the more complex fractures may have been treated with external fixation.

The Role of Arthroscopy. Arthroscopy has now been used for a number of years to assist in the reduction of intra-articular distal radius fractures but despite this there is no consensus on its utility. Advantages of arthroscopy include direct visualization of the articular surface with minimal soft tissue violation, which allows confirmation of joint reduction and exclusion of inadvertently placed intra-articular implants. However, technically and logistically there are disadvantages: a longer, more difficult procedure, greater expense, a long learning curve, and the risk of fluid extravasation, which may result in acute compartment syndrome.

Any benefit of arthroscopy to patient outcome has not been firmly established. Doi et al.[83] performed a randomized study comparing 34 patients with arthroscopy-assisted reduction, external fixation, and K-wires with 58 patients treated with ORIF and followed them for a minimum of 2 years. Radiologically, there was no difference in the residual step-off but a 0.5 mm difference in residual gap. This was statistically significant but its clinical significance must be in doubt. There was better metaphyseal alignment in the arthroscopic group. Better outcomes as measured by the Gartland and Werley and Green and O'Brien scores were reported in this group but this may be because of the improved metaphyseal alignment, which is difficult to attribute to the use of an arthroscope. In a later RCT,

20 fractures were treated with fluoroscopy alone and 20 with fluoroscopy and arthroscopy.[379] All fractures had a residual gap or step of 2 mm or more after closed reduction and were treated with external fixation and percutaneous pinning. The tourniquet time (and presumably, therefore, surgery time) was significantly prolonged in the arthroscopy group. The authors reported a mean of 0.45 mm less step or gap in the arthroscopy group and improved early outcome measures at 3 months. They concluded that the addition of arthroscopy improved the outcome of intra-articular distal radius fractures.

Salvage Procedures. In a small number of cases it may not be possible to restore articular congruity or metaphyseal alignment because of severe articular or metaphyseal comminution, poor bone quality, or any combination of the three. In these circumstances a salvage procedure may be required.

Distraction Plating. This technique involves bridging of the joint and metaphysis using a standard plate from the third metacarpal distally to the radial diaphysis proximal to the fracture. It has been described as an "internal fixator," using ligamentotaxis to obtain reduction and has been recommended for polytrauma patients who need to bear weight on the limb, for fractures caused by high-energy injury with extensive articular comminution and diaphyseal extension[126] and for osteoporotic patients with severely comminuted fractures.[296]

Technique. The plate is usually applied using minimally invasive techniques although an open approach may be used if necessary. Under tourniquet control, a 4-cm incision is made over the third metacarpal and the extensor tendons retracted. A similar-sized or slightly larger incision is made over the dorsum of the radius proximal to any diaphyseal comminution and the radius is exposed, taking care to protect the superficial radial nerve. A third small incision is made at the level of Lister tubercle and the EPL tendon is released from its groove. An elevator is then used to develop a plane deep to the extensor tendon. This incision can also be used to reduce the fracture or insert bone graft if necessary. A plate, usually containing 12 to 14 holes, is then passed from distal to proximal, and its position verified with fluoroscopy. Care should be taken to avoid entrapment of extensor tendons under the plate. One screw is inserted into the metacarpal and distraction applied to the fracture. The plate is then clamped to the proximal radius and the fracture reduction confirmed by fluoroscopy. Overdistraction should be avoided. The surgeon should then confirm that full forearm rotation and finger flexion are possible to exclude rotational deformity at the fracture or tendon entrapment. At least three screws proximally and distally are then inserted. The articular surface is then reduced if necessary through the middle incision and the fragments held with K-wires or screws. Bone graft is usually required as these fractures usually have a large metaphyseal void. Splintage is only required for a short period for pain relief following which the patient is encouraged to mobilize. The plate is removed after fracture union.

Outcome. Two reports of the outcome of this technique included 22[313] and 33 patients[296] with the latter study recruiting patients over 60 years of age. Both studies reported good restoration of both metaphyseal and articular alignment. The

DASH scores at 1 year were a mean of 15[313] and 32[296] respectively, but in the latter report had reduced to 11.5 at 2 years after injury. The severity of the fractures treated should be remembered when considering these results.

Double or Sandwich Plating. This technique is indicated in cases with both volar and dorsal comminution, which may cause severe instability. The use of a single plate may lead to loss of alignment in the opposite direction, for example, application of a volar plate may cause dorsal displacement (Fig. 32-30).[185] Articular displacement can be addressed prior to the insertion of the distal screws in the plate. Reports of this technique indicate that satisfactory radiographic reduction is usually achieved.[77,303] Functional results are variable with one study reporting 10 good or excellent, 14 fair, and 1 poor result according to the modified Green and O'Brien score at an average of 26 months after injury.[303] Day et al. reported a mean DASH score of 16 points in 10 patients at an average of 17 months after injury. Concerns about avascularity of fragments or delayed union are unfounded but the technique's disadvantages are the need for plate removal and the risk of tendon rupture.

Arthrodesis. Rarely, severe articular bone loss or incongruity cannot be corrected and in this situation, early radiocarpal or complete wrist arthrodesis should be considered. Such injuries are the result of high energy transfer and are most frequently caused by gunshot wounds, crush, or blast injuries.[112] When a decision is made that the fracture is irreparable, arthrodesis

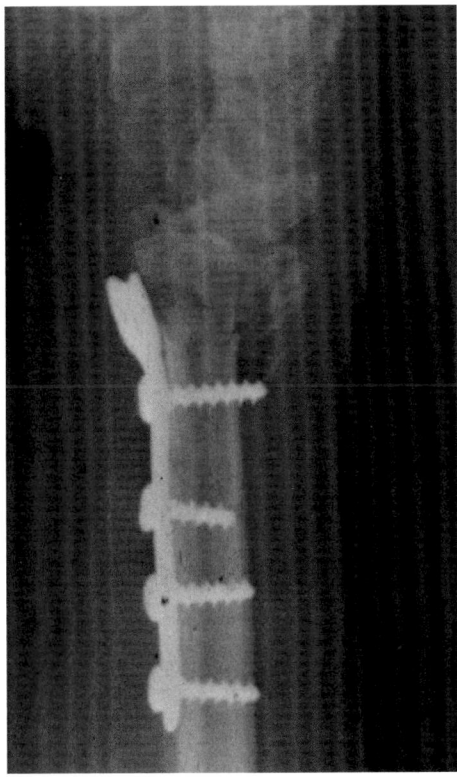

FIGURE 32-30 A poorly applied volar plate in the presence of both volar and dorsal comminution has resulted in a dorsal malunion.

should be performed primarily if the soft tissues allow or as a delayed primary procedure after satisfactory soft tissue coverage or healing is obtained. Early surgery will reduce the chance of posttraumatic stiffness in the hand and forearm.

Radiocarpal fusion has the advantage of retaining some wrist motion which occurs at the midcarpal and carpometacarpal joints. However in one study, 3 of 15 patients required conversion to total wrist fusion because of symptomatic midcarpal osteoarthritis occurring between 1 and 2 years after injury. Two patients required conversion to total wrist fusion because of nonunion of the radiocarpal fusion. At follow-up on 10 patients 8 years after surgery, there was sufficient residual pain in two cases to interfere with the normal activities of daily living. Grip strength was an average of 43% of the opposite side. There was an average of 50 degrees of a flexion extension arc but radial deviation was severely limited.[261]

For a complete wrist fusion, the midcarpal and carpometacarpal joints are included with the radiocarpal joints. Fusion is best performed in 10 to 20 degrees of wrist extension with slight ulnar deviation and this is most easily achieved with commercially available plates. Fusion rates are generally high and occur 3 to 4 months after surgery[112] with recovery of grip strength between 60% and 80%.

Partial Articular Fractures

Partial articular fractures of the distal radius are either volar shearing or volar lip (volar Barton's), dorsal shearing or dorsal lip (Barton's), or radial styloid (Chauffeur's) fractures and usually result from impaction of the scaphoid and lunate complex onto the distal radius. They are characterized as partial articular fractures because a part of the metaphysis remains intact and in continuity with the diaphysis of the radius and the intact part of the joint. The fracture line is oblique rendering it unstable but it can be anchored to the intact column of the radius using internal fixation.

Volar Shearing Fractures. These are the AO type B3 fractures and are categorized by the size and comminution of the volar fragment and whether the sigmoid notch is involved. They have long been recognized as being inherently unstable[24,93] and nonoperative treatment is therefore reserved for the elderly, frail patient, or the rare undisplaced fracture.

Operative treatment is with a palmar buttress plate with an emphasis on reduction of the articular surface, including the sigmoid notch. The plate should be slightly undercontoured to apply compression across the fracture against the intact dorsal cortex (Fig. 32-31). Care should be taken to place the plate sufficiently ulnar to support an ulnar-sided volar lip fracture which may be occult. The surgeon should examine the preoperative imaging carefully to exclude subtle fracture lines extending into the dorsal cortex which may otherwise be unrecognized risking dorsal malunion if an undercontoured plate is used.[185]

Most reports of the outcome of volar shearing fractures of the distal radius include a majority of cases with high-energy injury which may not reflect the true epidemiology of these injuries. Reported radiologic results are good provided the risk

of dorsal malunion is avoided.[5,177,185,255,347] Functional results are reported with a high proportion of excellent and good results in the older studies.[5,177] A more recent study reported a mean DASH score of 3.9 2 years after injury.[347] Bolmers et al.[35] reported much longer-term outcomes with a mean DASH score of 14 in 17 patients examined between 15 and 25 years after injury. The latter two studies found no significant differences in outcome between volar shearing fractures with or without a dorsal fracture line.

Dorsal Lip Fractures. Dorsal lip or dorsal marginal articular fractures are rare injuries and usually occur in association with a variety of other injuries and radiocarpal subluxation or dislocation (Fig. 32-32). Lozano-Calderon et al. identified four patterns of associated injury[226]:

1. Impaction of the majority of the articular surface with a simple volar metaphyseal fracture line.

2. Radiocarpal fracture dislocation with radiolunate ligament rupture.

3. Radiocarpal fracture dislocation with fracture of the volar margin of the lunate facet, the origin of the radiolunate ligament.

4. Central articular impaction with relative sparing of the volar half of the joint and the radial styloid.

They are frequently the result of high-energy injury and tend to occur in younger patients. Careful examination of the carpus is mandatory to exclude scaphoid fracture or carpal ligamentous injury.

Treatment of these injuries is usually surgical with a dorsal, volar, or combined approach depending on the characteristics of the injury. A study of 20 patients reported an average DASH score of 15 at 30 months, but more than half of the patients had unsatisfactory results with the modified Mayo risk score. The authors concluded that this is a severe injury in which permanent impairment should be anticipated.[226]

Radial Styloid Fractures. Radial styloid fractures are the commonest type of partial articular fracture. They may occur in isolation, in association with scaphoid fracture, scapholunate injury, radiocarpal dislocation, or with a more complex distal radius fracture. The latter is described in the section in this chapter on displaced articular fractures.

Isolated Radial Styloid Fractures. These are usually undisplaced and generally benign injuries but careful examination of the carpus is mandatory to exclude scaphoid fracture or carpal ligamentous injury. If undisplaced they may be treated in a cast or splint for pain relief and the wrist mobilized when symptoms allow. Intervention is indicated where there is a significant articular step or gap when surgery is usually required. If possible treatment should be percutaneous with manipulative reduction and fixation using pins, screws, or headless screws. If reduction cannot be achieved percutaneously then open reduction is necessary. Radial buttress plating may be necessary in this situation.

Helm and Tonkin reported the results of surgical treatment in 14 radial styloid fractures of which most were caused by high-energy injury. Four had associated carpal injury with

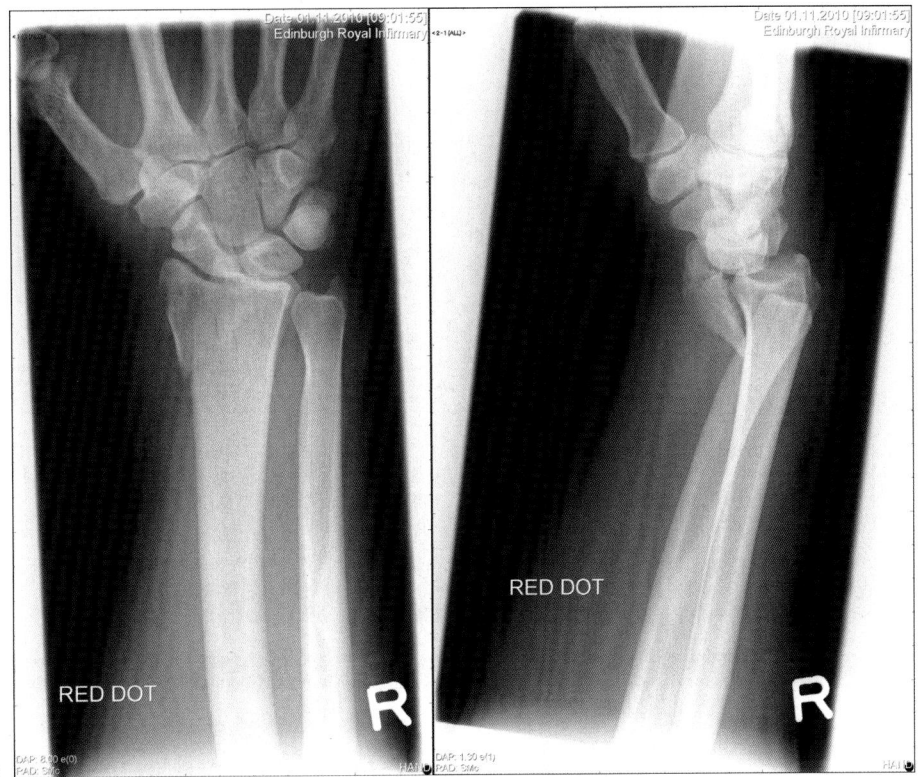

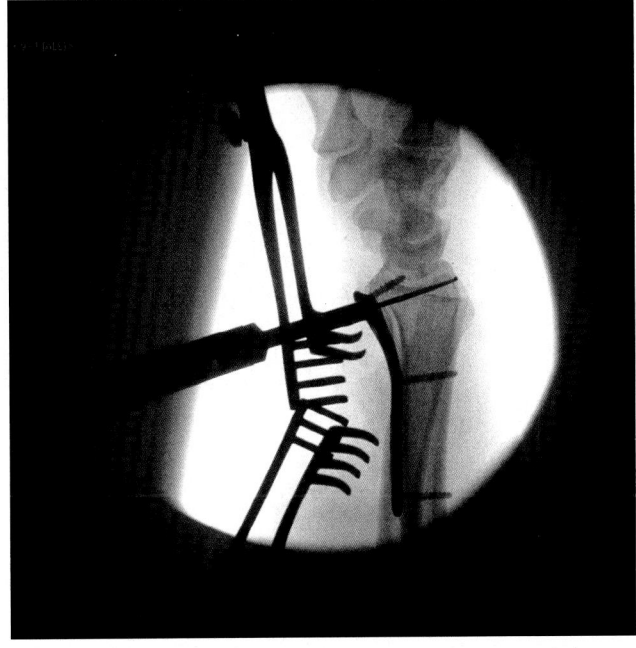

FIGURE 32-31 A: A volar shearing fracture of the distal radius. **B:** A palmar plate is being applied slightly undercontoured. Screws are inserted and tightened sequentially to compress the fracture against the intact dorsal cortex.

three scaphoid fractures and one transscaphoid, transstyloid perilunate fracture dislocation. Fixation of the radial styloid was with headless screws and K-wires and in one case a T plate. The authors reported good or excellent functional results.[153]

Radial Styloid and Scaphoid Fractures. Simultaneous fracture of the distal radius and carpal bones is uncommon. Hove[162] reported on 2,330 distal radius fractures and 390 scaphoid fractures with only 12 cases of combined fractures. Scaphoid fractures can occur with any type of distal radius fracture but

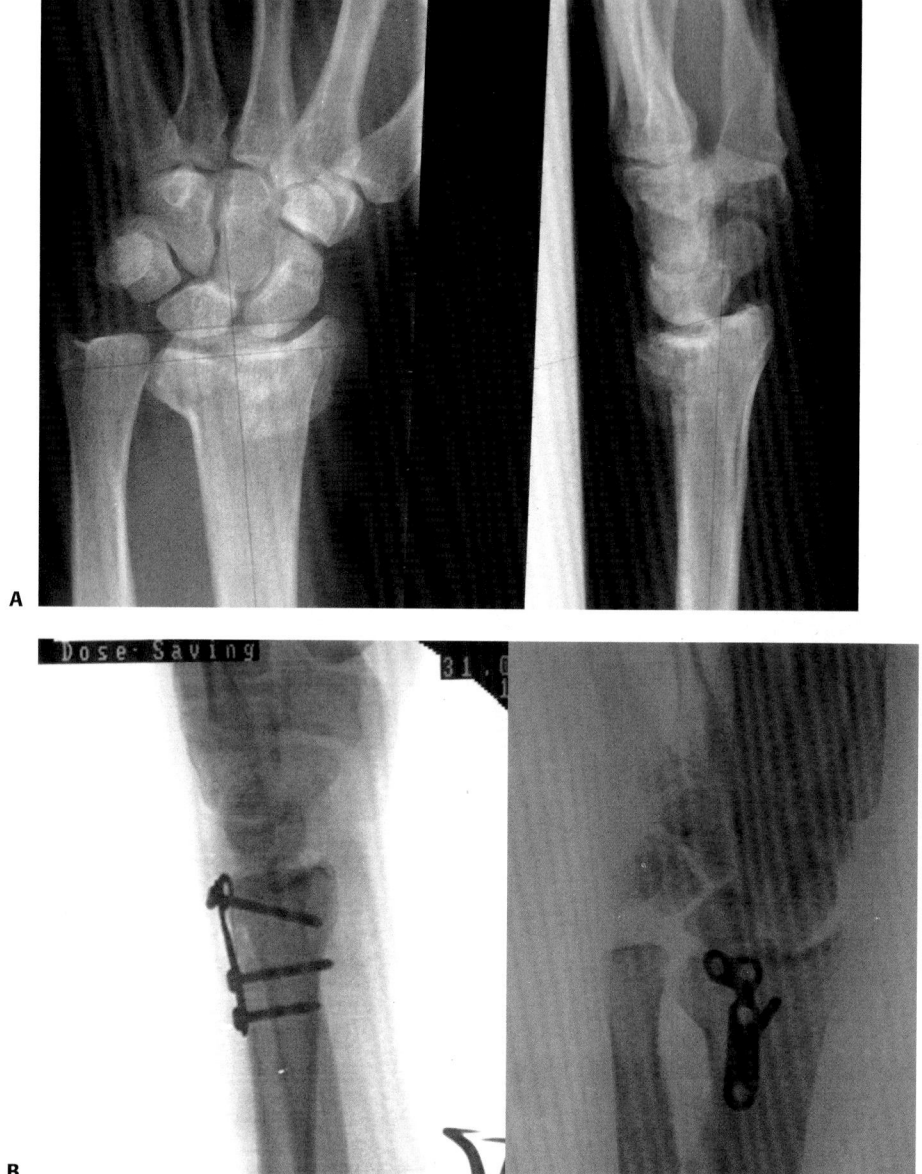

FIGURE 32-32 A: A dorsal lip fracture of the distal radius with carpal subluxation **B:** The fracture has been reduced and held with a small dorsal plate and the carpus is relocated.

are significantly more common in partial articular fractures.[197] The same authors report that the commonest associated carpal bone fracture is the scaphoid. Combined fractures were commoner in younger men with high-energy injuries and the authors stress the importance of CT imaging where combined fractures are suspected.

Treatment of combined fractures generally depends on the severity of the distal radius fracture and any displacement of the scaphoid fracture. Older reports suggest that nonoperative management yields reasonable results,[162,275] but more recent reports recognize a shift in strategy with increasing severity of the distal radius fracture. Of 10 patients Rutgers et al. treated 8 with surgery to both the distal radius and scaphoid. Of the two

treated nonoperatively initially one required ORIF of the scaphoid 6 weeks later. Low pain levels, good ranges of movement, and consistent return to previous employment were reported at a mean review time of 40 months and a minimum review time of 1 year. The authors recommend that if surgery is required for the distal radius fracture then the scaphoid fracture should also be fixed. They concluded that early aggressive internal fixation of both fractures combined with early rehabilitation led to satisfactory outcomes for low level of complications.[316]

Fractures of the Distal Ulna

Fractures of the distal ulna are a common association with distal radius fractures. They may involve the ulnar shaft, neck, head, or ulnar styloid, or a combination of several of these. Although common there is not much guidance in the current literature as to their management.

Extra-Articular Distal Ulnar Fractures

Extra-articular fractures of the distal ulna associated with distal radius fractures are either diaphyseal or in the neck or distal part of the ulna. The latter are defined as being within 5 cm of the dome of the ulna.[224] They have been reported as occurring in 5.6% of displaced distal radius fractures.[34]

Many of these fractures will be realigned once the distal radius is reduced in which case cast immobilization is sufficient (Fig. 32-33). However, if the ulna remains malaligned or unstable after distal radius stabilization, then ORIF is required. Malalignment has been defined as more than 10 degrees of

angulation and instability as more than 50% translation with forearm rotation.[51]

ORIF can be achieved by a number of different methods.[51,110,213,263,301] Although most of these studies include extra-articular fractures only one concentrates exclusively on neck or distal ulnar fractures without articular involvement.[51] This was a prospective nonrandomized study of 61 unstable or malaligned fractures of the distal ulna with associated distal radius fractures, all of which were internally fixed. The patients were all over 64 years of age. Twenty-nine patients were treated with ORIF and 32 with closed reduction and cast management. At an average review period of 34 months there were no significant differences in the radiologic or functional outcome.[51] For the older patient it seems that nonoperative management is satisfactory but there is

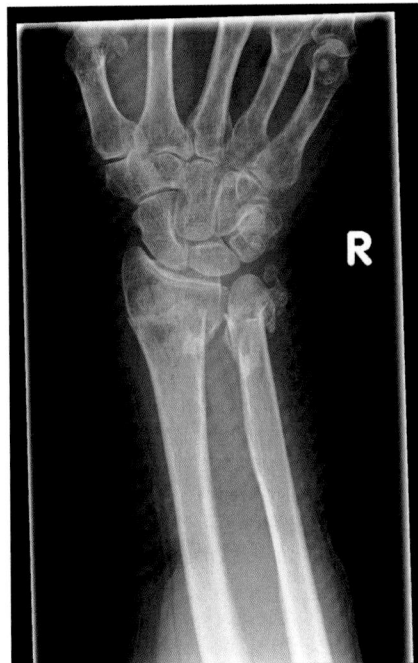
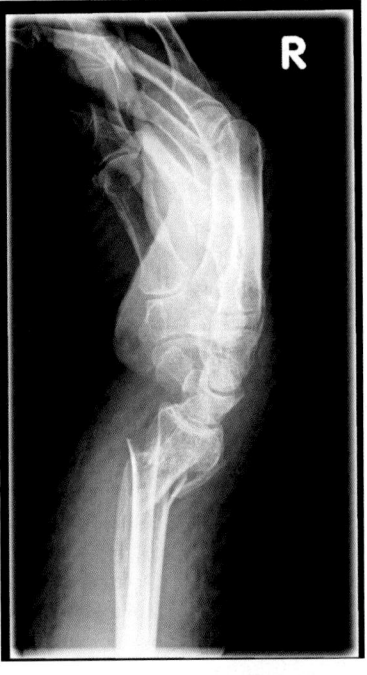

FIGURE 32-33 **A:** An unstable extra-articuar fracture of the distal radius with a comminuted fracture of the ulnar neck. **B:** After fixation of the distal radius the ulnar fracture is out to length with acceptable alignment and does not require fixation. Both fractures went on to heal in this position.

A

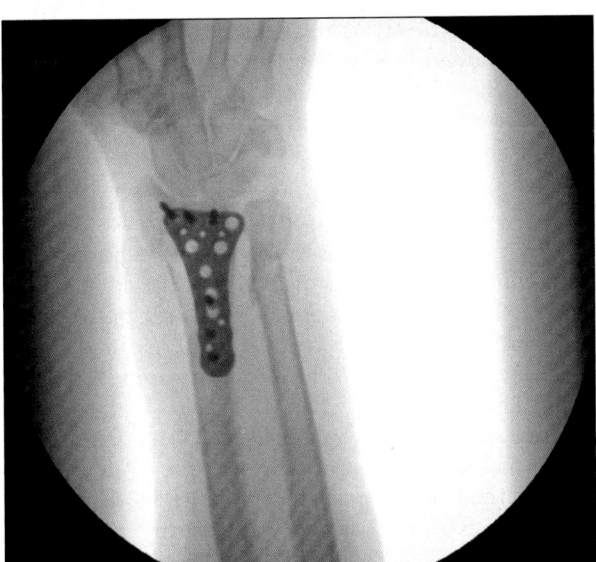
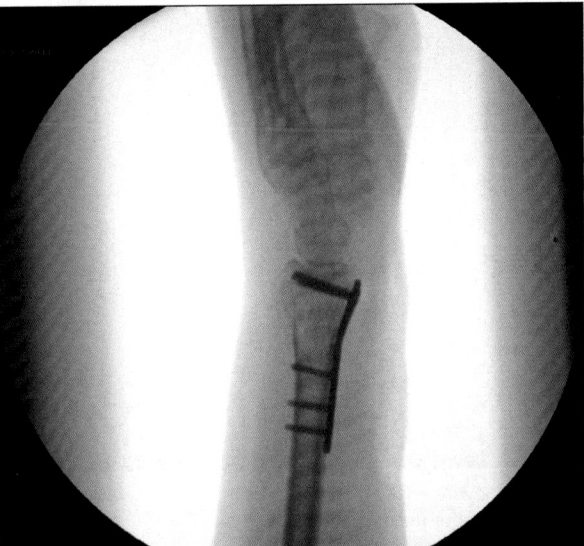

B

no available comparison of treatment methods in younger patients.

The results of ORIF of extra-articular fractures are generally good. Ring et al. reported on 24 patients, 21 of whom had extra-articular fractures. They used condylar blade plate fixation and reported good restoration of alignment and function, with 21 of their patients achieving good or excellent results according to the modified Gartland and Werley score. One fracture failed to unite and seven plates required removal.[301] Dennison reported on five distal ulnar fractures treated with locking plates which achieved excellent and good results with the modified Gartland and Werley score. Two patients had transient dorsal ulnar nerve symptoms.[79]

For the older patient it seems that nonoperative management of extra-articular distal ulnar fracture associated with distal radius fracture is satisfactory. If ORIF is deemed necessary it will achieve union with few complications and good functional result.

Intra-Articular Distal Ulnar Fractures

Intra-articular distal ulnar fractures may occur in isolation[338] or in association with distal radius fractures when they may occur with ulnar neck or styloid fractures. Treatment should follow the general principles of the treatment of intra-articular fractures as residual displacement is likely to cause a block to forearm rotation (Fig. 32-34).[338] Where there is significant displacement ORIF with headless screws or K-wires may be necessary, supplemented with plating where appropriate.

There are no reports of series of displaced intra-articular ulnar head fractures associated with distal radius fracture, but Namba et al. documented 14 patients with intra-articular ulnar fractures in association with distal radius fractures. The patients were all older than 55 years with an average age of 74 years and the ulnar fractures were treated nonoperatively after fixa-

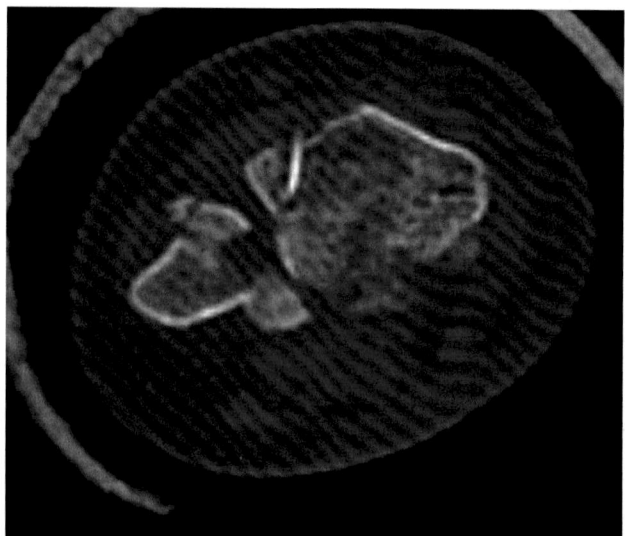

FIGURE 32-34 A severe intra-articular fracture of the ulnar head in association with a distal radius fracture. Without ORIF this would result in a block to forearm rotation.

tion of the distal radius fractures with plates. All had stable DRUJs perioperatively. At a mean of 18 months' review all had healed. Five had some residual ulnar angulation and five had mild radiographic arthrosis in the distal radioulnar joint but all had good or excellent results using the modified Gartland and Werley score. The authors concluded that bone union with satisfactory results can be achieved by nonoperative management, especially in older patients who may have osteoporotic bone.[263] Rarely, there may be severe comminution both within the joint and in the metaphysis when fixation is not feasible. This may be treated initially with restoration of alignment and cast management with the option of a salvage procedure at a later date. Acute salvage procedures have been described using ulnar head replacement,[133] resection of the ulnar head, and soft tissue interposition[328] or an acute Sauvé–Kapandji procedure,[159] but no author has demonstrated superiority of these techniques over later reconstruction.

Ulnar Styloid Fractures

Ulnar styloid fractures are the most common ulnar-sided injury associated with distal radius fractures being reported to occur in 40% to 60% of distal radius fractures.[114,190,243,277,370] Despite their frequency there remains controversy about their role in functional outcome after distal radius fracture.

There is conflicting evidence about the effect of an ulnar styloid fracture on the outcome. Older publications examine ulnar styloid fractures in association with a nonoperatively managed distal radius fracture. Frykman considered that ulnar styloid fracture had sufficient prognostic importance to include it in his classification.[114] Oskarsson et al. examined 158 patients with nonoperatively treated distal radius fractures, 70 of whom had an ulnar styloid fracture. The authors concluded that an ulnar styloid fracture was a more important predictor of outcome than articular involvement.[277] This was supported by Stoffelen et al.[356] who found a poorer prognosis in the presence of an ulnar styloid fracture.

However, other studies using nonoperative management of the distal radius fracture showed no prognostic value of an ulnar styloid fracture.[309,353] More recent studies evaluated a series of distal radius fractures treated with volar plating and ulnar styloid fractures without intraoperative distal radioulnar joint instability. None showed any correlation between functional outcomes and the presence, level, or displacement of an ulnar styloid fracture.[45,190,192,321,401,402] Kim et al.[190] concluded that an unrepaired ulnar styloid fracture does not affect wrist function or stability.

Ulnar Styloid Fracture with Distal Radioulnar Joint Instability. The stabilizing ligaments of the distal radioulnar joint (radioulnar, TFCC) insert on to the base of the ulnar styloid which may lead to concern in basal fractures that DRUJ instability is present. This is reported as occurring in 5% to 23% of distal radius fractures[115,150,184,190,210] but is likely to be less as these are selected series of unstable distal radius fractures. There is a recognized possibility of DRUJ instability with basal styloid nonunion and the importance of assessing DRUJ instability in all distal radius fractures has been emphasized.[150] Open fractures, more than 6 mm of ulnar variance, basal fracture with significant displacement, radial translation on initial radiographs, and initial fracture displacement have all been implicated as predictors of DRUJ instability.[115,210,243,298] Although suspicion of DRUJ instability should be heightened by the presence of these predictors it is generally recommended that DRUJ stability should be tested after stabilization of a distal radius fracture. This is achieved by the examiner grasping both the radius and ulna between their thumb and index finger and applying dorsal and volar pressure. The test is positive if there is more movement than on the opposite side with no firm endpoint.

If DRUJ instability is detected it can be expected to lead to a worse outcome, especially in younger patients.[224] There is no consensus on how this should be treated except when a basal ulnar styloid fracture coexists when most authorities agree that ORIF should be used to stabilize the DRUJ.

The styloid fragment is approached through a longitudinal incision over extensor carpi ulnaris with care being taken to protect the sensory branches of the ulnar nerve. Supination of the wrist may be required to reduce the fragment and fixation may then be achieved with a small cannulated screw if the fragment is large, or alternatively, K-wires and tension banding. Stability of the DRUJ should then be confirmed.

MANAGEMENT OF EXPECTED ADVERSE OUTCOMES AND UNEXPECTED COMPLICATIONS

Complications of distal radius fractures are relatively common and are reported to occur in a wide range from 5% to 31% of mixed series of fractures.[69,81,246] Some of these complications are associated with treatment of the fracture and are reported elsewhere in this chapter. This section will concentrate on fracture-specific complications.

Nerve Injury
Median Nerve

The commonest nerve injury associated with distal radius fracture is median nerve injury presenting as CTS. It has been reported as occurring in between 3% and 17% of fractures.[15,69,114,246,354] Suggested contributory causes of early CTS after distal radius fracture are swelling and hematoma extending into the carpal canal or deep to the fascia at the level of the fracture,[219,230,280] direct nerve contusion,[202,257] hematoma block,[69,202] and the Cotton-Loder position.[230] Later CTS has been attributed to callus formation and malunion.[15,69,219,280,354]

Itsubo et al. recognized that the onset of CTS after distal radius fracture can vary from 1 day to 25 years.[167,354] They grouped the onset intervals into three:

1. Acute—within 1 week of fracture (27.4%).

2. Subacute—1 to 12 weeks after fracture (44.3%).

3. Delayed—more than 12 weeks after fracture (28.3%).

The acute onset group was younger and contained significantly more males, high-energy injuries, and AO type C injuries. In contrast the other two groups had more older women with lower-energy injuries and extra-articular fractures. Residual deformity after reduction was evenly distributed between the three groups. A further group could be added—the transient CTS where symptoms resolve after reduction.[15]

It is important to recognize the development of acute CTS after distal radius fracture as failure to treat the condition can lead to permanent median nerve dysfunction. It is defined by its development within hours of fracture injury and reduction and its progressive worsening. It is thought to be caused by increased pressure in the carpal tunnel. Dyer et al. examined 50 patients who had carpal tunnel decompression for acute CTS and ORIF of their fracture, and using multivariant analysis identified women less than 48 years of age with more than 35% fracture translation as being at significant increased risk of developing acute CTS. The authors suggested that further study was required before considering prophylactic carpal tunnel decompression in this group and emphasized the need for vigilance in diagnosing acute CTS after distal radius fracture.[87]

Subacute or delayed onset CTS occurs in older patients with lower-energy injury, with malunion being a possible contributory factor.[15,167,354] Late CTS also has a negative influence on functional outcome after distal radius fracture.[31] Decompression is successful in the majority of patients,[230,354] but it should be noted that compression may occur proximal to the wrist crease at the level of the fracture and release should be extended to this area.[219]

Ulnar Nerve

Ulnar nerve injury is less common than median injury with prevalence reported as being 0.5% to 4.2%.[15,21] It is thought that the mobility of the ulnar nerve at the wrist and in the forearm protects it from injury.[63] Reported risk fractures are instability of the DRUJ,[63,345] open fractures, high-energy injury, and severe fracture displacement. Most of these injuries are neurapraxias which recover spontaneously. Exploration is recommended where there is complete ulnar palsy with an open wound or concurrent acute CTS.[345]

Tendon Injury

Tendon injury occurs with distal radius fractures treated both operatively and nonoperatively. The commonest tendon involved is EPL which is usually reported as occurring in less than 1% of fractures[161,246,354] but has been reported in up to 5% of fractures.[69,307,334]

A number of mechanisms for EPL injury after distal radius fracture have been proposed and may be either fracture- or hardware-related. Hardware-related ruptures most commonly occur with volar or dorsal plating and are discussed in the relevant sections of this chapter.

Both mechanical and biologic causes have been suggested for fracture-related EPL rupture. Attritional causes cited theorize that an intact extensor retinaculum holds the tendon on to a spike of sharp bone, a roughened area of the distal radius, or a nonunion of Lister tubercle.[152,350] Some authors have postulated a vascular cause with ischemia of a segment of the tendon because of narrowing of the third extensor compartment with an already poorly vascularized area becoming avascular and mechanical obstruction preventing the normal volume of synovial fluid.[156] This theory is supported by the ultrasonic finding of thickening of the EPL sheath after distal radius fracture.[279]

EPL ruptures have been reported as occurring more commonly in undisplaced or minimally displaced distal radius fractures[307] and at various times after injury. It is likely that fracture-related ruptures occur earlier after injury at an average of around 6 weeks whilst later ruptures may be more likely to be related to attritional problems on hardware. White et al.[391] reported that EPL rupture occurred at an average of 9 weeks after initial injury in nonoperatively managed patients and at an average of 20 months after plating.

If the patient has symptoms causing a functional problem after EPL rupture then tendon transfer, usually with extensor indicis proprius, should be considered. This is reported as achieving satisfactory outcomes with low DASH scores,[391] a high proportion of excellent and good results,[161] minimal loss of thumb extension, and restoration of around 70% of grip and tip pinch strength by 8 weeks after surgery.[125]

Fracture-related flexor tendon injuries are much rarer possibly because the muscle belly of pronator quadratus acts as a cushioning layer between the flexor tendons and bone. Before the early 1990s only 12 cases of flexor tendon rupture had been reported in the world literature. However, a literature search for flexor tendon rupture in distal radius fracture in the last 25 years records 19 studies specifically relating to flexor tendon rupture, mainly FPL, after volar plating indicating that this is a hardware-related problem.

Malunion

Malunion of fractures of the distal radius (Fig. 32-35) remains common although it is frequently not reported as a complication of distal radius fracture. When reported the prevalence is difficult to assess as there is considerable controversy around the definition of malunion. The reported rates of malunion are also affected by the selective nature of some studies in their recruitment of stable and unstable fractures and their methods of treatment, both of which influence the prevalence of malunion. The effect of malunion on functional outcome is also debatable but treatment of malunion should not be considered because of radiologic deformity alone but only in the symptomatic patient. A possible exception to this is in severe articular malunion where symptoms may not arise until there is irreversible degeneration within the joint. In these circumstances some authorities recommend osteotomy in cases with severe articular displacement in the absence of symptoms.[242,294,302]

Typical symptoms of malunion are as follows.

1. Pain—ulnar sided
   —carpal
   —radiocarpal
2. Weakness of grip
3. Reduced range of movement, especially rotation
4. Deformity

Pain is a common symptom of distal radius malunion and can be located in the DRUJ, the carpal area or the radiocarpal

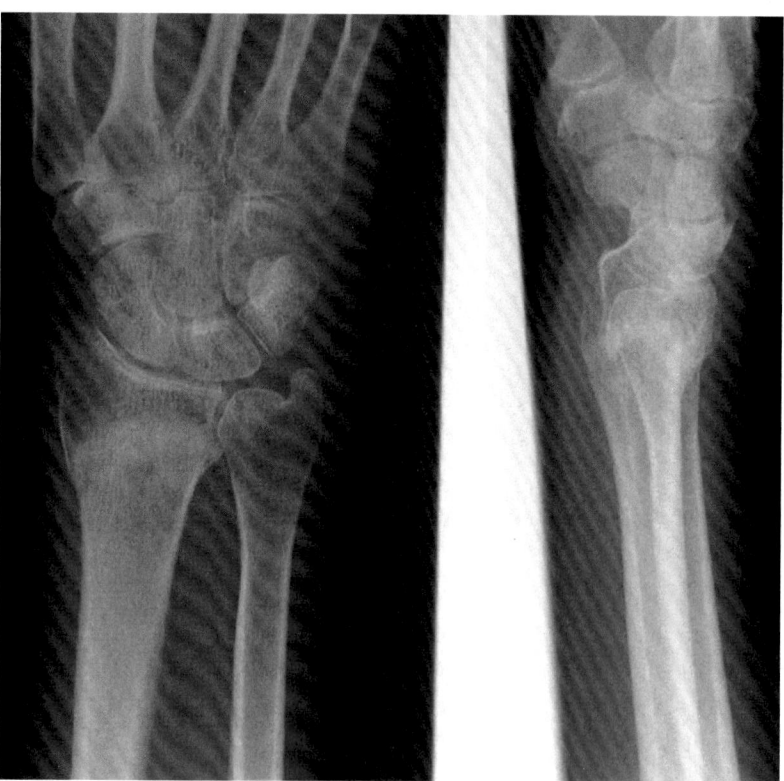

FIGURE 32-35 Malunion of a distal radius fracture with dorsal tilt, radial shortening, and carpal malalignment.

joint. DRUJ pain is common[253] and probably caused by incongruency of the sigmoid notch because of the tilt of the radius, intra-articular malunion, or damage to the cartilage of the ulnar head. Carpal pain is caused by the altered mechanics of the malaligned carpus,[30,143,285,361] is typically felt over the dorsum of the hand, and may develop gradually after fracture healing.[362] Radiocarpal pain is usually attributable to intra-articular malalignment or developing osteoarthritis in the radiocarpal joint. It is important to differentiate between the three areas of pain to direct treatment appropriately.

A reduced range of movement is also a common complaint after distal radius malunion, most frequently reduced forearm rotation caused by malalignment or incongruity of the DRUJ from dorsal or volar tilt, radial shortening, or intra-articular pathology. Wrist flexion may be reduced with dorsal malunion and extension with volar malunion. Weak grip strength may be because of pain or the mechanical disadvantage of the adaptive carpal collapse or malalignment. Later CTS may also develop as malunion of the distal radius.[15,280]

Treatment of Malunion

In the fit independent patient the treatment of symptomatic malunion is surgical.

Timing. The timing of surgical treatment has recently been questioned and highlights a dilemma for the surgeon. It is usual practice that correction of malunion be delayed as this allows a clear definition of residual problems and may prevent unnecessary surgery.[103] However, delay leads to an increased period of disability and more difficulty in defining the plane of deformity at surgery. Delay may also lead to soft tissue contracture and more challenging correction of the deformity with the potential for more added ulnar procedure. Jupiter and Ring examined 20 patients who had undergone distal radial osteotomy for a variety of deformities. Half had surgery within 14 weeks of fracture with an average of 8 weeks delay and 10 had later correction at a minimum of 30 weeks and an average of 40 weeks. At review at an average of 4 years for the early or "nascent" malunions and 34 months for the late malunions the authors demonstrated easier correction, less graft donor site morbidity, more rapid healing, and better outcomes in the early group.[179] A similar more recent study found fewer benefits although the early group required less bone grafting.[286] The former group concluded that early osteotomy should be considered in patients with high functional demand; the latter recommended early osteotomy if the patient presented early with symptoms but a period of review before coming to a decision on later presenting patients.

Contraindications to distal radial osteotomy include significant osteoarthritis of the radiocarpal joint when fusion may be necessary, intra-articular osteotomy in the presence of less than 2 mm of displacement, and the presence of complex regional pain syndrome.[44] Technique positioning is similar to that for ORIF with the patient supine and the affected arm abducted on the side table. A tourniquet is used. The approach and technique then depend on the anatomy of the deformity.

Dorsal Extra-Articular Malunion. Dorsal malunion usually requires a dorsal approach. The size of the incision is determined by the technique of stabilization used. For plating a dorsal longitudinal approach is required. The EPL tendon is released from its groove and the radius exposed subperiosteally. Alternatively, a minimally invasive technique using nonbridging external fixation may be used.[253] This requires a 3-cm transverse or skin crease incision at the level of the deformity with a longitudinal incision in the extensor retinaculum. The technique requires less dissection as access is only required for the saw blade. Some surgeons may utilize a volar approach if a volar locking plate is to be used.

Either a closing or an opening wedge may be used. A closing wedge osteotomy has the advantage of bone-to-bone contact and more stability although with modern implants the latter is less important. However there is no residual bone defect so bone grafting is not required. The disadvantage of a closing wedge is its failure to correct any radial shortening leading to the frequent need for ulnar-sided procedures.[382] An opening wedge osteotomy is more frequently used as it generates additional radial length. It can be tailored to correct both frontal and sagittal deformity (Fig. 32-36). The disadvantages of this technique are less stability and the need for bone graft.

Many types of fixation have been described to stabilize distal radial osteotomy. Dorsal plating has been the most popular[42,44,103,225,294] (Fig. 32-36) although some more recent reports have described the use of volar locked plates for dorsal deformity.[154,236,273] Cited advantages over dorsal plating are fewer tendon problems than dorsal plates and the use of morselized bone grafting as the volar locked plate does not need structural support[154] and in some cases no bone graft,[236] but these advantages have not yet been proven.

The use of nonbridging external fixation to stabilize the osteotomy (Fig. 32-37) has a number of potential advantages. These include a minimally invasive technique, easy control and correction of the distal fragment, the use of nonstructural cancellous bone graft, and the ease of removal of the implant which does not require hospital admission.[22,253]

Percutaneous pin stabilization of distal radial osteotomies has been used previously but does not give sufficient stability for a reliable result. The evolving technique of intramedullary nailing has also been reported to be successful.[47]

The consensus view on the outcome of osteotomy for a dorsal extra-articular malunion is that the procedure improves both radiologic and functional outcomes but rarely to normal.[44,103,207,225] All authors agree that prevention of malunion is preferable.

The technique is reliable in improving the radiologic outcome although volar tilt is not consistently restored with plating techniques.[42,44,103,225] Volar tilt is reported as being reliably restored and maintained using nonbridging external fixation, perhaps because of the control obtained by the distal pins.[253] Functional outcomes show consistent improvement in both objective and patient-related outcome measures,[154,179,207,253] but a number of authors caution that results can deteriorate in the longer term as distal radial osteotomy does not prevent

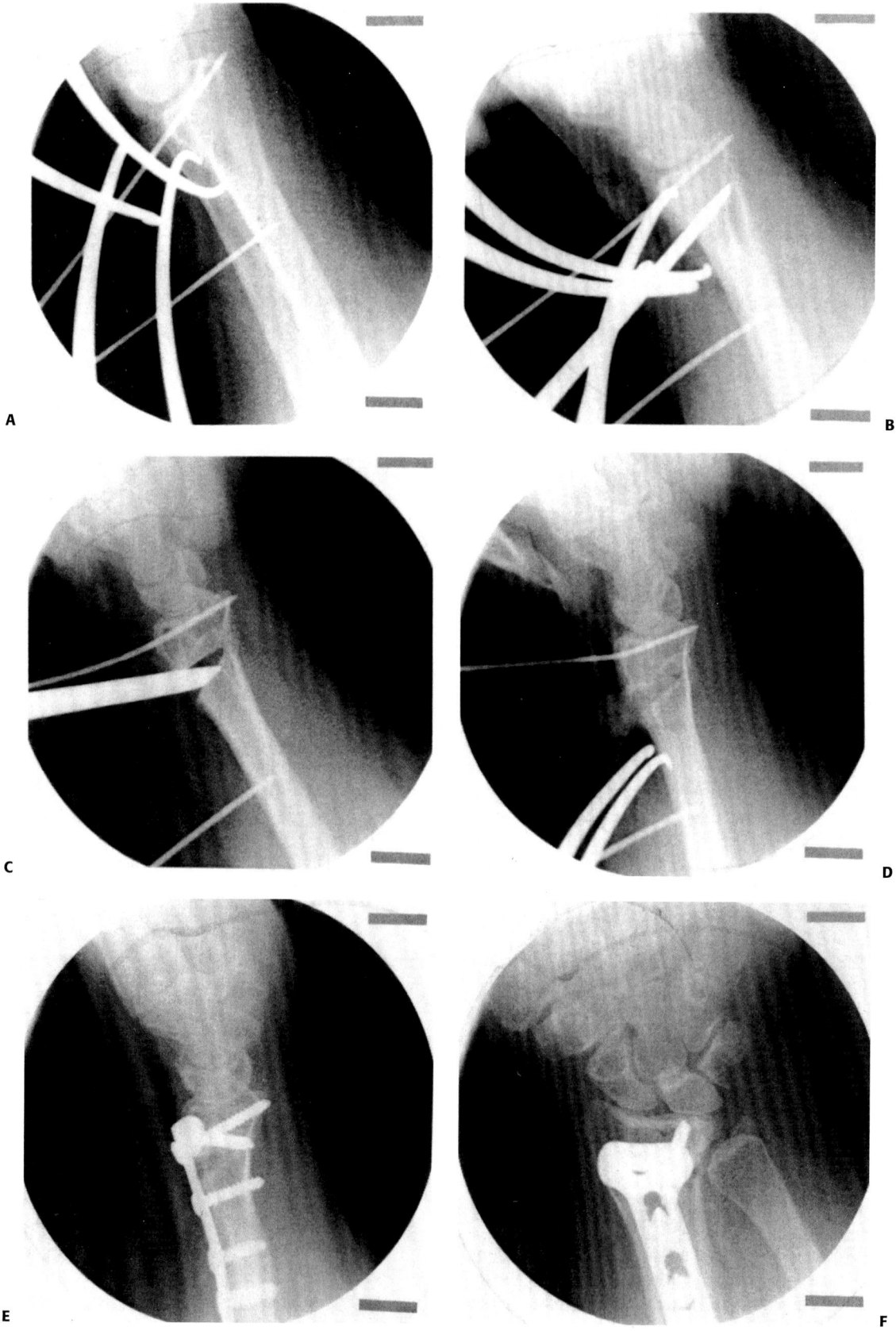

FIGURE 32-36 Technique of osteotomy for a dorsal malunion. Pins are placed parallel to the joint and perpendicular to the shaft **(A)**. An oscillating saw is used to cut the dorsal cortex **(B)**, whereas the palmar cortex is left intact. The fragment is levered into position **(C)**, and the bone graft is placed **(D)** and a dorsal plate is applied **(E, F)**.

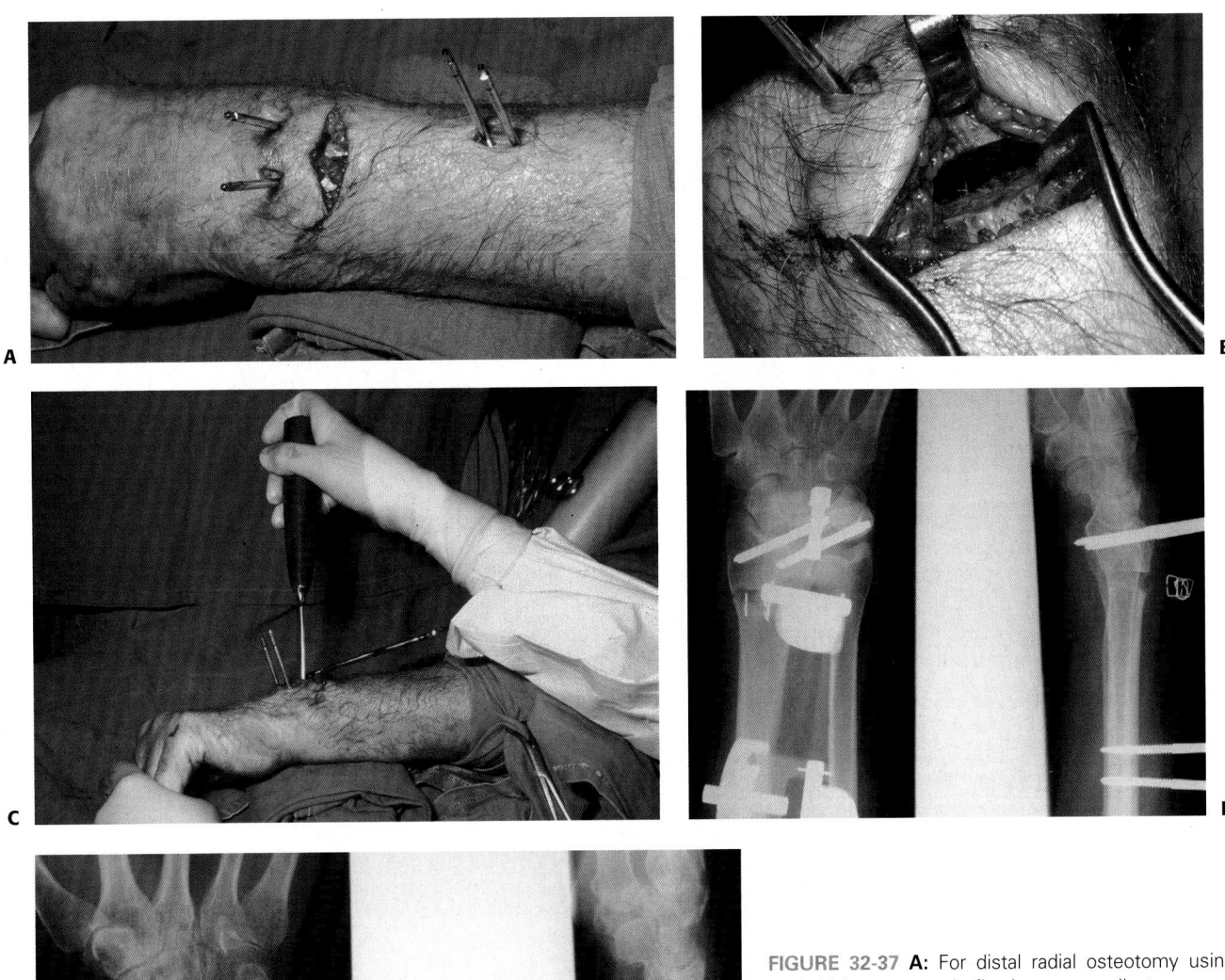

FIGURE 32-37 A: For distal radial osteotomy using nonbridging external fixation a small transverse skin incision is sufficient. A longitudinal incision is then made through the extensor retinaculum. **B:** After insertion of the fixator pins the osteotomy is made at the site of deformity. **C:** Correction is performed using an osteotome as a lever. The pins are only used for fine adjustments to avoid excessive force on them. **D:** The postoperative radiographs show cancellous bone graft in the defect and a good correction of the deformity shown in Figure 38. **E:** The external fixator is removed in the outpatient department at about 6 weeks when healing has taken place.

progression of osteoarthritis.[103,225] Complication rates are generally high with substantial reoperation rates in some series.[44,103,179,225]

Volar Extra-Articular Malunion. Volar malunion of the distal radius is less common than dorsal malunion, probably because the prevalence of volar displacement is less and because there is a general recognition that volar displaced fractures are unstable and undergo primary fixation.

The approach is volar and plating is the treatment of choice. Volar malunion is frequently a translational deformity with little angular deformity or bone loss. Where this is the case an oblique sliding osteotomy can be performed and bone grafting is not required (Fig. 32-38).[367] If an angular deformity is present an opening wedge osteotomy and bone graft is required.[329] Good radiographic and functional results have been reported with both techniques although residual DRUJ symptoms limit its success.[329,367]

Intra-Articular Malunion. Intra-articular malunion of the distal radius may have serious consequences with early onset of degenerative changes, particularly if associated with joint subluxation. Despite this there were few reports of intra-articular osteotomy until recently possibly because of concerns about the difficulty of the technique and potential complications. The advent of improved imaging may have promoted interest in the technique.

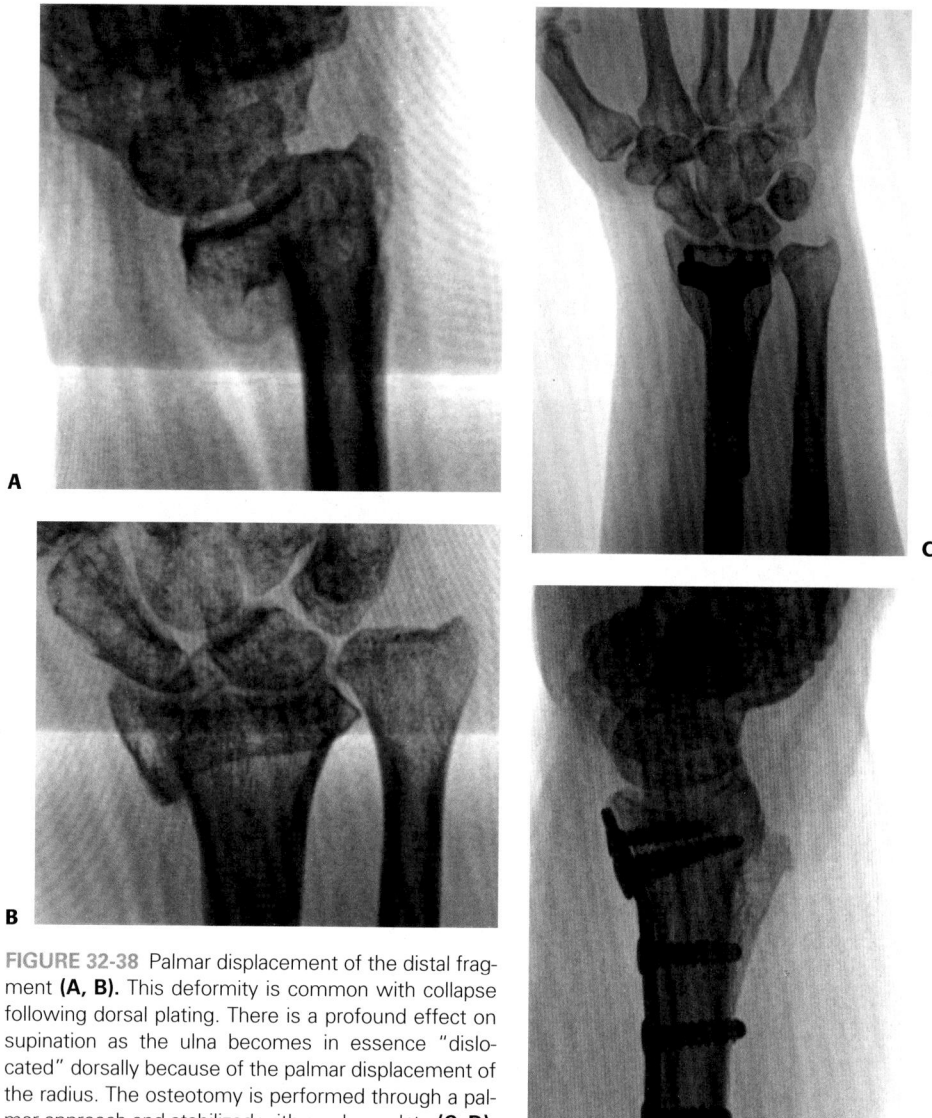

FIGURE 32-38 Palmar displacement of the distal fragment **(A, B).** This deformity is common with collapse following dorsal plating. There is a profound effect on supination as the ulna becomes in essence "dislocated" dorsally because of the palmar displacement of the radius. The osteotomy is performed through a palmar approach and stabilized with a palmar plate **(C, D).**

Indications for surgery are a residual step-off or gap of more than 2 mm especially if associated with extra-articular malunion or joint subluxation (Fig. 32-39). Surgery should not be considered in lower-demand patients or those with advanced osteoarthritis. Most authorities do not feel that it is necessary for the patient to be symptomatic as awaiting symptoms inevitably means progression of arthritis which may preclude a reconstructive procedure.[294,302]

The approach is dictated by the location of the malunion and both dorsal and volar approaches may be necessary. On the dorsal side the joint may be visualized by a transverse capsulotomy; on the volar side the joint should be seen through the osteotomy as a volar capsulotomy is contraindicated. The original fracture line is re-created using an osteotome and fixation is usually by small plates or wires (Fig. 32-39C). Bone grafting is required for any residual metaphyseal defect.

Marx and Axelrod reported an early series of four patients treated with intra-articular osteotomy and demonstrated excellent and good results, an average grip strength of 86%, and no advancing arthrosis at an average of 23 months postoperatively. The authors concluded that intra-articular osteotomy was the treatment of choice for intra-articular malunion.[242] More recently larger series have been reported. Both studies reported significant improvements in ranges of movement and grip strength with an average DASH score of 11 in one[44] and 19 of 23 good or excellent results in another.[302] The authors of the latter study concluded that the procedure rarely restored normal function but useful function could be obtained.

Ulnar-Sided Procedures. There are a number of ulnar-sided procedures available ranging from excisional hemiarthroplasty of the DRUJ to an excision of the distal ulna with or without replacement.[116] Ulnar-sided procedures are indicated for persistent pain, rotational contracture, or instability of the

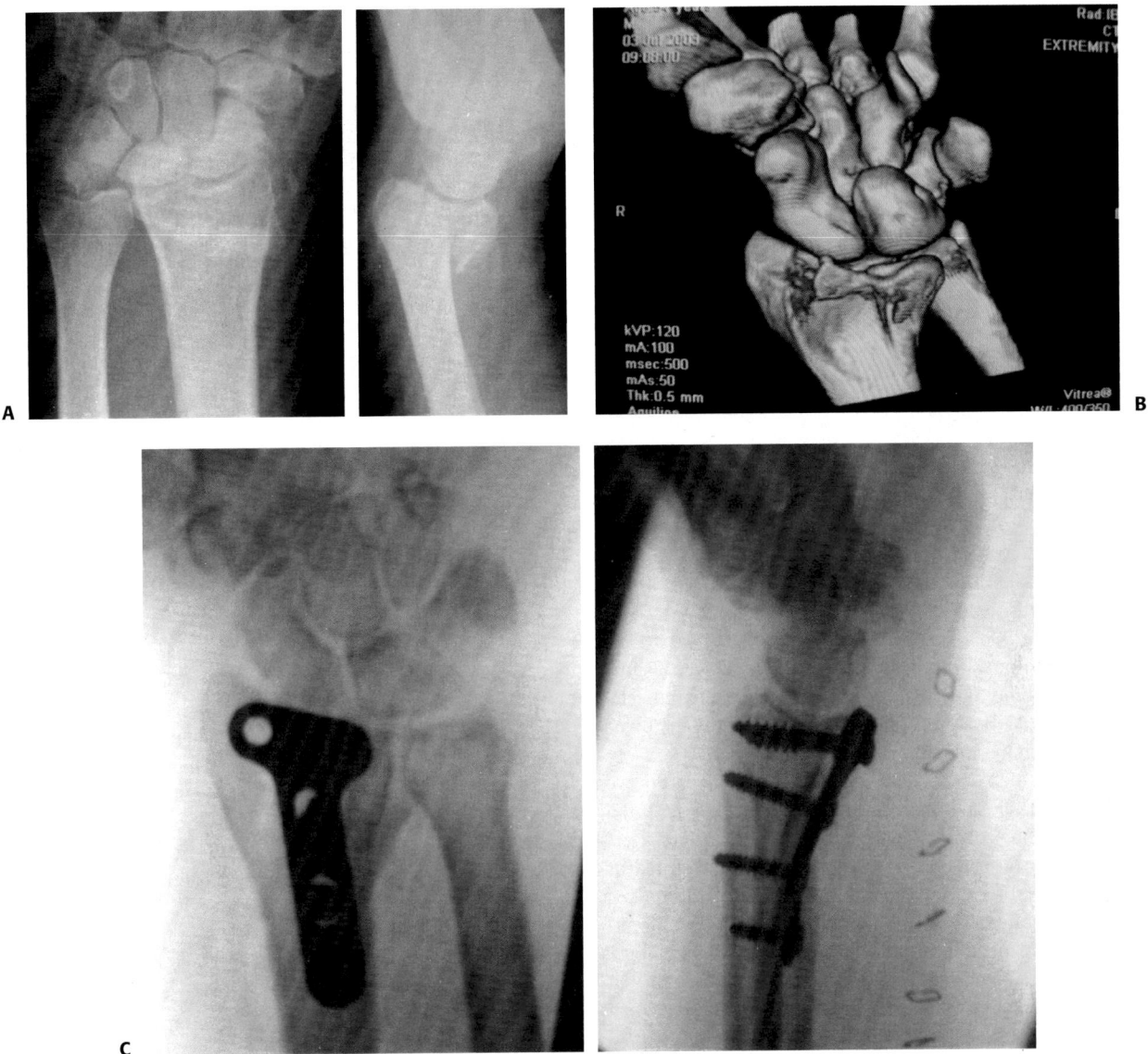

FIGURE 32-39 A: A displaced intra-articular fracture of the distal radius with volar subluxation of the joint 8 weeks after injury. **B:** A CT scan demonstrates the deformity. **C:** An intra-articular osteotomy was performed through a volar approach. The displacement and subluxation have been corrected.

DRUJ and may be performed in conjunction with distal radial osteotomy, at a later stage, or in isolation if there is no malunion of the distal radius. After distal radial osteotomy the range of forearm rotation should always be assessed. If rotation remains significantly compromised then an ulnar-sided procedure should be considered.

Bower's Procedure. This is a hemiresection interposition arthroplasty of the DRUJ and is indicated for a symptomatic DRUJ without an ulnar positive variance. This technique involves excision of a substantial portion of the ulnar head leaving the ulnar styloid, TFCC, and an ulnar column of cortex intact. It has the advantage of retaining the connection between the ulnar column and the radius leaving support on the ulnar side of the carpus from the ulnar styloid and TFCC. To gain full benefit the TFCC must be intact and sufficient bone must be

excised. It will not succeed where there is radial shortening as resection of the ulnar head allows some radioulnar convergence which may cause ulnocarpal impingement. In this situation the procedure should be combined with ulnar shortening.[37]

The outcome of the Bower's procedure is usually reported for mixed conditions and not specifically for distal radius fracture. Improvement in pain, function, and patient satisfaction is usually reported.[37,287]

Sauvé–Kapandji Procedure. The Sauvé–Kapandji procedure also maintains support on the ulnar side of the radiocarpal joint by retaining the ulnar head and fusing it with screws to the sigmoid notch (Fig. 32-40). To regain rotation a segment of ulna is excised at the level of the ulnar neck. If there is radial shortening the ulnar head must be aligned with the sigmoid notch prior to fusion. Sufficient bone must be excised to

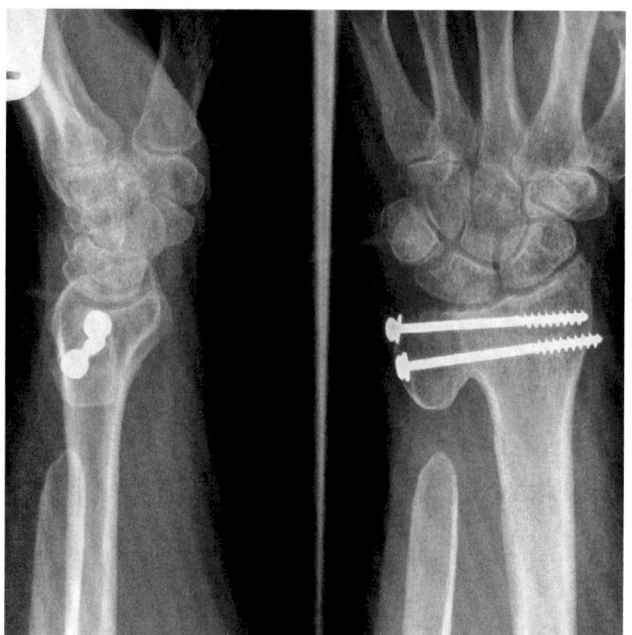

FIGURE 32-40 A Sauvé–Kapandji procedure.

prevent the osteotomy healing but this must be balanced against the risk of instability of the stump if too much is excised. The recommended length of excision is 10 to 15 mm plus any ulnar positive variance present.[49,75,123,361]

The outcome of this procedure is generally agreed to improve pain and function but not predictably. George et al.[123] reported mean DASH scores of 23 ranging from 0 to 60 at an average of 4 years postoperatively. Rotation is reliably restored or improved but in some cases remains painful with symptoms of clicking or instability at the osteotomy site.[49,123,361] Disappointing numbers of patients return to their preinjury employment, especially if manual laborers.[49,361] It should be recognized that this is a salvage technique and may not restore a painfree wrist.

Darrach's Procedure. Darrach's procedure is excision of the distal end of the ulnar and was first described for malunion

of the distal radius by William Darrach in 1912. The recommended level of excision is at the proximal end of the sigmoid notch.[123,247] Mixed results are reported with the main problem being radioulnar convergence which occurs with loss of the buttress at the DRUJ and causes scalloping in the radius at the level of the stump.[27] George et al.[123] reported a mean DASH score of 23 after Darrach's procedure with a range from 4 to 61. Grawe et al.[132] examined 27 patients in the longer term and found a mean score of 17 using the QuickDASH score. The range of rotation is reliably restored.[123,132,258]

Two studies have compared the Darrach's procedure with the Sauvé–Kapandji procedure with one of these also including Bower's procedure. Minami et al.[258] found significantly less pain relief, deterioration in grip strength, and fewer patients returning to work after Darrach's compared to Sauvé–Kapandji and Bower's with increased wrist instability, although they recognized that the Darrach's group was older. George et al.[123] found no significant differences between the Darrach's procedure and the Sauvé–Kapandji procedure in younger patients. It is generally recommended that Darrach's procedure should be reserved for older, frailer patients.

Ulnar Shortening. Ulnar shortening is indicated where there is symptomatic ulnocarpal impingement after a distal radius fracture, the commonest reason for ulnar positive variance.[116] If there is an accompanying angular malunion of the radius then up to 7 mm of radial length can be restored by distal radial osteotomy, but if larger length discrepancy needs to be corrected ulnar shortening is required. If the radius has shortened without angular deformity an isolated ulnar shortening is the procedure of choice. Where there is degenerative change evident in the DRUJ an added Bower's procedure may be necessary.

Ulnar shortening osteotomy is performed using parallel transverse cuts, a step cut, or an oblique osteotomy. A transverse osteotomy is simplest but requires the use of a compression device to stabilize the osteotomy during plating.[116] Compression plating is then used (Fig. 32-41). Immobilization is not required if the plating is secure.

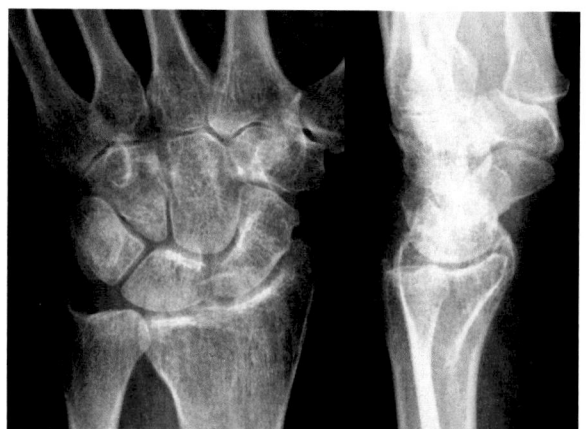
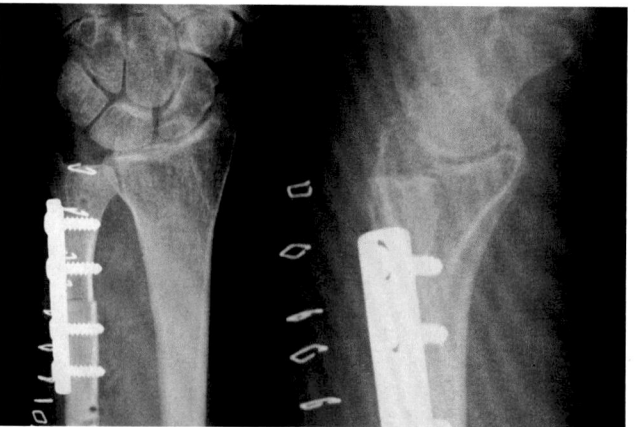

FIGURE 32-41 A distal radius fracture has healed without angular deformity but with radial shortening **(A)**. In this situation an isolated ulnar shortening procedure was performed using a transverse cut and a 4 hole plate **(B)**. The normal radio-ulnar relationship has been restored.

Ulnar shortening has been reported to result in patient satisfaction in most cases[113] with improvement in QuickDASH scores reported in one study from 43 preoperatively to 11 postoperatively at an average of almost 3 years after surgery.[349] The technique has a low complication rate with the commonest complication being nonunion. Step cut and oblique osteotomies are more complex and were proposed initially to reduce the nonunion rate but this benefit has not yet been demonstrated.[113]

Ulnar Head Replacement. Ulnar head replacement after distal radius fracture is a salvage procedure usually reserved for painful radioulnar impingement following failed Darrach or Sauvé–Kapandji procedures. Restoration of stability with the prosthesis depends on adequate soft tissues being available to stabilize the head of the implant in the sigmoid notch. Distal radial malunion should be corrected prior to replacement. Both short- and long-term results of this procedure are encouraging with restoration of lasting stability and few complications.[376,397]

Nonunion

Nonunion of the distal radius is rare occurring in well under 1% of fractures[21] and may occur in the presence of extensive metaphyseal comminution.[292] The diagnosis is made in the presence of continuing pain and increasing deformity. It is usually treated with plating and bone grafting to which most nonunions are amenable even with small distal fragments.[89,292,293] Wrist fusion should be reserved for cases where plating and bone grafting fail.

Complex Regional Pain Syndrome (CRPS)

CRPS is a serious and often debilitating complication of a number of injuries but is most commonly seen after distal radius fracture. Its etiology is unknown and it is characterized by a number of symptoms and signs including pain, swelling, color and temperature change, and joint contracture. The subject is considered in detail in Chapter 25.

CONTROVERSIES AND FUTURE DIRECTIONS

Fracture of the distal radius remains the commonest fracture treated by orthopedic trauma surgeons, but despite this there is no consensus about the treatment of more complex cases with metaphyseal instability or intra-articular displacement. More work is required to define more accurately those cases that require surgical management. It is essential to eliminate bias toward surgery from our studies and concentrate on patient benefit.

Over the next decade the most challenging aspect of distal radius fractures will be the increasing numbers of older patients presenting with the injury. To meet this challenge future research should focus on defining those older patients who will benefit from more invasive treatment.

REFERENCES

1. Abbaszadegan H, Jonsson U. Regional anesthesia preferable for Colles' fracture. Controlled comparison with local anesthesia. *Acta Orthop Scand.* 1990;61:348–349.
2. Abramo A, Kopylov P, Geijer M, et al. Open reduction and internal fixation compared to closed reduction and external fixation in distal radial fractures: a randomized study of 50 patients. *Acta Orthop.* 2009;80:478–485.
3. Adams BD. Effects of radial deformity on distal radioulnar joint mechanics. *J Hand Surg Am.* 1993;18:492–498.
4. Agee JM. Distal radius fractures. Multiplanar ligamentotaxis. *Hand Clin.* 1993;9:577–585.
5. Aggarwal AK, Nagi ON. Open reduction and internal fixation of volar Barton's fractures: a prospective study. *J Orthop Surg (Hong Kong).* 2004;12:230–234.
6. Ahlborg HG, Josefsson PO. Pin-tract complications in external fixation of fractures of the distal radius. *Acta Orthop Scand.* 1999;70:116–118.
7. Ahmed LA, Schirmer H, Bjornerem A, et al. The gender- and age-specific 10-year and lifetime absolute fracture risk in Tromso, Norway. *Eur J Epidemiol.* 2009;24:441–448.
8. Aktekin CN, Altay M, Gursoy Z, et al. Comparison between external fixation and cast treatment in the management of distal radius fractures in patients aged 65 years and older. *J Hand Surg Am.* 2010;35:736–742.
9. Allain J, le GP, Le MS, et al. Trans-styloid fixation of fractures of the distal radius. A prospective randomized comparison between 6- and 1-week postoperative immobilization in 60 fractures. *Acta Orthop Scand.* 1999;70:119–123.
10. Amorosa LF, Vitale MA, Brown S, et al. A functional outcomes survey of elderly patients who sustained distal radius fractures. *Hand (N Y).* 2011;6:260–267.
11. Andersen DJ, Blair WF, Steyers CM Jr, et al. Classification of distal radius fractures: an analysis of interobserver reliability and intraobserver reproducibility. *J Hand Surg Am.* 1996;21:574–582.
12. Andersen JK, Hogh A, Gantov J, et al. Colles' fracture treated with non-bridging external fixation: a 1-year follow-up. *J Hand Surg Eur Vol.* 2009;34:475–478.
13. Anderson R, O'Neil G. Comminuted fractures of the distal end of the radius. *Surg Gynaecol Obstet.* 1944;738:434–440.
14. Anzarut A, Johnson JA, Rowe BH, et al. Radiologic and patient-reported functional outcomes in an elderly cohort with conservatively treated distal radius fractures. *J Hand Surg Am.* 2004;29:1121–1127.
15. Aro H, Koivunen T, Katevuo K, et al. Late compression neuropathies after Colles' fractures. *Clin Orthop Relat Res.* 1988;217–225.
16. Arora R, Lutz M, Deml C, et al. A prospective randomized trial comparing nonoperative treatment with volar locking plate fixation for displaced and unstable distal radial fractures in patients sixty-five years of age and older. *J Bone Joint Surg Am.* 2011;93:2146–2153.
17. Arora R, Lutz M, Zimmermann R, et al. [Limits of palmar locking-plate osteosynthesis of unstable distal radius fractures]. *Handchir Mikrochir Plast Chir.* 2007;39:34–41.
18. Asadollahi S, Keith PP. Flexor tendon injuries following plate fixation of distal radius fractures: a systematic review of the literature. *J Orthop Traumatol.* 2013;14:227–234.
19. Atroshi I, Brogren E, Larsson GU, et al. Wrist-bridging versus non-bridging external fixation for displaced distal radius fractures: a randomized assessor-blind clinical trial of 38 patients followed for 1 year. *Acta Orthop.* 2006;77:445–453.
20. Azzopardi T, Ehrendorfer S, Coulton T, et al. Unstable extra-articular fractures of the distal radius: a prospective, randomised study of immobilisation in a cast versus supplementary percutaneous pinning. *J Bone Joint Surg Br.* 2005;87:837–840.
21. Bacorn RW, Kurtzke JF. Colles' fracture; a study of two thousand cases from the New York State Workmen's Compensation Board. *J Bone Joint Surg Am.* 1953;35-A:643–658.
22. Baillon R, Gris M, Tollet P, et al. [Corrective osteotomy using Hoffmann II external fixators for extra-auricular malunion of the distal radius]. *Acta Orthop Belg.* 2001;67:500–504.
23. Baratz ME, Des JJ, Anderson DD, et al. Displaced intra-articular fractures of the distal radius: the effect of fracture displacement on contact stresses in a cadaver model. *J Hand Surg Am.* 1996;21:183–188.
24. Barton JR. Views and treatment of an important injury of the wrist. *Medi Examiner.* 1838;1:365–368.
25. Batra S, Gupta A. The effect of fracture-related factors on the functional outcome at 1 year in distal radius fractures. *Injury.* 2002;33:499–502.
26. Beck C III. Fracture of the carpal end of the radius, with fissure or fracture of the lower end of the ulna, and other associated injuries. *Ann Surg.* 1901;34:249–267.
27. Bell MJ, Hill RJ, McMurtry RY. Ulnar impingement syndrome. *J Bone Joint Surg Br.* 1985;67:126–129.
28. Bengner U, Johnell O. Increasing incidence of forearm fractures. A comparison of epidemiologic patterns 25 years apart. *Acta Orthop Scand.* 1985;56:158–160.
29. Beumer A, McQueen MM. Fractures of the distal radius in low-demand elderly patients: closed reduction of no value in 53 of 60 wrists. *Acta Orthop Scand.* 2003;74:98–100.
30. Bickerstaff DR, Bell MJ. Carpal malalignment in Colles' fractures. *J Hand Surg Br.* 1989;14:155–160.
31. Bienek T, Kusz D, Cielinski L. Peripheral nerve compression neuropathy after fractures of the distal radius. *J Hand Surg Br.* 2006;31:256–260.
32. Bini A, Surace MF, Pilato G. Complex articular fractures of the distal radius: the role of closed reduction and external fixation. *J Hand Surg Eur Vol.* 2008;33:305–310.
33. Biyani A. Over-distraction of the radio-carpal and mid-carpal joints following external fixation of comminuted distal radial fractures. *J Hand Surg Br.* 1993;18:506–510.
34. Biyani A, Simison AJ, Klenerman L. Fractures of the distal radius and ulna. *J Hand Surg Br.* 1995;20:357–364.
35. Bolmers A, Luiten WE, Doornberg JN, et al. A comparison of the long-term outcome of partial articular (AO Type B) and complete articular (AO Type C) distal radius fractures. *J Hand Surg Am.* 2013;38:753–759.
36. Bong MR, Egol KA, Leibman M, et al. A comparison of immediate postreduction splinting constructs for controlling initial displacement of fractures of the distal radius: a prospective randomized study of long-arm versus short-arm splinting. *J Hand Surg Am.* 2006;31:766–770.
37. Bowers WH. Distal radioulnar joint arthroplasty. Current concepts. *Clin Orthop Relat Res.* 1992;275:104–109.
38. Brady O, Rice J, Nicholson P, et al. The unstable distal radial fracture one year post Kapandji intrafocal pinning. *Injury.* 1999;30:251–255.
39. Braun RM, Gellman H. Dorsal pin placement and external fixation for correction of dorsal tilt in fractures of the distal radius. *J Hand Surg Am.* 1994;19:653–655.
40. Brogren E, Hofer M, Petranek M, et al. Relationship between distal radius fracture malunion and arm-related disability: a prospective population-based cohort study with 1-year follow-up. *BMC Musculoskelet Disord.* 2011;12:9.

41. Brogren E, Petranek M, Atroshi I. Incidence and characteristics of distal radius fractures in a southern Swedish region. *BMC Musculoskelet Disord.* 2007;8:48.
42. Brown JN, Bell MJ. Distal radial osteotomy for malunion of wrist fractures in young patients. *J Hand Surg Br.* 1994;19:589–593.
43. Buhr AJ, Cooke AM. Fracture patterns. *Lancet.* 1959;1:531–536.
44. Buijze GA, Prommersberger KJ, Gonzalez del PJ, et al. Corrective osteotomy for combined intra- and extra-articular distal radius malunion. *J Hand Surg Am.* 2012;37:2041–2049.
45. Buijze GA, Ring D. Clinical impact of United versus nonunited fractures of the proximal half of the ulnar styloid following volar plate fixation of the distal radius. *J Hand Surg Am.* 2010;35:223–227.
46. Capo JT, Accousti K, Jacob G, et al. The effect of rotational malalignment on X-rays of the wrist. *J Hand Surg Eur Vol.* 2009;34:166–172.
47. Capo JT, Hashem J, Orillaza NS, et al. Treatment of extra-articular distal radial malunions with an intramedullary implant. *J Hand Surg Am.* 2010;35:892–899.
48. Capo JT, Rossy W, Henry P, et al. External fixation of distal radius fractures: effect of distraction and duration. *J Hand Surg Am.* 2009;34:1605–1611.
49. Carter PB, Stuart PR. The Sauve-Kapandji procedure for post-traumatic disorders of the distal radio-ulnar joint. *J Bone Joint Surg Br.* 2000;82:1013–1038.
50. Catalano LW III, Cole RJ, Gelberman RH, et al. Displaced intra-articular fractures of the distal aspect of the radius. Long-term results in young adults after open reduction and internal fixation. *J Bone Joint Surg Am.* 1997;79:1290–1302.
51. Cha SM, Shin HD, Kim KC, et al. Treatment of unstable distal ulna fractures associated with distal radius fractures in patients 65 years and older. *J Hand Surg Am.* 2012;37:2481–2487.
52. Chang HC, Poh SY, Seah SC, et al. Fragment-specific fracture fixation and double-column plating of unstable distal radial fractures using AO mini-fragment implants and Kirschner wires. *Injury.* 2007;38:1259–1267.
53. Changulani M, Okonkwo U, Keswani T, et al. Outcome evaluation measures for wrist and hand: which one to choose? *Int Orthop.* 2008;32:1–6.
54. Checketts RG. Pin track infections and the principles of pin track care. In: DeBastiani A, Apley GA, Goldberg DE, eds. *Orthofix External Fixation in Trauma and Orthopaedics.* Berlin: Springer; 2000:97–103.
55. Chen CE, Juhn RJ, Ko JY. Treatment of distal radius fractures with percutaneous pinning and pin-in-plaster. *Hand (N Y).* 2008;3:245–250.
56. Chia B, Catalano LW III, Glickel SZ, et al. Percutaneous pinning of distal radius fractures: an anatomic study demonstrating the proximity of K-wires to structures at risk. *J Hand Surg Am.* 2009;34:1014–1020.
57. Christensen OM, Christiansen TC, Krasheninnikoff M, et al. Plaster cast compared with bridging external fixation for distal radius fractures of the Colles' type. *Int Orthop.* 2001;24:358–360.
58. Chung KC, Kotsis SV, Kim HM. Predictors of functional outcomes after surgical treatment of distal radius fractures. *J Hand Surg Am.* 2007;32:76–83.
59. Chung KC, Shauver MJ, Birkmeyer JD. Trends in the United States in the treatment of distal radial fractures in the elderly. *J Bone Joint Surg Am.* 2009;91:1868–1873.
60. Chung KC, Shauver MJ, Yin H, et al. Variations in the use of internal fixation for distal radial fracture in the United States medicare population. *J Bone Joint Surg Am.* 2011;93:2154–2162.
61. Chung KC, Squitieri L, Kim HM. Comparative outcomes study using the volar locking plating system for distal radius fractures in both young adults and adults older than 60 years. *J Hand Surg Am.* 2008;33:809–819.
62. Chung KC, Watt AJ, Kotsis SV, et al. Treatment of unstable distal radial fractures with the volar locking plating system. *J Bone Joint Surg Am.* 2006;88:2687–2694.
63. Clarke AC, Spencer RF. Ulnar nerve palsy following fractures of the distal radius: clinical and anatomical studies. *J Hand Surg Br.* 1991;16:438–440.
64. Clayton RA, Gaston MS, Ralston SH, et al. Association between decreased bone mineral density and severity of distal radial fractures. *J Bone Joint Surg Am.* 2009;91:613–619.
65. Cobb AG, Houghton GR. Local anaesthetic infiltration versus Bier's block for Colles' fractures. *Br Med J (Clin Res Ed).* 1985;291:1683–1684.
66. Colles A. On the fracture of the carpal extremity of the radius. Edinb Med Surg J. 1814; 10:181. *Clin Orthop Relat Res.* 2006;445:5–7.
67. Cooley H, Jones G. A population-based study of fracture incidence in southern Tasmania: lifetime fracture risk and evidence for geographic variations within the same country. *Osteoporos Int.* 2001;12:124–130.
68. Cooney WP, Bussey R, Dobyns JH, et al. Difficult wrist fractures. Perilunate fracture-dislocations of the wrist. *Clin Orthop Relat Res.* 1987;136–147.
69. Cooney WP III, Dobyns JH, Linscheid RL. Complications of Colles' fractures. *J Bone Joint Surg Am.* 1980;62:613–619.
70. Cotton FJ III. The pathology of fracture of the lower extremity of the radius. *Ann Surg.* 1900;32:194–218.
71. Cotton FJ VIII. The pathology of fracture of the lower extremity of the radius. *Ann Surg.* 1900;32:388–415.
72. Court-Brown CM, Aitken S, Hamilton TW, et al. Nonoperative fracture treatment in the modern era. *J Trauma.* 2010;69:699–707.
73. Court-Brown CM, Caesar B. Epidemiology of adult fractures: A review. *Injury.* 2006;37:691–697.
74. Cummings SR, Black DM, Rubin SM. Lifetime risks of hip, Colles', or vertebral fracture and coronary heart disease among white postmenopausal women. *Arch Intern Med.* 1989;149:2445–2448.
75. Daecke W, Martini AK, Schneider S, et al. Amount of ulnar resection is a predictive factor for ulnar instability problems after the Sauve-Kapandji procedure: a retrospective study of 44 patients followed for 1-13 years. *Acta Orthop.* 2006;77:290–297.
76. Davis TR, Buchanan JM. A controlled prospective study of early mobilization of minimally displaced fractures of the distal radial metaphysis. *Injury.* 1987;18:283–285.
77. Day CS, Kamath AF, Makhni E, et al. "Sandwich" plating for intra-articular distal radius fractures with volar and dorsal metaphyseal comminution. *Hand (N Y).* 2008;3:47–54.
78. De Smet L. The DASH questionnaire and score in the evaluation of hand and wrist disorders. *Acta Orthop Belg.* 2008;74:575–581.
79. Dennison DG. Open reduction and internal locked fixation of unstable distal ulna fractures with concomitant distal radius fracture. *J Hand Surg Am.* 2007;32:801–805.
80. Dias JJ, Wray CC, Jones JM, et al. The value of early mobilisation in the treatment of Colles' fractures. *J Bone Joint Surg Br.* 1987;69:463–467.
81. Diaz-Garcia RJ, Oda T, Shauver MJ, et al. A systematic review of outcomes and complications of treating unstable distal radius fractures in the elderly. *J Hand Surg Am.* 2011;36:824–835.
82. Dicpinigaitis P, Wolinsky P, Hiebert R, et al. Can external fixation maintain reduction after distal radius fractures? *J Trauma.* 2004;57:845–850.
83. Doi K, Hattori Y, Otsuka K, et al. Intra-articular fractures of the distal aspect of the radius: arthroscopically assisted reduction compared with open reduction and internal fixation. *J Bone Joint Surg Am.* 1999;81:1093–1110.
84. Dowling JJ, Sawyer B Jr. Comminuted Colles' fractures. Evaluation of a method of treatment. *J Bone Joint Surg Am.* 1961;43-A:657–668.
85. Drobetz H, Kutscha-Lissberg E. Osteosynthesis of distal radial fractures with a volar locking screw plate system. *Int Orthop.* 2003;27:1–6.
86. Dupuytren G. *On the Injuries and Diseases of Bones.* 2012:119–120. Available from: http://books.google.co.uk/books/about/On_the_injuries_and_diseases_of_bones.html?id=2XYFAAAAQAAJ&redir_esc=y
87. Dyer G, Lozano-Calderon S, Gannon C, et al. Predictors of acute carpal tunnel syndrome associated with fracture of the distal radius. *J Hand Surg Am.* 2008;33:1309–1313.
88. Earnshaw SA, Aladin A, Surendran S, et al. Closed reduction of colles fractures: comparison of manual manipulation and finger-trap traction: a prospective, randomized study. *J Bone Joint Surg Am.* 2002;84-A:354–358.
89. Eglseder WA Jr, Elliott MJ. Nonunions of the distal radius. *Am J Orthop (Belle Mead NJ).* 2002;31:259–262.
90. Egol K, Walsh M, Tejwani N, et al. Bridging external fixation and supplementary Kirschner-wire fixation versus volar locked plating for unstable fractures of the distal radius: a randomised, prospective trial. *J Bone Joint Surg Br.* 2008;90:1214–1221.
91. Egol KA, Paksima N, Puopolo S, et al. Treatment of external fixation pins about the wrist: a prospective, randomized trial. *J Bone Joint Surg Am.* 2006;88:349–354.
92. Egol KA, Walsh M, Romo-Cardoso S, et al. Distal radial fractures in the elderly: operative compared with nonoperative treatment. *J Bone Joint Surg Am.* 2010;92:1851–1857.
93. Ellis J. Smith's and Barton's fractures. A method of treatment. *J Bone Joint Surg Br.* 1965;47:724–727.
94. Emmett JE, Breck LW. A review and analysis of 11,000 fractures seen in a private practice of orthopaedic surgery, 1937-1956. *J Bone Joint Surg Am.* 1958;40-A:1169–1175.
95. Esposito J, Schemitsch EH, Saccone M, et al. External fixation versus open reduction with plate fixation for distal radius fractures: a meta-analysis of randomised controlled trials. *Injury.* 2013;44:409–416.
96. Fanuele J, Koval KJ, Lurie J, et al. Distal radial fracture treatment: what you get may depend on your age and address. *J Bone Joint Surg Am.* 2009;91:1313-9.
97. Fernandez DL, Jupiter JB. *Epidemiology, Mechanism, Classification. Fractures of the distal radius.* 1st ed. New York, NY: Springer-Verlag; 1996:23–52.
98. Figl M, Weninger P, Liska M, et al. Volar fixed-angle plate osteosynthesis of unstable distal radius fractures: 12 months results. *Arch Orthop Trauma Surg.* 2009;129:661–669.
99. Finsen V, Rod O, Rod K, et al. The relationship between displacement and clinical outcome after distal radius (Colles') fracture. *J Hand Surg Eur Vol.* 2013;38:116–126.
100. Fischer T, Koch P, Saager C, et al. The radio-radial external fixator in the treatment of fractures of the distal radius. *J Hand Surg Br.* 1999;24:604–609.
101. Fitzpatrick SK, Casemyr NE, Zurakowski D, et al. The effect of osteoporosis on outcomes of operatively treated distal radius fractures. *J Hand Surg Am.* 2012;37:2027–2034.
102. Flinkkila T, Raatikainen T, Hamalainen M. AO and Frykman's classifications of Colles' fracture. No prognostic value in 652 patients evaluated after 5 years. *Acta Orthop Scand.* 1998;69:77–81.
103. Flinkkila T, Raatikainen T, Kaarela O, et al. Corrective osteotomy for malunion of the distal radius. *Arch Orthop Trauma Surg.* 2000;120:23–26.
104. Flinkkila T, Ristiniemi J, Hyvonen P, et al. Nonbridging external fixation in the treatment of unstable fractures of the distal forearm. *Arch Orthop Trauma Surg.* 2003;123:349–352.
105. Flinkkila T, Sirnio K, Hippi M, et al. Epidemiology and seasonal variation of distal radius fractures in Oulu, Finland. *Osteoporos Int.* 2011;22:2307–3212.
106. Foldhazy Z, Tornkvist H, Elmstedt E, et al. Long-term outcome of nonsurgically treated distal radius fractures. *J Hand Surg Am.* 2007;32:1374–1384.
107. Forgon M, Mammel E. [External fixator application in the therapy of radius fractures disposed to redislocation "in loco typico" (author's transl)]. *Magy Traumatol Orthop Helyreallito Seb.* 1982;25:63–71.
108. Forward DP, Davis TR, Sithole JS. Do young patients with malunited fractures of the distal radius inevitably develop symptomatic post-traumatic osteoarthritis? *J Bone Joint Surg Br.* 2008;90:629–637.
109. Forward DP, Lindau TR, Melsom DS. Intercarpal ligament injuries associated with fractures of the distal part of the radius. *J Bone Joint Surg Am.* 2007;89:2334–2340.
110. Foster BJ, Bindra RR. Intrafocal pin plate fixation of distal ulna fractures associated with distal radius fractures. *J Hand Surg Am.* 2012;37:356–359.
111. Franck WM, Dahlen C, Amlang M, et al. [Distal radius fracture–is non-bridging articular external fixator a therapeutic alternative? A prospective randomized study]. *Unfallchirurg.* 2000;103:826–833.
112. Freeland AE, Sud V, Jemison DM. Early wrist arthrodesis for irreparable intra-articular distal radial fractures. *Hand Surg.* 2000;5:113–118.
113. Fricker R, Pfeiffer KM, Troeger H. Ulnar shortening osteotomy in posttraumatic ulnar impaction syndrome. *Arch Orthop Trauma Surg.* 1996;115:158–161.
114. Frykman G. Fracture of the distal radius including sequelae–shoulder-hand-finger syndrome, disturbance in the distal radio-ulnar joint and impairment of nerve function. A clinical and experimental study. *Acta Orthop Scand.* 1967;108(suppl).
115. Fujitani R, Omokawa S, Akahane M, et al. Predictors of distal radioulnar joint instability in distal radius fractures. *J Hand Surg Am.* 2011;36:1919–1925.

116. Gaebler C, McQueen MM. Ulnar procedures for post-traumatic disorders of the distal radioulnar joint. *Injury*. 2003;34:47–59.
117. Gartland JJ Jr, Werley CW. Evaluation of healed Colles' fractures. *J Bone Joint Surg Am*. 1951;33-A:895–907.
118. Gavaskar AS, Muthukumar S, Chowdary N. Fragment-specific fixation for complex intra-articular fractures of the distal radius: results of a prospective single-centre trial. *J Hand Surg Eur Vol*. 2012;37:765–771.
119. Gay RE, Amadio PC, Johnson JC. Comparative responsiveness of the disabilities of the arm, shoulder, and hand, the carpal tunnel questionnaire, and the SF-36 to clinical change after carpal tunnel release. *J Hand Surg Am*. 2003;28:250–254.
120. Geissler WB, Fernandez DL. Percutaneous and limited open reduction of the articular surface of the distal radius. *J Orthop Trauma*. 1991;5:255–264.
121. Geissler WB, Freeland AE, Savoie FH, et al. Intracarpal soft-tissue lesions associated with an intra-articular fracture of the distal end of the radius. *J Bone Joint Surg Am*. 1996;78:357–365.
122. Gelberman RH, Szabo RM, Mortensen WW. Carpal tunnel pressures and wrist position in patients with Colles' fractures. *J Trauma*. 1984;24:747–749.
123. George MS, Kiefhaber TR, Stern PJ. The Sauve-Kapandji procedure and the Darrach procedure for distal radio-ulnar joint dysfunction after Colles' fracture. *J Hand Surg Br*. 2004;29:608–613.
124. Giannoudis PV, Tzioupis C, Papathanassopoulos A, et al. Articular step-off and risk of post-traumatic osteoarthritis. Evidence today. *Injury*. 2010;41:986–995.
125. Giessler GA, Przybilski M, Germann G, et al. Early free active versus dynamic extension splinting after extensor indicis proprius tendon transfer to restore thumb extension: a prospective randomized study. *J Hand Surg Am*. 2008;33:864–868.
126. Ginn TA, Ruch DS, Yang CC, et al. Use of a distraction plate for distal radial fractures with metaphyseal and diaphyseal comminution. Surgical technique. *J Bone Joint Surg Am*. 2006;88(Suppl 1 Pt 1):29–36.
127. Graafmans WC, Ooms ME, Bezemer PD, et al. Different risk profiles for hip fractures and distal forearm fractures: a prospective study. *Osteoporos Int*. 1996;6:427–431.
128. Gradl G, Gradl G, Wendt M, et al. Non-bridging external fixation employing multiplanar K-wires versus volar locked plating for dorsally displaced fractures of the distal radius. *Arch Orthop Trauma Surg*. 2013;133:595–602.
129. Grafstein E, Stenstrom R, Christenson J, et al. A prospective randomized controlled trial comparing circumferential casting and splinting in displaced Colles fractures. *CJEM*. 2010;12:192–200.
130. Graham CA, Gibson AJ, Goutcher CM, et al. Anaesthesia for the management of distal radius fractures in adults in Scottish hospitals. *Eur J Emerg Med*. 1997;4:210–212.
131. Gravier R, Flecher X, Parratte S, et al. [Trans-styloid and intrafocal pinning for extra-articular extension fractures of the distal radius: prospective randomized postoperative comparison with simple intra-focal pinning]. *Rev Chir Orthop Reparatrice Appar Mot*. 2006;92:657–662.
132. Grawe B, Heincelman C, Stern P. Functional results of the Darrach procedure: a long-term outcome study. *J Hand Surg Am*. 2012;37:2475–2480.
133. Grechenig W, Peicha G, Fellinger M. Primary ulnar head prosthesis for the treatment of an irreparable ulnar head fracture dislocation. *J Hand Surg Br*. 2001;26:269–271.
134. Green DP, O'Brien ET. Open reduction of carpal dislocations: indications and operative techniques. *J Hand Surg Am*. 1978;3:250–265.
135. Green DP, O'Brien ET. Classification and management of carpal dislocations. *Clin Orthop Relat Res*. 1980;149:55–72.
136. Grewal R, MacDermid JC. The risk of adverse outcomes in extra-articular distal radius fractures is increased with malalignment in patients of all ages but mitigated in older patients. *J Hand Surg Am*. 2007;32:962–970.
137. Grewal R, MacDermid JC, King GJ, et al. Open reduction internal fixation versus percutaneous pinning with external fixation of distal radius fractures: a prospective, randomized clinical trial. *J Hand Surg Am*. 2011;36:1899–1906.
138. Grewal R, MacDermid JC, Pope J, et al. Baseline predictors of pain and disability one year following extra-articular distal radius fractures. *Hand (N Y)*. 2007;2:104–111.
139. Grewal R, Perey B, Wilmink M, et al. A randomized prospective study on the treatment of intra-articular distal radius fractures: open reduction and internal fixation with dorsal plating versus mini open reduction, percutaneous fixation, and external fixation. *J Hand Surg Am*. 2005;30:764–772.
140. Gruber G, Gruber K, Giessauf C, et al. Volar plate fixation of AO type C2 and C3 distal radius fractures, a single-center study of 55 patients. *J Orthop Trauma*. 2008;22:467–472.
141. Gummesson C, Ward MM, Atroshi I. The shortened disabilities of the arm, shoulder and hand questionnaire (QuickDASH): validity and reliability based on responses within the full-length DASH. *BMC Musculoskelet Disord*. 2006;7:44.
142. Gupta A. The treatment of Colles' fracture. Immobilisation with the wrist dorsiflexed. *J Bone Joint Surg Br*. 1991;73:312–315.
143. Gupta A, Batra S, Jain P, et al. Carpal alignment in distal radial fractures. *BMC Musculoskelet Disord*. 2002;3:14.
144. Habernek H, Weinstabl R, Fialka C, et al. Unstable distal radius fractures treated by modified Kirschner wire pinning: anatomic considerations, technique, and results. *J Trauma*. 1994;36:83–88.
145. Hakimi M, Jungbluth P, Windolf J, et al. Functional results and complications following locking palmar plating on the distal radius: a retrospective study. *J Hand Surg Eur Vol*. 2010;35:283–288.
146. Handoll HH, Vaghela MV, Madhok R. Percutaneous pinning for treating distal radial fractures in adults. *Cochrane Database Syst Rev*. 2007;CD006080.
147. Hargreaves DG, Drew SJ, Eckersley R. Kirschner wire pin tract infection rates: a randomized controlled trial between percutaneous and buried wires. *J Hand Surg Br*. 2004;29:374–376.
148. Harley BJ, Scharfenberger A, Beaupre LA, et al. Augmented external fixation versus percutaneous pinning and casting for unstable fractures of the distal radius–a prospective randomized trial. *J Hand Surg Am*. 2004;29:815–824.
149. Harness NG, Ring D, Zurakowski D, et al. The influence of three-dimensional computed tomography reconstructions on the characterization and treatment of distal radial fractures. *J Bone Joint Surg Am*. 2006;88:1315–1323.
150. Hauck RM, Skahen J III, Palmer AK. Classification and treatment of ulnar styloid nonunion. *J Hand Surg Am*. 1996;21:418-22.
151. Hayes AJ, Duffy PJ, McQueen MM. Bridging and non-bridging external fixation in the treatment of unstable fractures of the distal radius: a retrospective study of 588 patients. *Acta Orthop*. 2008;79:540–547.
152. Helal B, Chen SC, Iwegbu G. Rupture of the extensor pollicis longus tendon in undisplaced Colles' type of fracture. *Hand*. 1982;14:41–47.
153. Helm RH, Tonkin MA. The chauffeur's fracture: simple or complex? *J Hand Surg Br*. 1992;17:156–159.
154. Henry M. Immediate mobilisation following corrective osteotomy of distal radius malunions with cancellous graft and volar fixed angle plates. *J Hand Surg Eur Vol*. 2007;32:88–92.
155. Hershman SH, Immerman I, Bechtel C, et al. The effects of pronator quadratus repair on outcomes after volar plating of distal radius fractures. *J Orthop Trauma*. 2013;27:130–133.
156. Hirasawa Y, Katsumi Y, Akiyoshi T, et al. Clinical and microangiographic studies on rupture of the E.P.L. tendon after distal radial fractures. *J Hand Surg Br*. 1990;15:51–57.
157. Hogel F, Mair S, Eberle S, et al. Distal radius fracture fixation with volar locking plates and additional bone augmentation in osteoporotic bone: a biomechanical study in a cadaveric model. *Arch Orthop Trauma Surg*. 2013;133:51–57.
158. Hollevoet N, Verdonk R. Outcome of distal radius fractures in relation to bone mineral density. *Acta Orthop Belg*. 2003;69:510–514.
159. Horii E, Ohmachi T, Nakamura R. The primary Sauve-Kapandji procedure–for treatment of comminuted distal radius and ulnar fractures. *J Hand Surg Br*. 2005;30:60–66.
160. Horne JG, Devane P, Purdie G. A prospective randomized trial of external fixation and plaster cast immobilization in the treatment of distal radial fractures. *J Orthop Trauma*. 1990;4:30–34.
161. Hove LM. Delayed rupture of the thumb extensor tendon. A 5-year study of 18 consecutive cases. *Acta Orthop Scand*. 1994A;65:199–203.
162. Hove LM. Simultaneous scaphoid and distal radial fractures. *J Hand Surg Br*. 1994B;19:384–388.
163. Hove LM, Krukhaug Y, Revheim K, et al. Dynamic compared with static external fixation of unstable fractures of the distal part of the radius: a prospective, randomized multicenter study. *J Bone Joint Surg Am*. 2010;92:1687–1696.
164. Howard PW, Stewart HD, Hind RE, et al. External fixation or plaster for severely displaced comminuted Colles' fractures? A prospective study of anatomical and functional results. *J Bone Joint Surg Br*. 1989;71:68–73.
165. Hudak PL, Amadio PC, Bombardier C. Development of an upper extremity outcome measure: the DASH (disabilities of the arm, shoulder and hand) [corrected]. The Upper Extremity Collaborative Group (UECG). *Am J Ind Med*. 1996;29:602–608.
166. Ilyas AM. Intramedullary fixation of distal radius fractures. *J Hand Surg Am*. 2009; 34:341–346.
167. Itsubo T, Hayashi M, Uchiyama S, et al. Differential onset patterns and causes of carpal tunnel syndrome after distal radius fracture: a retrospective study of 105 wrists. *J Orthop Sci*. 2010;15:518–523.
168. Ivers RQ, Cumming RG, Mitchell P, et al. Risk factors for fractures of the wrist, shoulder and ankle: the Blue Mountains Eye Study. *Osteoporos Int*. 2002;13:513–518.
169. Jakob M, Rikli DA, Regazzoni P. Fractures of the distal radius treated by internal fixation and early function. A prospective study of 73 consecutive patients. *J Bone Joint Surg Br*. 2000;82:340–344.
170. Jaremko JL, Lambert RG, Rowe BH, et al. Do radiographic indices of distal radius fracture reduction predict outcomes in older adults receiving conservative treatment? *Clin Radiol*. 2007;62:65–72.
171. Jenkins NH, Jones DG, Johnson SR, et al. External fixation of Colles' fractures. An anatomical study. *J Bone Joint Surg Br*. 1987;69:207–211.
172. Jenkins NH, Jones DG, Mintowt-Czyz WJ. External fixation and recovery of function following fractures of the distal radius in young adults. *Injury*. 1988;19:235–238.
173. Jenkins NH, Mintowt-Czyz WJ. Mal-union and dysfunction in Colles' fracture. *J Hand Surg Br*. 1988;13:291–293.
174. Jeudy J, Steiger V, Boyer P, et al. Treatment of complex fractures of the distal radius: a prospective randomised comparison of external fixation 'versus' locked volar plating. *Injury*. 2012;43:174–179.
175. Johnson PG, Szabo RM. Angle measurements of the distal radius: a cadaver study. *Skeletal Radiol*. 1993;22:243–246.
176. Johnston GH, Friedman L, Kriegler JC. Computerized tomographic evaluation of acute distal radial fractures. *J Hand Surg [Am]*. 1992;17:738–744.
177. Jupiter JB, Fernandez DL, Toh CL, et al. Operative treatment of volar intra-articular fractures of the distal end of the radius. *J Bone Joint Surg Am*. 1996;78:1817–1828.
178. Jupiter JB, Marent-Huber M. Operative management of distal radial fractures with 2.4-millimeter locking plates. A multicenter prospective case series. *J Bone Joint Surg Am*. 2009;91:55–65.
179. Jupiter JB, Ring D. A comparison of early and late reconstruction of malunited fractures of the distal end of the radius. *J Bone Joint Surg Am*. 1996;78:739–748.
180. Kaempffe FA, Walker KM. External fixation for distal radius fractures: effect of distraction on outcome. *Clin Orthop Relat Res*. 2000;380:220–225.
181. Kanis JA, Johnell O, Oden A, et al. Long-term risk of osteoporotic fracture in Malmo. *Osteoporos Int*. 2000;11:669–674.
182. Kapandji A. [Intra-focal pinning of fractures of the distal end of the radius 10 years later]. *Ann Chir Main*. 1987;6:57–63.
183. Kato N, Nemoto K, Arino H, et al. Ruptures of flexor tendons at the wrist as a complication of fracture of the distal radius. *Scand J Plast Reconstr Surg Hand Surg*. 2002;36:245–248.
184. Kazemian GH, Bakhshi H, Lilley M, et al. DRUJ instability after distal radius fracture: a comparison between cases with and without ulnar styloid fracture. *Int J Surg*. 2011;9:648–651.
185. Keating JF, Court-Brown CM, McQueen MM. Internal fixation of volar-displaced distal radial fractures. *J Bone Joint Surg Br*. 1994;76:401–405.

186. Kelsey JL, Browner WS, Seeley DG, et al. Risk factors for fractures of the distal forearm and proximal humerus. The Study of Osteoporotic Fractures Research Group. *Am J Epidemiol.* 1992;135:477–489.
187. Kendall JM, Allen P, Younge P, et al. Haematoma block or Bier's block for Colles' fracture reduction in the accident and emergency department–which is best? *J Accid Emerg Med.* 1997;14:352–356.
188. Kennedy C, Kennedy MT, Niall D, et al. Radiological outcomes of distal radius extra-articular fragility fractures treated with extra-focal Kirschner wires. *Injury.* 2010;41:639–642.
189. Kihara H, Palmer AK, Werner FW, et al. The effect of dorsally angulated distal radius fractures on distal radioulnar joint congruency and forearm rotation. *J Hand Surg Am.* 1996;21:40–47.
190. Kim JK, Koh YD, Do NH. Should an ulnar styloid fracture be fixed following volar plate fixation of a distal radial fracture? *J Bone Joint Surg Am.* 2010;92:1–6.
191. Kim JK, Koh YD, Kook SH. Effect of calcium phosphate bone cement augmentation on volar plate fixation of unstable distal radial fractures in the elderly. *J Bone Joint Surg Am.* 2011;93:609–614.
192. Kim JK, Yun YH, Kim DJ, et al. Comparison of united and nonunited fractures of the ulnar styloid following volar-plate fixation of distal radius fractures. *Injury.* 2011;42:371–375.
193. Kitay A, Swanstrom M, Schreiber JJ, et al. Volar plate position and flexor tendon rupture following distal radius fracture fixation. *J Hand Surg Am.* 2013;38:1091–1096.
194. Klein W, Dee W. [Initial experiences with a new wrist joint fixator in treatment of distal radius fractures]. *Handchir Mikrochir Plast Chir.* 1992;24:202–209.
195. Knight D, Hajducka C, Will E, et al. Locked volar plating for unstable distal radial fractures: clinical and radiological outcomes. *Injury.* 2010;41:184–189.
196. Knirk J, Jupiter J. Intraarticular fractures of the distal end of the radius in young adults. *J Bone Joint Surg.* 1986;68A:647–659.
197. Komura S, Yokoi T, Nonomura H, et al. Incidence and characteristics of carpal fractures occurring concurrently with distal radius fractures. *J Hand Surg Am.* 2012;37:469–476.
198. Kongsholm J, Olerud C. Carpal tunnel pressure in the acute phase after Colles' fracture. *Arch Orthop Trauma Surg.* 1986;105:183–186.
199. Konstantinidis L, Helwig P, Strohm PC, et al. Clinical and radiological outcomes after stabilisation of complex intra-articular fractures of the distal radius with the volar 2.4 mm LCP. *Arch Orthop Trauma Surg.* 2010;130:751–757.
200. Kopylov P, Johnell O, Redlund-Johnell I, et al. Fractures of the distal end of the radius in young adults: a 30-year follow-up. *J Hand Surg Br.* 1993;18:45–49.
201. Koval KJ, Harrast JJ, Anglen JO, et al. Fractures of the distal part of the radius. The evolution of practice over time. Where's the evidence? *J Bone Joint Surg Am.* 2008;90:1855–1861.
202. Kozin SH, Wood MB. Early soft-tissue complications after fractures of the distal part of the radius. *J Bone Joint Surg Am.* 1993;75:144–153.
203. Kreder HJ, Agel J, McKee MD, et al. A randomized, controlled trial of distal radius fractures with metaphyseal displacement but without joint incongruity: closed reduction and casting versus closed reduction, spanning external fixation, and optional percutaneous K-wires. *J Orthop Trauma.* 2006;20:115–121.
204. Kreder HJ, Hanel DP, Agel J, et al. Indirect reduction and percutaneous fixation versus open reduction and internal fixation for displaced intra-articular fractures of the distal radius: a randomised, controlled trial. *J Bone Joint Surg Br.* 2005;87:829–836.
205. Kreder HJ, Hanel DP, McKee M, et al. Consistency of AO fracture classification for the distal radius. *J Bone Joint Surg Br.* 1996A;78:726–731.
206. Kreder HJ, Hanel DP, McKee M, et al. Xray film measurements for healed distal radius fractures. *Journal of Hand Surgery.* 1996B;21A:31–39.
207. Krukhaug Y, Hove LM. Corrective osteotomy for malunited extra-articular fractures of the distal radius: a follow-up study of 33 patients. *Scand J Plast Reconstr Surg Hand Surg.* 2007;41:303–309.
208. Krukhaug Y, Ugland S, Lie SA, et al. External fixation of fractures of the distal radius: a randomized comparison of the Hoffman compact II non-bridging fixator and the Dynawrist fixator in 75 patients followed for 1 year. *Acta Orthop.* 2009;80:104–108.
209. Kwon BC, Choi SJ, Song SY, et al. Modified carpal stretch test as a screening test for detection of scapholunate interosseous ligament injuries associated with distal radial fractures. *J Bone Joint Surg Am.* 2011;93:855–862.
210. Kwon BC, Seo BK, Im HJ, et al. Clinical and radiographic factors associated with distal radioulnar joint instability in distal radius fractures. *Clin Orthop Relat Res.* 2012;470:3171–3179.
211. Landgren M, Jerrhag D, Tagil M, et al. External or internal fixation in the treatment of non-reducible distal radial fractures? *Acta Orthop.* 2011;82:610–613.
212. Lauritzen JB, Schwarz P, Lund B, et al. Changing incidence and residual lifetime risk of common osteoporosis-related fractures. *Osteoporos Int.* 1993;3:127–132.
213. Lee SK, Kim KJ, Park JS, et al. Distal ulna hook plate fixation for unstable distal ulna fracture associated with distal radius fracture. *Orthopedics.* 2012;35:e1358–e1364.
214. Lee YS, Wei TY, Cheng YC, et al. A comparative study of Colles' fractures in patients between fifty and seventy years of age: percutaneous K-wiring versus volar locking plating. *Int Orthop.* 2012;36:789–794.
215. Lenoble E, Dumontier C, Goutallier D, et al. Fracture of the distal radius. A prospective comparison between trans-styloid and Kapandji fixations. *J Bone Joint Surg Br.* 1995;77:562–567.
216. Lester GE, Anderson JJ, Tylavsky FA, et al. Update on the use of distal radial bone density measurements in prediction of hip and Colles' fracture risk. *J Orthop Res.* 1990;8:220–226.
217. Leung F, Tu YK, Chew WY, et al. Comparison of external and percutaneous pin fixation with plate fixation for intra-articular distal radial fractures. A randomized study. *J Bone Joint Surg Am.* 2008;90:16–22.
218. Leung KS, Shen WY, Leung PC, et al. Ligamentotaxis and bone grafting for comminuted fractures of the distal radius. *J Bone Joint Surg Br.* 1989;71:838–842.
219. Lewis MH. Median nerve decompression after Colles's fracture. *J Bone Joint Surg Br.* 1978;60-B:195–196.
220. Lilienfeldt A. Ueber den klassischen Radiusbruch. *Arch Klin Chir.* 1885;27:475.
221. Lin C, Sun JS, Hou SM. External fixation with or without supplementary intramedullary Kirschner wires in the treatment of distal radial fractures. *Can J Surg.* 2004;47:431–437.
222. Lindau T, Arner M, Hagberg L. Intraarticular lesions in distal fractures of the radius in young adults. A descriptive arthroscopic study in 50 patients. *J Hand Surg Br.* 1997;22:638–643.
223. Linscheid RL, Dobyns JH, Beabout JW, et al. Traumatic instability of the wrist: diagnosis, classification, and pathomechanics. *J Bone Joint Surg Am.* 2002;84-A:142.
224. Logan AJ, Lindau TR. The management of distal ulnar fractures in adults: a review of the literature and recommendations for treatment. *Strategies Trauma Limb Reconstr.* 2008;3:49–56.
225. Lozano-Calderon SA, Brouwer KM, Doornberg JN, et al. Long-term outcomes of corrective osteotomy for the treatment of distal radius malunion. *J Hand Surg Eur Vol.* 2010;35:370–380.
226. Lozano-Calderon SA, Doornberg J, Ring D. Fractures of the dorsal articular margin of the distal part of the radius with dorsal radiocarpal subluxation. *J Bone Joint Surg Am.* 2006;88:1486–1493.
227. Lucas-Championnière J. *Precis du traitement des fractures par le massage et la mobilisation.* Paris: G Steinheil; 1900.
228. Ludvigsen TC, Johansen S, Svenningsen S. [Unstable fractures of the distal radius. External fixation or percutaneous pinning?]. *Tidsskr Nor Laegeforen.* 1996;116:3093–3097.
229. Lundy D, Quisling S, Lourie G, et al. Tilted lateral radiographs in the evaluation of intra-articular distal radius fractures. *J Hand Surg Am.* 1999;24A:249–256.
230. Lynch AC, Lipscomb PR. The carpal tunnel syndrome and Colles' fractures. *JAMA.* 1963;185:363–366.
231. MacDermid JC, Donner A, Richards RS, et al. Patient versus injury factors as predictors of pain and disability six months after a distal radius fracture. *J Clin Epidemiol.* 2002;55:849–854.
232. MacDermid JC, Richards RS, Donner A, et al. Responsiveness of the short form-36, disability of the arm, shoulder, and hand questionnaire, patient-rated wrist evaluation, and physical impairment measurements in evaluating recovery after a distal radius fracture. *J Hand Surg Am.* 2000;25:330–340.
233. MacDermid JC, Turgeon T, Richards RS, et al. Patient rating of wrist pain and disability: a reliable and valid measurement tool. *J Orthop Trauma.* 1998;12:577–586.
234. Mackenney PJ, McQueen MM, Elton R. Prediction of instability in distal radial fractures. *J Bone Joint Surg Am.* 2006;88:1944–1951.
235. Mah ET, Atkinson RN. Percutaneous Kirschner wire stabilisation following closed reduction of Colles' fractures. *J Hand Surg Br.* 1992;17:55–62.
236. Mahmoud M, El SS, Kamal M. Correction of dorsally-malunited extra-articular distal radial fractures using volar locked plates without bone grafting. *J Bone Joint Surg Br.* 2012;94:1090–1096.
237. Malgaigne JF. *A Treatise on Fractures.* Philadelphia, PA: JB Lippincott; 1859.
238. Mallmin H, Ljunghall S. Incidence of Colles' fracture in Uppsala. A prospective study of a quarter-million population. *Acta Orthop Scand.* 1992;63:213–215.
239. Marcheix PS, Dotzis A, Benko PE, et al. Extension fractures of the distal radius in patients older than 50: a prospective randomized study comparing fixation using mixed pins or a palmar fixed-angle plate. *J Hand Surg Eur Vol.* 2010;35:646–651.
240. Marsh JL, Buckwalter J, Gelberman R, et al. Articular fractures: does an anatomic reduction really change the result? *J Bone Joint Surg Am.* 2002;84-A:1259–1271.
241. Marsh JL, Slongo TF, Agel J, et al. Fracture and dislocation classification compendium - 2007: Orthopaedic Trauma Association classification, database and outcomes committee. *J Orthop Trauma.* 2007;21:S1–S133.
242. Marx RG, Axelrod TS. Intraarticular osteotomy of distal radial malunions. *Clin Orthop Relat Res.* 1996;152–157.
243. May MM, Lawton JN, Blazar PE. Ulnar styloid fractures associated with distal radius fractures: incidence and implications for distal radioulnar joint instability. *J Hand Surg Am.* 2002;27:965–971.
244. McAuliffe TB, Hilliar KM, Coates CJ, et al. Early mobilisation of Colles' fractures. A prospective trial. *J Bone Joint Surg Br.* 1987;69:727–729.
245. McFadyen I, Field J, McCann P, et al. Should unstable extra-articular distal radial fractures be treated with fixed-angle volar-locked plates or percutaneous Kirschner wires? A prospective randomised controlled trial. *Injury.* 2011;42:162–166.
246. McKay SD, MacDermid JC, Roth JH, et al. Assessment of complications of distal radius fractures and development of a complication checklist. *J Hand Surg Am.* 2001;26:916–922.
247. McKee MD, Richards RR. Dynamic radio-ulnar convergence after the Darrach procedure. *J Bone Joint Surg Br.* 1996;78:413–418.
248. McQueen M, Caspers J. Colles fracture: does the anatomical result affect the final function? *J Bone Joint Surg Br.* 1988;70:649–651.
249. McQueen MM. Redisplaced unstable fractures of the distal radius. A randomised, prospective study of bridging versus non-bridging external fixation. *J Bone Joint Surg Br.* 1998;80:665–669.
250. McQueen MM, Hajducka C, Court-Brown CM. Redisplaced unstable fractures of the distal radius: a prospective randomised comparison of four methods of treatment. *J Bone Joint Surg Br.* 1996;78:404–409.
251. McQueen MM, MacLaren A, Chalmers J. The value of remanipulating Colles' fractures. *J Bone Joint Surg Br.* 1986;68:232–233.
252. McQueen MM, Simpson D, Court-Brown CM. Use of the Hoffman 2 compact external fixator in the treatment of redisplaced unstable distal radial fractures. *J Orthop Trauma.* 1999;13:501–505.
253. McQueen MM, Wakefield A. Distal radial osteotomy for malunion using non-bridging external fixation: good results in 23 patients. *Acta Orthop.* 2008;79:390–395.
254. Medoff RJ. Essential radiographic evaluation for distal radius fractures. *Hand Clin.* 2005;21:279–288.
255. Mehara AK, Rastogi S, Bhan S, et al. Classification and treatment of volar Barton fractures. *Injury.* 1993;24:55–59.
256. Mehling I, Muller LP, Delinsky K, et al. Number and locations of screw fixation for volar fixed-angle plating of distal radius fractures: biomechanical study. *J Hand Surg Am.* 2010;35:885–891.
257. Melone CP Jr. Articular fractures of the distal radius. *Orthop Clin North Am.* 1984;15:217–236.

258. Minami A, Iwasaki N, Ishikawa J, et al. Treatments of osteoarthritis of the distal radioulnar joint: long-term results of three procedures. *Hand Surg.* 2005;10:243–248.
259. Mirza A, Jupiter JB, Reinhart MK, et al. Fractures of the distal radius treated with cross-pin fixation and a nonbridging external fixator, the CPX system: a preliminary report. *J Hand Surg Am.* 2009;34:603–616.
260. Mrkonjic A, Geijer M, Lindau T, et al. The natural course of traumatic triangular fibrocartilage complex tears in distal radial fractures: a 13-15 year follow-up of arthroscopically diagnosed but untreated injuries. *J Hand Surg Am.* 2012;37:1555–1560.
261. Nagy L, Buchler U. Long-term results of radioscapholunate fusion following fractures of the distal radius. *J Hand Surg Br.* 1997;22:705–710.
262. Naidu SH, Capo JT, Moulton M, et al. Percutaneous pinning of distal radius fractures: a biomechanical study. *J Hand Surg Am.* 1997;22:252–257.
263. Namba J, Fujiwara T, Murase T, et al. Intra-articular distal ulnar fractures associated with distal radial fractures in older adults: early experience in fixation of the radius and leaving the ulna unfixed. *J Hand Surg Eur Vol.* 2009;34:592–597.
264. Ng CY, McQueen MM. What are the radiological predictors of functional outcome following fractures of the distal radius? *J Bone Joint Surg Br.* 2011;93:145–150.
265. Nguyen TV, Center JR, Sambrook PN, et al. Risk factors for proximal humerus, forearm, and wrist fractures in elderly men and women: the Dubbo Osteoporosis Epidemiology Study. *Am J Epidemiol.* 2001;153:587–595.
266. Nishiwaki M, Tazaki K, Shimizu H, et al. Prospective study of distal radial fractures treated with an intramedullary nail. *J Bone Joint Surg Am.* 2011;93:1436–1441.
267. Nordvall H, Glanberg-Persson G, Lysholm J. Are distal radius fractures due to fragility or to falls? A consecutive case-control study of bone mineral density, tendency to fall, risk factors for osteoporosis, and health-related quality of life. *Acta Orthop.* 2007;78: 271–277.
268. O'Connor D, Mullett H, Doyle M, et al. Minimally displaced Colles' fractures: a prospective randomized trial of treatment with a wrist splint or a plaster cast. *J Hand Surg Br.* 2003;28:50–53.
269. Older TM, Stabler EV, Cassebaum WH. Colles fracture: evaluation and selection of therapy. *J Trauma.* 1965;5:469–476.
270. Ombredanne L. *L'osteosynthese Temporaire Chez Les Enfants.* Paris: Masson et cie; 1929.
271. O'Neill TW, Cooper C, Finn JD, et al. Incidence of distal forearm fracture in British men and women. *Osteoporos Int.* 2001;12:555–558.
272. Orces CH, Martinez FJ. Epidemiology of fall related forearm and wrist fractures among adults treated in US hospital emergency departments. *Inj Prev.* 2011;17:33–36.
273. Osada D, Kamei S, Takai M, et al. Malunited fractures of the distal radius treated with corrective osteotomy using volar locking plate and a corticocancellous bone graft following immediate mobilisation. *Hand Surg.* 2007;12:183–190.
274. Oshige T, Sakai A, Zenke Y, et al. A comparative study of clinical and radiological outcomes of dorsally angulated, unstable distal radius fractures in elderly patients: intrafocal pinning versus volar locking plating. *J Hand Surg Am.* 2007;32:1385–1392.
275. Oskam J, De Graaf JS, Klasen HJ. Fractures of the distal radius and scaphoid. *J Hand Surg Br.* 1996;21:772–774.
276. Oskam J, Kingma J, Bart J, et al. K-wire fixation for redislocated Colles' fractures. Malunion in 8/21 cases. *Acta Orthop Scand.* 1997;68:259–261.
277. Oskarsson GV, Aaser P, Hjall A. Do we underestimate the predictive value of the ulnar styloid affection in Colles fractures? *Arch Orthop Trauma Surg.* 1997;116:341–344.
278. Owen RA, Melton LJ, III, Johnson KA, et al. Incidence of Colles' fracture in a North American community. *Am J Public Health.* 1982;72:605–607.
279. Owers KL, Lee J, Khan N, et al. Ultrasound changes in the extensor pollicis longus tendon following fractures of the distal radius–a preliminary report. *J Hand Surg Eur Vol.* 2007;32:467–471.
280. Paley D, McMurtry RY. Median nerve compression by volarly displaced fragments of the distal radius. *Clin Orthop Relat Res.* 1987;139–147.
281. Palvanen M, Kannus P, Parkkari J, et al. The injury mechanisms of osteoporotic upper extremity fractures among older adults: a controlled study of 287 consecutive patients and their 108 controls. *Osteoporos Int.* 2000;11:822–831.
282. Papadonikolakis A, Shen J, Garrett JP, et al. The effect of increasing distraction on digital motion after external fixation of the wrist. *J Hand Surg Am.* 2005;30:773–779.
283. Park C, Ha YC, Jang S, et al. The incidence and residual lifetime risk of osteoporosis-related fractures in Korea. *J Bone Miner Metab.* 2011;29:744–751.
284. Park DH, Goldie BS. Volar plating for distal radius fractures–do not trust the image intensifier when judging distal subchondral screw length. *Tech Hand Up Extrem Surg.* 2012;16:169–172.
285. Park MJ, Cooney WP III, Hahn ME, et al. The effects of dorsally angulated distal radius fractures on carpal kinematics. *J Hand Surg Am.* 2002;27:223–232.
286. Pillukat T, Schadel-Hopfner M, Windolf J, et al. [The malunited distal radius fracture - early or late correction?]. *Handchir Mikrochir Plast Chir.* 2013;45:6–12.
287. Pillukat T, van SJ. [The hemiresection-interposition arthroplasty of the distal radioulnar joint]. *Oper Orthop Traumatol.* 2009;21:484–497.
288. Ploegmakers JJ, Mader K, Pennig D, et al. Four distal radial fracture classification systems tested amongst a large panel of Dutch trauma surgeons. *Injury.* 2007;38:1268–1272.
289. Pool C. Colles's fracture. A prospective study of treatment. *J Bone Joint Surg Br.* 1973;55:540–544.
290. Porter M, Stockley I. Fractures of the distal radius. Intermediate and end results in relation to radiologic parameters. *Clin Orthop Relat Res.* 1987;220:241–252.
291. Pouteau C. *Oeuvres Posthumes de M. Pouteau.* http://books google sh/books/about/Oeuvres_posthumes_de_m_Pouteau html?id=0hm3HTopvSgC. 1783.
292. Prommersberger KJ, Fernandez DL. Nonunion of distal radius fractures. *Clin Orthop Relat Res.* 2004;419:51–56.
293. Prommersberger KJ, Fernandez DL, Ring D, et al. Open reduction and internal fixation of un-united fractures of the distal radius: does the size of the distal fragment affect the result? *Chir Main.* 2002;21:113–123.
294. Prommersberger KJ, Ring D, Gonzalez del PJ, et al. Corrective osteotomy for intra-articular malunion of the distal part of the radius. Surgical technique. *J Bone Joint Surg Am.* 2006;88(Suppl 1 Pt 2):202–211.
295. Rayhack JM. The history and evolution of percutaneous pinning of displaced distal radius fractures. *Orthop Clin North Am.* 1993;24:287–300.
296. Richard MJ, Katolik LI, Hanel DP, et al. Distraction plating for the treatment of highly comminuted distal radius fractures in elderly patients. *J Hand Surg Am.* 2012;37:948–956.
297. Richard MJ, Wartinbee DA, Riboh J, et al. Analysis of the complications of palmar plating versus external fixation for fractures of the distal radius. *J Hand Surg Am.* 2011;36:1614–1620.
298. Richards RS, Bennett JD, Roth JH, et al. Arthroscopic diagnosis of intra-articular soft tissue injuries associated with distal radial fractures. *J Hand Surg Am.* 1997;22:772–776.
299. Rikli DA, Regazzoni P. Fractures of the distal end of the radius treated by internal fixation and early function. A preliminary report of 20 cases. *J Bone Joint Surg Br.* 1996;78:588–592.
300. Ring D, Kadzielski J, Fabian L, et al. Self-reported upper extremity health status correlates with depression. *J Bone Joint Surg Am.* 2006;88:1983–1988.
301. Ring D, McCarty LP, Campbell D, et al. Condylar blade plate fixation of unstable fractures of the distal ulna associated with fracture of the distal radius. *J Hand Surg Am.* 2004;29:103–109.
302. Ring D, Prommersberger KJ, Gonzalez del PJ, et al. Corrective osteotomy for intra-articular malunion of the distal part of the radius. *J Bone Joint Surg Am.* 2005;87:1503–1509.
303. Ring D, Prommersberger K, Jupiter JB. Combined dorsal and volar plate fixation of complex fractures of the distal part of the radius. *J Bone Joint Surg Am.* 2005;87(Suppl 1):195–212.
304. Robertsson GO, Jonsson GT, Sigurjonsson K. Epidemiology of distal radius fractures in Iceland in 1985. *Acta Orthop Scand.* 1990;61:457–459.
305. Rodriguez-Merchan EC. Plaster cast versus percutaneous pin fixation for comminuted fractures of the distal radius in patients between 46 and 65 years of age. *J Orthop Trauma.* 1997;11:212–217.
306. Rogachefsky RA, Ouellette EA, Sun S, et al. The use of tricorticocancellous bone graft in severely comminuted intra-articular fractures of the distal radius. *J Hand Surg Am.* 2006;31:623–632.
307. Roth KM, Blazar PE, Earp BE, et al. Incidence of extensor pollicis longus tendon rupture after nondisplaced distal radius fractures. *J Hand Surg Am.* 2012;37:942–947.
308. Roumen RM, Hesp WL, Bruggink ED. Unstable Colles' fractures in elderly patients. A randomised trial of external fixation for redisplacement. *J Bone Joint Surg Br.* 1991;73:307–311.
309. Roysam GS. The distal radio-ulnar joint in Colles' fractures. *J Bone Joint Surg Br.* 1993;75:58–60.
310. Rozental TD, Blazar PE. Functional outcome and complications after volar plating for dorsally displaced, unstable fractures of the distal radius. *J Hand Surg Am.* 2006; 31:359–365.
311. Rozental TD, Blazar PE, Franko OI, et al. Functional outcomes for unstable distal radial fractures treated with open reduction and internal fixation or closed reduction and percutaneous fixation. A prospective randomized trial. *J Bone Joint Surg Am.* 2009; 91:1837–1846.
312. Rozental TD, Bozentka DJ, Katz MA, et al. Evaluation of the sigmoid notch with computed tomography following intra-articular distal radius fracture. *J Hand Surg Am.* 2001;26:244–251.
313. Ruch DS, Ginn TA, Yang CC, et al. Use of a distraction plate for distal radial fractures with metaphyseal and diaphyseal comminution. *J Bone Joint Surg Am.* 2005;87:945–954.
314. Ruch DS, Yang C, Smith BP. Results of palmar plating of the lunate facet combined with external fixation for the treatment of high-energy compression fractures of the distal radius. *J Orthop Trauma.* 2004;18:28–33.
315. Ruch DS, Yang CC, Smith BP. Results of acute arthroscopically repaired triangular fibrocartilage complex injuries associated with intra-articular distal radius fractures. *Arthroscopy.* 2003;19:511–516.
316. Rutgers M, Mudgal CS, Shin R. Combined fractures of the distal radius and scaphoid. *J Hand Surg Eur Vol.* 2008;33:478–483.
317. Sahu A, Charalambous CP, Mills SP, et al. Reoperation for metalwork complications following the use of volar locking plates for distal radius fractures: a United Kingdom experience. *Hand Surg.* 2011;16:113–118.
318. Sakano H, Koshino T, Takeuchi R, et al. Treatment of the unstable distal radius fracture with external fixation and a hydroxyapatite spacer. *J Hand Surg Am.* 2001;26:923–930.
319. Saleh M, Scott BW. Pitfalls and complications in leg lengthening. *Seminars in Orthopaedics.* 1992;7:207–222.
320. Sammer DM, Fuller DS, Kim HM, et al. A comparative study of fragment-specific versus volar plate fixation of distal radius fractures. *Plast Reconstr Surg.* 2008;122:1441–1450.
321. Sammer DM, Shah HM, Shauver MJ, et al. The effect of ulnar styloid fractures on patient-rated outcomes after volar locking plating of distal radius fractures. *J Hand Surg Am.* 2009;34:1595–1602.
322. Sarmiento A, Pratt GW, Berry NC, et al. Colles' fractures. Functional bracing in supination. *J Bone Joint Surg Am.* 1975;57:311–317.
323. Saw N, Roberts C, Cutbush K, et al. Early experience with the TriMed fragment-specific fracture fixation system in intraarticular distal radius fractures. *J Hand Surg Eur Vol.* 2008;33:53–58.
324. Schmalholz A. Epidemiology of distal radius fracture in Stockholm 1981-82. *Acta Orthop Scand.* 1988;59:701–703.
325. Schmalholz A. Closed rereduction of axial compression in Colles' fracture is hardly possible. *Acta Orthop Scand.* 1989;60:57–59.
326. Schonnemann JO, Hansen TB, Soballe K. Randomised study of non-bridging external fixation compared with intramedullary fixation of unstable distal radial fractures. *J Plast Surg Hand Surg.* 2011;45:232–237.
327. Schuit AJ, Schouten EG, Westerterp KR, et al. Validity of the Physical Activity Scale for the Elderly (PASE): according to energy expenditure assessed by the doubly labeled water method. *J Clin Epidemiol.* 1997;50:541–546.
328. Seitz WH Jr, Raikin SM. Resection of comminuted ulna head fragments with soft tissue reconstruction when associated with distal radius fractures. *Tech Hand Up Extrem Surg.* 2007;11:224–230.
329. Shea K, Fernandez DL, Jupiter JB, et al. Corrective osteotomy for malunited, volarly displaced fractures of the distal end of the radius. *J Bone Joint Surg Am.* 1997;79:1816–1826.

330. Shih JT, Lee HM, Hou YT, et al. Arthroscopically-assisted reduction of intra-articular fractures and soft tissue management of distal radius. *Hand Surg.* 2001;6:127-35.

331. Short WH, Palmer AK, Werner FW, et al. A biomechanical study of distal radial fractures. *J Hand Surg Am.* 1987;12:529–534.

332. Sigurdardottir K, Halldorsson S, Robertsson J. Epidemiology and treatment of distal radius fractures in Reykjavik, Iceland, in 2004. Comparison with an Icelandic study from 1985. *Acta Orthop.* 2011;82:494–498.

333. Silman AJ. Risk factors for Colles' fracture in men and women: results from the European Prospective Osteoporosis Study. *Osteoporos Int.* 2003;14:213–218.

334. Skoff HD. Postfracture extensor pollicis longus tenosynovitis and tendon rupture: a scientific study and personal series. *Am J Orthop (Belle Mead NJ).* 2003;32:245–247.

335. Smith DW, Henry MH. The 45 degrees pronated oblique view for volar fixed-angle plating of distal radius fractures. *J Hand Surg Am.* 2004;29:703–706.

336. Smith DW, Henry MH. Volar fixed-angle plating of the distal radius. *J Am Acad Orthop Surg.* 2005;13:28–36.

337. Smith RW. *A Treatise on Fracture in the Vicinity of Joints and on Certain Forms of Accidental and Congenital Dislocations.* Dublin: Hodges and Smith; 1847.

338. Solan MC, Rees R, Molloy S, et al. Internal fixation after intra-articular fracture of the distal ulna. *J Bone Joint Surg Br.* 2003;85:279–280.

339. Solgaard S. Classification of distal radius fractures. *Acta Orthop Scand.* 1985;56:249–252.

340. Solgaard S. Function after distal radius fracture. *Acta Orthop Scand.* 1988;59:39–42.

341. Solgaard S, Bunger C, Sllund K. Displaced distal radius fractures. A comparative study of early results following external fixation, functional bracing in supination, or dorsal plaster immobilization. *Arch Orthop Trauma Surg.* 1990;109:34–38.

342. Solgaard S, Petersen VS. Epidemiology of distal radius fractures. *Acta Orthop Scand.* 1985;56:391–393.

343. Sommerkamp TG, Seeman M, Silliman J, et al. Dynamic external fixation of unstable fractures of the distal part of the radius. A prospective, randomized comparison with static external fixation. *J Bone Joint Surg Am.* 1994;76:1149–1161.

344. Soong M, Got C, Katarincic J, et al. Fluoroscopic evaluation of intra-articular screw placement during locked volar plating of the distal radius: a cadaveric study. *J Hand Surg Am.* 2008;33:1720–1723.

345. Soong M, Ring D. Ulnar nerve palsy associated with fracture of the distal radius. *J Orthop Trauma.* 2007;21:113–116.

346. Souer JS, Lozano-Calderon SA, Ring D. Predictors of wrist function and health status after operative treatment of fractures of the distal radius. *J Hand Surg Am.* 2008;33:157–163.

347. Souer JS, Ring D, Jupiter JB, et al. Comparison of AO Type-B and Type-C volar shearing fractures of the distal part of the radius. *J Bone Joint Surg Am.* 2009;91:2605–2611.

348. Sprot H, Metcalfe A, Odutola A, et al. Management of distal radius fractures in emergency departments in England and Wales. *Emerg Med J.* 2013;30:211–213.

349. Srinivasan RC, Jain D, Richard MJ, et al. Isolated ulnar shortening osteotomy for the treatment of extra-articular distal radius malunion. *J Hand Surg Am.* 2013;38:1106–1110.

350. Stahl S, Wolff TW. Delayed rupture of the extensor pollicis longus tendon after nonunion of a fracture of the dorsal radial tubercle. *J Hand Surg Am.* 1988;13:338–341.

351. Stein AH Jr, Katz SF. Stabilization of comminuted fractures of the distal inch of the radius: percutaneous pinning. *Clin Orthop Relat Res.* 1975;174–181.

352. Stewart HD, Innes AR, Burke FD. Functional cast-bracing for Colles' fractures. A comparison between cast-bracing and conventional plaster casts. *J Bone Joint Surg Br.* 1984;66:749–753.

353. Stewart HD, Innes AR, Burke FD. Factors affecting the outcome of Colles' fracture: an anatomical and functional study. *Injury.* 1985A;16:289–295.

354. Stewart HD, Innes AR, Burke FD. The hand complications of Colles' fractures. *J Hand Surg Br.* 1985B;10:103–106.

355. Stoffelen D, Broos P. Minimally displaced distal radius fractures: do they need plaster treatment? *J Trauma.* 1998;44:503–505.

356. Stoffelen D, De SL, Broos P. The importance of the distal radioulnar joint in distal radial fractures. *J Hand Surg Br.* 1998;23:507–511.

357. Stoffelen DV, Broos PL. Kapandji pinning or closed reduction for extra-articular distal radius fractures. *J Trauma.* 1998;45:753–757.

358. Strohm PC, Muller CA, Boll T, et al. Two procedures for Kirschner wire osteosynthesis of distal radial fractures. A randomized trial. *J Bone Joint Surg Am.* 2004;86-A:2621–2628.

359. Sugun TS, Ozaksar K, Gurbuz Y. Screw prominence of locking plating in distal radius fractures. *J Hand Surg Am.* 2012;37:2646–2647.

360. Synn AJ, Makhni EC, Makhni MC, et al. Distal radius fractures in older patients: is anatomic reduction necessary? *Clin Orthop Relat Res.* 2009;467:1612–1620.

361. Taleisnik J. The Sauve-Kapandji procedure. *Clin Orthop Relat Res.* 1992;110–123.

362. Taleisnik J, Watson HK. Midcarpal instability caused by malunited fractures of the distal radius. *J Hand Surg Am.* 1984;9:350–357.

363. Tan V, Bratchenko W, Nourbakhsh A, et al. Comparative analysis of intramedullary nail fixation versus casting for treatment of distal radius fractures. *J Hand Surg Am.* 2012;37:460–468.

364. Tanabe K, Nakajima T, Sogo E, et al. Intra-articular fractures of the distal radius evaluated by computed tomography. *J Hand Surg Am.* 2011;36:1798–1803.

365. Tang JB, Shi D, Gu YQ, et al. Can cast immobilization successfully treat scapholunate dissociation associated with distal radius fractures? *J Hand Surg Am.* 1996;21:583–590.

366. Tarallo L, Mugnai R, Zambianchi F, et al. Volar plate fixation for the treatment of distal radius fractures: analysis of adverse events. *J Orthop Trauma.* 2013;27:740–745.

367. Thivaios GC, McKee MD. Sliding osteotomy for deformity correction following malunion of volarly displaced distal radial fractures. *J Orthop Trauma.* 2003;17:326–333.

368. Thompson PW, Taylor J, Dawson A. The annual incidence and seasonal variation of fractures of the distal radius in men and women over 25 years in Dorset, UK. *Injury.* 2004;35:462–466.

369. Trumble TE, Schmitt SR, Vedder NB. Factors affecting functional outcome of displaced intra-articular distal radius fractures. *J Hand Surg Am.* 1994;19:325–340.

370. Tsukazaki T, Iwasaki K. Ulnar wrist pain after Colles' fracture. 109 fractures followed for 4 years. *Acta Orthop Scand.* 1993;64:462–464.

371. Tumia N, Wardlaw D, Hallett J, et al. Aberdeen Colles' fracture brace as a treatment for Colles' fracture. A multicentre, prospective, randomised, controlled trial. *J Bone Joint Surg Br.* 2003;85:78–82.

372. Tyllianakis ME, Panagopoulos A, Giannikas D, et al. Graft-supplemented, augmented external fixation in the treatment of intra-articular distal radial fractures. *Orthopedics.* 2006;29:139–144.

373. Uchikura C, Hirano J, Kudo F, et al. Comparative study of nonbridging and bridging external fixators for unstable distal radius fractures. *J Orthop Sci.* 2004;9:560–565.

374. van der Linden W, Ericson R. Colles' fracture. How should its displacement be measured and how should it be immobilized? *J Bone Joint Surg Am.* 1981;63:1285–1288.

375. van Leerdam RH, Souer JS, Lindenhovius AL, et al. Agreement between Initial Classification and Subsequent Reclassification of Fractures of the Distal Radius in a Prospective Cohort Study. *Hand (N Y).* 2010;5:68–71.

376. van Schoonhoven J, Muhldorfer-Fodor M, Fernandez DL, et al. Salvage of failed resection arthroplasties of the distal radioulnar joint using an ulnar head prosthesis: long-term results. *J Hand Surg Am.* 2012;37:1372–1380.

377. van Staa TP, Dennison EM, Leufkens HG, et al. Epidemiology of fractures in England and Wales. *Bone.* 2001;29:517–522.

378. van Vugt R, Geerts RW, Werre AJ. Osteosynthesis of distal radius fractures with the Micronail. *Eur J Trauma Emerg Surg.* 2010;36:471–476.

379. Varitimidis SE, Basdekis GK, Dailiana ZH, et al. Treatment of intra-articular fractures of the distal radius: fluoroscopic or arthroscopic reduction? *J Bone Joint Surg Br.* 2008;90:778–785.

380. Vidal J, Buscayret C, Fischbach C, et al. [New method of treatment of comminuted fractures of the lower end of the radius: "ligamentary taxis"]. *Acta Orthop Belg.* 1977;43:781–789.

381. Voigt C, Plesz A, Jensen G, et al. [Volar locking plating for distal radial fractures. Is osteoporosis associated with poorer functional results and higher complications rates?]. *Chirurg.* 2012;83:463–471.

382. Wada T, Tatebe M, Ozasa Y, et al. Clinical outcomes of corrective osteotomy for distal radial malunion: a review of opening and closing-wedge techniques. *J Bone Joint Surg Am.* 2011;93:1619–1626.

383. Wagner WF Jr, Tencer AF, Kiser P, et al. Effects of intra-articular distal radius depression on wrist joint contact characteristics. *J Hand Surg Am.* 1996;21:554–560.

384. Wakefield AE, McQueen MM. The role of physiotherapy and clinical predictors of outcome after fracture of the distal radius. *J Bone Joint Surg Br.* 2000;82:972–976.

385. Wardrope J, Flowers M, Wilson DH. Comparison of local anaesthetic techniques in the reduction of Colles' fracture. *Arch Emerg Med.* 1985;2:67–72.

386. Washburn RA, McAuley E, Katula J, et al. The physical activity scale for the elderly (PASE): evidence for validity. *J Clin Epidemiol.* 1999;52:643–651.

387. Washburn RA, Smith KW, Jette AM, et al. The Physical Activity Scale for the Elderly (PASE): development and evaluation. *J Clin Epidemiol.* 1993;46:153–162.

388. Wei DH, Raizman NM, Bottino CJ, et al. Unstable distal radial fractures treated with external fixation, a radial column plate, or a volar plate. A prospective randomized trial. *J Bone Joint Surg Am.* 2009;91:1568–1577.

389. Werber KD, Raeder F, Brauer RB, et al. External fixation of distal radial fractures: four compared with five pins: a randomized prospective study. *J Bone Joint Surg Am.* 2003;85-A:660–666.

390. Westphal T, Piatek S, Schubert S, et al. Outcome after surgery of distal radius fractures: no differences between external fixation and ORIF. *Arch Orthop Trauma Surg.* 2005;125:507–514.

391. White BD, Nydick JA, Karsky D, et al. Incidence and clinical outcomes of tendon rupture following distal radius fracture. *J Hand Surg Am.* 2012;37:2035–2040.

392. Wilcke MK, Abbaszadegan H, Adolphson PY. Patient-perceived outcome after displaced distal radius fractures. A comparison between radiological parameters, objective physical variables, and the DASH score. *J Hand Ther.* 2007;20:290–298.

393. Wilcke MK, Abbaszadegan H, Adolphson PY. Wrist function recovers more rapidly after volar locked plating than after external fixation but the outcomes are similar after 1 year. *Acta Orthop.* 2011;82:76–81.

394. Wilcke MT, Abbaszadegan H, Adolphson PY. Evaluation of a Swedish version of the patient-rated wrist evaluation outcome questionnaire: good responsiveness, validity, and reliability, in 99 patients recovering from a fracture of the distal radius. *Scand J Plast Reconstr Surg Hand Surg.* 2009;43:94–101.

395. Wong TC, Chiu Y, Tsang WL, et al. Casting versus percutaneous pinning for extra-articular fractures of the distal radius in an elderly Chinese population: a prospective randomised controlled trial. *J Hand Surg Eur Vol.* 2010;35:202–208.

396. Xie X, Barenholdt O. Bone density and geometric properties of the distal radius in displaced and undisplaced Colles' fractures: quantitative CT in 70 women. *Acta Orthop Scand.* 2001;72:62–66.

397. Yen SN, Dion GR, Bowers WH. Ulnar head implant arthroplasty: an intermediate term review of 1 surgeon's experience. *Tech Hand Up Extrem Surg.* 2009;13:160–164.

398. Youm Y, McMurthy RY, Flatt AE, et al. Kinematics of the wrist. I. An experimental study of radial-ulnar deviation and flexion-extension. *J Bone Joint Surg Am.* 1978;60:423–431.

399. Young BT, Rayan GM. Outcome following nonoperative treatment of displaced distal radius fractures in low-demand patients older than 60 years. *J Hand Surg Am.* 2000;25:19–28.

400. Younger AS, Curran P, McQueen MM. Backslabs and plaster casts: which will best accommodate increasing intracompartmental pressures? *Injury.* 1990;21:179–181.

401. Zenke Y, Sakai A, Oshige T, et al. The effect of an associated ulnar styloid fracture on the outcome after fixation of a fracture of the distal radius. *J Bone Joint Surg Br.* 2009;91:102–107.

402. Zenke Y, Sakai A, Oshige T, et al. Treatment with or without internal fixation for ulnar styloid base fractures accompanied by distal radius fractures fixed with volar locking plate. *Hand Surg.* 2012;17:181–190.

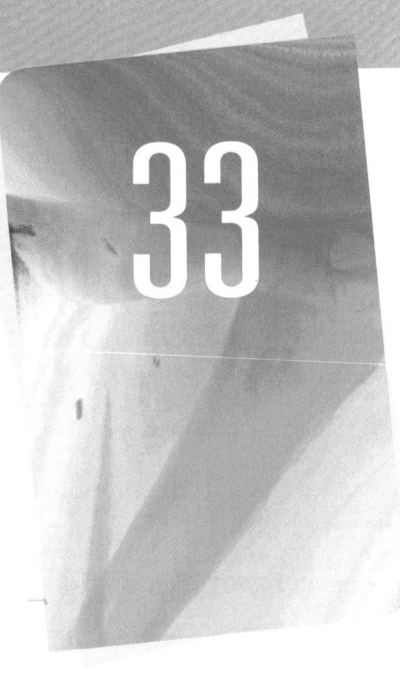

33

DIAPHYSEAL FRACTURES OF THE RADIUS AND ULNA

Philipp N. Streubel and Rodrigo F. Pesántez

INTRODUCTION TO DIAPHYSEAL FRACTURES OF THE RADIUS AND ULNA

The forearm plays an important role in positioning of the hand in space by flexion and extension of the elbow and wrist as well as pronation and supination through the proximal and distal radioulnar joints. Fractures of the ulnar and radial shaft can therefore result in significant dysfunction if treated inadequately.

This chapter will address fractures of the ulnar and radial shaft, including Galeazzi and Monteggia fracture dislocations. Radial shaft fractures are defined as those occurring between the radial neck proximally and the junction of the metaphysis and diaphysis distally, approximately 3 cm proximal to the distal articular surface. Ulnar shaft fractures are defined as those occurring between the distal aspect of the coronoid proximally and the ulnar neck distally.

Epidemiology of Diaphyseal Fractures of the Radius and Ulna

Forearm shaft fractures are often referred to as being frequent fractures. However, only limited data on the epidemiology of these fractures have been reported in the literature. Several epidemiologic studies on forearm fractures include fracture occurring along the whole extent of the ulna and radius. Distal radius fractures are known as one of the most frequent fractures of the upper extremity and hence account for the vast majority of fractures occurring in the forearm.[14,28,131,162] Diaphyseal forearm fractures on the contrary have been reported to be 10 times less frequent than distal radius fractures.[90]

The incidence of distal radius fractures has increased over the past decades. However, the frequency of forearm shaft fractures appears to be stable over time.[14] The average yearly incidence in adults has been reported to be 1.35 per 10,000 population, ranging from 0 to 4 per 10,000 population depending on age and gender. This is relatively infrequent compared to that of humerus shaft (0 to 10), femur (0 to 37), and tibia (0 to 21).[176] Four-fifths of forearm shaft fractures occur in children. Above the age of 20, the yearly incidence of forearm shaft fractures remains below 2 per 10,000 people, predominating in males throughout all age groups.[3,14]

Clinical studies on forearm fractures, without exception, show that forearm fractures predominantly occur in male patients. The proportion of males ranges from 63% to 91%.[13,27,48,60,71,73,108,109] The mean age ranges from 24 to 37 years, and the vast majority of forearm fractures occur during the first four decades of life.[13,27,32,36,48,49,60,64,71,73,74,108,109,113,119,135,156,163,166,179] Over half of all forearm shaft fractures occur in males within the ages of 15 and 39 years. This age group accounts for 80% of forearm fractures in males. As for femur and tibia shaft fractures, forearm shaft fractures have the highest incidence in males aged 15 to 40 years. In females, a lower incidence of forearm shaft fractures can be observed throughout life. A peak incidence has been reported in the seventh decade of life.[28,176] The distribution of forearm fractures is type B (see Chapter 3).

Among US high school athletes the incidence of forearm fractures is 4 per 10,000 athlete exposures, defined as one ath-lete participating in one practice or competition. The incidence is highest in male football and female soccer players at 6 per 10,000 athlete exposures and lowest for volleyball at 1 per 10,000 athlete exposures.[183]

Motor vehicle accidents account for an important frac-tion of forearm shaft fractures. It is estimated that 4% of restrained front seat passengers involved in a motor vehi-cle collision suffer a fracture of the upper extremity. In this setting, forearm fractures account for one quarter of upper extremity fractures, a fraction that is equal to that of wrist and hand fractures.[149]

Monteggia fractures account for 13% and Galeazzi fractures for 23% of forearm fractures.[27]

ASSESSMENT OF DIAPHYSEAL FRACTURES OF THE RADIUS AND ULNA

Mechanism of Injury of Diaphyseal Fractures of the Radius and Ulna

The vast majority of forearm shaft fractures occur in young males with good bone stock. Injuries therefore most frequently occur in the setting of high-energy trauma such as motor vehi-cle accidents or sports injuries.[20,39,52,105,109,120,146]

The force applied by trauma can be applied either directly or indirectly onto the diaphysis of the radius and/or ulna. Direct injury frequently results from gunshot injuries or from blunt injury to the forearm. In both instances, injury to the soft tissues can be substantial (Figs. 33-1 and 33-2). Isolated ulnar shaft fractures almost invariably occur as a consequence

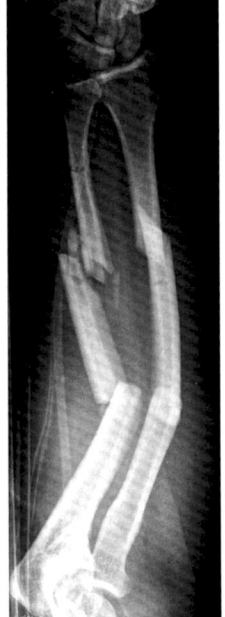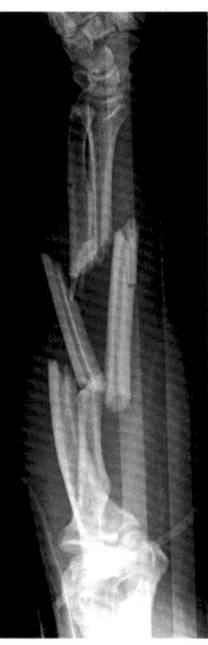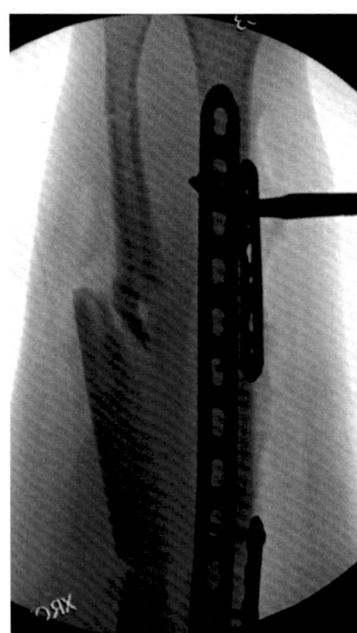

A, B   C

FIGURE 33-1 A and B: Segmental both-bone forearm fracture. Severe fracture of the forearm after direct blunt trauma with marked soft tissue injury. Note the widening of the interosseous space between the intermediate fracture segments suggesting concomitant longitudinal interosseous mem-brane disruption.

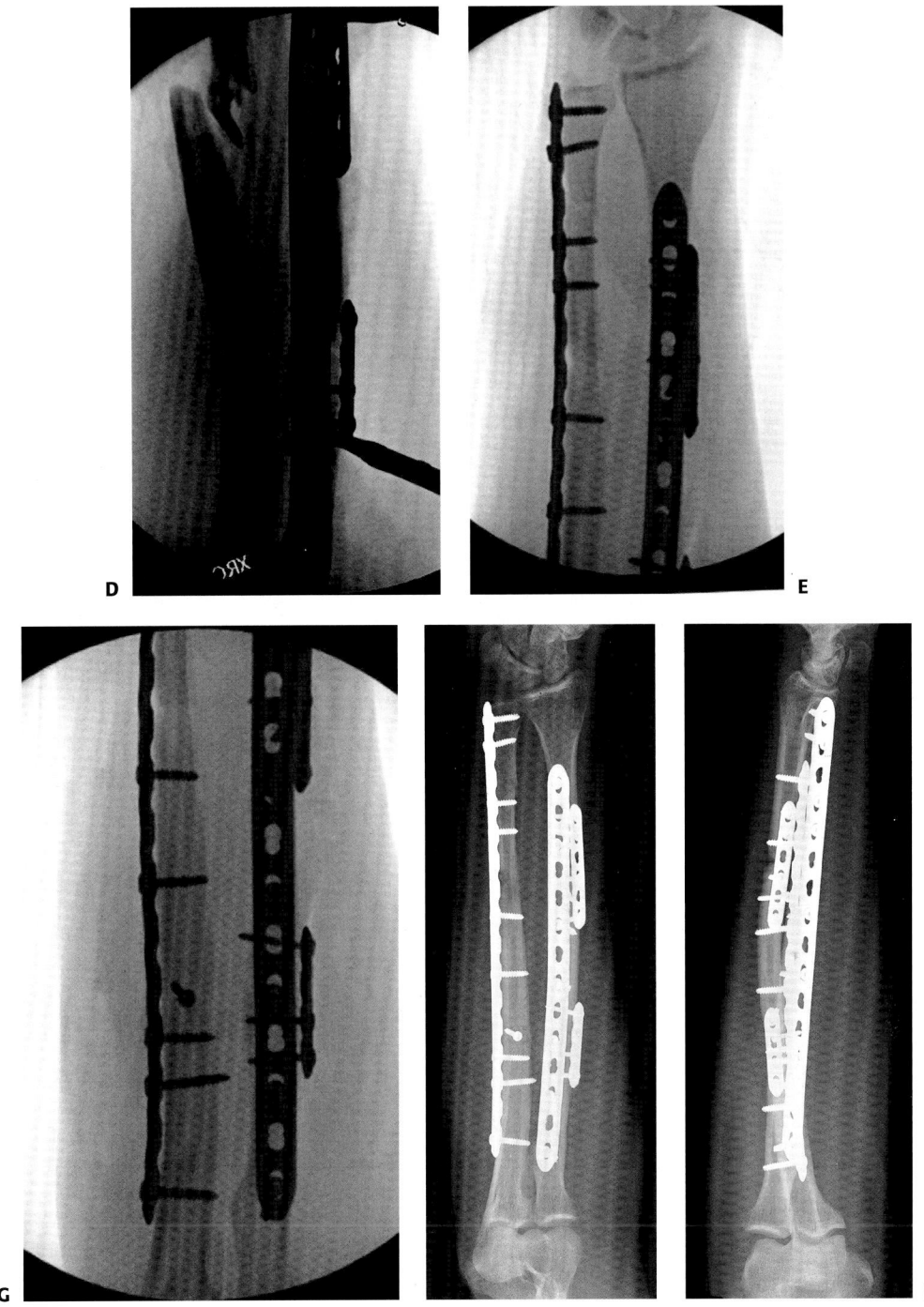

FIGURE 33-1 (*continued*) **C–F:** Intraoperative fluoroscopic images. Initial fixation of the radius was performed because of a more simple fracture pattern. Two separate 2.7-mm plates were used for each fracture and augmented with a long 3.5-mm plate. A single 16-hole 3.5-mm plate was used for fixation of the ulna. **G and H:** Follow-up images 6 weeks after surgery.

of direct injury to the ulnar shaft as the arm is raised to protect the body from a blow,[170] hence the descriptive term "night stick fractures" (Fig. 33-3). In this instance, given the subcutaneous location of the ulnar shaft, fractures may occur with only minor energy and exhibit a less significant soft tissue injury. However, the thinner overlying soft tissue envelope

makes these fractures more prone to being open, especially when severely displaced.

Indirect trauma on the other hand occurs either as bending or torsional forces. Bending forces can result in both-bone forearm fractures that are located at similar segments along the diaphysis of the ulna and radius (Fig. 33-4). In addition,

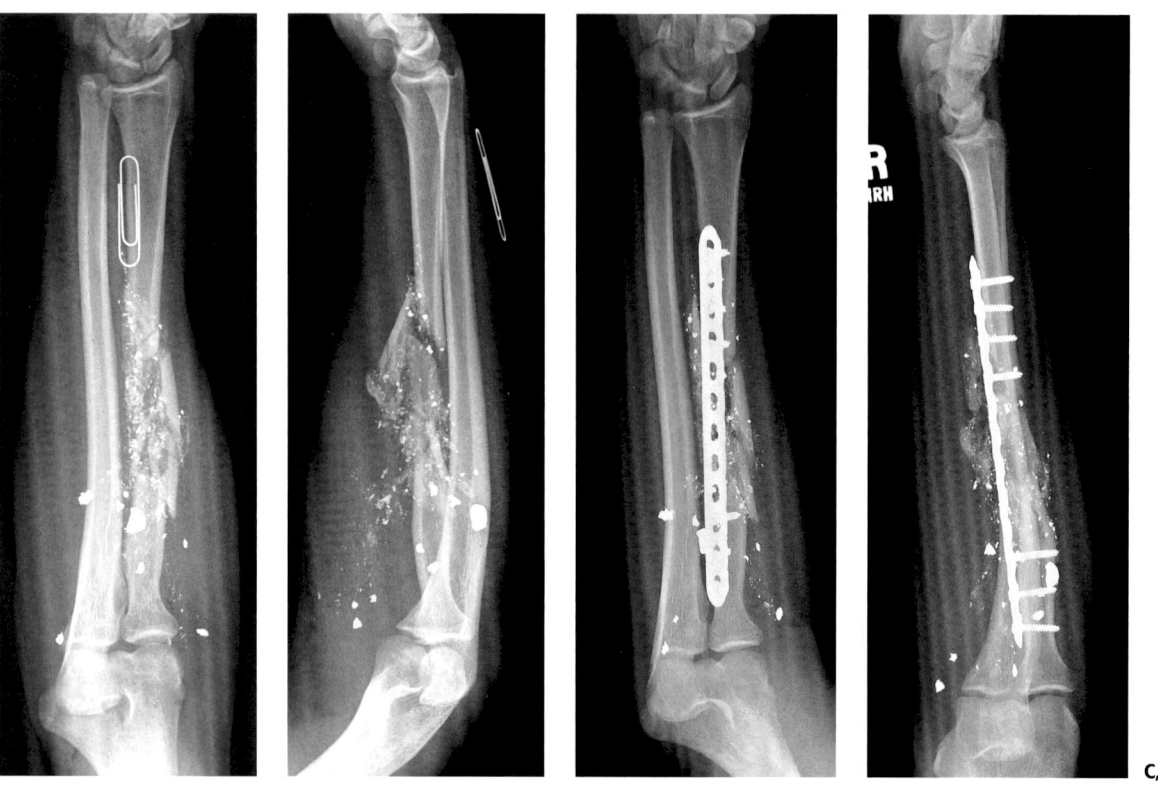

A, B

C, D

FIGURE 33-2 A and B: Gunshot fracture of the radial shaft. Note the marked comminution at the midproximal radial shaft. A paper clip marks the entry site with the fragmented projectile lodged in the soft tissues. **C and D:** Postoperative radiographs 2 weeks after fracture fixation with a bridging plate.

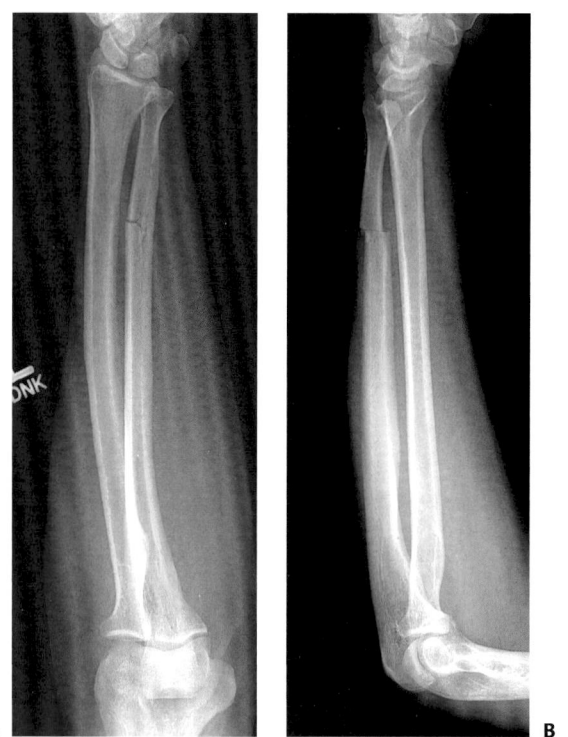

A

B

FIGURE 33-3 A and B: Nightstick fracture. Minimally displaced isolated ulna shaft fracture. Treatment consisted of a short arm brace for 6 weeks leading to uneventful healing.

bending forces can result in Monteggia fracture dislocation, in which the proximal ulna is fractured and the radiocapitellar and proximal radioulnar joints (PRUJs) dislocate in the direction of the ulnar deformity (Figs. 33-5, 33-9 and 33-12). Torsional forces with axial loading, such as those occurring during a fall with a hyperpronated forearm and wrist extension, can lead to both-bone forearm fractures at different levels or to Galeazzi fractures (Figs. 33-6 and 33-7). With this mechanism a fracture is generated through the radial shaft and progresses distally rupturing the interosseous membrane and finally injuring the triangular fibrocartilage complex (TFCC), thereby rendering the distal radioulnar joint unstable.[6,8,57,120] Whereas hyperpronation of the wrist is considered to generate Monteggia fractures with anterior dislocation of the radial head, Monteggia fractures with a posterior radial head dislocation are believed to occur as a consequence of a hypersupination injury and a fall onto the outstretched hand.[57]

Signs and Symptoms of Diaphyseal Fractures of the Radius and Ulna

With a fracture of the forearm there will be a history of a lower-energy injury such as a fall on to the outstretched hand or direct blow or of a higher-energy injury such as a fall from a height or a road traffic accident. The patient will complain of pain and swelling in the forearm and where there is displacement may also complain of a visible deformity. Neurologic injury should be suspected if there are neurologic symptoms. A history of

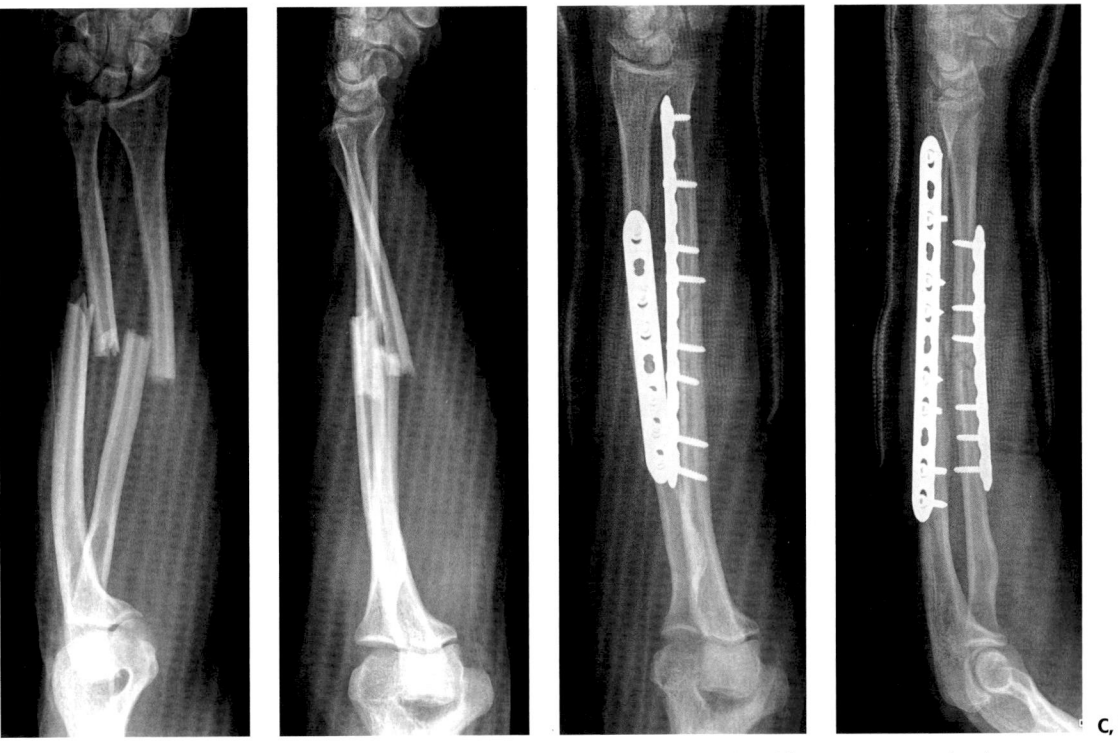

FIGURE 33-4 A and B: Both-bone forearm fracture. Note that both displaced fractures occurred at the same level of the ulna and radius. A nondisplaced fracture of the distal ulnar shaft is present. **C and D:** Postoperative radiographs after open reduction and internal fixation. Compression at the fracture site was achieved with dynamic plating.

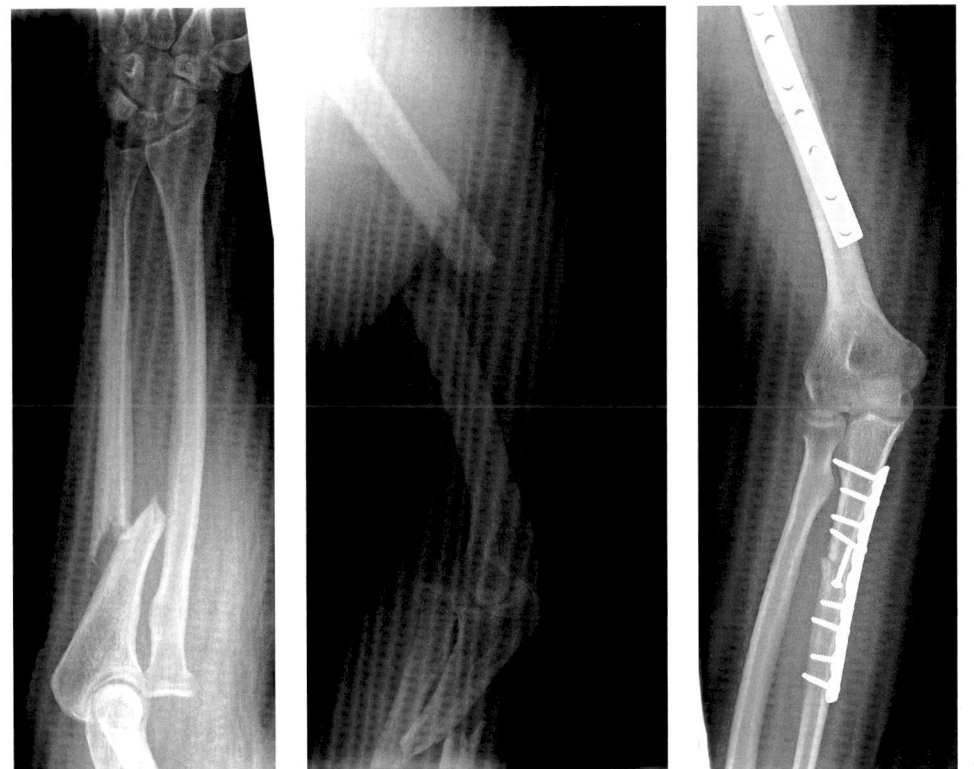

FIGURE 33-5 A: Monteggia fracture dislocation. Note an apex anterior deformity of the ulnar shaft with anterior dislocation of the radial head. **B:** This patient had a concomitant humerus shaft fracture.

(continues)

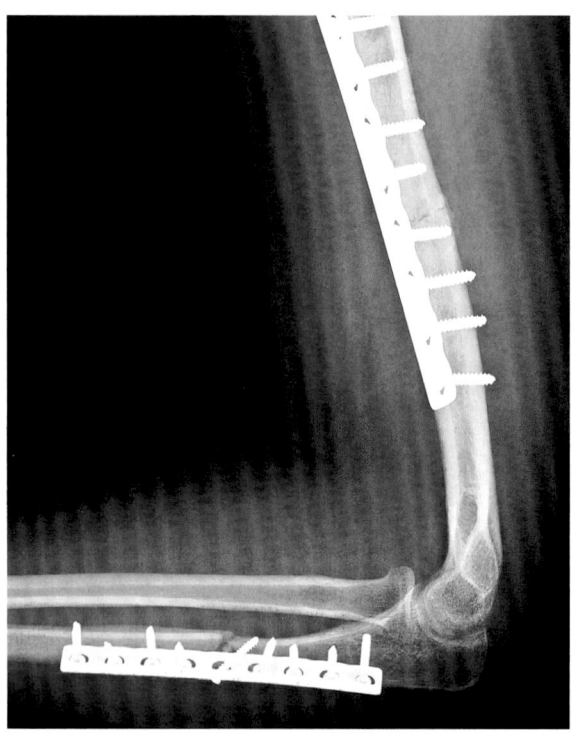

FIGURE 33-5 (*continued*) **C and D:** Postoperative radiographs after open reduction internal fixation of both the ulna and humerus. Reduction of the radiocapitellar and proximal radioulnar joint was achieved with reduction of the ulnar fracture.

distant pain suggests an associated injury in the ipsilateral limb or elsewhere.

On examination there will be swelling in the forearm and deformity in cases with displacement. The skin should be inspected to rule out any open wounds, which most commonly occur on the ulnar side. In the absence of neurologic injury, tenderness at the area of the fracture is invariable in the conscious patient and is useful in raising clinical suspicion in the undisplaced fracture without deformity. A thorough neurologic examination should be performed to exclude peripheral nerve injury. The examiner should remember to look for the symptoms and signs of acute compartment syndrome which may occur after forearm fractures (see Chapter 29).

Associated Injuries with Diaphyseal Fractures of the Radius and Ulna

Approximately one-third of forearm shaft fractures treated surgically occur as isolated injuries.[27] The remaining fractures occur in the presence of at least one additional injury. Associated injuries can be grouped into those occurring adjacent to the forearm shaft fracture, those occurring in other sites of the musculoskeletal system, and those affecting other organ systems. Injuries occurring locally surrounding the diaphyses of the radius and ulna range from minor contusion of the soft tissue sleeve in isolated minimally displaced ulna (nightstick) fractures to marked soft tissue injury in both-bone fractures and fracture dislocations. With

(*text continues on page 1130*)

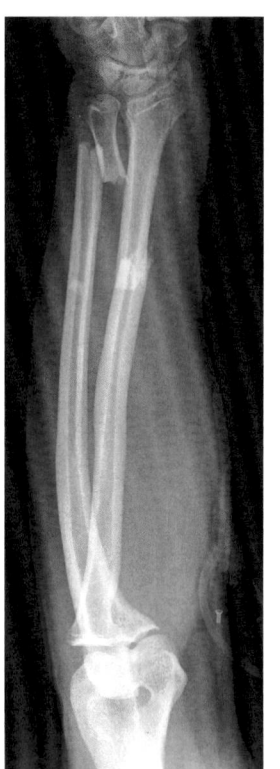 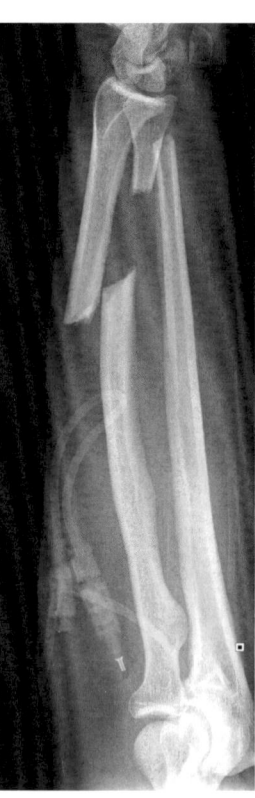 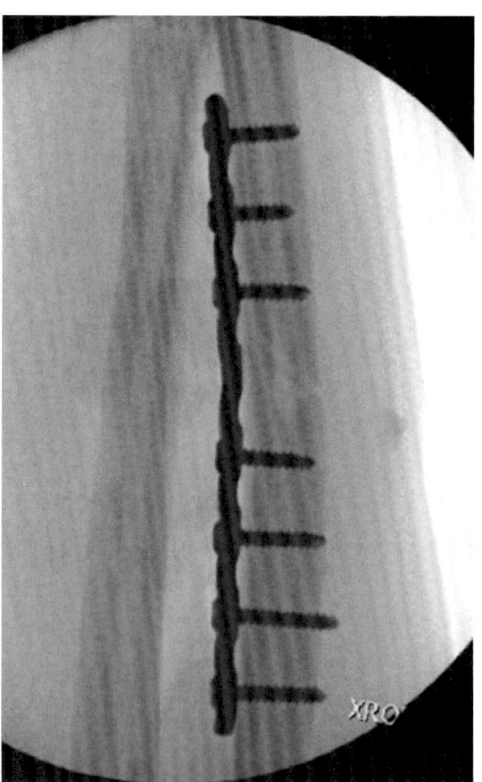

FIGURE 33-6 A and B: Both-bone forearm fracture. The mechanism of injury of this fracture was likely torsional in nature, leading to fracture of the shafts of both the ulna and radius at different levels. A concomitant radial styloid fracture is present.

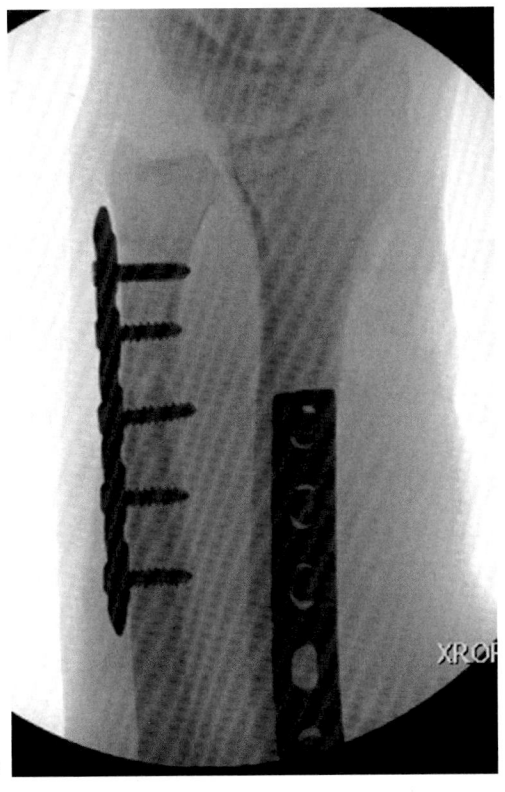

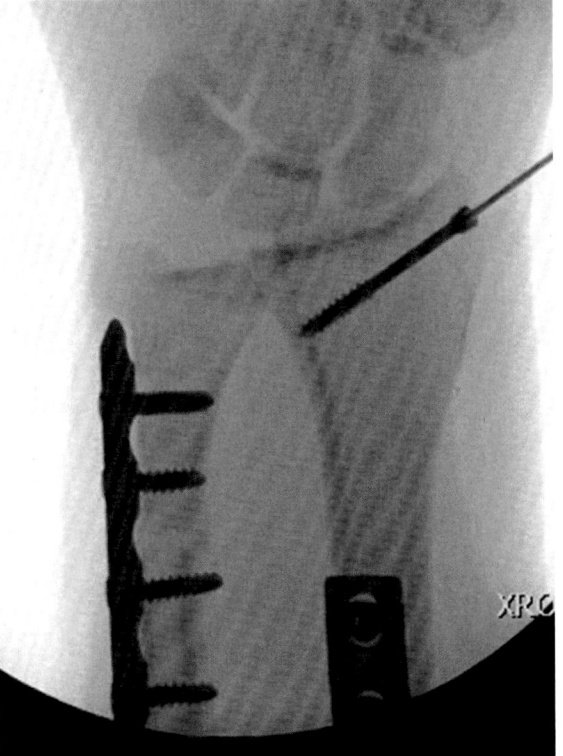

D   **E**

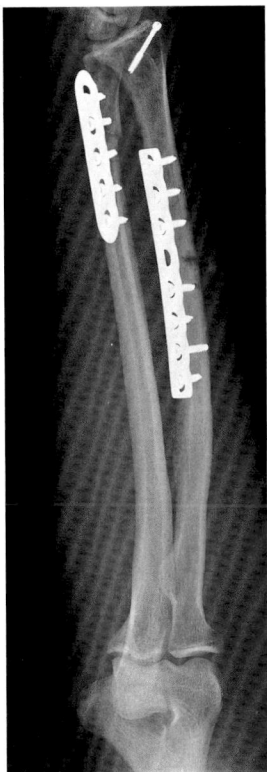

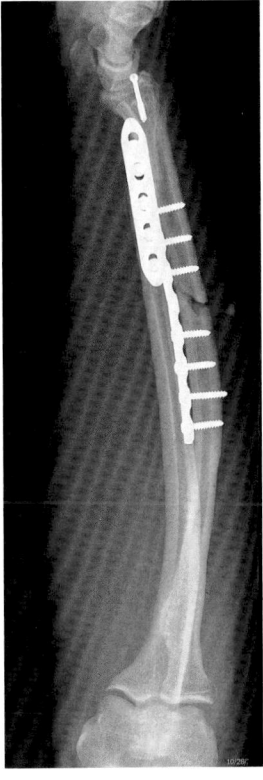

FIGURE 33-6 (*continued*) **C, D and E:** Intraoperative fluoroscopic images. Fixation of the radius and ulna was achieved with 3.5-mm plates and screws. Alternatively, a lag screw could have been placed through the oblique fracture of the radius. The radial styloid was fixed with a headless compression screw. **F and G:** Postoperative radiographs.

F   **G**

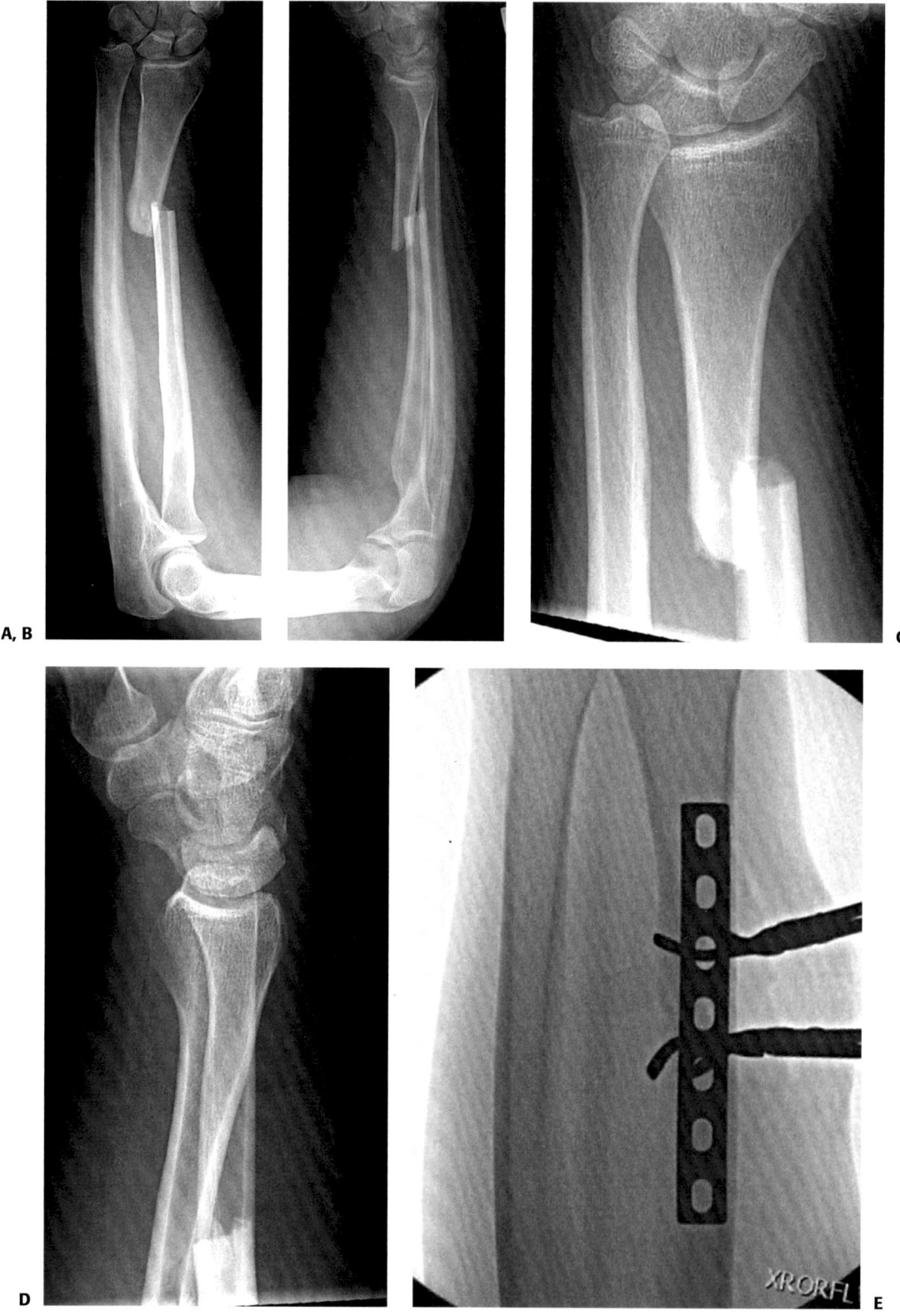

A, B

C

D

E

FIGURE 33-7 **A–D:** Galeazzi fracture dislocation. Note a displaced fracture of the distal radial shaft with pronounced shortening of the radius and an avulsion fracture of the ulnar styloid.

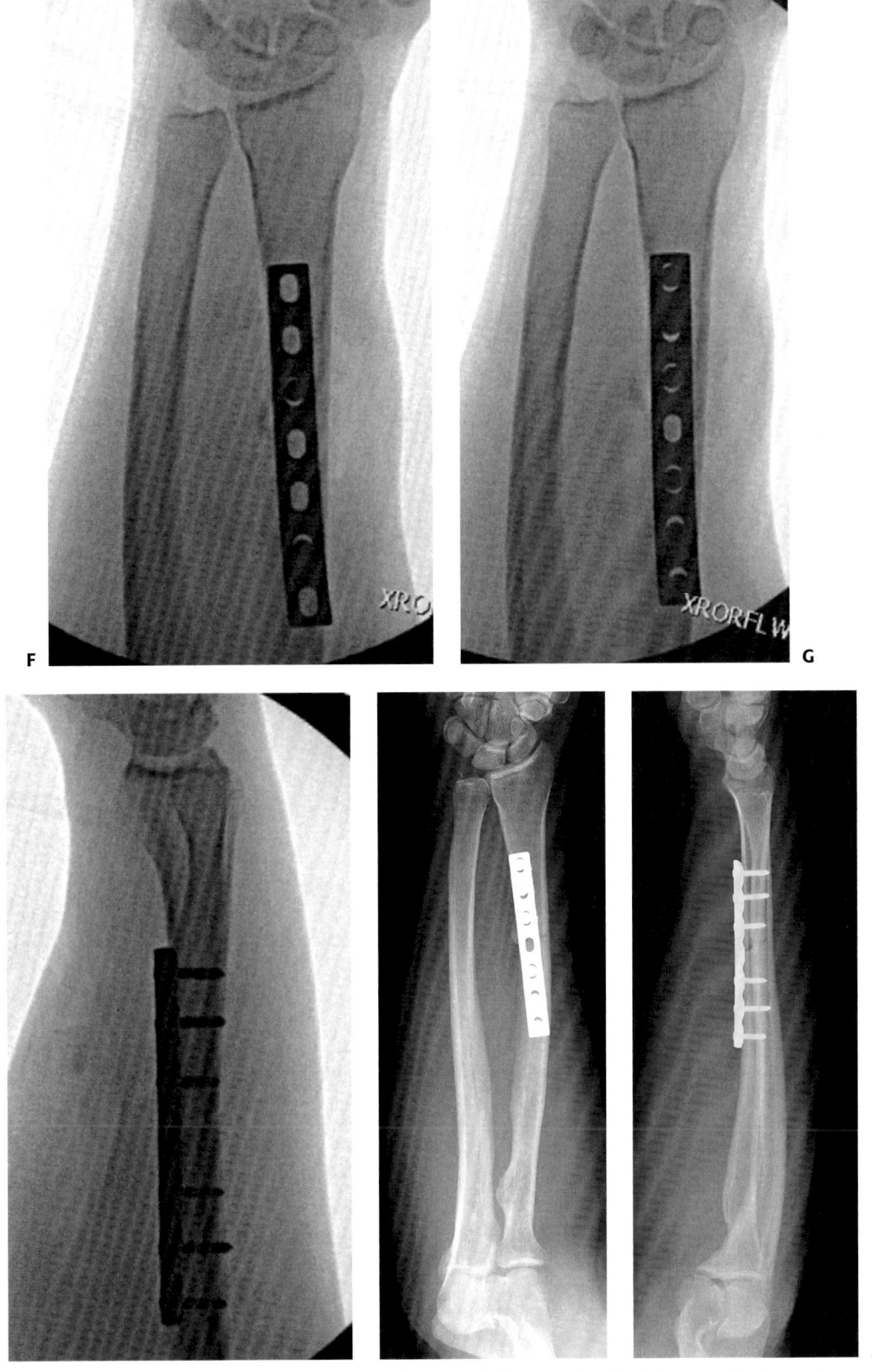

FIGURE 33-7 (*continued*) **E–H:** Intraoperative fluoroscopic images showing fracture reduction onto the plate held by lobster clamps. Fixation is achieved with dynamic plate compression and a total of six cortices being engaged by screws on each side of the fracture.

(*continues*)

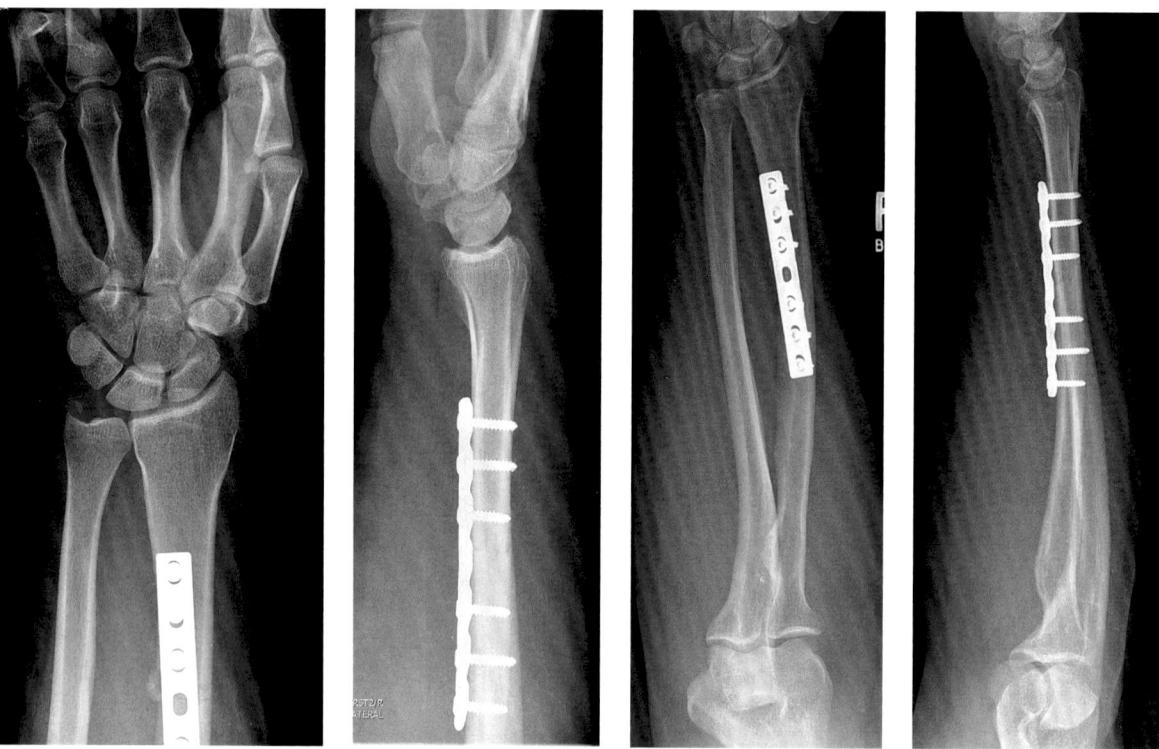

K, L

M, N

FIGURE 33-7 *(continued)* **I–L:** Postoperative radiographs 2 weeks after surgery. **M and N:** Radiographs at 3 months after surgery showing a healed fracture.

increasing energy, a greater extent of fracture comminution and displacement is seen, which in turn increases the risk of injury to the surrounding muscles. Direct trauma to the forearm causes blunt injury to the soft tissue sleeve, while fracture displacement will lead to laceration of the soft tissues by the sharp edges of the fracture and may injure the interosseous membrane, muscles, neurovascular structures, and skin. Rupture of the interosseous membrane occurs along the path connecting both shaft fractures in both-bone forearm fractures or the fracture and associated, either proximal or distal, radioulnar joint disruption in fracture dislocations. Monteggia fractures exhibit disruption of the interosseous membrane from the fracture site at the proximal half of the ulnar shaft to the PRUJ. The radial head dislocates in the direction of the deformity of the apex of the ulnar fracture, thereby disrupting the annular ligament. Occasionally, the radial head may buttonhole through the joint capsule, displacing but leaving the annular ligament intact.[145] Galeazzi fracture dislocations most frequently present with a fracture of the distal half of the radius with an associated dislocation of the DRUJ. In this setting, disruption of the interosseous membrane occurs from the fracture site to the distal radioulnar joint. Associated injury of the TFCC usually occurs, occasionally leading to further disruption of the fifth and sixth extensor compartments of the wrist. Ring et al.[155] established that in the setting of isolated radial shaft fractures, an associated distal radioulnar joint injury is present in 10 out of 36 cases.

Although the exact incidence of elbow dislocations in the setting of both-bone forearm fractures is not known, this constellation has been reported in several case reports[37,83,99,144]

(Fig. 33-8). Similarly, radial head fractures may present at the same time as diaphyseal forearm fractures.[52]

The frequency of open fractures ranges from less than 10% in isolated radial shaft fractures to 43% of fractures affecting both forearm bones.[20,27,39,52,65,104,105,109,155] Open fractures most frequently are type I according to the Gustilo classification.[61] They occur as a skin disruption from within, in which the sharp fracture edges pierce through the skin in an inside-out fashion. Displaced ulnar shaft fractures are at particular risk of being open given the subcutaneous location of this bone. Crush injuries and high-velocity gunshot wounds account for type III open fractures and are frequently accompanied by marked contamination, severe disruption of the muscular envelope, and injury to the neurovascular structures.[89,107]

Whereas some regional variation is reported in the literature,[108] around one-half of forearm shaft fractures occur in the setting of multisystem trauma.[20,27] Associated injuries most frequently affect either the upper or lower extremities. Upper extremity injuries occur in up to 26% of forearm fractures and include humeral shaft fractures, proximal humerus fractures, elbow dislocation (Fig. 33-8), wrist injuries[39,105,155] (Fig. 33-6), glenoid fractures,[59] and contralateral forearm fractures.[27,52,191] Distal biceps ruptures have been reported[85] as well as traumatic rotator cuff tears.[59]

Concomitant lower extremity fractures may occur, often affecting the tibial plateau, fibula, patella, femur,[20,59] tibia and ankle,[105] pelvis, and acetabulum.[39]

The most frequent nonskeletal injury is closed head injury[20,27,105,155] and peripheral neurologic injuries. In one series on forearm fractures, closed head injuries occurred in one quarter of patients.[27] Forearm fractures can occur in the presence of injuries to the brachial plexus and radial, posterior interosseous, ulnar, and median nerves.[20,105,154] Radial nerve injuries may occur either as a transection of the nerve from the forearm shaft fracture or as a consequence of an ipsilateral humerus shaft fracture.[107] Neurologic injury has been reported in 38% of forearm fractures caused by low-velocity gunshot wounds. Of these, 43% resulted in permanent nerve palsy. Ulnar artery disruption was reported in only 3% of these cases.[106]

Forearm fracture may occur in patients with abdominal and pelvic trauma with associated aortic transection, kidney lacera-

tion, and pelvic fractures.[59,109] Goldfarb et al.[59] reported 1 out of 23 patients included in a clinical study on both-bone forearm fractures who had suffered an aortic dissection and kidney laceration after a motor vehicle accident.

Imaging and Other Diagnostic Studies for Diaphyseal Fractures of the Radius and Ulna

Forearm fractures are routinely diagnosed with posteroanterior (PA) and lateral radiographs of the forearm. These images should show the forearm from the elbow to the wrist. A

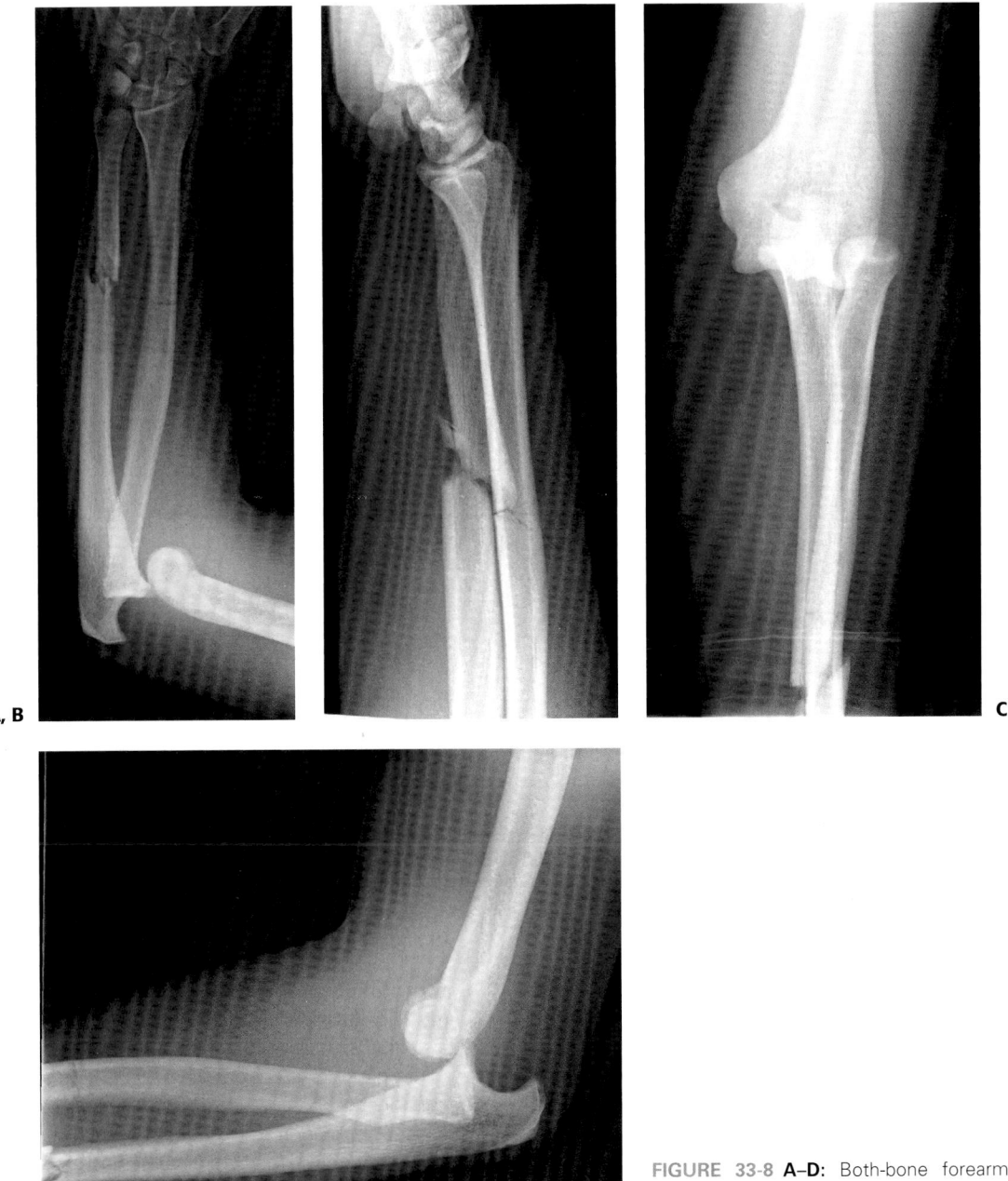

FIGURE 33-8 **A–D:** Both-bone forearm fracture with associated posterior elbow dislocation. (*continues*)

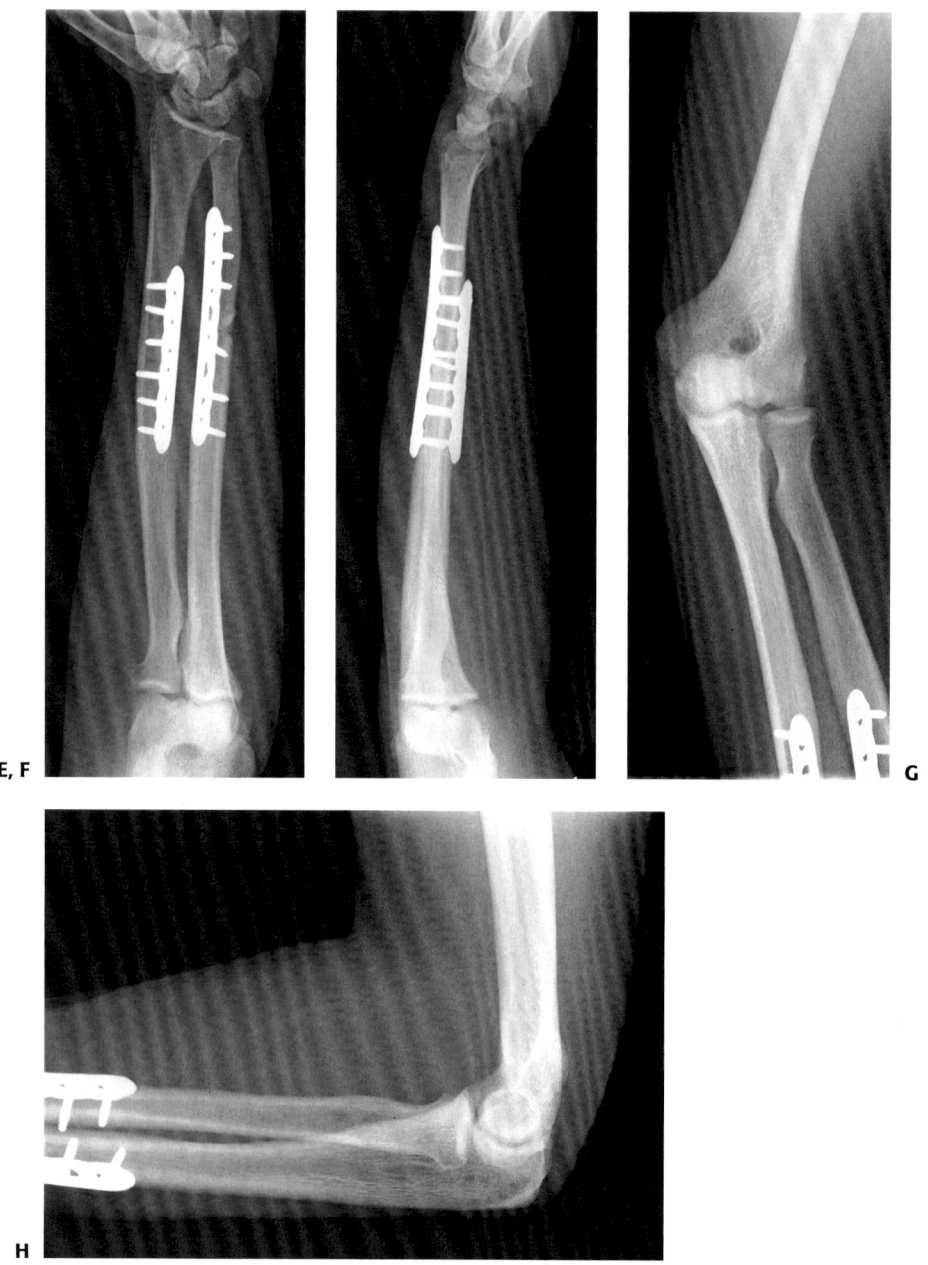

FIGURE 33-8 (*continued*) **E–H:** After initial closed reduction of the elbow, open reduction internal fixation was performed. At 3 months after surgery fracture healing was observed. Ossification of the medial collateral ligament of the elbow could be seen radiographically, without limiting the patient's range of motion.

standard PA view of the forearm is taken with the elbow in 90 degrees of flexion, the shoulder abducted, and the forearm in neutral rotation. A standard lateral radiograph is taken with the elbow flexed to 90 degrees and the forearm in neutral rotation (Fig. 33-9). This allows for two views that are orthogonal to each other. In some instances, additional oblique views may be helpful in case overlap of the ulna and radius on the lateral view do not clearly allow detailed fracture assessment.

The position of the bicipital tuberosity of the proximal radius can aid in assessing the amount of pronation or supina-

tion of the proximal fragment. The tuberosity view is taken with the elbow bent 90 degrees, the lateral and medial epicondyles equidistant from the plate, and the x-ray tube angulated 20 degrees posteriorly from the normal AP trajectory. Depending on the morphology of the biceps tuberosity on this view the amount of pronation or supination of the proximal radius can be determined with the help of a reference image, so that distal segment rotational alignment can be adjusted.[46]

Dedicated radiographs of the elbow and wrist are also recommended to rule out associated injuries to these joints[187]

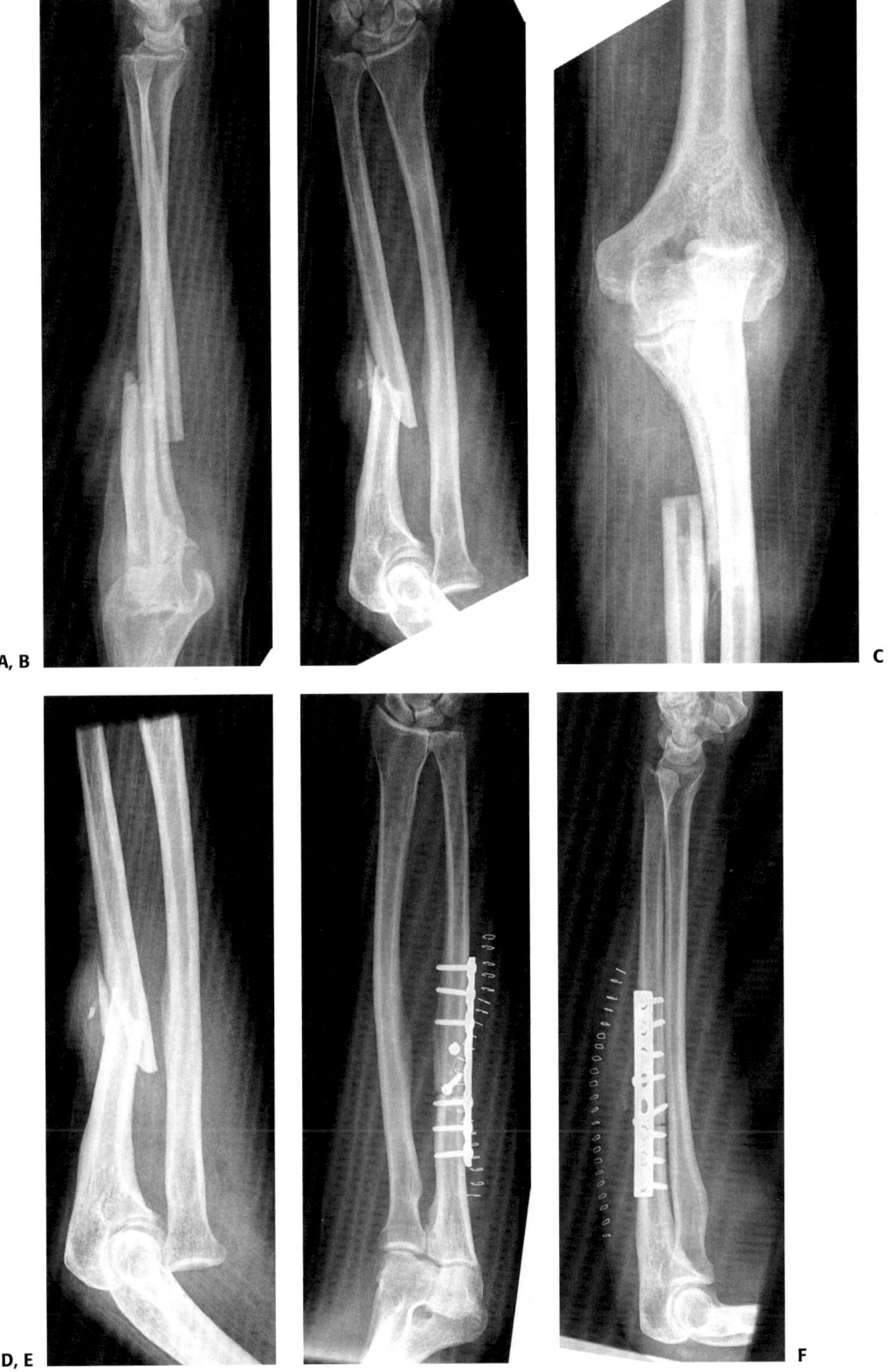

A, B

C

D, E

F

FIGURE 33-9 A–D: Monteggia fracture dislocation. **E and F:** Fixation was performed using two lag screws through the oblique fracture of the ulna and a neutralization plate. Secondary reduction of the radiocapitellar and proximal radioulnar joint was achieved.

(Figs. 33-7C, D and 33-8C, D). This is of special importance in isolated fractures of the ulna or radius to rule out Monteggia and Galeazzi fracture dislocations, respectively. However, even in both-bone forearm fractures, dislocation of the DRUJ, PRUJ, and elbow may occur. Unrecognized fractures of the proximal and distal ends of the ulna and radius, as well as injuries to the carpus and distal humerus may also be identified. AP and lateral elbow radiographs are required to demonstrate alignment of the axis of the radial neck and the humeral capitellum, which will confirm reduction of the PRUJ. PA and lateral wrist radiographs should show the ulnar head located within the sigmoid notch of the radius. Ulnar variance (see Chapter 32) should be quantified for objective assessment of the DRUJ. Dorsal displacement of the distal ulna and a change in ulnar variance of more than 5 mm suggests an injury to the DRUJ.[155] This is supported by biomechanical data that has shown all stabilizers of the DRUJ to be ruptured with 5 mm of ulnar positive variance.[126] Because of the variability of ulnar variance, contralateral wrist radiographs can be useful to determine the patient's normal anatomy. Additional radiographic signs for disruption of the DRUJ are fracture of the base of the styloid, widening of the DRUJ on the PA view, and dislocation of the ulna seen on the lateral view[57,125] (Fig. 33-7).

Computed tomography and magnetic resonance imaging are rarely required for the assessment of acute forearm fractures. Computed tomography is useful in confirming the radiographic and clinical suspicion of a nonunion. Furthermore, it can be useful in the presence of rotational fracture malunions and instability at the DRUJ[16] (Fig. 33-10). Magnetic resonance imaging can be used to diagnose injuries to the DRUJ and associated TFCC as well as to delineate disruption of the interosseous membrane.[189] Ultrasound has been described to assess the integrity of the interosseous membrane.[47,189]

Classification of Diaphyseal Fractures of the Radius and Ulna

As in most extremities, fractures of the forearm are described according to their location, pattern, displacement, and associated soft tissue disruption. From a therapeutic perspective, the following are answered when assessing a fracture of the forearm.

1. What bone(s) is (are) fractured?
2. In what location is the fracture (proximal, middle, distal third)

3. What is the fracture pattern (simple transverse, simple oblique, comminuted)?
4. Is there instability at the distal or proximal radioulnar joint?
5. Is the fracture open or closed?
6. Is a previous implant present?
7. Is a previous deformity present?
8. Is the bone stock normal?

No single classification takes into account all the above variables. In most instances forearm shaft fractures are classified according to location (proximal, middle, and distal third) or fracture comminution.[27,114] Open fractures are classified according to Gustilo's classification,[61,62] whereas Monteggia and Galeazzi fractures have their own subclassifications.[9,92,146]

The AO/OTA classification is the most widely used fracture classification of fractures of the forearm. Since forearm fractures affect the diaphysis of the forearm they are identified by the number 22 (2 for forearm, 2 for shaft).[114] Type A fractures are simple fractures, type B are wedge fractures, and type C are complex (highly comminuted or segmental) fractures. Type A and B fractures involve either the ulna (type A1, B1), the radius (type A2, B2), or both bones (type A3, B3). Type C fractures involve both bones, with a simple fracture of the radius and segmental comminution of the ulna in type C1, a simple fracture of the ulna and segmental comminution of the radius in type C2, and segmental comminution of both bones in type C3. Monteggia fractures are classified as type A1.3 and B1.3, depending on whether the ulnar fracture is simple (A1.3) or wedged (B1.3). Furthermore, Monteggia fracture dislocations in which both the radius and ulna are fractured are classified as type A3.2 or B3.2. Conversely, Galeazzi fracture dislocations are classified as type A2.3 and B2.3 depending on whether the radial fracture is simple (A2.3) or wedged (B2.3). Galeazzi fracture dislocations in which both the radius and ulna are fractured are classified as type A3.3 or B3.3.[114] Although the AO/OTA system has been widely adopted as the universal classification system for fractures, its utility in the management of forearm fractures is restricted mainly to research purposes because of the complexity of its nomenclature and low reliability[88,128] (Fig. 33-11).

Isolated ulna fractures are classified as stable or unstable. Stable fracture are those with less than 50% of displacement

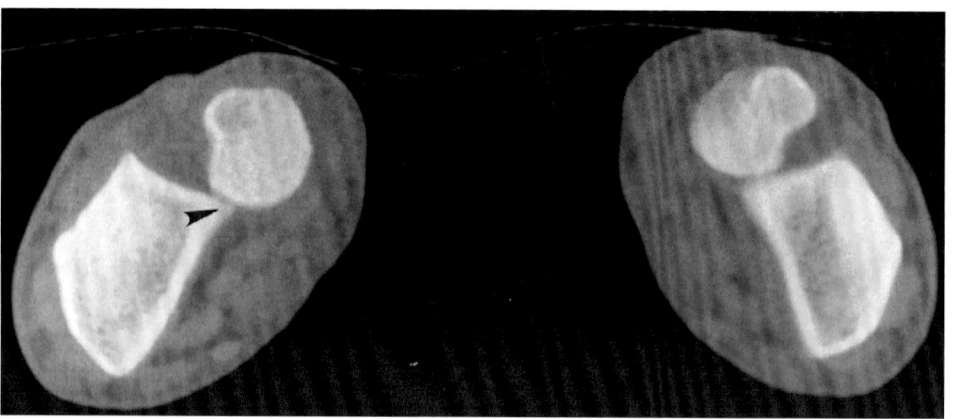

FIGURE 33-10 Computed axial tomogram showing volar subluxation of the right distal radioulnar joint (*arrow*) and volar translation of the distal ulna in relation to the radius because of incomplete reduction of a fracture of the distal radial diaphysis. There is little contact remaining between the dorsal articular surface of the distal ulna and the volar lip of the distal radial articular surface.

and less than 10 degrees of angulation.[42] This simple classification method has been widely accepted for decision making between operative and nonoperative management of these isolated fractures.[22,132,134,167,169,170,194]

Monteggia Fracture-Dislocation

Monteggia fracture-dislocations (or lesions) consist of a proximal radial dislocation and a fracture of the ulna.[9] They are classified according to Bado[9] based on the direction of the apex of the ulnar fracture and the direction of the proximal radial dislocation (Fig. 33-12):

Type 1: Anterior dislocation of the radial head, fracture of the ulnar diaphysis at any level with anterior angulation.

Type 2: Posterior or posterolateral dislocation of the radial head, fracture of the ulnar diaphysis with apex posterior angulation.

Type 3: Lateral or anterolateral dislocation of the radial head, fracture of the ulnar metaphysis. This occurs almost exclusively in children,[9] but isolated cases in adults have been described.[24]

(text continues on page 1139)

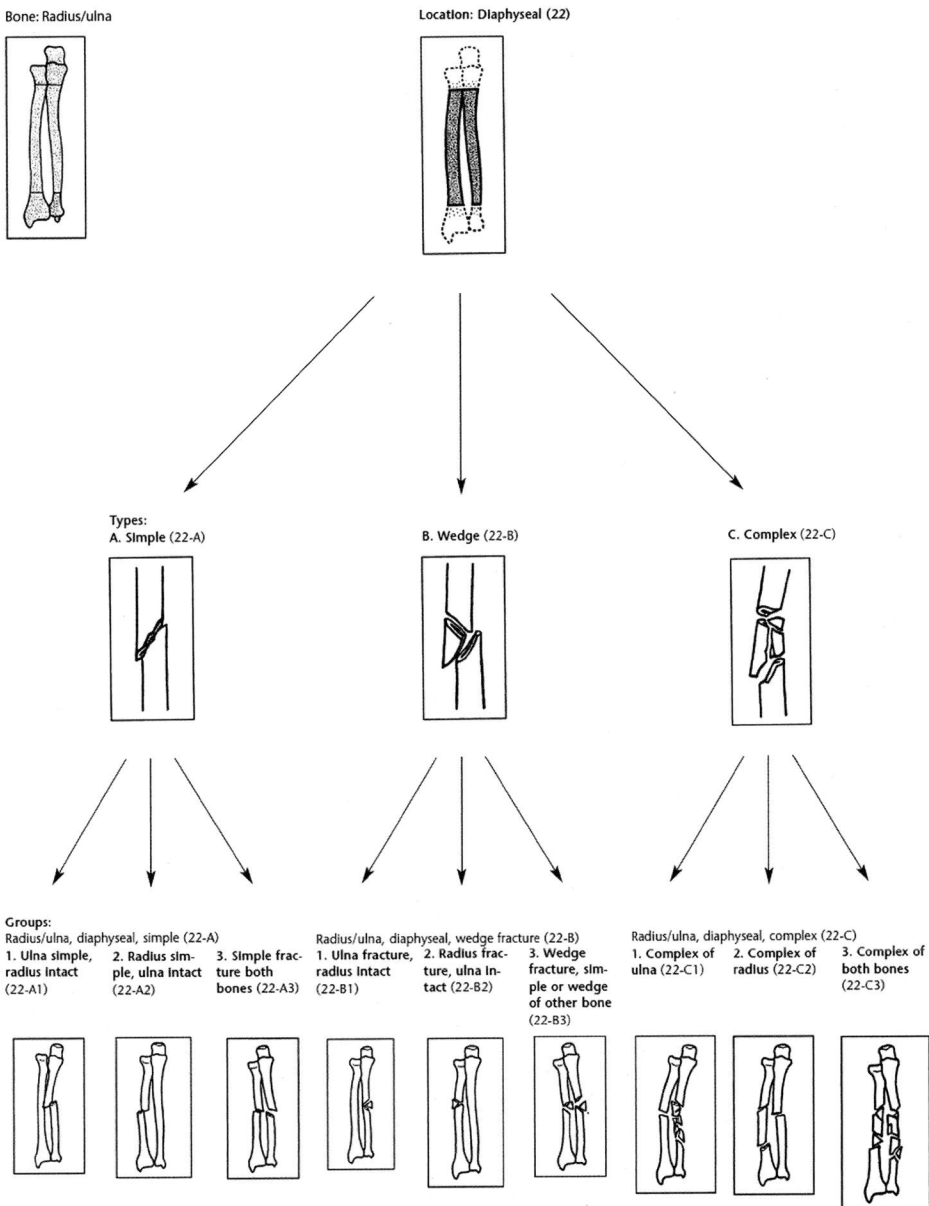

FIGURE 33-11 Shaft fractures of the forearm according to the unified AO/OTA classification. Forearm shaft fractures are identified by the number 22 (2 for forearm, 2 for shaft). Type A fractures are simple fractures, type B are wedge fractures, and type C are complex (highly comminuted or segmental) fractures. See text for further detail. (From Marsh JL, Slongo TF, Agel J, et al. Fracture and dislocation classification compendium—2007: Orthopaedic Trauma Association classification, database and outcomes committee. *J Orthop Trauma.* 2007;21(10 Suppl):S1–S133.) *(continues)*

Subgroups and qualifications:
Radius/ulna, diaphyseal, simple fracture of ulna (22-A1)
1. Oblique (22-A1.1)   2. Transverse (22-A1.2)   3. With dislocation of radial head
                                                                                     (Monteggia) (22-A1.3)

A1

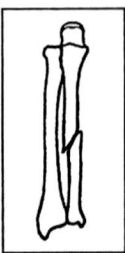   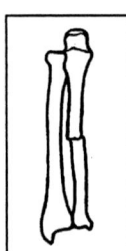   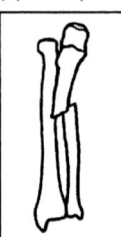

Radius/ulna, diaphyseal, simple fracture of radius (22-A2)
1. Oblique (22-A2.1)   2. Transverse (22-A2.2)   3. With dislocation of distal radio-
                                                                                     ulnar joint (Galeazzi) (22-A2.3)

A2

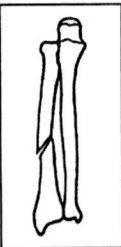   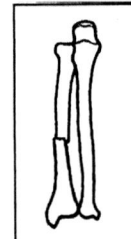   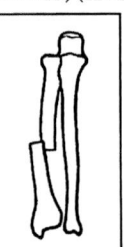

Radius/ulna, diaphyseal, simple fracture of both bones (22-A3)
(1) without dislocation
(2) with dislocation of radial head (Monteggia)
(3) with dislocation of distal radioulnar joint (Galeazzi)
(based on level of radial fracture)
1. Radius, proximal zone (22-A3.1)   2. Radius, middle zone (22-A3.2)   3. Radius, distal zone (22-A3.3)

A3

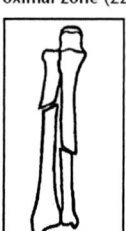   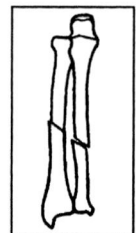   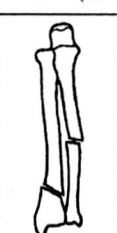

FIGURE 33-11 (continued)

Radius/ulna, diaphyseal, wedge fracture of ulna (22-B1)

1. Intact wedge (22-B1.1)   **2. Fragmented wedge (22-B1.2)**   **3. With dislocation of radial head (Monteggia) (22-B1.3)**

B1
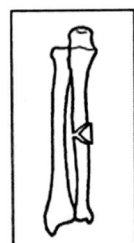 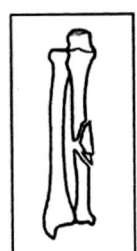 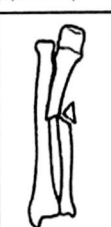

Radius/ulna, diaphyseal, wedge fracture of radius (22-B2)

1. Intact wedge (22-B2.1)   **2. Fragmented wedge (22-B2.2)**   **3. With dislocation of distal radio-ulnar joint (Galeazzi) (22-B2.3)**

B2
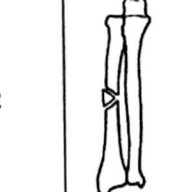 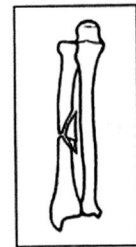 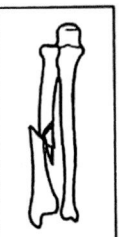

Radius/ulna, diaphyseal, wedge of 1, simple or wedge of other (22-B3)
(1) without dislocation
(2) with dislocation of radial head (Monteggia)
(3) with dislocation of distal radioulnar joint (Galeazzi)

1. Ulna wedge, simple fracture radius (22-B3.1)   **2. Radial wedge, simple fracture of ulna (22-B3.2)**   **3. Radial and ulnar wedge (22-B3.3)**

B3
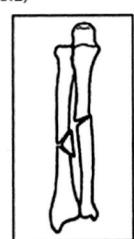 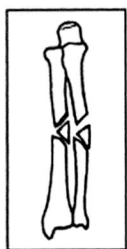

FIGURE 33-11 (*continued*)

(*continues*)

Radius/ulna, diaphyseal, complex fracture of ulna (22-C1)
1. Bifocal, radius intact (22-C1.1)
(1) without dislocation
(2) with radial head dislocated
(Monteggia)

2. Bifocal with radial fracture (22-C1.2)
(1) radius simple
(2) radius wedge

3. Irregular of ulna (22-C1.3)
(1) radius intact
(2) radius simple
(3) radius wedge

C1

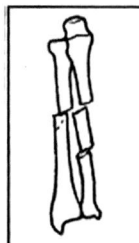
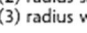
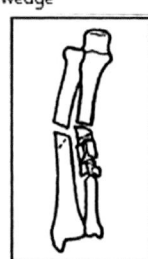

Radius/ulna, diaphyseal, complex fracture of radius (22-C2)
1. Bifocal, ulna intact (22-C2.1)
(1) without dislocation
(2) with dislocation of distal radioulnar joint (Galeazzi)

2. Bifocal, ulna fracture (22-C2.2)
(1) simple ulna
(2) wedge ulna

3. Irregular (22-C2.3)
(1) ulna intact
(2) ulna simple
(3) ulna wedge

C2

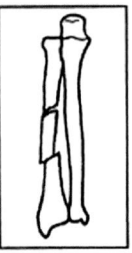
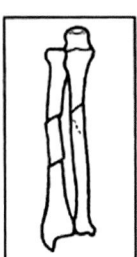
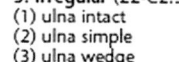
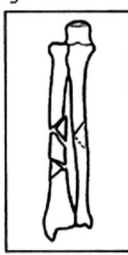

Radius/ulna, diaphyseal, complex of both bones (22-C3)
1. Bifocal (22-C3.1)

2. Bifocal of 1, irregular of other (22-C3.2)
(1) bifocal radius, irregular ulna
(2) bifocal ulna, irregular radius

3. Irregular (22-C3.3)

C3

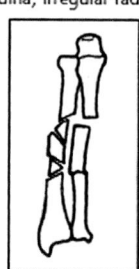
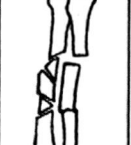
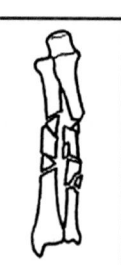

FIGURE 33-11 (*continued*)

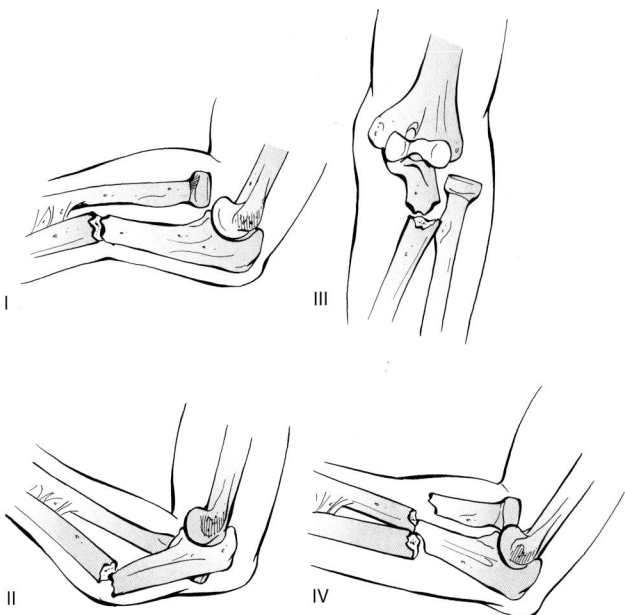

FIGURE 33-12 Bado's classification of Monteggia fractures. Type I: An anterior dislocation of the radial head with associated anteriorly angulated fracture of the ulna shaft. Type II: Posterior dislocation of the radial head with a posteriorly angulated fracture of the ulna. Type III: A lateral or anterolateral dislocation of the radial head with a fracture of the ulnar metaphysis. Type IV: Anterior dislocation of the radial head with a fracture of the radius and ulna.

Type 4: Anterior dislocation of the radial head with a fracture of the proximal third of the ulna and fracture of the radius at the same level. These occur exclusively in adult patients.[9]

Several fracture "equivalents" have been described in the literature, affecting either the proximal ulna and radius and are hence beyond the scope of this chapter.[9]

Understanding the deformity of the ulna and the direction of dislocation of the radial head is important for fracture reduction. In most instances, reduction of the ulnar fracture leads to reduction of the radial head. Whereas type 1 fractures are considered the most frequent type in children,[152] type 2 account for up to 80% of Monteggia fracture dislocations in adults.[139,140,151] Importantly, type 2 Monteggia fractures are frequently associated with radial head or coronoid fractures, therefore representing a more complex injury, potentially affecting elbow stability.[151] Jupiter et al. noted that although the most frequent site of ulnar fracture in type 2 Monteggia fractures is at the proximal shaft, it may occur at the proximal epiphysis or metaphysis. Type 2 Monteggia fractures were therefore further subclassified into four different patterns as follows.[92]

2A: Very proximal ulna fracture through the coronoid

2B: Fracture at the junction of the proximal metaphysis and diaphysis of the ulna

2C: Diaphyseal ulnar fracture

2D: Complex fracture involving the ulna from the olecranon into the diaphysis

Galeazzi Fractures

Galeazzi fractures consist of a fracture of the radial shaft with dislocation of the distal radioulnar joint. They are subclassified according to the distance of the radial fracture from the articular surface. Type 1 fractures occur within 7.5 cm of the articular surface of the distal radius and type 2 more proximally. The relevance of this classification lies in that type 1 are associated with a significantly higher rate of instability of the DRUJ, frequently requiring open repair of this joint.[146] DRUJ dislocations associated with Galeazzi fractures can additionally be classified as simple or complex. Simple dislocations readily reduce after radial alignment has been restored, whereas complex dislocations are those in which the DRUJ is irreducible after anatomic reduction of the radial shaft fracture.[23] Interposition of the extensor carpi ulnaris (ECU) or extensor digiti minimi (EDM) between the distal radius and ulna have been described as causes for DRUJ irreducibility.[2,26,124,146,182]

Open Fractures

As for other bones, open forearm fractures are classified according to Gustilo.[61,62] Type 1 fractures are those with a laceration of less than 1 cm and a clean wound. These are most frequently caused by an inside-out mechanism in which the displaced forearm shaft fracture pierces through the skin. Minimal comminution is usually present. Low-velocity gunshot wounds are an additional mechanism of injury for this fracture type. Type 2 fractures have a laceration of more than 1 cm, with minimal contamination. These are usually caused in an outside-in fashion.[62] Type 3 fractures are open segmental fractures or those that involve skin disruption of more than 10 cm. They are further subclassified into 3A (fractures in which sufficient and adequate soft tissue envelope is present to allow bony coverage), 3B (fractures in which soft tissue loss has occurred that requires some type of soft tissue reconstructive procedure to allow bony coverage), and 3C (fractures with associated vascular injury that places at risk distal perfusion, thereby requiring vascular repair). In forearm fractures type 3C fractures by definition have disruption of flow through both the radial and ulnar arteries.

Outcome Measures for Diaphyseal Fractures of the Radius and Ulna

Results after forearm fractures are assessed mainly based on complications, pain, range of motion, and radiographic alignment and evidence of healing.[4,6,7,9,10,19,20,27,32,36,39,57,64,69] In addition, grip and pinch strength dynamometry, as well as range of motion in elbow and wrist flexion extension and forearm pronation supination are recorded.[171]

Fracture healing is determined as fracture bridging seen on at least three out of four cortices on AP and lateral radiographs. Anderson et al.[4] classified fractures healing within 6 months of surgery as unions, those healing after 6 months without additional intervention as delayed unions, and those that failed to heal after 6 months or required additional unplanned surgical intervention to achieve healing as nonunions.

Infection is frequently subdivided into superficial, deep, and osteomyelitis. Superficial infections involve the skin and subcutaneous tissue, whereas deep infections are present below the fascia involving the fracture site and the implant.[27] Infection is most frequently defined based on clinical signs of local infection, including erythema, hyperthermia, edema, and drainage. Furthermore, laboratory values including elevated erythrocyte sedimentation rate (ESR), C-reactive protein (CRP), leukocytosis, and positive cultures are used to confirm the clinical suspicion. Osteomyelitis is defined as infections that yield positive bone cultures after surgical intervention.[27]

Anderson et al. devised an outcome scale by which results were based on final range of motion. An excellent rating was given to patients with less than 10 degrees loss of flexion–extension and less than 25 percent loss of pronation–supination. Patients with a satisfactory result achieved union with less than 20 degrees loss of flexion–extension and less than 50% loss of pronation–supination. Unsatisfactory results were those with union with more than 30 degrees loss of flexion–extension and greater than 50 percent loss of pronation–supination. A failure of treatment is determined by nonunion with or without loss of motion.[4,20] Grace and Eversmann devised a similar outcomes tool in which an excellent result was given to a healed fracture with at least 90% of normal rotation determined by the uninjured contralateral side. A good result is defined as a healed fracture with 80 to 89% of normal rotation. An acceptable result is a healed fracture and 60 to 79% of normal rotation. Finally, an unacceptable result is defined as nonunions or fractures with less than 60% of normal forearm rotation. In the absence of an uninjured and normal contralateral side, normal pronation supination is considered to be 80-0-80.[60]

More recently, clinical studies on forearm fractures have included the use of a patient-specific outcomes measure, the Disability of the Arm, Shoulder and Hand (DASH) questionnaire.[20,39,52,71,191] Whereas this scale has not been validated specifically for forearm fractures, it has been widely validated for several conditions of the upper extremity and has been formally translated and validated in several languages. The DASH is a standardized questionnaire that assesses upper extremity function based on pain symptoms and physical, emotional, and social domains. It contains 30 questions, including 21 on physical function, 6 on symptoms, and 3 evaluating social function. Each question is answered with one of five possible multiple choice answers. A high DASH score indicates more severe disability.[81]

PATHOANATOMY AND APPLIED ANATOMY RELATING TO DIAPHYSEAL FRACTURES OF THE RADIUS AND ULNA

The anatomy of the forearm is complex and requires a detailed understanding to avoid neurovascular injury during surgical treatment.

Osseous Plane

The osseous component of the forearm separates the anterior from the posterior aspect and is composed of the radius, ulna, and interosseous membrane (Fig. 33-13).

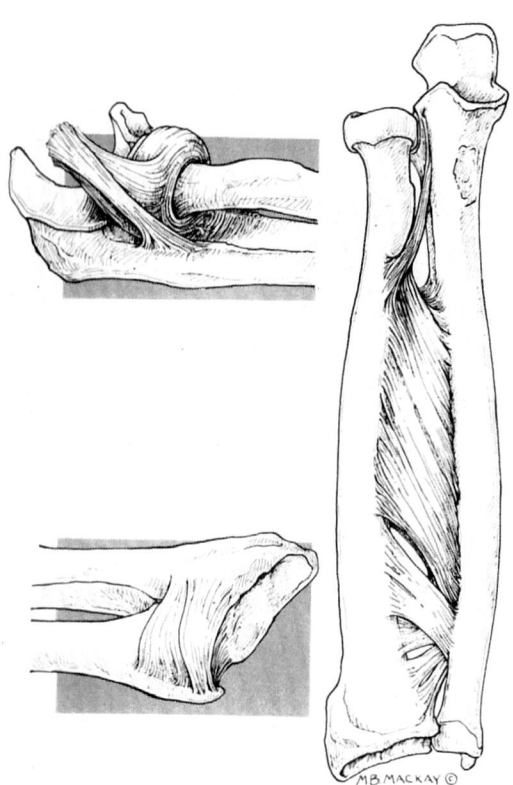

FIGURE 33-13 Line diagram showing the soft tissue connections of the radius and the ulna to each other. The proximal radioulnar joint is stabilized by the annular ligament. The distal radioulnar joint is stabilized by the dorsal and volar radioulnar ligaments and the triangular fibrocartilage complex. (From Richards RR. Chronic disorders of the forearm. *J Bone Joint Surg.* 1996;78:916–930.)

Radius

The adult radius measures on average 25 cm in length (range 21 to 29 cm). At the junction of the proximal and middle third, the radius measures on average 13 mm in the AP dimension and 16 mm in the medial–lateral dimension. At the junction of the middle and distal thirds, the diameter of the radius is 12 mm in the AP dimension and 15 mm in the medial–lateral dimension. The proximal radius comprises the radial head, neck, and biceps tuberosity. The radial head articulates with the radial notch (lesser sigmoid notch) of the proximal ulna. The shaft of the radius extends distal to the biceps tuberosity. It is located on the lateral aspect of the forearm in supination and dorsally in pronation. It has a prismatic triangular shape that broadens from proximal to distal. It has two curvatures, one medial, the major radial bow, and one lesser anterior curvature. Distally, the radius broadens to articulate with the carpus. Medially, the distal radius articulates with the ulnar head through the sigmoid notch.

The major radial bow extends from the bicipital tuberosity to the ulnar aspect of the articular surface of the distal radius. Schemitsch and Richards studied the importance of restoring the major radial bow after operative fixation of forearm fractures. The maximum radial bow on the uninjured side was found to be located on average at 60% of the distance between the biceps tuberosity and ulnar side of the distal articular surface. At this point, the maximum distance from the line connecting the biceps tuberosity and the ulnar aspect of the distal articular surface to the medial aspect of the radial shaft was on an average 15.3 mm. A higher deviation from this distance after operative fixation was related to a reduction in the normal range of rotation.[171]

The nutrient artery to the radius enters the shaft on the volar aspect at an average of 9 cm distal to the radial head (range 6 to 12 cm). Proximal and distal cancellous bone in the metaphyses of the radius extends on an average 4 cm distal to the proximal articular surface and 5 cm proximal to the distal articular surface, respectively. The isthmus of the radial endomedullary canal is located in over 90% of cases at the midpoint of the radius.[161]

Ulna

The ulna acts as the axis around which the radius rotates during pronation–supination[110] (Fig. 33-14). Effectively, the axis of rotation of the radius is located on the line connecting the center of the radial head and the head of the ulna. The proximal ulna comprises the olecranon and coronoid that form the trochlear notch (greater sigmoid notch) that articulates with the distal humerus. The radial notch (lesser sigmoid notch) is located on the lateral aspect of the proximal ulna, just distal to the trochlear notch. This concavity serves as the articulating surface for the radial head and as the insertion both anteriorly and posteriorly for the annular ligament.

The ulnar shaft is located on the medial aspect of the forearm, with a minimal anterior concavity. It has a broader prismatic shape proximally, becoming rounded and thinner distally. Posteriorly, the ulna has a clearly defined ridge proximally that separates the insertion of the flexor carpi ulnaris (FCU) medially and anteriorly and ECU laterally and posteriorly.

Before reaching the wrist, the ulnar shaft broadens again to form the head and styloid process. Distally and laterally, the ulnar head articulates with the sigmoid notch of the radius. Distally, the ulna serves as an insertion point for the TFCC.

Interosseous Space

The ulna and radius create a space between their proximal and distal articulations that is somewhat oval in shape. The greatest distance between the two bones is seen in full supination. The space is occupied mainly by the interosseous membrane that establishes a distinct barrier between the anterior and posterior compartments. The interosseous membrane has a marked thickening with fibers running obliquely from proximal radial to distal ulnar known as the interosseous ligament or central band of the interosseous membrane. This structure is 3.5 cm wide and its fibers are oriented in an oblique fashion, approximately 20 degrees to the axis of the forearm.[130] In the presence of a radius fracture, it acts as a constraint against radial shortening.[172] Hotchkiss et al.[79] determined that the central band is responsible for 71% of the longitudinal stiffness of the interosseous membrane after radial head resection (Fig. 33-15).

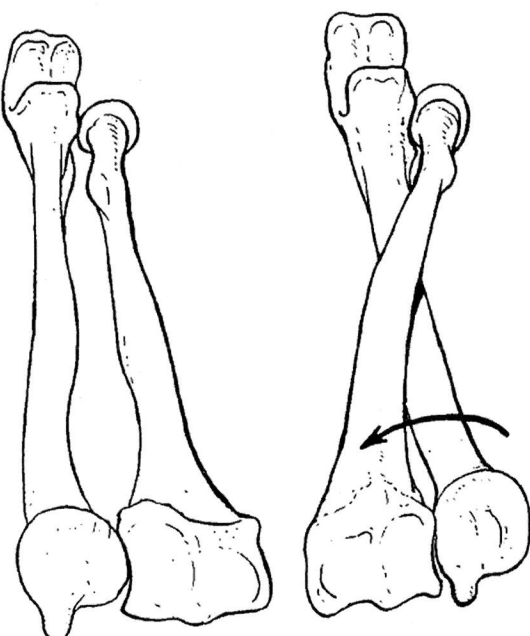

FIGURE 33-14 During pronosupination, the radius rotates about the ulna (*arrow*). The complex curvature of the radius and ulna allows approximately 150 degrees of rotation. (From Lindscheid RL. Biomechanics of the distal radioulnar joint. *Clin Orthop Relat Res.* 1992;275:46–55.)

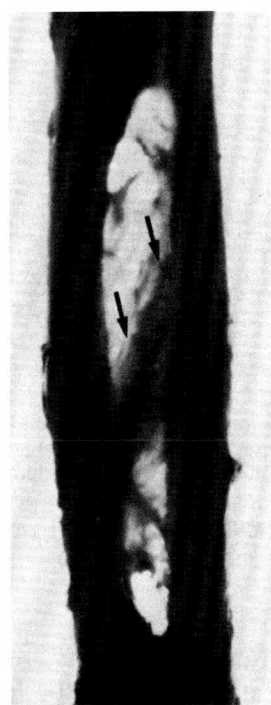

FIGURE 33-15 Backlit photograph of a forearm specimen. The central band of the interosseous membrane is indicated by *arrows*. (From Hotchkiss RN, An KN, Sowa DT, et al. An anatomic and mechanical study of the interosseous membrane of the forearm: pathomechanics of proximal migration of the radius. *J Hand Surg Am.* 1989;14:256–261.)

Triangular Fibrocartilage Complex (TFCC)

The TFCC serves as the medial continuation of the distal articular surface of the radius as well as a static stabilizer of the distal radioulnar joint. It consists of an articular disc, the dorsal radioulnar ligament (DRUL), and palmar radioulnar ligament (PRUL), the meniscus homologue, the ulnar collateral ligament, and the sheath of the ECU.[129,137] The articular disc extends from the distal rim of the sigmoid notch, along the ulnar edge of the lunate facet, blending in the periphery with the PRUL and DRUL. The PRUL and DRUL are the primary stabilizers of the DRUJ. They originate from the dorsal and palmar aspect of the sigmoid notch and converge in a triangular fashion toward the base of the ulnar styloid.[80]

Proximal Radioulnar Joint

The radial head articulates with the radial notch of the proximal ulna. This joint is stabilized by the annular ligament which originates from the anterior and posterior limits of the radial notch (lesser sigmoid notch) of the proximal ulna. It blends with fibers from the lateral collateral ligament of the elbow.

Muscles

The muscular plane of the forearm can be grossly divided into anterior and posterior muscles.

Anterior Muscles

The anterior muscle group can be divided into three layers: superficial, intermediate, and deep. From lateral to medial, muscles from the superficial layer comprise the pronator teres (PT), flexor carpi radialis (FCR), palmaris longus, and FCU. The intermediate layer is composed of the flexor digitorum superficialis (FDS). Three muscles form the deep layer: flexor pollicis longus (FPL) laterally, flexor digitorum profundus (FDP) medially, and pronator quadratus (PQ) distally.

The FCU and medial half of the FDP are innervated by the ulnar nerve. All remaining muscles of the anterior compartment are innervated by the median nerve or its branch, the anterior interosseous nerve. Specifically, the anterior interosseous nerve innervates the FPL, lateral half of the FDP, and PQ (Fig. 33-16).

Posterior Muscles

The posterior muscle group can be divided into two layers: superficial and deep. From lateral to medial, the superficial muscles are brachioradialis, extensor carpi radialis longus (ECRL), extensor carpi radialis brevis (ECRB), extensor digitorum, EDM, ECU, and anconeus. Proximally, the deep layer is composed of the supinator muscle and distally from lateral to medial by the abductor pollicis longus (APL), extensor pollicis brevis (EPB), extensor pollicis longus (EPL), and extensor indicis proprius (EIP). All posterior muscles are innervated by the radial nerve or its branch, the posterior interosseous nerve (Fig. 33-17).

Forearm muscles are encased in four compartments: superficial volar, deep volar, dorsal, and mobile wad. The superficial volar compartment comprises FCU, FDS, FCR, and PT. The deep volar compartment is made up by FDP and PQ. The dorsal compartment includes supinator, ECU, extensor digitorum communis (EDC), EDM, APL, EPL, EPB, and EIP. The mobile wad comprises brachioradialis, ECRL, and ECRB.

Deforming Forces

In the intact forearm, rotational muscle forces acting on the radius are balanced in a position of forearm pronation. Depending on the fracture location, the net deforming forces will tend to either pronate or supinate the proximal and distal radial segments. The main supinating forces are the supinator and biceps muscles. The main pronating forces are the PT and PQ. Besides exerting rotational forces on the radius, the supinator and both pronator muscles decrease the distance between the radius and ulna thereby shortening the interosseous space. The greatest rotational deformity of the radius can be expected in fractures that are distal to the supinating forces and proximal to the pronating forces. A radius fracture distal to the insertion of the supinator muscle and proximal to the PT will therefore lead to unopposed supination of the proximal segment and pronation of the distal segment, with a resultant severe rotational deformity. Fractures distal to the PT insertion will exhibit a less severe deformity, as the PT will counteract some of the supination forces of biceps and supinator.

Nerves
Median Nerve

The median nerve reaches the antecubital fossa of the anterior proximal forearm together with the brachial artery medial to the biceps tendon. The antecubital fossa is represented by a line between the epicondyles proximally, and the biceps tendon and brachioradialis laterally. The floor of the antecubital fossa is the brachialis muscle, the roof is the bicipital aponeurosis. Together with its branch, the anterior interosseous nerve (AIN), the median nerve passes first between the two heads of the PT and then between the two heads of the FDS underneath the sublimis bridge. The AIN travels between FPL laterally and FDP medially, innervating these muscles and continuing distally on the anterior surface of the interosseous membrane. The AIN then innervates the PQ and ends in the capsule of the wrist joint. The main trunk of the median nerve travels distally deep to the FDS. At the level of the wrist it wraps around the lateral margin of the FDS and assumes a position that is superficial to the tendon of the FDS and medial to the tendon of the FCR, entering in this position into the carpal tunnel. Six centimeters proximal to the wrist it gives off the palmar cutaneous branch which travels deep and slightly radial to the palmaris longus tendon.

Ulnar Nerve

The ulnar nerve enters the forearm through the cubital tunnel underneath Osborne's ligament between the olecranon and the medial epicondyle. It passes underneath the two heads of the FCU travelling on the deep aspect of this muscle together

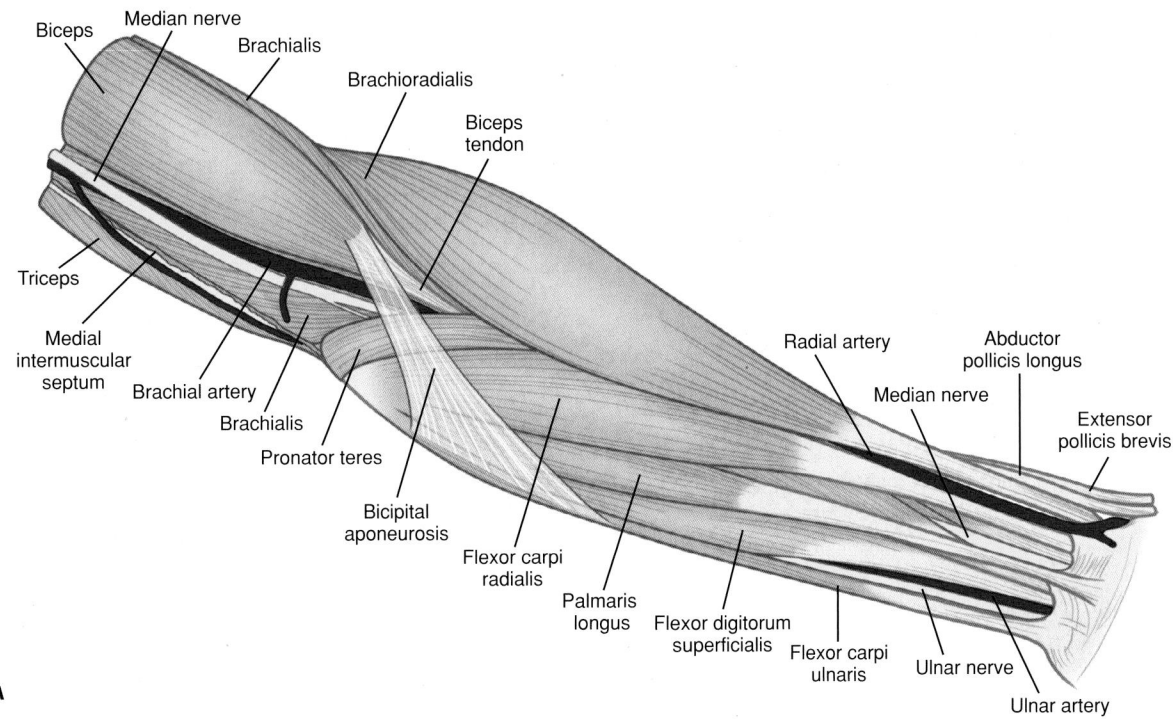

A

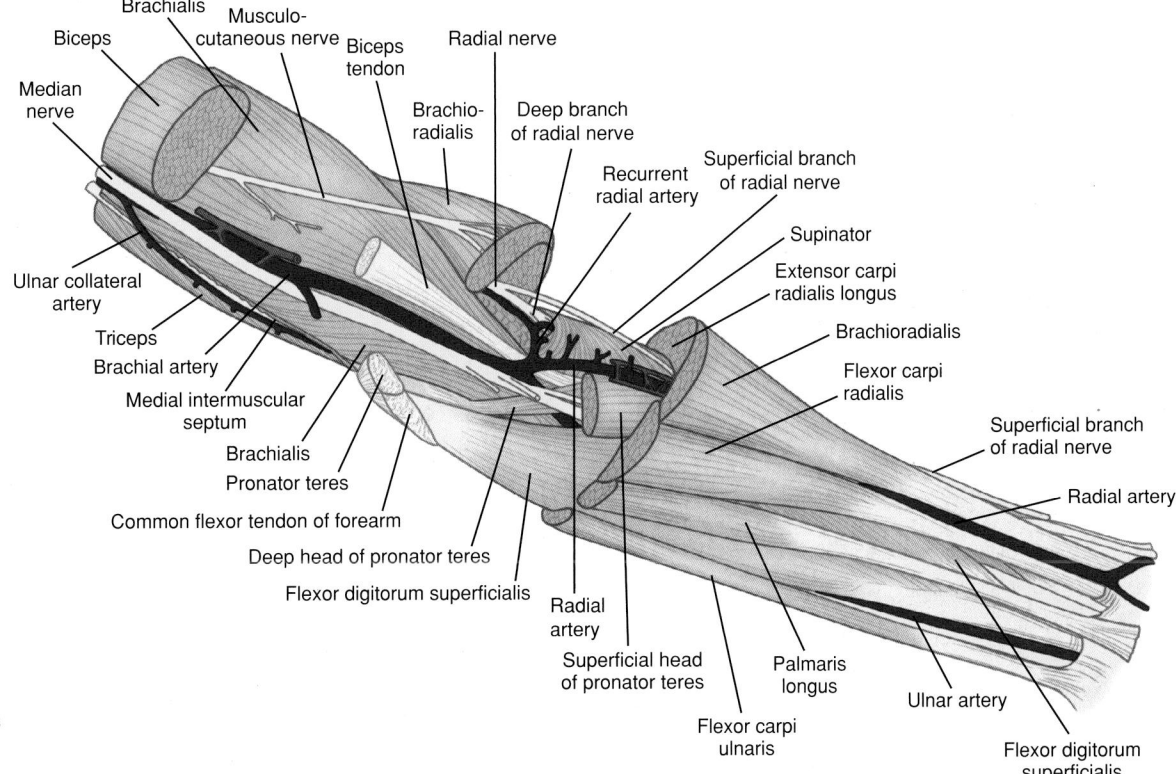

B

FIGURE 33-16 Anatomy of the anterior aspect of the forearm. **A:** Superficial layer of the forearm muscles. Note the position of the radial artery between brachioradialis and flexor carpi radialis distally. **B:** Intermediate layer of the proximal forearm deep to extensor carpi radialis longus, brachioradialis, flexor carpi radialis, palmaris longus, and flexor carpi ulnaris. The recurrent radial artery acts as a tether against ulnar translation of the radial artery during proximal dissection. The radial artery and superficial branch of the radial nerve continue distally on the undersurface of brachioradialis. Note the median nerve passing between the superficial and deep heads of the pronator teres continuing distally deep to the flexor digitorum superficialis.

(continues)

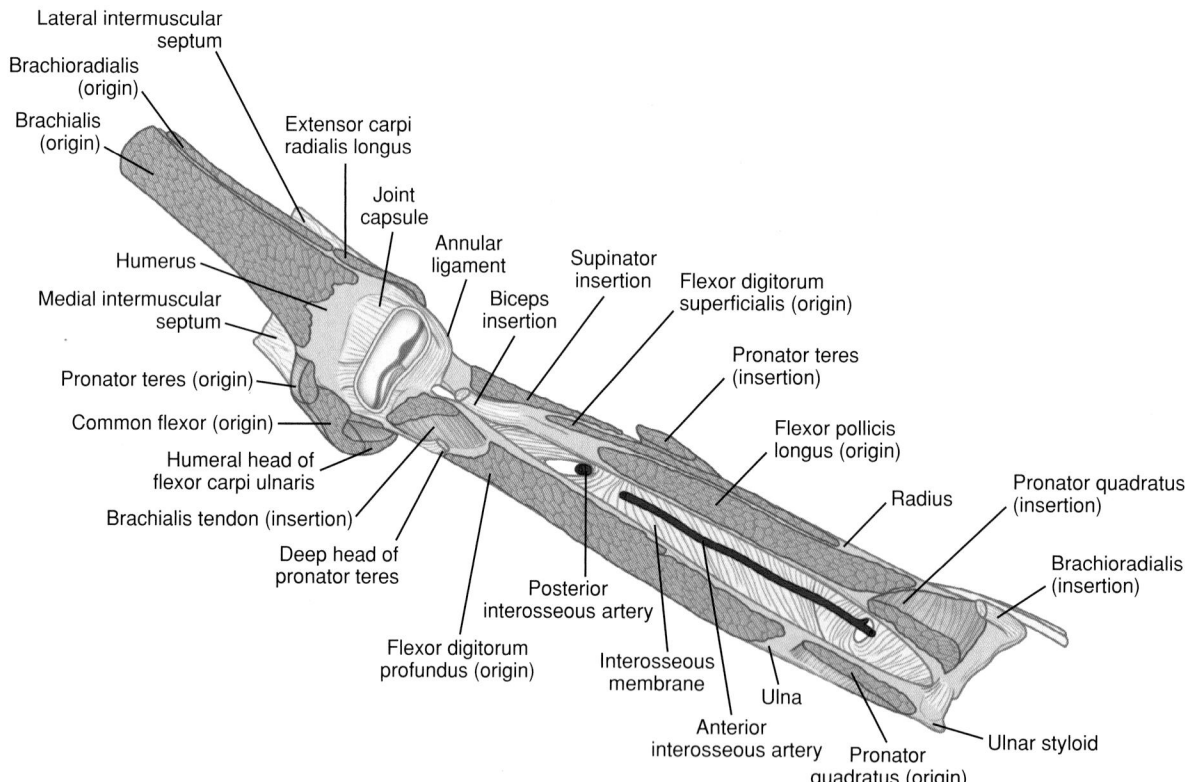

C

D

FIGURE 33-16 (*continued*) **C:** Deep layer of the forearm. The deep branch of the radial nerve passes under the proximal arch of the supinator muscle (arcade of Frohse). The ulnar artery and nerve and median nerve travel superficial to the flexor digitorum profundus. **D:** Muscular footprints on the anterior aspect of the forearm. The interosseous arteries are seen lying on the anterior and posterior surface of the interosseous membrane.

with the ulnar artery until it reaches the wrist. In the forearm it innervates the FCU and ulnar half of the FDP.

Radial Nerve

The radial nerve enters the forearm between the brachioradialis and brachialis muscles, innervating these two muscles and ECRL. At the level of the elbow it branches into the superficial branch, which continues deep to the brachioradialis distally to reach the skin of the lateral dorsum of the hand. The deep branch innervates ECRB and supinator muscle passing through the latter into the posterior compartment of the forearm. At this level or distally, the deep branch continues as the posterior interosseous nerve (PIN) traveling on the posterior surface of the interosseous membrane innervating ED, EDM, ECU, EPB, EPL, APL, and EIP.

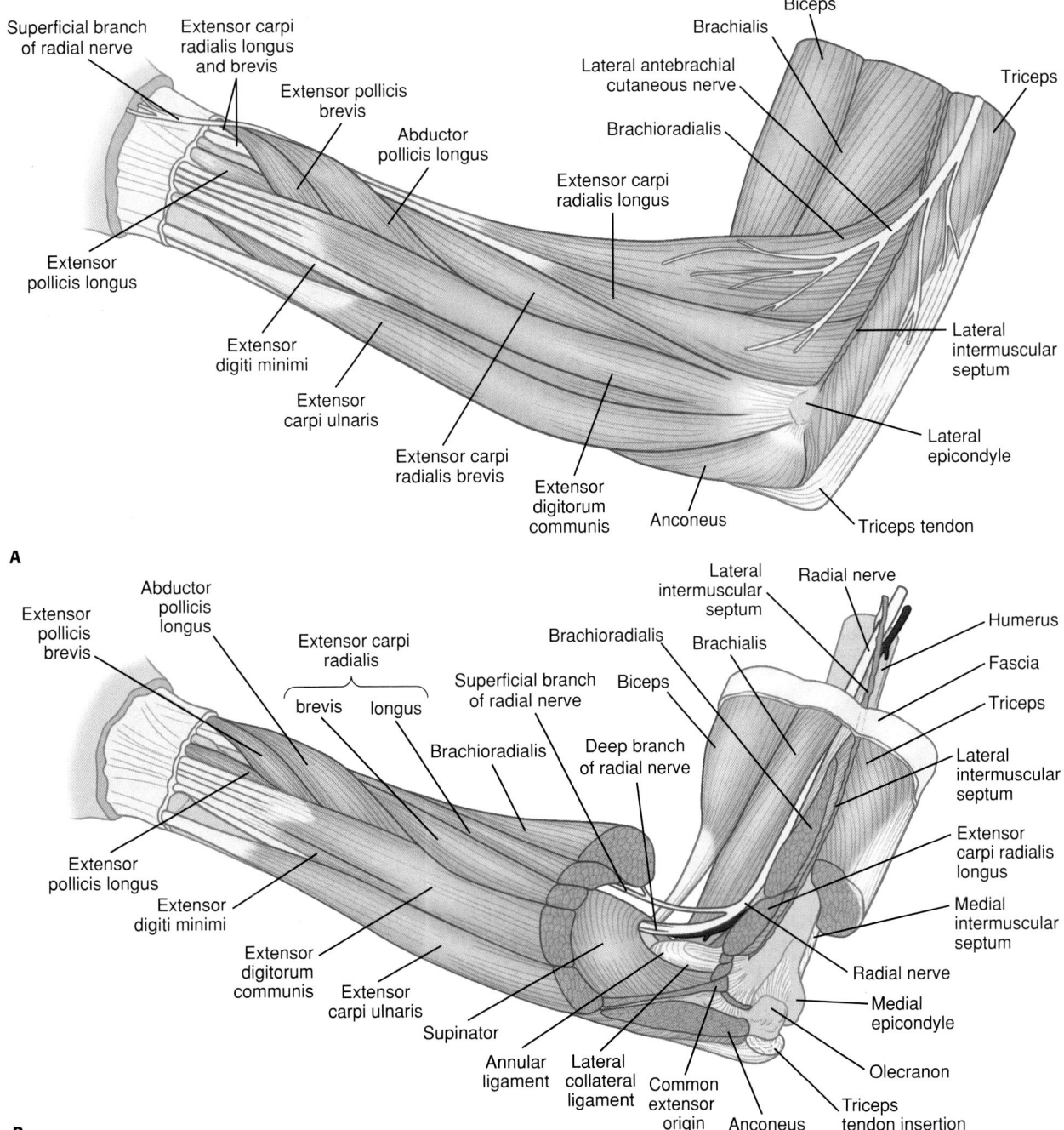

FIGURE 33-17 Anatomy of the posterior aspect of the forearm. **A:** Superficial layer of muscles. Note the outcropper muscles (abductor pollicis longus and extensor pollicis brevis) emerging distally between extensor carpi radialis brevis and extensor digitorum communis). **B:** The radial nerve branches into superficial and deep branches at the level of the elbow. Note the superficial branch travelling distally deep to brachioradialis. The deep branch passes through the arcade of Frohse becoming the posterior interosseous nerve after emerging from the supinator muscle.

(continues)

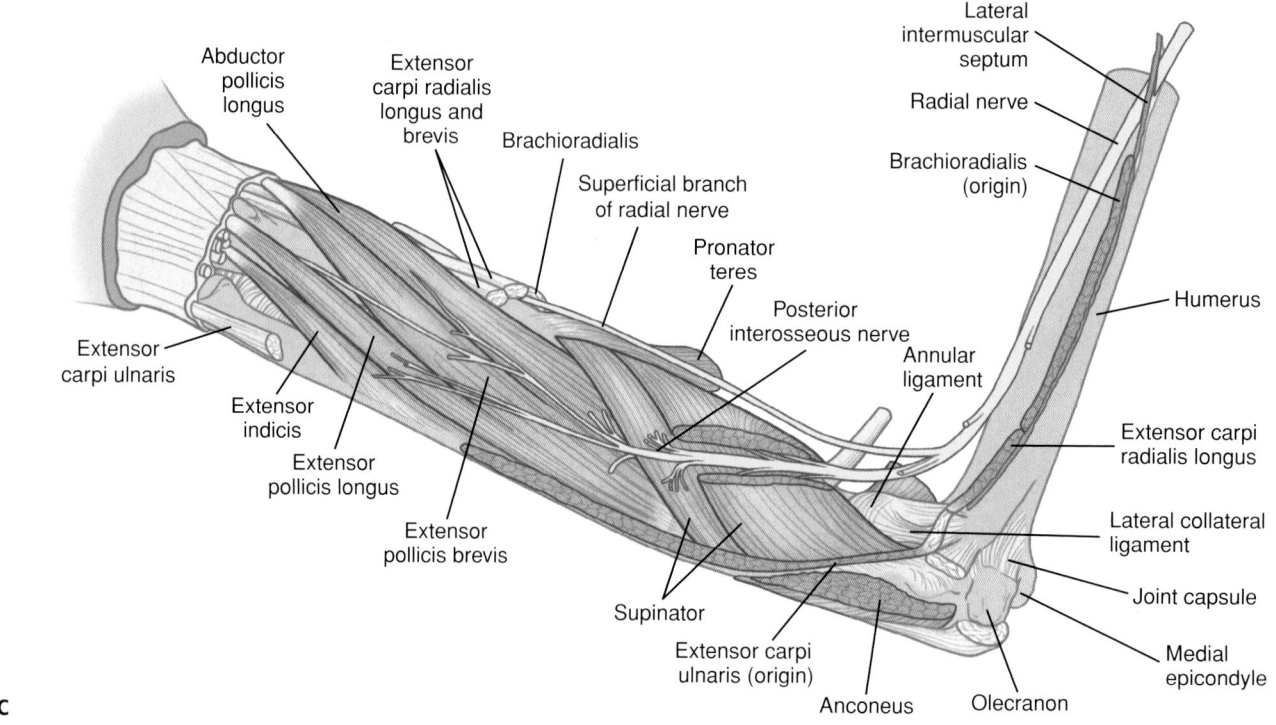

C

FIGURE 33-17 *(continued)* **C:** Deep layer. Note the course of the deep branch of the radial nerve through supinator and the branching pattern of the posterior interosseous nerve.

Arteries

The brachial artery reaches the forearm between the median nerve medially and the biceps tendon laterally. It branches into radial and ulnar and common interosseous arteries at the level of the antecubital fossa. The first branch of the radial artery is the radial recurrent artery (recurrent leash of Henry). This artery travels laterally and proximally, superficial to the supinator muscle to anastomose with the terminal branch of the profunda brachii artery between the brachialis and brachioradialis muscles. The radial artery continues distally along the proximal border of the PT onto the undersurface of the brachioradialis muscle. Proximal to the wrist it assumes a position between the FCR medially and brachioradialis laterally. It reaches the wrist deep to the APL tendon toward the floor of the anatomic snuff box.

The ulnar artery passes deep to FDS to join the ulnar nerve on the deep surface of the FCU. The common interosseous artery travels straight posterior toward the proximal border of the interosseous membrane where it divides into an anterior and a posterior interosseous artery. Each interosseous artery travels along the anterior and posterior surface of the interosseous membrane.

TREATMENT OPTIONS FOR DIAPHYSEAL FRACTURES OF THE RADIUS AND ULNA

General Considerations of Diaphyseal Fractures of the Radius and Ulna

The main goal of treatment of fractures of the shaft of the ulna and radius is to recover painless function of the forearm and upper extremity. Pain-free function is dependent on fracture healing;

range of motion of the elbow, forearm, and wrist; and avoidance of complications. Fracture healing depends on patient characteristics, type of injury, and surgeon-controlled variables. Patient factors such as smoking and diabetes may decrease the likelihood of fracture union. Injuries with extensive soft tissue loss and contamination are at a higher risk for nonunion. Finally, selection of the appropriate treatment modality and its correct execution will provide the optimal environment for the fracture to heal. Given the delicate interplay between the radius and ulna during forearm pronation–supination, there is little room for residual deformity. Furthermore, significant comminution, extensive soft tissue dissection, and prolonged immobilization will increase the probability of posttraumatic stiffness. Complications such as infection, and unrecognized compartment syndrome with secondary contracture will negatively influence outcome.

Principles of Treatment of Diaphyseal Fractures of the Radius and Ulna

As for most fractures, treatment of forearm fractures should follow these four key criteria.

1. Obtain adequate reduction
2. Achieve and maintain fracture reduction
   while
3. Preserving biology
   and allowing
4. Early range of motion.

Although the basic tenet of diaphyseal fracture reduction is restoration of length, alignment and rotation without the absolute necessity of anatomic reduction, this does not hold true for shaft fractures of the forearm. The geometric relationship of the ulna and radius allow for the unique motion of pronation and supination rendering the forearm a functional joint.[148] Anatomic reduction of the ulna and radius is therefore desirable whenever achievable to adequately restore the spatial relationship between these bones. Once adequate reduction has been achieved, stability is required to maintain reduction and allow early range of motion and allow healing to occur. Given the importance of reduction, stability, and early range of motion, nonoperative treatment of forearm fractures in adults is limited only to stable ulna fractures. In essentially all other instances, including both-bone fractures and fracture dislocations (Galeazzi and Monteggia), operative treatment is warranted.

Nonoperative Treatment of Diaphyseal Fractures of the Radius and Ulna

Nonoperative treatment of fractures involving the forearm is mainly limited to isolated fractures affecting the distal two-thirds of the ulna with less than 50% of displacement and less than 10 degrees of angulation.[170] Cadaver studies have shown that ulnar shaft fractures with displacement of greater than 50% have concomitant interosseous membrane disruption leading to fracture instability.[42,134] When treated nonoperatively, displaced isolated ulna fractures affecting the proximal third of the shaft have been shown to lead to higher rates of loss of forearm rotation, higher rates of nonunion, and poorer outcomes.[22,30,169] Furthermore, isolated displaced fractures of the proximal ulna shaft frequently occur in association with a PRUJ dislocation (Monteggia fracture). Anatomic reduction and rigid fixation is mandated in this setting to allow stable reduction of the PRUJ. Finally, up to 10 degrees of angulation can be tolerated without leading to a significant reduction in forearm rotation.[115]

Nonoperative treatment of displaced radius shaft fractures and fractures involving the radius and ulna shaft has shown to lead to high rates of unsatisfactory results.[82,95,138] Furthermore, prolonged healing time can be expected with nonoperative treatment of isolated radius shaft fractures.[190] Because of the deforming forces acting on the radius and ulna and the importance of restoring the normal anatomy of the ulna and radius, operative treatment is considered the indicated treatment modality for unstable fractures of the forearm, including displaced isolated ulna fractures, displaced isolated radius fractures, both-bone forearm fractures, and fracture dislocations (Monteggia and Galeazzi). In this setting nonoperative treatment should only be pursued when operative fixation is contraindicated.[167–169]

For stable isolated ulna shaft fractures, below-elbow immobilization is considered the treatment of choice since it compares favorably to long arm casting and to ace bandaging.[7,54] Immobilization may be obtained either with a short arm cast or with a below-elbow brace.[33]

Indications/Contraindications

Techniques. Initial immobilization for 3 weeks in a molded long arm cast has been recommended.[168,194] The cast is applied on the day of injury in longitudinal gravity traction using finger traps. A well-molded cast is then applied with the elbow bent

TABLE 33-1	Forearm Fracture
Nonoperative Treatment	
Indications	**Relative Contraindications**
Stable isolated ulna fracture (less than 50% of displacement)	Both-bone forearm fracture
Less than 10 degrees of angulation	Fracture dislocations (Galeazzi, Monteggia)
Distal two-thirds of the ulna	Displaced isolated radial shaft fracture
	Unstable isolated ulna fracture
	Isolated proximal third ulna shaft fracture

to 90 degrees and the forearm in neutral rotation. The cast is checked 48 hours after application and changed to a prefabricated ulnar fracture brace within 3 weeks of injury. The brace consists of two low-density polyethylene shells with a molded interosseous groove that theoretically provides increased fracture stability through compressive hydrostatic pressure along the interosseous membrane. The brace extends from the antecubital fossa to just proximal to the wrist crease. A layer of stockinette is applied directly onto skin and each shell is applied onto the volar and dorsal aspect of the forearm, snapped into place, and tightened with two Velcro straps. As swelling subsides, straps are adjusted to maintain adequate tightness at the fracture site (Fig. 33-18). Early range of motion of fingers, wrist, elbow, and shoulder are encouraged. Radiographic and clinical assessment is performed 1 week after initial brace application to confirm adequate alignment and brace tolerance by the patient. Monthly radiographic and clinical evaluation then follows until healing has occurred.[168,194]

Alternatively, below-the-elbow bracing or splinting may be performed in the acute setting as well. Close serial radiographic follow-up in weekly intervals during the first 3 weeks after injury should however occur to allow early identification of secondary displacement.[7,42,54,141]

Outcomes. High rates of healing can be expected with nonoperative treatment of isolated ulnar shaft fractures.[69] In the largest study on functional bracing of isolated ulnar shaft fractures, Sarmiento et al. reported 96.5% of good and excellent results and a healing rate of 99%. However 35% of patients were lost during follow-up.[169] Similar results have been reported by other authors.[7,33,54,132] De Boeck et al. reported a healing rate of 93% after short arm casting. Conversion to operative fixation because of complete fracture displacement was required in only one fracture.[33] In a randomized controlled trial, Atkin et al. found optimal outcomes with 8 weeks of immobilization of isolated ulnar shaft fractures in a short arm cast. Ace bandage immobilization achieved unsatisfactory rates of pain control and was associated with high rates of fracture displacement. Long arm cast immobilization on the other hand led to high rates of elbow stiffness.[7] Similar results were found by Gebuhr et al.[54] who observed significantly higher satisfaction and wrist range of motion after immobilization of

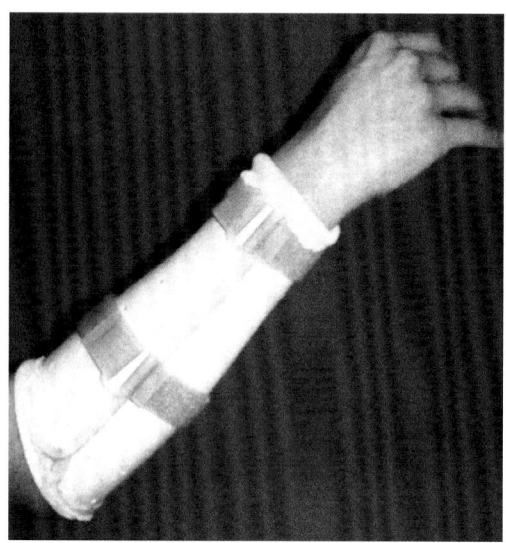

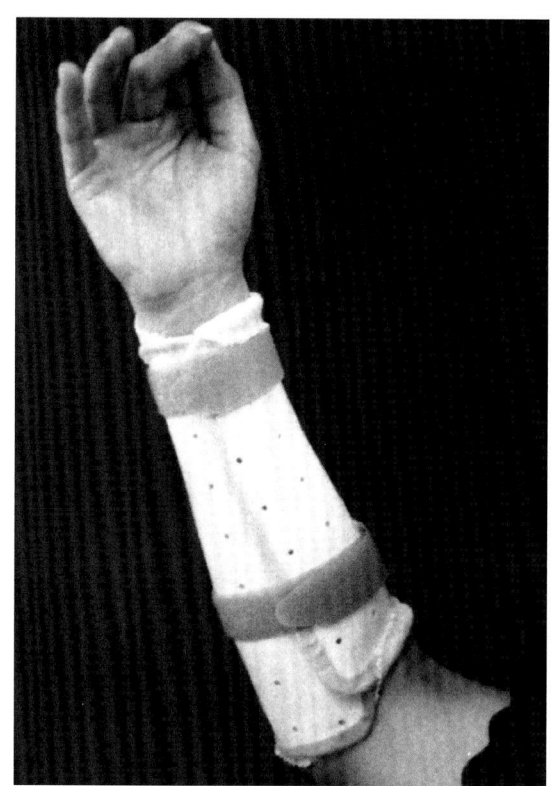

FIGURE 33-18 **A and B:** A functional brace fabricated for a nondisplaced ulnar shaft fracture. This allows motion at the wrist and elbow while stabilizing the fracture site.

A

B

isolated ulnar shaft fractures in a prefabricated functional brace, compared to long arm casting. Pollock et al. on the other hand observed a shorter time to fracture healing in 59 isolated ulna shaft fractures treated either without or for a period of immobilization of less than 2 weeks compared to 12 fractures that were treated with a long arm plaster cast. Nonunion occurred in 8% of fractures treated with long arm immobilization compared to none in the group with minimal immobilization. In a small case series of 10 patients, de Jong and de Jong[34] also achieved healing in all fractures and negligible loss of forearm rotation after treatment without immobilization and early exercises.

Operative Treatment of Diaphyseal Fractures of the Radius and Ulna

Operative treatment represents the rule rather than the exception in the treatment of forearm shaft fractures. Indications for operative treatment of forearm shaft fractures are essentially all fractures except undisplaced fractures or isolated stable ulna shaft fractures. The purpose of operative treatment is to achieve anatomic reduction and obtain stable fixation to allow early range of motion while healing occurs. Careful soft tissue management is important to minimize disruption of bone viability and optimize the chances for healing to occur.

Open reduction and internal fixation (ORIF) with plates and screws is the most widely used method of treatment for unstable forearm fractures. Fracture reduction is achieved with direct visualization of the fracture, allowing removal of interposed soft tissues and manipulation. Historically, intramedullary nailing of the forearm has been performed with the use of solid nails. Good outcomes are reported for pediatric forearm fractures.

Less favorable results have been shown for adult forearm fractures, since adequate reduction is difficult to achieve and only marginal rotational stability is provided. Intramedullary nailing using interlocking nails has been proposed for several years and has recently gained new interest, since it allows fracture fixation with only minimal soft tissue disruption (Table 33-2).

Surgical Approaches

Whether forearm fractures are treated via percutaneous or open surgical methods, access to the radius and ulna shafts occur

TABLE 33-2	Forearm Fracture
Operative Treatment	
Indications	**Relative Contraindications**
Both-bone forearm fracture	Severe contamination (may require staged procedure)
Proximal third displaced isolated ulna fracture	Physiologically unstable patient not tolerating operative procedure
Fracture dislocation (Galeazzi, Monteggia)	Dysvascular crush injury with low likelihood of limb salvage
Displaced isolated radial shaft fracture	
Unstable isolated ulna fracture (e.g., angulation greater >10 degrees)	
Pathologic fracture	

through the same soft tissue windows. Given the subcutaneous location of the ulna, the direct approach to this bone is universally used. The radius is approached either volarly in fractures of the mid- and distal diaphysis, or dorsally for fracture of the proximal and mid third.[78]

Ulna. The dorsomedial ridge of the ulna is easily palpated under the subcutaneous soft tissues. With the patient in the supine position, the incision may be performed with the elbow flexed on a hand table, thereby holding the forearm in a vertical position. The skin incision is centered over the fracture site and over the subcutaneous ulna. Once the skin is incised the ulnar

ridge is again palpated and identified. The underlying fascia is then incised and the interval between ECU and FCU developed. This is a true internervous plane, since the ECU is innervated by the PIN and the FCU by the ulnar nerve. Plates are placed either onto the dorsal aspect of the ulna underneath ECU or the volar aspect under FCU. Plate placement on the subcutaneous border of the ulna should be avoided as it will become symptomatic and place soft tissue healing at risk (Fig. 33-19).

Radius

Volar Approach of Henry. Exposure of the radius from the bicipital tuberosity to the distal articular surface of the radius

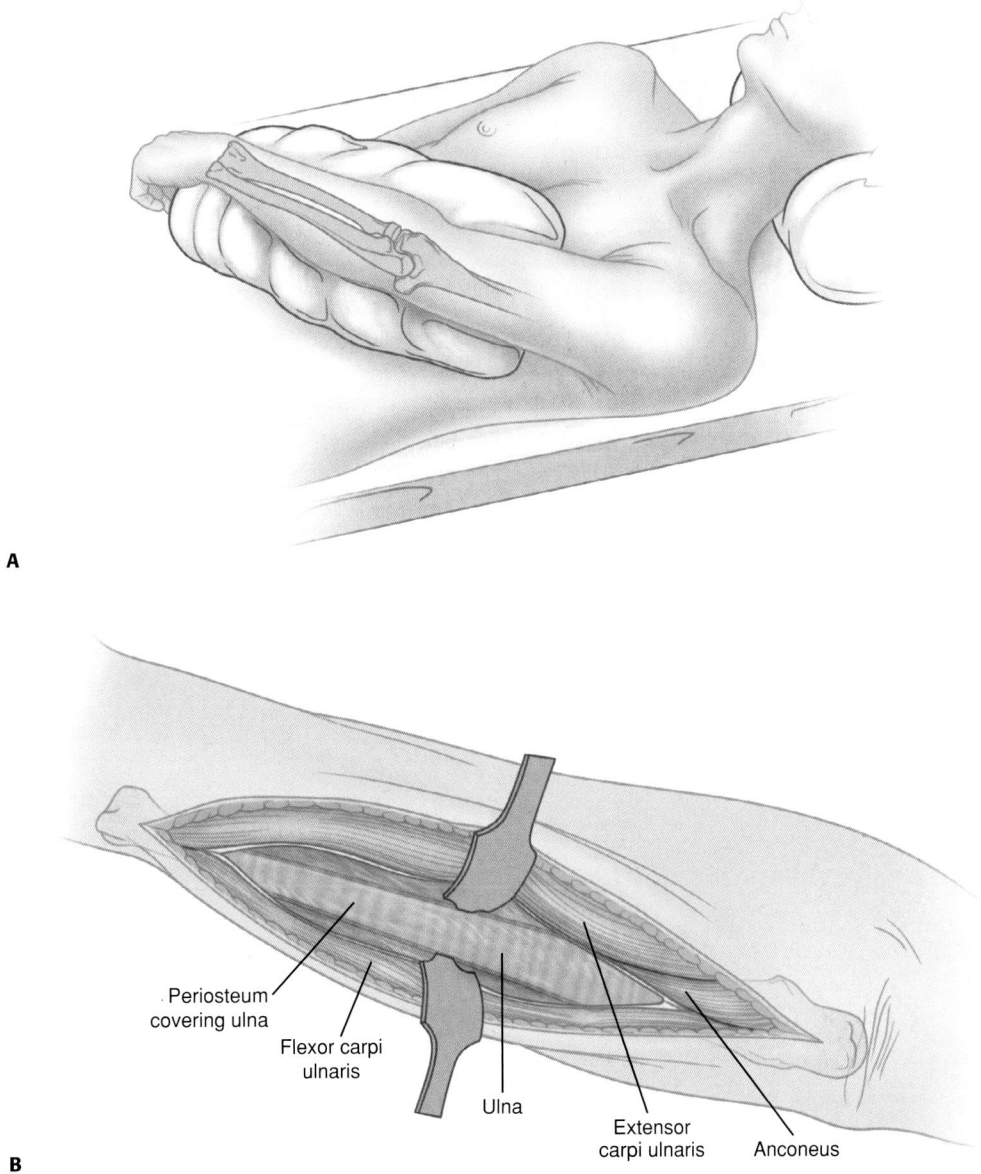

A

B

FIGURE 33-19 Surgical approach to the ulna. **A:** With the patient supine the forearm may be placed across the patient's chest or alternatively using a hand table and having the elbow flexed and the finger pointed towards the ceiling, especially when planning additional fixation of the radius. **B:** The ulna is exposed through the interval between extensor carpi ulnaris dorsally and flexor carpi ulnaris anteriorly.

(continues)

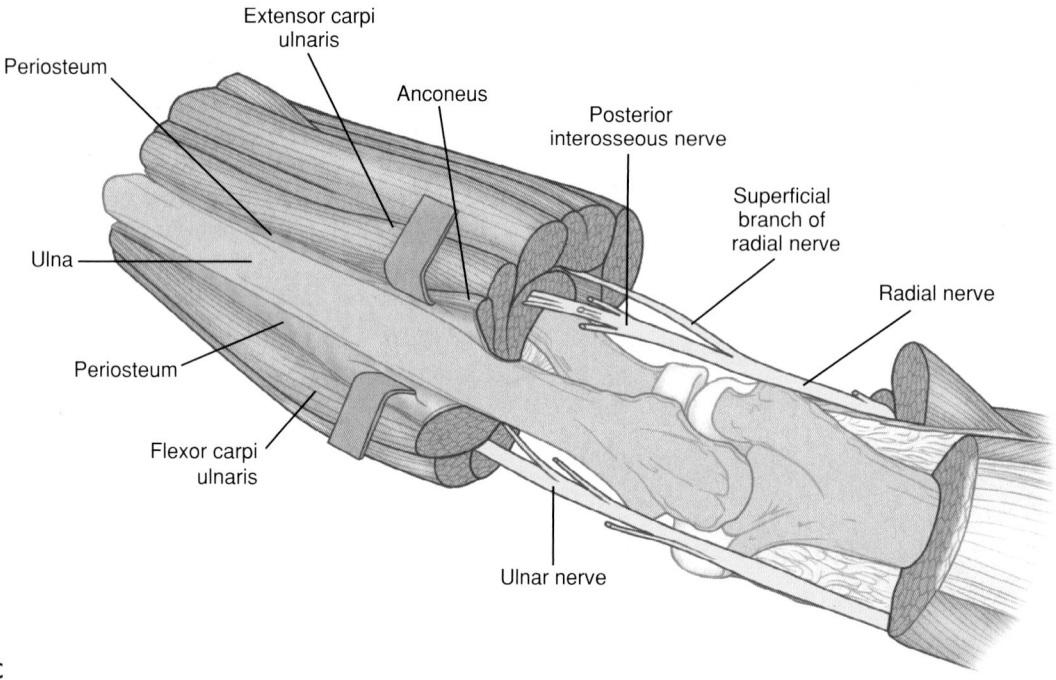

FIGURE 33-19 (*continued*) **C:** Location of the ulnar and radial nerve in the proximal aspect of the forearm.

can be achieved using the anterior approach[72] (Fig. 33-20). However, exposure of the proximal end of the radius is limited by the distal biceps tendon as it wraps around into the bicipital tuberosity. Proximal radius fractures are therefore preferentially approached through a dorsal approach.

Superficial dissection: The skin incision is performed on a line connecting the lateral aspect of the biceps tendon proximally with the radial styloid distally. This places the incision on the ulnar border of the brachioradialis muscle. Dissection proceeds between brachioradialis and the PT proximally and brachioradialis and FCR distally. The approach proceeds through a true internervous interval since the brachioradialis is innervated by the radial nerve and both PT and FCR are innervated by the median nerve. In the proximal and middle third of the forearm, the radial artery and its two venae comitantes

(*text continues on page 1153*)

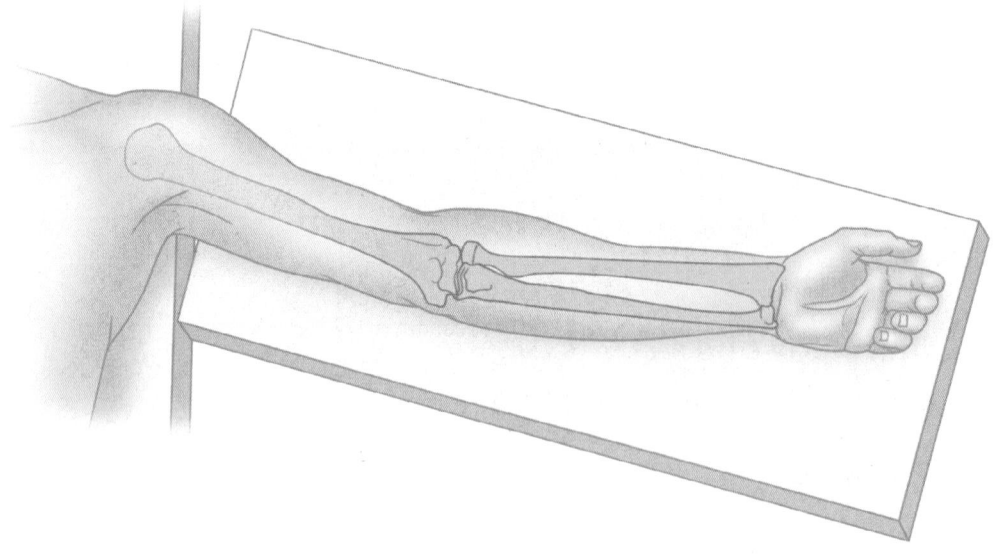

FIGURE 33-20 Anterior (Henry) approach to the radius. **A:** The patient is positioned in the supine position with the forearm supinated on a hand table.

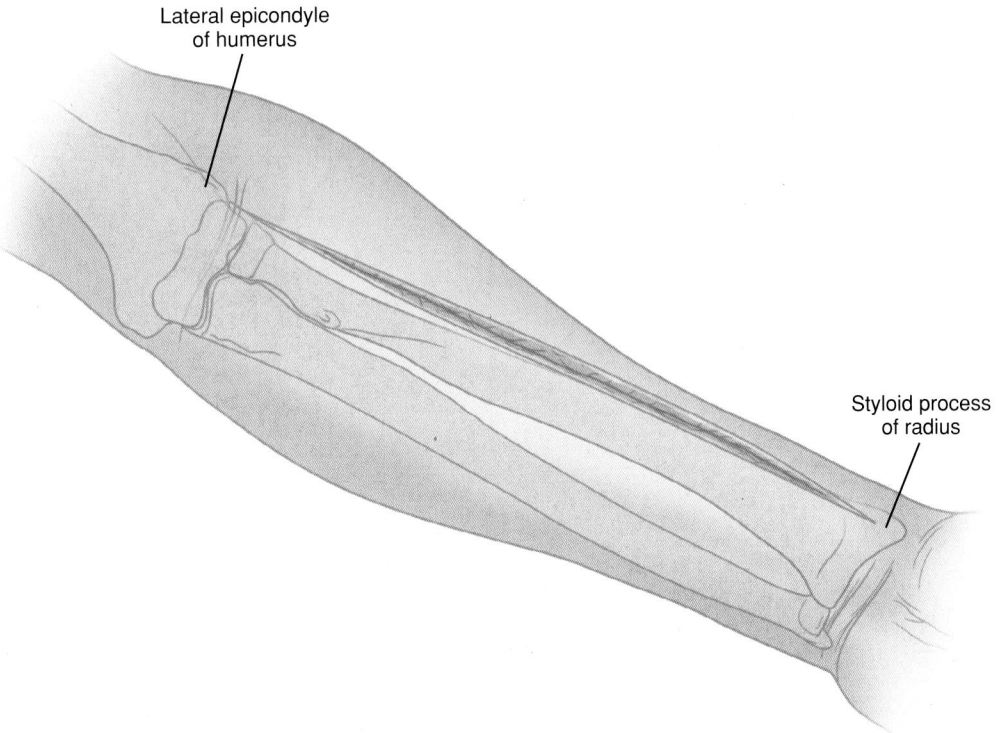

B

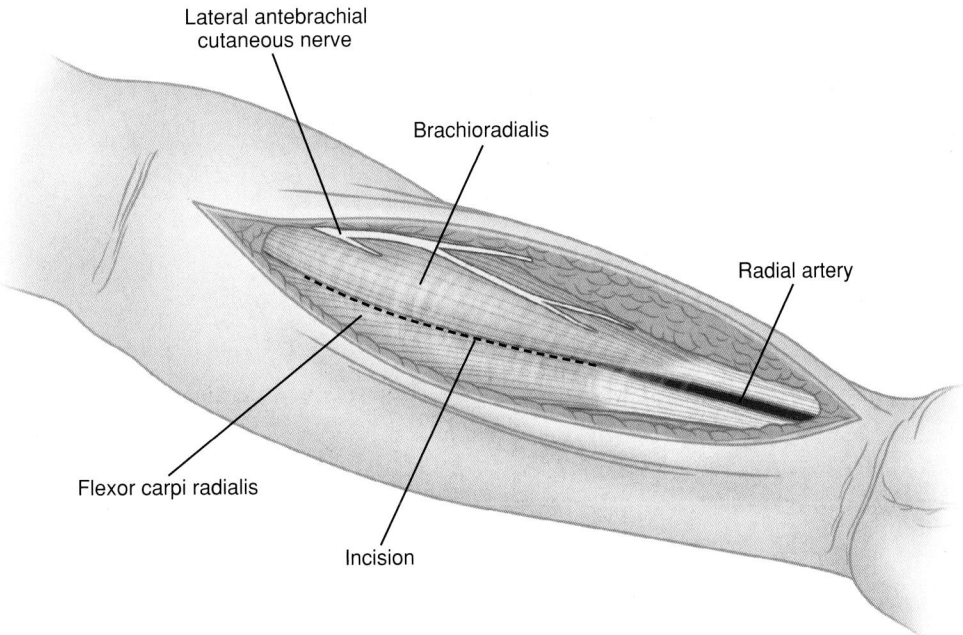

C

FIGURE 33-20 (*continued*) **B:** An incision is performed along a line from the lateral aspect of the distal biceps tendon proximally to the radial styloid distally. **C:** The interval between brachioradialis and flexor carpi radialis is identified in the midshaft. Distally, the interval between radial artery and brachioradialis is used.

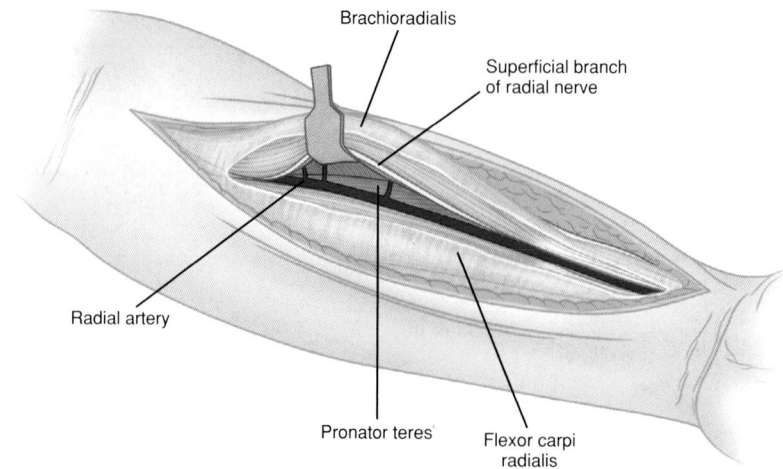

D

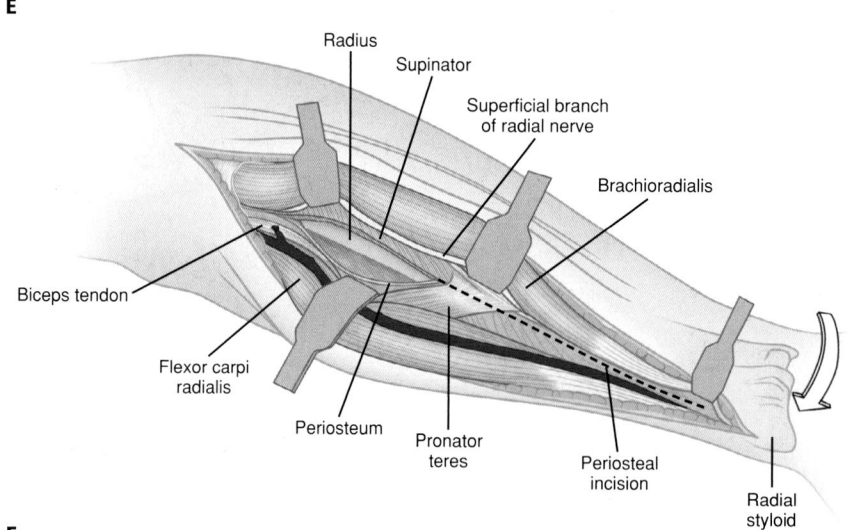

E

F

FIGURE 33-20 (*continued*) **D:** The interval between radial artery and brachioradialis is developed proximally by ligating branches from the radial artery to brachioradialis. The superficial branch of the radial nerve will be located on the undersurface of brachioradialis. **E:** From distal to proximal the radial shaft is covered by pronator quadratus, flexor digitorum superficialis, pronator teres, and supinator. Note that to gain proximal access to the radius the recurrent radial artery has to be ligated. **F:** Alternating between forearm pronation and supination will improve visualization of muscular insertions to allow bony exposure.

run underneath the brachioradialis muscle, assuming a position between the FCR and brachioradialis in the distal third. To allow ulnar retraction of the radial artery and veins along with the FCR, several vascular branches to the brachioradialis have to be identified and either coagulated or ligated. The superficial sensory branch of the radial nerve, on the other hand, is retracted laterally along with brachioradialis as it runs under this muscle lateral to the radial vascular bundle.

Deep Dissection. Access to the proximal third of the radial shaft is gained by releasing the supinator muscle from the radius. In order to protect the PIN, the forearm is fully supinated, thereby rotating the PIN into a posterior position. The supinator muscle is then released from its radial origin. If access to proximal end of the radius is required, the bicipital bursa is incised lateral to the distal biceps tendon. This will avoid injury to the brachial artery and its bifurcation located medial to this tendon. Ligation of the radial recurrent artery may be required to allow medial retraction of the proximal aspect of the radial artery. Retraction around the radial neck should be avoided to prevent injury to the PIN. The middle third of the radial shaft is accessed by pronating the forearm and incising the radial origins of the PT and FDS distal to the supinator muscle. Complete detachment of the PT and FDS should be avoided if possible. The distal third of the radius is accessed by sweeping the FPL ulnarly and exposing the underlying PQ muscle. By supinating the forearm, the PQ can be released from its radial origin and reflected ulnarly. To allow complete elevation of the PQ, its distal border is sharply incised along the watershed line of the distal radius, just proximal to the volar wrist capsule.

Posterior Approach to the Radius (Thompson). The posterior approach to the radius is a prolongation of Kaplan's interval at the elbow. It allows exposure of the dorsum of the radius and is most frequently used for proximal and midthird fractures. The incision is performed on a line from the lateral epicondyle toward Lister tubercle. Proximally, the approach gains access to the radius between ECRB medially and EDC laterally. Distally, access is gained between ECRB and EPL. This does not represent a true internervous plane, since ECRB is innervated by the deep branch of the radial nerve and EDC and EPL by the PIN, which branches off the deep branch of the radial nerve. The interval between ECRB and EDC is clearly identifiable distally as APL and EPB emerge through this interval from deep to superficial and ulnar to radial. To complete the interval between ECRB and EDC, the approach is therefore best completed in a distal to proximal fashion. Isolating the APL and EPB tendons with vascular loops or a Penrose drain can help in assuring adequate orientation of the interval between ECRB and EDC. More proximally, the interval between the origin of ECRB and EDC cannot be clearly identified. Furthermore, the origin of ECRB is covered by the origin of ECRL. Careful elevation of the ECRL origin is required to gain access to ECRB origin.[29] After splitting the interval between ECRB and EDC, the supinator muscle can be identified wrapping around the proximal radius. The PIN is identified at the distal edge of the supinator muscle. If access to the radial head and neck is not desired, the supinator muscle is elevated off its radial origin with the forearm in maximal supi-

nation. If on the other hand access to the radial head and neck is required, the supinator muscle is split in line with the course of the PIN. The ventral capsule and annular ligament are then incised in line with the axis of the radius. Distal to the crossing of EPB and APL, exposure proceeds between ECRB radially and EPL ulnarly. This approach gives direct access to the entire radius except where APL and EPB cross the bone. At this level, retraction of these muscles and submuscular sliding of plates are required to gain full access to the radial shaft. Because of the risk of tendon irritation at this level, distal third radius fractures are best approached through an anterior approach (Fig. 33-21).

Open Reduction with Plate and Screw Fixation

ORIF with plates and screws is considered the gold standard of operative treatment of forearm fractures.[127] Open reduction allows removal of soft tissue interposed at the fracture site and anatomic reduction of the fracture, thereby allowing restoration of the radial bow and the normal spatial arrangement of the ulna and radius. In Galeazzi and Monteggia fracture dislocations, anatomic reduction of the radius and ulna respectively will in most instances lead to stable reduction of the associated dislocated radioulnar joints. Finally, if required, bone grafting can be performed. Plate and screw fixation provides immediate fracture stability, obviating the need for postoperative immobilization and allowing early range of motion.[4,13,27,32,36,48,49,60,64,65,71,73,74,107,108,109,113,119,135,156,163,166,179,185]

Excellent healing rates for open reduction with plate and screw fixation have been reported by most clinical studies.[4,13,27,32,36,48,49,60,64,65,71,73,74,107–109,113,119,135,156,163,166,179,185] In 1965 Sargent and Teipner reported on 29 forearm shaft fractures that were treated with double plating using third tubular plates. Bone graft was not used and no postoperative immobilization was required. A 100% healing rate was achieved.[166] In a subsequent study, Teipner and Mast showed a 100% healing rate using single compression plates in 48 patients, compared with 98% in 55 patients treated with double third tubular plates. The authors concluded that single compression plating offers equal healing rates, whereas reducing fracture stripping and reducing surgical time.[185] Anderson et al.[4] reported a healing rate of 98% for radius shaft fractures and 96% for ulna shaft fractures using compression plating in a total of 330 diaphyseal forearm fractures. Chapman et al. achieved fracture healing in 98% of 129 forearm shaft fracture treated with either 3.5 or 4.5 mm compression plates and screws.[27] Multiple subsequent studies have consistently shown healing rates of above 90%.[13,32,36,48,49,60,64,65,71,73,74,107,108,109,113,119,135,156,163,179]

Compression plating is therefore established as the standard method of fixation of forearm shaft fractures. Early studies on compression plating used 4.5 mm plates and screws.[4,36,60] Subsequently, 3.5 mm plates were introduced with equally high healing rates and less periprosthetic fractures.[13,27,65,73,107,135,163,185] Introduction of locking plates and screws aimed at improving the biologic environment for fracture healing have not shown any clinical benefit over standard compression plates.[48,49,64,71,74,107,163]

(text continues on page 1157)

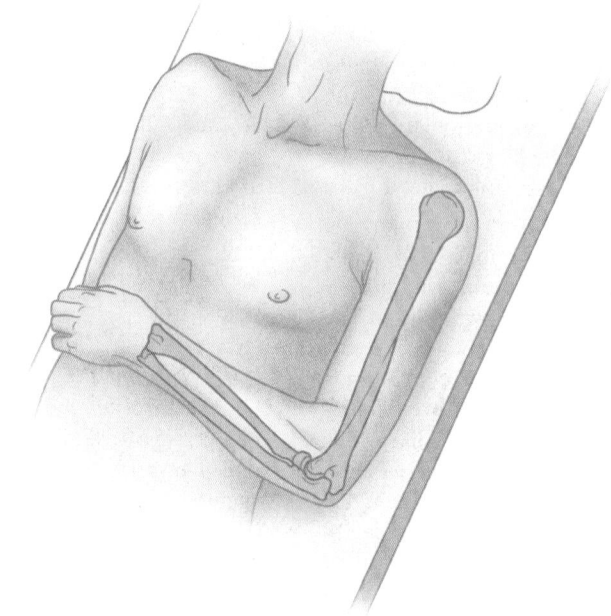

A

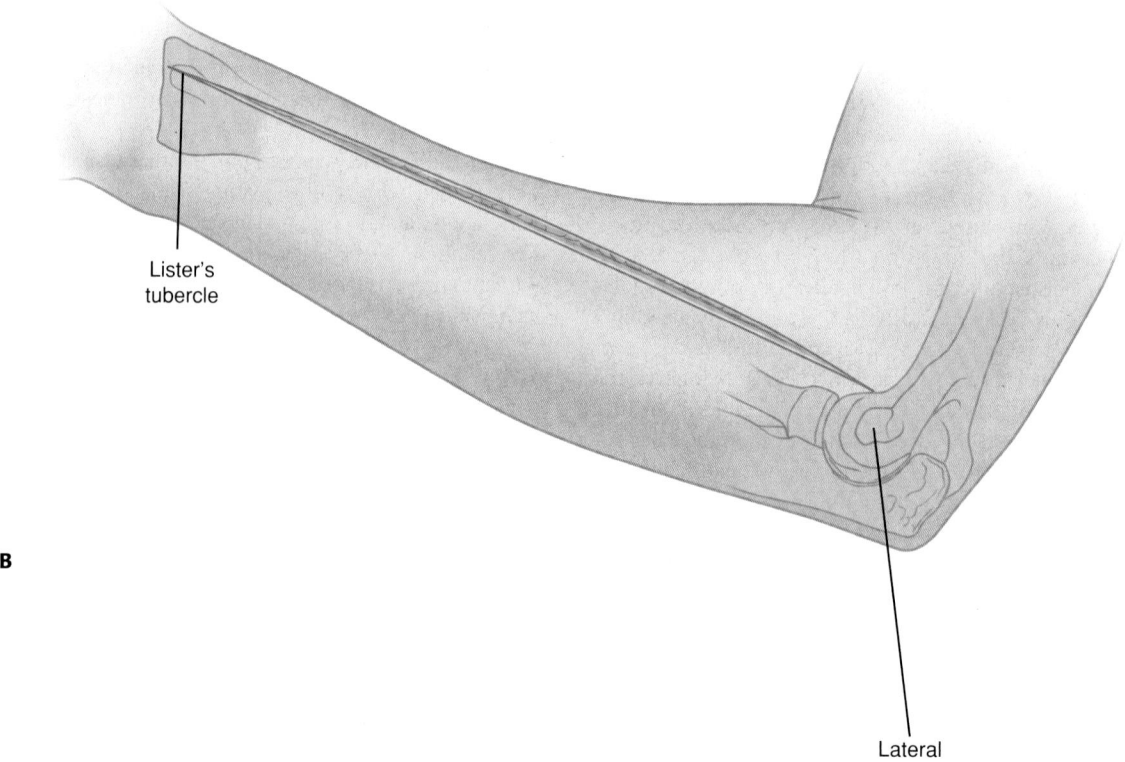

Lister's
tubercle

Lateral
epicondyle

B

FIGURE 33-21 Posterior (Thompson) approach to the radius. **A:** The patient is positioned in the supine position with the forearm pronated either across the chest or on a hand table. **B:** An incision is performed along a line from the lateral epicondyle of the humerus proximally toward Lister tubercle distally.

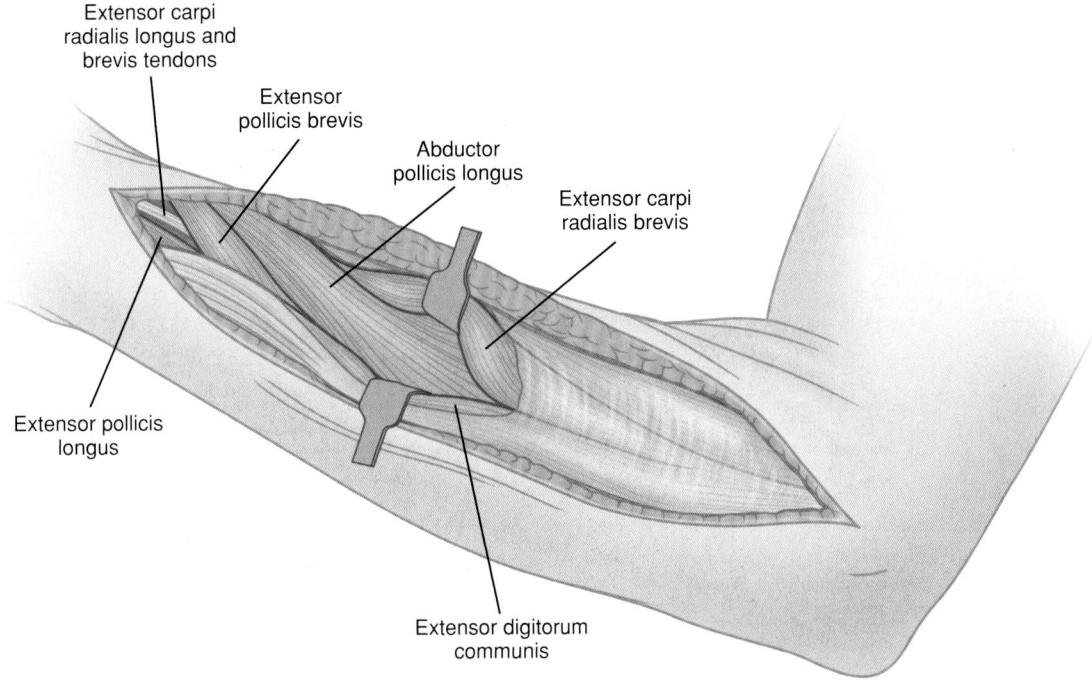

C

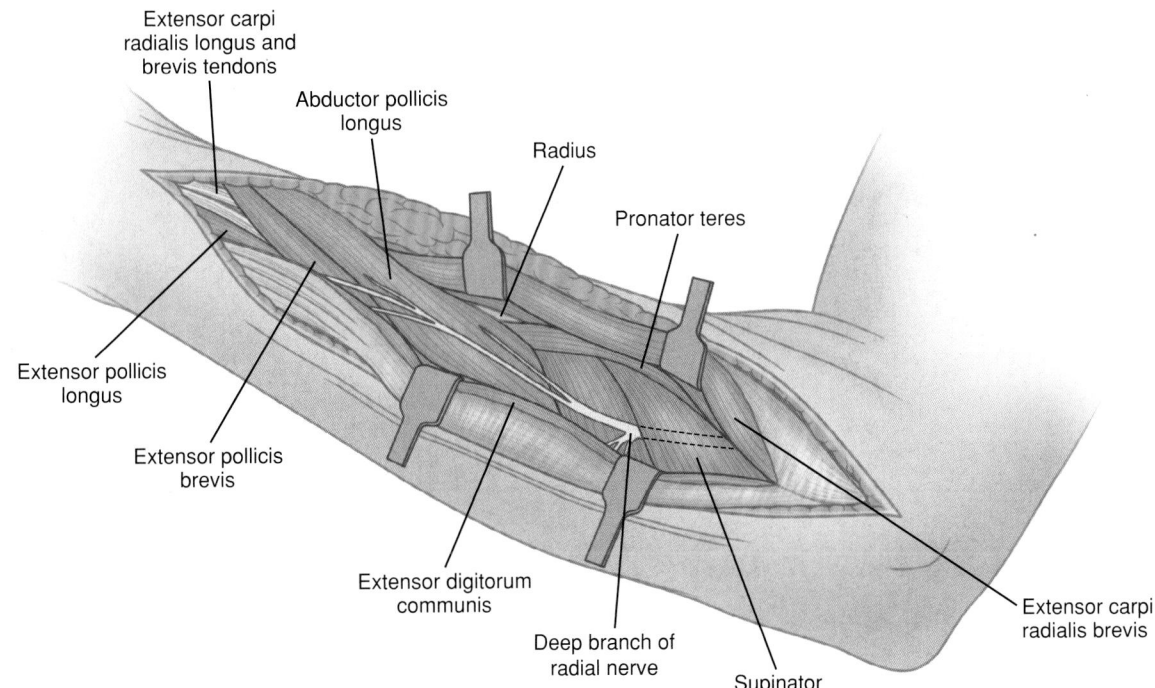

D

FIGURE 33-21 (*continued*) **C:** The interval between extensor carpi radialis brevis and extensor digitorum communis is easiest identified distally as it is split by the passage of the outcroppers (abductor
pollicis longus and extensor pollicis brevis). **D:** The interval is completed proximally by incising the
common extensor origin. The supinator is identified deep to the extensor origin. The posterior interosseous nerve can be identified emerging from the distal edge of supinator.

(continues)

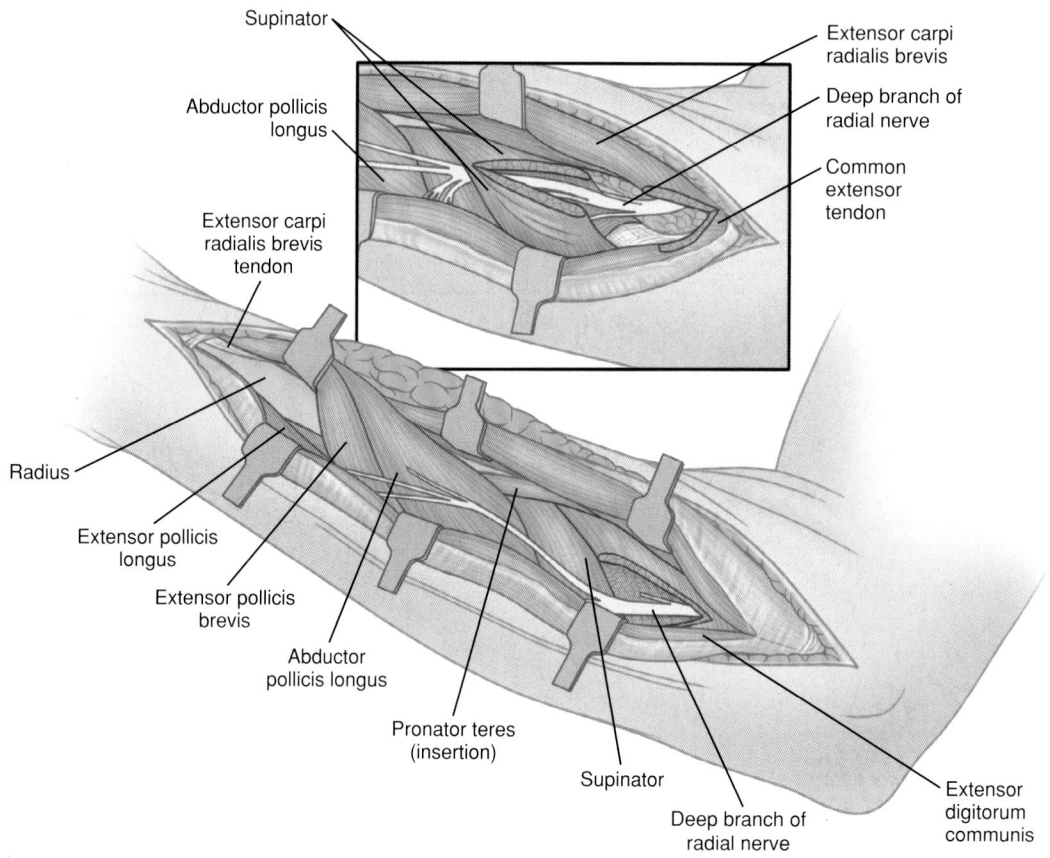

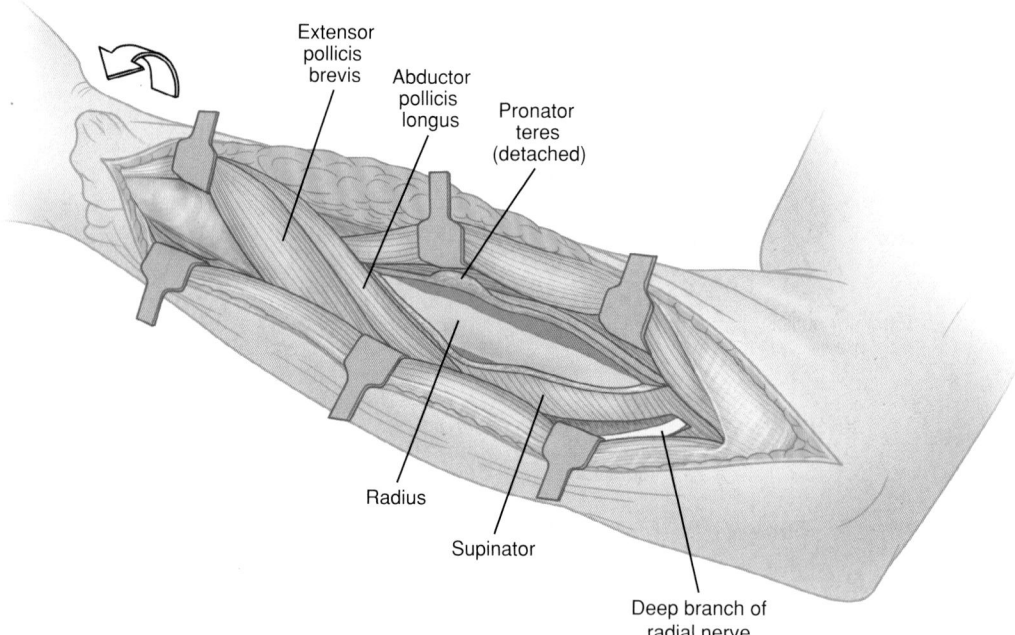

FIGURE 33-21 (*continued*) **E:** To fully expose the deep branch of the radial nerve the supinator muscle is split. This may be required to gain access to very proximal fractures of the radius. **F:** Alternatively, in fractures that are located distal to the neck of the radius the supinator is elevated from the radius without unroofing the deep branch of the radial nerve. This is best achieved by supinating the forearm. Note that distally the dorsal aspect of the radius can be exposed between the extensor carpi radialis brevis and extensor pollicis longus. The dorsal aspect of the second to most distal fifth of the radius remains covered by the outcropper muscles.

Preoperative Planning. The goal of operative treatment of any fracture is to achieve bony healing while avoiding complications and to allow return to a preinjury level of function. Preoperative planning plays a key role in optimizing conditions for fracture management. This includes defining surgical timing, patient positioning, the type of anesthesia, the surgical approach, a stepwise sequence of fracture reduction and fixation, postoperative wound management, and rehabilitation.

Preoperative planning relies on a detailed understanding of the fracture and associated injuries. Associated injuries requiring prioritized management will affect the timing of treatment of forearm fractures. Whereas isolated fractures in fit patients are usually treated within 72 hours of injury, in the polytraumatized patient operative fixation may be delayed for several days to weeks. Historically, open fractures are treated in a more urgent manner, with debridement within 6 hours of injury. The decision on the timing of definitive fixation and the need for a staged procedure will depend on the amount of contamination and soft tissue loss, patient comorbidities, and hemodynamic status.

Planning of definitive fracture fixation requires AP and lateral views of the forearm, wrist, and elbow to achieve a thorough understanding of the fracture and the presence of instability of either the DRUJ or PRUJ. Because of overlap of the radius and ulna on the lateral view, oblique radiographs may aid in defining whether the fracture pattern is simple or if comminution is present. This will determine the type of reduction and stabilization that will be used and the sequence in which fracture fixation will be performed. In most instances the bone with the more simple fracture pattern will be reduced and fixed first as this will aid in reduction of the other fractured bone, especially when comminution is present. The large majority of forearm fractures will be managed with 3.5 mm compression plates, which are available in most operating rooms. Simple fractures are fixed using compression but oblique fractures will in most instances require a lag screw and neutralization plate. Transverse fractures are stabilized with dynamic compression by eccentric drilling and screw fixation through dynamic compression plate holes. Butterfly fragments may be fixed using smaller 2, 2.4, or 2.7 mm screws in a lag mode (Fig. 33-22), while comminuted fractures will in most instances be fixed with a bridge plate (Fig. 33-2).[192] Long distal radius plates may be useful for the treatment of distal radial shaft fractures (Fig. 33-23), while precontoured proximal ulnar plates may aid in fixation of proximal ulnar shaft fractures (Fig. 33-24). Segmental fractures may benefit from temporary fixation using smaller plates and screws (Fig. 33-1). Foreseeing the need for special implants during preoperative planning will allow intraoperative availability of these implants.

Fracture location will determine what type of approach will be performed on the radius. Distal half fractures will most likely be fixed through a volar approach, while proximal half fractures are best managed using a dorsal approach.

Most surgeons recommend the use of a tourniquet. This allows a bloodless field with improved visualization of the soft tissue planes and reducing blood loss. Increased tourniquet time may however significantly increase postoperative pain.[133] ORIF of forearm shaft fractures may be performed without

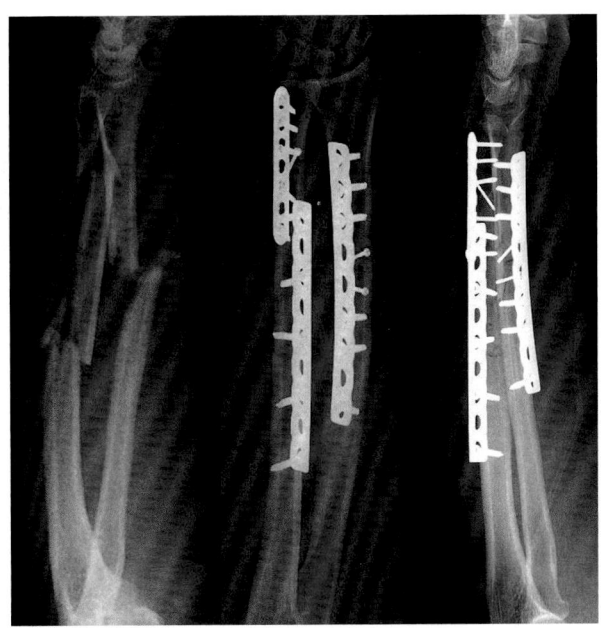

FIGURE 33-22 A segmentally comminuted ulnar fracture stabilized with two plates. A smaller plate was used for distal ulnar shaft fracture as it permitted fixation with more screws and offered a lower profile plate fit. Lag screws have been used for the butterfly fragments. (From Wright RD. Forearm fractures. In: Gardner MJ, Henley MB, eds. *Harborview illustrated tips and tricks in fracture surgery.* Philadelphia, PA: Lippincott Williams and Wilkins; 2010:98–106.)

tourniquet. This may lead to an increase in surgical time during the initial exposure, as hemostasis has to be achieved in this part of the procedure. Higher blood loss may also be expected although in most cases is only marginal. Benefits include less postoperative pain and decreased risk of hematoma formation. Intraoperatively, the radial artery may be more easily identified as its pulsations are easily palpable (Table 33-3).

Positioning. After undergoing general anesthesia, patients are positioned supine and the operative arm is placed on a radiolucent arm board. A nonsterile tourniquet is applied at the arm and the field prepped to the level of the mid arm. In the event of concomitant injuries being present at the operative upper extremity alternative positioning may be indicated. Concomitant humerus shaft fractures approached through a deltopectoral approach can be placed in the beach chair position and the forearm placed on a padded Mayo stand, with the use of a sterile tourniquet if desired.

Surgical Approaches. The ulna is almost universally approached through an ulnar approach between ECU and FCU. Plate positioning can be done either dorsally or volarly. Radius fractures of the distal half are approached through a volar Henry approach, whereas proximal half fractures are best approached through a dorsal Thompson approach.

Technique. In both-bone forearm fractures the sequence of fixation is usually determined by the amount of fracture comminution. If both fractures are simple, either fracture may be fixed first. However, because of the straight geometry of the ulna, it is frequently fixed initially, thereby facilitating radial shaft reduction and fixation. During surgical exposure, normal anatomy

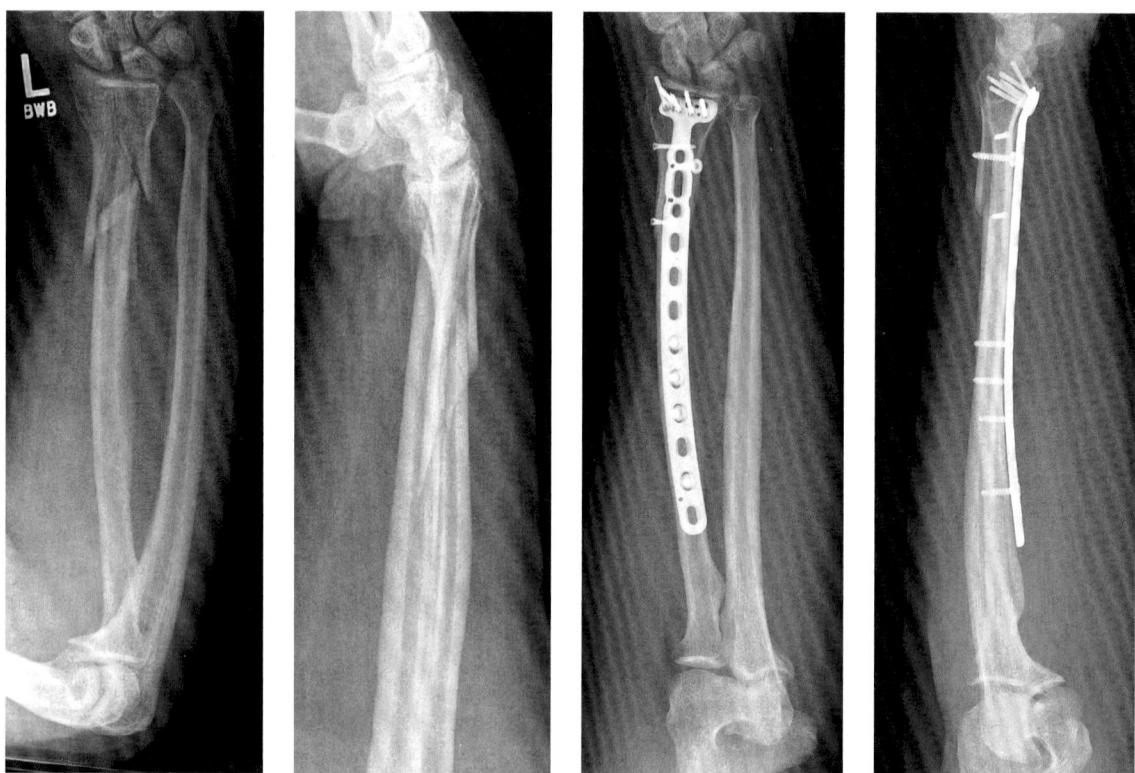

A, B   C, D

FIGURE 33-23 **A and B:** Distal radius shaft fracture. This likely represents a Galeazzi fracture. Marginal radial shortening and the presence of an avulsion fracture of the ulnar styloid suggest possible disruption of the TFCC. **C and D:** Postoperative radiographs. Fixation was achieved with a long distal radius plate that allowed angle stable fixation from the distal radial epiphysis to the middle third of the radial shaft.

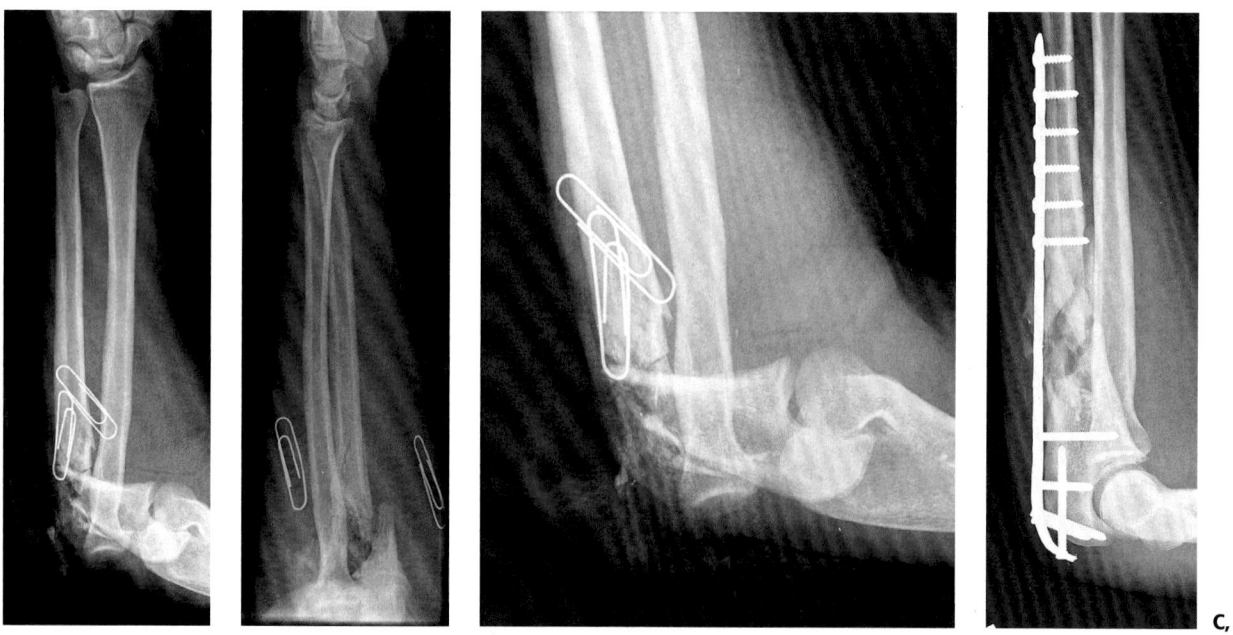

A, B   C, D

FIGURE 33-24 **A–C:** Comminuted gunshot fracture to the proximal ulna with marked comminution and posterior dislocation of the radial head (Monteggia). **D:** Open reduction and internal plate and screw fixation was achieved in a bridging mode, restoring alignment of the proximal radius and capitellum by regaining ulnar length and alignment. A proximal ulna plate was used to facilitate plate apposition and screw placement into the proximal ulna.

TABLE 33-3 ORIF of Forearm Shaft Fractures

Preoperative Planning Checklist

- OR Table: Standard table with radiolucent arm board.
- Anesthesia: General anesthesia. Avoid axillary block to allow clinical monitoring of postoperative compartment syndrome.
- Position/positioning aids: Patient supine, forearm placed on radiolucent arm board.
- Fluoroscopy location: Mini C-arm or standard C-arm coming in from the side.
- Equipment: 3.5 mm plates and screws for most fractures. 2, 2.4, and 2.7 mm screws and plates for complex fractures aiding in temporary fixation.
- Tourniquet: In most instances nonsterile tourniquet on the arm, inflated to 250 mm Hg. Tourniquet time should be kept below 2 hours to reduce postoperative pain. Fractures may be treated without a tourniquet. A sterile tourniquet is recommended when associated fractures are treated during the same operative procedure, e.g., humerus fracture.

may be severely distorted because of displaced fracture fragments injuring the surrounding soft tissue planes. Furthermore, marked swelling may be present, often distorting the normal dissection planes. When using the Henry approach, the FCR is easily identified distally. If a tourniquet is not used, the radial artery can be palpated just radial to the tendon. The artery is then followed proximally, thereby identifying the branches into the brachioradialis muscle. Once these branches are ligated or coagulated, the plane between brachioradialis and FCR/radial artery can be easily identified. Once FPL and FDS are retracted ulnarly, the fracture can be easily palpated. In most instances PT and PQ are elevated subperiosteally and sufficiently to allow adequate fracture exposure and implant positioning. Similarly, during the dorsal Thompson approach, the interval between ECRB and EDC is easiest identified distally at the outcropping of APL and EPB. The interval is then followed proximally and the fracture site identified by palpation. Elevation of the supinator or its splitting after identification of PIN is performed according to fracture location. Ulnar exposure follows the ulnar approach as described earlier. As for the radius, the fracture site should be exposed by preserving as much of the attached soft tissues as possible. Plate positioning will require either dorsal or volar subperiosteal dissection of the ECU or FCU respectively. This should be decided before fracture exposure to avoid stripping of both surfaces of the bone. Frequently, exposure of both bones before fixation will grant easier access to the fracture site to remove interposed tissues. This is of special relevance in simple fracture patterns. Once the fracture has been debrided, the least comminuted fracture is reduced and fixed.

It is generally recommended that screws should engage at least six cortices on each side of the fracture. Over the last decade several authors have studied the effect of number of screws at each side of the fracture. Biomechanical data has shown that similar construct stability can be obtained by using longer plates and fewer screws.[87,165,186] Use of fewer screws does however reduce the torsional and bending stiffness of the construct.[45] Clinically,

Crow et al. reported on 78 forearm fractures that were managed with plate and screw fixation using screw fixation engaging less than six cortices. Despite a nonunion rate of 9%, no hardware failures were reported.[32] Similarly, Lindvall and Sagi reported no hardware complications when using two screws with fixation into four cortices on each side of the 75 diaphyseal shaft fractures. One radius and one ulna nonunion occurred. The authors concluded that fixation of forearm fractures with standard length compression plates and four cortices of screw fixation can yield a stable construct for management of these fractures.[109] Most importantly, however, the use of only two screws on each side of the fracture requires excellent purchase of every screw, since loosening on only one screw will lead to rotational instability of the construct and likely catastrophic failure which is a particular risk in osteoporotic bone in the older patient. It is therefore advisable to obtain fixation with three screws on each side of the fracture into an intact shaft segment.[150]

Transverse Fractures. Reduction of simple transverse fractures is easiest performed by using a lobster claw or pointed reduction forceps. Application of force is thereby minimized and accurate fragment manipulation and reduction facilitated. In most instances, the distal and proximal fracture segment can be accurately keyed in, thereby anatomically reducing the fracture. Forearm supination or pronation can aid in achieving reduction. As mentioned, plate length should allow for placement of three screws on each side of the fracture. In most instances either a six- or a seven-hole plate will achieve this goal in simple transverse fractures. When using a six-hole plate, attention has to be paid to plate positioning to avoid screw placement into the fracture site. Prebending the plate to a slight concavity facing the bone surface, with the apex located at the fracture site, will provide compression along the near and far cortices of transverse fractures. While the fracture is held reduced the selected plate is laid over the fracture site and the planned position visualized. By removing the clamps for plate positioning, reduction is at this point frequently lost. Fixation of the plate to one of the fragments at the visualized position will greatly aid in proceeding with renewed reduction and definitive fixation. Alternatively, the plate may be held in position with two clamps while reducing the fracture (Fig. 33-7E). This technique, however, may be cumbersome and difficult to hold while screws are placed. Once the plate has been fixed to the shaft on one side and the fracture reduced a single clamp will hold the opposite shaft fragment reduced. At this time, fluoroscopy may be used to confirm adequate fracture reduction and plate placement. The opposite shaft fragment is then fixed to the plate with a screw going through an eccentrically drilled hole, thereby achieving interfragmentary compression. The remaining screws on the side of the initially stabilized shaft segment are then placed in a neutral position, whereas an additional compression screw hole may be drilled in the opposite shaft segment. Prior to final screw seating, the initial compression screw will have to be loosened and the second compression screw tightened, thereby providing further compression at the fracture site. The first compression screw is then retightened and a third neutral screw placed. Alternatively, a tension device may be used to achieve compression at the fracture site. Once one shaft segment has been fixed to the plate, the tension device exerts compression at the fracture site by pulling the end of the plate on the opposite shaft segment while using an independent screw as a post. All remaining screws are then placed in a neutral position. As for dynamic compression plating, prebending of the plate is required when using a tension device to provide compression across the near and far cortices.

Oblique Fractures. In simple oblique fractures, fixation may be achieved using either compression plating as described above or by using lag screws and a neutralization plate. If compression plating is used, the plate should be first fixed to the shaft segment that will create an acute angle between the plate and the obliquity of the fracture. This will force the opposite shaft segment to be wedged into this acute angle when compression is applied. Application follows the same sequence as for transverse fractures. Plate prebending is not required.

Frequently oblique fractures can be reduced using pointed reduction clamps. A lag screw is then placed in an orientation perpendicular to the obliquity of the fracture (Fig. 33-25). The near cortical hole is drilled to the size of the outer diameter of the threads of the planned screw size, whereas the far cortex is drilled to the size of the core of the screw threads. For a 3.5 mm cortical screw, the near cortex is drilled with a 3.5 mm drill bit, whereas the far cortex is drilled with a 2.5 mm drill bit. The near cortical hole is then countersunk and the screw length measured. Fixation at this point will allow removal of

clamps and application of a neutralization plate that will allow placement of three screws on each side of the fracture to capture a total of six cortices on each shaft segment. Precontouring is not required and screws are applied in a neutral position, as no further compression can be obtained once a lag screw has been placed. Alternatively, the lag screw may be applied through a plate hole. To achieve this, a plate of appropriate length is selected. The plate is fixed to one of the shaft segments in a position that will allow adequate lag screw placement and again achieve fixation into six cortices on each shaft segment. The opposite shaft segment is then reduced to the plate with a lobster claw forceps, and a lag screw placed through the appropriate screw hole, perpendicular to the fracture site. The remaining screws are then placed in a neutral position.

Comminuted Fractures. Comminuted fractures may be fixed with multiple lag screws if the fragments are sufficiently large. For smaller fragments, 2 or 2.4 mm screws may be used. Fracture fragments are anatomically reduced and fixed to the neighboring shaft segment with a lag screw technique. Careful fragment manipulation is required to preserve soft tissue attachments and maintain fragment viability. If fragment manipulation risks excessive soft tissue stripping, the fracture site may be bridged with a plate that is fixed to the proximal and distal shaft segments. In this setting it is especially useful to obtain anatomic reduction of the other forearm bone to allow partial secondary reduction of the comminuted segment. When both the ulna and radius are comminuted, the ulna is approached first.

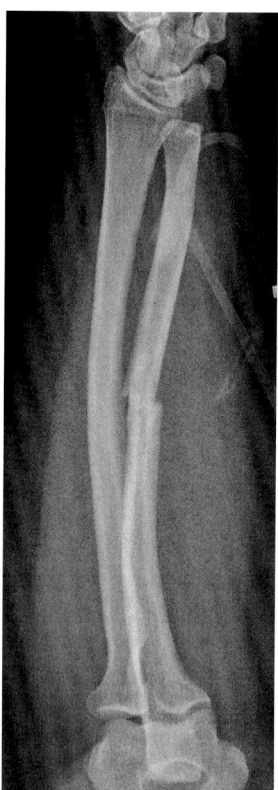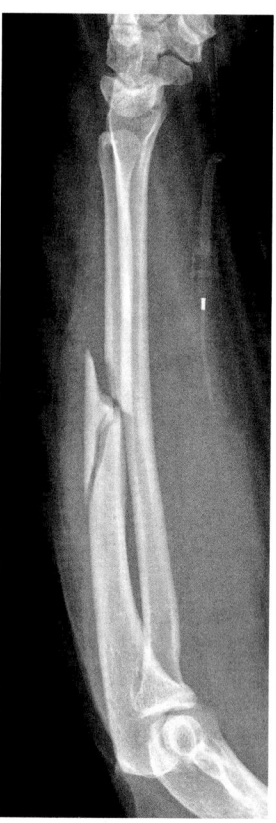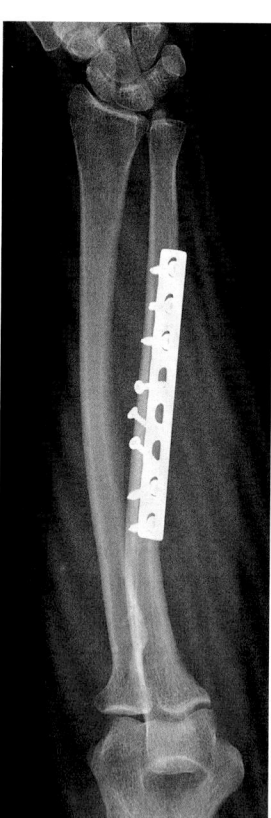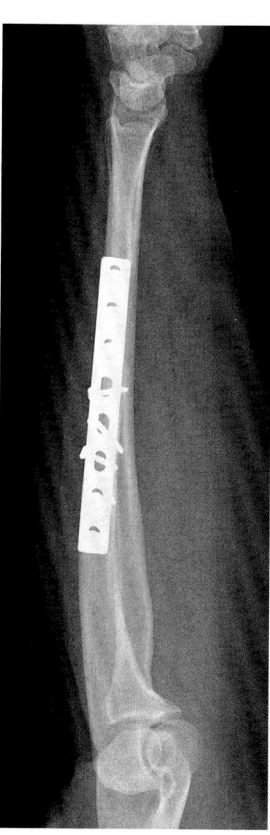

A, B   **C, D**

FIGURE 33-25 A and B: Isolated ulna midshaft fracture with a large butterfly fragment. **C and D:** Fixation was obtained with three interfragmentary lag screws and a neutralization plate.

Restoration of adequate length can be judged by the alignment and absence of excessive gapping between comminuted fracture fragments. Rotation should be judged by viewing a lateral view of the olecranon that shows a lateral view of the ulnar styloid at the wrist (Fig. 33-25D). A plate length is selected that will allow bridging of the fracture site, while providing screw fixation with three bicortical screws in each shaft segment. Temporary fixation of the bridging plate to the proximal and distal shaft segments should be followed with fluoroscopic assessment of reduction. It should be kept in mind that with a single screw on each shaft segment only angulation will be correctable. Change in rotation and length will require change of one of the two screws. Once adequate alignment, rotation, and length are verified the remainder of the screws is inserted. Once ulnar fixation has been achieved the radius is similarly fixed. Restitution of the radial bow may be difficult to achieve in comminuted fractures. When using a volar approach, one has to keep in mind that the ends of the plate will sit on the concave aspect of the radial bow, whereas the central plate segment bridging the fracture will lie on the concavity of the radius. Contouring of the plate may aid in restoring the normal concavity of the radius. As for the ulna temporary screw fixation should be followed by fluoroscopic verification of alignment, rotation, and length. Clinically, full pronation and supination confirm that adequate fracture reduction has been achieved.

Segmental Fractures. Segmental fractures may present as two simple fractures along the ulna and/or the radius. As for single simple fractures, oblique fractures may be managed with lag screw fixation, whereas transverse fractures will require compression plate fixation. The latter may add a significant challenge if compression of more than one fracture is to be achieved through a single plate. The use of short small fragment plates and screws to fix each transverse fracture independently followed by reinforcement of the construct with a long 3.5-mm plate may provide adequate stability and fixation for healing to occur (Fig. 33-1).

Once fracture fixation has been completed the wounds are irrigated and, if used, the tourniquet is released to obtain hemostasis. This will reduce the risk of subsequent hematoma. The skin is then closed with interrupted nonabsorbable monofilament suture stitches. In most instances wound closure can be obtained without undue skin tension. If excessive tension prevents closure of both skin incisions the ulnar incision is closed first to provide coverage of the more subcutaneously located ulna and plate. The radial incision may be covered with a nonadhesive dressing or negative pressure wound therapy. Final wound coverage may be achieved 5 to 7 days later, either with primary closure or more frequently with partial thickness skin grafting. A soft dressing is applied to encourage early range of motion of the elbow and wrist.

Bone grafting continues to be a topic of debate. Whereas some surgeons advocate routine grafting of comminuted fractures, including open fractures,[4,27,60] others have shown reproducible healing rates in the absence of grafting[13,32,48,49,64,71,73,74,107–109,113,119,135,163,166,179] (Table 33-4).

Postoperative Care. Patients undergoing operative fixation of forearm fractures are admitted overnight for clinical monitoring of compartment syndrome. In the obtunded patient, intracompartmental pressure monitoring should be used if clinical suspicion of compartment syndrome is present. If adequate pain control is achieved during the first postoperative day, patients are discharged home and instructed to report back if they experience a progressive increase in pain. Elevation of the operative extremity is recommended over the first 72 hours after surgery to reduce swelling and improve pain. Early range of motion of the elbow, wrist, and fingers is encouraged as well as active pronation and supination. Early range of motion after plate and screw fixation of forearm fractures leads to significantly better functional outcomes than prolonged postoperative immobilization. This effect is most marked in both-bone forearm fractures and open fractures.[60]

Sutures are removed at 2 weeks. Lifting with the affected extremity is limited to 2.27 kg (5 lb) until radiographic healing of the fracture is visible. This occurs on an average between 8 and 24 weeks after fixation, with open fractures taking a significantly longer time to unite.[27,107,109,135]

Patients are informed before surgery that hardware removal is not routinely recommended. Except for plates placed subcutaneously on the ulna, hardware is rarely symptomatic. Furthermore, removal of hardware may lead to nerve injury, infection, wound hematoma, and re-fracture. On average hardware removal may lead to 3.4 weeks of time off work and may lead to an increase in the surgical scar.[4,11,12,27,35,36,75,101,103,118,125,142,147,158,171,175]

Potential Pitfalls and Preventive Measures. The most important part of treating forearm shaft fractures is restoring function by restoring normal anatomical relationships and form of the forearm by means of re-establishing length, alignment, rotation, and radial bow.

Restoration of the radial bow is related to functional outcome, especially in regaining pronation and supination.[171] Intraoperative assessment of unhindered pronation and supination and careful radiographic assessment of reduction and fixation either with fluoroscopy or full length x-rays should be performed. Comparative radiographs of the opposite uninjured side can help in further clarifying any remaining doubt of the achieved reduction, especially in complex forearm fractures.

TABLE 33-4 ORIF of Forearm Shaft Fractures

Surgical Steps

- Upper extremity exsanguination by gravity or elastic bandage, insufflation of tourniquet to 250 mm Hg.
- Fracture exposure: ulnar approach for ulna, Henry approach for proximal half of radius shaft, Thompson approach for proximal half of radius
- Debridement, reduction, and fixation of the less comminuted fracture with minimal soft tissue disruption
- Release of tourniquet, control of hemostasis
- Closure with interrupted monofilament nonabsorbable suture
- Application of soft dressing

At the end of each case, especially in single-bone forearm fractures, examination of the stability of proximal and distal radioulnar joints is important to rule out occult instability of these joints.

Good surgical technique is paramount to reduce excessive soft tissue trauma and achieve adequate fixation. Residual gapping at the fracture site can occur if implants are inadequately selected and implanted in an incorrect sequence (Table 33-5).

Treatment-Specific Outcomes. A summary of outcomes after open plate and screw fixation of forearm shaft fractures is presented in Table 33-6.[4,13,27,36,48,60,64,65,71,73,74,107–109,135,166,185]

Behnke et al. compared the treatment of both-bone forearm fractures in 27 patients who underwent plate and screw fixation in both ulna and radius with 29 patients who underwent IM nailing of the ulna and plate and screw fixation of the radius. All except one radius in each group healed and there were no differences with regards to final range of motion and time to union.[13] Ozkaya et al. compared both-bone fractures in 22 patients treated with only plate and screw fixation and 20 patients who underwent intramedullary nailing only. All fractures healed. No differences were recorded with regards to operative time, the Grace and Eversmann score, or the DASH score. Since all fractures treated with intramedullary nailing were reduced closed, blood loss was reported as none, compared to a mean 60 cm^3 (range 20 to 240 cm^3) after open reduction and plate fixation, a difference that was found to be statistically significant. Furthermore, fractures treated with IM nailing healed on average in

10 weeks, a time frame that was significantly shorter than the average 14 weeks of healing reported after plate fixation. The major disadvantage of intramedullary nailing was the need for postoperative immobilization that ranged from splinting for 2 to 3 weeks to long arm cast immobilization until radiographic healing could be visualized.[135]

Intramedullary Nailing

Intramedullary nailing of forearm shaft fractures has been described for over a century.[173] Early implants were solid small-diameter nails including Kirschner wires, Steinmann and Rush pins, and larger V and U rods.[159,160,178] Because of the wide variability of medullary canal sizes at the radius and ulna, small-diameter nails were frequently the only implantable nail, requiring adjuvant prolonged cast immobilization to maintain reduction.[102,178] U and V rods introduced by Küntscher had the advantage of allowing interference fit because of the compressibility of the slotted nail design. In the forearm, however, this frequently led to nail entrapment and fracture distraction.[181] Improved results were obtained with the use of square and triangular nails that improved rotational stability at the fracture site while allowing restitution of the radial bow.[161,181] In 1986, Street reintroduced the concept that Schöne had described in 1913, of introducing a square nail into an intramedullary canal that had been reamed to a round cross area slightly smaller than the maximum diameter of the nail. Rotational stability was thereby obtained by interference of the corners of the nail into the round endomedullary canal. Street observed that with this implant design, nonunions decreased from 17% with Kirschner wire fixation and 11% with Rush nailing to only 3%.[181] More recently, hybrid fixation, using IM nailing for the ulna and ORIF of the radius for both-bone forearm fractures, has been reported with similar outcomes as ORIF of both.[13]

Currently available implants for intramedullary nailing of forearm shaft fracture include elastic titanium nails and intramedullary rods. Elastic nails rely entirely on interference fit based on the principle of three-point fixation. With this technique a bowed nail is in contact with the endomedullary canal at each end and at the lateral aspect of the bow. Maximization of stability is obtained with placement of two nails, providing resistance to bending forces and axial loads in simple fractures. However, rotational stability is not provided, so additional cast immobilization is required. Elastic nailing is recommended for pediatric fracture fixation where immobilization is better tolerated.[164] In the adult population, elastic nailing is not considered a favorable method of treatment.

Two types of intramedullary rods are currently available in the United States for the management of adult forearm shaft fractures. Both allow locking of the nail to the bone segment adjacent to the entry portal. They differ in the method by which rotational stability is provided at the tip of the nail. One design has a paddle-shaped blade tip that achieves an interference fit at the proximal aspect of the radius and distal segment of the ulna. The other design allows interlocking with screws distal to the entry site. Despite the advantage of theoretically allowing improved rotational stability of forearm shaft fractures, even with modern interlocking nails, some type of immobilization is

---

TABLE 33-5	ORIF of Forearm Shaft Fractures

Potential Pitfalls and Preventions

Pitfall	Preventions
Malreduction	Start with the more simple fracture by "keying" in fragments under direct visualization
	In comminuted fractures confirm correct alignment clinically by rotating the forearm and radiographically by checking radial bow and rotational alignment of proximal and distal radial segments
Postoperative gapping at simple fracture site	Prebend compression plates for transverse fractures
	If using dynamic plate compression for oblique fractures apply the plate first onto the shaft segment that will create an acute angle between the plate and the fracture line
	Careful lag screw technique. Place independent lag screws orthogonal to the plane between the fracture line and the cortical surface
	Follow correct sequence of screw placement. Do not lag the fracture after plate fixation on both sides of the fractures. Do not apply dynamic plate compression after lag screw placement

TABLE 33-6 Summary of Outcomes of Plate and Screw Fixation of Forearm Fractures

First Author	Patients (n)	Age (yr) Mean (range)	Fractures (n)	Open Fractures (n, %)	Implant	Healed (%)	Infection	Nerve Injury (%)	Synostosis (%)	Functional Measure	Result
Sargent[166]	21	32 (14–78)	29	19	Double-third tubular plate	100			5	No	
Dodge[36]	65	24 (13–59)	93	17	4.5-mm DCP	98	3%			No	
Anderson[4]	244		330	15	4.5-mm DCP	97	3%	2	1	Anderson	E or S: 85%
Grace[60]	64	24 (15–66)		25	AO and slotted plate	97	3%	5		No	
Teipner[185]	55		84		Double plate	97	4%			No	
	48		70		Compression plate	100	0%			No	
Hadden[65]	108			24	3.5-mm DCP	97	6%	7	6	No	
Chapman[27]	88	33 (13–79)	129	33	Mainly 3.5-mm DCP	97	2%	1	1	Anderson	E or S: 91%
Hertel[73]	131	38 (16–63)	206	22	3.5-mm DCP	96	1%	0	1	No	
Fernandez[48]	71	33 (14–69)	104	23	PC-Fix	100	1%			No	
Haas[64]	272	34 (11–94)	387	21	PC-Fix	96	2%		1	No	
Hertel[74]	52	37 (11–87)	83	17	PC-Fix	95	1%			No	
Leung[107]	47		66	19	3.5-mm LC-DCP	100	2%	5		Anderson Pain	E or S: 100% No pain: 98%
	45		59	17	PC-Fix	100	2%			Anderson Pain	E or S: 100% No pain: 86%
Leung[108]	32	35 (12–70)	45	3	3.5-mm LCP	100	3%			Anderson Pain	E or S: 100% No pain: 94%
Lindvall[109]	53	33 (13–82)	75	30	3.5-mm LC-DCP	97	0%			No	
Ozkaya[135]	22	32 (18–69)		9	3.5-mm DCP	100	0 deep	0		Grace and Eversmann DASH: Mean (range)	E or G: 82%; A: 18% 15 (4–30)
	20	33 (18–70)		5	Locked IM nail	100	0 deep	0		Grace and Eversmann DASH: Mean (range)	E or G: 90%; A: 10% 13 (3–25)
Henle[71]	53		84		3.5-mm LCP	92				DASH (mean)	14.9
Behnke[13]	27	32 (12–70)	54	22	3.5-mm DCP	96	0%	11	4	Grace and Eversmann	E: 67%, G: 7%, A: 19%, UA: 3%
	29	32 (15–62)	58	14	Hybrid (DCP radius, locked IM nail ulna)	96	0%	4		Grace and Eversmann	E: 59%, G: 17%, A: 21%, UA: 3%

DCP, dynamic compression plate; PC-Fix, point contact fixator; LC-DCP, limited contact dynamic compression plate; LCP, locking compression plate; IM, intramedullary; E, excellent; S, satisfactory; G, good; A, acceptable; UA, unacceptable; DASH, Disabilities of the arm, shoulder, and hand questionnaire.

required until early callus formation is seen radiographically.[31] The benefits of a minimally invasive technique using intramedullary fixation should therefore be carefully weighed against the detriment of limb immobilization.

Indications/Contraindications

Intramedullary nailing of forearm fractures is indicated for unstable forearm fractures. Interference fit nailing can be achieved in fractures with at least 5 cm of intact proximal or distal bone. For interlocking nails at least 2.5 cm of intact distal or proximal ulna and 2.5 cm of proximal and 4 cm of distal radius are recommended.[31]

Although plate and screw fixation is considered the gold standard for treatment of forearm shaft fractures, intramedullary nailing may be considered in some fracture types. These include segmental fractures, open fractures, and those with a poor soft tissue envelope, polytrauma, and osteopenic bone. The benefit of nailing for these fractures is theoretical and has not been shown by scientific data.

A contraindication for intramedullary nailing is obliteration of the medullary canal with a medullary diameter of less than 3 mm at the isthmus being a relative contraindication. In smaller medullary canals, more aggressive reaming will be required to allow placement of a nail of 3 mm diameter, potentially jeopardizing bone viability and risking thermal necrosis. In addition, small-diameter medullary canals place the fracture at risk of additional comminution during reaming and may lead to nail incarceration if insufficient reaming is performed.

Preoperative Planning. Scaled preoperative AP and lateral forearm radiographs of both the injured and the noninjured contralateral side should be available for preoperative planning. Preoperative selection of nail length is estimated by measuring the distance from the olecranon to the ulnar styloid on a radiograph of the uninjured side (Table 33-7). The ulnar nail should be 1 cm shorter than this distance, whereas the radial nail should be 3 cm shorter. A further option to determine nail length is the use of implant-specific radiographic templates. Intraoperatively, the nail may be overlaid on the fractured forearm, while traction is applied to re-establish normal length and implant size is assessed under fluoroscopic vision. Finally, if the ulnar nail length has been selected with the use of the intramedullary reamer, the radial nail is chosen 2 cm shorter.[31] Nail diameter is determined by measuring the isthmus, which ranges from 2 to 7 mm. Depending on the type of implant used, nail diameters come in sizes ranging from 3 to 5 mm. The final nail diameter should be 0.5 to 1 mm smaller than the diameter of the isthmus after reaming. Reaming is therefore required in medullary canals that measure 3.5 mm or less.

Positioning. The patient is placed supine with a radiolucent armboard at the side and a pneumatic tourniquet at the level of the arm. An image intensifier is required for the procedure.

Surgical Approach(es). If an open nailing technique is chosen, the radius is exposed using the volar approach for fractures of the distal half, and the dorsal approach for fractures affecting the proximal half. The ulnar fracture is accessed via an ulnar approach.

Technique. For the radius a longitudinal incision just lateral to Lister tubercle is performed. Careful blunt dissection should proceed after skin incision to avoid injuring the sensory branch of the radial nerve. A low ridge between ECRB and ECRL is identified. This starting point is selected to reduce irritation and the subsequent risk of rupture of the EPL. An entry hole is created by drilling at 45 degrees to the distal radial articular surface and in line with the medullary canal (Fig. 33-26A).[193] As a depth of 1 to 1.5 cm is reached, the drill is further aligned with the axis of the diaphysis and further advanced to a final depth of 2 to 4 cm.[181] For the ulna, a 1-cm longitudinal incision over the tip of the olecranon is performed. The triceps insertion is splint and a starting point on the proximal ulna is created 5 to 8 mm from the dorsal cortex and 5 mm from the lateral cortex. This allows insertion of a straight nail despite the lateral bow of the ulna, while avoiding the articular surface of the greater sigmoid notch. The use of a drill guide during establishment of the starting points both at the distal radius and proximal ulna is recommended to avoid injury to the soft tissues. The ulnar nerve is at special risk during creation of the proximal ulna starting point. If an open reduction is performed, the medullary canal is reamed through the fracture site both proximally and distally (Fig. 33-26B). Reaming of the whole length of the medullary canal is recommended especially in the distal segment of the ulna, as cancellous bone present at this level may interfere with nail advancement and lead to fracture distraction. Obtaining a starting point with a retrograde technique is not recommended for either the radius or the ulna. In the radius, retrograde creation of the distal starting point from within the medullary canal will lead to disruption of the distal articular surface. On the other hand a proximal starting point created in a retrograde fashion from within the medullary canal of the ulna will create a curved nail path because of the lateral offset of the medullary canal with regards to the proximal ulna. Seating of a straight nail will then lead to fracture malalignment.[181] In the setting of both-bone forearm fractures, the radius and ulna are reamed before fixation is started to allow easier access to the medullary canal.

Before stabilizing the radius, the nail geometry should be adjusted to mimic the lateral bow of the diaphysis. This step is not only important when using straight nails but also when using prebent nails, as the bow may not adequately align with the patient's anatomy. The use of a nail bender is very useful in allowing adjustments to the nail's geometry during surgery (Fig. 33-26C).

TABLE 33-7 **Intramedullary Nailing of Forearm Shaft Fractures**

Preoperative Planning Checklist

- OR Table: standard table with radiolucent side table
- Position: supine
- Fluoroscopy location: standard C-arm entering from the side
- Tourniquet: Tourniquet at the arm may be used
- Planned nail size: Measure nail size from preoperative radiographs

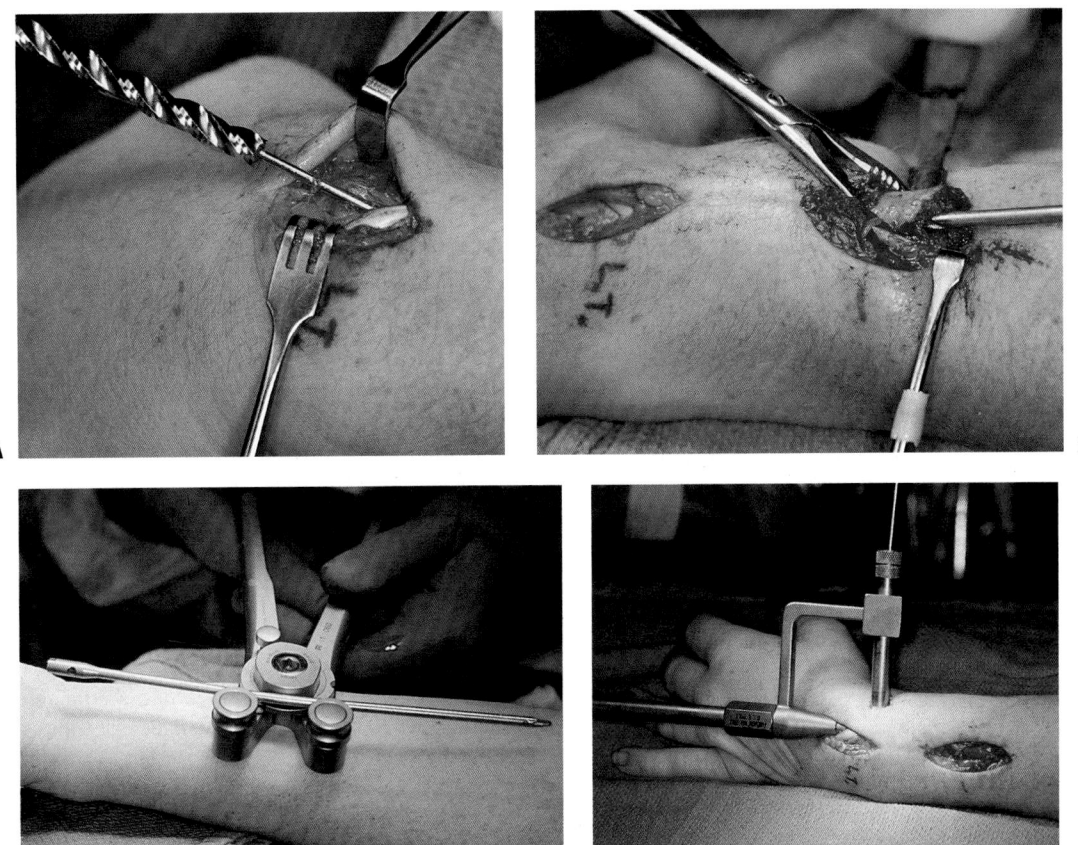

FIGURE 33-26 Intramedullary nailing of the radius **A:** The entry point is just lateral to Lister tubercle, protecting EPL. To enlarge the entry portal, the surgeon introduces a 6-mm cannulated reamer over the 2-mm trocar wire. Note the 45-degree angle to the articular surface of the distal radius. **B:** To prepare the canal at the fracture site, the surgeon uses a power reamer during open nailing. **C:** A nail bender is used to contour the radial nail. **D:** A 1.5-cm incision is made to insert the driving-end interlocking screw. Drill and screw guides must be placed onto the bone to avoid injury to the radial nerve. (From Zinar DM. Forearm fractures: intramedullary nailing. In: Wiss DA, ed. *Fractures*. Philadelphia, PA: Lippincott Williams and Wilkins; 2006:157–168.)

Final seating is usually started with the ulnar nail. However, the less comminuted fracture should be nailed first as it will allow a more accurate reduction of the fracture and will guide subsequent assessment of fracture alignment of the other bone. With currently available implants, interlocking of the near end of the nail is performed with the aiming jig, whereas the far end of the nail is locked using a perfect circles technique under fluoroscopic vision (Fig. 33-26D). Interlocking of the nail at the proximal end of the radius should keep in mind the potential risk of injury to the PIN (Table 33-8).

Postoperative Care. It is generally recommended that additional immobilization of forearm fractures managed with intramedullary nails is maintained with a long arm splint or cast until early radiographic healing can be observed. This may take approximately 6 weeks.[31] Thereafter, patients are allowed to use the affected extremity without weight bearing until solid radiographic healing has been achieved.

Potential Pitfalls and Preventative Measures. The main challenge with intramedullary nailing of forearm fractures

is obtaining an anatomic fracture reduction. Careful bending of the nail will allow accurate restoration of the radial bow (Fig. 33-27). Careful canal preparation is required to avoid fracture gapping and nail incarceration. One of the most severe intraoperative complications is injury to the posterior interosseous nerve during interlocking at the proximal end of the radius. To reduce this risk, a straight lateral entry at less than 3 cm from the radial head with the forearm in neutral rotation should be chosen for proximal radial interlocking[184] (Table 33-9).

Treatment-Specific Outcomes. Gao et al. reported on 32 fractures of the forearm in 18 patients managed with an interlocking intramedullary nail. Healing was achieved in all fractures. Mean time to union was 10 weeks in patients managed with closed nailing, whereas those that required fracture exposure before nailing healed on average after 15 weeks. Mean forearm rotation was from 62 degrees of pronation to 80 degrees of supination. Functional outcome was rated as excellent or good in 13 patients, acceptable in 3, and unacceptable in 2. Complications included radioulnar synostosis in one

| TABLE 33-8 | **Intramedullary Nailing of Forearm Fractures** |

Surgical Steps

- If closed reduction is planned start with obtaining starting point for the ulna and radius
- If open reduction is planned, the fracture is exposed first, followed by reaming and obtaining starting points
- The starting point is created proximally for the ulna and distally for the radius
- The surgical approach to the radius is dorsal for proximal half and volar for distal half. The ulna is approached with an ulnar approach.
- Shaft segments are reamed to 0.5 to 1 mm above final nail diameter
- Nail advancement is performed for the more simple fracture first to allow secondary alignment of the other fracture
- Ensure adequate apposition of the fracture surfaces, avoiding fracture gapping
- Perform near interlocking using aiming jig followed by far interlocking if required using perfect circle technique
- Confirm full pronation supination of the forearm and flexion–extension of the elbow and wrist
- Confirm adequate reduction and implant placement under fluoroscopic vision (Fig. 33-27).
- Wound irrigation, closure, immobilization in a long arm splint.

patient and two patients with painful distal ulnar interlocking screws. Four superficial infections occurred, all in the patients requiring open reduction.[52] Lee et al. reported on 38 forearm fractures treated in 27 adult patients with interlocking nails. Healing was achieved in all except one fracture at a mean of 14 weeks. No infections or radioulnar synostoses were observed and the functional outcome was graded as excellent or good in 92% of patients.[105] Visna et al. achieved healing in all 78 patients with 118 forearm fractures treated with an interlocking intramedullary nail system. Average time to union was 14 weeks. Delayed healing occurred in four cases. Complications included one superficial infection, three incomplete radioulnar synostoses, and one compartment syndrome.[188] Similar healing rates of 94% and 93% have been reported by Moerman

| TABLE 33-9 | **Intramedullary Nailing of Forearm Fractures** |

Potential Pitfalls and Prevention

Pitfall	Prevention
Fracture gapping	Confirm adequate fracture apposition before far interlocking if performed
Nail incarceration	Appropriate sizing of the nail with canal overreaming of at least 0.5 mm
Inadequate reduction	Ensure adequate nail contouring prior to final seating
Posterior interosseous nerve injury	Lateral entry for proximal interlocking of the radius at less than 3 cm from the radial head

et al.[123] and Street.[181] Weckbach et al. prospectively studied 32 patients treated with interlocking intramedullary nailing for 40 forearm shaft fractures. Healing was achieved in all except one patient. Additional complications included one nonunion and two radioulnar synostoses. No infections occurred.[191] Ozkaya et al. compared the results of 22 patients undergoing ORIF and 20 patients undergoing IM nailing of forearm fractures. At final follow-up similar DASH scores were recorded. No significant difference with regards to surgical duration was observed.[135]

Monteggia Fracture Dislocation

Monteggia fracture dislocations represent approximately 1% to 2% of forearm fractures.[25,145] Simple Monteggia fracture-dislocations affecting the proximal ulnar shaft with isolated radial head dislocation can be addressed with ORIF using plate and screws, usually yielding satisfactory outcomes.[145] In this setting, reduction and fixation of the ulnar shaft follows the same principles as discussed for both-bone forearm fractures. However, because of the frequent proximal location of the ulnar shaft fractures, precontoured proximal ulna plates may be helpful (Fig. 33-24). The surgical procedure may be performed with the patient supine and the forearm placed across the patient's chest or with the patient in the lateral decubitus position and the arm placed over a bolster.[43] The ulna is then exposed through a posterior approach and the plate placed onto the posterior surface of the proximal ulna to counter bending forces.[43,92,151] Since the TFCC and the interosseous membrane distal to the ulnar fracture remain intact, once reduction of the ulna has been achieved the PRUJ is generally reduced spontaneously into a stable configuration.[43,145]

However, Monteggia fracture-dislocations may yield a high rate of unsatisfactory results and complications, even after surgical treatment, when more complex injuries are present.[5,18,111,139,140] Korner et al.[97] and Egol et al.[44] observed that Monteggia lesions with associated proximal radius or coronoid fractures were associated with poorer outcomes. Reynders et al. reported 46% fair or poor results in 76 Monteggia lesions in adults. According to the Bado classification, good or excellent results were the norm in type 1 and type 3 Monteggia lesions. Fair or poor results were most frequently seen in type 2 and type 4 fractures. Involvement of the olecranon process was found to lead to poorer outcomes and persistent radial head dislocation was present in 7 cases (9%).[147] Similarly, Reckling found his best results in Bado type 1 fractures, with fair results as the rule for type 2, 3, and 4 fractures.[145] Givon et al., on the contrary, found Bado type 1 fractures to be at higher risk for poor outcomes, especially in type 1 equivalents with fracture of the proximal radius. In their study, involvement of the olecranon did not affect outcomes.[58] Jupiter et al. reported 45% fair or poor results after operative treatment of Bado type 2 Monteggia fracture dislocations. Of note, 10 of the 13 included cases had an associated radial head fracture, and the proximal ulna, including the coronoid, was frequently involved. Of the radial head fractures, seven underwent radial head excision, one was replaced with a silicone implant, and three managed with ORIF.[92] In a subsequent study, Ring et al. reported the results of 48 adult

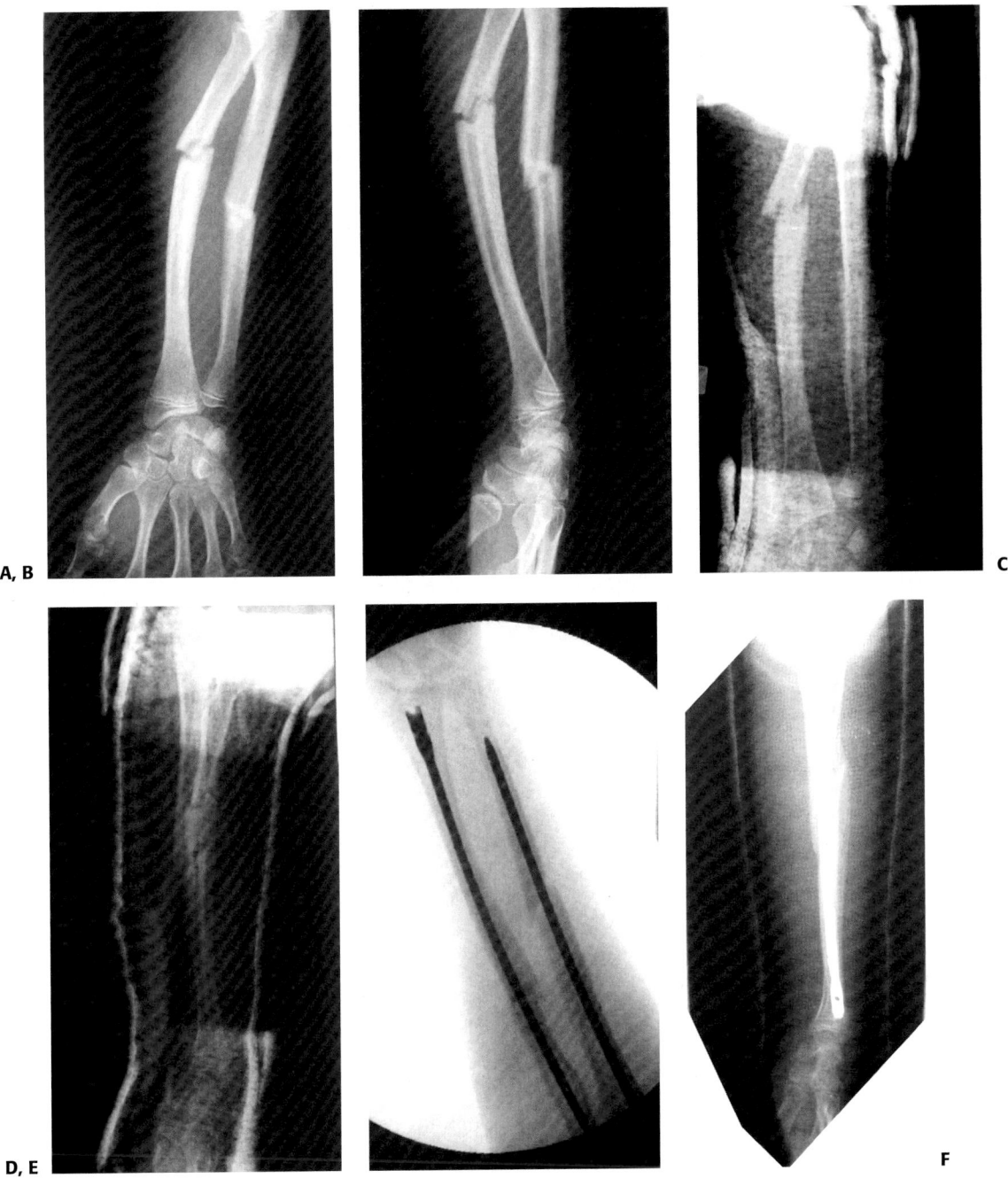

FIGURE 33-27 AP **(A)** and lateral **(B)** radiographs of preoperative radius and ulna, preoperative AP **(C)**, and lateral **(D)** radiograph after closed reduction of a bone bone forearm fracture. Postoperative AP **(E)** and lateral **(F)** radiographs after closed nailing. (From Zinar DM. Forearm fractures: intramedullary nailing. In: Wiss DA, ed. *Fractures*. Philadelphia, PA: Lippincott Williams and Wilkins; 2006:157–168.)

patients treated for a Monteggia fracture over a 10-year period. Fractures were classified as Bado type 1 in 7, type 2 in 38, type 3 in 1, and type 4 in 2 cases. A radial head fracture was present in 68% of type 2 lesions, one-third of which had an associated coronoid fracture. Nine patients required a reoperation, all of which had a Bado type 2 lesion. Indications for reoperation included loosening of ulnar fixation, radial head resection, and painful hardware. Additional complications included radioul-nar synostosis in three patients, posterolateral rotatory instability in one patient, and distal radioulnar joint instability in one patient. Overall, final results were graded as excellent or good in 40 patients (83%). Poor and fair results were found in four patients with a Bado type 2 lesion, in one patient with a Bado type 1 injury, and one patient with a Bado type 4 fracture. Poor outcomes occurred in the presence of coronoid or ulnar malre-duction, radial head fracture, or radioulnar synostosis.

In the setting of complex Monteggia fracture dislocations, careful reconstruction of the proximal ulna including the olecranon and coronoid may be required. Furthermore, fractures of the proximal radius will increase the likelihood of poor outcomes. If spontaneous reduction of the radial head does not occur after adequate reduction of the ulna, buttonholing of the proximal radius through the annular ligament or the anconeus muscle should be suspected.[145] Where there is an irreducible radial head or an associated proximal radius fracture, including proximal radial shaft, neck or head, an independent radial approach should be performed. In the past a combined approach to the proximal ulna and radius has been recommended,[21] but this approach places the elbow at unnecessary risk of a radioulnar synostosis.[151] A detailed discussion of the Monteggia lesions affecting the proximal ulna and radius is provided in Chapter 34.

Galeazzi Fracture Dislocations

An isolated radial shaft fracture with associated disruption of the DRUJ is commonly known as a Galeazzi fracture dislocation. Other eponyms for this injury include "fracture of necessity," Piedmont fracture, and reverse Monteggia fracture.[51,57,82] Forearm fractures that involve only the radial shaft occur in up to 75% of cases. The remaining 25% of radial shaft fractures present as a Galeazzi lesion with an associated dissociation of the DRUJ and disruption of the interosseous membrane distal to the fracture site.[155] According to Rettig and Raskin[146] isolated radial shaft fractures located within 7.5 cm of the lunate facet of the distal radius are at increased risk for DRUJ disruption. Disruption of the DRUJ may however also occur in the presence of both-bone forearm fractures and isolated ulna fractures.[9,43,57,120,145] Galeazzi fractures represent around 7% of adult forearm fractures.[125]

The principles of management of Galeazzi fractures follow those of both-bone forearm fractures. In adults, poor results can be universally expected with nonoperative treatment of these injuries because of inadequate control of deforming forces of the PQ, brachioradialis, and thumb abductors and extensors.[15,57,66–68,82] Anatomic reduction and stable fixation is required to restore the normal relationship between the radius and ulna to allow unrestricted forearm rotation and to avoid delayed arthritic changes in the DRUJ.[57,82,120]

Plate and screw fixation is the preferred mode of fracture stabilization (Fig. 33-7). Operative treatment is performed with the patient supine and the forearm placed on a radiolucent side table. The radial shaft is approached either via a volar or a dorsal approach. In most instances the fracture will be located in the distal half of the radius, making the volar the most frequently used approach. However, some authors have reported a higher use of the dorsal Thompson approach to reduce a theoretical risk of reduced pronation associated with the volar approach.[125] Reduction and fixation is obtained according to the fracture geometry. In most instances, anatomic reduction of the radial shaft will lead to stable reduction of the DRUJ.[182] When adequate reduction of the DRUJ is obtained after fixation of the radial shaft, the DRUJ should be assessed for stability. A stable DRUJ will remain reduced when anteroposterior

translation is applied. An unstable DRUJ on the other hand will allow dislocation of the DRUJ, even with the forearm in supination. Stable injuries are routinely immobilized for 3 to 6 weeks in a long arm splint or cast.[57,125] However, Gwinn et al. recently reported on an early motion protocol for selected Galeazzi fractures. When the DRUJ was found to be clinically and radiographically stable after radial shaft fixation, patients could safely be allowed to start immediate elbow motion, followed by progressive forearm rotation starting 2 weeks after surgery.[63] An unstable DRUJ caused by a soft tissue injury at this level may be treated with pinning of the DRUJ using Kirschner wires with or without open repair of the TFCC.[112] Pinning of the DRUJ is best performed with two 2-mm Kirschner wires placed 1 cm apart, with the distal most wire just proximal to the sigmoid notch.[97,180] Adequate postoperative immobilization should be provided. Inadvertent rotation of the forearm may lead to pin breakage at the DRUJ.[121] An unstable DRUJ with an associated fracture of the base of the ulnar styloid is best addressed with ORIF of this fragment.[121]

If DRUJ reduction is not achieved after ORIF of the radius, either inadequate fracture reduction has been performed or interposition of soft tissue or bony fragments may be present at the DRUJ. Interfering structures may include ECU, EDC, and EDQ tendons, periosteum, or an avulsed foveal fragment.[2,17,70,84,86,94,136] In this instance, an open reduction of the DRUJ will be required. Stabilization of the DRUJ with primary repair of the TFCC may be performed. Postoperatively, immobilization for 3 to 6 weeks in a long arm cast is recommended. Galeazzi fractures with dorsal dislocation are immobilized in supination, whereas those with volar dislocation are immobilized in pronation.[1,23,57,112,125] Some authors advocate immobilization in neutral after repair.[121] Intraoperative assessment of the position in forearm rotation that provides the most stable DRUJ is selected for immobilization.

If anatomic reduction of the radius and DRUJ is obtained, satisfactory results can be obtained in 80% to 92% of the cases.[100,117,124] Excellent results have been reported with primary repair of associated DRUJ instability in 95% of patients.[121] However, inadequate reduction of the radius and persistent incongruity of the DRUJ can lead to significant morbidity.[57,82,120]

Open Fractures

The frequency of open fractures ranges between 10% in isolated forearm shaft fractures to 43% of both-bone forearm fractures.[20,27,39,52,65,104,105,109,155] Of open forearm shaft fractures less than 10% are type IIIB or C according to the Gustilo classification, and the majority are type I.[41,61,122] Type I and II account for almost 80% of open forearm fractures.[122]

Satisfactory results have been reported with irrigation and debridement and definitive fixation within 24 hours of injury in 90% of type I, II, and IIIA open fractures.[41] Poorer results can be expected with more severe soft tissue injuries such as seen in grade IIIB and C fractures.[41,122] Jones studied a group of 18 patients with high-energy open forearm fractures. Seven patients had a type IIIA, eight a type IIIB, and three a type IIIC open fracture. All patients underwent irrigation and debridement and immediate plate and screw fixation followed by redebridement at 24- to 48-hour intervals as required. Bone grafting was performed in five patients at 8 to 10 weeks after the initial injury. Delayed reconstructive procedures including tendon transfer, arthrodesis, scar revision, and nerve reconstruction were required in eight patients. Minor wound complications occurred in three patients. One patient had a deep infection requiring repeat surgical intervention, one patient with a type IIIC fracture and prolonged warm ischemia required eventual amputation, and one patient required a second grafting procedure. Good or excellent results were obtained in 12 patients (66%).[89] Moed et al. studied 50 patients with 20 type I, 19 type II, and 11 type III open forearm fractures. All fractures were treated with irrigation and debridement and immediate ORIF. Complications included two deep infections and six nonunions. Excellent or good results were obtained in 85% of cases. Because of the relatively high rate of nonunions, the authors recommended bone grafting in comminuted fractures in which interfragmentary compression could not be obtained.[122]

Low-velocity gunshot injuries frequently cause isolated open fractures of the ulna or radius. As in their closed counterparts, non- or minimally displaced isolated ulna and radius fractures may be treated with immobilization, while displaced both-bone forearm fractures are best treated with immediate irrigation and debridement and ORIF (Figs. 33-2 and 33-24). Lenihan et al. studied 37 patients with such injuries. Only six (16%) affected both the ulna and radius. Fourteen were isolated ulna and seventeen isolated radius fractures. Twenty-three fractures were non- or minimally displaced. Almost 40% of patients had a nerve palsy before treatment. All except one nondisplaced and six displaced fractures were treated with casting, whereas the remainder underwent ORIF. All fractures healed, no infections occurred, and two patients developed a compartment syndrome. Sixty percent of nerve injuries resolved spontaneously. Poor results were observed in six patients, five of which had been in both-bone fractures treated with cast immobilization.[106]

Most open forearm fractures can be treated with irrigation and debridement and immediate ORIF using plates and screws. The optimal type and duration of antibiotic management is still being debated. Commonly accepted regimens include immediate intravenous Gram-positive coverage for all open fractures. Concomitant Gram-negative coverage is recommended for type 3 fractures. Additional anaerobic coverage with penicillin or clindamycin has been advised for combat injuries and those occurring with contamination in the farm environment. Type 1, 2, and 3A open fractures can be adequately managed with a single wash out and immediate ORIF and closure provided there is no doubt about tissue viability or contamination. Whereas immediate fixation may be performed in 3B fractures, repeat irrigation and debridement may be required at 72-hour intervals until a definitive soft tissue coverage can be obtained, usually with some type of tissue transfer (Fig. 33-28). Type 3C fractures are managed with fixation followed by vascular repair in most instances.

In selected cases in which massive soft tissue disruption with marked contamination is present, thereby precluding definitive plate and screw implantation, external fixation may be used. As for ORIF, understanding of the anatomy of the forearm is key for accurate and safe placement of external fixator pins.[53] Pins should be placed in a location that will not interfere with definitive plate and screw placement because of

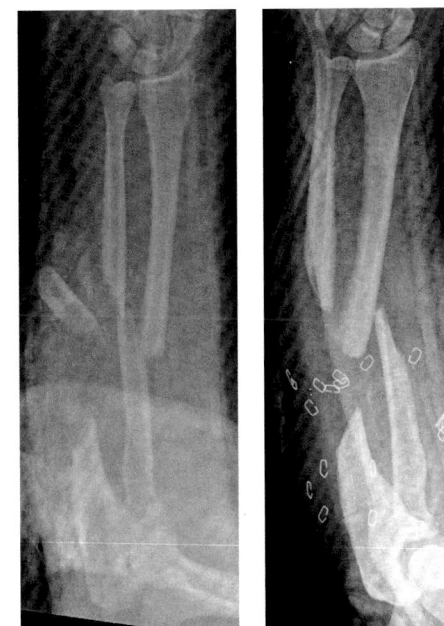
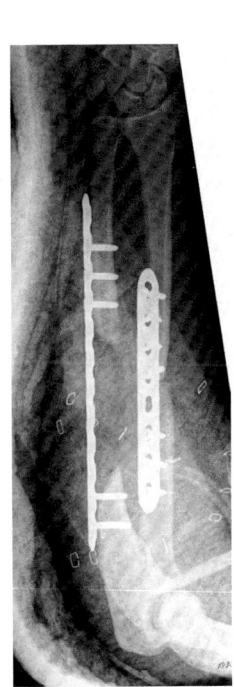
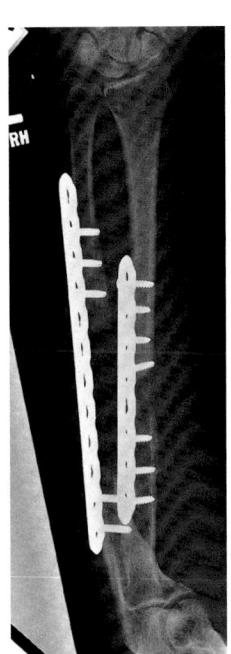
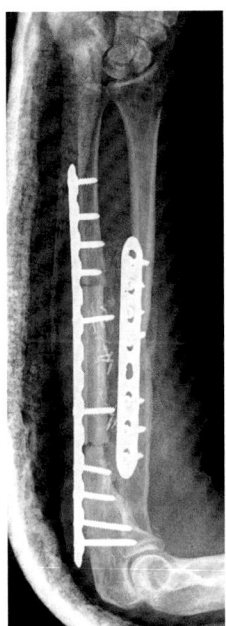

A, B
C, D

FIGURE 33-28 **A and B:** Type 3B open segmental fracture of the ulna and radius. Severe stripping of the intermediate fracture segment of the ulna was resected. A soft tissue flap was required to obtain adequate coverage and allow initial fixation **(C and D). E:** A vascularized fibula graft was used to bridge the fracture defect.

potential contamination of the surgical field by pin tracks. With the patient supine, using a radiolucent side table, two 3-mm Schantz pins are placed into each main shaft segment with the help of an image intensifier. Ulnar pins are placed by palpation of the subcutaneous border of this bone. Pins are then introduced through stab incisions in the interval between ECU and FCU. Because of radial shift of the muscles during pronation, this position is chosen during pin placement to reduce overlying soft tissues. Radial pins are inserted using the interval described for Thompson's dorsal approach. For the proximal half of the radius, pins are placed between the ECRB and EDC, while at the midshaft pins are placed in the interval between ECRB and EPL. Blunt spreading of the soft tissue after skin incision and the use of a soft tissue sleeve will aid in protecting the superficial branch of the radial nerve. At the distal radius, a distal dorsal pin can be placed proximal to Lister tubercle. This is easily palpated in most instances. A longitudinal skin incision followed by spreading of the soft tissues and pin insertion with a soft tissue sleeve will help protect the surrounding tendons. Associated soft tissue injuries may be covered with wet to dry dressings or managed with negative pressure wound therapy. Careful pin site care is required to avoid pin track infection and secondary loosening and possible osteomyelitis. Pins are covered with saline-soaked gauze. Any remaining tension between the pins and skin should be relieved with a skin cut perpendicular to the tension lines. After initial pin placement, pins may remain covered by the sterile dressing for 5 days, followed by twice daily pin site care.[50]

Schuind et al. reported on 93 patients with acute fractures of the diaphysis of the forearm treated by a Hoffmann external fixator in a half frame configuration. After a mean time of 13 weeks of external fixation a healing rate of 91.5% was observed. One re-fracture occurred after frame removal.[174] Smith and Cooney reported on the use of external fixation in complex upper extremity injuries in 40 patients, 32 of which were forearm fractures with both bones fractured in 27, the ulna in 4, and the radius in 1. All were open fractures: 29 Gustilo type III, 2 Gustilo type II, and 1 Gustilo type I. Associated vascular injuries were present in 13 and neurologic injuries in 11 cases. External fixation was maintained for 13 weeks on average but immobilization for a mean of 32 weeks. Sixteen of the thirty-two fractures were treated by ORIF with plates 3 to 5 days after frame removal. The authors reported the outcome of 28 of the 32 forearm fractures with excellent results in 14%, good in 57%, fair in 21%, and poor in 7%. Nonunion developed in 16% of cases and they were treated by ORIF with plates and bone grafting. Combining delayed union and nonunion requiring later treatment, 52% of patients required a second intervention.[177]

MANAGEMENT OF EXPECTED ADVERSE OUTCOMES AND UNEXPECTED COMPLICATIONS OF DIAPHYSEAL FRACTURES OF THE RADIUS AND ULNA

Infection

Infection has been reported to occur in between 0% and 3% of forearm fractures. Anderson et al. reported an infection rate of 3% in 330 fractures of the forearm treated with plate and screw

TABLE 33-10 **Forearm Fracture**
Common Adverse Outcomes and Complications
Infection
Malunion
Nonunion
Radioulnar synostosis
Re-fracture
Compartment syndrome

fixation. Of the seven infections, three cleared with antibiotic treatment and achieved a good result. One patient required antibiotic treatment and hardware removal after fracture healing with resection of sequestra and suction/irrigation. Out of a total of nine nonunions in the whole series, three additional patients developed a septic nonunion that required subsequent surgery. Interestingly, all infections occurred in closed fractures, with *Staphylococcus aureus* being the most frequent infecting organism.[4] Several studies have reported no infection after ORIF of forearm shaft fractures.[13,109,135] The highest infection rate was reported by Hadden et al.[65] with 6% of 108 patients having a deep infection after ORIF of forearm shaft fractures.

In most instances infection is recognized by erythema, increased temperature, and swelling. Whereas these signs are usually seen during the early uneventful postoperative period, increasing pain and malaise may further prompt suspicion. Additional factors include fever and purulent drainage, under which circumstances there is little doubt about the diagnosis of infection. Superficial infections can in most instances be treated with a 10-day course of oral antibiotic. In uncomplicated fractures, Gram-positive coverage with a first generation cephalosporin or penicillinase resistant β-lactam such as oxacillin leads to uneventful resolution.[52,64,73,108,188] In contrast deep infections require repeat interventions for irrigation and debridement. Careful debridement of devitalized or infected soft tissue and bone should be performed. Hardware should be retained if stable until fracture healing has been achieved. Intraoperative cultures should be obtained and broad-spectrum intravenous antibiotic coverage started. Antibiotics are adjusted according to culture growth and frequently continued for at least 6 weeks. In the presence of segmental bone loss, placement of antibiotic-loaded cement beads or spacer can be useful in achieving high local antibiotic concentrations. Resolution of infection can be monitored with laboratory markers such as CRP to assist in the timing of definitive reintervention for bone grafting and fixation.

Nonunion

Nonunion rates after screw and plate fixation range between 0% and 10%.[4,13,27,32,36,48,49,60,64,65,71,73,74,107–109,113,119,135,156,163,166,179,185] Nonunions lead to a significant delay in functional recovery and are frequently associated with poor final outcomes.[4]

Nonunions are generally secondary to inadequate biomechanics, inadequate biology, or both. Errors in achieving the adequate biomechanical environment for fractures to heal can be multiple. Fracture gapping after 3.5-mm screw and plate application because of inadequately followed principles of fixation will prevent primary bone healing and possibly result in nonunion.[60] Selection of an implant that does not provide sufficient stability, such as third tubular plates, may lead to excessive motion at the fracture site, which in simple fractures may lead to nonunion. Too much rigidity in a construct may lead to inadequate healing when bridge plating is performed. Factors affecting the biomechanics of fracture healing include selection of a plate of inadequate length, inadequate plate placement, and screw insertion too close to the fracture site when using compression plating only.[4] The second reason for nonunions is inadequate biology. High-energy injuries with open fractures, severe comminution, and excessive soft tissue stripping increase the risk of poor vascularity at the fracture site inhibiting healing. Furthermore, around one-third of nonunions occur in the presence of a deep surgical site infection.[4]

When treating suspected nonunions of the forearm the surgeon should wait for 6 months to adequately monitor the fracture and ensure that there is no radiographic progress to healing. In our experience absence of healing in three subsequent radiographs taken at monthly intervals after 3 months of injury reliably predict that healing will not occur without repeat intervention. If the patient is asymptomatic, further watchful waiting may be advised but the patient should be informed that the hardware is at risk of fatigue failure.

When planning the treatment of nonunions, infection should always be ruled out as a possible cause. In most instances a failure in the initial fixation mode can be observed and established as the likely cause for nonunion.[153] A careful assessment of forearm rotation and elbow and wrist range of motion is necessary to determine whether any malreduction is present. Comparative radiographs of the contralateral uninjured arm may provide additional useful information on the normal anatomy. Standard preparation of the forearm as well as the ipsilateral iliac crest should be performed in case autologous bone graft is required. Alternatively, the distal femur may be prepared for grafting from the lateral femoral condyle. Careful nonunion exposure should be performed under a bloodless field to reduce profuse bleeding frequently seen from scar tissue. Careful dissection is required to avoid iatrogenic injury to neurovascular structures. Once the fracture site is identified, hardware is removed and the underlying membrane tissue sent for culture. Soft tissue stripping should be kept to a minimum. The nonunion site is carefully debrided down to viable bone. In most instances bone grafting is not required and fixation may proceed following the standard principles for reduction and plate and screw application. In the presence of bone loss autologous iliac crest or lateral femoral condyle bone graft is harvested. Infected nonunions require excision of nonviable bone as described for deep infections. Intravenous antibiotic treatment and local antibiotic therapy may be used to achieve control of the infection. If soft tissue coverage is poor, soft tissue transfer may be indicated, followed by staged refixation and bone grafting.

Healing rates after surgical treatment of forearm nonunions have been reported to be as high as 100%. Kloen et al. reported on 47 patients with 51 forearm nonunions which were treated with ORIF alone in 30 cases, grafting alone in 7 cases, and a combination of ORIF and autologous bone grafting in 20 cases. All healed after a median of 7 months. Functional results were graded as excellent in 62%, satisfactory in 17%, and unsatisfactory in 21% of patients.[95] In a similar study, dos Reis et al. reported on compression plating and autologous bone grafting of 31 patients with forearm nonunions. All except one patient achieved bony healing at a mean of 3.5 months after surgery. Good functional outcome was reported in 26 patients (84%).[38] Ring et al. on the other hand reported on the use of ORIF and nonstructural autograft of nonunions with segmental defects. All of the 35 patients achieved bony union within 6 months of surgery. Functional outcomes were rated excellent in 5 patients, satisfactory in 18, unsatisfactory in 11, and poor in 1.[153] Less favorable outcomes have been reported for open intramedullary nailing of forearm nonunions. Hong et al.[77] reported almost 50% of unsatisfactory or failed results using this technique on 26 forearm nonunions.

Prasarn et al. reported on 15 patients operated over a 16-year period for infected nonunions of the forearm using a standard approach of debridement, definitive fixation after 7 to 14 days, tricortical iliac crest bone grafting for segmental defects, leaving wounds open to heal by secondary intention, 6 weeks of cultures, specific antibiotics, and early active range of motion exercises. All patients achieved bony healing in the absence of infection at a mean of 13 weeks.[143]

Radioulnar Synostosis

Complete radioulnar synostosis with a solid bony bridge occurs in 1% to 6% of forearm fractures.[4,65] Hadden et al. reported 6 patients with synostosis in a series of 108 patients with forearm fractures. All synostoses occurred in patients with a closed head injury.[65] Chapman et al. reported a single case of synostosis developing after operative treatment of forearm fractures in 88 patients. The affected patient had an associated closed head injury and had been treated with a 4.5-mm DCP plate for a Monteggia fracture. Haas et al. reported 2 patients who developed radioulnar synostosis out of 272 patients with forearm fractures treated using a minimal contact internal fixator. Both synostoses occurred in patients with high-energy fractures and required surgical release.[64]

Both-bone fractures affecting the radius and ulna at the same location in the forearm, along with significant comminution have been found to be associated with this complication.[4] When bone grafting is performed, care should be taken to avoid placement on the side of the interosseous membrane.[60]

According to Jupiter and Ring, proximal radioulnar synostosis can be classified as follows:

A. Distal to the bicipital groove

B. Involving the radial head on PRUJ

C. Extending to the distal aspect of the humerus

After simple excision of radioulnar synostosis in 18 patients, using an interposition fat graft in 8, the synostosis recurred in only one patient who had a closed head injury during the initial accident. Complications included one ulnar fracture, a broken pin from a hinged external fixator, and dislodgement of a fat graft. Final postoperative forearm rotation was on average 139 degrees in the 16 patients who did not have a recurrence.[91]

Nerve Palsy

The most frequently injured nerve during operative treatment of forearm fractures is the radial nerve or its terminal motor branch, the PIN. Anderson et al. reported on five PIN palsies, all of which occurred after proximal radius fixation through a posterior Thompson approach. Four palsies recovered within 4 weeks, whereas one required 6 months to fully recover.[4] Treatment of permanent nerve injury includes direct nerve repair and tendon transfers.[76] Occasionally, loss of flexor pollicis longus function can be noted after plating of the radius through the anterior approach. This is likely due to traction neurapraxia of the AIN, which commonly resolves with observation.[93]

Implant Removal and Re-Fracture

Less than 10% of plates require removal after ORIF of forearm fractures.[4] Ulnar plates are at the highest risk for ongoing symptoms because of the subcutaneous location of this bone (Fig. 33-29). Plates should therefore be placed either on the dorsal or volar aspect of this bone to allow some muscle coverage. Some patients describe recurrent deep pain at the surgical site, especially related to changes in the weather and temperature, associating this pain to the presence of surgical hardware. Removal of hardware should however not be performed without taking into account the several risks involved with this procedure. Re-fracture rates have been reported to be as high as 18%, with fractures occurring either through the original fracture site or through one of the empty screw holes.[4] Re-fracture through the original fracture site may be avoided by delaying hardware removal by 12 to 18 months and providing external protection in the form of a splint or prefabricated brace for 4 to 6 weeks.[4] Fractures through screw holes usually occur after a more severe injury and may occur several months after hardware removal.[75] Forearm fractures managed with 4.5-mm plates and screws are at higher risk for developing fractures through the screw holes. Early series using these implants reported re-fracture rates of 22% after removal, whereas some later series have shown no fracture after removal of 3.5-mm compression plates and screws.[27] Finally re-fractures may occur even in the presence of the original plate and screws These re-fractures usually occur through the most distal or most proximal screw hole after significant trauma.[101]

Several series have reported numerous complications that may occur after hardware removal. These include infection and nerve injury in up to 21% of cases. Additional costs should also be considered, as the hospital stay may range from 3 to 168 hours with associated absence from work averaging 3.4 weeks.[4,11,12,27,35,36,75,101,103,118,125,142,157,158,171,175]

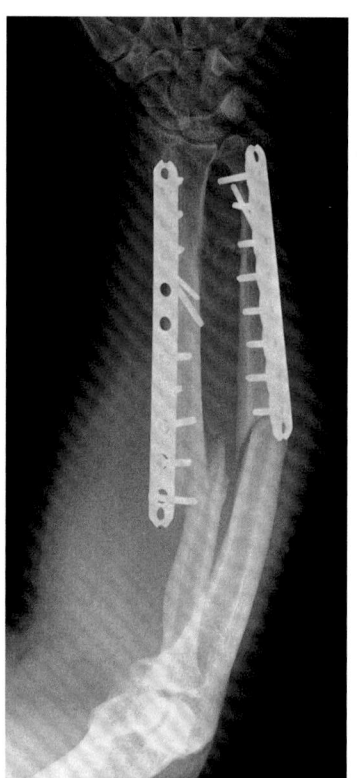 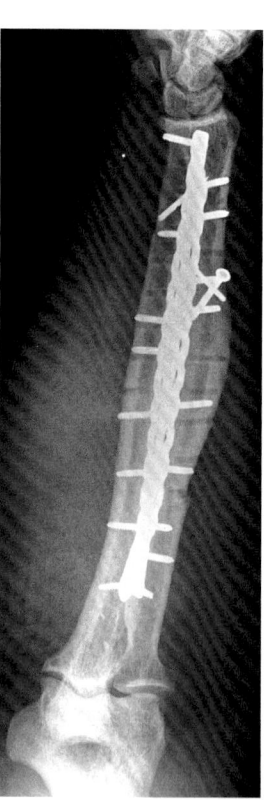 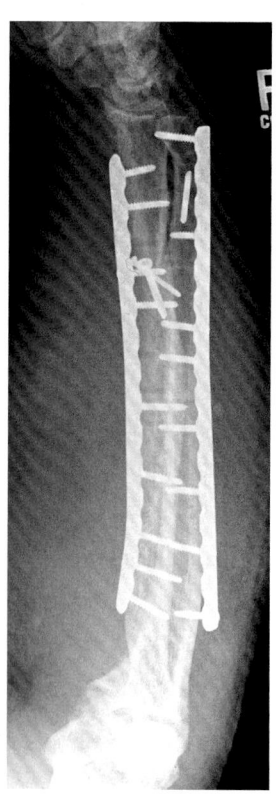

A, B   **C**

FIGURE 33-29 A: Peri-implant both-bone forearm fracture after a high-energy fall. Open reduction and internal fixation with plates and screws had been performed 3 years earlier. **B and C:** Long plates were used for both the radius and ulna to stabilize the fracture and splint the potential weak point of screw holes from the previous construct.

Acute Compartment Syndrome

Compartment syndrome of the forearm is a potentially devastating complication of radial and ulna shaft fractures. The incidence of forearm compartment syndrome is 2% after ORIF.[107] Compartment syndrome most frequently affects the anterior compartment of the leg, followed by the volar compartment of the forearm.[40,55,56] Young men are at especially high risk for developing this complication. A high level of suspicion should be present for this complication, even in fractures caused by seemingly minor trauma. We recommend overnight admission for patients undergoing surgical fixation of these fractures. In the presence of increased suspicion, intracompartmental monitoring should be performed. Emergent compartment release should be performed, if required, to reduce the risk of additional complications.[40,116] A curvilinear volar incision and a straight dorsal incision provide adequate access to forearm compartments for their release.[55] A detailed discussion of acute compartment syndrome is provided in Chapter 29.

AUTHOR'S PREFERRED TREATMENT FOR DIAPHYSEAL FRACTURES OF THE RADIUS AND ULNA

With the patient supine and a nonsterile tourniquet on the arm, radial fractures are exposed through a volar approach for distal half to distal two-third fractures, whereas proximal third fractures are exposed via a dorsal Thompson approach. The ulna is exposed through a standard ulnar approach. The tourniquet is not routinely inflated to reduce postoperative pain and the theoretical risk of reperfusion edema, especially in longer cases. In both-bone forearm fractures, the less comminuted fracture is exposed and fixed first, followed by exposure of the other bone. This allows realignment not only of the fracture but also of the soft tissues, thereby improving orientation during exposure. Forearm shaft fractures are treated almost without exception with nonlocking plate and screw fixation using 3.5 mm implants. Dynamic plate compression, lag screw fixation with neutralization plating, and bridge plating are used according to the fracture geometry. A total of three bicortical screws are used as the norm, proximal and distal to the fracture site (Fig. 33-30). For fractures of the distal or proximal ends of the ulna or radius precontoured plates or smaller implants may be required (Figs. 33-24 and 33-31). Examination of the DRUJ and PRUJ for instability is performed once definitive stabilization has been achieved. Full pronation supination and elbow and wrist flexion–extension should be present as well.

Monteggia fractures are approached with the patient supine, a nonsterile tourniquet on the arm, and the upper extremity placed over the patient's chest during exposure. This is the

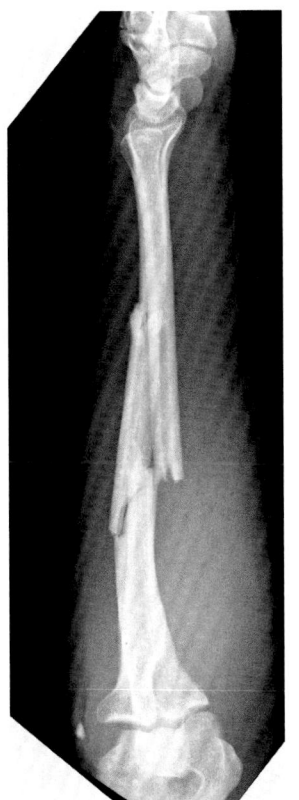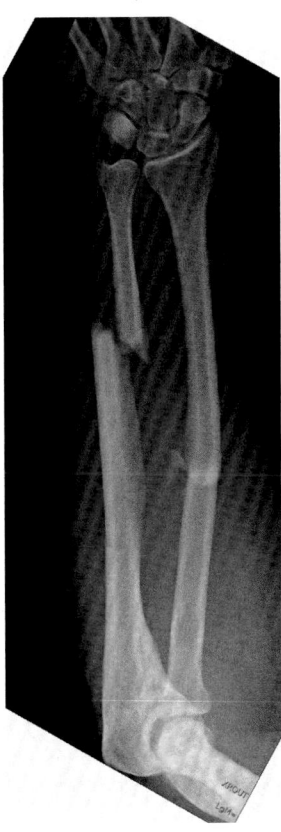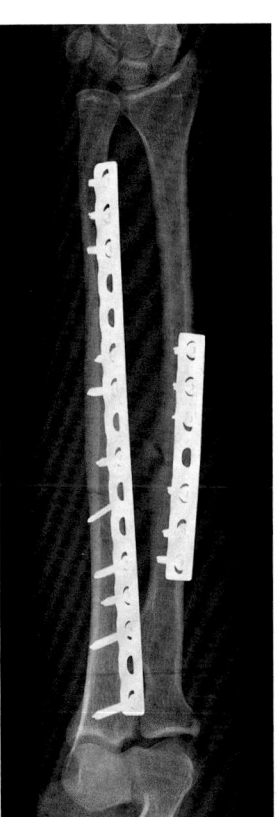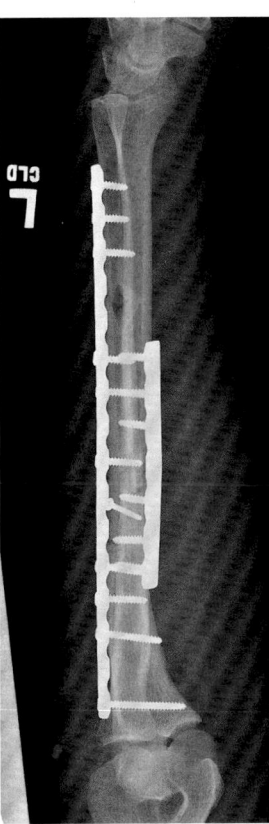

A, B   **C, D**

FIGURE 33-30 A and B: Both-bone forearm fracture with segmental component of the ulna. **C and D:** A single long plate was used for the ulna. Fixation was obtained to a minimum of six cortices on each end of the fracture.

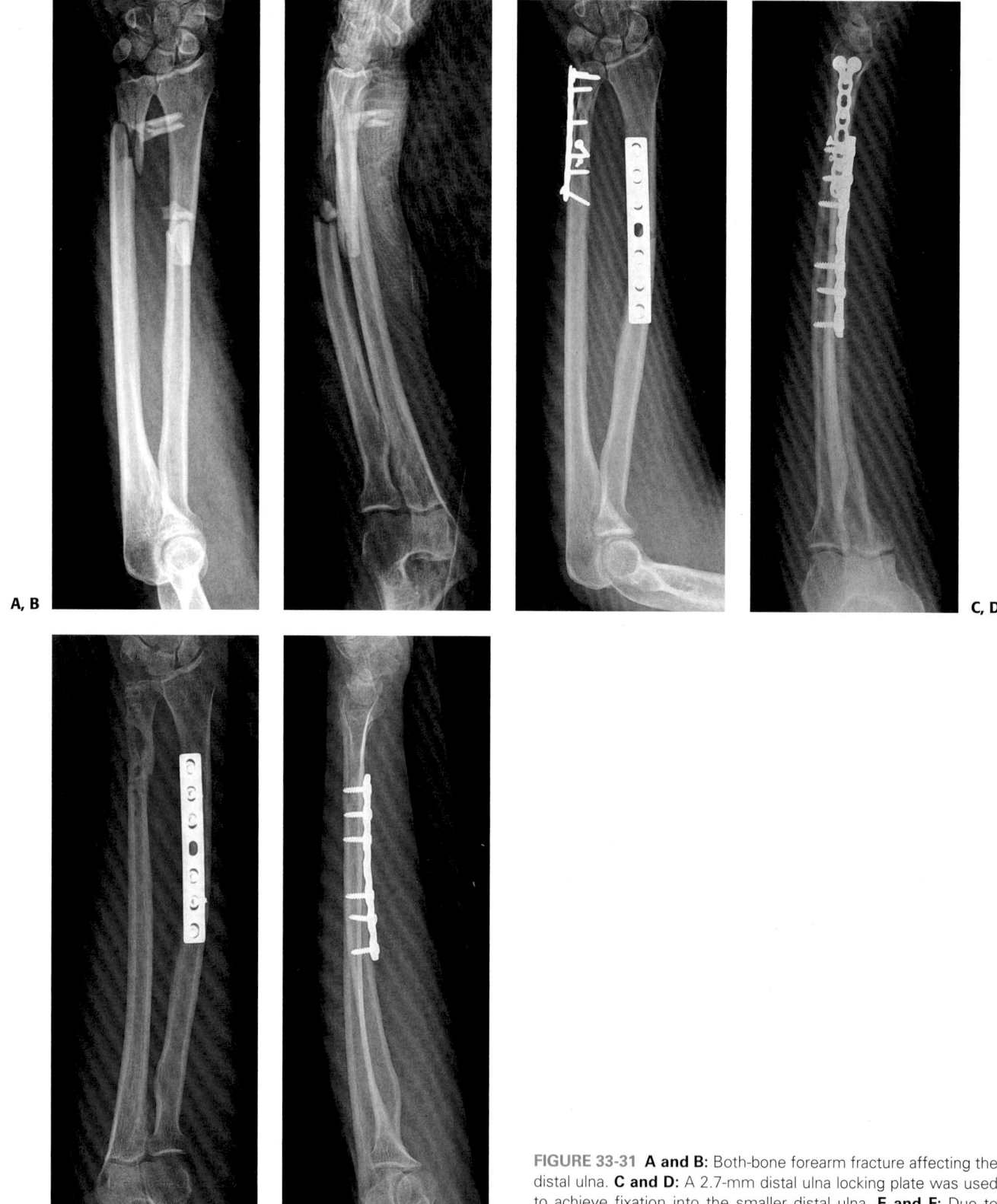

A, B

C, D

E

F

FIGURE 33-31 A and B: Both-bone forearm fracture affecting the distal ulna. **C and D:** A 2.7-mm distal ulna locking plate was used to achieve fixation into the smaller distal ulna. **E and F:** Due to symptoms, the ulnar plate was removed once healing had been achieved.

routine position for all elbow-related injuries, thereby standardizing anatomic orientation. This is of special importance when associated injuries to the proximal ulna or radius have to be addressed. In simple Monteggia fractures involving only the ulnar shaft fracture, a posterior approach is selected. An incision directly over the olecranon tip is avoided with the incision being directed radially at the level of the olecranon and redirected centrally more proximally. If the fracture affects the proximal ulnar metaphysis a proximal ulna plate is selected. Otherwise, a standard 3.5-mm plate is used and contoured as required. Care is taken not to penetrate the articular surface when proximal screws are placed. Once provisional fixation after anatomic ulnar reduction has been achieved, adequate reduction of the PRUJ is fluoroscopically confirmed. Final screw placement is then performed and the elbow checked for full elbow flexion–extension and forearm rotation. Careful examination of the DRUJ is also performed at this point.

Galeazzi fracture dislocations are addressed in a similar manner to radial shaft fractures in both-bone forearm fractures. Once anatomic reduction of the radius has been achieved, the DRUJ is examined. If reduction is not obtained or a "spongy" reduction is palpated, soft tissue interposition is suspected and the DRUJ exposed. At this point repair of the TFCC may be performed. If the DRUJ continues to be unstable after reduction of the radial shaft fracture, DRUJ translation is examined at different positions of forearm rotation. The position that allows the least amount of translation is selected and two 2 mm Kirschner wires are placed from the ulna into the radius. The most distal pin is placed just proximal to the distal ulnar facet of the radius. The second pin is placed 1 cm proximal to the first pin. Pins are then bent and cut and the forearm immobilized in a long arm splint without changing forearm rotation.

SUMMARY, CONTROVERSIES, AND FUTURE DIRECTIONS IN DIAPHYSEAL FRACTURES OF THE RADIUS AND ULNA

ORIF with nonlocking plate and screw fixation of forearm shaft fractures achieves a high rate of union and satisfactory functional outcomes. Although other treatment modalities, including locking plate fixation and intramedullary nailing have been extensively studied, no advantage has been shown over conventional screws and plates. External fixation is required in only rare exceptional circumstances.

Outcomes after forearm shaft fractures depend on adequate restoration of the relationship between the ulna and radius to allow unrestricted forearm rotation and elbow and wrist flexion extension. Whereas bony geometry is a key aspect to restoring forearm function, identification and appropriate management of instability of the proximal and distal radioulnar joints is essential to achieve good outcomes. High-energy fractures with associated injuries to the proximal ulna and radius and disruption of the soft tissue sleeve continue to pose a challenge, as they are related to higher rates of complications and poorer outcomes.

REFERENCES

1. Adams BD, Berger RA. An anatomic reconstruction of the distal radioulnar ligaments for posttraumatic distal radioulnar joint instability. *J Hand Surg Am.* 2002;27(2):243–251.
2. Alexander AH, Lichtman DM. Irreducible distal radioulnar joint occurring in a Galeazzi fracture—case report. *J Hand Surg Am.* 1981;6(3):258–261.
3. Alffram PA, Bauer GC. Epidemiology of fractures of the forearm. A biomechanical investigation of bone strength. *J Bone Joint Surg Am.* 1962;44-A:105–114.
4. Anderson LD, et al. Compression-plate fixation in acute diaphyseal fractures of the radius and ulna. *J Bone Joint Surg Am.* 1975;57(3):287–297.
5. Arenas AJ, et al. Anterior interosseous nerve injury associated with a Monteggia fracture-dislocation. *Acta Orthop Belg.* 2001;67(1):77–80.
6. Atesok KI, Jupiter JB, Weiss AP. Galeazzi fracture. *J Am Acad Orthop Surg.* 2011;19(10):623–633.
7. Atkin DM, et al. Treatment of ulnar shaft fractures: a prospective, randomized study. *Orthopedics.* 1995;18(6):543–547.
8. Aulicino PL, Siegel JL. Acute injuries of the distal radioulnar joint. *Hand Clin.* 1991;7(2):283–293.
9. Bado JL. The Monteggia lesion. *Clin Orthop Relat Res.* 1967;50:71–86.
10. Bansal H. Intramedullary fixation of forearm fractures with new locked nail. *Indian J Orthop.* 2011;45(5):410–416.
11. Beaupre GS, Csongradi JJ. Refracture risk after plate removal in the forearm. *J Orthop Trauma.* 1996;10(2):87–92.
12. Bednar DA, Grandwilewski W. Complications of forearm-plate removal. *Can J Surg.* 1992;35(4):428–431.
13. Behnke NM, et al. Internal fixation of diaphyseal fractures of the forearm: a retrospective comparison of hybrid fixation versus dual plating. *J Orthop Trauma.* 2012;26(11):611–616.
14. Bengner U, Johnell O. Increasing incidence of forearm fractures. A comparison of epidemiologic patterns 25 years apart. *Acta Orthop Scand.* 1985;56(2):158–160.
15. Bhan S, Rath S. Management of the Galeazzi fracture. *Int Orthop.* 1991;15(3):193–196.
16. Bindra RR, et al. Quantification of the radial torsion angle with computerized tomography in cadaver specimens. *J Bone Joint Surg Am.* 1997;79(6):833–837.
17. Biyani A, Bhan S. Dual extensor tendon entrapment in Galeazzi fracture-dislocation: a case report. *J Trauma.* 1989;29(9):1295–1297.
18. Biyani A, Olscamp AJ, Ebraheim NA. Complications in the management of complex Monteggia-equivalent fractures in adults. *Am J Orthop (Belle Mead NJ).* 2000;29(2):115–118.
19. Bolton H, Quinlan AG. The conservative treatment of fractures of the shaft of the radius and ulna in adults. *Lancet.* 1952;2(6737):700–705.
20. Bot AG, et al. Long-term outcomes of fractures of both bones of the forearm. *J Bone Joint Surg Am.* 2011;93(6):527–532.
21. Boyd HB. Surgical exposure of the ulna and proximal third of the radius through one incision. *Surg Gynecol Obstet.* 1940;71:86–88.
22. Brakenbury PH, Corea JR, Blakemore ME. Non-union of the isolated fracture of the ulnar shaft in adults. *Injury.* 1981;12(5):371–375.
23. Bruckner JD, Lichtman DM, Alexander AH. Complex dislocations of the distal radioulnar joint. Recognition and management. *Clin Orthop Relat Res.* 1992;(275):90–103.
24. Bryan RS. Monteggia fracture of the forearm. *J Trauma.* 1971;11(12):992–998.
25. Burwell HN, Charnley AD. Treatment of forearm fractures in adults with particular reference to plate fixation. *J Bone Joint Surg Br.* 1964;46:404–425.
26. Cetti NE. An unusual cause of blocked reduction of the Galeazzi injury. *Injury.* 1977;9(1):59–61.
27. Chapman MW, Gordon JE, Zissimos AG. Compression-plate fixation of acute fractures of the diaphyses of the radius and ulna. *J Bone Joint Surg Am.* 1989;71(2):159–169.
28. Chung KC, Spilson SV. The frequency and epidemiology of hand and forearm fractures in the United States. *J Hand Surg Am.* 2001;26(5):908–915.
29. Cohen MS, et al. Lateral epicondylitis: anatomic relationships of the extensor tendon origins and implications for arthroscopic treatment. *J Shoulder Elbow Surg.* 2008;17(6):954–960.
30. Corea JR, Brakenbury PH, Blakemore ME. The treatment of isolated fractures of the ulnar shaft in adults. *Injury.* 1981;12(5):365–370.
31. Crenshaw AH, Zinar DM, Pickering RM. Intramedullary nailing of forearm fractures. *Instr Course Lect.* 2002;51:279–289.
32. Crow BD, Mundis G, Anglen JO. Clinical results of minimal screw plate fixation of forearm fractures. *Am J Orthop (Belle Mead NJ).* 2007;36(9):477–480.
33. De Boeck H, et al. Treatment of isolated distal ulnar shaft fractures with below-elbow plaster cast. A prospective study. *Arch Orthop Trauma Surg.* 1996;115(6):316–320.
34. de Jong Ta, de Jong PCM. Ulnar-shaft fracture needs no treatment A pilot study of 10 cases. *Acta Orthop Scand.* 1989;60(3):263–264.
35. Deluca PA, Lindsey RW, Ruwe PA. Refracture of bones of the forearm after the removal of compression plates. *J Bone Joint Surg Am.* 1988;70(9):1372–1376.
36. Dodge HS, Cady GW. Treatment of fractures of the radius and ulna with compression plates. *J Bone Joint Surg Am.* 1972;54(6):1167–1176.
37. Domingo A, et al. Elbow dislocations associated with ipsilateral radial shaft fractures: a case report and review of the literature. *J Trauma.* 2008;64(1):221–224.
38. dos Reis FB, et al. Outcome of diaphyseal forearm fracture-nonunions treated by autologous bone grafting and compression plating. *Ann Surg Innov Res.* 2009;3:5.
39. Droll KP, et al. Outcomes following plate fixation of fractures of both bones of the forearm in adults. *J Bone Joint Surg Am.* 2007;89(12):2619–2624.
40. Duckworth AD, et al. Acute compartment syndrome of the forearm. *J Bone Joint Surg Am.* 2012;94(10):e63.
41. Duncan R, et al. Immediate internal fixation of open fractures of the diaphysis of the forearm. *J Orthop Trauma.* 1992;6(1):25–31.
42. Dymond IW. The treatment of isolated fractures of the distal ulna. *J Bone Joint Surg Br.* 1984;66(3):408–410.

43. Eathiraju S, Mudgal CS, Jupiter JB. Monteggia fracture-dislocations. *Hand Clin.* 2007;23(2):165–177, v.
44. Egol KA, et al. Does a Monteggia variant lesion result in a poor functional outcome?: A retrospective study. *Clin Orthop Relat Res.* 2005;438:233–238.
45. ElMaraghy AW, et al. Influence of the number of cortices on the stiffness of plate fixation of diaphyseal fractures. *J Orthop Trauma.* 2001;15(3):186–191.
46. Evans EM. Rotational deformity in the treatment of fractures of both bones of the forearm. *The Journal of Bone & Joint Surgery.* 1945;27(3):373–379.
47. Failla JM, Jacobson J, van Holsbeeck M. Ultrasound diagnosis and surgical pathology of the torn interosseous membrane in forearm fractures/dislocations. *J Hand Surg Am.* 1999;24(2):257–266.
48. Fernandez Dell' Oca AA, Masliah Galante R. Osteosynthesis of diaphyseal fractures of the radius and ulna using an internal fixator (PC-Fix). A prospective study. *Injury.* 2001;32(Suppl 2):B44–B50.
49. Fernandez Dell'Oca AA, et al. Treating forearm fractures using an internal fixator: a prospective study. *Clin Orthop Relat Res.* 2001;(389):196–205.
50. Ferreira N, Marais LC. Prevention and management of external fixator pin track sepsis. *Strategies Trauma Limb Reconstr.* 2012;7(2):67–72.
51. Galeazzi R. Über ein besonderes Syndrom bei Verletzungen im Bereich der Unterarmknochen. *Arch Orthop Unfallchir.* 1935;35:557–562.
52. Gao H, et al. Internal fixation of diaphyseal fractures of the forearm by interlocking intramedullary nail: short-term results in eighteen patients. *J Orthop Trauma.* 2005;19(6):384–391.
53. Gausepohl T, et al. The anatomical base of unilateral external fixation in the upper limb. *Injury.* 2000;31(Suppl 1):11–20.
54. Gebuhr P, et al. Isolated ulnar shaft fractures. Comparison of treatment by a functional brace and long-arm cast. *J Bone Joint Surg Br.* 1992;74(5):757–759.
55. Gelberman RH, et al. Compartment syndromes of the forearm: diagnosis and treatment. *Clin Orthop Relat Res.* 1981;(161):252–261.
56. Ghobrial TF, Eglseder WA Jr, Bleckner SA. Proximal ulna shaft fractures and associated compartment syndromes. *Am J Orthop (Belle Mead NJ).* 2001;30(9):703–707.
57. Giannoulis FS, Sotereanos DG. Galeazzi fractures and dislocations. *Hand Clin.* 2007;23(2):153–163, v.
58. Givon U, et al. Monteggia and equivalent lesions. A study of 41 cases. *Clin Orthop Relat Res.* 1997;(337):208–215.
59. Goldfarb CA, et al. Functional outcome after fracture of both bones of the forearm. *J Bone Joint Surg Br.* 2005;87(3):374–379.
60. Grace TG, Eversmann WW Jr. Forearm fractures: treatment by rigid fixation with early motion. *J Bone Joint Surg Am.* 1980;62(3):433–438.
61. Gustilo RB, Anderson JT. Prevention of infection in the treatment of one thousand and twenty-five open fractures of long bones: retrospective and prospective analyses. *J Bone Joint Surg Am.* 1976;58(4):453–458.
62. Gustilo RB, Mendoza RM, Williams DN. Problems in the management of type III (severe) open fractures: a new classification of type III open fractures. *J Trauma.* 1984;24(8):742–746.
63. Gwinn DE, O'Toole RV, Eglseder WA. Early motion protocol for select Galeazzi fractures after radial shaft fixation. *J Surg Orthop Adv.* 2010;19(2):104–108.
64. Haas N, et al. Treatment of diaphyseal fractures of the forearm using the Point Contact Fixator (PC-Fix): results of 387 fractures of a prospective multicentric study (PC-Fix II). *Injury.* 2001;32(Suppl 2):B51–B62.
65. Hadden WA, Reschauer R, Seggl W. Results of AO plate fixation of forearm shaft fractures in adults. *Injury.* 1983;15(1):44–52.
66. Hagert CG. The distal radioulnar joint in relation to the whole forearm. *Clin Orthop Relat Res.* 1992;(275):56–64.
67. Hagert CG. Distal radius fracture and the distal radioulnar joint–anatomical considerations. *Handchir Mikrochir Plast Chir.* 1994;26(1):22–26.
68. Hagert E, Hagert CG. Understanding stability of the distal radioulnar joint through an understanding of its anatomy. *Hand Clin.* 2010;26(4):459–466.
69. Handoll HH, Pearce P. Interventions for treating isolated diaphyseal fractures of the ulna in adults. *Cochrane Database Syst Rev.* 2012;6:CD000523.
70. Hanel DP, Scheid DK. Irreducible fracture-dislocation of the distal radioulnar joint secondary to entrapment of the extensor carpi ulnaris tendon. *Clin Orthop Relat Res.* 1988(234):56–60.
71. Henle P, et al. Problems of bridging plate fixation for the treatment of forearm shaft fractures with the locking compression plate. *Arch Orthop Trauma Surg.* 2011;131(1):85–91.
72. Henry AK. *Extensile exposure applied to limb surgery.* Second ed. 1973, Edinburgh: Churchill Livingstone.
73. Hertel R, et al. Plate osteosynthesis of diaphyseal fractures of the radius and ulna. *Injury.* 1996;27(8):545–548.
74. Hertel R, et al. Biomechanical and biological considerations relating to the clinical use of the Point Contact-Fixator–evaluation of the device handling test in the treatment of diaphyseal fractures of the radius and/or ulna. *Injury.* 2001;32(Suppl 2):B10–B14.
75. Hidaka S, Gustilo RB. Refracture of bones of the forearm after plate removal. *J Bone Joint Surg Am.* 1984;66(8):1241–1243.
76. Hirachi K, et al. Clinical features and management of traumatic posterior interosseous nerve palsy. *J Hand Surg Br.* 1998;23(3):413–417.
77. Hong G, et al. Treatment of diaphyseal forearm nonunions with interlocking intramedullary nails. *Clin Orthop Relat Res.* 2006;450:186–192.
78. Hoppenfeld S, deBoer P, Buckley R. *Surgical Exposures in Orthopaedics: The Anatomic Approach.* 4th ed. Philadelphia, PA: Lippincott Williams and Wilkins; 2009.
79. Hotchkiss RN, et al. An anatomic and mechanical study of the interosseous membrane of the forearm: pathomechanics of proximal migration of the radius. *J Hand Surg Am.* 1989;14(2 Pt 1):256–261.
80. Huang JI, Hanel DP. Anatomy and biomechanics of the distal radioulnar joint. *Hand Clin.* 2012;28(2):157–163.
81. Hudak PL, Amadio PC, Bombardier C. Development of an upper extremity outcome measure: the DASH (disabilities of the arm, shoulder and hand) [corrected]. The Upper Extremity Collaborative Group (UECG). *Am J Ind Med.* 1996;29(6):602–608.
82. Hughston JC. Fracture of the distal radial shaft; mistakes in management. *J Bone Joint Surg Am.* 1957;39-A(2):249–264; passim.
83. Hung SC, et al. Monteggia type I equivalent lesion: diaphyseal ulna and radius fractures with a posterior elbow dislocation in an adult. *Arch Orthop Trauma Surg.* 2003;123(6):311–313.
84. Itoh Y, et al. Extensor tendon involvement in Smith's and Galeazzi's fractures. *J Hand Surg Am.* 1987;12(4):535–540.
85. Jaeblon TD. A case of ipsilateral both bone forearm fracture and acute distal biceps rupture. *J Orthop Trauma.* 2011;25(11):e104–e106.
86. Jenkins NH, Mintowt-Czyz WJ, Fairclough JA. Irreducible dislocation of the distal radioulnar joint. *Injury.* 1987;18(1):40–43.
87. Johnston SA, et al. A biomechanical comparison of 7-hole 3.5 mm broad and 5-hole 4.5 mm narrow dynamic compression plates. *Vet Surg.* 1991;20(4):235–239.
88. Johnstone DJ, Radford WJ, Parnell EJ. Interobserver variation using the AO/ASIF classification of long bone fractures. *Injury.* 1993;24(3):163–165.
89. Jones JA. Immediate internal fixation of high-energy open forearm fractures. *J Orthop Trauma.* 1991;5(3):272–279.
90. Jonsson B, et al. Forearm fractures in Malmo, Sweden. Changes in the incidence occurring during the 1950s, 1980s and 1990s. *Acta Orthop Scand.* 1999;70(2):129–132.
91. Jupiter JB Ring D. Operative treatment of post-traumatic proximal radioulnar synostosis. *J Bone Joint Surg Am.* 1998;80(2):248–257.
92. Jupiter JB, et al. The posterior Monteggia lesion. *J Orthop Trauma.* 1991;5(4):395–402.
93. Keogh P, Khan H, Cooke E, et al. Loss of flexor pollicis longus function after plating of the radius. Report of six cases. *J Hand Surg Br.* 1997;22:375–376.
94. Kikuchi Y, Nakamura T. Irreducible Galeazzi fracture-dislocation due to an avulsion fracture of the fovea of the ulna. *J Hand Surg Br.* 1999;24(3):379–381.
95. Kloen P, Wiggers JK, Buijze GA. Treatment of diaphyseal non-unions of the ulna and radius. *Arch Orthop Trauma Surg.* 2010;130(12):1439–1445.
96. Knight RA, Purvis GD. Fractures of both bones of the forearm in adults. *J Bone Joint Surg Am.* 1949;31A(4):755–764.
97. Korner J, et al. [Monteggia injuries in adults: Critical analysis of injury pattern, management, and results]. *Unfallchirurg.* 2004;107(11):1026–1040.
98. Korompilias AV, et al. Distal radioulnar joint instability (Galeazzi type injury) after internal fixation in relation to the radius fracture pattern. *J Hand Surg Am.* 2011;36(5):847–852.
99. Kose O, Durakbasa MO, Islam NC. Posterolateral elbow dislocation with ipsilateral radial and ulnar diaphyseal fractures: a case report. *J Orthop Surg (Hong Kong).* 2008;16(1):122–123.
100. Kraus B, Horne G. Galeazzi fractures. *J Trauma.* 1985;25(11):1093–1095.
101. Labosky DA, Cermak MB, Waggy CA. Forearm fracture plates: to remove or not to remove. *J Hand Surg Am.* 1990;15(2):294–301.
102. Lambrinudi C. Intra-medullary Kirschner Wires in the Treatment of Fractures: (Section of Orthopaedics). *Proc R Soc Med.* 1940;33(3):153–157.
103. Langkamer VG, Ackroyd CE. Removal of forearm plates. A review of the complications. *J Bone Joint Surg Br.* 1990;72(4):601–604.
104. Langkamer VG, Ackroyd CE. Internal fixation of forearm fractures in the 1980s: lessons to be learnt. *Injury.* 1991;22(2):97–102.
105. Lee YH, et al. Interlocking contoured intramedullary nail fixation for selected diaphyseal fractures of the forearm in adults. *J Bone Joint Surg Am.* 2008;90(9):1891–1898.
106. Lenihan MR, et al. Fractures of the forearm resulting from low-velocity gunshot wounds. *J Orthop Trauma.* 1992;6(1):32–35.
107. Leung F, Chow SP. A prospective, randomized trial comparing the limited contact dynamic compression plate with the point contact fixator for forearm fractures. *J Bone Joint Surg Am.* 2003;85-A(12):2343–2348.
108. Leung F, Chow SP. Locking compression plate in the treatment of forearm fractures: a prospective study. *J Orthop Surg (Hong Kong).* 2006;14(3):291–294.
109. Lindvall EM, Sagi HC. Selective screw placement in forearm compression plating: results of 75 consecutive fractures stabilized with 4 cortices of screw fixation on either side of the fracture. *J Orthop Trauma.* 2006;20(3):157–162; discussion 162-3.
110. Linscheid RL. Biomechanics of the distal radioulnar joint. *Clin Orthop Relat Res.* 1992;(275):46–55.
111. Llusa Perez M, et al. Monteggia fractures in adults. Review of 54 cases. *Chir Main.* 2002;21(5):293–297.
112. Macule Beneyto F, et al. Treatment of Galeazzi fracture-dislocations. *J Trauma.* 1994;36(3):352–355.
113. Malecki P, et al. [Results of treating forearm bone shaft fractures with a 3.5 mm self compressive plate]. *Chir Narzadow Ruchu Ortop Pol.* 1997;62(5):393–399.
114. Marsh JL, et al. Fracture and dislocation classification compendium - 2007: Orthopaedic Trauma Association classification, database and outcomes committee. *J Orthop Trauma.* 2007;21(10 Suppl):S1–S133.
115. Matthews LS, et al. The effect on supination-pronation of angular malalignment of fractures of both bones of the forearm. *J Bone Joint Surg Am.* 1982;64(1):14–17.
116. McQueen MM, Gaston P, Court-Brown CM. Acute compartment syndrome. Who is at risk? *J Bone Joint Surg Br.* 2000;82(2):200–203.
117. Mestdagh H, et al. Long-term results in the treatment of fracture-dislocations of Galeazzi in adults. Report on twenty-nine cases. *Ann Chir Main.* 1983;2(2):125–133.
118. Mih AD, et al. Long-term follow-up of forearm bone diaphyseal plating. *Clin Orthop Relat Res.* 1994;(299):256–258.
119. Mikek M, et al. Fracture-related and implant-specific factors influencing treatment results of comminuted diaphyseal forearm fractures without bone grafting. *Arch Orthop Trauma Surg.* 2004;124(6):393–400.
120. Mikic ZD. Galeazzi fracture-dislocations. *J Bone Joint Surg Am.* 1975;57(8):1071–1080.
121. Mikic ZD. Treatment of acute injuries of the triangular fibrocartilage complex associated with distal radioulnar joint instability. *J Hand Surg Am.* 1995;20(2):319–323.
122. Moed BR, et al. Immediate internal fixation of open fractures of the diaphysis of the forearm. *J Bone Joint Surg Am.* 1986;68(7):1008–1017.
123. Moerman J, et al., Intramedullary fixation of forearm fractures in adults. *Acta Orthop Belg.* 1996;62(1):34–40.
124. Mohan K, et al. Internal fixation in 50 cases of Galeazzi fracture. *Acta Orthop Scand.* 1988;59(3):318–320.

125. Moore TM, et al. Results of compression-plating of closed Galeazzi fractures. *J Bone Joint Surg Am.* 1985;67(7):1015–1021.

126. Moore TM, Lester DK, Sarmiento A. The stabilizing effect of soft-tissue constraints in artificial Galeazzi fractures. *Clin Orthop Relat Res.* 1985;(194):189–194.

127. Moss JP, Bynum DK. Diaphyseal fractures of the radius and ulna in adults. *Hand Clin.* 2007;23(2):143–151, v.

128. Newey ML, Ricketts D, Roberts L. The AO classification of long bone fractures: an early study of its use in clinical practice. *Injury.* 1993;24(5):309–312.

129. Nishikawa S, Toh S. Anatomical study of the carpal attachment of the triangular fibrocartilage complex. *J Bone Joint Surg Br.* 2002;84(7):1062–1065.

130. Noda K, et al. Interosseous membrane of the forearm: an anatomical study of ligament attachment locations. *J Hand Surg Am.* 2009;34(3):415–422.

131. Nordqvist A, Petersson CJ. Incidence and causes of shoulder girdle injuries in an urban population. *J Shoulder Elbow Surg.* 1995;4(2):107–112.

132. Oberlander MA, Seidman GD, Whitelaw GP. Treatment of isolated ulnar shaft fractures with functional bracing. *Orthopedics.* 1993;16(1):29–32.

133. Omeroglu H, et al. The effect of using a tourniquet on the intensity of postoperative pain in forearm fractures. A randomized study in 32 surgically treated patients. *Int Orthop.* 1998;22(6):369–373.

134. Ostermann PA, et al. Bracing of stable shaft fractures of the ulna. *J Orthop Trauma.* 1994;8(3):245–248.

135. Ozkaya U, et al. [Comparison between locked intramedullary nailing and plate osteosynthesis in the management of adult forearm fractures]. *Acta Orthop Traumatol Turc.* 2009;43(1):14–20.

136. Paley D, Rubenstein J, McMurtry RY. Irreducible dislocation of distal radial ulnar joint. *Orthop Rev.* 1986;15(4):228–231.

137. Palmer AK, Werner FW. The triangular fibrocartilage complex of the wrist–anatomy and function. *J Hand Surg Am.* 1981;6(2):153–162.

138. Patrick J. A study of supination and pronation, with especial reference to the treatment of forearm fractures. *J Bone Joint Surg Am.* 1946;28(4):737–748.

139. Pavel A, et al. The posterior monteggia fracture: a clinical study. *J Trauma.* 1965;5:185–199.

140. Penrose JH. The Monteggia fracture with posterior dislocation of the radial head. *J Bone Joint Surg Br.* 1951;33-B(1):65–73.

141. Pollock FH, et al. The isolated fracture of the ulnar shaft. Treatment without immobilization. *J Bone Joint Surg Am.* 1983;65(3):339–342.

142. Pomerance J. Plate removal after ulnar-shortening osteotomy. *J Hand Surg Am.* 2005;30(5):949–953.

143. Prasarn ML, Ouellette EA, Miller DR. Infected nonunions of diaphyseal fractures of the forearm. *Arch Orthop Trauma Surg.* 2010;130(7):867–873.

144. Ramesh S, Lim YJ. Complex elbow dislocation associated with radial and ulnar diaphyseal fractures: a rare combination. *Strategies Trauma Limb Reconstr.* 2011;6(2):97–101.

145. Reckling FW. Unstable fracture-dislocations of the forearm (Monteggia and Galeazzi lesions). *J Bone Joint Surg Am.* 1982;64(6):857–863.

146. Rettig ME, Raskin KB. Galeazzi fracture-dislocation: a new treatment-oriented classification. *J Hand Surg Am.* 2001;26(2):228–235.

147. Reynders P, et al. Monteggia lesions in adults. A multicenter Bota study. *Acta Orthop Belg.* 1996;62(Suppl 1):78–83.

148. Richard MJ, Ruch DS, Aldridge JM 3rd. Malunions and nonunions of the forearm. *Hand Clin.* 2007;23(2):235–243, vii.

149. Richter M, et al. Upper extremity fractures in restrained front-seat occupants. *J Trauma.* 2000;48(5):907–912.

150. Ring D. Be skeptical. Be cautious. *J Orthop Trauma.* 2006;20(3):162–163.

151. Ring D, Jupiter JB, Simpson NS. Monteggia fractures in adults. *J Bone Joint Surg Am.* 1998;80(12):1733–1744.

152. Ring D, Waters PM. Operative fixation of Monteggia fractures in children. *J Bone Joint Surg Br.* 1996;78(5):734–739.

153. Ring D, et al. Ununited diaphyseal forearm fractures with segmental defects: plate fixation and autogenous cancellous bone-grafting. *J Bone Joint Surg Am.* 2004;86-A(11):2440–2445.

154. Ring D, et al. Comminuted diaphyseal fractures of the radius and ulna: does bone grafting affect nonunion rate? *J Trauma.* 2005;59(2):438–441; discussion 442.

155. Ring D, et al. Isolated radial shaft fractures are more common than Galeazzi fractures. *J Hand Surg Am.* 2006;31(1):17–21.

156. Ross ER, et al. Retrospective analysis of plate fixation of diaphyseal fractures of the forearm bones. *Injury.* 1989;20(4):211–214.

157. Rosson JW, Shearer JR. Refracture after the removal of plates from the forearm. An avoidable complication. *J Bone Joint Surg Br.* 1991;73(3):415–417.

158. Rumball K, Finnegan M. Refractures after forearm plate removal. *J Orthop Trauma.* 1990;4(2):124–129.

159. Rush LV, Rush HL. A technique for longitudinal pin fixation of certain fractures of the ulna and of the femur. *The Journal of Bone & Joint Surgery.* 1939;21(3):619–626.

160. Rush LV, Rush HL. The technique of longitudinal pin fixation of fractures of the forearm. *Miss Doct.* 1949;27(6):284–288.

161. Sage FP. Medullary fixation of fractures of the forearm. A study of the medullary canal of the radius and a report of fifty fractures of the radius treated with a prebent triangular nail. *J Bone Joint Surg Am.* 1959;41-A:1489–1516.

162. Sahlin Y. Occurrence of fractures in a defined population: a 1-year study. *Injury.* 1990;21(3):158–160.

163. Saikia K, et al. Internal fixation of fractures of both bones forearm: Comparison of locked compression and limited contact dynamic compression plate. *Indian J Orthop.* 2011;45(5):417–421.

164. Salai M, et al. [Closed intramedullary nailing of forearm fractures in young patients]. *Harefuah.* 1998;134(2):106–108, 158-9.

165. Sanders R, et al. Minimal versus maximal plate fixation techniques of the ulna: the biomechanical effect of number of screws and plate length. *J Orthop Trauma.* 2002;16(3):166–171.

166. Sargent JP, Teipner WA. Treatment of forearm shaft fractures by double-plating; a preliminary report. *J Bone Joint Surg Am.* 1965;47(8):1475–1490.

167. Sarmiento A, Cooper JS, Sinclair WF. Forearm fractures. Early functional bracing—A preliminary report. *J Bone Joint Surg Am.* 1975;57(3):297–304.

168. Sarmiento A, Latta LL. *Functional bracing of diaphyseal ulnar fractures, in Functional Fracture Bracing. A Manual.* Lippincott Williams & Wilkins.

169. Sarmiento A. et al. Isolated ulnar shaft fractures treated with functional braces. *J Orthop Trauma.* 1998;12(6):420–423; discussion 423-4.

170. Sauder DJ, Athwal GS. Management of isolated ulnar shaft fractures. *Hand Clin.* 2007;23(2):179–184, vi.

171. Schemitsch EH, Richards RR. The effect of malunion on functional outcome after plate fixation of fractures of both bones of the forearm in adults. *J Bone Joint Surg Am.* 1992;74(7):1068–1078.

172. Schneiderman G, et al. The interosseous membrane of the forearm: structure and its role in Galeazzi fractures. *J Trauma.* 1993;35(6):879–885.

173. Schöne G. Behandlung von Vorderarmfrakturen mit Bolzung. *Münch Med Wochenschr.* 1913;60:2327.

174. Schuind F, Andrianne Y, Burny F. Treatment of forearm fractures by Hoffman external fixation. A study of 93 patients. *Clin Orthop Relat Res.* 1991;(266):197–204.

175. Schweitzer G. Refracture of bones of the forearm after the removal of compression plates. *J Bone Joint Surg Am.* 1990;72(1):152.

176. Singer BR, et al. Epidemiology of fractures in 15,000 adults: the influence of age and gender. *J Bone Joint Surg Br.* 1998;80(2):243–248.

177. Smith DK, Cooney WP. External fixation of high-energy upper extremity injuries. *J Orthop Trauma.* 1990;4(1):7–18.

178. Soeur R. Intramedullary pinning of diaphyseal fractures. *J Bone Joint Surg Am.* 1946;28:309–331.

179. Stevens CT, ten Duis HJ. Plate osteosynthesis of simple forearm fractures: LCP versus DC plates. *Acta Orthop Belg.* 2008;74(2):180–183.

180. Stewart RL. In: Stannard JP, Schmidt AH, Kregor PJ, eds. *Forearm fractures, in Surgical treatment of orthopaedic trauma.* New York: Thieme; 2007:340–363.

181. Street DM. Intramedullary forearm nailing. *Clin Orthop Relat Res.* 1986;(212):219–230.

182. Strehle J, Gerber C. Distal radioulnar joint function after Galeazzi fracture-dislocations treated by open reduction and internal plate fixation. *Clin Orthop Relat Res.* 1993;(293):240–245.

183. Swenson DM, et al. Epidemiology of US high school sports-related fractures, 2005–2009. *Clin J Sport Med.* 2010;20(4):293–299.

184. Tabor OB Jr, et al. Iatrogenic posterior interosseous nerve injury: is transosseous static locked nailing of the radius feasible? *J Orthop Trauma.* 1995;9(5):427–429.

185. Teipner WA, Mast JW. Internal fixation of forearm diaphyseal fractures: double plating versus single compression (tension band) plating–a comparative study. *Orthop Clin North Am.* 1980;11(3):381–391.

186. Tornkvist H, Hearn TC, Schatzker J. The strength of plate fixation in relation to the number and spacing of bone screws. *J Orthop Trauma.* 1996;10(3):204–208.

187. Trousdale RT, Linscheid RL. Operative treatment of malunited fractures of the forearm. *J Bone Joint Surg Am.* 1995;77(6):894–902.

188. Visna P, et al. Interlocking nailing of forearm fractures. *Acta Chir Belg.* 2008;108(3):333–338.

189. Wallace AL. Magnetic resonance imaging or ultrasound in assessment of the interosseous membrane of the forearm. *J Bone Joint Surg Am.* 2002;84-A(3):496–497.

190. Wallny TA, et al. [Functional fracture treatment of the forearm]. The indications and results. *Chirurg.* 1997;68(11):1126–1131.

191. Weckbach A, Blattert TR, Weisser C. Interlocking nailing of forearm fractures. *Arch Orthop Trauma Surg.* 2006;126(5):309–315.

192. Wright RD. Forearm fractures. In: Gardner MJ, Henley MB, eds. *Harborview illustrated tips and tricks in fracture surgery.* Philadelphia, PA: Lippincott Williams and Wilkins; 2010:98–106.

193. Zinar DM. Forearm fractures: intramedullary nailing. In: Wiss DA, ed. *Fractures.* Philadelphia, PA: Lippincott Williams and Wilkins; 2006:157–168.

194. Zych GA, Latta LL, Zagorski JB. Treatment of isolated ulnar shaft fractures with prefabricated functional fracture braces. *Clin Orthop Relat Res.* 1987;(219):194–200.

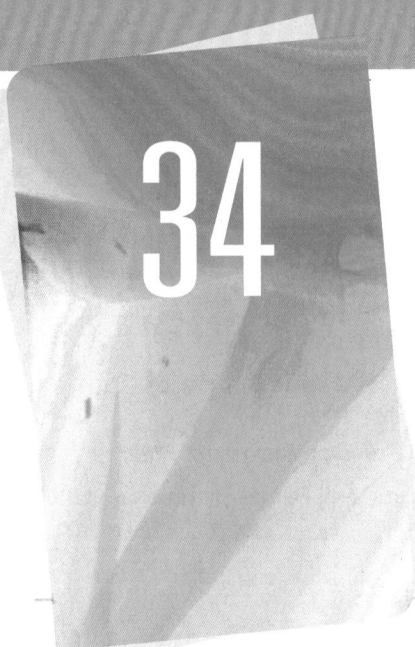

34 ELBOW FRACTURES AND DISLOCATIONS

Daphne M. Beingessner, J. Whitcomb Pollock, and Graham J.W. King

INTRODUCTION TO SIMPLE ELBOW DISLOCATION

A simple elbow dislocation is one in which there are no associated fractures. The elbow joint is the second most commonly dislocated joint in the adult population with a reported rate of 5.21 per 100,000 person-years in the US population.[105] Nearly half of simple dislocations are the result of sports with males at highest risk during football and females during gymnastics and skating. Adolescent males are the highest-risk group. The elbow is typically stable after a closed manipulative reduction in this injury; however, older patients or those with high-energy mechanisms may be at risk for residual instability that requires operative intervention.[31] A good functional outcome is typically reported by these patients, but some patients report residual subjective stiffness and pain. Less than 10% of patients report residual instability.[2]

ASSESSMENT OF SIMPLE ELBOW DISLOCATION

Mechanisms of Injury for Simple Elbow Dislocations

Simple elbow dislocations are typically the result of a fall on an outstretched hand. O'Driscoll described a valgus, axial, and posterolateral force that results in the typical posterolateral dislocation of the elbow joint (Fig. 34-1).[81] The soft tissue injury is thought to begin on the lateral side of the elbow with disruption of the lateral collateral ligament (LCL) and then proceeds through the capsule to the medial side with the medial collateral ligament (MCL) being injured last. The MCL may remain intact in some injuries. Less commonly, simple dislocation may be the result of a varus, axial, and posteromedial force where the injury proceeds from medial to lateral, but this mechanism typically results in a small anteromedial coronoid fracture, and this injury is discussed later in the chapter.[31]

Associated Injuries with Simple Elbow Dislocation

By definition, simple elbow dislocations are not associated with fractures. However, they typically are accompanied by signifi-cant disruption of the collateral ligaments, elbow capsule, and forearm flexor and extensor muscle origins.[53] Although rare, injury to the brachial artery has been described in closed simple dislocations and nerve palsies are possible. The ulnar nerve is the most commonly injured nerve following elbow dislocation, but entrapment of the median nerve in the joint after reduction has been described.[66]

Signs and Symptoms of Simple Elbow Dislocation

Patients typically present with an obvious deformity and pain about the affected elbow. Some patients may self-reduce or spontaneously reduce and will present with pain, swelling, and ecchymosis but no deformity. With the elbow flexed to 90 degrees, the medial and lateral epicondyles and the olecranon process should form an isosceles triangle; and if they do not, the elbow is likely dislocated or subluxated, with the elbow "jumping a runner" in the medial or lateral direction. The elbow should be evaluated for open wounds. A complete peripheral neurologic examination should be performed for both motor and sensory functions. Radial and ulnar pulses should be compared to the opposite side. If they are decreased, arm–arm indices are useful to help determine if there is a vascular injury.

Imaging and Other Diagnostic Studies for Simple Elbow Dislocations

Anteroposterior, lateral, and oblique radiographs are used to diagnose elbow dislocation and help to rule out associated fractures. Computed tomography (CT) scanning is rarely needed but can be useful if there is a questionable associated fracture. MRI is not needed unless there is concern for ulnar nerve entrapment in the joint since the pathology of the soft tissue injury associated with elbow dislocations has been well established.

Classification of Simple Elbow Dislocations

Simple elbow dislocations are often described based on the direction of dislocation. The majority of dislocations

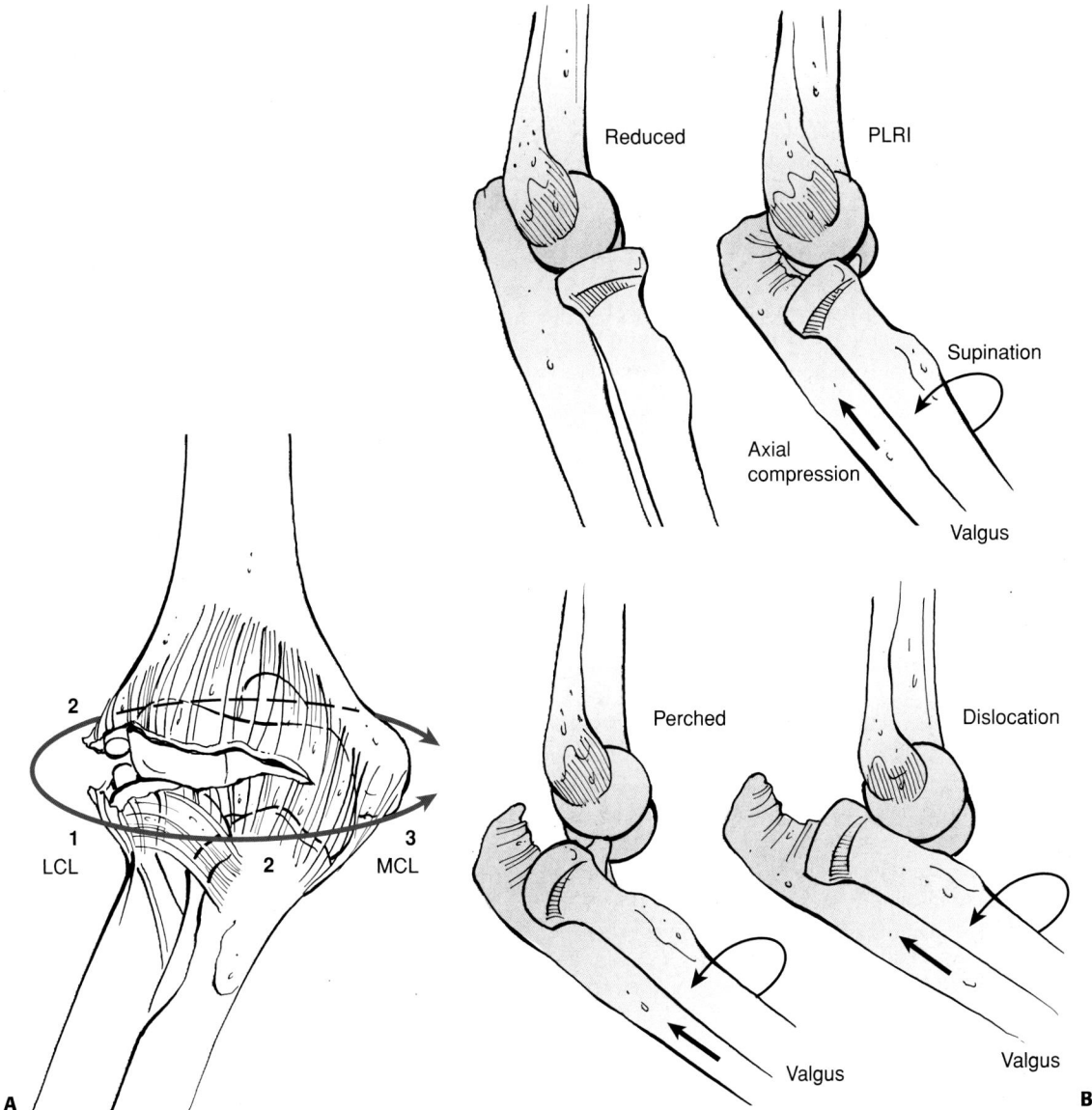

FIGURE 34-1 A, B: Elbow dislocations are thought to occur with a progression from lateral to medial. Complete dislocation is usually associated with disruption of the medial and lateral collateral ligaments and anterior capsule.

are posterior or posterolateral. However, anterior, medial, lateral, and divergent dislocations are possible. They can also be classified as acute, subacute (less than 6 weeks), or chronic.

Outcome Measures for Simple Elbow Dislocations

Several scoring systems have been used to evaluate the outcomes of simple elbow dislocation. Most recent publications have evaluated outcomes using the Disabilities of the Arm, Shoulder and Hand Questionnaire (DASH) and the Oxford Elbow Questionnaire.

PATHOANATOMY AND APPLIED ANATOMY RELATING TO SIMPLE ELBOW DISLOCATIONS

Elbow stability is provided by the soft tissue structures surrounding the joint as well as by bony articulations of the joint itself. The soft tissue restraints can be divided into both static and dynamic stabilizers. The static stabilizers include the joint capsule and the LCLs and MCLs. The normal joint capsule is thin but does contribute to stability with the elbow in full extension and flexion. The LCL has three components, the radial collateral ligament, annular ligament, and the lateral ulnar collateral ligament. It is the primary varus and posterolateral rotational stabilizer of the elbow. The radial head is surrounded by the annular ligament which attaches to the anterior and posterior margins of the radial notch of the proximal ulna. The radial collateral ligament arises from the lateral epicondyle and blends with the annular ligament. The lateral ulnar collateral ligament is posterior to the radial collateral ligament and attaches to the crista supinatoris of the proximal ulna, just distal to the annular ligament. The MCL consists of the anterior and posterior bundles. The anterior bundle is the key valgus stabilizer of the elbow, arising from the anterior-inferior aspect of the medial epicondyle to insert on the sublime tubercle of the proximal ulna. The posterior bundle provides a secondary restraint to valgus load and also resists ulnar rotation.

The dynamic restraints include the biceps, brachialis, and triceps which provide compressive stability to the elbow due to their joint reactive forces and are particularly important when the static stabilizers have been injured. The common extensor muscles provide varus stability and the common flexor muscles provide valgus stability. Pronation will stabilize the LCL-deficient elbow while supination decreases stability in this setting.[32]

Patients with simple elbow dislocations routinely have disruption of both the MCL and LCL and the elbow capsule.[81] The muscular origins may be disrupted as well; typically the injury to the lateral common extensor origin is more extensive than the medial common flexor origin. Although the MCL was once thought to be the most important stabilizer of the elbow joint, this is only true in patients that routinely load their elbow in valgus such as throwing athletes. Since most activities of daily living exert a varus force on the elbow than a valgus force, residual instability is usually due to incompetence of the LCL in the majority of patients. Sometimes when the elbow dislocates, the radial head causes an impression fracture of the posterior capitellum which can contribute to recurrent instability.

SIMPLE ELBOW DISLOCATION TREATMENT OPTIONS

Nonoperative Treatment of Simple Elbow Dislocations

The majority of simple elbow dislocations can be treated nonoperatively with closed manipulative reduction, evaluation of stability, and an early rehabilitation program (Fig. 34-2).

Indications/Contraindications (Table 34-1)

TABLE 34-1	Simple Elbow Dislocation	
	Nonoperative Treatment	
Indications	**Relative Contraindications**	
Closed elbow dislocation	Open dislocation	
	Vascular injury	
	Instability after closed reduction	

Techniques

A closed manipulative reduction of the elbow is usually performed in the emergency room or the operating room. Adequate conscious sedation with appropriate relaxation and monitoring of vital signs is important. The medial and lateral epicondyles are palpated and their relationship to the olecranon is determined in order to first correct and medial/lateral displacement in the coronal plane. The elbow is typically flexed to approximately 30 degrees, and traction is placed through the forearm while stabilizing the humerus. Direct pressure over the olecranon may help to guide it over the distal humerus and into joint. Supination of the forearm may be helpful to gain the reduction. The reduction maneuver should employ a steady slow force in order to avoid iatrogenic fracture of the distal humerus or proximal forearm.

After reduction, the elbow is taken through an arc of flexion–extension in pronation, neutral, and supination in order to evaluate for residual instability. Since the lateral sided soft tissue injuries are typically more severe, pronation of the forearm often improves stability. If the elbow redislocates when flexed to less than 30 degrees, operative treatment should be considered. However, in the majority of cases, the elbow will be stable after closed reduction, particularly after muscle tone returns in the arm. Most patients will have varus–valgus instability given the pathoanatomy of elbow dislocation, but this plane of instability alone is not an indication for operative treatment. The elbow is then immobilized in a light plaster splint with the forearm in pronation, neutral, or supination (depending on the position of maximal stability) and the elbow at 90 degrees of flexion. Radiographs are performed to ensure a congruous reduction has been achieved and to evaluate for the presence of fractures not visualized on the prereduction radiographs. Isometric exercises should be encouraged while immobilized in the splint to promote muscle activation and improved dynamic stability. The patient is seen within a week to ensure maintenance of the reduction and to begin active range of motion of the elbow.

After 1 week the splint is removed. The patient is examined for stability again and asked to actively extend and flex the elbow. Patients will typically move only within their stable arc and are unlikely to redislocate if they had a stable reduction and examination initially. A rehabilitation program is initiated encouraging active and active-assisted motion. A collar and cuff is used between exercises. Rarely, a hinged splint with an extension block can be used in those occasional patients with residual instability past 30 degrees of extension where compliance with avoiding this position is of concern. The patient is seen weekly for the first 3 weeks to decrease the extension block by 10 degrees per week. Radiographs are performed to confirm concentric reduction at each visit. The patient is then seen again at 6 weeks and may resume most normal activities and start a light strengthening program, avoiding varus or valgus loading until 12 weeks. Immobilization greater than 3 weeks should be avoided as this has been demonstrated to cause an increased incidence of stiffness and poorer functional outcomes.

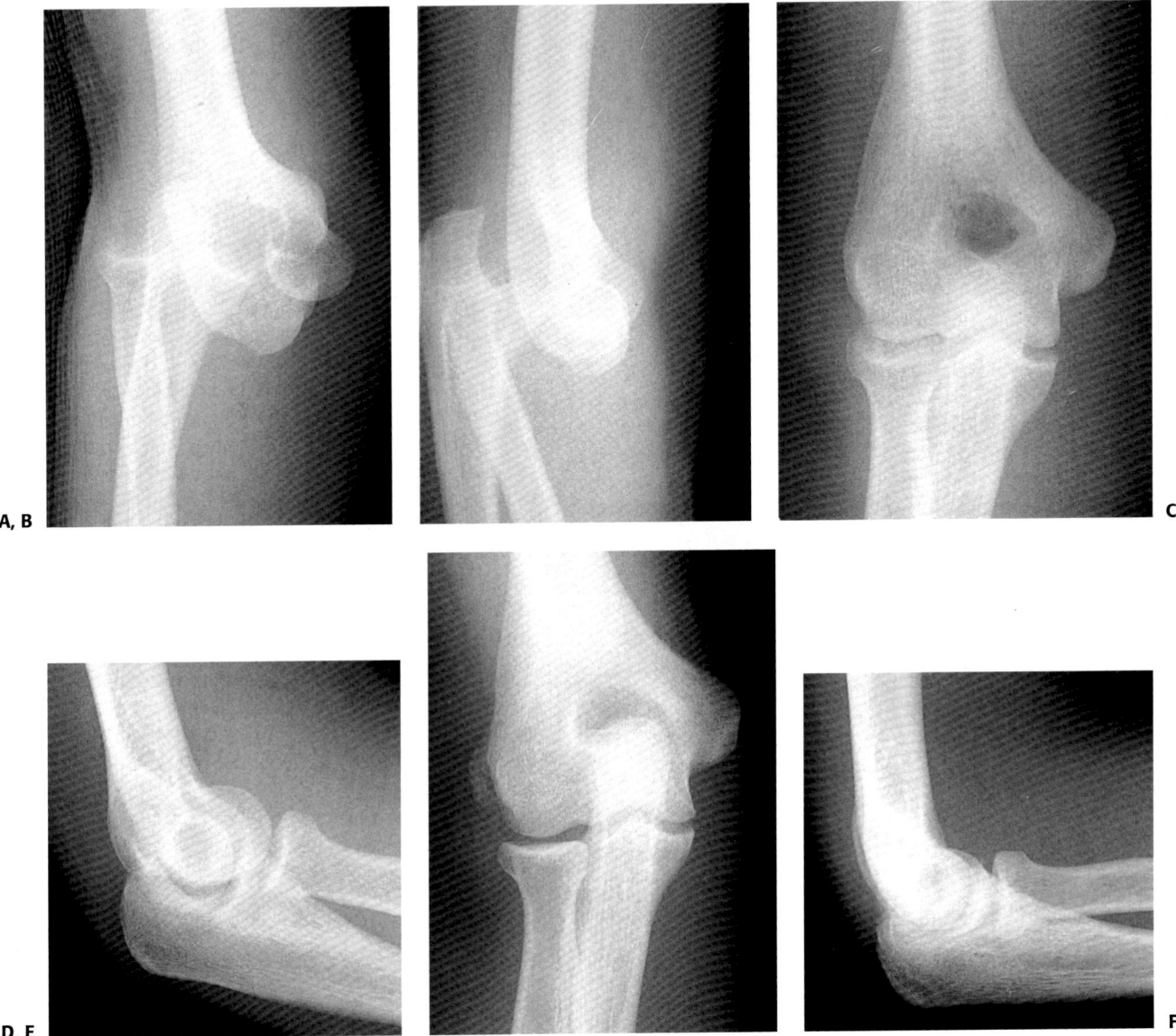

FIGURE 34-2 A, B: A healthy 22-year-old male fell sustaining a simple elbow dislocation. **C, D:** A closed reduction was performed under conscious sedation in the emergency room and postreduction examination revealed a stable elbow through a full arc of motion. **E, F:** Follow-up at 3 months demonstrated some ossification of the lateral ligament complex with a concentric elbow joint and full range of motion.

Some patients may have subtle residual mild posterolateral subluxation following a closed reduction. Coonrad et al.[22] described the "drop sign," an increase in the static ulnohumeral distance in unstressed postreduction lateral radiographs of dislocated elbows. In those patients, an active motion protocol should be employed. It consists of avoiding varus stress at all times by exercising with the elbow at the side while sitting or standing. Active motion is performed with the forearm pronated through the full range of motion. Supination is performed with the forearm flexed to 90 degrees or greater. This protocol takes advantage of the effects of the dynamic elbow stabilizers. Wolff and Hotchkiss[116] also describe performing the exercises with an overhead protocol which allows the effects of gravity to improve stability.

Outcomes

Several studies have reported good to excellent outcomes in the majority of patients after simple elbow dislocation. However, these injuries are not entirely benign. Josefsson et al.[52] reported on a series of 52 patients followed for an average of 24 years. More than half of the patients had mild residual symptoms. Nineteen patients reported loss of motion but the majority of patients did not have late arthritis. Recently, Anakwe et al.[2] reported outcomes of 110 patients with simple elbow dislocation at an average of 7.3 years after injury. The mean DASH Score was 6.7 points (the DASH is a disability score where a higher score is worse, 0 = a perfect arm, and 100 = completely disabled) and the mean Oxford Elbow Score was 90.3 points (0 = poor, 100 = good).

Fifty-six percent of patients reported residual subjective stiffness, and 62% of patients reported residual pain. Eight percent of patients reported residual instability although no patient required operative intervention for their instability. Reduced elbow flexion and female sex were predictors of a lower outcome score. Eygendaal et al.[34] evaluated 50 patients with closed simple dislocations with a mean follow-up of 9 years. Twenty-four patients had medial instability on stress radiographs, and 21 had degenerative changes. Medial instability was correlated with radiographic degeneration and a worse overall clinical result. Mehlhoff et al.[72] evaluated 50 patients at an average of 34.4 months. Sixty percent of patients reported residual symptoms including flexion contracture in 15%, residual pain in 45%, and pain on valgus stress in 35%. Prolonged immobilization after injury was associated with a worse result with increasing duration of immobilization leading to increased flexion contracture and more severe residual pain: In general, prolonged immobilization is to be avoided in this setting.

Operative Treatment of Simple Elbow Dislocations

Indications/Contraindications

The main indication for operative management of simple elbow dislocations is an inability to maintain a concentric elbow joint after closed reduction or a recurrent dislocation. Elbows which are so unstable that prolonged immobilization will be required should also be considered for early surgical management to avoid excessive stiffness. Open dislocations, vascular disruption (Fig. 34-3), and irreducible dislocations are also indications for operative treatment but these are rare injuries. Throwing athletes may benefit from direct repair of the MCL.[88]

Surgical Procedure

Preoperative Planning. Operative treatment may include open reduction with direct repair of ligaments, capsule, and muscle origins. Application of a static or hinged external fixation may occasionally be required to protect a tenuous soft tissue repair. Cross-pinning of the joint can be considered in patients that cannot tolerate an external fixator or when a fixator is unavailable. Temporary bridge plating of the elbow can also be considered to manage residual instability when application of an external fixator may be contraindicated such as in noncompliant or morbidly obese patients (Table 34-2).

Positioning. The patient is placed supine on the operating table with a radiolucent arm table on the affected side. Since both medial and lateral deep surgical approaches may be necessary, a preoperative examination of the shoulder should be performed to be sure that there is adequate external rotation of the shoulder in order to approach the medial side of the elbow. In the setting of significant shoulder stiffness, an alternative choice is to position the arm across the chest or use a lateral decubitus position. The C-arm is brought in from the head of the patient for both anteroposterior and lateral fluoroscopy. A sterile tourniquet should be available, but its use is optional.

Surgical Approach. A posterior midline incision is employed and a full thickness lateral flap is elevated on the deep fascia. In some dislocations, there is visible disruption of the lateral fascia and muscular origins from the injury itself. However, if there is not, then a fascial incision is made through the Kocher interval between the anconeus and extensor carpi ulnaris (ECU) for exposure of the LCL. If the medial structures require repair, full thickness elevation of the medial flap is performed and the ulnar nerve is identified and protected but not transposed. The MCL may be approached through the traumatic muscle disruption. The flexor pronator mass can be further elevated off the ulna to aid exposure as required. An alternative approach is to make paired medial and lateral skin incisions in the setting where the quality of the posterior skin is not suitable.

Technique: Soft Tissue Repair. Disruption of the LCL and extensor origins off of the posterolateral aspect of the distal humerus with capsular disruption is typically encountered.[71] The joint is inspected for chondral debris and injury and thoroughly irrigated.

The LCL can be repaired using transosseous bone tunnels or suture anchors (Fig. 34-4).[39] A single drill hole is placed at the center of the flexion–extension axis located at the center of the arc of curvature of the capitellum. Two drill holes are then placed on the posterior column of the lateral supracondylar ridge in patients with good bone or one drill hole placed anteriorly and one posteriorly to the supracondylar ridge in patients with poorer quality bone. Shuttle sutures are placed through these drill holes. Locking Krackow stitches are placed in the LCL while a second suture is placed in the extensor fascia. The sutures are tensioned while maintaining the forearm in pronation and the elbow at 90 degrees of flexion. Avoid over tensioning of the lateral ligaments if the MCL is deficient as medial gaping of the elbow can occur.[39] The elbow is then taken through a range of motion using gravity extension in pronation, supination, and neutral rotation and reduction is verified both clinically and

---

TABLE 34-2 **ORIF of Simple Elbow Dislocation**

Preoperative Planning Checklist

- OR Table: Radiolucent
- Position/positioning aids: Supine with arm table or lateral decubitus
- Fluoroscopy location: From head
- Equipment: Suture anchors, large external fixator, hinged external fixator, large fragment locking set with screws
- Tourniquet (sterile/nonsterile): Sterile preferred

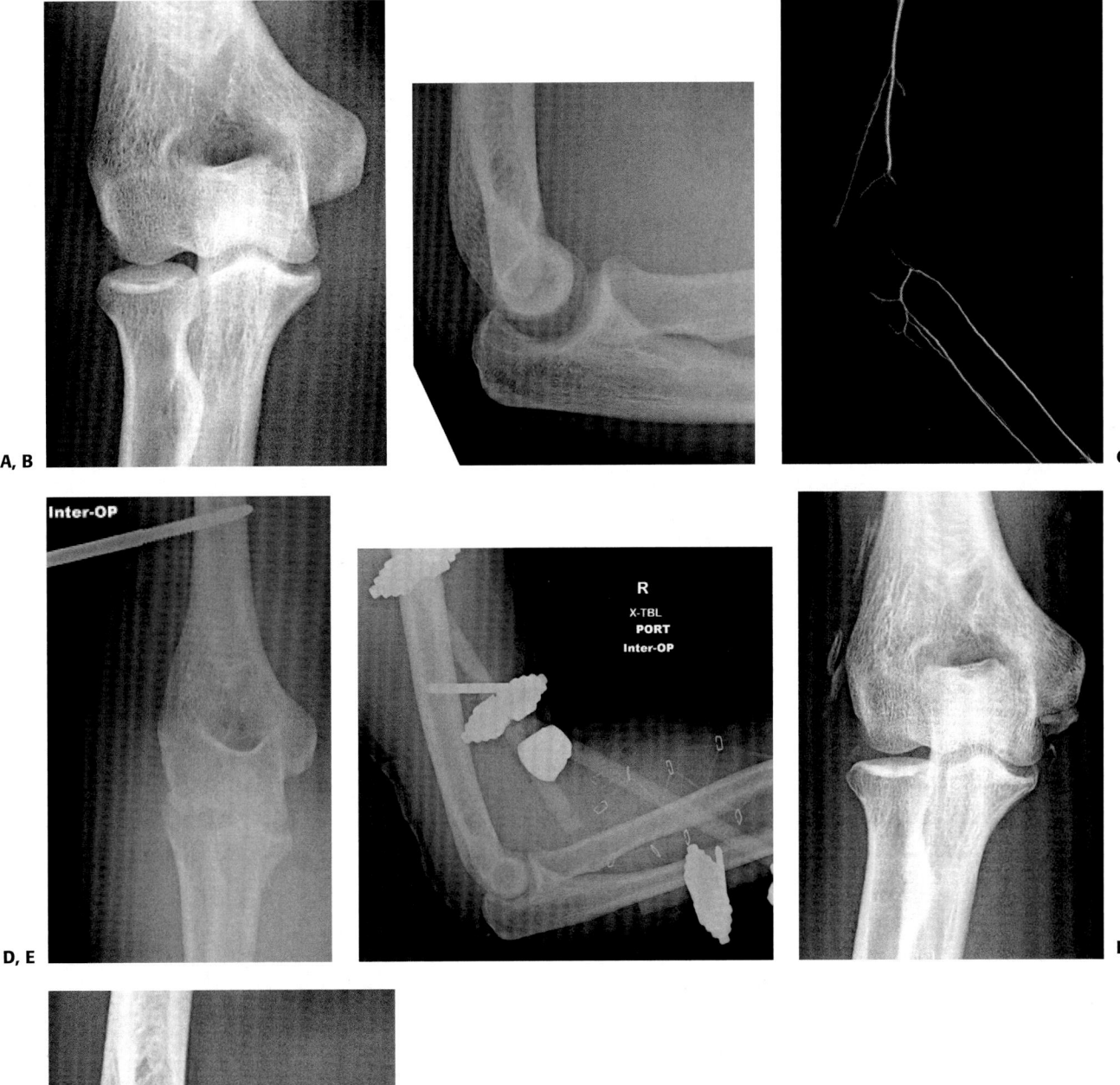

FIGURE 34-3 A 15-year-old male sustained a simple elbow dislocation while skiing. He self-reduced on the hill but presented with elbow subluxation **(A, B)**. (Note the increased ulnotrochlear space) and a decreased radial pulse. CT angiogram demonstrated transection of his brachial artery **(C)**. After vascular bypass and forearm fasciotomy, the elbow was placed into an external fixator to protect the vascular repair. The fixator was removed after 3 weeks. No ligament repair was done as the elbow was relatively stable following reduction and the open wound was anterior **(D, E)**. Follow-up at 3 months demonstrated some ossification of his collateral ligaments with a full range of motion, stable elbow, and intact vascular repair **(F, G)**.

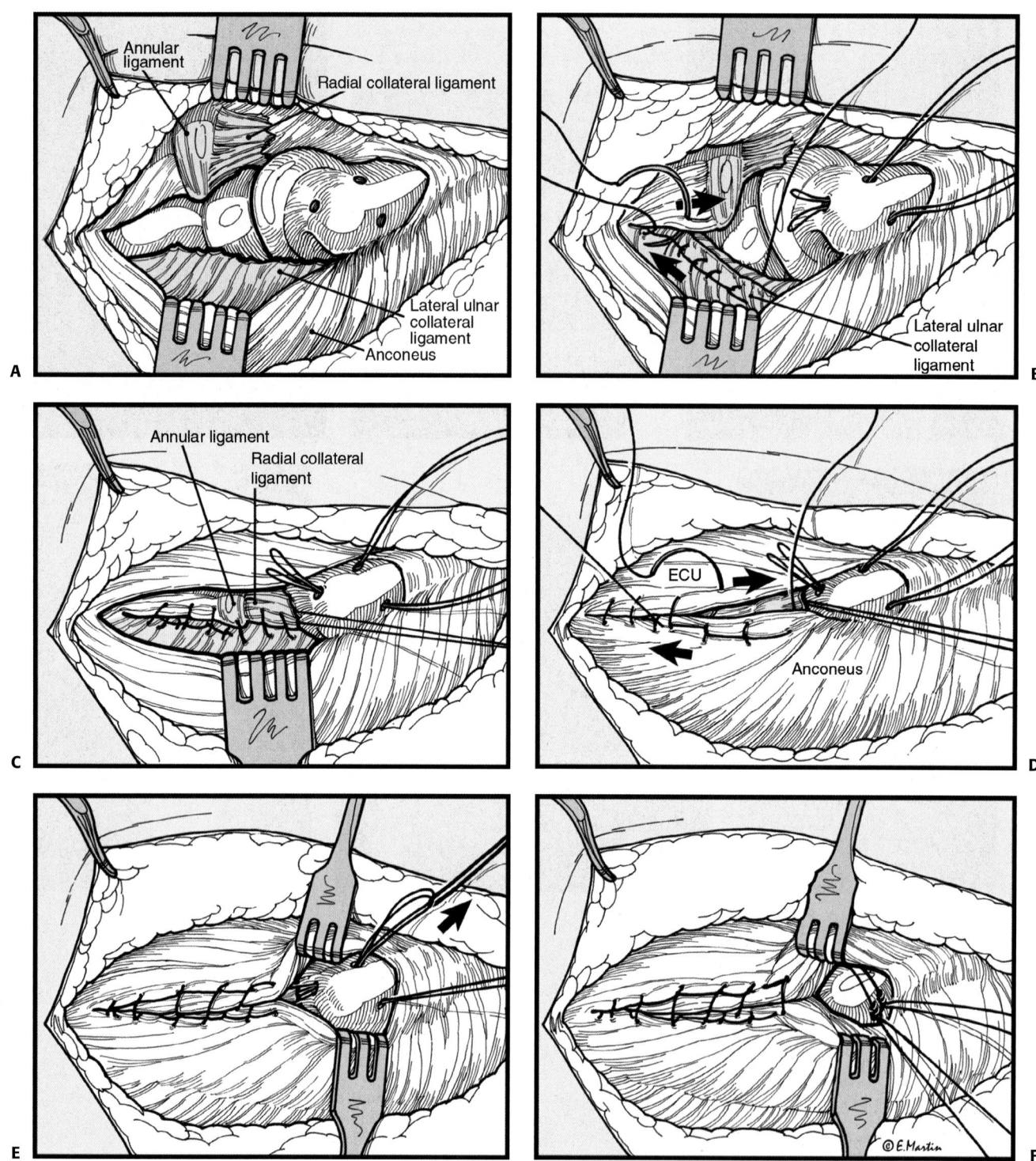

FIGURE 34-4 Repair of the LCL is performed using transosseous bone tunnels placed at the center of the capitellum and exiting anterior and posterior to the lateral epicondyle. Locking Krackow sutures are placed in the LCL, and then the common extensor origin is also repaired. Suture retrievers are used to pass the sutures through the bone tunnels which are then tensioned and tied across the bone bridge **(A–F).** In young patients with good-quality bone, both tunnels can be placed posterior to the epicondyle to simplify the procedure. (Illustration by Elizabeth Martin, ©2011. Reprinted with permission from Green's Operative Hand Surgery, 6th ed, Churchill Livingstone, Inc.)

fluoroscopically. Care should be taken not to "hold" the elbow in joint during this examination so that residual instability can be recognized. In the vast majority of cases, a medial ligament repair is not required and the surgery is complete.

In the unusual setting that the elbow remains unstable in spite of repair of the lateral structures, the medial side of the elbow is approached with care taken to protect the ulnar nerve. Repair of the MCL is performed using drill holes located at the anterior-inferior aspect of the medial epicondyle and two holes more proximally.[82] The flexor–pronator muscles are also repaired if they have been avulsed. Suture anchors can also be employed.

If the elbow is still unstable, then a static or hinged external fixator should be placed or, as a last resort, the elbow should be transfixed with a screw or robust Steinman pin. In the setting of a noncompliant patient, head-injured patient, or morbid obesity, a locking large fragment bridge plate can be used to temporarily fix the elbow using a triceps-splitting approach.[78]

The wound should be irrigated and closed in layers. Because an early motion protocol is desirable, suture rather than staple closure of skin is preferred for wound edge security.

Technique: External Fixation. There are many external fixation systems available and familiarity with the system on hand is important. A hinged fixator will allow for range of motion exercises to be performed while the external fixator is in place and should be considered if the surgeon has access to this and the experience to apply it. Static fixators are easier to apply and are more widely available. There are no studies comparing the outcome of static or dynamic fixators in the setting of simple elbow dislocations.

The key to all hinged devices is an understanding of the axis of elbow rotation. If the axis pin is malaligned, maltracking or even dislocation of the elbow may occur during motion. Device-specific instructions should be followed when applying these fixators and care must be taken not to damage the ulnar nerve when inserting the axis pin or the radial nerve when inserting the humeral pins. Elbow motion is initiated postoperatively within the first week. The frame is left in place for approximately 4 to 6 weeks, depending on a number of factors including the stability of the elbow, associated pin tract problems, etc.

If a hinged external fixator is not available or the surgeon is unfamiliar with its use, placement of a static external fixator is an alternative method that can be used. The elbow is placed at 90 degrees of flexion with the joint concentrically reduced. Two pins are placed in the humeral shaft laterally and two pins are placed in the ulnar shaft laterally in a position that allows for forearm rotation. Open pin placement is recommended to avoid injury to the radial nerve. Imaging is employed to ensure the pins are not placed too deep to avoid injury to the ulnar nerve. A static frame is assembled with the elbow joint reduced. The external fixator is left in place for approximately 4 weeks and then a range of motion protocol is initiated as outlined above for closed treatment.

Technique: Cross-Pins or Screws. In patients with residual instability where an external fixator is not available or in patients that are not candidates for an external fixator, a cross-screw technique may be employed. It should be emphasized that this technique is rarely required and should be reserved for use only as a salvage procedure. The elbow is concentrically reduced and a screw or pin is placed from the posterior aspect of the ulna, across the joint, exiting on the posterior border of the humerus. The screw or pin size should be consistent with the patent's size and compliance so that breakage does not occur (Fig. 34-5). Several screw threads should protrude from the posterior humeral border for the ease of extraction should the screw break. A 4.5-mm cortical screw or shaft screw is appropriate. The elbow is placed into a cast for 3 to 4 weeks, and the screw is then removed, and a motion protocol is started as above. Alternatively a robust Steinman pin can be utilized driven from the subcutaneous border of the ulna and out the posterior humerus.

Technique: Bridge Plate. In patients with residual instability that are not candidates for an external fixator, a temporary bridge plate may be employed. Indications are conditions where maintenance of reduction is challenging such as morbid obesity and patients with neurologic injuries such as spasticity or flaccid paralysis. After repair of the collateral ligaments as previously described a narrow 4.5-mm large fragment locking plate is bent to 90 degrees. A triceps-splitting approach is employed proximally to identify and protect the radial nerve. The triceps can be left attached to the olecranon. Three to four locking screws are placed in the ulna and the distal humerus avoiding the articulation and fossae. The plate is removed at 4 weeks, and a posterior capsulectomy and an elbow manipulation can be considered at the time of plate removal to increase the recovery of motion (Table 34-3).

TABLE 34-3	ORIF of Simple Elbow Dislocation

Surgical Steps

- Posterior midline incision
- Approach lateral side first
- Inspect and clean joint
- Repair LCL and extensor muscle origin to the lateral epicondyle of the humerus and repair fascia
- Test for stability using gravity extension
- If still unstable, repair MCL and flexor–pronator origin
- If still unstable, apply hinged or static external fixator
- Consider cross-pin or cross-screw as a salvage
- Temporary bridge plating can also be employed

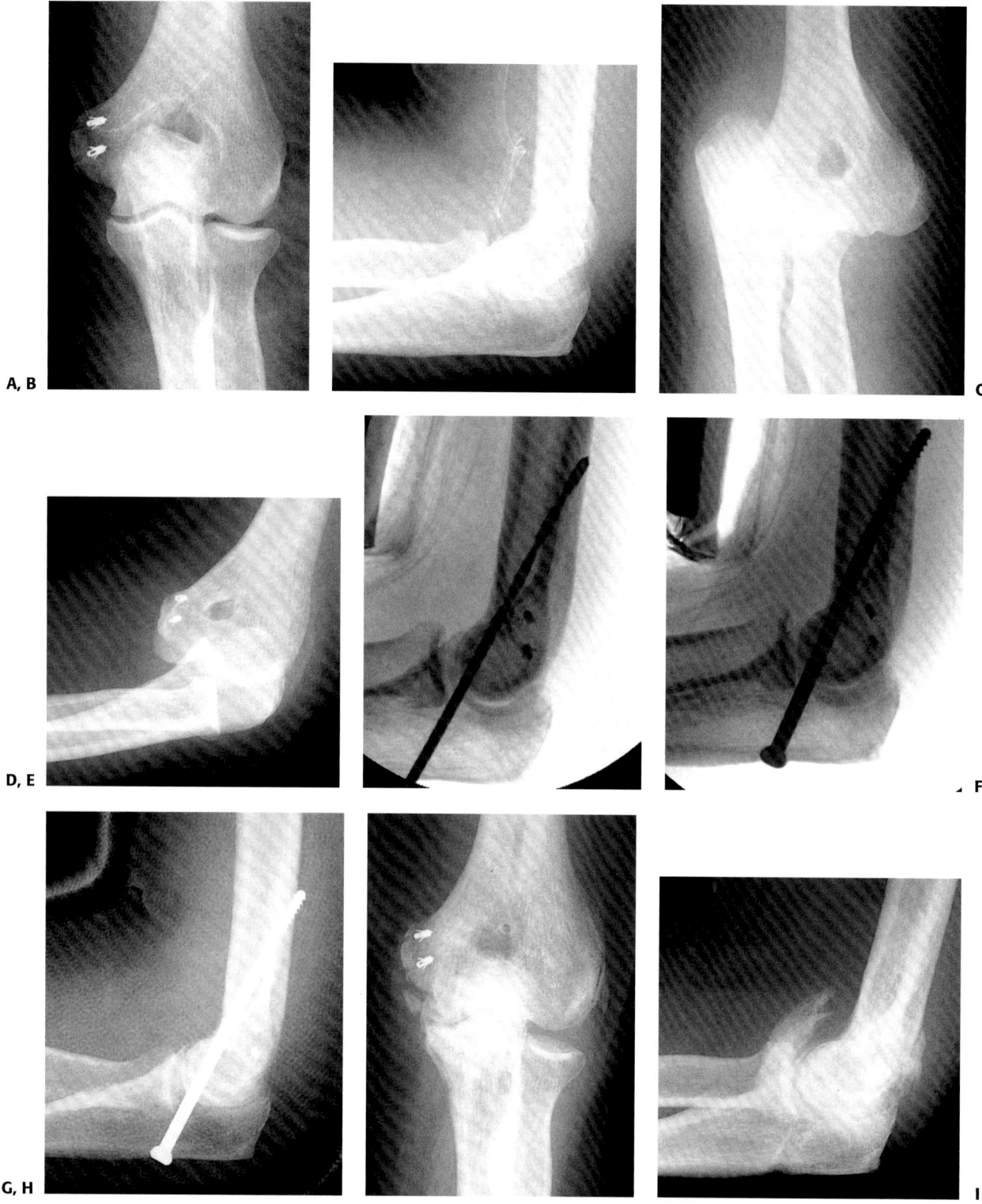

FIGURE 34-5 A 75-year-old male sustained an open elbow dislocation treated with irrigation and debridement of the medial wound and medial ligament repair **(A, B)**. He was presented to clinic 4 weeks later with increased pain, and radiographs demonstrated a redislocation likely due to the lack of repair of the lateral ligament resulting in posterolateral rotatory subluxation **(C, D)**. The patient was a poor candidate for extensive surgery due to multiple medical comorbidities. He was treated with a closed reduction and transarticular placement of a 4.5-mm screw **(E, F)**. He was casted until screw removal 6 weeks later **(G)**. Final follow-up revealed restricted range of motion with fixed varus alignment but a functional extremity **(H, I)**.

Postoperative Care. The patient is placed into a well-padded light splint with the elbow at 90 degrees of flexion and the forearm in pronation. Antibiotics are given for 24 hours. Ideally, the dressing will be removed and motion begun 48 hours after surgery unless static joint fixation has been required. The incision is covered and sutures are not removed before 14 days. The elbow should not be immobilized for longer than 1 week.

The precise rehabilitation protocol will depend on the integrity of the ligaments or any ligament repairs and the intraoperative evaluation for residual elbow instability. A safe arc of motion should be defined fluoroscopically under anesthesia so this can be taken into account when performing early motion. Active motion is preferred over passive motion as this tends to stabilize the elbow. If the MCL is intact and the LCL requires protection, then the forearm should be rehabilitated with the forearm in pronation with prosupination only performed at 90 degrees or greater of flexion.[107] Varus positioning of the arm should be avoided in patients with LCL injuries and repairs. Less commonly, if the MCL has been injured but not repaired and the LCL is competent, then flexion–extension of the elbow should be performed with the forearm maintained in supination. If both the MCL and LCL have been injured, active range of motion should be initiated with the forearm in neutral position. Extension is allowed only to the extent that allows congruent tracking intraoperatively. As muscle tone and stability improves, further extension is permitted.

Passive stretching of the elbow is not performed until ligament healing is progressing, typically beginning 6 weeks postoperatively. Static progressive splints are not routinely applied but can be employed to improve the range of motion as can turnbuckle splinting if motion goals are not being achieved. Light strengthening may be started 6 weeks postop with a formal strengthening program initiated at 3 months.

Potential Pitfalls and Preventative Measures. Symptomatic instability is uncommon after simple elbow dislocations treated operatively. However, inadequate or failed repair of the lateral structures may lead to persistent subluxation. Mild subluxation may be treated with an active motion or overhead rehabilitation protocol as previously described but frank dislocation may require repeat operative fixation or salvage procedures. Early recognition of this problem is important as late treatment of a stiff subluxated elbow is very difficult and may require extensive reconstruction including elbow release and LCL and MCL reconstruction.

Early postoperative motion is mandatory to prevent stiffness. Some patients may require elbow release or excision of heterotopic bone to restore motion. The use of indomethacin continues to be controversial and has not been proven to prevent heterotopic ossification around the elbow. Given the low incidence of heterotopic ossification with simple elbow dislocations and the lack of proven efficacy, indomethacin is not recommended by the authors.

Nerve palsies are uncommon but the ulnar and radial nerves are at risk with placement of an external fixator, with medial ligament repair or with extensive retraction of soft tissue structures. Direct visualization of the bone to ensure the nerve is not damaged by placement of the pin is recommended (Table 34-4).

Treatment-Specific Outcomes. Open treatment of unstable elbow dislocations is not commonly required. However, when necessary, the outcomes are generally satisfactory. In one group of 17 patients with persistent dislocation, 15 underwent open reduction and ligament repair and 2 had a closed reduction with cross-pinning of the joint.[31] Three patients had a hinged external fixator applied. There was one redislocation treated with the addition of a hinge, and four patients had residual subluxation treated with active motion and bracing. All patients eventually achieved a concentric stable reduction. These techniques may be successful as much as 30 weeks from injury without need for ligament reconstruction although early recognition is preferable.[56]

MANAGEMENT OF EXPECTED ADVERSE OUTCOMES AND UNEXPECTED COMPLICATIONS IN SIMPLE ELBOW DISLOCATIONS (TABLE 34-5)

TABLE 34-4 Simple Elbow Dislocation

Potential Pitfalls and Preventions

Pitfall	Preventions
Residual instability	Anatomic repair of ligaments with the elbow concentrically reduced while repairs are tightened Active motion protocol avoiding varus stress at all times
Elbow stiffness	Early range of motion Secure repair
Nerve palsy	Direct visualization of bone during pin placement Gentle retraction

TABLE 34-5 Simple Elbow Dislocation

Common Adverse Outcomes and Complications

Elbow stiffness and heterotopic ossification → Initiate early motion

Redislocation → Careful follow-up, recognize, and treat surgically

Residual subluxation → Active motion protocol, proceed with operative treatment if persists

AUTHOR'S PREFERRED METHOD OF TREATMENT FOR SIMPLE ELBOW DISLOCATIONS (FIG. 34-6)

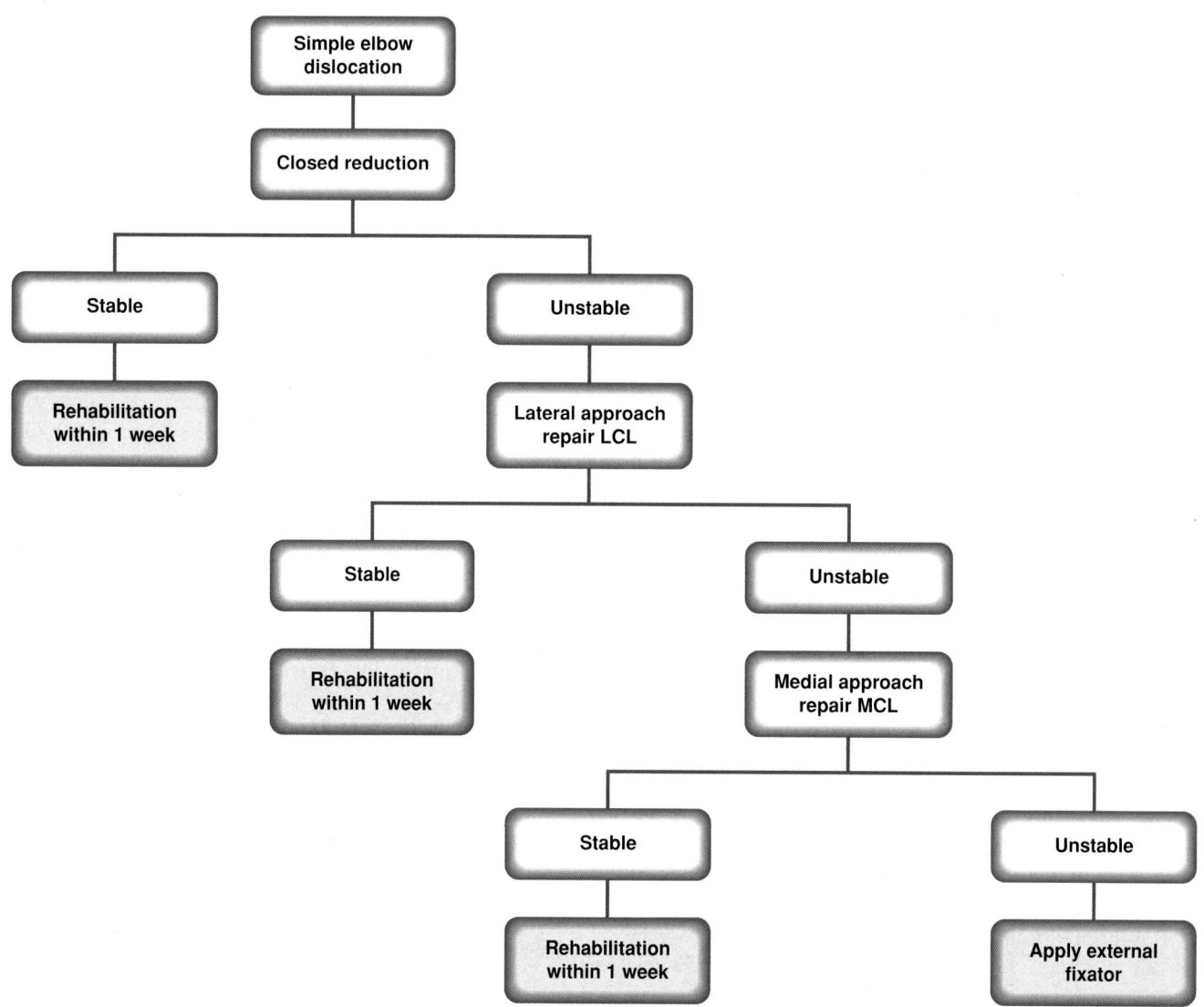

FIGURE 34-6 Author's preferred treatment.

SUMMARY, CONTROVERSIES, AND FUTURE DIRECTIONS IN SIMPLE ELBOW DISLOCATIONS

Simple elbow dislocations are common injuries that generally do well with closed manipulative reduction and early motion. Although thought to be relatively benign injuries, a large percentage of patients may have persistent subjective stiffness and mild residual pain; early discussion with the patient about outcomes is important. Throwing athletes may benefit from direct repair of an acute MCL injury. Similarly, high-energy injuries or those in the elderly may be more unstable and careful follow-up is mandatory to recognize and promptly treat persistent instability.

INTRODUCTION TO RADIAL HEAD FRACTURES

Radial head fractures are the most common fractures of the elbow with an estimated incidence of 2.5 to 2.9 per 10,000 people per year.[1] Radial head fractures are more common in women than men and most frequently occur between the ages of 20 and 60 years.[30] Undisplaced and minimally displaced radial head fractures typically occur as isolated injuries while more displaced and comminuted fractures commonly have associated injuries to the collateral ligaments and may have associated fractures of the coronoid, capitellum, or proximal ulna. In high-energy trauma, dislocations of the elbow and/or forearm can also occur. Disruption of the interosseous membrane and distal radial ulnar joint ligaments may result in axial instability of the forearm, termed the Essex–Lopresti lesion. The majority of radial head and neck fractures are minimally displaced and are isolated injuries. These fractures typically have a good functional outcome with nonsurgical treatment. The optimal management of displaced radial head fractures has not been established.

ASSESSMENT OF RADIAL HEAD FRACTURES

Mechanisms of Injury for Radial Head Fractures

Most radial head fractures occur as the result of low-energy mechanisms such as a trip and fall on an outstretched hand. Sporting activities as well as motor vehicle collisions cause higher-energy fractures typically with greater displacement and a higher incidence of concomitant injuries. Mechanisms of fracture vary but include three common patterns: (1). A valgus load causes impaction of the radial head into the capitellum, commonly with rupture of the MCL. (2). Posterolateral rotatory subluxation of the radial head with respect to the capitellum causes a partial articular shear fracture of the anterior portion of the radial head often with rupture of the LCL. (3). An axial forearm load causes impaction of the radial head into the capitellum with more severe trauma producing a fracture of the coronoid or rupture of the interosseous membrane and distal radioulnar joint ligaments; the so-called Essex–Lopresti injury.

Associated Injuries with Radial Head Fractures

Tears of the LCLs and/or MCLs are most commonly associated with radial head fractures. Dislocations of the elbow and fractures of the coronoid, capitellum, olecranon, and proximal ulna are also frequent. Rupture of the interosseous membrane while uncommon is best diagnosed and treated early as late reconstruction is challenging and often unsatisfactory.[33]

Signs and Symptoms of Radial Head Fractures

Patients present with complaints of pain, swelling, and stiffness of the elbow and forearm. Ecchymosis may develop several days later. Tenderness laterally over the radial head is expected; however, tenderness over the lateral epicondyle may indicate the presence of an associated LCL injury while similar tenderness over the medial epicondyle or sublime tubercle may suggest MCL disruption. The alignment of the elbow is assessed to rule out an associated dislocation or Monteggia fracture-dislocation. A careful examination of range of motion is performed since loss of forearm rotation is one of the primary indications for surgical intervention in the setting of displaced fractures. If pain precludes a proper evaluation of forearm rotation, the surgeon can aspirate the hemarthrosis and inject local anesthetic or re-evaluate the patient several days later when they are more comfortable. A loss of terminal extension is expected as a consequence of the hemarthrosis which accompanies all radial head fractures. The presence of clicking or crepitus with forearm rotation should be noted. The shoulder and wrist are examined for associated injuries. In particular, the distal radial ulnar joint should be palpated and balloted for both tenderness and instability.

Imaging and Other Diagnostic Studies for Radial Head Fractures

Anteroposterior and lateral radiographs are typically sufficient to diagnose most displaced radial head fractures. Undisplaced fractures may initially be difficult to diagnose, and they may only be suspected by the presence of an anterior and posterior fat pad sign from the concomitant hemarthrosis. A radiocapitellar view which places the radial head in profile can be a helpful adjunct to standard radiographs. Bilateral wrist radiographs should be performed in patients with wrist pain to evaluate for the presence of associated axial instability. CT can be helpful to better characterize the size, location, and displacement of radial head fractures. It is also useful to assess concomitant injuries of the coronoid, capitellum and to look for the presence of associated osteochondral fragments. While magnetic resonance imaging may be useful to define the presence of associated collateral ligament injuries, it is not commonly required for the management of acute radial head fractures.[57]

Classification of Radial Head Fractures

Numerous classifications have been described for fractures of the radial head. Mason described a Type I fracture as a fissure or marginal sector fracture without displacement; Type II as a marginal sector fracture with displacement; and a Type III as a comminuted fracture involving the whole head.[69] A Type IV injury was subsequently described which includes any radial head fracture associated with an elbow dislocation. The most popular classification is the Broberg and Morrey modification of the original Mason classification.[16] A Type I fracture is undisplaced or displaced less than 2 mm and involves less than 30% of the articular surface. A Type II fracture is displaced greater than 2 mm and involves greater than 30% of the articular surface. A Type III fractures is comminuted. Van Reit further modified this classification describing the Mayo–Mason classification whereby a suffix is added to the original modified Mason classification for concomitant soft tissue injuries, fractures, or dislocations of the elbow and forearm.[110]

Outcome Measures for Radial Head Fractures

Several scoring systems are commonly used to evaluate the outcomes of radial head fractures: The Broberg and Morrey Elbow Score, the American Shoulder and Elbow Surgeons elbow assessment system, the Mayo Elbow Performance Index, the Patient-rated Elbow Evaluation, the SF-36, and the DASH scoring system.

PATHOANATOMY AND APPLIED ANATOMY RELATING TO RADIAL HEAD FRACTURES

The radial head consists of a concave dish which articulates with the capitellum and a flattened articular margin which articulates with the lesser sigmoid (radial) notch of the ulna.

The nonarticular margin comprises about one-third of the diameter and is more rounded and often devoid of cartilage. A "safe zone" for placement of a plate on the nonarticular margin of the proximal radius has been defined, best identified during surgery by positioning the forearm in neutral rotation and placing the plate 10-degree anterior to the mid-axial line (Fig. 34-7).[19,104] The radial head is not circular but is somewhat elliptical in shape. Furthermore, the radiocapitellar dish is also elliptical and typically offset from the neck of the radius.[60,112] An understanding of the complex geometric shape of the radial head is required when repairing more comminuted fractures and when performing radial head replacement. Vascular supply of the radial head is supplied by branches of the radial recurrent artery and a branch of the ulnar artery which form a pericervical arterial ring. A branch of the interosseous artery supports the neck and the nutrient artery provides intraosseous blood supply.[63]

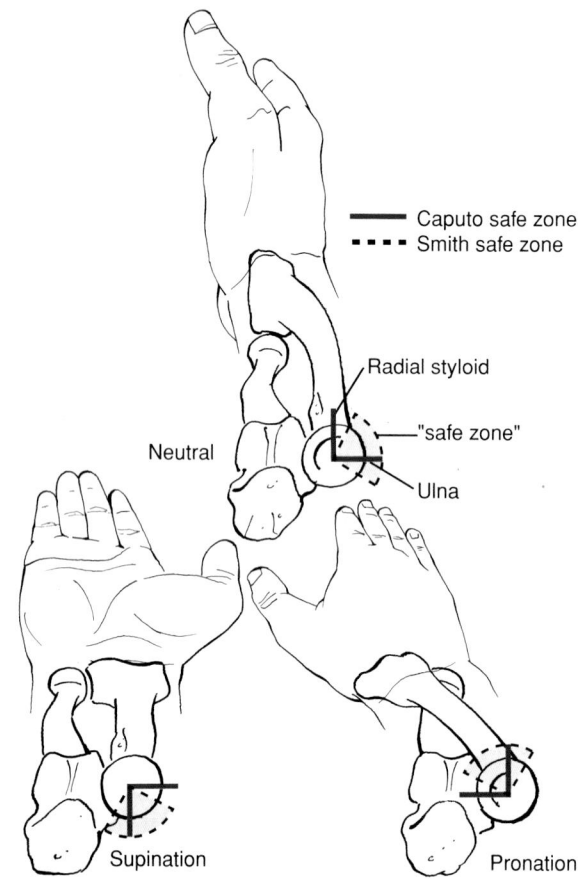

FIGURE 34-7 The nonarticular portion of the radial head is the area where plates can be applied without interfering with forearm rotation. Smith and Hotchkiss defined it based on lines bisecting the radial head in full supination, full pronation, and neutral. Implants can be placed as far as halfway between the middle and posterior lines and the anterior and middle lines. Caputo et al. recommended using the radial styloid and Lister's tubercle as guides. Alternatively the plate can be placed just anterior to the mid-axial line with the forearm in neutral rotation.

RADIAL HEAD FRACTURE TREATMENT OPTIONS

Nonoperative Treatment of Radial Head Fractures

Indications/Contraindications

Patients with undisplaced or minimally displaced radial head fractures without a block to forearm rotation should be treated nonsurgically. In the setting where there is a block to forearm rotation in a patient with radiographically undisplaced or minimally displaced fracture, the patient should be re-evaluated several days after injury when the elbow is less painful. Alternatively, aspiration of the hemarthrosis and injection of local anesthetic can be used to check for the presence of a mechanical block to rotation. A chondral flap of capitellar cartilage can be the cause of limited rotation and cannot be detected on imaging, typically noted at surgery.[19] It is unclear as to how large and how displaced a radial head fracture can be and still have a good outcome with nonsurgical management. While it has been suggested that partial articular fractures of the radial head which are displaced more than 2 mm and involve more than 30% of the articulation should be considered for open reduction and internal fixation, there are no comparative randomized clinical trials demonstrating an improved outcome relative to nonsurgical management. Displaced radial head fractures which have crepitus with forearm rotation may also be considered a relative indication for surgery (Table 34-6).

Techniques

Radial head fractures treated nonoperatively are immobilized for 2 or 3 days for comfort and then active motion is encouraged with the use of a sling or collar and cuff between exercises. Aspiration of the hemarthrosis can be considered for initial pain relief; however, it has not been shown to improve outcome so is not routinely indicated.[47] Careful radiographic and clinical follow-up is required to monitor for fracture displacement and recovery of motion.

Outcomes

Undisplaced or minimally displaced radial head fractures can be managed nonoperatively with good long-term results in the majority of patients.[46] The outcome of nonoperative management for displaced fractures of the radial head is variable in the literature with some series reporting mainly good outcomes and

TABLE 34-6	**Radial Head Fractures**	
Nonoperative Treatment		
Indications	**Relative Contraindications**	
Undisplaced fracture	Block to forearm rotation	
Displaced fracture without motion impairment	Incarcerated intra-articular fragment	
	Concomitant injuries requiring surgical management	

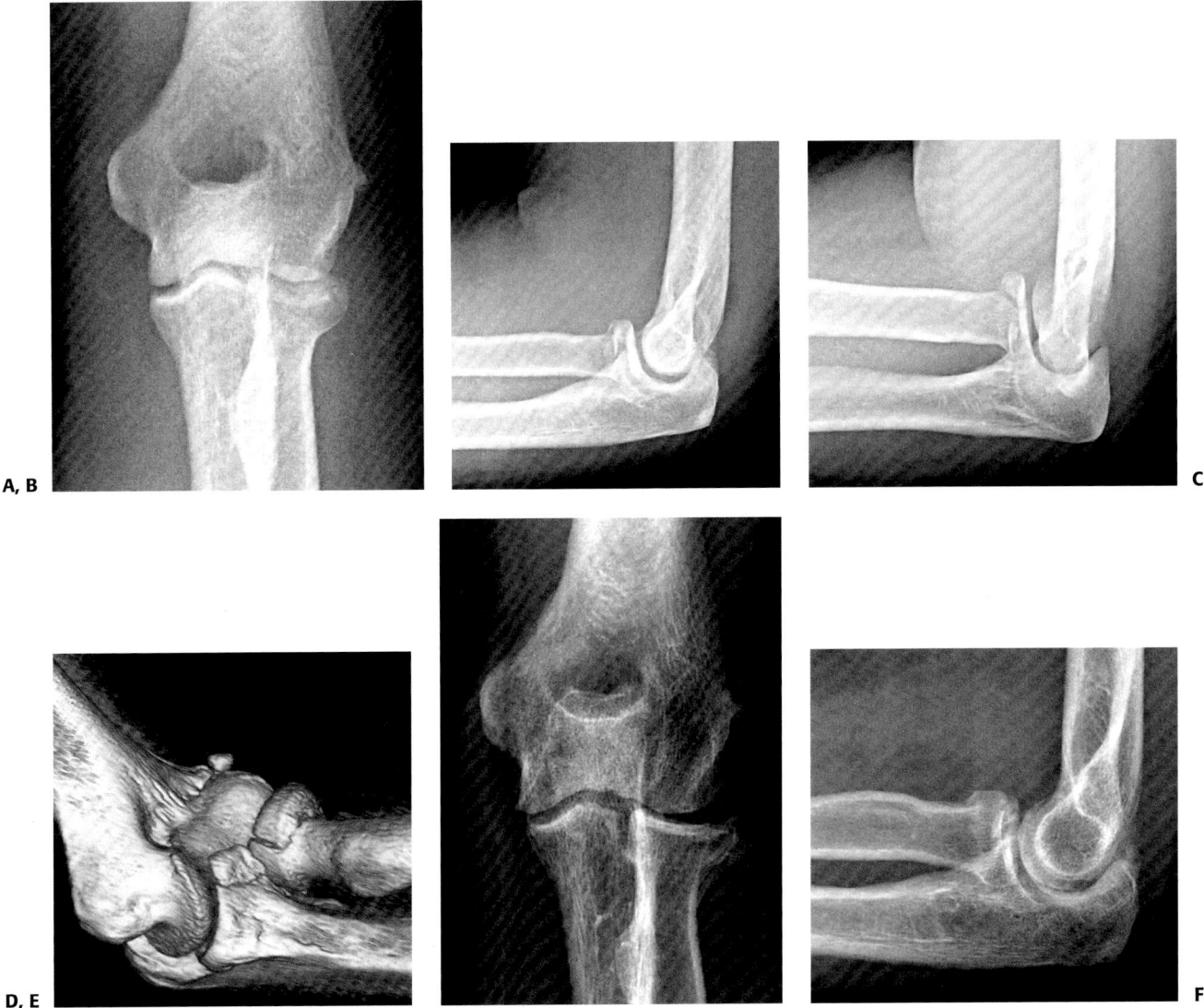

FIGURE 34-8 A–C: Anteroposterior, lateral, and oblique radiographs of a 53-year-old woman who sustained a slip and fall. **D:** CT scan shows an undisplaced coronoid fracture and a minimally displaced radial head fracture. **E, F:** One year postop, the patient had minimal pain and a near full range of motion in spite of radiographic malunion.

others reporting mixed results (Fig. 34-8). Mason reported that 9 of 15 patients had some pain following nonoperative treatment for fractures involving greater than 25% of the joint surface at an average of 11-year follow-up.[69] He advocated excision of the radial head for displaced radial head fractures. Radin and Riseborough reported better motion in patients with displaced radial head fractures managed with radial head excision than that achieved with nonoperative treatment.[86] Burton reported that only two of nine patients with displaced radial head fractures managed nonoperatively had good results; he recommended radial head excision in such cases.[18] Khalfayan et al.[58] reported on 26 patients with Mason Type II radial head fractures at an average of 18 months following either open reduction and internal fixation or nonoperative treatment with early motion. The operatively treated group had 90% good or excellent results

while the nonoperatively treated group had 44% good or excellent results. Pain, functional limitations, and osteoarthritis were more frequent in the nonoperatively treated group. Akesson et al.[1] reported on the outcome of 49 patients with moderately displaced Mason II fractures. At 19-year follow-up, the incidence of osteoarthritis was high at 82%; however, only six patients had an unsatisfactory result requiring a subsequent radial head excision and only 9 of the 49 patients had subjective complaints.

Operative Treatment of Radial Head Fractures

Indications/Contraindications

Patients with displaced radial head fractures with a block to motion, those who have concomitant injuries which require surgical intervention such as unstable fracture-dislocations, or those with retained intra-articular loose bodies are best treated surgically. Treatment options include radial head fragment excision, radial head excision, open reduction and internal fixation, and radial head arthroplasty.

Fragment excision is indicated in patients with a block to forearm motion by a small (less than 25% of the articular diameter) nonreconstructable displaced articular fracture of the radial head. The excision of large fragments of the radial head can cause painful clicking and contribute to instability in the setting of concomitant bony and ligament injuries as a consequence of loss of concavity–compression stability of the radiocapitellar joint.[8]

Radial head excision may be considered for isolated displaced fractures of the radial head that are not amenable to internal fixation. Given the documented high incidence of concomitant soft tissue injuries in patients with comminuted radial head fractures, primary excision of the radial head is infrequently performed. If excision is planned, a careful examination under anesthesia is mandatory to evaluate for the presence of elbow or forearm instability. Even in the presence of intact collateral ligaments, radial head excision has been documented to alter load transfer and kinematics across the elbow; however, the benefit of routine replacement of the radial head versus radial head excision has not been evaluated in randomized clinical trials.

The indications for open reduction and internal fixation remain controversial. Clear indications include displaced, noncomminuted fractures of the radial head limit forearm rotation, or radial head fractures fixed as a component of the surgical repair of an elbow fracture-dislocation. It has been suggested that fractures displaced greater than 2 mm and involving greater than 30% of the articular surface (a Type II fracture in the modified Mason classification) might be best treated with surgery; however, this remains unproven. The best candidates for internal fixation are younger patients with good-quality bone with three or fewer fragments.[91] The management of partial articular fractures tends to be more successful than complete fractures of the radial head and neck likely due to both improved stability with partial articular fractures and compromised vascularity with complete fractures of the radial neck. Low-profile tripod screw fixation has been shown to provide improved results relative to plate fixation; however, screw fixation alone is only indicated for radial neck fractures without comminution.[102]

Radial head arthroplasty is preferred in the setting of unreconstructable comminuted radial head fractures due to the high incidence of associated ligamentous and bony injuries. Radial head arthroplasty should not be performed in the setting of gross wound contamination, if the radial neck cannot be reconstructed to accept an implant, or if the capitellum is deficient or missing from an associated injury.

Fragment Excision

Preoperative Planning. Displaced fragments can be removed either arthroscopically or using standard open surgical techniques. A decision between an arthroscopic or open surgical approach is based on surgeon experience and the presence of concomitant injuries requiring treatment. Fragment excision is most commonly performed when fixation is planned but

---

TABLE 34-7 **Arthroscopic Excision of Radial Head Fragment(s)**

Preoperative Planning Checklist

- OR Table: Standard
- Position/positioning aids: Lateral decubitus, prone or supine
- Fluoroscopy: Operative side
- Equipment: 4.5-mm arthroscope, shavers, electrocautery, pituitary rongeurs
- Tourniquet (sterile/nonsterile): Sterile
- Instruments: Pituitary rongeurs/graspers

---

cannot be executed due to comminution, small fragment size, or osteopenia. The open surgical approaches for fragment excision will usually be the same as those chosen for open reduction and internal fixation.

Arthroscopic fragment removal requires surgeon experience with arthroscopy of the elbow. Supine, prone, or lateral decubitus arthroscopy can be performed depending on the surgeon's preference. Standard 4.5-mm arthroscope, motorized shavers, electrocautery devices, and pituitary rongeurs are required. Arthroscopic portals vary depending on the location of the fragment(s) (Table 34-7).

Positioning. Lateral decubitus on beanbag with arm positioner preferred by senior author.

Surgical Approach(es). Begin with an evaluation of joint stability using fluoroscopy. Insufflate the articulation with 20 cm³ of normal saline to make instrument insertion safer. Use proximal anterolateral, mid-anterolateral, and proximal anteromedial portals for anterior arthroscopy, posterocentral and mid-posterolateral portals for posterior arthroscopy, and a distal posterolateral portal for lateral arthroscopy. After the skin incision, use blunt dissection to enter the joint and safely insert the arthroscope and instruments.

Technique. Improve visualization by using shaver and electrocautery devices as required. Localize loose radial head fragment(s) and remove using a pituitary rongeur or grasper (Table 34-8).

Postoperative Care. Immediate active motion in a soft dressing is permitted if there are no associated injuries. Concomitant ligament injuries will direct the rehabilitation plan as outlined in the section on the operative treatment of elbow dislocations.

TABLE 34-8 **Arthroscopic Excision of Radial Head Fragment(s)**

Surgical Steps

- Evaluate elbow stability
- Insufflate joint
- Insert arthroscope
- Localize and remove radial head fragment(s)

TABLE 34-9 Arthroscopic Excision of Radial Head Fragment(s)

Potential Pitfalls and Preventions

Pitfall	Preventions
Excision of large radial head fragment leading to instability or clicking	Measure fragment size on CT preoperatively and at arthroscopy
Poor visualization at arthroscopy	Wait 5 d before arthroscopy Use tourniquet
Neurovascular injury	Check location and stability of ulnar nerve Careful portal placement Joint distention Elbow arthroscopic experience
Failure to remove loose fragments	CT imaging preoperatively to localize fragment(s) Full arthroscopic evaluation of the elbow

TABLE 34-10 Open Radial Head Excision

Preoperative Planning Checklist

- OR Table: Standard
- Position/positioning aids: Arm across chest or on arm table
- Fluoroscopy location: Operative side
- Equipment: Microsagittal saw, radial head arthroplasty system
- Tourniquet (sterile/nonsterile): Sterile

Potential Pitfalls and Preventative Measures. Avoid excision of larger radial head fragments, particularly in the setting of concomitant instability. The procedure should be abandoned and an open surgical approach performed if articular visualization is not adequate. Wait 5 days post injury to reduce intraoperative bleeding and improve visualization. Carefully examine for the location of the ulnar nerve preoperatively to avoid injury to a congenitally subluxating ulnar nerve. If an arthroscopic pump is used, keep the pressure low and ensure good fluid outflow to avoid excessive joint swelling (Table 34-9).

Treatment-Specific Outcomes. The outcome of patients undergoing open fragment excision of the radial head is variable in the limited available literature. There are no series reporting the outcome of arthroscopic fragment removal. Some authors have reported up to 80% good or excellent results in patients treated with open fragment excision.[51,77,115] However, Carstam reported that only half of their patients managed with fragment excision had good or excellent results. Avoid fragment excision in the setting of associated ligament and osseous injuries as the radial head is an important secondary stabilizer in this situation.

Radial Head Excision

Preoperative Planning. Excision of unreconstructable radial head fractures is not commonly performed in the setting of acute trauma due to a high incidence of associated injuries. The radial head may be removed for the treatment of malunions and nonunions. If radial head excision is contemplated, a careful inspection of the preoperative imaging is required to rule out associated fractures. The stability of the elbow should be evaluated fluoroscopically with varus, valgus, rotational, and axial stress tests before and after radial head excision. A radial head arthroplasty should be available for use if the elbow is determined to be unstable in any of these planes. The radial head can be removed using standard open surgical approaches as well as

arthroscopically using the techniques described in the previous section for radial head fragment excision (Table 34-10).

Positioning. The radial head can be excised with the arm placed across the chest with the surgeon standing or using an arm table with the surgeon sitting.

Surgical Approach. A direct lateral or a posterior skin incision is utilized. A posterior incision is longer but is more cosmetic, avoids cutaneous nerves and allows for an extensile approach to repair other structures if required. A Kocher approach between the ECU and anconeus is used when the LCL is ruptured and a common extensor tendon-splitting approach is preferred when the lateral ulnar collateral ligament is intact (Fig. 34-9).

Technique. Perform a fluoroscopic examination to rule out concomitant ligament injuries using varus, valgus, rotational, and axial stress tests. Use a common extensor-splitting approach when the LCL is intact, which is typical in the setting of a planned radial head excision. Divide the common extensor tendon and annular ligament at the mid-portion of the radial head. Iatrogenic lateral instability is avoided if dissection is maintained anterior to the mid-axis of the radial head. Maintain the

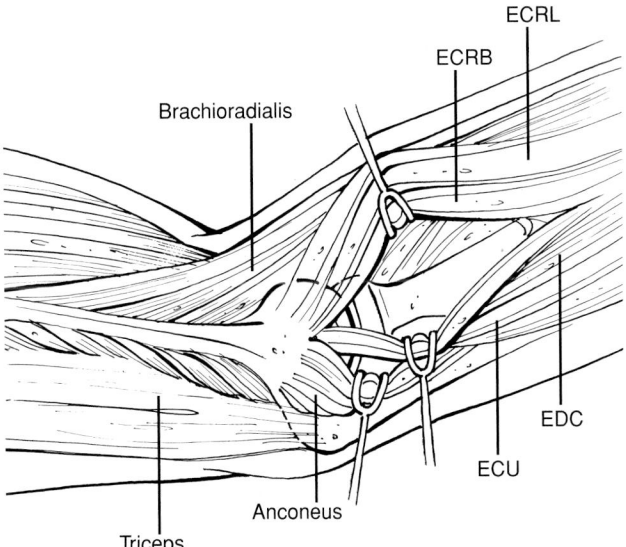

FIGURE 34-9 A Kocher approach between the anconeus and the extensor carpi ulnaris is preferred if the lateral collateral ligament is disrupted to facilitate ligament repair. A more anterior approach splitting the common extensor tendon at the mid-portion of the radial head is preferred when the ligaments are intact.

TABLE 34-11	Open Radial Head Excision

Surgical Steps

- Evaluate elbow and forearm stability using fluoroscopy
- Lateral or posterior skin incision
- Common extensor tendon-splitting approach
- Excise radial head at head–neck junction
- Remove all fragments of radial head
- Reevaluate elbow and forearm stability using fluoroscopy
- Repair annular ligament and extensor split

forearm in pronation while approaching the radial head and neck to protect the posterior interosseous nerve.[23] Further exposure can be achieved if needed by detaching the anterior portion of the radial collateral ligament off the lateral epicondyle and the extensor carpi radialis longus and brevis off the lateral supracondylar ridge. Do not dissect distal to the biceps tuberosity without visualizing the posterior interosseous nerve. Section the radial head perpendicular to the neck at the junction of the radial head and neck. Ensure that the stump of the proximal radius does not impinge with the lesser sigmoid notch of ulna during forearm rotation. Reconstruct the excised fragments of radial head to ensure all fragments are accounted for. Perform a fluoroscopic evaluation of the elbow to look for retained fragments and to reevaluate elbow and forearm stability. Repair the annular ligament and extensor split (Table 34-11).

Postoperative Care. Immediate active motion in a soft dressing is permitted if there are no associated injuries. Concomitant ligament injuries will direct the rehabilitation plan as outlined in the section on the operative treatment of elbow dislocations.

Potential Pitfalls and Preventative Measures. Do not excise the radial head without replacement in the setting of associated collateral ligament injuries, concomitant elbow dislocation, interosseous membrane disruption, or coronoid fractures due to the high incidence of persistent instability. Perform a careful fluoroscopic examination intraoperatively. Convert to a radial head arthroplasty if there is significant instability after radial head excision. Maintain the forearm in pronation and retract gently to protect the posterior interosseous nerve during the surgical approach. Avoid placing retractors around the anterior radial neck due to the risk of nerve compression (Table 34-12).

Treatment-Specific Outcomes. Given the high incidence of associated ligamentous injuries with more complex radial head fractures, our understanding of the key role of the radial head as a stabilizer in ligament deficient elbows, and its importance in load transfer across the elbow, primary excision of unreconstructable radial head fractures is less commonly performed. Long-term outcome studies have shown a high incidence of radiographic arthritis, an increase in the carrying angle, and proximal radial migration; however, the functional outcome with radial head excision for isolated fractures has been good in the majority of patients.[4,48,99] Since the outcome of late radial head excision is generally good, early radial head excision should probably be avoided.[15] Radial head excision should be avoided in patients with fracture-dislocations of the elbow.

TABLE 34-12	Open Radial Head Excision

Potential Pitfalls and Preventions

Pitfall	Preventions
Elbow or forearm instability	Fluoroscopic evaluation before and after radial head excision Replace radial head where possible Avoid radial head excision if concomitant ligamentous or osseous injuries
Posterior interosseous nerve injury	Maintain forearm in pronation during surgical approach Do not place retractors anterior to radial neck Do not dissect distal to biceps tuberosity
Retained fragment(s) of radial head	Reassemble radial head to check if all fragments removed Fluoroscopic evaluation of elbow

Open Reduction and Internal Fixation

Preoperative Planning. Early surgery is preferred when managing radial head fractures operatively; however, urgent fixation is not required unless there is persistent subluxation following a closed reduction, a progressive neurologic deficit, or an open injury. Small diameter (1.5- or 2-mm) screws should be available. Some surgeons prefer differential pitch bone screws. Cannulated (2.5- or 3-mm) screws are helpful when performing internal fixation of fractures of the radial neck. Small plates or radial head-specific periarticular locking plates should be available when treating complete articular fractures of the radial head and neck. Some radial head fractures that appear amenable to internal fixation will in fact have greater comminution than demonstrated by plain radiographs or CT. The surgeon should be prepared to proceed with arthroplasty if unexpected comminution or damage is found. In these situations, the availability of a radial head implant in the operating room and consent for placement is advisable when open reduction and internal fixation is planned (Table 34-13).

TABLE 34-13	ORIF of Radial Head and Neck Fractures

Preoperative Planning Checklist

- OR Table: Standard
- Position/positioning aids: Supine, arm across chest or on arm table; lateral decubitus an alternative
- Fluoroscopy location: Operative side
- Equipment: 0.035, 0.045 K-wires, 1.5- and 2-mm screws, 2.5-mm cannulated screws, periarticular locking plates, radial head arthroplasty system
- Tourniquet (sterile/nonsterile): Sterile

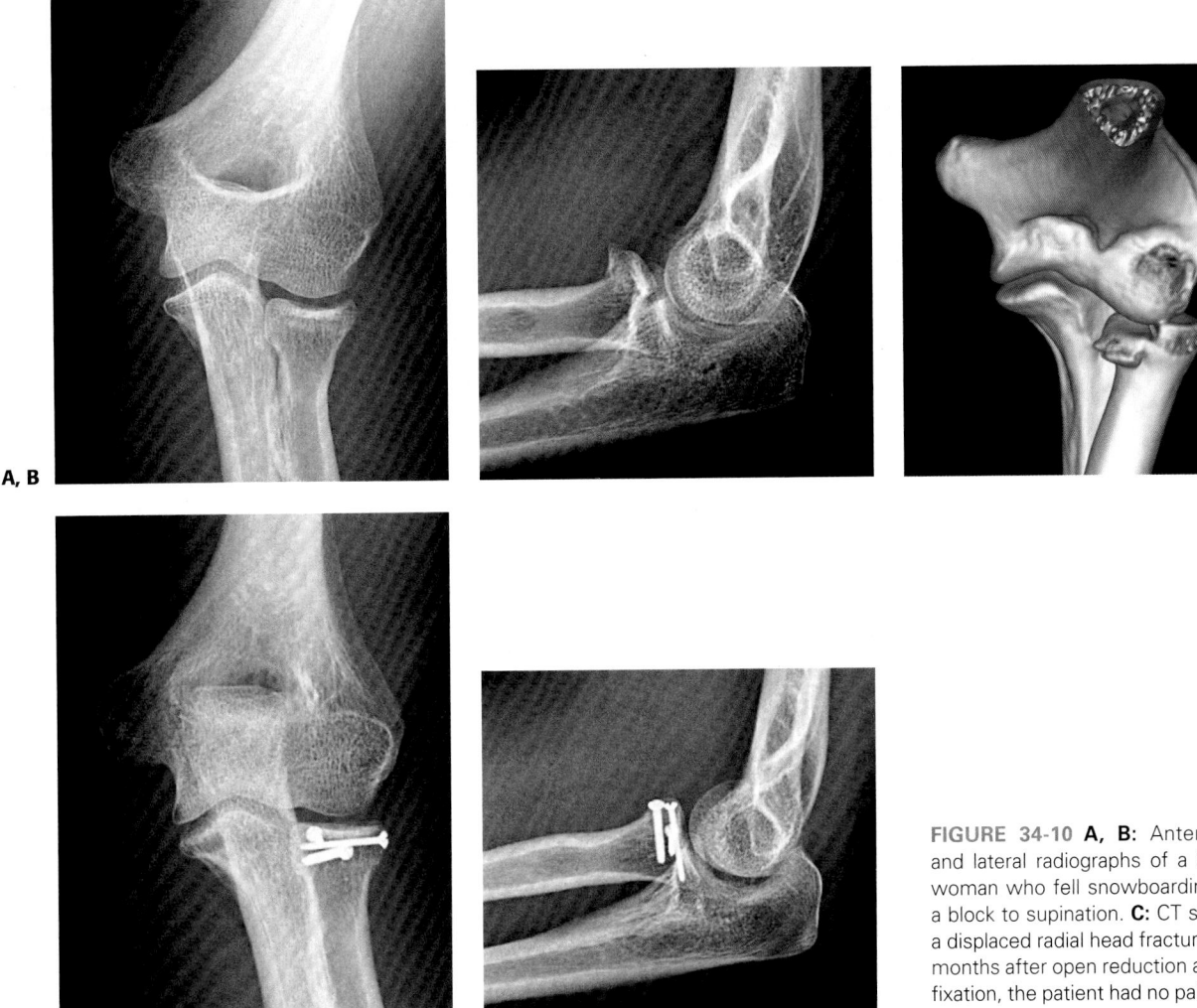

A, B

C

D

E

FIGURE 34-10 **A, B:** Anteroposterior and lateral radiographs of a 33-year-old woman who fell snowboarding and had a block to supination. **C:** CT scan shows a displaced radial head fracture. **D, E:** Six months after open reduction and internal fixation, the patient had no pain and a full range of motion.

Positioning. The radial head can be fixed with the arm placed across the chest with the surgeon standing or using an arm table with the surgeon sitting. When treating concomitant proximal ulna and olecranon fractures, the lateral decubitus position may be preferred.

Surgical Approach(es). Same as for radial head excision.

Technique. Periosteal attachments of the fragments should be preserved to maintain any residual blood supply and stability. The fractures are manipulated and provisionally reduced using Kirschner wires (K-wires). For partial articular fractures 1.5- or 2-mm countersunk screws are placed from the displaced fragments into the intact column of the radius typically using the same tracts as the provisional K-wire fixation (Fig. 34-10). In the setting of noncomminuted fractures of the radial neck, cross-cannulated screw fixation is performed using 2.5-mm screws. Cannulated fixation techniques are preferred as standard screws tend to deflect off the cortex of the radial neck when placed at an oblique angle of approach (Fig. 34-11). Low-profile nonlocking plates or periarticular fixed angle locking plates may be used in younger patients with more com-

minuted radial head and neck fractures; however, secondary plate removal is often required to treat rotational stiffness (Fig. 34-12). Plates should be placed on the nonarticular portion of the radial head which presents itself laterally with the forearm in neutral rotation (Fig. 34-7). In some circumstances where there are no periosteal attachments to the fragments, the radial head can be assembled on the back table, fixed to the plate and then the plate is attached to the radial neck. A careful fluoroscopic evaluation is performed to check the congruity of the reduction and to ensure optimal placement of internal fixation.

A side-to-side repair of the annular ligament and anterior portion of the radial collateral ligament with the overlying common extensor tendon is performed if an EDC-splitting approach is used. In the setting where the LCL is detached to facilitate exposure or is avulsed from the lateral epicondyle by the injury, transosseous sutures are preferred over suture anchors as this technique allows the tissues to be drawn toward the epicondyle for optimal tensioning (Fig. 34-4, Table 34-14).

Postoperative Care. Immediate active motion in a soft dressing is permitted if there are no associated injuries.

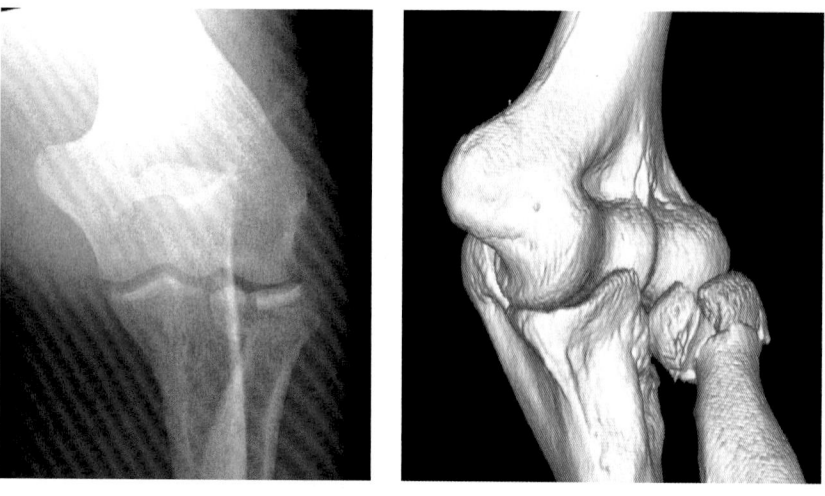
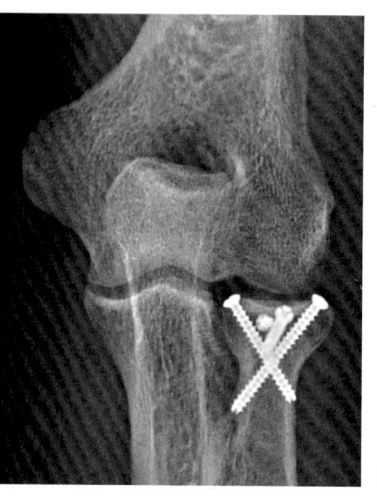

FIGURE 34-11 A: Anteroposterior radiograph of a 30-year-old man with a displaced radial head fracture and a block to rotation. **B:** CT scan shows pattern of fracture. **C:** Six months postop ORIF with cannulated "tripod" screws, the patient had minimal pain and a full forearm rotation.

FIGURE 34-12 A, B: Anteroposterior and lateral radiographs of a 56-year-old man with a proximal radius and ulna fracture. **C, D:** Two years after locking plate fixation of the radius and ulna, the patient had an occasional ache and lacked 20 degrees of supination and extension.

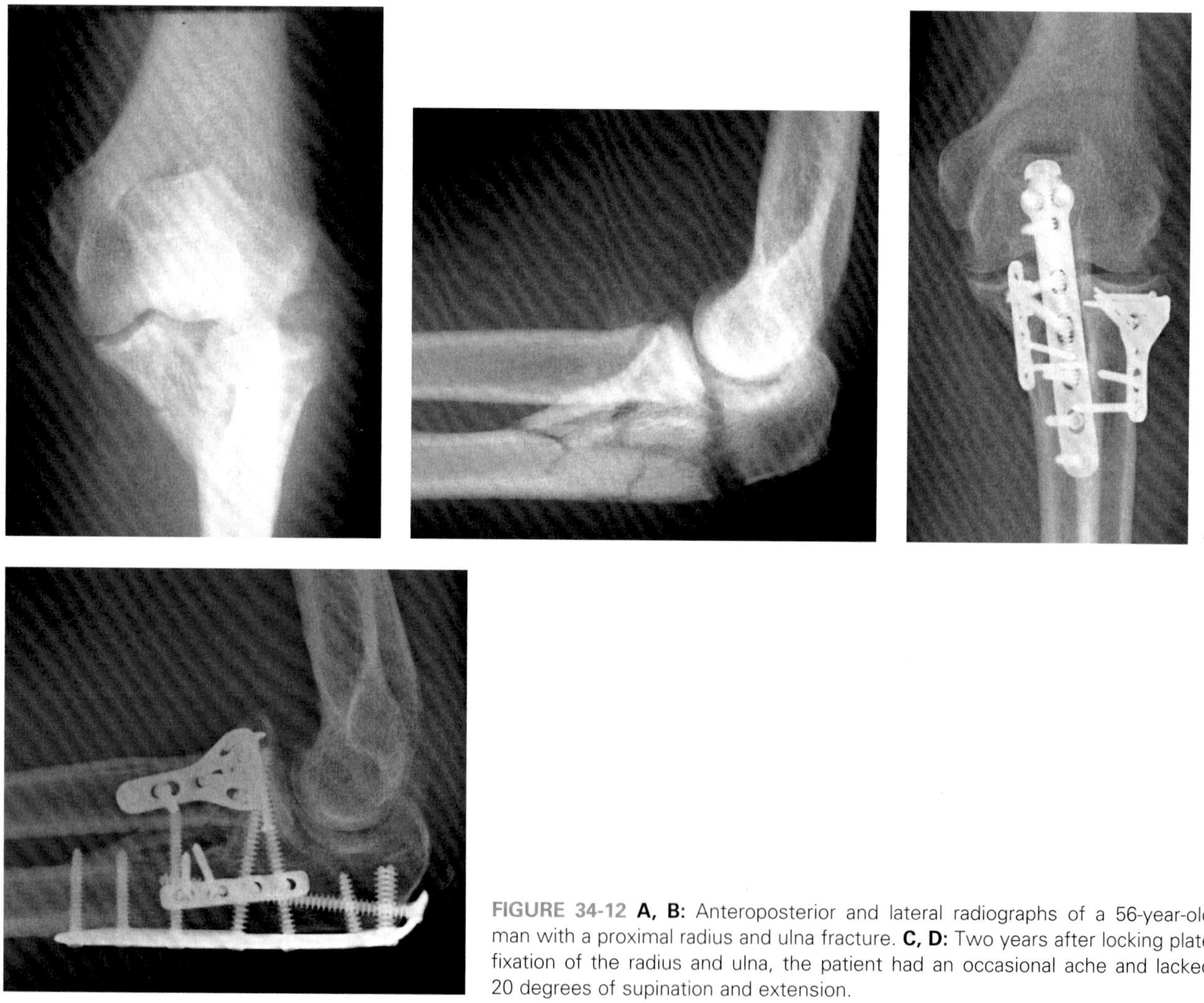

TABLE 34-14 **ORIF of Radial Head and Neck Fractures**

Surgical Steps

- Expose proximal radius
- Divide annular ligament
- Provisional reduction of fragments with K-wires
- Fixation with countersunk screws or plate as indicated

Concomitant ligament injuries will direct the rehabilitation plan as outlined in the section on the operative treatment of elbow dislocations. Strengthening is performed after fracture healing is secure, typically at 6 to 8 weeks postoperatively.

Some surgeons employ indomethacin 25 mg three times daily for a 3-week period in an effort to prevent heterotopic ossification. The effectiveness of this approach, however, has not been proven scientifically and complications such as delayed and/or nonunions, gastrointestinal side effects and allergies can occur with these medications. Radiation should be avoided as it has been demonstrated to increase the incidence of nonunions when employed for acute distal humeral fractures.[44]

Potential Pitfalls and Preventative Measures. The surgeon should not accept tenuous fixation of radial head fractures as clinical failure is common in such circumstances. If an anatomic reduction with stable internal fixation cannot be achieved, a radial head replacement should be considered. Maintain the forearm in pronation to protect the posterior interosseous nerve during the surgical approach. Avoid overzealous retraction anterior to the radial neck due to the risk of nerve compression (Table 34-15).

Treatment-Specific Outcomes. Open reduction and stable internal fixation of displaced radial head fractures yields good results in the majority of patients.[59,65,91] Partial articular fractures have better results than complete articular fractures. More comminuted fractures, especially those with more than three fragments or concomitant elbow instability have poorer outcomes; radial head arthroplasty should be strongly considered.[21,91] Patients treated with radial head excision have been reported to have poorer outcomes and a higher rate of osteoarthritis than those treated with ORIF.[14,49,65] At an average of 17 years postoperatively, Lindenhovius et al. reported a lower severity of arthritis and a reduced incidence of elbow dislocations in patients that had ORIF compared to those who had a radial head excision. Countersunk screws have a lower incidence or stiffness than ORIF with plates for patients with fractures of the radial neck.[79,102]

Radial Head Arthroplasty

Preoperative Planning. A modular metallic radial head arthroplasty system should always be available when operating on displaced radial head fractures because comminution is often more severe than predicted by plain radiographs or CT. In

TABLE 34-15 **Radial Head and Neck Fractures**

Potential Pitfalls and Preventions

Pitfall	Preventions
Fixation failure	Avoid fixation of small osteoporotic fractures Use locking plates Place screws through tracts of K-wires to avoid fragmentation of small fractures Ensure stable ligament repairs to avoid elbow subluxation which leads to fixation failure Use radial head arthroplasty if fixation is tenuous
Stiffness	Early motion Avoid plate fixation
Posterior interosseous nerve injury	Avoid dissection distal to biceps tuberosity Do not place retractors anterior to radial neck Maintain forearm in pronation during surgical approach
Avascular necrosis	Preserve periosteal attachments of fragments Rigid internal fixation to allow for fragment union and revascularization

the setting of neck comminution, small plates or cerclage wires should be available to allow for neck reconstruction and the use of a standard prosthesis. Alternatively a long stem bipolar prosthesis should be available in the uncommon situation where reconstruction of the radial neck to accept a standard prosthesis is not possible (Table 34-16).

Positioning. The radial head can be replaced with the arm placed across the chest with the surgeon standing or using an arm table with the surgeon sitting. When treating concomitant proximal ulna and olecranon fractures, the lateral decubitus position may be preferred.

Surgical Approach. Same as for radial head excision as outlined previously.

TABLE 34-16 **Radial Head Arthroplasty**

Preoperative Planning Checklist

- OR Table: Standard
- Position/positioning aids: Supine with arm across chest or arm table; lateral decubitus an alternative
- Fluoroscopy location: Operative side
- Equipment: Modular metallic radial head implant system, cerclage wires, and small plating systems in setting of concomitant neck fractures
- Tourniquet: Sterile

Technique. The annular ligament must be sectioned to adequately expose the radial head and neck and to facilitate the prosthesis insertion. The exact replacement technique will depend on the prosthesis system to be employed. After removing any loose fragments, section the radial neck at the junction of the radial head and neck or at the level of the fracture using an oscillating saw. Most radial head systems are modular to improve size matching with the native radial head and neck. Reassemble the excised fragments of radial head on the back table to ensure all fragments are removed from the elbow and to determine the optimal diameter and thickness of the radial head prosthesis to be employed. The native radial head is somewhat elliptical and is offset relative to the radial neck. Most commercially available implants are axisymmetric and nonanatomic; some employ a bipolar articulation. The optimal diameter of a radial head implant is not known but the articular dish of the implant should likely approximate the articular dish of the native radial head. The optimal implant diameter is typically the minor diameter of the elliptical native radial head, most commonly 2 mm smaller than the maximum diameter. An implant whose diameter is too large may cause an erosion of the lateral trochlea, prevents optimal closure of the annular ligament and may contribute to residual instability. When in between sizes, a smaller prosthesis is chosen both in diameter as well as thickness.

Measurement of radial head thickness should be performed using the excised fragments of the radial head where available. Over-lengthening (over-stuffing) with the placement of a radial head prosthesis that is too thick may be associated with the development of pain, stiffness, and capitellar wear.[13]

Place a Homan retractor around the posterior aspect of the radial neck and lever it against the ulna to translate the proximal radius laterally to prepare the radial canal and to insert the assembled modular prosthesis. If a smooth stem prosthesis is to be used choose a stem 1 mm smaller than the maximum-sized diameter neck rasp to allow the stem to move slightly in the neck such that the articular surface of the implant tracks optimally with the capitellum.

After placing the trial implants, the radial head should articulate at the level of the proximal radial ulnar joint which is typically 2 mm distal to the tip of the coronoid.[25] A careful evaluation for congruent tracking of the radial head implant on the capitellum both visually and fluoroscopically is required. Radiographic parameters are not very useful to detect over-lengthening of the radial head.[5,38,96] The medial ulnohumeral joint space should be parallel; over-lengthening causes the medial ulnohumeral joint to open laterally. However, this may not be evident until there is 6- to 8-mm over-lengthening of the radial head insert. Following insertion of the definitive radial head prosthesis, careful repair of the annular ligament and any concomitant osseous and ligament injuries are required to maintain elbow stability (Table 34-17).

Postoperative Care. Immediate active motion in a soft dressing is permitted if there are no associated injuries. Concomitant ligament injuries will direct the rehabilitation plan as outlined in the section on the operative treatment of elbow dislocations.

TABLE 34-17 **Radial Head Arthroplasty**

Surgical Steps

- Expose radial head and neck
- Use oscillating saw to section radial neck at the head–neck junction or at the level of the fracture
- Reassemble excised radial head fragments to measure diameter and thickness
- Use Homan retractor placed posterior to the radial neck to gently lever the proximal radius laterally to allow access to radial neck
- Rasp radial neck and select stem size 1 mm smaller than rasp
- Trial reduction
  - Check sizing of implant
  - Ensure congruent tracking of radial head on capitellum visually and with fluoroscopy
  - Evaluate radial length
- Insert radial head prosthesis
- Repair annular ligament and any concomitant osseous and ligament injuries

---

Potential Pitfalls and Preventative Measures. Incorrect implant sizing is a common problem following radial head arthroplasty. Unfortunately radiographic parameters are unreliable intraoperatively making the use of the excised radial head and the relationship of the radial head to the proximal ulna the most useful sizing tools. Do not use the distance between the capitellum and radial neck cut to size the implant as partial and complete LCL tears are common and this may lead to over-lengthening of the radial head implant.

Contralateral radiographs can be helpful to make the diagnosis of radial head over-lengthening postoperatively and to assist in planning preoperatively if the radial head has previously been removed. A measurement technique has been developed based on contralateral radiographs which can accurately quantify radial head implant length within 1 mm.[5]

Radial neck fractures can occur with overzealous retraction, reaming, and prosthesis insertion. Meticulous surgical technique should prevent this complication in most circumstances. Repair of the radial neck with cerclage wires usually allows successful prosthesis insertion.

Stiffness is prevented by encouraging early active motion. Indomethacin can be used in an effort to prevent heterotopic ossification in patients without contraindications; however, its effectiveness remains unproven.

Posterior interosseous nerve injuries can be avoided by maintaining the forearm in pronation during the surgical approach and avoidance of Homan retractors placed anterior to the radial neck.

Capitellar wear or erosions can occur, particularly with over-lengthening of a radial head prosthesis or maltracking of the implant.[13] Management can include revision or removal of the implant if the elbow is stable. Mechanical failure of the prosthesis can arise from failure to link the modular implant correctly, or a failure of the coupling mechanism such as a screw or polyethylene in the setting of a bipolar device. Revision should be corrective. Polyethylene wear with secondary osteolysis and implant loosening can also develop with a bipolar implant and

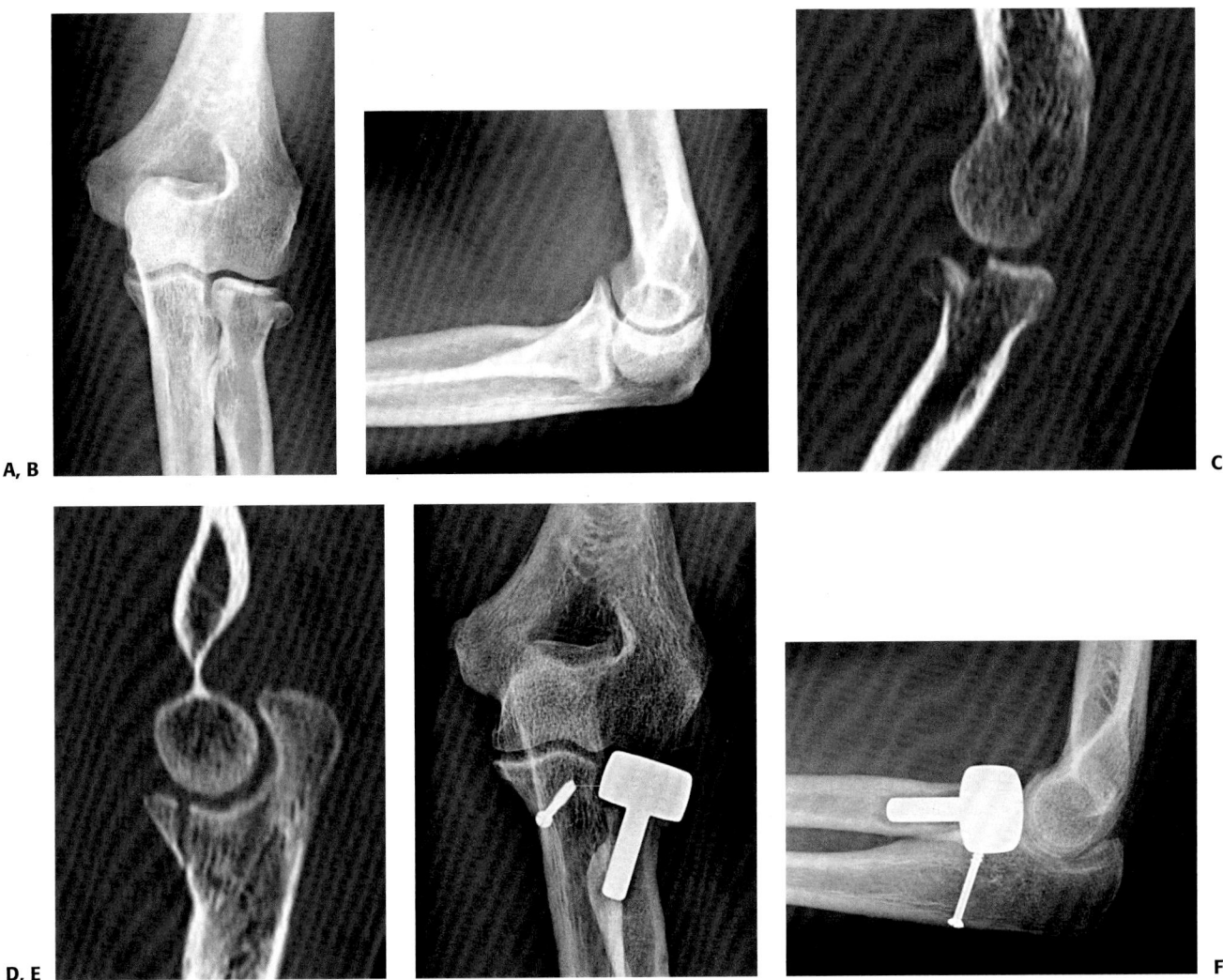

A, B

C

D, E

F

FIGURE 34-13 Anteroposterior and lateral radiographs of a 50-year-old woman who fell from a height **(A, B).** CT scan shows a comminuted, displaced radial head fracture and undisplaced coronoid fracture **(C, D).** Two years postop ORIF coronoid, radial head replacement, and LCL repair. The patient had no pain and a near full range of motion. The lucent lines around the smooth uncemented stem did not progress after 1 year **(E, F).**

is more problematic; prosthesis removal or revision should be considered as appropriate.[17,84] Nonprogressive radiolucent lines around smooth stemmed implants are common and are not usually associated with the presence of residual symptoms (Fig. 34-13).[35] Progressive lucency around a smooth-stemmed implant should raise the possibility of infection or residual instability which should be confirmed and managed. Implants with ingrowth stems which are loose may be symptomatic and require revision or removal (Table 34-18).[37]

Treatment-Specific Outcomes. The outcome of metallic radial head replacements in the medium term is good with a variety of implant designs.[17,26,42,94,98] Radiolucent lines around the stems of uncemented smooth stem components are commonly seen but do not correlate with patient symptoms.[35] However, radiolucent lines around rough ingrowth stems may indicate loosening and are often associated with pain, a com-

mon reason for reoperation.[37,111] Proximal radius stress shielding has been noted when using fully grit blasted uncemented stems. An uncemented smooth stem bipolar radial head replacement has shown good early results with no evidence of polyethylene wear.[118] Progressive osteolysis due to polyethylene wear debris has been reported at longer follow-up with cemented bipolar radial head replacements.[84] Early results with pyrocarbon implants have reported some catastrophic failures at the head–neck junction.[98]

MANAGEMENT OF EXPECTED ADVERSE OUTCOMES AND UNEXPECTED COMPLICATIONS IN RADIAL HEAD FRACTURES

Osteoarthritis is common following fractures of the radial head. Even minimally displaced fractures have a high incidence of

TABLE 34-18 **Radial Head Arthroplasty**

Potential Pitfalls and Preventions

Pitfall	Preventions
Incorrect implant size	Measure size of excised RH diameter and thickness
	Evaluate articulation of implant with respect to proximal radioulnar joint and coronoid
	Fluoroscopic evaluation of the ulnohumeral joint and implant alignment
Radial neck fracture	Gentle retraction of radial neck
	Avoid use of press fit stem that is too large
Stiffness	Early motion
	Possible use of indomethacin
Posterior interosseous nerve palsy	Maintain forearm in pronation during surgical approach
	Avoid dissection distal to biceps tuberosity
	Do not lever on retractors anterior to radial neck
Prosthesis failure	Ensure modular implant is securely coupled
	Avoid use of bipolar implants in younger more active patients were polyethylene wear may be more of a concern
	Ensure secure press fit of uncemented ingrowth stems

arthritis at long-term follow-up, likely as a consequence of traumatic articular damage at the time of injury as well as residual articular incongruity. Radial head replacement can be considered if the capitellar cartilage is relatively well preserved; however, radial head excision is preferred in the setting where the capitellar cartilage or bone has advanced disease. If there is post-traumatic arthritis of the radiocapitellar joint associated with residual elbow instability, radial head excision is contraindicated. A uni-compartmental radiocapitellar arthroplasty should be considered; however, these implants are relatively new, and their outcome remains unknown. Total elbow arthroplasty may be required to manage post-traumatic arthritis that involves the ulnohumeral joint.

Stiffness is common following radial head fractures. It can be isolated to a loss of flexion–extension or forearm rotation. The most common cause is capsular contracture; however, mechanical causes such as prominent hardware or retained cartilaginous or osseous fragments can also be responsible. The development of post-traumatic heterotopic ossification should also be considered. In the setting of capsular contracture passive stretching under the supervision of a therapist as well as the use of static progressive splinting is often successful. Turnbuckle splinting can also be employed. Patients with persistent stiffness following radial head fractures can be treated with

standard techniques of open or arthroscopic debridement and capsular release.

Malunions are common with nonsurgical management of displaced radial head fractures; however, in most cases patients have minimal, if any, symptoms. In some cases patients present restricted rotation, pain, clicking, or crepitus. Secondary degenerative changes of the capitellum and radial head can occur. Management options can include an intra- or extra-articular osteotomy of the radial head in younger patients without secondary degenerative changes of the capitellum.[93] Most patients presenting with symptomatic malunions have significant chondral damage to the radial head and/or capitellum and are therefore best treated by radial head excision or radial head arthroplasty.[101] Nonunions of radial neck fractures can occur with nonsurgical management; however, these may be asymptomatic. Nonunions following internal fixation are typically due to compromised vascularity and often do not respond to revision open reduction and internal fixation and grafting. Radial head excision or replacement is recommended in most circumstances.

Chronic valgus or axial instability is most commonly seen in patients who have had a radial head excision without replacement. This problem can typically be prevented by fixation or replacement of the radial head. Management of late valgus instability includes replacement of the radial head as well as an MCL reconstruction. Chronic varus and posterolateral rotatory instability (PLRI) can also occur in patients with radial head fractures due to deficient healing of the LCL. The absence of a radial head to provide concavity compression of the lateral column or properly tension the lateral ligaments exacerbates underlying instability. Reconstruction of the LCL using a tendon graft is preferred in the presence of a native radial head or prosthesis to help tension the graft and improve stability.

Early recognition and prevention of axial forearm instability is preferred. Unfortunately, most patients present late following radial head excision. While 2 to 3 mm of proximal migration of the radial head is expected after radial head excision with intact ligaments of the distal radial ulnar joint and interosseous membrane, marked proximal migration can occur with disruption of these stabilizing structures. The optimal management for chronic Essex–Lopresti injuries is unknown. Treatment options include a one-bone forearm, replacement of the radial head with an immediate or staged ulnar shortening, or techniques of interosseous membrane reconstruction combined with a radial head prosthesis (Table 34-19).[68]

TABLE 34-19 **Radial Head Fractures**

Common Adverse Outcomes and Complications

Post-traumatic arthritis

Stiffness

Symptomatic nonunion, malunion, or avascular necrosis

Elbow and/or forearm instability

AUTHOR'S PREFERRED METHOD OF TREATMENT FOR RADIAL HEAD FRACTURES (FIG. 34-14)

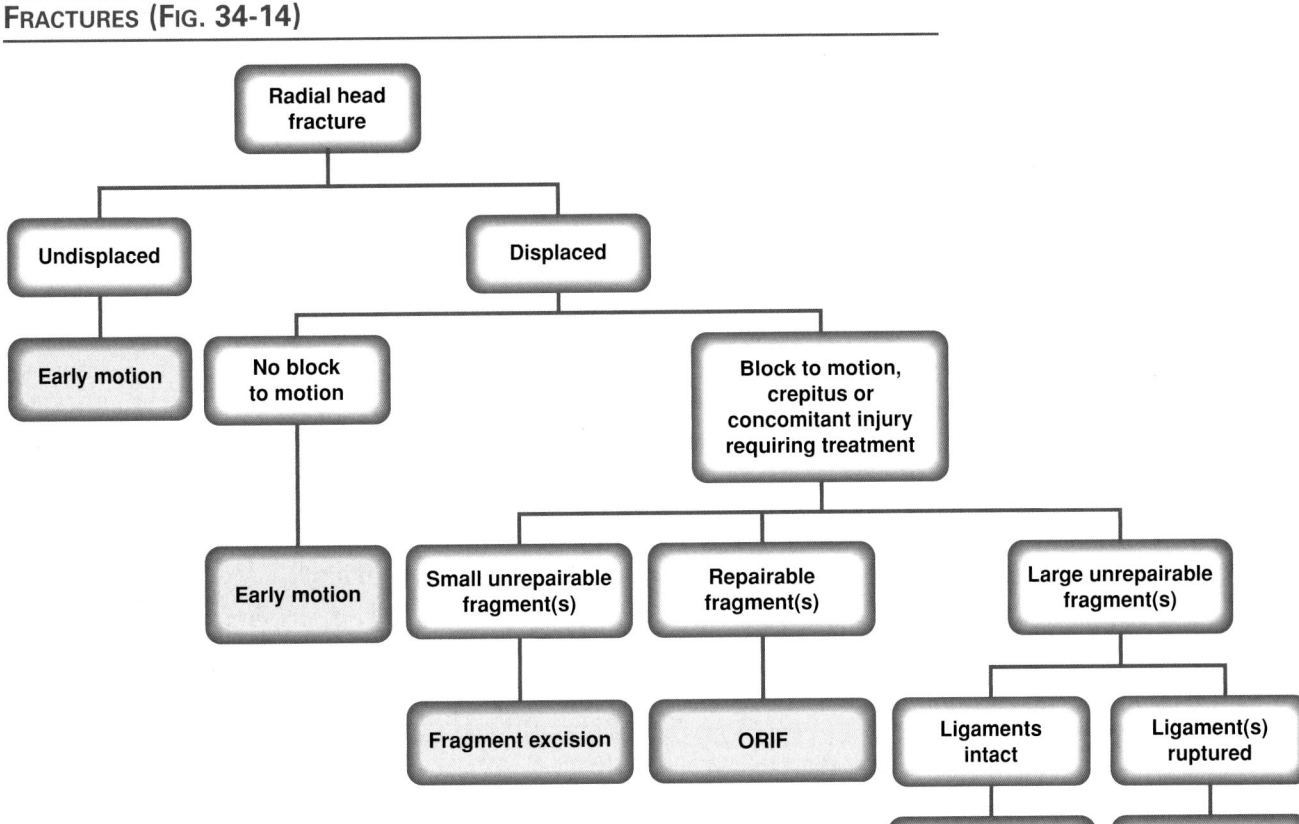

FIGURE 34-14 Author's preferred treatment.

SUMMARY, CONTROVERSIES, AND FUTURE DIRECTIONS IN RADIAL HEAD FRACTURES

Radial head fractures are common; however, the majority are minimally displaced or undisplaced and can be treated successfully nonoperatively. Advances in imaging, fixation devices, and newer prosthetic designs have improved the outcome of displaced fractures; however, the indications for surgery remain unclear. Randomized clinical trials are needed to provide a scientific rationale for the management of displaced radial head fractures without a block to motion. Radial head excision is uncommonly performed for acute radial head fractures due to a significant incidence of concomitant ligament injuries and the advent of reliable prosthetic arthroplasty.

INTRODUCTION TO CORONOID FRACTURES

Isolated fractures of the coronoid are uncommon with the majority having associated fractures of the radial head or proximal ulna, collateral ligament injuries, or concomitant dislocations. Fractures of the coronoid occur in 2% to 15% of patients with ulnohumeral dislocations.[114] The pattern and

size of the coronoid fracture and the extent of concomitant osseous and ligament injuries dictate the optimal treatment strategy.

Coronoid fractures have traditionally been classified using the Regan–Morrey classification system.[87] This classification system focuses on the height of the fracture in the coronal plane. Type I fractures are small coronoid tip fractures. Type II fractures involve less than 50% of the total coronoid height and Type III fractures involve greater than 50%. The classification is modified based on the presence or absence of an associated fracture-dislocation, with Type A defining an isolated fracture and Type B defining an associated dislocation.

O'Driscoll et al.[80] introduced a more comprehensive classification system that included fracture size, anatomic location, and mechanism of injury. This system is divided into three types. Type I fractures involve the coronoid tip and are divided into two subtypes based on size. Subtype I are tip fractures less than 2 mm, while subtype II are larger than 2 mm, but less than 50% of the coronoid height. Type II fractures involve the anteromedial facet and are divided into three subtypes. Subtype I involves the rim only, subtype II involves

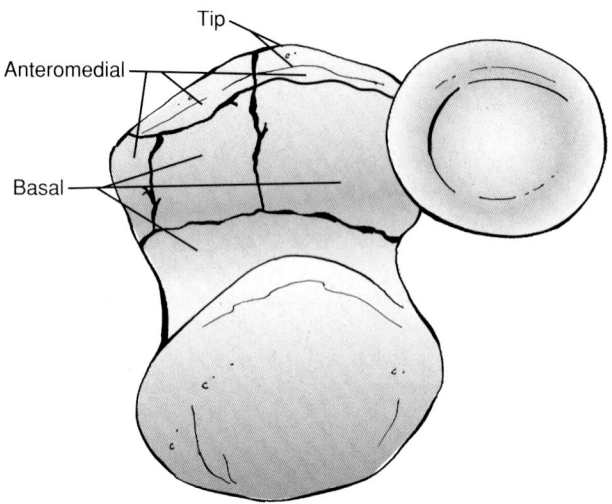

FIGURE 34-15 The O'Driscoll classification of coronoid fractures includes Type I, fractures of the tip, Type II, fractures involving the anteromedial facet, and Type III, basal fractures. Type I fractures are most commonly associated with terrible triad fracture-dislocations, Type II are associated with varus posteromedial rotatory instability, and Type III are associated with olecranon and proximal ulna fracture-dislocations.

the rim and tip, and subtype III involves the rim, and sublime tubercle, with or without involvement of the tip. Type III fractures include the coronoid base and consist of two subtypes. Subtype I comprises body and basal fractures while subtype II includes the former in addition to a transolecranon fracture (Fig. 34-15).

O'Driscoll Type I coronoid tip fractures are typically associated with fractures of the radial head and a concomitant elbow dislocation, the "terrible triad" injury of the elbow. These injuries typically occur with a PLRI mechanism, shearing off the anterolateral radial head and coronoid tip while dislocating. Type II anteromedial coronoid fractures are seen with posteromedial rotatory instability (PMRI) and are almost always have a concomitant avulsion of the LCL. Type III basal coronoid fractures are most commonly associated with fractures of the olecranon and proximal ulna and have a more direct posterior injury mechanism. They typically have larger fractures of the radial head and less ligamentous injuries. The management of coronoid fractures is best understood by considering the patterns of injury rather than focusing on the isolated treatment of the coronoid.

INTRODUCTION TO TERRIBLE TRIAD INJURIES OF THE ELBOW

Terrible triad injuries consist of a fracture of the radial head and coronoid and an elbow dislocation. These injuries may be challenging to treat and suboptimal clinical outcomes have been commonly described in the past. Advances in our knowledge of elbow biomechanics and improvements in implants have resulted in improved patient outcomes.

ASSESSMENT OF TERRIBLE TRIAD INJURIES

Mechanisms of Injury for Terrible Triad Injuries

Terrible triad injuries are thought to occur by posterolateral rotatory displacement of the ulna, resulting in elbow subluxation or dislocation (Fig. 34-1).[81] The proposed mechanism is a fall onto an outstretched arm, with supination, valgus, and axial-directed force. The trochlea causes a shear fracture of the coronoid and is accompanied by an LCL injury and/or radial head fracture.

Associated Injuries with Terrible Triad

Ipsilateral upper extremity injuries have been reported in 10% to 20% of patients with fracture-dislocations of the elbow with the majority involving fractures of the wrist.[27,54] Associated injuries of the head, chest, abdomen, pelvis, or lower extremities are seen in patients with higher-energy trauma. Neurovascular injuries are uncommon.

Signs and Symptoms of Terrible Triad Injuries

A detailed neurovascular examination must be performed before and after reduction of a dislocated elbow. Soft tissue status and the condition of the skin should be carefully assessed. The elbow should be palpated for signs of tenderness over the collateral ligament insertions. The shoulder, wrist, and distal radioulnar joint should be examined. Radiographic signs of these fractures are often subtle stressing the importance of detailed physical examination.

Imaging of Terrible Triad Injuries

Once the initial evaluation is complete, standard radiographs (AP and lateral views) are required to determine the direction of the dislocation and to identify associated fractures. Radiographs of the shoulder, forearm, and wrist are ordered as clinically indicated. Radiographs are repeated following a gentle closed reduction of the elbow dislocation under conscious sedation. The radiocapitellar joint can be widened with LCL disruption and the radial head can be subluxated posteriorly. CT may help to better evaluate radial head fracture patterns and demonstrate osteochondral fragments within the joint. Three-dimensional CT reconstructions have been shown to improve interobserver agreement on the classification and treatment of coronoid fractures relative to two-dimensional CT.[64] CT can also assist with selecting the surgical approach and type of internal fixation required.

Classification of Terrible Triad Injuries

Terrible triad injuries are subclassified by the pattern of radial head and coronoid fractures. The most common coronoid fractures seen in terrible triad injuries are Types I and II.[29] The radial head fracture classifications were outlined in the previous section.

Outcome Measures for Terrible Triad Injuries

Several scoring systems have been used to evaluate the outcomes of terrible triad injuries including the DASH Questionnaire, the Mayo Elbow Performance Score, and the Patient-rated Elbow Evaluation.

PATHOANATOMY AND APPLIED ANATOMY RELATING TO TERRIBLE TRIAD INJURIES

The primary stabilizers of the elbow joint are the coronoid, MCL, and LCL. The secondary constraints are the capsule, the radiocapitellar articulation, and the common extensor and flexor origins.[74] The radial head is a secondary valgus stabilizer while the coronoid is primary stabilizer to varus stress and an important stabilizer to axial, posteromedial and posterolateral rotatory forces.[7,75,83,100]

Biomechanical studies of a terrible triad model demonstrate that ligament repair and radial head arthroplasty can restore near normal elbow kinematics and stability if the coronoid fracture is small (Type I). However, larger coronoid fractures, such as Regan and Morrey Types II and III resulted in vertical and coronal plane instability, even in the setting of ligament repair and radial head repair or replacement.[9]

TERRIBLE TRIAD INJURIES TREATMENT OPTIONS

Nonoperative Treatment of Terrible Triad Injuries

Indications/Contraindications

Terrible triad injuries of the elbow are usually treated surgically due to residual instability precluding a congruous reduction and early motion. If the radial head and coronoid fractures are small and the elbow is congruously reduced following a closed reduction, nonoperative treatment should be considered. Fracture fragments which are interposed within the articulation and the presence of residual instability are contraindications to nonoperative treatment. Radial head fractures which are displaced and causing a block to forearm rotation are also contraindications for nonsurgical management (Table 34-20).

Technique

A closed manipulative reduction of the elbow is usually performed in the emergency room or the operating room. After

TABLE 34-20	Terrible Triad Injuries

Nonoperative Treatment

Indications	Relative Contraindications
Concentric elbow following closed reduction of dislocation	Nonconcentric elbow reduction
Undisplaced radial head fracture or displaced radial head fracture without a block to rotation	Displaced radial head fracture interfering with forearm rotation
Regan and Morrey subtype Type I coronoid fracture, undisplaced subtype II and III coronoid fractures	Displaced Regan and Morrey subtype Type II and III coronoid fractures. Fracture fragment interposed in articulation

reduction, the elbow is taken through an arc of flexion–extension in pronation, neutral, and supination in order to evaluate for residual instability. Since the lateral sided soft tissue injuries are typically more severe in terrible triad injuries, pronation of the forearm often improves stability. If the elbow redislocates between 0 and 30 degrees of flexion, operative treatment should be considered. Terrible triad injuries treated nonoperatively are immobilized in a light splint at 90 degrees of flexion for 7 to 10 days for comfort and to allow muscle tone to return to the elbow. Prolonged treatment in excessive flexion to maintain joint reduction should be avoided. Isometric contraction of the elbow muscles is encouraged while in the postreduction splint. After splint removal the patient is re-examined for stability and asked to actively extend and flex the elbow. Patients will typically move only within their stable arc and are unlikely to redislocate if they had a stable reduction and examination initially. Abduction of the arm and elbow from the chest and passive range of motion exercises are avoided as this produces a varus stress on their elbow. A 90-degree resting splint is used between exercises, typically the forearm in pronated which is usually the most stable position in the setting of more extensive lateral than medial sided soft tissue injury. Full extension in supination is not typically permitted for 4 weeks to limit the potential for elbow subluxation. Weekly radiographic and clinical follow-up is required to monitor for fracture displacement and recovery of motion. Persistent joint subluxation or redislocation is an indication for surgical management. At 6 weeks the resting splint is discontinued and gentle stretching may be initiated to manage residual stiffness. Varus or valgus loading as well as strengthening are avoided until 12 weeks. Static progressive splinting can be used to improve elbow motion.

Outcomes

There is little information regarding the nonoperative treatment of terrible triad injuries of the elbow. Nonoperative treatment has been associated with less desirable outcomes including stiffness, late instability, and arthrosis.[45,90] More recently, Guitton and Ring reported that three of the four patients treated nonoperatively had good results. The authors concluded that nonsurgical treatment could be considered for small and minimally displaced fractures of the coronoid and radial head with good elbow alignment.[43]

Operative Treatment of Terrible Triad Injuries

Indications/Contraindications

The majority of patients with terrible triad injuries require surgical management to achieve a stable congruous reduction of the elbow allowing early motion. Residual subluxation of the elbow following a closed reduction or residual instability precluding early motion is an indication for surgery. Displaced radial head fractures blocking motion or incarcerated fracture fragments in the articulation are also indications for surgery. Surgery may occasionally be contraindicated in patients whose medical comorbidities place them at an unacceptable risk as well as patients with nonfunctional upper extremities due to neurologic or other impairments.

Open Reduction and Internal Fixation

A systematic approach is important to address the critical components of this injury. This includes fixation or replacement of the radial head, fixation of the coronoid fragment, and repair of the LCL. The elbow is then evaluated intraoperatively for residual instability to determine if MCL repair is required or rarely if an external fixator is needed.

Preoperative Planning (Table 34-21)

TABLE 34-21   ORIF of Terrible Triad Injuries

Preoperative Planning Checklist

- OR Table: Radiolucent arm table
- Position/positioning aids: Supine with arm table or arm across chest
- Fluoroscopy location: Operative side
- Equipment: Suture anchors, 0.035, 0.045 K-wires, 1.5- and 2-mm screws, 2.5-mm cannulated screws, periarticular locking plates, radial head arthroplasty system, large external fixator, hinged external fixator, large fragment locking set with screws

Positioning. Terrible triad injuries can be repaired with the arm placed across the chest with the surgeon standing or using an arm table with the surgeon sitting. The use of a rolled-up sheet placed underneath the elbow can be helpful to approach the medial elbow when the arm is placed across the chest.

Surgical Approach. A posterior midline elbow skin incision is typically employed when managing terrible triad injuries of the elbow as it allows lateral, medial, and posterior access to the elbow. Alternatively separate lateral, medial, and posterior skin incisions can be employed as needed. A Kocher approach is preferred to allow repair of the LCL which typically is avulsed off the lateral epicondyle in terrible triad injuries.[71]

The optimal surgical approach to repair the coronoid has not been determined with various lateral, anterior, and medial options reported. In many cases the coronoid can be accessed and repaired from a lateral surgical exposure, particularly if a radial head replacement is required. A flexor pronator split can be used for Regan and Morrey Type I and II coronoid fractures (Fig. 34-16).[103] A Taylor and Scham approach may be preferred for the Type III basal fractures and when a medial plate is required.[108] This approach involves detaching the entire flexor pronator mass from the medial epicondyle and supracondylar ridge and provides excellent exposure to the entire coronoid and MCL. Our preferred surgical approach is to use the interval between the two heads of the flexor carpi ulnaris (FCU).[97] This also provides adequate access to the sublime tubercle and MCL. Meticulous release and mobilization of motor branches of the ulnar nerve can help improve distal exposure. Proximal articular branches may need to be sacrificed in order to obtain adequate exposure. Elevating the flexor–pronator muscles from distal to proximal helps isolate the sublime tubercle and identify and protect the anterior bundle of the MCL when it is intact. The authors routinely perform an in situ release of the ulnar nerve; transposition of the ulnar nerve should be considered if there are preoperative ulnar nerve symptoms or if further mobilization is needed to allow coronoid fixation.

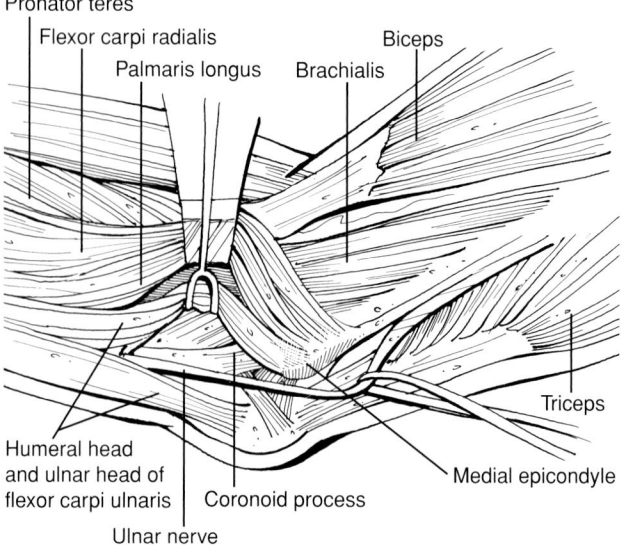

FIGURE 34-16 There are three medial approaches to fix the coronoid. A flexor pronator split, using the floor of the ulnar nerve which splits the two heads of the flexor carpi ulnaris, and elevation of the entire flexor carpi ulnaris of the ulna.

Technique. A fluoroscopic assessment of the elbow under anesthesia is important to determine the extent of collateral ligament injury and the magnitude of elbow instability. After performing a lateral or posterior elbow skin incision, an extended Kocher approach is used to provide a more complete exposure of the elbow and facilitate repair of the LCL. When extending the exposure a cuff of fascia should be left attached to the supracondylar ridge to assist with closure. In order to protect the posterior interosseous nerve, the forearm should be pronated and the distal extent of the exposure should not exceed 2 cm from the radio-capitellar joint.[23] The coronoid can be accessed through the radial head fracture or by hinging the elbow open through the lateral ligament injury. Coronoid fractures too small or comminuted to be amenable to screw fixation can be repaired using sutures passed around the coronoid process and anterior capsule through transosseous tunnels on the dorsal ulna.[40,70] Small tip fractures of the coronoid, less than 10% may be left unrepaired if a secure repair of the concomitant injuries is achieved.[11] If the radial head is nonreconstructable, resection will improve exposure of the coronoid. An anatomic reduction of the coronoid fracture fragments is performed and tentatively held with K-wires from a cannulated screw system. Once the coronoid is reduced the K-wires are systematically replaced with cannulated screws.[70] Use of an anterior cruciate ligament or similar targeting device can assist with accurate screw placement.

Coronoid fixation is followed by ORIF or replacement of the radial head. Partial or complete excision of the radial head is not recommended in the setting of terrible triad injuries as it has been shown to result in instability and arthrosis.[45] The decision between repair and replacement of the radial head has been described previously, understanding that secure fixation is needed in the setting of these more complex injuries especially with concomitant elbow instability. The LCL is usually ruptured at the origin on the lateral epicondyle. An isometric, anatomic repair of the LCL is essential to restore stability (Fig. 34-4). The isometric point corresponds to the center of the capitellum when viewing from the lateral side.

If the coronoid cannot be accessed from the lateral surgical approach, a medial surgical approach is performed as described above to repair the coronoid and MCL (Fig. 34-16). Reduction and fixation is performed with transosseous sutures, posterior to anterior cannulated screws or a buttress plate (Fig. 34-17). Rarely reconstruction of the coronoid is not possible due to bone lost or severe comminution and a structural bone graft is indicated.[92] Various options have been described, including iliac crest,[61] resected radial head,[109] allografts, and a fragment of the ipsilateral proximal olecranon.[73]

The elbow should be examined under fluoroscopy for evidence of residual instability with the forearm in pronation, neutral, and supination after repair of the coronoid, radial head, and LCL. If the elbow is still unstable, the MCL should be repaired. Static or dynamic external fixation can be used to protect complex osteoporotic fractures of the coronoid when stable fixation is not achieved and in the uncommon circumstance in patients who demonstrate residual instability in spite of repair of the radial head, coronoid, and both collateral ligaments.[70] Hinged external fixation is often useful in revision situations. Temporary cross-screw or bridge plate fixation of the elbow can also be considered as described previously (Table 34-22).

Postoperative Care. The integrity of the osseous and ligament repairs and the examination under anesthesia for stability at the conclusion of the operation will direct the rehabilitation plan as outlined in the section on the operative treatment

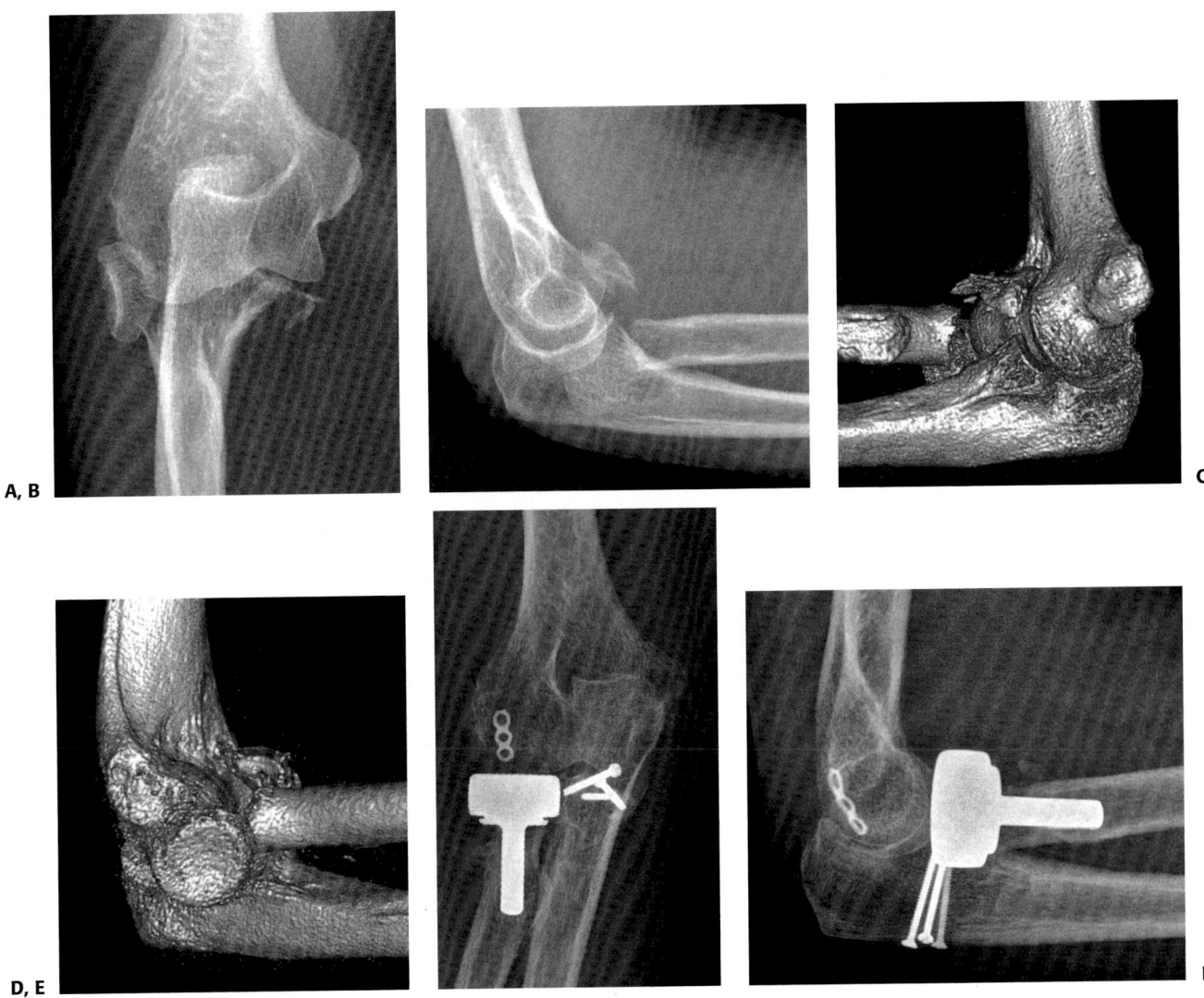

A, B

C

D, E

F

FIGURE 34-17 A 59-year-old female sustained a fall from two stairs onto her right outstretched arm. Radiographs following a closed reduction of an elbow dislocation demonstrate a displaced coronoid and radial head fracture with residual elbow subluxation. **A, B:** The 3D CT demonstrates significant comminution of both the coronoid and radial head fracture. **C, D:** Six months following radial head arthroplasty, transosseous LCL repair, and ORIF of the coronoid with cancellous bone graft taken from the radial head. Radiographs demonstrate a congruous elbow with mild heterotopic ossification. **E, F:** The patient achieved a functional range of motion.

TABLE 34-22	**Operative Repair of Terrible Triad Injuries**

Surgical Steps

- Fluoroscopic examination of elbow under anesthesia
- Lateral surgical approach to elbow through posterior midline or lateral skin incision
- Deep Kocher approach
- Fix coronoid from lateral surgical approach if possible using posterior to anterior screws if larger fragment or suture fixation of anterior capsule if smaller fragment(s)
- Fix or replace radial head
- Repair LCL and common extensor muscles using transosseous sutures or suture anchors
- Re-evaluate elbow stability using fluoroscopy
- Perform medial surgical approach if unable to fix coronoid fracture from lateral surgical approach if residual instability is present following repair of coronoid, radial head, and LCL
- Use floor of ulnar nerve approach to access coronoid and MCL
- Perform in situ release or transpose ulnar nerve
- Fix coronoid with posterior to anterior screws or buttress plate
- Repair MCL and common flexor muscles using transosseous sutures or suture anchors
- Re-evaluate elbow stability using fluoroscopy
- If the elbow is still unstable apply external fixator or temporary bridge plate

TABLE 34-23	**Terrible Triad Injuries**

Potential Pitfalls and Preventions

Pitfall	Preventions
Residual insta-bility	Repair or replacement of the radial head, fixation of larger coronoid fractures, and secure anatomic repair of collateral ligaments Active motion protocol avoiding varus stress at all times Employ external fixation or temporary bridge plate fixation if concerns about residual instability
Elbow stiffness	Early range of motion
Nerve palsy	Protect ulnar nerve during medial surgical approaches Direct visualization of bone during external fixator pin placement Gentle nerve and soft tissue handling

of elbow dislocations. In general, a stiff stable elbow is preferred over a loose incongruous one.

Potential Pitfalls and Preventative Measures. Symptomatic instability is uncommon after operative repair of terrible triad injuries. However, inadequate or failed repair of the lateral structures can lead to persistent subluxation. Mild subluxation may be treated with an active motion or overhead rehabilitation protocol, as previously described, but frank dislocation may require repeat operative fixation or salvage procedures. Early recognition of this problem is critical as late treatment of a stiff subluxated elbow may require extensive surgical management including elbow release and LCL and MCL reconstruction. Failure of radial head or coronoid fixation may also cause residual instability. The judicious use of static or dynamic external fixation or temporary bridge plate fixation should be considered in the setting of tenuous bony or soft tissue repairs, in patients with morbid obesity and those who are unable to be compliant with postoperative care such as patients in an intensive care unit.

Early postoperative motion is preferable to prevent stiffness; however, occasionally delayed mobilization is required due to poor soft tissues or tenuous fixation. Some patients may require elbow release or excision of heterotopic bone to restore motion. The use of indomethacin, while preferred by the authors in patients without contraindications to this medication, continues to be controversial and has not been proven to prevent heterotopic ossification around the elbow.

Ulnar nerve symptoms are common with medial surgical approaches to the coronoid and the radial nerve is at risk with plate fixation of the radial neck and with placement of an external fixator (Table 34-23).

Treatment-Specific Outcomes. Doornberg et al.[24] retrospectively studied 26 terrible triad injuries of the elbow. They reported good to excellent outcomes when stable fixation of the coronoid was achieved and unsatisfactory outcomes when stable fixation was not achieved. Pugh et al.[85] reviewed 36 terrible triad injuries that were treated with ORIF of the coronoid fracture and/or repair of the anterior capsule, repair or replacement of the radial head, and repair of the lateral ligament. In addition, repair of the MCL and/or application of a hinged external fixator were used for patients who demonstrated residual instability. They achieved 78% good to excellent results with a mean flexion–extension arc of 112 degrees and forearm rotation of 136 degrees. Ring et al.[90] reported poor results due to instability, arthrosis, and stiffness in 7 of 11 patients with terrible triad injuries who did not have the internal fixation of the coronoid.

MANAGEMENT OF EXPECTED ADVERSE OUTCOMES AND UNEXPECTED COMPLICATIONS IN TERRIBLE TRIAD INJURIES (TABLE 34-24)

TABLE 34-24	**Terrible Triad Injuries**

Common Adverse Outcomes and Complications

Elbow stiffness and heterotopic ossification → Initiate early motion

Redislocation → Careful follow-up and recognize and treat surgically

Residual subluxation → Active motion protocol, proceed with operative treatment if persists

AUTHOR'S PREFERRED METHOD OF TREATMENT FOR TERRIBLE TRIAD INJURIES (FIG. 34-18)

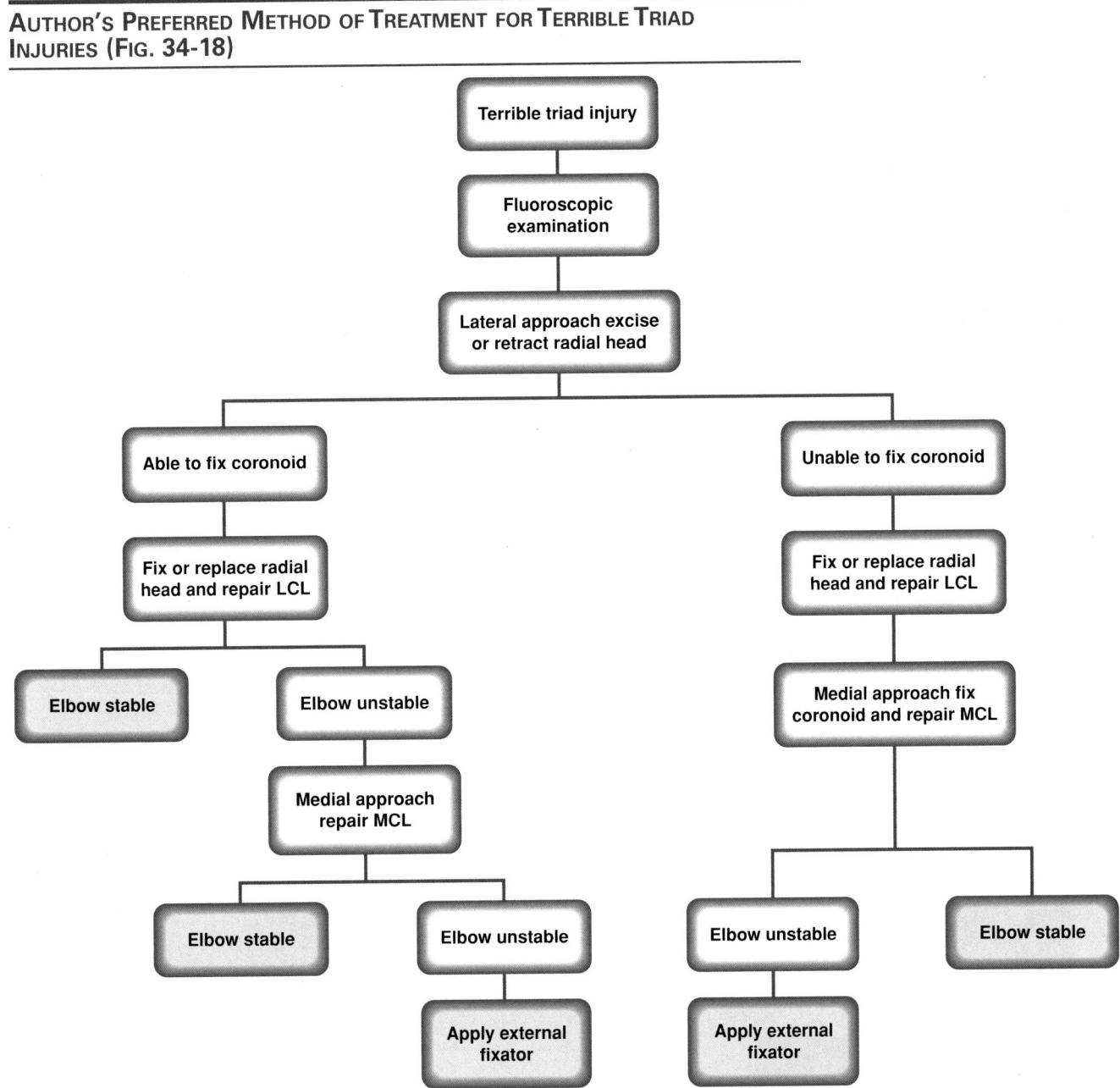

FIGURE 34-18 Authors preferred treatment.

SUMMARY, CONTROVERSIES, AND FUTURE DIRECTIONS IN TERRIBLE TRIAD INJURIES

While the outcome of terrible triad injuries has improved, a reliably good outcome continues to be difficult to achieve. Current challenges with the management of terrible triad injuries are the ability to achieve stable internal fixation of both coronoid and radial head fractures. While there are good radial head implants available for the management of unreconstructable radial head fractures, there is currently no available coronoid implant which makes the management of the comminuted coronoid difficult. The optimal surgi-

cal approach to the coronoid remains unknown as does the management of the ulnar nerve. The role of suture fixation of small coronoid fragments and repair of the MCL remains controversial. While some authors prefer articulated external fixation in the setting of residual instability, these devices are difficult to apply to precisely replicate the axis of motion and our experience has been mixed. We now prefer static external fixation or an internal bridge plate. Future studies are needed to determine the role of indomethacin in preventing heterotopic ossification in patients with terrible triad injuries.

INTRODUCTION TO POSTEROMEDIAL ROTATORY INSTABILITY (PMRI) OF THE ELBOW

Anteromedial fractures of the coronoid (AMC) and varus PMRI were first described by O'Driscoll et al.[80] in 2003. While these fractures are uncommon relative to coronoid fractures associated with terrible triad injuries, they are often subtle and may be missed, often leading to suboptimal outcomes due to a poor "natural history." Advances in our understanding of the mechanism of this injury and the biomechanics of treatment should lead to improved outcomes.

ASSESSMENT OF POSTEROMEDIAL ROTATORY INSTABILITY OF THE ELBOW

Mechanisms of Injury for Posteromedial Rotatory Instability of the Elbow

The anteromedial coronoid fracture (O'Driscoll Type II) has been postulated to occur by pronation, varus, and axially directed forces. It is commonly accompanied by avulsion injuries to the LCL and posterior bundle of the MCL, resulting in PMRI. Injury to the anterior bundle of the MCL can also occur with AMC fractures.[80]

Associated Injuries with Posteromedial Rotatory Instability of the Elbow

Given the limited reports available on AMC fractures the incidence of associated injuries is not known. While partial or complete injuries of the LCL are common the incidence of injury to the posterior bundle of the MCL is unclear. Unlike terrible triad injuries, the radial head is usually not fractured in patients with anteromedial coronoid fractures and this is a key to its recognition (Fig. 34-19). An anteromedial coronoid fracture should be suspected in any patient who appears to have a coronoid fracture when a radial head fracture is not present. While some patients present with a frank dislocation, the majority of patients do not: In such individuals a history of dislocation, "clunking" or instability with spontaneous reduction can often be elicited.

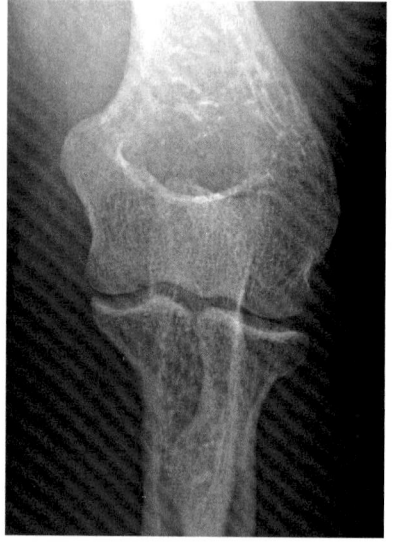
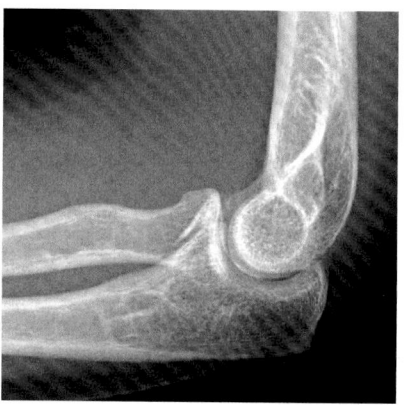
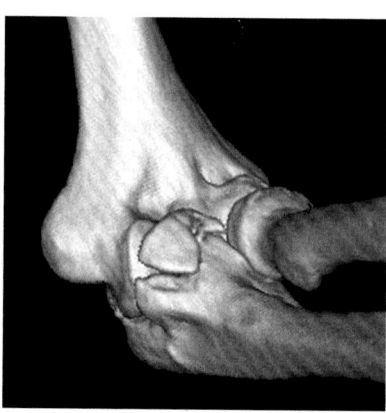

A, B

C

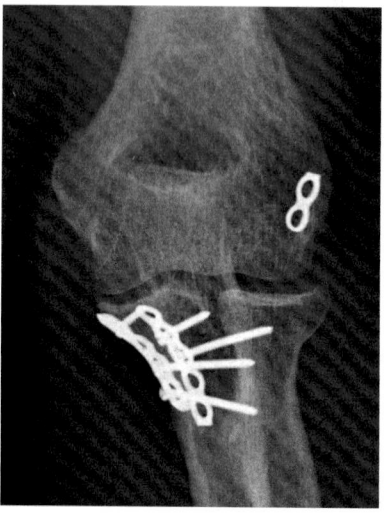
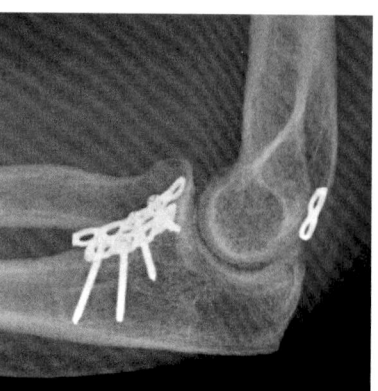

D

E

FIGURE 34-19 A 39-year-old woman following a fall on ice. The AP and lateral views demonstrate a subtle coronoid fracture without a radial head fracture. The patient had crepitus and pain with attempted motion with the arm abducted from the side. **A, B:** The 3D CT provides further detail of the subtype II anteromedial coronoid fracture. **C:** AP and lateral radiographs 1 year following transosseous LCL repair and buttress plate fixation of the anteromedial facet **(D, E).**

Signs and Symptoms of Posteromedial Rotatory Instability of the Elbow

A detailed neurovascular examination must be performed before and after reduction of a dislocated elbow if present. Soft tissue status and the condition of the skin should be carefully assessed. The elbow should be carefully palpated for signs of tenderness, particularly over the LCL. A patient may complain of crepitus with elbow motion with the arm abducted from the side (which produces a varus stress). This symptom is secondary to maltracking due to varus PMRI.

Imaging of Posteromedial Rotatory Instability of the Elbow

Standard radiographs (AP and lateral views) of the elbow are performed. Radiographs of the shoulder, forearm, and wrist are ordered as clinically indicated. Radiographs are repeated following the reduction of an associated elbow dislocation. Findings can be subtle, such as loss of a parallel medial ulnohumeral joint line, or varus malalignment of the elbow.[97] The radiocapitellar joint may be widened with LCL disruption and a "flake" fragment from the lateral condyle may be visible. CT scans with three-dimensional reconstruction improve the recognition and understanding of the pattern of anteromedial coronoid fractures and are recommended routinely in the evaluation of these injuries.[64]

Classification of Anteromedial Coronoid Fractures

O'Driscoll et al.[80] described three anteromedial coronoid fracture subtypes. Subtype I involves the anteromedial rim only, subtype II involves the rim and tip, and subtype III involves the rim, and sublime tubercle, with or without involvement of the tip.

Outcome Measures for Posteromedial Rotatory Instability of the Elbow

Several scoring systems have been used to evaluate the outcomes of anteromedial coronoid fractures including the DASH Questionnaire and the Mayo Elbow Performance Index.

PATHOANATOMY AND APPLIED ANATOMY RELATING TO POSTEROMEDIAL ROTATORY INSTABILITY OF THE ELBOW

A biomechanical study focusing on anteromedial coronoid fractures demonstrated that the size of the anteromedial facet fracture and the presence of a concomitant LCL injury appear to be important determinants of the need for open reduction and internal fixation. The LCL and the anteromedial coronoid are key varus stabilizers of the elbow. The authors reported that even small anteromedial coronoid fractures affect elbow kinematics, particularly with varus stress. LCL repair alone was not able to restore stability with anteromedial coronoid facet fractures larger than 2.5 mm.[83] Involvement of the sublime tubercle, (Subtype III) results in concomitant valgus instability due to disruption of the ulnar insertion of the MCL.

POSTEROMEDIAL ROTATORY INSTABILITY TREATMENT OPTIONS

Nonoperative Treatment of Posteromedial Rotatory Instability of the Elbow

Indications/Contraindications

The role of nonoperative treatment of PMRI of the elbow is unclear. If the anteromedial coronoid fracture is small and undisplaced, and the elbow is congruously reduced, nonoperative treatment should be considered. A fluoroscopic examination with stress views can be helpful to guide treatment; gross instability should be managed with surgery. CT should be performed to confirm the fracture pattern and joint congruity. Fracture fragments which are interposed within the articulation and the presence of articular subluxation are contraindications to nonoperative treatment (Table 34-25).

Technique

Anteromedial coronoid fractures, treated nonoperatively, are immobilized at 90 degrees of flexion for 7 to 10 days for comfort and to allow muscle tone to return to the elbow. Isometric contraction of the elbow muscles is encouraged while in the splint. After splint removal, the patient is asked to actively extend and flex the elbow. Patients will typically move only within their stable arc. Crepitus during motion suggests incongruity of the ulnohumeral joint and the need for examination under anesthesia and probable surgical repair. Abduction of the elbow away from the chest causes a varus moment on the elbow and should be avoided. A 90-degree resting splint with the forearm in neutral rotation is used between exercises. While pronation stabilizes the LCL deficient elbow, supination stabilizes the coronoid deficient elbow; hence neutral rotation is selected for flexion and extension exercises and for immobilization. Weekly radiographic and clinical follow-up is required to monitor for fracture displacement and recovery of motion. Joint subluxation or dislocation is an indication for surgical management. At 6 weeks the resting splint is discontinued and gentle stretching may be initiated to manage residual stiffness. Varus or valgus loading as well as strengthening are avoided until 12 weeks. Static progressive splinting can be used to improve elbow motion.

TABLE 34-25	Posteromedial Rotatory Instability Treatment
Nonoperative Treatment	
Indications	**Relative Contraindications**
Concentric elbow	Nonconcentric elbow
Small undisplaced anteromedial coronoid fracture	Displaced anteromedial coronoid fracture
	Fracture fragment interposed in articulation

Outcomes

There is little information regarding outcome of nonoperative PMRI of the elbow. Doornberg and Ring reported on 18 patients with anteromedial facet fractures with an average follow-up of 26 months. Of these, three patients had nonoperative treatment, and two had an excellent outcome and one fair.[28] Fragment malunion may lead to persistent subluxation and secondary osteoarthritis for which there is currently no good reconstructive option.

Operative Treatment of Posteromedial Rotatory Instability of the Elbow

Indications/Contraindications

The majority of patients with PMRI require surgical management to achieve a stable elbow allowing early motion. Residual subluxation or crepitus with motion suggests dynamic incongruity and are indications for surgery.

Open Reduction and Internal Fixation

Restoration of varus posteromedial rotatory stability is achieved by internal fixation of the coronoid and repair of the LCL. The sublime tubercle is fixed or the MCL is repaired if injured. An external fixator is used to manage residual instability or to protect tenuous internal fixation.

Preoperative Planning (Table 34-26)

TABLE 34-26 | **ORIF of Posteromedial Rotatory Instability of the Elbow**

Preoperative Planning Checklist

- OR Table: Radiolucent arm board
- Position/positioning aids: Supine with arm table or arm across chest
- Fluoroscopy location: Operative side
- Equipment: Suture anchors, 0.035, 0.045 K-wires, 1.5- and 2.0-mm screws, 2.5-mm cannulated screws, periarticular radial head and coronoid plates, radial head arthroplasty system, large external fixator, hinged external fixator, large fragment locking set with screws

---

Positioning. Posteromedial rotatory instability injuries of the elbow are best approached using an arm table with the surgeon sitting. A prerequisite for this positioning is sufficient external rotation of the shoulder to allow a medial surgical approach. Alternatively the injury can be repaired with the arm placed across the chest with the surgeon standing. A rolled-up sheet placed underneath the elbow can be helpful for medial exposure.

Surgical Approach. A posterior midline elbow skin incision is typically employed when managing PMRI as it allows lateral and medial access to the elbow as required. Alternatively separate lateral and medial skin incisions can be employed. The optimal surgical approach to repair the anteromedial coronoid has not been determined as outlined in the previous section

on terrible triad injuries. Our preferred surgical approach for anteromedial coronoid fractures is to use the interval between the two heads of the FCU.[97] This approach also provides adequate access to the sublime tubercle and MCL. Meticulous release and mobilization of motor branches of the ulnar nerve help improve distal exposure. The flexor–pronator muscles are elevated from distal to proximal to isolate the sublime tubercle and identify and protect the anterior bundle of the MCL. The authors routinely perform an in situ release of the ulnar nerve; transposing the nerve if there are preoperative ulnar nerve symptoms or if further mobilization is needed to allow coronoid fixation.

Deep lateral surgical approaches to the radial head and LCL have been described previously. In the setting of PMRI a Kocher approach is preferred to allow repair of the LCL which typically is avulsed off the lateral epicondyle.

Technique. An initial fluoroscopic assessment of the elbow under anesthesia is important to determine the extent of collateral ligament injury and magnitude of elbow instability. The anteromedial coronoid fracture is fixed first. After performing a medial or posterior elbow skin incision the ulnar nerve is released and protected for the remainder of the case. A transposition is performed if the nerve is tethered or interferes with coronoid exposure. After splitting the FCU the anterior portion is elevated off the ulna from distal to proximal protecting the insertion of the MCL on the sublime tubercle when it remains intact. To visualize the tip of the coronoid (a subtype II fracture), the flexor pronator muscles are detached from the medial epicondyle and medial supracondylar ridge leaving a small cuff of fascia for later repair. After reduction and preliminary fixation with K-wires, posterior to anterior cannulated screws, anterior to posterior screws, or buttress plate fixation is used for definitive repair. Suture fixation of coronoid tip fragments is not recommended

---

TABLE 34-27 | **Operative Repair of Posteromedial Rotatory Instability of the Elbow**

Surgical Steps

- Fluoroscopic examination of elbow under anesthesia
- Medial surgical approach to elbow through posterior midline or medial skin incision
- Split flexor carpi ulnaris and perform an in situ release of ulnar nerve; transpose if needed
- Use floor of ulnar nerve approach to coronoid
- Elevate flexor pronator muscles off ulna from distal to proximal, preserving the MCL insertion on the sublime tubercle
- Fix coronoid with posterior to anterior screws or buttress plate
- Use suture fixation of anterior capsule and small tip fragment(s)
- Repair MCL if injured and reattach flexor–pronator mass
- Re-evaluate elbow stability using fluoroscopy
- Perform lateral Kocher approach and repair LCL if required using transosseous sutures or suture anchors
- Re-evaluate elbow stability using fluoroscopy
- If elbow still unstable or coronoid fixation is tenuous, apply external fixator or temporary bridge plate

---

because the anteromedial rim requires stable internal fixation to prevent varus collapse. A buttress plate is preferred if the fragments are large enough.

If secure, coronoid fixation is achieved; a repeat fluoroscopic examination is performed and the elbow gently stressed in varus to determine if the LCL needs to be addressed. If only mild varus laxity is present, the LCL may be left untreated and a ligament-specific rehabilitation protocol is employed as described earlier. If the coronoid fixation is tenuous or the patient has residual varus instability, a lateral surgical approach to the elbow is performed using a posterior incision or a separate lateral incision and the LCL is repaired.

Static or dynamic external fixation can be used to protect complex osteoporotic fractures of the coronoid when stable fixation is not achieved and in patients who demonstrate residual instability in spite of repair of the coronoid and collateral ligaments.[85] Temporary cross-screw or bridge plate fixation of the elbow can also be considered as described previously (Table 34-27).

Postoperative Care. The elbow is placed into a well-padded light posterior splint with the elbow at 90 degrees of flexion and the forearm in neutral rotation. Ideally, the dressing is removed and motion begun 48 hours after surgery unless static joint fixation has been required. The elbow can be immobilized for up to 14 days if there is concern about the quality of the soft tissues or the stability of the fractures, quality of the ligament repairs, or stability of the elbow achieved at the end of the surgical procedure. An active motion protocol is then begun as outlined above for nonoperative treatment of anteromedial coronoid fractures including active and active-assisted exercises with the arm at the side avoiding varus stress at all times. The patient may actively flex and extend the elbow in the position of forearm rotation where they were most stable during the examination under anesthesia at the conclusion of the operative repair, most commonly neutral rotation. They may perform forearm rotation exercises at 90 degrees of flexion or greater. Passive stretching may be started 6 weeks postop with a formal strengthening program initiated at 3 months.

Potential Pitfalls and Preventative Measures. Symptomatic instability is uncommon after operative repair of PMRI of the elbow. However, inadequate or failed repair of the lateral structures or collapse of the coronoid fixation may lead to persistent subluxation. Early recognition and treatment of this problem is crucial to salvage a good outcome. The judicious use of static external fixation or temporary bridge plate fixation should be considered.

Early postoperative motion is preferable to prevent stiffness; however, sometimes delayed mobilization is required due to tenuous fixation with a plan for a subsequent contracture release to restore functional motion. Ulnar nerve symptoms are common with medial surgical approaches to the coronoid and prophylactic in situ release or transposition should be considered (Table 34-28).

Treatment-Specific Outcomes. Reports on the outcome of operative treatment of anteromedial coronoid fractures are limited. Doornberg and Ring completed a retrospective review of 67 fracture-dislocations of the elbow.[27] Eleven of those patients demonstrated varus posteromedial instability, all of which had anteromedial facet fractures of the coronoid. In a separate study, Doornberg and Ring reported on 18 patients with anteromedial facet fractures with an average follow-up of 26 months.[28] Of these, six patients had malalignment of the anteromedial facet, and all developed varus subluxation, arthrosis of the elbow, and a fair or poor functional result. The remaining 12 patients, with secure anatomical fixation of the anteromedial coronoid fracture, had good or excellent elbow function. Based on this limited information, repair of the LCL and ORIF of most anteromedial coronoid fractures is recommended.[27,28,83]

MANAGEMENT OF EXPECTED ADVERSE OUTCOMES AND UNEXPECTED COMPLICATIONS IN POSTEROMEDIAL ROTATORY INSTABILITY (TABLE 34-29)

TABLE 34-28 Posteromedial Rotatory Instability of the Elbow

Potential Pitfalls and Preventions

Pitfall	Preventions
Residual instability	Secure repair of larger anteromedial coronoid fractures and collateral ligament(s) Active motion protocol avoiding varus stress at all times Employ external fixation or temporary bridge plate fixation if concerns about residual instability
Elbow stiffness	Early range of motion
Nerve palsy	Protect ulnar nerve during medial surgical approaches Direct visualization of bone during external fixator pin placement Gentle nerve and soft tissue retraction

TABLE 34-29 Posteromedial Rotatory Instability of the Elbow

Common Adverse Outcomes and Complications

Elbow stiffness and heterotopic ossification → Initiate early motion.

Elbow subluxation or dislocation → Achieve stable fixation of the anteromedial coronoid and LCL. Use external fixator to protect repairs if tenuous. Careful follow-up to recognize instability and treat surgically.

Elbow arthritis → Achieve and anatomic reduction of the coronoid fracture and avoid residual instability.

AUTHOR'S PREFERRED METHOD OF TREATMENT FOR POSTEROMEDIAL ROTATORY INSTABILITY (FIG. 34-20)

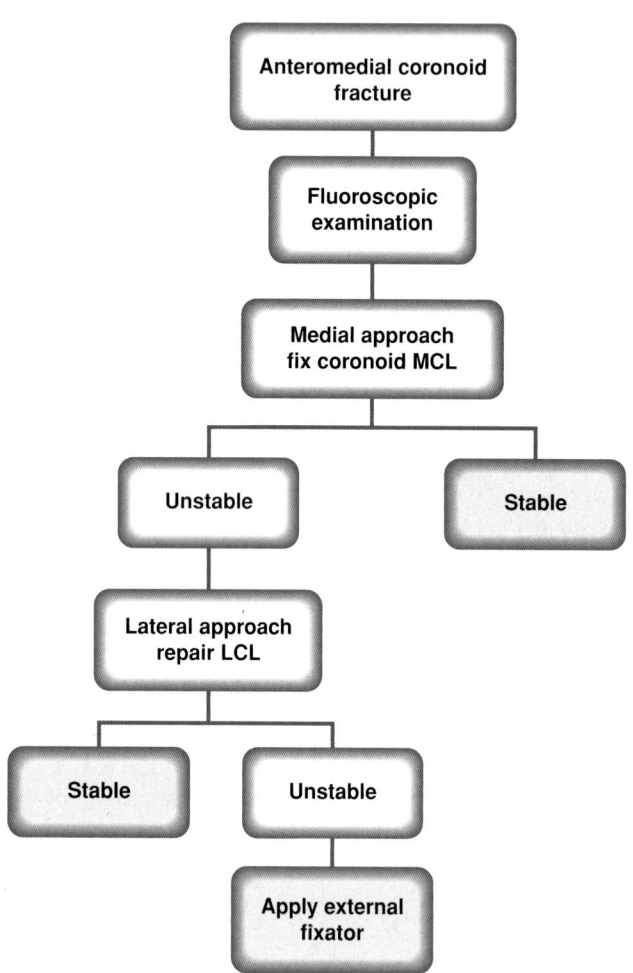

FIGURE 34-20 Author's preferred treatment.

SUMMARY, CONTROVERSIES, AND FUTURE DIRECTIONS IN POSTEROMEDIAL ROTATORY INSTABILITY

The optimal management of PMRI remains unclear. This entity can easily be missed because, relative to many elbow injuries, the history, physical examination, and radiographic findings can be subtle. Unfortunately if this instability pattern is not identified and the elbow remains subluxated, the outcome is often poor. Current challenges with the management of anteromedial coronoid fractures are the ability to achieve stable internal fixation and the lack of available coronoid prostheses to reconstruct the coronoid when it is deficient. The optimal surgical approach and technique of internal fixation of the coronoid remains unknown as does the management of the ulnar nerve. Furthermore the role of nonoperative treatment of these injuries needs to be better defined.

INTRODUCTION TO PROXIMAL ULNA FRACTURES

Proximal ulna fractures are common adult injuries that account for approximately 10% of fractures around the elbow. Proximal ulna fractures comprise a broad spectrum of injuries that include not only olecranon fractures but also transolecranon fracture-dislocations and the posterior Monteggia lesion.[55,89] As such, there is no single treatment or technique that is best suited for all injuries. However, these injury patterns are all intra-articular fractures of the proximal ulna that, in most cases, require anatomic alignment and secure fixation to allow for early elbow motion and to optimize functional outcome.

ASSESSMENT OF PROXIMAL ULNA FRACTURES

Mechanisms of Injury for Posterior Ulna Fractures

Proximal ulna fractures may result from either direct or indirect elbow trauma. Olecranon fractures typically result from a direct blow to the olecranon. More complex fracture-dislocation patterns may be the result of a more indirect injury such as a fall onto the outstretched hand. Transolecranon fracture-dislocations are typically the result of higher-energy trauma such as a fall from a height, assaults, or motor vehicle collisions. Although posterior Monteggia lesions may also result from high-energy trauma, they are typically lower-energy injuries that occur in more osteopenic bone and result from a ground-level fall.

Associated Injuries with Proximal Ulna Fractures

Given the subcutaneous location of the olecranon, open fractures are not uncommon and have a reported rate of 2% to 30% of fractures. Transolecranon fracture-dislocations may be associated with injuries to the coronoid process or segmental fractures of the ulna. Posterior Monteggia lesions may be associated with coronoid process fractures (26%), radial head fractures (68%), ipsilateral upper extremity injuries (24%), and injuries to the collateral ligaments.

Signs and Symptoms of Proximal Ulna Fractures

Although typically isolated upper extremity injuries, 20% of proximal ulna fractures are associated with polytrauma, and a complete examination of the patient for systemic injuries is important.[117] The affected extremity should be evaluated for shoulder, forearm, wrist, or hand injuries. The arm should be examined for open wounds and abrasions that typically occur over the dorsal surface of the proximal ulna. There is typically swelling about the elbow with fluid accumulation in the olecranon bursa. The elbow may have obvious deformity in the case of a fracture-dislocation. Examination of distal neurologic status with close attention to ulnar, median, and posterior interosseous nerve function is performed. Evaluation of vascular status and forearm compartments is necessary.

Imaging and Other Diagnostic Studies for Proximal Ulna Fractures

Anteroposterior, lateral, and radiocapitellar radiographs of the elbow are performed. In the case of a fracture-dislocation, radiographs should be performed after a closed reduction in order to better delineate the fracture components. A traction view is useful in these cases, especially if the elbow is unstable after closed reduction. The fracture components can be further evaluated in the operating room under general anesthesia using traction prior to fixation. CT may be useful to evaluate the pattern of associated coronoid or radial head fracture to aid with preoperative planning; however, it is not commonly required.

Classification of Proximal Ulna Fractures

Olecranon Fractures

The Mayo classification divides olecranon fractures into three groups based on fracture displacement and elbow stability (Fig. 34-21).[76] These groups include Type I (undisplaced), Type II (displaced but stable), and Type III (unstable). Each group is then subdivided into comminuted (A) or noncomminuted (B) fractures. This classification helps direct treatment with Type I generally being amenable to nonoperative management while Type II and III fractures generally require operative treatment.

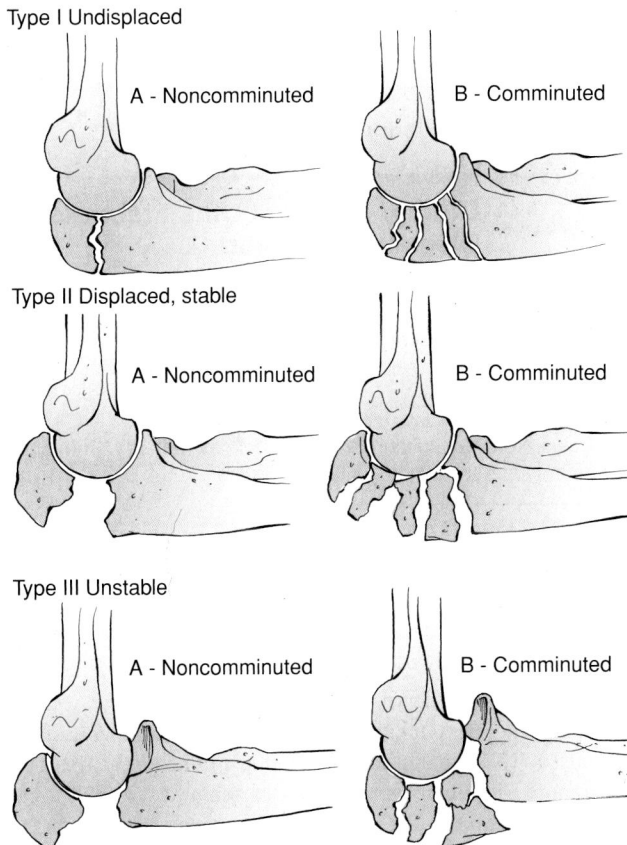

Type I Undisplaced

A - Noncomminuted   B - Comminuted

Type II Displaced, stable

A - Noncomminuted   B - Comminuted

Type III Unstable

A - Noncomminuted   B - Comminuted

FIGURE 34-21 The Mayo classification of olecranon fractures is based on the displacement of the fracture, subluxation of the articulation, and the presence of comminution.

Type B fractures are more suitably treated with plate fixation while Type A fractures may be treated with tension-band constructs if preferred.

Olecranon Fracture-Dislocations

Anterior fracture-dislocations of the olecranon have been termed "transolecranon fracture-dislocations".[89] These fractures are also represented by the Mayo Type III classification. An important feature of these injuries is that the proximal radioulnar joint is relatively preserved. Also, while fractures of the coronoid are not uncommon, the radial head and collateral ligaments are usually intact with this pattern. Although they may be multifragmentary, the coronoid fractures are typically single large anterior fragments or a fragment with a single longitudinal split.

Posterior fracture-dislocations are typically posterior Monteggia lesions (Bado Type II). Jupiter et al.[55] have classified these injuries into Type IIA (fracture at the level of the coronoid process with the coronoid as a separate fragment), IIB (fracture distal to the coronoid), IIC (fracture through the diaphysis), and IID (complex fracture extending from the olecranon to the diaphysis). Type IIA and Type IID fractures involve the proximal ulna and joint surface of the greater sigmoid notch. These fractures encompass a unique set of injuries including posterior angulation of the proximal ulna, a radial head fracture, a coronoid fracture, and collateral ligament injuries.[10,55] When this pattern is recognized, careful evaluation of radiographs should be carried out to define associated injuries. Traction films, fluoroscopy, and/or CT scanning are often useful. The coronoid fracture pattern is variable and may include a large anterior fragment, a small tip fragment, or both.

Outcome Measures for Proximal Ulna Fractures

Several studies evaluated the clinical and radiographic outcomes of proximal ulna fractures. The Broberg and Morrey Elbow Score in addition to the American Shoulder and Elbow Surgeons elbow assessment system, the Mayo Elbow Performance Index, the SF-36, and the DASH scoring system have been used.

PATHOANATOMY AND APPLIED ANATOMY RELATING TO PROXIMAL ULNA FRACTURES

The proximal ulna contributes to two articulations: The ulnohumeral joint and the proximal radioulnar joint. Both of these articulations may be involved with fractures and fracture-dislocations in this area. The greater sigmoid notch is covered with articular cartilage and comprises the ulnar articulation of the ulnohumeral joint. Radially, there is a small area of cartilage that articulates with the radial head at the proximal radioulnar joint. The greater sigmoid notch has a bare area that corresponds with the base of the coronoid. It is important during fixation of proximal ulna fractures to restore appropriate alignment to these articulations. In particular, avoidance of overcompression of the greater sigmoid notch in comminuted fractures is essential to prevent joint incongruity and the rapid progression of post-traumatic osteoarthritis.

The olecranon process prevents anterior subluxation of the ulna. Bell et al. demonstrated that valgus–varus angulation and ulnohumeral rotation progressively increase with sequential excision of up to 75% of the olecranon with gross instability occurring at greater than 87.5% of the olecranon.[12] The coronoid contributes to elbow stability, and injury to it has complex effects on elbow stability depending on the direction of loading and the location and size of fracture. In general, increasing coronoid fracture size leads to decreased stability of the elbow.[9]

The triceps tendon has a broad insertion onto the proximal ulna near the subcutaneous border. The medial head of the triceps has a tendon that is deep to the common tendon of the long and lateral heads but the insertion of the tendons is confluent. In addition to the ulnar attachment of the tendon proper, there is a triceps expansion that inserts onto the ECU fascia, the anconeus insertion, and the antebrachial fascia.[67]

PROXIMAL ULNA FRACTURE TREATMENT OPTIONS

Nonoperative Treatment of Proximal Ulna Fractures

Indications/Contraindications

Since these injuries involve an articular surface, the majority of proximal ulna fractures are treated operatively. However, a nondisplaced fracture or a minimally displaced fracture that remains reduced with the elbow flexed may be treated nonoperatively. Patients with significant medical comorbidities that are poor surgical candidates may be treated nonoperatively even with displaced fractures as long as there is no skin compromise or elbow instability. Displaced olecranon fractures involving 75% or less of the greater sigmoid notch in the elderly are the most common fractures which fulfill these criteria. This treatment may result in a fibrous union or a nonunion with some discomfort and limitation in both terminal extension and extensor strength. These limitations can be problematic for patients arising from a chair and ambulating with a walker (Table 34-30).

Techniques

Typically, the elbow is splinted for 2 to 3 weeks and then gentle active-assisted flexion is started avoiding active extension

TABLE 34-30 Proximal Ulna Fractures

Nonoperative Treatment

Indications	Relative Contraindications
Nondisplaced fracture	Displaced fracture in young active patient
Poor surgical candidate	Elbow instability
Displaced fracture in elderly patient with medical comorbidities	Associated fractures (radial head, coronoid)

against gravity or resistance for the first 6 weeks after injury. At 6 weeks, the patient can begin active motion against gravity with resistive exercises started at 3 months.

Outcomes

There is currently no literature on the outcomes of nonoperatively managed olecranon fractures. However, in our experience, in appropriately selected patients, this treatment method leads to acceptable results and a functional range of motion.

Operative Treatment of Proximal Ulna Fractures

Indications/Contraindications

The majority of proximal ulna fractures are treated surgically. Most fractures with displacement and those associated with dislocations or elbow instability as well as open fractures should be managed operatively.

Simple olecranon fractures without comminution or instability may be managed with tension-band wiring, plating, or an intramedullary rod. Comminuted fractures or those associated with elbow instability should be managed with plate fixation. In osteoporotic bone with significant comminution that precludes stable internal fixation, excision with triceps advancement may be used if the excised fragment comprises less than 75% of the olecranon, but this technique should be reserved for elderly, low-demand patients if possible.

Surgical Procedure—Olecranon Excision and Triceps Advancement

Preoperative Planning (Table 34-31)

TABLE 34-31 ORIF of Proximal Ulna Fractures—Olecranon Excision

Preoperative Planning Checklist

- OR Table: Radiolucent
- Position/positioning aids: Lateral, prone, or supine with arm over chest
- Fluoroscopy location: From head
- Equipment: No. 2 FiberWire or No. 2 Ticron suture, 2-mm drill
- Tourniquet (sterile/nonsterile): Sterile preferred

Positioning. The patient is placed supine on a radiolucent table. The arm is placed over the chest on a chest roll or on a radiolucent arm table. A sterile tourniquet should be available and used at the discretion of the surgeon.

Surgical Approach. A posterior midline incision is made and full thickness medial and lateral fasciocutaneous flaps are raised. The skin incision is placed just radial to the tip of the olecranon. The ulnar nerve should be identified so that it can be protected during the case but it is not necessary to dissect it free of the cubital tunnel. The interval between the ECU and FCU is developed and the subcutaneous border of the ulna is exposed. On the ulnar side, the FCU is elevated from the olecranon to visualize the joint. On the radial side, the anconeus

TABLE 34-32 Olecranon Excision and Triceps Advancement

Surgical Steps

- Olecranon fragments excised
- Nonabsorbable No. 2 suture (FiberWire, Ticron) placed in triceps tendon
- 2-mm drill holes placed in proximal ulna adjacent to the dorsal surface
- Suture placed through drill holes and tied avoiding dorsal prominence

TABLE 34-34 ORIF of Olecranon Fractures— Tension Banding

Preoperative Planning Checklist

- OR Table: Radiolucent
- Position/positioning aids: Lateral position, supine or prone, chest rolls, radiolucent arm board
- Fluoroscopy location: From the head of the table
- Equipment: 0.062 K-wires, 20-gauge stainless steel wire, pointed reduction clamps
- Tourniquet (sterile/nonsterile): Sterile tourniquet available

fascia is incised and the muscle can be elevated from the olecranon fragment for further visualization if needed.

Technique. The fracture is exposed and the fragments of the olecranon are identified and excised. Drill holes are then made in the ulna using a 2-mm drill bit starting adjacent to the dorsal surface and exiting on the shaft, just off the dorsal surface. Dorsal placement provides for improved extension strength relative to placement adjacent to the articular surface without sacrificing stability.[36] Care should be taken to protect the ulnar nerve. A running-locking nonabsorbable suture is then placed in the triceps over a broad area and passed through the drill holes and tied, avoiding dorsal placement of a prominent knot (Table 34-32).

Postoperative Care. The patient is placed into a long-arm splint in a semi-extended position to protect the skin incision. Sutures are removed in 2 weeks and active and active-assisted flexion and gravity-assisted extension are initiated. Active extension begins at 6 weeks and strengthening at 3 months postoperatively.

Potential Pitfalls and Preventative Measures. Careful attention to soft tissue dissection and incision placement is important. Elbow stability can be affected if more than 75% of the olecranon is excised and therefore this technique should only be used in carefully selected patients (Table 34-33).

Treatment-Specific Outcomes. Excision should be reserved for low-demand patients with poor bone quality. Attaching the triceps tendon directly adjacent to the joint will allow for a more congruent surface for motion. However, it may result in triceps weakness. Ferreira et al.[36] demonstrated a 30% decrease in triceps strength with a more anterior repair compared to a 24%

decrease in triceps strength with a more anterior repair. However, clinically it is unclear if this affects functional outcomes. Gartsman et al.[41] found no differences in strength between patients treated with internal fixation and those treated with excision. However, this trial was not randomized and selection bias may have contributed to this result. Excision should be reserved for those cases in which open reduction and internal fixation is likely to fail, or for intraoperative failure of osseous repair.

Surgical Procedure—Olecranon Tension-Band Wiring

Preoperative Planning. Radiographs are carefully examined to determine the fracture morphology. Tension-band technique is appropriate for stable elbows with noncomminuted fractures that are proximal to the coronoid (Table 34-34).

Positioning. The patient is placed lateral or prone on a radiolucent table. A radiolucent arm positioner is placed under the arm so that the elbow joint can be flexed and extended. The C-arm is brought in from the head of the table. The lateral and prone positions allow for easier access to fluoroscopy while hardware is being applied. The lateral position decreases risks, such as eye injury, associated with prone positioning, particularly in cases where operative time is prolonged. However, prone positioning gives the best exposure for fluoroscopy and may be useful in patients that have spine injuries. If the patient cannot tolerate lateral or prone positioning or a regional anesthetic is to be employed, a supine position with a bump may be used and the arm is placed over the chest. It may be more difficult to visualize and reduce more comminuted articular fractures in this position and imaging may be more difficult. Also, an assistant is usually required to hold the arm across the chest. In this case, the C-arm is brought in from the side of the table. Before draping, test images should be obtained to be sure high-quality images can be obtained during the procedure. A sterile tourniquet should be available and used at the discretion of the surgeon.

Surgical Approach. A posterior midline incision is made and full thickness medial and lateral fasciocutaneous flaps are raised. The skin incision is placed just radial to the tip of the olecranon for better coverage of hardware. The ulnar nerve should be identified so that it can be protected during the case, but it is not necessary to dissect it free of the cubital tunnel. The interval between the ECU and FCU is developed and the subcutaneous border of the ulna is exposed. On the ulnar side, the FCU is

TABLE 34-33 Proximal Ulna Fractures— Olecranon Excision

Potential Pitfalls and Preventions

Pitfall	Preventions
Elbow instability	Be sure fracture involves less than 75% of the articular surface
	Be sure there is no associated instability or other injuries preoperatively

elevated from the olecranon to visualize the joint. On the radial side, the anconeus fascia is incised and the muscle can be elevated from the olecranon fragment for further visualization if needed.

Technique. The fracture edges are exposed, cleaned, and the joint is inspected for damage to the trochlea or loose bodies. The fracture is reduced by extending the elbow. A drill hole is placed on the ulnar shaft both radially and ulnarly so that a pointed reduction clamp can be used to hold the reduction and apply compression on both sides with one tine in the drill hole and the other tine at the tip of the olecranon. A shoulder hook or dental pick can be used to hold the reduction of smaller fragments. Two 0.062-in K-wires are placed from the superior aspect of the olecranon exiting the anteromedial cortex and then are backed out a small amount to accommodate future impaction of the wires (Fig. 34-22). Avoid lateral placement as the K-wires can irritate the radial tuberosity and predispose to rotational stiffness and synostosis. Excessive length of the medial K-wire can injure the ulnar or median nerve. A drill hole is

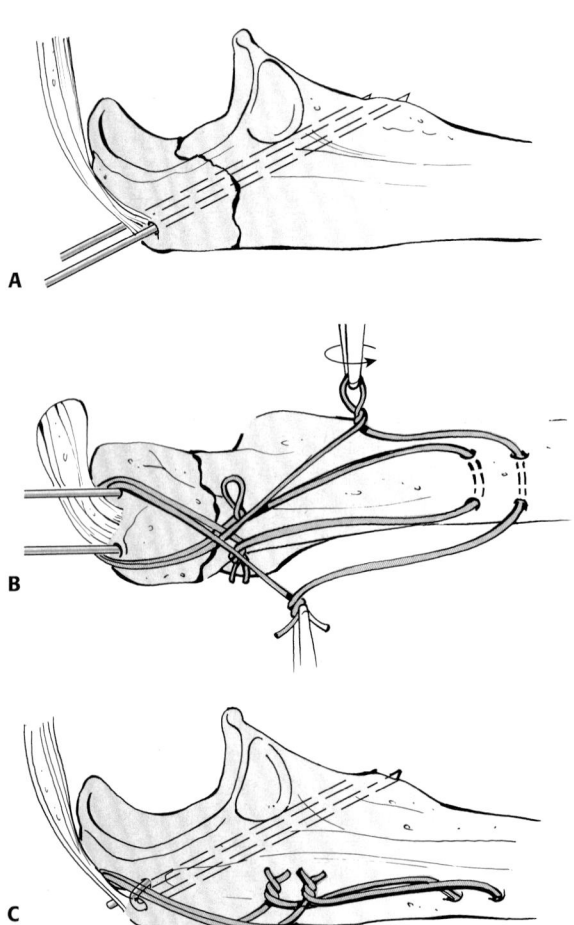

FIGURE 34-22 A: The fracture is reduced and secured with two 0.62-in K-wires drilled so as to engage the anteromedial cortex of the ulna. **B:** One or two 20-gauge stainless steel wires are placed underneath the triceps and through transverse drill holes placed distal to the fracture. The figure-of-eight wires are then tensioned evenly. **C:** The K- wires are bent 180 degrees and impacted underneath the triceps into the olecranon.

TABLE 34-35	ORIF of Olecranon Fractures— Tension Band

Surgical Steps

- Fracture edges cleaned and joint inspected
- Fracture reduced and held with pointed reduction clamps
- Two 0.062-in K-wires placed from tip of olecranon exiting the anteromedial ulnar cortex
- Drill hole placed in dorsal cortex distal to coronoid
- 20-gauge wire placed in a figure-of-eight fashion through drill hole and around wires
- Figure-of-eight wire tightened simultaneously radially and ulnarly
- K-wires impacted into tip of olecranon underneath triceps tendon

placed in the dorsal side of the ulna distal to the coronoid. Using an angiocath catheter, 20-gauge wire is used to create one or two figure-of-eight tension band(s) around the proximal end of the K-wires deep to the triceps and exiting through the distal drill hole. The wire is tensioned on both the ulnar and radial side simultaneously to create equal compression across the joint. The tips of the K-wires wires are bent and the wires are impacted into the olecranon tip through small incisions in the triceps. Alternatively, an intramedullary 4.5- or 6.5-mm screw may be used instead of the K-wires but care must be taken to not induce a deformity in the proximal segment secondary to a mismatch between the sigmoid shape of the ulna and the straight screw. The elbow is then taken through a full range of motion to be sure the fixation is secure, particularly in full flexion. The wound should be closed in a layered fashion, so early range of motion can begin while the sutures are still in place (Table 34-35).

Postoperative Care. The patient is placed into a semi-extended position in a long-arm splint. The splint and postoperative dressings are taken down 48 hours after surgery and the patient begins range of motion exercises including active and active-assisted flexion and gravity-assisted extension. Active exercises against gravity are started at 6 weeks with very gentle resistance progressing to full resistive exercises at 3 months or when the fracture has united.

Potential Pitfalls and Preventative Measures. Tension-band wiring can be successful in properly selected patients. To avoid loss of fixation, an anatomic reduction is necessary and this technique should be used only in simple fracture patterns. Hardware prominence requiring removal is common. To decrease the incidence of symptomatic hardware, the K-wires should be buried under the triceps and the cerclage wire knots should be buried as well. If the wires are left too prominent on the anteromedial aspect of the ulna, median and ulnar nerve injury is possible. Avoid wires that exit laterally in the region of the biceps tuberosity to prevent impingement or heterotopic ossification and subsequent synostosis (Table 34-36).

Treatment-Specific Outcomes. Outcomes of tension-band wiring for simple fractures are generally favorable. The most frequently reported problem with tension-band technique

TABLE 34-36 Olecranon Fractures— Tension-Band Wiring

Potential Pitfalls and Prevention

Pitfall	Preventions
Loss of fixation	Anatomic reduction Use only for simple fractures
Prominent hardware	Bury K-wire tips Bury cerclage wire knots
Biceps tuberosity impingement and synostosis	Avoid lateral placement of wires
Ulnar/median nerve injury	Avoid excessive length of the K-wires through the anteromedial cortex

is hardware prominence that requires removal. Villanueva et al.[113] reported on 37 consecutive olecranon fractures treated with tension-band wiring. Mean elbow extension was 7 degrees and flexion was 131 degrees with the majority reporting no or mild pain at 4-year follow-up. Mayo Elbow Performance Sores were rated as good or excellent in 86% of patients and patients had an average DASH score of 18. Almost one-third of patients developed arthritic changes and these were more commonly seen with associated fractures and/or elbow instability and at longer follow-up. More than half of the patients required hardware removal due to prominent or migrating K-wires which has been the most significant problem with this procedure.

Surgical Procedure—Olecranon Plating

Preoperative Planning. Plating of the olecranon is appropriate for fractures that are comminuted, associated with elbow instability such as transolecranon fracture-dislocations, or fractures that have extension down the shaft of the ulna such as posterior Monteggia injuries (addressed in a later section). Some surgeons routinely fix all olecranon fractures with a plate to avoid the high incidence of hardware complications from tension-band wiring (Fig. 34-23). Fractures proximal to the coronoid may be secured with periarticular nonlocking or locking precontoured plates or 2.7- or 3.5-mm reconstruction plates contoured around the tip of the olecranon. If the fracture extends distal to the coronoid, a reconstruction plate may not be strong enough, and a 3.5-mm LCDCP or equivalent strength precontoured plate should be used (Fig. 34-24, Table 34-37).

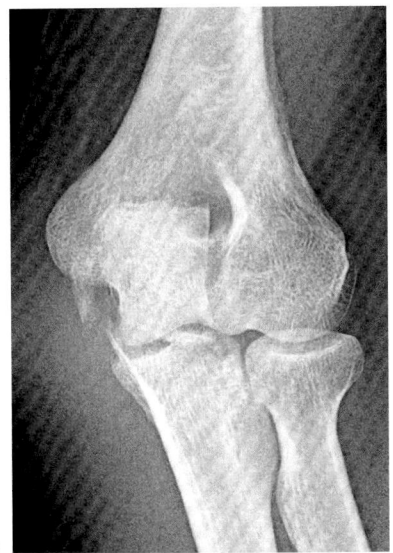
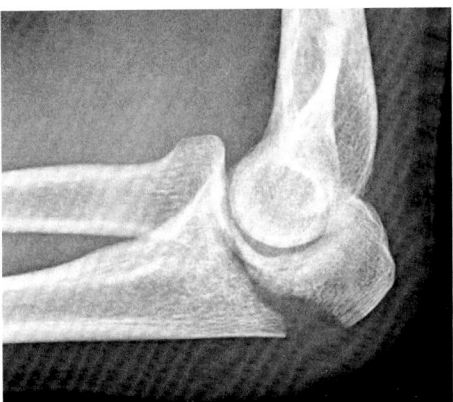
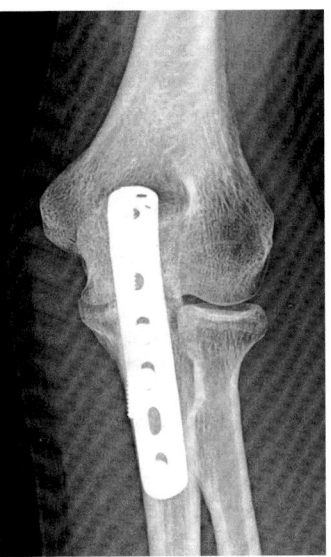

A, B

C

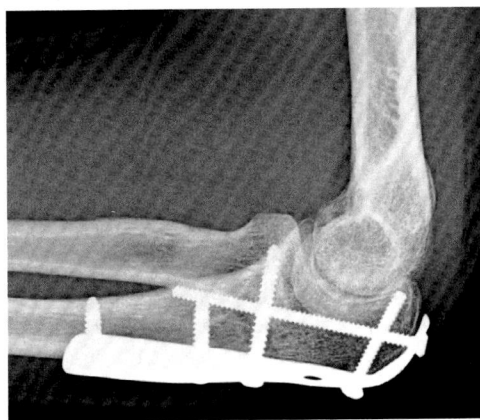

D

FIGURE 34-23 A, B: A 25-year-old female fell and sustained a simple olecranon fracture without dislocation. **C, D:** The fracture was treated with open reduction and plate fixation. At final follow-up, she had a healed fracture with asymptomatic hardware and a full range of motion.

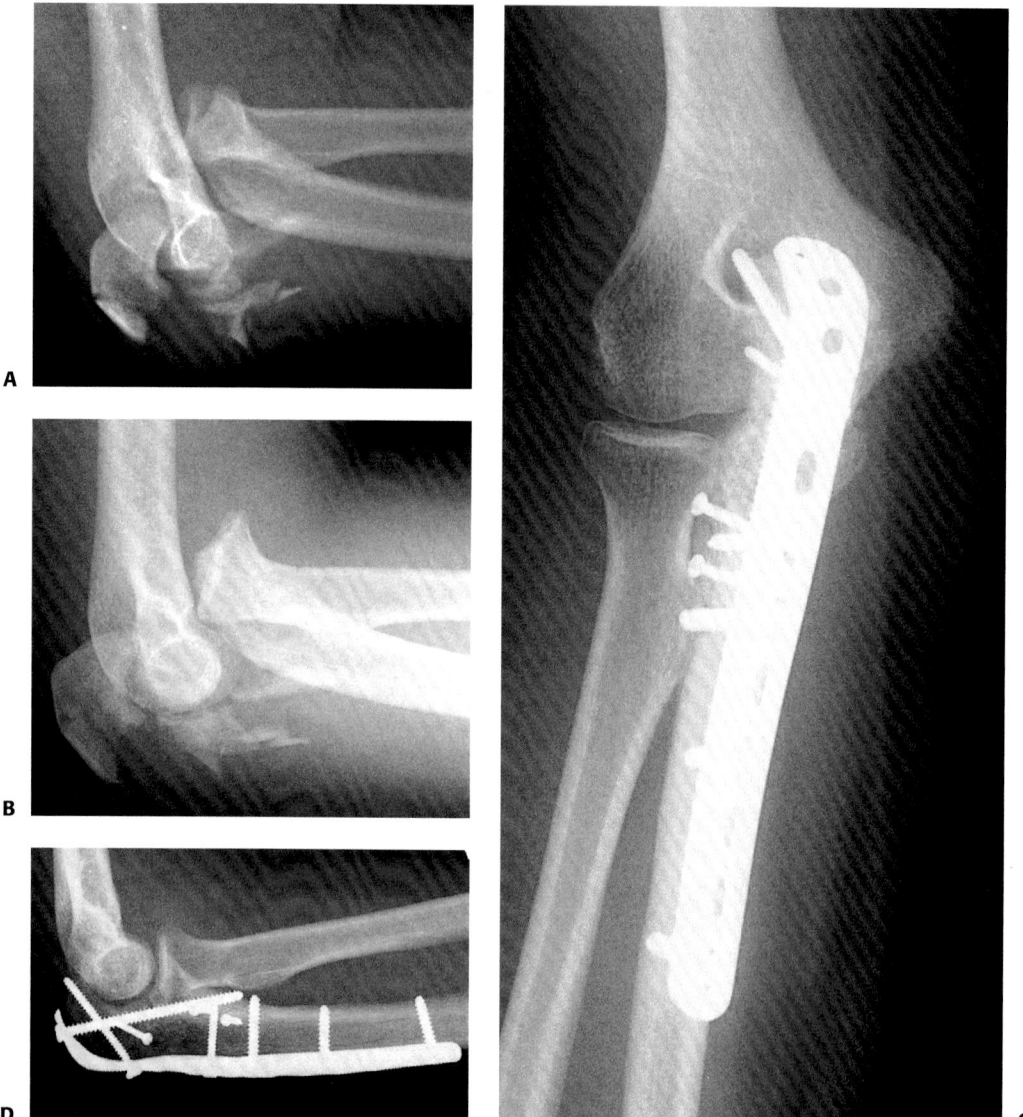

FIGURE 34-24 An 18-year-old female sustained a transolecranon fracture-dislocation in a motor vehicle accident. **A, B:** Plain radiographs demonstrate an anterior fracture-dislocation with an intact proximal radioulnar joint. **C, D:** She underwent operative fixation which included anatomic restoration of the comminuted joint, bone grafting the impacted central area, and plate fixation with a subchondral screw to support the elevated joint. Restoration of the sigmoid notch restored elbow stability. Final follow-up at 3 months demonstrated a stable elbow with a healed fracture and a well-aligned joint.

TABLE 34-37	ORIF of Proximal Ulna Fractures

Preoperative Planning Checklist

- OR Table: Radiolucent
- Position/positioning aids: Lateral, prone, or supine position, chest rolls, radiolucent arm board
- Fluoroscopy location: From the head of the table
- Equipment: Small fragment set, precontoured proximal ulna plates, 3.5-mm reconstruction plates, 2.7-mm reconstruction plates
- Tourniquet (sterile/nonsterile): Sterile available

Positioning. See previous section.

Surgical Approach. See previous section.

Technique. The fracture is reduced and clamped as above and held with provisional K-wires. A split is created in the triceps attachment to accommodate the proximal end of the plate. The plate should be held over the reduced fracture before making the split so it is made centrally over the olecranon tip. A precontoured plate or a plate contoured by the surgeon is placed around the tip of the olecranon extending distally along the ulnar border between the ECU and FCU. Due to the variable shape of the olecranon, some contouring of the proximal aspect of the plate is often required to ensure it is positioned against the bone. Fluoroscopy is recommended to check the position and contouring of the plate prior to placement of the screws. A short screw may be placed at the tip of the plate away from the lag hole to bring the plate to bone before applying the long subcortical screw. For noncomminuted fractures, a lag screw is placed from the tip of the plate exiting the anteromedial aspect of the ulna. For comminuted fractures, this screw should be placed in a nonlag fashion so the greater sigmoid notch is not overcompressed. Keeping the screw adjacent to the subchondral bone and placing it in a bicortical fashion will provide support to any comminution. The screw is directed medially so that there will be no impingement with the proximal radius. The shaft is secured with three screws. A final screw is placed into the tip of the olecranon for rotational control or to neutralize small proximal fragments. For fractures that are very proximal, care must be taken to capture the fragment in its entirety. If there is concern that the proximal fragment is comminuted or small, a "back-up" triceps suture can be placed to help secure the fragment and it can be tied to the proximal end of the plate or placed through a drill hole.[50] The elbow is examined clinically and fluoroscopically to be sure that there is no hardware in the proximal radioulnar joint or impinging on the biceps tuberosity. The wound is closed in layers to obtain as much deep coverage over the plate as possible (Table 34-38).

Postoperative Care. The rehabilitation protocol is the same as for tension-band wiring.

Potential Pitfalls and Preventative Measures. Although plating of olecranon fractures has generally good outcomes, attention to detail is important to avoid complications. Placement of the incision just radial to the tip of the olecranon, and not directly over it, will help to decrease wound complications. Skin flaps should be developed only as much as needed for adequate fracture reduction and hardware placement. The plate should be buried under the triceps proximally and if possible fascia should be closed over the plate distally to decrease hardware prominence.

Fixation of a small proximal fragment can fail if the implants do not adequately capture the fragment. The plate should be placed as proximal as possible and retrograde screws into the tip of the fragment can be placed for extra purchase. If needed, a "back-up" suture into the triceps can be placed and sewn to the proximal ulna through drill holes or attached to the plate.

The joint range of motion should be carefully examined at the conclusion of the case. Any crepitus in flexion and extension could indicate hardware in the ulnohumeral joint. Similarly, restrictions in rotation indicate potential hardware placement in the proximal radioulnar joint. By directing the long screw from the tip of the plate in an ulnar direction, this joint can be avoided while leaving room for further screws into the coronoid region to be placed safely (Table 34-39).

Treatment-Specific Outcomes. Plate fixation of olecranon fractures generally has good outcomes. Bailey et al.[6] demonstrated good outcomes with few complications and a relatively low incidence of hardware removal. Anderson et al.[3] demonstrated a high rate of union, low incidence of complications and 92% of patients in their series had good or excellent outcomes as measured by MEPI and DASH scores. Three of 32 patients had symptomatic hardware requiring removal.

Surgical Procedure—Posterior Monteggia Fractures

Posterior Monteggia lesions in adults are a spectrum of injuries involving the olecranon, coronoid, collateral ligaments, and radial head (Fig. 34-25). This section pertains to Jupiter Type IIA and IID Monteggia injuries that involve the elbow joint.

Preoperative Planning (Table 34-40)

TABLE 34-39 Proximal Ulna Fractures—Plating

Potential Pitfalls and Preventions

Pitfall	Preventions
Failure of fixation with small proximal fragments	Be sure plate is as proximal as possible "Back up" triceps suture to plate Capture with screws into the tip of the fragment
Hardware in Proximal Radioulnar Joint	Direct long tip screw ulnarly Careful examination radiographically and clinically prior to wound closure

TABLE 34-38 ORIF of Proximal Ulna Fracture—Plating

Surgical Steps

- Fracture reduced and held with pointed reduction clamp and K-wires
- Triceps split and plate placed onto bone
- Screw at tip of plate to bring plate to bone
- Apply fixation including a lag screw for noncomminuted fractures
- Protect tenuous fixation with suture through triceps for short proximal segments

TABLE 34-40 ORIF of Proximal Ulna Fractures—Posterior Monteggia Fractures

Preoperative Planning Checklist

- OR Table: Radiolucent
- Position/positioning aids: Lateral or prone position
- Fluoroscopy location: From head of table
- Equipment: Precontoured proximal ulna plates, LCDC plates, 2 minifragment straight plates and T-plates, 2- and 2.4-mm screws, radial head arthroplasty system, No. 2 nonabsorbable suture, suture anchors
- Tourniquet (sterile/nonsterile): Sterile preferred

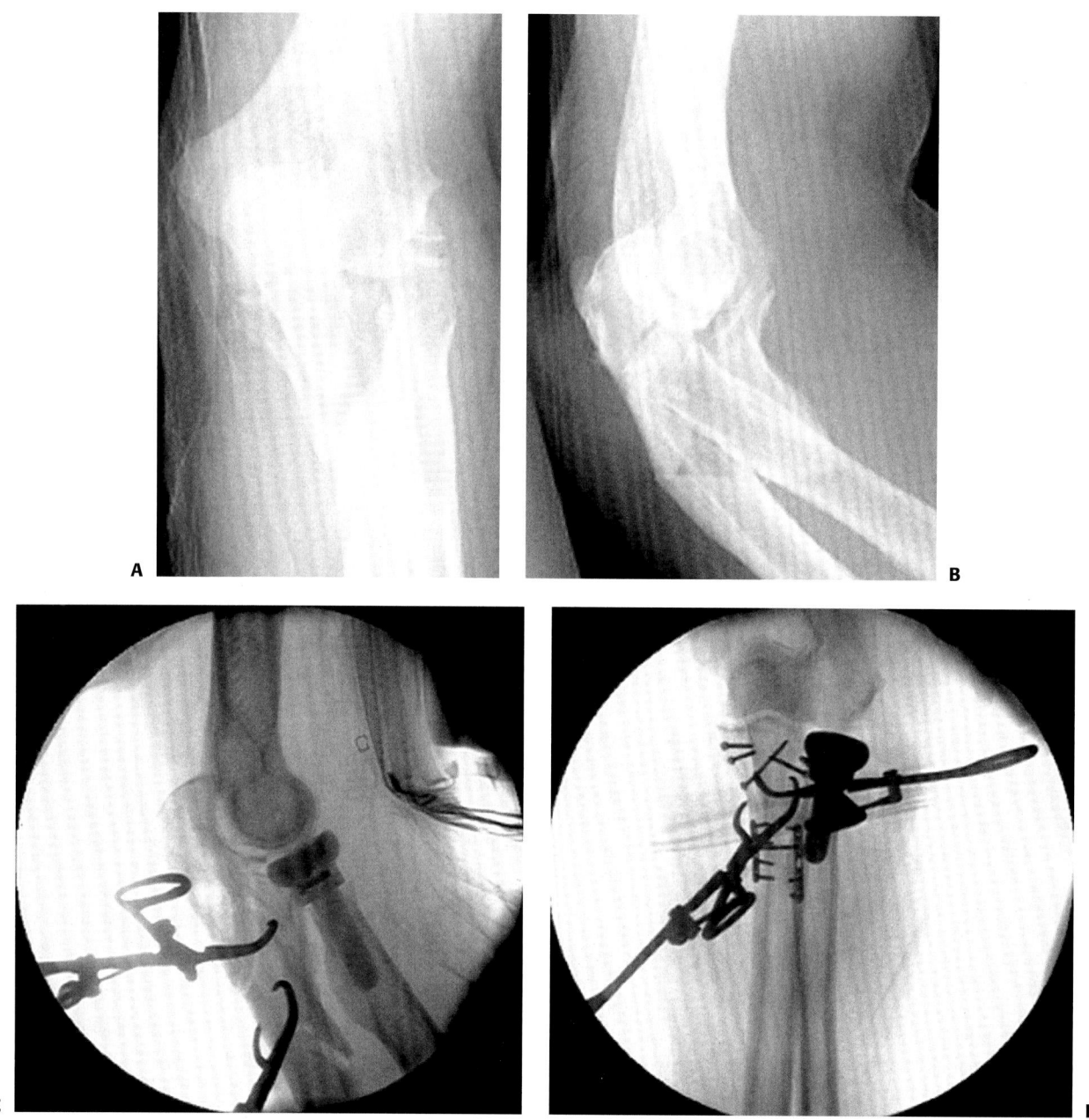

FIGURE 34-25 A 55-year-old male fell and sustained a posterior Monteggia fracture-dislocation. **A, B:** Radiographs demonstrated a proximal ulna fracture including a coronoid fracture, a radial head fracture, and disruption of the proximal radioulnar joint. **C:** Intraoperatively, the proximal ulna was provisionally reduced so that the radial head component could be properly sized. **D:** The definitive radial head prosthesis was then implanted, and the coronoid fracture was then reduced and held with small screws.

Positioning. See previous section. The lateral decubitus position is preferred.

Surgical Approach. A posterior midline incision is made and full thickness medial and lateral fasciocutaneous flaps are raised. The skin incision is curved radially around the tip of the olecranon for better coverage of hardware. The ulnar nerve should be identified so that it can be protected but it is not necessary to mobilize it. The interval between the ECU and FCU is

developed for exposure of the ulnar shaft. The trochlea, capitellum, and radial head are exposed by retracting the olecranon fragment proximally. The region of the lateral ligament complex origin on the lateral epicondyle of the humerus is palpated with a blunt instrument under the fascia, which is typically intact. If the epicondyle is devoid of soft tissue attachments, the fascia is incised so that a repair can be performed. The ECU and anconeus are elevated radially as required to expose the joint

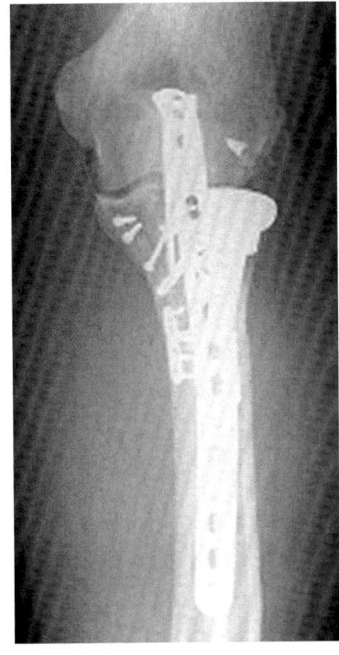
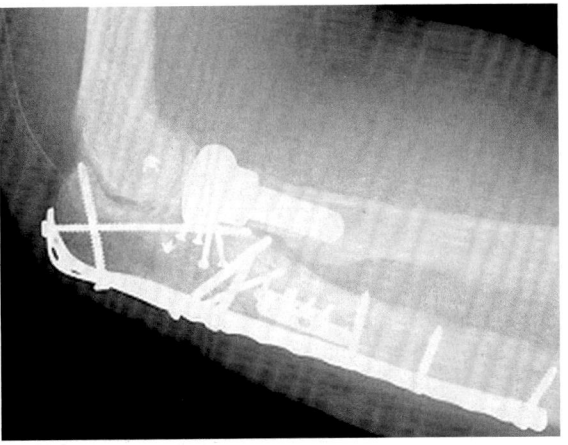

E   F

FIGURE 34-25 (*continued*) The olecranon and shaft were then neutralized with a long proximal ulna plate. Suture anchors were used to repair the collateral ligaments, and the elbow was stable after repair. **E, F:** The final construct demonstrated excellent alignment with a concentrically reduced elbow joint.

and shaft on the radial side and the FCU may be elevated laterally to expose the joint and shaft on the ulnar side.

Technique. The radial head is inspected to determine whether or not it can be repaired. If it is repairable, the fracture is fixed with small screws with or without plate supplementation depending on the fracture pattern. If the radial head is not repairable, the remaining head is resected and sized for a radial head arthroplasty. In order to determine appropriate height of the radial head implant, the coronoid, ulnar shaft, and olecranon components are temporarily reduced and held with clamps, hooks, and K-wires to be sure the correct height of implant is used. The height is checked with the trial implant using direct visualization as well as fluoroscopy to ascertain the relationship to the base of the coronoid. The olecranon and coronoid temporary fixation is then removed and the definitive radial implant is placed.

The fractured ulnar shaft is then reduced. Lag screws or small plates are used to provisionally hold the reduction. An anterior or anteromedial oblique fragment is often present which aligns with the coronoid more proximally and accurate reduction of this fragment is important. Restoring accurate length and alignment of the ulnar shaft is mandatory for maintenance of elbow stability. Due to the variable apex dorsal angulation of the proximal ulna, application of straight uncontoured plates may contribute to malreduction of the radiocapitellar joint.

The coronoid is then repaired with small plates, screws, or sutures depending on the fragment size. Small fragments are repaired using number 2 nonabsorbable sutures placed in the anterior capsule and through drill holes in the coronoid. These sutures are passed through drill holes and tied on the dorsal surface of the ulna. This suture may be placed before reduction

of other ulnar components for ease of access and it also may be necessary in conjunction with plate fixation for comminuted coronoids that include large and small fragments. This suture is not tied until the remaining hardware has been placed to minimize the chance of suture laceration by screws or wires.

The olecranon fragment is then reduced. A stout plate of 3.5 LCDC thickness is applied to the dorsal aspect of the ulna to hold the reduction of the olecranon and shaft components. Reconstruction or tubular plates are not sufficient for fixation. Periarticular precontoured plates are useful to reduce surgical time and assist in ulnar alignment. A screw from the tip of the olecranon is placed exiting the anteromedial ulnar cortex if possible. Screws from this plate into the coronoid fragment, if it is large enough, also augment stability and should be placed if possible. If there is significant comminution of the coronoid that has been held with suture fixation and there is no adequate docking site for a screw, a locked plate may be helpful to gain proximal fixation with shorter screws avoiding screws in the region of the sutures coronoid. If coronoid sutures have been placed, they are then tied over the dorsal aspect of the plate.

There is often a small fragment of bone ulnarly that includes the sublime tubercle with the insertion of the MCL. If it is large enough, it may be repaired with a small plate. If not, suture anchors are used. The LCL may be avulsed off the lateral epicondyle; however, the overlying fascia may be intact. The lateral ligament and extensor muscle origins are repaired with suture anchors or transosseous bone tunnels into the lateral epicondyle.

The elbow is then taken through a full range of motion to evaluate for stability (Table 34-41).

<table>
<tr><td>

TABLE 34-41 **ORIF of Proximal Ulna Fracture—Posterior Monteggia Fractures**

Surgical Steps

- Repair or replacement of the radial head
- Repair of the ulnar shaft with minifragment plates or lag screws
- Repair of the coronoid fracture with minifragment plates, screws, or suture
- Olecranon fragment reduced and plate spanning olecranon and shaft components are placed
- MCL evaluated and repaired as needed
- LCL evaluated and repaired as needed

</td></tr>
</table>

Postoperative Care. The elbow is splinted at 90 degrees of flexion with the forearm in neutral rotation for 48 hours. The splint is then removed and the patient is started on range of motion exercises. These exercises include active and active-assisted flexion and extension. Concomitant ligament injuries will direct the rehabilitation plan as outlined in the section on the operative treatment of elbow dislocations. Active extension and extension against gravity begins at 6 weeks. Static progressive splinting may be used if the patient has stiffness and the fracture has healed. At 3 months, a strengthening regimen is instituted.

Potential Pitfalls and Preventative Measures. Recognition of the fracture pattern and associated injuries is the first step in restoring stability. Nonunion is not common; however, it is important that surgeon technique does not contribute to this problem. Appropriate choice of fixation is essential and adherence to basic fracture principles is essential. Plates for Monteggia injuries should be of sufficient strength to support the proximal shaft of the ulna and tubular and reconstruction plates are to be avoided when the fracture extends distal to the coronoid. Tension-band wiring is not appropriate in these cases.

Recurrent instability may occur if restoration of the ulnar anatomy is not achieved. The ulna has a serpentine shape with a variable apex dorsal angulation and application of straight uncontoured plates may contribute to malreduction.[95] Precontoured plates may help with restoration of alignment, particularly in comminuted fractures. Alternatively, radiographs of the opposite extremity can help to determine the correct shape and length of the ulna to allow for more accurate contouring of implants if precontoured plates are not available. Also, since the fascia overlying the lateral ligament is often intact, an extensive LCL injury can be missed. Therefore it is imperative that the surgeon assesses for ligament injuries and repairs them when found.

Elbow stiffness and heterotopic ossification are possible. Sufficient fixation stability is mandatory to allow for early range of motion. The use of prophylaxis for heterotopic ossification remains controversial. Radiation has been shown to lead to an increased nonunion rate in the setting of distal humeral fractures and is not recommended (Table 34-42).

TABLE 34-42 **Proximal Ulna Fractures—Posterior Monteggia Fractures**

Potential Pitfalls and Preventions

Pitfall	Preventions
Instability	Accurate restoration of ulnar length, dorsal angulation, and serpentine shape. Repair of lateral ligament complex
Loss of fixation and nonunion	Appropriate choice of implant for fracture pattern with avoidance of tension-band constructs
Elbow stiffness	Secure fixation to allow for early range of motion

Treatment-Specific Outcomes. Posterior Monteggia fractures are complex injuries to manage. Complications may include nonunion, heterotopic ossification, recurrent subluxation, elbow stiffness, and post-traumatic arthritis. Konrad et al.[62] followed patients for an average of 9 years and satisfactory results were found in 34 of 47 patients. Factors predicting a poor outcome included fractures involving the radial head, coronoid, and complications requiring further surgery with 26% of patients requiring a secondary surgery within 12 months of the initial procedure. Strauss et al.[106] reported that patients with posterior Monteggia fractures that had a concomitant ulnohumeral dislocation had worse outcome. Beingessner et al.[10] evaluated a series of 16 patients with Type IID Monteggia fractures. All fractures united and there were no patients with recurrent instability. Three patients developed elbow stiffness with associated heterotopic ossification, one patient had prominent hardware, one had loss of radial head fixation but no subluxation, and one developed pronator syndrome. However, the majority of patients had good results with anatomic repair of all injured structures.

MANAGEMENT OF EXPECTED ADVERSE OUTCOMES AND UNEXPECTED COMPLICATIONS IN PROXIMAL ULNA FRACTURES (TABLE 34-43)

TABLE 34-43 **Proximal Ulna Fracture**

Common Adverse Outcomes and Complications

Prominent and symptomatic hardware → Careful technique of implant placement, hardware removal as needed

Heterotopic ossification and elbow stiffness → Secure fixation to allow for early range of motion

Nonunion and malunion → Adherence to proper fracture principles and techniques

Failure of fixation and elbow instability → Understand the fracture pattern and address each component

AUTHOR'S PREFERRED METHOD OF TREATMENT FOR PROXIMAL ULNA FRACTURES

We prefer to treat both simple and complex olecranon fractures with plate fixation since it is reliable and with improved implant designs hardware is typically not sufficiently symptomatic to require removal (Fig. 34-26A). In patients with significant osteopenia and poor bone quality, triceps advancement is used; however, this technique is rarely needed and significantly debilitated patients or those with very low functional demands can do well with nonoperative treatment as long as there is no associated elbow instability. We prefer a fragment-specific approach to Monteggia fractures including repair of all injured structures as outlined above (Fig. 34-26B).

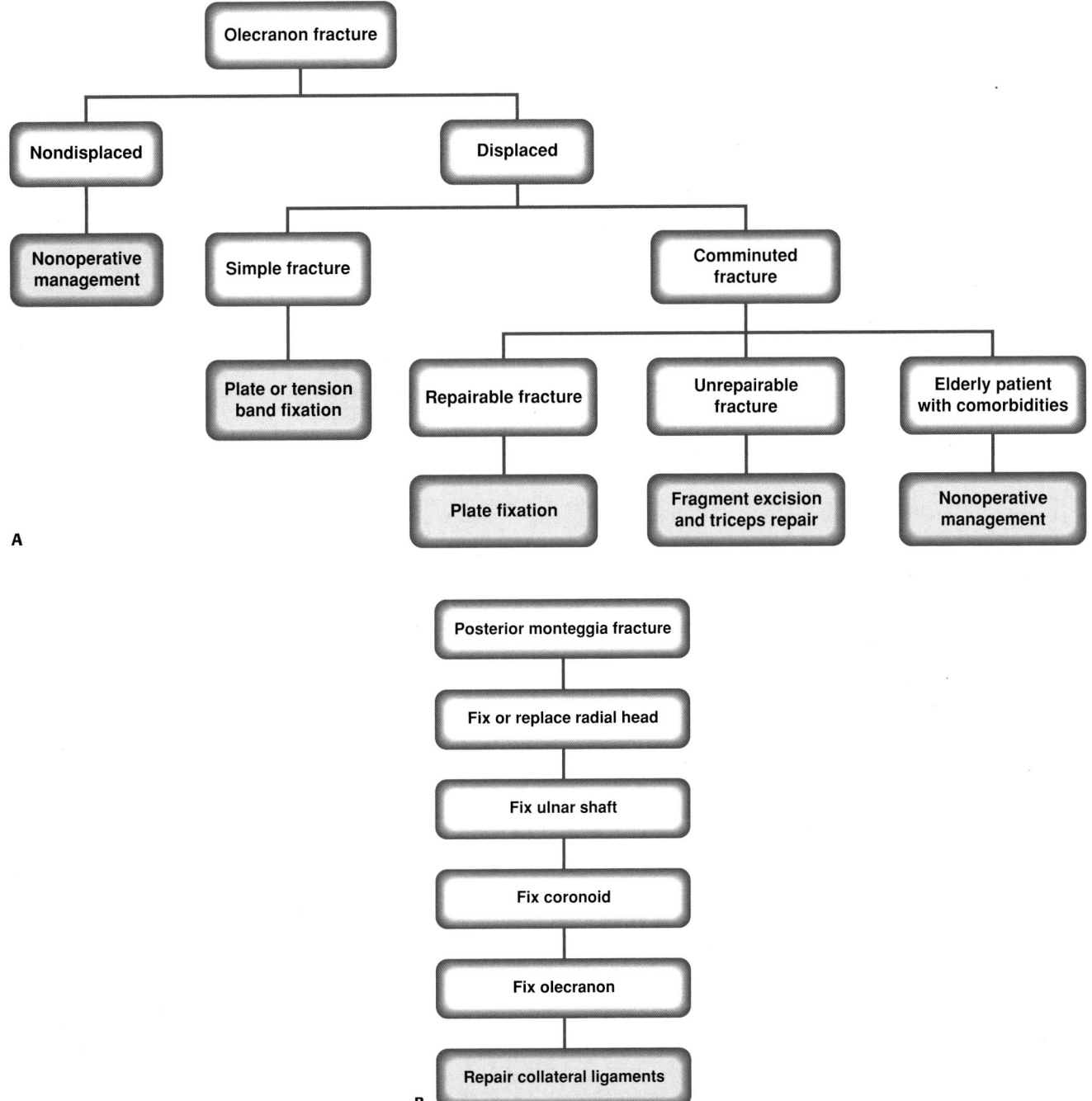

FIGURE 34-26 **A, B:** Author's preferred treatment.

Summary, Controversies, and Future Directions in Proximal Ulna Fractures

Proximal ulna fractures include a spectrum of fractures from simple olecranon fractures to complex fracture-dislocations. An accurate understanding of the injury pattern will lead to appropriate fixation choices for these injuries. The development of periarticular implants and the judicious use of fragment fixation with small plates have led to an improved outcome for these often difficult fractures.

REFERENCES

1. Akesson T, Herbertsson P, Josefsson PO, et al. Primary nonoperative treatment of moderately displaced two-part fractures of the radial head. *J Bone Joint Surg Am.* 2006; 88(9):1909–1914.
2. Anakwe RE, Middleton SD, Jenkins PJ, et al. Patient-reported outcomes after simple dislocation of the elbow. *J Bone Joint Surg Am.* 2011;93(13):1220–1226.
3. Anderson ML, Larson AN, Merten SM, et al. Congruent elbow plate fixation of olecranon fractures. *J Orthop Trauma.* 2007;21(6):386–393.
4. Antuna SA, Sanchez-Marquez JM, Barco R. Long-term results of radial head resection following isolated radial head fractures in patients younger than forty years old. *J Bone Joint Surg Am.* 2010;92(3):558–566.
5. Athwal GS, Rouleau DM, MacDermid JC, et al. Contralateral elbow radiographs can reliably diagnose radial head implant overlengthening. *J Bone Joint Surg Am.* 2011;93(14):1339–1346.
6. Bailey CS, MacDermid J, Patterson SD, et al. Outcome of plate fixation of olecranon fractures. *J Orthop Trauma.* 2001;15(8):542–548.
7. Beingessner DM, Dunning CE, Gordon KD, et al. The effect of radial head excision and arthroplasty on elbow kinematics and stability. *J Bone Joint Surg Am.* 2004; 86A(8):1730–1739.
8. Beingessner DM, Dunning CE, Gordon KD, et al. The effect of radial head fracture size on elbow kinematics and stability. *J Orthop Res.* 2005;23(1):210–217.
9. Beingessner DM, Dunning CE, Stacpoole RA, et al. The effect of coronoid fractures on elbow kinematics and stability. *Clin Biomech (Bristol, Avon).* 2007;22(2):183–190.
10. Beingessner DM, Nork SE, Agel J, et al. A fragment-specific approach to Type IID Monteggia elbow fracture-dislocations. *J Orthop Trauma.* 2011;25(7):414–419.
11. Beingessner DM, Stacpoole RA, Dunning CE, et al. The effect of suture fixation of type I coronoid fractures on the kinematics and stability of the elbow with and without medial collateral ligament repair. *J Shoulder Elbow Surg.* 2007;16(2):213–217.
12. Bell TH, Ferreira LM, McDonald CP, et al. Contribution of the olecranon to elbow stability: an in vitro biomechanical study. *J Bone Joint Surg Am.* 2010;92(4):949–957.
13. Birkedal JP, Deal DN, Ruch DS. Loss of flexion after radial head replacement. *J Shoulder Elbow Surg.* 2004;13(2):208–213.
14. Boulas HJ, Morrey BF. Biomechanical evaluation of the elbow following radial head fracture. Comparison of open reduction and internal fixation vs. excision, silastic replacement, and non-operative management. *Chir Main.* 1998;17(4):314–320.
15. Broberg MA, Morrey BF. Results of delayed excision of the radial head after fracture. *J Bone Joint Surg Am.* 1986;68(5):669–674.
16. Broberg MA, Morrey BF. Results of treatment of fracture-dislocations of the elbow. *Clin Orthop.* 1987;(216):109–119.
17. Burkhart KJ, Mattyasovszky SG, Runkel M, et al. Mid- to long-term results after bipolar radial head arthroplasty. *J Shoulder Elbow Surg.* 2010;19(7):965–972.
18. Burton AE. Fractures of the head of the radius. *Proc R Soc Med.* 1942;35:764–765.
19. Caputo AE, Mazzocca AD, Santoro VM. The nonarticulating portion of the radial head: anatomic and clinical correlations for internal fixation. *J Hand Surg Am.* 1998; 23(6):1082–1090.
20. Carstam N. Operative treatment of fractures of the upper end of the radius. *Acta Orthop Scand.* 1950;59:502–523.
21. Chen X, Wang SC, Cao LH, et al. Comparison between radial head replacement and open reduction and internal fixation in clinical treatment of unstable, multi-fragmented radial head fractures. *Int Orthop.* 2011;35(7):1071–1076.
22. Coonrad RW, Roush TF, Major NM, et al. The drop sign, a radiographic warning sign of elbow instability. *J Shoulder Elbow Surg.* 2005;14(3):312–317.
23. Diliberti T, Botte MJ, Abrams RA. Anatomical considerations regarding the posterior interosseous nerve during posterolateral approaches to the proximal part of the radius. *J Bone Joint Surg Am.* 2000;82(6):809–813.
24. Doornberg J, Ring D, Jupiter JB. Effective treatment of fracture-dislocations of the olecranon requires a stable trochlear notch. *Clin Orthop Relat Res.* 2004;(429): 292–300.
25. Doornberg JN, Linzel DS, Zurakowski D, et al. Reference points for radial head prosthesis size. *J Hand Surg Am.* 2006;31(1):53–57.
26. Doornberg JN, Parisien R, van Duijn PJ, et al. Radial head arthroplasty with a modular metal spacer to treat acute traumatic elbow instability. *J Bone Joint Surg Am.* 2007; 89(5):1075–1080.
27. Doornberg JN, Ring D. Coronoid fracture patterns. *J Hand Surg Am.* 2006;31(1): 45–52.
28. Doornberg JN, Ring DC. Fracture of the anteromedial facet of the coronoid process. *J Bone Joint Surg Am.* 2006;88(10):2216–2224.
29. Doornberg JN, van Duijn J, Ring D. Coronoid fracture height in terrible-triad injuries. *J Hand Surg Am.* 2006;31(5):794–797.
30. Duckworth AD, Clement ND, Jenkins PJ, et al. The epidemiology of radial head and neck fractures. *J Hand Surg Am.* 2012;37(1):112–119.
31. Duckworth AD, Ring D, Kulijdian A, et al. Unstable elbow dislocations. *J Shoulder Elbow Surg.* 2008;17(2):281–286.
32. Dunning CE, Zarzour ZD, Patterson SD, et al. Muscle forces and pronation stabilize the lateral ligament deficient elbow. *Clin Orthop.* 2001;(388):118–124.
33. Essex-Lopresti P. Fractures of the radial head with distal radio-ulnar dislocation. *J Bone Joint Surg Br.* 1951;33B:244–247.
34. Eygendaal D, Verdegaal SH, Obermann WR, et al. Posterolateral dislocation of the elbow joint. Relationship to medial instability. *J Bone Joint Surg Am.* 2000;82(4):555–560.
35. Fehringer EV, Burns EM, Knierim A, et al. Radiolucencies surrounding a smooth-stemmed radial head component may not correlate with forearm pain or poor elbow function. *J Shoulder Elbow Surg.* 2009;18(2):275–278.
36. Ferreira LM, Bell TH, Johnson JA, et al. The effect of triceps repair techniques following olecranon excision on elbow stability and extension strength: an in vitro biomechanical study. *J Orthop Trauma.* 2011;25(7):420–424.
37. Flinkkila T, Kaisto T, Sirnio K, et al. Short- to mid-term results of metallic press-fit radial head arthroplasty in unstable injuries of the elbow. *J Bone Joint Surg Br.* 2012; 94(6):805–810.
38. Frank SG, Grewal R, Johnson J, et al. Determination of correct implant size in radial head arthroplasty to avoid overlengthening. *J Bone Joint Surg Am.* 2009;91(7):1738–1746.
39. Fraser GS, Pichora JE, Ferreira LM, et al. Lateral collateral ligament repair restores the initial varus stability of the elbow: an in vitro biomechanical study. *J Orthop Trauma.* 2008;22(9):615–623.
40. Garrigues GE, Wray WH III, Lindenhovius AL, et al. Fixation of the coronoid process in elbow fracture-dislocations. *J Bone Joint Surg Am.* 2011;93(20):1873–1881.
41. Gartsman GM, Sculco TP, Otis JC. Operative treatment of olecranon fractures. Excision or open reduction with internal fixation. *J Bone Joint Surg Am.* 1981;63(5):718–721.
42. Grewal R, MacDermid JC, Faber KJ, et al. Comminuted radial head fractures treated with a modular metallic radial head arthroplasty. Study of outcomes. *J Bone Joint Surg Am.* 2006;88(10):2192–2200.
43. Guitton TG, Ring D. Nonsurgically treated terrible triad injuries of the elbow: report of four cases. *J Hand Surg Am.* 2010;35(3):464–467.
44. Hamid N, Ashraf N, Bosse MJ, et al. Radiation therapy for heterotopic ossification prophylaxis acutely after elbow trauma: a prospective randomized study. *J Bone Joint Surg Am.* 2010;92(11):2032–2038.
45. Heim U. Combined fractures of the radius and the ulna at the elbow level in the adult. Analysis of 120 cases after more than 1 year. *Rev Chir Orthop Reparatrice Appar Mot.* 1998;84(2):142–153.
46. Herbertsson P, Josefsson PO, Hasserius R, et al. Uncomplicated Mason type-II and III fractures of the radial head and neck in adults. A long-term follow-up study. *J Bone Joint Surg Am.* 2004;86-A(3):569–574.
47. Holdsworth BJ, Clement DA, Rothwell PN. Fractures of the radial head—the benefit of aspiration: a prospective controlled trial. *Injury.* 1987;18(1):44–47.
48. Iftimie PP, Calmet GJ, de Loyola GF, et al. Resection arthroplasty for radial head fractures: long-term follow-up. *J Shoulder Elbow Surg.* 2011;20(1):45–50.
49. Ikeda M, Sugiyama K, Kang C, et al. Comminuted fractures of the radial head. Comparison of resection and internal fixation. *J Bone Joint Surg Am.* 2005;87A:76–84.
50. Izzi J, Athwal GS. An off-loading triceps suture for augmentation of plate fixation in comminuted osteoporotic fractures of the olecranon. *J Orthop Trauma.* 2012;26(1):59–61.
51. Jones SG. Fractures of the head and neck of the radius – separation of upper radial epiphysis. *New England J Med.* 1935;212:914–917.
52. Josefsson PO, Johnell O, Gentz CF. Long-term sequelae of simple dislocation of the elbow. *J Bone Joint Surg Am.* 1984;66(6):927–930.
53. Josefsson PO, Johnell O, Wendeberg B. Ligamentous injuries in dislocations of the elbow joint. *Clin Orthop.* 1987;(221):221–225.
54. Josefsson PO, Nilsson BE. Incidence of elbow dislocation. *Acta Orthop Scand.* 1986;57(6):537–538.
55. Jupiter JB, Leibovic SJ, Ribbans W, et al. The posterior Monteggia lesion. *J Orthop Trauma.* 1991;5(4):395–402.
56. Jupiter JB, Ring D. Treatment of unreduced elbow dislocations with hinged external fixation. *J Bone Joint Surg Am.* 2002;84-A(9):1630–1635.
57. Kaas L, Turkenburg JL, van Riet RP, et al. Magnetic resonance imaging findings in 46 elbows with a radial head fracture. *Acta Orthop.* 2010;81(3):373–376.
58. Khalfayan EE, Culp RW, Alexander AH. Mason type II radial head fractures: operative versus nonoperative treatment. *J Orthop Trauma.* 1992;6(3):283–289.
59. King GJ, Evans DC, Kellam JF. Open reduction and internal fixation of radial head fractures. *J Orthop Trauma.* 1991;5(1):21–28.
60. King GJ, Zarzour ZD, Patterson SD, et al. An anthropometric study of the radial head: implications in the design of a prosthesis. *J Arthroplasty.* 2001;16(1):112–116.
61. Kohls-Gatzoulis J, Tsiridis E, Schizas C. Reconstruction of the coronoid process with iliac crest bone graft. *J Shoulder Elbow Surg.* 2004;13(2):217–220.
62. Konrad GG, Kundel K, Kreuz PC, et al. Monteggia fractures in adults: long-term results and prognostic factors. *J Bone Joint Surg Br.* 2007;89(3):354–360.
63. Koslowsky TC, Schliwa S, Koebke J. Presentation of the microscopic vascular architecture of the radial head using a sequential plastination technique. *Clin Anat.* 2011; 24(6):721–732.
64. Lindenhovius A, Karanicolas PJ, Bhandari M, et al. Interobserver reliability of coronoid fracture classification: two-dimensional versus three-dimensional computed tomography. *J Hand Surg Am.* 2009;34(9):1640–1646.
65. Lindenhovius AL, Felsch Q, Ring D, et al. The long-term outcome of open reduction and internal fixation of stable displaced isolated partial articular fractures of the radial head. *J Trauma.* 2009;67(1):143–146.
66. Linscheid RL, Wheeler DK. Elbow dislocations. *JAMA.* 1965;194(11):1171–1176.

67. Madsen M, Marx RG, Millett PJ, et al. Surgical anatomy of the triceps brachii tendon: anatomical study and clinical correlation. *Am J Sports Med.* 2006;34(11):1839–1843.
68. Marcotte AL, Osterman AL. Longitudinal radioulnar dissociation: identification and treatment of acute and chronic injuries. *Hand Clin.* 2007;23(2):195–208.
69. Mason ML. Some observations on fracture of the head of the radius with a review of one hundred cases. *Br J Surg.* 1954;42:123–132.
70. McKee MD, Pugh DM, Wild LM, et al. Standard surgical protocol to treat elbow dislocations with radial head and coronoid fractures. Surgical technique. *J Bone Joint Surg Am.* 2005;87A(suppl 1):22–32.
71. McKee MD, Schemitsch EH, Sala MJ, et al. The pathoanatomy of lateral ligamentous disruption in complex elbow instability. *J Shoulder Elbow Surg.* 2003;12(4):391–396.
72. Mehlhoff TL, Noble PC, Bennett JB, et al. Simple dislocation of the elbow in the adult. Results after closed treatment. *J Bone Joint Surg Am.* 1988;70(2):244–249.
73. Moritomo H, Tada K, Yoshida T, et al. Reconstruction of the coronoid for chronic dislocation of the elbow. Use of a graft from the olecranon in two cases. *J Bone Joint Surg Br.* 1998;80(3):490–492.
74. Morrey BF, An KN. Articular and ligamentous contributions to the stability of the elbow joint. *Am J Sports Med.* 1983;11(5):315–319.
75. Morrey BF, Tanaka S, An KN. Valgus stability of the elbow. A definition of primary and secondary constraints. *Clin Orthop.* 1991;175(265):187–195.
76. Morrey BF. Current concepts in the treatment of fractures of the radial head, the olecranon, and the coronoid. *Instr Course Lect.* 1995;44:175–185.
77. Murray RC. Fractures of the head and neck of the radius. *Br J Surg.* 1940;27:106–118.
78. Neuhaus V, Alqueza A, Mudgal CS. Open reduction and temporary internal fixation of a subacute elbow dislocation. *J Hand Surg Am.* 2012;37(5):1011–1014.
79. Neumann M, Nyffeler R, Beck M. Comminuted fractures of the radial head and neck: is fixation to the shaft necessary? *J Bone Joint Surg Br.* 2011;93(2):223–228.
80. O'Driscoll SW, Jupiter JB, Cohen MS, et al. Difficult elbow fractures: pearls and pitfalls. *Instr Course Lect.* 2003;52:113–134.
81. O'Driscoll SW, Morrey BF, Korinek S, et al. Elbow subluxation and dislocation. A spectrum of instability. *Clin Orthop.* 1992;(280):186–197.
82. Pichora JE, Fraser GS, Ferreira LF, et al. The effect of medial collateral ligament repair tension on elbow joint kinematics and stability. *J Hand Surg Am.* 2007;32(8):1210–1217.
83. Pollock JW, Brownhill J, Ferreira L, et al. The effect of anteromedial facet fractures of the coronoid and lateral collateral ligament injury on elbow stability and kinematics. *J Bone Joint Surg Am.* 2009;91(6):1448–1458.
84. Popovic N, Lemaire R, Georis P, et al. Midterm results with a bipolar radial head prosthesis: radiographic evidence of loosening at the bone-cement interface. *J Bone Joint Surg Am.* 2007;89(11):2469–2476.
85. Pugh DM, Wild LM, Schemitsch EH, et al. Standard surgical protocol to treat elbow dislocation with radial head and coronoid fractures. *J Bone Joint Surg Am.* 2004;86A(6):1122–1130.
86. Radin EL, Riseborough EJ. Fractures of the radial head. A review of eighty-eight cases and analysis of the indications for excision of the radial head and non-operative treatment. *J Bone Joint Surg Am.* 1966;48(6):1055–1064.
87. Regan W, Morrey B. Fractures of the coronoid process of the ulna. *J Bone Joint Surg Am.* 1989;71(9):1348–1354.
88. Richard MJ, Aldridge JM III, Wiesler ER, et al. Traumatic valgus instability of the elbow: pathoanatomy and results of direct repair. *J Bone Joint Surg Am.* 2008;90(11):2416–2422.
89. Ring D, Jupiter JB, Sanders RW, et al. Transolecranon fracture-dislocation of the elbow. *J Orthop Trauma.* 1997;11(8):545–550.
90. Ring D, Jupiter JB, Zilberfarb J. Posterior dislocation of the elbow with fractures of the radial head and coronoid. *J Bone Joint Surg Am.* 2002;84A(4):547–551.
91. Ring D, Quintero J, Jupiter JB. Open reduction and internal fixation of fractures of the radial head. *J Bone Joint Surg Am.* 2002;84-A(10):1811–1815.
92. Ring D. Fractures of the coronoid process of the ulna. *J Hand Surg Am.* 2006;31(10):1679–1689.
93. Rosenblatt Y, Young C, MacDermid JC, et al. Osteotomy of the head of the radius for partial articular malunion. *J Bone Joint Surg Br.* 2009;91(10):1341–1346.
94. Rotini R, Marinelli A, Guerra E, et al. Radial head replacement with unipolar and bipolar SBi system: a clinical and radiographic analysis after a 2-year mean follow-up. *Musculoskelet Surg.* 2012;96(suppl 1):S69–S79.
95. Rouleau DM, Faber KJ, Athwal GS. The proximal ulna dorsal angulation: a radiographic study. *J Shoulder Elbow Surg.* 2010;19(1):26–30.
96. Rowland AS, Athwal GS, MacDermid JC, et al. Lateral ulnohumeral joint space widening is not diagnostic of radial head arthroplasty overstuffing. *J Hand Surg Am.* 2007;32(5):637–641.
97. Sanchez-Sotelo J, O'Driscoll SW, Morrey BF. Medial oblique compression fracture of the coronoid process of the ulna. *J Shoulder Elbow Surg.* 2005;14(1):60–64.
98. Sarris IK, Kyrkos MJ, Galanis NN, et al. Radial head replacement with the MoPyC pyrocarbon prosthesis. *J Shoulder Elbow Surg.* 2012;21(9):1222–1228.
99. Schiffern A, Bettwieser SP, Porucznik CA, et al. Proximal radial drift following radial head resection. *J Shoulder Elbow Surg.* 2011;20(3):426–433.
100. Schneeberger A, Sadowski MM, Jacob HAC. Coronoid process and radial head as posterolateral rotatory stabilizers of the elbow. *J Bone Joint Surg Am.* 2004;86A(5):975–982.
101. Shore BJ, Mozzon JB, MacDermid JC, et al. Chronic posttraumatic elbow disorders treated with metallic radial head arthroplasty. *J Bone Joint Surg Am.* 2008;90(2):271–280.
102. Smith AM, Morrey BF, Steinmann SP. Low profile fixation of radial head and neck fractures: surgical technique and clinical experience. *J Orthop Trauma.* 2007;21(10):718–724.
103. Smith GR, Altchek DW, Pagnani MJ, et al. A muscle-splitting approach to the ulnar collateral ligament of the elbow. Neuroanatomy and operative technique. *Am J Sports Med.* 1996;24(5):575–580.
104. Smith GR, Hotchkiss RN. Radial head and neck fractures: anatomic guidelines for proper placement of internal fixation. *J Shoulder Elbow Surg.* 1996;5(2 Pt 1):113–117.
105. Stoneback JW, Owens BD, Sykes J, et al. Incidence of elbow dislocations in the United States population. *J Bone Joint Surg Am.* 2012;94(3):240–245.
106. Strauss EJ, Tejwani NC, Preston CF, et al. The posterior Monteggia lesion with associated ulnohumeral instability. *J Bone Joint Surg Br.* 2006;88(1):84–89.
107. Szekeres M, Chinchalkar SJ, King GJ. Optimizing elbow rehabilitation after instability. *Hand Clin.* 2008;24(1):27–38.
108. Taylor TK, Scham SM. A posteromedial approach to the proximal end of the ulna for the internal fixation of olecranon fractures. *J Trauma.* 1969;9(7):594–602.
109. van Riet RP, Morrey BF, O'Driscoll SW. Use of osteochondral bone graft in coronoid fractures. *J Shoulder Elbow Surg.* 2005;14(5):519–523.
110. van Riet RP, Morrey BF. Documentation of associated injuries occurring with radial head fracture. *Clin Orthop Relat Res.* 2008;466(1):130–134.
111. van Riet RP, Sanchez-Sotelo J, Morrey BF. Failure of metal radial head replacement. *J Bone Joint Surg Br.* 2010;92(5):661–667.
112. van Riet RP, Van Glabbeek F, Neale PG, et al. The noncircular shape of the radial head. *J Hand Surg Am.* 2003;28(6):972–978.
113. Villanueva P, Osorio F, Commessatti M, et al. Tension-band wiring for olecranon fractures: analysis of risk factors for failure. *J Shoulder Elbow Surg.* 2006;15(3):351–356.
114. Wells J, Ablove RH. Coronoid fractures of the elbow. *Clin Med Res.* 2008;6(1):40–44.
115. Wexner SD, Goodwin C, Parkes JC, et al. Treatment of fractures of the radial head by partial excision. *Orthop Rev.* 1985;14:83–86.
116. Wolff AL, Hotchkiss RN. Lateral elbow instability: nonoperative, operative, and postoperative management. *J Hand Ther.* 2006;19(2):238–243.
117. Wolfgang G, Burke F, Bush D, et al. Surgical treatment of displaced olecranon fractures by tension band wiring technique. *Clin Orthop Relat Res.* 1987;(224):192–204.
118. Zunkiewicz MR, Clemente JS, Miller MC, et al. Radial head replacement with a bipolar system: a minimum 2-year follow-up. *J Shoulder Elbow Surg.* 2012;21(1):98–104.

35

DISTAL HUMERUS FRACTURES

George S. Athwal

INTRODUCTION TO DISTAL HUMERUS FRACTURES

Distal humerus fractures remain some of the most challenging injuries to manage. They are commonly multifragmented, occur in osteopenic bone, and have complex anatomy with limited options for internal fixation. Treatment outcomes are often associated with elbow stiffness, weakness, and pain. A painless, stable, and mobile elbow joint is desired as it allows the hand to conduct the activities of daily living, most notably personal hygiene and feeding. Therefore, starting with a highly traumatized distal humerus and finishing with a stable, mobile, and pain- free joint requires a systematic approach. Thought is required in determining the operative indications, managing the soft tissues, selecting a surgical approach, obtaining an anatomic articular reduction, and creating a fixation construct that is rigid enough to tolerate early range of motion.

In 1913, Albin Lambotte[110] challenged the leading opinions of conservative management for distal humerus fractures and advocated an aggressive approach, which consisted of open reduction and internal fixation (ORIF). He described the principles of osteosynthesis and believed anatomic restoration of anatomy correlated with a better return to function. Unfortunately, surgical outcomes in that era were plagued with a high risk of infection and hardware failure. In 1937, Eastwood[46] described the technique of closed reduction under a general anesthetic and brief immobilization in a collar and cuff. He reviewed 14 patients treated with this technique and reported that 12 returned to their original occupation. He stated "a perfect anatomical reduction is not necessary in order to obtain a good result." Evans,[52] in 1953, termed this mode of treatment "bag of bones" and believed that although it may be appropriate for the elderly patient, it was not ideal for the young active patient.

The controversy between operative and nonoperative management continued for decades to follow. Riseborough and Radin,[186] in 1969, reported that operative treatment was unpredictable and often associated with poor outcomes, and therefore, they recommended nonsurgical management. Similarly, Brown and Morgan,[25] in 1971, reported satisfactory results with nonoperative management of 10 patients with distal humerus fractures. Their patients were managed with early active motion and at final follow-up had an average arc of motion of 98 degrees.

In the last quarter century, improved outcomes have been reported with surgery for distal humerus fractures. The principles set out by the Arbeitsgemeinschaft für Osteosynthesefragen—Association for the Study of Internal Fixation (AO-ASIF) group, including anatomic articular reduction and rigid internal fixation, allow for healing and early postoperative motion.[64,108,125,130,161,189,195] The last decade has seen advances in the understanding of elbow anatomy, improvements in surgical approaches, new innovative fixation devices, and an evolution of postoperative rehabilitation protocols.

In younger patients, ORIF of distal humerus fractures using modern fixation principles is considered the standard of treatment. In elderly patients, restoration of the anatomy and obtaining rigid internal fixation may be difficult because of poor bone quality and comminution of the articular surface and metaphysis. In cases where rigid internal fixation cannot be achieved to allow early range of motion, resultant prolonged immobilization often leads to poor outcomes. Other complications associated with potentially poor outcomes include malunion, nonunion, contracture, avascular necrosis, heterotopic ossification (HO), hardware failure, and symptomatic prominent hardware. In the elderly patient, the prolonged rehabilitation, propensity for stiffness, and increased reoperation rate associated with ORIF may convert a previously independent individual into a role of dependence.[190]

Primary total elbow arthroplasty (TEA) has evolved to become a viable treatment option for elderly patients with articular fragmentation, comminution, and osteopenia.[11,57,59,60,98,99,112,132,134,145] Most recently, there has been a renewed interest in distal humerus hemiarthroplasty for the treatment of distal humerus fractures,[2,3,14,28,83,166] including fractures of the capitellum and trochlea.

Partial articular fractures of the distal humerus are a distinct group of fractures that are different than distal humerus fractures. These fractures typically involve the capitellum and/or trochlea with variable involvement of other periarticular structures such as the epicondyles, the radial head, the medial collateral ligament (MCL), or the lateral collateral ligament (LCL) complex. These injuries are distal and do not extend proximal to the olecranon fossa to involve either column. Isolated fractures of the capitellum are rare[43,190,222] and isolated fractures of the trochlea are even more rare.[43,55]

Epidemiology of Distal Humerus Fractures
Extra-Articular and Complete Articular Fractures
Approximately 7% of all adult fractures involve the elbow; of these, approximately one-third involve the distal humerus.[8,162,191] Distal humerus fractures, therefore, comprise approximately 2% of all fractures. They have a bimodal age distribution,[162,163,189,190] with peak incidences occurring between the ages of 12 and 19 years, usually in males, and those aged 80 years and older, characteristically in females (Fig. 35-1). In young adults, the fractures are typically caused by high-energy injures, such as motor vehicular collisions, falls from height, sports, industrial accidents, and firearms. In contrast, greater than 60% of distal humerus fractures in the elderly occur from low-energy injuries, such as a fall from a standing height.[163,189]

Robinson et al.[189] reviewed a consecutive series of 320 patients with distal humerus fractures over a 10-year period. They calculated an overall incidence in adults of 5.7 cases per 100,000 in the population per year with a nearly equivalent male-to-female ratio. The most common mechanism of injury was a simple fall from a standing height (Table 35-1) and the most common fracture pattern was an extra-articular fracture accounting for just under 40% of all fractures. Bicolumn or complete intra-articular fractures were the second most common, accounting for 37%.

The overall incidence of distal humerus fractures is increasing, mimicking the increasing incidence in hip, proximal humerus, and wrist fractures.[90,100,101] Palvanen et al.[162] studied trends in

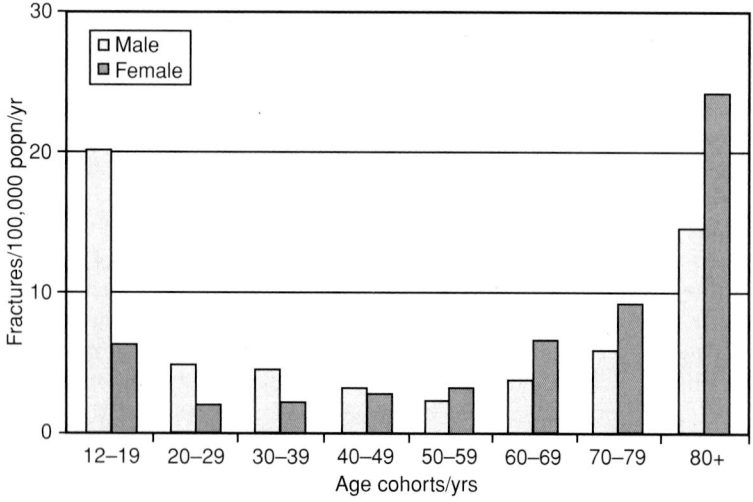

FIGURE 35-1 The age- and gender-related incidence of distal humerus fractures. (Data from Robinson CM, Hill RM, Jacobs N, et al. Adult distal humeral metaphyseal fractures: epidemiology and results of treatment. *J Orthop Trauma.* 2003;17(1):38–47.)

TABLE 35-1	**Mechanism of Injury in 320 Distal Humeral Fractures**				
Mechanism of Injury	Number of Fractures (*Number Open*)	Average Age in Yrs (Range)	Males	Females	M:F Ratio
Simple fall	219 (*12*)	57 (12–99)	86	133	0.6:1
Fall from a height	5 (*2*)	27 (14–41)	3	2	1.5:1
RTA	42 (*7*)	33.2 (14–77)	27	15	1.8:1
Sport	41 (*2*)	22.9 (13–44)	34	7	4.9:1
Other	13 (*0*)	39.2 (14–92)	9	4	2.3:1
Total	320 (*23*)	48.4 (12–99)	159	161	1:1

RTA, road traffic accident.

Data from Robinson CM, Hill RM, Jacobs N, et al. Adult distal humeral metaphyseal fractures: epidemiology and results of treatment. *J Orthop Trauma.* 2003;17(1):38–47.

osteoporotic distal humerus fractures in Finnish women. They reported a two-fold increase in the age-adjusted incidence of distal humerus fractures from 1970 (12/100,000) to 1995 (28/100,000), and predicted an additional three-fold increase by 2030. An aging population with increasing life expectancy combined with the fact that most of these fractures require surgical treatment is likely to result in increased health care expenditures. The identification and implementation of preventative strategies may help offset some of the economic impact of this injury. The mainstay of current fracture prevention strategy is to screen for osteopenia and osteoporosis with bone mineral density measurements and then to treat with medication therapy.[90] Other authors argue that a more important prevention strategy is to decrease the risk of falling. Falling is the greatest single risk factor for fracture[100,101] and can be predicted based on clinical risk factors, such as age, weight, smoking, previous fracture, and mother's hip fracture.[21]

Partial Articular Fractures

The reported annual incidence of partial articular fractures of the distal humerus is 1.5 per 100,000 population with a marked female predominance.[222]

ASSESSMENT OF DISTAL HUMERUS FRACTURES

Mechanisms of Injury and Associated Injuries with Distal Humerus Fractures

Extra-Articular and Complete Articular Fractures

The majority of distal humerus fractures occur in one of two ways, low energy falls or high energy trauma.[189] The most common cause is a simple fall in the forward direction.[163] In general, 70% of patients that sustain an elbow fracture fall directly on to the elbow because they are unable to break their fall with an outstretched arm.[163] High-energy injuries are the cause of most distal humerus fractures in younger adults. Motor vehicle collisions, sports, falls from height, and industrial accidents predominate. These mechanisms are also associated with a higher likelihood of accompanying injuries such as open frac-

tures, soft tissue injuries, other fractures in 16% of cases,[53] and polytrauma (Table 35-2).

Partial Articular Fractures

Fractures of the capitellum and trochlea are typically caused by coronal shear forces. The capitellum is thought to be particularly susceptible to shear forces because its centre of rotation is more anterior in reference to the humeral shaft. The most common mechanism of injury is a simple fall on the outstretched hand from a standing height. In women, there is a bimodal distribution with peaks under the age of 19 and above 80 years. The increased prevalence of this injury in women over the age of 60 years is believed to be because of the increased elbow-carrying angle in women and osteoporosis.[65,222] In men there is a unimodal distribution with a peak incidence under the age of 19 with the mechanism of injury typically being high energy,

TABLE 35-2	**The Relationship between Injury Mechanism and Soft Tissue Injury**						
—	—	—	Gustilo Grade				
Mechanism of Injury	Closed	Open (%)	I	II	IIIa	IIIb
Simple fall	207	12 (5%)	4	4	4	0
Fall from height	3	2 (40%)	0	0	2	0
MVC	35	7 (17%)	2	4	0	1
Sport	39	2 (5%)	0	2	0	0
Other	13	0	0	0	0	0
Total	**297**	**23 (7%)**	**6**	**10**	**6**	**1**

MVC, motor vehicle collision.

Data from Robinson CM, Hill RM, Jacobs N, et al. Adult distal humeral metaphyseal fractures: epidemiology and results of treatment. *J Orthop Trauma.* 2003;17(1):38–47.

such as motor vehicle collisions or falls from height. Other associated injuries, such as ligament tears and radial head fractures, occur in up to 20% of cases.[43,181,190,221,222]

Signs and Symptoms of Distal Humerus Fractures

The history should determine the mechanism of injury, the energy level, and the time since injury. In patients with high-energy injuries, vigilance is required in identifying systemic injures and associated fractures. The pain from polytrauma and other concurrent issues such as inebriation and drug uses may make identification of all injuries difficult; patients and their families should be pre-emptively counseled on the possibility of delayed identification of occult injuries.

Elderly patients, who comprise the majority of patients with distal humerus fractures, should be evaluated for the precipitants of the characteristic fall as they may have undiagnosed cardiac arrhythmias, cerebrovascular disease, polypharmacy, or alcohol dependence. Special attention is directed toward identifying comorbidities and reversible illnesses that may impact upon the treatment recommendations and perioperative risk. Mental status, the ability to cooperate with rehabilitation, ambulatory status, and the requirement of walking aides should be assessed. In addition, the preinjury functional abilities, demands, any limitations related to the upper extremities, as well as the patient handedness, each may affect the treatment decision-making.

A thorough physical examination should be conducted in all cases, particularly with high-energy trauma to identify systemic injuries and associated fractures. The injured extremity should be circumferentially examined for abrasions, bruising, swelling, fracture blisters, skin tenting, and open wounds. Open distal humerus fractures are common[133,140,189] and should be treated with a standard open fracture protocol involving removal of gross contamination, covering of the wound with a sterile dressing, splinting, antibiotics, tetanus, possible wound culture, and early surgical irrigation and debridement.

A neurologic examination must be performed and accurately documented preoperatively and postoperatively. Gofton et al.[64] reported that 26% of patients with distal humerus fractures had an associated incomplete ulnar neuropathy at the time of presentation. Vascular injuries, although rare in distal humerus fractures, should be assessed by examining the distal pulses, skin turgor, capillary refill, and color. Pulse diminution or other positive findings should trigger further examined with a brachial–brachial Doppler pressure index, which has been shown to be as specific and sensitive as arteriography in detecting brachial artery injuries.[49,136,188] The normal brachial–brachial Doppler pressure index is approximately 0.95 and it rarely falls below 0.85.[49,136,188] Patients with abnormal studies should be referred for vascular surgery consultation. Patients with excessive pain after high-energy trauma should be examined for compartment syndrome of the forearm. Compartment pressures should be conducted when the clinical examination is inconclusive.[22] If compartment syndrome is diagnosed clinically or by pressure measurement, urgent surgical fasciotomies are required.[135]

Specific to elderly patients, when considering elbow arthroplasty the contraindications must be addressed. Absolute con-

traindications to elbow arthroplasty include active infection and inadequate soft tissue coverage. The patient history requires probing questions to rule out common infections, such as urinary tract infections and active diabetic ulcers. Open wounds in low-energy distal humerus fractures are not an absolute contraindication to elbow arthroplasty, as they are typically small and clean. Such wounds, therefore, may undergo irrigation and debridement followed by staged elbow arthroplasty.

Imaging and Other Diagnostic Studies for Distal Humerus Fractures

Standard anteroposterior and lateral radiographs of the elbow are usually sufficient for diagnosis, classification, and surgical templating. However, initial radiographs obtained in plaster or a splint may obscure the fracture pattern and should be repeated. In some cases where fracture shortening, rotation, and angulation distorts the images, gentle traction views with appropriate analgesia or conscious sedation may improve the yield of the radiographs.

Computed tomography (CT) with three-dimensional reconstructions substantially improves the identification and visualization of fracture patterns.[24] While CT is not required for all cases, it is recommended for certain situations. In patients where a less invasive approach for ORIF is contemplated, such as a paratricipital approach rather than an olecranon osteotomy, a CT scan can assist with decision-making and in identifying the locations of fracture fragments intraoperatively. In elderly patients with highly comminuted fractures, a CT scan may be useful in deciding whether an attempt should be made at ORIF versus proceeding directly to arthroplasty. When considering hemiarthroplasty for distal humerus fractures, a CT scan will confirm the articular fragmentation and the characteristics of the condylar fractures.

Classification of Distal Humerus Fractures
Extra-Articular and Complete Articular Fractures
Early classification schemes for fractures of the distal humerus were based on the anatomic location of the fracture and its

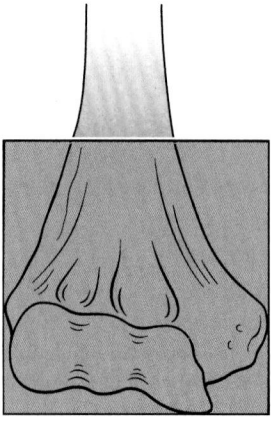

FIGURE 35-2 A distal humerus fracture is defined as a fracture with an epicenter that is located within a square whose base is the distance between the epicondyles on an anteroposterior radiograph.

appearance, using terms such as supracondylar, intracondylar, epicondylar, Y-type, and T-type. In 1990, Muller[150] defined the anatomic boundaries of a distal humerus fracture as one with an epicenter that occurs within a square whose base is the distance between the medial and lateral epicondyles on an anteroposterior radiograph (Fig. 35-2). The AO group devised the first comprehensive classification of distal humerus fractures which was then adopted by the Orthopaedic Trauma Association (OTA) in

1996.[56] In 2007, the AO Classification Supervisory Committee and the OTA Classification, Database and Outcomes Committee updated the compendium to its present form.[123]

The AO/OTA classification is an alphanumeric system that assigns the first two digits of 13 to distal humerus fractures and classifies them based on the location and degree of articular involvement (Fig. 35-3). The system then further subclassifies fractures based on fracture line orientation, displacement

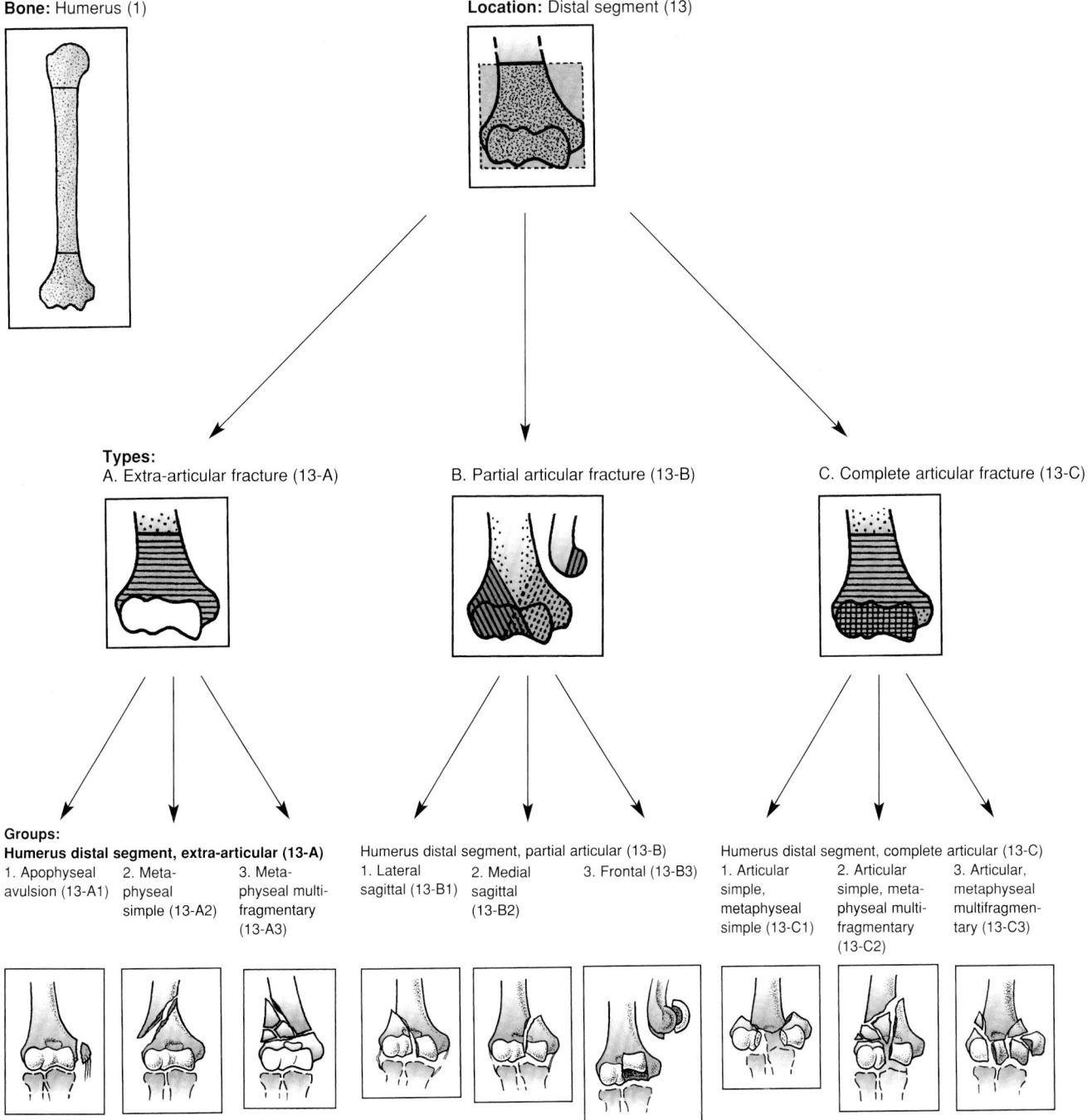

FIGURE 35-3 The AO/OTA classification of distal humerus fractures.[56,150]

(continues)

Subgroups and qualifications:
Humerus, distal, extra-articular apophyseal avulsion (13-A1)

1. Lateral epicondyle (13-A1.1)

2. Medial epicondyle, nonincarcerated (13-A1.2)
(1) nondisplaced
(2) displaced
(3) fragmented

3. Medial epicondyle, incarcerated (13-A1.3)

 A1

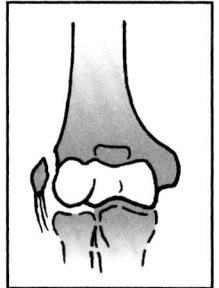

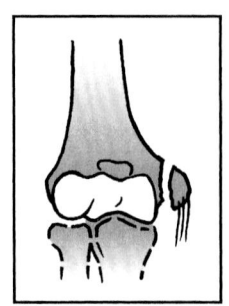

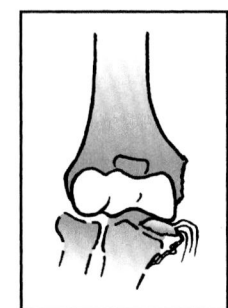

Humerus, distal, extra-articular metaphyseal simple (13-A2)

1. Oblique downward and inward (13-A2.1)

2. Oblique downward and outward (13-A2.2)

3. Transverse (13-A2.3)
(1) transmetaphyseal

(2) juxtaepiphyseal with posterior displacement (Kocher I)

(3) juxtaepiphyseal with anterior displacement (Kocher II)

A2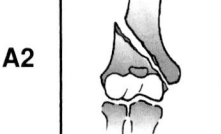

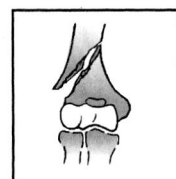

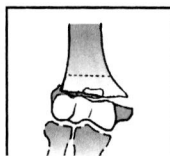

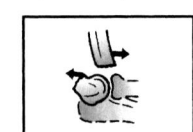

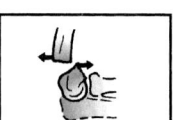

Humerus, distal, extra-articular metaphyseal multifragmentary (13-A3)

1. With intact wedge (13-A3.1)
(1) lateral
(2) medial

2. With fragmented wedge (13-A3.2)
(1) lateral
(2) medial

3. Complex (13-A3.3)

 A3

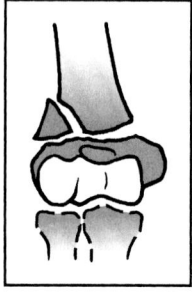

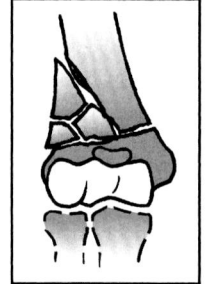
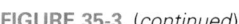

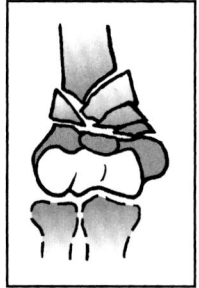

FIGURE 35-3 (continued)

direction, and degree of fragmentation.[123] Type A fractures are extra-articular and may involve the epicondyles or occur at the distal humerus metaphyseal level. Although these fractures receive less attention in the literature than the more complex intra-articular type C fractures, they do account for one-quarter of all distal humerus fractures.[189]

Type B fractures are termed partial articular as there remains some continuity between the humeral shaft and the articular segment. Type B fractures include unicondylar fractures and sagittal plane or shear fractures of the articular surface involving the capitellum, trochlea, or both. Single column fractures involve either the medial or lateral column, are intra-articular, and account for approximately 15% of all distal humerus fractures.[95,107,189] These fractures may also be classified by the Milch system,[139] which is based on whether the lateral portion of the trochlea remains attached to the humeral shaft. In a Milch type I

Humerus, distal, partial articular, lateral sagittal (13-B1)

1. Capitellum (13-B1.1)
(1) through the capitellum (Milch I)
(2) between capitellum and trochlea

2. Transtrochlear simple (13-B1.2)
(1) medial collateral ligament intact
(2) medial collateral ligament ruptured
(3) metaphyseal simple (classic Milch II) lateral condyle
(4) metaphyseal wedge
(5) metaphysio-diaphyseal

3. Transtrochlear multifragmentary (13-B1.3)
(1) epiphysio-metaphyseal
(2) epiphysio-metaphysio-diaphyseal

B1

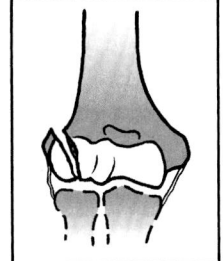 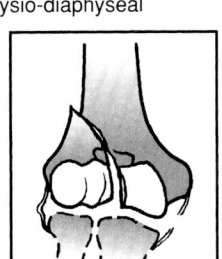 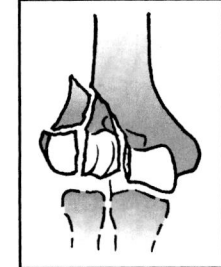

Humerus, distal, partial articular, medial sagittal (13-B2)

1. Transtrochlear simple, through medial side (Milch I) (13-B2.1)

2. Transtrochlear simple, through the groove (13-B2.2)

3. Transtrochlear multifragmentary (13-B2.3)
(1) epiphysio-metaphyseal
(2) epiphysio-metaphysio-diaphyseal

B2

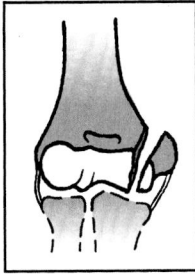 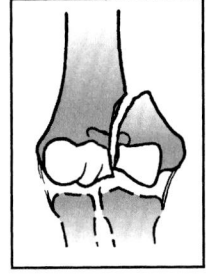 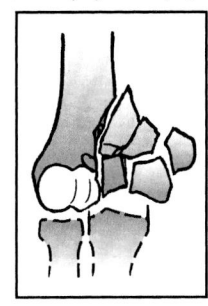

Humerus, distal, partial articular, frontal (13-B3)

1. Capitellum (13-B3.1)
(1) incomplete (Kocher-Lorenz)
(2) complete (Hahn-Steinthal 1)
(3) with trochlear component (Hahn-Steinthal 2)
(4) fragmented

2. Trochlea (13-B3.2)
(1) simple
(2) fragmented

3. Capitellum and trochlea (13-B3.3)

B3

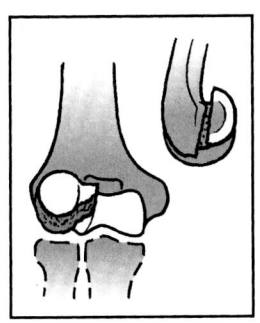 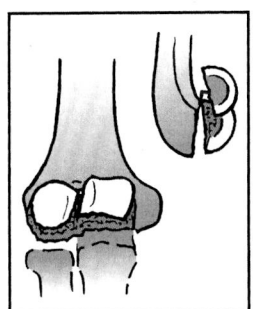

FIGURE 35-3 (continued)

(continues)

Humerus, distal complete, articular simple, metaphyseal simple (13-C1)

1. With slight displacement (13-C1.1)
(1) Y-shaped
(2) T-shaped
(3) V-shaped

2. With marked displacement (13-C1.2)
(1) Y-shaped
(2) T-shaped
(3) V-shaped

3. T-shaped epiphyseal (13-C1.3)

 C1

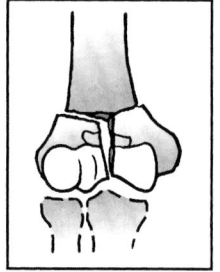 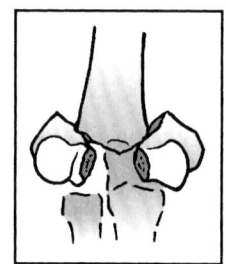 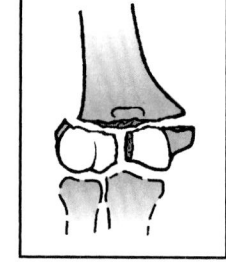

Humerus, distal, complete articular simple metaphyseal multifragmentary (13-C2)

1. With intact wedge (13-C2.1)
(1) metaphyseal lateral
(2) metaphyseal medial
(3) metaphysio-diaphyseal lateral
(4) metaphysio-diaphyseal medial

2. With a fragmented wedge (13-C2.2)
(1) metaphyseal lateral
(2) metaphyseal medial
(3) metaphysio-diaphyseal lateral
(4) metaphysio-diaphyseal medial

3. Complex (13-C2.3)

 C2

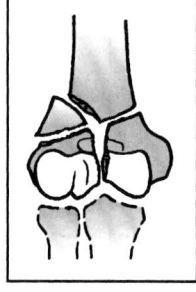 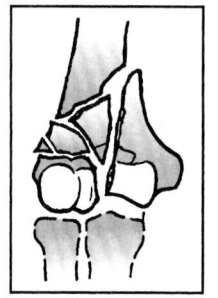 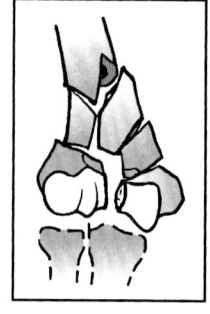

Humerus, distal, complete multifragmentary (13-C3)

1. Metaphyseal simple (13-C3.1)

2. Metaphyseal wedge (13-C3.2)
(1) intact
(2) fragmented

3. Metaphyseal complex (13-C3.3)
(1) localized
(2) extending into diaphysis

C3

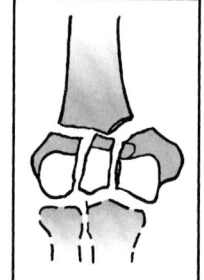 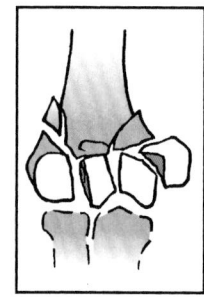 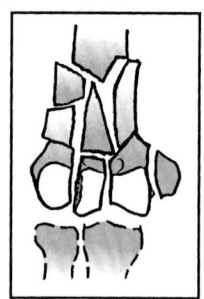

FIGURE 35-3 (*continued*)

fracture, the medial or lateral column can be fractured but the lateral eminence of the trochlea remains attached to the humeral shaft. In a Milch type II fracture, the lateral eminence of the trochlea is apart of the column fracture.

A "divergent" single column fracture has also been described which occurs predominantly in younger patients that are predisposed to this injury because of a septal aperture (fenestration) in the olecranon fossa.[63,107] This fracture pattern is theorized to occur after an axial load is applied to the olecranon, which is then driven into the trochlea. A fracture occurs that splits the trochlea and propagates proximally between the columns to eventually exit either medially or laterally creating a "high" single column fracture.

Type C fractures are termed complete articular, meaning there is no continuity between the articular segments and the humeral shaft. Type C fractures have historically been called

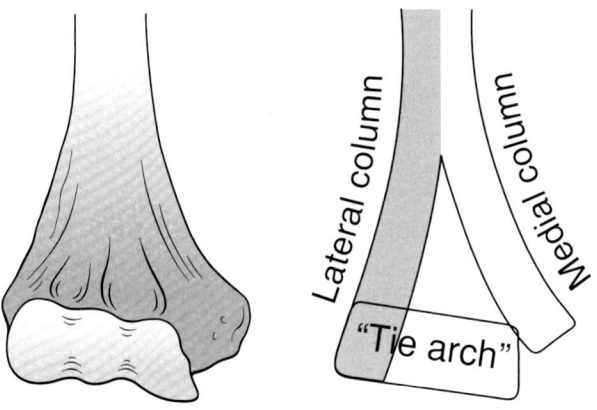

FIGURE 35-4 The medial and lateral columns support the articular segment. The distalmost part of the lateral column is the capitellum and the distalmost part of the medial column is the nonarticular medial epicondyle. The trochlea is the medial part of the articular segment and is intermediate in position between the capitellum and the medial epicondyle. The articular segment functions architecturally as a tie arch.

intracondylar fractures and the AO/OTA system further subclassifies them into simple (C1), simple articular with metaphyseal fragmentation (C2), and fragmentation of the articular surface and metaphyseal zone (C3). This system is widely used in the literature and trauma databases, and helps to standardize research protocols and treatment outcomes. Unfortunately, the classification system does have weaknesses as it does not account for factors such as the distal fragment height and amount of displacement, both of which may influence treatment.[77,183] The classification also does little to assist with the decision-making process between ORIF and arthroplasty and finally it has been criticized as being overly complex.

The Mehne and Matta classification of distal humerus fractures is also popular.[39,93] It is based on Jupiter's model[93] in which the distal humerus is composed of two divergent columns that support an intercalary articular segment (Fig. 35-4), which is similar to the AO concept of condyles. The classification has three main categories: Intra-articular, extra-articular intracapsular, and extracapsular. The intra-articular group is further subdivided in to bicolumn, single column, and articular fractures. The extra-articular intracapsular group consists of high and low transcolumn fractures, and the extracapsular group has medial and lateral epicondyle fractures (Fig. 35-5). This classification system has the same criticisms as the AO/OTA system with high complexity and moderate intra- and inter-rater reliability.[93] The classification also does not consider the specific types of articular fracture and the degree of fragment displacement. It is the author's opinion that the AO/OTA classification is preferred because it is more intuitive, it is ubiquitous, and because it is the official classification of the OTA.

Partial Articular Fractures (B3)

In 1853, Hahn[71] described an isolated capitellar fracture, which now bears his name along with Steinthal's,[209] who described the injury in 1898. The Hahn-Steinthal or conventional type I

fracture[27] involves the capitellar articular surface along with the subchondral bone (Fig. 35-6). The Kocher-Lorenz[104,117] or conventional type II fracture[27] is rare and consists of the capitellar articular surface along with a thin shell of subchondral bone. Bryan and Morrey[27] modified this classification and added type III fractures which are comminuted capitellar fractures. A fourth fracture pattern was added by McKee et al.,[126] which consisted of a type I fracture with medial extension to include the lateral half of the trochlea.

The AO/OTA comprehensive classification of fractures[123] classifies articular distal humerus fractures as type B3 (Fig. 35-3). Type B3 fractures are then further subclassified into capitellar, trochlear, and combined fractures.

Ring et al.[181] further examined articular shear fractures of the distal humerus and described them as a spectrum of injury. They observed that apparent isolated capitellar fractures on plain radiographs may turn out to be much more complex injuries when further imaged with CT. The authors identified five unique fracture patterns that progress in complexity (Fig. 35-7).

Dubberley et al.[43] recently reported another classification for capitellar and trochlear fractures, which was correlated to clinical outcome. The Dubberley et al.[43] classification has three types with a modifier for distal posterolateral column comminution. A type I fracture involves primarily the capitellum with or without the lateral trochlear ridge. A type II fracture involves the capitellum and most of the trochlea as one piece, while in the type III fracture the capitellum and trochlea are separate pieces. The authors found that as the complexity of the articular fractures increased, the outcomes worsened.

Outcome Measures for Distal Humerus Fractures

The outcome measurement tools for distal humerus fractures include scoring systems, range of motion, strength, rate of secondary surgeries, and complications.[119] Elbow-specific scoring systems that are typically used are the Mayo Elbow Performance Score (MEPS) and the Patient-Rated Elbow Evaluation (PREE). Rarely, the American Shoulder and Elbow Surgeons Elbow Form (ASES-e) is utilized, which has a section for patient responses and a section for physician's assessment of elbow function. The Disabilities of the Arm, Shoulder and Hand (DASH) score is frequently used and provides a global rating of upper extremity function. The outcome data related to the various treatment options for distal humerus fractures will be presented in the technique-specific sections below.

PATHOANATOMY AND APPLIED ANATOMY RELATING TO DISTAL HUMERUS FRACTURES

The elbow is anatomically a trocho-ginglymoid joint, meaning that it has trochoid (rotatory) motion through the radiocapitellar and proximal radioulnar joints and ginglymoid (hinge-like) motion through the ulnohumeral joint. An understanding of the complex bony anatomy of the elbow, the soft tissue stabilizers, and the adjacent neurovascular structures is imperative when surgically treating distal humerus fractures.

I. Intra-articular fractures
A. Single column

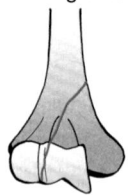 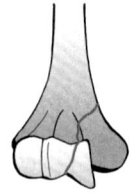 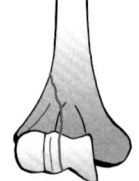 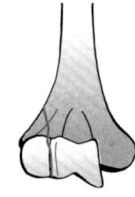 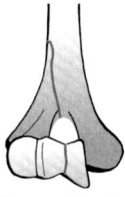

High medial column fracture (Milch type II) | Low medial column fracture (Milch type I) | High lateral column fracture (Milch type II) | Low lateral column fracture (Milch type I) | Divergent single column fracture

B. Bicolumn

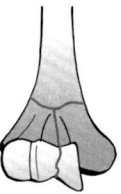 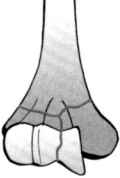 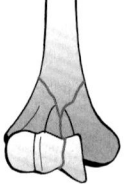 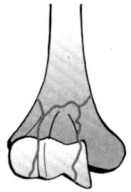 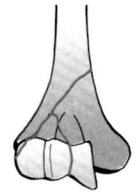 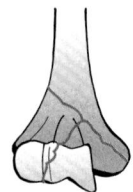

Bicolumn high T-fracture | Bicolumn low T-fracture | Bicolumn Y-fracture | Bicolumn H-fracture | Bicolumn medial lambda fracture | Bicolumn lateral lambda fracture

C. Articular surface fractures (capitellum, trochlea, or both)

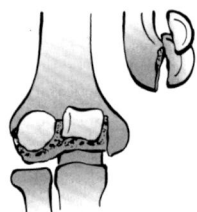

II. Extra-articular intracapsular fractures

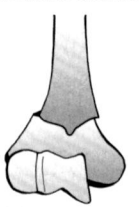 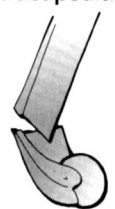 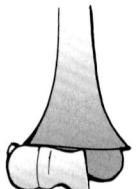 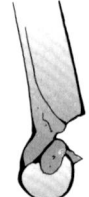 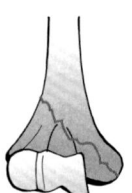 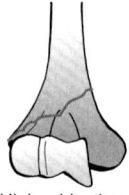

High flexion transcolumn fracture (anteroposterior view) | High flexion transcolumn fracture (lateral view) | Low extension transcolumn fracture (anteroposterior view) | Low extension transcolumn fracture (lateral view) | High abduction fracture | High adduction fracture

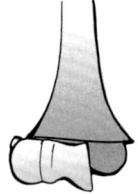 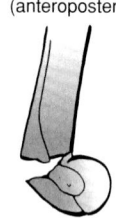 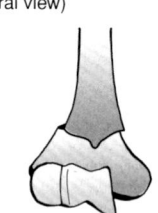 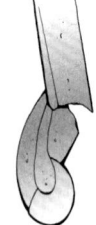

Low flexion transcolumn fracture (anteroposterior view) | Low flexion transcolumn fracture (lateral view) | High extension transcolumn fracture (anteroposterior view) | High extension transcolumn fracture (lateral view)

III. Extracapsular fractures

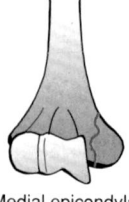 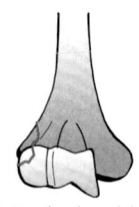

Medial epicondylar fracture | Lateral epicondylar fracture

FIGURE 35-5 The Mehne and Matta classification of distal humerus fractures.[93]

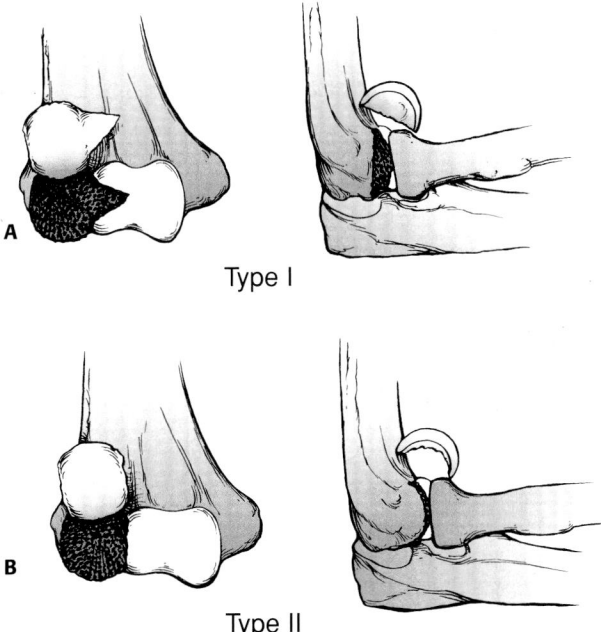

Type I

Type II

FIGURE 35-6 The Hahn-Steinthal (type I) fracture of the capitellum involves the articular surface and a large portion of the subchondral bone **(A).** The Kocher-Lorenz (type II) fracture involves the articular surface of the capitellum with a thin layer of subchondral bone **(B).**[71,209]

The distal humeral shaft is triangular-shaped in cross section with its apex directed anteriorly. As the shaft approaches the distal humerus it bifurcates into two divergent cortical columns, termed the medial and lateral columns. The medial column diverges approximately 45 degrees from the humeral shaft in

the coronal plane and terminates as the medial epicondyle. The lateral column, in the coronal plane, diverges at approximately 20 degrees from the shaft. As the lateral column extends distally it curves anteriorly creating a 35- to 40-degree angle with the shaft in the sagittal plane (Fig. 35-8). In the coronal plane, the trochlea is more distal than the capitellum resulting in a valgus alignment of 4 to 8 degrees. Overall, when including the ulna, the elbow has a valgus angle in extension of 10 to 17 degrees, termed the carrying angle. Axially, the distal humerus articular surface is internally rotated 3 to 8 degrees; therefore, as the elbow flexes it also internally rotates resulting in slight varus alignment.

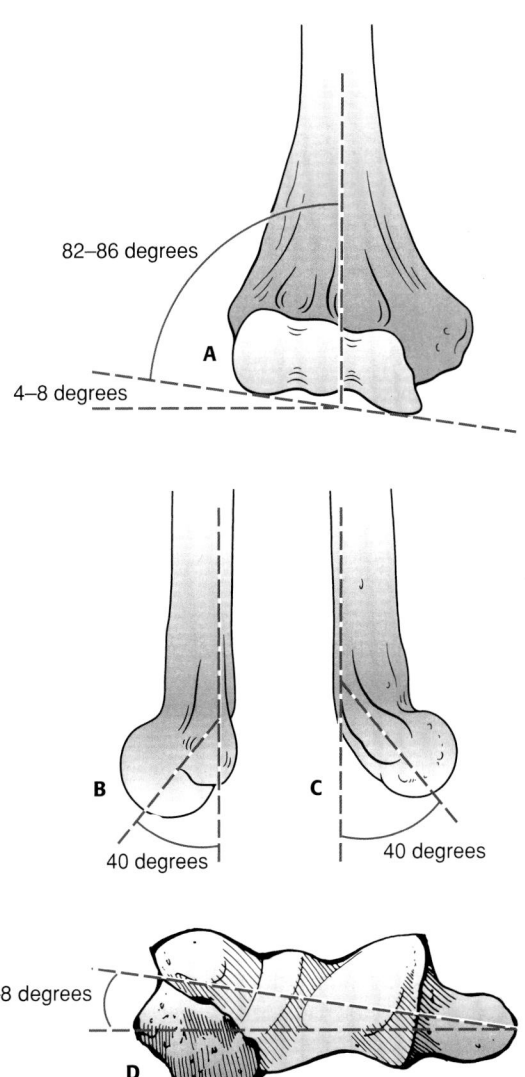

FIGURE 35-8 The distal humerus articular surface is aligned in 4 to 8 degrees of valgus relative to the shaft **(A)** and is angulated 35 to 40 degrees anteriorly in the sagittal plane. The medial epicondyle is the termination of the medial column and remains on the axis of the shaft in the sagittal view **(B),** while the lateral epicondyle follows the capitellum into flexion **(C).** Axially, the entire distal humerus articular surface is internally rotated 3 to 8 degrees **(D).**

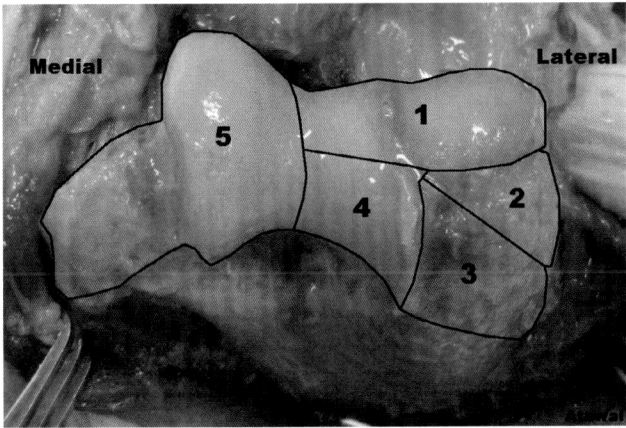

FIGURE 35-7 The Ring et al.[181] classification of distal humerus articular fractures has five patterns. A type I fracture involves the capitellum and the lateral portion of the trochlea. This fracture pattern has previously been described as a conventional type IV fracture. A type II fracture is described as a type I fracture that may be comminuted but includes a fracture of the lateral epicondyle. A type III fracture is a type II fracture that has comminution behind the capitellum with impaction of bone posteriorly. A type IV fracture is a type III fracture with an additional fracture of the posterior trochlea. A type V fracture is a type IV fracture that includes fracture of the medial epicondyle.

The posterior aspect of the lateral column is relatively flat and wide, well suited for application of a posterolateral plate. The lateral column terminates in the capitellum anteriorly. The articular surface of the capitellum starts at the most distal aspect of the lateral column and encompasses an arc of approximately 180 degrees in the sagittal plane. Posterior fixation can be applied distally on the lateral column because of the absence of cartilage; however, lengths of screws directed anteriorly into the capitellum must be carefully scrutinized to prevent perforation into the radiocapitellar joint.

The trochlea, which is Greek for pulley, is the intervening segment of bone between the terminal ends of the medial and lateral columns that articulates with the greater sigmoid notch of the ulna. It is covered by articular cartilage anteriorly, inferiorly, and posteriorly, creating an arc of almost 270 degrees. The trochlea is shaped like a spool with a central sulcus which articulates with the central ridge of the greater sigmoid notch of the proximal ulna.

Superior to the trochlea and between the medial and lateral columns lies the olecranon fossa posteriorly and the coronoid fossa anteriorly. These fossae lie adjacent to each other and are separated by a thin bony septum. Occasionally, this septum is absent and a septal aperture exists. The olecranon fossa is matched to the olecranon and accepts it during extension; similarly, the coronoid fossa is matched to the coronoid and accepts it during flexion. The tolerances of the fossae to accommodate their respective bony processes are narrow; therefore, screw placement through the fossae should be avoided as it may lead to impingement and decreased elbow range of motion. In distal humerus fractures with excessive metaphyseal comminution requiring supracondylar shortening, recreation of the fossae with a burr will improve range of motion.

In addition to the bony structures, there are several important soft tissue structures that require consideration when treating distal humerus fractures. The LCL complex consists of the radial collateral ligament, the lateral ulnar collateral ligament (LUCL), and the annular ligament. The annular ligament attaches to the anterior and posterior margins of the lesser sigmoid notch while the radial collateral ligament originates from an isometric point on the lateral epicondyle and fans out to attach to the annular ligament (Fig. 35-9). The LUCL also arises from the isometric point on the lateral epicondyle and attaches to the crista supinatoris of the proximal ulna. The LCL complex functions as an important restraint to varus and posterolateral rotatory instability.[45,88] The LCL complex is vulnerable to injury during application of a direct lateral plate; therefore, exposure of the lateral aspect of the distal lateral column should not extend past the equator of the capitellum.

The MCL consists of an anterior bundle, posterior bundle, and transverse ligament. The anterior bundle is of prime importance in elbow stability (Fig. 35-10). It originates from the anteroinferior aspect of the medial epicondyle, inferior to the axis of rotation, and inserts on the sublime tubercle of the coronoid. The MCL functions as an important restraint to valgus and posteromedial rotatory instability.[10,151] It is susceptible to injury at its origin during placement of a medial plate that curves around the medial epicondyle to lie on the ulnar aspect of the trochlea.

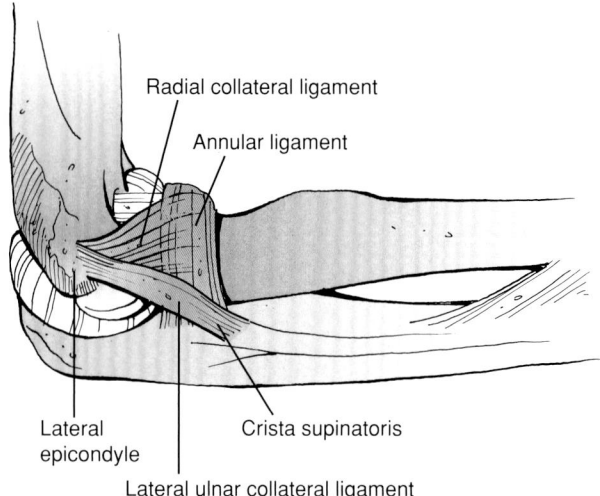

FIGURE 35-9 The lateral collateral ligament complex is an important restraint to varus and posterolateral rotatory instability and consists of the radial collateral ligament, the lateral ulnar collateral ligament, and the annular ligament. The annular ligament attaches to the anterior and posterior margins of the lesser sigmoid notch while the radial collateral ligament originates from an isometric point on the lateral epicondyle and fans out to attach to the annular ligament. The lateral ulnar collateral ligament also arises from the isometric point on the lateral epicondyle and attaches to the crista supinatoris of the proximal ulna.

The ulnar, radial, and median nerves cross the elbow and knowledge of their precise locations is required to safely manage distal humerus fractures (Fig. 35-11). The ulnar nerve pierces the medial intermuscular septum in the middle third of the arm to travel alongside the medial head of triceps. The arcade of Struthers, a musculofascial band present in 70% of the population,[206] is a potential area of nerve compression located approximately 8 cm proximal to the medial epicondyle. As the nerve approaches the

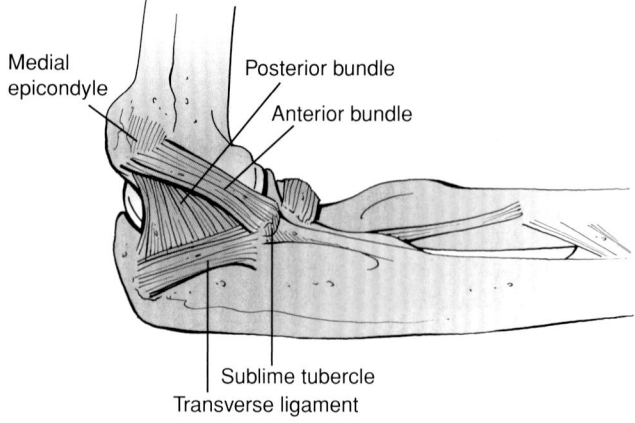

FIGURE 35-10 The medial collateral ligament functions as an important restraint to valgus and posteromedial rotatory instability. It consists of an anterior bundle, posterior bundle, and transverse ligament. The anterior bundle is of prime importance in elbow stability and it originates from the anteroinferior aspect of the medial epicondyle, and inserts on the sublime tubercle of the coronoid.

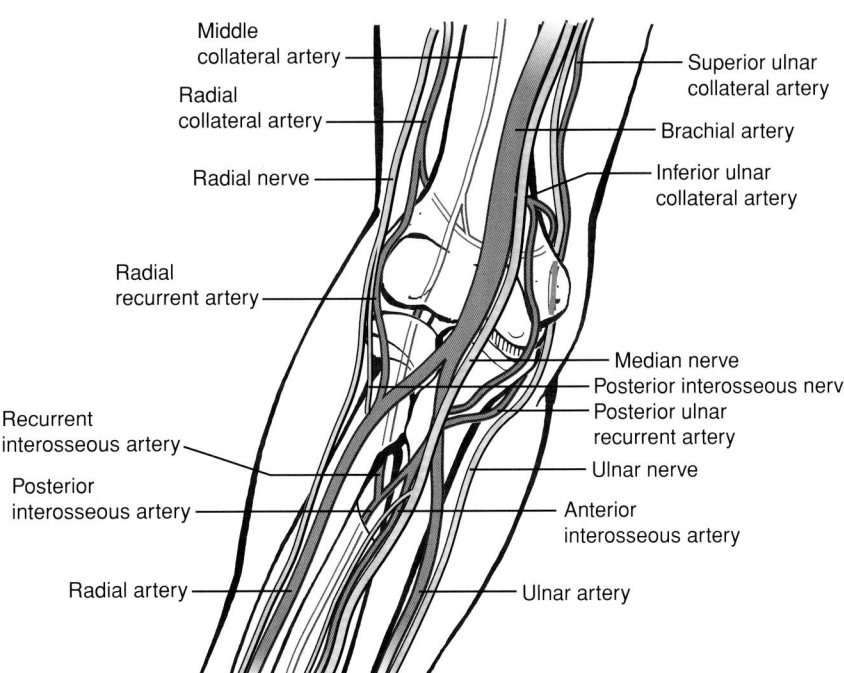

FIGURE 35-11 Three peripheral nerves, the median, ulnar, and radial, cross the elbow joint along with a robust collateral blood supply.

elbow it travels behind the medial epicondyle to enter the cubital tunnel, a fibro-osseous groove bordered by the medial epicondyle superiorly, olecranon laterally, and Osborne's ligament medially. When the nerve exits the cubital tunnel it travels between the two heads of the flexor carpi ulnaris (FCU) muscle.

The radial nerve circles around the posterior aspect of the midhumeral shaft in the spiral groove. On average, the nerve enters the spiral groove 20 cm proximal to the medial epicondyle (74% of the length of the humerus) and exits approximately 14 cm proximal to the lateral epicondyle (51% of the length of the humerus).[62] Along the lateral aspect of the humerus, two branches come off the nerve (nerve to the medial head of triceps and anconeus, and the lateral brachial cutaneous nerve) before it pierces the lateral intermuscular septum approximately 10 cm (36% of the length of the humerus) proximal to the lateral epicondyle.[62] The nerve then lies between brachialis and brachioradialis where it bifurcates into the posterior interosseous nerve and the radial sensory nerve. The radial nerve is vulnerable to injury during exposure of distal humerus fractures with proximal shaft extension and during application of long posterolateral or direct lateral plates.

The median nerve travels with the brachial artery between the biceps and brachialis muscles in the anteromedial aspect of the arm. The nerve passes under the bicipital aponeurosis to enter the medial antecubital fossa, medial to the biceps tendon and brachial artery. The nerve then passes between the heads of pronator teres. During fixation of distal humerus fractures, the median nerve is relatively protected from direct injury by the robust brachialis muscle.

There is a consistent blood supply to the adult elbow which can be organized into three vascular arcades: Medial, lateral, and posterior.[228] The lateral arcade is formed by the interosseous recurrent, radial recurrent, and radial collateral arteries

and supplies the capitellum, radial head, lateral epicondyle, and lateral aspect of the trochlea. The medial arcade is formed by the superior and inferior ulnar collaterals and the anterior and posterior ulnar recurrent arteries and supplies the medial epicondyle and the medial aspect of the trochlea. The posterior arcade is formed by the medial collateral artery and contributions from the medial and lateral arcades and supplies the olecranon fossa and supracondylar area.

DISTAL HUMERUS FRACTURE TREATMENT OPTIONS

Nonoperative Treatment of Distal Humerus Fractures (Extra-Articular and Complete Articular Fractures)

Indications/Contraindications for Nonoperative Treatment

Nonoperative management of distal humerus fractures in young patients is rarely recommended and it is generally reserved for patients deemed medically unfit to undergo surgery (Fig. 35-12). Patients with nondisplaced fractures may also be managed with a trial of nonoperative management. These patients should be followed for the first 3 to 4 weeks with weekly serial radiographs to ensure displacement or angulation does not occur. Surgical fixation of these fractures, however, enhances stability, allows immediate motion, and obviously decreases the risk of delayed fracture displacement. Other circumstances are elderly patients with unrepairable distal humerus fractures where arthroplasty is the most reasonable option; however, it is contraindicated because of soft tissue compromise, such as skin loss. Once the soft tissue issues have been dealt with, delayed arthroplasty can be done if patients are sufficiently symptomatic.

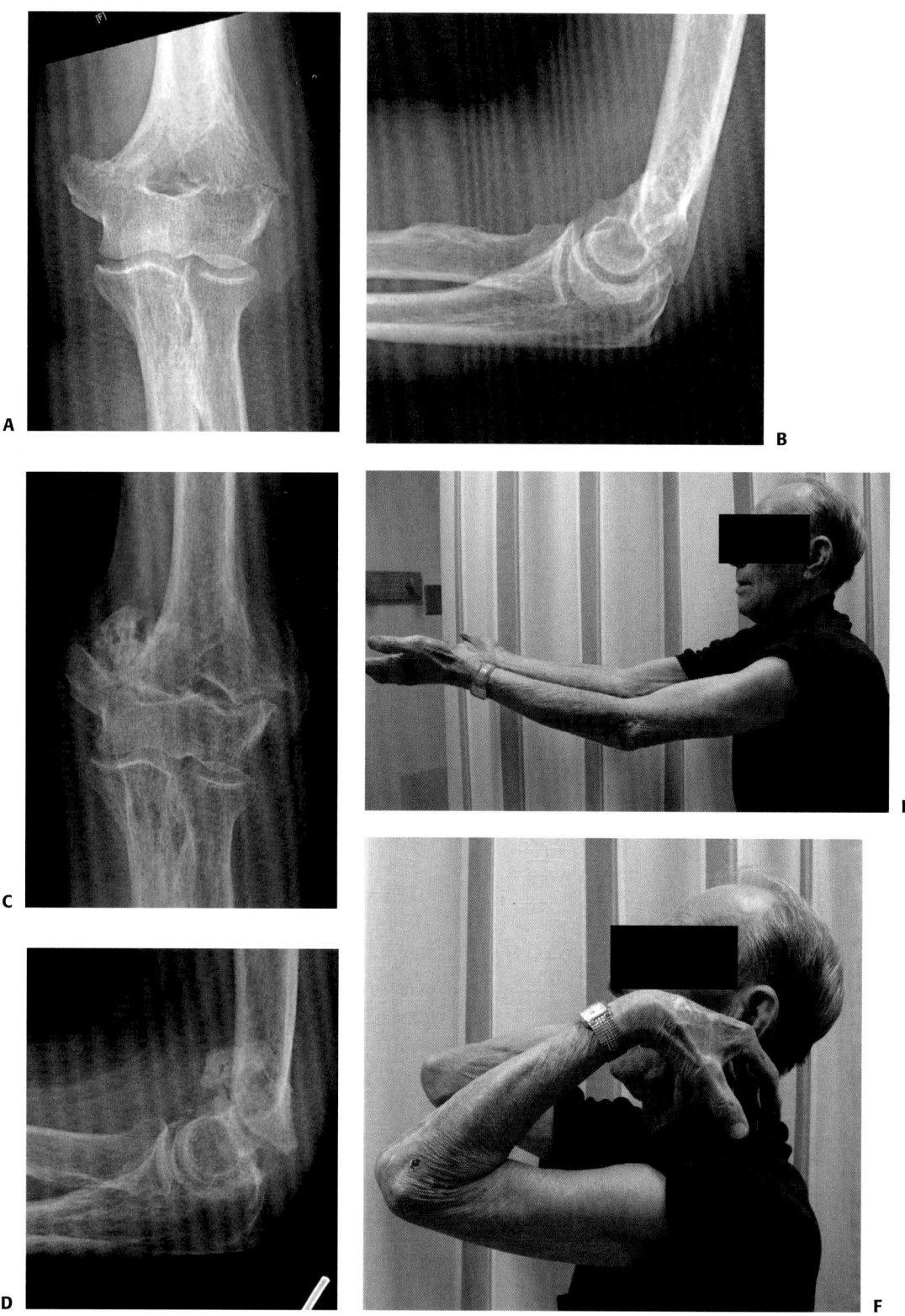

FIGURE 35-12 Radiographs of an 88-year-old man with a transcolumn fracture (AO/OTA A2) deemed medically unfit for surgery because of severe congestive heart failure and inoperable coronary artery disease **(A, B)**. The patient was treated with a collar and cuff and early range of motion. Radiographs at 1-year follow-up **(C, D)**. The patient has no pain with a functional range of motion **(E, F)**.

Techniques

Nonoperative management techniques include above-elbow casting, olecranon traction, and collar and cuff treatment, the so called "bag of bones" method. The traction method involves the placement of a transolecranon traction pin that is attached to weights through a pulley system.[103] Traction is applied for 3 to 4 weeks, until there is sufficient early callous to allow cast bracing. The major disadvantages of this method are the complications associated with prolonged bed rest. Patients who are typically treated nonoperatively, the frail elderly, have significant medical comorbidities that put them at high risk of bed rest-related complications, such as deep venous thrombosis, pulmonary embolism, and decubitus ulcers. The technique is largely of historical significance and has little use in modern distal humerus fracture care.

Collar and cuff treatment had been used for centuries before it was first reported in modern medical literature in 1937 by Eastwood.[46] He described a closed reduction followed by application of a collar and cuff with the elbow between 90 and 120 degrees of flexion. The elbow is hung freely to allow gravity-assisted reduction via a ligamentotaxis-type effect. Shoulder motion and active elbow flexion are initiated at 2 weeks and progressed.

Outcomes

In 1969, Riseborough and Radin[186] compared operative to nonoperative management in 29 patients with intra-articular distal humerus fractures. They reported better range of motion and less pain with nonoperative management, consisting of skeletal traction or manipulation and casting. The surgically treated group was plagued with early fracture displacement because of hardware failure from nonrigid fixation constructs. Brown and Morgan[25] in 1971 reported their results with nonoperative management of intra-articular distal humerus fractures in 10 patients at a mean follow-up of 2.5 years (range, 9 months to 4 years). At follow-up, the mean flexion was 128 degrees, the mean extension was 30 degrees, and the mean arc of motion was 100 degrees. Seven patients described no symptoms while three complained of elbow aches in cold and damp weather. In the present day, nonoperative management in active patients has been abandoned because of improved surgical techniques that have led to better outcomes.

Nonoperative Treatment of Partial Articular Fractures (B3)

Closed reduction and casting is a described method for the treatment of displaced capitellar fractures.[157,176] The reduction maneuver involves placing the elbow into full extension and forearm supination, which usually results in the capitellum spontaneously reducing. If still displaced, manual pressure over the capitellum and a slight varus force to the elbow may assist with the reduction. If successful, the elbow is flexed so the radial head captures the capitellar fragment and then fluoroscopy is used to confirm the reduction. The elbow is immobilized in an above-elbow plaster for 3 weeks with weekly radiographs to confirm maintenance of the reduction. If this technique is used, the author recommends postoperative CT imaging to confirm an anatomic reduction.

Operative Treatment

Distal humerus fractures are generally complex injuries with associated fragmentation, bony instability, osteopenia, and soft tissue injury. The risk of functional impairment is relatively high when these injuries are managed nonoperatively. Contemporary literature would support improved patient outcomes and lower complication rates when these injuries are managed with surgery. ORIF of these injuries is considered gold standard. However, ORIF may not be attainable in elderly patients with osteopenia, comminution, and articular fragmentation or in patients with pre-existing conditions of the elbow such as rheumatoid arthritis (RA). In such cases where rigid internal fixation cannot be achieved to allow early range of motion, elbow arthroplasty has been shown to be a reliable treatment option with good patient outcomes.

Timing of Surgery

Surgical fixation of distal humerus fractures requires preoperative planning, specialized implants, instruments, and surgical expertise. Medically fit and stabilized patients with noncompromised soft tissues may be best managed with early surgery within 48 to 72 hours.[86] Early surgery may lead to decreased complications such as HO and stiffness. Polytrauma patients who are unstable or those with identified modifiable risk factors should be medically optimized preoperatively. In cases with injured soft tissues, such as excessive swelling, bruising, fracture blisters, or abrasions, delay of surgery may be most appropriate. Generally, patients admitted to the intensive care unit can be managed with a well-padded splint that is checked daily and removed every 2 to 3 days to examine the soft tissues for compromise and pressure points. In some cases, prolonged secondary surgical procedures may be contraindicated for several weeks because of medical issues. In these patients static external fixation may be of benefit to stabilize the extremity for pain control, transfers, hygiene, and wound care. Ideally, external fixator pins should be placed as far away as possible from planned internal fixation implants to decrease the likelihood of infection. Although no literature exists to define a suitable delay, surgery should be conducted within 2 or 3 weeks. Delay beyond this time interval is possible; however, ORIF is made more difficult with increased surgical time, difficult fracture reductions because of partial healing and callous, increased bleeding, and the increased risk of HO.

Open Reduction Internal Fixation of Distal Humerus Fractures (Extra-Articular and Complete Articular Fractures)

Indications/Contraindications. Anatomic reduction and rigid internal fixation is considered the gold standard for most displaced intra-articular distal humerus fractures (AO/OTA types

B and C). Rigid internal fixation allows fracture healing to occur anatomically while permitting early range of motion to maximize functional recovery. The traumatized elbow is particularly prone to stiffness; therefore, early motion is vital, but not at the expense of fracture displacement. In cases where sufficient fracture stability cannot be obtained to allow early motion, anatomic reconstruction of the articular surface and overall elbow alignment take precedence. An anatomically aligned stiff elbow with a healed articular surface can be subsequently managed with contracture release, but a fracture with hardware failure and articular nonunion or fragmentation may be difficult to manage with revision surgery.

Surgical treatment is also recommended for displaced or angulated extra-articular fractures (transcolumn) of the distal humerus (AO/OTA types A2 and A3). Closed reduction and percutaneous Kirschner wire (K-wire) fixation has been described for treatment of these injuries in adults.[92] The technique in adults is similar to the technique used in pediatric supracondylar fractures with crossing K-wires inserted medially and laterally. In adults, this technique may be modified to exchange the K-wires for 3.5- or 4.5-mm cannulated screws. Closed reduction and percutaneous fixation has several disadvantages when used in adults. The fixation is semi-rigid and therefore requires supplementary splinting for up to 6 weeks, which may lead to elbow stiffness. The K-wires are also inadequate for elderly patients with osteopenic bone. In general, the crossing K-wire or cannulated screw technique is not recommended for adult patients with AO/OTA type A2 or A3 fractures.

ORIF is the preferred fixation technique for transcolumn fractures (AO/OTA types A2 and A3). These fractures can be exposed through a paratricipital approach or a limited triceps split. Exposure of the articular surface, as obtained from an olecranon osteotomy, is not required for these extra-articular fractures. Bicolumnar fixation is recommended with orthogonal or parallel plating techniques. When the transcolumn fracture line is just proximal to the articular segment, the pattern can be referred to as a "low" transcolumn fracture. Low transcolumn fractures have limited bone available for distal fixation; therefore, bicolumn plating is necessary with plates applied as distal as possible with as many screws as possible in the distal fragment. Commercially available precontoured plates have extra screw holes distally to allow high-density screw insertion into the distal articular segment. In certain low-transcolumn fractures in the elderly with severe osteopenia or pre-existing arthritis, TEA may be the most appropriate form of treatment. Elbow arthroplasty will be discussed later in this chapter.

The commonly used classification systems do not account for fracture displacement, fracture angulation, or the severity of the soft tissue injury. These factors should be considered when deciding upon surgical management. In general, medically fit patients with distal humerus fractures with displacement or angulation meet the indications for surgical intervention.

Preoperative Planning. The goals in surgical treatment of distal humerus fractures are similar to those used for any periarticular fracture. The objectives are to obtain anatomic restoration of the articular surface and recreation of joint alignment with rigid internal fixation, stable enough to allow early range of motion.

Anteroposterior and lateral radiographs of the elbow out of plaster are usually sufficient to determine the fracture pattern. If the radiographs are difficult to interpret or poorly demonstrate the articular fracture, a CT scan is preferred, with three-dimensional reconstructions, over traction radiographs requiring patient sedation. A CT scan can identify difficult fracture patterns such as coronal fractures of the capitellum or trochlea, "low" fracture types, and segmental articular fractures (for example, a fracture between the medial trochlea and the medial epicondyle, producing a free medial trochlear fragment). Three-dimensional images can also be manipulated to subtract the radius and ulna to allow unobstructed visualization of articular comminution. In elderly patients with comminuted fractures where ORIF may not be possible and elbow arthroplasty is considered, a CT scan may assist with the preoperative decision-making.

While awaiting surgery, patients are placed in a well-padded elbow splint and are encouraged to elevate the arm, ice the elbow, and to maintain hand and finger range of motion. On the day of surgery, the skin and soft tissues are re-examined and the neurologic status is redocumented. Patients generally receive a general anesthetic with an upper extremity regional block for postoperative pain control and therapy. Preoperatively, prophylactic antibiotics are administered intravenously.

Positioning. The patient is positioned supine with a bolster placed under the ipsilateral scapula and the elbow is supported by another bolster made of wrapped sterile sheet on the patient's chest (Fig. 35-13). The surgeon and assistant stand on the side of the injury while the scrub nurse and instruments are on the contralateral side, allowing the nurse to assist with arm positioning as required. A sterile tourniquet is used and the iliac crest is prepped and draped if bone grafting is anticipated. Portable (mini) fluoroscopy is used for all cases and is positioned on the operative side.

In circumstances when there is no surgical assistant available, a commercially available articulated arm positioner is preferred (Fig. 35-13C). The patient can also be positioned in the lateral decubitus fashion on a beanbag with a small axillary bolster. The elbow is then flexed over an elbow arthroscopy positioner and the scrub nurse and instrumentation are positioned on the same side. In the rare circumstance of bilateral fractures, when a second surgical team is available, the patient may be positioned prone with the elbows flexed over a positioner to allow simultaneous surgery.

Surgical Approaches. The principles of internal fixation start with the selection of an appropriate surgical approach. The chosen approach should be accommodating to intraoperative findings, which may alter the surgical procedure. For example, a paratricipital approach may be used to initially access a noncomminuted intra-articular fracture (AO/OTA type C1 or C2); however, if the fracture proves difficult to reduce or if more comminution is present than expected, the approach can be converted to an olecranon osteotomy. Similarly, an olecranon osteotomy should not be the index approach for an elderly

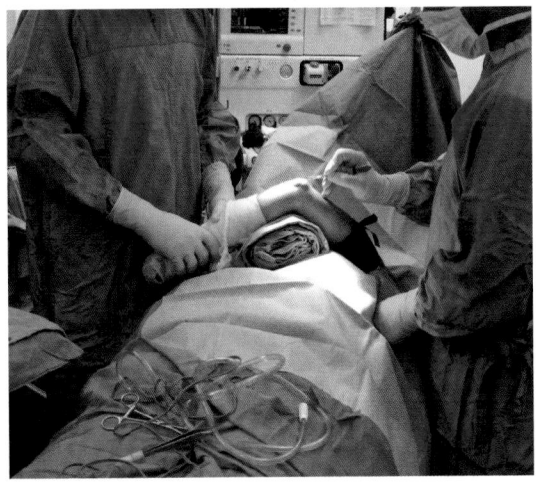

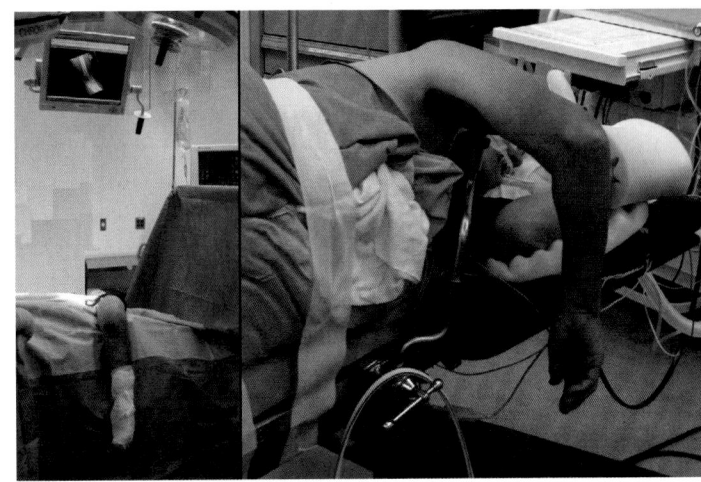

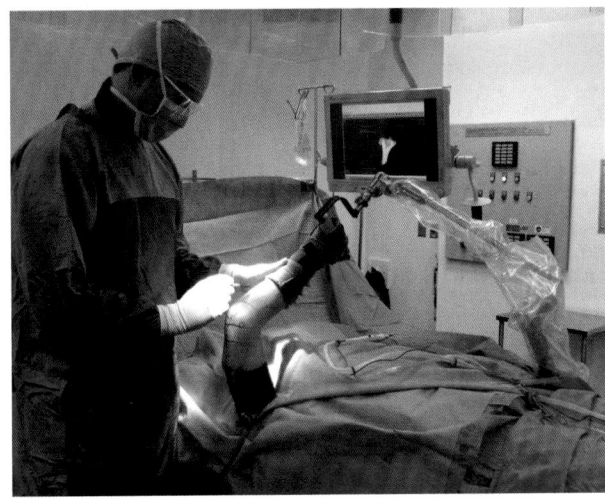

FIGURE 35-13 The patient may be positioned supine with a bolster placed under the ipsilateral scapula **(A)** or lateral decubitus on a bean-bag with the elbow flexed over an arthroscopy positioner **(B).** In circumstances when there is no surgical assistant available, a commercially available articulated arm positioner can also be used **(C).**

patient with a highly comminuted distal humerus fracture, which may be intraoperatively deemed unrepairable, necessitating TEA. AO/OTA type B1 (lateral column) fractures can be surgically approached by Kocher's interval with proximal extension to expose the lateral column. AO/OTA type B2 (medial column) fractures can be approached via a Hotchkiss approach with proximal extension to expose the medial column. Single column fractures (medial and lateral) may also be exposed by the paratricipital approach, which allows visualization of the posterior aspects of both columns and the posterior aspect of the articular surface. In cases where there is extensive articular comminution (AO/OTA types B1.3 and B2.3) an olecranon osteotomy may be required for improved visualization of the fracture and improved access for fixation (Fig. 35-14).

There are several surgical approaches described for exposure and fixation of distal humerus fractures. They can be classified based on direction; posterior, lateral, medial, and anterior, and then further subclassified based on their specific anatomic intervals (Table 35-3). The ideal approach to a specific fracture pattern should provide sufficient exposure to allow anatomic reconstruction of the fracture and the application of the required internal fixation with minimal soft tissue or bony disruption, to allow early mobilization. The selection of a sur-

gical approach depends on multiple factors including fracture pattern, extent of articular involvement, associated soft tissue injury, rehabilitation protocols, and surgeon preference.[169]

Skin incisions about the elbow may be placed posterior, lateral, medial, or anterior depending on the surgical approach selected. Most posterior approaches benefit from a posterior longitudinal skin incision which involves the elevation of full-thickness fasciocutaneous medial and lateral flaps.[42] The posterior skin incision can be straight or curved around the olecranon, medially or laterally, depending on surgeon preference. It is the author's preference to conduct a relatively straight posterior skin incision that curves gently around the medial aspect of the olecranon (Fig. 35-15A). The lateral approaches can be accessed via a direct lateral skin incision or by a posterior longitudinal skin incision with elevation of a lateral fasciocutaneous flap. Similarly, the medial approaches can be accessed via a direct medial skin incision or by a posterior longitudinal skin incision with elevation of a medial fasciocutaneous flap. There are several advantages to a direct midline posterior longitudinal skin incision, including access to both medial and lateral deep approaches and a decreased risk of cutaneous nerve injury.[42] The disadvantage of selecting a posterior longitudinal skin incision for isolated medial or lateral

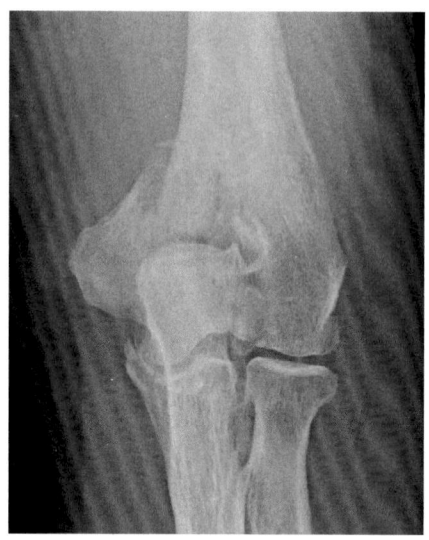
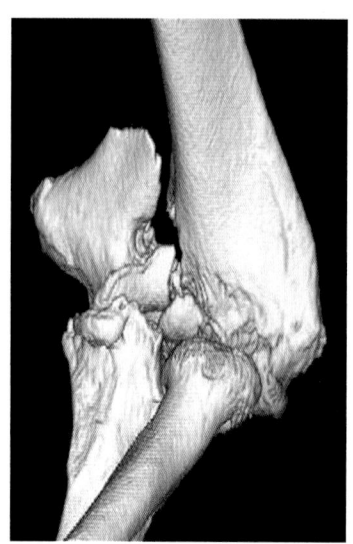
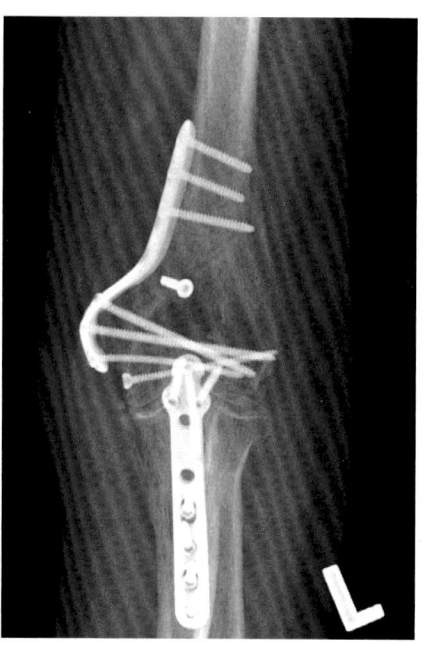

A, B

C

FIGURE 35-14 A 73-year-old woman with a comminuted intra-articular fracture of the medial column (AO/OTA type B1.3) treated with ORIF via an olecranon osteotomy **(A–C)**.

approaches is the increased risk of flap complications such as seromas and rarely necrosis.

Posterior Approaches to the Distal Humerus. There are several posterior approaches and they can be broadly classified into three general types: Olecranon osteotomy, paratri-cipital (triceps-on), and triceps-off type approaches (such as the triceps splitting, triceps reflecting, and the triceps tongue approaches). The selection of a particular type of posterior approach depends on several factors including the degree of articular visualization required for anatomic reduction and

TABLE 35-3	Surgical Approaches to the Distal Humerus				
Direction	**Surgical Approach**	**Indications**	**Contraindications**	**Advantages**	**Disadvantages**
Posterior	Olecranon osteotomy[36,78,118,180]	ORIF distal humerus and articular fractures (AO/OTA types B & C)	Avoid if possibility of TEA	Best visualization of the articular surface for reduction and fixation	Nonunion and hardware prominence—related to osteotomy Limited visualization of anterior articular surfaces
	Paratricipital[7,198]	ORIF extra-articular and simple intra-articular fractures (AO/OTA types C1 & C2) TEA	Comminuted intra-articular fractures	Avoids disruption of the extensor mechanism, no postoperative restrictions related to approach required	Limited visualization of the articular surfaces
	Triceps splitting[29,68]	ORIF extra-articular and intra-articular fractures TEA	Anterior coronal shear fractures of capitellum or trochlea Prior olecranon osteotomy approach	Avoids complications associated with olecranon osteotomy	Limited visualization of anterior articular surfaces Risk of triceps insufficiency
	Triceps reflecting[26]	TEA ORIF intra-articular fractures	Anterior coronal shear fractures of capitellum or trochlea Prior olecranon osteotomy approach Traumatic triceps tendon tear	Avoids complications associated with olecranon osteotomy	Limited visualization of anterior articular surfaces Risk of triceps insufficiency

TABLE 35-3 **Surgical Approaches to the Distal Humerus** (continued)

Direction	Surgical Approach	Indications	Contraindications	Advantages	Disadvantages
	TRAP[156]	ORIF intra-articular fractures TEA	Anterior coronal shear fractures of capitellum or trochlea Prior olecranon osteotomy approach Traumatic triceps tendon tear	Avoids complications associated with olecranon osteotomy Preserves nerve supply to anconeus	Limited visualization of anterior articular surfaces Risk of triceps insufficiency
	Van Gorder[219]	ORIF intra-articular fractures TEA	Anterior coronal shear fractures of capitellum or trochlea Prior olecranon osteotomy approach	Avoids complications associated with olecranon osteotomy	Limited visualization of anterior articular surfaces Risk of triceps insufficiency
Lateral	Kocher[105]	Lateral column fractures Lateral epicondyle fractures Capitellum ± lateral trochlear ridge fractures Fixation of associated radial head and neck fractures	Medial articular fractures (trochlea)	Good access to capitellum, and lateral column structures Improved access to medial joint by releasing LCL Good access to origin and insertion of LCL	No access to medial column
	EDC split	Lateral column fractures Lateral epicondyle fractures Capitellum ± lateral trochlear ridge fractures Fixation of associated radial head fractures	Medial articular fractures (trochlea)	Good access to capitellum, and lateral column structures Improved access to medial joint by releasing LCL	No access to medial column
	Kaplan[102]	Capitellum ± lateral trochlear ridge fractures Fixation of associated radial head fractures	Medial articular fractures (trochlea) Lateral collateral ligament injuries	Avoids disrupting extensor origin on lateral epicondyle LCL is safe	No access to medial column Difficult access to lateral epicondyle for ORIF fracture or LCL repair Limited access to radial neck for fixation
Medial	Hotchkiss over-the-top[81]	Medial epicondyle and medial column fractures Trochlear fractures	Associated MCL tears requiring repair Complex medial and lateral articular fractures	Good access to medial column and anteromedial joint capsule	Difficult access to MCL for repair
	Taylor and Scham[215]	Medial epicondyle and medial column fractures Trochlear fractures MCL tears and coronoid fractures	Complex medial and lateral articular fractures	Good visualization of trochlea Good access to MCL for repair and coronoid for ORIF	Reflection of flexors of medial ulna and medial epicondyle
Anterior	Henry	Vascular injury Median nerve laceration	Requirement for plate fixation of columns or fixation of articular surface	Good access to brachial artery and median nerve	Limited access to medial and lateral columns

ORIF, open reduction and internal fixation; TEA, total elbow arthroplasty; TRAP, triceps reflecting anconeus pedicle; LCL, lateral collateral ligament; EDC, extensor digitorum communis; MCL, medial collateral ligament.

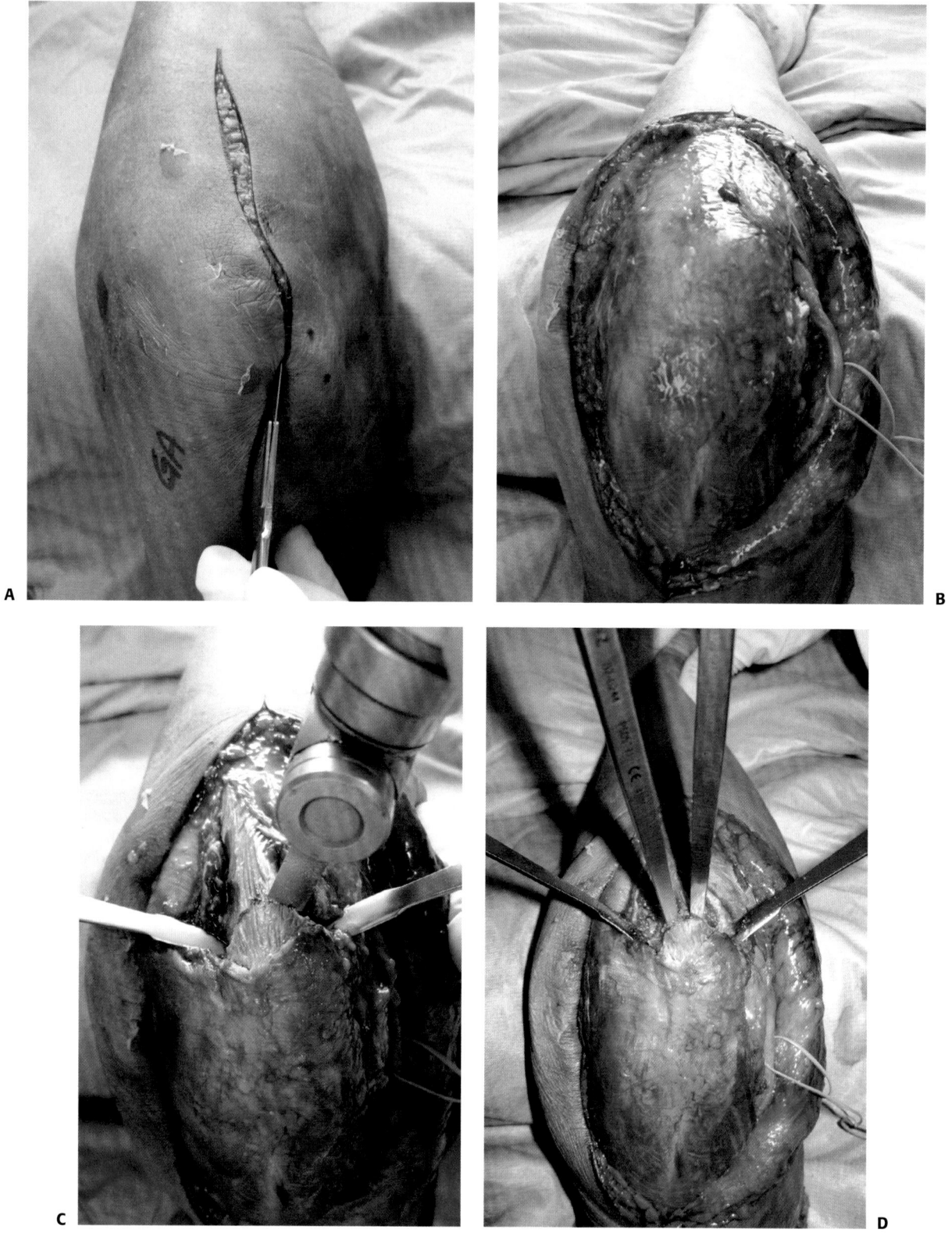

FIGURE 35-15 An olecranon osteotomy is approached via a longitudinal posterior skin incision **(A)**. The ulnar nerve is exposed and may be prepared for anterior subcutaneous transposition **(B)**. The subcutaneous border of the proximal ulna is exposed and the nonarticular portion of the greater sigmoid notch (the bare area) between the olecranon articular facet and the coronoid articular facet is clearly identified. This is accomplished by dissection along the medial and lateral sides of the olecranon to enter into the ulnohumeral joint. Medial and lateral retractors are then placed into the ulnohumeral joint and an apex distal chevron osteotomy entering into the bare area is marked on the subcutaneous border of the ulna. A microsagittal saw is used to complete two-thirds of the osteotomy **(C)** and two osteotomes, placed into each arm of the chevron, apply controlled leverage to fracture the remaining third **(D)**.

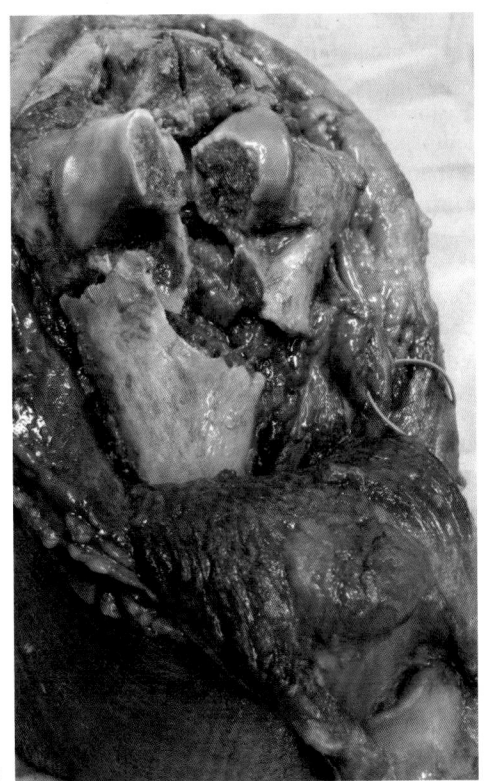

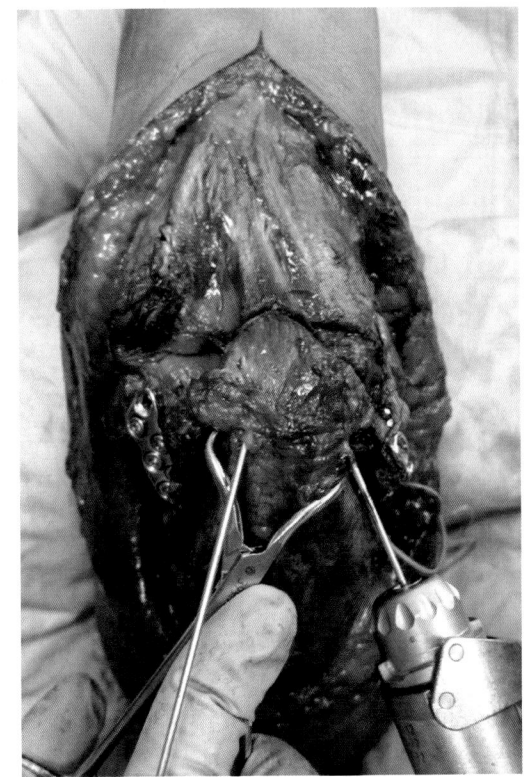

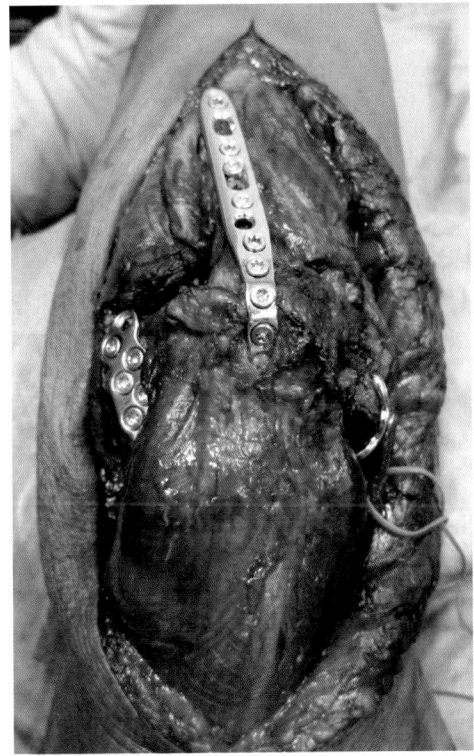

FIGURE 35-15 (*continued*) Once conducted, the olecranon fragment along with the triceps tendon and musculature can be bluntly dissected off the posterior aspect of the distal humerus **(E)**. At the completion of the case, provisional fixation of the olecranon fragment is done with crossing K-wires **(F)** followed by definitive compression plating **(G)**.

internal fixation, the appropriateness of primary arthroplasty, patient factors (elderly, low demand), fracture characteristics (articular comminution), and any associated injuries (i.e., triceps laceration or olecranon fracture) that may make one approach more favourable.

Olecranon Osteotomy. The olecranon osteotomy was first described by MacAusland[118] and has undergone several modifications.[30,58,180] When compared to other posterior approaches, osteotomy of the olecranon provides the best visualization of the distal humerus articular surface,[225] which is its main advantage.

The main disadvantages of the approach are the complications associated with an osteotomy, including nonunion, malunion, and hardware irritation. Olecranon osteotomies are most commonly used for AO/OTA type C fractures, which require superior visualization of the articular fragments for anatomic reduction and internal fixation. An osteotomy can also be used for partial articular fractures (AO/OTA type B), especially if they are comminuted. Relative contraindications to an osteotomy are very anterior articular fractures (AO/OTA type B3) which can be difficult to visualize through an osteotomy and if a TEA is planned as it may lead to problems with implant stability and osteotomy healing and fixation.

As for all posterior approaches, the ulnar nerve requires identification and protection to avoid iatrogenic nerve injury during fracture manipulation and fixation (Fig. 35-15B). It remains unclear whether the ulnar nerve should be transposed or replaced in the cubital tunnel at the conclusion of the procedure. Wiggers et al.[224] demonstrated that the occurrence of postoperative ulnar neuropathy was independent of whether or not the ulnar nerve was transposed at the time of fracture fixation. Conversely, Chen et al.[32] reported a four times increase in the rate of postoperative ulnar neuropathy after transposition. Presently, as there exists no level 1 evidence for or against transposition, it is my preference to conduct a formal anterior subcutaneous ulnar nerve transposition at the conclusion of the procedure.

Once the subcutaneous border of the proximal ulna is exposed, the nonarticular portion of the greater sigmoid notch (the "bare area") between the olecranon articular facet and the coronoid articular facet should be clearly identified. This is done by subperiosteally dissecting along the medial and lateral sides of the olecranon to enter into the ulnohumeral joint. Dissection should not proceed distally as it places the collateral ligament insertions at risk. Medial and lateral retractors are then placed into the ulnohumeral joint to protect the soft tissues and to allow direct visualization of the "bare area." An apex distal chevron osteotomy entering into the bare area is then marked on the subcutaneous border of the ulna (Fig. 35-15C). A microsagittal saw is used to complete two-thirds of the osteotomy. To avoid unpredictable propagation of the osteotomy, multiple perforations are carefully created through the remaining third using a K-wire. Two osteotomes, placed into each arm of the chevron, apply controlled leverage to the olecranon fragment causing fracture of the remaining third (Fig. 35-15D). The fractured surface of the olecranon improves fragment interdigitation and facilitates anatomic reduction and stability during the repair. A chevron-shaped osteotomy provides rotation stability, increased surface area for healing, and protects the collateral ligament insertions.[167] A transverse olecranon osteotomy is also an option as it is technically simpler and can be performed more rapidly.[58,80] Following the osteotomy, the olecranon fragment along with the triceps tendon and musculature can be bluntly dissected off the posterior aspect of the distal humerus (Fig. 35-15E). Typically, the anconeus muscle must be divided in order to reflect the triceps posteriorly which causes its denervation.[156] Anconeus muscle denervation can be avoided by reflecting the anconeus muscle posteriorly along with the olecranon fragment and triceps.[16] Once the osteotomy (Fig. 35-15F, G) is

conducted, flexion of the elbow is used to maximize visualization of distal humerus articular surface.

Fixation of the olecranon osteotomy can be achieved with tension band wiring,[124] screw/tension band constructs, or with compression plating.[64] The author's preferred method of fixation is compression plating.[78] When using this method, the plate is pre-fixed to the olecranon and then removed before conducting the osteotomy. This facilitates osteotomy reduction at the completion of the operative procedure. A 6.5- or 7.3-mm intramedullary compression screw may also be used for osteotomy fixation; however, care should be taken during screw insertion as malreduction is possible when the distal screw threads deflect into the normal varus bow of the ulna.[66]

Paratricipital Approach (Triceps-On). The paratricipital (bilaterotricipital, triceps sparing, or triceps-on) approach was first reported by Alonso-Llames[7] in 1972 for the management of pediatric supracondylar fractures. The approach involves the creation of surgical windows along the medial and lateral sides of the triceps muscle and tendon without disrupting its insertion on the olecranon.[198]

The approach starts with an extensile posterior skin incision and mobilization of the ulnar nerve. Along the medial side of the triceps, the interval between the triceps muscle and the medial intermuscular septum is developed (Fig. 35-16A) and the triceps muscle is elevated off the posterior aspect of the humerus (Fig. 35-16B). Laterally, the triceps is elevated off the lateral intermuscular septum and the posterior humerus in conjunction with the anconeus muscle (Fig. 35-16).[7,198] Distally, the paratricipital approach allows visualization of the medial and lateral columns, the olecranon fossa, and the posterior aspect of the trochlea. A modification of the paratricipital approach involves the creation of a third surgical window in Boyd's interval between the anconeus and lateral olecranon.[14] The third surgical window allows improved visualization of the distal humerus articular surface.

The paratricipital approach has several advantages including avoidance of an olecranon osteotomy; therefore, the risks of nonunion and symptomatic olecranon hardware are avoided. In addition, the triceps tendon insertion is not disrupted, allowing early active range of motion. This approach also preserves the innervation and blood supply of the anconeus muscle,[198] which provides dynamic posterolateral stability to the elbow. Finally, if further articular exposure is required, the paratricipital approach can be converted into an olecranon osteotomy. If further proximal exposure is required for associated fractures of the humeral shaft, the lateral side of the paratricipital approach can be converted into the Gerwin et al.[62] approach. This approach involves reflection of the triceps muscle unit from lateral to medial to expose 95% of the posterior humeral shaft and the radial nerve.

The disadvantage of the paratricipital approach is the limited visualization of the articular surface of the distal humerus; therefore, the approach is usually inadequate for fixation of type C3 fractures. The several advantages of this approach certainly indicate its use for AO/OTA types A2, A3, B1, B2, and possibly C1 and C2 fractures.[124,170,198]

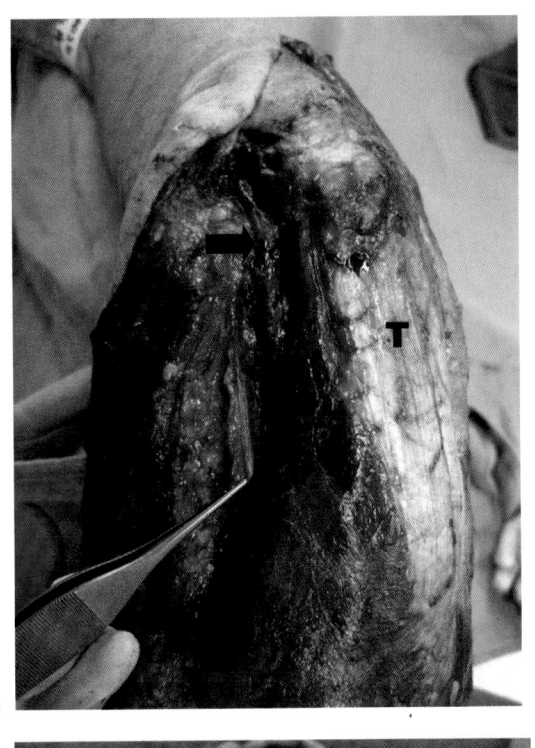

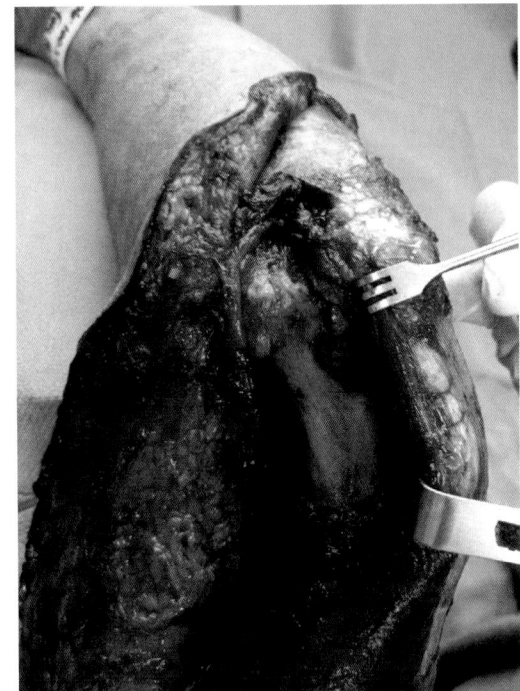

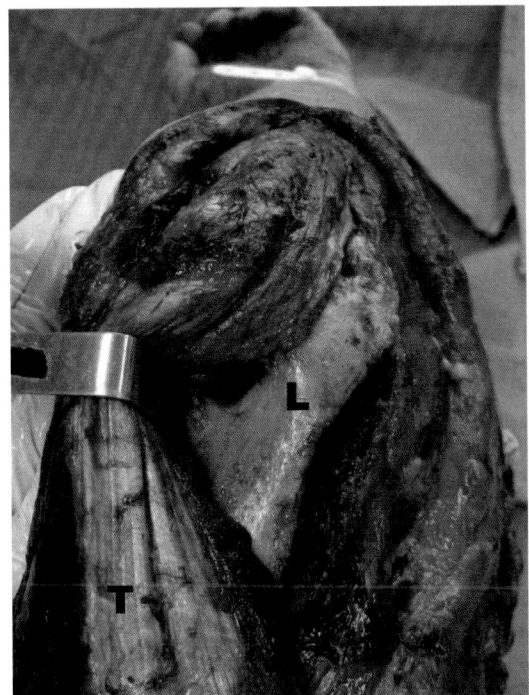

FIGURE 35-16 The paratricipital approach is done through a longitudinal posterior skin incision. Medially **(A),** the ulnar nerve (*black arrow*) is identified. The medial intermuscular septum (forceps) is excised and the triceps muscle is elevated off the posterior aspect of the distal humerus **(B).** Laterally, the triceps muscle is elevated off the posterolateral aspect of the distal humerus allowing exposure of the lateral column, olecranon fossa, and posterior aspect of the trochlea **(C).** L, lateral column; T, triceps.

In distal humerus fractures deemed unrepairable, where the intent is to proceed directly to TEA, the paratricipital approach is preferred because it avoids the problems associated with osteotomies and extensor mechanism healing in triceps detaching approaches. The approach is also useful in cases where an initial attempt at ORIF is planned and there is a possibility of an intraoperative conversion to TEA, should fixation be deemed unsuccessful.

Triceps Splitting Approach. The triceps splitting approach described by Campbell[29] involves a midline split through the triceps tendon. The medial and lateral columns are exposed with subperiosteal dissection starting from the midline and moving outward (Fig. 35-17). Visualization of the articular surface of the distal humerus is challenging and can be improved by partial excision of the olecranon tip and flexion of the elbow. This approach can be extended proximally to the level of the radial

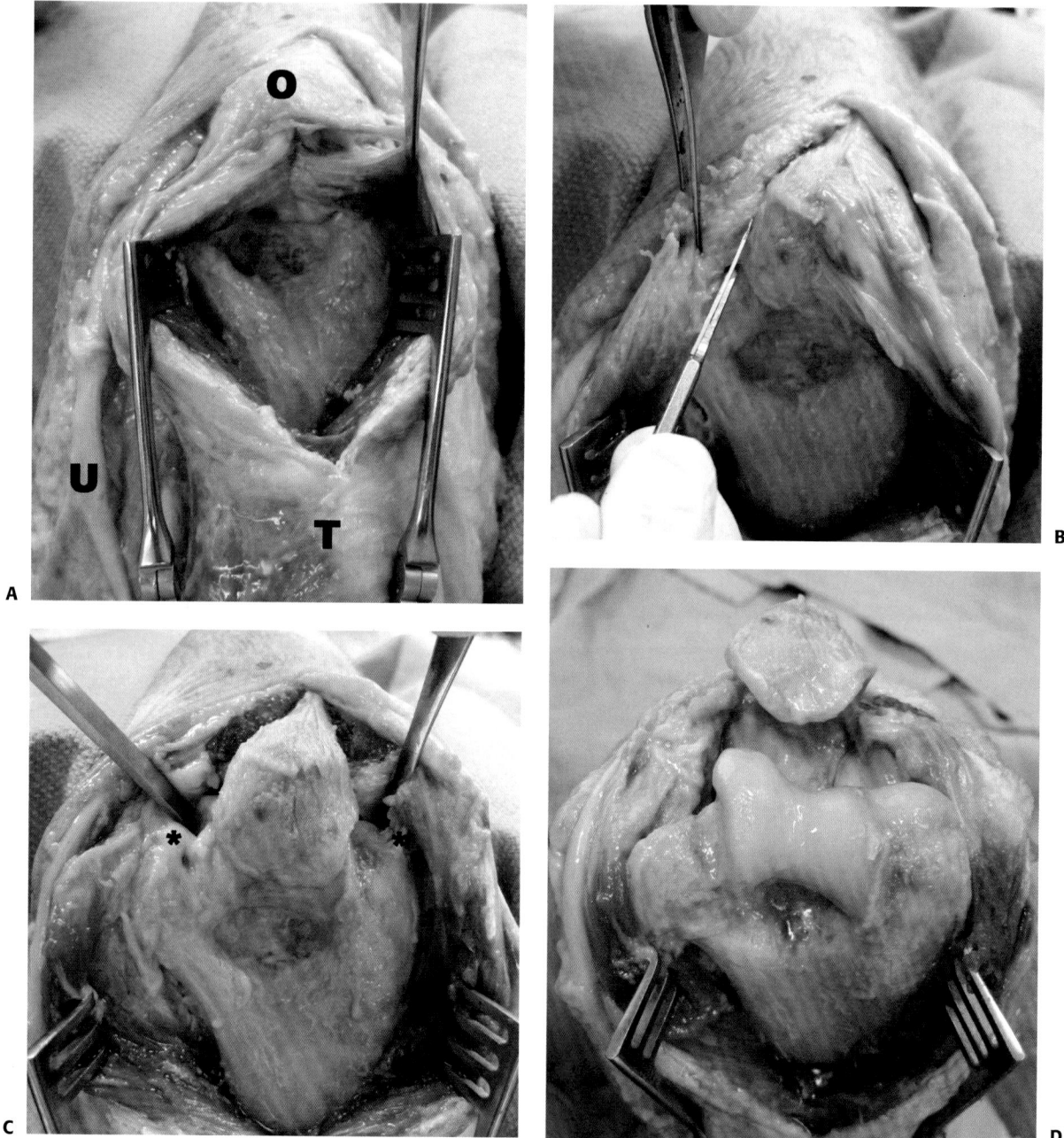

FIGURE 35-17 The triceps split approach described by Campbell involves a midline split through the triceps tendon and medial head **(A)**. The approach can be extended distally by splitting the triceps insertion on the olecranon and raising medial and lateral full-thickness fasciotendinous flaps **(B, C)**. To gain further exposure of the posterior trochlea, the elbow is flexed and the olecranon tip may be excised. For ORIF, the medial and lateral collateral ligaments are preserved (*asterisk*), however, to obtain further exposure for TEA, they may be released **(D)**. O, olecranon; U, ulnar nerve; T, triceps.

nerve as it crosses the humeral shaft in the spiral groove. To expand the approach distally, the split can be extended through the triceps insertion to the subcutaneous border of the ulna. The triceps insertion on the olecranon is split midline, with release of Sharpey fibers creating medial and lateral fasciotendinous sleeves. At the conclusion of the procedure, the triceps tendon is repaired to the olecranon via transosseous nonabsorbable braided sutures.

The advantages of the triceps splitting approach are its relative technical ease and the ability to convert from ORIF to TEA with few consequences. The disadvantages of the approach include limited visibility of the articular surface, and the requirement of postoperative protection of the triceps repair to decrease the risk of extensor mechanism disruption. In order to improve triceps healing, Gschwend et al.[68] modified the approach to incorporate a flake of olecranon bone. McKee et al.[133] compared the extensor mechanism strength of patients treated with an olecranon osteotomy versus a triceps splitting approach and found no statistical significant difference, concluding that both approaches are effective.

Triceps Reflecting Anconeus Pedicle (TRAP) Approach. The TRAP approach involves completely detaching the triceps from the proximal ulna with the anconeus muscle.[156] The approach

is done through a longitudinal posterior skin incision after identification of the ulnar nerve. Kocher's interval is used to elevate the anconeus muscle and develop the distal lateral portion of the flap (Fig. 35-18A). The medial portion of the flap is created by subperiosteal dissection from the subcutaneous border of the ulna. The anconeus flap is then reflected proximally to expose the triceps insertion which is also sharply released (Fig. 35-18B). The entire triceps–anconeus flap is then reflected

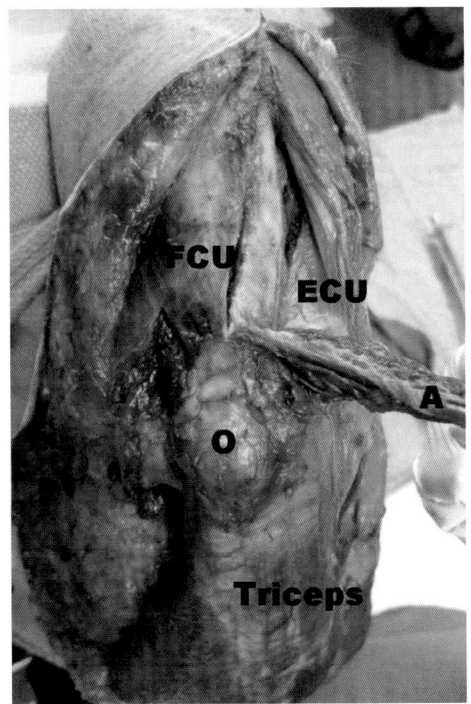
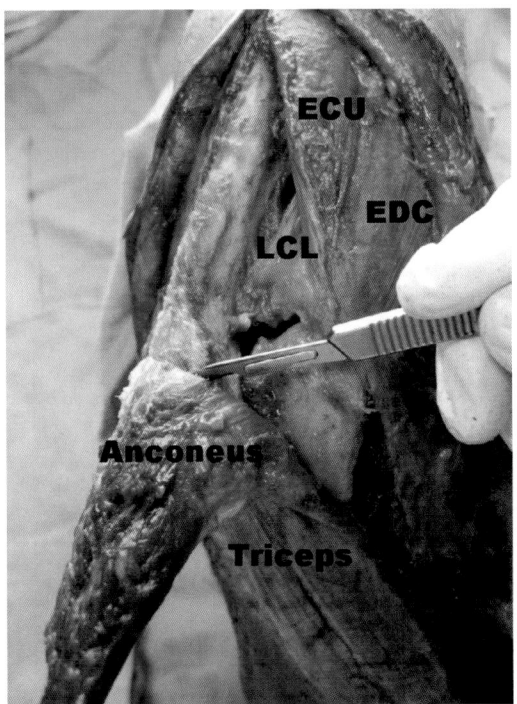
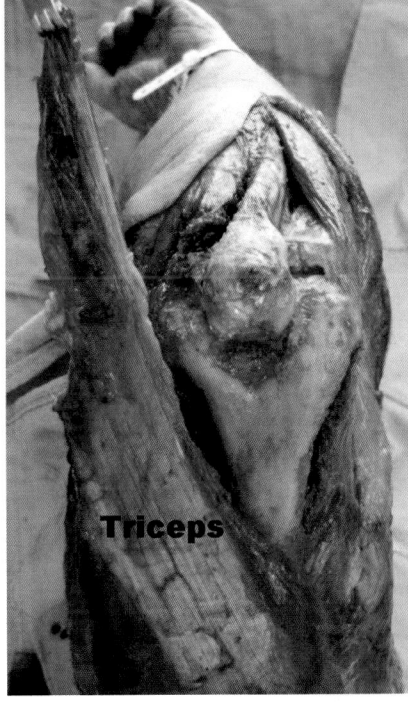

FIGURE 35-18 The triceps reflecting anconeus pedicle (TRAP) approach is done through a longitudinal posterior skin incision after identification of the ulnar nerve. The interval between anconeus and extensor carpi ulnaris is used to elevate the anconeus muscle and develop the distal lateral portion of the flap. The medial portion of the flap is created by subperiosteal dissection from the subcutaneous border of the ulna. The anconeus flap is then reflected proximally **(A)** to expose the triceps insertion which is also sharply released **(B).** The entire triceps–anconeus flap is then reflected proximally releasing the triceps muscle from the posterior aspect of the distal humerus **(C).** O, olecranon; FCU, flexor carpi ulnaris; ECU, extensor carpi ulnaris; LCL, lateral collateral ligament; A, anconeus; EDC, extensor digitorum communis.

proximally releasing the triceps muscle from the posterior aspect of the distal humerus (Fig. 35-18C). This approach provides good exposure to the posterior elbow joint while protecting the neurovascular supply to the anconeus muscle. The TRAP approach also avoids the complications of an olecranon osteotomy and allows the use of the trochlear sulcus as a template to assist with articular reduction of the distal humerus. The major disadvantage of this approach is that the triceps is completely released from its insertion; therefore, there is a risk of triceps dehiscence and extensor weakness.

Van Gorder Approach (Triceps Tongue). The Van Gorder approach involves division of the triceps tendon at its musculotendinous junction.[219] The approach is most commonly used for TEA and rarely for ORIF of distal humerus fractures. Transection of the triceps is done in the shape of a "V" so that a "V to Y" plasty can be done if lengthening of the extensor

mechanism is required. As the triceps is completely divided in this approach, it has the same risks as the TRAP approach. This approach is indicated for ORIF of distal humerus fractures when there is an associated complete or high-grade partial triceps tendon laceration.

Lateral Approaches to the Distal Humerus. Lateral approaches to the elbow can be accessed via a direct lateral skin incision or by a posterior longitudinal skin incision with elevation of a lateral fasciocutaneous flap. The approaches that will be discussed are the Kocher, Kaplan, and the extensor digitorum communis (EDC) split. Access to the radiocapitellar joint can also be obtained through a lateral epicondylar osteotomy or via a concurrent fracture of the lateral epicondyle.

The Kocher, Kaplan, and EDC split approaches are used to treat capitellar and radial head fractures. Proximal extension of these approaches can be used to access the lateral column, to

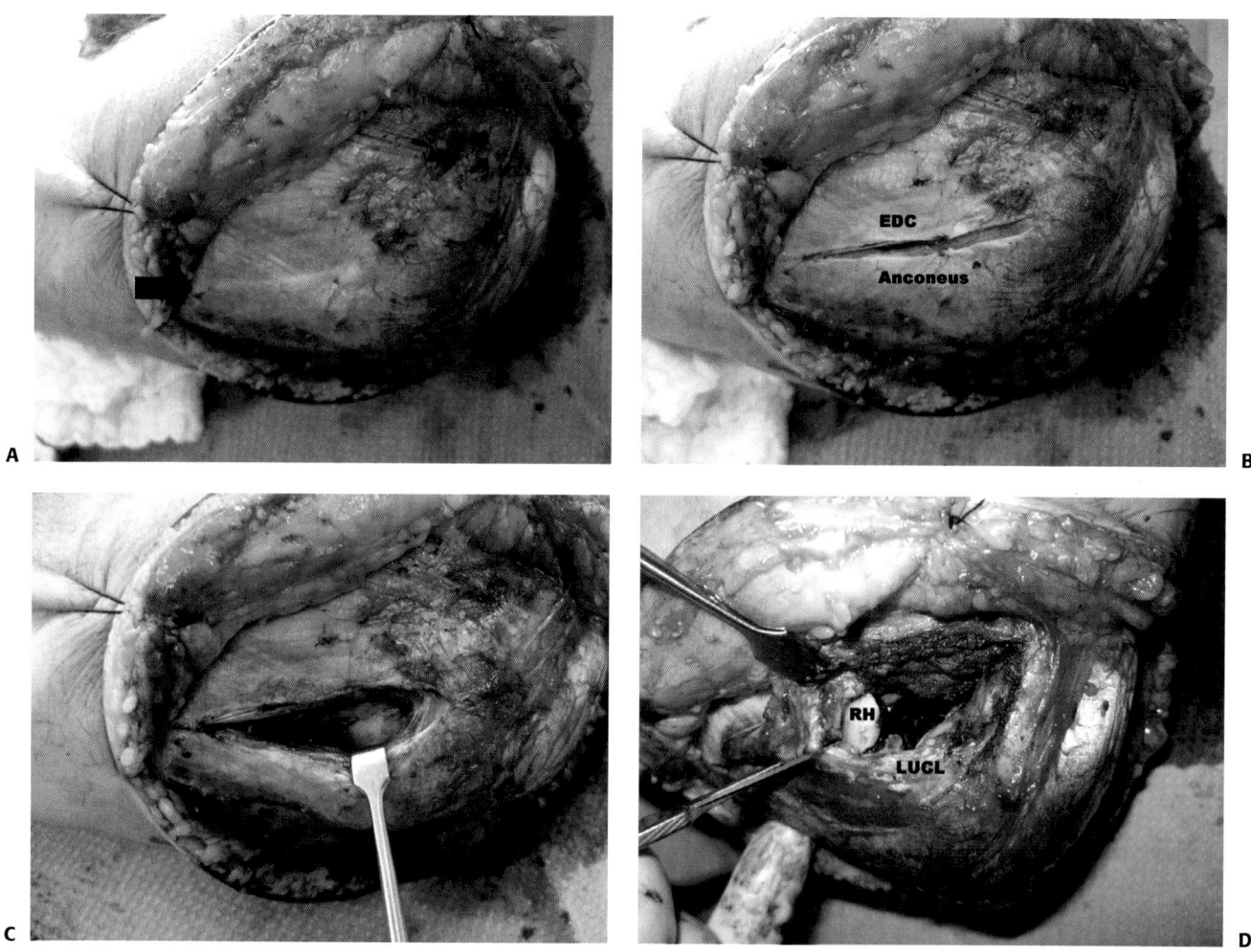

FIGURE 35-19 Kocher's approach[105] to the anterolateral elbow joint uses the interval between extensor carpi ulnaris (ECU) and anconeus **(A).** This interval can be identified by a thin fat stripe (*black arrow*). The interval is developed by bluntly undermining the anconeus muscle which will allow identification of the elbow joint capsule and the capsular thickening that is the lateral ulnar collateral ligament (LUCL) **(B, C).** The posterior portion of the common extensor tendon origin will have to be elevated off the LUCL to allow an arthrotomy to be made anterior to the ligament **(D).** RH, radial head; EDC, extensor digitorum communis.

treat partial articular lateral column fractures and some trans-column fractures.

The Kocher approach involves identification of the interval between extensor carpi ulnaris (ECU) and anconeus.[105] This interval can be identified by a thin fat stripe or by the perforating branches of the recurrent posterior interosseous artery (Fig. 35-19A). The interval is developed by bluntly undermining the anconeus muscle which will allow identification of the elbow joint capsule and the capsular thickening that is the LUCL (Figs. 35-19B and C). Some of the common extensor tendon origin will have to be elevated off the LUCL to allow an arthrotomy to be made anterior to the ligament (Fig. 35-19D). The forearm is pronated during the approach, which moves the posterior interosseous nerve more anterior and distal. The radial neck is exposed by incising the annular ligament. This approach can be extended proximally by releasing the extensor carpi radialis longus (ECRL) and the brachioradialis off the anterolateral supracondylar ridge. To expose the posterolateral elbow joint and posterior aspect of the lateral column, another arthrotomy is made posterior to the LUCL and the triceps is elevated off the posterior lateral column.

An easier, and some believe safer, approach to the radiocapitellar joint is the EDC split. This approach involves creation of a lateral elbow arthrotomy at the equator of the radiocapitellar joint (Fig. 35-20). The site of the arthrotomy is chosen by palpating the capitellum and radial head to determine the mid-equator. The structures below the equator include the LUCL and the posterolateral joint capsule which should not be incised as they are important elbow stabilizers. The arthrotomy, therefore, is made in-line with the tendon fibers of EDC at the equator of the radiocapitellar joint and may be extended proximally along the anterolateral aspect of the lateral column. Dissection below the mid-equator is avoided as it may disrupt the LUCL.

The Kaplan approach uses the interval between ECRL and EDC to access the radiocapitellar joint.[102] The approach provides good exposure of the radial head and capitellum and remains anterior to the LCL insertion. The forearm should be pronated during distal extension of the approach to maximize the distance to the posterior interosseous nerve.[38]

Medial Approaches to the Distal Humerus. Medial approaches to the elbow can be accessed by a direct medial skin incision or by a posterior longitudinal skin incision with elevation of a medial fasciocutaneous flap. When using a direct medial skin incision, care should be taken in identifying and protecting the branches of the medial antebrachial cutaneous nerve. The medial approaches can be used to treat isolated partial articular medial column fractures, trochlear fractures, coronoid fractures, and fractures of the medial epicondyle.

Hotchkiss described the medial "over-the-top" approach, which starts with identification and transposition of the ulnar nerve.[81,167] The medial supracondylar ridge is identified and the flexor–pronator origin is released off the ridge to the level of the medial epicondyle. At the medial epicondyle, the flexor origin is split distally in-line with its fibers. Dissection directly inferior to the medial epicondyle is avoided as it may disrupt the anterior bundle of the MCL.

The medial coronoid, the anterior bundle of the MCL, and the posteromedial ulnohumeral joint can be accessed through an approach that starts at the floor of the cubital tunnel. The humeral head of the FCU, palmaris longus, flexor carpi radialis, and pronator teres are bluntly elevated off the anterior bundle of the MCL and joint capsule in a posterior to anterior direction. Once exposed, an arthrotomy is made anterior to the anterior bundle of the MCL to enter the anterior aspect of the ulnohumeral joint. The posteromedial aspect of the ulnohumeral joint is accessed by dividing the posterior and transverse

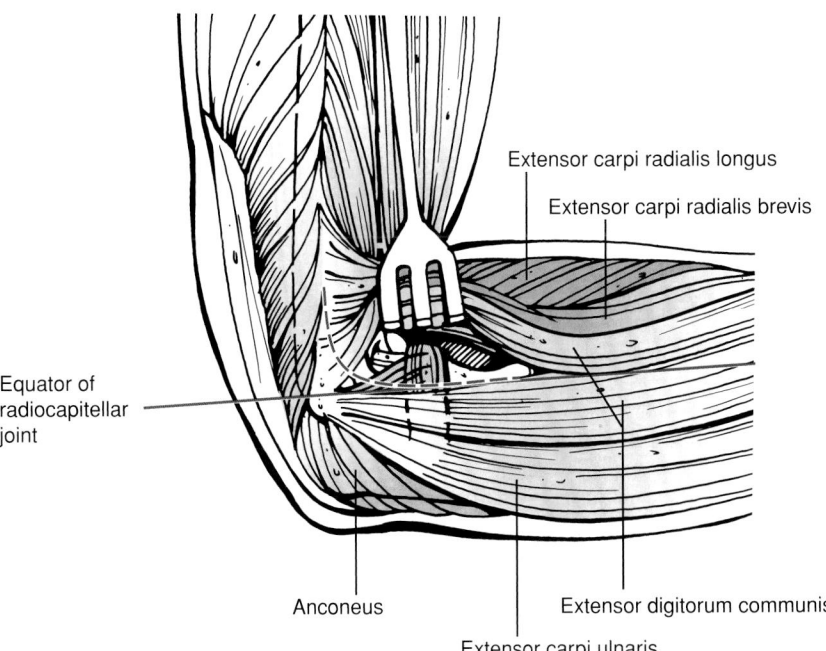

FIGURE 35-20 The extensor digitorum communis (EDC) split approach. The EDC tendon is split anterior to the mid-equator of the radiocapitellar joint to avoid injury to the lateral ulnar collateral ligament.

Extensor carpi radialis longus

Extensor carpi radialis brevis

Equator of radiocapitellar joint

Anconeus

Extensor digitorum communis

Extensor carpi ulnaris

bundles of the MCL. Taylor and Scham[215] described a similar approach with the only difference being that the ulnar head of FCU is elevated anteriorly with the other flexors.

Surgical Technique

Surgical Technique for AO/OTA Types A and C Fractures (Extra-Articular and Complete Articular Fractures). An extensile posterior skin incision is used with elevation of full-thickness medial and lateral fasciocutaneous flaps. The ulnar nerve is exposed, tagged, and prepared for anterior subcutaneous transposition, which will be done at the completion of the procedure.

In patients with comminuted intra-articular AO/OTA type C3 fractures, I prefer a chevron-shaped osteotomy through the bare area, which is then fixated with a precontoured olecranon plate (*please see section on Olecranon Osteotomy*). The plate is preapplied to the olecranon before the osteotomy; this facilitates olecranon reduction and plate application at the end of the operative procedure. For simple articular fractures (AO/OTA type C1 and C2) and extra-articular fractures (AO/OTA type A2 and A3), I prefer the paratricipital approach[7] (Fig. 35-16). This approach allows bicolumn exposure and plating with preservation of the triceps mechanism. Simple intra-articular fractures can be reduced indirectly by anatomic reduction of the supracondylar level fracture. The articular reduction can be assessed with elbow flexion and direct visualization of the posterior aspect of the trochlea or with fluoroscopy. The articular reduction may also be visualized directly by creation of a third surgical window in Boyd's interval, between the anconeus muscle and the lateral olecranon.[14]

The paratricipital approach is also preferred for cases where the reparability of the fracture will be determined intraoperatively. If the fracture is deemed fixable, it may be carried out through the paratricipital approach or the approach can be converted to an olecranon osteotomy. In cases where the fracture is deemed irreparable, a TEA may be done via the same approach.

For AO/OTA type C fractures, once the distal humerus articular surface is adequately exposed, the fracture hematoma is evacuated and the raw fracture surfaces are cleaned of loose debris. The origins of the common flexor and extensor tendons are preserved on the epicondyles as are the collateral ligament origins. The fracture fragments can be manipulated manually or with small diameter K-wires used as joy sticks. I typically prefer K-wires for manipulation and provisional reduction of fracture fragments (Fig. 35-21A to D). Usually, I place one K-wire through the fractured surface of the medial trochlea, aiming toward the medial epicondyle, running along the trochlear axis. This K-wire is then pulled out through the medial epicondyle until its tip lies flush and perpendicular to the fracture surface of the medial trochlea. A similar K-wire is placed through the lateral articular fragment. These wires are then used to individually manipulate the fracture fragments, to reduce and interdigitate them. A large pointed reduction tenaculum is used to hold the reduction and to provide compression until the medial K-wire can be drilled into the lateral fragment and the lateral K-wire drilled into the medial fragment. This provides provisional fixation of the articular segment.

Definitive fixation of the articular segment can be done with one or two centrally placed screws along the capitellar–trochlear axis (Fig. 35-22) or by screws placed through plates that are applied in a parallel fashion (Fig. 35-23). Ideally, intrafragmentary compression is best, however, not at the expense of shortening the trochlea in the medial–lateral plane. The trochlea is particularly susceptible to shortening when central comminution exists and lag screw fixation is used. In these instances, fully threaded (nonoverdrilled) position screws rather than lag screws should be used to stabilize the articular segment. Once the provisional articular reduction is obtained with transfixing K-wires, I typically place a single fully threaded standard screw (2.7, 3, or 3.5 mm) along the axis of the articular segment to maintain the reduction (Fig. 35-21E). This screw is usually inserted medial to lateral with its starting point located in the centre of the trochlea. A small diameter axis screw is used to minimize its effect on other screws that will eventually be used to fixate the articular segment through plates to the diaphysis. When using small diameter screws, my preference is not to use titanium as the resistance encountered during screw insertion in good quality bone has been known to shear off the screw heads.

Small articular fracture segments that cannot be incorporated into the greater fixation construct should be independently fixated. These small articular fractures may be located anteriorly and can be exposed by internally rotating the appropriate column fragment. Supplementary implants should be available to address these small osteochondral fragments such as mini-fragment plates, headless compression screws, countersunk small diameter screws, threaded K-wires, and/or bioabsorbable pins. These supplementary implants require strategic placement such that they do not interfere with trochlear fixation and bicolumnar plate application that will link the articular segment to the diaphysis.

The articular segment (AO/OTA type A fractures and AO/OTA type C fractures after articular fixation) requires rigid attachment to the medial and lateral columns or distal humerus shaft. This can be accomplished by orthogonal,[77,94,200] parallel,[193,194] or triple plating.[64,124] No clinical superiority of either method has been reported when comparing orthogonal to parallel plating techniques. Surgeons should be familiar with all plating techniques, including parallel, orthogonal, and triple plating, as some fractures will lend themselves to one technique over another. Generally, I prefer the technique of parallel plating; however, it does have its disadvantages. Thin and active patients may complain of hardware irritation from a prominent lateral plate. Therefore, in cases with a "high" lateral supracondylar level fracture, a posterolateral plate may be preferable (Fig. 35-24).

Orthogonal plating involves the placement of plates on both columns at approximately 90-degree angles (Fig. 35-24). Usually, the lateral plate is placed as distal as possible along the posterior aspect of the lateral column. The lateral plate should be contoured with a bend that matches the posterior curvature of the lateral column. To achieve maximum distal fixation, the end of the plate should lie just proximal to the posterior articular surface of the capitellum. Placement of the plate further distal may lead to impingement of the radial head against the plate in

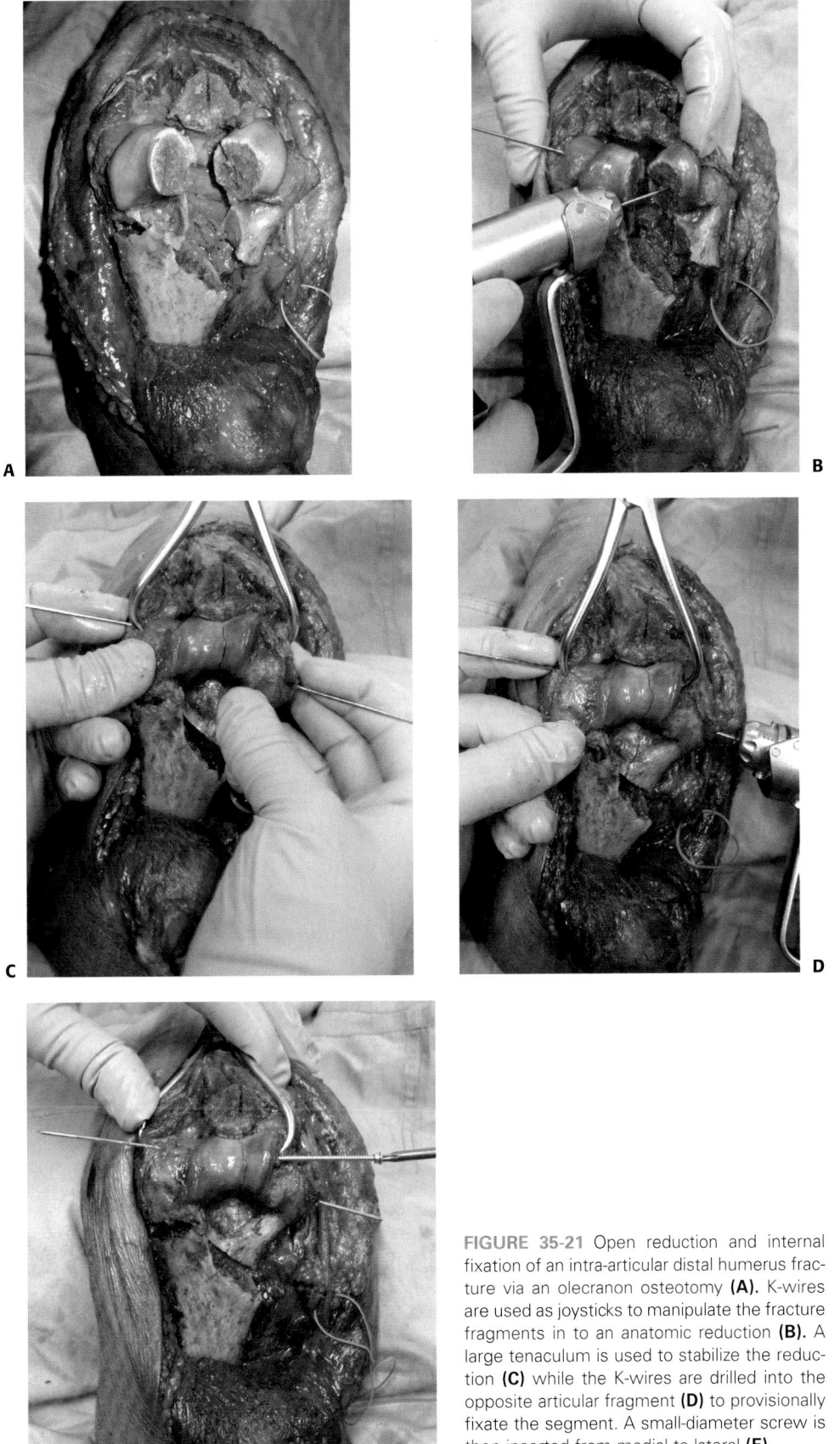

FIGURE 35-21 Open reduction and internal fixation of an intra-articular distal humerus fracture via an olecranon osteotomy **(A)**. K-wires are used as joysticks to manipulate the fracture fragments in to an anatomic reduction **(B)**. A large tenaculum is used to stabilize the reduction **(C)** while the K-wires are drilled into the opposite articular fragment **(D)** to provisionally fixate the segment. A small-diameter screw is then inserted from medial to lateral **(E)**.

(continues)

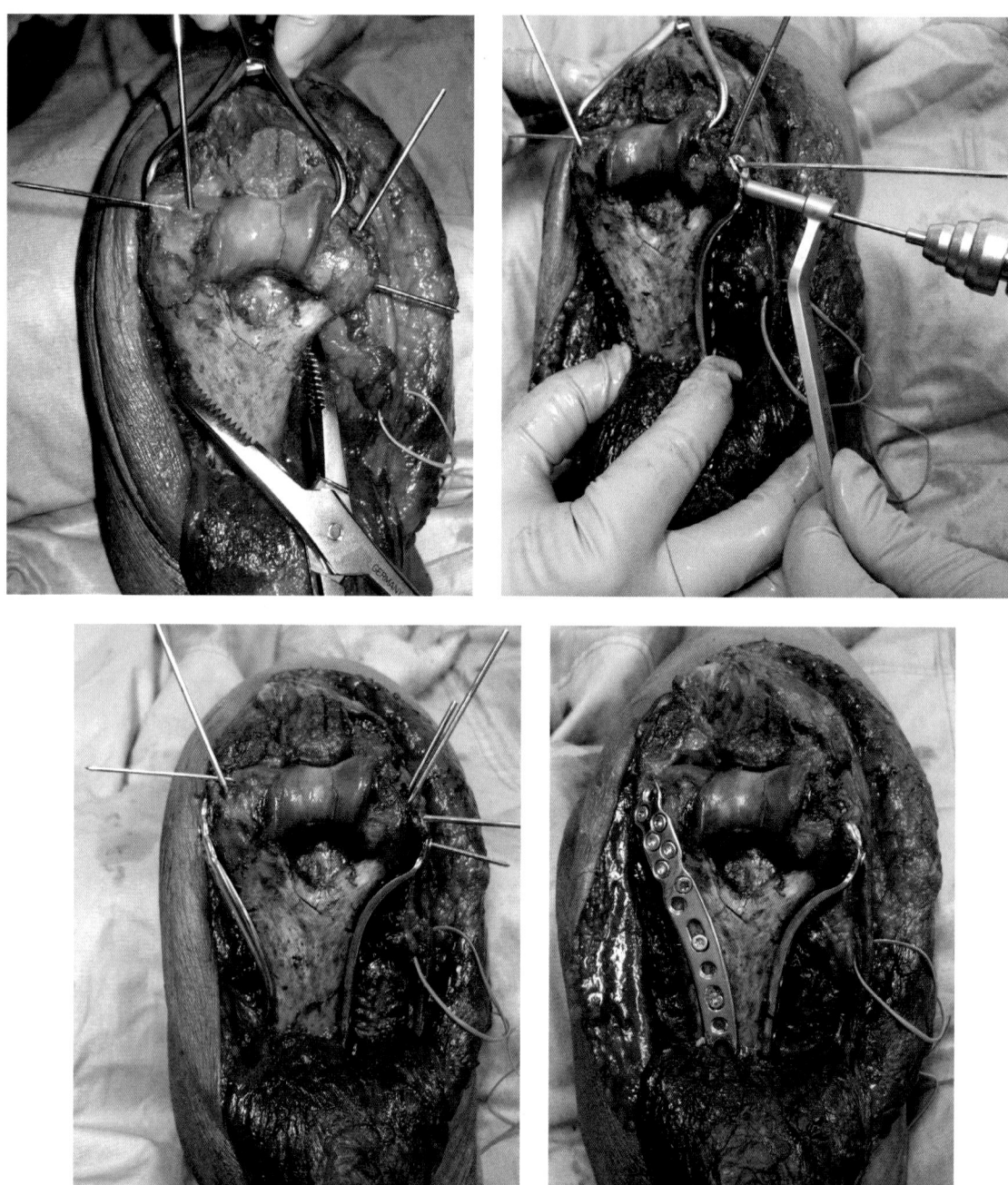

FIGURE 35-21 (*continued*) After the articular segment is fixated, it is reduced to the shaft and provisionally stabilized with long bicortical K-wires inserted up each column **(F)**. Definitive articular segment to shaft fixation is obtained with bicolumn plating in a parallel or orthogonal fashion **(G–I)**. Ideally, as many screws as possible are inserted through the plates into the articular segment; the screws should be as long as possible and they should engage as many articular fragments as possible. Screws should not be placed through the olecranon fossa as they may lead to impingement and decreased range of motion.

extension, resulting in pain and limited range of motion. Ideally, the lateral plate should be a 3.5-mm dynamic compression plate or equivalent. The medial plate is usually applied on the medial supracondylar ridge with contouring to curve around the medial epicondyle. The plate is typically a 3.5-mm reconstruction plate to allow easier bending; however, a 3.5-mm dynamic compression plate or a newer fracture-specific precontoured plate may be preferred.

Parallel plating also uses two plates; however, the plates are placed relatively parallel to each other on their respective

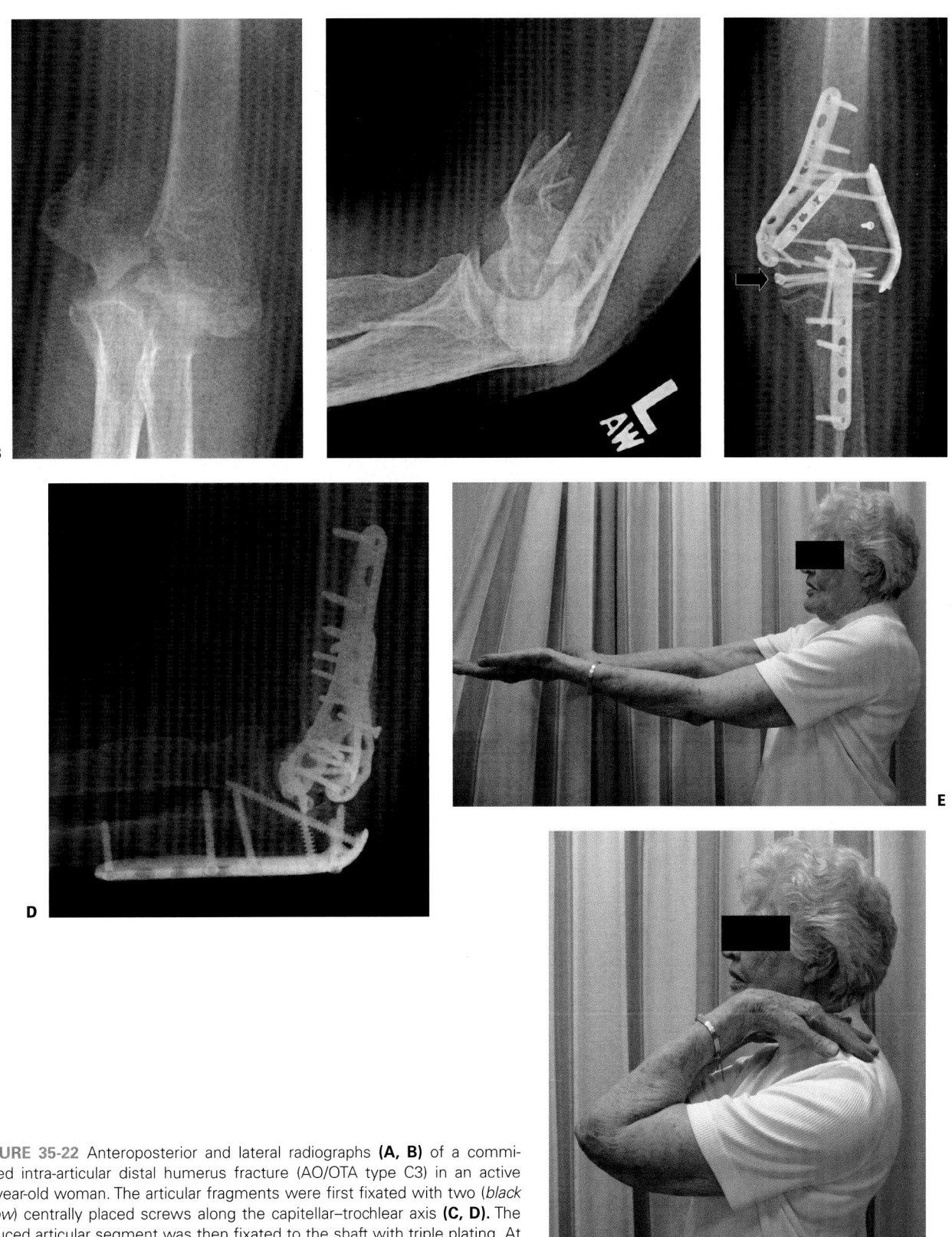

FIGURE 35-22 Anteroposterior and lateral radiographs **(A, B)** of a comminuted intra-articular distal humerus fracture (AO/OTA type C3) in an active 85-year-old woman. The articular fragments were first fixated with two (*black arrow*) centrally placed screws along the capitellar–trochlear axis **(C, D).** The reduced articular segment was then fixated to the shaft with triple plating. At 12 months follow-up, the fractures have healed and the patient has functional range of motion **(E, F).**

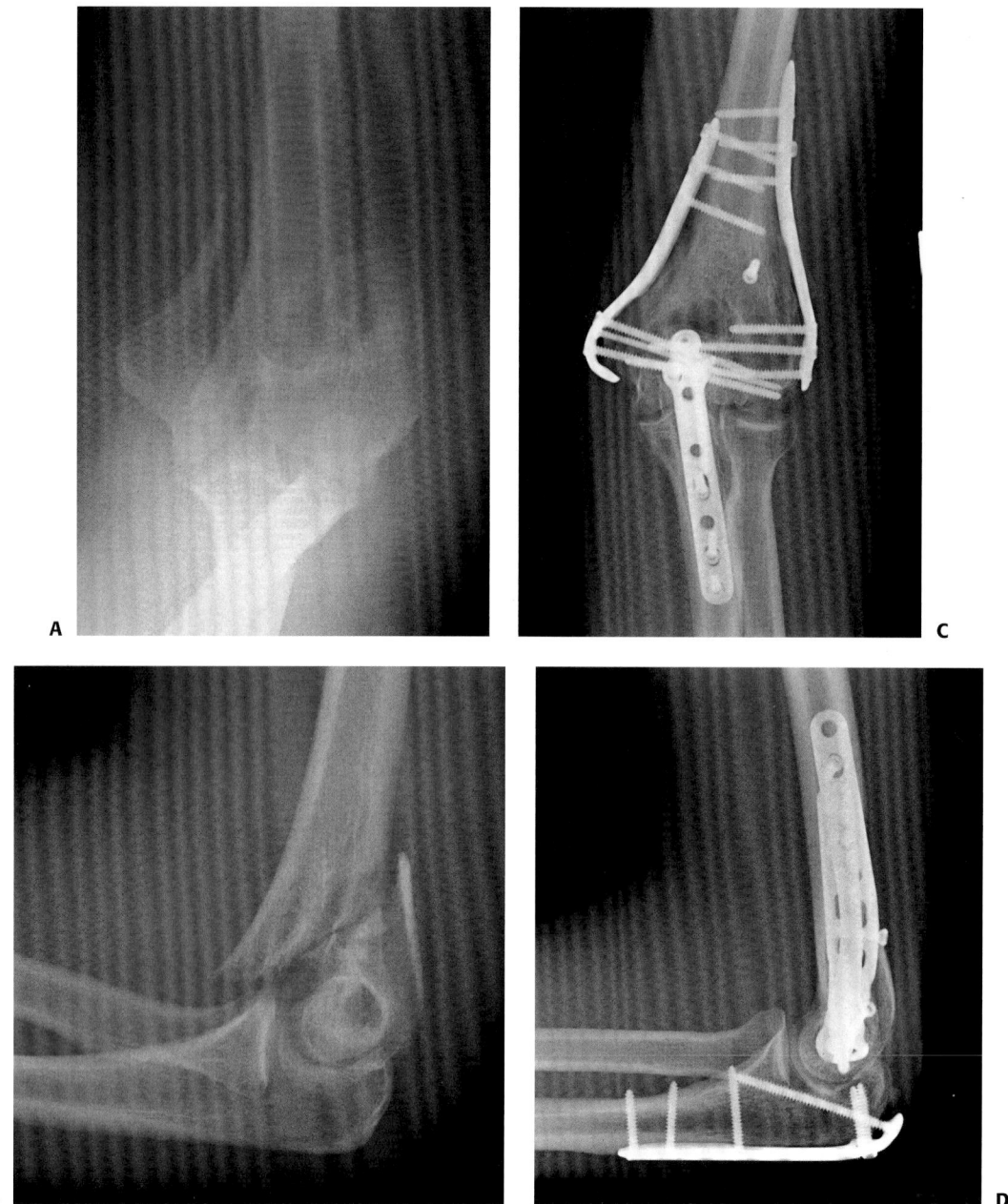

FIGURE 35-23 A bicolumn (AO/OTA type C1) fracture **(A, B)** treated with ORIF via an olecranon osteotomy. The distal humerus articular segment is fixated with three medial and three lateral screws placed through parallel plates **(C, D)**.

supracondylar ridges (Fig. 35-25). Screws into the articular segment are preferentially placed through the plates to link the articular segment to the humeral shaft. Ideally, the longest possible screws should be inserted through the plate, to capture as many articular fragments as possible, and to engage fragments that are secured to the opposite column.[154,155,193] This technique may be difficult to achieve and not always possible to perform. For example, longer screws can deflect and bend as they pass one another, causing displacement of tenuously stabilized osteochondral fragments.

My preference is that longitudinal K-wires are used to temporarily fix the reconstructed articular segment to the shaft to allow columnar plate application (Fig. 35-21F). Precontoured plates are then provisionally applied to the medial and lateral columns with K-wires placed distally and serrated bone reduction clamps proximally. Then, as many screws as possible are inserted through the plates into the articular segment (Fig. 35-21G); ideally the screws should be as long as possible and engage as many articular fragments as possible. Screws should not be placed through the olecranon fossa as they may lead

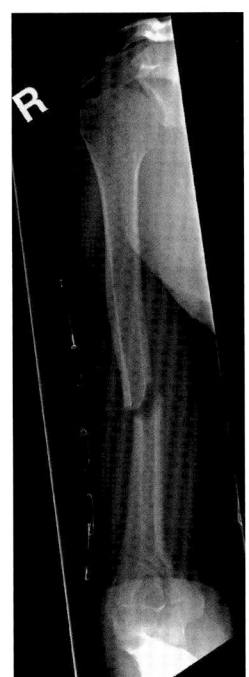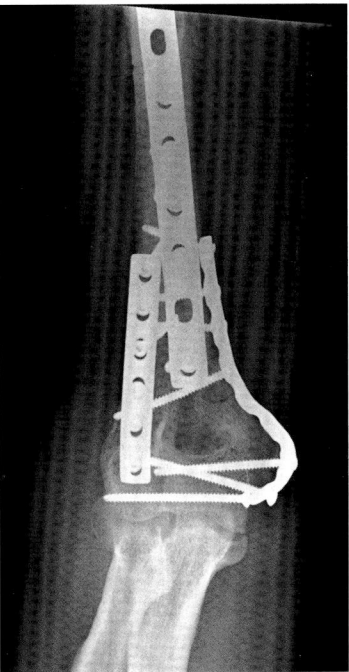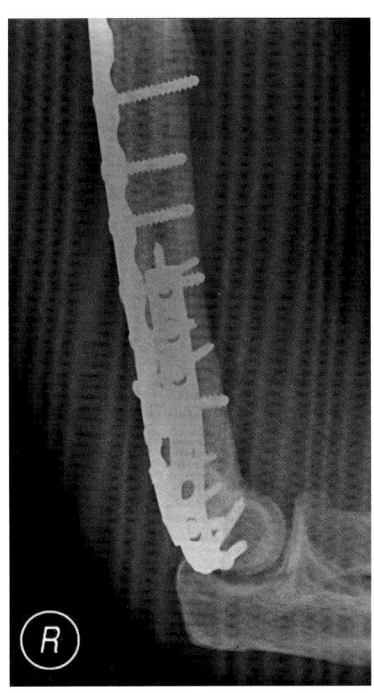

A, B

C

FIGURE 35-24 An AP injury radiograph **(A)** demonstrating a displaced intra-articular distal humerus fracture in association with an ipsilateral humeral shaft fracture. The fractures were exposed via a paratricipital approach extended proximally in to a Gerwin et al. approach. The patient's distal humerus fracture was fixated with orthogonal 3.5-mm dynamic compression plates **(B, C)** that were intra-operatively contoured. This technique has been popularized by the AO group and involves the placement of plates at 90-degree angles to each other. Usually, the lateral plate is placed as distal as possible along the posterior aspect of the lateral column. The medial plate is placed over the medial supracondylar ridge and curved around the medial epicondyle. R, "right" for right arm x-ray.

to impingement. The plates are then fixated to the humeral shaft with the first diaphyseal screws inserted in an eccentric fashion to provide supracondylar fracture compression. Ideally, the plates should end at different levels on the humeral shaft to minimize the stress riser effect (Figs. 35-21H and I). Once ORIF of the distal humerus fracture is complete, the elbow is placed through a range of motion to ensure there is no impingement or instability.

Metaphyseal bone loss may be present in high-energy comminuted distal humerus fractures. This bone loss can be addressed with supracondylar shortening or bridge plating with autologous bone graft or allograft. Supracondylar shortening involves removing the comminuted fragments of metaphyseal bone and compressing the reconstructed articular segment to the distal humeral shaft. Typically, the distal end of the shaft will require reshaping to increase the contact area between it and the articular segment.[152] If absolute rigid fixation cannot be achieved to allow early range of motion, triple plating should be considered as recommended by Gofton[6] and Jupiter and Mehne.[93] Triple plating can also be useful for fixation of coronal plane fractures (Fig. 35-22).

Several precontoured plating systems are available for fixation of distal humerus fractures. Although these plates are marketed as precontoured, they generally still require some contouring to match distal humeral anatomy. Newer precontoured locking plates are also available and are of two types, fixed angle locking and variable angle locking. These plates may offer enhanced fix-

ation in osteopenic bone; however, this has not yet been shown to be clinically superior. The disadvantages of the fixed angle locking plates are the screws have predetermined trajectories, which may not accommodate all fracture patterns in all patients. In some plate designs, the predetermined screw trajectory aims toward the articular surface, which may predispose to joint penetration if screws are placed too long.

Open Reduction Internal Fixation of Distal Humerus Fractures (Partial Articular Fractures)

Surgical Technique for AO/OTA Types B1 and B2 Fractures. In general, the fixation principles and techniques used for AO/OTA type C (bicolumn) fractures are applicable to type B1 and B2 (single column) fractures. These fractures may be fixed with multiple screws or with single column plating.[95] Single column plating has the advantage of providing an anti-glide construct at the proximal fracture line between the column and humeral shaft (Fig. 35-14). In certain highly comminuted partial–articular fractures in elderly patients with osteopenia, TEA may also be an appropriate treatment option. Elbow arthroplasty will be discussed later in this chapter.

Surgical Technique for ORIF of Partial Articular Fractures
Surgical Technique for Capitellum Fractures ± Lateral Trochlear Ridge (AO/OTA Type B3.1). Fractures of the capitellum with or without involvement of the lateral ridge of the trochlea

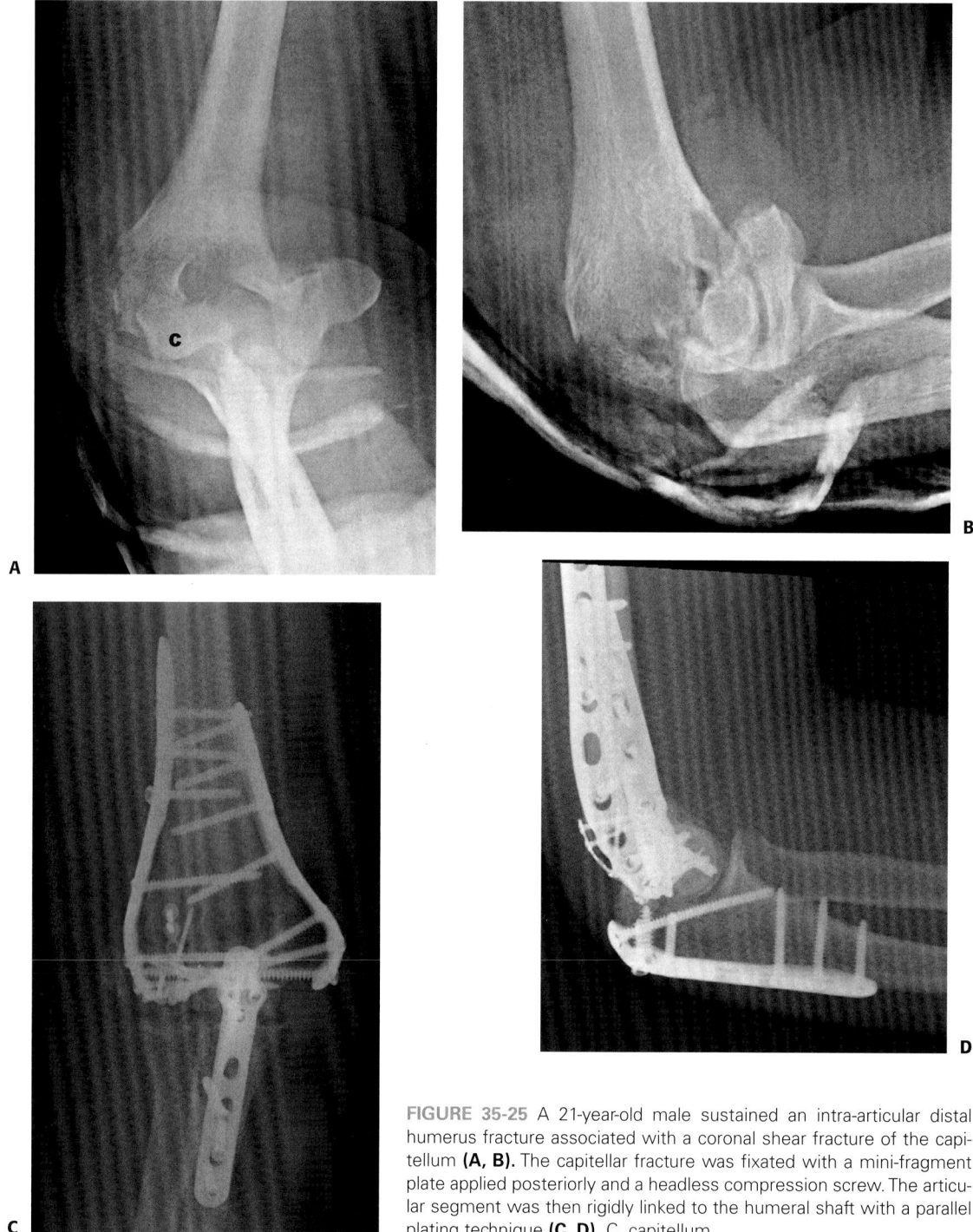

FIGURE 35-25 A 21-year-old male sustained an intra-articular distal humerus fracture associated with a coronal shear fracture of the capitellum **(A, B).** The capitellar fracture was fixated with a mini-fragment plate applied posteriorly and a headless compression screw. The articular segment was then rigidly linked to the humeral shaft with a parallel plating technique **(C, D).** C, capitellum.

can be approached through an extensile posterior skin incision or a direct lateral skin incision. The advantages of a posterior longitudinal skin incision are that it allows access both medially and laterally and it decreases the risk of cutaneous nerve injury.[42] The deep lateral approach is via Kocher's interval[105] between anconeus and ECU. The arthrotomy is made anterior to the LUCL and is extended proximally along the anterior aspect of the lateral supracondylar ridge, which then allows access to the

fractured capitellum. The fragment is typically anteriorly displaced and is reduced by elbow extension, forearm supination, and by application of a gentle varus force. Once an anatomic reduction is obtained the fragment is provisionally fixated with smooth small diameter K-wires. Permanent rigid internal fixation is obtained by countersunk screws[138,202] placed anterior to posterior through the articular surface (Fig. 35-26), or by screws placed into the capitellum in a retrograde fashion from

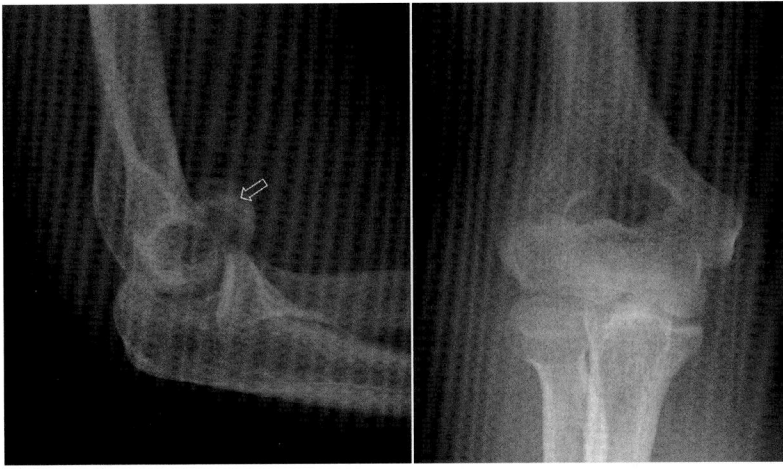 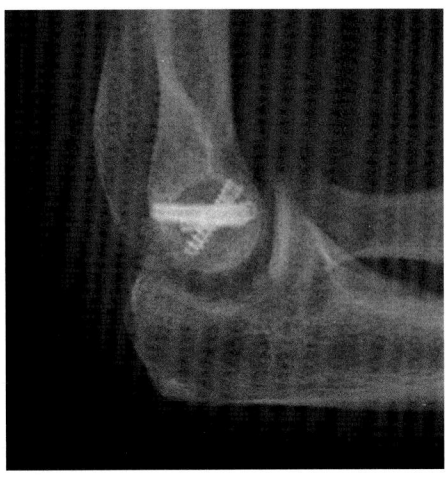

A **B**

FIGURE 35-26 Fracture of the capitellum and the lateral ridge of the trochlea **(A).** The double arc sign[126] is evident on the lateral radiograph (*arrow*). One arc represents the subchondral bone of the capitellum and the other arc represents the lateral ridge of the trochlea. This patient underwent open reduction and internal fixation with three headless compression screws inserted anterior to posterior **(B).**

the posterior aspect of the lateral column, or by a combined method (Fig. 35-27). The placement of posterior to anterior screws has been shown to be biomechanically more stable and has the added clinical benefit of not violating the articular surface.[48] In cases where rigid internal fixation is obtained, early active range of motion can be initiated.

When there is comminution or impaction of the posterior aspect of the lateral column (Ring et al.[181] type III and Dubberley et al.[43] type B), it may prevent anatomic reduction of the anterior capitellar fracture. These impaction fractures may require disimpaction and possibly bone grafting to fill the bony defects. In case with severe posterior comminution that may compromise anterior articular fixation, supplemental posterior lateral column plating may be required. Capitellar fractures that involve the lateral epicondyle (Ring et al. type II) may be exposed by using the lateral epicondylar fracture as an osteotomy, reflecting the epicondylar fragment with the origin of the LCL distally (Fig. 35-28). After fixation of the capitellum, the lateral epicondyle fracture may be fixated with screws or a plate, if large enough. If the fragment is too small to fixate, it is treated as a lateral ligament tear with repair through bone tunnels.

Rigid internal fixation of the Kocher-Lorenz[117,126] or conventional type II osteochondral fractures is difficult as the fragments are thin and may be comminuted. Treatment options for these fractures include attempted fixation with bioabsorbable pins, excision of the fragment, osteochondral grafts, or capitellar arthroplasty.

Surgical Technique for Capitellum and Trochlea Fractures (AO/OTA Type B3.3). Capitellar fractures that involve a large portion of the trochlea also require anatomic reduction and rigid internal fixation. Generally, these fractures require improved exposure of the medial trochlea and several surgical approach options exist. The LCL origin on the lateral epicondyle can be released to allow the elbow to be hinged open laterally. By releasing the

anterior and posterior joint capsules the distal humerus articular surface is booked open on the intact MCL. A similar approach utilizes a lateral epicondylar fracture, which may be reflected distally to hinge open the elbow joint. In addition, medial joint exposure can be obtained by a separate medial approach, such as the flexor–pronator split or the Hotchkiss medial "over-the-top" approach. Finally, an olecranon osteotomy can be used to obtain optimum distal humerus articular exposure.

Once exposed, these fractures are rigidly secured with small diameter headless compression or standard countersunk screws inserted antegrade, or with standard screws inserted retrograde. Fractures that are comminuted or have epicondylar involvement may benefit from additional plate application. Bone grafting may also be required for fractures that are comminuted or impacted.

Isolated trochlear fractures (AO/OTA type B3.2) are rare and should be treated with ORIF. Fixation may be done antegrade through the cartilage or retrograde from posterior through a medial deep approach.

Surgical Technique for Arthroscopic Reduction and Percutaneous Fixation. Arthroscopic reduction and percutaneous cannulated screw fixation is a described technique for treatment of isolated fractures of the capitellum.[109] The indications are narrow and include an acute, noncomminuted, simple, isolated fracture of the capitellum. Relative contraindications are associated comminution, posterolateral impaction, delayed presentation, and associated instability.

The technique is demanding and a prerequisite is experience with elbow arthroscopy. Generally, the set up involves arthroscopic equipment and instruments, intraoperative fluoroscopy, and cannulated screw instrumentation. The patient is positioned lateral decubitus with the affected elbow flexed over an arthroscopic elbow positioner. A sterile tourniquet is used and a C-arm fluoroscopy unit is positioned such that appropriate intraoperative images can be obtained during

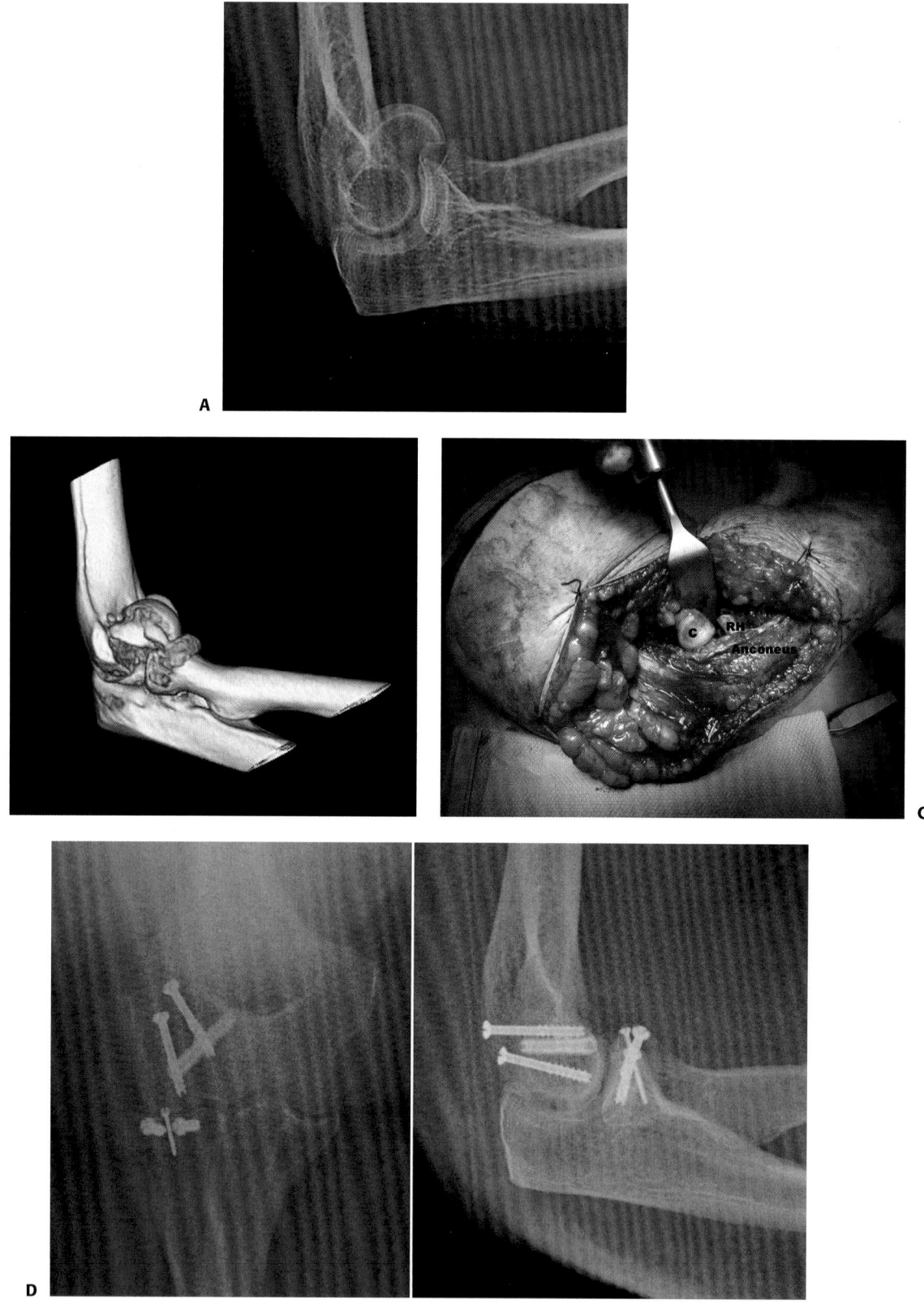

FIGURE 35-27 Fracture of the capitellum and lateral ridge of trochlea associated with a radial head fracture **(A, B).** Through a posterior longitudinal skin incision, Kocher's interval was used to approach the fractures for open reduction and internal fixation **(C, D).** C, capitellum; RH, radial head.

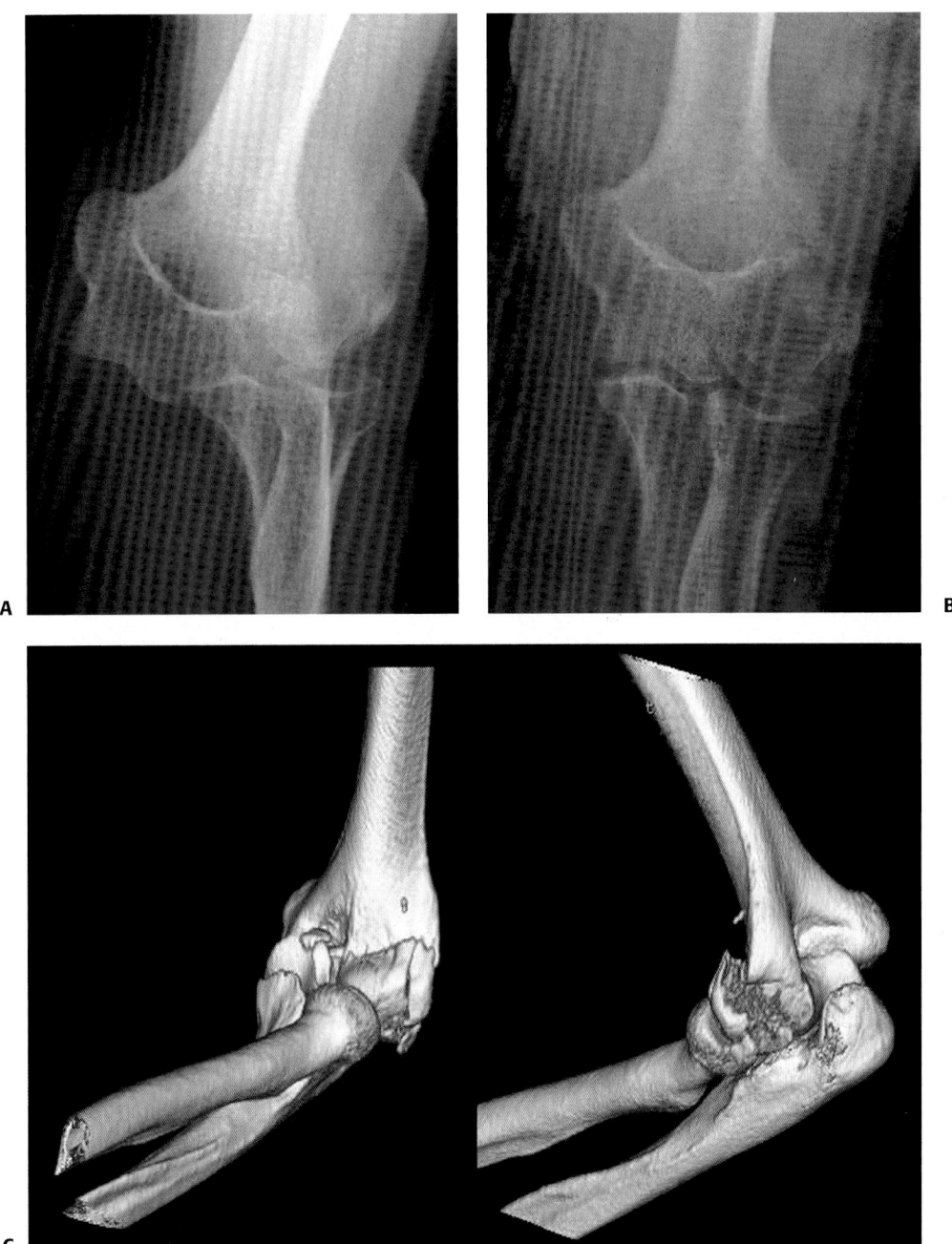

FIGURE 35-28 Posterolateral dislocation of the elbow associated with a capitellar fracture, lateral epicondyle fracture, and comminution and impaction of the posterior aspect of the lateral column **(A–C).**

(*continues*)

arthroscopy. The standard arthroscopy portals are marked and the elbow joint is entered anteriorly. The hemarthrosis is evacuated and the displaced capitellar fracture visualized. It is the author's preference to now switch the camera to view the radiocapitellar joint from posterior. Through the posterolateral radiocapitellar portal, the radial head and the fracture bed of the capitellum will be visiable. A closed reduction is now conducted as outlined in the previous section on closed reduction and casting. The articular reduction, once obtained,

will be visible from the posterolateral portal (Fig. 35-29) and can also be confirmed by viewing from anterior. Following an anatomic reduction, percutaneous cannulated screws can be placed posterior to anterior into the capitellum using fluoroscopic assistance.

The outcome studies on arthroscopic reduction and percutaneous screw fixation are few. Kuriyama et al.[109] described a case report of two patients and Hardy et al.[72] of one patient, all with good outcomes and healing at short term follow-up.

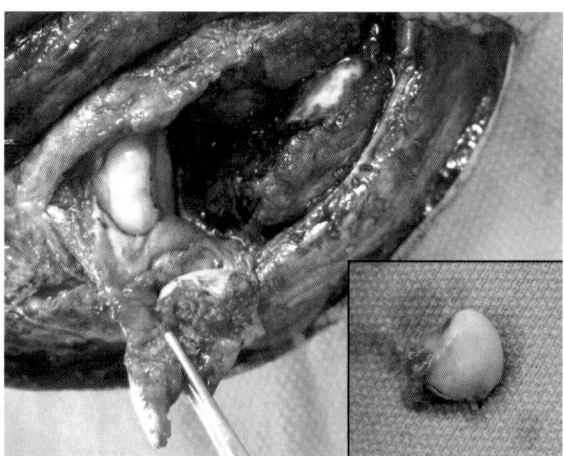

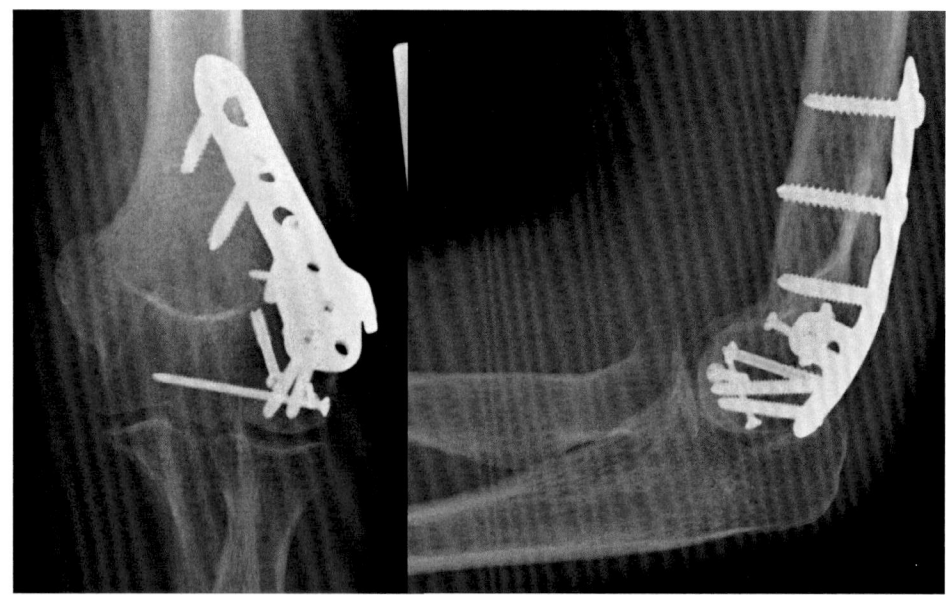

FIGURE 35-28 *(continued)* The lateral epicondyle fracture with the lateral collateral ligament (forceps) was reflected distally **(D)**, allowing access to the free capitellar fragment *(inset)*. Because of the posterior comminution, a posterolateral plate was required to support the articular segment **(E).**

Implant Biomechanics for ORIF. Controversy exists on which implant designs and plate configurations confer the greatest amount of stability when treating distal humerus fractures. Jacobson et al.[89] tested five different distal humerus plating constructs in cadaveric specimens. They reported that a medially applied 3.5-mm reconstruction plate along with an orthogonally applied posterolateral 3.5-mm dynamic compression plate provided the greatest sagittal plane stiffness, and equivalent frontal plane and torsion stiffness, when compared to other constructs which included parallel and triple plating. Helfet and Hotchkiss[75] also found that orthogonal plating provided greater rigidity and fatigue resistance when compared to a single "Y" plate or crossed screws.

In contrast, Schemitsch et al.[197] found that parallel plating with a medial 3.5-mm reconstruction plate and a lateral "J" plate had the greatest construct rigidity when compared to four other plate configurations, including orthogonal plating with 3.5-mm reconstruction plates. Self et al.[200] found that parallel plating trended toward having greater rigidity and load to failure than orthogonal plating; however, the differences did not reach statistical significance. Arnander et al.,[12] however, found that two 3.5-mm reconstruction plates applied in a parallel fashion did have statistically significant increased stiffness and strength in the sagittal plane when compared to two 3.5-mm reconstruction plates applied orthogonally.

Locking plates have several theoretical advantages, especially when used in patients with severe osteopenia. Schuster et al.[199] demonstrated that locking 3.5-mm reconstruction plates applied orthogonally had superior cyclic failure properties when compared to conventional nonlocked plates applied in a similar fashion in cadavers with low bone mineral density. Stoffel et al.[210] compared the mechanical stability of two different commercially available precontoured locking distal humeral plating systems. They reported significantly higher stability in

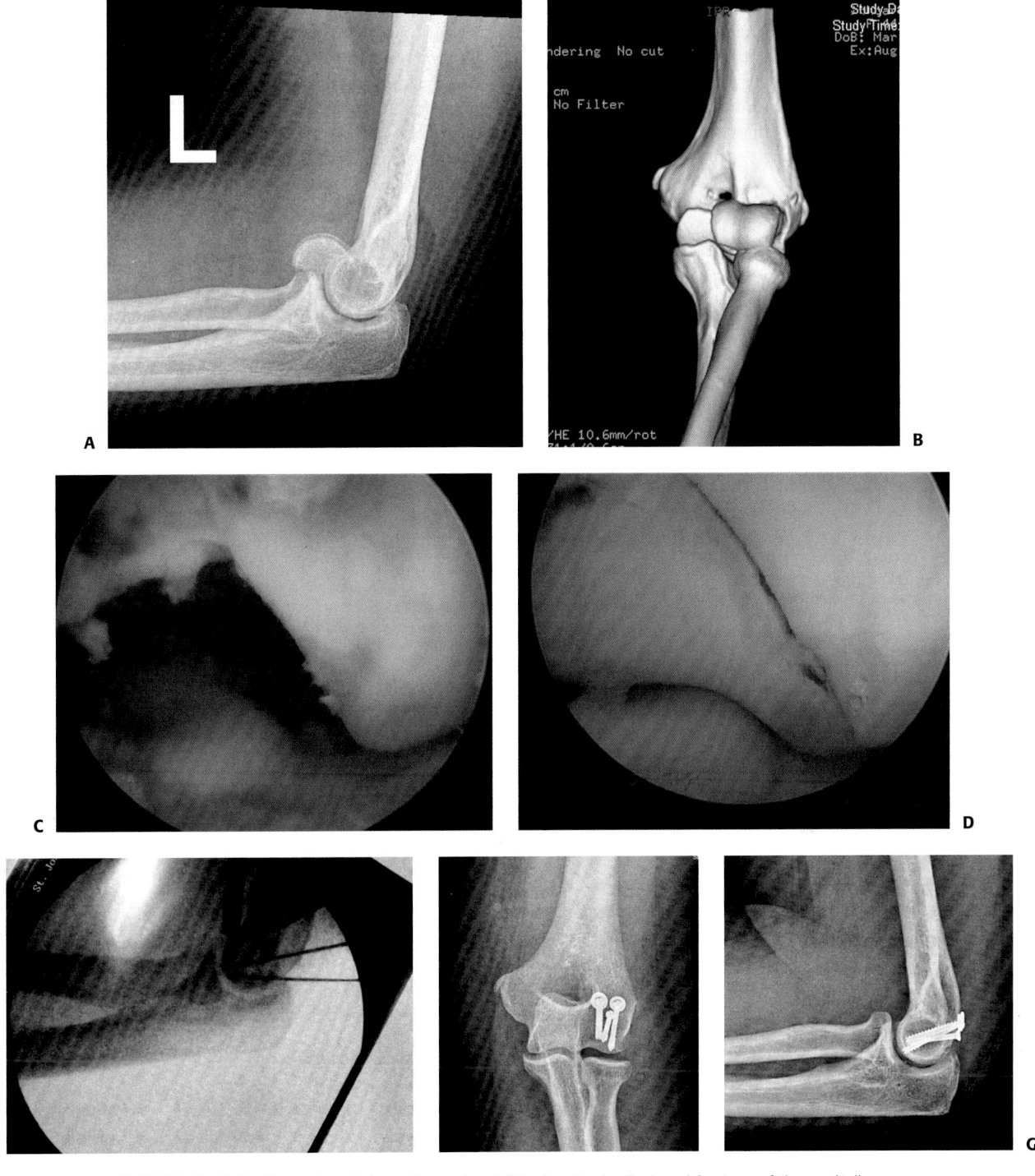

FIGURE 35-29 Radiograph and three-dimensional CT of a simple displaced fracture of the capitellum and lateral trochlea **(A, B)**. An arthroscopic reduction with percutaneous cannulated screw fixation was done. Viewing from the posterolateral portal, the radial head, proximal radioulnar joint, and the fracture bed of the capitellum are visible **(C)**. After a reduction maneuver, the fracture reduction is assessed arthroscopically **(D)** and fluoroscopically **(E)**. At 1-year follow-up after screw fixation, radiographs **(F, G)** demonstrate anatomic healing.

compression, external rotation, and a greater ability to resist axial plastic deformation in the parallel plate system versus the orthogonal plate system. It should be noted that no clinical difference has yet been demonstrated between parallel and orthogonal plating, and more likely than not, both are acceptable as long as the principles of rigid internal fixation are met.

On the contrary, there is no debate in the use of 1/3 tubular plates, which have been shown to have insufficient strength and are susceptible to breakage.[80,154,155,216] These plates should not be used in the primary two-plate construct; however, they may be used as a supplementary third plate.

Postoperative Care. Patients are placed in a well-padded plaster extension splint applied anteriorly and are encouraged to keep the arm elevated to minimize swelling. Active hand range of motion is started immediately. Elbow range of motion is started between days 2 and 7 postoperatively, depending on the status of the incision. Generally, active-assisted and active range of motion are encouraged (flexion, extension, pronation,

and supination) for patients with a paratricipital approach or an olecranon osteotomy fixated with a plate. Passive extension is reserved for patients who underwent an extensor mechanism disrupting approach. Typically, a night extension splint is used for the first 6 weeks. At 6 weeks post operation, passive stretching and static progressive splinting are used if required. Strengthening may begin at 12 weeks, provided there is evidence of radiographic union.

Potential Pitfalls and Preventative Measures. Surgical reconstruction of a comminuted intra-articular distal humerus fracture requires a systematic approach, starting with the appropriate exposure and concluding with stable fixation in order to initiate early motion. Potential pitfalls include an ineffective exposure such as using a paratricipital approach to visualize and conduct ORIF on a highly comminuted distal humerus articular segment. Advanced approaches, such as an olecranon osteotomy or another extensor mechanism releasing approach, should be considered for effective visualization. The

TABLE 35-4   Potential Pitfalls and Preventions for ORIF of Distal Humerus Fractures

Distal Humerus Fracture Potential Pitfalls and Preventions

Pitfall	Prevention
Missed skin tenting, excessive swelling, fracture blisters	Application of a well-padded splint while awaiting surgery Re-check skin, soft tissues, and neurovascular status immediately before surgery
Unrecognized coronal shear fractures and articular comminution (fracture line between medial trochlea and medial epicondyle)	CT scan for complex fracture patterns (preferred) or traction radiographs Appropriate surgical approach for visualization Have supplementary fixation available (headless compression screws, threaded K-wires, and/or bioabsorbable pins)
Failure to recognize bone loss in open fractures	CT scan for complex fracture patterns Be prepared for bone grafting by adding it to the surgical consent form and by prepping and draping the iliac crest. Understand technique of supracondylar shortening
Ineffective surgical exposure	Critically examine fracture pattern and choose an approach that balances required visualization for ORIF vs. complications Understand extensile options
Irreparable distal humerus fracture with comminution and osteopenia in an elderly patient	Be prepared for total elbow arthroplasty, add to consent, and have the system available Conduct a surgical approach that is conducive for elbow arthroplasty
Radial nerve injury with placement of a long lateral plate	Understand radial nerve anatomy Radial nerve identification and protection for "high" lateral column fractures
Inadequate fixation of "low" transcolumn fractures	Place as many screws as possible into the distal articular segment Use fracture-specific plates that allow high-density distal screw placement
Screws placed across the olecranon fossa causing impingement	Use fluoroscopy to ensure all hardware is extra-articular and of appropriate length Check elbow range of motion to ensure there is no impingement Visually confirm the absence of intra-articular or impinging screws
Supracondylar nonunion	Compress the articular segment to the shaft with plate compression technique Be prepared to bonegraft or conduct supracondylar shortening in cases with bone loss
Ulnar neuropathy	Identify and protect ulnar nerve during surgical approach and ORIF Preoperative neurologic examination to document pre-existing nerve injuries

choice of plates with insufficient strength, such as semi-tubular plates, has been shown to increase the rate of implant failure, nonunion, and malunion. This is no longer an issue with commercially available fracture-specific contoured plating systems, which tend to have plates of sufficient strength. Other potential pitfalls include intra-articular screws, screws placed into the olecranon fossa resulting in impingement, decreasing the width of a comminuted trochlea fracture with lag screws, and radial nerve injury with placement of a long lateral plate. The above mentioned complications are preventable with awareness and sound surgical technique. Please see Table 35-4 for other potential pitfalls and their preventions.

Treatment-Specific Outcomes

Outcomes of ORIF of Extra-Articular and Complete-Articular Fractures. When the principles of anatomic restoration of the joint surface, bicolumn plating, and rigid internal fixation to allow early range of motion are employed, good outcomes can be expected for patients with intra-articular distal humerus fractures.[6,13,41,47,57,67,69,82,159,160,161,190,193,205,216,229] When[15,50,113,115,175] averaging the outcomes of 21 series published between 2002 and 2012 (Table 35-5), 85% of patients experienced good to excellent outcomes at a mean follow-up of 50 months. Doornberg et al.[41] have shown that the rate of good to excellent outcomes is durable in the long term (12 to 30 years). Patients who sustain isolated intra-articular fractures of the distal humerus can expect some loss of elbow range of motion, although, functional range of motion (30 to 130 degrees) is usually attained. As would be expected, patients who sustain distal humerus fractures in association with polytrauma or severe soft tissue injuries can anticipate worse outcomes.

Gofton et al.[64] reported the patient-rated outcomes and physical impairments after orthogonal plating of AO/OTA type C distal humerus fractures in 23 patients. The SF-36 scores of patients at final follow-up compared to age- and sex-matched controls showed no significant differences. Patients rated their overall satisfaction at 93% and on functional assessment indicated a 10% subjective loss of function when comparing the affected to unaffected limb. The mean score on the DASH questionnaire was 12, which is very close to the overall normative score of 10.1.[84] The isometric strength of the affected elbow was significantly reduced in all ranges, although, grip and pinch strength were not statistically different between affected and unaffected limbs. McKee et al.[130] also found decreased strength in the affected elbows and rated it at approximately 75% of normal. The mean DASH score was 20 points, indicating a mild residual impairment. Two of the eight parameters of the SF-36, physical function, and role-physical, demonstrated small but significant differences between age-matched controls.

Outcomes of ORIF of Partial Articular Fractures. The outcomes after ORIF of capitellar fractures with or without involvement of the lateral trochlear ridge have been shown to be predictably good.[34,43,54,65,87,120,138,172,179,181,196,202] More complex fracture patterns with involvement of the anterior trochlea also have a relatively good prognosis[43,126,181,208]; however, Dubberley et al.[43] have shown that the outcomes do deteriorate with increasing fracture complexity.

Total Elbow Arthroplasty for Distal Humerus Fractures

Indications/Contraindications. Nonoperative treatment of distal humerus fractures, although appropriate for some elderly patients, often leads to loss of motion and unsatisfactory functional outcomes. Open reduction and rigid internal fixation is considered gold standard; however, it may not be attainable in elderly patients with osteopenia, comminution, and articular fragmentation or in patients with pre-existing conditions of the elbow such as RA (Fig. 35-30). In cases where rigid internal fixation cannot be achieved to allow early range of motion, resultant prolonged immobilization often leads to poor outcomes.[4] TEA for such fractures is a reliable treatment option with good outcomes.[11,57,60,74,97,98,99,112,147,149,173]

Absolute contraindications to TEA for distal humerus fractures include active infection and insufficient soft tissue coverage. The most important relative contraindication to elbow replacement for trauma is the younger active patient who is more appropriate for ORIF. Elderly patients with low-energy Gustilo and Anderson grade I open fractures are not an absolute contraindication to elbow arthroplasty. Generally, the wounds are punctures that are small and clean. However, if there has been a time delay until open fracture management or the cleanliness of a wound is questioned, a staged procedure with initial irrigation and debridement followed by splinting and antibiotics until definitive surgery is deemed appropriate.

Distal humerus hemiarthroplasty is another surgical option for unreconstructible partial articular fractures (Fig. 35-31). In cases with severe articular destruction with preserved columns and collateral ligaments, hemiarthroplasty presents an attractive option that resurfaces the damaged articulation. The theoretical advantage of a hemiarthroplasty is the absence of polyethylene wear debris and the associated osteolysis; however, it is a technically demanding procedure and no literature exists to support its use over TEA. Further studies are required to determine the role of distal humerus hemiarthroplasty in elbow trauma.

Preoperative Planning. TEA is a technically demanding procedure and should be done by an experienced upper limb or trauma surgeon. As with ORIF, anteroposterior and lateral radiographs of the elbow out of plaster are usually sufficient to determine the fracture pattern. If the feasibility of ORIF is questioned in an elderly patient, a CT scan may assist with the preoperative decision making.

Preoperatively, elbow radiographs should be templated to ensure implants of the appropriate size and lengths are available. Associated fractures or unique fracture patterns that may complicate elbow arthroplasty must be examined for, including proximal ulnar shaft fractures, olecranon fractures, and proximal fracture extension into the humeral diaphysis. While awaiting surgery, patients are placed in a well-padded elbow splint and are encouraged to elevate the arm, ice the elbow, and to maintain hand and finger range of motion. On the day of surgery, the skin and soft tissues are re-examined and the neurologic status is redocumented.

Positioning. Patients generally receive a general anesthetic with an upper extremity regional block for postoperative

TABLE 35-5 **Summary of Outcomes of AO/OTA Type C (Intra-Articular) Distal Humerus Fractures**

Author	Year	Number of Fractures	Average Age of Patients (Range)	Percentage of Open Fractures	Surgical Approach	Average Follow-up in Months (Range)	Outcome Assessment Used	Percentage with Excellent or Good Outcomes	Percentage with Satisfactory or Poor Outcomes
Pajarinen[161]	2002	18	44 (16–81)	28	OO[a]	25 (10–41)	OTA	56	44
Ozdemir[159]	2002	34	38 (20–78)	15	OO	82 (24–141)	Jupiter	62	38
Gupta[69]	2002	55	39 (18–65)	11	13 OO 42 TS	48 (24–108)	Aitken	93	7
Robinson[189]	2003	119	53 (13–99)	15	OO	19 (5–32)	n/a	n/a	n/a
Gofton[64]	2003	23	45 (14–89)	30	OO[a]	45 (14–89)	DASH, PRUNE, ASES-e, SF-36	93	7
Yang[229]	2003	17	41 (16–69)	29	OO	17 (13–38)	MEPS	88	12
Frankle[57]	2003	12	74 (65-86)	0	10 OO; 2 TS	57 (24–78)	MEPS	67	33
Allende[6]	2004	40	42 (16–77)	25	31 OO; 9 TR	47 (13–94)	Jupiter, OTA	85	15
Aslam[13]	2004	26	56 (18–82)	12	OO	35 (24–48)	Broberg/ Morrey	70	30
Soon[205]	2004	12	43 (21–80)	0	5 OO; 7 TS	11 (2–21)	MEPS	92	8
Huang[82]	2005	19	72 (65–79)	5	OO	97 (60–174)	Cassebaum, MEPS	100	0
Ozer[160]	2005	11	58 (16–70)	27	TRAP	26 (14–40)	OTA	91	9
Sanchez-Sotelo[b193]	2007	34	58 (16–99)	41	17 TRAP 5 OO 8 PT 2 BM 2 TT	24 (12–60)	MEPS	84	16
Doornberg[41]	2007	30	35 (13–64)	30	20 OO	19 yrs (12–30 yrs)	DASH ASES-e MEPS	87	13
Ek[47]	2008	7	41 (12–73)	14	BM	35 (6–78)	MEPS, SF-36 DASH	100	0
Greiner[b67]	2008	12	55 (21–83)	42	OO[a]	10 (6–14)	MEPS DASH	100	0
Athwal[15]	2009	32	56 (19–88)	31	18 OO 12 TRAP 1 PT 1 TT	27 (12–54)	MEPS DASH	69	31
Liu[115]	2009	32	69 (62–79)	n/a	OO	24.5 (14–60)	MEPS	100	0
Li[113]	2011	56	50 (18–70)	23	OO	30 (6–70)	ROM	n/a	n/a
Puchwein[175]	2011	22	43 (15–88)	27	19 OO[a]	69 ± 33	Cassebaum Jupiter Quick-DASH	82	18
Erpelding[b,50]	2012	17	47 (18–85)	21	PT	27 (5–82)	MEPS DASH	92	8
Total/Mean	—	628	50	21		47		85	15

[a]Olecranon osteotomy performed in most cases.
[b]Most fracture type C.

OO, olecranon osteotomy; TS, triceps split; n/a, not applicable; PRUNE, patient rated ulnar nerve evaluation; TR, triceps reflecting; TRAP, triceps reflecting anconeus pedicle; PT, paratricipital; BM, Bryan-Morrey; TT, triceps tongue; ROM, range of motion.

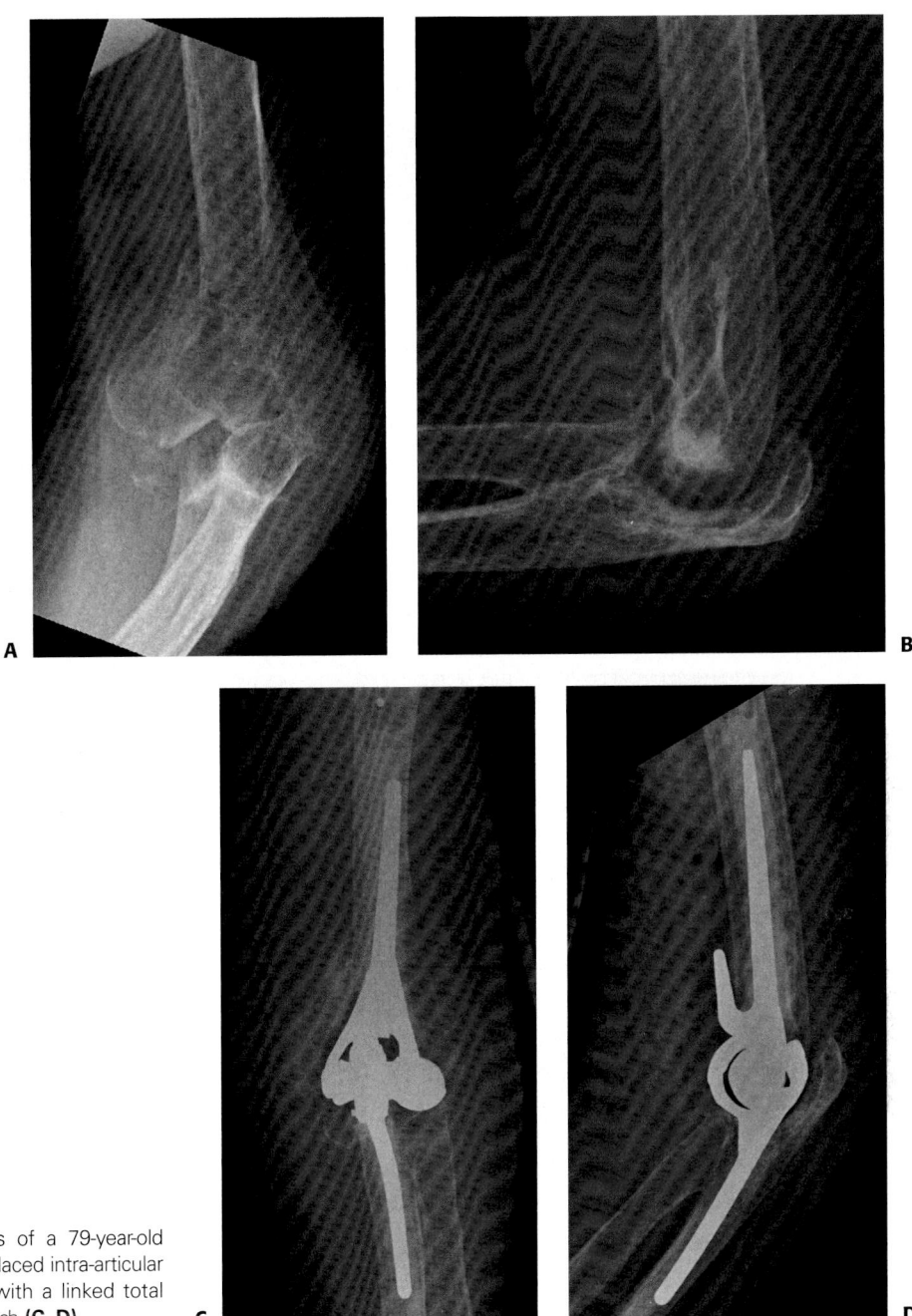

FIGURE 35-30 AP and lateral radiographs of a 79-year-old woman with rheumatoid arthritis and a displaced intra-articular medial column fracture **(A, B)** managed with a linked total elbow arthroplasty via a paratricipital approach **(C, D).**

pain control and therapy. The patient is positioned supine with a bolster placed under the ipsilateral scapula and the elbow is supported by another bolster made of wrapped sterile sheet on the patient's chest (Fig. 35-13). The surgeon and assistant stand on the side of the injury while the scrub nurse and arthroplasty instruments are on the contralateral side, allowing the nurse to assist with arm positioning as required. A sterile tourniquet is used. Before starting the operative procedure and inflating the tourniquet, prophylactic antibiotics are administered intravenously.

Surgical Approach(es). In general, posterior approaches are preferred in the exposure of distal humerus fractures in preparation for elbow arthroplasty. Although all posterior approaches may be used for arthroplasty, some have advantages over others. The paratricipital approach has the advantage of maintaining complete integrity of the extensor mechanisms while its disadvantage is that it increases the complexity of the procedure because it provides less visualization of the proximal ulna. The triceps splitting, triceps reflecting, and triceps dividing approaches all provide good visualization of the elbow joint; however, they all disrupt the triceps insertion in one way or another, and therefore require postoperative protection. Conducting a TEA through an olecranon osteotomy is possible, however, not encouraged. Ulnar component fixation

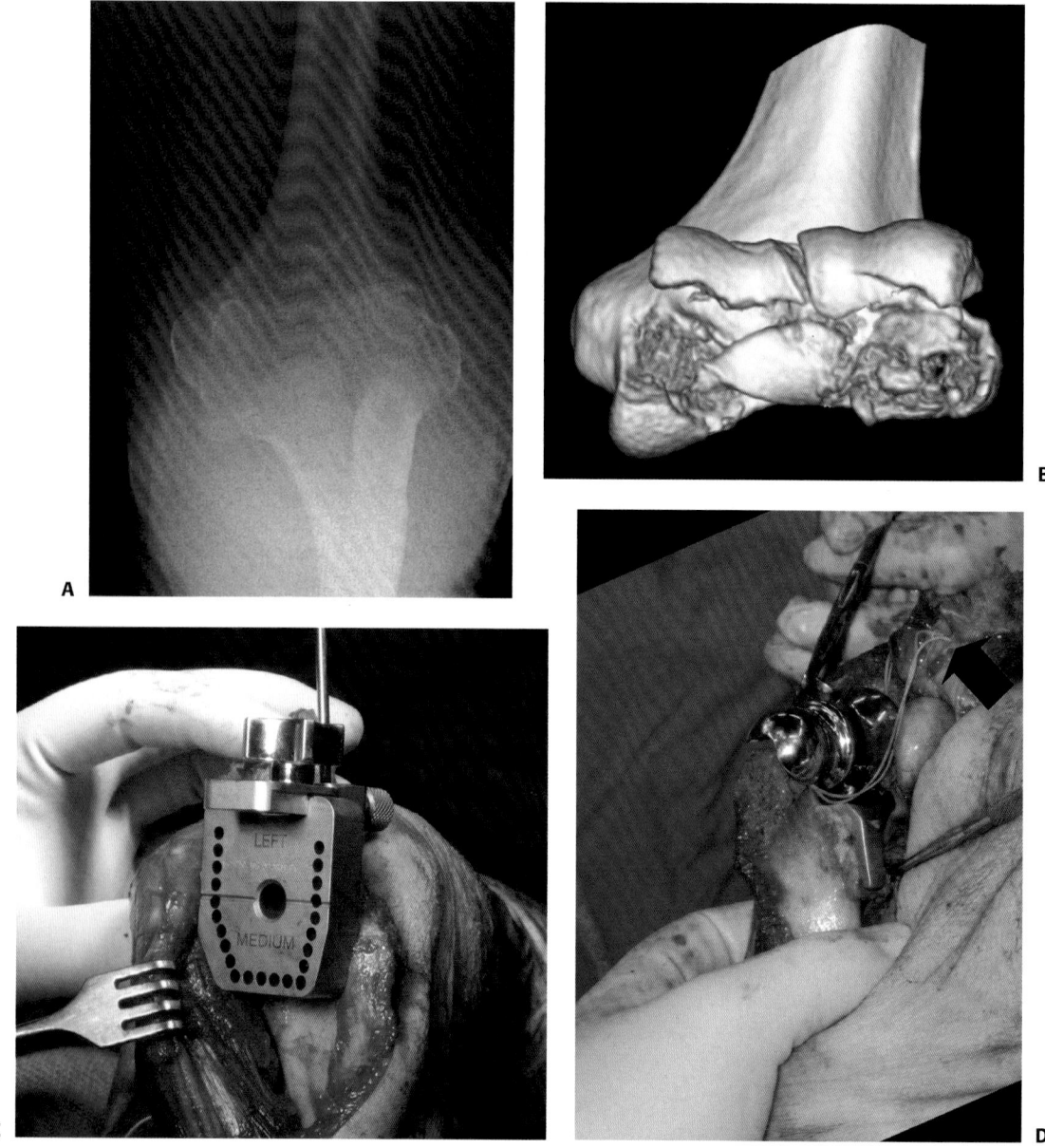

FIGURE 35-31 Fractures of the capitellum, trochlea, and lateral epicondyle **(A)** with associated osteo-chondral fragmentation **(B)** in a 78-year-old active woman. As the fracture was deemed unrepairable intraoperatively, hemiarthroplasty was done via an approach that hinged open the elbow on the intact medial collateral ligament **(C, D)**.

may be compromised with certain implant designs. There are also concerns with osteotomy healing after disruption of the intramedullary blood supply by ulnar component cementation.

My preferred approach for fractures deemed unreparable preoperatively, where the surgical plan is to proceed directly to TEA, is the paratricipital approach. This is also my preferred approach if an attempt at ORIF is planned for less comminuted articular fractures. In circumstances with high articular comminution in the elderly, where a complete attempt at ORIF is planned, with the intraoperative bailout being a TEA, I prefer the triceps split approach. The triceps split approach affords the

best visualization of the joint for a complete attempt at ORIF, while still leaving the option open for a TEA if rigid internal fixation cannot be achieved.

Another approach commonly used for TEA is the Bryan-Morrey approach.[26] The approach has been termed "triceps-sparing" which has led to confusion. The approach does not "spare" the triceps, but rather detaches the triceps tendon in continuity with the ulnar periosteum and anconeus creating a large reflection or sleeve. The ulnar nerve is first identified and protected, and then the triceps insertion and the ulnar periosteum are sharply reflected off the proximal ulna in a medial

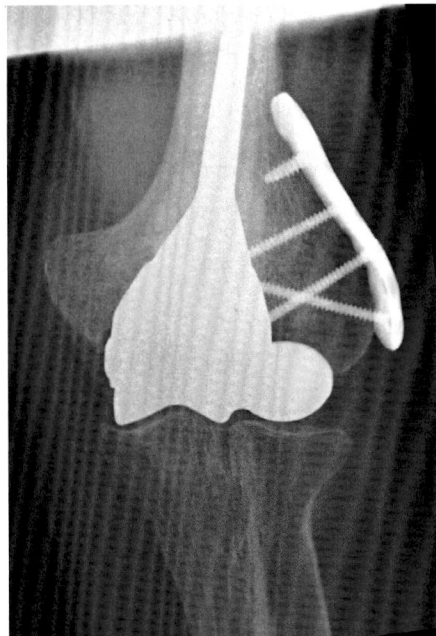
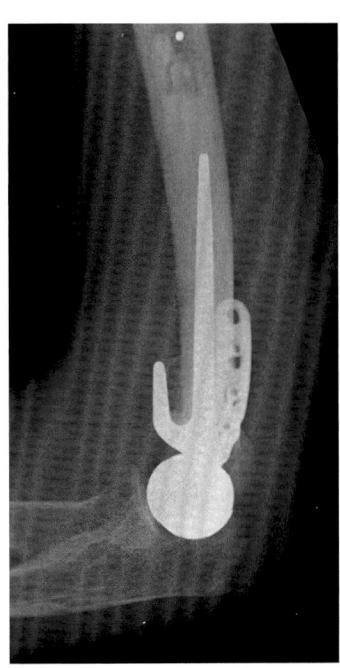

FIGURE 35-31 (*continued*) The lateral epicondyle fracture was fixated with sutures through the axis of the implant (*arrow*) and with a precontoured unicortical plate **(E, F)**.

E

F

to lateral direction (Fig. 35-32). The sleeve of tissue created incorporates the anconeus muscle. As with the triceps splitting approach, careful and solid repair of the triceps tendon is required via transosseous sutures. It is my preference not to use approaches that detach the extensor mechanism during arthro-

plasty for fracture; however, the Bryan-Morrey approach does allow better visualization of the joint, specifically the proximal ulna for ulnar component preparation and insertion.

Technique. Generally, a linked design of TEA should be used in the setting of distal humerus fracture. Unlinked designs

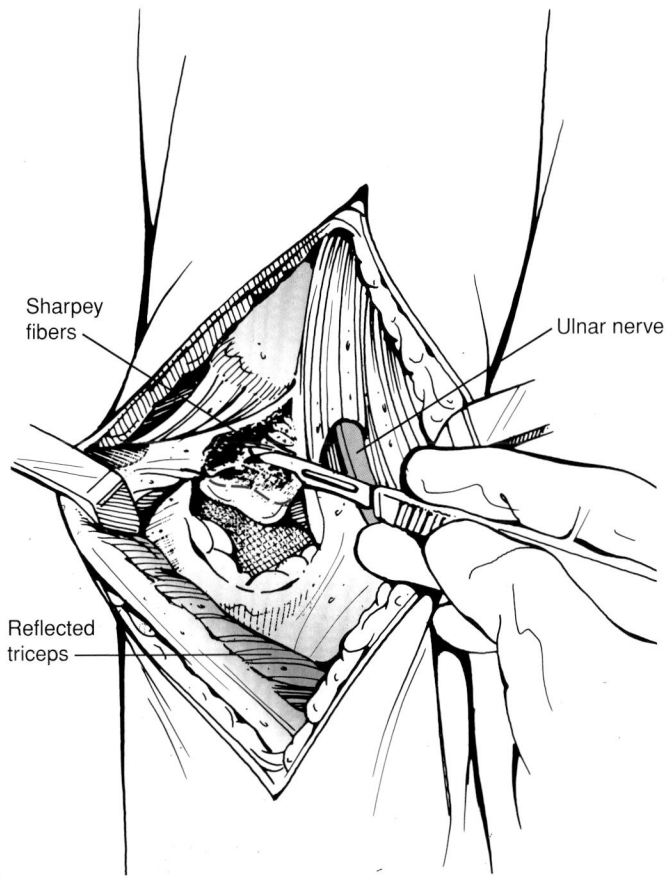

Sharpey fibers

Ulnar nerve

Reflected triceps

A

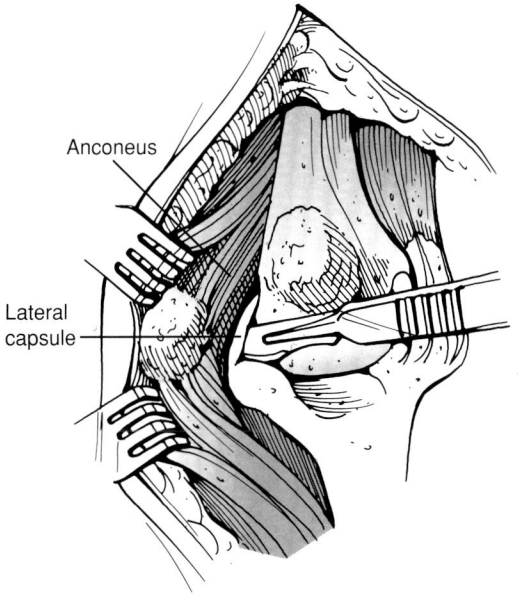

Anconeus

Lateral capsule

B

FIGURE 35-32 The Bryan-Morrey[26] approach is commonly used for total elbow arthroplasty. A posterior longitudinal skin incision is used and the ulnar nerve is identified and protected. The ulnar periosteum, triceps insertion, and anconeus muscle are sharply reflected off the proximal ulna in a medial **(A)** to lateral **(B)** direction. To access the articular surfaces for arthroplasty, the collateral ligaments are released.

may be used; however, great care must be taken in anatomically reducing and rigidly fixing the medial and lateral columns. Anatomic fixation of the columns allows appropriate tensioning of the MCLs and LCLs, which are required for unlinked implant stability.

The key steps for insertion of a linked elbow arthroplasty are discussed via a paratricipital approach. McKee et al.[131] have shown that condylar resection during TEA does not affect strength or functional outcome; therefore, through the medial arthrotomy while protecting the ulnar nerve, the MCL is released and the medial fracture fragments are excised. Similarly, through the lateral arthrotomy the LCL complex is released and the lateral fracture fragments are excised. The distal humeral shaft with the remaining metaphyseal bone can now be delivered from under the triceps and ulna. The humerus is then prepared following the steps outlined in the technical manual of the implant being used. Usually, the metaphyseal cutting blocks are not required, as the fractured condyles have already been excised. The keys to judging correct humeral component rotation are to examine the trefoil shape of the distal humerus shaft, as the posterior cortex is typically externally rotated about 14 degrees relative to the elbow flexion–extension axis.[192] Reaming and broaching of the humeral canal is done as described in the technical manual and the canal is sized for a cement restrictor. The length of the humerus and the level of the joint line must also be re-created. This is done by placing the resected condyles onto the remaining humeral shaft to measure the location of the joint line. The tension in the soft tissues can also be used to judge appropriate humeral component length, once trial components are in place. Most humeral components are designed with an anterior flange that accepts a bone graft, which can be prepared from resected bone fragments.

Preparation of the ulna with the paratricipital approach requires strategic retractor and arm positioning. The proximal ulna is delivered medial to the humeral shaft to avoid excessive tension on the ulnar nerve. The forearm is then rotated 90 degrees, the elbow is flexed, and a rake retractor is used to draw back the triceps insertion to allow exposure of the greater sigmoid notch. The tip of the olecranon may be excised to improve visualization of the greater sigmoid notch. The ulna is prepared as per the manufacturer's recommendations. As with the humerus, particular attention should be taken to ensure correct ulnar component placement. The correct rotation of the ulnar component can be determined by ensuring the axis of rotation bisects the radial head and by ensuring the axis is parallel to the flat surface on the proximal dorsal ulna.[44]

It is recommended that antibiotic laden bone cement be used and cement restrictors for the humeral and ulnar canals.[53] Cement is inserted into the humerus first with a small diameter nozzle and then into the ulna. The ulnar cement is manually pressurized and the component is inserted followed by pressurization of the humeral cement and humeral component insertion. Excess bone cement is removed and the components are held still until the cement has cured. In cases with extremely small ulnar canals, an extra small cement injection nozzle may be required. The humeral and ulnar components can be cemented together as described or separately. Once cured, a wedge of bonegraft fashioned from the resected articular segment is placed underneath the anterior flange of the humeral component. The components are then linked and the elbow is taken through a range of motion to ensure there is no impingement. Conversely, the implants can be linked just after insertion and the elbow placed into extension until the cement cures.

Postoperative Care. After the surgical procedure, the elbow is splinted in extension with an anteriorly applied slab of plaster. The arm is elevated for 24 hours and active hand range of motion is started immediately. Elbow range of motion is started between days 7 and 10 days postoperatively, depending on the status of the incision and soft tissues. Generally, unrestricted active range of motion is encouraged (flexion, extension, pronation, and supination) for patients with a paratricipital approach while patients with a triceps split approach are restricted to gravity-assisted extension for 6 weeks to protect the triceps repair.

Potential Pitfalls and Preventative Measures. TEA for fracture should be conducted by an experienced trauma or upper extremity surgeon. The operative procedure requires a systematic approach, starting with the correct indications, the appropriate surgical approach, and adherence to the technical steps to ensure correct implantation and alignment. Potential pitfalls (Table 35-6) include an ineffective exposure, such as using an olecranon osteotomy to approach an unreconstructable distal humerus fracture in an elderly patient. Typically, for distal humerus fractures undergoing arthroplasty, a triceps-on approach is preferred. Other potential pitfalls are incorrect implant selection and alignment. In general, a linked TEA is preferred for the management of distal humerus fractures. Although unlinked designs may be used, they are technically challenging as anatomic fixation of the epicondylar fractures and repair of the ligaments would be required to ensure implant stability. Misalignment of the implants must also be prevented. Sabo et al.[192] identified that in cases of distal humeral bone loss, where anatomic landmarks for alignment are absent, the flat posterior humeral cortical line can be used to refer correct humeral component rotation. Typically, the anatomic elbow flexion–extension axis is rotated 14 degrees internally relative to the posterior humeral cortex. The above mentioned pitfalls are preventable with awareness and good surgical technique.

Treatment-Specific Outcomes. The outcomes of TEA for distal humerus fractures at short-term and midterm follow-up have been reproducibly good (Table 35-7).[9,11,31,57,60,74,97,98,99,112,147,149,173] Most studies have used the Coonrad-Morrey implant (Zimmer, Warsaw IN), which is linked and described as semi-constrained because of its "sloppy" hinge.

In a retrospective study, Frankle et al. compared ORIF to elbow arthroplasty in women over the age of 65 years with AO/OTA type C distal humerus fractures. They reported improved outcomes in the arthroplasty group at short-term follow-up. The small sample size and selection bias, however, confounds the interpretation of the results because eight patients in the

TABLE 35-6 **Potential Pitfalls and Preventions of Total Elbow Arthroplasty for Distal Humerus Fractures**

Total Elbow Arthroplasty for Distal Humerus Fracture
Potential Pitfalls and Preventions

Pitfall	Prevention
Missed skin tenting, excessive swelling, fracture blisters	Application of a well-padded splint while awaiting surgery Re-check skin, soft tissues, and neurovascular status immediately before surgery
Ineffective surgical exposure	Choose an approach that balances required visualization for arthroplasty vs. complications; recommend leaving triceps attached to olecranon Understand extensile options
Inadequate exposure of ulna	Resect tip of olecranon to improve access to ulna
Incorrect humeral component height (re-creation of joint line/axial position of the flexion–extension axis)	Loosely reapproximate resected epicondylar fragments to the humeral shaft to judge the location of the elbow flexion–extension axis
Incorrect humeral component rotation	The humeral component should typically be 14 degrees internally rotated as compared to the flat posterior humeral cortex
Malposition ulna	The rotational axis of the ulnar component should bisect the radial head, and should be parallel to the ulnar flatspot
Osseous impingement	The elbow should be placed through a range of motion to ensure there is no bony impingement with the implant. The tip of the olecranon or coronoid may require resection
Ulnar neuropathy	Identify and protect ulnar nerve during surgical approach and during arthroplasty Preoperative neurologic examination to document pre-existing nerve injuries

TABLE 35-7 **Summary of Outcomes of Total Elbow Arthroplasty for the Management of Distal Humerus Fractures[190]**

Author	Year	Number of Patients	Average Age of Patients (Range)	Surgical Approach	Average Follow-up in Months	Range of Motion (Arc)	Outcome Assessment Used	Percentage with Excellent or Good Outcomes	Complications
Gambirasio[59]	2001	10	85 (57–95)	Bryan-Morrey	18	101	MEPS	100%	1 HO, 1 CRPS
Garcia[60]	2002	16	73 (61–95)	Triceps split	36	101	MEPS, DASH	100%	1 UN, 1 HO
Frankle[57]	2003	12	72 (65–88)	Bryan-Morrey	45	113	MEPS	100%	2 UN, 1 UP, 1 H, 1 DS
Kamineni[98]	2004	43	69 (34–92)	Bryan-Morrey	84	107	MEPS	93%	7 HO, 4 BW, 3 UIF, 1 HIF, 5 H, 1 DS
Lee[112]	2006	7	73 (55–85)	Bryan-Morrey	25	89	MEPS	100%	—
Kalogrianitis[97]	2008	9	73 (45–86)	Triceps split	42	118	MEPS, LES	88%	1 SS
Prasad[173]	2008	15	78 (61–89)	Triceps tongue	56	93	MEPS	85%	1 CRPS, 1 AS-U
Chalidis[31]	2009	11	79 (75–86)	Bryan-Morrey	33	107	MEPS	100%	1 UN, 1 PF
Antuna[9]	2012	16	76 (57–89)	Paratricipital (14) Olecranon osteotomy (2)	57	90	DASH, VAS, Patient subjective assessment	69%	8 UN, 3 DS
Total/Mean	—	139	75	—	44	102	—	93%	—

MEPS, Mayo Elbow Performance Score; HO, heterotopic ossification; CRPS, complex regional pain syndrome; DASH, Disabilities of the Arm, Shoulder and Hand; UN, ulnar nerve palsy; UP, uncoupled prosthesis; H, wound hematoma or dehiscence; DS, deep infection; BW, bushing wear; UIF, ulnar implant fracture; HIF, humeral implant fracture; LES, Liverpool Elbow Score; SS, superficial infection; AS-U, aseptic loosening ulna; PF, periprosthetic fracture.

arthroplasty group had RA and none had RA in the ORIF group. McKee et al.[132] conducted a randomized prospective study comparing ORIF to elbow arthroplasty in elderly patients with comminuted distal humerus fractures. Outcomes were assessed with the MEPS and DASH score. Twenty-one patients were initially randomized into the two treatment groups; however, five patients randomized to ORIF were intraoperatively converted to arthroplasty. At 2 years follow-up, the MEPS was significantly better in the TEA group; however, the DASH score was not significantly different between groups. The reoperation rate between the arthroplasty and the ORIF groups was also not significantly different.

At the present time, there are no mid-term or long-term studies comparing the outcomes and complications of ORIF to TEA for the treatment of complex distal humerus fractures in the elderly. It is probable that the revision surgery rate would increase over time in patients treated with elbow arthroplasty, when compared to patients undergoing ORIF, because of polyethylene wear, aseptic loosening, periprosthetic fracture, and infection.

Hemiarthroplasty for Distal Humerus Fractures

Hemiarthroplasty is another surgical option for unreconstructible distal humerus fractures. This procedure has been described in the past[137,201,211] and has recently experienced a renewed interest.[2,28,83,212] Two commercially available elbow arthroplasty systems have humerus implants that replicate the distal humeral articular surface, the Sorbie-Questor (Wright Medical Technology, Arlington, TN) and the Latitude (Tornier, Stafford, TX), and therefore can be used for hemiarthroplasty (Fig. 35-33). The added benefit of the Latitude hemiarthroplasty is that it can be converted to a linked or unlinked TEA. This is beneficial if intraoperative hemiarthroplasty stability cannot be achieved necessitating conversion to TEA. Other systems that have nonanatomic humeral components, such as the Kudo[2,3]

(Biomet Inc., Warsaw, IN, USA), have also been used for hemiarthroplasty. The use of nonanatomic components, however, is not recommended.

Indications/Contraindicaitons. The indications for distal humerus hemiarthroplasty are virtually identical to TEA. The theoretical advantage of a hemiarthroplasty is the absence of polyethylene wear debris and the associated osteolysis and aseptic loosening which are common modes of failure with total elbow arthroplasties. Hemiarthroplasty, therefore, may function as an "in between" in those patients with unreconstructible distal humerus fractures who are deemed too young or too active for TEA. It should be noted, however, that the believed benefits of hemiarthroplasty are completely speculative and no literature exists to support its use over TEA.

Hemiarthroplasty of the distal humerus resurfaces the articular segments of the trochlea and capitellum. For it to function optimally to allow elbow stability and range of motion, it relies on the integrity of the primary and secondary elbow stabilizers.[83,153] Therefore, when considering hemiarthroplasty, the medial and lateral columns must be reconstructible (Fig. 35-34), the radial head and coronoid must be intact, and the MCLs and LCLs must be repairable or intact on their respective condyles.[14,83]

The contraindications to distal humerus hemiarthroplasty are similar to those for TEA. Additional contraindications include deficient medial or lateral column bone, deficient MCLs or LCLs, or fractures of the radial head or coronoid that cannot be rigidly stabilized. Chondral damage to the greater sigmoid notch or radial head are also relative contraindications as patients may experience postoperative arthritic pain and limited motion. In the above circumstances with deficient bone or soft tissue, linked TEA should be considered.

Preoperative Planning. As with TEA, hemiarthroplasty is a technically demanding procedure and should only be

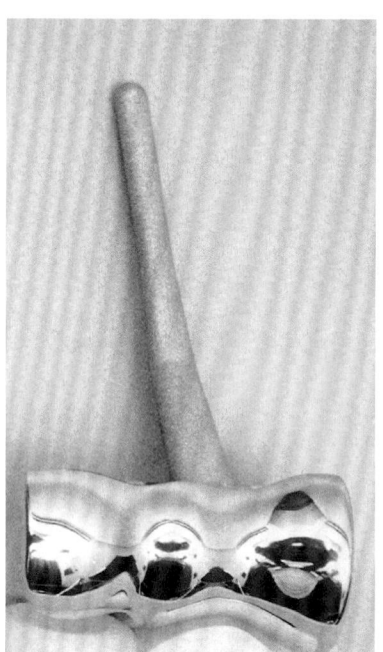
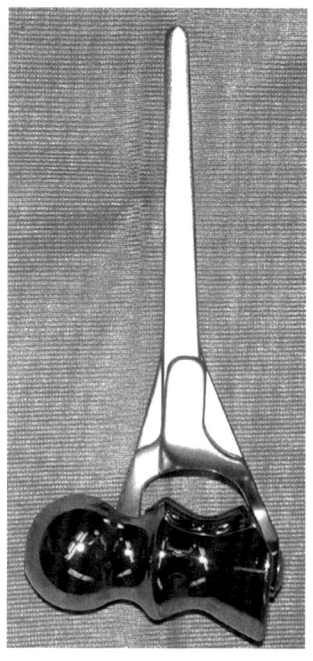

A **B**

FIGURE 35-33 The Sorbie-Questor (Wright Medical Technology, Arlington, TN) **(A)** and the Latitude (Tornier, Stafford, TX) total elbow system **(B)** are two commercially available arthroplasty systems that have humeral implants that replicate the distal humeral articular anatomy, and therefore can be used for hemiarthroplasty.

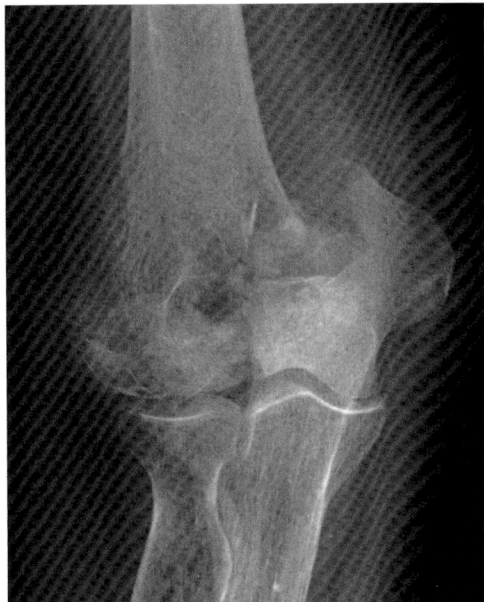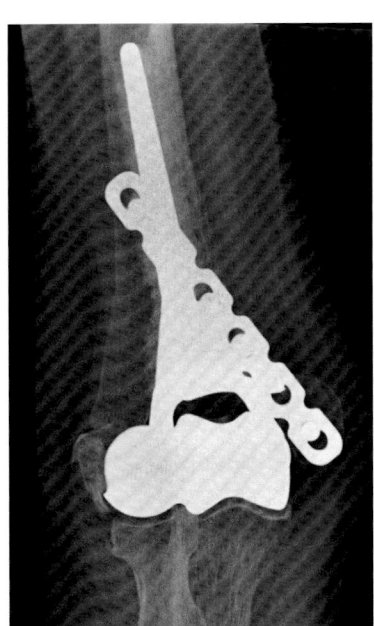

FIGURE 35-34 A distal humerus fracture **(A)** treated with hemiarthroplasty and plate fixation of the medial column and suture fixation of the lateral epicondyle **(B)**.

conducted by surgeons experienced in upper limb arthroplasty or complex trauma. Standard elbow radiographs are usually sufficient for assessing the fracture pattern and for implant templating. CT will confirm the articular fragmentation, will identify occult fractures (such as fractures of the coronoid and radial head), and may assist with ORIF of the columns.

Positioning and Surgical Approaches. Patients can be positioned supine or in the lateral decubitus fashion. A sterile tourniquet is used and the approach starts with a longitudinal posterior skin incision. The ulnar nerve is identified, released, and prepared for anterior subcutaneous transposition. The options available for exposure of the elbow for hemiarthroplasty include olecranon osteotomy, paratricipital approach, triceps split, triceps reflection, and triceps dividing approaches (please see section on surgical approaches). The most commonly used approaches for hemiarthroplasty are the olecranon osteotomy and the paratricipital approach. The olecranon osteotomy allows the best visualization of the joint; however, has a higher rate of complications if intraoperative conversion to a TEA is required. The paratricipital approach maintains integrity of the extensor mechanism, however, affords less visualization of the articular surfaces. For hemiarthroplasty, the paratricipital approach can be modified by maintaining the collateral ligament attachments on the epicondyles and working through the fracture interval.

Technique. Once the fracture is visualized, it should be carefully inspected to ensure ORIF is not possible. If hemiarthroplasty is deemed appropriate, sizing of the implant should be done next. The determination of correct humeral component size can be done in three ways, preoperative templating of contralateral elbow radiographs, piecing together the fractured trochlea and capitellum and comparing with the available trial implants, and by placing trial implants into the greater sigmoid

notch to select which one best aligns with the coronoid and radial head. The humeral canal is then entered by resecting the superior aspect of the olecranon fossa. The canal is reamed and broached to accept the chosen trial implant. The trial implant must be inserted to the correct depth to recreate the joint line. Local landmarks, such as the collateral ligament origins and the condyles, are used to gauge correct implant length. Provisional fixation of one or both of the fractured columns with K-wires may also assist with determination of the correct implant length. Conservative bone cuts are then made using the available cutting blocks. If use of the cutting blocks is not feasible, conservative free-hand cuts are made and revised as necessary. The trial implant is then inserted into the humerus and the elbow is reduced and taken through a range of motion to ensure there is no restriction or impingement.

Once the appropriate orientation, length, and size of trial implant have been determined, the next step involves cementation of the true prosthesis and definitive fixation of the columnar fractures. This step can be done in one of several different orders: (1) the fractured columns can be definitively fixated in anatomic position with contoured plates/screws or with K-wires/tension bands augmented with sutures (Fig. 35-35) and then the implant cemented; (2) the implant can be cemented first in anatomic position followed by columnar fracture fixation; (3) the less comminuted column is definitively fixated first to allow easier fracture reduction and to assist with correct implant orientation and length. The implant is inserted and once the cement has hardened, the other column undergoes ORIF to the humeral shaft and stable implant. When conducting this procedure through an olecranon osteotomy, all the above methods are feasible; however, if using a paratricipital approach only the latter two are possible.

Prior to definitive implant insertion, a humeral cement restrictor is inserted and the canal is lavaged and dried. Antibiotic

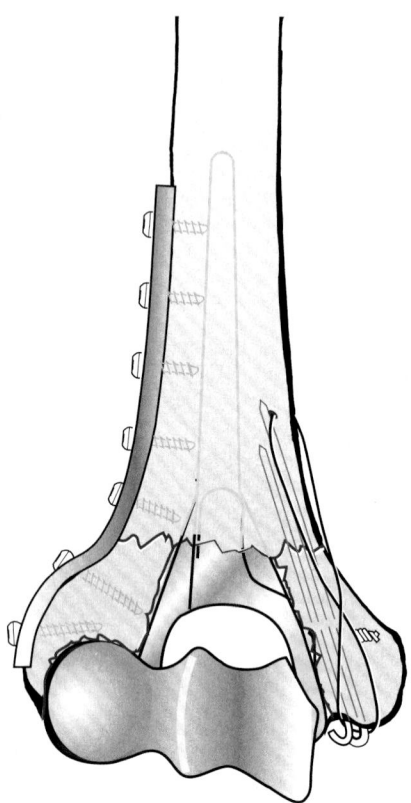

FIGURE 35-35 Medial and lateral column fixation in hemiarthroplasty for distal humerus fractures may be accomplished by plates and screws, sutures, and tension band constructs.

cement is inserted via a thin nozzled pressurization gun. All excess cement is removed, especially around the medial and lateral column fracture surfaces. Once the implant has been cemented and columnar ORIF is complete, the elbow is placed through a range of motion and stability is checked. Postoperatively, the elbow is splinted for 2 to 3 days and then early active assisted range of motion is initiated.

Potential Pitfalls and Preventative. Hemiarthroplasty for distal humerus fractures is a technically challenging procedure. It is recommended that only experienced surgeons undertake this procedure. Potential pitfalls include nonanatomic epicondylar reduction with poor collateral ligament tension, nonrigid fixation of condyles, humeral component malrotation, incorrect humeral component length relationship, and incorrect articular sizing. All of the aforementioned pitfalls are technique-dependent and will likely adversely affect patient outcomes. This procedure, therefore, should only be conducted by experienced surgeons.

Treatment-Specific Outcomes. There is little information in the literature pertaining to the outcomes of distal humerus hemiarthroplasty for trauma.[2,3,28,83,166,201] Adolfsson and Nestorson reported on eight cases using the nonanatomic Kudo (Biomet Inc., Warsaw, IN, USA) humeral prosthesis.[2,3] At a mean of 4 years follow-up, the MEPSs were good or excellent in all patients. The mean elbow range of motion was 31 to

126 degrees and all patients described having no pain. Radiographic signs of ulnar erosion were present in three patients, but did not correlate to functional outcomes. Parsons et al.[166] also reported on four patients undergoing hemiarthroplasty for acute fractures using the anatomic Sorbie-Questor implant (Wright Medical Technology, Arlington, TN). At early follow-up, they reported a mean ASES score of 83.5 and a mean elbow flexion of 130 degrees and an extension of 16 degrees. Unfortunately, these two short-term follow-up studies are all that is available in the literature; therefore, further studies are required to determine if distal humeral hemiarthroplasty for acute trauma is feasible in the long term.

SPECIAL CIRCUMSTANCES AND MANAGEMENT OF EXPECTED ADVERSE OUTCOMES AND UNEXPECTED COMPLICATIONS OF DISTAL HUMERUS FRACTURES

Open Distal Humerus Fractures

Approximately 7% of distal humerus fracture are open[189] and they are classified according to the system of Gustilo and Anderson.[70] The principles of open fracture treatment have remained unchanged for the last 3 decades. The priorities are wound irrigation and debridement, intravenous antibiotics, tetanus coverage, fracture stabilization, and appropriate soft tissue management.[70,158] The common complications associated with open fractures include infection, nonunion, hardware failure, and wound problems.

The grade of open fracture varies with the mechanism of injury. Most blunt mechanisms of injury lead to grade I punctures while blast or gun shots lead to grade III wounds.[189] Typically, most grade I puncture wounds are located posteriorly or posterolaterally on the elbow and are commonly associated with lacerations of the triceps tendon or muscle.[133,189] In cases of an intra-articular fracture with a triceps tendon laceration, the Van Gorder (triceps tongue) or triceps splitting approaches are preferred as they prevent a second disruption of the extensor mechanism with an olecranon osteotomy.

Typically, in open injuries contaminated or devascularized bone and soft tissues are excised. This rule, however, does not hold absolutely true when dealing with large segments of articular surface. The risk of infection with retaining the fragments must be weighed against the risk of post-traumatic arthritis and the potential need for secondary bone grafting or allograft reconstruction if the fragments are removed. Generally, an attempt should be made to preserve all articular segments with thorough cleansing and meticulous removal of all foreign material and contamination.

McKee et al.[133] reviewed 26 patients who underwent ORIF of open distal humerus fractures. According to the system of Gustilo and Anderson, 50% were grade I, 35% were grade II, and 15% were grade III. At follow-up, 15 patients (57%) had good to excellent outcomes based on the MEPS and the mean DASH score was 24 indicating minimal to moderate disability. The mean elbow arc of flexion–extension motion was 97 degrees (range, 55 to 140 degrees). The overall infection rate was 11% (three patients) with only one patient sustaining a deep infection requiring operative debridement. Four patients (15%) were diagnosed with delayed union (>16 weeks) with two patients going on to require bone grafting. Min et al.,[140] in a case-controlled study, compared closed to open AO/OTA type C fractures in 28 patients. At final follow-up, patients with open fractures were found to have significantly worse functional outcomes.

Nonunion of Distal Humerus Fractures

Nonunions occur in approximately 6% (range, 0% to 25%) of distal humerus fractures treated by modern doubling plating techniques.[6,13,47,57,64,67,69,82,106,130,133,160,161,190,193,205,216] Nonunions typically occur at the supracondylar level, are rarely intra-articular, and are usually related to inadequate fixation.[5,76,128,164,184,203,204] Other risk factors for nonunion include "low" fracture types with limited distal bone for screw purchase, extensive comminution, and severe osteopenia. Patients typically present with pain, stiffness, and functional limitation. If there is associated failure of fixation, patient may also present with abnormal motion caused by a mobile nonunion.

In patients presenting with nonunion after ORIF of distal humerus fractures, it is important to establish the cause of the nonunion. All patients should undergo infection screening blood work (complete blood count with differential, erythrocyte sedimentation rate, and C-reactive protein levels). Injury and postoperative radiographs should be examined critically to determine the initial fracture pattern and the adequacy of initial ORIF. Examining postoperative radiographs in a serial fashion may reveal the cause of failure.

Treatment options for distal humerus nonunions include splinting, revision ORIF, and elbow arthroplasty. Splinting with externally applied bone stimulators, such as ultrasound, may be effective if fixation failure has not occurred. If surgical treatment is deemed necessary, a CT scan may be beneficial in examining the quality and quantity of the remaining distal humerus bone.

Revision ORIF should be the procedure of choice in healthy active patients. Revision procedures are technically demanding because of the altered anatomy, presence of failed hardware, excessive scarring, and generally poor bone quality. Because of these issues, an olecranon osteotomy is the preferred approach to allow the best access to the joint.[5,76,128,184] The goals of surgery are to obtain an anatomic articular reduction, rigid bicolumn fixation, and to stimulate bone healing with autologous bone graft. Additional procedures that are usually required with revision ORIF of distal humerus fractures are anterior and posterior capsulectomy to address elbow stiffness and ulnar nerve neurolysis and transposition.[76,128,184] The outcomes of revision ORIF are generally satisfactory[5,76,128,184] with bony union occurring in greater than 90% of patients.

In some nonunions, revision ORIF is not feasible, whether it is because of extensive bone loss or post-traumatic arthrosis. In these cases, TEA is a reliable treatment option.[51,129,141,142] Patients who have a healed prior olecranon osteotomy can be approached via a paratricipital approach, Bryan-Morrey (triceps reflecting) approach, or by a triceps split. Patients with a nonunion of an olecranon osteotomy are approached through

the osteotomy site. After elbow arthroplasty, the olecranon is fixated with a K-wire/tension band construct, plate/screws, or with excision of the fragment and triceps advancement.[122] Other treatment options for distal humerus nonunions include arthrodesis,[177] resection arthroplasty, allograft distal humerus replacement,[1,37,217,218] vascularized bone grafting,[19] and Ilizarov methods.[23]

Elbow Stiffness and Heterotopic Ossification of Distal Humerus Fractures

Patients typically achieve functional range of motion after ORIF of distal humerus fractures. Risk factors for elbow stiffness and HO are head injury, polytrauma, severe soft tissue injury, delay to surgical intervention, prolonged postoperative immobilization, and open fractures.[61,86,96,124,165,182,183,193]

The reported incidence of HO after surgical treatment of distal humerus fractures varies from 0% to 49%.[6,13,47,67,69,160,193,205] The majority of patients with HO do not experience any significant functional deficits; therefore, resection is not always necessary. HO about the elbow can be classified by the system of Hastings and Graham[73] (Table 35-8). The incidence of elbow stiffness and contracture is difficult to determine as almost all patients who undergo ORIF have some limitation in motion. The distinction between an elbow contracture and a normal postoperative outcome is dependent on several variables, including patient's expectations, activity level, age, and occupation. Morrey,[146,148] in an effort to identify the etiology of elbow contractures, has classified them as intrinsic, extrinsic, and combined. Intrinsic causes involve the articular surface while extrinsic causes include capsular contracture and HO.

Primary prevention should be used by all surgeons to limit post-traumatic elbow contracture. For patients at high risk of HO, such as those with head injuries, postoperative indomethacin and/or radiation is recommended. For the treatment of elbow contractures, initial management should be nonoperative with physiotherapy, splints, and braces. Static progressive splinting under the direction of a physiotherapist has been reported as an effective method of regaining elbow range of motion.[40]

When splints and braces fail to obtain functional range of motion, the elbow may be treated surgically using either open

TABLE 35-8 The Hastings Classification of Heterotopic Ossification

Class	Sub-Type	Description
I	—	Radiographic heterotopic ossification without functional limitation
II	A	Limitation of flexion/extension
	B	Limitation of forearm pronation/supination
	C	Limitation in both planes
III	—	Bony ankylosis of either the elbow or forearm

or arthroscopic techniques. Generally, arthroscopy has a limited role in the treatment of contractures after distal humerus ORIF because of the often extensive internal fixation hardware that requires open removal. Open contracture releases may be done via a medial "over-the-top" exposure, a lateral column procedure, or a combined approach.[146,148,214] The preoperative assessment of patients includes identification of prior surgical incisions, examination of the ulnar nerve, and clear localization of the pathology to determine the most appropriate surgical approach. The procedure typically involves ulnar nerve release, capsulectomy, debridement of the olecranon, coronoid and radial fossae, excision of symptomatic HO, and finally removal of internal fixation hardware. Postoperatively, patients are managed with continuous passive motion devices and static progressive splints. The routine use of indomethacin for HO prophylaxis after contracture release remains controversial.

The surgical excision of symptomatic HO should be delayed until its growth has ceased and it has become corticated. Preoperative or early postoperative single dose radiation treatment has been recommended to decrease HO recurrence; however, there is little literature to support its use. The excision of HO is associated with significantly better gains in range of motion than release of soft tissue-only contractures.[165]

Wound Complications and Infection in Distal Humerus Fractures

Superficial wound infections are relatively common after ORIF of distal humerus fractures. Elbows should be examined to ensure there are no deep fluid collections which may indicate infected hematomas or seromas. The management of superficial infections consists of oral antibiotics, dressing changes, and close observation.

Deep infections after ORIF of distal humerus fractures have a reported rate between 0% and 10%.[6,13,47,57,64,67,69,82,106,108,130,133,160,161,183,193,205,216] Management consists of surgical debridement and organism-specific intravenous antibiotics. Intraoperatively, fracture fixation is assessed to ensure it is stable. If stable, the patient is managed serial surgical debridements as required and intravenous antibiotics until healing. If fracture stability is lost, staged revision ORIF is required along with intravenous antibiotics until healing.

Wound necrosis is also a complication that can occur after ORIF of distal humerus fractures. This is managed with surgical debridement to viable tissue. The remaining soft tissue defect is assessed to determine whether primary closure is possible or if coverage is required. Coverage options depend on several variables, including size and depth of the defect, exposed hardware or vital structures, patient comorbidities, and potential donor site morbidity.[33,91] Consultation with a plastic or soft tissue reconstructive surgeon is recommended.

Ulnar Neuropathy in Distal Humerus Fractures

The ulnar nerve is the most commonly affected nerve in patients with distal humerus fractures. Injury can occur at the time of fracture, intraoperatively, or postoperatively. At the time of fracture, the nerve may be injured by a direct impact or indirectly by traction caused by wide displacement of the fracture fragments. Intraoperatively, injury may occur by traction, manipulation of the nerve, or by injury to its blood supply causing ischemia. Postoperatively, neuritis may occur by nerve "kinking" in flexion or extension, exuberant scarring, or by irritation against fixation hardware.

Patients with preoperative neuropathy should undergo ulnar nerve exploration during the surgical procedure. The nerve should be decompressed and examined with loop magnification to ensure it is intact. If partially or completely lacerated, the nerve should undergo immediate microsurgical repair. If the nerve is intact, a complete neurolysis should be done. The decision whether or not to transpose the nerve remains controversial.

In a retrospective study of 107 patients to determine the incidence and predisposing factors for the onset of postoperative ulnar neuropathy, Wiggers et al.[224] identified neuropathy in 17 (16%) patients with the only risk factor being the type of fracture. The authors found that columnar fractures had a greater risk of postoperative ulnar neuropathy than capitellar or trochlear fractures, and this effect was independent of whether or not the nerve was transposed at the time of surgery. Chen et al.[32] in a multicenter retrospective study compared the rate of ulnar neuropathy in patients with and without ulnar nerve transposition during ORIF of distal humerus fractures. The authors found that patients who underwent intraoperative ulnar nerve transposition had almost four times the incidence of post-operative ulnar neuropathy. The authors, therefore, recommended against ulnar nerve transposition.

Ulnar neuropathy that presents postoperatively, in a transposed nerve, can be managed with initial observation. The management of postoperative neuropathy in a nerve left in situ remains controversial; anecdotally, some recommend observation while others recommend acute decompression with anterior transposition. It is the author's practice to conduct a complete release and anterior subcutaneous transposition in all surgically treated distal humerus fractures.

The outcome of ulnar neuropathy with an intact nerve is good; patients have a high rate of satisfaction, good return of intrinsic muscle strength, and a return of hand functionality.[127] Although the prognosis is generally good after ulnar neuropathy, patients do not return to completely normal.[18,127]

Olecranon Osteotomy Complications in Distal Humerus Fractures

An olecranon osteotomy affords the best visualization of the articular surface of the distal humerus, and therefore is a valuable approach for comminuted articular fractures. An olecranon osteotomy should be conducted in a systematic way to avoid complications such as inadvertent fracture propagation, incorrect osteotomy location, and malreduction. Complications associated with olecranon osteotomies have been reported to occur in 0% to 31% of cases.[6,13,36,57,64,69,78,205,229]

Nonunion or delayed union of olecranon osteotomies have been reported in up to 10% of cases.[6,13,36,57,64,78,190,205,229] In many cases, the olecranon osteotomy requires more time to heal than the distal humerus fracture[58], perhaps because of the ulna's unique blood supply.[226] The theorized risk factors for nonunion include use of a tension band technique, a transverse osteotomy, and single screw fixation, although, the literature does not support this. Three recent studies[36,78,180] on the outcomes of olecranon osteotomy looked at a total of 129 patients. All patients underwent an apex distal chevron osteotomy, although, the types of fixation varied (plates, single medullary screws, and tension band constructs). There were no nonunions, one delayed union, three patients who had early hardware failure required revision ORIF, and 18 patients (14%) had hardware removal specifically for irritation.

The management of olecranon nonunions includes ruling out infective causes and then revision plate ORIF with autologous bone grafting. In some cases when revision ORIF is not feasible because of the small size of the fragment or associated poor bone quality, the fragment may be excised with advancement of the triceps insertion.[122,220] Delayed unions of the olecranon are managed expectantly with consideration given to external bone stimulation devices.

Prominent symptomatic hardware is common after fixation of olecranon osteotomies. Patients may experience local pain, tenderness, or an inability to rest the elbow hard surfaces. These symptoms can be addressed by hardware removal after the olecranon is completely healed.

Total Elbow Arthroplasty Complications in Distal Humerus Fractures

Complications of TEA include infection and wound healing, neuropathies, triceps insufficiency, instability, osteolysis and loosening, mechanical failure, periprosthetic fracture, and stiffness.

The rate of deep infection in TEA ranges from 2% to 5%. The rate has been noted to be declining over time.[2,11,35,59,60,98,112,144,171,178] The rate of infection can be minimized by meticulous surgical technique, use of perioperative antibiotics, sterile tourniquets, and antibiotic laden cement. The consequences of deep infection can be devastating. The treatment will often include organism-specific intravenous antibiotics and surgical debridements with possible staged reconstruction. Organisms such as Staphylococcus epidermidis are particularly difficult to eradicate, and resection arthroplasty may be the consequence.

Ulnar neuropathy is common in traumatic conditions of the elbow. The probability of persistent ulnar neuropathy after TEA for trauma is high and is reported to occur in up to 28% of patients, with permanent dysfunction in up to 10%.[11,17,35,59,74,97,98,173,178,187] Ulnar nerve exposure, complete neurolysis, and anterior transposition is recommended, although, transposition also has risks, such as devascularization. The surgical approach used for elbow arthroplasty is also influential as the extended Kocher approach has a higher risk of postoperative ulnar nerve palsy.[79,116]

Triceps insufficiency is a common problem after TEA performed via an extensor mechanism disrupting approach, and is reported in up to 11% of patients.[143,168,174,178,223] Surgical exposures that utilize a triceps-on approach such as the paratricipital

approach, although more technically challenging, may avoid this complication. When using a triceps disrupting approach this complication can be minimized by solid anatomic repair of the triceps insertion and postoperative protection of the repair by avoiding active extension for 6 weeks. Many patients, such as those that use ambulatory aids or self-propelled wheelchairs, require a strong intact triceps mechanism. These patients may be best suited for the paratricipital approach. Patients who develop extensor mechanism insufficiency and who rely on active extension may benefit from extensor mechanism revision repair or reconstruction with auto- or allograft.

Instability after TEA is a problem associated with unlinked designs. These designs rely on correct implant positioning, preserved bony architecture, and intact soft tissue stabilizers. Typically, unlinked designs are not used for distal humerus fracture because of disrupted bony and soft tissue stabilizers; however, they may be used if these structures are anatomically repaired. Newer unlinked designs have several advantages, they have greater contact surface area in the ulnohumeral articulation providing increased constraint, some have the option of a radial head arthroplasty which provides additional stability, and others have the ability to convert to a linked implant. If intraoperative instability exists in an unlinked arthroplasty after repair of the bony structures and soft tissues, then conversion to a linked prosthesis should be performed.

Bearing wear in a TEA is inevitable. Many implants allow for change of the bearing surface without revision of the components. Accelerated wear rates have been found in younger patients, in patients with post-traumatic conditions, and in cases with persistent postoperative malalignment or deformity.[85,111,121,141] The problem with polyethylene wear is the host reaction that causes osteolysis, which can lead to aseptic loosening and loss of bone stock.

TEA implants can also undergo fatigue fracture.[17] Metal fatigue most commonly affects titanium implants because of their notch sensitivity. Implants at risk are those with insufficient bony support of their metaphyseal segments because of fractured or resected condyles or osteolysis. These at-risk implants experience high cantilever bending forces at the junction of the poorly supported metaphyseal segment and the well-fixed diaphyseal segment.

Periprosthetic fractures can occur intraoperatively and postoperatively. Risk factors for intraoperative fractures include osteopenic bone, excessive diaphyseal bowing with use of long stem implants, overly aggressive reaming and revision cases. Fixation of condylar fractures when using a linked system is not required; however, shaft fractures require reduction and stabilization with some combination of long stem components with cerlage wires, allograft struts, or plate and screw fixation. Postoperative periprosthetic fractures can occur secondary to trauma or through pathologic bone weakened by osteolysis. Periprosthetic fractures with unstable components will likely require revision arthroplasty in the medically fit patient. Periprosthetic fractures with stable components may be managed with immobilization or ORIF. Allograft strut grafts are useful adjuncts in these situations especially in those with bone loss.

AUTHOR'S PREFERRED TREATMENT FOR DISTAL HUMERUS FRACTURES (FIG. 35-36)

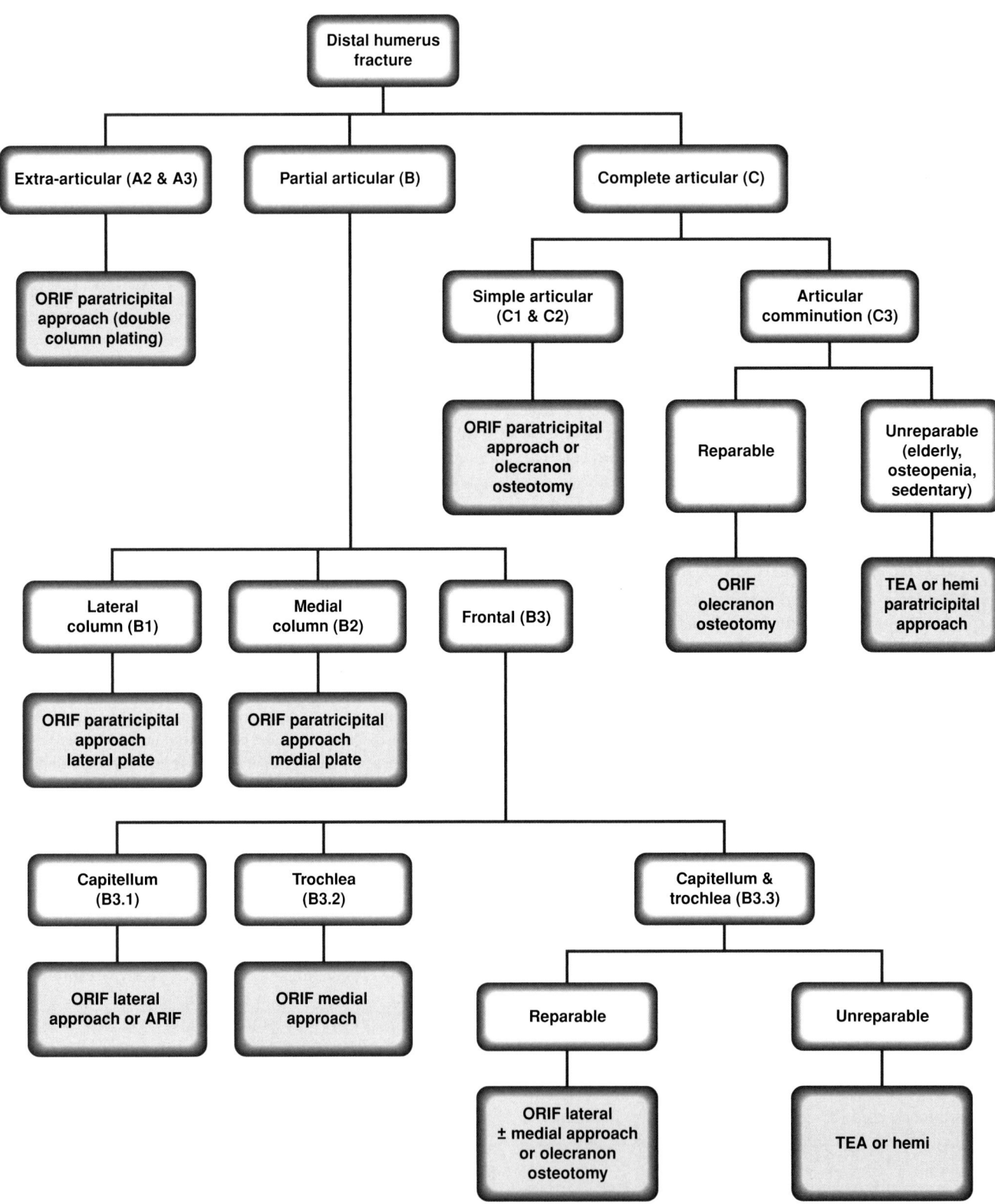

Figure 35-36 Authors Preferred Treatment Algorithm for Distal Humerus Fractures.

My preferred surgical approach for ORIF of A2, A3, B1, B2, C1, and C2 fractures is the paratricipital approach. For C1 and C2 fractures, and all C3 fractures, which are deemed fixable, and cannot be addressed via this less invasive approach, I prefer the olecranon osteotomy.

The paratricipital approach is also preferred for cases where the reparability of the fracture will be determined intraoperatively. If the fracture is deemed fixable, it may be conducted via the paratricipital approach or the approach can be converted to an olecranon osteotomy. In cases where the fracture is deemed irreparable, a TEA may be done via the original paratricipital approach.

For ORIF, surgeons should be familiar with all plating techniques, including parallel, orthogonal, and triple plating, as some fractures will lend themselves to one technique over another. Generally, I prefer the technique of parallel plating. The fixation principles and techniques used for AO/OTA type C (bicolumn) fractures are applicable to type A2 and A3 fractures. B1 and B2 (single column) fractures may be fixed with multiple screws; however, my preference is to use an ipsilateral single column plate.

Irreparable distal humerus fractures in an age-appropriate patient may be managed with a linked TEA. My preference is to resect the condyles and to conduct the replacement through a paratricipital approach. My indications for hemiarthroplasty for distal humerus fractures are narrow; typically, the fractures have a high degree of articular comminution with relatively simple non-comminuted columnar fracture in a more active elderly patient.

CONTROVERSIES/FUTURE DIRECTIONS IN DISTAL HUMERUS FRACTURES

Several implant-related advancements have been made over the last few years. The use of precontoured and locking plates has become ubiquitous; however, no clinical advantages have been reported. Further study is required to determine if their additional cost leads to improved patient outcomes, especially in today's fiscally responsible health care environment.

TEA has certainly demonstrated predictably good outcomes in short- to medium-term follow-up; however, as with all total joints the survivorship decreases over time. The role of hemiarthroplasty, therefore, requires further investigation to determine if it effectively functions as an intermediate to total joint replacement.

ACKNOWLEDGMENTS

I would like to thank Drs. C. Michael Robinson, Graham J.W. King, Marc Prud'homme-Foster, and Kenneth J. Faber for their assistance with the preparation of this chapter.

REFERENCES

1. Ackerman G, Jupiter JB. Non-union of fractures of the distal end of the humerus. *J Bone Joint Surg Am.* 1988;70(1):75–83.
2. Adolfsson L, Hammer R. Elbow hemiarthroplasty for acute reconstruction of intraarticular distal humerus fractures: a preliminary report involving 4 patients. *Acta Orthop.* 2006;77(5):785–787.
3. Adolfsson L, Nestorson J. The Kudo humeral component as primary hemiarthroplasty in distal humeral fractures. *J Shoulder Elbow Surg.* 2012;21(4):451–455.
4. Aitken GK, Rorabeck CH. Distal humeral fractures in the adult. *Clin Orthop Relat Res.* 1986;(207):191–197.
5. Ali A, Douglas H, Stanley D. Revision surgery for nonunion after early failure of fixation of fractures of the distal humerus. *J Bone Joint Surg Br.* 2005;87(8):1107–1110.
6. Allende CA, Allende BT, Allende BL, et al. Intercondylar distal humerus fractures–surgical treatment and results. *Chir Main.* 2004;23(2):85–95.
7. Alonso-Llames M. Bilaterotricipital approach to the elbow. Its application in the osteosynthesis of supracondylar fractures of the humerus in children. *Acta Orthop Scand.* 1972;43(6):479–490.
8. Anglen J. Distal humerus fractures. *J Am Acad Orthop Surg.* 2005;13(5):291–297.
9. Antuna SA, Laakso RB, Barrera JL, et al. Linked total elbow arthroplasty as treatment of distal humerus fractures. *Acta Orthop Belg.* 2012;78(4):465–472.
10. Armstrong AD, Dunning CE, Faber KJ, et al. Single-strand ligament reconstruction of the medial collateral ligament restores valgus elbow stability. *J Shoulder Elbow Surg.* 2002;11(1):65–71.
11. Armstrong AD, Yamaguchi K. Total elbow arthroplasty and distal humerus elbow fractures. *Hand Clin.* 2004;20(4):475–483.
12. Arnander MW, Reeves A, MacLeod IA, et al. A biomechanical comparison of plate configuration in distal humerus fractures. *J Orthop Trauma.* 2008;22(5):332–336.
13. Aslam N, Willett K. Functional outcome following internal fixation of intraarticular fractures of the distal humerus (AO type C). *Acta Orthop Belg.* 2004;70(2):118–122.
14. Athwal GS, Goetz TJ, Pollock JW, et al. Prosthetic replacement for distal humerus fractures. *Orthop Clin North Am.* 2008;39(2):201–212.
15. Athwal GS, Hoxie SC, Rispoli DM, et al. Precontoured parallel plate fixation of AO/OTA type C distal humerus fractures. *J Orthop Trauma.* 2009;23(8):575–580.
16. Athwal GS, Morrey BF. Revision total elbow arthroplasty for prosthetic fractures. *J Bone Joint Surg Am.* 2006;88(9):2017–2026.
17. Athwal GS, Rispoli DM, Steinmann SP. The anconeus flap transolecranon approach to the distal humerus. *J Orthop Trauma.* 2006;20(4):282–285.
18. Bartels RH, Grotenhuis JA. Anterior submuscular transposition of the ulnar nerve. For post-operative focal neuropathy at the elbow. *J Bone Joint Surg Br.* 2004;86(7):998–1001.
19. Beredjiklian PK, Hotchkiss RN, Athanasian EA, et al. Recalcitrant nonunion of the distal humerus: treatment with free vascularized bone grafting. *Clin Orthop Relat Res.* 2005;(435):134–139.
20. Bilic R, Kolundzic R, Anticevic D. Absorbable implants in surgical correction of a capitellar malunion in an 11-year-old: a case report. *J Orthop Trauma.* 2006;20(1):66–69.
21. Black DM, Steinbuch M, Palermo L, et al. An assessment tool for predicting fracture risk in postmenopausal women. *Osteoporos Int.* 2001;12(7):519–528.
22. Boody AR, Wongworawat MD. Accuracy in the measurement of compartment pressures: a comparison of three commonly used devices. *J Bone Joint Surg Am.* 2005;87(11):2415–2422.
23. Brinker MR, O'Connor DP, Crouch CC, et al. Ilizarov treatment of infected nonunions of the distal humerus after failure of internal fixation: an outcomes study. *J Orthop Trauma.* 2007;21(3):178–184.
24. Brouwer KM, Lindenhovius AL, Dyer GS, et al. Diagnostic accuracy of 2- and 3-dimensional imaging and modeling of distal humerus fractures. *J Shoulder Elbow Surg.* 2012;21(6):772–776.
25. Brown RF, Morgan RG. Intercondylar T-shaped fractures of the humerus. Results in ten cases treated by early mobilisation. *J Bone Joint Surg Br.* 1971;53(3):425–428.
26. Bryan RS, Morrey BF. Extensive posterior exposure of the elbow. A triceps-sparing approach. *Clin Orthop Relat Res.* 1982;(166):188–192.
27. Bryan RS, Morrey BF. Fractures of the distal humerus. In: Morrey BF, ed. *The Elbow and its Disorders.* Philadelphia, PA: WB Saunders; 1985:302–339.
28. Burkhart KJ, Nijs S, Mattyasovszky SG, et al. Distal humerus hemiarthroplasty of the elbow for comminuted distal humeral fractures in the elderly patient. *J Trauma.* 2011;71(3):635–642.
29. Campbell WC. Incision for exposure of the elbow joint. *Am J Surg.* 1932;15:65–67.
30. Cassebaum WH. Open reduction of T & Y fractures of the lower end of the humerus. *J Trauma.* 1969;9(11):915–925.
31. Chalidis B, Dimitriou C, Papadopoulos P, et al. Total elbow arthroplasty for the treatment of insufficient distal humeral fractures. A retrospective clinical study and review of the literature. *Injury.* 2009;40(6):582–590.
32. Chen RC, Harris DJ, Leduc S, et al. Is ulnar nerve transposition beneficial during open reduction internal fixation of distal humerus fractures? *J Orthop Trauma.* 2010;24(7):391–394.
33. Choudry UH, Moran SL, Li S, et al. Soft-tissue coverage of the elbow: an outcome analysis and reconstructive algorithm. *Plast Reconstr Surg.* 2007;119(6):1852–1857.
34. Clough TM, Jago ER, Sidhu DP, et al. Fractures of the capitellum: a new method of fixation using a maxillofacial plate. *Clin Orthop Relat Res.* 2001;(384):232–236.
35. Cobb TK, Morrey BF. Total elbow arthroplasty as primary treatment for distal humeral fractures in elderly patients. *J Bone Joint Surg Am.* 1997;79(6):826–832.
36. Coles CP, Barei DP, Nork SE, et al. The olecranon osteotomy: a six-year experience in the treatment of intraarticular fractures of the distal humerus. *J Orthop Trauma.* 2006;20(3):164–171.
37. Dean GS, Holliger EH 4th, Urbaniak JR. Elbow allograft for reconstruction of the elbow with massive bone loss. Long term results. *Clin Orthop Relat Res.* 1997;(341):12–22.
38. Diliberti T, Botte MJ, Abrams RA. Anatomical considerations regarding the posterior interosseous nerve during posterolateral approaches to the proximal part of the radius. *J Bone Joint Surg Am.* 2000;82(6):809–813.
39. Doornberg J, Lindenhovius A, Kloen P, et al. Two- and three-dimensional computed tomography for the classification and management of distal humeral fractures. Evaluation of reliability and diagnostic accuracy. *J Bone Joint Surg Am.* 2006;88(8):1795–1801.
40. Doornberg JN, Ring D, Jupiter JB. Static progressive splinting for posttraumatic elbow stiffness. *J Orthop Trauma.* 2006;20(6):400–404.

41. Doornberg JN, van Duijn PJ, Linzel D, et al. Surgical treatment of intra-articular fractures of the distal part of the humerus. Functional outcome after twelve to thirty years. *J Bone Joint Surg Am.* 2007;89(7):1524–1532.
42. Dowdy PA, Bain GI, King GJ, et al. The midline posterior elbow incision. An anatomical appraisal. *J Bone Joint Surg Br.* 1995;77(5):696–699.
43. Dubberley JH, Faber KJ, Macdermid JC, et al. Outcome after open reduction and internal fixation of capitellar and trochlear fractures. *J Bone Joint Surg Am.* 2006;88(1):46–54.
44. Duggal N, Dunning CE, Johnson JA, et al. The flat spot of the proximal ulna: a useful anatomic landmark in total elbow arthroplasty. *J Shoulder Elbow Surg.* 2004;13(2):206–207.
45. Dunning CE, Zarzour ZD, Patterson SD, et al. Ligamentous stabilizers against posterolateral rotatory instability of the elbow. *J Bone Joint Surg Am.* 2001;83-A(12):1823–1828.
46. Eastwood WJ. The T-shaped fracture of the lower end of the humerus. *J Bone Joint Surg Am.* 1937;19:364–369.
47. Ek ET, Goldwasser M, Bonomo AL. Functional outcome of complex intercondylar fractures of the distal humerus treated through a triceps-sparing approach. *J Shoulder Elbow Surg.* 2008;17(3):441–446.
48. Elkowitz SJ, Polatsch DB, Egol KA, et al. Capitellum fractures: a biomechanical evaluation of three fixation methods. *J Orthop Trauma.* 2002;16(7):503–506.
49. Ergunes K, Yilik L, Ozsoyler I, et al. Traumatic brachial artery injuries. *Tex Heart Inst J.* 2006;33(1):31–34.
50. Erpelding JM, Mailander A, High R, et al. Outcomes following distal humeral fracture fixation with an extensor mechanism-on approach. *J Bone Joint Surg Am.* 2012;94(6):548–553.
51. Espiga X, Antuna SA, Ferreres A. Linked total elbow arthroplasty as treatment of distal humerus nonunions in patients older than 70 years. *Acta Orthop Belg.* 2011;77(3):304–310.
52. Evans EM. Supracondylar-Y fractures of the humerus. *J Bone Joint Surg Br.* 1953;35-B(3):371–375.
53. Faber KJ, Cordy ME, Milne AD, et al. Advanced cement technique improves fixation in elbow arthroplasty. *Clin Orthop Relat Res.* 1997;(334):150–156.
54. Faber KJ. Coronal shear fractures of the distal humerus: the capitellum and trochlea. *Hand Clin.* 2004;20(4):455–464.
55. Foulk DA, Robertson PA, Timmerman LA. Fracture of the trochlea. *J Orthop Trauma.* 1995;9(6):530–532.
56. Fracture and dislocation compendium. Orthopaedic trauma association committee for coding and classification. *J Orthop Trauma.* 1996;10(Suppl 1):1–154.
57. Frankle MA, Herscovici D Jr, DiPasquale TG, et al. A comparison of open reduction and internal fixation and primary total elbow arthroplasty in the treatment of intraarticular distal humerus fractures in women older than age 65. *J Orthop Trauma.* 2003;17(7):473–480.
58. Gainor BJ, Moussa F, Schott T. Healing rate of transverse osteotomies of the olecranon used in reconstruction of distal humerus fractures. *J South Orthop Assoc.* 1995;4(4):263–268.
59. Gambirasio R, Riand N, Stern R, et al. Total elbow replacement for complex fractures of the distal humerus. An option for the elderly patient. *J Bone Joint Surg Br.* 2001;83(7):974–978.
60. Garcia JA, Mykula R, Stanley D. Complex fractures of the distal humerus in the elderly. The role of total elbow replacement as primary treatment. *J Bone Joint Surg Br.* 2002;84(6):812–816.
61. Garland DE, O'Hollaren RM. Fractures and dislocations about the elbow in the head-injured adult. *Clin Orthop Relat Res.* 1982(168):38–41.
62. Gerwin M, Hotchkiss RN, Weiland AJ. Alternative operative exposures of the posterior aspect of the humeral diaphysis with reference to the radial nerve. *J Bone Joint Surg Am.* 1996;78(11):1690–1695.
63. Glanville EV. Perforation of the coronoid-olecranon septum. Humero-ulnar relationships in Netherlands and African populations. *Am J Phys Anthropol.* 1967;26(1):85–92.
64. Gofton WT, Macdermid JC, Patterson SD, et al. Functional outcome of AO type C distal humeral fractures. *J Hand Surg Am.* 2003;28(2):294–308.
65. Grantham SA, Norris TR, Bush DC. Isolated fracture of the humeral capitellum. *Clin Orthop Relat Res.* 1981;(161):262–269.
66. Grechenig W, Clement H, Pichler W, et al. The influence of lateral and anterior angulation of the proximal ulna on the treatment of a Monteggia fracture: an anatomical cadaver study. *J Bone Joint Surg Br.* 2007;89(6):836–838.
67. Greiner S, Haas NP, Bail HJ. Outcome after open reduction and angular stable internal fixation for supra-intercondylar fractures of the distal humerus: preliminary results with the LCP distal humerus system. *Arch Orthop Trauma Surg.* 2008;128(7):723–729.
68. Gschwend N, Simmen BR, Matejovsky Z. Late complications in elbow arthroplasty. *J Shoulder Elbow Surg.* 1996;5(2 Pt 1):86–96.
69. Gupta R, Khanchandani P. Intercondylar fractures of the distal humerus in adults: a critical analysis of 55 cases. *Injury.* 2002;33(6):511–515.
70. Gustilo RB, Anderson JT. Prevention of infection in the treatment of one thousand and twenty-five open fractures of long bones: retrospective and prospective analyses. *J Bone Joint Surg Am.* 1976;58(4):453–458.
71. Hahn NF. Fall von einer besonderes varietat der frakturen des ellenbogens. *Zeitsch Wundartze Geburtshlefer.* 1853;6:185.
72. Hardy P, Menguy F, Guillot S. Arthroscopic treatment of capitellum fracture of the humerus. *Arthroscopy.* 2002;18(4):422–426.
73. Hastings H 2nd, Graham TJ. The classification and treatment of heterotopic ossification about the elbow and forearm. *Hand Clin.* 1994;10(3):417–437.
74. Hastings H 2nd, Theng CS. Total elbow replacement for distal humerus fractures and traumatic deformity: results and complications of semiconstrained implants and design rationale for the Discovery Elbow System. *Am J Orthop.* 2003;32(9 Suppl):20–28.
75. Helfet DL, Hotchkiss RN. Internal fixation of the distal humerus: a biomechanical comparison of methods. *J Orthop Trauma.* 1990;4(3):260–264.
76. Helfet DL, Kloen P, Anand N, et al. Open reduction and internal fixation of delayed unions and nonunions of fractures of the distal part of the humerus. *J Bone Joint Surg Am.* 2003;85-A(1):33–40.
77. Helfet DL, Schmeling GJ. Bicondylar intraarticular fractures of the distal humerus in adults. *Clin Orthop Relat Res.* 1993;(292):26–36.
78. Hewins EA, Gofton WT, Dubberly J, et al. Plate fixation of olecranon osteotomies. *J Orthop Trauma.* 2007;21(1):58–62.
79. Hodgson SP, Parkinson RW, Noble J. Capitellocondylar total elbow replacement for rheumatoid arthritis. *J R Coll Surg Edinb.* 1991;36(2):133–135.
80. Holdsworth BJ, Mossad MM. Fractures of the adult distal humerus. Elbow function after internal fixation. *J Bone Joint Surg Br.* 1990;72(3):362–365.
81. Hotchkiss RN. Elbow contractures. In: Green DP, Hotchkiss RN, Pederson WC, eds. *Green's Operative Hand Surgery.* Vol 1. Philadelphia, PA: Churchill Livingstone; 1999:673–674.
82. Huang TL, Chiu FY, Chuang TY, et al. The results of open reduction and internal fixation in elderly patients with severe fractures of the distal humerus: a critical analysis of the results. *J Trauma.* 2005;58(1):62–69.
83. Hughes JS. Distal humeral hemiarthroplasty. In: Yamaguchi K, King GJ, McKee MD, O'Driscoll SW, eds. *Advanced Reconstruction Elbow.* Rosemont: American Academy of Orthopaedic Surgeons; 2006:219–228.
84. Hunsaker FG, Cioffi DA, Amadio PC, et al. The American academy of orthopaedic surgeons outcomes instruments: normative values from the general population. *J Bone Joint Surg Am.* 2002;84-A(2):208–215.
85. Ikavalko M, Belt EA, Kautiainen H, et al. Souter arthroplasty for elbows with severe destruction. *Clin Orthop Relat Res.* 2004(421):126–133.
86. Ilahi OA, Strausser DW, Gabel GT. Post-traumatic heterotopic ossification about the elbow. *Orthopedics.* 1998;21(3):265–268.
87. Imatani J, Morito Y, Hashizume H, et al. Internal fixation for coronal shear fracture of the distal end of the humerus by the anterolateral approach. *J Shoulder Elbow Surg.* 2001;10(6):554–556.
88. Imatani J, Ogura T, Morito Y, et al. Anatomic and histologic studies of lateral collateral ligament complex of the elbow joint. *J Shoulder Elbow Surg.* 1999;8(6):625–627.
89. Jacobson SR, Glisson RR, Urbaniak JR. Comparison of distal humerus fracture fixation: a biomechanical study. *J South Orthop Assoc.* 1997;6(4):241–249.
90. Jarvinen TL, Sievanen H, Khan KM, et al. Shifting the focus in fracture prevention from osteoporosis to falls. *BMJ.* 2008;336(7636):124–126.
91. Jensen M, Moran SL. Soft tissue coverage of the elbow: a reconstructive algorithm. *Orthop Clin North Am.* 2008;39(2):251–264.
92. Jones KG. Percutaneous pin fixation of fractures of the lower end of the humerus. *Clin Orthop Relat Res.* 1967;50:53–69.
93. Jupiter JB, Mehne DK. Fractures of the distal humerus. *Orthopedics.* 1992;15(7):825–833.
94. Jupiter JB, Neff U, Holzach P, et al. Intercondylar fractures of the humerus. An operative approach. *J Bone Joint Surg Am.* 1985;67(2):226–239.
95. Jupiter JB, Neff U, Regazzoni P, et al. Unicondylar fractures of the distal humerus: an operative approach. *J Orthop Trauma.* 1988;2(2):102–109.
96. Jupiter JB, O'Driscoll SW, Cohen MS. The assessment and management of the stiff elbow. *Instr Course Lect.* 2003;52:93–111.
97. Kalogrianitis S, Sinopidis C, El Meligy M, et al. Unlinked elbow arthroplasty as primary treatment for fractures of the distal humerus. *J Shoulder Elbow Surg.* 2008;17(2):287–292.
98. Kamineni S, Morrey BF. Distal humeral fractures treated with noncustom total elbow replacement. *J Bone Joint Surg Am.* 2004;86-A(5):940–947.
99. Kamineni S, Morrey BF. Distal humeral fractures treated with noncustom total elbow replacement. Surgical technique. *J Bone Joint Surg Am.* 2005;87(Suppl 1Pt 1):41–50.
100. Kannus P, Niemi S, Parkkari J, et al. Why is the age-standardized incidence of low-trauma fractures rising in many elderly populations? *J Bone Miner Res.* 2002;17(8):1363–1367.
101. Kannus P. Preventing osteoporosis, falls, and fractures among elderly people. Promotion of lifelong physical activity is essential. *BMJ.* 1999;318(7178):205–206.
102. Kaplan EB. Surgical approaches to the proximal end of the radius and its use in fractures of the head and neck of the radius. *J Bone Joint Surg Am.* 1941;23:86.
103. Keon-Cohen BT. Fractures at the elbow. *J Bone Joint Surg Am.* 1966;48A:1623–1639.
104. Kocher T. Beitrage zur kenntniss einger praktisch wishctiger fraktur formen. Mitheil a Klin u Med Inst and Schweiz Basal, reihe. 1896:767.
105. Kocher T. *Textbook of Operative Surgery.* 3rd ed. London: Adam and Charles Black; 1911.
106. Korner J, Lill H, Muller LP, et al. Distal humerus fractures in elderly patients: results after open reduction and internal fixation. *Osteoporos Int.* 2005;16(Suppl 2):S73–S79.
107. Kuhn JE, Louis DS, Loder RT. Divergent single-column fractures of the distal part of the humerus. *J Bone Joint Surg Am.* 1995;77(4):538–542.
108. Kundel K, Braun W, Wieberneit J, et al. Intraarticular distal humerus fractures. Factors affecting functional outcome. *Clin Orthop Relat Res.* 1996;(332):200–208.
109. Kuriyama K, Kawanishi Y, Yamamoto K. Arthroscopic-assisted reduction and percutaneous fixation for coronal shear fractures of the distal humerus: report of two cases. *J Hand Surg Am.* 2010;35(9):1506–1509.
110. Lambotte A. *Chirurgie Operatoire des Fractures.* Paris: Masson et Cie; 1913.
111. Lee BP, Adams RA, Morrey BF. Polyethylene wear after total elbow arthroplasty. *J Bone Joint Surg Am.* 2005;87(5):1080–1087.
112. Lee KT, Lai CH, Singh S. Results of total elbow arthroplasty in the treatment of distal humerus fractures in elderly Asian patients. *J Trauma.* 2006;61(4):889–892.
113. Li SH, Li ZH, Cai ZD, et al. Bilateral plate fixation for type C distal humerus fractures: experience at a single institution. *Int Orthop.* 2011;35(3):433–438.
114. Liberman N, Katz T, Howard CB, et al. Fixation of capitellar fractures with the Herbert screw. *Arch Orthop Trauma Surg.* 1991;110(3):155–157.
115. Liu JJ, Ruan HJ, Wang JG, et al. Double-column fixation for type C fractures of the distal humerus in the elderly. *J Shoulder Elbow Surg.* 2009;18(4):646–651.

116. Ljung P, Jonsson K, Rydholm U. Short-term complications of the lateral approach for non-constrained elbow replacement. Follow-up of 50 rheumatoid elbows. *J Bone Joint Surg Br.* 1995;77(6):937–942.
117. Lorenz H. Zur kenntnis der fractural capitulum humeri (Eminentiae Capitatae). *Dtsche Ztrschr f Chir.* 1905;78:531–545.
118. MacAusland WR. Ankylosis of the elbow: with report of four cases treated by arthroplasty. *JAMA.* 1915;64:312–318.
119. MacDermid JC. Outcome evaluation in patients with elbow pathology: issues in instrument development and evaluation. *J Hand Ther.* 2001;14(2):105–114.
120. Mahirogullari M, Kiral A, Solakoglu C, et al. Treatment of fractures of the humeral capitellum using Herbert screws. *J Hand Surg Br.* 2006;31(3):320–325.
121. Mansat P, Morrey BF. Semiconstrained total elbow arthroplasty for ankylosed and stiff elbows. *J Bone Joint Surg Am.* 2000;82(9):1260–1268.
122. Marra G, Morrey BF, Gallay SH, et al. Fracture and nonunion of the olecranon in total elbow arthroplasty. *J Shoulder Elbow Surg.* 2006;15(4):486–494.
123. Marsh JL, Slongo TF, Agel J, et al. Fracture and dislocation classification compendium—2007: Orthopaedic Trauma Association classification, database and outcomes committee. *J Orthop Trauma.* 2007;21(10 Suppl):S1–S133.
124. McCarty LP, Ring D, Jupiter JB. Management of distal humerus fractures. *Am J Orthop.* 2005;34(9):430–438.
125. McKee M, Jupiter J, Toh CL, et al. Reconstruction after malunion and nonunion of intra-articular fractures of the distal humerus. Methods and results in 13 adults. *J Bone Joint Surg Br.* 1994;76(4):614–621.
126. McKee MD, Jupiter JB, Bamberger HB. Coronal shear fractures of the distal end of the humerus. *J Bone Joint Surg Am.* 1996;78(1):49–54.
127. McKee MD, Jupiter JB, Bosse G, et al. Outcome of ulnar neurolysis during post-traumatic reconstruction of the elbow. *J Bone Joint Surg Br.* 1998;80(1):100–105.
128. McKee MD, Jupiter JB. A contemporary approach to the management of complex fractures of the distal humerus and their sequelae. *Hand Clin.* 1994;10(3):479–494.
129. McKee MD, Jupiter JB. Semiconstrained elbow replacement for distal humeral nonunion. *J Bone Joint Surg Br.* 1995;77(4):665–666.
130. McKee MD, Kim J, Kebaish K, et al. Functional outcome after open supracondylar fractures of the humerus. The effect of the surgical approach. *J Bone Joint Surg Br.* 2000;82(5):646–651.
131. McKee MD, Pugh DM, Richards RR, et al. Effect of humeral condylar resection on strength and functional outcome after semiconstrained total elbow arthroplasty. *J Bone Joint Surg Am.* 2003;85-A(5):802–807.
132. McKee MD, Veillette CJ, Hall JA, et al. A multicenter, prospective, randomized, controlled trial of open reduction–internal fixation versus total elbow arthroplasty for displaced intra-articular distal humeral fractures in elderly patients. *J Shoulder Elbow Surg.* 2009;18(1):3–12.
133. McKee MD, Wilson TL, Winston L, et al. Functional outcome following surgical treatment of intra-articular distal humeral fractures through a posterior approach. *J Bone Joint Surg Am.* 2000;82-A(12):1701–1707.
134. McKee MD. *Randomized Trial of ORIF versus Total Elbow Arthroplasty for Distal Humerus Fractures.* AAOS San Diego; 2007.
135. McQueen MM, Gaston P, Court-Brown CM. Acute compartment syndrome. Who is at risk? *J Bone Joint Surg Br.* 2000;82(2):200–203.
136. Meissner M, Paun M, Johansen K. Duplex scanning for arterial trauma. *Am J Surg.* 1991;161(5):552–555.
137. Mellen RH, Phalen GS. Arthroplasty of the elbow by replacement of the distal portion of the humerus with an acrylic prosthesis. *J Bone Joint Surg Am.* 1947;29:348–353.
138. Mighell M, Virani NA, Shannon R, et al. Large coronal shear fractures of the capitellum and trochlea treated with headless compression screws. *J Shoulder Elbow Surg.* 2010;19(1):38–45.
139. Milch H. Fractures and fracture dislocations of the humeral condyles. *J Trauma.* 1964;4:592–607.
140. Min W, Ding BC, Tejwani NC. Comparative functional outcome of AO/OTA type C distal humerus fractures: open injuries do worse than closed fractures. *J Trauma Acute Care Surg.* 2012;72(2):E27–E32.
141. Moro JK, King GJ. Total elbow arthroplasty in the treatment of posttraumatic conditions of the elbow. *Clin Orthop Relat Res.* 2000;(370):102–114.
142. Morrey BF, Adams RA. Semiconstrained elbow replacement for distal humeral nonunion. *J Bone Joint Surg Br.* 1995;77(1):67–72.
143. Morrey BF, Bryan RS. Complications of total elbow arthroplasty. *Clin Orthop Relat Res.* 1982;(170):204–212.
144. Morrey BF, Bryan RS. Infection after total elbow arthroplasty. *J Bone Joint Surg Am.* 1983;65(3):330–338.
145. Morrey BF. Fractures of the distal humerus: role of elbow replacement. *Orthop Clin North Am.* 2000;31(1):145–154.
146. Morrey BF. Post-traumatic contracture of the elbow. Operative treatment, including distraction arthroplasty. *J Bone Joint Surg Am.* 1990;72(4):601–618.
147. Morrey BF. Surgical treatment of extraarticular elbow contracture. *Clin Orthop Relat Res.* 2000;(370):57–64.
148. Morrey BF. The posttraumatic stiff elbow. *Clin Orthop Relat Res.* 2005;(431):26–35.
149. Muller LP, Kamineni S, Rommens PM, et al. Primary total elbow replacement for fractures of the distal humerus. *Oper Orthop Traumatol.* 2005;17(2):119–142.
150. Muller M. *The Comprehensive Classification of Fractures of Long Bones.* Berlin: Springer-Verlag; 1990.
151. O'Driscoll SW, Morrey BF, Korinek S, et al. Elbow subluxation and dislocation. A spectrum of instability. *Clin Orthop Relat Res.* 1992;(280):186–197.
152. O'Driscoll SW, Sanchez-Sotelo J, Torchia ME. Management of the smashed distal humerus. *Orthop Clin North Am.* 2002;33(1):19–33.
153. O'Driscoll SW. Elbow instability. *Hand Clin.* 1994;10(3):405–415.
154. O'Driscoll SW. Optimizing stability in distal humeral fracture fixation. *J Shoulder Elbow Surg.* 2005;14(1 Suppl S):186S–194S.
155. O'Driscoll SW. Supracondylar fractures of the elbow: open reduction, internal fixation. *Hand Clin.* 2004;20(4):465–474.
156. O'Driscoll SW. The triceps-reflecting anconeus pedicle (TRAP) approach for distal humeral fractures and nonunions. *Orthop Clin North Am.* 2000;31(1):91–101.
157. Ochner RS, Bloom H, Palumbo RC, et al. Closed reduction of coronal fractures of the capitellum. *J Trauma.* 1996;40(2):199–203.
158. Olson SA, Rhorer AS. Orthopaedic trauma for the general orthopaedist: avoiding problems and pitfalls in treatment. *Clin Orthop Relat Res.* 2005;(433):30–37.
159. Ozdemir H, Urguden M, Soyuncu Y, et al. [Long-term functional results of adult intra-articular distal humeral fractures treated by open reduction and plate osteosynthesis]. *Acta Orthop Traumatol Turc.* 2002;36(4):328–335.
160. Ozer H, Solak S, Turanli S, et al. Intercondylar fractures of the distal humerus treated with the triceps-reflecting anconeus pedicle approach. *Arch Orthop Trauma Surg.* 2005;125(7):469–474.
161. Pajarinen J, Bjorkenheim JM. Operative treatment of type C intercondylar fractures of the distal humerus: results after a mean follow-up of 2 years in a series of 18 patients. *J Shoulder Elbow Surg.* 2002;11(1):48–52.
162. Palvanen M, Kannus P, Niemi S, et al. Secular trends in the osteoporotic fractures of the distal humerus in elderly women. *Eur J Epidemiol.* 1998;14(2):159–164.
163. Palvanen M, Kannus P, Parkkari J, et al. The injury mechanisms of osteoporotic upper extremity fractures among older adults: a controlled study of 287 consecutive patients and their 108 controls. *Osteoporos Int.* 2000;11(10):822–831.
164. Papaioannou N, Babis GC, Kalavritinos J, et al. Operative treatment of type C intra-articular fractures of the distal humerus: the role of stability achieved at surgery on final outcome. *Injury.* 1995;26(3):169–173.
165. Park MJ, Kim HG, Lee JY. Surgical treatment of post-traumatic stiffness of the elbow. *J Bone Joint Surg Br.* 2004;86(8):1158–1162.
166. Parsons M, O'Brien, RJ, Hughes JS. Elbow hemiarthroplasty for acute and salvage reconstruction of intra-articular distal humerus fractures. *Techniques in Shoulder and Elbow Surgery.* 2005;6(2):87–97.
167. Patterson SD, Bain GI, Mehta JA. Surgical approaches to the elbow. *Clin Orthop Relat Res.* 2000;(370):19–33.
168. Pierce TD, Herndon JH. The triceps preserving approach to total elbow arthroplasty. *Clin Orthop Relat Res.* 1998;(354):144–152.
169. Pollock JW, Athwal GS, Steinmann SP. Surgical exposures for distal humerus fractures: a review. *Clin Anat.* 2008;21(8):757–768.
170. Pollock JW, Faber KJ, Athwal GS. Distal humerus fractures. *Orthop Clin North Am.* 2008;39(2):187–200.
171. Potter D, Claydon P, Stanley D. Total elbow replacement using the Kudo prosthesis. Clinical and radiological review with five- to seven-year follow-up. *J Bone Joint Surg Br.* 2003;85(3):354–357.
172. Poynton AR, Kelly IP, O'Rourke SK. Fractures of the capitellum–a comparison of two fixation methods. *Injury.* 1998;29(5):341–343.
173. Prasad N, Dent C. Outcome of total elbow replacement for distal humeral fractures in the elderly: a comparison of primary surgery and surgery after failed internal fixation or conservative treatment. *J Bone Joint Surg Br.* 2008;90(3):343–348.
174. Prokopis PM, Weiland AJ. The triceps-preserving approach for semiconstrained total elbow arthroplasty. *J Shoulder Elbow Surg.* 2008;17(3):454–458.
175. Puchwein P, Wildburger R, Archan S, et al. Outcome of type C (AO) distal humeral fractures: follow-up of 22 patients with bicolumnar plating osteosynthesis. *J Shoulder Elbow Surg.* 2011;20(4):631–636.
176. Puloski S, Kemp K, Sheps D, et al. Closed reduction and early mobilization in fractures of the humeral capitellum. *J Orthop Trauma.* 2012;26(1):62–65.
177. Rashkoff E, Burkhalter WE. Arthrodesis of the salvage elbow. *Orthopedics.* 1986;9(5):733–738.
178. Ray PS, Kakarlapudi K, Rajsekhar C, et al. Total elbow arthroplasty as primary treatment for distal humeral fractures in elderly patients. *Injury.* 2000;31(9):687–692.
179. Richards RR, Khoury GW, Burke FD, et al. Internal fixation of capitellar fractures using Herbert screws: a report of four cases. *Can J Surg.* 1987;30(3):188–191.
180. Ring D, Gulotta L, Chin K, et al. Olecranon osteotomy for exposure of fractures and nonunions of the distal humerus. *J Orthop Trauma.* 2004;18(7):446–449.
181. Ring D, Gulotta L, Jupiter JB. Unstable nonunions of the distal part of the humerus. *J Bone Joint Surg Am.* 2003;85-A(6):1040–1046.
182. Ring D, Jupiter JB, Gulotta L. Articular fractures of the distal part of the humerus. *J Bone Joint Surg Am.* 2003;85-A(2):232–238.
183. Ring D, Jupiter JB. Complex fractures of the distal humerus and their complications. *J Shoulder Elbow Surg.* 1999;8(1):85–97.
184. Ring D, Jupiter JB. Operative release of complete ankylosis of the elbow due to heterotopic bone in patients without severe injury of the central nervous system. *J Bone Joint Surg Am.* 2003;85-A(5):849–857.
185. Ring D, Jupiter JB. Operative treatment of osteochondral nonunion of the distal humerus. *J Orthop Trauma.* 2006;20(1):56–59.
186. Riseborough EJ, Radin EL. Intercondylar T fractures of the humerus in the adult. A comparison of operative and non-operative treatment in twenty-nine cases. *J Bone Joint Surg Am.* 1969;51(1):130–141.
187. Rispoli DM, Athwal GS, Morrey BF. Neurolysis of the ulnar nerve for neuropathy following total elbow replacement. *J Bone Joint Surg Br.* 2008;90(10):1348–1351.
188. Roberts RM, String ST. Arterial injuries in extremity shotgun wounds: requisite factors for successful management. *Surgery.* 1984;96(5):902–908.
189. Robinson CM, Hill RM, Jacobs N, et al. Adult distal humeral metaphyseal fractures: epidemiology and results of treatment. *J Orthop Trauma.* 2003;17(1):38–47.
190. Robinson CM. Fractures of the distal humerus. In: Bucholz RW HJ, Court-Brown C, Tornetta P, Koval KJ, eds. *Rockwood and Green's Fractures in Adults.* 6th ed. Philadelphia, PA: Lippincott Williams & Wilkins; 2005:1051–1116.
191. Rose SH, Melton LJ 3rd, Morrey BF, et al. Epidemiologic features of humeral fractures. *Clin Orthop Relat Res.* 1982;(168):24–30.

192. Sabo MT, Athwal GS, King GJ. Landmarks for rotational alignment of the humeral component during elbow arthroplasty. *J Bone Joint Surg Am*. 2012;94(19):1794–1800.

193. Sanchez-Sotelo J, Torchia ME, O'Driscoll SW. Complex distal humeral fractures: internal fixation with a principle-based parallel-plate technique. *J Bone Joint Surg Am*. 2007;89(5):961–969.

194. Sanchez-Sotelo J, Torchia ME, O'Driscoll SW. Complex distal humeral fractures: internal fixation with a principle-based parallel-plate technique. Surgical technique. *J Bone Joint Surg Am*. 2008;90(Suppl 2):31–46.

195. Sanders RA, Raney EM, Pipkin S. Operative treatment of bicondylar intraarticular fractures of the distal humerus. *Orthopedics*. 1992;15(2):159–163.

196. Sano S, Rokkaku T, Saito S, et al. Herbert screw fixation of capitellar fractures. *J Shoulder Elbow Surg*. 2005;14(3):307–311.

197. Schemitsch EH, Tencer AF, Henley MB. Biomechanical evaluation of methods of internal fixation of the distal humerus. *J Orthop Trauma*. 1994;8(6):468–475.

198. Schildhauer TA, Nork SE, Mills WJ, et al. Extensor mechanism-sparing paratricipital posterior approach to the distal humerus. *J Orthop Trauma*. 2003;17(5):374–378.

199. Schuster I, Korner J, Arzdorf M, et al. Mechanical comparison in cadaver specimens of three different 90-degree double-plate osteosyntheses for simulated C2-type distal humerus fractures with varying bone densities. *J Orthop Trauma*. 2008;22(2):113–120.

200. Self J, Viegas SF, Buford WL Jr, et al. A comparison of double-plate fixation methods for complex distal humerus fractures. *J Shoulder Elbow Surg*. 1995;4(1 Pt 1):10–16.

201. Shifrin PG, Johnson DP. Elbow hemiarthroplasty with 20-year follow-up study. A case report and literature review. *Clin Orthop Relat Res*. 1990;(254):128–133.

202. Singh AP, Vaishya R, Jain A, et al. Fractures of capitellum: a review of 14 cases treated by open reduction and internal fixation with Herbert screws. *Int Orthop*. 2010;34(6):897–901.

203. Sodergard J, Sandelin J, Bostman O. Mechanical failures of internal fixation in T and Y fractures of the distal humerus. *J Trauma*. 1992;33(5):687–690.

204. Sodergard J, Sandelin J, Bostman O. Postoperative complications of distal humeral fractures. 27/96 adults followed up for 6 (2-10) years. *Acta Orthop Scand*. 1992;63(1):85–89.

205. Soon JL, Chan BK, Low CO. Surgical fixation of intra-articular fractures of the distal humerus in adults. *Injury*. 2004;35(1):44–54.

206. Spinner M, Kaplan EB. The relationship of the ulnar nerve to the medial intermuscular septum in the arm and its clinical significance. *Hand*. 1976;8(3):239–242.

207. Spinner RJ, Morgenlander JC, Nunley JA. Ulnar nerve function following total elbow arthroplasty: a prospective study comparing preoperative and postoperative clinical and electrophysiologic evaluation in patients with rheumatoid arthritis. *J Hand Surg Am*. 2000;25(2):360–364.

208. Stamatis E, Paxinos O. The treatment and functional outcome of type IV coronal shear fractures of the distal humerus: a retrospective review of five cases. *J Orthop Trauma*. 2003;17(4):279–284.

209. Steinthal D. Die isolirte fraktur der eminenthia capetala in ellenbogengelenk. *Zentralb Chir*. 1898;15:17.

210. Stoffel K, Cunneen S, Morgan R, et al. Comparative stability of perpendicular versus parallel double-locking plating systems in osteoporotic comminuted distal humerus fractures. *J Orthop Res*. 2008;26(6):778–784.

211. Street DM, Stevens PS. A humeral replacement prosthesis for the elbow: results in ten elbows. *J Bone Joint Surg Am*. 1974;56(6):1147–1158.

212. Swoboda B, Scott RD. Humeral hemiarthroplasty of the elbow joint in young patients with rheumatoid arthritis: a report on 7 arthroplasties. *J Arthroplasty*. 1999;14(5):553–559.

213. Tachihara A, Nakamura H, Yoshioka T, et al. Postoperative results and complications of total elbow arthroplasty in patients with rheumatoid arthritis: three types of nonconstrained arthroplasty. *Mod Rheumatol*. 2008;18(5):465–471.

214. Tan V, Daluiski A, Simic P, et al. Outcome of open release for post-traumatic elbow stiffness. *J Trauma*. 2006;61(3):673–678.

215. Taylor TK, Scham SM. A posteromedial approach to the proximal end of the ulna for the internal fixation of olecranon fractures. *J Trauma*. 1969;9(7):594–602.

216. Tyllianakis M, Panagopoulos A, Papadopoulos AX, et al. Functional evaluation of comminuted intra-articular fractures of the distal humerus (AO type C). Long term results in twenty-six patients. *Acta Orthop Belg*. 2004;70(2):123–130.

217. Urbaniak JR, Aitken M. Clinical use of bone allografts in the elbow. *Orthop Clin North Am*. 1987;18(2):311–321.

218. Urbaniak JR, Black KE Jr. Cadaveric elbow allografts. A six-year experience. *Clin Orthop Relat Res*. 1985;(197):131–140.

219. Van Gorder GW. Surgical approach in supracondylar "T" fractures of the humerus requiring open reduction. *J Bone Joint Surg Am*. 1940;22:278.

220. Veillette CJ, Steinmann SP. Olecranon fractures. *Orthop Clin North Am*. 2008;39(2):229–236.

221. Ward WG, Nunley JA. Concomitant fractures of the capitellum and radial head. *J Orthop Trauma*. 1988;2(2):110–116.

222. Watts AC, Morris A, Robinson CM. Fractures of the distal humeral articular surface. *J Bone Joint Surg Br*. 2007;89(4):510–515.

223. Weiland AJ, Weiss AP, Wills RP, et al. Capitellocondylar total elbow replacement. A long-term follow-up study. *J Bone Joint Surg Am*. 1989;71(2):217–222.

224. Wiggers JK, Brouwer KM, Helmerhorst GT, et al. Predictors of diagnosis of ulnar neuropathy after surgically treated distal humerus fractures. *J Hand Surg Am*. 2012;37(6):1168–1172.

225. Wilkinson JM, Stanley D. Posterior surgical approaches to the elbow: a comparative anatomic study. *J Shoulder Elbow Surg*. 2001;10(4):380–382.

226. Wright TW, Glowczewski F. Vascular anatomy of the ulna. *J Hand Surg Am*. 1998;23(5):800–804.

227. Yamaguchi K, Adams RA, Morrey BF. Infection after total elbow arthroplasty. *J Bone Joint Surg Am*. 1998;80(4):481–491.

228. Yamaguchi K, Sweet FA, Bindra R, et al. The extraosseous and intraosseous arterial anatomy of the adult elbow. *J Bone Joint Surg Am*. 1997;79(11):1653–1662.

229. Yang KH, Park HW, Park SJ, et al. Lateral J-plate fixation in comminuted intercondylar fracture of the humerus. *Arch Orthop Trauma Surg*. 2003;123(5):234–238.

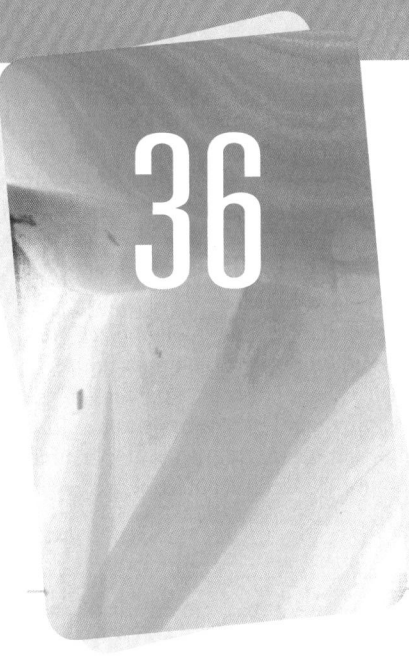

36

HUMERAL SHAFT FRACTURES

Christos Garnavos

INTRODUCTION TO HUMERAL SHAFT FRACTURES

Epidemiology and other social parameters related to diaphyseal humeral fractures have not been extensively studied as those related to fractures occurring in other parts of the human skeleton, such as the proximal femur or the distal radius. Nevertheless, the available bibliographical resources report that the general incidence of humeral shaft fractures remain in the area to 1% to 2% of all fractures occurring in the human body[30,55,142] and 14% of all fractures of the humerus.[175]

The first description of a diaphyseal humeral fracture goes back to ancient Egypt and has been recorded on the Edwin Smith Papyrus, the world's oldest surviving surgical text that was written in Egyptian hieratic script around the 17th century BC.[288] The papyrus was discovered by Edwin Smith in the 1860s and it was recently decoded by James P. Allen of the Metropolitan Museum of Art in New York. The author of the papyrus described the fracture of the humerus and proposed conservative treatment: "Thou shouldst place him prostrate on his back, with something folded between his two shoulder-blades; thou shouldst spread out his shoulders, in order to stretch apart his upper arm until that break falls into its place. Thou shouldst make for him two splints of linen, (and) thou shouldst apply one of them to the inside of his arm, (and) the other of them to the underside of his arm. Thou shouldst bind it with cloth, (and) treat afterward with honey every day until he recovers."

It is obvious that little has changed in the treatment of diaphyseal humeral fractures since ancient times, as humeral fractures heal within a short time. During the treatment patients are mobile whereas shoulder and elbow joints compensate for some malalignment. However, patients in modern times demand faster union rates and earlier return to preinjury activities while preserving functionality and motion of nearby joints. Therefore, over the last few decades, we have witnessed significant advances in the field of surgical management of diaphyseal humeral fractures.

Epidemiologic Data Related to Humeral Shaft Fractures

Up to the age of 60 years, diaphyseal humeral fractures occur equally in men and women and the incidence does not seem to increase with age. After the age of 60 years 80% are

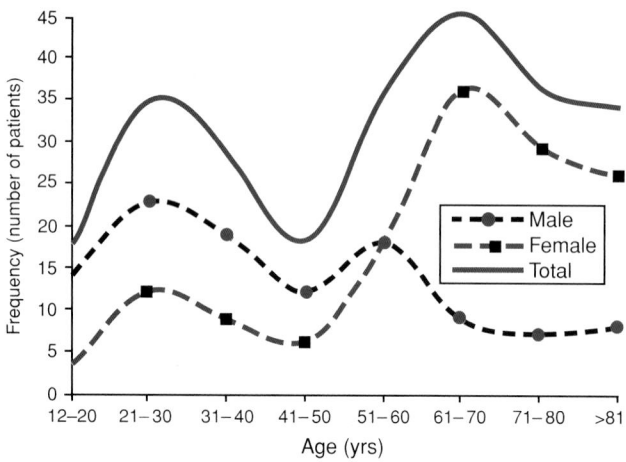

FIGURE 36-1 Age and gender distribution of fractures of the humeral shaft in 249 patients from Edinburgh. (From Tytherleigh-Strong G, Walls N, McQueen MM. The epidemiology of humeral shaft fractures. *J Bone Joint Surg Br.* 1998;80(2):249–253, with permission.)

women[303] and humeral shaft fractures become more frequent (Fig. 36-1).[74,145,278,303] The epidemiology of humeral fractures is discussed in Chapter 3.

The most common reason for a humeral shaft fracture is a fall, followed by motor vehicle accident.[74,145,238,300,303] Other causes that account for less than 10% of humeral shaft fractures include sporting activities, working accidents, fall from a height, violence, and bone pathology. Pathologic and open fractures of the humeral shaft are uncommon (6% to 8% and 2% to 5% of all diaphyseal humeral fractures, respectively).[74,303] Kim et al.[145] studied the annual incidence of humeral fractures in the United States on the basis of the Nationwide Emergency Department Sample and they estimated that the number of humeral fractures is increasing over the years and in 2030 will be almost double compared with 2008.

ASSESSMENT OF HUMERAL SHAFT FRACTURES

Mechanisms of Injury for Humeral Shaft Fractures

The mechanisms of injury for the occurrence of diaphyseal humeral fractures vary and mainly depend on geographical and social parameters. While most studies agree that a ground-level fall is the commonest cause followed by a road traffic accident (RTA),[74,139,145,238,300,303] socioeconomic and geographical conditions influence the prevalence of humeral shaft fractures. According to Kim et al.[145] the ratio of a simple fall to an RTA is 9/1 in the United States, while Tytherleigh-Strong et al.[294] reported that the same ratio is 3.5/1 in the United Kingdom and Reboso et al.[229] reported this ratio for Spain as 1.2/1. While Kim et al. and Reboso et al. found that simple falls and RTAs account for more than 90% of all diaphyseal humeral fractures in USA and Spain respectively, in other countries falls from a height or sporting activities play an important role in the pathogenesis of the injury. So, in Sweden and the United Kingdom, falls from a height and sports account for 8% and 5% to 7% of humeral shaft fractures, respectively, and it is

reported that patients with fractures caused by low-energy trauma tended to be older women and those with high-energy fractures were younger men.[238,303]

Associated Injuries with Humeral Shaft Fractures

Severe injuries of the humeral diaphysis and neighboring anatomical structures threaten the function of the upper limb and may require an individualized and difficult approach for a satisfactory outcome. Not infrequently, these injuries result in restrictions in the range of motion (ROM) of the upper limb joints or neurologic symptoms. Disability from associated injuries may be substantial.

Nerve Injury

The commonest associated injury to a closed diaphyseal humeral fracture is the injury of the radial nerve (10% to 12% of all closed humeral shaft fractures).[74,208,265,275] The clinical manifestation is the inability to dorsiflex the wrist and digits while numbness occurs on the dorsoradial aspect of the hand and the dorsal aspect of the radial 3½ digits (Fig. 36-2).

There has been a lot of controversy regarding the need for immediate exploration of the nerve when there are clinical symptoms of radial nerve palsy. Shao et al. reviewed all papers between 1964 and 2004 in both English and German that included at least 10 patients with the combination of humeral shaft fracture and radial nerve palsy. They concluded that a policy of initial expectant treatment should be preferred to early nerve exploration.[275] They also proposed that the overall waiting time for the nerve to recover should not be longer than 6 months. Bumbasirević et al. studied 117 cases of diaphyseal humeral fractures associated with radial nerve palsy. They did

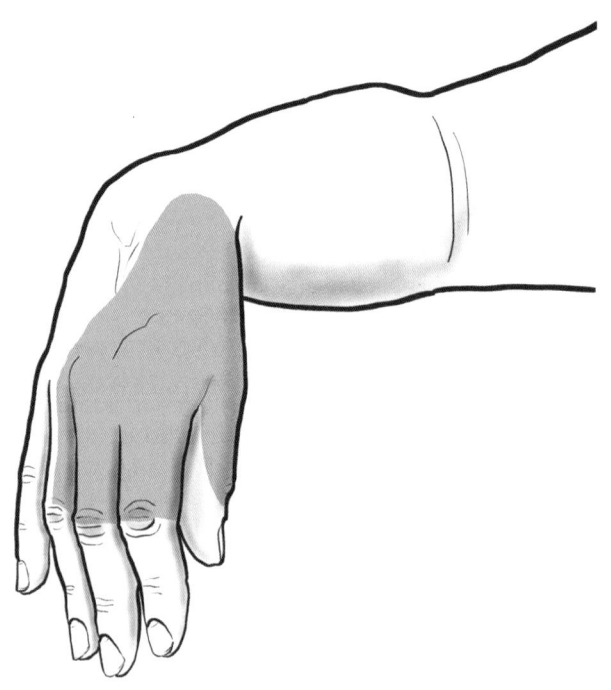

FIGURE 36-2 The clinical picture of a radial nerve palsy.

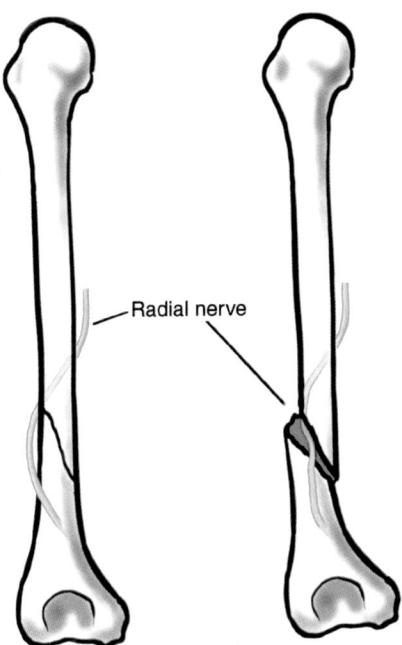

FIGURE 36-3 The Holstein-Lewis fracture.

not recommend early exploration of the nerve but proposed secondary intervention by 10 to 12 weeks from injury in the absence of clinical or electromyographic signs of recovery.[32] Venouziou et al. performed early exploration of the radial nerve and internal fixation of the accompanying humeral fractures in 18 patients with radial nerve palsy and concluded that in cases of high-energy trauma the radial nerve can sustain neurotmesis or severe contusion. They recommended that patients should be informed about the poor prognosis and the probability of tendon transfers.[309] Other indications for early exploration of the nerve include concomitant vascular injury, gunshot wounds, open fractures or severe soft tissue injury, and sharp or penetrating injury.[77,242,275] In 1963, Holstein and Lewis[123] associated a special type of fracture of the distal humerus, a simple displaced spiral fracture, with the distal end deviating toward the radial side occurring in about 7% of all humeral shaft fractures, with an increased rate of radial nerve palsy (Fig. 36-3). They reported a high incidence of entrapment of the nerve within this type of fracture and recommended radial nerve exploration in the presence of clinical symptoms. Subsequent studies confirmed an increased risk of radial nerve injury with this type of fracture but supported the expectant policy even in the presence of clinical symptoms, as their findings indicated that the radial nerve usually recovers spontaneously regardless of the pattern and location of the humeral shaft fracture.[75,275]

Heckler and Bamberger[114] surveyed practice tendencies in USA by sending a questionnaire to 2,650 physicians regarding their practice in cases of humeral shaft fracture associated with radial nerve palsy. From 558 responses, the authors concluded that most physicians agreed that the incidence of recovery is high and observation is justified. There was also a consensus that the nerve should be explored when operative intervention is indicated for the fracture and in cases of open fractures.

Injuries of ulnar and median nerves associated with humeral shaft fractures are not as frequent as injuries of the radial nerve, and relevant information is limited. Noble et al.[208] found that the ulnar and median nerves had been injured in 2.4% and 1.3% respectively in a population of 444 patients with diaphyseal humeral fractures. Omer[215] studied nerve injuries of the upper extremity from any cause (high-velocity gunshot injuries, fracture dislocations, lacerations, etc.) and reported high rates of spontaneous recovery, similar for all nerves, especially in closed injuries. In the absence of more information a similar policy to that for radial nerve injury should be adopted in cases of ulnar or median nerve injury associated with humeral shaft fracture.

Concomitant Dislocation of the Ipsilateral Shoulder

Fracture of the humeral diaphysis and a concomitant dislocation of the ipsilateral shoulder is an infrequent combination that has been reported in the literature in around 11 case reports since 1990. Sasashige et al.[266] described two cases of such a combination, one with anterior and the other with posterior shoulder dislocation, and stressed the high index of suspicion that is required, especially in the case of a posterior dislocation, in order not to miss shoulder injury.

It has been generally accepted that the shoulder dislocation should be reduced immediately under anesthetic, while the management of the diaphyseal humeral fracture remains a matter of controversy. Both nonoperative and operative management have been proposed, all with good outcomes (Fig. 36-4).[42,152]

Other Soft Tissue Injuries of the Ipsilateral Shoulder

Other soft tissue injuries of the ipsilateral shoulder in patients with diaphyseal humeral fractures can be overlooked. However, these injuries can cause problems with the patient's rehabilitation and outcome and also could influence the effectiveness of the humeral fracture treatment, especially in cases treated with antegrade intramedullary nailing. O'Donnell et al.[209] investigated the ipsilateral shoulder after humeral shaft fracture with MRI scans and found that 63.6% had evidence of abnormality such as bursitis of the subacromial space, partial or complete tear of the rotator cuff, inflammatory changes in the acromioclavicular joint, and fracture of the coracoid process. The authors concluded that these injuries may contribute to pain and dysfunction of the shoulder following treatment, and antegrade nailing could be only partly responsible for these symptoms postoperatively.

Floating Elbow

A combination of injuries that involve both the humeral diaphysis and the middle to proximal parts of the radius and ulna with or without significant concomitant injury of the soft tissues around the elbow joint is often the result of high-energy trauma, creating an unstable intermediate articulation, the so-called floating elbow. Although this injury is more common in the pediatric population, it has been studied in adults as well with a few retrospective case series studies over the last 30 years.

Rogers et al.[249] presented one of the biggest series in the literature (19 patients) of floating elbow injury. Eleven patients

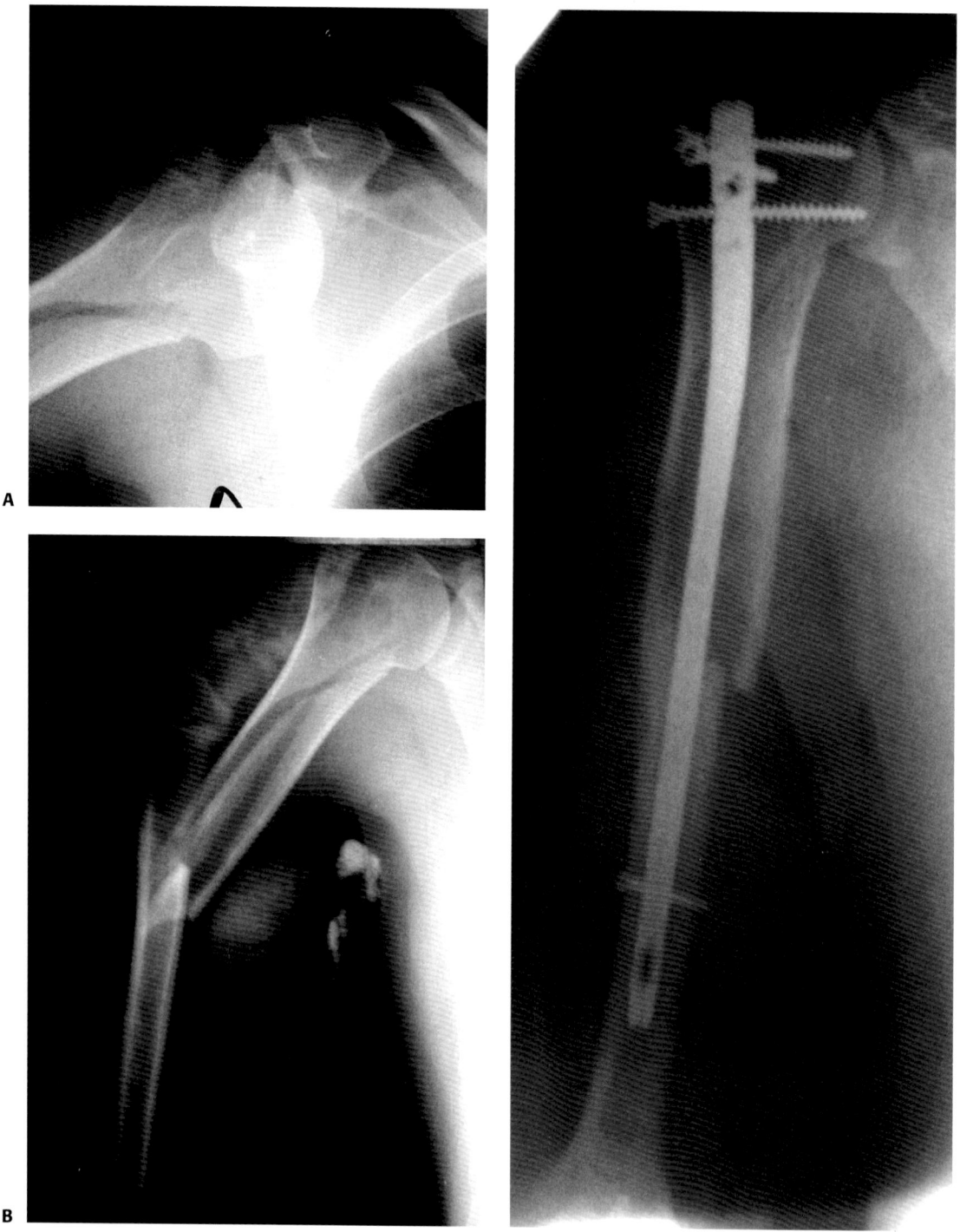

FIGURE 36-4 A: A case of fracture of the proximal humeral diaphysis with associated anterior dislocation of the ipsilateral shoulder. There is fracture of the greater tuberosity as well. **B:** Immediate reduction of the dislocated shoulder under sedation. **C:** Definitive management with intramedullary nailing 2 days later.

did not have concomitant elbow joint injuries while in ten at least one of the components of the injury was open, indicating the severity of this infrequent combination. The management of the injuries varied but, as a general rule, displaced forearm fractures were treated with internal fixation while undisplaced

forearm fractures were treated with a cast. Half of the humeral fractures were treated operatively with plating or percutaneous pinning for closed fractures and external fixators for the open fractures, while conservative treatment was followed in the remainder. Apart from one, all the intra-articular fractures of the elbow were managed with internal fixation. The results revealed many significant complications such as seven humeral and one radial nonunions, three deep infections, one case of myositis ossificans, 11 cases of severe neurovascular problems with incomplete recovery in most cases, and two amputations. The main conclusion of the study was that patients with closed injuries did better than those with open injuries and patients treated with open reduction and internal fixation (ORIF) did significantly better than those treated conservatively. This was confirmed by Langer and Foster 1 year later in a smaller series of nine patients with "floating" elbow injuries. They reported satisfactory outcomes only in those who underwent surgery for all fractures.[158] Although it seems logical that concomitant neurovascular injury would be an adverse prognostic factor for patients who have sustained floating elbow injury, Yokoyama et al.[322] stated that the functional outcome of such patients is irrelevant to the existence of open fractures or neurovascular injuries. Solomon et al.[281] debated the previous statement and supported that sustaining a nerve injury is a poor prognostic factor for patients with "floating" elbow injuries.

Apart from the typical injury of the concomitant fractures of the diaphysis of the humerus, radius, and ulna, there have been sporadic reports that describe variations of floating elbow injuries, such as combinations of additional soft tissue injury to the elbow (e.g., concomitant dislocation) or additional fractures (mainly of the humeral condyles). The common denominator of all reports is that floating elbow is a severe injury that warrants surgical management and meticulous postoperative rehabilitation with a high complication rate and not infrequent suboptimal results (Fig. 36-5).

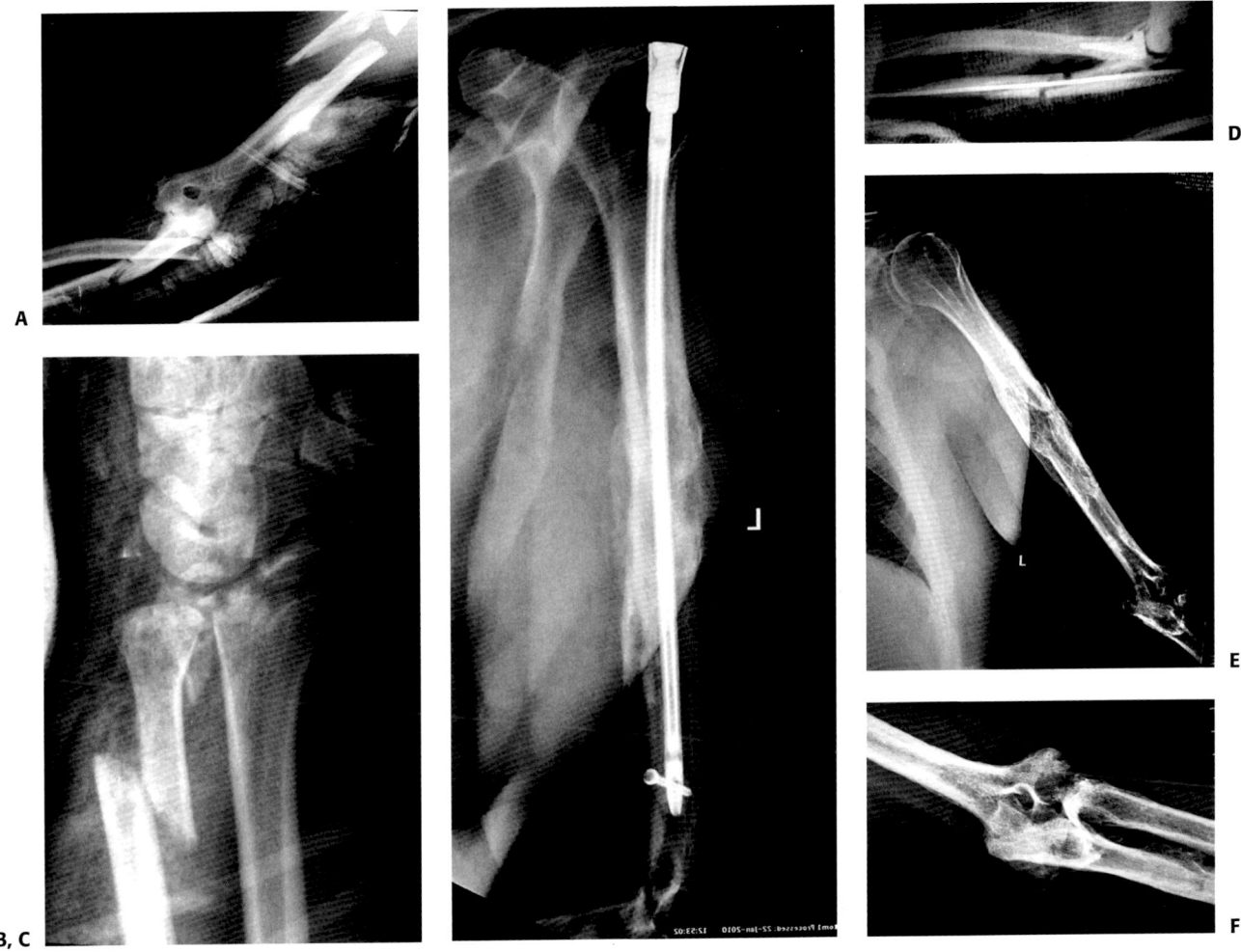

FIGURE 36-5 A: Severe "floating" elbow injury. Fracture of the humeral and ulna diaphysis, open fracture of the radial head, and elbow dislocation. **B:** Ipsilateral fractures of the distal radius and ulna and fractures/dislocations of the carpal bones. **C:** After resuscitating the patient (who also suffered a severe pelvic injury) and provisional stabilization of the arm with splints, the humerus was fixed with intramedullary nailing. **D:** The elbow dislocation was reduced, the radial head replaced, and the ulna was stabilized with a long pin, that was fixing its fractured distal diaphysis as well. **E:** Eighteen months later the nail was removed to reveal a well-healed humeral fracture. **F:** Unfortunately, deep infection developed at the elbow that required removal of the radial head prosthesis. It settled with IV antibiotics but left a stiff and painful elbow. The patient declined further surgical assistance.

Signs and Symptoms of Humeral Shaft Fractures

The alert patient can provide a detailed description of the accident that can characterize the injury as being of high or low velocity and turn our attention to specific elements that may require either immediate care or additional investigations. The majority of humeral shaft fractures occur as a result of ground-level falls or minor twisting injuries in older osteoporotic patients while the precipitating cause in younger individuals is often higher-energy injury and includes RTA, industrial accident, fall from a height, sports, and throwing injuries.[76,150,265] The possibility of a fracture through pathologic bone should be also borne in mind in cases with a history of minimal trauma, and thorough investigation of the patient's past medical history is of paramount importance. Additional information should be sought about comorbidities, medication, previous surgery, and habits that could interfere with anesthetic, fracture healing, or rehabilitation, such as smoking, alcoholism, or drug abuse.

In nonpolytrauma patients the most striking clinical symptom is the excruciating pain at the fracture site. The patient's upper arm appears swollen and often obviously deformed. The patient supports the injured arm with the opposite hand and tries to avoid any manipulation or movement of the ipsilateral shoulder and elbow joints. While the patient is reluctant to allow any examination of the injured arm by the physician, an effort should be made to exclude injury in other areas of the upper limb, or anywhere else in the body, such as head, neck, chest, or abdominal injury. The arm and axilla must be thoroughly inspected in the case of a wound that allows communication of the bone with the environment. In the most frequent scenario of closed fracture, attention is then paid to the neurovascular status of the arm. Radial and ulna arteries are palpated at the wrist and the hand is assessed for the adequacy of capillary refill. The neurologic status of the arm is then assessed. Although clinical examination should be performed for all main peripheral nerves, special attention should be paid to the functionality of the radial nerve, as because of its anatomical relationship to the humerus, it is more frequently injured. Dorsiflexion of the wrist and the interphalangeal joint of the thumb along with sensory examination of the dorsum of the hand can reveal potential injury of the radial nerve and any findings–negative or positive—should be recorded. The ipsilateral elbow, forearm, wrist, and hand are palpated for sensitivity and inspected for pathologic signs such as edema, bruises, wounds, or discoloration.

In cases of polytraumatized patients it may be difficult or impossible to obtain any information from the patient. Therefore, the physician must collect data about the accident and the patient's preinjury status from witnesses, paramedics, or relatives. Usually, the injury of the arm has low priority in relation to other injuries and the patient should be managed according to Advanced Trauma Life Support (ATLS) guidelines. Upon stabilization of the patient and after exclusion of life- or limb-threatening pathology, attention is directed to the injured arm. If the patient is co-operative the clinical examination will proceed as described above. With unconscious or distressed patient the examination can be difficult and impor-

tant parameters such as assessment of neurologic status of the arm may be impossible. This may be a problem because if a nerve palsy is subsequently detected the surgeon will not know whether the nerve injury resulted from a manipulation of the fracture or a surgical intervention. The rest of the clinical examination must be meticulous; thorough circumferential inspection should reveal the existence of wound(s) and raise the possibility of an open fracture, whereas discoloration of the arm can indicate a vascular problem, and deformities pinpoint other sites of injury. The examining physician must be alert that in polytraumatized patients there is an increased incidence of injuries in other areas of the arm (floating elbow) or around the shoulder joint (shoulder dislocation, coexisting fracture of the proximal humerus), and that patients with closed fractures that occurred in high-velocity injuries may develop acute compartment syndrome.

Imaging and Other Diagnostic Studies for Humeral Shaft Fractures

Any patient with a suspected humeral shaft fracture should undergo x-ray investigation in two planes at 90 degrees to each other. The ipsilateral shoulder and elbow joints must be included in the x-ray image, in order to exclude either fracture extension or an associated injury to the joint. The majority of humeral diaphyseal fractures will not require further imaging and the two good-quality plain films will be adequate for fracture assessment and treatment planning. In the event of doubts about fracture morphology or the existence of associated injuries in the vicinity of the humerus or elsewhere, further x-rays centered on the shoulder, elbow, forearm, or the wrist and hand may be ordered. If x-rays reveal or raise a suspicion of a possible proximal or distal intra-articular fracture, more detailed investigation with a CT scan may be necessary.

Clinical signs of vascular injury can be initially investigated with a pulse oximeter or a Doppler and in cases of severe injuries with angiogram (Fig. 36-6). If, following the stabilization of a humeral shaft fracture, there are clinical signs of nerve injury, ultrasonography can be useful in the detection of the injury and its extent.[299]

Nerve conduction studies and electromyography (EMG) can be used for the assessment of the functional status of a nerve and its recovery rate and are used mostly after radial nerve palsy. However, these investigations do not significantly influence the decision regarding the management of the fracture.

Classification of Humeral Shaft Fractures
Bone Injury

Classification systems have been introduced in orthopedic practice as valuable tools that could provide information about the severity of the injury, indicate treatment options, and predict outcomes. Categorization of fracture patterns with classification systems contributes toward better organization of research projects and more comprehensive analysis of their results.

In 1990 the AO group presented the AO/Müller classification for long-bone fractures.[203] The classification was revised in 1996 by the Orthopaedic Trauma Association (OTA) and was

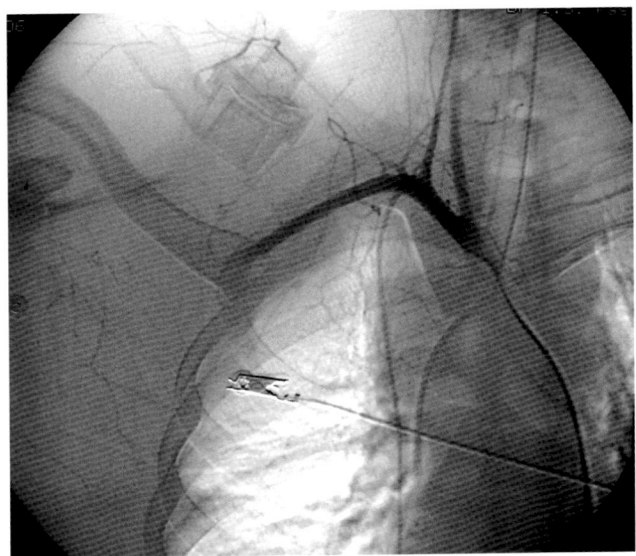

FIGURE 36-6 Angiogram showing traumatic rupture of the subclavian artery. Complete sternoclavicular separation can also be seen.

TABLE 36-1	**Garnavos Classification**	
Topography		**Morphology**

Topography	Morphology
P: Proximal	**S:** Simple (no butterflies)
M: Middle	**t:** Transverse or oblique
D: Distal	**s:** Spiral
j: Extension toward the joint	**I:** Intermediate (one or two sizable butterflies)
	C: Complex (three or more any size butterflies or big comminution)

demic communication. However, over the years, it has received criticism for being complicated, with low inter- and intraobserver variation agreement and reliability.[136,205,291,293] The latest version (2007) became more complex without being validated for users' agreement and other important parameters such as treatment selection, outcomes, and ease of use in everyday clinical practice.[180] Recently, we presented a new, simple classification system for diaphyseal long-bone fractures that could facilitate clinical communication, assist in the choice of treatment method, and predict complications and outcome (Table 36-1 and Fig. 36-8).[91] The system divides the diaphysis of each long bone (femur, tibia, humerus, radius, ulna) into three zones of equal length. The proximal zone is assigned the capital letter P (for proximal), the middle zone the capital letter M (for middle), and the distal zone the capital letter D (for distal). The capital letters P, M, D describe the location of a fracture. When a fracture extends to more than one zone or occurs in the transition area between two zones the location is described appropriately by two or three initials from proximal to distal. Fractures are morphologically described as simple (S), intermediate (I), or complex (C), with these letters following the letter(s) defining the location. Simple fractures are those with no comminution (clear-cut fractures) and are further separated into transverse or slightly oblique (t) and spiral (s). One or two minor bony chips should not change the definition of a fracture as simple. Intermediate fractures have one or two sizable bony fragments, whereas complex fractures have >3 sizable bony fragments or greater comminution. We proposed that while the

further improved and expanded in 2007 to include all fractures of the human skeleton (Chapter 2).[180] The comprehensive classification of humeral diaphyseal fractures according to Fracture and Dislocation Classification Compendium 2007 is presented in Figure 36-7. The system designates the humerus as a bone (1), divided into three parts: Proximal (11), diaphyseal (12), and distal (13). The diaphyseal segment is further divided into three types: Simple fractures (12-A) consisting of two main fragments—proximal and distal, wedge fractures (12-B) where there are one or more intermediate fragments with contact between the main fragments after reduction, and complex fractures (12-C) where there is more comminution and no contact of the main proximal and distal fragments after reduction. The types are further divided into three groups depending on the morphology, from "benign" (1) to "difficult" (3), and each group into three subgroups that define the proximal, middle, or distal zone of the diaphysis, where the fracture happened.

Since its introduction the AO/Müller classification system has been regarded as an invaluable tool for research and aca-

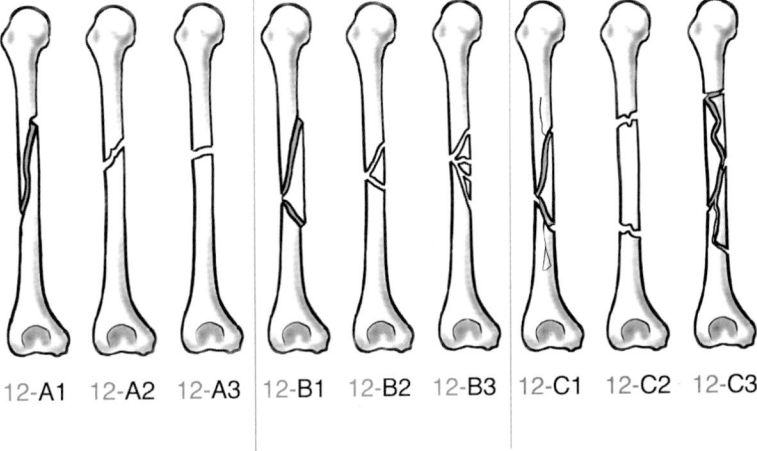

12-A1   12-A2   12-A3   12-B1   12-B2   12-B3   12-C1   12-C2   12-C3

FIGURE 36-7 AO/OTA classification of diaphyseal humeral fractures.

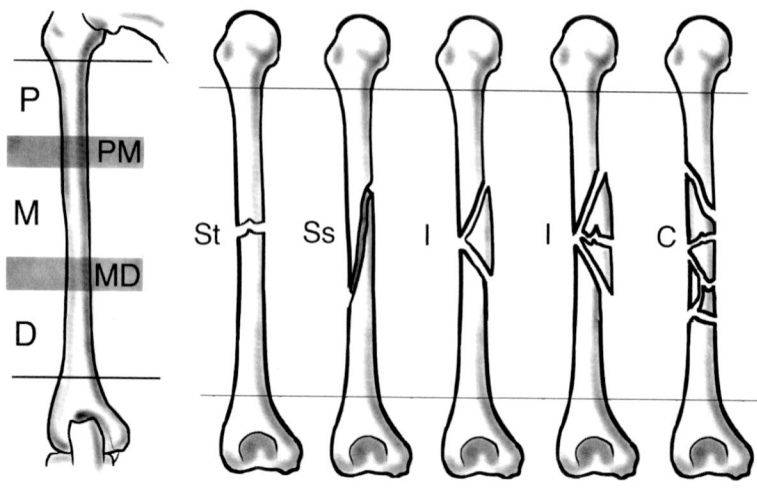

FIGURE 36-8 Garnavos classification of diaphyseal humeral fractures.

AO/OTA classification should be used for scientific projects and research the newly proposed classification could become a useful tool for everyday clinical practice and communication.

Soft Tissue Injury

The severity of soft tissue injury is of paramount importance for treatment selection and outcome of a diaphyseal humeral fracture (Chapter 2). Open fractures have been classified since 1976 by Gustilo and Anderson into three grades.[106,107] Grade I is an inside-out puncture wound to the skin caused by the fracture as result of a low-energy injury. Grade II is caused by higher velocity and the wound is greater than 1 cm without extensive soft tissue damage, flaps, or avulsions. Grade III is a severe injury with extensive soft tissue damage that is further divided into three subgroups: (A) with adequate soft tissue coverage, (B) with significant soft tissue loss with periosteal stripping and bone exposure that will require flap coverage, and (C) with vascular injury that will require repair.

The Open Fracture Study Group of the OTA recently produced a proposal about a new classification for open fractures.[216] The Study Group identified factors in the literature that had been used clinically to evaluate open fractures of the upper extremity, lower extremity, and pelvis. This list of factors was reviewed by a seven-member panel of orthopedic traumatologists, each of whom independently examined and prioritized each factor for inclusion or exclusion in the new open fracture classification scheme. The results of this analysis were discussed by an "open fracture work group" and a new open fracture classification system was proposed. This proposal was further revised after being tested through a process of clinical data collection. The proposed New Classification of Open Fractures is presented in Table 36-2.

Tscherne and Gotzen[301] classified the soft tissue damage in closed fractures, as it can play an important role in the course of treatment and the outcome of the injury (Table 36-3).

Outcome Measures for Humeral Shaft Fractures

Outcome assessment following the management of diaphyseal humeral fractures must consider parameters related to bone and soft tissue healing as well as the restoration of function of the ipsilateral shoulder and elbow joints. Functional assessment of the nearby joints is even more important in cases of complications such as nonunion or neurologic problems.

The process of bone healing is typically assessed with plain x-rays and clinical examination at 4- to 6-week intervals until fracture union. Widely accepted radiologic signs for fracture union are the identification of bridging callus on two orthogonal views or in three of the four cortices.[317] More specifically, for

---

TABLE 36-2 **OTA/OFS Group Classification of Open Fractures**

Skin
1. Can be approximated
2. Cannot be approximated
3. Extensive degloving

Muscle
1. No muscle in area, no appreciable muscle necrosis, some muscle injury with intact muscle function
2. Loss of muscle but the muscle remains functional, some localized necrosis in the zone of injury that requires excision, intact muscle–tendon unit
3. Dead muscle, loss of muscle function, partial or complete compartment excision, complete disruption of a muscle–tendon unit, muscle defect does not approximate

Arterial
1. No injury
2. Artery injury without ischemia
3. Artery injury with distal ischemia

Contamination
1. None or minimal contamination
2. Surface contamination (easily removed, not embedded in bone or deep soft tissues)
3. a. Embedded in bone or deep soft tissues
   b. High-risk environmental conditions (barnyard, fecal dirty water, etc.)

Bone Loss
1. None
2. Bone missing or devascularized but still some contact between proximal and distal fragments
3. Segmental bone loss

fractures of the humeral diaphysis, Sarmiento et al.[265] defined fracture union as the osseous bridging between the main fragments, observed on at least one radiograph if there is no pain at the fracture site. CT scan can offer more detailed information and confirm delayed or nonunion but should be reserved for patients whose fracture healing is not progressing, as assessed by standard x-ray imaging and physical examination.[14]

Functional recovery of shoulder and elbow joints can be affected either by the initial injury or by the treatment and is assessed with scoring systems. Perhaps the most popular scoring system to assess post-traumatic shoulder recovery has been proposed by Constant and Murley[52] in 1987. The Constant-Murley score is a 100-point functional shoulder assessment tool in which higher scores reflect increased function. It includes pain score (15 points), functional assessment (20 points), Range of Motion (ROM) (40 points), and strength measures (25 points) (Table 36-4). A weakness of this system is that it

---

TABLE 36-3 Tscherne and Gotzen Classification of Soft Tissue Damage in Closed Fractures

Grade 0: Minimal soft tissue damage, indirect violence, simple fracture pattern

Grade I: Superficial abrasion of contusion caused by pressure from within, mild to moderate fracture pattern

Grade II: Deep contaminated abrasions associated with localized skin or muscle contusion, impending compartment syndrome, severe fracture

Grade III: Extensive skin contusion or crush, underlying severe muscle, decompensated compartment syndrome, associated major vascular injury, severe fracture

---

TABLE 36-4 The Constant-Murley Score for Assessing the Recovery of the Soulder Joint Following Trauma

Pain 15/100 points	Severe pain	0		
	Moderate pain	5		
	Minimal pain	10		
	No pain	15		
Motion 40/100 points	**Forward flexion 10 points**		**Abduction 10 points**	
	0–30	0	0–30	0
	31–60	2	31–60	2
	61–90	4	61–90	4
	91–120	6	91–120	6
	121–150	8	121–150	8
	151–180	10	151–180	10
	External rotation 10 points (hand not allowed to touch the head)		**Internal rotation 10 points**	
	Not reaching the head	0	End of the thumb to lateral thigh	0
	Hand behind head with elbow forward	2	End of the thumb to buttock	2
	Hand behind head with elbow back	2	End of the thumb to lumbosacral junction	4
	Hand on top of head with elbow forward	2	End of the thumb to L3 (waist)	6
	Hand on top of head with elbow back	2	End of the thumb to T 12	8
	Full elevation from on top of head	2	End of the thumb to T 7(interscapular)	10
Strength 25/100 points	Strength of abduction against resistance at the level of the scapula with the forearm pronated. The score is allocated on a sliding scale up to 25 points.			
Function 20/100 points	Ability to work	0 to 4 points		
	Recreational activities	0 to 4 points		
	Ability to sleep	0 to 2 points		
	Ability to work at the level:			
	Of the waist	2 points		
	Of the xiphoid	4 points		
	Of the neck	6 points		
	Of the head	8 points		
	Above the head	10 points		

requires a large amount of objective data collection by the clinician which may affect interobserver reliability.

Other popular shoulder scores used for assessing the efficacy of treatment after injury are the following:

The American Shoulder and Elbow Surgeons Self-Report Form for the Shoulder (ASES-s)

This is a 100-point standardized shoulder assessment form, 50 points of which are provided from a patient self-report in the form of Visual Analog Scales (VASs) for pain and instability and a questionnaire about the ability to perform daily living activities.[146] The physician assessment section includes an area to collect demographic information and assesses ROM, specific physical signs, strength, and stability.

The Oxford Shoulder Score

This system relies on the patient's subjective assessment of pain and impairment of daily living activities to provide the assessment.[63] A clinical follow-up visit is therefore not necessary. The Oxford Shoulder Questionnaire adds up to a total score with a maximum value of 60, of which four pain-related questions make up 33 points while the remaining 27 points are derived from eight questions related to daily activities. It should be noted that the highest scores are attributed to the worst outcomes.

Elbow function after trauma is usually assessed with flexion and extension lag. Popular scoring systems assessing the elbow joint recovery following trauma are the following:

The Mayo Elbow Performance (MEP) Index

This is probably the most popular scoring system for assessment of the recovery of the elbow joint following trauma.[198] This system assesses motion in terms of flexion and extension. Neither strength nor deformity is included in the content of the scale. Function and motion are weighted less heavily than pain (Table 36-5).

TABLE 36-5	The Mayo Elbow Performance (MEP) Index for Assessing the Recovery of the Elbow Joint Following Trauma	
Pain (max points 45)	None	45
	Mild	30
	Moderate	15
	Severe	0
Motion (max points 20)	Arc of motion >100 degrees	20
	Arc of motion >50 and <100 degrees	15
	Arc of motion <50 degrees	5
Stability (max points 10)	Stable	10
	Moderate stability	5
	Grossly unstable	0
Function (max points 25)	Can comb hair	5
	Can eat	5
	Can perform hygiene	5
	Can put on shirt	5
	Can put on shoe	5

TABLE 36-6	The QuickDASH Scoring System Assesses the Symptoms and Functional Status of the Whole Injured Arm

1: No difficulty; 2: Mild difficulty; 3: Moderate difficulty
4: Severe difficulty; 5: Unable

1. Open jar		1	2	3	4	5
2. Pain intensity		1	2	3	4	5
3. Tingling intensity		1	2	3	4	5
4. Sleep		1	2	3	4	5
5. Socialize		1	2	3	4	5
6. Wash back		1	2	3	4	5
7. Forceful recreation		1	2	3	4	5
8. Heavy chores		1	2	3	4	5
9. Carry a bag		1	2	3	4	5
10. Use knife		1	2	3	4	5
11. Limited in work		1	2	3	4	5

The American Shoulder and Elbow Surgeons Self-Report Form for the Elbow (ASES-e)

This scoring system was developed by the American Shoulder and Elbow Research Committee.[146] The patient self-evaluation section contains VASs for pain and a series of questions relating to function of the extremity. The physician assessment section has four parts: Motion, stability, strength, and physical findings. Higher scores indicate worse function.

Apart from scoring systems dedicated to the functional assessment of either the shoulder or the elbow joints, the Disabilities of the Arm, Shoulder and Hand (DASH) system (joint initiative of the American Academy of Orthopedic Surgeons [AAOS], the Council of Musculoskeletal Specialty Societies [COMSS], and the Institute for Work & Health [Toronto, Ontario]) assesses the symptoms and functional status of the whole injured arm.[127] The DASH is a 30-item questionnaire with a five-item response option for each item. The test has a maximum score of 100, where higher scores reflect greater disability. The DASH index is a valid and reliable tool for assessing recovery after multiple injuries of the upper extremity. The Quick-DASH (Table 36-6) is a shortened version of the DASH scoring system. It consists of 11 items to measure physical function and symptoms in people with any or multiple musculoskeletal disorders of the upper limb. Similar to the DASH, each item has five response options. The final score ranges between 0 (no disability) and 100 (the greatest possible disability). Only one missing item can be tolerated, and, if two or more items are missing, the score cannot be calculated.

PATHOANATOMY AND APPLIED ANATOMY RELATING TO HUMERAL SHAFT FRACTURES

The humeral diaphysis extends from the surgical neck of the humerus, just below the greater and lesser tuberosities to the supracondylar ridge at the elbow.[91,104] A cross section of the humeral shaft is round proximally and changes gradually to be triangular distally, with the medullary canal becoming narrower at the distal part. For descriptive reasons the bone can be divided into three equal parts in length, the proximal, middle, and distal thirds. The surface of the humerus can be also divided into three longitudinal parts; anterolateral, anteromedial, and posterior. Each area is defined by bony ridges that extend from the tuberosities to the supracondylar region. Knowledge of the polymorphy of the cross section and the surface anatomy of the humeral diaphysis can facilitate internal fixation as plates fit better on flat surfaces while introduction of a retrograde nail can be troublesome if the narrower triangular shape of the distal humerus is overlooked. Important osseous landmarks of the humeral diaphysis are the deltoid tuberosity (point of insertion of the deltoid muscle) on the anterolateral surface at the junction of the proximal and middle thirds of the diaphysis and the spiral groove in the middle/posterior aspect that contains the radial nerve and the profunda brachii artery.

The humerus is covered by a thick envelope of soft tissues that include strong muscles and a rather complicated arrangement of neurovascular structures (Fig. 36-9). Muscles that surround the humerus from proximal to distal include the deltoid, pectoralis major, teres major, latissimus dorsi, coracobrachialis, brachialis, brachioradialis, and the triceps brachii. Knowledge of the course and the site of insertion of each muscle can explain the displacement that occurs in diaphyseal fractures and also can facilitate preoperative planning and fixation technique. A typical example is the displacement in abduction of the proximal humeral fragment in cases of fractures occurring proximal to the insertion of pectoralis major because of the pull of the deltoid muscle. The muscles surrounding the humeral diaphysis form two compartments, the anterior and posterior that are separated by fascial membranes (septa). The anterior compartment contains the flexors of the elbow (biceps, brachialis, and coracobrachialis) and the posterior contains the triceps brachialis

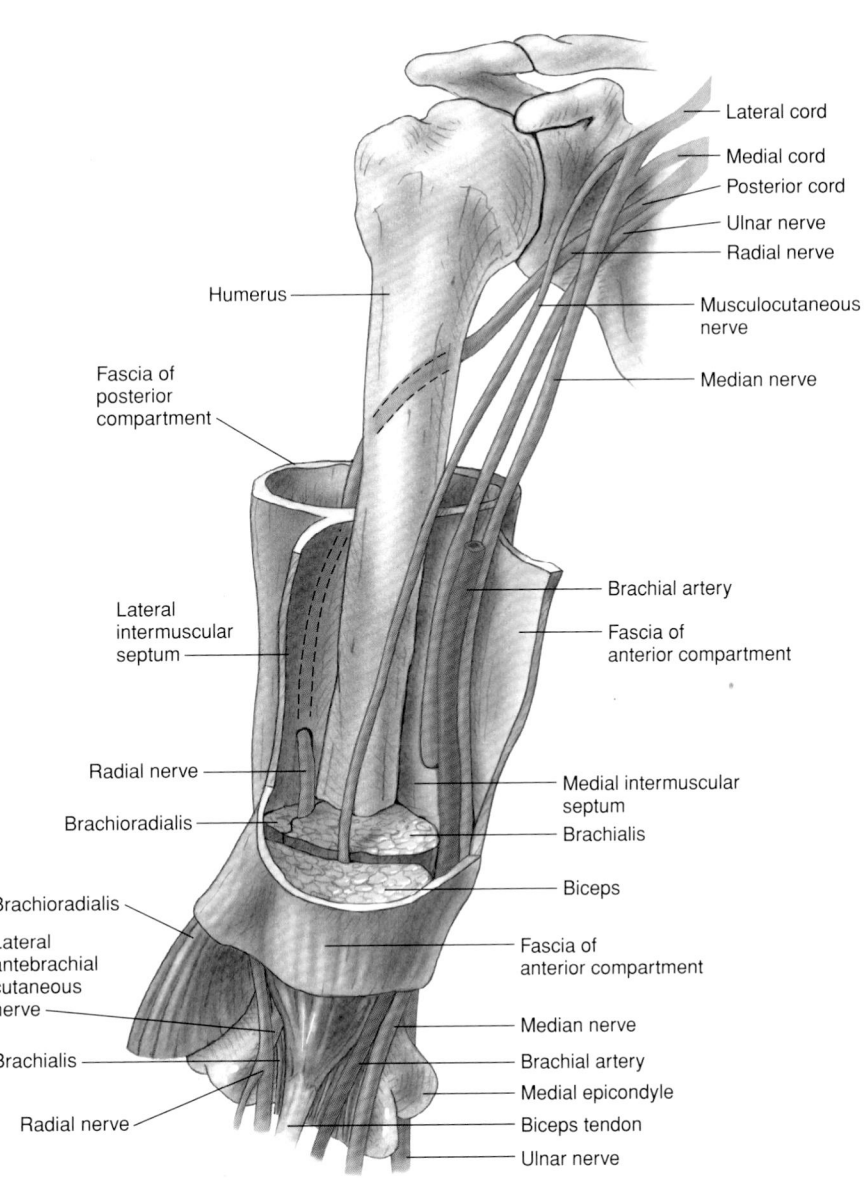

FIGURE 36-9 The neurovascular anatomy of the upper arm.

with its three heads (long, lateral, and medial). The radial nerve enters the posterior compartment and runs between the long and lateral heads of the triceps, enters the spiral groove which is posterior to the deltoid tuberosity, and runs its course postero-laterally adjacent to the bone before it exits the spiral groove on the lateral aspect of the humerus approximately 10 to 15 cm proximal to the lateral epicondyle.[105]

It is important to note when planning surgical procedures at the distal humerus that as the radial nerve exits the spiral groove and becomes anterior, the distance from the articular surface of the distal humerus is never less than 7.5 cm.[304] The median nerve and the brachial artery have a common course on the medial aspect of the anterior compartment and at the level of the elbow lie between the pronator teres and the biceps tendon. The musculocutaneous nerve also lies within the anterior compartment and crosses the distal humerus longitudinally, lateral to the median nerve and brachial artery. It can be endangered during anteroposterior (AP) distal interlocking in antegrade nailing or in the distal window of Minimally Invasive Plate Osteosynthesis (MIPO). The proximal part of the ulna nerve runs in proximity to the median nerve within the anterior compartment but at the arcade of Struthers, approximately 8 cm from the medial epicondyle, it enters into the posterior compartment and runs medially toward the cubital tunnel.[230]

Although the proximal humerus is dealt with in Chapter 37 knowledge of its surgical anatomy is necessary for the management of humeral shaft fractures. Penetration of the rotator cuff is the standard approach for antegrade nailing, while proximal locking screws penetrate the deltoid and/or the subscapularis. Surgeons must be aware that the supraspinatus tendon is relatively avascular near its insertion into the greater tuberosity and therefore, it is recommended that the entry portal for antegrade nailing should be created toward its musculotendinous area.[116]

The axillary nerve runs around the proximal humerus, circumferentially, from posterior to anterior at a distance of 4 to 7 cm from the tip of the acromion and it can be injured either from an extended lateral approach to the proximal diaphysis or from the drill bit and the screws used for proximal interlocking of an intramedullary nail.[302] Likewise, the anterior and posterior circumflex arteries of the humeral head could be injured from the drill or the proximal locking screws of an antegrade nail.

HUMERAL SHAFT FRACTURE TREATMENT OPTIONS

Nonoperative Treatment of Humeral Shaft Fractures

Indications/Contraindications

It is generally accepted that acute, closed, uncomplicated fractures of the humeral diaphysis that occur in ambulatory, co-operative patients have high rates of union with good functional results, if treated nonoperatively.[68,188,219] However, as for any treatment, the indications and contraindications for applying nonoperative treatment in fractures of the humeral diaphysis are constantly reviewed and subject to change, as surgical techniques are improving and the socioeconomic environment favors treatment options that can offer a faster recovery and earlier return to normal activities.

A review of studies on the nonoperative treatment of diaphyseal fractures of the humerus published in the first decade of the 21st century was performed to define modern indications and contraindications for nonoperative treatment. Closed, acute, and isolated fractures were primary indications for nonoperative treatment in all studies. Sarmiento et al.[265] reviewed 620 patients who had sustained humeral shaft fractures and were treated with functional bracing. Apart from the primary indications they also treated fractures that were open (155, 25%), segmental (6, 1%), associated with dislocation of the ipsilateral shoulder (12, 2%) and with primary radial nerve palsy (67, 11%). Patients who had suffered a nerve injury because of penetrating trauma or a high-velocity gunshot wound were excluded. Koch et al.[150] reported that they treated patients with multiple injuries, open fractures, and cases with associated radial nerve palsy nonoperatively but do not recommend nonoperative treatment for patients with additional fractures of the ipsilateral arm. Toivanen et al. excluded multiply injured patients or pathologic fractures from nonoperative treatment. Interestingly they noted that there was a high rate of nonunion after conservative treatment when the fracture was located at the proximal third of the diaphysis (54%) and in AO type A fractures (23%).[297] Similarly Ekholm et al.[76] treated 78 patients who had sustained an acute, isolated, non-pathologic humeral shaft fracture, but excluded patients with multiple fractures, pathologic fractures, periprosthetic fractures, and previous fractures of the same humerus. In the study period there were nine patients (10%) with primary radial nerve palsy but only five of these were treated nonoperatively. Although the authors reported good results overall, they recognized that there was a trend toward an increased number of nonunions in patients with OTA type A fractures if compared with type B and C fractures. This finding was confirmed in a review of 18 studies of humeral shaft fractures treated with functional bracing. The authors found an overall union rate of 94.5%, but an average nonunion rate of 15.4% in type A fractures, in the five articles that reported the prevalence of nonunion with regard to AO classification.[219] This raises the possibility that patients who suffer a type A humeral shaft fracture could have better results if treated operatively.

Rutgers and Ring[259] excluded open fractures, polytrauma patients, and periprosthetic fractures from nonoperative treatment and noted that noncompliant patients are hard to manage with nonoperative treatment. They also made a comment about a trend toward nonunion in long oblique fractures of the proximal third, confirmed in a subsequent study from the same institute.[243] The same observation was made in an earlier study by Castella et al.[35] Pehlivan[223] reviewed 21 young, compliant patients who had sustained acute, closed, and isolated fractures of the distal part of the humerus and were treated nonoperatively. Having excluded from the treatment protocol multitrauma, open fractures, or fractures with neurovascular injuries all fractures united uneventfully. Decomas and Kaye[65] recently tried to identify risk factors associated with failure of nonoperative treatment of diaphyseal humeral fractures. Their

TABLE 36-7	Indications, Relative Indications, and Relative Contraindications for Nonoperative Management of Diaphyseal Humeral Fractures		
Strong Indication	**Relative Indications**		**Relative Contraindications**
Acute/closed/isolated fracture in a Cooperative and Ambulatory patient	Type A fracture (AO classification) Proximal third, long oblique fracture Segmental fracture Open fracture without neurovascular injury Noncompliant patient		Multiple injuries Vascular injury Additional injuries to the ipsilateral arm Persisting or increasing nerve dysfunction Bilateral fractures Pathologic fracture Nonunited fracture

conclusions were in agreement with the previous data that short oblique fractures and fractures occurring at the proximal third of the diaphysis are at greater risk for nonunion.

It should be noted that primary radial nerve injury in closed fracture should not be considered a contraindication for nonoperative treatment.[76,150,265] While all studies regarded additional injury to the ipsilateral arm as a contraindication for nonoperative treatment,[76,150,223,259,265,297] one study proposed that fractures with concomitant shoulder dislocation can be treated nonoperatively.[265] Finally, regarding behavioral and morphologic characteristics, it is worth mentioning that noncompliant patients may not be suitable for nonoperative treatment of a humeral shaft fracture[223,259] and, despite older reports, none of the most recent studies referred to obesity or women with large breasts as contraindications for nonoperative treatment.

Using this information an updated list of the indications and contraindications for nonoperative management of humeral shaft fractures has been created, which requires evaluation in future studies (Table 36-7).

Techniques

Nonoperative treatment of diaphyseal humeral fractures can be accomplished with various techniques such as skeletal traction, Velpeau bandage, a sling and body bandage, abduction cast or splint, coaptation splint or U-slab, hanging arm cast, and functional bracing. Of these, skeletal traction and the abduction cast have been abandoned as their application is troublesome and cannot be easily tolerated by patients. Velpeau bandage, a sling and body bandage, U-slabs, and hanging casts are still in use, but over the last 2 to 3 decades functional bracing, as described by Sarmiento et al.,[264] has dominated the nonoperative management of humeral shaft fractures. However, functional braces may not be immediately available and temporary immobilization of the arm is usually necessary. Therefore, a basic knowledge of alternative splinting techniques is required.

Sling/Swathe and Velpeau Bandage. A sling and swathe is an easy, inexpensive technique that can offer rapid immobilization of the arm. A sling supports the weight of the arm while a swathe immobilizes the arm against the chest. Padding should be placed in the axilla to provide some comfort to the patient. Velpeau bandage is a similar technique, except that the bandaging around the arm and the patient's torso is more restrictive, the patient's elbow is flexed, and the forearm lies against the chest (Fig. 36-10A). Both techniques are difficult for the patient to tolerate for more than few days and should be replaced by functional bracing as soon as possible.

U-Slab/Coaptation Splint. A U-slab is commonly used for temporary immobilization of humeral shaft fractures, especially if they are located in the middle or distal humerus (Fig. 36-10B). The arm is covered with a stockinette and wool bandage and a strip of plaster is applied from the axilla to the medial side of the arm, around the olecranon, and turned upward on the lateral side of the arm up to the level of the acromion. It is secured in this position with an elastic bandage. The disadvantage of this splint is that it loosens easily and slips downward

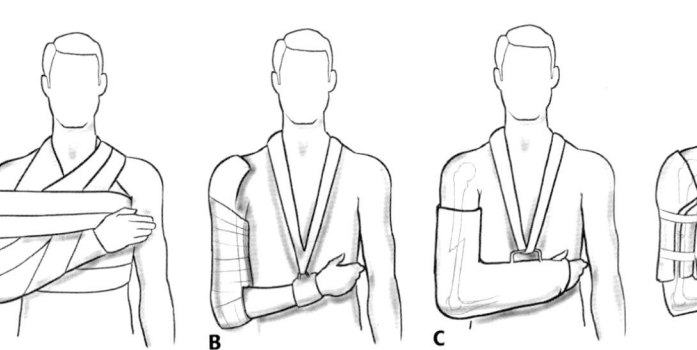

FIGURE 36-10 **A:** Velpeau bandage. **B:** U-slab. **C:** Hanging cast. **D:** Functional brace.

requiring frequent adjustment or replacement. As with the Velpeau bandage technique, the U-slab should be replaced by functional bracing as soon as possible.

Hanging Cast. Hanging casts have been used for many decades for the management of humeral shaft fractures, especially in cases with shortening and displacement (Fig. 36-10C). Most frequently these are simple, oblique, or spiral fractures in the middle third of the humerus. In cases of transverse fractures with shortening, a hanging cast can be applied to reduce the humerus to the proper length and alignment. However, this technique requires close supervision because if neglected it can distract the fracture and contribute to healing problems. The hanging cast technique requires a full arm cast, with the plaster extending from above the fracture to the wrist, with the elbow flexed to 90 degrees, and the forearm in the neutral position. The patient should be instructed to keep the arm in a "hanging" position for as long as possible to allow gravity to restore humeral length and alignment. Most surgeons use hanging casts routinely for 1 week to 10 days to achieve fracture reduction and then continue with functional bracing.

Functional Bracing. Since it was first described in 1977 by Sarmiento et al.[264] functional bracing has been the most popular definitive technique for the nonoperative management of humeral shaft fractures. Immediately after the accident the arm may be temporarily immobilized with one of the techniques described above. The duration of this temporary immobilization should not exceed 7 to 10 days. At that time the patient is examined in the outpatient department and, if the acute symptoms and edema have subsided, is provided with a prefabricated brace that consists of two plastic sleeves that fit on opposite sides of the arm, either medial and lateral or anterior and posterior. They are held together with adjustable Velcro straps (Fig. 36-10D). Tightening of the straps creates a "custom made" well-fitted splint that applies pressure to the muscle belly surrounding the humerus and immobilizes the fracture. Patients are provided with a collar-and-cuff sling but they are instructed to move their elbow every day to avoid stiffness of the joint. They are also taught how to adjust the plastic sleeves and tighten the Velcro straps in the case of loosening or loss of position of the brace. Pendulum movements of the arm are encouraged from the beginning. Patients are instructed to avoid abduction and active elevation exercises or resting the injured arm on the arm of a chair, a table, or their lap, because leaning on the elbow of a fractured extremity during the early stages of healing may cause varus angulation. After application of the brace regular review is required for examination and radiographic evaluation of the healing progress. The patient is advised to increase shoulder and elbow exercises during the recovery period.

Outcomes

Functional bracing, as described by Sarmiento et al. is widely used by orthopedic practitioners for the management of acute diaphyseal humeral fractures.[264,265] Sarmiento et al.[265] have also presented the largest series of 620 patients treated with functional bracing with adequate follow-up. Apart from closed,

uncomplicated fractures, open fractures (155, 25%) and closed fractures associated with radial nerve palsy (67, 11%) were included. Open fractures with concomitant nerve injury and polytrauma patients were not treated by functional bracing. The authors reported a low (2.6%) nonunion rate (1.5% in closed fractures and 5.8% in open fractures). The healing time was on average 9.5 weeks for closed fractures and 14 weeks for open fractures. There were no significant differences regarding healing times for fractures located in any of the proximal, middle, or distal parts of the humerus or for fractures with differing patterns (transverse, oblique, comminuted, or segmental). Bearing in mind that up to 20 degrees anterior or posterior angular deformity and 15 degrees of varus,[15,147] can be tolerated well by the arm, the authors reported an average of 9 degrees of varus angulation in transverse fractures, 4 degrees in oblique fractures, and 8 degrees in comminuted fractures. The occurrence of valgus deformity was insignificant, while more than 80% of the patients had less than 15 degrees of anterior or posterior angulation. Regarding functional recovery 88.6% of the patients lost less than 10 degrees of motion of the shoulder joint, while 92% of the patients lost less than 10 degrees of motion of the elbow as compared with the opposite side. Over the last 3 decades there have been several studies with substantial number of patients that confirm and validate the effectiveness of functional bracing in the management of diaphyseal humeral fractures.[15,76,82,131,150,223,259,263,315,323] The average healing time in all these studies was 93.5% (77.4% to 100%) while time to union was reported from 6.5 to 22 weeks (average 10.7 weeks).

Within the first decade of the 21st century, there have been further valuable observations. Fjalestad et al.[82] reported that of 67 diaphyseal humeral fractures that were treated with functional bracing, 61 (91%) united but a detailed functional assessment revealed that 21 patients (38%) experienced significant loss of external rotation of the ipsilateral shoulder joint. In an effort to explain this finding the authors performed CT in a selected group of patients and found that rotational malunion may be responsible for functional deficiency after nonoperative treatment and they proposed early application of the functional brace to avoid this problem. Sarmiento et al. had previously reported that in a series of 72 patients, 26 (45%) had lost from 5 to 45 degrees of external rotation of the shoulder and suggested that this happened because of shrinkage of the shoulder capsule. At the time, this clinical parameter was not considered significant.[263] Loss of shoulder joint motion with the use of functional bracing for the treatment of humeral shaft fractures has also been reported by others. Koch et al. found that only 28 out of 48 patients (58.3%) regained symmetrical and normal range of shoulder motion.[150] Pehlivan[223] followed up 21 patients and reported that when the brace was removed, restriction of movement occurred in the shoulder that improved with use of the extremity. Rosenberg and Soudry[253] reported that 9 of the 15 consecutive patients who had sustained diaphyseal humeral fractures and were treated with functional bracing were unable to return to their previous activities because of shoulder impairment. Furthermore, 13 of the 15 patients experienced noticeable shoulder pain (6 of them admitted VAS values higher than five).

Functional bracing has been considered particularly useful for fractures located at the distal third of the humeral diaphysis.[131,223,263] Sarmiento et al.[263] were able to review 65 patients who had sustained 54 closed and 11 open fractures of the distal humeral diaphysis. Twelve patients with associated radial nerve palsy had recovered partially or completely at the latest follow-up. Union rate was 96% (with only one nonunion in the group of open fractures) while angular deformities were recorded as 4 degrees of maximum median angulation in 80% of the patients, 3 to 22 degrees of posterior angulation in 39% of the patients, and 1 to 30 degrees of anterior angulation in 41% of the patients. The authors also recorded 2 to 15 mm of shortening in 36% of the patients. Twenty-six patients (45%) lost 5 to 45 degrees of external rotation of the shoulder joint while abduction and forward flexion were also impaired from 10 to 60 degrees and 5 to 20 degrees in nine (15.5%) and eight (13%) patients respectively. Elbow joint motion was affected in 15 patients (26%) who experienced 5 to 25 degrees of reduced flexion while 14 patients (24%) had 5 to 25 degrees of limited extension. Pehlivan[223] presented similar results after treating a small group of patients, who suffered a fracture of the distal humeral diaphysis, with functional bracing. The author raised concerns about difficulties with fracture reduction and the risk of axial deviation at the fracture site, as 8 out of 21 patients (38%) experienced significant varus angulation.

Although the overall effectiveness of functional bracing is not disputed, recent studies have raised questions about more specific issues. Toivanen et al.[297] noted that fractures located in the proximal part of the humerus had a higher nonunion rate (6 out of 13 united) than fractures located either in the middle (48 out of 59 united) or the distal third (18 out of 21 united). A similar finding was reported by Rutgers and Ring[259] who also noticed that the ununited proximal third fractures had a long-oblique pattern. Castellá et al.[35] reviewed humeral nonunions that occurred after nonoperative management and noticed that a significant proportion had occurred in a specific fracture pattern (hemi-transverse medial fracture with a long and sharp lateral butterfly) located at the junction of the proximal and middle thirds of the diaphysis. Likewise, Ring et al. found that spiral/oblique fractures that involve the middle or proximal third of the diaphysis are more likely not to unite with functional bracing.[243] Ekholm et al.[76] observed that AO type A fractures had a higher nonunion rate than other types of fractures when treated with functional bracing. It seems that apart from the latter study the literature does not support the general impression that simple transverse fractures of the humerus are slow to heal nonoperatively.[219] It should be noted that two studies prior to 2000 suggested that fractures located in the middle or distal third of the humerus were at greater risk for nonunion,[264,315] while other studies do not regard fracture location as a key predictor of fracture union.[76,82,253]

Operative Treatment of Humeral Shaft Fractures

Indications/Contraindications

Indications for operative reduction and fixation of diaphyseal humeral fractures were first defined by Bandi[16] and included

TABLE 36-8	Indications and Relative Indications for Operative Management of Diaphyseal Humeral Fractures
Indications	**Relative Indications**
Inability to maintain satisfactory reduction by closed means	Open fractures
Multiple injuries	Segmental fractures
Bilateral fractures	Noncompliant patients
Floating elbow	Obesity or large breasts
Intra-articular fracture extension	Periprosthetic fractures
Progressive nerve palsy or nerve palsy after closed manipulation	Type A fracture in the middle third of the humerus
Significant vascular injury	Long oblique fracture of the proximal humerus
Neurologic deficit after penetrating injury	
Nonunion	
Pathologic fractures	

diaphyseal fractures in an unacceptable position after conservative treatment, open fractures, transverse fractures, comminuted fractures with radial nerve palsy and pseudoarthrosis. By 1996 the previous list was enriched with segmental fractures, pathological fractures, bilateral fractures, floating elbow, polytrauma cases, neurologic loss after penetrating injury, associated vascular injury, and intra-articular fracture extension while some of the previous indications, such as open fractures or fractures associated with radial nerve palsy, were reassessed.[327] Over the last 10 to 20 years surgeons have paid attention to the details and secondary characteristics of fracture patterns and although the basic list of indications for operative treatment has not changed, more "relative" indications have been added (Table 36-8).

Inability to maintain satisfactory reduction by closed means is one of the main indications for surgical treatment. With nonoperative treatment angular deformity of more than 15 to 20 degrees in any direction and rotational malalignment of more than 30 degrees should not be accepted unless the patient is willing to accept visible deformity. The maximum humeral shortening that can be accepted is not precisely known. Although it has been reported that humeral shortening up to 5 cm can pass unnoticed, it sounds more reasonable to limit shortening to no more than 2 to 3 cm.[188,323]

Patients with multiple injuries should benefit from surgery, as these patients lie recumbent for many days or weeks and are prone to malunion.[19,163] These patients are likely to undergo surgery for other injuries and therefore, they will inevitably undergo anesthesia which is considered to be one of the disadvantages of operative treatment of humeral shaft fractures in isolated injury. Furthermore, nursing care, cleanliness, and comfort are facilitated with surgical treatment.

Bilateral humeral fractures or fractures associated with other injuries of the ipsilateral arm (floating elbow, combined fractures/dislocations of the proximal humerus and humeral shaft) constitute indications for operative management of all injuries to allow early mobilization of joints and rapid recovery of independence and comfort. Furthermore, if the joints ipsilateral to the humeral shaft fracture are injured, surgical treatment will permit earlier initiation of physiotherapy and avoidance of joint stiffness.[31,86,93,158,168,249] Segmental fractures of the humeral diaphysis with minimal displacement could be managed nonoperatively but this can be difficult if the middle fragment is displaced.[93,168]

Progressive neurologic deficit, nerve palsy after manipulation, or significant vascular laceration after penetrating trauma will require exploration and repair of the injured structures.[36,50,51,256,312] Secure stabilization of the fracture is then mandatory to protect the repair and allow frequent wound inspections and changing of dressings without disturbing the surgical site or risking damage from mobile bone fragments. Likewise, humeral shaft fractures associated with brachial plexus injury should be stabilized operatively to allow rapid mobilization of the entire arm and prevent nonunion, as the arm loses a part of its muscular support because of neurologic deficit.[188] Pathological fractures should be stabilized operatively for palliative care if the patient's life expectancy is more than 6 months and their general condition allows operative treatment.[11,144,213]

Open fractures are heterogeneous injuries. Depending on the severity, as classified by Gustilo and Anderson,[106] (Chapter 10) open humeral fractures can be treated with different treatment methods. For example, grade I fractures can be managed well with functional bracing, grade II can be treated either conservatively or operatively depending on the wound contamination, and grade III fractures should be treated operatively.[199,256,265,272]

Noncooperative and indigent patients constitute another relative indication for operative treatment. Sarmiento et al.[265] mentioned that indigent patients were frequently lost to follow-up and proposed that these patients should not be treated with functional bracing. However, indigent and noncompliant patients may not follow the rehabilitation program after operative fixation of their fractures and therefore, may be at equal risk of suffering postoperative complications.

Obese patients and ladies with large breasts may benefit from the operative stabilization of their humeral shaft fracture as, because of their body mass, they have greater risk of malunion or nonunion.[103,132] However, it could be argued that angular deformity should be less visible within a substantive soft tissue envelope and that these patients may be at greater risk for complications from the anesthesia or the sizeable wounds.[138] It is my opinion that patients with increased body mass should be treated individually bearing in mind their comorbidities, after thorough discussion with the anesthetist and the patient.

Periprosthetic fracture is a relative indication for immediate operative management, as there seems to be a consensus that if the prosthesis is stable, conservative management can be attempted. In cases with a loose prosthesis or failure of conservative management operative treatment is necessary with revision of the prosthesis to a cemented longer stem, plating, and strut grafts.[66,260]

Transverse or oblique midshaft fractures or long-oblique proximal shaft fractures should be included nowadays in the list of relative indications for surgical management, as it has been reported that these fractures have high risk of nonunion if treated conservatively.[35,219,243]

Old age and osteoporosis are not included in the list of indications or relative indications for operative management of humeral shaft fractures because there is no strong evidence that osteoporosis significantly influences the healing process. However, older people often cannot tolerate bracing and can be noncompliant. Therefore, the decision about the best treatment option for osteoporotic people with fractures of the humeral diaphysis must be based on careful assessment of the fracture characteristics and the patient's comorbidities and personality.

Plate Osteosynthesis

Preoperative Planning. Winston Churchill said during World War II that "failing to plan is planning to fail." Preoperative planning is a mandatory step that has to precede any surgical procedure to minimize intraoperative problems and maximize the possibility of a successful outcome. It should be stressed that initially the patient should be fully informed about the procedure and the postoperative rehabilitation course. Consultation with the anesthetist should take place concentrating on the patient's comorbidities and technical issues that could interfere with anesthesia (such as patient positioning or placement of the endotracheal tube away from the injured side).

At least two x-ray views of the whole humerus should be available, one neutral AP and one oblique-lateral. The length of the humerus should be measured from the available x-rays, taking into account the magnification, and depending on fracture extension and location the surgeon should estimate the length of the plate that will be required for the fixation of the fracture. If the fracture is close to the proximal or the distal metaphysis, there should be consideration of the adequacy of the implant to fix the shorter segment and in doubtful situations there should be alternative fixation options readily available. Whenever fracture lines extend toward the shoulder or elbow joints further x-ray views, centered in the suspected area, must be obtained. If there are still doubts about the integrity of the joints, a CT scan should be performed.

The surgeon must be certain that the appropriate operating room with a suitable orthopedic table that can accommodate the planned procedure is available. The practice of accurate preoperative drawing of the fracture and the fixation technique now appears old-fashioned in the digital era and radiographic films are replaced by computer images. Relevant software programs that allow digital picture modification, measurement, and drawing are becoming available allowing preoperative planning to move from paper to screen.[110]

In any case, the surgeon must decide in advance how the fracture will be approached, must be familiar with the anatomy and able to predict difficulties (such as structures at risk) that could be met during the operation. Preoperative drawings of fracture reduction and fixation can be a good approximation of the type and size of implant that will be needed and the tools that will be required (such as reduction forceps), so the surgeon should be able to check suitability, compatibility, and availability of the necessary tools and implants. A complete preoperative planning of plate fixation should also consider the type and order of screw insertion. Finally, the surgeon should make

TABLE 36-9	Preoperative Planning Checklist for Plate Fixation of Diaphyseal Humeral Fracture

1. Operating Theater

Operating Room Table
- Regular orthopedic
- Radiolucent arm support
- Forearm extension
- Other

X-ray
- C-arm
  Left
  Right
- Plain films

4. Implants
- Large fragment locking set
- Large fragment standard set
- Small fragment locking set
- Small fragment standard set
- K-wires
- Cerclage wires
- Other

2. Position/Positioning Aids
- Supine
- Prone
- Beach chair
- Lateral (right side up)
- Lateral (left side up)
- Positioning aids

3. Equipment
- Battery drill
- Bone graft instruments
- Large bone reduction tools
- Other

5. Other

certain that the image intensifier will be on the site and working as there may be the need for intraoperative x-ray imaging.

The development of a checklist that can be provided in advance to the operating room personnel (Table 36-9) leads to better organization of the operating procedure and the immediate availability of the necessary equipment.

Positioning. Patient positioning depends on the surgical approach. More specifically, plating fractures of the middle and proximal humeral diaphysis is usually performed via an anterolateral approach with the patient in the supine position with some padding underneath the scapula to support the torso and elevate the limb. The arm lies on a radiolucent arm board, abducted 45 to 60 degrees which will facilitate intraoperative x-ray imaging, if necessary. Fractures located at the proximal humeral diaphysis can be plated using the proximal part of the anterolateral approach with the operating table inclined headend up by 20 to 30 degrees in the so-called "beach chair" position. The arm is adducted with the injured arm protruding from the operating table and the forearm is positioned on a forearm support. The inclined position makes proximal extension of the approach easier and if the operating table is not too broad and the arm of the image intensifier is sufficiently curved, the image intensifier can be positioned on the opposite side of the table and be readily available at any time without interfering with the operating field. Fractures located in the middle third of the humeral diaphysis can be approached by a straight anterolateral incision with the patient supine and the arm abducted on a radiolucent extension. Fractures at the distal humeral diaphysis are better approached with the patient prone, because with this position the whole arm can be brought free of the operating table on a radiolucent extension, allowing good visualization with the image intensifier.

Alternatively, the posterior approach can be performed equally well with the patient in the lateral position with the shoulder flexed and abducted and the elbow flexed over a support but intraoperative imaging may be more challenging in this position. For the minimal invasive plate osteosynthesis (MIPO) procedure the patient lies supine with the arm on a radiolucent table as in traditional plating of a fracture located in the middle of the humerus. The only difference is that the arm must be adducted to facilitate the insertion of the plate through the proximal humerus.

Surgical Approaches for (ORIF). The most frequently used approaches are the anterolateral (for middle and proximal diaphyseal fractures) and the posterior (for distal diaphyseal humeral fractures or for exploration of the radial nerve). However, a direct lateral approach has also been described (mostly used for the exploration of the radial nerve) and a medial approach for the exploration of the neurovascular structures on the medial side. Recently, approaches have also been described for MIPO of diaphyseal humeral fractures.[124,172,188,195,270,326]

Anterolateral Approach. The surgeon can use any part of this approach depending on the fracture location. The skin incision starts at the tip of the coracoid process and runs distally in line with the deltopectoral groove to the lateral aspect of the humerus at the deltoid insertion (Fig. 36-11A). From there, the incision continues distally following the lateral border of the biceps until about 5 cm proximal to the flexion crease of the elbow joint.

At the proximal part of the approach division of the superficial fascia will reveal the cephalic vein which runs within the deltopectoral groove. The humerus is then approached by retracting the deltoid laterally and the pectoralis major medially (Fig. 36-11B). Care must be taken not to apply excessive

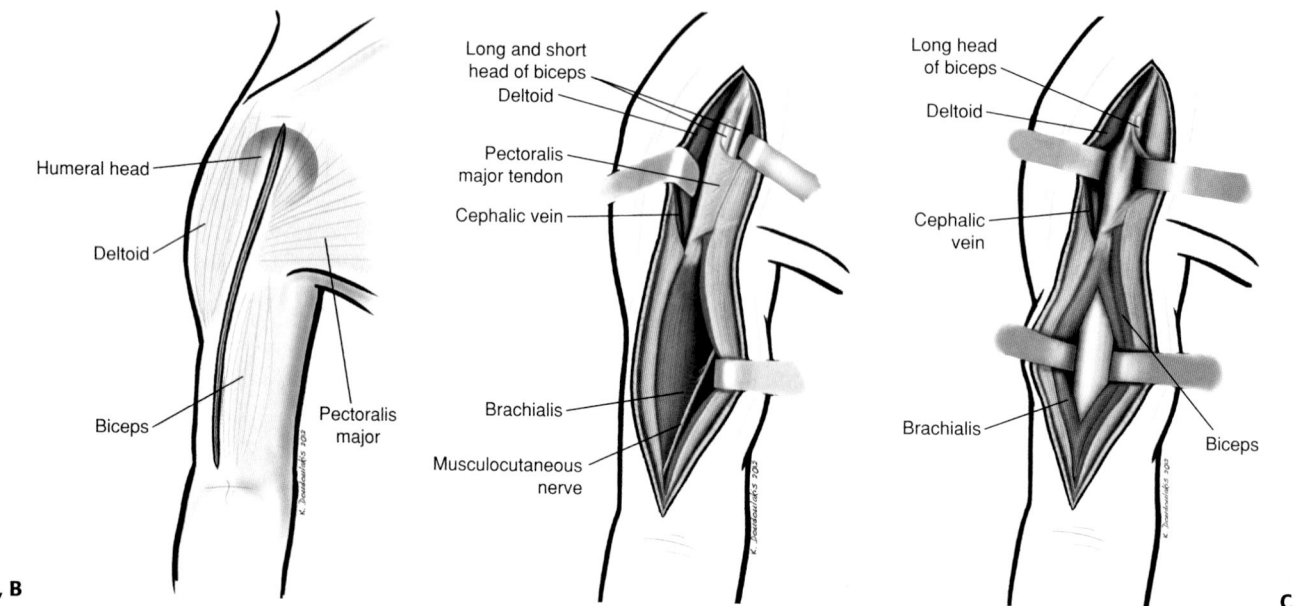

FIGURE 36-11 Anterolateral approach to the right humerus. **A:** Incision. **B:** Retraction of the deltoid laterally and the long head of biceps medially will reveal the tendon of pectoralis major proximally and brachialis more distal. **C:** Partial detachment of the tendon of pectoralis major and split of brachialis will expose the anterolateral humeral shaft.

retraction to the deltoid as this may cause compression injury to the axillary nerve and paralyze the anterior half of the muscle. The periosteum lateral to the tendon of the long head of biceps is then incised and the insertion of the pectoralis major is detached from the lateral aspect of the bicipital groove. The anterior circumflex artery will be encountered during the deep dissection and should be ligated.

In the middle third the deep fascia is incised in line with the skin incision and the biceps is mobilized medially to expose the brachialis muscle that covers the anterior humerus. The brachialis is split longitudinally in the midline to expose the anterior humeral diaphysis. A midline incision in brachialis protects the innervation of the muscle provided by the radial nerve laterally and musculocutaneous nerve medially (Fig. 36-11C). Exposure can be facilitated by flexion of the elbow. The radial nerve is protected more proximally by the lateral half of the brachialis muscle. Closer to the elbow the radial nerve on the lateral aspect and the musculocutaneous nerve medially should be protected as the approach continues between the brachialis medially and the brachioradialis laterally.

Posterior Approach. The posterior approach exposes the distal two-thirds of the posterior humeral shaft from the olecranon fossa to the junction of the proximal and middle thirds of the humerus. The patient is positioned in the prone or lateral position with the arm abducted 90 degrees on a radiolucent support. The incision is longitudinal in the midline of the posterior aspect of the arm from the tip of the olecranon to about 5 to 10 cm distal to the acromion (Fig. 36-12A). The dissection begins at the proximal end of the incision where the interval between the long and lateral head of the triceps is identified and developed by blunt dissection. The common tendon of the

triceps muscle should be incised sharply in the midline, as it runs distally and inserts into the olecranon. Retraction of the lateral head of triceps laterally and the long head medially, at the proximal part of the incision, will reveal the radial nerve and the profunda brachii artery as they run together in the spiral groove (Fig. 36-12B). The medial head of the triceps is deep to the lateral and long heads and originates just distal to the spiral groove. Longitudinal midline dissection will reveal the periosteum of the posterior humeral shaft. Incision of the periosteum and its retraction will give access to the distal humerus and also will protect the radial, ulnar, and the lateral brachial cutaneous nerves (Fig. 36-12C).

A variation of the standard posterior approach is the "triceps-sparing" or "paratricipital" approach that provides good exposure to the distal humerus posteriorly, avoids injury to the triceps muscle with less risk of denervating a portion of the triceps or the anconeus, and therefore, may improve postoperative elbow function. Although most commonly used at the elbow proximal extension of this exposure is possible, particularly on the lateral side, by mobilizing the radial nerve and elevating the triceps off the humerus.

In a cadaveric study the location of the radial nerve was defined during the posterior approach to the humerus.[274] The posterior anatomic location of the radial nerve was found to be 39 ± 2.1 mm from the point of confluence between the long and lateral heads of the triceps and the triceps aponeurosis. This information should assist surgeons in identifying the radial nerve especially if they are not familiar with the specific anatomic area.

Lateral Approach. The lateral approach extends from the deltoid insertion along the humeral diaphysis to the lateral

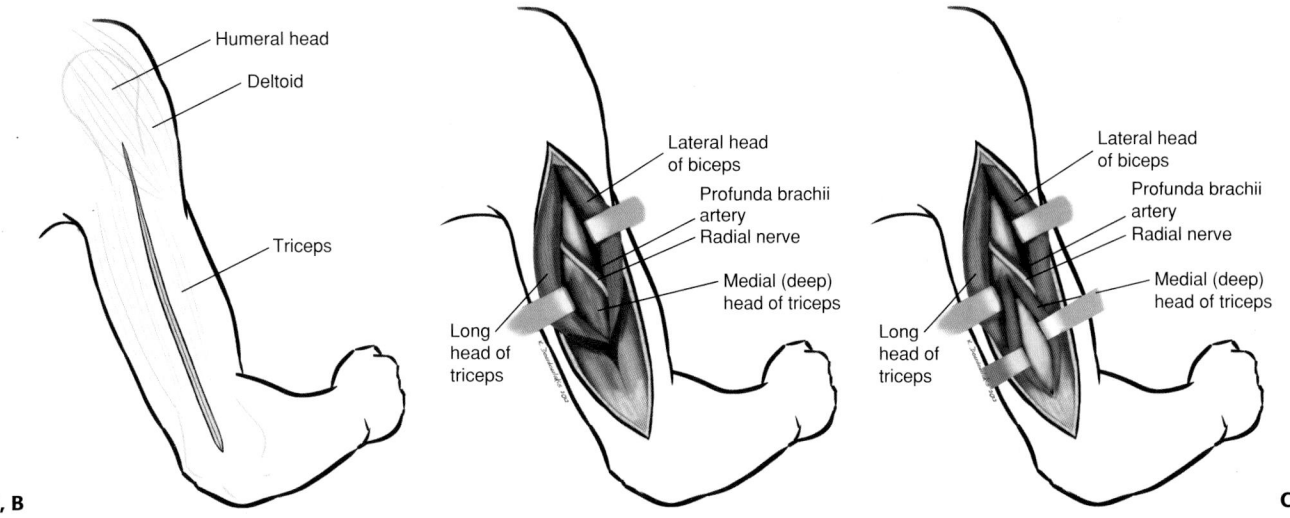

FIGURE 36-12 Posterior approach to the distal humerus. **A:** Skin incision. **B:** Development of the interval between the long and lateral heads of triceps will reveal the radial nerve as it emerges within the spiral groove. **C:** Longitudinal midline dissection of the medial head of triceps will reveal the periosteum of the posterior humeral shaft.

epicondyle and can be extended proximally either anteriorly along the anterior border of the deltoid or posteriorly in a triceps-splitting exposure. The patient is positioned supine, and the humerus is approached through the interval between the lateral intermuscular septum and the triceps. The radial nerve can be found within the fat immediately adjacent to the triceps as it emerges from behind the humerus and can be followed between the brachialis and brachioradialis in the anterior compartment of the arm (Fig. 36-13). It can be mobilized by releasing the lateral intermuscular septum and its retraction will expose the distal two-thirds of the humerus.

Anteromedial Approach. This approach is rarely chosen for routine fracture fixation but provides access to the brachial artery and median and ulnar nerves and is mainly used in cases of injury to these important neurovascular structures.[50,140] The surgical incision runs along the medial margin of the biceps and is directed to the medial epicondyle. The subcutaneous tissue is incised in line with the skin incision. The ulnar nerve is identified underneath the superficial fascia and is retracted posteromedially. The median nerve and brachial artery are identified and retracted anterolaterally. Within the surgical field there are many small branches of the artery that require ligation. The medial intermuscular septum can

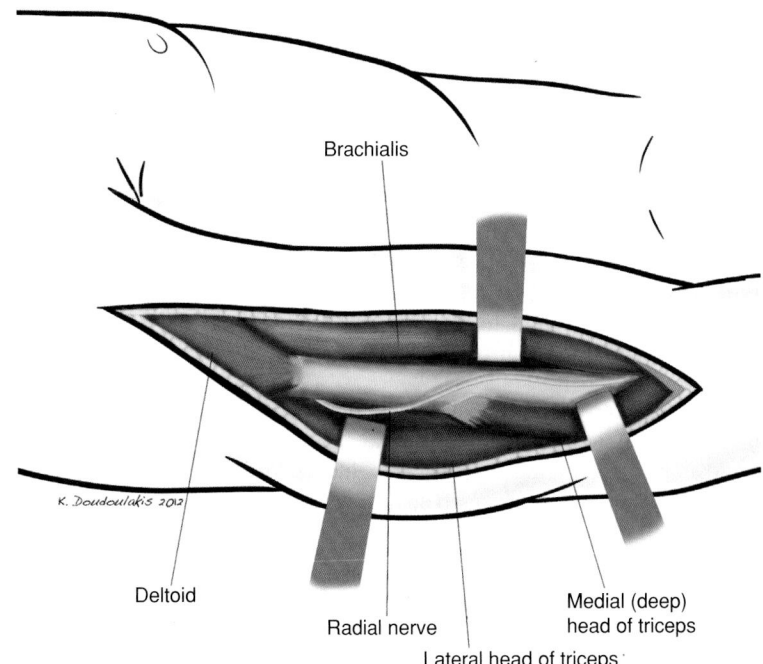

FIGURE 36-13 The lateral approach to the humeral diaphysis.

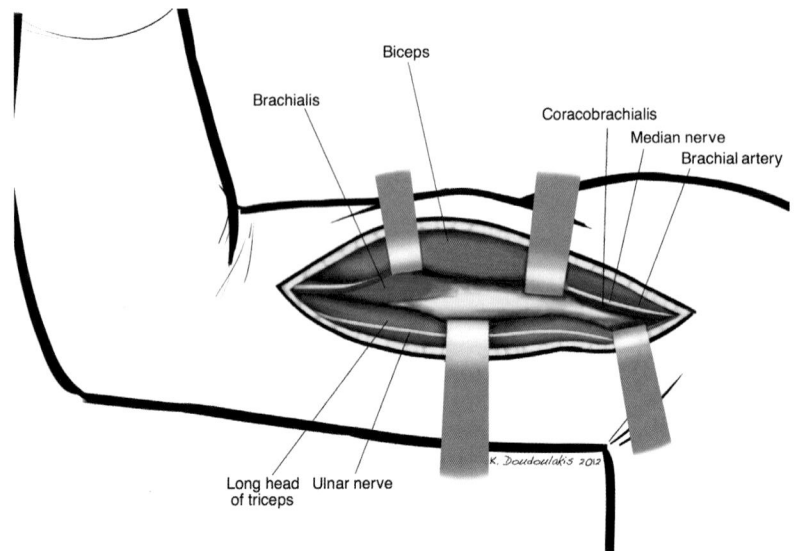

Brachialis

Biceps

Coracobrachialis

Median nerve

Brachial artery

Long head of triceps   Ulnar nerve

K. Doudoulakis 2012

FIGURE 36-14 The anteromedial approach to the humeral diaphysis.

be partially resected to improve bone exposure and facilitate plate application. The triceps is stripped from the shaft and reflected posteriorly as required, and the coracobrachialis is reflected anteriorly (Fig. 36-14). Apart from the excellent exposure of the medially located neurovascular structures, this approach is good cosmetically as the scar is well hidden on the medial side of the arm. However, because there are so many neurovascular structures that have to be identified and protected and proximal extension is difficult, the approach is rarely used.

Technique for Open Reduction and Internal Fixation.

Regardless of fracture location and surgical approach, ORIF of a diaphyseal humeral fracture follows the guidelines set by AO/ASIF many years ago.[202] It is of paramount importance that, during dissection, care should be taken not to devitalize any bony fragments by avoiding excessive soft tissue or periosteal stripping. Reduction of fracture fragments to their anatomical position is not obligatory if this could cause devascularization that could lead to necrosis and bone healing problems. Therefore, accurate reduction that requires direct manipulation of the fracture fragments should be done mainly for the reduction of the main fragments and with minimal soft tissue stripping. Other fracture fragments should be reduced indirectly which can be accomplished with the use of either manual traction or an external fixator or distractor. Reduction of the fracture, once obtained, can be temporarily maintained with reduction forceps or K-wires. If the temporary reduction is maintained with the use of reduction forceps, if possible, the plate should be applied to the bone first and used as an indirect reduction tool because it may not be possible to apply it to the bone with reduction forceps in situ. Alternatively, if K-wires are used for maintaining a temporary reduction, care should be taken to insert the wires so that they do not interfere with the placement of the plate.

For diaphyseal humeral fractures the traditional 4.5-mm narrow dynamic compression plate (DCP) or the more recent limited contact dynamic compression plate (LC-DCP) is used.[250] There should be a minimum of three to four holes

proximal and distal to the fracture (Fig. 36-15A, B). In simple fractures an 8- to 10-hole plate should be sufficient, while in comminuted fractures it is recommended that the plate should span the area of comminution (bridging plate) requiring longer plates. In the past, the 4.5-mm DCP was used in the humerus, as its configuration permitted insertion of staggered screws. However, for patients with a narrow humerus the 4.5-mm narrow DCP is preferred, as its screws can be inserted divergently and achieve a similar effect. LC-DCP plates can also be used as they are easier to contour and offer the additional advantages of decreased stress shielding and preservation of blood supply of the periosteum because of the limited plate–bone contact.[224]

Depending on the fracture site, the plate may need to be precontoured which is easiest with the use of special flexible templates that most manufacturers provide. If reduction has not been achieved prior to plate application the plate is applied to the bone on one side of the fracture and the other side is aligned with its longitudinal axis. It is then provisionally secured to the bone with reduction clamps and fixed in this position with one screw. The next step is to reduce the fracture by aligning the bone on the other side of the fracture with the plate. If the alignment is satisfactory, the unsecured end of the plate is clamped to the bone. Care should be taken with the use of reduction clamps not to injure any of the neurovascular structures, which in the humerus may be close to the bone. Alignment is confirmed, either visually or with the image intensifier, and the remainder of the screws can be inserted. In cases with a simple fracture pattern the plate should be applied in compression, with the use of either self-compressing holes in a DCP or lag screws. The final reduction and the plate and screw lengths are confirmed with the image intensifier prior to wound closure. If the fixation involved the exploration of a nerve that was nearby or crossing the plate (for instance, the radial nerve during the posterior approach), the exact relationship of the nerve to the plate must be confirmed and recorded to avoid inadvertent placement of the plate on the nerve and reduce the risk of accidental nerve damage during plate removal at any time in the future (Table 36-10).

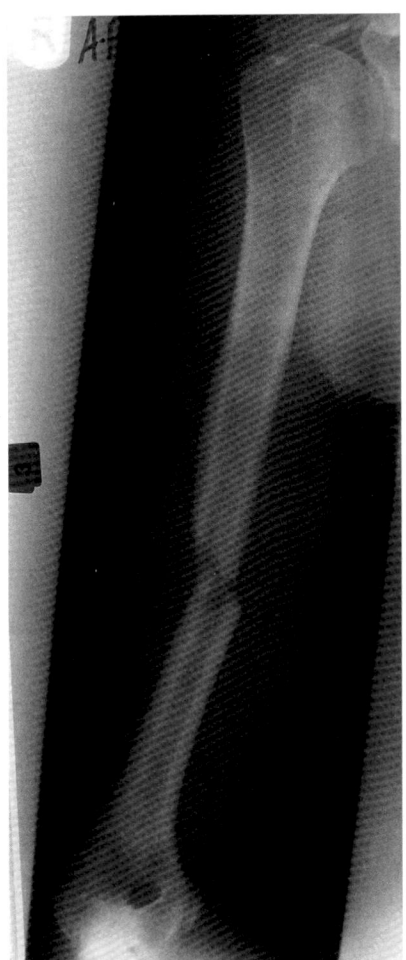

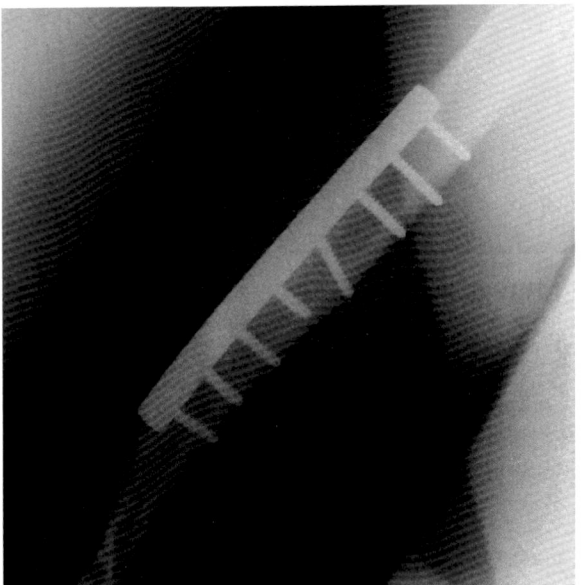

FIGURE 36-15 A: Transverse fracture of the mid-distal humeral diaphysis. **B:** Fixation with traditional plating technique.

TABLE 36-10	Surgical Steps for Open Reduction and Internal Fixation of Diaphyseal Humeral Fracture

Surgical Steps
- Expose the humeral diaphysis through the selected approach
- Identify and protect neurovascular structures that are nearby or cross the surgical field
- Avoid soft tissue or periosteal stripping
- Reduce the fracture manually by traction
- Apply external fixator or distractor across the fracture to maintain reduction if required
- Reduce the fracture and provisionally stabilize with reduction forceps or K-wires. Use the plate as indirect reduction tool
  - Avoid iatrogenic damage to the nerves and vessels with the reduction forceps
- Implant of choice is the 4.5-mm narrow dynamic compression plate or the 4.5-mm low-contact plate
- Secure the plate provisionally with one or two screws in each main fragment, check reduction and alignment, then proceed to insert the remainder of the screws
- Avoid screws in areas of comminution
- Confirm fracture reduction and plate/screw length with image intensifier prior to wound closure

The number of screws required on either side of the fracture remains controversial and, among other parameters, depends on the fracture pattern and location, the length of the plate, and the bone quality. Although there have not been substantive studies to investigate this issue, most surgeons would agree that, without a lag screw, at least four screws (eight cortices) proximally and distally to the fracture are required while the presence of a solid lag screw could reduce the number of screws to three (six cortices) proximally and three screws (six cortices) distally. Fracture comminution, poor screw purchase, poor bone quality, or other negative factors should prompt longer plate application with more screws.[193]

Locking compression plates (LCPs), in which screws with threaded heads can be screwed into the plate holes to create a fixed-angle implant, appeared at the beginning of the 21st century. Regarding the use of LCPs in the treatment of diaphyseal humeral fractures an initial biomechanical study did not demonstrate any obvious biomechanical benefit in comparison with nonlocking plates.[211] However, subsequent biomechanical studies not only reported that locking plates provide improved mechanical performance over nonlocking plates in osteoporotic cadaveric fracture models[62] but also that only two locking screws for each main bony segment provide adequate stability.[109] The clinical studies by Ring et al.[245] and

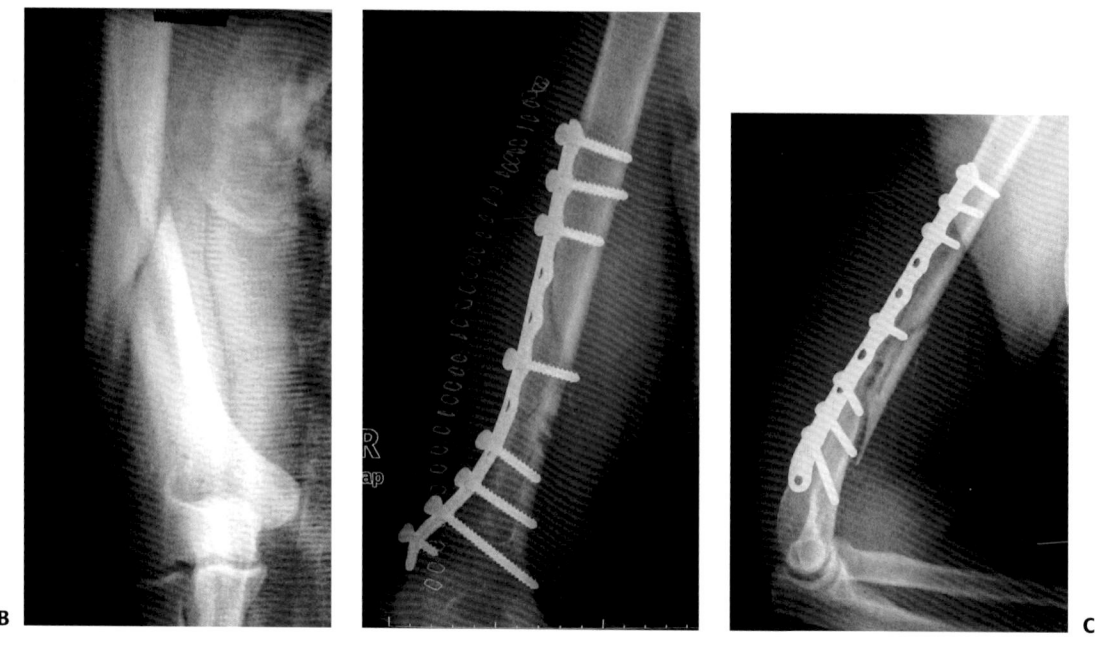

A, B
C

FIGURE 36-16 **A:** Fracture of the distal humeral diaphysis. **B, C:** Fixation with a posterolateral plate that allows screw fixation of the lateral column.

Spitzer et al.[284] confirmed the usefulness of locking plates in the management of difficult fractures and nonunions of the humeral diaphysis.

Fractures of the distal humeral diaphysis, close to the metaphyseal area, have received special attention because of the "difficult" anatomy of the elbow and the many nearby neurovascular structures (Fig. 36-16). Levy et al. recognized that traditional centrally located posterior plates often encroach on the olecranon fossa, limiting distal osseous fixation. They proposed the use of a modified tibial plate that could allow posterior plating of the distal humeral diaphysis and angled to fit along the lateral column.[161] Prasarn et al. addressed the same problem with the application of a lateral 2.7-mm or 3.5-mm pelvic reconstruction plate which reduced and fixed the fracture provisionally. This plate was contoured to extend along the lateral column proximally up to the humeral shaft and fixed in position with the necessary bicortical and lag screws. Having the fracture provisionally reduced and stabilized, a second more rigid plate was then applied posterolaterally.[233] Spitzer et al. tried a "hybrid" plate containing 3.5-mm locking holes on one end and 4.5-mm locking holes on the other end in metadiaphyseal fractures of the proximal and distal humerus. They applied the side of the plate with the smaller diameter screws toward the metaphysis to obtain more screws within the short bone segment, and they reported excellent results. Although interesting, all these proposals need further validation.[284]

Surgical Approaches for Minimally Invasive Plate Osteosynthesis (MIPO).
Within the first decade of the 21st century percutaneous plate fixation of humeral shaft fractures using two or three small incisions has been reported, similar to the technique described for lower limb long-bone fractures.[6,282]

The technique is mostly used for fractures located around the middle portion of the humerus and uses two incisions, one proximal and one distal. The proximal incision is 3 to 5 cm in length and lies between the lateral border of the proximal part of the biceps and the medial border of the deltoid. The distal incision is also 3 to 5 cm in length and is made along the lateral border of the biceps 5 cm proximal to the elbow crease. The interval between biceps and brachialis is identified and care is taken to avoid injury to the musculocutaneous nerve (Fig. 36-17A). The brachialis is split longitudinally in the midline. The musculocutaneous nerve is retracted with the medial half of the brachialis while the radial nerve is protected by the lateral half of the brachialis. A cadaveric study by Apivatthakakul et al.[7] confirmed previous data that the musculocutaneous nerve is at risk by a "small" distal approach and the authors advise full supination of the forearm and an open approach to identify and protect the nerve. Recently, some studies have reported placement of the plate laterally with two or three incisions. The proximal incision is made 3 to 5 cm below the acromion and the distal 2 to 3 cm between the brachioradialis and brachialis muscles at the distal humerus. A middle window has been proposed at the level of the middle segment of the humerus to facilitate the passage of the plate between the biceps and triceps muscles. Leaving a thin layer of muscle beneath the plate is recommended to avoid direct contact between the radial nerve and the plate.[134,282]

Technique for Minimally Invasive Plate Osteosynthesis.
After the soft tissue preparation is completed in the proximal and distal windows an extraperiosteal tunnel is opened along the surface of the humerus to prepare the insertion of the plate. Apivatthakakul et al.[8] proposed that after the exit of the tunneling instrument from the near window, the selected plate

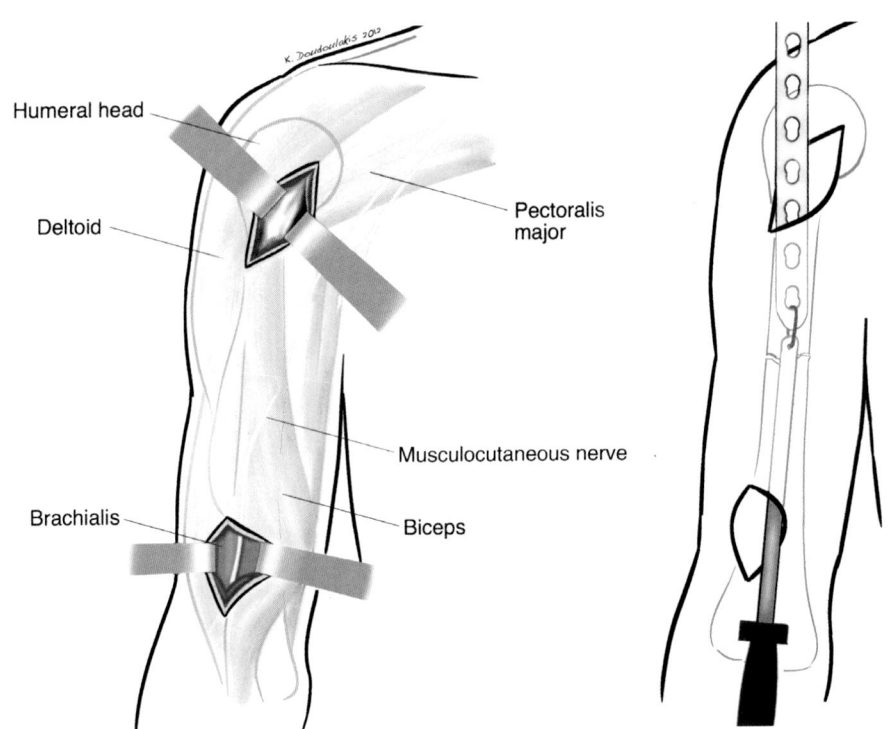

FIGURE 36-17 The anterior approach for minimally invasive plate osteosynthesis. **A:** The proximal and distal windows. **B:** Insertion of the plate is facilitated with the use of a tunneling instrument. **A**

should be tied with a suture to a hole at the tip of the tunneling instrument. Withdrawal of the tunneling instrument will pull the plate toward the far window, along the track that it has created (Fig. 36-17B). When the position of the plate is confirmed with the image intensifier, it is secured in one of the two main fragments with a bicortical screw. Under constant x-ray and visual control to avoid axial and rotational malalignment, the plate is aligned with the other main fragment and is secured with a bicortical screw. After verification of the correct positioning of the plate and the fracture reduction including restoration of length and rotational alignment of the humerus, the remaining proximal and distal screws are inserted. Final reduction and plate and screw lengths are confirmed with image intensifier prior to wound closure (Table 36-11).

Utilization of a lateral placement of the plate with the MIPO technique follows the same basic steps of the anterior approach. However, extra care should be taken to protect the radial nerve which is vulnerable with this approach.[134,282]

Postoperative Care. Postoperatively, patients treated by either ORIF or MIPO should have their arm placed in a collar and cuff support. Those with stable internal fixation can begin physiotherapy 2 to 3 days after the operation with shoulder and elbow movements, as tolerated. While most surgeons do not allow other than simple ROM exercises for 3 to 4 weeks, Tingstad et al.[296] reported no significant differences in malunion and union rates in patients who progressed with immediate weightbearing of the arm and those who did not, following plating of a diaphyseal humeral fracture. Regarding the MIPO procedure Apivatthakakul et al. suggested that when the fixation has been accomplished by only

TABLE 36-11 Surgical Steps for Minimally Invasive Plate Osteosynthesis of Diaphyseal Humeral Fracture

Surgical Steps
- Expose the proximal and distal "windows" through the selected approach (anterior/lateral)
- Identify and protect neurovascular structures that are nearby or cross the surgical field (musculocutaneous nerve anteriorly, radial nerve laterally)
- Reduce the fracture manually by traction
- Apply external fixator or distractor across the fracture to maintain reduction
- Create an extraperiosteal tunnel alongside the surface of the humerus
- Use the tunneling instrument to align and position the plate on the humerus
  - Avoid iatrogenic damage to the nerves and vessels with the tunneling instrument or the plate
- Implant of choice is the 4.5-mm narrow dynamic compression plate or the 4.5-mm low-contact plate
- Secure the plate provisionally with one screw in one main fragment, reduce fracture, and secure the plate with a screw to the other main fragment. Check reduction and alignment, then proceed to insertion of the remainder of the screws
- Check screw insertion and screw length with the image intensifier regularly
- Avoid screws in areas of comminution
- Confirm fracture reduction and plate/screw lengths with image intensifier prior to wound closure

two screws in any fragment, flexion and extension of the elbow and pendulum exercises of the shoulder should be allowed, but rotation of the arm should start after the appearance of visible callus formation, usually after 6 weeks.[8]

Potential Pitfalls and Preventative Measures. One of the major issues that can affect treatment outcome with ORIF of a diaphyseal humeral fracture, before even fracture reduction and fixation, is the stripping and devitalization of bone fragments during the surgical approach. It is imperative that the bone fragments, especially free large bony segments, should be protected during dissection, and unnecessary bone stripping must be avoided. Another pitfall that could delay or inhibit bone healing is the inadequate reduction of the fracture. Although fracture reduction does not have to be anatomical in the humerus, lack of bone contact or a gap at the fracture site has a poor prognosis for union. Bone defects up to 2 to 3 cm should be dealt with shortening, as the arm can accommodate small discrepancies without functional consequences. Larger bone defects should be bridged with bone grafting, preferably autologous. The fixation technique must provide adequate stability with the plate being strong (4.5 mm DCP) and long enough to allow at least four holes and three to four screws in each main fragment although not every screw hole has to be filled. Additional screws (e.g., lag screws) that enhance stability can be used. As a general principle, the chosen plate for the fixation should be positioned symmetrically to allow an equal number of screws on both sides of the fracture. Therefore, ORIF of distal humeral fractures could require screw placement in one or both condyles or even double plating to provide the necessary stability to the fracture. Iatrogenic injury to neurovascular structures and most particularly to the radial nerve as it runs around the humerus must be avoided by identifying and protecting the neurovascular structures in most approaches. Apart from direct injury to the radial nerve during dissection, it should be noted that cerclage wiring or drills and screws inserted from the opposite cortex can also injure the nerve (Table 36-12).

MIPO shares many of the pitfalls described for the open plating technique, such as problems from inadequate reduction, fixation, and intraoperative neurovascular injury. Although reduction of a transverse fracture is a straightforward step during open plating it can be difficult with the closed technique. Transverse fractures must be brought out to length otherwise they will unite with an angular deformity. The musculocutaneous nerve must be identified and protected in the distal anterior window before splitting the brachialis. MIPO should not be used for fractures associated with radial nerve palsy preoperatively because the risk of further injury to the nerve is substantial. Pointed retractors must not be used because the tips can injure the radial nerve either on the medial side of the proximal incision or on the lateral side of the distal incision. AP drilling and bicortical screw insertion should be avoided in the middle third of the humerus because of the high risk of radial nerve injury (Table 36-13).

Treatment-Specific Outcomes. The efficacy of a treatment method is evaluated by careful review of a number of

TABLE 36-12	Potential Pitfalls and Preventions for Plating Diaphyseal Humeral Fractures with Open Reduction and Internal Fixation
Pitfalls	**Preventions**
Excessive soft tissue and periosteal stripping	Familiarity with the anatomy of the arm Careful dissection
Unacceptable fracture reduction	Adequate surgical exposure Use the image intensifier 2–3 cm of shortening is acceptable in the humerus Bone graft for larger gaps
Unstable fixation	4.5 mm dynamic compression plate 3–4 screws in each main fragment Use lag screws, if feasible Incorporate the condyles in the fixation or double plate distal humeral fractures
Iatrogenic neurovascular injury	Careful dissection Identify and protect nearby nerves/vessels Avoid excessive retraction Avoid cerclage wiring Be careful with drills and screws from the opposite cortex

parameters, which include the nature of intervention (aggressive/minimal), intraoperative and immediate postoperative incidents and adverse events, iatrogenic hazards, potential problems and complications during the rehabilitation period, the time needed for the patient to achieve the best outcome, and the quality of life at the end of treatment. These must be under constant review to assess not only the effectiveness of a specific treatment method but also to allow comparison with alternative treatment options.

Open Reduction and Internal Fixation. Plating has been regarded as the surgical treatment of choice for diaphyseal humeral fractures. It is associated with a high, uncomplicated union rate, minimal shoulder or elbow morbidity, and rapid return to previous activities. It can be used in periarticular fractures and has been successfully used in open fractures.[19,86,104,185,188,191,267,307] Outcomes of plating have been published in many studies during 70s and 80s. However, development of new techniques for plating "difficult" fractures, modern implants (e.g., locking plates), and MIPO have been evolving in recent years and will be reviewed in this section.

An important target of all treatment methods for fractures is fracture union. The union rate of ORIF of humeral shaft fractures exceeded 95% in most clinical studies over the last few decades.[19,86,115,191,307] Complications were infrequent and included radial nerve palsy (2% to 5%, usually neurapraxia)

TABLE 36-13	**Potential Pitfalls and Preventions for Plating Diaphyseal Humeral Fractures with the MIPO Technique**
Pitfalls	**Preventions**
Unacceptable fracture reduction	Use the image intensifier Bring the fracture out to length with traction Slight shortening of comminuted fractures is acceptable
Unstable fixation	4.5-mm dynamic compression plate 2–4 screws in each main fragment
Iatrogenic nerve injury	Identify and protect the musculocutaneous nerve with the anterior approach and the radial nerve with the lateral approach Avoid excessive retraction and pointed retractors Avoid anteroposterior drilling and bicortical screw insertion in the middle third of the humerus
CRIF in the presence of radial nerve palsy	Exclude by good clinical examination prior to surgery

and infection (1% to 2% for closed fractures, 2% to 5% for open fractures). However, at the turn of the century, Paris et al.[220] tempered the enthusiasm for the technique when they reported a large series of 156 patients (21 with polytrauma) who were treated with ORIF. The union rate was 87% with eight postoperative transient radial nerve palsies, two deep infections, and 10 implant-related revisions. While 88% of the patients were satisfied with their outcome, only 54% obtained complete anatomical and functional recovery. Niall et al.[206] restored the reputation of the technique by treating 49 diaphyseal humeral fractures (15 polytrauma injuries) with plating, 96% of which united in an average of 9 weeks. There were no major complications and all patients without significant comorbidities regained a full range of shoulder and elbow movements and returned to previous activities. Idoine et al.[129] found a 94.7% union rate at an average of 16.9 weeks in a large series of 96 polytrauma patients with humeral shaft fractures. The authors used an anterior approach but in two-thirds of the patients the plate was applied on the medial side of the humerus by retracting the biceps laterally. 3.5 mm plates were used in most cases because the authors stated that there was not enough biomechanical evidence to justify the use of larger, stiffer plates. However, they experienced four implant failures within 3 months of surgery along with two infections and two incidences of iatrogenic injury to the lateral antebrachial cutaneous nerve. Bearing in mind that the patients were polytraumatized the functional results can be considered satisfactory, as 80.2% regained within 10 degrees of the full range of shoulder motion barring flexion where only 60.5% regained an almost

full range. All patients regained elbow ROM to within 10 degrees compared to the contralateral elbow while the median DASH score was 23.8 (0 to 79). Levy et al.[161] used a modified 4.5-mm tibial head buttress plate to treat 12 patients with distal third diaphyseal humeral fractures. They proposed that such a plate design accommodates the anatomy of the distal humerus better and provides more stable fixation. Prasarn et al.[233] described the addition of a 2.7/3.5 mm pelvic reconstruction plate laterally that can serve as a reduction tool prior to the insertion of a precontoured extra-articular distal humeral locking plate with a "hockey stick" distal configuration, similar to that described previously by Levy et al.[161] They treated 15 patients with the dual plate fixation and only one patient complained of tenderness over the distal posterolateral humerus and underwent implant removal. A further study exploited the potential advantages provided by modern implants and tried a "hybrid" locking plate, that could provide 4 to 5 mm screws for the longer fragment segment and 3.5 mm screws for the shorter one, in a cohort of 24 patients with proximal and distal metaphyseal recent fractures and nonunions.[284] All recent fractures (14) united in an average of 19.5 weeks (13 to 26) with one iatrogenic transient radial nerve palsy as the sole complication. The patients managed a mean of 145 degrees of forward elevation of the shoulder and 138 degrees of total elbow ROM.

Apart from case series, the outcome of treating humeral shaft fractures with plating has been investigated in studies that compared the technique with alternative treatment methods. Three studies have compared plating with intramedullary nailing.[38,41,187] The results of the comparison will be discussed below but the outcomes of plating are of the interest to this discussion. In all three studies a total of 92 patients were treated with plating. The union rate was 92.4% (85/92) and the average time to union was similar for the two studies that provided the relevant information (10.4 weeks for Chapman et al. and 8.9 weeks for Changulani et al.). One incident of iatrogenic transient radial nerve palsy and three to five infections occurred in each of those two studies respectively. All three studies reported satisfactory clinical outcomes. Similar results of the ORIF technique were reported in two studies that compared traditional plating with the newly introduced MIPO.[135,214] From 46 fractures that were included in the two studies and treated with traditional plating 43 united with an average time to union of 16.7 and 21.3 weeks for Oh et al. and Jiang et al., respectively. It is important to mention that the latter study reported five incidences of postoperative radial nerve palsy, that all recovered spontaneously from 12 to 52 weeks. Otherwise, both studies confirm the good radiologic and functional outcomes of ORIF in the treatment of humeral shaft fractures.

An under-reported outcome of plating diaphyseal humeral fractures is the ability of patients to immediately bear weight on their injured arm. Tingstad et al.[296] investigated this parameter by studying 83 humeral diaphyseal fractures (70 in polytrauma patients) which were treated in a 10-year period with ORIF, 86% with 4.5-mm DC plates. The postoperative weight-bearing status of the involved humerus was decided on the basis of the presence or absence of a lower extremity injury that required restricted weightbearing and not on the basis of the humeral fracture pattern or comminution. Apart from a high union rate (94%) and low complication rate, the main outcome from this study was that ORIF of a diaphyseal humeral fracture followed by immediate weightbearing through the involved humerus is a safe procedure.

Review of older and more modern studies of the treatment of diaphyseal humeral fractures with ORIF revealed that the reported outcomes can be categorized in two groups:

• Principal outcomes that are provided by all studies and offer the basis for evaluation, comparison, and conclusions. These include fracture union rate, time to union, and complications. Restoration of joint motion and functional results fall within an intermediate grey zone with some studies providing adequate information and others not.

• Nonprincipal outcomes, such as duration of the operation, blood loss, timing of initiation and duration of physiotherapy, hospitalization, return to previous activities, and patient-related outcomes, are not provided by many studies. However, these outcomes can offer substantial information that could significantly influence the overall opinion regarding the quality and efficacy of a treatment method and should be reported in modern studies. Otherwise critical evaluation of the effectiveness of any treatment will be incomplete.

Minimally Invasive Plate Osteosynthesis (MIPO). Adopted from the technique initially introduced for femoral and tibial fractures, the MIPO has also been utilized for the treatment of diaphyseal humeral fractures. The humerus, however, has complicated anatomy and MIPO has been considered risky for the neurovascular structures and in particular for the radial and musculocutaneous nerves. Although there has been skepticism about the use of the technique in the humerus, studies that have appeared in the last few years have dealt with the problematic technical issues to develop a useful and safe MIPO technique suitable for humeral shaft fractures.

Livani and Belangero[172] reported the use of MIPO in the treatment of 15 patients with humeral shaft fractures, 8 of which were polytraumatized. They used 4.5 mm DC plates with two screws in each main fragment and they reported only one screw loosening. They also encountered one superficial infection and one nonunion. The healing time for the united fractures ranged from 8 to 12 weeks and all but two patients regained full range of elbow motion. Subsequent studies also included small number of patients apart from one by Concha et al. that included 35 patients.[8,49,134,135,148,231,324] All these studies had good outcomes with few complications. More specifically, four of these studies described the management of a total of 60 humeral shaft fractures between them with an anterior minimally invasive technique.[49,135,148,231,324] They all used 4.5 mm plates. Union rate was 96.6% (58/60) in an average of 15 weeks (11 to 32). As one of the theoretical advantages of MIPO in the humerus is the reduced operating time in comparison with ORIF, this parameter was provided by three of the four studies that reported very similar operating times (117.5, 127.6, and 113.8 minutes, respectively).[135,148,324] Two of the studies

provided information about the blood loss that was 170 mL and 490 mL on average.[135,148] Significant complications did not occur in these studies and the patients were instructed to start movements of their injured arm as early as tolerated. All patients regained an excellent ROM of their shoulder and elbow. Concha et al.[49] presented the largest series of 35 patients, 15 of which were polytraumatized. They used MIPO with two screws on each side of the fracture. Union rate was 91.5% (32/35) at an average of 12 weeks (8 to 16). The authors reported some complications that included two infections and three cases of varus malunion of more than 15 degrees. They also reported that only 20/32 patients had full extension of the elbow and 20/32 patients obtained 130 degrees of flexion. While it was concluded that MIPO is a safe and efficient procedure for humeral shaft fracture treatment, with high union and low complication rate, it was noted that elbow flexion contracture could be a problem and might indicate the need for a formal elbow rehabilitation protocol.

Ji et al.[134] used the MIPO technique to treat distal humeral shaft fractures via a lateral approach as they found the anterior approach unsuitable for proximal and middle third fractures because of the anatomical restrictions of the anterior surface of the distal humerus. They initially tried the approach in 14 cadaveric arms and subsequently treated 23 humeral shaft fractures with 4.5 mm LCPs. All fractures showed bridging callus at an average time of 6.3 weeks (4 to 11). The only information about the clinical recovery was that "the function and ROM of the shoulder and elbow joints were satisfactory" but one patient developed a postoperative radial nerve palsy. Spagnolo et al.[282] had similarly good outcomes with the use of MIPO (4.5 mm LCP) in 16 patients with humeral shaft fractures and the lateral approach. The authors described the lateral approach to the humerus with three windows: One proximal, through the deltoid for the insertion of the plate, a second in the middle for facilitating the passage between the biceps and triceps muscles, and the third distally for the direct visualization of the radial nerve and the distal end of the plate. All fractures healed at 14.9 weeks on average (11 to 20). Good functional recovery was reported with excellent UCLA scores in 62.5% and good in 37.5%, and excellent Mayo scores in all of the patients. There were no neurovascular complications. According to these two studies the lateral approach is advantageous because it can accommodate fractures of the proximal and distal humerus without significant risks of injury to the radial nerve if precautions are taken such as the supination of the forearm during the procedure, visualization of the radial nerve (as proposed by Spagnolo et al.), and no screw insertion close to the nerve.

As the main reason for caution with the use of MIPO for humeral shaft fractures is the risk of neurologic damage from the plate and screws, ultrasound has been used to investigate the relationship between the radial nerve and the implants.[172] In a group of 19 patients who had undergone MIPO fixation of humeral shaft fracture, it was found that regardless of the location of the fracture (middle or distal thirds of the humeral diaphysis), the radial nerve is in close proximity to the implants (plate or screws). This distance was measured between 1.6 and 19.6 mm (mean 9.3 mm) for midshaft fractures and between 1 and 8.1 mm (mean 4 mm) for distal fractures. In a cadaveric study the danger zone for locking screw placement in MIPO of humeral shaft fractures was examined and the authors concluded that the danger zone for the musculocutaneous and radial nerves could be determined as a percentage of the humeral length.[7] The danger zone for the musculocutaneous nerve averaged 18.37% to 42.67% of the humeral length from the lateral epicondyle. The danger zone for the radial nerve averaged 36.35% to 59.2% of the humeral length, and the most dangerous screws that penetrated or touched the radial nerve lay 47.22% to 53.21% of the humeral length from the lateral epicondyle. An AP locking screw placed percutaneously endangered both the musculocutaneous and radial nerves.

Both studies revealed that despite clinical evidence that the MIPO technique is safe in the treatment of diaphyseal humeral fractures, the risk for injury to radial and musculocutaneous nerves is substantial and should not be underestimated.

Intramedullary Nailing

Preoperative Planning. Preoperative planning for intramedullary nailing of a diaphyseal humeral fracture is no different from what was described previously for plating. However, it should be reiterated that the patient must be fully informed about the nature, expected outcomes, and potential complications of the operation while the anesthetist should be fully involved in the whole process of preoperative assessment and planning, because each surgical technique (e.g.,

antegrade or retrograde nailing) requires a different anesthetic approach.

The main preoperative planning starts with at least two x-ray views of the whole humerus, one neutral AP and one lateral. In most cases, no further imaging studies should be required. Preoperative measurement of the humeral length and the width of the narrowest part of the intact humeral canal (taking into account the magnification on the x-ray) will help to determine the desired nail length and diameter. Whenever fracture lines extend toward the shoulder or elbow joints further x-ray views, centered in the suspected area, may be needed. If there are still doubts about the integrity of the joints, a CT scan should be performed.

Preoperative checking of operating room facilities and other actions that can facilitate the procedure, such as the drawing of the fixation, confirming implants and tools availability, and image intensifier working status, have been described in the relevant section regarding ORIF. As with ORIF, a checklist will allow better organization of the operating procedure and ensure immediate availability of the necessary equipment (Table 36-14).

Positioning. Intramedullary nailing of diaphyseal fractures of the humerus can be performed either via the humeral head (antegrade nailing) or via the supracondylar area of the distal humerus (retrograde nailing). Each technique requires different patient positioning.

Antegrade Nailing. The patient is positioned supine with a padded support under the shoulder. The patient's torso is on the operating table, while the injured arm overhangs the main table.

TABLE 36-14	**Preoperative Planning Checklist for Intramedullary Nailing of Diaphyseal Humeral Fractures**

1. Operating Theater

Operating Room Table
- Regular orthopedic
- Radiolucent arm support
- Forearm extension
- Other

X-ray
- C-arm
  Left
  Right
- Plain films

4. Implants
- Long nails complete set
- Short nails complete set
- Locking screws
- K-wires
- Other

2. Position/Positioning Aids
- Supine
- Prone
- Beach chair
- Lateral (right side up)
- Lateral (left side up)
- Positioning aids

3. Equipment
- Battery drill
- Guidewires of same length
- Humeral reamers
- Distal targeting device
- Bone graft instruments
- Large bone reduction tools
- Other

5. Other

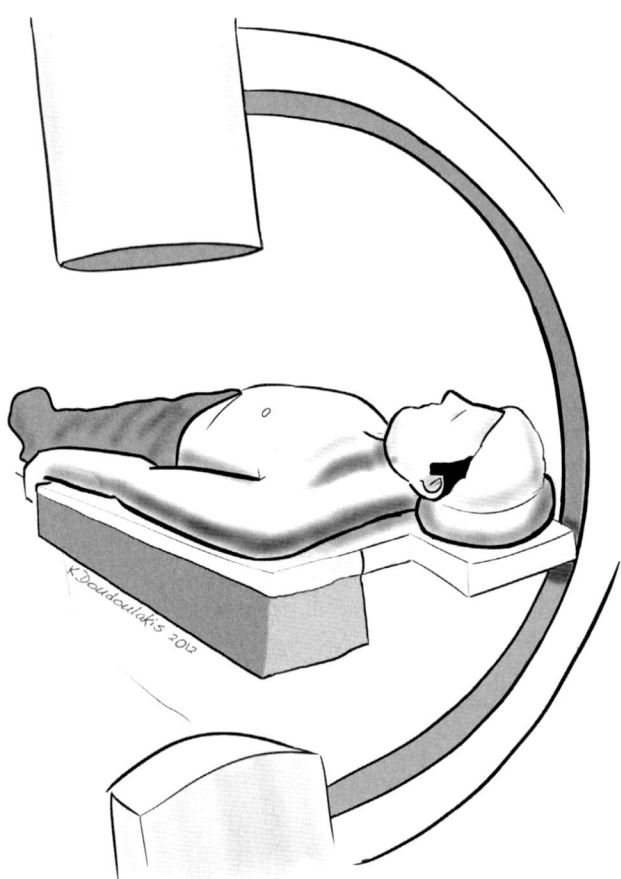

FIGURE 36-18 Positioning the patient for antegrade nailing.

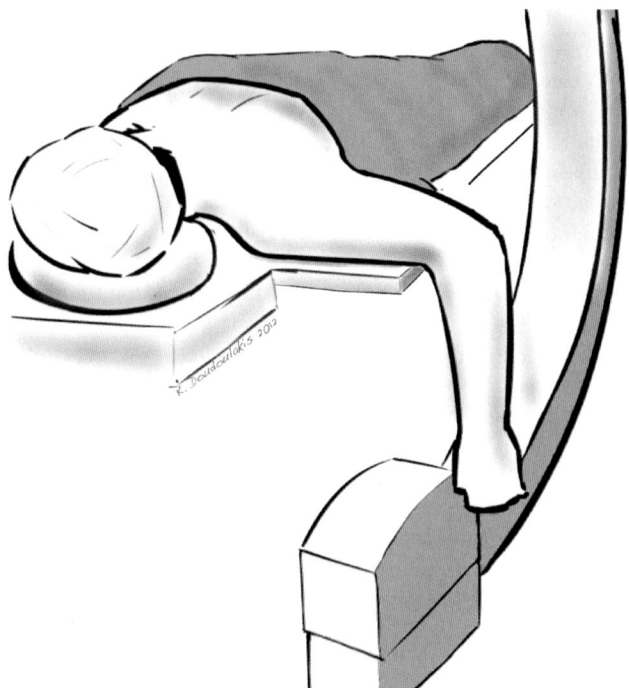

FIGURE 36-19 Positioning the patient for retrograde nailing.

Some surgeons prefer the "beach chair" position with the arm hanging on the side or supported by a forearm support while others prefer the patient supine or slightly inclined upward with the whole arm supported on a radiolucent arm support. The elbow, the humerus and the shoulder are within the sterile field. The location of the image intensifier varies, depending not only on personal preference but also on the width of the operating table and the concavity of the C-arm. I prefer the C-arm on the opposite side (Fig. 36-18), as it does not crowd the operating area. The anesthetist must be familiar with the procedure because the uninjured arm must be positioned next to the patient on the operating table and is not easily accessible. This problem is solved with line extensions that allow drug injection from a distance. If it is anticipated that the image intensifier will be on the opposite side, the compatibility of the C-arm curvature with the width of the operating table must be checked in advance to confirm that imaging of the overhanging injured arm is feasible. Care should also be taken to assemble the operating table in advance to avoid obstacles such as the leg of the table that may obstruct use of the image intensifier.

Retrograde Nailing. The patient can be positioned either prone or in the lateral decubitus position. Prone positioning is generally preferred as it offers unobstructed viewing of the whole humerus. The image intensifier remains on the same side as the injured arm. The arm is positioned on a radiolucent support that

must allow at least 100- to 110-degree elbow flexion, to facilitate insertion of the nail (Fig. 36-19). Correct rotational alignment is achieved in this position without further manipulation of the arm. If the general condition of the patient or any other reason does not allow prone positioning, it is possible to perform retrograde nailing of the humerus on the lateral decubitus position. However, visualization of the humerus with the C-arm is more difficult. It is of paramount importance to ensure preoperatively that good images of the humerus and shoulder can be obtained.

Surgical Approaches

Antegrade Nailing. A 2- to 3-cm incision is made from the anterolateral edge of the acromion obliquely forward and the deltoid muscle is split longitudinally along its fibers to reveal the subacromial bursa and the rotator cuff (Fig. 36-20). Before incising the cuff the location of the entry portal of the nail should be verified with a blunt instrument and a single AP view on the image intensifier to minimize the possibilities of a poorly placed incision that will cause unnecessary damage to the rotator cuff (Fig. 36-21). This location ideally should be on the sulcus or toward its medial border. The rotator cuff is then incised in the direction of the supraspinatus fibers. Direct visualization of the humeral head is not necessary and should be avoided. The long head of biceps tendon can be palpated and protected. In most cases, the correct entry portal will bring the awl in direct contact with the acromion. The direction of the awl should be slightly oblique aiming toward the medial cortex of the humerus. In the infrequent case of a broad acromion the arm can be placed in a "downward hanging" position to access the humeral head anterior to the acromion or with the use of a small bone hook or lever the humeral head can be pulled

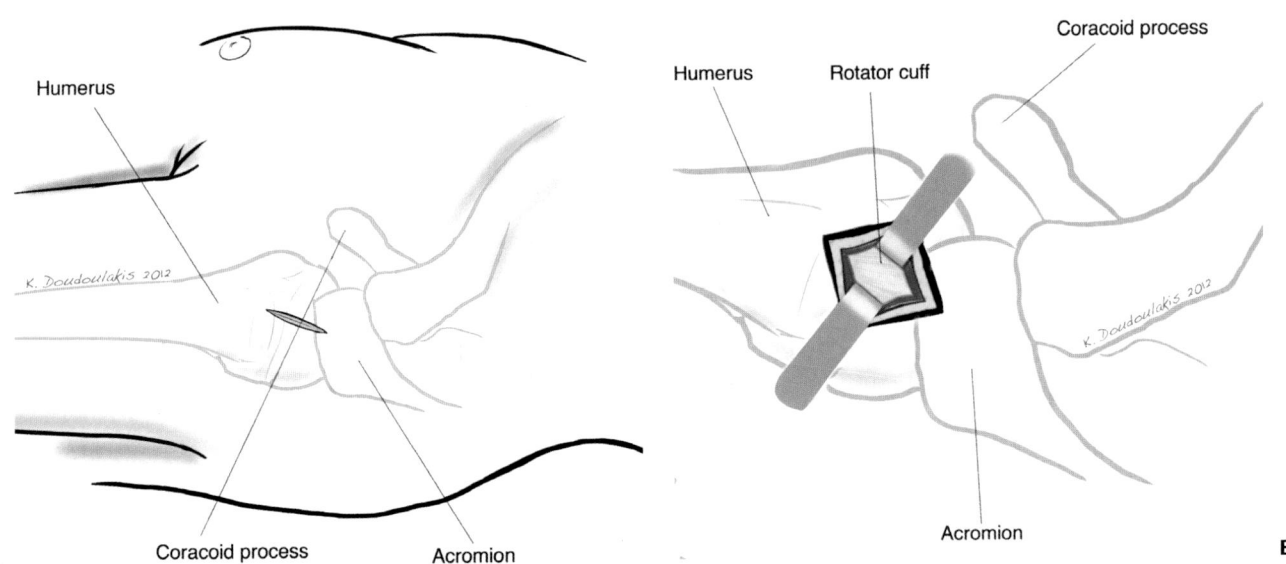

FIGURE 36-20 The approach for the antegrade nailing. **A:** Skin incision. **B:** Exposure of the rotator cuff.

laterally. Adduction of the arm to facilitate the access to the humeral head is usually unsuccessful, as the thorax does not allow sufficient adduction in the neutral position. Elevation of the arm to avoid the acromion moves the humeral head posteriorly and may also displace the fracture.

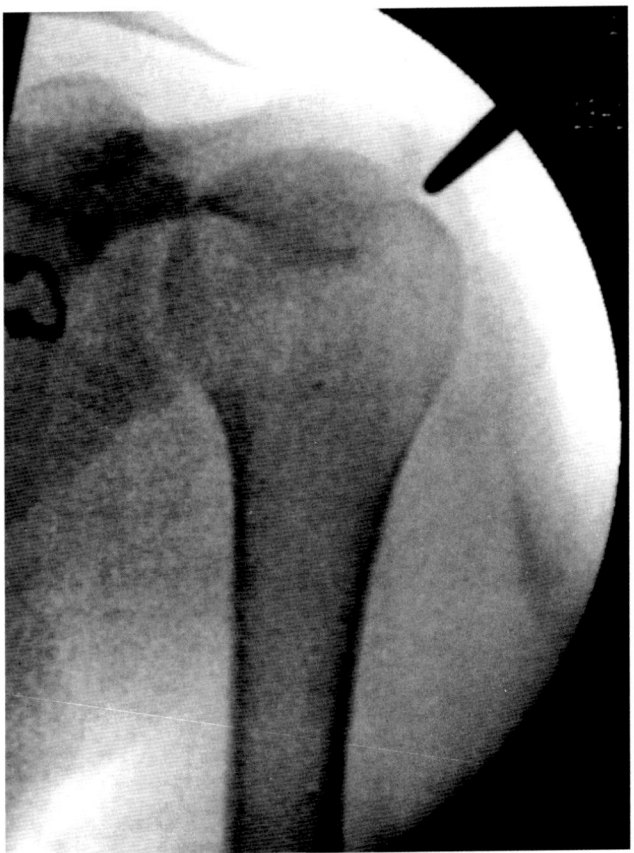

FIGURE 36-21 Verification of the entry portal of the nail with a blunt instrument before incising the rotator cuff.

These technical difficulties along with concerns about damage to the rotator cuff generated proposals for alternative approaches to the humeral head or "sophisticated" nail designs that aimed to bypass these problems. Stannard et al.[285] described a lateral entry point just distal to the insertion of the rotator cuff and used an articulated nail that could accommodate such an eccentric introduction. Dimakopoulos et al.[70] proposed a similar entry portal and used a rigid nail to treat a series of 29 patients with diaphyseal humeral fractures without any major complications regarding the approach. Others approached the humeral head through the rotator cuff interval with a rather extensive exposure of the proximal humerus.[221,258] Despite the theoretical advantages of these approaches to the humeral head, they have not become popular. With the use of the lateral approach there are a number of possible reasons: Firstly the fear of iatrogenic fracture either on the medial humeral cortex or around the entry portal, secondly the difficulty of treating proximal humeral diaphyseal fractures, and finally the increased cost of the articulated nail and fears about the difficulties with removal. Regarding the approach through the rotator cuff interval, it seems that the extensive exposure of the proximal humerus compromises the concept of minimal invasiveness of the intramedullary nailing technique.

Retrograde Nailing. The patient is positioned prone, with the arm on a radiolucent support, as described for posterior plating (Fig. 36-19). The skin incision is 4 to 5 cm, longitudinal from the tip of the olecranon, extending in a proximal direction (Fig. 36-22). The fascia over the triceps tendon is incised longitudinally and the underlying tendon and muscle are split with blunt dissection in line with the skin incision until the olecranon fossa can be seen. As there are no vulnerable structures in the area, there are no variations of this approach.

Technique

Antegrade Nailing. The entry portal for standard antegrade nailing is opened with the hand awl (Fig. 36-23A). More medial

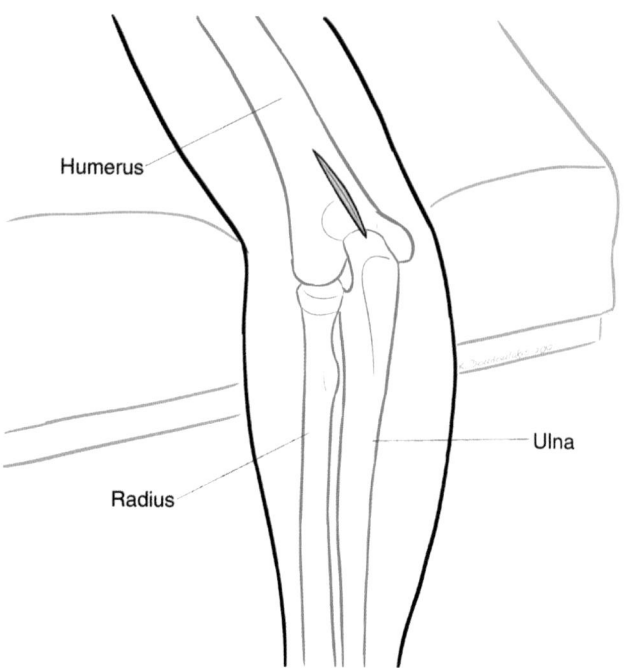

FIGURE 36-22 The skin incision for retrograde nailing.

location of the entry portal would facilitate nail insertion but it is usually not possible because of the presence of the acromion. The hand awl must penetrate the humeral head for at least 4 to 5 cm to create the pathway for the guidewire in the case of a cannulated nail or for a solid nail. Most humeral nails are cannulated and a guidewire is used to facilitate the passage of the nail through the fracture site by closed means (Fig. 36-23B). The correct alignment of the arm is obtained by traction, supination of the forearm, and 90 degrees of elbow flexion applied and maintained by the assis-

tant (Fig. 36-23C). A lateral view at the fracture site cannot be easily obtained in the humerus so the passage of the guidewire to the distal fragment can be confirmed with rotation of the arm by 40 to 50 degrees or allowing some angulation at the fracture site. Careful reaming of the humeral canal follows when required. Each nail manufacturer provides instructions for the selection of the most suitable nail size although it is prudent to ream to 1 to 1.5 mm larger than the nail. After the insertion of the nail to its final position it must be locked to provide adequate stability to the fracture and allow immediate mobilization (Fig. 36-23D–G).

The complex anatomy and unique biomechanical properties of the arm have created significant controversy regarding the "locking" feature of humeral nails. Use of drills and screws for the standard locking technique has an increased risk of neurovascular and/or musculotendinous injury. Furthermore, distal locking of an antegrade nail with the "freehand" technique is considered difficult because of the combination of three factors.

1. A round and "slippery" distal humeral cortex
2. The small diameter of the locking nail hole
3. Difficult imaging

Apart from risking iatrogenic injury to vulnerable soft tissues, all these factors potentially increase radiation exposure, prolong operating time, and result in high rates of targeting failure. All these factors generated the making of humeral nails (that I call "bio" nails) that offer alternative options for distal interlocking but provide inferior biomechanical stability to the fracture site when compared with nails that use locking bolts distally (that I call "fixed" nails) (Figs. 36-24A–C and 36-25A–E).[25,61,96,97,325] However, if we consider that functional bracing does not rigidly immobilize a humeral shaft fracture, it seems that the optimal stability that is provided by locking bolts in the humerus may not be vital for the healing process of humeral diaphyseal fractures. Nevertheless, the necessity of finding a new balance between stability

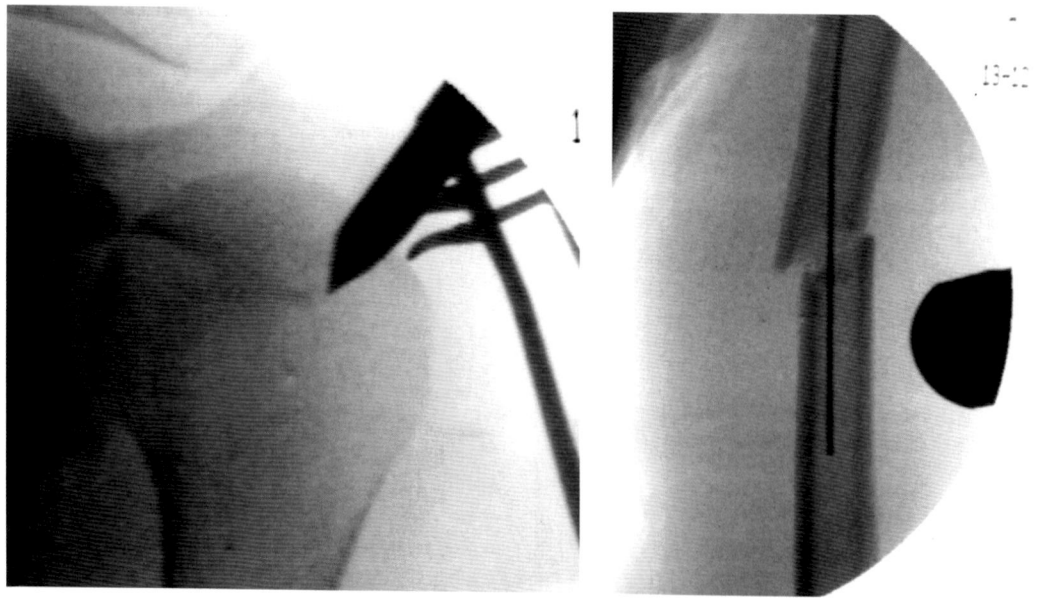

FIGURE 36-23 Antegrade nailing of a proximal diaphyseal humeral fracture. **A:** Opening the entry portal with the hand awl. **B:** Passage of the guidewire to the distal fragment.

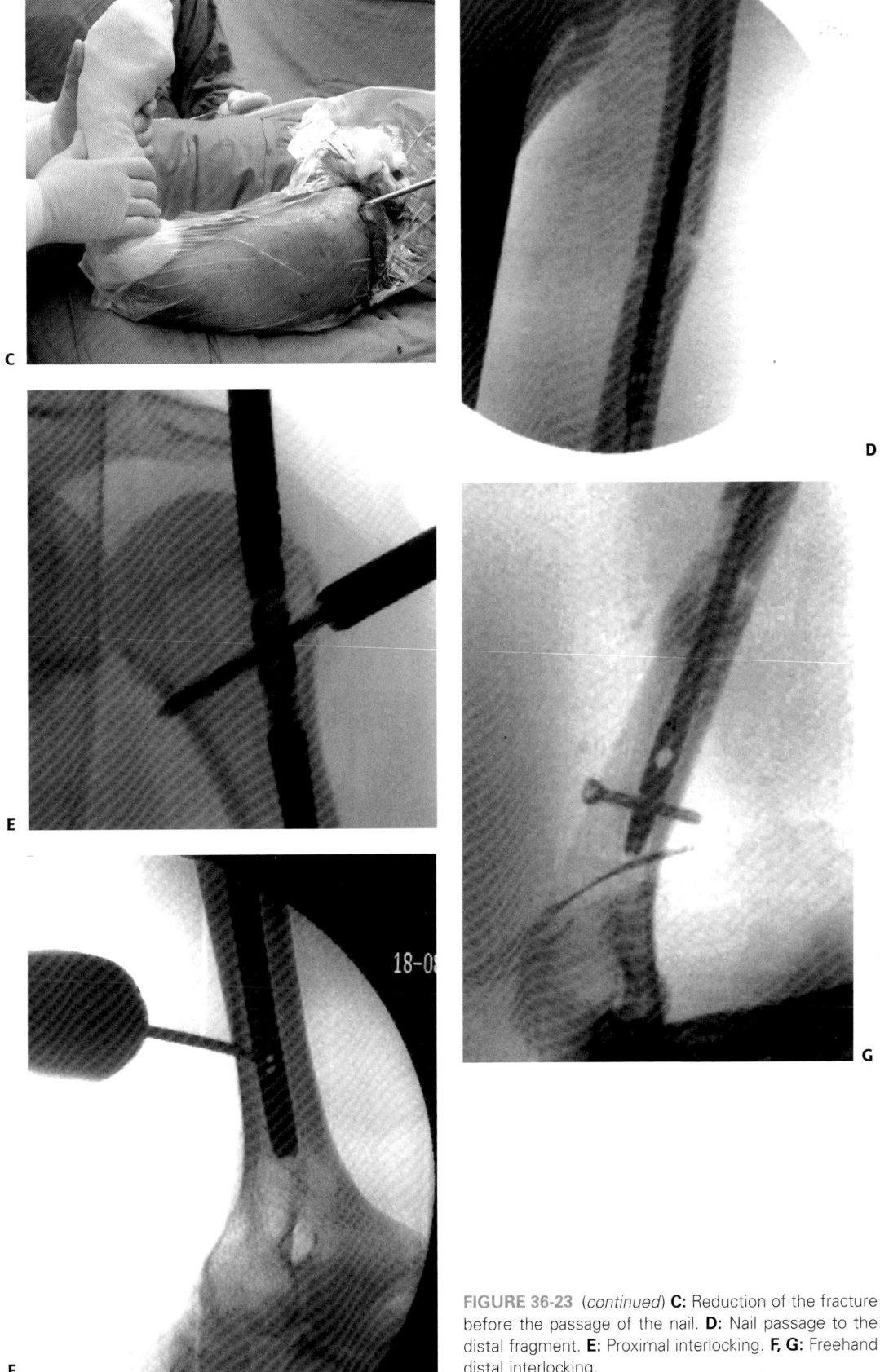

FIGURE 36-23 (*continued*) **C:** Reduction of the fracture before the passage of the nail. **D:** Nail passage to the distal fragment. **E:** Proximal interlocking. **F, G:** Freehand distal interlocking.

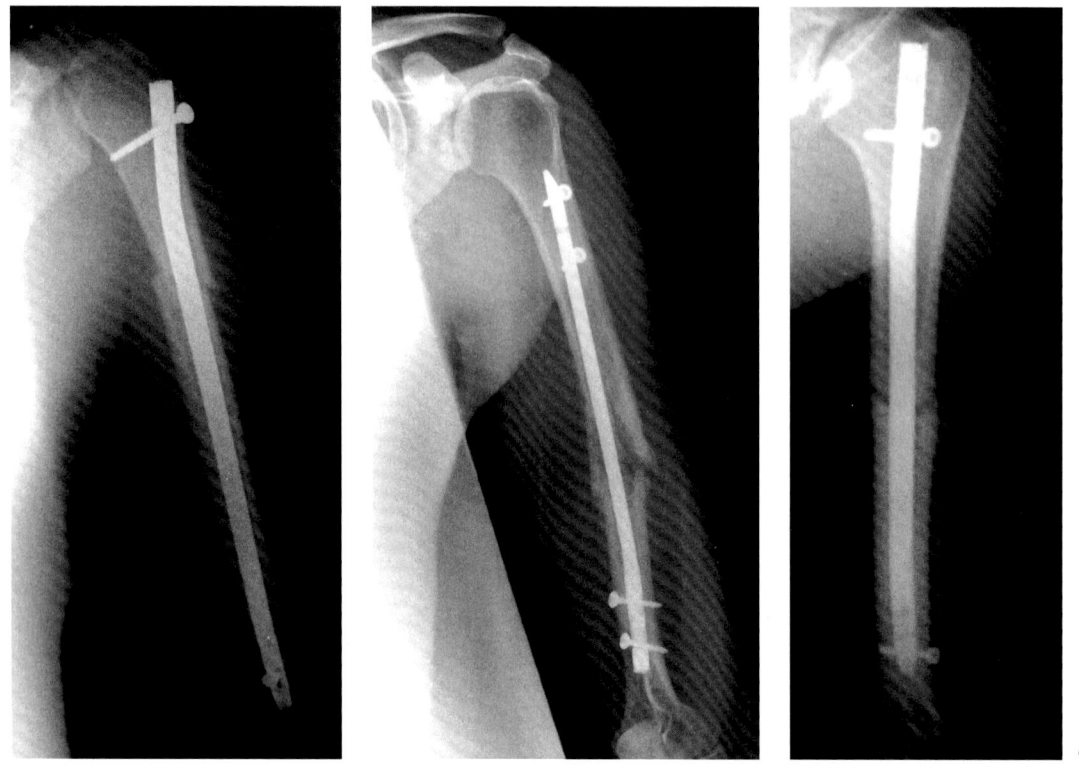

FIGURE 36-24 'Fixed" nails. **A:** Russell-Taylor nail. **B:** Unreamed Humeral nail. **C:** T2 nail.

and biology in fracture treatment has been emphasized recently[225] but until this is achieved, the debate between supporters of "fixed" and "bio" humeral nailing continues. "Fixed" nailing supporters claim that optimal stability provided by the locking bolts allows faster rehabilitation and results in higher fracture union rates. The opponents claim that "bio" nailing eliminates neurovascular complications, reduces radiation, and reduces operating time, while the fracture healing process is not influenced.[88,92,95,96,269]

After implantation of the nail, the locking process follows. While proximal interlocking for antegrade nails and distal interlocking for retrograde nails is uniformly straightforward through reliable targeting devices, distal interlocking of antegrade nailing or proximal interlocking of retrograde nailing each depends on the nail design. "Fixed" nails are locked with locking screws which are usually inserted with the "freehand" technique (Fig. 36-23F, G). Because of the difficulties with targeting some manufacturers provide long targeting devices but their success has not been consistent, possibly because of their long length and the narrow screw holes of humeral nails.[93,97,197] Distal locking of "bio" antegrade nails or proximal locking for "bio" retrograde nails varies. Nail expansion (Seidel nail) or inflation (Fixion nail), activation of diverging rods (Marchetti nail), or a special design (True-Flex nail, Garnavos nail), have all been tried in an effort to improve the performance of intramedullary nailing in the humerus (Fig. 36-25A–E).

At the end of the procedure the rotator cuff should be repaired. The deltoid muscle is sutured with one or two absorbable stitches and the superficial layers are closed as usual. Suction drainage is not necessary (Table 36-15).

TABLE 36-15 | **Surgical Steps for Antegrade Intramedullary Nailing of Diaphyseal Humeral Fracture**

Surgical Steps
- Expose the subacromial bursa and the rotator cuff
- 1-cm stab incision to the rotator cuff
- Open the entry portal of the nail with a hand awl
- Reduce the fracture under image intensifier control
- Pass the guidewire through the fracture to the distal fragment
- Ream the canal, if necessary
  - Start reaming when the reamer is within the humeral head
  - Avoid injuring the radial nerve with the reamer whenever the fracture is located at the middle/distal humeral diaphysis
  - On withdrawal, stop reaming while the reamer is still within the humeral head
  - Meticulous washing out the reaming by-products from underneath the rotator cuff
- Introduce the selected nail to its final position
  - Maintain fracture reduction during the insertion of the nail
  - Do not allow destruction at the fracture site
  - Do not allow protrusion of the nail from the humeral head
- Lock the nail proximally with the use of a targeting device and distally according to the type of the nail ("fixed" or "bio")
  - Long targeting devices are not reliable
  - Never leave a nail unlocked
  - Avoid neurologic injury with the use of locking screws

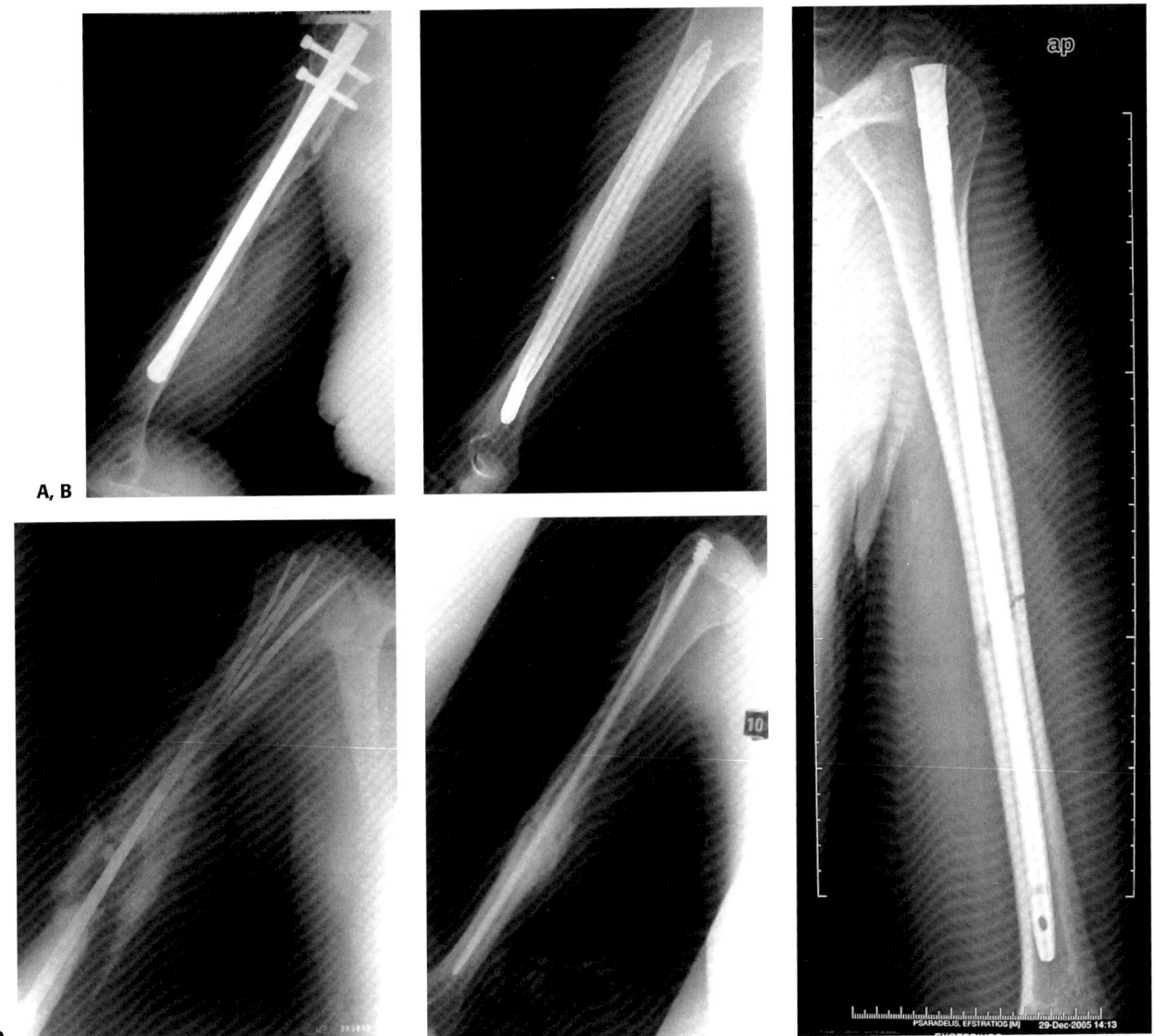

FIGURE 36-25 "Bio" nails. **A:** Seidel nail. **B:** Fixion nail. **C:** Marchetti-Vincenzi nail. **D:** True-Flex nail. **E:** Garnavos nail.

Retrograde Nailing. The entry portal for retrograde nailing must accommodate the eccentric insertion of the nail into a narrow canal. It is usually formed by multiple drill holes which are connected with an osteotome and its dimensions should be at least 10 mm by 20 to 25 mm (Fig. 36-26A). It is important to smooth the edges of the entry hole and de-roof the bone at its proximal end with a burr to facilitate the insertion of the nail. Reduction of the fracture is then performed either with gentle manipulation or with the use of a reduction rod ("joystick") under image intensifier control. If the nail is cannulated a guidewire is inserted and passed through the fracture site to the proximal fragment. As with antegrade nailing, reaming of the humeral canal is a controversial issue. However, as there are not any vulnerable structures in the posterior distal humerus, gentle reaming of the narrow distal humeral canal can be performed to ease

the insertion of the nail. Care should be taken not to create an iatrogenic fracture at the supracondylar area either with aggressive reaming or with careless introduction of the intramedullary nail. The appropriate size of nail is introduced and advanced toward the proximal humerus (Fig. 36-26B, C). The proximal and distal interlocking procedures have been described above for antegrade nailing (Fig. 36-26D–F). The fascia of the triceps tendon is repaired and approximation of the fat tissue and the skin is performed as usual. Suction drainage is optional (Table 36-16).

Postoperative Care. Thromboprophylaxis or antibiotics should not be necessary for uncomplicated, isolated, closed fractures. Postoperatively, patients should have their arm on a collar and cuff support. Passive flexion and abduction exercises of the shoulder and flexion and extension exercises

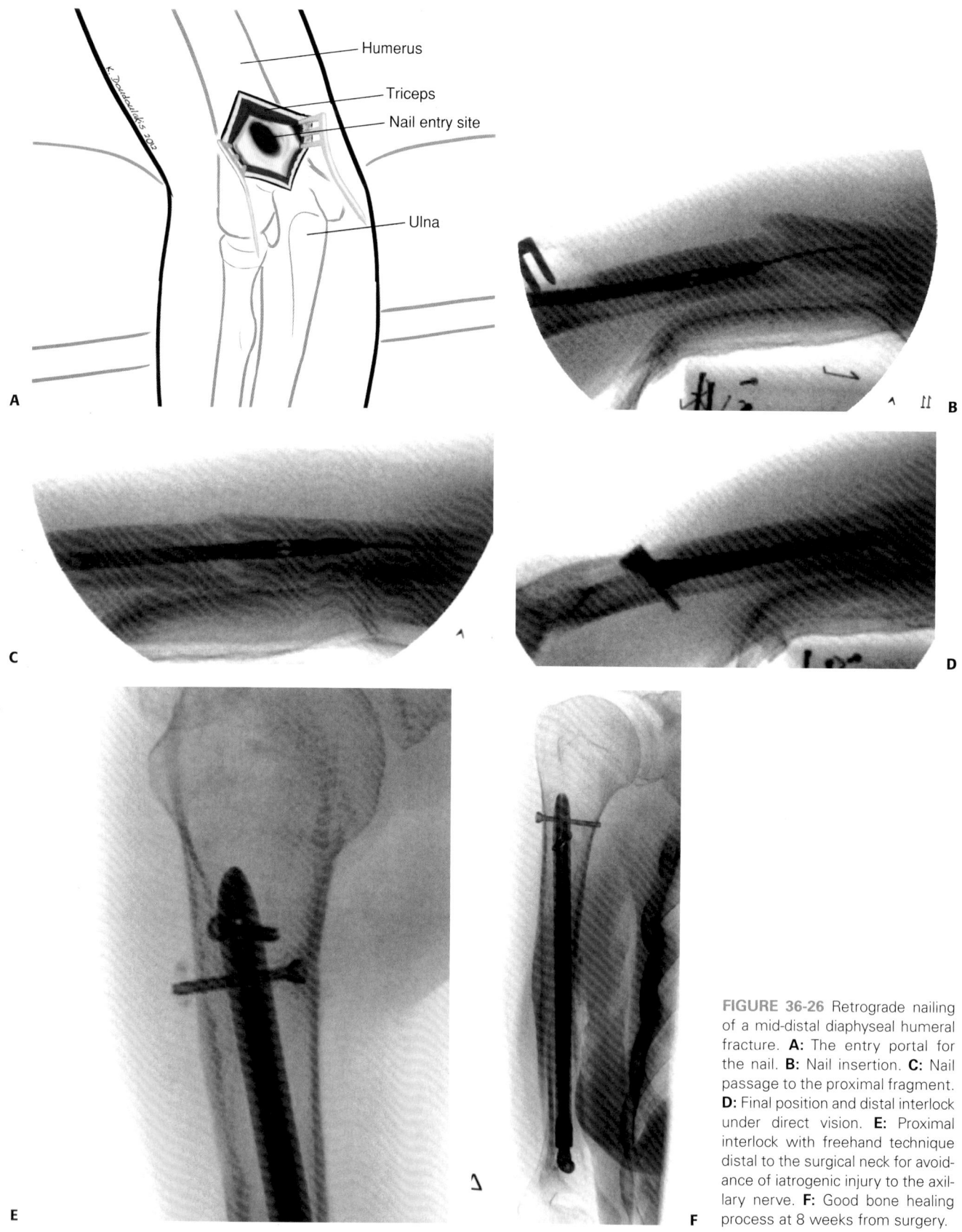

FIGURE 36-26 Retrograde nailing of a mid-distal diaphyseal humeral fracture. **A:** The entry portal for the nail. **B:** Nail insertion. **C:** Nail passage to the proximal fragment. **D:** Final position and distal interlock under direct vision. **E:** Proximal interlock with freehand technique distal to the surgical neck for avoidance of iatrogenic injury to the axillary nerve. **F:** Good bone healing process at 8 weeks from surgery.

TABLE 36-16	Surgical Steps for Retrograde Intramedullary Nailing of Diaphyseal Humeral Fracture

Surgical Steps
- Expose the posterior supracondylar humeral cortex
- Open a 1 × 2 cm entry portal by connecting multiple drill holes with an osteotome
- Reduce the fracture under image intensifier control
- Pass the guidewire through the fracture to the distal fragment
- Ream the canal, if necessary
  - Take care not to create a fracture at the supracondylar area with the reamers. Hand reaming is preferred
  - Avoid injuring the radial nerve with the reamer whenever the fracture is located at the middle/distal humeral diaphysis
  - Meticulous washing out of the reaming by-products
- Introduce the selected nail to its final position
  - Take care not to create a fracture at the supracondylar area
  - Maintain fracture reduction during the insertion of the nail
  - Do not allow destruction at the fracture site
- Lock the nail distally with the use of a targeting device and proximally according to the type of the nail ("fixed" or "bio")
  - Long targeting devices are not reliable
  - Never leave a nail unlocked
  - Avoid neurologic injury from the use of locking screws

of the elbow can commence on the second postoperative day. More active exercises should start after 10 to 15 days and rotational exercises should be instructed when soft callus is visible on radiographs.[92,168,251,269] "Fixed" nailing is preferred for patients unable to walk to allow the use of crutches with an axillary support as soon as pain allows, generally within 2 to 3 weeks from surgery. Patients unable to walk who have been treated with "bio" nailing should postpone loading and the use of crutches until radiographic signs of fracture healing are evident.[269] The physiotherapy program should be modified in patients with multiple injuries to accommodate the patient's general condition and accompanying comorbidities.[92]

In all cases the aim is to mobilize the shoulder and elbow joints as early as possible following the nailing procedure. Routine follow-up consists of radiographic and clinical assessment in the outpatient clinic at 4 to 6 week intervals until fracture healing. Thereafter, the follow-up visits must continue at 2 to 3 month intervals until the completion of functional recovery of the arm.

Potential Pitfalls and Preventative Measures (Table 36-17). Intramedullary nailing requires unobstructed imaging of the operating field with the image intensifier; so the location of the image intensifier in relation to the patient, the surgeon, the assistant, and the scrub nurse is of paramount importance. The patient's positioning should allow viewing without any metal items obscuring the image. If the image intensifier is located on the opposite site of the operated arm, it should provide images of the whole humerus without obstacles (e.g., the leg of the operating table).

TABLE 36-17	Potential Pitfalls and Preventative Measures for Intramedullary Nailing of Diaphyseal Humeral Fractures

General Pitfalls	Preventions
Problems with the image intensifier	Position the patient in such a way that metal items will not obstruct the viewing
	If the image intensifier remains on the same side as the injured arm, allocate precisely the position of the assistant and scrub nurse and avoid contamination of the operating field by its volume
	If the image intensifier remains on the opposite side of the injured arm (antegrade nailing) take care that it can pass underneath the operating table without obstacles (such as the table leg)
Not locking "fixed" nails distally in antegrade nailing or proximally in retrograde nailing	"Bio" nails are better than unlocked "fixed" nails
	Never try to incarcerate "fixed" nails within the humeral canal to avoid locking screws

Antegrade Nailing Pitfalls	Preventions
Unnecessary violation of the rotator cuff	Select the location of the rotator cuff incision carefully. It should not be >1 cm
"Blind" insertion of locking screws nearby important neurovascular structures	Open approach for screws close to vulnerable soft tissues

Retrograde Nailing Pitfall	Preventions
Underestimate the danger for supracondylar iatrogenic fracture	Open a sizable entry portal
	Enlarge the distal humeral canal with careful hand reaming
	Flex the elbow >100 degrees during nail insertion

A frequent pitfall with the antegrade nailing is unnecessary damage to the rotator cuff. This can be avoided by carefully selecting the location of the rotator cuff incision and minimizing the size of the incision to avoid problems with shoulder movement and postoperative shoulder pain.

Locking screws should be carefully used in both antegrade and retrograde nailing to avoid iatrogenic soft tissue damage. If the design of the nail allows the choice of "safe" screws, these screws should be preferred; screws that are close to vulnerable soft tissues should be inserted with small but adequate incisions that will allow direct visualization of the area and identification of neurovascular structures.

"Fixed" nails require locking screws. If the surgeon is not comfortable with the freehand insertion of locking screws, then a "bio" nail should be used. Unlocked "fixed" nails increase the possibility of fracture healing problems. In addition, if the surgeon attempts to insert a very tight "fixed" nail within the humeral canal in an effort to avoid locking screws there is a significant risk of causing fracture comminution or the creation of a new fracture (Fig. 36-27).

The most important pitfall during retrograde nailing is the underestimation of the danger of creating a fracture at the supracondylar area either during the reaming or during the insertion of the nail. The reasons for this devastating complication include the narrow distal humeral canal, the hardness of the bone in the area, and the eccentric introduction of the tools and implants within the humeral canal because of the presence of the olecranon. Preventative measures include the opening of a wide/long entry portal, use of hand reamers to enlarge the distal humeral canal, and flexion of the elbow during nail insertion as much as possible (>100 degrees) to minimize the olecranon interference.

Treatment-Specific Outcomes. Since the Seidel nail, considered by many as the first intramedullary rod specifically made for the treatment of diaphyseal humeral fractures, was introduced around 1990, much has changed regarding the theoretical and practical aspects of intramedullary nailing of the humerus. Initial enthusiasm was followed by skepticism and

fears that intramedullary nailing of the humerus might not be as successful as the same technique when applied in the diaphyseal fractures of the long bones of the leg.[17,59,120,130,133,240,247,308]

The use of flexible intramedullary rods for the treatment of diaphyseal humeral fractures has continued despite reports about high complication rates and significant problems with functional recovery of shoulder and elbow joints.[31,112,287] Liebergall et al.[163] and Chen et al.[43] used Ender nails in 25 and 118 diaphyseal humeral fractures respectively. There were some implant-related complications such as proximal migration and impingement of a small number of nails, but both studies reported an excellent union rate (92% and 96% respectively), a low complication rate, and good functional recovery of the neighboring joints. However, Liebergall et al. used bracing or a plaster as added protection for 3 to 6 weeks while Chen et al. used no external protection and started mobilization with physiotherapy immediately after surgery. In a later study Ender nails were compared with dynamic compression plating and interlocking nails.[40] Patients treated with the flexible intramedullary rods had a shorter mean operation time, less mean blood loss, and a shorter mean hospital stay. The rates of union and general complications were comparable. Although the authors state that all patients followed uniform rehabilitation program with an arm sling postoperatively, immediate pendulum and elbow movements, and active shoulder exercises 3 weeks postoperatively, they unfortunately do not provide detailed information about restoration of shoulder and elbow motion or functional recovery of the patients. They concluded that all three methods are reliable within their limitations in the management of diaphyseal humeral fractures. Pinning of the humeral diaphysis with multiple Rush pins in 200 patients was presented by Gadegone and Salphale.[89] Open reduction was necessary in 14 patients. There were eight pin migrations into the shoulder and one into the elbow, four postoperative radial nerve palsies, and 10 cases with notable malrotation of the fracture. However, only four nonunions occurred (union rate of 98%) and 92% of the patients had excellent-to-good ROM of the shoulder and elbow. The authors concluded that fixation of humeral shaft fractures with Rush pins can be a good treatment option bearing in mind the cost of the implant. Chaarani,[37] proposed the use of a single antegrade Rush pin for the management of distal diaphyseal humeral fractures with the Rush pin being impacted into the lateral humeral condyle. Thirty-seven patients were treated with this method. All fractures united in an average of 5.7 weeks although the earliest stated union time of 2 weeks casts some doubt on the method of assessing fracture union. The only problems were two postoperative transient nerve palsies and a varus deformity of up to 13 degrees in 11 patients. The patients regained full shoulder and almost full elbow movements.

Despite the encouraging results from the use of flexible intramedullary pins in the treatment of diaphyseal humeral fractures, it is generally accepted that operative management of fractures should, in general, provide more stability to the fracture site. A stable environment promotes fracture union and allows early mobilization and return to activities without the need for close medical supervision. This has resulted in ongoing

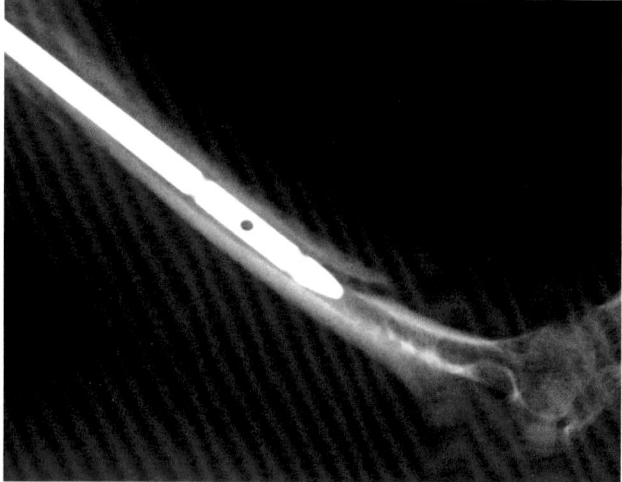

FIGURE 36-27 New fracture at the tip of a "fixed" nail that was inserted deliberately tight to avoid distal locking with screws.

investigation of nailing of diaphyseal humeral fractures with many studies indicating the need to modify both the technique of lower limb nailing and the design of lower limb nails to accommodate the unique anatomical and biomechanical characteristics of the humerus.[2,56,79,83,85,98,121,170,194,226]

In the previous section describing the technique of intramedullary nailing, "fixed" (distal end locked with screws) and "bio" (distal end locked without screws) were defined to allow better understanding of the biomechanical and biologic differences between the two groups. The terms "fixed" and "bio" refer to nail design in contrast to the terms "static" and "dynamic" or "locked" and "unlocked" that refer to the surgical technique. Modabber and Jupiter[196] proposed that humeral rods should be grouped into "rigid" and "flexible" based on the stiffness of humeral rods used at the time. Hackethal nails, Ender nails, and Rush rods were included in the "flexible" group while nails such as the Seidel and the Russell-Taylor nail were included in the "rigid" group. This grouping is not meaningful today, as the use of traditional "flexible" rods is less popular. Furthermore, most modern "rigid" types of nails are made of titanium and therefore, are not as rigid as older nails that were made of stainless steel.

A "fixed" nail that has been in use since the mid 1990s is the unreamed humeral nail (UHN). Blum et al.[24] presented satisfactory outcomes from using the UHN with both antegrade and retrograde techniques in 84 diaphyseal humeral fractures. Operating time was less than 90 minutes in 85% of the cases and union rate 91.2% in an average of 13 weeks. A number of complications occurred and included the need for open reduction, fissuring, or additional fracture during retrograde nailing, difficult distal interlocking, transient secondary radial nerve palsy, and the need for additional hardware to enhance fracture stability. While most patients regained shoulder motion and functionality, 3.7% had poor shoulder function after antegrade nailing and 1.8% had poor elbow function after retrograde nailing. Subsequent studies with the UHN had similar outcomes.[67,81,251,261] Although the UHN offers a mechanism that enables compression of specific fracture types (AO/OTA A2 or A3), most authors do not describe the use of this mechanism, suggesting that compression may not be considered necessary. Mückley et al.[208] reported good outcomes with the use of another "fixed" humeral nail (T2) which is cannulated and also allows compression of the fracture. The series consisted of 36 fractures treated with both the antegrade and retrograde techniques. Only one fracture did not unite and complications included fracture during nail insertion in 2 of the 14 retrograde cases and one breakage of a locking screw because of overbending when using the compression mechanism. Functional recovery was satisfactory with an average Constant score of 88 for the shoulders and an average Morrey score of 97 for the elbows. There were no significant differences in the functional outcomes of the shoulder and the elbow between antegrade and retrograde techniques.

Stannard et al.[285] reported on an articulated, and thus flexible, "fixed" nail (Flexnail) that used a more lateral entry portal just distal to the insertion of the rotator cuff into the greater tuberosity, to avoid iatrogenic injury to the rotator cuff. The Flexnail is inserted with articulations which become rigid with

the use of a stiffening mechanism when the nail is in its final position. It can be then locked proximally and distally with screws. The nail can also accommodate retrograde insertion. The authors followed up 41 patients who underwent antegrade (19) and retrograde (22) nailings for diaphyseal humeral fracture with the Flexnail. Complications included one deep infection, two nonunions, and two nail breakages, all of which occurred in fractures treated with smaller 7.5-mm diameter nails. Thirty-nine fractures united within 12 weeks on average. Nine of the ten patients who had some loss of motion of the shoulder and elbow joints had undergone retrograde nailing. Despite the lateral insertion, 20 patients had shoulder pain; three of four patients with moderate-to-severe shoulder pain had undergone retrograde nailing. The authors concluded that this type of nail was an option for locked intramedullary nailing of the humerus but in smaller diameter canals other methods of treatment should be considered. Few complications and better functional outcomes with the retrograde use of Flexnail were reported by Müller et al.[201] Matityahu and Eglseder[186] used the Flexnail to treat 43 diaphyseal humeral fractures in multiply injured patients, 27 with the antegrade and 16 with the retrograde technique. They encountered seven nonunions, five of them with the retrograde technique. The authors recommended the use of flexible nailing with the antegrade technique in polytrauma cases where plate fixation may be problematic. The two nail breakages reported by Stannard et al.[285] and the fracture at the insertion site during removal reported by Müller et al.[201] suggest that the flexibility of the nail may be difficult to restore after longer periods of implantation. This raises concern about the ease of removal of these devices.

"Bio" nails appeared in the late 1980s because of distal locking difficulties and the fear of injury to neurovascular structures with locking screws. The Seidel nail is regarded as the first "bio" nail, providing distal locking effect with expansion of distal fins.[273] Although there are studies with satisfactory results from the use of Seidel nail,[229,237] its use has been associated with several problems and complications mainly related to its bulky proximal design, rigidity (stainless steel), and the distal locking mechanism that, apart from its questionable effectiveness, was a problem at the time of nail removal because of bone formation around the expanded fins.[153,290,295,318] Other "bio" nails, such as the antegrade True-Flex and the retrograde Marchetti-Vicenzi nails appeared in the early 1990s. These nails provide distal interlock by tight contact with the endosteum or by long, flexible, expanding fins respectively.[95,125,184,269,294]. The exclusive retrograde insertion of the Marchetti Vicenzi nail helps to avoid rotator cuff problems. Three studies reported satisfactory outcomes from treating substantive number of patients with humeral shaft fractures with the Marchetti-Vicenzi nail.[125,184,294] Fracture union rate exceeded 95% with average healing times of 19, 11, and 16 weeks respectively with good functional outcomes. In the series by Martinez et al.,[184] which was the largest including 143 patients, shoulder function was excellent in 66.4%, moderate in 30%, and poor in 3.5%, and elbow function was excellent in 62.2%, moderate in 33.5%, and poor in 4.2%. Complications included penetration of the shoulder by the nails in five cases, intraoperative fracture at the insertion site in two cases, and fracture during nail removal in one case. They also reported 16 cases of varus or valgus of more than 10 degrees and five cases of anterior/posterior malunions of more than 10 degrees.[184] Simon et al.[276] presented good results from the use of the Marchetti-Vicenzi nail but focused on its problematic removal after fracture union. They stated that all 20 attempted removals were difficult procedures while one was impossible and in seven cases supracondylar fractures occurred at removal. The Halder nail had similarities with Marchetti-Vicenzi nail, as it could be used only with the retrograde technique and provided interlocking at its far end with the deployment and expansion of three wires within the humeral head.[111] It was used to treat 39 acute diaphyseal humeral fractures that united within 6 to 8 weeks. Ninety-five percent of the patients were virtually pain-free and 90% could do simple household tasks at 3 weeks from surgery. However, at the end of 1 year, mean shoulder abduction was 115 degrees while seven patients suffered >13 degrees elbow extension loss. Similar to the Marchetti-Vicenzi nail there were three incidences of breakage of the expanding wires and five penetrations of the humeral head by the nail and/or the wires. It should be noted that one of the co-authors of the study was unable to replicate these results in his own centre and reported an unacceptably high rate of fixation failure, nonunion, and need for removal in 21 patients.[313]

At the beginning of the new century Franck et al.[88] published their experience with a novel "bio," noncannulated humeral nail (Fixion) that could provide distal interlocking by expansion within the humeral canal with the use of a pump and saline. The authors used the Fixion nail in 25 acute osteoporotic fractures (18 antegrade and 7 retrograde) and reported bone healing in an average of 16 weeks while all patients regained their pre-existing shoulder and elbow ranges of motion without any significant complications. The same group had previously reported similarly good outcomes from the use of the same nail in 23 metastatic humeral fractures.[87] Further studies also reported satisfaction with the use of Fixion nail.[34,137,174] However, a more recent study has reported more complications with the Fixion nail.[176] Although only eight patients with acute humeral shaft fractures were treated, there were two nonunions, two intraoperative implant failures, and two postoperative radial nerve palsies. The authors concluded that they could not replicate the advantages of the nail as described in previous studies. Although the Fixion nail is also being used in the treatment of fractures of the lower limb recent reports are less favorable.[218,227,279]

The latest development regarding "bio" nails is the "Garnavos" humeral nail, a cannulated, square rod with concave sides that provides distal interlocking by a tight fit within the humeral canal.[92] If a tight fit cannot be achieved either because of sizing error, excessive comminution, or a short humeral fragment, locking screws can be used distally and the nail is converted to a "fixed" type. Additional features of the nail are modularity, with two different "cups" for antegrade or retrograde insertion and the avoidance of proximal locking screws during the antegrade technique. Garnavos et al. reported good results and few complications from the use of the nail in 63 acute humeral shaft fractures but further validation of the nail is necessary.

Despite the vast number of different humeral nails, comparative studies are scarce. The first study comparing two different nails was organized by Scheerlinck and Handelberg. A "fixed" UHN and a "bio" (Marchetti-Vicenzi) nail, inserted with the antegrade and retrograde techniques respectively, were used for the management of 52 diaphyseal humeral fractures.[269] Anesthetic time was longer in the UHN group (107.7 vs. 89.2 minutes). Iatrogenic fracture occurred three times in each nail group. There were four cases of protrusion of the UHN at the insertion point while in two cases the pins of the Marchetti-Vicenzi nail perforated the greater tuberosity. One patient developed a transitory radial nerve paresis. In 43 evaluated patients there were three nonunions (two in the Marchetti-Vicenzi group and one in the UHN group). Primary fracture healing within 3 months was achieved in 88% of the reviewed patients in the Marchetti-Vicenzi group compared with 66.7% in the UHN group. Functional evaluation at 2 years revealed that Marchetti-Vicenzi nail resulted in better shoulder function and similar elbow function compared with the antegrade UHN. In a prospective, randomized study 44 antegrade nailed cases were compared with 45 retrograde nailed cases using the same "fixed" nail in 89 acute fractures of the middle third of the humeral diaphysis.[45] The only statistically significant difference perioperatively was a longer operating time for retrograde nailing. Fracture union rate was similar (95% and 93% respectively) and time to healing did not differ significantly (10.8 and 12 weeks respectively). Although the average Neer score was similar in both groups the antegrade group needed a significantly longer time for shoulder functional recovery. Similarly, for elbow joints, the average postoperative MEP score (96.3 vs. 94.8) did not differ significantly between the two approaches, but the retrograde approach needed a significantly longer time for elbow functional recovery. However, all patients, except those with associated injuries, resumed their pretrauma occupations or activities. Bearing in mind significant and insignificant differences in the two treatment groups the authors recommended that retrograde nailing should be used in patients with a wide medullary canal or pre-existing shoulder problems and antegrade nailing should be used in patients with young age or a small medullary canal.

Plating or Nailing. Antegrade "fixed" nailing (with the Russell-Taylor nail) has been compared with standard plating techniques in three studies since 2000.[38,41,187] Surprisingly, the three studies produced diverging results. Chapman et al. reported on 84 humeral diaphyseal fractures treated with either open reduction and plating (46) or intramedullary nailing (38). They found equivalence in time to fracture healing but intramedullary nailing was significantly associated with shoulder pain and stiffness. Plating was significantly associated with elbow stiffness especially in distal third fractures but not with elbow pain. The authors concluded that both intramedullary nailing and compression plating provide predictable methods for achieving fracture stabilization and ultimate healing.[41] In the same year a prospective randomized study of 44 fractures treated with either plating or intramedullary nailing found a significantly higher rate of complications in the nailing group including shoulder impingement. The authors suggested that plating remained the best treatment for unstable fractures of the humeral shaft because intramedullary nailing was technically more demanding and had a higher rate of complications.[181] In contrast, Changulani et al.[38] found a higher rate of complications with plating and concluded that nailing is a better surgical option for the management of diaphyseal fractures of the humerus.

Further evidence was provided by Heineman et al.[118,119] when they updated their own synchronous meta-analysis examining the dilemma of plating or nailing for humeral shaft fractures. While in the initial meta-analysis the authors concluded that pooling of the data failed to provide a firm conclusion because of the heterogeneity of implant types and fracture patterns, the addition of 34 patients from a recent study by Putti et al.,[236] changed the conclusions in favor of plating. More recently, Kurup et al.[155] reviewed five relevant studies and concluded that intramedullary nailing is associated with an increased risk of shoulder impingement, with an increase in restriction of shoulder movement and also increased need for removal of metalwork while there was insufficient evidence to determine if there were any differences including functional outcome.

A recent study compared the more modern "fixed" UHN and Expert humeral nail with plate fixation in a substantive group of 91 patients who had sustained humeral shaft fractures. The results were in favor of plating and the authors proposed that nails should be used in pathologic fractures, in morbidly obese and osteopenic patients, and large segmental fractures of the humerus.[69] In 2012 Chen et al.[44] reviewed the catalogues of a USA social insurance program to identify patients who had sustained a humeral shaft fracture between 1993 and 2007 and were treated with ORIF or nailing. They identified 451 patients (172 with plates and 279 with nails) who had complete 1-year follow-up data. Analysis of the findings regarding operating time, reoperation rate, and 1-year mortality revealed that nailing has a shorter mean operative time and the two surgical techniques had no significant differences in terms of risk of secondary procedures and 1-year mortality.

Shoulder joint impairment is the main problem with antegrade nailing. In a study designed to compare the functional outcomes of the shoulder joint in 73 patients, 44 patients underwent antegrade nailing and 29 ORIF with a DCP.[84] There was no statistically significant difference in shoulder pain, functional scores, or isometric strength parameters between the two groups. Shoulder joint motion and strength did not recover to normal after humeral shaft fracture and the authors concluded that antegrade nailing, if performed properly, should not be considered responsible for shoulder joint impairment. However, a more recent study by Li et al.[162] disputed these findings and showed that patients who underwent nailing, apart from having lower shoulder functional scores and a decreased range of shoulder motion, also had a greater degree of malrotation of the humeral fracture than patients who underwent plating.

It appears that the available data regarding the comparison of plating with intramedullary nailing for the humeral shaft fractures have not produced conclusive results possibly because of the small number of acute fractures that are treated operatively, the ongoing appearance of new implants and techniques, and the long learning curve required for the new techniques. It may be

some time before definitive evidence establishes which technique is better for the management of humeral diaphyseal fractures.

External Fixation

Indications and Preoperative Planning. External fixation has a limited role in the management of acute humeral diaphyseal fractures and is mainly used in open fractures with extensive soft tissue and bone loss, during the damage control approach in multiple injured patients and in nonunions especially if they are infected.[47,48,192] Ruland also included as indications fractures of the distal humerus, bilateral humeral fractures, the post-traumatic paralysis of the radial nerve, fractures associated with vascular injuries, burns, and fractures with soft tissue interposition.[256] In general, external fixation should be used for provisional stabilization of diaphyseal humeral fractures and should be substituted with the definitive treatment in due course (Fig. 36-28).[141,256]

In the acute setting external fixation is an emergency procedure used to save either the limb or the patient's life. Under these circumstances, there may be insufficient time for planning, especially if it is expected that definitive fixation of the fracture will follow. However, especially in some cases of multiple injured patients, it may not be feasible to return to the operating room for definitive fixation and the external fixator may be the definitive treatment. For this reason, even in the acute setting of a damage control situation, surgeons must try to apply the external fixation efficiently, bearing in mind that there may not be another opportunity to correct problems related to fracture reduction and limb alignment. Preoperative preparation must include adequate imaging of the fractured humerus, as the surgeon must be aware of the integrity of the proximal and distal parts of the bone where the pins of the external fixator will be inserted.

Complete and detailed preoperative planning is needed in cases where the external fixation is performed as an elective procedure; for example, for treatment of a nonunion of a humeral fracture. The planning must include the removal of previously inserted implants with provision of suitable instruments for removal, organization of the necessary equipment, and tools for the surgical debridement, decortication, and harvesting of bone graft. Availability of allograft or bone substitutes should also be ensured. Finally, there should always be an alternative plan in case of unexpected problems. Table 36-18 shows a preoperative planning checklist for acute or elective external fixation of a diaphyseal humeral fracture.

Surgical Technique and Postoperative Care. The patient is positioned supine with the arm on a radiolucent support. In the acute setting two or three pins are inserted above and below the fracture under image intensifier control for confirmation of fracture alignment and correct placement of the pins. If any of the pins is close to neurovascular structures, open placement of the pin is advised. Adherence to proper surgical technique and regular review of the fracture healing process will allow adjustments of the fixator to improve alignment or provide compression whenever indicated. As pin track infection is one of the anticipated problems postoperatively, daily pin track care should be undertaken.

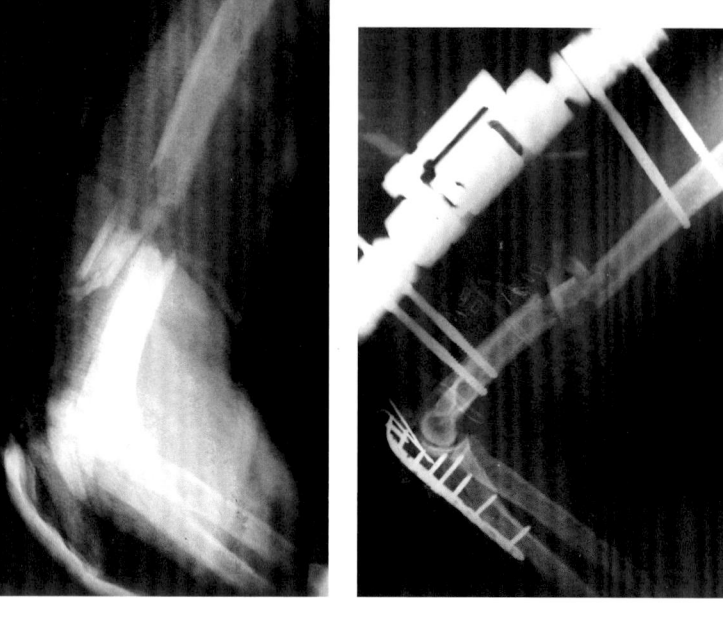
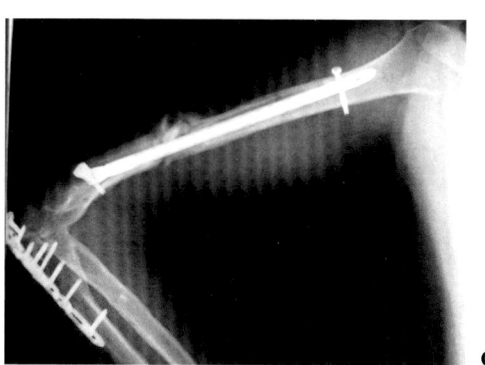
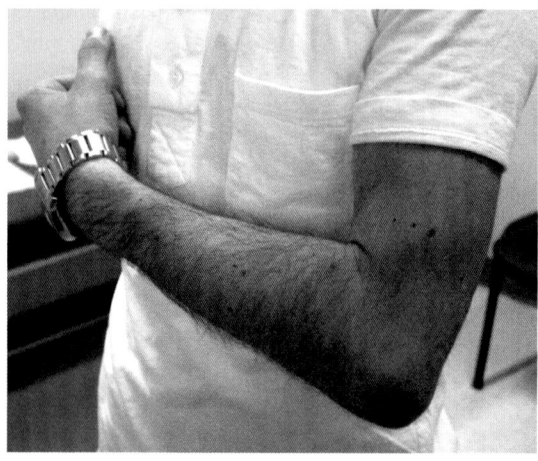
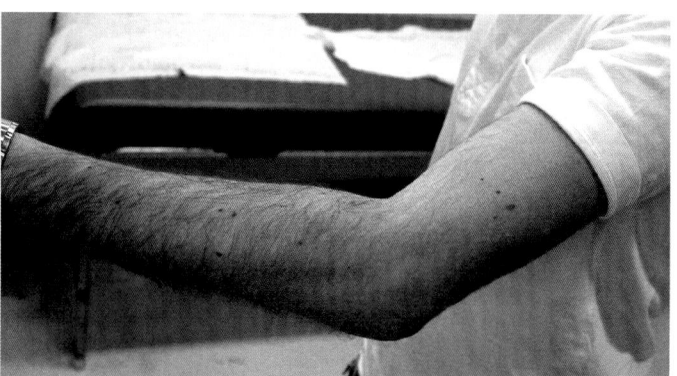

A, B

C

D

E

FIGURE 36-28 A: Severe open fracture (IIIb according to Gustilo and Anderson classification) of the distal humeral diaphysis and the olecranon. **B:** Immediate plating of the olecranon and external fixation to the humerus. **C:** Conversion to "fixed" intramedullary nailing and autologous grafting 4 weeks later. **D, E:** Clinical picture at 2 months post nailing. The final ROM was 20 to 115 degrees.

Treatment-Specific Outcomes. On reviewing outcomes of the management of humeral shaft fractures with external fixation it must be remembered that most studies deal with complex cases (e.g., open fractures or multitrauma patients) that are prone to complications and adverse outcomes. Mostafavi and Tornetta[199] and Marsh et al.[179] evaluated 18 and 15 such patients respectively. Almost half of the patients in both studies developed pin track infections, while there were two refractures after the removal of the fixator, four nonunions, and three malunions. Mostafavi and Tornetta[199] also reported good to excellent function in only 12 of the 18 patients. Nonunion occurred in four out of seven diaphyseal humeral fractures that were treated with external fixation by Choong and Griffiths.[47] Somewhat better results were reported by Ruland[256] in a mixed group of 16 closed and open fractures of the humeral shaft that were treated with external fixation.

Outcomes from the use of external fixation in less complicated humeral shaft fractures are better. Catagni et al.[36] undertook a retrospective review of 84 acute diaphyseal humeral fractures that were treated with external fixation. Only four were open injuries. There was an average operative time of 30 minutes (18 to 50) and the hospital stay for the isolated humeral fractures was 3.5 days. All fractures healed by 6 months from the accident while 80% of the patients achieved excellent or good shoulder functional outcome based on the Constant score and 93% obtained excellent or good elbow functional outcome. The only complication recorded was superficial pin track infection in 12%. Similarly good results have been presented by de Azevedo et al.[64] who applied external fixation in 58 acute fractures (45 open and 13 closed).

Despite the encouraging results from these more recent studies, modern plating and nailing techniques are more popu-

TABLE 36-18	**Preoperative Planning Checklist for External Fixation of Diaphyseal Humeral Fractures**

1. Operating Theater

Operating Table
- Regular orthopedic
- Radiolucent arm support
- Forearm extension
- Other

X-ray
- C-arm location
  Left
  Right
- Plain films

2. Position/Positioning Aids
- Supine
- Beach chair
- Positioning aids

3. Equipment
- Battery drill
- Bone graft instruments
- Large bone reduction tools
- Tools for the removal of existing implants

4. Implants and Tools
- Monolateral external fixation
- Hybrid external fixation
- "Sarmiento" rings
- Humeral external fixation pins
- Large fragment standard set
- Small fragment standard set
- K-wires
- Other

5. Other

lar while nonoperative treatment is still considered an excellent option for the treatment of uncomplicated humeral diaphyseal fractures. Nevertheless, external fixation has a role in the management of open fractures and in damage control for multiple trauma patients. However, even in these cases most surgeons would wish to replace the external fixation with another definitive form of fixation when circumstances allow. Suzuki et al.[289] tried to verify the safety, efficacy, and best timing for the removal of the "temporary" external fixator and insertion of a definitive implant. They revised unilateral external fixation to plating within 2 weeks of injury in 17 patients who had sustained multiple trauma and severe open fractures. Two infected nonunions occurred while the other fractures healed at an average time of 11.1 weeks. They concluded that immediate external fixation with planned conversion to plate fixation within 2 weeks is a safe and effective approach for the management of humeral shaft fractures in selected patients with multiple injuries or severe soft tissue injuries that preclude early definitive treatment.

MANAGEMENT OF EXPECTED ADVERSE OUTCOMES AND UNEXPECTED COMPLICATIONS IN HUMERAL SHAFT FRACTURES

Adverse outcomes and complications after diaphyseal humeral fractures can be separated into two categories, those that occur with all treatment methods and those that are related to specific surgical or nonsurgical techniques (Table 36-19).

General Adverse Outcomes and Complications Related to Humeral Shaft Fractures

Nonunion

The prevalence of nonunion for diaphyseal humeral fractures has been reported as 1% to 10% after non-surgical and 10% to 15% after surgical management.[122,259,265] Increased incidence of nonunion post

surgery may reflect a selection bias, as more "benign" fractures are managed conservatively and more "difficult" fractures are treated operatively. Fractures that are open, segmental, transverse, highly comminuted, with significant displacement, bone loss, or in patients with multiple injuries have a higher risk of nonunion.[4] Factors like smoking, diabetes, medications (such as nonsteroidal anti-inflammatory drugs), malnutrition, and noncompliance with physicians' instructions may contribute to healing compromise. Other conditions that inhibit fracture healing are pre-existing shoulder or elbow stiffness and local infection.[4] Nonunion following operative treatment is often

TABLE 36-19	**Common Adverse Outcomes and Complications of Humeral Shaft Fractures**

A. General
- Nonunion
- Infection
- Secondary neurologic injury

B. Implant-specific
- Plating
  - Loss of fixation
- Nailing
  - Injury to arteries, muscles, or tendons by the locking screws
  - Nail protrusion and impingement (antegrade)
  - Shoulder dysfunction (antegrade)
  - "backing out" of proximal locking screws (antegrade)
  - Fracture at the supracondylar area during insertion (retrograde)
  - Complications attributed to each specific nail design
- External fixation
  - Pin track infection
  - Re-fracture after removal of the fixator

the result of technical error (such as inadequate fixation or fracture site distraction) or mechanical failure.[22,85,86,188] Therefore, the incidence of nonunion can be reduced with appropriate evaluation and assessment of the risk factors, careful selection of patients who would benefit from a specific treatment method, attention to the surgical technique, and proper implant selection.

The management of nonunion of a diaphyseal humeral fracture is based on providing mechanical stability while stimulating biology at the nonunion site, because most humeral shaft nonunions are atrophic.[139,217,222,244,305,321] The most popular management for a humeral shaft nonunion has been ORIF with autologous bone grafting.[1,4,20,113,126,164,181,217,232,244] Patients with atrophic nonunion should be warned about the need for using autograft, allograft, bone morphogenetic proteins (BMPs), or the necessity for shortening if there is a bone defect.[94,100,232,284,306] The traditional technique starts with wide exposure of the nonunion site and removal of previously inserted implants. Surgical debridement with removal of all dead bony fragments and fibrous tissue must be performed until healthy bleeding bone appears on both sides of the nonunion. The plate must be strong (4.5-mm DCP broad or narrow) with at least four screws above and four below the nonunion site (Figs. 36-29 and 36-30). With insertion of a lag screw it is possible to reduce

the number of the screws to three on each side of the plate. Over recent years locking plates have been used increasingly, especially in osteoporotic patients.[58,204,245,284]

Hierholzer et al.[122] compared autologous iliac crest bone graft with demineralized bone matrix (DBM) in two groups of patients who had developed atrophic humeral nonunions and were treated with ORIF. Having achieved 100% and 97% union rates respectively, the authors concluded that DBM can be used for standard graft augmentation in the treatment of humeral nonunions and delayed unions to avoid harvesting iliac bone graft and its associated donor site morbidity.[9,71] Allografts have also been used successfully in the management of diaphyseal humeral nonunions.[171,178,306]

Complications that can occur after plating and grafting a diaphyseal humeral nonunion include persistence of the nonunion (up to 20%),[60,246] infection (3% to 10%),[1,126,164,178] and postoperative transient radial nerve palsy (0% to 17%).[1,60,126,164] Results regarding functional outcomes vary from excellent or good[126,178,217,246] to poor[1,39] and this dissimilarity possibly reflects the many factors involved such as the duration of nonunion, the number and invasiveness of previous operations, and the quality of the rehabilitation program.

Intramedullary nailing has been also used for the management of humeral shaft nonunion. While there have been

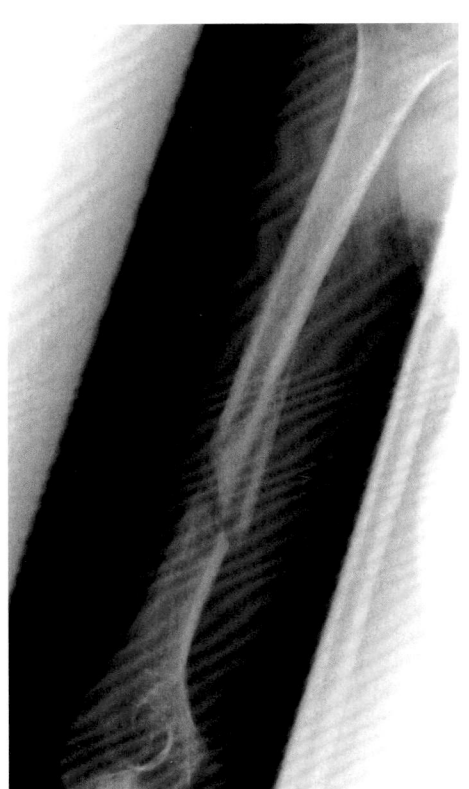
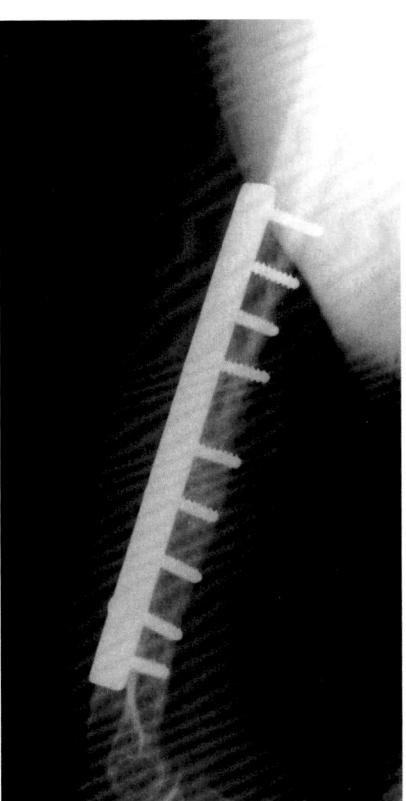
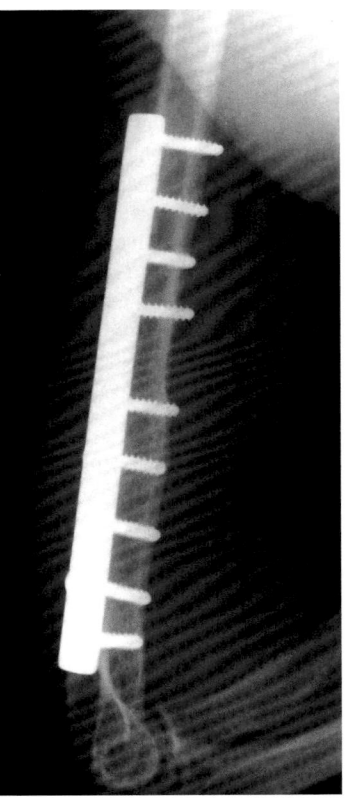

A, B

C

FIGURE 36-29 **A:** Nonunited fracture after 6 months of functional bracing. **B:** Early postoperative x-ray showing open reduction internal fixation and autologous bone grafting. Note the middle lag screw and four screws on each side of the nonunion. **C:** Confirmation of excellent bone healing process 6 months later.

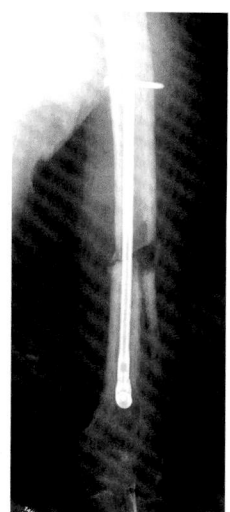
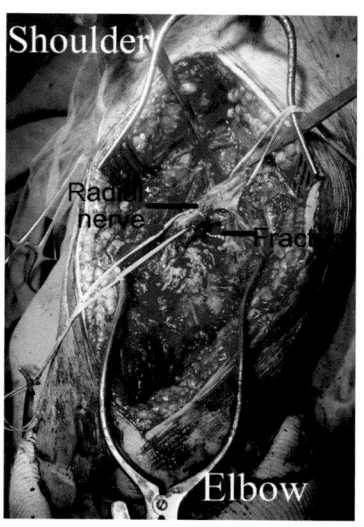
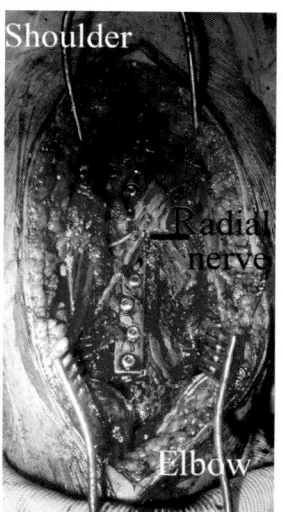
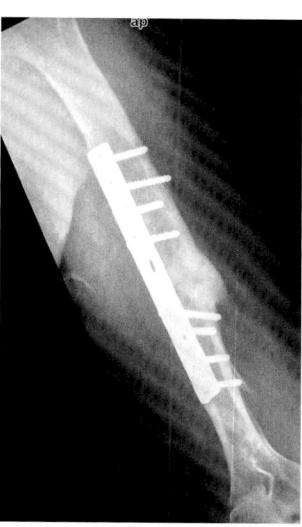

A, B   **C, D**

FIGURE 36-30 A: Nonunited fracture in a polytrauma patient who was treated with intramedullary nailing 4 months after the accident and the nailing operation. **B:** Intraoperative picture (posterior approach) the nail has been removed, the radial nerve identified, and the nonunion debrided. **C:** The plate and bone graft has been applied and all screws tightened. **D:** Six months later, sound union of the fracture.

reports with favorable results from the use of "fixed" nailing with or without bone grafting,[143,166,171] other studies did not achieve high nonunion rates.[85,189,310] Disappointed with their results Dujardin et al.[73] stated that "rather than abandoning the technique, it would be advisable to conduct further research to determine what factors are determinants in its failures." Recently there has been an effort to improve the role of nailing in the management of humeral shaft nonunions by using supplementary implants or introducing technical improvements. "Fixed" nailing and grafting were supplemented with interfragmentary wires to treat nonunions of the humeral diaphysis with an overall union rate of 96.9%, minimal complications, and good functional outcomes.[171] Apard et al.[5] used the compression feature provided by the nail that was in situ to successfully treat seven patients with humeral shaft nonunion. Fenton et al.[80] used an intramedullary nail with a compression mechanism to achieve healing in 12 patients with humeral shaft nonunion. However, not all diaphyseal humeral nonunions can be compressed and not all humeral nails provide a compression mechanism. In addition, dynamization for delayed fracture healing process is not effective in the upper limb and the use of reaming is controversial in the humerus.[96] Bearing these factors in mind Garnavos et al.[94] proposed that the advantages of "fixed" nailing could be exploited in cases of delayed unions (3 to 6 months from the accident) with the adjuvant contribution of concentrated bone marrow, introduced percutaneously in the nonunion site. In five cases of delayed union the use of this technique was successful in achieving union.

External fixators are not popular in the treatment of humeral nonunions because of the complex humeral anatomy, fear of pin track complications, or patients' adverse comments about the fixator. Nevertheless, Lavini et al. treated 20 atrophic diaphyseal humeral nonunions with unilateral external fixation, decortica-

tion, and bone grafting while seven patients with hypertrophic nonunion were treated with unilateral external fixation only. All nonunions healed at an average time of 4.9 months with only six superficial pin track infections.[159] Mariconda et al.[177] also had good results with the use of unilateral external fixation in the management of 12 patients with nonunion of the humeral shaft but failed to show any benefit from the supplementary use of platelet gel. Ilizarov external fixation has been used more frequently than unilateral fixators for the management of all nonunion types (atrophic, hypertrophic, and infected) with good results and few complications (Fig. 36-31).[149,157,222,298]

Other Techniques. The use of an intramedullary fibular graft for the treatment of humeral shaft nonunions has been proposed to offer a reliable solution for "difficult" humeral nonunions.[60,140,311,321] Vascular bone grafts, in general, have been used sporadically for the management of persistent nonunions with some success. However, the technique is only recommended in selective cases of recalcitrant nonunion by experienced plastic and/or orthopedic surgeons, because of the extensive dissection and the small number of cases that require such management.[160]

The use of electrical bone stimulators in the treatment of nonunited long-bone fractures remains controversial. However, bone stimulators should not be used when the nonunion is the result of poor technique.[102,277]

Comparative Studies. Atalar et al.[10] presented a retrospective comparison of 21 cases of compression plating, 36 cases of circular external fixation, and 24 cases of unilateral external fixation, for the treatment of atrophic humeral shaft nonunions. There was one case of persistent nonunion in each group and between three and five neurologic complications from the radial and ulnar nerves in each group of which 11

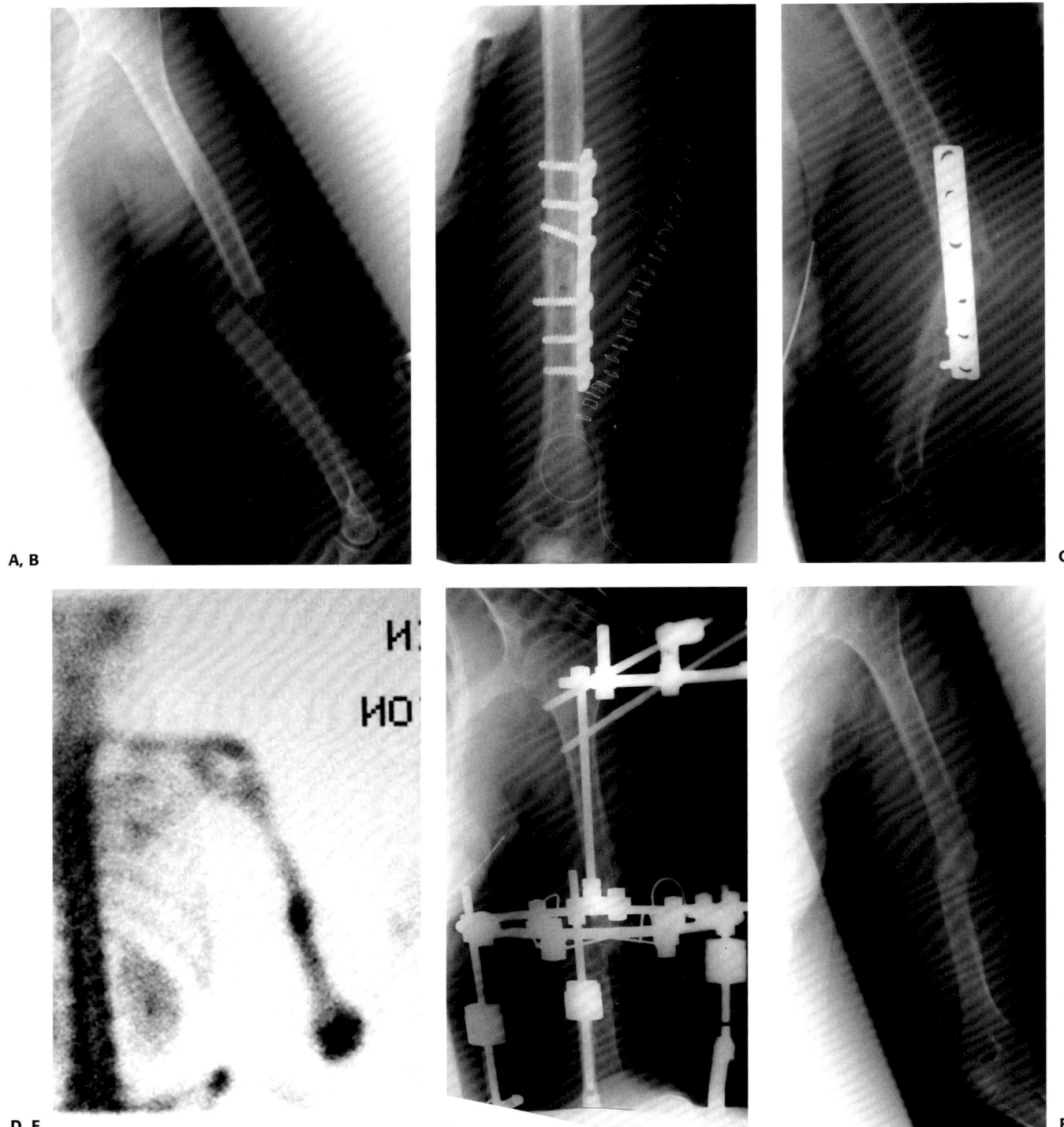

A, B

C

D, E

F

FIGURE 36-31 A: A transverse fracture of the middle third of the humeral diaphysis, treated with functional bracing, as appeared on the follow-up 3 months post accident. **B:** Open reduction and internal fixation with a six-hole plate. **C:** Three months later the fixation became painful, while the arm was swollen and warm. The x-ray showed loss of reduction and nonunion. **D:** The bone scan confirmed the clinical diagnosis of infected nonunion. **E:** The plate was removed, the nonunion site debrided thoroughly, IV antibiotics were administered and Ilizarov type external fixator applied. **F:** Six months later the infection was eradicated and the fracture healed.

recovered spontaneously. The total complication rate was 24% for the plating group, 31% for the circular fixation group, and 25% for the unilateral fixation group. These differences were not considered statistically significant. There were no statistical differences in union times or the DASH score between the three groups. The conclusion highlighted that, if performed properly, both forms of external fixation and plating can produce good results in the management of humeral shaft nonunions. Rubel et al. compared single to dual plating in 18 and 19 patients respectively with humeral shaft nonunions.[254] There was a total 92% union rate and the authors concluded that although the dual plating construct is mechanically stiffer, there does not seem to be any detectable benefit from its use. Martinez et al. treated 50 patients who had developed atrophic humeral shaft nonunion, 24 with "fixed" UHN and autologous bone graft, and 26 with plating and autologous bone graft. While they achieved 100% union rate and had minimal complications with both methods, they concluded that nailing achieves earlier union with fewer complications.[182] The same group some years later presented good results of double plating and bone grafting in a series of 22 patients with diaphyseal humeral nonunion.[183]

Infection

Infection is a devastating complication that usually develops either after open fractures or after operative treatment, related to the size of the open wound, soft tissue stripping, devitalization of bony fragments, and duration of surgery. The prevalence of infection is low in the humerus because of the excellent blood supply and adequate soft tissue coverage. When deep infection develops after surgical intervention the general principles of treatment of infection must be followed by establishing the diagnosis, defining the responsible micro-organism with cultures, administration of intravenous antibiotics, and surgical debridement of the infected wound. Augmenting standard techniques with the addition of an antibiotic impregnated, osteoconductive bone substitute can provide a very high local concentration of antibiotics at the infection site. Eradication of infection in 23 of 25 cases of infected humeral diaphyseal infections was reported using this method.[192]

If there has been previous surgical intervention and the fixation is stable, the implant should be left in situ; otherwise the implant should be removed and replaced by external fixation that can be used either as temporary or as definitive treatment (Fig. 36-31). High rates of eradication of the infection and fracture union have been reported with the combined use of unilateral fixators or Ilizarov frames, wound debridement, and antibiotics.[18,29,157] However, complications encountered in the management of infected humeral nonunions are not infrequent and include pin track infections and cases of persistently infected nonunion. Other complications include neurologic injury, fractures after the removal of the fixator, and suboptimal functional results.[29,108,157] Despite the challenges and complications of surgical management, it is generally accepted that deep humeral infections should not be treated conservatively.[108] The management of infected fractures is dealt with in more detail in Chapter 26.

Secondary Neurologic Injury

Secondary nerve injury can occur because of medical intervention that can be anything from a simple manipulation to a more invasive surgical procedure. Unfortunately, information in the literature about these injuries is limited as they are infrequent and may be under-reported. Shao et al.[275] reviewed 30 articles dealing with the management of radial nerve injury and were unable to find sufficient data to justify recommendations about the management of secondary radial nerve palsy. However, Böstman et al.[28] treated 16 cases of secondary radial nerve palsy that developed after closed manipulation of a humeral shaft fracture and proposed expectant treatment as the principal initial policy. Gregory[104] also recommended observation, while Schatzker[268] advocated immediate exploration because of the possibility of the nerve being trapped within the fracture when a later exploration would be more difficult in the presence of new bone formation.

Secondary nerve palsy that develops after surgery is usually transient, although it has been reported that it can be permanent in 2% to 3% of patients.[220,280] To avoid this complication, surgeons must be familiar with the anatomy of the arm and, during surgical procedures, nearby nerves should be identified and protected. Care should be taken to avoid excessive tension on the soft tissues during retraction. Although there have been reports regarding the danger of neurologic injury from the locking screws of intramedullary nails[26,79,170,257] or external fixator pins[48] their prevalence is unknown.

Expectant treatment of secondary nerve palsy remains the preferred choice unless there is an obvious technical mistake.[316] If the nerve does not recover by 4 to 6 months, there should be consideration of exploration of the nerve and repair or tendon transfers. Although controversial, it has been reported that tendon transfer provides better and earlier functional recovery in comparison to nerve repair.[154]

Implant-Specific Adverse Outcomes and Complications Related to Humeral Shaft Fractures

Loss of fixation happens more frequently with plating than with nailing or external fixation (Table 36-19).[129,220] Suboptimal surgical technique, weak implants, and poor bony purchase mainly because of osteoporosis have been recognized as the main reasons for this problem.[109,246]

Intramedullary nailing has more implant-specific complications.[79,170] Dysfunction and pain at the shoulder has been regarded as the most common problem of antegrade intramedullary nailing of diaphyseal humeral fractures.[79,247,287] However, many authors believe that nailing alone may not be responsible for this problem.[76,84,96,253,314] Nevertheless, iatrogenic injury to the rotator cuff could be avoided with the implementation of the retrograde technique or other approaches that spare the rotator cuff.[70,221] Other complications that originate from the use of locking screws include neurologic damage and other soft tissue complications such as injury to arteries, muscles, and tendons.[26,78,167,241,257] Injury to the long head of the biceps and the axillary nerve can be reduced by avoiding the proximal antero-posterior locking screw that many antegrade nails provide. Retrograde "fixed" nails reduce but do not abolish the incidence of injury to vulnerable soft tissues around the shoulder girdle.[173] Another problem of antegrade nailing is protrusion of the nail and impingement at the acromion.[2,79,128,229] However, it is now recognized that antegrade nails must be embedded within the humeral head and protrusion and impingement should be regarded as technical error. Another under-reported problem of antegrade nailing is backing out of the proximal screws, because of the poor purchase within the cancellous bone of the head, especially in osteoporotic patients.[56,67,170] To overcome this problem some nails provide either locking proximal screws or a polyethylene augmentation that covers the proximal screw holes and keeps the screws in situ. Specific to retrograde humeral nailing is the complication of iatrogenic fracture at the supracondylar area during the insertion of the nail.[24,79,81,165,170] This problem can be reduced by flexing the elbow beyond 100 degrees during nail insertion, opening a wide entry portal, de-roofing of the entry portal, reaming the distal humeral canal, and the use of a nonrigid nail.[96] Sporadic complications of "fixed" nails include heat-induced segmental necrosis of the diaphysis and heterotopic ossification of the deltoid, both attributed to the reaming process[212,239,271] and fracture at the tip of the nail (Fig. 36-27).[190] "Bio" nails that provide stability without the use of locking screws have

specific complications. The diverging pins of the Marchetti-Vicenzi humeral nail can penetrate the humeral head,[184,276,294] while its removal can be difficult or even impossible.[184,276] For the Fixion and True-Flex nails implant-specific sporadic complications include intraoperative failures and rotational instability.[95,99,176,218]

Specific problems that complicate external fixation in the management of diaphyseal humeral fractures are pin track infection and re-fracture after the removal of the fixator.[36,179,199,256] Meticulous pin track care and care after removal of the fixator could reduce the incidence of these complications.

AUTHOR'S PREFERRED TREATMENT FOR HUMERAL SHAFT FRACTURES

My preferred method of operative treatment for diaphyseal humeral fractures is intramedullary nailing (Fig. 36-32). The technique offers the significant advantages of being minimally invasive and respecting the biology while it can accommodate all humeral shaft fractures. Unfortunately, it should be admitted that humeral nailing, in general, has not so far reproduced the results that have established the technique as

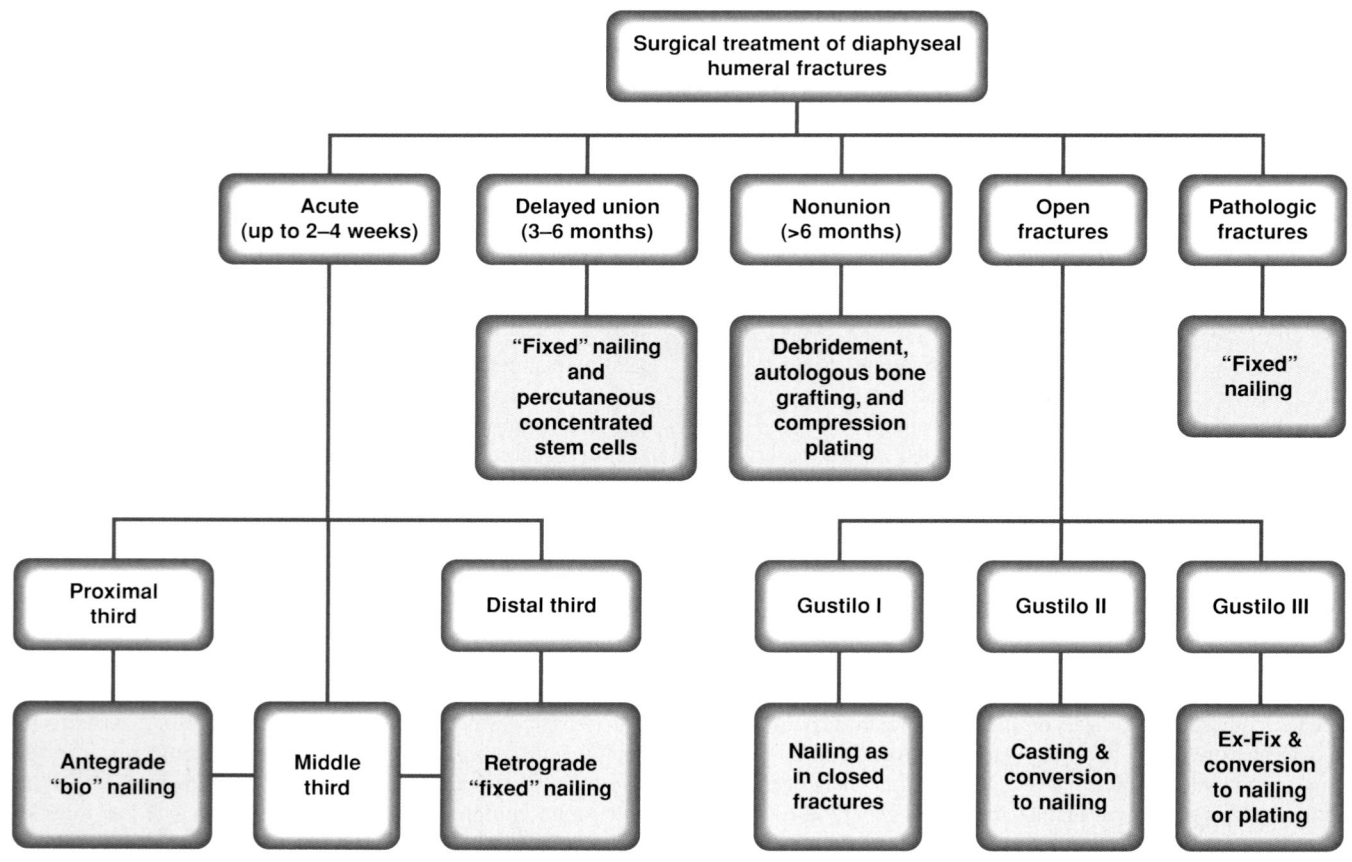

FIGURE 36-32 The author's preferred treatment for diaphyseal humeral fractures with indications for surgery.

the "gold standard" treatment for femoral and tibial diaphyseal fractures[6,7,16,58,72,143,163,242,284,296,314] possibly because of the complexity of the humeral anatomy and the unique biomechanical characteristics of the arm. In addition, there has been no consensus regarding the fundamental principles of the surgical technique of humeral nailing (e.g., selection of antegrade or retrograde technique, reamed or unreamed nailing, avoidance of complications) or the important technical aspects (such as biomechanical requirements of the humeral nail or nail selection criteria).[96]

In an effort to improve the efficacy and outcomes of intramedullary nailing of diaphyseal humeral fractures I have proposed that humeral nails must be differentiated in two categories based on their biomechanical properties: "fixed" nails that use screws for interlocking their end opposite to the entry portal and "bio" nails that provide interlocking distal to the insertion site without screws.[97] Important considerations that differentiate humeral nailing from the nailing of the femur and tibia and should be taken into account to justify the use of "bio" nailing in the humerus are the following:

1. The humerus is a non–weight-bearing bone
2. Because of the wide ROM of the shoulder and elbow joints, the humerus can tolerate certain degrees of axial and rotational malalignment
3. A few centimeters of humeral shortening can pass unnoticed
4. Freehand locking is more difficult and risky in the humerus
5. Functional bracing of a humeral shaft fracture does not provide strong axial or rotational stability to the fracture site but is still an effective treatment for humeral diaphyseal fractures

All of these parameters enhance the role of "bio" nailing in the management of humeral shaft fractures. However, it is my opinion that both "fixed" and "bio" nails are reliable implants for the humerus but that each type of nail must be used correctly. "Fixed" nails provide optimum stability with the proximal and distal locking screws and, if their design allows, the site of insertion (antegrade or retrograde technique) depends on surgeon preference. The stability provided by "bio" nails depends on their distal locking facility. Stability can be achieved in the Seidel nail if the distal expanding fins engage the endosteum, in the Marchetti-Vincenzi nail if the pins are long enough to diverge and embed into the humeral head, and in the Fixion nail if its expanded body fits tightly in the distal canal. The benefit of "bio" nailing, my preferred technique, is the avoidance of distal locking screws, a procedure that is time-consuming and difficult in the humerus, endangers the radial and lateral cutaneous nerves in antegrade nailing, and the axillary nerve in retrograde nailing.[23,26,151,170,173,197,257]

Iatrogenic injury of the rotator cuff has been considered responsible for suboptimal clinical outcomes and shoulder joint discomfort after antegrade humeral nailing.[79,247,315] However, apart from ongoing efforts to find less traumatic approaches to the proximal humerus or invent new implants that avoid violating the rotator cuff,[70,221,285] it is my opinion that the consequences from the approach through the rotator cuff can be eliminated if[96,97]:

1. The entry portal is created as medially as possible (to approach the humeral head through the musculotendinous rather than the tendinous area of the rotator cuff).
2. The incision in the rotator cuff is made with a sharp blade and is not more than 1 cm. It is important to be precise about the location of the entry portal and avoid more than one incision.
3. Reaming is totally avoided. Although relevant studies are missing, it is logical to assume that sharp reamers create further damage to the rotator cuff during insertion and withdrawal. Furthermore, the reaming products can lodge in the rotator cuff and may contribute to shoulder joint problems postoperatively. In addition, reaming risks injury to the radial nerve by the reamer if a comminuted fracture is located at the middle third of the humerus.
4. Meticulous repair of the rotator cuff is performed at the end of the operation.

There is supportive evidence that antegrade intramedullary nailing, if performed correctly, may not be responsible for shoulder joint complications.[82,84,92,150,200,211,220,253,263,285]

Iatrogenic injury of vulnerable soft tissues (axillary nerve, circumflex artery, long head of biceps, deltoid) around the proximal humerus by the proximal locking screws in antegrade nailing and "fixed" retrograde nailing[3,27,78,167,173,235] can be reduced by the use of necessary screws only and avoidance of an AP proximal locking screw if possible. Alternative proximal locking options for antegrade nailing that aim to reduce the problems from the proximal locking screws have been proposed but have not been validated with further studies.[92,95] Problems from the proximal locking screws during antegrade nailing in middle and distal diaphyseal humeral fractures can be eliminated with the use of the retrograde technique. In these cases the nail can be shorter so that the proximal locking screws can be inserted just below the surgical neck of the humerus and avoid injury to the axillary nerve.[96] Another good reason for choosing the retrograde technique for fractures located at the mid-distal humeral diaphysis is the biomechanical evidence that nailing from short to longer bone segments can improve the mechanical properties of the fixation construct because of better nail/bone interface purchase.[169] This information is more valid for "bio" nails without distal locking screws and supports the use of retrograde nailing in more distal fractures.

In retrograde nailing, the entry portal must be wide enough to accommodate the eccentric insertion of the nail. The narrow humeral canal at the distal humerus can be enlarged with staged reaming because in this area there are no vulnerable soft tissues that can be harmed by the reamers. However, extra care is needed for the avoidance of fissuring or fractures at the supracondylar area, and meticulous washing out of the reaming debris must be performed at the end of the procedure.[24,96]

My last recommendation regarding the use of intramedullary nailing for the management of diaphyseal humeral fractures refers to the timing of surgery. As I do not favor humeral reaming and dynamization cannot be applied effectively in the arm, union of a humeral fracture relies a lot on the fracture hematoma. Therefore, the chances of uncomplicated healing for humeral shaft fractures are maximized if nailing is performed in fresh fractures, which in my practice is up to 2 to 4 weeks from accident. In cases where the fracture union progress seems delayed or can be characterized as delayed (3 to 6 months), I use "fixed" intramedullary nailing and percutaneous autologous concentrated stem cells at the fracture site.[94]

Established nonunion of a humeral shaft fracture is usually atrophic and in my opinion requires surgical debridement, autologous corticocancellous bone grafting, and rigid fixation that can be provided effectively by compression plating.

I treat open fractures without significant contamination with a U-slab and antibiotics for a few days (maximum 10 to 12 days), until the wound allows definitive treatment with intramedullary nailing. For open fractures with severe contamination and soft tissue compromise, I use external fixation with conversion to nailing or plating with the timing of the conversion depending on the extent and location of the soft tissue injury.

For pathologic fractures I also use intramedullary nailing (usually "fixed") that offers a reliable, quick, and atraumatic solution that serves as palliative treatment.[92,95]

SPECIAL CONSIDERATIONS

Open Fractures

Despite reports that open humeral fractures are not amenable to treatment with functional bracing,[223,243,259,297] there have been studies that present good results with nonoperative treatment.[15,76,150,263,315,323] Sarmiento et al. in two studies treated 11 and 155 open fractures respectively with functional bracing.[263,265] The authors reported excellent healing rates (10/11 and 146/155 respectively) with no infections. Zagorski et al.[323] treated 43 open diaphyseal humeral fractures with functional bracing, 35 of which were gunshot injuries. The patients underwent operative exploration, debridement, intravenous antibiotics, and provisional immobilization with a plaster splint. All wounds were left open to heal by secondary intention. Bracing was initiated at the time of the first change of dressings at 2 to 3 days after injury. Following this protocol, only one nonunion developed in this substantive series of open fractures.

For most physicians, the treatment regime for open humeral shaft fracture depends on the severity of the injury, as has been classified by Gustilo and Anderson[106] (Chapter 2). Grade I fractures can be managed well with functional bracing, grade II fractures can be treated either conservatively or operatively depending on the wound contamination, and grade III fractures should be treated operatively.[51,199,265,272] The preferred method of treatment for severely open humeral shaft fractures is external fixation either as definitive treatment or as temporary stabilization that is converted to plating or nailing, as soon as the condition of the injured soft tissues allows.[72,256,289]

Immediate plating has been used in the management of open humeral shaft fractures.[19,220] However, until recently, there was insufficient evidence about its performance as many reports were of sporadic cases mixed with closed fractures.[19,220] Recently, Connolly et al.[51] documented good results from traditional plating techniques in 46 patients with open humeral

fractures. Apart from six cases of delayed union all other fractures healed uneventfully at a mean time of 18.4 weeks (12 to 26). Idoine et al.[129] reported equally good results after treating 20 open humeral shaft fractures (within a cohort of 46 multitrauma patients) with immediate plating. Immediate intramedullary nailing has also been used successfully for the treatment of open humeral fractures.[57,251,272] However, similarly to plating, the literature lacks adequate evidence regarding the use of the technique in open humeral fractures.

Osteoporotic Fractures

Although it was generally believed that osteoporosis alone does not interfere with the healing process of a fractured bone, more recent data challenged this assumption and introduced doubts that could influence the management of fragility fractures in the future.[54,207,292] The choice of implant and technique for the management of osteoporotic humeral shaft fractures when surgical treatment is indicated is always difficult. The main reason is the weak bone and potential loss of screw purchase resulting in fixation failure.[53,252] Intramedullary nailing has been considered a reliable option for the management of humeral fractures and nonunions in the elderly because the intramedullary rod is a load-sharing implant.[88,94,226,251] Locking plates, in which screws with threaded heads can be screwed into the plate hole to create a fixed-angle implant, seem to be advantageous in osteoporotic fractures and nonunions in general and more specifically in the humerus.[62,109,211,245,284] Complicated osteoporotic cases may require a combination of implants to provide optimum stability that will allow an effective and uncomplicated rehabilitation program (Fig. 36-33A–D). Gardner et al.[90] found no biomechanical differences in hybrid constructs (combining locking and nonlocking screws in the same plate) as compared with fully locked plates which may help to reduce the cost, bearing in mind that locking screws are more expensive than the traditional ones.

Pathological Fractures

Sarahrudi et al.[262] proposed that patients in the advanced stage of metastatic disease are better treated with intramedullary nailing while ORIF should be kept for metaphyseal fractures and for those patients with a solitary metastasis in the humerus or those with a better prognosis. However, most studies propose intramedullary nailing as the treatment of choice in metastatic fractures of the humeral diaphysis because this allows splintage wand protection of the whole humerus.[11,176,228,234,283] As, in general fracture healing is not expected, nail augmentation and filling of the areas of bone loss with cement or other substances has been proposed.[156,234,255] Taking advantage of the minimal invasiveness of the MIPO technique and the extensive coverage of the humeral shaft that such a plate provides, Choo et al.[46] described the management of a metastatic lesion of the distal humerus with MIPO plating creating a new indication for this technique.

Periprosthetic Fractures

Periprosthetic fractures of the humerus are rare but will become more frequent, as the number of shoulder and elbow arthroplasties increase and people live longer.[12,13,260,286,319] Periprosthetic humeral fractures can occur perioperatively or postoperatively. Common risk factors include perioperative technical errors

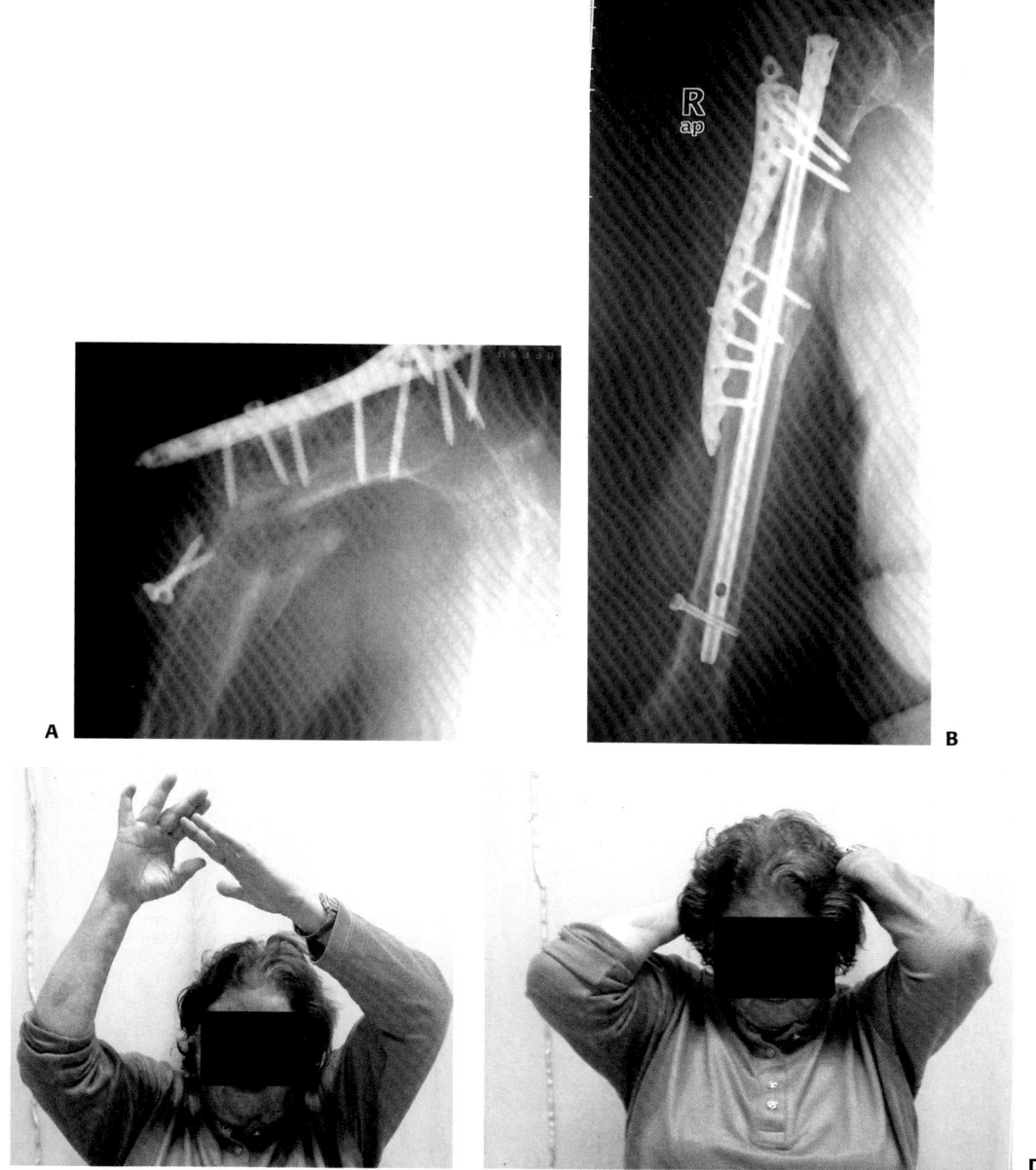

FIGURE 36-33 A: Sixty-eight-year-old female patient with a proximal diaphyseal humeral fracture at the tip of a plate that was used for the fixation of a proximal humeral fracture 8 months ago. **B:** After the removal of the plate the new, grossly osteoporotic fracture, was treated with a combination of intramedullary nailing (to splint the whole humerus internally) and locking plating. The plate was taken from the distal tibia set, because it could provide locking screws that could go around the nail, as well as unicortical screws that could compress the nail against the endosteum and increase the stability of the fixation. **C, D:** Clinical result at 6 months post operation. The patient expressed her satisfaction from the treatment and did not attend the next follow-up appointment.

during primary or revision arthroplasty, over-reaming the humeral canal, and other general factors such as rheumatoid arthritis, osteoporosis, revision surgery, and osteolysis or loosening of the prosthesis. Wright and Cofield[320] classified periprosthetic humeral fractures after a shoulder arthroplasty. Type A are those that start at the tip of the prosthesis and extend proximally; type B are around the tip of the prosthesis; and type C are located distal to the tip of the prosthesis. Likewise, O'Driscoll and Morrey classified periprosthetic humeral and ulna fractures that occur after elbow joint arthroplasty. Type I are periarticular/metaphyseal fractures at the level of the condyles/olecranon, type II fractures at the level of the stem of the prosthesis, and type III beyond the tip of the prosthesis in the diaphysis (Mayo classification).[210]

Treatment options for periprosthetic humeral fractures depend on the stability of the prosthesis, the location of the fracture, and the bone quality.[66] In general, nonoperative treatment can be attempted for undisplaced fractures in the presence of a stable prosthesis. Surgery can be reserved for failures of conservative treatment which is more frequent with types B and C for shoulder arthroplasty and type III for elbow arthroplasty. Nonoperative treatment can also be attempted in the case of displaced fracture but only with a stable prosthesis. If the prosthesis is loose or unstable it must be removed and replaced by a longer one, either cemented or not. The new stem must bypass the fracture by at least two cortical diameters and if cemented, care should be taken not to allow the cement to protrude at the fracture site and prevent bone healing. Augmentation of the revision prosthesis with a side plate and/or cerclage wire(s) is usually necessary for stabilization of the fracture. Complications that can occur during or after these procedures include infection, neurologic problems, loss of fixation, hardware failure, and delayed union or nonunion of the fracture.[13,33,210]

SUMMARY, CONTROVERSIES, AND FUTURE DIRECTIONS RELATED TO HUMERAL SHAFT FRACTURES

Nonoperative treatment, mainly in the form of functional bracing, remains the preferred treatment method for acute diaphyseal humeral fractures despite the progress of surgical techniques over the last decades because of the following:

- The ease of nonoperative management (simple splinting, ambulatory patient, no hospitalization).

- The complex anatomy and unique biomechanical characteristics of the arm that make surgical intervention demanding.

- The lack of consensus about:

  - indications for and timing of surgical intervention.

  - nailing issues, such as the indications for antegrade or retrograde, reamed or unreamed, static or dynamic, "fixed" or "bio" techniques.

While surgical techniques and implants are emerging and improving (locking plates, MIPO, new nail designs, and less traumatic approaches), we witness an enduring and fascinating debate among the supporters of each treatment method.[101] Research is ongoing and future directions are unclear but, in general, the trend is toward less invasive techniques that can provide high fracture union rates while minimizing complications, faster and better shoulder and elbow joint functional recovery, and prompt return to everyday activities. Future research may reveal that the treatment of diaphyseal humeral fractures depends more on fracture characteristics (pattern, location, timing of injury) and patient's details (age, comorbidities, occupation, etc.) rather than the surgeon's preference.

ACKNOWLEDGMENT

The author would like to thank Dr. K. Doudoulakis MD, for his invaluable contribution with the drawings of the chapter.

REFERENCES

1. Abalo A, Dosseh ED, Adabra K, et al. Open reduction and internal fixation of humeral non-unions: Radiological and functional results. *Acta Orthop Belg.* 2011;77(3): 299–303.
2. Ajmal M, O'Sullivan M, McCabe J, et al. Antegrade locked intramedullary nailing in humeral shaft fractures. *Injury.* 2001;32(9):692–694.
3. Albritton MJ, Barnes CJ, Basamania CJ, et al. Relationship of the axillary nerve to the proximal screws of a flexible humeral nail system: An anatomic study. *J Orthop Trauma.* 2003;17(6):411–414.
4. Anglen JO, Archdeacon MT, Cannada LK, et al. Avoiding complications in the treatment of humeral fractures. *J Bone Joint Surg Am.* 2008;90(7):1580–1589.
5. Apard T, Ducellier F, Hubert L, et al. Isolated interfragmentary compression for non-union of humeral shaft fractures initially treated by nailing: A preliminary report of seven cases. *Injury.* 2010;41(12):1262–1265.
6. Apivatthakakul T, Arpornchayanon O, Bavornratanavech S. Minimally invasive plate osteosynthesis (MIPO) of the humeral shaft fracture. Is it possible? A cadaveric study and preliminary report. *Injury.* 2005;36(4):530–538.
7. Apivatthakakul T, Patiyasikan S, Luevitoonvechkit S. Danger zone for locking screw placement in minimally invasive plate osteosynthesis (MIPO) of humeral shaft fractures: A cadaveric study. *Injury.* 2010;41(2):169–172.
8. Apivatthakakul T, Phornphutkul C, Laohapoonrungsee A, et al. Less invasive plate osteosynthesis in humeral shaft fractures. *Oper Orthop Traumatol.* 2009;21(6):602–613.
9. Arrington ED, Smith WJ, Chambers HG, et al. Complications of iliac crest bone graft harvesting. *Clin Orthop Relat Res.* 1996;329:300–309.
10. Atalar AC, Kocaoglu M, Demirhan M, et al. Comparison of three different treatment modalities in the management of humeral shaft nonunions (plates, unilateral, and circular external fixators). *J Orthop Trauma.* 2008;22(4):248–257.
11. Atesok K, Liebergall M, Sucher E, et al. Treatment of pathological humeral shaft fractures with unreamed humeral nail. *Ann Surg Oncol.* 2007;14(4):1493–1498.
12. Athwal GS, Morrey BF. Revision total elbow arthroplasty for prosthetic fractures. *J Bone Joint Surg Am.* 2006;88(9):2017–2026.
13. Athwal GS, Sperling JW, Rispoli DM, et al. Periprosthetic humeral fractures during shoulder arthroplasty. *J Bone Joint Surg Am.* 2009;91(3):594–603.
14. Axelrad TW, Einhorn TA. Use of clinical assessment tools in the evaluation of fracture healing. *Injury.* 2011;42(3):301–305.
15. Balfour GW, Mooney V, Ashby ME. Diaphyseal fractures of the humerus treated with a ready-made fracture brace. *J Bone Joint Surg Am.* 1982;64(1):11–13.
16. Bandi W. [Indication to and technic for osteosynthesis in the shoulder]. *Helv Chir Acta.* 1964;31:89–100.
17. Barnes CE, Shuler TE. Complications associated with the Seidel nail. *Orthop Rev.* 1993; 22(6):699–706.
18. Bassiony AA, Almoatasem AM, Abdelhady AM, et al. Infected non-union of the humerus after failure of surgical treatment: Management using the Orthofix external fixator. *Ann Acad Med Singapore.* 2009;38(12):1090–1094.
19. Bell MJ, Beauchamp CG, Kellam JK, et al. The results of plating humeral shaft fractures in patients with multiple injuries. The Sunnybrook experience. *J Bone Joint Surg Br.* 1985;67(2):293–296.
20. Bernard de Dompsure R, Peter R, Hoffmeyer P. Uninfected nonunion of the humeral diaphyses: Review of 21 patients treated with shingling, compression plate, and autologous bone graft. *Orthop Traumatol Surg Res.* 2010;96(2):139–146.
21. Bhandari M, Devereaux PJ, McKee MD, et al. Compression plating versus intramedullary nailing of humeral shaft fractures–a meta-analysis. *Acta Orthop.* 2006;77(2): 279–284.
22. Bhattacharyya T, Levin R, Vrahas MS, et al. Nonsteroidal anti-inflammatory drugs and nonunion of humeral shaft fractures. *Arthritis Rheum.* 2005;53(3):364–367.
23. Blum J, Engelmann R, Küchle R, et al. Intramedullary nailing of humeral head and humeral shaft Fractures. *Eur J Trauma Emerg Surg.* 2007;33:149–158.
24. Blum J, Janzing H, Gahr R, et al. Clinical performance of a new medullary humeral nail: Antegrade versus retrograde insertion. *J Orthop Trauma.* 2001;15(5):342–349.
25. Blum J, Karagul G, Sternstein W, et al. Bending and torsional stiffness in cadaver humeri fixed with a self-locking expandable or interlocking nail system: A mechanical study. *J Orthop Trauma.* 2005;19(8):535–542.
26. Blyth MJ, Macleod CM, Asante DK, et al. Iatrogenic nerve injury with the Russell-Taylor humeral nail. *Injury.* 2003;34(3):227–228.
27. Bono CM, Grossman MG, Hochwald N, et al. Radial and axillary nerves. Anatomic considerations for humeral fixation. *Clin Orthop Relat Res.* 2000;373:259–264.
28. Böstman O, Bakalim G, Vainionpaa S, et al. Radial palsy in shaft fracture of the humerus. *Acta Orthop Scand.* 1986;57(4):316–319.
29. Brinker MR, O'Connor DP, Crouch CC, et al. Ilizarov treatment of infected nonunions of the distal humerus after failure of internal fixation: An outcomes study. *J Orthop Trauma.* 2007;21(3):178–184.
30. Brinker MR, O'Connor DP. The incidence of fractures and dislocations referred for orthopaedic services in a capitated population. *J Bone Joint Surg Am.* 2004;86-A(2): 290–297.
31. Brumback RJ, Bosse MJ, Poka A, et al. Intramedullary stabilization of humeral shaft fractures in patients with multiple trauma. *J Bone Joint Surg Am.* 1986;68(7): 960–970.
32. Bumbasirević M, Lesic A, Bumbasirević V, et al. The management of humeral shaft fractures with associated radial nerve palsy: A review of 117 cases. *Arch Orthop Trauma Surg.* 2010;130(4):519–522.
33. Campbell JT, Moore RS, Iannotti JP, et al. Periprosthetic humeral fractures: Mechanisms of fracture and treatment options. *J Shoulder Elbow Surg.* 1998;7(4):406–413.
34. Capelli RM, Galmarini V, Molinari GP, et al. The Fixion expansion nail in the surgical treatment of diaphyseal fractures of the humerus and tibia. Our experience. *Chir Organi Mov.* 2003;88(1):57–64.

35. Castellá FB, Garcia FB, Berry EM, et al. Nonunion of the humeral shaft: Long lateral butterfly fracture–a nonunion predictive pattern? *Clin Orthop Relat Res.* 2004;424:227–230.
36. Catagni MA, Lovisetti L, Guerreschi F, et al. The external fixation in the treatment of humeral diaphyseal fractures: Outcomes of 84 cases. *Injury.* 2010;41(11):1107–1111.
37. Chaarani MW. Antegrade Rush nailing for fractures of the distal humerus. A case series. *J Bone Joint Surg Br.* 2007;89(7):940–942.
38. Changulani M, Jain UK, Keswani T. Comparison of the use of the humerus intramedullary nail and dynamic compression plate for the management of diaphyseal fractures of the humerus. A randomised controlled study. *Int Orthop.* 2007;31(3):391–395.
39. Chantelot C, Ferry S, Lahoude-Chantelot S, et al. [Surgery for pseudarthrosis of humeral shaft fractures: A retrospective series of 21 cases]. *Chir Main.* 2005;24(2):84–91.
40. Chao TC, Chou WY, Chung JC, et al. Humeral shaft fractures treated by dynamic compression plates, Ender nails and interlocking nails. *Int Orthop.* 2005;29(2):88–91.
41. Chapman JR, Henley MB, Agel J, et al. Randomized prospective study of humeral shaft fracture fixation: Intramedullary nails versus plates. *J Orthop Trauma.* 2000;14(3):162–166.
42. Chen CH, Lai PL, Niu CC, et al. Simultaneous anterior dislocation of the shoulder and fracture of the ipsilateral humeral shaft. Two case reports. *Int Orthop.* 1998;22(1):65–67.
43. Chen CM, Chiu FY, Lo WH. Treatment of acute closed humeral shaft fractures with Ender nails. *Injury.* 2000;31(9):683–685.
44. Chen F, Wang Z, Bhattacharyya T. Outcomes of nails versus plates for humeral shaft fractures: A medicare cohort study. *J Orthop Trauma.* 2013;27(2):68–72.
45. Cheng HR, Lin J. Prospective randomized comparative study of antegrade and retrograde locked nailing for middle humeral shaft fracture. *J Trauma.* 2008;65(1):94–102.
46. Choo SK, Woo SJ, Oh HK. Minimally invasive plate osteosynthesis for metastatic pathologic humeral fractures. *Orthopedics.* 2012;35(2):e290–e293.
47. Choong PF, Griffiths JD. External fixation of complex open humeral fractures. *Aust N Z J Surg.* 1988;58(2):137–142.
48. Clement H, Pichler W, Tesch NP, et al. Anatomical basis of the risk of radial nerve injury related to the technique of external fixation applied to the distal humerus. *Surg Radiol Anat.* 2010;32(3):221–224.
49. Concha JM, Sandoval A, Streubel PN. Minimally invasive plate osteosynthesis for humeral shaft fractures: Are results reproducible? *Int Orthop.* 2010;34(8):1297–1305.
50. Connolly J. Management of fractures associated with arterial injuries. *Am J Surg.* 1970;120(3):331.
51. Connolly S, McKee MD, Zdero R, et al. Immediate plate osteosynthesis of open fractures of the humeral shaft. *J Trauma.* 2010;69(3):685–690.
52. Constant CR, Murley AH. A clinical method of functional assessment of the shoulder. *Clin Orthop Relat Res.* 1987;214:160–164.
53. Cornell CN. Internal fracture fixation in patients with osteoporosis. *J Am Acad Orthop Surg.* 2003;11(2):109–119.
54. Cortet B. Bone repair in osteoporotic bone: Postmenopausal and cortisone-induced osteoporosis. *Osteoporos Int.* 2011;22(6):2007–2010.
55. Court-Brown CM, Caesar B. Epidemiology of adult fractures: A review. *Injury.* 2006;37(8):691–697.
56. Cox MA, Dolan M, Synnott K, et al. Closed interlocking nailing of humeral shaft fractures with the Russell-Taylor nail. *J Orthop Trauma.* 2000;14(5):349–353.
57. Crates J, Whittle AP. Antegrade interlocking nailing of acute humeral shaft fractures. *Clin Orthop Relat Res.* 1998;350:40–50.
58. Crawford CH 3rd, Seligson D. Atrophic nonunion of humeral diaphysis treated with locking plate and recombinant bone morphogenetic protein: Nine cases. *Am J Orthop (Belle Mead NJ).* 2009;38(11):567–570.
59. Crolla RM, de Vries LS, Clevers GJ. Locked intramedullary nailing of humeral fractures. *Injury.* 1993;24(6):403–406.
60. Crosby LA, Norris BL, Dao KD, et al. Humeral shaft nonunions treated with fibular allograft and compression plating. *Am J Orthop (Belle Mead NJ).* 2000;29(1):45–47.
61. Dalton JE, Salkeld SL, Satterwhite YE, et al. A biomechanical comparison of intramedullary nailing systems for the humerus. *J Orthop Trauma.* 1993;7(4):367–374.
62. Davis C, Stall A, Knutsen E, et al. Locking plates in osteoporosis: A biomechanical cadaveric study of diaphyseal humerus fractures. *J Orthop Trauma.* 2012;26(4):216–221.
63. Dawson J, Fitzpatrick R, Carr A. Questionnaire on the perceptions of patients about shoulder surgery. *J Bone Joint Surg Br.* 1996;78(4):593–600.
64. de Azevedo MC, de Azevedo GM, Hayashi AY, et al. Treatment of post-traumatic humeral fractures and complications using the osteoline external fixator: A treatment option. *Rev Bras Ortop.* 2011;46(4):390–397.
65. Decomas A, Kaye J. Risk factors associated with failure of treatment of humeral diaphyseal fractures after functional bracing. *J La State Med Soc.* 2010;162(1):33–35.
66. Dehghan N, Chehade M, McKee MD. Current perspectives in the treatment of periprosthetic upper extremity fractures. *J Orthop Trauma.* 2011;25(suppl 2):S71–S76.
67. Demirel M, Turhan E, Dereboy F, et al. Interlocking nailing of humeral shaft fractures. A retrospective study of 114 patients. *Indian J Med Sci.* 2005;59(10):436–442.
68. Denard A Jr, Richards JE, Obremskey WT, et al. Outcome of nonoperative vs. operative treatment of humeral shaft fractures: A retrospective study of 213 patients. *Orthopedics.* 2010;33(8).
69. Denies E, Nijs S, Sermon A, et al. Operative treatment of humeral shaft fractures. Comparison of plating and intramedullary nailing. *Acta Orthop Belg.* 2010;76(6):735–742.
70. Dimakopoulos P, Papadopoulos AX, Papas M, et al. Modified extra rotator-cuff entry point in antegrade humeral nailing. *Arch Orthop Trauma Surg.* 2005;125(1):27–32.
71. Dimitriou R, Mataliotakis GI, Angoules AG, et al. Complications following autologous bone graft harvesting from the iliac crest and using the RIA: A systematic review. *Injury.* 2011;42(suppl 2):S3–S15.
72. Dougherty PJ, Silverton C, Yeni Y, et al. Conversion from temporary external fixation to definitive fixation: Shaft fractures. *J Am Acad Orthop Surg.* 2006;14(10 Spec No.):S124–S127.
73. Dujardin FH, Mazirt N, Tobenas AC, et al. [Failure of locked centro-medullary nailing in pseudarthrosis of the humeral diaphysis]. *Rev Chir Orthop Reparatrice Appar Mot.* 2000;86(8):773–780.
74. Ekholm R, Adami J, Tidermark J, et al. Fractures of the shaft of the humerus. An epidemiological study of 401 fractures. *J Bone Joint Surg Br.* 2006;88(11):1469–1473.
75. Ekholm R, Ponzer S, Tornkvist H, et al. The Holstein-Lewis humeral shaft fracture: Aspects of radial nerve injury, primary treatment, and outcome. *J Orthop Trauma.* 2008;22(10):693–697.
76. Ekholm R, Tidermark J, Tornkvist H, et al. Outcome after closed functional treatment of humeral shaft fractures. *J Orthop Trauma.* 2006;20(9):591–596.
77. Elton SG, Rizzo M. Management of radial nerve injury associated with humeral shaft fractures: An evidence-based approach. *J Reconstr Microsurg.* 2008;24(8):569–573.
78. Evans PD, Conboy VB, Evans EJ. The Seidel humeral locking nail: An anatomical study of the complications from locking screws. *Injury.* 1993;24(3):175–176.
79. Farragos AF, Schemitsch EH, McKee MD. Complications of intramedullary nailing for fractures of the humeral shaft: A review. *J Orthop Trauma.* 1999;13(4):258–267.
80. Fenton P, Qureshi F, Bejjanki N, et al. Management of non-union of humeral fractures with the Stryker T2 compression nail. *Arch Orthop Trauma Surg.* 2011;131(1):79–84.
81. Fernandez FF, Matschke S, Hulsenbeck A, et al. Five years' clinical experience with the unreamed humeral nail in the treatment of humeral shaft fractures. *Injury.* 2004;35(3):264–271.
82. Fjalestad T, Strømsøe K, Salvesen P, et al. Functional results of braced humeral diaphyseal fractures: Why do 38% lose external rotation of the shoulder? *Arch Orthop Trauma Surg.* 2000;120(5-6):281–285.
83. Flinkkila T, Hyvonen P, Lakovaara M, et al. Intramedullary nailing of humeral shaft fractures. A retrospective study of 126 cases. *Acta Orthop Scand.* 1999;70(2):133–136.
84. Flinkkila T, Hyvonen P, Siira P, et al. Recovery of shoulder joint function after humeral shaft fracture: A comparative study between antegrade intramedullary nailing and plate fixation. *Arch Orthop Trauma Surg.* 2004;124(8):537–541.
85. Flinkkila T, Ristiniemi J, Hamalainen M. Nonunion after intramedullary nailing of humeral shaft fractures. *J Trauma.* 2001;50(3):540–544.
86. Foster RJ, Dixon GL Jr, Bach AW, et al. Internal fixation of fractures and nonunions of the humeral shaft. Indications and results in a multi-center study. *J Bone Joint Surg Am.* 1985;67(6):857–864.
87. Franck WM, Olivieri M, Jannasch O, et al. An expandable nailing system for the management of pathological humerus fractures. *Arch Orthop Trauma Surg.* 2002;122(7):400–405.
88. Franck WM, Olivieri M, Jannasch O, et al. Expandable nail system for osteoporotic humeral shaft fractures: Preliminary results. *J Trauma.* 2003;54(6):1152–1158.
89. Gadegone WM, Salphale YS. Antegrade Rush nailing for fractures of humeral shaft: An analysis of 200 cases with an average follow-up of 1 year. *Eur J Orthop Surg Traumatol.* 2008;18:93–99.
90. Gardner MJ, Griffith MH, Demetrakopoulos D, et al. Hybrid locked plating of osteoporotic fractures of the humerus. *J Bone Joint Surg Am.* 2006;88(9):1962–1967.
91. Garnavos C, Kanakaris NK, Lasanianos NG, et al. New classification system for long-bone fractures supplementing the AO/OTA classification. *Orthopedics.* 2012;35(5):e709–e719.
92. Garnavos C, Lasanianos N, Kanakaris NK, et al. A new modular nail for the diaphyseal fractures of the humerus. *Injury.* 2009;40(6):604–610.
93. Garnavos C, Lasanianos N. Intramedullary nailing of combined/extended fractures of the humeral head and shaft. *J Orthop Trauma.* 2010;24(4):199–206.
94. Garnavos C, Mouzopoulos G, Morakis E. Fixed intramedullary nailing and percutaneous autologous concentrated bone-marrow grafting can promote bone healing in humeral shaft fractures with delayed union. *Injury.* 2010;41(6):563–567.
95. Garnavos C, Seaton J, Lunn PG. The treatment of selected fractures of the humeral shaft with the True-Flex nail. *Injury.* 1998;29(4):269–275.
96. Garnavos C. Diaphyseal humeral fractures and intramedullary nailing: Can we improve outcomes? *Indian J Orthop.* 2011;45(3):208–215.
97. Garnavos C. Humeral nails: When to choose what and how to use. *Curr Orthop.* 2005;19:294–304.
98. Garnavos C. Intramedullary nailing for humeral shaft fractures: The misunderstood poor relative. *Current Orthop.* 2001;15:68–75.
99. Garnavos C. Preliminary clinical experience with a new fluted humeral nail. *Injury.* 1994;25(4):241–245.
100. Giannoudis PV, Kanakaris NK, Dimitriou R, et al. The synergistic effect of autograft and BMP-7 in the treatment of atrophic nonunions. *Clin Orthop Relat Res.* 2009;467(12):3239–3248.
101. Gill I, Siddiqi RA, Ricketts D. Comments on "Humeral nailing revisited" by Rommens et al. [Injury 2008;39:1319–1328]. *Injury.* 2010;41(6):e17; author reply e18–e19.
102. Goldstein C, Sprague S, Petrisor BA. Electrical stimulation for fracture healing: Current evidence. *J Orthop Trauma.* 2010;24(suppl 1):S62–S65.
103. Green E, Lubahn JD, Evans J. Risk factors, treatment, and outcomes associated with nonunion of the midshaft humerus fracture. *J Surg Orthop Adv.* 2005;14(2):64–72.
104. Gregory PR. Fractures of the humeral shaft. In: Bucholz RW, Heckman JD, eds. *Rockwood and Green's Fractures in Adults.* 5th ed. Philadelphia, PA: Lippincott Williams & Wilkins; 2001:973–996.
105. Guse TR, Ostrum RF. The surgical anatomy of the radial nerve around the humerus. *Clin Orthop Relat Res.* 1995;320:149–153.
106. Gustilo RB, Anderson JT. Prevention of infection in the treatment of one thousand and twenty-five open fractures of long bones: Retrospective and prospective analyses. *J Bone Joint Surg Am.* 1976;58(4):453–458.
107. Gustilo RB, Mendoza RM, Williams DN. Problems in the management of type III (severe) open fractures: A new classification of type III open fractures. *J Trauma.* 1984;24(8):742–746.
108. Haidukewych GJ, Sperling JW. Results of treatment of infected humeral nonunions: The Mayo Clinic experience. *Clin Orthop Relat Res.* 2003;414:25–30.

109. Hak DJ, Althausen P, Hazelwood SJ. Locked plate fixation of osteoporotic humeral shaft fractures: Are two locking screws per segment enough? *J Orthop Trauma.* 2010;24(4): 207–211.

110. Hak DJ, Rose J, Stahel PF. Preoperative planning in orthopedic trauma: Benefits and contemporary uses. *Orthopedics.* 2010;33(8):581–584.

111. Halder SC, Chapman JA, Choudhury G, et al. Retrograde fixation of fractures of the neck and shaft of the humerus with the 'Halder humeral nail'. *Injury.* 2001;32(9): 695–703.

112. Hall RF Jr, Pankovich AM. Ender nailing of acute fractures of the humerus. A study of closed fixation by intramedullary nails without reaming. *J Bone Joint Surg Am.* 1987; 69(4):558–567.

113. Healy WL, White GM, Mick CA, et al. Nonunion of the humeral shaft. *Clin Orthop Relat Res.* 1987;219:206–213.

114. Heckler MW, Bamberger HB. Humeral shaft fractures and radial nerve palsy: To explore or not to explore…That is the question. *Am J Orthop (Belle Mead NJ).* 2008;37(8):415–419.

115. Hee HT, Low BY, See HF. Surgical results of open reduction and plating of humeral shaft fractures. *Ann Acad Med Singapore.* 1998;27(6):772–775.

116. Hegedus EJ, Cook C, Brennan M, et al. Vascularity and tendon pathology in the rotator cuff: A review of literature and implications for rehabilitation and surgery. *Br J Sports Med.* 2010;44(12):838–847.

117. Heim D, Herkert F, Hess P, et al. Surgical treatment of humeral shaft fractures–the Basel experience. *J Trauma.* 1993;35(2):226–232.

118. Heineman DJ, Bhandari M, Nork SE, et al. Treatment of humeral shaft fractures–meta-analysis reupdated. *Acta Orthop.* 2010;81(4):517.

119. Heineman DJ, Poolman RW, Nork SE, et al. Plate fixation or intramedullary fixation of humeral shaft fractures. *Acta Orthop.* 2012;81(2):216–223.

120. Hems TE, Bhullar TP. Interlocking nailing of humeral shaft fractures: The Oxford experience 1991 to 1994. *Injury.* 1996;27(7):485–489.

121. Herbst U, Ruettger K, Mockwitz J. Experiences with the Russell-Taylor nail in humeral shaft fractures-an analysis of postoperative results and complications. *Osteo Trauma Care.* 2003;11:13–20.

122. Hierholzer C, Sama D, Toro JB, et al. Plate fixation of ununited humeral shaft fractures: Effect of type of bone graft on healing. *J Bone Joint Surg Am.* 2006;88(7):1442–1447.

123. Holstein A, Lewis GM. Fractures of the humerus with radial-nerve paralysis. *J Bone Joint Surg Am.* 1963;45:1382–1388.

124. Hoppenfeld S, deBoer P. *Surgical Exposures in Orthopedics.* Philadelphia, PA: J.B. Lippincott; 1984.

125. Hossain S, Roy N, Ayeko C, et al. Shoulder and elbow function following Marchetti-Vicenzi humeral nail fixation. *Acta Orthop Belg.* 2003;69(2):137–141.

126. Hsu TL, Chiu FY, Chen CM, et al. Treatment of nonunion of humeral shaft fracture with dynamic compression plate and cancellous bone graft. *J Chin Med Assoc.* 2005;68(2):73–76.

127. Hudak PL, Amadio PC, Bombardier C. Development of an upper extremity outcome measure: The DASH (disabilities of the arm, shoulder and hand) [corrected]. The Upper Extremity Collaborative Group (UECG). *Am J Ind Med.* 1996;29(6):602–608.

128. Iacobellis C, Agro T, Aldegheri R. Locked antegrade intramedullary nailing of humeral shaft fractures. *Musculoskelet Surg.* 2012;96(2):67–73.

129. Idoine JD 3rd, French BG, Opalek JM, et al. Plating of acute humeral diaphyseal fractures through an anterior approach in multiple trauma patients. *J Orthop Trauma.* 2012;26(1):9–18.

130. Ingman AM, Waters DA. Locked intramedullary nailing of humeral shaft fractures. Implant design, surgical technique, and clinical results. *J Bone Joint Surg Br.* 1994;76(1): 23–29.

131. Jawa A, McCarty P, Doornberg J, et al. Extra-articular distal-third diaphyseal fractures of the humerus. A comparison of functional bracing and plate fixation. *J Bone Joint Surg Am.* 2006;88(11):2343–2347.

132. Jensen AT, Rasmussen S. Being overweight and multiple fractures are indications for operative treatment of humeral shaft fractures. *Injury.* 1995;26(4):263–264.

133. Jensen CH, Hansen D, Jorgensen U. Humeral shaft fractures treated by interlocking nailing: A preliminary report on 16 patients. *Injury.* 1992;23(4):234–236.

134. Ji F, Tong D, Tang H, et al. Minimally invasive percutaneous plate osteosynthesis (MIPPO) technique applied in the treatment of humeral shaft distal fractures through a lateral approach. *Int Orthop.* 2009;33(2):543–547.

135. Jiang R, Luo CF, Zeng BF, et al. Minimally invasive plating for complex humeral shaft fractures. *Arch Orthop Trauma Surg.* 2007;127(7):531–535.

136. Johnstone DJ, Radford WJ, Parnell EJ. Interobserver variation using the AO/ASIF classification of long bone fractures. *Injury.* 1993;24(3):163–165.

137. Jovanovic A, Pirpiris M, Semirli H, et al. Fixion nails for humeral fractures. *Injury.* 2004;35(11):1140–1142.

138. Jupiter JB, Ring D, Rosen H. The complications and difficulties of management of nonunion in the severely obese. *J Orthop Trauma.* 1995;9(5):363–370.

139. Jupiter JB, von Deck M. Ununited humeral diaphyses. *J Shoulder Elbow Surg.* 1998; 7(6):644–653.

140. Jupiter JB. Complex non-union of the humeral diaphysis. Treatment with a medial approach, an anterior plate, and a vascularized fibular graft. *J Bone Joint Surg Am.* 1990; 72(5):701–707.

141. Kamhin M, Michaelson M, Waisbrod H. The use of external skeletal fixation in the treatment of fractures of the humeral shaft. *Injury.* 1978;9(3):245–248.

142. Kanis JA, Johnell O, Oden A, et al. Epidemiology of osteoporosis and fracture in men. *Calcif Tissue Int.* 2004;75(2):90–99.

143. Kesemenli CC, Subasi M, Arslan H, et al. Treatment of humeral diaphyseal nonunions by interlocked nailing and autologous bone grafting. *Acta Orthop Belg.* 2002;68(5): 471–475.

144. Kim JH, Kang HG, Kim JR, et al. Minimally invasive surgery of humeral metastasis using flexible nails and cement in high-risk patients with advanced cancer. *Surg Oncol.* 2011;20(1):e32–e37.

145. Kim SH, Szabo RM, Marder RA. Epidemiology of humerus fractures in the United States: Nationwide emergency department sample, 2008. *Arthritis Care Res (Hoboken).* 2012;64(3):407–414.

146. King GJ, Richards RR, Zuckerman JD, et al. A standardized method for assessment of elbow function. Research Committee, American Shoulder and Elbow Surgeons. *J Shoulder Elbow Surg.* 1999;8(4):351–354.

147. Klenerman L. Fractures of the shaft of the humerus. *J Bone Joint Surg Br.* 1966;48(1): 105–111.

148. Kobayashi M, Watanabe Y, Matsushita T. Early full range of shoulder and elbow motion is possible after minimally invasive plate osteosynthesis for humeral shaft fractures. *J Orthop Trauma.* 2010;24(4):212–216.

149. Kocaoglu M, Eralp L, Tomak Y. Treatment of humeral shaft non-unions by the Ilizarov method. *Int Orthop.* 2001;25(6):396–400.

150. Koch PP, Gross DF, Gerber C. The results of functional (Sarmiento) bracing of humeral shaft fractures. *J Shoulder Elbow Surg.* 2002;11(2):143–150.

151. Kolonja A, Vecsei N, Mousani M, et al. Radial nerve injury after antegrade and retrograde locked intramedullary nailing of humerus. *Osteo Trauma Care.* 2002;10: 192–196.

152. Kontakis GM, Galanakis IA, Steriopoulos KA. Dislocation of the shoulder and ipsilateral fracture of the humeral shaft: Case reports and literature review. *J Trauma.* 1995;39(5):990–992.

153. Kontakis GM, Papadokostakis GM, Velivassakis EG, et al. Bone formation blocking closure of the expanded distal fins during removal of a Seidel humeral nail. *Acta Orthop Belg.* 2005;71(4):491–492.

154. Kruft S, von Heimburg D, Reill P. Treatment of irreversible lesion of the radial nerve by tendon transfer: Indication and long-term results of the Merle d'Aubigne procedure. *Plast Reconstr Surg.* 1997;100(3):610–616; discussion 617–618.

155. Kurup H, Hossain M, Andrew JG. Dynamic compression plating versus locked intramedullary nailing for humeral shaft fractures in adults. *Cochrane Database Syst Rev.* 2011;CD005959.

156. Laitinen M, Nieminen J, Pakarinen TK. Treatment of pathological humerus shaft fractures with intramedullary nails with or without cement fixation. *Arch Orthop Trauma Surg.* 2011;131(4):503–508.

157. Lammens J, Bauduin G, Driesen R, et al. Treatment of nonunion of the humerus using the Ilizarov external fixator. *Clin Orthop Relat Res.* 1998;353:223–230.

158. Lange RH, Foster RJ. Skeletal management of humeral shaft fractures associated with forearm fractures. *Clin Orthop Relat Res.* 1985;195:173–177.

159. Lavini F, Renzi Brivio L, Pizzoli A, et al. Treatment of non-union of the humerus using the Orthofix external fixator. *Injury.* 2001;32(suppl 4):SD35–SD40.

160. Leung YF, Ip SP, Ip WY, et al. Accessory radial collateral vascular bone graft for the management of nonunion of humeral shaft fracture after intramedullary nailing. *J Plast Reconstr Aesthet Surg.* 2008;61(12):1524–1527.

161. Levy JC, Kalandiak SP, Hutson JJ, et al. An alternative method of osteosynthesis for distal humeral shaft fractures. *J Orthop Trauma.* 2005;19(1):43–47.

162. Li Y, Wang C, Wang M, et al. Postoperative malrotation of humeral shaft fracture after plating compared with intramedullary nailing. *J Shoulder Elbow Surg.* 2011;20(6):947–954.

163. Liebergall M, Jaber S, Laster M, et al. Ender nailing of acute humeral shaft fractures in multiple injuries. *Injury.* 1997;28(9-10):577–580.

164. Lin CL, Fang CK, Chiu FY, et al. Revision with dynamic compression plate and cancellous bone graft for aseptic nonunion after surgical treatment of humeral shaft fracture. *J Trauma.* 2009;67(6):1393–1396.

165. Lin J, Hou SM, Hang YS, et al. Treatment of humeral shaft fractures by retrograde locked nailing. *Clin Orthop Relat Res.* 1997;342:147–155.

166. Lin J, Hou SM, Hang YS. Treatment of humeral shaft delayed unions and nonunions with humeral locked nails. *J Trauma.* 2000;48(4):695–703.

167. Lin J, Hou SM, Inoue N, et al. Anatomic considerations of locked humeral nailing. *Clin Orthop Relat Res.* 1999;368:247–254.

168. Lin J, Hou SM. Locked nailing of severely comminuted or segmental humeral fractures. *Clin Orthop Relat Res.* 2003;406:195–204.

169. Lin J, Inoue N, Valdevit A, et al. Biomechanical comparison of antegrade and retrograde nailing of humeral shaft fracture. *Clin Orthop Relat Res.* 1998;351:203–213.

170. Lin J, Shen PW, Hou SM. Complications of locked nailing in humeral shaft fractures. *J Trauma.* 2003;54(5):943–949.

171. Lin WP, Lin J. Allografting in locked nailing and interfragmentary wiring for humeral nonunions. *Clin Orthop Relat Res.* 2010;468(3):852–860.

172. Livani B, Belangero WD. Bridging plate osteosynthesis of humeral shaft fractures. *Injury.* 2004;35(6):587–595.

173. Logters TT, Wild M, Windolf J, et al. Axillary nerve palsy after retrograde humeral nailing: Clinical confirmation of an anatomical fear. *Arch Orthop Trauma Surg.* 2008; 128(12):1431–1435.

174. Lorich DG, Geller DS, Yacoubian SV, et al. Intramedullary fixation of humeral shaft fractures using an inflatable nail. *Orthopedics.* 2003;26(10):1011–1014.

175. Lovald S, Mercer D, Hanson J, et al. Complications and hardware removal after open reduction and internal fixation of humeral fractures. *J Trauma.* 2011;70(5):1273–1277; discussion 1277-1278.

176. Mallick E, Hazarika S, Assad S, et al. The Fixion nailing system for stabilising diaphyseal fractures of the humerus: A two-year clinical experience. *Acta Orthop Belg.* 2008; 74(3):308–316.

177. Mariconda M, Cozzolino F, Cozzolino A, et al. Platelet gel supplementation in long bone nonunions treated by external fixation. *J Orthop Trauma.* 2008;22(5):342–345.

178. Marinelli A, Antonioli D, Guerra E, et al. Humeral shaft aseptic nonunion: Treatment with opposite cortical allograft struts. *Chir Organi Mov.* 2009;93(suppl 1):S21–S28.

179. Marsh JL, Mahoney CR, Steinbronn D. External fixation of open humerus fractures. *Iowa Orthop J.* 1999;19:35–42.

180. Marsh JL, Slongo TF, Agel J, et al. Fracture and dislocation classification compendium—2007: Orthopaedic Trauma Association classification, database and outcomes committee. *J Orthop Trauma.* 2007;21(suppl 10):S1–S133.

181. Marti RK, Verheyen CC, Besselaar PP. Humeral shaft nonunion: Evaluation of uniform surgical repair in fifty-one patients. *J Orthop Trauma.* 2002;16(2):108–115.

182. Martinez AA, Cuenca J, Herrera A. Treatment of humeral shaft nonunions: Nailing versus plating. *Arch Orthop Trauma Surg.* 2004;124(2):92–95.

183. Martinez AA, Cuenca J, Herrera A. Two-plate fixation for humeral shaft non-unions. *J Orthop Surg (Hong Kong).* 2009;17(2):135–138.

184. Martinez AA, Malillos M, Cuenca J, et al. Marchetti nailing of closed fresh humeral shaft fractures. *Chir Main.* 2004;23(5):237–242.

185. Mast JW, Spiegel PG, Harvey JP Jr, et al. Fractures of the humeral shaft: A retrospective study of 240 adult fractures. *Clin Orthop Relat Res.* 1975;112:254–262.

186. Matityahu A, Eglseder WA Jr. Locking flexible nails for diaphyseal humeral fractures in the multiply injured patient: A preliminary study. *Tech Hand Up Extrem Surg.* 2011;15(3):172–176.

187. McCormack RG, Brien D, Buckley RE, et al. Fixation of fractures of the shaft of the humerus by dynamic compression plate or intramedullary nail. A prospective, randomised trial. *J Bone Joint Surg Br.* 2000;82(3):336–339.

188. McKee MD, Larsson S. Humeral shaft fractures. In: Bucholz RW, Court-Brown CM, Heckman JD, Tornetta P III, eds. *Rockwood and Green's Fractures in Adults.* 7th ed. Philadelphia, PA: Lippincott Williams & Wilkins; 2010:999–1038.

189. McKee MD, Miranda MA, Riemer BL, et al. Management of humeral nonunion after the failure of locking intramedullary nails. *J Orthop Trauma.* 1996;10(7):492–499.

190. McKee MD, Pedlow FX, Cheney PJ, et al. Fractures below the end of locking humeral nails: A report of three cases. *J Orthop Trauma.* 1996;10(7):500–504.

191. McKee MD, Seiler JG, Jupiter JB. The application of the limited contact dynamic compression plate in the upper extremity: An analysis of 114 consecutive cases. *Injury.* 1995;26(10):661–666.

192. McKee MD, Wild LM, Schemitsch EH, et al. The use of an antibiotic-impregnated, osteoconductive, bioabsorbable bone substitute in the treatment of infected long bone defects: Early results of a prospective trial. *J Orthop Trauma.* 2002;16(9):622–627.

193. McKee MD. Fractures of the shaft of the humerus. In: Bucholz RW, Heckman JD, Court-Brown CM, eds. *Rockwood and Green's Fractures in Adults.* 6th ed. Philadelphia, PA: Lippincott Williams & Wilkins; 2006.

194. Meekers FS, Broos PL. Operative treatment of humeral shaft fractures. The Leuven experience. *Acta Orthop Belg.* 2002;68(5):462–470.

195. Mills WJ, Hanel DP, Smith DG. Lateral approach to the humeral shaft: An alternative approach for fracture treatment. *J Orthop Trauma.* 1996;10(2):81–86.

196. Modabber MR, Jupiter JB. Operative management of diaphyseal fractures of the humerus. Plate versus nail. *Clin Orthop Relat Res.* 1998;347:93–104.

197. Moran MC. Distal interlocking during intramedullary nailing of the humerus. *Clin Orthop Relat Res.* 1995;317:215–218.

198. Morrey BF, An KN, Chao EYS. Functional evaluation of the elbow. In: Morrey BF, ed. *The Elbow and its Disorders.* 2nd ed. Philadelphia, PA: Saunders; 1993:86–97.

199. Mostafavi HR, Tornetta P 3rd. Open fractures of the humerus treated with external fixation. *Clin Orthop Relat Res.* 1997;337:187–197.

200. Mückley T, Diefenbeck M, Sorkin AT, et al. Results of the T2 humeral nailing system with special focus on compression interlocking. *Injury.* 2008;39(3):299–305.

201. Müller CA, Henle P, Konrad G, et al. [The AO/ASIF Flexnail: A flexible intramedullary nail for the treatment of humeral shaft fractures]. *Unfallchirurg.* 2007;110(3):219–225.

202. Müller ME, Allgöwer M, Schneider R, et al. *Manual of Internal Fixation. Techniques Recommended by the AO-ASIF Group.* 3rd ed. Berlin: Springer-Verlag; 1991.

203. Müller ME, Nazarian S, Koch P, Schatzker J, Heim U. *The Comprehensive Classification of Fractures of Long Bones.* 1st ed. Berlin, Heidelberg, New York, NY: Springer-Verlag; 1990.

204. Nadkarni B, Srivastav S, Mittal V, et al. Use of locking compression plates for long bone nonunions without removing existing intramedullary nail: Review of literature and our experience. *J Trauma.* 2008;65(2):482–486.

205. Newey ML, Ricketts D, Roberts L. The AO classification of long bone fractures: An early study of its use in clinical practice. *Injury.* 1993;24(5):309–312.

206. Niall DM, O'Mahony J, McElwain JP. Plating of humeral shaft fractures–has the pendulum swung back? *Injury.* 2004;35(6):580–586.

207. Nikolaou VS, Efstathopoulos N, Kontakis G, et al. The influence of osteoporosis in femoral fracture healing time. *Injury.* 2009;40(6):663–668.

208. Noble J, Munro CA, Prasad VS, et al. Analysis of upper and lower extremity peripheral nerve injuries in a population of patients with multiple injuries. *J Trauma.* 1998;45(1):116–122.

209. O'Donnell TM, McKenna JV, Kenny P, et al. Concomitant injuries to the ipsilateral shoulder in patients with a fracture of the diaphysis of the humerus. *J Bone Joint Surg Br.* 2008;90(1):61–65.

210. O'Driscoll SW, Morrey BF. Periprosthetic fractures about the elbow. *Orthop Clin North Am.* 1999;30(2):319–325.

211. O'Toole RV, Andersen RC, Vesnovsky O, et al. Are locking screws advantageous with plate fixation of humeral shaft fractures? A biomechanical analysis of synthetic and cadaveric bone. *J Orthop Trauma.* 2008;22(10):709–715.

212. Ochsner PE, Baumgart F, Kohler G. Heat-induced segmental necrosis after reaming of one humeral and two tibial fractures with a narrow medullary canal. *Injury.* 1998;29(suppl 2):B1–B10.

213. Ofluoglu O, Erol B, Ozgen Z, et al. Minimally invasive treatment of pathological fractures of the humeral shaft. *Int Orthop.* 2009;33(3):707–712.

214. Oh CW, Byun YS, Oh JK, et al. Plating of humeral shaft fractures: Comparison of standard conventional plating versus minimally invasive plating. *Orthop Traumatol Surg Res.* 2012;98(1):54–60.

215. Omer GE Jr. Injuries to nerves of the upper extremity. *J Bone Joint Surg Am.* 1974; 56(8):1615–1624.

216. Orthopaedic Trauma Association: Open Fracture Study Group. A new classification scheme for open fractures. *J Orthop Trauma.* 2010;24(8):457–464.

217. Otsuka NY, McKee MD, Liew A, et al. The effect of comorbidity and duration of nonunion on outcome after surgical treatment for nonunion of the humerus. *J Shoulder Elbow Surg.* 1998;7(2):127–133.

218. Ozturk H, Unsaldi T, Oztemur Z, et al. Extreme complications of Fixion nail in treatment of long bone fractures. *Arch Orthop Trauma Surg.* 2008;128(3):301–306.

219. Papasoulis E, Drosos GI, Ververidis AN, et al. Functional bracing of humeral shaft fractures. A review of clinical studies. *Injury.* 2010;41(7):e21–e27.

220. Paris H, Tropiano P, Clouet D'orval B, et al. [Fractures of the shaft of the humerus: Systematic plate fixation. Anatomic and functional results in 156 cases and a review of the literature]. *Rev Chir Orthop Reparatrice Appar Mot.* 2000;86(4):346–359.

221. Park JY, Pandher DS, Chun JY, et al. Antegrade humeral nailing through the rotator cuff interval: A new entry portal. *J Orthop Trauma.* 2008;22(6):419–425.

222. Patel VR, Menon DK, Pool RD, et al. Nonunion of the humerus after failure of surgical treatment. Management using the Ilizarov circular fixator. *J Bone Joint Surg Br.* 2000;82(7):977–983.

223. Pehlivan O. Functional treatment of the distal third humeral shaft fractures. *Arch Orthop Trauma Surg.* 2002;122(7):390–395.

224. Perren SM, Klaue K, Pohler O, et al. The limited contact dynamic compression plate (LC-DCP). *Arch Orthop Trauma Surg.* 1990;109(6):304–310.

225. Perren SM. Evolution of the internal fixation of long bone fractures. The scientific basis of biological internal fixation: Choosing a new balance between stability and biology. *J Bone Joint Surg Br.* 2002;84(8):1093–1110.

226. Petsatodes G, Karataglis D, Papadopoulos P, et al. Antegrade interlocking nailing of humeral shaft fractures. *J Orthop Sci.* 2004;9(3):247–252.

227. Phillips AW, Patel AD, Donell ST. Explosion of Fixion humeral nail during cremation: Novel "complication" with a novel implant. *Injury Extra.* 2006;37:357–358.

228. Piccioli A, Maccauro G, Rossi B, et al. Surgical treatment of pathologic fractures of humerus. *Injury.* 2010;41(11):1112–1116.

229. Pogliacomi F, Devecchi A, Costantino C, et al. Functional long-term outcome of the shoulder after antegrade intramedullary nailing in humeral diaphyseal fractures. *Chir Organi Mov.* 2008;92(1):11–16.

230. Polatsch DB, Melone CP Jr, Beldner S, et al. Ulnar nerve anatomy. *Hand Clin.* 2007; 23(3):283–289.

231. Pospula W, Abu Noor T. Percutaneous fixation of comminuted fractures of the humerus: Initial experience at Al Razi hospital, Kuwait. *Med Princ Pract.* 2006;15(6):423–426.

232. Prasarn ML, Achor T, Paul O, et al. Management of nonunions of the proximal humeral diaphysis. *Injury.* ;41(12):1244–1248.

233. Prasarn ML, Ahn J, Paul O, et al. Dual plating for fractures of the distal third of the humeral shaft. *J Orthop Trauma.* 2011;25(1):57–63.

234. Pretell J, Rodriguez J, Blanco D, et al. Treatment of pathological humeral shaft fractures with intramedullary nailing. A retrospective study. *Int Orthop.* 2010;34(4):559–563.

235. Prince EJ, Breien KM, Fehringer EV, et al. The relationship of proximal locking screws to the axillary nerve during antegrade humeral nail insertion of four commercially available implants. *J Orthop Trauma.* 2004;18(9):585–588.

236. Putti AB, Uppin RB, Putti BB. Locked intramedullary nailing versus dynamic compression plating for humeral shaft fractures. *J Orthop Surg (Hong Kong).* 2009;17(2):139–141.

237. Ramos L, Santos JA, Devesa F, et al. Interlocking nailing with the Seidel nail in fractures of the humeral diaphysis in Paget's disease: A report on two cases. *Acta Orthop Belg.* 2004;70(1):64–68.

238. Reboso MLE AA, Valdes GD, Aguirrw-Jaime A. Epidemiological review of humeral shaft fractures in adults. Retrospective study. *Rev Ortp Traumatol.* 2001;45:10–16.

239. Remiger AR, Miclau T, Lindsey RW, et al. Segmental avascularity of the humeral diaphysis after reamed intramedullary nailing. *J Orthop Trauma.* 1997;11(4):308–311.

240. Riemer BL, Butterfield SL, D'Ambrosia R, et al. Seidel intramedullary nailing of humeral diaphyseal fractures: A preliminary report. *Orthopedics.* 1991;14(3):239–246.

241. Riemer BL, D'Ambrosia R. The risk of injury to the axillary nerve, artery, and vein from proximal locking screws of humeral intramedullary nails. *Orthopedics.* 1992;15(6): 697–699.

242. Ring D, Chin K, Jupiter JB. Radial nerve palsy associated with high-energy humeral shaft fractures. *J Hand Surg Am.* 2004;29(1):144–147.

243. Ring D, Chin K, Taghinia AH, et al. Nonunion after functional brace treatment of diaphyseal humerus fractures. *J Trauma.* 2007;62(5):1157–1158.

244. Ring D, Jupiter JB, Quintero J, et al. Atrophic ununited diaphyseal fractures of the humerus with a bony defect: Treatment by wave-plate osteosynthesis. *J Bone Joint Surg Br.* 2000;82(6):867–871.

245. Ring D, Kloen P, Kadzielski J, et al. Locking compression plates for osteoporotic nonunions of the diaphyseal humerus. *Clin Orthop Relat Res.* 2004;425:50–54.

246. Ring D, Perey BH, Jupiter JB. The functional outcome of operative treatment of ununited fractures of the humeral diaphysis in older patients. *J Bone Joint Surg Am.* 1999;81(2):177–190.

247. Robinson CM, Bell KM, Court-Brown CM, et al. Locked nailing of humeral shaft fractures. Experience in Edinburgh over a two-year period. *J Bone Joint Surg Br.*1992; 74(4):558–562.

248. Rodríguez-Merchán EC. Compression plating versus hackethal nailing in closed humeral shaft fractures failing nonoperative reduction. *J Orthop Trauma.* 1995;9(3):194–197.

249. Rogers JF, Bennett JB, Tullos HS. Management of concomitant ipsilateral fractures of the humerus and forearm. *J Bone Joint Surg Am.* 1984;66(4):552–556.

250. Rommens PM, Blum J, White RR. Humerus shaft. In: Rüedi TP MW, ed. *AO Principles of Fracture Management.* New York, NY: Thieme; 2000:291–305.

251. Rommens PM, Kuechle R, Bord T, et al. Humeral nailing revisited. *Injury.* 2008; 39(12):1319–1328.

252. Rosen H. The treatment of nonunions and pseudarthroses of the humeral shaft. *Orthop Clin North Am.* 1990;21(4):725–742.

253. Rosenberg N, Soudry M. Shoulder impairment following treatment of diaphyseal fractures of humerus by functional brace. *Arch Orthop Trauma Surg.* 2006;126(7):437–440.

254. Rubel IF, Kloen P, Campbell D, et al. Open reduction and internal fixation of humeral nonunions: A biomechanical and clinical study. *J Bone Joint Surg Am.* 2002;84-A(8):1315–1322.

255. Ruggieri P, Mavrogenis AF, Bianchi G, et al. Outcome of the intramedullary diaphyseal segmental defect fixation system for bone tumors. *J Surg Oncol.* 2011;104(1): 83–90.

256. Ruland WO. Is there a place for external fixation in humeral shaft fractures? *Injury.* 2000;31(suppl 1):27–34.

257. Rupp RE, Chrissos MG, Ebraheim NA. The risk of neurovascular injury with distal locking screws of humeral intramedullary nails. *Orthopedics.* 1996;19(2):593–595.

258. Russo R, Cautiero F, Lombardi LV, et al. Telegraph antegrade nailing in the treatment of humeral fractures with rotator interval split technique. *Chir Organi Mov.* 2009;93 (suppl 1):S7–S14.

259. Rutgers M, Ring D. Treatment of diaphyseal fractures of the humerus using a functional brace. *J Orthop Trauma.* 2006;20(9):597–601.

260. Sanchez-Sotelo J, O'Driscoll S, Morrey BF. Periprosthetic humeral fractures after total elbow arthroplasty: Treatment with implant revision and strut allograft augmentation. *J Bone Joint Surg Am.* 2002;84-A(9):1642–1650.

261. Sanzana ES, Dummer RE, Castro JP, et al. Intramedullary nailing of humeral shaft fractures. *Int Orthop.* 2002;26(4):211–213.

262. Sarahrudi K, Wolf H, Funovics P, et al. Surgical treatment of pathological fractures of the shaft of the humerus. *J Trauma.* 2009;66(3):789–794.

263. Sarmiento A, Horowitch A, Aboulafia A, et al. Functional bracing for comminuted extra-articular fractures of the distal third of the humerus. *J Bone Joint Surg Br.* 1990; 72(2):283–287.

264. Sarmiento A, Kinman PB, Galvin EG, et al. Functional bracing of fractures of the shaft of the humerus. *J Bone Joint Surg Am.* 1977;59(5):596–601.

265. Sarmiento A, Zagorski JB, Zych GA, et al. Functional bracing for the treatment of fractures of the humeral diaphysis. *J Bone Joint Surg Am.* 2000;82(4):478–486.

266. Sasashige Y, Kurata T, Masuda Y, et al. Dislocation of the shoulder joint with ipsilateral humeral shaft fracture: Two case reports. *Arch Orthop Trauma Surg.* 2006;126(8): 562–567.

267. Schatzer J TM. Fractures of the humerus. In: Schatzer J TM, ed. *The Rationale for Operative Fracture Care.* Berlin: Springer-Verlag; 1996:83–94.

268. Schatzker J. Fractures of the humerus. In: Schatzker J, Tile M, eds. *The Rationale of Operative Fracture Care.* 3rd ed. Berlin Heidelberg New York, NY: Springer; 2005.

269. Scheerlinck T, Handelberg F. Functional outcome after intramedullary nailing of humeral shaft fractures: Comparison between retrograde Marchetti-Vicenzi and unreamed AO antegrade nailing. *J Trauma.* 2002;52(1):60–71.

270. Schemitsch EH BMTM. Fractures of the humeral shaft. In: Browner BD JJ, Levine AM, Trafton PG, Krettek C, eds. *Skeletal Trauma.* Philadelphia, PA: Saunders; 2008:1593–1622.

271. Schmidt AH, Templeman DC, Grabowski CM. Antegrade intramedullary nailing of the humerus complicated by heterotopic ossification of the deltoid: A case report. *J Orthop Trauma.* 2001;15(1):69–73.

272. Schoots IG, Simons MP, Nork SE, et al. Antegrade locked nailing of open humeral shaft fractures. *Orthopedics.* 2007;30(1):49–54.

273. Seidel H. Humeral locking nail: A preliminary report. *Orthopedics.* 1989;12(2): 219–242.

274. Seigerman DA, Choung EW, Yoon RS, et al. Identification of the radial nerve during the posterior approach to the humerus: A cadaveric study. *J Orthop Trauma.* 2012;26(4):226–228.

275. Shao YC, Harwood P, Grotz MR, et al. Radial nerve palsy associated with fractures of the shaft of the humerus: A systematic review. *J Bone Joint Surg Br.* 2005;87(12): 1647–1652.

276. Simon P, Jobard D, Bistour L, et al. Complications of Marchetti locked nailing for humeral shaft fractures. *Int Orthop.* 1999;23(6):320–324.

277. Simonis RB, Good C, Cowell TK. The treatment of non-union by pulsed electromagnetic fields combined with a Denham external fixator. *Injury.* 1984;15(4):255–260.

278. Singer BR, McLauchlan GJ, Robinson CM, et al. Epidemiology of fractures in 15,000 adults: The influence of age and gender. *J Bone Joint Surg Br.* 1998;80(2):243–248.

279. Smith MG, Canty SJ, Khan SA. Fixion–an inflatable or deflatable nail? *Injury.* 2004; 35(3):329–331.

280. Sodergard J, Sandelin J, Bostman O. Postoperative complications of distal humeral fractures. 27/96 adults followed up for 6 (2–10) years. *Acta Orthop Scand.* 1992;63(1): 85–89.

281. Solomon HB, Zadnik M, Eglseder WA. A review of outcomes in 18 patients with floating elbow. *J Orthop Trauma.* 2003;17(8):563–570.

282. Spagnolo R, Pace F, Bonalumi M. Minimally invasive plating osteosynthesis technique applied to humeral shaft fractures: The lateral approach. *Eur J Orthop Surg Traumatol.* 2010;20:205–210.

283. Spencer SJ, Holt G, Clarke JV, et al. Locked intramedullary nailing of symptomatic metastases in the humerus. *J Bone Joint Surg Br.* 2010;92(1):142–145.

284. Spitzer AB, Davidovitch RI, Egol KA. Use of a "hybrid" locking plate for complex metaphyseal fractures and nonunions about the humerus. *Injury.* 2009;40(3):240–244.

285. Stannard JP, Harris HW, McGwin G Jr, et al. Intramedullary nailing of humeral shaft fractures with a locking flexible nail. *J Bone Joint Surg Am.* 2003;85-A(11):2103–2110.

286. Steinmann SP, Cheung EV. Treatment of periprosthetic humerus fractures associated with shoulder arthroplasty. *J Am Acad Orthop Surg.* 2008;16(4):199–207.

287. Stern PJ, Mattingly DA, Pomeroy DL, et al. Intramedullary fixation of humeral shaft fractures. *J Bone Joint Surg Am.* 1984;66(5):639–646.

288. Sullivan R. The identity and work of the ancient Egyptian surgeon. *J R Soc Med.* 1996; 89(8):467–473.

289. Suzuki T, Hak DJ, Stahel PF, et al. Safety and efficacy of conversion from external fixation to plate fixation in humeral shaft fractures. *J Orthop Trauma.* 2010;24(7):414–419.

290. Svend-Hansen H, Skettrup M, Rathcke MW. Complications using the Seidel intramedullary humeral nail: Outcome in 31 patients. *Acta Orthop Belg.* 1998;64(3):291–295.

291. Swiontkowski MF, Agel J, McAndrew MP, et al. Outcome validation of the AO/OTA fracture classification system. *J Orthop Trauma.* 2000;14(8):534–541.

292. Tarantino U, Cerocchi I, Scialdoni A, et al. Bone healing and osteoporosis. *Aging Clin Exp Res.* 2011;23(suppl 2):62–64.

293. Taylor JK. AO fracture classification logos, as evocative signposts. *J Orthop Trauma.* 1996;10(2):146.

294. Tennant S, Thomas M, Murphy JP, et al. The Marchetti-Vincenzi humeral nail–a useful device in fresh fractures. *Injury.* 2002;33(6):507–510.

295. Thomsen NO, Mikkelsen JB, Svendsen RN, et al. Interlocking nailing of humeral shaft fractures. *J Orthop Sci.* 1998;3(4):199–203.

296. Tingstad EM, Wolinsky PR, Shyr Y, et al. Effect of immediate weightbearing on plated fractures of the humeral shaft. *J Trauma.* 2000;49(2):278–280.

297. Toivanen JA, Nieminen J, Laine HJ, et al. Functional treatment of closed humeral shaft fractures. *Int Orthop.* 2005;29(1):10–13.

298. Tomic S, Bumbasirevic M, Lesic A, et al. Ilizarov frame fixation without bone graft for atrophic humeral shaft nonunion: 28 patients with a minimum 2-year follow-up. *J Orthop Trauma.* 2007;21(8):549–556.

299. Toros T, Karabay N, Ozaksar K, et al. Evaluation of peripheral nerves of the upper limb with ultrasonography: A comparison of ultrasonographic examination and the intraoperative findings. *J Bone Joint Surg Br.* 2009;91(6):762–765.

300. Tsai CH, Fong YC, Chen YH, et al. The epidemiology of traumatic humeral shaft fractures in Taiwan. *Int Orthop.* 2009;33(2):463–467.

301. Tscherne H, Gotzen L. *Fractures with Soft Tissue Injuries.* Berlin, Germany: Springer-Verlag; 1984.

302. Tubbs RS, Tyler-Kabara EC, Aikens AC, et al. Surgical anatomy of the axillary nerve within the quadrangular space. *J Neurosurg.* 2005;102(5):912–914.

303. Tytherleigh-Strong G, Walls N, McQueen MM. The epidemiology of humeral shaft fractures. *J Bone Joint Surg Br.* 1998;80(2):249–253.

304. Uhl RL, Larosa JM, Sibeni T, et al. Posterior approaches to the humerus: When should you worry about the radial nerve? *J Orthop Trauma.* 1996;10(5):338–340.

305. Valchanou VD, Michailov P. High energy shock waves in the treatment of delayed and nonunion of fractures. *Int Orthop.* 1991;15(3):181–184.

306. Van Houwelingen AP, McKee MD. Treatment of osteopenic humeral shaft nonunion with compression plating, humeral cortical allograft struts, and bone grafting. *J Orthop Trauma.* 2005;19(1):36–42.

307. Vander Griend R, Tomasin J, Ward EF. Open reduction and internal fixation of humeral shaft fractures. Results with AO plating techniques. *J Bone Joint Surg Am.* 1986;68(3):430–433.

308. Varley GW. The Seidel locking humeral nail: The Nottingham experience. *Injury.* 1995; 26(3):155–157.

309. Venouziou AI, Dailiana ZH, Varitimidis SE, et al. Radial nerve palsy associated with humeral shaft fracture. Is the energy of trauma a prognostic factor? *Injury.* 2011;42(11): 1289–1293.

310. Verbruggen JP, Stapert JW. Failure of reamed nailing in humeral non-union: An analysis of 26 patients. *Injury.* 2005;36(3):430–438.

311. Vidyadhara S, Vamsi K, Rao SK, et al. Use of intramedullary fibular strut graft: A novel adjunct to plating in the treatment of osteoporotic humeral shaft nonunion. *Int Orthop.* 2009;33(4):1009–1014.

312. Walker M, Palumbo B, Badman B, et al. Humeral shaft fractures: A review. *J Shoulder Elbow Surg.* 2011;20(5):833–844.

313. Wallace A. Problems with Halder nail fixation of humeral fractures. *Injury.* 2003; 34(3):245; author reply 246.

314. Wallny T, Sagebiel C, Westerman K, et al. Comparative results of bracing and interlocking nailing in the treatment of humeral shaft fractures. *Int Orthop.* 1997;21(6): 374–379.

315. Wallny T, Westermann K, Sagebiel C, et al. Functional treatment of humeral shaft fractures: indications and results. *J Orthop Trauma.* 1997;11(4):283–287.

316. Wang JP, Shen WJ, Chen WM, et al. Iatrogenic radial nerve palsy after operative management of humeral shaft fractures. *J Trauma.* 2009;66(3):800–803.

317. Whelan DB, Bhandari M, McKee MD, et al. Interobserver and intraobserver variation in the assessment of the healing of tibial fractures after intramedullary fixation. *J Bone Joint Surg Br.* 2002;84(1):15–18.

318. Wong MW, Chow DH, Li CK. Rotational stability of Seidel nail distal locking mechanism. *Injury.* 2005;36(10):1201–1205.

319. Worland RL, Kim DY, Arredondo J. Periprosthetic humeral fractures: Management and classification. *J Shoulder Elbow Surg.* 1999;8(6):590–594.

320. Wright TW, Cofield RH. Humeral fractures after shoulder arthroplasty. *J Bone Joint Surg Am.* 1995;77(9):1340–1346.

321. Wright TW, Miller GJ, Vander Griend RA, et al. Reconstruction of the humerus with an intramedullary fibular graft. A clinical and biomechanical study. *J Bone Joint Surg Br.* 1993;75(5):804–807.

322. Yokoyama K, Itoman M, Kobayashi A, et al. Functional outcomes of "floating elbow" injuries in adult patients. *J Orthop Trauma.* 1998;12(4):284–290.

323. Zagorski JB, Latta LL, Zych GA, et al. Diaphyseal fractures of the humerus. Treatment with prefabricated braces. *J Bone Joint Surg Am.* 1988;70(4):607–610.

324. Zhiquan A, Bingfang Z, Yeming W, et al. Minimally invasive plating osteosynthesis (MIPO) of middle and distal third humeral shaft fractures. *J Orthop Trauma.* 2007; 21(9):628–633.

325. Zimmerman MC, Waite AM, Deehan M, et al. A biomechanical analysis of four humeral fracture fixation systems. *J Orthop Trauma.* 1994;8(3):233–239.

326. Zlotolow DA, Catalano LW 3rd, Barron OA, et al. Surgical exposures of the humerus. *J Am Acad Orthop Surg.* 2006;14(13):754–765.

327. Zuckerman JD, Koval KJ. Fractures of the shaft of the humerus. In: Rockwood A, Green DP, Bucholz RW, Heckman JD, eds. *Rockwood and Green's Fractures in Adults.* Philadelphia, PA: Lippincott-Raven; 1996:1025–1053.

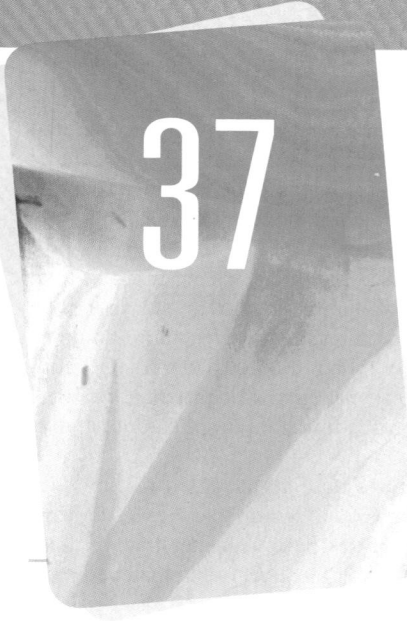

37

PROXIMAL HUMERAL FRACTURES

Philipp N. Streubel, Joaquin Sanchez-Sotelo, and Scott P. Steinmann

INTRODUCTION

Proximal humeral fractures, defined as fractures occurring at or proximal to the surgical neck of the humerus, lead to 185,000 emergency department visits in the United States alone[202] and affect 2.4% of women over the age of 75 years.[233] It is the commonest fracture affecting the shoulder girdle in adults[292] and its incidence is rising. Studies of approximately 50 years ago showed that proximal humeral fractures comprised 4% of all fractures and approximately one-half of all humerus fractures.[182,343] The current fracture epidemiology described in Chapter 3 shows that nowadays proximal humeral fractures account for almost 7% of all fractures and make up 80% of all humeral fractures. In patients above the age of 65 years proximal humeral fractures are the second most frequent upper extremity fracture, and the third most common nonvertebral osteoporotic fracture after proximal femur and distal radius fractures, accounting for >10% of fractures in this patient population.[18,19,58,233,256] This is illustrated in Tables 3-8 and 3-11.

In the adult population, proximal humeral fractures have a unimodal distribution.[77,202] The incidence of proximal humeral fractures fluctuates with age. Extrapolation of the data shown in Chapter 3 shows that the incidence of proximal humeral fractures in males and females aged 20 to 29 years is 7.5 and 9.1/10^5/year, respectively and that the incidences in the 80 to 89 years population are 390 and 512/10^5/year. Comparison with data from the same area 15 years earlier[77] shows similar incidences in the 20- to 29-year patients but a 197% increase in the incidence of proximal humeral fractures in 80- to 89-year females. Of interest is the fact that there has been a 358% increase in the incidence of proximal humeral fractures in 80- to 89-year males suggesting that improved male health has resulted in more osteoporotic fractures. Females are more commonly affected than males and it has been demonstrated that 15% to 30% of fractures occur in males[24] but it seems likely that this proportion will rise.

The incidence has been shown to increase exponentially at a rate of over 40% every 5 years at age 40 in females and age 60 in males.[202,222,343] The calculated annual incidence has been stated to be 36/10⁵/year for males and 78/10⁵/year for females[202,247] but the 2010/11 data presented in Chapter 3 confirms that the incidence is increasing and was recorded as being 61/10⁵/year in males and 120/10⁵/year in females. It seems likely that the average age of patients who present with proximal humeral fractures is also rising. In 2002 the average age of patients with proximal humeral fractures was 63 years[233] but Table 3-3 shows the average age to be 66 years in 2010/11. Men who present with proximal humeral fractures are on average 8 to 10 years younger than women.[301] The average age of patients with displaced two-part surgical neck fractures is 72 years, and the vast majority of patients are 50 years or older.[78]

As has already been pointed out proximal humerus fractures have become progressively more frequent over the past few decades. Among Finnish women 80 years of age or older the frequency of proximal humeral fractures increased from 88/10⁵/year fractures in 1970 to 298/10⁵/year in 2007.[193] In Finnish patients aged 60 years or older, low-energy proximal humeral fractures increased from 32/10⁵/year in 1970 to 105/10⁵/year in 2002.[308] In the United States, the number of patients presenting with proximal humeral fractures is expected to reach 275,000 by 2030.[202]

The vast majority of proximal humeral fractures are treated nonoperatively.[24,202,343] However, surgical treatment is becoming more frequent, with fracture reconstruction increasing at a higher rate than prosthetic replacement.[24] There is a high regional variation in fracture incidence, ranging from 0.57 to 4.97 per 1,000 Medicare enrollees across the United States, with an overall higher incidence in the East Coast compared to the rest of the country.[24] The rate of surgically treated fractures shows similar variability, ranging from less than 10% to 40% or more. Interestingly, in regions with lower incidence of fractures, surgical treatment is more likely.[24]

White females have the highest risk of suffering a proximal humerus fracture.[65,153,197] As with other osteoporosis-related fractures, additional risk factors for proximal humeral fractures include low bone mass and an increased risk of falls.[24] Furthermore patients with poor vision, use of hearing aid, diabetes mellitus, depression, alcohol consumption, use of anticonvulsive medication, and a maternal history of hip fracture have been identified as being at increased risk of sustaining a proximal humeral fracture.[17,65,153,197,233,289] A personal history of spinal or upper or lower extremity fracture has also been found to be more prevalent in patients with proximal humeral fractures than in controls.[301] Fractures are more frequent during winter months, possibly because of an increased risk of falls both outside and at home, where most fractures occur.[247] Hormonal replacement therapy and calcium intake have been found to be protective factors.[65,182,197]

Although most studies support good outcomes of nonoperative treatment of nondisplaced fractures, a recent prospective study has shown that marked functional impairment may occur even in nondisplaced proximal humeral fractures with over two-thirds of patients having chronic pain.[58] This is of relevance taking into account that elderly patients with

two-part proximal humeral fractures are generally considered healthy, with over 90% living at home and taking care of their own dressing and personal hygiene.[78] The impact of lost quality of life in this patient population may therefore be considerable.

Overall, patients with proximal humerus are more fit than patients suffering proximal femur fractures, but less than those with distal radius fractures.[77] However, more complex fractures are found in more frail and older patients. As a consequence, up to one-third of patients with proximal humeral fractures may require hospital admission, despite nonoperative treatment.[247]

Proximal humeral fractures pose an increased risk for subsequent distal radius and proximal femur fractures.[182] Patients with proximal humeral fractures have a greater than 5 times risk of suffering a hip fracture within 1 year than matched pairs without proximal humeral fractures.[69,301] An increased risk for hip fracture however continues over the years, with a lifetime risk of suffering a hip fracture after a proximal humeral fracture of 16%, which is identical to that after distal radius fractures and 1.5 times higher than that of nonfractured patients.[230] Patients with proximal humeral fractures carry a 2.5-fold risk of a subsequent spinal fracture, a 2.8-fold risk of a subsequent upper extremity fractures and a 2-fold risk of a subsequent lower extremity fractures.[301]

When analyzing individuals 45 years or older, patients with proximal humeral fractures have a higher mortality rate than age-matched controls. This risk has been found to be more marked in subjects at the younger extreme of this group and is likely related to increased comorbidity as a possible underlying cause for fracture.[361]

Mechanisms of Injury for Proximal Humerus Fractures

Approximately half of all proximal humeral fractures occur at home with the majority occurring as a consequence of falls on level ground.[202,222,247] In individuals 60 years or older, over 90% of proximal humeral fractures result from a fall from a standing height.[78] In younger individuals there is a higher incidence of proximal humeral fractures occurring outside the home, as a result of higher-energy trauma, such as a fall from a height, motor vehicle accidents (MVAs), sports, or assaults.[77,202,247,380] Analysis of the proximal humeral fractures presented in Chapter 3 shows that 9.4% were caused by falls from a height, MVAs, sports, or assaults. The average age of this group was 42.5 years and 71% were males.

The proximal humerus can fracture as a consequence of three main loading modes: compressive loading of the glenoid onto the humeral head, bending forces at the surgical neck, and tension forces of the rotator cuff at the greater and lesser tuberosities. When the glenoid impacts on the humeral head during a fall in individuals with normal bone, the proximal humeral epiphysis appears to be able to resist local compressive loads. The energy is then transferred further distally, where the weaker metaphyseal bone may yield, resulting in a surgical neck fracture. In individuals with osteoporotic bone, weaker epiphyseal bone may yield simultaneously with the surgical neck, thereby leading to more complex multifragmentary fractures. In isolated greater tuberosity fractures, and in the exceptionally rare isolated lesser tuberosity fracture the mechanism of fracture is usually a dislocation of the glenohumeral joint with tension failure of the fragment secondary to the pull of the rotator cuff on the tuberosities.[222] Tension forces may also play a role in multifragmentary fractures, where tuberosity fractures are caused in combination with compression of the humeral head. These tension forces play a further role in displacement because of the unopposed pull of the rotator cuff muscles on the tuberosities, once they have become unstable.

Apart from bone quality fracture configuration is influenced by the amount of kinetic energy conveyed to the shoulder, and by the position of the upper limb during injury. High-energy fractures in normal bone result in marked comminution of the surgical neck area with extension into the proximal humeral shaft with the integrity of the proximal humeral epiphysis usually being preserved. When falling onto the outstretched hand with the shoulder in flexion, abduction, and internal rotation the glenoid forces the humeral head into valgus, hinging around the inferomedial aspect of the stronger calcar bone.[99] In the event that the patient falls directly onto the shoulder the deforming force on the humeral head will create a varus deformity which, due to the natural retroversion of the humeral head will most probably cause a posterior rotational deformity of the head segment.

Associated Injuries with Proximal Humeral Fractures

The great majority of proximal humeral fractures occur as isolated injuries.[68,77] However, since they occur primarily in frail elderly patients and young patients involved in higher-energy trauma, associated injuries may occur. In one of the largest series of proximal humeral fractures, in patients between the ages of 10 and 99 years, Court-Brown et al. found that 90% of fractures were isolated injuries. Ninety-seven of 1,015 patients (9.6%) had other musculoskeletal injuries, including distal radius fractures in 3% and proximal femur fractures in 2% of cases. One-third of associated distal radius fractures were in the same arm as the proximal humerus fracture. Contralateral distal radial fractures occurred in less than 1% of cases and only 0.3% of patients were considered to have major trauma with an Injury Severity Score of 15 or more.[77] Interestingly, a subsequent study from the same institution showed that along with distal radius and proximal femur fractures, elderly patients with proximal humeral fractures were at high risk of having associated fractures, with 16% of proximal humerus fracture occurring simultaneously with another fracture.[68]

In polytrauma patients, proximal humeral fractures frequently exhibit marked comminution extending into the humeral shaft.[104,190] Furthermore, in the presence of fracture dislocations, glenoid rim and neck fractures and avulsion fractures of the coracoid may occur.[190] Other injuries such as subarachnoid hemorrhage, craniofacial fractures, hemothorax, and closed liver injuries have also been described.[136]

Unlike polytrauma in the younger patient population, standing falls account for 80% of multiple fractures in elderly patients 65 years or older.[68] Sixteen percent of elderly patients with proximal humeral fractures present with an additional fracture. Seven percent of proximal humeral fractures in this patient group occur concomitantly with proximal femur fractures with a further 2% occurring with distal radius and pelvic fractures and 1% with scapula and finger fractures.[68] As in high-energy fractures, associated glenoid rim and coracoid fractures may occur in elderly patients (Fig. 37-1).

The association of arterial injuries with proximal humeral fractures is rare and is reported in the literature as isolated case reports. Vascular injury mainly affects the axillary artery and can occur either as a traumatic dissection due to kinking because of direct trauma by the medially displaced shaft (Fig. 37-2) or as an avulsion of one of the circumflex arteries.[148] Fracture displacement, age older than 50 years and brachial plexus injury are risk factors for vascular injury.[262] Early recognition is important as upper extremity amputation may be required in up to 21% of cases.[262]

Electromyographic evidence of neurologic injury can be present in as many as 67% of proximal humeral fractures. The most frequently affected nerves are the axillary nerve (58%) and suprascapular nerve (48%), with combined neurologic lesions being frequent.[404] Although neurologic injuries most frequently occur in displaced proximal humeral fractures caused by high-energy trauma, up to one-third can occur as a consequence of a standing fall.[165,404] As with vascular injuries, the axillary nerve can be injured by medial displacement of the humeral shaft segment. Combined nerve injuries, as a consequence of traction injuries of the brachial plexus, can also occur ranging from neurapraxia to complete nerve transections. Approximately 50% of neurologic injuries occur in the presence of an arterial injury.[165]

The association of rotator cuff tears with proximal humeral fractures has been found to increase with age.[421] However it should be remembered that because of age-related rotator cuff degeneration, a high proportion of tears may be present before injury and are diagnosed incidentally during fracture assessment. Full-thickness tears have been found in only 6% of proximal humerus patients under 60 years of age compared to 30% in those patients above 60 years of age.[236] Some studies have shown rotator cuff tears in as many as 50% of proximal humeral fractures, reaching 61% in patients 60 years or older.[109,128,233,282,351,419] It remains unclear whether rotator cuff integrity may play a role in fracture displacement and whether it affects outcome.[282,419] Tears believed to have been caused as a consequence of acute trauma most frequently occur along the rotator cuff interval between the tendons of supraspinatus and subscapularis. Partial- and full-thickness substance tears have also been described.[116,128]

Gunshot injuries to the shoulder may result in proximal humeral fractures. Injuries may range from isolated simple surgical neck fractures to severely comminuted fractures with neurovascular injury and soft tissue loss (Fig. 37-3).

(text continues on page 1346)

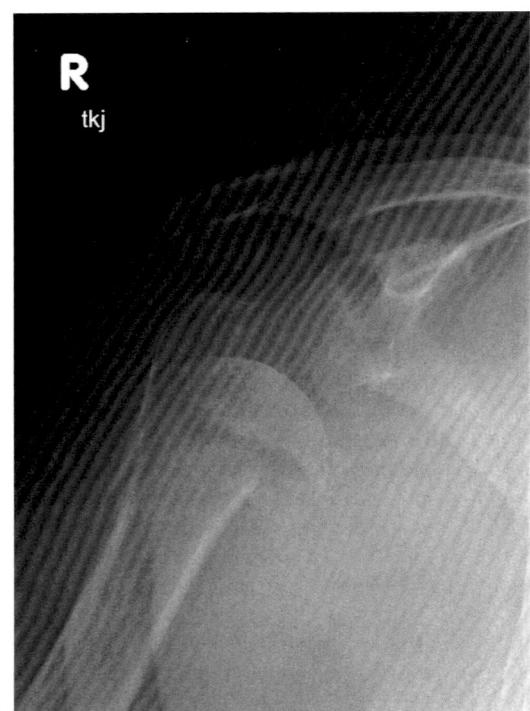

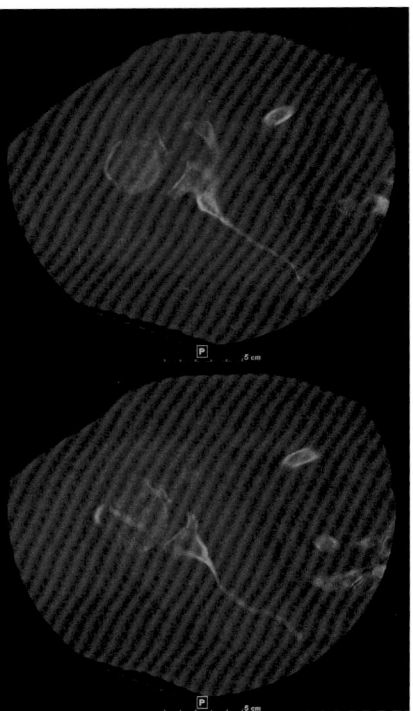

FIGURE 37-1 Eighty-seven-year old patient who sustained a complex proximal humerus fracture. **A:** AP view of the right shoulder showing four-part valgus-impacted proximal humerus fracture. **B:** Axial CT images. An avulsion fracture of the coracoid and anterior rim fracture of the glenoid can be seen.

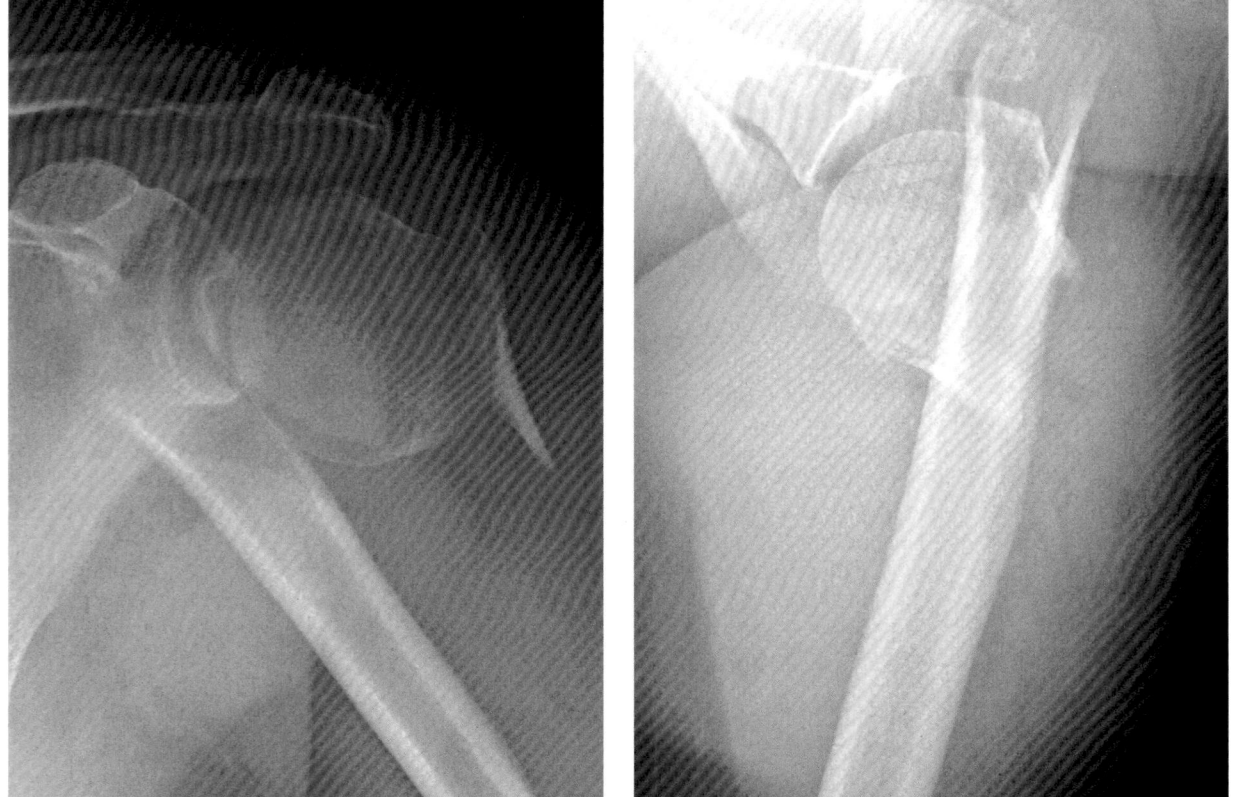

FIGURE 37-2 Sixty-eight-year old female with a proximal humerus fracture and absent distal pulses. **A:** AP view of the left shoulder showing marked medial displacement of the humeral shaft. **B:** Axillary view of the left shoulder shows anterior displacement of the humeral shaft segment.

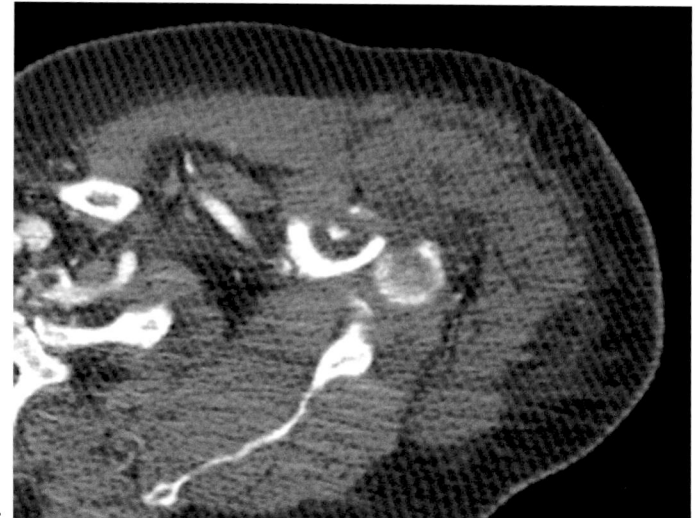

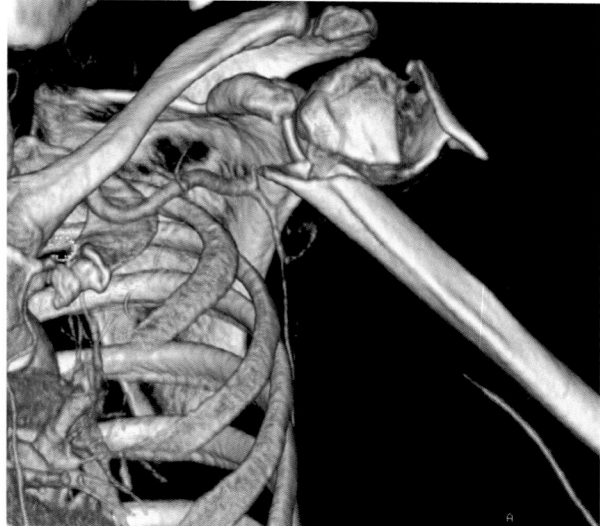

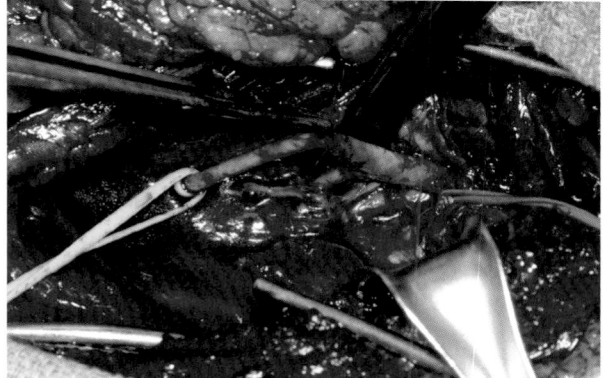

FIGURE 37-2 (*continued*) **C:** CT angiography. Axial cuts show interruption of flow of the axillary artery at the level of the proximal medial spike of the displaced humeral shaft. **D:** 3D reconstruction showing interrupted flow distal to occlusion of the axillary artery by the humeral shaft spike. **E:** Intraoperative image showing axillary artery contusion and thrombosis.

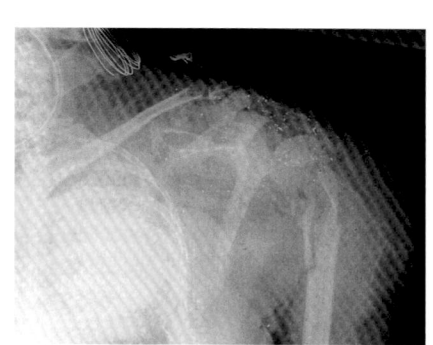

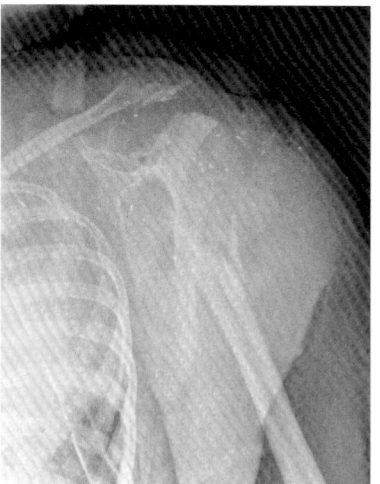

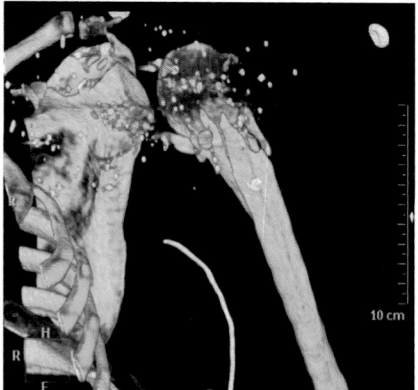

FIGURE 37-3 Thirty-eight-year old female who suffered a severe injury to her left shoulder during a failed suicide attempt with a shotgun. **A and B:** AP and lateral views of the left shoulder show marked comminution of the proximal shoulder and fracture of the acromion and glenoid with presence of multiple pellets in the soft tissues. **C:** 3D reconstruction of the left shoulder confirming the injuries seen on plain radiographs.

Signs and Symptoms of Proximal Humeral Fractures

Alert patients with isolated proximal humeral fractures complain of localized shoulder pain and limitation of movement in the affected extremity. In the polytraumatized patient, proximal humeral fractures may go unnoticed clinically as attention is directed toward more life-threatening injuries. Furthermore due to the bulk of the deltoid, fracture deformity is not readily identifiable as in other anatomic locations. Proximal humeral fractures in polytraumatized patients are usually detected during the secondary survey following ATLS guidelines.

Clinical examination usually shows soft tissue swelling and in many cases a large ecchymosis is readily apparent, especially in elderly patients. Loss of the normal convex contour of the shoulder can be seen in more severe fracture patterns and in fracture dislocations. However in the acute phase local soft tissue signs may be absent, particularly in overweight patients. Open fractures are rare but should be ruled out by confirming skin integrity. Open wounds are most commonly seen on the medial aspect of the upper arm adjacent to the axilla because pectoralis major pulls the proximal humerus anteromedially.

Neurovascular injury is unusual but has to be excluded by careful clinical examination. Axillary nerve sensation should be examined as this is the most frequently affected nerve. Hypoesthesia over the lateral aspect of the proximal arm suggests an axillary nerve injury. Theoretically motor function of the axillary nerve can be assessed by palpating the deltoid as the patient attempts to actively extend, abduct, and flex the shoulder but pain often precludes this.

The biceps, brachioradialis, and triceps reflexes should be examined in every patient.

The radial pulse and capillary refill of the fingers should be assessed and compared to the contralateral side. Because of the rich collateral circulation of the upper extremity, only minor clinical findings may occur after vascular injury. A weak or asymmetric pulse should therefore result in further investigation even in minimally displaced fractures.

Imaging and Other Diagnostic Studies for Proximal Humerus Fractures
Radiographs

The initial assessment of proximal humeral fractures should include a standard shoulder trauma radiograph series consisting of three views: An anteroposterior (AP) view of the shoulder perpendicular to the plane of the scapula (the Grashey view), a Neer (scapula Y) view, and an axillary view (Figs. 37-4 and 37-5).

The Grashey AP view of the shoulder is taken in neutral arm rotation with the torso rotated 30 to 45 degrees bringing the side opposite to the injured shoulder forward (Fig. 37-6). The x-ray beam is thereby aimed perpendicular to the plane of the scapula, imaging the glenoid in profile and avoiding overlap between the glenoid and the humeral head. The Neer view is taken with the patient facing toward the cassette and the x-ray source located posteriorly. With the affected shoulder located against the cassette the patient's torso is rotated 60 degrees bringing the side opposite to the injured shoulder toward the source. The scapula is thereby imaged perpendicular to the Grashey view (Fig. 37-7).

The axillary view is taken with the arm in neutral rotation and abducted as much as possible, with the patient supine and the x-ray beam projected from the axilla onto the cassette which is located on top of the shoulder (Fig. 37-8). Ideally the glenoid and coracoid process should be visible. Frequently, pain

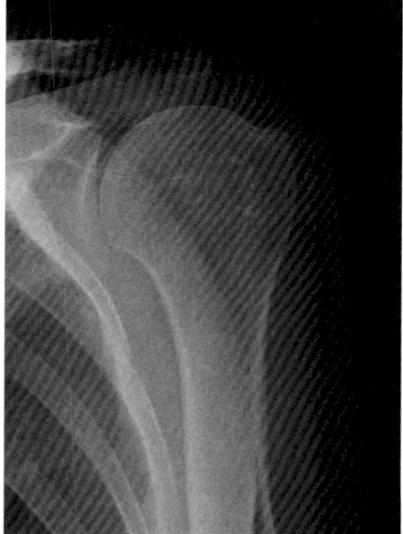 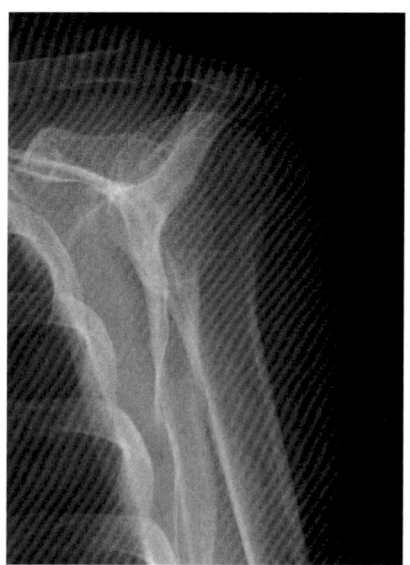 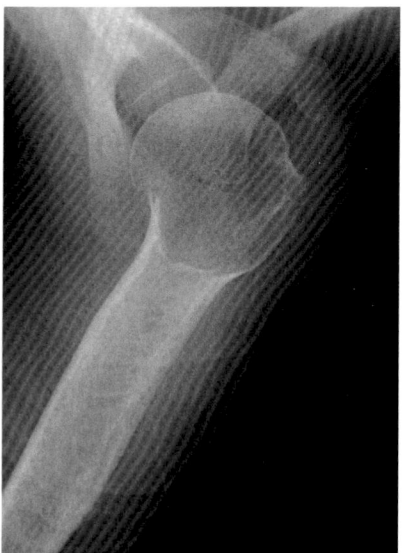

A, B   **C**

FIGURE 37-4 Radiographic trauma series. **A:** AP Grashey view of the left shoulder. Note the tangential view of the glenoid articular surface. **B:** Neer lateral (Y) view of the left shoulder. **C:** Axillary view. Note how the humeral head is centered on the glenoid in the transverse plane.

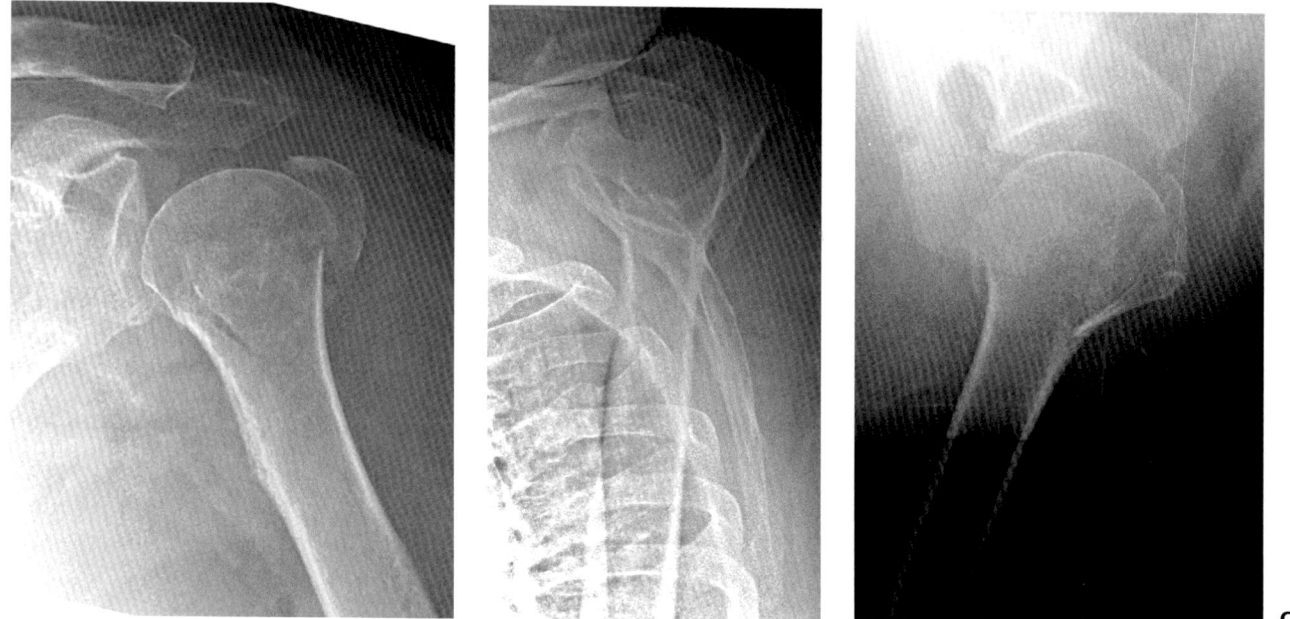

A, B

C

FIGURE 37-5 Valgus-impacted proximal humerus fracture. **A:** AP Grashey view. **B:** Neer lateral (Y) view. **C:** Axillary view.

does not allow sufficient abduction to obtain a useful axillary view. A modified Velpeau axillary view is then performed. This view is obtained with the x-ray beam being projected down perpendicularly onto a cassette. The patient is asked to lean back, to place the shoulder between the x-ray source and the cassette. This can be done with the upper extremity in a sling (Fig. 37-9). The combination of these views offers a detailed assessment of the fracture. As the Grashey and Neer views offer a perpendicular view of the fracture it is therefore important to maintain the arm in the same rotation during both views. By

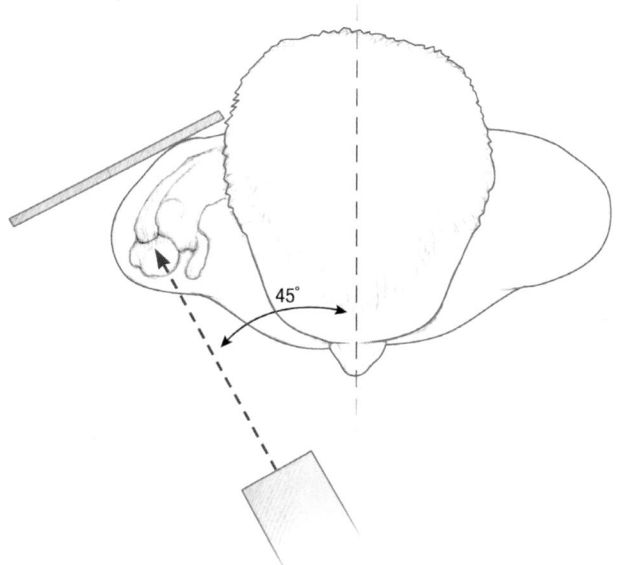

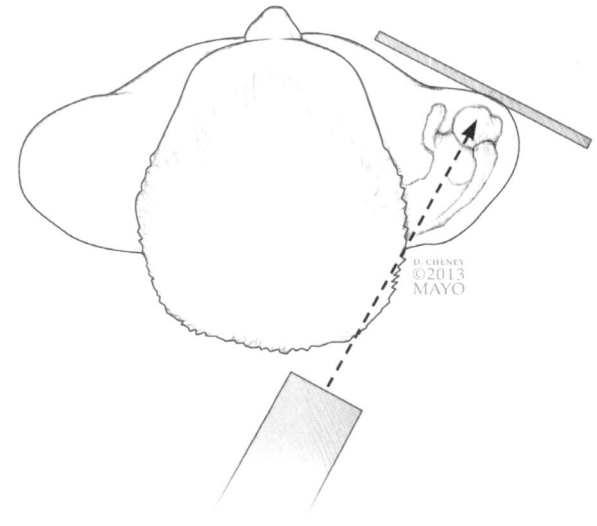

FIGURE 37-6 AP Grashey view of the shoulder. The patient's torso is rotated 30–45 degrees bringing the side opposite to the injured shoulder forward. The x-ray beam is thereby aimed perpendicular to the plane of the scapula, imaging the glenoid in profile and avoiding overlap between the glenoid and the humeral head.

FIGURE 37-7 Neer view (lateral Y) of the shoulder. With the affected shoulder located against the cassette the patient's torso is rotated 60 degrees bringing the side opposite to the injured shoulder toward the source. This gives a view that is perpendicular to Grashey view.

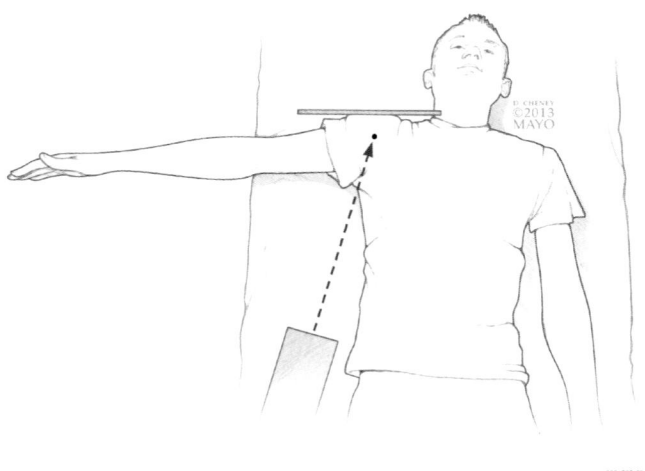

FIGURE 37-8 Axillary view of the shoulder. The arm is abducted as much as possible, with the patient supine and the x-ray beam projected from the axilla onto the cassette located on top of the shoulder.

taking Grashey and Neer views with the arm hanging gravity will provide traction which facilitates the understanding of fracture morphology. A formal traction view taken while the distal arm is actively pulled may be helpful if there is fracture comminution, especially at the metadiaphyseal junction. The axillary

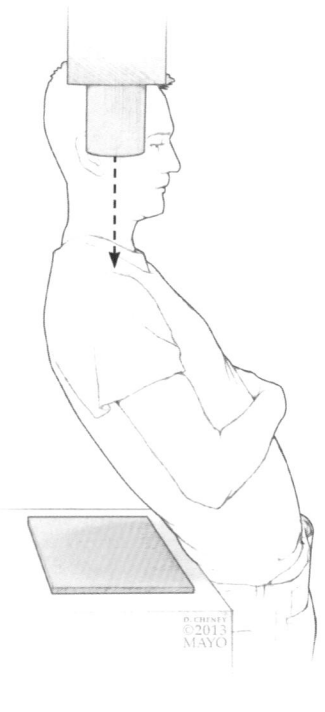

FIGURE 37-9 Velpeau axillary view of the shoulder. The x-ray beam is projected down perpendicularly onto a cassette. The patient is asked to lean back, to place the shoulder between the x-ray source and the cassette. This can be done with the upper extremity in a sling.

view is important to assess the relationship of the humeral head and glenoid to look for glenohumeral dislocation.

Computed Tomography

Computed tomography (CT) of proximal humeral fractures is helpful in providing further understanding of fracture configuration.[16] It also allows a more detailed understanding of the degree of osteopenia, the presence and location of bone impaction, and the extent of fracture comminution. Modern spiral multidetector CT scanners obtain axial images in 0.6-mm increments of 1-mm thick slices. Coronal and sagittal reformatted images are usually performed at 2-mm increments with 2-mm thick slices and therefore have a lower resolution than axial images. As with Grashey and Neer radiographs, coronal and sagittal CT reconstructions are performed perpendicular and parallel to the glenoid, respectively. Axial images can confirm displacement of the lesser and greater tuberosity fragments in the transverse plane, while confirming the spatial relationship between the humeral head and the glenoid (Fig. 37-10A).

Coronal reconstruction images give more detail about the alignment of the humeral head and they allow assessment of comminution at the level of the humeral calcar, the integrity of the inferomedial hinge, and extent of metaphyseal fracture extension (Fig. 37-10B). Sagittal reconstructions help in determining whether there is a flexion or extension deformity of the proximal humerus with regard to the shaft. Furthermore, in this plane, using a soft tissue window, fatty atrophy of the rotator cuff muscles may be analyzed, which may be of value in patients with questionable preinjury rotator cuff pathology (Fig. 37-10C).

Three-dimensional (3D) reconstruction images can be helpful in analyzing fracture configuration. Axial images and sagittal and coronal reconstructions may intersect the fracture fragments in an oblique fashion depending on the amount of arm rotation and the orientation of the fracture thereby limiting interpretation of the images. 3D reconstructions improve the spatial understanding of fracture morphology. Ideally 3D reconstructions should be performed with and without scapular subtraction. In the absence of the scapula, the proximal humerus can be analyzed from every angle. Having the scapula present however helps in establishing intraoperative reference points and deforming forces. One has to keep in mind that 3D reconstructions offer a surface view of the fracture that on its own does not allow assessment of impaction and bony deficiencies occurring within the fractured proximal humerus (Fig. 37-11). Furthermore, 3D reconstruction images are obtained by averaging images between the slices. The quality of 3D reconstruction is therefore dependent on the slice thickness of the axial CT scan images.

Magnetic Resonance Imaging

Magnetic resonance imaging (MRI) plays only a marginal role in the diagnosis of proximal humeral fractures. MRI may be helpful in confirming a nondisplaced fracture in a patient with shoulder trauma, normal radiographic findings, and clinical symptoms. Increased signal is usually seen in the T2 sequence

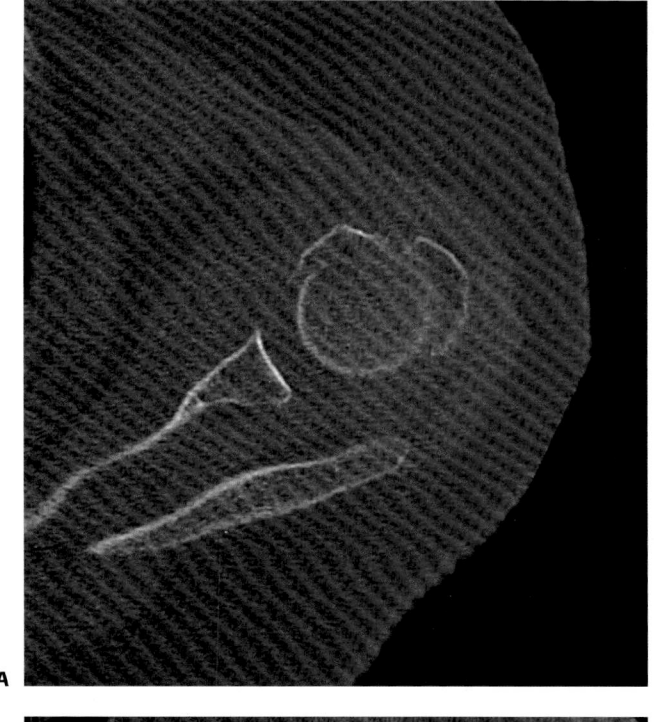

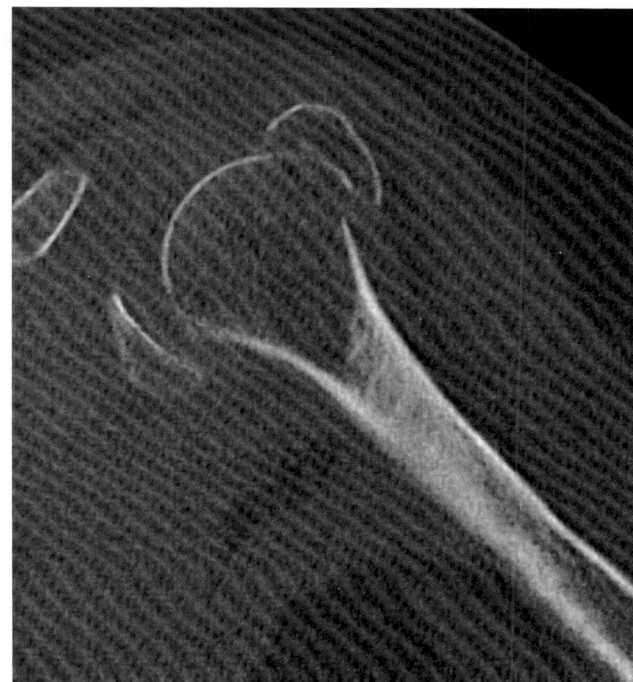

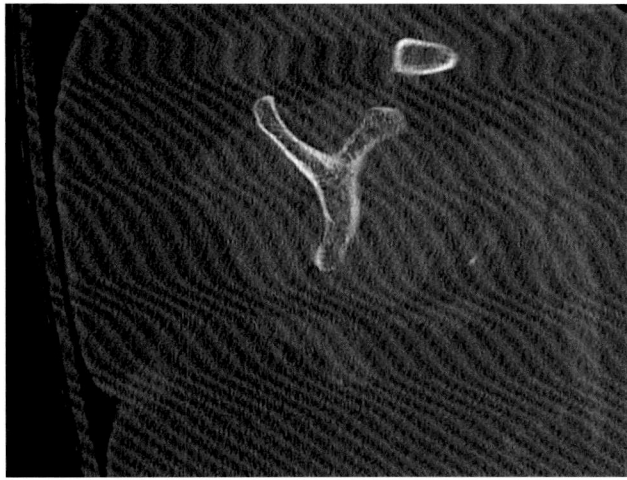

FIGURE 37-10 CT scan. **A:** Axial cuts through the proximal humerus. The lesser and greater tuberosities can be seen displaced toward the periphery. The humeral head is centered on the glenoid. **B:** Oblique coronal CT reconstruction. Note valgus impaction of the humeral head with disruption of the greater tuberosity. The medial hinge between the humeral head and the proximal metaphysis is intact. **C:** Oblique sagittal CT reconstruction. Cut through the junction of the scapular body, scapular spine, and coronoid. Note the absence of atrophy of the rotator cuff muscles.

and may be located through any of the common fracture sites. Furthermore, in fracture dislocations MRI will allow assessment of the glenoid labrum and rotator cuff and identify nondisplaced occult glenoid rim fractures. Studies have also suggested that MRI can be useful in assessing the integrity of the medial periosteal hinge to indicate whether there is vascularity of the humeral head in multifragmentary fractures.[405] Further studies have also analyzed the use of Gadolinium-enhanced MRI for the direct assessment of humeral head perfusion.[43,173] MRI can also be useful in determining whether a proximal humeral fracture may be pathologic.

Other Imaging Techniques

Vascular imaging is required when there is a suspicion of a vascular injury. Several imaging methods are available. Although bi-planar angiography used to be considered the gold standard for the assessment of vascular injuries, CT angiography has become the diagnostic modality of choice as it allows rapid evaluation of the vascular system, while simultaneously allowing assessment of the bone and soft tissues[265] (Fig. 37-2 C and D).

Ultrasound has been shown to be a useful modality for the diagnosis of occult proximal humeral fractures.[346] It may also have a role in the diagnosis of rotator cuff tears in nondisplaced fractures. Ultrasound is however dependent on the skill of the operator. In addition it may not be possible to achieve maximal internal rotation because of pain, this being required to perform rotator cuff ultrasound.[395] Vascular Doppler ultrasound can be useful in the early assessment of a suspected vascular injury.

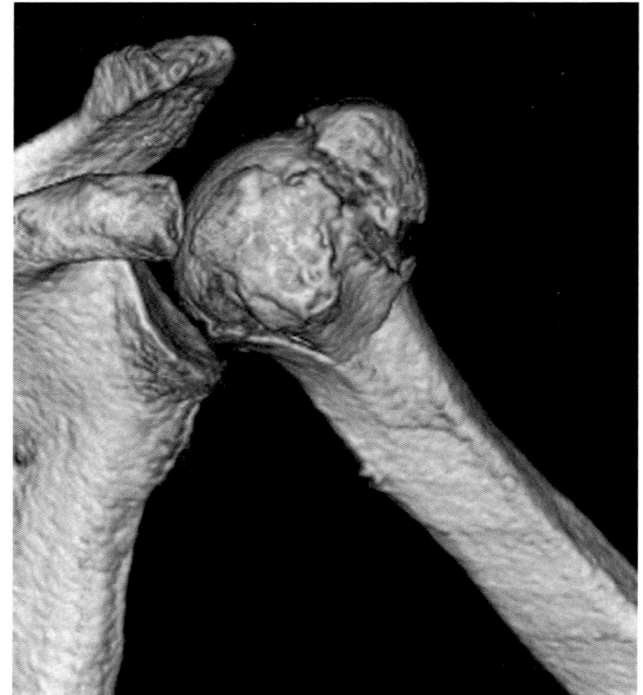

A

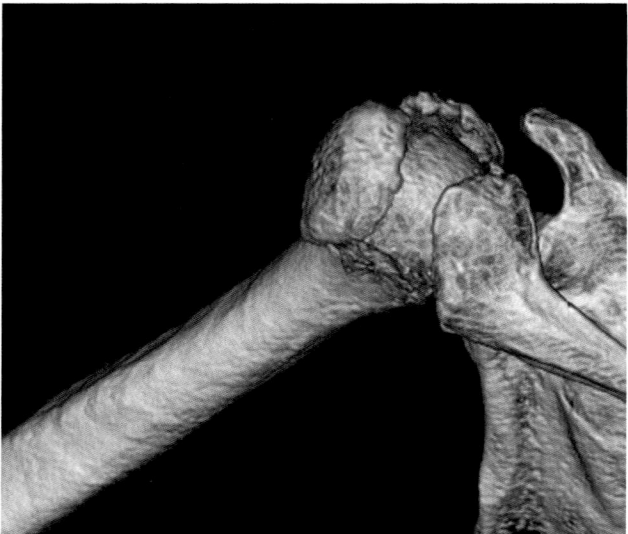

B

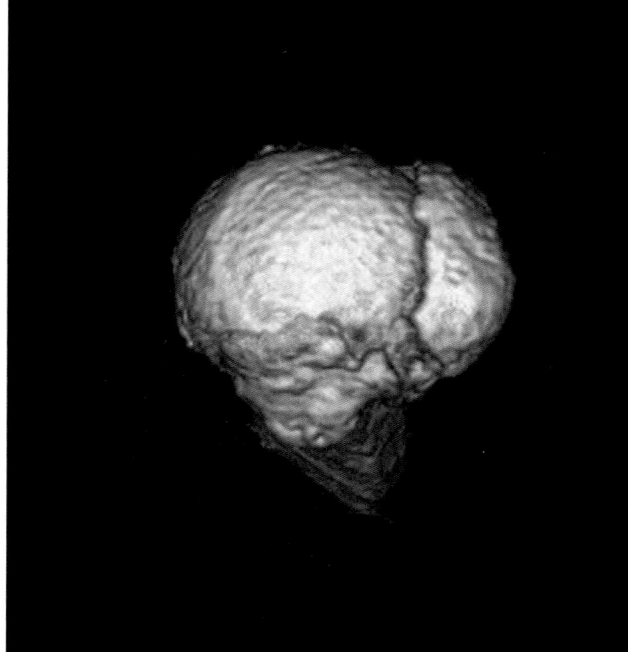

C

FIGURE 37-11 CT three-dimensional surface rendering. **A:** Anterior view of the fracture seen in Figures 37-5 and 37-10. Valgus impaction of the humeral head can be seen with peripheral displacement of the tuberosities. Note the typical location of the cleavage line between the greater and lesser tuberosities just lateral to the bicipital groove. **B:** Posterosuperior view. Absence of posteromedial comminution at the proximal metaphysis is seen in this specific fracture. **C:** Superior view with subtraction of the scapula.

Bone mineral densitometry with dual energy x-ray absorptiometry (DXA) may be appropriate in elderly patients with proximal humeral fractures or in those patients with risk factors for osteoporosis. As discussed earlier, fragility proximal humeral fractures in the elderly are associated with an increased risk of subsequent osteoporotic fractures. Bone density scanning should be the first step toward enrolling osteoporotic patients in a fracture prevention program.

Proximal Humeral Fracture Classification

In 1934 Codman stated that the fracture lines of the proximal humerus reproducibly occurred between four major fragments these being the humeral head, the greater tuberosity, the lesser tuberosity, and the humeral shaft just proximal to the insertion of the pectoralis major tendon (Fig. 37-12). Codman described 16 different fracture combinations in his seminal work and his classification set the foundation for our understanding of proximal humeral fractures[71] (Fig. 37-13). Although several proximal humerus fracture classification systems have been described since Codman the two most widely used are the Neer classification and the AO/OTA classification, both of which focus mainly on displaced fractures.[99,257,284,390]

Neer Classification

In 1970, Neer introduced the concept of fracture segments instead of fragments. In doing so it was emphasized that proximal humeral fractures can reproducibly yield up to four anatomic segments with or without additional fracture lines, rather than single fragments. Displaced fractures were arbitrarily defined as those in which a segment was translated by at least 1 cm or angulated by a minimum of 45 degrees. The resulting four segment classification offers a descriptive system of proximal humeral fractures, with the main purpose of conceptualizing the pathoanatomy of proximal humeral fractures and the terminology to identify each category.[287] Fractures of less than 1 cm of displacement and less than 45 degrees of angulation are considered nondisplaced and are commonly called one-part fractures. The terminology for displaced fractures takes into account the number of displaced segments and the key segment that displaces. Specifically two-part fractures are named after the site of displacement as two-part greater tuberosity, two-part lesser tuberosity, two-part surgical neck, and two-part anatomic neck fractures. Isolated greater tuberosity fractures displace posteromedially by the unopposed pull of the supraspinatus and infraspinatus tendons. Lesser tuberosity fractures displace medially by the pull of the subscapularis tendon. Two-part surgical neck fractures frequently exhibit anteromedial displacement of the proximal humeral shaft because of the

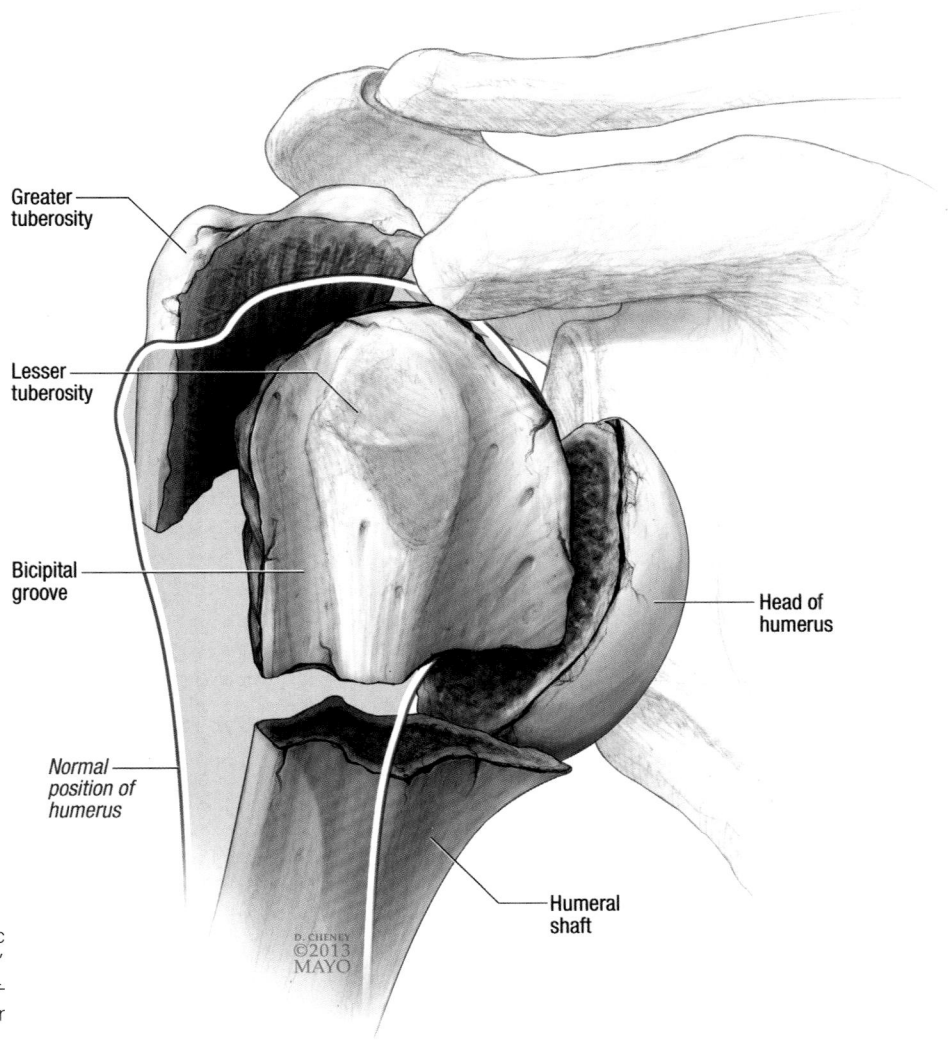

FIGURE 37-12 Depiction of the classic cleavage plane between the four "parts" of the proximal humerus (greater tuberosity, head of the humerus, lesser tuberosity, and shaft).

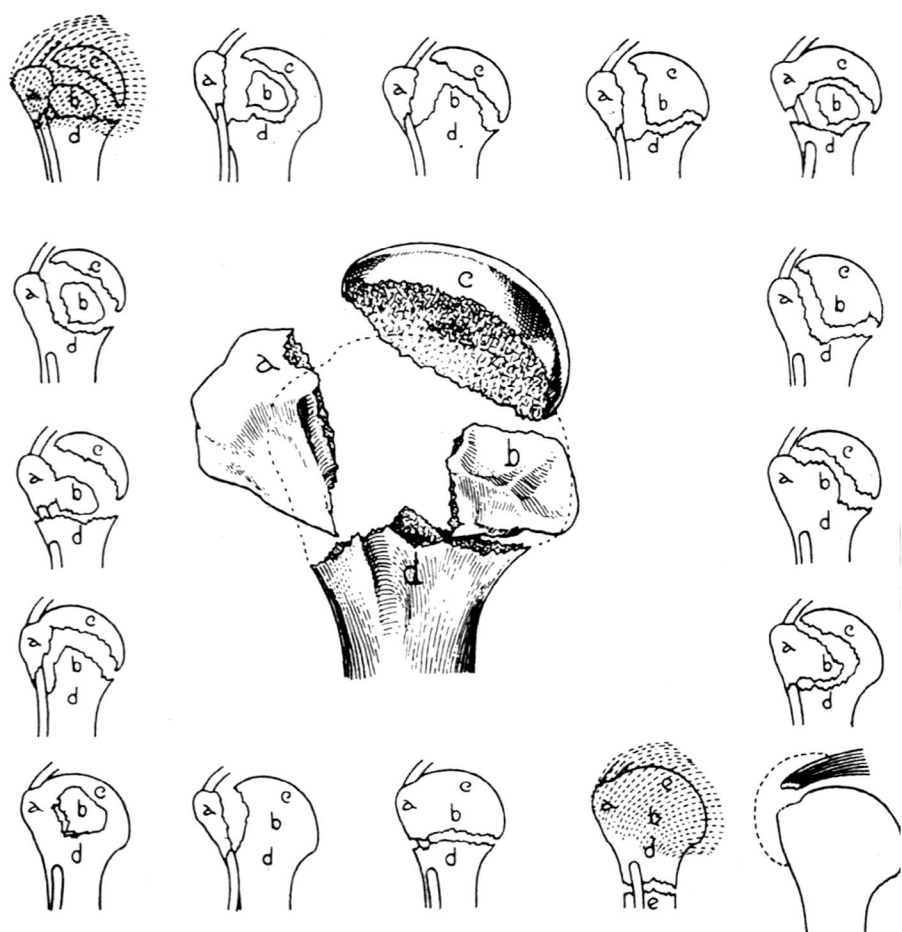

FIGURE 37-13 Codman's original depiction of proximal humerus fractures. Fractures were described as occurring between the greater tuberosity (a), humeral head (c), lesser tuberosity (b) or shaft (d). From Codman[71].

pull of the pectoralis major. Although theoretically five different types of three-part proximal humeral fractures could exist, Neer found that these fractures invariably occurred with a fracture through the surgical neck and a concomitant fracture of either the greater or the lesser tuberosity. The intact tuberosity and the pulling forces of its attached rotator cuff tendon determine three-part fracture displacement. In three-part greater tuberosity fractures the head segment is internally rotated by action of the subscapularis muscle. In three-part lesser tuberosity fractures the head segment is externally rotated and abducted by the action of the supraspinatus and infraspinatus muscles. Four-part fractures exhibit displacement of all segments. As with two-part fractures, the greater tuberosity is displaced posteromedially and the lesser tuberosity anteromedially. The humeral head exhibits valgus or varus tilt with or without displacement.

Fractures combined with a glenohumeral dislocation are classified as fracture dislocations. In true fracture dislocations, the humeral head segment is displaced, either anterior or posterior to the glenoid rim, with rupture of the joint capsule. Fractures involving the articular surface, such as head-splitting and impaction fractures, are included in the group of fracture dislocations[284,287] (Fig. 37-14).

Siebenrock and Gerber assessed the reliability of the Neer classification among shoulder surgeons. The mean kappa coefficient for inter- and intraobserver reliability was 0.40 and 0.60, respectively.[363] Similar results with poor to fair reliability have been found by other authors.[117,221,254,362] Some studies suggest that reliability increases with surgeon experience and the use of CT imaging and 3D image rendering.[29,50,117,221] However other studies have not shown that CT scanning increases reliability.[117,254,371]

AO/OTA Classification

The AO/OTA classification is based on fracture location and the presence of impaction, angulation, translation, or comminution of the fracture, as well as whether a dislocation is present (Fig. 37-15). These fractures are classified as belonging to the 11 bone segment (1 for humerus, 1 for proximal segment) and they are subclassified into types, groups, and subgroups. Finally each subgroup fracture is assigned a level of severity.[280]

Type A fractures are extra-articular unifocal fractures associated with a single fracture line, type B are extra-articular bifocal fractures associated with two fracture lines, and type C are articular fractures which involve the humeral head or anatomic neck. Type A fractures are grouped into greater tuberosity

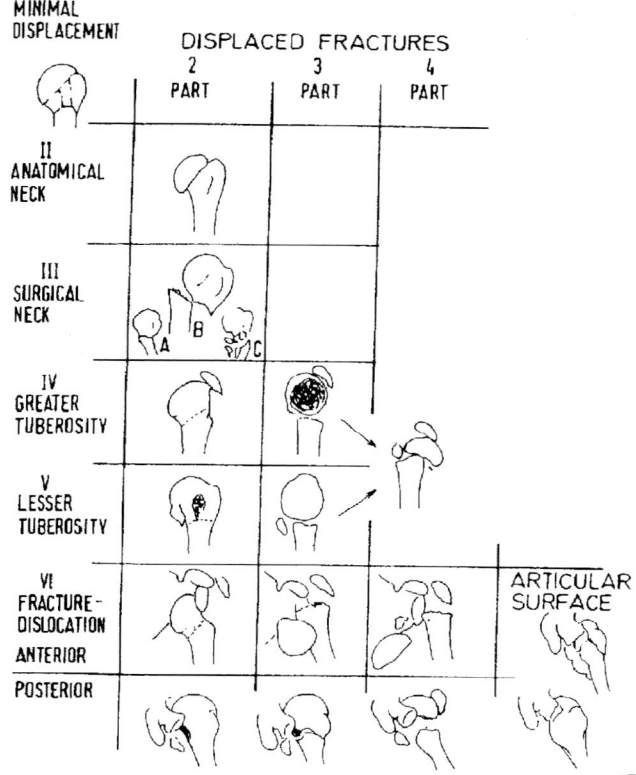

MINIMAL
DISPLACEMENT

DISPLACED FRACTURES

2 PART   3 PART   4 PART

II ANATOMICAL NECK

III SURGICAL NECK

IV GREATER TUBEROSITY

V LESSER TUBEROSITY

VI FRACTURE-DISLOCATION
ANTERIOR
POSTERIOR

ARTICULAR SURFACE

FIGURE 37-14 Neer's four-part proximal humerus fracture classification. From Neer.[287]

fractures (A1), surgical neck fractures with metaphyseal impaction (A2), and surgical neck fractures without metaphyseal impaction (A3). Type B fractures are grouped into surgical neck fractures with metaphyseal impaction and a displaced fracture of either the greater or the lesser tuberosity (B1), nonimpacted surgical neck fractures with a displaced fracture of either the greater or the lesser tuberosity (B2), and surgical neck fracture with a displaced fracture of either the greater or the lesser tuberosity and glenohumeral dislocation (B3). Type C fractures are grouped into anatomic neck fractures with slight displacement (C1), anatomic neck fractures with marked displacement (C2), and anatomic neck fractures with glenohumeral dislocation (C3). Each fracture type is further subgrouped according to displacement, valgus or varus angulation of the humeral head, comminution, and the presence and direction of glenohumeral joint dislocation. Fractures can thereby be assigned 1 of 52 different fracture types.

Although this classification system theoretically provides a comprehensive method of describing proximal humeral fractures, it is complex which reduces its clinical usefulness. Siebenrock and Gerber assessed the reliability of the AO classification among shoulder surgeons. The mean kappa coefficient for interobserver reliability was 0.53 when fractures were classified into one of three types (A to C) and 0.42 when fractures were classified into one of nine groups (A1 to C3). Mean kappa coefficient for intraobserver reliability was 0.58 for types and

0.48 for groups.[363] Similar results have been shown by other authors.[254,371] The addition of CT scanning does not appear to increase these values.[254,371]

Both, Neer and AO/OTA classifications provide a nomenclature to describe fracture morphology. Although treatment may be guided by the fracture type a classification that correlates with outcome has not as yet been devised. Specifically, decision making between operative fixation and humeral head replacement continues to be controversial. As a general rule fractures in which the vascularity of the humeral head has been severely compromised are theoretically best treated with arthroplasty, whereas those in which perfusion of the head is at least partially preserved should benefit from operative fixation. Four-part fractures and fracture dislocations are considered to have the highest risk for humeral head necrosis. An exception to this are four-part valgus-impacted fractures, in which displacement of the tuberosities is present, but the head is tilted into valgus in relation to the humeral shaft and there is no translation. Overall favorable outcomes can be expected with operative fixation of these fractures.[187,326] Court-Brown et al.[76] further showed that impacted valgus fractures (AO/OTA B1.1) could be safely managed nonoperatively.

Risk of Avascular Necrosis

The arcuate artery from the anterolateral ascending branch of the anterior circumflex humeral artery (ACHA) has historically been considered to provide the main arterial supply to the humeral head.[147] Fractures through the anatomic neck have therefore been considered to permanently disrupt perfusion of the humeral head. However more recent literature has shown that branches from the posterior circumflex humeral artery (PCHA) to the posteromedial proximal humeral metaphysis provide equally important blood perfusion to the humeral head.[46,95,227,266,267] Coudane et al.[75] showed, with arteriography, that in patients with complex proximal humeral fractures the PCHA was preserved in 85% of cases as opposed to only 20% of the ACHA.

In complex proximal humeral fractures, the posteromedial branches from the PCHA therefore become the main supply to the head. Several morphologic fracture features have been proposed to estimate the possibility of the disruption of this blood supply and hence to assess the risk of avascular necrosis (AVN). These features include varus displacement of the head,[377] the size of metaphyseal fracture extension of the humeral head and the medial displacement of the humeral shaft in relation to the humeral head.[170] Hertel et al. studied 100 intracapsular proximal humeral fractures, in which at least one component of the fracture was proximal to the anatomic neck, undergoing operative treatment. Several fracture characteristics, as possible predictors for humeral head ischemia, were studied and shown to correlate with intraoperative assessment of humeral head perfusion. Distal metaphyseal extension of the head fragment of 8 mm or less, disruption of the medial hinge between the humeral head and the shaft at the level of the calcar, and fractures through the anatomic neck were independent predictors for humeral head ischemia.[170] Although this study has been widely used to help in decision making between fixation and replacement of proximal humeral fractures, a follow-up

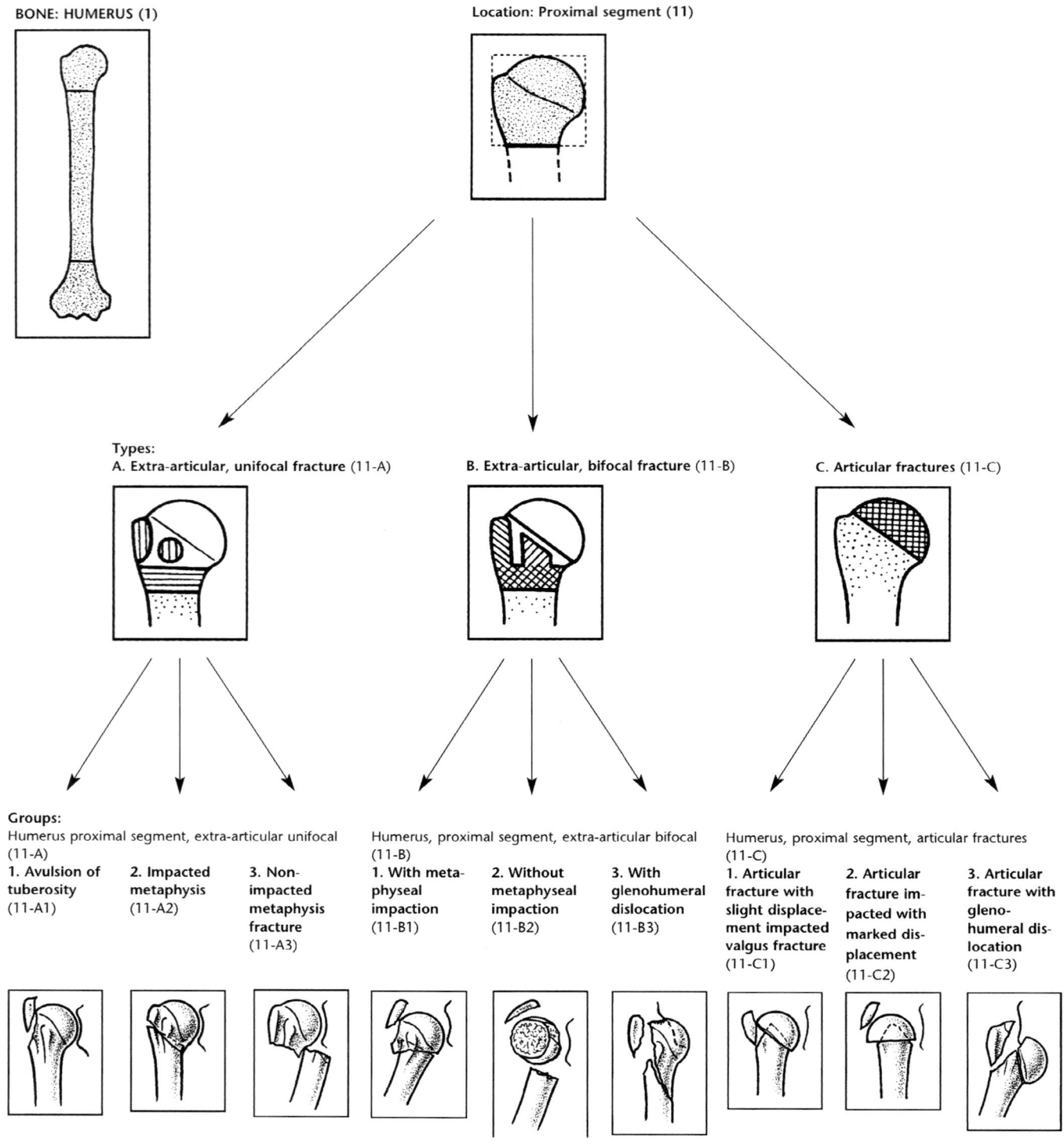

FIGURE 37-15 AO/OTA classification for proximal humerus fractures.[257,280]

study from the same authors found a poor correlation between intraoperative ischemia and development of AVN.[20] This discrepancy is further supported by a study of Croby et al., in which tetracycline was administered to 19 patients with three- and four-part fractures of the proximal humerus during 5 days preceding operative treatment. Humeral head biopsies were obtained from hemiarthroplasty surgery and analyzed using fluoroscopic microscopy. Fluorescence was observed in all specimens suggesting that vascular supply was not disrupted in any of the fracture patterns.[81]

Fracture Frequency

In 2001 Court-Brown et al.[77] published a comprehensive study on the distribution of proximal humerus fracture types. Over a 5-year period the senior author classified a total of 1,027 consecutive proximal humeral fractures based on standard radiographs. Nondisplaced or minimally displaced one-part fractures comprised half (49%) of all fractures. Two-part fractures occurred in 37% of cases. Surgical neck fractures represented three quarters of these and 28% of the whole group. Two-part greater tuberosity fractures occurred in almost 10% of cases with one-half occurring in the absence of an anterior glenohumeral dislocation and the other half in association with a dislocation. Two-part anatomic neck fractures were exceedingly rare and occurred in only 0.3% of proximal humeral fractures. Lesser tuberosity fractures only occurred in association with a posterior fracture dislocation and comprised only 0.2% of fractures. The vast majority of three-part fractures were greater tuberosity fractures comprising 9% of all fractures. Lesser tuberosity three-part fractures and three-part fracture dislocations occurred in 0.3% and 0.2%, respectively. Four-part fractures comprised only 3% of fractures, of which one-third were true fracture dislocations. Fractures involving the articular surface occurred in 0.7% of cases. Proximal humerus fractures can therefore be approximately distributed in the following manner. Half are nondisplaced or minimally displaced, one-quarter are two-part surgical neck fractures, one-tenth are three-part greater tuberosity fractures, one-tenth are two part greater tuberosity fractures or fracture dislocations, and every 30th proximal humerus fracture will be a four-part fracture. The remaining fractures can be considered to be exceedingly rare.[77]

Outcome Measures for Proximal Humerus Fractures

In the early 1900s, E. Amory Codman, who is frequently cited as the father of shoulder surgery, introduced his "end result idea." It was his belief that every treated patient should be followed long enough to determine whether treatment had been effective or not.[70] Although his idea did initially face strong resistance, outcome assessment has become the backbone of clinical research, audit, and clinical governance.[86]

Numerous measures have been used to assess outcomes after proximal humeral fracture. Historically and to the present date, results are most frequently reported on the basis of radiographic assessment[3,5,6,12,14,15,33,49,51,59,60,61,67,90,96,102,114,136,139, 140,141,160,161,162,174,177,188,190,191,201,208,209,211,220,225,232,237,241,250,258,259, 260,261,268,277,288,291,293,296,298,299,303,304,309,312,314,315,317,318,319,323,327,339, 345,353,354,358,359,377,378,383,384,388,397,400,402,406,420,423,426] and the occurrence of complications.[45,59,114,160,161,174,191,201,208,209,211,232,258,259,260,268,277,303, 309,318,319,353,358,377,378,383,384,388,397,400,420] Other frequently reported measures include pain,[42,140,162,209,211,225,237,250,303,339,348,394,402,416,426] strength,[42,162,250] range of motion,[6,12,137,162,206,220,225,237,241,250,258, 259,291,307,354,358,377,388,402,418,424,427] and patient satisfaction.[241,259,261, 315,348,359,418,427]

Radiographic Assessment

Radiographic follow-up is usually performed at set intervals these frequently being 6 weeks and 3, 6, and 12 months after injury or surgery. Follow-up radiographs should be obtained with the same projection that was used initially to allow for accurate comparison. Healing is determined by observing bridging callus, especially in fractures treated nonoperatively or with a lower rigidity construct. However when rigid fixation is used, callus formation is not readily apparent and bridging trabeculae are sought on radiographs to determine whether healing has occurred.

Fracture alignment is assessed on intraoperative or immediate postoperative images and compared on subsequent outpatient reviews. The most frequently considered measures are tuberosity displacement and head-shaft angle[53,114] Furthermore hardware position within the proximal humerus is frequently assessed to evaluate possible cutout, failure, or loosening.[3,5,6,12,14,15,33,49,51,59,60,61,67,90,96,102,114,136,139,140,141,160,161,162,174,177, 188,190,191,201,208,209,211,220,225,232,237,241,250,258,259,260,261,268,277,288,291,293,296, 298,299,303,304,309,312,314,315,317,318,319,323,327,339,345,353,354,358,359,377,378,383,384, 388,397,400,402,406,420,423,426]

AVN of the humeral head is the most frequently evaluated radiographic long-term outcome after nonreplacement reconstruction of proximal humeral fractures. Several degrees of severity of AVN are frequently reported, ranging from isolated changes in the trabecular organization to collapse of the humeral head with loss of sphericity.[20,82,114] Changes in trabecular organization have been described as increased radiodensity with cystic and sclerotic regions and coarse trabeculae.[20,82]

Serial radiographic assessment is a key component of long-term follow-up of arthroplasty for proximal humeral fractures. Implant loosening is monitored by assessing the appearance of progressive radiolucent lines between the implant and the bone. Furthermore osteolysis, with increased cavitation of bone adjacent to the implant, places the implant at increased risk of loosening and failure. In reverse total shoulder arthroplasty assessment of glenoid notching is required, as it may lead to glenoid component loosening and failure.[61,369]

Complications

The most frequently reported complications after proximal humeral fractures are nonunion, malunion, implant failure, humeral head collapse, infection, post-traumatic arthritis, hardware penetration, axillary nerve dysfunction, revision surgery, and mortality. Multiple definitions exist for each of these. Clinical, radiographic, and laboratory criteria are used to diagnose and monitor these complications.[45,59,114,161,160,174,191,201,208,209,211,318,319, 232,258,259,260,268,277,303,309,353,358,377,378,383,384,388,397,400,420]

Pain

Pain is a key component of patient satisfaction. It is frequently quantified using a visual analog scale (VAS) and reported as a value from 0 to 10.[42,140,162,209,211,225,237,250,303,339,348,394,402,416,426]

Range of Motion

Active and passive forward elevation, abduction, external rotation, and internal rotation are frequently reported.[53] The use of a standardized technique with a goniometer is important to achieve reproducible measurements.

Strength

Strength is frequently reported as a measure of the weight that can be lifted in a specific plane. The use of a dynamometer to assess strength in 90 degrees of abduction is often reported.[42,49,59,114,191,208,209,211,229,258,259,303,353,357,383,384,402] A 25-year-old male with a normal shoulder is expected to lift 25 lb in this plane. Lower values are expected for females and older people.[42,73,162,250]

Functional Outcomes Scales

Although each of the criteria that have been outlined help in determining certain aspects of the outcomes of proximal humeral fractures, they do not allow a quantitative assessment at a given point in time. Furthermore, they do not permit a summarized assessment of the overall function of the shoulder. Over the last decades several outcomes scales have been developed that summarize the results of the assessment of several aspects of shoulder function.[7,23,70,73,86,87,103,142,143,162,183,234,235,249,328,330,372,391,399,413,417] Scores can then be obtained after applying an algorithm or by grouping responses.[86] Several function scales rely mostly on criteria that are obtained by an evaluator.[86,103,284] These include range of motion, strength, specific clinical signs, radiographic alignment, and healing. Other scales focus on the subjective patient perception of shoulder function and pain. These are frequently questionnaires that are answered directly by the patient and inquire about multiple activities in which different aspects of shoulder function are involved.[23,87,183,234,249,330,417] Finally, some shoulder scores use a combined approach in which both evaluator-based and patient-based outcomes are included.[73,328]

In addition to outcomes scales that focus on the shoulder or upper extremity, modern functional assessment frequently includes evaluation of overall patient health. Although scales that assess patient function in a broader spectrum may be less accurate in measuring changes in shoulder function, they play an important role in measuring the impact of a specific shoulder condition on the overall health and quality of life of the patient.[391,399,413]

Currently Used Outcomes Scales

Over 150 clinical studies on proximal humeral fractures are referenced in the National Library of Medicine (PubMed) for the period 2009 to 2012. The shoulder scale most widely used for outcomes assessment was the Disabilities of the Arm, Shoulder, and Hand (DASH)[6,31,33,52,57,58,90,119,126,140,159,164,177,188,190,194,208,229,288,298,299,300,303,307,317,337,353,354,388,406,420] followed by the Constant-Murley Scale,[42,49,59,114,191,208,209,211,229,258,259,303,353,357,383,384,402] the American Shoulder and Elbow Surgeons (ASES) scale,[114,137,160,161,220,237,241,291,293,307,348,354,359,416,418,426] Neer criteria,[52,106,201,209,211,250,277,306] the University of California Los Angeles (UCLA) Shoulder Score,[11,14,164,232,268,293,359,416] the Oxford Shoulder Scale (OSS),[45,48,156,229,307,318,424] and the Simple Shoulder Test (SST).[42,293,359,406,416,418] Other scales used during this time period include Quick-DASH,[34] Shoulder Pain and Disability Index (SPADI),[358] Subjective shoulder value (SSV) or Single Assessment Numerical Evaluation (SANE),[21,59,137,258,259,303] and University of Pennsylvania (Penn) shoulder score.[137,327]

Although used less frequently global quality of life assessment tools were also used, mainly in prospective clinical trials. The most frequently used tool was EuroQol 5D,[57,58,90,229,298,299,300,348,416] followed by SF36[48,90,119,188,190,307,322,383] and the Short Musculoskeletal Function Assessment (SMFA).[190]

DASH and Quick-DASH. The DASH questionnaire is a patient-based, self-administered outcome instrument developed to measure symptoms and disability of the upper extremity. It evaluates six domains: daily activities, symptoms, social function, work function, sleep, and confidence. It consists of 30 questions regarding the level of difficulty in performing a set of activities. Each question is rated on a Likert scale from 1 (no difficulty) to 5 (unable to do). Lower values represent higher function.[183]

The Quick-DASH is an 11-item questionnaire derived from the DASH through item reduction using a concept-retention approach, in which the domains from the original instrument were retained while the amount of items of each domain were reduced. As for DASH, higher scores represent higher disability. Like the DASH, Quick-DASH has two optional modules, one for function at work and one for function during sports and performing arts.[23]

Constant-Murley Score. The Constant-Murley Score has a subjective patient-based component and an objective evaluator-based component. Subjective parameters include pain and shoulder function based on the ability to perform activities of daily living. For pain, scoring ranges from 0 for "severe" pain to 15 for no pain. A total of 20 points can be obtained with regard to shoulder function. The evaluator-based assessment includes active shoulder range of motion and strength. Range-of-motion is quantified by scores for elevation and external and internal rotation. A maximum of 10 points are scored when at least 151 degrees of elevation can be reached. A total of 10 points can be obtained for external rotation and internal rotation, respectively and are quantified according to rotational maneuvers that place the hand into defined positions with regard to the head, neck, and trunk. A total of 25 points can be scored for strength and are obtained by a 25-year-old male who is able to lift at least 25 lb to 90 degrees of abduction. Proportional values are assigned for the lifted weight and adjusted for age and gender. The maximum score is 100 points, with higher values representing higher function.[73]

ASES Standardized Shoulder Assessment Form. The ASES Standardized Shoulder Assessment Form consists of an evaluator-based and a patient-based subjective component. The patient-based component assesses pain, instability, and activities of daily living. Pain is determined with the use of a 10-cm VAS to quantify pain from 0 (no pain at all) to 10 (pain as bad as it can be). A similar VAS is used for instability. Activities of daily living are assessed with 10 questions that are answered on a four-point ordinal scale ranging from 0 (unable to do the activity) to 3 (no difficulty in performing the activity). The evaluator-based component includes range of motion, several shoulder specific clinical signs, strength, and instability. The score is obtained from the patient-based component with the following formula: (10−points on VAS for pain) × 5 + 5/3 × (total points for activities of daily living).[328]

Neer Criteria. In 1970 Neer published his criteria for the evaluation of results of proximal humeral fractures. They include four variables: (1) pain, (2) function, (3) range of motion, and (4) anatomy. Pain represents a total of 35 points, ranging from "totally disabled" (0 points) to "none" (35 points). Function represents 30 points and comprises strength, reach, and stability, each yielding up to 10 points. Range of motion represents 25 points, and is comprised of flexion (up to 6 points), extension (up to 3 points), abduction (up to 6 points), external rotation (up to 5 points), and internal rotation (up to 5 points). Anatomy represents 10 points, ranging from 0 to 10 points with regard to rotation, angulation, articular congruity, tuberosity displacement, hardware failure, heterotopic ossification, nonunion, and AVN of the humeral head. A maximum score of 100 can thereby be obtained. Results are classified as excellent for 90 points or more, satisfactory for 80 to 89 points, unsatisfactory for 70 to 79 points and failure for 69 points or less.[284]

UCLA. The original UCLA shoulder scale was first published by Amstutz et al.[7] for the assessment of shoulder arthroplasty. The scale was subsequently modified by Ellman et al.[103] for the evaluation of rotator cuff surgery. It evaluates pain, function, range of motion, strength, and patient satisfaction. Pain and function can yield a maximum of 10 points, whereas the remaining items can score a maximum of 5 points each, leading to a maximum overall score of 35 for an asymptomatic and normal shoulder.

Oxford Shoulder Scale. The Oxford Shoulder Score is a patient-based questionnaire that includes 12 questions with regard to pain and activities of daily living. Each question can be answered on a Likert scale from 0 to 5. The total score ranges from 0 to 60 with lower scales reflecting better outcomes.[87]

Simple Shoulder Test. The SST includes 11 questions regarding shoulder function and pain. Each question is answered with a yes/no option. Affirmative questions are then counted and reflect the final score.[249]

Shoulder Pain and Disability Index. The SPADI is a patient-based questionnaire that includes 13 questions assessing the domains of pain and disability. Each question is answered using a VAS. Results are presented as a percentage of the maximum achievable score. Higher scores reflect more pain and disability.[330]

Subjective Shoulder Value and Single Assessment Numerical Evaluation. Gerber et al.[143] introduced SSV as a means to assess outcomes after surgery for massive rotator cuff tear surgery. It consists of a single question asking the patient to estimate the function of the affected shoulder as a percentage of function of an entirely normal shoulder. The same question was further validated by Williams et al.[417] as the SANE in a cohort of patients undergoing surgery for shoulder instability.

University of Pennsylvania Shoulder Score. The PENN shoulder scale is a 100-point shoulder-specific self-reported patient-based questionnaire consisting of three subscales: pain, satisfaction, and function. Pain and satisfaction are rated using a 10-point Likert scale. Pain is assessed at different levels of activity (at rest, normal activities, and strenuous activities) and can achieve a maximum of 10 points each. Satisfaction can reach a maximum of 10 points. Function is assessed using a total of 20 questions, each answered on a scale from 0 to 3. Function can thereby reach a maximum of 60 points. The maximum total score is 100 points with higher scores representing higher function.[234,235]

Validity, Responsiveness, Reproducibility

As with any gauging tool, outcomes scales require a certain set of criteria to be able to provide accurate measurements. Outcomes measurement tools should be valid, reliable, and sensitive to change. For a scale to be valid it needs to be developed in a manner that assesses what is important to the patient. Furthermore, it needs to be easily obtainable and easy to evaluate.[142] Despite the abundance of shoulder assessment scales, many do not fulfill these criteria. Furthermore, scales are frequently used for conditions different than those for which they were developed and validated, raising concern about their accuracy.[86] This is the case in proximal humeral fractures. To our knowledge, only one study has to date specifically evaluated an upper extremity outcomes scales for proximal humeral fractures. Slobogean et al. studied the validity and reliability of the DASH and EQ-5D in patients with proximal humeral fractures. Both showed strong reliability with an intraclass correlation coefficient (ICC) of 0.77 for EQ-5D and 0.93 for DASH. Construct validity was determined with strong correlation between EQ-5D and DASH.[372] These results are extremely helpful and allow researchers and clinicians to continue using these scales to assess the outcomes of proximal humeral fractures.

PATHOANATOMY AND APPLIED ANATOMY

Bone

The proximal humerus consists of the humeral head, the greater and lesser tuberosities, and the humeral shaft (Fig. 37-16). The region of transition between the articular cartilage and surrounding bone is defined as the anatomic neck, whereas the region immediately inferior to the tuberosities is termed the surgical neck. Several studies have analyzed the anatomy of the proximal humerus and have shown considerable variation between individuals. The mean radius of curvature of the humeral head is 25 mm, ranging from 23 to 29 mm. The humeral head height, defined as the perpendicular distance from the plane of the anatomic neck to the surface of the humeral head consistently is approximately three-fourths of the radius of curvature of the humeral head.[313] Although the head size varies the surface arc covered by hyaline cartilage is approximately 160 degrees.[313] In the coronal plane, the angle between the anatomic neck and the humeral shaft averages 41 degrees, ranging from 30 to 50 degrees.[313,331] In the axial plane, the posterior angle of the anatomic neck of the humerus with relation to the epicondylar axis averages 17 degrees and ranges from 5 degrees of anteversion to 50 degrees of retroversion.[36] In the coronal plane, the geometric center of the humeral head is located 4 to 14 mm medial to the axis of the humeral shaft.

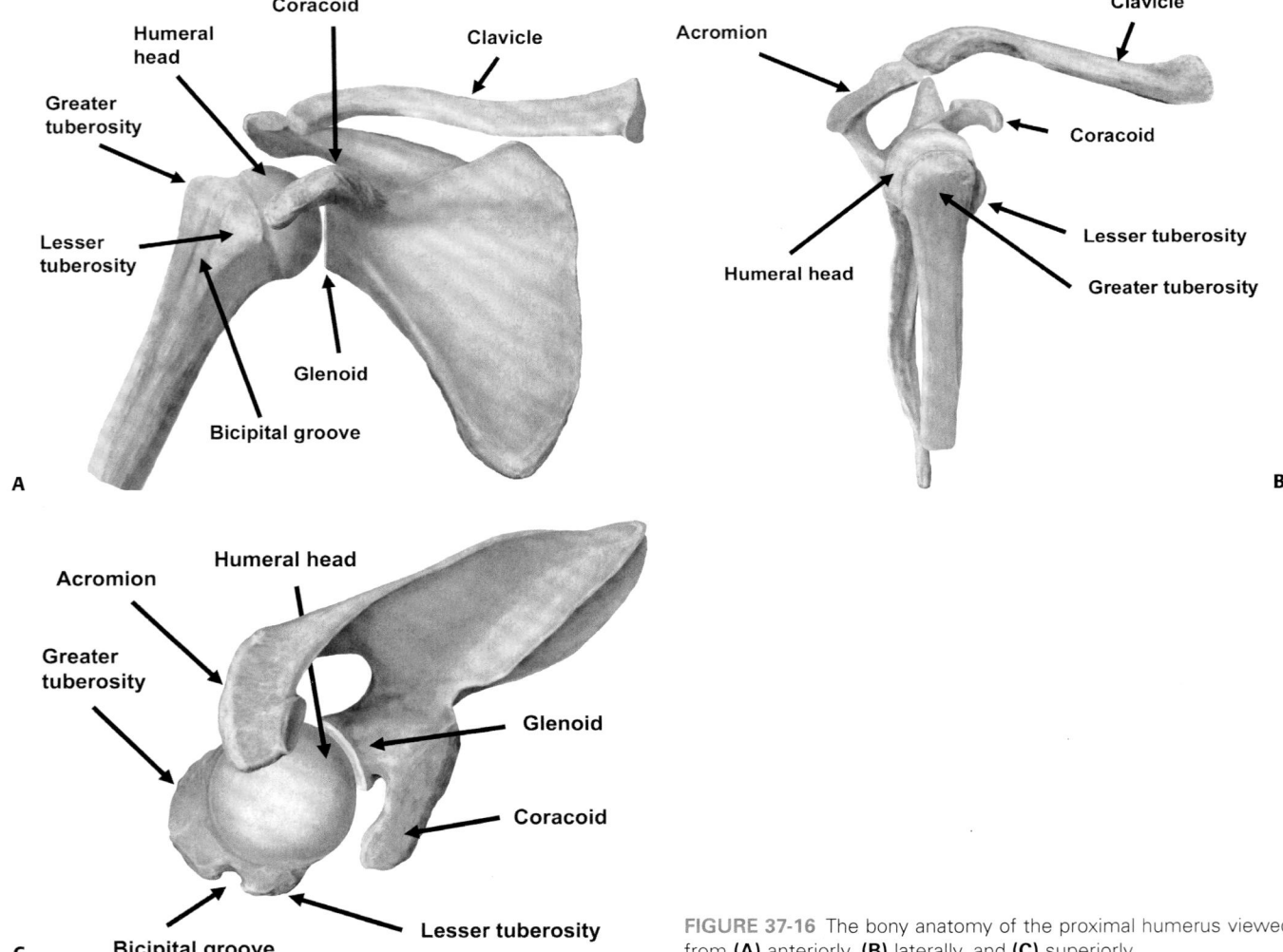

FIGURE 37-16 The bony anatomy of the proximal humerus viewed from **(A)** anteriorly, **(B)** laterally, and **(C)** superiorly.

In the sagittal plane the center of the humeral head can be located from 4 mm anterior to 14 mm posterior to the axis of the humeral shaft. The humeral canal diameter averages 12 mm and ranges from 10 to 14 mm.[313]

The greater tuberosity lies laterally on the proximal humerus and is the insertion point for the supraspinatus tendon superiorly, the infraspinatus tendon posterosuperiorly and the teres minor tendon posteriorly.[272] The greater tuberosity is located on average 9 mm distal to the most proximal aspect of the humeral head (range: 6 to 10 mm). This head to tuberosity distance is important in facilitating adequate rotator cuff function. Too short a distance leads to insufficient rotator cuff tension and subacromial impingement, whereas a very low tuberosity may lead to excessive tendon strain and failure. Inability to reconstitute the correct head tuberosity distance has been shown to give poor results in both arthroplasty and fracture reduction.[184]

The lesser tuberosity is situated anteriorly in the proximal humerus. It is the insertion site of the subscapularis muscle. The lesser and greater tuberosities are separated by the bicipital groove, which serves as the track for the long head of the biceps to travel from its supraglenoid insertion inside the glenohumeral joint to the anterior aspect of the arm. The bicipital groove has a spiral trajectory from superior and laterally toward the midline inferiorly. Proximally, the bicipital groove consistently lies 7 mm anterior to the intramedullary (IM) axis of the humerus and serves as a reliable reference point to establish humeral head retroversion.[8] The bicipital groove is covered by the transverse ligament and the insertion of the coracohumeral ligament. The bone surrounding the bicipital groove is strong cortical bone and is therefore fractured only in cases of high-energy trauma or severe osteopenia. It is therefore a useful landmark for fracture reduction (Fig. 37-17).

Vascularity

Perfusion of the upper extremity is mainly from the axillary artery and its branches. Perfusion of the proximal humerus arises from the axillary artery where it passes between the pectoralis minor and teres major muscles. At this level, the axillary artery gives off the humeral circumflex arteries (Fig. 37-18). The ACHA runs horizontally behind the conjoined tendon over the anterior aspect of the surgical neck of the humerus to anastomose

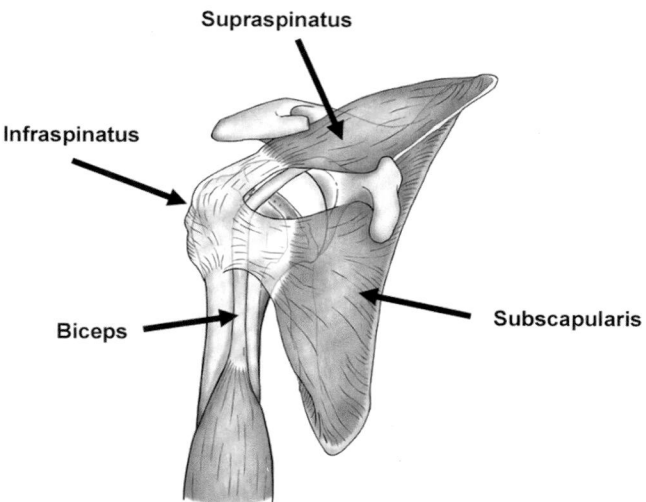

FIGURE 37-17 Anatomy of the rotator cuff and biceps.

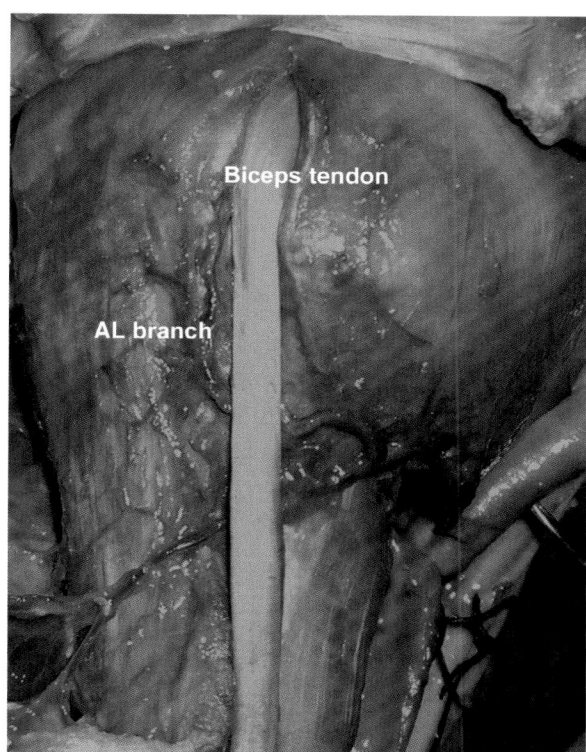

FIGURE 37-19 Vascularity of the proximal humerus, anterior view. Note the proximity of the ramus ascendens (AL branch) of the ACHA and the biceps tendon. From Hettrich et al.[173]

laterally with the PCHA. At the level of the biceps tendon the ACHA gives off a branch that ascends behind the long head of the biceps on the surface of the bicipital groove proximally (Fig. 37-19). Within 5 mm of the articular surface it penetrates the cortical bone, becoming the arcuate artery which provides vascularity to most of the humeral head[46,147] (Fig. 37-20).

The PCHA arises as a larger branch at the same level as the ACHA at the lower margin of the subscapularis muscle. It travels posteriorly with the axillary nerve giving off several branches that pierce the posteromedial aspect of the proximal humeral metaphysis providing vascularity to the humeral head. The PCHA finally crosses the quadrilateral space winding around the surgical neck and anastomosing anteriorly with the ACHA. While some authors have found the arcuate artery from the anterolateral ascending branch of the ACHA to be the main arterial supply to the humeral head,[147] several studies have shown branches from the PCHA to the posteromedial head to be at least equally important[46,95,227,266,267] (Figs. 37-20 and 37-21).

Muscles

Several muscles play a role in proximal humeral fractures. The rotator cuff muscles play an important role in displacement of the proximal fracture segment, whereas pectoralis major is responsible for displacing the shaft segment (Fig. 37-22). Furthermore understanding of the deltoid anatomy and the interval between deltoid and pectoralis major is important to safely achieve fracture exposure.

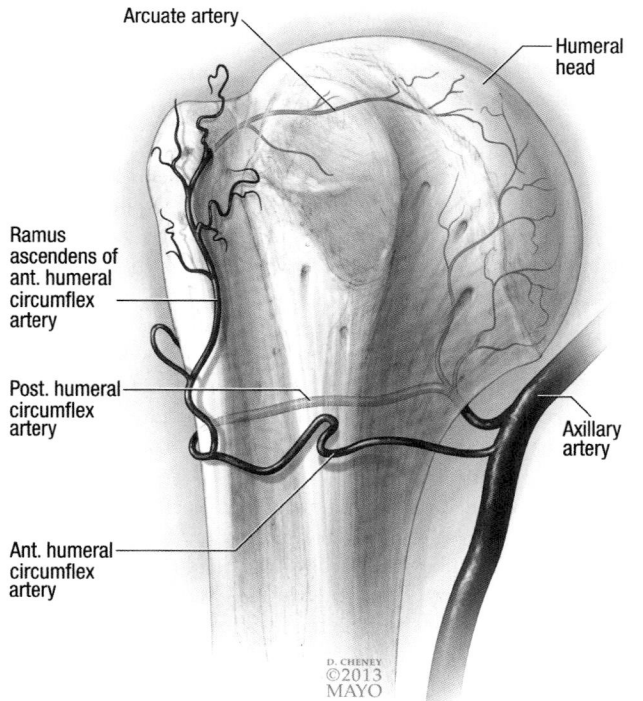

FIGURE 37-18 Vascular supply of the humeral head. The anterior circumflex humeral artery (ACHA) and posterior circumflex humeral artery (PCHA) branch off of the axillary artery. The ramus ascendens of the ACHA ends as the arcuate artery in the superolateral aspect of the proximal humerus. The PCHA provides multiple metaphyseal branches to the posteromedial aspect of the proximal humerus.

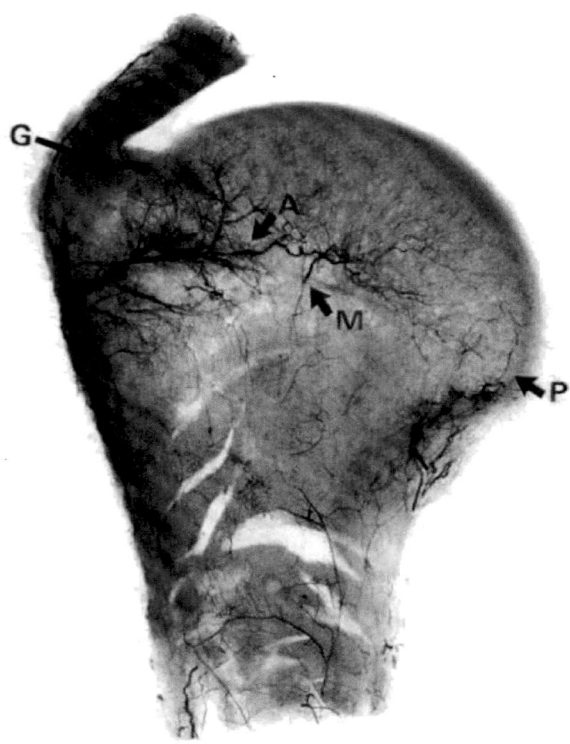

FIGURE 37-20 Vascularity of the proximal humerus, Spalteholz technique coronal section. Note intraosseous branching of the arcuate artery form the ACHA **(A)** and from metaphyseal branches of the PCHAP. From Brooks et al.[46]

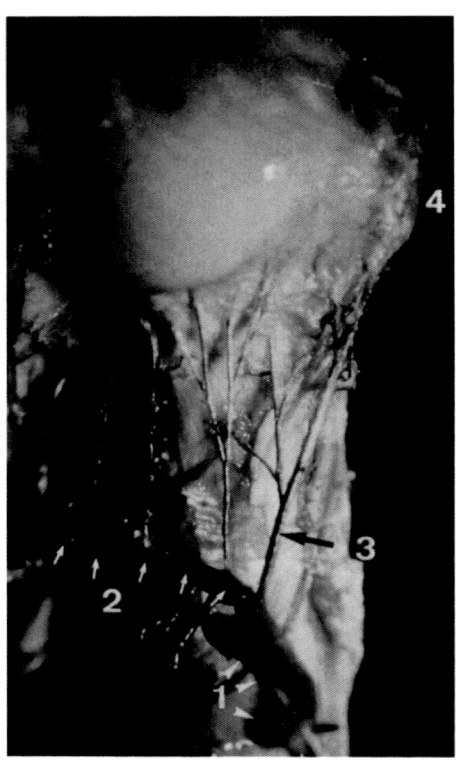

FIGURE 37-21 Vascularity of the proximal humerus. The axillary artery (1-white arrow heads) is pulled anteriorly. Note the larger size of the PCHA (2-small white arrows) in comparison to the ACHA (3-large black arrow).

The rotator cuff is composed of the subscapularis anteriorly, the supraspinatus superiorly, and the infraspinatus and teres minor posteriorly. The subscapularis muscle originates from the subscapularis fossa on the anterior surface of the scapular body and inserts into the lesser tuberosity. The supra- and infraspinatus muscles originate from the posterior surface of the scapular body above and below the scapular spine, respectively. The teres minor muscle originates from the lateral border of the scapular body. These three muscles insert onto the greater tuberosity of the proximal humerus. The supraspinatus inserts superiorly, the infraspinatus posterosuperiorly, and the teres minor posteriorly.[272] These muscles play a key role in shoulder function, and are essential to preserve a rotational fulcrum during activation of the deltoid. The subscapularis muscle is innervated by the upper and lower subscapular nerves which originate from the posterior cord of the brachial plexus. It derives its perfusion from the subscapular artery which is the largest branch of the axillary artery. The supra- and infraspinatus muscles are innervated by the suprascapular nerve which originates from the upper trunk of the brachial plexus. Blood supply is provided by the suprascapular artery which comes from the thyrocervical trunk which originates from the subclavian artery. The teres minor is innervated by the axillary artery and perfused by the posterior humeral circumflex and the circumflex scapular arteries which originate from the subscapular artery.

The rotator interval is a triangular region delineated at the apex medially by the coracoid process, the supraspinatus superiorly, the subscapularis inferiorly and the bicipital groove laterally. It contains the coracohumeral and superior glenohumeral ligaments which play a key role in shoulder stability. In proximal humeral fractures rotator cuff tears may start through the rotator cuff interval. In arthroplasty reconstruction of proximal humeral fractures, separation of the lesser and greater tuberosities may be safely performed through the rotator interval to avoid damage to the rotator cuff.

The long head of the biceps originates at the supraglenoid tubercle, traveling over the humeral head across the rotator interval into the intertubercular groove. During its course through the intertubercular groove the tendon is covered by the transverse humeral ligament. Muscle fibers of the long head join those of the short head at the level of the middle third of the humerus. Due to its location, the long head of the biceps can serve as a useful landmark for orientation particularly in comminuted fractures. The tendon can be identified in the proximal third of the arm and traced proximally to locate the intertubercular groove and tuberosities.

The deltoid originates on the anterior aspect of the lateral third of the clavicle, the periphery of acromion, and the lateral third of the scapular spine. It is commonly described as consisting of three segmental units, anterior, middle and posterior, which respectively provide shoulder flexion, abduction and

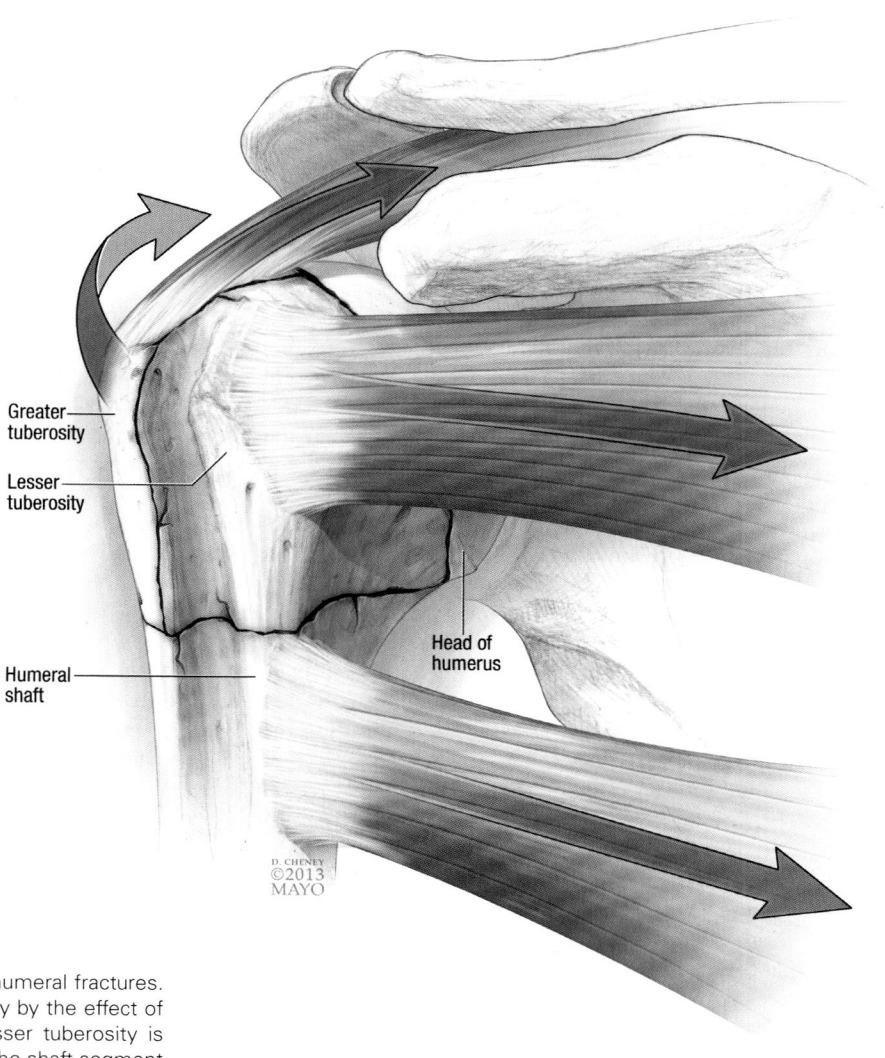

Greater tuberosity

Lesser tuberosity

Head of humerus

Humeral shaft

D. CHENEY
©2013
MAYO

FIGURE 37-22 Deforming forces of proximal humeral fractures. The greater tuberosity is pulled posteromedially by the effect of the supra- and infraspinatus tendons. The lesser tuberosity is pulled anteriorly by the subscapularis tendon. The shaft segment is pulled anteromedially by the pectoralis major tendon.

e3281922-01

extension. The anterior deltoid originates from the clavicle and the anterior aspect of the acromion.[204] A fibrous raphe extending from the anterolateral corner of the acromion distally separates the anterior from the middle deltoid. The deltoid fibers converge laterally inserting onto the deltoid tuberosity of the humerus in a trapezoidal fashion. The insertion measures 5 to 7 cm in length with a width of 22 mm proximally and 13 mm distally.[204,329] Distally, interconnections of the deltoid and its fascia with the lateral intermuscular septum and the brachialis muscle allow for partial release of the deltoid during surgical approach without the need for repair.[329] The deltoid muscle is innervated by the axillary nerve. Blood supply to the deltoid is provided by the PCHA.

The pectoralis major muscle has two heads, the clavicular and the sternocostal. The clavicular portion originates on the anterior surface of the clavicle, medial to the deltoid insertion. The sternocostal head originates from the anterior surface of the sternum, the superior six costal cartilages and the fascia of

the external oblique muscle. Both muscles and tendons converge laterally to insert onto the lateral aspect of the bicipital groove of the humerus. The pectoralis major is innervated by the lateral and medial pectoral nerves that originate from the lateral and medical cords of the brachial plexus, respectively. The blood supply is derived from the pectoral branch of the thoracoacromial trunk originating from the axillary artery.

The cephalic vein runs in the deltopectoral interval. It serves as a useful landmark to identify the interval between the deltoid and pectoralis major muscles to allow safe access to the anterior aspect of the shoulder. More tributaries to the cephalic vein arise from the deltoid than from the pectoralis major.[320] Some surgeons therefore recommend lateral retraction of the vein during the deltopectoral approach. Proximally the cephalic vein passes through the deltopectoral triangle just caudal to the clavicle to join the axillary vein. Perivascular fat can be found at the deltopectoral triangle, which can serve as a useful landmark to safely identify the cephalic vein. The course of the vein through the deltopectoral interval arches with a medial concavity and therefore most surgeons recommend medial retraction of the vein to minimize tension during retraction.

Nerves

Several nerves are at risk of damage from manipulation of the proximal humerus or surgery. The axillary nerve can be injured by the initial injury, or secondarily by percutaneous fixation. The axillary nerve is one of the terminal branches of the posterior cord of the brachial plexus. Its motor fibers innervate the teres minor and deltoid muscles; the sensory component innervates the skin overlying the lateral aspect of the proximal arm. At the level of the proximal humerus, the axillary nerve passes from anterior to posterior, accompanied by the posterior circumflex artery, inferior to the anatomic neck through the quadrilateral space surrounded by teres major superiorly, the long head of the triceps medially, teres major inferiorly, and the humeral shaft laterally. After giving off the branch to the teres minor, it passes anteriorly on the undersurface of the deltoid at a distance ranging from 2 to 7 cm distal to the acromion.[55,133,192] This distance has been found to be inversely proportional to the length of the deltoid.[213] It crosses the anterior deltoid raphe between the anterior and middle deltoid in the form of a single terminal branch allowing for preservation of the innervation of the anterior deltoid when the nerve is isolated during the deltoid-splitting approach.[133,134]

The musculocutaneous nerve is at risk from medial retraction when performing the deltopectoral approach. The musculocutaneous nerve originates from the lateral cord of the brachial plexus. The most proximal motor branch to the coracobrachialis muscle is located about 3 to 4 cm distal to the tip of the coracoid, being less than 5 cm in 75% of cases.[66] The musculocutaneous nerve then enters the coracobrachialis at a mean distance of 5.6 cm inferior to the coracoid process.[66,115,425] Farther distally, it pierces the biceps at an average of 10 cm

distal to the coracoid. It then travels between biceps and the underlying brachialis muscle innervating both muscles. It ends as the lateral antebrachial cutaneous nerve providing sensation to the lateral aspect of the forearm.[425]

FRACTURE TREATMENT OPTIONS

Nonoperative Treatment of Proximal Humeral Fractures

Nonoperative treatment continues to be used for the majority of proximal humeral fractures.[198,217,396] The majority of proximal humeral fractures are nondisplaced or minimally displaced and nonoperative treatment is indicated. The use of nonoperative treatment can be determined by assessing fracture stability. Fracture stability can be assessed both radiographically and clinically. Radiographically, stable fractures exhibit impaction or interdigitation between bone fragments (Fig. 37-23). Most frequently impaction occurs between the humeral head and the shaft at the level of the surgical neck (Fig. 37-24). Furthermore, in four-part valgus-impacted fractures, the humeral head is tilted into valgus thereby impacting the anatomic neck into the surrounding metaphysis (Figs. 37-5, 37-10, and 37-11). While the greater and lesser tuberosities are fractured, their periosteal sleeve remains intact thereby avoiding displacement by the pull of the rotator cuff muscles.

Clinically, fracture stability may be assessed by palpating the proximal humerus just distal to the acromion with one hand, while rotating the arm at the elbow with the other. If the proximal humerus is felt to move as a unit with the distal segment, the fracture is considered stable. Crepitation may be palpated and if it is it suggests bony contact. Lack of crepitation and absence of synchronous motion between the distal and proximal segments on the other hand suggest fracture displacement. Although this examination may be possible in some patients

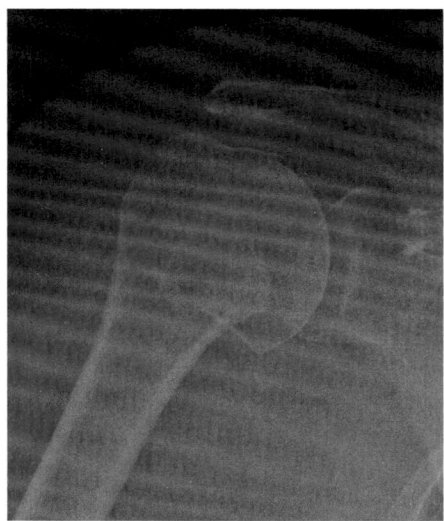
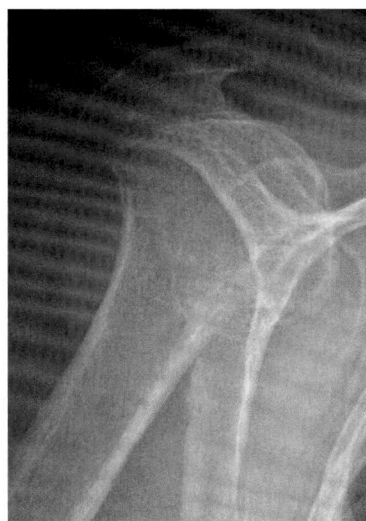
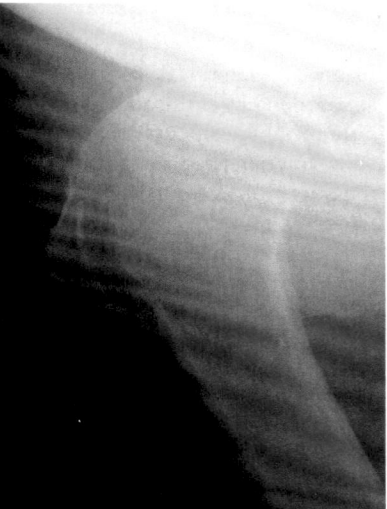

A, B   **C**

FIGURE 37-23 Stable proximal humeral fractures through the anatomic neck. **(A–C)** Case 1: **A:** AP view. **B:** Neer Y view. **C:** Axillary view.

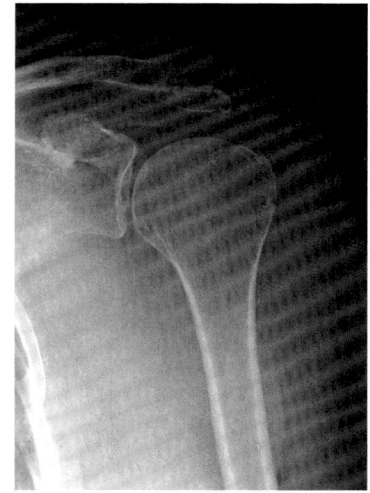
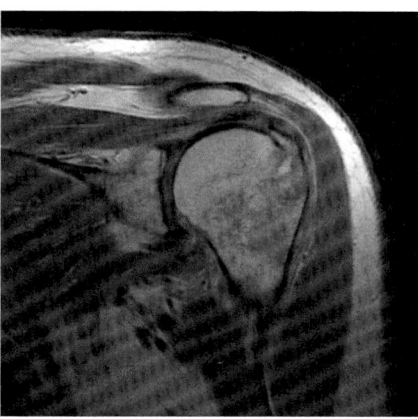
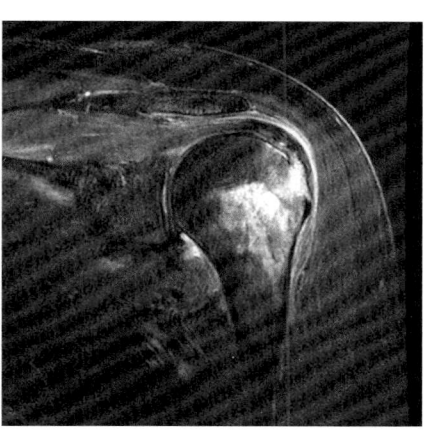

D, E   F

FIGURE 37-23 (*continued*) **D–F** Case 2: **D:** AP view. **E:** MRI coronal view, T1-weighted image. **F:** MRI coronal view, T2-weighted image. Note increased signal along the anatomic neck of the humerus and integrity of the rotator cuff.

surgeons should be aware that pain, obesity, and the presence of other injuries may preclude its use in many patients. Clinical and radiographic follow-up are required in the early phase of nonoperative treatment to monitor fracture displacement (Fig. 37-25).

Indications/Contraindications

The indications and contraindications for nonoperative management are shown in Table 37-1. Nonoperative treatment is considered as the standard of treatment for nondisplaced, mini-

mally displaced, and stable proximal humeral fractures. Several criteria for nonoperative treatment have been described in the past centering around patient age and mental and health status.

Techniques

Several immobilization techniques have been described for nonoperative treatment of proximal humeral fractures. Immobilization of the arm to the chest using a simple collar and cuff sling, Gilchrist or Velpeau type shoulder immobilizer is generally

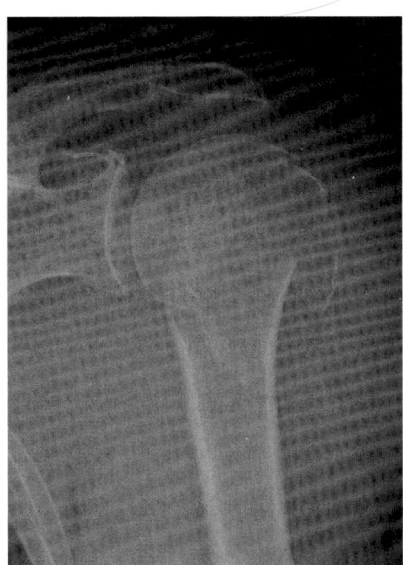
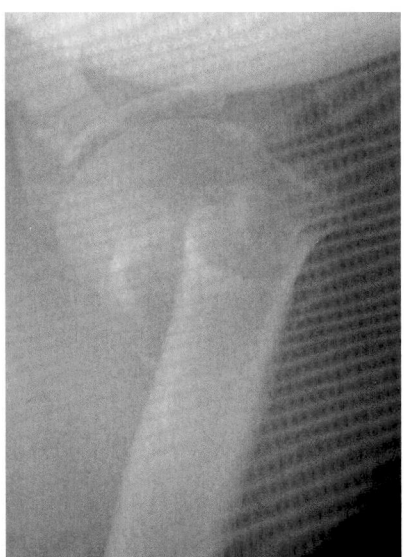
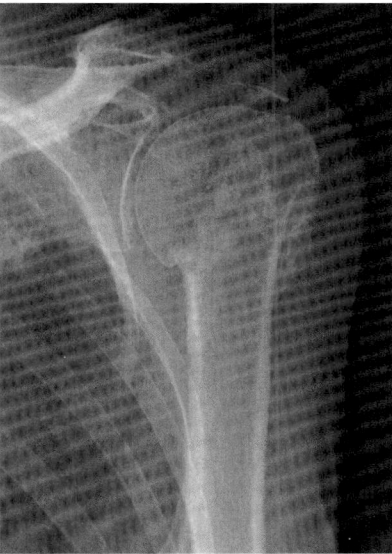

A, B   C

FIGURE 37-24 Nonoperative treatment of proximal humerus fractures. **A–E:** 78-year-old female with two-part surgical neck fracture. **A and B:** AP and axillary views of the left shoulder. Note impaction of the shaft into the proximal humerus. The axillary view shows apex anterior angulation at the fracture site with partial anterior displacement of the shaft fragment. Complete displacement is however prevented by impaction and interdigitation of the fracture fragments.

(*continues*)

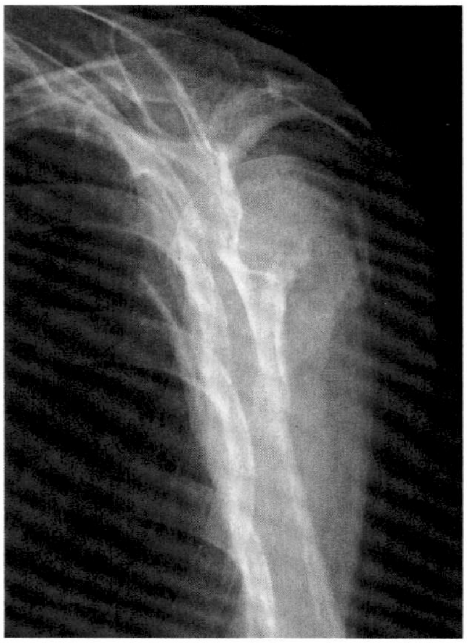

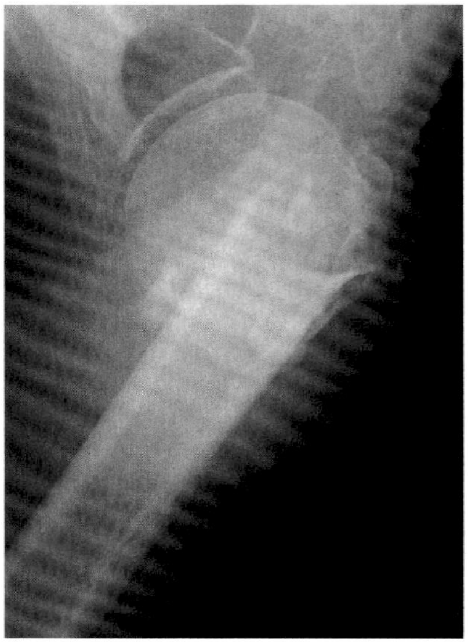

D, E

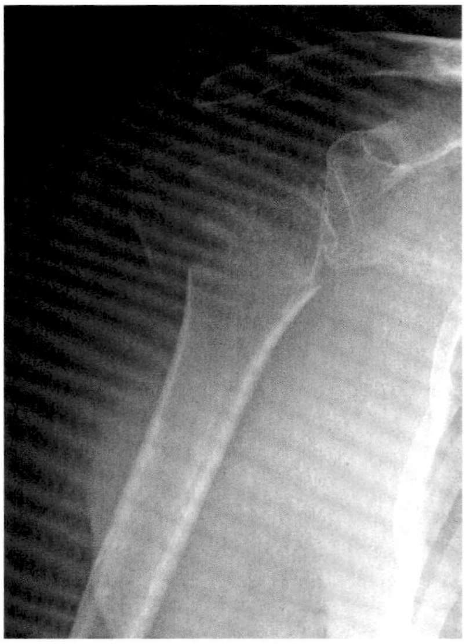

F

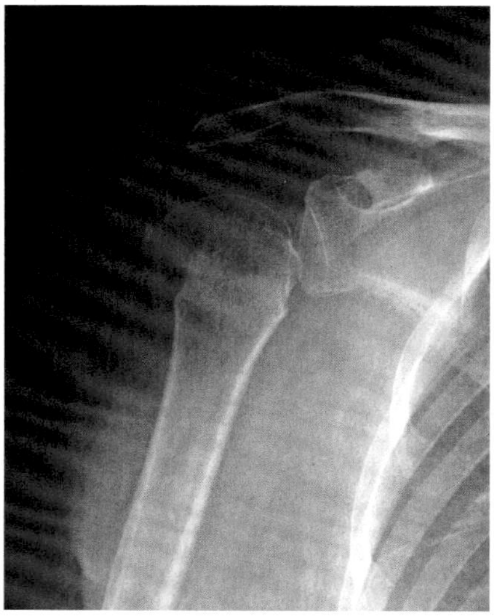

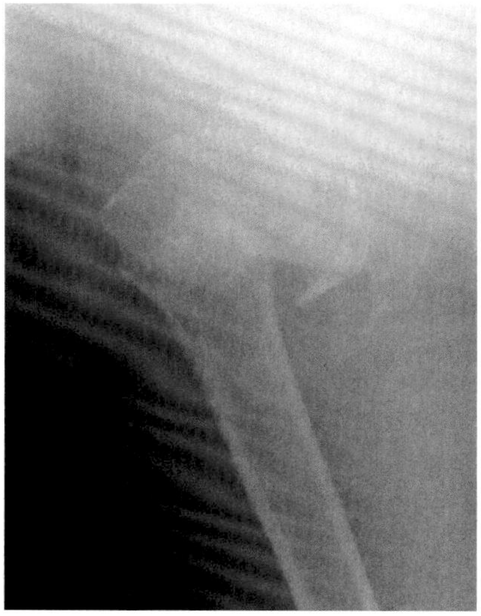

G, H

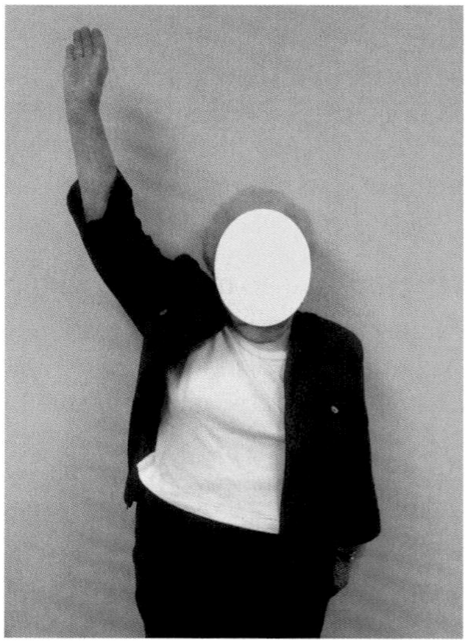

I

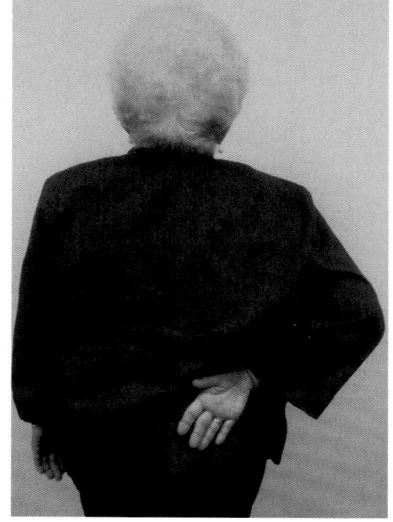

J

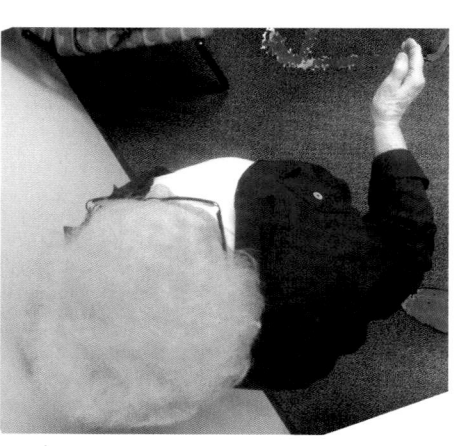

K

FIGURE 37-24 (continued) **C, D, and E:** AP, Neer and axillary views at 4 months after injury. Note early bony healing of the fracture. There has been no change in fracture alignment. **F–K:** 89-year-old female with a four-part valgus-impacted proximal humerus fracture. **F:** AP view on the day of injury. **G and H:** AP and axillary views at 3 months after nonoperative treatment. Note residual posterior displacement of the greater tuberosity. **I:** Forward elevation at 3 months after injury. **J:** Internal rotation at 3 months after injury. **K:** External rotation at 3 months after injury.

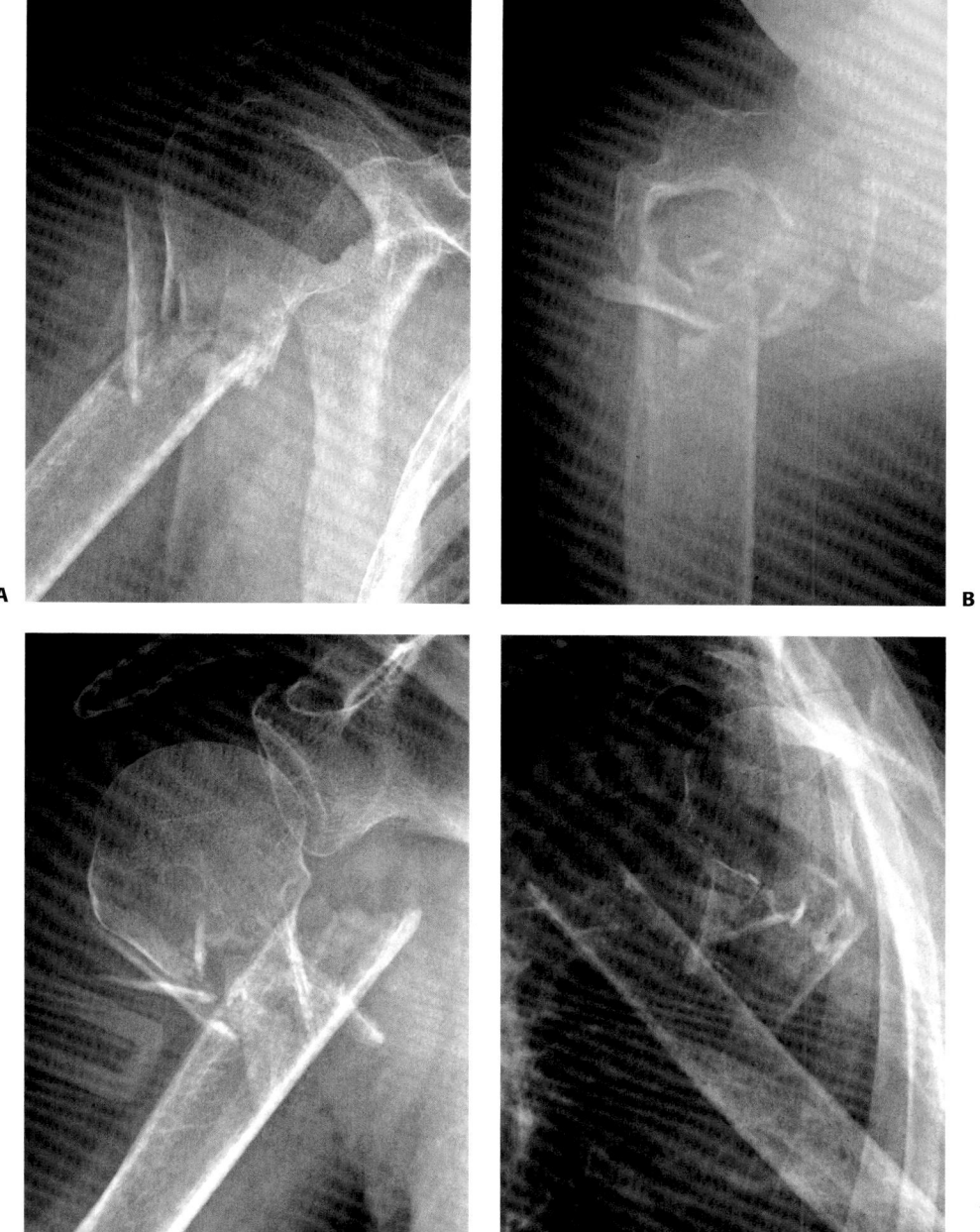

FIGURE 37-25 Two-part surgical neck fracture. **A and B:** AP and axillary views of the right shoulder. Note comminution at the metadiaphyseal junction. Alignment and bony contact between the proximal segment and the shaft is however preserved. **C and D:** AP and axillary views taken 2 weeks after the initial injury seen in **A** and **B:** Immobilization in a sling had been established for nonoperative treatment. Note marked displacement of the proximal shaft secondary to pull of the pectoralis major tendon. The patient had noted a dramatic decrease of pain 2 day prior to these images being taken.

TABLE 37-1	**Non-Operative Treatment**
Indications	**Relative Contraindications**
Stable nondisplaced or minimally displaced fractures	Displaced fractures with loss of bony contact
Patients not fit for surgery	
Elderly patients with low functional demand	

well tolerated by patients.[114,341] Due to the pull of the pectoralis major tendon on the proximal shaft segment, placement of a pad in the axilla may help in aligning the fracture. Regardless of the type of nonoperative treatment method, close follow-up is required to confirm acceptable alignment and fracture stability. Weekly radiographs should be performed during the first month of treatment, followed by biweekly radiographs until 6 weeks after injury or initial callus formation is visible. Final radiographs are taken at 3 months to confirm union.

Shoulder immobilization is used during the first 4 to 6 weeks after injury. From the beginning, patients are instructed to perform active range-of-motion exercises of the wrist and hand. Pain usually subsides within 2 weeks after injury to allow passive range-of-motion exercises of the shoulder. These should be performed four to six times per day with the help of an assistant. An initial session with a physical therapist can aid in instructing the patient and his or her assistant on how to perform the exercises. Fracture stability will guide the arc of allowable motion. Ideally, patients should be able to achieve 90 degrees of forward elevation and rotation from the hand placed on the chest to neutral with the hand pointing straight forward. During the first 2 to 3 weeks, passive range-of-motion exercises are best tolerated in the supine position. As the patient adapts to these exercises, they can be continued in the sitting or standing position. In addition, Codman pendulum exercises can be performed for passive range-of-motion exercises of the shoulder. The patient is instructed to lean forward while standing. The upper extremity is then allowed to freely dangle from the shoulder assisted by gravity. As much as 90 degrees of forward shoulder elevation can thereby be achieved. The upper extremity is then passively moved by turning the trunk in a circular manner letting the arm dangle like a pendulum. As bony union is achieved, active-assisted range-of-motion exercises are started at 6 weeks, with strengthening exercises starting 3 months after the injury according to radiographic and clinical healing.

Outcomes

Stable nondisplaced or minimally displaced proximal humeral fractures can be reliably treated nonoperatively. A high union rate with satisfactory functional outcome can be achieved.[198,217,396] Predictors for outcomes have been found to be age, the American Society of Anesthesia (ASA) classification and the AO/OTA fracture classification.[15]

Nonoperative treatment has been further advocated for several displaced fractures. Court-Brown et al. studied 131 two-part surgical neck fractures in patients with a mean age of 73 years for females and 69 for males. At 1-year follow-up, patients under the age of 50 consistently achieved higher functional scores and regained the ability to return to shopping and housework. Nonoperative treatment yielded results similar to those of surgical treatment even in fractures with translation of 66% or more.[78]

Court-Brown et al. further assessed nonoperative treatment of four-part valgus-impacted fractures in elderly patients. Good or excellent results were achieved in 81% of patients according to Neer's criteria. Interestingly, patients subjectively rated their results above the objective evaluation of the physician. No difference was found in patients with and without greater tuberosity displacement. Function only decreased in the presence of combined surgical neck and greater tuberosity displacement and was mainly related to loss of flexion and abduction power.[76] Hanson et al. evaluated the outcomes of nonoperative treatment in 75 one-part, 60 two-part, 23 three-part fractures, and 2 four-part or head-splitting fractures. Four patients required surgery due to displacement and five required arthroscopic subacromial decompression due to impingement. At 1 year after the fracture, the injured shoulders averaged an 8.2 point loss of Constant score and a 10.2 point loss of DASH scores

compared to the contralateral shoulder. The highest variability in outcomes was found in patients with two-part fractures.[159]

Kristiansen et al.[224] randomized a group of two-, three-, and four-part fractures to either closed treatment or external fixation. Of 11 fractures treated nonoperatively, nonunion occurred in 2 surgical neck fractures and 2 greater tuberosity fractures, and 2 patients developed AVN of the humeral head after 1 year. Of 13 patients treated with external fixation that were followed for 1 year, one deep infection occurred, two fractures did not unite, and AVN was seen in one case. The median Neer score was 79 after external fixation and 60 after nonoperative treatment. Satisfactory or excellent results were achieved in only four patients in the nonoperative group compared to eight in the external fixation group.

Several studies have shown results contradicting those of Kristiansen et al. Court-Brown et al. did not find an improvement in outcomes in displaced two-part fracture treated surgically versus those treated nonoperatively.[78] Furthermore, in a randomized controlled study comparing nonoperative treatment with tension band fixation of three- and four-part fractures, Zyto et al. found higher Constant scores after nonoperative than after operative treatment. While no differences were found with regard to pain, range of motion, strength, and activities of daily living subscales, a higher proportion of complications were found after operative treatment, including infection, AVN, nonunion, post-traumatic arthritis, pulmonary embolus, and Kirschner-wire (K-wire) penetration.[428] Similar results were found by Fjalestad et al., who found no differences in Constant scores when randomizing patients to either nonoperative treatment or locking plate fixation of three- and four-part proximal humeral fractures.[114] Another recent randomized controlled trial could not establish significant differences in Constant and Simple Shoulder Test scores in patients undergoing either nonoperative treatment or hemiarthroplasty for four-part fractures. Although the surgically treated group had better pain scores at 3 months after surgery, no differences were seen at 1 year.[42] Sanders et al. compared the results of three-part fractures treated with locking plate fixation to a matched nonsurgical control group.[348] Better range of motion was found after nonoperative treatment, while no differences were found in patient satisfaction and in the ASES self-assessment score. Over half of operatively managed patients required additional treatment compared to only 11% in the nonoperative group. Similar results were found by Olerud et al. in a prospective randomized study comparing locked plate fixation with nonoperative treatment of three-part fractures.[299] Complications in the operative group included screw perforation of the articular surface in 17%. Reoperation was required in 30% of patients. Malunion was however observed in 86% of patients treated nonoperatively.

Using CT imaging, Foruria et al. observed fracture healing in 98% of fractures and excellent or satisfactory results as determined by Neer criteria in 75% of fractures treated nonoperatively. Patients with valgus impaction and a greater tuberosity fragment and those with varus impaction had the greatest loss of function as determined by both ASES and DASH scores.[119] Jakob et al.[187] and Court-Brown et al.,[76] however had previously published favorable outcomes in valgus-impacted fractures.

Hodgson et al. studied the timing of physical therapy for two-part proximal humeral fractures. The authors found that at 16 weeks after injury patients who started physical therapy within 1 week achieved greater function and less pain than those immobilized for a period of 3 weeks. Although functional differences at 52 weeks were not statistically significant, residual shoulder disability was slower to resolve, even 2 years after injury in patients with prolonged immobilization.[179,244]

Despite the overall favorable outcomes published in the literature for nonoperative treatment of nondisplaced fractures, recent data suggests that marked functional impairment may occur, with over two-thirds of patients disclosing chronic pain.[58] However, based on the published literature, nonoperative treatment appears to provide outcomes that are comparable to those of either operative fixation or hemiarthroplasty, even in displaced three- and four-part fractures.[42,78,114,224,299,348,428] Several randomized controlled trials assessing nonoperative treatment are currently under way and will further help in determining the ideal treatment option for proximal humeral fractures.[48,90,156,229]

Operative Treatment of Proximal Humeral Fractures

Surgical Approaches

Two surgical approaches are commonly used to perform open reduction and internal fixation (ORIF). These are the deltopectoral approach and the deltoid-splitting approach.

Deltopectoral Approach. The deltopectoral approach is considered the workhorse for reconstructive shoulder surgery. It is classically described as an incision starting over the coracoid process and advanced along the deltopectoral groove with subsequent identification and lateral reflection of the cephalic vein.[181] In the authors' experience, an incision starting over the

clavicle directed over 1 to 2 cm lateral to the coracoid process toward a point at the midline of the anterior arm 2 cm distal from the axillary crease will allow improved exposure (Fig. 37-26). The deltopectoral interval is not always apparent, especially in patients with muscle atrophy or previous surgery. To identify the cephalic vein a full-thickness skin flap is developed medially at the proximal extent of the incision to about 1 to 2 cm medial to the coracoid process. At this level a fat triangle is invariably found with its base at the clavicle. The cephalic vein can be readily identified traveling from this triangle distally. Most textbooks recommend dissecting the interval by retracting the cephalic vein laterally, based on the fact that lateral tributary veins are more frequent than their medial counterparts. However, mobilizing the cephalic vein medially allows for improved exposure by avoiding proximal tethering of the cephalic vein when lateral retraction of the deltoid is required (Fig. 37-26). Once the deltopectoral interval has been developed the subdeltoid space is identified and freed from hypertrophic bursal tissue. At this point, depending on the time elapsed since injury, fracture hematoma, fibrous scar tissue, or early callus formation is encountered. Careful soft tissue management is required to avoid devascularization of the fracture fragments. Of particular importance is identification of the long head of the biceps on the anterior aspect of the proximal shaft as this will facilitate fracture identification and reduction and plate placement. The biceps tendon is easily identified by digital palpation just medial to the insertion of the pectoralis major tendon (Fig. 37-26). Because of its proximity to the ascending branch of the ACHA extensive dissection of this tendon should be avoided. However, the biceps tendon may have been injured with the fracture and a tenodesis may be required to remove a possible source of pain. Furthermore, the presence of the biceps tendon may make fracture reduction more difficult.

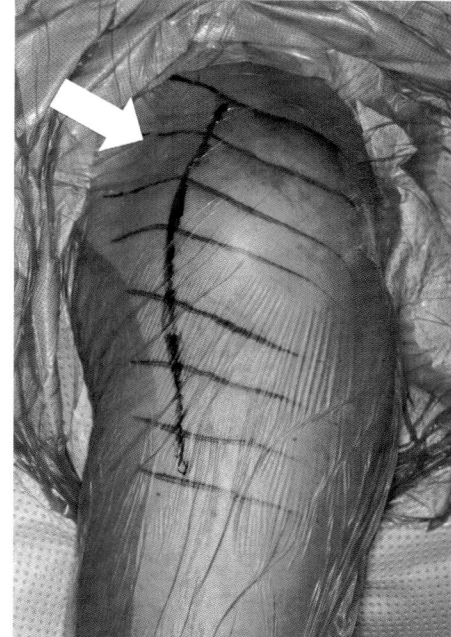 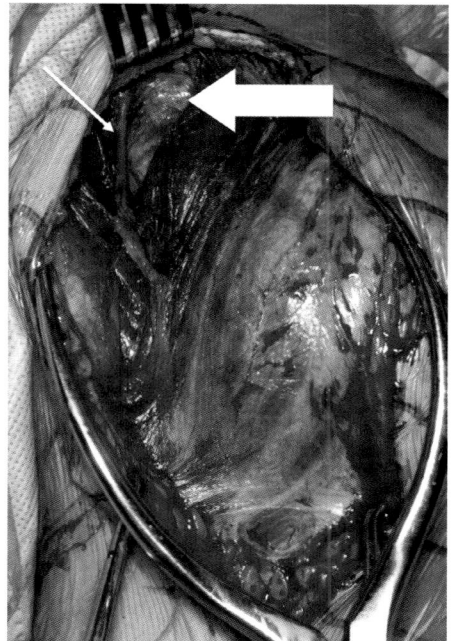

FIGURE 37-26 Deltopectoral approach. **A:** Image shows anterior aspect of the shoulder to the left. Incision is marked out 1 cm lateral to the coracoid (*arrow*). This point is connected to a point at the level of the axillary crease dividing the arm in 60% lateral and 40% medial. The incision starts at the level of the clavicle proximally and distally for approximately 10 cm. **B:** A fat triangle can be identified just distal to the clavicle helping identification of the deltopectoral interval. The interval is usually 1 cm medial to the coracoid (*large arrow*). The cephalic vein (*small arrow*) is retracted medially after coagulating lateral tributaries.

(*continues*)

A

B

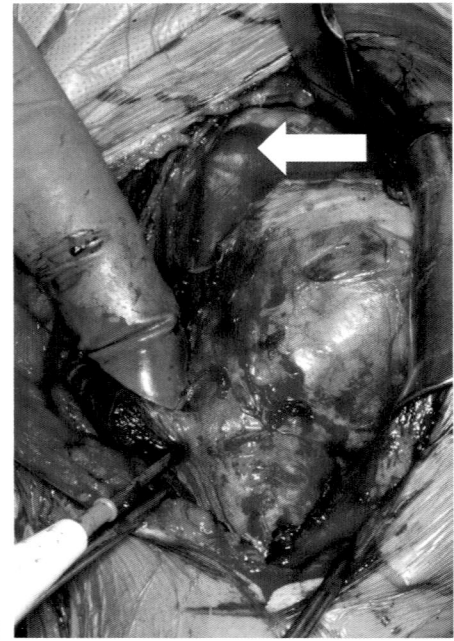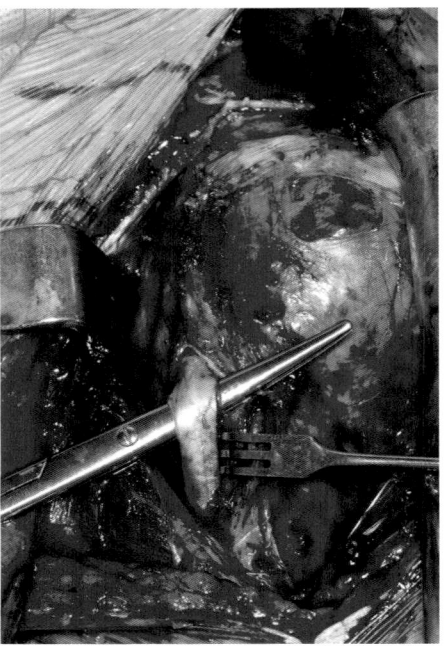

FIGURE 37-26 (*continued*) **C:** The coracoid helps orientation (*arrow*). The pectoralis major (between left index finger and cautery tip) is identified. The long head of the biceps will be located just medial to it. **D:** The long head of the biceps is identified aiding in orientation and exposure of the fracture of the proximal humerus.

Deltoid-Splitting Approach. The deltoid-splitting approach is favored by several authors since it allows a direct approach through the fracture site between the greater and lesser tuberosities.[131,132,133] To perform this approach a longitudinal incision or a shoulder strap incision is performed and the raphe between the anterior and middle deltoid identified.[333] This interval is divided using a vertical 4 cm incision starting at the anterolateral corner of the acromion.[132,226,375] The axillary nerve can be identified by digital palpation on the undersurface of the deltoid traveling from posterior to anterior at an average of 5 cm distal to the acromion. A stay suture is placed at the inferior aspect of the split to avoid inadvertent propagation distally thereby protecting the axillary nerve (Fig. 37-27). Since the nerve crosses the anterior raphe as a single branch innervation of the anterior deltoid can be preserved by protecting it during dissection.[131,132,133,333] Once identified, the raphe may be further split distal to the nerve to allow access to the lateral shaft for plate placement. Alternatively, a minimally invasive approach, using only the split above the nerve and percutaneously placed screws can be used.

The deltoid-splitting approach has two major disadvantages. In anteroinferior fracture dislocations, the humeral head fragment may not be accessible through this approach. In addition, the terminal anterior branch of the axillary nerve may be inadvertently damaged thereby leading to potential deltoid dysfunction.

Plate and Screw Fixation

ORIF is the most frequently used method of surgical treatment of proximal humeral fractures.[24] Direct exposure of the fracture site offers the advantages of allowing direct fragment

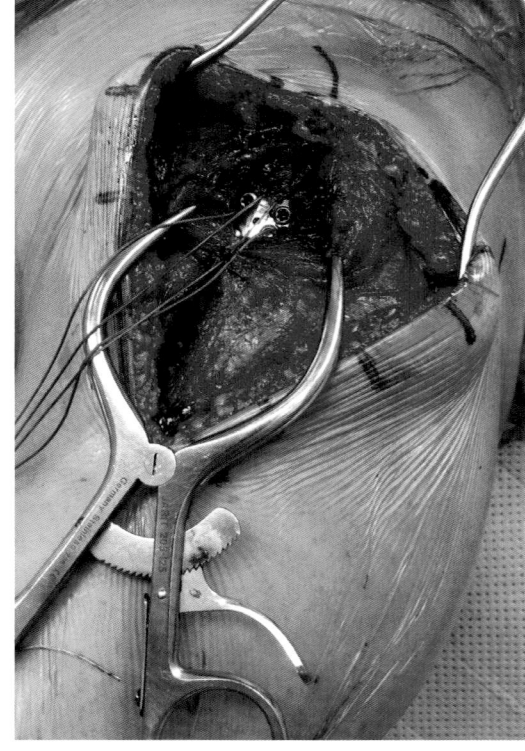

FIGURE 37-27 Deltoid split. Anterolateral approach starting at the tip of the acromion. Note stay suture 5 cm from the acromion tip to avoid splitting of the deltoid and subsequent damage to the anterior branch of the axillary nerve. Sutures exiting the split can be seen. These provide additional fixation between the rotator cuff tendons and the implanted locking plate.

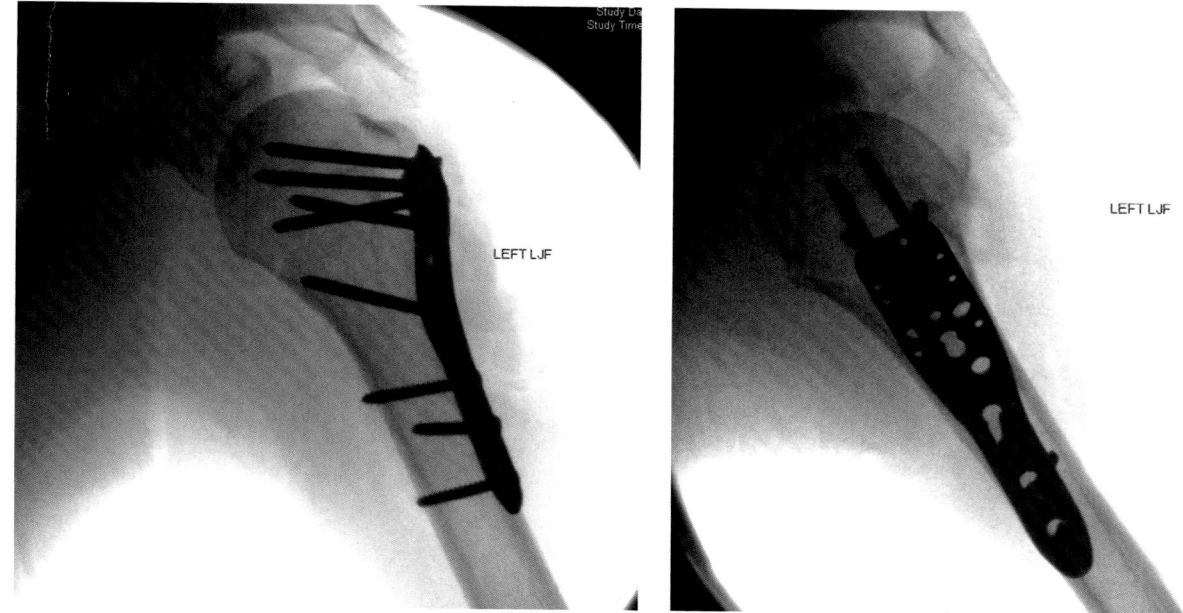

FIGURE 37-28 Intraoperative views of plate and screw fixation of a proximal humerus fracture. **A:** AP view. **B:** Lateral view of the proximal humerus. Note that the screw tips are kept short of the subchondral bone to prevent secondary perforation.

manipulation and visualization of reduction and implant position. However, surgical dissection may jeopardize fracture biology thereby potentially interfering with healing and increasing the risk of AVN of the humeral head.[223,387] Careful soft tissue management and judicious debridement should therefore be followed. Despite the advantage of direct visualization and access to the fracture site, ORIF requires a clear understanding of fracture geometry and deforming forces to aid in fracture manipulation in a manner similar to that of closed reduction techniques. Furthermore, ORIF should be performed with the assistance of fluoroscopic vision to verify fracture reduction and allow adequate hardware placement (Fig. 37-28).

The most widely used approach for ORIF is the deltopectoral approach. This approach has the advantage of allowing the surgeon to work through an internervous plane with a wide exposure. Furthermore, this approach allows the surgeon to convert from ORIF to hemiarthroplasty if required. The deltopectoral approach however requires significant soft tissue dissection to gain access to the lateral aspect of the proximal humerus for fracture reduction and plate placement. While several factors may affect humeral head vascularity after a proximal humerus fracture, the extensive surgical dissection required for ORIF through a deltopectoral approach has been suggested to play a role.[223,387] An extended anterolateral deltoid-splitting approach has gained increasing popularity over the last decade as a less invasive and more biologically sound approach.[131,133,134] While some debate exists regarding the clinical benefits of the anterolateral approach,[168,420] it does allow a more direct access to the greater tuberosity[133] and to the area between the greater and lesser tuberosities, just lateral to the bicipital groove.[99] This allows for a more direct manipulation of the humeral head, as well as allowing plate and screw placement in line with the inci-

sion. However, the potential for injury to the anterior branch of the axillary nerve is its main disadvantage, as it may lead to anterior deltoid dysfunction.

Multiple methods of ORIF have been developed since the advent of operative treatment of proximal humeral fractures. The most widely used methods have historically been tension band wiring and plate and screw fixation.[3,4,5,6,12,14,26,31,32,47,49,52,56,62,67, 74,80,85,86,91,92,96,101,105,107,108,110,111,112,114,116,118,121,123,127,130,131,132,133,134, 139,140,151,152,155,158,160,162,164,166,167,168,169,171,172,174,176,177,178,185,190,191,199, 200,201,203,206,208,209,210,211,215,216,223,226,228,229,231,232,238,350,252,253,354,260, 261,263,268,273,279,288,295,296,299,300,302,303,304,305,407,309,311,312,316,322,327,332,337, 338,339,340,342,345,347,348,349,353,355,356,360,366,370,373,374,375,376,377,378,384,385,386, 388,397,398,400,403,406,412,415,422,423,426,428] Tension band wiring relies on incorporating the rotator cuff to neutralize the deforming forces. Wire or suture fixation through the entheses of the rotator cuff has the advantage of not relying on weak osteoporotic bone which is frequently seen in patients with these fractures but on stronger tendinous tissue.[12]

Over the last 50 years compression plate and screw fixation has become the standard of care for treatment of several diaphyseal fractures as well as fractures of the distal humerus. Several studies have reported satisfactory healing rates and functional outcomes after conventional plate and screw fixation of proximal humeral fractures, especially in younger patient populations.[108,273,350,355,415,422] Favorable outcomes have been reported even with minimal hardware using a combination of nonlocking third tubular plate fixation and suture tension band fixation for three- and four-part fractures.[169] Other studies have however reported high rates of infection, humeral head necrosis, and subacromial impingement.[223,306,392,412] Furthermore, high rates of postoperative displacement and varus collapse have been reported, especially in elderly patients and three- and four-part fractures.[171,176] The inability of conventional plates and screws to resist varus deforming forces in the proximal humerus, particularly if the bone is osteoporotic, has led to locking plate fixation being used for these fractures. Unlike conventional screws and plates, locking plate technology allows for angular stability between the screws and plate. Biomechanical data has shown that constructs using locking plates are significantly stronger and more resilient than those using nonlocking screws, blade plates, and IM nails.[100,244,366,356] Several clinical studies have shown high rates of healing and excellent functional recovery with proximal humerus locking plates.[5,32,110,112,216,226,260,309,316,228,360] This has led to multiple precontoured proximal humerus plates becoming available in the market. Plate designs vary in terms of the number of proximal screws and their arrangement, as well as the ability to place screws at different angles with regard to the plate[31,32,105,110,208,338,347,406]

Preoperative Planning. As for any type of treatment, planning for ORIF of proximal humeral fractures requires a detailed understanding of fracture configuration. This is best achieved with a standard radiographic trauma series and CT scanning with 3D surface renderings. In many instances, preoperative assessment of fracture morphology and patient-related factors for AVN can reliably establish if the fracture will require reconstruction or replacement of the humeral head. Frequently, however, the final decision will be made intraoperatively. It is therefore recommended that, especially in complex fractures, a prosthesis be available at the time of ORIF. If ORIF is the planned procedure, a deltoid-splitting approach may be used. In equivocal cases, a deltopectoral approach is however recommended.

A preoperative planning checklist is given in Table 37-2. Careful patient positioning and preoperative verification of adequate radiographic imaging are important to allow for accurate intraoperative assessment of fracture reduction and hardware placement. Clearance of the humeral head and glenoid from underlying radiopaque structures should be assured. EKG leads, side rails, and tubing may interfere with obtaining an unobstructed radiographic view of the fracture during surgery.

A detailed understanding of the implant is important to allow adequate plate and screw placement. Too proximal plate placement should be avoided, as it will lead to subacromial impingement. The plate should be placed to allow for two screws to be directed from the plate toward the inferomedial aspect of the humeral head. Furthermore, the plate should be positioned in such a way that it does not impinge on the long head of the biceps. Varying distances from the bicipital groove will be recommended depending on the selected implant.

Plate length should be selected on the basis of the comminution at the metadiaphyseal level. While there is no biomechanical data regarding how many diaphyseal screws should be used we routinely use three bicortical screws. In fractures with extensive diaphyseal extension customized plates may have to be specifically ordered to achieve this goal.

Positioning. Adequate patient positioning will allow unhindered fracture reduction, fluoroscopic visualization, and implant placement. Fluoroscopic AP and lateral views are per-

TABLE 37-2	**Open Reduction and Internal Fixation**

Preoperative Planning Checklist

- OR Table: Standard (beach chair) or radiolucent table (supine)
- Position/positioning aids:
  Beach chair: Head holder/shoulder positioner, hip positioner at thigh. Waist flexed 45 degrees, knees bent 30 degrees.
  Supine: Bump under ipsilateral scapula, rotating the trunk 30 degrees toward the injured side. Use of a plexiglass sheet under patients torso and protruding 30 cm of lateral border of the table underneath the injured shoulder may aid in positioning, especially on narrow radiolucent tables and with large patients.[129]
  Shoulders draped free to the level of medial scapular border
- Fluoroscopy location:
  Beach chair: At head of patient, coming in line with long axis of the bed.
- Supine on radiolucent table (Jackson): Entering perpendicular to table from opposite to operative extremity.
- Equipment:
  Large- and small-pointed reduction clamps (Weber)
  Power wire driver and drill
  Proximal humerus plating system (locking and nonlocking screws)
  2.5-mm terminally threaded Kirschner wires
  2.5/4.0 mm Schantz pins
  3.5 cannulated screw set
  Small drill or wire sleeve
  Small bone hook
  Blunt narrow periosteal elevator, bone tamp
  Mallet

formed before draping to confirm adequate visualization and accurately identify anatomic landmarks and fracture fragments.

ORIF can be performed in the beach chair position or supine on a radiolucent table.

Beach Chair Position. The beach chair position is most easily obtained with a special shoulder positioner that includes a head holder (Fig. 37-29). The shoulder should be accessible to the level of the medial border of the scapula posteriorly and the angle of the jaw superiorly. The bed is flexed 45 degrees at the waist and the knees bent 30 degrees. The C-arm is positioned at the head of the patient entering along the side of the table. Draping of the iliac crest should be performed if autograft is required (Fig. 37-29).

In the beach chair position, the use of a specialized arm holder may be of help in positioning the upper extremity during imaging, fracture manipulation and plate placement. This is particularly useful if the procedure is performed with only one assistant (Fig. 37-30). Alternatively, a padded Mayo stand can be used.

Supine Position. In the supine position, the torso may be tilted 30 degrees toward the injured side using a bump or wedge. A 70 × 40 × 1 cm plexiglass sheet may be placed under the patient's torso so that it protrudes about 30 cm under the injured extremity. This allows the patient's flank to be placed in line with the lateral border of the table, while supporting

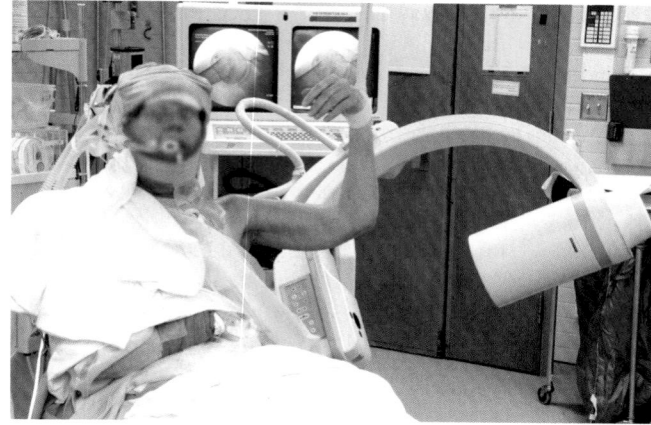

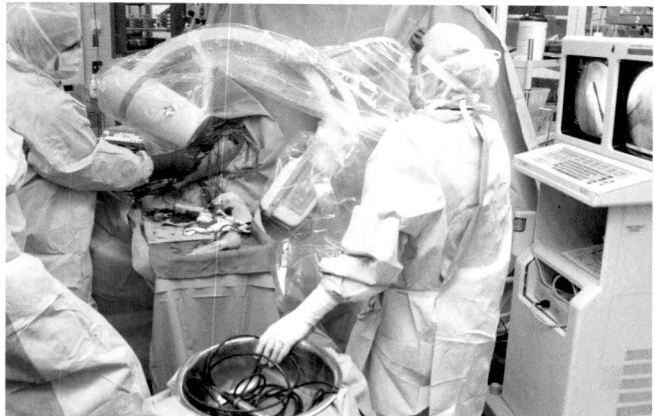

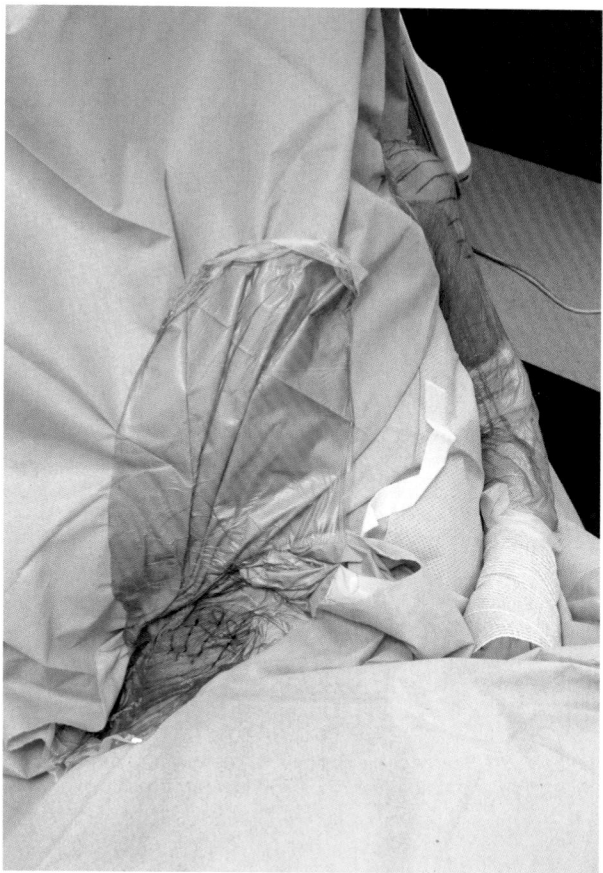

FIGURE 37-29 Patient positioning. Beach chair. **A:** A head holder is required to safely maintain control of the head during surgery. Intraoperative imaging can be obtained with a mini-C-arm (as seen) or a standard C-arm. **B and C:** If iliac crest bone graft is required as in this surgical neck nonunion, the contralateral iliac crest is prepared and draped. Intraoperative imaging can be obtained with a mini-C-arm (as seen) or a standard C-arm.

the arm during surgery.[129] When the supine position is used on a radiolucent tabletop such as the Jackson OSI, the C-arm is ideally brought in perpendicular to the table from the opposite side. When a cantilever-type radiolucent table is used, the image intensifier is best placed parallel to the operating table.

Surgical Approach. Either the deltopectoral approach or a deltoid-splitting approach may be used.

Technique. The surgical technique is outlined in Table 37-3. Once the fracture site has been identified, the fracture lines should be exposed by limited periosteal elevation to allow assessment of fracture reduction. Careful preservation of the soft tissues is important for two reasons. Firstly it will reduce the risk of AVN and nonunion and secondly it will facilitate fracture reduction, by leaving intact periosteal sleeves to guide fragment position. The ultimate goal of proximal fracture fixation is to achieve stability of the reduced fragments. This is achieved by reducing the medial aspect of the surgical or anatomic neck and by approximating the tuberosities around the humeral head. Once this is achieved the hardware will function by sharing the load with the reconstructed proximal humerus, rather than having to support and bear the weight on its own.

TABLE 37-3 **Open Reduction and Internal Fixation**

Surgical Technique

- Verify adequate fluoroscopic visualization of AP and lateral views
- Expose proximal humerus
- Identify and tag tuberosities through cuff tendons
- Reduce humeral head
- Reduce tuberosities
- Manipulate shaft to reduce surgical neck
- Obtain temporary fixation with pins and transtendinous sutures
- Confirm reduction
- Place plate lateral to biceps groove and sufficiently inferior to avoid subacromial impingement
- Place two proximal screws
- Place single shaft screw
- Verify correction of apex anterior angulation at surgical neck
- Place second shaft screw
- Complete proximal and distal fixation
- Thread tuberosity sutures through plate holes and tie
- Confirm adequate screw length, stability, and absence of impingement with live fluoroscopy
- Irrigate and close

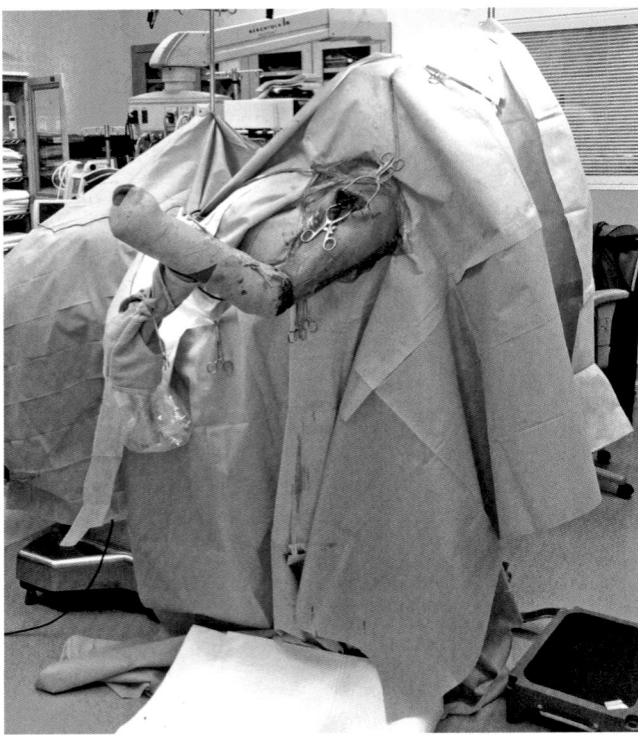

FIGURE 37-30 Beach chair position for deltoid-splitting approach. The use of an arm holder can aid in intraoperative positioning.

Once preliminary fixation has been achieved, AP and lateral views are obtained by turning the arm in a 90-degree arc. Reduction of the medial proximal humeral metaphysis should be carefully confirmed as well as the correction of an apex anterior deformity at the level of the surgical neck. A plate is then selected to allow at least three screws to be placed into the distal shaft segment. The plate position is also selected to avoid subacromial impingement[135] and to allow two screws to be placed into inferomedial aspect of the humeral head. In the sagittal plane, the plate is placed posterior to the biceps tendon to avoid impingement with this structure and to allow adequate positioning of screws into the humeral head (Fig. 37-33). Once final plate placement has been defined, two locking screws are placed into the proximal segment. Rotational alignment is again verified and a single screw is placed into the shaft segment. At this point, angular correction will still be possible through rotation around this single shaft screw. Final verification of adequate reduction of angulation of the surgical neck is performed on the lateral view and a second shaft screw is placed. Subsequently, a minimum of five or six screws are routinely placed into the proximal segment. Screw placement should be performed by drilling through the near cortex only and then using a depth gauge as a sound until subchondral bone is palpated. This avoids inadvertent perforation of the articular surface, theoretically reducing the possibility of secondary screw penetration.[26] While biomechanical studies have suggested that

Identifying the biceps tendon will aid in locating the bicipital groove and correlating its position with the fracture morphology as shown on the preoperative images. Reduction of the tuberosities is achieved by placing strong sutures through the distal tendons of the rotator cuff for fragment manipulation. The greater tuberosity is controlled by two separate sutures placed into the infra- and supraspinatus tendons, while the lesser tuberosity is controlled with a suture placed through the subscapularis tendon (Fig. 37-31). Reduction of the humeral head is obtained by correcting varus–valgus angulation. In three- and four-part valgus-impacted fractures, the humeral head has to be disimpacted from the lateral proximal humeral metaphysis (Fig. 37-32). This should be done with gentle manipulation using an elevator though the split between the greater and lesser tuberosities, while longitudinal traction on the arm is applied. Once the position of the head has been corrected, the tuberosities can be reduced to their anatomic positions. In three-part greater tuberosity fractures, manipulation of the subscapularis allows for correction of an internal rotation deformity of the humeral head, while an elevator may be used to correct a flexion deformity. Temporary K-wire fixation is frequently used for initial stabilization of the fracture fragments. These may follow patterns similar to those of percutaneous pin fixation and should be outside of the planned position of the plate. In two-part proximal humeral fractures a K-wire placed into the shaft segment anterior to the biceps tendon can be helpful as a temporary anchor to tension the rotator traction sutures and provide preliminary fixation.

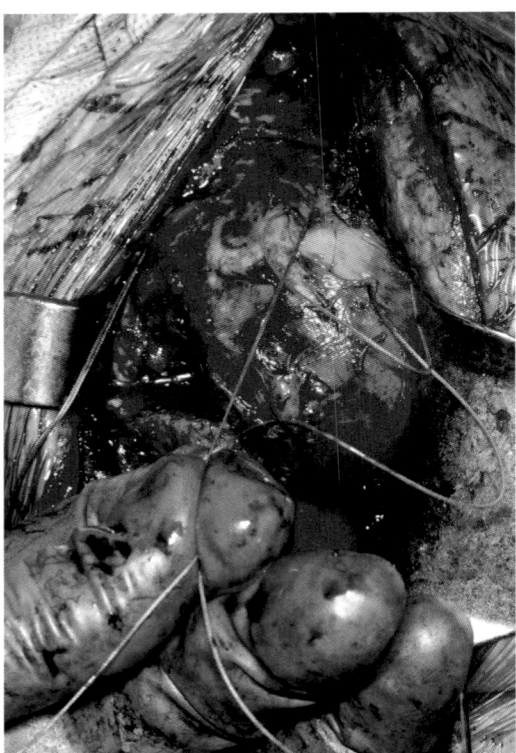

FIGURE 37-31 Sutures through the rotator cuff tendons can aid in obtaining control of the proximal fragments. Incorporation of sutures into the final construct may provide additional stability.

the screw tips be placed in subchondral bone to achieve great-est stability,[243] it is recommended that shorter screws be used to decrease the risk of late head penetration and glenoid dam-age[191] (Fig. 37-28).

Several reduction techniques have been described to achieve adequate fracture reduction. One of these involves the use of a 2- or 2.7-mm K-wire placed through the most proximal hole of the plate into the humeral head. The K-wire is then used to manipulate the head until adequate alignment has been achieved and the plate fixed onto the proximal segment.[332] This technique requires a good understanding of where to place the K-wire as it will define plate position in both the craniocaudal dimension and in the sagittal plane. Nonlocking screws can be

used to pull the shaft segment onto the plate, thereby aiding in correcting any residual malalignment and achieving cortical plate apposition.

Once the plate and screws have been placed transtendinous sutures are tied onto the plate to provide additional fixation (Fig. 37-34). Most modern plate designs offer special holes for this purpose. The fracture is then taken through functional range of motion of the shoulder to confirm stability and absence of impingement. Under live fluoroscopy, screw position should be carefully checked to rule out humeral head perforation.

The use of IM fibular strut grafting has been described to improve stability of varus-impacted fractures in which the medial calcar may not be reliably reconstructed. Several techniques have

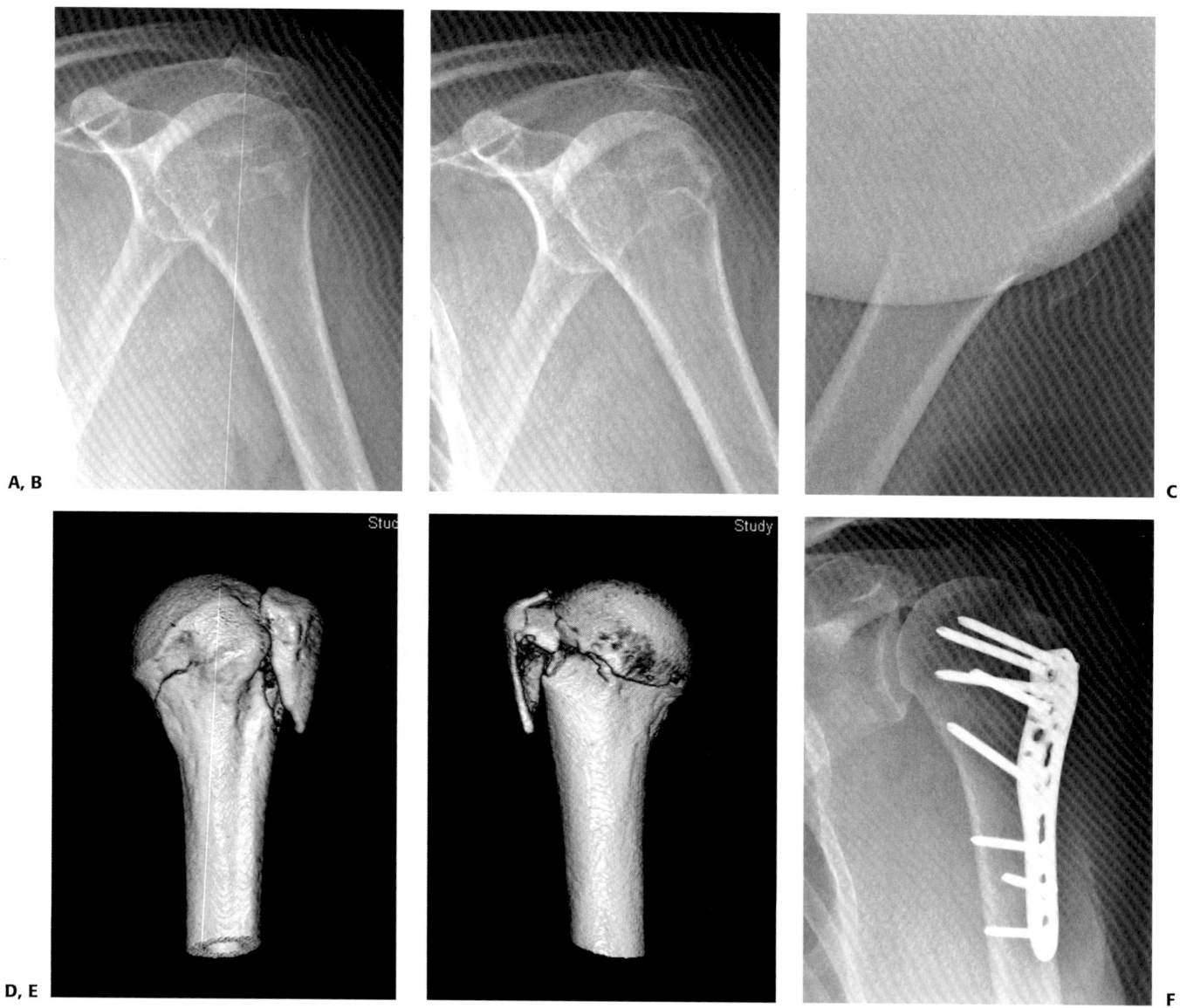

A, B
C
D, E
F

FIGURE 37-32 Three-part greater tuberosity proximal humerus in a 42-year-old female. **A, B, C:** Subtle displacement at the inferomedial aspect of the humeral neck differentiates this injury from a two-part greater tuberosity fracture. **D and E:** 3D reconstructions confirming fracture geometry.

(continues)

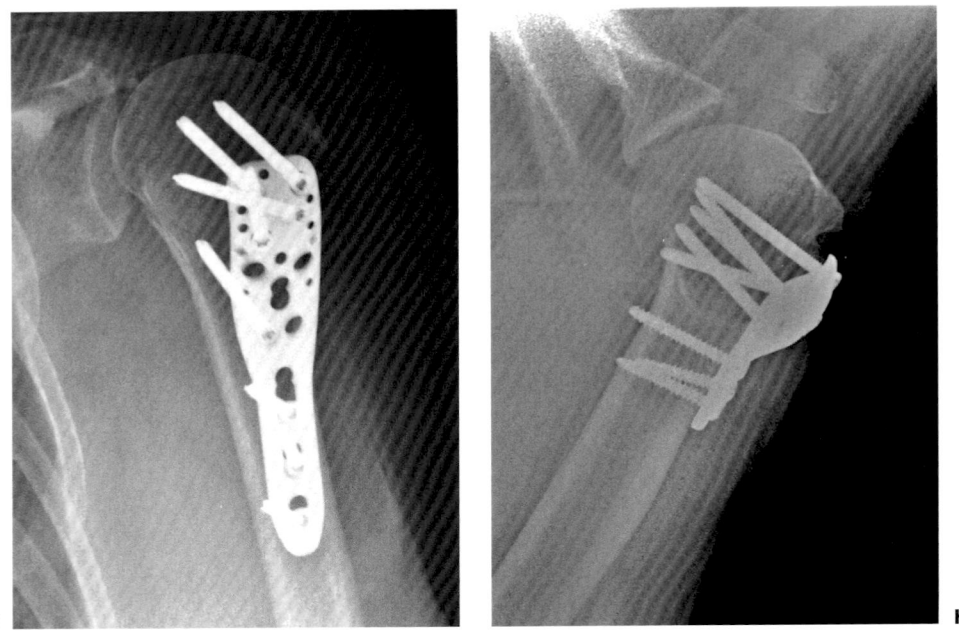

G

H

FIGURE 37-32 (*continued*) **F–H:** Final reduction and fixation. Note residual impaction of the lateral anatomic neck.

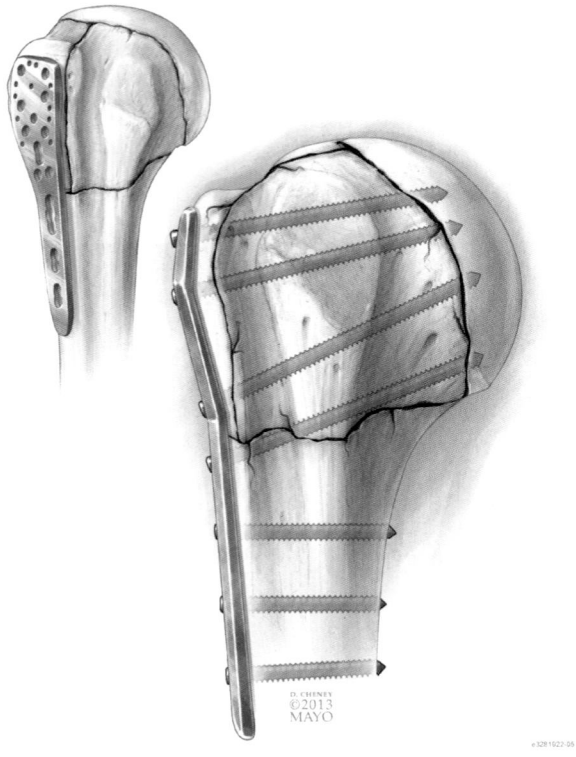

FIGURE 37-33 Ideal plate placement. Multiple plate designs are available. Plate position should avoid impingement onto the bicipital groove and allow placement of three bicortical screws at the level of the humeral shaft and proximal screw(s) into the medial calcar region of the proximal humerus.

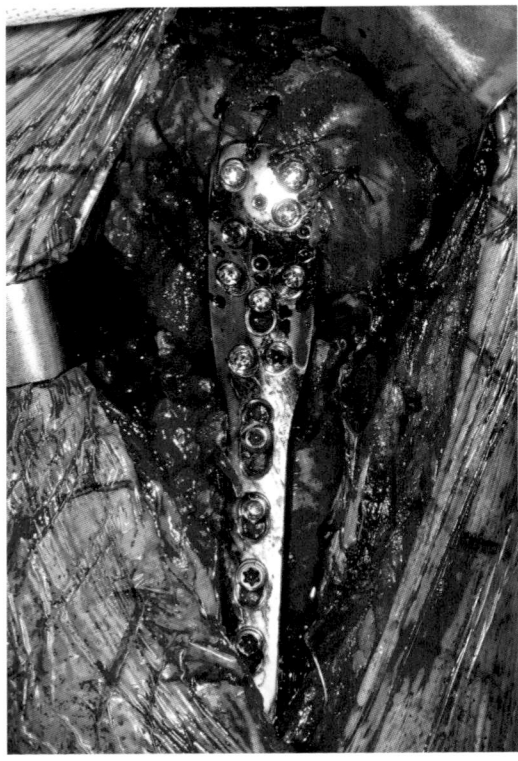

FIGURE 37-34 Final plate placement through a deltopectoral approach. Note transtendinous sutures threaded through the plate to reinforce the construct.

been described, with the common goal being to create a buttress at the inferior aspect of the anatomic neck to prevent delayed varus collapse[13,64,130,288] (Fig. 37-35).

If a minimally invasive approach is selected using a deltoid split, distal screw fixation into the humeral shaft is achieved through stab incisions. These should be placed in such a manner that injury to the axillary nerve is avoided. This has also to be taken into account for screw placement into the inferior aspect of the proximal segment, as screw trajectory may

be in line with the axillary nerve.[338,349,375] Special aiming jigs have been developed to aid with plate insertion and safe screw placement.[338,349]

Postoperative Care. Patients are followed at 2 weeks, 6 weeks, and 3 months after surgery. Patients are immobilized for 6 weeks in a sling while active range-of-motion exercises of the elbow, wrist, and hand are encouraged. Depending on the fracture pattern and stability that was achieved, passive range

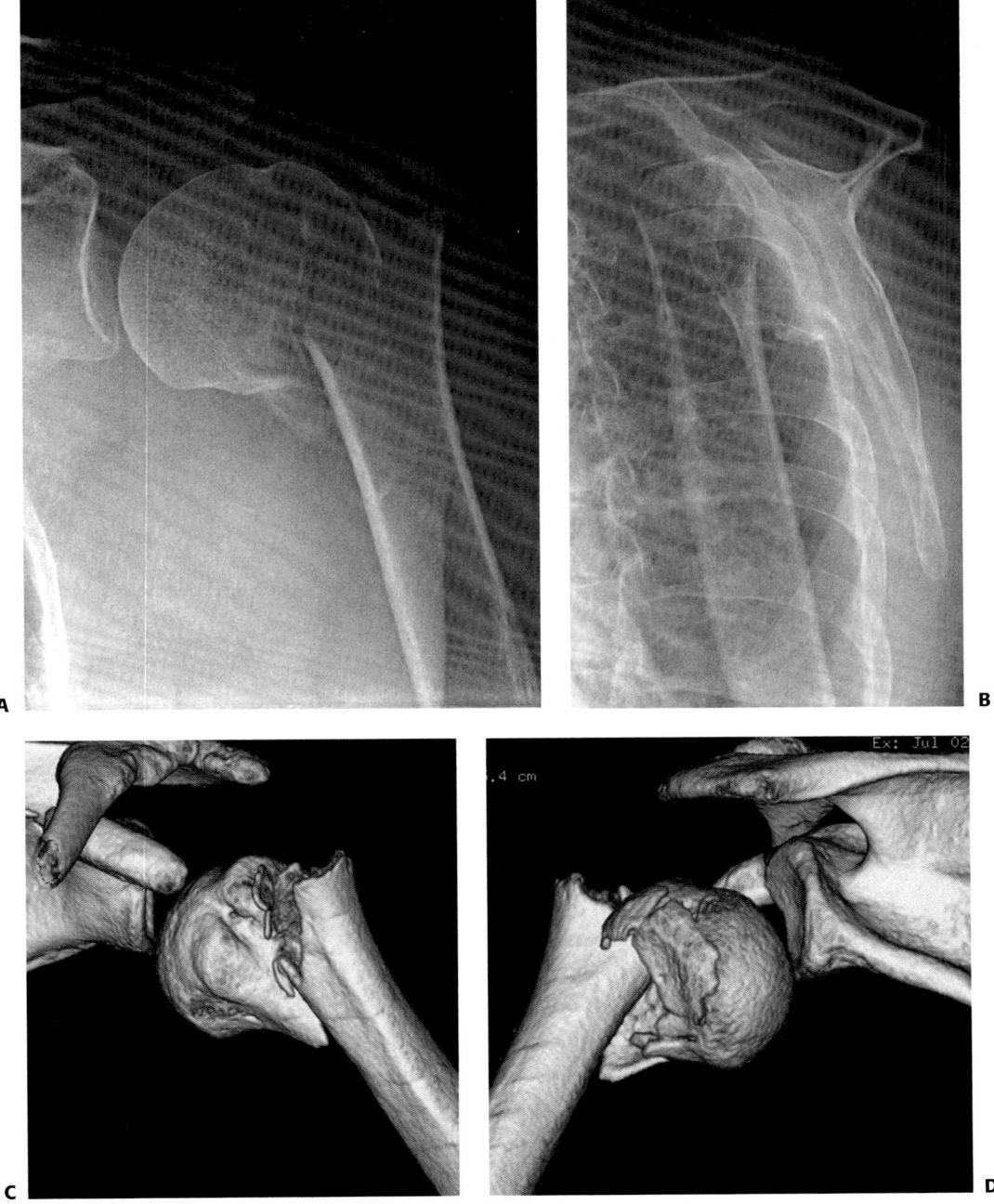

FIGURE 37-35 A, B, C: Thirty-two-year old male with a high-energy two-part surgical neck fracture of the proximal humerus. **D:** Posteromedial comminution is present, raising concern about possible delayed displacement after fixation.

(*continues*)

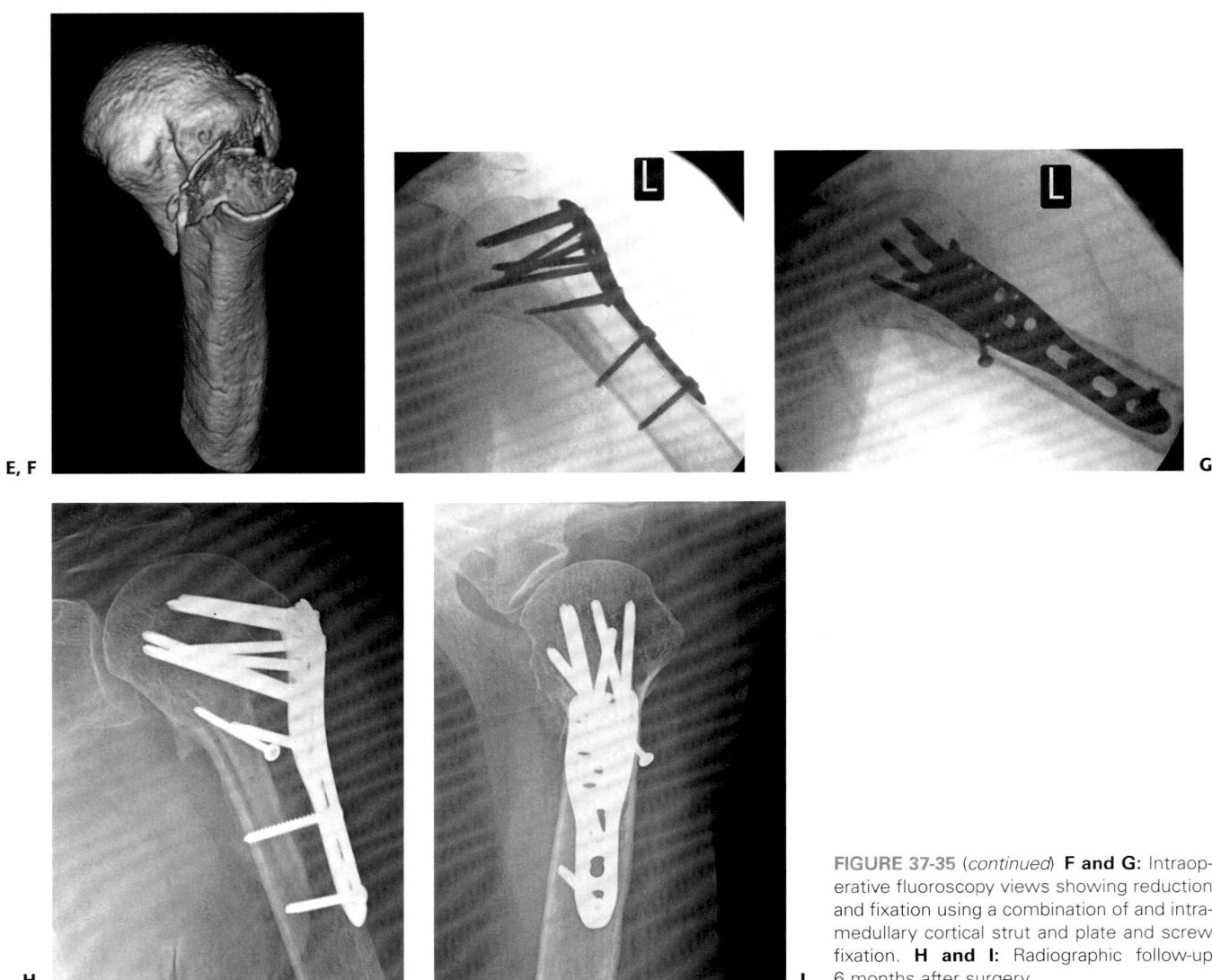

FIGURE 37-35 (*continued*) **F and G:** Intraoperative fluoroscopy views showing reduction and fixation using a combination of and intramedullary cortical strut and plate and screw fixation. **H and I:** Radiographic follow-up 6 months after surgery.

of motion is started between 2 and 4 weeks after surgery with forward elevation, external rotation, and pendulum exercises. If healing has adequately progressed both clinically and radiographically at 6 weeks active-assisted range of motion is started.

Potential Pitfalls and Preventive Measures. These are listed in Table 37-4. Despite their theoretical advantages, recent data has shown that locking plates can carry a significant rate of complications including screw back out, screw cut out, plate failure, malunion, and nonunion[52,67,101,263,305,342,388,373,378,397] which frequently require reoperation.[62,105,178] Several factors have been associated with loss of reduction with locking plates, including preoperative varus deformity, advanced age, smoking, varus malreduction, failure to incorporate the rotator cuff to the construct with tension bands, and inadequate medial support.[4,135,218,232,239,268,279,302,303,304,305,378,360,377]

Südkamp et al. found that over half of complications associated with proximal humeral locking plate fixation occurred intraoperatively. Primary screw perforation of the humeral head was the most common complication. The frequency of screw penetration was increased in cases of fracture collapse and secondary penetration[388] (Fig. 37-36). Careful selection of screw length is therefore advised. Furthermore inadvertent head penetration while drilling should be avoided as this creates a path for easier head perforation.[67]

Gardner et al.[135] demonstrated the impact that the absence of medial support has on subsequent loss of reduction, increased rate of screw perforation, and overall loss of height by critical retrospective appraisal of radiographs of proximal humeral fractures treated with locked plates. The importance of the medial support was also demonstrated in a study by Yang et al. who showed that in a prospective observational study of 64 consecutive patients treated with a locking proximal humerus plate, those with an intact medial support had significantly better functional outcomes at 1 year (Constant score of 81 [medial support] vs. 65 [no medial support], $p = 0.002$).[423]

TABLE 37-4 **Open Reduction and Internal Fixation**

Potential Pitfalls and Preventions

Pitfall	Preventions
Vascular disruption of the proximal humerus	Careful dissection. Atraumatic manipulation of the humeral head, especially in four-part fractures. Minimize medial retraction around the humeral neck.
Malreduction	Sequential confirmation of adequate reduction in two planes under fluoroscopic vision.
Subacromial impingement	Verify plate placement using guides and fluoroscopic vision. Confirm placement after preliminary fixation and before definitive screw placement. Achieve adequate tuberosity reduction.
Head screw perforation/penetration	Avoid self-drilling screws. Drill through lateral cortex only, use depth gauge as sound, stopping at subchondral bone. Select a screw 4 mm shorter than measured.
Loss of fixation	Achieve reduction of medial humeral metaphysis. Confirm adequate placement in the sagittal plane to enable correct screw placement into humeral head. Achieve adequate reduction of tuberosities. Incorporate sutures around rotator cuff tendons into plate construct. Select appropriate screw length and number both into the head and into the shaft. Assure adequate engagement of locking screw into plate.
Glenoid erosion from perforating/ penetrating screws	Intraoperatively, detailed assessment of screws in humeral head under "live" dynamic fluoroscopic view. Postoperatively, careful monitoring of head subsidence and possible cut out. Early screw removal if penetrating.
Axillary nerve injury	If using deltoid split, place stay sutures to avoid inadvertent distal propagation of window. During percutaneous screw placement avoid high risk holes. Verify plate placement underneath the axillary nerve before initial screw placement.

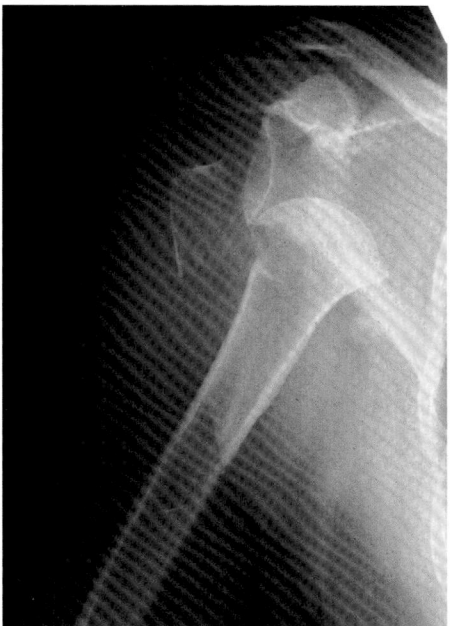
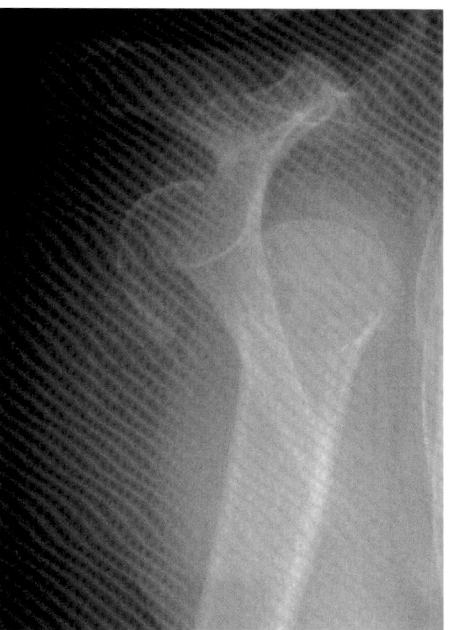

A   B

FIGURE 37-36 A–I: Thirty-six-year old male with four-part valgus-impacted fracture dislocation of the right proximal humerus managed with open reduction and locking plate fixation.

(continues)

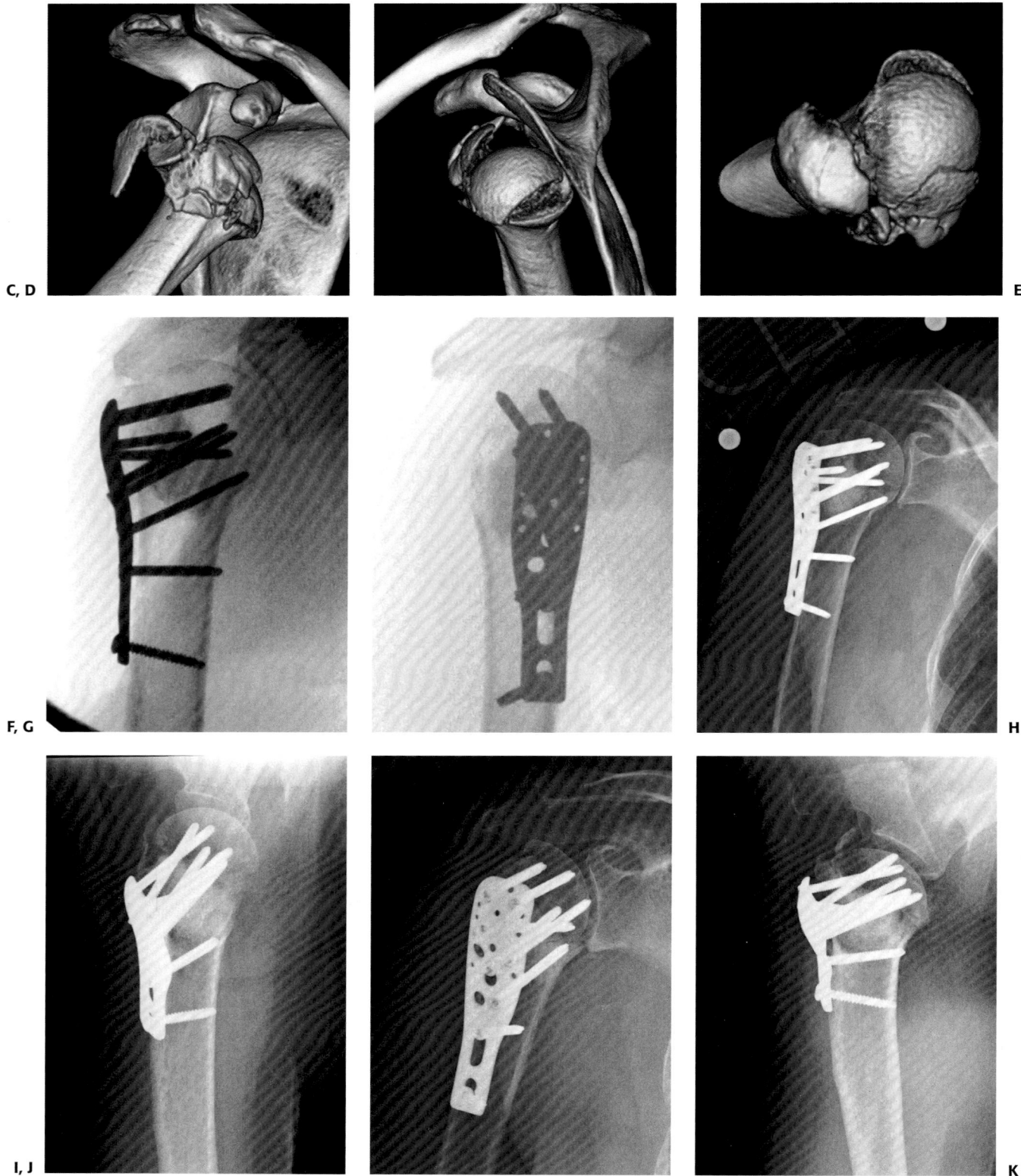

FIGURE 37-36 (*continued*) **J–M:** At 8 months head collapse leads to secondary screw penetration. **N–Q:** After removal of hardware progressive head collapse occurs with severe humeral head necrosis.

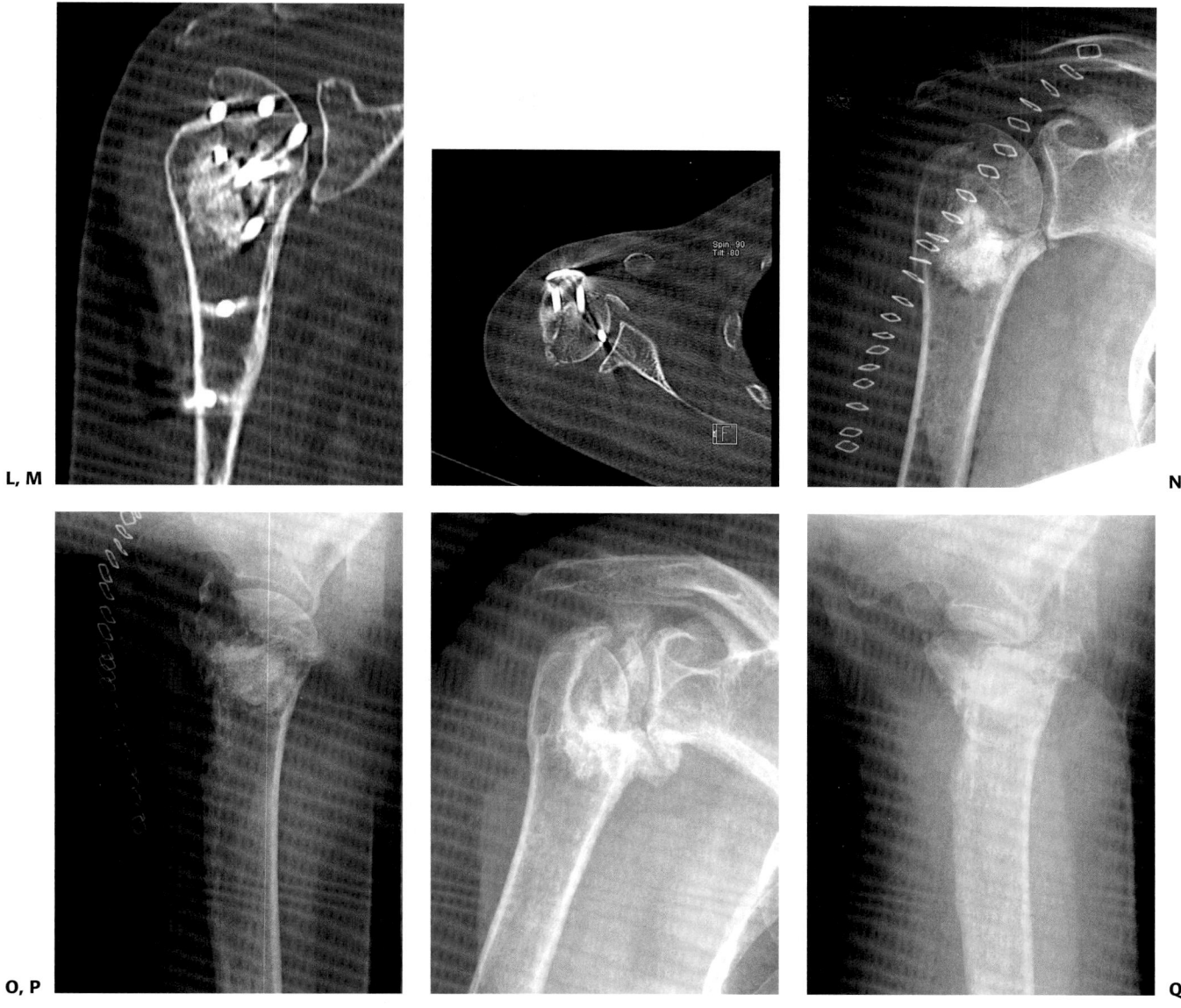

L, M

N

O, P

Q

FIGURE 37-36 (*continued*)

Treatment-Specific Outcomes. Tables 37-5 and 37-6 detail the outcomes for plate and screw fixation of proximal humeral fractures in a number of studies. Table 37-5 shows the results in a number of published studies and Table 37-6 shows the main complications in the same studies. It shows that despite the advent of locking plates, complications after plate and screw fixation of proximal humerus fracture continue to be high. Complications of varus collapse and hardware loosening of conventional screws and plates appear to have been replaced by screw penetration and cutout in locked plates.[388,389] Several studies report good-to-excellent outcomes after locked plate fixation,[52,114,151,209,226,388,406,426] but others report only fair results.[178,279,300] Interestingly, some studies have shown no advantage of locked plate fixation over nonoperative treatment of displaced proximal humeral fractures with regard to range

of motion and functional scores.[299,348] Similar outcomes have also been reported for treatment using intamedullary nail fixation,[151] whereas others have shown significantly better ASES scores, pain scores, and strength after locked plate fixation, with the disadvantage of higher complication rates.[426] Furthermore, similar results have been reported between ORIF and hemiarthroplasty in complex proximal humeral fractures, as long as adequate reduction and stable fixation is achieved after ORIF.[21] Other authors have however found significantly higher Constant scores after locked plate fixation than after hemiarthroplasty.[378] According to the most recent Cochrane Review, little evidence exists to support ORIF versus other treatment modalities in displaced proximal humeral fractures.[157]

Several ongoing studies are comparing the results of ORIF with nonoperative treatment as well as arthroplasty.[48,156,229,403]

| TABLE 37-5 | Published Results of the Treatment of Proximal Humeral Fractures with Plates. Where Possible the Fracture Types are Defined by the Neer Classification with Two-, Three- and Four-Part Fractures and Fracture Dislocation (FD) and Head-Splitting (HS) Fractures |

Authors	Technique	Fracture Type (Neer parts) 2 3 4 FD HS	Age (years) Mean (Range)	Follow-up (months) Mean (Range)	Outcome Scores	Results
Esser[202,233]	Plate	0 17 8 6	55 (19–62)	74 (12–144)	ASES	92% Ex/Good
Hessmann et al.[171]	Plate	50 37 11 5	(30–80)	34 (24–72)	Constant	69% Ex/Good
Hinterman et al.[176]	Blade plate	0 31 7	72 (52–92)	41 (29–54)	Constant	79% Ex/Good
Wijgman et al.[415]	Plate/ wire	0 22 11 27	48 (19–79)	120 (48–264)	Constant	87% Ex/Good
Wanner et al.[412]	Plate	10 33 17	62 (17–89)	17 (6–42)	Constant	Fair (average)
Machani et al.[253]	Locking plate	19 37 6	61 (19–76)	19 (11–39)	HSS	60% Ex/Good
Meier et al.[263]	Plate	4 13 19	69 (23–88)	22 (13–28)	Constant	Fair (average)
Hirschmann et al.[178]	Locking plate	31 47 41	68	12	Constant	Fair (average)
Moonot et al.[279]	Locking plate	0 20 12	60 (18–87)	11 (3–24)	Constant	Fair (average)
Laflamme et al.[226]	Locking plate	17 10 0 (Valgus fractures)	64 (38–88)	19 (12–34)	Constant/ UCLA	Good (average)
Helwig et al.[164]	Locking plate	34 38 8 7	64 (16–93)	27 (12–73)	Constant/ UCLA/DASH	60% Ex/Good
Brunner et al.[52]	Locking plate	45 66 35 7 4	65 (19–94)	84% for 1 year	Constant	Good (average)
Südkamp et al.[388]	Locking plate	187	63	83% for 1 year	Constant	Good (average)
Gradl et al.[151]	Locking plate	26 30 16 4	63	12 (12–14)	Constant/DASH	Good (average)
Olerud et al.[300]	Locking plate	50 0 0	75 (55–93)	24	Constant/DASH	Fair (average)
Yang et al.[423]	Locking plate	8 32 24	62	18 (14–38)	Constant	48% Ex/Good
Zhu et al.[426]	Locking plate	26 0 0	51	36	Constant/ASES	Excellent (average)
Röderer et al.[340]	Locking plate	107	66 (18–91)	10 (6–12)	IADL	
Olerud et al.[299]	Locking plate	0 27 0	72 (56–92)	24 minimum	Constant/DASH/ EG-5D	Fair (average)
Voigt et al.[406]	Locking plate	0 48 8	74 (60–87)	86% for 1 year	Constant/SST/ DASH	Good (average)
Konrad et al.[209]	Locking plate	153	65	86% for 1 year	Constant/Neer	Excellent (average)
Fjalestad et al.[114]	Locking plate	0 13 12	72 (60–86)	12	Constant/ASES	Good (average)
Fankhauser et al.[110]	Locking plate	AO/OTA A (4) B(15) C(9)	64 (28–82)	12	Constant	Good (average)

These will help to guide the orthopedic surgeon in the treatment of proximal humeral fractures.

Tension Band Fixation

Tension band fixation has been used in the treatment of proximal humeral fractures for several decades.[285] Several techniques of tension band fixation have been described in the literature using steel wire or either absorbable monofilament or nonabsorbable braided suture.[74,85,92,162,169,185,231,295,311,428] While tension band fixation is most frequently used as an adjunct to plates and screw fixation, IM nailing, and arthroplasty,[12,74,85,169,219,310,407] satisfactory clinical outcomes can be obtained when used as the sole fixation method.[74,85,92,162,169,185,231,295,311,428]

The main goal of tension band fixation is the neutralization of tension forces generated by the rotator cuff at the level of the tuberosities, and bending at the level of the surgical neck. Based on the load-sharing properties of tension band fixation, neutralization of tension forces on the surface of the proximal humerus will generate compression between fragments during motion, thereby promoting healing and allowing early rehabilitation. As described by Hertel, the humeral head can be conceptualized as a thin shell of subchondral bone with negligible bony structure inside its volume. Stabilization of this fragment in multifragmentary proximal humeral fractures relies mainly on peripheral loading of the rim of the head onto the surrounding tuberosities, in the same manner an empty eggshell can be

TABLE 37-6 — The Complications Published in the Papers Detailed in Table 37-5

%

Authors	Technique	Revision Surgery	AVN	Implant Loosening	Joint Penetration	Infection Deep	Infection Super	Nerve Injury	Nonunion	OA	Dislocation	Malunion	Subacromial Impingement
Esser[202,233]	Plate	0	0	4									16
Hessmann et al.[171]	Plate	9	4			3		1	1			15	
Hinterman et al.[176]	Blade plate	21	5			3				8		8	
Wijgman et al.[415]	Plate/wire	0	37										3
Wanner et al.[412]	Plate	12	3	5							2		3
Meier et al.[263]	Plate	28	0	25			6					3	
Machani et al.[253]	Locking plate	0	0	13		10	8	3					
Hirschmann et al.[178]	Locking plate	22	3	4			1		2				12
Moonot et al.[279]	Locking plate	13	3	9				3	3			6	3
Laflamme et al.[226]	Locking plate	7	0									33	
Helwig et al.[164]	Locking plate	0	17	16	13	6			1				3
Brunner et al.[52]	Locking plate	25	8	40		1	1	3					2
Südkamp et al.[388]	Locking plate	19	4	12	21	2	1	2					
Gradl et al.[151]	Locking plate	13	3	7	8							12	
Olerud et al.[300]	Locking plate	16	0	19	28	2							2
Yang et al.[423]	Locking plate	13	3	5	8	3							3
Zhu et al.[426]	Locking plate	19	0		19								
Röderer et al.[340]	Locking plate	33	5	9	19				3				
Olerud et al.[299]	Locking plate	30	10	39	29	7			4				7
Voigt et al.[406]	Locking plate	21	10		27							17	
Konrad et al.[209]	Locking plate	16	1	23	15	1	1	1					
Fjalestad et al.[114]	Locking plate	16	8	4	28			12					
Fankhauser et al.[110]	Locking plate	8	8	8	4			8				12	12

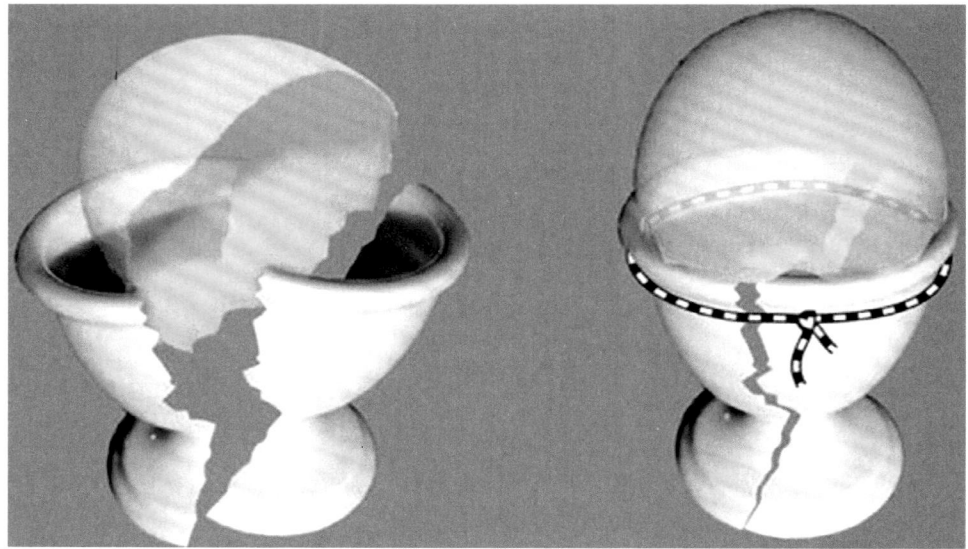

A   B

FIGURE 37-37 From Hertel[169]. In proximal humerus fractures, the tuberosities hold the humeral head in a manner similar to an egg cup holding the shell of an egg. By restoring stability between the two broken shells of the cup (greater and lesser tuberosity fragments-**A**), the head can theoretically be held without major fixation to the head being required **(B)**.

held in an egg cup.[169] In most instances in which the anatomic neck of the proximal humerus is affected, the tuberosities are separated, and hence the egg cup is broken. The purpose of tension band fixation is to create a cohesive egg cup by linking the tuberosities against each other thereby allowing support to the humeral head (Fig. 37-37).[169]

The main challenge is to place the sutures or wires of the tension band through tissue that will resist loading of the proximal humerus during early rehabilitation. While some authors have described transosseous placement of wires or sutures, this may fail, especially in elderly, osteoporotic patients. Placement of sutures into the stronger distal segment of the rotator cuff tendons should provide more secure fixation.

The main advantage of tension band fixation is the minimal amount of hardware that is required. This can potentially reduce the risk of implant-related subacromial impingement. Furthermore, if used as the sole method of fixation, no risk of penetration into the humeral head exists. However, compared to percutaneous techniques, tension band fixation requires open fracture exposure, thereby theoretically increasing the risk of soft tissue damage.

Preoperative Planning. A preoperative planning checklist is shown in Table 37-7. It summarizes the important aspects of preoperative planning. Preoperative planning of tension band fixation not only requires an understanding of the concepts explained in the section on plate fixation but it also requires a clear understanding of the fragmentation of tuberosities and humeral shaft to determine the ideal placement of sutures and wires. As a load-sharing construction, tension band fixation is ideally used in fractures with minimal comminution of the main fracture parts. Several studies however suggest that in four-part valgus-impacted fractures, the head segment can

be left unreduced, while the tuberosities are fixed onto the humeral shaft. Furthermore, comminution of the surgical neck may be managed by impacting the shaft into the humeral head and then proceeding with tension band fixation.

Positioning. Positioning for tension band wire fixation follows the same principles as for plate and screw fixation.

Surgical Approach. Most authors recommend a deltoid-splitting approach for the fixation of two-part greater tuberosity fractures, whereas either a deltopectoral or deltoid-splitting approach can be used for other two-part fractures as well as three- and four-part fractures.

TABLE 37-7	**Tension Band Fixation**

Preoperative Planning Checklist

- OR Table: Standard (beach chair) or radiolucent table (supine)
- Position/positioning aids:
  Beach chair: Head holder/shoulder positioner, hip positioner at thigh. Waist flexed 45 degrees, knees bent 30 degrees.
  Supine: Bump under ipsilateral scapula, rotating the trunk 30 degrees toward opposite side.
  Shoulder draped free to the level of medial scapular border.
- Fluoroscopy location:
  At head of patient, coming in line with long axis of the bed.
- Equipment:
  Power drill
  Heavy suture/wire: Nonabsorbable (#5 polyester, #2 polyethylene; 20-gauge steel wire); absorbable (#2 PDS)
  Large-pointed reduction clamps
  14 gauge colpotomy or spinal needle
  Blunt narrow periosteal elevator, bone tamp
  Mallet

Technique. Several techniques have been described in the literature. Hawkins et al. described tension band wiring for the management of three-part fractures using a deltopectoral approach. After reduction and temporary clamp fixation of the displaced tuberosity fragment onto the head a 14-gauge colpotomy needle is used to pass parallel 20-gauge stainless steel wires through the subscapularis tendon and lesser tuberosity toward the medial aspect of the greater tuberosity posteriorly. The needle thereby penetrates the lateral aspect of the head segment. Each wire is then passed in a figure-of-eight pattern through a separate humeral shaft cortical hole and tied.[162,428]

Ochsner and Ilchman[295] described a tension band technique replacing stainless steel with heavy resorbable polydioxanone (PDS) suture, the theoretical advantage being that future hardware removal was not required. According to their technique, the greater and lesser tuberosities are tagged with separate sutures through their respective rotator cuff tendons and fixed distally through separate cortical holes in the proximal shaft segment.

Flatow et al. described the use of heavy nonabsorbable suture fixation of the greater tuberosity in displaced two-part greater tuberosity fractures. Using a deltoid-splitting approach the greater tuberosity fragment is identified and mobilized. Multiple traction sutures are placed through the rotator cuff for fragment manipulation. The frequently associated rotator cuff tear is repaired and traction sutures placed through cortical bone tunnels in the proximal shaft, thereby reducing the fracture.[116] A similar technique is used for three-part greater tuberosity fractures, in which, using a deltopectoral approach, the head segment is reduced onto the shaft and fixed with heavy nonabsorbable polyester or polyethylene multifilament sutures through the subscapularis and lesser tuberosity proximally and separate cortical holes medial to the biceps tendon distally. The greater tuberosity is then reduced and fixed as described above.[311]

Cornell et al. modified Hawkins' technique by impacting the humeral head segment into the shaft and fixing it with a 6.5-mm screw from the shaft into the subchondral bone in the center of the head. Two tension band constructs are then created with 18-gauge stainless steel wire as described by Hawkins.[74,162]

Darder et al. used a tension band technique in addition to modified K-wires for the treatment of four-part fractures.[85] Three-millimeter K-wires with a 1 mm orifice at one of the ends to allow threading of the tension band wire are placed through the greater and lesser tuberosities into the humeral canal once reduction has been obtained. The tension band wire is then brought through each K-wire and through a cortical hole in the proximal humeral shaft.[85]

A more recent study by Dimakopoulos et al. used transosseous suture fixation for four-part valgus-impacted and three-part greater and lesser tuberosity fractures and two-part greater tuberosity fractures. The procedure was performed through a deltoid split. A total of six sutures were pulled through drill holes established with a 2.7-mm drill bit through each of the fracture parts.[92]

Postoperative Care. Rehabilitation after tension band fixation starts with pendulum exercises for the first 6 weeks

after surgery. Active-assisted range of motion is started thereafter and transitioned to strengthening at 3 months, if clinical and radiographic healing has been established.

Potential Pitfalls and Preventive Measures. A list of potential pitfalls and preventative measures is given in Table 37-8. Complications after tension band fixation include painful steel wire, AVN of the humeral head, infection, and transient axillary neurapraxia. Hawkins reported 2 patients with AVN after the treatment of 14 patients with three-part proximal humeral fractures.[162] Flatow et al. reported one transient neurapraxia in 12 patients undergoing tension band fixation of two-part greater tuberosity fractures through a deltoid-splitting approach. A stay suture had not been placed in this patient, but full recovery was achieved by 9 months after surgery.[116] Ochsner and Ilchmann had two deep infections in 22 patients undergoing tension band fixation with either steel wire or PDS suture. One infection, requiring a subsequent arthrodesis, occurred in 10 patients who underwent fixation with steel wire, while one infection, that resolved with surgical debridement, occurred in 12 patients fixed with PDS suture. A 50% AVN rate was observed. This was unrelated to the type of material used for fixation and was determined primarily by the initial fracture pattern.[295] Other authors have found no AVN when treating two- or three-part fractures.[311] In the largest series on tension band fixation published to date, Dimakopoulos et al. found an AVN rate of 7%. Nonunion occurred in 2% of cases, while malunion was seen in 5%.[92]

Treatment-Specific Outcomes. Hawkins et al. reported that 8 of 15 patients achieved a good result based on Hawkins criteria. Average active elevation and external rotation were 126 degrees and 29 degrees, respectively, ranging from 60 to 170 degrees and from 15 to 60 degrees, respectively.[162] Based on subjective criteria, Flatow et al. reported 12 good or excellent outcomes after the treatment of 12 two-part greater tuberosity fractures, all of which healed.[116] Park showed excellent or satisfactory outcomes based on Neer criteria in 89% of patients treated with tension band fixation who had two-part greater

TABLE 37-8	**Fracture**
Potential Pitfalls and Preventions	
Pitfall	**Preventions**
Construct failure	Multiple suture placement Use of braided heavy nonabsorbable suture
Axillary nerve palsy	Use deltopectoral approach if possible If deltoid split is used, carefully identify the axillary nerve and protect it throughout the procedure. Use a stay suture to avoid inadvertent distal splitting of the deltoid split into the nerve
Painful hardware	Use of suture instead of steel wire

tuberosity or surgical neck, or three-part greater tuberosity fractures. There were no differences in functional outcomes according to fracture classification.[311]

Zyto et al.[428] did not show improved outcomes after tension band fixation compared to nonoperative treatment in displaced three- and four-part proximal humeral fractures Ilchmann et al.[185] found similar results for three-part fractures, while improved function was observed with operative fixation in the case of four-part fractures.[185] In a series of 165 patients with two-, three-, and four-part proximal humeral fractures, Dimakopoulos et al. observed a mean Constant score of 91 5 years after braided nonabsorbable suture tension band fixation. This represented 94% of the function of the contralateral shoulder.[92]

Closed Reduction and Percutaneous Fixation

Closed reduction with percutaneous fixation of proximal humeral fractures has the theoretical advantage of minimizing soft tissue trauma, thereby promoting healing and reducing the risk of AVN of the humeral head. Two-part, three-part, and valgus-impacted four-part fractures of the proximal humerus can be treated with closed reduction and percutaneous fixation (CRPF) by surgeons that have a thorough understanding of the radiographic morphology of the proximal humerus, as assessment of fracture reduction will rely entirely on fluoroscopic imaging. Furthermore, a detailed understanding of the structures at risk of iatrogenic injury is required. These include the cephalic vein and long head of the biceps anteriorly and the axillary nerve on the medial, posterior, lateral, and anterior aspects of the surgical neck.[344] Rowles and McGrory showed in a cadaveric study that, when using a standard pin placement technique, the biceps tendon and cephalic vein may be pierced in 30% and 10% of cases, respectively. Furthermore, pins are located at an average of 3 mm from the anterior branch of the axillary nerve.[344] Similar findings have been confirmed by other authors.[192] Pin placement along established safe windows is therefore required to minimize the risk of iatrogenic neurovascular injury.

Bone quality plays an important role in achieving adequate fixation with CRPF and to avoid pin migration and construct failure.[207,264] Several authors have observed a correlation between pin migration and construct failure with increased age.[113,194] In two-part surgical neck fractures with comminution of the calcar, pin fixation may be insufficient to withstand varus deforming forces and should therefore be avoided. The size of tuberosity fractures and the absence of comminution should be such that percutaneous manipulation can be reliably performed and adequate fixation with pins and screws achieved. Four-part valgus-impacted fractures can be managed with CRPF because of the special morphologic characteristics of this fracture. In this fracture the head has been pushed into valgus, thereby pushing the tuberosities peripherally, and leaving an intact medial hinge between the humeral head and calcar.[187] Furthermore, the tuberosities have a periosteal connection with the humeral shaft. Integrity of the medial hinge and periosteal continuity, in the absence of gross tuberosity migration, are important for CRPF to be successful.

Preoperative Planning. A preoperative planning checklist is given in Table 37-9. Successful CRPF requires a good understanding of fracture morphology and considerable operative experience. AP, axillary, and lateral Y scapula views are essential to understand the fracture pattern. CT images with 3D reconstructions are valuable to clearly establish the amount of fragment involvement and the degree of displacement and comminution. Depending on the fracture pattern, the surgeon should decide whether he or she feels that the best possible result can be offered with CRPF. Patients should be counseled about the risks associated with this specific technique, including axillary nerve injury, pin tract infection and pin migration. A clear understanding of these risks and the requirement for close follow-up for radiographic monitoring are essential for optimal patient compliance. Finally patient age and any risk factors for poor bone stock should be taken into account as they will reduce pin stability and may necessitate either the use of adjuvant stabilization or the use of a different surgical technique.

Positioning. CRPF can be performed in the beach chair position or supine on a radiolucent table. The beach chair position is facilitated by using a special shoulder or head holder. The shoulder should be accessible to the level of the medial border of the scapula posteriorly and the angle of the jaw superiorly. The bed is flexed 45 degrees at the waist and 30 degrees at the knees. In the supine position, the torso is tilted 30 degrees toward the injured side using a bump or wedge, allowing access to the medial border of the scapula and extension of the arm for fracture reduction. Adequate patient positioning will allow

---

TABLE 37-9	**Closed Reduction and Percutaneous Fixation**

Preoperative Planning Checklist

- OR Table: Standard (beach chair) or radiolucent table (supine)
- Position/positioning aids:
  Beach chair: Head holder/shoulder positioner, hip positioner at thigh. Waist flexed 45 degrees, knees bent 30 degrees.
  Supine: Bump under ipsilateral scapula, rotating the trunk 30 degrees toward opposite side.
  Shoulders draped free to the level of medial scapular border.
- Fluoroscopy location:
  Beach chair: At head of patient, coming in line with long axis of the bed.
  Supine: Entering perpendicular to table from opposite to operative extremity.
- Equipment:
  Radiation reduction gloves
  Power wire driver and drill
  2.5-mm terminally threaded Kirschner wires
  3.5-mm cannulated screw set (fully threaded)
  Small drill or wire sleeve
  Small bone hook
  Blunt narrow periosteal elevator, bone tamp
  Mallet

unhindered fracture reduction, fluoroscopic visualization, and implant placement. For the beach chair position, the C-arm is positioned at the head of the patient, while it is placed perpendicular to the table coming in from the opposite side for the supine position. Fluoroscopic AP, axillary, and Y-lateral views are performed before draping to confirm adequate visualization and accurately identify the anatomic landmarks and fracture fragments. It is furthermore recommended that closed reduction maneuvers are trialed before draping to confirm adequate patient positioning.

Surgical Approach. In two-part surgical neck fractures, the procedure may be performed entirely with closed reduction techniques. More complex fractures require strategically placed percutaneous instruments to achieve fragment reduction. An anterior reduction portal is obtained with a 1- to 2-cm skin incision just lateral to the biceps tendon that can be reliably positioned under fluoroscopic guidance on the lateral third of the humerus at the level of the surgical neck.[324] After the skin and deltoid fascia have been incised, the underlying deltoid is bluntly dissected in line with its fibers. Digital palpation can aid in identifying the long head of the biceps. In four-part fractures, the humeral head can be accessed through the split between the greater and lesser tuberosities just lateral to the bicipital groove. The tuberosities may also be manipulated through this incision. A lateral incision just distal to the acromion will allow a small bone hook to be introduced to aid reduction of a medially and posteriorly displaced greater tuberosity. Further reduction may be improved with the use of a ball spike pusher. The axillary nerve may be palpated on the undersurface of the deltoid, through either incision aiding in the safe placement of instruments and implants.

TABLE 37-10 Closed Reduction and Percutaneous Fixation

Surgical Technique

- Take AP external rotation and axillary fluoroscopic views of unaffected shoulder for intraoperative referencing.
- Confirm adequate visualization of fracture in AP, axillary and Neer views, before draping.
- Perform reduction maneuvers before draping, confirming adequate positioning
- After draping identify and draw major landmarks on skin, including expected location of axillary nerve
- Perform close reduction of surgical neck fracture component
- Establish anterior reduction portal if required
- Create distal entry portals for retrograde pins and dissect bluntly onto bone
- Over wire sleeve, transfix surgical neck fracture with two lateral pins and one anterior if required
- Fluoroscopically confirm adequate reduction and fixation
- Reduce tuberosities and fix with pins
- Confirm reduction and fixation
- Replace pins for cannulated screws if planned
- Cut pins short to leave subcutaneously
- Close reduction portal
- Immobilize in sling

Technique. The surgical technique is outlined in Table 37-10. While the technique for closed and percutaneous reduction follows an established pattern, several percutaneous fixation methods have been described in the literature. We will describe the most widely published technique involving fixation using terminally threaded 2.5-mm K-wires placed in several planes.[102,186,187,319,393] Because of concerns about pin migration and insufficient construct stiffness the addition of a mechanism that allows linkage between pins has been studied.[33,59] The purpose is to anchor the pins to avoid migration and provide angular stability to improve implant stiffness. Furthermore, pin guidance through predetermined trajectories has been suggested to improve pin positioning within the strongest bone inside the humeral head.[35,51,94,188,325]

Two-Part Fractures. Two-part surgical neck fractures are reduced by manipulating the distal segment into 80 to 90 degrees of abduction to match the deformity of the proximal segment. Manipulation of the distal segment requires longitudinal traction to oppose the fracture surfaces, and posterior pressure to correct apex anterior angulation. Correction of rotation is then undertaken under fluoroscopic guidance. Rotation is judged by obtaining a perfect profile view of the proximal humerus. With the elbow bent at 90 degrees, the distal segment is aligned with the forearm in 30 degrees of external rotation in relation to the imaging plane. Manipulation of the proximal segment may be performed with the use of percutaneously placed 2.5-mm K-wires or 4.0 Schantz pins. Inability to achieve reduction by closed means may suggest interposition of the long head of the biceps in the fracture site. An anterior percutaneous portal as described above allows palpation of the biceps tendon and release from the fracture site if necessary. Furthermore, a periosteal elevator may be used to shoehorn the proximal segment over the shaft. This maneuver should be done with great care to avoid comminution at the fracture site. Once adequate reduction has been achieved, fracture fixation is obtained with the use of 2.5 mm terminally threaded K-wires. The surgical neck component is usually transfixed with a minimum of three K-wires directed from distal to proximal, placed in two planes at different angulations. Three pins are routinely used, one from anterior to posterior and two from lateral to medial. Anterior pins increase torsional stiffness of the construct and should be added if two lateral pins are deemed to provide insufficient stability.[281] However, anterior pins risk perforating the long head of the biceps or cephalic vein and should therefore be used carefully.[344] Based on biomechanical data, two pins from the tuberosities into the medial proximal humeral cortex can increase construct rigidity compared to retrograde lateral pins alone.[97] To avoid injury to the axillary nerve, lateral pins should enter the humeral cortex at a point at least twice the distance from the upper aspect of the head to the inferior head margin with the wire angulated approximately 45 degrees to the cortical surface. After blunt dissection, to further reduce the risk of neurologic injury, pins should be placed through a sleeve, into the

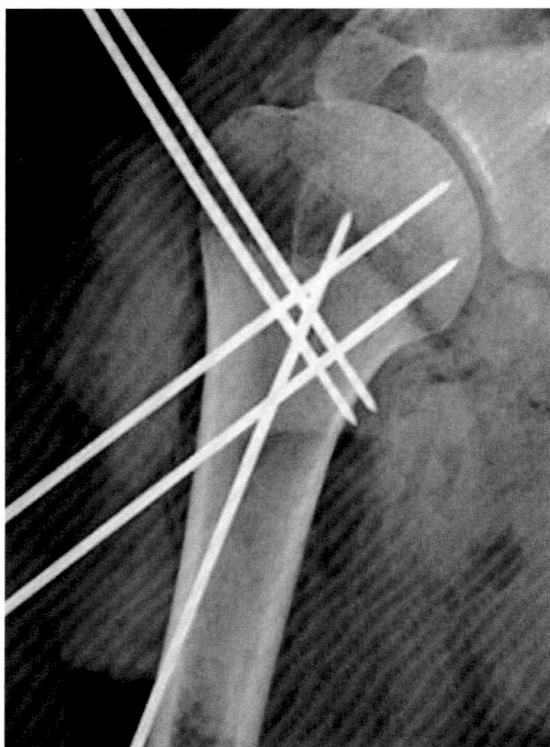

FIGURE 37-38 Typical pin configuration for closed reduction and percutaneous fixation. From Rowles et al.[344]

humeral head in 30 degrees of retroversion. To maximize stability, pins should diverge both at the fracture site and inside the humeral head, and be advanced to the level of the subchondral bone, avoiding penetration of the articular surface[186,196,344] (Fig. 37-38).

Pin placement should be carefully checked fluoroscopically, in both the AP and axillary views with maximum internal and external rotation. Pins directed into the posterior aspect of the humeral tuberosity are at greatest risk of penetrating the articular surface without being detected on fluoroscopy. An AP image with the shoulder in 60 degrees of external rotation has been shown to reliably exclude this.[205]

Three-Part Fractures. Since the great majority of three-part fractures involve a separate greater tuberosity fragment, the head segment is internally rotated. The humeral shaft and head segment are therefore aligned at the surgical neck by placing the arm into adduction and internal rotation. Apex anterior deformity is corrected with a posterior force and K-wires placed as for two-part surgical neck fractures. The arm is then placed into neutral rotation and abduction. A percutaneously placed bone hook is used to secure the greater tuberosity and to reduce it into the correct position. Engagement of the fragment at the rotator cuff insertion site is recommended to reduce the risk of fragmentation. Fixation is achieved with two K-wires placed from the tuberosity and directed into the medial cortex of the proximal humerus. To avoid injury to the axillary nerve at that level, the tip of the K-wire should exit the medial cortex at least 2 cm distal to the most distal aspect of the humeral head.[344] If desired, definitive fixation may be completed by either cutting the wires subcutaneously or by replacing them with cannulated screws.[326] Since interfragmentary compression is not absolutely necessary for fixation, and may increase the risk of secondary fragmentation, fully threaded screws are recommended. This improves stability.

Valgus-Impacted Four-Part Fractures. Reduction of valgus-impacted four-part fractures begins with correcting the lateral tilt of the humeral head. With the shoulder in adduction, a blunt elevator is introduced through the anterior reduction portal. Access to the head is gained through the split between the greater and lesser tuberosities, almost invariably 5 mm behind the bicipital groove. Once coronal alignment of the head has been corrected, the head is fixed with two pins from the distal lateral humeral cortex into the humeral head. By reducing the humeral head, the greater tuberosity will usually regain its anatomic position, tethered by the bridging periosteum distally and the rotator cuff proximally.[326] The greater tuberosity is then fixed either with K wires or cannulated screws (Fig. 37-39). These should be directed into the head proximally and into the shaft distally. The arm is then brought into 70 degrees of abduction and internal rotation to obtain an axillary view of the shoulder to visualize the profile of the anterior proximal humerus. The lesser tuberosity is then controlled with a bone hook and reduced under fluoroscopic guidance into its anatomic position. Provisional fixation with a K wire followed by fixation with an AP screw is obtained. The arm is then mobilized under fluoroscopic visualization to confirm adequate stability. The lateral pins are cut to allow subcutaneous placement.

Postoperative Care. Patients are followed weekly both clinically and radiographically to monitor fracture healing and detect any possible pin migration or skin problems. Patients are immobilized for 3 to 4 weeks in a sling, while active range-of-motion exercises of the elbow, wrist, and hand are encouraged. Passive range of motion is started thereafter with forward elevation, external rotation and pendulum exercises. If healing has adequately progressed at 6 weeks the pins are removed under local anesthesia and active range of motion is started.

Potential Pitfalls and Preventative Measures. A list of potential pitfalls and preventative measures is given in Table 37-11. In elderly patients and in patients with osteoporosis the pins may not gain sufficient bone stability putting the construct at risk of failure. Comminution of the greater tuberosity is a contraindication to CRPF as it will not provide reliable stability with pin or screw fixation alone. A limited open approach using a cerclage suture may be more useful. Calcar comminution in two-part surgical neck fractures may place the construct at risk of varus collapse. IM nailing or locked plate fixation may be preferable in this circumstance. If there is a vascular injury open reduction and fixation should be performed. In patients in whom close postoperative follow-up is unlikely to occur CRPF is contraindicated as weekly radiographs are required.

Careful pin placement is required to avoid iatrogenic injury to the axillary nerve, biceps tendon, cephalic vein, and humeral articular cartilage.

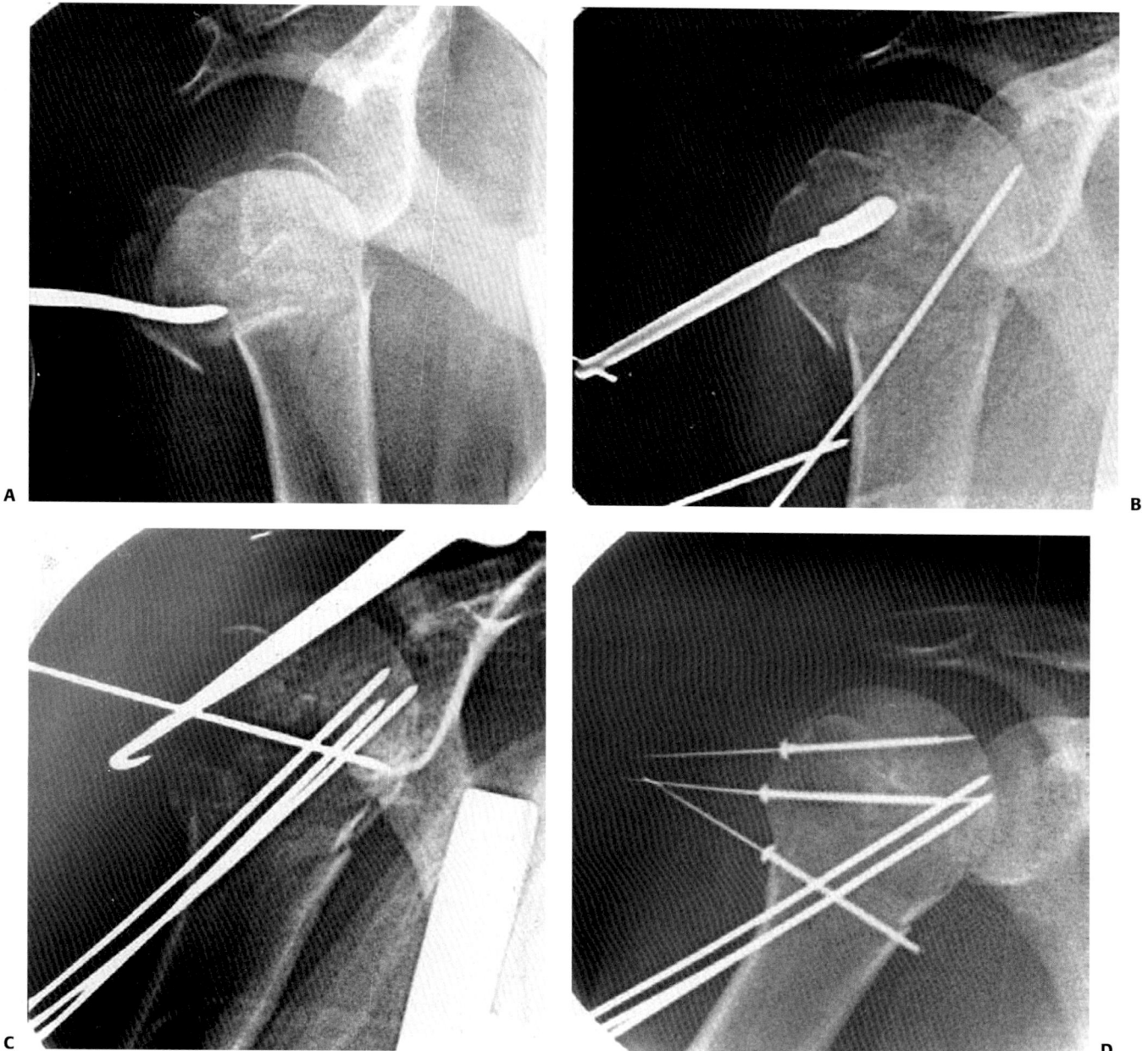

FIGURE 37-39 Valgus-impacted proximal humerus fracture treated with percutaneous reduction and pinning. **A and B:** A periosteal elevator is introduced between the greater and lesser tuberosity fragments to elevate the humeral head. Provision fixation with one pin is provided. **C:** A bone hook is used to reduce the greater tuberosity. **D:** Final reduction and fixation with the use of multiple cannulated screws. From Resch et al.[326]

Treatment-Specific Outcomes. CRPF has received increased attention over the past few years. Table 37-12 summarizes the outcomes of the technique in the literature whereas Table 37-13 details the complications of the technique. While overall satisfactory outcomes have been reported, malunion and AVN rates of up to 22 and 26%, respectively have been reported (Table 37-13). Furthermore, premature pin removal, due to migration, has been reported to be required in up to 40% of cases.[51] Outcomes have been correlated with both patient age

and the underlying fracture type, with four-part valgus-impacted fractures having lower functional outcomes scores than three- and two-part fractures.[35,161] Only two comparative studies have been published in the English literature and both compare standard CRPF with CRPF employing augmentation with an external pin linking mechanism. In both studies, linkage lead to significantly lower pin migration and higher functional scores, even in older patients.[33,59] Brunner et al. reported on the use of

(*text continues on page 1390*)

TABLE 37-11 **Closed Reduction and Percutaneous Fixation**

Potential Pitfalls and Preventions

Pitfall	Preventions
Axillary nerve injury	Mark possible location of axillary nerve on skin referencing measurements performed fluoroscopically. Confirm axillary nerve position with digital palpation through reduction portal. Use blunt dissection and sleeve for pin placement. Place pins according to recommended guidelines (see text).
Construct failure (pin migration)	Avoid CRPF in elderly patients. Use terminally threaded pins. Select fractures without tuberosity or calcar comminution. Place pins in a divergent manner spreading their distance both at the fracture site and inside the head.
Humeral head pin penetration	Establish three-dimensional direction of pins Verify pin placement under live fluoroscopic visualization
Pin site infection	Cut pins short for tip to be located 5 mm subcutaneously Avoid active shoulder range of motion while pins in place

TABLE 37-12 **Published Results of the Treatment of Proximal Humeral Fractures with Closed Reduction and Percutaneous Fixation (CRPF) and a Number of Variants. Where Possible the Fracture Types are Defined by the Neer Classification with Two-, Three- and Four-Part Fractures and Fracture Dislocations (FD)**

Authors	Technique	Fracture Type (Neer parts) 2 3 4 FD	Age (years) Mean (Range)	Follow-up (months) Mean (Range)	Outcome Scores	Results
Kocialkowski and Wallace[207]	CRPF	22	61 (13–91)	19 (6–16)	Neer	38% Ex/Good
Jakob et al.[187]	CRPF	0 0 19	49 (24–81)	4 (2–10)	Neer	74% Ex/Good
Jaberg et al.[186]	CRPF	32 8 5 3	63 (17–85)	36 (24–84)	Neer	70% Ex/Good
Fenichel et al.[423]	CRPF	24 26 0	50 (21–78)	30 (12–48)	Constant	70% Ex/Good
Keener et al.[196]	CRPF	19 37 6	61 (19–76)	35 (12–77)	Constant/ ASES	58% Ex/Good
Blonna et al.[33]	CRPF	30 9 3	62 (27–83)	25 (12–45)	Constant/ DASH	Means 70/21
Carbone et al.[59]	CRPF	0 15 11	78 (68–89)	24	Constant	52 (average)
Harrison et al.[161]	CRPF	5 12 10	59 (42–67)	84 (37–128)	ASES	82 (average)
Resch et al.[326]	CRPF ± cannulated screws	0 9 18	54 (25–68)	24 (18–47)	Constant	Good (average)
Kayalar et al.[194]	CRPF ± retrograde IM K wires	5 13 0	48 (14–89)	23 (8–60)	DASH	18 (average)
Seyhan et al.[357]	CRPF ± antegrade IM K wires	36 0 0	52 (41–86)	38 (30–60)	Constant	83% Ex/Good
Bogner et al.[35]	Humerusblock	0 32 16	80 (70–96))	34 (6–81)	Constant	88% Ex/Good
Brunner et al.[51]	Humerusblock	25 22 11	70 (32–95)	15 (12–28)	Constant	77% Ex/Good
Blonna et al.[33]	Hybrid	24 18 7	67 (37–91)	25 (12–40)	Constant/ DASH	Means 78/16
Joeckell[78]	ButtonFix	8 4 5	69 (16–89)	18 (12–20)	Constant	76% contralateral shoulder
Carbone[59]	MIROS	0 17 11	81 (76–85)	24	Constant	60 (average)

TABLE 37-13 The Complications Published in the Papers Detailed in Table 37-12

Authors	Technique	Revision Surgery	AVN	Implant Loosening	Joint Penetration	Infection (%) Deep	Infection (%) Super	Nerve Injury	Nonunion	OA	Dislocation	Malunion
Kocialkowski and Wallace[207]	CRPF	9	5	41			23	5	5			0
Jakob et al.[187]	CRPF		26									0
Jaberg et al.[186]	CRPF	17	21	10		2	8		4			0
Fenichel et al.[423]	CRPF	6	0	14			10					
Keener et al.[196]	CRPF		4	4			4					17
Blonna et al.[33]	CRPF		2	4			4					17
Carbone et al.[59]	CRPF		8	27		4	15					0
Harrison et al.[161]	CRPF			26								
Resch et al.[326]	CRPF ± cannulated screws	7	7	4								19
Kayalar et al.[194]	CRPF ± retrograde IM K wires	6		39					1			22
Seyhan et al.[357]	CRPF ± antegrade IM K wires		0				6					0
Bogner et al.[35]	Humerusblock	10	8	10								0
Brunner et al.[51]	Humerusblock	40	4	14	26							0
Blonna et al.[33]	Hybrid	4	2	2		2	4		2			2
Joeckell[78]	ButtonFix	6	6	6								0
Carbone[59]	MIROS		7	4			4					0

the "Humerusblock" device, for distal lateral linking of the pins. While pin migration was eliminated, pin perforation into the humeral head occurred in 26% of cases.[51]

While some studies support the use of CRPF in elderly patients in conjunction with linking implants,[51,59] we recommend the use of this technique in younger patients with adequate bone stock. Close radiographic follow-up should be obtained for early detection of pin perforation and pin migration.

Intramedullary Nailing

IM fixation is an attractive alternative for the treatment of proximal humeral fractures given its theoretical biomechanical advantages in osteoporotic bone and by allowing stabilization with minimal surgical invasion.[172]

Several IM devices have been used to treat proximal humeral fractures. The use of multiple solid, small diameter nails, such as Enders nails or Evans staples, has been described for IM fixation in an antegrade fashion with an insertion point through the humeral head.[22,84,358,409] Similar implants, namely prebent K-wires, have also been used with a retrograde insertion from the lateral cortex into the proximal humeral head.[102,393] These implants allow for gross alignment of displaced surgical neck fractures and may be used in conjunction with cerclage fixation of additional tuberosity fractures.[85,310]

Modern proximal humeral IM nailing however is performed with the use of antegrade locking nails that vary between 8 and 12 mm in proximal diameter. These nails incorporate features derived from those used in the lower extremity to allow for greater construct rigidity and strength (Fig. 37-40). Several nails are available on the market, offering several different interlocking options and the option to incorporate suture fixation through the rotator cuff tendons.[1,321]

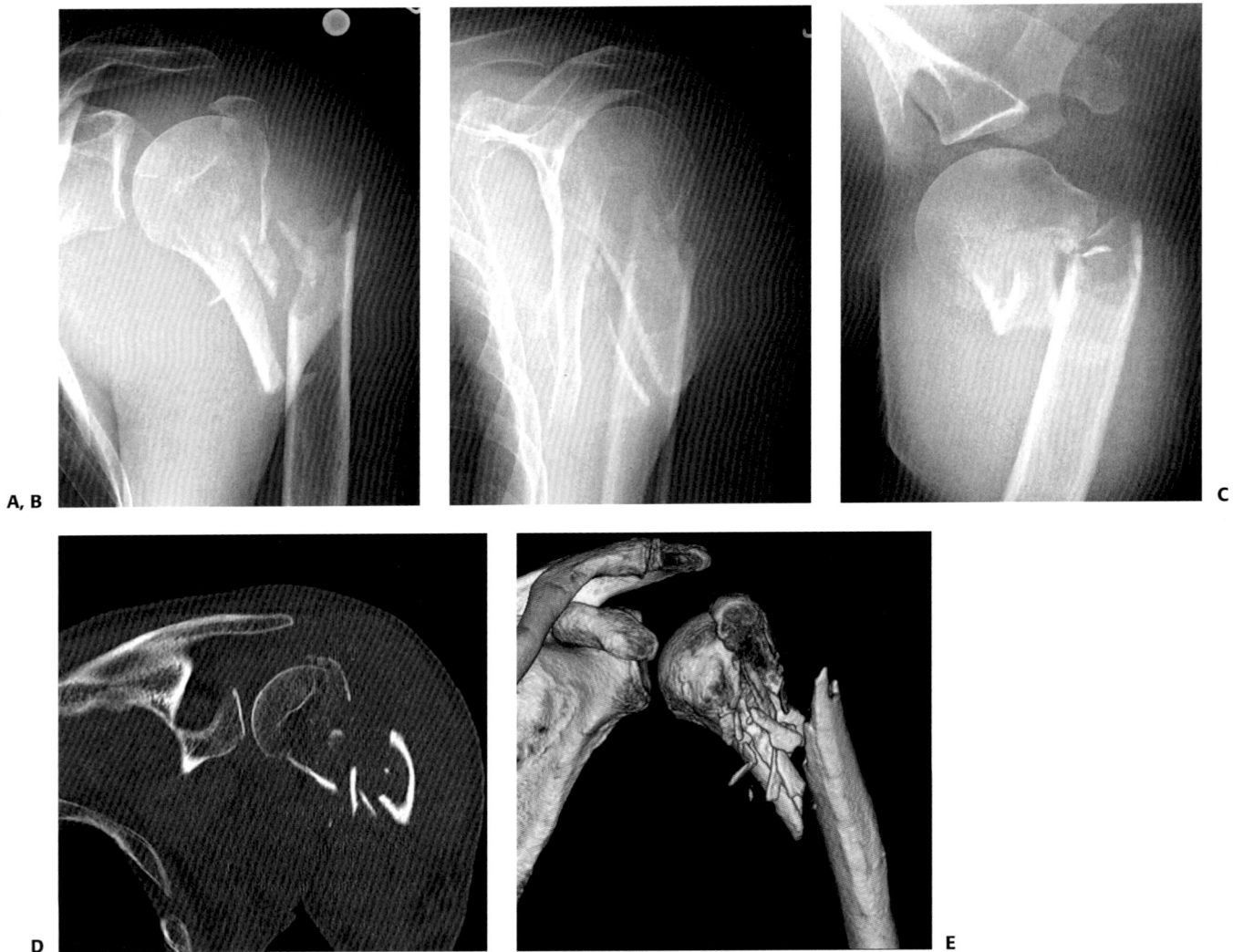

FIGURE 37-40 Intramedullary nailing of proximal humerus fractures. **A–J:** Twenty-five-year-old male with a high-energy proximal humerus fracture with comminution at the surgical neck and extension into the humeral shaft.

The main indications for proximal humerus interlocking IM nailing are displaced two-part surgical neck fractures, especially those with extension into the humeral diaphysis, and pathologic fractures.[1,271,321] Three-part greater tuberosity fractures may also be amenable to fixation with IM nailing.[1,122,150,195,246,271] While IM nailing of four-part fractures has been reported, poorer outcomes can be expected in this patient group.[1,150] IM nailing

is not recommended in varus four-part fractures with lateral displacement of the humeral head and in head-splitting fractures.[271]

While IM nailing is the treatment of choice in two-part surgical neck fractures with marked comminution or distal diaphyseal extension, caution should be exercised in the latter, especially in the presence of preoperative nerve palsy. Nerve

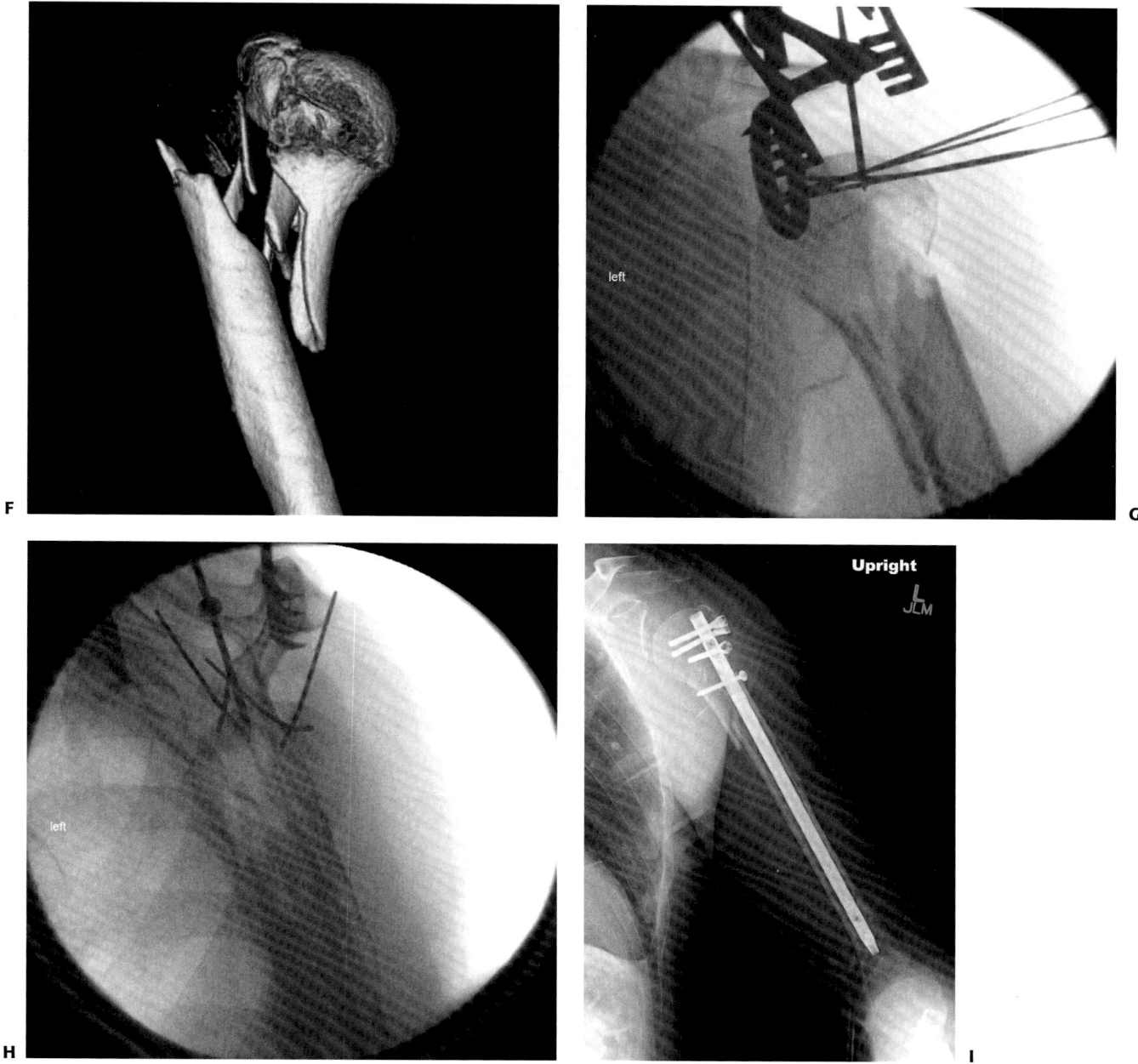

F

G

H

I

FIGURE 37-40 (continued) Valgus impaction of the head is present with minor displacement of the greater tuberosity. Fixation is obtained with a modern intramedullary nail allowing multidirectional proximal interlocking and incorporation of transtendinous sutures through the cuff into the final construct. **K–M:** Fifty-seven-year-old female with a two-part surgical neck fracture treated with intramedullary nailing. **N:** At only 6 days after fixation catastrophic failure has occurred. Possibly due to inadequate intraoperative imaging a too anterior entry point was selected leading to suboptimal stability.

(continues)

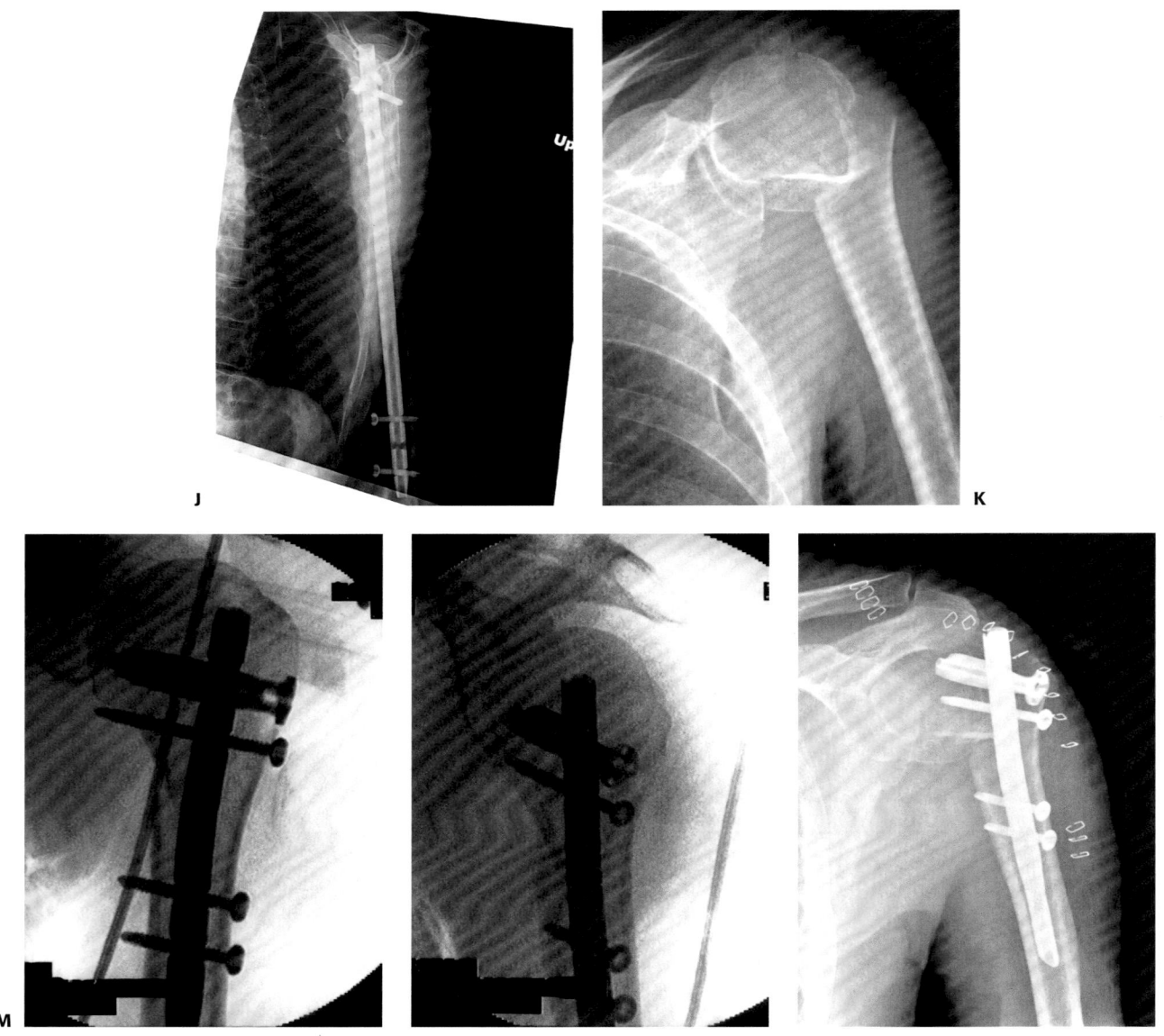

FIGURE 37-40 (*continued*)

entrapment at the fracture site may lead to catastrophic neurologic injury during reaming and nail placement.

Preoperative Planning. A checklist for preoperative planning is given in Table 37-14. Preoperative planning for IM nailing of proximal humeral fractures follows the same guidelines as for other treatment modalities. Imaging of the contralateral uninjured shoulder is recommended for preoperative templating of fracture fixation. Placing the nail template over the uninjured humerus will help in determining the starting point.

Availability of other fixation or reconstruction methods is recommended in case optimal outcomes cannot be achieved with IM nailing. Nails come in different diameters and lengths. Preoperative templating using both the injured and the unaffected contralateral side will be required for accurate implant selection.

TABLE 37-14 **Intramedullary Nailing**

Preoperative Planning Checklist

- OR Table: Standard table with beach chair positioner or radiolucent table
- Position/positioning aids: For beach chair: Head holder/shoulder positioner; for supine: Lateral Plexiglas extension (see text)
- Fluoroscopy location: For beach chair: Entering from the head, in line with the patient. Supine: Entering perpendicular to table from opposite to operative extremity. Confirm adequate visualization of fracture in AP and Y lateral views (Neer)
- Equipment:
  Kirschner wires/Steinmann pins/Schantz pins
  Intramedullary Nail set: Guidewire, starter awl, reamers, aiming jig, screwdrivers, etc.

Positioning. Careful patient positioning is required to facilitate fracture reduction, fluoroscopic visualization, and implant placement. Unlike ORIF of proximal humeral fractures, IM nailing does not allow shoulder abduction once the starting point has been created. An intraoperative axillary view is hence not possible. Imaging therefore requires a Neer lateral Y view and a Grashey AP view of the shoulder to be obtained by rotating the C-arm while keeping the shoulder adducted.

As with the other surgical techniques, positioning can be done in either the beach chair or supine position. Slight extension of the shoulder is required to obtain adequate clearance of the humeral entry site from the anterolateral acromion. This may be somewhat easier to achieve in the beach chair position. In the beach chair position the C-arm enters the surgical field from the head of the patient, parallel to the patient's body. AP and lateral views are obtained by rotating the C-arm around the long axis of the humerus. In the supine position the patient is placed on a radiolucent table with a Plexiglas board placed as a lateral extension as described for ORIF. The C-arm enters perpendicular to the long axis of the table from the side of the uninjured extremity. A bump is placed under the scapula of the injured side to roll the patient's torso 30 degrees toward the uninjured side. A Grashey view is thereby obtained by rolling the C-arm back 60 degrees, whereas a Y lateral view is obtained by rolling the C-arm forward 30 degrees. Adequate imaging should be confirmed before draping.

Surgical Approach. The key to IM nailing of the proximal humerus is to gain optimal access into the humeral head in a location that allows maintenance of reduction once final seating of the nail has been achieved. The exact entry point will vary depending on nail design and patient anatomy. Nails with a proximal lateral bend will have an entry point closer to the footprint of the rotator cuff and theoretically will damage less articular surface. Straight nails on the other hand will enter the humeral head via a split in the musculotendinous junction of the rotator cuff into articular surface of the humeral head. Straight nails will avoid compromising the footprint of the rotator cuff, by splitting the supraspinatus musculotendinous junction more medially, but will damage a greater area of articular cartilage.

For nails with a proximal lateral bend, a 3-cm incision is performed from the anterolateral corner of the acromion distally. For straight nails a more medial incision, in line with the acromioclavicular joint may be preferable. A proximal deltoid split is performed in line with the muscle fibers. Once the subdeltoid bursa has been incised and resected, the underlying rotator cuff is exposed. In more complex fractures a formal deltoid-splitting approach may be used paying close attention not to injure the axillary nerve. Alternatively, the middle deltoid may be detached subperiosteally from the acromion as a full-thickness flap of fascia and muscle. The anterior branch of the axillary nerve should be identified with digital palpation along the undersurface of the deltoid to confirm safe placement of pins for temporary stabilization as well as definitive proximal interlocking.

After partial resection of the subacromial bursa the underlying supraspinatus tendon will be exposed. The biceps tendon

is identified as a key landmark to assist in fracture reduction and establishing the proximal entry site. Once adequate fracture reduction has been obtained (see below), the supraspinatus tendon is split in line with its fibers 1 to 1.5 cm posterior to the biceps tendon. Depending on the type of nail, the tendon will be split either close to the footprint of the rotator cuff or at the level of the musculotendinous junction. Tendon edges are tagged with nonabsorbable suture for subsequent retraction and should be carefully protected during surgery.

Technique. The surgical technique is outlined in Table 37-15. For two-part surgical neck fractures, a Schantz pin, or two 2.5-mm K-wires directed from the lateral cortex into the head segment outside of the planned path of the nail will aid in fracture manipulation. Alignment of the distal segment is corrected with traction, rotation, and a posteriorly directed force onto the proximal humeral shaft. Once adequate reduction has been obtained and confirmed fluoroscopically, the starting point is selected using the C-arm. The AP view should show the starting point in a position that will not affect fracture reduction once final seating has been obtained. In the lateral Y view the entry point should be approximately 1 to 1.5 cm posterior to the anterior margin of the greater tuberosity. Trajectory of the guide pin should be from the starting point toward the center of the medullary canal at the level of the calcar. The entry hole is then created with an awl or a starting drill, using a soft tissue sleeve to protect the surrounding rotator cuff tendon. Depending on the type of implant a nail may then be inserted either directly or over a guidewire, with or without prior reaming. Due to the width of the proximal humeral canal and the need for a short nail in most instances, no cortical chatter will be obtained during reaming. Some mismatch between the shaft and nail can be expected. For three- and four-part fractures reduction of the head and tuberosities is required before nail insertion. Temporary fixation is achieved with K-wires outside of the predicted nail path. The placement of heavy nonabsorbable

---

TABLE 37-15 Intramedullary Nailing

Surgical Technique

- Confirm adequate imaging
- Expose subdeltoid space through deltoid split
- Identify the biceps tendon and understand your fragments
- Reduce fracture using a combination of
  1. Traction sutures into rotator cuff
  2. Steinmann or Schantz pins or Kirschner wires
  3. Shaft manipulation
- Confirm reduction fluoroscopically in two views
- Establish entry hole under two- view fluoroscopy
- Prepare nail as required per implant specific technique
- Introduce nail and verify position under fluoroscopy
- Place proximal fixation
- Complete distal fixation
- Incorporate tuberosity sutures into construct
- Confirm adequate screw length with live fluoroscopy
- Close

sutures around the bone tendon junction is useful to manipulate displaced tuberosities, obtain temporary stabilization and provide structural reinforcement to the final construct when tied to interlocking screws. It is important to keep in mind that fracture reduction, especially between the head and shaft has to be achieved before nail preparation and seating, since this will determine the spatial relationship between these two segments. During preparation of the starting point in three-part greater tuberosity fractures and four-part fractures, the fracture between the greater tuberosity and head segment has to be kept reduced as instrumentation will tend to separate the fragments, leading to inadvertent loss of fracture reduction during final nail seating and poorer outcomes.[2]

The nail is inserted by hand, until it lies at least 10 mm deep to the articular surface. Fracture alignment, nail depth, and rotation should be reassessed fluoroscopically. Depending on the type of nail selected, proximal interlocking implants are directed either toward the head or in a manner that ensures that the tuberosities are captured. While it is frequently stated that screws placed into the humeral should be just short of the subchondral bone, it may be safer to select screws that are 5 mm shorter than measured to avoid delayed screw penetration. As with ORIF, measurement of screw length should be performed by drilling the lateral cortex only and then advancing the depth gauge advanced to the level of subchondral bone. This will avoid head penetration with the drill, thereby reducing the risk of late screw protrusion. In three- and four-part fractures, nail insertion depth should not exceed 3 cm, as this is likely to lead to inadequate fixation of the tuberosities by the proximal locking screws. While incorporation of rotator cuff traction sutures into the final construct is advisable whenever possible, it is required if there is tuberosity comminution, as bony fixation with screws will be unreliable.

After proximal locking has been performed the proximal humerus should be reassessed fluoroscopically to see if there is a fracture gap that may be corrected by impacting the distal segment proximally with gentle blows against the elbow. The distal segment is finally interlocked with one screw in the dynamic hole. This allows further collapse at the surgical neck to facilitate union.

Due to the risk of iatrogenic injury to the axillary nerve during nailing, it is important to determine the relationship of the locking holes and the axillary and radial nerves. Modern implants are designed to place proximal and distal locking holes in a safe window away from these nerves. In smaller patients or in the presence of abnormal anatomy, this safe window may however be altered.

The cuff split is closed with nonabsorbable sutures. The deltoid split is closed with absorbable sutures. If the deltoid was detached, osseous tunnels are drilled into the acromion for reattachment with heavy nonabsorbable sutures. Full-thickness stitches into the deltoid are required to allow for strong repair.

Postoperative Care. Patients are placed into a postoperative sling and pendulum exercises are started on the first postoperative day. Active range-of-motion exercises of the elbow, wrist and hand are encouraged. Passive forward elevation and external rotation is allowed depending on the fracture stability that has been achieved and the bone quality. It is recommended to err toward slow progression of motion to reduce the risk of secondary fracture displacement. Most frequently passive range-of-motion exercises are continued until the sixth postoperative week. Active-assisted range of motion is then started, with transition to strengthening exercises occurring at 3 months.

Potential Pitfalls and Preventative Measures. A list of potential pitfalls and appropriate preventative measures is given in Table 37-16. Regardless of the type of implant used, IM nailing violates the rotator cuff and this may lead to secondary symptoms.[291,426] Proximal humerus nails with a lateral bend may increase the risk the damage to the footprint of the rotator cuff, which may lead to postoperative shoulder pain. Straight nails have been advocated as they disrupt the rotator cuff at the level of the musculotendinous junction which theoretically leads to less rotator cuff problems.

Correct entry point placement is crucial to avoid displacement of a well-reduced fracture during nail seating. Fluoroscopic confirmation in both the coronal and sagittal planes of the starting pin should precede entry portal establishment. Understanding of implant geometry and preoperative templating using the unaffected contralateral extremity helps in avoiding intraoperative fracture displacement and also improves biomechanical stability by optimizing implant position.

Nail insertion depth and rotation should be checked before interlocking to allow for optimal implant placement.

Treatment-specific Outcomes. Antegrade nailing of displaced proximal humeral fractures has gained popularity because it is minimally invasive and satisfactory outcomes have been reported in many case series. However the main concern

---

TABLE 37-16 Intramedullary Nailing

Potential Pitfalls and Preventions

Pitfall	Preventions
Primary intraoperative fracture displacement	Obtain fracture reduction before preparing nail entry site. Determine correct starting point based on preoperative template Careful fluoroscopic confirmation of fracture reduction and adequate entry site in AP and Y-lateral views.
Postoperative shoulder pain	Careful sharp incision of rotator cuff, perpendicular to footprint. Judicious soft tissue retraction during reaming and nail insertion. Avoid impingement by adequately seating the nail at least 10 mm below the articular surface.
Glenohumeral screw protrusion	Select final head screw length 5 mm shorter than measured when directed toward articular surface.

with antegrade locked IM nailing is the violation of the rotator cuff with the risk of subsequent shoulder pain.[291,426]

The most frequent complication after locked IM nailing of proximal humeral fractures is backing out of the proximal screws.[2,83,150,195,248] In one large case series of 115 patients treated with the Targon Proximal Humerus Nail (Aesculap, Tuttlingen, Germany), the most frequent complication after a mean follow-up of 8.7 months was backing out of one or more screws. This occurred in almost one-quarter of patients and required surgical removal of the screws to facilitate resolution of symptoms.[271] Other complications include glenohumeral screw protrusion, osteonecrosis of the humeral head, nonunion, malunion, and tuberosity displacement.[150,246,321,381]

Hemiarthroplasty

Hemiarthroplasty, also known as humeral head replacement, is indicated when the humeral head is deemed to be unreconstructable or when its biologic viability is likely to be severely compromised. Comminuted head-splitting fractures and head depression fractures involving more than 40% of the articular surface are frequently considered to be unreconstructable. Predictors of head ischemia are further considered in the decision-making process between operative fixation and replacement. Hertel and Bastian found that fractures through the anatomic neck of the humerus carried an increased risk of head ischemia. Furthermore, a metaphyseal extension of the humeral head of less than 8 mm, loss of the medial hinge and displacement of the humeral head further predicted loss of humeral head perfusion at the time of surgery. While these criteria are frequently used to argue in favor of replacement surgery, intraoperative ischemia has not been correlated with clinically significant AVN of the humeral head when fixation is chosen for treatment. Furthermore, some authors have found that AVN after proximal humerus fixation is associated with results that are comparable to those of hemiarthroplasty.[378]

The main challenge associated with hemiarthroplasty is the unpredictability of outcomes. Results published in the literature follow a bimodal distribution, in which some patients attain a result that is close to the uninjured extremity, whereas others achieve adequate pain control with only fair function. Several factors play a key role in achieving optimal results. Adequate reduction of the tuberosities and restitution of the correct head-to-tuberosity height are paramount to provide the biomechanical conditions for the reconstruction to function properly. Furthermore, adequate fixation of the tuberosities has to be obtained to achieve tuberosity healing and maintain function in the long term. Finally, glenoid erosion may lead to delayed shoulder pain in the mid to long term.

Unpredictability of outcomes after hemiarthroplasty for proximal humerus fractures may be further affected by the relatively low frequency with which this procedure is performed. According to a recent meta-analysis, surgeons perform on average three hemiarthroplasties for proximal humeral fractures per year, with case frequency per surgeon ranging from 0.21 to 9.6 per year.[212] This calculation is obtained from surgeons involved in academic centers and it is therefore likely that many pro-cedures are performed with an even lower frequency in the overall orthopedic surgeon population.

Preoperative Planning. A preoperative planning checklist is given in Table 37-17. As with any proximal humerus fracture standard trauma shoulder radiographs are required. A CT scan with sagittal, coronal, and 3D reconstructions is also desirable to achieve full understanding of fracture geometry and rule out associated injuries. The bone window should be used to assess fracture configuration and determine the morphology of the humeral head fragment. Furthermore, measurement of the greater tuberosity fragment and establishing the involvement of the medial calcar will aid in determining depth of stem placement. Associated fractures of the glenoid or acromion should be ruled out. The soft tissues in both axial and sagittal reconstructions should be analyzed to determine cuff muscle degeneration.[149] Advanced atrophy or fatty infiltration suggesting pre-existing rotator cuff pathology should be considered as a relative indication for proceeding with reverse total shoulder arthroplasty instead of hemiarthroplasty.

As with any method of treatment, the surgeon should have sufficient experience and skills to treat a proximal humeral fracture with an arthroplasty prosthesis. Referral to a shoulder specialist or traumatologist with experience in the treatment of these difficult fractures should be undertaken to achieve the best possible outcome.

In most fractures intraoperative fracture assessment will determine whether reconstruction with reduction and fixation is possible or whether arthroplasty will be required. Furthermore, the decision between hemiarthroplasty and reverse total

---

TABLE 37-17 **Hemiarthroplasty**

Preoperative Planning Checklist

- OR Table: Standard table (beach chair)
- Anesthesia: General with interscalene block
- Position/positioning aids:
  Head holder/shoulder positioner, hip positioner at thigh. Waist flexed 60 degrees, knees bent 30 degrees, reverse Trendelenburg.
  Shoulders draped free to level of medial scapular border, mid third of the clavicle and mandibular angle.
  Articulated arm holder may aid in the presence of a single assistant.
  If arm draped free: Padded Mayo stand.
- Fluoroscopy location:
  At head of patient, coming in line with long axis of the bed.
- Equipment:
  Deltoid retractor (e.g., Browne retractor)
  Power drill
  2-mm drill bit
  #2 braided non absorbable suture
  Ruler
  Cement, antibiotic powder (Vancomycin + Tobramycin), methylene blue
  Shoulder implant system (reamers, broaches, head sizers, retroversion guide etc.)

shoulder arthroplasty may be made intraoperatively. It is therefore desirable to have instruments and implants available to allow intraoperative flexibility of final decision making. Several arthroplasty systems are available that use the same stem regardless of whether hemiarthroplasty or reverse total shoulder arthroplasty will be performed. This will reduce the amount of instrumentation as well as intraoperative time.

Shoulder arthroplasty can be performed with regional or general anesthesia. If general anesthesia will be used, a preoperative interscalene block will aid in postoperative pain management.

Positioning. Patients undergoing arthroplasty of the shoulder are placed in the beach chair position. Special attention is given to being able to fully adduct the shoulder and achieve extension during reaming and cementing of the humerus. The patient should be positioned such that the medial border of the scapular is accessible posteriorly, the middle third of the clavicle anteriorly and the angle of the mandible superiorly. Several beach chair positioners are available with a posterior cutout at the level of the shoulder and a special superior segment that allow stabilization of the patient's head. If two assistants are available, the operative arm is draped free. During the operative procedure, the distal aspect of the upper extremity can be positioned on the Mayo stand and abduction adjusted by elevating or lowering its position. If only one assistant is available, an articulated arm positioner is recommended. Bony prominences should be carefully padded. If surgical time is expected to be prolonged, a urinary catheter is recommended.

Surgical Approaches. Hemiarthroplasty is performed through the deltopectoral approach. A 10-cm incision is performed from the clavicle distally. At the level of the coracoid the incision should pass 1 cm lateral to it. At the height of the axillary fold the incision should end at a point located between the medial 40% and lateral 60% of the medial to lateral arm width. Proximally a medial skin flap is elevated just superficial to the deltoid muscle. The cephalic vein can be identified at the fat triangle located between the deltoid, clavicle and pectoralis major, approximately 1 cm medial to the coracoid process. The cephalic vein is then dissected either medially or laterally, while the branches are coagulated. The subdeltoid space is then released with blunt dissection. Fracture hematoma is evacuated. If intact, the clavipectoral fascia is incised along the lateral border of the conjoint tendon, carefully preserving the underlying subscapularis tendon. For improved exposure, 1 cm of the coracoacromial ligament may be removed and 1 to 2 cm of the pectoralis major tendon may be released distally.

Technique. The surgical technique is outlined in Table 37-18. Once the subdeltoid space has been released a deltoid retractor is inserted and the fracture site exposed. To extract the humeral head, the biceps tendon is identified distal to the fracture site and followed proximally. The bicipital groove is then identified. In most fractures requiring hemiarthroplasty a fracture line is present just lateral to the bicipital groove. This allows access to the joint cavity. The humeral head can then be removed and saved for subsequent bone grafting. The wound is irrigated to remove any clots from the fracture site. The greater tuberosity

TABLE 37-18 **Hemiarthroplasty**
Surgical Technique
• Expose proximal humerus
• Identify and tag tuberosity fragments
• Release rotator interval
• Identify and extract humeral head
• Use for bone graft
• Confirm rotator cuff integrity and healthy glenoid surface
• Prepare humeral canal
• Measure depth of insertion that allows balanced tuberosity reduction
• Place shaft sutures
• Cement humeral component in adequate retroversion and length
• Place humeral head
• Obtain graft from humeral head and place around proximal humeral stem
• Reduce tuberosities around stem and tie
• Confirm stability and range of motion
• Place drain
• Close wound
• Immobilize in sling

is then tagged with four large caliber (#2 or #5) braided nonabsorbable sutures that are placed through the posterior rotator cuff just proximal to its bony insertion. The lesser tuberosity is then tagged with two traction sutures through the distal subscapularis tendon. If the rotator interval is found to be intact, it is incised to the level of the glenoid. The long head of biceps is cut at its insertion onto the superior glenoid labrum and tagged for later tenodesis. The glenoid is then assessed to rule out any traumatic injury or pre-existing chondral damage. Associated glenoid fractures should be stabilized accordingly. Rarely, pre-existing osteoarthritis may require placement of a glenoid component. The humeral shaft is then prepared according to the technique described for the particular implant. In most instances, the humeral canal is reamed with progressively larger reamers until cortical contact is obtained. It is recommended to use the reamer as a sound by gently advancing the reamer with back and forth rotation of the reamer around its longitudinal axis. Aggressive rotation of the reamer in one single direction is discouraged to avoid a possible torsional fracture of the humeral shaft. Once the final reamer has been advanced, the proximal humerus is broached following the manufacturer's guidelines. A fracture-specific stem should be used. These implants have a lean proximal geometry that allows for bone grafting around the proximal humeral metaphysis to improve tuberosity healing. A number of implants have a textured proximal metaphyseal segment to promote bony ingrowth.

The biceps tendon is then followed distally to identify the bicipital grove at the level of the proximal humeral shaft and two 2-mm drill holes are placed 1 cm apart and 1 cm from the proximal fracture edge into the humeral shaft. Two large caliber nonresorbable sutures are passed through these holes. A trial stem is then introduced that will allow a cement mantle of at least 1 mm between the implant and humeral shaft. Routine cementation of humeral stems for the management of proximal humeral fractures is recommended since this will allow both axial as well as rotational stability of the stem. One of the key aspects of hemiarthroplasty is to determine the correct height of the prosthesis. Several methods have been described to achieve this:

1. The trial stem is inserted with a head closely resembling the size of the extracted native head. The native head is examined to evaluate the presence of a metaphyseal extension that will be missing on the humeral shaft. This "gap" should be visible at the moment of seating of the humeral stem. Conversely, the head may have fractured proximal to the inferior aspect of the anatomic neck, thereby leaving a fragment of head attached to the humeral shaft. Resecting the head remnant at the anatomic neck will provide a medial reference point onto which the prosthetic head can be lowered.

2. The depth of stem insertion should allow reduction of the greater tuberosity into a gap formed between the prosthetic head and shaft laterally.

3. The head to tuberosity height should be between 5 and 9 mm.

4. Under fluoroscopic vision, the so-called gothic arch formed by the lateral border of the scapular body and the medial aspect of the proximal humeral shaft should be restituted with adequate stem placement.

To adequately establish humeral stem insertion it is recommended that a combination of these methods be used. Once the appropriate stem height has been determined, the depth of insertion should be marked on the trial stem with regard to an identifiable reference point on the humeral shaft. Most implants provide reference marks that are matched on the definitive implant. While cumbersome to use, most systems provide external jigs that can aid in inserting the stem to the appropriate depth. The humeral canal is then irrigated and a cement restrictor introduced 1 cm distal to the expected position of the tip of the stem to avoid distal cement migration and improve cement pressurization. The canal is then irrigated and dried and filled in a retrograde fashion with cement. Due to the low rate of humeral loosening, some surgeons recommend cementing only the proximal segment between the stem and the proximal humeral shaft, sufficient to allow rotational and axial stability of the implant. Cement removal is theoretically easier if revision is required. Antibiotics may be added to the cement to reduce the risk of infection. Methylene blue can be added to provide a color contrast with native bone which aids in cement removal should revision be required in the future. The stem is then inserted in 30 degrees of retroversion to the desired depth following the previously determined depth mark and reference point. Excessive cement is carefully removed to avoid interposition between fracture fragments. Once the cement has hardened, a trial head is placed and the tuberosities provisionally reduced to reassess stem height and address glenohumeral tracking. If this is deemed appropriate, the greater tuberosity sutures are brought around the medial aspect of the humeral stem. Most modern prostheses provide a slot through which the sutures can be threaded. The most superior and inferior sutures of the greater tuberosity are then passed from deep to superficial through the insertion of the distal subscapularis tendon. The remaining two greater tuberosity sutures are brought directly around the stem and the humeral head is impacted onto the stem. Cancellous bone graft obtained from the morselized humeral head is placed between the humeral stem and tuberosities and the greater tuberosity sutures tied to their respective tails. The greater tuberosity is then reduced and stabilized around the stem. The sutures from the greater tuberosity that have been passed through the subscapularis tendon are tied to their respective tails, thereby reducing the lesser tuberosity and fixing the greater and lesser tuberosities around the stem. Finally, each suture placed through drill holes in the shaft is passed through the anterior and posterosuperior cuff, respectively and tied, thereby providing an additional vertical anchor of the tuberosities into the humeral shaft. Two additional stitches may be placed at the level of the rotator interval. The long head of the biceps may be incorporated into the vertical fixation stitches or may be formally tenodesed to the pectoralis major tendon (Fig. 37-41). The wound is then irrigated and the deltopectoral interval closed with interrupted absorbable sutures. The subcutaneous tissues and skin are then closed. A drain may be used.

In exceptional occasions, pre-existing osteoarthritis of the glenohumeral joint may require total shoulder arthroplasty. The glenoid component should be placed prior to final humeral stem placement.

Postoperative Care. Patients routinely stay at least one night in hospital. If a wound drain is used it is removed within 24 hours of surgery. Passive range-of-motion exercises are started on the first postoperative day. They are limited to neutral rotation and 90 degrees of forward elevation. Patients are followed up clinically and radiographically at 2 weeks, 6 weeks, and 3 months. Active-assisted range-of-motion exercises are started at 6 weeks and strengthening exercises at 3 months. With regard to long-term follow-up patients should have radiographs at 1 year, 2 years, 5 years, and every 5 years thereafter or sooner if symptoms arise. Standard antibiotic prophylaxis for invasive procedures is recommended for life. There are no weight-bearing restrictions

Potential Pitfalls and Preventive Measures. Potential pitfalls and appropriate preventative measures are listed in Table 37-19. Shoulder hemiarthroplasty requires accurate reconstruction of the proximal humerus for the rotator cuff to stabilize and power the shoulder for adequate function. Poor function after fracture hemiarthroplasty is often related to complications related to the tuberosities.[39,89,269]

Tuberosity malunion leads to an inadequate head to tuberosity height, thereby altering the biomechanics of the shoulder. Placing the humeral head too proud leads to a tuberosity that is too distal with regard to the humeral head. The rotator cuff is thereby placed under increased tension and may subsequently rupture. Furthermore, increased stresses may occur between the prosthetic head and glenoid surface, potentially leading to early glenoid erosion. Too deep humeral stem placement will

(text continues on page 1402)

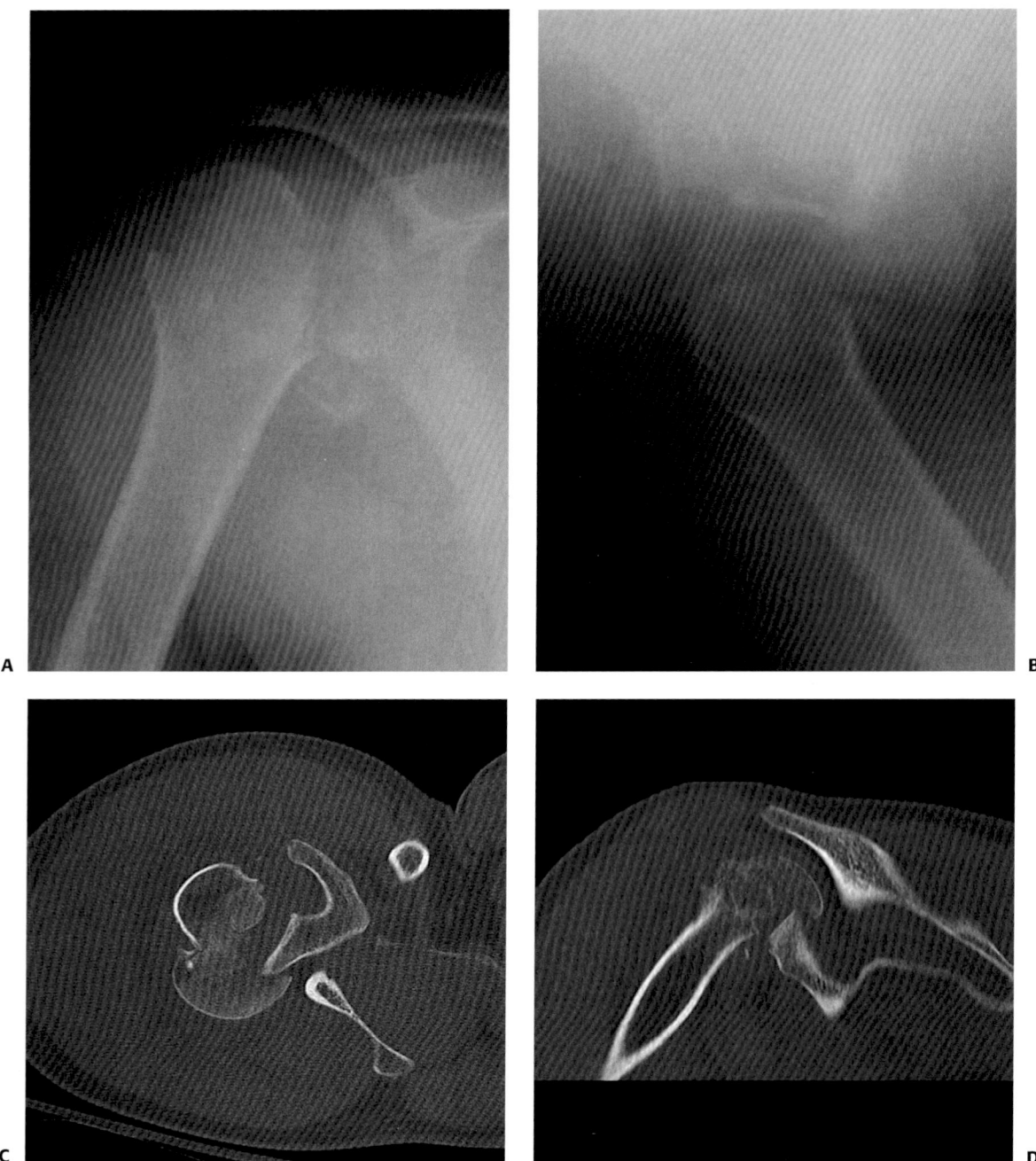

FIGURE 37-41 Hemiarthroplasty. Posterior four-part fracture dislocation in a 47-year-old male. **A, B:** Radiographic AP and axillary views of the shoulder. **C–H:** CT scan images showing axial **(C)** cuts, coronal **(D, E)** reconstructions and three-dimensional surface renderings **(F–H)**. **I:** Intraoperative images showing tag sutures to control the greater tuberosity and allow subsequent fixation around the final implant. **J–L:** Final implant placement and bone grafting. **M:** Definitive suture fixation as depicted in **(N)**. **O, P:** Radiographic follow-up at 1 year after surgery.

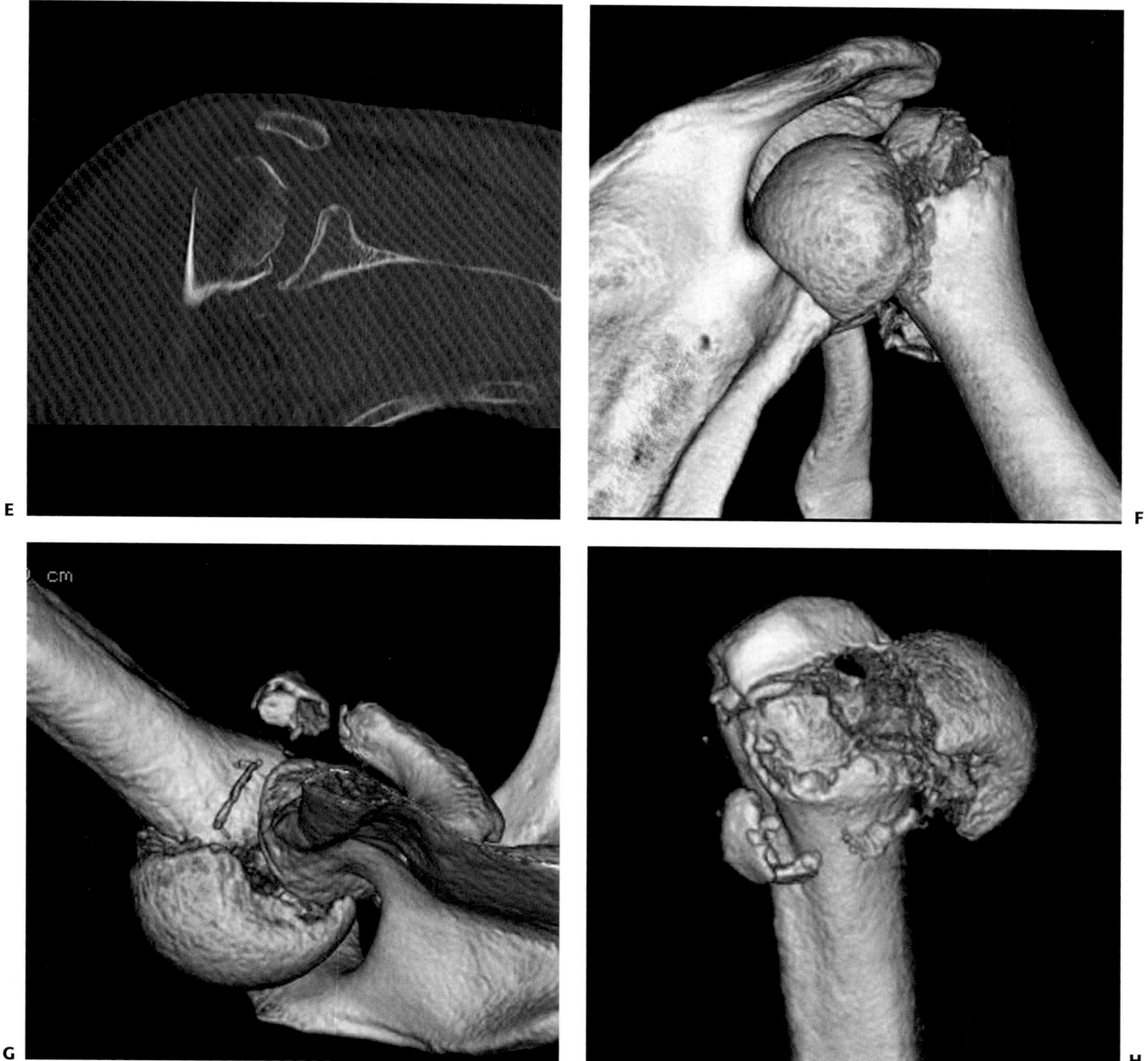

FIGURE 37-41 (continued)

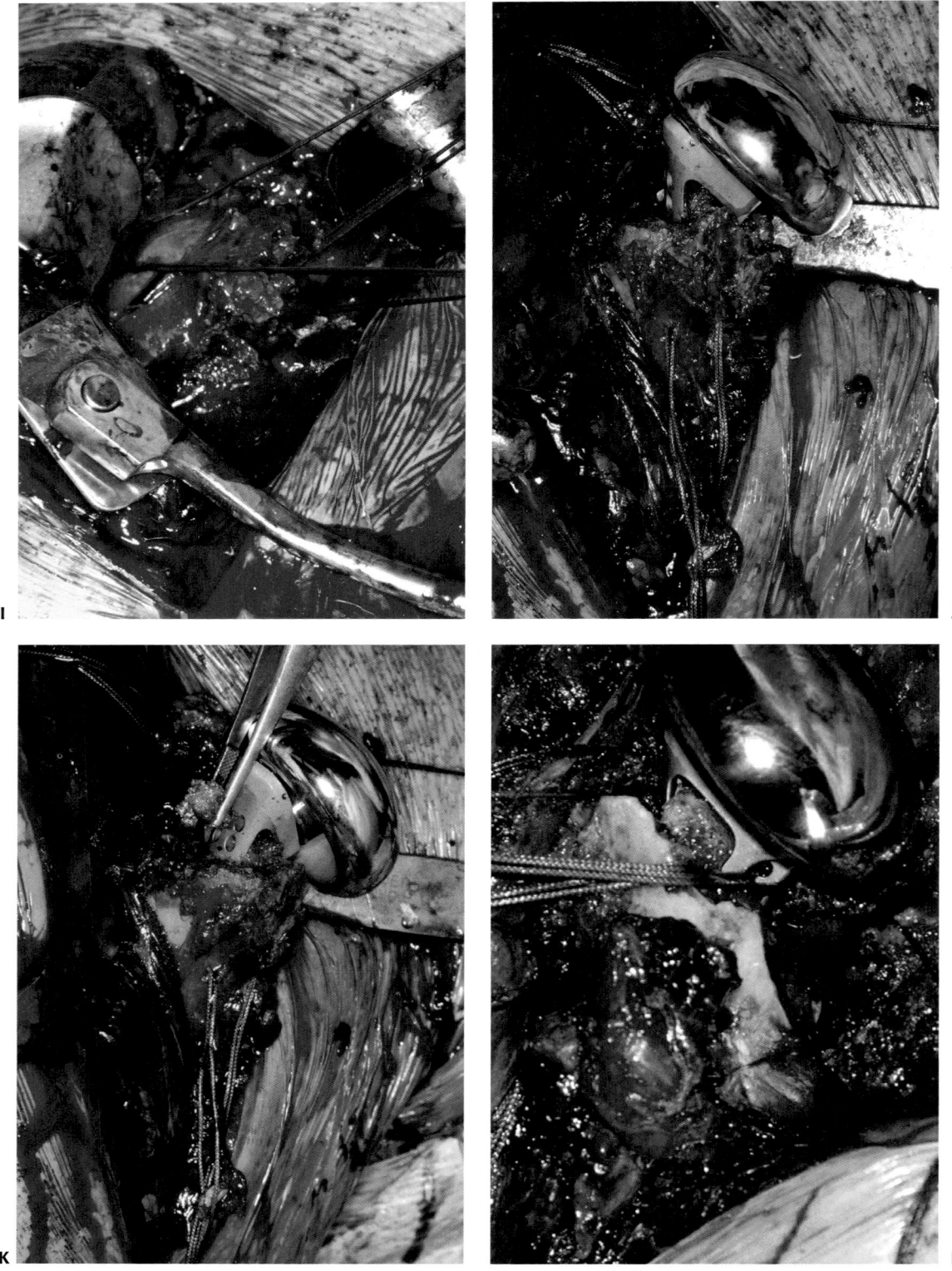

FIGURE 37-41 (*continued*)

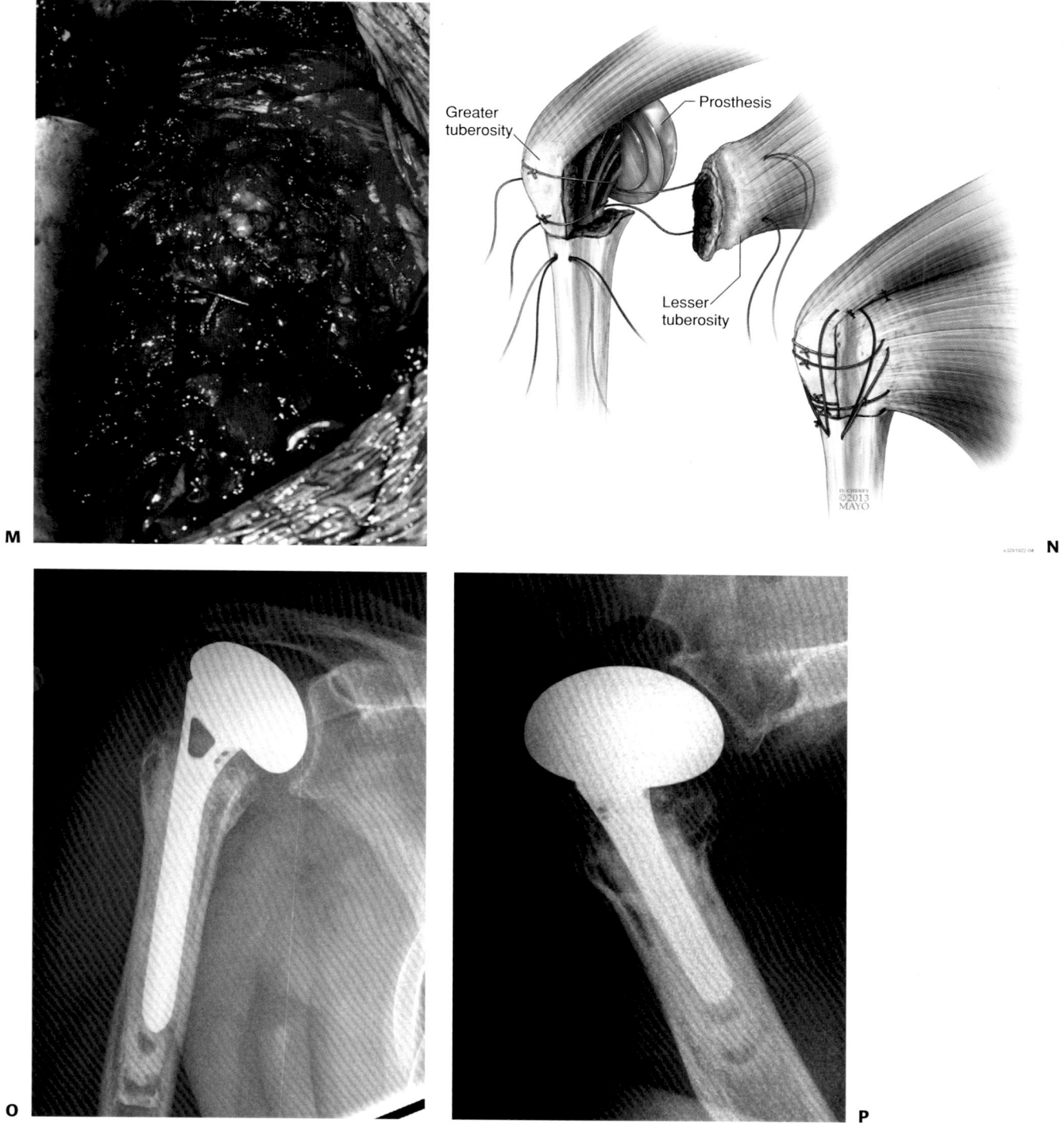

Greater tuberosity

Prosthesis

Lesser tuberosity

M

N

O

P

FIGURE 37-41 (*continued*)

TABLE 37-19 **Hemiarthroplasty**

Potential Pitfalls and Preventions

Pitfall	Preventions
Tuberosity malunion	Establish correct stem insertion depth Adequate tendon release Stable suture fixation from tendon insertion around humeral stem Avoid over-tightening of sutures
Tuberosity nonunion	Stable suture fixation from tendon insertion around humeral stem Bone grafting Conservative progression of physical therapy
Instability	Stable suture fixation of lesser tuberosity Establish adequate stem retroversion
"Overstuffing"	Establish correct stem insertion depth Select appropriate head size

lead to a tuberosity that is too high with regard to the humeral head. This will lead to subacromial impingement and shoulder dysfunction. Carefully determining the correct depth of insertion of the humeral stem is therefore critical to avoid tuberosity malposition.

Long-term function depends on achieving healing of the tuberosities to the shaft. Stable fixation of the tuberosities should therefore be obtained with the addition of bone graft around the proximal aspect of the humeral stem. Furthermore, while physical therapy is important to regain motion, exercises should be progressed cautiously so as to not overstress the construct and risk failure of fixation with subsequent tuberosity migration or nonunion. Finally, selection of too large a humeral head component should be avoided as this will lead to a limited range of motion and may also result in early glenoid erosion. Careful matching of the prosthetic component with the size of the native head should be done, with a tendency to err toward the smaller prosthetic head.

Treatment-Specific Outcomes. Hemiarthroplasty continues to be the preferred option for the operative treatment of unreconstructable proximal humeral fractures. The results of a number of studies of hemiarthroplasty are given in Tables 37-20 and 37-21. Reliable pain control is achieved as reported by studies with up to 10 years of follow-up.[89,212,214,269,274,335] Although several studies show good-to-excellent results in up to 90% of patients, others show that a large subset of patients, while achieving adequate pain control, have only fair functional results.[212,214,269,274,335] Forward elevation after hemiarthroplasty for proximal humeral fractures averages 110 degrees, ranging from 20 to 180 degrees.[9,89] Despite a large variability in function, prosthetic revision rates are low, with survival reported as high as 97% at 1 year, 95% at 5 years, and 94% at 10 years.[9,335] However functional outcomes at an average follow-up of 10 years show unsatisfactory results in over half of patients.[9]

Comparative studies between ORIF and hemiarthroplasty have shown conflicting results with regard to functional outcome. One study showed that similar functional outcomes can be expected after locked plate fixation of proximal humeral fractures with nonischemic humeral heads and hemiarthroplasty,

TABLE 37-20 **Published Results of the Treatment of Proximal Humeral Fractures with Hemiarthroplasty. Where Possible the Fracture Types are Defined by the Neer Classification with Two-, Three-, and Four-Part Fractures and Fracture Dislocation (FD) and Head-Splitting (HS) Fractures**

Authors	Fracture Type (Neer parts) 2 3 4 FD HS	Age (years) Mean (Range)	Follow-up (months) Mean (Range)	Outcome Scores	Results
Moeckel et al.[274]	0 5 13 4	70 (49–87)	36 (29–46)	HSS	91% Ex/Good
Robinson et al.[335]		66 (30–90)	76 (24–156)	Constant	Fair (average)
Mighell et al.[269]	1 22 41 28 8	66 (39–89)	36 (12–89)	ASES	Fair (average)
Demirhan et al.[89]	0 2 15 15	58 (37–83)	35 (8–80)	Constant	47% Ex/Good
Antuña et al.[9]	0 3 32 13 5	66 (23–89)	124 (60–264)	Neer	47% Ex/Good
Gallinet et al.[126]	0 8 13	74 (49–95)	17 (6–55)	Constant	39 (average)
Esen et al.[106]	0 7 25 6 4	70 (59–81)	79 (48–118)	Constant/Neer	86% Ex/Good
Bastian and Hertel[21]		66 (38–87)	60 (40–88)	Constant	70 (median)
Pijls et al.[315]	0 4 25 1	72 (55–91)	37 (13–62)	Constant	68 (average)
Olerud et al.[298]	0 0 27	76 (58–90)	27	Constant	48 (average)
Noyes et al.[293]	100% 3 or 4 part	61 (31–79)	49 (5–100)	Constant	50 (average)
Boyle et al.[45]		72 (27–96)	60	Oxford	32 (average)
Spross et al.[383]	8 14	76 (55–92)	36 (12–83)	Constant	54 (average)
Boons et al.[42]	0 0 25	76	12	Constant	65 (average)

Authors	Revision Surgery	HO	Implant Loosening	Joint Penetration	Infection Deep	Infection Super	Nerve Injury	Nonunion	Fracture	Dislocation	Malunion	Subacromial Impingement
												%
Moeckel et al.[274]	9	41								5		5
Robinson et al.[335]	8	0	3		1			3			21	
Mighell et al.[269]	6	25					3				6	3
Demirhan et al.[89]	0	0									17	
Antuña et al.[9]	0	0	10		3				10			
Gallinet et al.[126]	0	0				5	5		5	14		
Esen et al.[106]	7	0	5				5					
Bastian and Hertel[21]	20	0	6							3		
Pijls et al.[315]	3	0										
Olerud et al.[298]	11	0	19									
Noyes et al.[293]												
Boyle et al.[45]												
Spross et al.[383]	5	5						5				
Boons et al.[42]	4	0										

when intraoperative head vascularity is absent.[21] Other studies have shown that ORIF achieves significantly better functional outcomes than hemiarthroplasty. Solberg et al. found significantly higher Constant scores after locked-plate fixation (68.6 points) than after hemiarthroplasty (60.6 points). Interestingly, while AVN of the humeral head, lead to functional scores that were significantly lower than internally fixed fractures without AVN, the results were similar to those after hemiarthroplasty.[378]

Complications associated with hemiarthroplasty include nonunion of the tuberosities in 18% of patients.[212,378] Infection occurs in 0.6% to 1.6% of cases, with some studies reporting infection in up to 8% of cases.[212,378] While heterotopic ossification occurs in up to 8.8% of cases, it does not limit function.[212]

Reverse Total Shoulder Arthroplasty

While it is possible to obtain clinical results that are similar to those of a normal shoulder with hemiarthroplasty the literature indicates that functional results are frequently disappointing.[9,39] For this reason many surgeons now use reverse total shoulder arthroplasty, rather than hemiarthroplasty, for the treatment of proximal humeral fractures. Reverse total shoulder arthroplasty has become the implant of choice for the management of several conditions associated with significant rotator cuff dysfunction such as cuff tear arthropathy, massive irreparable rotator cuff tears with painful pseudoparesis and glenohumeral joint arthritis with advanced rotator cuff pathology.[38,411,414] Because of concerns about possible tuberosity malposition and nonunion, reverse total shoulder arthroplasty has therefore been proposed as an alternative for the management of acute complex proximal humeral fractures.[53,61,126,137,237,241,323,402,424]

By placing a hemisphere onto the glenoid surface and a concave tray onto the humeral stem, reverse shoulder arthroplasty allows for rotation to occur at the glenohumeral joint through activation of the deltoid, without the need for a functional rotator cuff/tuberosity unit. Furthermore medialization of the center of glenohumeral rotation improves the lever arm of the deltoid, thereby theoretically optimizing its biomechanics for shoulder elevation. Reverse total shoulder arthroplasty therefore not only offers an alternative for the management of complex acute proximal humeral fractures, but also for the management of proximal humerus malunion or nonunion where the normal anatomy of the tuberosities cannot be reliably restored.[251,258,259,401,418] It has been suggested that rehabilitation after reverse total shoulder arthroplasty is quicker than after hemiarthroplasty, since the inherent implant stability and the fact that tuberosity healing is not important allows patients to regain an earlier active range of motion.[146]

Shoulder elevation and abduction can be achieved in the absence of a functional rotator cuff, but glenohumeral rotation may be limited. While the anterior and the posterior deltoid allow for some rotation of the native glenohumeral joint, this ability is lost in reverse total shoulder arthroplasty due to medialization of the center of rotation. It is therefore recommended that the tuberosities be incorporated into reverse total shoulder arthroplasty construct for internal and external rotations of the shoulder to occur by action of the subscapularis and teres minor muscles, respectively.[146,367,369,414]

TABLE 37-22	**Reverse Shoulder Arthroplasty**
Preoperative Planning Checklist (in Addition to Items Described for Hemiarthroplasty)	
• Equipment • Glenoid retractors • Reverse total shoulder arthroplasty system	

Preoperative Planning. A preoperative planning checklist for reverse shoulder arthroplasty is shown in Table 37-22. The preoperative planning for reverse total shoulder arthroplasty involves the same principles outlined for hemiarthroplasty. However because of the requirement for a glenoid component, a more focused assessment of the glenoid is required. One of the most frequent complications of reverse total shoulder arthroplasty is glenoid notching, which occurs when chronic medial impingement between the humeral component and the glenoid neck leads to progressive bone loss that can result in loosening of the glenoid component.[61,53,290,368] Placement of the glenoid baseplate should therefore be aimed at maximizing inferomedial clearance by achieving some inferior overhang between the glenosphere and the glenoid neck. Furthermore, inferior tilt of the baseplate has been associated with improved biomechanical loading of the implant-bone interface and favorable clinical outcomes.[155,368] Finally, the use of a lateral offset glenosphere can reduce the amount of medial glenohumeral impingement.[154] While the normal glenoid is usually unaffected by a proximal humerus fracture, a clear understanding of the patient's glenoid anatomy is key to achieving adequate implant positioning. In most instances, glenoid reaming will be performed parallel to the glenoid surface in the axial plane and with slight inferior inclination in the frontal plane. Pre-existing posterior or anterosuperior wear should be carefully assessed on radiographs and CT scans to allow intraoperative adjustment thereby ensuring central seating of the central peg of the baseplate in the glenoid vault.

Positioning. Patient positioning is the same as detailed for hemiarthroplasty.

Surgical Approaches. Reverse shoulder arthroplasty can be performed either through a deltopectoral approach or through a superolateral deltoid-splitting approach. If there is cuff tear arthropathy, the superolateral approach has the advantage of being associated with less instability compared to the deltopectoral approach, as the subscapularis tendon is left intact.[276] This advantage is however not present in proximal humeral fractures requiring arthroplasty, since access to the humeral canal is allowed by the displaced tuberosities. The deltopectoral approach has been shown to provide more reliable glenoid component positioning, with lower rates of glenoid loosening and glenoid notching.[275] The deltopectoral approach is therefore recommended for proximal humeral fractures.

Technique. The technique of using a reverse shoulder arthroplasty to treat a proximal humeral fracture is outlined in Table 37-23. Implantation of a reverse total shoulder arthroplasty

TABLE 37-23 **Reverse Shoulder Arthroplasty**

Surgical Technique

- Expose proximal humerus
- Find long head of the biceps distally and follow proximally to intertubercular groove for fracture fragment identification
- Transect long head of biceps at the level of surgical neck and tag distal segment for later tenodesis
- Identify and tag lesser tuberosity
- Release rotator interval
- Identify and extract humeral head and prepare for bone graft
- Place four braided nonabsorbable sutures around greater tuberosity through rotator cuff tendon
- Prepare glenoid
  - Use proximal biceps stump to circumferentially resect glenoid labrum
  - Identify inferior border of glenoid by releasing origin of triceps
  - Ream glenoid to place baseplate in 10 degrees of inferior tilt
  - Place and fix baseplate
  - Place and fix glenosphere
- Prepare humeral canal
  - Ream
  - Place trial stem with tray and reduce onto glenosphere
  - Apply traction onto arm while pushing tray and stem against glenosphere
  - Measure depth of insertion
  - Drill two 2-mm holes on anterior aspect of humerus shaft 1 cm apart and 1 cm distal to proximal fracture edge and pass two braided nonabsorbable sutures
  - Place cement restrictor 1 cm distal to expected stem tip position
  - Retrograde insert cement
  - Introduce stem in 30 degrees of retroversion to pre-established depth
  - After cement hardening place tray and reduce onto glenosphere
  - Select final tray according to desired tension
  - Place greater tuberosity sutures around humeral stem
  - Pass two greater tuberosity sutures through subscapularis around lesser tuberosity
  - Place definitive tray and reduce joint
  - Place bone graft around proximal stem
  - Reduce and tie greater tuberosity around stem
  - Reduce and tie lesser tuberosity around stem
  - Pass transosseous humeral shaft sutures through anterior and posterosuperior rotator cuff, respectively
  - Incorporate long head of the biceps for tenodesis
- Confirm stability and range of motion
- Place drain
- Close wound
- Immobilize in sling

is initially similar to hemiarthroplasty. Once the tuberosities have been tagged, the humeral head extracted and the long head of the biceps cut, the glenoid is exposed with the use of two glenoid retractors. The labrum is then circumferentially released from the glenoid. Exposure of the glenoid in proximal humeral fractures is usually straightforward, due to absence of the humeral head and separation of the tuberosities. Care should be taken to fully expose the inferior border of the glenoid to allow as inferior placement of the baseplate as possible. Partial release of the triceps insertion from the infraglenoid tubercle is usually required.

A central guide pin is placed in such a manner that the baseplate will be positioned centrally in the AP plane, caudally in the frontal plane and with 10 degrees of inferior tilt. After reaming and fixation of the baseplate, the glenosphere is placed.

Humeral preparation is then completed as for hemiarthroplasty and the proposed trial stem is inserted in 10 to 30 degrees of retroversion with the thinnest humeral tray. The humeral component is then reduced onto the glenoid and the distal humerus pulled, while pushing the humeral stem onto the glenosphere allowing the humeral shaft to telescope around the stem. Unlike hemiarthroplasty, final stem insertion is not aimed at reconstituting an adequate head to tuberosity height, but rather to obtaining adequate tension of the deltoid to avoid instability. Once maximum tension of the soft tissues is achieved the depth of insertion of the humeral stem is determined and marked. The definitive stem is then cemented to the set depth using standard cementing techniques and maintaining retroversion. Once the cement has hardened, the components are again reduced using the smallest trial insert. Final insert thickness is then increased until adequate soft tissue tension is obtained as determined by tightness of the conjoined tendon and deltoid muscle. Tuberosity fixation is then prepared as described for hemiarthroplasty. The definitive tray and insert are then placed and the components reduced. The tuberosities are then tied as described for hemiarthroplasty. Because of the geometry of reverse shoulder arthroplasty and changes in the alignment of the shoulder, anatomic reduction of the tuberosities is not always possible, or required. However, contact between the tuberosities and shaft should be established and the area bone grafted to achieve union (Fig. 37-42).

Postoperative Care. Patients routinely stay in hospital for at least one night. A similar postoperative protocol as described for hemiarthroplasty is used. Some authors advocate early active-assisted range of motion as pain allows.[146] Due to the importance of obtaining tuberosity healing for rotation, it is however recommended that surgeons use a more conservative approach of passive range of motion for the first 6 weeks after surgery, followed by subsequent active-assisted range-of-motion exercises for 6 weeks and strengthening exercises at 3 months if required. Weight bearing is limited to less than 20 lb for life.

(*text continues on page 1412*)

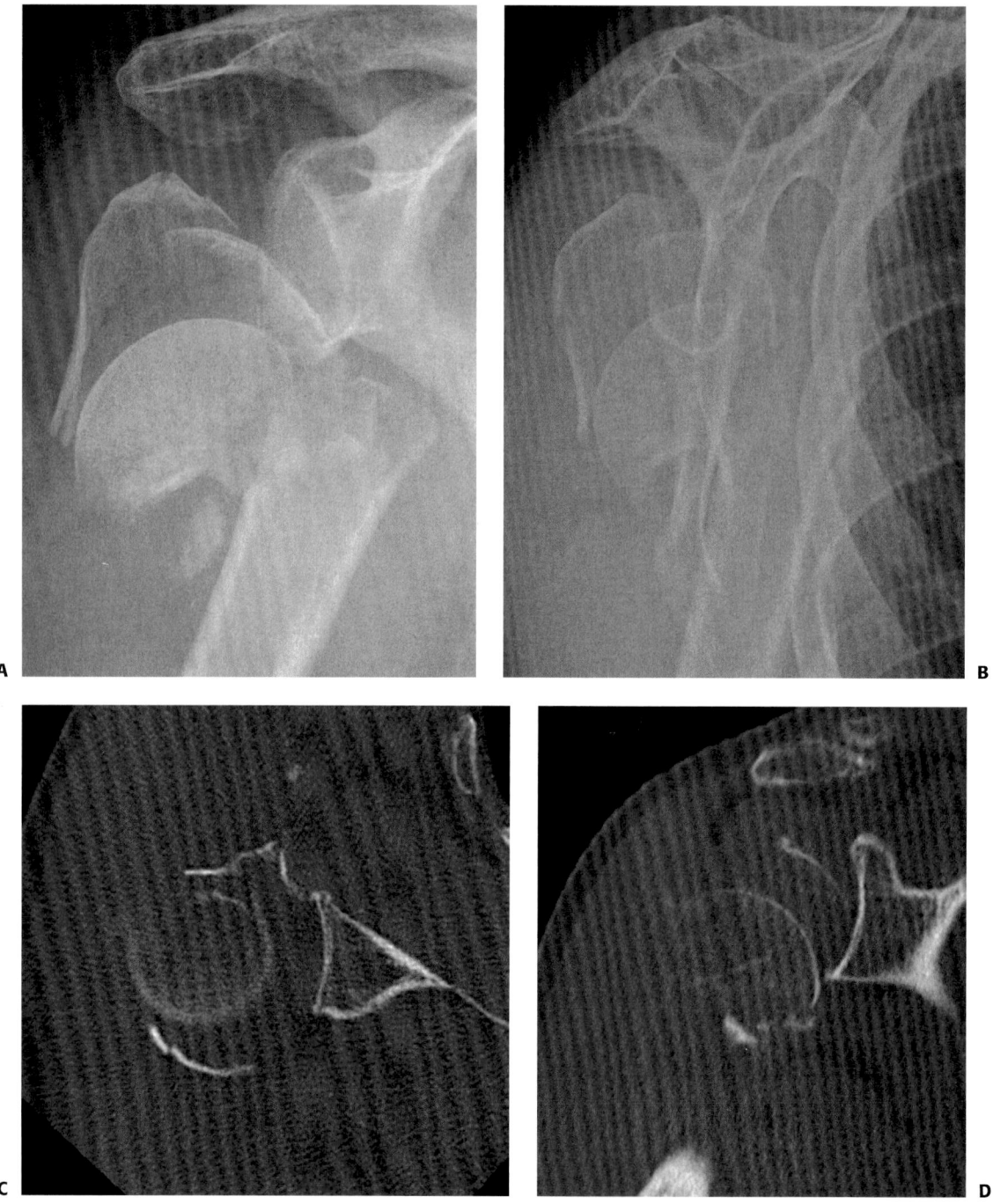

FIGURE 37-42 A–F: Reverse total shoulder arthroplasty. Four-part head split proximal humerus fracture in an 80-year-old female.

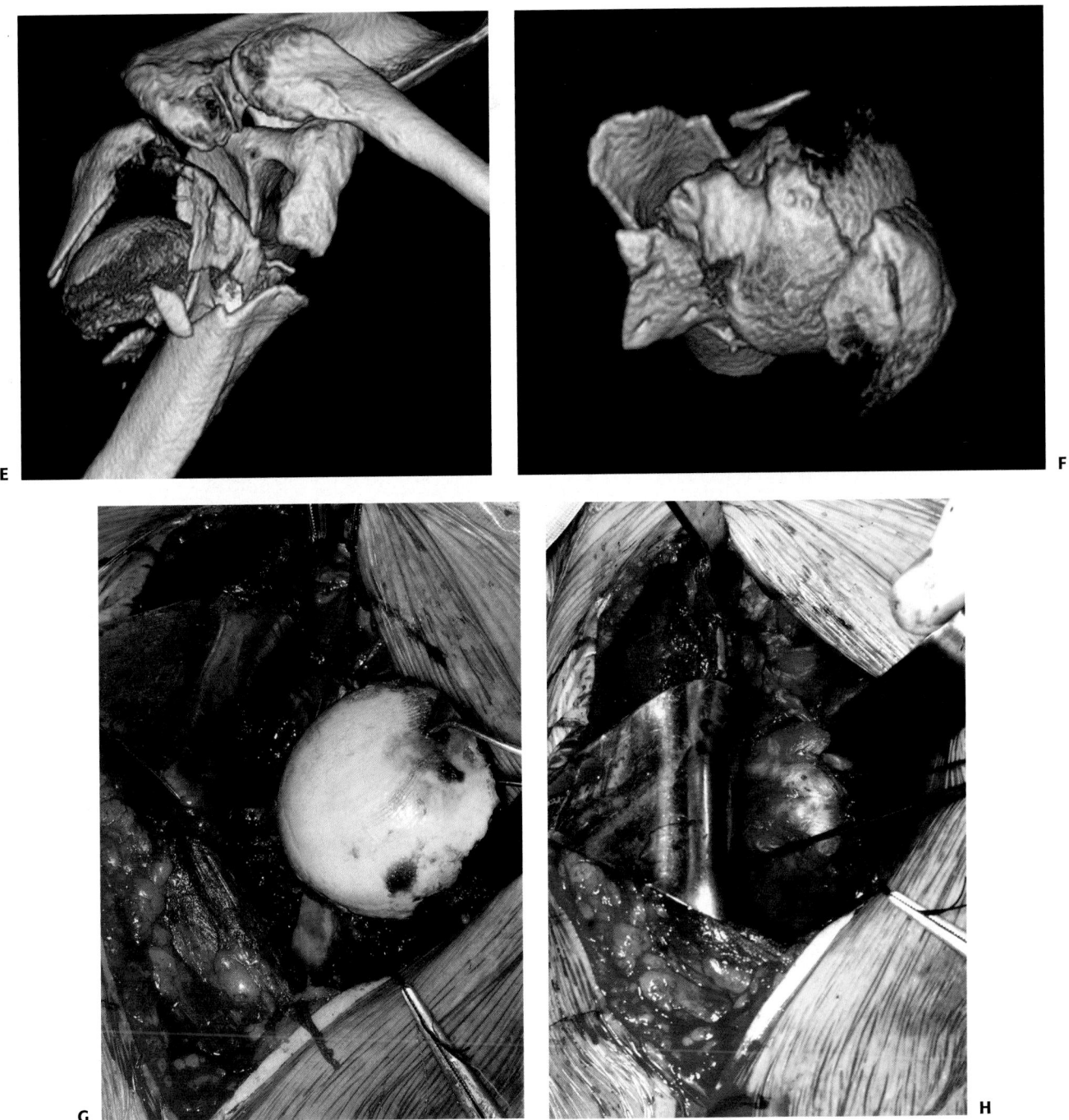

FIGURE 37-42 (*continued*) **G:** Intraoperative image showing extraction of the humeral head fragment.
H: Tagging of the greater tuberosity.   (*continues*)

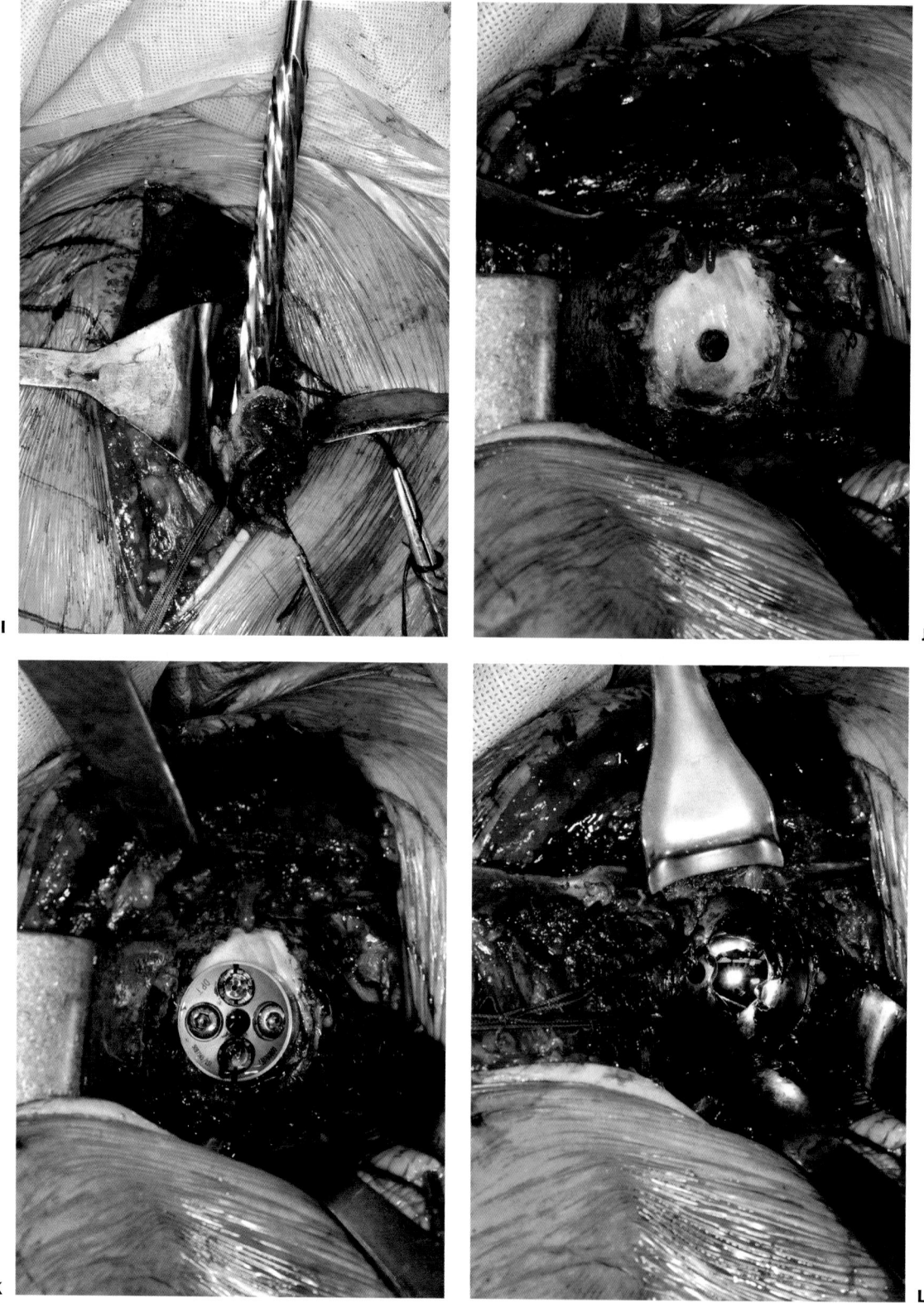

FIGURE 37-42 (*continued*) **I:** Reaming of the humeral canal. **J:** Reaming of the glenoid. **K and L:** Placement of the baseplate and glenosphere.

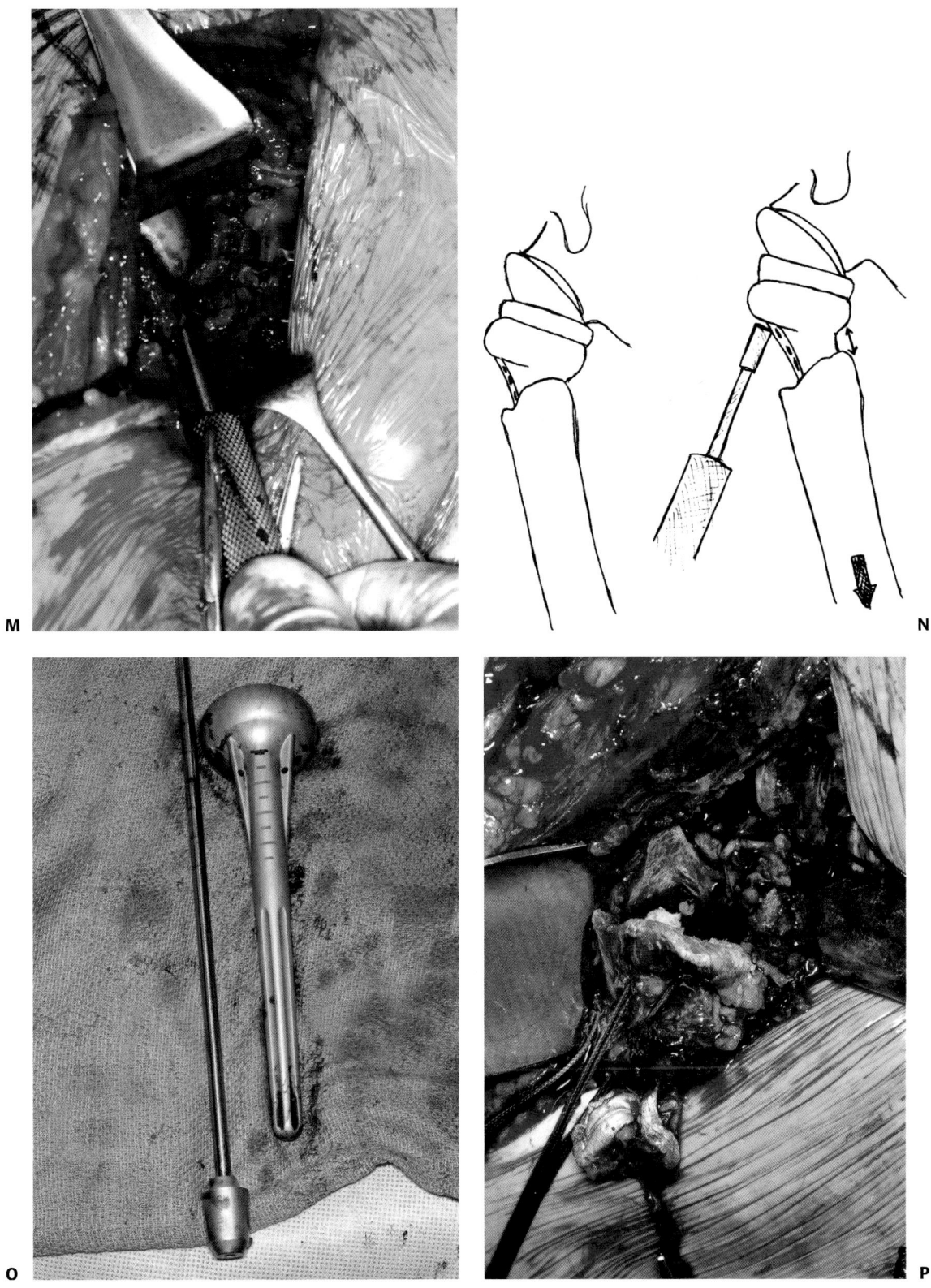

FIGURE 37-42 (*continued*) **M and N:** Assessment of humeral length and depth of stem cementation. While the elbow is pulled distally, the proximal humeral trial component is pushed against the implanted glenosphere. The resulting stem depth is marked. (Part N: Courtesy of Juan Pablo Simone, MD.) **O:** Depth of insertion marked on trial stem and corresponding cement restrictor. **P:** Cement in place. Note the use of methylene blue and placement of two diaphyseal sutures.

(*continues*)

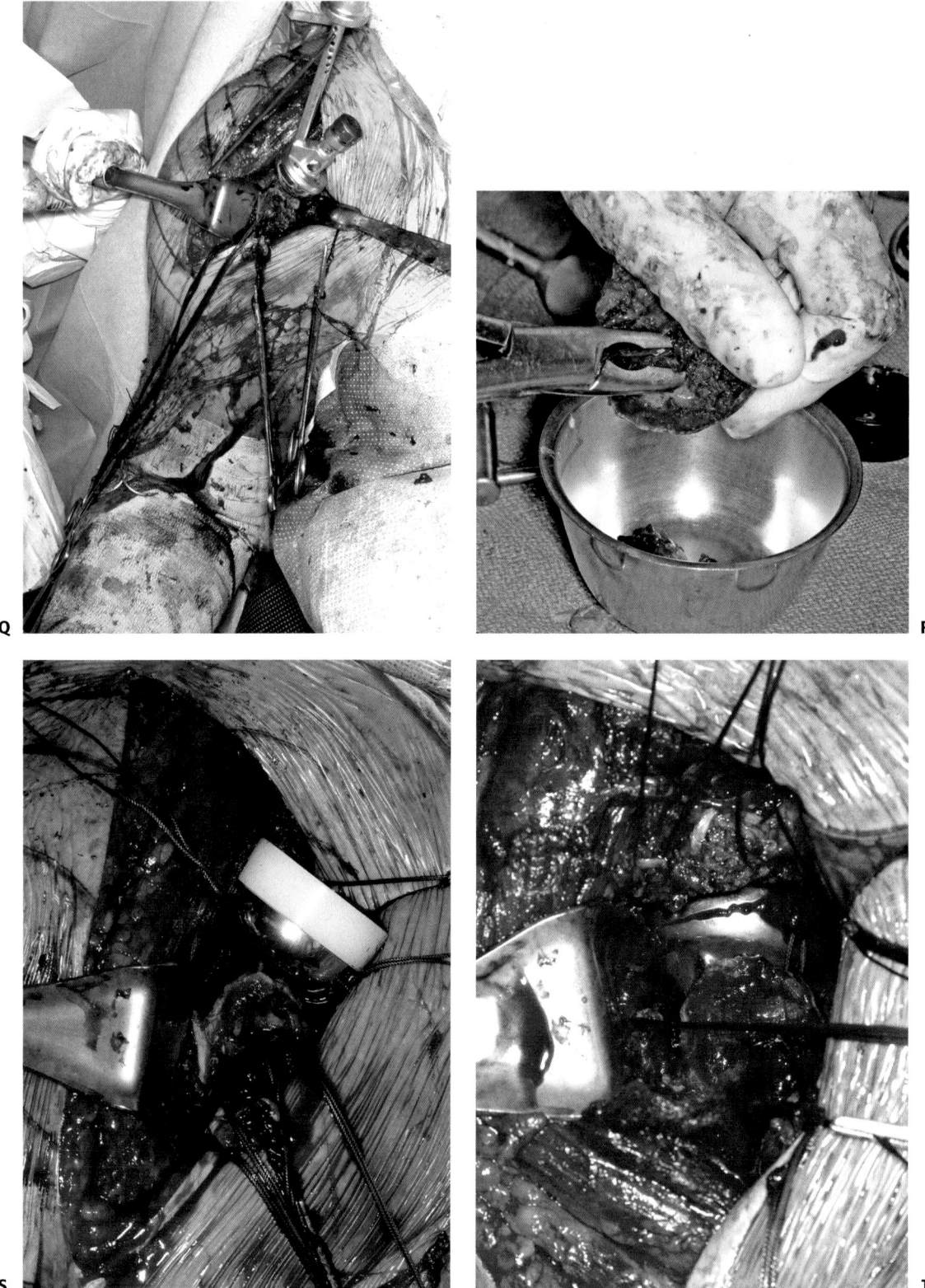

Q

R

S

T

FIGURE 37-42 (*continued*) **Q:** Cementation of final stem in 30 degrees of retroversion using the axis of the forearm as a reference (note the proximal guide pin). **R:** Bone graft is obtained from the resected humeral head. **S:** Proximal humeral polyethylene insert in place. **T:** Preliminary tuberosity reduction.

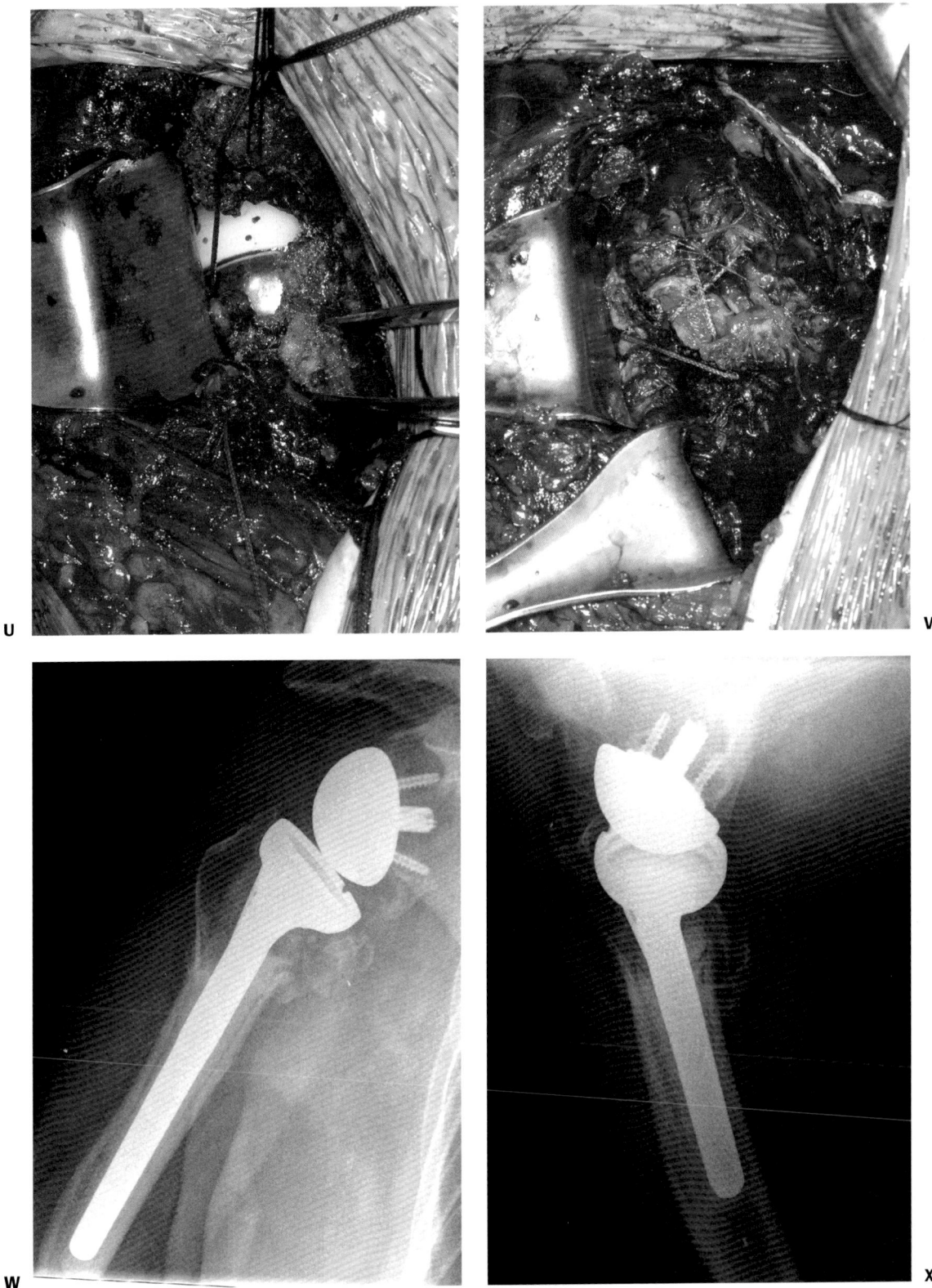

FIGURE 37-42 (*continued*) **U:** Grafting between stem and tuberosities. **V:** Final reduction of tuberosities. **W and X:** Radiographic follow-up 5 months after surgery.

TABLE 37-24 **Reverse Total Shoulder Arthroplasty**

Potential Pitfalls and Preventions

Pitfall	Preventions
Glenoid notching	Adequate inferior exposure of the glenoid to allow inferior glenoid baseplate and glenosphere placement Use of a lateralized glenosphere
Wound hematoma	Careful hemostasis Drain placement Avoid anticoagulation
Instability	Obtain adequate soft tissue tension Use of large glenosphere

Potential Pitfalls and Preventive Measures. A list of potential pitfalls and their prevention is given in Table 37-24. The three main complications associated with reverse total shoulder arthroplasty are wound hematoma and instability in the short-term and glenoid notching, with glenoid component loosening, in the mid to long term.[53,61,323,414]

The incidence of glenoid notching in proximal humeral fractures ranges from 10% to 53%.[53,61] As described, glenoid notching is best avoided with inferior placement of the glenosphere to allow inferomedial clearance of the proximal humerus during adduction. This can be achieved by positioning the baseplate inferiorly on the glenoid. Some systems allow for eccentric positioning of the glenosphere onto the baseplate, thereby permitting a more inferior glenosphere placement.[88] The use of lateralized glenospheres, especially those with a circumference larger than half a sphere, can allow increased medial clearance.[154]

Wound hematoma is the most frequent early postoperative complication after reverse total shoulder arthroplasty.[414] It is therefore recommended to use careful hemostasis during the procedure. A postoperative drain is used for the early postoperative period.

Instability has been shown to be a frequent complication after reverse total shoulder arthroplasty for proximal humeral fractures.[323] Adequate soft tissue tension is required to achieve inherent stability between the humeral concavity and the glenosphere. Theoretically, larger glenospheres should be more stable but these are frequently not implantable in this predominantly smaller elderly female population.

Treatment-Specific Outcomes. Results after reverse total shoulder arthroplasty have been found to frequently be similar to those of hemiarthroplasty, especially during the first 6 postoperative months.[45,126,424] As with hemiarthroplasty, functional scores and range of motion are frequently unpredictable.[237,241] However decline in function over time appears to be more marked after hemiarthroplasty with reverse total shoulder arthroplasty showing improved function 5 years after surgery.[45,137].

In a comparative study of 40 patients with proximal humeral fractures treated with either hemiarthroplasty or reverse total

shoulder arthroplasty, those in the hemiarthroplasty group reported better internal and external rotations. Those in the total shoulder group demonstrated better shoulder abduction, forward elevation, and functional scores. Tuberosity malunion was found in three patients with hemiarthroplasties, whereas 15 patients with reverse arthroplasty developed scapular notching.[126] In a different comparative study of 10 patients with a mean age of 76 years similar functional scores were found between patients undergoing reverse total shoulder arthroplasty and those undergoing hemiarthroplasty. Similar forward elevation and external rotation were found in both the groups.[424]

Cazeneuve et al. reported on 36 patients who had undergone reverse total shoulder arthroplasty. The average age was 75 years with a range of 58 to 92 years. After 7 years of follow-up function of the replaced shoulder was 67% of that of the contralateral shoulder. The complications included four dislocations, one infection, and two cases of complex regional pain syndrome. A total of three components (two glenoid components and one humeral stem) were found to be loose. The most frequent radiographic complications were scapular notching which occurred in 19 patients (53%).[61] Bufquin et al. reported on 43 patients with reverse total shoulder arthroplasty for proximal humeral fractures in patients ranging from 65 to 97 years of age. After a mean follow-up of 2 years, forward elevation and external rotation averaged 97 degrees and 30 degrees, respectively. However a large variation in results was reported with values ranging from 35 to 160 degrees for elevation and 0 to 80 degrees for external rotation. At final follow-up 10 cases (25%) showed scapular notching.[53]

Support for reverse total shoulder arthroplasty for the treatment of acute proximal humeral fractures continues to be scarce in the literature. While some studies show promising results, cautious use of reverse total shoulder arthroplasty should be advised because of the high rate of complications that has been reported. The ideal candidate for reverse total shoulder arthroplasty in a patient with a complex proximal humerus fracture is a low demand elderly patient with pre-existing rotator cuff pathology and glenoid pathology.

MANAGEMENT OF ADVERSE OUTCOME AND COMPLICATIONS

There are numerous complications of proximal humeral fractures that have been described, but most are rare. Complications may occur as an inevitable consequence of a more severe injury or as a result of treatment. The latter may be because of errors in treatment selection or in the surgery that was undertaken. Implant-specific operative complications have been described in the previous sections and will not be discussed further here.

Boileau et al. retrospectively analyzed 203 patients who presented with sequelae of proximal humeral fractures and were subsequently treated with an unconstrained modular prosthesis.[37] They identified 137 (67.5%) cases of humeral head collapse or necrosis, 25 (12.3%) cases of irreducible dislocations or fracture dislocations, 22 (10.8%) cases of nonunion and 19 (9.4%) severe tuberosity malunions. The study did not include all complications of proximal humeral fractures but it highlighted the problems associated with osteonecrosis of the humeral head, nonunion, and tuberosity malunion in particular. These three complications are considered in detail together with an overview of other complications and their treatment.

Osteonecrosis

Humeral Head

Osteonecrosis of the humeral head occurs as a consequence of impaired blood supply of the articular surface and subchondral bone, which undergo involutional change, leading to articular collapse and fibrosis. This condition may or may not be symptomatic,[415] and the head may collapse completely, or there may be partial involvement, with or without articular collapse.[20,170]

This complication may be an inevitable complication of the injury, because of the severe damage to the blood supply of the humeral head. Three- and four-part fractures and fracture dislocations are therefore at higher risk than are one- and two-part fractures. It may also occur as a consequence of operative treatment, because of excessive fracture manipulation and stripping of soft tissues, which contain the residual vascularity to the articular segment. Some individuals may also be predisposed to this complication, either because of their poor physiologic state secondary to their medical comorbidities and drug treatment, or through smoking and alcohol abuse. The pathophysiology of this condition is incompletely understood at present and other unknown factors may also be important. It does not invariably develop even if the head is completely denuded of blood supply,[20,145,170] whereas some cases appear to occur after a relatively innocuous injury.

The presentation is usually with pain, stiffness, and loss of function, typically after a latent period, where function has been satisfactory. Radiologically, the changes vary from patchy humeral head sclerosis, to complete humeral head resorption and collapse. The differential diagnosis is from post-traumatic osteoarthrosis, in which the degree of collapse is usually less severe, and from chronic joint sepsis, which, if clinically suspected, should be excluded by bacteriologic examination of a joint aspirate. CT and especially MRI are useful in the evaluation of the extent and severity of head involvement.

In some cases, the osteonecrosis may not be associated with severe symptoms, and nonoperative treatment is advisable.[415] Core decompression may occasionally be indicated for patients who have early radiologic changes,[278] but most patients have advanced collapse and are symptomatic by the time they present.[144] Hemiarthroplasty is indicated where symptoms are debilitating and function is poor.[93,40] This technique is much more likely to be successful if there is no associated malunion that requires treatment.[144] If there are reciprocal glenoid changes, a total joint arthroplasty may be more successful in relieving pain and restoring motion.[93]

Where there is a severe associated tuberosity malunion or cuff tear, reverse shoulder arthroplasty may provide better function, although comparative studies have not yet been performed to evaluate this.[259,418]

Tuberosity

Osteonecrosis may also occur in one or both tuberosities after fracture, regardless of the viability of the humeral head. Resorption, sclerosis and collapse may be seen after fracture of the greater tuberosity (the "disappearing tuberosity") and may also occur in the lesser tuberosity. It may occur after two-, three-, or four-part fractures and may follow nonoperative treatment, internal fixation, or arthroplasty. This complication is predictable, because until a fractured tuberosity unites, it only receives blood supply through residual periosteal attachments and its cuff attachments, which are often relatively avascular in elderly patients. The patient usually has debilitating shoulder pain and loss of function, with clinical signs of rotator cuff weakness and dysfunction. Subclinical forms probably occur frequently, and the precise pathology has not yet been fully elucidated. At present, there is no known treatment for this complication.

Nonunion

Nonunion of the head to the shaft of the proximal humerus is a rare but debilitating complication.[79] The normal time for clinical union of a proximal humeral fracture is typically 4 to 8 weeks. It is therefore logical to define nonunion to be present if a fracture site is still mobile 16 weeks postinjury, although 6 months has been used in some studies. In the only study to have evaluated the epidemiology of this complication, the overall reported incidence was 1.1%, although this rose to 8% if metaphyseal comminution was present and 10% if there was significant translation of the surgical neck.[79] Nonunion was shown to very rare in varus-impacted proximal humeral fractures. Nonunion of one or both tuberosities to the head is less common and is considered together with tuberosity malunions later in the chapter.

Although nonunion may occur for no obvious reason, in most instances there are identifiable patient-, fracture-, or treatment-related risk factors: Common patient-related factors include osteoporosis, poor physiologic state, medical comorbidities and drug treatment, heavy smoking, and alcohol abuse.[163,352,408] Inflammatory or degenerative shoulder conditions associated with preinjury shoulder stiffness, may also predispose to nonunion.[171] The fractures most at risk of nonunion are two-, three-, or four-part displaced fractures, where there is minimal residual cortical contact between the humeral head and shaft, and in those where there is marked metaphyseal comminution.[79] The complete disruption of the periosteal sleeve leads to mechanical instability, and soft tissue interposition of periosteum, muscle, and the tendinous portion of the long head of biceps may also inhibit callus formation.[124,125,283] It has been suggested that nonoperative treatment with hanging casts, which distract the fracture, and overzealous shoulder mobilization may predispose to nonunion.[286] Poor surgical technique with extensive soft tissue stripping and a mechanically unstable fracture reduction and fixation may also cause nonunion.

In clinical practice the diagnosis of a nonunion is seldom a problem. Pain, stiffness, and loss of function in the arm are the most constant complaints. The pain tends to be severe and debilitating and is aggravated by use of the arm and shoulder, because most movement occurs at the site of the nonunion. This is not amenable to splinting, and the use of a sling further compromises shoulder function. On examination, the patient often has a "pseudoparalysis" of the deltoid, rotator cuff, and periscapular muscles, with a flail arm. Attempted movement of the shoulder is painful and any motion occurs at the fracture site rather than the glenohumeral joint. Radiologically, there is resorption and widening of the fracture line, often with massive bone resorption.

Further investigation should include CT to confirm the nonunion and assess the state of the humeral head articular cartilage, the degree of separation, union of any associated tuberosity fractures, and the feasibility of reduction and fixation of the fracture. If surgical reconstruction has been previously performed, infection should be excluded at the site of the nonunion by culture of an aspirate performed under ultrasound control.[93]

Sustained pain relief and restoration of function after the development of this complication can only be provided by operative treatment. This is technically challenging, because of capsular contractures and scarring from previous surgery, bone loss, distorted anatomy, and osteopenia of the humeral head.[124,125] Unfortunately, many patients with established nonunions are too elderly, frail, or medically unfit to undergo this type of surgery and the prolonged shoulder rehabilitation program thereafter. Pain management and activity modification are all that can be offered to these patients.

All medically fit patients should be offered a surgical reconstruction. Attempts have been made to classify these according to their anatomic site and the degree of bone loss.[63] In practice, the principal decision is whether the nonunion is amenable to ORIF or whether a humeral head replacement is required. The decision as to which form of treatment is most appropriate is individualized, but absence of infection, adequate humeral head bone stock, lack of severe tuberosity malunion, and absence of degenerative change or collapse of the articular surface are mandatory if ORIF is undertaken.

Open Reduction and Internal Fixation

The exposure is similar to that used for primary ORIF. The nonunion is exposed and taken down by excision of the fibrous union and pseudocapsule and removal of any devitalized bone fragments. Arthrolysis of a stiff joint may be required, which aids in subsequent rehabilitation and limits force transmission at the nonunion site.[163] However, care must be taken to avoid devitalization by excessive soft tissue stripping to expose the nonunion. It is essential to ensure that the bone ends are bleeding and the medullary canal is clear of fibrous debris.

If there is minimal bone loss, the bone ends may be reduced in a relatively anatomic fashion. This is unusual, and more commonly there is extensive metaphyseal bone loss because of the

"windscreen-wiper" effect of the shaft at the site of the mobile synovial nonunion. Satisfactory viable bone contact can usually only be achieved by impaling the relatively narrow bayonet of the shaft into the sheath of the wide humeral head metaphysis. The nonunion site is typically grafted with either corticocancellous strips of iliac crest bone graft, an IM bone plug, or a fibular strut graft.[410] This may result in significant humeral shortening, but this is usually well tolerated. If maintenance of length is deemed to be important in a younger patient, this requires more extensive grafting of the metaphyseal defect, using autograft augmented with fibular strut grafting.

Provisional fixation is achieved with K-wires and definitive plate fixation is then performed. A locking proximal humeral plate is the ideal implant in this situation, given the relatively poor proximal humeral bone stock. Postoperative rehabilitation follows the guidelines given for primary fixation.

The treatment of any associated tuberosity fractures depends on whether they are healed and their degree of displacement. Ununited fragments may be amenable to reduction and stabilization using the osteosuturing techniques previously described, whereas healed, minimally displaced tuberosity fragments do not require adjuvant treatment. Tuberosity osteotomy may occasionally be used if there is a severe malunion, but this should be avoided if at all possible because of the risk of subsequent nonunion of the fragment.

Most series that have reported on head-conserving reconstruction of established nonunions have reported a high success rate in achieving union, often with a good eventual functional outcome. However, a high rate of postoperative complications is to be expected, which may require further surgery, and the functional recovery time is usually prolonged.

Humeral Head Arthroplasty

This technique is preferred if there is poor humeral head and metaphyseal bone stock and cavitation, severe tuberosity malunion or displaced nonunion, or collapse and degenerative change of the humeral articular surface. The main aim of the treatment is pain relief, and the eventual poor functional recovery is often worse than for a primary arthroplasty. Although hemiarthoplasty is most commonly used, total shoulder replacement may be indicated if there is glenoid articular surface wear or defects. The functional outcome is poor when osteotomy of the tuberosities is performed, and this should be avoided if possible.[37,39] It has been suggested that reverse shoulder arthroplasty may improve the shoulder function in patients with nonunions associated with severe tuberosity malunions,[37] although comparative studies have not yet been reported.

Most studies that have reported on the use of arthroplasty to treat nonunion suggest that the procedure may be effective in reducing or eliminating pain but there is a high rate of complications which often require further surgery and are associated with a disappointing functional recovery.[10,37,163,283] It remains to be seen in future clinical studies whether the use of reverse shoulder arthroplasty will improve the outcomes obtained with conventional arthroplasty in the treatment of this challenging complication.[41] At present, an arthroplasty should only be considered for patients who have poorly controlled pain and have nonunions that are not amenable to reduction and internal fixation.

Malunion

Some degree of malunion is inevitable in displaced proximal humeral fractures that are treated nonoperatively. It may occur after surgery through intraoperative malreduction or through inadequate fixation that allows secondary redisplacement. Two types of malunion are distinguishable and often coexist. Malunion of the head on the shaft either through impaction, translation, rotation, or angulatory deformity is common and is well tolerated in most patients. Malunion of one of both tuberosities is also common and well tolerated in older patients with limited functional expectations. However, in physiologically younger patients, the altered shoulder mechanics produced by the defunctioning and tearing of the rotator cuff tendons and mechanical impingement of the displaced tuberosity fragments often produces an unacceptable degree of pain and functional compromise. Where the two conditions coexist, it is therefore most often the tuberosity malunion that is symptomatic.

A symptomatic malunion will typically give rise to shoulder pain, which is usually localized over the anterior deltoid. The pain is usually aggravated by use of the arm and particularly by forward flexion, abduction, and internal rotation. This frequently results in impairment of the patient's ability to perform normal daily activities and leisure pursuits. It is important to try to distinguish the cause of symptoms on physical examination, because rotator cuff impingement and tears, post-traumatic shoulder stiffness, acromioclavicular joint dysfunction, biceps tendinopathy, and complex region pain syndromes may all contribute to the symptoms. In addition to specific clinical testing of these structures, a good response to subacromial local anesthetic tends to localize symptoms to the subacromial space. If infection is suspected, appropriate hematologic studies and bacteriologic examination of a joint aspirate are warranted.

The complex anatomy of most malunions is best appreciated using CT with 3D reconstructions. MRI may be useful in evaluating the state of the rotator cuff and capsule, but interpretation of images is frequently hampered by the distorted anatomy. It may be useful in detecting radiologically occult early osteonecrosis. As with nonunion, attempts have been made to classify this complication[27,37] but most often treatment is individualized on the basis of the patient's physiologic status and level of symptoms, the anatomy of the injury, and the likelihood of success from a surgical reconstructive procedure.

The results of corrective surgery are unpredictable, and for older patients a trial of nonoperative treatment is advisable. A shoulder rehabilitation program, pain management, and activity modification may reduce the symptoms to acceptable levels and improve function. The patients who remain symptomatic despite this treatment and request surgery should be carefully counseled about the likely limited gains from surgery, as well as the significant risk of complications. The technical details of the operative treatment according to the anatomic pattern of malunion are discussed below.

Two-Part Greater Tuberosity Malunion or Displaced Nonunion

Isolated malunions and nonunions of the greater tuberosity are relatively common but are usually debilitating only in younger, physically active patients. The deforming forces of the attached cuff muscles cause the tuberosity to retract posterosuperomedially but the articular surface is unaffected. The posterior displacement may produce a bony block to external rotation, while superior displacement may block abduction and lead to subacromial impingement. Tuberosity malposition can also produce cuff dysfunction, attrition, and tears.[364] Arthroscopic assessment may provide useful information and the condition may occasionally be amenable to arthroscopic mobilization and fixation if there is a relatively mobile nonunion.[138]

Surgical reconstruction is usually performed using a deltoid-splitting approach to gain access to the displaced tuberosity, which is usually fixed and immobile. The fragment is mobilized by excision of the fibrous nonunion or osteotomy of a malunion. An extensive posterior capsular release or excision and a rotator interval dissection are often required to mobilize the fragment sufficient for it to be reduced to its decorticated native bed. Fixation is achieved using either interosseous sutures or screw fixation, as for an acute fracture. It is important to test the repair by fully internally rotating the arm, to ensure the repair is not unduly tight. An acromioplasty and subacromial decompression should be performed if the subacromial space is narrowed, to reduce the risk of later impingement. If the repair is tight, the arm is immobilized for 4 weeks in neutral or slight external rotation, to reduce the risk of failure of the repair. The postoperative treatment protocol is otherwise identical to the treatment of an acute fracture. There are a few reports of the results of treatment of greater tuberosity malunions,[27] which report substantial pain relief and functional improvement but with prolonged recovery times.

Two-Part Lesser Tuberosity Malunion or Displaced Nonunion

Two-part lesser tuberosity fractures are frequently diagnosed late or missed at initial presentation.[98,240,294,297] The displaced fragment may block internal rotation or cause subscapularis weakness, and occasionally this may be amenable to arthroscopic treatment.[175] The fragment is exposed through a deltopectoral approach and mobilized with capsular releases as for malunion of the greater tuberosity. Reduction and fixation of an associated articular fracture can be performed with heavy interosseous sutures or screws, dependent on the fragment size.

Two-Part Surgical Neck Malunion

An isolated surgical neck malunion is seldom a cause of severe disability unless the humeral head heals with a varus deformity sufficient to cause secondary cuff impingement or dysfunction.[25,93,364,365,379] The deformity is characteristically a complex angulatory (varus or rarely valgus) and internal rotational malunion, with translation of the shaft anteromedially.[28,93,364,365]

Operative treatment is seldom indicated except in younger patients who are still symptomatic after a prolonged shoulder rehabilitation program. If clinically indicated, osteotomy to correct the deformity and locking plate fixation are performed.[25,379] Open capsular release is usually performed if there is significant associated post-traumatic stiffness and the osteotomy is usually bone grafted. The results from this technique are satisfactory in most reported series.[25,379]

Three- and Four-Part Malunions

In a minority of cases where there is no osteonecrosis and the deformity is less severe, soft tissue release and an osteotomy of the fracture fragments, followed by internal fixation, may be attempted. A successful outcome can only be achieved if there is a good correction of both osseous and soft tissue abnormalities.[27,28] However, most symptomatic malunions are complex 3D deformities, which can usually only be treated by prosthetic replacement. The integrity of the glenoid articular surface determines whether humeral hemiarthroplasty or total shoulder arthroplasty is performed. The chief indication is for pain relief and the functional gains are often minimal. Extensive capsular excision is usually required, and any associated rotator cuff tears should be repaired.

In some cases of tuberosity malposition, a greater tuberosity osteotomy can be avoided by using a small stem that is shifted in the medullary canal to compensate for the tuberosity malposition or by the use of an eccentric modular humeral head. If the normal relationship between the tuberosities and the humeral head cannot be achieved, either a tuberosity osteotomy and conventional arthroplasty, or a reverse shoulder arthroplasty should be performed. There may also be a role for the use of a resurfacing humeral hemiarthroplasty in selected cases, as this does not require the use of an IM stem for fixation. Three quarters of the humeral head must remain after reaming for this technique to be used, to allow secure fixation and prosthetic bone ingrowth.

The available case series literature for treatment of complex multipart malunions is scarce, but the results of arthroplasty are inferior to those of prosthetic treatment of similar acute fractures. In particular, the requirement for tuberosity osteotomy is associated with a poor prognosis.[37] Pain relief is usually achieved, but shoulder range of motion and strength are often limited.[10,27,28,37,44,93,120,255,394] The results of the use of reverse shoulder arthroplasty for the treatment of severe malunion are still largely unknown in the longer term, although this is a promising new technique and the results of comparative outcome studies are awaited.[41]

Other Complications

Post-Traumatic Shoulder Stiffness

The causes of post-traumatic shoulder stiffness are often multifactorial. Although capsular contracture is usually the main cause of refractory stiffness, other factors may include fracture malunion, complex regional pain syndrome, thoracic outlet syndrome, mechanical impingement of implants, and rotator cuff dysfunction from impingement or tears. These factors are poorly described in the contemporary literature but may nevertheless be contributory to persistent stiffness after fracture.

The most characteristic finding is of restriction of movement in a "capsular pattern," with generalized stiffness but selectively greater loss of shoulder abduction and external rotation. The initial treatment is nonoperative with shoulder rehabilitation to attempt to regain movement by selective stretching exercises. Most patients improve to a degree on this regime, and recovery of movement is often protracted over the first year after injury. A plateau in recovery is usually heralded by the presence of a firm "woody" feel on terminal stretching exercises, suggesting a mechanical block to movement. Distension arthrography is useful in stretching and rupturing the capsule in idiopathic adhesive capsulitis, but it is the authors' experience that this procedure is less effective in the post-traumatic shoulder.

In malunited fractures, it is important to distinguish whether the stiffness is because of soft tissue contracture or the malunion itself. An examination under anesthesia under fluoroscopy followed by an arthroscopic examination of the shoulder is often required to distinguish these conditions. If the malunion is considered to be the cause of the stiffness, it is unlikely that a soft tissue release will be effective and consideration must be given to corrective osteotomy as described previously.

In patients with refractory post-traumatic stiffness without malunion, a manipulation under anesthesia is usually performed. This procedure is contraindicated in patients with uncertain fracture healing and in patients with severe osteoporosis, where there is a substantial risk of humeral shaft fracture during manipulation. If manipulation is unsuccessful in regaining sufficient movement, it should be followed by arthroscopic release of capsular tissue from the rotator interval, circumferential intra-articular capsular releases, subacromial decompression, and removal of impinging metal work.[54,180,242] It is important to check for restoration of movement at each stage of the release and to measure the final on-table range of movement at the end of the procedure. The use of a continuous passive movement machine with regional anesthesia may be useful in retaining movement in the early postoperative period. Prolonged physiotherapy is often required thereafter to consolidate the improved range of movement.

Infection

Infection is relatively rare in the shoulder even after surgical repair using open methods. This is because of the rich vascularity of the region and the good soft tissue cover.[72,189] The precise prevalence of this complication is difficult to evaluate, because most reported case series of operative treatment are retrospective. Although infection is usually a postsurgical complication, it may occasionally develop after nonoperative treatment. This is more likely in thin, debilitated patients, either from infection of the fracture hematoma, or in those with displaced surgical neck fractures from pressure on the anterior soft tissues.

Most infections are encountered after surgery and the risk is likely to be increased in thin and debilitated patients, in those patients with a more severe soft tissue injury and a more severe grade of fracture or if there is prolonged surgical time, poor surgical technique, or operator inexperience. It is important to distinguish superficial from deep infections. Superficial infections are common, confined to the skin and subcutaneous layer, and do not form a purulent collection. Superficial pin track infections are a particularly common complication of percutaneous pinning of fractures.[186,207] In contrast, deep infections often form a sinus with a deep purulent collection that extends to the implant. These fail to resolve without further surgical treatment. Ultrasound and MRI may be useful in assessing for the presence of a deep collection.

Superficial infections with a bacteriologically proven growth of pathogenic organisms invariably resolve with antibiotic therapy. It is often difficult to distinguish between a superficial infection and a wound hematoma, especially if cultures are equivocal. Broad-spectrum antibiotic therapy and topical dressings are frequently given empirically following discharge from hospital, and most superficial infections resolve on this regimen. More severe superficial infections should be treated with parenteral antibiotics, guided by wound cultures. An ultrasound guided aspirate is useful in distinguishing a deep purulent infection from a sterile wound hematoma. Large sterile wound hematomas require surgical drainage, as wound dehiscence may otherwise occur, with the risk of subsequent bacterial colonization and deep infection.

Deep infections may occur either early or as a delayed complication, as with any implant-related infection. Early sepsis with a stable implant should be treated with a protocol of repeated surgical irrigation and debridement and with prolonged parenteral and then oral antibiotic therapy. The sepsis may be refractory to this treatment protocol, and in these circumstances a radical debridement with implant removal may be required to eradicate the infection, thereby allowing later revision surgery.

Late deep infection may occur several years after a humeral head arthroplasty. It may follow a transient bacteremia, and the organism may be of low virulence or be antibiotic resistant.[242,382] Debridement, metal work removal, spacer insertion, and antibiotic therapy may help to suppress or eradicate infection. Delayed reimplantation may be possible if the infection can be eradicated.[242,382]

AUTHORS' PREFERRED METHOD

General Treatment Philosophy of Proximal Humerus Fractures

The great majority of proximal humeral fractures are treated nonoperatively. This includes essentially all nondisplaced fractures as well as most valgus-impacted fractures, especially in patients with lower functional expectations. In patients with higher baseline shoulder function and intrinsically higher expectations, surgical treatment may be recommended for most displaced fractures.[30,157,270] Finally, patients with severely displaced and complex proximal humeral fractures are encouraged in most instances to undergo surgery.

In the subset of patients undergoing surgical treatment, we believe that fracture reduction and fixation should be performed in the great majority of cases. In the ideal setting anatomic reduction, with adequate fixation will lead to reestablishing the normal biomechanical relationship between the rotator cuff and a viable humeral head, potentially yielding a close to preinjury level of function. While humeral head necrosis will in most instances adversely affect outcome, partial necrosis may provide an acceptable outcome that is comparable to that of head replacement. We do not feel that based on the current literature, an accurate prediction can be made on what fractures will result in severe humeral head collapse. Results after shoulder hemiarthroplasty have been shown to be highly unpredictable and data on reverse total shoulder arthroplasty is still limited. We therefore consider that every effort should be made to reconstruct the proximal humerus with emphasis being placed on achieving anatomic reduction and stable fixation of the tuberosities. Shoulder arthroplasty is considered in fractures in which a high suspicion of head nonviability is suspected because of severe displacement of the fracture through the anatomical neck without metaphyseal extension, disruption of the medial hinge and frank dislocation from the glenoid. We believe that in technically unreconstructable fractures with fragmentation of the articular surface, arthroplasty should also be considered. In younger patients, hemiarthroplasty is the chosen treatment method. However, in elderly patients, reverse shoulder arthroplasty has become our treatment of choice.

Except for two-part surgical neck fractures, which may be treated with IM nailing, the authors' preferred method of head preserving reconstruction of the proximal humerus is open reduction internal fixation with a locking screw construct. A deltopectoral approach is used for most open reconstructions, especially arthroplasties. A deltoid split is occasionally used for two-part greater tuberosity fractures and three-part greater tuberosity fractures and is the routine approach when IM nail fixation is planned.

Treatment of Individual Injury Patterns of Proximal Humerus Fracture
Nondisplaced or Minimally Displaced One-Part Fractures

These injuries are almost invariably treated nonoperatively with initial immobilization in a sling. Weekly radiographs and clinical assessment are performed for the first 3 weeks. Elbow, wrist, and hand mobilization begins immediately. Passive range-of-motion exercises are begun at 3 weeks if no change in fracture position has been confirmed. Active-assisted range-of-motion exercises are begun at 6 weeks and strengthening is started at 3 months when bony healing has been confirmed radiologically.

Greater Tuberosity Fractures

Neer's criteria of displacement being defined as 1cm of translation or 45 degrees of angulation[284,287] have guided surgeons in their management of proximal humeral fractures for many years and historically these were the criteria that many surgeons applied to the treatment of greater tuberosity fractures.[116,284] However more recently the currently accepted threshold for surgical treatment of greater tuberosity fractures in active patients has become 5 mm with some authors suggesting that greater tuberosity fractures with 3 mm of displacement should be treated surgically in younger patients who have to undertake heavy overhead activity, such as athletes and laborers.[196,245,306,364]

Displacement of the greater tuberosity is poorly tolerated because of its key role in shoulder function.[39,184] In two-part greater tuberosity fractures the greater tuberosity is displaced posteromedially by the pull of supraspinatus, infraspinatus, and teres minor. Displacement of more than 5 mm has been shown to cause symptomatic malunion[364] and to limit abduction and external rotation. As the tuberosity displaces medially it leads to subacromial impingement, which limits abduction, and with posterior displacement abutment of the greater tuberosity against the posterior glenoid will result in limited external rotation. It is in fact likely that shortening of the rotator cuff muscles and altered muscle pull occurs with only minimal greater tuberosity displacement.

Favorable outcomes can be expected when displaced two-part greater tuberosity fractures heal without residual displacement after operative fixation. Flatow et al.[116] reported the results of 12 displaced two-part greater tuberosity fractures that were treated by heavy suture fixation and rotator cuff repair through an anterolateral deltoid-splitting approach. All fractures healed without displacement and the authors reported 100% excellent or good results. Similar results have been reported by other authors.[92,311] We therefore advocate operative fixation of greater tuberosity fractures which are displaced by more than 5 mm in active patients.

Two-Part Greater Tuberosity Fractures and Fracture Dislocations

In older, frail patients (usually older than 80 years) with limited functional expectations, a substantial degree of displacement can be accepted without recourse to operative treatment. These patients often have a poor outcome from surgical reduction and fixation, because of their poor bone quality and pre-existing cuff dysfunction, which precludes stable fixation. Although they will often have signs of continued cuff dysfunction from the tuberosity nonunion or malunion, their functional outcome will usually be adequate for their needs.

Operative treatment is advised for physiologically younger patients, who are typically younger than 65 years, active patients with fractures, which are either primarily displaced by more than 5 mm or become displaced by this amount within the first 2 weeks after injury. Selected older patients, usually aged between 65 and 80 years, with fragment displacement of 1 cm or more are offered operative reconstruction. When there is a tuberosity fragment of greater than 2.5 cm open reduction through a limited deltoid-splitting approach and internal fixation using partially threaded cancellous 3.5-mm screws is performed. It is important to insert screws to transfix the fragment to both the humeral head and the medial cortex of the metaphysis. Meticulous repair of any associated rotator cuff injury is also performed.

When the fragment is smaller than 2.5 cm or if it is heavily comminuted, the injury is treated in the same manner as a rotator cuff avulsion. The injury may be treated either with an arthroscopic technique or an open approach. Fixation is obtained either with suture anchors in a double row pattern or by the use of transosseous sutures.[116,245] Alternatively, a small T-plate may be fixed laterally onto the proximal humerus with three screws and the horizontal component of the plate used to anchor sutures for tuberosity fixation. This may be of particular use in very osteopenic bone.

Associated Bankart lesions are rare and most frequently occur in younger patients.[334] If after tuberosity fixation, the shoulder is found to be unstable when tested intraoperatively, the bony or labral glenoid rim avulsion is repaired.

Two-Part Lesser Tuberosity Fractures and Fracture Dislocations

Isolated lesser tuberosity fractures typically occur in younger or middle-aged patients and are displaced. Nonoperative treatment of these injuries risks later functional incapacity, because of subscapularis dysfunction. It is the authors' policy to treat all these fractures operatively in medically fit patients. ORIF is performed through a standard deltopectoral approach. If there is a single large fragment, definitive internal fixation is performed using partially threaded 3.5-mm cancellous screws, inserted through the lesser tuberosity.[336] Judging accurate screw length (typically between 40 and 50 mm) is an important technical aspect of the procedure, to gain bicortical purchase. If there is comminution associated with a fragment which is 2.5 cm or less screw fixation risks secondary comminution and may not provide sufficient stability. For these patients, the reduction is maintained by transosseous sutures, placed through the bone–tendon junction and through the metaphysis located deep to the fracture bed and lateral to it.[336] Frequently, the long head of the biceps is found to be medially dislocated and injured by the fracture fragment. A biceps tenodesis may therefore be considered.

In the minority of patients where the lesser tuberosity fracture is associated with a locked posterior dislocation, an attempt is initially made to obtain closed reduction of the dislocation under anesthesia. Where this is not possible, an open reduction is performed through an extended deltoid-splitting approach. After reduction of the shoulder has been obtained, the stability of the shoulder is assessed throughout a full range of internal and external rotations with the arm at the side and in 90 degrees of abduction. If the shoulder is acutely unstable because of reengagement of a reverse Hill–Sachs lesion on the posterior glenoid beyond neutral rotation, the reverse Hill–Sachs lesion is either elevated and bone-grafted or, if there is a larger defect, filled with piece of shaped femoral head allograft, which is secured with two countersunk 3.5-mm partially threaded cancellous screws or headless compression screws. The lesser tuberosity is then reattached anatomically, using the same techniques as for other isolated two-part fractures, using either two 3.5-mm partially threaded cancellous screws or transosseous sutures.

Two-Part Surgical Neck Fractures

Almost all fractures in which the shaft is impacted into the surgical neck are treated nonoperatively. A substantial degree of translation of these two fragments is usually tolerated, as long as there is residual cortical contact and impaction. Occasionally, if there is severe varus angulation of the head fragment in a physiologically younger individual (typically younger than 65 years), operative disimpaction, anatomic reduction, and plate fixation will be performed to reduce the risk of later impingement of the greater tuberosity in the narrowed subacromial space and dysfunction of the rotator cuff from its shortened lever arm. In physiologically younger patients, displaced and comminuted surgical neck fractures are managed with ORIF using a locking plate.

An attempt is made to reduce the fracture anatomically whenever possible. It is important to restore continuity of the medial calcar support to prevent acute fixation failure using either structural graft or a low inferomedial screw, which is inserted through the plate. Occasionally, if there is extensive metaphyseal comminution in an older patient, the risk of metaphyseal nonunion is high. If there is extensive metaphyseal comminution shortening and impaction of the shaft fragment within the head is performed to produce a more stable configuration before the plate application. If the bone quality of the humeral head is very poor, a short proximal humeral locked IM nail will often provide more secure fixation than a plate. However, if possible, a locking plate is preferred for definitive fixation to minimize the risk of later rotator cuff dysfunction which is associated with nailing.

Three- and Four-Part Fractures

Fractures that occur in physiologically older patients should be treated nonoperatively if there is residual cortical continuity of the humeral head fragment on the shaft, the tuberosities are not too widely displaced, and the humeral head appears viable. Although the outcome is often imperfect, after union these patients will usually have a pain-free shoulder, which has sufficient function for their everyday needs.

Operative treatment is offered to physiologically younger patients, where it is thought that the risk of nonunion, cuff dysfunction, or osteonecrosis is high or where operative treatment is likely to provide a significant improvement in shoulder function over nonoperative treatment. In practice, this means that surgery to prevent nonunion or cuff dysfunction is often offered to patients with fractures in which the humeral shaft and tuberosities have significantly displaced from the humeral head. The risk of osteonecrosis is determined by the fracture configuration, with wide displacement of the head from the shaft with probable loss of the medial periosteal and capsular hinge, and the absence of a medial metaphyseal spike particularly associated with a higher risk of this complication. There are substantial functional gains from internal fixation for fractures in which the humeral head has displaced from its normal 130-degree head-shaft orientation to occupy an extreme position of varus (90-degree head–shaft angle) or valgus (180-degree head-shaft angle) or where there is marked humeral head articular surface incongruity from displaced marginal articular fragments attached to the tuberosities.

ORIF is performed whenever possible, and preoperative CT can provide an indication of the likelihood that this will be feasible. The goal is to attempt anatomic or near-anatomic reconstruction. Definitive internal fixation is performed, using a proximal humeral locking plate.

The patient is always preoperatively counseled that if the fracture is deemed to be unreconstructable, an arthroplasty will be performed. In young patients a cemented humeral head replacement will be performed, while a reverse total shoulder arthroplasty will be performed in the older patients.

REFERENCES

1. Adedapo AO, Ikpeme JO. The results of internal fixation of three- and four-part proximal humeral fractures with the Polarus nail. *Injury.* 2001;32(2):115–121.
2. Agel J, Jones CB, Sanzone AG, et al. Treatment of proximal humeral fractures with Polarus nail fixation. *J Shoulder Elbow Surg.* 2004;13(2):191–195.
3. Aggarwal S, Bali K, Dhillon MS, et al. Displaced proximal humeral fractures: An Indian experience with locking plates. *J Orthop Surg Res.* 2010;5:60.
4. Agudelo J, Schürmann M, Stahel P, et al. Analysis of efficacy and failure in proximal humeral fractures treated with locking plates. *J Orthop Trauma.* 2007;21(10):676–681.
5. Aksu N, Göğüs A, Kara AN, et al. Complications encountered in proximal humeral fractures treated with locking plate fixation. *Acta Orthop Traumatol Turc.* 2010;44(2):89–96.
6. Altman GT, Gallo RA, Molinero KG, et al. Minimally invasive plate osteosynthesis for proximal humeral fractures: functional results of treatment. *Am J Orthop (Belle Mead NJ).* 2011;40(3):E40–E47.
7. Amstutz HC, Sew Hoy AL, Clarke IC. UCLA anatomic total shoulder arthroplasty. *Clin Orthop Relat Res.* 1981;(155):7–20.
8. Angibaud L, Zuckerman JD, Flurin PH, et al. Reconstructing proximal humeral fractures using the bicipital groove as a landmark. *Clin Orthop Relat Res.* 2007;458:168–174.
9. Antuña SA, Sperling JW, Cofield RH. Shoulder hemiarthroplasty for acute fractures of the proximal humerus: A minimum five-year follow-up. *J Shoulder Elbow Surg.* 2008;17(2):202–209.
10. Antuña SA, Sperling JW, Sánchez-Sotelo J, et al. Shoulder arthroplasty for proximal humeral nonunions. *J Shoulder Elbow Surg.* 2002;11(2):114–121.
11. Babhulkar A, Shyam AK, Sancheti PK, et al. Hemiarthroplasty for comminuted proximal humeral fractures. *J Orthop Surg (Hong Kong).* 2011;19(2):194–199.
12. Badman B, Frankle M, Keating C, et al. Results of proximal humeral locked plating with supplemental suture fixation of rotator cuff. *J Shoulder Elbow Surg.* 2011;20(4):616–624.
13. Bae JH, Oh JK, Chon CS, et al. The biomechanical performance of locking plate fixation with intramedullary fibular strut graft augmentation in the treatment of unstable fractures of the proximal humerus. *J Bone Joint Surg Br.* 2011;93(7):937–941.
14. Bahrs C, Badke A, Rolauffs B, et al. Long-term results after non-plate head-preserving fixation of proximal humeral fractures. *Int Orthop.* 2010;34(6):883–889.
15. Bahrs C, Rolauffs B, Dietz K, et al. Clinical and radiological evaluation of minimally displaced proximal humeral fractures. *Arch Orthop Trauma Surg.* 2010;130(5):673–679.
16. Bahrs C, Rolauffs B, Südkamp NP, et al. Indications for computed tomography (CT-) diagnostics in proximal humeral fractures: A comparative study of plain radiography and computed tomography. *BMC Musculoskelet Disord.* 2009;10:33.
17. Baron JA, Barrett J, Malenka D, et al. Racial differences in fracture risk. *Epidemiology.* 1994;5(1):42–47.
18. Baron JA, Barrett JA, Karagas MR. The epidemiology of peripheral fractures. *Bone.* 1996;18(suppl 3):209S–213S.
19. Baron JA, Karagas M, Barrett J, et al. Basic epidemiology of fractures of the upper and lower limb among Americans over 65 years of age. *Epidemiology.* 1996;7(6):612–618.
20. Bastian JD, Hertel R. Initial post-fracture humeral head ischemia does not predict development of necrosis. *J Shoulder Elbow Surg.* 2008;17(1):2–8.
21. Bastian JD, Hertel R. Osteosynthesis and hemiarthroplasty of fractures of the proximal humerus: Outcomes in a consecutive case series. *J Shoulder Elbow Surg.* 2009;18(2):216–219.
22. Baumfeld JA, O'Driscoll SW, Steinmann SP. Treatment of Two-Part Humeral Surgical Neck Fractures (OTA Code 11-A3) with the Evans Staple, in Orthopedic Trauma Association Annual Meeting 2003: Salt Lake City, Utah.
23. Beaton DE, Wright JG, Katz JN. Development of the QuickDASH: Comparison of three item-reduction approaches. *J Bone Joint Surg Am.* 2005;87(5):1038–1046.
24. Bell JE, Leung BC, Spratt KF, et al. Trends and variation in incidence, surgical treatment, and repeat surgery of proximal humeral fractures in the elderly. *J Bone Joint Surg Am.* 2011;93(2):121–131.
25. Benegas E, Zoppi Filho A, Ferreira Filho AA, et al. Surgical treatment of varus malunion of the proximal humerus with valgus osteotomy. *J Shoulder Elbow Surg.* 2007;16(1):55–59.
26. Bengard MJ, Gardner MJ. Screw depth sounding in proximal humeral fractures to avoid iatrogenic intra-articular penetration. *J Orthop Trauma.* 2011;25(10):630–633.

27. Beredjiklian PK, Iannotti JP, Norris TR, et al. Operative treatment of malunion of a fracture of the proximal aspect of the humerus. *J Bone Joint Surg Am.* 1998;80(10): 1484–1497.
28. Beredjiklian PK, Iannotti JP. Treatment of proximal humerus fracture malunion with prosthetic arthroplasty. *Instr Course Lect.* 1998;47:135–140.
29. Bernstein J, Adler LM, Blank JE, et al. Evaluation of the Neer system of classification of proximal humeral fractures with computerized tomographic scans and plain radiographs. *J Bone Joint Surg Am.* 1996;78(9):1371–1375.
30. Bhandari M, Matthys G, McKee MD, Evidence-Based Orthopaedic Trauma Working Group. Four part fractures of the proximal humerus. *J Orthop Trauma.* 2004;18(2): 126–127.
31. Bigorre N, Talha A, Cronier P, et al. A prospective study of a new locking plate for proximal humeral fracture. *Injury.* 2009;40(2):192–196.
32. Bjorkenheim JM, Pajarinen J, Savolainen V. Internal fixation of proximal humeral fractures with a locking compression plate: A retrospective evaluation of 72 patients followed for a minimum of 1 year. *Acta Orthop Scand.* 2004;75(6):741–745.
33. Blonna D, Castoldi F, Scelsi M, et al. The hybrid technique: Potential reduction in complications related to pins mobilization in the treatment of proximal humeral fractures. *J Shoulder Elbow Surg.* 2010;19(8):1218–1229.
34. Blonna D, Rossi R, Fantino G, et al. The impacted varus (A2.2) proximal humeral fracture in elderly patients: is minimal fixation justified? A case control study. *J Shoulder Elbow Surg.* 2009;18(4):545–552.
35. Bogner R, Hübner C, Matis N, et al. Minimally-invasive treatment of three- and four-part fractures of the proximal humerus in elderly patients. *J Bone Joint Surg Br.* 2008;90(12):1602–1607.
36. Boileau P, Bicknell RT, Mazzoleni N, et al. CT scan method accurately assesses humeral head retroversion. *Clin Orthop Relat Res.* 2008;466(3):661–669.
37. Boileau P, Chuinard C, Le Huec JC, et al. Proximal humerus fracture sequelae: Impact of a new radiographic classification on arthroplasty. *Clin Orthop Relat Res.* 2006;442:121–130.
38. Boileau P, Gonzalez JF, Chuinard C, et al. Reverse total shoulder arthroplasty after failed rotator cuff surgery. *J Shoulder Elbow Surg.* 2009;18(4):600–606.
39. Boileau P, Krishnan SG, Tinsi L, et al. Tuberosity malposition and migration: Reasons for poor outcomes after hemiarthroplasty for displaced fractures of the proximal humerus. *J Shoulder Elbow Surg.* 2002;11(5):401–412.
40. Boileau P, Trojani C, Walch G, et al. Shoulder arthroplasty for the treatment of the sequelae of fractures of the proximal humerus. *J Shoulder Elbow Surg.* 2001;10(4): 299–308.
41. Boileau P, Watkinson D, Hatzidakis AM, et al. Neer Award 2005: The Grammont reverse shoulder prosthesis: Results in cuff tear arthritis, fracture sequelae, and revision arthroplasty. *J Shoulder Elbow Surg.* 2006;15(5):527–540.
42. Boons HW, Goosen JH, van Grinsven S, et al. Hemiarthroplasty for humeral four-part fractures for patients 65 years and older: a randomized controlled trial. *Clin Orthop Relat Res.* 2012;470(12):3483–3491.
43. Boraiah S, Dyke JP, Helfet DL, et al. *Quantitative Assessment of the Vascularity of the Proximal Humerus using Gadolinium Enhanced MRI, in Annual Meeting of the American Academy of Orthopaedic Surgeons 2009:* Las Vegas, NV.
44. Bosch U, Skutek M, Fremerey RW, et al. Outcome after primary and secondary hemiarthroplasty in elderly patients with fractures of the proximal humerus. *J Shoulder Elbow Surg.* 1998;7(5):479–484.
45. Boyle MJ, Youn SM, Frampton CM, et al. Functional outcomes of reverse shoulder arthroplasty compared with hemiarthroplasty for acute proximal humeral fractures. *J Shoulder Elbow Surg.* 2013;22(1):32–37.
46. Brooks CH, Revell WJ, Heatley FW. Vascularity of the humeral head after proximal humeral fractures. An anatomical cadaver study. *J Bone Joint Surg Br.* 1993;75(1): 132–136.
47. Brorson S, Frich LH, Winther A, et al. Locking plate osteosynthesis in displaced 4-part fractures of the proximal humerus. *Acta Orthop.* 2011;82(4):475–481.
48. Brorson S, Olsen BS, Frich LH, et al. Effect of osteosynthesis, primary hemiarthroplasty, and non-surgical management for displaced four-part fractures of the proximal humerus in elderly: A multi-centre, randomised clinical trial. *Trials.* 2009;10:51.
49. Brorson S, Rasmussen JV, Frich LH, et al. Benefits and harms of locking plate osteosynthesis in intraarticular (OTA Type C) fractures of the proximal humerus: A systematic review. *Injury.* 2012;43(7):999–1005.
50. Brunner A, Honigmann P, Treumann T, et al. The impact of stereo-visualisation of three-dimensional CT datasets on the inter- and intraobserver reliability of the AO/OTA and Neer classifications in the assessment of fractures of the proximal humerus. *J Bone Joint Surg Br.* 2009;91(6):766–771.
51. Brunner A, Weller K, Thormann S, et al. Closed reduction and minimally invasive percutaneous fixation of proximal humeral fractures using the Humerusblock. *J Orthop Trauma.* 2010;24(7):407–413.
52. Brunner F, Sommer C, Bahrs C, et al. Open reduction and internal fixation of proximal humeral fractures using a proximal humeral locked plate: A prospective multicenter analysis. *J Orthop Trauma.* 2009;23(3):163–172.
53. Bufquin T, Hersan A, Hubert L, et al. Reverse shoulder arthroplasty for the treatment of three- and four-part fractures of the proximal humerus in the elderly: A prospective review of 43 cases with a short-term follow-up. *J Bone Joint Surg Br.* 2007;89(4):516–520.
54. Burkhart SS. Arthroscopic subscapularis tenolysis: A technique for treating refractory glenohumeral stiffness following open reduction and internal fixation of a displaced three-part proximal humerus fracture. *Arthroscopy.* 1996;12(1):87–91.
55. Burkhead WZ Jr, Scheinberg RR, Box G. Surgical anatomy of the axillary nerve. *J Shoulder Elbow Surg.* 1992;1(1):31–36.
56. Burton DJ, Wells G, Watters A, et al. Early experience with the PlantTan Fixator Plate for 2 and 3 part fractures of the proximal humerus. *Injury.* 2005;36(10):1190–1196.
57. Cai M, Tao K, Yang C, et al. Internal fixation versus shoulder hemiarthroplasty for displaced 4-part proximal humeral fractures in elderly patients. *Orthopedics.* 2012;35(9):e1340–e1346.
58. Calvo E, Morcillo D, Foruria AM, et al. Nondisplaced proximal humeral fractures: High incidence among outpatient-treated osteoporotic fractures and severe impact on upper extremity function and patient subjective health perception. *J Shoulder Elbow Surg.* 2011;20(5):795–801.
59. Carbone S, Tangari M, Gumina S, et al. Percutaneous pinning of three- or four-part fractures of the proximal humerus in elderly patients in poor general condition: MIROS(R) versus traditional pinning. *Int Orthop.* 2012;36(6):1267–1273.
60. Cazeneuve JF, Cristofari DJ. Long term functional outcome following reverse shoulder arthroplasty in the elderly. *Orthop Traumatol Surg Res.* 2011;97(6):583–589.
61. Cazeneuve JF, Cristofari DJ. The reverse shoulder prosthesis in the treatment of fractures of the proximal humerus in the elderly. *J Bone Joint Surg Br.* 2010;92(4):535–539.
62. Charalambous CP, Siddique I, Valluripalli K, et al. Proximal humeral internal locking system (PHILOS) for the treatment of proximal humeral fractures. *Arch Orthop Trauma Surg.* 2007;127(3):205–210.
63. Checchia SL, Doneux P, Miyazaki AN, et al. Classification of non-unions of the proximal humerus. *Int Orthop.* 2000;24(4):217–220.
64. Chow RM, Begum F, Beaupre LA, et al. Proximal humeral fracture fixation: Locking plate construct +/− intramedullary fibular allograft. *J Shoulder Elbow Surg.* 2012;21(7):894–901.
65. Chu SP, Kelsey JL, Keegan TH, et al. Risk factors for proximal humerus fracture. *Am J Epidemiol.* 2004;160(4):360–367.
66. Clavert P, Lutz JC, Wolfram-Gabel R, et al. Relationships of the musculocutaneous nerve and the coracobrachialis during coracoid abutment procedure (Latarjet procedure). *Surg Radiol Anat.* 2009;31(1):49–53.
67. Clavertt P, Adam P, Bevort A, et al. Pitfalls and complications with locking plate for proximal humerus fracture. *J Shoulder Elbow Surg.* 2010;19(4):489–494.
68. Clement ND, Aitken S, Duckworth AD, et al. Multiple fractures in the elderly. *J Bone Joint Surg Br.* 2012;94(2):231–236.
69. Clinton J, Franta A, Polissar NL, et al. Proximal humeral fracture as a risk factor for subsequent hip fractures. *J Bone Joint Surg Am.* 2009;91(3):503–511.
70. Codman EA. Committee for Standardization of Hospitals [of the American College of Surgeons]. Minimum standard for hospitals. *Bull Am Coll Surg.* 1924;8(4).
71. Codman EA. *The Shoulder: Rupture of the Supraspinatus Tendon and Other Lesions in or About the Subacromial Bursa.* Boston, MA: Thomas Todd Co; 1934.
72. Connor, PM, Flatow EL. Complications of internal fixation of proximal humeral fractures. *Instr Course Lect.* 1997;46:25–37.
73. Constant CR, Murley AH. A clinical method of functional assessment of the shoulder. *Clin Orthop Relat Res.* 1987;(214):160–164.
74. Cornell CN, Levine D, Pagnani MJ. Internal fixation of proximal humeral fractures using the screw-tension band technique. *J Orthop Trauma.* 1994;8(1):23–27.
75. Coudane H, Fays J, De La Selle H, et al. Arteriography after complex fractures of the upper extremity of the humerus bone: A prospective study - preliminary results, in 13th Congress of the European Society for Surgery of the Shoulder and Elbow1999: The Hague, Netherlands.
76. Court-Brown CM, Cattermole H, McQueen MM. Impacted valgus fractures (B1.1) of the proximal humerus. The results of non-operative treatment. *J Bone Joint Surg Br.* 2002;84(4):504–508.
77. Court-Brown CM, Garg A, McQueen MM. The epidemiology of proximal humeral fractures. *Acta Orthop Scand.* 2001;72(4):365–371.
78. Court-Brown CM, Garg A, McQueen MM. The translated two-part fracture of the proximal humerus. Epidemiology and outcome in the older patient. *J Bone Joint Surg Br.* 2001;83(6):799–804.
79. Court-Brown CM, McQueen MM. Nonunions of the proximal humerus: their prevalence and functional outcome. *J Trauma.* 2008;64(6):1517–1521.
80. Court-Brown CM, McQueen MM. Open reduction and internal fixation of proximal humeral fractures with use of the locking proximal humerus plate. *J Bone Joint Surg Am.* 2009;91(11):2771; author reply 2771–2772.
81. Crosby LA, Finnan RP, Anderson CG, et al. Tetracycline labeling as a measure of humeral head viability after 3- or 4-part proximal humerus fracture. *J Shoulder Elbow Surg.* 2009.
82. Cruess RL. Steroid-induced avascular necrosis of the head of the humerus. Natural history and management. *J Bone Joint Surg Br.* 1976;58(3):313–317.
83. Cuny C, Scarlat MM, Irrazi M, et al. The Telegraph nail for proximal humeral fractures: A prospective four-year study. *J Shoulder Elbow Surg.* 2008;17(4):539–545.
84. Cuomo F, Flatow EL, Maday MG, et al. Open reduction and internal fixation of two- and three-part displaced surgical neck fractures of the proximal humerus. *J Shoulder Elbow Surg.* 1992;1(6):287–295.
85. Darder A, Darder A, Sanchis V, et al. Four-part displaced proximal humeral fractures: Operative treatment using Kirschner wires and a tension band. *J Orthop Trauma.* 1993;7(6):497–505.
86. Dawson J, Carr A. Outcomes evaluation in orthopaedics. *J Bone Joint Surg Br.* 2001;83(3):313–315.
87. Dawson J, Fitzpatrick R, Carr A. Questionnaire on the perceptions of patients about shoulder surgery. *J Bone Joint Surg Br.* 1996;78(4):593–600.
88. De Biase CF, Delcogliano M, Borroni M, et al. Reverse total shoulder arthroplasty: radiological and clinical result using an eccentric glenosphere. *Musculoskelet Surg.* 2012;96(suppl 1):S27–S34.
89. Demirhan M, Kilicoglu O, Altinel L, et al. Prognostic factors in prosthetic replacement for acute proximal humeral fractures. *J Orthop Trauma.* 2003;17(3):181–188; discussion 188–189.
90. Den Hartog D, Van Leishout EM, Tuinebreijer WE, et al. Primary hemiarthroplasty versus conservative treatment for comminuted fractures of the proximal humerus in the elderly (ProCon): A multicenter randomized controlled trial. *BMC Musculoskelet Disord.* 2010;11:97.
91. Dietz SO, Hartmann F, Schwarz T, et al. Retrograde nailing versus locking plate osteosynthesis of proximal humeral fractures: A biomechanical study. *J Shoulder Elbow Surg.* 2012;21(5):618–624.
92. Dimakopoulos P, Panagopoulos A, Kasimatis G. Transosseous suture fixation of proximal humeral fractures. *J Bone Joint Surg Am.* 2007;89(8):1700–1709.

93. Dines DM, Warren RF, Altchek DW, et al. Posttraumatic changes of the proximal humerus: Malunion, nonunion, and osteonecrosis. Treatment with modular hemiarthroplasty or total shoulder arthroplasty. *J Shoulder Elbow Surg.* 1993;2(1):11–21.
94. Duda GN, Epari DR, Babst R, et al. Mechanical evaluation of a new minimally invasive device for stabilization of proximal humeral fractures in elderly patients: A cadaver study. *Acta Orthop.* 2007;78(3):430–435.
95. Duparc F, Muller JM, Freger P. Arterial blood supply of the proximal humeral epiphysis. *Surg Radiol Anat.* 2001;23(3):185–190.
96. Duralde XA, Leddy LR. The results of ORIF of displaced unstable proximal humeral fractures using a locking plate. *J Shoulder Elbow Surg.* 2010;19(4):480–488.
97. Durigan A Jr, Barbieri CH, Mazzer N, et al. Two-part surgical neck fractures of the humerus: Mechanical analysis of the fixation with four Shanz-type threaded pins in four different assemblies. *J Shoulder Elbow Surg.* 2005;14(1):96–102.
98. Earwaker J. Isolated avulsion fracture of the lesser tuberosity of the humerus. *Skeletal Radiol.* 1990;19(2):121–125.
99. Edelson G, Kelly I, Vigder F, et al. A three-dimensional classification for fractures of the proximal humerus. *J Bone Joint Surg Br.* 2004;86(3):413–425.
100. Edwards SL, Wilson NA, Zhang LQ, et al. Two-part surgical neck fractures of the proximal part of the humerus. A biomechanical evaluation of two fixation techniques. *J Bone Joint Surg Am.* 2006;88(10):2258–2264.
101. Egol KA, Ong CC, Walsh M, et al. Early complications in proximal humeral fractures (OTA Types 11) treated with locked plates. *J Orthop Trauma.* 2008;22(3):159–164.
102. El-Alfy BS. Results of the percutaneous pinning of proximal humeral fractures with a modified palm tree technique. *Int Orthop.* 2011;35(9):1343–1347.
103. Ellman H, Hanker G, Bayer M. Repair of the rotator cuff. End-result study of factors influencing reconstruction. *J Bone Joint Surg Am.* 1986;68(8):1136–144.
104. El-Sayed MM. Surgical management of complex humerus head fractures. *Orthop Rev (Pavia).* 2010;2(2):e14.
105. Erhardt JB, Roderer G, Grob K, et al. Early results in the treatment of proximal humeral fractures with a polyaxial locking plate. *Arch Orthop Trauma Surg.* 2009;129(10):1367–1374.
106. Esen E, Doğramaci Y, Gültekin S, et al. Factors affecting results of patients with humeral proximal end fractures undergoing primary hemiarthroplasty: A retrospective study in 42 patients. *Injury.* 2009;40(12):1336–1341.
107. Esser RD. Open reduction and internal fixation of three- and four-part fractures of the proximal humerus. *Clin Orthop Relat Res.* 1994;(299):244–251.
108. Esser RD. Treatment of three- and four-part fractures of the proximal humerus with a modified cloverleaf plate. *J Orthop Trauma.* 1994;8(1):15–22.
109. Fallatah S, Dervin GF, Brunet JA, et al. Functional outcome after proximal humeral fractures treated with hemiarthroplasty. *Can J Surg.* 2008;51(5):361–365.
110. Fankhauser F, Boldin C, Schippinger G, et al. A new locking plate for unstable fractures of the proximal humerus. *Clin Orthop Relat Res.* 2005;(430):176–181.
111. Farmer KW, Wright TW. Three- and four-part proximal humeral fractures: open reduction and internal fixation versus arthroplasty. *J Hand Surg Am.* 2010;35(11): 1881–1884; quiz 1884.
112. Fazal MA, Haddad FS. Philos plate fixation for displaced proximal humeral fractures. *J Orthop Surg (Hong Kong).* 2009;17(1):15–18.
113. Fenichel I, Oran A, Burstein G, et al. Percutaneous pinning using threaded pins as a treatment option for unstable two- and three-part fractures of the proximal humerus: A retrospective study. *Int Orthop.* 2006;30(3):153–157.
114. Fjalestad T, Hole MØ, Hovden IA, et al. Surgical treatment with an angular stable plate for complex displaced proximal humeral fractures in elderly patients: A randomized controlled trial. *J Orthop Trauma.* 2012;26(2):98–106.
115. Flatow EL, Bigliani LU, April EW. An anatomic study of the musculocutaneous nerve and its relationship to the coracoid process. *Clin Orthop Relat Res.* 1989;(244):166–171.
116. Flatow EL, Cuomo F, Maday MG, et al. Open reduction and internal fixation of two-part displaced fractures of the greater tuberosity of the proximal part of the humerus. *J Bone Joint Surg Am.* 1991;73(8):1213–1218.
117. Foroohar A, Tosti R, Richmond JM, et al. Classification and treatment of proximal humeral fractures: Inter-observer reliability and agreement across imaging modalities and experience. *J Orthop Surg Res.* 2011;6:38.
118. Foruria AM, Carrascal MT, Revilla C, et al. Proximal humerus fracture rotational stability after fixation using a locking plate or a fixed-angle locked nail: The role of implant stiffness. *Clin Biomech (Bristol, Avon).* 2010;25(4):307–311.
119. Foruria AM, de Gracia MM, Larson DR, et al. The pattern of the fracture and displacement of the fragments predict the outcome in proximal humeral fractures. *J Bone Joint Surg Br.* 2011;93(3):378–386.
120. Frich LH, Sojbjerg JO, Sneppen O. Shoulder arthroplasty in complex acute and chronic proximal humeral fractures. *Orthopedics.* 1991;14(9):949–954.
121. Friess DM, Attia A. Locking plate fixation for proximal humeral fractures: a comparison with other fixation techniques. *Orthopedics.* 2008;31(12).
122. Fuchtmeier B, Bröckner S, Hente R, et al. The treatment of dislocated humeral head fractures with a new proximal intramedullary nail system. *Int Orthop.* 2008;32(6): 759–765.
123. Gaheer RS, Hawkins A. Fixation of 3- and 4-part proximal humeral fractures using the PHILOS plate: Mid-term results. *Orthopedics.* 2010;33(9):671.
124. Galatz LM, Iannotti JP. Management of surgical neck nonunions. *Orthop Clin North Am.* 2000;31(1):51–61.
125. Galatz LM, Williams GR Jr, Fenlin JM Jr, et al. Outcome of open reduction and internal fixation of surgical neck nonunions of the humerus. *J Orthop Trauma.* 2004;18(2): 63–67.
126. Gallinet D, Clappaz P, Garbulo P, et al. Three or four parts complex proximal humeral fractures: Hemiarthroplasty versus reverse prosthesis: a comparative study of 40 cases. *Orthop Traumatol Surg Res.* 2009;95(1):48–55.
127. Gallo RA, Hughes T, Altman G. Percutaneous plate fixation of two- and three-part proximal humeral fractures. *Orthopedics.* 2008;31(3):237–242.
128. Gallo RA, Sciulli R, Daffner RH, et al. Defining the relationship between rotator cuff injury and proximal humeral fractures. *Clin Orthop Relat Res.* 2007;458:70–77.
129. Gardner MJ. Proximal humeral fractures. In: Gardner MJ, Dunbar R, Henley M, Nork S, eds. *Harborview Illustrated Tips and Tricks in Fracture Surgery.* Philadelphia, PA: Lippincott Williams & Wilkins; 2010:42–53.
130. Gardner MJ, Boraiah S, Helfet DL, et al. Indirect medial reduction and strut support of proximal humeral fractures using an endosteal implant. *J Orthop Trauma.* 2008;22(3):195–200.
131. Gardner MJ, Boraiah S, Helfet DL, et al. The anterolateral acromial approach for fractures of the proximal humerus. *J Orthop Trauma.* 2008;22(2):132–137.
132. Gardner MJ, Griffith MH, Dines JS, et al. A minimally invasive approach for plate fixation of the proximal humerus. *Bull Hosp Jt Dis.* 2004;62(1-2):18–23.
133. Gardner MJ, Griffith MH, Dines JS, et al. The extended anterolateral acromial approach allows minimally invasive access to the proximal humerus. *Clin Orthop Relat Res.* 2005;(434):123–129.
134. Gardner MJ, Voos JE, Wanich T, et al. Vascular implications of minimally invasive plating of proximal humeral fractures. *J Orthop Trauma.* 2006;20(9):602–607.
135. Gardner MJ, Weil Y, Barker JU, et al. The importance of medial support in locked plating of proximal humeral fractures. *J Orthop Trauma.* 2007;21(3):185–191.
136. Garnavos C, Lasanianos N. Intramedullary nailing of combined/extended fractures of the humeral head and shaft. *Journal of orthopaedic trauma.* 2010;24(4):199–206.
137. Garrigues GE, Johnston PS, Pepe MD, et al. Hemiarthroplasty versus reverse total shoulder arthroplasty for acute proximal humeral fractures in elderly patients. *Orthopedics.* 2012;35(5):e703–e708.
138. Gartsman GM, Taverna E. Arthroscopic treatment of rotator cuff tear and greater tuberosity fracture nonunion. *Arthroscopy.* 1996;12(2):242–244.
139. Gavaskar AS, Muthukumar S, Chowdary N. Biological osteosynthesis of complex proximal humeral fractures: Surgical technique and results from a prospective single center trial. *Arch Orthop Trauma Surg.* 2010;130(5):667–672.
140. Geiger EV, Maier M, Kelm A, et al. Functional outcome and complications following PHILOS plate fixation in proximal humeral fractures. *Acta Orthop Traumatol Turc.* 2010;44(1):1–6.
141. Georgousis M, Kontogeorgakos V, Kourkouvelas S, et al. Internal fixation of proximal humeral fractures with the polarus intramedullary nail. *Acta Orthop Belg.* 2010;76(4):462–467.
142. Gerber C. Integrated scoring systems for the functional assessment of the shoulder. In: Matsen FAI, Fu FH, Hawkins RJ, eds. *The Shoulder: A Balance of Mobility and Stability.* Rosemont, IL: American Academy of Orthopaedic Surgeons; 1993:531–550.
143. Gerber C, Fuchs B, Hodler J. The results of repair of massive tears of the rotator cuff. *J Bone Joint Surg Am.* 2000;82(4):505–515.
144. Gerber C, Hersche O, Berberat C. The clinical relevance of posttraumatic avascular necrosis of the humeral head. *J Shoulder Elbow Surg.* 1998;7(6):586–590.
145. Gerber C, Lambert SM, Hoogewoud HM. Absence of avascular necrosis of the humeral head after post-traumatic rupture of the anterior and posterior humeral circumflex arteries. A case report. *J Bone Joint Surg Am.* 1996;78(8):1256–1259.
146. Gerber C, Pennington SD, Nyffeler RW. Reverse total shoulder arthroplasty. *J Am Acad Orthop Surg.* 2009;17(5):284–295.
147. Gerber C, Schneeberger AG, Vinh TS. The arterial vascularization of the humeral head. An anatomical study. *J Bone Joint Surg Am.* 1990;72(10):1486–1494.
148. Gorthi V, Moon YL, Jo SH, et al. Life-threatening posterior circumflex humeral artery injury secondary to fracture-dislocation of the proximal humerus. *Orthopedics.* 2010:200–202.
149. Goutallier D, Postel JM, Gleyze P, et al. Influence of cuff muscle fatty degeneration on anatomic and functional outcomes after simple suture of full-thickness tears. *J Shoulder Elbow Surg.* 2003;12(6):550-4.
150. Gradl G, Dietze A, Arndt D, et al. Angular and sliding stable antegrade nailing (Targon PH) for the treatment of proximal humeral fractures. *Arch Orthop Trauma Surg.* 2007; 127(10):937–944.
151. Gradl G, Dietze A, Kääb M, et al. Is locking nailing of humeral head fractures superior to locking plate fixation? *Clin Orthop Relat Res.* 2009;467(11):2986–2993.
152. Greiner S, Kääb MJ, Haas NP, et al. Humeral head necrosis rate at mid-term follow-up after open reduction and angular stable plate fixation for proximal humeral fractures. *Injury.* 2009;40(2):186–191.
153. Griffin MR, Ray WA, Fought PL, et al. Black-white differences in fracture rates. *Am J Epidemiol.* 1992;136(11):1378–1385.
154. Gutiérrez S, Comiskey CA 4th, Luo ZP, et al. Range of impingement-free abduction and adduction deficit after reverse shoulder arthroplasty. Hierarchy of surgical and implant-design-related factors. *J Bone Joint Surg Am.* 2008;90(12):2606–2615.
155. Gutierrez S, Walker M, Willis M, et al. Effects of tilt and glenosphere eccentricity on baseplate/bone interface forces in a computational model, validated by a mechanical model, of reverse shoulder arthroplasty. *J Shoulder Elbow Surg.* 2011;20(5):732–739.
156. Handoll H, Brealey S, Rangan A, et al. Protocol for the ProFHER (PROximal Fracture of the Humerus: Evaluation by Randomisation) trial: A pragmatic multi-centre randomised controlled trial of surgical versus non-surgical treatment for proximal fracture of the humerus in adults. *BMC Musculoskelet Disord.* 2009;10:140.
157. Handoll HH, Ollivere BJ. Interventions for treating proximal humeral fractures in adults. *Cochrane Database Syst Rev.* 2010;(12):CD000434.
158. Handschin AE, Cardell M, Contaldo C, et al. Functional results of angular-stable plate fixation in displaced proximal humeral fractures. *Injury.* 2008;39(3):306–313.
159. Hanson B, Neidenbach P, de Boer P, et al. Functional outcomes after nonoperative management of fractures of the proximal humerus. *J Shoulder Elbow Surg.* 2009;18(4):612–621.
160. Hardeman F, Bollars P, Donnelly M, et al. Predictive factors for functional outcome and failure in angular stable osteosynthesis of the proximal humerus. *Injury.* 2012;43(2):153–158.
161. Harrison AK, Gruson KI, Zmistowski B, et al. Intermediate outcomes following percutaneous fixation of proximal humeral fractures. *J Bone Joint Surg Am.* 2012;94(13): 1223–1228.
162. Hawkins RJ, Bell RH, Gurr K. The three-part fracture of the proximal part of the humerus. Operative treatment. *J Bone Joint Surg Am.* 1986;68(9):1410–1414.

163. Healy WL, Jupiter JB, Kristiansen TK, et al. Nonunion of the proximal humerus. A review of 25 cases. *J Orthop Trauma.* 1990;4(4):424–431.

164. Helwig P, Bahrs C, Epple B, et al. Does fixed-angle plate osteosynthesis solve the problems of a fractured proximal humerus? A prospective series of 87 patients. *Acta Orthop.* 2009;80(1):92–96.

165. Hems TE, Mahmood F. Injuries of the terminal branches of the infraclavicular brachial plexus: Patterns of injury, management and outcome. *J Bone Joint Surg Br.* 2012;94(6):799–804.

166. Hepp P, Lill H, Bail H, et al. Where should implants be anchored in the humeral head? *Clin Orthop Relat Res.* 2003;(415):139–147.

167. Hepp P, Theoplod J, Osterhoff G, et al. Bone quality measured by the radiogrammetric parameter "cortical index" and reoperations after locking plate osteosynthesis in patients sustaining proximal humeral fractures. *Arch Orthop Trauma Surg.* 2009;129(9):1251–1259.

168. Hepp P, Theopold J, Voigt C, et al. The surgical approach for locking plate osteosynthesis of displaced proximal humeral fractures influences the functional outcome. *J Shoulder Elbow Surg.* 2008;17(1):21–28.

169. Hertel R. Fractures of the proximal humerus in osteoporotic bone. *Osteoporos Int.* 2005;16(suppl 2):S65–S72.

170. Hertel R, Hempfing A, Steihler M, et al. Predictors of humeral head ischemia after intracapsular fracture of the proximal humerus. *J Shoulder Elbow Surg.* 2004;13(4):427–433.

171. Hessmann M, Baumgaertel F, Gehling H, et al. Plate fixation of proximal humeral fractures with indirect reduction: Surgical technique and results utilizing three shoulder scores. *Injury.* 1999;30(7):453–462.

172. Hessmann MH, Hansen WS, Krummenauer F, et al. Locked plate fixation and intramedullary nailing for proximal humeral fractures: A biomechanical evaluation. *J Trauma.* 2005;58(6):1194–1201.

173. Hettrich CM, Boraiah S, Dyke JP, et al. Quantitative assessment of the vascularity of the proximal part of the humerus. *J Bone Joint Surg Am.* 2010;92(4):943–948.

174. Hettrich CM, Neviaser A, Beamer BS, et al. Locked plating of the proximal humerus using an endosteal implant. *J Orthop Trauma.* 2012;26(4):212–125.

175. Hinov V, Wilson F, Adams G. Arthroscopically treated proximal humeral fracture malunion. *Arthroscopy.* 2002;18(9):1020–1023.

176. Hintermann B, Trouillier HH, Schafer D. Rigid internal fixation of fractures of the proximal humerus in older patients. *J Bone Joint Surg Br.* 2000;82(8):1107–1112.

177. Hirschmann MT, Fallegger B, Amsler F, et al. Clinical longer-term results after internal fixation of proximal humeral fractures with a locking compression plate (PHILOS). *J Orthop Trauma.* 2011;25(5):286–293.

178. Hirschmann MT, Quarz V, Audigé L, et al. Internal fixation of unstable proximal humeral fractures with an anatomically preshaped interlocking plate: A clinical and radiologic evaluation. *J Trauma.* 2007;63(6):1314–1323.

179. Hodgson SA, Mawson SJ, Saxton JM, et al. Rehabilitation of two-part fractures of the neck of the humerus (two-year follow-up). *J Shoulder Elbow Surg.* 2007;16(2):143–145.

180. Holloway GB, Schenk T, Williams GR, et al. Arthroscopic capsular release for the treatment of refractory postoperative or post-fracture shoulder stiffness. *J Bone Joint Surg Am.* 2001;83-A(11):1682–1687.

181. Hoppenfeld S, deBoer P, Buckley R. The shoulder. In: Hoppenfeld S, deBoer P, Buckley R, eds. *Surgical Exposures in Orthopaedics: The Anatomic Approach.* Lippincott Williams & Wilkins; 2009;2–71.

182. Horak J, Nilsson BE. Epidemiology of fracture of the upper end of the humerus. *Clin Orthop Relat Res.* 1975;(112):250–253.

183. Hudak PL, Amadio PC, Bombardier C. Development of an upper extremity outcome measure: The DASH (disabilities of the arm, shoulder and hand) [corrected]. The Upper Extremity Collaborative Group (UECG). *Am J Ind Med.* 1996;29(6):602–608.

184. Iannotti JP, Gabriel JP, Schneck SL, et al. The normal glenohumeral relationships. An anatomical study of one hundred and forty shoulders. *J Bone Joint Surg Am.* 1992;74(4):491–500.

185. Ilchmann T, Ochsner PE, Wingstrand H, et al. Non-operative treatment versus tension-band osteosynthesis in three- and four-part proximal humeral fractures. A retrospective study of 34 fractures from two different trauma centers. *Int Orthop.* 1998;22(5):316–320.

186. Jaberg H, Warner JJ, Jakob RP. Percutaneous stabilization of unstable fractures of the humerus. *J Bone Joint Surg Am.* 1992;74(4):508–515.

187. Jakob RP, Miniaci A, Anson PS, et al. Four-part valgus impacted fractures of the proximal humerus. *J Bone Joint Surg Br.* 1991;73(2):295–298.

188. Jöckel JA, Brunner A, Thormann S, et al. Elastic stabilisation of proximal humeral fractures with a new percutaneous angular stable fixation device (ButtonFix((R))): a preliminary report. *Arch Orthop Trauma Surg.* 2010;130(11):1397–1403.

189. Johansson O. Complications and failures of surgery in various fractures of the humerus. *Acta Chir Scand.* 1961;120:469–478.

190. Jones CB, Sietsema DL, Williams DK. Locked plating of proximal humeral fractures: Is function affected by age, time, and fracture patterns? *Clin Orthop Relat Res.* 2011;469(12):3307–3316.

191. Jost B, Spross C, Grehn H, et al. Locking plate fixation of fractures of the proximal humerus: Analysis of complications, revision strategies and outcome. *J Shoulder Elbow Surg.* 2013;22(4):542–549.

192. Kamineni S, Ankem H, Sanghavi S. Anatomical considerations for percutaneous proximal humeral fracture fixation. *Injury.* 2004;35(11):1133–1136.

193. Kannus P, Palvanen M, Niemi S, et al. Rate of proximal humeral fractures in older Finnish women between 1970 and 2007. *Bone.* 2009;44(4):656–659.

194. Kayalar M, Toros T, Bal E, et al. The importance of patient selection for the treatment of proximal humeral fractures with percutaneous technique. *Acta Orthop Traumatol Turc.* 2009;43(1):35–41.

195. Kazakos K, Lyras DN, Galanis V, et al. Internal fixation of proximal humeral fractures using the Polarus intramedullary nail. *Arch Orthop Trauma Surg.* 2007;127(7):503–508.

196. Keener JD, Parsons BO, Flatow EL, et al. Outcomes after percutaneous reduction and fixation of proximal humeral fractures. *J Shoulder Elbow Surg.* 2007;16(3):330–338.

197. Kelsey JL, Browner WS, Seeley DG, et al. Risk factors for fractures of the distal forearm and proximal humerus. The Study of Osteoporotic Fractures Research Group. *Am J Epidemiol.* 1992;135(5):477–489.

198. Keser S, Bölükbasi S, Bayar A, et al. Proximal humeral fractures with minimal displacement treated conservatively. *Int Orthop.* 2004;28(4):231–234.

199. Khunda A, Stirrat AN, Dunlop P. Injury to the axillary artery, a complication of fixation using a locking plate. *J Bone Joint Surg Br.* 2007;89(11):1519–1521.

200. Kilic B, Uysal M, Cinar BM, et al. Early results of treatment of proximal humeral fractures with the PHILOS locking plate]. *Acta Orthop Traumatol Turc.* 2008;42(3):149–153.

201. Kim SH, Lee YH, Chung SW, et al. Outcomes for four-part proximal humeral fractures treated with a locking compression plate and an autologous iliac bone impaction graft. *Injury.* 2012;43(10):1724–1731.

202. Kim SH, Szabo RM, Marder RA. Epidemiology of humerus fractures in the United States: Nationwide emergency department sample, 2008. *Arthritis Care Res (Hoboken).* 2012;64(3):407–414.

203. Kirchhoff C, Braunstein V, Kirchhoff S, et al. Outcome analysis following removal of locking plate fixation of the proximal humerus. *BMC Musculoskelet Disord.* 2008;9:138.

204. Klepps S, Auerbach J, Calhon O, et al. A cadaveric study on the anatomy of the deltoid insertion and its relationship to the deltopectoral approach to the proximal humerus. *J Shoulder Elbow Surg.* 2004;13(3):322–327.

205. Klepps SJ, Miller SL, Lin J, et al. Determination of radiographic guidelines for percutaneous fixation of proximal humeral fractures using a cadaveric model. *Orthopedics.* 2007;30(8):636–641.

206. Kobayashi M, Watanabe Y, Matsushita T. Early full range of shoulder and elbow motion is possible after minimally invasive plate osteosynthesis for humeral shaft fractures. *J Orthop Trauma.* 2010;24(4):212–216.

207. Kocialkowski A, Wallace WA. Closed percutaneous K-wire stabilization for displaced fractures of the surgical neck of the humerus. *Injury.* 1990;21(4):209–212.

208. Königshausen M, Kübler L, Godry H, et al. Clinical outcome and complications using a polyaxial locking plate in the treatment of displaced proximal humeral fractures. A reliable system? *Injury.* 2012;43(2):223–231.

209. Konrad G, Audigé L, Lambert S, et al. Similar outcomes for nail versus plate fixation of three-part proximal humeral fractures. *Clin Orthop Relat Res.* 2012;470(2):602–609.

210. Konrad G, Bayer J, Hepp P, et al. Open reduction and internal fixation of proximal humeral fractures with use of the locking proximal humerus plate. Surgical technique. *J Bone Joint Surg Am.* 2010;92(suppl 1 pt 1):85–95.

211. Konrad G, Hirschmüller A, Audigé L, et al. Comparison of two different locking plates for two-, three- and four-part proximal humeral fractures–results of an international multicentre study. *Int Orthop.* 2012;36(5):1051–1058.

212. Kontakis G, Koutras C, Tosounidis T, et al. Early management of proximal humeral fractures with hemiarthroplasty: A systematic review. *J Bone Joint Surg Br.* 2008;90(11):1407–1413.

213. Kontakis GM, Steriopoulos K, Damilakis J, et al. The position of the axillary nerve in the deltoid muscle. A cadaveric study. *Acta Orthop Scand.* 1999;70(1):9–11.

214. Kontakis GM, Tosounidis TI, Christoforakis Z, et al. Early management of complex proximal humeral fractures using the Aequalis fracture prosthesis: A two- to five-year follow-up report. *J Bone Joint Surg Br.* 2009;91(10):1335–1340.

215. Korkmaz MF, Aksu N, Göğüş A, et al. The results of internal fixation of proximal humeral fractures with the PHILOS locking plate]. *Acta Orthop Traumatol Turc.* 2008;42(2):97–105.

216. Koukakis A, Apostolou CD, Taneja T, et al. Fixation of proximal humeral fractures using the PHILOS plate: early experience. *Clin Orthop Relat Res.* 2006;442:115–120.

217. Koval KJ, Gallagher MA, Marsicano JG, et al. Functional outcome after minimally displaced fractures of the proximal part of the humerus. *J Bone Joint Surg Am.* 1997;79(2):203–207.

218. Krappinger D, Bizzotto N, Riedmann S, et al. Predicting failure after surgical fixation of proximal humeral fractures. *Injury.* 2011;42(11):1283–1288.

219. Krishnan SG, Bennion PW, Reineck JR, et al. Hemiarthroplasty for proximal humeral fracture: Restoration of the Gothic arch. *Orthop Clin North Am.* 2008;39(4):441–450, vi.

220. Krishnan SG, Reineck JR, Bennion PD, et al. Shoulder arthroplasty for fracture: Does a fracture-specific stem make a difference? *Clin Orthop Relat Res.* 2011;469(12):3317–3323.

221. Kristiansen B Andersen UL, Olsen CA, et al. The Neer classification of fractures of the proximal humerus. An assessment of interobserver variation. *Skeletal Radiol.* 1988;17(6):420–422.

222. Kristiansen B, Barfod G, Bredesen J, et al. Epidemiology of proximal humeral fractures. *Acta Orthop Scand.* 1987;58(1):75–77.

223. Kristiansen B, Christensen SW. Plate fixation of proximal humeral fractures. *Acta Orthop Scand.* 1986;57(4):320–323.

224. Kristiansen B, Kofoed H. Transcutaneous reduction and external fixation of displaced fractures of the proximal humerus. A controlled clinical trial. *J Bone Joint Surg Br.* 1988;70(5):821–824.

225. Kryzak TJ, Sperling JW, Schleck CD, et al. Hemiarthroplasty for proximal humeral fractures in patients with Parkinson's disease. *Clin Orthop Relat Res.* 2010;468(7):1817–1821.

226. Laflamme GY, Rouleau DM, Berry GK, et al. Percutaneous humeral plating of fractures of the proximal humerus: Results of a prospective multicenter clinical trial. *J Orthop Trauma.* 2008;22(3):153–158.

227. Laing PG. The arterial supply of the adult humerus. *J Bone Joint Surg Am.* 1956;38-A(5):1105–1116.

228. Lau TW, Leung F, Chan CF, et al. Minimally invasive plate osteosynthesis in the treatment of proximal humeral fracture. *Int Orthop.* 2007;31(5):657–664.

229. Launonen AP, Lepola V, Flinkkilä, et al. Conservative treatment, plate fixation, or prosthesis for proximal humeral fracture. A prospective randomized study. *BMC Musculoskelet Disord.* 2012;13:167.

230. Lauritzen JB, Schwarz P, McNair P, et al. Radial and humeral fractures as predictors of subsequent hip, radial or humeral fractures in women, and their seasonal variation. *Osteoporos Int.* 1993;3(3):133–137.
231. Lee CK, Hansen HR. Post-traumatic avascular necrosis of the humeral head in displaced proximal humeral fractures. *J Trauma.* 1981;21(9):788–791.
232. Lee CW, Shin SJ. Prognostic factors for unstable proximal humeral fractures treated with locking-plate fixation. *J Shoulder Elbow Surg.* 2009;18(1):83–88.
233. Lee SH, Dargent-Molina P, Breart G. Risk factors for fractures of the proximal humerus: results from the EPIDOS prospective study. *J Bone Miner Res.* 2002;17(5):817–825.
234. Leggin BG, Iannotti J. Shoulder outcome measurement. In: Iannotti JP, Williams GR, eds. *Disorders of the Shoulder: Diagnosis and Management.* Philadelphia, PA: Lippincott, Williams & Wilkins; 1999:1024–1040.
235. Leggin BG, Michener LA, Shaffer MA, et al. The Penn shoulder score: Reliability and validity. *J Orthop Sports Phys Ther.* 2006;36(3):138–151.
236. Lehman C, Cuomo F, Kummer FJ, et al. The incidence of full thickness rotator cuff tears in a large cadaveric population. *Bull Hosp Jt Dis.* 1995;54(1):30–31.
237. Lenarz C, Sishhani Y, McCrum C, et al. Is reverse shoulder arthroplasty appropriate for the treatment of fractures in the older patient? Early observations. *Clin Orthop Relat Res.* 2011;469(12):3324–3331.
238. Leonard M, Mokotedi L, Alao U, et al. The use of locking plates in proximal humeral fractures: Comparison of outcome by patient age and fracture pattern. *Int J Shoulder Surg.* 2009;3(4):85–89.
239. Lescheid J, Zdero R, Shah S, et al. The biomechanics of locked plating for repairing proximal humeral fractures with or without medial cortical support. *J Trauma.* 2010;69(5):1235–1242.
240. Leslie A, Cassar-Pullicino VN. Avulsion of the lesser tuberosity with intra-articular injury of the glenohumeral joint. *Injury.* 1996;27(10):742–745.
241. Levy JC, Badman B. Reverse shoulder prosthesis for acute four-part fracture: tuberosity fixation using a horseshoe graft. *J Orthop Trauma.* 2011;25(5):318–324.
242. Levy O, Webb M, Even T, et al. Arthroscopic capsular release for posttraumatic shoulder stiffness. *J Shoulder Elbow Surg.* 2008;17(3):410–414.
243. Liew AS, Johnson JA, Patterson SD, et al. Effect of screw placement on fixation in the humeral head. *J Shoulder Elbow Surg.* 2000;9(5):423-6.
244. Lill H, Hepp P, Korner J, et al. Proximal humeral fractures: How stiff should an implant be? A comparative mechanical study with new implants in human specimens. *Arch Orthop Trauma Surg.* 2003;123(2-3):74–81.
245. Lin CL, Hong CK, Jou IM, et al. Suture anchor versus screw fixation for greater tuberosity fractures of the humerus–a biomechanical study. *J Orthop Res.* 2012;30(3): 423–428.
246. Lin L. Effectiveness of locked nailing for displaced three-part proximal humeral fractures. *J Trauma.* 2006;61(2):363–374.
247. Lind T, Kroner K, Jensen J. The epidemiology of fractures of the proximal humerus. *Arch Orthop Trauma Surg.* 1989;108(5):285–287.
248. Linhart W, Ueblacker P, Grossterlinden L, et al. Antegrade nailing of humeral head fractures with captured interlocking screws. *J Orthop Trauma.* 2007;21(5):285–294.
249. Lippitt SB, Harryman DT, Matsen FA. A practical tool for evaluation of function: the simple shoulder test. In: *The Shoulder: A Balance of Mobility and Stability.* Rosemont, IL: American Academy of Orthopaedic Surgery; 1993.
250. Liu J, Li SH, Cai ZD, et al. Outcomes, and factors affecting outcomes, following shoulder hemiarthroplasty for proximal humeral fracture repair. *J Orthop Sci.* 2011;16(5):565–572.
251. Lollino N, Paladini P, Campi F, et al. Reverse shoulder prosthesis as revision surgery after fractures of the proximal humerus, treated initially by internal fixation or hemiarthroplasty. *Chir Organi Mov.* 2009;93(suppl 1):S35–S39.
252. Lupo R, Rapisarda SA, Lauria S, et al. Plates with angular stability: Our personal experience in surgical treatment of fractures of the proximal extremity of the humerus. *Chir Organi Mov.* 2008;91(2):97–101.
253. Machani B, Sinopidis C, Brownson P, et al. Mid term results of PlantTan plate in the treatment of proximal humeral fractures. *Injury.* 2006;37(3):269–276.
254. Majed A, Macleod I, Bull AM, et al. Proximal humeral fracture classification systems revisited. *J Shoulder Elbow Surg.* 2011;20(7):1125–1132.
255. Mansat P, Guity MR, Bellumore Y, et al. Shoulder arthroplasty for late sequelae of proximal humeral fractures. *J Shoulder Elbow Surg.* 2004;13(3):305–312.
256. Maravic M, Le Bihan C, Landais P, et al. Incidence and cost of osteoporotic fractures in France during 2001. A methodological approach by the national hospital database. *Osteoporos Int.* 2005;16(12):1475–1480.
257. Marsh JL, Slongo TF, Agel G, et al. Fracture and dislocation classification compendium - 2007: Orthopaedic Trauma Association classification, database and outcomes committee. *J Orthop Trauma.* 2007;21(suppl 10):S1–S133.
258. Martinez AA, Bejarano C, Carbonel I, et al. The treatment of proximal humerus nonunions in older patients with the reverse shoulder arthroplasty. *Injury.* 2012.
259. Martinez AA, Calvo A, Bejarano C, et al. The use of the Lima reverse shoulder arthroplasty for the treatment of fracture sequelae of the proximal humerus. *J Orthop Sci.* 2012;17(2):141–147.
260. Martinez AA, Cuenca J, Herrera A. Philos plate fixation for proximal humeral fractures. *J Orthop Surg (Hong Kong).* 2009;17(1):10–14.
261. Matziolis D, Kaeaeb M, Zandi SS, et al. Surgical treatment of two-part fractures of the proximal humerus: Comparison of fixed-angle plate osteosynthesis and Zifko nails. *Injury.* 2010;41(10):1041–1046.
262. McLaughlin JA, Light R, Lustrin I. Axillary artery injury as a complication of proximal humeral fractures. *J Shoulder Elbow Surg.* 1998;7(3):292–294.
263. Meier RA, Messmer P, Regazzoni P, et al. Unexpected high complication rate following internal fixation of unstable proximal humeral fractures with an angled blade plate. *J Orthop Trauma.* 2006;20(4):253–260.
264. Mellado JM, Calmet J, García Forcada IL, et al. Early intrathoracic migration of Kirschner wires used for percutaneous osteosynthesis of a two-part humeral neck fracture: A case report. *Emerg Radiol.* 2004;11(1):49–52.
265. Merchant N, Scalea T, Stein D. Can CT angiography replace conventional bi-planar angiography in the management of severe scapulothoracic dissociation injuries? *The American surgeon.* 2012;78(8):875–882.
266. Meyer C, Alt V, Hassanin H, et al. The arteries of the humeral head and their relevance in fracture treatment. *Surg Radiol Anat.* 2005;27(3):232–237.
267. Meyer C, Alt V, Kraus R, et al. The arteries of the humerus and their relevance in fracture treatment. *Zentralbl Chir.* 2005;130(6):562–567.
268. Micic ID, Kim SC, Shin DJ, et al. Analysis of early failure of the locking compression plate in osteoporotic proximal humeral fractures. *J Orthop Sci.* 2009;14(5):596–601.
269. Mighell MA, Kolm GP, Collinge CA, et al. Outcomes of hemiarthroplasty for fractures of the proximal humerus. *J Shoulder Elbow Surg.* 2003;12(6):569–577.
270. Misra A, Kapur R, Maffulli N. Complex proximal humeral fractures in adults–a systematic review of management. *Injury.* 2001;32(5):363–372.
271. Mittlmeier TW, Stedfeld HW, Ewert A, et al. Stabilization of proximal humeral fractures with an angular and sliding stable antegrade locking nail (Targon PH). *J Bone Joint Surg Am.* 2003;85-A(suppl 4):136–146.
272. Mochizuki T, Sugaya H, Uomizu M, et al. Humeral insertion of the supraspinatus and infraspinatus. New anatomical findings regarding the footprint of the rotator cuff. *J Bone Joint Surg Am.* 2008;90(5):962–969.
273. Moda SK, Chadha NS, Sangwan SS, et al. Open reduction and fixation of proximal humeral fractures and fracture-dislocations. *J Bone Joint Surg Br.* 1990;72(6): 1050–1052.
274. Moeckel BH, Dines DM, Warren RF, et al. Modular hemiarthroplasty for fractures of the proximal part of the humerus. *J Bone Joint Surg Am.* 1992;74(6):884–889.
275. Molé D, Favard L. Excentered scapulohumeral osteoarthritis. *Rev Chir Orthop Reparatrice Appar Mot.* 2007;93(suppl 6):37–94.
276. Molé D, Wein F, Dézaly C, et al. Surgical technique: the anterosuperior approach for reverse shoulder arthroplasty. *Clin Orthop Relat Res.* 2011;469(9):2461–2468.
277. Monga P, Verma R, Sharma VK. Closed reduction and external fixation for displaced proximal humeral fractures. *J Orthop Surg (Hong Kong).* 2009;17(2):142–145.
278. Mont MA, Maar DC, Urquhart MW, et al. Avascular necrosis of the humeral head treated by core decompression. A retrospective review. *J Bone Joint Surg Br.* 1993;75(5):785–788.
279. Moonot P, Ashwood N, Hamlet M. Early results for treatment of three- and four-part fractures of the proximal humerus using the PHILOS plate system. *J Bone Joint Surg Br.* 2007;89(9):1206–1209.
280. Muller ME, et al. *The Comprehensive Classification of Fractures of Long Bones.* New York, NY: Springer; 1990.
281. Naidu SH, Bixler B, Capo JT, et al. Percutaneous pinning of proximal humeral fractures: A biomechanical study. *Orthopedics.* 1997;20(11):1073–1076.
282. Nanda R, Goodchild L, Gamble A, et al. Does the presence of a full-thickness rotator cuff tear influence outcome after proximal humeral fractures? *J Trauma.* 2007;62(6): 1436–1439.
283. Nayak NK, Schickendantz MS, Regan WD, et al. Operative treatment of nonunion of surgical neck fractures of the humerus. *Clin Orthop Relat Res.* 1995;(313):200–205.
284. Neer CS 2nd. Displaced proximal humeral fractures. I. Classification and evaluation. *J Bone Joint Surg Am.* 1970;52(6):1077–1089.
285. Neer CS 2nd. Displaced proximal humeral fractures. II. Treatment of three-part and four-part displacement. *J Bone Joint Surg Am.* 1970;52(6):1090–1103.
286. Neer CS. Four-segment classification of displaced proximal humeral fractures. *Instructional Course Lecture. Instructional Course Lecture.* Rosemont, IL: American Academy of Orthopaedic Surgeons; 1975.
287. Neer CS 2nd. Four-segment classification of proximal humeral fractures: purpose and reliable use. *J Shoulder Elbow Surg.* 2002;11(4):389–400.
288. Neviaser AS, Hettrich CM, Beamer BS, et al. Endosteal strut augment reduces complications associated with proximal humeral locking plates. *Clin Orthop Relat Res.* 2011;469(12):3300–3306.
289. Nguyen TV, Center JR, Sambrook PN, et al. Risk factors for proximal humerus, forearm, and wrist fractures in elderly men and women: The Dubbo Osteoporosis Epidemiology Study. *Am J Epidemiol.* 2001;153(6):587–595.
290. Nicholson GP, Strauss EJ, Sherman SL. Scapular notching: Recognition and strategies to minimize clinical impact. *Clin Orthop Relat Res.* 2011;469(9):2521–2530.
291. Nolan BM, Kippe MA, Wiater JM, et al. Surgical treatment of displaced proximal humeral fractures with a short intramedullary nail. *J Shoulder Elbow Surg.* 2011.
292. Nordqvist A, Petersson CJ. Incidence and causes of shoulder girdle injuries in an urban population. *J Shoulder Elbow Surg.* 1995;4(2):107–112.
293. Noyes MP, Kleinhenz B, Markert RJ, et al. Functional and radiographic long-term outcomes of hemiarthroplasty for proximal humeral fractures. *J Shoulder Elbow Surg.* 2011;20(3):372–377.
294. O'Donnell TM, McKenna JV, Kenny P, et al. Concomitant injuries to the ipsilateral shoulder in patients with a fracture of the diaphysis of the humerus. *J Bone Joint Surg Br.* 2008;90(1):61–65.
295. Ochsner PE, Ilchmann T. [Tension band osteosynthesis with absorbable cords in proximal comminuted fractures of the humerus]. *Unfallchirurg.* 1991;94(10):508–510.
296. Ockert B, Braunstein V, Kirchhoff C, et al. Monoaxial versus polyaxial screw insertion in angular stable plate fixation of proximal humeral fractures: Radiographic analysis of a prospective randomized study. *J Trauma.* 2010;69(6):1545–1551.
297. Ogiwara N, Aoki M, Okamura K, et al. Ender nailing for unstable surgical neck fractures of the humerus in elderly patients. *Clin Orthop Relat Res.* 1996;(330):173–180.
298. Olerud P, Ahrengart L, Ponzer S, et al. Hemiarthroplasty versus nonoperative treatment of displaced 4-part proximal humeral fractures in elderly patients: A randomized controlled trial. *J Shoulder Elbow Surg.* 2011;20(7):1025–1033.
299. Olerud P, Ahrengart L, Ponzer S, et al. Internal fixation versus nonoperative treatment of displaced 3-part proximal humeral fractures in elderly patients: A randomized controlled trial. *J Shoulder Elbow Surg.* 2011;20(5):747–755.
300. Olerud P, Ahrengart L, Söderqvist A, et al. Quality of life and functional outcome after a 2-part proximal humeral fracture: a prospective cohort study on 50 patients treated with a locking plate. *J Shoulder Elbow Surg.* 2010;19(6):814–822.

301. Olsson C, Nordqvist A, Petersson CJ. Increased fragility in patients with fracture of the proximal humerus: A case control study. *Bone*. 2004;34(6):1072–1077.
302. Osterhoff G, Baumgartner D, Favre P, et al. Medial support by fibula bone graft in angular stable plate fixation of proximal humeral fractures: An in vitro study with synthetic bone. *J Shoulder Elbow Surg*. 2011;20(5):740–746.
303. Osterhoff G, Hoch A, Wanner GA, et al. Calcar comminution as prognostic factor of clinical outcome after locking plate fixation of proximal humeral fractures. *Injury*. 2012;43(10):1651–1656.
304. Osterhoff G, Ossendorf C, Wanner GA, et al. The calcar screw in angular stable plate fixation of proximal humeral fractures–a case study. *J Orthop Surg Res*. 2011;6:50.
305. Owsley KC, Gorczyca JT. Fracture displacement and screw cutout after open reduction and locked plate fixation of proximal humeral fractures [corrected]. *J Bone Joint Surg Am*. 2008;90(2):233–240.
306. Paavolainen P, Björkenheim JM, Slätis P, et al. Operative treatment of severe proximal humeral fractures. *Acta Orthop Scand*. 1983;54(3):374–379.
307. Padua R, Padua L, Galluzzo M, et al. Position of shoulder arthroplasty and clinical outcome in proximal humeral fractures. *Musculoskelet Surg*. 2011;95(suppl 1):S55–S58.
308. Palvanen M, Kannus P, Niemi S, et al. Update in the epidemiology of proximal humeral fractures. *Clin Orthop Relat Res*. 2006;442:87–92.
309. Papadopoulos P, Karataglis D, Stavridis SI, et al. Mid-term results of internal fixation of proximal humeral fractures with the Philos plate. *Injury*. 2009;40(12):1292–1296.
310. Park JY, An JW, Oh JH. Open intramedullary nailing with tension band and locking sutures for proximal humeral fracture: Hot air balloon technique. *J Shoulder Elbow Surg*. 2006;15(5):594–601.
311. Park MC, Murthi AM, Roth NS, et al. Two-part and three-part fractures of the proximal humerus treated with suture fixation. *J Orthop Trauma*. 2003;17(5):319–325.
312. Parmaksizoğlu AS, Kabukçuoğlu Y, Ozkaya U, et al. Locking plate fixation of three- and four-part proximal humeral fractures. *Acta Orthop Traumatol Turc*. 2010;44(2):97–104.
313. Pearl ML, Volk AG. Coronal plane geometry of the proximal humerus relevant to prosthetic arthroplasty. *J Shoulder Elbow Surg*. 1996;5(4):320–326.
314. Pijls BG, Werner PH, Eggen PJ. Alternative humeral tubercle fixation in shoulder hemiarthroplasty for fractures of the proximal humerus. *J Shoulder Elbow Surg*. 2010;19(2):282–289.
315. Pijls BG, Werner PH, Eggen PJ. Primary uncemented hemiarthroplasty for severe fractures of the proximal humerus. *J Orthop Trauma*. 2011;25(5):279–285.
316. Plecko M, Kraus A. Internal fixation of proximal humeral fractures using the locking proximal humerus plate. *Oper Orthop Traumatol*. 2005;17(1):25–50.
317. Poeze M, Lenssen AF, Van Empel JM, et al. Conservative management of proximal humeral fractures: Can poor functional outcome be related to standard transscapular radiographic evaluation? *J Shoulder Elbow Surg*. 2010;19(2):273–281.
318. Popescu D, Fernandez-Valencia JA, Rios M, et al. Internal fixation of proximal humeral fractures using the T2-proximal humeral nail. *Arch Orthop Trauma Surg*. 2009;129(9):1239–1244.
319. Pospula W, Abu Noor T. Hackethal bundle nailing with intramedullary elastic nails in the treatment of two- and three-part fractures of the proximal humerus: Initial experience at Al Razi Hospital, Kuwait. *Med Princ Pract*. 2009;18(4):284–288.
320. Radkowski CA, Richards RS, Pietrobon R, et al. An anatomic study of the cephalic vein in the deltopectoral shoulder approach. *Clin Orthop Relat Res*. 2006;442:139–142.
321. Rajasekhar C, Ray PS, Bhamra MS. Fixation of proximal humeral fractures with the Polarus nail. *J Shoulder Elbow Surg*. 2001;10(1):7–10.
322. Rancan M, Dietrich M, Lamdark T, et al. Minimal invasive long PHILOS(R)-plate osteosynthesis in metadiaphyseal fractures of the proximal humerus. *Injury*. 2010;41(12):1277–1283.
323. Reitman RD, Kerzhner E. Reverse shoulder arthoplasty as treatment for comminuted proximal humeral fractures in elderly patients. *Am J Orthop (Belle Mead NJ)*. 2011;40(9):458–461.
324. Resch H, Beck E, Bayley I. Reconstruction of the valgus-impacted humeral head fracture. *J Shoulder Elbow Surg*. 1995;4(2):73–80.
325. Resch H, Hubner C, Schwaiger R. Minimally invasive reduction and osteosynthesis of articular fractures of the humeral head. *Injury*. 2001;32(suppl 1):SA25–SA32.
326. Resch H, Povacz P, Frölich R, et al. Percutaneous fixation of three- and four-part fractures of the proximal humerus. *J Bone Joint Surg Br*. 1997;79(2):295–300.
327. Ricchetti ET, Warrender WJ, Abboud JA. Use of locking plates in the treatment of proximal humeral fractures. *J Shoulder Elbow Surg*. 2010;19(suppl 2):66–75.
328. Richards RR, An KN, Bigliani LU, et al. A standardized method for the assessment of shoulder function. *J Shoulder Elbow Surg*. 1994;3(6):347–352.
329. Rispoli DM, Athwal GS, Sperling JW, et al. The anatomy of the deltoid insertion. *J Shoulder Elbow Surg*. 2009;18(3):386–390.
330. Roach KE, Budiman-Mak E, Songsiridej N, et al. Development of a shoulder pain and disability index. *Arthritis Care Res*. 1991;4(4):143–149.
331. Robertson DD, Yuan J, Bigliani LU, et al. Three-dimensional analysis of the proximal part of the humerus: Relevance to arthroplasty. *J Bone Joint Surg Am*. 2000;82-A(11):1594–1602.
332. Robinson CM, Inman D, Phillips SA. The Plate-Joystick technique to reduce proximal humeral fractures and nonunions with a varus deformity through the extended deltoid-splitting approach. *J Orthop Trauma*. 2011;25(10):634–640.
333. Robinson CM, Kahn L, Akhtar A, et al. The extended deltoid-splitting approach to the proximal humerus. *J Orthop Trauma*. 2007;21(9):657–662.
334. Robinson CM, Kelly M, Wakefield AE. Redislocation of the shoulder during the first six weeks after a primary anterior dislocation: risk factors and results of treatment. *J Bone Joint Surg Am*. 2002;84-A(9):1552–1559.
335. Robinson CM, Page RS, Hill RM, et al. Primary hemiarthroplasty for treatment of proximal humeral fractures. *J Bone Joint Surg Am*. 2003;85-A(7):1215–1223.
336. Robinson CM, Teoh KH, Baker A, et al. Fractures of the lesser tuberosity of the humerus. *J Bone Joint Surg Am*. 2009;91(3):512–520.
337. Robinson CM, Wylie JR, Ray AG, et al. Proximal humeral fractures with a severe varus deformity treated by fixation with a locking plate. *J Bone Joint Surg Br*. 2010;92(5):672–678.
338. Röderer G, Abouelsoud M, Gebhard F, et al. Minimally invasive application of the non-contact-bridging (NCB) plate to the proximal humerus: An anatomical study. *J Orthop Trauma*. 2007;21(9):621–627.
339. Röderer G, Erhardt J, Graf M, et al. Clinical results for minimally invasive locked plating of proximal humeral fractures. *J Orthop Trauma*. 2010;24(7):400–406.
340. Röderer G, Erhardt J, Kuster M, et al. Second generation locked plating of proximal humeral fractures–a prospective multicentre observational study. *Int Orthop*. 2011;35(3):425–432.
341. Rommens PM, Heyvaert G. Conservative treatment of subcapital humerus fractures. A comparative study of the classical Desault bandage and the new Gilchrist bandage. *Unfallchirurgie*. 1993;19(2):114–118.
342. Rose PS, Adams CR, Torchia ME, et al. Locking plate fixation for proximal humeral fractures: Initial results with a new implant. *J Shoulder Elbow Surg*. 2007;16(2):202–207.
343. Rose SH, Melton LJ, Morrey BF, et al. Epidemiologic features of humeral fractures. *Clin Orthop Relat Res*. 1982;(168):24–30.
344. Rowles DJ, McGrory JE. Percutaneous pinning of the proximal part of the humerus. An anatomic study. *J Bone Joint Surg Am*. 2001;83-A(11):1695–1699.
345. Ruchholtz S, Hauk C, Lewan U, et al. Minimally invasive polyaxial locking plate fixation of proximal humeral fractures: A prospective study. *J Trauma*. 2011;71(6):1737–1744.
346. Rutten MJ, Jager GJ, de Wall Malefijt MC, et al. Double line sign: A helpful sonographic sign to detect occult fractures of the proximal humerus. *European radiology*. 2007;17(3):762–767.
347. Sadowski C, Riand N, Stern R, et al. Fixation of fractures of the proximal humerus with the PlantTan Humerus Fixator Plate: Early experience with a new implant. *J Shoulder Elbow Surg*. 2003;12(2):148–151.
348. Sanders RJ, Thissen LG, Teepen JC, et al. Locking plate versus nonsurgical treatment for proximal humeral fractures: Better midterm outcome with nonsurgical treatment. *J Shoulder Elbow Surg*. 2011;20(7):1118–1124.
349. Saran N, Bergeron SG, Benoit B, et al. Risk of axillary nerve injury during percutaneous proximal humerus locking plate insertion using an external aiming guide. *Injury*. 2010;41(10):1037–1040.
350. Savoie FH, Geissler WB, Vander Griend RA. Open reduction and internal fixation of three-part fractures of the proximal humerus. *Orthopedics*. 1989;12(1):65–70.
351. Schai PA, Hintermann B, Koris MJ. Preoperative arthroscopic assessment of fractures about the shoulder. *Arthroscopy*. 1999;15(8):827–835.
352. Scheck M. Surgical treatment of nonunions of the surgical neck of the humerus. *Clin Orthop Relat Res*. 1982;(167):255–259.
353. Schliemann B, Siemoneit J, Theisen C, et al. Complex fractures of the proximal humerus in the elderly–outcome and complications after locking plate fixation. *Musculoskelet Surg*. 2012;96(suppl 1):S3–S11.
354. Schulte LM, Matteini LE, Neviaser RJ. Proximal periarticular locking plates in proximal humeral fractures: Functional outcomes. *J Shoulder Elbow Surg*. 2011;20(8):1234–1240.
355. Sehr JR, Szabo RM. Semitubular blade plate for fixation in the proximal humerus. *J Orthop Trauma*. 1988;2(4):327–332.
356. Seide K, Triebe J, Faschingbauer M, et al. Locked vs. unlocked plate osteosynthesis of the proximal humerus - a biomechanical study. *Clin Biomech (Bristol, Avon)*. 2007;22(2):176–182.
357. Seyhan M, Kocaoglu B, Nalbantoglu U, et al. Technique of Kirschner wire reduction and fixation of displaced two-part valgus angulated proximal humeral fractures at the surgical neck. *J Orthop Trauma*. 2012;26(6):e46–e50.
358. Sforzo CR, Wright TW. Treatment of acute proximal humeral fractures with a polarus nail. *J Surg Orthop Adv*. 2009;18(1):28–34.
359. Shah N, Iqbal HJ, Brookes-Fazakerley S, et al. Shoulder hemiarthroplasty for the treatment of three and four part fractures of the proximal humerus using Comprehensive(R) Fracture stem. *Int Orthop*. 2011;35(6):861–867.
360. Shahid R, Mushtaq A, Northover J, et al. Outcome of proximal humeral fractures treated by PHILOS plate internal fixation. Experience of a district general hospital. *Acta Orthop Belg*. 2008;74(5):602–608.
361. Shortt NL, Robinson CM. Mortality after low-energy fractures in patients aged at least 45 years old. *J Orthop Trauma*. 2005;19(6):396–400.
362. Sidor ML, Zuckerman JD, Lyon T, et al. The Neer classification system for proximal humeral fractures. An assessment of interobserver reliability and intraobserver reproducibility. *J Bone Joint Surg Am*. 1993;75(12):1745–1750.
363. Siebenrock KA, Gerber C. The reproducibility of classification of fractures of the proximal end of the humerus. *J Bone Joint Surg Am*. 1993;75(12):1751–1755.
364. Siegel JA, Dines DM. Proximal humerus malunions. *Orthop Clin North Am*. 2000;31(1):35–50.
365. Siegel JA, Dines DM. Techniques in managing proximal humeral malunions. *J Shoulder Elbow Surg*. 2003;12(1):69–78.
366. Siffri PC, Peindl RD, Coley ER, et al. Biomechanical analysis of blade plate versus locking plate fixation for a proximal humerus fracture: Comparison using cadaveric and synthetic humeri. *J Orthop Trauma*. 2006;20(8):547–554.
367. Simovitch RW, Helmy N, Zumstein MA, et al. Impact of fatty infiltration of the teres minor muscle on the outcome of reverse total shoulder arthroplasty. *J Bone Joint Surg Am*. 2007;89(5):934–939.
368. Simovitch RW, Zumstein MA, Lohri E, et al. Predictors of scapular notching in patients managed with the Delta III reverse total shoulder replacement. *J Bone Joint Surg Am*. 2007;89(3):588–600.
369. Sirveaux F, Favard L, Oudet D, et al. Grammont inverted total shoulder arthroplasty in the treatment of glenohumeral osteoarthritis with massive rupture of the cuff. Results of a multicentre study of 80 shoulders. *J Bone Joint Surg Br*. 2004;86(3):388–395.
370. Siwach R, Singh R, Rohilla RK, et al. Internal fixation of proximal humeral fractures with locking proximal humeral plate (LPHP) in elderly patients with osteoporosis. *J Orthop Traumatol*. 2008;9(3):149–153.

371. Sjödén GO, Movin T, Günter P, et al. Poor reproducibility of classification of proximal humeral fractures. Additional CT of minor value. *Acta Orthop Scand.* 1997;68(3):239–242.

372. Slobogean GP, Noonan VK, O'Brien PJ. The reliability and validity of the Disabilities of Arm, Shoulder, and Hand, EuroQol-5D, Health Utilities Index, and Short Form-6D outcome instruments in patients with proximal humeral fractures. *J Shoulder Elbow Surg.* 2010;19(3):342–348.

373. Smith AM, Mardones PM, Sperling JW, et al. Early complications of operatively treated proximal humeral fractures. *J Shoulder Elbow Surg.* 2007;16(1):14–24.

374. Smith AM, Sperling JW, Cofield RH. Complications of operative fixation of proximal humeral fractures in patients with rheumatoid arthritis. *J Shoulder Elbow Surg.* 2005;14(6):559–564.

375. Smith J, Berry G, Laflamme Y, et al. Percutaneous insertion of a proximal humeral locking plate: An anatomic study. *Injury.* 2007;38(2):206–211.

376. Smith M, Jacobs L, Banks L, et al. Internal fixation of fractures of the proximal humerus with a humeral fixator plate (PlantTan Plate): A two year follow-up. *Acta Orthop Belg.* 2008;74(6):735–746.

377. Solberg BD, Moon CN, Franco DP, et al. Locked plating of 3- and 4-part proximal humeral fractures in older patients: The effect of initial fracture pattern on outcome. *J Orthop Trauma.* 2009;23(2):113–119.

378. Solberg BD, Moon CN, Franco DP, et al. Surgical treatment of three and four-part proximal humeral fractures. *J Bone Joint Surg Am.* 2009;91(7):1689–1697.

379. Solonen KA, Vastamaki M. Osteotomy of the neck of the humerus for traumatic varus deformity. *Acta Orthop Scand.* 1985;56(1):79–80.

380. Sonderegger J, Simmen HP. [Epidemiology,treatment and results of proximal humeral fractures: Experience of a district hospital in a sports- and tourism area]. *Zentralbl Chir.* 2003;128(2):119–124.

381. Sosef N, Stobbe I, Hogervorst M, et al. The Polarus intramedullary nail for proximal humeral fractures: Outcome in 28 patients followed for 1 year. *Acta Orthop.* 2007;78(3):436–441.

382. Sperling JW, Cofield RH, Torchia ME, et al. Infection after shoulder arthroplasty. *Clin Orthop Relat Res.* 2001;(382):206–216.

383. Spross C, Platz A, Erschbamer M, et al. Surgical treatment of Neer Group VI proximal humeral fractures: Retrospective comparison of PHILOS(R) and hemiarthroplasty. *Clin Orthop Relat Res.* 2012;470(7):2035–2042.

384. Spross C, Platz A, Rufibach K, et al. The PHILOS plate for proximal humeral fractures–risk factors for complications at one year. *J Trauma Acute Care Surg.* 2012;72(3):783–792.

385. Sproul RC, Iyengar JJ, Devcic Z, et al. A systematic review of locking plate fixation of proximal humeral fractures. *Injury.* 2011;42(4):408–413.

386. Stern R. Re: Lessons learned from a case of proximal humeral locked plating gone awry. *J Orthop Trauma.* 2010;24(1):59; author reply 60.

387. Sturzenegger M, Fornaro E, Jakob RP. Results of surgical treatment of multifragmented fractures of the humeral head. *Arch Orthop Trauma Surg.* 1982;100(4):249–259.

388. Südkamp N, Bayer J, Hepp P, et al. Open reduction and internal fixation of proximal humeral fractures with use of the locking proximal humerus plate. Results of a prospective, multicenter, observational study. *J Bone Joint Surg Am.* 2009;91(6):1320–1328.

389. Südkamp NP, Audigé L, Lambert S, et al. Path analysis of factors for functional outcome at one year in 463 proximal humeral fractures. *J Shoulder Elbow Surg.* 2011;20(8):1207–1216.

390. Sukthankar AV, Leonello DT, Hertel RW, et al. A comprehensive classification of proximal humeral fractures: HGLS system. *J Shoulder Elbow Surg.* 2013.

391. Swiontkowski MF, Engelberg R, Martin DP, et al. Short musculoskeletal function assessment questionnaire: Validity, reliability, and responsiveness. *J Bone Joint Surg Am.* 1999;81(9):1245–1260.

392. Szyszkowitz R, Seggl W, Schleifer P, et al. Proximal humeral fractures. Management techniques and expected results. *Clin Orthop Relat Res.* 1993;(292):13–25.

393. Takeuchi R, Koshino T, Nakazawa A, et al. Saito T. Minimally invasive fixation for unstable two-part proximal humeral fractures: Surgical techniques and clinical results using j-nails. *J Orthop Trauma.* 2002;16(6):403–408.

394. Tanner MW, Cofield RH. Prosthetic arthroplasty for fractures and fracture-dislocations of the proximal humerus. *Clin Orthop Relat Res.* 1983;(179):116–128.

395. Teefey SA, Middleton WD, Yamaguchi K. Shoulder sonography. State of the art. *Radiol Clin North Am.* 1999;37(4):767–785, ix.

396. Tejwani NC, Liporace F, Walsh M, et al. Functional outcome following one-part proximal humeral fractures: A prospective study. *J Shoulder Elbow Surg.* 2008;17(2):216–129.

397. Thalhammer G, Platzer P, Oberleitner G, et al. Angular stable fixation of proximal humeral fractures. *J Trauma.* 2009;66(1):204–10.

398. Thanasas C, Kontakis G, Angoules A, et al. Treatment of proximal humeral fractures with locking plates: A systematic review. *J Shoulder Elbow Surg.* 2009;18(6):837–844.

399. The EuroQol Group. EuroQol–a new facility for the measurement of health-related quality of life. *Health Policy.* 1990;16(3):199–208.

400. Thyagarajan DS, Haridas SJ, Jones D, et al. Functional outcome following proximal humeral interlocking system plating for displaced proximal humeral fractures. *Int J Shoulder Surg.* 2009;3(3):57–62.

401. Tischer T, Rose T, Imhoff AB. The reverse shoulder prosthesis for primary and secondary treatment of proximal humeral fractures: a case report. *Arch Orthop Trauma Surg.* 2008;128(9):973–978.

402. Valenti P, Katz D, Kilinc A, et al. Mid-term outcome of reverse shoulder prostheses in complex proximal humeral fractures. *Acta Orthop Belg.* 2012;78(4):442–449.

403. Verbeek PA, van den Akker-Scheek I, Wendt KW, et al. Hemiarthroplasty versus angle-stable locking compression plate osteosynthesis in the treatment of three- and four-part fractures of the proximal humerus in the elderly: Design of a randomized controlled trial. *BMC Musculoskelet Disord.* 2012;13:16.

404. Visser CP, Coene LN, Brand R, et al. Nerve lesions in proximal humeral fractures. *J Shoulder Elbow Surg.* 2001;10(5):421–427.

405. Voigt C, Ewig M, Vosshenrich R, et al. Value of MRI in preoperative diagnostics of proximal humeral fractures compared to CT and conventional radiography. *Unfallchirurg.* 2010;113(5):378–385.

406. Voigt C, Geisler A, Hepp P, et al. Are polyaxially locked screws advantageous in the plate osteosynthesis of proximal humeral fractures in the elderly? A prospective randomized clinical observational study. *J Orthop Trauma.* 2011;25(10):596–602.

407. Voigt C, Hurschler C, Rechi L, et al. Additive fiber-cerclages in proximal humeral fractures stabilized by locking plates: No effect on fracture stabilization and rotator cuff function in human shoulder specimens. *Acta Orthop.* 2009;80(4):465–471.

408. Volgas DA, Stannard JP, Alonso JE. Nonunions of the humerus. *Clin Orthop Relat Res.* 2004;(419):46–50.

409. Wachtl SW, Marti CB, Hoogewoud HM, et al. Treatment of proximal humerus fracture using multiple intramedullary flexible nails. *Arch Orthop Trauma Surg.* 2000;120 (3-4):171–175.

410. Walch G, Badet R, Nové-Josserand L, et al. Nonunions of the surgical neck of the humerus: Surgical treatment with an intramedullary bone peg, internal fixation, and cancellous bone grafting. *J Shoulder Elbow Surg.* 1996;5(3):161–168.

411. Wall B, Nové-Josserand L, O'Connor DP, et al. Reverse total shoulder arthroplasty: A review of results according to etiology. *J Bone Joint Surg Am.* 2007;89(7):1476–1485.

412. Wanner GA, Wanner-Schmid E, Romero J, et al. Internal fixation of displaced proximal humeral fractures with two one-third tubular plates. *J Trauma.* 2003;54(3):536–544.

413. Ware JE Jr, Sherbourne CD. The MOS 36-item short-form health survey (SF-36). I. Conceptual framework and item selection. *Med Care.* 1992;30(6):473–483.

414. Werner CM, Steinmann PA, Gilbart M, et al. Treatment of painful pseudoparesis due to irreparable rotator cuff dysfunction with the Delta III reverse-ball-and-socket total shoulder prosthesis. *J Bone Joint Surg Am.* 2005;87(7):1476–1486.

415. Wijgman AJ, Roolker W, Patt TW, et al. Open reduction and internal fixation of three and four-part fractures of the proximal part of the humerus. *J Bone Joint Surg Am.* 2002;84-A(11):1919–1925.

416. Wild JR, DeMers A, French R, et al. Functional outcomes for surgically treated 3- and 4-part proximal humeral fractures. *Orthopedics.* 2011;34(10):e629–e633.

417. Williams GN, Gangel TJ, Arciero RA, et al. Comparison of the Single Assessment Numeric Evaluation method and two shoulder rating scales. Outcomes measures after shoulder surgery. *Am J Sports Med.* 1999;27(2):214–221.

418. Willis M, Min W, Brooks JP, et al. Proximal humeral malunion treated with reverse shoulder arthroplasty. *J Shoulder Elbow Surg.* 2012;21(4):507–513.

419. Wilmanns C, Bonnaire F. Rotator cuff alterations resulting from humeral head fractures. *Injury.* 2002;33(9):781–789.

420. Wu CH, Ma CH, Yeh JJ, et al. Locked plating for proximal humeral fractures: Differences between the deltopectoral and deltoid-splitting approaches. *J Trauma.* 2011;71(5):1364–1370.

421. Yamaguchi K, Ditsios K, Middleton WD, et al. The demographic and morphological features of rotator cuff disease. A comparison of asymptomatic and symptomatic shoulders. *J Bone Joint Surg Am.* 2006;88(8):1699–1704.

422. Yamano Y. Comminuted fractures of the proximal humerus treated with hook plate. *Arch Orthop Trauma Surg.* 1986;105(6):359–363.

423. Yang H, Li Z, Zhou F, et al. A prospective clinical study of proximal humeral fractures treated with a locking proximal humerus plate. *J Orthop Trauma.* 2011;25(1):11–17.

424. Young SW, Segal BS, Turner PC, et al. Comparison of functional outcomes of reverse shoulder arthroplasty versus hemiarthroplasty in the primary treatment of acute proximal humerus fracture. *ANZ J Surg.* 2010;80(11):789–793.

425. Zarkadas PC, Throckmorton TW, Steinmann SP. Neurovascular injuries in shoulder trauma. *Orthop Clin North Am.* 2008;39(4):483–490, vii.

426. Zhu Y, Lu Y, Shen J, et al. Locking intramedullary nails and locking plates in the treatment of two-part proximal humeral surgical neck fractures: A prospective randomized trial with a minimum of three years of follow-up. *J Bone Joint Surg Am.* 2011;93(2):159–168.

427. Zhu Y, Lu Y, Wang M, et al. Treatment of proximal humeral fracture with a proximal humeral nail. *J Shoulder Elbow Surg.* 2010;19(2):297–302.

428. Zyto K, Ahrengart L, Sperber A, et al. Treatment of displaced proximal humeral fractures in elderly patients. *J Bone Joint Surg Br.* 1997;79(3):412–417.

38 CLAVICLE FRACTURES

Michael D. McKee

INTRODUCTION TO CLAVICLE FRACTURES

Clavicle fractures are common injuries in young, active individuals, especially those who participate in activities or sports where high-speed falls (bicycling, motorcycles) or violent collisions (football, hockey) are frequent, and they account for approximately 2.6% of all fractures.[29–32,46,112,116,122,123,126] In contrast to most fractures, Robinson[155] reported in an epidemiologic study that the annual incidence in males was highest in the under 20 age group, decreasing with each subsequent age cohort (Fig. 38-1). The incidence in females was more constant, with peaks seen in the teenager (sports, motor vehicle accidents) and the elderly (osteoporotic fractures from simple falls). The annual incidence of fractures in their Scottish population was 29 per 100,000 persons per year.[155]

The majority of clavicular fractures (80% to 85%) occur in the midshaft of the bone, where the typical compressive forces applied to the shoulder and the narrow cross section of the bone combine and result in bony failure.[7–16,18–24,26–32,107,155,179] Distal third fractures are the next most common type (15% to 20%), and, although they can result from the same mechanisms of injury as that seen with midshaft fractures, they tend to occur in more elderly individuals from simple falls.[56,153,156,157,193] Medial third fractures are the rarest (0% to 5%), perhaps due to the difficulty in accurately imaging (and identifying) them.[167,185] One recent study of 57 such fractures reported that patients were typically men in their fifth decade and the usual mechanism of injury was from a motor vehicle accident.[185] These authors also noted a relatively high (20%) associated mortality from concomitant head and chest injuries.

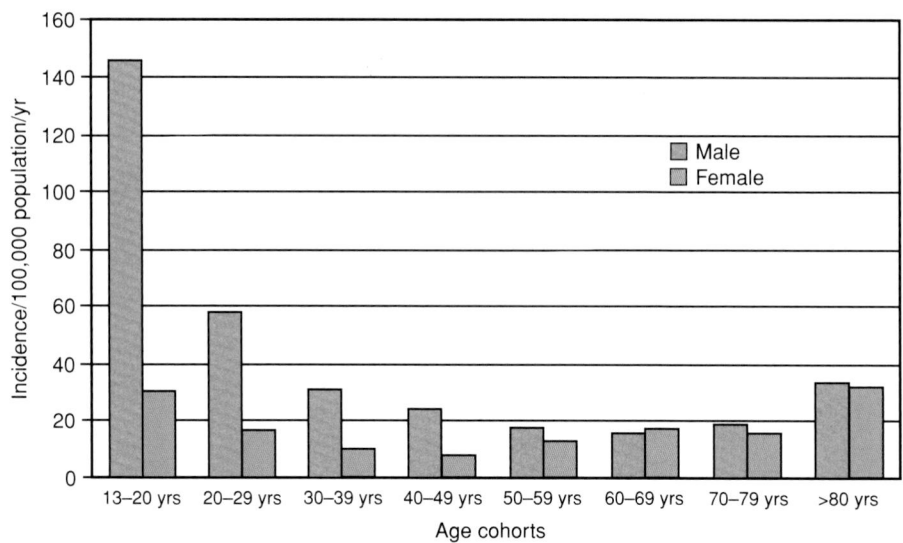

FIGURE 38-1 The epidemiology of clavicle fractures in Edinburgh, Scotland. (Adapted from Robinson CM, Court-Brown CM, McQueen MM, et al. Estimating the risk of nonunion following nonoperative treatment of a clavicle fracture. *J Bone Joint Surg Am.* 2004;86-A(7):1359–1365.)

Older studies suggested that a fracture of the shaft of the clavicle, even when significantly displaced, was an essentially benign injury with an inherently good prognosis when treated nonoperatively.[112–116] In a landmark 1960 study Neer[115] reported nonunion in only three of 2,235 patients with middle third fractures of the clavicle treated by a sling or a figure-of-eight bandage. Rowe[160] showed an overall incidence of nonunion of 0.8% in 566 clavicle fractures treated in a similar fashion. Thus, what was felt to be the most serious complication following clavicular fracture, nonunion, appeared to be extremely rare. Also, malunion of the clavicle (which occurred radiographically on a predictable basis in displaced fractures), was described as being of radiographic interest only, with little or no functional consequences. This thinking dominated the approach to clavicle fractures for decades.

More recently, there has been increasing evidence that the outcome of the nonoperatively treated (especially displaced or shortened) midshaft fracture is not as optimal as was once thought.[14,42,59,68,85,99,103,123–125] In 1997, Hill et al.[68] were the first to use patient-oriented outcome measures to examine 66 consecutive patients with displaced midshaft clavicle fractures and they found an unsatisfactory outcome in 31%, as well as a nonunion rate of 15%. In a meta-analysis of the literature from 1975 to 2005, Zlowodzki et al.[209] found that the nonunion rate for nonoperatively treated displaced midshaft clavicle fractures was 15.1%, exponentially higher than that previously described (Table 38-1). Other recent epidemiologic and prospective studies have supported these findings.[14,42,68,99,121,123,124,153–155] In addition, the malunion of the clavicle has been clearly shown by multiple authors to be a distinct clinical entity with characteristic signs and symptoms that can be significantly improved by corrective osteotomy.[7,9,21,24,41,84,102,103] Potential explanations for the increased complication rate seen following the nonoperative care of these fractures may be due to changing injury patterns (especially from "extreme" sports such as mountain bicycling, snowboarding, and all-terrain vehicle riding), increased expectations of the modern patient, comprehensive follow-up (including patient-oriented outcome measures) and focusing on adults (eliminating children with their inherently good prognosis and remodeling potential).[71,76,96,101,125,143,154,181,195,205]

Good results with a high union rate and a low complication rate have been reported from a variety of techniques for primary fixation of displaced fractures of the clavicle, dispelling some of the pessimism that surrounded prior studies where a poor understanding of soft tissue handling, a selection bias of patients, and inadequate implants combined to produce inferior results.[2,15,23,41,53,63,82,91,119,140–142] Zlowodzki's[209] systematic

---

TABLE 38-1 | **A Meta-Analysis of Nonoperative Treatment, Intramedullary Pinning, and Plate Fixation for Displaced Midshaft Fractures of the Clavicle (Published 1975–2005)**

Treatment Method	Percentage with Nonunion	Infections (Total)	Infections (Deep)	Fixation Failures
Nonoperative (n = 159)	15.1	0	0	0
Plating (n = 460)	2.2	4.6	2.4	2.2
Intramedullary pinning (n = 152)	2.0	6.6	0	3.9

Adapted from Zlowodzki M, Zelle BA, Cole PA, et al. Treatment of midshaft clavicle fractures: Systematic review of 2144 fractures: On behalf of the Evidence-Based Orthopaedic Trauma Working Group. *J Orthop Trauma,* 2005;19(7):504–507.

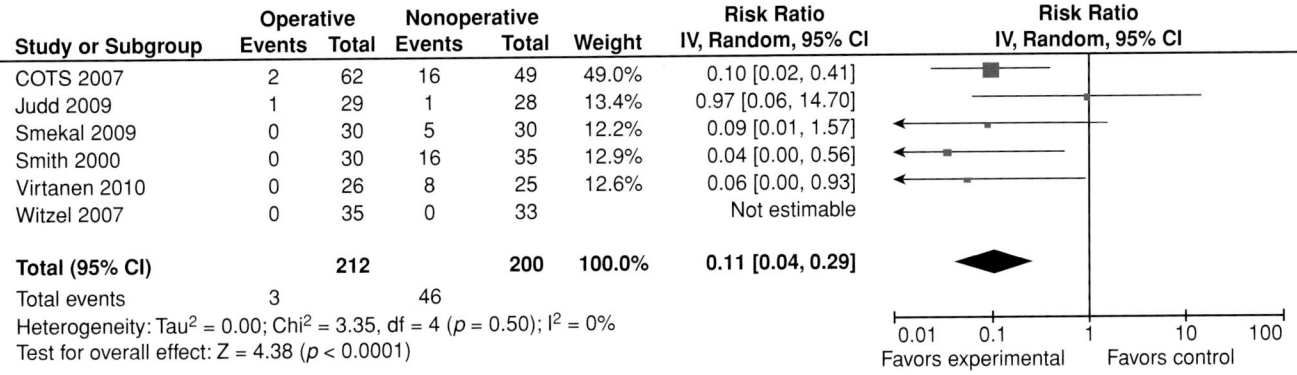

Study or Subgroup	Operative Events	Total	Nonoperative Events	Total	Weight	Risk Ratio IV, Random, 95% CI	Risk Ratio IV, Random, 95% CI
COTS 2007	2	62	16	49	49.0%	0.10 [0.02, 0.41]	
Judd 2009	1	29	1	28	13.4%	0.97 [0.06, 14.70]	
Smekal 2009	0	30	5	30	12.2%	0.09 [0.01, 1.57]	
Smith 2000	0	30	16	35	12.9%	0.04 [0.00, 0.56]	
Virtanen 2010	0	26	8	25	12.6%	0.06 [0.00, 0.93]	
Witzel 2007	0	35	0	33		Not estimable	
Total (95% CI)		**212**		**200**	**100.0%**	**0.11 [0.04, 0.29]**	
Total events	3		46				

Heterogeneity: Tau^2 = 0.00; Chi^2 = 3.35, df = 4 (p = 0.50); I^2 = 0%
Test for overall effect: Z = 4.38 (p < 0.0001)

0.01 0.1 1 10 100
Favors experimental   Favors control

FIGURE 38-2 A forest plot comparing the nonunion rate between nonoperative (control) and operative (experimental) groups from multiple randomized trials of clavicle fracture fixation for displaced midshaft fractures. Operative intervention results in a significantly decreased nonunion rate compared to nonoperative treatment (p = 0.002). The size of the squares is proportionate to the size of the study, and the diamond is the pooled data. (Adapted from: McKee RC, Whelan DB, Sche mitsch EH, et al. Operative versus nonoperative care of displaced midshaft clavicular fractures: A meta-analysis of randomized clinical trials. *J Bone Joint Surg Am.* 2012;94(8):675–684, with permission.)

review showed a relative risk reduction of 86% (from 15.1% to 2.2%) for nonunion with primary plate fixation compared to nonoperative treatment. In addition, a recent meta-analysis by McKee et al. of six randomized clinical trials of operative versus nonoperative care for displaced midshaft clavicle fractures demonstrated a reduction of nonunion and symptomatic malunion from 46/200 cases (23%) in the nonoperative group to 3/212 cases (1.4%) in the operative group (Fig. 38-2).[105]

While there is increasing interest in, and enthusiasm for, primary fixation of clavicle fractures, it is vital to remember that the majority of these fractures can and should be treated nonoperatively. The current research in this area should not provoke a swing of the operative pendulum into indiscriminate fixation of all clavicle injuries. Clinical and basic science research in this field adds objective information to this topic and is directed at prompting a thoughtful assessment of each injury based on these data and each case's individual merits such as the function and expectations of the patient, the location of the fracture, and the degree of displacement or comminution. Treatment is then based upon this assessment, the evidence-based facts now available, and a rational balance of the potential risks and benefits of surgery, rather than an extreme operative or nonoperative approach.

ASSESSMENT OF CLAVICLE FRACTURES

Mechanisms of Injury for Clavicle Fractures

A direct blow on the point of the shoulder is the commonest reported mechanism of injury that produces a midshaft fracture of the clavicle.[15,107,155,179] This can occur in a number of ways, including being thrown from a vehicle or bicycle, during a sports event, from the intrusion of objects or vehicle structure during a motor vehicle accident, or falling from a height (Fig. 38-3). A recent prospective trial of over 130 completely displaced midshaft fractures of the clavicle identified motor vehicle/motorcycle accidents, bicycling accidents, skiing/snowboarding

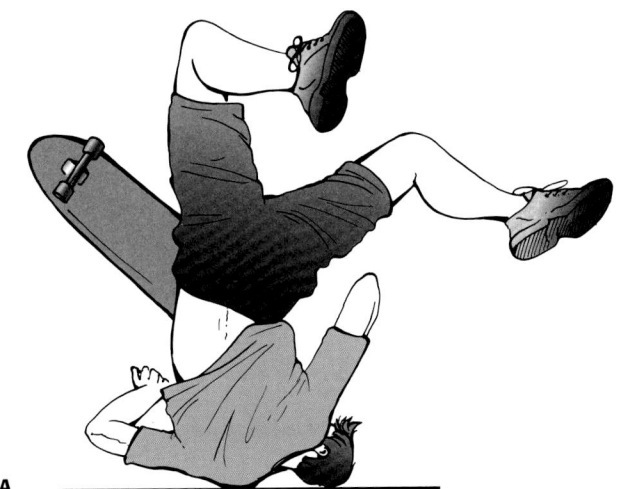

A

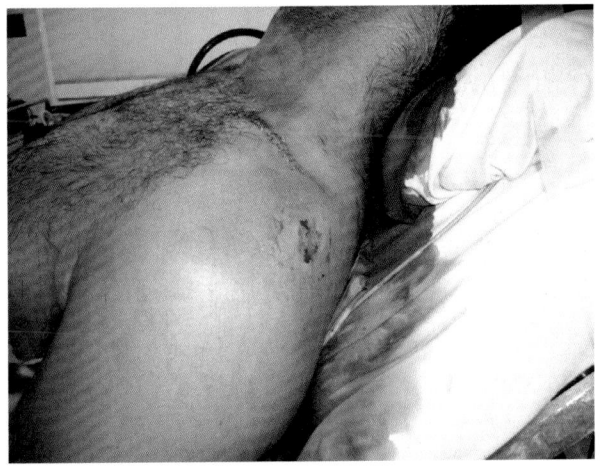

B

FIGURE 38-3 **A:** Mechanism of injury. Clavicle fractures are usually produced by a fall directly on the involved shoulder. **B:** Corresponding clinical photograph demonstrating posterior skin abrasion following displaced midshaft clavicle fracture.

falls or collisions, sports injuries, and falls as the most commonly involved mechanisms.[15] As the shoulder girdle is subjected to compression force directed from laterally, the main strut maintaining position is the clavicle and its articulations (Fig. 38-4). As the force exceeds the capacity of this structure to withstand it, failure can occur in one of the three ways. The acromioclavicular (AC) articulation may fail, the clavicle may break, or the sternoclavicular (SC) joint may dislocate. SC injuries are rare and typically associated with more posteriorly directed blows against the medial clavicle (posterior dislocations) or posteriorly directed blows to the distal shoulder girdle (levering the proximal clavicle into an anterior dislocation).[90,177] Presumably there are subtle nuances in the direction and magnitude of applied forces and local anatomy that dictate whether the failure occurs in the AC joint, or in the clavicle, and the magnitude of displacement that occurs. Most (85%) clavicle fractures occur in the midshaft of the bone where, as can be seen in a cross section, the bone is narrowest and enveloping soft tissue structures (which may help dissipate injury force) are most scarce.[29–32,153,155] It is typical to see a large abrasion or contusion on the posterior aspect of the shoulder in patients with displaced midshaft clavicular fractures, especially those who fall from bicycles, motorcycles, or other vehicles. This force vector may also contribute to the location of the injury: Midshaft fracture, distal fracture, or AC joint injury. The direction of the initial deforming force, and both gravitational and muscular forces on the clavicle are significant and result in the typical deformity seen after fracture, with the distal fragment being translated inferiorly, anteriorly, and medi-

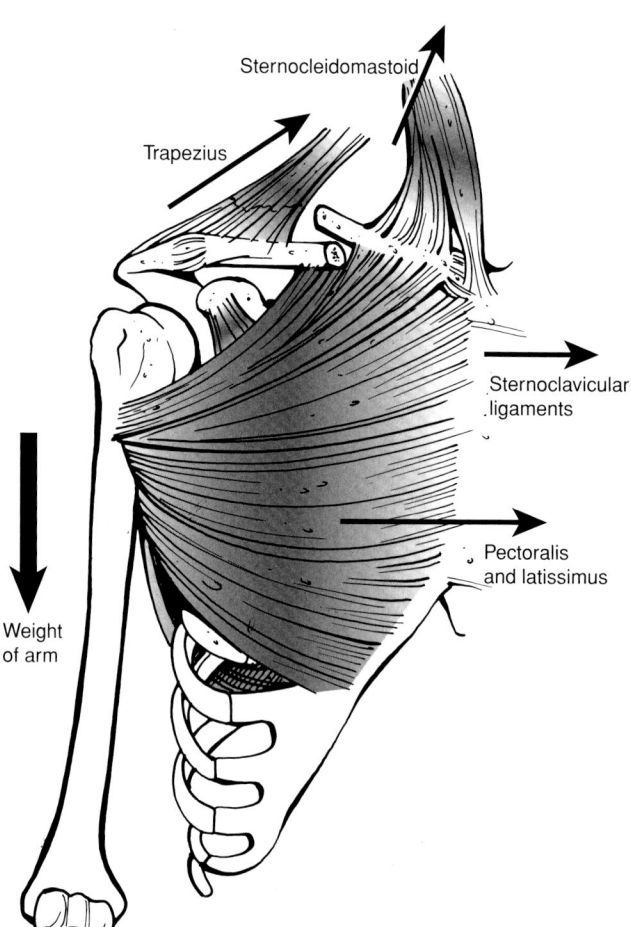

FIGURE 38-5 Muscular and gravitational forces acting on the fractured clavicle with resultant deformity. The distal fragment is translated anteriorly, medially, and inferiorly, and rotated anteriorly. This results in the scapula being protracted.

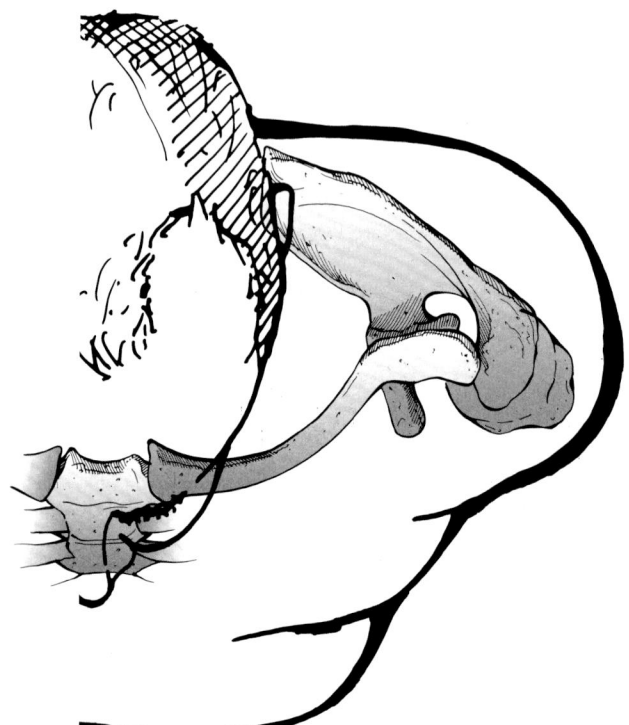

FIGURE 38-4 The strut function of the clavicle, the only bony articulation between the axial skeleton and the upper limb.

ally (shortened), and rotated anteriorly (Fig. 38-5). With recent advances in imaging techniques, there is an increasing level of information available regarding the complex three-dimensional deformity that can result from a displaced midshaft fracture of the clavicle (Fig. 38-6).[152]

Simple falls from a standing height are unlikely to produce a displaced fracture in a healthy young person, but can result in injury in elderly, osteoporotic individuals: These fractures are typically seen in the distal third of the clavicle. If the mechanism of injury is trivial and does not seem commensurate with the fracture depicted, then a careful investigation for a pathologic fracture should be performed (Fig. 38-7).[32,176]

Associated Injuries with Clavicle Fractures

Associated injuries are increasingly common in patients with fractures of the clavicle, compared to the incidence reported in older traditional studies.[39,43,44,101,181,207] There may be several reasons for this, including more liberal use of improved

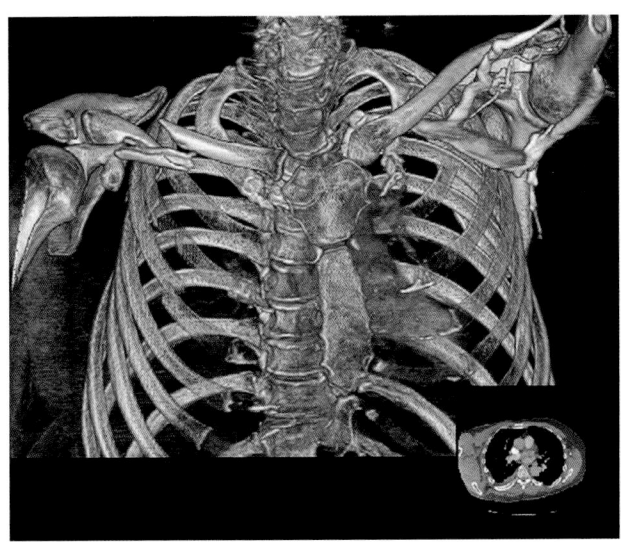

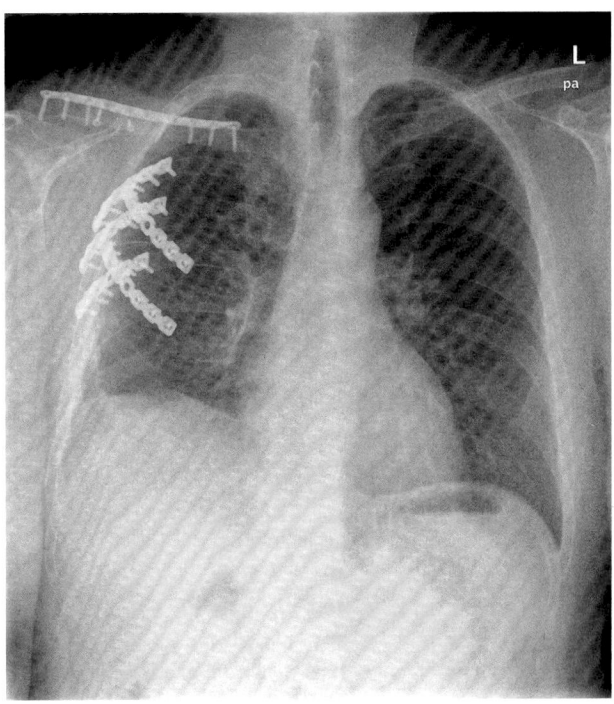

A   B

FIGURE 38-6 A: Preoperative three-dimensional CT scan of a patient with a displaced clavicle fracture and ipsilateral flail chest. This injury pattern represents a severe injury with significant instability of the entire forequarter. **B:** Following plate fixation of both the clavicle and multiple ipsilateral ribs, the flail segment became stable.

diagnostic techniques (i.e., CT scanning), the greater speed and violence of many modern sports (such as motocross and snowboarding) and the improved survivorship of patients with significant chest trauma who would have succumbed prior to the institution of comprehensive treatment of the trauma patient. In fact, several studies from Level 1 trauma centers have examined the characteristics of polytrauma patients with clavicle fractures, and have noted a high mortality rate (20% to 34%) from associated chest and head traumas.[101,181] Presumably these series of critically injured patients contain survivors who live to require treatment for the complications of their clavicle fractures who may not have survived without modern trauma care.

Patients who have sustained high-energy vehicular trauma are more likely to have associated injures to the thoracic cage, including ipsilateral rib fractures, scapular and/or glenoid fractures, proximal humeral fractures, and hemo/pneumothoraces (Fig. 38-8).[29,101,181] In addition to simply being good medicine, identification of these injuries is important for multiple reasons. Patients may require urgent treatment directed specifically at the associated injury (i.e., tube thoracostomy for pneumothorax), their presence may influence the treatment of the clavicle fracture (i.e., an associated displaced glenoid neck fracture, the so-called "floating shoulder," see below), or (as objective information on this entity increases) they may give an indication of the likelihood of a negative outcome for the clavicle fracture

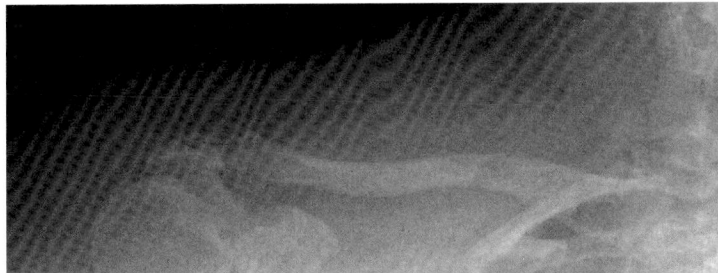

FIGURE 38-7 A 45-year-old previously well woman presented to the fracture clinic with shoulder pain following an episode of minor trauma. Radiographs revealed a fracture through a lytic lesion of the clavicle. This was the presentation of what subsequent investigation revealed to be a widely disseminated metastatic adenocarcinoma of unknown source.

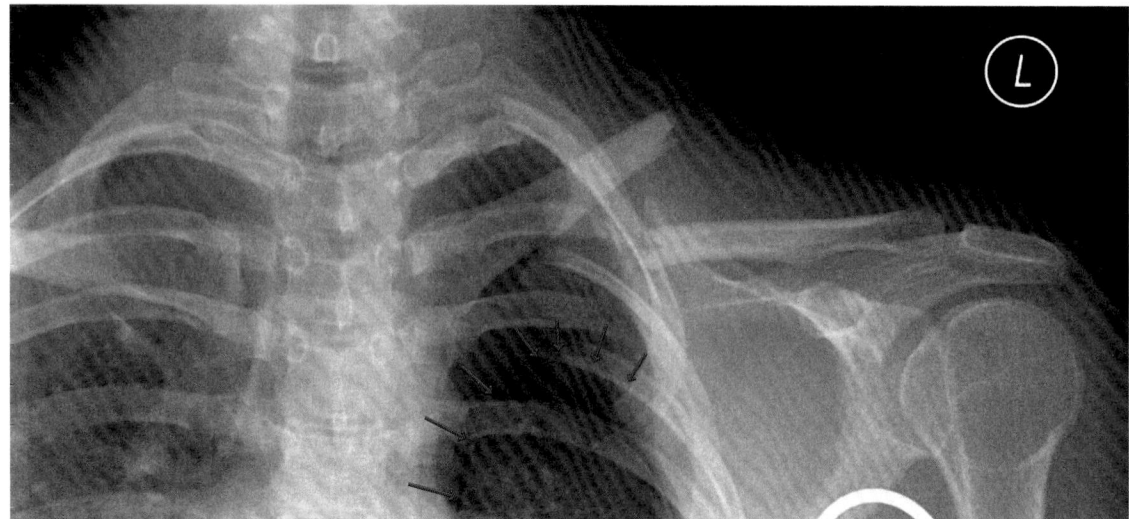

FIGURE 38-8 Anteroposterior radiograph of the clavicle in a 42-year-old man involved in a motor vehicle collision. Associated injuries include multiple ipsilateral upper rib fractures, an ipsilateral pneumothorax (*arrows* outlining collapsed lung), and multiple lower extremity fractures. This patient has four relative indications for operative fixation; (1) the severe displacement of the clavicle fracture, (2) the multiple upper rib fractures, which tend to destabilize the shoulder girdle, (3) the associated lower extremity fractures and the resultant need for immediate upper extremity use, and (4) the pneumothorax, which is indicative of the degree of trauma applied to the shoulder.

(malunion, nonunion) that may have implications regarding primary fixation (Fig. 38-9). There is also some evidence that multiple ipsilateral rib fractures are significant for a number of reasons: The degree of disruptive energy imparted to, and the resultant deformity and instability of, the chest and shoulder girdle may be associated with higher rates of poor outcome in the associated clavicle fracture. In addition, there is increasing interest in the primary fixation of mechanically unstable chest wall segments (or "flail chest") as a means of improving the respiratory outcome and ventilatory care of such patients (Fig. 38-6).[62,183]

The clavicle can also be injured from penetrating trauma including projectiles, blasts, and sword or machete blows (Fig. 38-10). In this situation, diagnosing and treating underlying chest and/or vascular injuries is critically important, and the clavicle can be treated on its own merits.[30,32,36,69,78,111,148,187] However, if a vascular repair has been performed, clavicular fixation (if possible) provides an optimally stable environment for healing.

Signs and Symptoms of Clavicle Fractures
History

The history should delineate a number of aspects to optimize the patient's care. In addition to the standard demographic data, the details of the mechanism of injury are important. A clavicle fracture caused by a simple low-energy fall is unlikely to be associated with other fractures or intrathoracic injuries, while a fracture that occurs as a result of severe vehicular trauma or a fall from a height should prompt a search for other injuries. In my experience, clavicle fractures that result from falls while bicycling often have multiple ipsilateral upper rib fractures. At a Level 1 trauma center, we studied 105 polytrauma patients

(multiple system injury and injury severity score greater than 16) with fractures of the clavicular shaft and found a mortality rate of 32%, mainly due to associated head and chest injuries.[101] This high incidence of associated head/chest injuries mandates careful clinical and radiographic investigation. The physical mechanism of injury is important: While the majority of fractures will result from a blow to the shoulder, failure of the bone can also occur from a traction-type injury. This usually occurs in an industrial or dockyard injury in which the involved arm is forcefully pulled away from the body as it is caught in machinery. It can also occur in vehicular trauma when the arm is pinned against or strikes a fixed object as the torso continues past it. This can lead to scapulothoracic dissociation, as the shoulder girdle fails in tension at the SC joint, the clavicle or the AC joint. This is evident on the radiographs when a completely displaced, distracted fracture site is seen (as opposed to the typical overlapping fracture fragments) (Fig. 38-11). The high incidence of neurologic and vascular traction injuries seen in this setting mandates further investigation (i.e., angiography), because they can be limb threatening.[30,39,58,111,136,207]

If the clavicular fracture has occurred with minimal trauma, one must be alert to the possibility of a pathologic fracture (Fig. 38-7). Metabolic processes that weaken bone (i.e., renal disease, hyperparathyroidism), benign or malignant tumors (i.e., myeloma, metastases), or pre-existing lesions (i.e., congenital pseudarthrosis of the clavicle) can result in pathologic fracture. In this setting, nonoperative treatment of the clavicle fracture is recommended initially, while intervention is directed toward diagnosis and treatment of the underlying condition. Once the primary diagnosis has been made and treatment initiated, the clavicle fracture is treated based on its individual aspects. Also,

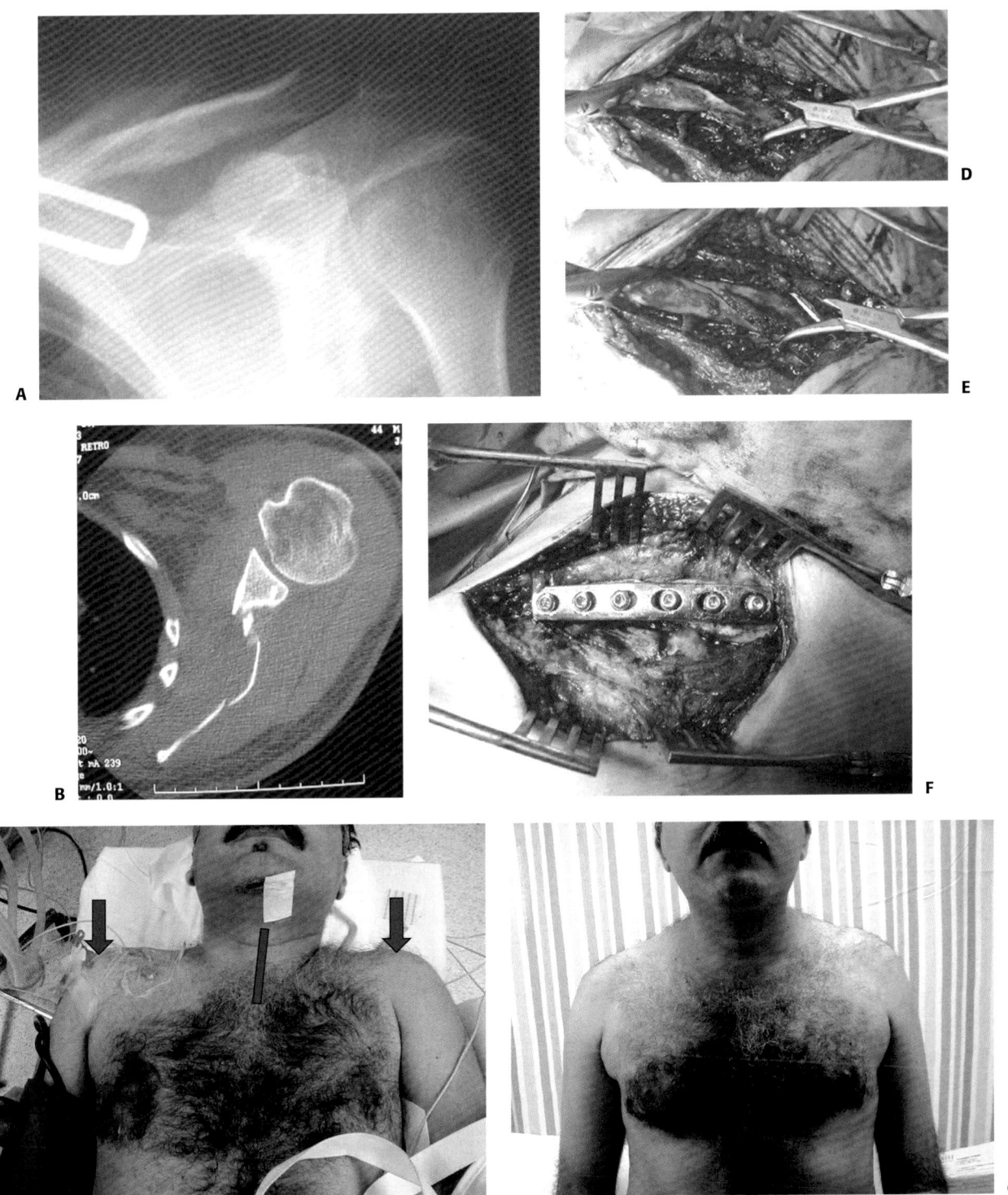

FIGURE 38-9 A "floating shoulder" injury. This patient was injured in a motor vehicle accident. **A:** An anteroposterior radiograph demonstrates a displaced, shortened left clavicle fracture. **B:** A CT scan of the shoulder reveals a comminuted glenoid neck fracture. **C:** There is significant clinical deformity. **D:** Intraoperatively, the fracture is reduced with the aid of reduction clamps, and an anterior fixation plate is applied **(E, F)**. Symmetry of the shoulder was restored by clavicle fixation alone, and it was not necessary to repair the glenoid fracture. **G:** There was an excellent clinical result with full restoration of motion and a Constant score of 95.

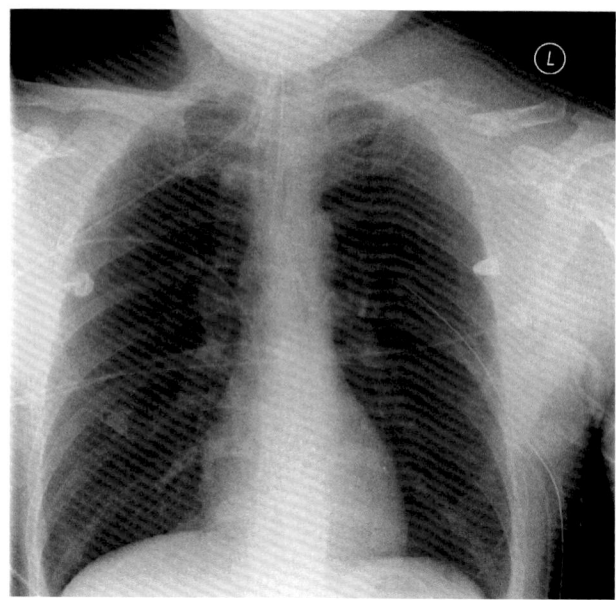

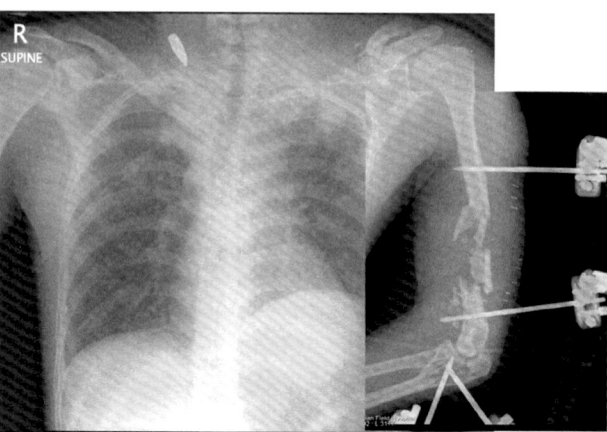

FIGURE 38-10 **A:** A comminuted clavicle fracture resulting from a low-velocity gunshot wound with an associated hemopneumothorax and a retained intrathoracic bullet, treated with tube thoracostomy. The degree of clavicular deformity and the associated injuries represent a relative indication for operative repair. **B:** Severe injuries in a 25-year-old soldier struck by a high-velocity bullet fired by an insurgent in Afghanistan. The AK-47 bullet fractured the humerus, struck the clavicle, shattering the midportion, lacerated the subclavian vein and artery (causing life-threatening hemorrhage) and came to rest in the soft tissues of the neck. In an austere operating environment, the clavicle fragments were resected and a vascular repair was performed.

repetitive or unusual loads may induce a stress fracture of the clavicle, typically in bodybuilders or weightlifters.[134,159,169]

In the past, when treatment of all clavicular shaft fractures was consistently nonoperative, a detailed history of lifestyle, occupation, and medical conditions was usually perfunctory at best, since these factors did little to influence decision making. However, there is now increasing evidence that operative intervention is superior in carefully selected cases of displaced clavicular shaft fracture, such that additional information gleaned from the history contributes to the risk/benefit analysis regarding possible

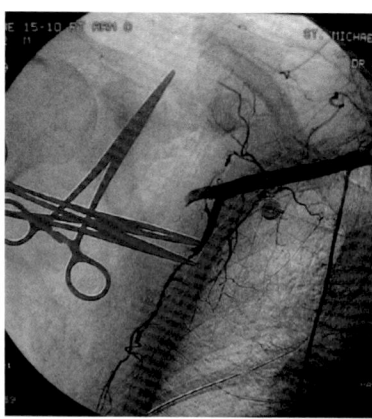

FIGURE 38-11 Emergency angiogram of a patient with a **scapulothoracic** dissociation and wide distraction of a very distal clavicle fracture. There is an associated axillary artery avulsion, a complete brachial plexus injury, and multiple ipsilateral upper extremity fractures.

surgery. Compliant patients in the 16 to 60 age group, who have active recreational lifestyles and/or physically demanding occupations (especially those that require throwing, repetitive overhead work, or recurrent lifting) are candidates for primary operative repair if they are medically fit and have completely displaced fractures with good bone quality.[15,108,140,190,209] Factors associated with noncompliance and a high rate of fixation failure, such as drug and alcohol abuse, untreated psychiatric conditions, homelessness, or uncontrolled seizure disorders are contraindications for primary operative repair of clavicle fractures.[10]

Physical Examination

When nonoperative treatment was chosen for the vast majority of clavicle fractures, there was little emphasis placed on a careful physical examination of the shoulder girdle. However, there are a number of findings that are important in surgical decision making. There is usually swelling, bruising, and ecchymosis at the fracture site, as well as deformity with displaced fractures. Visible deformity of the shoulder girdle, best seen when the patient is standing, is an important feature to recognize. The usual position seen with a completely displaced midshaft fracture of the clavicle has been described as shoulder "ptosis," with a droopy, medially driven, and shortened shoulder (Fig. 38-12).[64,74,136,150] In addition, the shoulder translates and rotates forward: This is a deformity that can best be seen by viewing the patient from above. Due to this malposition of the shoulder girdle, inspection of the patient from behind may reveal a subtle prominence of the inferior aspect of the scapula from scapular protraction as it moves with the distal fragment.

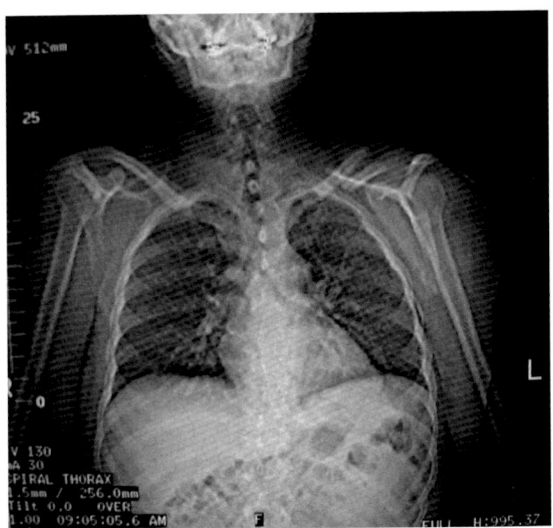
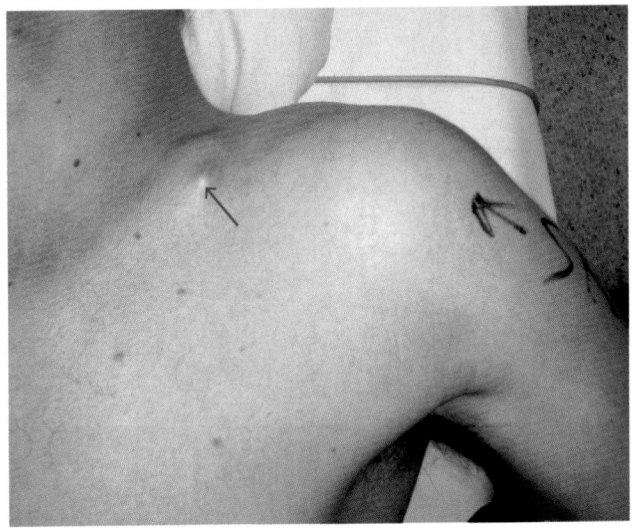

FIGURE 38-12 A: The "scout" portion of a CT scan in a polytrauma patient with a displaced clavicle fracture demonstrates the typical deformity which occurs with these injuries. **B:** The corresponding clinical photograph demonstrates blanching of the skin over the medial fragment (*arrow*).

Shortening of the clavicle should be measured clinically with a tape measure. A mark is made in the midline of the suprasternal notch and another is made at the palpable ridge of the AC joint: Measuring this length gives the difference between the involved and normal shoulder girdle.[172] The degree of shortening at the fracture site is very important in the decision making of operative versus nonoperative care, as it has been reported in multiple studies to be of prognostic significance (greater shortening, especially more than 1.5 to 2 cm, is associated with a worse prognosis). Radiographs, especially of long oblique fractures, tend to overestimate the degree of shortening which emphasizes the importance of a proper clinical examination.

A careful neurologic and vascular examination of the involved limb is mandatory, especially if surgical intervention is contemplated. If a deficit is not noted preoperatively, then it may be incorrectly attributed to the surgery which has prognostic, medical–legal, and treatment implications.[29–32]

Open Fractures

Surprisingly, given its subcutaneous nature and exposed position, open fractures of the clavicle are relatively rare. Most open fractures are associated with high-energy vehicular trauma, and recognition is important for a number of reasons: The fracture itself will require irrigation, debridement, and fixation, and there is a high incidence of associated injuries. Two large, recent series focused on open fractures of the clavicle. Taitsman et al.[181] described 20 patients with this injury; 15 had pulmonary injuries, 13 had head injuries, 8 had scapular fractures, 11 had facial trauma, and there was a variety of other injuries. In the largest published series to date, Gottschalk et al.[61] identified 53 open clavicle fractures from an active Level 1 trauma center over a 16-year period (roughly three cases per year, illustrating the rarity of this condition). They also reported many associated serious injuries, with the 26 patients with penetrating injuries having a high incidence of great vessel injury, while

the 21 patients with blunt trauma had a 52% rate of serious head injury. They stated that an open clavicle fracture should immediately raise suspicion for a serious concomitant injury, and that a prompt and thorough evaluation should be initiated. As far as treatment of the clavicle fracture itself is concerned, no specific recommendations are available in the literature, but general principles should be followed. Prophylactic antibiotics should be administered, and in general the instability associated with such a fracture will warrant operative stabilization as promptly as the patient's general condition permits.

Imaging and Other Diagnostic Studies for Clavicle Fractures

Simple anteroposterior (AP) radiographs are usually sufficient to establish the diagnosis of a clavicle fracture. The diagnosis may also be made from a single AP chest radiograph, which may be the only available film in an urgent trauma setting. The chest radiograph can also be used to evaluate the deformity of the involved clavicle relative to the normal side, and to look for associated skeletal injuries such as rib, glenoid, and scapular fractures. A measurement of length can be made on the chest radiograph comparing the injured to the uninjured side: Shortening of 2 cm or more represents a relative indication for primary fixation. To best delineate a clavicular fracture, as when one is determining whether operative intervention is warranted, a radiograph should be taken in the upright position (where gravity will demonstrate maximal deformity). Ideally, the radiographic beam for the AP radiograph of the clavicle should be angled 20 degrees superiorly to eliminate the overlap of the thoracic cage and show the clavicle in profile.[29–32,149,194] In addition, if the torso is internally rotated a similar 20 degrees (rotating internally when standing or by bumping up the opposite side while supine), the scapula and shoulder girdle are placed parallel to the cassette for a true AP film. CT scanning of midshaft clavicular fractures is rarely performed in the clinical setting, although

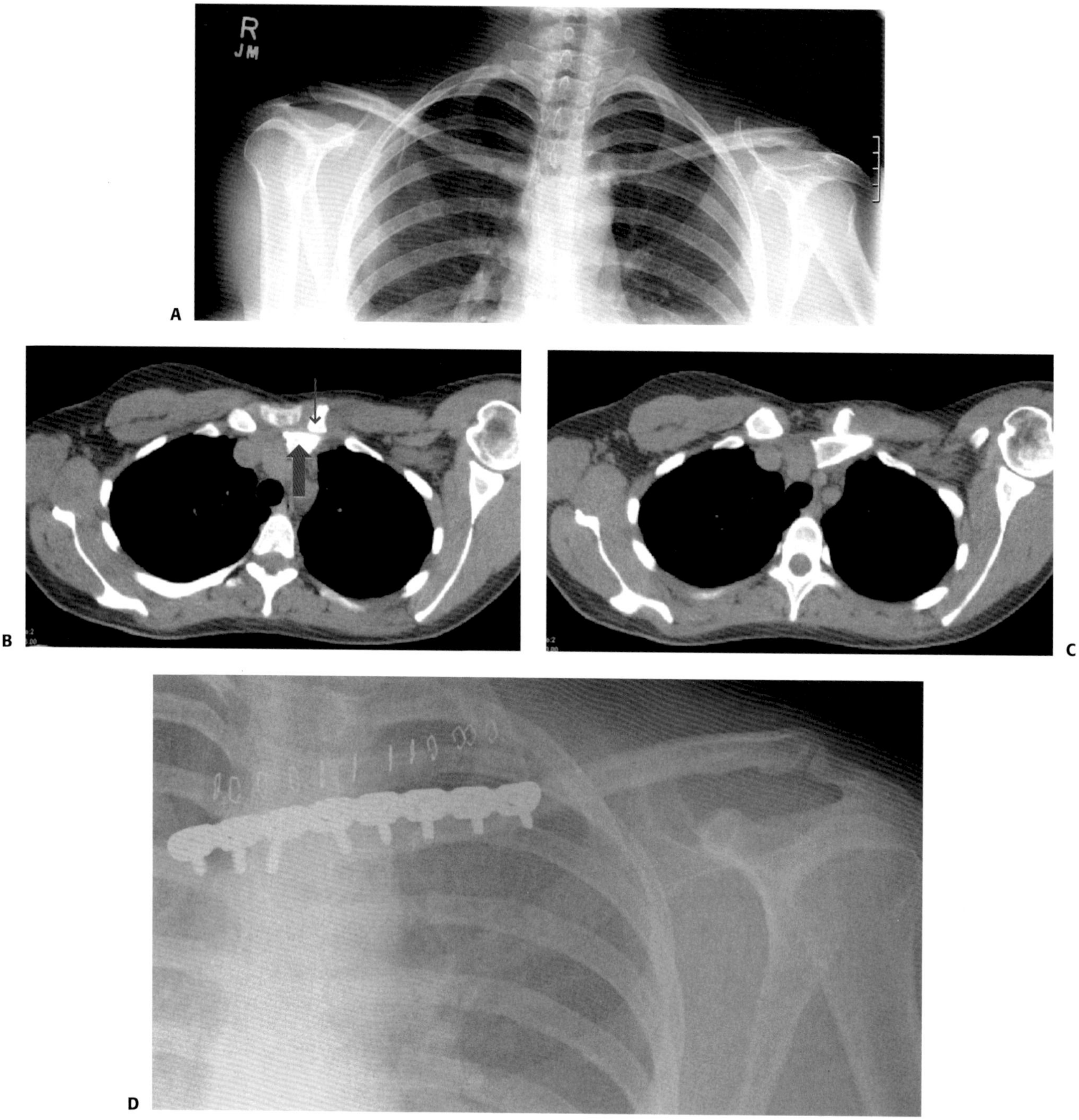

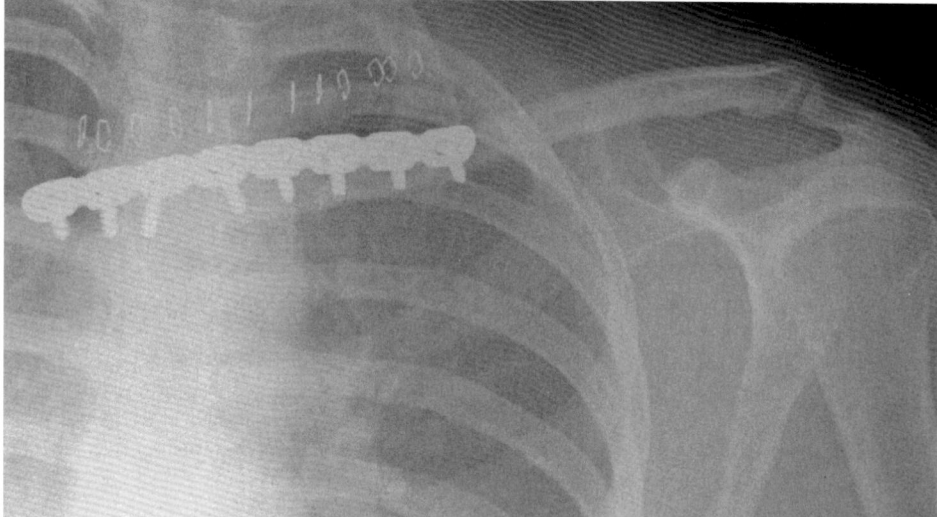

FIGURE 38-13 Fractures of the medial end of the clavicle are difficult to visualize with conventional radiography. This 32-year-old female equestrian sustained a medial clavicle fracture following a riding accident when her horse fell on her. The anteroposterior radiograph **(A)** reveals some asymmetry of the clavicles but it is difficult to define the exact nature of the injury due to the overlap of bony axial structures and the spinal column. **B:** A CT scan clearly demonstrates the medial fracture with a small residual medial fragment (*small arrow*) and posterior displacement of the shaft (*big arrow*), **(C)** impinging on the mediastinal structures. **D:** Plate fixation was performed, with extension of the plate onto the sternum due to the small size of the medial fragment. Once bony union has occurred (between 3 and 6 months), such a plate should be removed. (Case courtesy of Dr. Jeremy A. Hall.)

this imaging modality can demonstrate the complex three-dimensional deformity that affects the shoulder girdle with these injuries, including significant scapular angulation and protraction.[64] It is also useful for evaluating fractures of the medial third of the clavicle and the remainder of the shoulder girdle, such as the glenoid neck in cases of a "floating shoulder."[45,145,158]

Lateral clavicle fractures can be well visualized with AP radiographs. Centering the radiograph on the AC joint and angling the beam in a cephalic tilt of approximately 15 degrees (the Zanca view) helps delineate the fracture well, by removing the overlap of the upper portion of the thoracic cage.[30,32] To accurately delineate the degree of fracture displacement, these radiographs should be taken with the patient standing and the arm unsupported by slings, braces, or the uninjured arm. On occasion, it may be useful to obtain a stress view to determine the integrity of the coracoclavicular ligaments (as this can influence the choice of fixation): A 2.26- to 4.53 kg (5- to 10-lb) weight is suspended from the wrist of the affected arm and then radiographs are taken. CT scanning of lateral clavicle fractures is rarely required clinically; but can be useful in selected cases to determine intra-articular extension or displacement.

Fractures of the medial clavicle, especially those involving the SC joint, are notoriously difficult to accurately assess with plain radiographs. CT scanning is the radiographic procedure of choice when the anatomy of the fracture is unclear. This investigation can help distinguish between a medial epiphyseal fracture (common in individuals up to 25 years of age) and true SC dislocations (Fig. 38-13).[30,167,185,206]

Classification of Clavicle Fractures

A number of classification schemes have been proposed for fractures of the clavicle. These have traditionally been based on the position of the fracture, with the groups originally divided by Allman into proximal (Group I), middle (Group II), and distal (Group III) third fractures. This general grouping has the advantage of corresponding to the clinical approach to these fractures of most orthopedic surgeons.[30] Recognizing that this basic scheme does not take into effect factors that influence treatment and outcome, such as fracture pattern, displacement, comminution, and shortening, various authorities have refined the classification to include other variables. Due to their high rate of delayed union and nonunion, Neer divided distal clavicle fractures into three subgroups, based on their ligamentous attachments and degree of displacement (Type II was subsequently modified by Rockwood).[30,113]

Type I: Distal clavicle fracture with the coracoclavicular ligaments intact

Type II: Coracoclavicular ligaments detached from the medial fragment, with the trapezoidal ligament attached to the distal fragment

    IIA (Rockwood): Both conoid and trapezoid attached to the distal fragment

    IIB (Rockwood): Conoid detached from the medial fragment

Type III: Distal clavicle fracture with extension into the AC joint.

Ideally, a classification scheme should be reproducible with a low rate of inter- and intra-observer variability, should help direct treatment, can be used to predict outcome, should be useful in both the clinical and research realms, and should be simple enough to be practically useful yet robust enough to include all fracture patterns. While at the present time there is no classification scheme that has been rigorously tested to meet all these objectives, modern schemes based on prospective, comprehensive population-based studies are available. Nordqvist et al.[123] examined over 2,035 fractures of the clavicle over a 10-year period and essentially expanded on Allman's original scheme by adding subtypes based on fracture displacement, including a comminuted category for midshaft fractures. In a similar population-based study in Edinburgh, Robinson[155] evaluated over 1,000 consecutive fractures of the clavicle, and developed a classification scheme based on prognostic variables from the analysis of their data (Fig. 38-14). It continues the traditional scheme of dividing the clavicle into thirds, and adds variables that are of proven diagnostic value (intra-articular extension, displacement, and comminution). However, a feature of this scheme is that it reverses the traditional numbering scheme, describing medial fractures as Type I, middle third fractures as Type II, and distal third fractures as Type III. Since distal third fractures are firmly entrenched in the orthopedic lexicon as "Type II" fractures, this can lead to significant confusion. Despite this drawback, the Robinson classification is based on an extensive database that includes prospectively gathered, objective clinical data. For this reason, it is the classification I prefer to use clinically as it can help predict outcome and hence guide treatment, including the decision to operate and the fixation methods chosen. The AO/OTA Fracture and Dislocation Classification Compendium was updated in 2007 to include recent developments including a unified numbering scheme and measures to improve observer reliability (Fig. 38-15). The clavicle is designated as segment 15, and is divided into the standard medial metaphyseal, diaphyseal, and lateral metaphyseal fractures.[95] An important difference is that the metaphyseal fractures in this scheme are not one-third of the length of the bone but are shorter segments, according to the AO "rule of squares." For the all-important diaphysis, there are simple (15-B1), wedge (15-B2), and complex (15-B3) subtypes.

Outcome Measures for Clavicle Fractures

It has become apparent that outcome measures previously used for fractures in general, and clavicle fractures in particular, have not reliably demonstrated significant residual deficits following injury.[115,160] Gauging success or failure based on the isolated finding of the presence or absence of union on a post-injury radiograph was shown to be inadequate by Gossard.[59] They used patient-based questionnaires that revealed a 32% rate of patient dissatisfaction following the nonoperative treatment of displaced midshaft clavicle fractures, a significantly higher rate than expected from traditional (i.e., radiographic or surgeon-based) outcome measures. In addition, they showed that a significant proportion of patients (15%) were dissatisfied despite radiographic union, confirming the existence of symptomatic clavicular malunion for the first time in a large series. McKee et al.[99] used

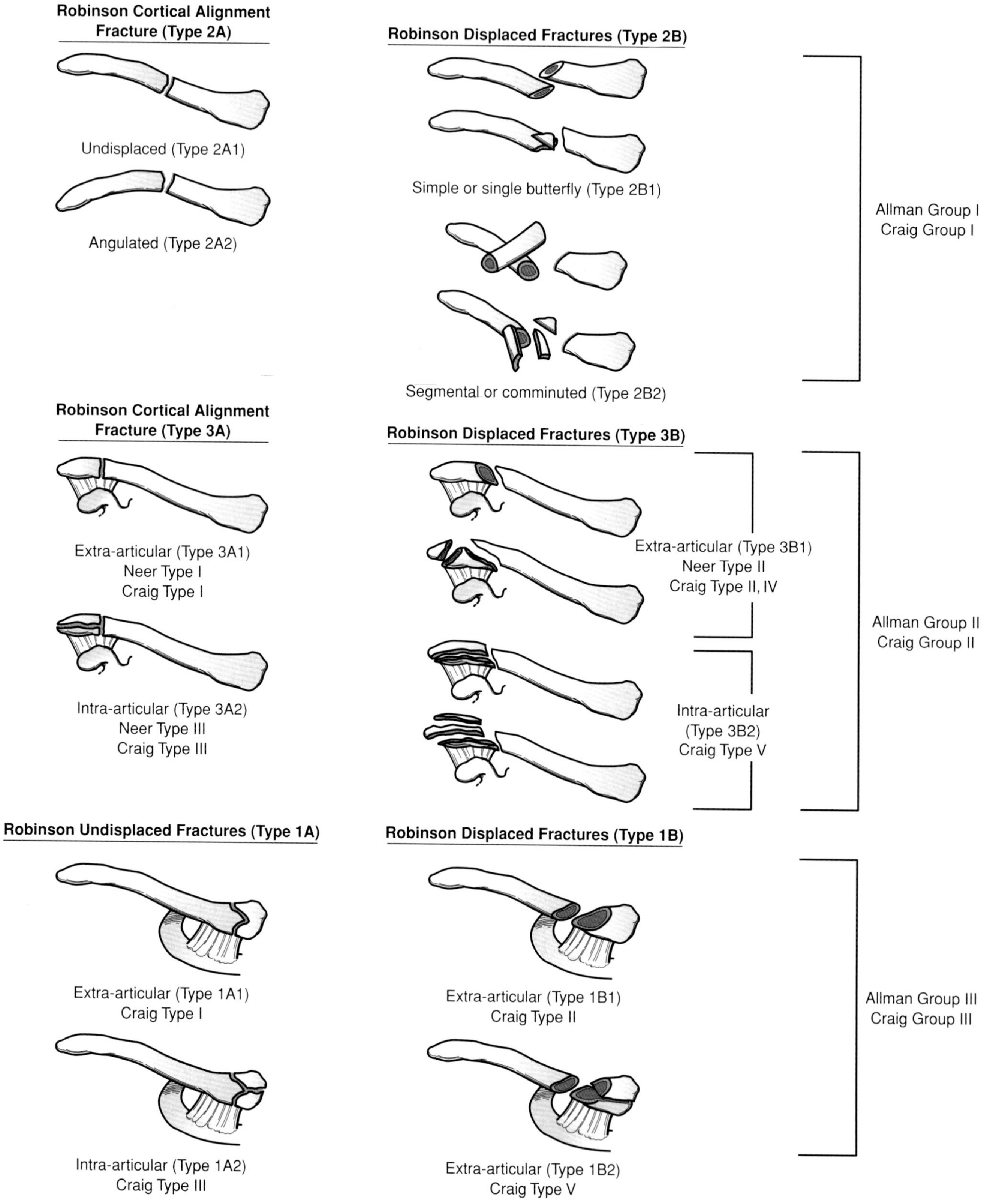

Robinson Cortical Alignment Fracture (Type 2A)

Undisplaced (Type 2A1)

Angulated (Type 2A2)

Robinson Displaced Fractures (Type 2B)

Simple or single butterfly (Type 2B1)

Segmental or comminuted (Type 2B2)

Allman Group I
Craig Group I

Robinson Cortical Alignment Fracture (Type 3A)

Extra-articular (Type 3A1)
Neer Type I
Craig Type I

Intra-articular (Type 3A2)
Neer Type III
Craig Type III

Robinson Displaced Fractures (Type 3B)

Extra-articular (Type 3B1)
Neer Type II
Craig Type II, IV

Intra-articular
(Type 3B2)
Craig Type V

Allman Group II
Craig Group II

Robinson Undisplaced Fractures (Type 1A)

Extra-articular (Type 1A1)
Craig Type I

Intra-articular (Type 1A2)
Craig Type III

Robinson Displaced Fractures (Type 1B)

Extra-articular (Type 1B1)
Craig Type II

Extra-articular (Type 1B2)
Craig Type V

Allman Group III
Craig Group III

FIGURE 38-14 Robinson classification scheme of clavicle fractures.

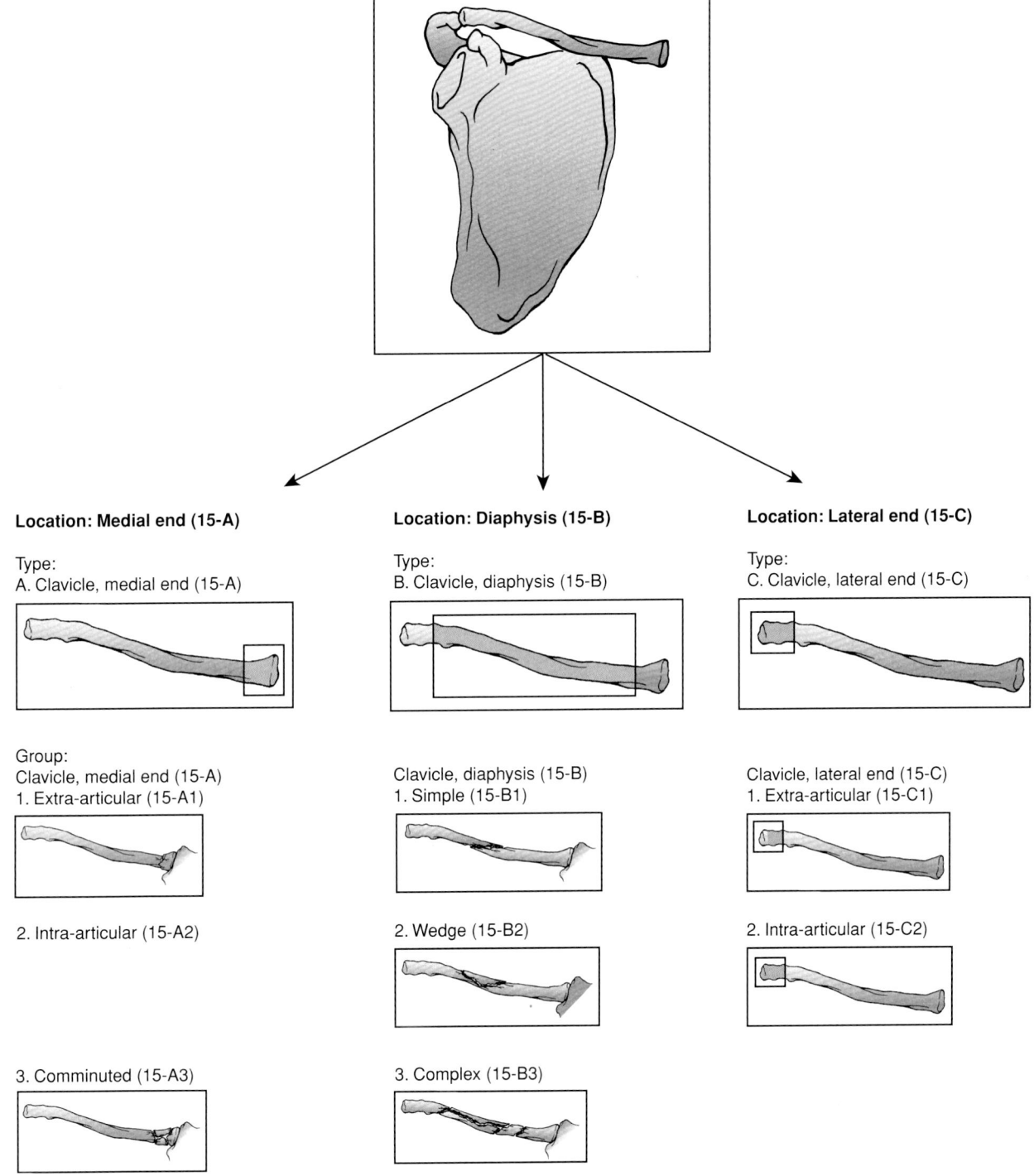

Location: Medial end (15-A)

Type:
A. Clavicle, medial end (15-A)

Group:
Clavicle, medial end (15-A)
1. Extra-articular (15-A1)

2. Intra-articular (15-A2)

3. Comminuted (15-A3)

Location: Diaphysis (15-B)

Type:
B. Clavicle, diaphysis (15-B)

Clavicle, diaphysis (15-B)
1. Simple (15-B1)

2. Wedge (15-B2)

3. Complex (15-B3)

Location: Lateral end (15-C)

Type:
C. Clavicle, lateral end (15-C)

Clavicle, lateral end (15-C)
1. Extra-articular (15-C1)

2. Intra-articular (15-C2)

FIGURE 38-15 AO/OTA classification scheme of clavicle fractures.

machine-based objective strength measurements on patients with clavicular malunion to demonstrate strength deficits of up to 30% that were not apparent on the traditional manual strength testing against the physicians resisting arm.

Similar findings in other areas have prompted extensive research into the evaluation of outcome. A number of modern, validated, responsive, consistent outcome measures are now available for the evaluation following shoulder girdle injuries.

Most clinical research studies examining patient outcome in this anatomic area use a comprehensive set of outcome measures including a patient-oriented general health status measurement such as the SF-36 or MFA, a patient-oriented limb-specific outcome measure such as the Disabilities of the Arm, Shoulder, and Hand (DASH), a surgeon-based outcome score such as the Constant shoulder score or UCLA shoulder score, and a radiographic measure. With regard to the radiographic measurements, there is

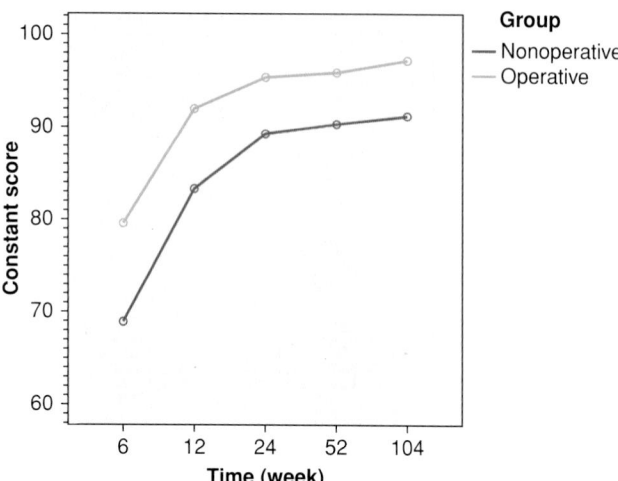

FIGURE 38-16 Constant shoulder scores of patients following operative versus nonoperative treatment of a displaced midshaft fracture of the clavicle at 2 years are similar to 1-year scores, indicating that function plateaus after 1-year post injury. (Adapted from: Schemitsch LA, Schemitsch EH, Veillette C, et al. Function plateaus by one year in patients with surgically treated displaced midshaft clavicle fractures. *Clin Orthop Relat Res.* 2011;469(12:3351–3355, with permission.)

increasing focus on standardizing technique so as to obtain consistent results. There are now data available from multiple studies on the effect of a clavicle fracture on these outcome measures that help the attending surgeon with treatment and prognostication (see below).[15,85,103,143,155]

Another previously unanswered yet important question regarding outcome following clavicle fracture was the length of follow-up required to determine the time of maximal recovery, or when a patient "plateaued" following injury. While most scientific journals require a minimum follow-up of 2 years for outcome studies, this can be extremely difficult to obtain in the

"trauma population," which tends to be predominantly young, male, and transient. A recent study by Schemitsch et al.[164] demonstrated that outcome measures such as the DASH or Constant score do not change appreciably after 1 year in patients with midshaft clavicle fractures (Fig. 38-16). This finding has important implications. Clinically, following either operative or nonoperative treatment, patients can be told that their functional outcome is unlikely to change significantly from their status at 1 year post injury. Researchers can plan for a single year of follow-up post-intervention, with the knowledge that the expense and effort of longer monitoring is unnecessary as changes in outcome measures past this point are minimal. In addition, economists can use the 1-year data from such studies for definitive calculations of the long-term cost-effectiveness of various treatment methods.[137]

PATHOANATOMY AND APPLIED ANATOMY RELATING TO CLAVICLE FRACTURES

Bony Anatomy of the Clavicle

The clavicle is a relatively thin bone, widest at its medial and lateral expansions where it articulates with the sternum and acromion, respectively (Fig. 38-17). It has two distinct curves: The larger, obvious curve is in the coronal plane giving the bone its characteristic S shape (medial end convex anterior and lateral end concave anterior).[107] There is also a more subtle superior curve delineated in a cadaver study by Huang et al.[70] This milder superior bow had its apex laterally a mean of 37 mm from the acromial articulation, with a mean magnitude of 5 mm. The medial superior surface of the clavicle was found to be flat. This article also described the fit of a precontoured clavicular plate to 100 pairs of cadaver clavicles. The authors found that there were significant sex and racial differences in the fit of the plate from best (black male clavicles) to worst (white female clavicles). This article helps explain why intraoperatively it often

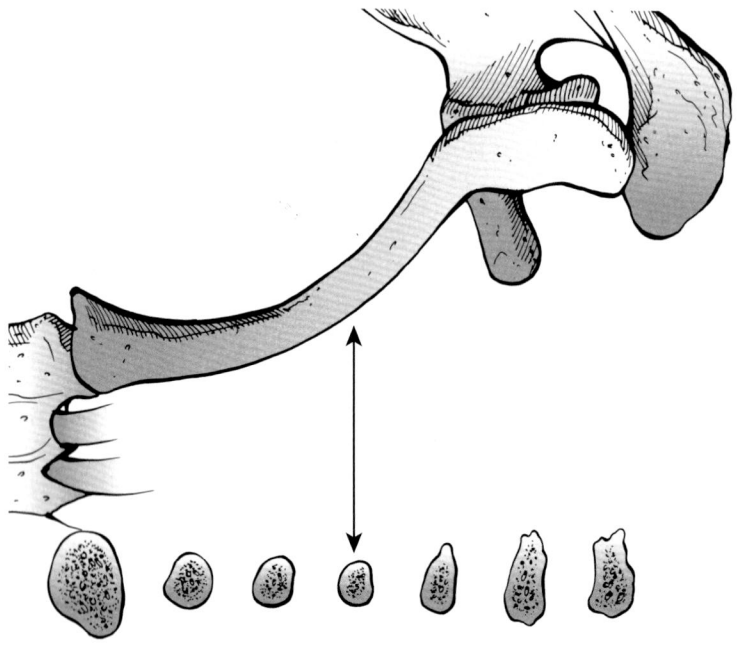

FIGURE 38-17 The cross-sectional and topographic anatomy of the clavicle. The clavicle is narrowest in its midportion, explaining the high incidence of fractures in this area.

is necessary to adjust or contour even "anatomic" plates for the clavicle to achieve an optimal fit.[70] The bone in the relatively thin diaphysis is typically hard cortical bone best suited for cortical screws, whereas the medial and lateral expansions are softer cancellous bone where larger pitch cancellous screws can be inserted without tapping.

Ligamentous Anatomy of the Clavicle

Medial

There is relatively little motion at the SC joint, and the supporting soft tissue structures are correspondingly thick. Medially the clavicle is secured to the sternum by the SC capsule, and although there are not easily demonstrable "ligaments," the thickening of the posterior capsule has been determined to be the single most important soft tissue constraint to anterior or posterior translation of the medial clavicle. There is also an interclavicular ligament which runs from the medial end of one clavicle, gains purchase from the superior aspect of the sternum at the sternal notch, and attaches to the medial end of the contralateral clavicle. Acting as a tension wire at the base of the clavicle, this ligament helps prevent inferior angulation or translation of the clavicle. In addition, there are extremely stout ligaments that originate on the first rib and insert on the undersurface or the inferior aspect of the clavicle.[19] A small fossa inferomedially, the rhomboid fossa, has been described as an attachment point for these ligaments, which primarily resist translation of the medial clavicle.

Lateral

The coracoclavicular ligaments are the trapezoid (more lateral) and conoid (more medial) which are stout ligaments that arise from the base of the coracoid and insert onto the small osseous ridge of the inferior clavicle (trapezoid) and the clavicular conoid tubercle (conoid). These ligaments are very strong and provide the primary resistance to superior displacement of the lateral clavicle. Their integrity, or lack thereof, plays an important role in the decision making and fixation selection in the treatment of displaced lateral third clavicle fractures. Clavicle fractures in this location will often have an avulsed inferior fragment to which these ligaments are attached, especially in younger individuals. Inclusion of these fragments in surgical fixation selection enhances the stability of the operative repair. The capsule of the AC joint is thickened superiorly and is primarily responsible for resisting AP displacement of the joint. It is important to repair this structure, which is usually reflected surgically as part of the deep myofascial layer, when operating on the lateral end of the clavicle. If one is inserting a hook plate for fixation of a very distal fracture, a small defect can be made in the posterolateral aspect of the capsule for insertion of the hook portion into the posterior subacromial space.[23,42,83,98,193]

Muscular Anatomy of the Clavicle

The clavicle is not as important as the scapula in terms of muscle origin, but still serves as the attachment site of several large muscles. Medially, the pectoralis major muscle originates from the clavicular shaft anteroinferiorly, and the sternocleidomastoid originates superiorly. The pectoralis origin merges with the origin of the anterior deltoid laterally, while the trapezius

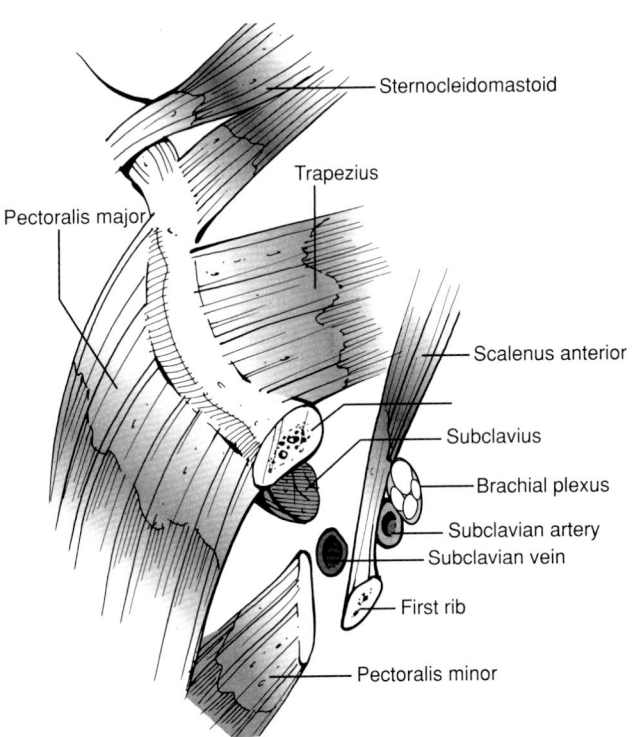

FIGURE 38-18 Applied anatomy of the clavicle. Anterosuperiorly, the pectoralis major muscle and fascia envelope the medial 60% of the clavicle while the lateral 40% is covered by the deltoid muscle and its fascia. Posterosuperiorly, the trapezius muscle attaches to the clavicle.

insertion blends superiorly with the deltoid origin at the lateral margin (Fig. 38-18). Muscle attachment plays a significant role in the deformity which results after fracture: The medial clavicular fragment is elevated by the unopposed pull of the sternocleidomastoid muscle, while the distal fragment is held inferiorly by the deltoid and medially by the pectoralis major. The undersurface of the clavicle is the insertion site of the subclavius muscle, which is of little significance functionally but serves as a soft tissue buffer in the subclavicular space superior to the brachial plexus and subclavian vessels. The platysma or "shaving muscle" is variable in terms of thickness and extent, but usually envelopes the anterior and superior aspects of the clavicle and runs in the subcutaneous tissues, extending superiorly to the mandible and the deeper facial muscles. It is divided during the surgical approach, and is typically included in the closure of the superficial, or skin/subcutaneous layer.

Neurovascular Anatomy of the Clavicle

The supraclavicular nerves originate from cervical roots C3 and C4 and exit from a common trunk behind the posterior border of the sternocleidomastoid muscle. There are typically three major branches (anterior, middle, and posterior) that cross the clavicle superficially from medial to lateral, and are at risk during surgical approaches. If they are divided, an area of numbness is typically felt inferior to the surgical incision, although this tends to improve with time. A more difficult problem can be the development of a painful neuroma in the scar which, although rare, can negatively affect an otherwise good surgical outcome. For this reason, some authorities recommend identification and protection of these nerves during operative repair.[75,76,174] More vital neurovascular structures lie inferior to the clavicle. The subclavian vein runs directly below the subclavius muscle and above the first rib, where it is readily accessible (for central venous access) and vulnerable (to inadvertent injury). More posteriorly lie the subclavian artery and the brachial plexus, separated from the vein and clavicle by the additional layer of the scalenus anterior muscle medially. The plexus is closest to the clavicle in its midportion, where the greatest care needs to be taken in not violating the subclavicular space with drills, screws, or instruments. A recent study by Sinha et al.[171] used reconstructed three-dimensional CT arteriograms of the head, neck, and shoulder to better define the relationship between these vascular structures and the clavicle. Their goal was to define "safe zones," in terms of distance and direction, for potential drill penetration during plate and screw fixation of the clavicle. They divided the clavicle into medial, middle, and distal thirds, and found that the subclavian vessels were closest at the medial end, with the vein directly apposed to the posterior cortex of the medial clavicle in some cases. In the middle third, the artery and vein were a mean of 17 and 13 mm from the clavicle, respectively, at an approximate angle of 60 degrees to the horizontal (i.e., the vessels were posterior-inferior to the clavicle, Figs. 38-19 and 38-20). Laterally, the distances were greater, with the artery and vein a mean of 63 and 76 mm, respectively form the clavicle. Using these findings, the authors made a number of recommendations regarding surgical technique: Extreme caution must be used when manipulating medial clavicular fracture fragments, and superior plating may be safer than anterior plating in this area. Also, they felt that anterior plating had less potential for vessel injury from drill or screw penetration, as compared to superior plating, in the more common middle third fractures. They felt the risk of iatrogenic vessel injury was

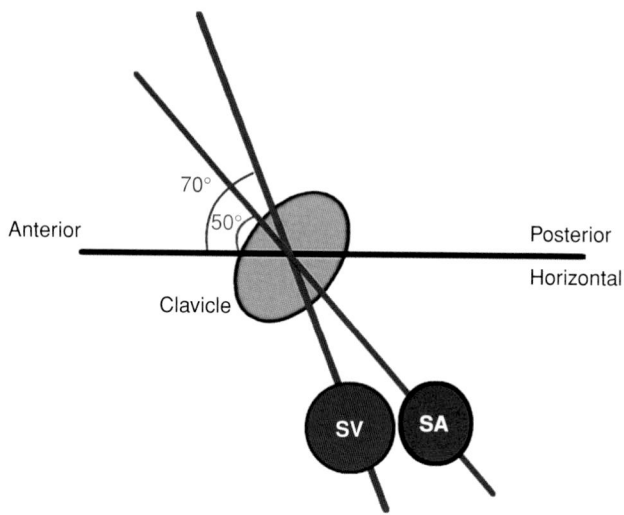

FIGURE 38-20 Schematic illustration indicating the location of the subclavian artery and vein in relation to the middle third of the clavicle, and the angle from the horizontal of potential drill/screw penetration to be avoided. (Adapted from Sinha A, Edwin J, Sreeharsha B, Bhalaik V, Brownson P. A radiological study to define safe zones for drilling during plating of clavical fractures. *J Bone Joint Surg Br.* 2001;93-B:1247–1252, with permission.)

much less in the fixation of distal third fractures. Despite the proximity of these vital structures, iatrogenic injury is surprisingly rare in clavicle fracture fixation (see below).

CLAVICLE FRACTURE TREATMENT OPTIONS

A recent review article focusing on evidence-based medicine outlined treatment approaches to displaced midshaft fractures of the clavicle.[104] This resource summarizes the available objective evidence about recommendations for the optimal treatment of these injuries (Table 38-2). The grades of recommendation are as follows.

Grade A: Good evidence (high-quality prospective, randomized clinical trials (RCTs) with consistent findings) recommending for or against intervention

Grade B: Fair evidence (lesser quality RCTs, prospective comparative studies, case-control series) recommending for or against intervention

Grade C: Poor-quality evidence (case series or expert opinions) recommending for or against intervention

Grade I: There is insufficient or conflicting evidence not allowing a recommendation for or against intervention

While there is an abundance of manuscripts detailing the treatment of clavicle fractures, most tend to be retrospective reviews, although there are an increasing number of prospective and/or randomized trials being published.[15,59,74,154] My personal recommendations for treatment must be considered in light of the evidence available in Tables 38-1 and 38-2.

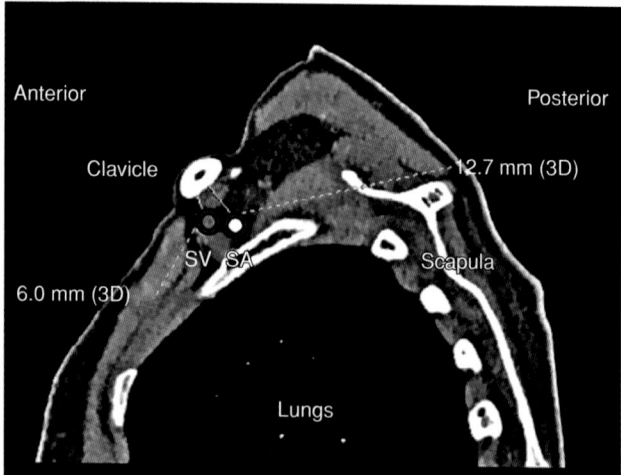

FIGURE 38-19 The relationship of the subclavian artery (SA) and vein (SV) to the midshaft of the clavicle. (Adapted from: Sinha A, Edwin J, Sreeharsha B, Bhalaik V, Brownson P. A radiological study to define safe zones for drilling during plating of clavical fractures. *J Bone Joint Surg Br.* 2001;93-B:1247–1252, with permission.)

TABLE 38-2	Recommendations for the Optimal Treatment of Displaced Midshaft Fractures of the Clavicle		
Statement		**Grade**[a]	**References**
Young active patients with completely displaced midshaft fractures of the clavicle will have superior results with primary fracture fixation.		B	15,174,209
Anteroinferior plating may reduce the risk of symptomatic hardware compared to superior plating.		C	27,91
There is no difference in outcome between a regular sling and a figure-of-eight bandage when nonoperative treatment is selected.		B	3,178
There is no difference in outcome between plating and intramedullary nailing of displaced midshaft clavicle fractures.		I	7,26,63,73, 140,209
Factors associated with poor outcome following nonoperative treatment of displaced midshaft clavicle fractures include shortening, and increasing fracture comminution.		A	14,59,102,125, 154,174,209

[a]Grade of recommendation.

Nonoperative Treatment of Clavicle Fractures

The earliest reported attempt at closed reduction of a displaced midshaft fracture of the clavicle was recorded in the "Edwin Smith" papyrus dating from the 30th century BC. Hippocrates described the typical deformity resulting from this injury, and emphasized the importance of trying to correct it.[1] It is usually possible to obtain an improvement in position of the fracture fragments by placing the patient supine, with a roll or sandbag behind the shoulder blades to let the anterior displacement and rotation of the distal fragment correct with gravity, followed by superior translation and support of the affected arm. Unfortunately, it is difficult or impossible to maintain the reduction achieved. For this reason, over the millennia that followed the first description of treatment of this fracture, there have been hundreds of descriptions of different devices designed to maintain the reduction, including splints, body jackets, casts, braces, slings, swathes, and wraps.[1,3,16,31,59,97] At the present time, there is no convincing evidence that any of these devices reliably maintains the fracture reduction or improves clinical, radiographic, or functional outcomes. For many years the standard of care in North America was the "figure-of-eight" bandage: Andersen et al.[3] examined its utility in a prospective, randomized, controlled clinical trial comparing it to a simple sling in 60

patients. They could demonstrate no functional or radiographic difference between the two groups, and in general the patients preferred the sling (2/27 dissatisfied with the sling compared to 9/34 dissatisfied with the figure-of-eight bandage, $p = 0.09$). In a retrospective review of 140 patients treated nonoperatively, Stanley and Norris did not find any difference between a standard sling and a figure-of-eight bandage, a finding confirmed by other authors.[138,139,178] Also, a figure-of-eight bandage that is over-tightened can result in a temporary lower trunk brachial plexus palsy and for this reason my practice, if nonoperative care is selected, is to apply a simple, conventional sling with a padded neckpiece, and no attempt at reduction is made.

Outcomes—Nonoperative Treatment

Traditionally, clavicle fractures have been treated nonoperatively but recent studies have shown that the union rate for displaced midshaft fractures of the clavicle may not be as favorable as previously described. In a prospective series of 868 patients with clavicle fractures treated nonoperatively, Robinson et al.[154] reported a significantly higher nonunion rate (21%) in displaced comminuted midshaft fractures. An analysis of this paper by Brinker et al.[14] suggested a nonunion rate varying between 20% and 33% for displaced comminuted fractures in males. Hill et al.[68] studied 66 consecutive displaced midshaft clavicle fractures and found a 15% nonunion rate and a 31% rate of patient dissatisfaction with nonoperative care. Based on their data, they concluded that displacement of the fracture fragments of greater than 2 cm was associated with an unsatisfactory result. A meta-analysis of studies of clavicle fractures from 1975 to 2005 revealed that displaced midshaft clavicle fractures treated nonoperatively had a nonunion rate of 15.1%. This meta-analysis also showed that primary plate fixation was, contrary to prevailing opinion, a safe and reliable procedure.[209] Nowak et al.[125,126] examined the late sequelae in 208 adult patients with clavicle fractures at 10 years post injury. Interestingly, 96 (46%) still had symptoms despite the fact that only 15 (7%) had an established nonunion. McKee et al.[99] reported on a series of patients who has nonoperative treatment of a displaced midshaft clavicle fracture a mean of over 4 years earlier. Objective muscle strength testing revealed significant strength deficits, especially of shoulder abduction and flexion which help explain some of the patient dissatisfaction seen despite bony union.

While it is unclear why such a dramatic difference exists in outcome between previous reports on clavicle fractures and contemporary studies, one possibility may be the inclusion of children in the older reports, which, due their inherent healing abilities and remodeling potential, may artificially improve the overall results. Also, patient-oriented outcome measures, as used by Hill et al. and McKee et al. have been shown to reveal functional deficits in the upper extremity that have not been detected traditionally.[15,68,99] A focus on radiographic outcomes would not reveal such problems. Patient expectations and injury patterns are changing. Several studies that examined clavicular shaft fractures in polytrauma patients found that the presence of a clavicle fracture was associated with a 20% to 30% mortality rate (mainly from concomitant chest and head injuries), and that survivors displayed a significant level of residual disability in the involved

TABLE 38-3	Cosmesis Following Operative Versus Nonoperative Care of Clavicular Fractures		
Complaint	Operative (*n* = 62)	Nonoperative (*n* = 49)	*p* Value
"Droopy" shoulder	0	10	**0.001**
Bump/Asymmetry	0	22	**0.001**
Scar	3	0	0.253
Sensitive/painful fracture site	9	10	0.891
Hardware irritation/ prominence	11	0	**0.001**
Incisional numb- ness	18	0	**0.001**
Satisfied with appearance of shoulder	52	26	**0.001**

shoulder.[101,184] Thus, there is a surviving patient population (with clavicle fractures) that has an intrinsically worse prognosis where long-term sequelae may be more common.

Although it is not typically an orthopedic priority, cosmesis is important to patients, and an unsightly scar has been a traditional deterrent to operative treatment of clavicular fractures.[29,30,32,115,118,128,142] However, to a body image conscious patient (predominantly young, male population), a droopy shoulder is also of significant cosmetic concern. In a recent RCT comparing operative and nonoperative treatments, despite the incidence of hardware prominence and incisional complications (numbness, sensitivity) in the operative group, more patients in this group answered "yes" to the question "Are you satisfied with the appearance of your shoulder?" than in the nonoperative group (52/62 vs. 26/49, *p* = 0.001, Table 38-3). This study also showed superior surgeon-based (Constant score) and patient-based (DASH) upper extremity outcomes.[15]

In contradistinction to older case series, recent studies on the primary plate fixation of acute midshaft clavicle fractures have reported high success rates with union rates ranging from 94% to 100% and low rates of infection and surgical complications. A recent meta-analysis of plate fixation for 460 displaced fractures revealed a nonunion rate of only 2.2%. With improved implants, prophylactic antibiotics, and better soft tissue handling one can conclude that plate fixation is reliable and reproducible.[15,82,140,141,209]

Operative Treatment of Clavicle Fractures
Indications/Contraindications

There are numerous large series that describe relatively good results following nonoperative treatment of clavicle fractures, and it is my opinion that the majority of clavicle fractures can, and should, be treated in this fashion.[3,43,49,78,115,160] However, there are serious deficiencies in these papers including the inclusion of children (who have an intrinsically good result and

remodeling potential), large numbers of patients lost to follow-up, and radiographic and/or surgeon-based outcomes that are insensitive to residual deficits. Recent evidence from prospective and randomized clinical trials has suggested that there is a subset of individuals who benefit from primary operative care (Fig. 38-21).[15,59,74,105,140,154,169,173,192,201] Operative repair in this setting should be reserved for medically well, physically active patients who stand to benefit the most from a rapid restoration of normal anatomy and stable fixation. There are multiple potential indications for primary operative fixation, outlined in Table 38-4. The majority of modern prospective studies examining the potential benefits of primary clavicle fracture fixation have been in adult patients, with 16 years of age the typical (arbitrary) lowest age of inclusion. Thus, it is unclear if adolescent patients, in general, would benefit from operative repair to a similar degree as adult patients. However, adolescent patients can develop symptomatic malunion following nonoperative treatment of displaced midshaft fractures of the clavicle, although nonunion remains rare as one would expect. Vander Have et al.[189] performed a retrospective study on 43 adolescent patients (mean age: 15.4 years) with displaced midshaft clavicle fractures, 17 of whom underwent primary plate fixation, and 25 of whom were treated nonoperatively. They found that complications in the plate group were minor, and a more rapid return to function with a shorter time to union resulted. Five patients in the nonoperative group, with a mean of 26 mm of shortening, developed a symptomatic malunion, with four patients choosing corrective osteotomy. It is clear that some adolescent patients with significantly displaced midshaft clavicle fractures have suboptimal results following closed

TABLE 38-4	Relative Indications for Primary Fixation of Midshaft Clavicle Fractures

Fracture-Specific
1. Displacement >2 cm
2. Shortening >2 cm
3. Increasing comminution (>3 fragments)
4. Segmental fractures
5. Open fractures
6. Impending open fractures with soft tissue compromise
7. Obvious clinical deformity (usually associated with 1 and 2 above)
8. Scapular malposition and winging on initial examination

Associated Injuries
1. Vascular injury requiring repair
2. Progressive neurologic deficit
3. Ipsilateral upper extremity injuries/fractures
4. Multiple ipsilateral upper rib fractures
5. "Floating shoulder"
6. Bilateral clavicle fractures

Patient Factors
1. Polytrauma with requirement for early upper extremity weight-bearing/arm use
2. Patient motivation for rapid return of function (e.g., elite sports or the self-employed professional)

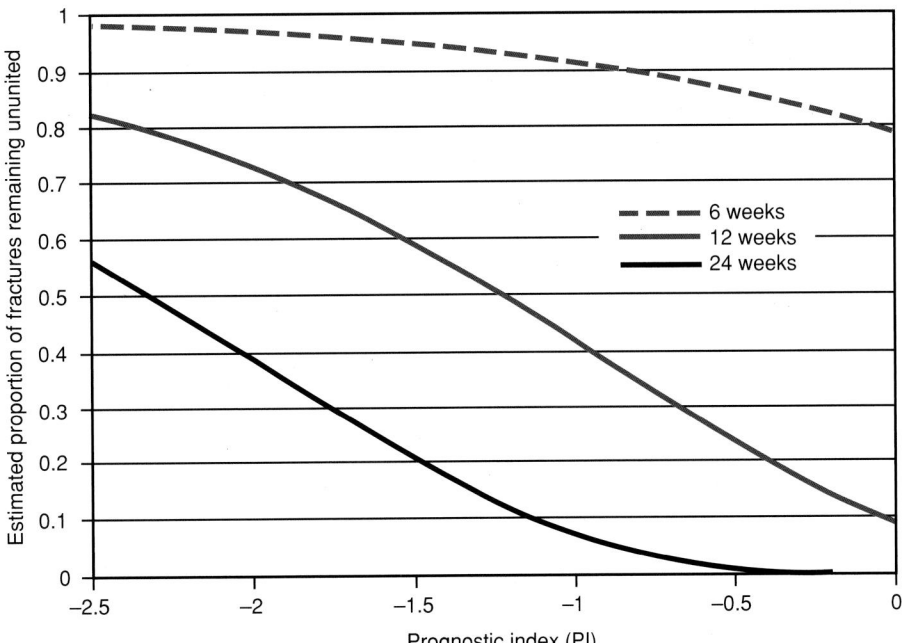

FIGURE 38-21 Probability of nonunion at various time points following a midshaft clavicle fracture. The PI (Prognostic index) becomes more negative with each of the following factors: Increasing age, increasing comminution, increasing displacement, and female sex. (Adapted from Robinson CM, Court-Brown CM, McQueen MM, et al. Estimating the risk of nonunion following nonoperative treatment of a clavicle fracture. *J Bone Joint Surg Am.* 2004;86-A(7):1359–1365.)

treatment, and that plate fixation is a safe and reliable fixation method with a low complication rate in this group. Prospective, randomized studies of operative versus nonoperative treatment in this specific group are required to determine the exact role, if any, for primary operative repair of these fractures. At present, the consensus is that operative intervention should be reserved for older, larger adolescents with severely displaced fractures.[17]

External Fixation

There are reports in the literature of various techniques of external fixation for clavicle fractures.[35,165,186] This method takes advantage of the intrinsic healing ability of the clavicle and allows restoration of length and translation without the scarring or morbidity of a surgical approach. In addition, there is no retained hardware at the conclusion of treatment. Schuind[165] reported on a series of 20 patients treated with external fixation for clavicular injuries, many of whom had local soft tissue compromise; union occurred in all. Tomic et al.[186] described the treatment of 12 patients with nonunion of the clavicular shaft by application of a modified Ilizarov device. Union was achieved in 11 of 12 patients with an increase in the mean Constant score from 30 preoperatively to 69 postoperatively. It is clear that this technique is technically possible to perform, and may be useful in certain specific situations. Unfortunately, the practical difficulties associated with the position and prominence of the fixation pins, coupled with a lack of patient acceptance in the North American population, has resulted in minimal use of this technique (Table 38-5).

Intramedullary Pinning

Preoperative Planning. Intramedullary (IM) pinning of fractures of the shaft of the clavicle has several advantages. These are similar to the benefits seen with IM fixation of long bone fractures in other areas, although this technique had not been as consistently successful in the clavicle as series in the femur or tibia have reported.[8,30,48,51,63,73,106] Advantages include a smaller, more cosmetic skin incision, less soft tissue stripping at the fracture site, decreased hardware prominence following fixation, technically straightforward hardware removal, and a possibly lower incidence of refracture or fracture at the end of the implant. Recently, modifications to the technique have included a radiographically guided completely "closed" technique.[26] Since, at the present time, there is no consistently reliable way to "lock" an IM clavicle pin, complications include those common to all unlocked IM devices, namely failure to control axial length and rotation, especially with increasing fracture comminution and decreasing intrinsic fracture stability. In addition, a biomechanical study of clavicular osteotomies by Golish et al.[57] comparing 3.5-mm compression plates to 3.8- or 4.5-mm IM pins showed that the plated constructs were superior in resisting displacement in a number of different testing modes (maximal load, cyclical

TABLE 38-5	**External Fixation of Clavicle Fractures: Preoperative Planning Checklist**
OR table	Radiolucent table
Position	Semisitting with small pad between scapulae
Fluoroscopy location	C-arm is placed ipsilateral and enters from the side
Equipment	External or ring fixator of surgeon's choice
Special considerations	This is a complex technique requiring a subspecialty skill level and is not well tolerated by some patients

TABLE 38-6	Intramedullary Fixation of Clavicle Fractures: Preoperative Planning Checklist
OR table	Radiolucent table
Position	Semisitting with small pad between scapulae
Fluoroscopy location	C-arm is placed ipsilateral, and enters from the side
Equipment	Intramedullary pins, reamers, inserters, and any attachment guides or jigs
Special considerations	At present, this technique is reserved for simple fractures such as transverse or short oblique patterns without significant comminution

stress) compared to both IM pin constructs. Therefore, based on clinical and biomechanical evidence, at the present time this technique is, in general, reserved for simple fracture patterns (transverse and short oblique fractures) (Table 38-6).

Patient Positioning. The technique includes positioning the patient in a semisitting position on a radiolucent table, with an image intensifier on the ipsilateral side. By rotating the image 45 degrees caudal and 45 degrees cephalad orthogonal views of the clavicle can be obtained. A small pad is placed between the scapulae to allow the shoulder to "fall back," aiding in reduction, as the typical clavicle fracture deformity results in protraction of the shoulder girdle. The arm may be free-draped if a difficult reduction is anticipated (i.e., as with significant shortening), but in general this is not necessary. The head is turned to the opposite side and taped in place.

Surgical Approach/Technique. A small incision is then made over the posterior-lateral corner of the clavicle 2 to 3 cm medial to the AC joint (Fig. 38-22). The posterior clavicle at this point is identified and the canal breached with a drill consistent with the planned fixation device. A reduction of the fracture is then performed, either through a small open incision or, as experience increases, in a completely closed fashion using a percutaneous reduction clamp on the medial fragment and a "joystick" in the distal fragment. Alternatively, the fixation device can be inserted using a "retrograde" technique where it is passed out from the fracture site through the lateral fragment. The fracture is then reduced and the IM device is inserted into the medial fragment under direct vision. It is important to accurately reduce length and rotation, although the latter can be quite difficult if done closed and no visual clues from the fracture configuration are available. A small incision may be necessary to reduce vertically oriented comminuted fragments and "tease" then back into alignment. Following this, the canal is drilled to the appropriate size to accept the planned IM device. Options include headed pins, partially threaded pins or screws, cannulated screws, and smooth wires. Although some series report favorable results with smooth wires, the North American experience with small diameter smooth pin fixation includes breakage and migration and is, in general, dismal.[87,93,109,120] Smooth wires are contraindicated for fracture fixation about the shoulder in general and the clavicle in particular. It is important not to distract the fracture site with the fixation device, which can occur as the pin is inserted into the unyielding opposite cortex as the S-shaped clavicle comes into contact with the end of the straight pin. If this occurs, the pin must be withdrawn slightly or a shorter pin is used. The head of the pin or screw can be left prominent to facilitate early removal through a small posterior incision, or can be left flush with the bone to decrease soft tissue irritation (Fig. 38-23).

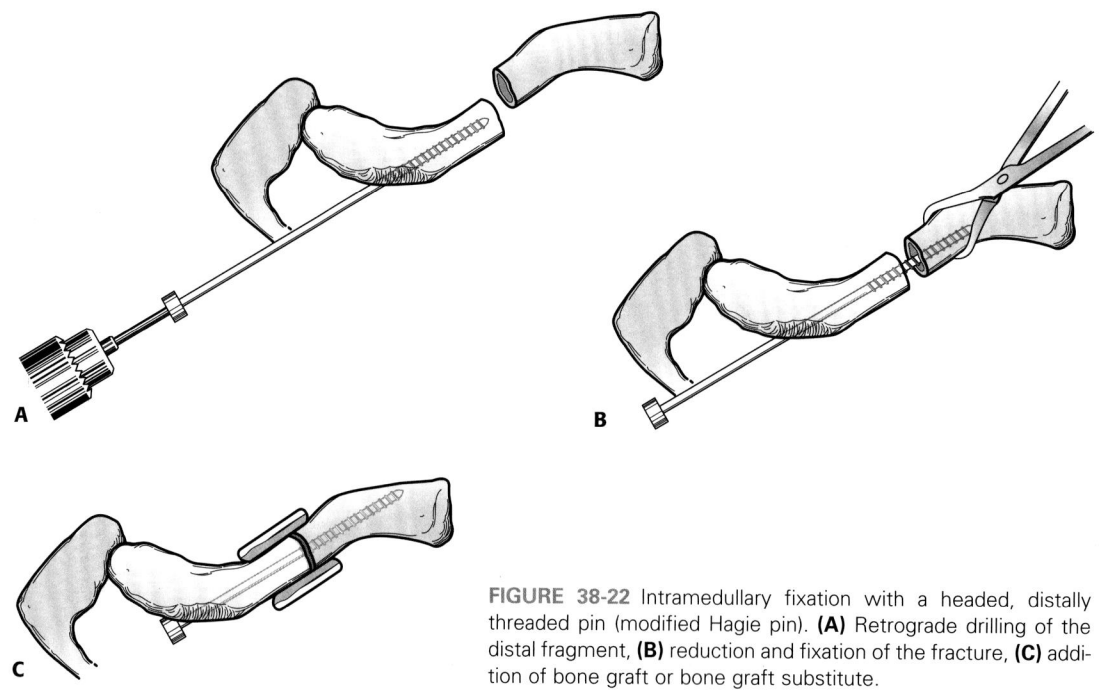

FIGURE 38-22 Intramedullary fixation with a headed, distally threaded pin (modified Hagie pin). **(A)** Retrograde drilling of the distal fragment, **(B)** reduction and fixation of the fracture, **(C)** addition of bone graft or bone graft substitute.

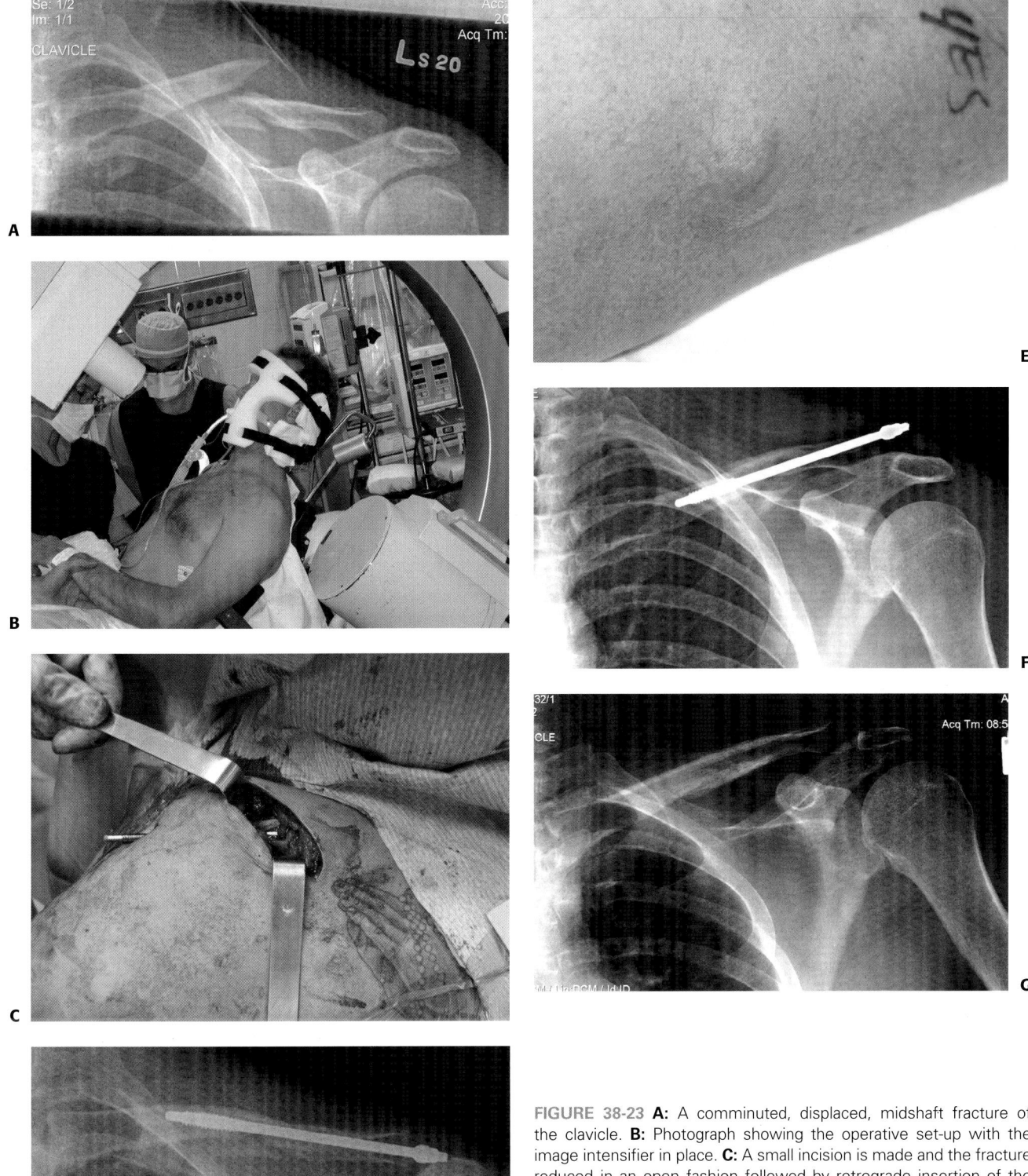

FIGURE 38-23 A: A comminuted, displaced, midshaft fracture of the clavicle. **B:** Photograph showing the operative set-up with the image intensifier in place. **C:** A small incision is made and the fracture reduced in an open fashion followed by retrograde insertion of the pin. **D:** Postoperative radiograph revealing reduction of the fracture. **E:** Skin irritation over prominent pin. **F:** Radiograph demonstrating bony union. **G:** Follow-up radiograph following uneventful union and pin removal. (Case courtesy of, and copyright by, Dr. David Ring).

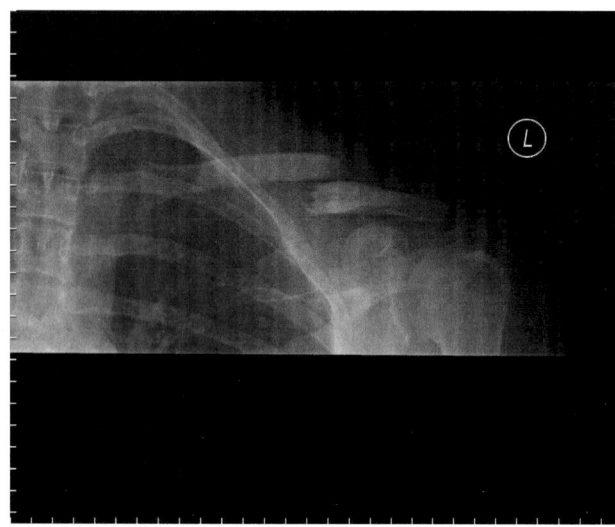
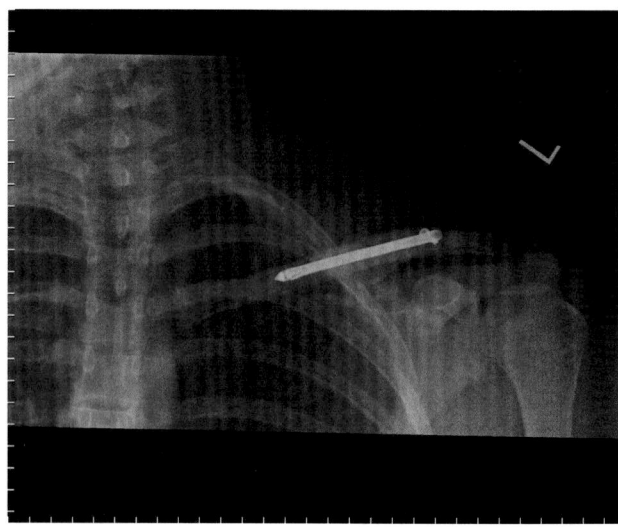

FIGURE 38-24 A: A completely displaced transverse fracture of the midshaft of the clavicle treated with a lockable, large diameter intramedullary nail. **B:** While this device represents an advance in the treatment of these injuries, more outcome data is required prior to implementation in unstable fracture patterns. (Case courtesy of Dr. Aaron Nauth).

Postoperative Protocol. Some authors advocate leaving the pin in a prominent position subcutaneously for easy access in the clinic at the time of early (7 to 8 weeks postoperative) hardware removal. This step depends on the type of fixation device used and the philosophy of the treating surgeon. The incisions are closed in a fashion similar to that used for plate fixation, although they are typically smaller. If the surgeon is confident with the stability of the repair, early motion is instituted similar to that performed following plate fixation.

Potential Pitfalls and Preventative Measures

Outcome. While there are many theoretical advantages to IM fixation, it would appear that the results of this method with currently available implants are more unpredictable than the results reported for plate fixation. Biomechanically, IM devices appear to be inferior in resisting displacement when compared to plate fixation.[60] Two clinical studies comparing IM fixation to nonoperative treatment failed to show any advantage in the IM fixation group. Grassi et al. described a high complication rate with IM fixation including eight infections, three "refractures," two delayed unions and two nonunions with hardware failure in 40 patients.[63] Judd et al.,[74] in a randomized trial, failed to show an advantage of IM fixation over nonoperative care in 57 patients, with nearly half the operative group losing some degree of reduction. A recent study by Strauss et al.[180] described a complication rate of 50%, (including three cases of skin necrosis) in 16 patients treated with Hagie pin fixation. They recommended against the continued use of this device. A meta-analysis by Zlowodzki et al.[209] did not reveal any significant differences between plate and IM fixation, although this analysis was hampered by the lack of any direct comparative studies. Conversely, Chuang et al.[26] described 100% union with no significant complications in a group of 34 patients with an acute midshaft fractures of the clavicle treated with an IM cannulated screw. Also, these studies examine the clinical outcomes

of implants that, in general, are essentially unlocked, have poor rotational or axial control, and are not suitable for unstable or comminuted fractures. Newer devices are now available that have the potential to improve on traditional IM implants with locking capability (Fig. 38-24): Further studies will elucidate if their theoretical advantages are borne out in clinical practice. See also "Controversies: Method of Fixation," below.

Open Reduction and Plate Fixation

Preoperative Planning. While this section will describe the author's technique of operative repair of a midshaft clavicle fracture, it is important to remember that the majority of midshaft fractures can be treated nonoperatively. A careful physical examination (see above) is mandatory to rule out other injuries, which may influence the anesthetic choice (i.e., an ipsilateral pneumothorax), or the surgery itself (compromised skin or deficient soft tissue, neurovascular injury). The skin in this area is typically bruised, with extensive swelling, following a displaced midshaft fracture. Since the difficulty of reduction and fixation does not increase until approximately 2 weeks following injury, it may be prudent to delay operative intervention (as one would in other areas) until the soft tissue in the vicinity of the planned surgical approach is more robust. Radiographs of the injured clavicle are usually sufficient. The surgeon should observe the severity of the displacement, the number of fracture fragments, and the location of the main fracture line (Fig. 38-25). There is often a vertically oriented anterosuperior fragment, which may benefit from lag screw fixation and minifragment screws should be available as this fragment may be quite narrow. Also, the number of screws that potentially can be placed into the distal fragment can be determined preoperatively, so that the appropriate size of plate can be available. Older series describing fixation of clavicle fractures have described poor results when inadequate fixation such as

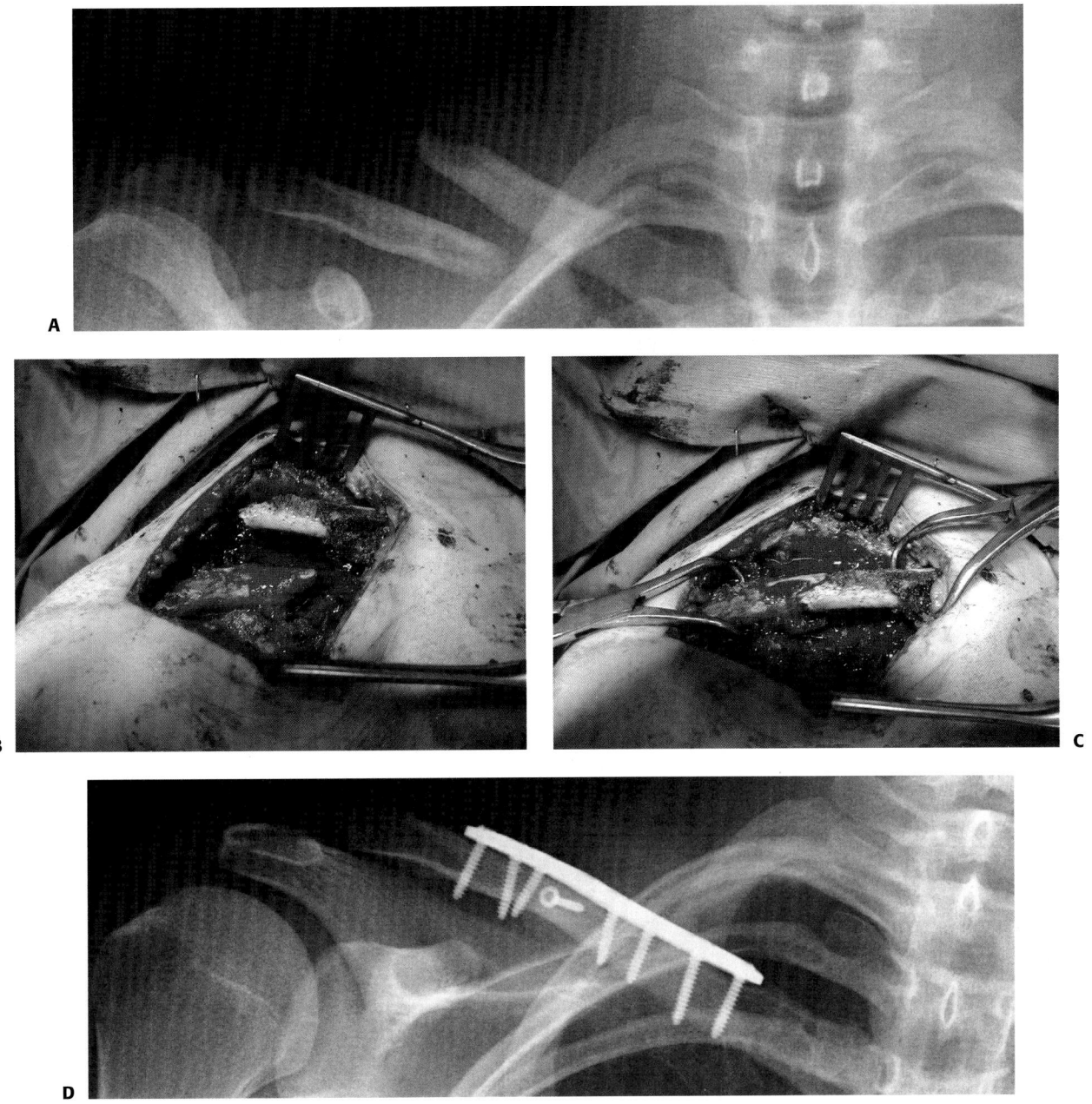

FIGURE 38-25 **A:** Anteroposterior radiograph of a displaced midshaft clavicle fracture. Note the difference in diameter of the proximal and distal fragments at the fracture site, suggesting that a significant degree of rotation has occurred. **B:** Intraoperative photograph of a displaced fracture, **(C)** reduced anatomically with small fragment reduction forceps. **D:** Postoperative radiograph after open reduction and internal fixation with an anterior to posterior lag screw followed by fixation with an anatomic plate.

cerclage wires alone or plates of inadequate size or length are used (Figs. 38-26 and 38-27).[114,115,142,160] A fixation set that includes plates which are precontoured, or "anatomic," to fit the S shape of the clavicle is ideal. Although these plates may require some intraoperative adjustments, they typically save significant time associated with the extensive contouring required to make a straight plate fit the bone. They help to decrease the soft tissue irritation that occurs when the end of a straight plate protrudes past the end of the bone as the clavicle curves away.

Currently, there are two common surgical approaches applicable to the fixation of clavicle fractures, each with its own advantages and disadvantages. They are as follows.

Anteroinferior. Several groups have published large series on the advantages of anteroinferior plating of acute clavicle fractures.[27,82,170] Advantages of this technique include an easier screw trajectory with less likelihood of serious neurovascular injury with inadvertent overpenetration of the drill (although

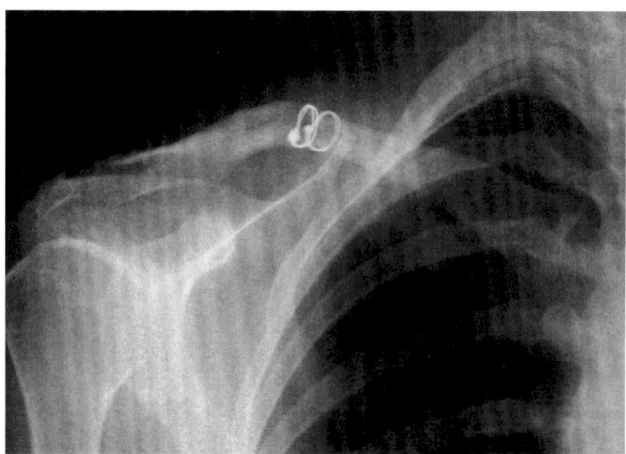

FIGURE 38-26 Cerclage wiring in isolation is inadequate to control the deforming forces at the site of a displaced clavicle fracture. It results in all of the risks of surgical intervention with few of the benefits, and is to be avoided.

the incidence of iatrogenic nerve injury is very low), and the ability to insert longer screws in the wider AP dimension of the clavicle, and decreased hardware prominence. It is also technically easier to contour a small-fragment compression plate along the anterior border as opposed to the superior surface. However, the advent of precontoured plates has largely negated this particular advantage. Collinge et al.[27] reported on the use of this technique in 58 patients and described 1 fixation failure, 1 nonunion, 3 infections, and only 2 hardware removals. Potential disadvantages of this technique include the lack of general familiarity with the approach, and that the plate tends to

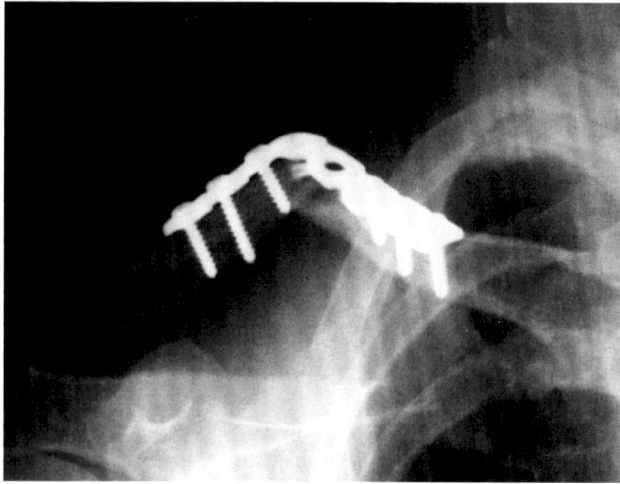

FIGURE 38-27 Anteroposterior radiograph of a 35-year-old man who weighed over 200 pounds (200 lb), whose clavicle nonunion was fixed with a 3.5-mm pelvic reconstruction plate. Early mechanical failure occurred through deformation of the plate. This type of plate may be suitable for smaller, low-demand individuals but has a higher failure rate when used in larger, more physically active patients, especially given the current availability of stronger, precontoured plates.

obscure the fracture site radiographically. Also, although there remains some controversy on the matter, biomechanical studies have in general shown that the most advantageous position for plate placement is the superior surface.

Anterosuperior. Anterosuperior plating can reasonably be considered the most popular operative method for fixation of the clavicle.[11,12,15,26,33] Its advantages include a general familiarity with this approach in most surgeons' hands, the ability to extend it simply to both the medial and lateral ends of the clavicle, and the benefit of clear radiographic views of the clavicle postoperatively. Its disadvantages include the trajectory of screw placement (from superior to inferior) that can be difficult, and inadvertent "plunging" with the drill can place the underlying lung and neurovascular structures at risk. Also, the clavicle is fairly narrow in its superoinferior dimension, and typically the length of screws inserted range from 14 to 16 mm in females to 16 to 18 mm in males (Table 38-7).

Patient Positioning. The patient is positioned in the "beach-chair" semisitting position on a regular operating room (OR) table with an attached foot piece to support the legs. It has not been routinely necessary to use special tables or positioners. The head is placed on a round support and, if general anesthesia is to be used, the endotracheal tube is taped to the opposite side. The arm does not need to be free-draped for isolated injuries and is usually padded and strapped to the patients' side. It is helpful to place a small pad behind the involved shoulder to elevate it and then check to ensure that the anticipated superior drill trajectory is free from obstruction. This is less of a concern if an anterior-inferior plate application is chosen.

Surgical Approach (Anterosuperior). A superior approach and plating is my preferred technique because of its simplicity, the well-proven clinical record of superior plate application, and several biomechanical studies that have suggested that the optimal location for plate placement is superior.[60,72]

TABLE 38-7	Open Reduction and Plate Fixation of Clavicle Fractures: Preoperative Planning Checklist
OR table	A regular or radiolucent table may be used at the surgeon's discretion
Position	Semisitting with small pad between scapulae—this aids in reduction of the fracture
Fluoroscopy location	Fluoroscopy is not mandatory, and is used at the discretion of the surgeon if a difficult reduction is anticipated. If used, the C-arm is place ipsilaterally, and enters from the side
Equipment	Precontoured plates, small fragment fixation set, drill
Special considerations	Most fractures are amenable to plate fixation, and this procedure is within the skill set of most orthopedic surgeons

It is possible that anterior–inferior plating leads to less plate irritation than placement of the plate on the superior surface of the clavicle. In the one direct comparison (nonrandomized) between the two techniques, Lim et al.[91] reported a significantly better pain visual analog scale for patients in the anterior/inferior fixation group ($p = 0.05$). This finding awaits confirmation from further studies.

An oblique skin incision is made centered superiorly over the fracture site. The subcutaneous tissue and platysma muscle are kept together as one layer and extensively mobilized, especially proximally and distally. As experience with the technique increases, a smaller incision using "minimally invasive" principles can be employed. Care is taken to identify, isolate, and protect any visible, larger branches of the supraclavicular nerves; smaller ones may need to be divided. It is usually wise to warn patients that they may experience some numbness inferior to the incision which will typically improve with time. The myofascial layer over the clavicle is incised and elevated in one continuous layer. Therefore, at the conclusion of the procedure, fracture site and plate coverage are enhanced by having two soft tissue layers (skin/subcutaneous tissue, myofascial layer) to close. Care is taken to preserve the soft tissue attachments to any major fragments, especially the vertically oriented fragment of the anterosuperior clavicle that is often seen. It is not necessary to completely denude these fragments in order to reduce them.

Technique. The main fracture line and major fragments are clearly identified and cleaned of debris and hematoma, and a fixation strategy is formulated. If there is a free fragment of sufficient size to be structurally important (one-third of the clavicle circumference or greater), it can be reduced to the proximal or distal clavicle that it arose from and fixed with a lag screw, simplifying the fracture to a simple pattern (Fig. 38-28). The proximal and distal fragments are then reduced with the aid of reduction forceps; they can be held temporarily with a K-wire or, ideally, with a lag screw. A precontoured plate of sufficient length is then applied to the superior surface. If a lag screw has been placed, it is usually sufficient to secure the fracture with three bicortical screws (six cortices) both proxi-

mally and distally. If it is not possible to place a lag screw, then four screws should be inserted both proximally and distally. If the main fracture line is of a stable configuration, compression holes can be used to apply compression. If the fracture is comminuted or of an unstable pattern, then the plate should be applied in a "neutral" mode. Care must be taken not to violate the subclavicular space and the vital structures therein. If there is any concern intraoperatively about violation of the pleural space, a Valsalva maneuver should be performed to identify any leakage of air.

In general, surgical intervention is selected for only young active patients with high-quality bone, and for this reason screw purchase is usually excellent, especially in the cortical area. Although there has been increasing interest in the use of locking plate technology in this area, there have been few reports on this technique in the clavicle. Celestre et al.[20] reported that a superiorly placed locking plate was biomechanically superior to a conventional compression plate, although there is little clinical information regarding locking plate use at the present time. One small retrospective series[78] described their use in recalcitrant clavicular nonunions: All 11 fractures eventually healed. I have not found that locking plates are routinely necessary for the fixation of clavicle fractures, and I have no experience with them. Following fixation, it is important to close both soft tissue layers with interrupted, nonabsorbable sutures. Postoperative radiographs are taken in the recovery room.

Postoperative Care. The surgery can typically be done on an outpatient basis. Postoperatively, the arm is placed in a standard sling for comfort and gentle pendulum exercises are allowed, and the patient is seen in the fracture clinic at 10 to 14 days postoperatively. The wound is checked and radiographs are taken. The sling is discontinued, and unrestricted range-of-motion exercises are allowed, but no strengthening, resisted exercises, or sporting activities are allowed. At 6 weeks postoperatively, radiographs are taken to ensure bony union. If they are acceptable, the patient is allowed to begin resisted and strengthening activities. If delayed union is evident, then more aggressive activities are avoided. It is generally advised

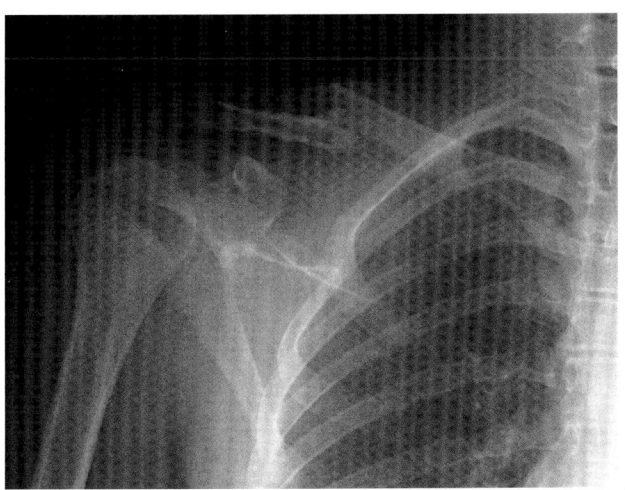

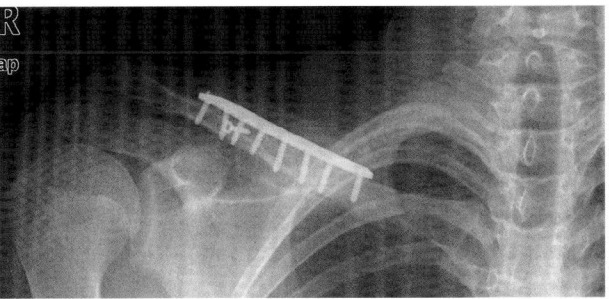

FIGURE 38-28 A: A displaced midshaft fracture of the clavicle in a 16-year-old boy, with abrasion and tenting of the skin, approximately 2.5-cm shortening, and an obvious clinical deformity. **B:** The intervening fragments were fixed with a lag screw followed by plate fixation. Prompt anatomic healing occurred, as might be expected in an adolescent.

that contact (football, hockey) and/or unpredictable (mountain biking, snowboarding) sports be avoided for 12 weeks postoperatively. However, compliance in this predominately young, male population is variable and many individuals return to such activities earlier than recommended.

The clavicle has relatively poor soft tissue coverage, and hardware prominence following plate fixation is a clinical concern. Previously, prior to the advent of plates specifically designed for the clavicle, it was often necessary to contour a straight compression plate to fit the bone by twisting it on its long axis so that it faced the bone as the underlying clavicle curved away from it.[100,108] In addition to making screw placement difficult, this led to undue prominence of the ends of the plate and a high incidence of subsequent plate removal. With the current availability of stronger, curved, low-profile plates symptomatic prominence of the plates is much lower and routine plate removal is not typically required.

Outcome—Plate Fixation. Older reports described a high rate of complications and hardware failure with primary plate fixation of the clavicle. However, with the development of improved implants, prophylactic antibiotics, and better soft tissue handling and techniques plate fixation has become a reliable and reproducible technique which can reasonably be considered the gold standard at the present time (see also "Controversies: Method of Fixation," below). Recent studies on the primary plate fixation of acute midshaft clavicle fractures have reported high success rates with union from 94% to 100%. Infection and surgical complication rates are low, under 10%, and functional outcome is superior to nonoperative treatment. A meta-analysis of plate fixation for 460 displaced fractures revealed a nonunion rate of only 2.2%.[14–16] In the most recently published randomized trial comparing operative versus nonoperative treatment, Virtanen et al.[192] reported union of all 28 fractures in the plate fixation group, with a low complication rate. In the largest similar trial reported to date, the union rate in the plate fixation group was reported to be over 95%, with the commonest complication being hardware irritation and the requirement for plate removal. While plating remains the most popular method of clavicle fixation, the position of plate placement is controversial, with some authorities recommending plate placement on the superior surface of the clavicle, while others recommend the anterior/inferior surface.[10,15,27,31,82,208] At the present time, there is no published direct comparison between the two techniques. What is apparent is that plate fixation, for a selected subgroup of individuals with completely displaced fractures of the midshaft clavicle, is a safe, reproducible, and reliable technique with a union rate of 95% and a low complication rate.

Potential Pitfalls and Preventative Measures— Operative Treatment

- Patient selection is critical: Operative intervention is reserved for young, healthy, physically active patients with good bone quality and completely displaced fractures (typically with visible deformity) who stand to benefit most from operative fixation with an intrinsically low complication rate (Fig. 38-29).

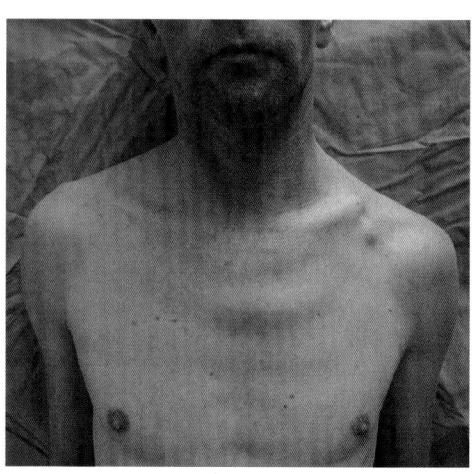

FIGURE 38-29 The typical clinical deformity following a displaced left midshaft clavicular fracture with a short, droopy, "ptotic" shoulder with anterior translation and rotation of the distal fragment and limb.

- Noncompliance and substance abuse (be it alcohol, illicit drugs, or prescription narcotics) are contraindications to surgical intervention. No clavicular fixation is strong enough to withstand an unprotected fall down stairs or a physical altercation in the immediate postoperative period.[49,140,141] The rates of hardware failure, nonunion, and reoperation are significantly higher in such individuals.

- It is critical to develop, protect, and securely close the two soft tissue layers. The superficial layer is the skin and subcutaneous tissue and the deep layer is the deltotrapezial myofascial layer. This helps protect against deep infection and ensures plate coverage if there is a superficial infection.

- Comminuted fragments, especially the often seen vertically displaced anterior-superior fragment, should be gently "teased" back into position, maintaining its soft tissue attachments. They can be secured with mini- or small-fragment screws. Reduction is important but not at the cost of denuding all of the soft tissue attachment (Fig. 38-30).

- While typically it is not necessary to dissect in the subclavicular space to place protective retractors, it is very important not to "plunge" into this area with drills or taps. If a lung injury is suspected intraoperatively, the wound is filled with saline and the anesthetist performs a Valsalva maneuver. The presence of air escape indicates pleural injury and should prompt a chest radiograph and consultation for pleural drainage (catheter or chest tube).

- A plate of size and strength commensurate with the patients' size and compliance should be used. In general, 3.5-mm compression plates or precontoured plates are ideal, especially for larger individuals (>150 lb) or those who will rehabilitate aggressively.

- IM fixation is reserved for simple fracture patterns (transverse and short oblique fractures).

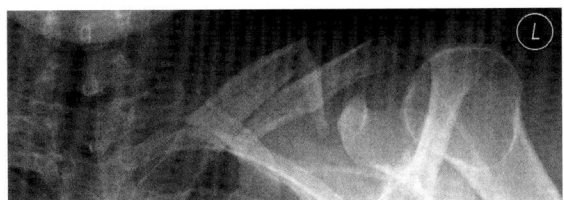
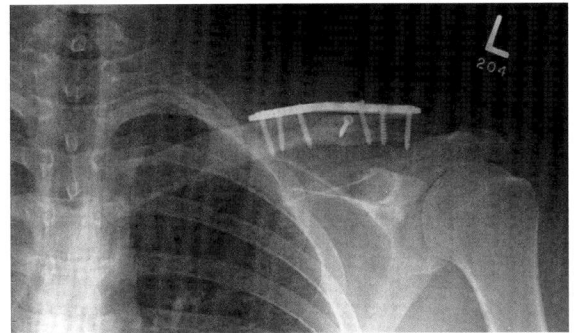

A   B

FIGURE 38-30 A: Anteroposterior radiograph with 20-degree cephalad tilt demonstrating a completely displaced midshaft clavicle fracture with shortening. There are often vertically oriented fracture fragments that arise from the anterosuperior surface of the clavicle at the site of displaced midshaft fractures, giving many fractures a "Z" pattern. If possible, they should be gently teased back into place and fixed with small or minifragment screws, followed by plate fixation. It is important not to denude the fragment when attempting to fix it. Reduction is performed by reducing the vertical intercalated fragment to the distal fragment and securing it with a 2.7-mm lag screw. The distal assembly is then reduced to the proximal fragment with the aid of two towel clip reduction forceps, followed by plate fixation with a precontoured plate. **B:** Postoperative radiograph revealing restoration of length and anatomic reduction.

• Reduce the risk of refracture by avoiding routine plate removal: If required, wait a minimum of 2 years following fracture union before performing hardware removal (Table 38-8).

Plate or Hook Plate Fixation of Displaced Fractures of the Lateral Clavicle

Preoperative Planning. A careful examination of the skin over the lateral clavicle and planned operative site is important. As with midshaft fractures, temporizing until the soft tissue status improves may be prudent. The major technical challenges in these injuries are purchase in the distal fragment and resisting the primary displacing forces, which draw the proximal fragment superiorly and the distal fragment (secured by the AC and coracoclavicular ligaments to the coracoid and scapula) inferiorly.[4,23,42,77,83,130] In addition, the cancellous bone of the distal fragment may be inferior in quality to that of the shaft, and there may be unrecognized comminution. The treating surgeon should template the fracture preoperatively to determine the number of screws that will have purchase in the distal fragment. There are a number of precontoured "anatomic" plates available for this purpose. If it is anticipated that there will be insufficient distal purchase then alternative fixation strategies

TABLE 38-8	**Potential Pitfalls and Prevention—Operative Treatment**
Pitfall	**Prevention**
Poor patient selection	Young, active patients with displaced fractures benefit from primary fixation: Poor bone quality, medical comorbidities, and noncompliance negatively affect outcome. Substance abusers have a dramatically higher complication and reoperation rate. Nonoperative care is preferred in these individuals
Deep wound infection with exposed hardware	A two layer closure, consisting of a deep myofascial layer and a superficial skin/subcutaneous tissue layer, will help decrease or eliminate this potential complication
Plate breakage	Use a strong plate consistent with the size, demands, and compliance of the patient. Most precontoured plates approach the biomechanical strength of a compression plate. Avoid 3.5-mm reconstruction type plates, especially in larger individuals
Hardware irritation	Use a precontoured plate, especially in an individual of smaller stature
Loss of reduction and shortening	Avoid unlocked or small diameter intramedullary devices in complex or comminuted fracture patterns. Obtain lag screw fixation if possible, and a minimum of six cortices on either side of the fracture site, when using plate and screw fixation
Nonunion after operative fixation	Avoid excessive soft tissue stripping at the fracture site. Small comminuted fragments should be teased into the best position possible and secured with screws or suture. Soft tissue attachments are preserved

need to be considered. These can include augmenting fixation into the coracoid process or achieving purchase to or under the acromion. In this instance the use of a hook plate (a pre-contoured plate with a projection or "hook" that is inserted posteriorly in the subacromial space) can be extremely useful, especially with very distal fractures.[51,56,98]

Patient Positioning. Patients are positioned in the "beach-chair" or semisitting position, similar to the position used for midshaft fractures. A small pad or bump is placed behind the involved shoulder to elevate it into the surgical field. The head is placed on a round support and rotated out of the way of the operative field. Recently, frames and supports designed to give greater exposure of the shoulder (i.e., for shoulder arthroscopy) have become popular. This type of operative set-up can also be used, and may facilitate intraoperative radiography. It is not usually necessary to free-drape the involved arm, although this can be done if there is any difficulty anticipated with the reduction (i.e., if the fracture is severely displaced or greater than 2 to 3 weeks old).

Surgical Approach. The surgical approach is similar to that used for superior plating of the clavicle. A skin incision placed directly superiorly over the distal clavicle, extending approximately 1 cm past the AC joint is made. The skin and subcutaneous layer is developed, and the deltotrapezial myofascial layer is incised directly over the distal clavicle and reflected anteriorly and posteriorly. The AC joint is identified. This can be done by inserting an 18-gauge needle into the joint from the superior aspect, and an arthrotomy can be avoided. It is possible to use an anterior/inferior approach for plate fixation of distal clavicle fractures although in my experience this involves a significant amount of detachment of the deltoid and it is not possible to convert easily to coracoclavicular screw augmentation or hook plate fixation.[204]

Technique. The fracture site is identified and cleaned of debris and hematoma. The fracture is reduced and it may be held with either a K-wire or a lag screw. Elevating the distal fragment to meet the proximal fragment may aid in reduction. If the main fracture line is in the coronal plane, it may be possible to lag the fracture from anterior to posterior through a small anterior stab incision separate from the primary incision. Once the fracture is reduced and provisionally stabilized, the optimal type of plate is chosen. Anatomic plates that fit the distal clavicle are now available, and placing four bicortical, fully threaded, cancellous screws in the distal fragment should be the goal (Fig. 38-31). Following fixation, the surgeon must judge whether the number and quality of distal fragment screws are sufficient to provide stability until union occurs. If fixation is judged to be inadequate, there are several options at this point. Since the primary deforming force at the fracture site is superior displacement of the proximal fragment, it is possible to augment fixation by securing the proximal fragment to the coracoid with a longer screw inserted through one of the plate holes (Fig. 38-32). This screw, typically 30 to 40 mm long, helps secure the proximal fragment to the coroacoid and prevents this superior displacement. Since there is some intrinsic motion between the clavicle and the coracoid and scapula, with time this screw either loosens or it may break, but it will give 6 to 8 weeks of stability to secure fracture healing before doing so. Alternatively, it may be necessary to augment fixation by using a hook plate with fixation under the acromion to prevent superior migration of the proximal fragment. This technique is selected when there is insufficient bony purchase in the distal fragment with conventional screws.[53,56,98] This may be readily apparent during preoperative planning (Fig. 38-33), or may only be realized intraoperatively. The advantage of subacromial fixation is that conventional plating can be rapidly converted to this technique intraoperatively. The AC joint is identified,

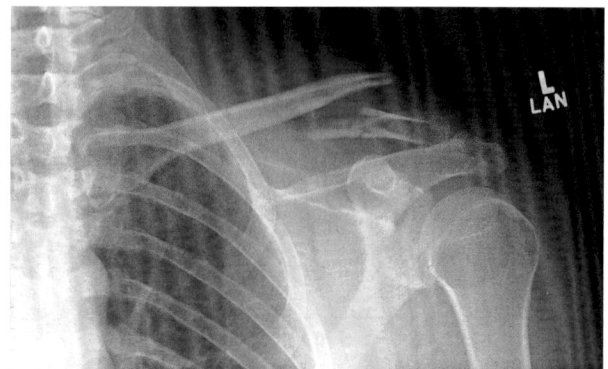
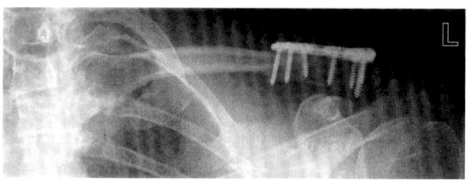

FIGURE 38-31 Anteroposterior radiograph of a displaced distal clavicle fracture in a 38-year-old physician following a fall off a mountain bike at high speed **(A)**. Although the fracture was closed, there was significant bruising and swelling over the shoulder. The degree of displacement of this fracture suggests a high likelihood that of delayed union or nonunion would result with nonoperative treatment. After the soft tissue swelling had subsided 10 days post injury, operative fixation was performed with a plate specifically designed for the distal clavicle, allowing for the placement of four screws in the small distal fragment **(B)**. The fracture healed uneventfully and the patient was able to return to work within a week of the surgery. A final follow-up radiograph **(C)** following hardware removal for local soft tissue irritation, a common problem in this area, shows solid union.

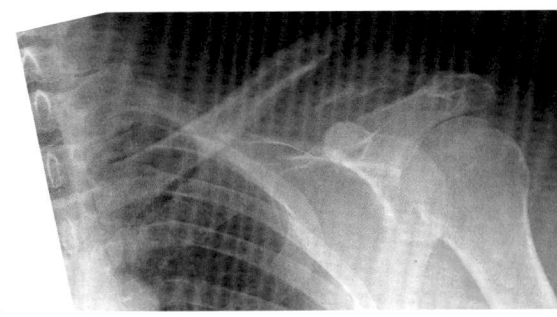

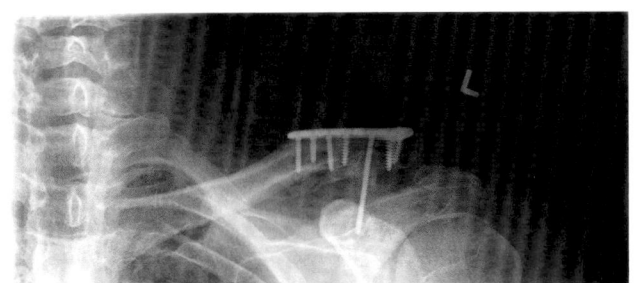

FIGURE 38-32 A: It is possible to augment fixation in distal clavicle fractures with poor-quality bone or a very small distal fragment by placing a screw through the plate into the coracoid process, which helps resist the forces that displace the fracture (superior displacement of the proximal fragment, inferior displacement of the distal fragment). Since there is 10 to 15 degrees of rotational motion between the clavicle and the coracoid, this fixation will eventually loosen (as it has in this case) or break **(B)**. However, typically it provides augmented fixation for 6 to 8 weeks postoperatively, which is usually enough for the fracture to heal.

and the posterior edge of the distal clavicle is dissected free. An entrance into the subacromial space is then made with a pair of heavy curved scissors that will create the path of the "hook" extension of the plate. It is important that this space is made posteriorly, so that there will be no impingement of the rotator cuff in the critically tight anterior subacromial space. Once this path has been created, the hook is placed in it and the plate reduced to the shaft of the clavicle. Several different hook depths and lengths are currently available for this plate, and trial reductions can be performed to determine the optimal plate type. Alternatively, the plate can be "walked down" onto the clavicular shaft by sequential placement of the screws from distal to proximal. This can be a very effective technique of fracture reduction as this maneuver "levers" the distal fragment to the proximal fragment. On occasion, it may be necessary to contour the shaft of the plate to prevent over-reduction of the fracture; however, if excessive contouring appears to be required, a more likely explanation is that the fracture is not reduced and that there is residual superior angulation. It is possible to securely repair even very distal fractures (that are essentially AC joint fracture-dislocations) with this technique. Minimal, if any, purchase is required in the distal fragment.

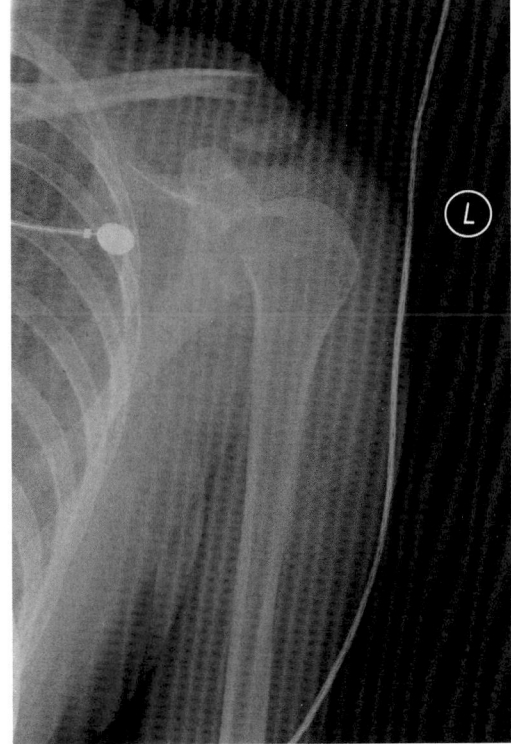

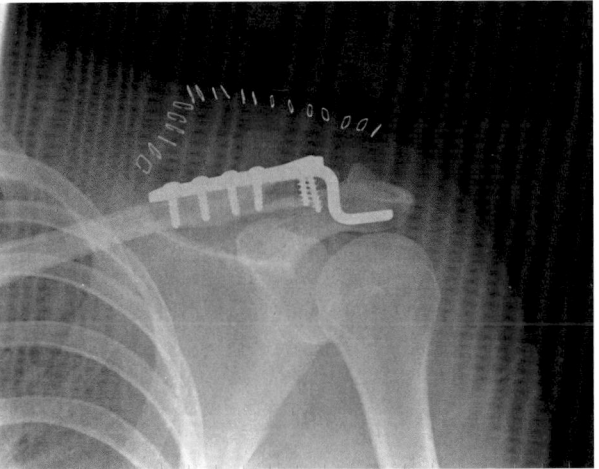

FIGURE 38-33 A: Anteroposterior radiograph of a very distal clavicle fracture in a 22-year-old female pedestrian struck by a street car. The fracture was open with significant soft tissue damage, near transection of the superior deltoid and trapezius, and severe instability of the shoulder girdle. It can be anticipated that conventional plating may be inadequate given the small size of the distal fragment and the associated shoulder girdle instability. **B:** The radiograph following irrigation and debridement, hook plate fixation, and deltoid/trapezial muscle repair. Early motion was initiated and an excellent result ensued.

Unlike static fixation across the AC joint which is doomed to loosening or fatigue failure, hook plate fixation allows some motion between the bones. A cadaver study revealed that this technique most closely reflected the biomechanics of the native AC joint, namely secure enough to provide reliable fixation yet physiologically flexible.[98] Following fixation, the wound is thoroughly irrigated and a two-layer closure similar to that for midshaft fractures is performed.

Postoperative Care. The arm is placed in a sling and the patient is allowed early active motion in the form of pendulum exercises. At 10 to 14 days postoperatively the wound is checked and the stitches are removed. The sling is then discarded and full range-of-motion exercises are instituted; sling protection can be extended if the quality of fixation is questionable. At 6 to 8 weeks, if radiographs are favorable, resisted and strengthening exercises are instituted. Return to full contact or unpredictable sports (i.e., mountain biking) is usually discouraged until 12 weeks postoperatively. While hardware removal is typically optional for those with conventional plates, it can be anticipated that a high percentage of individuals with hook plate fixation will require plate removal to regain terminal shoulder flexion and abduction (see Hardware Removal). This is usually performed at a minimum of 6 months postoperatively.

Potential Pitfalls and Preventative Measures

- The rate of delayed union and nonunion for completely displaced distal clavicle fractures treated nonoperatively is approximately 40%.

- Even minimally displaced fractures may take an excessive period of time to heal, or may develop a fibrous union. However, without displacement, they are often not symptomatic enough to warrant surgical intervention.

- The technical challenge faced during operative treatment of distal clavicle fractures is the fixation of the distal fragment; the surgeon should be prepared to deal with unexpected comminution or poor screw purchase in the distal fragment using anatomic plates, coracoclavicular fixation, or hook plates.

- Hook plate fixation is an effective alternative to conventional plate fixation when faced with inadequate distal purchase. To avoid subacromial impingement, the hook should be placed posteriorly.

- A high percentage of patients treated with hook plate fixation will require plate removal to regain full range of shoulder motion.

- Rigid transacromial fixation has a high rate of loosening and fatigue failure due to the intrinsic motion at the AC joint and is therefore not routinely recommended.

Outcomes. There are a number of studies that define the outcome of nonoperatively treated fractures of the distal clavicle.[23,121,132,153,157] The largest and most comprehensive is by Robinson et al.[153] who examined a cohort of 127 nonoperatively treated patients with follow-up of 101 these individuals. The mean Constant score was 93 points, although this excluded

14 patients (14%) with symptoms severe enough to warrant delayed surgical intervention. Interestingly, although 21 patients (21%) had a radiographic nonunion, they were minimally symptomatic and their outcome scores (Constant, SF-36) were no different than those in patients with uneventful union. They concluded that nonoperative treatment achieved good results in middle-aged and elderly patients, with only a small percentage (14%) requiring delayed surgery. These results were mirrored by Rokito et al.[157] who compared 14 patients treated operatively for displaced distal third fractures with 16 nonoperatively treated patients and found no difference in ASES, Constant, or UCLA shoulder scores despite the fact that 7 (of 16) patients in the nonoperative group developed a radiographic nonunion. In a systematic review of 425 patients (21 studies), Oh et al.[132] described a nonunion rate of 33% in the 60 patients treated nonoperatively, but noted that little functional deficit occurred. It is clear from these studies that although the nonunion rate is relatively high following the nonoperative treatment of displaced distal third clavicle fractures, functional deficit (especially in middle-aged and elderly patients) is minimal and conservative care should, at present, be considered acceptable in most cases. The same study by Oh et al. described the outcome following various surgical interventions in 365 patients, and recommended that coracoclavicular fixation was preferred due to its low complication rate (4.8%) compared to hook plate fixation (40.7%) or K-wire tension banding (20.0%). IM fixation was also associated with a low complication rate (2.4%) but the number of cases amenable to this type of fixation is limited. In direct comparisons of surgical techniques, Tan et al.[182] reported equivalent union rates between hook plate fixation and small fragment T plate fixation (100%), but that more patients in the hook plate group had residual shoulder pain that required hardware removal (15/23, 74%) for relief. Klein et al.[80] compared early versus late distal clavicle fracture repair with hook plate fixation (22 patients) and superior locked plate application (16 patients). They found a high rate of success (union in 36/38 patients), but that fractures repaired early (<4 weeks) had better outcomes than the delayed group (ASES score 78 vs. 65), with a lower complication rate (7% early vs. 36% delayed). Unfortunately, there are few prospective or randomized trials examining distal clavicle fractures. In the absence of high-quality evidence, we must rely on available information that would suggest that the majority of these injuries should be treated nonoperatively initially, especially in middle-aged or elderly individuals.[23,80,121,132,153,169] Operative intervention is reserved for severely displaced fractures, high-demand patients, or for failures of nonoperative care: In these cases a variety of methods (hook plate repair, coracoclavicular fixation, tension-band wiring, etc.) can have a high degree of success.[34,42,53,80,132,182,193,204]

Medial Clavicle Fractures

There are very few reports on medial fractures of the clavicle, a rare entity. Low et al.[92] reported the successful treatment of five cases of completely displaced medial clavicle fractures using internal fixation (plates and/or screws). They stressed the importance of preoperative imaging as this area is difficult to visualize with plain radiographs. In a similar series, this was emphasized by Oe et al.,[129] who reported on 10 cases of medial clavicular fracture. The medial clavicular epiphysis is the last long bone epiphysis to fuse in the body, and may persist in patients until 25 to 30 years of age. Therefore, medial clavicular fractures are often epiphyseal fracture-subluxations or fracture-dislocations. This can be defined by the preoperative CT scan. There is little in the way of evidence-based medicine to dictate treatment, with the majority of information on this entity contained in small retrospective case series. Fractures that are significantly displaced may warrant operative repair, especially if there is posterior displacement. The primary technical difficulty with these injuries is the fixation in the medial fragment. The surgical approach is similar to that made to the shaft. It is important to remember that the subclavian vessels are in close proximity to the bone medially. Following identification, debridement, and reduction of the fracture, it can be temporarily held reduced with K-wires. Definitive plate fixation can then be performed in a variety of ways. If the medial fragment is large enough, then standard plate and screw fixation can be performed; a plate with an expanded end section (as in a distal clavicle plate from the contralateral side) may augment multiple screw purchase. There is a significant expansion of the medial clavicle (Fig. 38-17) and this allows for placement of longer (22 to 24 mm) cancellous screws. If there is insufficient purchase, than the plate can be extended across the joint onto the sternum. This construct will eventually loosen due to motion at the SC joint, but will typically stabilize the fracture long enough (3 months) for union to occur, at which the point the plate should be removed. Rarely, fixation with a hook plate intrasternally or retrosternally may be required. This is a highly specialized technique and cardiovascular support should be available in the event of inadvertent injury to the vascular structures found retrosternally. Fixation of the fracture using smooth wires or pins alone is contraindicated, due to the potential for migration and visceral injury.

Management of the "Floating Shoulder"

The combination of ipsilateral fractures of the clavicle and scapular neck has traditionally been called the "floating shoulder," which has been considered to be an unstable injury that may require operative fixation.[45,145,158,188,191,198,200] In fact, this injury pattern can be considered to be a subgroup of the "double disruption of the superior shoulder suspensory complex (SSSC)," a concept introduced by Goss.[58,136] This describes the bone and soft tissue circle, or ring, of the glenoid, coracoid process, coracoclavicular ligaments, clavicle (especially its distal part), AC joint, and acromion. This complex is extremely important biomechanically, as it maintains the anatomic relationship between the upper extremity and the axial skeleton. The clavicle is the only bony connection between the two, and the scapula is suspended from it by the coracoclavicular and AC ligaments. Thus, any injury that disrupts this ring at two or more locations is considered inherently unstable and one whose cumulative effect may be greater than the sum of its individual constituents.[203] Long-term functional problems have been reported following significantly displaced injuries of this nature, including shoulder weakness and stiffness, impingement syndrome, neurovascular compression, and pain.[30,43,45,65–67,88,145,158,188,191,198,200] Such injuries have been considered relative indications for operative intervention (Fig. 38-9). Combined scapular (or glenoid neck) and clavicle fractures are the commonest type of double disruptions of the SSSC, and there remains considerable controversy over optimal treatment.

A study by Leung and Lam[88] described good or excellent to results in 14 of 15 patients with this injury pattern following fixation of both the clavicle and glenoid fractures. However, Herscovici et al.[66] described excellent results in seven of nine patients who had their floating shoulder treated with reduction and fixation of the clavicular fracture only. These findings were confirmed in a study by Rikli et al.[150] who performed clavicle fixation is isolation in 11 patients with combined clavicle and glenoid fractures. They described an average final Constant score in the operated shoulders of 95% of the unaffected side. These studies support the concept, in selected cases, of clavicular fracture reduction and fixation alone. It is postulated that reduction of the clavicle helps to reduce and stabilize the glenoid fracture, eliminating the requirement for operative fixation of the glenoid. This is an important point, since open reduction and internal fixation of the glenoid can be a difficult and complex procedure with a high complication rate, especially if the surgeon lacks experience in this anatomic area.

There are also reports that support nonoperative management of this injury. Ramos et al.[145] described the results of nonoperative treatment in 16 patients with ipsilateral fractures of the clavicle and glenoid. Eleven patients had a complete recovery to near-normal status, although one had a significant malunion of the glenoid neck and three had significant shoulder asymmetry. Edwards et al.[43] reported good results ("pleased" or "satisfied") in 16 of 20 patients with floating shoulder injuries treated nonoperatively. There were four patients who were "dissatisfied" or "unhappy" with their outcome. While the outcome assessment of these patients was suboptimal it would appear that nonoperative treatment may be considered, especially for minimally displaced fractures. Interestingly, two of the four patients with poor results had severely displaced clavicular fractures. In a clinical study, Williams et al.[198] evaluated 9 of 11 patients with a floating shoulder treated nonoperatively and found five excellent, one good, and three fair results. They found that the worse clinical results were strongly associated with 3 cm or more of medial displacement of the glenoid, and recommended nonoperative care for lesser amounts of glenoid displacement. Similarly, van Nort et al.[188] performed a questionnaire review including 31 of 35 floating shoulder patients treated nonoperatively and found that only 3 required late operative reconstruction for clavicular malunion or nonunion. They found that results in the nonoperative group (a mean Constant score 76) deteriorated with increasing degrees of glenoid displacement. Interestingly, they also found that three of the four patients who had their clavicle fracture fixed primarily had a poor result due to scapular malunion. They believed that this failure of indirect glenoid reduction following clavicular reduction and fixation was due to associated ligamentous injuries that caused a dissociation of the two structures.

There is some limited biomechanical evidence to support the intuitive clinical finding that increasing degrees of fracture displacement in floating shoulder injuries corresponds to poorer results if left unreduced. Williams et al.[200] performed a cadaver biomechanical study by establishing a scapular neck fracture and investigating the effect of an ipsilateral clavicle fracture, a coracoacromial ligament injury, and an AC ligament injury. They found that substantial instability (lack of resistance to a medially directed force) only occurred after associated ligamentous disruption. Although there are limitations to this study (such as the uniaxial direction of the applied deforming force), it remains one of the only biomechanical studies on this topic.

Unfortunately, given the variable and sporadic nature of this injury, there is a paucity of prospective, randomized, or comparative trials upon which to base treatment recommendations. What is clear is that earlier recommendations for routine operative fixation for all floating shoulder injuries were too liberal, and that poor results occur regularly with badly displaced fractures that are treated nonoperatively. In addition, the aggressiveness of treatment must be commensurate with the risk of intervention and the expected functional demands of the patient. Thus, an operative approach may be indicated in a young healthy individual who works overhead for a living whereas the same fracture pattern may be treated nonoperatively in an elderly, low-demand patient with multiple medical comorbidities. Further research in this area may help identify currently unknown factors that may predict outcome and hence guide treatment.[79] Currently, standard operative indications include the following.

1. A clavicle fracture that warrants, in isolation, fixation
2. Glenoid displacement of greater than 2.5 to 3 cm
3. Displaced intra-articular glenoid fracture extension
4. Patient-associated indications (i.e., polytrauma with a requirement for early upper extremity weight bearing)
5. Severe glenoid angulation, retroversion, or anteversion >40 degrees (Goss Type II)
6. Documented ipsilateral coracoacromial and/or AC ligament disruption or its equivalent (coracoid fracture, i.e., AC joint disruption)

If operative intervention is chosen, then anatomic reduction and internal fixation of the clavicle is typically performed first, and the shoulder then reimaged. If there is indirect reduction of the glenoid such that its alignment is within acceptable parameters, then no further intervention is required apart from close follow-up. If the glenoid remains in an "unacceptable" position, then fixation of the glenoid neck, typically performed through a posterior approach, is indicated (see "Fractures of the Scapula, Chapter 39"). Also, Oh et al. reported the failure of isolated clavicle fixation in two cases of floating shoulder. If this method is chosen in this setting, the clavicle may experience greater loads than with isolated fractures, and the size and length of the fixation device selected should be commensurate with these anticipated loads (Table 38-9).[131]

TABLE 38-9 **Management of Expected Adverse Outcomes and Unexpected Complications**

Clavicle Fractures Common Complications	Prevention	Treatment
Infection	Careful technique, short operative times, prophylactic antibiotics	Irrigation, debridement, local and intravenous antibiotics, maintain fixation if stable, remove if loose
Nonunion	Primary fixation reduces nonunion rate in selected cases	Plate or IM pin fixation, add iliac crest bone graft or osteoinductive bone substitute if atrophic
Malunion	Primary fixation reduces symptomatic malunion rate in selected cases	Corrective osteotomy and plate fixation
Neurovascular injury	Careful technique to avoid iatrogenic injury (see text)	Treatment of established injury difficult, and usually expectant. Prevention is the key (see text)
Hardware failure	Use a plate strong enough for size, activity level, and compliance of patient. Precontoured plates ideal, 3.5-mm reconstruction plates should be avoided	If fracture site stable and not displaced, it may heal with observation. Most cases will require revision ORIF with stronger plate, ± iliac crest bone graft to promote healing
Hardware prominence	Use a precontoured plate, especially in smaller individuals	Hardware removal, minimum 2 years post implantation
Refracture	Avoid plate removal, if necessary, for 2 years after fixation	If minimally displaced, may heal with nonoperative Rx. If displaced or unstable, repeat ORIF indicated
Scapular winging	Due to residual clavicular malposition (malunion, nonunion). Primary fixation lessens incidence	Corrective clavicular surgery with plate or IM pin may be indicated if symptoms severe

MANAGEMENT OF EXPECTED ADVERSE OUTCOMES AND UNEXPECTED COMPLICATIONS IN CLAVICLE FRACTURES

Infection in Clavicle Fractures

Infection had traditionally been one of the most feared complications following fixation of displaced clavicular fractures, and earlier series described an unacceptably high rate of deep infection.[2,31,54,115] However, significant improvements have been made in a number of areas that are well recognized to decrease infection, including perioperative antibiotics, selective operative timing with regard to soft tissue conditions, better soft tissue handling, two-layer soft tissue closure, and fixation which is superior biomechanically.[15,82,91,117,140,141,162,166] In a recent meta-analysis that examined operative series from 1975 to 2005, Zlowodzki et al.[209] reported a superficial infection rate of 4.4%, and a deep infection rate of only 2.2%; these figures are significantly improved compared to earlier studies. When infection does occur, if it is superficial, then it is usually possible to temporize with local wound care and systemic antibiotics until fracture union has occurred. At that point, plate removal, debridement, and thorough irrigation have a high success rate in infection eradication.

Deep infection with unstable implanted hardware is a more complex problem. If it appears that there is progressive bone formation, then temporizing until union occurs followed by hardware removal and debridement may be successful. If there is no obvious progress toward union, then operative intervention is indicated. Hardware removal followed by radical debridement of infected bone and dead or devitalized tissue and subsequent irrigation is performed. At this point there are several options. If the patient is healthy without comorbidities (as is usually the case) and the infecting organism is a sensitive one, then immediate reconstruction with plating, bone grafting, and local antibiotics may be warranted. Alternatively, especially with polymicrobial infections or resistant organisms (i.e., methicillin-resistant *Staphylococcus aureus*), local antibiotic impregnated polymethylmethacrylate cement beads, or an antibiotic impregnated bone substitute are implanted into any residual dead space following debridement, and systemic antibiotics are administered until clinical and hematologic markers indicate the infection has been eradicated. Delayed reconstruction can then be performed. If there is a significant soft tissue deficiency, then the assistance of a plastic surgeon who can perform soft tissue coverage, typically with a rotational pectoralis major flap, is ideal.[184,199]

Nonunion in Clavicle Fractures

Traditionally, the rate of nonunion of the clavicle has been described as being less than 1% of all fractures. This was based on two sentinel studies, one by Neer in 1960 that described 3 nonunions in 2235 patients, and one by Rowe in 1968 in which only 4 of 566 patients developed nonunion after a fracture of the clavicle.[115,160] More recently, however, the nonunion rate following closed treatment of completely displaced midshaft fractures of the clavicle has been describe as being exponentially higher, in the 15% to 20% range.[15,68,154,209] The reason for this difference is unclear but probably includes more complete follow-up in

recent studies, the exclusion of children (with their inherently good natural history), changing mechanisms of injury (mountain biking, all-terrain vehicles, parachuting), and the modern patients' intolerance of prolonged immobilization. In addition, several prospective population-based studies have been helpful in elucidating factors associated with the development of nonunion (Fig. 38-21). Robinson et al.[154] identified increasing age, female sex, fracture displacement, and comminution as risk factors for nonunion in midshaft fractures. Lateral third fractures had higher nonunion rates as patient age and fracture displacement increased.[153] Nowak et al.[125] prospectively followed 208 patients with radiographically verified clavicle fractures and, 9 to 10 years post injury, found that 96 (46%) still had sequelae. They identified no bony contact between the fracture fragments as the strongest predictor for sequelae. Nonunion occurred in 15 patients (7%). Zlowodzki et al.[209] performed a meta-analysis of all series of displaced midshaft fractures from 1975 to 2005 and identified 22 published manuscripts. They found that, for the specific entity of completely displaced midshaft fractures of the clavicle the nonunion rate with nonoperative treatment was 15.1%, while the nonunion rate following operative treatment was 2.2%. This represents a relative risk reduction (for nonunion) of 86% (95 CI 71% to 93%). This meta-analysis, in addition to recent prospective studies examining primary operative fixation of clavicle fractures, definitively terminated the postulation that primary fixation was associated with a higher, not lower, nonunion rate (Table 38-1). This observation was based on early operative studies with poor patient selection, inadequate fixation (Figs. 38-26 and 38-27) and inferior soft tissue management. Undoubtedly there are other factors that contribute to the incidence of nonunion (i.e., associated fractures, soft tissue interposition, rotation at the fracture site) that have yet to be clarified.[144,178,195,197] Therefore, at the present time, factors associated with the development of nonunion include complete fracture displacement (no contact between the main proximal and distal fragments), shortening of greater than 2 cm, advanced age, more severe trauma (both in terms of mechanism of injury and associated fractures), and refracture. Primary operative fixation however is not associated with a higher nonunion rate.

Nonunion is defined as the lack of radiographic healing at 6 months post injury (Fig. 38-34). While a significant percentage of distal nonunions may be asymptomatic, especially in the elderly,[122] the majority of midshaft nonunions in young active individuals will be symptomatic enough to require treatment.[5,13,40,50,89,94,110,127,133,163]

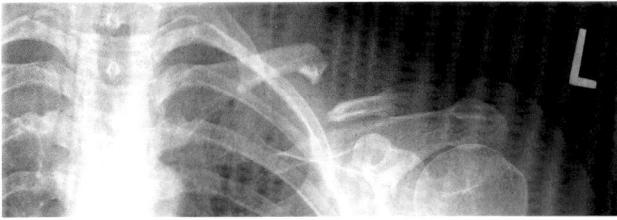

FIGURE 38-34 An atrophic nonunion of the clavicle. The degree of bone loss demonstrated in this case suggests that an intercalary graft may be required to restore length and obtain union.

A variety of methods have been described for the treatment of an established clavicular nonunion that is symptomatic enough to warrant operative intervention.[11,12,30,32,33,40,50,75,76,94,197,203] Successful nonunion repair usually decreases pain and improves function. Described methods range from noninvasive techniques such as electrical stimulation and low-intensity ultrasound to minimally invasive techniques (isolated bone grafting, screw fixation) to formal open reduction and internal fixation with iliac crest bone grafting. Apart from isolated case reports, or cases described in larger series of standard treatments, there is very little objective evidence to support the use of electrical stimulation or ultrasound in this area.[13,30,32] In rare cases where there is minimal deformity or shortening, a stable hypertrophic nonunion with good soft tissue coverage and no infection, and a biologically favorable host (i.e., no smoking or diabetes), such techniques may occasionally be successful in promoting union. However, the majority will require mechanical stabilization and biologic stimulation.

There are two main techniques used to achieve union, plate fixation, and IM screw or pin fixation. The gold standard treatment against which other methods must be compared is open reduction and internal fixation with a compression plate and iliac crest bone graft. Reported success rates with this technique are high if appropriate size and length plates are used. Manske and Szabo (10/10 healed), Eskola et al. (20/22 healed), Jupiter and Leffert (16/19 healed), Boyer and Axelrod (7/7 healed), Olsen et al. (16/17 healed), and Bradbury et al. (31/32 healed) all describe excellent results with a low complication rate.[11,12,50,75,94,133] It is important to note that the forces generated by deformity correction and the longer healing time will mean that the operative construct for a nonunion will require greater stability for a longer period of time than that for an acute fracture. Multiple authors stress that short four-hole plates, weak 1/3 tubular plates, or even 3.5-mm pelvic reconstruction plates in larger (>200 lb) patients are inadequate for this type of fixation, and have higher failure rates (Fig. 38-27). A small fragment compression plate, a precontoured "anatomic" plate or their equivalent with a minimum of three bicortical screws in each fragment is recommended (see Authors Preferred Technique, below).[11,12,30,32,33,40,50,75,76,94]

There are many theoretical advantages to IM pinning with open bone grafting for the treatment of clavicular nonunions. A smaller incision with better cosmesis, less soft tissue stripping, decreased hardware irritation, and easier hardware removal (often under a local anesthetic) are proposed benefits compared to plate fixation. There are several reports describing good results including Boehme et al. (20/21 healed) and Enneking et al. (13/14 healed).[8,48] In the only comparative study of fixation techniques for clavicle nonunion, Wu[203] described union in 9 of 11 patients treated with plate fixation and 16 of 18 of those treated with IM fixation. However, Johnston and Wilkins reported pin failure in two of four patients treated in this fashion, and the two failed IM fixations in the series by Wu both healed with subsequent plate fixation.[197,203] In addition to IM fixation being weaker biomechanically and not controlling length and rotation as well as a plate, others have reported difficulty with pin migration and breakage using this

technique.[79,93,109,120] A randomized, prospective study comparing plate and IM fixation is required to define their respective roles in this setting.

Severe bone loss and/or poor bone quality, typically associated with multiple failed operative procedures and infection, can complicate the reconstruction of recalcitrant clavicular nonunions. The final treatment option in such circumstances is clavicular excision, or claviculectomy (either partial or total).[30,32,202] Considering the important strut effect of the clavicle for upper extremity function, and the availability of modern treatment options, this must be considered a salvage procedure. While reasonable results with retention of a full range of motion and relief of pain have been described in selected cases with severe preoperative pathology, a significant decrease in strength (especially overhead) and a loss of shoulder girdle stability typically result.

My preferred surgical treatment for a midshaft nonunion of the clavicle is open reduction and internal fixation with a precontoured anatomic clavicular plate with the addition of an iliac crest bone graft or an osteoinductive bone graft substitute. Patient positioning and draping is similar to that used for the fixation of acute midshaft fractures, with the exception of having an iliac crest bone graft site prepared (typically the contralateral side) if bone grafting is anticipated (see below). The surgical approach is similar to that used for a fracture, taking care to reflect and preserve the myofascial layer for later closure, and the superior surface of the clavicle at the nonunion site is identified. The ends of the nonunion are identified, and judicious soft tissue dissection is performed around them to allow correction of deformity. This usually involves bringing the distal fragment out to length and translating it superiorly and posteriorly. The distal fragment is often rotated anteriorly, and derotating it brings the flat superior surface directly superiorly, facilitating plate placement on the superior surface. The sclerotic ends of the proximal and distal fragments are identified and a rongeur is used to clear them back to bleeding bone. It is rarely necessary to resect excessive bone to do this. The medullary canals are then re-established with a drill to allow the free egress of osteoprogenitor cells to the nonunion site. Reduction forceps are then placed on the proximal and distal fragments and a reduction is performed. Remembering that there is a slight apex superior bow to the native clavicle, excess superior callus is rongeured away to allow the plate to fit on the superior surface of the clavicle. Any excess callus removed in the approach, debridement or deformity correction is saved, morcellized and inserted into the fracture site at the conclusion of the procedure. If possible, the nonunion is then fixed with an anterior to posterior small- or minifragment lag screw (Fig. 38-35). The chance of success of this helpful step can be increased by recognizing the orientation of the nonunion line during the approach and debridement. Lag screw fixation helps hold the reduction while the plate is applied and also increases the construct stability. If this is not possible than a 2-mm K-wire can be inserted to hold the reduction while a precontoured clavicle plate is applied to the superior surface. I typically use an eight-hole plate. This allows for one or even two empty holes at the nonunion site (often necessary due to

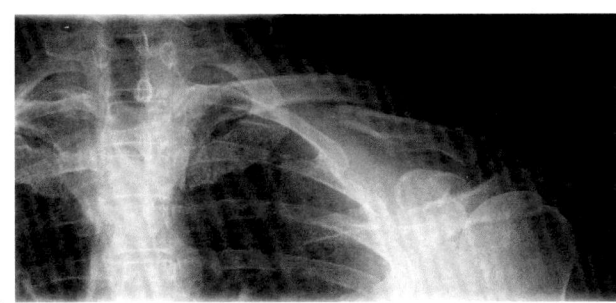
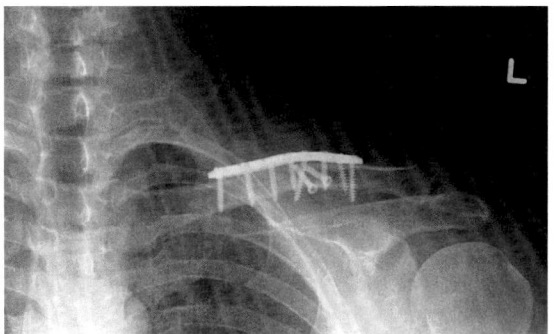

FIGURE 38-35 **A:** An atrophic nonunion 14 months following nonoperative care of a completely displaced fracture of the clavicle. **B:** Successful repair with correction of deformity, plate fixation, and addition of bone morphogenetic protein to the nonunion site. The oblique nature of the nonunion in the coronal plane facilitated initial fixation with two anterior to posterior lag screws.

bony configuration or lag screw interference) while providing for three bicortical screws both proximal and distal, which I consider to be the absolute minimum for fixation. If the nonunion is transverse in nature the first screws on each side are inserted in a compression mode, and tightened after the provisional K-wire has been removed. Although they are available, I have not found it routinely necessary to use locking screws or plates in the clavicle.

If the nonunion is hypertrophic (the minority) then the morcellized autograft from the local bone is applied to the nonunion site and a standard closure, as for a fracture case, is performed. Thorough irrigation and hemostasis is achieved before closure, and drains are not used.

If the nonunion is atrophic, then either morcellized autograft from the iliac crest or an osteoinductive bone substitute, such as a bone morphogenic protein, is packed in and around the nonunion site. Bone substitutes with little osteoinductive capability, such as calcium phosphates or sulfates, allograft, or demineralized bone, are to be avoided. A structural or intercalary graft may be required in certain cases where there has been excessive loss of length or failed previous surgery. Shortening can often be determined preoperatively by comparing the length of the clavicle radiographically to the measured clinical length. If there appears to be significant bone loss then an intercalary graft, as per the technique of Jupiter and Ring,[76] can be employed. Postoperative care is similar to that following malunion reconstruction or acute fracture fixation.

Malunion in Clavicle Fractures

Traditionally, it was believed that malunion of the clavicle (which was ubiquitous with displaced fractures) was of radiographic interest only, and success in the clinical setting was defined as fracture union. However, more recently, a number of investigators have described a fairly consistent pattern of patient symptomatology (with orthopedic, neurologic, "functional," and cosmetic features) following malunion of displaced midshaft fractures of the clavicle.[7,21,64,74,84,103,136,150] While all of the factors that contribute to the development of this condition are unclear; it is typically diagnosed in young, active patients with significant degrees of shortening at the malunion site (Fig. 38-36). As could be reasonably anticipated, shortening of the shoulder girdle (with the typical inferior displacement and anterior rotation of the distal fragment) results in a variety of biomechanical and anatomic abnormalities that translate

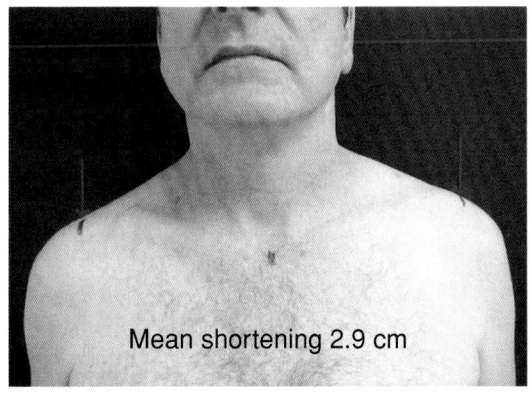
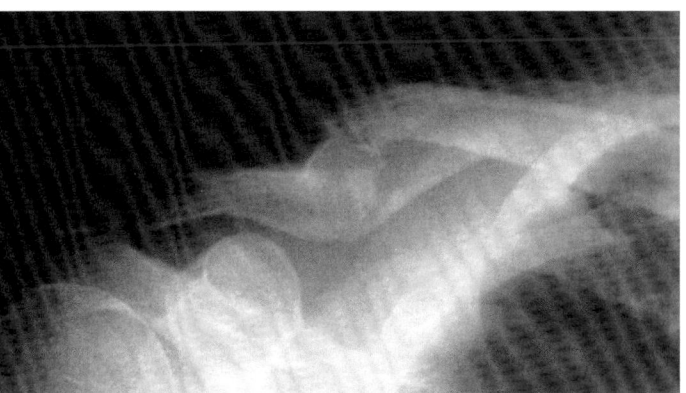

Mean shortening 2.9 cm

FIGURE 38-36 Typical clinical features of clavicle malunion **(A)** with corresponding radiograph **(B)**. Note the shoulder asymmetry, and the difference in the position of the AC joints (*arrows*).

Shoulder strength

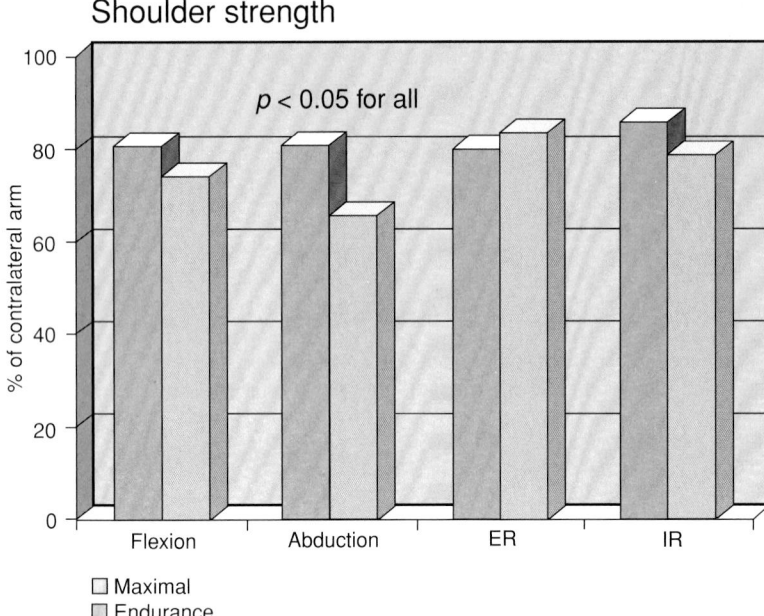

FIGURE 38-37 Objectively measured shoulder strength following nonoperative treatment of a displaced midshaft fracture of the clavicle (maximal, endurance) compared to the normal contralateral side.[99] Patients were a minimum of 14 months post injury, with a mean of 54 months. ER = ecternal rotation; IR = internal rotation. (Adapted from: McKee MD, Pedersen EM, Jones C, et al. Deficits following nonoperative treatment of displaced midshaft clavicular fractures. *J Bone Joint Surg AM*. 2006; 88(1):35–40, with permission.)

directly into patient complaints. Orthopedically, shortening of the muscle-tendon units that traverse the malunion site results in a sense of weakness and rapid fatigability, with a loss of endurance strength. It has been previously shown that there are significant, objective, deficits in maximal strength and endurance (especially of abduction) following the healing of displaced midshaft fractures of the clavicle treated nonoperatively (Fig. 38-37).[99,172] Narrowing and displacement of the thoracic outlet (the inferior border of which is the clavicle) result in numbness and paraesthesias, usually in the C8 to T1 nerve root distribution, exacerbated by provocative overhead activities. Due to their deformity, patients complain of the appearance of their shoulder and difficulty with backpacks, hiking packs, military gear, and shoulder straps: This has been termed a deficit in "functional cosmesis." Patients with this condition also complain of upper back pain and periscapular aching, especially with repetitive activity. There is objective evidence that the displacement of the distal fragment (to which the scapula is attached) results in malalignment of the scapulothoracic joint and a form of scapular winging; this produces periscapular muscle spasm and fatigue pain.[64,146]

It would appear that the predominant risk factor for the development of this condition is shortening at the malunion site. Gossard[59] found that shortening of 2 cm or more was associated with poor functional outcome and a high rate of patient dissatisfaction. McKee et al.[103] described a series of 15 patients with a symptomatic clavicular malunion who had a mean amount of shortening of 2.9 cm and Bosch et al.[9] described an "extension osteotomy" in 4 patients with shortening of 0.9 to 2.2 cm. In a retrospective study, Eskola et al.[49] reported on 83 patients with displaced fractures and found that shortening of 1.2 cm or more was associated with increased pain at final follow-up. However, this point remains controversial. In retrospective reviews, Nordqvist et al.[124] (225 midshaft clavicle

fractures) and Oroko et al.[135] (41 midshaft clavicle fractures) could not demonstrate a relationship between shortening and a poor outcome. It is probable that length is just one component of a complex three-dimensional deformity that, combined with the intrinsic variability of human response to skeletal injury, explains why some individuals with a malunion function well and others determinedly seek operative correction. For patients with a symptomatic malunion who have failed a course of physiotherapy for muscle strengthening, the options are to accept the disability or have a corrective osteotomy.

Operative intervention is reserved for patients with signs and symptoms of malunion that are specific to the condition and sufficiently severe to warrant surgery. A vague and generalized ache about the shoulder (especially in a patient with medical–legal or compensation issues) and a radiographic malunion is not necessarily an indication for surgery. Patients selected for surgery are typically young, active, and healthy with good bone stock. The primary goal of surgery is to correct the deformity, and preoperative planning is important (Fig. 38-38). Careful measurement both clinically and radiographically defines the degree of length to be restored. A posteroanterior thorax or chest radiograph that includes both clavicles has been shown to be a reliable way of comparing length to the opposite (normal) clavicle.[172] Inferior displacement and anterior rotation of the distal fragment is corrected by having the plate applied to the superior surface flush both medially and laterally; some contouring of the plate may be required in the anterosuperior plane as there is a slight caudal bow to the clavicle.

Patient positioning and the surgical approach are similar to those used for acute fracture fixation or nonunion repair.[102] The exception is that in certain cases it is prudent to have an iliac crest bone graft site prepared (see below). In general, it has not been routinely necessary to insert an intercalary graft to restore length. It is usually possible to identify the position of the

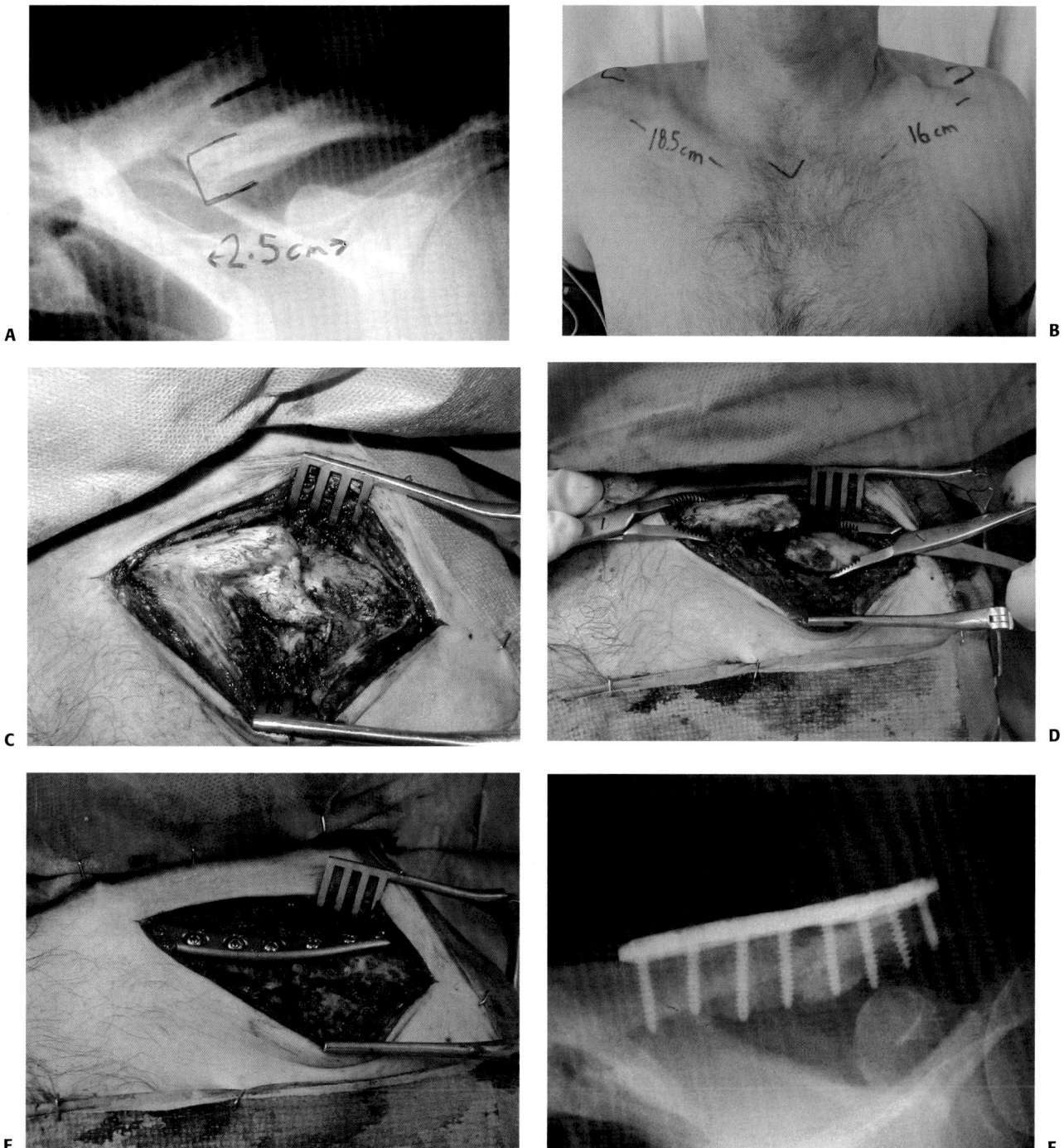

FIGURE 38-38 **A:** Anteroposterior radiograph of a symptomatic clavicle malunion with 2.5 cm of shortening. **B:** The corresponding clinical photograph showing the measurement of clavicular length from the sternal notch to the acromioclavicular joint. **C:** An intraoperative photograph of the malunion site demonstrating the typical displacement of the distal fragment with medial, inferior, and anterior translation. This also demonstrates the abundant local bone which is usually present at the malunion site. While it is difficult to appreciate, there is anterior rotation of the distal fragment as well. **D:** An intraoperative photograph following osteotomy of the malunion, recreating the original fracture line and rongeuring of excess callus (which will be used to graft the osteotomy site), and distracting the fragments to their correct length and position. It is typically not necessary to perform an intercalary bone graft, as there is rarely absolute bone loss, and the original proximal and distal fragments can be re-established using a combination of a microsagittal saw and osteotomes. **E:** An intraoperative photograph following reduction and plate fixation using an anatomic precontoured plate. **F:** An anteroposterior radiograph following union. The patient's preoperative symptoms resolved fully.

proximal and distal fragments in most patients. The malunion site is cleared, and a mark is made in the bone proximally and distally and the length is measured. This enables the surgeon to calculate how much length has been gained by remeasuring the distance between the two marks at the conclusion of the osteotomy. Next, the osteotomy to recreate the original fracture and proximal and distal fragments is made with a combination of a microsagittal saw and osteotomes. Care is taken not to violate the subclavicular space. Following the osteotomy, the proximal and distal fragments are grasped with a reduction forceps and gently distracted to the desired position. It is not routinely necessary to free-drape the arm for traction. For difficult cases, a minidistractor can be used to correct length and maintain position while fixation is applied. Care must be taken not to overdistract the fragments as neurologic injury may result.[151] Depending on the configuration of the bone ends, after the osteotomy is performed it is often possible to fashion an interdigitating or step cut contour to improve intrinsic stability and increase the bony surface area for healing. The medullary canals are re-established with a drill, and the osteotomy is temporarily secured with a K-wire. It is then measured for correction of deformity and length. On occasion, an absolute bone deficit may be encountered, such that reduction of the fragments does not restore length. Options at this point include accepting some shortening or using an intercalary graft. This situation can be anticipated preoperatively when the measured clinical shortening (i.e., 3 cm) is significantly greater than the degree of shortening seen on the radiograph of the involved clavicle. Once deformity correction is confirmed, definitive fixation is performed. There are several precontoured "anatomic" plates designed for clavicular fixation that are ideal for this purpose.[70] If a lag screw can be placed across the osteotomy then three additional screws both proximally and distally are usually sufficient. If not, four screws proximally and distally are recommended. Additional local bone can be morcellized and added to the osteotomy site. Wound closure and postoperative care are the same as that for acute fracture fixation or nonunion repair.

Neurovascular Injury in Clavicle Fractures

Despite the proximity of the brachial plexus and subclavian vessels, neurovascular injury is surprisingly rare, given the number of severely displaced clavicular shaft fractures seen in practice.[6,10,18,22,34,38,55,69,147,151,161,187] In general, neurovascular injuries associated with clavicle fractures can be divided into three groups: Acute injuries, delayed injuries, and iatrogenic injuries.

Acute Injuries

A careful vascular and neurologic examination is critical with any clavicular injury, especially those associated with high-energy trauma. If the signs of vascular injury are present, an angiogram is indicated. In addition to being diagnostic, with the refinement of interventional techniques such as embolization and stenting, the procedure can also be therapeutic (Fig. 38-39). While direct impalement of bony fragments can occur, most neurovascular injuries occur from excessive traction, which in its most severe form is termed scapulothoracic dissociation. The unique feature of these injuries is that the associated clavicular fracture is typically distracted, rather than shortened. This can be a limb or life-threatening injury. A study by Ebraheim et al. reported 3 deaths in 15 patients, and Zelle et al. described 3 deaths and 6 amputations in 22 patients in their series from a major European trauma center.[39,207] If limb salvage is to be performed, shoulder girdle stabilization (typically plate fixation of the clavicle fracture) is indicated to create an optimal healing environment for the soft tissue structures.

There have also been case reports of direct neurologic injury from clavicular fracture fragments. In this situation operative decompression of the brachial plexus by reduction and fixation of the clavicle fracture is indicated.[6,10,34,55,69,147,161]

Delayed Injuries

Delayed injuries tend to occur due to encroachment upon the thoracic outlet, either from displacement of the borders (i.e., from clavicular displacement due to malunion or nonunion), or encroachment from inferior clavicular callus formation. This phenomenon can be especially severe in patients with a concomitant head injury (Fig. 38-40). In the case reports describing this entity, debridement of local callus with realignment and fixation of the clavicle injury is indicated.[26,47,147] The timing of this intervention is controversial, but in general it should be performed as promptly as the patient's general condition allows. The commonest reason for brachial plexus irritation following clavicular fracture is the chronic thoracic outlet syndrome (TOS) that results from clavicular malunion (see above). In this setting, operative treatment should be directed toward re-establishing the preinjury dimensions of the thoracic outlet through a corrective clavicular osteotomy.[7,9,21,103] Simply removing the "bump" around the fracture site, or conventional treatments for TOS such as first rib resection have a high failure rate. This is due to the fact that the fundamental anatomical problem is the change in position, orientation, and contour of the thoracic outlet from the displacement of the distal clavicular segment, rather than from local impingement of callus or normal structures (i.e., the first rib). Connolly and Ganjianpour[28] reported the case of a patient with TOS following a clavicular malunion that was treated with first rib resection to no avail, while corrective clavicular osteotomy resulted in prompt resolution of symptoms. McKee et al.[103] reported resolution of TOS symptoms in 16 patients who underwent corrective clavicular osteotomy to treat a malunion. Chronic encroachment upon the thoracic outlet leading to TOS is probably the commonest form of neurovascular "injury" following displaced clavicular fractures.

Iatrogenic Injury

Despite the proximity of the brachial plexus, catastrophic injury from intraoperative penetration by drills or taps is very rare. Shackford and Connolly[168] reported a case of subclavian pseudoaneurysm formation with distal embolization from

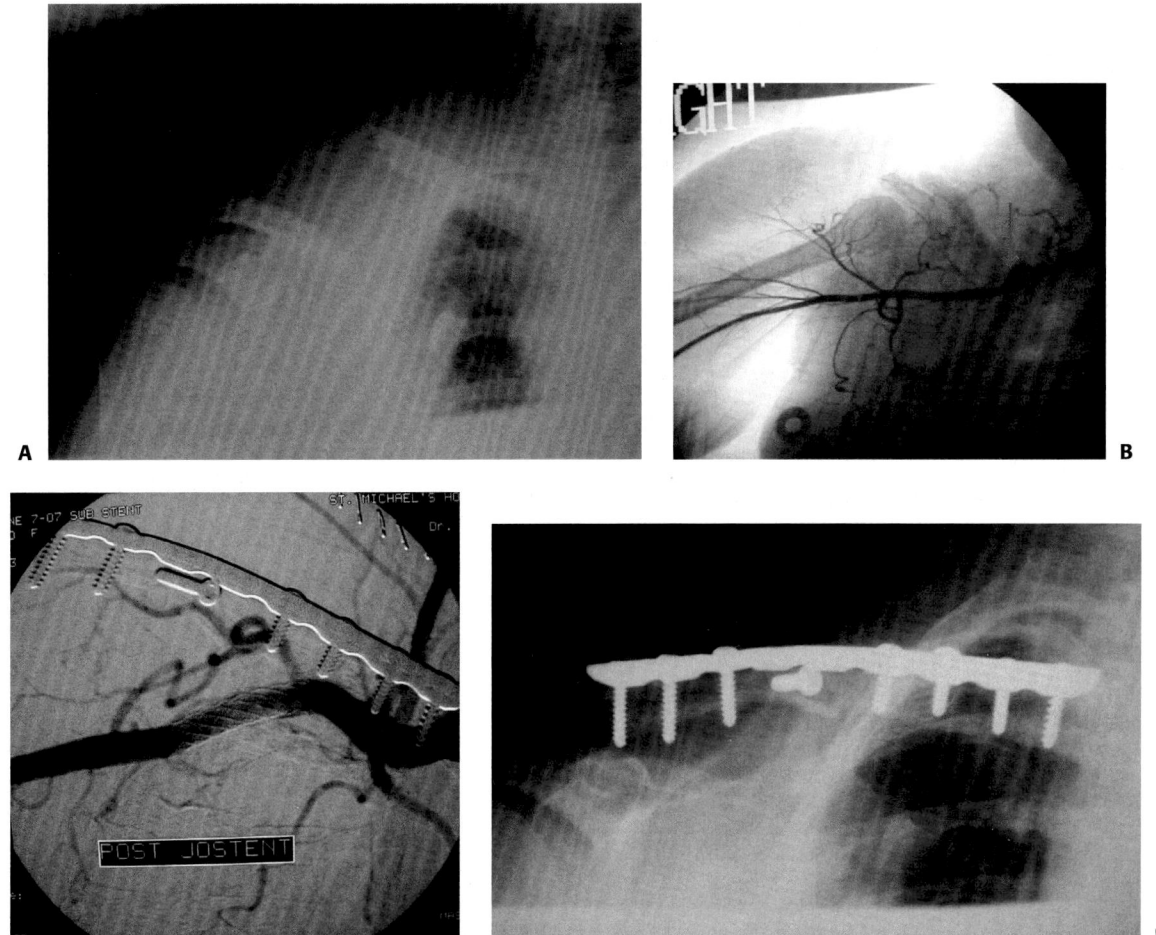

FIGURE 38-39 A: Anteroposterior radiograph of a morbidly obese 57-year-old nurse who sustained a severely displaced midshaft fracture of the clavicle in a fall from a standing height. She also had a partial brachial plexus injury and a partial laceration of the subclavian artery with pseudoaneurysm formation (*arrow*), demonstrated on the preoperative angiogram **(B)**. The patient was treated with immediate stenting of the resultant pseudoaneurysm, followed by plate fixation of the fracture with a 3.5-mm limited contact dynamic compression plate **(C)**. The indications for fixation included reducing the severe displacement and creating an optimal environment for neurologic and vascular healing. Uneventful bony and soft tissue healing ensued **(D)**.

screw penetration after plate fixation of a clavicular nonunion, and Casselman[18] described a similar case. Iatrogenic injury can occur, but is thought to occur in specific situations where distraction can occur. Ring and Holovacs[151] described three cases of brachial plexus palsy after IM fixation of clavicle fractures. They postulated that the distraction of the fracture site (a prerequisite for reduction and pin insertion) and the delayed presentation (patients were diagnosed several weeks after their injury) led to a traction injury of the brachial plexus. Fortunately, all three palsies recovered completely with nonoperative care. It would appear that distraction of a shortened clavicular fracture, especially one that presents or is treated some weeks or months following initial injury, creates a risk for a traction-type injury to the adjacent brachial plexus. Overdistraction at the fracture site or any violation of the subclavicular space is to

be avoided during operative repair of clavicular injuries. Fortunately, with the information presently available, these injuries are usually transient in nature and a full recovery with time can usually be expected.

Hardware Failure in Clavicle Fractures

This complication occurs when the stress placed upon the implant exceeds its biomechanical strength, typically due to early overuse from noncompliance, implant/patient size mismatch, or delayed union or nonunion. This complication can be prevented by proper surgical technique (i.e., avoiding extensive soft tissue stripping, stable fixation) and the use of implants commensurate with the patient's size and compliance (i.e., avoiding the use of 3.5-mm pelvic reconstruction plates). These technical details are described in "Plate Fixation" (above). The incidence of hardware

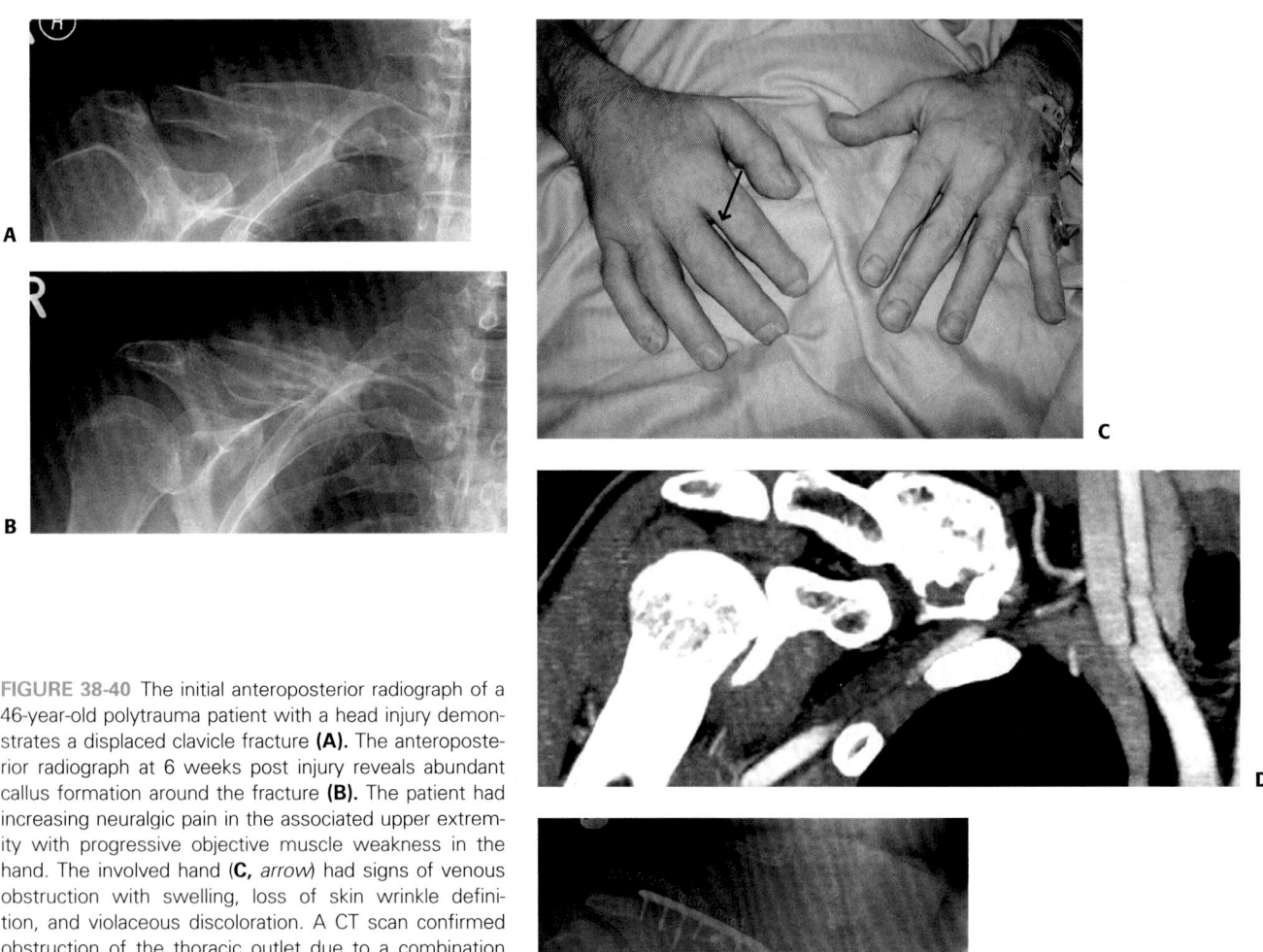

FIGURE 38-40 The initial anteroposterior radiograph of a 46-year-old polytrauma patient with a head injury demonstrates a displaced clavicle fracture **(A)**. The anteroposterior radiograph at 6 weeks post injury reveals abundant callus formation around the fracture **(B)**. The patient had increasing neuralgic pain in the associated upper extremity with progressive objective muscle weakness in the hand. The involved hand (**C,** *arrow*) had signs of venous obstruction with swelling, loss of skin wrinkle definition, and violaceous discoloration. A CT scan confirmed obstruction of the thoracic outlet due to a combination of severe shortening and displacement of the fracture site and exuberant callus formation **(D)**. This patient was treated with operative corrective of the deformity, complete resection of the supraclavicular callus, and judicious resection of infraclavicular callus followed by plate fixation. A prompt resolution of symptoms, complete neurologic recovery, and uncomplicated fracture union ensued **(E)**.

failure should decrease as improved implants (in terms of strength, materials and contour) become available.

Hardware Prominence in Clavicle Fractures

Local irritation from prominent hardware remains a clinical concern following the operative treatment of clavicle fractures, given its relatively scanty soft tissue coverage. The incidence of hardware removal ranges from less than 5% to essentially 100% in some series (i.e., where pin removal is a planned second stage of the procedure). The use of bulky, straight plates in thin or small individuals is associated with greater degrees of local irritation. It is probable that the incidence of plate removal can be minimized by using a precontoured plate. In addition, proponents of anterior-inferior plating suggest that this technique results in less prominence and irritation, although this remains to be proven. With regard to plate fixation in general, it is clear that routine plate removal is not recommended or desirable in the majority of cases following ORIF. Asymptomatic plates can and should be left in situ with a low rate of long-term complications, similar to retained plates in other areas in the upper extremity such as the forearm or humerus. Plates that provoke local irritation sufficient to warrant operative intervention should be removed only after 2 years have elapsed since fracture union to minimize the risk of refracture (as in the forearm). Collision athletes should have their plates removed at the end of a season to further decrease refracture risk. Anecdotally, many patients who have symptomatology at 1 year and desire plate removal find that by 2 years post injury the symptoms have ameliorated to the point where intervention is not desired. In general, small diameter or unlocked IM devices are removed because of the high degree of backing out and prominence as the fracture consolidates. This can be performed earlier than plate removal due to the intrinsic differences in healing patterns between these implants. It is unclear if more modern lockable

IM devices will have a lower removal rate, although that is certainly one of their theoretical advantages.

Refracture in Clavicle Fractures

True refracture after healing of a fracture of a clavicle is surprisingly rare. It has been my experience that many individuals who have claimed to have sustained multiple fractures of the clavicle have in fact a nonunion of their initial fracture that has never healed completely. Recurrent episodes of trauma prompt medical attention, and new radiographs are misinterpreted as showing a "refracture." The few cases that are reported describe a higher nonunion rate following "refracture". Regardless of the exact etiology, patients with this condition should be counseled about the high rate of unsatisfactory outcome and that they may benefit from fixation.[15,30,32]

Given the increasing popularity of operative fixation of displaced clavicle fractures, and the patient population involved, it is not surprising that fractures at the end of a plate used for fixation of a prior clavicle fracture are being encountered. This typically happens from recurrent high-energy trauma. Large prospective series are not available and recommendations are based on only a few cases. In general, a fracture in the upper extremity that occurs at the end of a stable implanted diaphyseal plate has a poor natural history and a high chance of delayed union or nonunion. It is my experience that these fractures, if displaced, generally require repeat fixation. Attempts should be made to fix the fracture and span the area of bone previously repaired (Fig. 38-41). If the fracture is minimally displaced, a trial of nonoperative care with the arm at rest in a sling is reasonable.

Scapular Winging in Clavicle Fractures

Scapular winging has a variety of etiologies, and there are a number of case reports describing this condition following the nonoperative treatment of displaced midshaft fractures of the clavicle. Rasyid et al.[146] reported two cases of winging of the scapula, one from a "neglected" fracture of the clavicle with 2-cm of shortening. A recent paper by Ristevski et al.[152] examined 18 patients with symptomatic clavicular malunion and evidence of scapular winging clinically (Fig. 38-42) The authors performed CT scanning of all patients and were the first to be able to describe and quantify a consistent pattern of scapular malalignment. The patients had a mean clavicular shortening of 2.1 cm, and the acromion was found to translate with the distal clavicular fragment medially, inferiorly, and anteriorly. The average acromial translation was 2.4 cm. The posterior aspects of the scapula were found to translate less (superior angle, 1 cm; inferior angle, 0.6 cm). This gives the typical clinical appearance of a shortened, protracted shoulder seen in clavicle malunion or nonunion (Fig. 38-43). The main function of the clavicle is as a strut to position the scapula in its correct location. Since the scapula is the base upon which the arm and hand function, a malunion or nonunion of the clavicle alters the position of the scapula such that the mechanical advantage of the associated muscles is affected. The negative mechanical effects of this shoulder position are well documented, with a mean decrease in rotational strength ranging from 13% to 24% in one study.[175] While it is difficult to prove a direct link between scapular malalignment and poor outcome following nonoperative treatment of displaced fractures of the clavicle, it is hypothesized that the early fatigability, weakness, spasm, and pain from the shoulder girdle musculature may be related to scapular malposition.

While the relationship between scapular malalignment and outcome may be unclear at present it may help explain some of the variability in outcome seen with clavicle fractures. While we use the measurement of clavicular shortening as a surrogate for overall displacement, it is clear that significant degrees of scapular malposition (and inherent symptomatology) can result from translation and rotation of the distal clavicular fragment and scapula with minimal "shortening" seen on standard radiographs. Prospective studies to analyze the degree of scapular malalignment in the acute setting of a clavicle fracture would help determine whether a correlation exists between this malalignment and outcome, and could aid in surgical decision making.

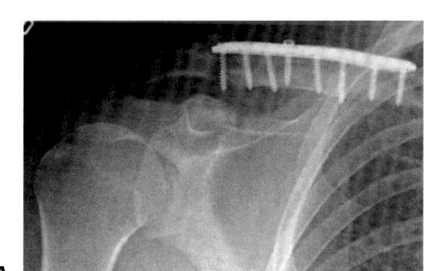
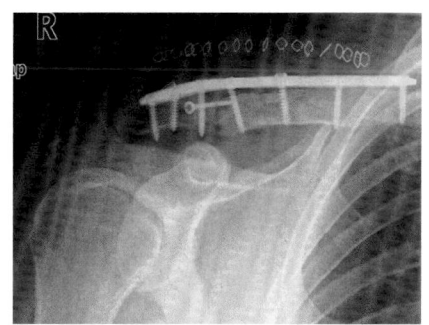

FIGURE 38-41 A 40-year-old professional motorcycle racer had plate fixation of a midshaft clavicle nonunion that developed following a displaced midshaft fracture. The nonunion healed uneventfully, but 2 years later, following another high-velocity crash, he sustained a fracture at the lateral end of the plate **(A)**. This fracture also developed into a nonunion, and required repeat fixation with a longer plate **(B)**. This is a potential risk for individuals with plate fixation of the clavicle who continue to participate in high-risk activities.

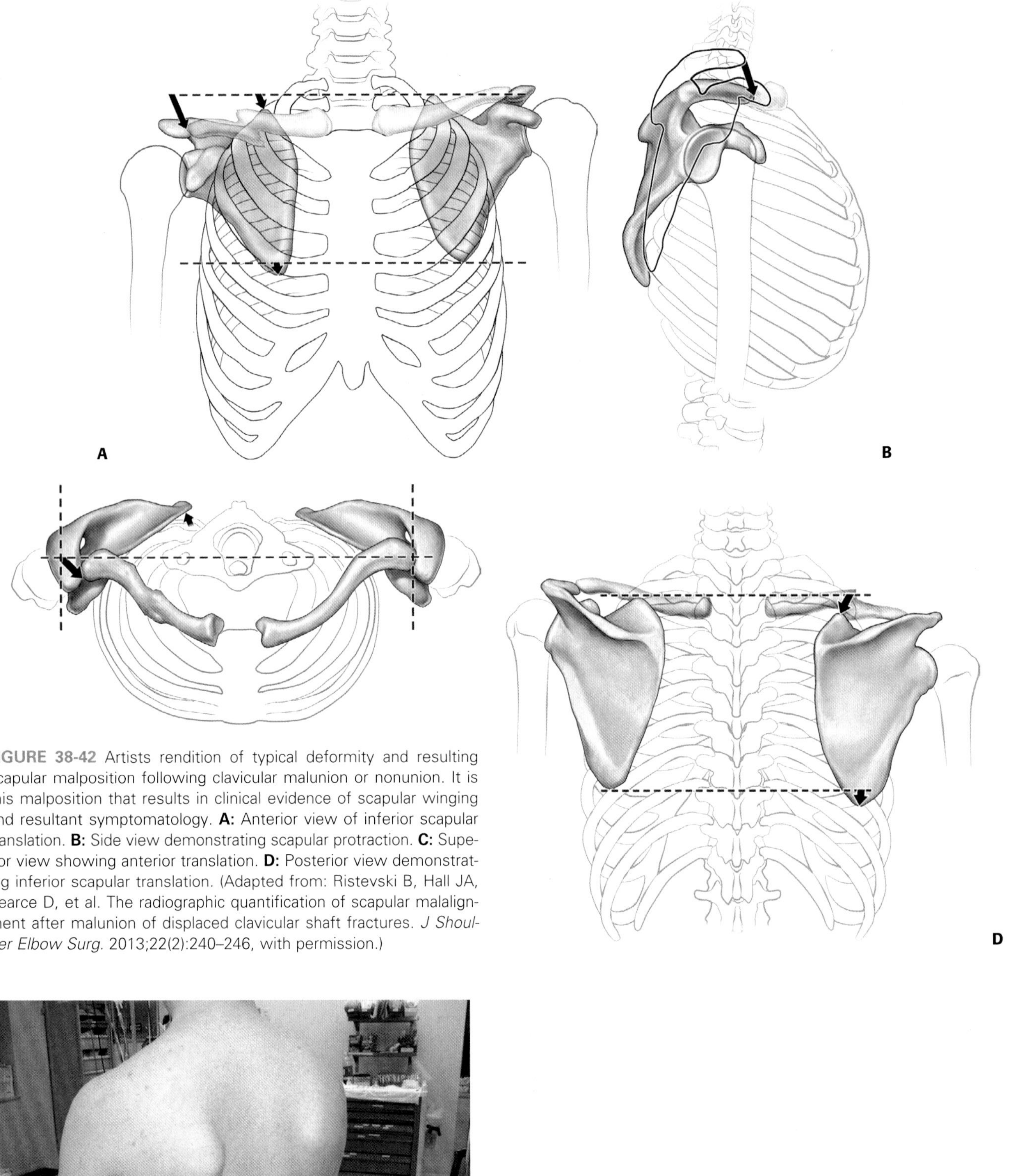

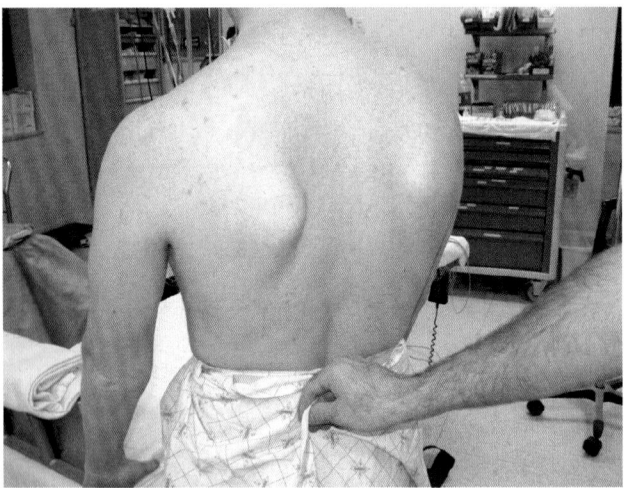

FIGURE 38-42 Artists rendition of typical deformity and resulting scapular malposition following clavicular malunion or nonunion. It is this malposition that results in clinical evidence of scapular winging and resultant symptomatology. **A:** Anterior view of inferior scapular translation. **B:** Side view demonstrating scapular protraction. **C:** Superior view showing anterior translation. **D:** Posterior view demonstrating inferior scapular translation. (Adapted from: Ristevski B, Hall JA, Pearce D, et al. The radiographic quantification of scapular malalignment after malunion of displaced clavicular shaft fractures. *J Shoulder Elbow Surg.* 2013;22(2):240–246, with permission.)

FIGURE 38-43 A clinical photograph of scapular winging of the left shoulder associated with a midshaft clavicle malunion with 3-cm shortening. There is a characteristic protrusion of the inferior angle of the scapula, produced as the scapula rotates and translates anteriorly with the distal clavicular fragment.

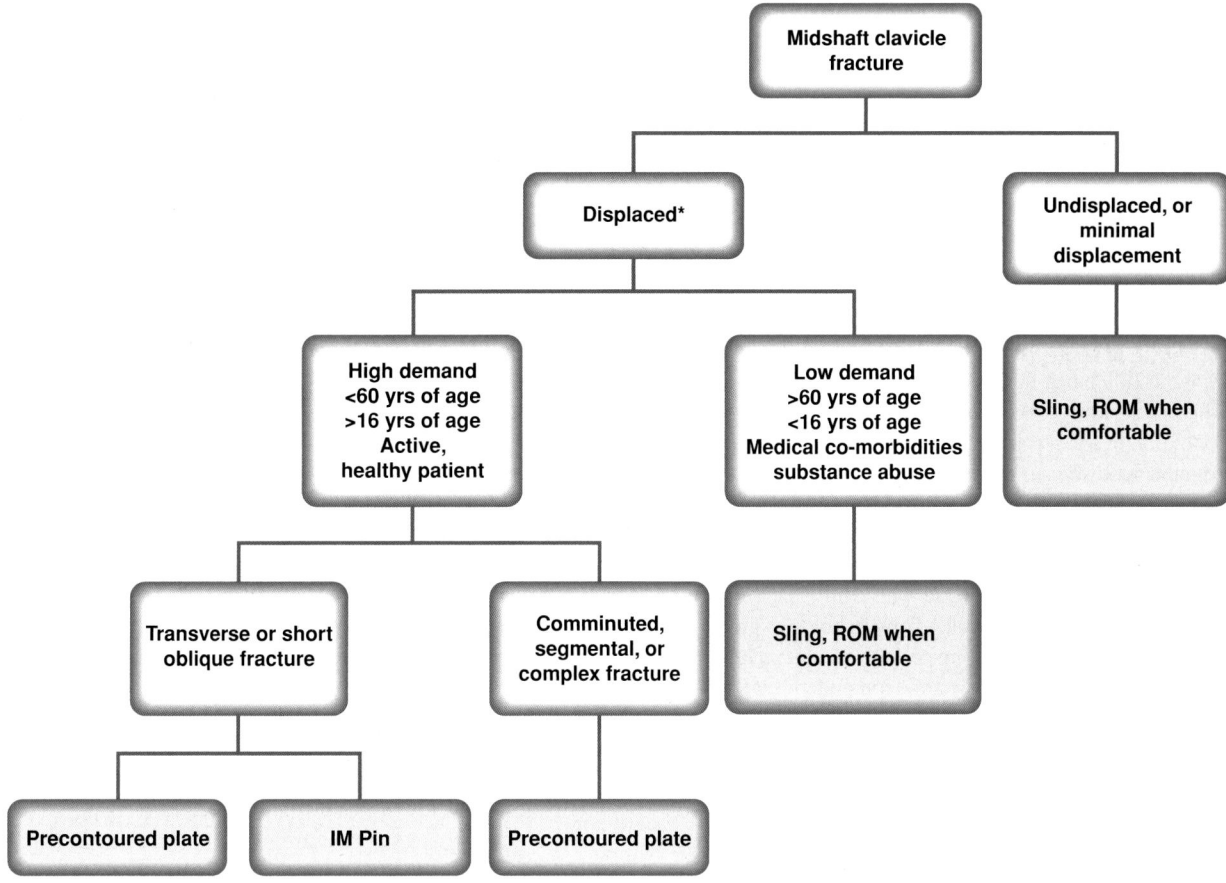

*Displaced: 1.5-cm shortening, obvious clinical deformity, associated rotational deformity, and scapular winging.

FIGURE 38-44 Clavicle: Author's Preferred Treatment.

AUTHOR'S PREFERRED METHOD OF TREATMENT FOR CLAVICLE FRACTURES

The above figure describes the author's preferred method of treatment of clavicle fractures (Fig. 38-44).

CONTROVERSIES AND FUTURE DIRECTIONS IN CLAVICLE FRACTURES

Patient Selection for Operative Intervention for Clavicle Fractures

Recent studies have made it clear that there is a subset of patients, especially those with shortened, displaced fractures who would benefit from primary operative repair of clavicular injuries.[15,68,154] However, these early interventions are not without risk and consume significant health care resources. In addition, there are patients who would seem to have prognostic factors for a poor outcome following a clavicular fracture (i.e., displacement of greater than 2 cm) and yet heal promptly (albeit in a "displaced" position) with minimal symptomatology and full function of the involved shoulder. While some of the explanation for this is undoubtedly due to the inherent variability of patient response to musculoskeletal injury, there may be other factors that are not clearly define or understood at present. For example, while most studies use the magnitude of shortening when defining fracture displacement, this alone is a relatively simplistic linear measurement of what is typically a complex three-dimensional deformity. Since most of the major muscle groups of the shoulder have a scapular origin it may be that the final position of the scapula relative to the trunk and upper arm (which is difficult to measure, see Scapular Winging) may be the dominant factor in determining prognosis.[64] While the prognostic index published by Robinson et al.[154] is a dramatic advance in providing objective information and facilitating our ability to predict outcome, there are still significant improvements that can be made so that intervention can be selected specifically for those patients for whom the risk/benefit ratio of surgery is favorable. It is also clear that patient noncompliance, especially when associated with substance abuse, is a clear contraindication for surgery. Bostman et al.,[10] in a study of 103 consecutive adults with acute, displaced midshaft fractures of the clavicle, stated that "Patient noncompliance with the postoperative regimen could be suspected to have a major cause of the failures."

Method of Fixation for Clavicle Fractures

There has been increasing interest in direct comparative studies examining the outcome of various IM nails versus plates for displaced fractures of the midshaft clavicle. This includes two prospective randomized trials, two retrospective comparative studies, and one meta-analysis.[25,37,52,81,86] In a prospective study, Ferran et al.[52] randomized 32 patients to Rockwood pin fixation (17 patients) or small fragment compression plate fixation (15 patients) and found 100% union in both groups with no difference in Constant scores at final follow-up (pin group mean score 92, plate group mean score 89, p = 0.365). They concluded that both techniques were effective, although there was a high rate of hardware removal (100% of pins and 53% of plates), and their study could be criticized for its small numbers. Lee et al. performed a similar study (Knowles pins vs. plate fixation) in 62 patients over the age of 50 years, and although there was no difference in functional outcome (Constant score 85 in the pin group vs. 84 in the plate group), there were fewer complications, decreased OR time and hospital stays, and less symptomatic hardware in the pin group. Kleweno et al.[81] performed a retrospective review of 40 patients treated operatively for completely displaced, simple pattern (transverse or wedge type) midshaft fractures of the clavicle and were able to follow up 18 treated with Rockwood pins and 14 treated with plates. They reported five complications in the pin group and five adverse events in the plate group with no documented differences in functional outcome, and concluded that pinning was a suitable option for simple pattern fractures. Chen et al.[25] reported on a 141 patients treated with flexible titanium elastic nails (TENs, 57 patients) or small fragment pelvic reconstruction plates (plate, 84 patients). They reported no significant difference between the two groups with regard to complications, although the TEN group had shorter operative times and less blood loss than the plate group, with better DASH scores (mean 8 point difference) early at 6 months. There was no difference at 2 years, with excellent DASH and Constant scores (mean 96 in both groups) in both groups. They concluded that TEN fixation was an excellent option but it should be stressed that they restricted its use to simple fracture patterns in a group of patients typically much smaller than the North American population. At the present time, TEN nailing has not been widely reported in the North American literature, and caution must be used in its application. Duan et al.[37] conducted a meta-analysis of these studies and concluded that the evidence failed to show a difference in treatment effects between plating and IM pin fixation, although there were more hardware complications with plating. They also stress that more high-quality, multicenter comparative studies are required for firm conclusions to be made.

Timing of Surgical Intervention for Clavicle Fractures

Conventional thinking has been that nonoperative treatment is appropriate for most if not all fractures of the clavicle, even severely displaced injuries, with the assumption that the reconstructive repair of those that developed nonunion or symptomatic malunion would produce results similar to that of primary operative repair of the original fracture. Since these injuries are nonarticular, and the reported "success" rate of reconstruction is high, this approach seems to have inherent merit. However, there is recent evidence that while operative reconstruction of malunion or nonunion is a reliable procedure, with increas-

ing refinement of outcome measures and objective muscle strength testing it is apparent that there are residual deficits compared to what primary operative repair can provide. Potter et al.[143] examined a cohort of 15 patients who had undergone late reconstruction with plate fixation for clavicular nonunion or malunion ("delayed group") at a mean of 63 months post injury and compared them to a similar cohort of 15 patients who had primary plate fixation of a clavicle fracture a mean of 0.5 months after injury ("acute group"). The groups were similar in age, sex, original fracture characteristics, and mechanism of injury. They found that there were subtle but significant differences between the two groups with regard to shoulder scores (Constant score 89 in the delayed group, and 95 in the acute group, p = 0.02), and the delayed group demonstrated inferior endurance strength in the involved shoulder. They concluded that while late reconstruction is a reliable and reproducible procedure, there were subtle decreases in outcome compared to acute fixation, and they recommended that this information be used in decision making when counseling patients with displaced midshaft fractures of the clavicle. Rosenberg et al.[158] reported similar results in a group of 13 patients who had late reconstruction for clavicular malunion and nonunion. While osseous healing occurred in all cases there was a mean 20-point deficit in Constant score (61 vs. 81, p = 0.01) in the affected shoulders. The authors felt that "lasting functional impairment" was possible even with objective success. With time, substantial adaptive changes (muscle atrophy, soft tissue contracture, bone loss) occur in the shoulder girdle of individuals with clavicular malunion or nonunion that will compromise the outcome of late reconstructive surgery to some degree when compared to the results of primary fixation. This is useful, objective information to use when evaluating the risk/benefit ratio of early operative intervention.

CLAVICLE FRACTURE SUMMARY

There are now available a number of high-quality, prospective, and randomized studies that define the role of primary operative intervention for fractures of the clavicle. While the majority of clavicle fractures will heal with nonoperative care (a simple sling is probably best) and a prompt return of near normal shoulder function can be expected, there is a subset of fractures that benefit from operative intervention. Poor prognostic signs that have been defined include increasing fracture displacement (especially shortening), fracture comminution, and an increasing number of fracture fragments, especially in older patients. A meta-analysis of randomized clinical trials comparing operative versus nonoperative treatment for displaced midshaft fractures of the clavicle has revealed some consistent findings: Plate fixation is a reliable technique with a low nonunion rate, nonoperative treatment results in a nonunion rate of 20% to 25%, malunion remains a problem in nonoperatively treated patients, and primary fixation results in modest (10 points on a 100-point scale) improvement, in general, in the operative group. Anterior-inferior plate placement may have some advantages over superior plate positioning with respect to soft tissue irritation. IM fixation has many theoretical advantages and a high rate of success in skilled hands, although results in the literature remain inconsistent. Although the difference is small, primary plate fixation provides significantly improved results in terms of strength and shoulder scores compared to delayed reconstruction. Malunion of the clavicle is a definite clinical entity that benefits from corrective osteotomy, which can usually be performed without a bone graft. Scapular winging from scapular malposition is a consistent, definable, and common finding following the failure of primary nonoperative care and the development of a nonunion or a symptomatic malunion, and it can lead to significant patient symptomatology. Future studies that are randomized, prospective, and comparative are needed to refine the indications for primary operative repair, investigate the role that scapular malposition plays, and determine the ideal method of fixation.

REFERENCES

1. Adams FL. *The Genuine Works of Hippocrates*. New York, NY: William Wood and Co.; 1886.
2. Ali Khan MA, Lucas HK. Plating of fractures of the middle third of the clavicle. *Injury*. 1978;9(4):263–267.
3. Andersen K, Jensen PO, Lauritzen J. Treatment of clavicular fractures. Figure-of-eight bandage versus a simple sling. *Acta Orthop Scand*. 1987;58(1):71–74.
4. Ballmer FT, Gerber C. Coracoclavicular screw fixation for unstable fractures of the distal clavicle. A report of five cases. *J Bone Joint Surg Br*. 1991;73(2):291–294.
5. Ballmer FT, Lambert SM, Hertel R. Decortication and plate osteosynthesis for nonunion of the clavicle. *J Shoulder Elbow Surg*. 1998;7(6):581–585.
6. Barbier O, Malghem J, Delaere O, et al. Injury to the brachial plexus by a fragment of bone after fracture of the clavicle. *J Bone Joint Surg Br*. 1997;79(4):534–536.
7. Basamania CJ. Claviculoplasty. *J Shoulder Elbow Surg*. 1999;8(5):540. [Abstracts: Seventh International Conference on Surgery of the Shoulder, 1999.]
8. Boehme D, Curtis RJ Jr, DeHaan JT, et al. Nonunion of fractures of the mid-shaft of the clavicle. Treatment with a modified Haigie intramedullary pin and autogenous bone-grafting. *J Bone Joint Surg Am*. 1991;73(8):1219–1226.
9. Bosch U, Skutek M, Peters G, et al. Extension osteotomy in malunited clavicular fractures. *J Shoulder Elbow Surg*. 1998;7(4):402–405.
10. Bostman O, Manninen M, Pihlajamaki H. Complications of plate fixation in fresh displaced midclavicular fractures. *J Trauma*. 1997;43(5):778–783.
11. Boyer MI, Axelrod TS. Atrophic nonunion of the clavicle: Treatment by compression plate, lag-screw fixation and bone graft. *J Bone Joint Surg Br*. 1997;79(2):301–303.
12. Bradbury N, Hutchinson J, Hahn D, et al. Clavicular nonunion: 31/32 healed after plate fixation and bone grafting. *Acta Orthop Scand*. 1996;67(4):367–370.
13. Brighton CT, Pollack SR. Treatment of recalcitrant nonunion with a capacitively coupled electrical field: A preliminary report. *J Bone Joint Surg Am*. 1985;67(4):577–585.
14. Brinker MR, Edwards TB, O'Connor DP. Letter to the editor. *J Bone Joint Surg Am*. 2005;87 A(3):677–678.
15. Canadian Orthopaedic Trauma Society. Nonoperative treatment compared with plate fixation of displaced midshaft fractures. A multicenter, randomized clinical trial. *J Bone Joint Surg Am*. 2007;89(1):1–10.
16. Carley S. Towards evidence based emergency medicine: Best BETS from the Manchester Royal Infirmary. Collar and cuff or sling after fracture of the clavicle. *J Accid Emerg Med*. 1999;16(2):140.
17. Carry PM, Koonce R, Pan Z, et al. A survey of physician opinion: Adolescent midshaft clavicle fracture treatment preferences among POSNA members. *J Pediatr Orthop*. 2011;31(1):44–49.
18. Casselman F, Vanslembroek K, Verougstraete L. An unusual case of thoracic outlet syndrome. *J Trauma*. 1997;43(1):142–143.
19. Cave AJ. The nature and morphology of the costoclavicular ligament. *J Anat*. 1961; 95:170–179.
20. Celestre P, Roberston C, Mahar A, et al. Biomechanical evaluation of clavicle fracture plating techniques: Does a locking plate provide improved stability? *J Orthop Trauma*. 2008;22(4):241–247.
21. Chan KY, Jupiter JB, Leffert RD, et al. Clavicle malunion. *J Shoulder Elbow Surg*. 1999;8(4):287–290.
22. Chen CE, Liu HC. Delayed brachial plexus neurapraxia complicating malunion of the clavicle. *Am J Orthop*. 2000;29(4):321–322.
23. Chen CH, Chen WJ, Shih CH. Surgical treatment for distal clavicle fractures with coracoclavicular ligament disruption. *J Trauma*. 2002;52(1):72–78.
24. Chen DJ, Chuang DC, Wei FC. Unusual thoracic outlet syndrome secondary to fractured clavicle. *J Trauma*. 2002;52(2):398–399.
25. Chen YF, Wei HF, Zhang C, et al. Retrospective comparison of titanium elastic nail (TEN) and reconstruction plate repair of displaced midshaft clavicular fractures. *J Shoulder Elbow Surg*. 2012;21(4):495–501.
26. Chuang TY, Ho WP, Hsieh PS, et al. Closed reduction and internal fixation for acute midshaft clavicular fractures using cannulated screws. *J Trauma*. 2006;60(6):1320–1321.
27. Collinge C, Devinney S, Herscovici D, et al. Anterior-inferior plate fixation of middle-third fractures and nonunions of the clavicle. *J Orthop Trauma*. 2006;20(10):680–686.
28. Connolly JF, Ganjianpour M. Thoracic outlet syndrome treated by double osteotomy of a clavicular malunion: A case report. *J Bone Joint Surg Am*. 2002;84-A(3):437–440.
29. Craig EV. Fractures of the clavicle. In: Rockwood CA, Green DP, Bucholz RW, Heckman JD, eds. *Rockwood and Green's Fractures in Adults*. Philadelphia, PA: Lippincott-Raven; 1996:1109–1161.
30. Craig EV. Fractures of the clavicle. In: Rockwood CA, Matsen FA, eds. *The Shoulder*. 3rd ed. Philadelphia, PA: WB Saunders; 1998:428–482.
31. Craig EV. Fractures of the clavicle. In: Rockwood CA, Matsen FA, eds. *The Shoulder*. Philadelphia, PA: WB Saunders; 1990:367–412.
32. Crenshaw AH. Fractures of the shoulder girdle, arm, and forearm. In: Willis CC, ed. *Campbell's Operative Orthopaedics*. 8th ed. St. Louis, MO: Mosby-Yearbook Inc; 1992:989–995.
33. Davids PH, Luitse JS, Strating RP, et al. Operative treatment for delayed union and nonunion of mid-shaft clavicular fractures: AO reconstruction plate fixation and early mobilization. *J Trauma*. 1996;40(6):985–986.
34. Della Santa D, Narakas A, Bonnard C. Late lesions of the brachial plexus after fracture of the clavicle. *Ann Chir Main Memb Super*. 1991;10(6):531–540.
35. Demiralp B, Atesalp AS, Sehirlioglu A, et al. Preliminary results of the use of Ilizarov fixation in clavicular non-union. *Arch Orthop Trauma Surg*. 2006;126(6):401–405.
36. Dickson JW. Death following fractured clavicle. *Br Med J*. 1952;2:666.
37. Duan X, Zhong G, Cen S, et al. Plating versus intramedullary pin or conservative treatment for midshaft fracture of clavicle: A meta-analysis of randomized controlled trials. *J Shoulder Elbow Surg*. 2011;20(6):1008–1015.
38. Dutta A, Malhotra SK, Kumar V. A fractured clavicle and vascular compression: A non-orthopedic indication of figure-of-eight bandage. *Anesth Analg*. 2003;96(3):910.
39. Ebraheim NA, An HS, Jackson WT, et al. Scapulothoracic dissociation. *J Bone Joint Surg Am*. 1988;70(3):428–432.
40. Ebraheim NA, Mekhail AO, Darwich M. Open reduction and internal fixation with bone grafting of clavicular nonunion. *J Trauma*. 1997;42(4):701–704.
41. Edelson JG. The bony anatomy of clavicular malunions. *J Shoulder Elbow Surg*. 2003;12(2):173–178.
42. Edwards DJ, Kavanagh TG, Flannery MC. Fractures of the distal clavicle: A case for fixation. *Injury*. 1992;23(1):44–46.
43. Edwards SG, Whittle AP, Wood GW. Nonoperative treatment of ipsilateral fractures of the scapula and clavicle. *J Bone Joint Surg Am*. 2000;82(6):774–780.
44. Edwards SG, Wood GW, Whittle AP. Factors associated with short form-36 outcome in nonoperative treatment for ipsilateral fractures of the clavicle and scapula. *Orthopedics*. 2002;25(7):733–738.
45. Egol KA, Connor PM, Karunakar MA, et al. The floating shoulder: Clinical and functional results. *J Bone Joint Surg Am*. 2001;83(8):1188–1194.
46. Eiff MP. Management of clavicle fractures. *Am Fam Physician*. 1997;55(1):121–128.
47. England JD, Tiel RL. AAEM case report 33: Costoclavicular mass syndrome. American Association of Electrodiagnostic Medicine. *Muscle Nerve*. 1999;22(3):412–418.
48. Enneking TJ, Hartlief MT, Fontijine WP. Rushpin fixation for midshaft clavicular non-unions: Good results in 13/14 cases. *Acta Orthop Scand*. 1999;70(5):514–516.
49. Eskola A, Vainionpaa S, Myllynen P, et al. Outcome of clavicular fracture in 89 patients. *Arch Orthop Trauma Surg*. 1986;105(6):337–338.
50. Eskola A, Vainionpaa S, Myllynen P, et al. Surgery for ununited clavicular fracture. *Acta Orthop Scand*. 1986;57(4):366–367.
51. Fann CY, Chiu FY, Chuang TY, et al. Transacromial Knowles pin in the treatment of Neer type 2 distal clavicle fractures. A prospective evaluation of 32 cases. *J Trauma*. 2004;56(5):1102–1105.
52. Ferran NA, Hodgson P, Vannet N, et al. Locked intramedullary fixation versus plating for displaced and shortened mid-shaft clavicle fractures: A randomized clinical trial. *J Shoulder Elbow Surg*. 2010;19(6):783–789.
53. Flinkkila T, Ristiniemi J, Hyvonen P, et al. Surgical treatment of unstable fractures of the distal clavicle: A comparative study of Kirschner wire and clavicular hook plate fixation. *Acta Orthop Scand*. 2002;73(1):50–53.
54. Fowler AW. Treatment of fractured clavicle. *Lancet*. 1968;1:46–47.
55. Fujita K, Matsuda K, Sakai Y, et al. Late thoracic outlet syndrome secondary to malunion of the fractured clavicle: Case report and review of the literature. *J Trauma*. 2001;50(2):332–345.
56. Goldberg JA, Bruce WJ, Sonnabend DH, et al. Type 2 fractures of the distal clavicle: A new surgical technique. *J Shoulder Elbow Surg*. 1997;6(4):380–382.
57. Golish SR, Oliviero JA, Francke EI, et al. A biomechanical study of plate versus intramedullary devices for midshaft clavicle fixation. *J Orthop Surg Res*. 2008;3(1):28.
58. Goss TP. Scapular fractures and dislocations: Diagnosis and treatment. *J Am Acad Orthop Surg*. 1995;3(1):22–33.
59. Gossard JM. Closed treatment of displaced middle-third fractures of the clavicle gives poor results [Letter to the editor]. *J Bone Joint Surg Br*. 1998;80(3):558.
60. Goswami T, Markert RJ, Anderson CG, et al. Biomechanical evaluation of a pre-contoured clavicle plate. *J Shoulder Elbow Surg*. 2008;17(5):815–818.
61. Gottschalk HP, Dumont G, Khanani S, et al. Open clavicle fractures: Patterns of trauma and associated injuries. *J Orthop Trauma*. 2012;26(2):107–109.
62. Granetzny A, Abd El-Aal M, Emam E, et al. Surgical versus conservative treatment of flail chest. Evaluation of the pulmonary status. *Interact Cardiovasc Thorac Surg*. 2005;4(6):583–587.
63. Grassi FA, Tajana MS, D'Angelo F. Management of midclavicular fractures: Comparison between nonoperative treatment and open intramedullary fixation in 80 patients. *J Trauma*. 2001;50(6):1096–1100.
64. Hall JA, Farrugia M, Potter J, et al. The radiographic quantification of scapular winging following malunion of displaced clavicular shaft fractures [abstract]. COA Abstract Supplement, June 1, 2007; 43.
65. Hashiguchi H, Ito H. Clinical outcome of the treatment of floating shoulder by osteosynthesis for clavicular fracture alone. *J Shoulder Elbow Surg*. 2003;12(6):589–591.
66. Herscovici D Jr, Fiennes AG, Allgower M, et al. The floating shoulder: Ipsilateral clavicle and scapular neck fractures. *J Bone Joint Surg Br*. 1992;74(3):362–364.
67. Herscovici D Jr, Sanders R, DiPasquale T, et al. Injuries of the shoulder girdle. *Clin Orthop Relat Res*. 1995;318:54–60.

68. Hill JM, McGuire MH, Crosby LA. Closed treatment of displaced middle-third fractures of the clavicle gives poor results. *J Bone Joint Surg Br.* 1997;79(4):537–539.

69. Howard FM, Shafer SJ. Injuries to the clavicle with neurovascular complications. A study of fourteen cases. *J Bone Joint Surg Am.* 1965;47(7):1335–1346.

70. Huang JI, Toogood P, Chen MR, et al. Clavicular anatomy and the applicability of precontoured plates. *J Bone Joint Surg Am.* 2007;89(10):2260–2265.

71. Hudak PL, Amadio PC, Bombardier C. Development of an upper extremity outcome measure: The DASH. The Upper Extremity Collaborative Group (UECG). *Am J Ind Med.* 1996;29(6):602–608.

72. Iannotti MR, Crosby LA, Stafford P, et al. Effects of plate location and selection on the stability of midshaft clavicle osteotomies: A biomechanical study. *J Shoulder Elbow Surg.* 2002;11(5):457–462.

73. Jubel A, Andermahr J, Schiffer G, et al. Elastic stable intramedullary nailing of midclavicular fractures with a titanium nail. *Clin Orthop Relat Res.* 2003;408:279–285.

74. Judd DB, Pallis MP, Smith E, et al. Acute operative stabilization versus nonoperative management of clavicle fractures. *Am J Orthop.* 2009;38(7):341–345.

75. Jupiter JB, Leffert RD. Non-union of the clavicle. Associated complications and surgical management. *J Bone Joint Surg Am.* 1987;69(5):753–760.

76. Jupiter JB, Ring D. Fractures of the clavicle. In: Iannotti JP, Williams GR, eds. *Disorders of the Shoulder: Diagnosis and Management.* Philadelphia, PA: Lippincott Williams & Wilkins; 1999.

77. Kao FC, Chao EK, Chen CH, et al. Treatment of distal clavicle fracture using Kirschner wires and tension-band wires. *J Trauma.* 2001;51(3):522–525.

78. Khan SA, Shamshery P, Gupta V, et al. Locking compression plate in long standing clavicular nonunions with poor bone stock. *J Trauma.* 2008;64(2):439–441.

79. Kim KC, Rhee KJ, Shin HD, et al. Can the glenopolar angle be used to predict outcome and treatment of the floating shoulder? *J Trauma.* 2008;64(1):174–178.

80. Klein SM, Badman BL, Keating CJ, et al. Results of surgical treatment for unstable distal clavicular fractures. *J Shoulder Elbow Surg.* 2010;19(7):1049–1055. doi: 10.1016/j.jse.2009.11.056.

81. Kleweno CP, Jawa A, Wells JH, et al. Midshaft clavicular fractures: Comparison of intramedullary pin and plate fixation. *J Shoulder Elbow Surg.* 2011;20(7):1114–1117.

82. Kloen P, Sorkin AT, Rubel IF, et al. Anteroinferior plating of midshaft clavicular nonunions. *J Orthop Trauma.* 2002;16(6):425–430.

83. Kona J, Bosse JM, Staeheli JW, et al. Type II distal clavicle fractures: A retrospective review of surgical treatment. *J Orthop Trauma.* 1990;4(2):115–120.

84. Kuhne JE. Symptomatic malunions of the middle clavicle. *J Shoulder Elbow Surg.* 1999;8(5):539. [Abstracts: Seventh International Conference on Surgery of the Shoulder, 1999.]

85. Ledger M, Leeks N, Ackland T, et al. Short malunions of the clavicle: An anatomic and functional study. *J Shoulder Elbow Surg.* 2005;14(4):349–354.

86. Lee YS, Lin CC, Huang CR, et al. Operative treatment of midclavicular fractures in 62 elderly patients: Knowles pin versus plate. *Orthopedics.* 2007;30(11):959–964.

87. Leppilahti J, Jalovaara P. Migration of Kirschner wires following fixation of the clavicle–report of 2 cases. *Acta Orthop Scand.* 1999;70(5):517–519.

88. Leung KS, Lam TP. Open reduction and internal fixation of ipsilateral fractures of the scapular neck and clavicle. *J Bone Joint Surg Am.* 1993;75(7):1015–1018.

89. Leupin S, Jupiter JB. LC-DC plating with bone graft in posttraumatic nonunions in the middle third of the clavicle. *Swiss Surg.* 1998;4(2):89–94.

90. Lewonowski K, Bassett GS. Complete posterior sternoclavicular epiphyseal separation. A case report and review of the literature. *Clin Orthop Relat Res.* 1992;281:84–88.

91. Lim M, Kang J, Kim K, et al. Anterior inferior reconstruction plates for the treatment of acute midshaft clavicle fractures. In: Proceedings from the 20th Annual Meeting of the Orthopaedic Trauma Society; Salt Lake City, Utah, 2003.

92. Low AK, Duckworth DG, Bokor DJ. Operative outcome of displaced medial-end clavicle fractures in adults. *J Shoulder Elbow Surg.* 2008;17(5):751–754.

93. Lyons FA, Rockwood CA Jr. Migration of pins used in operations on the shoulder. *J Bone Joint Surg Am.* 1990;72(8):1262–1267.

94. Manske DJ, Szabo RM. The operative treatment of mid-shaft clavicular non-unions. *J Bone Joint Surg Am.* 1985;67(9):1367–1371.

95. Marsh JL, Slongo TF, Agel J, et al. Fracture and dislocation classification compendium-2007: Orthopaedic Trauma Association classification, database and outcomes committee. *J Orthop Trauma.* 2007;21(10):S1–S33.

96. Matsumoto K, Miyamoto K, Sumi H, et al. Upper extremity injuries in snowboarding and skiing: A comparative study. *Clin J Sport Med.* 2002;12(6):354–359.

97. McCandless DN, Mowbray MA. Treatment of displaced fractures of the clavicle. Sling versus figure-of-eight bandage. *Practitioner.* 1979;223:266–267.

98. McConnell AJ, Yoo DJ, Zdero R, et al. Methods of operative fixation of the acromioclavicular joint: A biomechanical comparison. *J Orthop Trauma.* 2007;21(4):248–253.

99. McKee MD, Pedersen EM, Jones C, et al. Deficits following nonoperative treatment of displaced midshaft clavicular fractures. *J Bone Joint Surg Am.* 2006;88(1):35–40.

100. McKee MD, Seiler JG, Jupiter JB. The application of the limited contact dynamic compression plate in the upper extremity: An analysis of 114 consecutive cases. *Injury.* 1995;26(10):661–666.

101. McKee MD, Stephen DJ, Kreder HJ, et al. Functional outcome following clavicle fractures in polytrauma patients. *J Trauma.* 2000;47(3):616.

102. McKee MD, Wild LM, Schemitsch EH. Midshaft malunion of the clavicle. Surgical technique. *J Bone Joint Surg Am.* 2004;86-A(1):37–43.

103. McKee MD, Wild LM, Schemitsch EH. Midshaft malunions of the clavicle. *J Bone Joint Surg Am.* 2003;85(5):790–797.

104. McKee MD. What is the Optimal Treatment of Displaced Midshaft Clavicle Fractures? In: Wright JG, ed. *Evidence Based Orthopaedics.* Saunders Elsevier, 2009.

105. McKee RC, Whelan DB, Schemitsch EH, et al. Operative versus nonoperative care of displaced midshaft clavicular fractures: A meta-analysis of randomized clinical trials. *J Bone Joint Surg Am.* 2012;94(8):675–684.

106. Moore TO. Internal pin fixation for fracture of the clavicle. *Am Surg.* 1951;17(7):580–583.

107. Moseley HF. The clavicle: Its anatomy and function. *Clin Orthop Relat Res.* 1968;58:17–27.

108. Mullaji AB, Jupiter JB. Low-contact dynamic compression plating of the clavicle. *Injury.* 1994;25(1):41–45.

109. Naidoo P. Migration of a Kirschner wire from the clavicle into the abdominal aorta. *Arch Emerg Med.* 1991;8(4):292–295.

110. Naidu SH, Heppenstall RB, Brighton CT, et al. Clavicle non-union: Results of treatment with electricity, AO dynamic compression plating and autogenous bone grafting, and excision of the non-union in 43 patients. *Orthop Trans.* 1994;18:1072.

111. Natali J, Maraval M, Kieffer E, et al. Fractures of the clavicle and injuries of the subclavian artery. Report of 10 cases. *J Cardiovasc Surg (Torino).* 1975;16(5):541–547.

112. Neer CS. Fractures of the Clavicle. In: Rockwood CA, Green DP, eds. *Fractures in Adults.* 2nd ed. Philadelphia, PA: JB Lippincott; 1984:707–713.

113. Neer CS. Fractures of the distal clavicle with detachment of the coracoclavicular ligaments in adults. *J Trauma.* 1963;3:99–110.

114. Neer CS. Fractures of the distal third of the clavicle. *Clin Orthop Relat Res.* 1968;58:43–50.

115. Neer CS. Nonunion of the clavicle. *J Am Med Assoc.* 1960;172:1006–1011.

116. Neviaser JS. The treatment of fractures of the clavicle. *Surg Clin North Am.* 1963;43:1555–1563.

117. Neviaser RJ, Neviaser JS, Neviaser TJ, et al. A simple technique for internal fixation of the clavicle. A long term evaluation. *Clin Orthop Relat Res.* 1975;109:103–107.

118. Neviaser RJ. Injuries to the clavicle and **acromioclavicular** joint. *Orthop Clin North Am.* 1987;18(3):433–438.

119. Ngarmukos C, Parkpian V, Patradul A. Fixation of fractures of the midshaft of the clavicle with Kirschner wires. Results in 108 patients. *J Bone Joint Surg Br.* 1998;80(1):106–108.

120. Nordback I, Markkula H. Migration of Kirschner pin from clavicle into ascending aorta. *Acta Chir Scand.* 1985;151(2):177–179.

121. Nordqvist A, Petersson C, Redlund-Johnell I. The natural course of lateral clavicle fracture. 15 (11–21) year follow-up of 110 cases. *Acta Orthop Scand.* 1993;64(1):87–91.

122. Nordqvist A, Petersson C. The incidence of fractures of the clavicle. *Clin Orthop Relat Res.* 1994;300:127–132.

123. Nordqvist A, Petersson CJ, Redlund-Johnell I. Mid-clavicle fractures in adults: End result study after conservative treatment. *J Orthop Trauma.* 1998;12(8):572–576.

124. Nordqvist A, Redlund-Johnell I, von Scheele A, et al. Shortening of clavicle after fracture. Incidence and clinical significance, a 5-year follow-up of 85 patients. *Acta Orthop Scand.* 1997;68(4):349–351.

125. Nowak J, Holgersson M, Larsson S. Can we predict long-term sequelae after fractures of the clavicle based on initial findings? A prospective study with nine to ten years follow-up. *J Shoulder Elbow Surg.* 2004;13(5):479–486.

126. Nowak J, Mallmin H, Larsson S. The aetiology and epidemiology of clavicular fractures. A prospective study during a two-year period in Uppsala, Sweden. *Injury.* 2000;35(5):353–358.

127. O'Connor D, Kutty S, McCabe JP. Long-term functional outcome assessment of plate fixation and autogenous bone grafting for clavicular non-union. *Injury.* 2004;35(6):575–579.

128. O'Rourke IC, Middleton RW. The place and efficacy of operative management of fractured clavicle. *Injury.* 1975;6(3):236–240.

129. Oe K, Gaul L, Hierholzer C, et al. Operative management of periarticular medial clavicle fractures-report of 10 cases. *J Trauma.* 2011.

130. Ogden JA. Distal clavicular physeal injury. *Clin Orthop Relat Res.* 1984;188:68–73.

131. Oh CW, Kyung HS, Kim PT, et al. Failure of internal fixation of the clavicle in the treatment of ipsilateral clavicle and glenoid neck fractures. *J Orthop Sci.* 2001;6(6):601–603.

132. Oh JH, Kim SH, Lee JH, et al. Treatment of distal clavicle fracture: A systematic review of treatment modalities in 425 fractures. *Arch Orthop Trauma Surg.* 2011;131(4):525–533.

133. Olsen BS, Vaesel MT, Sojbjerg JO. Treatment of midshaft clavicular nonunion with plate fixation and autologous bone grafting. *J Shoulder Elbow Surg.* 1995;4(5):337–344.

134. Ord RA, Langdon JD. Stress fracture of the clavicle. A rare late complication of radical neck dissection. *J Maxillofac Surg.* 1986;14(5):281–284.

135. Oroko PK, Buchan M, Winkler A, et al. Does shortening matter after clavicular fractures? *Bull Hosp Jt Dis.* 1999;58(1):6–8.

136. Owens BD, Goss TP. The floating shoulder. *J Bone Joint Surg Br.* 2006;88B(11):1419–1424.

137. Pearson AM, Tosteson AN, Koval KJ, et al. Is surgery for displaced, midshaft clavicle fractures in adults cost-effective? Results based on a multicenter randomized, controlled trial. *J Orthop Trauma.* 2010;24(7):426–433.

138. Pedersen MS, Kristiansen B, Thomsen F, et al. [Conservative treatment of clavicular fractures]. *Ugeskr Laeger.* 1993;155(47):3832–3834.

139. Petracic B. [Efficiency of a rucksack bandage in the treatment of clavicle fractures]. *Unfallchirurgie.* 1983;9(1):41–43.

140. Poigenfurst J, Rappold G, Fischer W. Plating of fresh clavicular fractures: Results of 122 operations. *Injury.* 1992;23(4):237–241.

141. Poigenfurst J, Reiler T, Fischer W. [Plating of fresh clavicular fractures. Experience with 60 operations]. *Unfallchirurgie.* 1988;14(1):26–37.

142. Post M. Current concepts in the treatment of fractures of the clavicle. *Clin Orthop Relat Res.* 1989;245:89–101.

143. Potter JM, Jones C, Wild LM, et al. Does delay matter? The restoration of objectively measured shoulder strength and patient-oriented outcome after immediate fixation versus delayed reconstruction of displaced midshaft fractures of the clavicle. *J Shoulder Elbow Surg.* 2007;16(5):514–518.

144. Pyper JB. Non-union of fractures of the clavicle. *Injury.* 1978;9(4):268–270.

145. Ramos L, Mencia R, Alonso A, et al. Conservative treatment of ipsilateral fractures of the scapula and clavicle. *J Trauma.* 1997;42(2):239–242.

146. Rasyid HN, Nakajima T, Hamada K, et al. Winging of the scapula caused by disruption of "sternoclaviculoscapular linkage": Report of 2 cases. *J Shoulder Elbow Surg.* 2000;9(2):144–147.

147. Reichenbacher D, Siebler G. Early secondary lesions of the brachial plexus–A rare complication following clavicular fracture. *Unfallchirurgie.* 1987;13(2):91–92.

148. Renger RJ, de Bruijn AJ, Aarts HC, et al. Endovascular treatment of a pseudoaneurysm of the subclavian artery. *J Trauma.* 2003;55(5):969–971.

149. Riemer BL, Butterfield SL, Daffner RH, et al. The abduction lordotic view of the clavicle: A new technique for radiographic visualization. *J Orthop Trauma.* 1991;5(4):392–394.

150. Rikli D, Regazzoni P, Renner N. The unstable shoulder girdle: Early functional treatment utilizing open reduction and internal fixation. *J Orthop Trauma.* 1995;9(2):93–97.

151. Ring D, Holovacs T. Brachial plexus palsy after intramedullary fixation of a clavicular fracture. A report of three cases. *J Bone Joint Surg Am.* 2005;87(8):1834–1837.

152. Ristevski B, Hall JA, Pearce D, et al. The radiographic quantification of scapular malalignment after malunion of displaced clavicular shaft fractures. *J Shoulder Elbow Surg.* 2012;22(2):240–246.

153. Robinson CM, Cairns DA. Primary nonoperative treatment of displaced lateral fractures of the clavicle. *J Bone Joint Surg Am.* 2004;86-A(4):778–782.

154. Robinson CM, Court-Brown CM, McQueen MM, et al. Estimating the risk of nonunion following nonoperative treatment of a clavicle fracture. *J Bone Joint Surg Am.* 2004;86-A(7):1359–1365.

155. Robinson CM. Fractures of the clavicle in the adult. Epidemiology and classification. *J Bone Joint Surg Br.* 1998;80(3):476–484.

156. Rockwood CA. Fractures of the outer clavicle in children and adults. *J Bone Joint Surg Br.* 1982;64:642.

157. Rokito AS, Zuckerman JD, Shaari JM, et al. A comparison of nonoperative and operative treatment of type II distal clavicle fractures. *Bull Hosp Jt Dis.* 2003;61(1–2):32–39.

158. Rosenberg N, Neumann L, Wallace AW. Functional outcome of surgical treatment of symptomatic nonunion and malunion of midshaft clavicle fractures. *J Shoulder Elbow Surg.* 2007;16(5):510–513.

159. Roset-Llobet J, Sala-Orfila JM. Sports-related stress fracture of the clavicle: A case report. *Int Orthop.* 1998;22(4):266–268.

160. Rowe CR. An atlas of anatomy and treatment of midclavicular fractures. *Clin Orthop Relat Res.* 1968;58:29–42.

161. Rumball KM, Da Silva VF, Preston DN, et al. Brachial-plexus injury after clavicular fracture: Case report and literature review. *Can J Surg.* 1991;34(3):264–266.

162. Russo R, Visconti V, Lorini S, et al. Displaced comminuted midshaft clavicle fractures: Use of Mennen plate fixation system. *J Trauma.* 2007;63(4):951–954.

163. Sakellarides H. Pseudarthrosis of the clavicle: A report of twenty cases. *J Bone Joint Surg Am.* 1961;43:130–138.

164. Schemitsch LA, Schemitsch EH, Veillette C, et al. Function plateaus by one year in patients with surgically treated displaced midshaft clavicle fractures. *Clin Orthop Relat Res.* 2011;469(12):3351–3355.

165. Schuind F, Pay-Pay E, Andrianne Y, et al. External fixation of the clavicle for fracture or non-union in adults. *J Bone Joint Surg Am.* 1988;70(5):692–695.

166. Schwarz N, Hocker K. Osteosynthesis of irreducible fractures of the clavicle with 2.7 mm ASIF plates. *J Trauma.* 1992;33(2):179–183.

167. Seo GS, Aoki J, Karakida O, et al. Nonunion of a medical clavicular fracture following radical neck dissection: MRI diagnosis. *Orthopedics.* 1999;22(10):985–986.

168. Shackford SR, Connolly JF. Taming of the screw: A case report and literature review of limb-threatening complications after plate osteosynthesis of a clavicular nonunion. *J Trauma.* 2003;55(5):840–843.

169. Shellhaas JS, Glaser DL, Drezner JA. Distal clavicular stress fracture in a female weight lifter: A case report. *Am J Sports Med.* 2004;32(7):1755–1758.

170. Shen WJ, Liu TJ, Shen YS. Plate fixation of fresh displaced midshaft clavicle fractures. *Injury.* 1999;30(7):497–500.

171. Sinha A, Edwin J, Sreeharsha B, et al. A radiological study to define safe zones for drilling during plating of clavicle fractures. *J Bone Joint Surg Br.* 2011;93(9):1247–1252.

172. Smekal V, Deml C, Irenberger A, et al. Length determination in midshaft clavicle fractures: Validation of measurement. *J Orthop Trauma.* 2008;22(7):458–462

173. Smekal V, Irenberger A, Struve P, et al. Elastic stable intramedullary nailing versus nonoperative treatment of displaced midshaft clavicular fractures-a randomized, controlled, clinical trial. *J Orthop Trauma.* 2009;23(2):106–112.

174. Smith CA, Rudd J, Crosby LA. Results of operative versus non-operative treatment for 100% displaced mid-shaft clavicle. In: Proceedings from the 16th annual open meeting of the American shoulder and elbow surgeons; Orlando, Florida, March 18, 2000, 41.

175. Smith J, Dietrich CT, Kotajarvi BR, et al. The effect of scapular protraction on isometric shoulder rotation strength in normal subjects. *J Shoulder Elbow Surg.* 2006;15(3):339–343.

176. Spar I. Total claviculectomy for pathological fractures. *Clin Orthop Relat Res.* 1977;129:236–237.

177. Spencer EE, Kuhn JE. Biomechanical analysis of reconstructions for sternoclavicular joint instability. *J Bone Joint Surg Am.* 2004;86-A(1):98–105.

178. Stanley D, Norris SH. Recovery following fractures of the clavicle treated conservatively. *Injury.* 1988;19(3):162–164.

179. Stanley D, Trowbridge EA, Norris SH. The mechanism of clavicular fracture. A clinical and biomechanical analysis. *J Bone Joint Surg Br.* 1988;70(3):461–464.

180. Strauss EJ, Egol KA, France MA, et al. Complications of intramedullary Hagie pin fixation for acute midshaft clavicle fractures. *J Shoulder Elbow Surg.* 2007;16(3):280–284.

181. Taitsman L, Nork SE, Coles CP, et al. Open clavicle fractures and associated injuries. *J Orthop Trauma.* 2006;20(6):396–399.

182. Tan HL, Zhao JK, Qian C, et al. Clinical results of treatment using a clavicular hook plate versus a T-plate in neer type II distal clavicle fractures. *Orthopedics.* 2012;35(8):e1191–e1197.

183. Tanaka H, Yukioka T, Yamaguti Y, et al. Surgical stabilization of internal pneumatic stabilization? A prospective randomized study of management of severe flail chest patients. *J Trauma.* 2002;52(4):727–732.

184. Tarar MN, Quaba AA. An adipofascial turnover flap for soft tissue cover around the clavicle. *Br J Plast Surg.* 1995;48(3):161–164.

185. Throckmorton T, Kuhn JE. Fractures of the medial end of the clavicle. *J Shoulder Elbow Surg.* 2007;16(1):49–54.

186. Tomic S, Bumbasirevic M, Lesic A, et al. Modification of the Ilizarov external fixator for aseptic hypertrophic nonunion of the clavicle: An option for treatment. *J Orthop Trauma.* 2006;20(2):122–128.

187. Tse DH, Slabaugh PB, Carlson PA. Injury to the axillary artery by a closed fracture of the clavicle. A case report. *J Bone Joint Surg Am.* 1980;62(8):1372–1374.

188. van Noort A, te Slaa RL, Marti RK, et al. The floating shoulder. A multicentre study. *J Bone Joint Surg Br.* 2001;83(6):795–798.

189. Vander Have KL, Perdue AM, Caird MS, et al. Operative versus nonoperative treatment of midshaft clavicle fractures in adolescents. *J Pediatr Orthop.* 2010;30(4):307–312.

190. Verborgt O, Pittoors K, Van Glabbeek F, et al. Plate fixation of middle-third fractures of the clavicle in the semi-professional athlete. *Acta Orthop Belg.* 2005;71(1):17–21.

191. Veysi VT, Mittal R, Agarwal S, et al. Multiple trauma and scapula fractures: So what? *J Trauma.* 2003;55(6):1145–1147.

192. Virtanen KJ, Remes V, Pajarinen J, et al. Sling compared with plate osteosynthesis for treatment of displaced midshaft clavicular fractures: A randomized clinical trial. *J Bone Joint Surg Am.* 2012;94(17):1546–1553.

193. Webber MC, Haines JF. The treatment of lateral clavicle fractures. *Injury.* 2000;31(3):175–179.

194. Weinberg B, Seife B, Alonso P. The apical oblique view of the clavicle: Its usefulness in neonatal and childhood trauma. *Skeletal Radiol.* 1991;20(3):201–203.

195. White RR, Anson PS, Kristiansen T, et al. Adult clavicle fractures: Relationship between mechanism of injury and healing. *Orthop Trans.* 1989;13:514–515.

196. Wick M, Muller EJ, Kollig E, et al. Midshaft fractures of the clavicle with a shortening of more than 2 cm predispose to nonunion. *Arch Orthop Trauma Surg.* 2001;121(4):207–211.

197. Wilkins RM, Johnston RM. Ununited fractures of the clavicle. *J Bone Joint Surg Am.* 1983;65(6):773–778.

198. Williams GR Jr., Silverberg DA, Iannotti JP, et al. Non-operative treatment of ipsilateral clavicle and glenoid neck fractures. American shoulder and elbow surgeons 15th Open Meeting, Anaheim, CA: 1999.

199. Williams GR, Koffler K, Pepe M, et al. Rotation of the clavicular portion of the pectoralis major for soft-tissue coverage of the clavicle. An anatomical study and case report. *J Bone Joint Surg Am.* 2000;82(12):1736–1742.

200. Williams GR, Naranja J, Klimkiewicz J, et al. The floating shoulder: A biomechanical basis for classification and management. *J Bone Joint Surg Am.* 2001;83-A(8):1182–1187.

201. Witzel K. Intramedullary osteosynthesis in fractures of the mid-third of the clavicle in sports traumatology. *Z Orthop Unfall.* 2007;145(5):639–642.

202. Wood VE. The results of total claviculectomy. *Clin Orthop Relat Res.* 1986;207:186–190.

203. Wu CC, Shih CH, Chen, WJ et al. Treatment of clavicular aseptic nonunion: Comparison of plating and intra medullary nailing techniques. *J Trauma.* 1998;45(3):512–516.

204. Yamaguchi H, Arakawa H, Kobayashi M. Results of the Bosworth method for unstable fractures of the distal clavicle. *Int Orthop.* 1998;22(6):366–368.

205. Yian EH, Ramappa AJ, Arneberg O, et al. The Constant score in normal shoulders. *J Shoulder Elbow Surg.* 2005;14(2):128–133.

206. Zaslav KR, Ray S, Neer CS 2nd. Conservative management of a displaced medial clavicular physeal injury in an adolescent athlete. A case report and literature review. *Am J Sports Med.* 1989;17(6):833–836.

207. Zelle BA, Pape HC, Gerich TG, et al. Functional outcome following scapulothoracic dissociation. *J Bone Joint Surg Am.* 2004;86-A(1):2–8.

208. Zenni EJ Jr., Krieg JK, Rosen MJ. Open reduction and internal fixation of clavicular fractures. *J Bone Joint Surg Am.* 1981;63(1):147–151.

209. Zlowodzki M, Zelle BA, Cole PA, et al. Treatment of acute midshaft clavicle fractures: Systematic review of 2144 fractures: On behalf of the Evidence-Based Orthopaedic Trauma Working Group. *J Orthop Trauma,* 2005;19(7):504–507.

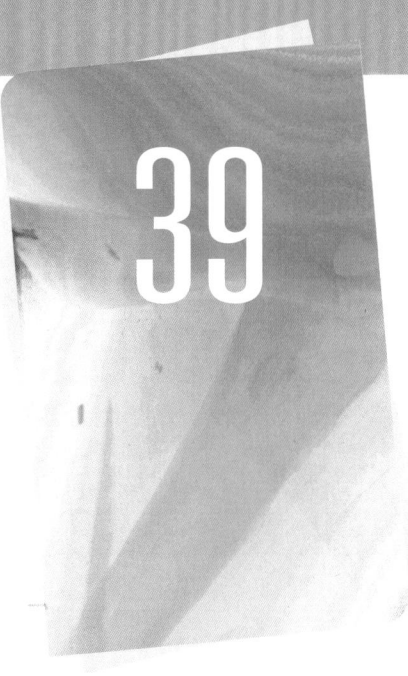

39 | SCAPULAR FRACTURES

Jan Bartoníček

INTRODUCTION TO SCAPULA FRACTURES

Scapula fractures occur relatively infrequently. According to various studies, they account for 0.4% to 0.9% of all fractures and for about 3% to 5% of all fractures of the shoulder girdle.[38,157,159] The reason for such low incidences is that the scapula is well protected against injury by a robust muscular envelope, the surrounding bones (clavicle, humerus), and its mobility and location on the elastic chest wall. Scapula fractures result mostly from high-energy trauma and, therefore, are often found in polytrauma patients. They are, as a rule, unilateral. Bilateral or open fractures are rare.[85] Scapula fractures occur predominantly in men (72%) with the mean age of 44 years.[191]

Until recently, little attention had been paid to these fractures. Of late, however, interest in scapula fractures has grown and the debate increasingly focuses on their operative treatment.[31,35,51,90,94,102,119,120,128,137,138,192,200]

ANATOMY RELATING TO SCAPULA FRACTURES

The scapula, together with the clavicle, comprises the shoulder girdle. The scapula is attached to the axial skeleton solely by the clavicle, or, more specifically, by the acromioclavicular (AC) and sternoclavicular (SC) joints. The scapula is enveloped in multiple layers of muscles and is separated from the chest wall by thin gliding fibrofatty tissue, allowing its smooth excursion over the chest wall. Thanks to its relatively free connection with the axial skeleton, the scapula is mobile but at the same time provides an efficient support to the humeral head. As a result, compression forces are optimally transmitted from the upper limb to the shoulder girdle, without compromising stability and mobility of the glenohumeral joint.

Scapula Architecture

The basic part of the scapula is the body, which is triangular, when viewed anteroposteriorly, with its base situated superiorly and its apex inferiorly. The triangle is bounded by its three borders (superior, medial, and lateral) and three angles (superior, inferior, and lateral). Although the bone at the former two angles is relatively thin, the lateral angle gets gradually thicker to form the scapular neck, bearing the articular surface—the glenoid fossa. The hook-shaped coracoid process curves forward from the superior surface of the scapular neck. On the posterior

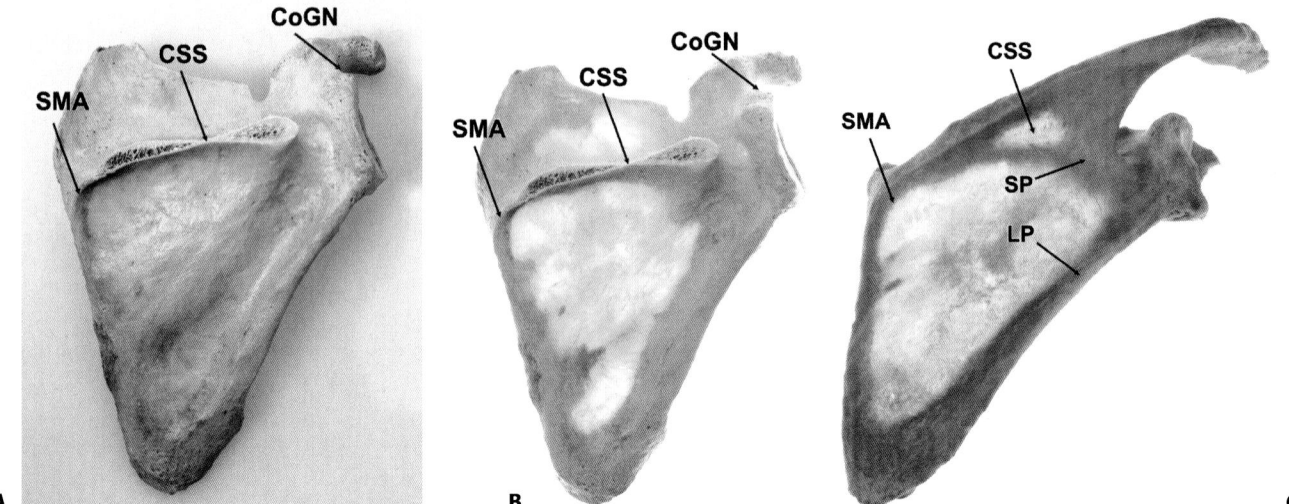

FIGURE 39-1 Anatomy and internal architecture of the right scapula: **A:** Posterior aspect of scapula after resection of scapular spine. **B:** The same specimen transilluminated. **C:** Posteroinferior aspect of transilluminated scapula. SMA, spinomedial angle; CSS, the thinner center of scapular spine; CoGN, coracoglenoidal notch; SP, spinal pillar; LP, lateral pillar.

surface of the scapular body there arises a prominent plate of bone—the scapular spine—gradually becoming more elevated and ending in a flattened bony process—the acromion—curving forward.

The distribution of the bony mass of the scapula is highly uneven, with areas of thick bone and areas that are almost translucent.[26,181,188] When held up to the light, the scapula shows the highest concentration of bony mass in the glenoid, the scapular neck, including the base of the coracoid process and the lateral border of the scapular body (Fig. 39-1).

Extending between the glenoid and the scapular body are two bony pillars that transmit compression forces from the glenoid fossa.[108] The lateral pillar, part of which is the lateral border, connects the inferior border of the glenoid with the inferior angle. The spinal pillar arises from the central part of the glenoid and continues medially to become part of the base of the scapular spine. Its course can be seen better by viewing the scapula from the front against the light. From the posterior view it is evident that the two pillars connected by a markedly thinner medial border of the scapular body are the basic load-bearing structure of the scapular body. This triangle constitutes the *biomechanical body of the scapula,* as the superior angle and the adjacent part of the supraspinous fossa form merely an appendage, which serves as a surface of insertion or origin of muscles, but does not transmit compression forces from the glenoid. Therefore, it is necessary to distinguish between the *anatomical and biomechanical bodies of the scapula.*[181]

The weakest area of the circumference of the biomechanical body of the scapula is the connection of the scapular spine and the medial border of the scapula, the *spinomedial angle.* In the majority of scapula body fractures one of the main fracture lines passes through this region. Another area of weak bone is in the central part of the scapular spine where fracture lines can also be seen fairly frequently.

Superior Shoulder Suspensory Complex

The superior shoulder suspensory complex (SSSC) was defined by Goss.[70] The SSSC is a bony and soft tissue ring composed of the glenoid process, coracoid process, coracoclavicular (CC) ligament, lateral clavicle, AC joint, and acromion (Fig. 39-2). This ring is connected by two bony struts. The superior strut consists of the middle third of the clavicle, whereas the inferior strut is the junction of the most lateral portion of the scapular body and the most medial portion of the scapular neck. Goss subdivided the whole complex into three units: The clavicular–AC joint–acromial strut; the junction of the glenoid, coracoid, and acromion with the scapular body; and the clavicular–coracoclavicular ligamentous–coracoid linkage. The complex as a whole maintains a normal stable relationship between the scapula and upper extremity and the axial skeleton, allows limited motion to occur through the AC joint and the CC ligament and provides a firm point of attachment for several soft tissue structures.

Muscles of the Scapula

In total, 18 muscles are attached to the scapula. Only three of them, namely the subscapularis, supraspinatus, and infraspinatus, originate from the broad surface of the scapula in their respective fossae. Other muscles insert into, or originate from, the borders of the scapula or its processes.

The muscles of the scapula may be divided into two systems. The first, the scapuloaxial system connects the scapula with the axial skeleton, particularly the vertebral column and the chest wall. This system controls movement of the scapula over the chest wall. The second, the scapulobrachial system is

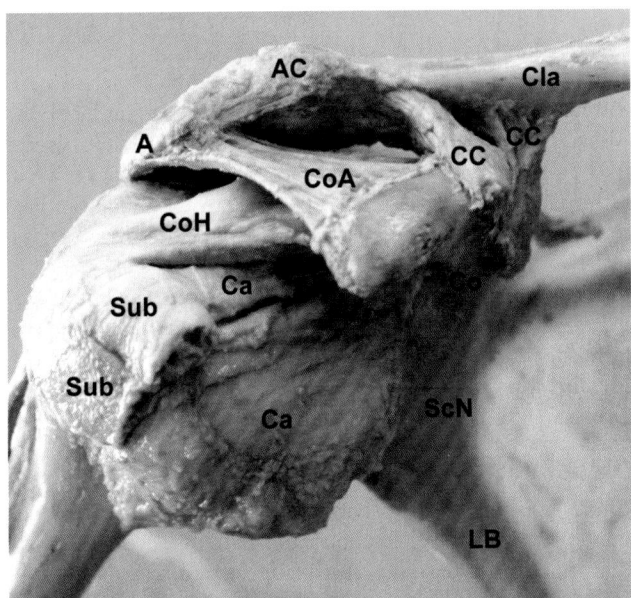

FIGURE 39-2 Superior shoulder suspensory complex (SSSC), anterior aspect of the right scapula. A, acromion; AC, acromioclavicular joint; Ca, articular capsule of glenohumeral joint; Cla, clavicle; Co, coracoid process; CoA, coracoacromial ligament; CoH, coracohumeral ligament; CC, coracoclavicular ligament; LB, lateral border of scapular body; ScN, scapular neck; Sub, insertion of subscapularis tendon into lesser tuberosity.

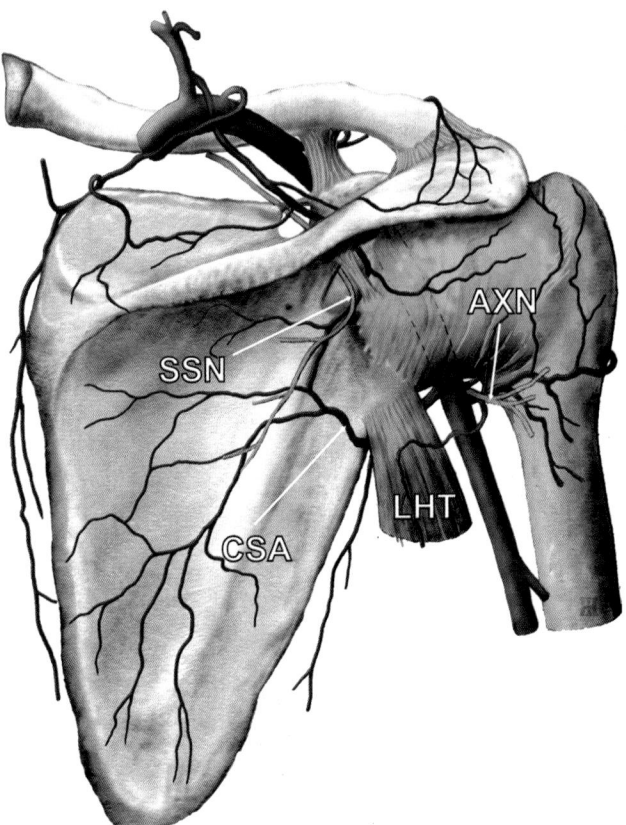

FIGURE 39-3 Course of suprascapular neurovascular bundle on posterior aspect of the right scapula. AXN, axillary nerve; CSA, circumflex suprascapular artery; LHT, long head of triceps; SSN, suprascapular nerve accompanied by suprascapular artery.

formed by the muscles originating from the scapula and attaching to the bones of arm, that is, the humerus, proximal radius, and proximal ulna. Its task is to control movements between the scapula and arm.

The scapula, thereby, integrates activity of the two groups of muscles and provides optimal support for the humeral head during motion.

Blood Vessels and Nerves of the Scapula

A number of blood vessels and nerves pass in the region of the scapula. However, only the suprascapular nerve and vessels and the scapular circumflex artery are intimately related to it.

The suprascapular nerve arises from the supraclavicular part of the brachial plexus. Together with the suprascapular vessels, it travels posteriorly through the scapular notch and then along the bottom of the supraspinatous fossa, covered by the supraspinatus muscle belly. At the bottom of the fossa, the trunk sends motor branches medially to the supraspinatus, and to the upper portion of the infraspinatus. The main suprascapular nerve descends around the base of the lateral border of the scapular spine, through the spinoglenoid notch, to the infraspinous fossa, passing under the spinoglenoid ligament. Then it runs medially and splits into several motor branches to supply the distal portion of the infraspinatus (Fig. 39-3).

The scapular circumflex artery curves around the lateral border of the scapular body to the posterior surface of the scapula about 3 cm distal to the inferior border of the glenoid. It passes through the teres minor and usually splits into two

branches, one entering the anterior surface of the infraspinatus and the other anastomosing in the spinoglenoid groove with the suprascapular artery.

INJURY ASSESSMENT OF SCAPULA FRACTURES

A knowledge of injury mechanisms, and careful clinical and radiologic examinations are essential to determine the proper diagnosis.

Mechanisms of Injury for Scapula Fractures

The mechanism of scapula fractures varies. Most often the fracture is caused by a direct blow to the scapula, during a traffic accident, or a fall from height, or by the fall of a heavy object on the shoulder.[12,30] The fracture pattern depends on the shape of the object, the energy of the blow, and the force vector.

Scapula fractures may be caused by the humeral head, either by its direct impact on the surrounding processes of the scapula, or as a result of its dislocation over the rim of the glenoid fossa. In cases of a direct impact, the fracture pattern is determined by the position of the arm at the time of injury.[14] With the arm in abduction, the humeral head is driven against the inferior glenoid, which separates off, together with some, or all, of the lateral border of the scapula. With the arm in adduction, a blow on the elbow along the axis of the humerus proximally dislocates the humeral head, which hits the acromion or the coracoid.[73,106] Anterior dislocation of the humeral head may result in separation of the anteroinferior rim of the glenoid fossa, whereas posterior dislocation may cause a fracture of the posterior rim of the glenoid fossa.[66]

Scapula fractures may also be caused by a violent muscle contracture, mostly as a result of electrical injury, or epileptic seizure.[91] Typical of this mechanism are compression fractures of the scapular body, fractures of the glenoid, or avulsion of the part of the bone carrying a muscle attachment. Avulsion fracture of the coracoid caused by pull of the CC ligament is described in AC dislocation.[112,116] Scapula fractures resulting from gunshot injuries or pathologic fractures (bone cyst, osteodystrophy, tumor metastasis) are quite rare. Fatigue fractures of the coracoid have been described in athletes and fatigue fractures of the scapular spine and the acromion are described in cases of insufficiency of the rotator cuff.[29,78,171]

Associated Injuries with Scapula Fractures

Most scapular injuries are caused by medium- to high-energy violence. As a result, these fractures are often associated with other injuries and may be found not infrequently in polytrauma patients. These associated injuries are of different severity and affect both the shoulder girdle and other parts of the body. Some of them occur commonly with scapula fractures, for example, rib fractures, whereas others are rare, such as a fracture of the scapular body penetrating through the chest wall.[170]

Isolated scapula fractures are less frequent. In the relevant literature, their incidence ranges between 14% and 33% of all scapula fractures,[9,12,24,86,110,119,135,174,180] although Thompson[178] recorded only 1.8% of such single injuries in a group of 56 patients.

Fractures of the ribs are the most frequent injuries associated with scapula fractures which is not surprising in view of its location on the rib cage.[9,12,57,82,98,174,180,187] Their frequency ranges from 27%[98] up to 65%.[180] Such a wide range may have several explanations. The study by Imatani[98] was published in 1975, when rib fractures were diagnosed only by radiographs. By contrast, in all patients in the Tuček's[180] group a CT scan was obtained, capturing the surrounding ribs. Another reason may be an increase in the number of high-energy traumas with a much higher incidence of associated injuries, including rib fractures.

Injuries to the thoracic cavity and lungs, such as pneumothorax, hemothorax, emphysema, and lung contusion, have been reported in 16% to 67% of cases.[82,136,166,170,174,187]

Injuries to the shoulder girdle, that is to the clavicle, proximal humerus, and AC joint occur in between 8% and 47% of cases of scapula fracture.[12,119,180] The reason for the wide range may be that some authors focused merely on clavicular fractures, whereas others also included AC joint dislocation.

Head injuries, that is cerebral contusion, intracerebral hemorrhage, and fractures of the skull occur in 10% to 42% of all cases of scapula fracture.[12,110,135,174,180]

Other injuries occur at variable rates in groups of patients described by individual authors. Certain groups show a higher share of pelvic injuries, sometimes up to 20%.[174] In contrast, Tuček recorded only one fracture of the acetabulum in 25 cases. Thompson[178] described injuries to major blood vessels in the shoulder region (brachial, subclavian, and axillary arteries) in 10% of cases. In addition to blood vessels, injuries may involve also the brachial plexus. Scapula fractures may be associated, additionally, with other injuries to the skeleton including fractures of thoracic, or lumbar, vertebrae, distal humerus, forearm, femoral shaft, proximal tibia, tibial shaft, ankle, metatarsals, or even subtalar dislocations.[180]

Mortality in scapula fractures is reported to vary between 2% and 14%.[9,35,174,178,191]

Signs and Symptoms of Scapula Fractures

Clinical examination of patients with scapular injuries depends on the patient's general condition. In polytrauma patients, where the priority is to save life, the treatment of a scapula fracture, even if identified during primary examination, may be postponed to a later time. An exception is an open scapula fracture. In a number of polytrauma patients, scapula fractures are often found coincidentally on a radiograph or a CT scan of the chest.[176]

Patients in a less severe general condition who are able to communicate may undergo standard clinical examination. As scapula fractures are often associated with other injuries, it is essential first to make a thorough comprehensive examination of the patient and only then to focus on the shoulder. Where one fracture of a shoulder girdle is found, for example, that of the clavicle, it is necessary to exclude other potential injuries in the same area.

Patient's medical history: A knowledge of the exact mechanism of the injury and the patient's subjective complaints are essential to a successful diagnosis.

Visual assessment: Careful examination is performed of the shoulder and the entire chest, including the axilla. The shoulder may be deformed by a clavicle fracture, an AC dislocation, a shoulder dislocation, a displaced scapula fracture, or by significant swelling. The skin should be examined as a skin abrasion may indicate a site of impact.

Palpation: A large part of the skeleton of the shoulder girdle may be examined by palpation, that is, the clavicle, SC joint, AC joint, the acromion and scapular spine, the tip of the coracoid, and the humeral head; in less muscular individuals also the inferior angle and medial border of the scapula. Palpation may reveal crepitus, or pathologic mobility. It is also important to palpate the axilla and the adjacent chest. As the fracture may be combined with a lesion of the brachial plexus or vascular injury, it is important to examine distal neurovascular function.

Range of motion: Examination of the range of motion, mainly the active motion, in scapula fractures is limited by pain. If possible, passive motion in the glenohumeral joint is carefully examined.

Periphery: A thorough assessment of other parts of the ipsilateral extremity should be undertaken to exclude associated injuries.

Imaging and Other Diagnostic Methods for Scapula Fractures

Radiologic examination is essential for the diagnosis of scapula fractures, the determination of the fracture patterns, and the method of treatment. Other imaging methods may include MRI and ultrasound scanning, although they are indicated only exceptionally and their contribution is limited.[134] As scapula fractures often occur in polytrauma patients, the radiodiagnostic algorithm described below has to be adjusted to the patient's general condition.

Radiology

Anteroposterior radiograph of the entire shoulder girdle covering the whole scapula, the whole clavicle, AC and SC joints, and proximal humerus is part of the basic examination in a suspected scapula fracture. It provides general information about the whole shoulder girdle. Scapula fractures are often associated with a clavicular fracture, less frequently with a proximal humeral fracture or AC dislocation. This projection is usually not sufficient to determine the fracture pattern and displacement of fragments. Therefore, in cases of a suspected scapula fracture it should be combined with both Neer projections.

Neer I projection, the true anteroposterior radiograph of the scapula, is used to assess the glenohumeral joint space, displacement of the glenoid in relation to the lateral border of the scapula, and to measure the glenopolar angle (GPA).[20]

Neer II projection, also called Y-view, is a true lateral scapula projection. This projection allows assessment of scapular body fractures in terms of translation, angulation, and overlap of fragments, particularly of the lateral border. In addition, it displays clearly the relationship between the acromion and the lateral clavicle, and can be used to identify any avulsion of the anterior rim of the glenoid.

A chest radiograph in polytrauma patients is often the first examination in which a diagnosis of a scapula fracture is suspected. It is important mostly for assessment of the position of both scapulae in relation to the spine (scapulothoracic dissociation).

Other special projections, axillary in particular, are recommended by some authors as complementary views, to diagnose fractures of the glenoid, acromion, and coracoid.[31,72,102] However, for most patients with a scapular or rib fracture an axillary projection is painful. In addition, it should not be a substitute for CT examination.

CT Scans

CT examination has fundamentally changed the radiodiagnostics of scapula fractures.[16,29,43,133,175] It is always indicated when radiographic examination does not reveal the exact fracture pattern, involvement of the articular surface, or displacement.

CT transverse sections are very useful in the assessment of the glenoid fossa. They may also reveal undisplaced fractures of the scapular processes, especially those of the coracoid and acromion. However, they do not provide a three-dimensional image of the fracture anatomy.

Two-dimensional CT reconstructions (2D CT), mainly in the frontal plane, are used to assess the glenoid articular surface, especially in fractures of the base of the coracoid process involving the glenoid fossa.

Three-dimensional CT reconstructions (3D CT) are the only way to obtain a reliable determination of the fracture pattern, particularly in fractures of the scapular body and neck, although they do not show fine fracture lines, especially in minimally displaced fragments. Reconstructions should be made in several basic views, preferably with subtraction of ribs, clavicle, and proximal humerus. The *posterior view* (Fig. 39-4B) allows assessment of the course of fracture lines with regard to the scapular spine. The *anterior view* (Fig. 39-4A) is important in

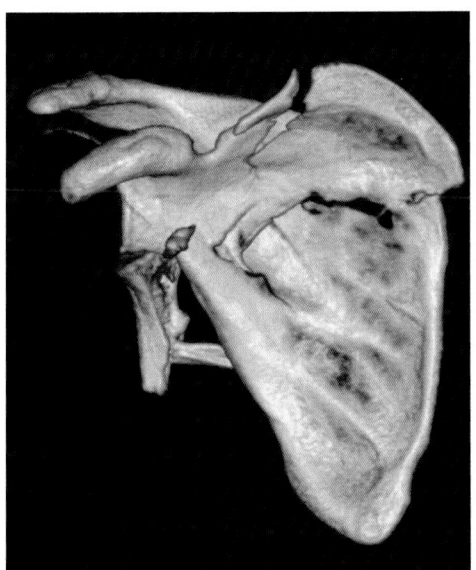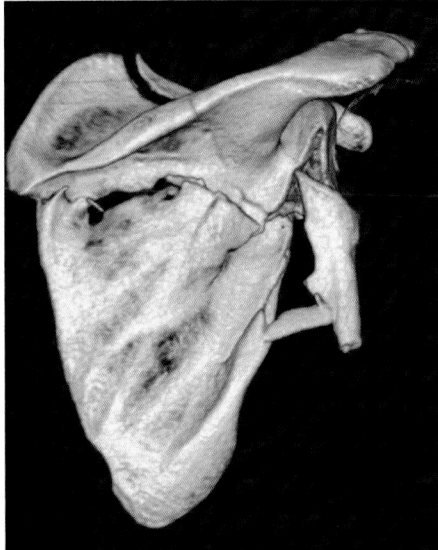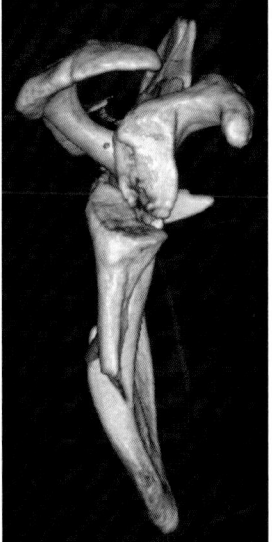

A, B

C

FIGURE 39-4 Three standardized views of the scapula in 3D CT reconstructions. **A:** Anterior aspect. **B:** Posterior aspect. **C:** Lateral aspect.

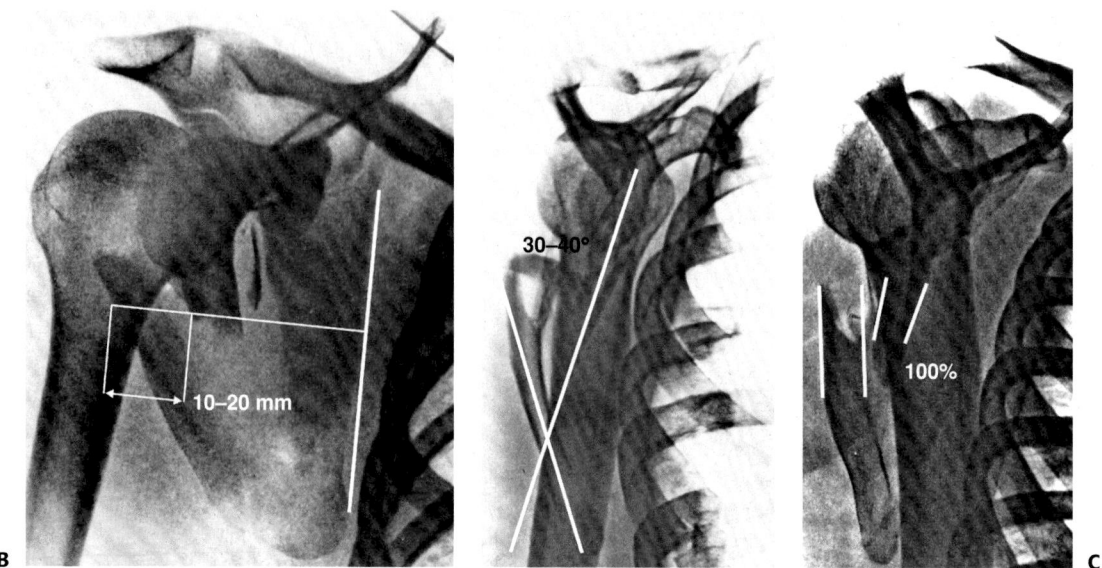

FIGURE 39-5 Measurement of displacement of fractures of the scapular body or scapular neck. **A:** Mediolateral displacement. **B:** Angular displacement. **C:** Translational displacement.

fractures of the scapular neck and helps to identify the different fracture lines in injuries of the anatomical and surgical necks of the scapula. Glenoid fractures require *a lateral view,* always with subtraction of the humeral head. In fractures of the lateral border of the scapular body, this view helps to assess its shortening, angulation, and translation, or the shape and displacement of small intermediate fragments (Fig. 39-4C).

Measurements of Angulation, Translation, Medialization, and GPA

These measurements quantify different types and directions of displacement of fragments, particularly of the lateral border of the scapula, and support management decisions (Fig. 39-5). Measurements may be made using both the Neer projections and 3D CT reconstructions.[4,35] Anavian et al.[6] have proved that displacement of some extra-articular fractures may progress during the postinjury period, which may require a further radiologic assessment after a short time.

Medialization of the main fragments of the lateral border of the scapula is measured in the Neer I projection on the anterior view (Fig. 39-5A) and in 3D CT reconstructions. Cole[31,34,35] considers medialization of 10 to 20 mm to be an indication for operative treatment. However, the term medialization is not quite correct.[156,201] In most cases there occurs lateral displacement of the infraglenoid part of the scapular body by the pull of muscles as the intact clavicle maintains a constant distance between the glenoid and the sternum. Zuckerman et al.[201] described, in scapula fractures, a slight lateral displacement of the glenoid with regard to the other side. The displacement of fragments is more accurately expressed by the term mediolateral displacement.

Angulation of the main fragments of the lateral border of the scapula may be evaluated in the Neer II projection (Fig. 39-5B), or in the lateral view based on 3D CT reconstructions. Cole[31,34,35]

considers angulation of more than 30 to 45 degrees as an indication for operative treatment.

Translation of the main fragments of the lateral border of the scapula is also measured by the Neer II view (Fig. 39-5C). A strong indication for operative treatment is considered to be translation of fragments by 100%.[14,31,34,35]

GPA, defined by Bestard et al.,[20] is the angle subtended by two lines, one connecting the most cranial with the most caudal point of the glenoid and one connecting the most cranial point of the glenoid with the most caudal part of the scapula (Fig. 39-6). The normal GPA is 30 to 46 degrees. In recent studies, some authors used the GPA as a radiologic predictor of the functional outcome after nonoperative treatment of scapula fractures.[24,44,111,117,155,163] Romero et al.[163] reported that a GPA of less than 20 degrees was associated with a poor functional outcome whereas another study[111] encountered worse functional outcomes in patients with a GPA of less than 30 degrees. Labler et al.[117] considered a GPA of less than 30 degrees to be an indirect indication of injury to the surrounding ligaments. A detailed analysis of various studies, however, shows that GPA measurement has not been standardized. In addition, it cannot be used in all fractures of the scapular body and neck. Despite these reservations, the GPA is, unlike medialization, angulation, and translation, the only radiologic measurement where correlation between its value and the functional outcome has been reported,[24,44,111,117,155,163] with a value of less than 20 degrees being likely to compromise function.

Classification of Scapula Fractures

Since the time of Petit, classification has developed over time[13] but there is still no generally accepted classification of scapula fractures. Currently there are several different classifications.[1,14,42,53,54,69,83,96,97,132,179,192]

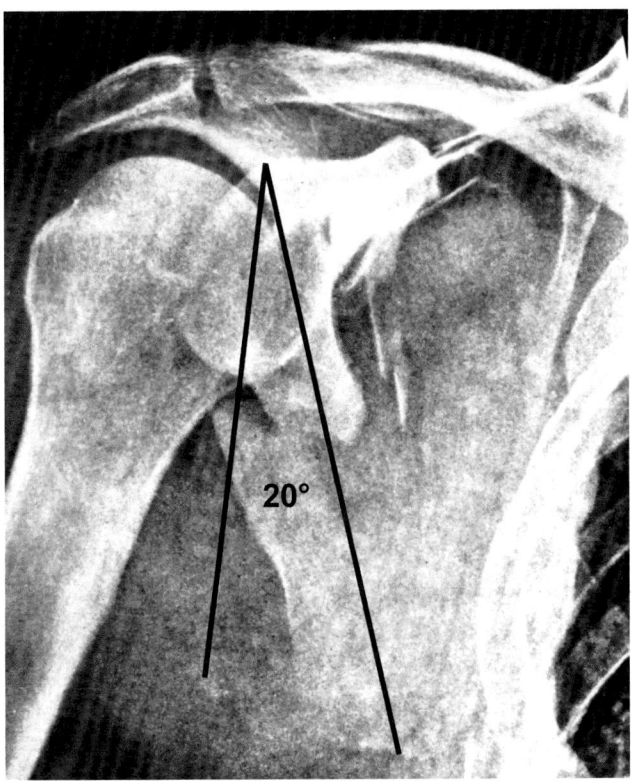

FIGURE 39-6 Glenopolar angle. The GPA is defined as the angle between the line connecting the superior and inferior poles of the glenoid and the line connecting the superior pole of the glenoid and the center of the inferior angle of scapula. A GPA of less than 20 degrees is one of the criteria for operative treatment.

Overview of Present Classifications

In 1975, Tscherne and Christ[179] divided scapula fractures into five basic patterns:

1. Fractures of processes
2. Fractures of the scapular body
3. Fractures of the scapular neck
4. Fractures of the glenoid fossa
5. Combined and comminuted fractures

In 1991, Ada and Miller[1] published a similar anatomical alphanumerical classification based on an analysis of conventional radiographs of 113 scapula fractures:

I. Fractures of processes: IA—acromion fractures, IB—scapular spine fractures, IC—coracoid process fractures

II. Fractures of the neck: IIA—fracture of the surgical neck, II B—transspinous fractures of the neck, IIC—fractures of the neck inferior to the scapular spine

III. Fractures of the glenoid

IV. Fractures of the body

In 1992, Euler et al.[53] developed an anatomical classification based on 153 scapula fractures, of which only 18, mostly fractures of the glenoid, were treated operatively. This classification was revised by Euler and Rüedi[54] in 1996, using an alphanumeric code analogous to the Müller/AO classification.

A. Body fractures

B. Fractures of processes (B1—spine, B2—coracoid, and B3—acromion)

C. Neck fractures (C1—anatomical neck, C2—surgical neck, C3—surgical neck with clavicular and/or acromial fracture, or rupture of CC and/or coracoacromial [CA] ligaments)

D. Intra-articular fractures (D1—glenoid rim fractures, D2—glenoid fossa fractures with inferior fossa fragment, with horizontal scapula split, with glenocoracoid block, comminuted fractures of the glenoid fossa, and D3—combined fractures of glenoid fossa and scapular neck, or body)

E. Scapula fractures combined with humeral head fractures

In 1996, the OTA (Orthopaedic Trauma Association) presented an alphanumerical classification that grouped fractures of individual anatomical parts of the scapula according to the principles of the Müller/AO classification.[151]

In 1984, and again in 1995, Ideberg[96,97] published a classification of glenoid fractures, based on analysis of conventional AP and lateral radiographs of 338 scapula fractures. He recognized five types: (1) Anterior glenoid rim fracture, (2) inferior glenoid fracture involving part of the neck, (3) superior glenoid fracture extending through the base of the coracoid process, (4) horizontal fracture involving both the scapular neck and body, the fracture line always running inferior to the spine of the scapula, and (5) horizontal fracture as in type IV, but with additional complete or incomplete neck fracture.

In 1992, Goss[69] modified the Ideberg classification, without specifying the radiographic examination technique or the number of his cases. Using Roman numerals instead of the Arabic ones, he converted the Ideberg's type I to Ia—fracture of anterior rim and type Ib—fracture of posterior rim. Type V was divided into three subtypes—type Va (combination of types II and IV), type Vb (combination of types III and IV), and type Vc (combination of types II, III, and IV). Type VI was also added.

In 1998, Mayo et al.[132] revised the Ideberg classification and changed the numerical order of individual types. The revision was based on a group of 27 patients who had surgery for a glenoid fracture. In several patients, 3D CT reconstruction was used and found to be more valuable than either routine radiographs of the scapula or 2D CT reconstructions.

Controversies of Present Classifications

The weakness of classifications of scapula fractures is the difficulty in accurate interpretation of the imaging. Different types of scapula fractures were identified primarily on the basis of plain radiographs. In view of the complicated anatomy of the scapula and its position on the chest, standard views are not easy to obtain and their unambiguous interpretation and determination of the type of fracture was difficult or impossible. CT was used only minimally, correlation of radiologic and intraoperative findings was not mentioned, because only a minimum of analyzed cases were treated operatively. Thus, almost no author was able to verify whether the identification of the types of fractures on the basis of plain radiographs was accurate.

Another disadvantage of the current classifications is the oversimplified schematic drawings of fracture lines mostly on the anterior surface of the scapula[69,151,152] as it is not always possible to determine the course of a fracture line in relation to the scapular spine. Simplistic schematic drawings of the scapular shape, mainly of the relationship of the upper part of the glenoid to the coracoid base, are also misleading[151,152] The coracoid arises directly from the superior pole of the glenoid and the upper surface of the neck is reduced to a small notch only a few millimeters deep. However, the illustrations in most classifications show the origin of the coracoid shifted markedly medially which makes the upper surface of the anatomical neck of the scapula seem significantly longer. As a result, the drawings of fracture lines running in this region are not realistic.

The current classifications also describe certain fracture patterns whose existence is questionable, or that are misinterpreted.

Scapular neck fractures: A number of authors use only the term "fracture of the scapular neck," without specifying its type.[33,75,102,162] Schematic drawings in the OTA classification, published in 2007, include only a fracture of the anatomical neck. Fracture of the surgical neck is missing.[152]

Analyses of 3D CT reconstructions and intraoperative findings have proved that most fractures, interpreted on the basis of plain radiographs as fractures of the scapular neck, were actually fractures of the scapular body (Fig. 39-7).

Another problem is terminology. Ada and Miller[1] classified transverse infraspinous fractures as type IIC fractures of the neck inferior to the scapular spine. This fracture line does not separate the glenoid from the scapular body, but splits the scapular body into two parts. In spite of this, some authors have taken over this incorrect term and further contributed to the confusion in scapula fracture classification.[71,133]

These issues cast doubt on the existing statistical data on incidence rates of individual types of scapula fractures and on the outcomes of clinical studies dealing with fractures of the scapular body and neck, and floating shoulder.

Glenoid fractures: Euler and Rüedi,[53,54] Goss,[69] and the OTA classification[151,152] described comminuted fractures of the entire glenoid fossa. However, their existence is questionable, as no 3D CT reconstruction of such a fracture has been published so far.

The so-called transverse fractures of the glenoid, that is, type 5(V) of the Ideberg,[97] Goss,[69] or Mayo et al.[132] classifications, are in fact fractures of the inferior glenoid involving the lateral border of the scapular body. The fracture line in these fractures runs through the infraspinous part of the scapular body and not through the supraspinous part as it may seem from the accompanying drawings. These classifications also present a fracture of the superior pole of the glenoid fossa as a transverse fracture of the glenoid. However, these are intra-articular fractures of the coracoid base that may involve the superior border, or superior angle, of the scapula.

Importance of Internal Architecture of Scapula for Fracture Classification

Currently, 3D CT reconstructions are increasingly used to characterize scapula fractures.[16,35,133] In addition, the volume of information related to operative treatment of these fractures is growing. This allows a more exact determination of the course of fracture lines in individual cases and their distribution in relation to the anatomical parts of the scapula.[8,181]

The scapular spine is essential to the distribution of fracture lines. The posterior view shows the separation of the anatomical body of the scapula into two parts. The supraspinous thin portion of the anatomical body constitutes, together with the acromion and the coracoid, the "upper scapula" serving for attachment of muscles and ligaments. The lower, infraspinous portion of the anatomical body, that is, the biomechanical body of the scapula receives compression forces transmitted from the glenoid by two pillars, the spinal and the lateral one, as

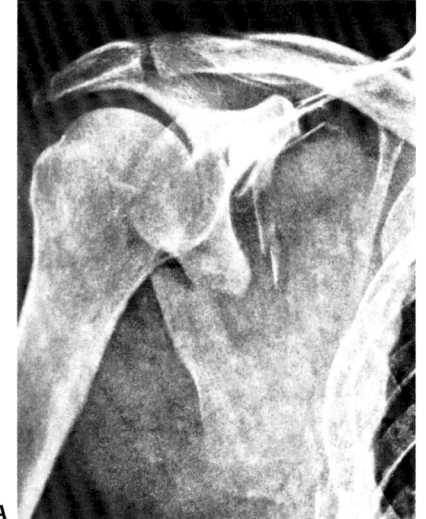 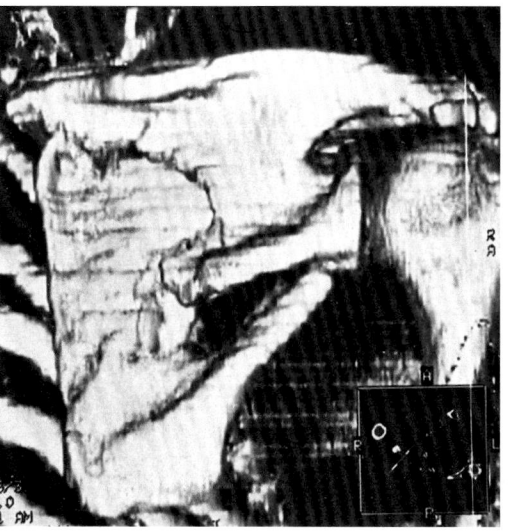

FIGURE 39-7 A common mistake in interpretation of shoulder radiograph. **A:** An AP radiograph of the injured right shoulder is often interpreted as a fracture of scapular neck. **B:** The posterior aspect of scapula on 3D CT reconstruction of the same patient demonstrates the actual type of fracture, that is, a two-part fracture of the scapular body.

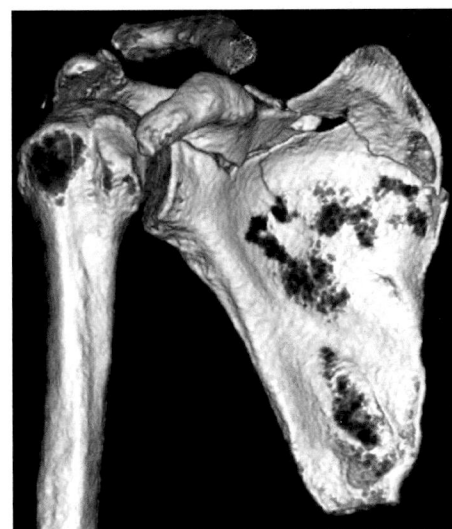 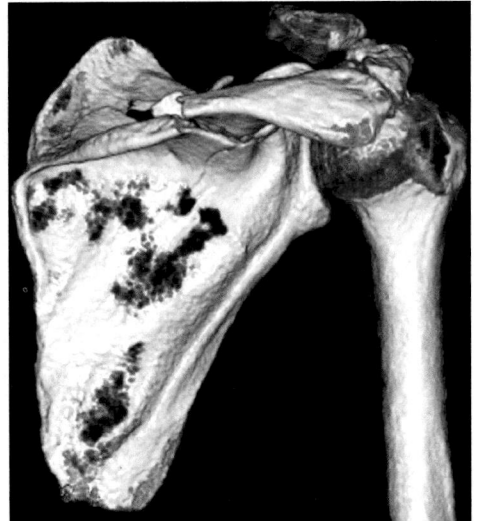

FIGURE 39-8 Fractures of the scapular processes (fractures of "upper" scapula) in 3D CT reconstruction. **A:** Anterior aspect. **B:** Posterior aspect. Both views demonstrate an intra-articular fracture of the coracoid base, a fracture of the superior angle, a fracture of the scapular spine, and a fracture of acromion. (Courtesy Prof. Zwipp.)

described earlier. The scapular spine is actually a barrier preventing the propagation of fracture lines from the infraspinous to the supraspinous body and vice versa. This is supported by clinical experience as fractures of the anatomical body are less common than fractures of the biomechanical body.

As revealed by Armitage et al.[8] in their study as well as by 3D CT reconstruction of cases,[14,16] barring a few exceptions, fracture lines propagate from the infraspinous to the supraspinous fossae through the weaker areas, that is, through the spinomedial angle, or through the central thin part of the scapular spine.[8,181]

Comprehensive Anatomical Classification

This classification is based on classifications developed by Tscherne and Christ,[179] Ada and Miller,[1] and Euler and Rüedi.[54] However, the basic groups of this classification include only the fracture lines whose existence has been verified by 3D CT reconstructions or intraoperatively.

- Fractures of the processes
- Fractures of the scapular body
- Fractures of the scapular neck
- Fractures of the glenoid
- Combined fractures of the scapula

Process Fractures. These fractures may be caused by a direct blow to the upper part of the scapula, a direct impact of the dislocated humeral head, or pull of muscles and ligaments. They include also fractures of the superior border and the superior angle of the scapula. As these fractures often occur simultaneously, they may be called fractures of "the upper scapula" (Fig. 39-8).

A1—fractures of the superior border and the superior angle

A2—fractures of the acromion and the lateral part of the scapular spine

A3—fractures of the coracoid process

There is no exact dividing line between fractures of the scapular spine and of the acromion and therefore they are included in one group. Fractures of the acromion and of the lateral part of the scapular spine and fractures of the coracoid process may be further subdivided.[55,91,99,115,144–147]

Body Fractures. These fractures may be divided, in terms of severity, into two groups:

B1—fractures of the anatomical body

B2—fractures of the biomechanical body

In fractures of the anatomical body, fracture lines pass from the supraspinous fossa through the scapular spine to the infraspinous fossa, whereas in fractures of the biomechanical body they run only within the infraspinous fossa (Fig. 39-9).

Neck Fractures. These fractures may be defined as those separating the glenoid from the scapular body.[42,58] The following three basic fractures of the scapular neck may be distinguished according to the course of the fracture line and the shape of the glenoid fragment (Figs. 39-10 and 39-11).

C1—fracture of the anatomical neck separates only the glenoid from the scapular body. The fracture line starts proximally between the upper rim of the glenoid and the coracoid base, that is, in the coracoglenoid notch (Fig. 39-11A).

C2—fracture of the surgical neck (Fig. 39-11B) starts in the scapular notch and passes through the spinoglenoid notch, that is, lateral to the scapular spine base. The lateral fragment is formed by the glenoid and the coracoid. Surgical neck fractures are divided into stable and unstable ones. Instability is caused by rupture of the CC and CA ligaments, or by avulsion of that part of the coracoid process to which these ligaments are attached.

C3—transspinous fracture of the scapular neck is rare and little known. The fracture line starts medial to the scapular

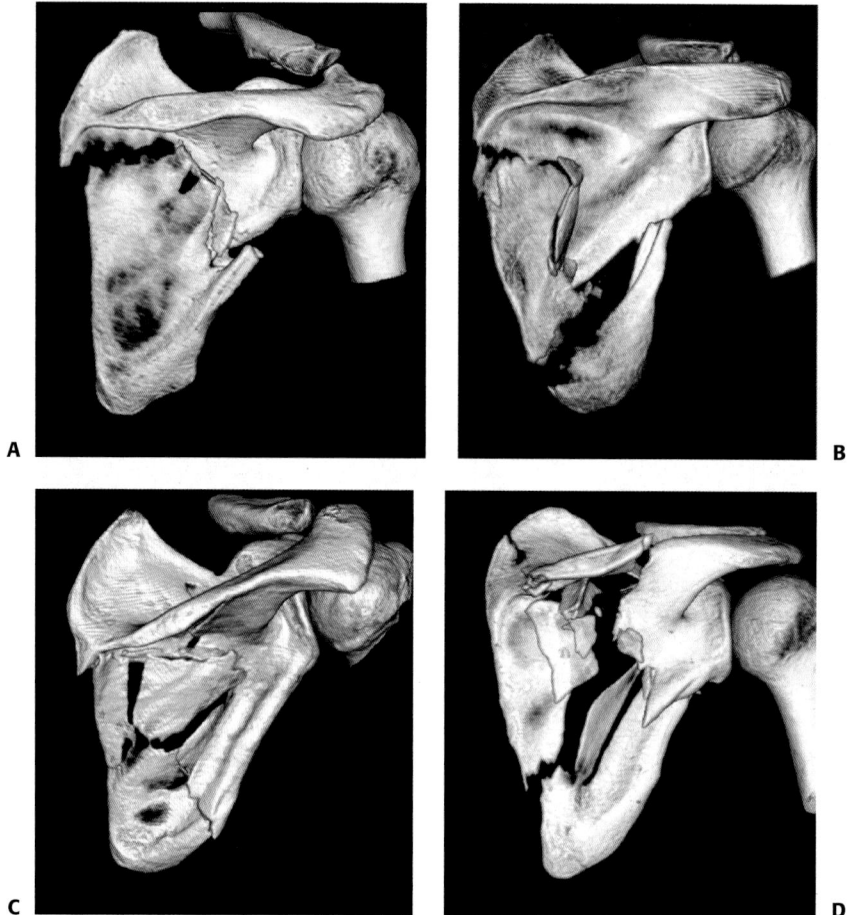

FIGURE 39-9 Fractures of the scapular body. **A:** A two-part fracture of the biomechanical body, **(B)** a three-part fracture of the biomechanical body, **(C)** a comminuted fracture of the biomechanical body involving the base of the scapular spine, **(D)** a comminuted fracture of the anatomical body.

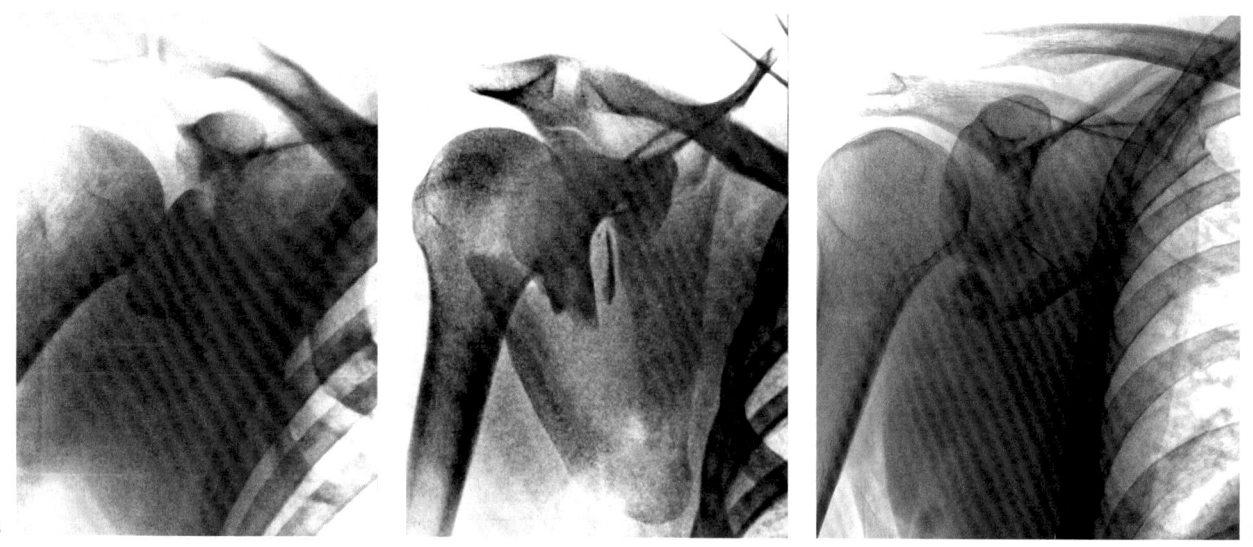

FIGURE 39-10 Fractures of the scapular neck in an AP shoulder radiograph. **A:** Fracture of the anatomical neck. **B:** Fracture of the surgical neck. **C:** A transspinous neck fracture.

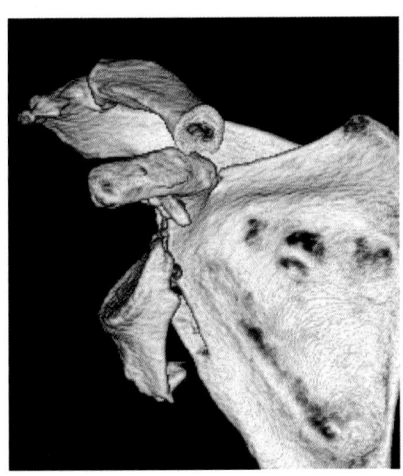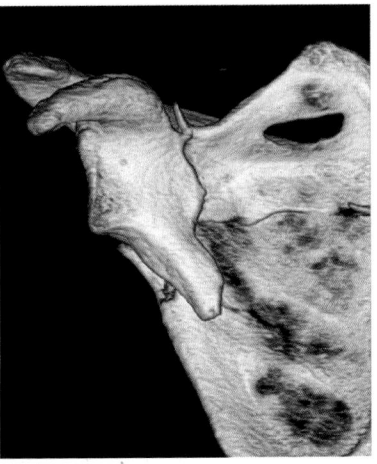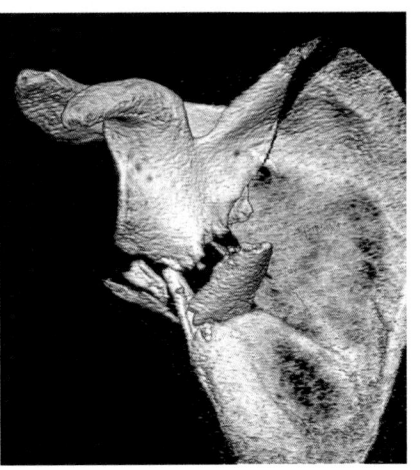

A, B

C

FIGURE 39-11 Fractures of the scapular neck in 3D CT reconstruction—anterior aspect. **A:** A fracture of the anatomical neck. The fracture line passes through the coracoglenoid notch, lateral to the coracoid process. **B:** Fracture of the surgical neck The fracture line passes through the suprascapular notch medial to coracoid process. The glenoid fragment bears the coracoid process. **C:** A transspinous neck fracture. The fracture line passes medial to the suprascapular notch. The glenoid fragment bears the coracoid process, acromion, and the lateral part of the scapular spine.

notch and passes through the centre of the scapular spine (Fig. 39-11C). The lateral fragment is formed by the glenoid, the coracoid, and the lateral part of the scapular spine, including the acromion.

Glenoid Fossa Fractures. These intra-articular fractures may be divided according to the part of the glenoid that is affected (Fig. 39-12).

If they are displaced, congruence and stability of the glenohumeral joint are compromised, depending on the location, size, and degree of displacement of the separated fragment.

D1—fractures of the superior glenoid are caused by avulsion of the coracoid base, including part of the articular surface. Part of the fragment may be a portion of the superior border of the scapula, variable in size. The fracture line always passes superior to the scapular spine (Fig. 39-12A).

D2—avulsion of the anteroinferior rim of the glenoid occurs in association with anterior dislocation of the humeral head (Fig. 39-12B). The size of fragment(s) varies.

D3—fractures of the inferior glenoid affect the one to two distal thirds of the glenoid fossa, together with a part of the lateral

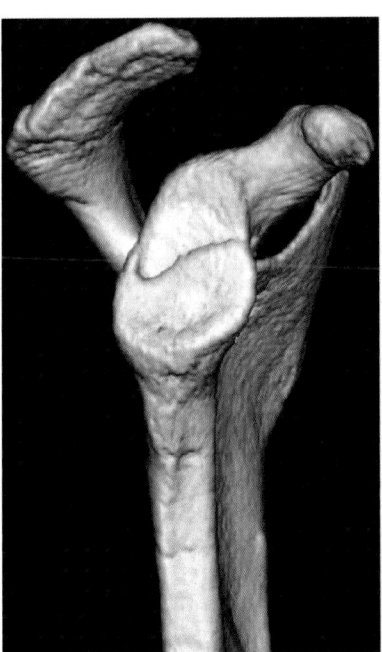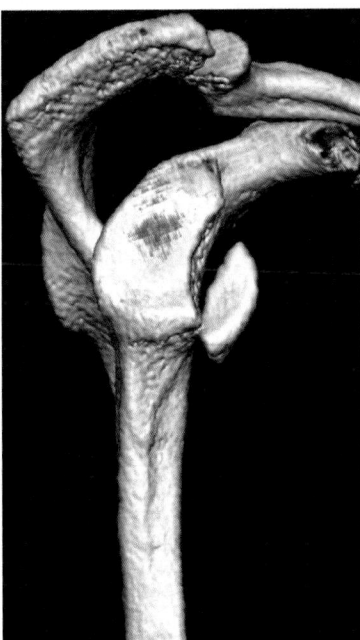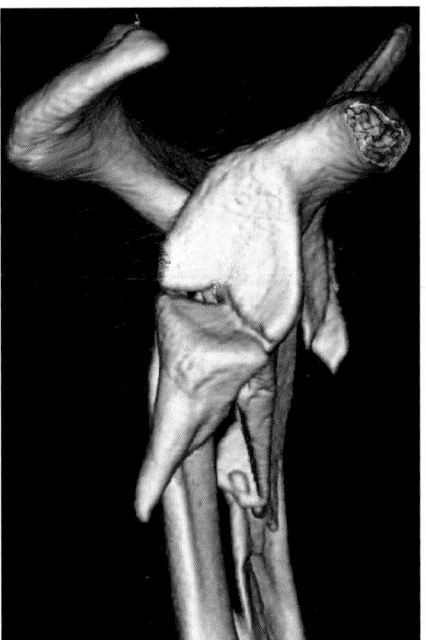

A, B

C

FIGURE 39-12 Types of glenoid fractures in 3D CT reconstruction, right scapula. **A:** Superior glenoid fracture. **B:** Fracture of anterior glenoid rim. **C:** Inferior glenoid fracture.

border of the scapula, of variable length. The fracture line extends as far as the lateral pillar of the scapula, at a variable distance from the inferior rim of the glenoid (Fig. 39-12C). In most of these fractures, however, there are also additional fracture lines involving the scapular body.

D4—fractures of the posterior rim of the glenoid are very rare, occurring in association with the posterior dislocation of the humeral head.

Combined Fractures. This miscellaneous group may be divided into two subgroups.

The first subgroup includes a combination of the four basic scapula fracture patterns. The most common fractures of this subgroup are combined fractures of the scapular body and the distal glenoid.

The second subgroup comprises combinations of one or two basic scapula fractures with injuries to other bones, or joints, of the shoulder girdle. A specific type of combined fracture is the so-called floating shoulder, that is, an unstable fracture of the surgical neck of the scapula combined with a fracture of the shaft of the clavicle.

Scapulothoracic Dissociation

Scapulothoracic dissociation is a traction (avulsion) injury of the muscular apparatus of the scapula, characterized by lateral displacement of the scapula, with a wide range of concomitant injuries, including those of the shoulder girdle, while the skin is usually intact.[3,65,118,198]

TREATMENT OF SCAPULA FRACTURES

The aim of treatment of scapula fractures is to restore a full, pain-free range of motion of the shoulder and to prevent the development of late complications, including malunion, nonunion, osteoarthritis of the glenohumeral joint, lesions of the rotator cuff, and chronic pain. Specifically, it implies restoration of the congruence and stability of the glenohumeral joint in glenoid fractures; restoration of the anatomical form and alignment of the scapular body and the glenoid in fractures of the scapular neck and body; and prevention of painful nonunion, or impingement of humeral head, resulting from malunion of fractures of the acromion or coracoid processes.

Treatment Options for Scapula Fractures

There is a general consensus that all nondisplaced fractures of the scapula should be treated nonoperatively. Until recently, nonoperative treatment had also been used in most displaced extra-articular fractures of the scapular neck and body, based on repeated reports of good outcomes of this treatment.[98,124,166,193,197] However, the authors evaluated their results without taking into account individual types of injury often with very short review periods of a few months. The only indications for operation were usually displaced glenoid fractures.

Of late, the situation has started to change, mainly in view of a number of studies evaluating the long-term results of nonoperatively treated displaced scapular neck and body fractures.[1,9,77,140,155,163] These studies have revealed that a number of patients with malunion of the scapular body or neck suffer from

pain, disability, limited range of motion, and sometimes even damage to the rotator cuff, proven by MRI. Views on treatment have also changed following the introduction of CT scanning, and especially 3D reconstructions. Although the debate has not delivered clear conclusions, a number of authors prefer operative treatment for displaced scapula fractures, mainly those of the body and neck. Other authors, on the other hand believe that nonoperative treatment is best based on some reported good outcomes. An analysis of retrospective studies was made by two groups of authors.[119,200]

Zlowodzki et al.[200] analyzed 520 scapula fractures from 22 case series and reported that

- 80% of the glenoid fractures were treated operatively and excellent-to-good results were achieved in 82% of them.

- 80% of isolated fractures of the scapular body were treated nonoperatively and excellent or good results were achieved in 86% of them.

- 83% of all nonarticular fractures of the scapular neck were treated nonoperatively and excellent-to-good results were achieved in 77% of them.

Lantry et al.[119] reviewed the results of 243 scapula fractures treated operatively in 17 studies and reported that

- 48% of patients sustained a fracture of the glenoid fossa, 7% a fracture of the glenoid rim, 26% a fracture of the scapular neck, 8% a process fracture, 26% of patients sustained an ipsilateral fracture of the clavicle, or an AC dislocation.

- the indication for surgery in glenoid fractures was displacement of 4 to 10 mm, most often 5 mm.

- 4.2% of patients developed postoperative infective complications, 2.4% sustained suprascapular nerve injury, and 7.1% of cases required removal of the hardware for local problems or breakage of the implant.

- 163 patients were evaluated in terms of their functional outcomes, using different scoring systems, with excellent-to-good results achieved in 83% of cases, and fair or poor results in 17% of patients, with an average follow-up of 50 months.

The authors of both reviews stated that there were significant differences between individual studies and that the validity of the presented data was often questionable. Prospective multicentre studies were recommended.

Outcome Measurements

Different shoulder scoring systems are in use to evaluate functional outcomes: American Shoulder and Elbow Surgeons score,[160] Constant score,[37] DASH score,[95] Herscovici score,[89] Neer score,[139] Rowe score,[164] Oxford questionnaire,[40] Short Form 36 score,[189] Simple Shoulder Test,[125] University of California Los Angeles score,[50] or subjective scores based on the surgeon's assessment.[80] The details of these are reviewed in Chapter 37.

Nonoperative Treatment of Scapula Fractures

Nonoperative treatment is indicated in all undisplaced fractures. It should also be used in intra- or extra-articular displaced fractures when the patient's general, or local, condition does not allow operation.

Nonoperative treatment consists of pain relief and about 2 weeks of sling immobilization. It is then possible to start passive range-of-motion exercises with the aim of achieving a full passive range of motion within 1 month of the injury.[35] A full active range of motion should be restored during the second month. In the third month, strengthening of the rotator cuff muscles and parascapular muscles may be started.

The potential disadvantages of nonoperative treatment include deformity of the scapula and incongruity and instability of the glenohumeral joint.

Recent Results of Nonoperative Treatment

Over the past 12 years, a number of studies have evaluated the outcome of nonoperative treatment of scapula fractures by means of the different scoring systems listed above. This allowed a more objective assessment of functional outcomes. However, with few exceptions, the problem of these studies remains the verification of the types of fractures being evaluated.

Romero et al.[163] in 2001 evaluated the results of nonoperative treatment of scapular neck fractures in 19 patients with a mean age of 42 years (21 to 61) and a mean follow-up of 8 years (2 to 21), using the Constant–Murley score. The authors found functional problems in patients with a GPA less than 20 degrees. Pace et al.[155] described nine patients with glenoid neck fractures, with pain in the shoulder in seven cases associated with a subacromial bursitis, diagnosed by MRI. The mean age of patients was 34 years (21 to 64) and the mean follow-up 58 months (24 to 96). The authors attributed the pain to malunion of the scapula. Bozkurt et al.[24] reported the outcomes of conservative treatment of scapular neck fractures (surgical neck 12, anatomical neck 6) in 18 patients with a mean age of 43 years (23 to 62) and a mean follow-up of 25 months. The authors found a positive correlation between the Constant–Murley score and GPA.

The outcome of conservative treatment of scapular neck fractures in 13 patients with a mean age of 45 years and a mean follow-up of 5.5 years (1.6 to 12) was reported by Van Noort et al.[184] GPA was always more than 20 degrees, and the Constant–Murley score indicated good and excellent results in all the patients. Gosens et al.[68] in 2009 analyzed a total of 22 patients with a scapular body fracture treated conservatively, with a mean age of 49 years (7 to 67) and a mean follow-up of 63 months (41 to 85). In 14 patients it was the sole injury, but 8 patients had polytrauma. Based on DASH, SST, and SF 36 scores, the authors found worse results in the polytrauma patients.

Good results of nonoperative treatment after a mean review time of 65 months were reported in 50 patients with a mean age of 44 years (20 to 82) at the time of injury.[169] The mean follow-up was 65 months (13 to 120). Fractures of the scapular neck and body accounted for 82%, glenoid fractures for 10%, and fractures of processes for 8%. Regardless of the fracture type and using the Constant score, 23% of results were considered excellent, 51% good, 20% fair, and 6% poor. Restriction of range of motion had no impact on the functional outcome.

Dimitroulias et al.[44] in 2011 evaluated 32 patients with a mean age of 47 years (21 to 84), each with a displaced fracture of the scapular body. The mean follow-up was 15 months (6 to 33). The fracture type was verified by 3D CT reconstruction. The mean GPA value on the affected side was 9 degrees less than that on the intact side. The mean change in the DASH score of 10.2 was considered of minimal clinical importance but a high ISS and the presence of rib fractures compromised the outcome.

Operative Treatment of Scapula Fractures

Operative treatment of scapula fractures is currently the subject of an intense debate with the number of its advocates increasing. A standard operative method is open reduction and internal fixation,[11,14,18,74,80,101,126] although there are also some reports in the literature on treatment of certain types of scapula fractures (acromion, glenoid) by arthroscopically assisted internal fixation[19,27,64,93,165,173,177] or partial resection.[81]

Indications/Contraindications

The main indication for operative treatment of the glenoid fractures is displacement, that is, a gap, or step-off, $\geq$3 to 10 mm, with the simultaneous involvement of 20% to 30% of the articular surface (Fig. 39-13) and/or persisting subluxation of the humeral head.[35] The aim of operation is to restore congruity and stability of the glenohumeral joint.

In displaced fractures of the processes, particularly the coracoid, acromion, and scapular spine, the aim is to achieve healing in an anatomical position, as healing in displacement may cause impingement syndrome and compromise the rotator cuff. Nonunion of processes of the scapula is often painful because of muscle pull. Displacement of fragments of more than 1 cm has been cited as an indication for operative treatment in fractures of the acromion or coracoid.[7]

In displaced extra-articular fractures of the scapular body and neck, the aim is restoration of the original alignment of

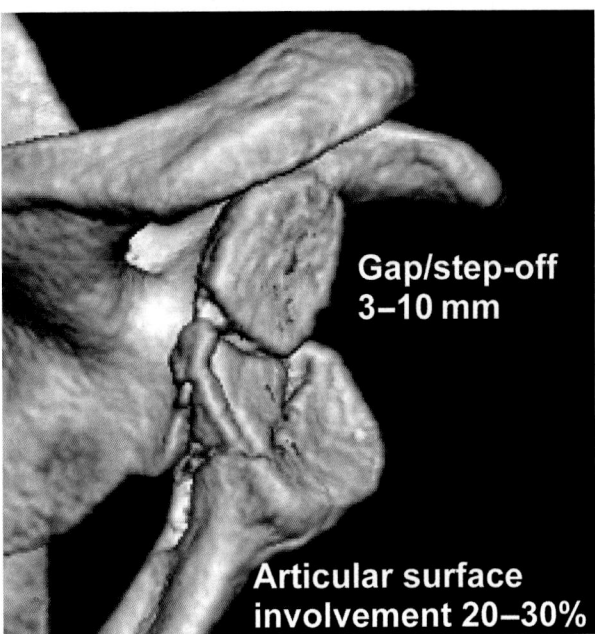

Gap/step-off 3–10 mm

Articular surface involvement 20–30%

FIGURE 39-13 Criteria for operative treatment of intra-articular fractures of the scapula.

the glenoid with the scapular body (GPA), primarily by reconstruction of the length and integrity of the lateral border. This will restore the normal orientation of the glenoid in relation to the scapular body and the humeroscapular rhythm (shoulder imbalance), as well as the normal course of muscles, particularly those of the rotator cuff. For normal mobility of the scapula it is also important to restore the congruence between its anterior surface and the chest wall and, if necessary, to remove fragments of the scapula impacted in the chest wall. Current indications for operative treatment are fractures of the scapular body and neck with the following types of displacement.[14,31–33,35]

- 100% translation of fragments of the lateral border
- 30- to 40-degree angulation of main fragments of the lateral border
- Mediolateral displacement of the glenoid in relation to the lateral border of the scapular body of more than 1 to 2 cm
- GPA less than 20 degrees

These criteria are not absolute. It is necessary to take into account all other injuries, mainly those of the chest, the patient's age, physical condition, skin integrity of the shoulder and consider all potential risks.

Surgical Approaches

Most scapula fractures are exposed from the Judet posterior, or the anterior deltopectoral, approach. Some authors recommend the Dupont–Evrard posterolateral, or the superior approach of Goss.

Judet Posterior Approach. This surgical approach, described by Robert Judet[105] in 1964, is currently used in various modifications.[17,46,104,141,150] The Judet approach provides an excellent exposure of the entire infraspinous fossa, lateral and medial borders of the scapula, the scapular spine, the scapular neck, and the posterior and inferior rims of the glenoid.

Indication. The Judet approach is indicated as a universal exposure in fractures of the scapular body, scapular neck, posteroinferior glenoid, and in combinations of these fractures.

Patient Positioning and Draping. The patient is placed in a semiprone position on the intact side with supports in the region of the lumbar spine and chest. Reference structures are marked on the skin, that is, contours of the scapular body, the scapular spine, and acromion. The extremity must be draped free to allow its manipulation during surgery.

Incision and Dissection. Judet typically retracted the skin flap together with the portion of the deltoid arising from the scapular spine. In the author's modification, the Judet approach has three phases. The first phase consists of a boomerang skin incision along the scapular spine and the medial border of the scapula. A skin flap is then raised and the posterior border of the deltoid identified. In the next phase, the posterior deltoid is detached from the scapular spine and turned back laterally and distally. Finally, the infraspinatus is mobilized and retracted proximally (Fig. 39-14).

The skin incision is made from the posterior border of the acromion along the scapular spine to the spinomedial angle, where it curves following the medial border of the scapula and

continues to the inferior angle of the scapula. Subcutaneous fibrofatty tissue is incised down to, but not through, the common fascia of the deltoid and infraspinatus. A skin flap is raised, retracted laterodistally and held in this position by two sutures.

A prerequisite for a careful mobilization of the deltoid is identification of its posterior edge, which is not always easy. The spinal portion of the deltoid and the medial portion of the infraspinatus are covered by a common fascia passing from the medial part of the infraspinatus to the posterior edge of the deltoid (Fig. 39-14A). After identification of the posterior border of the deltoid, the common fascia is split by a T-shaped incision, with one part of the incision following the posterior edge of the deltoid and the other running perpendicular to it (Fig. 39-14B). This incision exposes both the posterior border of the deltoid and the medial half of the infraspinatus. Subsequently, the spinal portion of the deltoid is carefully released from the scapular spine as far as the posterior rim of the acromion and retracted laterally and distally. This will display the entire posterior surface of the infraspinatus.

Before releasing the infraspinatus, it is necessary to identify the interval between its lateral border and the teres minor (Fig. 39-14C), exposing the scapular circumflex vessels perforating teres minor (Fig. 39-14D). These lie some 3 to 4 cm distal to the lower rim of the glenoid and pass round the lateral border of the scapula to its posterior surface. These blood vessels must be ligated and cut. Only then can the infraspinatus be detached from the scapular spine, the medial border, the lateral border, the inferior angle, and from the infraspinous fossa. When retracting the infraspinatus proximally, care should be taken to avoid injury to the neurovascular bundle of the muscle which can be seen in the spinoglenoid notch (Fig. 39-14D).

Limited Approaches. In some cases it is possible to make only medial and lateral windows without mobilizing the whole infraspinatus. On the lateral side it is sufficient to detach the infraspinatus from the lateral border of the scapula only; on the medial side it is typically released in the spino-medial angle.

Reinsertion of Muscles and Wound Closure. After completion of the internal fixation, the infraspinatus is carefully reinserted to the inferior angle of the scapula, preferably using the infraspinatus fascia. The spinal portion of the deltoid is then carefully reattached and the subcutaneous tissues and skin closed.

Extended Judet Approach. In 2008, the author[17] described a combination of the Judet and the sabre-cut approaches. This combined approach allows treatment of any associated fracture of the lateral clavicle, or AC dislocation, via a single incision.

Posterosuperior Approach. This approach uses the horizontal part of the Judet incision.[59,113] It is indicated in isolated fractures of the posterior rim of the glenoid, the scapular spine, and the acromion. The incision extends along the posterior border of the acromion and the lateral part of the scapular spine. After detachment of the spinal, and partially of the acromial, portions of the deltoid from the scapula, the muscle can be retracted distally, allowing exposure of the tendon of the infraspinatus. The infraspinatus tendon and

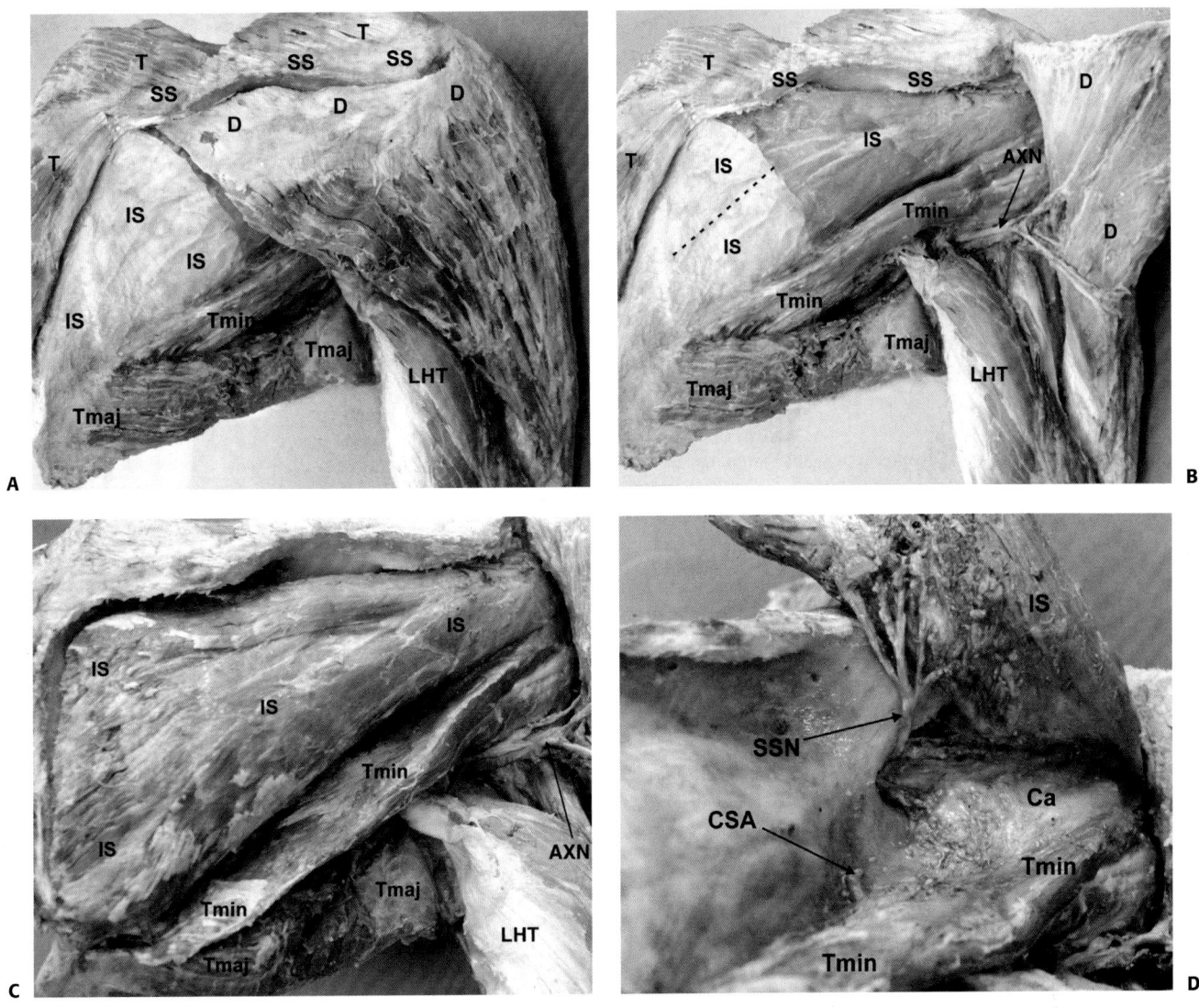

FIGURE 39-14 Judet approach—anatomical dissection. **A:** Posterior aspect of the right scapula. Note that the fascia of the infraspinatus continues into the deltoid fascia. **B:** The spinous portion of deltoid is released from the scapular spine and reflected laterally; the *dotted line* indicates the incision into the infraspinatus fascia. **C:** Identification of the interval between infraspinatus and teres minor. **D:** The released infraspinatus is retracted superiorly. Care must be taken not to overdistract the suprascapular neurovascular bundle. D, deltoid; IS, infraspinatus and its fascia; SS, scapular spine; T, trapezius, Tmin, teres minor; Tmaj, teres major; LHT, long head of triceps; AXN, axillary nerve; SSN, suprascapular nerve; CSA, circumflex scapular artery, Ca, articular capsule of glenohumeral joint.

posterior capsule of the shoulder are incised or osteotomized from the greater tuberosity and the resultant flap retracted medially. This exposes the posterior surface of the glenoid and the scapular neck. When necessary, this approach may be extended to the Judet approach.

Mini-Invasive Posterior Approach. Gauger and Cole[62] described a mini-invasive approach that is based on the principles of the Judet approach but is performed from two separate shorter incisions.

Dupont–Evrard Posterolateral Approach. The Dupont–Evrard approach, described in 1932, provides direct

exposure of the lateral border of the scapula in the interval between the infraspinatus and the teres minor.[45] Its main disadvantage is that it exposes only the lateral border of the scapula and cannot be extended, if necessary. Modifications of this approach have been described in the literature, differing only in respect of the type of the skin incision.[25,103,109,142,185,196]

Deltopectoral Approach. This classical approach is indicated in fractures of the anteroinferior rim of the glenoid and of the coracoid process. It is described in Chapter 37.

Superior Approach. This approach was described by Goss[74] as a complementary approach in fractures of the superior part of the glenoid. The skin incision runs over the superior aspect of the shoulder. The trapezius is split within the angle between the clavicle, acromion, and the scapular spine, to expose the underlying supraspinatus. Splitting of the supraspinatus in the line of its fibers exposes the superior surface of the glenoid.

Operative Technique, Postoperative Treatment

The operative technique of scapula fractures has been described by many authors.[14,15,32,34,52,74,80,101,126,141] However, their procedures differ in a number of details.

Implants. Scapula fractures can be fixed by small- and mini-implants, including 3.5- or 2.7-mm cortical screws, 3.5- or 2.7-mm reconstruction plates, a 3.5-mm semitubular plate, a 3.5-mm T-plate, or a 2.7-mm L- or T-shaped plate. Some authors recommend anatomically shaped plates, designed specifically for the scapula[52] whereas others prefer locking plates.[3,35] Cannulated screws are useful in internal fixation of fractures of the coracoid process and miniscrews (2.4 and 2 mm) may be used in fixation of small fragments of the glenoid fossa or intermediate fragments of the lateral border of the scapula.

Reduction and Fixation. The scapula is a bone with an uneven distribution of bony mass. Therefore, only certain areas offer sufficient anchorage for implants, primarily the lateral border of the scapular body, the scapular spine, and the scapular neck with the glenoid although it may also be necessary to fix fractures in less suitable locations, for example, in the spinomedial, or inferior angles. The scapula heals very well, with rapid callus formation. As most scapula fractures are operated on after a delay of several days, it is sometimes necessary to clear the fracture site of callus prior to reduction.

In *fractures of the scapular body and neck* it is essential to restore the integrity of the biomechanical body and in particular the lateral border of the scapula. Therefore, the first step is to stabilize fractures of the lateral border.

Displaced fractures of the body cause shortening of the lateral border of the scapula. Reduction may be achieved by means of two Schanz pins driven into each of the main fragments, used as joysticks, or by a small external fixator.[31,35] Another option is reduction using two bone hooks. For easier manipulation, it is helpful to have the hook tips inserted into holes drilled in the lateral border of the scapula by a 2.5-mm drill bit, or to manipulate 3.5-mm cortical screws inserted into these holes. The chosen locations of the holes should allow their subsequent use for attachment of the plate.

In unstable oblique fractures of the lateral border of the body, reduction may be maintained by the technique of the "lost" K-wire inserted as an intramedullary peg into a track drilled into each of the main fragments (Fig. 39-15).[14,15] If larger intermediate fragments are separated from the lateral border of the scapula, they have to be fixed with screws to restore the integrity of the lateral border.

Final fixation may be completed with a 2.7- or 3.5-mm reconstruction plate or in some cases with a 3.5-mm semitubular plate. In simple fractures of the lateral border it is sufficient to use 2+2 plate fixation, that is, two screws in each of the two fragments. In fractures of the lateral border with intermediate fragments, a 3+3 fixation is preferred. It may also be necessary to fix a fracture in the spinomedial angle, preferably with a 2.7-mm reconstruction plate. The inferior angle of the scapula may be fixed using a 2.7-mm reconstruction plate or a 3.5-mm T-plate.

Fractures of the scapular spine that are part of fractures of the anatomical body, or transspinous fractures of the neck, are best fixed by either a 2.7-mm reconstruction plate or a pre-shaped semitubular plate.

Scapular neck fractures are in most cases fixed using a combination of implants, for example, a 2.7- or 3.5-mm reconstruction plate, a 3.5-mm semitubular plate, or a 3.5-mm T-plate. When inserting screws into a glenoid fragment, care should be taken to avoid intra-articular penetration. Fixation of the lateral border is complemented with a plate placed on the posterior

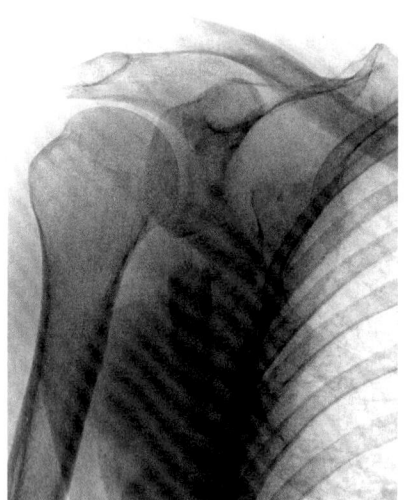
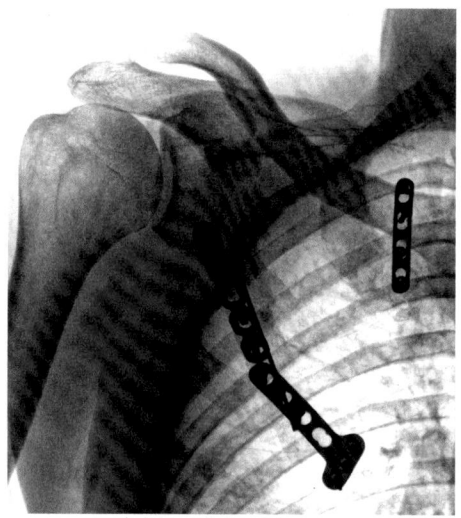
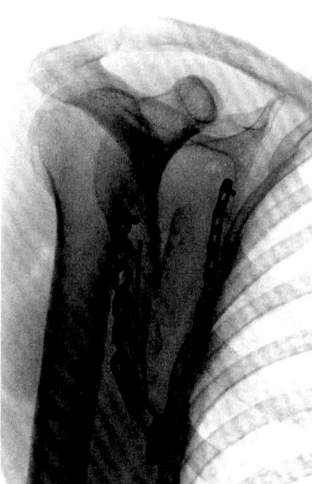

FIGURE 39-15 Technique of lost K-wire. **A:** A three-part fracture of the biomechanical body of the scapula. **B:** AP radiograph after surgery. **C:** Oblique radiograph after surgery. Both radiographs show that the K-wire has been inserted as an intramedullary peg.

surface of the neck, or by 3.5-mm cortex screws inserted into the glenoid fragment from the scapular spine.[126] Care should be used to avoid injury to the neurovascular structures in the spinoglenoid notch.

Glenoid fractures are treated according to the type of injury. An avulsed fragment of the anterior rim of the glenoid is fixed depending on its size with lag screws and washers or with a small plate. Similar procedures may be applied to fractures of the posterior rim. Reduction and fixation of the superior pole, that is, intra-articular fractures of the coracoid, may be difficult because of the pull of the muscles attached to the coracoid. These fractures may be fixed using cannulated lag screws with washers inserted through the coracoid into the glenoid or the scapular neck.

Fractures of the inferior glenoid are usually associated with fractures of the scapular body. If the joint capsule and labrum are not ruptured, incision of the capsule should run parallel to the posterior rim of the glenoid and labrum. This allows both palpation and a visual check of the glenoid fossa reduction. Reduction and fixation depend on the shape of the inferior joint fragment. This variable fragment may carry either a small, or a large, part of the lateral border. In both cases, it is necessary to clean the fracture surfaces carefully. Reduction and fixation of a short fragment is usually easier. A long fragment may be reduced by means of two screws inserted into the scapular neck close to the fracture line. Screws are compressed together by small Spanish forceps. Reduction of a long fragment must be accurate along the whole length of the fracture line. This is the only guarantee of an anatomical reduction of the joint surface. If there is another separate, usually smaller, fragment, it has to be anatomically reduced and fixed by small lag screws. The main two fragments may be fixed using various techniques, most often by a combination of different plates, that is, a 3.5-mm T-plate, 3.5-mm reconstruction or semitubular plates, or 2.7-mm L-shaped or straight plates, and lag screws.

Postoperative Treatment. Postoperatively, the arm is immobilized in a sling. Drainage is removed by 48 hours after surgery. Radiographs of the shoulder are obtained using Neer I and II views. After discharge, the patient is reviewed 2 weeks after operation to assess wound healing and remove sutures. Radiographs are taken at 6 weeks (Neer I and II views), 3 months (Neer I view), 6 months (Neer I view, if necessary), and 1 year after operation (Neer I and II views). Scapula fractures heal as a rule in 6 to 8 weeks.

Correct rehabilitation is very important for the final outcome. Passive range-of-motion exercises of the shoulder should begin on the first postoperative day and continue for about 6 weeks using a CPM machine if available. Active range-of-motion exercises start at approximately 4 to 5 weeks postoperatively, depending on the extent of the surgical approach and presence of other injuries. The range of motion is assessed at 6 weeks and, if unsatisfactory, the shoulder is examined under general anesthesia and careful manipulation performed if necessary. Active resistance exercises may be started approximately 8 weeks after operation. All restrictions are lifted around 3 months postoperatively. Between the third and twelfth months, the range of motion usually improves only slightly. The final subjective, objective, and radiologic outcomes of the operation cannot be assessed before 1 year after the operation at the earliest.

Results

There are many studies in the literature that evaluate the outcome of operative treatment of scapula fractures. Their validity and comparisons between studies are questionable for a number of reasons. Firstly, most case series are heterogeneous in terms of fracture pattern. Authors often evaluate both extra- and intra-articular fractures together. Homogeneity of the case series cannot even be guaranteed by separate evaluation of intra- or extra-articular fractures. For instance, fractures of the anterior rim of the glenoid are different from and require a different surgical approach from those of the inferior glenoid, which are usually associated with fractures of the scapular body.

Secondly, data on individual types of fractures should be interpreted with caution. Most such reported fractures were diagnosed only by means of standard radiographs. A further problem is the low number of patients in individual case series and the relative lack of experience of the treating surgeons, and the long period over which patients are recruited. The presence of associated injuries to the shoulder girdle, the brachial plexus, or the ribs may influence the outcome. In addition, the methods of evaluation of functional outcomes are also heterogeneous with different authors using different scoring systems. There are no prospective studies, or comparative studies examining surgically and nonsurgically treated fractures.

Hardegger et al.[80] in 1984 evaluated 34 of 37 patients treated surgically for a scapula fracture. Their mean age was 42 years (17 to 85) with a mean follow-up of 6.5 years (1.5 to 18). Fractures included four process fractures, 11 fractures of the glenoid rim, 12 fractures of the glenoid fossa, three fractures of the surgical neck, two fractures of the anatomical neck, and five combined scapula fractures. The authors evaluated range of motion, pain, and muscle strength. In 21 patients (64%) full function of the shoulder was restored, and in 79% of patients the result was evaluated as excellent or good.

Bauer et al.[18] in 1995 evaluated the results of surgery in 20 patients with a scapula fracture. The mean age was 36 years, (16 to 69) and the mean follow-up was 6 years (1 to 11). This series included two fractures of the scapular body, six process fractures, six fractures of the neck (surgical and anatomical), and six glenoid fractures. Evaluation on the basis of the Constant score showed 75% very good and good results, 20% fair results, and 5% poor results.

Herrera et al.[87] in 2009 treated 22 patients with a scapula fracture treated surgically 3 and more weeks after injury. Fourteen of 16 patients available for review were evaluated by means of the DASH and Short Form 36 scores. The mean follow-up was 27 months (12 to 72). Nine cases were intra-articular and five cases extra-articular fractures. The mean DASH score was 14. Of all 16 patients, 13 resumed their normal activities without restriction.

A number of authors have reported the results of fixation of glenoid fractures. Kavanagh et al.[109] in 1993 described nine patients with glenoid fossa fractures. The mean age was 35 years (22 to 49) and the mean follow-up was 4 years (2 to 10). The authors evaluated range of motion and reported that the mean abduction was 167 degrees (110 to 180). A study of 22 cases of glenoid fractures of Ideberg types II to V, with a follow-up of 5 to 23 years revealed a median Constant score which was 94% of the opposite shoulder. In four patients it was less than 50%. In two cases, internal fixation failed and one patient developed a deep infection.[167]

In another study of 14 glenoid fractures of Ideberg types II to V, with the mean age of patients of 35 years (23 to 53) all cases had excellent or good results.[122] The mean follow-up was 30 months (18 to 68). Mayo et al.[132] in 1998 evaluated the results of 27 surgically treated glenoid fractures with a mean follow-up of 2 years. The mean age of patients was 29 years (15 to 64), the mean follow-up was 43 months (25 to 75). Anatomical reduction was achieved in 89% of cases. Results were based on the Shoulder rating score and were excellent in 22%, good in 60%, and fair in 11% of cases. Seven percent of results were poor.

More recently Heim et al.[86] evaluated 11 patients with a mean age of 34 years (22 to 49), of whom 10 sustained a scapular neck or body fracture and 1 patient a fracture of the scapular neck and glenoid. All the patients were operated on via the Judet approach. The mean follow-up was 24 months (6 to 53). Evaluation was based on the UCLA score; eight patients had excellent-to-good results, two patients fair results, and one patient a poor result.

Khallaf et al.[110] in 2005 operated on 14 patients with a mean age of 34 years (19 to 44) and a displaced fracture of the scapular neck although according to the description and radiographs published they were fractures of the scapular neck and body. The Judet approach was used. The mean follow-up was 20 months (6 to 30). Using the UCLA shoulder score there were excellent in 86% and good results in 14% of cases. A further study[104] in 2009 evaluated 37 patients with a mean age of 30 years (16 to 68) with fractures of the scapular body and neck fixed using the Judet approach. The review period was a minimum of 1 year. In 17 cases the fracture also involved the clavicle, which was always treated operatively. No infection or internal fixation failure was recorded. The reported range of motion averaged 158 degrees (range 90 to 180 degrees). Esenkaya and Ünay[52] in 2011 treated 11 fractures of the scapular body or neck in nine patients with a mean age of 37 years (19 to 52) and a mean follow-up of 40 months (12 to 77). The result, evaluated according to the Herscovici score, was excellent in all the patients.

Bartoníček and Frič[14] evaluated 22 patients with a mean age of 35 years (19 to 56) and a mean follow-up of 26 months (19 to 56). All the patients were operated on by the same surgeon using the Judet approach. In 17 patients an infraspinous fracture of the scapular body (biomechanical body) was recorded and in five cases this fracture was combined with a fracture of the inferior glenoid. The mean Constant score was 94. In 21 patients the results were evaluated as excellent or very good (Constant score 95 to 100). One poor result was recorded in a patient with an injury to the brachial plexus.

A radiographic review of 84 fractures of the scapular body, or neck, with or without articular involvement was reported by Cole et al.[34] Surgery was performed by a single surgeon via the Judet approach. The mean age of the patients was 45 years (18 to 76) and the mean follow-up was 23.5 months (6 to 70). All fractures healed, but with three malunions. Neither infection nor wound dehiscence was reported.

Anavian et al.[7] examined 26 patients with 27 fractures of the processes of scapula treated operatively. The mean age was 36 years (18 to 67) and the mean review period was 11 months (2 to 42). Acromion fracture patterns included six acromion base fractures and seven fractures lateral to the base. Coracoid fracture patterns included 11 fractures of the coracoid base and 3 fractures distal to the base. The results were evaluated by means of the DASH and SF 36 scores. All fractures healed and all patients had recovered full range of motion without pain.

Treatment of Individual Fracture Types for Scapula Fractures

In selecting the appropriate treatment it is important to know the exact type and displacement of the fracture and the age, functional expectations, and general condition of the patient.

Process Fractures

Process fractures include those involving the coracoid, acromion and the scapular spine, and the superior angle and the superior border of the scapula.[73] All of these parts of the scapula serve only for attachment of muscles and ligaments, and are not involved in the transmission of compressive forces from the glenoid to the scapular body. Fractures of processes are avulsion fractures caused by the pull of muscles and ligaments, by a direct blow and stress fractures.[21,66,78,91,143]

Fractures of processes often occur in various combinations, such as fractures of the acromion and the coracoid,[73,123,199] fractures of the acromion and the scapular spine or rarely in all the four processes simultaneously (fractures of the upper scapula). Fractures of the acromion, scapular spine, and coracoid are usually associated with a fracture of the humeral head, clavicle, AC dislocation,[28,99,116] rupture of the tendon of the long head of biceps, or injuries to the suprascapular nerve or brachial plexus.[145]

Clinically the most important are fractures of the coracoid, acromion, and the lateral part of the scapular spine. Malunion may compromise the subacromial and subcoracoid spaces and cause impingement and the pull of muscles on a nonunited fragment may cause pain.[23,61]

Fractures of the Acromion and the Lateral Scapular Spine. These fractures may be divided according to the course of the fracture line[145] or the type of displacement.[115] The fracture line usually passes out with the AC joint. It may be difficult to distinguish between a fracture and an os acromiale. Acromion fractures may be associated with an extensive rotator cuff tear when the radiographs may show proximal migration of the humeral head. In such cases imaging of the rotator cuff is necessary.

Undisplaced fractures may be treated conservatively. Immobilization in a sling for 3 weeks is often sufficient. Passive mobilization may begin immediately after the injury, and active exercises after the fracture union. If displaced fractures compromise the subacromial space, they should be reduced and stabilized.[7,67,73] Fixation may be performed using cerclage wiring, lag screws, or a plate.[190] Hsu[93] describes an arthroscopically assisted fixation. If the avulsed acromial fragment is small, it should be excised.

Coracoid Fractures. Coracoid fractures may be isolated, but mostly they are associated with other injuries to the scapula or the shoulder such as fractures of the glenoid, the surgical neck of the scapula or the acromion,[199] AC dislocation,[112] lateral clavicle fractures, dislocation of the humeral head, or a rotator cuff tear.[106]

Coracoid fractures are divided according to the location of the fracture line. Eyres et al.[55] described five types, Goss[73] three, and Ogawa[144,147] only two. The Ogawa type I is a fracture of the coracoid base, with the fracture line passing posterior to the insertion of the CC ligament into the coracoid. Ogawa does not distinguish between extra- and intra-articular fractures of the coracoid base. In Ogawa type II, which is an avulsion fracture of the coracoid tip, the fracture line passes anterior to the insertion of CC ligament. Type I is more frequent.

The author has modified the Goss classification and divided coracoid fractures into three basic types. Type I is an avulsion fracture of the coracoid tip. The fracture line passes anterior to the attachment of the CC ligament. The tip is displaced distally by the pull of the conjoined tendon of the coracobrachialis and the short head of biceps. Type I fractures may result in a painful nonunion or exceptionally they may prevent reduction of a dislocated humeral head. In types II and III, the fracture line runs posterior to the attachment of the CC ligament. Type II is an extra-articular fracture of the coracoid base. Type III includes intra-articular fractures of the coracoid or fractures of the superior pole of the glenoid extending as far as the superior border of the scapula. There is a direct relation between the size of the separated articular surface of the glenoid fossa and extension of the fracture line as far as the superior border or superior angle of the scapula. Types II and III occur more frequently than type I. Fracture types II and III are equivalent to a CC ligament rupture and may compromise the integrity of the SSSC. In addition, type III displaced fractures compromise the congruence of the glenoid fossa.

There is no consensus in the literature about the treatment of coracoid fractures.[7,130,147] Some authors prefer conservative treatment for undisplaced or minimally displaced fractures. The aim of treatment of displaced fractures is to prevent progression to a painful nonunion (type I), displacement and instability in associated injuries to the AC joint, floating shoulder in associated fractures of the surgical neck of scapula, or glenoid incongruence (types II and III). For these reasons it is preferable, especially in younger active individuals, to treat displaced fractures operatively by open reduction and fixation with screws, or, if necessary, with a small plate in fractures of the coracoid base[112] In type I fractures it is better to excise the small fragment and reattach the conjoined tendon.[73]

Fracture of the Superior Border, or Superior Angle, of the Scapula. Fractures of the superior border or superior angle of the scapula occur rarely in isolation mostly being part of fractures of the upper scapula.[146,195] Fractures of the superior border of the scapula are often associated with intra-articular fractures of the coracoid base. Isolated fractures may be displaced by the pull of the levator scapulae on the superior angle. Despite displacement, these fractures are treated conservatively.

Body Fractures

Fractures of the scapular body are often confused with fractures of the scapular neck and vice versa. In terms of severity, they may be divided into fractures of the anatomical body and fractures of the biomechanical body.[14,181] Fractures of the biomechanical body are more common. In terms of the number of border fragments, they may be divided into two-, three-, and multifragment fractures.[14] Fractures of the anatomical body are less common and almost all of them are comminuted. This demonstrates that these are high-energy injuries, as they also involve the strong scapular spine. Both groups may be combined with fractures of the surgical neck of the scapula, fractures of the clavicle, or AC dislocations.

Fractures of the scapular body compromise the alignment between the glenoid and the lateral border of the scapular body without affecting the relation between the glenoid, coracoid, and acromion. Diagnosis of scapular body fractures and an exact determination of the fracture pattern are impossible without 3D CT reconstructions.

Until recently these fractures were treated conservatively. Currently there is a growing number of articles documenting very good outcomes from operative treatment of displaced scapular body fractures.[14,34,35,52]

AUTHOR'S PREFERRED METHOD OF TREATMENT FOR SCAPULA BODY FRACTURES

Significantly displaced fractures of the scapular body are indications for operative treatment via the Judet approach (Fig. 39-16). The first and most important goal is restoration of the integrity of the lateral border of the body and, consequently, the relationship between the border and glenoid. Where necessary, internal fixation is performed in the spinomedial and inferior angles of the scapula. In the presence of an associated fracture of the clavicle, internal fixation of the scapula should be performed first and then followed by internal fixation of the clavicle.[14,15]

Neck Fractures

There are many publications on fractures of the glenoid neck in relation to unsatisfactory outcomes of conservative treatment and also in connection with the floating shoulder[41,71,88,121,155,163,184] and also some case reports.[10,110,186] Malunion of the scapular neck changes the GPA and relations in the subacromial and subcoracoid space.

Anatomical Neck Fractures. This type of fracture has been mentioned by many authors,[18,42,71,80,101] although it is quite rare. Anatomical neck fractures are unstable. The glenoid fragment is displaced distally with the humeral head by the pull of the long head of triceps, and the subacromial space becomes wider.

There are only four radiologically documented cases of anatomical neck fractures. Two cases were published by Hardegger

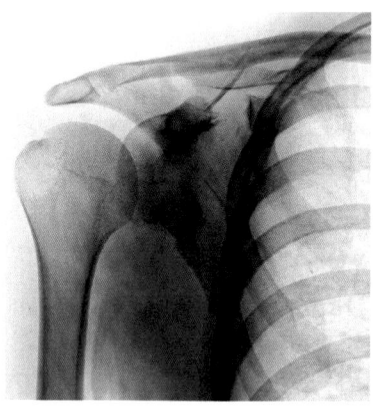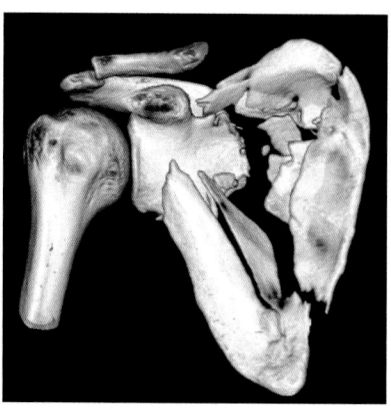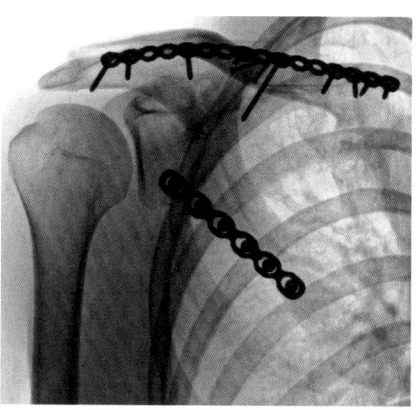

A, B   C

FIGURE 39-16 Reduction and fixation of a comminuted fracture of the anatomical body of the scapula. **A:** AP radiograph after injury, (**B**) 3D reconstruction of injured scapula, anterior aspect, (**C**) anatomical reduction and fixation of lateral border with 3.5-mm reconstruction plate and scapular spine with 2.7-mm reconstruction plate.

et al.,[80] one case by Arts and Louette,[10] and one case by Jeong,[102] who included also 3D CT reconstruction. The author himself recorded two cases, in one of which 3D CT reconstruction was performed. In all six cases fracture displacement was the indication for operative treatment, using the Judet approach. Fixation was performed with two plates, lag screws, or a combination of both.

Surgical Neck Fractures. Surgical neck fractures are the most frequently discussed of all scapular neck fractures.[71,92,126,184] Surgical neck fractures are stable if they are not associated with rupture of the CC and CA ligaments. Magerl[126] described two degrees of instability. Type I includes injuries consisting of rupture of only the CA ligament, combined with anterior displacement of the glenoid. In type II, both ligaments are ruptured and the glenoid is displaced anteriorly, distally, and medially by the pull of the muscles attached to the coracoid. The CC space is wider and the relation between the acromion and the coracoid is compromised. Extra-articular fracture of the coracoid base is equivalent to rupture of the CC and CA ligaments.[71] In this case, however, distal displacement of the glenoid is less marked, because the neck is not displaced by the muscles attached to the coracoid. Surgical neck fractures may be combined with a fracture of the scapular body or with a clavicular fracture.

Diagnosis of surgical neck fractures based on a radiograph alone is difficult in most cases. 3D CT reconstruction is very helpful in determining the fracture pattern.

Displacement of fractures of the surgical neck of the scapula is currently increasingly regarded as an indication for operative treatment. Fixation may be performed via the Judet approach, using plates or a combination of a plate and transspinous screws.

Transspinous Fractures of the Scapular Neck. Transspinous fracture of the neck is almost unknown. Gagey et al.[58] were the first to publish a drawing as late as in 1984 and called it "fracture transpinale." Ada and Miller classified a fracture with a fracture line similar to a type IIB scapular neck fracture.[1]

Cole[33] published a 3D CT reconstruction of a transspinous fracture of the scapular neck which he called a scapular neck fracture. The author of this chapter recorded two cases of transspinous fracture of the neck of which one was in combination with a clavicular fracture.

A definite diagnosis of a transspinous fracture is only possible with the use of 3D CT reconstruction. Displaced fractures can be reduced and fixed to the spinal and lateral pillars from the Judet approach, preferably using plates.

AUTHOR'S PREFERRED METHOD OF TREATMENT FOR SCAPULA NECK FRACTURES

In younger, physically active patients all three types of scapular neck fractures, if displaced, are indications for operative treatment via the Judet approach using plates and lag screws (Fig. 39-17).

Glenoid Fractures

The goal of treatment of glenoid fractures is to restore congruity and stability to the glenohumeral joint. Undisplaced, minimally displaced, or displaced fractures of the glenoid rim with a small fragment may be treated conservatively.[114] Larger, displaced fragments may be reduced and fixed operatively.[2,109,122,167] The main indication for operative treatment of glenoid fractures is currently considered to be displacement of more than 3 to 10 mm with a simultaneous involvement of 20% to 30% of the articular surface.

Fractures of the Superior Glenoid. Fractures of the superior glenoid are intra-articular fractures of the coracoid base. Displacement is caused primarily by the pull of the muscles attached to the coracoid. Significant displacement of the fragment results in malalignment of the coracoid which may compromise the subcoracoid space and lead to the

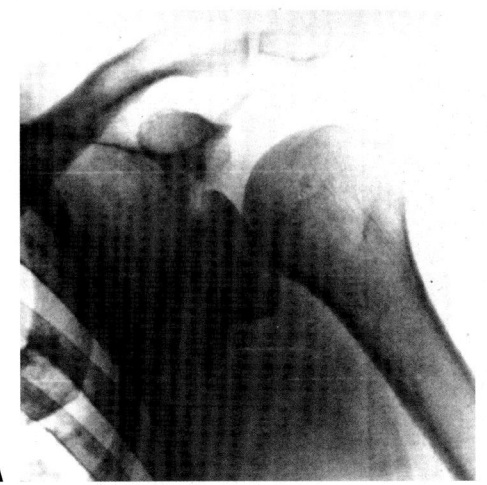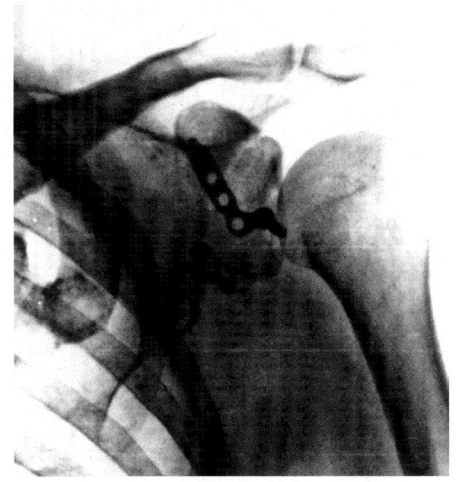

FIGURE 39-17 Reduction and fixation of fracture of an anatomical scapular neck fracture. **A:** Postinjury AP radiograph with typical displacement of the glenoid fragment. **B:** Reduction and fixation with two 3.5-mm plates and a wire loop.

development of coracoid impingement.[63] Fixation is usually performed via the deltopectoral approach, using lag screws, or a small plate.

Fracture of the Anteroinferior Rim of the Glenoid.
Fractures of the anteroinferior rim of the glenoid are associated with anterior dislocation of the glenohumeral joint. The size of the avulsed fragments varies. There are differing opinions on the treatment of these fractures. Most authors recommend operative treatment especially in cases with bigger fragments or a persisting subluxation of the humeral head.[2,27,153,168,177] However, Maquieira et al.[127] published very good results in 14 patients with a fracture of the anteroinferior glenoid rim with fragments of more than 5 mm in size and displacement of more than 2 mm, who underwent conservative treatment and were followed up for an average of 5.5 years. Open reduction and fixation with cannulated screws, a small plate, or bone anchors are performed via the deltopectoral approach. Some authors also describe arthroscopic treatment.

Fractures of the Posterior Rim of the Glenoid.
These rare fractures, resulting from posterior dislocation of the glenohumeral joint, are treated similarly to fractures of the anterior rim of the glenoid. Where reduction and fixation are indicated, they may be performed either by an open procedure from the posterosuperior approach or arthroscopically.

Fracture of the Inferior Glenoid.
Fracture of the inferior glenoid separates the distal one- to two-thirds of the glenoid fossa. These fractures are caused by a direct impact of the abducted humeral head on the lower half of the glenoid and typically occur in cyclists, or motorcyclists.[14] The fracture line extends as far as the lateral pillar of the scapula and mostly involves the scapular body (Fig. 39-18). Mayo et al.,[132] Schandelmaier et al.,[167] Cole,[33,34] Jones et al.,[104] and Bartoníček and Cronier[14] recommend treating displaced fractures via the posterior Judet approach.

AUTHOR'S PREFERRED METHOD OF TREATMENT FOR GLENOID FRACTURES

Displaced fractures of the glenoid, mainly those of its anterior rim and of its lower part, are indications for surgery, mainly in younger or physically active patients. Surgical fixation of a larger avulsion of the anterior rim restores congruity and stability to the glenohumeral joint.

Fractures of the inferior glenoid and fractures of the scapular body may be treated from the posterior Judet approach which allows a simultaneous reconstruction of both the articular surface and the biomechanical body of the scapula. The posterolateral approach provides only a limited exposure of the inferior glenoid and lateral border of the scapula and is not suitable for treatment of these cases. Internal fixation is performed using a combination of lag screws and plates, depending on the fracture anatomy (Fig. 39-19). Stable internal fixation allows rehabilitation to start immediately after operation.

Combined Fractures
Combined fractures of the scapula may be divided into two groups. The first group includes fractures resulting from a combination of the four basic patterns of scapula fractures. The second group comprises combinations of one or more basic patterns of scapula fractures associated with injuries to other bones, or joints, of the shoulder girdle.

Floating Shoulder. Floating shoulder results from ipsilateral fractures of the scapular neck and the clavicle. It is a rare injury, frequently discussed in the literature mainly in terms of its anatomy and management.[43,48,49,60,84,89,100,117,121,148,149,154,158,161,182,183,194]

Floating shoulder results from violation of the integrity of the SSSC. Double disruption of the SSSC, or its single disruption in combination with a fracture of one or both struts, creates a potentially unstable anatomical situation. This may have

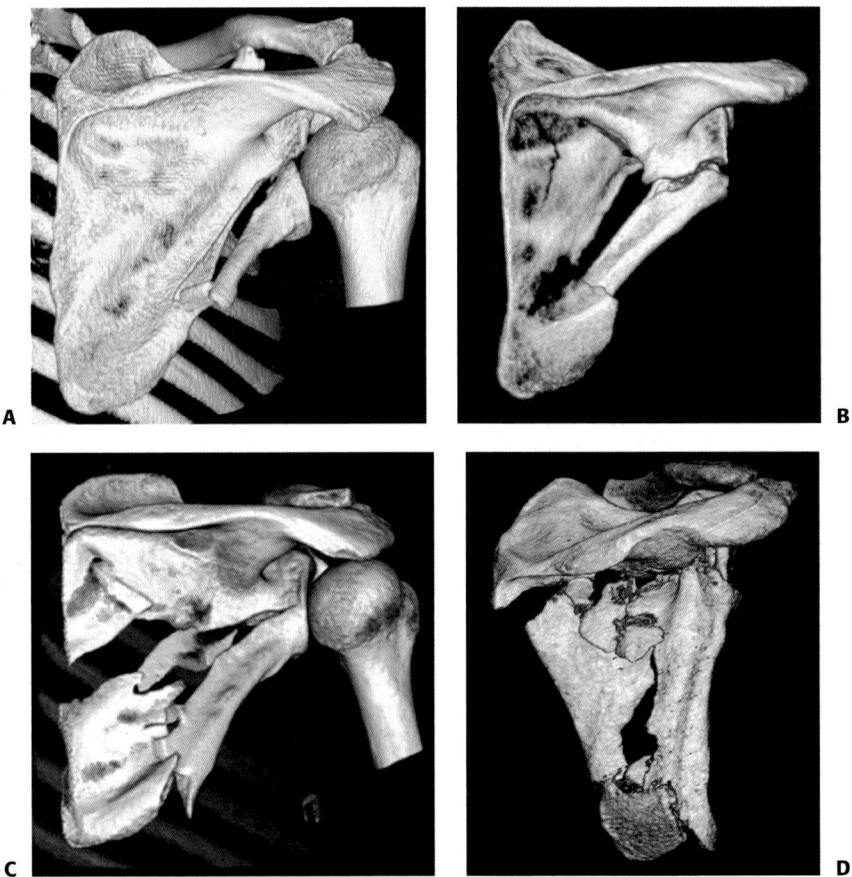

FIGURE 39-18 Different types of inferior glenoid fractures. **A:** The intra-articular fragment is formed by the inferior half of the glenoid fossa and by a short part of the lateral border. **B:** The intra-articular fragment is formed by the inferior third of the glenoid fossa and the whole lateral border. The fracture involves the center of the infraspinous fossa; the medial border of the scapular body is intact. **C:** The intra-articular fragment is formed by the inferior third of glenoid fossa. The inferior angle of the scapula forms a separate fragment. **D:** The intra-articular fragment is formed by the inferior half of the glenoid fossa and the whole lateral border. The whole biomechanical body is involved.

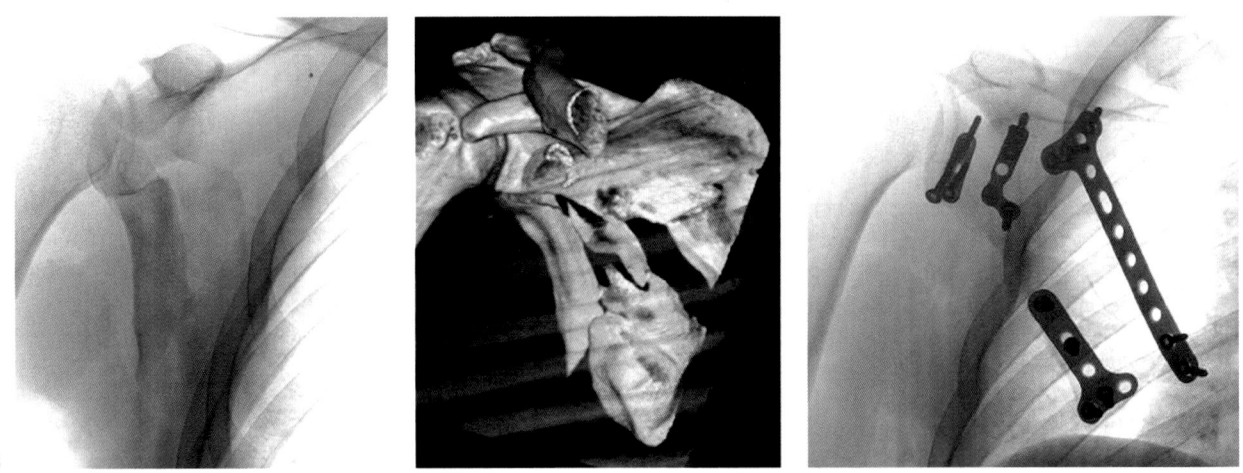

FIGURE 39-19 Reduction and fixation of the inferior glenoid and biomechanical body. **A:** AP radiograph of the injured right scapula, (**B**) 3D CT reconstruction, anterior aspect. For the posterior aspect see Figure 39-18C. **C:** Anatomical reduction and fixation with four 3.5-mm plates.

clinical consequences such as delayed union, nonunion, or malunion. Combination of a fracture of the glenoid neck with another SSSC disruption, for example, an associated fracture of the middle third of the clavicle, may produce a "floating shoulder." Floating shoulder was defined by Herscovici et al.[89] as "ipsilateral midclavicular and scapular neck fractures," implying a clavicle fracture medial to the attachment of the CC ligament.

Williams et al.[194] pointed out that Goss did not include the CA ligament in the structures of the bone–soft tissue ring. DeFranco and Patterson[43] considers this ligament as an important stabilizer in the SSSC. Williams et al.[194] also stated that midshaft clavicular and surgical neck fractures alone cannot produce a floating shoulder. Scapular neck fragments are attached to the clavicle by the CC ligament. In the presence of an ipsilateral fracture of clavicular shaft and surgical neck, the glenoid has lost its attachment to the axial skeleton. However, it is still attached to the acromion by the CA ligament and by the osseoligamentous chain consisting of the CC ligament, distal clavicular fragment, and the AC capsular ligaments. As a result, a floating shoulder may develop only after disruption of the CC and CA ligaments.

Analysis of studies on the floating shoulder revealed a number of problematic issues. Most authors included in their case series not only patients with a midshaft clavicular fracture, but also those with a fracture of the lateral or even medial clavicle and patients with AC dislocation. In all case series, fractures of the scapular neck were diagnosed only by standard radiographs and not by 3D CT reconstruction. Analysis of the radiographs in these studies, however, showed that they were mainly fractures of the scapular body rather than fractures of the scapular neck. DeFranco and Patterson[43] and Owens,[154] therefore, recommend 3D CT reconstructions to properly define the fracture pattern. In addition, most authors do not describe injuries to individual ligaments constituting the SSSC complex.

All these deficiencies are reflected in the studies that report good results for both conservative and operative treatment. Some authors perform only internal fixation of the clavicle with the aim of diminishing displacement of the scapular neck. The concept that reduction of the clavicular fracture will also reduce the scapula fracture is in many cases illusory (Fig. 39-20). When better results are reported after internal fixation of the clavicle it has to be taken into account that stabilization of the clavicle allows an intensive rehabilitation of shoulder girdle much sooner than with conservative treatment which may have an impact on the final result. Oh et al.[149] described two cases of failure of plating of the clavicle in the treatment of ipsilateral clavicle and glenoid neck fractures. Very good results after simultaneous internal fixation of the clavicle and the scapula were described by Labler et al.,[117] Egol et al.,[49] and Leung and Lam.[121]

The condition of floating shoulder requires careful review on the basis of new studies with identification of the individual types of this injury and their displacement by 3D CT reconstruction.

Scapulothoracic Dissociation

Scapulothoracic dissociation is a rare, severe, high-energy injury characterized by a wide range of concomitant injuries including those to the shoulder girdle (SC dislocation, clavicle fracture, AC dislocation), tears of the levator scapulae, rhomboids, trapezius, latissimus dorsi, pectoralis minor and deltoid muscles, vascular injuries to subclavian or axillary artery, and partial or complete avulsion of brachial plexus. There is massive soft tissue swelling in the shoulder region while the skin is usually intact. It is caused by a violent lateral distraction or rotational displacement of the shoulder girdle when the upper extremity is caught on a fixed object while the body is moving at high speed.[3,65,75,118,198] The mortality is reported to be 11%.[198]

The diagnosis is not easy and is based on clinical examination and radiologic findings. The injury may be suspected clinically in the presence of a palpable gap between the medial border of the scapula and the spinous processes. It is important to perform an anteroposterior chest radiograph to show lateral displacement of the scapula. In a hemodynamically stable patient arteriography may determine the extent and localization of the vascular injury.

The treatment of scapulothoracic dissociation depends on the severity of associated injuries and the general condition of the patient. Zelle et al.[198] proposed a system for classifying the

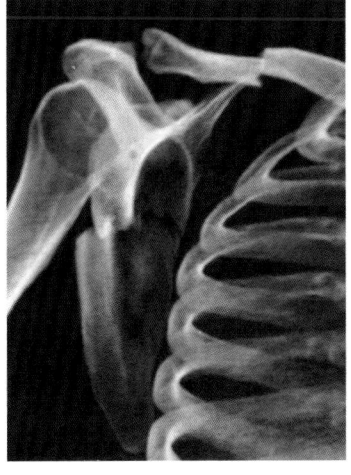
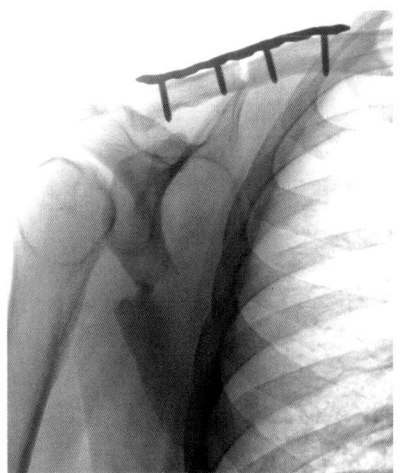

FIGURE 39-20 Combined fracture of the scapular body and clavicle. This fracture is often presented as a floating shoulder. **A:** 3D CT reconstruction of the right scapula after injury. **B:** Reduction and fixation of clavicle failed to reduce the fracture of scapular body.

TABLE 39-1	Zelle's System for Classifying the Severity of Scapulothoracic Dissociation
Type	**Clinical Findings**
1	Musculoskeletal injury alone
2A	Musculoskeletal injury with vascular injury
2B	Musculoskeletal injury with incomplete neurologic impairment of the upper extremity
3	Musculoskeletal injury with incomplete neurologic impairment of the upper extremity and vascular injury
4	Musculoskeletal injury with complete brachial plexus avulsion

Adapted from Zelle BA, Pape HC, Gerich TG, et al. Functional outcome following scapulothoracic dissociation. *J Bone Joint Surg Am.* 2004;86-A:2–7.

severity of scapulothoracic dissociation (Table 39-1). Treatment should focus on the neurovascular injury. Surgical repair should be performed, if necessary. However, there is an extensive collateral network around the shoulder which may substitute for the injured major blood vessel. Vascular repair in patients with a complete brachial plexus palsy is somewhat questionable. Neurologic repair is also controversial. Zelle et al.[198] demonstrated that the extent of the brachial plexus injury is the most important predictor of the functional outcome. Patients with partial plexus injuries had a better prognosis. All patients with a complete brachial plexus injury had either an amputation or poor shoulder function. He recommended an immediate above-elbow amputation if upper extremity function is not recoverable. This solution seems to result in better functional outcomes and lower rates of complications.

The best treatment of associated shoulder girdle injuries is unclear. Goss[75] recommended internal fixation of clavicular fractures and stabilization of disrupted AC or SC joints to protect the brachial plexus, subclavian, and axillary vessels, to improve conditions for bone healing and to restore stability to the shoulder girdle.

COMPLICATIONS OF SCAPULA FRACTURES AND THEIR TREATMENT

Both conservative and operative treatments of scapula fractures have a number of early and late complications, leading ultimately to pain, limitation of the range of motion, reduction of muscle strength, or instability of the shoulder.

Complications of Nonoperative Treatment for Scapula Fractures

Malunion is the most common complication of nonoperative treatment of scapula fractures.[36,79,131,137] Healing of extra-articular fractures in a nonanatomical position changes the relationship between the glenoid and the scapular body and consequently the

course of the muscles of the rotator cuff. This has an impact on their function. Subjectively, it is manifested by feelings of weakness, pain, and stiffness. Pace et al.[155] described in these cases late degenerative changes of the rotator cuff. Malunion may also result in impingement syndrome.[63] Fractures of the glenoid that have healed in displacement result in incongruity, instability, or both, and subsequently in degenerative joint disease.[167]

Malunion is treated by osteotomy and reorientation of the scapular neck and/or body.[36] In intra-articular malunion, one successful case of osteotomy of the glenoid fossa has been described by Haraguchi et al.[79] Prominence of a malunited bony fragment may be painful. The solution is excision of the projecting part of the bone.[130]

Delayed union was described by Curtis et al.[39] in a 15-year-old sportsman with a nondisplaced fracture of the scapular neck.

Nonunions of the scapular body are rare.[56,76,107,137] In 2009, only 15 had been reported in the English literature, all of them treated conservatively.[129] Nonunion of the acromion has also been reported.[75] The solution is internal fixation or excision of the ununited fragment.

Injury to the suprascapular nerve can occur in fractures of the scapular neck when the suprascapular nerve becomes entrapped in the fracture line[37]. This injury is manifested by atrophy of the infraspinatus.[22,47,172]

Rib nonunion may be a rare cause of chronic pain after a scapula fracture. In the four reported cases, the situation was successfully treated by internal fixation.[5]

Complications of Operative Treatment for Scapula Fractures

Complications of operative treatment may be divided into intraoperative, early postoperative, and late postoperative ones.

Intraoperative complications include injuries to the suprascapular nerve, malreduction, and intra-articular perforation by screws. In an analysis of 212 cases, Lantry et al.[119] found injury to the suprascapular nerve in 2.4%. It is difficult to distinguish whether the injury was caused by the original trauma or during surgery. Reduction of the fragments may be hard to achieve in comminuted fractures of the scapular body, or in significantly displaced fractures of the scapular neck, particularly if surgery is delayed. Screws can be placed into the joint particularly during internal fixation of the scapular neck or of the lateral border of the scapula.

Early postoperative complications include first of all hematoma, and infection, either superficial or deep.[2,80,167] According to Lantry et al.,[119] the infection rate is quite high at 4.2%. Hematoma may require evacuation. Most cases of superficial infection may be treated with antibiotics and local care but deep infection requires debridement of the surgical wound, and, where necessary, removal of the implant.

A relatively common complication is a limited range of motion of the shoulder, requiring manipulation if it persists for more than 6 weeks after surgery.[2,167]

Late complications are reported quite frequently. Failure of internal fixation frequently requires reoperation,[80,119,167] as does nonunion.[129] Oh et al.[149] described two cases of failure of plate fixation of the clavicle in the treatment of ipsilateral clavicle and glenoid neck fractures. The authors concluded that where a scapular neck fracture remains displaced even after internal fixation of the clavicle, its reduction and fixation are necessary.

Residual incongruity as a result of nonanatomical reduction was described by Mayo.[132] Hardegger[80] reported reoperation for joint instability. Two cases of heterotopic ossification have been described, in one of which there was compression of the axillary nerve requiring surgical decompression.[109,119] Heim et al.[86] reported postoperative scapular widening. Acromial impingement after internal fixation of the glenoid can be treated by acromioplasty.[167] Prominence of implants, requiring their removal, is a problem mainly in fractures of the acromion, scapular spine, or associated clavicular fractures.[34,119] One report also describes late infection 11 months after operation, requiring hardware removal.[167] In addition, one breakage of a plate was recorded after several years in a healed scapula fracture.[167]

Posttraumatic degenerative disease after scapula fractures is reported to occur in 1.9% of cases. If symptomatic it can be managed by arthrodesis[2,80,119] but the current treatment of choice is shoulder arthroplasty.

SUMMARY, CONTROVERSIES, AND FUTURE DIRECTIONS IN SCAPULA FRACTURES

The basic problem of the current studies on scapula fractures is that radiology does not always allow proper determination of the fracture pattern leading to unsatisfactory classification, inaccurate determination of fragment displacement, and heterogeneous and nonvalid outcome measurements. Small numbers of scapula fractures are treated in any single department, which results in limited experience of operative treatment for any one treating surgeons. Randomized studies with mid- and long-term results are not available.

Plain radiographs should be supplemented by 3D CT reconstructions, allowing exact determination of the fracture pattern and a classification must be developed that reflects clinical reality. Indications for conservative, or operative, treatment have to be based on objective evaluation of fragment displacement. Special attention should be given to associated injuries. Evidence-based studies must concentrate on single fracture types, mainly comparing the results of conservative and operative treatments and use validated and specific outcome instruments.

REFERENCES

1. Ada JR, Miller ME. Scapula fractures. Analysis of 113 cases. *Clin Orthop Rel Res.* 1991;269:174–180.
2. Adam FF. Surgical treatment of displaced fractures of the glenoid cavity. *Inter Orthop (SICOT).* 2002;26:150–153.
3. Althausen PL, Lee MA, Finkemeier CG. Scapulothoracic dissociation: Diagnosis and treatment. *Clin Orthop Relat Res.* 2003;416:237–244.
4. Anavian J, Conflicitti JM, Khanna G, et al. A reliable radiographic measurement technique for extra-articular scapular fractures. *Clin Orthop Rel Res.* 2011;469:3371–3378.
5. Anavian J, Guthrie T, Cole PA. Surgical management of multiple painful rib nonunions in patient with a history of severe shoulder girdle trauma: A case report and literature review. *J Orthop Trauma.* 2009;23:600–604.
6. Anavian J, Khanna G, Plocher EK, et al. Progressive displacement of scapula fractures. *J Trauma.* 2010;69:156–161.
7. Anavian J, Wijdicks CA, Schroder L, et al. Surgery for scapula process fractures. *Acta Orthop.* 2009;80:344–350.
8. Armitage BM, Wijdicks CA, Tarkin IS, et al. Mapping of scapular fractures with three-dimensional computed tomography. *J Bone Joint Surg Am.* 2009;91-A:2222–2228.
9. Armstrong CP, van der Spuy J. The fractured scapula: Importance and management based on a series of 62 patients. *Injury.* 1984;15:324–329.
10. Arts V, Louette L. Scapular neck fractures; an update of the concept of floating shoulder. *Injury.* 1999;30:146–148.
11. Aulicino PL, Reinert C, Kornberg M, et al. Displaced intra-articular glenoid fractures treated by open reduction and internal fixation. *J Trauma.* 1986;26:1137–1141.
12. Baldwin KD, Ohman-Strickland P, Mehta S, et al. Scapular fractures: A marker for concomitant injury? A retrospective review of data in the national trauma database. *J Trauma.* 2008;65:430–435.
13. Bartoníček J, Cronier P. History of the treatment of scapular fractures. *Arch Orthop Trauma Surg.* 2010;130:83–92.
14. Bartoníček J, Frič V. Scapular body fractures: Results of the operative treatment. *Inter Orthop (SICOT).* 2011;35:747–753.
15. Bartoníček J, Frič V, Tuček M. Intra-operative reduction of the scapular body—A technical trick. *J Orthop Trauma.* 2009;23:294–298.
16. Bartoníček J, Frič V, Tuček M. Radiodiagnostika zlomenin lopatky. [Radiographic evaluation of scapula fractures]. *Rozhl Chir.* 2009;88:84–88.
17. Bartoníček J, Tuček M, Luňáček L. Judetův zadní přístup k lopatce [Judet posterior approach to the scapula]. *Acta Chir Orthop Traumatol Čech.* 2008;75:429–435.
18. Bauer G, Fleischmann W, Dussler E. Displaced scapular fractures: Indication and long-term results of open reduction and internal fixation. *Arch Orthop Trauma Surg.* 1995;114:215–219.
19. Bauer T, Abadie O, Hardy P. Arthroscopic treatment of glenoid fractures. *Arthroscopy.* 2006;22:569–576.
20. Bestard EA, Schvene HR, Bestard EH. Glenoplasty in the management of recurrent shoulder dislocation. *Contemp Orthop.* 1986;12:47–55.
21. Binazzi R, Assiso J, Vaccari V, et al. Avulsion fractures of the scapula: Report of eight cases. *J Trauma.* 1992;33:785–789.
22. Boerger TO, Limb D. Suprascapular nerve injury at the spinoglenoid notch after glenoid neck fracture. *J Shoulder Elbow Surg.* 2000;9:236–237.
23. Böhm P. Pseudoarthrosis of the spine of the scapula – case report of a minimally invasive osteosynthesis technique. *Acta Orthop Scand.* 1998;69:645–647.
24. Bozkurt M, Can F, Kirdemir V, et al. Conservative treatment of scapular neck fracture: The effect of stability and glenopolar angle on clinical outcome. *Injury.* 2005;36:1176–1181.
25. Brodsky JW, Tullos HS, Gartsman G. Simplified posterior approach to the shoulder joint. *J Bone Joint Surg [Am].* 1987;69-A:773–774.
26. Burke CS, Roberts CS, Nyland JA, et al. Scapular thickness - implications for fracture fixation. *J Shoulder Elbow Surg.* 2006;15:645–648.
27. Cameron SE. Arthroscopic reduction and internal fixation of an anterior glenoid fracture. *Arthroscopy.* 1998;14:743–746.
28. Carr AJ, Broughton NS. Acromioclavicular dislocation associated with fracture of the coracoid process. *J Trauma.* 1989;29:125–126.
29. Chan CM, Chung CT, Lan HHC. Scapular fracture complicating suprascapular neuropathy: The role of computed tomography with 3D reconstruction. *J Chin Med Assoc.* 2009;72:340–342.
30. Coimbra R, Conroy C, Tominaga GT, et al. Causes of scapular fractures differ from other shoulder injuries in occupants seriously injured during motor vehicle crashes. *Injury.* 2010;41:151–155.
31. Cole PA. Scapula fractures. *Orthop Clin N Amer.* 2002;33:1–18.
32. Cole PA. Scapula fractures: Open reduction internal fixation. In: Wiss DA, ed. *Master techniques in orthopaedic surgery.* Philadelphia, PA: Lippincott Williams & Wilkins; 2006:15–36.
33. Cole PA, Marek DJ. Shoulder girdle injuries. In: Standard JP, Schmidt AH, Gregor PJ, eds. *Surgical treatment of orthopaedic trauma.* New York, NY: Stuttgart, Thieme; 2007:207–237.
34. Cole PA, Gauger EM, Herrera DA, et al. Radiographic follow-up of 84 operatively treated scapula neck and body fractures. *Injury.* 2012;43:327–333.
35. Cole PA, Gauger EM, Schroder LK. Management of scapular fractures. *J Am Acad Orthop Surg.* 2012;20:130–141.
36. Cole PA, Talbot M, Schroder LK, et al. Extra-articular malunions of the scapula: A comparison of functional outcome before and after reconstruction. *J Orthop Trauma.* 2011;25:649–656.
37. Constant CR, Murley AHG. A clinical method of functional assessment of the shoulder. *Clin Orthop Rel Res.* 1987;214:160–164.
38. Court-Brown Ch, McQueen MM, Tornetta P. *Trauma (shoulder girdle).* Philadelphia, PA: Lippincott Williams & Wilkins; 2006:68–88.
39. Curtis C, Sharma V, Micheli L. Delayed union of a scapular fracture – an unusual cause of persistent shoulder pain. *Med Sci Sport Exercise.* 2007;12:2095–2098.
40. Dawson J, Carr A. Questionnaire on the perceptions of patients about shoulder surgery. *J Bone Joint Surg.* 1996;78-B:593–600.
41. de Beer J, Berghs BM, van Rooyen KS, et al. Displaced scapular neck fracture: A case report. *J Shoulder Elbow Surg.* 2004;13:123–125.
42. Decoulx P, Minet P, Lemerle. Fractures de l'omoplate. *Lille Chirurgical.* 1956;11:217–227.
43. DeFranco MJ, Patterson BM. The floating shoulder. *J Am Acad Orthop Surg.* 2006;14:499–509.
44. Dimitroulias A, Molinero KG, Krenk DE, et al. Outcomes of nonoperatively treated displaced scapular body fractures. *Clin Orthop Rel Res.* 2011;469:1459–1465.
45. Dupont R, Evrard H. Sur une voie d'accès postérieure de l'omoplate. *J Chir (Paris).* 1932;39:528–534.
46. Ebraheim NA, Mekhail AO, Padanilum TG, et al. Anatomic considerations for a modified posterior approach to the scapula. *Clin Orthop Rel Res.* 1997;344:136–143.
47. Edeland HG, Zachrisson BE. Fracture of the scapular notch associated with lesion of the suprascapular nerve. *Acta Orthop Scand.* 1975;46:758.
48. Edwards SG, Whittle AP, Wood GW. Nonoperative treatment of ipsilateral fractures of the scapula and clavicle. *J Bone Joint Surg Am.* 2000;84-A:774–780.
49. Egol KA, Connor PM, Karunakar MA, et al. The floating shoulder: Clinical and functional results. *J Bone Joint Surg Am.* 2001;83-A:1188–1194.

50. Ellman H, Hanker G, Bayer M. Repair of the rotator cuff. End-result study of factors influencing reconstruction. *J Bone Joint Surg.* 1986;68-A:1136–1144.
51. Esenkaya I. Surgical treatment of scapular fractures. *Acta Chir Orthop Traumatol Turc.* 2003;37:33–40.
52. Esenkaya I, Ünay K. Anatomical frame plate osteosynthesis in Ada-Miller Type 2 or 4 scapular fractures. *Acta Chir Orthop Traumatol Turc.* 2011;45:151–161.
53. Euler E, Habermeyer P, Kohler W, et al. Skapulafrakturen - Klassifikation und Differential therapie. *Orthopäde.* 1992;21:158–162.
54. Euler E, Rüedi T. Skapulafraktur. In: Habermeyer P, Schweiberer L eds. *Schulterchirurgie.* München: Urban und Schwarzenberg; 1996.
55. Eyres KS, Brooks A, Stanley D. Fractures of the coracoid process. *J Bone Joint Surg.* 1995;77-B:425–428.
56. Ferraz IC, Papadimitriou NG, Sotereanos DG. Scapular body nonunion: A case report. *J Shoulder Elbow Surg.* 2002;11:98–100.
57. Findlay RT. Fractures of the scapula and ribs. *J Am Surg.* 1937;38:489–494.
58. Gagey O, Curey JP, Mazas F. Les fractures récentes de l'omoplate. A propos de 43 cas. *Rev Chir Orthop.* 1984;70:443–447.
59. Gagey O, Spraul JM, Vinh TS. Posterolateral approach of the shoulder: Assessment of 50 cases. *J Shoulder Elbow Surg.* 2001;10:47–51.
60. Ganz R, Noesberger B. Die Behandlung der Scapula-Frakturen. *H Unfallheilkunde.* 1975;126:59–62.
61. Garcia-Elias M, Salo JM. Nonunion of a fractured coracoid process after dislocation of the shoulder. *J Bone Joint Surg.* 1985;67-B:722–723.
62. Gauger EM, Cole PA. A minimally invasive approach to scapula neck and body fractures. *Clin Orthop Rel Res.* 2011;469:3390–3399.
63. Gerber C, Terrier F, Ganz R. The role of the coracoid process in the chronic impingement syndrome. *J Bone Joint Surg.* 1985;67-B:703–708.
64. Gigante A, Marinelli M, Verdenelli A, et al. Arthroscopy-assisted reduction and percutaneous fixation of a multiple glenoid fracture. *Knee Surg Sports Traumatol Arthroscopy.* 2003;11:112–115.
65. Goldstein LJ, Watson JM. Traumatic scapulothoracic dissociation: Case report and literature review. *J Trauma.* 2000;48:533–535.
66. Goodrich A, Crosland E, Pye J. Acromion fractures associated with posterior shoulder dislocation. *J Orthop Trauma.* 1998;12:521–522.
67. Gorczyca JT, Davis RT, Hartford JM, et al. Open reduction and internal fixation after displacement of a previously nondisplaced acromial fracture in a multiply injured patient: Case report and review of literature. *J Orthop Trauma.* 2001;15:369–373.
68. Gosens T, Speigner B, Minekus J. Fracture of the scapular body: Functional outcome after conservative treatment. *J Shoulder Elbow Surg.* 2009;18:443–448.
69. Goss TP. Fractures of the glenoid cavity. *J Bone Joint Surg Am.* 1992;74-A:299–305.
70. Goss TP. Double disruption of the superior shoulder suspensory complex. *J Orthop Trauma.* 1993;7:99–106.
71. Goss TP. Fractures of the glenoid neck. *J Shoulder Elbow Surg.* 1994;3:42–52.
72. Goss TP. Scapula fractures and dislocations: Diagnosis and treatment. *J Am Acad Orthop Surg.* 1995;3:22–33.
73. Goss TP. The scapula: Coracoid, acromial and avulsion fractures. *Am J Orthop.* 1996;25:106–115.
74. Goss TP. Open reduction and internal fixation of glenoid fractures. In: Craig EV, ed. *Master Techniques in Orthopaedic Surgery.* Philadelphia, PA: Lippincot Williams & Wilkins; 2004:461–480.
75. Goss TP. Fractures of the scapula. In: Rockwood CA, Matsen FA, Wirth MA, et al., eds. *The Shoulder.* 3rd ed. Philadelphia, PA: Saunders; 2004;413–454.
76. Gupta R, Sher J, Williams GR, et al. Non-union of the scapular body. *J Bone Joint Surg Am.* 1998;80-A:428–430.
77. Guttentag IJ, Rechtine GR. Fractures of the scapula: A review of the literature. *Orthop Rev.* 1988;17:147–158.
78. Hall RJ, Calvert PT. Stress fracture of the acromion: An unusual mechanism and review of the literature. *J Bone Joint Surg.* 1995;77-B:153–154.
79. Haraguchi N, Toga H, Sekiguchi Y, et al. Corrective osteotomy for malunited fracture of the glenoid cavity. *Clin Orthop Rel Res.* 2002;404:269–274.
80. Hardegger F, Simpson LA, Weber BG. The operative treatment of scapular fractures. *J Bone Joint Surg Br.* 1984;66-B:725–731.
81. Harmon PH, Baker DR. Fracture of the scapula with displacement. *J Bone Joint Surg.* 1943;25:834–838.
82. Harris RD, Harris JH. The prevalence and significance of missed scapular fractures in blunt chest trauma. *Am J Roentgenol.* 1988;151:747–750.
83. Harvey E, Audigé L, Hersovici D, et al. Development and validation of the new international classification for scapula fractures. *J Orthop.* Trauma on line.
84. Hashiguchi H, Ito H. Clinical outcome of the treatment of floating shoulder by osteosynthesis for clavicular fracture alone. *J Shoulder Elbow Surg.* 2003;12:589–591.
85. Heatly MD, Breck LW. Bilateral fracture of the scapula. *Am J Surgery.* 1946;71:256–259.
86. Heim KA, Lantry JM, Burke ChS, et al. Early results of scapular fractures treated operatively at a level one trauma center. *Europ J Trauma.* 2008;34:55–59.
87. Herrera DA, Anavian J, Tarkin IS, et al. Delayed operative management of fractures of the scapula. *J Bone Joint Surg.* 2009;91-B:619–626.
88. Herscovici D. Open reduction and internal fixation of ipsilateral fractures of the scapular neck and clavicle. *J Bone Joint Surg Am.* 1994;76-A:1112–1113.
89. Herscovici D, Fiennes AGTW, Allgöwer M, et al. The floating shoulder: Ipsilateral clavicle and scapular neck fractures. *J Bone Joint Surg Br.* 1992;74-B:362–364.
90. Hersovici D, Roberts CS. Scapula fractures: To fix or not to fix? *J Orthop Trauma.* 2006;20:227–229.
91. Heyse-Moore GH, Stoker DJ. Avulsion fractures of the scapula. *Skeletal Radiol.* 1982;9:27–32.
92. Hitzrot JM, Bolling RW. Fractures of the neck of the scapula. *Ann Surg.* 1916;63:215–236.
93. Hsu JE, Lee CS. Arthroscopic reduction and internal fixation of a displaced fracture of the acromion: Case report and arthroscopic technique. *Cur Orthop Practice.* 2011;22:564–566.
94. Hubbard D. Scapula fractures. *Cur Opin Orthop.* 2004;14:254–256.
95. Hudak PL, Amadio PC, Bombardier C. Development of an upper extremity outcome measure: The DASH (disabilities of arm, shoulder and hand): The upper extremity collaborative group (UECG). *Am J Ind Med.* 1996;29:602–608.
96. Ideberg R. Fractures of the scapula involving glenoid fossa. In: Bateman JE, Welsh RP, eds. *Surgery of the Shoulder.* Philadelphia, PA: Decker. 1984:63.
97. Ideberg R, Grevsten S, Larsson S. Epidemiology of scapular fractures. *Acta Orthop Scand.* 1995;66:395–397.
98. Imatani RJ. Fractures of the scapula: A review of 53 cases. *J Trauma.* 1975;15:473–478.
99. Ishizuki M, Yamaura I, Isobe Y, et al. Avulsion fracture of the superior border of the scapula. *J Bone Joint Surg Am.* 1981;63-A:820–822.
100. Izadpanah K, Jaeger M, Maeir, et al. The floating shoulder—clinical and radiological results after intramedullary stabilization of the clavicle in cases with minor displacement of the scapular neck. *J Trauma Acute Care Surg.* 2012;72:E8–E13.
101. Izadpanah M. Osteosynthese bei den Scapulafrakturen. *Arch Orthop-Unfall Chir.* 1975;83:153–164.
102. Jeong GK, Zuckerman JD. Scapula fractures. In: Zuckerman JD, Koval KJ, eds. *Shoulder Fractures.* New York, NY: Thieme; 2005:199–222.
103. Jerosch J, Greig M, Peuker ET, et al. The posterior subdeltoid approach: A modified access to the posterior glenohumeral joint. *J Shoulder Elbow Surg.* 2001;10:265–268.
104. Jones CB, Cornelius JP, Sietsema, DL, et al. Modified Judet approach and minifragment fixation of scapular body and glenoid neck fractures. *J Orthop Trauma.* 2009;23:558–564.
105. Judet R. Traitement chirurgical des fractures de l'omoplate. *Acta Orthop Belg.* 1964;30:673–678.
106. Kälicke T, Andereya S, Gekle J, et al. Coracoid pseudarthrosis caused by anterior shoulder dislocation with concomitant coracoid fracture. *Unfallchirurg.* 2002;105:843–844.
107. Kaminsky SB, Pierce VD. Nonunion of a scapula body fracture in a high school football player. *Am J Orthop.* 2002;31:456–457.
108. Karelse A, Kegels L, De Wilde L. The pillars of the scapula. *Clin Anat.* 2005;20:392–399.
109. Kavanagh BF, Bradway JK, Cofield RH. Open reduction and internal fixation of displaced intra-articular fractures of the glenoid fossa. *J Bone Joint Surg Am.* 1993;75-A:479–484.
110. Khallaf F, Mikami A, Al-Akkad M. The use of surgery in displaced scapular neck fractures. *Med Princ Pract.* 2006;15:443–448.
111. Kim KC, Rhee KJ, Shin HD, et al. Can the glenopolar angle be used to predict outcome and treatment of the floating shoulder? *J Trauma.* 2008;64:174–178.
112. Kim KC, Rhee KJ, Shin HD, et al. Displaced fracture of the coracoid process associated with acromioclavicular dislocation: A two-bird-one-stone-solution. *J Trauma.* 2009;67:403–405.
113. Kligman M, Roffman M. Posterior approach for glenoid fracture. *J Trauma.* 1997;42:733–735.
114. Kligman M, Roffman M. Glenoid fracture: Conservative treatment versus surgical treatment. *J South Orthop Assoc.* 1998;7:1–5.
115. Kuhn JE, Blasier RB, Carpenter JE. Fractures of the acromion process: A proposed classification system. *J Orthop Trauma.* 1994;8:6–13.
116. Kurdy NMG, Shah SV. Fracture of the acromion associated with acromioclavicular dislocation. *Injury.* 1995;26:636–637.
117. Labler L, Platz A, Weishaupt D, et al. Clinical and functional results after floating shoulder injuries. 2004;57:595–602.
118. Lange RH, Noel SH. Traumatic lateral scapular displacement: An expanded spectrum of associated neurovascular injury. *J Orthop Trauma.* 1993;7:361–366.
119. Lantry JM, Roberts CS, Giannoudis PV. Operative treatment of scapular fractures: A systematic review. *Injury.* 2008;39:271–283.
120. Lapner PC, Uhthoff HK, Papp S. *Scapula fractures Orthop Clin N Am.* 2008;39:459–474.
121. Leung KS, Lam TP. Open reduction and internal fixation of ipsilateral fractures of the scapula neck and clavicle. *J Bone Joint Surg Am.* 1993;75-A:1015–1017.
122. Leung KS, Lam TP, Poon KM. Operative treatment of displaced intra-articular glenoid fractures. *Injury.* 1993;24:324–328.
123. Lim KE, Wang CR, Chin KC, et al. Concomitant fracture of the coracoid and acromion after direct shoulder trauma. *J Orthop Trauma.* 1996;10:437–439.
124. Lindholm A, Leven H. Prognosis in fractures of the body and neck of the scapula: A follow-up study. *Acta Chir Scand.* 1974;140:33–36.
125. Lipitt SB, Harryman DT, Matsen FA. A practical tool for evaluating function: The simple shoulder test. In: Matsen FA, Fu FH, Hawkins RJ, eds. *The Shoulder: A Balance of Mobility and Stability.* Rosemont, IL: American academy of orthopaedic surgeons; 1993;501–518.
126. Magerl F. Osteosynthesen im Bereich der Schulter. *Helv Chir Acta.* 1974;41:225–232.
127. Maquieira GJ, Espinosa N, Gerber C, et al. Non-operative treatment of large anterior glenoid rim fractures after traumatic anterior dislocation of the shoulder. *J Bone Joint Surg Br.* 2007;89-B:1347–1351.
128. Mara G, Stover M. Glenoid and scapular body fractures. *Cur Opin Orthop.* 1999;10:238–288.
129. Marek DJ, Sechriest VF, Swiontkowski MF, et al. Case report: Reconstruction of a recalcitrant scapular neck nonunion and literature review. *Clin Orthop Relat Res.* 2009;467:1370–1376.
130. Martín-Herrero T, Rodríguez-Merchán C, Munuera-Martínez L. Fractures of the coracoid process: Presentation of seven cases and review of the literature. *J Trauma.* 1990;30:1597–1599.
131. Martin SD, Weiland AJ. Missed scapular fracture after trauma. A case report and a 23-year follow-up report. *Clin Orthop Relat Res.* 1994;(299):259–262.
132. Mayo KA, Benirschke SK, Mast JW. Displaced fractures of the glenoid fossa. *Clin Orthop Relat Res.* 1998;346:122–130.
133. McAdams TR, Blevins FT, Martin TP, et al. The role of plain films and computed tomography in the evaluation of scapular neck fractures. *J Orthop Trauma.* 2002;16:7–11.
134. McCrady BM, Schaefer MP. Sonographic visualization of a scapular body fracture: A case report. *J Clin Ultrasound.* 2011;39:466–468.
135. McGinnis M, Denton JR. Fractures of scapula: A retrospective study of 40 fractured scapulas. *J Trauma.* 1989;29:1488–1493.
136. McLennen JG, Ungersma J. Pneumothorax complicating fractures of the scapula. *J Bone Joint Surg Am.* 1982;64-A:598–599.

137. Michael D, Zazal MA, Cohen B. Nonunion of a fracture of the body of the scapula: Case report and literature review. *J Shoulder Elbow Surg.* 2001;10:385–386.

138. Nau T, Petras N, Vécsei V. Fractures of the scapula – classification and treatment principles. *Osteo Trauma Care.* 2004;12:174–179.

139. Neer CS. Displaced proximal humeral fractures. Part I. Classification and evaluation. *J Bone Joint Surg Am.* 1970;52-A:1077–1089.

140. Nordqvist A, Petersson C. Fractures of the body, neck, or spine of the scapula. *Clin Orthop Rel Res.* 1992;283:139–144.

141. Nork SE, Barei DP, Gardner MJ, et al. Surgical exposure and fixation of displaced type IV, V, and VI glenoid fractures. *J Orthop Trauma.* 2008;22:487–493.

142. Norwood LA, Matiko JA, Terry G. Posterior shoulder approach. *Clin Orthop Rel Res.* 1985;201:167–172.

143. Ogawa K, Ikegami H, Takeda T, et al. Defining impairment and treatment of subacute and chronic fractures of the coracoid process. *J Trauma.* 2009;67:1040–1045.

144. Ogawa K, Inokuchi S, Matsui K. Fracture of the coracoid process. *Acta Orthop Scand.* 1990;61:7–8.

145. Ogawa K, Naniwa T. Fractures of the acromion and the lateral scapular spine. *J Shoulder Elbow Surg.* 1997;6:544–548.

146. Ogawa K, Yoshida A. Fractures of the superior border of the scapula. *Int Orthop.* 1997;21:371–373.

147. Ogawa K, Yoshida A, Takahashi M, et al. Fractures of the coracoid process. *J Bone Joint Surg Br.* 1997;78-B:17–19.

148. Oh CW, Jeon IH, Kyung HS, et al. The treatment of double disruption of the superior shoulder suspensory complex. *Inter Orthop (SICOT).* 2002;26:145–149.

149. Oh CW, Kyung HS, Kim PT, et al. Failure of internal fixation of the clavicle in the treatment of ipsilateral clavicle and glenoid neck fractures. *J Orthop Sci.* 2001;6:601–603.

150. Ombremskey WT, Lyman JR. A modified Judet approach to the scapula. *J Orthop Trauma.* 2004;18:696–699.

151. Orthopaedic Trauma Association. Fracture and dislocation compendium. Scapula fractures. *J Orthop Trauma.* 1996;(suppl 1):S81–S84.

152. Orthopaedic Trauma Association Fracture and dislocation compendium. Scapula fractures. *J Orthop Trauma.* 2007;(suppl 1):S68–S71.

153. Osti M, Gohm A, Benedetto KP. Results of open reconstruction of anterior glenoid rim fractures following shoulder dislocation. *Arch Orthop Trauma Surg.* 2009;129:1245–1249.

154. Owens BD, Goss TP. The floating shoulder. *J Bone Joint Surg Br.* 2006;88-B:1419–1424.

155. Pace AM, Stuart R, Brownlow H. Outcome of glenoid neck fractures. *J Shoulder Elbow Surg.* 2005;14:585–590.

156. Patterson JM, Galatz L, Streubel PN, et al. CT evaluation of extra-articular glenoid neck fractures: Does the glenoid medialize or does the scapula lateralize? *J Orthop Trauma.* 2012;26:360–363.

157. Plagemann H. Zur Diagnostik und Statistik der Frakturen vor und nach Verwertung der Röntgendiagnostik. *Beitr Chir.* 1911;73:688–738.

158. Ramos L, Mencia R, Alonso A, et al. Conservative treatment of ipsilateral fractures of the scapula and clavicle. *J Trauma.* 1997;42:239–242.

159. Reggio AW. Fractures of the shoulder girdle. In: Wilson PD, ed. *Experience in the Management of Fractures and Dislocations, Based on an Analysis of 4390 Cases.* Philadelphia, PA: Lippincott Williams & Wilkins; 1938:370–374.

160. Richards RR, An K-N, Bigliani LU, et al. A standardized method for assessment of shoulder function. *J Shoulder Elbow Surg.* 1994;3.347–352.

161. Rikli D, Regazzoni P, Renner N. The unstable shoulder girdle: Early functional treatment utilizing open reduction and internal fixation. *J Orthop Trauma.* 1995;9:93–97.

162. Ring D, Jupiter J. Injuries to the shoulder girdle. In: Browner BD, Jupiter J, Levine AM, et al., eds. *Skeletal Trauma.* 3rd ed. Philadelphia, PA: Sanders; 2003:1625–1654.

163. Romero J, Schai O, Imhoff AB. Scapular neck fracture: The influence of permanent malalignment of the glenoid neck on clinical outcome. *Arch Orthop Trauma Surg.* 2001; 121:313–316.

164. Rowe CR. Evaluation of the shoulder. In: Rowe, ed. *The Shoulder.* New York, NY: Churchill Livingstone; 1988:631–637.

165. Russo R, Vernaglia, Lombardi L, et al. Arthroscopic treatment of isolated fracture of the posterolateral angle of the acromion. *Arthroscopy.* 2007;23:798.

166. Scavenius M, Sloth C. Fractures of the scapula. *Acta Orthop Belg.* 1996;62:129–131.

167. Schandelmaier P, Blauth M, Schneider C, et al. Fractures of the glenoid treated by operation. *J Bone Joint Surg Br.* 2002;84-B:173–177.

168. Scheibel M, Magosh P, Lichtenberg S, et al. Open reconstruction of anterior glenoid rim fractures. *Knee Surg Traumatol Arthrosc.* 2004;12:568–573.

169. Schofer MD, Sehrt AC, Timmesfeld N, et al. Fractures of the scapula: Long-term results after conservative treatment. *Arch Orthop Trauma Surg.* 2009;129:1511–1519.

170. Schwartzbach CC, Seoudi H, Ross AE, et al. Fracture of the scapula with intrathoracic penetration in a skeletally mature patient. A case report. *J Bone Joint Surg Am.* 2006;88-A:2735–2738.

171. Shindle MK, Wanich T, Pearle AD, et al. Atraumatic scapular fractures in the setting of chronic rotator cuff tear arthropathy: A report of two cases. *J Shoulder Elbow Surg.* 2008;17:e4–e8.

172. Solheim LF, Roaas A. Compression of the scapular nerve after fracture of the scapular notch. *Acta Orthop Scand.* 1978;49:338.

173. Sugaya H, Kon Y, Tsuchiaya A. Arthroscopic repair of glenoid fractures using suture anchors. *J Arthrosc Rel Surg.* 2005;21:635e1–635e5.

174. Tadros AM, Lunsjo K, Czechowski J, et al. Usefulness of different imaging modalities in the assessment of scapular fractures caused by blunt trauma. *Acta Radiol.* 2007;48: 71–75.

175. Tadros AM, Lunsjo K, Czechowski J, et al. Multiple-region scapular fractures had more severe chest injury than single-region fractures: A prospective study of 107 blunt trauma patients. *J Trauma.* 2007;63:889–893.

176. Tadros AMA, Lunsjo K, Czechowski J, et al. Causes of delayed diagnosis of scapular fractures. *Injury.* 2008;39:314–318.

177. Tauber M, Moursy M, Eppel M, et al. Arthroscopic screw fixation of large anterior glenoid fractures. *Knee Surg Sports Traumatol Arthrosc.* 2008;6:326–332.

178. Thompson DA, Flynn TC, Miller PW, et al. The significance of scapular fractures. *J Trauma.* 1985;25:974–977.

179. Tscherne H, Christ M. Konservative und operative Therapie der Schulterblattbrüche. *H Unfallheilkunde.* 1975;126:52–57.

180. Tuček M, Bartoníček J. Přidružená poranění u zlomenin lopatky [Associated injuries of scapula fractures]. *Rozhl Chir.* 2010;89(5):288–292.

181. Tuček M, Bartoníček J, Frič V. Kostní anatomie lopatky: Její význam pro klasifikaci zlomenin těla lopatky [Osseous anatomy of scapula: Its importance for classification of scapular body]. *Ortopedie.* 2011;5(3):104–109.

182. van Noort A, te Slaa RL, Marti RK, et al. The floating shoulder. A multicentre study. *J Bone Joint Surg Br.* 2001;83-B:795–798.

183. van Noort A, van der Werken C. The floating shoulder. *Injury.* 2006;37:218–227.

184. van Noort A, van Kampen A. Fractures of the scapula surgical neck: Outcome after conservative treatment in 13 cases. *Arch Orthop Trauma Surg.* 2005;125:696–700.

185. van Noort A, van Loon CJM, Rinjberg WJ. Limited posterior approach for internal fixation of a glenoid fracture. *Arch Orthop Trauma Surg.* 2004;124:140–144.

186. van Wellen PAJ, Casteleyn PP, Opdecam P. Traction-suspension therapy for unstable glenoid neck fracture. *Injury.* 1992;23:57–58.

187. Veysi VT, Mittal R, Agarwal S, et al. Multiple trauma and scapula fractures: So what? *J Trauma.* 2003;55:1145–1147.

188. von Schroeder HP, Kuiper SD, Botte MJ. Osseous anatomy of the scapula. *Clin Orthop Rel Res.* 2001;83:131–139.

189. Ware JE, Kosinski M, Keller SD. *SF-36 physical and mental health summary scales: A user's manual.* Boston: New England Medical Center, Health Assessment Lab; 1994.

190. Weber D, Sadri H, Hoffmeyer P. Isolated fracture of the posterior angle of the acromion: A case report. *J Shoulder Elbow Surg.* 2000;9:534–535.

191. Weening B, Walton C, Cole PA, et al. Lower mortality in patients with scapular fractures. *J Trauma.* 2005;59:1477–1481.

192. Wiedemann E. Frakturen der Scapula. *Unfallchirurg.* 2004;107:1124–1133.

193. Wilber MC, Evans EB. Fractures of the scapula. An analysis of forty cases and review of the literature. *J Bone Joint Surg Am.* 1977;59-A:358–362.

194. Williams GR Jr, Naranja J, Klimkiewicz J, et al. The floating shoulder: A biomechanical basis for classification and management. *J Bone Joint Surg.* 2001;83-A:1182–1187.

195. Williamson DM, Wilson-McDonald J. Bilateral avulsion fractures of the cranial margin of the scapula. *J Trauma.* 1988;28:713–714.

196. Wirth MA, Butters KP, Rockwood CA Jr. The posterior deltoid-splitting approach to the shoulder. *Clin Orthop Relat Res.* 1993;296:92–98.

197. Zdravkovic D, Damholt VV. Comminuted and severely displaced fractures of the scapula. *Acta Arthop Scand.* 1974;45:60–65.

198. Zelle BA, Pape HC, Gerich TG, et al. Functional outcome following scapulothoracic dissociation. *J Bone Joint Surg Am.* 2004;86-A:2–7.

199. Zilberman Z, Rejovitzky R. Fracture of the coracoid process of the scapula. *Injury.* 1981;13:203–206.

200. Zlowodzki M, Bhandari M, Zelle BA, et al. Treatment of scapula fractures: Systematic review of 520 fractures in 22 case series. *J Orthop Trauma.* 2006;20:230–233.

201. Zuckerman SL, Song Y, Ombreskey WT. Understanding the concept of medialization in scapula fractures. *J Orthop Trauma.* 2012;26:350–357.

40

GLENOHUMERAL INSTABILITY

Andrew Jawa and Eric T. Ricchetti

BACKGROUND ON GLENOHUMERAL INSTABILITY

Definition of Glenohumeral Instability

Glenohumeral *instability* is defined as the symptomatic and pathologic condition in which the humeral head does not remain centered in the glenoid fossa. Although the definition is simple, it includes a wide spectrum of diseases which has become larger with more nuances as our understanding of the pathoanatomy and clinical presentation evolves.

Importantly, instability is not the same as *laxity*, which is a physical examination finding that is a property of normal joints. Laxity is defined as the degree to which the humeral head passively translates, relative to the glenoid, with the application of a load. By definition, it is asymptomatic. It varies with age, gender, and congenital factors.[74,248,347] In addition, there is a wide spec-trum of laxity among normal individuals.[119,118] *Hyperlaxity* may contribute to instability, but the two are separate concepts.[248]

Classification of Glenohumeral Instability

A number of classification systems have been developed to define glenohumeral instability, but with a rapidly evolving understanding of the pathology, many are incomplete and none are universal. As such, a descriptive classification of instability has become the standard rather than one based on reproducibility and high intra- and interobserver reliability.

Descriptive Classification

Glenohumeral instability is currently defined by six characteristics: Severity (*subluxation vs. dislocation*), etiology (*traumatic, microtraumtic, atraumatic, neuromuscular*), chronicity (*acute vs.*

TABLE 40-1	Descriptive Classification of Shoulder Instability

Severity	Volition
Subluxation	Voluntary
Dislocation	Involuntary
Etiology	Direction
Traumatic	Anterior
Microtraumatic	Posterior
Atraumatic	Inferior
Neuromuscular	Superior
Chronicity	Bidirectional
Acute	Multidirectional
Chronic	
Frequency	
Initial	
Recurrent	

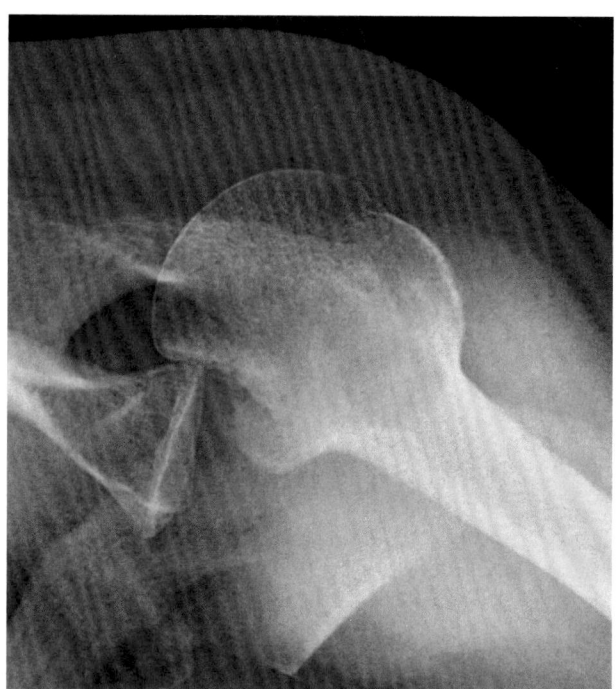

FIGURE 40-1 Axillary view of a chronic subacromial posterior dislocation with the humeral head "locked" or "fixed" on the posterior glenoid. Note the position of the humeral head directly below the acromion.

chronic), frequency (*initial vs. recurrent*), volition (*voluntary vs. involuntary*), and direction (*anterior, posterior, inferior, superior, bidirectional, multidirectional (MDI)*). Each of these terms can be used in a description of a patient's instability episode. For example, an instability event may be described as a recurrent, acute, traumatic, involuntary, anterior dislocation of the glenohumeral joint (Table 40-1).

Severity. A *dislocation* is defined as a complete symptomatic dissociation of the articular surfaces of the humeral head and glenoid *without* spontaneous reduction. The need for a manual reduction (or a confirmatory radiograph) is required to define a dislocation. A *subluxation* is a symptomatic dissociation of the articular surfaces *with* spontaneous reduction. The degree or dissociation varies and includes complete separation.[256]

Symptomology is the key feature for both. The symptom felt is typically *apprehension,* the feeling of the humeral head translating out of the glenoid fossa. Pain may also be a symptom, but, without apprehension, other diagnoses should be considered.

Etiology. There are currently four defined etiologies of instability: *Traumatic, neuromuscular, atraumatic,* and *microtraumatic.* Traumatic causes include injuries such as falls or motor vehicle accidents in which a large external force is the major contributor to the instability. This etiology should be distinguished from neuromuscular causes like seizures and strokes in which the imbalance of the glenohumeral muscular stabilizers leads to instability. Atraumatic instability, by definition, is not associated with a single traumatic episode. Microtraumatic instability is a controversial theoretical category in which repetitive symptomatic and asymptomatic microtrauma lead to chronic joint changes and subsequent instability. Microtraumatic instability is sometimes called *acquired* instability. As discussed later, atraumatic or microtraumatic instability is often associated with *posterior, bidirectional,* and *multidirectional* instability and underlying hyperlaxity. *Congenital* predisposition to instability may be related to glenoid dysplasia, or systemic syndromes like Ehlers–Danlos. Often these patients have atraumatic or microtraumatic instability.

Frequency and Chronicity. The *frequency* of instability is defined as either an *initial* or *recurrent* episode. The event may be either a subluxation or a dislocation. The *chronicity* of instability is a spectrum with no clear definition for what defines *acute* versus *chronic.* Typically the terms are used to describe a dislocation (vs. subluxation). As such, acute is best defined as a time from the episode to presentation in which a closed reduction is likely to succeed (3 to 6 weeks).[56,126,311] *Chronic* dislocations are typically *locked* or *fixed,* meaning the humeral head is impaled on the edge of the glenoid making reduction difficult (Fig. 40-1). The terms *locked, chronic,* and *fixed* have sometimes been used interchangeably and the exact definition can be confusing.[126,311] As such, it is best to define the timeframe as well as the humeral head pathology.

Volition. *Voluntary* instability, in which the patient can dislocate at will, is often atraumatic and can be associated with psychiatric problems or secondary gain. Rowe designated these patients "habitual dislocators."[233,308] This group should be distinguished from patients who have no underlying psychological issues, but who have learned the position(s) of instability. They can reproduce their instability, but are symptomatic and try to avoid these positions. These patients seek medical advice because they typically have an *involuntary* component that they cannot control. Last, there is a rare group of patients who can dissociate their humeral head and glenoid at will, but are neither symptomatic nor desire secondary gain. By definition, they do not have instability because they have exceptional control over their glenohumeral joint.[97]

Direction

The directions of instability have increased with the growing recognition of patient pathology and presentation. *Anterior, posterior, superior, inferior,* and *multi-* or *bidirectional*[25] instability have all been described. Confusion certainly exists in defining the direction of instability because there can be overlap or misdiagnosis.

Anterior unidirectional instability is, by far, the most common.[183,254] There are a number of named types of anterior dislocations that likely represent a spectrum of direction. Nonetheless, they have been described and need to be mentioned though there are few implications for treatment. The typical anterior dislocation, representing about two-thirds of anterior dislocations, is called a *subcoracoid* dislocation as the humeral head is located below the coracoid process (Fig. 40-2).[49] *Subglenoid* dislocations, in which the humeral head is inferior to the glenoid, represents about one-third of dislocations (Fig. 40-3). Often this type of dislocation is associated with a greater tuberosity fracture.[49] The remaining two types, *subclavicular,* in which the humeral head is medial to the glenoid and inferior to the clavicle, and *intrathoracic,* in which the humeral head lies within the thorax, are very uncommon.[49,71,361]

Posterior instability, as discussed later in the epidemiology section, represents less than 10% of instability. Several types of dislocations have been named, but the terminology is uncommonly used as it has little or no implication for treatment. The terms *subacromial* (most common), *subspinous,* and *subglenoid* have all been used to describe the position of the posterior dislocation, though the exact definitions are not clear (Fig. 40-1). Posterior *subluxation,* however, is more common than frank dislocation and commonly associated with an *inferior* component—making the instability *bi-* or *multidirectional.*[25]

A directly *inferior* dislocation is also known as *luxatio erecta* (Fig. 40-4). This is an uncommon traumatic injury in which

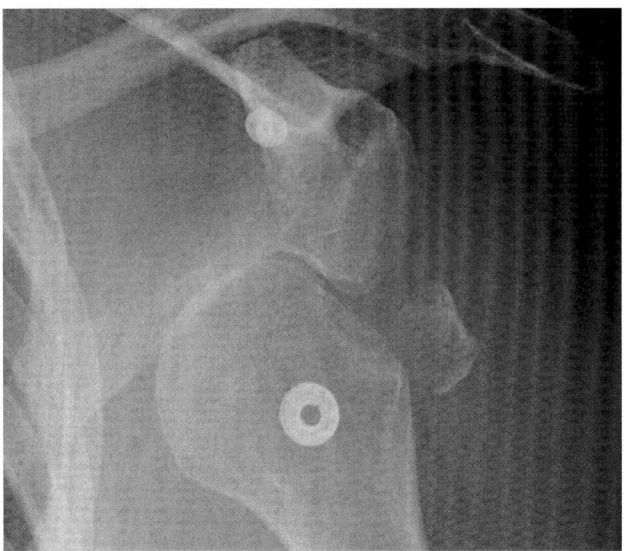

FIGURE 40-3 AP view of a subglenoid dislocation. Note the associated greater tuberosity fracture.

the humeral head is directly inferior to the glenoid and the humerus is locked in 100 to 160 degrees of abduction.[81,86,109,206] More typically, inferior instability is an atraumatic subluxation associated with a posterior or MDI component (Fig. 40-5).[233]

Superior dislocations are extremely high-energy injuries that have only been described in case reports.[69] This type should be distinguished from superior humeral head migration associated with chronic rotator cuff arthropathy (Fig. 40-6).

MDI is inconsistently defined in the literature.[212] We use the simplest definition: Instability in two or more directions. Some authors do distinguish between bidirectional instability

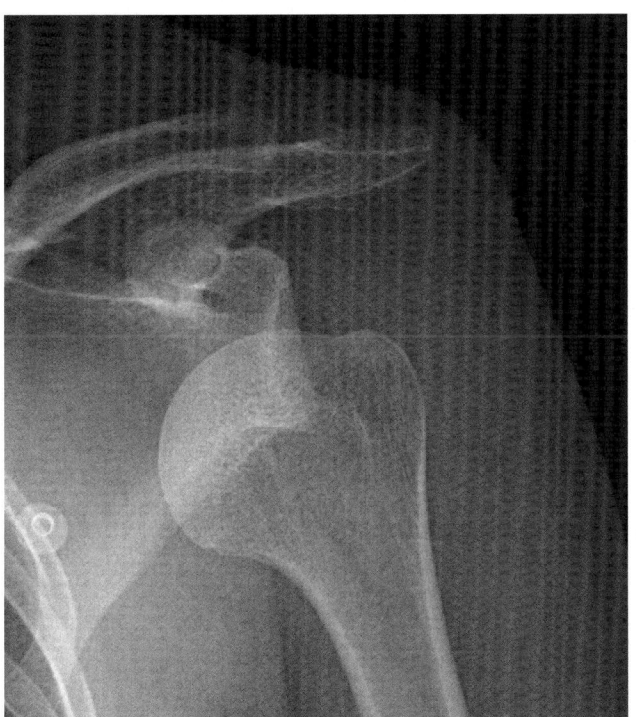

FIGURE 40-2 AP view of a subcoracoid dislocation.

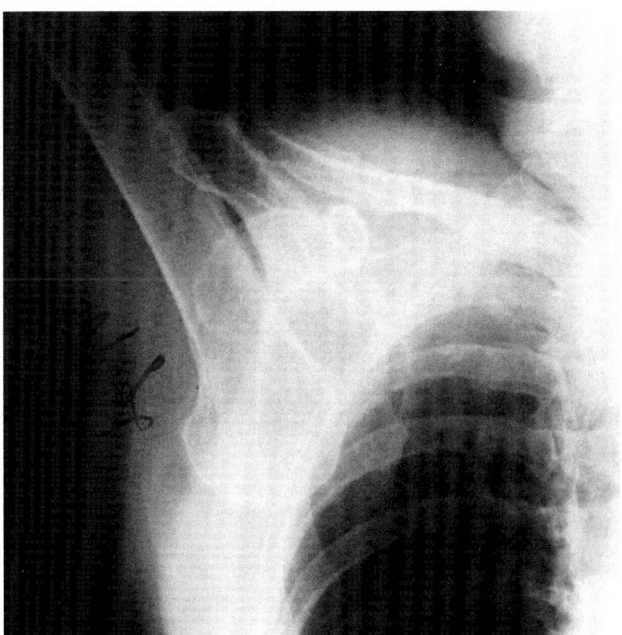

FIGURE 40-4 Locked inferior dislocation of the glenohumeral joint, also known as *luxatio erecta.*

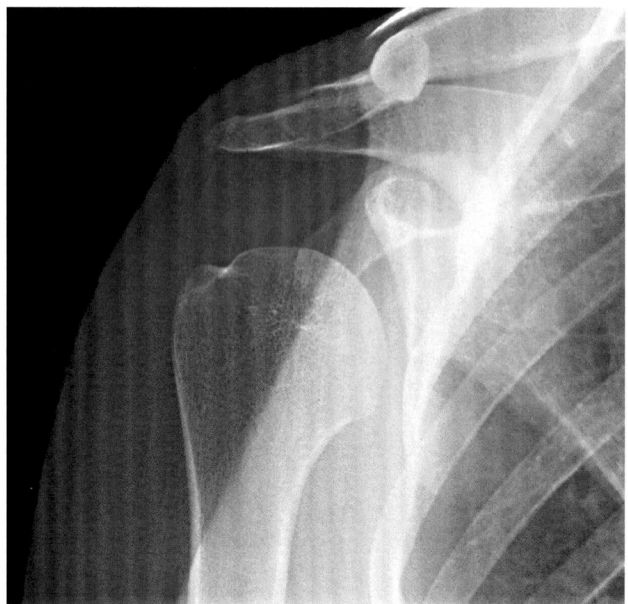

FIGURE 40-5 Inferior subluxation of the humeral head seen in a patient with atraumatic multidirectional instability.

(typically anteroinferior or posteroinferior)[25] and global MDI instability as management can be affected.

Common Patterns of Instability

Because the six criteria create a large number of permutations in the classification of instability, we discuss below the most

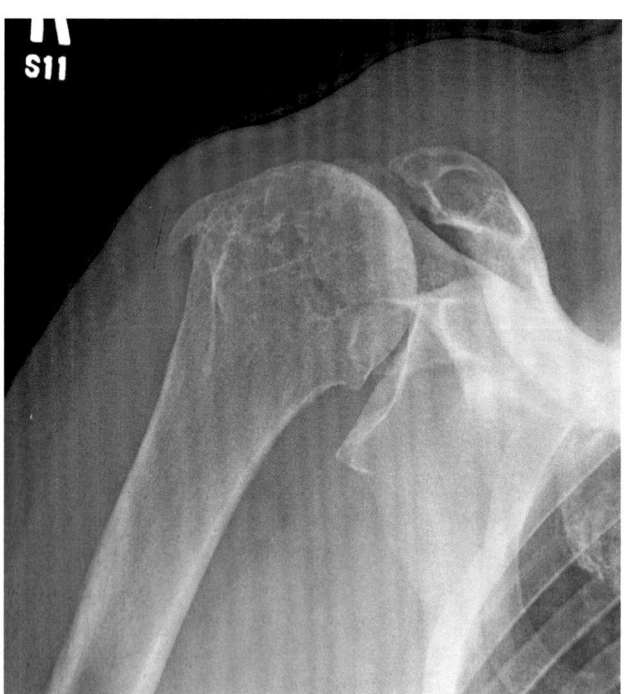

FIGURE 40-6 Superior migration of the humeral head associated with a chronic massive rotator cuff tear. This superior displacement should be distinguished from a superior dislocation which is caused by a rare, acute, high-energy injury mechanism.

common patterns seen clinically. The epidemiology, pathoanatomy, and clinical presentation are expanded upon later in the text.[233]

Traumatic Anterior Dislocation. The typical patient is a young male less than 30 years of age. This pattern is also seen in older patients, but with a higher incidence of associated injuries (especially rotator cuff injuries).[236] The pathoanatomy is often a capsule-labral avulsion (Bankart lesion), but others are described in detail below. Recurrence is most common in the younger population and often requires surgery.[299]

Recurrent Anterior Subluxation. This pattern is uncommon, but is also under-recognized. It has been described in the high-level athlete or military population. Repetitive stresses such as pitching, stretching the static stabilizers (e.g., capsule), and fatigue of the dynamic stabilizers (e.g., rotator cuff) precipitates apprehension or pain.[310]

Acute and Chronic Traumatic Posterior Dislocation. Posterior dislocations are uncommon and are seen in high-energy motor vehicle accidents, seizures (especially during alcohol withdrawal), or electric shock. Acute dislocations have been reported to be missed up to 50% of the time[126,215] and hence become chronic.

Recurrent Posterior Subluxation

Acquired Recurrent Posterior Subluxation. This is the most common form of recurrent posterior subluxation. Patients may have a completely atraumatic form, acquire the instability through macrotrauma with a definable causative event, or acquire instability by repetitive microtrauma that leads to deformation of the static stabilizers (e.g., capsule) over time. There is an overlap with inferior instability and even ultimately with MDI.[25,89] These patients also respond well to rehabilitation.

Volitional Recurrent Posterior Subluxation. Voluntary recurrent instability comes in two forms: Habitual dislocaters (those who dislocate or subluxate for secondary gain and psychological need)[308] and patients without psychiatric issues, but who are able to recreate their position of instability. In both groups, these patients can selectively inhibit certain muscle groups to create posterior instability.[259] However, in the latter, the patients also have a symptomatic involuntary component that they cannot control. These patients respond well to therapy. The habitual dislocaters do poorly with all treatment.

Dysplastic Recurrent Posterior Subluxation. Congenital causes such as localized posterior glenoid hypoplasia[72] or increased retroversion can lead to recurrent instability, but these conditions are rare (Fig. 40-7). These abnormalities do not necessitate instability, but may predispose patients to it.[95]

Multidirectional Instability. MDI is not fully understood, but is simply defined as involuntary instability (dislocation or subluxation) in two or more directions. However, the inconsistency in the literature of the characteristic findings makes a more specific definition difficult.[212] The etiology

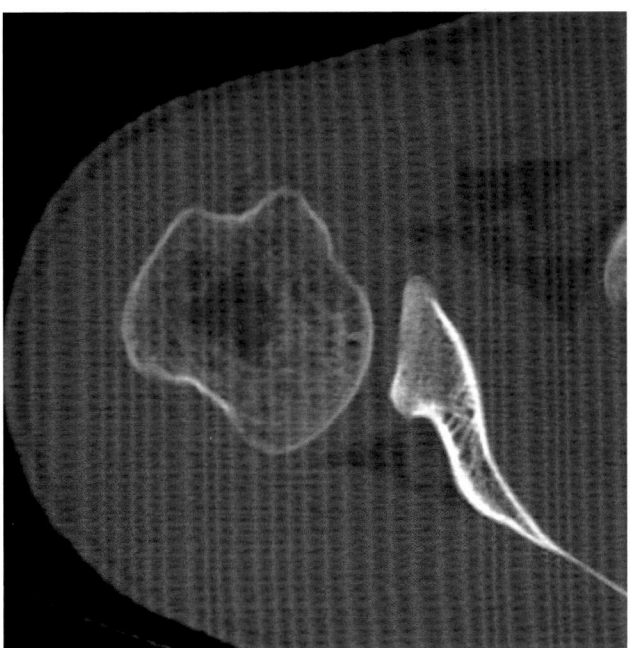

FIGURE 40-7 Posterior glenoid hypoplasia seen on a CT scan in a patient with recurrent posterior instability. Note the posterior subluxation of the humeral head.

is either atraumatic or acquired with repetitive microtrauma. Altered proprioception and scapular dyskinesis have also been associated with MDI. Importantly, there is sometimes confusion between hyperlaxity and instability leading to misdiagnosis. Patients with instability are symptomatic, and patients with hyperlaxity may be predisposed to instability[97,248] MDI patients often do well with rehabilitation, but can be successfully treated with a capsular shift if nonoperative measures fail.

Other Classifications

Orthopaedic Trauma Association. The Orthopaedic Trauma Association (OTA) in their 2007 Fracture and Dislocation Compendium included a classification for shoulder dislocations.[208] In this system, the shoulder region is "10." The first digit ("1") specifies the shoulder girdle whereas the second digit ("0") specifies dislocation. A letter is used to identify the specific joint (A, glenohumeral; B, sternoclavicular; C, acromioclavicular; D, scapulothoracic), followed by another number to describe the direction (1, anterior; 2, posterior; 3, lateral (theoretical); 4, medial (theoretical); 5, other (inferior-luxatio erecta)).

For example, an anterior glenohumeral dislocation would be classified as "10-A1." The system is excellent for defining an acute event and for recording it in a database. However, the system is not comprehensive enough to define other key factors in treatment including severity (*subluxation vs. dislocation*), etiology (*traumatic vs. atraumatic/acquired vs. neuromuscular*), chronicity (*acute vs. chronic*), frequency (*initial vs. recurrent*), and volition (*voluntary vs. involuntary*).

Epidemiology of Glenohumeral Instability

The glenohumeral joint is the most commonly dislocated joint in the body representing 45% of all dislocations.[164] Reported instability rates range from 11.2 to 23.9/100,000 person-years[241,324,374] and likely underestimate the true incidence as the data is defined by patients seeking medical attention. The data does not include patients with self-reduced dislocations or subluxations who did not present to emergency departments.

The best and most current data comes from the study by Zacchilli and Owens in 2010 finding an incidence of 23.9/100,000 person-years in patients presenting to emergency departments in the United States.[374] A total of 8,940 dislocations were seen over a 4-year period between 2002 and 2006. Men, compared to women, had an incidence rate ratio of 2.64, with 71.8% of dislocations occurring in men. There was no difference based on race. The peak incidence of dislocation (47.8/100,000 person-years) occurred between ages 20 and 29 years with 46.8% of all dislocations occurring in patients between 15 and 29 years of age. There is a bimodal distribution, however, with a second peak incidence rate between 80 and 89 years of age. Most dislocations (58.8%) occurred during a fall, whereas 48.3% occurred during sports activities (Fig. 40-8). Importantly, this data did not exclude recurrent dislocations.[374]

The risk of recurrent anterior instability is highest among young male patients.[132,306] The reported rates have varied considerably in the literature from 30%[323] to 90%[272] mainly because of lack of follow-up and the retrospective nature of most studies. Robinson et al.[299] in their prospective observational cohort study found patients between 15 and 35 years of age developed recurrent instability in 55.7% of shoulders within the first 2 years after dislocation. The rate increased to 66.8% by the fifth year. As previous reports documented, young males were at greatest risk for recurrent anterior instability (Table 40-2). In addition, Marans et al. reported in 21 patients with open physes that the risk of recurrent instability was 100% regardless of gender.[205]

There is a paucity of epidemiologic work for posterior instability. Robinson et al. performed the best retrospective review of traumatic posterior dislocations[301] finding a prevalence of 1.1/100,000 patient years or 5% of all dislocations.[374] Like anterior dislocations, there is a bimodal distribution with peaks in male patients between 20 and 49 years of age and over 70 years of age. Up to 70% are caused by a traumatic accident with the remainder caused by seizures. Recurrent instability is seen in 18% of shoulders in the first year with risk factors including seizure etiology, a large humeral head defect, and age less than forty.

Little is known about the epidemiology of subluxations (anterior, posterior, or MDI) in the general population as most patients do not present for medical attention. However, some of this data has been captured in the military population, which is intrinsically younger and more active than the general population. Over a 10-month period, all new traumatic shoulder instability events in the United States Military Academy were evaluated.[254] Among 4,141 students, 117 experienced new traumatic shoulder instability events with 11 experiencing multiple events. Interestingly, only 18 events were dislocations (15.4%) whereas 99 were subluxations (84.6%). Of the 99 subluxations,

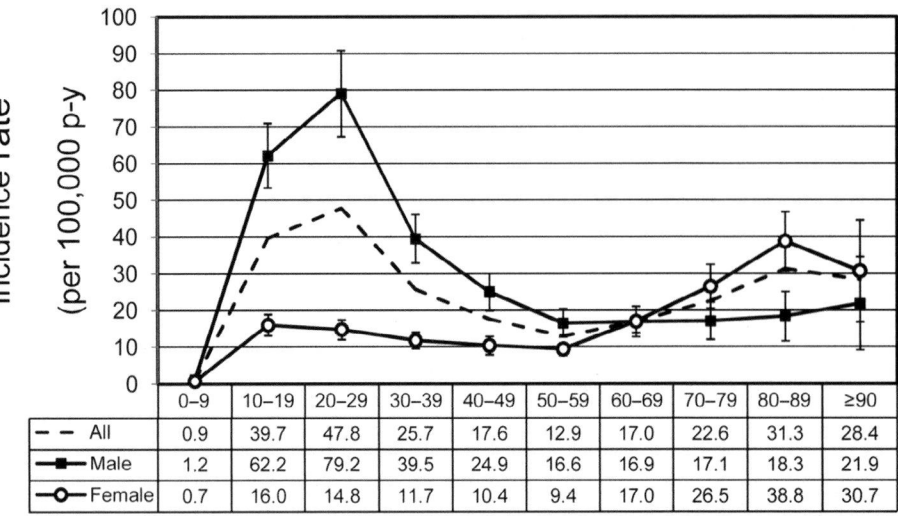

Shoulder dislocation
Incidence rate by age and gender

	0–9	10–19	20–29	30–39	40–49	50–59	60–69	70–79	80–89	≥90
– – All	0.9	39.7	47.8	25.7	17.6	12.9	17.0	22.6	31.3	28.4
Male	1.2	62.2	79.2	39.5	24.9	16.6	16.9	17.1	18.3	21.9
Female	0.7	16.0	14.8	11.7	10.4	9.4	17.0	26.5	38.8	30.7

FIGURE 40-8 Total weighted NEISS estimates of all shoulder dislocations in the United States between 2002 and 2006 by age and sex, demonstrating a bimodal distribution with peaks among males between the ages of 20 and 29 years and females between the ages of 80 and 89 years. p-y, person-years. The vertical bars denote the 95% confidence interval. (From Zacchilli MA, Owens BD. Epidemiology of shoulder dislocations presenting to emergency departments in the United States. *J Bone Joint Surg Am.* 2010;92(3):542–549).

TABLE 40-2 **Age and Sex-Specific Estimated Probability of Recurrent Instability within the First 2 Years After a Primary Glenohumeral Dislocation**

Age (yrs)	Males	Females
15	0.86	0.54
16	0.84	0.51
17	0.81	0.48
18	0.78	0.45
19	0.75	0.42
20	0.72	0.40
21	0.69	0.37
22	0.66	0.34
23	0.62	0.32
24	0.59	0.30
25	0.56	0.28
26	0.53	0.26
27	0.50	0.24
28	0.47	0.22
29	0.43	0.20
30	0.41	0.19
31	0.39	0.17
32	0.36	0.16
33	0.34	0.15
34	0.31	0.14
35	0.29	0.13

Reproduced from Robinson CM, Howes J, Murdoch H, et al. Functional outcome and risk of recurrent instability after primary traumatic anterior shoulder dislocation in young patients. *J Bone Joint Surg Am.* 2006;88(11):2326-3336.

45 (45.5%) were primary events, whereas 54 (54.5%) were recurrent. The majority of the 117 events were anterior (80.3%), whereas 12 (10.3%) were posterior, and 11 (9.4%) were MDI. Contact and noncontact injuries were responsible for 44 and 41% of the instability events, respectively. Data was unavailable for the remaining 15%. We are unaware of any other literature reliably examining the epidemiology of MDI.

The direction of dislocation was only recorded in one of the six primary epidemiologic studies[183,241,253,254,324,374] on shoulder instability and therefore, our current understanding is limited. In their study of 216 dislocations, Kroner et al. found anterior and posterior dislocations (subluxations were not recorded) to represent 97.2 and 2.8% of events, respectively.[183] No inferior dislocations were noted.

Anatomy and Pathoanatomy Relating to Glenohumeral Instability

Anatomy of Glenohumeral Stability

Joint stability is maintained by both static and dynamic elements. The static stabilizers include the bony anatomy, the glenoid labrum, negative intra-articular pressure, adhesion–cohesion, capsuloligamentous structures, and the rotator cuff. The dynamic stabilizers include the rotator cuff muscles, the biceps tendon, the deltoid, scapular motion, and proprioception.

Static Constraints

Bone. The glenoid face is pear-shaped with the inferior two-thirds roughly a circle (Fig. 40-9).[141] The average width and height are 24 and 35 mm, respectively.[55] The glenoid covers only a maximum of 25% to 30% of the humeral head[315] and therefore the glenohumeral joint has limited intrinsic bony stability. This stability is enhanced by a slight concavity of the glenoid—both through a slightly conforming bony anatomy and the thinning of the cartilage in the center of the glenoid ("the bare area").[353] However, because mobility is critical to the shoulder joint, the radius of curvature of the glenoid surface is greater (less curved) than the humeral head by 2.3 mm to prevent impingement of the head at the periphery of the glenoid.[142]

The glenoid also has a slight (5 to 10 degrees) superior inclination relative to the vertical axis of the scapular body.[17,314] This inclination may play a role in preventing inferior instability of the glenohumeral joint as patients with MDI are more likely to have a downward facing glenoid.[17]

Labrum. The labrum is a wedge-shaped dense fibrous structure of packed collagen fibers circumferentially surrounding the glenoid. Its purpose is to deepen the glenoid fossa and to create more surface area.[344] Anatomically, the labrum and cartilage together effectively deepen the glenoid by 80% helping to prevent the head from rolling over the glenoid edge.[190] In addition, the labrum indirectly confers stability by allowing for the attachment of the glenohumeral ligaments as discussed below (Fig. 40-10).[58]

It is important to note that recent studies demonstrated that if the labrum could be removed with the ligament attachment sites maintained, glenohumeral stability in the midrange of motion decreased, but was unaltered at the end-range[290] when the capsuloligamentous structures were taut.[190] In other words, an isolated labral lesion (without capsular injury) is not sufficient to cause gross instability, but can lead to a nonconcentric humeral head position.

Intra-Articular Pressure. The osmotic action of the synovium to remove fluid creates a negative intra-articular pressure in the

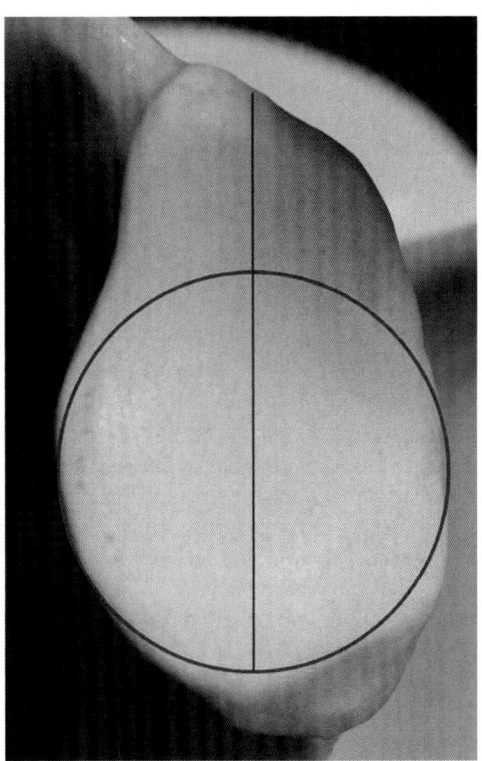

FIGURE 40-9 The glenoid face is pear shaped with the inferior two-thirds roughly a circle. The diameter of the red circle is exactly two-thirds the blue line, the height of the glenoid.

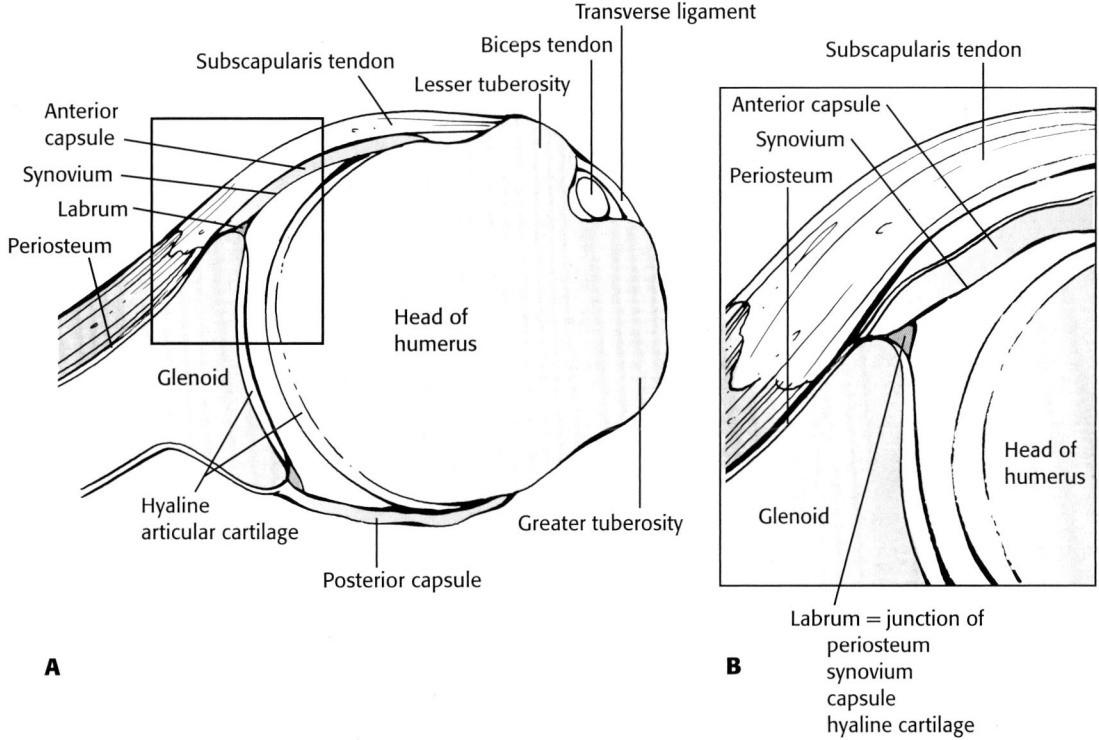

FIGURE 40-10 **A:** Cross-sectional anatomy of a normal shoulder. Note the close relationship between the subscapularis tendon and the anterior capsule. **B:** A magnified view of the anterior joint is essentially devoid of fibrocartilage and is composed of tissues from nearby hyaline cartilage, capsule, synovium, and periosteum.

joint.[195] When the capsule is vented with an 18-gauge needle, the force necessary to translate the humeral head decreases by almost 50%, particularly in the inferior direction.[99] Traumatic capsular tears or an enlarged rotator interval, sometimes seen after a dislocation, may result in decreased pressure and increased instability.[114]

Adhesion–Cohesion. The glenohumeral joint normally only contains 1 cc of synovial fluid that nourishes the articular surface. This fluid also provides a minor stabilizing mechanism through adhesion–cohesion. Through intermolecular forces, the fluid allows for the sliding of cartilage surfaces and confers a static restraint to separation.[143,145] The clinical effect, like intra-articular pressure, is small.

Capsule and Ligament. The capsuloligamentous structures are the primary static stabilizers of the glenohumeral joint. However, unlike in the elbow or knee where the ligaments are isometric during motion, the ligaments and capsule in the shoulder are generally lax and only provide stability at the extremes of motion under tension.[118] The normal glenohumeral joint capsule is loose and redundant to allow for range of motion. Depending on the position of the shoulder, certain capsuloligamentous structures will tighten and act as a restraint against humeral head translation.[252] These glenohumeral ligaments are expanded upon below (Fig. 40-11).

The Superior Glenohumeral Ligament. The superior glenohumeral ligament (SGHL) originates from the anterior superior aspect of the glenoid (anterior and inferior to the biceps origin) and extends to the anterior aspect of the humeral head to the superior edge of the lesser tuberosity. It crosses over the capsule

of the rotator interval between the supraspinatus and the subscapularis and lies deep to the coracohumeral ligament (CHL). It is the most consistent of all the glenohumeral ligaments and is present in over 90% of shoulders.[246]

Some biomechanical studies differ in explaining the primary and secondary roles of the ligament.[246] The SGHL, however, clearly limits inferior humeral head translation and external rotation in the adducted arm.[17] In addition, it limits posterior humeral head translation with the arm in forward flexion, adduction, and internal rotation[17,354] Basmajian further makes the point that the SGHL works in conjunction with the superior tilt of the glenoid to provide passive restraint to inferior humeral head translation.[17]

The Middle Glenohumeral Ligament. The middle glenohumeral ligament (MGHL) is less consistent than the SGHL with variable origins.[77] It can arise from the supraglenoid tubercle, anterosuperior aspect of the labrum, or the scapular neck and insert variably on the anterior humeral head medial and inferior to the lesser tuberosity. In up to one-third of shoulders it may be absent or significantly attenuated, potentially contributing to anterior instability.[77] The MGHL is maximally taut in external rotation and about 45 degrees of abduction,[346] functioning as a primary stabilizer of anterior translation and a secondary stabilizer to external rotation in abduction. It may also act as a secondary stabilizer to inferior translation in adduction.[354] In abduction, beyond 45 degrees, the role of the IGHL becomes more important.

The Inferior Glenohumeral Ligament Complex. The inferior glenohumeral ligament complex (IGHLC) consists of three

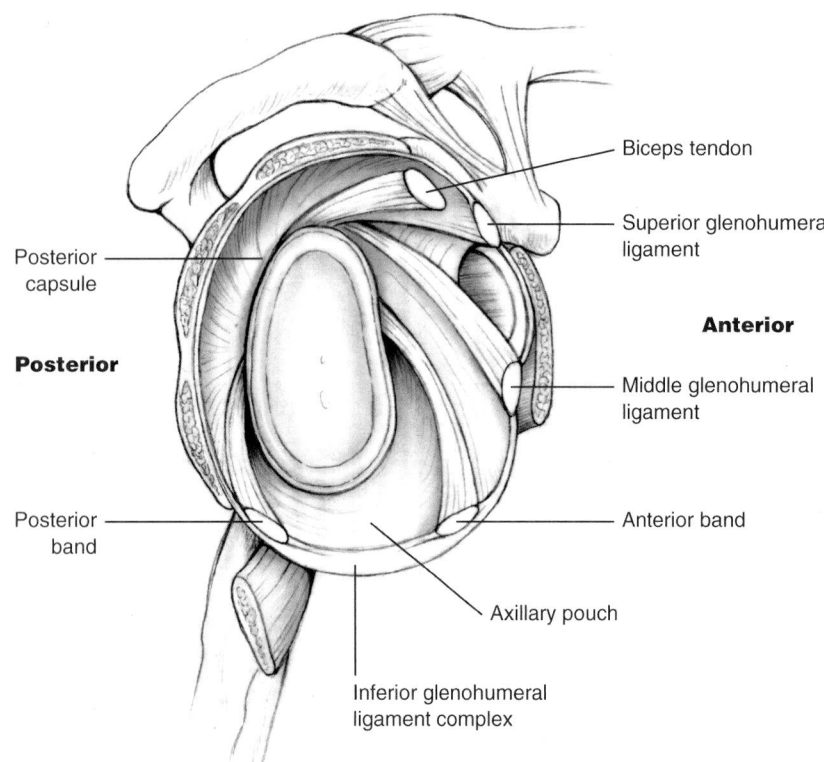

FIGURE 40-11 The capsuloligamentous anatomy of the glenohumeral joint. (From Iannotti JP. *Disorders of the Shoulder: Diagnosis and Management.* 2nd ed. Lippincott Williams and Wilkins; 2006 with permission.)

different components: The anterior band, the axillary pouch, and the posterior band, with the anterior band the thickest at 2.8 mm.[243] The ligament originates from the anteroinferior–posteroinferior labrum and extends to the inferior aspect of the lesser tuberosity and around the anatomic neck of the humerus. It is intimately associated with the joint capsule.[245] Compared to the MGHL, the anterior part of the IGHLC is tensioned in further abduction and external rotation and in this position has been demonstrated to be the primary stabilizer against anterior and inferior translation of the humeral head.[244] In addition, in 90 degrees of abduction and internal rotation, the posterior band along with the capsule is the primary stabilizer to posterior translation.[243] In adduction, the IGHLC is a secondary stabilizer to inferior translation.[354] The IGHLC is the most important ligament clinically.

The Coracohumeral Ligament and The Rotator Interval. In contrast to the glenohumeral ligaments, the coracohumeral ligament originates from outside the joint. It arises from the lateral aspect of the coracoid process, passes within the interval between the subscapularis and the supraspinatus tendons blending with the capsule, and attaching in two bands to the lesser and greater tuberosities, respectively.[161] The CHL is a constant structure. Together with the SGHL, the CHL and the capsule collectively form the roof of the rotator interval. The CHL plays the same role as the SGHL,[120,161] limiting external rotation and inferior translation when the arm is adducted. It is also a secondary stabilizer to posterior instability.[120]

The Coracoacromial Ligament. The coracoacromial ligament connects two points of the scapula, originating from the lateral aspect of the coracoid and attaching to the anterior portion of the acromion. Though, at rest, it does not directly restrain the humeral head, its resection increases anterior humeral translation in slight abduction and implies a stabilizing effect to the joint.[328,329] In addition, the ligament is a constraint to superior escape of the humeral head in the setting of massive rotator cuff tears.[116]

The Posterior Capsule. The capsule extending from the posterior band of the IGHLC to the biceps insertion is termed the posterior capsule. It is extremely thin and does not have additional ligamentous support.[243] It helps to limit posterior translation when the shoulder is flexed, adducted, and internally rotated.[243,244]

The Rotator Cuff. The rotator cuff plays a minor role in static stability likely through the barrier and tenodesis effect of the muscles and tendon. In abduction, the subscapularis limits anterior humeral head translation whereas the infraspinatus and teres minor play a role in limiting posterior translation.[150,151,232,252]

Dynamic Stabilizers

The Rotator Cuff. The muscles of the rotator cuff individually fire to counterbalance each other and the forces created by the other muscles in the shoulder girdle. For example, the subscapularis and the infraspinatus are often contracting at the same time to balance each other and maintain the center position of the humeral head in the glenoid.[140,314] In this manner,

rotator cuff muscles dynamically stabilize the glenohumeral joint.[31,186] As mentioned earlier, contraction of the rotator cuff compresses the humeral head against the glenoid, increasing the role of the labrum for stability and the force needed to translate the head. This compression–concavity effect is well founded in the literature and is a key aspect of dynamic stability by the rotator cuff and other muscles in the shoulder girdle.[192,352] Last, in their function to rotate and elevate the humerus, the cuff muscles can dynamically tighten the capsule and ligaments. Each ligament, as discussed above, provides a different checkrein to translation in varying degrees of rotation and adduction–abduction.[198,354]

The Biceps Tendon. The role that the long head of the biceps (LHB) tendon plays in the stabilization of the glenohumeral joint is controversial, but some studies indicate that both passively and dynamically the LHB helps limit anterior, posterior, and inferior translation of the humeral head, especially in adduction.[147,152,169]

Other Dynamic Stabilizers. The deltoid and the scapular stabilizers all likely play some role in the normal stabilization of the glenohumeral joint, but the extent and the exact mechanism of each is not well defined in our current science. For instance, glenoid positioning changes with the motion of the scapula such that protraction by the serratus anterior helps to prevent posterior instability.[356] In addition, scapular positioning affects the tension of the glenohumeral capsuloligamentous structures. This mechanism is seen when firing of the trapezius retracts the scapula, increasing the inclination of the glenoid, tightening the superior capsuloligamentous structures, and theoretically preventing against inferior instability.[150,152,354,356]

Proprioception. Other factors such as capsular and muscular proprioception likely play a role. Mechanoreceptors have been found in the capsule and labrum and likely provide positional feedback of humeral head and joint positioning.[31] A number of studies have noted altered proprioception in patients with MDI and in patients after a traumatic dislocation.[16,31]

Pathoanatomy of Glenohumeral Instability

Labrum, Capsule, and Ligament

Bankart Lesion. The disruption between the anterior inferior labrum and the glenoid, as seen in traumatic anterior instability, was termed the "essential lesion" by Bankart in 1938.[15] Subsequently it has been dubbed the "Bankart lesion." This disruption is critical in the development of recurrent instability because it serves as the anchor for the IGHLC, which is the primary static stabilizer against anterior and inferior humeral translation in abduction and external rotation. Second, the concavity–compression effect (described above) formed through the combination of dynamic humeral head compression and the increased glenoid concavity by the labrum is disrupted (Fig. 40-12).[339]

Importantly, an isolated labral lesion is likely not enough to lead to gross instability and needs to include detachment of the capsuloligamentous complex. Further, additional capsular deformation or stretch is likely necessary for recurrent instability.[330,339] If the IGHLC detaches with a small piece of

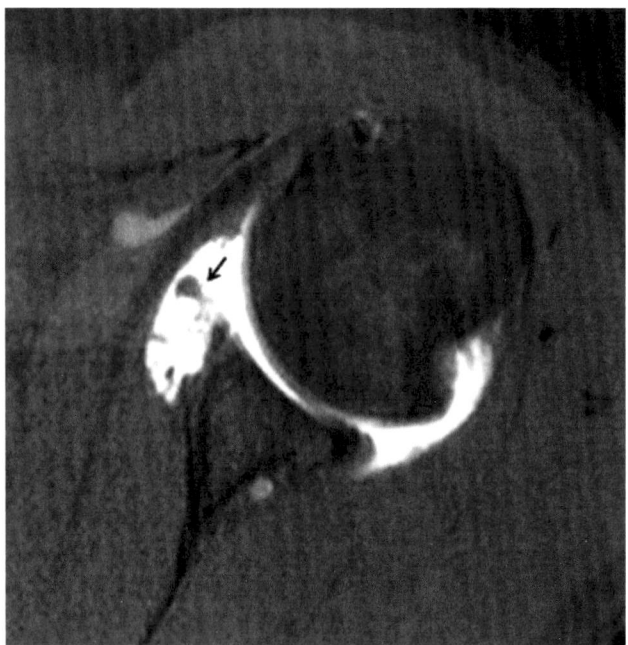

FIGURE 40-12 An axial cut of a T2-weighted MR arthrogram with a classic Bankart lesion (*arrow*).

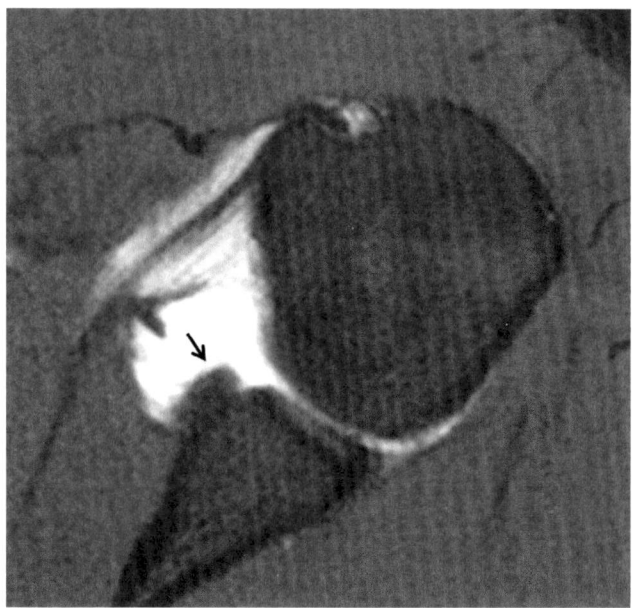

FIGURE 40-13 An axial cut of a T2-weighted MR arthrogram with a chronic ALPSA lesion (*arrow*) characterized by medial displacement of the labrum with surrounding fibrous scar tissue.

avulsed glenoid, the lesion is called a bony Bankart. A bony Bankart lesion can also be a "shear" fracture.

Posterior labral pathology is also noted in the recurrent posterior instability. In fact, there can be a large spectrum of posterior labral pathology ranging from a marginal crack without labral detachment (the "Kim" lesion) to chondral–labral erosion to a detached posterior labral flap (reverse Bankart).[5,37,174,359]

Anterior Labral Ligamentous Periosteal Sleeve Avulsion. In chronic situations, the labrum and the attached periosteum of the anterior glenoid can heal in a medialized position (Fig. 40-13). Nevaisser coined the term anterior labral ligamentous periosteal sleeve avulsion (ALPSA) in 1993 in his description of the lesion.[238] Because of the chronicity, ALPSA lesions are technically more difficult to treat and the outcomes have been shown to be inferior to treatment of more acute capsuloligamentous tears (i.e., Bankart lesions).[257]

Superior Labrum Anterior Posterior Tears. Though the origin of the IGHLC to the labrum is below the equator of the glenoid, the labral detachment may extend superiorly and include the biceps attachment. Snyder et al. labeled these as superior labrum anterior posterior tears (SLAP) which are generally seen in higher energy trauma.[221,327,348] Importantly, the labrum above the equator of the glenoid is normally more loosely attached to the glenoid.

Humeral Avulsion of Glenohumeral Ligaments. Though recognized almost 70 years ago by Nicola, the humeral avulsion of glenohumeral ligament (HAGL) lesion has been more recently described and classified.[8,42,239,240,294] This injury is a traumatic rupture of the IGHLC at its humeral attachment (Fig. 40-14). Typically it occurs with the arm in hyperabduction and external rotation and often results in instability. The

majority is anterior (>90%), but there are six described variations: (1) anterior, (2) anterior bony avulsion, (3) concurrent anterior glenoid-sided avulsion ("floating anterior HAGL"), (4) posterior, (5) posterior bony avulsion, (6) floating posterior HAGL. The avulsion of the posterior IGHLC is a rare cause or recurrent posterior instability.

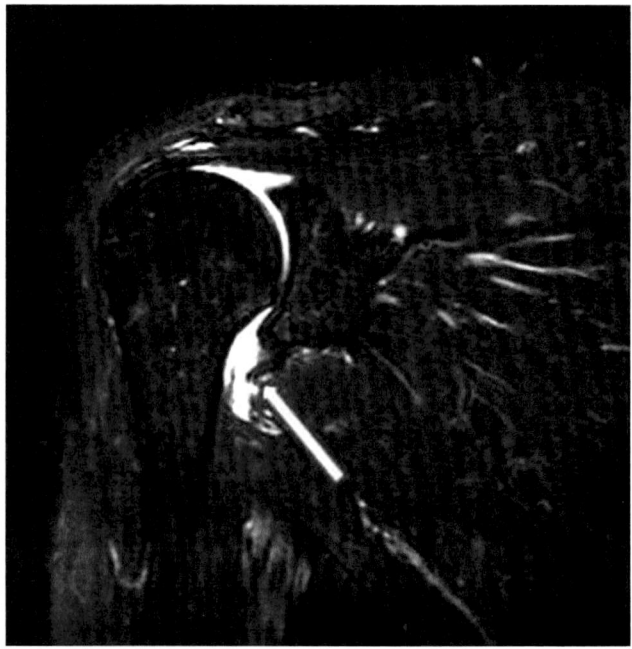

FIGURE 40-14 A coronal cut of a T2-weighted MRI showing a humeral avulsion of the glenohumeral ligament from the humeral neck, or HAGL lesion.

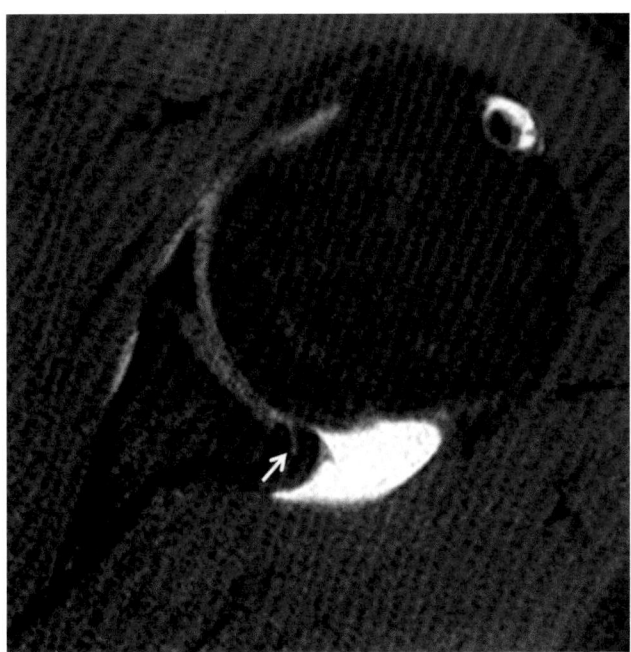

FIGURE 40-15 An axial cut of a T2-weighted MR arthrogram with a patulous posterior capsule and posterior labral tear (*arrow*).

Other Capsular Pathoanatomy. Though the pathoanatomy of a Bankart lesion is inherently capsuloligamentous, capsular pathology can occur in the absence of a labral injury or an "essential lesion." Most commonly, a single or recurrent dislocation can cause tearing and stretching of ligaments which can lead to increased joint volume and further instability.[28]

This type of pathology has been implicated in MDI and posterior instability. With these patterns, the capsule is often noted to be "patulous" as it has stretched over time or torn with repetitive microtrauma and healed in an elongated position (Fig. 40-15).[268,270] The stretching of the posterior band of the IGHL, specifically, plays an important role and has been shown to correlate with posterior translation of the humeral head.[219] However, in some anatomic experiments, posterior dislocations do not occur until an additional anterior structure (rotator interval, anterior capsule, or subscapularis) is released. This "circle" concept of instability, however, is controversial.[278,281] Repetitive overhead sports (swimming, volleyball, tennis, baseball) have been associated with this pathology.

Insufficiency or redundancy can also be specifically seen in the anterior-superior capsule (rotator interval). With this pathology, excessive inferior translation may be seen with external rotation and may be manifested by a positive sulcus sign on physical examination.[282]

Last, capsular insufficiency may be seen in an acute trauma, which is quite rare, or after multiple failed surgeries, which is more common. Iatrogenic injury is particularly seen in open surgeries and following thermal capsulorrhaphy.

Rotator Cuff. As discussed later, rotator cuff tears are uncommon in patients under 40 years of age with glenohumeral instability, but can be seen in high-energy injuries. Supraspinatus and subscapularis tears are the most common

in traumatic events. Subscapularis deficiency, however, should always be evaluated after a failed stabilization procedure, especially after open repairs. Though supraspinatus tears decrease the dynamic stabilization of the joint, subscapularis insufficiency plays a far greater role in instability with loss of tenodesis, compression–concavity, and the direct barrier to anterior dislocation.[1,140,152,198,352]

Bone

Glenoid. Alterations of version can, but do not always, lead to instability. There is no apparent disparity in version between anterior dislocaters and normal subjects, though most anterior dislocations are traumatic.[67] However, some patients with significantly retroverted, hypoplastic glenoids are predisposed to recurrent posterior instability (Fig. 40-7).[105,129,365] Posterior glenoid rim fractures or chronic bone loss are sometimes a cause of posterior instability.[358]

The pathoanatomy in traumatic anterior instability is most often bone loss of the anterior-inferior glenoid either from an acute fracture/bony Bankart or chronic bony erosion (Fig. 40-16) from multiple dislocations. In both events, the glenoid concavity and surface area are decreased significantly, decreasing the load to dislocation. Gerber and Nyffler found that if the length of the defect was greater than the radius of a best-fit circle of the bottom two-thirds of the glenoid, the force to dislocation was decreased by 70%.[97] Burkhart and Debeer coined the phrase the "inverted pair" referring to what the glenoid looks like with chronic anterior inferior bone loss viewing from a superior arthroscopic portal.[44] Measuring the bone loss is discussed below, but clinical and biomechanical studies indicate that arthroscopic repair is contraindicated with bone loss greater than 25% because of the high failure rates.[44,277]

Humeral Head. A compression fracture of the posterosuperolateral humeral head, also known as a Hill–Sachs lesion, is a sequela of an anterior dislocation. The lesion is created with the arm in abduction and external rotation with the posterior humeral head crushed on the anterior glenoid rim.[228] With recurrent dislocations, the defect may enlarge[170,228] small defects do not often affect treatment. However, with a very large lesion, a progressively enlarging lesion with recurrent dislocations, or with concomitant glenoid bone loss, the relevance of the Hill–Sachs becomes increasingly important in the pathoanatomy of recurrent instability (Fig. 40-16).[268,270] Interestingly, Hill–Sachs deformities are not often seen in atraumatic instability.

Engaging Hill–Sachs lesions are defined as defects which are parallel to the long axis of the glenoid rim in positions of function (abduction and external rotation) and therefore "engage" or contribute to glenohumeral instability. *Nonengaging* lesions are not parallel to the rim and therefore do not effect stability in positions of function. The type of lesion is determined by the position of the arm during dislocation.[44,268,270]

For posterior dislocations, the initial size of a "reverse" Hill–Sachs on the anterior humeral head is an important predictor of who may have recurrent instability (Fig. 40-1). If there is a delay in reduction for weeks, which is not atypical, the lesion enlarges because of rotation of the arm and erosion of bone.

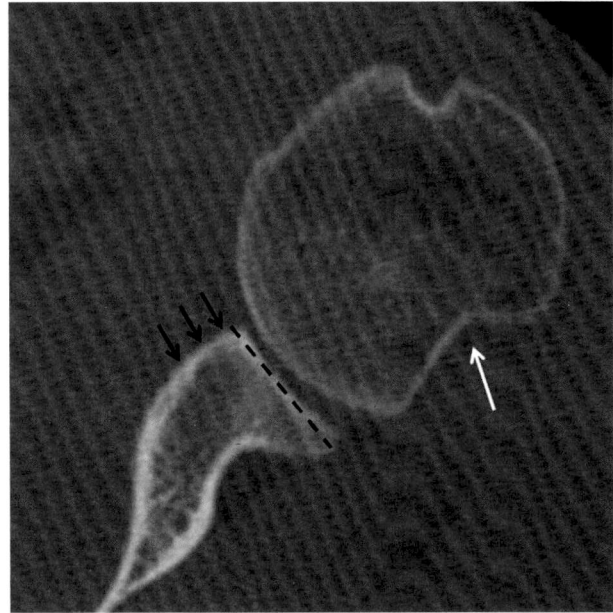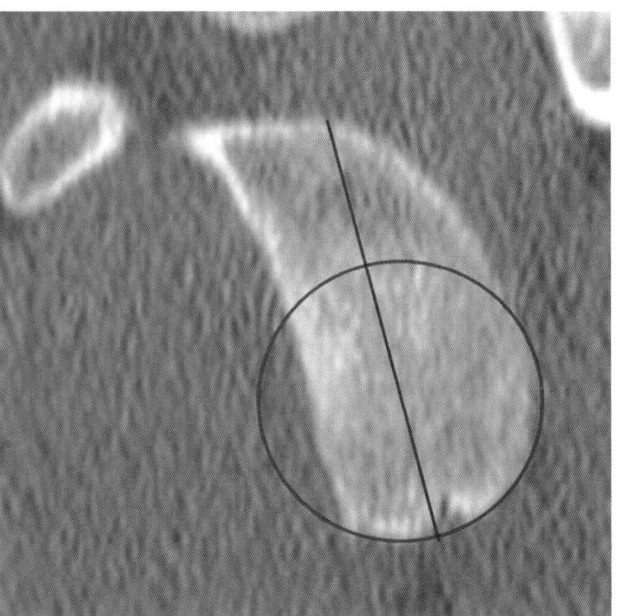

A **B**

FIGURE 40-16 **A:** An axial cut of a CT scan showing chronic anterior glenoid bone loss (*black arrows*) and a large Hill–Sachs lesion (*white arrow*). The dashed line represents the plane of the sagittal reconstruction **(B)** which demonstrates anterior inferior bone loss with a best-fit circle of the inferior two-thirds of the glenoid.

In addition, it may become corticated. Lesions greater than 40% of the head appear to have worse outcomes than smaller defects.[263] Importantly, however, there is no standard method to measure these lesions.

ASSESSMENT OF GLENOHUMERAL INSTABILITY

Mechanisms of Injury for Glenohumeral Instability

For some patients, particularly those with recurrent subluxations or MDI the mechanism of instability may be completely atraumatic or the result of repetitive microtrauma. However, most patients with instability have an initial known traumatic episode requiring manual reduction. An estimate of the ratio of traumatic to atraumatic instability is unknown as many with atraumatic instability do not initially seek medical attention.

Anterior instability occurs through an indirect mechanism with arm abduction, extension, and external rotation with the humeral head challenging the anterior capsule and ligaments, glenoid rim, and rotator cuff. Rarely is the episode a direct blow. For younger patients, athletic injuries are common[254,374] whereas for older patients, falls are more typical.[127] Less common types of anterior instability (e.g., intrathoracic) are typically extremely high energy.

Posterior instability occurs through the indirect mechanism of flexion, adduction, and internal rotation with an axial load (e.g., fall on an outstretched arm). Patients may suffer either a posterior dislocation from a single traumatic event or may develop recurrent subluxations from repetitive microtrauma in this position. This repetitive trauma can be seen with American football players, for instance, who keep their arms outstretched in blocking.

Neuromuscular events (e.g., alcohol withdrawal, seizures or electric shock) account for 30% of all posterior dislocations and lead to instability through violent muscle contraction.[301]

In these cases, the internal rotators (latissimus dorsi, pectoralis major, subscapularis) overwhelm the less strong external rotators (teres minor, infraspinatus) forcing the humeral head over the edge of the glenoid fossa.

Other forms of instability include *luxatio erecta,* a purely inferior dislocation. This uncommon dislocation occurs with extreme hyperabduction in which the proximal humerus levers against the acromion and dislocates inferiorly. These dislocations are often associated with greater tuberosity fractures or rotator cuff tears. Superior dislocations are extremely rare, but occur with extreme upward force through an adducted arm.

Associated Injuries with Glenohumeral Instability

Significant injuries can be associated with shoulder instability with most occurring during an initial traumatic episode and relatively few associated with atraumatic and MDI. All types of injuries have been reported. Tearing of the ligamentous and capsular restraints is the most common injury and the key pathoanatomy for recurrent dislocation. However, other associated injuries need to be recognized and cannot be missed as they have implications for prognosis and the ideal treatment for the patient. These injuries differ with the direction of instability.

Anterior Instability

The Hill–Sachs lesion, described in detail above, is the most common associated injury with anterior instability (Fig. 40-16). The incidence approaches 100% in patients with recurrent dislocations and 40% to 90%[47,309] after a single dislocation. With repeated events, the lesion often enlarges and may become clinically symptomatic and further contribute to recurrent instability.[228]

Acute fractures at the time of dislocation should be considered and recognized as they affect early management. Specifically, there should be a high suspicion for a nondisplaced neck fracture that may displace with reduction. Atoun et al. reported this association is especially prevalent in first-time dislocators older than 40 with a greater tuberosity fracture and no recognized neck fracture. A fracture of the greater tuberosity fracture was present in 20% of cases. Outcomes, whether with fixation or hemiarthroplasty, are generally poor.[10] Treating clinicians should avoid repeated closed reductions and should have a low threshold for reduction in the operating room with full muscle relaxation.

Greater tuberosity fractures (Fig. 40-3) are the most common and are three times more prevalent in patients older than 30 compared to younger.[131] Further, combining greater tuberosity fractures with ultrasound-proven rotator cuff tears, Robinson et al. found a prevalence of 33.4% in a large population-based study of anterior shoulder dislocations.[302] Interestingly, an associated fracture decreases the risk of recurrent instability.[131,132]

Rotator cuff tears alone are also commonly seen and the incidence increases with age with some reports describing a tear rate of 40% in patients over 40 years of age.[266] Patients over 60 years of age had a rate as high as 80%.[302] Patients present with weakness and even stiffness, specifically in external rotation and abduction. Also, subscapularis rupture can be a reason for persistent instability in older patients.[235,236]

Sometimes rotator cuff tears are misdiagnosed as a neurologic injury, specifically to the axillary nerve.[235] However, up to 25% of patients have both a neurologic and a rotator cuff injury, much higher than previously considered.[302] This is particularly true for female patients for unclear reasons.[302] Early identification of these injuries is critical to best outcomes and therefore for patients older than 40 years of age consideration should be given to ordering an MRI or ultrasound.

Neurologic injury is common (13% to 65%) because the glenohumeral joint is in close proximity to the brachial plexus.[64] An axillary nerve injury is the most common (73%), but often it is not clinically relevant. In a number of studies, up to one-third of patients have EMG evidence of injury, but only 5% having clinically detectable or relevant symptoms.[32,302,340] This injury occurs because of traction as well as direct pressure on the nerve as it travels inferior to the subscapularis and below the capsule of the glenohumeral joint. Patients with isolated nerve injuries tend to be younger and male, whereas those with multiple-nerve lesions are more likely to be older than 60 and female.[302] Unfortunately, the ability to recover from neurologic injury decreases with age leaving some older patients quite debilitated.

Because sensory testing alone can be misleading with patients having normal axillary nerve sensation and EMG documented nerve injury, the neurologic examination must include motor (isometric contraction of the deltoid) testing. If a neurologic injury is not recovering in the first 6 weeks, electrophysiologic examination should be performed as a baseline. Prognosis is worse if no recovery is seen in 3 months, but signs of recovery may take upward of 6 months.[32,64,302] The timing of surgical intervention is unclear, however intervention at 3 months can be considered if there is no recovery.[303] Last, in high-energy settings with a combined shoulder dislocation and brachial plexus injury, consideration should be given to evaluating the cervical spine and nerve root avulsions with the need for early surgical intervention.

Vascular injuries are rare and are typically seen in older patients who have more fragile vessels. Injury to the axillary artery and vein are the most common injuries characteristically effecting the second part of the vessels, directly behind the pectoralis major.[6] The artery is relatively fixed at the lateral margin of pectoralis minor and becomes taut with abduction and external rotation which makes it prone to injury with dislocation or reduction. Occlusion of the artery and vein is more common with luxatio erecta (inferior dislocation).[166] Injury with reduction is seen with the elderly, specifically in chronic dislocations with attempted reduction.[91] Signs and symptoms include a dysvascular arm or expanding hematoma. Ligation has poor outcomes.[177] Urgent consultation with a vascular surgeon is mandatory.

Posterior Instability

Based on the best, limited evidence, upward of 65% of posterior dislocations have associated injuries.[263,301] Fractures are the most common seen in 21% to 34% of cases with neck fractures the most prevalent (19%), followed by lesser tuberosity (14%) and greater tuberosity fractures (8%).[301] Importantly, many of the neck fractures are nondisplaced and may be missed or become displaced in an attempted reduction. Reverse Hill–Sachs lesions are seen in 29% to 86% of posterior dislocations (Fig. 40-1).[317] Articular cartilage damage is often greater than with true Hill–Sachs lesions.

Rotator cuff tear injuries are relatively uncommon compared to anterior dislocations with tears seen in 13% of cases.[263,301] Interestingly, cuff tears are almost five times more common in the absence of a fracture or reverse Hill–Sachs.[263,301]

Signs and Symptoms of Glenohumeral Instability

Presentation of Acute Instability

History. Some patients with acute instability present to the emergency room usually with an unreduced dislocation from a traumatic event. However, many patients with a subluxation episode or a self-reduced dislocation likely do not present.

Acute dislocations are typically extremely painful caused by the inciting event and the subsequent spasm of muscle attempting to stabilize the joint. Often the patient can clearly describe the mechanism of injury and shoulder position during dislocation. At other times, this information may be better obtained from an eyewitness. Though anterior dislocations represent the vast majority of acute trauma, suspicion of a posterior dislocation should be raised with a history of a high-energy trauma or strong muscle contraction as seen with a seizure or electric shock. As with any injury, previous episodes, and prior treatments should all be noted. Hand dominance, occupation, activity level, and general health history should also be obtained along with a general trauma survey of the patient.

A high level of suspicion for a posterior dislocation is needed since upward of 50% of these injuries are missed because of inadequate radiologic evaluation, concomitant fractures, multiple injuries, or an unresponsive, intubated, or sedated patient.

Rarely, a patient with volitional instability will present to the emergency room for secondary gain. Suspicion should be raised if the story is vague, the mechanism does not coincide with their radiographs or physical findings, or the patient has an inappropriate affect such as minimal pain, or indifference to typically painful reduction maneuvers.

Physical Examination. Inspection of the shoulder may reveal localized swelling, or a gross deformity. In thin patients, fullness is often noted in the anterior or posterior shoulder depending on the direction of instability. For anterior dislocations, the humeral head may be palpable or prominent beneath the skin and the lateral edge and posterolateral corner of the acromion may appear prominent. For posterior dislocations, a striking deformity may be absent, though sometimes a posterior fullness can be noted with anterior flattening and a corresponding prominence of the coracoid anteriorly. Notably, posterior dislocations are rare in comparison to their anterior counterpart.

A complete shoulder examination is often limited by pain; however, before any attempt at shoulder manipulation, a complete neurovascular examination of the upper extremity must be performed and documented. As noted above in the *associated injuries* section, one electrodiagnostic study reported a 60% rate of axillary nerve injury with anterior dislocations.[64] Deltoid strength and axillary nerve sensation should be carefully examined. The musculocutaneous nerve is the next most commonly injured nerve and careful attention to contraction of the biceps or brachialis is important along with testing of sensation in the lateral antebrachial cutaneous distribution on the lateral aspect of the forearm. Although quite rare, vascular injuries following shoulder dislocations have also been reported therefore the brachial, radial, and ulnar pulse should always be examined.[194]

Shoulder motion examination will be limited; however, the position of the patient's arm and their motion limitation may provide insight into both the severity and the direction of the instability. Patients with an anterior dislocation typically will have a limitation to internal rotation and abduction. Patients with a posterior dislocation will often demonstrate limitations in external rotation and abduction with limited passive elevation to 90 degrees. With the rare instance of *luxatio erecta,* the patient's arm may be locked in a fully abducted position.[371]

After a reduction is performed and verified radiographically, the examination may be limited by guarding. Testing Postreduction range of motion is not advised or should be very limited if the patient is awake. In addition, testing may lead to another dislocation. A thorough neurovascular examination should be reperformed.

Presentation of Nonacute Instability

History. Patients who present to the office have a much broader range of signs and symptoms of instability. Some may present to the office for definitive care after being treated at a local emergency room for an acute shoulder dislocation. Others may present with symptoms of recurrent instability and/or symptoms of apprehension. Some may only present with a vague history of pain with an unclear pattern or direction(s) or instability. Because of this variability in presentation, the importance of an accurate and complete history cannot be overemphasized.

For all types of patients with instability, a standard history should have a checklist of important factors to consider. Background factors include age, handedness, sporting activity, and family history of instability. Next, the circumstances around the initial event need to be elucidated including traumatic/atraumatic event, position of the arm, and documented emergency room reduction. Prior radiographs, especially of the shoulder in the dislocated position, are invaluable. Subsequent history should then be noted including number of documented recurrences, degree of trauma with the recurrences, unilateral or bilateral instability, dislocation during sleep, previous surgeries, presence of pain and location, sensory or strength issues, and whether the instability is voluntary. If a patient can dislocate the shoulder voluntarily, concerns for secondary gain and psychological issues should be raised. However, there should be a distinction between patients who habitually dislocate or subluxate and have a psychogenic component to their instability and those who learn the position of subluxation and can recreate it for examiners. Typically the latter patients try to avoid the provocative position because of discomfort.

Characteristic History of Anterior Instability. Patients with recurrent anterior instability almost always had an initial traumatic dislocation with their arm in abduction and external rotation subjected to a large degree of force. Common injuries include a fall during skiing, blocking in basketball, or an arm tackle in football. These events create tearing or avulsion of the inferior capsule and labrum. Also, it should be noted that as instability becomes more chronic, the force needed for both dislocation and reduction decreases, with many episodes requiring only self-reduction.

Characteristic History of Posterior Instability. The characteristic history for atraumatic instability includes a patient in their late teens or twenties with apprehension, pain, or even weakness in a provocative position–typically flexion, adduction, and internal rotation. An inciting traumatic event is uncommon, but certain activities consistently create the symptoms. As noted above, many patients can recreate the position of instability, but generally avoid this. Activities of daily living are not affected, but participation in sports can be troublesome. The symptoms may progress, however, to daily life. The disability is variable.

Characteristic History of Multidirectional Instability. Patients with MDI may present in a variety of ways. Some present similarly to those with posterior instability with many having a primary posterior component, complicating the diagnosis. Patients often present in their second or third decades with vague complaints of weakness, pain, and decreasing athletic performance without a specific inciting event. This is commonly seen in sports with the potential for repetitive microtrauma like gymnastics and swimming. An inciting event sometimes can be identified after which the symptoms progressed and affected activities of daily living. Many MDI patients, though not all, have hypermobile joints and a subgroup may have Ehlers–Danlos or other syndromes resulting in ligamentous laxity.

Physical Examination. The goal of the physical examination is to confirm an impression created by a detailed history. Specifically, the goal is to confirm if the suspected arm position and application of force is consistent in creating apprehension. Though the goal is to not dislocate the shoulder in the examination, it can sometimes happen and should obviously be avoided. Therefore, some of the findings may be subtle, and the ultimate diagnosis may be difficult to establish.

In patients who have suffered a recent instability episode, associated symptoms may be severe enough to preclude an adequate examination. Basic examination to document glenohumeral joint reduction (radiographic) and neurologic status may be all that can be accomplished during the initial visit. A more thorough evaluation may need to be postponed to a later date when the majority of the pain has subsided. A detailed neurologic examination of the upper extremity must be performed and documented during all clinical evaluations.

The physical examination should begin with inspection. Any abnormalities such as asymmetry, muscular atrophy, scapular winging, or ecchymosis should be noted. Even early on, at the first visit after a closed reduction, deltoid atrophy can be seen and may represent an axillary nerve injury. Scapular dyskinesis is often associated with instability, as either a cause or result (Fig. 40-17). Careful attention to scapular motion should be noted. Scars indicating previous surgery should be also noted.

Next, the cardinal motions of the shoulder should be measured: Forward elevation in the plane of the scapula, external rotation with the arm in adduction, and internal rotation with use of the spinal levels as a reference (i.e., internal rotation to T10). In addition, external and internal rotation in abduction should be noted which can often be increased (>90) in MDI instability. These measurements should always be compared to the contralateral side and differences between active and passive range of motion should be noted.

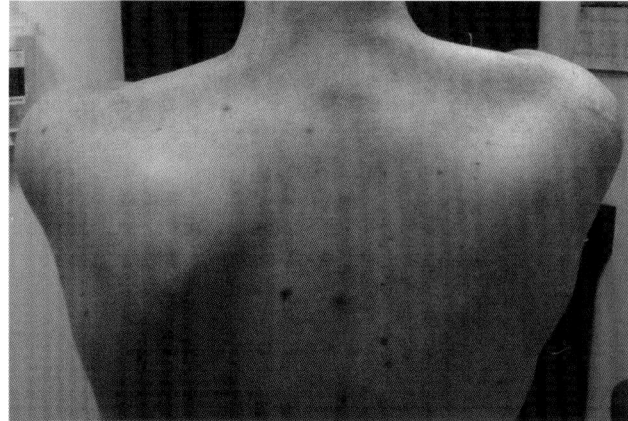

FIGURE 40-17 A patient with recurrent right shoulder instability with scapular dyskinesis and asymmetric motion. Note right posterior incision from a failed capsulorrhaphy.

Chronic or missed anterior dislocations typically will have a limitation to internal rotation and abduction. Patients with posterior dislocations will often demonstrate limitations in external rotation and abduction. Also, lack of supination of the forearm has been noted in patients with a chronic posterior dislocation.

General strength testing is performed with specific maneuvers to identify rotator cuff weakness. This is particularly important for an older individual because the association between rotator cuff tears and shoulder dislocations increases significantly with age.

Five physical signs of generalized ligamentous laxity according to the Beighton scale should be noted.[18] These include passive dorsiflexion of the little finger beyond 90 degrees; passive apposition of the thumb to the ipsilateral forearm; active hyperextension of the elbow beyond 10 degrees; active hyperextension of the knee beyond 10 degrees; and forward flexion of the trunk with the knees fully extended with the palms resting flat on the floor. Each positive test is one point and the first four are performed bilaterally. A score of ≥4 points (out of a possible 9) is diagnostic of generalized joint laxity (Fig. 40-18).

All of these examinations precede glenohumeral laxity and apprehension testing, which should be done last as it can make patients feel the most uncomfortable. The examination begins

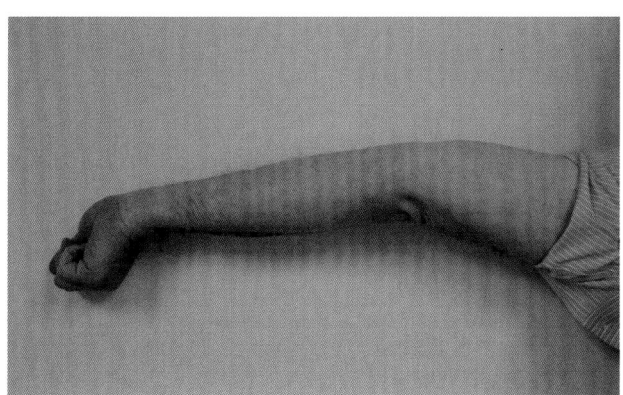
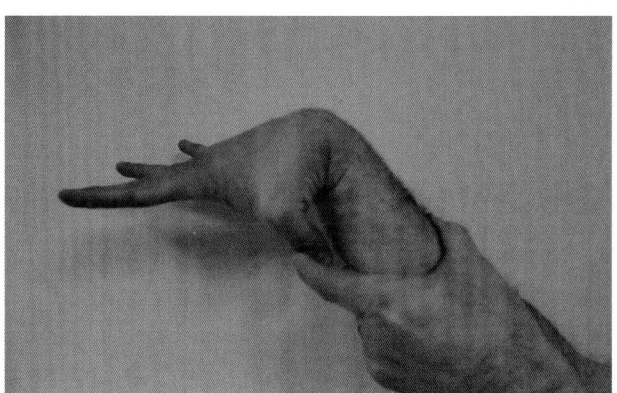

FIGURE 40-18 Examples of a patient with generalized ligamentous laxity.

with asking the patient to recreate the position of instability. This gives more information than most tests. This clearly determines if the instability is anterior if the position is abduction and external rotation versus cross-body adduction for posterior instability.

General Tests for Laxity

Drawer Test. One of the most common examinations of laxity is the "drawer" test. This maneuver is generally performed with the patient sitting with the examiner behind the patient.

With the forearm on the patient's lap, the acromion is stabilized with one hand, whereas the other hand manipulates the humeral head for anterior and posterior translation (Fig. 40-19).

For normal shoulders, this translation is smooth with a firm endpoint assessing the static restraints. If the translation is excessive, the patient has increased *laxity,* but not necessarily instability. If the maneuver reproduces the clinical symptoms of apprehension or pain, a presumed diagnosis of instability (anterior or posterior) may be established if consistent with the

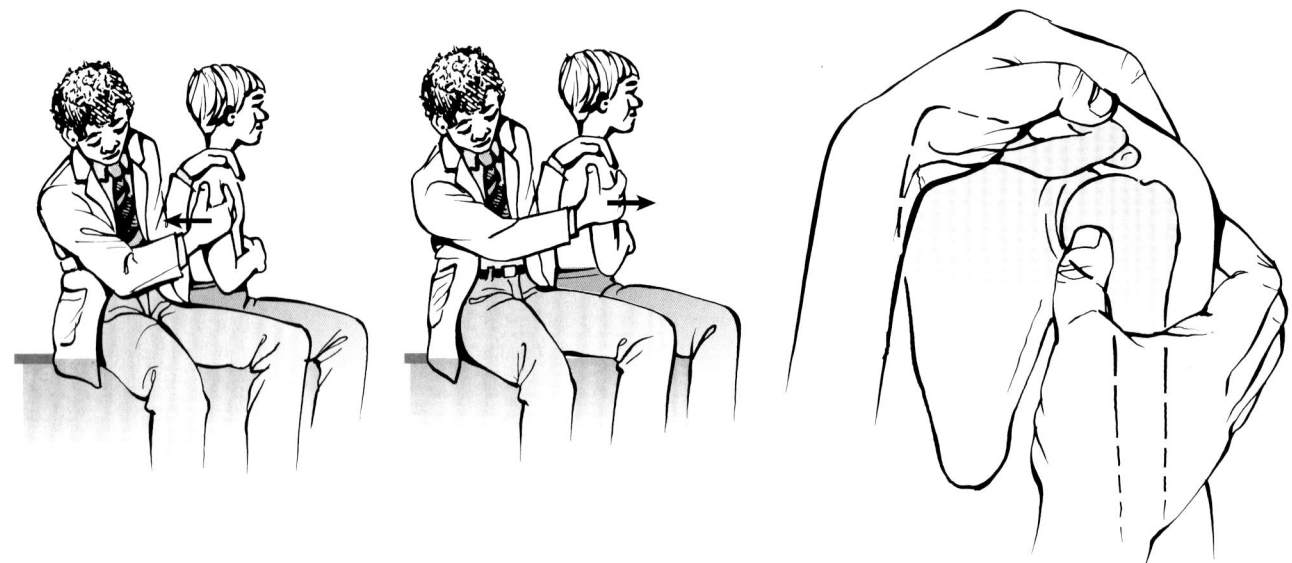

A

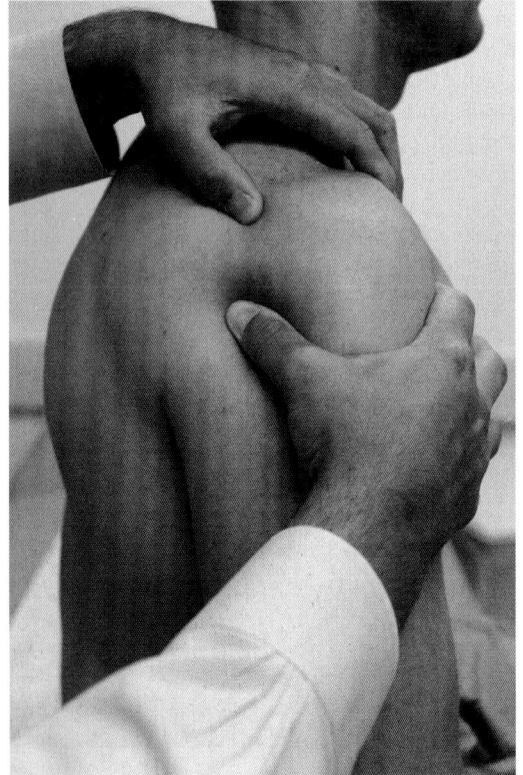

B

FIGURE 40-19 The Drawer Test. While stabilizing the scapula with one hand, the other hand grasps the humeral head. A gentle pressure is then applied toward the center of the glenoid. At the same time, the humeral head is manually translated in the anterior and in the posterior direction. (**A** and **B**) Illustration and clinical photo of the Drawer Test.

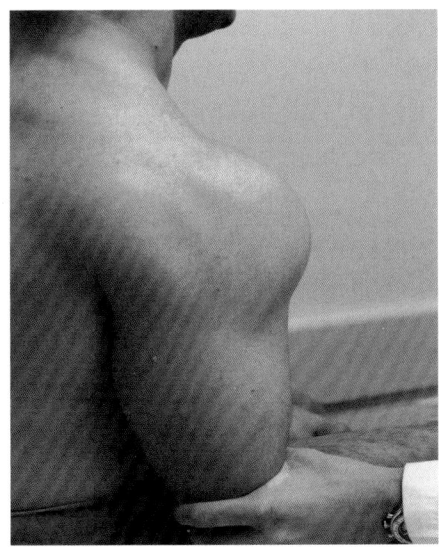
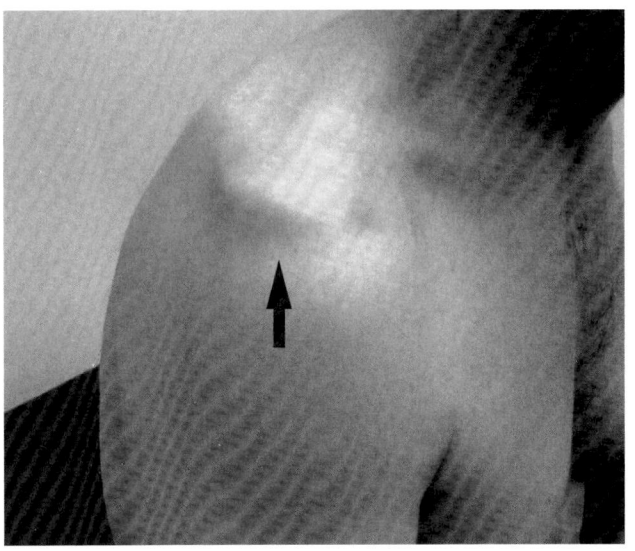

FIGURE 40-20 The sulcus test for inferior instability of the shoulder. With the patient in the sitting position, a downward traction is placed on the adducted arm **(A)**. With a positive test **(B)**, excessive inferior translation produces a dimple (*arrow*) on the lateral aspect of the acromion. By performing this test with the arm in external rotation, the maneuver can also be used to test the integrity of the rotator interval structures.

history and other examination findings. This is a reliable test when the patient is able to relax the shoulder muscle sufficiently and allow the maneuver to be performed without tension.[76,94]

Load and Shift Test. A variant of the drawer test is the load and shift test.[94,322] The patient is placed supine with arm abducted to 60 degrees. An axial pressure is applied to the humeral head to press the humeral head against the glenoid with the forearm in neutral position. Similar to the drawer test, the humeral head is then grasped and translated in either the anterior or posterior direction to assess for laxity and pain. Translation of the head to the glenoid rim is graded 1+; translation over the rim with spontaneous reduction is graded 2+; and dislocation without spontaneous reduction is grade 3+.[3] The test may recreate the symptoms of instability.

Sulcus Test. In the sulcus test, the patient is seated with their arm relaxed at their side and the arm is then pulled downward. A positive test reveals a "sulcus" or hollow area below the acromion. By placing the shoulder in external rotation, the sulcus test can also be used to estimate the laxity of the rotator interval structures (the coracohumeral and the SGHLs) as this maneuver places these structures under tension. The test is measured by noting the translation of the humeral head away from the acromion. Less than 1 cm of translation is graded as 1+; 1 to 2 cm is 2+; greater than 2 cm is 3+. Importantly, the sulcus sign is generally used to test for inferior laxity and is considered positive for inferior instability if the patient also has apprehension or even pain. It is often positive in many patients with MDI or posterior instability (Fig. 40-20).[233]

Gagey Hyperabduction Test. Gagey and Gagey[84] recently described another test of inferior laxity and instability. In this test, the examiner stands behind the patient with their forearm pushed down against the shoulder girdle whereas using the

other hand to gently passively abduct the patient's arm. The patient's elbow is flexed to 90 degrees (Fig. 40-21). Patients who can be abducted over 105 degrees have increased laxity whereas those with symptoms of apprehension suggest a diagnosis of inferior instability. Normal abduction should be 85 to 90 degrees. This test was positive in 85% of patients with known instability treated with anterior-inferior capsulorrhaphy. It is typically positive with MDI and should be performed for

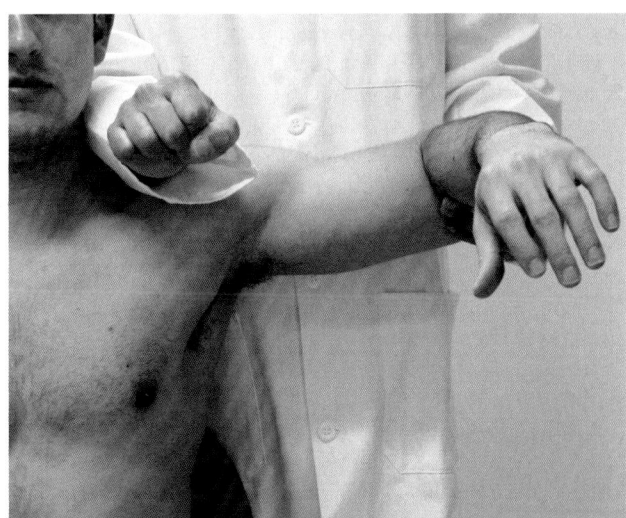

FIGURE 40-21 The Gagey abduction test for inferior laxity. The examiner stands behind the patient with their forearm pushed down against the shoulder girdle using the other hand to gently passively abduct the patient's arm. Normal abduction is about 90 degrees as seen in this patient. Abduction over 105 degrees reflects increased laxity, whereas symptoms of apprehension suggest a diagnosis of inferior instability.

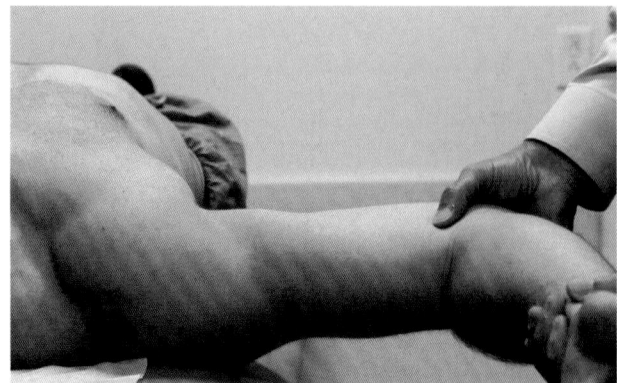 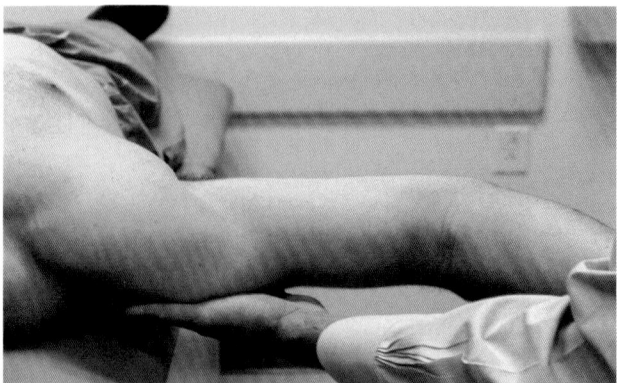

A   **B**

FIGURE 40-22 The apprehension and the fulcrum tests for anterior instability. In the apprehension test, the shoulder is abducted and externally rotated such that it is in a position vulnerable to dislocation with the patient in supine position **(A).** Symptomatic patients will report the sensation of apprehension or "getting ready to dislocate." In the fulcrum test, this sensation of instability is accentuated by placing an anteriorly directed force on the posterior humeral head **(B).**

all patients with posterior instability as there is frequently a bidirectional component.

Specific Examinations for Anterior Instability

Apprehension Tests. The "apprehension" test, originally described by Rowe and Zarins,[310] can be performed with the patient supine or sitting with the examiner behind the patient. From a position of 90 degrees of abduction and neutral rotation, the shoulder is externally rotated until it reaches its maximal limit or until the feeling of apprehension is reported by the patient (Fig. 40-22). It may be necessary to hold the arm in this position for 1 to 2 minutes to fatigue the subscapularis before apprehension is felt from capsular insufficiency. Although pain may be used as an indicator for instability, it is typically not as specific or as reliable as apprehension in documenting anterior instability.[76,331] In the *relocation* test as described by Jobe et al.,[158] a posteriorly directed force is placed on the anterior aspect of the shoulder to eliminate the feeling of apprehension (Fig. 40-23).

A variation of this test in which an anterior-directed pressure is added to the humeral head is called the *crank* test (Fig. 40-24). The *fulcrum* test is performed with the patient supine with the shoulder off the edge of the examination table and the arm in 90 degrees of abduction. The examiner places one hand behind the shoulder which acts as a fulcrum as the examiner's other hand is used to gently extend and externally rotate the patients arm. A test is positive if apprehension is felt by the patient (Fig. 40-22).

Finally, the *surprise* test is another variation of the apprehension test where the examination starts with a posteriorly directed force on the anterior shoulder. As this force is stabilizing the glenohumeral joint, the patient does not experience apprehension even when the shoulder is placed in abduction and maximal external rotation. By abruptly removing this force, the patient will suddenly experience apprehension or pain. Although all these maneuvers can detect anterior instability, a recent study has suggested that the surprise test may be the most sensitive.[199]

Studies have found the specificity of the anterior apprehension, relocation, and surprise tests to be above 90%.[199] The anterior drawer test, on the other hand, is less specific. The sensitivity of all these tests range from approximately 50% to 70%.[76] In addition, when pain is used instead of the feeling of apprehension both the sensitivity and specificity are poor.[156]

Specific Examinations for Posterior Instability. Posterior instability is best tested with the patient sitting or standing

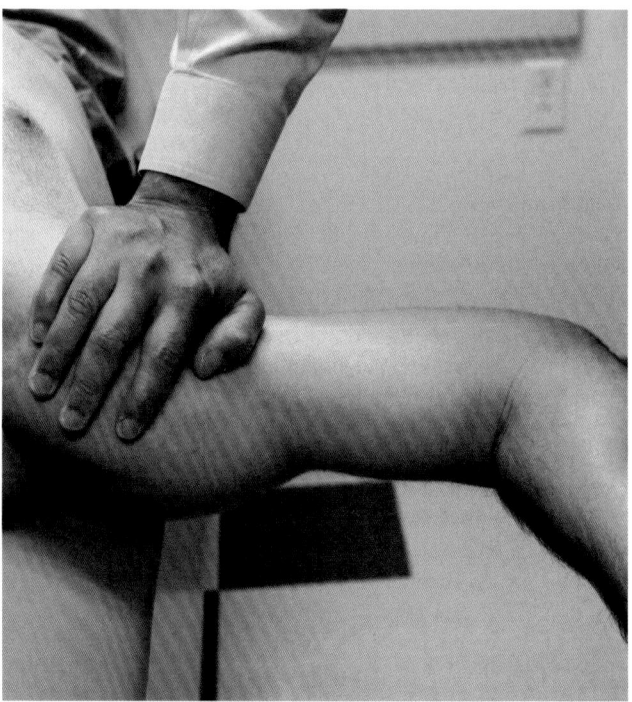

FIGURE 40-23 The relocation test for anterior instability. With the patient supine, the shoulder is abducted and externally rotated such that it is in a position vulnerable to dislocation. With a positive relocation test, the apprehension is reduced with a posteriorly directed force on the shoulder.

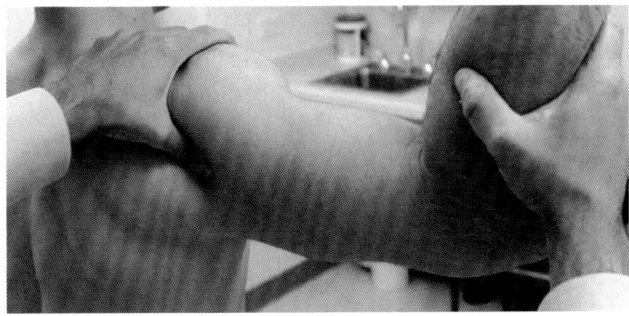

FIGURE 40-24 The crank test for anterior instability. The shoulder is abducted and externally rotated such that it is in a position vulnerable to anterior dislocation with the patient in sitting position. With an anteriorly directed force on the posterior humeral head, the instability is accentuated to cause the sensation of apprehension or "getting ready to dislocate."

for easy visualization of the posterior musculature and bony contours. With very unstable patients, a posteriorly dislocated head can be seen with adduction and internal rotation. Most patients can demonstrate their subluxation and the position of apprehension.

The main provocative maneuver is the *jerk* test. With the arm elevated to 90 degrees and internally rotated (Fig. 40-25)[176] an axial load is placed such that the humeral head is compressed against the glenoid and the scapula is stabilized by the examiner's other hand. This can be easily accomplished by pushing axially against the flexed elbow. By gradually adducting the shoulder, the humeral head may subluxate or even dislocate posteriorly and produce a sudden jerk. When the shoulder is returned to its original position, the humeral head will abruptly reduce back onto the glenoid and produce another jerk. The findings from this test can be quite dramatic in patients with posterior instability, but can be difficult to create if the patient is not fully relaxed. Some authors have suggested a painful test has a worse prognosis with nonoperative treatment.[176]

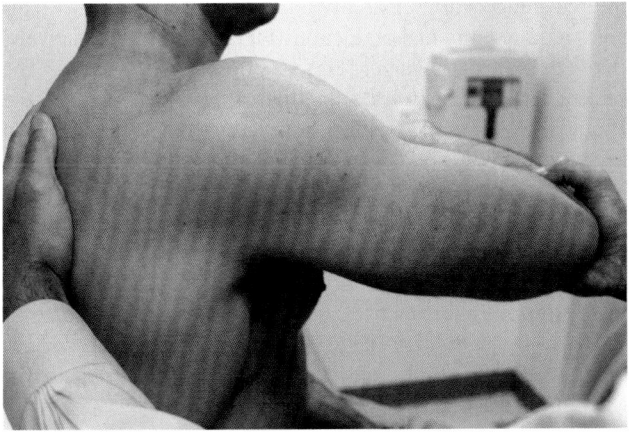

FIGURE 40-25 The jerk test for posterior instability. With the patient in either sitting or supine position, the arm is abducted and internally rotated. An axial load is then placed on the humerus while the arm is moved horizontally across the body. With a positive test, a sudden jerk occurs when the humeral head slides off of the back of the glenoid and when it is reduced back onto the glenoid.

Specific Examinations for Multidirectional Instability. There is no specific test for MDI, but inferior instability, by definition, is a major aspect of the pathology. Therefore, specific tests of inferior laxity such as the sulcus sign and the Gagey hyperabduction test may be symptomatic along with other laxity tests (drawer and load and shift). Importantly, signs of hyperlaxity may be present in other joints or the contralateral shoulder, but may not be symptomatic. Because scapular dyskinesis has been observed as either a cause or result of MDI, asymmetry of the scapula in both the resting state and with forward motion should be noted.

Imaging and Other Diagnostic Studies for Glenohumeral Instability

The Grashey View

Because of the oblique position of the scapula on the thorax, in a routine anteroposterior (AP) radiograph of the entire shoulder, the shadow of the humeral head will overlap with the glenoid fossa. This view is difficult to interpret with respect to the glenohumeral joint (Fig. 40-26A).

A "true" anterior–posterior radiograph of the glenohumeral joint is obtained when the x-ray beam is parallel to the glenoid fossa, roughly perpendicular to the scapular body (Fig. 40-26B). The x-ray beam is angled 35 to 45 degrees oblique to the sagittal plane of the body, centered on the coracoid process with the plate flat on the scapula. In this view, described by Grashey in 1923,[104] there is no overlap between the glenoid and the humeral head. In normal shoulders, a concave contour of the glenoid fossa should match the convex articular surface of the humeral head. If any overlap is seen between the glenoid and the humeral head, a dislocation should be suspected (Fig. 40-27). Although anterior dislocations are usually readily apparent, posterior dislocations can be very subtle on the AP radiograph. Inferior glenoid fractures can also be seen on this view, though the injury is best seen on the West-point axillary view described later. In addition, it has been noted by several authors that the loss of 5 mm of the inferior sclerotic line of the glenoid on the Grashey view is moderately sensitive (50% to 60%), but highly specific to anterior rim defects associated with recurrent anterior instability (Fig. 40-28).[14,154]

Axillary Views

An AP radiograph of the glenohumeral joint must be accompanied by an orthogonal view to document the location of the humeral head relative to the glenoid fossa. An axillary view is preferable because it can clearly display the bony anatomy and whether the humeral head is located. The view unambiguously shows the direction and magnitude of humeral head displacement and some associated fractures of both the humeral head and glenoid can be seen.

The *standard axillary* radiograph is obtained by placing the cassette on the superior aspect of the shoulder and directing the x-ray beam between the thorax and the abducted arm (Fig. 40-29A). For patients who cannot abduct the arm, two additional techniques have also been described. The *trauma axillary lateral* is performed with the patient supine with the

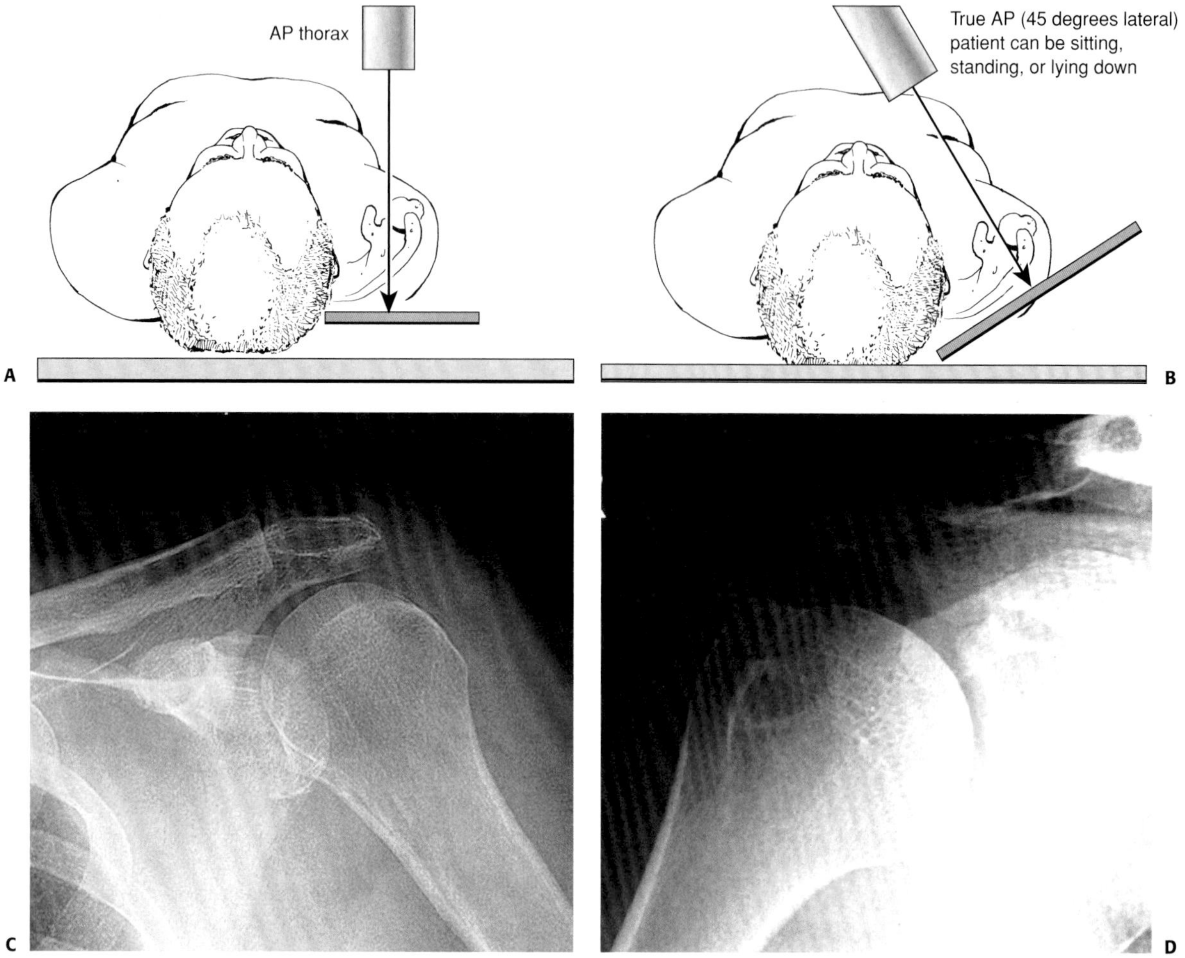

AP thorax

True AP (45 degrees lateral)
patient can be sitting,
standing, or lying down

A

B

C

D

FIGURE 40-26 Technique for obtaining anteroposterior (AP) thorax **(A)** and true AP **(B)** radiographs of the shoulder. In an AP view, the radiograph actually represents an oblique view of the shoulder joint. In a true AP view, the x-ray beam is parallel to the joint so that there is minimal overlap between the humeral head and the glenoid surface. The radiographic views of the shoulder AP **(C)** and shoulder true AP **(D)** are demonstrated.

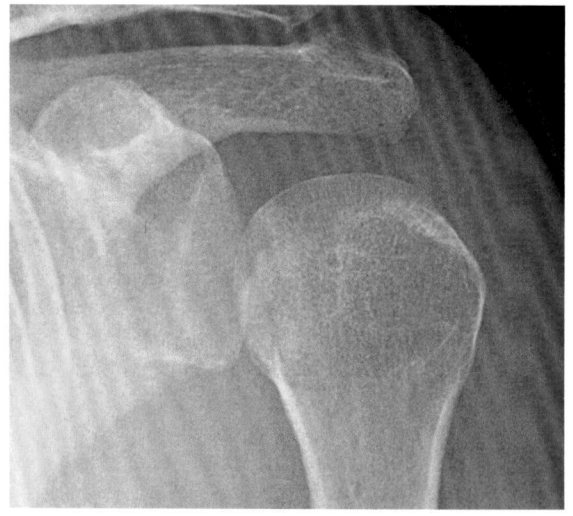

FIGURE 40-27 AP shoulder radiograph of a posterior dislocation. Note the widened space between the anterior glenoid rim and the humeral head.

injured slinged arm held by a foam wedge or pillow. This view requires minimal abduction (Fig. 40-29B). Alternatively, the *Velpeau axillary lateral* (Fig. 40-30) is performed with the patient leaning backward with their arm in a sling until the shoulder is over a horizontal cassette at the lower back. The x-ray beam is directed superior to inferior.[33]

The *West Point axillary* provides a tangential view of the anterior glenoid and is particularly useful in the identification of glenoid rim fractures which are missed on the *standard axillary* and its trauma modifications. It is taken with the patient in a prone position with the cassette placed on the superior aspect of the shoulder. The x-ray beam is directed 25 degrees downward from the horizontal and inward toward the axilla (Fig. 40-31).[304]

The Scapular Y View

The scapular Y view is a second orthogonal view to the Grashey view; however, it is difficult to understand the bony anatomy specifically with regards to the location of humeral head in relation to the glenoid fossa.

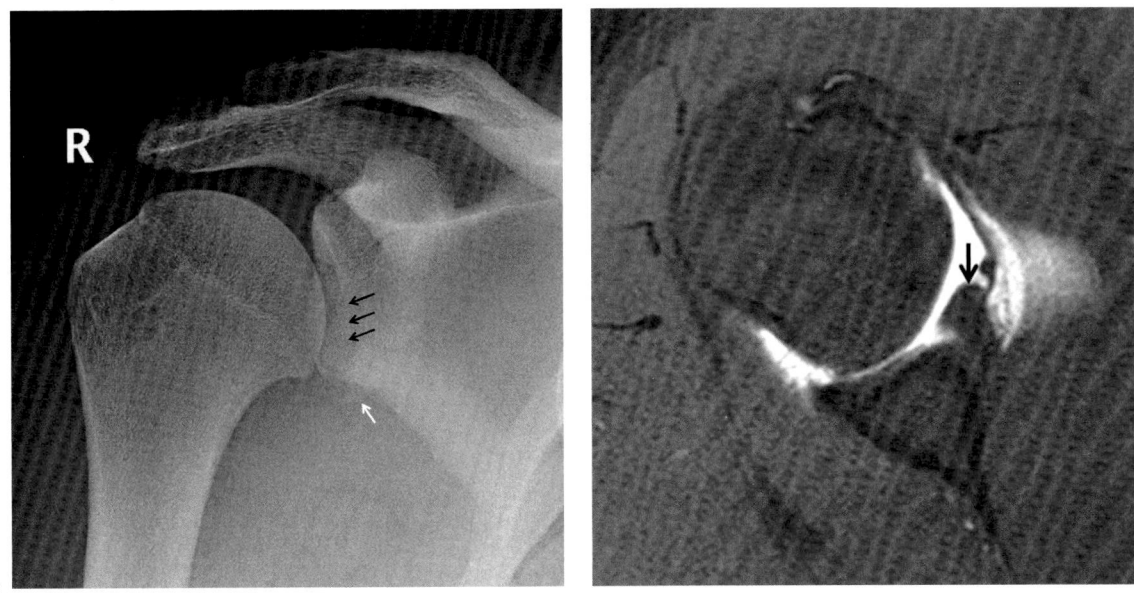

FIGURE 40-28 A: Grashey view with loss of the anterior sclerotic line (*black arrows*) which is moderately sensitive, but highly specific for anterior rim fractures of the inferior glenoid (*white arrow*). **B:** Corresponding MRI showing a bony Bankart lesion.

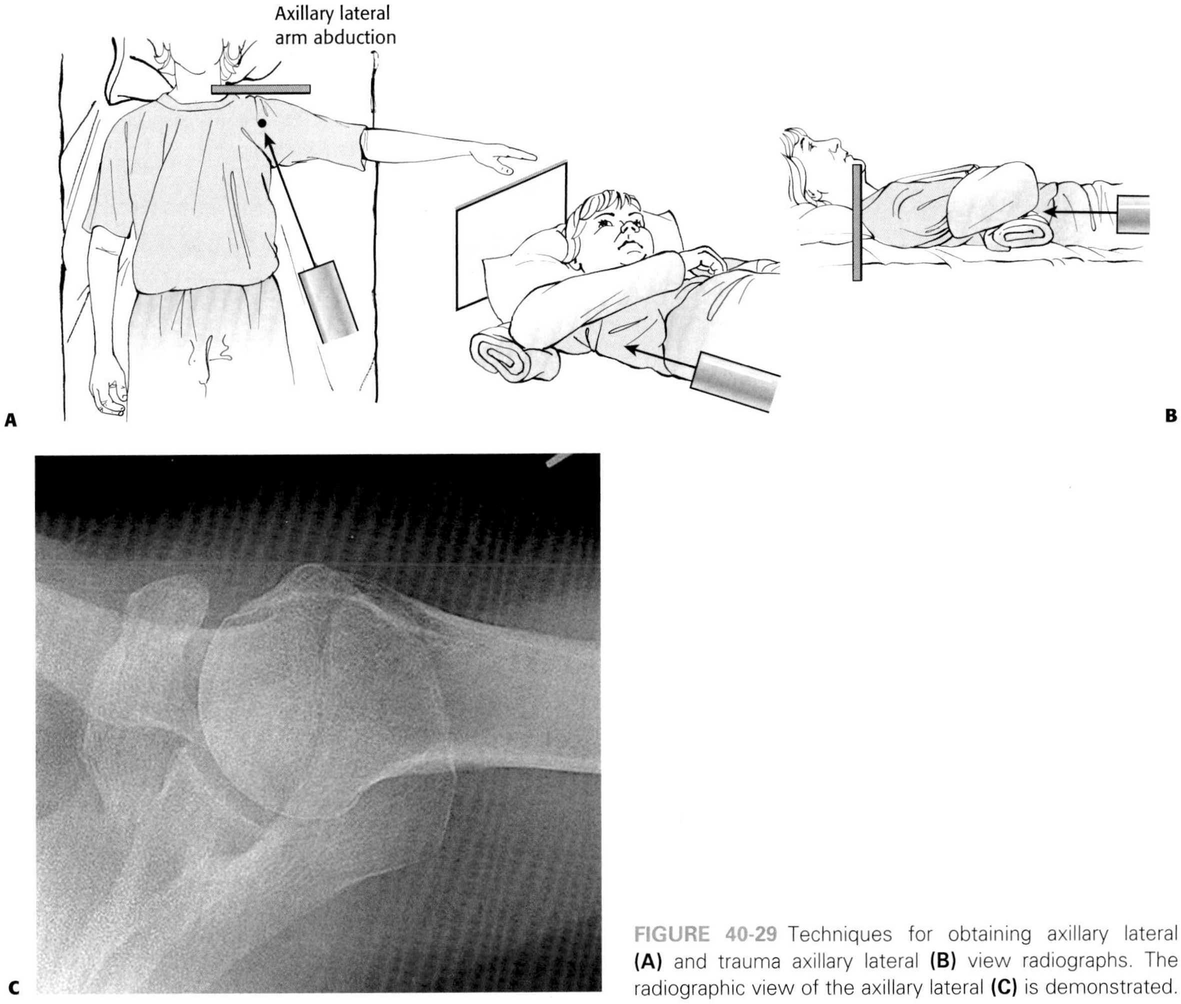

FIGURE 40-29 Techniques for obtaining axillary lateral **(A)** and trauma axillary lateral **(B)** view radiographs. The radiographic view of the axillary lateral **(C)** is demonstrated.

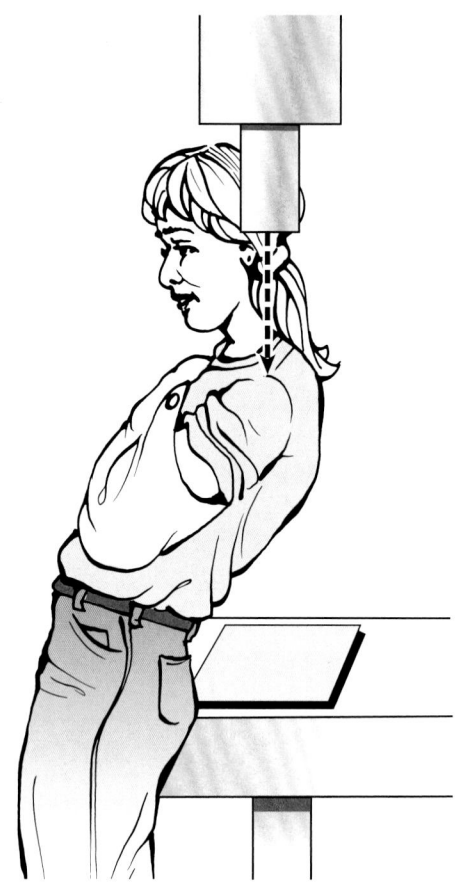

FIGURE 40-30 Positioning of the patient for the Velpeau axillary lateral view radiograph.

The radiograph is obtained by placing the cassette on the anterolateral aspect of the shoulder and directing the x-ray beam medial to lateral, parallel to the spine of the scapula (Fig. 40-32).[227] The x-ray shadows outline the scapula as the letter "Y"—hence the name of this view. The two upper limbs of the letter Y represent the scapula spine and the coracoid process, respectively, whereas the inferior limb of the Y represents the scapular body. The glenoid fossa is located in the center of the Y where all the limbs intersect and where the humeral head should be centered.

The Apical Oblique View

Sometimes referred to as the *Garth* view, the apical oblique view clearly reveals the anterior inferior and posterior superior glenoid rims. Acute anterior inferior fractures or chronic bone loss associated with recurrent instability can be seen on this view. Additionally, Hill–Sachs deformities are seen as the posterolateral humeral head is well defined.

In this view, the patient is upright with the cassette flat against the scapula. Like the Grashey view, the x-ray beam is directed orthogonal to the scapula to get a "true" AP of the joint. In addition, a 45-degree caudal tilt is used so the beam is directed downward and medial to lateral[87,88] (Fig. 40-33).

The Stryker Notch View

The Stryker notch view is the best to characterize the Hill–Sachs defect and the posterior-superior humeral head (Fig. 40-34).[115] The film is taken with the patient supine with the cassette under the shoulder. The palm of the hand rests on the patient's

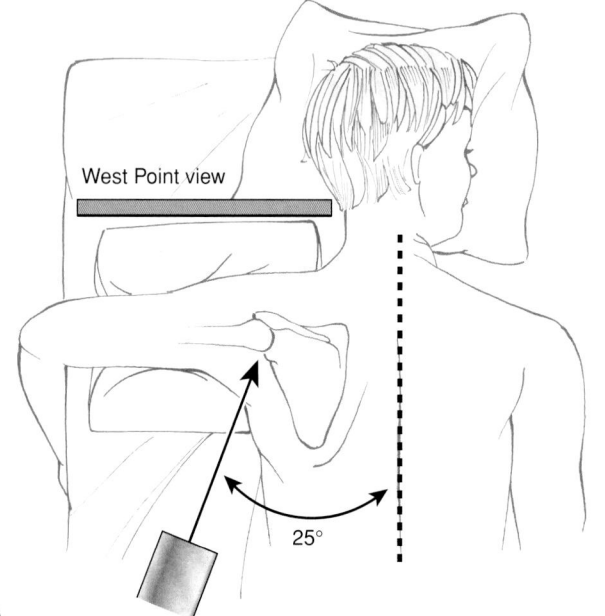

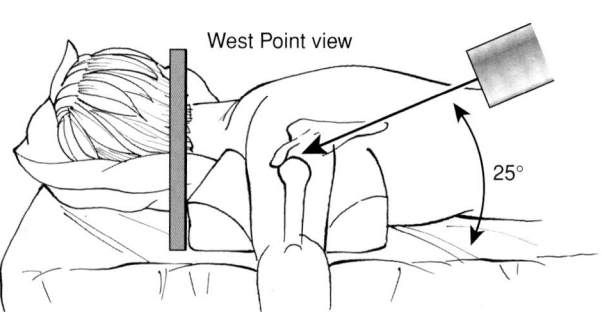

FIGURE 40-31 West Point view for the identification of a glenoid rim lesion. This radiograph is taken with the patient in the prone position. The beam is angled approximately 25 degrees from the midsagittal plane **(A)** to provide a tangential view of the glenoid. In addition, the beam is angled 25 degrees downward **(B)** to highlight the anterior and posterior aspects of the glenoid.

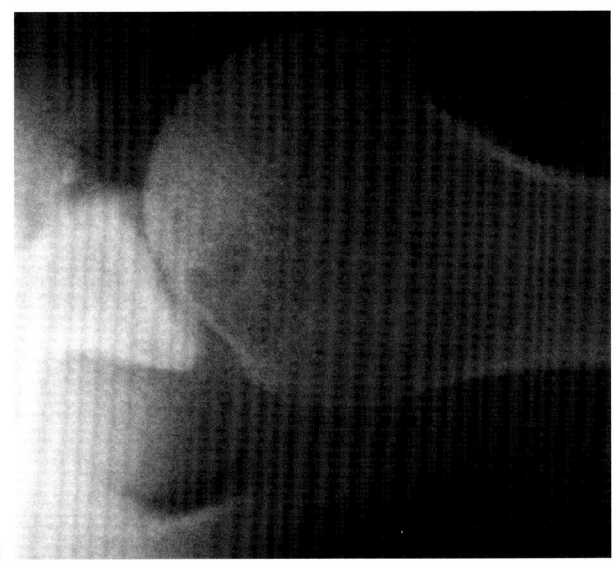

C

FIGURE 40-31 (*continued*) In this fashion, the entire glenoid rim can be clearly visualized **(C).**

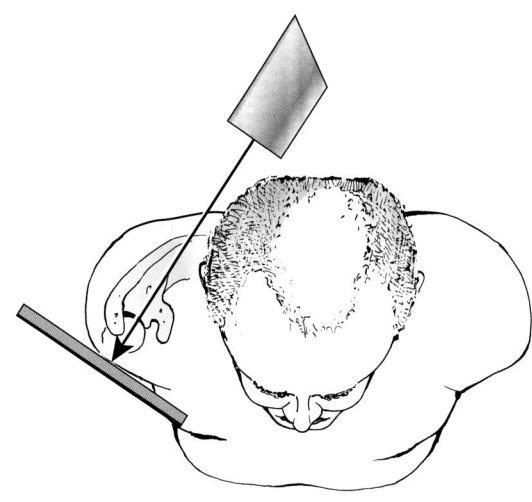

FIGURE 40-32 Technique for obtaining a scapula lateral, also known as the "Y," view radiograph. With the cassette placed on the anterior lateral aspect of the shoulder, the x-ray beam is directed parallel to the plane of the scapula.

head with the arm forward flexed such that the bent elbow is over the face and pointed straight upward. The x-ray beam is angled approximately 10 degrees caudal relative to a vertical line orthogonal to the patient's torso. The beam is centered over the coracoid.

Computed Tomography and Magnetic Resonance Imaging

Computed tomography (CT) and magnetic resonance imaging (MRI) are often necessary for full understanding of the pathogenesis of glenohumeral instability. A CT scan may be useful in the

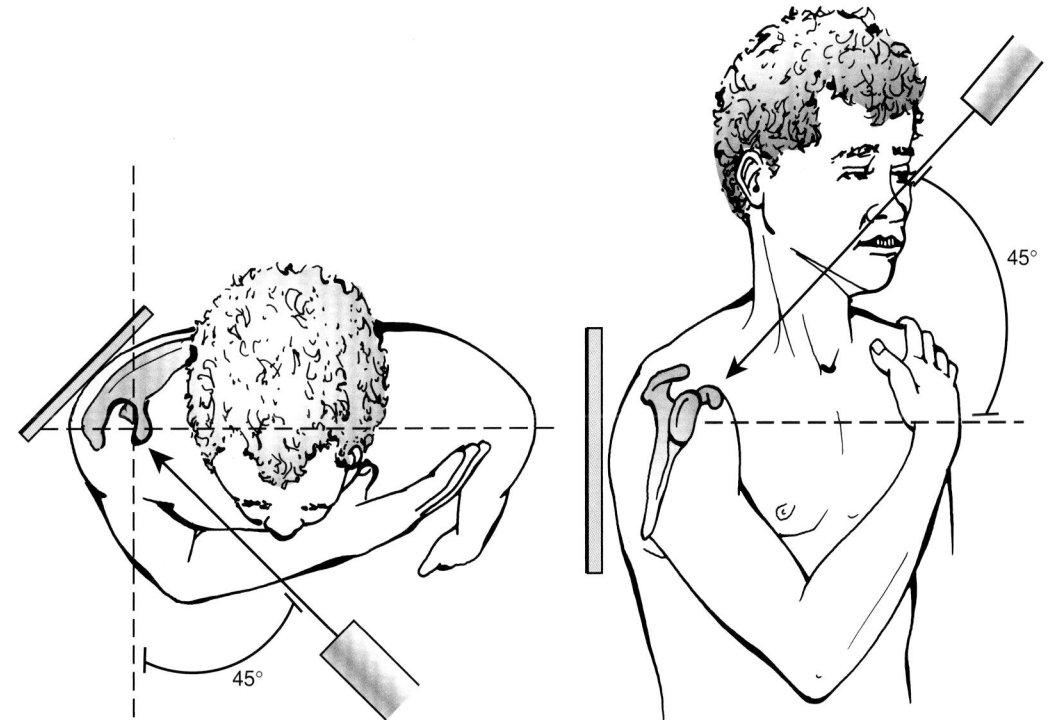

A

B

FIGURE 40-33 Apical oblique view for the identification of a glenoid rim lesion. This radiograph is taken with the beam angled approximately 45 degrees **(A)** to provide a "true AP" view of the glenoid. In addition, the beam is angled 45 degrees downward **(B)** to highlight the anterior inferior aspect of the glenoid.

(continues)

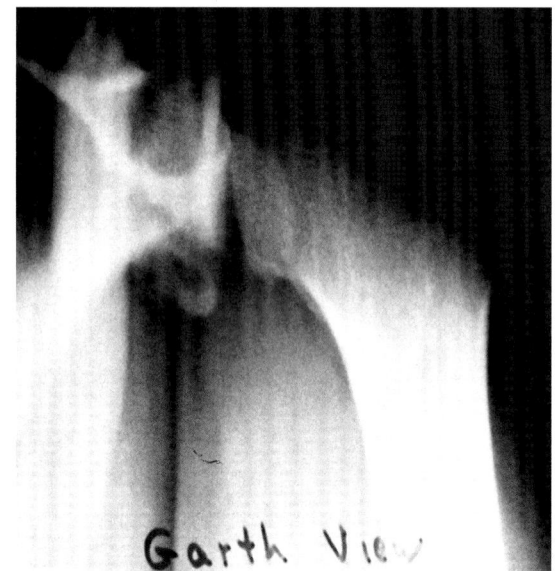

C

FIGURE 40-33 (*continued*) As such, a bony defect in the anterior inferior aspect of the glenoid **(C)** can be easily visualized. (Modified from Garth WP, Slappey CE, Ochs CW. Roentgenographic demonstration of instability of the shoulder: The apical oblique projection. A technical note. *J Bone Joint Surg* 1984;66-A:1450–1453.)

acute setting when limited quality radiographs or other circumstances do not clearly demonstrate glenohumeral joint pathology. In addition, CT is necessary to determine the size and displacement of a suspected glenoid fracture or the presence of proximal humerus fractures as routine radiographs can be difficult to interpret. In the acute setting, there is limited need for an MRI.

In the subacute (first office visit of a first time dislocater) or a nonacute setting, if consideration is given to surgical treatment, MRI (in comparison to CT) is considered the standard of reference for the determination of pathoanatomy because the

majority of injuries are capsuloligamentous. MRI is also necessary to evaluate for rotator cuff tears and humeral avulsions of the glenohumeral ligaments (HAGL). Importantly, MR arthrography (the injection of contrast into the joint) has been shown to be more sensitive than conventional MRI in the detection of labral, capsule, and rotator cuff tears and is the investigation of choice for soft tissue pathology.[50,191]

Many of the studies comparing MR arthrography to conventional MRI, however, were performed in the 1990s with lower resolution (non 3-Tesla) scanners.[50] More recent studies confirm a high sensitivity and specificity for both MR arthrography and conventional MRI, but still favor MR arthrography.[250] In MR arthrography, labral and rotator cuff tears all had sensitivities >95% and specificities of nearly 100%; conventional 3-T MRI had similar specificities,[250] but lower sensitivities in the 80% to 90% range.[162,202]

As discussed later in this section, CT scan with three-dimensional reconstructions is the ideal study for the evaluation of bony pathology: Acute fracture, anterior-inferior glenoid humeral bone loss, and Hill–Sachs deformities. The addition of contrast dye for CT arthrography allows for the visualization of soft tissue pathology such as rotator cuff tears and capsular lesions. The sensitivity of CT arthrography approaches conventional MRI in evaluating labral tears (80% to 90%) with specificities in the 90% range. However, CT arthrography still falls short of MR arthrography.[50,349] In addition, extracapsular soft tissue is not well seen[249] and the quality of imaging still varies considerably between institutions.

Defining Glenoid Bone Loss

Radiographs are moderately sensitive for identifying glenoid bone loss,[21,26,88] but have little value in measuring clinically relevant loss. CT scans with three-dimensional reconstructions and modeling are the gold standard as MRI may underestimate the degree of bone loss.[148] With these scans and contralateral imaging of the shoulder, a best-fit circle of the inferior two-

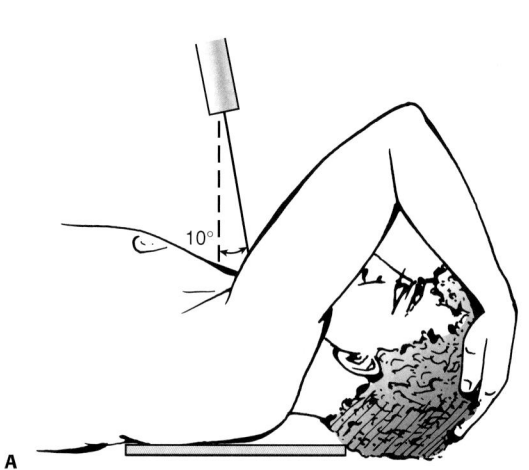

A

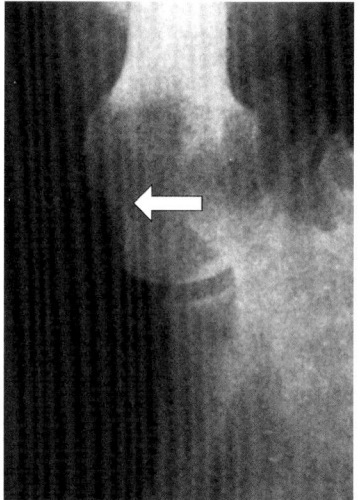

B

FIGURE 40-34 Stryker notch view for humeral head defects. The patient is in the supine position with the arm flexed to 120 degrees so that the hand can be placed on top of the head **(A)**. The x-ray beam is then angled approximately 10 degrees. The radiograph **(B)** can clearly reveal the presence of any osseous defects (*arrow*). (Modified from Hall RH, Isaac F, Booth CH. Dislocations of the shoulder with special reference to accompanying small fractures. *J Bone Joint Surg* 1959;41:489–494.)

thirds of the normal shoulder can be superimposed onto the effected side to estimate the amount of bone loss.[26,200] The average diameter of this circle for a normal glenoid is approximately 24 mm.[141] Numerous methods have been used for the estimation of bone loss, but the simplest involves using the diameter to calculate this percentage (Fig. 40-35).[200]

$$\% \text{ Bone loss} = \frac{(\text{Radius of best fit circle}) - (\text{Distance from center to anterior defect})}{\text{Diameter of best fit circle}}$$

According to Lo et al.,[200] an anterior defect of 7.5 mm corresponds to approximately 25% of total bone loss. Importantly, small differences in the size of the best-fit circle along with the angle in which the sagittal reconstructions are made relative to the scapular body may make a significant difference in the measurements.

Defining the Hill–Sachs Defect

The Hill–Sachs lesion, especially if it is large, can sometimes be visualized on routine radiographs especially the "true" AP radiographs of the shoulder as well as a standard axillary view. A true AP view with full internal rotation of the arm can allow better visualization, however, none of these views are fully sensitive. The Stryker–Notch view is the most sensitive in identifying the Hill–Sachs and is regarded as the best view to gauge its relative size.[115] Ultimately, however, CT scans and three-dimensional imaging and reconstructions are ideal: However, there is no universally standard way to measure the size or significance. Many methods have used percentage of total articular surface as a gauge of the defect, but unlike the developments in measuring glenoid bone loss, better methods are still required.

Diagnostic Arthroscopy

Ultimately, if there is any question of the diagnosis, or the amount of glenoid or humeral bone loss, a diagnostic arthroscopy is an ideal tool for clarification. Lo et al. described a method of quantifying glenoid bone loss by measuring glenoid width with the "bare area" as a reference point. This relatively constant spot is defined by absent cartilage in the center of the native glenoid.[199] In addition, the size, engagement, and clinical relevance of the Hill–Sachs can be determined.

AUTHOR'S PREFERRED DIAGNOSTIC WORK-UP

Acute Instability

In the emergency room, with a reduced dislocation, we prefer a true AP or Grashey view to evaluate the concentricity of the joint and signs of glenoid or proximal humerus fracture; an apical oblique or Garth view to better view a glenoid fracture; and a Velpeau or trauma axillary to clearly determine the reduction of the joint. None of these views require the patient to remove the sling. If there is any question of joint reduction, a CT scan is performed—though this is uncommon.

Nonacute Instability

The evaluation of the patient with recurrent instability in the office setting requires the same views as in the acute setting, but a Stryker–Notch view is added to evaluate for the Hill–Sachs defect. If there is little concern for bone loss based on the history and radiographs, a high-resolution conventional MRI is our preferred study to not only evaluate for a capsular tear but for other pathology such as a HAGL or a rotator cuff tear. Given the high quality of current MRI scanners as well as the invasive nature and the additional cost of arthrography, MR arthrography is not routinely used.

If bone loss is a major concern, a CT scan is ordered. With the improvement of CT arthrograms, however, this may be the single ideal study, however, the quality of the imaging differs between institutions. Consideration of patient age, the additional radiation of CT scans, and the invasive nature is always considered before pursuing this study.

Last, if there is any question of the degree of bone loss, the engagement of the Hill–Sachs, the quality of tissue or the presence of other intra-articular pathology, a diagnostic arthroscopy is performed.

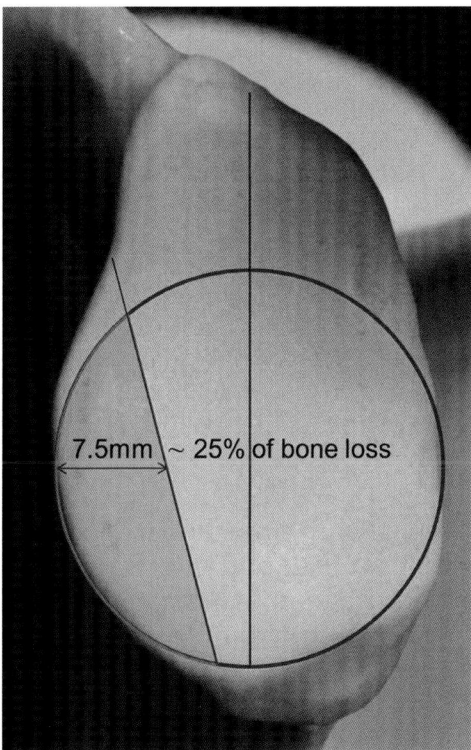

FIGURE 40-35 Using the best-fit circle of the inferior two-thirds of the glenoid, total glenoid bone loss can be estimated with the equation in the text. The average glenoid diameter is 24 mm and 7.5 mm of anterior bone loss corresponds to approximately 25% of total loss.

OUTCOME MEASURES FOR GLENOHUMERAL INSTABILITY

General health and general shoulder scores such as the Medical Outcomes Study 36-item Short Form (SF-36) and American

Shoulder and Elbow Surgeons (ASES) score, respectively, have been used to measure instability outcomes. However, these scores are not ideal and subsequently there are two specific glenohumeral instability scores that have been developed: the Western Ontario Shoulder Instability Index (WOSI) and the Oxford Instability Score.

The Rowe score was described by Carter Rowe in his classic 1978 article evaluating long-term results of Bankart repairs.[307] This unvalidated score has a maximum of 100 points and rates patient outcome based on three domains about the shoulder: Stability (50 points), motion (20 points), and function (30 points). Because this was the first score to be developed, it has a number of weaknesses. First, the various weights of the three items are arbitrary and unsupported. Second, how the three domains are evaluated is unclear. For instance, it is not clear if the motion measurements are active or passive and how the three motions (external rotation, forward elevation, and internal rotation) are combined to make up the 20 points. For these reasons, this score should only be used for historical comparison in addition to a modern validated outcome score.

The WOSI is a validated score that was established in 1998.[178] The test consists of 21 questions with 4 domains: Physical symptoms (10 questions); sports, recreation, and work (4 questions); lifestyle (4 questions); and emotions (3 questions). The score ranges from 0 to 2100 with a lower score representing a better outcome. A percentage score is calculated per the following formula:

$$\frac{2100 - \text{raw score}}{2100 \times 100}$$

The estimate for a minimal clinically important difference (MCID) is 220 points or 10.4%. For moderate and large differences, the estimates are 469 (22.3%) and 527 (25%), respectively. The WOSI has been shown to be more responsive to measuring shoulder instability than the following scores in order: Rowe, DASH, Constant, ASES, UCLA, and SF-12.

The Oxford Shoulder Instability Questionnaire was developed in 1999 by Dawson et al.[62] This is a 12-item questionnaire with each item scored from 1 to 5 with the higher numbers reflecting greater severity. The numbers are combined to form a score from 12 to 60 with a lower number as a better score. The questions were developed by interviewing 20 patients with shoulder instability and then iteratively retesting the questions on different groups at different times. Construct validity has been further tested with prospective studies with comparison to other shoulder scores with moderate agreement.

The WOSI or Oxford score are reliable and reproducible tools for the use in a modern study evaluating shoulder instability.

COMMON SURGICAL APPROACHES OF GLENOHUMERAL INSTABILITY

Open Anterior Approach of Glenohumeral Instability

The skin incision varies depending on the procedure. If the surgery is mainly on the glenoid side, a very cosmetic incision is placed on the anterior axillary crease, which is identified with arm adduction, starting just distal to the coracoid process (Fig. 40-36A). If work will be done on the humeral side, the skin incision can be directed more laterally from the coracoid. After the skin incision and subcutaneous dissection, the interval between the anterior deltoid and the pectoralis major muscle is identified. This area, also referred to as the deltopectoral interval, is defined by the cephalic vein which must be dissected and retracted away from the surgical field (Fig. 40-36B). The cephalic drains the anterior part of the deltoid and therefore it is easier to take the vein laterally, however, the surgeon should limit the amount of retraction on the vein to prevent tearing. This interval is typically slightly medial to the skin incision.

A self-retainer placed below the deltoid and pectoralis allows visualization of the underlying clavipectoral fascia which can be incised just at the lateral edge of the coracobrachialis muscle fibers (Fig. 40-36C). Bringing the arm into flexion and slight abduction relaxes the deltoid and can help with exposure. At this point, though some experienced surgeons place a self-retaining retractor beneath the conjoined tendon, we believe this is not advisable given the risk of musculocutaneous nerve injury. The musculocutaneous nerve enters on average 5 cm from the tip of the coracoid. However, in our experience, it can be as close as 1 cm.[372]

A blunt handheld retractor, such as a Green retractor, can pull the conjoined tendon medially giving exposure to the subscapularis muscle and tendon. Some surgeons release part of the lateral conjoined for improved exposure, though we have no experience with this. Typically, there is a bursa overlying the muscle and tendon that needs to be excised. The axillary nerve is often easily palpable and visualized slightly medially and inferiorly at the subscapularis. It should be protected with a handheld retractor.

Management of the subscapularis for exposure to the underlying capsule is arguably the most important aspect of the exposure. The overlying subscapularis muscle and tendon may be split in line with its fibers or it can be incised 1 cm medial to its insertion at the lesser tuberosity (Fig. 40-36D) and reflected medially. The key is defining the plane between the subscapularis and capsule medially, deep to the muscular part of the subscapularis because the tendon and capsule merge laterally.

At this point, the capsule can be incised a number of ways depending on surgeon preference and the goal of the surgery. When performing an open capsulorrhaphy, we prefer a "T" incision with a horizontal incision at the center of the joint with a vertical incision medial and parallel to the glenoid rim.

Open Posterior Approach of Glenohumeral Instability

The skin incision is placed just medial to the posterolateral corner of the acromion, extending to the axillary crease. Traditional approaches have released the deltoid muscle from its origin on the acromion. However, access can be achieved by splitting the deltoid which is easiest at the middle and posterior thirds, often identified by a fatty stripe. This split also typically starts at the posterolateral corner of the acromion to the upper border of the teres minor—approximately 10 cm (Fig. 40-37). The theoretical advantage of this modification is the preservation of strength and function of the posterior deltoid.

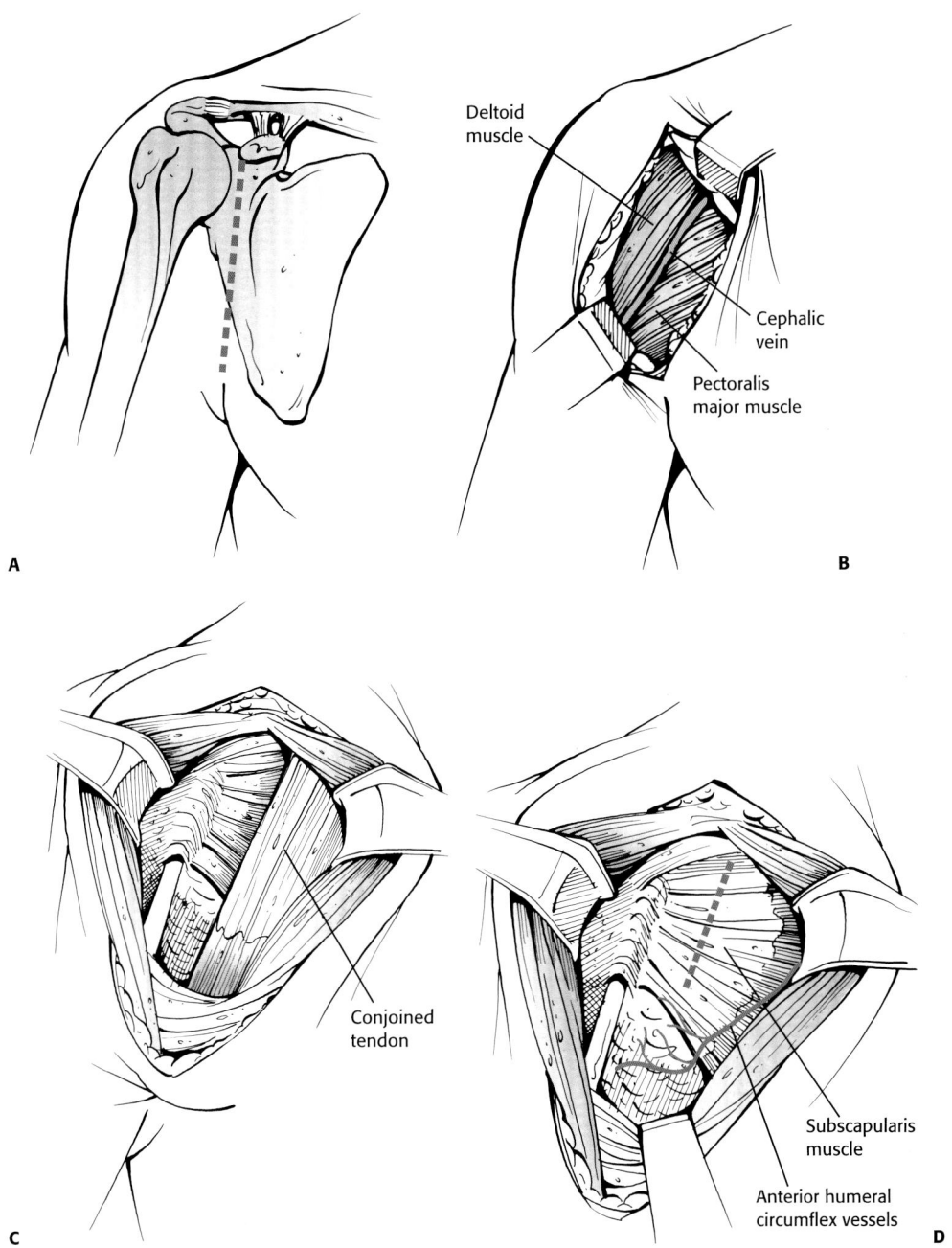

FIGURE 40-36 Anterior approach to the shoulder. **A:** The incision extends from the coracoid to the axillary fold. **B:** The deltopectoral interval is identified and developed, taking the cephalic vein laterally with the deltoid. **C:** The conjoined tendon and subscapularis are identified. **D:** A subscapularis tenotomy is made vertically, separating the subscapularis tendon from the underlying capsule.

Sometimes, in patients whose deltoid muscle contains significant bulk and resting tone, adequate exposure of the shoulder may not be possible by simply splitting the muscle. In these rare circumstances, the posterior deltoid is released from its origin on the acromion, and then reattached at the end of the procedure using bone tunnels.

The infraspinatus is identified by its bipennate nature and its broad posterior insertion onto the greater tuberosity. The teres minor is inferior and has a more narrow insertion.

Generally the infraspinatus tendon is lax, and can simply be retracted superiorly instead of releasing it. The teres minor muscle fibers are then retracted inferiorly to gain exposure to the posterior capsule. External rotation can help relax these muscles. Alternatively, there is a fat stripe between upper and lower portions of the teres that can be split, allowing exposure to the midpoint of the joint capsule.

The posterior capsule is isolated from the musculature medially with the sweep of a finger or blunt instrument. Laterally,

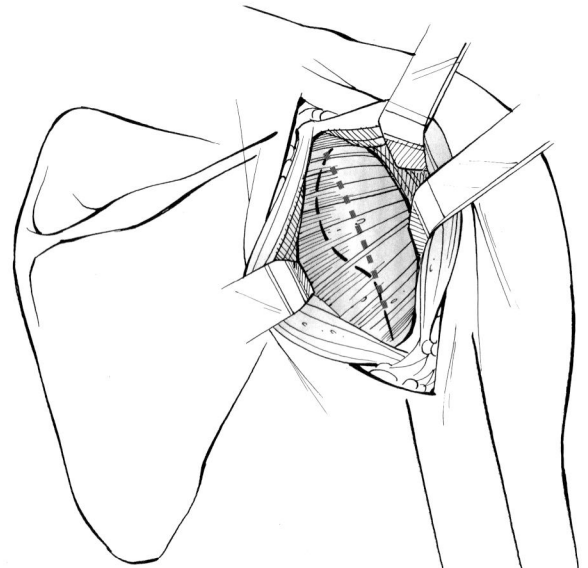

FIGURE 40-37 The posterior approach to the shoulder. After the skin incision, the deltoid muscle can be split along its fibers from the acromion to the upper border of the teres minor. Underlying rotator cuff tendons can then be split to gain access to the shoulder capsule and joint.

however, meticulous sharp dissection is required to separate the tendinous portion of the muscles from the capsule.

If exposure is difficult, the infraspinatus muscle can be isolated with a Penrose drain placed for traction. The tendon can then be incised 0.5 cm from its insertion and reflected medially. Excessive medial reflection should be avoided to prevent injury to the suprascapular nerve. Care must be taken when

handling the teres minor because the axillary nerve and the posterior humeral circumflex vessels lie just inferior in the quadrilateral space.

Once the posterior capsule is isolated, it is incised to expose the joint. The capsulotomy incisions vary with each procedure and technique, as described below.

Arthroscopic Approach and Portal Placement

The typical subcutaneous bony structures marked out on the skin prior to surgery include the scapular spine, acromion, clavicle, acromioclavicular joint, and coracoid process (Fig. 40-38). From these landmarks, initial portal placement can be defined. Although shoulder arthroscopy can be performed in either the lateral decubitus position or the beach chair position, arthroscopic portal placement is similar for the two different surgical approaches. Arthroscopic stabilization procedures typically utilize multiple intra-articular portals, including standard anterior and posterior portals, as well as accessory portals like the accessory superolateral portal.

The primary posterior portal is defined by the natural soft spot that exists between the humeral head and glenoid posteriorly (Fig. 40-38)—typically around 1 to 2 cm medial and 2 to 3 cm distal to the posterolateral corner of the acromion.

The primary anterior portal is typically made next (Fig. 40-38). This portal enters the glenohumeral joint through the triangular space defined by the long head of the biceps tendon superiorly, the upper border of the subscapularis tendon inferiorly, and the anterosuperior glenoid and labrum medially (Fig. 40-39). The site and angle of entry for this portal on the skin is best determined with the use of a spinal needle. This

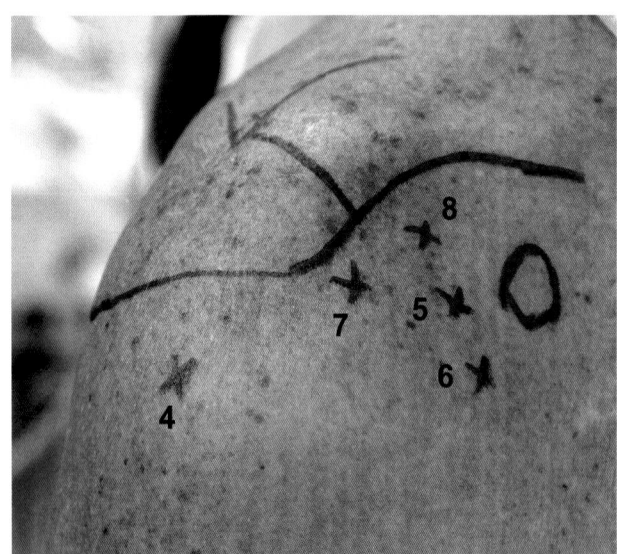

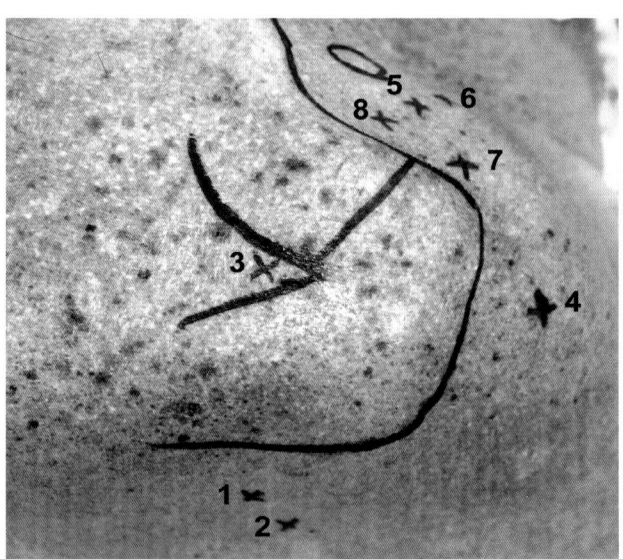

FIGURE 40-38 Anterior **(A)** and superior **(B)** views of the right shoulder, with the subcutaneous borders of the scapular spine, acromion, acromioclavicular joint, clavicle, and coracoid process outlined. The numbered Xs represent possible arthroscopic portal sites: 1, primary posterior; 2, posteroinferior; 3, supraspinatus or Neviaser; 4, lateral subacromial; 5, primary anterior; 6, anteromedial; 7, accessory superolateral; 8, anterior acromioclavicular.

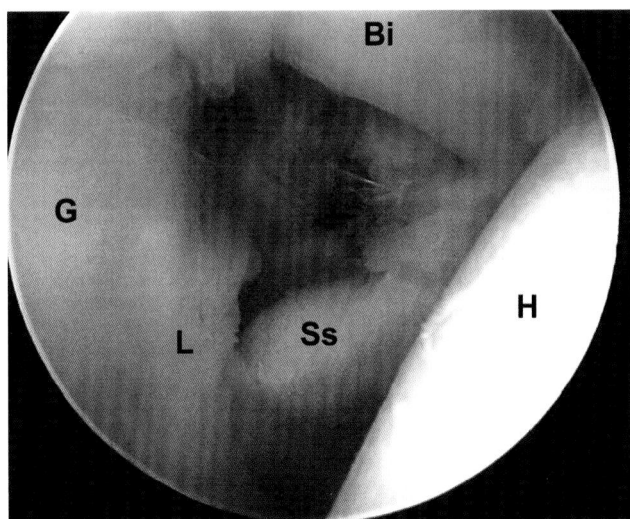

FIGURE 40-39 Arthroscopic view from the primary posterior portal in a right shoulder, showing the anterior triangular space through which the primary anterior portal is directed. This space is defined by the long head of the biceps tendon (Bi) superiorly, the upper border of the subscapularis inferiorly (Ss), and the anterosuperior glenoid (G) and labrum (L) medially. The site and angle of entry for this portal is best determined with use of a spinal needle. H, humeral head.

provides confirmation that portal placement will allow appropriate access to all necessary structures before making the skin incision. The superior–inferior position of this portal will also vary, depending on its intended use. This portal should be placed just above the upper border of the subscapularis tendon, often called an anteromedial portal, to allow appropriate access to the anteroinferior labrum during arthroscopic labral repair.

An anteroinferior portal has also been described, if needed, to allow for inferior enough anchor placement during arthroscopic repair of the anteroinferior labrum.[61] The portal is made lower than the typical anterior portal, passing through the subscapularis tendon to access the 5 or 6 o'clock position on the glenoid.

An accessory superolateral portal is frequently used for arthroscopic stabilization procedures, and is made through the rotator interval.[61,188] This portal is commonly used for visualization of the anterior glenoid during anterior labral repair.

The supraspinatus portal or Neviaser portal may occasionally be utilized for labral repairs, particularly repairs of the superior labrum.[237] This portal is defined on the skin where the scapular spine meets the medial border of the acromion, just posterior to the acromioclavicular joint (Fig. 40-38). A spinal needle can be placed at this spot, passing through the supraspinatus muscle belly, and brought into the glenohumeral joint along the superior aspect of the glenoid and labrum.

For posterior arthroscopic stabilization procedures like posterior labral repair, one or more accessory posterior portals may be utilized. An accessory posteroinferior portal, often called the 7 o'clock portal, can be made for inferior anchor placement during arthroscopic posterior labral repair.[60] Typically the skin incision for this portal is several centimeters inferior and lat-

eral to the standard posterior viewing portal (Fig. 40-38). For anchor placement along the posterosuperior glenoid, it may be necessary to make a portal of Wilmington.[218] The skin incision for this portal is approximately 1 cm anterior and 1 cm lateral to the posterolateral corner of the acromion.

If the subacromial space needs to be accessed, typically because of the presence of rotator cuff pathology, the primary posterior portal can be used to enter and visualize this space. Alternatively, a lateral portal is made approximately 2 to 3 cm distal to the lateral edge of the acromion, along the anterior aspect of the bone.

TREATMENT OPTIONS FOR GLENOHUMERAL INSTABILITY

Anterior Instability

As discussed above, anterior instability is the most common direction of glenohumeral instability, occurring most commonly from a traumatic injury in males less than 30 years of age. First-time dislocation events can typically be managed nonoperatively, with closed reduction followed by shoulder rehabilitation. The decision to proceed with surgical intervention usually arises from the development of recurrent instability.

Because of the high risk of recurrence, the ideal treatment for young and active patients with an acute shoulder dislocation is debated. Some authors have recommended immediate surgical stabilization of the shoulder in specific high-risk patient groups,[160,300,362] although others have found that surgical stabilization is necessary in only a minority of patients and recommend against immediate surgery.[312] Ultimately, the decision to proceed with nonoperative versus operative management should be made on a case-by-case basis, based on the patient's age, activity level, presenting history, and type and severity of pathology.

Nonoperative and Closed Treatment

Indications/Contraindications

Acute Anterior Dislocations. An acute anterior dislocation of the glenohumeral joint can be treated with closed reduction in almost all cases and should proceed as soon as possible. Ideally, closed reduction should be performed within the first several hours after the dislocation event, as the shoulder can become more difficult to reduce closed the longer it has been out. Shoulder dislocations that are greater than a day old may still be possible to close reduce, but the likelihood of success decreases and the risk of complications, such as fracture, increases. A dislocation that is more than a week old may have developed soft tissue contractures that no longer make close reduction possible.

Chronic Anterior Dislocations. If a patient has a chronic anterior dislocation (>3 to 6 weeks), closed reduction may no longer be possible and may be contraindicated because of the risk of fracture or neurovascular injury. In these situations, nonoperative management may be an appropriate choice. Chronic dislocations are seen most commonly in elderly patients or those whose comorbidities, especially dementia, may make them unaware that they have sustained a significant injury.

These patients are often low demand, and may have reasonably good function and minimal pain in the affected shoulder. With a functional contralateral arm and limited demand, nonoperative management may be the best treatment option for these elderly patients and severe comorbidities or dementia.

Recurrent Anterior Instability. Nonoperative management for recurrent anterior instability may be considered in patients too medically ill to undergo an operation, those patients with no prior treatment, or in patients wishing to avoid surgery. The mainstay of nonoperative treatment has been physical therapy. Therapy is focused on strengthening the dynamic stabilizers of the shoulder; including the rotator cuff, deltoid, pectoralis major, and scapular stabilizing muscles; to provide stability for the compromised glenohumeral joint. However, there is no data we are aware of that supports the theoretical benefit of therapy (Table 40-3).

TABLE 40-3   Anterior Instability

Nonoperative Treatment

Indications	Relative Contraindications
First-time acute dislocation	Irreducible first-time acute dislocation
Recurrent instability without prior treatment	Recurrent instability failing nonoperative management
Recurrent atraumatic instability	Open injuries
Chronic dislocation with good function and no pain	Chronic dislocation with poor function and pain
Patient medically unstable for surgery	
Unstable epilepsy	

Closed Reduction

Preoperative Planning. Obtaining adequate muscle relaxation is essential to successfully reducing a shoulder dislocation in a closed fashion, regardless of the technique utilized. Some level of anesthesia is usually required to achieve muscle relaxation and pain control prior to reduction. However, some acute dislocations can be reduced without the use of medication if performed immediately after the injury before muscle spasm has developed. Intravenous analgesic and sedation agents are usually used, but require careful patient monitoring because of the possibility of respiratory depression from excessive sedation. Appropriate backup for airway protection should be available. This is usually possible in the emergency room setting, but if adequate respiratory support is not available, the reduction should be performed in the operating room with formal anesthesia. The used of formal anesthesia in the operating room may also be necessary if adequate muscle relaxation cannot be obtained without deeper levels of sedation. The surgeon should also be prepared for open reduction if closed reduction fails in the operating room, although this is very rare.

Three randomized trials, along with other lower level studies, have compared the use of intravenous agents for analgesia and muscle relaxation to a intra-articular injection of lidocaine into the glenohumeral joint. Collectively, these studies have shown high rates of success with intra-articular lidocaine with fewer adverse events, a shorter hospital stay, and adequate pain relief[53,66,209,222,251] (Table 40-4).

TABLE 40-4   Closed Reduction of an Anterior Dislocation

Preoperative Planning

- Adequate sedation and muscle relaxation
- Appropriate airway protection available
- Radiolucent table or bed
- Patient positioning in the room to allow for fluoroscopy
- Orthosis for arm immobilization should be available postreduction

Positioning. Patient positioning is dependent on the particular closed reduction technique, as described below. The patient can be placed supine, either completely flat or in a beach-chair position, or prone. The use of a radiolucent table can be helpful to allow for easier use and positioning of fluoroscopy. Fluoroscopy should be positioned to obtain both AP and axillary views. This can be achieved by bringing the machine in from the opposite side of the bed or from the same side from a cephalad position.

Techniques. A simple traction–countertraction closed reduction technique, as described originally by Hippocrates, is used very commonly (Fig. 40-40).[128,185] In the original method, reduction is performed by a single person, who provides countertraction by placing a foot against the chest wall, just inferior to the axilla, while pulling gentle traction on the arm. In most instances, assistance is available to allow this technique to be performed in a more elegant manner. The patient lies supine and countertraction is provided by a sheet wrapped around the waist of an assistant and around the upper thorax of the patient (Fig. 40-40). The surgeon can then stand on the side of the dislocated shoulder with a second sheet wrapped around his or her waist and around the forearm of the patient with the elbow flexed to 90 degrees. Against the assistant's countertraction, slow and steady traction is applied to the patient's arm with the second sheet to distract the humeral head away from the glenoid and disengage it from the glenoid rim. The surgeon can pull traction without the use of a sheet, but the sheet keeps the surgeon's hands free to internally rotate, externally rotate, abduct, or adduct the patient's arm, or provide direct pressure on the humeral head as needed to assist with "unlocking" the dislocation.

The Stimson technique also utilizes slow, steady traction on the arm to achieve reduction.[335] The patient is placed prone with the affected arm hanging free over a table, allowing the table to provide a stable base against which a gentle downward traction is placed on the arm (Fig. 40-41). Traction can be applied manually or by attaching weights to the wrist. Usually 5 lb is sufficient for most patients, but more may be needed depending on patient size. Slow, steady traction provided by the attached weights results in fatigue and relaxation of the shoulder musculature that disengages the humeral head and

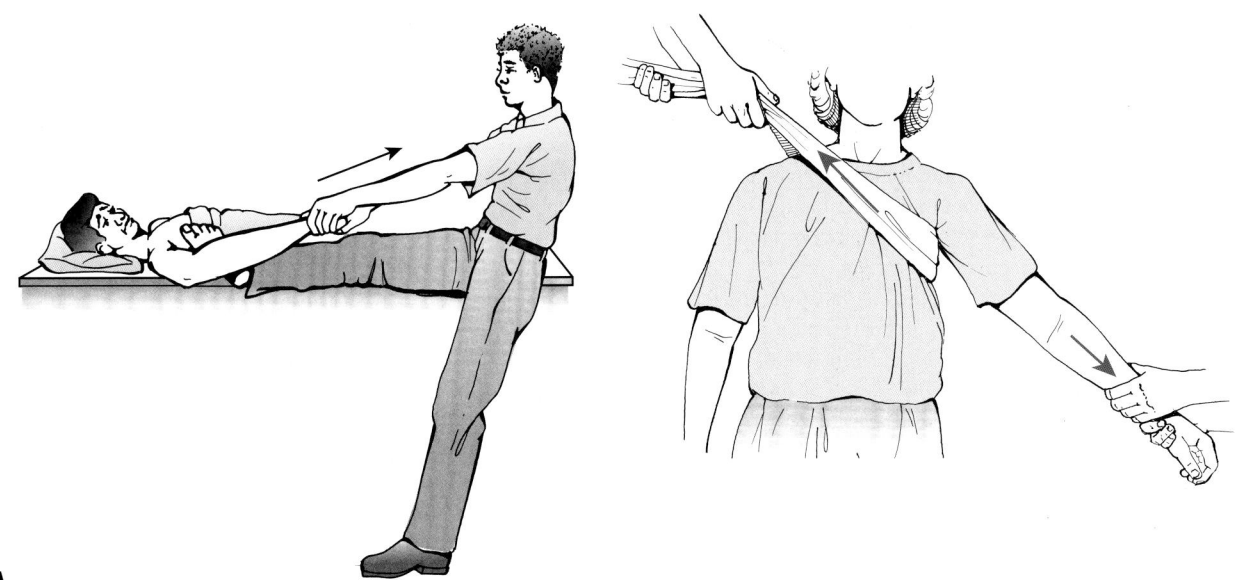

A   **B**

FIGURE 40-40 Closed shoulder reduction using traction–countertraction. The original Hippocratic method **(A)** uses gentle traction on the arm against countertraction provided by placing the foot on the chest wall. Care must be taken to avoid placing the foot in the axilla, as it can cause damage to neurovascular structures. With the help of an assistant, this technique can be performed using a sheet wrapped around the upper thorax to provide countertraction **(B).**

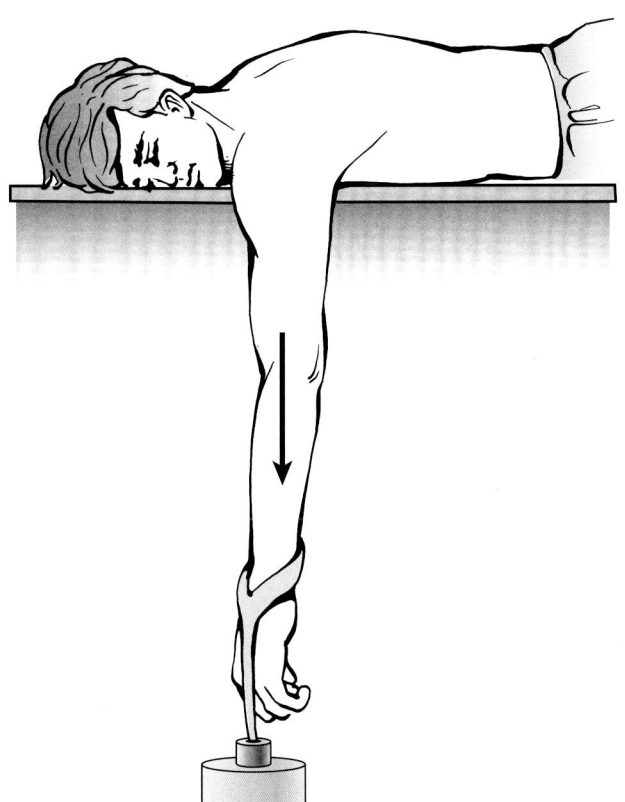

FIGURE 40-41 The Stimson technique for closed shoulder reduction. With the patient lying prone, weight is hung from the wrist to provide traction to the shoulder joint. This steady traction leads to fatigue and relaxation in the shoulder musculature, resulting in joint reduction.

reduces the shoulder after traction is released. This method usually takes up to 15 to 20 minutes to produce its effect; however, the patient should be monitored closely to avoid a prolonged period of time in this position that could result in traction injury to a nerve.

The Milch technique can also be utilized to close reduce an anterior dislocation, but relies on shoulder position more so than traction.[220] The maneuver can be performed with the patient in either a supine or prone position. The arm is slowly abducted while stabilizing the humeral head with the opposite hand. The shoulder is then slowly externally rotated, causing the humeral head to spontaneously reduce when the shoulder has reached approximately 90 degrees of abduction and 90 degrees of external rotation. The opposite hand that is stabilizing the humeral head can also be used to provide posterior pressure to help guide the humeral head back into the joint. This method has been reported to have a high rate of success with minimal complications and can be performed without premedication.[85,247]

A recent trial compared the success of the Milch versus the Stimson techniques for reduction in nonsedated patients. The authors found significantly better success rates and time to reduction for the Milch technique. Importantly, earlier reductions and low levels of pain at presentation were predictive of greater success.[4]

Postoperative Management. Once closed reduction is complete, anatomic reduction of the glenohumeral joint must be confirmed with fluoroscopy or plain radiographs. Grashey and axillary views should be obtained and will also demonstrate any associated fractures. Postreduction documentation of the neurovascular status of the arm should also be performed and compared to the pre-reduction examination for any changes.

The arm is immobilized for a period of time following closed reduction to avoid recurrent instability. There has been conflicting information on the length, type, and position of immobilization required for the shoulder. Earlier studies have reported decreased rates of recurrent instability in patients whose shoulders were immobilized for greater than 3 weeks.[164,179,336] In contrast, several more recent studies have not reported an association between the duration of immobilization and the development of recurrent instability.[132,133,262] A recent systematic review of Level I and II studies evaluating the length of immobilization time following a primary anterior shoulder dislocation found no significant difference in rate of recurrent instability in patients younger than 30 years of age immobilized for 1 week or less (41%) versus 3 weeks or longer (37%).[262]

The position of immobilization has received significant attention recently. In an initial MRI study, Itoi et al. demonstrated that the position of the anterior labrum after closed reduction of a traumatic anterior shoulder dislocation was more anatomic when the arm was positioned in slight external rotation.[153] In a subsequent randomized controlled trial, the authors demonstrated a significantly lower rate of recurrent instability at minimum 2-year follow-up (26% vs. 42%) for first time traumatic anterior dislocations immobilized in external rotation for 3 weeks compared to those immobilized in internal rotation.[146] However, other authors have not shown an advantage for immobilization in external rotation. Liavaag et al. performed a randomized controlled trial comparing immobilization for 3 weeks in external versus internal rotation in patients with first time traumatic anterior dislocations.[197] At minimum 2-year follow-up, there was no significant difference in the rate of recurrent instability between groups (30.8% for external rotation vs. 24.7% for internal rotation). It appears that immobilization in external rotation does not clearly show a benefit over a traditional sling.

To restore function as promptly as possible, a brief period of immobilization should be followed by mobilization and rehabilitation. Shoulder rehabilitation is focused both on regaining range of motion and strengthening of the shoulder. The dynamic stabilizers of the shoulder; including the rotator cuff, deltoid, pectoralis major, and scapular stabilizing muscles are strengthened to provide stability for the compromised glenohumeral joint.[46,100,185]

Pitfalls and Solutions (Table 40-5)

Outcomes. The most common complication after a successful closed reduction is the development of recurrent instability. As noted above, risk factors have been identified for the development of recurrent instability, such as age, gender, activity level, compliance, and associated injuries (rotator cuff tears, fractures, bone defects, etc.), with the risk of recurrent anterior instability highest among highly active, young male patients.

Operative Treatment of Anterior Instability

Indications/Contraindications

Acute Anterior Dislocatons. The indications for surgical intervention for an acute anterior dislocation include an irreducible or unstable injury, dislocations associated with a displaced proximal humerus fracture, and open injuries. Irreducible or unstable injuries may be caused by a bony cause (proximal humerus fracture, glenoid fracture, large Hill–Sachs defect), a large rotator cuff tear, or soft tissue interposition in the glenohumeral joint by torn rotator cuff tissue or the long head of the biceps tendon.[40,57,112,144,341]

Chronic Anterior Dislocations. As discussed above, nonoperative management may be indicated with certain chronic dislocations in elderly patients if they are demented, too sick for surgery, or if the shoulder has good function and no pain. Otherwise, if the patient is stable for surgery and poor function and pain are present, surgery is indicated. The choice of procedure, as discussed below, depends on the bone and soft tissue injuries that are present. If large Hill–Sachs and/or glenoid bone defects are present because of a long-standing dislocation, these may require reconstruction with bone grafts or treatment with shoulder arthroplasty.[98]

Recurrent Anterior Instability. Surgical treatment of recurrent anterior instability is indicated when nonoperative management has failed. Stabilization of the shoulder may be performed arthroscopically, or through an open anterior approach, with or without bony reconstruction (humeral and/or glenoid), as discussed below. Arthroscopic procedures have the benefit of evaluating the entire glenohumeral joint prior to treatment, which may uncover additional pathology that requires surgical repair, such as posterior or superior labral tears[293] (Table 40-6).

TABLE 40-5 **Closed Reduction of an Anterior Dislocation**

Potential Pitfalls and Solutions

Pitfall	Solutions
Displacement of fracture	ORIF Hemiarthroplasty or reverse total shoulder arthroplasty
Acute instability or irreducibility	Open or arthroscopic procedure discussed below
Recurrent instability	Open or arthroscopic procedure discussed below

---

TABLE 40-6 **Anterior Instability**

Operative Treatment

Indications	Contraindications
Irreducible or unstable first time acute dislocation	Reducible, first time acute dislocation
Recurrent instability failing nonoperative management	Recurrent instability without prior treatment
Open injuries	Patient medically unstable for surgery
Chronic dislocation with poor function and pain	Chronic dislocation with good function and no pain
Dislocation associated with displaced proximal humerus fracture	Unstable epilepsy

Open Reduction of an Anterior Dislocation. If a stable closed reduction is unsuccessful, open reduction with or without additional procedures must be performed. In the acute setting, open reduction may be all that is needed to stabilize the joint; however, other soft tissue surgery may be required, such as capsulolabral repair or rotator cuff repair, if tears are present. Soft tissue interposition in the glenohumeral joint, either from torn rotator cuff tissue or the long head of the biceps tendon, should also be addressed if present with repair or tenodesis, respectively.[40,57,112,144,341]

In the chronic setting, significant bone loss is more likely to be present in the humeral head and/or glenoid and additional surgery may be needed to address the bone defects, as discussed below.[98]

Preoperative Planning (Table 40-7)

TABLE 40-7 **Open Anterior Reduction of an Anterior Dislocation**

Preoperative Planning

- Radiolucent or beach-chair table
- Patient positioning in the room to allow for fluoroscopy
- Standard open shoulder instruments
- Additional equipment, as needed, for potential bony or soft tissue repairs (suture anchors, small fragment set, etc.)
- Orthosis for arm immobilization should be available postreduction

---

Positioning. Our standard setup is the beach-chair position with an articulated arm holder. A supine position may also be used. Fluoroscopy should be positioned to obtain both AP and axillary views as noted above.

Surgical Approach and Technique. A standard deltopectoral approach (Fig. 40-36) is used with the long head of the biceps tendon as a guide to find the lesser tuberosity and the rotator interval. In situations requiring no additional repairs, the biceps tendon can be followed proximally and the rotator interval released to gain access to the glenohumeral joint. A finger can be placed through the interval and into the joint to help manually pull the humeral head laterally with traction to disimpact the head. Sometimes a bone hook can be utilized to help pull lateral traction, but care should be taken to not damage the cartilage of the humeral head. The shoulder can be internally or externally rotated as needed to assist with unlocking the humeral head. Once the humeral head is disimpacted, it can be brought posteriorly with digital pressure to help reduce the shoulder. Stability of the reduction should be tested in abduction and by bringing the arm into external rotation. Positioning of the arm postoperatively, as with closed reductions, is determined by the assessment of intraoperative stability. Most shoulders are stable after reduction; however, if gross instability is present, an open capsular repair should be performed as described below.

If reduction cannot be performed through the rotator interval alone, then the subscapularis tendon should be taken down to completely access the glenohumeral joint as discussed earlier in the chapter. If a significant humeral head defect is present following reduction, humeral head disimpaction may be considered. A disimpaction procedure is an option if the humeral head bone stock is good, the impacted cartilage can be salvaged, the defect is <40%, and the dislocation is less than 3 weeks old.[9,279] Chronic dislocations suffer from disuse osteopenia. The technique involves elevating an impaction fracture to restore humeral head anatomy. A cortical window is created opposite the defect, through which bone tamps can be inserted to disimpact the fracture in a retrograde fashion.[165] It may also be performed percutaneously.[289] Once elevated, the humeral head void is filled with cancellous allograft (our preferred choice), iliac crest, or another bone substitute product.[165,216,289]

Postoperative Management. The postoperative management is the same as with closed reduction. However, if the subscapularis tendon is taken down as part of the surgery, rehabilitation is significantly slower to allow for healing of the tendon with no external rotation beyond neutral for 6 weeks.

Pitfalls and Solutions (Table 40-8)

TABLE 40-8 **Open Anterior Reduction of an Anterior Dislocation**

Potential Pitfalls and Solutions

Pitfalls	Solutions
Displacement of fracture	ORIF Hemiarthroplasty or reverse total shoulder arthroplasty
Irreducible dislocation	Subscapularis takedown for complete glenohumeral joint access
Intraoperative instability	Bony or soft tissue repair as indicated (described below)
Axillary nerve injury	Direct repair Observation

Outcomes. There is limited data on the outcomes of simple open reduction of an anterior dislocation.[112] Often, whether the dislocation is acute or chronic, associated pathology is present that requires surgical intervention in addition to the open reduction.

Humeral head disimpaction in the setting of anterior shoulder instability has only been reported in a handful of cases, including one case of chronic dislocation.[216,289] Re et al. evaluated the results of four patients who underwent humeral head disimpaction as part of an open instability procedure.[289] No complications or recurrent instability was noted at greater than 1-year follow-up. Three patients also underwent open anterior capsulolabral reconstruction and the fourth underwent a Latarjet procedure.

Open Anterior Procedures for Chronic Anterior Dislocations. As discussed above, significant bone loss may be present in the humeral head and/or glenoid that require additional surgery following open reduction in the setting of a chronic dislocation. Soft tissue injuries, including rotator cuff tears and labral tears, may also require repair in this setting to stabilize the joint. Anterior glenoid defects of 25% or more should be addressed with a bone reconstruction procedure (Latarjet procedure, iliac crest bone graft, allograft bone graft), whereas Hill–Sachs defects involving 25% or more of the humeral head may be addressed with allograft reconstruction or partial resurfacing.[9,224,276,279] Shoulder arthroplasty may be necessary for even larger defects, especially in older patients with Hill–Sachs defects involving 40% to 45% or more of the humeral head an indication for complete humeral head replacement.[9,80,274,279]

Preoperative Planning (Table 40-9)

TABLE 40-9 Open Anterior Procedures for Chronic Anterior Dislocations

Preoperative Planning

- Beach-chair table with pneumatic arm holder
- Fluoroscopy may be needed to check direction and length of screws or confirm joint reduction
- Standard open shoulder instruments
- Additional equipment, as needed, for potential bony or soft tissue procedures, or shoulder arthroplasty (suture anchors, small fragment set, etc.)
  - Fresh frozen allograft for glenoid defect
  - Size-matched fresh frozen allograft for humeral head defect
  - Screws for fixation of glenoid and/or humeral head graft
  - Arthroplasty equipment (partial resurfacing, standard and/or reverse replacement sets)
- Suture anchors for rotator cuff or labral repair
- Orthosis for arm immobilization should be placed after surgery

---

Positioning. The beach-chair position is used as described above.

Surgical Approach. A standard deltopectoral approach is used for these procedures.

Technique. The techniques for reconstruction of the anterior capsulolabral structures, or for reconstruction of bony defects of the glenoid and humeral head are the same as those utilized in the management of recurrent anterior instability and are described in the sections below. Most commonly, a subscapularis tenotomy is performed to access the glenohumeral joint for these procedures. In contrast to a reduced joint, however, significant adhesions and soft tissue contractures may be present in the setting of a chronic, unreduced dislocation. The soft tissue plane between the conjoined tendon and the subscapularis tendon, for example, may be scarred together because of the anteriorly dislocated humeral head. Careful dissection is necessary in developing this plane to avoid neurovascular injury. When the glenohumeral joint is exposed, the chronic dislocation must first be unlocked and mobilized to allow for joint reduction and the necessary soft tissue or bony reconstructions. This may require extensive capsular releases around the joint, particularly posteriorly, where the capsule may be significantly contracted in a chronic anterior dislocation. In addition, the long head of the biceps tendon is often pathologic or limits visualization of the joint and therefore we typically excise the intra-articular portion and tenodese the remainder to the pectoralis major tendon with nonabsorbable suture.

Arthroplasty. As noted above, shoulder arthroplasty may be necessary for larger humeral head defects, or if advanced degenerative changes are present.[9,80,274,279] Hemiarthroplasty is usually performed in younger patients below the age of 50 and patients with good glenoid cartilage. Total shoulder arthroplasty is indicated in older patients with significant glenoid degenerative changes. In the elderly patient, reverse total shoulder arthroplasty may be necessary if the rotator cuff is deficient, or if there is concern for persistent instability with a standard shoulder replacement.

Key technical considerations in arthroplasty include management of the subscapularis and version of the humeral component. Both subscapularis peel and lesser tuberosity osteotomy are acceptable options; however, a robust repair is critical to prevent further instability. The prosthesis version should match the patients' anatomical version which varies dramatically with an average of 19 degrees of retroversion.[296] Attention should be paid to not overly anteroverting the component, which is the natural tendency because of, sometimes, inadequate exposure.

Postoperative Management. For bone reconstruction and arthroplasty procedures, the patient's shoulder is protected in an orthosis for 6 weeks with no active shoulder use during this time. At 6 weeks, active shoulder use is allowed and range of motion stretching is begun. Strengthening is started 3 months after surgery.

Pitfalls and Solutions (Table 40-10)

TABLE 40-10 Open Anterior Procedures for Chronic Anterior Dislocations

Potential Pitfalls and Solutions

Pitfalls	Solutions
Axillary nerve injury	Direct repair Observation
Osteopenic head or significant degenerative changes	Consider arthroplasty
Pull-out of transosseous sutures during subscapularis repair	Drill through the bicipital groove
Fracture of lesser tuberosity osteotomy	Use small screw (2.0 or 2.7 mm) Consider anchors or transosseous suture

---

Outcomes. There is limited data on the outcomes of surgical treatment of chronic anterior shoulder dislocations. Rouhani and Navali reported on eight cases of open reduction with anterior capsulolabral repair for chronic anterior dislocation.[305] Mean follow-up was 1 year, with one fair, three good, and four excellent results, and a mean Rowe and Zarin's score of 86. Two patients had persistent anterior subluxation of the humeral head. Goga reviewed a series of 10 patients that underwent coracoid transfer to the anterior glenoid and temporary acromiohumeral K-wire fixation (4 weeks) for treatment of a chronic anterior dislocation.[101] Minimum follow-up was 2 years, with two fair, five good, and three excellent results, and no recurrent dislocations. Pin site infections occurred in 8/10 patients, but resolved with pin removal. Finally, Flatow et al.[80] reviewed a series of 10 patients who underwent surgery for a chronic anterior dislocation. One patient underwent coracoid transfer for an anterior glenoid defect, but had persistent anterior subluxation and underwent a revision soft tissue reconstruction to stabilize the shoulder. The other nine patients underwent shoulder arthroplasty (one hemiarthroplasty, eight total shoulder arthroplasties). Humeral component retroversion was increased as needed for stability, and three cases required anterior glenoid bone grafting to support the glenoid component. The hemiarthroplasty was lost to follow-up, whereas mean follow-up was 3.9 years in the other cases. There were four satisfactory and four excellent results, and no recurrent dislocations.

Open Soft Tissue Procedures for Recurrent Anterior Instability.

Open anterior shoulder stabilization consisting of a capsulolabral (Bankart) repair has traditionally been considered the "gold standard" for surgical treatment of recurrent anterior instability, with many studies reporting good-to-excellent outcomes in the vast majority of patients.[20,75,137,157,159,196,229,258,273,295,291,364] However, with the increased use of arthroscopic techniques and the continual development of arthroscopic instrumentation and suture anchors, outcomes of arthroscopic capsulolabral (Bankart) repair have been reported to be equivalent to the open procedure in selected patients.[7,38,75,163,173,203,265,283,332,342350] Therefore, provided that the surgery is performed with adequate expertise, the choice between open and arthroscopic capsulolabral repair does not appear to significantly affect the overall outcome.

Situations where an open technique may be preferred include revision surgery or other cases where anatomy is altered or deformity is present.[223] Repair of a humeral avulsion of glenohumeral ligaments (HAGL lesion) may also require open repair.[42,93,367] Importantly, patient selection for open versus arthroscopic repair is critical to outcomes. Balg et al. has created an instability severity index score which reliably identifies patients who have a high risk of recurrent instability after arthroscopic management. The risk factors include: Patients under the age of 20 (2 points); involvement in contact sports or those with forced overhead activity (1 point); shoulder hyperlaxity (1 point); a Hill–Sachs lesion present on the AP radiograph in external rotation (2 points); and loss of the sclerotic inferior glenoid contour (2 points).[14] A score of 6 points or less predicted a recurrence risk after arthroscopic repair of 10%. Patients with more than 6 points had a recurrence risk of 70%.

Preoperative Planning (Table 40-11)

TABLE 40-11 **Open Anterior Soft Tissue Repair**

Preoperative Planning

- Beach-chair table with pneumatic arm holder
- Fluoroscopy is not needed
- Standard open shoulder instruments
- Suture anchors for labral or capsular repair, as needed
- Orthosis for arm immobilization should be placed after surgery

---

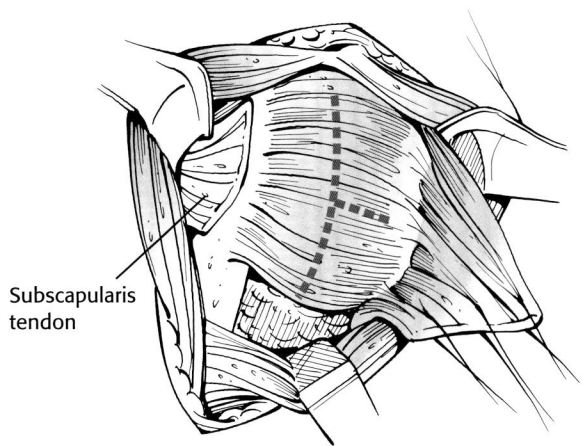

FIGURE 40-42 "T"-shaped capsulotomy with superior and inferior flaps for glenohumeral joint exposure. The vertical incision can be placed laterally near the humeral neck or medially along the glenoid rim.

Positioning. The beach-chair position is used as described above.

Surgical Approach. A standard deltopectoral approach is used for the procedure.

Technique

Open Anterior Capsulolabral (Bankart) Repair. Capsulolabral repair can be performed with a subscapularis tenotomy or through a subscapularis split, as described above. The capsule is then exposed and must be incised to access the glenohumeral joint and torn labrum. This can be performed in several ways depending on surgeon preference. A single transverse incision can be made in line with the subscapularis division, or a vertical incision can be combined with the transverse incision to create a "T"-shaped capsulotomy with superior and inferior flaps (Fig. 40-42). The vertical incision can be placed laterally near the humeral neck or medially along the glenoid rim. Tag sutures should be placed through the split superior and inferior capsule with either technique.

A humeral head retractor, such as a Fukuda retractor, is placed between the humeral head and posterior rim of the glenoid to displace the humeral head posteriorly. One or two single-prong or multi-prong glenoid retractors are placed along the anterior glenoid neck to allow for adequate medial exposure. The detached labrum is then elevated from the glenoid neck if required, to mobilize the tissue. The torn labrum is typically healed in an inferomedial position and must be adequately freed up to restore the tissue to its original anatomic location. The glenoid neck and rim are next abraded with a rasp or high-speed burr to healthy, bleeding bone to establish a healing bed for the labral repair.

Labral repair is then performed with suture anchors, or bone tunnels. Three or four suture anchors are typically needed to span the 3 o'clock-to-6 o'clock (or 9 to 6 on a left shoulder) position along the anteroinferior glenoid (Fig. 40-43). Specifically, the anchors should be placed on the face on the glenoid and not too anterior. Heavy, #2 nonabsorbable sutures are passed through the torn labrum and capsuloligamentous tissue

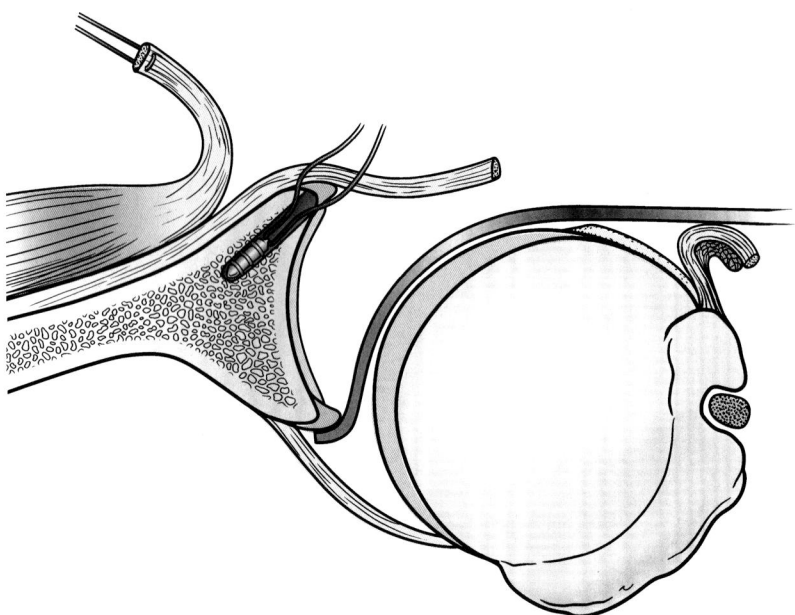

FIGURE 40-43 Drill hole for suture anchor placement in open Bankart repair. Holes should be placed right at the anterior glenoid articular margin.

for labral repair and capsulorrhaphy. If a small, avulsion-type glenoid rim fragment is also present, such as in a bony Bankart injury, this can also be incorporated with the torn soft tissue into the repair. The suture is typically passed through the tissue inferior to the anchor, or around it if a bony tunnel is used, both to re-establish the torn labrum along its anatomic location and to perform the desired capsulorrhaphy. The degree of capsular laxity noted intraoperatively dictates the amount of capsular shift that is performed. The capsule should not be overtightened to avoid stiffness of the glenohumeral joint, which can lead to increased joint contact forces and restriction of motion.[351] The sutures should be tied off of the joint surface, along the capsule, to prevent the knots from lying within the joint and causing mechanical symptoms. The arm is usually positioned in approximately 30 degrees of abduction and external rotation to avoid overtightening the repair.

The sutures are not cut after being tied, so that the limbs can be used to imbricate the superior flap of the split capsule to the repair site. The superior flap is shifted inferiorly to overlap with the inferior flap that was already shifted superiorly and tied down as a part of the Bankart repair (Fig. 40-44). The amount that the superior flap is shifted and the location the sutures are passed through and tied down on this flap are dictated by the degree of capsular laxity that is present.

After capsulolabral repair is complete, the subscapularis is closed. If a tenotomy is performed, the tendon can be repaired back to the lateral stump with interrupted, heavy, #2 nonabsorbable sutures. A subscapularis split can be closed with interrupted #0 or #1 absorbable sutures.

Open Repair of HAGL Lesion. If a HAGL lesion is noted at the time of open labral repair, this must also be addressed. The lesion is typically found in the inferior pouch of the shoulder, between the 6 o'clock and 8 o'clock position on the humeral neck.[8,36,93] The injury may be exposed using a subscapularis tenotomy or a mini-open technique in which some or all of

the subscapularis tendon is preserved.[8,24,93] After preparing a healthy, bleeding bone bed, the avulsed glenohumeral ligament is repaired back to its attachment site with suture anchors or drill holes through bone.

Postoperative Management. The patient's shoulder is protected in an abduction splint for 6 weeks with no active shoulder use during this time. Passive range-of-motion exercises,

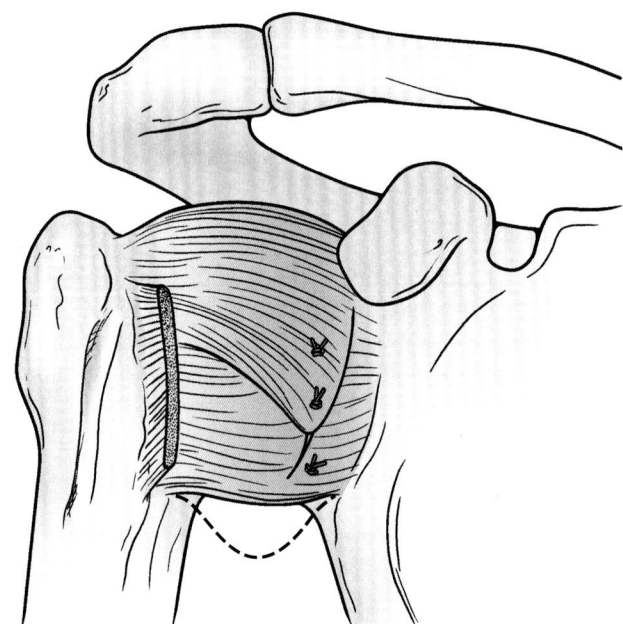

FIGURE 40-44 Capsular closure with open Bankart repair. The superior flap is shifted inferiorly to overlap with the inferior flap that was already shifted superiorly and tied down as a part of the Bankart repair. The amount that the superior flap is shifted and the location the sutures are passed through and tied down on this flap are dictated by the degree of capsular laxity that is present.

including forward flexion and external rotation stretching, can be started within the first 6 weeks of surgery based on surgeon preference. At 6 weeks, active shoulder use is allowed and range of motion stretching is advanced to active exercises in all planes. Strengthening is started 3 months after surgery, with a return to contact activities at 5 to 6 months postoperatively.

Pitfalls and Solutions (Table 40-12)

TABLE 40-12 Open Anterior Soft Tissue Repair

Potential Pitfalls and Solutions

Pitfalls	Solutions
Axillary nerve injury	Avoid being too inferior in the surgical approach Avoid excessive humeral head distraction
Inadequate shift of associated capsular laxity	Intraoperative assessment of shoulder range-of-motion after repair
Excessive capsular shift	Appropriate arm position during repair (approximately 30 degrees of abduction and external rotation) Intraoperative assessment of shoulder range-of-motion after repair
Unrecognized HAGL lesion	HAGL repair, open or arthroscopic
Unrecognized anterior glenoid bone loss	Open bony procedure (Bristow–Latarjet, auto- or allograft)
Fixation failure	Minimum of three suture anchors for anteroinferior repair or tunnels through bony Firm placement of suture anchors in subchondral bone, seated below articular margin
Improper anchor placement	Placement of anchors on the face of the glenoid and not too anterior Placement of anchors between 3 and 6 o'clock (right). Avoid superior anchors

Outcomes

Open Anterior Capsulolabral (Bankart) Repair. Using the suture anchor method, good-to-excellent results have been reported in 88% to 94% of patients, with recurrent dislocation rates of 0% to 9.7% at short- to midterm follow-up.[20,75,159,196,273,295] Even in athletes with high functional demands, the open Bankart procedure has been associated with good-to-excellent results in 92% to 97% of patients, with recurrent instability rates of 0% to 4%, and return to preinjury level of competition in 68% to 89% of patients.[157,229,258]

In a long-term follow-up study, Pelet et al. evaluated 30 patients at a mean of 29 years after open Bankart repair using a bone tunnel technique.[264] Recurrent dislocation occurred in three patients (10%), with one undergoing a revision open stabilization. Radiographic evidence of glenohumeral arthritis was present in 40% of patients, with five patients (16.6%) undergoing total shoulder arthroplasty at a mean of 26.6 years after

Bankart repair because of symptomatic arthritis. Of the remaining patients, there was 1 poor, 4 fair, and 20 good results. Mean loss of shoulder external rotation was 24 degrees, and mean loss of internal rotation was 19 degrees. Outcome scores (Constant, Rowe modified, ASES) in the operative shoulder were significantly lower than the contralateral side. All patients said they would recommend the surgery.[264]

Open Repair of HAGL Lesions. Data on open repair of HAGL lesions has been limited to small studies or case reports.[8,24,36] Arciero and Mazzocca reported no cases of recurrent instability in eight patients who underwent mini-open repair, whereas Bhatia et al. also reported no episodes of recurrent instability with a mini-open technique.[8,24]

Arthroscopic Soft Tissue Procedures for Recurrent Anterior Instability.
Recent data has demonstrated that, for most patients, there are equivalent outcomes between arthroscopic and open capsulolabral (Bankart) repair.[7,38,75,163,173,203,265,283,332,342,350,375] Reported complication rates may also be lower with the arthroscopic technique.[255] These findings, in combination with the increased use and development of arthroscopic methods, have led to a national trend toward arthroscopic shoulder stabilization, with the use of open capsulolabral repair declining.[255] Importantly, a certain group of high-risk patients may not benefit from arthroscopic repair and require an open procedure. Balg and Boileau[14] identified these risk factors in their instability severity score (discussed above).

Arthroscopic treatment of other instability-related lesions may also be performed with or without Bankart repair, if indicated. HAGL lesion may be amenable to arthroscopic suture anchor repair,[42,93,367] and arthroscopic remplissage can also be considered. Remplissage is the term used to describe arthroscopic posterior capsulodesis and infraspinatus tenodesis, in which the posterior capsule and infraspinatus are anchored into the surface of a Hill–Sachs defect to prevent engagement of the lesion.[65,182,279,284] Although the indication for the procedure is still evolving, it is often performed in the presence of a moderate to large Hill–Sachs defect associated with anterior glenoid bone loss that is not large enough for an open bony procedure (<25%).[9,279]

Preoperative Planning (Table 40-13)

TABLE 40-13 Arthroscopic Soft Tissue Repair

Preoperative Planning

- Beach-chair table with pneumatic arm holder, or lateral decubitus position with arm traction
- Fluoroscopy is not needed
- Standard arthroscopic shoulder instruments; 5 and 8 mm cannulas
- Suture anchors for labral or capsular repair
- Orthosis for arm immobilization should be placed after surgery

Positioning. The beach-chair or lateral decubitus position is used as described above.

Surgical Approach. The standard arthroscopic technique describe above is utilized.

Technique

Arthroscopic Anterior Capsulolabral (Bankart) Repairs.
After initial evaluation of the glenohumeral joint through the posterior portal to define the tear, an anterior portal is established just above the upper border of the subscapularis tendon. This portal is utilized for instrumentation and anchor placement during labral repair, and should be made low enough to provide complete access to the anteroinferior labrum. We prefer to visualize from an anterior position during the procedure; therefore, an accessory superolateral portal is next established through the rotator interval and the arthroscope is placed in this portal with the use of switching sticks.

Arthroscopic labral repair utilizes the same steps as the open technique. The detached labrum is first elevated from the glenoid neck to mobilize the tissue. This can be performed with an arthroscopic tissue elevator and shaver, passed through the anterior portal. The glenoid neck and rim are next abraded with an arthroscopic rasp or burr to healthy, bleeding bone to establish a healing bed for the labral repair. Suture anchors are then sequentially placed through the anterior portal along the anterior glenoid articular margin. As with the open technique, three or four anchors are needed to span the 3 o'clock-to-6 o'clock position along the anteroinferior glenoid (Fig. 40-45). Typically, the most inferior anchor is placed first at the 6 o'clock position and the suture from this anchor is passed and tied down. The same steps are then repeated with the other anchors as they are placed, moving superiorly up the anterior glenoid rim. Suture passage is performed with a shuttle-relay device passed through the anterior portal. The torn labrum and capsule are captured with this device, and the posterior portal can be used to grab the wire or suture from the device to shuttle the suture from the anchor back through the captured tissue. As with the open technique, care is taken to pass the suture through tissue inferior to the anchor site, both to re-establish the torn labrum along its anatomic location and to perform the desired capsulorrhaphy. If a small glenoid rim fragment is also present, such as in a bony Bankart injury, this can also be incorporated with the torn soft tissue into the repair. The degree of capsular laxity noted intraoperatively dictates the amount of capsular shift that is performed, but typically less capsular tissue is shifted as the suture anchors are placed more superiorly. The sutures should again be tied off of the joint surface, along the capsule, to prevent the knots from lying within the joint and causing mechanical symptoms.

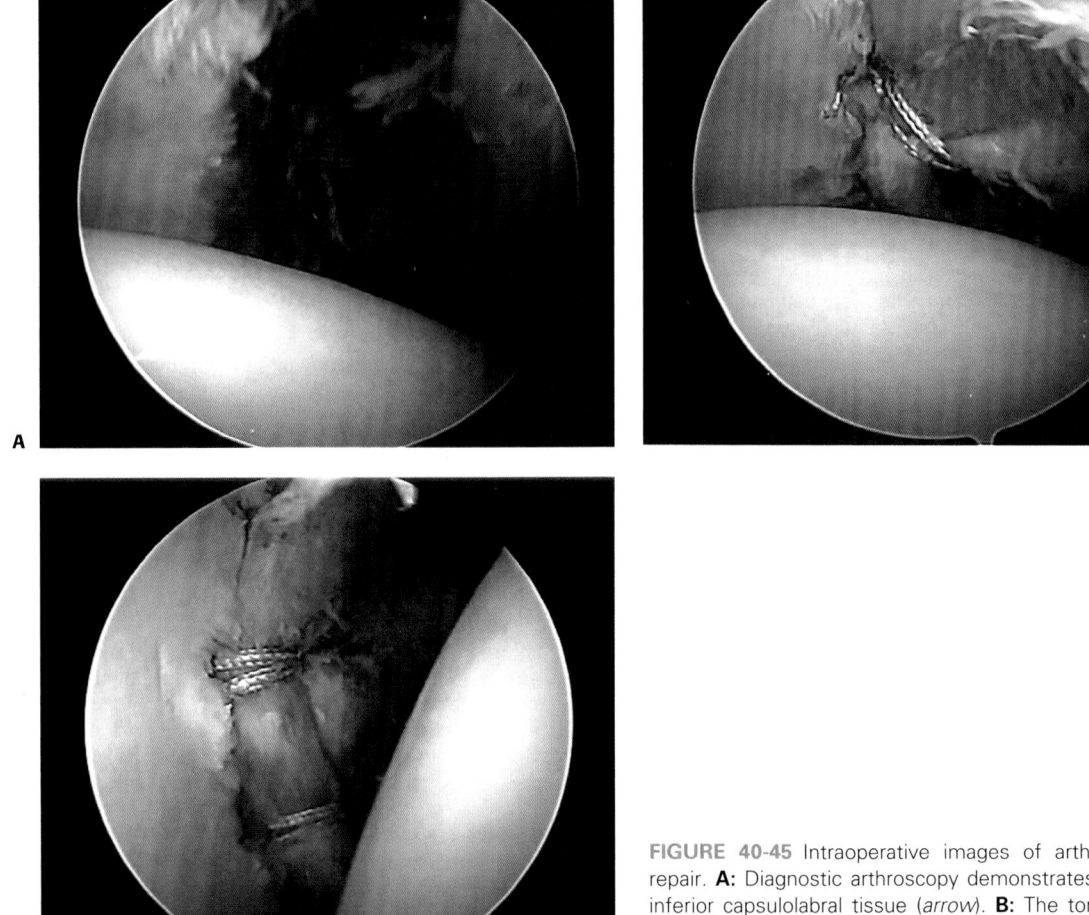

FIGURE 40-45 Intraoperative images of arthroscopic Bankart repair. **A:** Diagnostic arthroscopy demonstrates the torn antero-inferior capsulolabral tissue (*arrow*). **B:** The torn labrum is reattached to the glenoid rim using suture anchors, with the initial anchors placed inferiorly. **C:** Completed Bankart repair.

Newer, knotless anchors are now also being used in arthroscopic labral repair. With these anchors, a free heavy, nonabsorbable suture is typically first passed through the torn capsule and labrum using standard techniques and then incorporated into the knotless anchor while the anchor is being placed.

Arthroscopic Repair of HAGL Lesions. If a HAGL lesion is noted at the time of arthroscopy, it may also be possible to address with arthroscopic suture anchor repair. Accessory portals, such as an anteroinferior or posteroinferior portal, may be necessary to obtain the proper angle of anchor insertion.[23] Suture passage through the avulsed glenohumeral ligament is also performed using a shuttle-relay device. In general, however, an open repair is recommended if a HAGL lesion is diagnosed preoperatively.

Remplissage. Remplissage is typically performed with the arthroscope in one of the anterior portals. As with the other arthroscopic repairs, suture anchors are utilized for the technique. One or two anchors are placed through a posterior portal, either with a cannula or percutaneously, into the Hill–Sachs lesion. This portal should be placed to obtain the proper angle of anchor insertion. Suture passage through the posterior capsule and infraspinatus tendon is also performed using a shuttle-relay device. Sutures are passed in a horizontal mattress fashion and then visualized and tied down in the subacromial/subdeltoid space, creating the posterior capsulodesis and infraspinatus tenodesis and filling the Hill–Sachs defect.

Postoperative Management. The protocol is the same as that for an open capsulolabral repair.

Pitfalls and Solutions. These pitfalls are the same as with an open repair, with the notable exceptions below (Table 40-14).

TABLE 40-14 Arthroscopic Soft Tissue Repair

Potential Pitfalls and Solutions

Pitfalls	Solutions
Nerve injury	Avoid excessive humeral head distraction if using arm traction
Chondrolysis	Avoid thermal capsulorrhaphy and intra-articular pain pumps

Outcomes

Arthroscopic Anterior Capsulolabral (Bankart) Repairs. Good-to-excellent results have been reported in the vast majority of patients undergoing arthroscopic Bankart repair, including high-demand patients, such as collegiate and professional overhead athletes.[7,38,48,75,173,163,203,265,283,332,342,350,375] At relatively short-term follow-up, rates of recurrent instability have been reported from 0% to 10% in most patients, and 12.5% to 16.5% for high-demand athletes.[48,75,173,210,342] At midterm follow-up of 2 to 6 years, recurrent instability rates have been reported as 4% to 7%.[171,189,300] Risk factors for recurrent instability following arthroscopic anterior capsulolabral repair include glenoid and/or humeral bone loss, inferior laxity, or MDI instability, use of three or less suture anchors for repair, and the presence of an anterior labroligamentous periosteal sleeve avulsion (ALPSA lesion).[35,288] In addition, the instability severity scale (discussed above) was developed by Balg and Boileau[14] to help predict patients with higher risks of recurrence after arthroscopic repairs.

As discussed above, recent data has demonstrated equivalent outcomes between arthroscopic and open capsulolabral (Bankart) repair, including several randomized controlled trials.[7,38,75,163,173,203,265,283,332,342,350,375] Petrera et al. performed a meta-analysis to compare the results of open versus arthroscopic Bankart repair for recurrent traumatic anterior instability.[265] Only studies directly comparing the two techniques and using suture anchors for repair in both methods were included. Six studies met inclusion criteria (two Level I, four Level III), with 267 patients in the open group (mean follow-up 29.9 months) and 234 in the arthroscopic group (mean follow-up 30.2 months). The rates of recurrent instability (6.7% open vs. 6.0% arthroscopic) and reoperation (6.6% open vs. 4.7% arthroscopic) were not significantly different. Interestingly, recurrent instability (2.9% vs. 9.2%) and reoperation (2.2% vs. 9.2%) were both significantly lower in the arthroscopic group if only studies later than 2002 were included. Functional scores could not be compared because of the different outcome measures used across studies. Importantly, all six studies had strict inclusion criteria and this data cannot be extrapolated to more high risk patients such as patients with significant humeral bone loss, for example.

In a long-term follow-up study, Zaffagnini et al. compared the results of open versus arthroscopic Bankart repair at 10 to 17 years.[375] No significant differences were seen in outcomes in 33 patients undergoing open repair (mean follow-up 15.7 years) and 49 patients undergoing arthroscopic repair (mean follow-up 13.7 years), including recurrent instability (9% open vs. 12.5% arthroscopic). Radiographic findings of glenohumeral arthritis were also not significantly different between groups (18.2% moderate to severe changes in open group vs. 12.2% in arthroscopic group).

With increasing technology and expertise in arthroscopy, a number of studies have recently reported on the use of arthroscopic surgery in shoulders that were traditionally addressed with open techniques. Patients who have previously failed an instability procedure have undergone arthroscopic revision Bankart repair with reasonable outcomes.[38,234] Arthroscopic Bankart repair has also been shown to produce successful results in the setting of smaller amounts of glenoid bone loss, with incorporation of a glenoid rim fragment into the repair, if present.[228,271,337,338]

Arthroscopic Repair of HAGL Lesions. As with open repair, data on arthroscopic repair of HAGL lesions has been limited to small studies or case reports.[78,93,180,367] Kon et al. and Field et al. both reported no cases of recurrent instability in small patient series at short-term follow-up.[78,180]

Remplissage. Small series on arthroscopic remplissage, typically performed in combination with arthroscopic Bankart repair, have reported good outcomes with a low rate of recurrent instability.[34,242,260,284,376] There have been some reports of loss of shoulder external rotation with the procedure because of the capsulodesis and tenodesis effect.[65,121] Boileau et al.[34] reported on a series of 47 patients with recurrent instability that underwent arthroscopic Bankart repair and remplissage for a large, engaging Hill–Sachs lesion without substantial glenoid bone loss. At mean 2-year follow-up, 87% good-to-excellent results were reported, with only one case of recurrent instability and 90% of patients returning to sports, including 68% at the same level. In comparison with the contralateral shoulder, mean loss of external rotation was 8 degrees with the arm at the side, and 9 degrees in abduction, with no patient expressing dissatisfaction with this loss of motion.

Bony Procedures for Recurrent Anterior Instability.

Significant bone loss along the anterior glenoid or from a large Hill–Sachs defect, either in the primary or revision setting, is an indication for a bony procedure for surgical treatment of recurrent anterior instability, as a soft tissue only repair in this setting is associated with a high rate of failure.[44,200,228,267] Studies have attempted to determine this critical level of bone loss and although different measurement techniques have been utilized, reported defects of greater than 21% to 30% of the surface area of the glenoid, and a Hill–Sachs defect involving 25% or more of the humeral head or one that engages the anterior glenoid rim with abduction and external rotation, have been identified as indications for bony reconstruction of the glenoid and/or humeral head.[9,44,107,149,224,230,267,276,279] Although substantial bone loss is more commonly seen along the glenoid than the humeral head, the combined bone loss on both sides of the joint should be taken into consideration in surgical decision-making.[267,341,370]

Typically, glenoid bone loss of 25% of the surface area of the glenoid is an indication for bony reconstruction of this defect, which is most commonly anteroinferior.[267,279] Several different bone augmentation techniques have been described; including the Latarjet procedure, use of iliac crest autograft, or use of structural allograft. All function to fill the glenoid defect with a structural bone graft taken from another site. Theoretically, any of these procedures can work if the bone and soft tissue deficiency is adequately addressed. However, the Latarjet procedure, involving transfer of the coracoid process to the anteroinferior glenoid, has been the most well studied and popular of these techniques.[134–136] Use of iliac crest or allograft may be necessary if bone loss exceeds what can be reconstructed with a coracoid transfer. Reconstruction of a large Hill–Sachs defect can be performed with allograft bone or a partial resurfacing implant.[9,224,276,279]

Preoperative Planning (Table 40-15)

| TABLE 40-15 | **Open Bony Procedures for Recurrent Anterior Instability** |

Preoperative Planning

- Beach-chair table with pneumatic arm holder
- Fluoroscopy may be needed to check bone graft placement, or direction and length of screws
- Standard open shoulder instruments
- Additional equipment, as needed, for potential bony or soft tissue procedures (suture anchors, small fragment set, etc.)
  - Fresh frozen allograft for glenoid defect
  - Size-matched fresh frozen allograft for humeral head defect
  - Screws for fixation of glenoid and/or humeral head graft
- Suture anchors for labral repair
- Orthosis for arm immobilization should be placed after surgery

---

Positioning. The beach-chair position is used as described above.

Surgical Approach. Although cases necessitating bony reconstruction require an open deltopectoral approach, an initial arthroscopic evaluation of the glenohumeral joint may still be necessary to confirm or determine that bony reconstruction of a glenoid and/or Hill–Sachs defect is required.

Technique

Latarjet Procedure. Before entering the glenohumeral joint, the coracoid is exposed for osteotomy. The pectoralis minor tendon is released from the medial aspect of the coracoid, and the bone is exposed proximally to its base. Coracoid osteotomy can be performed with an osteotome or angled, oscillating saw with the cut made starting along the superior surface of the bone, just anterior to the coracoclavicular ligaments near the coracoid base, in a medial-to-lateral direction (Fig. 40-46). The coracoacromial ligament is then released, leaving a 1-cm stump of the ligament attached to the coracoid process laterally. The conjoined tendon (coracobrachialis and short head of the biceps) remains attached to the osteotomized coracoid, and it is mobilized to allow for placement along the anteroinferior glenoid. Care should be taken to avoid injury to the musculocutaneous nerve during mobilization.

The glenohumeral joint is next exposed similar to an open Bankart repair. The glenoid rim and neck in the area of the defect are debrided of any soft tissue and lightly decorticated with a high-speed burr to establish a bed of healthy, bleeding

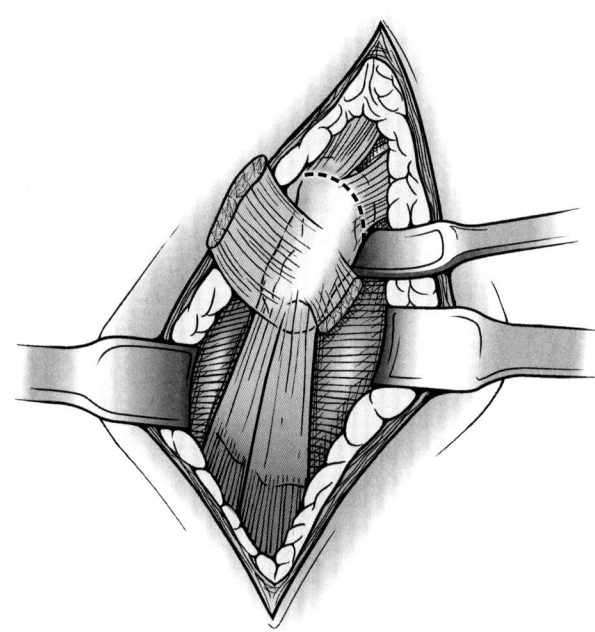

FIGURE 40-46 Coracoid exposure and osteotomy for Latarjet procedure. Coracoid osteotomy can be performed with an osteotome or angled, oscillating saw, with the cut made starting along the superior surface of the bone, just anterior to the coracoclavicular ligaments near the coracoid base, in a medial-to-lateral direction. A 1-cm stump of the coracoacromial ligament is left attached to the coracoid.

bone for osseous union. The same procedure is performed on the coracoid surface that will be placed into the defect site. Superior and inferior drill holes are then made through the coracoid graft for screw fixation. The bone is placed in the glenoid defect (typically below the glenoid equator for an antero-inferior lesion), flush with the glenoid rim. The position can be held with temporary K-wire fixation. The superior hole in the coracoid is then used to drill through the glenoid bicortically,

followed by screw placement. The same steps are then repeated to place the inferior screw (Fig. 40-47). Partially threaded, 4.0-mm cancellous or 3.5-mm cortical screws can be used for coracoid fixation in a "lag" fashion, and typically measure 30 to 36 mm in length.

Differences in placement of the coracoid transfer and subsequent soft tissue repair have been described.[276] The inferior surface can be placed against the glenoid defect site, with the

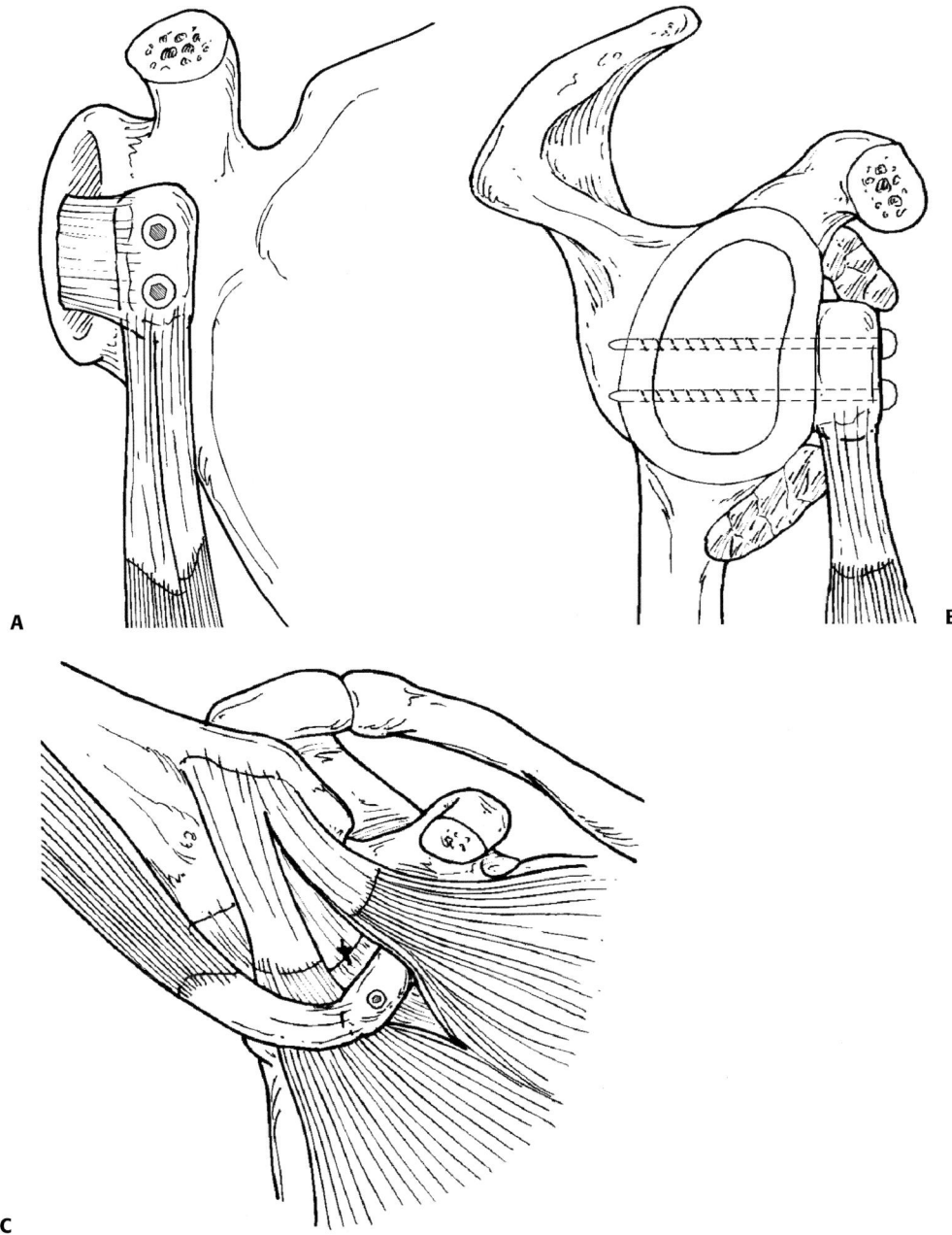

FIGURE 40-47 Anteroposterior **(A)** and **(B)** lateral views following fixation of the coracoid graft to the anterior glenoid. **C:** The stump of the coracoacromial ligament is repaired to the lateral capsular flap made during capsular incision. Note the sling effect created by placement of the coracoid graft through the split in the subscapularis. The inferior third of the subscapularis is maintained in an inferior position, further stabilizing the glenohumeral joint. From ElAttrache NS, Harner CD. *Surgical Techniques in Sports Medicine.* Wolters Kluwer Health; 2006.

stump of the coracoacromial ligament directed laterally. The lateral capsular flap made during capsular incision can then be repaired to the coracoacromial ligament stump, creating an intra-articular graft (Fig. 40-47C). The graft can be made extra-articular by repairing the native capsule to the native glenoid rim using suture anchors or bone tunnels, which must be placed prior to fixation of the coracoid graft. Burkhart et al. described extra-articular graft placement using suture anchors for the capsular repair, and also placed the medial surface of the coracoid graft against the glenoid defect site (Fig. 40-48).[45] This technique creates a longer articulating surface in the anterior-to-posterior direction when compared with placing the inferior surface of the coracoid into the defect site. However, the width of bone for screw placement is narrowed and care should be taken to avoid fracture of the graft.

In theory, stabilization of the glenohumeral joint occurs by three mechanisms with the Latarjet procedure: (1) A bony effect by correcting the anterior glenoid deficiency; (2) a muscular ("sling") effect created by maintaining the inferior third of the subscapularis in an inferior position by the conjoined tendon (Fig. 40-47C); and (3) a capsular effect by the capsular repair or repair of the coracoacromial ligament to the capsule at the end of the procedure.

Iliac Crest Autograft or Allograft Glenoid Reconstruction. The anterior glenoid bone defect is exposed and prepared similarly to the Latarjet procedure. A tricortical iliac crest autograft is obtained and sized to fit the bone defect. A graft that is 3 cm long and 2 cm deep is usually of adequate size. The inner table of the iliac crest has a similar contour to the glenoid surface and is, therefore, faced laterally when secured to the native glenoid. Graft position and fixation is performed similar to the Latarjet procedure, with partially threaded, 4.0-mm cancellous or 3.5-mm cortical screws utilized. The graft can be made

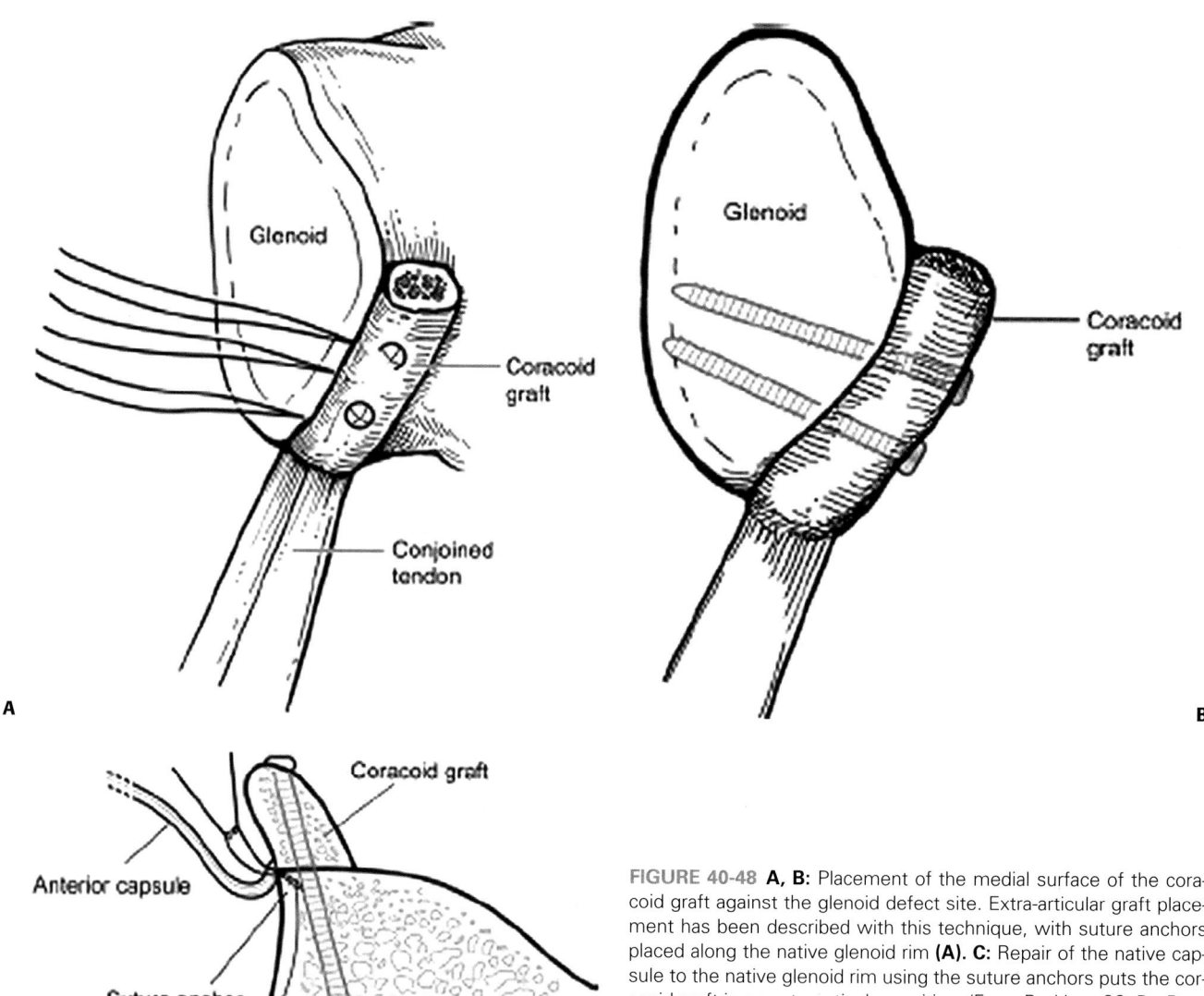

FIGURE 40-48 A, B: Placement of the medial surface of the coracoid graft against the glenoid defect site. Extra-articular graft placement has been described with this technique, with suture anchors placed along the native glenoid rim **(A). C:** Repair of the native capsule to the native glenoid rim using the suture anchors puts the coracoid graft in an extra-articular position. (From Burkhart SS, De Beer JF, Barth JR, Cresswell T, Roberts C, Richards DP. Results of modified Latarjet reconstruction in patients with anteroinferior instability and significant bone loss. *Arthroscopy.* 2007;23(10):1033–1041, with permission)

intra-articular or extra-articular based on the capsular repair. Repair of the lateral capsular flap with sutures secured around the screw heads creates an intra-articular graft, whereas repairing the native capsule to the native glenoid rim leaves the graft extra-articular.

Fresh or fresh-frozen allograft may be used similar to iliac crest autograft, while avoiding the morbidity of graft harvest. Glenoid allograft provides an ideal match to native anatomy, but may be difficult to obtain.[280]

Reconstruction of Hill–Sachs Defect. To access the Hill–Sachs defect through a standard deltopectoral approach, a subscapularis tenotomy is performed, as described above. The humeral head is then dislocated from the glenohumeral joint and the Hill–Sachs defect exposed with simultaneous adduction, extension, and maximal external rotation of the arm. An oscillating saw is used to contour the bone into a wedge-shaped defect to accept an allograft. The length, width, and height of the prepared area are then measured and the allograft bone is cut to the matching size. A fresh or fresh-frozen humeral head or femoral head allograft can be used as a graft source, but care must be taken to obtain a graft that is appropriately sided and sized for the patient. The allograft bone is then fitted into the defect and further contoured as needed to create a smooth articular transition between native and allograft bone. The graft is then fixed to native bone using two, 3.0 or 3.5-mm cannulated screws with countersunk heads (Fig. 40-49). Anterior capsulolabral repair or glenoid bone grafting is performed after reconstruction of the Hill–Sachs lesion if both procedures are necessary.

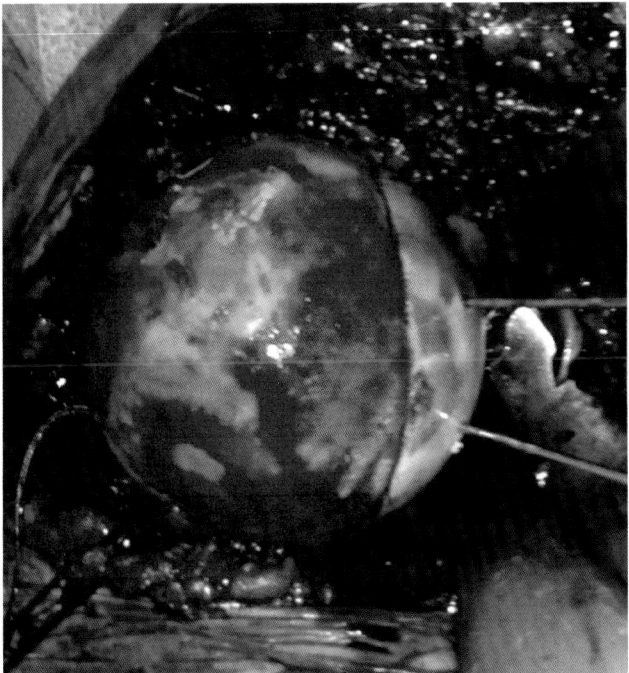

FIGURE 40-49 After appropriate contouring of the defect and graft, the allograft bone is fitted into the Hill–Sachs defect and provisionally held in place with guidewires. Cannulated screws can be placed over the guidewires for definitive graft fixation.

Postoperative Management. The protocol is the same as that for an open capsulolabral repair.

Pitfalls and Solutions (Table 40-16)

TABLE 40-16	Open Bony Procedures for Recurrent Anterior Instability
Potential Pitfalls and Solutions	
Pitfalls	**Solutions**
Axillary nerve injury	Avoid being too inferior in the surgical approach Avoid excessive humeral head distraction
Musculocutaneous nerve injury	Adequate mobilization of conjoint tendon during coracoid transfer
Avoid lateral overhang of glenoid bone graft	Use temporary K-wires to judge graft placement
Prominent hardware	Screws in glenoid graft placed away from the articular surface Screws in humeral graft adequately countersunk
Fixation failure	Two screws needed for fixation of humeral head or glenoid bone graft
Intraoperative fracture of graft	Avoid using too small a graft
Inadequate bony reconstruction	Avoid using too small a graft

Outcomes

Latarjet Procedure. Long-term studies of the Latarjet procedure have shown good-to-excellent clinical results in 86% to 97% of the patients, with reported recurrent instability rates of 7% to 13.6%.[2,134–136,138,139,325] The procedure has been associated with the development of glenohumeral joint arthrosis, with radiographic evidence of arthropathy seen in as many as 71% of the patients, although the majority of the changes are mild.[2,134–136,138,139,325] Hovelius et al. have extensively reported on the procedure over several long-term studies.[134–136,138,139] In a prospective study of 118 shoulders followed for a mean of 15.2 years, the authors reported good or excellent results in 86% of patients, with 98% of patients satisfied or very satisfied with the procedure.[136] Redislocation occurred in 3.4% of patients, with one patient requiring revision surgery, and recurrent subluxations occurred in 10.2% of patients. Mean loss of external rotation at the side was 10.7 degrees. In a subsequent study, the same patient cohort was evaluated for radiographic development of arthrosis at 15-year follow-up.[135] Bony healing of the graft was seen in 85% of patients, with moderate-to-severe arthropathy at the glenohumeral joint in 14% of patients, and mild arthropathy in 35%. A lower percentage of moderate-to-severe arthropathy was seen when the graft was placed medial to the glenoid rim, and when the screw and graft were parallel to the joint line, but this difference was not significant.

Recently a large analysis noted better outcomes in Latarjet patients compared to Bankart patients at mean 17-year follow-up.[138] This included revision surgery because of recurrent instability (1% vs. 5.6%, $p = 0.08$), rate of recurrent instability (13.4% vs. 28.7%, $p = 0.017$), patient satisfaction (97% vs. 90%, $p = 0.0.01$), mean WOSI score (88 vs. 79, $p = 0.002$), and mean loss of external rotation with the arm at the side (11 degrees vs. 19 degrees, $p = 0.012$).

Finally, a recent systematic review examined complication and reoperation rates following original or the modified version of the Bristow or Latarjet procedure.[108] A total of 1,904 cases across 45 studies (all Level IV) were reviewed, and recurrent dislocation and subluxation rates were 2.9% and 5.8%, respectively. Most dislocations occurred in the first year postoperatively, but only 7% of patients required reoperation.

Iliac Crest Bone Graft. Long-term studies of the use of iliac crest bone graft with older techniques have shown good-to-excellent results in 75% to 85% of the patients.[41,285,287] Reported rates of recurrent instability have ranged from 4% to 33%.[41,181,285,287] Radiographic evidence of joint arthrosis has also been reported in 33% to 89% of patients at long-term follow-up.[181,285,287] Studies utilizing more modern methods of graft fixation and contouring to the native articular surface have shown good results and a low rate of recurrent instability.[19,113,168,319,355] Warner et al. reported on the use of tricortical iliac crest autograft for significant anterior glenoid bone defects in a series of 11 patients with recurrent instability.[355] At mean 33-month follow-up, all grafts had incorporated and there were no cases of recurrent instability.

The use of allograft for anterior glenoid reconstruction has only been reported in small series.[168,280,360] Weng et al. reported on the use of femoral head allograft in nine patients with recurrent instability and large anterior glenoid bone defects.[360] Minimum follow-up was 4.5 years, with all grafts incorporating and a mean Rowe score of 84. One redislocation occurred in one patient, and one subluxation occurred in another, both following grand mal seizures, with no further instability developing.

Reconstruction of Hill–Sachs Defect. Clinical outcomes on reconstruction of large Hill–Sachs defects have been limited to small studies or case reports.[110,224,231,343,369] Miniaci and Gish reported on the use of a humeral head allograft in 18 patients with prior failed instability surgery and a Hill–Sachs lesion involving more than 25% of the humeral head.[224] At minimum 2-year follow-up, there were no cases of recurrent instability, with a mean Constant score of 78.5, and 89% of patients had return to work. Interestingly, in our limited experience, many of the patients requiring reconstruction have uncontrolled seizure disorders leading to recurrent instability and humeral head bone loss.

Posterior Instability

As discussed above, posterior instability is relatively uncommon accounting for less than 2% to 12% of overall instability.[37] Seizures, motor vehicle accidents, substance abuse, systemic disease (e.g., Ehlers–Danlos), and psychiatric illness all have been associated with posterior instability.[298] Management should be discussed by the type of instability: Acute dislocation (<3 weeks) which is rare, chronic dislocation which is even more uncommon, and recurrent instability which is the most

common form. The use of 3 weeks is arbitrary, but as discussed below, attempted closed reduction becomes less successful around this time.

The pathogenesis of recurrent instability may start with an acute dislocation; however, it typically starts with subluxation and an atraumatic or microtraumatic etiology as discussed above. Last, it should be noted that because recurrent posterior instability is relatively uncommon, few surgeons encounter it often though it is now being recognized with increasing frequency. Errors in diagnosis and management are common and evidence-based management is lacking. Almost all the reported literature are case series and the definitions of posterior instability are unclear.

Nonoperative and Closed Treatment
Indications/Contraindications
Acute Posterior Dislocations. Unless a patient is severely infirm and unable to tolerate an attempt at closed reduction, intervention (closed or open) should always be considered. There are few other indications to leave an acute dislocation unreduced and treated nonoperatively. Similarly, a reduced dislocation that has persistent subluxation or instability because of a large glenoid fracture should always be considered for surgical intervention. This is discussed in more detail in the scapular fracture chapter.

Chronic Posterior Dislocations. If a patient has a chronic dislocation (>3 to 6 weeks), attempt at closed reduction without full muscle relaxation should not be attempted because of the risk of fracture and neurovascular injury (Fig. 40-1). The typical history is a violent dislocation during a motor vehicle accident or a seizure. The patient may be unaware of the injury or intubated and sedated, and the injury can go unrecognized for a long period of time. Though surgical management is standard for patients who are infirm or have reasonably good function and minimal pain, nonoperative treatment may be the appropriate choice. All patients with a posterior dislocation will have limited motion—specifically anterior elevation and external rotation, but sometimes it can be as high as 60% to 85% of normal.[357] In agreement with others, we have observed some patients to have minimal pain. Therefore with a functional contralateral arm and limited demand, nonoperative treatment may be the best treatment. For patients with epilepsy, the seizures need to be controlled before any surgery is considered. If the seizures are frequent and uncontrollable, consideration should also be given to nonoperative treatment.

Recurrent Posterior Instability. For recurrent posterior instability, vigorous nonoperative management is the mainstay as the pathogenesis is incompletely understood and the results of posterior repair are unpredictable. Many shoulders are managed with strengthening, education, neuromuscular rehabilitation, and even psychological counseling for patients with voluntary instability. Strengthening is focused on the dynamic stabilizers, specifically the rotator cuff, posterior deltoid and the periscapular muscles. Surgery is only considered for involuntary recurrent instability after failed nonoperative treatment. Physical therapy, however, is more likely to be successful in the absence of a large reverse labral lesion or bony defect. The success rate of an exercise program in patients with disabling symptoms was as high as 68% in one study.[82] Many of these patients were improved, but still had some recurrences of instability. Conversely, some studies show that patients who fail therapy have a surgical success rate as high as 90% (Table 40-17).[82]

TABLE 40-17 Posterior Instability	
Nonoperative Treatment	
Indications	**Contraindications**
Recurrent atruamatic instability	Acute dislocation
Infirm patient	Acute destabilizing glenoid fracture
Chronic dislocation with good function	Open injuries
Unstable epilepsy	

Closed Reduction. Many posterior dislocations are locked and initially missed with the exact timing of the injury sometimes unclear. In addition, 30% to 40% of dislocations have an associated fracture[301] and for these reasons, closed reduction requires complete muscle relaxation and fluoroscopy. In our institution, all of these dislocations are taken to the operating room for closed reduction and are not reduced in the emergency room. In the OR, postreduction stability can be assessed, real-time fluoroscopy can be used to help guide the reduction and prevent the catastrophic creation of a humeral neck or head fracture. If after a first careful attempt at reduction is unsuccessful, consideration for open or arthroscopic reduction and stabilization is suggested and easily performed in the OR.

With a moderately sized humeral head defect (>20% to 25%) an attempt at closed reduction has a higher risk of recurrent instability. Some authors use this as a relative indication for open management,[263] whereas others, including ourselves, have had success with closed treatment. Close attention to detail and gentle maneuvers are required along with assessment of postreduction stability. Recurrent instability beyond neutral arm rotation should be considered an indication for an operative stabilizing procedure, as discussed below.

Importantly, there is no clear timeframe to define an "acute" versus "chronic" dislocation; however, reduction appears to be more difficult after 3 weeks and it is often cited as the division between the two.[126] Known nondisplaced fractures, in our opinion, should be treated open to decrease the risk of displacement.

Preoperative Planning. We always prepare for an open procedure in case a closed reduction is not successful. Some authors have discussed using arthroscopy-assisted reduction using standard portals: we have no experience with this (Table 40-18).

TABLE 40-18 Closed Reduction of a Posterior Dislocation
Preoperative Planning
• Radiolucent or beach-chair table
• Supine or beach-chair angled in the room to allow for fluoroscopy
• Lateral position with bean-bag if arthroscopy is considered
• Fluoroscopy coming in from the head parallel to the table for supine and beach-chair positioning.
• Fluoroscopy coming in from the foot for lateral positioning.
• Preparation for open or arthroscopic procedure (see below)
• Orthosis in neutral arm rotation should be available postoperatively

Positioning. In the OR, the patient can be placed in a beach-chair position or supine on a radiolucent table. If consideration is given to arthroscopy and the preferred position for this technique is lateral (as opposed to beach-chair), lateral position with a bean bag should be used.

Fluoroscopy should be used to get orthogonal views. This is most easily done with the machine coming cephalad on the side of dislocated shoulder with the C rotating to get an axillary and AP or Grashey view (Fig. 40-50). This C-arm positioning works for supine and beach-chair, but works best from the foot

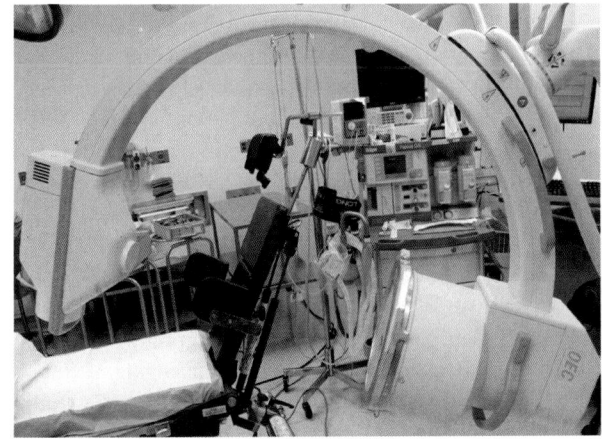
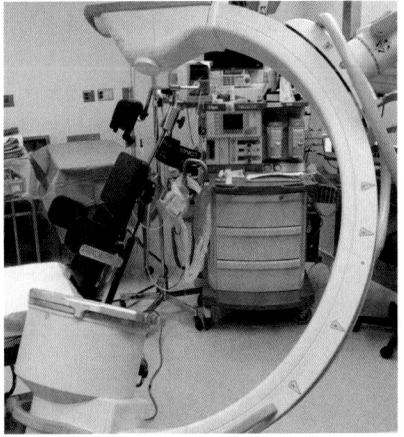

FIGURE 40-50 Intraoperative positioning in the beach-chair position with the C-arm coming over the top for both a **(A)** true AP and **(B)** axillary view.

for lateral positioning. Positions *must* include potential access to anterior and posterior shoulder.

Technique. The reduction maneuver is forward flexion with the arm in adduction and internal rotation. As an assistant places gentle cross-body traction, gentle digital pressure is placed on the posterior humeral head. In addition, gentle internal and external rotation can be used to disimpact the reverse Hill–Sachs lesion. Once the head is disimpacted, the head should be brought anteriorly and externally rotated. Aggressive external rotation against resistance can lead to a shearing fracture of the humeral head or neck. Stability of the joint should be tested in adduction with gentle range of motion under fluoroscopy. Specifically, stability in internal rotation should be checked. Postreduction, the arm should be placed in neutral rotation with a bump under the sling or a "gun-slinger orthosis" splint. Consideration should be given to further open procedures if instability is encountered at a neutral arm position or beyond.

Postoperative Management. The patient is kept 3 to 6 weeks in a sling in a neutral position. We prefer a longer timeframe to allow the posterior capsule to heal. Elbow, wrist, and hand motions are encouraged during this time. A strengthening program is started once the splint or orthosis is discontinued. Persistent instability after nonoperative management will require operative intervention as discussed below.

Pitfalls and Solutions (Table 40-19)

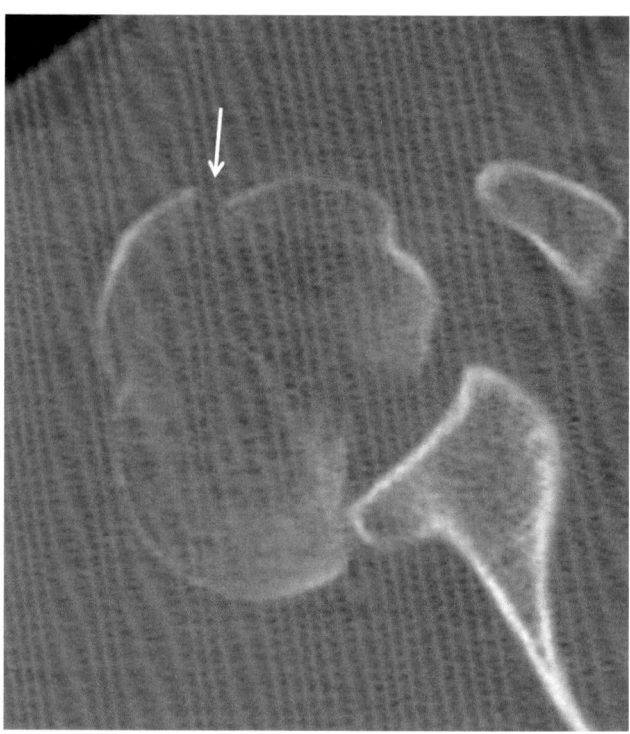

FIGURE 40-51 Acute posterior dislocation. Note the fracture (*arrow*) that could further displace with attempted closed reduction.

TABLE 40-19	**Closed Reduction of a Posterior Dislocation**

Potential Pitfalls and Solutions

Pitfalls	Solutions
Displacement of fracture	ORIF Hemiarthroplasty
Acute instability	External rotation orthosis Open anterior procedure (below) Arthroscopic capsulorrhaphy
Recurrent instability	Open or arthroscopic procedure discussed below

Outcomes. Patients with a successful closed reduction, even with initial instability in internal rotation, have been reported to have excellent outcomes with near full motion and limited pain in both the short and long terms. The most common complication after this injury is recurrent instability, occurring in approximately 15% to 20% of patients and typically within the first year.[301] Predisposing factors for recurrent instability are size of the humeral defect, dislocation because of seizure, and age less than 40. The risk is lower in patients following a MVA or with a traumatic incident—specifically if the patient is older and has a small anterior humeral head defect. There are small but persistent deficits of shoulder function by outcomes scores, though most series report generally good function.[263,297,301]

Operative Treatment of Posterior Instability

Indications/Contraindications

Acute Posterior Dislocations. In the acute setting, the indications for surgery are irreducible or unstable dislocations, dislocation-associated fracture of the proximal humerus, open injuries, a significant glenoid fracture contributing to instability, or a reverse Hill–Sachs >20% to 25%. Most, if not all proximal humerus fractures identified preoperatively should be treated with open reduction with or without fixation because of the high risk of displacement and catastrophic consequences if a forceful closed reduction is performed (Fig. 40-51).

Chronic Posterior Dislocations. The indications for nonoperative treatment or "skillful neglect" were discussed above. However, for all other patients, the results of operative intervention are generally superior to nonoperative care. The choice of procedure, as discussed below, depends on the size of the humeral head defect and patient factors.

Recurrent Posterior Instability. For recurrent instability, surgical stabilization is indicated if nonoperative treatment has failed. These procedures may be performed arthroscopically, or through an open posterior approach with or without a bony procedure (glenoid osteotomy or posterior bone block procedure). Arthroscopic procedures have the benefit of evaluating the entire joint before treatment and limiting patient morbidity, but these procedures are technically challenging. Arthroscopic repairs are contraindicated in the setting of glenoid abnormalities (e.g., glenoid retroversion) that need to be addressed. In addition, many patients with posterior instability have inferior or bidirectional instability which also needs to be addressed (Table 40-20).

TABLE 40-20 Posterior Instability

Operative Treatment

Indications	Contraindications
Failed nonoperative treatment for recurrent instability	Unstable epilepsy
Failed closed reduction	Infirm patient
Dislocation >3–6 wks	
Reverse Hill–Sachs >20–25%	
Significant glenoid defect	
Proximal humerus fracture	

Open Anterior Reduction of a Posterior Dislocation[51]. If a stable closed reduction is unsuccessful, the patient has a defect >20% to 25% of the humeral head, or the patient has had a dislocation for >3 weeks, an open reduction with or without additional procedures such as disimpaction of the reverse Hill–Sachs defect is indicated. If, however, the humeral head defect is greater than 40%, other anterior techniques that address the lesion are indicated because of the extremely high risk of recurrent dislocation. These techniques, including subscapularis transfer, lesser tuberosity transfer, or hemiarthroplasty, are discussed later in the setting of chronic posterior dislocations.

Preoperative Planning. Despite the chronicity of a dislocation, an anterior approach is the work-horse for open reduction because it is a safe and standard approach. A surgeon should also be prepared for a posterior approach if the anterior approach is unsuccessful, but this is uncommon. In addition, the surgeon should be prepared for a disimpaction of a small reverse Hill–Sachs defect if necessary. Fluoroscopy or intraoperative radiographs should be considered to confirm reduction and to evaluate fracture displacement. The setup is similar to the closed reduction setup of posterior dislocations (Table 40-21).

Positioning. Our standard setup is in beach-chair position with an articulated arm holder as in all our open anterior procedures. As with closed reductions, both a lateral and supine position can be used. The lateral position also allows for arthroscopy (if preferred laterally) and for a posterior approach. A supine position is the simplest, but does not allow for a posterior approach if required. In addition, the lateral or supine positions are poor for an arthroplasty procedure, if required.

TABLE 40-21 Open Anterior Reduction of a Posterior Dislocation

Preoperative Planning

- Refer to setup for closed reduction of a posterior dislocation
- Standard open shoulder instruments
- Narrow, long tamps and cancellous allograft are needed for the disimpaction procedure (if considered)
- An oscillating saw and curved ostetomes are needed for the lesser tuberosity osteotomy
- A small fragment set and power should be available

Surgical Approach and Technique. A standard deltopectoral approach is used with the biceps tendon as a guide to find the lesser tuberosity. The tendon is best found distally, medial to the pectoralis major insertion. In the setting of a posterior dislocation, the axillary nerve is precariously close medially and is very taut. The nerve should be palpated or seen before any surgical releases are attempted. In simple situations, the biceps tendon can be followed and the rotator interval released to gain access to the joint. A finger can be placed through the interval and into the joint to manually pull the humeral head laterally to disimpact the head with the arm in an adducted and slightly flexed position. Once the humeral head is disimpacted, it can be brought anteriorly with digital pressure and the arm can be externally rotated, aiding in reduction. Stability of the reduction should be tested in adduction, as with bringing the arm into internal rotation. Positioning of the arm postoperatively, is determined by this intraoperative stability.

If a reduction cannot be performed through the interval, then the subscapularis can be released (and subsequently repaired) in the standard techniques described above for anterior instability. The humeral head can be reduced manually or by lateral traction with a bone hook. Care should be taken to not damage the cartilage.

Last, if the humeral head defect is large, humeral head disimpaction or subscapularis transfer should be considered (discussed below). A disimpaction procedure should only be considered if the humeral head bone stock is good, the impacted cartilage can be salvaged, the defect is <40%, and the dislocation is less the 3 weeks. Chronic dislocations suffer from disuse osteopenia.

A cortical window is created with internal rotation of the humeral head in the greater tuberosity, though in reality it is difficult to preserve the cortical bone. A large tamp is introduced to disimpact the fracture. The head needs to be externally rotated to check elevation progress. The humeral head void is filled with cancellous allograft (our preferred choice), iliac crest, or another bone substitute product (Fig. 40-52).

Postoperative Management. Postoperative treatment is similar to that in closed management. A brace in neutral position is used for 6 weeks.

Pearls and Pitfalls (Table 40-22)

TABLE 40-22 Open Anterior Reduction of a Posterior Dislocation

Potential Pitfalls and Solutions

Pitfalls	Solutions
Displacement of fracture	ORIF Hemiarthroplasty
Acute instability	External rotation orthosis Subscapularis transfer (below) Posterior approach and capsular repair
Irreducible dislocation	Posterior approach
Axillary nerve injury	Direct repair Observation

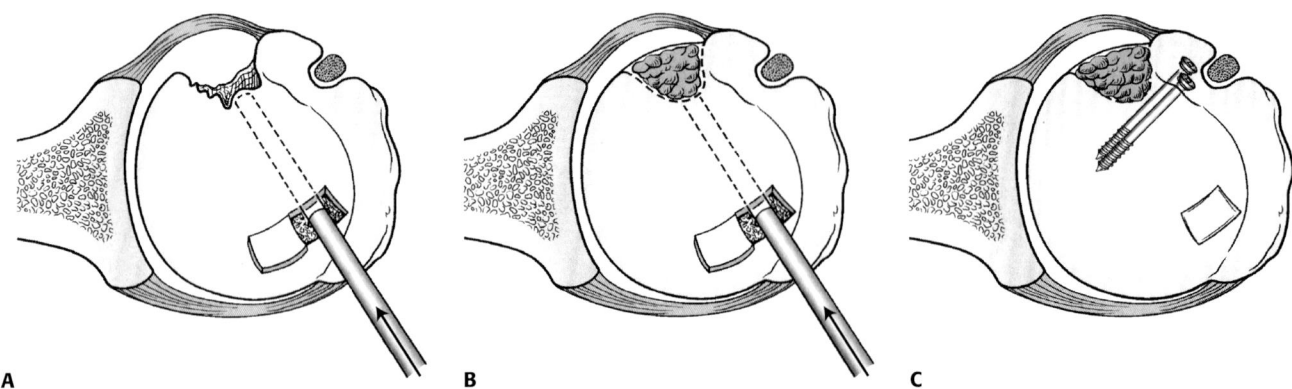

A **B** **C**

FIGURE 40-52 Disimpaction of an acute reverse Hill Sachs defect using a cortical window opposite to the lesion **(A)**, to pack cancellous bone graft into the defect **(B)**. Sometimes the disimpaction is supported by screws **(C)**.

Outcomes. There is limited data on the outcomes of simple open reduction. All the literature includes additional subscapularis transfer or capsulorrhaphy. However, in our limited experience, the open and closed reductions have similar and generally excellent outcomes. In addition, subscapularis transfer or capsulorrhaphy is not often required.[56] The chance of recurrence is likely similar.[70,126] There are only a few series looking at disimpaction in isolation: They reveal that success correlates with good bone stock.[167]

Open Anterior Procedures for Chronic Posterior Dislocations. Following (open reduction or gentle attempt at closed reduction) the humeral head stability is tested with adduction and internal rotation. As the size of the reverse Hill–Sachs increases, so does the degree of instability. With instability in neutral, an adjunctive stabilization procedure should be considered. With defects smaller than 20% of the humeral head, a subscapularis transfer with (modified McLaughlin) or without the lesser tuberosity (McLaughlin) is recommended. For patients with a 20% to 40% defect, an osteoarticular allograft should be considered. In most cases, an arthroplasty is needed for defects larger than 40%. In addition, as the time from injury increases, so does the disuse osteopenia and the need for an arthroplasty. Preparation for an arthoplasty should therefore, always be considered. The guidelines are based mainly on expert observation with no evidence-based studies available.

Preoperative Planning (Table 40-23)

TABLE 40-23	**Open Anterior Procedures for Chronic Posterior Dislocations**

Preoperative Planning

- Beach-chair table with pneumatic arm holder
- Fluoroscopy may be needed to check direction and length of screws
- Equipment is the same as an open anterior stabilization
  - Small oscilllating saw needed for lesser tuberosity transfer
  - Size-matched fresh frozen allograft of the humeral head
  - Headless screws needed for fixation of allograft
  - Arthroplasty equipment should always be available
- External rotation orthosis should be available

Positioning. The beach-chair position is used as described above.

Surgical Approach. A standard deltopectoral approach is used for all these stabilizations.

Technique

Subscapularis Transfer. The approach is the same as described above for open reduction. The biceps is identified at the lateralmost aspect of the subscapularis insertion on the lesser tuberosity. From here, the subscapularis tendon, along with the underlying capsule are reflected from the tuberosity as a sleeve and tagged. The joint is exposed and the head reduced as described above. Careful attention should be paid to the axillary nerve which is very taut in posterior dislocations. The scar tissue is debrided and the joint inspected. If the bony defect is less than 20% of the humeral head surface and the remaining cartilage is in good condition, the tendon can be transferred into the defect. The subscapularis tendon and capsule are transferred into the defect and held in position with #2 nonabsorbable transosseous sutures. We prefer to release the biceps from the supraglenoid tubercle and tenodese it to the superior aspect of the pectoralis major tendon. This allows us to pass the drill holes through the bicipital groove which generally has excellent bone quality. Anchors can also be used to secure the tendon, but this is not our preference as bone tunnels are cheaper and generally stronger (Fig. 40-53A). The humeral head should be tested for stability. If instability still exists, or the remaining cartilage in poor condition, consideration should be given to the other procedures.

Lesser Tuberosity Transfer. A modification of this procedure was described by Hawkins and Neer (Fig. 40-53B) in which the lesser tuberosity is osteotomized with the attached tendon and transferred into the bony defect.[126,215] In this technique, we always release the biceps tendon from the supraglenoid tubercle by opening the rotator interval. We tenodese the tendon to the superior pectoralis major tendon and then perform the osteotomy with a 10-mm oscillating saw followed by a curved osteotome. It is critical to keep the bony piece thick to hold screws and to fill the defect. After the joint is reduced and evaluated, and the defect debrided to bleeding cancellous bone,

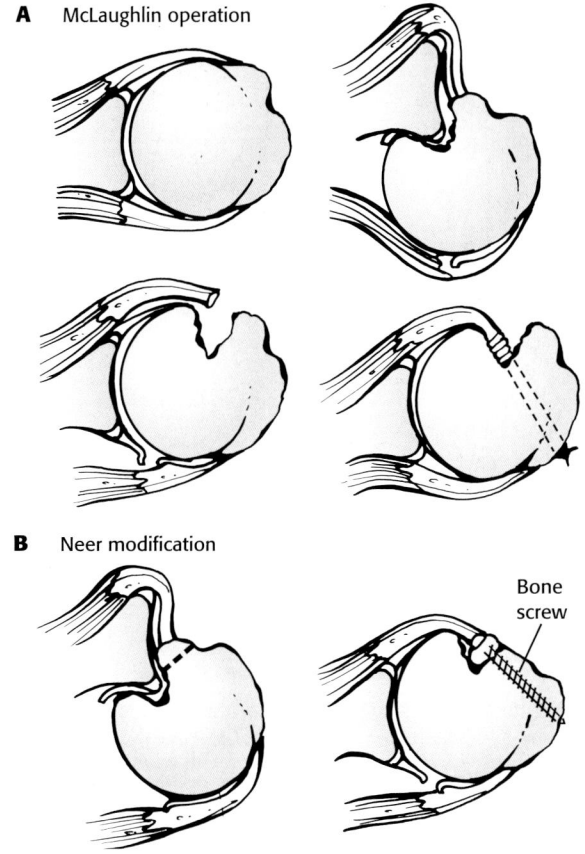

A McLaughlin operation

B Neer modification

Bone screw

FIGURE 40-53 A: The McLaughlin operation. In the presence of a large anterior humeral head lesion, the subscapularis tendon can be transferred into the defect. **B:** A subsequent modification by Neer transfers the lesser tuberosity with the attached subscapularis tendon.

the osteotomy can be secured to the defect with two cancellous screws as originally described. Transosseous sutures can augment fixation (Fig. 40-54).

Allograft Reconstruction. The approach is similar to described above.[96] We prefer a lesser tuberosity osteotomy for exposure as well as a backup procedure if we have difficulty with the allograft. The edges of the defect are sharply cut with an oscillating saw or osteotome. The defect is measured and the humeral head allograft is cut 2 mm larger to allow for a press fit then contoured as needed. Once the head is well seated, headless screws (or countersunk headed screws) are used for fixation. The shoulder is taken through a range of motion to check stability. The subscapularis or lesser tuberosity osteotomy is repaired with five large nonabsorbable transosseous sutures through the bicipital groove (Fig. 40-55).

Arthroplasty. If the articular cartilage is in poor condition or the humeral head defect is greater than 40%, a hemiarthroplasty or total shoulder arthroplasty should be used.[92,297] Hemiarthroplasty can be used in younger patients below the age of 50 and patients with good glenoid cartilage. Total shoulder replacements should be considered for the others. We perform a lesser tuberosity osteotomy. The head is externally rotated and brought out of the wound where a humeral head cut is made in the anatomic version. Some have discussed anteroverting the humeral head in cases of a locked dislocation to prevent further instability. We prefer not to distort the bony anatomy, which may have implications for long term glenoid wear (bony or prosthetic) or glenoid component loosening. Instead we balance the soft tissue by plicating any lax posterior capsule with figure-of-eight nonabsorbable #2 stitches. A glenoid component is placed if the cartilage is poor or the patient is older. The

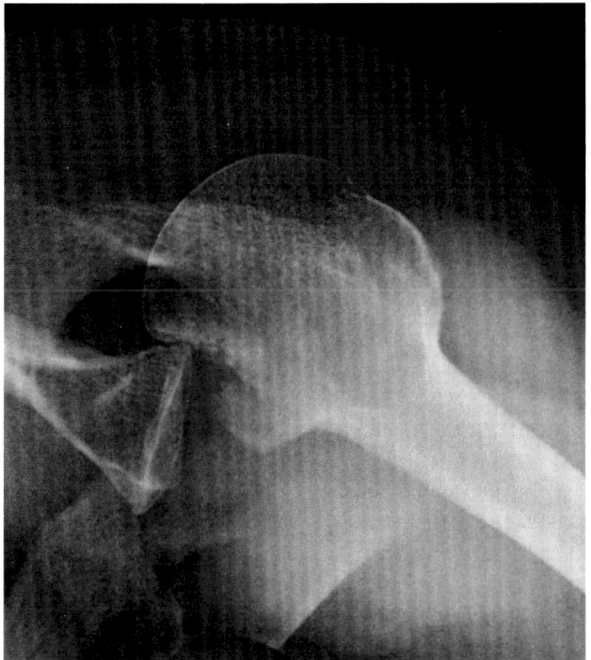

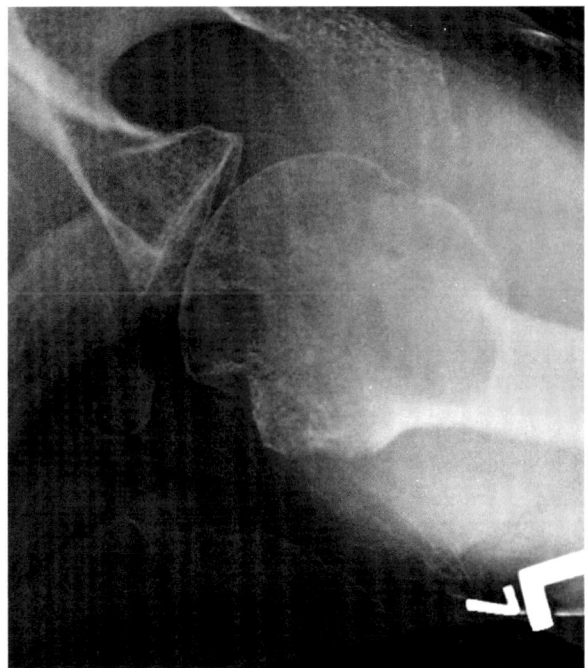

FIGURE 40-54 A: Chronic posterior dislocation with <20% defect treated with **(B)** a lesser tuberosity transfer using suture and bone tunnels.

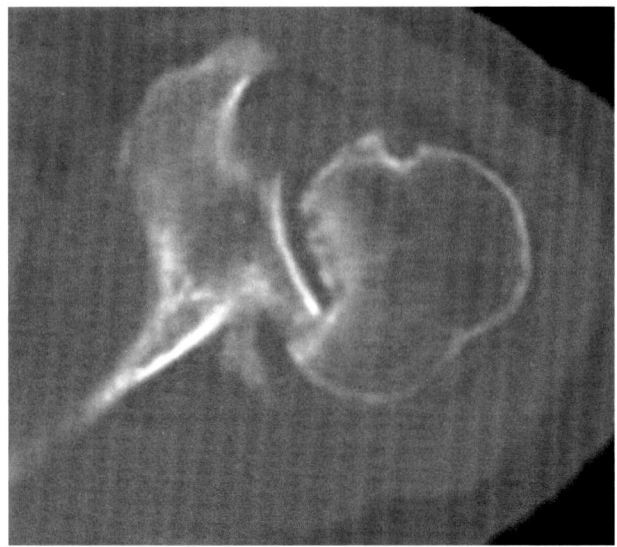

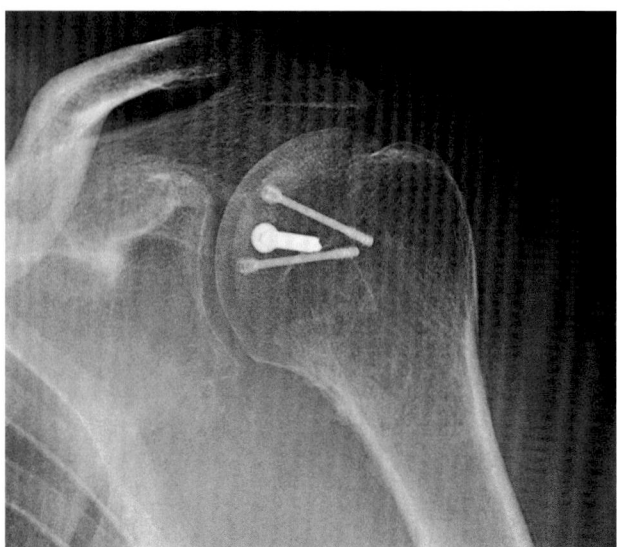

A   **B**

FIGURE 40-55 **A:** Chronic posterior dislocation. Note large reverse Hill–Sachs defect (40% of head) and heterotopic bone from chronic displacement. **B:** Treated with humeral head allograft and headless screws.

lesser tuberosity is repaired with transosseous sutures through the bicipital groove.

Postoperative Management. For all of the above procedures, including arthroplasty, the patient is kept in an orthosis keeping the arm in neutral for 6 weeks to allow the posterior capsule and the subscapularis to heal. We do not allow external rotation beyond neutral as some advocate for fear of disrupting the subscapularis repair. At 6 weeks, full gentle range of motion is allowed with strengthening at 3 months.

Pitfalls and Solutions (Table 40-24)

TABLE 40-24 Open Anterior Procedures for Chronic Posterior Dislocations

Potential Pitfalls and Solutions

Pitfalls	Solutions
Axillary nerve injury	Note displacement of nerve on initial approach
Osteopenic head	Consider arthroplasty
Pull-out of transosseous sutures	Drill through the bicipital groove
Fracture of lesser tuberosity bone	Use small screw (2.0 or 2.7 mm) Consider anchors or transosseous suture

Outcomes

Subscapularis and Lesser Tuberosity Transfer. Only a few studies have been published for subscapularis transfer procedures, but most have reported stable shoulders with congruent motion in the majority of patients who were treated with this operation.[51,79,215] Typically forward flexion remains

full, although external rotation does have some limitation to approximately 45 degrees as described in a number of reports.

Allograft Reconstruction. Allograft reconstruction is safe with satisfactory results.[51,68] Gerber first described his results with four patients at 5 years.[96] Three patients had excellent results whereas one suffered AVN considered to be related to the patient's alcohol intake. He advocated this procedure in young patients to restore normal anatomy and shoulder biomechanics. Further, if an arthroplasty is needed subsequently, it is easier to perform after allograft reconstruction than after subscapularis transfer.

Arthroplasty. There are limited reports on the use of arthroplasty for chronic posterior dislocations, but the results are mixed. Cheng reported satisfactory results in seven patients with no failures.[52] Checcia, however, reported three failures of hemiarthroplasty in eight patients and four failures of five total shoulders. The cause of the failures vary including anterior and posterior instability, nerve injury, limited range of motion, and bony glenoid wear.[51]

Open Posterior Capsulorrhaphy for Recurrent Instability

Preoperative Planning (Table 40-25)

TABLE 40-25 Open Posterior Capsulorrhaphy or Labral Repair

Preoperative Planning

- Bean bag for lateral position or beach-chair table with arm holder
- Fluoroscopy is not needed
- Standard open shoulder instruments
- Custom external orthosis should be premade and fitted prior to surgery

Positioning. The patient can be placed prone with the shoulder off the operating room table to allow for full scapular and humeral motion. However, lateral decubitus with the patient supported by a full-length bean bag is preferred by many surgeons. We prefer the beach-chair position because it gives us access to both the anterior and posterior aspect of the shoulder if needed. However, patients have to be placed quite vertical and for larger patients, this can be difficult.

Surgical Approach. The posterior approach is as detailed above in the surgical approach section.

Technique. The capsule is incised transversely at the midpoint from the medial to lateral direction (away from the suprascapular nerve) followed by a vertical incision 5 mm from its humeral insertion (Fig.40-56A). The incision must be extended inferiorly enough to address any inferior redundancy. Typically the release to the 6 o'clock position is enough, but with a very lax inferior capsule, it needs to be released all the way around the humeral neck to the anterior inferior side.

The corners are tagged with traction sutures and a humeral head retractor such as a Fukuda is then easily placed into the joint without damage to the cartilage. The posterior labrum is inspected for a lesion. If a lesion is found, the posterior glenoid neck should be decorticated with a rasp or burr and anchors should be placed—typically three or more (Fig. 40-56B). Sutures are passed around the labrum and tied with the knots on the external surface of the capsule/labrum—acting as a buttress. Before tying, the arm is abducted in the plane of the scapula to 20 degrees and neutral rotation.

Attention is then turned to the posteroinferior capsular shift. The inferior capsular flap is then shifted laterally and superiorly, reducing any inferior redundancy, with no. 2

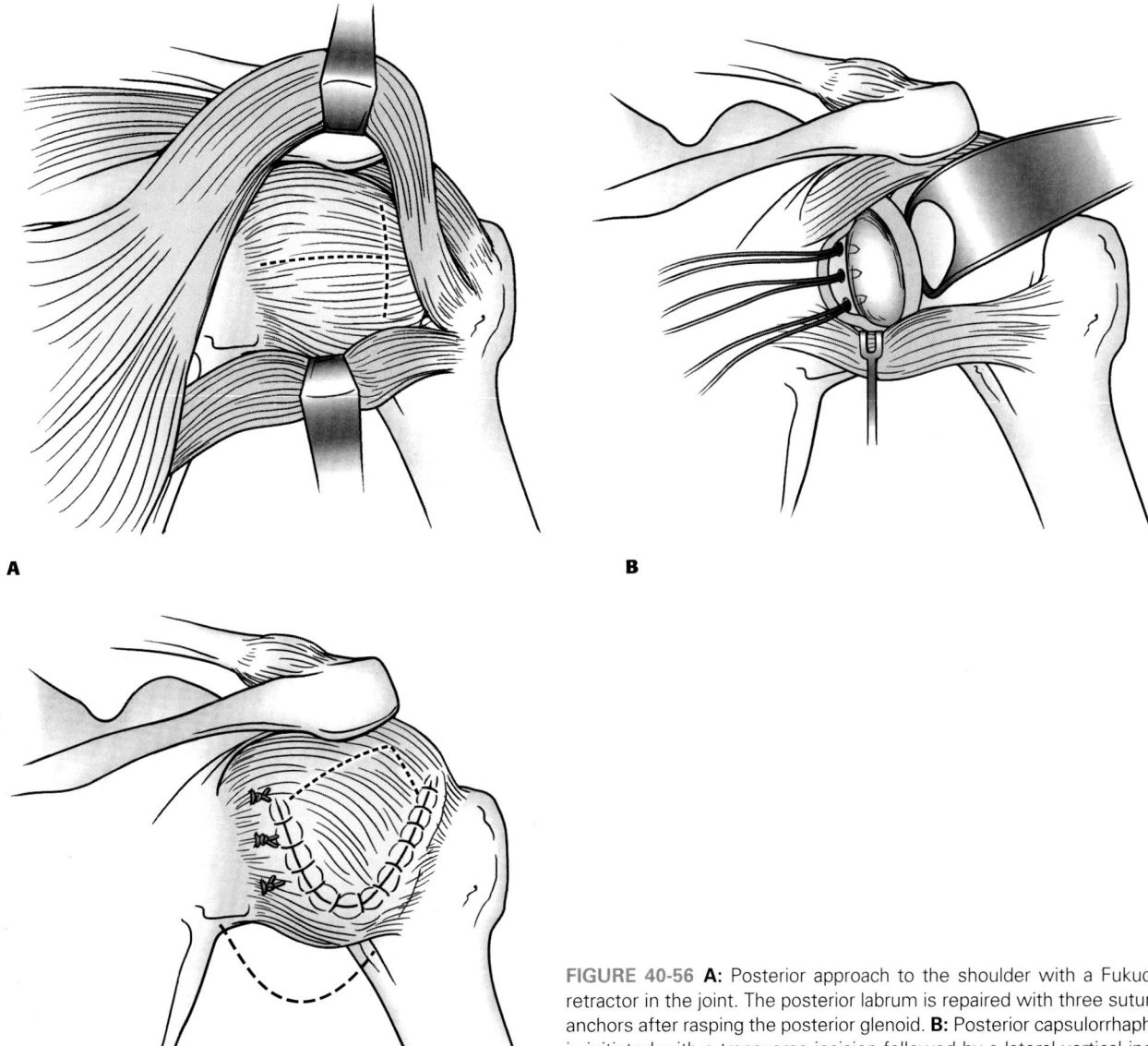

A

B

C

FIGURE 40-56 **A:** Posterior approach to the shoulder with a Fukuda retractor in the joint. The posterior labrum is repaired with three suture anchors after rasping the posterior glenoid. **B:** Posterior capsulorrhaphy is initiated with a transverse incision followed by a lateral vertical incision. **C:** The inferior flap is advanced superiorly and laterally and the superior flap is advanced laterally and inferiorly.

nonabsorable sutures passed and tied laterally. The superior flap is then shifted inferiorly to a point of tension. The interval between the flaps is reinforced with nonabsorbable sutures. At this point, if the infraspinatus tendon is felt to be excessively loose, it can also be slightly shortened by imbricating upon itself (Fig. 40-56C).

Postoperative Management. The patient is put into an orthosis in 20 degrees of abduction and 10 degrees of external rotation for 6 weeks. This orthosis generally needs to be made and fitted ahead of surgery. Inferior traction should be avoided along with internal rotation especially during bathing. A gentle range-of-motion program is started. Forward flexion is initially started with the patient supine along with gentle internal rotation. Strengthening is started at 3 months and return to contact sports at 6 months.

Pitfalls and Solutions (Table 40-26)

TABLE 40-26 Open Posterior Cappsulorraphy and Labral Repair

Potential Pitfalls and Solutions

Pitfalls	Solutions
Axillary nerve injury	Avoid being too inferior in the surgical approach
Missed labral tear	Inspection of the joint
Inadequate shift of associated inferior redundancy	Adequate inferior capsular releases around the humeral neck
Suprascapular nerve injury	Minimize medial retraction
Adequate shift	Abduction and external rotation of the arm prior to capsular shift
Overtightening	Avoid excessive external rotation prior to tying the suture

Outcomes. The results of posterior capsulorrhaphy are generally good according to a small group of recent retrospective case series. These studies have reported good-to-excellent results in 90% to 100% of the patients treated with a primary posterior inferior shift for recurrent posterior instability. The rate drops to 80% when revision cases were included. The recurrence rate of instability has been reported to be between 0% and 23%.[27,83,125,225,292,366] Age older than 37 and chondral injury discovered at the time of the procedure have been associated with worse long-term outcomes.

In a 2005 study by Bottoni et al., looking strictly at patients with the less common traumatic (vs. atraumatic) cause for instability, both open and arthroscopic procedures led to excellent outcomes, but the results favored the arthroscopic procedure in terms of functional scores.[37]

Arthroscopic Posterior Capsulorrhaphy for Recurrent Instability

Preoperative Planning (Table 40-27)

TABLE 40-27 Arthroscopic Posterior Capsulorrhaphy

Preoperative Planning

- Same as for anterior arthroscopic capsulorrhaphy (discussed above)
- Custom external orthosis should be premade and fitted prior to surgery

Positioning. The setup is identical for arthroscopic anterior stabilization as described above with the use of either beach-chair or lateral decubitus position. Again, we prefer a lateral decubitus position because we believe it allows more inferior and posterior visualization.

Surgical Approach. The surgical approach is similar to a standard arthroscopy with the notable exception that visualization, though it initially starts with posterior camera insertion, changes to anterior superior visualization through the rotator interval. In addition, the initial posterior camera position should start slightly more lateral to allow for the second inferior posterior cannula and a better angle for anchor placement.

Technique

Posterior Capsulorrhaphy. After switching to an anterior viewing portal, the posterior pathology can be identified which can involve labral detachments, labral tears, capsular tears at the labrum, an enlarged posteroinferior capsule, and chondral injury (Fig. 40-57).

A larger cannula is needed to pass a curved suture passing device. The posterior glenoid is prepared with a burr, rasp, or shaver. If the labrum and capsule are detached, which is not typical, these both should be mobilized prior to repair and 3-5 anchors can be inserted sequentially starting at the 5 or 6 o'clock position (Fig. 40-58).

In addition, a capsular plication can be performed to reduce redundancy of the posteroinferior capsule. First, a suture passing device is passed through the full thickness of the capsule at

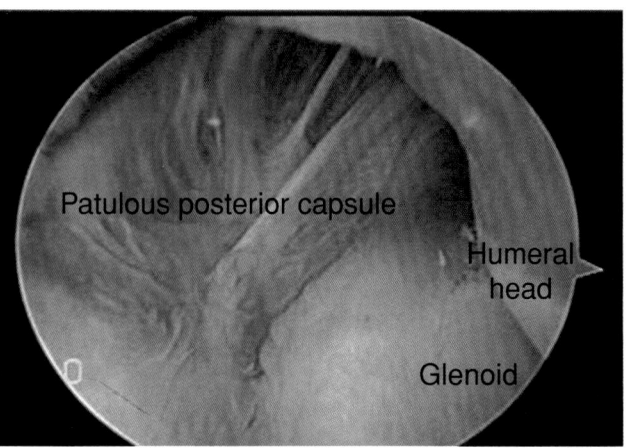

FIGURE 40-57 Anterior-superior view of a patulous posterior capsule in recurrent posterior instability.

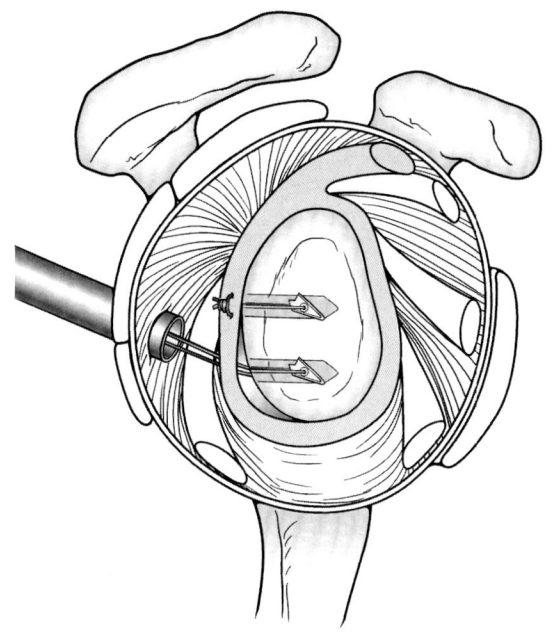

FIGURE 40-58 Diagram of posterior labral repair with anchors.

the 6 o'clock position. A second pass is made under the labrum to create a "pleat." A monofilament suture is placed and can be used as a tie or shuttle for a no. 2 nonabsorbable braided suture. The suture is tied with the goal to decrease the posterior redundancy. The steps are repeated superiorly along the posterior capsule until the redundant capsule is sufficiently reduced and tightened (Fig. 40-59).

Rotator Interval Closure. The rotator interval can be closed in addition to the capsular plication if there is still remaining laxity or it is considerably widened. It is controversial, however, whether this procedure is necessary or helpful. Using a posterior viewing portal, a #2 nonabsorbable suture is introduced with a spinal needle just anterior to the supraspinatus through the SGHL (and CHL, though it is not identified). The suture is retrieved through the anterior cannula with a suture retrieving device that has been passed through the MGHL just above the subscapularis. A knot is tied outside the joint in the subacromial space (Fig. 40-60).

Postoperative Management. The protocol is the same as that for an open capsulorrhaphy.

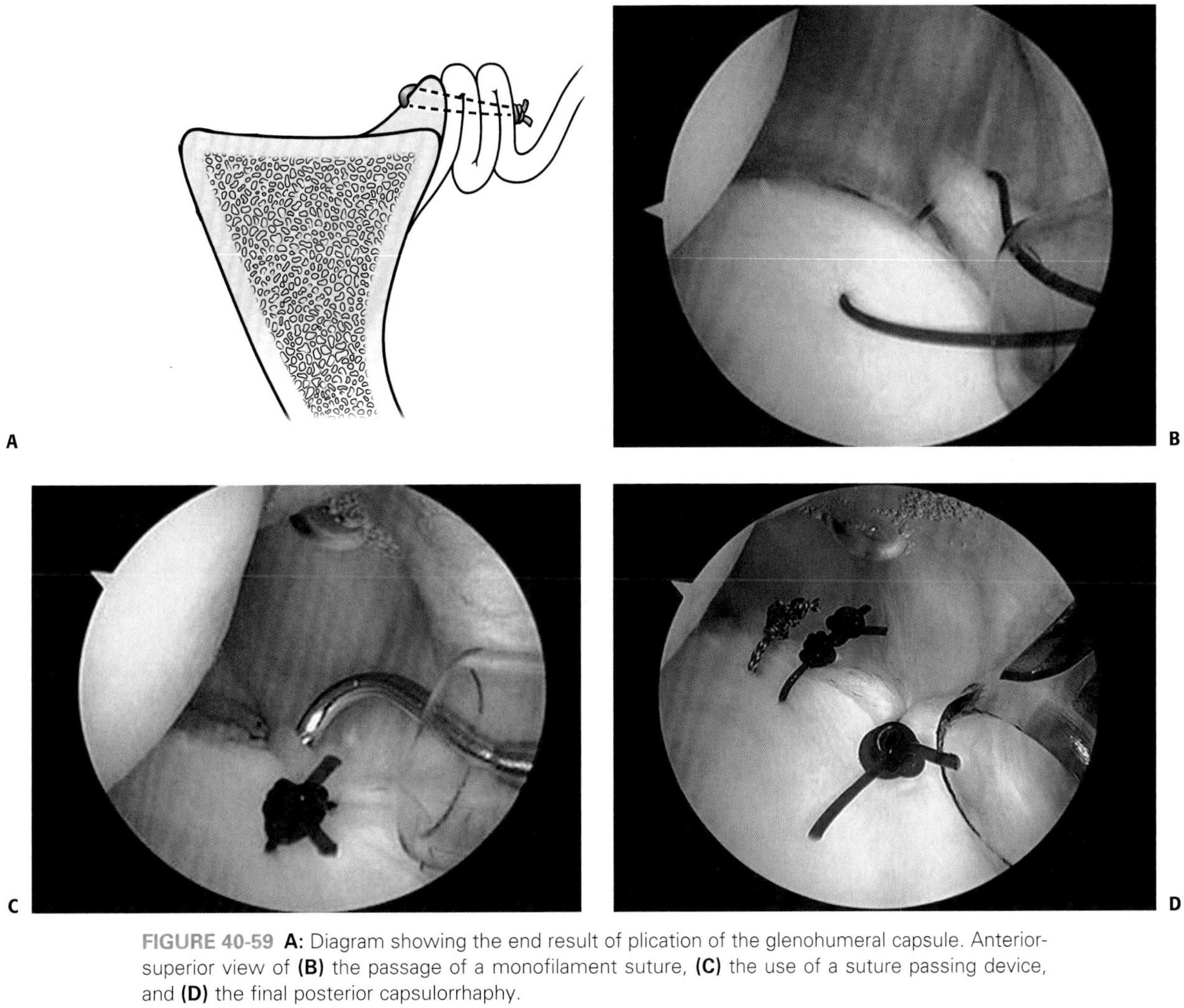

FIGURE 40-59 A: Diagram showing the end result of plication of the glenohumeral capsule. Anterior-superior view of **(B)** the passage of a monofilament suture, **(C)** the use of a suture passing device, and **(D)** the final posterior capsulorrhaphy.

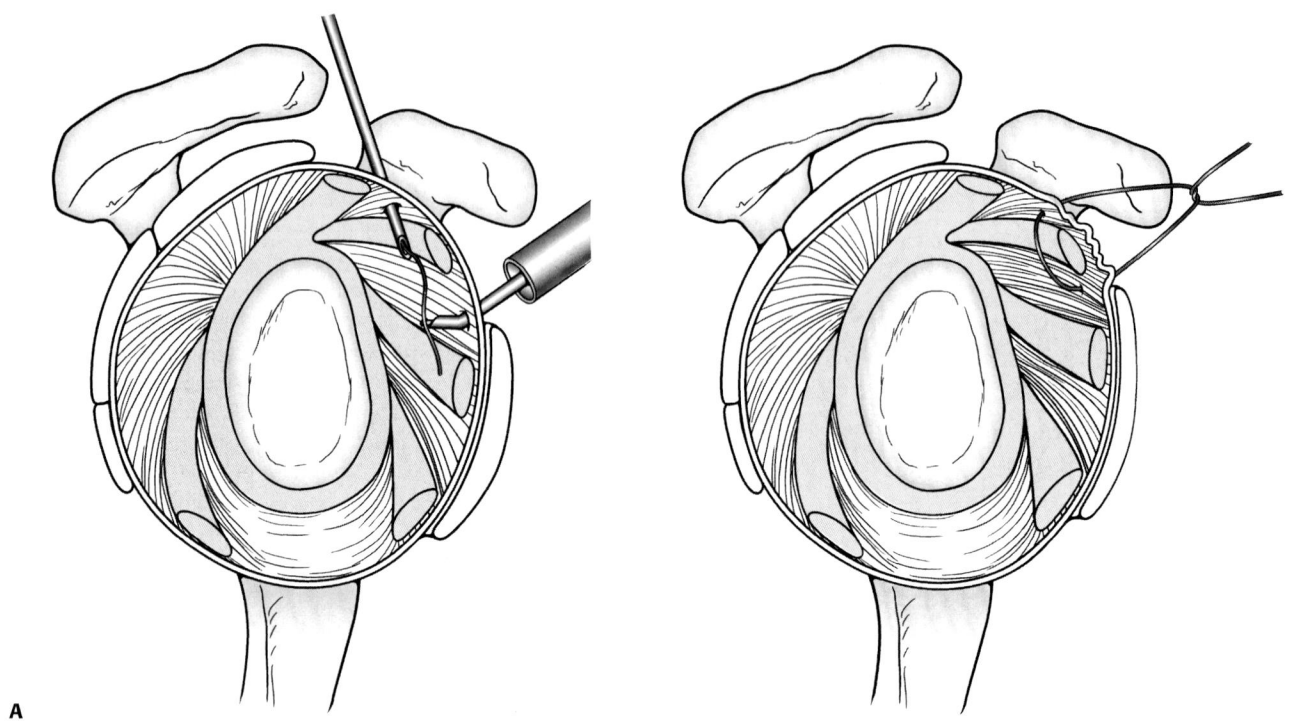

FIGURE 40-60 **A:** Diagram showing the passage of suture for the **(B)** closure of the rotator interval.

Pitfalls and Solutions (Table 40-28)

TABLE 40-28	**Arthroscopic Posterior Capsulorrhaphy**

Potential Pitfalls and Solutions

Pitfalls	Solutions
Undertightening	Convert to open procedure if there is excessive laxity
	Additional rotator interval closure
Unrecognized glenoid hypoplasia or erosion	Preoperative CT and MRI
	Convert to open bony procedure
Unrecognized labral tear (Kim lesion)	Use of anchors instead of simple plication
Very thin posterior capsule	Incorporate the infraspinatus in the repair
Unrecognized posterior HAGL	HAGL repair open or arthroscopic
Unrecognized posterior bone loss	Open bony augmentation

Outcomes. The literature for arthroscopic posterior repairs is difficult to interpret because isolated labral repairs and capsular plication are often combined. In addition, although some series report symptoms of recurrence as a failure, others do not as patients have a decrease in the subjective sense of instability.

Overall, however, these repairs have resulted in successful stabilization. Authors have reported good-to-excellent results in 75% to 97% of the patients at short to midterm follow up.[11,37,174,193,214,275,286,318,363,368] Rates of recurrent instability in these studies have ranged from 0% to 25%.[37,275,363] One recent study confirmed that frank posterior dislocations after surgery were very rare; however, clinically significant posterior subluxations may be more common.[39,318] In this study, 11% of the patients failed clinical stability tests and 8% pursued revision surgery for persisting pain, instability, or decreased function.[39] A contemporary study in 2008 by Savoie et al. reported recurrent instability in only 2/92 patients with a 97% success rate. With evolving techniques, the results continue to improve.[318]

Posterior Bony Augmentation or Glenoid Osteotomy. Posterior bony augmentation with or without glenoid osteotomy should be approached with caution given the high complication rate. Unlike anterior instability, the degree of bone loss or retroversion necessitating these procedures are based mainly on expert opinion rather than clinical or biomechanical reports. However, bone loss exceeding 25% or retroversion >20 degrees, are often used as indications for bone grafting or osteotomy, respectively. Failure of extensive nonoperative management and even previous attempts at surgery such as a posterior capsulorrhaphy, is often necessary before these bony procedures are considered. Preoperative planning with a CT to determine bone loss and retroversion is mandatory.

Preoperative Planning (Table 40-29)

TABLE 40-29	**Open Posterior Bony Augmentation or Glenoid Osteotomy**

Preoperative Planning

- Same as open capsular shift
- Prone or lateral position should be considered for the use of iliac graft (vs. scapular spine)
- Small or large fragment set and power equipment
- Sharp osteotomes

Positioning. Prone positioning with exposure of the iliac crest works well; however, lateral decubitus or beach-chair positioning can be used as described above. We favor a lateral position on a full-body bean bag.

Surgical Approach. A standard posterior approach is used as described above for a posterior capsulorrhaphy.

Technique

Bone Augmentation. The joint is exposed in the same manner as a posterior capsulorrhaphy with a transverse midcapsular incision. However, with bony augmentation, a vertical capsular incision should be made just lateral to the glenoid to both allow exposure to the posterior glenoid and to allow for enough capsule to repair to the posterior part of the bone block (intra-articular bone block) or to allow a capsular shift to the native glenoid with anchors (extra-articular bone block). We prefer an extra-articular bone block with a capsular shift. A 3- × 2- × 1-cm bone graft is obtained from the posterior iliac crest. The suprascapular nerve needs to be identified and protected as it lies only 1 to 2 cm medial to the glenoid rim. The posterior glenoid neck is prepared with a burr or rasp and the corticocancellous graft is placed with two lag screws. We prefer 3.5 partially threaded screws. It is critical that the graft does not overlap laterally. We then use three double-loaded anchors at the glenoid-graft margin to perform a capsular shift overlapping the capsular flaps as described above.

Opening-Wedge Glenoid Osteotomy. The joint is exposed similar to the capsular shift as described above with the vertical capsular incision on the glenoid side. It is important to leave a medial capsular flap as anchors cannot be used with the osteotomy for the capsular shift. An opening wedge osteotomy is performed at the posterior scapular neck. The opening wedge can be stabilized with a bone graft from the iliac crest or scapular spine. Surgical exposure of the scapular neck must be performed with caution as the suprascapular nerve lies in close proximity and is susceptible to injury during the procedure (Fig. 40-61).

Before performing the osteotomy, a straight blunt instrument is inserted into the joint so that it rests on the anterior and posterior glenoid rim to fully understand the version. The osteotomy is made approximately 1 cm from the glenoid rim, where a drill can be used to determine width of the glenoid and to help guide the direction of the osteotome. A sharp wide osteotome or oscillating saw is then advanced parallel to the blunt instrument, but should not exit anteriorly. The bone is gently opened later-ally to create an opening wedge osteotomy, hinging on the intact anterior cortex. An 8- × 30-mm bone graft placed firmly holds the wedge open. Screws are typically not needed. A posterior capsular shift is performed without anchors.

Postoperative Management. The standard posterior capsulorrhaphy protocol is used.

Pitfalls and Solutions (Table 40-30)

TABLE 40-30	**Open Posterior Bony Augmentation or Glenoid Osteotomy**

Potential Pitfalls and Solutions

Pitfalls	Solutions
Suprascapular nerve injury	Identify the nerve
Anterior coracoid abutment	Avoid excessive external rotation during capsular shift
Violating anterior cortex	Use drill bit to measure depth
Avoid lateral overhang of bone block	Use temporary K-wires to judge graft placement
Intra-articular fracture	Place K-wire or drill bit parallel to joint to guide osteotome
Limited capsular tissue for shift	Vertical capsular incision 5 mm lateral to glenoid

Outcomes. Case series of glenoid osteotomy and bone block procedures have mostly produced only satisfactory or poor results.[22] Rates of recurrent instability after the procedures have been reported to be between 12% and 50%.[95,103,122] In addition, these procedures are also associated with a variety of complications including anterior subluxation or instability, coracoid impingement, glenohumeral arthrosis, and intra-articular glenoid fracture.[95,103,122] Graichen et al. reported unusually good results in 82% of their 32 patients who were treated with an osteotomy procedure.[103] However, Meuffels et al.[217] in 2010 showed extremely poor long-term results of a bone-block procedure with nearly half of the 11 patients having regretted their decision for surgery. Based on this data and our experience we believe there is a very limited role for this procedure.

Multidirectional Instability

Nonoperative Treatment

Indications and Contraindications. As discussed above, there is no one single pathologic lesion that leads to MDI. Instead, many have hypothesized that the observed abnormalities of the static stabilizers (redundant inferior capsule and rotator interval) put an increased burden on the dynamic stabilizers (the rotator cuff, the shoulder girdle musculature) that may fail with an acute traumatic event or repetitive microtrauma. A number of observations support this concept including glenohumeral proprioceptive deficits as well as abnormal coordination of muscle contraction in MDI. The result is scapular dyskinesis, weakness, pain, and ultimately instability.

Nonoperative treatment, therefore, focuses on improving the coordination of the dynamic stabilizers to improve the

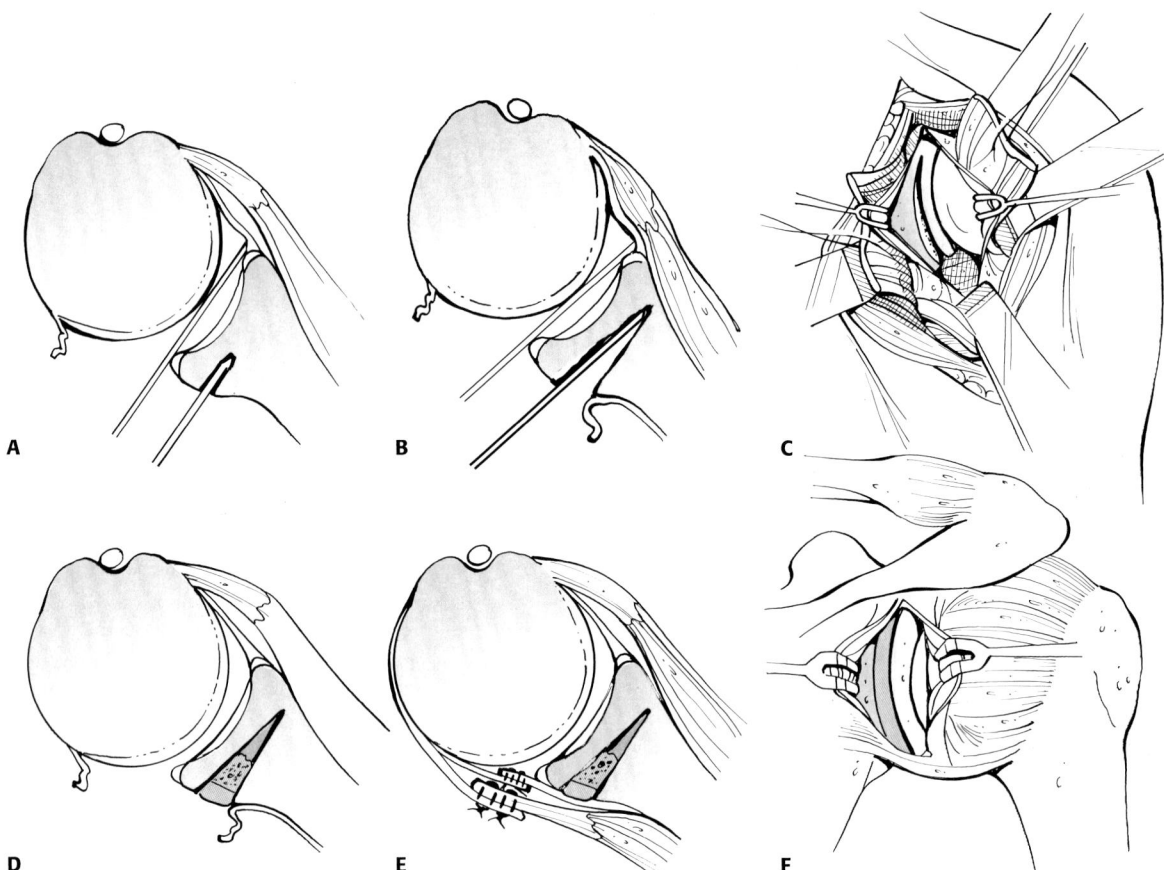

FIGURE 40-61 Posterior glenoid osteotomy. **A:** An osteotome is placed in the joint to use as a parallel guide. A second osteotome is then used to begin the osteotomy. **B:** The osteotome is advanced approximately 90% the distance across the glenoid, being sure to leave an anterior hinge of bone. **C:** The osteotome is removed. **D:** The osteotomy is then bone grafted to maintain the desired change in version. **E:** The posterior capsule and infraspinatus are repaired. **F:** Note the change in version which is maintained by the bone graft.

scapulothoracic motion, to strengthen the rotator cuff, and to improve the glenohumeral proprioception. All patients diagnosed with MDI should have a physical therapy program for a minimum of 6 months before surgical intervention is considered. There is generally no contraindication to this strategy.

Outcomes. A number of studies have shown good success with a strengthening protocol for MDI. Burkhead and Rockwood,[46] for instance, found that 80% of patients with atraumatic shoulder instability were successfully treated with a specific set of exercises to strengthen the shoulder musculature. Patients with a traumatic etiology, however, fared poorly with rehabilitation. This and other studies indicate that patients who do respond to therapy, demonstrated improvements within 3 months.[226]

On the other hand, a recent study by Misamore et al.[226] found that the long-term outcomes of young athletic patients with MDI treated with rehabilitation was poor: more than half did not respond. Therefore, if physical rehabilitation does not provide adequate improvement, patients often require surgical repair, specifically with an inferior capsular shift procedure.[12,59]

Operative Treatment

Indications and Contraindications. The nuances in establishing a clear diagnosis of MDI has contributed to the lack of consensus for the indications of surgical management. Much of this difficulty comes from the fact that patients may have a primary element of instability in one, two, or all three directions (inferior, posterior, or anterior). The treatment corresponds with the pathology.

Most surgeons do agree, however, that the primary treatment for patients with atraumatic MDI instability should be nonoperative with a shoulder rehabilitation program. Operative treatment is indicated only with failure of this program after 6 months or the rare acute traumatic form of MDI. Psychogenic instability (i.e., habitual dislocators) is a contraindication for surgery as well as patients who have demonstrated noncompliant behavior with the requisite nonoperative treatment. Some surgeons feel Ehlers–Danlos or other connective tissue disease is a relative contraindication with a high surgical failure rate. Allograft tissue should be considered to supplement the repair, if performed (Table 40-31).

TABLE 40-31 Multidirectional Instability

Operative Treatment

Indications	Contraindications
Failed nonoperative structured rehabilitation program after 6 mos	Psychogenic instability
Acute traumatic MDI with pan-labral pathology	Inability to comply with post-operative therapy Connective tissue disorder unless repair is augmented with allograft

Pitfalls and Solutions (Table 40-32)

TABLE 40-32 Anterior Approach for Inferior Capsulorrhaphy

Potential Pitfalls and Solutions

Pitfalls	Solutions
Axillary nerve injury	Identification of the nerve Protection with blunt retractors prior to capsulotomy
Inadequate inferior release	Release inferior subscapularis if exposure is inadequate Release to the posterior-inferior quadrant
Subscapularis failure	Attempt to preserve inferior tendon Release at the tendon and not near the muscular–tendon junction
Posterior instability	Repair with 30 degrees of abduction and external rotation
Missed labral tears	Examine inside the joint

Open Capsulorrhaphy. Once the decision for an operative stabilization has been established, the procedure may be performed arthroscopically or as an open procedure. Often referred to as an "inferior capsular shift," the procedure is designed to reduce the capsular volume on the side of the greatest instability as well as inferiorly and the opposite side. Therefore, open procedures are performed from either an anterior or posterior approach based on the pathology. Some surgeons preferentially utilize an anterior approach, because the capsule is thicker and it allows access to the rotator interval for further imbrication if necessary.

The "gold standard" for surgical management of MDI instability has been open stabilization, though this is rapidly changing with improved arthroscopic skill and techniques.

Deciding on a primary anterior or posterior approach (and capsulorrhaphy) is difficult. This decision should be based on the direction of greatest instability as ascertained from the history and physical examination. The examination with the patient under anesthesia can also provide insight, though, this rarely changes the operative approach.

Surgical Planning and Technique. Both the open anterior and posterior capsular shift techniques have been described above in detail. The key for both these procedures in the treatment of MDI is the placement of the vertical capsular incision. We prefer a humeral based incision for both the anterior and posterior shifts because we feel inferior redundancy is best eliminated with this technique.

Postoperative Care. Postoperative rehabilitation is slower for patients with MDI. Following surgical stabilization, the involved shoulder is immobilized in a sling for approximately 6 weeks. Passive motion is instituted at 4 weeks after the surgery. The limits of motion may vary depending on the stability of the repair. Shortly after the procedure, however, flexion, and external rotation are typically limited to 90 and 30 degrees, respectively. These limits are gradually increased to gain near full motion by 8 to 10 weeks. Upon removal of immobilization, active motion is instituted. Active strengthening exercises may be started by 10 to 12 weeks after the procedure. Patients are typically allowed full use of their shoulder by 6 months after the procedure; however, participation in high-demand activities and contact sports is deferred for at least 9 months in most patients.

Outcomes. There are a few reports describing the outcome of surgical treatment of MDI and they are inherently confounded by the lack of consensus on a definition and the variability of patient inclusion. Nonetheless, the few published reports show a high level of satisfaction and limited recurrence for open anterior stabilizations. Biomechanical analysis of the inferior capsular shift demonstrated near normal glenohumeral mechanics and contact pressures implying a low risk of long-term arthrosis.[351]

Neer and Foster reported good or excellent results in 78% of their 40 patients, with only one patient developing recurrent instability. Several subsequent studies have reported comparable findings with good-to-excellent results in over 90% of patients and recurrent instability in less than 10%.[12,59] Importantly, when the procedure is performed in a revision setting, the outcomes are less impressive.

Other studies utilized either an anterior or posterior approach based on the primary degree of instability. The results of these methods are equally satisfactory with good-to-excellent results in 85% to 94% of the patients,[54,117,207,269,334] with the rate of recurrent instability relatively low in two studies (4% to 9%). One study, however, reported recurrent instability in 26% of the patients, but with most of the failures occurring early—potentially pointing to a technical issue.[117]

Arthroscopic Capsulorrhaphy. Arthroscopic treatment of MDI has the advantage of evaluating the entire joint for other pathology and for having access to both the anterior and posterior sides. In addition, less trauma is created to the surrounding tissue. However, some have argued that a less extensive shift is possible arthroscopically because the technique is typically glenoid based where there is less tissue to mobilize compared to the humeral-based open shift.

Preoperative Planning (Table 40-33)

TABLE 40-33	Arthroscopic Capsulorrhaphy for MDI

Preoperative Planning

- Same as the arthroscopic setup described above for a posterior capsulorrhaphy
- Small glenoid anchors (2.4–3.0 mm)
- Both 5 and 8 mm cannulas will be used. The large cannula is needed for passage of a suture-passing device

Positioning. Either the lateral or beach-chair position can be used.

Technique. An examination under anesthesia should be performed to confirm the diagnosis and primary direction of instability. A diagnostic arthroscopy begins with a standard posterior portal. Pathology should be identified with specific attention paid to laxity and the quality of tissue of the inferior pouch, the rotator interval, the labrum and both the anterior and posterior capsules both on the glenoid and humeral sides. The posterior capsule can be extremely thin and difficult to effectively mobilize. Most patients with atraumatic MDI do not have a capsulolabral detachment, but this pathology can sometimes be seen. The most common finding is the presence of redundant anterior, inferior, and posterior capsules.

Similar to the arthroscopic posterior capsulorrhaphy described above, the lax capsule is managed with plication sutures or bioabsorbable anchor placement. For arthroscopic capsulorrhaphy in the anterior region, the arthroscope is typically placed through a posterior portal whereas the instruments and the sutures are managed through anterior portals. In contrast, for posterior capsulorrhaphy, the arthroscope is placed through the anterior portal and the instruments and the sutures are managed through posterior portals.

The capsulorrhaphy is performed with a curved suture passer that is passed through the full thickness of the capsule at the 6 o'clock position. A second pass is made under to the labrum to create a "pleat." A monofilament suture is placed and can be used as a tie or shuttle for a #2 nonabsorbable braided suture. The suture is tied with the knot away from the glenoid with the goal to decrease the capsular redundancy. It is important for the first stitch and its subsequent superior shift to be adequate to reduce the inferior laxity. It is difficult to correct capsular laxity if this shift is inadequate (Fig. 40-62).

The steps are repeated superiorly along the anterior and posterior capsules until the redundant capsule is sufficiently reduced and tightened. If the posterior capsule is thin, the infraspinatus can be incorporated. This can be done by passing a spinal needle through the tendon and passing a suture or suture shuttle to be retrieved by the suture passer placed through the capsule. The cannula is pulled back out of the joint into the subacromial space. A crochet hook is then placed through the cannula to blindly grab the suture passed through the tendon. The suture is then tied blindly in the subacromial space and the amount of capsular tightening is viewed inside the joint.

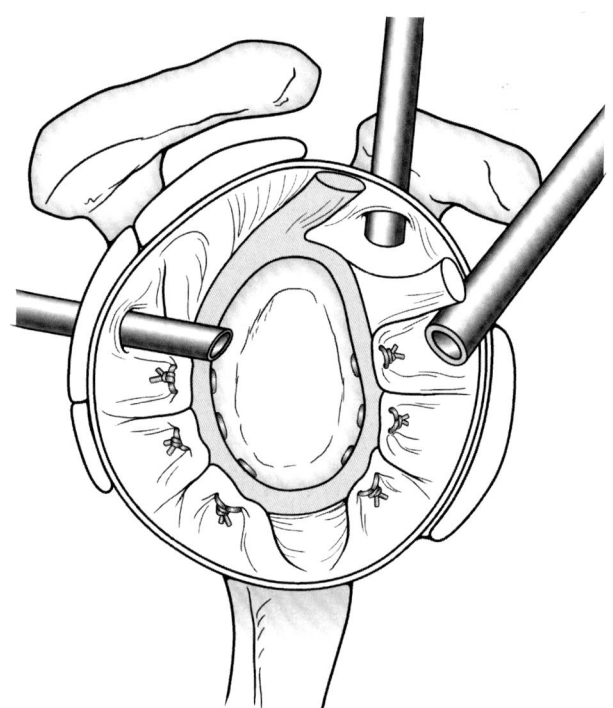

FIGURE 40-62 Diagram showing anterior and posterior arthroscopic glenoid-based capsulorrhaphy for MDI.

Rotator interval closure may be added to capsular plication in the setting of MDI instability to further limit humeral head translation. The technique is described above in the arthroscopic posterior capsulorrhaphy section (Fig. 40-60).

Postoperative Care. The postoperative protocol is similar to the open repair, but is individualized based on the primary direction of instability. If the primary laxity and repair is anterior, the protocol for the open anterior approach for MDI is used. Otherwise the posterior instability protocol is used with a custom orthosis in neutral rotation.

Pitfalls and Solutions (Table 40-34)

TABLE 40-34	Arthroscopic Capsulorrhaphy for MDI

Potential Pitfalls and Solutions

Pitfalls	Solutions
Thin posterior capsule	Incorporate infraspinatus tendon Use a bioabsorable anchor
Inadequate inferior exposure	Lateral position facilitates this exposure
Inadequate shift	A large initial superior shift at the 6 o'clock position is key

Outcomes. Only short-term follow-up studies are available for arthroscopic repair techniques.[89,90,213,345] Nonetheless, the results are very good and appear comparable to open repairs.

Treacy and Savoie had 88% good-to-excellent results and 12% recurrent instability using the suture technique described above.[345] Similarly, Gartsman et al. reported good-to-excellent results in 94% of patients with 35 months of follow-up.[90] These and other reports confirm this success rate with a recurrent instability generally less than 10%.[13,175]

COMPLICATIONS OF GLENOHUMERAL INSTABILITY (TABLE 40-35)

TABLE 40-35 Glenohumeral Instability
Complications
Incorrect diagnosis
Infection
Nerve injury
Hardware complications
Recurrence of instability
Loss of motion
Capsulorrhaphy arthropathy
Subscapularis failure

Incorrect Diagnosis of Glenohumeral Instability

Based on the literature, approximately 90% of instability is traumatic in the anterior direction.[254,324,374] Therefore, few surgeons will encounter atraumatic anterior, MDI or posterior instability regularly. Recognition of these often subtle presentations requires an understanding of the evolving theories explaining or classifying these diagnoses. For example, Hawkins and Hawkins reported on a small series of 46 patients in their referral practice with continuing difficulty after anterior instability procedures. They determine that 12 patients had unrecognized MDI or posterior instability.[123] Other reports have found similar findings.[211]

Other traumatic pathologies may also be missed leading to the incorrect procedure. Commonly missed pathologies include HAGL lesions,[367] rotator interval defects, residual capsular laxity, and bone loss for both the glenoid and humeral head.[44,111,367] Though, relatively uncommon, failure to recognize these pathologies and to subsequently treat the patient simply with a Bankart-type repair would likely lead to continued instability.

Infection

Regardless of the specific surgical approach, infection is an uncommon complication following a shoulder stabilization procedure. Review of all anterior shoulder stabilizations performed at the Mayo Clinic between 1980 and 2001 identified only six infections.[333] Similarly, a review of the recent literature on arthroscopic shoulder stabilizations has demonstrated an infection rate less than 0.25%.[111,171,363]

Recent attention has been given to prevalence of infection with the bacteria *Proprionibacterium acnes*, which is normal skin flora prevalent in the axilla.[261] It has been noted to lead to both indolent and grossly symptomatic infections in both open and arthroscopic shoulder procedures.[155,184] Suspicion needs to be high to identify the infection with a combination of lab values, aspiration, and extended culture times (10 to 14 days). Certain skin preparations and antibiotics are also better in preventing the infection including chlorhexidine and clindamycin, respectively.[155,316]

Nerve Injuries

For arthroscopic procedures, nerve dysfunction of almost all major upper extremity nerves has been reported related to the traction or compression by the arm holder, fluid distention of the joint, and fluid extravasation. Direct nerve injury to the axillary or musculocutaneous nerve is exceedingly rare. Almost all nerve injuries are neurapraxias that resolve with time. In the modern literature, the incidence of neurologic dysfunction, mild or otherwise, has been reported to be approximately 3%.[90,102,326]

For open procedures, nerve dysfunction has been reported to be as high as 8.2% in 282 patients who underwent an open anterior stabilization surgery.[130] Though most are neurapraxias, it points to the increased risk open surgery incurs because of the proximity of both the musculocutaneous and the axillary nerves. The musculocutaneous nerve is likely to be injured because of excessive retraction on the conjoined tendon especially with a self-retaining retractor. With the Latarjet procedure, both the axillary and musculocutaneous nerves are exposed and must be protected by an anterior humeral neck retractor. Shah et al.[321] reported a 10% nerve injury rate with this procedure, though most injuries resolved. Injury to the axillary nerve can occur during dissection of the shoulder capsule in the anterior inferior quadrant of the glenoid. Though traction is often the culprit, direct injury to the axillary nerve has been reported, and the likelihood of a spontaneous recovery is low.[201] Last, with anterior bone grafting procedures, the suprascapular nerve can be injured on the posterior side of the glenoid with placement of screws. Injury can be avoided with low placement of the graft and the use of oscillation when drilling.[204]

Hardware Complications

Hardware complications can be seen with specific techniques such as the Latarjet (Fig. 40-63).[373] However, small glenoid suture anchors are universal and are used for open and arthroscopic procedures for all directions of instability. Generally few complications are reported, but a few points should be noted. Metallic suture anchors should not be used in the glenoid because of the risk of migration, prominence, and chondral injury. Bioabsorbable suture anchors decrease the risk of hardware-related complications, but foreign body reaction has been reported.[43] Attention to countersinking the anchors below subchondral bone, and not just the cartilage, is critical as chondral injury can still occur.

Recurrence of Instability

Anterior Instability

The recurrence of instability is one of the most common complications after any instability procedure. However, the incidence

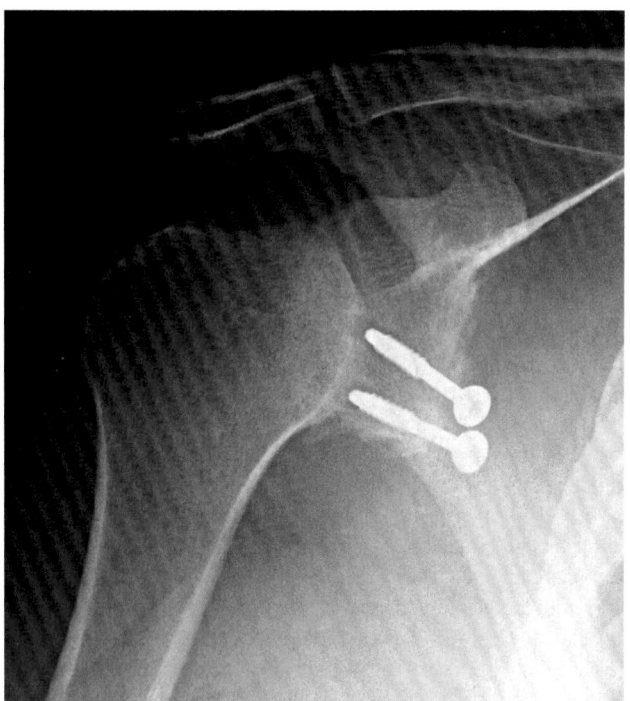

FIGURE 40-63 Failed Latarjet with loosening of the screws because of graft resorption and recurrent dislocation leading to humeral head erosion on the screw heads.

varies dramatically based on the technique and reasons for surgery. With modern techniques, the recurrence rates for both arthroscopic and open techniques are similar, ranging from 0% to 20%. Some believe open surgery still has a slightly lower rate of recurrence, especially with certain specific risk factors.

The reason for failure varies broadly to include inherent risk factors, incorrect diagnosis, incorrect surgical procedure or technical error, and unanticipated event such as repeat trauma.

Posterior Instability

Generally speaking, the results of posterior stabilization are inferior to those of anterior repair. The modern literature is promising and indicates a failure rate of about 0% to 23% with arthroscopic procedures having generally better results.[37,268,363,368] This can be attributed to a number of factors including a less clear diagnosis with significant overlap with MDI, the absence of an "essential" pathologic lesion to treat, and less experience by surgeons relative to anterior instability. Recurrence rates are certainly higher when previous surgery has been performed, but the common trend in the literature is failure to either address the inferior laxity or a deficient rotator interval.[275,281] Patients with posterior bone-block procedures have significantly worse outcomes with recurrence rates as high as 40%.[95,217]

Multidirectional Instability

The most recognized problem seen with MDI is the recurrence of instability; however, the rates for both open and arthroscopic repairs are acceptable. For open procedures, Neer and Foster, Pollock et al., and Bak et al. found a recurrence rate of

approximately 10% for open procedures.[12,233,269] Similarly, for arthroscopic procedures, a number of investigators have found satisfactory rates with comparable rates of recurrence.[90]

Loss of Motion

Open anatomic capsulolabral reconstruction procedures generally lead to a greater degree of stiffness than arthroscopic repairs.[75] Some of this stiffness is attributed to the relatively increased surgical trauma of open repairs as well as the increased ability to tighten the capsule. Stiffness for anterior arthroscopic repairs is reported to be 10% to 15% though the loss of motion is often less than 10 degrees, typically in external rotation.[75,106] Interestingly, the Latarjet procedure, though often considered motion limiting, does not lead to greater loss or motion compared to open Bankart repairs.[320]

Other common causes of stiffness following shoulder stabilization surgery include prolonged immobilization and poor compliance with the rehabilitation program. It is important to initiate a rehabilitation program that focuses on motion as soon as possible following the repair. The need for early motion, however, must be balanced against placing the underlying surgical construct at risk for failure. Three to four weeks of immobilization has been recommended by a number of investigations.[171,172]

Capsulorrhaphy Arthropathy

An overtightening of the anterior capsule leads to contracture and abnormal glenohumeral mechanics.[124] In turn, the altered mechanics lead to degenerative changes characterized by glenohumeral arthritis, eccentric posterior glenoid wear, or even posterior subluxation (Fig. 40-64). Most patients present late when advanced arthritic change necessitates an arthroplasty. Bigliani reported on a group of such patients who required arthroplasty at a mean of 16 years after their index instability surgery.[29] These arthroplasties are particularly difficult because of the internal rotation contractures from scarred anterior soft tissues and posterior glenoid wear. The outcomes for arthroplasty for capsulorrhaphy arthropathy, though good, are worse than for osteoarthritis and revisions are common given the younger age and active nature of the patients. In Bigliani's series 13 (77%) patients had satisfactory results, whereas 4 (33%) had poor results related to pain, limited motion, and subscapularis failure.

Subcapularis Failure

There is little or no risk of subscapularis failure in an arthroscopic repair as the tendinous insertion is not violated. However, in open procedures, the muscle and tendon are often taken down completely or are significantly violated. Sachs et al. reported on 30 patients with open Bankart repairs: Seven patients had an incompetent subscapularis with four having poor outcomes. Limiting early rehabilitation, especially external rotation, is key.[313] Management of a failed subscapularis is difficult as direct repair is often impossible. A pectoralis major muscle transfer can improve function, but there are some data that it might exacerbate instability as the direction of pull is relatively anterior compared to the normal subscapularis.[73]

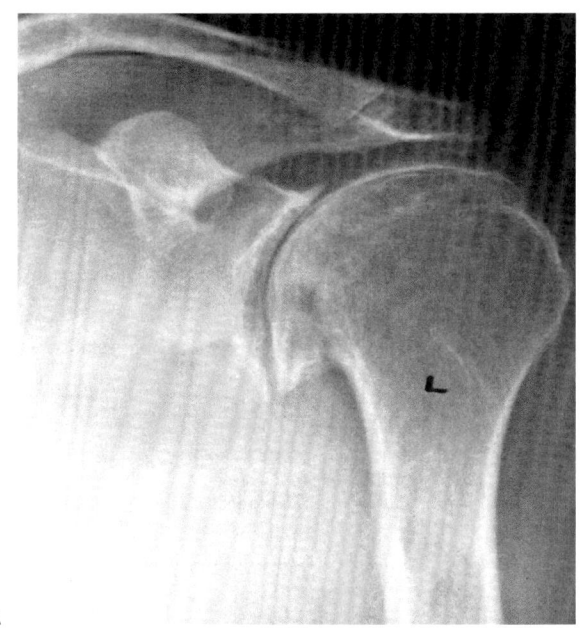
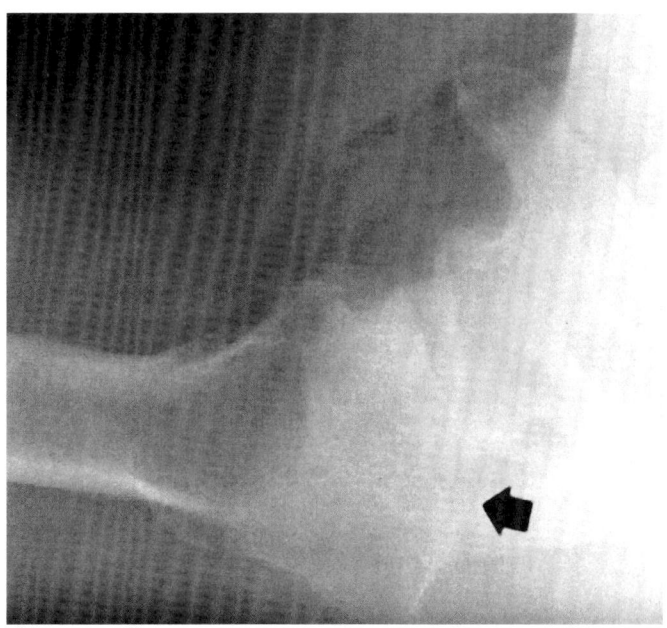

A

B

FIGURE 40-64 Capsulorrhaphy arthropathy after previous instability procedure. AP **(A)** and axillary **(B)** radiographs reveal large osteophytes and posterior subluxation with loss of joint space.

AUTHOR'S PREFERRED TREATMENT FOR GLENOHUMERAL INSTABILITY (FIGS. 40-65–40-67)

CONTROVERSIES AND FUTURE DIRECTIONS RELATED TO GLENOHUMERAL INSTABILITY

Treatment After Initial Traumatic Anterior Dislocation

We can currently treat glenohumeral instability arthroscopically with limited complications and low recurrence rates. Therefore, the optimal treatment of patients after an initial traumatic anterior dislocation is controversial. Early treatment from an acute injury is technically simpler when the tissue is pliable and acute tissue injury enhances healing. For patients with low rates of recurrent instability after an initial dislocation (such as older patients) (Table 40-2) the small risks of surgery may outweigh the benefits. Conversely, men less than 20 years of age with recurrence rates as high as 84% in the first 2 years may benefit from primary arthroscopic stabilization.[299,300]

A number of prospective observational studies and trials, as discussed above, have given us excellent data about the accurate risks of recurrent instability and complications for both operative and nonoperative treatment after primary traumatic anterior instability.[63,187,299,300] This data combined with decision-analysis modeling can help us decide the best treatment for individual patients based on their risk aversity. A recent article by Bishop et al.[30] looks at expected-value analysis to maximize patient outcome based on objective methods of determining patient values. They found that patients with a high rate of recurrent instability (i.e., young men) would benefit from stabilization after only one dislocation. Older patients and risk-averse patients would not.

Management of Bone Loss

Bone loss on both the glenoid and humeral side is increasingly recognized as a major contributor to recurrent instability and surgical treatment failure. Numerous methodologies of measuring glenoid bone loss have been created, but none are universal and the indications for treatment and the types of treatments have been evolving. There has been a renewed interest in bony procedures such as the Latarjet and even the use of allograft for both the glenoid and certain Hill–Sachs defects. However, there are a certain number of unknown questions that exist including:

1. When does a Hill–Sachs lesion need to be treated and how does glenoid bone loss effect this equation?

2. When is an open capsulorrhaphy indicated versus a bony procedure?

3. Given the high complication rates with a Latarjet, is there value in an initial arthroscopic approach for borderline cases or does this worsen outcomes if a bony procedure is subsequently performed?

4. Should the bone block be intra or extra-articular?

Many of these questions have preliminary answers, but none are fully elucidated.

The Role of Open Capsulorrhaphy

Last, I believe we are at an inflection point in terms of the techniques with which we treat instability. With the amazing arthroscopic skills of some, fewer surgeons performing open capsulorrhaphies, and a generation of new surgeons who may never have seen an open capsulorrhaphy, the way we manage instability is likely forever changed. The data seems to imply that arthroscopic procedures are as good or better than open

(*text continues on page 1566*)

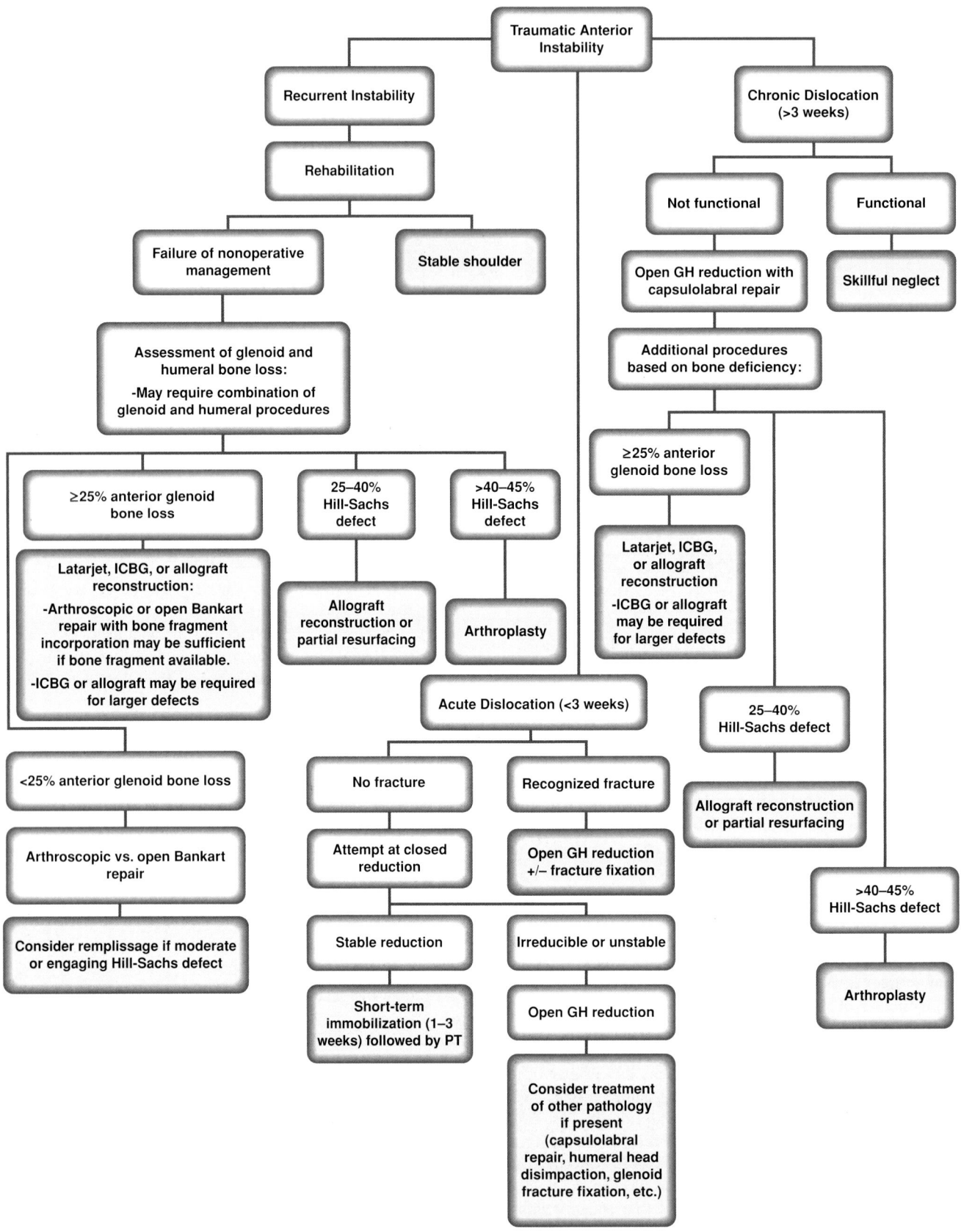

FIGURE 40-65 Anterior instability.

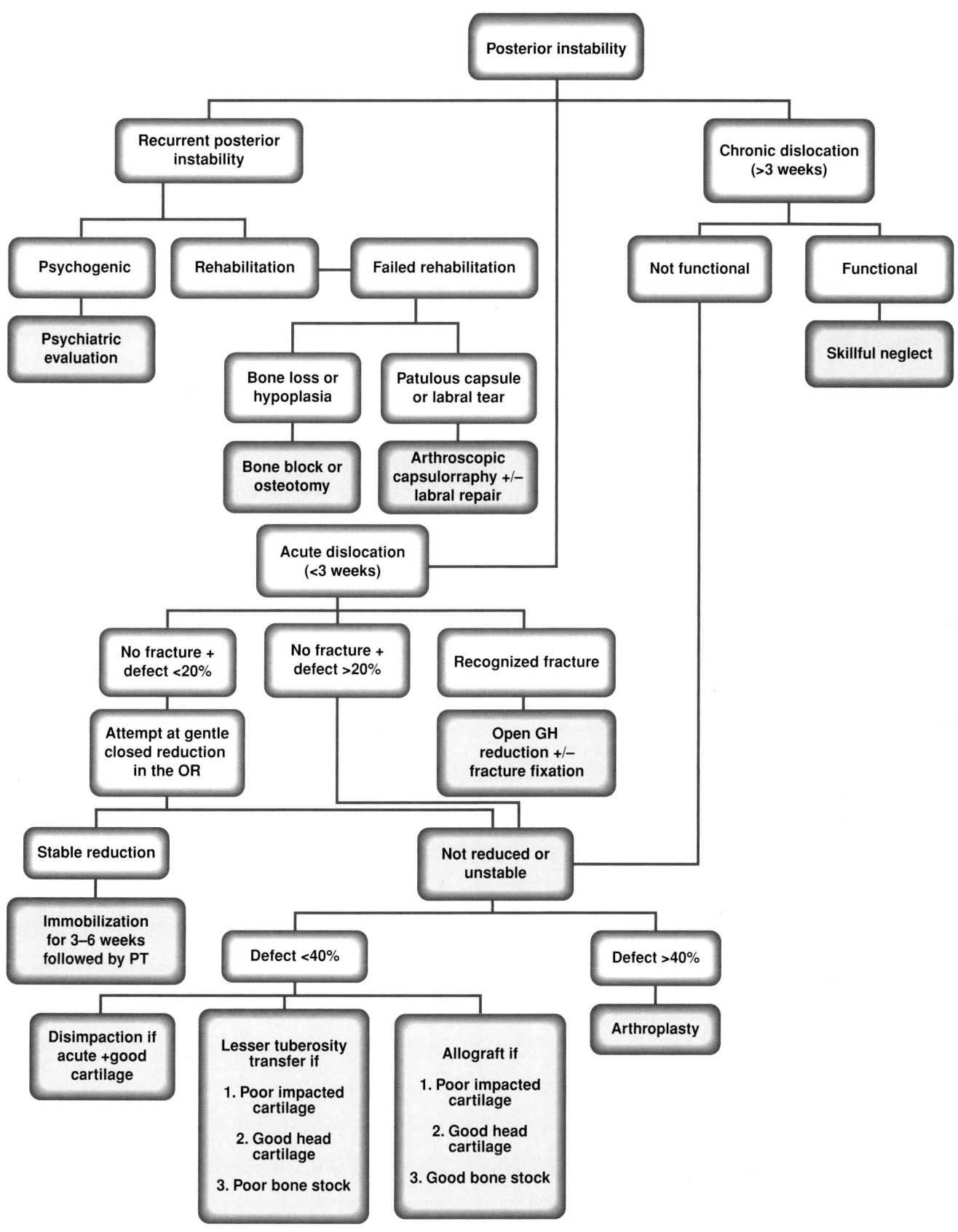

FIGURE 40-66 Posterior instability.

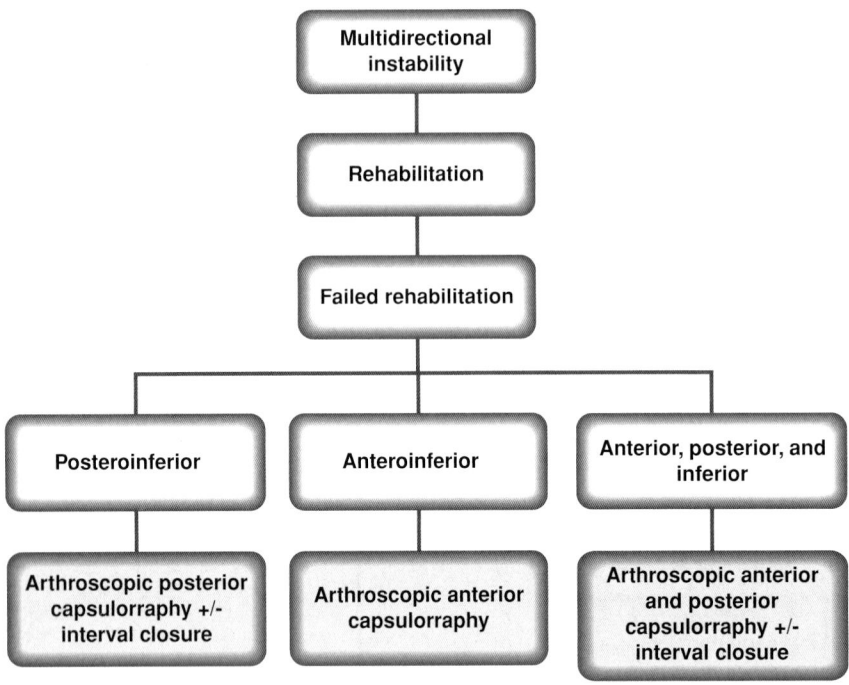

FIGURE 40-67 Multidirectional instability.

procedures for most cases. The risks are significantly lower as well. Besides open bony procedures, open capsulorraphies, much like Putti–Platt, will likely not be addressed significantly in future Rockwood editions to come. This may not be a good thing, but inevitable, nonetheless.

REFERENCES

1. Abboud JA, Soslowsky LJ. Interplay of the static and dynamic restraints in glenohumeral instability. *Clin Orthop Relat Res.* 2002;400:48–57.
2. Allain J, Goutallier D, Glorion C. Long-term results of the Latarjet procedure for the treatment of anterior instability of the shoulder. *J Bone Joint Surg Am.* 1998;80(6):841–852.
3. Altchek DW, Warren RF, Skyhar MJ, et al. T-plasty modification of the Bankart procedure for multidirectional instability of the anterior and inferior types. *J Bone Joint Surg Am.* 1991;73(1):105–112.
4. Amar E, Maman E, Khashan M, et al. Milch versus Stimson technique for nonsedated reduction of anterior shoulder dislocation: A prospective randomized trial and analysis of factors affecting success. *J Shoulder Elbow Surg.* 2012;21(11):1443–1449.
5. Amrami KK, Savcenko V, Dahm DL, et al. Radiologic Case Study. Reverse Bankart lesion with posterior labral tear. *Orthopedics.* 2002;25(7):720, 779–780.
6. Antal CS, Conforty B, Engelberg M, et al. Injuries to the axillary due to anterior dislocation of the shoulder. *J Trauma.* 1973;13(6):564–566.
7. Archetti Netto N, Tamaoki MJ, Lenza M, et al. Treatment of Bankart lesions in traumatic anterior instability of the shoulder: A randomized controlled trial comparing arthroscopy and open techniques. *Arthroscopy.* 2012;28(7):900–908.
8. Arciero RA, Mazzocca AD. Mini-open repair technique of HAGL (humeral avulsion of the glenohumeral ligament) lesion. *Arthroscopy.* 2005;21(9):1152.
9. Armitage MS, Faber KJ, Drosdowech DS, et al. Humeral head bone defects: Remplissage, allograft, and arthroplasty. *Orthop Clin North Am.* 2010;41(3):417–425.
10. Atoun E, Narvani A, Even T, et al. Management of first time dislocations of the shoulder in patients over 40 years of age: The prevalence of iatrogenic fracture. *J Orthop Trauma.* 2013;27(4):190–193.
11. Bahk MS, Karzel RP, Snyder SJ. Arthroscopic posterior stabilization and anterior capsular plication for recurrent posterior glenohumeral instability. *Arthroscopy.* 2010;26(9):1172–1180.
12. Bak K, Spring BJ, Henderson JP. Inferior capsular shift procedure in athletes with multidirectional instability based on isolated capsular and ligamentous redundancy. *Am J Sports Med.* 2000;28(4):466–471.
13. Baker CL 3rd, Mascarenhas R, Kline AJ, et al. Arthroscopic treatment of multidirectional shoulder instability in athletes: A retrospective analysis of 2- to 5-year clinical outcomes. *Am J Sports Med.* 2009;37(9):1712–1720.
14. Balg F, Boileau P. The instability severity index score. A simple pre-operative score to select patients for arthroscopic or open shoulder stabilisation. *J Bone Joint Surg Br.* 2007;89(11):1470–1477.
15. Bankart A. The pathology and treatment of recurrent dislocation of the shoulder joint. *Br J Surg.* 1938;26:23.
16. Barden JM, Balyk R, Raso VJ, et al. Dynamic upper limb proprioception in multidirectional shoulder instability. *Clin Orthop Relat Res.* 2004;420420:181–189.
17. Basmajian JV, Bazant FJ. Factors preventing downward dislocation of the adducted shoulder joint. An electromyographic and morphological study. *J Bone Joint Surg Am.* 1959;41-A:1182–1186.
18. Beighton P, Horan F. Orthopaedic aspects of the Ehlers–Danlos syndrome. *J Bone Joint Surg Br.* 1969;51(3):444–453.
19. Beran MC, Donaldson CT, Bishop JY. Treatment of chronic glenoid defects in the setting of recurrent anterior shoulder instability: A systematic review. *J Shoulder Elbow Surg.* 2010;19(5):769–780.
20. Bernageau J, Patte D, Debeyre J, et al. (Value of the glenoid profile in recurrent luxations of the shoulder). *Rev Chir Orthop Reparatrice Appar Mot.* 1976;62:142.
21. Bernageau J, Patte D, Debeyre J, et al. (Value of the glenoid profile in recurrent luxations of the shoulder). *Rev Chir Orthop Reparatrice Appar Mot.* 1976;62:142.
22. Bessems JH, Vegter J. Glenoplasty for recurrent posterior shoulder instability. Good results in 13 cases followed for 1-16 years. *Acta Orthop Scand.* 1995;66(6):535–537.
23. Bhatia DN, de Beer JF. The axillary pouch portal: A new posterior portal for visualization and instrumentation in the inferior glenohumeral recess. *Arthroscopy.* 2007;23(11):1241.e1,1241.e5.
24. Bhatia DN, DeBeer JF, van Rooyen KS. The "subscapularis-sparing" approach: A new mini-open technique to repair a humeral avulsion of the glenohumeral ligament lesion. *Arthroscopy.* 2009;25(6):686–690.
25. Bigliani LU, Kurzweil PR, Schwartzbach CC, et al. Inferior capsular shift procedure for anterior-inferior shoulder instability in athletes. *Am J Sports Med.* 1994;22(5):578–584.
26. Bigliani LU, Newton PM, Steinmann SP, et al. Glenoid rim lesions associated with recurrent anterior dislocation of the shoulder. *Am J Sports Med.* 1998;26(1):41–45.
27. Bigliani LU, Pollock RG, McIlveen SJ, et al. Shift of the posteroinferior aspect of the capsule for recurrent posterior glenohumeral instability. *J Bone Joint Surg Am.* 1995;77(7):1011–1020.
28. Bigliani LU, Pollock RG, Soslowsky LJ, et al. Tensile properties of the inferior glenohumeral ligament. *J Orthop Res.* 1992;10(2):187–197.
29. Bigliani LU, Weinstein DM, Glasgow MT, et al. Glenohumeral arthroplasty for arthritis after instability surgery. *J Shoulder Elbow Surg.* 1995;4(2):87–94.
30. Blasier RB, Crall TS, Kocher MS. Operative versus nonoperative treatment after primary traumatic anterior glenohumeral dislocation: Expected-value decision analysis. *J Shoulder Elbow Surg.* 2011;20(7):1087–1094.
31. Blasier RB, Carpenter JE, Huston LJ. Shoulder proprioception. Effect of joint laxity, joint position, and direction of motion. *Orthop Rev.* 1994;23(1):45–50.
32. Blom S, Dahlback LO. Nerve injuries in dislocations of the shoulder joint and fractures of the neck of the humerus. A clinical and electromyographical study. *Acta Chir Scand.* 1970;136(6):461–466.
33. Bloom MH, Obata WG. Diagnosis of posterior dislocation of the shoulder with use of Velpeau axillary and angle-up roentgenographic views. *J Bone Joint Surg Am.* 1967;49(5):943–949.
34. Boileau P, O'Shea K, Vargas P, et al. Anatomical and functional results after arthroscopic Hill-Sachs remplissage. *J Bone Joint Surg Am.* 2012;94(7):618–626.

35. Boileau P, Villalba M, Hery JY, et al. Risk factors for recurrence of shoulder instability after arthroscopic Bankart repair. *J Bone Joint Surg Am.* 2006;88(8):1755–1763.
36. Bokor DJ, Conboy VB, Olson C. Anterior instability of the glenohumeral joint with humeral avulsion of the glenohumeral ligament. A review of 41 cases. *J Bone Joint Surg Br.* 1999;81(1):93–96.
37. Bottoni CR, Franks BR, Moore JH, et al. Operative stabilization of posterior shoulder instability. *Am J Sports Med.* 2005;33(7):996–1002.
38. Bottoni CR, Smith EL, Berkowitz MJ, et al. Arthroscopic versus open shoulder stabilization for recurrent anterior instability: A prospective randomized clinical trial. *Am J Sports Med.* 2006;34(11):1730–1737.
39. Bradley JP, Baker CL 3rd, Kline AJ, et al. Arthroscopic capsulolabral reconstruction for posterior instability of the shoulder: A prospective study of 100 shoulders. *Am J Sports Med.* 2006;34(7):1061–1071.
40. Bridle SH, Ferris BD. Irreducible acute anterior dislocation of the shoulder: Interposed scapularis. *J Bone Joint Surg Br.* 1990;72(6):1078–1079.
41. Brox JI, Finnanger AM, Merckoll E, et al. Satisfactory long-term results after Eden-Hybbinette-Alvik operation for recurrent anterior dislocation of the shoulder: 6–20 years' follow-up of 52 patients. *Acta Orthop Scand.* 2003;74(2):180–185.
42. Bui-Mansfield LT, Banks KP, Taylor DC. Humeral avulsion of the glenohumeral ligaments: The HAGL lesion. *Am J Sports Med.* 2007;35(11):1960–1966.
43. Burkart A, Imhoff AB, Roscher E. Foreign-body reaction to the bioabsorbable suretac device. *Arthroscopy.* 2000;16(1):91–95.
44. Burkhart SS, De Beer JF. Traumatic glenohumeral bone defects and their relationship to failure of arthroscopic Bankart repairs: Significance of the inverted-pear glenoid and the humeral engaging Hill-Sachs lesion. *Arthroscopy.* 2000;16(7):677–694.
45. Burkhart SS, De Beer JF, Barth JR, et al. Results of modified Latarjet reconstruction in patients with anteroinferior instability and significant bone loss. *Arthroscopy.* 2007;23(10):1033–1041.
46. Burkhead WZ Jr, Rockwood CA Jr. Treatment of instability of the shoulder with an exercise program. *J Bone Joint Surg Am.* 1992;74(6):890–896.
47. Calandra JJ, Baker CL, Uribe J. The incidence of Hill-Sachs lesions in initial anterior shoulder dislocations. *Arthroscopy.* 1989;5(4):254–257.
48. Carreira DS, Mazzocca AD, Oryhon J, et al. A prospective outcome evaluation of arthroscopic Bankart repairs: Minimum 2-year follow-up. *Am J Sports Med.* 2006;34(5):771–777.
49. Ceroni D, Sadri H, Leuenberger A. Anteroinferior shoulder dislocation: An auto-reduction method without analgesia. *J Orthop Trauma.* 1997;11(6):399–404.
50. Chandnani VP, Yeager TD, DeBerardino T, et al. Glenoid labral tears: Prospective evaluation with MRI imaging, MR arthrography, and CT arthrography. *AJR Am J Roentgenol.* 1993;161(6):1229–1235.
51. Checchia SL, Santos PD, Miyazaki AN. Surgical treatment of acute and chronic posterior fracture-dislocation of the shoulder. *J Shoulder Elbow Surg.* 1998;7(1):53–65.
52. Cheng SL, Mackay MB, Richards RR. Treatment of locked posterior fracture-dislocations of the shoulder by total shoulder arthroplasty. *J Shoulder Elbow Surg.* 1997;6(1):11–17.
53. Cheok CY, Mohamad JA, Ahmad TS. Pain relief for reduction of acute anterior shoulder dislocations: A prospective randomized study comparing intravenous sedation with intra-articular lidocaine. *J Orthop Trauma.* 2011;25(1):5–10.
54. Choi CH, Ogilvie-Harris DJ. Inferior capsular shift operation for multidirectional instability of the shoulder in players of contact sports. *Br J Sports Med.* 2002;36(4):290–294.
55. Churchill RS, Brems JJ, Kotschi H. Glenoid size, inclination, and version: An anatomic study. *J Shoulder Elbow Surg.* 2001;10(4):327–332.
56. Cicak N. Posterior dislocation of the shoulder. *J Bone Joint Surg Br.* 2004;86(3):324–332.
57. Connolly S, Ritchie D, Sinopidis C, et al. Irreducible anterior dislocation of the shoulder due to soft tissue interposition of subscapularis tendon. *Skeletal Radiol.* 2008;37(1):63–65.
58. Cooper DE, Arnoczky SP, O'Brien SJ, et al. Anatomy, histology, and vascularity of the glenoid labrum. An anatomical study. *J Bone Joint Surg Am.* 1992;74(1):46–52.
59. Cooper RA. The inferior capsular-shift procedure for multidirectional instability of the shoulder. 1992;74(10):1516–1521.
60. Davidson PA, Rivenburgh DW. The 7-o'clock posteroinferior portal for shoulder arthroscopy. *Am J Sports Med.* 2002;30(5):693–696.
61. Davidson PA, Tibone JE. Anterior-inferior (5 o'clock) portal for shoulder arthroscopy. *Arthroscopy.* 1995;11(5):519–525.
62. Dawson J, Fitzpatrick R, Carr A. The assessment of shoulder instability. The development and validation of a questionnaire. *J Bone Joint Surg Br.* 1999;81(3):420–426.
63. DeBerardino TM, Arciero RA, Taylor DC, et al. Prospective evaluation of arthroscopic stabilization of acute, initial anterior shoulder dislocations in young athletes. Two- to five-year follow-up. *Am J Sports Med.* 2001;29(5):586–592.
64. de Laat EA, Visser CP, Coene LN, et al. Nerve lesions in primary shoulder dislocations and humeral neck fractures. A prospective clinical and EMG study. *J Bone Joint Surg Br.* 1994;76(3):381–383.
65. Deutsch AA, Kroll DG. Decreased range of motion following arthroscopic remplissage. *Orthopedics.* 2008;31(5):492.
66. Dhinakharan SR, Ghosh A. Towards evidence based emergency medicine: Best BETs from the Manchester Royal Infirmary. Intra-articular lidocaine for acute anterior shoulder dislocation reduction. *Emerg Med J.* 2002;19(2):142–143.
67. Dias JJ, Mody BS, Finlay DB, et al. Recurrent anterior glenohumeral joint dislocation and torsion of the humerus. *Injury.* 1993;24(5):329–332.
68. Diklic ID, Ganic ZD, Blagojevic ZD, et al. Treatment of locked chronic posterior dislocation of the shoulder by reconstruction of the defect in the humeral head with an allograft. *J Bone Joint Surg Br.* 2010;92(1):71–76.
69. Downey EF Jr, Curtis DJ, Brower AC. Unusual dislocations of the shoulder. *AJR Am J Roentgenol.* 1983;140(6):1207–1210.
70. Duralde XA, Fogle EF. The success of closed reduction in acute locked posterior fracture-dislocations of the shoulder. *J Shoulder Elbow Surg.* 2006;15(6):701–706.
71. Eberson CP, Ng T, Green A. Contralateral intrathoracic displacement of the humeral head. A case report. *J Bone Joint Surg Am.* 2000;82(1):105–108.
72. Edelson JG. Localized glenoid hypoplasia. An anatomic variation of possible clinical significance. *Clin Orthop Relat Res.* 1995;321:189–195.
73. Elhassan B, Ozbaydar M, Massimini D, et al. Transfer of pectoralis major for the treatment of irreparable tears of subscapularis: Does it work? *J Bone Joint Surg Br.* 2008;90(8):1059–1065.
74. Emery RJ, Mullaji AB. Glenohumeral joint instability in normal adolescents. Incidence and significance. *J Bone Joint Surg Br.* 1991;73(3):406–408.
75. Fabbriciani C, Milano G, Demontis A, et al. Arthroscopic versus open treatment of Bankart lesion of the shoulder: A prospective randomized study. *Arthroscopy.* 2004;20(5):456–462.
76. Farber AJ, Castillo R, Clough M, et al. Clinical assessment of three common tests for traumatic anterior shoulder instability. *J Bone Joint Surg Am.* 2006;88(7):1467–1474.
77. Ferrari DA. Capsular ligaments of the shoulder. Anatomical and functional study of the anterior superior capsule. *Am J Sports Med.* 1990;18(1):20–24.
78. Field LD, Bokor DJ, Savoie FH 3rd. Humeral and glenoid detachment of the anterior inferior glenohumeral ligament: A cause of anterior shoulder instability. *J Shoulder Elbow Surg.* 1997;6(1):6–10.
79. Finkelstein JA, Waddell JP, O'Driscoll SW, et al. Acute posterior fracture dislocations of the shoulder treated with the Neer modification of the McLaughlin procedure. *J Orthop Trauma.* 1995;9(3):190–193.
80. Flatow EL, Miller SR, Neer CS 2nd. Chronic anterior dislocation of the shoulder. *J Shoulder Elbow Surg.* 1993;2(1):2–10.
81. Frank MA, Laratta JL, Tan V. Irreducible luxatio erecta humeri caused by an aberrant position of the axillary nerve. *J Shoulder Elbow Surg.* 2012;21(7):e6–e9.
82. Fronek J, Warren RF, Bowen M. Posterior subluxation of the glenohumeral joint. *J Bone Joint Surg Am.* 1989;71(2):205–216.
83. Fuchs B, Jost B, Gerber C. Posterior-inferior capsular shift for the treatment of recurrent, voluntary posterior subluxation of the shoulder. *J Bone Joint Surg Am.* 2000;82(1):16–25.
84. Gagey OJ, Gagey N. The hyperabduction test. *J Bone Joint Surg Br.* 2001;83(1):69–74.
85. Garnavos C. Technical note: Modifications and improvements of the Milch technique for the reduction of anterior dislocation of the shoulder without premedication. *J Trauma.* 1992;32(6):801–803.
86. Garrigues GE, Nagda SH, Yu J. Open luxatio erecta: A case report and literature review. *J Orthop Trauma.* 2011;25(4):e34–e37.
87. Garth WP Jr, Allman FL Jr, Armstrong WS. Occult anterior subluxations of the shoulder in noncontact sports. *Am J Sports Med.* 1987 Nov-Dec;15(6):579-85.
88. Garth WP Jr, Slappey CE, Ochs CW. Roentgenographic demonstration of instability of the shoulder: The apical oblique projection. A technical note. *J Bone Joint Surg Am.* 1984;66(9):1450–1453.
89. Gartsman GM, Roddey TS, Hammerman SM. Arthroscopic treatment of bidirectional glenohumeral instability: Two- to five-year follow-up. *J Shoulder Elbow Surg.* 2001;10(1):28–36.
90. Gartsman GM, Roddey TS, Hammerman SM. Arthroscopic treatment of multidirectional glenohumeral instability: 2- to 5-year follow-up. *Arthroscopy.* 2001;17(3):236–243.
91. Gates JD, Knox JB. Axillary artery injuries secondary to anterior dislocation of the shoulder. *J Trauma.* 1995;39(3):581–583.
92. Gavriilidis I, Magosch P, Lichtenberg S, et al. Chronic locked posterior shoulder dislocation with severe head involvement. *Int Orthop.* 2010;34(1):79–84.
93. George MS, Khazzam M, Kuhn JE. Humeral avulsion of glenohumeral ligaments. *J Am Acad Orthop Surg.* 2011;19(3):127–133.
94. Gerber C, Ganz R. Clinical assessment of instability of the shoulder. With special reference to anterior and posterior drawer tests. *J Bone Joint Surg Br.* 1984;66(4):551–556.
95. Gerber C, Ganz R, Vinh TS. Glenoplasty for recurrent posterior shoulder instability. An anatomic reappraisal. *Clin Orthop Relat Res.* 1987;216:70–79.
96. Gerber C, Lambert SM. Allograft reconstruction of segmental defects of the humeral head for the treatment of chronic locked posterior dislocation of the shoulder. *J Bone Joint Surg Am.* 1996;78(3):376–382.
97. Gerber C, Nyffeler RW. Classification of glenohumeral joint instability. *Clin Orthop Relat Res.* 2002;400:65–76.
98. Gerber C. Chronic, Locked Anterior, and Posterior Dislocations. In: Warner JJ, Iannotti JP, Flatow EL, eds. *Complex and Revision Problems in Shoulder Surgery.* 2nd ed. Philadelphia, PA: Lippincott Williams & Wilkins; 2005. p. 89-103.
99. Gibb TD, Sidles JA, Harryman DT 2nd, et al. The effect of capsular venting on glenohumeral laxity. *Clin Orthop Relat Res.* 1991;268:120–127.
100. Glousman R, Jobe F, Tibone J, et al. Dynamic electromyographic analysis of the throwing shoulder with glenohumeral instability. *J Bone Joint Surg Am.* 1988;70(2):220–226.
101. Goga IE. Chronic shoulder dislocations. *J Shoulder Elbow Surg.* 2003;12(5):446–450.
102. Goubier JN, Iserin A, Duranthon LD, et al. A 4-portal arthroscopic stabilization in posterior shoulder instability. *J Shoulder Elbow Surg.* 2003;12(4):337–341.
103. Graichen H, Koydl P, Zichner L. Effectiveness of glenoid osteotomy in atraumatic posterior instability of the shoulder associated with excessive retroversion and flatness of the glenoid. *Int Orthop.* 1999;23(2):95–99.
104. Grashey R. *Atlas Typischer Rontgenfilder.* Munich: Lehman; 1923.
105. Grasshoff H, Buhtz C, Gellerich I, et al. CT diagnosis in instability of the shoulder joint. *Rofo.* 1991;155(6):523–526.
106. Green MR, Christensen KP. Arthroscopic versus open Bankart procedures: A comparison of early morbidity and complications. *Arthroscopy.* 1993;9(4):371–374.
107. Greis PE, Scuderi MG, Mohr A, et al. Glenohumeral articular contact areas and pressures following labral and osseous injury to the anteroinferior quadrant of the glenoid. *J Shoulder Elbow Surg.* 2002;11(5):442–451.
108. Griesser MJ, Harris JD, McCoy BW, et al. Complications and re-operations after Bristow-Latarjet shoulder stabilization: A systematic review. *J Shoulder Elbow Surg.* 2013;22(2):286–292.
109. Groh GI, Wirth MA, Rockwood CA Jr. Results of treatment of luxatio erecta (inferior shoulder dislocation). *J Shoulder Elbow Surg.* 2010;19(3):423–426.
110. Grondin P, Leith J. Case series: Combined large Hill-Sachs and bony Bankart lesions treated by Latarjet and partial humeral head resurfacing: A report of 2 cases. *Can J Surg.* 2009;52(3):249–254.

111. Guanche CA, Quick DC, Sodergren KM, et al. Arthroscopic versus open reconstruction of the shoulder in patients with isolated Bankart lesions. *Am J Sports Med.* 1996;24(2):144–148.
112. Guha AR, Jago ER. Irreducible acute anterior shoulder dislocation. *Int J Clin Pract.* 2004;58(12):1184–1186.
113. Haaker RG, Eickhoff U, Klammer HL. Intraarticular autogenous bone grafting in recurrent shoulder dislocations. *Mil Med.* 1993;158(3):164–169.
114. Habermeyer P, Schuller U, Wiedemann E. The intra-articular pressure of the shoulder: An experimental study on the role of the glenoid labrum in stabilizing the joint. *Arthroscopy.* 1992;8(2):166–172.
115. Hall RH, Isaac F, Booth CR. Dislocations of the shoulder with special reference to accompanying small fractures. *J Bone Joint Surg Am.* 1959;41-A(3):489–494.
116. Hamada K, Fukuda H, Mikasa M, et al. Roentgenographic findings in massive rotator cuff tears. A long-term observation. *Clin Orthop Relat Res.* 1990;254:92–96.
117. Hamada K, Fukuda H, Nakajima T, et al. The inferior capsular shift operation for instability of the shoulder. Long-term results in 34 shoulders. *J Bone Joint Surg Br.* 1999;81(2):218–225.
118. Harryman DT 2nd, Sidles JA, Clark JM, et al. Translation of the humeral head on the glenoid with passive glenohumeral motion. *J Bone Joint Surg Am.* 1990;72(9):1334–1343.
119. Harryman DT, Sidles JA, Harris SL, et al. The effect of articular conformity and the size of the humeral head component on laxity and motion after glenohumeral arthroplasty. A study in cadavera. *J Bone Joint Surg Am.* 1995;77(4):555–563.
120. Harryman DT 2nd, Sidles JA, Harris SL, et al. The role of the rotator interval capsule in passive motion and stability of the shoulder. *J Bone Joint Surg Am.* 1992;74(1):53–66.
121. Haviv B, Mayo L, Biggs D. Outcomes of arthroscopic "remplissage": Capsulotenodesis of the engaging large Hill-Sachs lesion. *J Orthop Surg Res.* 2011;6:29.
122. Hawkins RH. Glenoid osteotomy for recurrent posterior subluxation of the shoulder: Assessment by computed axial tomography. *J Shoulder Elbow Surg.* 1996;5(5):393–400.
123. Hawkins RH, Hawkins RJ. Failed anterior reconstruction for shoulder instability. *J Bone Joint Surg Br.* 1985;67(5):709–714.
124. Hawkins RJ, Angelo RL. Glenohumeral osteoarthrosis. A late complication of the Putti-Platt repair. *J Bone Joint Surg Am.* 1990;72(8):1193–1197.
125. Hawkins RJ, Janda DH. Posterior instability of the glenohumeral joint. A technique of repair. *Am J Sports Med.* 1996;24(3):275–278.
126. Hawkins RJ, Neer CS 2nd, Pianta RM, et al. Locked posterior dislocation of the shoulder. *J Bone Joint Surg Am.* 1987;69(1):9–18.
127. Henry JH, Genung JA. Natural history of glenohumeral dislocation–revisited. *Am J Sports Med.* 1982;10(3):135–137.
128. Hippocrates. Injuries of the shoulder. Dislocations. *Clin Orthop Relat Res.* 1989;246:4–7.
129. Hirschfelder H, Kirsten U. Biometric analysis of the unstable shoulder. *Z Orthop Ihre Grenzgeb.* 1991;129(6):516–520.
130. Ho E, Cofield RH, Balm MR, et al. Neurologic complications of surgery for anterior shoulder instability. *J Shoulder Elbow Surg.* 1999;8(3):266–270.
131. Hovelius L. Anterior dislocation of the shoulder in teen-agers and young adults. Five-year prognosis. *J Bone Joint Surg Am.* 1987;69(3):393–399.
132. Hovelius L, Augustini BG, Fredin H, et al. Primary anterior dislocation of the shoulder in young patients. A ten-year prospective study. *J Bone Joint Surg Am.* 1996;78(11):1677–1684.
133. Hovelius L, Olofsson A, Sandstrom B, et al. Nonoperative treatment of primary anterior shoulder dislocation in patients forty years of age and younger. a prospective twenty-five-year follow-up. *J Bone Joint Surg Am.* 2008;90(5):945–952.
134. Hovelius L, Sandstrom B, Olofsson A, et al. The effect of capsular repair, bone block healing, and position on the results of the Bristow-Latarjet procedure (study III): Long-term follow-up in 319 shoulders. *J Shoulder Elbow Surg.* 2012;21(5):647–660.
135. Hovelius L, Sandstrom B, Saebo M. One hundred eighteen Bristow-Latarjet repairs for recurrent anterior dislocation of the shoulder prospectively followed for fifteen years: Study II-the evolution of dislocation arthropathy. *J Shoulder Elbow Surg.* 2006;15(3):279–289.
136. Hovelius L, Sandstrom B, Sundgren K, et al. One hundred eighteen Bristow-Latarjet repairs for recurrent anterior dislocation of the shoulder prospectively followed for fifteen years: Study I–clinical results. *J Shoulder Elbow Surg.* 2004;13(5):509–516.
137. Hovelius L, Thorling J, Fredin H. Recurrent anterior dislocation of the shoulder. Results after the Bankart and Putti-Platt operations. *J Bone Joint Surg Am.* 1979;61(4):566–569.
138. Hovelius L, Vikerfors O, Olofsson A, et al. Bristow-Latarjet and Bankart: A comparative study of shoulder stabilization in 185 shoulders during a seventeen-year follow-up. *J Shoulder Elbow Surg.* 2011;20(7):1095–1101.
139. Hovelius LK, Sandstrom BC, Rosmark DL, et al. Long-term results with the Bankart and Bristow-Latarjet procedures: Recurrent shoulder instability and arthropathy. *J Shoulder Elbow Surg.* 2001;10(5):445–452.
140. Howell SM, Kraft TA. The role of the supraspinatus and infraspinatus muscles in glenohumeral kinematics of anterior should instability. *Clin Orthop Relat Res.* 1991;263:128–134.
141. Huysmans PE, Haen PS, Kidd M, et al. The shape of the inferior part of the glenoid: A cadaveric study. *J Shoulder Elbow Surg.* 2006;15(6):759–763.
142. Iannotti JP, Gabriel JP, Schneck SL, et al. The normal glenohumeral relationships. An anatomical study of one hundred and forty shoulders. *J Bone Joint Surg Am.* 1992;74(4):491–500.
143. Iannotti JP, Williams GR. *Disorders of the shoulder: Diagnosis & management.* 2nd ed. Philadelphia, PA: Lippincott Williams & Wilkins; 2007.
144. Inao S, Hirayama T, Takemitsu Y. Irreducible acute anterior dislocation of the shoulder: Interposed bicipital tendon. *J Bone Joint Surg Br.* 1990;72(6):1079–1080.
145. Inokuchi W, Sanderhoff Olsen B, Sojbjerg JO, et al. The relation between the position of the glenohumeral joint and the intraarticular pressure: An experimental study. *J Shoulder Elbow Surg.* 1997;6(2):144–149.
146. Itoi E, Hatakeyama Y, Sato T, et al. Immobilization in external rotation after shoulder dislocation reduces the risk of recurrence. A randomized controlled trial. *J Bone Joint Surg Am.* 2007;89(10):2124–2131.
147. Itoi E, Kuechle DK, Newman SR, et al. Stabilising function of the biceps in stable and unstable shoulders. *J Bone Joint Surg Br.* 1993;75(4):546–550.
148. Itoi E, Lee SB, Amrami KK, et al. Quantitative assessment of classic anteroinferior bony Bankart lesions by radiography and computed tomography. *Am J Sports Med.* 2003;31(1):112–118.
149. Itoi E, Lee SB, Berglund LJ, et al. The effect of a glenoid defect on anteroinferior stability of the shoulder after Bankart repair: A cadaveric study. *J Bone Joint Surg Am.* 2000;82(1):35–46.
150. Itoi E, Motzkin NE, Morrey BF, et al. Bulk effect of rotator cuff on inferior glenohumeral stability as function of scapular inclination angle: A cadaver study. *Tohoku J Exp Med.* 1993;171(4):267–276.
151. Itoi E, Motzkin NE, Morrey BF, et al. The static rotator cuff does not affect inferior translation of the humerus at the glenohumeral joint. *J Trauma.* 1999;47(1):55–59.
152. Itoi E, Newman SR, Kuechle DK, et al. Dynamic anterior stabilisers of the shoulder with the arm in abduction. *J Bone Joint Surg Br.* 1994;76(5):834–836.
153. Itoi E, Sashi R, Minagawa H, et al. Position of immobilization after dislocation of the glenohumeral joint. A study with use of magnetic resonance imaging. *J Bone Joint Surg Am.* 2001;83-A(5):661–667.
154. Jankauskas L, Rudiger HA, Pfirrmann CW, et al. Loss of the sclerotic line of the glenoid on anteroposterior radiographs of the shoulder: A diagnostic sign for an osseous defect of the anterior glenoid rim. *J Shoulder Elbow Surg.* 2010;19(1):151–156.
155. Jawa A, Shi L, O'Brien T, et al. Prosthesis of antibiotic-loaded acrylic cement (PROSTALAC) use for the treatment of infection after shoulder arthroplasty. *J Bone Joint Surg Am.* 2011;93(21):2001–2009.
156. Jia X, Petersen SA, Khosravi AH, et al. Examination of the shoulder: The past, the present, and the future. *J Bone Joint Surg Am.* 2009;91(suppl 6):10–18.
157. Jobe FW, Giangarra CE, Kvitne RS, et al. Anterior capsulolabral reconstruction of the shoulder in athletes in overhand sports. *Am J Sports Med.* 1991;19(5):428–434.
158. Jobe FW, Kvitne RS, Giangarra CE. Shoulder pain in the overhand or throwing athlete. The relationship of anterior instability and rotator cuff impingement. *Orthop Rev.* 1989;18(9):963–975.
159. Jolles BM, Pelet S, Farron A. Traumatic recurrent anterior dislocation of the shoulder: Two- to four-year follow-up of an anatomic open procedure. *J Shoulder Elbow Surg.* 2004;13(1):30–34.
160. Jones KJ, Wiesel B, Ganley TJ, et al. Functional outcomes of early arthroscopic bankart repair in adolescents aged 11 to 18 years. *J Pediatr Orthop.* 2007;27(2):209–213.
161. Jost B, Koch PP, Gerber C. Anatomy and functional aspects of the rotator interval. *J Shoulder Elbow Surg.* 2000;9(4):336–341.
162. Jung JY, Yoon YC, Yi SK, et al. Comparison study of indirect MR arthrography and direct MR arthrography of the shoulder. *Skeletal Radiol.* 2009;38(7):659–667.
163. Karlsson J, Magnusson L, Ejerhed L, et al. Comparison of open and arthroscopic stabilization for recurrent shoulder dislocation in patients with a Bankart lesion. *Am J Sports Med.* 2001;29(5):538–542.
164. Kazar B, Relovszky E. Prognosis of primary dislocation of the shoulder. *Acta Orthop Scand.* 1969;40(2):216–224.
165. Kazel MD, Sekiya JK, Greene JA, et al. Percutaneous correction (humeroplasty) of humeral head defects (Hill-Sachs) associated with anterior shoulder instability: A cadaveric study. *Arthroscopy.* 2005;21(12):1473–1478.
166. Kelley SP, Hinsche AF, Hossain JF. Axillary artery transection following anterior shoulder dislocation: Classical presentation and current concepts. *Injury.* 2004;35(11):1128–1132.
167. Khayal T, Wild M, Windolf J. Reconstruction of the articular surface of the humeral head after locked posterior shoulder dislocation: A case report. *Arch Orthop Trauma Surg.* 2009;129(4):515–519.
168. Khazzam M, Kane SM, Smith MJ. Open shoulder stabilization procedure using bone block technique for treatment of chronic glenohumeral instability associated with bony glenoid deficiency. *Am J Orthop (Belle Mead NJ).* 2009;38(7):329–335.
169. Kido T, Itoi E, Konno N, et al. Electromyographic activities of the biceps during arm elevation in shoulders with rotator cuff tears. *Acta Orthop Scand.* 1998;69(6):575–579.
170. Kim DS, Yoon YS, Yi CH. Prevalence comparison of accompanying lesions between primary and recurrent anterior dislocation in the shoulder. *Am J Sports Med.* 2010;38(10):2071–2076.
171. Kim SH, Ha KI, Cho YB, et al. Arthroscopic anterior stabilization of the shoulder: Two to six-year follow-up. *J Bone Joint Surg Am.* 2003;85-A(8):1511–1518.
172. Kim SH, Ha KI, Jung MW, et al. Accelerated rehabilitation after arthroscopic Bankart repair for selected cases: A prospective randomized clinical study. *Arthroscopy.* 2003;19(7):722–731.
173. Kim SH, Ha KI, Kim SH. Bankart repair in traumatic anterior shoulder instability: Open versus arthroscopic technique. *Arthroscopy.* 2002;18(7):755–763.
174. Kim SH, Ha KI, Park JH, et al. Arthroscopic posterior labral repair and capsular shift for traumatic unidirectional recurrent posterior subluxation of the shoulder. *J Bone Joint Surg Am.* 2003;85-A(8):1479–1487.
175. Kim SH, Kim HK, Sun JI, et al. Arthroscopic capsulolabroplasty for posteroinferior multidirectional instability of the shoulder. *Am J Sports Med.* 2004;32(3):594–607.
176. Kim SH, Park JC, Park JS, et al. Painful jerk test: A predictor of success in nonoperative treatment of posteroinferior instability of the shoulder. *Am J Sports Med.* 2004;32(8):1849–1855.
177. Kirker JR. Dislocation of the shoulder complicated by rupture of the axillary vessels. *J Bone Joint Surg Br.* 1952;34-B(1):72–73.
178. Kirkley A, Griffin S, McLintock H, et al. The development and evaluation of a disease-specific quality of life measurement tool for shoulder instability. The Western Ontario Shoulder Instability Index (WOSI). *Am J Sports Med.* 1998;26(6):764–772.
179. Kiviluoto O, Pasila M, Jaroma H, et al. Immobilization after primary dislocation of the shoulder. *Acta Orthop Scand.* 1980;51(6):915–919.
180. Kon Y, Shiozaki H, Sugaya H. Arthroscopic repair of a humeral avulsion of the glenohumeral ligament lesion. *Arthroscopy.* 2005;21(5):632.

181. Konig DP, Rutt J, Treml O, et al. Osteoarthritis and recurrences after Putti-Platt and Eden-Hybbinette operations for recurrent dislocation of the shoulder. *Int Orthop.* 1997;21(2):72–76.

182. Koo SS, Burkhart SS, Ochoa E. Arthroscopic double-pulley remplissage technique for engaging Hill-Sachs lesions in anterior shoulder instability repairs. *Arthroscopy.* 2009;25(11):1343–1348.

183. Kroner K, Lind T, Jensen J. The epidemiology of shoulder dislocations. *Arch Orthop Trauma Surg.* 1989;108(5):288–290.

184. Kwon YW, Kalainov DM, Rose HA, et al. Management of early deep infection after rotator cuff repair surgery. *J Shoulder Elbow Surg.* 2005;14(1):1–5.

185. Kwon YW, Kulwicki KJ, Zuckerman JD. Glenohumeral Joint Subluxations, Dislocations, and Instability. In: Bucholz RW, Heckman JD, Court-Brown CM, et al., eds. *Rockwood and Green's Fractures in Adults.* 7th ed. Philadelphia, PA: Lippincott Williams & Wilkins; 2010:1165–1209.

186. Labriola JE, Lee TQ, Debski RE, et al. Stability and instability of the glenohumeral joint: The role of shoulder muscles. *J Shoulder Elbow Surg.* 2005;14(1 suppl S):32S–38S.

187. Larrain MV, Botto GJ, Montenegro HJ, et al. Arthroscopic repair of acute traumatic anterior shoulder dislocation in young athletes. *Arthroscopy.* 2001;17(4):373–377.

188. Laurencin CT, Deutsch A, O'Brien SJ, et al. The superolateral portal for arthroscopy of the shoulder. *Arthroscopy.* 1994;10(3):255–258.

189. Law BK, Yung PS, Ho EP, et al. The surgical outcome of immediate arthroscopic Bankart repair for first time anterior shoulder dislocation in young active patients. *Knee Surg Sports Traumatol Arthrosc.* 2008;16(2):188–193.

190. Lazarus MD, Sidles JA, Harryman DT 2nd, et al. Effect of a chondral-labral defect on glenoid concavity and glenohumeral stability. A cadaveric model. *J Bone Joint Surg Am.* 1996;78(1):94–102.

191. Lecouvet FE, Simoni P, Koutaissoff S, et al. Multidetector spiral CT arthrography of the shoulder. Clinical applications and limits, with MR arthrography and arthroscopic correlations. *Eur J Radiol.* 2008;68(1):120–136.

192. Lee SB, Kim KJ, O'Driscoll SW, et al. Dynamic glenohumeral stability provided by the rotator cuff muscles in the mid-range and end-range of motion. A study in cadavera. *J Bone Joint Surg Am.* 2000;82(6):849–857.

193. Lenart BA, Sherman SL, Mall NA, et al. Arthroscopic repair for posterior shoulder instability. *Arthroscopy.* 2012;28(10):1337–1343.

194. Lev-El A, Adar R, Rubinstein Z. Axillary artery injury in erect dislocation of the shoulder. *J Trauma.* 1981;21(4):323–325.

195. Levick JR. Joint pressure-volume studies: Their importance, design and interpretation. *J Rheumatol.* 1983;10(3):353–357.

196. Levine WN, Richmond JC, Donaldson WR. Use of the suture anchor in open Bankart reconstruction. A follow-up report. *Am J Sports Med.* 1994;22(5):723–726.

197. Liavaag S, Brox JI, Pripp AH, et al. Immobilization in external rotation after primary shoulder dislocation did not reduce the risk of recurrence: A randomized controlled trial. *J Bone Joint Surg Am.* 2011;93(10):897–904.

198. Lippitt S, Matsen F. Mechanisms of glenohumeral joint stability. *Clin Orthop Relat Res.* 1993(291):20–28.

199. Lo IK, Nonweiler B, Woolfrey M, et al. An evaluation of the apprehension, relocation, and surprise tests for anterior shoulder instability. *Am J Sports Med.* 2004;32(2):301–307.

200. Lo IK, Parten PM, Burkhart SS. The inverted pear glenoid: An indicator of significant glenoid bone loss. *Arthroscopy.* 2004;20(2):169–174.

201. Loomer R, Graham B. Anatomy of the axillary nerve and its relation to inferior capsular shift. *Clin Orthop Relat Res.* 1989;243:100–105.

202. Magee T. 3-T MRI of the shoulder: Is MR arthrography necessary? *AJR Am J Roentgenol.* 2009;192(1):86–92.

203. Mahirogullari M, Ozkan H, Akyuz M, et al. Comparison between the results of open and arthroscopic repair of isolated traumatic anterior instability of the shoulder. *Acta Orthop Traumatol Turc.* 2010;44(3):180–185.

204. Maquieira GJ, Gerber C, Schneeberger AG. Suprascapular nerve palsy after the Latarjet procedure. *J Shoulder Elbow Surg.* 2007;16(2):e13–e15.

205. Marans HJ, Angel KR, Schemitsch EH, et al. The fate of traumatic anterior dislocation of the shoulder in children. *J Bone Joint Surg Am.* 1992;74(8):1242–1244.

206. Marks TO, Kelsall NK, Southgate JJ. Bilateral luxatio erecta: Recognition and reduction. *Emerg Med Australas.* 2011;23(4):510–511.

207. Marquardt B, Potzl W, Witt KA, et al. A modified capsular shift for atraumatic anteriorinferior shoulder instability. *Am J Sports Med.* 2005;33(7):1011–1015.

208. Marsh JL, Slongo TF, Agel J, et al. Fracture and dislocation classification compendium—2007: Orthopaedic Trauma Association classification, database and outcomes committee. *J Orthop Trauma.* 2007;21(10 suppl):S1–S133.

209. Matsen FA 3rd, Lippitt SA, Bertlesen A, et al. Glenohumeral instability. In: Rockwood CA Jr, Matsen FA 3rd, Wirth MA, et al., eds. *The Shoulder.* 4th ed. Philadelphia, PA: Saunders Elsevier; 2009:617–770.

210. Mazzocca AD, Brown FM Jr, Carreira DS, et al. Arthroscopic anterior shoulder stabilization of collision and contact athletes. *Am J Sports Med.* 2005;33(1):52–60.

211. McAuliffe TB, Pangayatselvan T, Bayley I. Failed surgery for recurrent anterior dislocation of the shoulder. Causes and management. *J Bone Joint Surg Br.* 1988;70(5):798–801.

212. McFarland EG, Kim TK, Park HB, et al. The effect of variation in definition on the diagnosis of multidirectional instability of the shoulder. *J Bone Joint Surg Am.* 2003; 85-A(11):2138–2144.

213. McIntyre LF, Caspari RB, Savoie FH 3rd. The arthroscopic treatment of multidirectional shoulder instability: Two-year results of a multiple suture technique. *Arthroscopy.* 1997;13(4):418–425.

214. McIntyre LF, Caspari RB, Savoie FH 3rd. The arthroscopic treatment of posterior shoulder instability: Two-year results of a multiple suture technique. 1997;13(4):426–432.

215. McLaughlin HL. Posterior dislocation of the shoulder. *J Bone Joint Surg Am.* 1952; 24-A:3:584–590.

216. Mehta V. Humeral head plasty for a chronic locked anterior shoulder dislocation. *Orthopedics.* 2009;32(1):52.

217. Meuffels DE, Schuit H, van Biezen FC, et al. The posterior bone block procedure in posterior shoulder instability: A long-term follow-up study. *J Bone Joint Surg Br.* 2010;92(5):651–655.

218. Meyer M, Graveleau N, Hardy P, et al. Anatomic risks of shoulder arthroscopy portals: Anatomic cadaveric study of 12 portals. *Arthroscopy.* 2007;23(5):529–536.

219. Mihata T, Lee Y, McGarry MH, et al. Excessive humeral external rotation results in increased shoulder laxity. *Am J Sports Med.* 2004;32(5):1278–1285.

220. Milch H. Treatment of dislocation of the shoulder. *Surgery.* 1938;3:732–740.

221. Mileski RA, Snyder SJ. Superior labral lesions in the shoulder: Pathoanatomy and surgical management. *J Am Acad Orthop Surg.* 1998;6(2):121–131.

222. Miller SL, Cleeman E, Auerbach J, et al. Comparison of intra-articular lidocaine and intravenous sedation for reduction of shoulder dislocations: A randomized, prospective study. *J Bone Joint Surg Am.* 2002;84-A(12):2135–2139.

223. Millett PJ, Clavert P, Warner JJ. Open operative treatment for anterior shoulder instability: When and why? *J Bone Joint Surg Am.* 2005;87(2):419–432.

224. Miniaci A, Gish MW. Management of anterior glenohumeral instability associated with large Hill-Sachs defects. *Tech Shoulder Elbow Surg.* 2004;5(3):170–175.

225. Misamore GW, Facibene WA. Posterior capsulorrhaphy for the treatment of traumatic recurrent posterior subluxations of the shoulder in athletes. *J Shoulder Elbow Surg.* 2000;9(5):403–408.

226. Misamore GW, Sallay PI, Didelot W. A longitudinal study of patients with multidirectional instability of the shoulder with seven- to ten-year follow-up. *J Shoulder Elbow Surg.* 2005;14(5):466–470.

227. Moeller JC. Compound posterior dislocation of the glenohumeral joint. Case report. *J Bone Joint Surg Am.* 1975;57(7):1006–1007.

228. Mologne TS, Provencher MT, Menzel KA, et al. Arthroscopic stabilization in patients with an inverted pear glenoid: Results in patients with bone loss of the anterior glenoid. *Am J Sports Med.* 2007;35(8):1276–1283.

229. Montgomery WH 3rd, Jobe FW. Functional outcomes in athletes after modified anterior capsulolabral reconstruction. *Am J Sports Med.* 1994;22(3):352–358.

230. Montgomery WH Jr, Wahl M, Hettrich C, et al. Anteroinferior bone-grafting can restore stability in osseous glenoid defects. *J Bone Joint Surg Am.* 2005;87(9):1972–1977.

231. Moros C, Ahmad CS. Partial humeral head resurfacing and Latarjet coracoid transfer for treatment of recurrent anterior glenohumeral instability. *Orthopedics.* 2009;32(8).

232. Motzkin NE, Itoi E, Morrey BF, et al. Contribution of capsuloligamentous structures to passive static inferior glenohumeral stability. *Clin Biomech (Bristol, Avon).* 1998;13(1):54–61.

233. Neer CS 2nd, Foster CR. Inferior capsular shift for involuntary inferior and multidirectional instability of the shoulder. A preliminary report. *J Bone Joint Surg Am.* 1980;62(6):897–908.

234. Neri BR, Tuckman DV, Bravman JT, et al. Arthroscopic revision of Bankart repair. *J Shoulder Elbow Surg.* 2007;16(4):419–424.

235. Neviaser RJ, Neviaser TJ, Neviaser JS. Concurrent rupture of the rotator cuff and anterior dislocation of the shoulder in the older patient. *J Bone Joint Surg Am.* 1988;70(9):1308–1311.

236. Neviaser RJ, Neviaser TJ, Neviaser JS. Anterior dislocation of the shoulder and rotator cuff rupture. *Clin Orthop Relat Res.* 1993;291:103–106.

237. Neviaser TJ. Arthroscopy of the shoulder. *Orthop Clin North Am.* 1987;18(3):361–372.

238. Neviaser TJ. The anterior labroligamentous periosteal sleeve avulsion lesion: A cause of anterior instability of the shoulder. *Arthroscopy.* 1993;9(1):17–21.

239. Nicola T. Acute anterior dislocation of the shoulder. *J Bone Joint Surg Am.* 1949;31A(1):153–159.

240. Nicola T. Recurrent dislocation of the shoulder. *Am J Surg.* 1953;86(1):85–91.

241. Nordqvist A, Petersson CJ. Incidence and causes of shoulder girdle injuries in an urban population. *J Shoulder Elbow Surg.* 1995;4(2):107–112.

242. Nourissat G, Kilinc AS, Werther JR, et al. A prospective, comparative, radiological, and clinical study of the influence of the "remplissage" procedure on shoulder range of motion after stabilization by arthroscopic Bankart repair. *Am J Sports Med.* 2011;39(10):2147–2152.

243. O'Brien SJ, Neves MC, Arnoczky SP, et al. The anatomy and histology of the inferior glenohumeral ligament complex of the shoulder. *Am J Sports Med.* 1990;18(5):449–456.

244. O'Brien SJ, Schwartz RS, Warren RF, et al. Capsular restraints to anterior-posterior motion of the abducted shoulder: A biomechanical study. *J Shoulder Elbow Surg.* 1995;4(4):298–308.

245. O'Brien SJ, Warren RF, Schwartz E. Anterior shoulder instability. *Orthop Clin North Am.* 1987;18(3):395–408.

246. O'Connell PW, Nuber GW, Mileski RA, et al. The contribution of the glenohumeral ligaments to anterior stability of the shoulder joint. *Am J Sports Med.* 1990;18(6):579–584.

247. O'Connor DR, Schwarze D, Fragomen AT, et al. Painless reduction of acute anterior shoulder dislocations without anesthesia. *Orthopedics.* 2006;29(6):528–532.

248. O'Driscoll SW, Evans DC. Contralateral shoulder instability following anterior repair. An epidemiological investigation. *J Bone Joint Surg Br.* 1991;73(6):941–946.

249. Oh JH, Kim JY, Choi JA, et al. Effectiveness of multidetector computed tomography arthrography for the diagnosis of shoulder pathology: Comparison with magnetic resonance imaging with arthroscopic correlation. *J Shoulder Elbow Surg.* 2010;19(1):14–20.

250. Omoumi P, Teixeira P, Lecouvet F, et al. Glenohumeral joint instability. *J Magn Reson Imaging.* 2011;33(1):2–16.

251. Orlinsky M, Shon S, Chiang C, et al. Comparative study of intra-articular lidocaine and intravenous meperidine/diazepam for shoulder dislocations. *J Emerg Med.* 2002;22(3):241–245.

252. Ovesen J, Nielsen S. Anterior and posterior shoulder instability. A cadaver study. *Acta Orthop Scand.* 1986;57(4):324–327.

253. Owens BD, Dawson L, Burks R, et al. Incidence of shoulder dislocation in the United States military: Demographic considerations from a high-risk population. *J Bone Joint Surg Am.* 2009;91(4):791–796.

254. Owens BD, Duffey ML, Nelson BJ, et al. The incidence and characteristics of shoulder instability at the United States Military Academy. *Am J Sports Med.* 2007;35(7):1168–1173.

255. Owens BD, Harrast JJ, Hurwitz SR, et al. Surgical trends in Bankart repair: An analysis of data from the American Board of Orthopaedic Surgery certification examination. *Am J Sports Med.* 2011;39(9):1865–1869.
256. Owens BD, Nelson BJ, Duffey ML, et al. Pathoanatomy of first-time, traumatic, anterior glenohumeral subluxation events. *J Bone Joint Surg Am.* 2010;92(7):1605–1611.
257. Ozbaydar M, Elhassan B, Diller D, et al. Results of arthroscopic capsulolabral repair: Bankart lesion versus anterior labroligamentous periosteal sleeve avulsion lesion. *Arthroscopy.* 2008;24(11):1277–1283.
258. Pagnani MJ, Dome DC. Surgical treatment of traumatic anterior shoulder instability in American football players. *J Bone Joint Surg Am.* 2002;84-A(5):711–715.
259. Pande P, Hawkins R, Peat M. Electromyography in voluntary posterior instability of the shoulder. *Am J Sports Med.* 1989;17(5):644–648.
260. Park MJ, Tjoumakaris FP, Garcia G, et al. Arthroscopic remplissage with Bankart repair for the treatment of glenohumeral instability with Hill-Sachs defects. *Arthroscopy.* 2011;27(9):1187–1194.
261. Patel A, Calfee RP, Plante M, et al. Propionibacterium acnes colonization of the human shoulder. *J Shoulder Elbow Surg.* 2009;18(6):897–902.
262. Paterson WH, Throckmorton TW, Koester M, et al. Position and duration of immobilization after primary anterior shoulder dislocation: A systematic review and meta-analysis of the literature. *J Bone Joint Surg Am.* 2010;92(18):2924–2933.
263. Paul J, Buchmann S, Beitzel K, et al. Posterior shoulder dislocation: Systematic review and treatment algorithm. *Arthroscopy.* 2011;27(11):1562–1572.
264. Pelet S, Jolles BM, Farron A. Bankart repair for recurrent anterior glenohumeral instability: Results at twenty-nine years' follow-up. *J Shoulder Elbow Surg.* 2006;15(2):203–207.
265. Petrera M, Patella V, Patella S, et al. A meta-analysis of open versus arthroscopic Bankart repair using suture anchors. *Knee Surg Sports Traumatol Arthrosc.* 2010;18(12):1742–1747.
266. Pevny T, Hunter RE, Freeman JR. Primary traumatic anterior shoulder dislocation in patients 40 years of age and older. *Arthroscopy.* 1998;14(3):289–294.
267. Piasecki DP, Verma NN, Romeo AA, et al. Glenoid bone deficiency in recurrent anterior shoulder instability: Diagnosis and management. *J Am Acad Orthop Surg.* 2009;17(8):482–493.
268. Pollock RG, Bigliani LU. Recurrent posterior shoulder instability. Diagnosis and treatment. *Clin Orthop Relat Res.* 1993;291:85–96.
269. Pollock RG, Owens JM, Flatow EL, et al. Operative results of the inferior capsular shift procedure for multidirectional instability of the shoulder. *J Bone Joint Surg Am.* 2000;82-A(7):919–928.
270. Pollock RG, Wang VM, Bucchieri JS, et al. Effects of repetitive subfailure strains on the mechanical behavior of the inferior glenohumeral ligament. *J Shoulder Elbow Surg.* 2000;9(5):427–435.
271. Porcellini G, Campi F, Paladini P. Arthroscopic approach to acute bony Bankart lesion. *Arthroscopy.* 2002;18(7):764–769.
272. Postacchini F, Gumina S, Cinotti G. Anterior shoulder dislocation in adolescents. *J Shoulder Elbow Surg.* 2000;9(6):470–474.
273. Potzl W, Witt KA, Hackenberg L, et al. Results of suture anchor repair of anteroinferior shoulder instability: A prospective clinical study of 85 shoulders. *J Shoulder Elbow Surg.* 2003;12(4):322–326.
274. Pritchett JW, Clark JM. Prosthetic replacement for chronic unreduced dislocations of the shoulder. *Clin Orthop Relat Res.* 1987;216:89–93.
275. Provencher MT, Bell SJ, Menzel KA, et al. Arthroscopic treatment of posterior shoulder instability: Results in 33 patients. *Am J Sports Med.* 2005;33(10):1463–1471.
276. Provencher MT, Bhatia S, Ghodadra NS, et al. Recurrent shoulder instability: Current concepts for evaluation and management of glenoid bone loss. *J Bone Joint Surg Am.* 2010;92(suppl 2):133–151.
277. Provencher MT, Detterline AJ, Ghodadra N, et al. Measurement of glenoid bone loss: A comparison of measurement error between 45 degrees and 0 degrees bone loss models and with different posterior arthroscopy portal locations. *Am J Sports Med.* 2008;36(6):1132–1138.
278. Provencher MT, Dewing CB, Bell SJ, et al. An analysis of the rotator interval in patients with anterior, posterior, and multidirectional shoulder instability. *Arthroscopy.* 2008;24(8):921–929.
279. Provencher MT, Frank RM, Leclere LE, et al. The Hill-Sachs lesion: Diagnosis, classification, and management. *J Am Acad Orthop Surg.* 2012;20(4):242–252.
280. Provencher MT, Ghodadra N, LeClere L, et al. Anatomic osteochondral glenoid reconstruction for recurrent glenohumeral instability with glenoid deficiency using a distal tibia allograft. *Arthroscopy.* 2009;25(4):446–452.
281. Provencher MT, LeClere LE, King S, et al. Posterior instability of the shoulder: Diagnosis and management. *Am J Sports Med.* 2011;39(4):874–886.
282. Provencher MT, Mologne TS, Romeo AA, et al. The use of rotator interval closure in the arthroscopic treatment of posterior shoulder instability. *Arthroscopy.* 2009;25(1):109,10; author reply 110-1.
283. Pulavarti RS, Symes TH, Rangan A. Surgical interventions for anterior shoulder instability in adults. *Cochrane Database Syst Rev.* 2009;(4):CD005077.
284. Purchase RJ, Wolf EM, Hobgood ER, et al. Hill-Sachs "remplissage": An arthroscopic solution for the engaging Hill-Sachs lesion. *Arthroscopy.* 2008;24(6):723–726.
285. Rachbauer F, Ogon M, Wimmer C, et al. Glenohumeral osteoarthrosis after the Eden-Hybbinette procedure. *Clin Orthop Relat Res.* 2000;373:135–140.
286. Radkowski CA, Chhabra A, Baker CL 3rd, at al. Arthroscopic capsulolabral repair for posterior shoulder instability in throwing athletes compared with nonthrowing athletes. *Am J Sports Med.* 2008;36(4):693–699.
287. Rahme H, Wikblad L, Nowak J, et al. Long-term clinical and radiologic results after Eden-Hybbinette operation for anterior instability of the shoulder. *J Shoulder Elbow Surg.* 2003;12(1):15–19.
288. Randelli P, Ragone V, Carminati S, et al. Risk factors for recurrence after Bankart repair a systematic review. *Knee Surg Sports Traumatol Arthrosc.* 2012;20(11):2129–2138.
289. Re P, Gallo RA, Richmond JC. Transhumeral head plasty for large Hill-Sachs lesions. *Arthroscopy.* 2006;22(7):798.e1,798.e4.
290. Reeves B. Experiments on the tensile strength of the anterior capsular structures of the shoulder in man. *J Bone Joint Surg Br.* 1968;50(4):858–865.
291. Rhee YG, Ha JH, Cho NS. Anterior shoulder stabilization in collision athletes: Arthroscopic versus open Bankart repair. *Am J Sports Med.* 2006;34(6):979–985.
292. Rhee YG, Lee DH, Lim CT. Posterior capsulolabral reconstruction in posterior shoulder instability: Deltoid saving. *J Shoulder Elbow Surg.* 2005;14(4):355–360.
293. Ricchetti ET, Ciccotti MC, O'Brien DF, et al. Outcomes of arthroscopic repair of panlabral tears of the glenohumeral joint. *Am J Sports Med.* 2012;40(11):2561–2568.
294. Richards DP, Burkhart SS. Arthroscopic humeral avulsion of the glenohumeral ligaments (HAGL) repair. *Arthroscopy.* 2004;20(suppl 2):134–141.
295. Richmond JC, Donaldson WR, Fu F, et al. Modification of the Bankart reconstruction with a suture anchor. Report of a new technique. *Am J Sports Med.* 1991;19(4):343–346.
296. Robertson DD, Yuan J, Bigliani LU, et al. Three-dimensional analysis of the proximal part of the humerus: Relevance to arthroplasty. *J Bone Joint Surg Am.* 2000;82-A(11):1594–1602.
297. Robinson CM, Aderinto J. Posterior shoulder dislocations and fracture-dislocations. *J Bone Joint Surg Am.* 2005;87(3):639–650.
298. Robinson CM, Aderinto J. Recurrent posterior shoulder instability. *J Bone Joint Surg Am.* 2005;87(4):883–892.
299. Robinson CM, Howes J, Murdoch H, et al. Functional outcome and risk of recurrent instability after primary traumatic anterior shoulder dislocation in young patients. *J Bone Joint Surg Am.* 2006;88(11):2326–2336.
300. Robinson CM, Jenkins PJ, White TO, et al. Primary arthroscopic stabilization for a first-time anterior dislocation of the shoulder. A randomized, double-blind trial. *J Bone Joint Surg Am.* 2008;90(4):708–721.
301. Robinson CM, Seah M, Akhtar MA. The epidemiology, risk of recurrence, and functional outcome after an acute traumatic posterior dislocation of the shoulder. *J Bone Joint Surg Am.* 2011;93(17):1605–1613.
302. Robinson CM, Shur N, Sharpe T, et al. Injuries associated with traumatic anterior glenohumeral dislocations. *J Bone Joint Surg Am.* 2012;94(1):18–26.
303. Robinson LR. Traumatic injury to peripheral nerves. *Muscle Nerve.* 2000;23(6):863–873.
304. Rokous JR, Feagin JA, Abbott HG. Modified axillary roentgenogram. A useful adjunct in the diagnosis of recurrent instability of the shoulder. *Clin Orthop Relat Res.* 1972;82:84–86.
305. Rouhani A, Navali A. Treatment of chronic anterior shoulder dislocation by open reduction and simultaneous Bankart lesion repair. *Sports Med Arthrosc Rehabil Ther Technol.* 2010;2:15,2555-2-15.
306. Rowe CR. Prognosis in dislocations of the shoulder. *J Bone Joint Surg Am.* 1956;38-A(5):957–977.
307. Rowe CR, Patel D, Southmayd WW. The Bankart procedure: A long-term end-result study. *J Bone Joint Surg Am.* 1978;60(1):1–16.
308. Rowe CR, Pierce DS, Clark JG. Voluntary dislocation of the shoulder. A preliminary report on a clinical, electromyographic, and psychiatric study of twenty-six patients. *J Bone Joint Surg Am.* 1973;55(3):445–460.
309. Rowe CR, Sakellarides HT. Factors related to recurrences of anterior dislocations of the shoulder. *Clin Orthop.* 1961;20:40–48.
310. Rowe CR, Zarins B. Recurrent transient subluxation of the shoulder. *J Bone Joint Surg Am.* 1981;63(6):863–872.
311. Rowe CR, Zarins B. Chronic unreduced dislocations of the shoulder. *J Bone Joint Surg Am.* 1982;64(4):494–505.
312. Sachs RA, Lin D, Stone ML, et al. Can the need for future surgery for acute traumatic anterior shoulder dislocation be predicted? *J Bone Joint Surg Am.* 2007;89(8):1665–1674.
313. Sachs RA, Williams B, Stone ML, et al. Open Bankart repair: Correlation of results with postoperative subscapularis function. *Am J Sports Med.* 2005;33(10):1458–1462.
314. Saha AK. Dynamic stability of the glenohumeral joint. *Acta Orthop Scand.* 1971;42(6):491–505.
315. Saha AK. *Theory of shoulder mechanism: Descriptive and applied.* Springfield, IL: C. C. Thomas; 1961.
316. Saltzman MD, Nuber GW, Gryzlo SM, et al. Efficacy of surgical preparation solutions in shoulder surgery. *J Bone Joint Surg Am.* 2009;91(8):1949–1953.
317. Saupe N, White LM, Bleakney R, et al. Acute traumatic posterior shoulder dislocation: MR findings. *Radiology.* 2008;248(1):185–193.
318. Savoie FH 3rd, Holt MS, Field LD, et al. Arthroscopic management of posterior instability: Evolution of technique and results. *Arthroscopy.* 2008;24(4):389–396.
319. Scheibel M, Nikulka C, Dick A, et al. Autogenous bone grafting for chronic anteroinferior glenoid defects via a complete subscapularis tenotomy approach. *Arch Orthop Trauma Surg.* 2008;128(11):1317–1325.
320. Schmid SL, Farshad M, Catanzaro S, et al. The Latarjet procedure for the treatment of recurrence of anterior instability of the shoulder after operative repair: A retrospective case series of forty-nine consecutive patients. *J Bone Joint Surg Am.* 2012;94(11):e75.
321. Shah AA, Butler RB, Romanowski J, et al. Short-term complications of the Latarjet procedure. *J Bone Joint Surg Am.* 2012;94(6):495–501.
322. Silliman JF, Hawkins RJ. Classification and physical diagnosis of instability of the shoulder. *Clin Orthop Relat Res.* 1993;291:7–19.
323. Simonet WT, Cofield RH. Prognosis in anterior shoulder dislocation. *Am J Sports Med.* 1984;12(1):19–24.
324. Simonet WT, Melton LJ 3rd, Cofield RH, et al. Incidence of anterior shoulder dislocation in Olmsted County, Minnesota. *Clin Orthop Relat Res.* 1984;186:186–191.
325. Singer GC, Kirkland PM, Emery RJ. Coracoid transposition for recurrent anterior instability of the shoulder. A 20-year follow-up study. *J Bone Joint Surg Br.* 1995;77(1):73–76.
326. Sisco M, Dumanian GA. Anterior interosseous nerve syndrome following shoulder arthroscopy. A report of three cases. *J Bone Joint Surg Am.* 2007;89(2):392–395.
327. Snyder SJ, Karzel RP, Del Pizzo W, et al. SLAP lesions of the shoulder. *Arthroscopy.* 1990;6(4):274–279.
328. Soslowsky LJ, An CH, DeBano CM, et al. Coracoacromial ligament: In situ load and viscoelastic properties in rotator cuff disease. *Clin Orthop Relat Res.* 1996;330:40–44.

329. Soslowsky LJ, An CH, Johnston SP, et al. Geometric and mechanical properties of the coracoacromial ligament and their relationship to rotator cuff disease. *Clin Orthop Relat Res.* 1994;304:10–17.

330. Speer KP, Deng X, Borrero S, et al. Biomechanical evaluation of a simulated Bankart lesion. *J Bone Joint Surg Am.* 1994;76(12):1819–1826.

331. Speer KP, Warren RF, Pagnani M, et al. An arthroscopic technique for anterior stabilization of the shoulder with a bioabsorbable tack. *J Bone Joint Surg Am.* 1996;78(12):1801–1807.

332. Sperber A, Hamberg P, Karlsson J, et al. Comparison of an arthroscopic and an open procedure for posttraumatic instability of the shoulder: A prospective, randomized multicenter study. *J Shoulder Elbow Surg.* 2001;10(2):105–108.

333. Sperling JW, Cofield RH, Torchia ME, et al. Infection after shoulder instability surgery. *Clin Orthop Relat Res.* 2003;414:61–64.

334. Steinbeck J, Jerosch J. Surgery for atraumatic anterior-inferior shoulder instability. A modified capsular shift evaluated in 20 patients followed for 3 years. *Acta Orthop Scand.* 1997;68(5):447–450.

335. Stimson L. An easy method of reducing dislocations of the shoulder and hip. *Med Record.* 1900;57:356–357.

336. Stromsoe K, Senn E, Simmen B, et al. Recurrence frequency following traumatic shoulder dislocation. *Helv Chir Acta.* 1980;47(1-2):85–88.

337. Sugaya H, Moriishi J, Dohi M, et al. Glenoid rim morphology in recurrent anterior glenohumeral instability. *J Bone Joint Surg Am.* 2003;85-A(5):878–884.

338. Sugaya H, Moriishi J, Kanisawa I, et al. Arthroscopic osseous Bankart repair for chronic recurrent traumatic anterior glenohumeral instability. *J Bone Joint Surg Am.* 2005;87(8):1752–1760.

339. Taylor DC, Arciero RA. Pathologic changes associated with shoulder dislocations. Arthroscopic and physical examination findings in first-time, traumatic anterior dislocations. *Am J Sports Med.* 1997;25(3):306–311.

340. te Slaa RL, Wijffels MP, Brand R, et al. The prognosis following acute primary glenohumeral dislocation. *J Bone Joint Surg Br.* 2004;86(1):58–64.

341. Tietjen R. Occult glenohumeral interposition of a torn rotator cuff. A case report. *J Bone Joint Surg Am.* 1982;64(3):458–459.

342. Tjoumakaris FP, Abboud JA, Hasan SA, et al. Arthroscopic and open Bankart repairs provide similar outcomes. *Clin Orthop Relat Res.* 2006;446:227–232.

343. Tjoumakaris FP, Sekiya JK. Combined glenoid and humeral head allograft reconstruction for recurrent anterior glenohumeral instability. *Orthopedics.* 2008;31(5):497.

344. Townley CO. The capsular mechanism in recurrent dislocation of the shoulder. *J Bone Joint Surg Am.* 1950;32A(2):370–380.

345. Treacy SH, Savoie FH 3rd, Field LD. Arthroscopic treatment of multidirectional instability. *J Shoulder Elbow Surg.* 1999;8(4):345–350.

346. Turkel SJ, Panio MW, Marshall JL, et al. Stabilizing mechanisms preventing anterior dislocation of the glenohumeral joint. *J Bone Joint Surg Am.* 1981;63(8):1208–1217.

347. Uhthoff HK, Piscopo M. Anterior capsular redundancy of the shoulder: Congenital or traumatic? An embryological study. *J Bone Joint Surg Br.* 1985;67(3):363–366.

348. Waldherr P, Snyder SJ. SLAP-lesions of the shoulder. *Orthopade.* 2003;32(7):632–636.

349. Waldt S, Metz S, Burkart A, et al. Variants of the superior labrum and labro-bicipital complex: A comparative study of shoulder specimens using MR arthrography, multi-slice CT arthrography and anatomical dissection. *Eur Radiol.* 2006;16(2):451–458.

350. Wang C, Ghalambor N, Zarins B, et al. Arthroscopic versus open Bankart repair: Analysis of patient subjective outcome and cost. *Arthroscopy.* 2005;21(10):1219–1222.

351. Wang VM, Sugalski MT, Levine WN, et al. Comparison of glenohumeral mechanics following a capsular shift and anterior tightening. *J Bone Joint Surg Am.* 2005;87(6):1312–1322.

352. Warner JJ, Bowen MK, Deng X. Effect of joint compression on inferior stability of the glenohumeral joint. *J Shoulder Elbow Surg.* 1999;8(1):31–36.

353. Warner JJ, Bowen MK, Deng XH, et al. Articular contact patterns of the normal glenohumeral joint. *J Shoulder Elbow Surg.* 1998;7(4):381–388.

354. Warner JJ, Deng XH, Warren RF, et al. Static capsuloligamentous restraints to superior-inferior translation of the glenohumeral joint. *Am J Sports Med.* 1992;20(6):675–685.

355. Warner JJ, Gill TJ, O'hollerhan JD, et al. Anatomical glenoid reconstruction for recurrent anterior glenohumeral instability with glenoid deficiency using an autogenous tricortical iliac crest bone graft. *Am J Sports Med.* 2006;34(2):205–212.

356. Warner JJ, Micheli LJ, Arslanian LE, et al. Scapulothoracic motion in normal shoulders and shoulders with glenohumeral instability and impingement syndrome. A study using Moire topographic analysis. *Clin Orthop Relat Res.* 1992;285:191–199.

357. Warner JJP, Iannotti JP, Flatow EL. *Complex and revision problems in shoulder surgery.* 2nd ed. Philadelphia, PA: Lippincott Williams & Wilkins; 2005.

358. Weishaupt D, Zanetti M, Nyffeler RW, et al. Posterior glenoid rim deficiency in recurrent (atraumatic) posterior shoulder instability. *Skeletal Radiol.* 2000;29(4):204–210.

359. Wellmann M, Bobrowitsch E, Khan N, et al. Biomechanical effectiveness of an arthroscopic posterior bankart repair versus an open bone block procedure for posterior shoulder instability. *Am J Sports Med.* 2011;39(4):796–803.

360. Weng PW, Shen HC, Lee HH, et al. Open reconstruction of large bony glenoid erosion with allogeneic bone graft for recurrent anterior shoulder dislocation. *Am J Sports Med.* 2009;37(9):1792–1797.

361. West EF. Intrathoracic dislocation of the humerus. *J Bone Joint Surg Br.* 1949;31B(1):61.

362. Wheeler JH, Ryan JB, Arciero RA, et al. Arthroscopic versus nonoperative treatment of acute shoulder dislocations in young athletes. *Arthroscopy.* 1989;5(3):213–217.

363. Williams RJ 3rd, Strickland S, Cohen M, et al. Arthroscopic repair for traumatic posterior shoulder instability. *Am J Sports Med.* 2003;31(2):203–209.

364. Wirth MA, Blatter G, Rockwood CA Jr. The capsular imbrication procedure for recurrent anterior instability of the shoulder. *J Bone Joint Surg Am.* 1996;78(2):246–259.

365. Wirth MA, Seltzer DG, Rockwood CA Jr. Recurrent posterior glenohumeral dislocation associated with increased retroversion of the glenoid. A case report. *Clin Orthop Relat Res.* 1994;308:98–101.

366. Wolf BR, Strickland S, Williams RJ, et al. Open posterior stabilization for recurrent posterior glenohumeral instability. *J Shoulder Elbow Surg.* 2005;14(2):157–164.

367. Wolf EM, Cheng JC, Dickson K. Humeral avulsion of glenohumeral ligaments as a cause of anterior shoulder instability. *Arthroscopy.* 1995;11(5):600–607.

368. Wolf EM, Eakin CL. Arthroscopic capsular plication for posterior shoulder instability. *Arthroscopy.* 1998;14(2):153–163.

369. Yagishita K, Thomas BJ. Use of allograft for large Hill-Sachs lesion associated with anterior glenohumeral dislocation. A case report. *Injury.* 2002;33(9):791–794.

370. Yamamoto N, Itoi E, Abe H, et al. Contact between the glenoid and the humeral head in abduction, external rotation, and horizontal extension: A new concept of glenoid track. *J Shoulder Elbow Surg.* 2007;16(5):649–656.

371. Yamamoto T, Yoshiya S, Kurosaka M, et al. Luxatio erecta (inferior dislocation of the shoulder): A report of 5 cases and a review of the literature. *Am J Orthop (Belle Mead NJ).* 2003;32(12):601–603.

372. Yang ZX, Pho RW, Kour AK, et al. The musculocutaneous nerve and its branches to the biceps and brachialis muscles. *J Hand Surg Am.* 1995;20(4):671–675.

373. Young AA, Maia R, Berhouet J, et al. Open Latarjet procedure for management of bone loss in anterior instability of the glenohumeral joint. *J Shoulder Elbow Surg.* 2011;20(2 suppl):S61–S69.

374. Zacchilli MA, Owens BD. Epidemiology of shoulder dislocations presenting to emergency departments in the United States. *J Bone Joint Surg Am.* 2010;92(3):542–549.

375. Zaffagnini S, Marcheggiani Muccioli GM, Giordano G, et al. Long-term outcomes after repair of recurrent post-traumatic anterior shoulder instability: Comparison of arthroscopic transglenoid suture and open Bankart reconstruction. *Knee Surg Sports Traumatol Arthrosc.* 2012;20(5):816–821.

376. Zhu YM, Lu Y, Zhang J, et al. Arthroscopic Bankart repair combined with remplissage technique for the treatment of anterior shoulder instability with engaging Hill-Sachs lesion: A report of 49 cases with a minimum 2-year follow-up. *Am J Sports Med.* 2011;39(8):1640–1647.

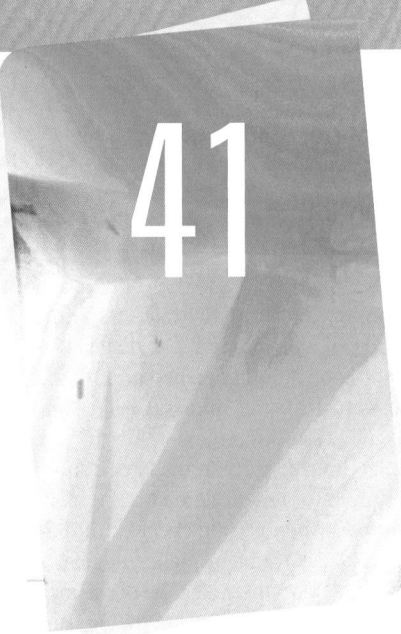

41

ACROMIOCLAVICULAR JOINT INJURIES

Cory Edgar, Anthony DeGiacomo, Mark J. Lemos and Augustus D. Mazzocca

INTRODUCTION TO ACROMIOCLAVICULAR JOINT INJURIES

Injuries to the acromioclavicular (AC) joint represent a spectrum of soft tissue disruptions that can result in mild, transient pain about the joint to significant displacement, chronic pain, and changes in shoulder biomechanics resulting in long-term disability. These injures most commonly occur in male patients <30 years and are associated with contact sports or athletic activity in which a direct blow to the lateral aspect of the shoulder occurs. The contact or collision athlete represents a "high-risk" individual, especially those who play sports like football, rugby, and hockey.[38,43,75,116] The management of these injuries has been discussed in academic forums since the time of Hippocrates and Galen, but there still appears to be no consensus regarding when operative management is necessary and which procedure produces the best functional outcome with the least morbidity.[88,97,120,127,136,141] This chapter will focus on the traumatic aspects of AC disorders through an in depth review of the local anatomy and applied

biomechanics of the joint. A classification based on the spectrum of injury is presented in addition to nonsurgical and surgical treatment options. However, there remains a lack of high-quality comparative studies from which treatment guidelines can be made and therefore an overview of approaches is presented.

From a historical perspective, the treatment of AC joint dislocations has been a subject of controversy from the earliest medical writings. For example, Hippocrates[1] (460–377 BC) wrote:

> "Physicians are particularly liable to be deceived in this accident (for as the separated bone protrudes, the top of the shoulder appears low and hollow), so that they may prepare as if for dislocation of the shoulder; for I have known many physicians otherwise not expert at the art who have done much mischief by attempting to reduce shoulders, thus supposing it as a case of dislocation."

Galen[1] (129–199 AD) had obviously paid close attention to Hippocrates, because he diagnosed his own AC dislocation received from wrestling in the Palaestra. This famous physician of the Greco-Roman period treated himself in the manner of Hippocrates (tight bandages to hold the projecting clavicle down while keeping the arm elevated). He abandoned the treatment after only a few days because it was so uncomfortable. It is appropriate that one of the earliest reported cases in the literature was related to sports, because athletic participation is certainly one of the most common causes of AC dislocations and the story highlights the low compliance rate of shoulder bracing.

The surgical treatment of AC joint injuries has evolved with our understanding of the local anatomy and the biomechanics of the joint, and demonstrates a clear historical progression. Samuel Cooper[127] is given credit for the initial report of the surgical management of a displaced, painful AC joint dislocation in 1861. In 1917, Cadenat[21] described transfer of the coracoacromial ligament, a procedure later popularized by Weaver and Dunn.[161] Multiple studies have been published using variations of this technique clouding the literature of its true efficacy. Interestingly, over the last 10 to 15 years there has been an increase in the number of publications of surgical treatment of AC joint dislocations with repairs or reconstruction procedures (Fig. 41-1). Presumably, it is related to a better understanding of the important anatomy. The rapid progression of orthopedic implant technology has also led to the application of improved surgical techniques and strategies. This has dramatically changed the way these injuries are surgically managed. Open reconstruction techniques have a common goal to reduce the AC joint to an anatomic position. This can be accomplished using traditional methods that provide a very rigid construct or a more anatomic approach, in which the goal is to provide a reconstruction that addresses the three-dimensional function of the AC joint complex.

It is clear that a "gold standard" for surgical stabilization of acute, painful AC joint dislocations has yet to be established.

ASSESSMENT OF ACROMIOCLAVICULAR JOINT INJURIES

Mechanisms of Injury of Acromioclavicular Joint Injury

There are numerous ways in which trauma to the shoulder girdle can result in AC joint injury. As with any traumatic injury the direction and magnitude of the force vector dictates the resultant injury pattern. Falling on an outstretched arm, locked in extension at the elbow, can drive the humeral head superior into the acromion typically resulting in low-grade AC joint injuries (Fig. 41-2). A medial directed force to the lateral shoulder that drives the acromion into and underneath the distal clavicle, as occurs, for example, when getting checked into the boards during a hockey game, can result in higher degrees of injury and subsequently more displacement.[127] One of the more commonly described patterns involves falling or being tackled onto the lateral aspect of the shoulder with the arm in an adducted position which produces a compressive (medial) and shear (vertical) force across the joint. This typically produces a higher degree of displacement because the force is enough to both the AC and coracoclavicular (CC) ligaments (Fig. 41-2). One common misconception is the clavicle "elevates" superior to the acromion. In actuality the shoulder girdle is suspended from the axial skeleton by the AC joint complex (the specific anatomy of which will be discussed in the next section). The injury force which drives the acromion medially and downward produces a progressive injury pattern; first disruption of the AC ligaments, followed by disruption of the CC ligaments, and finally disruption of the fascia overlying the clavicle that connects the deltoid and trapezius muscle attachments.[99] At this point, the upper extremity has lost its suspensory support from the clavicle and the scapula and associated glenohumeral articulation displaces inferiorly secondary to forces of gravity. Although there may be a slight upward displacement of the clavicle from the pull of the trapezius muscle, the character-

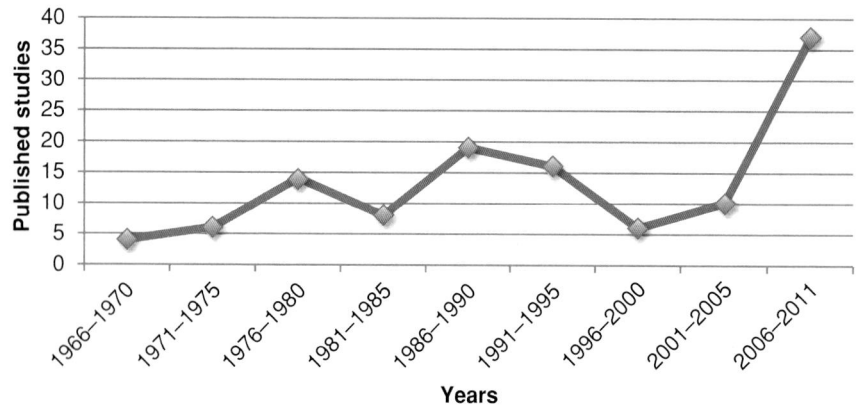

Outcomes studies reporting on surgical techniques (April 1966–October 2011)

FIGURE 41-1 Trends in reported surgical techniques to repair or reconstruct AC joint dislocations. (From Beitzel K, Cote MP, Apostolakos J, et al. Current concepts in the treatment of acromioclavicular joint dislocations. *Arthroscopy.* 2013;29(2):387–397.)

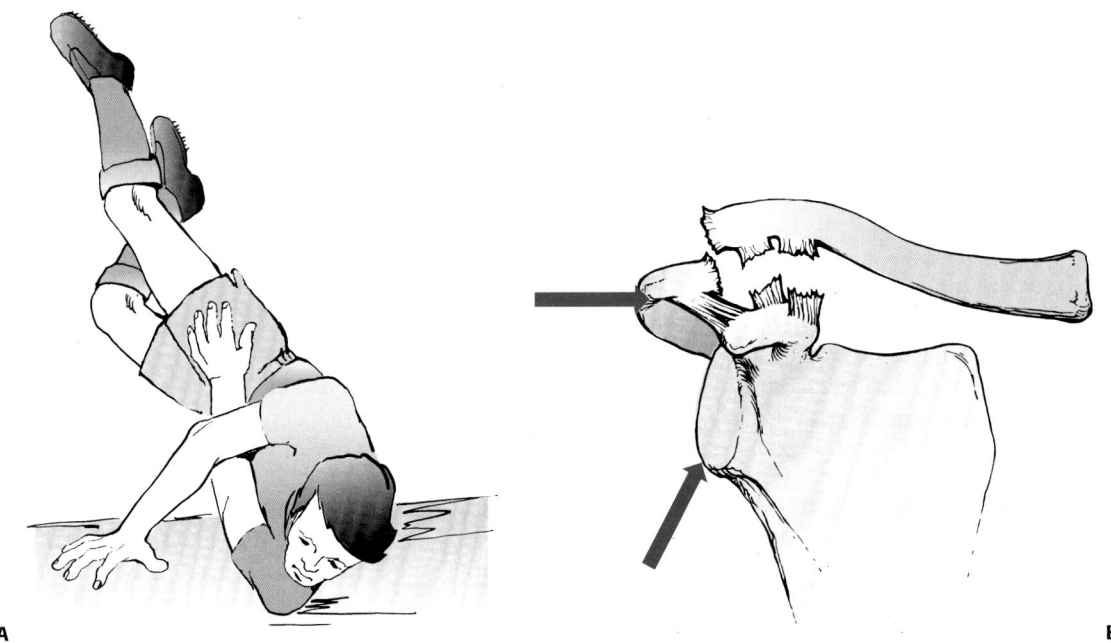

FIGURE 41-2 A: Most common position of injury; adducted arm with axial load to superior AC joint. **B:** Illustration of force directions that can cause displacement of the glenohumeral complex away from or into the AC suspensory complex causing injury to the ligaments; superior, inferior, and medial.

istic anatomic feature is actually inferior displacement of the shoulder and arm. Because the weight of the arm is no longer suspended from the clavicle, there may be a slight upward pull by the trapezius muscle on the clavicle. However, the major deformity seen in complete AC dislocation is a downward displacement of the shoulder (Fig. 41-3).

The mechanism of inferior dislocation of the clavicle under the coracoid is thought to be a very severe direct force onto the superior surface of the distal clavicle; along with abduction of the arm and retraction of the scapula,[100,127] this type of AC joint dislocation is exceedingly rare.

Associated Injuries with Acromioclavicular Joint Injury

Glenohumeral Intra-Articular Pathology

Only two studies have reported on the incidence of gleno-humeral pathology documented with arthroscopy during the

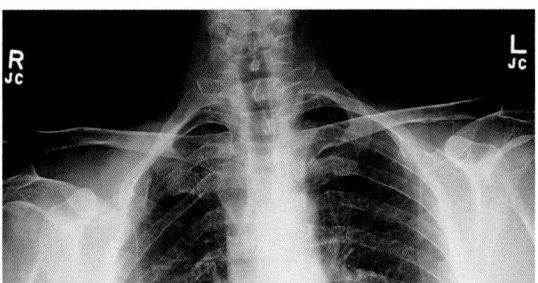

FIGURE 41-3 Radiograph example of Zanca view with bilateral AC joints visualized. Note the displaced AC joint on the right. This view allows for measurement and comparison of CC distance from injured to uninjured side, note the CC distance measured on the left (uninjured side).

treatment of high-grade AC joint dislocations. In a series of 77 patients with grade III to V injuries, arthroscopic evaluation determined 18.2% had a superior labral anterior to posterior (SLAP) lesion, one patient had a complete tear of the supraspi-natus and two patients had partial articular-sided cuff tears.[152] Treatment consisted of debridement of the partial cuff tears and type I SLAP tears, but all additional pathology was surgically repaired. Pauly et al.[117] noted a 15% (6/40) incidence of intra-articular pathology in their series of 40 consecutive patients undergoing arthroscopic-assisted reconstruction of grade III to V AC joint dislocations. They reported three patients with SLAP lesions and three patients with partial articular-sided cuff tears, usually in the supraspinatus. As there is overlapping innerva-tion to this region of the shoulder through the lateral pectoral and suprascapular nerves it may be difficult for the patient to completely localize their pain.[58] Currently there is no data to support getting a preoperative MRI arthrogram to aid in the diagnosis of a concomitant injury or surgical intervention to treat the pathology.

Fractures

Any fracture that disrupts the CC ligaments and AC joint cap-sule/ligaments effectually disrupts the suspension of the upper limb in the same manner as a grade III or greater AC separation. The most common fracture pattern is the distal or lateral clav-icle fracture that is discussed later in the chapter. Similarly the base or neck of the coracoid process can be fractured leaving the CC ligaments attached to the fracture fragment but present-ing as a high-grade AC separation.[78,80,85,160] Another uncommon combination is fracture of the clavicle shaft in conjunction with an AC joint separation, Wurtz et al.[166] reported on four patients with a fracture of the middle third of the clavicle and dislocation of the AC joint. In three cases with grade IV AC separations the AC joint was treated with either a CC screw or Steinmann pins across the AC joint and the clavicle fracture treated nonoperatively. The final case was treated nonoperatively. Patients were followed from 1 to 3 years and excellent motion and function was reported. In a patient less than age 30, concomitant injury to the medial clavicular epiphysis has been reported that required open reduction at the epiphyseal fracture to facilitate reduction of a posterior AC joint dislocation.[70,135,158]

Bipolar Injuries: AC and SC Joint Dislocations

An uncommon and frequently unrecognized injury to the sternoclavicular (SC) joint can occur in conjunction with AC joint dislocations and has been referred to as a "floating clavicle" or panclavicular dislocation. These bipolar injury patterns typically occur with high-energy trauma and may be associated with neurologic symptoms. All the reported cases describe anterior dislocation at the SC joint combined with a posterior dislocation of the AC joint.[45,57,73,133,135] Conservative management is described with success in the older or lower demand patients.[133] Techniques used to surgically treat these bipolar injuries have been varied. Bilateral (Balser) hook plates have recently been used with good success,[135] but more traditional methods of open reduction with capsular repair and in some cases augmentation with Kirschner wires has also been reported with success.[45,133]

Brachial Plexus Abnormalities

Meislin et al.[101] have reported a patient who developed a brachial plexus neurapraxia 8 years after sustaining a type III AC separation. A patient responded well to CC stabilization. Brachial plexus injuries associated with AC separations are not common. Sturm and Perry,[147] in a review of 59 patients with brachial plexus injuries, identified two patients with AC separations.

Coracoclavicular Ossification

CC ossification has been referred to as both ossification and calcification. It is secondary to intrinsic healing response within this area following injury to the CC ligaments. This has been observed and described since the 1940s and has never been associated with increased pain or dysfunction.[157] However, it is commonly observed radiographically in cases of chronic AC separations and often in cases with higher degrees of injury. The calcification can be formed heterotopically around the area of injury, or it can form a bridge between the coracoid and the clavicle. Usually, it has no effect on the functional outcome but must be removed to facilitate full reduction of the AC joint and CC distance at the time of operative intervention.

Osteolysis of the Distal Clavicle

Osteolysis of the distal clavicle is a radiographic finding that may or may not be associated with significant symptoms of pain at the AC joint with cross-arm adduction and overhead lifting. Traumatic distal clavicle osteolysis can be associated with low-grade AC separations in which an extended inflammatory response or repeated injury occurs, leading to the osteolysis observed on radiographs. Madsen[92] reported on seven patients with the complication known as posttraumatic osteolysis of the distal clavicle. He identified eight cases in the literature and seven of his own, all of which had some level of AC joint separation or repeated microtrauma to the area (i.e., pneumatic tool worker). Cahill[22] reported on 46 patients who were athletes with traumatic distal clavicle osteolysis (typically from weight lifting). With histologic analysis, he and others described the intense osteoblastic activity of the subchondral bone from surgical specimens of these osteolytic patients.[20,22,139] These observations confirmed the hypothesis that repeated microtrauma with a recurrent inflammatory process was part of the etiology. Additional microscopic studies have been reported by Murphy et al.[109] and Madsen[92] in which they describe demineralization, subchondral cysts, and erosion of the distal clavicle observed in pathology from intraoperative tissue samples. Griffiths and Glucksman[62] performed a biopsy 8 months after injury that showed patches of necrotic and reactive woven bone.

The radiographic findings are osteoporosis, osteolysis, and tapering of the distal clavicle. Usually, bony changes do not occur in the acromion. Changes usually occur only in the injured shoulder. If changes are noted in both shoulders, then other conditions should be considered, such as rheumatoid arthritis, hyperparathyroidism, and scleroderma. The differential diagnosis of a lesion in one shoulder should include Gorham's massive osteolysis, gout, and a neoplasm such as multiple myeloma. The use of technetium bone scans and a 35-degree cephalic tilt radiographic view to help make the diagnosis has been reported to help determine the activity of the bone resorption process.[22]

Scapulothoracic Dissociation

Scapulothoracic dissociation is a very rare but potentially devastating injury, especially if missed, that can occur through an AC separation.[102] Scapulothoracic dissociations are characterized by lateral displacement of the scapula resulting in a traction injury to the neurovascular structures of the shoulder. In more significant lateral displacement the patient can present with a severe vascular injury and brachial plexus injury. Disruption of the shoulder girdle occurs through either a high-grade AC separation, a displaced clavicle fracture, or a SC disruption. Scapulothoracic dissociations are often clinically subtle injuries in a patient with a distraction injury to the shoulder. A head injury may mask the acute determination of neurovascular injury. Therefore, it is important to consider this injury in the "unexaminable" (i.e., unconscious, head injured) patient with significant trauma and a high-grade AC separation. In the examinable patient a complaint of chest pain or pain in the periscapular and perithoracic region should elicit a chest radiograph as part of the work up. Clinical examination demonstrates the AC deformity as well as marked tenderness in the periscapular and perithoracic region. An anteroposterior (AP) chest radiograph demonstrates an increased distance between the medial scapular border and the midline on the affected side compared with the unaffected side, as well as other signs of thoracic trauma such as a pleural effusion. Magnetic resonance imaging of the thorax demonstrates increased signal in the periscapular and perithoracic muscles in addition to intrathoracic pathology.

Signs and Symptoms of Acromioclavicular Joint Injury

Clinical Presentation and History

As this injury is secondary to a traumatic event, the clinical history almost always involves a description of injury to the affected shoulder or upper extremity. As clinical deformity is a common finding and complaint, the patient should be examined, whenever possible, in the standing or sitting position to allow for accentuation of the deformity by gravity. Traditionally, a weighted stress view of the AC joint was performed in an attempt to create maximal distraction between the CC space and the AC joint. It is postulated that this maneuver allows indirect determination of the deltopectoral fascia integrity, therefore differentiating a type III injury from a type V. This has not been validated in any study using this technique in correlation with intraoperative findings. It is our opinion that this study does not increase the sensitivity of diagnosis, change the "grade" or classification of the AC joint injury, does not change treatment, and more importantly it is a very painful maneuver for the patient in an acute injury. Therefore we do not recommend its routine use.

The mechanism for AC joint injuries and distal clavicle fractures is direct trauma, caused by a fall or blow with the arm in the adducted position. The subcutaneous position of the joint, makes observation of the deformity quite apparent and after the pain resolves it is one of the most common clinical complaints. It should be noted that indirect injury to the AC joint could occur by falling on an adducted outstretched hand or elbow which causes the humerus to translate superiorly and impact the acromion.

The majority of AC joint injuries occurs in young to middle-aged males and is typically caused by a direct load to the lateral shoulder or a forced impaction of the humeral head superiorly into the acromion. The contact or collision athlete represents a "high-risk" individual and AC injuries are typically associated with sports like football, rugby, and hockey.[38,43,75,127] A recent report estimated that AC joint injuries accounted for 4.5% of all injuries, but 32% of all shoulder injuries in a population of NCAA football players followed for 5 years.[43] Interestingly, of the 748 injuries to the AC joint recorded, the vast majority (96%) were "low-grade" injuries, classified as type I or II sprains (according to the Rockwood classification system). Similar injury incidences were reported by Kaplan et al.,[75] AC joint injuries accounted for 41% of the shoulder injuries reported when players at the NFL combines were asked to recall collegiate injuries that forced them to miss playing time. The incidence among hockey players is less well studied but the rates appear similar. In one study of Finnish hockey players followed for a season, 12% of the 755 injuries within the upper extremity reported to insurance providers were AC joint sprains.[103]

Physical Examination

As with any shoulder examination, the patient should be completely exposed to allow for comparison with the uninjured shoulder. Commonly the patient describes pain originating from the anterior-superior aspect of the shoulder, but it may

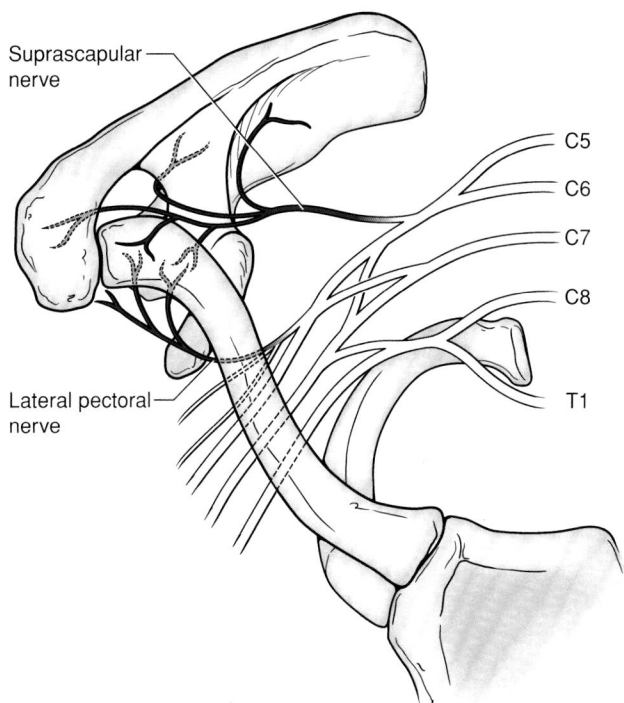

FIGURE 41-4 Illustration representing the overlapping innervation to the AC joint and glenohumeral joint via the anterior lateral pectoral nerve and the posterior suprascapular nerve. Artist rendition view from superior looking down onto the AC joint with scapula below.

be challenging to localize to a specific structure as the source. It should be noted that the lateral pectoral nerve, which also provides sensation to the anterior aspect of the shoulder and glenohumeral joint, provides the innervation of the AC joint capsule (Fig. 41-4).[58] Gerber et al.[58] evaluated patterns of pain and found that irritation to the AC joint produced pain over the AC joint, the anterolateral neck, and in the region in the anterolateral deltoid. Stimulation within the subacromial space produced pain slightly more lateral, in the region of the lateral acromion and lateral deltoid muscle, but did not produce pain in the neck or trapezius region.

The clinical triad of point tenderness at the AC joint, pain exacerbation with cross-arm adduction, and relief of symptoms by injection of a local anesthetic agent confirm injury to the AC joint. The cross-arm adduction test is performed with the arm elevated to 90 degrees and then adducted across the chest with the elbow bent at approximately 90 degrees. A positive test produces pain specifically at the AC joint. The reason that the cross-arm adduction test causes pain at the AC joint specifically is because of the compression across the AC joint with that motion. Walton et al.[159] recently documented the accuracy of clinical tests for determining whether pain is caused by AC joint injury. They describe using the Paxinos test (thumb pressure at the posterior AC joint) and a bone scan to accurately assess pain secondary to AC joint pathology. MRI scanning has been shown to be just as accurate.[146] O'Brien et al.[115] recommended the active compression test for diagnosis of AC joint abnormalities and labral pathology.

They reported 88% (55/62) of patients who had pain in the AC joint with the active compression test demonstrated abnormalities in the joint at the time of operative treatment, or had radiographic evidence of AC injury. The O'Brien test may be particularly helpful when attempting to differentiate symptoms of AC joint arthrosis from intra-articular lesions, especially those of the superior glenoid labrum. The test is performed with the arm elevated to 90 degrees, elbow in extension, adduction of 10 to 15 degrees, and a maximum pronation of the forearm with obligate internal rotation of the arm. The examiner applies a downward force resisted by the patient. Symptoms referred to the top of the shoulder and confirmed by examiner palpation suggest AC joint pathology. Localization of pain more distal to the rotator interval or anterior aspect of the shoulder suggests possible labral or biceps injury. The O'Brien maneuver, to determine superior labral pathology in isolation, is difficult to apply given its reported sensitivity is 63% and the specificity 73%.[58] Therefore, clinical history, exam, imaging findings or pathology should be used together. Often times we find utilizing Ultrasound Guided injections helpful for pain localization especially when attempting to differentiate intra-articular process from a painful AC joint.

Examination Findings Based on Injury Grade

Type I Injury. In a type I injury, there is minimal to moderate tenderness to palpation over the AC joint. In the acute patient, mild swelling over the AC joint may be present. Usually there is only minimal pain with arm movements, including adduction across the body. Tenderness is not present in the CC interspace. These patients respond very well to local anesthetic/corticosteroid injections for reduction of inflammation and acute pain relief. By definition, this grade does not demonstrate significant displacement visualized or quantifiable on radiography.

Type II Injury. By definition this grade has a higher degree of injury to the AC ligaments and capsule and consequently typically presents with moderate to severe pain with palpation of the joint. If the patient is examined shortly after injury, the outer end of the clavicle may be noted to be slightly superior to the acromion, and ecchymosis may be present. Adduction motion of the shoulder typically produces pain in the AC joint, as well as lateral pressure. A common complaint is difficulty sleeping. If the distal clavicle is grasped and the acromion stabilized, anterior–posterior motion of the clavicle in the horizontal plane can be evaluated after the acute inflammation has decreased. There should be little, if any, instability in the vertical plane (Fig. 41-5). Tenderness may be noted when the physician palpates anteriorly in the CC interspace. Radiographic evidence is subtle and would demonstrate small (<50% clavicle width) of superior clavicle displacement at AC joint if compared to contralateral side on a bilateral Zanca AC joint view.

Type III Injury. The patient with a type III injury characteristically presents with the upper extremity held adducted close to the body and supported in an elevated position to relieve the pain in the AC joint. By definition the AC joint capsule and ligaments are disrupted and the CC ligaments have significant injury that allows inferior translation of the limb and produces the characteristic shoulder droop sign (Fig. 41-6). Consequently, the clavicle may be prominent enough to tent the skin. Moderate pain is the rule, and any motion of the arm, particularly abduction, increases the pain.

Tenderness is noted at the AC joint, the CC interspace, and along the superior aspect of the lateral fourth of the clavicle. The entire length of the clavicular shaft should be palpated to detect an associated clavicle shaft fracture. The lateral clavicle is unstable in both the horizontal and vertical planes (Fig. 41-5). The key to the diagnosis of a type III injury is that the AC joint can be reduced with upward pressure under the elbow, or by having the patient actively shrug and reduce the joint; this is known as the "shrug test." A type III or reducible injury is thus differentiated from a type IV or V injury, which cannot be reduced if the deltotrapezial fascia is interposed.

Considerable controversy surrounds the gradation by radiography and thus it is important to utilize bilateral, or Zanca, views of the AC joints without weights. This allows for the measurements to be used for classification: (1) The amount of dis-

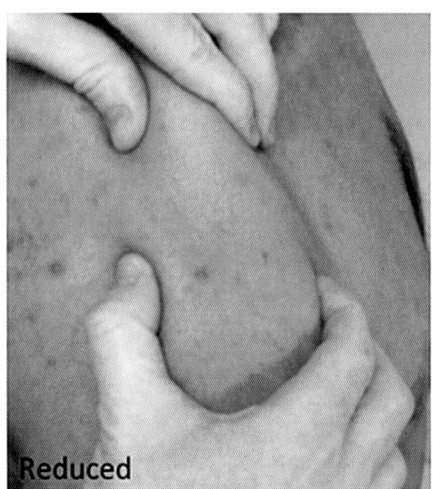 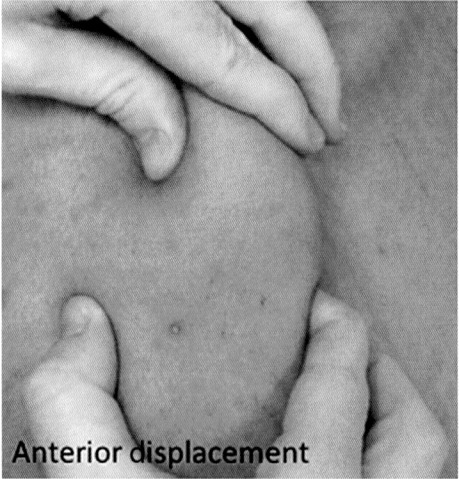

FIGURE 41-5 Clinical photo of a patient with type III AC joint dislocation with symptomatic instability with cross-arm adduction. Looking from lateral, examiner is grabbing the acromion with right hand and clavicle with the left, which is easily translated anterior and posterior approximately 3 to 5 cm.

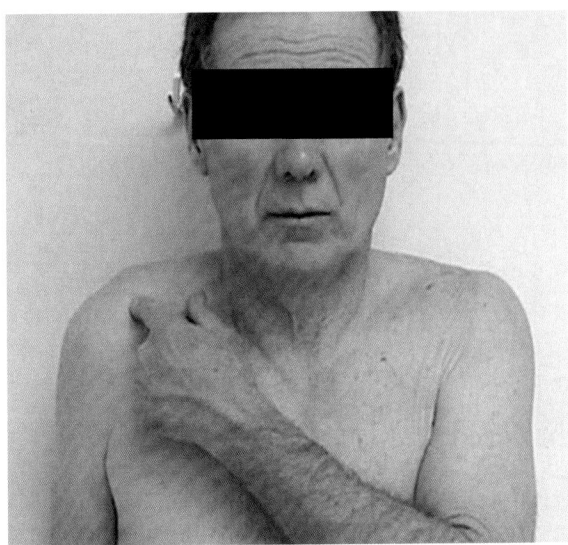

FIGURE 41-6 Clinical photo of a patient with a chronic type III (based on Zanca views) localizing his pain with activity to the deformity.

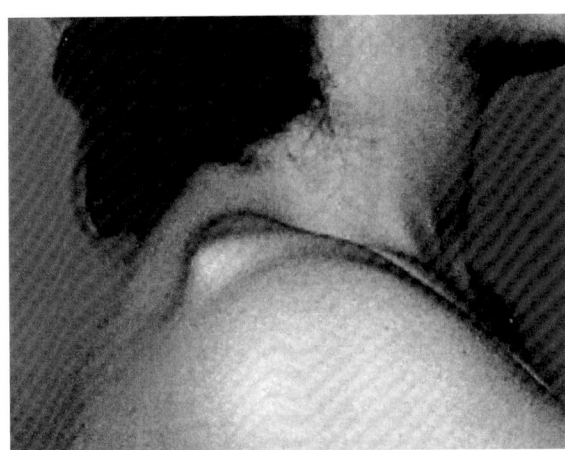

FIGURE 41-8 Patient with type IV AC joint injury. Note that the distal end of the clavicle is displaced posteriorly back into and through the trapezius muscle. (From Rockwood CA, Young DC. Disorders of the acromioclavicular joint. In: Rockwood CA, Matsen F III, eds. *The Shoulder*. Philadelphia, PA: WB Saunders; 1990:446.)

placement of distal clavicle above the acromion, this has been measured in percentage of clavicle width or a direct measurement in millimeter from superior clavicle to superior acromion. (2) The distance from undersurface of clavicle to superior cortex of the coracoid process (Fig. 41-7).

Type IV Injury. The patient with a type IV injury has essentially all the clinical findings of a type III injury. In addition, examination of the seated patient from above reveals that the outline of the displaced clavicle is inclined posteriorly compared with the uninjured shoulder. The clavicle usually is displaced so severely posteriorly that it becomes "buttonholed" through the trapezius muscle and tents the posterior skin (Fig. 41-8). Consequently, motion of the shoulder is more painful than in a type III injury. Often times in this injury pattern, the AC joint cannot be reduced manually. There is no evidence to support operating room reduction, but injection with lidocaine and attempted reduction if Acute is reasonable. It is important to remember with this injury pattern to examine the SC joint for an associ-

ated anterior dislocation, termed "bipolar" or "floating clavicle" injuries AC and SC dislocation can occur together, as discussed in a previous section within this chapter.

This type is best observed on the axillary radiograph. It will show the distal clavicle posterior to the glenoid and displaced posterior to the end of the acromion (Fig. 41-9).

Type V Injury. The type V injury is an exaggeration of the type III injury in which the distal end of the clavicle appears to be grossly superiorly displaced and tenting the skin (Fig. 41-10). This apparent deformity is the result of downward displacement of the upper extremity. The patient has more pain than with a type III injury, particularly over the distal half of the clavicle. This is secondary to the extensive muscle and soft tissue disruption around the clavicle that occurs with this injury. Often the shoulder musculature becomes weak secondary to

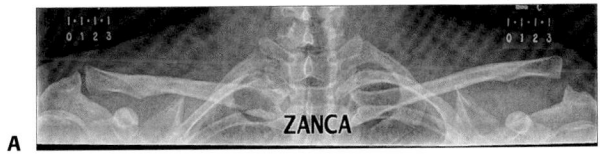

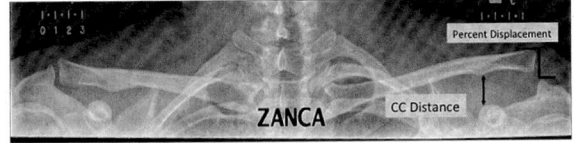

FIGURE 41-7 **A:** Radiographic quantification of AC joint displacement with Zanca radiograph with bilateral AC joints on one cassette for direct comparison, note the AC joint injury on the left side. **B:** Same Zanca radiograph with the two areas measured for quantifying the amount of displacement, CC (Coracoclavicular) distance and percentage displacement of distal clavicle above acromion.

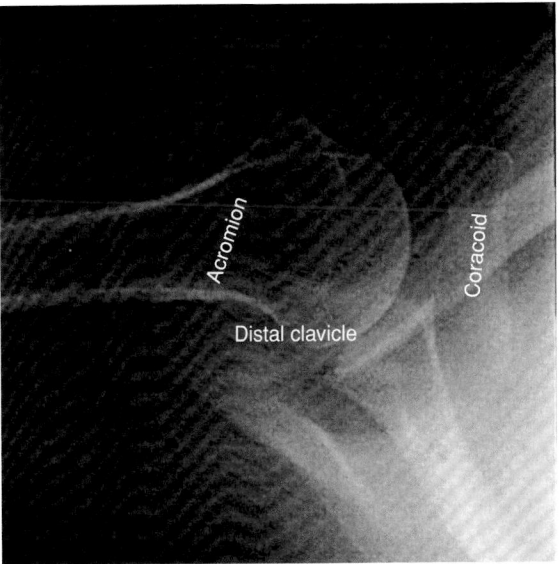

FIGURE 41-9 Axillary radiograph of a patient with a type IV AC joint injury. Note the posterior displacement of the clavicle.

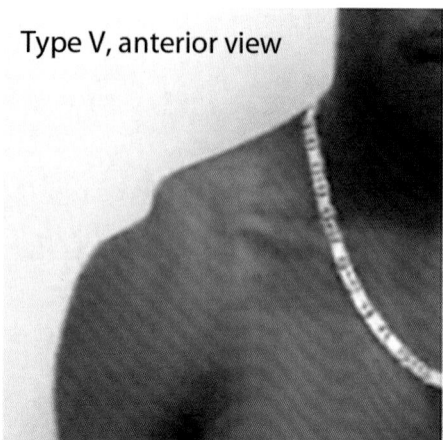

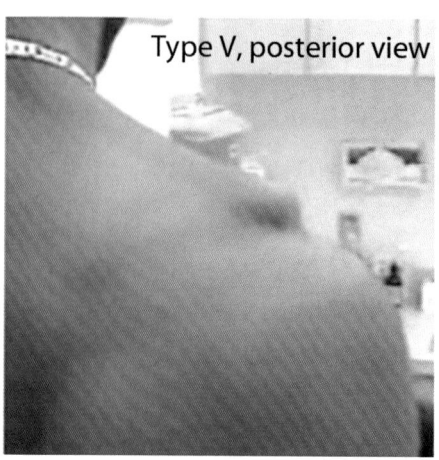

FIGURE 41-10 Clinical images of a football player with type V (radiographic) separation, picture taken from facing front and posterior to demonstrate skin tenting secondary to displacement through the deltotrapezial fascia.

disuse or as part of the injury pattern resulting in scapular dyskinesis. This can significantly impact the shoulder function and cause pain (Fig. 41-11).[65]

The radiographic assessment using the comparative Zanca view is important as this type represents a high degree of injury than the type III and thus larger distances between the clavicle and coracoid (CC distance) as well as the distance in displacement between the distal clavicle and coracoid (Fig. 41-7).

Type VI Injury. Type VI injuries are very rare. The superior aspect of the shoulder has a flat appearance, as opposed to the rounded contour of the normal shoulder. With palpation, the acromion is prominent, and there is a definite step to the superior surface of the coracoid process. Because of the degree of trauma required to produce a subcoracoid dislocation of the clavicle, there may be associated fractures of the clavicle and upper ribs or injury to the upper roots of the brachial plexus. These associated injuries may produce so much swelling of the shoulder that the disruption of the AC joint may not be recognized initially.[59,100,138] No vascular injuries were noted. However, all the adult cases reported by McPhee and Gerber and

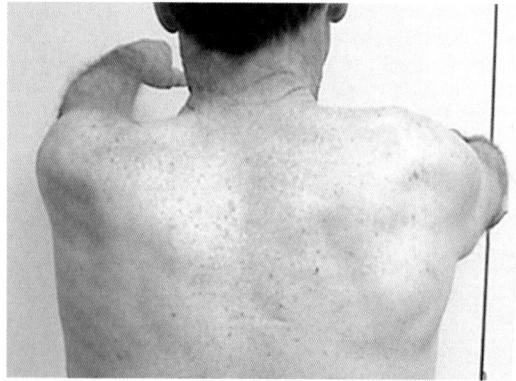

FIGURE 41-11 Clinical picture of a patient with a chronic type III AC joint dislocation with significant scapula dyskinesia. This is the same patient from Figure 41-6. Note the scapula position as the patient attempts to forward flex his arm.

Rockwood had transient paresthesias before reduction of the dislocation. After reduction, the neurologic deficits did resolve.

Imaging and Other Diagnostic Studies for Acromioclavicular Joint Injury

Good-quality radiographs of the AC joint require one-third to one-half the beam penetration required to image the glenohumeral joint. Radiographs of the AC joint taken using routine shoulder technique will be overpenetrated (i.e., dark), and small fractures may be overlooked. Therefore, the radiographic technician must be specifically requested to take radiographs of the "AC joint" rather than the "shoulder."

Anteroposterior Views

Routine AP views should be obtained with the patient standing or sitting and their back against the x-ray cassette, the arms hanging unsupported at the side. Because of significant individual variation in AC joint anatomy and because the CC interspace will vary with the angle of the x-ray beam and with the distance between the beam and the patient, both AC joints should be imaged simultaneously on one large (14- × 17-in) cassette. Large patients with shoulders too broad to be visualized on a single cassette should have radiographs made with two smaller (10- × 12-in) cassettes using identical technique.

The difficulty in evaluating AC joint injuries lies in the fact that with this projection, the distal clavicle and acromion are superimposed on the spine of the scapula. Subtle fractures of the distal clavicle are easily missed. Zanca[168] noted this during a review of 1,000 radiographs of patients with shoulder pain. Therefore, he recommended a 10- to 15-degree cephalic tilt view to project an unobscured image of the joint (Fig. 41-12). This cephalic tip not only allows for better exposure but also standardizes the distance between clavicle and coracoid which apparently increases with a more AP view secondary to x-ray parallax and bone contour (Fig. 41-12). This view is now routinely used in the evaluation of AC joint injuries and is particularly useful when there is suspicion of a small fracture or loose body on routine views (Fig. 41-7A,B).

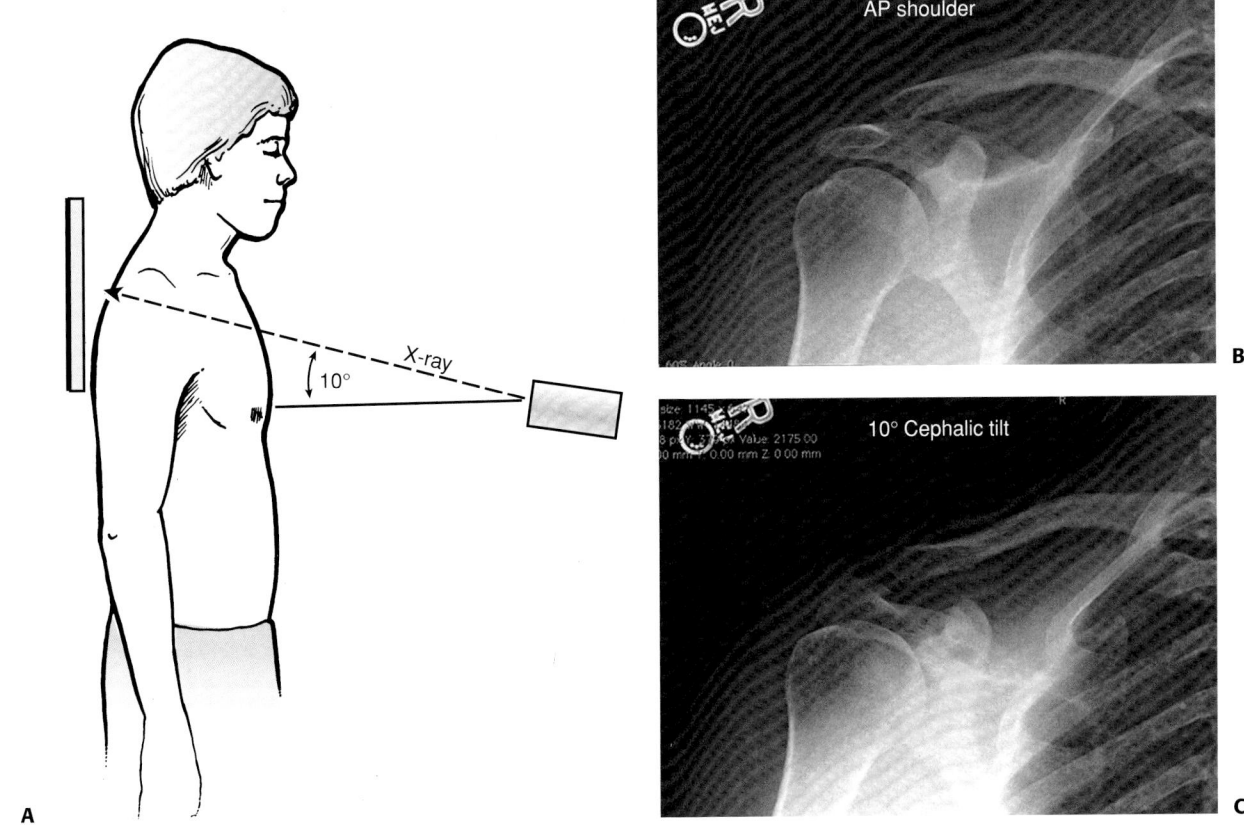

FIGURE 41-12 A: Illustration of the "Zanca view" which is shot with the x-ray beam placed 10 degrees cephalad to the perpendicular plane. **B:** Radiograph of shoulder perpendicular to floor. **C:** Radiograph done with Zanca view—10-degree cephalad tilt to demonstrate the effect of the view on the AC joint alignment and visualization of the CC distance.

Axillary Lateral View

As with any musculoskeletal injury, a radiograph in one plane is not sufficient to classify an AC joint injury. An axillary lateral view should be taken of the injured shoulder when an AC dislocation is suspected. The cassette should be placed on the superior aspect of the shoulder and medial enough to expose as much of the lateral third of the clavicle as possible. This will reveal any posterior displacement of the clavicle as well as any small fractures that may have been missed on the AP view within the coracoid (Fig. 41-9).

Stryker Notch View

A variant of an AC joint injury involves a fracture of the coracoid process. This injury should be suspected when there is an AC joint dislocation on the AP projection, but the CC distance is normal, or equal to that on the opposite, uninvolved side. A Stryker notch view taken appropriately puts the coracoid in profile and is the best view for evaluating this injury. This is performed with the patient supine and the arm elevated over the head with the palm behind the head. The humerus must be parallel to the longitudinal axis of the body, with the elbow pointed straight toward the ceiling (Fig. 41-13). This can be a difficult view to obtain in the acutely injured shoulder.[10]

Other Modalities

Schmid and Schmid[137] reported the use of ultrasonography in the diagnosis of 22 cases of type III AC dislocation. Ultrasound examination demonstrated visible instability of the distal clavicle, incongruity of the joint, hematoma formation, and visible ligament remnants in all cases. In the case of a painful type II or type III chronic injury the ultrasound study can delineate dynamic instability specifically in the anterior–posterior direction. This does help in surgical decision-making process, as unstable patients with chronic disruptions may be candidates for surgical repair. In the typical patient, sophisticated imaging modalities as ultrasonography, computed tomography (CT), and magnetic resonance imaging are not required. Plain radiography continues to be the most readily available, cost-effective method for routine investigation of injuries to the AC joint (Table 41-1).

Classification of Acromioclavicular Joint Injury

AC joint injuries are best classified according to the extent of damage inflicted by a given force. However, unlike other joints, the differential diagnosis of sprains of the AC joint is based on the severity of injury sustained by the capsular ligaments (AC ligaments) and extracapsular ligaments (CC ligaments), as well

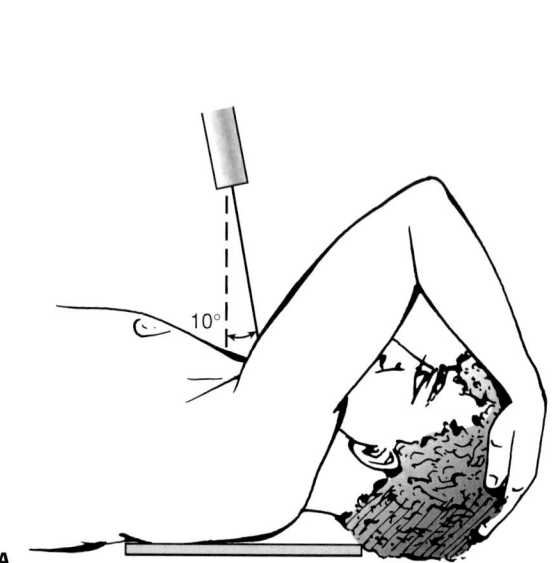

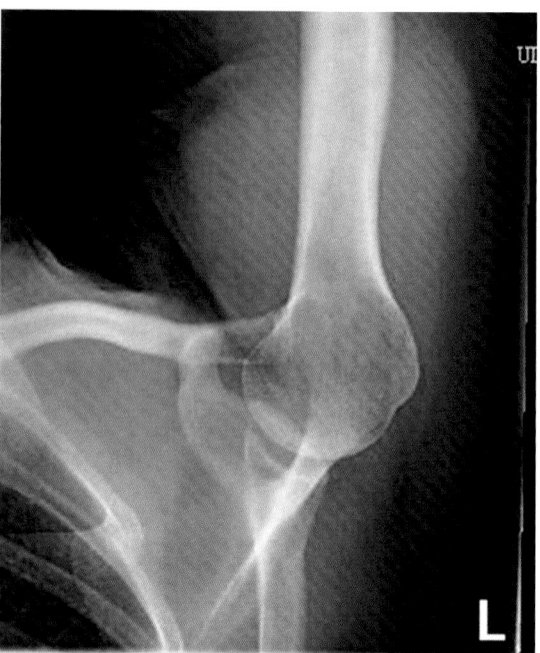

FIGURE 41-13 **A:** Illustration of positioning for the Stryker notch view. **B:** Stryker notch view radiograph of a patient. Note the view of the coracoid base where a fracture could be visualized.

TABLE 41-1	Summary of Clinical Presentation and Diagnostic Work up

Mechanism of Injury

Direct Trauma
- Force to lateral shoulder/acromion with adducted arm
- Medial and inferior force resulting in progression of injury
  - AC joint ligaments
  - CC ligaments
  - Deltotrapezial fascia
- Landing on outstretched arm or flexed elbow forcing humeral head into acromion
  - Usually results in AC joint/ligament injury
  - Can result in instability at AC joint (anterior–posterior direction) without CC ligament complex injury (minimal dislocation)

Nontraumatic or Chronic Overuse
- AC joint arthrosis—weight lifting, laborer (pneumatic jackhammer), repetitive overhead activity
- Repetitive low-grade AC joint injuries
- Medical cause: Rheumatoid arthritis, hyperparathyroidism, scleroderma, and rarely Gorham's osteolysis

Physical Examination
Diffuse Shoulder Pain—anterolateral neck, AC joint, anterolateral deltoid
Point tender at AC joint ± deformity (prominence)
    Positive cross-arm adduction test (arm flexed 90 degrees, adducted across chest) produces compression pain localized to AC joint
    O'Brien's active compression test with localized pain over AC joint
    Paxinos test (thumb pressure directed anterior at the posterior AC joint)
    Diagnostic analgesic injection—positive relief in pain/symptoms

Radiographic Findings
Zanca view to determine displacement with comparison to contralateral AC joint and CC distance
Zanca view: Beam placed 10–15 degrees cephalad and using 50% of the AP penetration strength
Axillary view—determine anterior/posterior position of distal clavicle in relation to acromion
Cross-arm stress view—Basmania view (AP with arm adducted)
Reducibility Stress Views—Active shrug maneuver with AP of shoulder or with patient applying upload directed load on elbow by lining on table while radiograph of AC joint (Goal: determine is deltotrapezial fascia interposed to prevent reduction)

as the supporting musculature (deltoid and trapezius muscles). Therefore, injuries to the AC joint are graded according to the amount of injury to the AC and CC ligaments. Injuries in this anatomic area have traditionally been referred to as "AC joint injuries," although they have varying degrees of disruption between the scapula and the clavicle, not limited to the one particular joint.

The strength of any classification system depends on its ability to guide treatment and predict prognosis. Rockwood et al.[127,163] developed the most widely accepted classification system, based on the original work of Tossy et al.[154] in 1963. It is an expanded, accurate classification system based on the anatomic severity of the injury. The modified classification is described below, summarized in Table 41-2, and illustrated in Figure 41-14.

In all reported cases of subcoracoid dislocation, the clavicle has become lodged behind an intact conjoined tendon. The AC ligaments are disrupted in either a subacromial or subcoracoid dislocation. The CC ligament, however, is intact in a subacromial dislocation and completely disrupted in a subcoracoid dislocation. Likewise, the integrity of the deltoid and trapezius muscle attachments depends on the degree of clavicular displacement.

Normal Joints

The width and configuration of the AC joint in the coronal plane may vary significantly from individual to individual. This should be remembered so that a normal variant is not mistaken as an injury. In a study of 100 radiographs of normal shoulders, Urist[157] found that nearly half (49%) of the AC joints were inclined superolateral to inferomedial, with the articular surface of the clavicle overriding the acromion; 27% were vertical and 3% were inclined superomedial to inferolateral, with the articular surface of the clavicle underriding the acromion. Another 21% of the joints were incongruent, with the clavicle lying either superior or inferior to the acromial articular surface.

The normal width of the AC joint in the coronal plane is 1 to 3 mm. Petersson and Redlund-Johnell[119] measured AC joint width radiographically in 151 normal individuals and drew several conclusions: The AC joint space normally diminishes with increasing age, a joint space of 0.5 mm in a patient older than 60 years is conceivably normal, and a joint space of greater than 7 mm in men and 6 mm in women is pathologic.

The CC interspace also exhibits significant individual variation. The average distance between the clavicle and the coracoid process ranges from 1.1 to 1.3 cm.[7] An increase in the CC distance of 50% over the normal side signifies a complete AC dislocation.[7] Complete dislocation has been seen with as little as a 25% increase in the CC distance.

Type I Injury. In a type I injury, the radiographs of the AC joint are normal, except for mild soft tissue swelling, as compared with the uninjured shoulder. There is no radiographic widening, no separation, and no deformity.

Type II Injury. In a type II injury, the lateral end of the clavicle may be slightly elevated. The AC joint, when compared

TABLE 41-2	**Summary Table of Tossy–Rockwood AC Joint Dislocation Classification**
Type I	A mild force to the point of the shoulder produces a minor strain to the fibers of the AC ligaments. The ligaments remain intact, and the AC joint remains stable.
Type II	A moderate force to the point of the shoulder is severe enough to rupture the ligaments of the AC joint. The distal end of the clavicle is unstable in the horizontal plane (i.e., anteroposterior), but vertical (i.e., superoinferior) stability is preserved by virtue of the (damaged but) intact coracoclavicular ligament. The scapula may rotate medially, producing a widening of the AC joint. There may be a slight, relative upward displacement of the distal end of the clavicle secondary to stretching of the coracoclavicular ligaments.
Type III	A severe force is applied to the point of the shoulder which tears the AC and coracoclavicular ligaments resulting in a complete AC dislocation. The distal clavicle appears to be displaced superiorly as the scapula and shoulder complex droop inferomedially. Radiographic findings include a 25–100% increase in the coracoclavicular space in comparison to the normal shoulder.[126]
Type IV	Posterior dislocation of the distal end of the clavicle, or a type IV AC dislocation, is relatively rare. The clavicle is posteriorly displaced into or through the trapezius muscle as the force applied to the acromion drives the scapula anteriorly and inferiorly. Posterior clavicular displacement may be so severe that the skin on the posterior aspect of the shoulder becomes tented. The literature concerning posterior AC dislocations consists mostly of small series and case reports.[69,93] Some[5,11,145] refer to this injury as a "posterior dislocation of the clavicle," and others[69,111] prefer the term "anterior dislocation of the AC joint."
Type V	Type V AC dislocation is a markedly more severe version of the type III injury. The distal clavicle has been stripped of all its soft tissue attachments (i.e., AC ligaments, coracoclavicular ligament, and the deltotrapezial muscle attachments) and lies subcutaneously. When combined with superior displacement of the clavicle owing to unopposed pull of the sternocleidomastoid muscle, the severe downward droop of the extremity produces a marked disfiguration of the shoulder. Radiographically, the coracoclavicular space is increased greater than 100% in comparison to the opposite, normal shoulder.[126]
Type VI	Inferior dislocation of the distal clavicle, or type VI AC dislocation, is an exceedingly rare injury.[59,100,129] Gerber and Rockwood's[59] series of three patients is the largest one reported in the literature. The injury is often the result of severe trauma and is frequently accompanied by multiple injuries. The mechanism of dislocation is thought to be severe hyperabduction and external rotation of the arm, combined with retraction of the scapula. The distal clavicle occupies either a subacromial or a subcoracoid location.

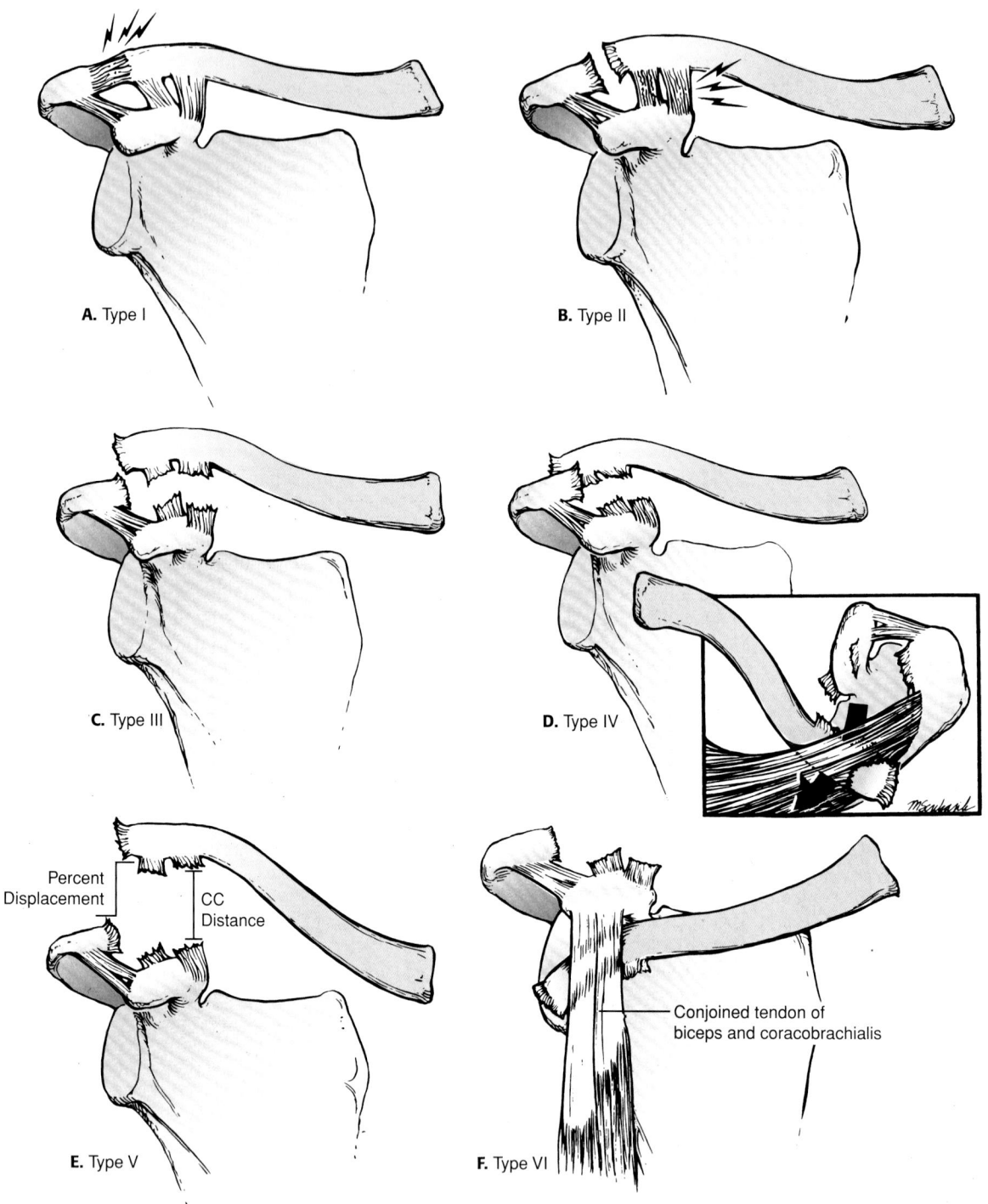

A. Type I

B. Type II

C. Type III

D. Type IV

Percent
Displacement

CC
Distance

E. Type V

Conjoined tendon of
biceps and coracobrachialis

F. Type VI

FIGURE 41-14 Schematic drawings of the classification of ligamentous injuries to the AC joint. **A:** In the type I injury, a mild force applied to the point of the shoulder does not disrupt either the AC or the coracoclavicular ligaments. **B:** A moderate to heavy force applied to the point of the shoulder will disrupt the AC ligaments, but the coracoclavicular ligaments remain intact (type II). **C:** When a severe force is applied to the point of the shoulder both the AC and the coracoclavicular ligaments are disrupted (type III). **D:** In a type IV injury, not only are the ligaments disrupted, but the distal end of the clavicle is also displaced posteriorly into or through the trapezius muscle. **E:** A larger enough force applied to the point of the shoulder not only ruptures the AC and coracoclavicular ligaments but also disrupts the muscle attachments and creates a major separation between the clavicle and the acromion (type V). **F:** This is an inferior dislocation of the distal clavicle in which the clavicle is inferior to the coracoid process and posterior to the biceps and coracobrachialis tendons. The AC and coracoclavicular ligaments are also disrupted (type VI).

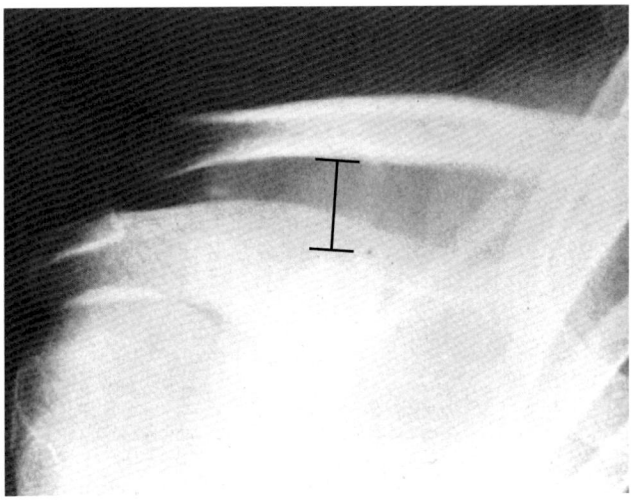
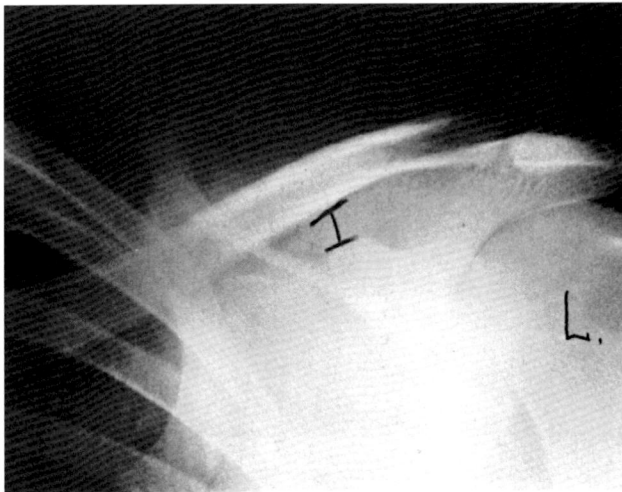

FIGURE 41-15 X-ray appearance of a grade III injury. Not only is the right AC joint displaced compared with the left, but also, more significantly, notice the great increase in the coracoclavicular interspace on the injured right shoulder compared with the normal left shoulder.

with the normal side, may appear to be widened. The widening probably results from a slight medial rotation of the scapula and slight posterior displacement of the clavicle due to trapezius muscle contraction. The CC space of the injured shoulder is the same as that of the normal shoulder.

Type III Injury. In type III AC dislocations, the joint is totally displaced. The lateral end of the clavicle is displaced completely above the superior border of the acromion and the CC interspace is significantly (25% to 100%) greater than in the normal shoulder (Fig. 41-15). Fractures may be noted involving the distal clavicle or the acromion process.

Rarely, complete AC dislocation will be accompanied by a fracture of the coracoid process rather than by disruption of the CC ligaments. Although the fracture of the coracoid process is difficult to visualize on routine radiographs, its presence should

be suspected because of the presence of a complete AC separation and a normal CC distance, as compared with the uninjured shoulder. The ideal radiograph for visualizing the coracoid fracture is the Stryker notch view (as described) (Fig. 41-16). A few unusual injury patterns uncommonly occur and are variations of type III dislocations. Most often, complete separation of the articular surfaces of the distal clavicle and acromion is accompanied by complete disruption of the AC and CC ligaments.

Children and adolescents may sustain a variant of complete AC dislocation. Radiographs reveal displacement of the distal clavicular metaphysis superiorly with a large increase in the CC interspace. These injuries are most often Salter–Harris type I or II injuries in which the epiphysis and the intact AC joint remain in their anatomic locations whereas the distal clavicular metaphysis is displaced superiorly through a dorsal

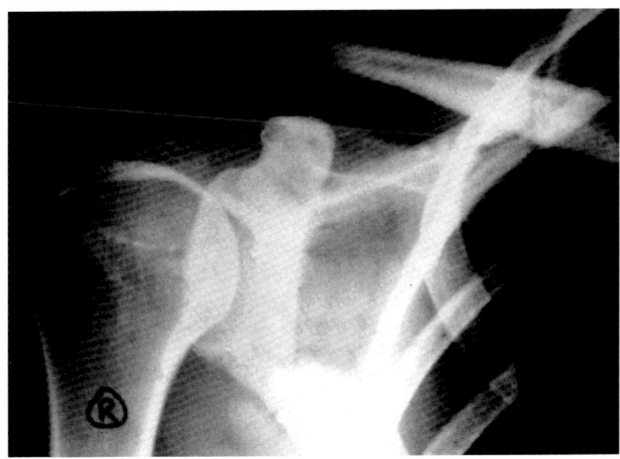
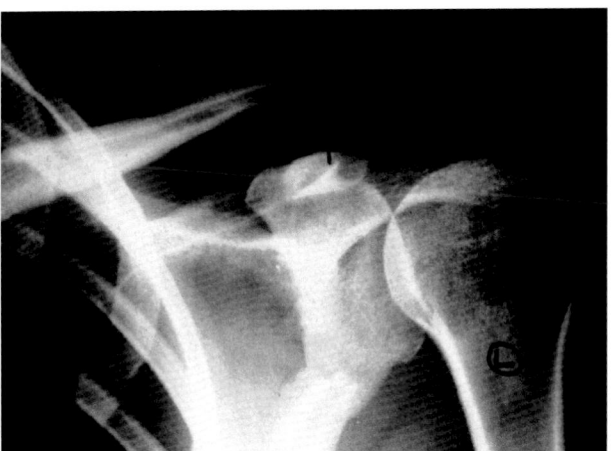

A   **B**

FIGURE 41-16 Radiographs of a patient with a type III variant injury involving the AC joint and a fracture of both the base and the tip of the coracoid. **A:** An anteroposterior radiograph of the injured right side. The coracoid injury is not visualized. **B:** A radiograph of the uninjured left side demonstrating that the coracoclavicular distance is equal on the injured and unaffected sides.

(continues)

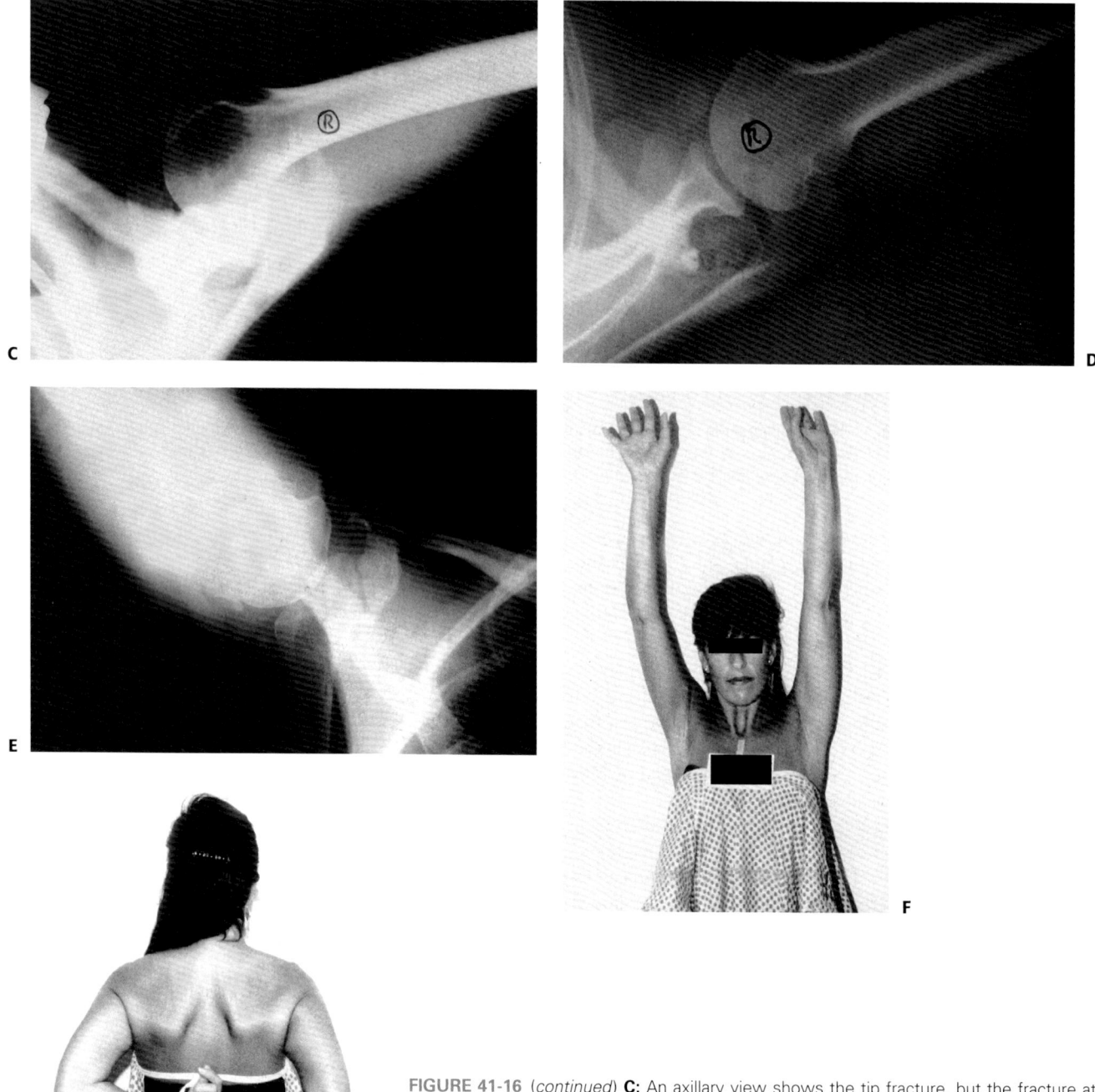

FIGURE 41-16 (*continued*) **C:** An axillary view shows the tip fracture, but the fracture at the base is not easily detected. **D:** The West Point view clearly shows the fracture at the tip of the coracoid process. **E:** The Stryker notch view clearly shows the fracture at the base of the coracoid. **F:** Nonoperative treatment in this case led to an excellent result as evidenced by full overhead elevation. **G:** The patient regained near-normal internal rotation.

rent in the periosteal sleeve (Fig. 41-17).[12,37,47,48,71] The lateral epiphysis of the clavicle is barely visible because it is thin and fuses over a short time period at approximately 19 years of age. Eidman et al.[47] reported on 25 AC injuries in children treated surgically. In all patients younger than 13 years of age, there was a lateral Salter–Harris clavicular fracture rather than a true AC dislocation. The importance of recognizing this injury is that the intact CC ligaments remain attached to the periosteal sleeve. Nonoperative management most often results in healing of the clavicular fracture and thus re-establishment of the integrity of the CC ligaments. Those authors who recommend surgical repair in selected instances emphasize the importance of repairing the dorsal rent in the periosteal sleeve.[47,48]

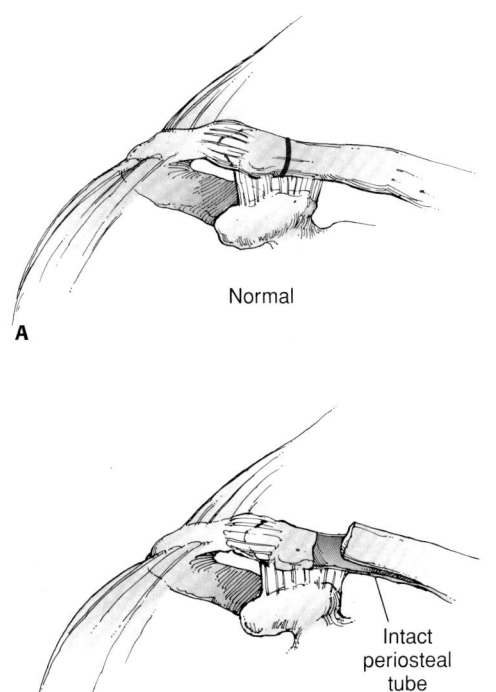

Normal

A

Intact
periosteal
tube

B Type III variant

FIGURE 41-17 A: In children and adolescents, the distal clavicular physis lies medial to the AC capsular reflection. Injuries in this age group are often type II Salter–Harris fractures involving the physis rather than AC dislocations. **B.** The coracoclavicular ligaments remain attached to the intact periosteal sleeve whereas the medial clavicular fragment displaces through a dorsal periosteal rent.

A variation of the type III injury involves complete separation of the AC articular surface combined with a fracture of the coracoid process.[25,81,95] This is an extremely uncommon injury. In most cases the CC ligaments have remained intact

and attached to the displaced coracoid process fracture, which most often occurs through the base.

Both operative and nonoperative methods of treatment have been described for combined AC dislocation and coracoid process fracture with intact CC ligaments. Results seem to be similar in both groups. Therefore, most authors recommend nonoperative treatment. Most often, the coracoid process fracture is extra-articular. However, we have encountered instances in which the coracoid fragment contains a significant portion of the glenoid fossa. The conjoined tendon rotates the coracoid process and glenoid inferolaterally and can result in substantial articular displacement. In this situation, open reduction and internal fixation may be necessary and is predicated on the amount of displacement of the articular fragment (Fig. 41-18).[128]

Type IV Injury. Although the radiographic findings associated with a type IV injury include a relative upward displacement of the clavicle from the acromion and an increase in the CC interspace, the most striking feature is the posterior displacement of the distal clavicle, as seen on the axillary lateral radiograph (Fig. 41-19). In patients with heavy, thick shoulders or in patients with multiple injuries in whom an axillary lateral view of the shoulder or a scapular lateral radiographic view cannot be taken, a CT scan may be of great value in helping to confirm clinical suspicions of a posteriorly dislocated AC joint.

Type V Injury. The characteristic radiographic feature of type V injuries is a marked increase (100% to 300%) in the CC distance. The clavicle appears to be grossly displaced superiorly away from the acromion (Fig. 41-20). However, radiographs reveal that the clavicle on the injured side is actually at approximately the same level as the clavicle on the normal side, and the scapula is displaced inferiorly.

Type VI Injury. There are two types of inferior AC dislocation: Subacromial and subcoracoid. In the subacromial type, radiographs reveal a decreased CC distance (i.e., less than the

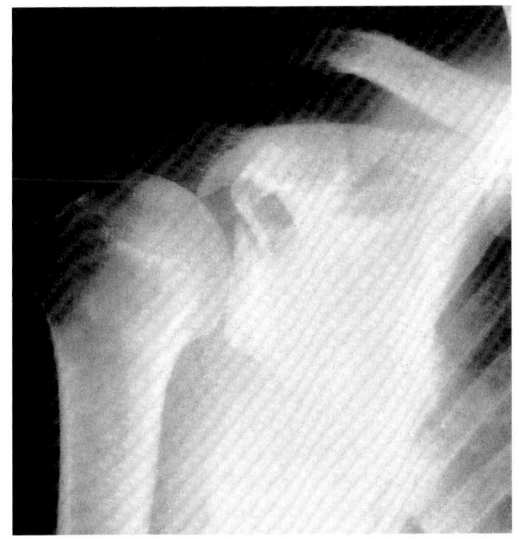

A

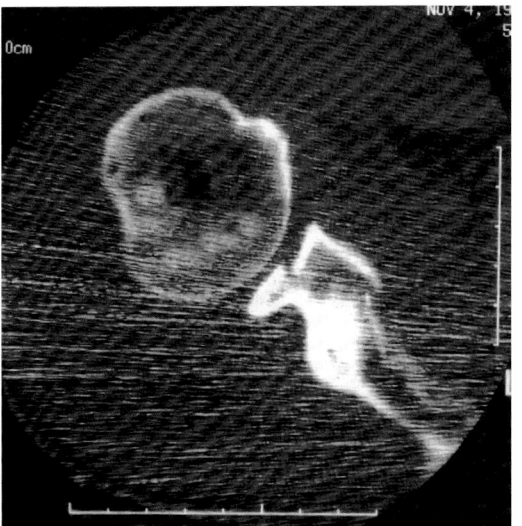

B

FIGURE 41-18 Coracoid fracture with intra-articular extension. **A:** Anteroposterior radiograph showing the fracture through the coracoid. **B:** A CT scan showing the glenoid displacement necessitating open reduction and internal fixation of the glenoid.

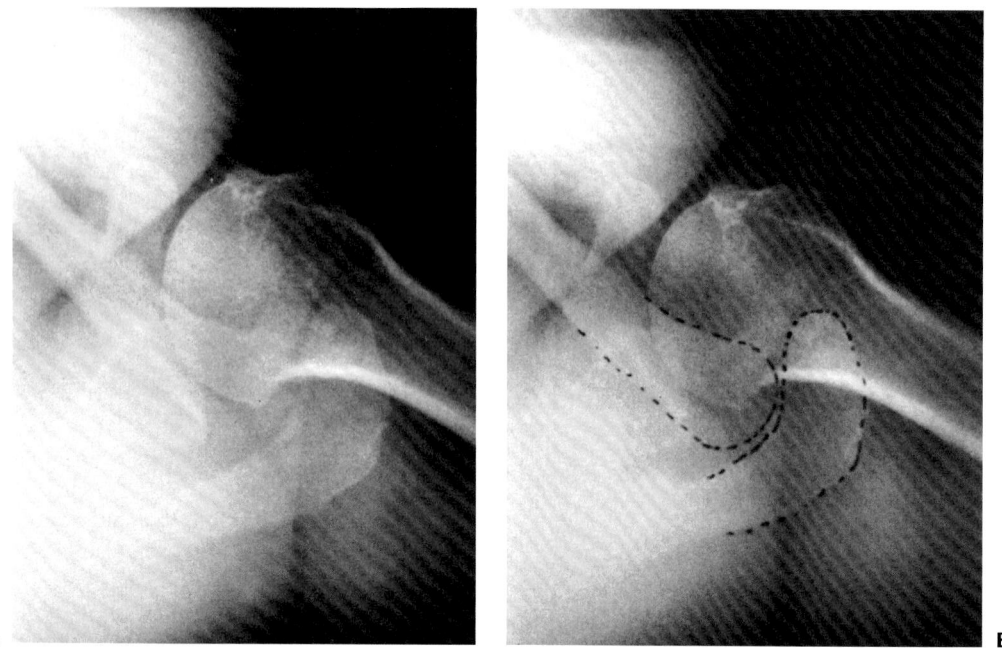

FIGURE 41-19 Type IV posterior dislocation of the AC joint. **A:** Axillary lateral radiograph of the right shoulder. **B:** Axillary view with the distal clavicle and acromion outlined.

normal side), and the distal clavicle is in a subacromial location. The subcoracoid dislocation is characterized by a reversed CC distance, with the clavicle displaced inferior to the coracoid process (Fig. 41-21). Because this injury usually is the result of severe trauma, it often is accompanied by multiple other fractures of the clavicle and ribs.

Outcome Measures for Acromioclavicular Joint Injury

The treatment of AC joint injures is an area of much controversy. The definition of injury pattern is based on the amount of separation or displacement observed on radiographs and classi-

fied by Rockwood.[126] Traditional treatment of all injury patterns involves an early period of rest, ice, and immobilization with a sling. However, the time needed to return to sport is not clear. Recent reports suggest 10 to 15 days for low-grade, type I and II, injures is all that is needed; however, return to pain-free play or the need for anesthetic injections to play was not evaluated in these reports.[2,4] However, clinical experience suggests the time to return to true pain-free sport with or without supplemental anesthetic injection may be longer. Among Australian Rules football and rugby players the use of local anesthetic injections for painful AC joint dislocations has been very successful with very limited side effects.[9] In this population, the

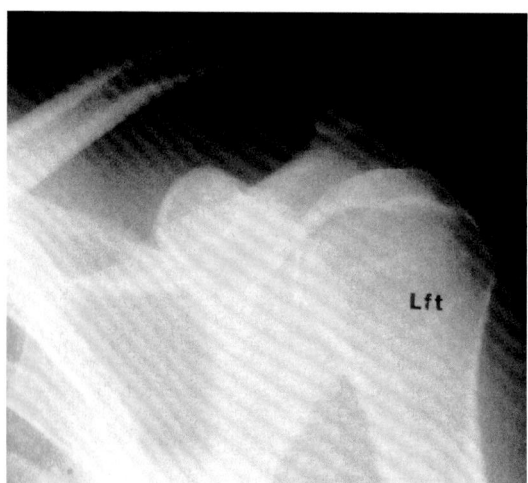

FIGURE 41-20 An anteroposterior radiograph of a type V dislocation shows the marked increase in the coracoclavicular interspace. The clavicle appears to be grossly displaced away from the acromion.

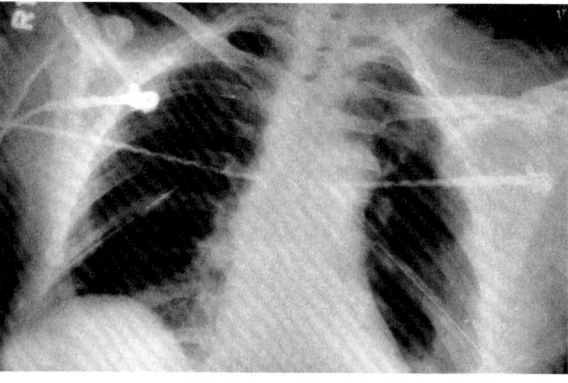

FIGURE 41-21 Type VI AC dislocation. The distal end of the **Left** clavicle is in the subcoracoid position. The high-energy trauma causing this injury is evidenced by the bilateral chest tubes in this patient. (From Rockwood CA, Young DC. Disorders of the acromioclavicular joint. In: Rockwood CA, Matsen F III, eds. *The Shoulder*. Philadelphia, PA: WB Saunders; 1990:447. Courtesy of RC. Erickson and D. Massillion.)

mean number of games using an injection to play was stratified among the various injuries treated: AC joint dislocations had the highest need, an average of 5.7 games.[9] Clinical practice demonstrates that these competitive athletes will return to play despite a painful joint, but if given the option of local treatment to help symptoms will readily accept it.

PATHOANATOMY AND APPLIED ANATOMY RELATING TO ACROMIOCLAVICULAR JOINT INJURIES

Applied Anatomy of the Acromioclavicular Joint

The AC joint, a diarthrodial joint, is located between the medial margin of the acromion and lateral end of the clavicle. Within the AC joint, there is a fibrocartilaginous disk of varying size and shape. In viewing the AC joint from the anterior–posterior direction, the inclination of the joint may be almost vertical, or it may be inclined downward and medially, with the clavicle overriding the acromion by an angle as much as 50 degrees (Fig. 41-22).[131] There may be an underriding type of inclination, with the clavicular facet under the acromion process. Approximately 50% of the time, the articular surface of the clavicle overrides the articular surface of the acromion resulting in incongruent articular surfaces. However, there is evidence to support that the articulating surfaces to impart some level biomechanical support and should be considered when surgical repair or reconstruction is performed.[19]

There are two types of fibrocartilaginous intra-articular disks—complete and partial (meniscoid). The disk varies greatly in size and shape,[41] and with age the meniscus undergoes degeneration until it is essentially no longer functional beyond the fourth decade.[41,118,130] The nerve supply to the AC joint is from branches of the axillary, suprascapular, and lateral pectoral nerves (Fig. 41-4).

Acromioclavicular Ligaments

The AC ligaments, consisting of anterior, posterior, superior, and inferior ligaments, surround the AC joint (Fig. 41-23). The fibers of the superior AC ligament, which are the strongest of the capsular ligaments, blend with the fibers of the deltoid and trapezius muscles, which are attached to the superior aspect of the clavicle and the acromion process. These muscle attachments are important in adding stability to the AC joint. The AC ligaments stabilize the joint in an AP direction (the horizontal plane).[40,130,157] Recent studies have shown that the distance from the lateral clavicle to the insertion of the superior AC ligament/capsule ranges from 5.2 to 7 mm in women and approximately 8 mm in men.[14,138] An AC resection that extends medial to the capsular insertion leads to instability in the horizontal plane.[13]

Coracoclavicular Ligament

The CC ligament is a very strong, heavy ligament whose fibers run from the outer, inferior surface of the clavicle to the base of the coracoid process of the scapula. The CC ligament has two components: The conoid and the trapezoid ligaments (Fig. 41-23). The trapezoid ligament measures from 0.8 to 2.5 cm in length and from 0.8 to 2.5 cm in width. The conoid ligament varies from 0.7 to 2.5 cm in length and from 0.4 to 0.95 cm in width.[130] The distance from the lateral clavicle to the most lateral fibers of the trapezoid ligament may measure as little as 10 mm.[14,67,68,124]

The conoid ligament, the more medial of the two ligaments, is cone shaped, with the apex of the cone attaching on the posteromedial side of the base of the coracoid process. The base of the cone attaches onto the conoid tubercle on the posterior undersurface of the clavicle. The conoid tubercle is located at the apex of the posterior clavicular curve, which is at the junction of the lateral third of the flattened clavicle with the medial two-thirds of the triangular shaft.

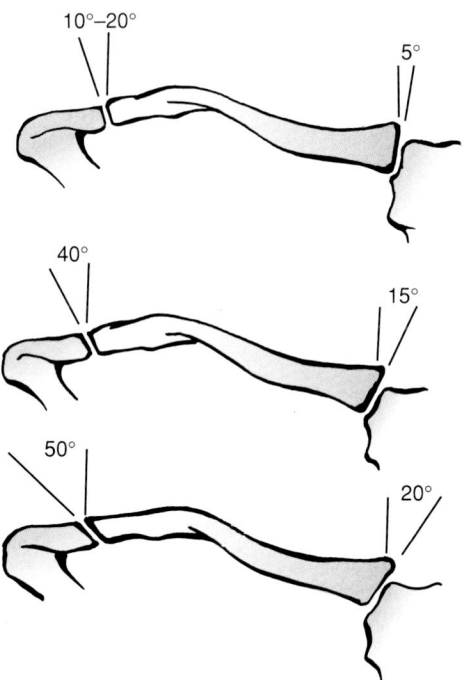

FIGURE 41-22 Variations of the inclination of the AC and the sternoclavicular joints. (Redrawn from DePalma AF. *Surgery of the Shoulder.* Philadelphia, PA: JB Lippincott; 1973.)

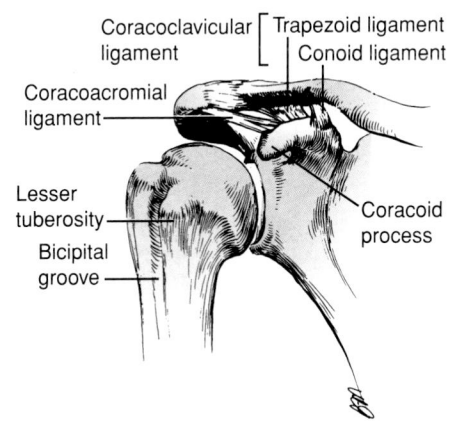

FIGURE 41-23 Normal anatomy of the AC joint.

The trapezoid ligament arises from the coracoid process, anterior and lateral to the attachment of the conoid ligament. This is just posterior to the attachment of the pectoralis minor tendon. The trapezoid ligament extends superiorly to a rough line on the undersurface of the clavicle.

Biomechanics of the Acromioclavicular Joint

The biomechanics of the AC joint involve static stability, dynamic stability, and AC joint motion. The only connection between the upper extremity and the axial skeleton is through the clavicular articulations at the AC and SC joints. Moreover, through anatomic dissections of the SC ligaments, he demonstrated how these ligaments prevent downward displacement of the distal end of the clavicle. Hence, in the erect position, the strong SC ligaments support the clavicles suspended away from the body, like the wings from the body of an airplane. Furthermore, just as the jet engines are suspended from the underside of the wings, the upper extremities are suspended from the distal clavicles through the CC ligament. Thus, the CC ligament is the prime suspensory ligament of the upper extremity.

AC joint stability is maintained predominantly by the surrounding ligamentous structures, specifically the CC ligaments (conoid and trapezoid) and the AC capsule and ligaments. Following excision of the AC joint capsule, Urist[157] demonstrated that the distal clavicle could be completely dislocated anteriorly and posteriorly away from the acromion process. However, vertical displacement of the clavicle, in relation to the acromion, occurs only after the CC ligaments are transected (Fig. 41-24). Fukuda et al.[52] performed load-displacement tests with a fixed displacement after sequential ligament sectioning to determine individual contributions of the various ligaments to AC stability. The contribution of the AC, trapezoid, and conoid ligaments was determined at small and large displacements. At small displacements, the AC ligaments were the primary restraint to both posterior (89%) and superior (68%) translation of the clavicle—the most common failure patterns seen clinically. At large displacements, the conoid ligament provided the primary restraint (62%) to superior translation, whereas the AC ligaments remained the primary restraint (90%) to posterior translation. At both large and small displacements, the trapezoid ligament served as the primary restraint to AC joint compression.

Studies have demonstrated that the trapezoid ligament has a greater role in resistance to posterior displacement of the clavicle and the conoid has a greater role in anterior displacement of the clavicle.[86,142] The role of the AC joint capsule and ligaments has been studied extensively with respect to distal clavicle resection.[17,40,49,50] Posterior abutment of the clavicle against the acromion is avoided with only 5 mm of bone removal. This

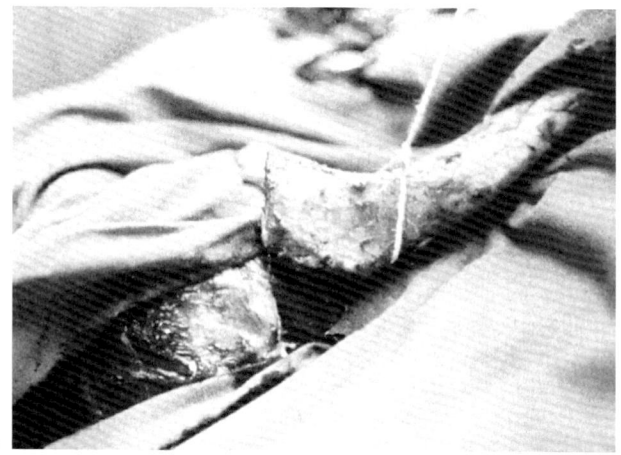

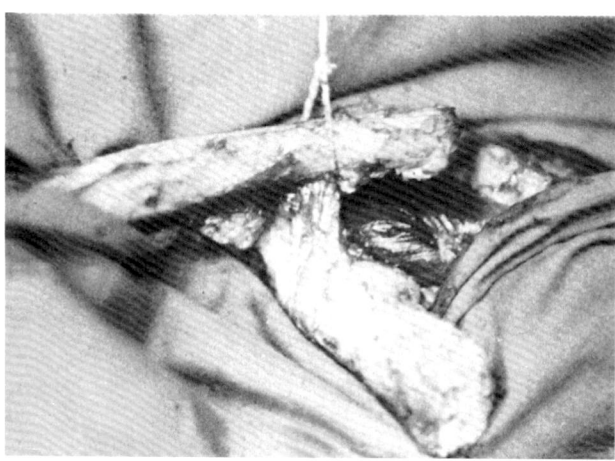

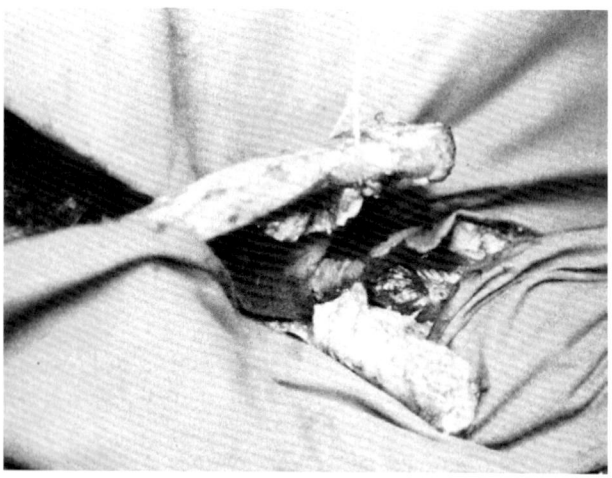

FIGURE 41-24 The importance of the AC and coracoclavicular ligaments for stability of the AC joint, demonstrated in a fresh cadaver. **A:** With the muscles and AC capsule and ligaments resected and with the coracoclavicular ligaments intact, the clavicle can be displaced anteriorly, as shown, or posteriorly from the articular surface of the acromion. **B:** However, because the coracoclavicular ligaments are intact, the clavicle cannot be displaced significantly upward. **C:** Following the transection of the coracoclavicular ligaments, the clavicle can be displaced completely above the acromion process. This suggests that the horizontal stability of the AC joint is accomplished by the AC ligaments, and vertical stability is obtained through the coracoclavicular ligaments.

preserves the capsule and ligaments, maintaining AP stability of the AC joint. Larger resections have been shown to result in excessive posterior translation.[13,79] Together, these experiments have led to the following conclusions regarding the AC joint:

- The horizontal stability is controlled by the AC ligament and capsule.
- The vertical stability is controlled by the CC ligaments.

The CC ligament helps to couple glenohumeral abduction/flexion to scapular rotation on the thorax. Full overhead elevation cannot be accomplished without combined and synchronous glenohumeral and scapulothoracic motion.[28,72,76] As the clavicle rotates upward, it dictates scapulothoracic rotation by virtue of its attachment to the scapula—the conoid and trapezoid ligaments.

Motion of the Acromioclavicular Joint

Motion of the AC joint has been a subject of debate. The clavicle rotates superiorly 40 to 50 degrees with elevation of the shoulder. Rockwood et al.[127] showed that there was only 5 to 8 degrees of rotation of the clavicle relative to the acromion. Although the clavicle rotates 40 to 50 degrees during full overhead elevation, this rotation is combined with simultaneous scapular rotation rather than with pure AC joint motion.[167] This "synchronous scapuloclavicular" motion was originally described by Codman[28] and more recently elucidated by Flatow.[49]

ACROMIOCLAVICULAR JOINT INJURY TREATMENT OPTIONS

Nonoperative Treatment of Acromioclavicular Joint Injuries

There is a general consensus supporting nonoperative treatment of Rockwood type I and type II AC joint injuries.[34,97] Both type I and type II AC joint injuries are treated in the acute setting with an initial period of immobilization. Although both type I and type II AC injuries are on the lower end of the spectrum, both types may remain symptomatic several years following injury.[35,106] Consequently, these lower grade AC joint injuries remain symptomatic for a variety of reasons, such as posttraumatic arthritis, posttraumatic osteolysis of clavicle, recurrent AP subluxation, torn capsular ligaments trapped within the joint, loose pieces of articular cartilage, or detached intra-articular meniscus. In a study by Mouhsine et al.,[106] 52% of patients with type I and type II injuries were found to be symptomatic at an average of 6 years from injury. Operative treatment of the persistently symptomatic type I and type II AC joint injuries is tailored toward addressing the mechanism behind the symptoms and will be discussed in more detail in the following operative section. In contradistinction to type I and type II AC joint injuries, greater controversy exists regarding the optimal treatment of type III AC joint injuries. Part of the controversy in managing type III AC joint injuries is due to the difficulty in differentiating type III from type V injuries of the AC joint. Furthermore, there has been an oscillating preference in treatment between operative and nonoperative means of handling these AC injuries. Type III AC joint injuries have a

completely torn AC and CC ligaments with 25% to 100% superior displacement in comparison to the contralateral shoulder. Type V AC joint injuries have, in addition to complete tears of the AC and CC ligaments, stripping of deltotrapezial fascia that results in greater than 100% superior displacement compared to the contralateral shoulder. With this similarity in the direction of displacement, there has been difficulty in determining not only the correct classification but also the correct treatment. During the 1930s to 1940s, conservative treatment of type III AC joint injuries was predominant. During the 1950s to 1970s, with advances in surgical technique, operative repair became the mainstay for managing these dislocated AC injuries. In a poll study by Powers and Bach[121] in 1974, the majority of residency programs across the United States treated type III AC joint injuries with open reduction with 60% using temporary AC fixation and 35% using CC fixation. In the early 1990s, Cox et al.[36] polled two groups of orthopedist—one group of specialized sports medicine orthopedists and a second group of chairmen of orthopedic residency programs. Both groups preferred nonoperative management of type III AC joint injuries at 86.4% in the sports medicine specialist group and 72.2% in the orthopedic residency programs. Recently, in 2007, Nissen and Chatterjee[112] polled members of the American Orthopaedic Society for Sports Medicine (AOSSM) and residency directors of orthopedic surgery programs who together had inclination toward nonoperative treatment of type III AC injuries. In light of higher levels of evidence, there is a couple of prospective randomized studies of nonoperative versus operative treatment for AC injuries.[3,84] In a prospective randomized study, Bannister et al.[3] had patients treated operatively with reduction and fixation by a CC screw or treated nonoperatively with a broad arm sling for 2 weeks followed by the same rehabilitation as the operative group. After 4 years of follow-up, the nonoperatively treated group demonstrated quicker regain of movement, quicker return to work and sports, and fewer poor results. However, subgroup analysis of AC dislocations with >2 cm of displacement showed better results in the operatively treated group. In a subsequent prospective randomized study, Larsen et al.[84] had patients randomized to nonoperative treatment with a sling or operative treatment using the Phemister procedure that consisted of reduction and fixation of the AC joint with two threaded 2-mm Kirschner wires crossing the joint space followed by suturing of the AC ligament, CC ligament, and surrounding muscle ruptures. From this study, the nonoperatively treated group demonstrated shorter rehabilitation time and the operatively treated group demonstrated higher amount of complications with about half of the operatively treated patients having problems with the metallic device or superficial infections. In comparison between the operative and nonoperative groups, there was no difference in clinical results.[84]

Polytrauma patients with AC joint injuries are given more profound consideration toward operative management. In a report by Gallay et al.,[54] they showed an AC joint injury, accompanying a polytrauma patient, has greater ramifications with regard to shoulder function as assessed by disease specific and general health outcomes. The type IV, V, and VI AC joint injuries, with attention to the soft tissue disruption and

TABLE 41-3	**Acromioclavicular Joint Injuries**

Nonoperative Treatment

Indications	Relative Contraindications
Type I AC joint injury	Chronic symptomatic injury
Type II AC joint injury	Chronic symptomatic injury
Type III AC joint injury	Failed nonoperative management, athlete, polytrauma, heavy laborers

persistently dislocated joint, are generally treated operatively and discussion of these treatments will be deferred to the next section of operative treatment (Table 41-3).

The nonoperative treatment of AC injuries consists of an immobilization device and the so-called skillful neglect.[127] Immobilization devices consisted of many variations including slings, adhesive tape strappings, braces, harnesses, traction techniques, and plaster casts.[126] Among these immobilization devices, the sling has been the more recently acknowledged and applied method of conservative treatment. In particular, the principle behind the immobilization device is to support the weight of the upper extremity with the intention of reducing the stress placed upon the ligaments of the joint.[34] Briefly, during the first week of treatment, the immobilization device, together with ice and analgesics, help reduce the pain and inflammation as a result of the AC joint injury. Similarly, to expedite the healing process, the patient is encouraged to use the injured upper extremity as tolerated. The amount of injury to the AC joint complex and gradation of dislocation does not change from the time of injury. Consequently, the goal of acute phase management is pain control. Following the initial period of immobilization, 1 to 2 weeks depending on grade of dislocation, strengthening exercises are commenced with particular focus on periscapular muscles that are important to shoulder biomechanics.[97] However, both heavy lifting and contact sports are avoided during the second phase of treatment with strengthening exercises.[97] Athletes who desire an earlier return to sports should be encouraged to use protective padding over the AC joint. An earlier return to sports that sustains a second injury to the AC joint, prior to complete ligament healing, can change a partially subluxated AC joint into a complete AC dislocation. Given this possible sequela, a forewarning must be provided to all athletes wishing to return to play at an earlier time.

Outcomes

Successful nonoperative treatment of types I to III AC joint injuries has been reported in the literature. Lower-grade energy injuries of the AC joint, classified as type I and II, are in majority treated by nonoperative methods and careful supervision. In the majority of type I and II AC joint injuries, Bjerneld et al.[11] showed that patients, at 6 years following injury, treated with a brief period of shoulder immobilization had excellent or good results. In this same study, patients with complete separation of the AC joint, also treated conservatively, showed good to excellent results. Although most patients achieve good outcomes with

nonoperative treatment of type I and II AC injuries, Mouhsine et al.[106] reported that only 52% of 33 consecutive patients, at a mean of 6.3 years from injury, remained completely asymptomatic. Even among type III AC injuries, several studies have demonstrated good outcomes with conservative measures. For instance, type III AC joint dislocations treated nonoperatively were evaluated in a study by Wojtys and Nelson,[165] with a mean follow-up of 2.6 years. In this study, patients returned to work on average 2.1 weeks from injury and the strength and endurance levels of the injured shoulder were comparable to the contralateral uninjured shoulder. Comparatively, the strength and endurance of the affected shoulder with a type III AC injury, conservatively treated, was found to be no different than the performance characteristics of the opposite normal shoulder at an average follow-up of 4.5 years.[151] In addition, patients treated conservatively had full range of motion and for this reason neither activities of daily living nor athletic participation was impaired. In a study by Dias[42] 44 patients with type III AC injury were followed for 5 years after injury. These patients were treated by a broad arm sling for 3 to 5 weeks followed by shoulder mobilization. Subjectively, the majority of patients reported only mild discomfort and no patients had discomfort that subsequently led to a change in occupation. In a follow-up study by Rawes and Dias,[123] 30 patients of the previously reported cohort (who were treated conservatively by a sling) maintained good outcomes at 12.5 years from the injury despite persistent dislocation of the AC joint.

Several studies have compared nonoperative treatment to operative treatment of AC injuries. In one of the earlier comparison studies, Galpin et al.[55] compared operative treatment, by a Bosworth CC screw, with nonoperative treatment of complete AC dislocations. The results of this study reported equal, if not superior, results in the nonoperatively treated group with regard to earlier return to activities, sports, and work. In both groups, despite the treatment, range of motion and strength were found to be equal. In a more recent study, Gstettner et al.[64] retrospectively reviewed patients with type III AC injury treated surgically with a hook plate in comparison to those treated conservatively at a mean follow-up of 34 months. Improved Constant Scores were found in the surgically treated group. In contradistinction, Calvo et al.[23] reported no significant difference in results between operative and nonoperative treatment of type III AC joint injury. In particular, the operatively treated AC injuries showed a significantly higher incidence of osteoarthritis and CC ligament ossification. Taft et al.[148] compared a group of patients treated nonoperatively with sling, taping, or a Kenny-Howard sling to a group treated operatively with AC or CC fixation. Subjective ratings of pain and stiffness and objective ratings of strength and range of motion were similar in both groups. There was a much higher complication rate in the operative group. Press et al.[122] found benefits to both operative and nonoperative treatment, but earlier return to work and sports with nonoperative treatment. There were no significant differences with respect to shoulder range of motion, manual muscle strength, and neurovascular findings between the two groups. In prospective randomized studies between operative and nonoperative treatment of type III AC joint injuries,[3,84] patients treated nonoperatively demonstrated a quicker return of function and sustained fewer complications than patients treated operatively. For this reason, the management of type I to III AC injuries, especially in the acute setting, is initially approached with a trial of conservative treatment.

Operative Treatment of Acromioclavicular Joint Injuries

Indications/Contraindications

The treatment goals for AC joint dislocations include a pain-free shoulder movement in a range of motion arc approaching normal. Various opinions exist regarding the optimal surgical treatment for these injuries. Operative intervention should be clearly discussed with each patient, as the objectives are different for each patient. Type I and II lesions are generally treated conservatively with a sling, ice, and a brief period of immobilization, typically lasting 3 to 7 days. Return to full motion, no or minimal pain, and full function with the ability of self-protection are prerequisites to return to competitive sports. If full function is achieved and only pain remains, a local anesthetic injection can be considered to allow return to sports if timing is crucial. However, no overall consensus exists on treatment for type III dislocations although a trend toward initial nonoperative treatment is presently favored in most cases.[125] An undetermined proportion of these conservatively treated patients will have persistent pain and an inability to return to their sport or job. Subsequent surgical stabilization, albeit delayed, has allowed return to sport or work in such cases. It is important to note that to date no high-quality prospective study has demonstrated surgical benefit for the treatment for type III injuries.[141,143,149] At our institution, acute type I, II, III, and V injuries are managed with a 6-week course of supervised rehabilitation to maximize rotator cuff strength and the stabilizing function of the periscapular muscles.[24,34] In our experience, patients who have failed a minimum 6 weeks of shoulder stabilization–directed physical therapy still have had good to excellent results with delayed surgical reconstruction using a tendon graft.[24] In light of the controversy and clear lack of evidence supporting acute surgical management of grade III AC separations, we recommend initial treatment with up to 6 weeks of nonoperative management.[24,34,155] It should be noted that altered shoulder biomechanics secondary to complete AC joint displacement was shown in a recent study of patients with type III injuries to result in scapular dyskinesis and, eventually, SICK scapula syndrome (scapular malposition, inferior medial border prominence, coracoid pain and malposition, and dyskinesis of scapular movement). This condition developed in 54% of patients with chronic type III AC dislocations in another study.[34,65] Overall, operative treatment is generally the accepted method for active healthy patients with complete AC joint injuries (types IV, V, and VI) because of the significant morbidity associated with the injury pattern that can lead to a persistently dislocated, unstable AC joint, with a change in scapular kinematics, and shoulder dysfunction.

Surgical Procedure—Historical/Classic Techniques

The surgical treatment for AC joint dislocations has a clear historical progression. Transarticular fixation of the AC joint with pins

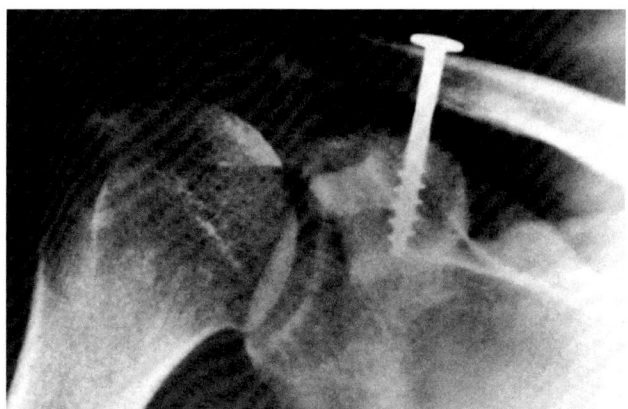

FIGURE 41-25 Postoperative anteroposterior radiograph of the shoulder with a Bosworth screw in place. Note that the AC joint has been reduced and the coarse lag threads of the screw are well seated into the coracoid process.

or wires was one of the first techniques to be described. Fixation was meant to enhance temporary reduction allowing the native soft tissue an opportunity to heal with the AC joint in a reduced position. However, reports of fixation failure, loss of reduction, and disastrous migration of hardware led to abandonment of this technique.[96,113] Similarly, the Bosworth "screw suspension" technique was introduced in 1941 as an extra-articular transient fixation device for acute, reducible AC joint dislocations (Fig. 41-25).[16] It was meant to provide enough stability to allow CC ligament healing or scar formation to occur. For several reasons, including the contrast between the rigid fixation provided by the screw and the intrinsic motion between the clavicle and (coracoid) scapula, hardware failure, migration, and coracoid fractures were reported with this construct. Taking a similar approach, alternative "CC suspension" constructs appeared in the literature; Dacron grafts, wires, and various types of sutures.[127,141] The concept was to allow for motion, with a less rigid construct, but provide enough fixation to hold the CC distance reduced and allow for AC- and CC-ligament healing. In 1972, Weaver and Dunn[161] published their technique of distal clavicle resection and transfer of the CA ligament to the distal clavicle to restore and reconstruct the CC ligaments and treat acute and chronic AC joint instability. Over the years, numerous modifications to this technique have been described.[127] This technique represents an open procedure, which uses the detached CA ligament as a retaining structure for the distal clavicle. The modification of this nonanatomic technique involves an additional suture construct for increased primary stability (Fig. 41-26).[161] This approach, along with various technical modifications, is still widely utilized to reconstruct the CC ligaments, although it is considered inferior biomechanically compared to the other techniques.[98,99,150] Historically, although good to excellent results of this procedure have been reported, 75%,[127] the initial strength of the CA ligament after transfer has been shown to be only 25% of the normal, intact CC ligaments, and it does not recreate horizontal plane stability.[87] In a recent cadaveric model, the ultimate load to failure of the modified Weaver–Dunn was found to be 39% less than control.[150] There can be an upward rate of 30% of recurrent instability with this technique, typically

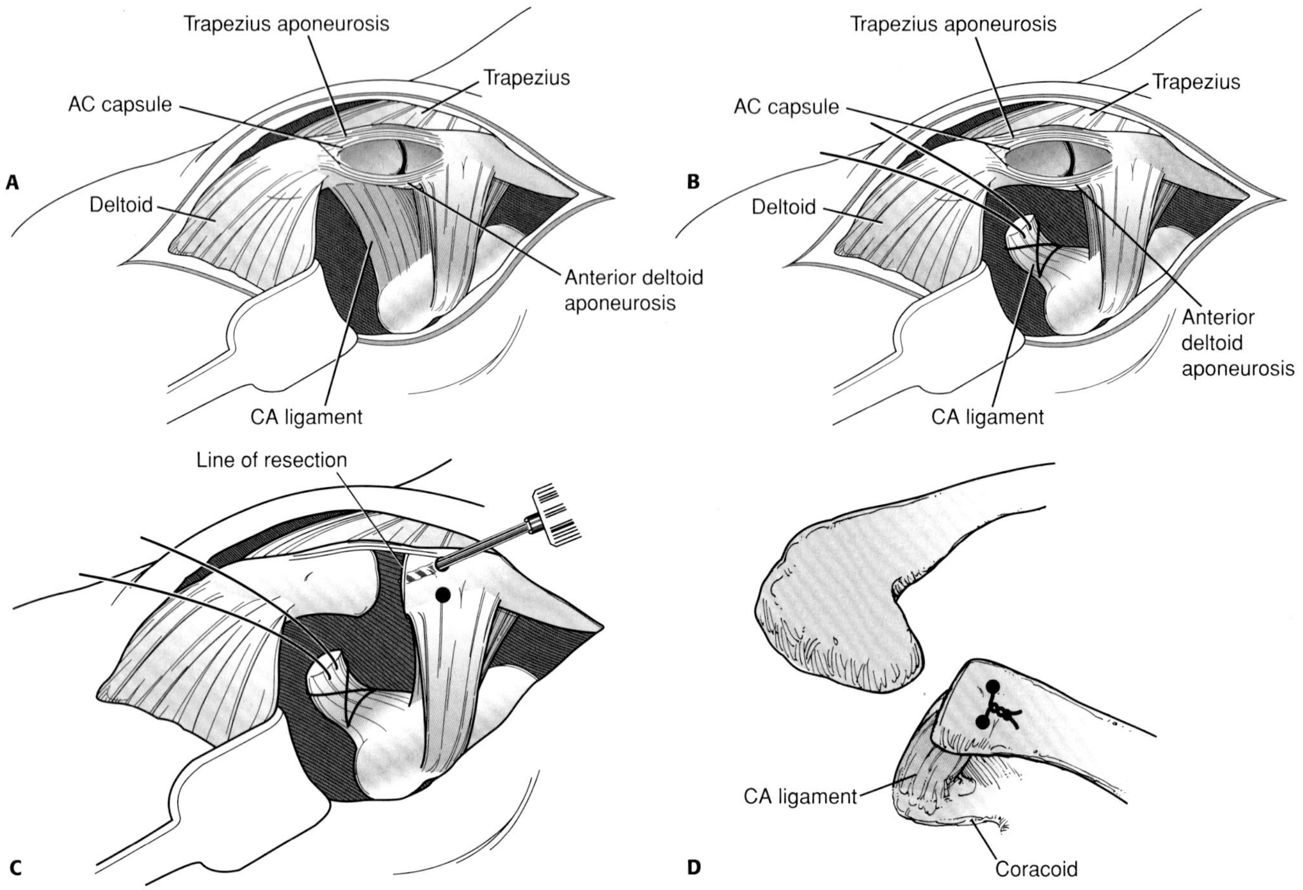

A

Trapezius aponeurosis

Trapezius

AC capsule

Deltoid

Anterior deltoid
aponeurosis

CA ligament

B

Trapezius aponeurosis

Trapezius

AC capsule

Deltoid

Anterior
deltoid
aponeurosis

CA ligament

C

Line of resection

D

CA ligament

Coracoid

FIGURE 41-26 Transfer of the acromial attachment of the coracoacromial ligament. **A:** A small portion of the anterior deltoid is reflected from the anterior acromion to expose the coracoacromial ligament. **B:** The ligament is released from the acromion and sutures are placed in the end. **C:** Two unicortical drill holes are placed in the posterosuperior surface of the distal clavicle, exiting through the medullary canal. **D:** The coracoacromial ligament is transferred to the medullary canal. The sutures are placed through the drill holes and tied over the top of the clavicle.

in the anterior–posterior direction at the AC joint.[98,99,162] From a biomechanical perspective, the importance of the AC ligaments in controlling superior and horizontal translations has been demonstrated.[52,79] Superior clavicle plates with lateral hooks or "AC hook plates" have been reported in the literature since the 1980s with mixed results.[140] There have been a few modifications to the plate to lower its profile or add "locking screw technology" but the concept remains the same. This type of fixation holds the CC distance in a reduced position by "hooking" under the acromion elevating the glenohumeral joint (Fig. 41-27). Most reported cases involving superior clavicle "hook" plates are used in patients with chronic dislocations often with concomitant AC joint arthrosis.[140] Rates of good or excellent results ranging between 60% and 94% have been reported, but complications of this technique include acromial fracture or erosion and hardware irritation necessitating removal of the plate or of the tab on the distal end articulating under the acromion. Recently reported was a retrospective study of chronic AC dislocations treated by a Weaver–Dunn procedure in which constructs augmented with PDS no. 1 braided suture

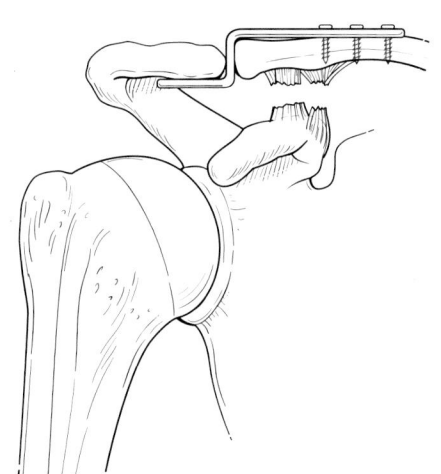

FIGURE 41-27 Superior clavicle hook plate. (With permission From Iannotti JP, Miniaci A, Williams G, Zuckerman DJ. *Disorders of the Shoulder: Sports Injuries.* Philadelphia, PA: Lippincott Williams & Wilkins; 2013.)

around the coracoid were compared to a hook plate (Synthes, Solothurn, Switzerland). Patients treated with the hook plate augmentation did not have increased AC joint stability after plate removal, and although not powered to detect significance there was a trend to lower Constant Scores in the hook plate group. More importantly, the hook plate group had more pain related to the plate and all required surgical removal.[15] Other complications associated with hook plates have been recently reported, including chronic irritation in the subacromial space resulting in a persistent pain syndrome, and plate removal[77] or sustained acromial osteolysis and fractures.[27] In the study reported by Kienast et al.,[77] there was an overall complication rate of 10.6% with a 2% redislocation rate. A similar study reported a 12% redislocation rate.

Anatomic Approaches

The first attempt at the reconstruction of the CC ligaments was reported in 1942 by Vargus, describing transfer of part of the conjoined tendon anterior to the clavicle. Anatomic reconstruction of the native CC ligaments and AC ligaments represents an improved understanding of the biomechanics in this area with the possibility of improved surgical outcomes. The anatomic coracoclavicular ligament reconstruction (ACCR) technique described here attempts to restore the biomechanics of the AC joint complex for the treatment of painful or unstable dislocations.[5,17,18,21,33]

Chronic Acromioclavicular Injuries

Patients with type I and II AC joint injuries may develop late degenerative changes.[9,35,106] The meniscus and articular cartilage often sustain an injury that leads to these degenerative changes. Chronic pain after type I and II injuries is treated with mild analgesics such as nonsteroidal anti-inflammatory medication, avoidance of painful activity or positions, and intra-articular injection with corticosteroid preparations. Many will resolve with this conservative treatment.

Patients with chronic type I injuries who do not respond to conservative care may require operative excision of the distal clavicle to provide relief of pain. This can be performed using an open or an arthroscopic technique.[51,56,107,144] The important aspect of either technique is preservation or repair of the AC joint capsule to maintain AP stability of the joint.[17] Resections should be limited to less than 10 mm of distal clavicle as to limit the disruption of the superior and posterior capsular/ligament structures. Violation of these structures can lead to residual anterior–posterior clavicle instability and pain.

In patients with chronic pain after type II AC sprains, the initial conservative regimen is the same as for type I injuries. If conservative, symptomatic treatment fails, surgery may be indicated. Isolated distal clavicle excision after a type II injury may fail because of AP instability of the distal clavicle and resultant posterior abutment of the clavicle on the scapular spine. Therefore, the patient should be examined carefully for increased AP translation of the clavicle relative to the acromion during preoperative examination. If excessive AP instability exists, distal clavicle excision should be combined with AC capsular reconstruction or coracoacromial ligament transfer.[161]

Chronic pain and instability after complete AC dislocations (types III, IV, and V) should not be treated with isolated distal

clavicle excision. This merely shortens the clavicle without stabilizing it and is often associated with persistent postoperative symptoms. Therefore, distal clavicle excision should be combined with stabilization in chronic, symptomatic, and complete AC injuries. The most popular reconstructive procedure is transfer of the acromial attachment of the coracoacromial ligament to the resected surface of the distal clavicle and concurrent CC stabilization. CC stabilization greatly increases the strength of the construct.[44,66,68,74,122]

AUTHOR'S PREFERRED TREATMENT FOR ACROMIOCLAVICULAR JOINT INJURIES

Acute Treatment

Initial treatment is with a sling placed to fully support and elevate the arm and to take tension off the injured ligaments. In lower-grade injuries shoulder activity can be initiated at 1 week and is typically pain free by 2 to 3 weeks. In higher-grade injuries formal physical therapy to address shoulder muscle weakness and periscapular strengthening is started at 2 weeks. Heavy stresses, lifting, and contact sports should be delayed until there is a full range of motion and no pain to joint palpation. This process can take upto 2 to 4 weeks and is dependent upon AC joint separation grade, patient pre-injury condition and...., as well as patient pain tolerance. All patients are given a trial of 6 to 8 weeks of nonoperative care until surgical intervention is considered unless neurologic or skin issues dictate earlier intervention. Contact sports can resume at 4 to 6 weeks and is dictated by pain with activity. To date no study has demonstrated a progression of AC separation with early return to sport but pain with collision sports is certainly a limitation and can be addressed by preactivity injections to the AC joint—with or without corticosteroids.

Anatomic reconstruction of the native CC ligaments and AC ligaments represents an improved understanding of the biomechanics in this area with the attempt to improve surgical outcomes. Although still controversial, the authors believe that all stabilizing structures of the AC joint complex should be reconstructed to achieve optimal result. The ACCR technique attempts to restore the biomechanics of the AC joint complex as treatment for painful or unstable dislocations. The rationale of this technique is to reconstruct both CC ligaments by anatomically fixing a tendon graft in two clavicle tunnels placed in the anatomic insertion site of the conoid and trapezoid ligaments. In addition, the AC ligaments are reconstructed with the remaining limb of the graft exiting the more lateral trapezoid tunnel. This technique has been previously reported during various stages of its development and this description represents the current version.[24,98,125]

Patient Positioning

The procedure is performed in the beach-chair position with the hip flexed to 60 to 70 degrees, and the patient positioned far lateral on the operating table to allow the arm to fall into extension. This facilitates exposure and mobilization of the shoulder for scapula reduction to the clavicle. A small towel bump is

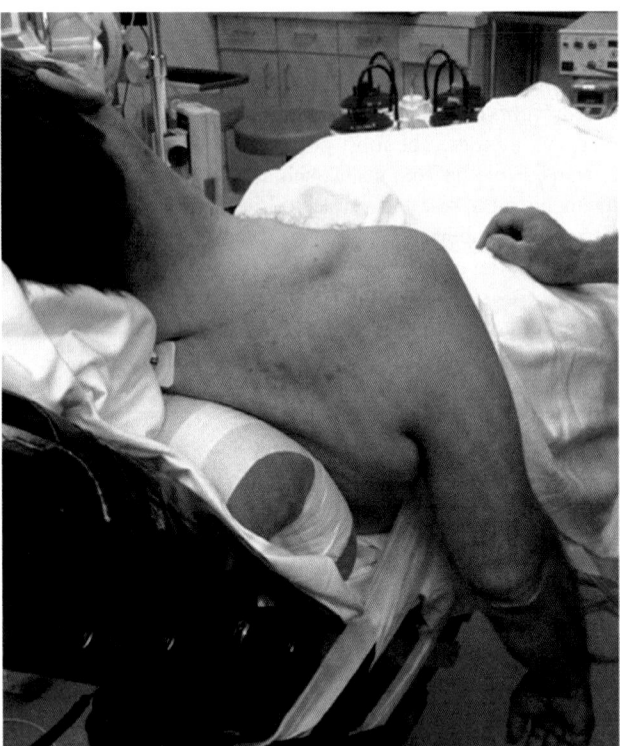

FIGURE 41-28 ACCR technique: Patient positioning. Note the far lateral position with shoulder free to extend, small scapula bump along medial scapula border, and head position extended and rotated away from operative side. (With permission from Iannotti JP, Miniaci A, Williams G, Zuckerman DJ. *Disorders of the Shoulder: Sports Injuries*. Philadelphia, PA: Lippincott Williams & Wilkins; 2013.)

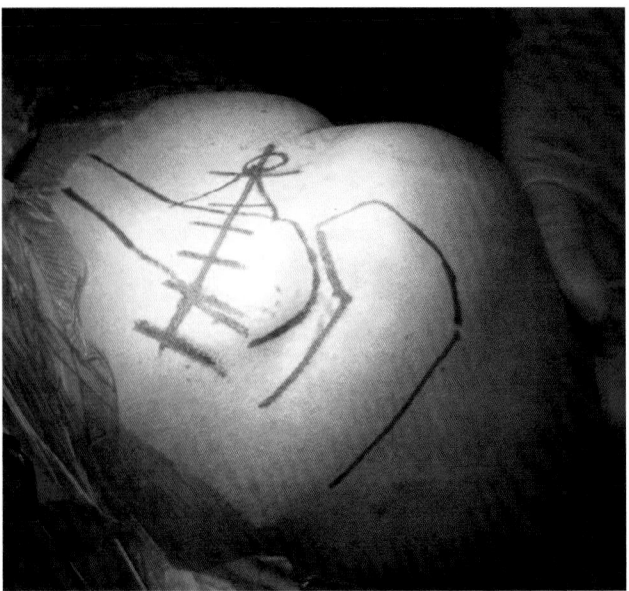

FIGURE 41-29 The vertical incision is made along Langer lines, centered on the clavicle approximately 3.5 cm medial to the AC joint, in a curvilinear fashion starting from the posterior clavicle to just medial of the coracoid process. (With permission from Iannotti JP, Miniaci A, Williams G, Zuckerman DJ. *Disorders of the Shoulder: Sports Injuries*. Philadelphia, PA: Lippincott Williams & Wilkins; 2013.)

placed along the medial border of the scapula to prevent protraction of the scapula. In addition, this elevates the torso away from the table thereby improving access to the clavicle for drilling the bone tunnels. Gently rotating the patient's head away from the operative field with some extension aids in exposure (Fig. 41-28). It is important not to be aggressive with this maneuver to limit excessive tension to the brachial plexus during the procedure. The patient is secured with a safety belt and 3-in cloth tape around the chest. It is important to drape a wide operative field; from the SC joint, to the nipple line, up the neck to the base of the ear, and extends several inches behind the posterior aspect of the clavicle. Before prepping, the miniature C-arm is prepositioned to allow imaging intraoperatively, if needed. Imaging can be obtained by advancing the image machine from above, in line with the AP image from the patient's head direction. In addition, a comparative Zanca view is made of the normal AC joint to act as a reference for the measurement of the intact CC distance.

Surgical Approach

We use a direct approach with a saber incision made over the clavicle approximately 3.5 cm medial to the AC joint. The incision starts posterior to the clavicle, crossing just medial to the tip of the coracoid process, and extending inferior enough to ensure visualization of the coracoid for graft passage (Fig. 41-29). The incision should be long enough to accommodate

AC joint visualization with Gelpi retractor perpendicular to the incision. This incision is medial to the approach typically used for the Weaver–Dunn reconstruction. Needle tip electrocautery is used to obtain hemostasis and carry the dissection down to the deltotrapezial fascia. Generous skin flaps are raised directly above the fascia to improve visualization. This is well tolerated about the shoulder because of the vascularity of the region. The deltotrapezial fascia is then elevated from the distal clavicle as full-thickness flaps (Fig. 41-30). The fascia is incised in line with the natural demarcation between the trapezius insertion to the posterior aspect of the clavicle and the deltoid origin on the anterior clavicle. Dissection of the fascia should extend far enough medially to expose the conoid ligament insertion, approximately 46.3 mm ± 5 mm from the distal end of the clavicle.[98,125,127] Skeletonizing the clavicle can be done sharply with an elevator or electrocautery, but maintaining full-thickness periosteal flaps is critical to obtaining a good closure (Fig. 41-31). Tagging stitches are placed in the flaps to aid in retraction and then facilitate accurate reapproximation at closure. It is important to note that the deltoid has an insertion on the undersurface of the clavicle and care should be given to ensure that the deltoid is not violated. This is done by carefully and slowly peeling the deltoid and trapezius off the clavicle with the periosteum, understanding the clavicle is a tubular structure and to follow the curve with the elevator inferior and not to transect the deltoid from the anterior edge. Gelpi retractors are used to retract the flaps parallel and perpendicular to the incision with alternating pressure to facilitate exposure of the AC joint or coracoid base. The distal end of the clavicle is exposed to allow for reduction and preservation of any AC

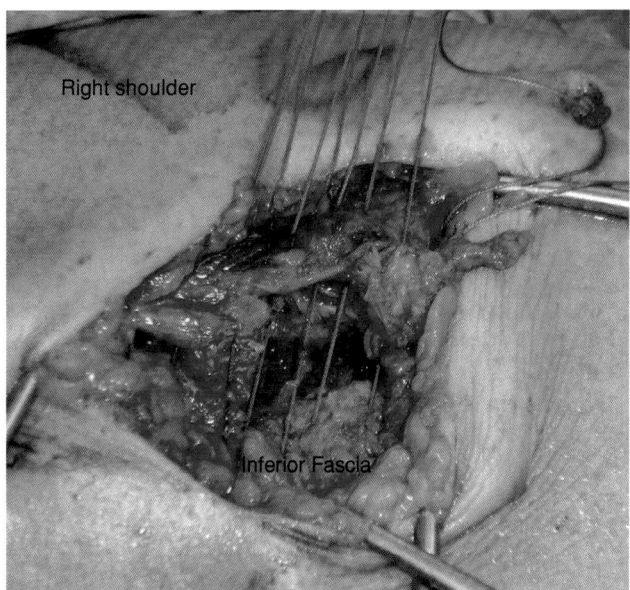

FIGURE 41-30 ACCR technique. Right shoulder taken from lateral looking medial. Skeletonizing of the clavicle is started with electrocautery, then thick subperiosteal flaps are raised sharply with elevator to ensure the trapezius and deltoid attachments are elevated off in a sleeve, superior and inferior. Tagging stitches can be placed to aid in tight closure of this layer as a critical step during closure. (With permission from Iannotti JP, Miniaci A, Williams G, Zuckerman DJ. *Disorders of the Shoulder: Sports Injuries*. Philadelphia, PA: Lippincott Williams & Wilkins; 2013.)

capsule/ligaments if possible. Reduction of the AC joint is accomplished by elevating the scapulohumeral complex to the clavicle by supporting the elbow and scapula. Visual inspection is usually adequate for assessing reduction; however, a mini C-arm can be used intraoperatively to confirm the reduction. An image of the uninjured shoulder can be saved or printed for comparative CC distance measurements. In chronic AC dislocations, there can be significant scar tissue inferior to the AC joint which needs to be removed to allow adequate reduction.

Bone Tunnel Placement

Placement of clavicle bone tunnels for graft reconstruction of the CC ligaments is designed to reproduce their anatomic positions in relation to the distal clavicle. Smooth guide pins for the 5-mm–cannulated reamer are placed at the anatomic location

corresponding to the conoid and trapezoid ligaments with a Cobb elevator or retractor inferior to the clavicle for protection. Guide pin placement for the conoid ligament tunnel is placed 45 mm medial to the distal clavicle and posterior to the midline of the clavicle in the coronal plane (Fig. 41-32). The bone density in fresh cadaveric specimens reveals the more lateral bone has less mineralization with softer bone for fixation. Thus, the surgeon should error on being slightly more medial to take advantage of improved bone density in this location. A secondary anatomic reference is the conoid tubercle, which can be palpated on the posterior surface of the clavicle. A second pin is placed lateral to the conoid pin by 20 mm and just anterior to the clavicle midline again in the coronal plane, this corresponds to the trapezoid ligament tunnel and should not be less than 15 mm from the end of the clavicle. Again it is important to be no less than 20 to 25 mm from the distal clavicle for bone quality and a minimum of 20-mm bone bridge between the tunnels to prevent fracture. Bone tunnels must also be placed at least 3 mm from the edge of the clavicle toward the midline. The objective is to ensure enough bone between the tunnel and the edge of the clavicle to prevent blowout fracture of the cortical bone edge during interference screw placement. For tunnel preparation, power reaming is used to create the tunnel but power is then shut off for reamer extraction, the "ream-in, pull-out" technique, to ensure the tunnel is not made eccentrically, optimizing fixation of the graft. In summary, the reamer is advanced in under power with care not to dive through the far cortex; the drill is stopped and then disconnected while it is pulled out. The goal is to make the tunnel as tight as possible and therefore graft passage should be somewhat difficult. In our experience, the complication of clavicle fracture has not been observed in patients or during cadaver experiments with tunnels 5 mm or less. A secure fit between the graft and tunnel is a critical aspect of the procedure. Interference fixation is obtained with implantable polyetheretherketone (PEEK) polymer screws, (an inert, MRI compatible material). These screws have a higher pull-out strength than bioabsorbable screws, but do not cut or rip the tissue as can occur with metal screws. The bone tunnels must be tapped prior to placement of the PEEK screws. This allows easier screw placement, minimizing graft "creep" with interference screw tightening, and decreases the torque needed to seat the screw, lowering stress on the bone tunnel. Oversizing of the tunnel impairs fixation and can be a cause of failure. In the

FIGURE 41-31 ACCR technique. Right shoulder, picture taken from posterior: Medial is left. Tunnel positions are measured and marked: Conoid (at least 45 mm from distal clavicle), using conoid tunnel mark as reference the trapezoid tunnel position is marked to ensure at least 25 mm of bone bridge between tunnels and at least 4 mm from the clavicle edge toward the midline (20 to 25 mm from distal clavicle). (With permission from Iannotti JP, Miniaci A, Williams G, Zuckerman DJ. *Disorders of the Shoulder: Sports Injuries*. (Philadelphia, PA: Lippincott Williams & Wilkins; 2013.)

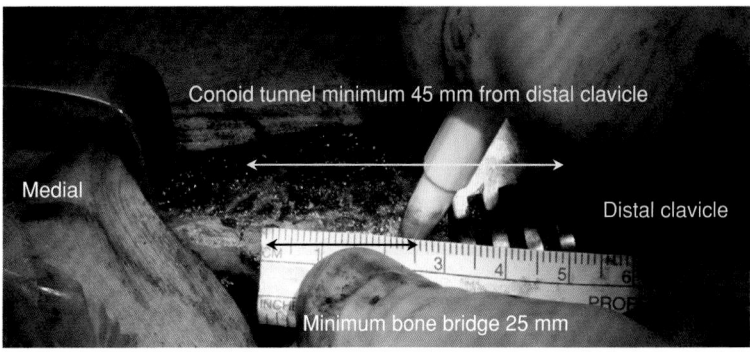

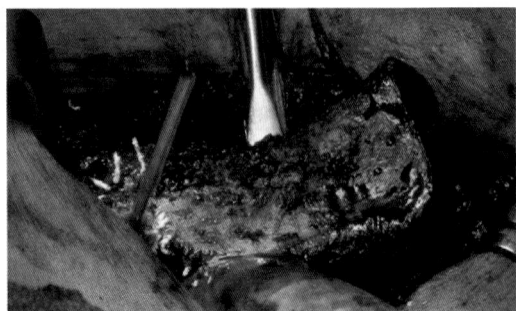

FIGURE 41-32 ACCR technique. Threaded guide pins for a 5.5-mm cannulated drill are placed corresponding to anatomic position. Care is taken to prevent fracture or cortical blowout by ensuring at least. 3-mm from cortical edge. (With permission from Iannotti JP, Miniaci A, Williams G, Zuckerman DJ. *Disorders of the Shoulder: Sports Injuries.* Philadelphia, PA: Lippincott Williams & Wilkins; 2013.)

event of cortical fracture that does not allow PEEK screw fixation, the graft limbs can be passed over the clavicle and then sutured together on top of the clavicle. In the specific situation of a type IV AC joint dislocation with significant posterior displacement of the clavicle, the bone tunnel positions can be adjusted more posterior to the midclavicle line. This provides an anterior force vector in the reconstruction that improves the reduction. However, the minimal bone bridge and cortical edge distances must still be maintained. If additional anterior reduction force is needed, the two ends of the graft should not be crossed before being shuttled through the clavicle bone tunnels (Fig. 41-33).

Graft Preparation and Passage

Graft options include a semitendinosus allograft or autograft. Anterior tibialis allograft is another suitable graft source but must be trimmed significantly because it is often quite thick. Semitendinosus allograft is our preferred graft for numerous reasons; simplification of patient positioning, no donor site

morbidity, decreased operative time, and consistency in the graft tissue size. To date, there has been no reported cases of infectious transmission in soft tissue only allografts.[6,46] Semitendinosus allograft typically comes in diameters ≥5 mm and minimum lengths of 230 mm, which is sufficient for this reconstructive technique. The minimal length needed to ensure graft available for AC ligament reconstruction is approximately 110 mm. The graft is prepared with a continuous running locked stitch of high-strength nonabsorbable suture. These sutures are then pulled tightly to help tubularize the flat end of the tendon while compressing the looped end, so that the tendon is of uniform diameter after preparation. Frayed graft ends are excised to allow easy passage. The graft is passed beneath the coracoid using either a shuttling stitch and a curved clamp such as the Satinsky aortic cross clamp or a curved suture passing device (Fig. 41-33). A no.2 high-strength nonabsorbable suture is passed with the graft to provide additional nonbiologic fixation. This suture will eventually be shuttled through the cannulation of the interference screw and when tied provides additional fixation during healing of the graft. The graft is passed from medial to lateral under direct visualization, to minimize the risk of injury to the underlying neurovascular structures.

After passing the graft and no.2 suture beneath the coracoid, the limbs of the graft are crossed in figure of eight fashion before being shuttled through the bone tunnels from inferior to superior direction (Fig. 41-33). A commercial or homemade suture passer is used to assist in graft placement through the bone tunnels, beginning with the conoid (posteromedial) tunnel. The graft is then cyclically loaded by pulling up on both ends to remove any slack, and seesawed back and forth to allow for easy passage. The graft is arranged so that a shorter limb of approximately 2 cm exits the conoid tunnel. The remaining length of the graft exits the trapezoid tunnel. This longer limb will be used later to reinforce the AC joint and recreate the superior and anterior AC ligaments (Fig. 41-33).

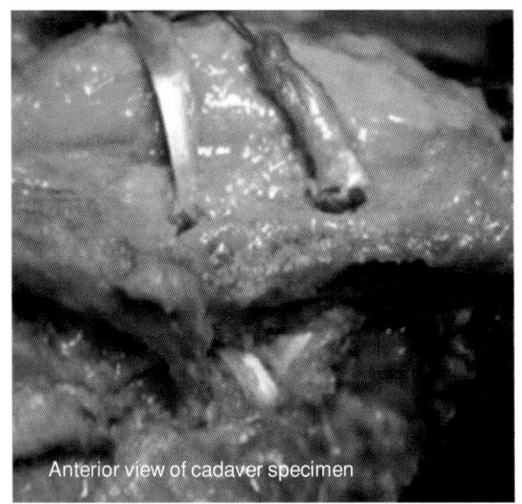

A

Anterior view of cadaver specimen

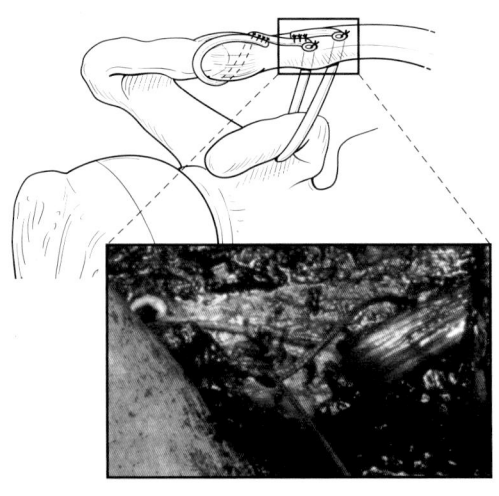

B

FIGURE 41-33 ACCR technique: Graft construct and medial fixation. **A:** Cadaver right shoulder looking from anterior at construct around coracoid base figure of eight pattern. **B:** Artist rendering of ACCR construct, magnification of medial construct.

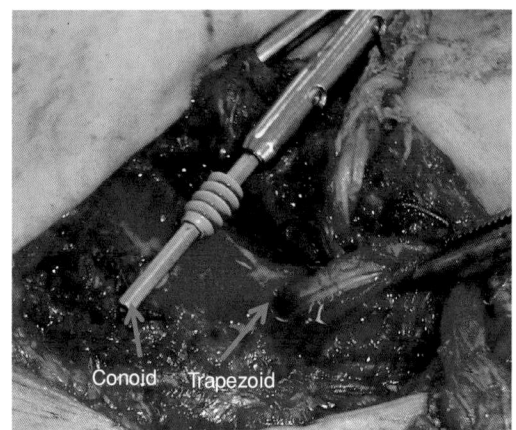
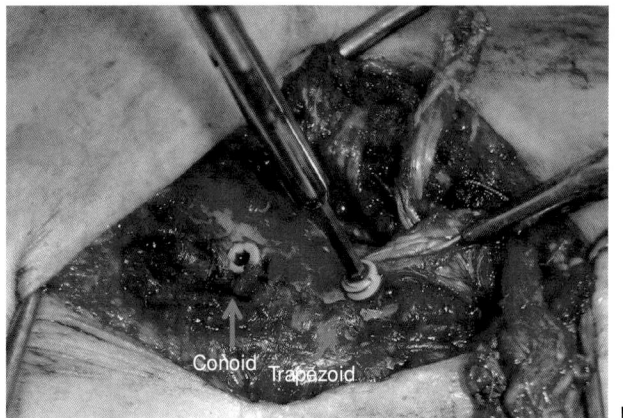

FIGURE 41-33 (*continued*) **C, D:** Intraoperative photo of right shoulder from above. Fixation of the graft into the bone tunnels. Bone tunnels are tapped prior to graft passage. Graft limbs are kept under tension while the PEEK screw is inserted. (With permission from Iannotti JP, Miniaci A, Williams G, Zuckerman DJ. *Disorders of the Shoulder: Sports Injuries.* Philadelphia, PA: Lippincott Williams & Wilkins; 2013.)

Acromioclavicular Joint Reduction and Graft Fixation

Reduction of the AC joint is accomplished by elevating the scapulohumeral complex to the clavicle by having an assistant push on the elbow. The quality of reduction can be assessed under direct visualization, but radiographic assessment may also be used. Measurement of the CC distance can be made intraoperatively and compared to the uninjured side prior to graft fixation. An anatomical reduction of the AC joint is critical. While an assistant maintains the reduction, the grafts are secured with interference screws. Interference fixation of the grafts within the bone tunnels is done with a 5.5- × 8-mm PEEK screw placed in the anterior aspect of the tunnel while tension is maintained on the graft (Fig. 41-33). One limb of the no.2 high-strength suture is passed with the graft beneath the coracoid and through the respective tunnels. It is then passed through the first interference screw used to fix the conoid portion of the reconstruction. Fixation of the posteromedial graft, corresponding to the conoid ligament tunnel, is done first. After interference screw placement, the other limb of the graft exiting the AP bone tunnel, representing the trapezoid ligament, is cyclically tensioned to remove any residual slack and held under maximal tension while the second interference screw is placed in the anterior aspect of the tunnel (Fig. 41-33). Prior to secure fixation and placement of the interference screw the other limb of the no. 2 high-strength nonabsorbable end suture is brought through the cannulation hole of the PEEK screw (Fig. 41-34). After fixation of the graft in both tunnels, both limbs of the no.2 suture are tied on the superior aspect of the clavicle. Secondary graft fixation is accomplished by suturing the shorter limb of graft exiting the posterior medial tunnel to the base of the long graft limb exiting anterior lateral tunnel to create a closed figure of eight loop (Fig. 41-34). The remnants of the AC joint capsule/ligaments are identified and repaired with figure of eight stitches using absorbable suture. This repair is augmented with the longer limb of graft exiting the anterior lateral bone tunnel. The graft should have enough length to be looped over the top of the AC joint to reinforce this repair and reconstruct the anterior AC ligaments, important for anterior–posterior stability (Fig. 41-35). We use a free needle and tie this as a horizontal mattress securing periosteum and remnants of the original AC ligament to make a band across the top part of the joint. With sufficient graft length, the posterior AC ligament repair is reinforced by looping the graft posterior and incorporating the trapezial fascia with high-strength nonabsorbable suture on the acromial side of the joint.

Closure

The deltotrapezial fascia closure is an important step; the large fascia flaps are closed tightly with interrupted high-strength nonabsorbable sutures. Approximation of the attachments of the anterior deltoid fascia and the trapezius fascia are brought together with inverted interrupted stitches so that the knots are tied on the inferior side of the flap (Fig. 41-35), to minimize skin irritation. Occasionally, simple sutures are used to bury or tie down knots that appear prominent. The deep dermal layer is closed with buried 3.0 vicryl sutures, and a running subcuticular stitch is used for skin closure. In addition to intraoperative C-arm imaging to confirm reduction, final postoperative radiographs are taken to quantify AC joint reduction and bone tunnel position.

Postoperative Management for ACCR Technique

During the first 6 to 8 weeks, patients wear a prefabricated (Lerman Shoulder Brace, DJO inc. Vista, CA.) or abduction brace. It is most important that the postoperative brace provides a reduction support and protects the surgical repair against the pull of gravity. The brace may be removed for grooming and supine range of motion exercises only. After 8 weeks, the graft has obtained sufficient stability to begin upright range of motion exercises. At 12 weeks, if there is a pain-free normal range of motion, strengthening exercises are begun. These should target the scapular stabilizers that help retract the scapula and thereby decrease loads across the AC joint. Weight training may begin at 3 to 5 months postoperatively. Full contact athletics are

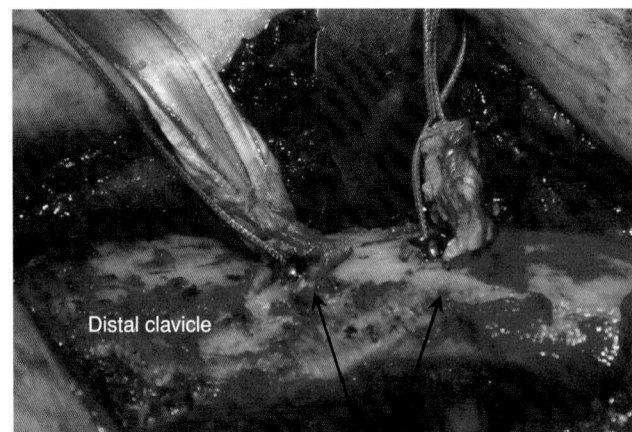

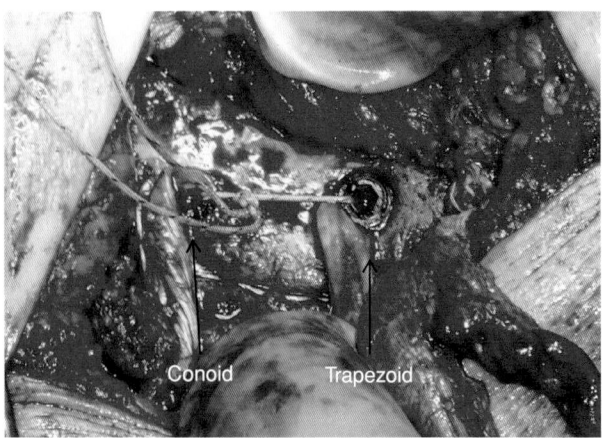

5.5-mm PEEK interference screw

FIGURE 41-34 ACCR technique. Fixation at CC ligament reconstruction. **A:** After graft is wrapped around the coracoid elbow in crossing fashion the two ends are brought up through there corresponding tunnels such that the conoid tunnel graft is shorter than the trapezoid tunnel graft. Length of the conoid tunnel graft should be sufficient to span the bone bridge between tunnels and an additional 20 to 30 mm to suture to the base of the trapezoid tunnel graft for fixation. The remaining graft length should be exiting from the trapezoid tunnel and sufficient to span the 30 mm to the AC joint and augment the AC capsule/ligament repair superiorly. **B:** No. 2 high-strength nonabsorbable end suture is brought through the cannulation hole of the PEEK screw and tied over the clavicle. (With permission from Iannotti JP, Miniaci A, Williams G, Zuckerman DJ. *Disorders of the Shoulder: Sports Injuries.* Philadelphia, PA: Lippincott Williams & Wilkins; 2013.)

allowed at 6 months but generally it requires 9 months to a year for patients to regain peak strength particularly with pressing activities, or lifting from the floor as in a dead lift.

Type III/V Variants

We treat all acute dislocations with an attempt at a nonoperative approach. They nearly always recover without incident, and rarely have any further sequelae. AC injuries associated with

fractures of the coracoid process are treated nonoperatively in most cases. The fractures usually occur at the tip or the base of the coracoid. As long as the deltotrapezial fascia is not disrupted to a large extent, and there is no severe coracoid displacement, they are treated in the same manner as a type III injury. If the fracture of the coracoid extends intra-articularly into the glenoid, we consider surgical repair. This depends largely on the amount of intra-articular displacement. We use 5 mm or more of glenoid

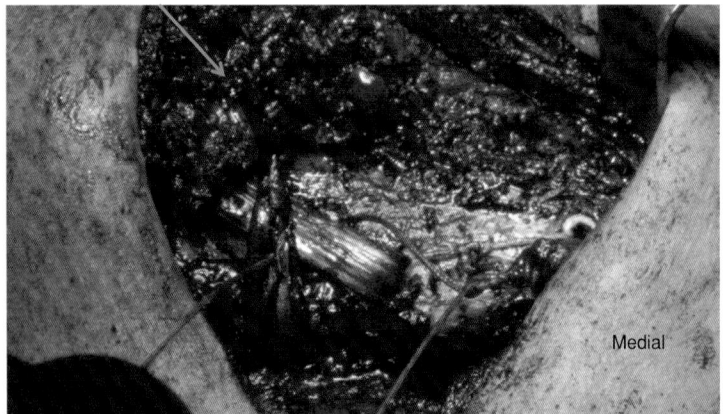

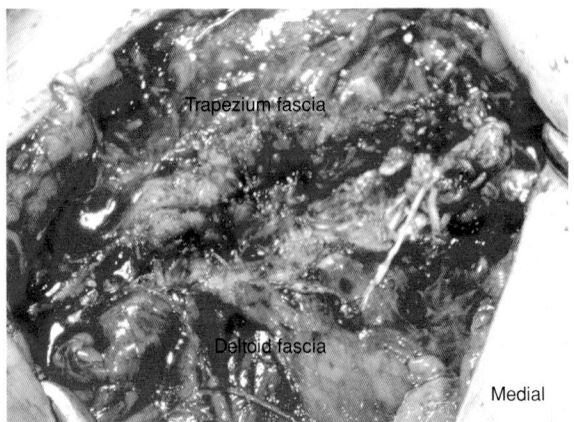

FIGURE 41-35 ACCR technique. AC ligament reconstruction and fascia repair. Right shoulder viewed from anterior. Integration of the graft at the AC capsule/ligament reconstruction. **A:** The long limb of the graft is taken lateral and posterior and used to augment posterior capsule repair. It is also incorporated into the trapezium fascia. The remnant is carried superior and used to augment the superior AC capsule repair. This is with nonabsorbable high-strength suture. **B:** Using "pants-over-vest" suture-repair technique, the deltoid–Trapezium fascia is repaired securely over the length of the clavicle. Note the repair is a critical part of the procedure and good tension and approximation of the fascia closure is vital. (With permission from Iannotti JP, Miniaci A, Williams G, Zuckerman DJ. *Disorders of the Shoulder: Sports Injuries.* Philadelphia, PA; Lippincott Williams & Wilkins; 2013.)

TABLE 41-4	**Surgical Pearls and Pitfalls**

- While exposing the clavicle, create thick, intact deltotrapezial flaps to assist closure at the end of the case
- Clear the medial and lateral margins of the coracoid to assist passage of suture and graft under it
- Use a Satinsky vascular clamp to pass the shuttle suture under the coracoid from medial to lateral
- Keep an adequate bone bridge between the drill holes in the clavicle to reduce the risk of fracture
- Clear tissue from drill holes on the undersurface of the clavicle to ease passage of the graft
- Push up on the elbow to reduce the acromion to the clavicle before securing the repair

displacement as our criterion for surgical treatment. A CT scan is performed to evaluate this fracture as the glenoid fracture extension is readily appreciated with this study.

Potential Pitfalls and Preventative Measures

A thorough understanding of CC and AC anatomy is essential to the safe and effective treatment of AC joint injuries. Table 41-4 lists some of the surgical tips that may help assist the surgeon during reconstruction of the AC joint as well as help to stay away from some of the common pitfalls associated with this procedure.

Indication for surgery is again one of the most difficult; we attempt to treat all patients nonoperatively. We allow for physical therapy to proceed for 4 weeks and then re-evaluate the patient. There are three studies that indicate early treatment (<6 weeks) leads to better return to sport (82 to 100%) compared to patients treated surgically but in a delayed (<6 weeks) fashion (77% to 78% return to sport).[8] Pain and function loss are the reasons for reconstruction not cosmetic, as often the reconstruction will loosen and a residual deformity will persist after over reduction in the operating room.

One of the most common mistakes in the operating room is to not expose the AC joint, remove calcified tissue or scar within the CC space to allow for adequate reduction which is monitored and verified intraoperatively with fluoroscopy. Clavicle fracture is a real intraoperative complication and bone tunnels must be <5.5 mm, with enough bone between hole and posterior cortex to ensure no fracture secondary to stress raiser. Lastly, do not underestimate the importance of the deltotrapezial fascia closure with suture purchase in large flaps with over reduction of the fascia over the clavicle for added strength and blood supply.[91]

Postoperative brace wear and a very slow controlled therapy program will ensure optimal success. Wound complications can occur, so close monitoring in the first few weeks is important. A brace that elevates the forearm up toward the AC joint is important to protect the repair construct and compliancy with brace wear is one of the most significant hurdles in postoperative management.

MANAGEMENT OF EXPECTED ADVERSE OUTCOMES AND UNEXPECTED COMPLICATIONS IN ACROMIOCLAVICULAR JOINT INJURIES

An inferiorly and medially directed force applied to the dorsum of the acromion most often results in injury to the AC articula-

tion, the SC articulation, or the shaft of the clavicle. However, combined injuries have been reported. Wurtz et al.[166] and Lancourt[83] have reported combined AC dislocation and clavicle fracture. Several reports exist of simultaneous dislocations of both the SC and AC ends of the clavicle or "bipolar" dislocations.[2,32,45,73,133] When this injury does occur, it is most often a posterior or type IV AC dislocation associated with an anterior SC dislocation. This underscores the importance of a thorough evaluation of any patient with an AC joint injury with particular attention being paid to the SC joint.

Many complications may result from operative treatment of AC dislocations. Besides general complications such as wound infection and osteomyelitis that might develop from the operative procedure, several other specific complications may occur (e.g., a fracture through a drill hole, loss of purchase of the internal fixation, metal failure, and migration of the fixation device to other parts of the body). The incidence of loss of reduction is significant. The weight of the entire upper extremity is supported through a limited available area for fixation. In addition, the potential planes of motion at the injured AC joint are numerous and result in complex loading of the reconstruction. For these reasons, we advocate longer postoperative immobilization than is commonly described.

Migration of Pins in Acromioclavicular Joint Injuries

Pins used to stabilize the AC joint have been reported to migrate into remote, life-threatening locations such as the lung, the spinal cord, the neck posterior to the carotid sheath, and the pleura or close to it.[53,90] Vessels in the thorax and neck have also been penetrated by pin migration injury (more historical at this point).

In most instances, pin migration can be prevented by bending a hook on the portion of the pin that protrudes from the acromion process. However, the pins can break, and then part of the pin is free to migrate. Patients must be prepared and forewarned of the possible necessity of pin removal and the complications of pins that are not removed.

Lyons and Rockwood[90] reviewed 37 reports of pin migration in operations about the shoulder, and recommended that pin use should be avoided in this area. When pins are utilized, they should be bent or have restraining devices to decrease the risk of migration. The patient should be informed of the risks. Close follow-up should be performed and the pins should be removed at the conclusion of therapy or whenever migration is noted. Pin migration may have devastating consequences, and there are reported deaths. (In general, pins should be avoided in this area.)

Failure of Soft Tissue Repairs in Acromioclavicular Joint Injuries

In the treatment of a ligamentous injury to the AC joint, simple repair of the CC and AC ligaments without the additional support of CC sutures, screws, or internal fixation, will likely fail. This is particularly true in chronic injury of the AC joint as there is often significant displacement between the clavicle and the coracoid. Transfer of the acromial attachment of the coracoacromial ligament onto or into the medullary canal of the distal clavicle (the Weaver–Dunn technique) alone is not strong enough in general. It must be supplemented with additional fixation as recommended in the treatment section.

Failure of soft tissue repairs can also result from suture breakage, suture anchor pullout, or screw breakage. If failure is noticed early in the postoperative period, reoperation to correct the problem is usually indicated. If failure occurs weeks to months after surgery, infection should be suspected and ruled out.

Recently Reported Complications with ACCR Technique

Open treatment of highly displaced or chronic AC joint dislocations by reconstructing the CC ligaments with allograft tendons is gaining popularity in the literature, but complications are possible. This is highlighted by the recent report of three cases of clavicle fracture following AC joint reconstruction by Turman et al.[156] In this report the incidence of clavicle fracture occurred in three of seven patients treated with CC ligament reconstruction: All patients had type V injuries, two patients had acute reconstructions (<6 month after injury), and one patient was treated

2 years after injury. The paper discusses clavicle bone tunnel diameter (all cases >5.5 mm) and the lack of AC joint ligament repair or reconstruction as a possible mode of failure. Increased anterior–posterior translation at the AC joint without AC ligament integrity has been demonstrated, this leads to increased forces on the native or reconstructed CC ligaments.[40,52,99] As a second mode of possible catastrophic failure, bone tunnel widening has been reported[167] and clavicle osseous anatomy and bone density relating to fracture risk for bone tunnel position and diameter. Our current recommendation to prevent this complication is to avoid >5.5 mm tunnels, minimize the graft, tap the clavicle tunnels before interference screw insertion and ensure at least 25 mm of bone between tunnels.

Complications Related to Nonabsorbable Tape or Suture

CC fixation using grafts or synthetic material has been associated with various complications. Goldberg et al.[61] described erosion of a Dacron graft through the distal clavicle in their series (Fig. 41-36). Moneim and Balduini[104] noted a coracoid

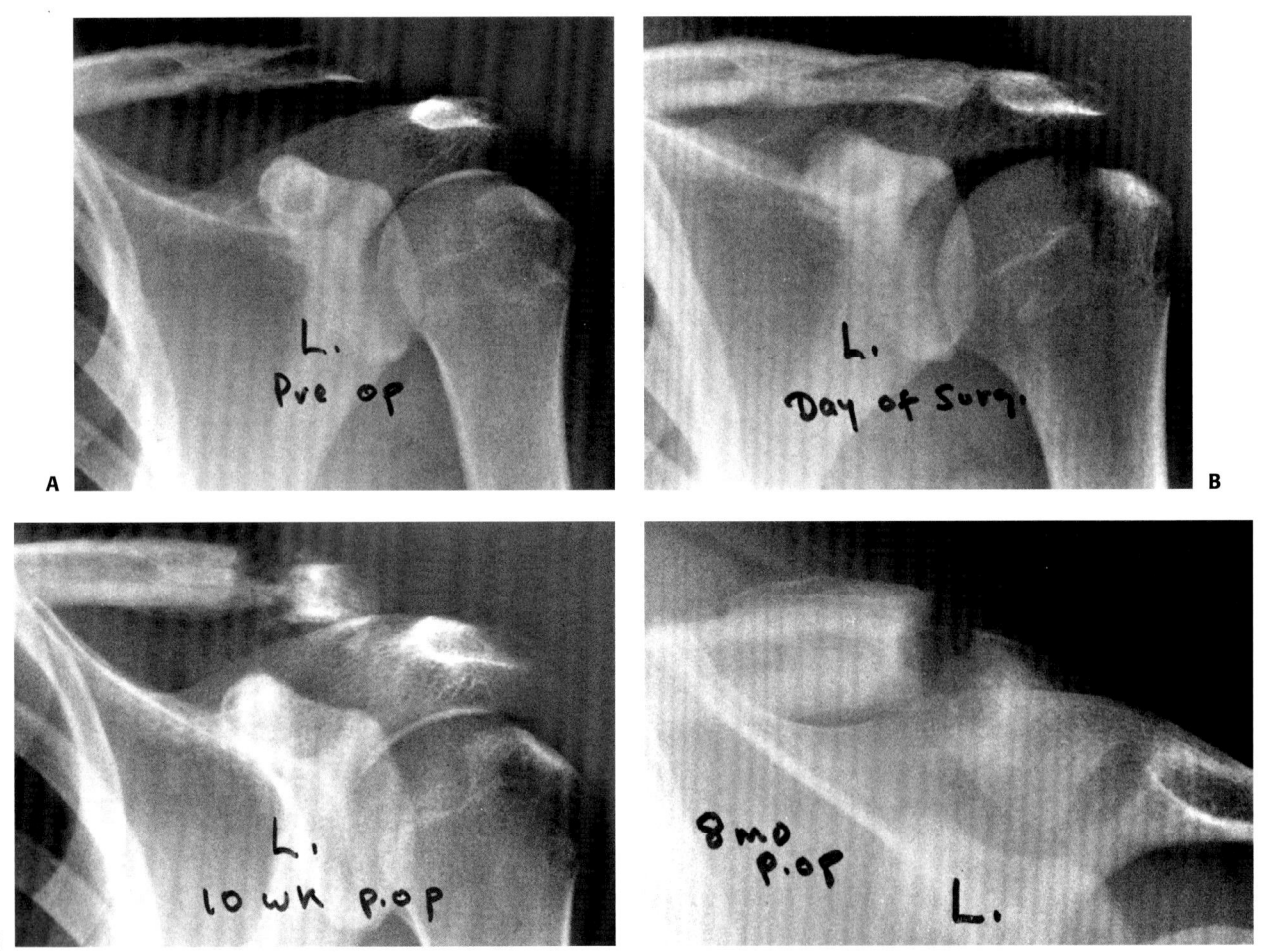

FIGURE 41-36 Complications from using cerclage material as a loop around the top of the clavicle and under the coracoid process for treatment of complete AC dislocations. **A:** Preoperative radiograph demonstrating the type III dislocation of the AC joint. **B:** The postoperative radiograph demonstrates near-anatomic reduction using a 6-mm soft Dacron vascular graft loop. **C:** Gradual erosion of the Dacron graft completely through the distal clavicle can be seen. **D:** Note the superior migration of the shaft of the clavicle.

fracture after reconstruction of the CC ligaments through two drill holes in the distal clavicle. Fractures of the distal clavicle secondary to the use of loop sutures between the coracoid and the distal clavicle have been reported.[94] Other complications include aseptic foreign body reactions and infections; Neault et al.[110] reported three cases in which nonabsorbable tape or suture was directly related to a postoperative infection. Two infections occurred within a year, but one 5 years after repair of a type III injury. Colosimo et al.[30] reported two cases of aseptic foreign body reactions to Dacron graft material 2 and 4 years after surgery. Microscopic examination revealed chronic inflammation with a foreign body giant cell reaction. Both patients improved after removal of the Dacron material and returned to work in 10 days.

Acromioclavicular Arthritis

Symptomatic arthritis of the AC joint may occur after surgical fixation. Weaver and Dunn[161] recommended distal clavicle excision and transfer of the coracoacromial ligament for both acute and chronic AC separations. In a review article, Cook and Heiner[31] recommend distal clavicle excision as part of the acute surgical management of patients with AC separations. They reported that postoperative degenerative changes in the AC joint may occur in as many as 24% of patients following AC joint injury and that primary excision of the distal clavicle was associated with little morbidity. Conversely, the vast majority of series reporting the results of surgical management of AC separations do not advocate primary excision of the distal clavicle.[8] Therefore, there is no consensus regarding primary distal clavicle excision and coracoacromial ligament transfer for acute AC injuries. It is our practice to preserve the AC joint articulation whenever possible. However, the scar formed within the dislocation space including the meniscus homologue needs to be removed to allow for reduction. If any distal clavicle is removed we attempt to remove it from the posterior edge of the clavicle as that is typically the location of abutment or impingement with the posterior edge of the acromion which may produce pain.

THE ROLE OF ARTHROSCOPY IN THE TREATMENT OF ACROMIOCLAVICULAR JOINT INJURIES

The first report of arthroscopy for acute AC joint injuries by Wolf and Pennington[164] described an all-arthroscopic technique of AC joint reconstruction. The coracoid was visualized through the subcoracoid recess in the anterior aspect of the joint. An anterior cruciate ligament guide is used to drill a hole through the clavicle and coracoid, and SecureStrand cable (Surgical Dynamics, Norwalk, CT) was used for fixation. They reported a series of four patients with no recurrence of deformity. Lafosse et al.[82] published an all-arthroscopic technique for CC ligament reconstruction, which releases the coracoacromial ligament from the undersurface of the acromion and transfers it to the inferior clavicle. Proponents of arthroscopic reconstruction claim the benefits of this more minimally invasive technique include minimal violation of the deltotrapezial

fascia, faster postoperative recovery, less pain, and fewer complications.

Although many different arthroscopic techniques have been proposed, few clinical outcome studies have been published. Chernchujit et al.[26] published a series of 13 patients who had an arthroscopic reconstruction following AC joint disruption using suture anchors and a titanium plate. These patients were followed for a mean of 18 months. Twelve patients returned to work without pain within 3 months of the operation and the average Constant Score at last follow-up was 95. Postoperative radiographs confirmed an anatomic reduction in 10 patients, residual subluxation in two patients, and redislocation of the joint in one patient. Given this, as well as evolving surgical techniques, an expanding role for arthroscopy in the management of these injuries may be seen in the future.

Arthroscopic-assisted techniques to reconstruct the anatomic position of the CC ligaments have gained popularity in the last several years after initial reported successes.[108,132,153] These techniques are being applied to reconstruction of type III and V AC joint dislocations acutely, and in chronic cases after failed conservative treatment. The use of suture-containing devices with cortical buttons is applied CC distance fixation, which if necessary can even be augmented with soft tissue graft and a separate AC joint capsule repair procedure, or when done very acutely (<1 week) allows for indirect reduction and scaring of the injured AC joint ligaments in a reduced position. These arthroscopic techniques allow for minimal soft tissue dissection, smaller incisions, and "safer" graft passage around the coracoid process as it is done under direct visualization. Comparing nonoperative to operative management of type III separations has not demonstrated significant improvement,[143] but newer techniques may provide more stability while still allowing physiologic clavicle motion important for function.

Saltzman et al. reported the latest progression in the refinement of this technique. They described the anatomic placement of two suture–button devices corresponding to the position of the ruptured trapezoid and conoid ligaments using two independent 3.5-mm clavicle and coracoid bone tunnels. Twenty-three patients were followed for an average of 30 months. The majority[132] were reported to be Rockwood type V dislocations, and all procedures were done acutely (<10 days) with a comprehensive outcome with visual analog scale, Constant Score, SF-36 score, and repeat radiographs were performed. However, seven patients were lost to follow-up and they were not included, two failures, one infection needing removal of implant, four patients lost to follow-up. Certainly, the technique is innovative and may lead to shorter rehabilitation and better functional outcomes when compared to nonoperative management, but this remains uncertain. A prospective study with a nonoperative control group is required. This technique is not without complications, including increased CC distance, osteolysis around the suture–button device, and migration of implants. The VAS, Constant Scores improved significantly after surgery, however, similar to previous reports, the AC joint alignment was radiographically unsatisfactory in eight cases. A clear disadvantage of this technique is the superior clavicular displacement in over 30% of cases at 24 months postoperatively, and a high incidence of pain over the superior clavicle button. Despite some of the limitations of this paper the authors report good results but caution that this is an advanced arthroscopic technique and that tunnel and button placement are of utmost importance to avoid postoperative failures or loss of reduction. Scheibel et al.[134] using an identical technique, published results on the arthroscopic stabilization of acute Rockwood type V AC dislocations in 28 of 37 consecutive patients available for final follow-up at an average of 26 months. Although there was a significant loss to follow-up they report good function, with ROM comparable to the uninjured side, no difference in strength, and maintenance of the CC distance reduction obtained intraoperatively. Complications included tenderness over the superior buttons in 11 patients (although none required removal). In addition, twenty-five patients (89%) demonstrated implant migration within the bone tunnels with mild osteolysis and enlargement of the tunnels. No significant loss of reduction was reported even with "stress" radiographs taken during evaluation.

As noted in a few reports, the metallic button design tends to see more "motion" at the bone–button interface as the motion between the clavicle and scapula occurs with shoulder abduction.[29,33,105,108,134] A recent study by Cohen et al.[29] noted a decrease in pain, increase in CC distance, and metallic button migration into the clavicle with a larger "second-generation" button in which the diameter was increased from 6.5 mm to 10 mm. A second report by Motta et al.[105] in which osteolysis and button migration was observed with 6-mm (first generation) prosthesis was eliminated in patients reconstructed with constructs containing 10-mm superior metallic buttons. Augmentation of a suture-suspension device with graft tissue provides increased initial stability and a load to failure that is similar to native CC ligaments. In a recently published technique, a suture–button device was utilized in part to facilitate this laboratory data.[39] The superior, larger diameter, "low profile" washer can centrally accommodate a graft which gives the construct strength approaching the normal anatomy, while accommodating motion between the clavicle and scapula. This technique was applied to 10 patients with acute and chronic high-grade injuries with a short-term follow-up of 6 months with good to excellent results, and no reported complications (infection, hardware, or graft failure) encountered to date. The authors did not specifically address the AC joint, except in a few of the chronic cases in which a distal clavicle excision up to 5 mm was performed. Complications at the level of the coracoid fixation following arthroscopically assisted techniques have also recently been reported in conjunction with noncompliance or trauma.[60] Gerhardt et al.[60] reported a case of coracoid base fracture in an older but very athletic female patient who failed fixation secondary to fracture within 1 week following allograft tendon augmented CC fixation with a 6-mm suture–button construct.

REFERENCES

1. Adams FL. *The Genuine Works of Hippocrates.* Vols 1 and 2. New York, NY: William Wood; 1886.
2. Arenas AJ, Pampliega T, Iglesias J. Surgical management of bipolar clavicular dislocation. *Acta Orthop Belg.* 1993;59:202–205.
3. Bannister GC, Wallace WA, Stableforth PG, et al. The management of acute acromioclavicular dislocation. A randomized prospective controlled trial. *J Bone Joint Surg.* 1989;71(5):848–850.
4. Bannister GC, Wallace WA, Stableforth PG, et al. A classification of acute acromioclavicular dislocation: A clinical, radiological, and anatomical study. *Injury.* 1992;23:194–196.
5. Barber FA. Complete posterior acromioclavicular dislocation: A case report. *Orthopedics.* 1987;10:493–496.
6. Barbour SA, King W. The safe and effective use of allograft tissue: An update. *Am J Sports Med.* 2003;31:791–797.
7. Bearden JM, Hughston JC, Whatley GS. Acromioclavicular dislocation: Method of treatment. *J Sports Med.* 1973;1:5–17.
8. Beitzel K, Cote MP, Apostolakos J, et al. Current concepts in the treatment of acromioclavicular joint dislocations. *Arthroscopy.* 2013;29(2):387–397.
9. Bergfeld JA, Andrish JT, Clancy WG. Evaluation of the acromioclavicular joint following first- and second-degree sprains. *Am J Sports Med.* 1978;6:153–159.
10. Bernard TNJ, Brunet ME, Haddad RJ. Fractured coracoid process in acromioclavicular dislocations: Report of four cases and review of the literature. *Clin Orthop.* 1983;175:227–232.
11. Bjerneld H, Hovelius L, Thorling J. Acromioclavicular separations treated conservatively. A 5-year follow-up study. *Acta Orthop Scand.* 1983;54:743–745.
12. Black GB, McPherson JAM, Reed MH. Traumatic pseudodislocation of the acromioclavicular joint in children: A 15-year review. *Am J Sports Med.* 1991;19:644–646.
13. Blazar PE, Iannotti JP, Williams GR. Anteroposterior instability of the distal clavicle after distal clavicle resection. *Clin Orthop.* 1998;(348):114–120.
14. Boehm TC. The relation of the coracoclavicular ligament insertion to the acromioclavicular joint. A cadaver study of relevance to lateral clavicle resection. *Acta Orthop Scand.* 2003;74(6):718–721.
15. Bostrom-Windhamre HA, von Heideken JP, Une-Larsson VE, et al. Surgical treatment of chronic acromioclavicular dislocations: A comparative study of Weaver-Dunn augmented with PDS-braid or hook plate. *J Shoulder Elbow Surg.* 2010;19(7):1040–1048.
16. Bosworth BM. Acromioclavicular separation: New method of repair. *Surg Gynecol Obstet.* 1941;73:866–871.
17. Branch TP, Burdette HL, Shahriari AS, et al. The role of the acromioclavicular ligaments and the effect of distal clavicle resection. *Am J Sports Med.* 1996;24:293–297.
18. Breslow MJ, Jazrawi LM, Bernstein AD, et al. Treatment of acromioclavicular joint separation: Suture or suture anchors? *J Shoulder Elbow Surg.* 2002;11(3):225–229.
19. Browne JE, Stanley RF, Tullos HS. Acromioclavicular joint dislocations: Comparative results following operative treatment with and without primary distal clavisectomy. *Am J Sports Med.* 1977;5:258–263.
20. Brunet ME, Reynolds MC, Cook SD, et al. Atraumatic osteolysis of the distal clavicle: Histologic evidence of synovial pathogenesis. A case report. *Orthopedics.* 1986;9(4):557–559.
21. Cadenat FM. The treatment of dislocations and fractures of the outer end of the clavicle. *Int Clin.* 1917;1:145–169.
22. Cahill BR. Osteolysis of the distal part of the clavicle in male athletes. *J Bone Joint Surg.* 1982;64(7):1053–1058.
23. Calvo E, Lopez-Franco M, Arribas IM. Clinical and radiologic outcomes of surgical and conservative treatment of type III acromioclavicular joint injury. *J Shoulder Elbow Surg.* 2006;15(3):300–305.
24. Carofino BC, Mazzocca AD. The anatomic coracoclavicular ligament reconstruction: Surgical technique and indications. *J Shoulder Elbow Surg.* 2010;19(2 suppl):37–46.
25. Carr AJ, Broughton NS. Acromioclavicular dislocation associated with fracture of the coracoid process. *J Trauma.* 1989;29:125–126.
26. Chernchujit B, Tischer T, Imhoff AB. Arthroscopic reconstruction of the acromioclavicular joint disruption: Surgical technique and preliminary results. *Arch Orthop Trauma Surg.* 2006;126:575–581.
27. Chiang CL, Yang SW, Tsai MY, et al. Acromion osteolysis and fracture after hook plate fixation for acromioclavicular joint dislocation: A case report. *J Shoulder Elbow Surg.* 2010; 19(4):e13–e15.
28. Codman EA. Rupture of the supraspinatus tendon and other lesions in or about the subacromial bursa. In: Codman EA, ed. *The Shoulder.* Boston, MA: Thomas Todd; 1934:32–65.
29. Cohen G, Boyer P, Pujol N, et al. Endoscopically assisted reconstruction of acute acromioclavicular joint dislocations using a synthetic ligament. Outcomes at 12 months. *Orthop Traumatol Surg Res.* 2011;97:145–151.
30. Colosimo AJ, Hummer CD 3rd, Heidt RS Jr. Aseptic foreign body reaction to Dacron graft material used for coracoclavicular ligament reconstruction after type III acromioclavicular dislocation. *Am J Sports Med.* 1996;24:561–563.
31. Cook DA, Heiner JP. Acromioclavicular joint injuries. *Orthop Rev.* 1990;14:510–516.
32. Cook F, Horowitz M. Bipolar clavicular dislocation: Report of a case. *J Bone Joint Surg.* 1987;69(1):145–147.
33. Costic RS, Labriola JE, Rodosky MW. Biomechanical rationale for development of anatomical reconstructions of coracoclavicular ligaments after complete acromioclavicular joint dislocations. *Am J Sports Med.* 2004;32:1929–1936.
34. Cote MP, Wojcik KE, Gomlinski G, et al. Rehabilitation of acromioclavicular joint separations: Operative and nonoperative considerations. *Clin Sports Med.* 2010;29(2):213–228.
35. Cox JS. The fate of the acromioclavicular joint in athletic injuries. *Am J Sports Med.* 1981;9:50–53.
36. Cox JS. Current method of treatment of acromioclavicular joint dislocations. *Orthopedics.* 1992;15:1041–1044.
37. Curtis RJ. Operative management of children's fractures of the shoulder region. *Orthop Clin North Am.* 1990;21:315–324.
38. Daly P, Sim FH, Simonet WT. Ice hockey injuries: A review. *Sports Med.* 1990;10:122–131.
39. DeBerardino TM, Pensak MJ, Ferreira J, et al. Arthroscopic stabilization of acromioclavicular joint dislocation using the AC graftrope system. *J Shoulder Elbow Surg.* 2010;19(2 suppl):47–52.
40. Debski RE, Parsons IM, Woo SL, et al. Effect of capsular injury on acromioclavicular joint mechanics. *J Bone Joint Surg Am.* 2001;83-A:1344–1351.
41. DePalma AF. The role of the disks of the sternoclavicular and the acromioclavicular joints. *Clin Orthop.* 1959;13:222–233.

42. Dias JJ, Steingold RF, Richardson RA, et al. The conservative treatment of acromioclavicular dislocation. Review after 5 years. *J Bone Joint Surg*. 1987;69(5):719–722.
43. Dragoo JL, Braun HJ, Bartlinski SE, et al. Acromioclavicular joint injuries in national collegiate athletic association football: Data from the 2004-2005 through 2008-2009 national collegiate athletic association injury surveillance system. *Am J Sports Med*. 2012;40(9): 2066–2071.
44. Dumontier C, Sautet A, Man M, et al. Acromioclavicular dislocations: Treatment by coracoacromial ligamentoplasty. *J Shoulder Elbow Surg*. 1995;4:130–134.
45. Echo BS, Donati RB, Powell CE. Bipolar clavicular dislocation treated surgically: A case report. *J Bone Joint Surg Am*. 1988;70(8):1251–1253.
46. Edgar CM, Zimmer S, Jones H, et al. Prospective comparison of auto and allograft hamstring tendon constructs for ACL reconstruction. *Clin Orthop Relat Res*. 2008;466(9): 2238–2246.
47. Eidman DK, Siff SJ, Tullos HS. Acromioclavicular lesions in children. *Am J Sports Med*. 1981;9:150–154.
48. Falstie-Jensen S, Mikkelsen P. Pseudodislocation of the acromioclavicular joint. *J Bone Joint Surg*. 1982;64(3):368–369.
49. Flatow EL. The biomechanics of the acromioclavicular, sternoclavicular, and scapulothoracic joints. *Instr Course Lect*. 1993;42:237–245.
50. Flatow EL, Cordasco FA, Bigliani LU. Arthroscopic resection of the outer end of the clavicle from a superior approach: A critical, quantitative, radiographic assessment of bone removal. *Arthroscopy*. 1992;8:55–64.
51. Flatow EL, Duralde XA, Nicholson GP, et al. Arthroscopic resection of the distal clavicle with a superior approach. *J Shoulder Elbow Surg*. 1995;4:41–50.
52. Fukuda K, Craig EV, An KN, et al. Biomechanical study of the ligamentous system of the acromioclavicular joint. *J Bone Joint Surg*. 1986;68(3):434–440.
53. Galatz LM, Williams GR. Acromioclavicular joint injuries. In: Bucholz RW, Heckman JD, Court-Brown C, eds. *Rockwood and Green's Fractures in Adults*. Vol 2. 6th ed. Philadelphia, PA: Lippincott Williams & Wilkins; 2006:1331–1364.
54. Gallay SH, Hupel TM, Beaton DE, et al. Functional outcome of acromioclavicular joint injury in polytrauma patients. *J Orthop Trauma*. 1998;12:159–163.
55. Galpin RD, Hawkins RJ, Grainger RW. A comparative analysis of operative versus nonoperative treatment of grade III acromioclavicular separations. *Clin Orthop*. 1985;193: 150–155.
56. Gartsman GM. Arthroscopic resection of the acromioclavicular joint. *Am J Sports Med*. 1993;21:71–77.
57. Gearen PF, Petty W. Panclavicular dislocation. Report of a case. *J Bone Joint Surg*. 1982;64(3):454–455.
58. Gerber C, Galantay RV, Hersche O. The pattern of pain produced by irritation of the acromioclavicular joint and the subacromial space. *J Shoulder Elbow Surg*. 1998;7(4):352–355.
59. Gerber C, Rockwood CA. Subcoracoid dislocation of the lateral end of the clavicle: A report of three cases. *J Bone Joint Surg Am*. 1987;69(6):924–927.
60. Gerhardt DC, Vanderwerf JD, Rylander LS, et al. Postoperative coracoid fracture after transcoracoid acromioclavicular joint reconstruction. *J Shoulder Elbow Surg*. 2011;20(5):e6–e10.
61. Goldberg JA, Viglione W, Cumming WJ, et al. Review of coracoclavicular ligament reconstruction using Dacron graft material. *Aust NZ J Surg*. 1987;57:441–445.
62. Griffiths CJ, Glucksman E. Post traumatic osteolysis of the clavicle: A case report. *Arch Emerg Med*. 1986;3:129–132.
63. Grutter PW, Petersen SA. Anatomical acromioclavicular ligament reconstruction: A biomechanical comparison of reconstructive techniques of the acromioclavicular joint. *Am J Sports Med*. 2005;33:1723–1728.
64. Gstettner C, Tauber M, Hitzl W, et al. Rockwood type III acromioclavicular dislocation: Surgical versus conservative treatment. *J Shoulder Elbow Surg*. 2008;17(2):220–225.
65. Gumina S, Carbone S, Postacchini F. Scapular dyskinesis and SICK scapula syndrome in patients with chronic type III acromioclavicular dislocation. *Arthroscopy*. 2009;25(1):40–45.
66. Guy DK, Wirth MA, Griffin JL, et al. Reconstruction of chronic and complete dislocations of the acromioclavicular joint. *Clin Orthop*. 1998;347:138–149.
67. Harris RI, Vu DH, Sonnabend DH, et al. Anatomic variance of the coracoclavicular ligaments. *J Shoulder Elbow Surg*. 2001;10(6):585–588.
68. Harris RI, Wallace AL, Harper GD, et al. Structural properties of the intact and the reconstructed coracoclavicular ligament complex. *Am J Sports Med*. 2000;28(1):103–108.
69. Hastings DE, Horne JG. Anterior dislocation of the acromioclavicular joint. *Injury*. 1979;10:285–288.
70. Havranek P. Injuries of distal clavicular physis in children. *J Pediatr Orthop*. 1989;9: 213–215.
71. Hawkins RJ, Warren RF, Noble JS. *Suture repair technique for acute and chronic acromioclavicular dislocations*. Rosemont, IL: American Academy of Orthopaedic Surgeons videotape series; 2005.
72. Inman VT, Saunders M, Abbott LC. Observations on the function of the shoulder joint. *J Bone Joint Surg*. 1944;26:1–30.
73. Jain AS. Traumatic floating clavicle: A case report. *J Bone Joint Surg Br*. 1984;66(4):560–561.
74. Jones HP, Lemos MJ, Schepsis AA. Salvage of failed acromioclavicular joint reconstruction using autogenous semitendinosus tendon from the knee. Surgical technique and cast report. *Am J Sports Med*. 2001;29(2):234–237.
75. Kaplan LD, Flanigan DC, Norwig J, et al. Prevalence and variance of shoulder injuries in elite collegiate football players. *Am J Sports Med*. 2005;33(8):1142–1146.
76. Kennedy JC, Cameron H. Complete dislocation of the acromioclavicular joint. *J Bone Joint Surg Br*. 1954;36-B(2):202–208.
77. Kienast B, Thietje R, Queitsch C, et al. Mid-term results after operative treatment of Rockwood grade III-V acromioclavicular joint dislocations with an AC-hook plate. *Eur J Med Res*. 2011;16(2):52–56.
78. Kim KC, Rhee KJ, Shin HD, et al. Displaced fracture of the coracoid process associated with acromioclavicular dislocation: A two-bird-one-stone solution. *J Trauma*. 2009;67(2):403–405.
79. Klimkiewicz JJ, Williams GR, Sher JS, et al. The acromioclavicular capsule as a restraint to posterior translation of the clavicle: A biomechanical analysis. *J Shoulder Elbow Surg*. 1999;8:119–124.
80. Kumar A. Management of coracoid process fracture with acromioclavicular joint dislocation. *Orthopaedics*. 1990;13:770–772.
81. Kumar S, Sethi A, Jain AK. Surgical treatment of complete acromioclavicular dislocation using the coracoacromial ligament and coracoclavicular fixation: Report of a technique in 14 patients. *J Orthop Trauma*. 1995;9:507–510.
82. Lafosse L, Baier GP, Leuzinger J. Arthroscopic treatment of acute and chronic acromioclavicular joint dislocation. *Arthroscopy*. 2005;21:1017–1028.
83. Lancourt JB. Acromioclavicular dislocation with adjacent clavicular fracture in a horseback rider: A case report. *Am J Sports Med*. 1990;18:321–322.
84. Larsen E, Bjerg-Nielsen A, Christensen P. Conservative or surgical treatment of acromioclavicular dislocation. A prospective, controlled, randomized study. *J Bone Joint Surg*. 1986;68(4):552–555.
85. Lasda NA, Murray DG. Fracture separation of the coracoid process associated with acromioclavicular dislocation: Conservative treatment–a case report and review of the literature. *Clin Orthop Relat Res*. 1978;134:222–224.
86. Lee KW, Debski RE, Chen CH, et al. Functional evaluation of the ligaments at the acromioclavicular joint during anteroposterior and superoinferior translation. *Am J Sports Med*. 1997;25:858–862.
87. Lee SJ, Nicholas SJ, Akizuki KH, et al. Reconstruction of the coracoclavicular ligament with tendon grafts: A comparative biomechanical study. *Am J Sports Med*. 2003;31:648–654.
88. Lemos MJ. The evaluation and treatment of the injured acromioclavicular joint in athletes. *Am J Sports Med*. 1998;26:137–144.
89. Lizaur A, Marco L, Cebrian R. Acute dislocation of the acromioclavicular joint. Traumatic anatomy and the importance of deltoid and trapezius. *J Bone Joint Surg Br*. 1994;76(4):602–606.
90. Lyons FA, Rockwood CA. Migration of pins used in operations on the shoulder. *J Bone Joint Surg*. 1990;72(8):1262–1267.
91. MacDonald PB, Alexander MJ, Frejuk J, et al. Comprehensive functional analysis of shoulders following complete acromioclavicular separation. *Am J Sports Med*. 1988; 16:475–480.
92. Madsen B. Osteolysis of the acromial end of the clavicle following trauma. *Br J Radiol*. 1963;36:822–828.
93. Malcapi C, Grassi G, Oretti D. Posterior dislocation of the acromioclavicular joint: A rare or an easily overlooked lesion? *Ital J Orthop Traumatol*. 1978;4:79–83.
94. Martell JR. Clavicular nonunion. Complication with the use of mersilene tape. *Am J Sports Med*. 1992;20:360–362.
95. Martin-Herrero T, Rodriguez-Merchan C, Munuera-Martinez L. Fracture of the coracoid process: Presentation of seven cases and review of the literature. *J Trauma*. 1993;30:1597–1599.
96. Mazet RJ. Migration of a Kirschner wire from the shoulder region into the lung: A report of two cases. *J Bone Joint Surg*. 1943;25A:477–483.
97. Mazzocca AD, Arciero RA, Bicos J. Evaluation and treatment of acromioclavicular joint injuries. *Am J Sports Med*. 2007;35:316–329.
98. Mazzocca AD, Santangelo SA, Johnson ST. A biomechanical evaluation of an anatomical coracoclavicular ligament reconstruction. *Am J Sports Med*. 2006;34:236–246.
99. Mazzocca AD, Spang JT, Rodriguez RR, et al. Biomechanical and radiographic analysis of partial coracoclavicular ligament injuries. *Am J Sports Med*. 2008;36(7):1397–1402.
100. McPhee IB. Inferior dislocation of the outer end of the clavicle. *J Trauma*. 1980;20: 709–710.
101. Meislin RJ, Zuckerman JD, Nainzadeh N. Type III acromioclavicular joint separation associated with late brachial plexus neurapraxia. *J Orthop Trauma*. 1992;6:370–372.
102. Merk BR, Minihane KP, Shah NA. Scapulothoracic dissociation with acromioclavicular separation: A case report of a novel fixation method. *J Orthop Trauma*. 2008;22(8):572–575.
103. Molsa J, Urho K, Pertti M, et al. Injuries to the upper extremity in ice hockey analysis of a series of 760 injuries. *Am J Sports Med*. 2003;31(5):751–757.
104. Moneim MS, Balduini FC. Coracoid fracture as a complication of surgical treatment by coracoclavicular tape fixation. A case report. *Clin Orthop*. 1982;168:133–135.
105. Motta P, Maderni A, Bruno L, et al. Case report: Suture rupture in acromioclavicular joint dislocations treated with flip buttons. *Arthroscopy*. 2011;27(2):294–298.
106. Mouhsine E, Garofalo R, Crevoisier X, et al. Grade I and II acromioclavicular dislocations: Results of conservative treatment. *J Shoulder Elbow Surg*. 2003;12(6):599–602.
107. Mumford EB. Acromioclavicular dislocation. *J Bone Joint Surg*. 1941;23:799–802.
108. Murena L, Vulcano E, Ratti C, et al. Arthroscopic treatment of acute acromioclavicular joint dislocation with double flip button. *Knee Surg Sports Traumatol Arthrosc*. 2009;17: 1511–1515.
109. Murphy OB, Bellamy R, Wheeler W, et al. Posttraumatic osteolysis of the distal clavicle. *Clin Orthop*. 1975;109:108–114.
110. Neault MA, Nuber GW, Marymont JV. Infections after surgical repair of acromioclavicular separations with nonabsorbable tape or suture. *J Shoulder Elbow Surg*. 1996;5:477–478.
111. Nieminen S, Aho AJ. Anterior dislocation of the acromioclavicular joint. *Ann Chir Gynaecol*. 1984;73:21–24.
112. Nissen CW, Chatterjee A. Type III acromioclavicular separation: Results of a recent survey on its management. *Am J Orthop*. 2007;36:89–93.
113. Norell H, Llewellyn RC. Migration of a threaded Steinmann pin from an acromioclavicular joint into the spinal canal. *J Bone Joint Surg*. 1965;47A:1024–1026.
114. Nuber GW, Bowen MK. Disorders of the acromioclavicular joint: pathophysiology, diagnosis, and management. In: Iannotti JP, Williams GR, eds. *Disorders of the Shoulder: Diagnosis and Management*. Philadelphia, PA: Lippincott Williams & Wilkins; 1999:739–764.
115. O'Brien SJ, Pagnani MJ, Fealy S, et al. The active compression test: A new and effective test for diagnosing labral tears and acromioclavicular joint abnormality. *Am J Sports Med*. 1998;26(5):610–613.
116. Pallis M, Cameron KL, Svoboda SJ, et al. Epidemiology of acromioclavicular joint injury in young athletes. *Am J Sports Med*. 2012;40(9):2072–2077.

117. Pauly S, Gerhardt C, Haas NP, et al. Prevalence of concomitant intraarticular lesions in patients treated operatively for high-grade acromioclavicular joint separations. *Knee Surg Sports Traumatol Arthrosc.* 2009;17(5):513–517.

118. Petersson CJ. Degeneration of the acromioclavicular joint. *Acta Orthop Scand.* 1983;54:434–438.

119. Petersson CJ, Redlund-Johnell I. Radiographic joint space in normal acromioclavicular joints. *Acta Orthop Scand.* 1983;54:431–433.

120. Post M. Current concepts in the diagnosis and management of acromioclavicular dislocations. *Clin Orthop.* 1985;200:234–247.

121. Powers JA, Bach PJ. Acromioclavicular separation: Closed or open treatment. *Clin Orthop.* 1974;104:213–233.

122. Press J, Zuckerman JD, Gallagher M, et al. Treatment of grade III acromioclavicular separations. Operative versus nonoperative management. *Bull Hosp Jt Dis.* 1997;56:77–83.

123. Rawes ML, Dias JJ. Long-term results of conservative treatment for acromioclavicular dislocation. *J Bone Joint Surg Br.* 1996;78(3):410–412.

124. Renfree KJ, Riley MK, Wheeler D, et al. Ligamentous anatomy of the distal clavicle. *J Shoulder Elbow Surg.* 2003;12(4):355–359.

125. Rios CG, Arciero RA, Mazzocca AD. Anatomy of the clavicle and coracoid process for reconstruction of the coracoclavicular ligaments. *Am J Sports Medicine.* 2007;35(5):811–817.

126. Rockwood CA. Injuries to the acromioclavicular Joint. In: Rockwood CA, Green DP, eds. *Fractures in Adults.* Vol 1. 2nd ed. Philadelphia, PA: JB Lippincott; 1984:860.

127. Rockwood CA, Williams GR, Young DC. Disorders of the acromio-clavicular joint. In: Rockwood CA, Matsen FA, eds. *The Shoulder.* 3rd ed. Philadelphia, PA: WB Saunders Co; 2004:521–586.

128. Rowe CR. In: Cave EF, ed. *Fractures and other injuries.* Chicago, IL: Year Book Medical; 1961.

129. Sage J. Recurrent inferior dislocation of the clavicle at the acromioclavicular joint. *Am J Sports Med.* 1982;10:145–146.

130. Salter EG, Nasca RJ, Shelley BS. Anatomical observations on the acromioclavicular joint and supporting ligaments. *Am J Sports Med.* 1987;15:199–206.

131. Salter EG, Shelley BS, Nasca R. A morphological study of the acromioclavicular joint in humans. *Anat Rec.* 1985;211:353.

132. Salzman GM, Walz L, Schoettle PB, et al. Arthroscopic anatomical reconstruction of the acromioclavicular joint. *Acta Orthop Belg.* 2008;74:397–400.

133. Sanders JO, Lyons FA, Rockwood CA. Management of dislocations of both ends of the clavicle. *J Bone Joint Surg.* 1990;72A:399–402.

134. Scheibel M, Droschel S, Gerhardt C, et al. Arthroscopically assisted stabilization of acute high-grade acromioclavicular joint separations. *Am J Sports Med.* 2011;39(7):1507–1516.

135. Schemitsch LA, Schemitsch EH, McKee MD. Bipolar clavicle injury: Posterior dislocation of the acromioclavicular joint with anterior dislocation of the sternoclavicular joint: A report of two cases. *J Shoulder and Elbow Surg.* 2011;20(1):e18–e22.

136. Schlegel TF, Burks RT, Marcus RL, et al. A prospective evaluation of untreated acute grade III acromioclavicular separations. *Am J Sports Med.* 2001;29(6):699–703.

137. Schmid A, Schmid F. [Use of arthrosonography in diagnosis of Tossy III lesions of acromioclavicular joints]. *Aktuel Traumatol.* 1988;18:957–962.

138. Schwarz N, Kuderna H. Inferior acromioclavicular separation: Report of an unusual case. *Clin Orthop.* 1988;234:28–30.

139. Schwarzkopf R, Ishak C, Elman M, et al. Distal clavicular osteolysis: A review of the literature. *Bull NYU Hosp Jt Dis.* 2008;66(2):94–101.

140. Sim E, Schwarz N, Hocker K, et al. Repair of complete acromioclavicular separations using the acromioclavicular-hook plate. *Clin Orthop.* 1995;314:134–142.

141. Simovitch R, Sanders B, Ozbaydar M, et al. Acromioclavicular joint injuries: Diagnosis and management. *J Am Acad Orthop Surg.* 2009;17(4):207–219.

142. Skjeldal S, Lundblad R, Dullerud R. Coracoid process transfer for acromioclavicular dislocation. *Acta Orthop Scand.* 1988;59:180–182.

143. Smith TO, Chester R, Pearse EO, et al. Operative versus nonoperative management following Rockwood grade III acromioclavicular separation; a meta-analysis of the current evidence base. *J Orthop Traumatol.* 2011;12(1):19–27.

144. Snyder S, Banas M, Karzel R. The arthroscopic Mumford procedure: An analysis of results. *Arthroscopy.* 1995;11:157–164.

145. Sondergard-Petersen P, Mikkelsen P. Posterior acromioclavicular dislocation. *J Bone Joint Surg Br.* 1982;64(1):52–53.

146. Strobel K, Pfirrmann CW, Zanetti M, et al. MRI features of the acromioclavicular joint that predict pain relief from intraarticular injection. *AJR Am J Roentgenol.* 2003;181(3):755–760.

147. Sturm JT, Perry JFJ. Brachial plexus injuries from blunt trauma—a harbinger of vascular and thoracic injury. *Ann Emerg Med.* 1987;16(4):404–406.

148. Taft TN, Wilson FC, Oglesby JW. Dislocation of the acromioclavicular joint. An end-result study. *J Bone Joint Surg Am.* 1987;69(7):1045–1051.

149. Tamaoki MJ, Belloti JC, Lenza M, et al. Surgical versus conservative interventions for treating acromioclavicular dislocation of the shoulder in adults. *Cochrane Database Syst Rev.* 2010;(8).

150. Thomas K, Litsky A, Jones G, et al. Biomechanical comparison of coracoclavicular reconstructive techniques. *Am J Sports Med.* 2011;39(4):804–810.

151. Tibone J, Sellers R, Tonino P. Strength testing after third-degree acromioclavicular dislocations. *Am J Sports Med.* 1992;20:328–331.

152. Tischer T, Salzmann GM, El-Azab H, et al. Incidence of associated injuries with acute acromioclavicular joint dislocations types III through V. *Am J Sports Med.* 2009;37(1):136–139.

153. Tomlinson DP, Altcheck DW, Davila J, et al. A modified technique of arthroscopically assisted AC joint reconstruction and preliminary results. *Clin Orthop Relat Res.* 2008;466:639–645.

154. Tossy J, Newton CM, Sigmond HM. 11 acromioclavicular separations: Useful and practical classification for treatment. *Clin Orthop Relat Res.* 1963;28:111–119.

155. Trainer G, Arciero RA, Mazzocca AD. Practical management of grade III acromioclavicular separations. *Clin J Sports Med.* 2008;18(2):162–166.

156. Turman KA, Miller CD, Miller MD. Clavicular fractures following coracoclavicular ligament reconstruction with tendon graft: A report of three cases. *J Bone Joint Surg Am.* 2010;92(6):1526–1532.

157. Urist MR. Complete dislocation of the acromioclavicular joint: The nature of the traumatic lesion and effective methods of treatment with an analysis of 41 cases. *J Bone Joint Surg.* 1946;28:813–837.

158. Wade AM, Barrett MO, Crist BD, et al. Medial clavicular epiphyseal fracture with ipsilateral acromioclavicular dislocation: A case report of panclavicular fracture dislocation. *J Orthop Trauma.* 2007;21(6):418–421.

159. Walton J, Mahajan S, Paxinos A, et al. Diagnostic values of tests for acromioclavicular joint pain. *J Bone Joint Surg Am.* 2004;86:807–812.

160. Wang K, Hsu K, Shih C. Coracoid process fracture combined with acromioclavicular dislocation and coracoclavicular ligament rupture: A case report and review of the literature. *Clin Orthop.* 1994;300:120–122.

161. Weaver JK, Dunn HK. Treatment of acromioclavicular injuries, especially complete acromioclavicular separation. *J Bone Joint Surg Am.* 1972;54(6):1187–1194.

162. Weinstein DM, McCann PD, McIlveen SJ, et al. Surgical treatment of complete acromioclavicular dislocations. *Am J Sports Med.* 1995;23:324–331.

163. Williams GR, Nguyen VD, Rockwood CR. Classification and radiographic analysis of acromioclavicular dislocations. *Appl Radiol.* 1989;12:29–34.

164. Wolf EM, Pennington WT. Arthroscopic reconstruction for acromioclavicular joint dislocation. *Arthroscopy.* 2001;17(5):558–563.

165. Wojtys EM, Nelson G. Conservative treatment of grade III acromioclavicular dislocations. *Clin Orthop.* 1991;268:112–119.

166. Wurtz LD, Lyons FA, Rockwood CA Jr. Fracture of the middle third of the clavicle and dislocation of the acromioclavicular joint. A report of four cases. *J Bone Joint Surg Am.* 1992;74(1):133–137.

167. Yoo JC, Choi NH, Kim S, et al. Distal clavicle tunnel widening after 389 coracoclavicular ligament reconstruction with semitendinous tendon: A case 390 report. *J Shoulder Elbow Surg.* 2006;15(2):256–259.

168. Zanca P. Shoulder pain: Involvement of the acromioclavicular joint: Analysis of 1000 cases. *AJR.* 1971;112:493–506.

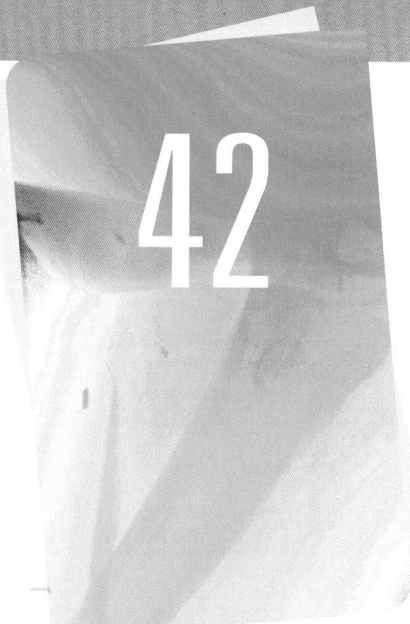

42 INJURIES TO THE STERNOCLAVICULAR JOINT

Anil K. Dutta, Aaron J. Bois, Michael A. Wirth, and Charles A. Rockwood, Jr

INTRODUCTION TO STERNOCLAVICULAR JOINT INJURIES

In Sir Astley Cooper's 1824 text, sternoclavicular (SC) injuries are discussed as injuries that can essentially be managed with a sling and swathe.[50] The first case reports of SC injury are attributed to Rodrigues[192] who described a patient with posterior dislocation presenting with signs of suffocation following a compression injury between a wall and a cart. Isolated 19th century reports in Europe were followed by those of American authors in the 1920s and 1930s.[55,64,140] SC joint injuries are uncommon and are usually relatively benign injuries. However, the more severe posterior injury patterns can represent true medical emergencies and require the orthopedic surgeon to be knowledgeable regarding the proper steps in diagnosis and treatment. Computed tomography (CT) remains the imaging modality of choice for diagnosing SC joint injuries. Early and prompt reduction is indicated for posterior dislocations and posterior physeal injuries. A variety of reconstructive techniques are available if needed, but are rarely required.

SURGICAL AND APPLIED ANATOMY OF THE STERNOCLAVICULAR JOINT

Surgical Anatomy of the Sternoclavicular Joint

The surgeon who is planning an operative procedure on or near the SC joint should be completely knowledgeable about the vast array of anatomic structures immediately posterior to the SC joint. There is a "curtain" of muscles (the sternohyoid, sternothyroid, and scaleni) posterior to the SC joint and the inner third of the clavicle, and this curtain blocks the view of the vital structures. Some of these vital structures include the innominate artery, innominate vein, vagus nerve, phrenic nerve, internal

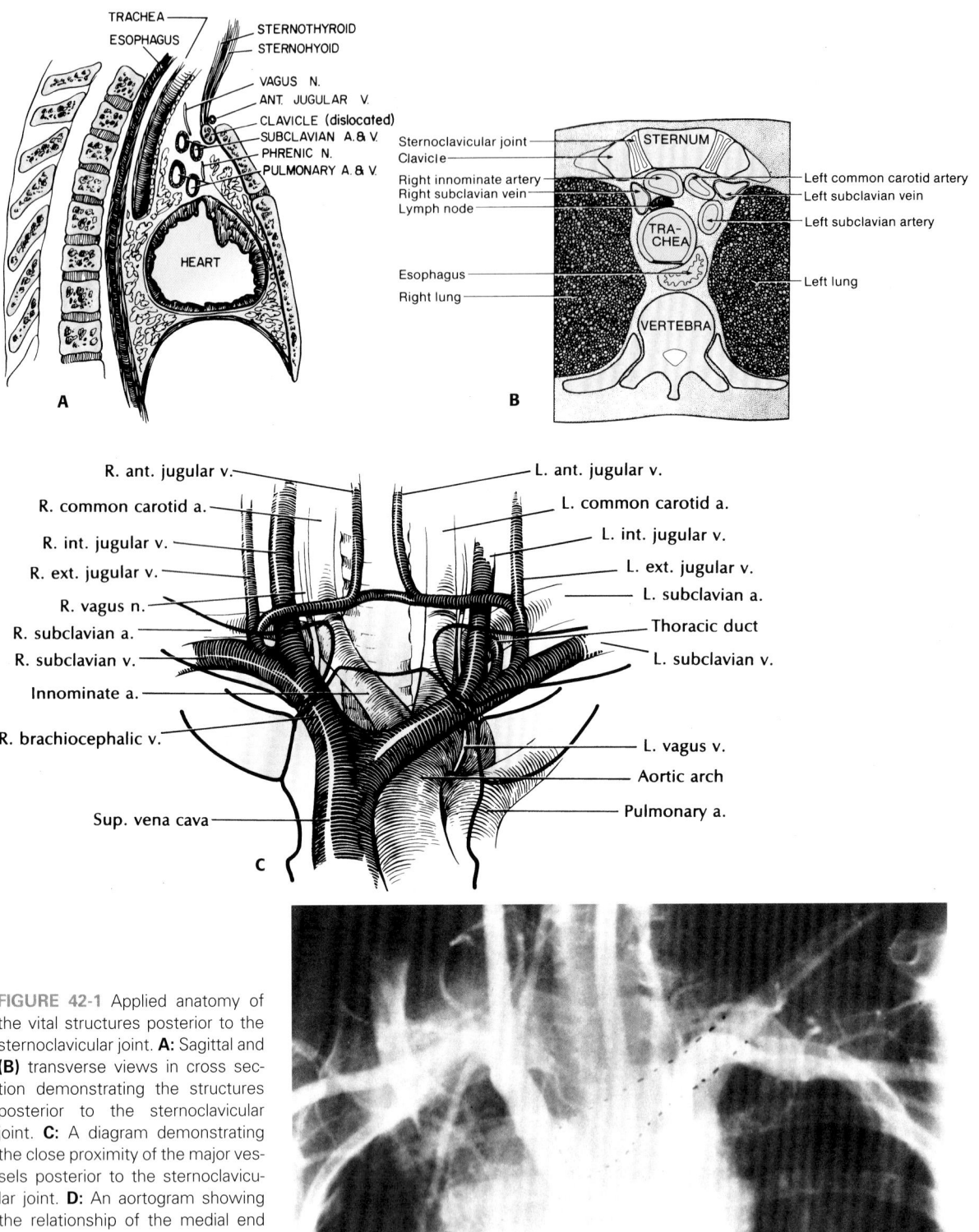

FIGURE 42-1 Applied anatomy of the vital structures posterior to the sternoclavicular joint. **A:** Sagittal and **(B)** transverse views in cross section demonstrating the structures posterior to the sternoclavicular joint. **C:** A diagram demonstrating the close proximity of the major vessels posterior to the sternoclavicular joint. **D:** An aortogram showing the relationship of the medial end of the clavicle to the major vessels in the mediastinum.

jugular vein, trachea, and esophagus (Fig. 42-1). It is important to remember that the arch of the aorta, the superior vena cava, and the right pulmonary artery are also very close to the SC joint. Another structure to be aware of is the anterior jugular vein, which is between the clavicle and the curtain of muscles.

Applied Anatomy of the Sternoclavicular Joint

The SC joint is a diarthrodial joint and is the only true articulation between the upper extremity and the axial skeleton. The articular surface of the clavicle is much larger than that of the sternum, and both are covered with hyaline cartilage.[59] The enlarged bulbous medial end of the clavicle is concave front to back and convex vertically, and therefore creates a saddle-type joint with the clavicular notch of the sternum.[95,190] The clavicular notch of the sternum is curved, and the joint surfaces are not congruent. Cave[45] demonstrated that in 2.5% of patients there is a small facet on the inferior aspect of the medial clavicle, which articulates with the superior aspect of the first rib at its synchondral junction with the sternum. Because less than half of the medial clavicle articulates with the upper angle of the sternum, the SC joint has the distinction of having the least amount of bony stability of the major joints of the body.

Ligaments of the Sternoclavicular Joint

There is so much joint incongruity that the integrity of the SC joint has to come from its surrounding ligaments: The intra-articular disc ligament, the extra-articular costoclavicular ligament (rhomboid ligament), the capsular ligament, and the interclavicular ligament.

Intra-Articular Disc Ligament. The intra-articular disc ligament is a very dense, fibrous structure that arises from the synchondral junction of the first rib and the sternum and passes through the SC joint. It divides the joint into two separate spaces.[95,190] The upper attachment is on the superior and posterior aspects of the medial clavicle. DePalma[57] has shown that the disc is perforated only rarely; the perforation allows a free communication between the two joint compartments. Anteriorly and posteriorly, the disc blends into the fibers of the capsular ligament. The disc acts as a checkrein against medial displacement of the inner clavicle. Histologic observations[71] have demonstrated that the sternal side of the disc is composed of fibrocartilage and dense connective tissue, whereas the clavicular side of the disc is composed of only fibrocartilage. Therefore, it is the clavicular side of the articular disc that has the function of resisting the compressive load to the clavicular surface.

Costoclavicular Ligament. The costoclavicular ligament, also called the rhomboid ligament, is short and strong and consists of an anterior and a posterior fasciculus.[17,44,95] Cave[44] reported that the average length is 1.3 cm, the maximum width is 1.9 cm, and the average thickness is 1.3 cm. Bearn[17] has shown that there is always a bursa between the two components of the ligament. Because of the two different parts of the ligament, it has a twisted appearance.[95] The costoclavicular ligament attaches below to the upper surface of the first rib adjacent to the portion comprising the synchondral junction with the sternum. It attaches above to the margins of the impression on the inferior surface of the medial end of the clavicle, sometimes known as the rhomboid fossa.[95,190] Cave has shown, in a study of 153 clavicles, that the attachment point of the costoclavicular ligament to the clavicle can be one of the three types: (a) a depression, the rhomboid fossa (30%); (b) flat (60%); or (c) an elevation (10%).

The fibers of the anterior fasciculus arise from the anteromedial surface of the first rib and are directed upward and laterally. The fibers of the posterior fasciculus are shorter and arise lateral to the anterior fibers on the rib and are directed upward

and medially. The fibers of the anterior and posterior components cross and allow for stability of the joint during rotation and elevation of the clavicle. The two-part costoclavicular ligament is in many ways similar to the two-part configuration of the coracoclavicular ligament on the outer end of the clavicle.

Bearn[17] has shown experimentally that the anterior fibers resist excessive upward rotation of the clavicle and that the posterior fibers resist excessive downward rotation. Specifically, the anterior fibers also resist lateral displacement, and the posterior fibers resist medial displacement.

Interclavicular Ligament. The interclavicular ligament connects the superomedial aspects of each clavicle with the capsular ligaments and the upper sternum. According to Grant,[93] this band may be comparable to the wishbone of birds. This ligament helps the capsular ligaments to produce "shoulder poise," that is, to hold up the shoulder. This can be tested by putting a finger in the superior sternal notch; with elevation of the arm, the ligament is quite lax, but as soon as both arms hang at the sides, the ligament becomes tight.

Spencer et al.[210] have shown experimentally that the costoclavicular and interclavicular ligaments have little effect on anterior or posterior translation of the SC joint. In an anatomic study Tubbs et al.[223] found that the interclavicular ligament prevented superior displacement of the clavicle with shoulder adduction and depression and failure occurred at 53.7 N.

Capsular Ligament. The capsular ligament covers the anterosuperior and posterior aspects of the joint and represents thickenings of the joint capsule.

According to the original work of Bearn,[17] this may be the strongest ligament of the SC joint, and it is the first line of defense against the upward displacement of the inner clavicle caused by a downward force on its distal end. The clavicular attachment of the ligament is primarily onto the epiphysis of the medial clavicle, with some secondary blending of the fibers into the metaphysis. The senior author has demonstrated this, as have Poland,[178] Denham and Dingley,[56] and Brooks and Henning.[32] Although some authors report that the intra-articular disc ligament greatly assists the costoclavicular ligament in preventing upward displacement of the medial clavicle, Bearn has shown that the capsular ligament is the most important structure in preventing upward displacement of the medial clavicle.[17] In experimental postmortem studies, he determined, after cutting the costoclavicular, intra-articular disc, and interclavicular ligaments, that they had no effect on clavicle poise. However, the division of the capsular ligament alone resulted in a downward depression on the distal end of the clavicle. Bearn's findings have many clinical implications for the mechanisms of injury of the SC joint.

Through a cadaver study Spencer et al.[210] measured anterior and posterior translation of the SC joint. Anterior and posterior translation was measured in intact specimens and following transection of randomly chosen ligaments about the SC joint. Cutting the posterior capsule resulted in significant increases in anterior and posterior translation. Cutting the anterior capsule produced significant increases in anterior translation. This study demonstrated that the posterior SC joint capsule is the

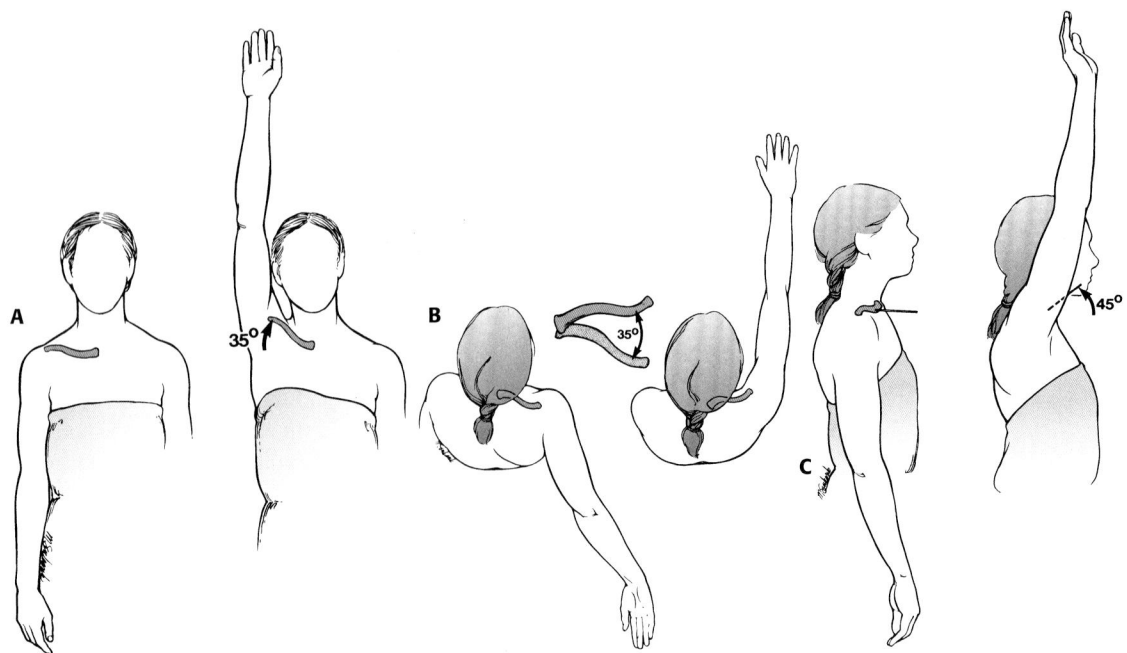

FIGURE 42-2 Motions of the clavicle at the sternoclavicular joint. **A:** With full overhead elevation the clavicle elevates 35 degrees. **B:** With adduction and extension, the clavicle displaces anteriorly and posteriorly 35 degrees. **C:** The clavicle rotates on its long axis 45 degrees, as the arm is elevated to the full overhead position.

most important structure for preventing both anterior and posterior translation of the SC joint, with the anterior capsule acting as an important secondary stabilizer.

The Subclavius Muscle

Reis et al.[184] studied the function of the subclavius muscle and found that the basic function of the subclavius was to stabilize the SC joint. They also stated that the subclavius could act as a substitute for the ligaments of the SC joint. We believe that this is an important study as it might explain why some people, after loss of the medial clavicle and the SC ligament, do not have instability of the medial end of the clavicle. It also gives a reason for leaving the subclavius muscle intact during operations on the SC joint.

Range of Motion of the Sternoclavicular Joint

The SC joint is freely movable and functions almost like a ball-and-socket joint with motion in almost all planes, including rotation.[26,141] In normal shoulder motion the clavicle, via motion through the SC joint, is capable of 30 to 35 degrees of upward elevation, 35 degrees of combined forward and backward movement, and 45 to 50 degrees of rotation around its long axis (Fig. 42-2). It is most likely the most frequently moved joint of the long bones in the body, because almost any motion of the upper extremity is transferred proximally to the SC joint.

Epiphysis of the Medial Clavicle

Although the clavicle is the first long bone of the body to ossify (fifth intrauterine week), the epiphysis at the medial end of the clavicle is the last of the long bones in the body to appear and the last epiphysis to close (Fig. 42-3). The medial clavicular epiphysis does not ossify until the 18th to 20th year, and it fuses with the shaft of the clavicle around the 23rd to 25th year.[93,95,178] Webb and Suchey,[234] in an extensive study of the physis of the medial clavicle in 605 males and 254 females at autopsy, reported that complete union may not be present until 31 years of age. This knowledge of the epiphysis is important, because many of the SC dislocations in young adults are injuries through the physeal plate.

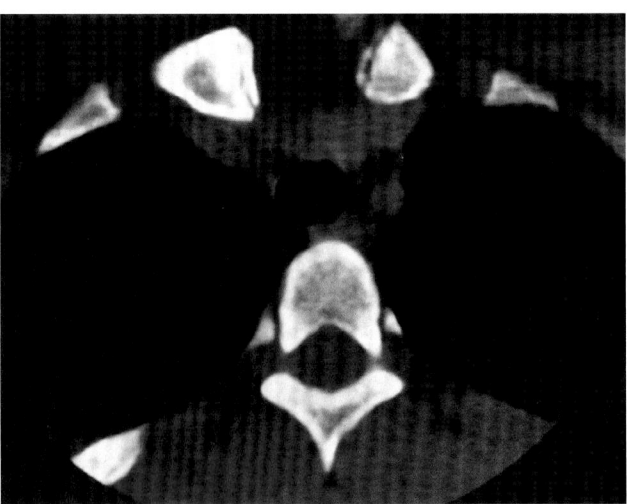

FIGURE 42-3 CT scan demonstrating the thin, wafer-like disc of the epiphysis of the medial clavicle.

PRINCIPLES OF DIAGNOSIS AND EVALUATION OF STERNOCLAVICULAR JOINT INJURIES

Mechanisms of Injury of the Sternoclavicular Joint

Either direct or indirect force can produce a dislocation of the SC joint. Because the SC joint is subject to practically every motion of the upper extremity and because the joint is small and incongruous, one would think that it would be the most commonly dislocated joint in the body. However, the supporting ligamentous structures are strong and so designed that it is, in fact, one of the least commonly dislocated joints. For this reason, a traumatic dislocation of the SC joint usually occurs only after tremendous forces, either direct or indirect, have been applied to the shoulder.

Direct Force

When a force is applied directly to the anteromedial aspect of the clavicle, the clavicle is pushed posteriorly behind the sternum and into the mediastinum (Fig. 42-4). This may occur in a variety of ways: An athlete lying on his/her back is jumped on and the knee of the jumper lands directly on the medial end of the clavicle; a kick is delivered to the front of the medial clavicle; a person lying supine is run over by a vehicle; or a person

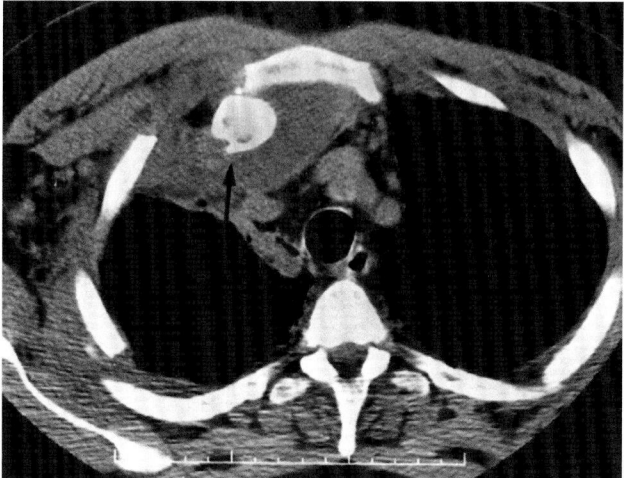

FIGURE 42-5 Computed axial tomogram of a posterior sternoclavicular joint dislocation that occurred when the driver's chest impacted the steering wheel during a motor vehicle accident.

is pinned between a vehicle and a wall (Fig. 42-5). Anatomically, it is essentially impossible for a direct force to produce an anterior SC dislocation.

Indirect Force

A force can be applied indirectly to the SC joint from the anterolateral or posterolateral aspects of the shoulder. This is the most common mechanism of injury to the SC joint. Mehta et al.[154] reported that three of four cases of posterior SC dislocations resulted from indirect force, and Heinig[103] reported that indirect force was responsible for eight of nine cases of posterior SC dislocations. If the shoulder is compressed and rolled forward, an ipsilateral posterior dislocation results; if the shoulder is compressed and rolled backward, an ipsilateral anterior dislocation results (Fig. 42-6).

Most Common Cause of Injuries

The most common cause of dislocation of the SC joint is vehicular accidents, followed by an injury sustained during participation in sports.[121,124,163,167,181,196,231] Omer,[167] in his review of patients from 14 military hospitals, found 82 cases of SC joint dislocations. He reported that almost 80% of these occurred as a result of vehicular accidents (47%) or in athletics (31%).

Incidence of Injury

The incidence of SC dislocation, based on the series of 1,603 injuries of the shoulder girdle reported by Cave et al.,[46] is 3% (specific incidences in the study were glenohumeral dislocations, 85%; acromioclavicular [AC] injuries, 12%; and SC injuries, 3%). In the series by Cave, and in our experience, dislocation of the SC joint is not as rare as posterior dislocation of the glenohumeral joint.

In a study of 3,451 injuries during alpine skiing, Kocher and Feagin,[124] showed that injuries involving the shoulder complex accounted for 39.1% of upper-extremity injuries and 11.4% of all alpine skiing injuries. Of the 393 injuries involving the shoulder complex, SC injuries accounted for 0.5%.

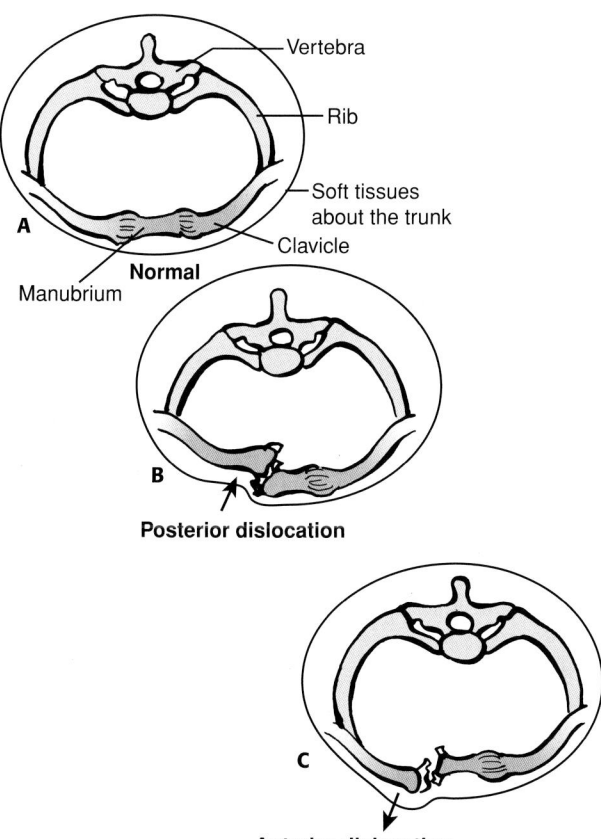

FIGURE 42-4 Cross sections through the thorax at the level of the sternoclavicular joint. **A:** Normal anatomical relations. **B:** Posterior dislocation of the SC joint. **C:** Anterior dislocation of the SC joint.

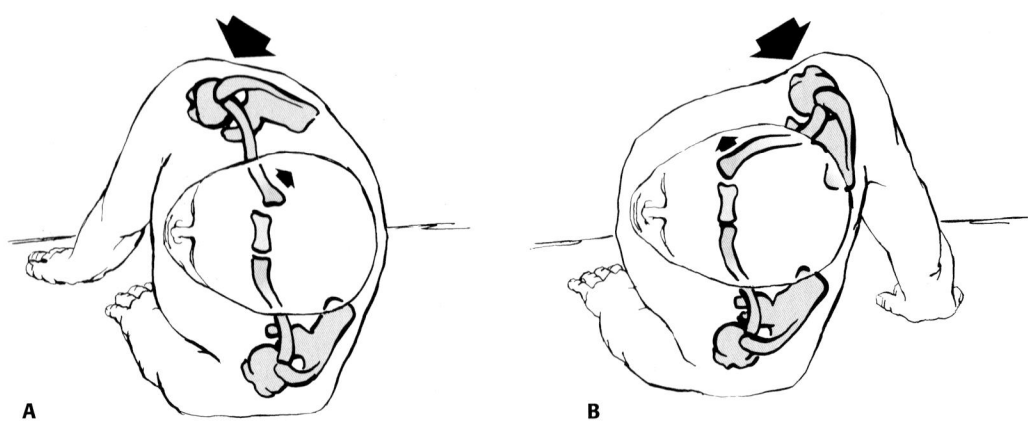

FIGURE 42-6 Mechanisms that produce anterior or posterior dislocation of the sternoclavicular joint. **A:** If the patient is lying on the ground and a compression force is applied to the posterolateral aspect of the shoulder, the medial end of the clavicle will be displaced posteriorly. **B:** When the lateral compression force is directed from the anterior position, the medial end of the clavicle is dislocated anteriorly.

The largest published series from a single institution is reported by Nettles and Linscheid[163] who studied 60 patients with SC dislocations (57 anterior and 3 posterior). Fery and Sommelet[79] found a ratio of 40 anterior to 8 posterior dislocations. Waskowitz[231] reviewed 18 cases of SC dislocations, none of which was posterior. However, in our series of 185 traumatic SC injuries, there was 135 patients with anterior dislocation and 50 patients with posterior dislocation.

Associated Injuries with the Sternoclavicular Joint

SC injury can be accompanied by significant trauma to the critical surrounding structures in the neck and thorax and/or by other musculoskeletal injuries. Significant concomitant injuries of the mediastinum must be considered to avoid catastrophic outcomes. These injuries almost always occur in the setting of posterior SC fractures and dislocations and include the following:

1. *Tracheal compression:* From the initial case report of Rodrigues[192] to multiple recent case reports, the trachea can be displaced by the posteriorly displaced medial aspect of the clavicle. Acute airway compromise or subacute dyspnea are key symptoms.[143,161]

2. *Pneumothorax:* Pleural violation by the clavicle has been noted with SC dislocation and should be especially considered in high-energy direct trauma.[172]

3. *Laceration/compression of the great vessels:* The great vessels of the mediastinum can be directly transected or compressed and multiple case reports of both arterial and venous injuries exist,[51,84,101,109,168,207,240] including the pulmonary artery,[240] brachiocephalic vein,[51] superior vena cava,[172] and innominate artery.[147] Compression of any of the great vessels without frank laceration can also occur[20,164,168] and may present as a thrombosis.[47]

4. *Esophageal perforation/rupture:* Cases of esophageal rupture are often described in relation to local sequelae. Howard[110] reported a case of rupture complicated by osteomyelitis of the clavicle. Wasylenko and Busse[232] reported on a fatal tracheoesophageal fistula.

5. *Plexus injury/compression:* A high index of suspicion should be maintained for brachial plexus injury which may occur concomitantly with the overall injury pattern or from the static posterior position of the clavicle after dislocation.[85] Careful evaluation of associated cervical spine injury should be completed as it cannot be assumed that neurological injury is located in the brachial plexus.[134]

Orthopedic Injuries Associated with the Sternoclavicular Joint

Bilateral Dislocations

In 1896, Hotchkiss[108] reported a bilateral traumatic dislocation of the SC joint. The senior author has treated four cases of bilateral SC dislocation. A recent case of bilateral posterior physeal fracture–dislocations treated operatively has been reported by Baumann et al.[16] Bilateral subluxation[91] and compression of the brachiocephalic vein from bilateral posterior dislocation has also been described.[67]

Dislocations of Both Ends of the Clavicle

When dislocation of both ends of the clavicle occurs, the SC dislocation is usually anterior.[97,172,199] To our knowledge the first reported case of dislocation of both ends of the clavicle was by Porral[180] in 1831. In 1923, Beckman[18] reported a single case and reviewed 15 cases that had been previously reported. With the exception of this single patient, all patients had been treated conservatively with acceptable function. Dieme et al.[62] reported 3 cases of "floating clavicle." In 1990, Sanders et al.[197] reported six patients who had a dislocation of both ends of the clavicle; two patients with lower demands did well following nonoperative management with only minor symptoms. The other four patients had persistent symptoms that were localized to the AC joint. Each of these patients had a reconstruction of the AC joint, which resulted in a painless, full range of motion, and a return to normal activity (Fig. 42-7). AC joint dislocation can also accompany medial clavicle physeal fracture/dislocation.[88] Wade et al.[230] reported a irreducible posterior inferior AC dislocation associated with

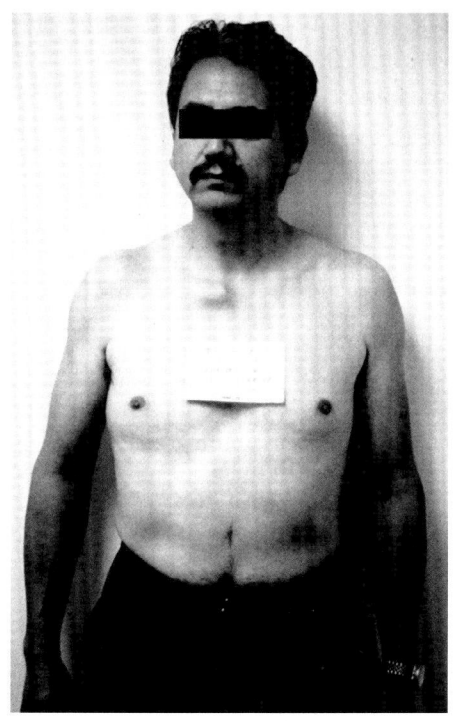

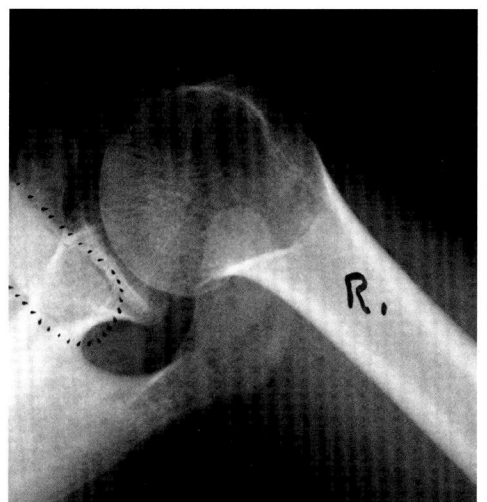

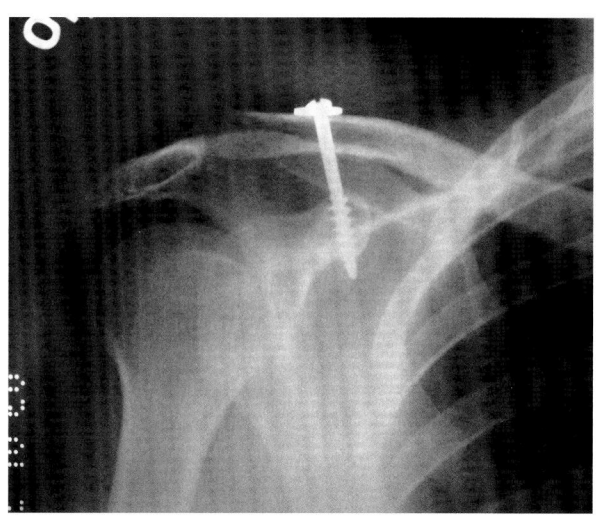

FIGURE 42-7 Dislocation of both ends of the clavicle. **A:** Clinical view demonstrating anterior dislocation of the right sternoclavicular joint. **B:** The axillary x-ray reveals posterior dislocation of the acromioclavicular joint. **C:** These injuries are generally treated by acromioclavicular joint repair/reconstruction with return of near normal function.

a medial epiphyseal fracture which required open reduction of the AC joint and exploration of the SC injury with a good result.

Combined Sternoclavicular Injury and Fractures and Dislocations of the Clavicle

Fracture of the midshaft of the clavicle with either anterior or posterior subluxation/dislocation of the SC joint has been noted. It is important to assess the AC joint and the SC joint in the face of the more obvious midshaft clavicle fracture to avoid a delay in diagnosis. Tanlin,[215] Arenas et al.,[4] Friedl and Fritz,[82] and Thomas and Friedman[216] have all reported on patients who had an anterior dislocation of the SC joint and a fracture of the midclavicle. Several authors have reported on a skeletally immature patient who had an ipsilateral clavicle fracture and a posterior physeal injury of the SC joint.[3,160,162,219]

Velutini and Tarazona[228] reported a bizarre case of posterior dislocation of the left medial clavicle, the first rib, and a section of the manubrium. Elliott[68] reported on a tripartite injury about the clavicle region in which the patient had an anterior subluxation of the right SC joint, a type II injury to the right AC joint, and a fracture of the right midclavicle. Pearsall and Russell[174] reported a patient who had an ipsilateral clavicle fracture, an anterior SC joint subluxation, and a long thoracic nerve injury. All of these injuries involving the SC joint and the clavicle were associated with severe trauma to the shoulder region.

Combined Sternoclavicular Dislocation and Scapulothoracic Dissociation

Tsai et al.[221] reported a patient with an SC dislocation associated with a scapulothoracic dissociation. This patient had also sustained a transection of the axillary artery and an avulsion of the median nerve. Following a vascular repair and an above the elbow amputation this patient was left with a complete brachial plexopathy.

History and Physical Examination of Sternoclavicular Joint Injuries

Elucidating the mechanism of injury can alert the initial treating physician to associated injuries and to the direction of dislocation. The patient should be questioned about pain in the adjacent AC joint and glenohumeral joint. The patient with a posterior dislocation usually has more pain than a patient with an anterior dislocation. The usually palpable medial end of the clavicle is displaced posteriorly and as a consequence the anterosuperior fullness of the chest normally produced by the clavicle is less prominent when compared with the unaffected side.[87] The corner of the sternum is easily palpated as compared with the normal SC joint. Venous congestion may be present in the neck or in the upper extremity.[94] Symptoms may also include a dry irritating cough and hoarseness.[69,176] Breathing difficulties, shortness of breath, or a choking sensation may be noted. Circulation to the ipsilateral arm may be decreased although the presence of pulses does not exclude vessel injury. The patient may complain of difficulty in swallowing or a tight feeling in the throat or may be in a state of complete shock or possibly have a pneumothorax. The distal neurologic examination may reveal diminished sensation or weakness secondary to brachial plexus compression. Complete nerve deficits suggest more severe injury patterns. The examination should include assessment of the Wynne-Davies signs[241] of generalized ligamentous laxity as these patients are predisposed to atraumatic anterior SC joint subluxation. As a cautionary note, we have seen a number of patients who clinically appeared to have an anterior dislocation of the SC joint, but on x-ray studies were shown to have complete posterior dislocation, reinforcing that one cannot always rely on clinical findings to differentiate between anterior and posterior dislocations.

Radiographic Assessment of the Sternoclavicular Joint Injuries

Anteroposterior Views

Occasionally, the routine anteroposterior (AP) or posteroanterior x-rays of the chest or SC joint suggest something is wrong with one of the clavicles, because it appears to be displaced as compared with the normal side. McCulloch et al.[151] reported that on nonrotated frontal radiographs, a difference in the relative craniocaudal positions of the medial clavicles of greater than 50% of the width of the heads of the clavicles suggests dislocation. It would be ideal to take a view at right angles to the AP plane, but because of the anatomy, it is impossible to obtain a true 90-degree cephalic-to-caudal lateral view. Lateral x-rays of the chest are at right angles to the AP plane, but they cannot be interpreted because of the density of the chest and the overlap of the medial clavicles with the first rib and the sternum. Regardless of a clinical impression that suggests an anterior or posterior dislocation, x-rays and preferably a CT scan must be obtained to confirm one's suspicions (Fig. 42-8).

Special Projected Views

There have been numerous special x-ray projections recommended for the SC joint.[74,78,103,105,117,129,186,200,220] While the serendipity view is frequently obtained as a front-line image for evaluation of the SC joint, the Heinig and Hobbs views are rarely obtained if CT is available. However, the Hobbs and Heinig views can be useful when suspicion is high on clinical examination and confirmation is needed before obtaining a CT, especially in the outpatient setting where delayed presentation often leads to misdiagnosis.

Heinig View. With the patient in a supine position, the x-ray tube is placed approximately 76.2 cm (30 in) from the involved SC joint and the central ray beam is directed tangential to the joint and parallel to the opposite clavicle. The cassette is

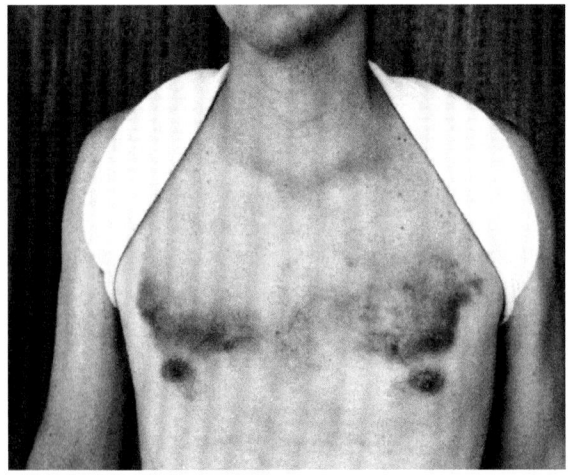
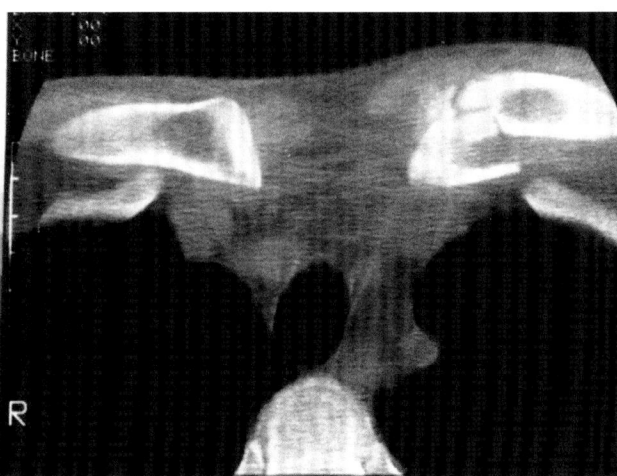

FIGURE 42-8 A: A 34-year-old patient was involved in a motorcycle accident and sustained an anterior blow to the chest. Note the symmetric anterior chest wall ecchymosis. **B:** Computed tomography reveals a left medial clavicle fracture without disruption of the sternoclavicular joint.

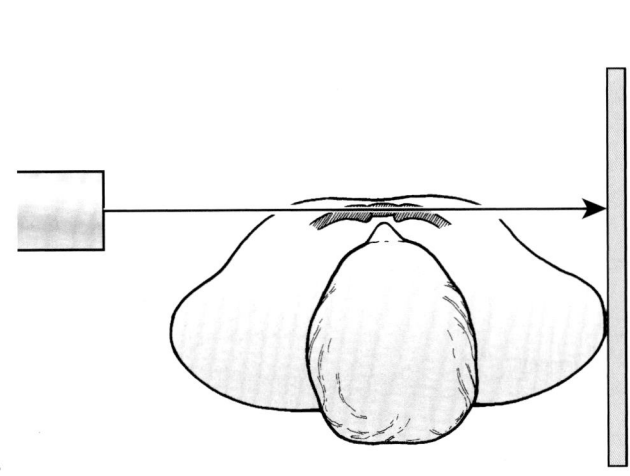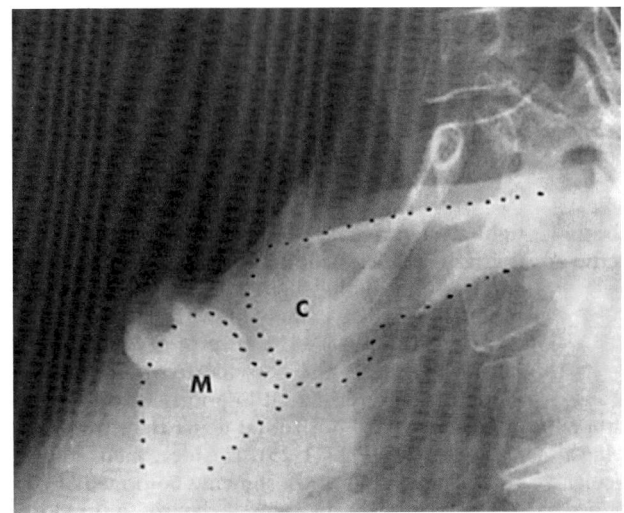

A

B

FIGURE 42-9 Heinig view. **A:** Positioning of the patient for x-ray evaluation of the sternoclavicular joint, as described by Heinig. **B:** Heinig view demonstrating a normal relationship between the medial end of the clavicle (*C*) and the manubrium (*M*).

placed against the opposite shoulder and centered on the manubrium (Fig. 42-9).

Hobbs View. In the Hobbs view, the patient is seated at the x-ray table, high enough to lean forward over the table. The cassette is placed on the table, and the lower anterior rib cage is against the cassette (Fig. 42-10). The patient leans forward so that the nape of his flexed neck is almost parallel to the table. The flexed elbows straddle the cassette and support the head and neck. The x-ray source is above the nape of the neck, and the beam passes through the cervical spine to project the SC joints onto the cassette.

Serendipity View. The "serendipity view" is rightfully named because that is the way it was developed. The senior

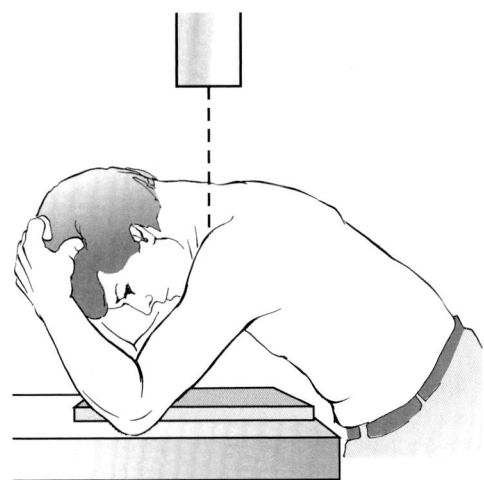

FIGURE 42-10 Hobbs view. Positioning of the patient for x-ray evaluation of the sternoclavicular joint, as recommended by Hobbs. (Modified from: Hobbs DW. Sternoclavicular joint: A new axial radiographic view. *Radiology* 1968;90:801–802.)

author accidentally noted that the next best thing to having a true cephalocaudal lateral view of the SC joint was a 40-degree cephalic tilt view. The patient is positioned supine squarely and in the center of the x-ray table. The tube is tilted at a 40-degree angle of the vertical and is centered directly on the sternum (Figs. 42-11 to 42-14). A nongrid 27.94- × 35.56-cm (11- × 14-in) cassette is placed squarely on the table and under the patient's upper shoulders and neck so that the beam aimed at the sternum will project both clavicles onto the film.

Special Imaging Techniques

Tomograms

Tomograms can be very helpful in distinguishing between an SC dislocation and a fracture of the medial clavicle. They are also helpful in questionable anterior and posterior injuries of the SC joint to distinguish fractures from dislocations and to evaluate arthritic changes.

In 1959, Baker[10] recommended the use of tomography, which was developed in the late 1920s, and said it was "far more valuable than routine radiographs and the fingertips of the examining physician." In 1975, Morag and Shahin[159] reported on the value of tomography, which they used in a series of 20 patients, and recommended that it should be used routinely to evaluate problems of the SC joint. From a study of normal SC joints, they pointed out the variation in the x-ray appearance in different age groups.

CT Scans. Without question, the CT scan is the best technique to study problems of the SC joint (Fig. 42-15). CT clearly distinguishes injuries of the joint from fractures of the medial clavicle and defines minor subluxations of the joint. One must remember to request CT scans of *both SC joints and the medial half of both clavicles* so the injured side can be compared with the normal side. Numerous authors have reported on the value of using a CT scan as the method of choice for radiographic evaluation of the SC joint.[37,52,53,60,61,63,131,135,142] While plain films may be suggestive of the nature of the injury, it is critical that a

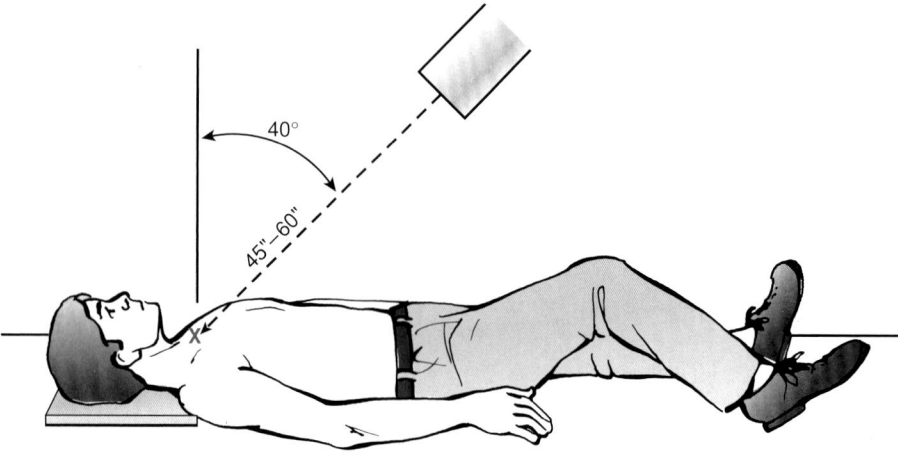

FIGURE 42-11 Serendipity view. Positioning of the patient to take the "serendipity" view of sternoclavicular joints. The x-ray tube is tilted 40 degrees from the vertical position and aimed directly at the manubrium. The nongrid cassette should be large enough to receive the projected images of the medial halves of both clavicles. In children the tube distance from the patient should be 114.3 cm (45 in); in thicker-chested adults the distance should be 152.4 cm (60 in).

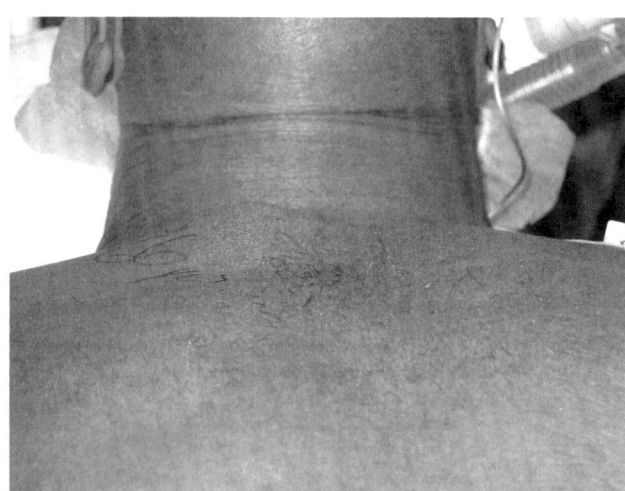

FIGURE 42-12 When viewed from around the level of the patient's knees, it is apparent that the left clavicle (patient's right) is dislocated anteriorly.

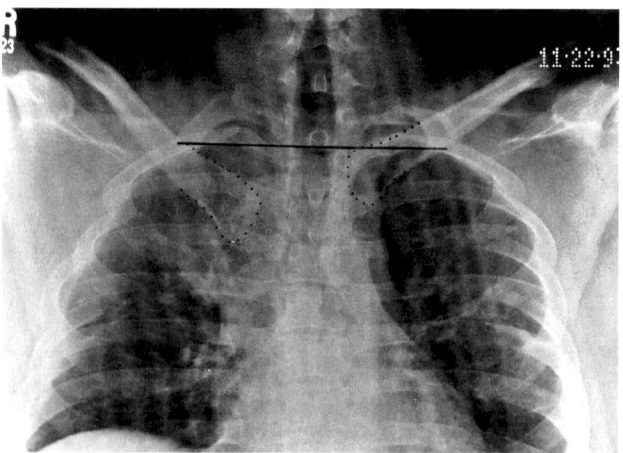

FIGURE 42-13 Posterior dislocation of the right medial clavicle as seen on 40-degree cephalic tilt serendipity x-ray. The right clavicle is inferiorly displaced as compared to the normal left clavicle.

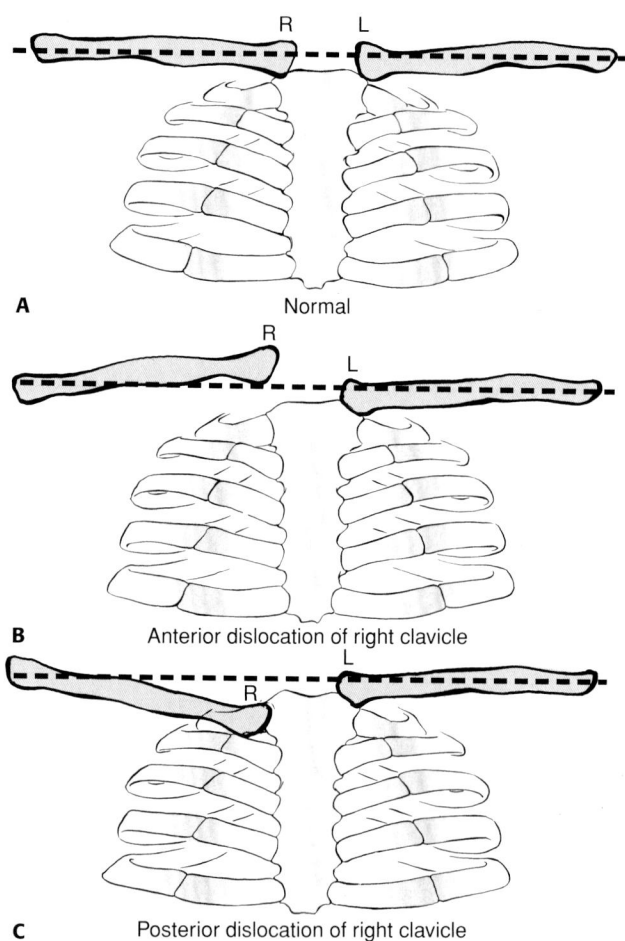

FIGURE 42-14 Interpretation of the cephalic tilt (serendipity view) x-ray films of the sternoclavicular joints. **A:** In the normal person, both clavicles appear on the same imaginary line drawn horizontally across the film. **B:** In a patient with an anterior dislocation of the right sternoclavicular joint, the medial half of the right clavicle is projected above the imaginary line drawn through the level of the normal left clavicle. **C:** If the patient has a posterior dislocation of the right sternoclavicular joint, the medial half of the right clavicle is displaced below the imaginary line drawn through the normal left clavicle.

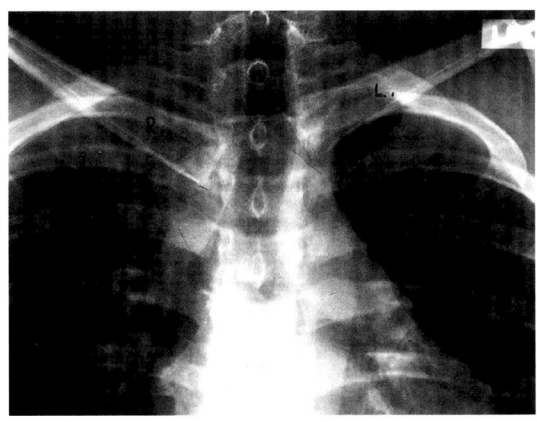
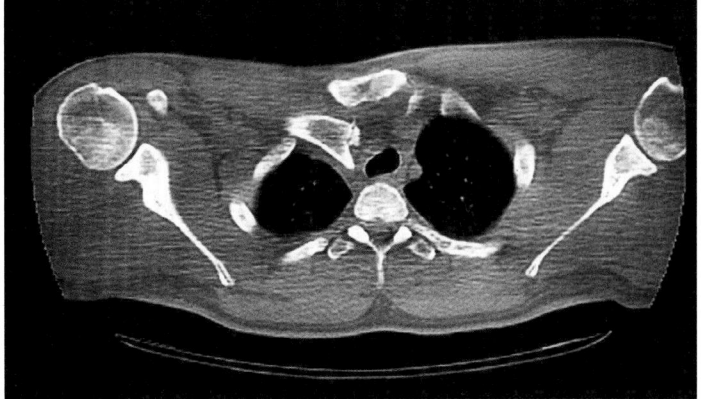

FIGURE 42-15 A: Routine anteroposterior (AP) x-ray of posteriorly dislocated right sternoclavicular joint. **B:** The AP view is suggestive of a posterior dislocation. However, the computed tomography (CT) scan clearly demonstrates the posteriorly displaced right medial clavicle. Note the displacement of the trachea.

CT scan is obtained for the superior specificity and sensitivity of CT in the diagnosis of SC joint pathology. Lucet et al.[142] used CT scans to evaluate the SC joints in 60 healthy subjects homogeneously distributed by sex and decade of life from 20 to 80 years old. They reported that 98% of the subjects had at least one sign of various abnormalities, such as sclerosis, osteophytes, erosion, cysts, and joint narrowing. The number of signs increased with age and the number of clavicular signs was greater than those in the sternum.

Tuscano et al.[224] obtained CT scans from 104 healthy subjects free from SC joint pathology and demonstrated that greater than 10% of patients show substantial asymmetry in the SC joints (i.e., SC joint space and distance between the manubrium and anterior margin of clavicular head), which may be interpreted as pathologic. These authors suggest exercising caution in attributing a disease state to asymmetry because of the frequency of this finding in the asymptomatic population. These findings become clinically useful in the setting of chronic subluxation or dislocation of the SC joint.

Magnetic Resonance Imaging. Brossman et al.[33] correlated magnetic resonance imaging (MRI) scans with anatomic sections in 14 SC joints from elderly cadavers. They concluded that MRI did depict the anatomy of the SC joint and surrounding soft tissues (Fig. 42-16). T2-weighed images were superior to T1-weighted images in depicting the intra-articular disc. Magnetic resonance arthrography allowed the delineation of perforations in the intra-articular disc. In children and young adults when there are questions of diagnosis between SC joint dislocation and physeal injury, the MRI scan can be used to determine if the epiphysis has displaced with the clavicle or is still adjacent to the manubrium.[86,98] Some have also advocated the use of MRI in young children to avoid radiation exposure in this age group.[132] Benitez et al.[19] evaluated 41 patients with SC trauma at an average of 9 months post injury and found an 80% incidence of articular disc injury and a 59% incidence of subluxation. MRI may be useful in this clinical scenario to better understand the in vivo mechanisms of injury of the SC joint and to elucidate causes of pain well after the traumatic event.

Ultrasound. Ultrasound can be used to observe abnormal contour in the joint, hematoma, and occlusion of vessels. Proper ultrasound technique requires a linear array probe placed parallel to the clavicle.[76] Pollock et al.[179] and more recently Blakeley et al.[25] reported the use of ultrasound in the diagnosis of posterior dislocation of the SC joint. An additional application of ultrasound may be the use of intraoperative sonography to confirm whether a closed reduction has been successful or not.[22,205] The ability of ultrasound to obtain the diagnosis of posterior SC dislocation has shown promise, but does require knowledge of ultrasound technology for the accurate and reliable diagnosis of SC joint pathology. In addition, sonography is dependent on operator experience and knowledge of regional anatomy. As such, a CT scan remains the gold standard and must be obtained to confirm the diagnosis of a SC joint dislocation and to assess the quality of closed reduction. In 2012, Sullivan et al.[213] described the use of an O-arm intraoperative CT system to verify reduction in two cases of posterior SC joint dislocation.

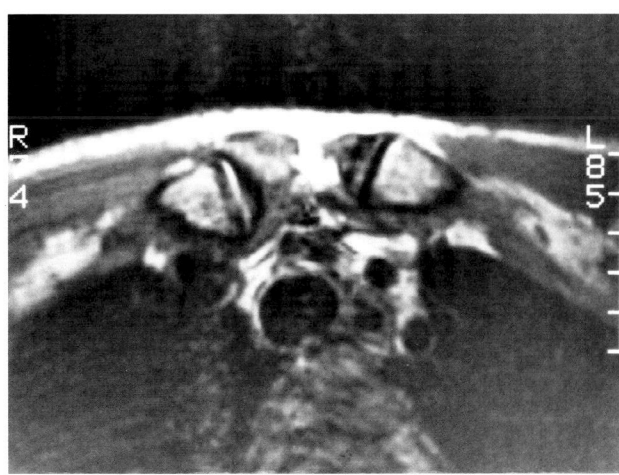

FIGURE 42-16 Magnetic resonance imaging (MRI) of the sternoclavicular joint. The epiphysis on both medial clavicles is clearly visible.

Lastly, duplex ultrasonography can be obtained for the diagnosis of thrombosis and vessel occlusion in cases where vascular insult is suspected.[47,101] However, CT angiography remains the gold standard vascular study to define the location and extent of vessel injury.

CT Angiography. The role for advanced vascular imaging cannot be understated and should be performed if vascular injury is present or suspected acutely, and for all chronic or late presentations. Multiple reports have shown the value of CT angiography in diagnosing vascular injury before taking the patient to the operating room.[20,67,101,106,147,157]

Classification and Differential Diagnosis

Two methods can be used to classify SC joint subluxations and dislocations; first, the anatomic position of the injury, and second, the etiology of the problem. The OTA classification is simply based on the direction of the dislocation and not on etiology.

OTA Classification

The anterior and posterior dislocations are well described (Fig. 42-17). A recent case report confirms the possibility of

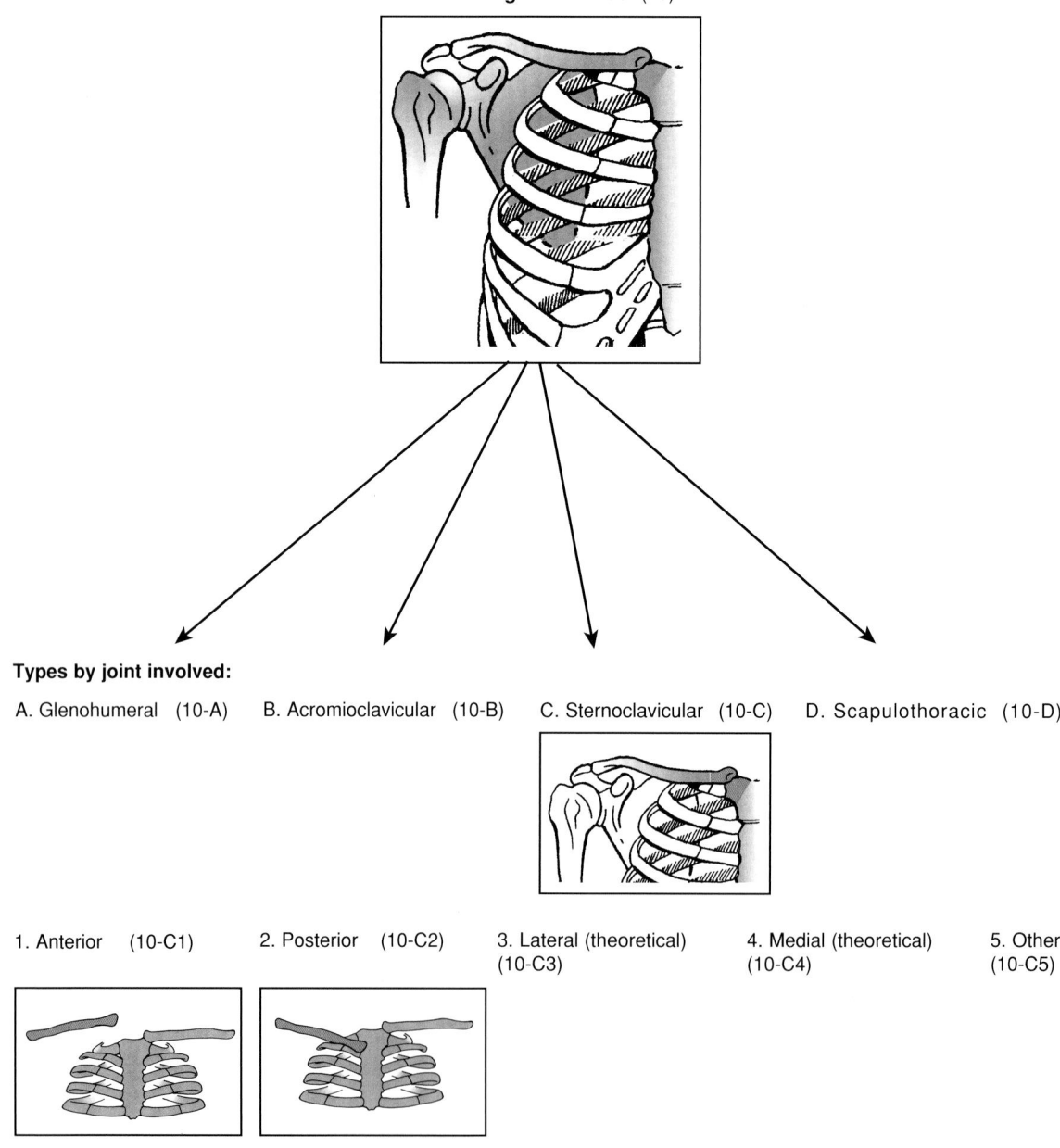

Dislocation region: Shoulder (10)

Types by joint involved:

A. Glenohumeral (10-A)   B. Acromioclavicular (10-B)   C. Sternoclavicular (10-C)   D. Scapulothoracic (10-D)

1. Anterior (10-C1)   2. Posterior (10-C2)   3. Lateral (theoretical) (10-C3)   4. Medial (theoretical) (10-C4)   5. Other (10-C5)

FIGURE 42-17 OTA classification of sternoclavicular injuries (From: Marsh JL, Slongo TF, Agel J, et al. Fracture and dislocation classification compendium–2007: Orthopaedic Trauma Association classification, database, and outcomes committee. *J Orthop Trauma.* 2007;21(10 suppl):S104–S107, with permission.)

a superior dislocation which occurred after an indirect force mechanism. The authors noted that only the interclavicular and intra-articular disc ligaments were ruptured.[137]

Anatomic Classification

Anterior Subluxation and Dislocation. Anterior dislocations are the most common. The medial end of the clavicle is displaced anteriorly or anterosuperiorly to the anterior margin of the sternum.

Posterior Dislocation. Posterior SC dislocations are uncommon. The medial end of the clavicle is displaced posteriorly or posterosuperiorly with respect to the posterior margin of the sternum.

Etiologic Classification

Atraumatic Problems

Spontaneous Subluxation or Dislocation. This condition typically occurs in women during the late teens or young adult life and usually occurs in patients who have generalized ligament laxity of other joints. While both SC joints can be affected,[91] usually one joint is more of a problem than the other (Fig. 42-18). In middle-aged women, spontaneous anterior or anterior/superior subluxation can occur and may be in association with condensing osteitis of the clavicle.[226] In some patients, the atraumatic anterior dislocation of the SC joint is painful and is associated with a snap or pop as the arm is elevated overhead, and another snap occurs when the arm is returned to the patient's side. Atraumatic posterior dislocation[149] and subluxation have also been reported.[150]

Traumatic Injuries

Sprains. In a mild sprain, all the ligaments are intact and the joint is stable. There may be local damage to the capsule and the joint may develop an effusion, but there is no increased translation of the clavicle or loss of congruity.

Subluxation. In a moderate sprain, there is subluxation of the SC joint. The capsular, intra-articular disc, and costoclavicular ligaments may be partially disrupted. The subluxation is usually anterior but posterior subluxation can occur.

Acute Dislocation. In a dislocated SC joint, the capsular and intra-articular ligaments are ruptured. Occasionally, the costoclavicular ligament is intact but stretched out enough to allow dislocation of the joint.

Chronic Dislocation. If the initial acute traumatic dislocation does not heal, mild to moderate forces may produce recurrent dislocations; this is rare.

The original dislocation may go unrecognized, it may be irreducible, or the physician may decide not to reduce certain dislocations.

Physeal Injury

Acute Physeal Fracture. The medial clavicular physis is the last physis to close and typically fuses around the age of 23 to 25. As such, most SC separations in childhood and adolescence are actually physeal fractures with displacement of the clavicle, not dislocation of the joint. The injury can be anterior or posterior.

Chronic Physeal Fracture. Like SC dislocations, physeal fractures of the SC joint are at risk for being missed on initial presentation and unfortunately a delayed presentation is not uncommon. Chronic dislocation is not specifically defined by any absolute time from injury, but as a general rule injuries that present 7 to 10 days after initial injury are categorized as chronic. This is because closed reduction is not likely to be an option and indeed successful closed reduction after 48 hours is rarely reported in the literature. After 7 to 10 days, scarring and adhesions increase the risk of vascular injury with attempted reduction and place the injury in a separate category of management as described later in this chapter.

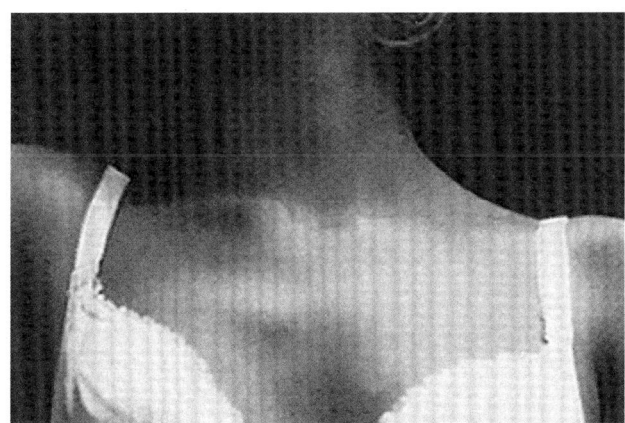 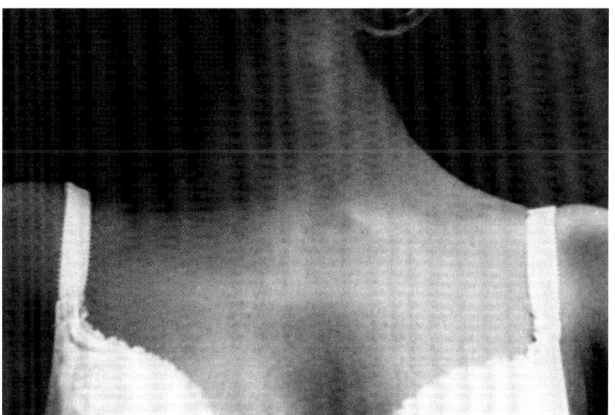

FIGURE 42-18 Spontaneous anterior subluxation of the sternoclavicular joint. **A:** With the arm in the overhead position, the medial end of the right clavicle spontaneously subluxates anteriorly without any trauma. **B:** When the arm is brought back down to the side, the medial end of the clavicle spontaneously reduces. Usually this is not associated with significant discomfort. (From: Rockwood CA, Matsen F III, eds. *The Shoulder.* Philadelphia, PA: WB Saunders, 1990, with permission.)

Other Conditions of the Sternoclavicular Joint Injuries

It is important to consider other pathologies particular to the SC joint during the diagnostic process. Infection may mimic trauma and should especially be considered in patients with history of IV drug abuse, immunocompromise, or indwelling subclavian catheters. Sternoclavicular hyperostosis is an inflammatory condition of the SC joint and medial ribs which results in new bone formation and even ankylosis of the SC joint. This condition is associated with Japanese ethnicity and dermatologic lesions in the palms and plantar regions. Three conditions which predominate in women are condensing osteitis, Friedrich's disease, and osteoarthritis.[237] Condensing osteitis of the medial clavicle typically occurs in women of late childbearing age and presents as a painful joint with sclerosis on radiographs, similar to condensing osteitis of the ilium and pubis seen in the same demographic group. Friedrich's disease is osteonecrosis of the medial clavicle. Osteoarthritis typically manifests in the postmenopausal years and can appear as a pseudosubluxation anteriorly.[30]

CURRENT TREATMENT OPTIONS FOR STERNOCLAVICULAR JOINT INJURIES

The majority of injuries to the SC joint can be successfully managed by nonoperative measures (observation or closed reduction). This includes most of the acute and chronic anterior subluxations and dislocations, the acute traumatic posterior subluxations and dislocations, and, remembering that the physis of the medial clavicle does not close until the 23rd to 25th year, the acute traumatic anterior and posterior physeal injuries of the medial clavicle.

In contrast, chronic posterior dislocations and acute irreducible posterior dislocations require an open surgical procedure. This is an area of consensus as it is critical to avoid the sequelae of the posterior intrusion of the clavicle on the mediastinum. Some authors also recommend open reduction and internal fixation of acute and chronic anterior dislocations; however, this remains controversial and is reserved for special circumstances.

Anterior Sternoclavicular Joint Injuries

Atraumatic Anterior Sternoclavicular Joint Instability

As with the classification of glenohumeral joint instability, the importance of distinguishing between traumatic and atraumatic instability of the SC joint must be recognized if complications are to be avoided with this condition. Rowe (personal communication, 1988) described several patients who had undergone one or more unsuccessful attempts to surgically stabilize the SC joint. In all cases the patient was able to voluntarily dislocate the clavicle after surgery.

We have seen a number of patients with spontaneous subluxation or dislocation of the SC joint. Many of these patients have the characteristic finding of generalized ligamentous laxity (i.e., hyperextension of the elbows, knees, and fingers as well as

hypermobility of the glenohumeral joints) (Fig. 42-19). Bilateral symptoms is a feature of atraumatic anterior subluxation. Certain activities or sports may also predispose to atraumatic instability.[65] About the only symptom such patients seem to complain about is that the medial end of the clavicle subluxes or dislocates anteriorly when they raise their arms over their head (Fig. 42-18)[191] and only occasionally complain of pain during the displacement. Because it is difficult to surgically stabilize the joint and prevent its subluxation/dislocation and allow pain-free range of motion, we manage the problem with skillful neglect.

In a review by Rockwood and Odor,[191] of 37 patients with spontaneous atraumatic subluxation, 29 were managed without surgery and 8 were treated (elsewhere) with surgical reconstruction. With an average follow-up of more than 8 years, all 29 patients treated nonoperatively were doing just fine without limitations of activity or lifestyle. The eight patients treated with surgery had increased pain, limitation of activity, alteration of lifestyle, persistent instability, and significant scars. In many instances, before reconstruction or resection, these patients had minimal discomfort, excellent range of motion, and only complained of a "bump" that slipped in and out of place with certain motions. Postoperatively, these patients still had the bump, along with scars and painful range of motion (Fig. 42-20).

Crosby and Rubino[54] reported a case of spontaneous atraumatic anterior dislocation secondary to pseudoarthrosis of the first and second ribs. Despite a 6-month course of

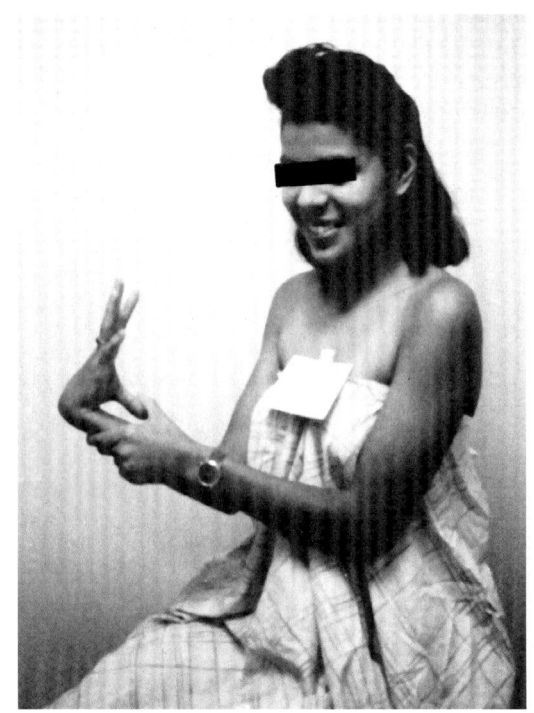

FIGURE 42-19 This patient has developed spontaneous subluxation of her sternoclavicular joint. She also has generalized ligamentous laxity of the wrists, fingers, and elbows.

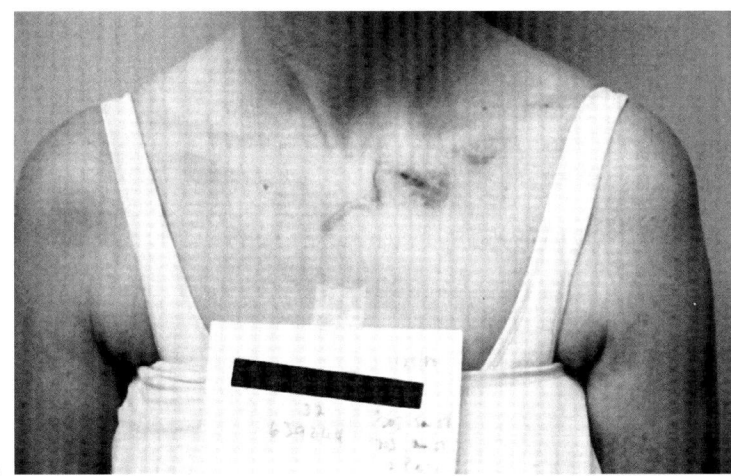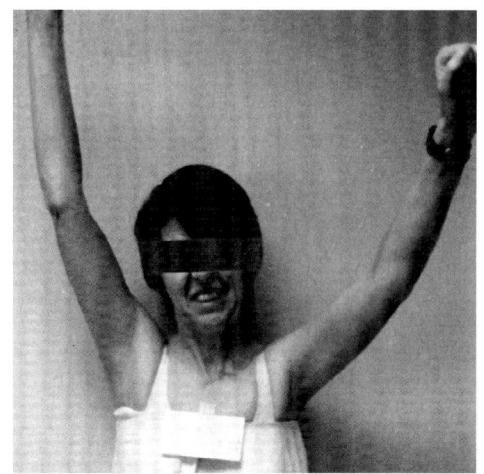

FIGURE 42-20 Patients treated with surgery for spontaneous, atraumatic subluxation of the sternoclavicular joint often have increased pain, limitation of activity, alteration of lifestyle, persistent instability of the joint, and a significant scar. **A:** Not only was the cosmetic scarring a problem **(B)** but also motion and pain were worse than before the reconstruction. (From: Rockwood CA, Matsen F III, eds. *The Shoulder*. Philadelphia, PA: WB Saunders, 1990, with permission.)

conservative treatment this 14-year-old girl was still painful. A computed tomographic scan of the chest with three-dimensional (3D) reconstruction was performed. The scan revealed a pseudoarthrosis anteriorly between the first and second ribs underlying the medial part of the clavicle. Resection of the anterior portions of the first and second ribs containing the pseudoarthrosis relieved her symptoms and allowed the patient to return to her normal activities. The authors recommended chest radiographs and a possible CT scan with 3D reconstruction to completely evaluate an underlying congenital condition if the subluxation is rigid and unresponsive to nonoperative care.

Traumatic Anterior Sternoclavicular Joint Injuries

Anterior Sprain/Subluxation. The treatment of sprain or subluxation is nonoperative. Application of ice is recommended for the first 12 hours, followed by heat for the next 24 to 48 hours. The joint may be subluxated anteriorly or posteriorly, which may be reduced by drawing the shoulders backward as if reducing and holding a fracture of the clavicle. For both anterior and posterior subluxations that are stable, a clavicle strap can be used to hold the reduction. A sling and swath can also be used to support the shoulder and to prevent motion of the arm. The patient should be protected from further injury for 4 to 6 weeks.

Anterior Dislocation

Method of Closed Reduction. In most instances, even knowing that the anterior dislocation will be unstable, we still try to reduce the anterior displacement. Muscle relaxants and narcotics are administered intravenously, and the patient is placed supine on a table with a stack of three or four towels between the shoulder blades. While an assistant gently applies downward pressure on the anterior aspect of both shoulders, the medial end of the clavicle is pushed backward where it belongs. On some occasions, rare as they may be, the medial clavicle will stay adjacent to the sternum. However, in most cases, either with the shoulders still held back or when they are relaxed, the anterior displacement promptly recurs. We explain to the patient that the joint is unstable and that the hazards of internal fixation are too great, and we prescribe a sling for a couple of weeks and allow the patient to begin using the arm as soon as tolerated.

Most of the anterior injuries that we have treated in patients 25 years of age or younger are not dislocations of the SC joint. Rather they are type I or II physeal injuries, which heal and remodel without operative treatment. Patients older than 25 years with anterior dislocations of the SC joint do have persistent prominence of the anterior clavicle. However, this does not seem to interfere with usual activities and, in some cases, has not interfered with heavy manual labor.

Postreduction Care of Anterior Dislocations. After reduction, to allow ligament healing, the shoulders should be held back for 4 to 6 weeks with a figure-of-eight dressing or one of the commercially available figure-of-eight straps used to treat fractures of the clavicle. If the reduction is unstable, the arm is placed into a sling for a week or so, and then the patient can begin to use the arm for gentle everyday activities.

Acute Anterior Dislocation. There still is some controversy regarding the treatment of acute anterior dislocation of the SC joint. A large series of SC injuries was published in 1988 by Fery and Sommelet.[79] They reported on 40 anterior dislocations, 8 posterior dislocations, and 1 unstable SC joint. Fifteen injuries were managed closed, 17 patients were managed operatively, and 17 patients were not treated. They had good and excellent results with both closed and operative treatment, but recommended that closed reduction should be initially undertaken. In 1990, de Jong and Sukul[55] reported the long-term results in 10 patients with traumatic anterior SC dislocations. All patients were treated nonoperatively with analgesics and immobilization. The results of treatment were good in seven patients, fair in two patients, and poor in one patient at an average follow-up of 5 years. In summary, most acute anterior dislocations are unstable following reduction, and many operative procedures have been described to repair or reconstruct the joint. At this time, the mixed results of these procedures have not clearly advanced a case for their use instead of observation.

Anterior Physeal Injuries of the Medial Clavicle. Many so-called dislocations of the SC joint in adolescents and young adults (≤ 25 years) are not dislocations but physeal injuries. Most of these injuries will heal without surgical intervention. In time, the remodeling process eliminates any bone deformity or displacement. Anterior physeal injuries can certainly be left alone without problems. If an anterior physeal injury is recognized, closed reduction, as described above for anterior dislocation of the SC joint, can be performed. The shoulders should be held back in a clavicular strap or figure-of-eight dressing for 3 to 4 weeks, even if the reduction is stable. Healing is prompt, and remodeling will occur at the site of the deformity.

Chronic Anterior Dislocation. Chronic or unreduced anterior dislocations can be reconstructed, but do not generally require such procedures. Most patients with an unreduced and permanent anterior dislocation of the SC joint have few symptoms, have nearly full range of motion, and can work and even perform manual labor with few limitations. Because the joint is so small and incongruous and because the results following attempted reconstruction are inconsistent, we recommend a plan of "skillful neglect."

If the patient has persistent symptoms of post-traumatic arthritis for 6 to 12 months following a dislocation or a previous arthroplasty, and if the symptoms can be completely relieved by injection of local anesthesia into the SC joint region, we perform an excision arthroplasty of the SC joint (Fig. 42-21). Occasionally, following conservative treatment of a subluxation of the SC joint, the pain lingers on and the symptoms of popping and grating persist. Joint exploration may be required as several authors have reported symptom relief following joint exploration, removal of the torn or degenerated intra-articular disc along with a capsulorrhaphy.[6,14,64] Many authors have included chronic or unreduced anterior dislocations with posterior dislocations in their series of operative results. This makes it difficult to understand the true benefits of surgery in this situation. Postoperatively, recurrent instability,[79] limitations of activity,[8] and pain[72] often occur and patient expectations should be adjusted accordingly.

Panzica et al.[170] recently reported the long-term operative results of 11 patients with anterior SC joint instability who were managed with either resection arthroplasty (6 patients) or ligament reconstruction (5 patients). Treatment occurred an average of 19.1 months after injury or diagnosis in the resection group and within 2 weeks of injury in the reconstruction group. The results of treatment were evaluated at a mean of 9.9 years using the ASES, DASH, and Constant-Murley outcome scores. The outcome evaluation and postoperative pain scores did not differ significantly between the two operative groups; however, overall results were worse in the reconstruction group when the SC joint reconstruction was not performed soon after injury and in the resection arthroplasty group if the costoclavicular ligament was not preserved or reconstructed.

In 2012, Van Tongel et al.[227] conducted a survey regarding treatment options in acute and chronic symptomatic anterior SC dislocation among three groups of orthopedic surgeons (from a general orthopedic society and from two societies with special interest in shoulder and elbow surgery). There were a

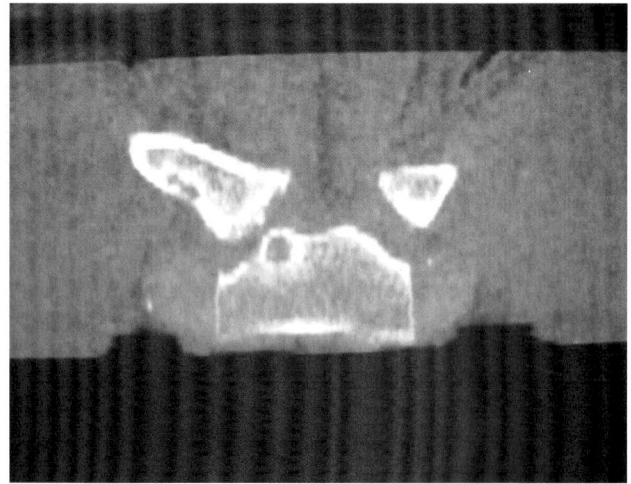
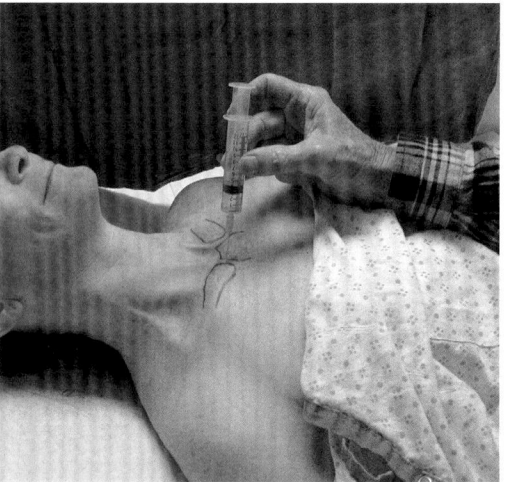

FIGURE 42-21 A: CT scan of the sternoclavicular joint. This 42-year-old patient had a symptomatic chronic anterior sternoclavicular joint dislocation. Note joint space narrowing, medial clavicle osteophytes, and manubrial cysts. **B:** This patient's symptoms were completely relieved by injection of local anesthesia into the sternoclavicular joint.

total of 212 respondents (212 of 753, or 28%). A majority of surgeons would not perform an open reduction in an acute situation if a closed reduction failed or redislocation occurred. Concerning the treatment for chronic symptomatic anterior SC dislocation, 60% of all respondents chose conservative treatment. However, the majority of surgeons (34 of 48, or 71%) from the American Shoulder and Elbow Society indicated they would perform open treatment (i.e., ligamentous reconstruction or medial claviculectomy) for a chronic symptomatic anterior SC dislocation.

Posterior Sternoclavicular Joint Injuries

Atraumatic Posterior Sternoclavicular Joint Instability

Spontaneous posterior subluxation or dislocation has only been noted in a few isolated case reports. We have never seen a spontaneous posterior subluxation or dislocation of the SC joint. Martin et al.[149] described a case of spontaneous atraumatic posterior dislocation in a 50-year-old previously healthy woman who awoke one morning with a painful SC joint. A CT scan confirmed the posterior dislocation. She later developed dysphagia, and a closed reduction was unsuccessful. At 1 year without any other treatment, she was back to playing golf and was asymptomatic. More recently, Martinez et al.[150] reported on the operative treatment of a 19-year-old woman with a symptomatic spontaneous posterior subluxation. The posteriorly displaced medial clavicle was stabilized with a figure-of-eight suture technique using a gracilis autograft. At follow-up the patient was pain free; however, a repeat CT scan demonstrated posterior subluxation of the medial clavicle with erosion of the clavicle and manubrium. In light of the recurrence of subluxation after reconstruction, the authors recommended conservative treatment of atraumatic posterior subluxation of the SC joint.

Traumatic Posterior Sternoclavicular Joint Injuries

Posterior Sprain/Subluxation. In mild sprains, the ligaments remain intact and the patient complains of moderate discomfort. The joint may be swollen and tender to palpation. Care must be taken to rule out the more significant posterior dislocation, which may have initially occurred and spontaneously reduced. When in doubt, it is best to protect the SC joint with a figure-of-eight bandage for 2 to 6 weeks. As with all injuries to the SC joint, it must be carefully evaluated by CT scan.

Posterior Dislocation. Posterior SC dislocation is considered a true orthopedic emergency as it can be a life-threatening injury. As a general rule, whenever a posterior dislocation of the SC joint is suspected, the physician must perform a very careful examination of the patient to rule out injury to the adjacent posterior structures such as the trachea, esophagus, brachial plexus, great vessels, and lungs. A careful physical examination, special radiographs, and CT scan of both medial clavicles are pertinent for proper diagnosis. Whenever vascular injuries are suspected, the CT scan will need to be combined with an arteriogram of the great vessels.

From a review of the earlier literature, it would appear that the treatment of choice for posterior SC dislocation was operative. However, since the 1950s, the treatment of choice has been closed reduction.[40,49,53,77,99,103,152,153,158,173,196,212] Closed reduction should be performed in an operating room with the capacity for cardiac bypass, with instruments prepared for sternotomy, and with the cardiothoracic team available.

For appropriate pain control, general anesthesia is usually required for reduction of a posterior dislocation of the SC joint. However, for the stoic patient, some authors have performed the reduction using intravenous narcotics and muscle relaxants.

Closed Reduction/Closed Treatment. Most posterior SC dislocations are successfully reduced closed if attempted within 48 hours of injury. Closed reduction after 48 hours is rarely reported but has been noted even at 10 days post injury.[97] The experience of the senior author at our institution is that most closed reductions are stable when performed acutely.[97] The most common techniques for closed reduction are described below.

Abduction Traction Technique. For the abduction traction technique,[58,77,119,148,152,158,187] the patient is placed supine with the injured shoulder near the edge of the table. A 3- to 4-inch thick sandbag is placed between the shoulders (Fig. 42-22). Lateral traction is applied to the abducted arm, which is then gradually brought back into extension. This may be all that is necessary to accomplish the reduction. The clavicle usually reduces with an audible pop or snap and can be noted visibly and by palpation and is almost always stable. Too much extension can bind the anterior surface of the dislocated medial clavicle on the back of the manubrium. Occasionally, it may be necessary to grasp the medial clavicle with one's fingers to dislodge it from behind the sternum. If this fails, the skin is prepared, and a sterile towel clip is used to grasp the medial clavicle to apply lateral and anterior traction to it.

Adduction Traction Technique (Buckerfield and Castle Technique). In this technique,[36] the patient is supine on the table with a 3- to 4-inch bolster between the shoulders. Traction is then applied to the arm in adduction, while a downward pressure is exerted on the shoulder (Fig. 42-23). The clavicle is levered over the first rib into its normal position. Buckerfield and Castle[36] reported that this technique was successful in seven patients when the abduction traction technique had failed.

Direct Reduction with Towel Clip. If the traction techniques described above are not successful, an assistant grasps or pushes down on the clavicle in an effort to dislodge it from behind the sternum. Occasionally, in a stubborn case, especially in a thick-chested person or a patient with extensive swelling, it is impossible to obtain a secure grasp on the clavicle with the fingers alone. The skin should then be surgically prepared and a sterile towel clip used to gain purchase on the medial clavicle percutaneously (Fig. 42-22). The towel clip should encircle the shaft of the clavicle as the dense cortical bone prevents

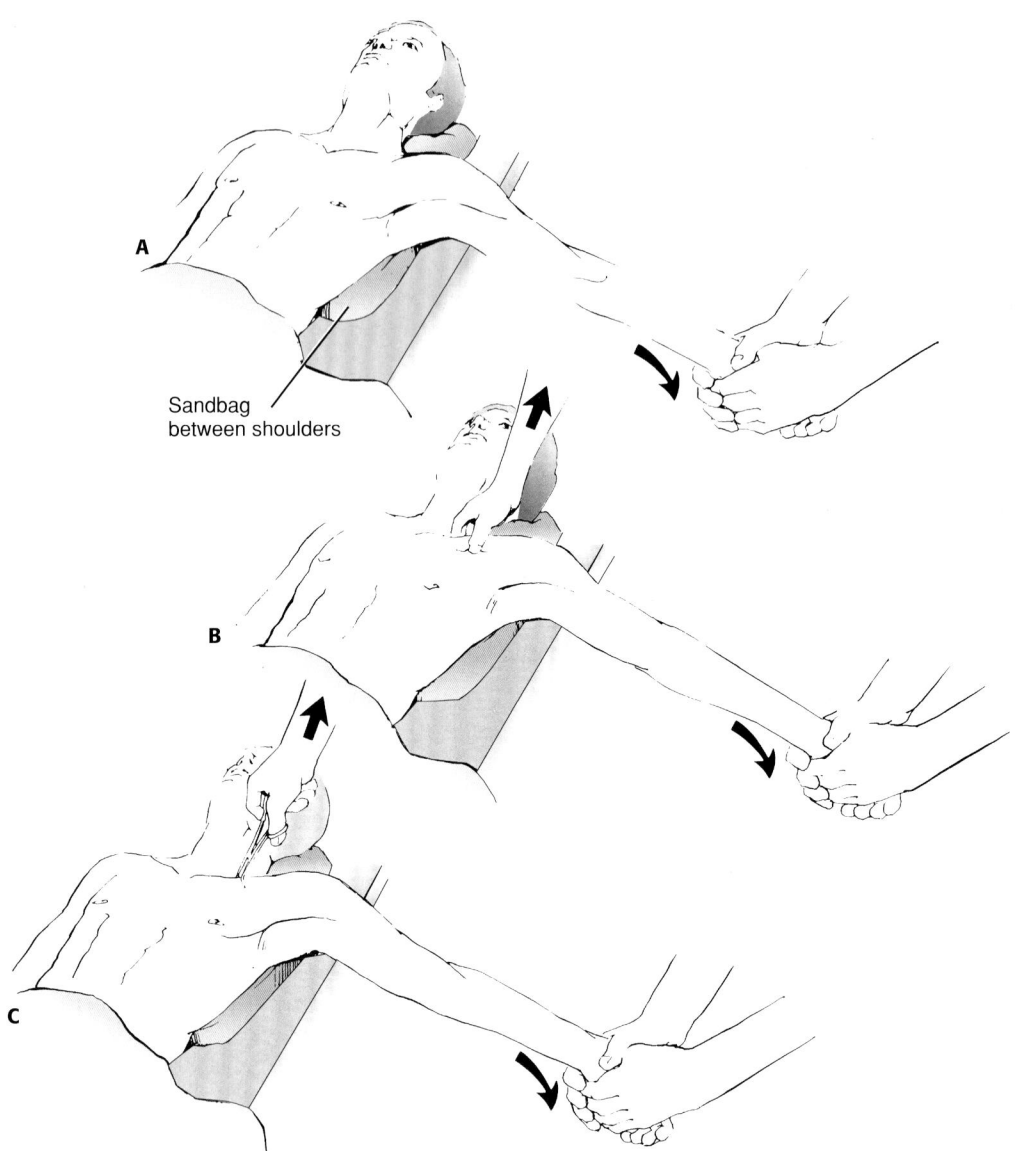

Sandbag
between shoulders

FIGURE 42-22 Technique for closed reduction of a posterior dislocation of the sternoclavicular joint. **A:** The patient is positioned supine with a sandbag placed between the two shoulders. Traction is then applied to the arm against countertraction in an abducted and slightly extended position. In anterior dislocations, direct pressure over the medial end of the clavicle may reduce the joint. **B:** In addition to the traction it may be necessary to manipulate the medial end of the clavicle with the fingers to dislodge it from behind the manubrium. **C:** In stubborn posterior dislocations, it may be necessary to sterilely prepare the medial end of the clavicle and use a towel clip to grasp around the medial clavicle to lift it back into position.

the purchase of the towel clip into the clavicle (Fig. 42-24). Then the combined traction through the arm plus the anterior lifting force on the towel clip will reduce the dislocation. Following the reduction, the SC joint is usually stable, even with the patient's arm at their side.

Postreduction Care of Posterior Dislocations. We always hold the shoulders back in a well-padded figure-of-eight clavicle strap for 3 to 4 weeks to allow for soft tissue and ligamen-

tous healing, even when the reduction is quite stable in the operating room.

Acute Posterior Physeal Injuries of the Medial Clavicle

Posterior physeal injuries, like posterior SC dislocations, should be reduced when they present acutely. The techniques for closed reduction are identical to those described for SC dislocations.

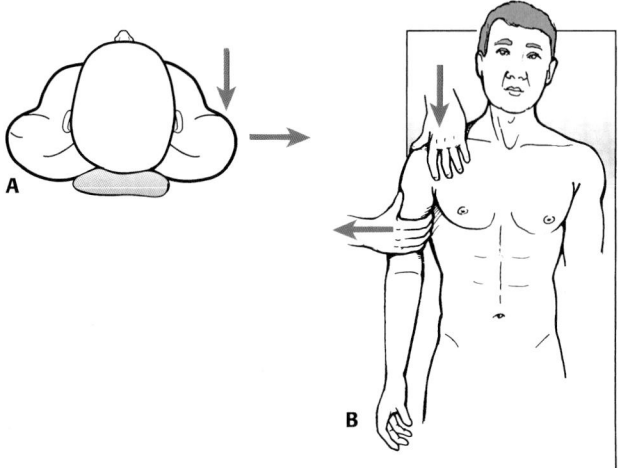

FIGURE 42-23 The Buckerfield–Castle technique. **A, B:** The patient is lying on the table with a bolster between the shoulders. Traction is applied to the arm in adduction while a downward force is applied on the shoulder.

After a stable reduction is achieved, the SC joint is protected with the shoulders held back in a figure-of-eight dressing or strap. Immobilization should continue for 3 to 4 weeks.

Closed reduction maneuvers have been reported with varied success.[28,32,36,42,56,72,97,107,111,130,136,212,233,236,242] New strategies can be employed to confirm reduction intraoperatively,[213] but in some cases redislocation may occur unexpectedly, even when the surgeon is confident of the intraoperative stability. Cases of late recurrence even after 1 week have been noted.[130] As such, it is important to note that confirmed intraoperative reduction may still require further imaging when clinical suspicion warrants.

The singular difference in treatment between posterior physeal separations and posterior SC dislocations occurs when a posterior physeal dislocation cannot be reduced by closed means and the patient is having *no significant symptoms*. In this scenario the displacement can in theory be observed while remodeling occurs.[243] Generally, this situation occurs when an attempted closed reduction is performed and postreduction CT shows residual posterior displacement or when a patient presents after 48 hours with no symptoms but with a confirmed posterior fracture separation on imaging. The patient may then be counseled regarding open treatment options (Fig. 42-25). Indeed, as with other physeal injuries, the potential for remodeling is significant and may extend until the 23rd to 25th year. The senior author[188] has demonstrated a similar mechanism to support conservative treatment of adolescent AC joint injuries or "pseudo-dislocations," in which there is a partial tear of the periosteal tube containing the distal clavicle. The coracoclavicular ligaments remain secured to the periosteal tube. Because of its high osteogenic potential, spontaneous healing and remodeling to the preinjury "reduced" position occurs within this periosteal conduit. The potential for late complications must be emphasized (see Chronic Posterior Physeal Injuries)

and patients should be monitored closely both clinically and radiographically at regular intervals for several years to confirm adequacy of the mediastinal space.

If the posterior displacement is symptomatic and cannot be reduced by closed means, the displacement must be reduced surgically and reconstructed as is required for posterior SC dislocations in adults. Waters et al.[233] reported successful operative treatment of 13 traumatic posterior SC fracture–dislocations in children and adolescents and other authors have also reported the successful open treatment of similar injuries in adolescents.[42,107,111,242,243] In 2010, Lafosse[130] reported a large multicenter series of 30 patients with posterior dislocations and posterior physeal separations. The success rate of closed reduction with posterior dislocation was 50% (5/10) and 0% with posterior physeal separations (0/4). These authors recommended open reduction for posterior physeal separations and suggested that closed reduction is hampered by the metaphyseal spike of the type II Salter–Harris fracture line. The emphasis on more aggressive open treatment of posterior physeal injuries underscores the need for vigilance in these patients and the need for more studies to evaluate the natural history of residual displacement in asymptomatic patients treated expectantly over time.

Chronic Posterior Dislocation

Complications accompanying unreduced posterior dislocations include late thoracic outlet syndrome, late and significant vascular problems, respiratory compromise, and dyspnea on exertion.[31,85,139,220] We have treated patients with a medial clavicle resection and reconstruction who have had complaints of swelling and arm discoloration, in addition to signs and symptoms of effort thrombosis and dysphagia secondary to a posteriorly displaced medial clavicle. In the adult, because of the potential problems that can be associated with the clavicle remaining displaced posteriorly into the mediastinum, an arthroplasty is performed as described in the author's preferred technique section with a figure-of-eight reconstruction (Fig. 42-26). Chronic posterior SC dislocation can be divided into late presentation (>48 hours) and late chronic (months to years after injury). As mentioned previously, after 48 hours closed reduction becomes much less likely to succeed and open reduction is usually necessary. Importantly, it is around 1 to 2 weeks post injury when the surrounding tissues scar to the posterior clavicle increasing the risk of vascular injury during the reduction maneuver.[147] In these cases, it is especially critical to obtain a CT angiogram preoperatively to assess the vascular status prior to surgery and be prepared for vascular and bypass surgical team presence in the operating room.

Late chronic posterior dislocations can present with consequences not initially present in the acute or subacute phase of the injury. Stankler[211] reported on two cases of nonoperative management of posterior dislocation, with one patient having mild symptoms of vascular congestion with activity, while the other developed an actual subclavian vein thrombosis 4.5 years later. Mehta et al.[154] presented a case report of a delayed subclavian artery occlusion 6 months post injury. Ege et al.[67] reported

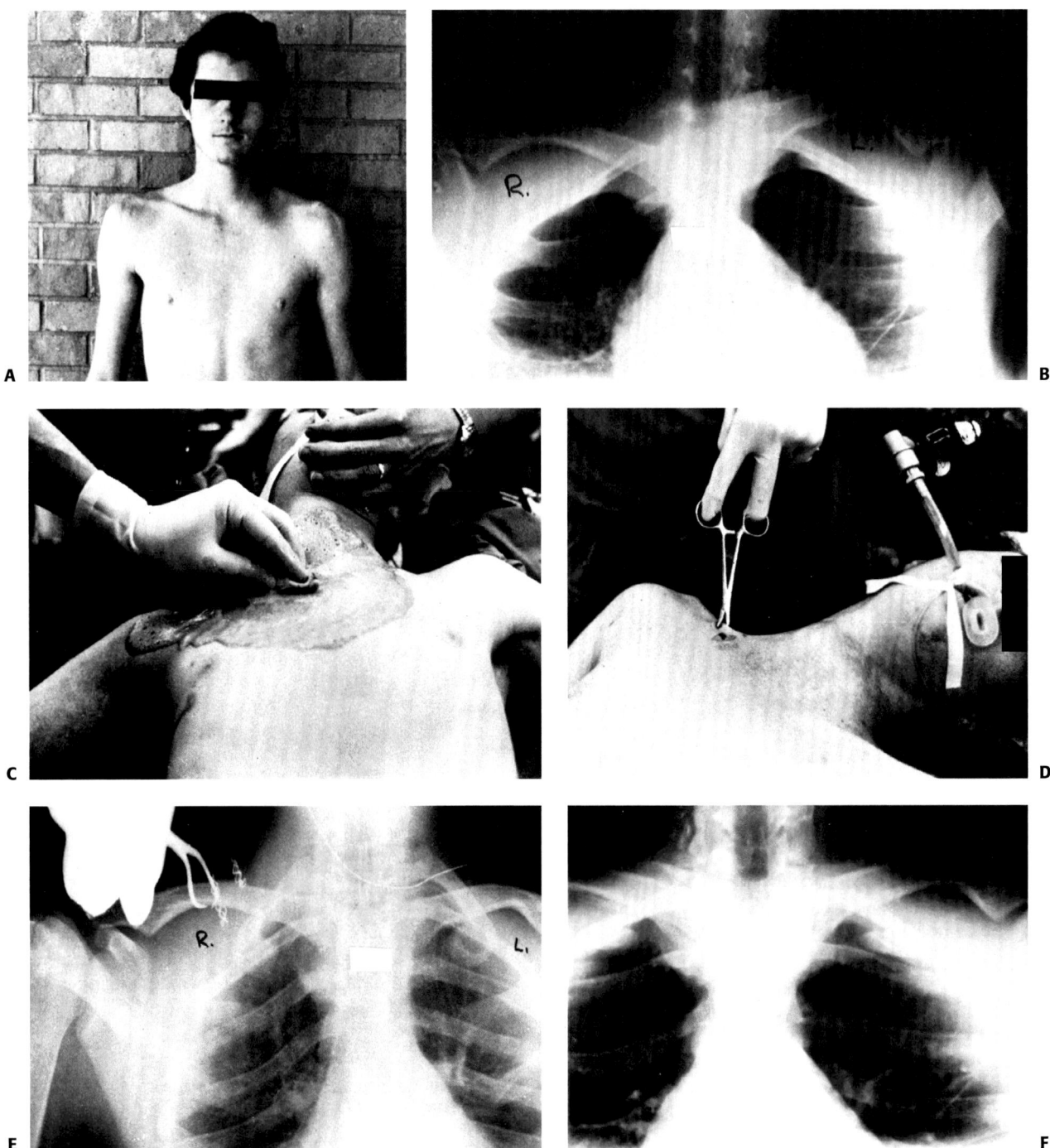

FIGURE 42-24 Posterior dislocation of the right sternoclavicular joint. **A:** A 16-year-old boy has a 48-hour-old posterior dislocation of the right medial clavicle that occurred from a direct blow to the anterior right clavicle. He noted the immediate onset of difficulty in swallowing and some hoarseness in his voice. **B:** A 40-degree cephalic tilt x-ray confirmed the posterior displacement of the right medial clavicle as compared with the left clavicle. Because of the patient's age, this was considered most likely to be a physeal injury of the right medial clavicle. **C:** Because the injury was 48 hours old, we were unable to reduce the dislocation with simple traction on the arm. The right shoulder was surgically cleansed so that a sterile towel clip could be used. **D:** With the towel clip placed securely around the clavicle and with continued lateral traction, a visible and audible reduction occurred. **E:** Postreduction x-rays showed that the medial clavicle had been restored to its normal position. The reduction was quite stable, and the patient's shoulders were held back with a figure-of-eight strap. **F:** The right clavicle has remained reduced. Note the periosteal new bone formation along the superior and inferior borders of the right clavicle. This is the result of a physeal injury, whereby the epiphysis remains adjacent to the manubrium while the clavicle is displaced out of a split in the periosteal tube.

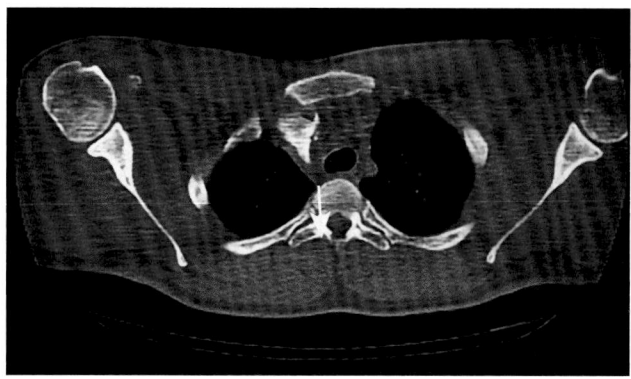

FIGURE 42-25 CT scan of a 19-year-old patient who was involved in a motor vehicle accident and presented with complaints of chest pain and a "choking sensation" that was exacerbated by lying supine. Note the physeal injury of the medial clavicle and compression of the trachea.

a case of bilateral chronic posterior dislocations which presented 2 years post injury and resulted in vascular compression on CT angiography. These symptoms resolved with resection of both clavicular heads. In addition to vascular consequences, multiple other sequelae from chronic unreduced retrosternal dislocations are noted in the section "Complications."[154] As such, operative treatment is strongly recommended for skeletally mature patients with posterior SC dislocations.

Chronic Posterior Physeal Injuries of the Medial Clavicle

In cases of late presentation or chronic posterior physeal injury with symptoms or with evidence of vascular compression on imaging, treatment is identical to chronic posterior SC disloca-

tions in adults. Open reduction is performed and the emphasis on preoperative vascular and/or cardiothoracic surgical collaboration is again paramount. However, controversy persists in young adults and adolescents who have no symptoms and present with chronic posterior physeal dislocations. In this situation, the physician can wait to see if the physeal plate remodeling process removes the posteriorly displaced bone.[189] Zaslav et al.[243] reported on a 13-year-old male with a late presentation of a posterior physeal injury. At 6-months post injury, the patient was asymptomatic and had complete remodeling on CT. In contrast, Emms et al.[70] reported on a subclavian thrombosis which occurred 2 years after an initial injury which was treated nonoperatively for what was originally diagnosed as a posterior subluxation. The patient had a new injury at 2 years which precipitated vascular symptoms 3 weeks later and on CT had evidence of a remodeled old medial physeal injury. The patient required a first rib resection to decompress the subclavian vein. Carbone et al.[41] reported on a similar case of superior vena cava obstruction after abnormal remodeling of a medial physeal fracture, and a second injury precipitated the occlusion. As such, close observation for the first 2 years, with serial vascular studies and/or serial CT scans, appears to be an important element of nonoperative care in the skeletally immature patient as most case reports of delayed complications occur in this time frame.[67,70,154,212]

Surgical Techniques for the Sternoclavicular Joint Injuries

Surgical Reconstructions

There are several procedures described to maintain the medial end of the clavicle in its normal articulation with the sternum (Table 42-1). In general, these techniques can be used

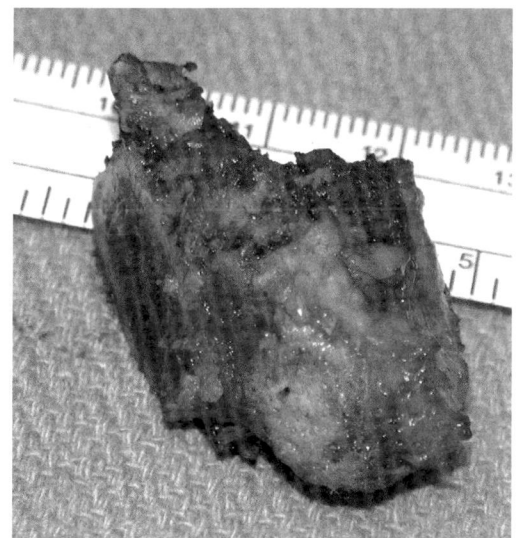

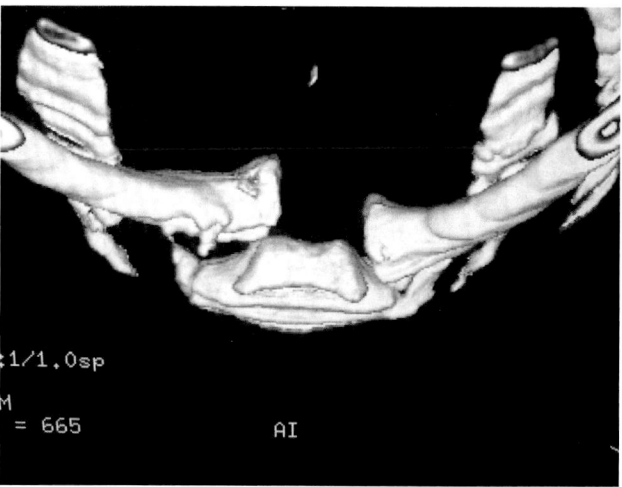

FIGURE 42-26 Chronic posterior sternoclavicular joint dislocation. **A:** An osteophyte projecting from medial clavicle corresponds to the area of capsular injury. **B:** 3D reconstruction CT scan demonstrating the osteophyte.

TABLE 42-1	**Surgical Techniques for Sternoclavicular Reconstruction**
1. Open excision with intramedullary ligament repair	Use intra-articular disc ligament as a transfer into medial clavicle, reinforced with local tissue repair[188]
2. Soft tissue graft used for figure-of-eight reconstruction	Reconstitute capsular ligaments with graft. Technique described using either semitendinosus[43,183] or plantaris tendon graft[7]
3. Subclavius tenodesis: Technique of Burrows	Use a slip of subclavius to reconstruct the costoclavicular ligament. Modification is to use graft (fascia lata) to recreate costoclavicular ligament[39]
4. Sternocleidomastoid reconstruction to first rib and clavicle	Use a partial slip of sternocleidomastoid through first rib and clavicle to recreate costoclavicular ligament[26]
5. Sternocleidomastoid to clavicle and manubrium	Use a partial slip of sternocleidomastoid to recreate capsular ligaments, no exposure of first rib[5,34]
6. Plate stabilization	*Balser Plate:* Inserted into manubrium, repair of local capsule, plate removal required[81]
	Ledge Plating: Standard 3.5-mm LC/DCP 6-hole plate placed anteriorly with medial two holes over manubrium[104]
	Locking Plate: 2-, 3.5-mm precontoured locking plates placed 90 degrees to each other[204]

to surgically reconstruct the SC joint in the setting of either anterior or posterior instability. This is because the fundamental objective of the operation is stabilization of the medial end of the clavicle to an adjacent structure, regardless of the initial direction of displacement. Much like the AC joint, the recent literature has focused on case reports of technique descriptions and modifications of existing surgeries. Given the rarity of the injury and even rarer necessity for surgery, there is no large experience with any of the techniques. However, certain basic principles should be adhered to in the midst of this creative atmosphere.

The operative procedure should be performed in a manner that disrupts as few of the anterior ligament structures as possible. If the procedure can be performed with the anterior ligaments intact, then the reduction may be stable with the shoulders held back in a figure-of-eight dressing. If all the ligaments are disrupted, a decision has to be made whether to try to stabilize the SC joint or to resect the medial 2.54 to 3.81 cm (1 to 1.5 in) of the clavicle and anatomically stabilize the remaining clavicle to the first rib. Resection alone cannot be performed in the setting of disrupted ligaments as doing so may worsen the instability of the residual medial clavicle, requiring even greater attention to the need for ligament reconstruction in such a scenario.[23]

Once faced with the need for reconstruction, the surgeon has to embrace a surgical strategy from the existing armamentarium. Procedures can be viewed from two different perspectives - tissue and stabilization routes. Tissue options include: (a) local ligaments and capsule, (b) tendon transfers (subclavius or sternocleidomastoid), or (c) grafts. Stabilization options include: (a) stabilize to the first rib, (b) stabilize to the manubrium, or (c) stabilize to the first rib and manubrium. Fixation is generally provided by soft tissue tensioning and suture, although augments with pins, plates, or screws have all been proposed.

Three broad technical philosophies have been characterized by Spencer et al.[210]: (a) intramedullary ligament transfer;

(b) costoclavicular ligament reconstruction; (c) SC ligament reconstruction. Spencer et al.[210] through a biomechanical analysis evaluated the three different reconstruction techniques in a cadaver model. The intramedullary ligament,[190] the subclavius tendon transfer,[39] and a semitendinosus graft placed in a figure-of-eight fashion through drill holes in the clavicle and manubrium were used to reconstruct the SC joint. Each of the three reconstruction methods was subjected to anterior or posterior translation to failure, and the changes in stiffness compared with the intact state were analyzed statistically. The figure-of-eight semitendinosus reconstruction showed superior initial mechanical properties to the other two techniques. The authors believed that this method reconstructs both the anterior and posterior joint capsules providing an initial stiffness that is closer to that of the intact SC joint. This technique has now been described with some success in young adults with refractory anterior and posterior instability.[8,43,183] A plethora of other techniques abound in the literature. Some of the literature from the 1960s and 1970s recommended stabilization of the SC joint with Kirschner wires (K-wires) or Steinmann pins.[32,35,56,58,69] These techniques have become largely historical due to their high complication rate as will be discussed later. Other authors have recommended the use of various types of suture wires across the joint,[11,38,82,100,118,166,177,182,212,214] reconstruction using local tendons,[7,12,26,144,146] or the use of a special plate.[102,104,175,193,204] Screw fixation across the joint, osteotomy of the medial clavicle, and resection of the medial end of the clavicle have also been advocated.[2,11,12,34,39,95,121,140,144,156,167,190,208]

Transfer of the sternocleidomastoid has been revisited in different forms. Booth and Roper[26] described transferring the sternal head of the tendon around the first rib and through the clavicle and back upon itself. Brown[34] used the clavicular head of the sternocleidomastoid as an anterior sling across the SC joint augmented with pins. Armstrong and Dias[5] have modified the use of the sternocleidomastoid by using only a slip of the sternal head and passing it through a medial clavicle bone tunnel. The graft is sutured to itself to recreate the anterior SC ligament without exposure of the first rib.

Thomas et al.[217] reported a safe surgical technique for stabilization of the SC joint with the use of suture material. Their technique involved tying the suture material on the superficial aspects of the medial clavicle and manubrium. This avoids the exposure of the first rib and avoids drilling through the inner cortex of the clavicle and manubrium. Abiddin et al.[1] has described a similar technique with the use of suture anchors in the manubrium and drill holes in the clavicle. In 2010, Rotini et al.[193] described using a hybrid fixation technique for a traumatic anterior SC joint dislocation. Suture anchors are first placed within the manubrium; transosseous sutures are then passed through the medial end of the clavicle and secured through holes of a "rotator cuff miniplate" that is stabilized on the medial clavicle.

While smooth pin and wire fixation is now taboo, fixation of the SC joint with other metal implants is still considered a valid option, although the implants do require removal. Franck et al.[81] reported an alternative therapy for traumatic SC instability using a plate for stabilization. A Balser plate was contoured to match the shape of the clavicle and the hook of the plate was used for sternal fixation. A retrosternal hook position was used for seven anterior dislocations and an intrasternal position was used for three posterior dislocations. For each patient the plate was attached to the clavicle with screws and the torn ligaments were repaired. All plates were removed by 3 months. At 1-year follow-up 9 of 10 patients had excellent results with no cases of redislocation. One patient developed a postoperative seroma that required surgical drainage, and one patient developed arthrosis. Using a similar technique, Hecox and Wood[104] described the use of a "ledge plate" for an unstable posterior SC joint dislocation. A standard 3.5-mm LC/DCP plate is contoured and fixed to the medial clavicle in a position that allows two holes of the plate to serve as a "ledge" over the manubrium.

Two other plate techniques have recently been described. Shuler and Pappas[204] used two, 3.5-mm locking reconstruction plates placed at 90 degrees across the SC joint for an unstable posterior dislocation. Pensey and Eglseder[175] described the use of combined suture anchor fixation and a long pelvic reconstruction plate that was contoured to the ipsilateral clavicle, manubrium, and contralateral clavicle for a posterior SC joint fracture–dislocation. No screws were placed in the manubrium, and fixation was achieved with three screws each in the right and left clavicle.

In 1997, Brinker et al.[31] described another technique of hardware fixation across the joint. The authors used two 75-mm cannulated screws to stabilize an unstable posterior dislocation of the SC joint. The screws were removed at 3 months, and at 10 months the patient had full range of motion without pain and returned to college level football.

Interpositional arthroplasty techniques have also emerged in recent years. Battaglia et al.[15] presented three cases of an Achilles tendon allograft and bone plug used to treat anterior instability in two patients and a medial clavicle fracture nonunion in one. The graft was fixed to a trough in the medial clavicle resection with screws, passed through bone tunnels in the manubrium and sutured upon itself. Meis et al.[155] reported using an intramedullary transfer of the sternocleidomastoid as an interposition for degenerative SC joint pain after resection.

Since 1982, various authors have recommended open reduction and internal fixation for *acute* injuries, as well as for chronic problems. In 1982, Pfister and associates[176,177] recommended open reduction and repair of the ligaments over nonoperative treatment. In 1988, Fery and Sommelet[79] reported 49 cases of SC joint dislocations. In these patients, if closed reduction was not successful, they performed open reduction. In symptomatic chronic unreduced dislocations, they either performed a myoplasty or excised the medial end of the clavicle if the articular surfaces were damaged. They were able to follow 55% of their patients, for an average of more than 6 years. They had 42% excellent results among the operative cases. Of those patients who were treated with closed reduction, 58% were satisfied. Ferrandez et al.[75] reported 18 subluxations and dislocations of the SC joint. Seven had moderate sprains and 11 had dislocations. Of the three patients with a posterior dislocation, all had symptoms of dysphagia. All of the subluxations were treated nonoperatively with excellent results. The remaining 10 patients with dislocations were treated with surgery (i.e., open reduction with suture of the ligaments and K-wires placed across the clavicle and the sternum). The wires were removed 3 to 4 weeks following surgery. At 1- to 4-year follow-up, most of the operative cases had a slight deformity. In two patients, migration of the K-wires was noted but was without clinical significance.

Eskola[72,73] strongly urged operative repair of chronic dislocations of the SC joint. In 1989, they reported on 12 patients treated for painful SC joints. The average time from injury was 1.5 years, and the average follow-up after surgery was 4.7 years. In five patients, the SC joint was stabilized with a palmaris longus or plantaris tendon graft placed between the first rib and the manubrium; in four patients, the medial 2.5 cm of the clavicle was resected without any type of stabilization; and in three patients, the clavicle was fixed to the first rib with a fascia lata graft. They reported good results in four patients, three treated with tendon grafts and one with a fascia lata graft. They had four fair results and four poor results in those patients who had only resection of the medial clavicle. There was little discussion of the patients' preoperative symptoms, work habits, or range of motion, or the degree of joint reduction following the surgery. In 1990, Tricoire et al.[220] reported six retrosternal dislocations of the medial end of the clavicle. They recommended reduction of these injuries to avoid the possible complications arising from protrusion of the clavicle into the mediastinum. SC capsulorrhaphy was performed in two patients and a subclavius tenodesis was used in the remaining four patients. All joints were temporarily stabilized with SC pins for 6 weeks. Results were satisfactory in all cases at a mean follow-up of 27 months.

Two recent systematic reviews of the available literature have been performed in 2011 to determine the ideal reconstruction technique for symptomatic, chronic anterior and irreducible or recurrent posterior SCJ dislocations.[90,218] The only available articles in the literature were Level IV retrospective case series and two biomechanical studies. In cases

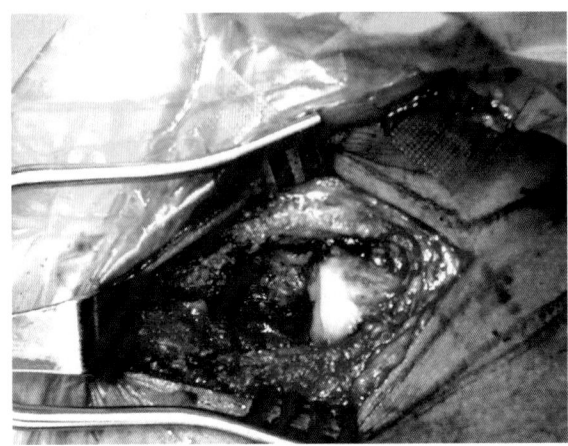

FIGURE 42-27 Resection of the right medial clavicle, retaining the costoclavicular ligament. White structure within the depth of the wound represents hyaline cartilage covering the clavicular notch of the manubrium (patient's head at top of image).

of failed closed reduction, the option for open reduction is always available, and the data have shown that its effectiveness is not negatively affected by the failed reduction attempt. If an open reduction is necessary there is evidence that repair of the joint capsule is sufficient surgical treatment; however, a tenodesis or ORIF are also effective and recommended treatments. In cases of chronic instability (anterior and posterior), reconstruction with tendon tissue woven in a figure-of-eight pattern through drill holes in the manubrium and clavicle is stronger than reconstruction with local tissue and is supported not only in biomechanical, but also clinical studies. Perhaps one of the most important factors that affect the success of treatment is the duration of time elapsed after the injury. The functional outcomes for patients with acute dislocations are significantly better than for those with chronic dislocations; therefore, accurate diagnosis and prompt treatment as close to the time of injury is optimal.

Resection of the Medial End of the Clavicle

McLaughlin,[153] Breitner and Wirth,[29] Pridie,[181] Bateman,[13,14] and Milch[156] have all recommended excision of the medial clavicle when degenerative changes are noted in the joint. If the medial end of the clavicle is to be removed because of degenerative changes, the surgeon should be careful not to damage the costoclavicular ligament (Fig. 42-27).

Recently, using the results of an anatomic study of 86 cadavers, Bisson et al.[24] recommended a safe resection length that

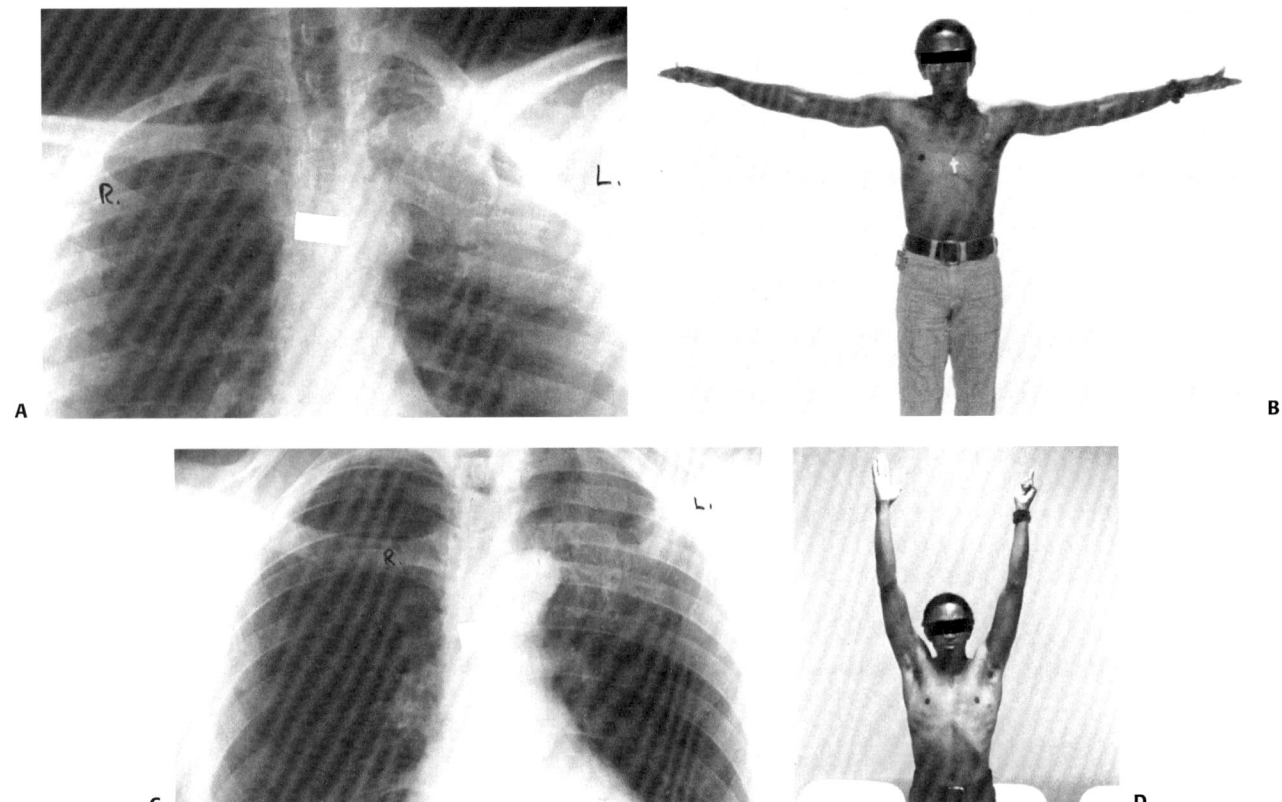

FIGURE 42-28 The effect of an arthrodesis of the sternoclavicular joint on shoulder function. **A:** As a result of a military gunshot wound to the left sternoclavicular joint, this patient had a massive bony union of the left medial clavicle to the sternum and the upper three ribs. **B:** Shoulder motion was limited to 90 degrees of flexion and abduction. **C:** Radiograph after resection of the bony mass and freeing up the medial clavicle. **D:** The motion of the left shoulder was essentially normal after the elimination of the sternoclavicular arthrodesis.

would result in no or minimal disruption of the costoclavicular ligament of 1 cm in men, and 0.9 cm in women.

Arthrodesis

Arthrodesis was once reported[185] in the treatment of a habitual dislocation of the SC joint. However, this procedure should *not* be done because it prevents the previously described normal elevation, depression, and rotation of the clavicle. The end result would be a severe restriction of shoulder movement (Fig. 42-28).

Postoperative Care

In most situations, the shoulders are held back with a figure-of-eight bandage for 4 to 6 weeks. When K-wires or Steinmann pins are used, the patient should avoid vigorous activities until

the pins are removed. The pins should be carefully monitored with radiographs until they are removed.

AUTHOR'S PREFERRED METHOD OF TREATMENT FOR STERNOCLAVICULAR JOINT INJURIES

Anterior Sternoclavicular Joint Injuries
Atraumatic Instability

The authors strongly recommend nonoperative treatment for spontaneous subluxation of the SC joint as surgical outcomes are not consistent and frequently worse or disabling compared to observation.

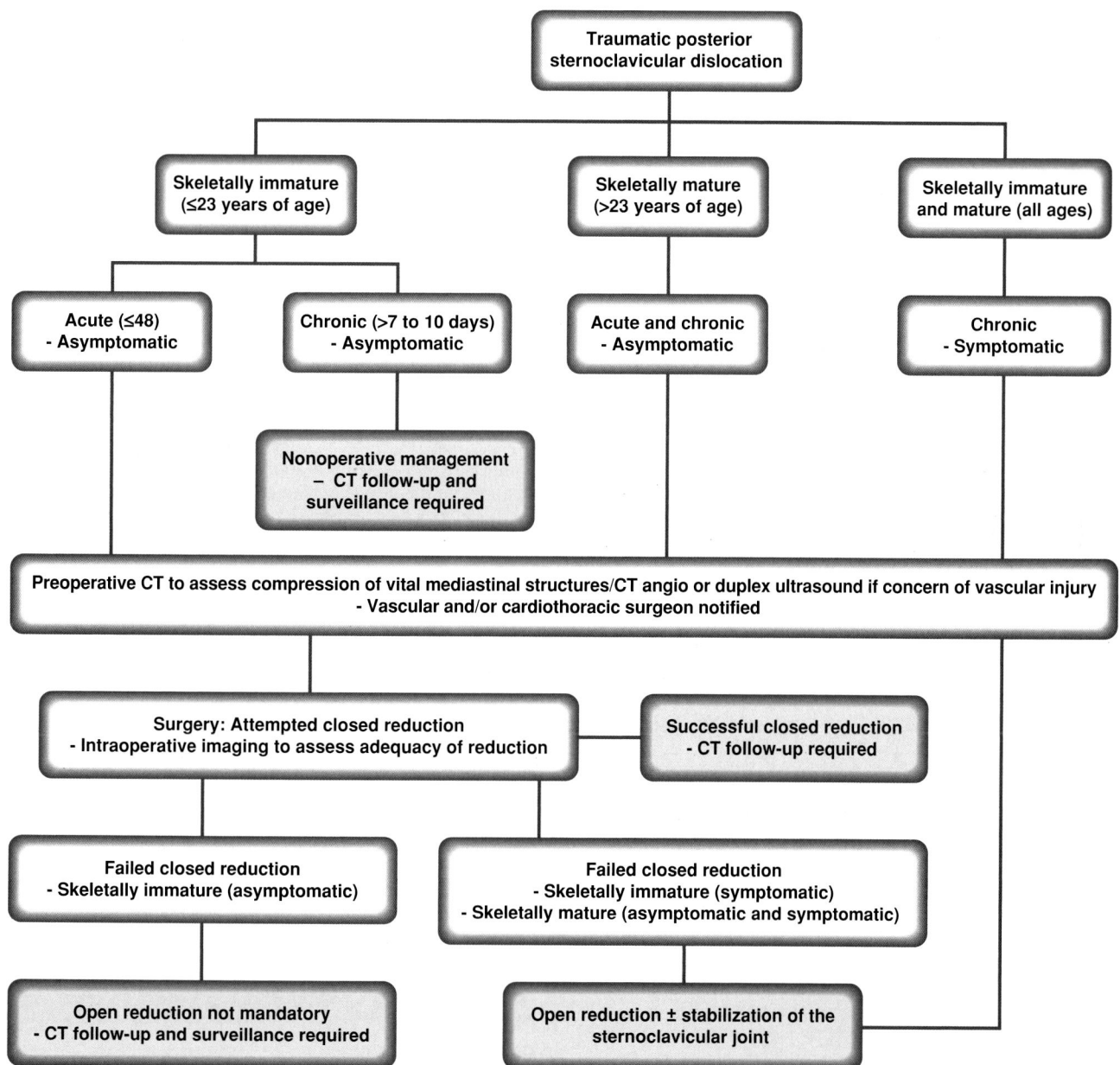

FIGURE 42-29 Treatment algorithm for traumatic posterior sternoclavicular joint dislocation.

Subluxation

For mild sprains we recommend the use of cold packs for the first 12 to 24 hours and a sling to rest the joint. Ordinarily, after 5 to 7 days, the patient can use the arm for everyday activities.

In addition to the cold pack, we may use a soft, padded figure-of-eight clavicle strap to gently hold the shoulders back to allow the SC joint to rest. The harness can be removed after a week or so. Then the arm is placed in a sling for about another week, or the patient is allowed to return gradually to everyday activities.

Dislocation

In general, we manage anterior dislocations of the SC joint in adults by either a closed reduction or by "skillful neglect." Most of the anterior dislocations are unstable, but we accept the deformity since we believe it is less of a problem than the potential problems of operative repair and internal fixation. In cases where symptoms persist and no other recourse exists outside of surgical management, the preferred technique is medial clavicle resection and figure-of-eight ligament reconstruction as described in the section below.

Posterior Sternoclavicular Joint Injuries

Subluxation

We recommend treatment with ice for 24 to 48 hours, and rest in a sling for 1 week. This is followed by range of motion as tolerated for the following 4 weeks but no contact sports during this time frame to allow healing and avoid recurrent posterior subluxation. It is important to emphasize that these patients should be monitored very closely as a missed diagnosis can have devastating consequences. If any doubt about SC stability emerges, liberal use of CT or MRI to confirm location is warranted.

Dislocation (Fig. 42-29)

After an appropriate history and physical examination (Table 42-2), radiographs and a CT scan should be obtained. If the patient has distention of the neck vessels, swelling or bluish discoloration of the arm, or difficulty swallowing or breathing, then the patient should be evaluated using a CT scan with con-

trast to assess the vascular structures. It is also important to determine if the patient has a feeling of choking or hoarseness. If any of these symptoms are present, indicating pressure on the mediastinal structures, the appropriate cardiovascular or thoracic specialist should be consulted urgently. The patient should always be consented for possible open reduction in the event a closed reduction fails.

Closed Reduction

We then proceed to the operating room urgently for closed reduction as outlined previously (Fig. 42-22). We prefer to start with the abduction traction technique. If reduction cannot be accomplished with the patient's arm in abduction, we will use the adduction technique of Buckerfield and Castle[36] that is described above (Fig. 42-23).

If these methods are not successful, we utilize the towel clip technique combined with downward pressure on the lateral clavicle and traction on the arm.

Open Surgical Procedures

Acute Repair of Posterior Dislocation

If all methods of closed reduction fail, an open reduction should be performed. It is critical that a thoracic surgeon and bypass team are immediately available when the patient is taken to the operating room to intervene if needed. The patient is positioned supine on a radiolucent operating table. The chest and abdomen along with the involved ipsilateral limb are prepped and draped free. A curvilinear incision is made over the SC joint with the horizontal limb in line with the clavicle and the vertical limb along the manubrium. Skin flaps are elevated and the periosteum is incised in a horizontal fashion. Care is taken to preserve the capsule for later repair and closure (Fig. 42-30). The posteriorly displaced clavicle is reduced with traction, towel clip elevation, and/or by gently leveraging the clavicle from posterior to anterior with a blunt retractor (Fig. 42-31). The posterior capsule along with the intra-articular disc ligament is then incorporated into a running locking suture using no. 2 Ethibond (Johnson & Johnson) (Fig. 42-32).

TABLE 42-2	Keys to Diagnosis of Posterior Sternoclavicular Dislocation

History of violent injury
Painful sternoclavicular joint
Difficulty in swallowing
Difficulty in breathing
Decreased range of motion of the upper extremity
Palpable step-off of the sternoclavicular joint
Positive "serendipity view"
Posterior displacement on computed tomography

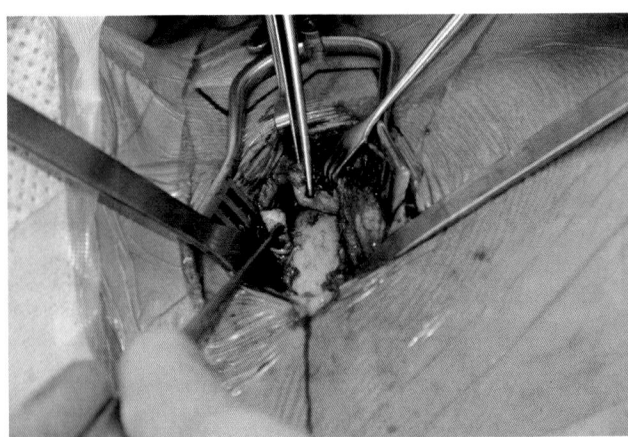

FIGURE 42-30 Initial elevation of periosteum and capsule (held in forceps) and exposure of the medial clavicle (clinical example of right posterior SC joint dislocation; patient's head at left of image).

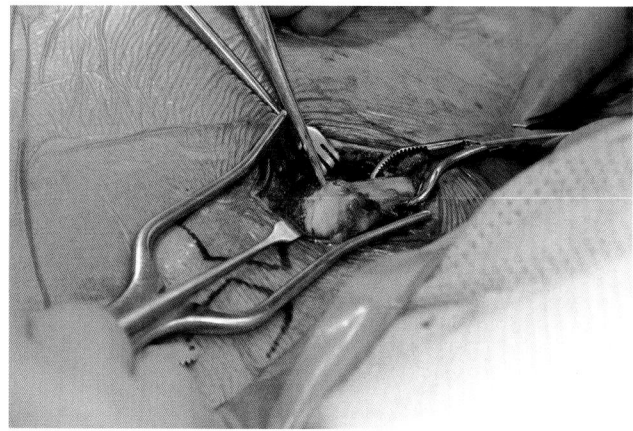

FIGURE 42-31 Elevation and open reduction of the medial clavicle with clamp (right SC joint, viewed superiorly; patient's head at bottom right of image).

Drill holes are then passed through the clavicle from anterior-to-posterior taking care to protect the neurovascular structures. A Hewson suture passer is used to shuttle sutures through the posterior cortex of the clavicle (Fig. 42-33). The defect in the posterior capsule is then repaired with interrupted permanent suture (Fig. 42-34). After the capsular defect is closed, the previously passed transosseous sutures are secured along the anterior cortex (Fig. 42-35). The remaining capsular sleeve is closed with absorbable sutures to complete the repair.

Acute Repair with Medial Clavicle Resection (Technique of Rockwood and Wirth)

The medial clavicle may need to be acutely resected in certain scenarios as described by the senior author.[190] Examples include severely damaged medial articulations, the need to decompress the posterior structures, and the necessity to provide improved access for the thoracic surgeon to the mediastinum. When operating on the SC joint, care must be taken to evaluate the residual stability of the medial clavicle. It is the same analogy as used when resecting the distal clavicle for an old AC joint problem. If the coracoclavicular ligaments are intact, an excision of the distal

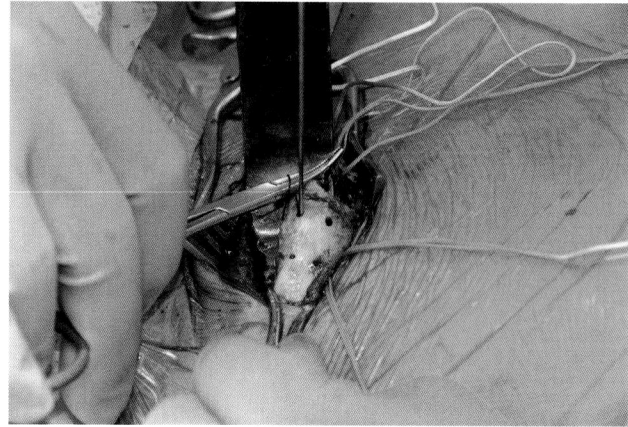

FIGURE 42-33 Drill holes through clavicle for the purpose of transosseous repair.

clavicle is indicated. In this case if the coracoclavicular ligaments are attenuated, then, in addition to excision of the distal clavicle, one must reconstruct the coracoclavicular ligaments. With an SC joint injury, if the costoclavicular ligaments are intact, the clavicle medial to the ligaments should be resected and beveled smooth. If the ligaments are torn, the clavicle must be stabilized to the first rib. If too much clavicle is resected, or if the clavicle is not stabilized to the first rib, residual joint instability and patient symptoms can result (Fig. 42-36). The patient is placed supine on the table, and three to four towels or a sandbag should be placed between the scapulae. The upper extremity should be draped out free so that lateral traction can be applied during the open reduction. In addition, a folded sheet around the patient's thorax should be left in place so that it can be used for countertraction when traction is applied to the involved extremity. An anterior incision is used that parallels the superior border of the medial 7.62 to 10.16 cm (3 to 4 in) of the clavicle and then extends downward over the sternum just medial to the involved SC joint (Fig. 42-37). During exposure of the SC joint it is crucial to leave the anterior capsular ligament intact. The reduction can usually be accomplished with traction and countertraction

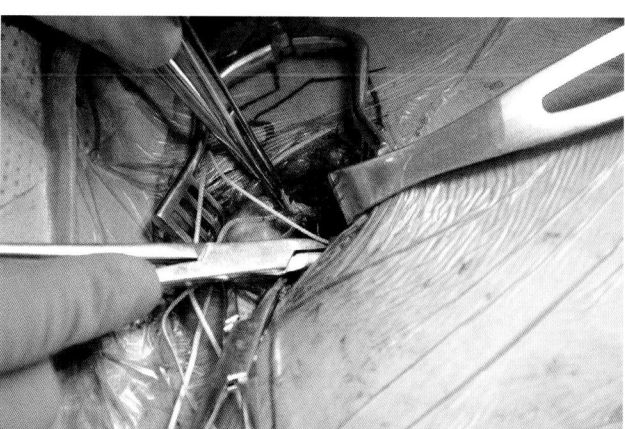

FIGURE 42-32 Grasping suture in the posterior capsule and intra-articular disc ligament.

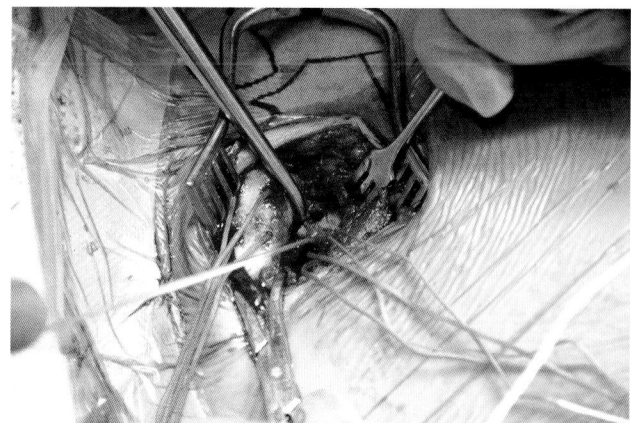

FIGURE 42-34 Repair of the posterior capsule defect with interrupted suture.

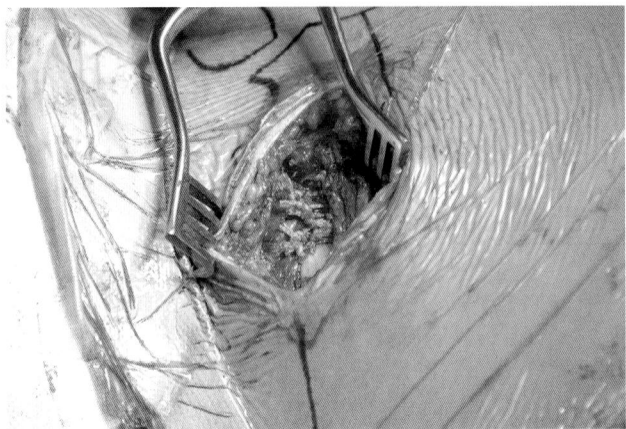

FIGURE 42-35 Completed repair after transosseous sutures secured.

while lifting up anteriorly on a clamp placed around the medial clavicle. Along with the traction and countertraction, it may be necessary to use an elevator to pry the clavicle back to its articulation with the manubrium.

When the reduction has been obtained, and with the shoulders held back, the reduction will be stable if the anterior capsule has been left intact. If the anterior capsule is damaged or is insufficient to prevent anterior displacement of the medial end of the clavicle, we recommend excision of the medial 2.54 to 3.81 cm (1 to 1.5 in) of the clavicle and securing the residual clavicle anatomically to the first rib with 1-mm Dacron tape. The medial clavicle is exposed by careful subperiosteal dissection (Fig. 42-38). When possible, any remnant of the capsular or intra-articular disc ligaments should be identified and preserved as these structures can be used to help stabilize the medial clavicle. The capsular ligament covers the anterosuperior and pos-

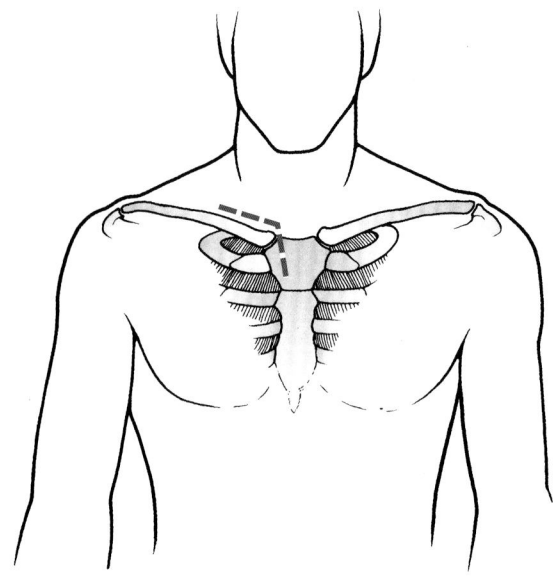

FIGURE 42-37 The proposed skin incision used for open reduction of a posterior sternoclavicular dislocation.

terior aspects of the joint and represents thickenings of the joint capsule. This ligament is primarily attached to the epiphysis of the medial clavicle and is usually avulsed from this structure with posterior SC dislocations. The intra-articular disc ligament is a very dense, fibrous structure and may be intact. It arises from the synchondral junction of the first rib and sternum and is usually avulsed from its attachment site on the medial clavicle. If the sternal attachment sites of the intra-articular and/or capsular ligaments are intact, a nonabsorbable no. 1 cottony Dacron suture is woven back and forth through the ligament(s) so that the ends of the suture exit through the avulsed free end of the tissue. The medial 2.54 to 3.81 cm (1 to 1.5 in) end of the clavicle is resected, being careful to protect the underlying vascular

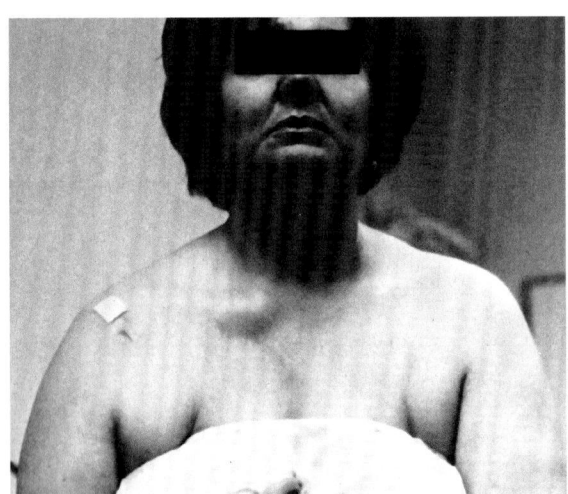

FIGURE 42-36 This postmenopausal, right-handed woman had a resection of the right medial clavicle because of a preoperative diagnosis of "possible tumor." The postoperative microscopic diagnosis was degenerative arthritis of the right medial clavicle. After surgery, the patient complained of pain and discomfort, marked prominence, and gross instability of the right medial clavicle.

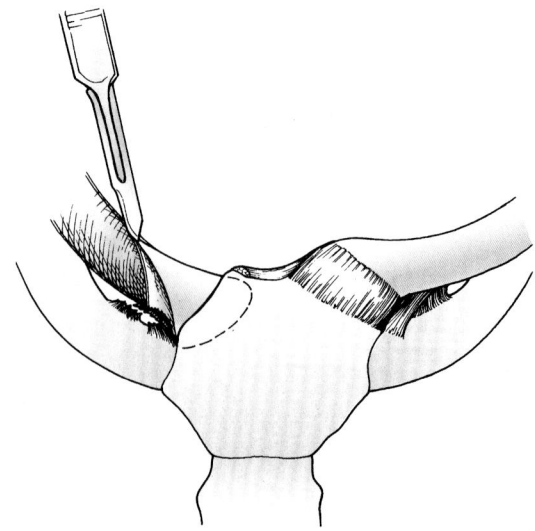

FIGURE 42-38 Subperiosteal exposure of the medial clavicle. Note the posteriorly displaced medial end of the clavicle.

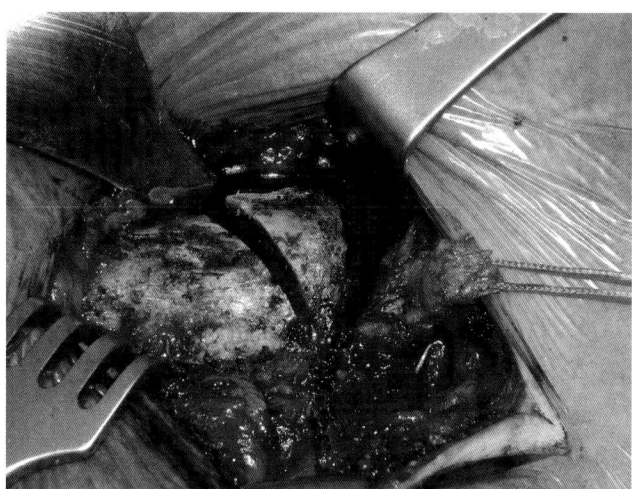

FIGURE 42-39 Resection of the right medial clavicle and identification of the intra-articular ligament tagged with suture (Courtesy of Charles E. Rosipal, MD and R. Michael Gross, MD).

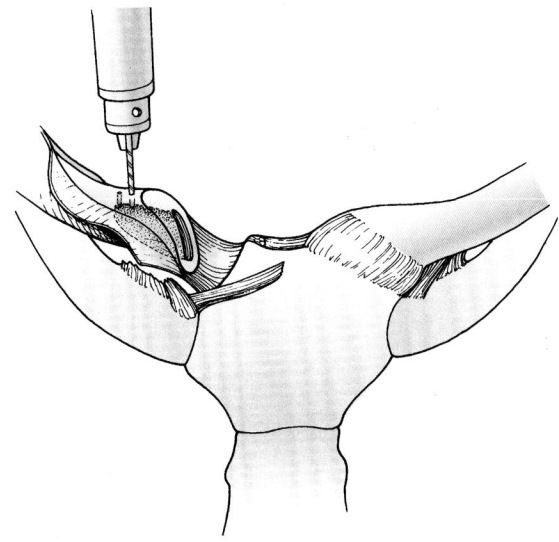

FIGURE 42-41 Drill holes are placed in the superior cortex of the clavicle, approximately 1 cm lateral to the osteotomy site.

structures, and being careful not to damage any of the residual costoclavicular (rhomboid) ligament. The vital vascular structures are protected by passing a curved Crego elevator or ribbon retractor around the posterior aspect of the medial clavicle to isolate them from the operative field during the bony resection.

Excision of the medial clavicle is facilitated by creating drill holes through both cortices of the clavicle at the intended site of clavicular osteotomy. Following this step, an air drill with a side-cutting bur is used to complete the osteotomy (Fig. 42-39). The anterior and superior corners of the clavicle are beveled smooth with an air bur for cosmetic purposes. The medullary canal of the medial clavicle is drilled and curetted to receive the transferred intra-articular disc ligament (Fig. 42-40). Two small drill holes are then placed in the superior cortex of the medial clavicle, approximately 1 cm lateral to the site of resection (Fig. 42-41). These holes communicate with the medullary canal and will be used to secure the suture in the transferred ligament. The free ends of the suture are passed into the medullary canal of the medial

clavicle and out the two small drill holes in the superior cortex of the clavicle (Fig. 42-42). While the clavicle is held in a reduced AP position in relation to the first rib and sternum, the sutures are used to pull the ligament tightly into the medullary canal of the clavicle (Fig. 42-43). The suture is tied over the cortical bone bridge of the superior clavicle, thus securing the transferred ligament into the clavicle (Fig. 42-44). The stabilization procedure is completed by passing multiple (five or six) 1-mm cottony Dacron sutures around the reflected periosteal tube, the clavicle, and any of the residual underlying costoclavicular ligament and periosteum on the dorsal surface of the first rib (Figs. 42-45 to 42-47). The intent of the sutures passed around the periosteal tube and clavicle and through the costoclavicular ligament and periosteum of the first rib is to anatomically restore the normal space between the clavicle and the rib. To place sutures around the clavicle and the first rib and pull them tight would decrease the space and

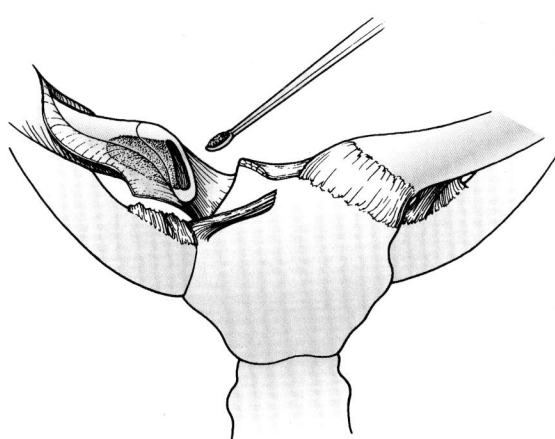

FIGURE 42-40 The medullary canal of the medial clavicle is curetted in preparation for receiving the transferred intra-articular ligament.

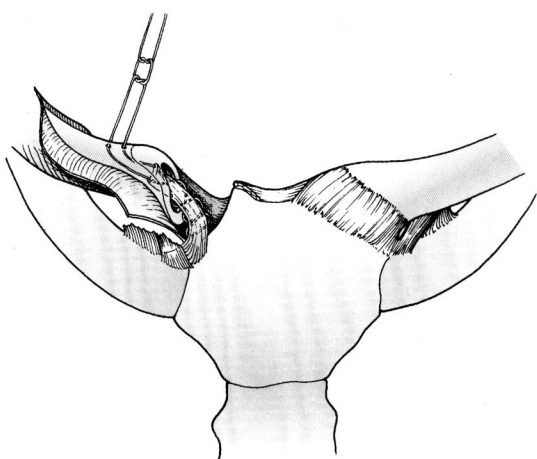

FIGURE 42-42 The free ends of the suture are passed into the medullary canal and out the two holes in the superior cortex.

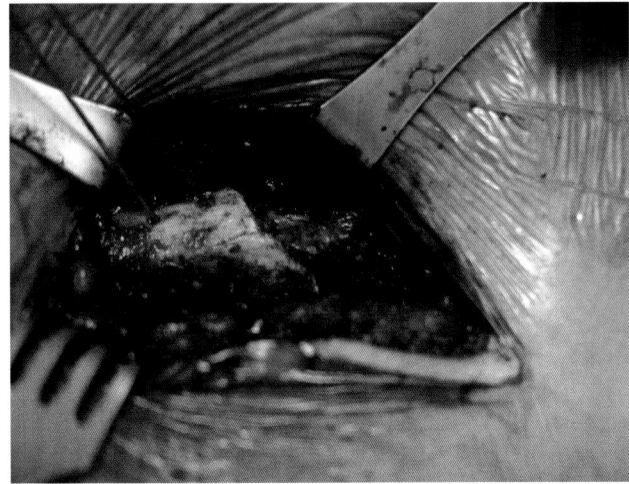

FIGURE 42-43 Passage of the intra-articular disc ligament into the medullary canal. (Courtesy of Charles E. Rosipal, MD and R. Michael Gross, MD).

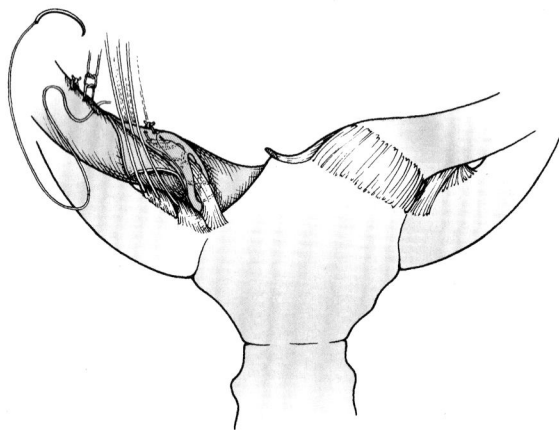

FIGURE 42-44 The transferred ligament is secured into the medial clavicle by tying the sutures exiting from the superior cortex of the clavicle.

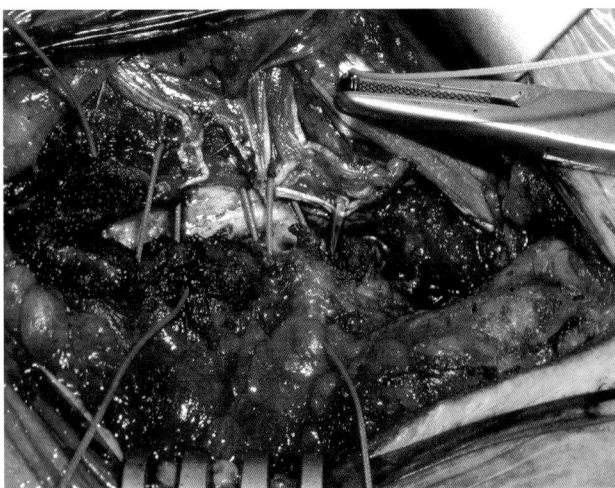

FIGURE 42-45 Passage of sutures through the clavicle and sutures through the periosteal sleeve (Courtesy of Charles E. Rosipal, MD and R. Michael Gross, MD).

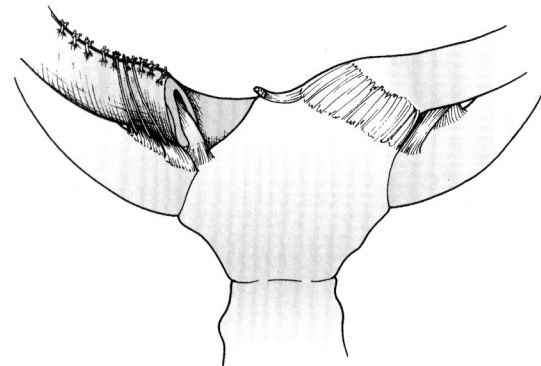

FIGURE 42-46 Closure of the periosteal sleeve around the medial clavicle and secure fixation of these structures to the costoclavicular ligament.

could lead to pain. We usually detach the clavicular head of the sternocleidomastoid, which temporarily eliminates the superior pull of the muscle on the medial clavicle. Postoperatively, the shoulders should be held back in a figure-of-eight dressing for 4 to 6 weeks to allow for healing of the soft tissues.

In 1997, Rockwood et al.[190] reported on a series of 23 patients who had undergone a resection of the medial end of the clavicle. The patients were divided into two groups: Group I, those who underwent resection of the medial end of the clavicle with maintenance or reconstruction of the costoclavicular ligament; and group II, those who had a resection without maintaining or reconstructing the costoclavicular ligament. The outcome in all but one of the seven patients in group II was poor, with persistence or worsening of preoperative symptoms. The only patient of this group with a successful result had a posterior epiphyseal separation in which the costoclavicular ligament remained attached to the periosteum, thus preventing instability. All of the eight patients in group I who had a

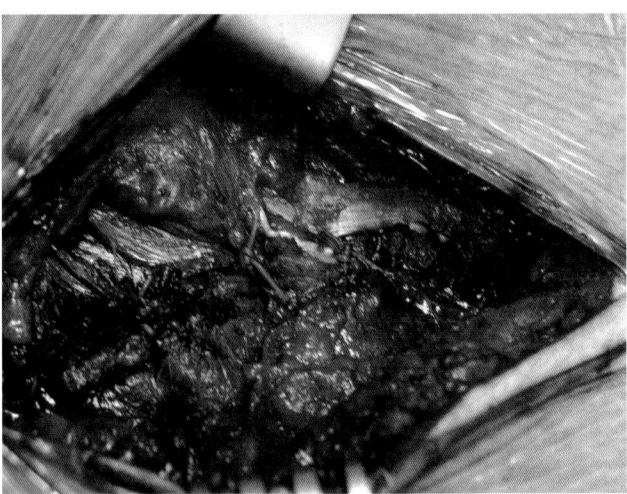

FIGURE 42-47 Intraoperative photograph showing Dacron sutures around the reflected periosteal tube, the clavicle, and the residual underlying costoclavicular ligament and periosteum on the dorsal surface of the first rib. (Courtesy of Charles E. Rosipal, MD and R. Michael Gross, MD.)

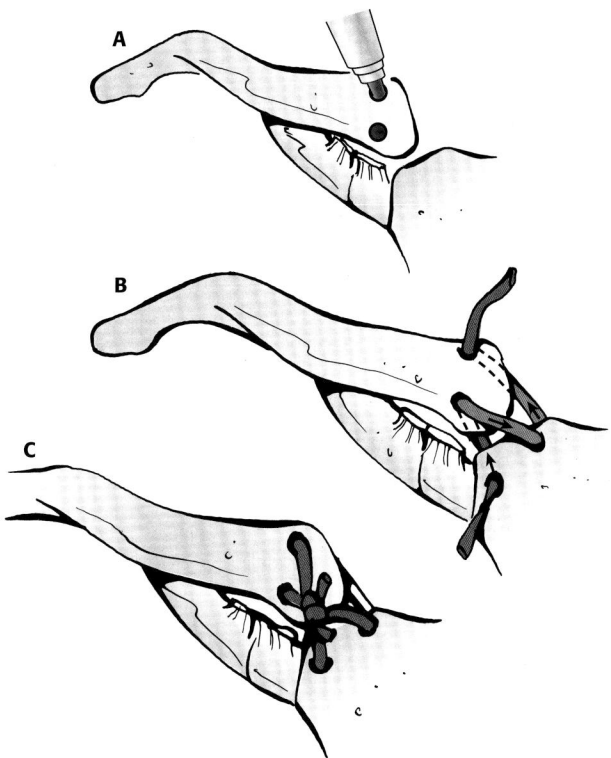

FIGURE 42-48 Semitendinosus figure-of-eight reconstruction. **A:** Drill holes are passed from anterior to posterior through the medial part of the clavicle and the manubrium. **B:** A free semitendinosus tendon graft is woven through the drill holes such that the tendon strands are parallel to each other posterior to the joint and cross each other anterior to the joint. **C:** The tendon ends are tied in a square knot and secured with suture. (Redrawn after Spencer EE, Kuhn JE. Biomechanical analysis of reconstructions for sternoclavicular joint instability. *J Bone Joint Surg* 2004;86 A(1):98–105.)

primary surgical resection of the medial end of the clavicle with maintenance of the costoclavicular ligaments had an excellent result. When the operation was performed as a revision of a previous procedure with reconstruction of the costoclavicular ligament, the results were less successful, but only one patient of seven was not satisfied with the outcome of treatment.

Open Surgical Reconstruction with Graft (Figure-of-Eight Tendon Graft)

In cases where acute repair is not possible due to late presentation or poor tissue quality, the authors' preferred technique for reconstruction of the SC joint is the figure-of-eight tendon graft described by Spencer and Kuhn.[209] We expose the SC joint as above for acute repair with careful preservation of the periosteal sleeve for later closure. Drill holes are created in both the clavicle and the manubrium. The graft of choice is semitendinosus allograft or autograft which is prepared with a running locking permanent suture to reinforce the tendon and prevent graft fraying. A Hewston suture passer is used to facilitate graft passage and the tendon is tensioned to itself and secured with multiple no. 2 Ethibond sutures (Ethicon, Johnson & Johnson) (Figs. 42-48 and 42-49).

Postreduction Care of Posterior Dislocations

If open reduction is required, a figure-of-eight dressing is used for 6 weeks and this is followed by a sling for another 6 weeks. During this time, the patient is instructed to avoid using the arm for any and all strenuous activities of pushing, pulling, or lifting. They should not elevate or abduct the arm more than 60 degrees during the 12-week period. They can use the involved arm to care for bodily needs, that is, eating, drinking, dressing, and toilet care. This prolonged immobilization will allow the soft tissues a chance to consolidate and stabilize the medial clavicle to the first rib. After 12 weeks, the patient is allowed to gradually use the arm for usual daily living activities, including over the head activities. *However, we do not recommend that the patients, after resection of the medial clavicle and ligament reconstruction, return to heavy laboring activities.*

Pearls and Pitfalls

We do not recommend the use of K-wires, Steinmann pins, or any other type of metallic pins to stabilize the SC joint. The complications can be very serious and are discussed in the section on complications.

Physeal Injuries of the Medial Clavicle

The treatment algorithm for posterior physeal injuries of the medial clavicle is essentially the same as for posterior dislocation. We perform the closed reduction maneuvers as described above. If unsuccessful, then an open reduction of the physeal injury is indicated. The open exposure is essentially the same as above for posterior SC acute repair and we repair the posterior capsule and costoclavicular ligament in the same fashion. If the medial epiphysis is large enough, sutures can be passed from the medial clavicle to the epiphysis to augment the soft tissue repair with bone fixation. After reduction, the shoulders are held back with a figure-of-eight strap or dressing for 3 to 4 weeks.

Before the epiphysis ossifies at the age of 18, one cannot be sure whether a displacement about the SC joint is a dislocation of the SC joint or a fracture through the physeal plate.[202,236] Despite the fact that there is significant displacement of the medial shaft with either a type I or type II physeal fracture, the periosteal tube remains in its anatomic position and the attaching ligaments are intact to the periosteum (i.e., the costoclavicular ligament inferiorly and the capsular and intra-articular disc ligaments medially) (Fig. 42-50).

Treatment of Combined SC Injuries

Bilateral dislocations are managed on the basis of the criteria for treatment of each individual dislocation separately. When patients have dislocations of both ends of the clavicle, the authors recommend stabilization of the AC joint with appropriate surgical techniques for type III, IV, V, and VI separations. The SC dislocation is generally left with nonoperative treatment with the exception of the unreduced posterior dislocation which is treated as per guidelines outlined earlier in this chapter. When the clavicle is fractured with an SC dislocation, the clavicle should be stabilized with internal fixation for posterior injuries and treated as appropriate for isolated clavicle

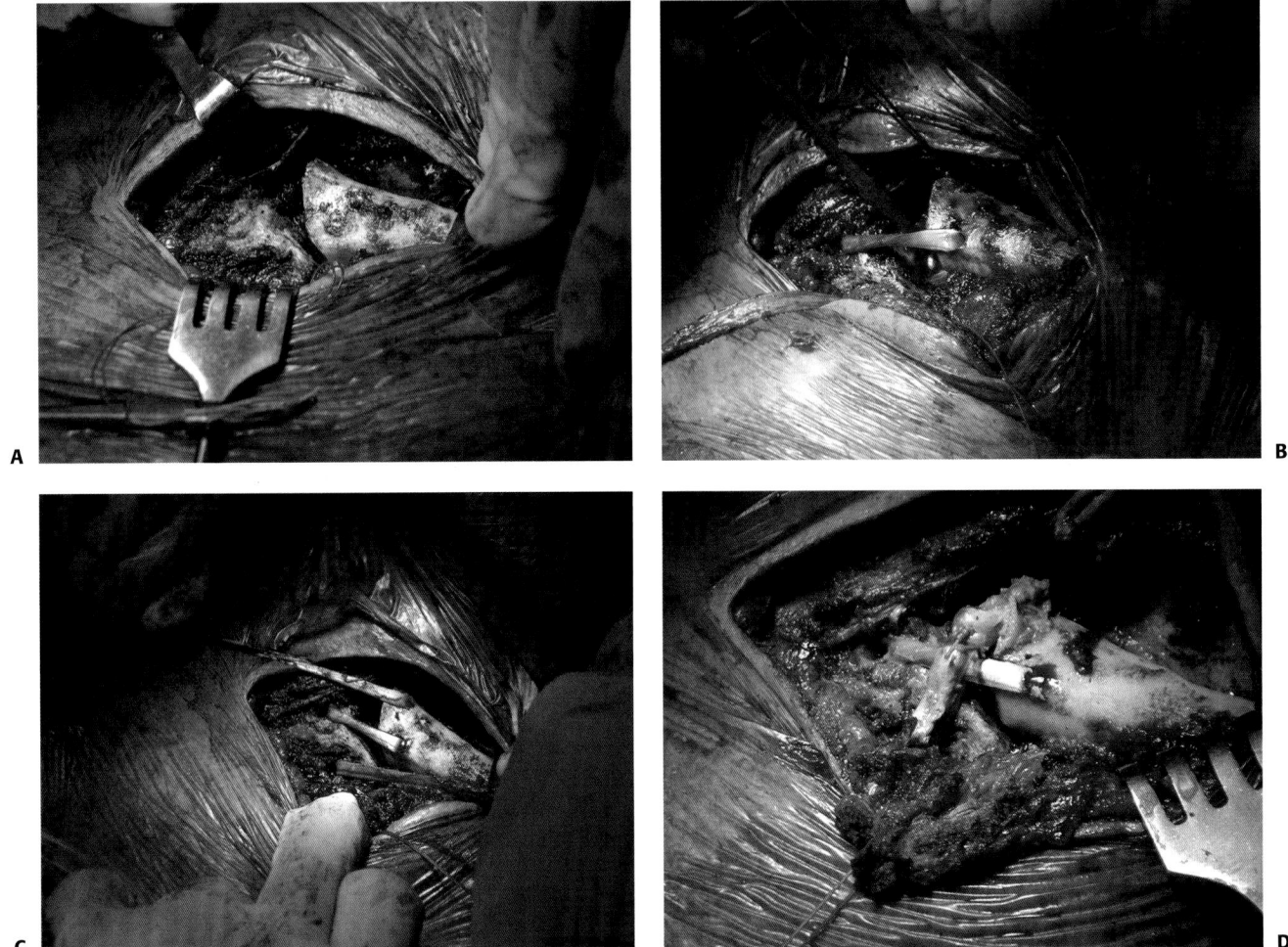

FIGURE 42-49 Semitendinosus figure-of-eight reconstruction. **A:** Reduction of the SC joint **(B)** passing the tendon graft through bone tunnels with suture passer. **C:** Tensioning of the graft. **D:** Completed figure-of-eight construct. (Courtesy Charles E. Rosipal, MD and T. Kevin O'Malley, MD.)

fractures when the SC dislocation is anterior. In the rare case of a scapulothoracic dissociation and SC dislocation, the criteria for management of SC dislocation in isolation can be applied.

COMPLICATIONS IN STERNOCLAVICULAR JOINT INJURIES

Nonoperative Complications in Sternoclavicular Joint Injuries

About the only complications that occur with anterior dislocation of the SC joint are cosmetic bumps or late degenerative changes.[237–239] The serious complications that occur at the time of dislocation of the SC joint are primarily limited to the posterior injuries (Fig. 42-51). Many complications have been reported secondary to the retrosternal dislocation: right pulmonary artery laceration[240]; transected internal mammary artery and lacerated brachiocephalic vein[51]; pneumothorax and laceration of the superior vena cava[172]; tracheal stenosis and respiratory distress[161,220]; venous congestion in the neck;

rupture of the esophagus with abscess and osteomyelitis of the clavicle[27]; pressure on the subclavian artery in an untreated patient[110,164,211]; late occlusion of the subclavian artery in an untreated patient[211]; obstruction of the subclavian vein caused by an unreduced type II Salter–Harris injury of the medial clavicular physis[70]; compression and thrombosis of the brachiocephalic vein[122]; myocardial conduction abnormalities[220]; compression of the right common carotid artery by a fracture-dislocation of the SC joint[110]; pseudoaneurysm of the right subclavian artery, brachial plexus compression[152]; hoarseness of the voice, onset of snoring, and voice changes from normal to falsetto with movement of the arm[27,118,158,196,225]; fatal tracheoesophageal fistula[232]; mediastinal compression[115]; and severe thoracic outlet syndrome with swelling and cyanosis of the upper extremity.[85,112]

Worman and Leagus,[240] in their excellent review of the complications associated with posterior dislocations of the SC joint, reported that 16 of 60 (26.7%) patients reviewed from the literature had suffered complications of the trachea, esophagus, or great vessels.[96,118,178]

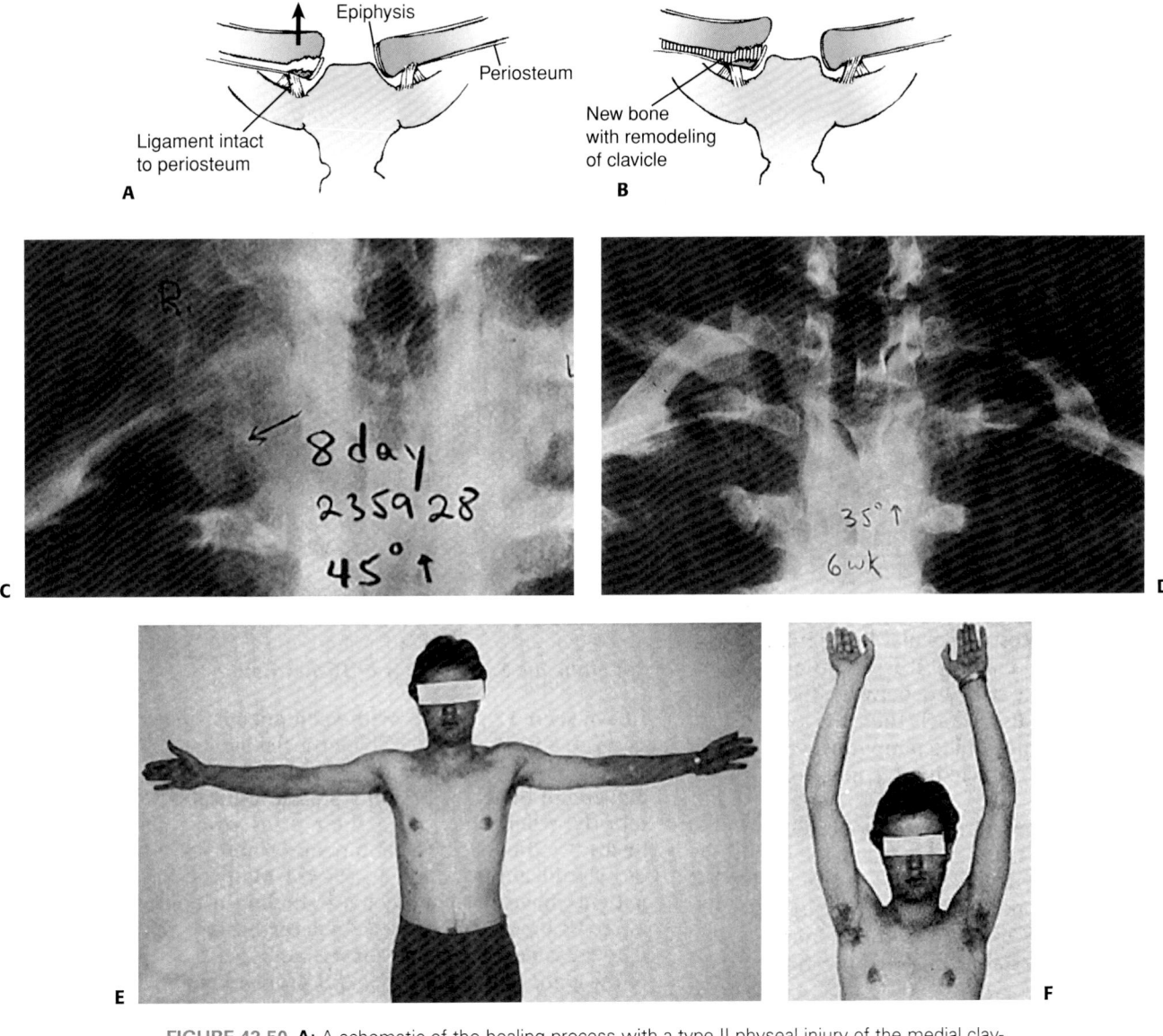

FIGURE 42-50 A: A schematic of the healing process with a type II physeal injury of the medial clavicle. The medial clavicle splits out of the periosteal tube, leaving a small fragment (Thurston-Holland sign) behind. The costoclavicular ligament is intact to the inferior periosteal tube. **B:** Through remodeling from the retained epiphysis and the periosteal tube, the fracture heals. **C:** A radiograph at 8 days reveals that the right medial clavicle is displaced superiorly from the left clavicle. The inferior medial corner of the clavicle is still located in its normal position adjacent to the epiphysis. **D:** A radiograph at 6 weeks reveals new bone formation along the inferior periosteal tube. Note the thin epiphyseal plate of the normal left medial clavicle. **E, F:** Clinically, at 8 weeks the physeal injury has healed and the patient has a full range of motion. (From: Rockwood CA, Matsen F III, eds. *The Shoulder*. Philadelphia, PA: WB Saunders, 1990, with permission.)

Complications Following Operative Procedures in Sternoclavicular Joint Injuries

The Use of Pins to Stabilize the Sternoclavicular Joint

There have been numerous reports of deaths and four near deaths from migrations of intact or broken K-wires or Steinmann pins into the heart, pulmonary artery, or aorta.[21,48,80,83,89,94,113,116,120,125,126,134,138,163,171,197,206,222] Numerous other authors have reported complications from pin migration into the pulmonary artery,[34,134,137] aorta,[165] heart,[66,114,194,198] subclavian artery,[203] mediastinum,[75,92,128,229] breast,[91] and endopelvic region between the iliac vessels and the right colon.[9]

In 1990, Lyons and Rockwood[145] published data on the migration of pins from the SC joint in 21 patients. They reported that pins from the SC joint had migrated into the chest, heart, mediastinum, subclavian vein, and lung. They recommended that large, small, smooth, threaded, bent, or straight pins *not*

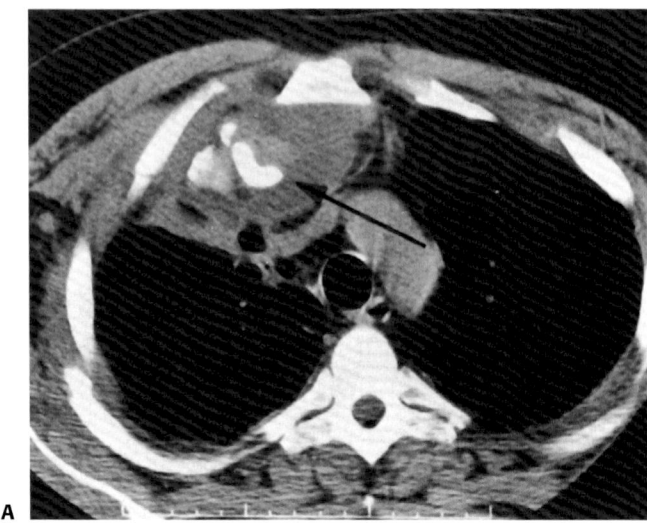

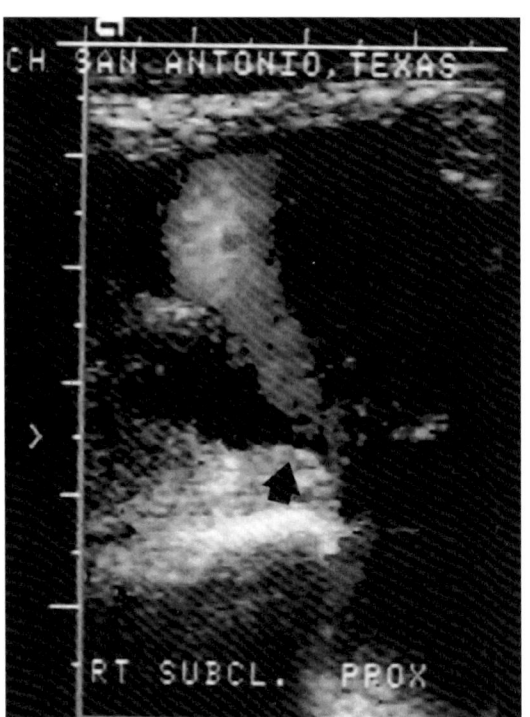

FIGURE 42-51 A: CT scan revealing a posterior fracture-dislocation of the sternoclavicular joint with significant soft tissue swelling and compromise of the hilar structures. **B:** Duplex ultrasound study revealing a large pseudoaneurysm of the right subclavian artery. Note the large neck of the pseudoaneurysm, which measured approximately 1 cm in diameter (*arrow*).

be used for fixation of the SC joint because of their potential to migrate into vital structures and even cause death. Further, they recommended that anytime pins were used to manage any problems about the shoulder, that is, clavicle fractures or injuries to the AC joint, that the pins be monitored very closely with x-rays and that they should always be removed (Fig. 42-52).

Residual Instability. After reduction of a posterior dislocation, there may be some increased laxity which should normalize with time. A case report of anterior subluxation after closed reduction of a posterior dislocation noted that the residual anterior instability resolved with observation.[198] Even with reconstructive procedures, the joint may remain subluxated or subjectively unstable with motion.[170] This is particularly true of patients who were treated surgically for atraumatic instability. Excessive resection of the medial clavicle without successful stabilization can create a challenging instability of the residual medial clavicle for which few options exist (Fig. 42-53). In such cases total claviculectomy may be the only option.[127] An islandized hemipectoralis muscle flap has also been suggested as a means for filling a large medial clavicular defect and may prove useful in these cases.[201]

THE STERNOCLAVICULAR JOINT INJURIES—THE PAST, PRESENT, AND FUTURE

Few surgeons have substantial experience with SC joint injuries as these injuries are rare. As a result, many injuries go unrecognized or are treated inappropriately. Only an occasional publication cites the SC joint and because of the rarity of the problem, it can almost be called the "forgotten joint." It is one of the strongest and most stable joints and when it

dislocates it is difficult to stabilize. It would be helpful if more surgeons report their management of this rare condition to improve the available literature regarding this injury. Despite the years of experience managing this injury, the ultimate stabilizing procedure for dislocations of the SC joint has yet to be published.

Most surgeons treat anterior SC joint dislocations nonoperatively as patients typically function well despite some instability. The question is—why shouldn't we be able to reduce and hold the SC joint in place until the ligaments are healed? Presently, it is accepted that these dislocations should not be stabilized with K-wires, Steinman pins, or similar devices. Simple pinning of the joint with or without repairing the ligaments usually results in pin migration to the chest, mediastinum, abdominal organs, or even to the spinal canal. Many deaths have been reported from intracardiac penetration of migrating pins. Recently the use of a combination clavicle plate with intrasternal hook has been reported, but long-term results are needed before this is a commonly accepted procedure.

Management of posterior dislocations of the SC joint is a challenge. Certainly, we must recognize the condition in adults because the continued displacement of the clavicle can cause erosion into the great vessels and mediastinum and can produce severe complications. If the clavicle is removed from the mediastinum the question is what do you do next? Do you try to stabilize the joint with a plate or do you resect the medial 2 cm and stabilize the residual clavicle to the first rib to prevent anterior/superior and/or continued posterior displacement?

While dislocations are a problem so are the patients with anterior/posterior spontaneous subluxation of the SC joint. Do you stabilize the joint, excise the medial clavicle or continue

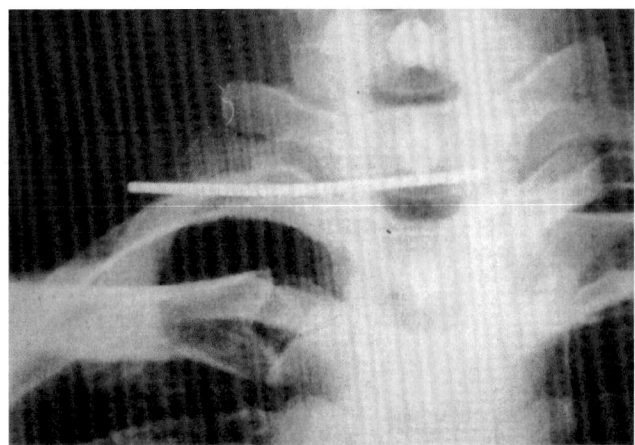

FIGURE 42-52 Migration of pins from the sternoclavicular joint. **A, B:** Migration of Steinmann pin into the spinal canal. **C:** Migration of Steinmann pin into the mediastinum.

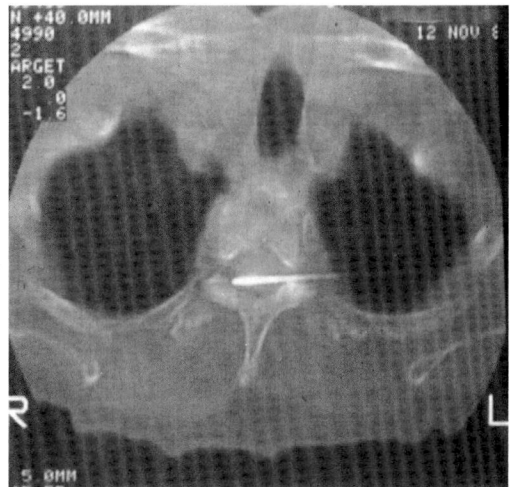

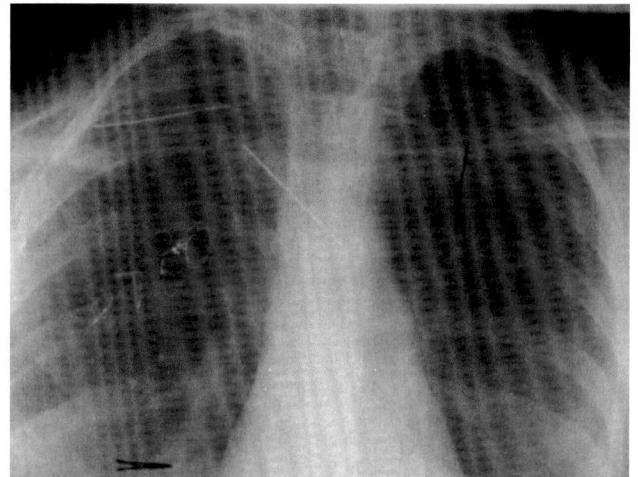

to observe the patient? So far, the literature reflects that this condition occurs in young people and the symptoms gradually disappear with aging. Again, if there were more publications on this complex problem then more orthopedists would understand it.

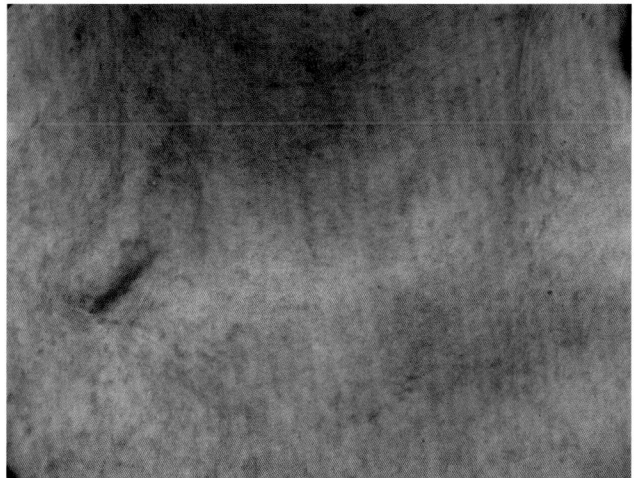

FIGURE 42-53 Excessive resection of the right medial clavicle resulting in residual instability of the medial clavicle with adduction.

So what can we look forward to in the diagnosis and treatment of traumatic and atraumatic conditions of the SC joint? Certainly the proliferation of techniques for surgical repair continues. New fixation techniques and new implants are showing efficacy in stabilizing the SC joint with acceptable functional outcomes. The reports of surgical repair must be taken with caution as these studies are rarely prospective or randomized and the concern for overly aggressive surgical treatment must be stated. An area of continued uncertainty remains the management of posterior physeal injuries in adolescents. The exact criteria for open treatment versus closed treatment remains controversial in these patients when they present with no *major* symptoms. It appears promising that in the future we will see an increase in publications that will educate orthopedic surgeons in the management of problems of the SC joint.

REFERENCES

1. Abiddin Z, Sinopidis C, Grocock CJ, et al. Suture anchors for treatment of sternoclavicular joint instability. *J Shoulder Elbow Surg.* 2006;15:315–318.
2. Allen AW. Living suture grafts in the repair of fractures and dislocations. *Arch Surg.* 1928;16:1007–1020.
3. Allen BF, Zielinski CJ. Posterior fracture through the sternoclavicular physis associated with a clavicle fracture: A case report and literature review. *Am J Ortho.* 1999;28(10): 598–600.
4. Arenas AJ, Pampliega T, Iglesias J. Surgical management of bipolar clavicular dislocation. *Acta Orthop Belg.* 1993;59(2):202–205.

5. Armstrong AL, Dias JJ. Reconstruction for instability of the sternoclavicular joint using the tendon of the sternocleidomastoid muscle. *J Bone Joint Surg Br.* 2008;90B:610–613.
6. Aumann U, Brüning W. Die Discopathie des sternoclaviculargelenkes. *Chirurg.* 1980;51:722–726.
7. Aure A, Hetland KR, Rokkum M. Chronic posterior sternoclavicular dislocation. *J Orthop Trauma.* 2012; 26:e33–e35.
8. Bae DS, Kocher MS, Waters PM, et al. Chronic recurrent anterior sternoclavicular joint instability: Results of surgical management. *J Pediatr Orthop.* 2006;26:71–74.
9. Ballas R, Bonnel F. Endopelvic migration of a sternoclavicular K-wire: Case report and review of the literature. *Orthop Traumatol Surg Res.* 2012; 98(1): 118–121.
10. Baker EC. Tomography of the sternoclavicular joint. *Ohio State Med J.* 1959;55:60.
11. Bankart ASB. An operation for recurrent dislocation (subluxation) of the sternoclavicular joint. *Br J Surg.* 1938;26:320–323.
12. Barth E, Hagen R. Surgical treatment of dislocations of the sternoclavicular joint. *Acta Orthop Scand.* 1983;54:746–747.
13. Bateman JE. *The Shoulder and Neck.* Philadelphia, PA: WB Saunders; 1972.
14. Bateman JE. *The Shoulder and Neck,* 2nd ed. Philadelphia, PA: WB Saunders; 1978.
15. Battaglia TC, Pannunzio ME, Abhinav CB, et al. Interposition arthroplasty with bone-tendon allograft: A technique for treatment of the unstable sternoclavicular joint. *J Orthop Trauma.* 2005;19:124–129.
16. Baumann M, Vogel T, Weise K, et al. Bilateral posterior sternoclavicular dislocation. *Orthopedics.* 2010;33(7):510.
17. Bearn JD. Direct observation on the function of the capsule of the sternoclavicular joint in clavicular support. *J Anat.* 1967;101:159–180.
18. Beckman T. A case of simultaneous luxation of both ends of the clavicle. *Acta Chir Scand.* 1923;56:156–163.
19. Benitez CL, Mintz DN, Potter HG. MR imaging of the sternoclavicular joint following trauma. *Clin Imaging.* 2004;28:59–63.
20. Bennett AN, Edwards E, Kiss Z, et al. Posterior sternoclavicular joint dislocation with brachiocephalic vein compression in an elite hockey player. *Injury Extra.* 2006;37: 422–424.
21. Bensafi H, Laffosse JM, Taam SA, et al. Tamponade following sternoclavicular dislocation surgical fixation. *Orthop Traumatol Surg Res.* 2010;96:314–318.
22. Benson LS, Donaldson JS, Carroll NC. Use of ultrasound in management of posterior sternoclavicular dislocation. *J Ultrasound Med.* 1991;10(2):115–118.
23. Bicos J, Nicholson GP. Treatment and results of sternoclavicular injuries. *Clin Sports Med.* 2003;22:359–370.
24. Bisson LJ, Dauphin N, Marzo JM. A safe zone for resection of the medial end of the clavicle. *J Shoulder Elbow Surg.* 2003;12(6):592–594.
25. Blakeley CJ, Harrison HL, Siow S, et al. The use of bedside ultrasound to diagnose posterior sterno-clavicular dislocation. *Emerg Med J.* 2011;28(6):542.
26. Booth CM, Roper BA. Chronic dislocation of the sternoclavicular joint: An operative repair. *Clin Orthop.* 1979;140:17–20.
27. Borowiecki B, Charow A, Cook W, et al. An unusual football injury (posterior dislocation of the sternoclavicular joint). *Arch Otolaryngol.* 1972;95:185–187.
28. Borrero E. Traumatic posterior displacement of the left clavicular head causing chronic extrinsic compression of the subclavian artery. *Physician Sports Med.* 1987;15:87–89.
29. Breitner S, Wirth CJ. [Resection of the acromial and sternal ends of the clavicle.] *Z Orthop.* 1987;125:363–368.
30. Brenner RA. Monarticular, noninfected subacute arthritis of the sternoclavicular joint. *J Bone Joint Surg.* 1959;41B:740–743.
31. Brinker MR, Bartz RL, Reardon PR, et al. A method for open reduction and internal fixation of the unstable posterior sternoclavicular joint dislocation. *J Orthop Trauma.* 1997;11:378–381.
32. Brooks AL, Henning GD. Injury to the proximal clavicular epiphysis. *J Bone Joint Surg.* 1972;54A:1347–1348.
33. Brossman J, Stabler A, Preidler KW, et al. Sternoclavicular joint: MR imaging—anatomic correlation. *Radiology.* 1996;198(1):193–198.
34. Brown JE. Anterior sternoclavicular dislocation: A method of repair. *Am J Orthop.* 1961;31:184–189.
35. Brown R. Backward and inward dislocation of sternal end of clavicle: Open reduction. *Surg Clin North Am.* 1927;7:1263.
36. Buckerfield C, Castle M. Acute traumatic retrosternal dislocation of the clavicle. *J Bone Joint Surg.* 1984;66A:379–385.
37. Burnstein MI, Pozniak MA. Computed tomography with stress maneuver to demonstrate sternoclavicular joint disease. *J Comput Assist Tomogr.* 1990;14(1):159–160.
38. Burri C, Neugebauer R. Carbon fiber replacement of the ligaments of the shoulder girdle and the treatment of lateral instability of the ankle joint. *Clin Orthop.* 1985; 196:112–117.
39. Burrows HF. Tenodesis of subclavius in the treatment of recurrent dislocation of the sternoclavicular joint. *J Bone Joint Surg Br.* 1951;33B:240–243.
40. Butterworth RD, Kirk AA. Fracture dislocation sternoclavicular joint: Case report. *Va Med Mon.* 1952;79:98–100.
41. Carbone P, Rose M, O'Daniel JA, et al. Posterior remodeling of medial clavicle causing superior vena cava impingement. *Am J Orthop.* 2011;40(6):297–300.
42. Carmichael KD, Longo A, Lick S, et al. Posterior sternoclavicular epiphyseal fracture-dislocation with delayed diagnosis. *Skeletal Radiol.* 2006;35:608–612.
43. Castropil W, Ramadan LB, Bitar AC, et al. Sternoclavicular dislocation-reconstruction with semitendinosus tendon autograft: A case report. *Knee Surg Sports Traumatol Arthrosc.* 2008;16:865–868.
44. Cave AJE. The nature and morphology of the costoclavicular ligament. *J Anat.* 1961; 95:170–179.
45. Cave EF. *Fractures and Other Injuries.* Chicago, IL: Year Book Medical; 1958.
46. Cave ER, Burke JF, Boyd RJ. *Trauma Management.* Chicago, IL: Year Book Medical; 1974:409–411.
47. Chotai PN, Ebraheim NA. Posterior sternoclavicular dislocation presenting with upper-extremity deep vein thrombosis. *Orthopedics.* 2012; 35(10):e1542–e1547.
48. Clark RL, Milgram JW, Yawn DH. Fatal aortic perforation and cardiac tamponade due to a Kirschner wire migrating from the right sternoclavicular joint. *South Med J.* 1974;67:316–318.
49. Collins JJ. Retrosternal dislocation of the clavicle. *J Bone Joint Surg.* 1972;54B:203.
50. Cooper AP. *The Lectures of Sir Astley Cooper on the Principles and Practices of Surgery.* Philadelphia, PA: E.L. Carey & A. Hart; 1935:559.
51. Cooper GJ, Stubbs D, Waller DA, et al. Posterior sternoclavicular dislocation: A novel method of external fixation. *Injury.* 1992;23:565–567.
52. Cope R. Dislocations of the sternoclavicular joint. *Skeletal Radiol.* 1993;22:233–238.
53. Cope R, Riddervold HO. Posterior dislocation of the sternoclavicular joint: Report on two cases, with emphasis on radiologic management and early diagnosis. *Skeletal Radiol.* 1988;17:247–250.
54. Crosby LA, Rubino LJ. Subluxation of the sternoclavicular joint secondary to pseudoarthrosis of the first and second ribs. *J Bone Joint Surg.* 2002;84A(4):623–626.
55. de Jong KP, Sukul DM. Anterior sternoclavicular dislocation: A long-term follo-up study. *J Orthop Trauma.* 1990;4:420–423.
56. Denham R Jr, Dingley AF Jr. Epiphyseal separation of the medial end of the clavicle. *J Bone Joint Surg.* 1967;49A:1179–1183.
57. DePalma AF. The role of the discs of the sternoclavicular and the acromioclavicular joints. *Clin Orthop.* 1959;13:222–233.
58. DePalma AF. *Surgery of the Shoulder.* 2nd ed. Philadelphia, PA: JB Lippincott; 1973: 328–340.
59. DePalma AF. Surgical anatomy of acromioclavicular and sternoclavicular joints. *Surg Clin North Am.* 1963;43:1541–1550.
60. Destouet JM, Gilula LA, Murphy WA, et al. Computed tomography of the sternoclavicular joint and sternum. *Radiology.* 1981;138:123–129.
61. Deutsch AL, Rexnick D, Mink JH. Computed tomography of the glenohumeral and sternoclavicular joints. *Orthop Clin North Am.* 1985;16(3):497–511.
62. Dieme C, Bousso A, Sane A, et al. Bipolar dislocation of the clavicle or floating clavicle. A report of 3cases. *Chir Main.* 2007;26:113–116.
63. Djerf K, Tropp H, Asberg B. Case report: Retrosternal clavicular dislocation in the sternoclavicular joint. *Clin Radiol.* 1998;53:75–76.
64. Duggan N. Recurrent dislocation of sternoclavicular cartilage. *J Bone Joint Surg Am.* 1931;13:365.
65. Echlin PS, Michaelson JE. Adolescent butterfly swimmer with bilateral subluxing sternoclavicular joints. *Br J Sports Med.* 2006;40:e12.
66. Durpekt R, Vojâcek J, Lischke R, et al. Kirschner wire migration from the right sternoclavicular joint to the heart: A case report. *Heart Surg Forum.* 2006;9:e840–e842.
67. Ege T, Canbaz S, Pekindil G, et al. Bilateral retrosternal dislocation and hypertrophy of medial clavicular heads with compression to brachiocephalic vein. *Int Angiol.* 2003;22(3):325–327.
68. Elliott AC. Tripartite injury of the clavicle. *S Afr Med J.* 1986;70:115.
69. Elting JJ. Retrosternal dislocation of the clavicle. *Arch Surg.* 1972;104:35–37.
70. Emms NW, Morris AD, Kaye JC, et al. Subclavian vein obstruction caused by an unreduced type II Salter Harris injury of the medial clavicular physis. *J Shoulder Elbow Surg.* 2002;11(3):271–273.
71. Emura K, Arakawa T, Terashima T, et al. Macroscopic and histological observations on the human sternoclavicular joint disc. *Anat Sci Int.* 2009; 84: 182–188.
72. Eskola A. Sternoclavicular dislocation—A plea for open treatment. *Acta Orthop Scand.* 1986;57:227–228.
73. Eskola A, Vainiopaa S, Vastamaki M, et al. Operation for old sternoclavicular dislocation. *J Bone Joint Surg.* 1989;71B:63–65.
74. Fedoseev VA. Method of radiographic study of the sternoclavicular joint. *Vestn Rentgenol Radiol.* 1977;3:88–91.
75. Ferrandez L, Yubero J, Usabiaga J, et al. Sternoclavicular dislocation, treatment and complications. *Ital J Orthop Traumatol.* 1988;14:349–355.
76. Ferri M, Finlay K, Popowich T, et al. Sonographic examination of the acromioclavicular and sternoclavicular joints. *J Clin Ultrasound.* 2005;33(7):345–355.
77. Ferry AM, Rook FW, Masterson JH. Retrosternal dislocation of the clavicle. *J Bone Joint Surg.* 1957;39A:905–910.
78. Fery A, Leonard A. Transsternal sternoclavicular projection: Diagnostic value in sternoclavicular dislocations. *J Radiol.* 1981;62:167–170.
79. Fery A, Sommelet J. Dislocation of the sternoclavicular joint: A review of 49 cases. *Int Orthop.* 1988;12:187–195.
80. Fowler AW. Migration of a wire from the sternoclavicular joint to the pericardial cavity (letter). *Injury.* 1981;13:261–262.
81. Franck WM, Jannasch O, Siassi M, et al. Balser plate stabilization: An alternate therapy for traumatic sternoclavicular instability. *J Shoulder Elbow Surg.* 2003;12(3):276–281.
82. Friedl W, Fritz T. Die PDS-Kordefixation der Sternockavikularen Luxation und Paraartikularen Klavikulafrakturen. *Unfallchirurg.* 1994;97:263–265.
83. Fueter-Töndury M. Drahtwanderung nach Osteosynthese. *Schweiz Med Wochenschr.* 1976;106:1890–1896.
84. Gale DW, Dunn ID, McPherson S, et al. Retrosternal dislocation of the clavicle: The "stealth" dislocation: A case report. *Injury.* 1992;23:563–564.
85. Gangahar DM, Flogaites T. Retrosternal dislocation of the clavicle producing thoracic outlet syndrome. *J Trauma.* 1978;18:369–372.
86. Garg S, Alshameeri ZA, Wallace WA. Posterior sternoclavicular joint dislocation in a child: A case report with review of literature. *J Shoulder Elbow Surg.* 2012; 21:e11–e16.
87. Garretson RB III, Williams GR Jr. Clinical evaluation of injuries to the acromioclavicular and sternoclavicular joints. *Clin Sports Med.* 2003;22:239–254.
88. Gaudernak T, Poigenfurst J. Simulatenous dislocation-fracture of both ends of the clavicle. *Unfallchirurgie.* 1991;17:362–364.
89. Gerlach D, Wemhoner SR, Ogbuihi S. On two cases of fatal heart tamponade due to migration of fracture nails from the sternoclavicular joint. *Z Rechtsmed.* 1984;93:53–60.
90. Glass ER, Thompson JD, Cole PA, et al. Treatment of sternoclavicular joint dislocations: A systematic review of 251 dislocations in 24 case series. *J Trauma.* 2011;70(5): 1294–1298.

91. Gleason BA. Bilateral, spontaneous, anterior subluxation of the sternoclavicular joint: A case report and literature review. *Mil Med.* 2006;171:790–792.
92. Grabski R. Unusual dislocation of a fragment of Kirschner wire after fixation of the sternoclavicular joint. *Wiad Lek.* 1987;40:630–632.
93. Grant JCB. *Method of Anatomy.* 7th ed. Baltimore, MD: Williams & Wilkins; 1965.
94. Grauthoff Von H, Klammer NI. Komplihationem durch Drahtvenderungen nach Kirschnerdracht-Sprakungen on der Klavikula. *Fortschr Geb Rontgenstr Nuklearmed Erganzungsband.* 1978;128:591–594.
95. Gray H. Osteology. In: Goss CM, ed. *Anatomy of the Human Body.* 28th ed. Philadelphia, PA: Lea & Febiger; 1966:324–326.
96. Greenlee DP. Posterior dislocation of the sternal end of the clavicle. *JAMA.* 1944; 125:426–428.
97. Groh GI, Wirth MA, Rockwood CA Jr. Treatment of traumatic posterior sternoclavicular dislocations. *J Shoulder Elbow Surg.* 2011;20(1):107–113.
98. Groh GI, Wirth MA. Management of traumatic sternoclavicular joint injuries. *J Am Acad Orthop Surg.* 2011;19(1):1–7.
99. Gunther WA. Posterior dislocation of the sternoclavicular joint: Report of a case. *J Bone Joint Surg.* 1949;31A:878–879.
100. Habernek H, Hertz H. [Origin, diagnosis and treatment of sternoclavicular joint dislocation.] *Aktuelle Traumatol.* 1987;17(1):23–28.
101. Hanby C, Pasque C, Sullivan JA. Medial clavicle physis fracture with posterior displacement and vascular compromise: The value of three-dimensional computed tomography and duplex ultrasound. *Orthopedics.* 2003;26:81–84.
102. Haug W. Retention Einer Seltenen Sternoclavicular Lluxationsfrktur Mittels Modifizierter Y-platte der AO. *Aktuel Traumatol.* 1986;16:39–40.
103. Heinig CF. Retrosternal dislocation of the clavicle: Early recognition, x-ray diagnosis, and management. *J Bone Joint Surg.* 1968;50A:830.
104. Hecox SE, Wood GW. Ledge plating technique for unstable posterior sternoclavicular dislocation. *J Orthop Trauma.* 2010;24:255–257.
105. Hobbs DW. Sternoclavicular joint: A new axial radiographic view. *Radiology.* 1968; 90:801–802.
106. Hoekzema N, Torchia M, Adkins M, et al. Posterior sternoclavicular joint dislocation. *Can J Surg.* 2008;51(1):e19–e20.
107. Hofwegen CV, Wolf B. Suture repair of posterior sternoclavicular physeal fractures: A report of two cases. *Iowa Orthop J.* 2008;28:49–52.
108. Hotchkiss LW. Double dislocation of the sternal end of the clavicle. *Ann Surg.* 1896;23:600.
109. Howard FM, Shafer SJ. Injuries to the clavicle with neurovascular complications: A study of fourteen cases. *J Bone Joint Surg.* 1965;47A:1335–1346.
110. Howard NJ. Acromioclavicular and sternoclavicular joint injuries. *Am J Surg.* 1939; 46:284–291.
111. Hsu HC, Wu JJ, Lo WH, et al. Epiphyseal fracture—retrosternal dislocation of the medial end of the clavicle: A case report. *Chin Med J.* 1993;52:198–202.
112. Jain S, Monbaliu D, Thompson JF. Thoracic outlet syndrome caused by chronic retrosternal dislocation of the clavicle. *J Bone Joint Surg.* 2002;84B:116–118.
113. Janssens de Varebeke B, Van Osselaer G. Migration of Kirschner's pin from the right sternoclavicular joint resulting in perforation of the pulmonary artery main trunk. *Acta Chir Belg.* 1993;93:287–291.
114. Jelesijevic V, Knoll D, Klinke F, et al. [Penetrating injuries of the heart and intrapericardial blood vessels caused by migration of a Kirschner pin after osteosynthesis.] *Acta Chir Iugosl.* 1982;29:274–276.
115. Jougon JB, Denis JL, Dromer CEH. Posterior dislocation of the sternoclavicular joint leading to mediastinal compression. *Ann Thorac Surg.* 1996;61:711–713.
116. Kahle M, Filler RL, Forster R. Luxations in the sternoclavicular joint. *Aktuelle Traumatol.* 1990;20:83–86.
117. Kattan KR. Modified view for use in roentgen examination of the sternoclavicular joints. *Radiology.* 1973;108:8.
118. Kennedy JC. Retrosternal dislocation of the clavicle. *J Bone Joint Surg.* 1949;31B:74–75.
119. Kennedy PT, Mawhinney HJD. Retrosternal dislocation of the sternoclavicular joint. *J R Coll Surg Edinb.* 1995;40:208–209.
120. Keferstein R, Frese J. Intrathoracic dislocation of a metal-piece after the use of wires in bone-surgery. *Unfallchirurgie.* 1980;6(1):56–61.
121. Key JA, Conwell HE, eds. *The Management of Fractures, Dislocations, and Sprains.* 5th ed. St. Louis, MO: CV Mosby; 1951:458–461.
122. Kiroff GK, McClure DN, Skelley JW. Delayed diagnosis of posterior sternoclavicular joint dislocation. *Med J Aust.* 1996;164(19):242–243.
123. Klein MA, Spreitzerm AM, Miro PA, et al. MR imaging of the abnormal sternoclavicular joint—a pictorial essay. *Clin Imaging.* 1997;21:138–143.
124. Kocher MS, Feagin JA Jr. Shoulder injuries during alpine skiing. *Am J Sports Med.* 1996;24:665–669.
125. Konstantinov B, Cherkes-Zade D. Case of injury to the aorta by a Kirschner pin during osteosynthesis of the sternoclavicular joint. *Ortop Travmatol Protez.* 1972;33:73–74.
126. Kremens V, Glauser F. Unusual sequela following pinning of medial clavicular fracture. *Am J Roentgenol Radium Ther Nucl Med.* 1956;76:1066–1069.
127. Krishnan SG, Schiffern SC, Pennington SD, et al. Functional outcomes after total claviculectomy as a salvage procedure. A series of six cases. *J Bone Joint Surg.* 2007; 89A:1215–1219.
128. Kumar P, Rees GM, Godbole R, et al. Intrathoracic migration of a Kirschner wire. *J R Soc Med.* 2002;95:198–199.
129. Kurzbauer R. The lateral projection in roentgenography of the sternoclavicular articulation. *AJR Am J Roentgenol.* 1946;56:104–105.
130. Laffosse JM, Espie A, Bonnevialle N, et al. Posterior dislocation of the sternoclavicular joint and epiphyseal disruption of the medial clavicle with posterior displacement in sports participants. *J Bone Joint Surg.* 2010;92B:103–109.
131. Laurencin CT, Senatus P, Patti J, et al. Dislocation of the sternoclavicular joint. Evaluation using paraxial computed tomographic reconstruction. *Orthop Rev.* 1993;22(1): 101–103.
132. Lehnert M, Maier B, Jakob H, et al. Fracture and retrosternal dislocation of the medial clavicle in a 12-year-old child: Case report, options for diagnosis, and treatment in children. *J Pediatr Surg.* 2005;40(11):e1–e3.
133. Lemire L, Rosman M. Sternoclavicular epiphyseal separation with adjacent clavicular fracture: A case report. *J Pediatr Orthop.* 1984;4:118–120.
134. Leonard JW, Gifford RW. Migration of a Kirschner wire from the clavicle into pulmonary artery. *Am J Cardiol.* 1965;16:598–600.
135. Levinsohn EM, Bunnell WP, Yuan HA. Computed tomography in the diagnosis of dislocations of the sternoclavicular joint. *Clin Orthop Relat Res.* 1979;140:12–16.
136. Lewonowski K, Bassett GS. Complete posterior sternoclavicular epiphyseal separation: A case report and review of the literature. *Clin Orthop Relat Res.* 1992;281:84–88.
137. Little NJ, Bismil Q, Chipperfield A, et al. Superior dislocation of the sternoclavicular joint. *J Shoulder Elbow Surg.* 2008;17:e22–e23.
138. Liu HP, Chang CH, Lin PJ, et al. Migration of Kirschner wire for the right sternoclavicular joint into the main pulmonary artery: A case report. *Chang Keng I Hsueh.* 1992; 15(1):49–53.
139. Louw JA, Louw JA. Posterior dislocation of the sternoclavicular joint associated with major spinal injury: A case report. *S Afr Med J.* 1987;71:791–792.
140. Lowman CL. Operative correction of old sternoclavicular dislocation. *J Bone Joint Surg Am.* 1928;10:740–741.
141. Lucas DB. Biomechanics of the shoulder joint. *Arch Surg.* 1973;107:425–432.
142. Lucet L, Le Loet X, Menard JF, et al. Computed tomography of the normal sternoclavicular joint. *Skeletal Radiol.* 1996;25:237–241.
143. Luhmann JD, Bassett GS. Posterior sternoclavicular epiphyseal separation presenting with hoarseness: A case report and discussion. *Pediatr Emerg Care.* 1998;14: 130–132.
144. Lunseth PA, Chapman KW, Frankel VH. Surgical treatment of chronic dislocation of the sternoclavicular joint. *J Bone Joint Surg.* 1975;57B:193–196.
145. Lyons F, Rockwood CA Jr. Current concepts review. Migration of pins used in operations of the shoulder. *J Bone Joint Surg.* 1990;72A:1262–1267.
146. Maguire WB. Safe and simple method of repair of recurrent dislocation of the sternoclavicular joint. *J Bone Joint Surg.* 1986;68B:332.
147. Marcus MS, Tan VJ. Cerebrovascular accident in a 19-year-old patient: A case report of posterior sternoclavicular dislocation. *Shoulder Elbow Surg.* 2011;20(7):e1–e4.
148. Marker LB, Klareskov B. Posterior sternoclavicular dislocation: An American football injury. *Br J Sports Med.* 1996;30(1):71–72.
149. Martin SD, Altchek D, Erlanger S. Atraumatic posterior dislocation of the sternoclavicular joint. *Clin Orthop.* 1993;292:159–164.
150. Martinez A, Rodriguez A, Gonzalez G, et al. Atraumatic spontaneous posterior subluxation of the sternoclavicular joint. *Arch Orthop Trauma Surg.* 1999;119:344–346.
151. McCulloch P, Henley BM, Linnau KF. Radiographic clues for high-energy trauma: Three cases of sternoclavicular dislocation. *AJR Am J Roentgenol.* 2001;176:1534.
152. McKenzie JMM. Retrosternal dislocation of the clavicle: A report of two cases. *J Bone Joint Surg.* 1963;45B:138–141.
153. McLaughlin H. *Trauma.* Philadelphia, PA: WB Saunders; 1959:291–292.
154. Mehta JC, Sachdev A, Collins JJ. Retrosternal dislocation of the clavicle. *Injury.* 1973;5:79–83.
155. Meis RC, Love RB, Keene JS, et al. Operative treatment of the painful sternoclavicular joint: A new technique using interpositional arthroplasty. *J Shoulder Elbow Surg.* 2006;15:60–66.
156. Milch H. The rhomboid ligament in surgery of the sternoclavicular joint. *J Int Coll Surg.* 1952;17:41–51.
157. Mirza AH, Alam K, Ali A. Posterior sternoclavicular dislocation in a rugby player as a cause of silent vascular compromise: A case report. *Br J Sports Med.* 2005;39(5):e28.
158. Mitchell WJ, Cobey MC. Retrosternal dislocation of the clavicle. *Med Ann Dist Columbia.* 1960;29:546–549.
159. Morag B, Shahin N. The value of tomography of the sternoclavicular region. *Clin Radiol.* 1975;26:57–62.
160. Mounasamy V, Fleming M, Birnbaum M. Ipsilateral posterior sternoclavicular dislocation and fracture of the medial third clavicle: A case report. *Eur J Orthop Surg Traumatol.* 2006;16:351–353.
161. Nakayama E, Tanaka T, Noguchi T, et al. Tracheal stenosis caused by retrosternal dislocation of the right clavicle. *Ann Thorac Surg.* 2007;83:685–687.
162. Nakazato T, Wada I, Tsuchiya D, et al. Clavicle fracture and posterior sternoclavicular dislocation in a newborn. *Ortho.* 2001;24(12):1169–1170.
163. Nettles JL, Linscheid R. Sternoclavicular dislocations. *J Trauma.* 1968;8:158–164.
164. Noda M, Shiraishi H, Mizuno K. Chronic posterior sternoclavicular dislocation causing compression of a subclavian artery. *J Shoulder Elbow Surg.* 1997;6(6):564–569.
165. Nordback I, Markkula H. Migration of Kirschner pin from clavicle into ascending aorta. *Acta Chir Scand.* 1985;151:177–179.
166. Nutz V. [Fracture dislocation of the sternoclavicular joint.] *Unfallchirurg.* 1986;89: 145–148.
167. Omer GE. Osteotomy of the clavicle in surgical reduction of anterior sternoclavicular dislocation. *J Trauma.* 1967;7:584–590.
168. Ono K, Inagawa H, Kiyota K, et al. Posterior dislocation of the sternoclavicular joint with obstruction of the innominate vein: Case report. *J Trauma.* 1998;44(2): 381–383.
169. Pang KP, Yung SW, Lee TS, et al. Bipolar clavicular injury. *Med J Malaysia.* 2003;58: 621–624.
170. Panzica M, Zeichen J, Hankemeier S, et al. Long-term outcome after joint reconstruction or medial resection arthroplasty for anterior SCJ instability. *Arch Orthop Trauma Surg.* 2010;130:657–665.
171. Pate JW, Wilhite J. Migration of a foreign body from the sternoclavicular joint to the heart: A case report. *Am Surg.* 1969;35:448–449.
172. Paterson DC. Retrosternal dislocation of the clavicle. *J Bone Joint Surg.* 1961;43B:90–92.
173. Peacock HK, Brandon JR, Jones OL. Retrosternal dislocation of the clavicle. *South Med J.* 1970;63:1324–1328.

174. Pearsall AW, Russell GV. Ipsilateral clavicle fracture, sternoclavicular joint subluxation, and long thoracic nerve injury: An unusual constellation of injuries sustained during wrestling. *Am J Sports Med.* 2000;28(6):904–908.
175. Pensy RA, Eglseder WA. Posterior sternoclavicular fracture-dislocation: A case report and novel treatment method. *J Shoulder Elbow Surg.* 2010;19:e5–e8.
176. Pfister U, Ode E. Die Luxation im sterno-clavicular-gelenk. *Unfallmed Arbeit.* 1983 (October).
177. Pfister U, Weller S. Luxation of the sternoclavicular joint. *Unfallchirurgie.* 1982;8:81–87.
178. Poland J. *Traumatic Separation of Epiphyses of the Upper Extremity.* London: Smith, Elder; 1898:135–143.
179. Pollock RC, Bankes MJK, Emery RJH. Diagnosis of retrosternal dislocation of the clavicle with ultrasound. *Injury.* 1996; 27(9):670–671.
180. Porral MA. Observation d'une double luxation de la clavicule droite. *J Univ Hebd Med Chir Prat.* 1831;2:78–82.
181. Pridie K. Dislocation of acromio-clavicular and sterno-clavicular joints. *J Bone Joint Surg.* 1959;41B:429.
182. Prime HT, Doig SG, Hooper JC. Retrosternal dislocation of the clavicle. *Am J Sports Med.* 1991;19:92–93.
183. Qureshi SA, Shah AK, Pruzansky ME. Using the semitendinosus tendon to stabilize sternoclavicular joints in a patient with Ehlers-Danlos syndrome: A case report. *Am J Orthop.* 2005;34:315–318.
184. Reis FP, de Camargo AM, Vitti M, et al. Electromyographic study of the subclavius muscle. *Acta Anat.* 1979;105:284–290.
185. Rice EE. Habitual dislocation of the sternoclavicular articulation: A case report. *J Okla State Med Assoc.* 1932;25:34–35.
186. Ritvo M, Ritvo M. Roentgen study of the sternoclavicular region. *AJR Am J Roentgenol.* 1947;53:644–650.
187. Rockwood CA Jr. Dislocation of the sternoclavicular joint. In: Rockwood CA Jr, Green DP, eds. *Fractures.* Vol 1. 1st ed. Philadelphia, PA: JB Lippincott; 1975:756–787.
188. Rockwood CA Jr. Injuries to the sternoclavicular joint. In: Rockwood CA Jr, Green DP, eds. *Fractures.* Vol 1. 2nd ed. Philadelphia, PA: JB Lippincott; 1984:910–948.
189. Rockwood CA Jr. The shoulder: Facts, confusions, and myths. *Int Orthop.* 1991;15:401–405.
190. Rockwood CA Jr, Groh GI, Wirth MA, et al. Resection arthroplasty of the sternoclavicular joint. *J Bone Joint Surg.* 1997;79A:387–393.
191. Rockwood CA Jr, Odor JM. Spontaneous atraumatic anterior subluxation of the sternoclavicular joint. *J Bone Joint Surg.* 1989;71A:1280–1288.
192. Rodrigues H. Case of dislocation, inwards, of the internal extremity of the clavicle. *Lancet.* 1843;1:309–310.
193. Rotini R, Guerra E, Bettelli G, et al. Sternoclavicular joint dislocation: A case report of a surgical stabilization technique. *Musculoskelet Surg.* 2010; 94(suppl 1):S91–S94.
194. Rubenstein ZR, Moray B, Itzchak Y. Percutaneous removal of intravascular foreign bodies. *Cardiovasc Intervent Radiol.* 1982;5:64–68.
195. Sadr B, Swann M. Spontaneous dislocation of the sternoclavicular joint. *Acta Orthop Scand.* 1979;50:269–74.
196. Salvatore JE. Sternoclavicular joint dislocation. *Clin Orthop.* 1968;58:51–54.
197. Sanders JO, Lyons FA, Rockwood CA Jr. Management of dislocations of both ends of the clavicle. *J Bone Joint Surg.* 1990;72A:399–402.
198. Schechter DC, Gilbert L. Injuries of the heart and great vessels due to pins and needles. *Thorax.* 1969;24:246–253.
199. Schemitsch LA, Schemitsch EH, McKee MD. Bipolar clavicle injury: Posterior dislocation of the acromioclavicular joint with anterior dislocation of the sternoclavicular joint: A report of two cases. *J Shoulder Elbow Surg.* 2011;20(1):e18–e22.
200. Schmitt WGH. Articulatis Sternoclavicularis: Darstellung in Einer Zweiter Ebene. *Rontgenpraxis.* 1981;34:262–267.
201. Schulman MR, Parsons BO, Lin H, et al. Islandized hemipectoralis muscle flap for sternoclavicular defect. *J Shoulder Elbow Surg.* 2007;16:e31–e34.
202. Selesnick FH, Jablon M, Frank C, et al. Retrosternal dislocation of the clavicle: Report of four cases. *J Bone Joint Surg Am.* 1984;66(2):287–291.
203. Sethi GK, Scott SM. Subclavian artery laceration due to migration of a Hagie pin. *Surgery.* 1976;80:644–646.
204. Shuler FD, Pappas N. Treatment of posterior sternoclavicular dislocation with locking plate osteosynthesis. *Orthopedics.* 2008;31(3):1–4.
205. Siddiqui AA, Turner SM. Posterior sternoclavicular dislocation: The value of intraoperative ultrasound. *Injury.* 2003;34:448–453.
206. Smolle-Juettner FM, Hofer PH, Pinter H, et al. Intracardiac malpositioning of a sternoclavicular fixation wire. *J Orthop Trauma.* 1992;6:102–105.
207. Southworth SR, Merritt TR. Asymptomatic innominate vein tamponade with retromanubrial clavicular dislocation: A case report. *Orthop Rev.* 1988;17:789–791.
208. Speed K. *A Textbook of Fractures and Dislocations.* 4th ed. Philadelphia, PA: Lea & Febiger; 1942:282–290.
209. Spencer EE, Kuhn JE. Biomechanical analysis of reconstructions for sternoclavicular joint instability. *J Bone Joint Surg.* 2004;86A(1):98–105.
210. Spencer EE, Kuhn JE, Huston LJ, et al. Ligamentous restraints to anterior and posterior translation of the sternoclavicular joint. *J Shoulder Elbow Surg.* 2002;11(1):43–47.
211. Stankler L. Posterior dislocation of clavicle: A report of 2 cases. *Br J Surg.* 1962;50:164–168.
212. Stein AH. Retrosternal dislocation of the clavicle. *J Bone Joint Surg.* 1957;39A:656–660.
213. Sullivan JP, Warme BA, Wolf BR. Use of an O-arm intraoperative computed tomography scanner for closed reduction of posterior sternoclavicular dislocations. *J Shoulder Elbow Surg.* 2012;21:e17–e20.
214. Tagliabue D, Riva A. Le lussazioni sterno-claveari. *Minerva Orthop.* 1985;36:876–871.
215. Tanlin Y. Ipsilateral sternoclavicular joint dislocation and clavicle fracture. *J Orthop Trauma.* 1996;10(7):506–507.
216. Thomas CB Jr, Friedman RJ. Ipsilateral sternoclavicular dislocation and clavicle fracture. *J Orthop Trauma.* 1989;3:355–357.
217. Thomas DP, Williams PR, Hoddinott HC. A 'safe' surgical technique for stabilization of the sternoclavicular joint: A cadaveric and clinical study. *Ann R Coll Surg Engl.* 2000;82:432–435.
218. Thut D, Hergan D, Dukas A, et al. Sternoclavicular joint reconstruction: A systematic review. *Bull NYU Hosp Jt Dis.* 2011;69(2):128–135.
219. Tompkins M, Bliss J, Villarreal R, et al. Posterior sternoclavicular disruption with ipsilateral clavicle fracture in a nine-year-old hockey player. *J Orthop Trauma.* 2010;24(4):e36–e39.
220. Tricoire JL, Colombier JA, Choiron P, et al. Retrosternal dislocation of the clavicle: A report of six cases. *Fr J Orthop Surg.* 1990;1:107–112.
221. Tsai DW, Swiontkowski MF, Kottra CL. A case of sternoclavicular dislocation with scapulothoracic dissociation. *AJR Am J Roentgenol.* 1996;167:332.
222. Tubbax H, Hendzel P, Sergeant P. Cardiac perforation after Kirschner wire migration. *Acta Chir Belg.* 1989;89:309–311.
223. Tubbs RS, Loukas M, Slappey JB, et al. Surgical and clinical anatomy of the interclavicular ligament. *Surg Radiol Anat.* 2007;29:357–360.
224. Tuscano D, Banerjee S, Terk MR. Variations in normal sternoclavicular joints: A retrospective study to quantify SCJ asymmetry. *Skeletal Radiol.* 2009;38:997–1001.
225. Tyler HDD, Sturrock WDS, Callow FM. Retrosternal dislocation of the clavicle. *J Bone Joint Surg.* 1963;45B:132–137.
226. van Holsbeeck M, van Melkebeke J, Dequeker J, et al. Radiographic findings of spontaneous subluxation of the sternoclavicular joint. *Clin Rheumatol.* 1992;11:376–381.
227. Van Tongel A, McRae S, Gilhen A, et al. Management of anterior sternoclavicular dislocation: A survey of orthopaedic surgeons. *Acta Orthop Belg.* 2012;78:164–169.
228. Velutini J, Tarazona P. Fracture of the minubrium with posterior displacement of the clavicle and first rib. *Int Orthop.* 1998;22:269–271.
229. Venissac N, Alifano M, Dahan M, et al. Intrathoracic migration of Kirschner pins. *Ann Thorac Surg.* 2000;69:1953–1955.
230. Wade AM, Barrett MO, Crist BD, et al. Medial clavicular epiphyseal fracture with ipsilateral acromioclavicular dislocation: A case report of panclavicular fracture dislocation. *J Orthop Trauma.* 2007;21:418–421.
231. Waskowitz WJ. Disruption of the sternoclavicular joint: An analysis and review. *Am J Orthop.* 1961;3:176–179.
232. Wasylenko MJ, Busse EF. Posterior dislocation of the clavicle causing fatal tracheoesophageal fistula. *Can J Surg.* 1981;24:626–627.
233. Waters PM, Bae DS, Kadiyala RK. Short-term outcomes after surgical treatment of traumatic posterior sternoclavicular fracture-dislocations in children and adolescents. *J Pediatr Orthop.* 2003;23(4):464–469.
234. Webb PA, Suchey JMM. Epiphyseal union of the anterior iliac crest and medial clavicle in a modern multiracial sample of American males and females. *Am J Phys Anthropol.* 1985;68:457–466.
235. Wettstein M, Borens O, Garofalo R, et al. Anterior subluxation after reduction of a posterior traumatic sterno-clavicular dislocation: A case report and a review of the literature. *Knee Surg Sports Traumatol Arthrosc.* 2004;12:453–456.
236. Winter J, Sterner S, Maurer D, et al. Retrosternal epiphyseal disruption of medial clavicle: Case and review in children. *J Emerg Med.* 1989;7:9–13.
237. Wirth MA, Rockwood CA. Chronic conditions of the acromioclavicular and sternoclavicular joints. In: Chapman MW, ed. *Operative Orthopaedics, Part XI.* 2nd ed. Philadelphia, PA: JB Lippincott; 1992:1683–1693.
238. Wirth MA, Rockwood CA. Complications following repair of the sternoclavicular joint. In: Bigliani LU, ed. *Complications of the Shoulder.* Baltimore, MD: Williams & Wilkins; 1993:139–153.
239. Wirth MA, Rockwood CA. Complications of treatment of injuries to the shoulder. In: Epps CH, ed. *Complications in Orthopaedic Surgery.* 3rd ed. Philadelphia, PA: JB Lippincott; 1994:229–253.
240. Worman LW, Leagus C. Intrathoracic injury following retrosternal dislocation of the clavicle. *Trauma.* 1967;7:416–423.
241. Wynne-Davies R. Familial joint laxity. *Proc R Soc Med.* 1971;64:689–690.
242. Yang J, Al-Etani H, Letts M. Diagnosis and treatment of posterior sternoclavicular joint dislocation in children. *Am J Ortho.* 1996;25(8):565–569.
243. Zaslav KR, Ray S, Neer CS. Conservative management of a displaced medial clavicular physeal injury in an adolescent athlete. *Am J Sports Med.* 1989;17(6):833–836.

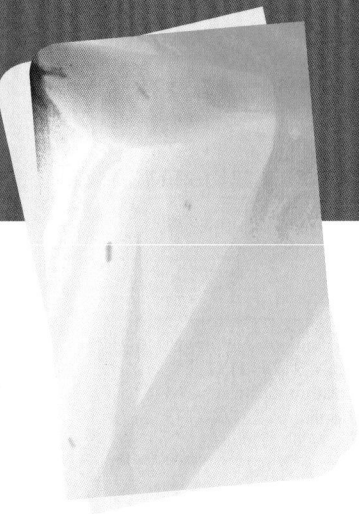

Index

Page numbers followed by an *f* indicate figure; page numbers followed by a *t* indicate tables.